INCLUDES NETTER'S ANATOMY ART

2 0 1 2

ICD-10-CM

D R A F T

Carol J. Buck
MS, CPC, CPC-H, CCS-P
Former Program Director
Medical Secretary Programs
Northwest Technical College
East Grand Forks, Minnesota

ELSEVIER

ELSEVIER
SAUNDERS

3251 Riverport Lane
St. Louis, Missouri 63043

2012 ICD-10-CM DRAFT, STANDARD EDITION

ISBN: 978-1-4557-3384-2

Notices

Knowledge and best practice in this field are constantly changing. As new research and experience broaden our understanding, changes in research methods, professional practices, or medical treatment may become necessary.

Practitioners and researchers must always rely on their own experience and knowledge in evaluating and using any information, methods, compounds, or experiments described herein. In using such information or methods they should be mindful of their own safety and the safety of others, including parties for whom they have a professional responsibility.

With respect to any drug or pharmaceutical products identified, readers are advised to check the most current information provided (i) on procedures featured or (ii) by the manufacturer of each product to be administered, to verify the recommended dose or formula, the method and duration of administration, and contraindications. It is the responsibility of practitioners, relying on their own experience and knowledge of their patients, to make diagnoses, to determine dosages and the best treatment for each individual patient, and to take all appropriate safety precautions.

To the fullest extent of the law, neither the Publisher nor the authors, contributors, or editors, assume any liability for any injury and/or damage to persons or property as a matter of products liability, negligence or otherwise, or from any use or operation of any methods, products, instructions, or ideas contained in the material herein.

ISBN: 978-1-4557-3384-2

Content Strategy Director: Jeanne R. Olson
Senior Content Development Specialist: Jenna Johnson
Publishing Services Manager: Pat Joiner-Myers
Senior Designer: Amy Buxton

Printed in the United States of America

Last digit is the print number: 9 8 7 6 5 4 3 2 1

CONTENTS

ICD-10-CM

SYMBOLS AND CONVENTIONS

The ICD-10-CM Tabular List contains illustrations, pictures, and items to assist you in understanding difficult terminology, diseases/conditions, or coding in a specific category. Items are always printed in ████████ ink so that the added material is not mistaken for official notations or instructions. ████████ ink is used for other annotations in the text. Your ideas on what other descriptions or illustrations should be in future editions of this text are always appreciated.

ICD-10-CM Tabular List Symbols

Throughout this text revisions and additions are indicated by the following symbols:

●   **Use Additional Character(s):** The colored dot cautions that the code requires additional character(s) to ensure the greatest specificity.

●   **Unacceptable Principal Diagnosis:** These codes have a black dot before them and give additional information or describe the circumstances affecting the health care encounter but are unacceptable as principal diagnosis in the FY2011 *Definitions of Medicare Code Edits* (MCE) for inpatient admission.

■   **Unspecified:** The square before a code indicates that although the code is valid as a principal (first-listed) diagnosis, it is not as specific as other codes without the symbol.

OGCR   The *Official Guidelines for Coding and Reporting* symbol includes the placement of a portion of a guideline as that guideline pertains to the code by which it is located. The complete OGCR are located in Part I.

▓   **Includes:** This note appears immediately under a three-character code title to further define or give examples of the content of the category and is highlighted in ████████ for easier reference.

Excludes Notes

The ICD-10-CM has two types of excludes notes. Each note has a different definition for use, but they are both similar in that they indicate that codes excluded from each other are independent of each other.

Excludes1

A type 1 Excludes note is a pure excludes. It means "NOT CODED HERE!" An Excludes1 note indicates that the code excluded should never be used at the same time as the code above the Excludes1 note. An Excludes1 is for use when two conditions cannot occur together, such as a congenital form versus an acquired form of the same condition.

Excludes2

A type 2 Excludes note represents "Not included here." An Excludes2 note indicates that the condition excluded is not part of the condition it is excluded from but a patient may have both conditions at the same time. When an Excludes2 note appears under a code, it is acceptable to use both the code and the excluded code together.

▓   **Code first:** The words indicate an instructional note that directs the coder to sequence the underlying condition before the manifestation. "Code first" is highlighted in ████████ for easier reference.

▓   **Use additional:** The words indicate an instructional note that another code may be needed and are highlighted in ████████ for easier reference.

Certain conditions have both an underlying etiology and multiple body system manifestations due to the underlying etiology. For such conditions the ICD-10-CM has a coding convention that requires the underlying condition be sequenced first, followed by the manifestation. Wherever such a combination exists, there is a "use additional code" note at the etiology code, and a "code first" note at the manifestation code. These instructional notes indicate the proper sequencing order of the codes, etiology followed by manifestation.

In most cases the manifestation codes will have in the code title, "in diseases classified elsewhere." Codes with this title are a component of the etiology/manifestation convention. The code title indicates that it is a manifestation code. "In diseases classified elsewhere" codes are never permitted to be used as first-listed or principal diagnosis codes. They must be used in conjunction with an underlying condition code and they must be listed following the underlying condition.

▓   **Code also:** A "code also" note instructs that two codes may be required to fully describe a condition but the sequencing of the two codes is discretionary, depending on the severity of the conditions and the reason for the encounter.

  7th characters and placeholder X: For codes less than 6 characters that require a 7th character a placeholder X should be assigned for all characters less than 6. The 7th character must always be the 7th character of a code.

🪙 🪙   Indicates complications and comorbidities and major complications and comorbidities according to the Inpatient Prospective Payment System (IPPS) rule published in the *Federal Register*.

❶   **First Listed:** The number 1 inside a circle appears before Z codes that are to be listed as the first code according to the OGCR.

①/②   **First Listed or Secondary:** The 1/2 inside a circle appears before a Z code to indicate that the code may be the first listed code or a secondary code.

❷   Secondary Only: The number 2 inside a circle appears before Z codes that are to be listed as a secondary code. These codes may not be listed as the first code.

HAC is a Hospital-Acquired Condition that, when present as a secondary diagnosis in an inpatient setting, is a higher cost, higher volume, or both, and results in a higher MS-DRG assignment according to the Inpatient Prospective Payment System (IPPS) published in the *Medicare Severity Diagnosis Related Groups (MS-DRGs), Definitions Manual* (FY 2012 IPPS).

Present on Admission: These code categories represent circumstances regarding the health care encounter or factors influencing health status that do not represent a current disease or injury or are always present on admission according to the *Medicare Severity Diagnosis Related Groups (MS-DRGs), Definitions Manual,* Version 28.0 R1.

Age conflict: The FY2011 *Definitions of Medicare Code Edits* (MCE) detects inconsistencies between a patient's age and diagnosis. For example, a 5-year-old patient with benign prostatic hypertrophy or a 78-year-old pregnant female.

The diagnosis is clinically and virtually impossible in a patient of the stated age. Therefore, either the diagnosis or the age is presumed to be incorrect. There are four age categories for diagnoses in the FY2011 *Definitions of Medicare Code Edits* (MCE):

N • Newborn. Age of 0 years; a subset of diagnoses intended only for newborns and neonates (e.g., fetal distress, perinatal jaundice).

P • Pediatric. Age range is 0-17 years inclusive (e.g., Reye's syndrome, routine child health exam).

M • Maternity. Age range is 12-55 years inclusive (e.g., diabetes in pregnancy, antepartum pulmonary complication).

A • Adult. Age range is 15-124 years inclusive (e.g., senile delirium, mature cataract).

♀♂ Sex conflict: FY2011 *Definitions of Medicare Code Edits* (MCE) detects inconsistencies between a patient's sex and any diagnosis or procedure on the patient's record. For example, a male patient with cervical cancer (diagnosis) or a female patient with a prostatectomy (procedure). In both instances, the indicated diagnosis or the procedure conflicts with the stated sex of the patient. Therefore, either the patient's diagnosis, procedure, or sex is presumed to be incorrect.

▸ Manifestation Code: Describes the manifestation of an underlying disease, not the disease itself, and therefore, should not be assigned as a principal diagnosis, according to the FY2011 *Definitions of Medicare Code Edits* (MCE).

NOTICE: At the time of publication of this text, Medicare Code Editor V28.0 was unavailable. Medicare Code Editor Version 27.0 was utilized; therefore users will note inconsistencies due to the fact that Medicare Code Editor V27.0 does not account for the 2012 ICD-10-CM code updates.

ICD-10-CM Tabular

Use Additional Character(s): The colored dot cautions you that the code requires additional digit(s) to ensure greatest specificity.

Volume 1, Tabular List

● **K22 Other diseases of esophagus**
  [Excludes2]   esophageal varices (I85.-)

■ **A02.20 Localized salmonella infection, unspecified**

Unspecified: These codes are for use when the information in the medical record is insufficient to assign a more specific code. For those categories for which an unspecified code is not provided, the "other specified" code may represent both other and unspecified.

Unacceptable Principal Diagnosis: These codes have a black dot before them and are not permitted as a first-listed or principal diagnosis. They must be assigned in conjunction with an underlying condition code, and they must be listed following the underlying condition.

● **B95.0 *Streptococcus, group A, as the cause of diseases classified elsewhere***

A48.3 Toxic shock syndrome
  Use additional code to identify the organism
  (B95, B96)

Use additional code: Located at the etiology code and directs you to assign a manifestation code.

Code first indicates the etiology code is to be first-listed before the manifestation code.

B39 Histoplasmosis
  Code first associated AIDS (B20)

Notes define terms or give coding instructions.

E34.0 Carcinoid syndrome
  Note: May be used as an additional code to identify functional activity associated with a carcinoid tumor.

Codes or index entries are for purposes of illustration only and may not be current.

OGCR Section I.C.6.B.5.

Neoplasm Related Pain Code G89.3 is assigned to pain documented as being related, associated or due to cancer, primary or secondary malignancy, or tumor. This code is assigned regardless of whether the pain is acute or chronic.

OGCR: The Official Guidelines for Coding and Reporting are placed near the codes to which they refer and are highlighted.

First Listed: This symbol appears before Z codes that are acceptable as first-listed diagnoses according to the OGCR.

❶ Z33.2 **Encounter for elective termination of pregnancy**

Excludes1   early fetal death with retention of dead fetus (O02.1)

late fetal death (O36.4)

spontaneous abortion (O03)

First or Secondary: This symbol appears before Z codes that are acceptable as first or secondary diagnoses.

Ⓥ Z21 **Asymptomatic human immunodeficiency virus [HIV] infection status**

Secondary Only: This symbol appears before Z codes that are acceptable only as secondary diagnoses.

❷ Z33.1 **Pregnant state, incidental**

I70.2 **Atherosclerosis of native arteries of the extremities**
Mönckeberg's (medial) sclerosis
Use additional code, if applicable, to identify chronic total occlusion of artery of extremity (I70.92)

code, if applicable, directs the coder to other conditions that may be appropriate to report.

I74 **Arterial embolism and thrombosis**

Includes   embolic infarction
embolic occlusion
thrombotic infarction
thrombotic occlusion

The word "and" should be interpreted to mean either "and" or "or" when it appears in a statement.

Codes or index entries are for purposes of illustration only and may not be current.

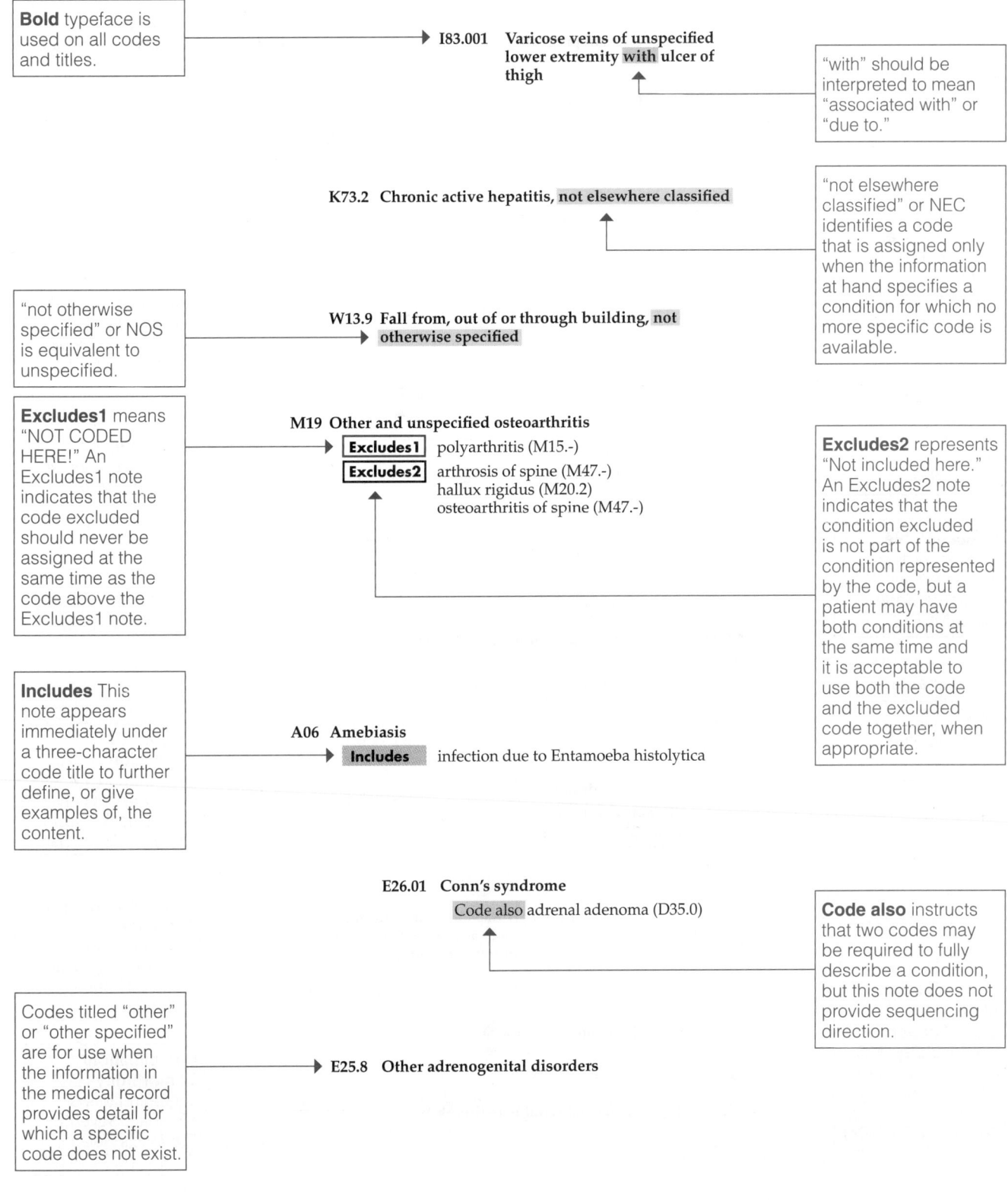

Bold typeface is used on all codes and titles.

I83.001 **Varicose veins of unspecified lower extremity with ulcer of thigh**

"with" should be interpreted to mean "associated with" or "due to."

K73.2 **Chronic active hepatitis, not elsewhere classified**

"not elsewhere classified" or NEC identifies a code that is assigned only when the information at hand specifies a condition for which no more specific code is available.

"not otherwise specified" or NOS is equivalent to unspecified.

W13.9 **Fall from, out of or through building, not otherwise specified**

Excludes1 means "NOT CODED HERE!" An Excludes1 note indicates that the code excluded should never be assigned at the same time as the code above the Excludes1 note.

M19 **Other and unspecified osteoarthritis**
  Excludes1 polyarthritis (M15.-)
  Excludes2 arthrosis of spine (M47.-)
         hallux rigidus (M20.2)
         osteoarthritis of spine (M47.-)

Excludes2 represents "Not included here." An Excludes2 note indicates that the condition excluded is not part of the condition represented by the code, but a patient may have both conditions at the same time and it is acceptable to use both the code and the excluded code together, when appropriate.

Includes This note appears immediately under a three-character code title to further define, or give examples of, the content.

A06 **Amebiasis**
  Includes infection due to Entamoeba histolytica

E26.01 **Conn's syndrome**
      Code also adrenal adenoma (D35.0)

Code also instructs that two codes may be required to fully describe a condition, but this note does not provide sequencing direction.

Codes titled "other" or "other specified" are for use when the information in the medical record provides detail for which a specific code does not exist.

E25.8 **Other adrenogenital disorders**

Codes or index entries are for purposes of illustration only and may not be current.

O00.2 Ovarian pregnancy **M**

Maternity DX (Diagnosis) for ages 12-55 according to the *Definitions of Medicare Code Edits* (MCE)

P02.20 Newborn (suspected to be) affected by unspecified morphological and functional abnormalities of placenta **N**

Newborn, Age 0, according to the *Definitions of Medicare Code Edits* (MCE)

L21.0 Seborrhea capitis
       Cradle cap **P**

Pediatric Age, 0-17, according to the *Definitions of Medicare Code Edits* (MCE)

G30.1 Alzheimer's disease with late onset **A**

Adult Age, 15-124, according to the *Definitions of Medicare Code Edits* (MCE)

B37.3 Candidiasis of vulva and vagina ♀

Females Only according to the *Definitions of Medicare Code Edits* (MCE)

C60.1 Malignant neoplasm of glans penis ♂

Males Only according to the *Definitions of Medicare Code Edits* (MCE)

● H16.8 Other keratitis

Unacceptable PDX according to the *Definitions of Medicare Code Edits* (MCE)

▶ H22 *Disorders of iris and ciliary body in diseases classified elsewhere*
       Code first underlying disease, such as:
          gout (M1A-, M10.-)

Manifestation according to the *Definitions of Medicare Code Edits* (MCE)

G14 Postpolio syndrome
     Includes   Postpolio myelitic syndrome
     Excludes1 sequelae of poliomyelitis (B91)

Present On Admission (POA) according to the *Medicare Severity Diagnosis Related Groups (MS-DRGs)*

T81.512 Adhesions due to foreign body accidentally left in body following kidney dialysis

Hospital-Acquired Condition according to the *Medicare Severity Diagnosis Related Groups (MS-DRGs)*

Major Complication/ Comorbidity (MCC) according to the *Medicare Severity Diagnosis Related Groups (MS-DRGs)*

R57.1 Hypovolemic shock

B25.1 Cytomegaloviral hepatitis

Complication/ Comorbidity (CC) according to the *Medicare Severity Diagnosis Related Groups (MS-DRGs)*

Codes or index entries are for purposes of illustration only and may not be current.

Alphabetic Index

Main terms are in **bold** typeface.

Aberrant (congenital) —*see also* Malposition, congenital
adrenal gland Q89.1

Etiology code first followed by the manifestation code in brackets. The code in brackets is always to be sequenced second.

Amyloid heart (disease) E85.4 *[I43]*

"see" indicates another term should be referenced.

Amylophagia —*see* Pica

Angiofibroma —*see also* Neoplasm, benign, by site

"*see also*" follows a main term and instructs that there is another main term that may also be referenced.

Appendicitis (pneumococcal) (retrocecal) K37
   with
      perforation or rupture K35.2
      peritoneal abscess K35.3

A default code is listed next to the main term and represents that condition most commonly associated with the main term. If a condition is documented in a medical record without any additional information, such as acute or chronic, the default code should be assigned.

Codes or index entries are for purposes of illustration only and may not be current.

PART I

Introduction

ICD-10-CM Official Guidelines for Coding and Reporting 2012
Narrative changes appear in bold text
Items underlined have been moved within the guidelines
since the 2011 version
Italics are used to indicate revisions to heading changes

The Centers for Medicare and Medicaid Services (CMS) and the National Center for Health Statistics (NCHS), two departments within the U.S. Federal Government's Department of Health and Human Services (DHHS) provide the following guidelines for coding and reporting using the International Classification of Diseases, 10th Revision, Clinical Modification (ICD-10-CM). These guidelines should be used as a companion document to the official version of the ICD-10-CM as published on the NCHS website. The ICD-10-CM is a morbidity classification published by the United States for classifying diagnoses and reason for visits in all health care settings. The ICD-10-CM is based on the ICD-10, the statistical classification of disease published by the World Health Organization (WHO).

These guidelines have been approved by the four organizations that make up the Cooperating Parties for the ICD-10-CM: the American Hospital Association (AHA), the American Health Information Management Association (AHIMA), CMS, and NCHS.

These guidelines are a set of rules that have been developed to accompany and complement the official conventions and instructions provided within the ICD-10-CM itself. The instructions and conventions of the classification take precedence over guidelines. These guidelines are based on the coding and sequencing instructions in the Tabular List and Alphabetic Index of ICD-10-CM, but provide additional instruction. Adherence to these guidelines when assigning ICD-10-CM diagnosis codes is required under the Health Insurance Portability and Accountability Act (HIPAA). The diagnosis codes (Tabular List and Alphabetic Index) have been adopted under HIPAA for all healthcare settings. A joint effort between the healthcare provider and the coder is essential to achieve complete and accurate documentation, code assignment, and reporting of diagnoses and procedures. These guidelines have been developed to assist both the healthcare provider and the coder in identifying those diagnoses and procedures that are to be reported. The importance of consistent, complete documentation in the medical record cannot be overemphasized. Without such documentation accurate coding cannot be achieved. The entire record should be reviewed to determine the specific reason for the encounter and the conditions treated.

1

The term encounter is used for all settings, including hospital admissions. In the context of these guidelines, the term provider is used throughout the guidelines to mean physician or any qualified health care practitioner who is legally accountable for establishing the patient's diagnosis. Only this set of guidelines, approved by the Cooperating Parties, is official.

The guidelines are organized into sections. Section I includes the structure and conventions of the classification and general guidelines that apply to the entire classification, and chapter-specific guidelines that correspond to the chapters as they are arranged in the classification. Section II includes guidelines for selection of principal diagnosis for non-outpatient settings. Section III includes guidelines for reporting additional diagnoses in non-outpatient settings. Section IV is for outpatient coding and reporting. It is necessary to review all sections of the guidelines to fully understand all of the rules and instructions needed to code properly.

ICD-10-CM Official Guidelines for Coding and Reporting

Section I. Conventions, general coding guidelines and chapter specific guidelines

A. Conventions for the ICD-10-CM
    1. The Alphabetic Index and Tabular List
    2. Format and Structure:
    3. Use of codes for reporting purposes
    4. Placeholder character
    5. 7th Characters
    6. Abbreviations
        a. Alphabetic Index abbreviations
        b. Tabular List abbreviations
    7. Punctuation
    8. Use of "and"
    9. Other and Unspecified codes
        a. "Other" codes
        b. "Unspecified" codes
    10. Includes Notes
    11. Inclusion terms
    12. Excludes Notes
        a. Excludes1
        b. Excludes2
    13. Etiology/manifestation convention ("code first", "use additional code" and "in diseases classified elsewhere" notes)
    14. "And"
    15. "With"
    16. "See" and "See Also"
    17. "Code also note"
    18. Default codes
B. General Coding Guidelines
    1. Locating a code in the ICD-10-CM
    2. Level of Detail in Coding
    3. Code or codes from A00.0 through T88.9, Z00-Z99.8
    4. Signs and symptoms
    5. Conditions that are an integral part of a disease process
    6. Conditions that are not an integral part of a disease process
    7. Multiple coding for a single condition
    8. Acute and Chronic Conditions
    9. Combination Code
    10. *Sequela* (Late Effects)
    11. Impending or Threatened Condition
    12. Reporting Same Diagnosis Code More than Once
    13. Laterality
    14. Documentation for BMI and Pressure Ulcer Stages
    15. Syndromes
    16. Documentation of Complications of Care

C. Chapter-Specific Coding Guidelines
    1. Chapter 1: Certain Infectious and Parasitic Diseases (A00-B99)
        a. Human Immunodeficiency Virus (HIV) Infections
        b. Infectious agents as the cause of diseases classified to other chapters
        c. Infections resistant to antibiotics
        d. Sepsis, Severe Sepsis, and Septic Shock
        e. Methicillin Resistant *Staphylococcus aureus* (MRSA) Conditions
    2. Chapter 2: Neoplasms (C00-D49)
        a. Treatment directed at the malignancy
        b. Treatment of secondary site
        c. Coding and sequencing of complications
        d. Primary malignancy previously excised
        e. Admissions/Encounters involving chemotherapy, immunotherapy and radiation therapy
        f. Admission/encounter to determine extent of malignancy
        g. Symptoms, signs, and abnormal findings listed in Chapter 18 associated with neoplasms
        h. Admission/encounter for pain control/management
        i. Malignancy in two or more noncontiguous sites
        j. Disseminated malignant neoplasm, unspecified
        k. Malignant neoplasm without specification of site
        l. Sequencing of neoplasm codes
        m. Current malignancy versus personal history of malignancy
        n. Leukemia, Multiple Myeloma, and Malignant Plasma Cell Neoplasms in remission versus personal history
        o. Aftercare following surgery for neoplasm
        p. Follow-up care for completed treatment of a malignancy
        q. Prophylactic organ removal for prevention of malignancy
        r. Malignant neoplasm associated with transplanted organ
    3. Chapter 3: Disease of the blood and blood-forming organs and certain disorders involving the immune mechanism (D50-D89)
    4. Chapter 4: Endocrine, Nutritional, and Metabolic Diseases (E00-E89)
        a. Diabetes mellitus
    5. Chapter 5: Mental, Behavioral and *Neurodevelopmental* disorders (F01 – F99)
        a. Pain disorders related to psychological factors
        b. Mental and behavioral disorders due to psychoactive substance use
    6. Chapter 6: Diseases of the Nervous System (G00-G99)
        a. Dominant/nondominant side
        b. Pain - Category G89
    7. Chapter 7: Diseases of the Eye and Adnexa (H00-H59)
        a. Glaucoma
    8. Chapter 8: Diseases of the Ear and Mastoid Process (H60-H95)
    9. Chapter 9: Diseases of the Circulatory System (I00-I99)
        a. Hypertension
        b. Atherosclerotic Coronary Artery Disease and Angina
        c. Intraoperative and Postprocedural Cerebrovascular Accident
        d. Sequelae of Cerebrovascular Disease
        e. Acute myocardial infarction (AMI)
  10. Chapter 10: Diseases of *the* Respiratory System (J00-J99)
        a. Chronic Obstructive Pulmonary Disease [COPD] and Asthma
        b. Acute Respiratory Failure
        c. Influenza due to certain identified influenza viruses
        d. Ventilator associated Pneumonia
  11. Chapter 11: Diseases of *the* Digestive System (K00-K95)
  12. Chapter 12: Diseases of *the* Skin and Subcutaneous Tissue (L00-L99)
        a. Pressure ulcer stage codes
  13. Chapter 13: Diseases of the Musculoskeletal System and Connective Tissue (M00-M99)
        a. Site and laterality
        b. Acute traumatic versus chronic or recurrent musculoskeletal conditions
        c. Coding of Pathologic Fractures
        d. Osteoporosis

GUIDELINES (ICD-10-CM)

GUIDELINES (ICD-10-CM)

Section I. Conventions, general coding guidelines and chapter specific guidelines

The conventions, general guidelines and chapter-specific guidelines are applicable to all health care settings unless otherwise indicated. The conventions and instructions of the classification take precedence over guidelines.

A. **Conventions for the ICD-10-CM**

The conventions for the ICD-10-CM are the general rules for use of the classification independent of the guidelines. These conventions are incorporated within the Alphabetic Index and Tabular List of the ICD-10-CM as instructional notes.

1. **The Alphabetic Index and Tabular List**

The ICD-10-CM is divided into the Alphabetic Index, an alphabetical list of terms and their corresponding code, and the Tabular List, a chronological list of codes divided into chapters based on body system or condition. The Alphabetic Index consists of the following parts: the Index of Diseases and Injury, the Index of External Causes of Injury, the Table of Neoplasms and the Table of Drugs and Chemicals.

See Section I.C2. General guidelines
See Section I.C.19. Adverse effects, poisoning, underdosing and toxic effects

2. **Format and Structure:**

The ICD-10-CM Tabular List contains categories, subcategories and codes. Characters for categories, subcategories and codes may be either a letter or a number. All categories are 3 characters. A three-character category that has no further subdivision is equivalent to a code. Subcategories are either 4 or 5 characters. Codes may be 3, 4, 5, 6 or 7 characters. That is, each level of subdivision after a category is a subcategory. The final level of subdivision is a code. Codes that have applicable 7th characters are still referred to as codes, not subcategories. A code that has an applicable 7th character is considered invalid without the 7th character.

The ICD-10-CM uses an indented format for ease in reference

3. **Use of codes for reporting purposes**

For reporting purposes only codes are permissible, not categories or subcategories, and any applicable 7th character is required.

4. **Placeholder character**

The ICD-10-CM utilizes a placeholder character "X". The "X" is used as a placeholder at certain codes to allow for future expansion. An example of this is at the poisoning, adverse effect and underdosing codes, categories T36-T50. Where a placeholder exists, the X must be used in order for the code to be considered a valid code.

5. **7th Characters**

Certain ICD-10-CM categories have applicable 7th characters. The applicable 7th character is required for all codes within the category, or as the notes in the Tabular List instruct. The 7th character must always be the 7th character in the data field. If a code that requires a 7th character is not 6 characters, a placeholder X must be used to fill in the empty characters.

6. **Abbreviations**

a. **Alphabetic Index abbreviations**

NEC "Not elsewhere classifiable"

This abbreviation in the Alphabetic Index represents "other specified". When a specific code is not available for a condition the Alphabetic Index directs the coder to the "other specified" code in the Tabular List.

NOS "Not otherwise specified"

This abbreviation is the equivalent of unspecified.

b. **Tabular abbreviations**

NEC "Not elsewhere classifiable"

This abbreviation in the Tabular List represents "other specified". When a specific code is not available for a condition, the Tabular List includes an NEC entry under a code to identify the code as the "other specified" code.

NOS   "Not otherwise specified"
This abbreviation is the equivalent of unspecified.

7. **Punctuation**
   [ ] Brackets are used in the Tabular List to enclose synonyms, alternative wording or explanatory phrases. Brackets are used in the Alphabetic Index to identify manifestation codes.
   ( ) Parentheses are used in both the Alphabetic Index and Tabular List to enclose supplementary words that may be present or absent in the statement of a disease or procedure without affecting the code number to which it is assigned. The terms within the parentheses are referred to as nonessential modifiers.
   :   Colons are used in the Tabular List after an incomplete term which needs one or more of the modifiers following the colon to make it assignable to a given category.

8. **Use of "and"**
   When the term "and" is used in a narrative statement it represents and/or.

9. **Other and Unspecified codes**
   a. **"Other" codes**
   Codes titled "other" or "other specified" are for use when the information in the medical record provides detail for which a specific code does not exist. Alphabetic Index entries with NEC in the line designate "other" codes in the Tabular List. These Alphabetic Index entries represent specific disease entities for which no specific code exists so the term is included within an "other" code.

   b. **"Unspecified" codes**
   Codes titled "unspecified" are for use when the information in the medical record is insufficient to assign a more specific code. For those categories for which an unspecified code is not provided, the "other specified" code may represent both other and unspecified.

10. **Includes Notes**
    This note appears immediately under a three-character code title to further define, or give examples of, the content of the category.

11. **Inclusion terms**
    List of terms is included under some codes. These terms are the conditions for which that code is to be used. The terms may be synonyms of the code title, or, in the case of "other specified" codes, the terms are a list of the various conditions assigned to that code. The inclusion terms are not necessarily exhaustive. Additional terms found only in the Alphabetic Index may also be assigned to a code.

12. **Excludes Notes**
    The ICD-10-CM has two types of excludes notes. Each type of note has a different definition for use but they are all similar in that they indicate that codes excluded from each other are independent of each other.

    a. **Excludes1**
    A type 1 Excludes note is a pure excludes note. It means "NOT CODED HERE!" An Excludes1 note indicates that the code excluded should never be used at the same time as the code above the Excludes1 note. An Excludes1 is used when two conditions cannot occur together, such as a congenital form versus an acquired form of the same condition.

    b. **Excludes2**
    A type 2 excludes note represents "Not included here". An excludes2 note indicates that the condition excluded is not part of the condition represented by the code, but a patient may have both conditions at the same time. When an Excludes2 note appears under a code, it is acceptable to use both the code and the excluded code together, when appropriate.

GUIDELINES (ICD-10-CM)

13. **Etiology/manifestation convention ("code first", "use additional code" and "in diseases classified elsewhere" notes)**

    Certain conditions have both an underlying etiology and multiple body system manifestations due to the underlying etiology. For such conditions, the ICD-10-CM has a coding convention that requires the underlying condition be sequenced first followed by the manifestation. Wherever such a combination exists, there is a "use additional code" note at the etiology code, and a "code first" note at the manifestation code. These instructional notes indicate the proper sequencing order of the codes, etiology followed by manifestation.

    In most cases the manifestation codes will have in the code title, "in diseases classified elsewhere." Codes with this title are a component of the etiology/ manifestation convention. The code title indicates that it is a manifestation code. "In diseases classified elsewhere" codes are never permitted to be used as first-listed or principal diagnosis codes. They must be used in conjunction with an underlying condition code and they must be listed following the underlying condition. See category F02, Dementia in other diseases classified elsewhere, for an example of this convention.

    There are manifestation codes that do not have "in diseases classified elsewhere" in the title. For such codes a "use additional code" note will still be present and the rules for sequencing apply.

    In addition to the notes in the Tabular List, these conditions also have a specific Alphabetic Index entry structure. In the Alphabetic Index both conditions are listed together with the etiology code first followed by the manifestation codes in brackets. The code in brackets is always to be sequenced second.

    An example of the etiology/manifestation convention is dementia in Parkinson's disease. In the Alphabetic Index, code G20 is listed first, followed by code F02.80 or F02.81 in brackets. Code G20 represents the underlying etiology, Parkinson's disease, and must be sequenced first, whereas codes F02.80 and F02.81 represent the manifestation of dementia in diseases classified elsewhere, with or without behavioral disturbance.

    "Code first" and "Use additional code" notes are also used as sequencing rules in the classification for certain codes that are not part of an etiology/ manifestation combination.

    See Section I.B.7. Multiple coding for a single condition.

14. **"And"**

    The word "and" should be interpreted to mean either "and" or "or" when it appears in a title.

15. **"With"**

    The word "with" should be interpreted to mean "associated with" or "due to" when it appears in a code title, the Alphabetic Index, or an instructional note in the Tabular List.

    The word "with" in the Alphabetic Index is sequenced immediately following the main term, not in alphabetical order.

16. **"See" and "See Also"**

    The "see" instruction following a main term in the Alphabetic Index indicates that another term should be referenced. It is necessary to go to the main term referenced with the "see" note to locate the correct code.

    A "see also" instruction following a main term in the Alphabetic Index instructs that there is another main term that may also be referenced that may provide additional Alphabetic Index entries that may be useful. It is not necessary to follow the "see also" note when the original main term provides the necessary code.

17. **"Code also note"**

    A "code also" note instructs that two codes may be required to fully describe a condition, but this note does not provide sequencing direction.

18. **Default codes**

    A code listed next to a main term in the ICD-10-CM Alphabetic Index is referred to as a default code. The default code represents that condition that is most commonly associated with the main term, or is the unspecified code for the condition. If a condition is documented in a medical record (for example, appendicitis) without any additional information, such as acute or chronic, the default code should be assigned.

B. General Coding Guidelines

1. Locating a code in the ICD-10-CM

To select a code in the classification that corresponds to a diagnosis or reason for visit documented in a medical record, first locate the term in the Alphabetic Index, and then verify the code in the Tabular List. Read and be guided by instructional notations that appear in both the Alphabetic Index and the Tabular List.

It is essential to use both the Alphabetic Index and Tabular List when locating and assigning a code. The Alphabetic Index does not always provide the full code. Selection of the full code, including laterality and any applicable 7th character can only be done in the Tabular List. A dash (-) at the end of an Alphabetic Index entry indicates that additional characters are required. Even if a dash is not included at the Alphabetic Index entry, it is necessary to refer to the Tabular List to verify that no 7th character is required.

2. Level of Detail in Coding

Diagnosis codes are to be used and reported at their highest number of characters available.

ICD-10-CM diagnosis codes are composed of codes with 3, 4, 5, 6 or 7 characters. Codes with three characters are included in ICD-10-CM as the heading of a category of codes that may be further subdivided by the use of fourth and/or fifth characters and/or sixth characters, which provide greater detail.

A three-character code is to be used only if it is not further subdivided. A code is invalid if it has not been coded to the full number of characters required for that code, including the 7th character, if applicable.

3. Code or codes from A00.0 through T88.9, Z00-Z99.8

The appropriate code or codes from A00.0 through T88.9, Z00-Z99.8 must be used to identify diagnoses, symptoms, conditions, problems, complaints or other reason(s) for the encounter/visit.

4. Signs and symptoms

Codes that describe symptoms and signs, as opposed to diagnoses, are acceptable for reporting purposes when a related definitive diagnosis has not been established (confirmed) by the provider. Chapter 18 of ICD-10-CM, Symptoms, Signs, and Abnormal Clinical and Laboratory Findings, Not Elsewhere Classified (codes R00.0 - R99) contains many, but not all codes for symptoms.

5. Conditions that are an integral part of a disease process

Signs and symptoms that are associated routinely with a disease process should not be assigned as additional codes, unless otherwise instructed by the classification.

6. Conditions that are not an integral part of a disease process

Additional signs and symptoms that may not be associated routinely with a disease process should be coded when present.

7. Multiple coding for a single condition

In addition to the etiology/manifestation convention that requires two codes to fully describe a single condition that affects multiple body systems, there are other single conditions that also require more than one code. "Use additional code" notes are found in the Tabular List at codes that are not part of an etiology/manifestation pair where a secondary code is useful to fully describe a condition. The sequencing rule is the same as the etiology/manifestation pair, "use additional code" indicates that a secondary code should be added.

For example, for bacterial infections that are not included in chapter 1, a secondary code from category B95, Streptococcus, Staphylococcus, and

Enterococcus, as the cause of diseases classified elsewhere, or B96, Other bacterial agents as the cause of diseases classified elsewhere, may be required to identify the bacterial organism causing the infection. A "use additional code" note will normally be found at the infectious disease code, indicating a need for the organism code to be added as a secondary code.

"Code first" notes are also under certain codes that are not specifically manifestation codes but may be due to an underlying cause. When there is a "code first" note and an underlying condition is present, the underlying condition should be sequenced first.

"Code, if applicable, any causal condition first", notes indicate that this code may be assigned as a principal diagnosis when the causal condition is unknown or not applicable. If a causal condition is known, then the code for that condition should be sequenced as the principal or first-listed diagnosis.

Multiple codes may be needed for **sequela**, complication codes and obstetric codes to more fully describe a condition. See the specific guidelines for these conditions for further instruction.

8. Acute and Chronic Conditions

If the same condition is described as both acute (subacute) and chronic, and separate subentries exist in the Alphabetic Index at the same indentation level, code both and sequence the acute (subacute) code first.

9. Combination Code

A combination code is a single code used to classify:
Two diagnoses, or
A diagnosis with an associated secondary process (manifestation)
A diagnosis with an associated complication
Combination codes are identified by referring to subterm entries in the Alphabetic Index and by reading the inclusion and exclusion notes in the Tabular List.

Assign only the combination code when that code fully identifies the diagnostic conditions involved or when the Alphabetic Index so directs. Multiple coding should not be used when the classification provides a combination code that clearly identifies all of the elements documented in the diagnosis. When the combination code lacks necessary specificity in describing the manifestation or complication, an additional code should be used as a secondary code.

10. *Sequela* (Late Effects)

A **sequela** is the residual effect (condition produced) after the acute phase of an illness or injury has terminated. There is no time limit on when a **sequela** code can be used. The residual may be apparent early, such as in cerebral infarction, or it may occur months or years later, such as that due to a previous injury. Coding of **sequela** generally requires two codes sequenced in the following order: The condition or nature of the **sequela** is sequenced first. The **sequela** code is sequenced second.

An exception to the above guidelines are those instances where the code for **sequela** is followed by a manifestation code identified in the Tabular List and title, or the **sequela** code has been expanded (at the fourth, fifth or sixth character levels) to include the manifestation(s). The code for the acute phase of an illness or injury that led to the **sequela** is never used with a code for the late effect.

See Section I.C.9. Sequelae of cerebrovascular disease
See Section I.C.15. Sequelae of complication of pregnancy, childbirth and the puerperium
*See Section I.C.19. **Application of 7th characters for Chapter 19***

11. Impending or Threatened Condition

Code any condition described at the time of discharge as "impending" or "threatened" as follows:
If it did occur, code as confirmed diagnosis.
If it did not occur, reference the Alphabetic Index to determine if the condition has a subentry term for "impending" or "threatened" and also reference main term entries for "Impending" and for "Threatened."

If the subterms are listed, assign the given code.

If the subterms are not listed, code the existing underlying condition(s) and not the condition described as impending or threatened.

12. **Reporting Same Diagnosis Code More than Once**

Each unique ICD-10-CM diagnosis code may be reported only once for an encounter. This applies to bilateral conditions when there are no distinct codes identifying laterality or two different conditions classified to the same ICD-10-CM diagnosis code.

13. **Laterality**

For bilateral sites, the final character of the codes in the ICD-10-CM indicates laterality. An unspecified side code is also provided should the side not be identified in the medical record. If no bilateral code is provided and the condition is bilateral, assign separate codes for both the left and right side.

14. **Documentation for BMI and Pressure Ulcer Stages**

For the Body Mass Index (BMI) and pressure ulcer stage codes, code assignment may be based on medical record documentation from clinicians who are not the patient's provider (i.e., physician or other qualified healthcare practitioner legally accountable for establishing the patient's diagnosis), since this information is typically documented by other clinicians involved in the care of the patient (e.g., a dietitian often documents the BMI and nurses often documents the pressure ulcer stages). However, the associated diagnosis (such as overweight, obesity, or pressure ulcer) must be documented by the patient's provider. If there is conflicting medical record documentation, either from the same clinician or different clinicians, the patient's attending provider should be queried for clarification.

The BMI codes should only be reported as secondary diagnoses. As with all other secondary diagnosis codes, the BMI codes should only be assigned when they meet the definition of a reportable additional diagnosis (see Section III, Reporting Additional Diagnoses).

15. **Syndromes**

Follow the Alphabetic Index guidance when coding syndromes. In the absence of Alphabetic Index guidance, assign codes for the documented manifestations of the syndrome.

16. **Documentation of Complications of Care**

Code assignment is based on the provider's documentation of the relationship between the condition and the care or procedure. The guideline extends to any complications of care, regardless of the chapter the code is located in. It is important to note that not all conditions that occur during or following medical care or surgery are classified as complications. There must be a cause-and-effect relationship between the care provided and the condition, and an indication in the documentation that it is a complication. Query the provider for clarification, if the complication is not clearly documented.

C. **Chapter-Specific Coding Guidelines**

In addition to general coding guidelines, there are guidelines for specific diagnoses and/or conditions in the classification. Unless otherwise indicated, these guidelines apply to all health care settings. Please refer to Section II for guidelines on the selection of principal diagnosis.

1. **Chapter 1: Certain Infectious and Parasitic Diseases (A00-B99)**

   a. **Human Immunodeficiency Virus (HIV) Infections**

      1) **Code only confirmed cases**

Code only confirmed cases of HIV infection/illness. This is an exception to the hospital inpatient guideline Section II, H.

In this context, "confirmation" does not require documentation of positive serology or culture for HIV; the provider's diagnostic statement that the patient is HIV positive, or has an HIV-related illness is sufficient.

2) Selection and sequencing of HIV codes

(a) Patient admitted for HIV-related condition

If a patient is admitted for an HIV-related condition, the principal diagnosis should be B20, **Human immunodeficiency virus [HIV] disease** followed by additional diagnosis codes for all reported HIV-related conditions.

(b) Patient with HIV disease admitted for unrelated condition

If a patient with HIV disease is admitted for an unrelated condition (such as a traumatic injury), the code for the unrelated condition (e.g., the nature of injury code) should be the principal diagnosis. Other diagnoses would be B20 followed by additional diagnosis codes for all reported HIV-related conditions.

(c) Whether the patient is newly diagnosed

Whether the patient is newly diagnosed or has had previous admissions/encounters for HIV conditions is irrelevant to the sequencing decision.

(d) Asymptomatic human immunodeficiency virus

Z21, Asymptomatic human immunodeficiency virus [HIV] infection status, is to be applied when the patient without any documentation of symptoms is listed as being "HIV positive," "known HIV," "HIV test positive," or similar terminology. Do not use this code if the term "AIDS" is used or if the patient is treated for any HIV-related illness or is described as having any condition(s) resulting from his/her HIV positive status; use B20 in these cases.

(e) Patients with inconclusive HIV serology

Patients with inconclusive HIV serology, but no definitive diagnosis or manifestations of the illness, may be assigned code R75, Inconclusive laboratory evidence of human immunodeficiency virus [HIV].

(f) Previously diagnosed HIV-related illness

Patients with any known prior diagnosis of an HIV-related illness should be coded to B20. Once a patient has developed an HIV-related illness, the patient should always be assigned code B20 on every subsequent admission/encounter. Patients previously diagnosed with any HIV illness (B20) should never be assigned to R75 or Z21, Asymptomatic human immunodeficiency virus [HIV] infection status.

(g) HIV Infection in Pregnancy, Childbirth and the Puerperium

During pregnancy, childbirth or the puerperium, a patient admitted (or presenting for a health care encounter) because of an HIV-related illness should receive a principal diagnosis code of O98.7-, Human immunodeficiency [HIV] disease complicating pregnancy, childbirth and the puerperium, followed by B20 and the code(s) for the HIV-related illness(es). Codes from Chapter 15 always take sequencing priority.

Patients with asymptomatic HIV infection status admitted (or presenting for a health care encounter) during pregnancy, childbirth, or the puerperium should receive codes of O98.7- and Z21.

(h) Encounters for testing for HIV

If a patient is being seen to determine his/her HIV status, use code Z11.4, Encounter for screening for human immunodeficiency virus [HIV]. Use additional codes for any associated high risk behavior.

If a patient with signs or symptoms is being seen for HIV testing, code the signs and symptoms. An additional counseling code Z71.7, Human immunodeficiency virus [HIV] counseling, may be used if counseling is provided during the encounter for the test.

When a patient returns to be informed of his/her HIV test results and the test result is negative, use code Z71.7, Human immunodeficiency virus [HIV] counseling.

If the results are positive, see previous guidelines and assign codes as appropriate.

b. Infectious agents as the cause of diseases classified to other chapters

Certain infections are classified in chapters other than Chapter 1 and no organism is identified as part of the infection code. In these instances, it is necessary to use an additional code from Chapter 1 to identify the organism. A code from category B95, Streptococcus, Staphylococcus, and Enterococcus as the cause of diseases classified to other chapters, B96, Other bacterial agents as the cause of diseases classified to other chapters, or B97, Viral agents as the cause of diseases classified to other chapters, is to be used as an additional code to identify the organism. An instructional note will be found at the infection code advising that an additional organism code is required.

c. Infections resistant to antibiotics

Many bacterial infections are resistant to current antibiotics. It is necessary to identify all infections documented as antibiotic resistant. Assign **a** code **from category** Z16, **Resistance to antimicrobial drugs,** following the infection code **only if the infection code does not identify drug resistance.**

d. Sepsis, Severe Sepsis, and Septic Shock

1) Coding of Sepsis and Severe Sepsis

(a) Sepsis

For a diagnosis of sepsis, assign the appropriate code for the underlying systemic infection. If the type of infection or causal organism is not further specified, assign code A41.9, Sepsis, unspecified **organism**.

A code from subcategory R65.2, Severe sepsis, should not be assigned unless severe sepsis or an associated acute organ dysfunction is documented.

(i) Negative or inconclusive blood cultures and sepsis
Negative or inconclusive blood cultures do not preclude a diagnosis of sepsis in patients with clinical evidence of the condition, however, the provider should be queried.

(ii) Urosepsis
The term urosepsis is a nonspecific term. It is not to be considered synonymous with sepsis. It has no default code in the Alphabetic Index. Should a provider use this term, he/she must be queried for clarification.

(iii) Sepsis with organ dysfunction
If a patient has sepsis and associated acute organ dysfunction or multiple organ dysfunction (MOD), follow the instructions for coding severe sepsis.

(iv) Acute organ dysfunction that is not clearly associated with the sepsis
If a patient has sepsis and an acute organ dysfunction, but the medical record documentation indicates that the acute organ dysfunction is related to a medical condition other than the sepsis, do not assign a code from subcategory R65.2, Severe sepsis. An acute organ dysfunction must be associated with the sepsis in order to assign the severe sepsis code. If the documentation is not clear as to whether an acute organ dysfunction is related to the sepsis or another medical condition, query the provider.

(b) Severe sepsis

The coding of severe sepsis requires a minimum of 2 codes: first a code for the underlying systemic infection, followed by a code from subcategory R65.2, Severe sepsis. If the causal organism is not documented, assign code A41.9, Sepsis, unspecified **organism**, for the infection. Additional code(s) for the associated acute organ dysfunction are also required.

Due to the complex nature of severe sepsis, some cases may require querying the provider prior to assignment of the codes.

2) Septic shock

(a) Septic shock **generally refers to** circulatory failure associated with severe sepsis, and therefore, it represents a type of acute organ dysfunction.

For all cases of septic shock, the code for the underlying systemic infection should be sequenced first, followed by code R65.21, Severe sepsis with septic shock **or code T81.12, Postprocedural septic shock.** Any additional codes for the other acute organ dysfunctions should also be assigned. **As noted in the sequencing instructions in the Tabular List, the code for septic shock cannot be assigned as a principal diagnosis.**

3) Sequencing of severe sepsis

If severe sepsis is present on admission, and meets the definition of principal diagnosis, the underlying systemic infection should be assigned as principal diagnosis followed by the appropriate code from subcategory R65.2 as required by the sequencing rules in the Tabular List. A code from subcategory R65.2 can never be assigned as a principal diagnosis.

When severe sepsis develops during an encounter (it was not present on admission) the underlying systemic infection and the appropriate code from subcategory R65.2 should be assigned as secondary diagnoses.

Severe sepsis may be present on admission but the diagnosis may not be confirmed until sometime after admission. If the documentation is not clear whether severe sepsis was present on admission, the provider should be queried.

4) Sepsis and severe sepsis with a localized infection

If the reason for admission is both sepsis or severe sepsis and a localized infection, such as pneumonia or cellulitis, a code(s) for the underlying systemic infection should be assigned first and the code for the localized infection should be assigned as a secondary diagnosis. If the patient has severe sepsis, a code from subcategory R65.2 should also be assigned as a secondary diagnosis. If the patient is admitted with a localized infection, such as pneumonia, and sepsis/severe sepsis doesn't develop until after admission, the localized infection should be assigned first, followed by the appropriate sepsis/severe sepsis codes.

5) Sepsis due to a postprocedural infection

(a) Documentation of causal relationship

As with all postprocedural complications, code assignment is based on the provider's documentation of the relationship between the infection and the procedure.

(b) Sepsis due to a postprocedural infection

For such cases, the postprocedural infection code, such as, T80.2, Infections following infusion, transfusion, and therapeutic injection, T81.4, Infection following a procedure, T88.0, Infection following immunization, or O86.0, Infection of obstetric surgical wound, should be coded first, followed by the code for the specific infection. If the patient has severe sepsis the appropriate code from subcategory R65.2 should also be assigned with the additional code(s) for any acute organ dysfunction.

(c) Postprocedural infection and postprocedural septic shock

In cases where a postprocedural infection has occurred and has resulted in severe sepsis and postprocedural septic shock, the code for the precipitating complication such as code T81.4, Infection following a procedure, or O86.0, Infection of obstetrical surgical wound should be coded first followed by code R65.21, Severe sepsis with septic shock and a code for the systemic infection.

6) Sepsis and severe sepsis associated with a noninfectious process (condition)

In some cases a noninfectious process (condition), such as trauma, may lead to an infection which can result in sepsis or severe sepsis. If sepsis or severe sepsis is documented as associated with a noninfectious condition, such as a burn or serious injury, and this condition meets the definition for principal diagnosis, the code for the noninfectious condition should be sequenced first, followed by the code for the resulting infection. If severe sepsis, is present a code from subcategory R65.2 should also be assigned with any associated organ dysfunction(s) codes. It is not necessary to assign a code from subcategory R65.1, Systemic inflammatory response syndrome (SIRS) of non-infectious origin, for these cases.

If the infection meets the definition of principal diagnosis it should be sequenced before the non-infectious condition. When both the associated non-infectious condition and the infection meet the definition of principal diagnosis either may be assigned as principal diagnosis.

Only one code from category R65, Symptoms and signs specifically associated with systemic inflammation and infection, should be assigned. Therefore, when a non-infectious condition leads to an infection resulting in severe sepsis, assign the appropriate code from subcategory R65.2, Severe sepsis. Do not additionally assign a code from subcategory R65.1, Systemic inflammatory response syndrome (SIRS) of non-infectious origin.

See Section I.C.18. SIRS due to non-infectious process

7) Sepsis and septic shock complicating abortion, pregnancy, childbirth, and the puerperium

See Section I.C.15. Sepsis and septic shock complicating abortion, pregnancy, childbirth and the puerperium

8) Newborn sepsis

See Section I.C.16. f. Bacterial sepsis of Newborn

e. Methicillin Resistant *Staphylococcus aureus* (MRSA) Conditions

1) Selection and sequencing of MRSA codes

(a) Combination codes for MRSA infection

When a patient is diagnosed with an infection that is due to methicillin resistant *Staphylococcus aureus* (MRSA), and that infection has a combination code that includes the causal organism (e.g., sepsis, pneumonia) assign the appropriate combination code for the condition (e.g., code A41.02, Sepsis due to Methicillin resistant Staphylococcus aureus or code J15.212, Pneumonia due to Methicillin resistant Staphylococcus aureus). Do not assign code B95.62, Methicillin resistant Staphylococcus aureus infection as the cause of diseases classified elsewhere, as an additional code because the combination code includes the type of infection and the MRSA organism. Do not assign a code from subcategory Z16.11, Resistance to penicillins, as an additional diagnosis.

*See Section C.1. for instructions on coding and sequencing of **sepsis and severe sepsis**.*

(b) Other codes for MRSA infection

When there is documentation of a current infection (e.g., wound infection, stitch abscess, urinary tract infection) due to MRSA, and that infection does not have a combination code that includes the causal organism, assign the appropriate code to identify the condition along with code B95.62, Methicillin resistant Staphylococcus aureus infection as the cause of diseases classified elsewhere for the MRSA infection. Do not assign a code from subcategory Z16.11, Resistance to penicillins.

(c) Methicillin susceptible Staphylococcus aureus (MSSA) and MRSA colonization

The condition or state of being colonized or carrying MSSA or MRSA is called colonization or carriage, while an individual person is described as being colonized or being a carrier. Colonization means that MSSA or MSRA is present on or in the body without necessarily causing illness. A positive MRSA colonization test might be documented by the provider as "MRSA screen positive" or "MRSA nasal swab positive".

Assign code Z22.322, Carrier or suspected carrier of Methicillin resistant Staphylococcus aureus, for patients documented as having MRSA colonization. Assign code Z22.321, Carrier or suspected carrier of Methicillin susceptible Staphylococcus aureus, for patient documented as having MSSA colonization. Colonization is not necessarily indicative of a disease process or as the cause of a specific condition the patient may have unless documented as such by the provider.

(d) MRSA colonization and infection

If a patient is documented as having both MRSA colonization and infection during a hospital admission, code Z22.322, Carrier or suspected carrier of Methicillin resistant Staphylococcus aureus, and a code for the MRSA infection may both be assigned.

2. **Chapter 2: Neoplasms (C00-D49)**
   General guidelines
   Chapter 2 of the ICD-10-CM contains the codes for most benign and all malignant neoplasms. Certain benign neoplasms, such as prostatic adenomas, may be found in the specific body system chapters. To properly code a neoplasm it is necessary to determine from the record if the neoplasm is benign, in-situ, malignant, or of uncertain histologic behavior. If malignant, any secondary (metastatic) sites should also be determined.

   Primary malignant neoplasms overlapping site boundaries
   A primary malignant neoplasm that overlaps two or more contiguous (next to each other) sites should be classified to the subcategory/code .8 ('overlapping lesion'), unless the combination is specifically indexed elsewhere. For multiple neoplasms of the same site that are not contiguous such as tumors in different quadrants of the same breast, codes for each site should be assigned.

   Malignant neoplasm of ectopic tissue
   Malignant neoplasms of ectopic tissue are to be coded to the site mentioned, e.g., ectopic pancreatic malignant neoplasms are coded to pancreas, unspecified (C25.9).

   The neoplasm table in the Alphabetic Index should be referenced first. However, if the histological term is documented, that term should be referenced first, rather than going immediately to the Neoplasm Table, in order to determine which column in the Neoplasm Table is appropriate. For example, if the documentation indicates "adenoma," refer to the term in the Alphabetic Index to review the entries under this term and the instructional note to "see also neoplasm, by site, benign." The table provides the proper code based on the type of neoplasm and the site. It is important to select the proper column in the table that corresponds to the type of neoplasm. The Tabular List should then be referenced to verify that the correct code has been selected from the table and that a more specific site code does not exist.

   See Section I.C.21. Factors influencing health status and contact with health services, Status, for information regarding Z15.0, codes for genetic susceptibility to cancer.

   a. **Treatment directed at the malignancy**
   If the treatment is directed at the malignancy, designate the malignancy as the principal diagnosis.
   The only exception to this guideline is if a patient admission/encounter is solely for the administration of chemotherapy, immunotherapy or radiation therapy, assign the appropriate Z51.— code as the first-listed or principal diagnosis, and the diagnosis or problem for which the service is being performed as a secondary diagnosis.

   b. **Treatment of secondary site**
   When a patient is admitted because of a primary neoplasm with metastasis and treatment is directed toward the secondary site only, the secondary neoplasm is designated as the principal diagnosis even though the primary malignancy is still present.

   c. **Coding and sequencing of complications**
   Coding and sequencing of complications associated with the malignancies or with the therapy thereof are subject to the following guidelines:

   1) **Anemia associated with malignancy**
   When admission/encounter is for management of an anemia associated with the malignancy, and the treatment is only for anemia, the appropriate code for the malignancy is sequenced as the principal or first-listed diagnosis followed by **the appropriate code for the anemia (such as** code D63.0, Anemia in neoplastic disease**).**

2) Anemia associated with chemotherapy, immunotherapy and radiation therapy

When the admission/encounter is for management of an anemia associated with an adverse effect **of the administration** of chemotherapy or immunotherapy and the only treatment is for the anemia, **the anemia code is sequenced first** followed by the appropriate codes for the neoplasm **and the adverse effect (T45.1X5, Adverse effect of antineoplastic and immunosuppressive drugs).**

When the admission/encounter is for management of an anemia associated with an adverse effect of radiotherapy, the anemia code should be sequenced first, followed by the appropriate neoplasm code and code Y84.2, Radiological procedure and radiotherapy as the cause of abnormal reaction of the patient, or of later complication, without mention of misadventure at the time of the procedure.

3) Management of dehydration due to the malignancy

When the admission/encounter is for management of dehydration due to the malignancy, and only the dehydration is being treated (intravenous rehydration), the dehydration is sequenced first, followed by the code(s) for the malignancy.

4) Treatment of a complication resulting from a surgical procedure

When the admission/encounter is for treatment of a complication resulting from a surgical procedure, designate the complication as the principal or first-listed diagnosis if treatment is directed at resolving the complication.

d. Primary malignancy previously excised

When a primary malignancy has been previously excised or eradicated from its site and there is no further treatment directed to that site and there is no evidence of any existing primary malignancy, a code from category Z85, Personal history of malignant neoplasm, should be used to indicate the former site of the malignancy. Any mention of extension, invasion, or metastasis to another site is coded as a secondary malignant neoplasm to that site. The secondary site may be the principal or first-listed with the Z85 code used as a secondary code.

e. Admissions/Encounters involving chemotherapy, immunotherapy and radiation therapy

1) Episode of care involves surgical removal of neoplasm

When an episode of care involves the surgical removal of a neoplasm, primary or secondary site, followed by adjunct chemotherapy or radiation treatment during the same episode of care, the code for the neoplasm should be assigned as principal or first-listed diagnosis.

2) Patient admission/encounter solely for administration of chemotherapy, immunotherapy and radiation therapy

If a patient admission/encounter is solely for the administration of chemotherapy, immunotherapy or radiation therapy assign code Z51.0, Encounter for antineoplastic radiation therapy, or Z51.11, Encounter for antineoplastic chemotherapy, or Z51.12, Encounter for antineoplastic immunotherapy as the first-listed or principal diagnosis. If a patient receives more than one of these therapies during the same admission more than one of these codes may be assigned, in any sequence.

The malignancy for which the therapy is being administered should be assigned as a secondary diagnosis.

3) Patient admitted for radiation therapy, chemotherapy or immunotherapy and develops complications

When a patient is admitted for the purpose of radiotherapy, immunotherapy or chemotherapy and develops complications such as uncontrolled nausea and vomiting or dehydration, the principal or first-listed diagnosis is Z51.0, Encounter for antineoplastic radiation therapy, or Z51.11, Encounter for antineoplastic chemotherapy, or Z51.12, Encounter for antineoplastic immunotherapy followed by any codes for the complications.

f. Admission/encounter to determine extent of malignancy

When the reason for admission/encounter is to determine the extent of the malignancy, or for a procedure such as paracentesis or thoracentesis, the primary malignancy or appropriate metastatic site is designated as the principal or first-listed diagnosis, even though chemotherapy or radiotherapy is administered.

g. Symptoms, signs, and abnormal findings listed in Chapter 18 associated with neoplasms

Symptoms, signs, and ill-defined conditions listed in Chapter 18 characteristic of, or associated with, an existing primary or secondary site malignancy cannot be used to replace the malignancy as principal or first-listed diagnosis, regardless of the number of admissions or encounters for treatment and care of the neoplasm.

See section I.C.21. Factors influencing health status and contact with health services, Encounter for prophylactic organ removal.

h. Admission/encounter for pain control/management

See Section I.C.6. for information on coding admission/encounter for pain control/management.

i. Malignancy in two or more noncontiguous sites

A patient may have more than one malignant tumor in the same organ. These tumors may represent different primaries or metastatic disease, depending on the site. Should the documentation be unclear, the provider should be queried as to the status of each tumor so that the correct codes can be assigned.

j. Disseminated malignant neoplasm, unspecified

Code C80.0, Disseminated malignant neoplasm, unspecified, is for use only in those cases where the patient has advanced metastatic disease and no known primary or secondary sites are specified. It should not be used in place of assigning codes for the primary site and all known secondary sites.

k. Malignant neoplasm without specification of site

Code C80.1, Malignant (primary) neoplasm, unspecified, equates to Cancer, unspecified. This code should only be used when no determination can be made as to the primary site of a malignancy. This code should rarely be used in the inpatient setting.

l. Sequencing of neoplasm codes

1) Encounter for treatment of primary malignancy

If the reason for the encounter is for treatment of a primary malignancy, assign the malignancy as the principal/first-listed diagnosis. The primary site is to be sequenced first, followed by any metastatic sites.

2) Encounter for treatment of secondary malignancy

When an encounter is for a primary malignancy with metastasis and treatment is directed toward the metastatic (secondary) site(s) only, the metastatic site(s) is designated as the principal/first-listed diagnosis. The primary malignancy is coded as an additional code.

3) Malignant neoplasm in a pregnant patient

When a pregnant woman has a malignant neoplasm, a code from subcategory O9A.1-, Malignant neoplasm complicating pregnancy, childbirth, and the puerperium, should be sequenced first, followed by the appropriate code from Chapter 2 to indicate the type of neoplasm.

4) Encounter for complication associated with a neoplasm

When an encounter is for management of a complication associated with a neoplasm, such as dehydration, and the treatment is only for the complication, the complication is coded first, followed by the appropriate code(s) for the neoplasm.

The exception to this guideline is anemia. When the admission/encounter is for management of an anemia associated with the malignancy, and the treatment is only for anemia, the appropriate code for the malignancy is sequenced as the principal or first-listed diagnosis followed by code D63.0, Anemia in neoplastic disease.

5) Complication from surgical procedure for treatment of a neoplasm
When an encounter is for treatment of a complication resulting from a surgical procedure performed for the treatment of the neoplasm, designate the complication as the principal/first-listed diagnosis. See guideline regarding the coding of a current malignancy versus personal history to determine if the code for the neoplasm should also be assigned.

6) Pathologic fracture due to a neoplasm
When an encounter is for a pathological fracture due to a neoplasm, **and** the focus of treatment is the fracture, a code from subcategory M84.5, Pathological fracture in neoplastic disease, should be sequenced first, followed by the code for the neoplasm.

If the focus of treatment is the neoplasm with an associated pathological fracture, the neoplasm code should be sequenced first, followed by a code from M84.5 for the pathological fracture.

m. Current malignancy versus personal history of malignancy
When a primary malignancy has been excised but further treatment, such as an additional surgery for the malignancy, radiation therapy or chemotherapy is directed to that site, the primary malignancy code should be used until treatment is completed.

When a primary malignancy has been previously excised or eradicated from its site, there is no further treatment (of the malignancy) directed to that site, and there is no evidence of any existing primary malignancy, a code from category Z85, Personal history of malignant neoplasm, should be used to indicate the former site of the malignancy.

See Section I.C.21. Factors influencing health status and contact with health services, History (of)

n. Leukemia, Multiple Myeloma, and Malignant Plasma Cell Neoplasms in remission versus personal history
The categories for leukemia, and category C90, Multiple myeloma and malignant plasma cell neoplasms, have codes **indicating whether or not the leukemia has achieved** remission. There are also codes Z85.6, Personal history of leukemia, and Z85.79, Personal history of other malignant neoplasms of lymphoid, hematopoietic and related tissues. If the documentation is unclear, as to whether the **leukemia has achieved** remission, the provider should be queried.

See Section I.C.21. Factors influencing health status and contact with health services, History (of)

o. Aftercare following surgery for neoplasm
See Section I.C.21. Factors influencing health status and contact with health services, Aftercare

p. Follow-up care for completed treatment of a malignancy
See Section I.C.21. Factors influencing health status and contact with health services, Follow-up

q. Prophylactic organ removal for prevention of malignancy
See Section I.C. 21, Factors influencing health status and contact with health services, Prophylactic organ removal

r. Malignant neoplasm associated with transplanted organ
A malignant neoplasm of a transplanted organ should be coded as a transplant complication. Assign first the appropriate code from category T86.-, Complications of transplanted organs and tissue, followed by code C80.2, Malignant neoplasm associated with transplanted organ. Use an additional code for the specific malignancy.

3. **Chapter 3: Disease of the blood and blood-forming organs and certain disorders involving the immune mechanism (D50-D89)**
Reserved for future guideline expansion

4. Chapter 4: Endocrine, Nutritional, and Metabolic Diseases (E00-E89)

a. Diabetes mellitus

The diabetes mellitus codes are combination codes that include the type of diabetes mellitus, the body system affected, and the complications affecting that body system. As many codes within a particular category as are necessary to describe all of the complications of the disease may be used. They should be sequenced based on the reason for a particular encounter. Assign as many codes from categories E08 – E13 as needed to identify all of the associated conditions that the patient has.

1) Type of diabetes

The age of a patient is not the sole determining factor, though most type 1 diabetics develop the condition before reaching puberty. For this reason type 1 diabetes mellitus is also referred to as juvenile diabetes.

2) Type of diabetes mellitus not documented

If the type of diabetes mellitus is not documented in the medical record the default is E11.-, Type 2 diabetes mellitus.

3) Diabetes mellitus and the use of insulin

If the documentation in a medical record does not indicate the type of diabetes but does indicate that the patient uses insulin, code E11, Type 2 diabetes mellitus, should be assigned. Code Z79.4, Long-term (current) use of insulin, should also be assigned to indicate that the patient uses insulin. Code Z79.4 should not be assigned if insulin is given temporarily to bring a type 2 patient's blood sugar under control during an encounter.

4) Diabetes mellitus in pregnancy and gestational diabetes

See Section I.C.15. Diabetes mellitus in pregnancy.
See Section I.C.15. Gestational (pregnancy induced) diabetes

5) Complications due to insulin pump malfunction

(a) Underdose of insulin due to insulin pump failure

An underdose of insulin due to an insulin pump failure should be assigned to a code from subcategory T85.6, Mechanical complication of other specified internal and external prosthetic devices, implants and grafts, that specifies the type of pump malfunction, as the principal or first-listed code, followed by code T38.3x6-, Underdosing of insulin and oral hypoglycemic [antidiabetic] drugs. Additional codes for the type of diabetes mellitus and any associated complications due to the underdosing should also be assigned.

(b) Overdose of insulin due to insulin pump failure

The principal or first-listed code for an encounter due to an insulin pump malfunction resulting in an overdose of insulin, should also be T85.6-, Mechanical complication of other specified internal and external prosthetic devices, implants and grafts, followed by code T38.3x1-, Poisoning by insulin and oral hypoglycemic [antidiabetic] drugs, accidental (unintentional).

6) Secondary diabetes mellitus

Codes under categories E08, Diabetes mellitus due to underlying condition, and E09, Drug or chemical induced diabetes mellitus, identify complications/manifestations associated with secondary diabetes mellitus. Secondary diabetes is always caused by another condition or event (e.g., cystic fibrosis, malignant neoplasm of pancreas, pancreatectomy, adverse effect of drug, or poisoning).

(a) Secondary diabetes mellitus and the use of insulin

For patients who routinely use insulin, code Z79.4, Long-term (current) use of insulin, should also be assigned. Code Z79.4 should not be assigned if insulin is given temporarily to bring a patient's blood sugar under control during an encounter.

(b) Assigning and sequencing secondary diabetes codes and its causes

The sequencing of the secondary diabetes codes in relationship to codes for the cause of the diabetes is based on the Tabular List instructions for categories E08 and E09. For example, for category E08, Diabetes mellitus due to underlying condition, code first the underlying condition; for category E09, Drug or chemical induced diabetes mellitus, code first the drug or chemical (T36-T65).

> **(i) Secondary diabetes mellitus due to pancreatectomy**
> For postpancreatectomy diabetes mellitus (lack of insulin due to the surgical removal of all or part of the pancreas), assign code E89.1, Postprocedural hypoinsulinemia. Assign a code from category E13 and a code from subcategory Z90.41-, Acquired absence of pancreas, as additional codes.

> **(ii) Secondary diabetes due to drugs**
> Secondary diabetes may be caused by an adverse effect of correctly administered medications, poisoning or **sequela** of poisoning.

See section I.C.19.e for coding of adverse effects and poisoning, and section I.C.20 for external cause code reporting.

5. **Chapter 5: Mental, Behavioral and *Neurodevelopmental* disorders (F01 – F99)**

   a. **Pain disorders related to psychological factors**
   Assign code F45.41, for pain that is exclusively **related to psychological disorders. As indicated by the Excludes 1 note under category G89, a code from category G89 should not be assigned with code F45.41**

   Code F45.42, Pain disorders with related psychological factors, should be used with a code from category G89, Pain, not elsewhere classified, if there is documentation of a psychological component for a patient with acute or chronic pain.
   See Section I.C.6. Pain

   b. **Mental and behavioral disorders due to psychoactive substance use**

      1) **In Remission**
      Selection of codes for "in remission" for categories F10-F19, Mental and behavioral disorders due to psychoactive substance use (categories F10-F19 with -.21) requires the provider's clinical judgment. The appropriate codes for "in remission" are assigned only on the basis of provider documentation (as defined in the Official Guidelines for Coding and Reporting).

      2) **Psychoactive Substance Use, Abuse And Dependence**
      When the provider documentation refers to use, abuse and dependence of the same substance (e.g. alcohol, opioid, cannabis, etc.), only one code should be assigned to identify the pattern of use based on the following hierarchy:
      - If both use and abuse are documented, assign only the code for abuse
      - If both abuse and dependence are documented, assign only the code for dependence
      - If use, abuse and dependence are all documented, assign only the code for dependence
      - If both use and dependence are documented, assign only the code for dependence.

      3) **Psychoactive Substance Use**
      As with all other diagnoses, the codes for psychoactive substance use (F10.9-, F11.9-, F12.9-, F13.9-, F14.9-, F15.9-, F16.9-) should only be assigned based on provider documentation and when they meet the definition of a reportable diagnosis (see Section III, Reporting Additional Diagnoses). The codes are to be used only when the psychoactive substance use is associated with a mental or behavioral disorder, and such a relationship is documented by the provider.

6. **Chapter 6: Diseases of the Nervous System (G00-G99)**

   a. **Dominant/nondominant side**
   Codes from category G81, Hemiplegia and hemiparesis, and subcategories, G83.1, Monoplegia of lower limb, G83.2, Monoplegia of upper limb, and G83.3, Monoplegia, unspecified, identify whether the dominant or nondominant side is affected. Should the affected side be documented, but not specified as

dominant or nondominant, and the classification system does not indicate a default, code selection is as follows:

- For ambidextrous patients, the default should be dominant.
- If the left side is affected, the default is non-dominant.
- If the right side is affected, the default is dominant.

b. Pain - Category G89

1) General coding information

Codes in category G89, Pain, not elsewhere classified, may be used in conjunction with codes from other categories and chapters to provide more detail about acute or chronic pain and neoplasm-related pain, unless otherwise indicated below.

If the pain is not specified as acute or chronic, post-thoracotomy, postprocedural, or neoplasm-related, do not assign codes from category G89.

A code from category G89 should not be assigned if the underlying (definitive) diagnosis is known, unless the reason for the encounter is pain control/management and not management of the underlying condition.

When an admission or encounter is for a procedure aimed at treating the underlying condition (e.g., spinal fusion, kyphoplasty), a code for the underlying condition (e.g., vertebral fracture, spinal stenosis) should be assigned as the principal diagnosis. No code from category G89 should be assigned.

(a) Category G89 Codes as Principal or First-Listed Diagnosis

Category G89 codes are acceptable as principal diagnosis or the first-listed code:

- When pain control or pain management is the reason for the admission/encounter (e.g., a patient with displaced intervertebral disc, nerve impingement and severe back pain presents for injection of steroid into the spinal canal). The underlying cause of the pain should be reported as an additional diagnosis, if known.
- When a patient is admitted for the insertion of a neurostimulator for pain control, assign the appropriate pain code as the principal or first-listed diagnosis. When an admission or encounter is for a procedure aimed at treating the underlying condition and a neurostimulator is inserted for pain control during the same admission/encounter, a code for the underlying condition should be assigned as the principal diagnosis and the appropriate pain code should be assigned as a secondary diagnosis.

(b) Use of Category G89 Codes in Conjunction with Site Specific Pain Codes

(i) Assigning Category G89 and Site-Specific Pain Codes

Codes from category G89 may be used in conjunction with codes that identify the site of pain (including codes from chapter 18) if the category G89 code provides additional information. For example, if the code describes the site of the pain, but does not fully describe whether the pain is acute or chronic, then both codes should be assigned.

(ii) Sequencing of Category G89 Codes with Site-Specific Pain Codes

The sequencing of category G89 codes with site-specific pain codes (including chapter 18 codes), is dependent on the circumstances of the encounter/admission as follows:

- If the encounter is for pain control or pain management, assign the code from category G89 followed by the code identifying the specific site of pain (e.g., encounter for pain management for acute neck pain from trauma is assigned code G89.11, Acute pain due to trauma, followed by code M54.2, Cervicalgia, to identify the site of pain).
- If the encounter is for any other reason except pain control or pain management, and a related definitive diagnosis has not been established (confirmed) by the provider, assign the code for the specific site of pain first, followed by the appropriate code from category G89.

2) Pain due to devices, implants and grafts

See Section I.C.19. Pain due to medical devices

3) Postoperative Pain

The provider's documentation should be used to guide the coding of postoperative pain, as well as *Section III. Reporting Additional Diagnoses* and *Section IV. Diagnostic Coding and Reporting in the Outpatient Setting.*

The default for post-thoracotomy and other postoperative pain not specified as acute or chronic is the code for the acute form.

Routine or expected postoperative pain immediately after surgery should not be coded.

(a) Postoperative pain not associated with specific postoperative complication

Postoperative pain not associated with a specific postoperative complication is assigned to the appropriate postoperative pain code in category G89.

(b) Postoperative pain associated with specific postoperative complication

Postoperative pain associated with a specific postoperative complication (such as painful wire sutures) is assigned to the appropriate code(s) found in Chapter 19, Injury, poisoning, and certain other consequences of external causes. If appropriate, use additional code(s) from category G89 to identify acute or chronic pain (G89.18 or G89.28).

4) Chronic pain

Chronic pain is classified to subcategory G89.2. There is no time frame defining when pain becomes chronic pain. The provider's documentation should be used to guide use of these codes.

5) Neoplasm Related Pain

Code G89.3 is assigned to pain documented as being related, associated or due to cancer, primary or secondary malignancy, or tumor. This code is assigned regardless of whether the pain is acute or chronic.

This code may be assigned as the principal or first-listed code when the stated reason for the admission/encounter is documented as pain control/pain management. The underlying neoplasm should be reported as an additional diagnosis.

When the reason for the admission/encounter is management of the neoplasm and the pain associated with the neoplasm is also documented, code G89.3 may be assigned as an additional diagnosis. It is not necessary to assign an additional code for the site of the pain.

See Section I.C.2 for instructions on the sequencing of neoplasms for all other stated reasons for the admission/encounter (except for pain control/pain management).

6) Chronic pain syndrome

Central pain syndrome (G89.0) and chronic pain syndrome (G89.4) are different than the term "chronic pain," and therefore codes should only be used when the provider has specifically documented this condition.

See Section I.C.5. Pain disorders related to psychological factors

7. Chapter 7: Diseases of the Eye and Adnexa (H00-H59)

a. Glaucoma

1) Assigning Glaucoma Codes

Assign as many codes from category H40, Glaucoma, as needed to identify the type of glaucoma, the affected eye, and the glaucoma stage.

2) Bilateral glaucoma with same type and stage

When a patient has bilateral glaucoma and both eyes are documented as being the same type and stage, and there is a code for bilateral glaucoma, report only the code for the type of glaucoma, bilateral, with the seventh character for the stage.

When a patient has bilateral glaucoma and both eyes are documented as being the same type and stage, and the classification does not provide a code for bilateral glaucoma (i.e. subcategories H40.10, H40.11 and H40.20) report only one code for the type of glaucoma with the appropriate seventh character for the stage.

3) Bilateral glaucoma stage with different types or stages

When a patient has bilateral glaucoma and each eye is documented as having a different type or stage, and the classification distinguishes laterality, assign the appropriate code for each eye rather than the code for bilateral glaucoma.

When a patient has bilateral glaucoma and each eye is documented as having a different type, and the classification does not distinguish laterality (i.e. subcategories H40.10, H40.11 and H40.20), assign one code for each type of glaucoma with the appropriate seventh character for the stage.

When a patient has bilateral glaucoma and each eye is documented as having the same type, but different stage, and the classification does not distinguish laterality (i.e. subcategories H40.10, H40.11 and H40.20), assign a code for the type of glaucoma for each eye with the seventh character for the specific glaucoma stage documented for each eye.

4) Patient admitted with glaucoma and stage evolves during the admission

If a patient is admitted with glaucoma and the stage progresses during the admission, assign the code for highest stage documented.

5) Indeterminate stage glaucoma

Assignment of the seventh character "4" for "indeterminate stage" should be based on the clinical documentation. The seventh character "4" is used for glaucomas whose stage cannot be clinically determined. This seventh character should not be confused with the seventh character "0", unspecified, which should be assigned when there is no documentation regarding the stage of the glaucoma.

8. **Chapter 8: Diseases of the Ear and Mastoid Process (H60-H95)**
   Reserved for future guideline expansion

9. **Chapter 9: Diseases of the Circulatory System (I00-I99)**

   a. **Hypertension**

      1) Hypertension with Heart Disease

Heart conditions classified to I50.- or I51.4-I51.9, are assigned to, a code from category I11, Hypertensive heart disease, when a causal relationship is stated (due to hypertension) or implied (hypertensive). Use an additional code from category I50, Heart failure, to identify the type of heart failure in those patients with heart failure.

The same heart conditions (I50.-, I51.4-I51.9) with hypertension, but without a stated causal relationship, are coded separately. Sequence according to the circumstances of the admission/encounter.

2) Hypertensive Chronic Kidney Disease

Assign codes from category I12, Hypertensive chronic kidney disease, when both hypertension and a condition classifiable to category N18, Chronic kidney disease (CKD), are present. Unlike hypertension with heart disease, ICD-10-CM presumes a cause-and-effect relationship and classifies chronic kidney disease with hypertension as hypertensive chronic kidney disease.

The appropriate code from category N18 should be used as a secondary code with a code from category I12 to identify the stage of chronic kidney disease.
See Section I.C.14. Chronic kidney disease.

If a patient has hypertensive chronic kidney disease and acute renal failure, an additional code for the acute renal failure is required.

3) Hypertensive Heart and Chronic Kidney Disease

Assign codes from combination category I13, Hypertensive heart and chronic kidney disease, when both hypertensive kidney disease and hypertensive heart disease are stated in the diagnosis. Assume a relationship between the hypertension and the chronic kidney disease, whether or not the condition is so designated. If heart failure is present, assign an additional code from category I50 to identify the type of heart failure.

The appropriate code from category N18, Chronic kidney disease, should be used as a secondary code with a code from category I13 to identify the stage of chronic kidney disease.
See Section I.C.14. Chronic kidney disease.

The codes in category I13, Hypertensive heart and chronic kidney disease, are combination codes that include hypertension, heart disease and chronic kidney disease. The Includes note at I13 specifies that the conditions included at I11 and I12 are included together in I13. If a patient has hypertension, heart disease and chronic kidney disease then a code from I13 should be used, not individual codes for hypertension, heart disease and chronic kidney disease, or codes from I11 or I12.

For patients with both acute renal failure and chronic kidney disease an additional code for acute renal failure is required.

4) Hypertensive Cerebrovascular Disease

For hypertensive cerebrovascular disease, first assign the appropriate code from categories I60-I69, followed by the appropriate hypertension code.

5) Hypertensive Retinopathy

Subcategory H35.0, Background retinopathy and retinal vascular changes, should be used with **a** code **from category** I10 – I15, **Hypertensive disease** to include the systemic hypertension. The sequencing is based on the reason for the encounter.

6) Hypertension, Secondary

Secondary hypertension is due to an underlying condition. Two codes are required: one to identify the underlying etiology and one from category I15 to identify the hypertension. Sequencing of codes is determined by the reason for admission/encounter.

7) Hypertension, Transient

Assign code R03.0, Elevated blood pressure reading without diagnosis of hypertension, unless patient has an established diagnosis of hypertension. Assign code O13.-, Gestational [pregnancy-induced] hypertension without significant proteinuria, or O14.-, Pre-eclampsia, for transient hypertension of pregnancy.

8) Hypertension, Controlled

This diagnostic statement usually refers to an existing state of hypertension under control by therapy. Assign the appropriate code from categories I10-I15, Hypertensive diseases.

9) Hypertension, Uncontrolled

Uncontrolled hypertension may refer to untreated hypertension or hypertension not responding to current therapeutic regimen. In either case, assign the appropriate code from categories I10-I15, Hypertensive diseases.

b. Atherosclerotic Coronary Artery Disease and Angina

ICD-10-CM has combination codes for atherosclerotic heart disease with angina pectoris. The subcategories for these codes are I25.11, Atherosclerotic heart disease of native coronary artery with angina pectoris and I25.7, Atherosclerosis of coronary artery bypass graft(s) and coronary artery of transplanted heart with angina pectoris.

When using one of these combination codes it is not necessary to use an additional code for angina pectoris. A causal relationship can be assumed in a patient with both atherosclerosis and angina pectoris, unless the documentation indicates the angina is due to something other than the atherosclerosis.

If a patient with coronary artery disease is admitted due to an acute myocardial infarction (AMI), the AMI should be sequenced before the coronary artery disease.

See Section I.C.9. Acute myocardial infarction (AMI)

c. Intraoperative and Postprocedural Cerebrovascular Accident

Medical record documentation should clearly specify the cause-and-effect relationship between the medical intervention and the cerebrovascular accident in order to assign a code for intraoperative or postprocedural cerebrovascular accident.

Proper code assignment depends on whether it was an infarction or hemorrhage and whether it occurred intraoperatively or postoperatively. If it was a cerebral hemorrhage, code assignment depends on the type of procedure performed.

GUIDELINES (ICD-10-CM)

d. Sequelae of Cerebrovascular Disease

1) Category I69, Sequelae of Cerebrovascular disease

Category I69 is used to indicate conditions classifiable to categories I60-I67 as the causes of **sequela** (neurologic deficits), themselves classified elsewhere. These "late effects" include neurologic deficits that persist after initial onset of conditions classifiable to categories I60-I67. The neurologic deficits caused by cerebrovascular disease may be present from the onset or may arise at any time after the onset of the condition classifiable to categories I60-I67.

2) Codes from category I69 with codes from I60-I67

Codes from category I69 may be assigned on a health care record with codes from I60-I67, if the patient has a current cerebrovascular disease and deficits from an old cerebrovascular disease.

3) Code Z86.73

Assign code Z86.73, Personal history of transient ischemic attack (TIA), and cerebral infarction without residual deficits (and not a code from category I69) as an additional code for history of cerebrovascular disease when no neurologic deficits are present.

e. Acute myocardial infarction (AMI)

1) ST elevation myocardial infarction (STEMI) and non ST elevation myocardial infarction (NSTEMI)

The ICD-10-CM codes for acute myocardial infarction (AMI) identify the site, such as anterolateral wall or true posterior wall. Subcategories I21.0-I21.2 and code I21.**3** are used for ST elevation myocardial infarction (STEMI). Code I21.4, Non-ST elevation (NSTEMI) myocardial infarction, is used for non ST elevation myocardial infarction (NSTEMI) and nontransmural MIs.

If NSTEMI evolves to STEMI, assign the STEMI code. If STEMI converts to NSTEMI due to thrombolytic therapy, it is still coded as STEMI.

For encounters occurring while the myocardial infarction is equal to, or less than, four weeks old, including transfers to another acute setting or a postacute setting, and the patient requires continued care for the myocardial infarction, codes from category I21 may continue to be reported. For encounters after the 4 week time frame and the patient **is still receiving** care related to the myocardial infarction, the appropriate aftercare code should be assigned, rather than a code from category I21. **For old or healed myocardial infarctions not requiring further care,** code I25.2, Old myocardial infarction, may be assigned.

2) Acute myocardial infarction, unspecified

Code I21.3, ST elevation (STEMI) myocardial infarction of unspecified site, is the default for unspecified acute myocardial infarction. If only STEMI or transmural MI without the site is documented, assign code I21.3.

3) AMI documented as nontransmural or subendocardial but site provided

If an AMI is documented as nontransmural or subendocardial, but the site is provided, it is still coded as a subendocardial AMI.

See Section I.C.21.3 for information on coding status post administration of tPA in a different facility within the last 24 hours.

4) Subsequent acute myocardial infarction

A code from category I22, Subsequent ST elevation (STEMI) and non ST elevation (NSTEMI) myocardial infarction, is to be used when a patient who has suffered an AMI has a new AMI within the 4 week time frame of the initial AMI. A code from category I22 must be used in conjunction with a code from category I21. The sequencing of the I22 and I21 codes depends on the circumstances of the encounter.

10. Chapter 10: Diseases of *the* Respiratory System (J00-J99)

a. Chronic Obstructive Pulmonary Disease [COPD] and Asthma

1) Acute exacerbation of chronic obstructive bronchitis and asthma

The codes in categories J44 and J45 distinguish between uncomplicated cases and those in acute exacerbation. An acute exacerbation is a worsening or a decompensation of a chronic condition. An acute exacerbation is not equivalent to an infection superimposed on a chronic condition, though an exacerbation may be triggered by an infection.

b. Acute Respiratory Failure

1) Acute respiratory failure as principal diagnosis

A code from subcategory J96.0, Acute respiratory failure, or subcategory J96.2, Acute and chronic respiratory failure, may be assigned as a principal diagnosis when it is the condition established after study to be chiefly responsible for occasioning the admission to the hospital, and the selection is supported by the Alphabetic Index and Tabular List. However, chapter-specific coding guidelines (such as obstetrics, poisoning, HIV, newborn) that provide sequencing direction take precedence.

2) Acute respiratory failure as secondary diagnosis

Respiratory failure may be listed as a secondary diagnosis if it occurs after admission, or if it is present on admission, but does not meet the definition of principal diagnosis.

3) Sequencing of acute respiratory failure and another acute condition

When a patient is admitted with respiratory failure and another acute condition, (e.g., myocardial infarction, cerebrovascular accident, aspiration pneumonia), the principal diagnosis will not be the same in every situation. This applies whether the other acute condition is a respiratory or nonrespiratory condition. Selection of the principal diagnosis will be dependent on the circumstances of admission. If both the respiratory failure and the other acute condition are equally responsible for occasioning the admission to the hospital, and there are no chapter-specific sequencing rules, the guideline regarding two or more diagnoses that equally meet the definition for principal diagnosis *(Section II, C.)* may be applied in these situations.

If the documentation is not clear as to whether acute respiratory failure and another condition are equally responsible for occasioning the admission, query the provider for clarification.

c. Influenza due to certain identified influenza viruses

Code only confirmed cases of influenza **due to certain identified influenza viruses (category J09)**. This is an exception to the hospital inpatient guideline Section II, H. (Uncertain Diagnosis).

In this context, "confirmation" does not require documentation of positive laboratory testing specific for avian or **other** novel H1N1 (H1N1 or swine flu) influenza **A**. However, coding should be based on the provider's diagnostic statement that the patient has avian influenza, **or other novel influenza A**.

If the provider records "suspected or possible or probable avian influenza," the appropriate influenza code from category J11, Influenza due to **unidentified** influenza virus, should be assigned. A code from category J09, Influenza due to certain identified influenza viruses, should not be assigned.

d. Ventilator associated Pneumonia

1) Documentation of Ventilator associated Pneumonia

As with all procedural or postprocedural complications, code assignment is based on the provider's documentation of the relationship between the condition and the procedure.

Code J95.851, Ventilator associated pneumonia, should be assigned only when the provider has documented ventilator associated pneumonia (VAP). An additional code to identify the organism (e.g., Pseudomonas aeruginosa, code B96.5) should also be assigned. Do not assign an additional code from categories J12-J18 to identify the type of pneumonia.

Code J95.851 should not be assigned for cases where the patient has pneumonia and is on a mechanical ventilator **and** the provider has not specifically stated that the pneumonia is ventilator-associated pneumonia. If the documentation is unclear as to whether the patient has a pneumonia that is a complication attributable to the mechanical ventilator, query the provider.

2) Ventilator associated Pneumonia Develops after Admission

A patient may be admitted with one type of pneumonia (e.g., code J13, Pneumonia due to Streptococcus pneumonia) and subsequently develop VAP. In this instance, the principal diagnosis would be the appropriate code from categories J12-J18 for the pneumonia diagnosed at the time of admission. Code J95.851, Ventilator associated pneumonia, would be assigned as an additional diagnosis when the provider has also documented the presence of ventilator associated pneumonia.

11. **Chapter 11: Diseases of *the* Digestive System (K00-K95)**

Reserved for future guideline expansion

12. **Chapter 12: Diseases of *the* Skin and Subcutaneous Tissue (L00-L99)**

   a. **Pressure ulcer stage codes**

   1) Pressure ulcer stages

Codes from category L89, Pressure ulcer, are combination codes that identify the site of the pressure ulcer as well as the stage of the ulcer.

The ICD-10-CM classifies pressure ulcer stages based on severity, which is designated by stages 1-4, unspecified stage and unstageable.

Assign as many codes from category L89 as needed to identify all the pressure ulcers the patient has, if applicable.

   2) Unstageable pressure ulcers

Assignment of the code for unstageable pressure ulcer (L89.--0) should be based on the clinical documentation. These codes are used for pressure ulcers whose stage cannot be clinically determined (e.g., the ulcer is covered by eschar or has been treated with a skin or muscle graft) and pressure ulcers that are documented as deep tissue injury but not documented as due to trauma. This code should not be confused with the codes for unspecified stage (L89.--9). When there is no documentation regarding the stage of the pressure ulcer, assign the appropriate code for unspecified stage (L89.--9).

   3) Documented pressure ulcer stage

Assignment of the pressure ulcer stage code should be guided by clinical documentation of the stage or documentation of the terms found in the Alphabetic Index. For clinical terms describing the stage that are not found in the Alphabetic Index, and there is no documentation of the stage, the provider should be queried.

   4) Patients admitted with pressure ulcers documented as healed

No code is assigned if the documentation states that the pressure ulcer is completely healed.

   5) Patients admitted with pressure ulcers documented as healing

Pressure ulcers described as healing should be assigned the appropriate pressure ulcer stage code based on the documentation in the medical record. If the documentation does not provide information about the stage of the healing pressure ulcer, assign the appropriate code for unspecified stage.

If the documentation is unclear as to whether the patient has a current (new) pressure ulcer or if the patient is being treated for a healing pressure ulcer, query the provider.

   6) Patient admitted with pressure ulcer evolving into another stage during the admission

If a patient is admitted with a pressure ulcer at one stage and it progresses to a higher stage, assign the code for the highest stage reported for that site.

13. **Chapter 13: Diseases of the Musculoskeletal System and Connective Tissue (M00-M99)**

   a. **Site and laterality**

Most of the codes within Chapter 13 have site and laterality designations. The site represents the bone, joint or the muscle involved. For some conditions where more than one bone, joint or muscle is usually involved, such as osteoarthritis, there is a "multiple sites" code available. For categories where no multiple site code is provided and more than one bone, joint or muscle is involved, multiple codes should be used to indicate the different sites involved.

1) Bone versus joint
For certain conditions, the bone may be affected at the upper or lower end, (e.g., avascular necrosis of bone, M87, Osteoporosis, M80, M81). Though the portion of the bone affected may be at the joint, the site designation will be the bone, not the joint.

b. Acute traumatic versus chronic or recurrent musculoskeletal conditions
Many musculoskeletal conditions are a result of previous injury or trauma to a site, or are recurrent conditions. Bone, joint or muscle conditions that are the result of a healed injury are usually found in chapter 13. Recurrent bone, joint or muscle conditions are also usually found in chapter 13. Any current, acute injury should be coded to the appropriate injury code from chapter 19. Chronic or recurrent conditions should generally be coded with a code from chapter 13. If it is difficult to determine from the documentation in the record which code is best to describe a condition, query the provider.

c. Coding of Pathologic Fractures
7th character A is for use as long as the patient is receiving active treatment for the fracture. Examples of active treatment are: surgical treatment, emergency department encounter, evaluation and treatment by a new physician. 7th character, D is to be used for encounters after the patient has completed active treatment. The other 7th characters, listed under each subcategory in the Tabular List, are to be used for subsequent encounters for treatment of problems associated with the healing, such as malunions, nonunions, and sequelae.

Care for complications of surgical treatment for fracture repairs during the healing or recovery phase should be coded with the appropriate complication codes.

See Section I.C.19. Coding of traumatic fractures.

d. Osteoporosis
Osteoporosis is a systemic condition, meaning that all bones of the musculoskeletal system are affected. Therefore, site is not a component of the codes under category M81, Osteoporosis without current pathological fracture. The site codes under category M80, Osteoporosis with current pathological fracture, identify the site of the fracture, not the osteoporosis.

1) Osteoporosis without pathological fracture
Category M81, Osteoporosis without current pathological fracture, is for use for patients with osteoporosis who do not currently have a pathologic fracture due to the osteoporosis, even if they have had a fracture in the past. For patients with a history of osteoporosis fractures, status code Z87.310, Personal history of (healed) osteoporosis fracture, should follow the code from M81.

2) Osteoporosis with current pathological fracture
Category M80, Osteoporosis with current pathological fracture, is for patients who have a current pathologic fracture at the time of an encounter. The codes under M80 identify the site of the fracture. A code from category M80, not a traumatic fracture code, should be used for any patient with known osteoporosis who suffers a fracture, even if the patient had a minor fall or trauma, if that fall or trauma would not usually break a normal, healthy bone.

14. Chapter 14: Diseases of Genitourinary System (N00-N99)

a. Chronic kidney disease

1) Stages of chronic kidney disease (CKD)
The ICD-10-CM classifies CKD based on severity. The severity of CKD is designated by stages 1-5. Stage 2, code N18.2, equates to mild CKD; stage 3, code N18.3, equates to moderate CKD; and stage 4, code N18.4, equates to severe CKD. Code N18.6, End stage renal disease (ESRD), is assigned when the provider has documented end-stage-renal disease (ESRD).

If both a stage of CKD and ESRD are documented, assign code N18.6 only.

2) Chronic kidney disease and kidney transplant status

Patients who have undergone kidney transplant may still have some form of chronic kidney disease CKD because the kidney transplant may not fully restore kidney function. Therefore, the presence of CKD alone does not constitute a transplant complication. Assign the appropriate N18 code for the patient's stage of CKD and code Z94.0, Kidney transplant status. If a transplant complication such as failure or rejection or other transplant complication is documented, see section I.C.19.g for information on coding complications of a kidney transplant. If the documentation is unclear as to whether the patient has a complication of the transplant, query the provider.

3) Chronic kidney disease with other conditions

Patients with CKD may also suffer from other serious conditions, most commonly diabetes mellitus and hypertension. The sequencing of the CKD code in relationship to codes for other contributing conditions is based on the conventions in the Tabular List.

See I.C.9. Hypertensive chronic kidney disease.
See I.C.19. Chronic kidney disease and kidney transplant complications.

15. Chapter 15: Pregnancy, Childbirth, and the Puerperium (O00-O9A)

a. General Rules for Obstetric Cases

1) Codes from chapter 15 and sequencing priority

Obstetric cases require codes from chapter 15, codes in the range O00-O9A, Pregnancy, Childbirth, and the Puerperium. Chapter 15 codes have sequencing priority over codes from other chapters. Additional codes from other chapters may be used in conjunction with chapter 15 codes to further specify conditions. Should the provider document that the pregnancy is incidental to the encounter, then code Z33.1, Pregnant state, incidental, should be used in place of any chapter 15 codes. It is the provider's responsibility to state that the condition being treated is not affecting the pregnancy.

2) Chapter 15 codes used only on the maternal record

Chapter 15 codes are to be used only on the maternal record, never on the record of the newborn.

3) Final character for trimester

The majority of codes in Chapter 15 have a final character indicating the trimester of pregnancy. The timeframes for the trimesters are indicated at the beginning of the chapter. If trimester is not a component of a code it is because the condition always occurs in a specific trimester, or the concept of trimester of pregnancy is not applicable. Certain codes have characters for only certain trimesters because the condition does not occur in all trimesters, but it may occur in more than just one.

Assignment of the final character for trimester should be based on the provider's documentation of the trimester (or number of weeks) for the current admission/encounter. This applies to the assignment of trimester for pre-existing conditions as well as those that develop during or are due to the pregnancy. The provider's documentation of the number of weeks may be used to assign the appropriate code identifying the trimester.

Whenever delivery occurs during the current admission, and there is an "in childbirth" option for the obstetric complication being coded, the "in childbirth" code should be assigned.

4) Selection of trimester for inpatient admissions that encompass more than one trimesters

In instances when a patient is admitted to a hospital for complications of pregnancy during one trimester and remains in the hospital into a subsequent trimester, the trimester character for the antepartum complication code should be assigned on the basis of the trimester when the complication developed, not the trimester of the discharge. If the condition developed prior to the current admission/encounter or represents a pre-existing condition, the trimester character for the trimester at the time of the admission/encounter should be assigned.

5) Unspecified trimester

Each category that includes codes for trimester has a code for "unspecified trimester." The "unspecified trimester" code should rarely be used, such as when the documentation in the record is insufficient to determine the trimester and it is not possible to obtain clarification.

6) *7th character for Fetus Identification*

Where applicable, a 7th character is to be assigned for certain categories (O31, O32, O33.3 - O33.6, O35, O36, O40, O41, O60.1, O60.2, O64, and O69) to identify the fetus for which the complication code applies.

Assign 7th character "0":
- For single gestations
- When the documentation in the record is insufficient to determine the fetus affected and it is not possible to obtain clarification.
- When it is not possible to clinically determine which fetus is affected.

b. Selection of OB Principal or First-listed Diagnosis

1) Routine outpatient prenatal visits

For routine outpatient prenatal visits when no complications are present, a code from category Z34, Encounter for supervision of normal pregnancy, should be used as the first-listed diagnosis. These codes should not be used in conjunction with chapter 15 codes.

2) Prenatal outpatient visits for high-risk patients

For routine prenatal outpatient visits for patients with high-risk pregnancies, a code from category O09, Supervision of high-risk pregnancy, should be used as the first-listed diagnosis. Secondary chapter 15 codes may be used in conjunction with these codes if appropriate.

3) Episodes when no delivery occurs

In episodes when no delivery occurs, the principal diagnosis should correspond to the principal complication of the pregnancy which necessitated the encounter. Should more than one complication exist, all of which are treated or monitored, any of the complications codes may be sequenced first.

4) When a delivery occurs

When a delivery occurs, the principal diagnosis should correspond to the main circumstances or complication of the delivery. In cases of cesarean delivery, the selection of the principal diagnosis should be the condition established after study that was responsible for the patient's admission. If the patient was admitted with a condition that resulted in the performance of a cesarean procedure, that condition should be selected as the principal diagnosis. If the reason for the admission/encounter was unrelated to the condition resulting in the cesarean delivery, the condition related to the reason for the admission/encounter should be selected as the principal diagnosis.

5) Outcome of delivery

A code from category Z37, Outcome of delivery, should be included on every maternal record when a delivery has occurred. These codes are not to be used on subsequent records or on the newborn record.

c. Pre-existing conditions versus conditions due to the pregnancy

Certain categories in Chapter 15 distinguish between conditions of the mother that existed prior to pregnancy (pre-existing) and those that are a direct result of pregnancy. When assigning codes from Chapter 15, it is important to assess if a condition was pre-existing prior to pregnancy or developed during or due to the pregnancy in order to assign the correct code.

Categories that do not distinguish between pre-existing and pregnancy-related conditions may be used for either. It is acceptable to use codes specifically for the puerperium with codes complicating pregnancy and childbirth if a condition arises postpartum during the delivery encounter.

d. Pre-existing hypertension in pregnancy

Category O10, Pre-existing hypertension complicating pregnancy, childbirth and the puerperium, includes codes for hypertensive heart and hypertensive chronic kidney disease. When assigning one of the O10 codes that includes

hypertensive heart disease or hypertensive chronic kidney disease, it is necessary to add a secondary code from the appropriate hypertension category to specify the type of heart failure or chronic kidney disease.
See Section I.C.9. Hypertension.

e. Fetal Conditions Affecting the Management of the Mother

1) Codes from categories O35 and O36

Codes from categories O35, Maternal care for known or suspected fetal abnormality and damage, and O36, Maternal care for other fetal problems, are assigned only when the fetal condition is actually responsible for modifying the management of the mother, i.e., by requiring diagnostic studies, additional observation, special care, or termination of pregnancy. The fact that the fetal condition exists does not justify assigning a code from this series to the mother's record.

2) In utero surgery

In cases when surgery is performed on the fetus, a diagnosis code from category O35, Maternal care for known or suspected fetal abnormality and damage, should be assigned identifying the fetal condition. Assign the appropriate procedure code for the procedure performed.

No code from Chapter 16, the perinatal codes, should be used on the mother's record to identify fetal conditions. Surgery performed in utero on a fetus is still to be coded as an obstetric encounter.

f. HIV Infection in Pregnancy, Childbirth and the Puerperium

During pregnancy, childbirth or the puerperium, a patient admitted because of an HIV-related illness should receive a principal diagnosis from subcategory O98.7-, Human immunodeficiency [HIV] disease complicating pregnancy, childbirth and the puerperium, followed by the code(s) for the HIV-related illness(es).

Patients with asymptomatic HIV infection status admitted during pregnancy, childbirth, or the puerperium should receive codes of O98.7- and Z21, Asymptomatic human immunodeficiency virus [HIV] infection status.

g. Diabetes mellitus in pregnancy

Diabetes mellitus is a significant complicating factor in pregnancy. Pregnant women who are diabetic should be assigned a code from category O24, Diabetes mellitus in pregnancy, childbirth, and the puerperium, first, followed by the appropriate diabetes code(s) (E08-E13) from Chapter 4.

h. Long term use of insulin

Code Z79.4, Long-term (current) use of insulin, should also be assigned if the diabetes mellitus is being treated with insulin.

i. Gestational (pregnancy induced) diabetes

Gestational (pregnancy induced) diabetes can occur during the second and third trimester of pregnancy in women who were not diabetic prior to pregnancy. Gestational diabetes can cause complications in the pregnancy similar to those of pre-existing diabetes mellitus. It also puts the woman at greater risk of developing diabetes after the pregnancy. Codes for gestational diabetes are in subcategory O24.4, Gestational diabetes mellitus. No other code from category O24, Diabetes mellitus in pregnancy, childbirth, and the puerperium, should be used with a code from O24.4.

The codes under subcategory O24.4 include diet controlled and insulin controlled. If a patient with gestational diabetes is treated with both diet and insulin, only the code for insulin-controlled is required.

Code Z79.4, Long-term (current) use of insulin, should not be assigned with codes from subcategory O24.4.

An abnormal glucose tolerance in pregnancy is assigned a code from subcategory O99.81, Abnormal glucose complicating pregnancy, childbirth, and the puerperium.

j. Sepsis and septic shock complicating abortion, pregnancy, childbirth and the puerperium

When assigning a chapter 15 code for sepsis complicating abortion, pregnancy, childbirth, and the puerperium, a code for the specific type of infection should be assigned as an additional diagnosis. If severe sepsis is present, a code from subcategory R65.2, Severe sepsis, and code(s) for associated organ dysfunction(s) should also be assigned as additional diagnoses.

k. Puerperal sepsis

Code O85, Puerperal sepsis, should be assigned with a secondary code to identify the causal organism (e.g., for a bacterial infection, assign a code from category B95-B96, Bacterial infections in conditions classified elsewhere). A code from category A40, Streptococcal sepsis, or A41, Other sepsis, should not be used for puerperal sepsis. If applicable, use additional codes to identify severe sepsis (R65.2-) and any associated acute organ dysfunction.

l. Alcohol and tobacco use during pregnancy, childbirth and the puerperium

1) Alcohol use during pregnancy, childbirth and the puerperium

Codes under subcategory O99.31, Alcohol use complicating pregnancy, childbirth, and the puerperium, should be assigned for any pregnancy case when a mother uses alcohol during the pregnancy or postpartum. A secondary code from category F10, Alcohol related disorders, should also be assigned to identify manifestations of the alcohol use.

2) Tobacco use during pregnancy, childbirth and the puerperium

Codes under subcategory O99.33, Smoking (tobacco) complicating pregnancy, childbirth, and the puerperium, should be assigned for any pregnancy case when a mother uses any type of tobacco product during the pregnancy or postpartum. A secondary code from category F17, Nicotine dependence, or code Z72.0, Tobacco use, should also be assigned to identify the type of nicotine dependence.

m. Poisoning, toxic effects, adverse effects and underdosing in a pregnant patient

A code from subcategory O9A.2, Injury, poisoning and certain other consequences of external causes complicating pregnancy, childbirth, and the puerperium, should be sequenced first, followed by the appropriate **injury,** poisoning, toxic effect, adverse effect or underdosing code, and then the additional code(s) that specifies the condition caused by the poisoning, toxic effect, adverse effect or underdosing.

See Section I.C.19. Adverse effects, poisoning, underdosing and toxic effects.

n. Normal Delivery, Code O80

1) Encounter for full term uncomplicated delivery

Code O80 should be assigned when a woman is admitted for a full-term normal delivery and delivers a single, healthy infant without any complications antepartum, during the delivery, or postpartum during the delivery episode. Code O80 is always a principal diagnosis. It is not to be used if any other code from chapter 15 is needed to describe a current complication of the antenatal, delivery, or perinatal period. Additional codes from other chapters may be used with code O80 if they are not related to or are in any way complicating the pregnancy.

2) Uncomplicated delivery with resolved antepartum complication

Code O80 may be used if the patient had a complication at some point during the pregnancy, but the complication is not present at the time of the admission for delivery.

3) Outcome of delivery for O80

Z37.0, Single live birth, is the only outcome of delivery code appropriate for use with O80.

o. The Peripartum and Postpartum Periods

1) Peripartum and Postpartum periods

The postpartum period begins immediately after delivery and continues for six weeks following delivery. The peripartum period is defined as the last month of pregnancy to five months postpartum.

2) Peripartum and postpartum complication

A postpartum complication is any complication occurring within the six-week period.

3) Pregnancy-related complications after 6 week period

Chapter 15 codes may also be used to describe pregnancy-related complications after the peripartum or postpartum period if the provider documents that a condition is pregnancy related.

4) Admission for routine postpartum care following delivery outside hospital

When the mother delivers outside the hospital prior to admission and is admitted for routine postpartum care and no complications are noted, code Z39.0, Encounter for care and examination of mother immediately after delivery, should be assigned as the principal diagnosis.

5) Pregnancy associated cardiomyopathy

Pregnancy associated cardiomyopathy, code O90.3, is unique in that it may be diagnosed in the third trimester of pregnancy but may continue to progress months after delivery. For this reason, it is referred to as peripartum cardiomyopathy. Code O90.3 is only for use when the cardiomyopathy develops as a result of pregnancy in a woman who did not have pre-existing heart disease.

p. Code O94, Sequelae of complication of pregnancy, childbirth, and the puerperium

1) Code O94

Code O94, Sequelae of complication of pregnancy, childbirth, and the puerperium, is for use in those cases when an initial complication of a pregnancy develops a sequelae requiring care or treatment at a future date.

2) After the initial postpartum period

This code may be used at any time after the initial postpartum period.

3) Sequencing of Code O94

This code, like all **sequela** codes, is to be sequenced following the code describing the sequelae of the complication.

q. Abortions

1) Abortion with Liveborn Fetus

When an attempted termination of pregnancy results in a liveborn fetus assign a code from subcategory O60.1, Preterm labor with preterm delivery, and a code from category Z37, Outcome of Delivery. The procedure code for the attempted termination of pregnancy should also be assigned.

2) Retained Products of Conception following an abortion

Subsequent encounters for retained products of conception following a spontaneous abortion or elective termination of pregnancy are assigned the appropriate code from category O03, Spontaneous abortion, or codes O07.4, Failed attempted termination of pregnancy without complication and Z33.2, Encounter for elective termination of pregnancy. This advice is appropriate even when the patient was discharged previously with a discharge diagnosis of complete abortion.

r. Abuse in a pregnant patient

For suspected or confirmed cases of abuse of a pregnant patient, a code(s) from subcategories O9A.3, Physical abuse complicating pregnancy, childbirth, and the puerperium, O9A.4, Sexual abuse complicating pregnancy, childbirth, and the puerperium, and O9A.5, Psychological abuse complicating pregnancy, childbirth, and the puerperium, should be sequenced first, followed by the appropriate codes (if applicable) to identify any associated current injury due to physical abuse, sexual abuse, and the perpetrator of abuse.

See Section I.C.19. Adult and child abuse, neglect and other maltreatment.

16. **Chapter 16:** *Certain Conditions Originating in the Perinatal Period* **(P00-P96)**
    For coding and reporting purposes the perinatal period is defined as before birth through the 28th day following birth. The following guidelines are provided for reporting purposes

    a. **General Perinatal Rules**

    1) **Use of Chapter 16 Codes**
    Codes in this chapter are <u>never</u> for use on the maternal record. Codes from Chapter 15, the obstetric chapter, are never permitted on the newborn record. Chapter 16 codes may be used throughout the life of the patient if the condition is still present.

    2) **Principal Diagnosis for Birth Record**
    When coding the birth episode in a newborn record, assign a code from category Z38, Liveborn infants according to place of birth and type of delivery, as the principal diagnosis. A code from category Z38 is assigned only once, to a newborn at the time of birth. If a newborn is transferred to another institution, a code from category Z38 should not be used at the receiving hospital.

    A code from category Z38 is used only on the newborn record, not on the mother's record.

    3) **Use of Codes from other Chapters with Codes from Chapter 16**
    Codes from other chapters may be used with codes from chapter 16 if the codes from the other chapters provide more specific detail. Codes for signs and symptoms may be assigned when a definitive diagnosis has not been established. If the reason for the encounter is a perinatal condition, the code from chapter 16 should be sequenced first.

    4) **Use of Chapter 16 Codes after the Perinatal Period**
    Should a condition originate in the perinatal period, and continue throughout the life of the patient, the perinatal code should continue to be used regardless of the patient's age.

    5) **Birth process or community acquired conditions**
    If a newborn has a condition that may be either due to the birth process or community acquired and the documentation does not indicate which it is, the default is due to the birth process and the code from Chapter 16 should be used. If the condition is community-acquired, a code from Chapter 16 should not be assigned.

    6) **Code all clinically significant conditions**
    All clinically significant conditions noted on routine newborn examination should be coded. A condition is clinically significant if it requires:
    - clinical evaluation; or
    - therapeutic treatment; or
    - diagnostic procedures; or
    - extended length of hospital stay; or
    - increased nursing care and/or monitoring; or
    - has implications for future health care needs

    Note: The perinatal guidelines listed above are the same as the general coding guidelines for "additional diagnoses", except for the final point regarding implications for future health care needs. Codes should be assigned for conditions that have been specified by the provider as having implications for future health care needs.

    b. **Observation and Evaluation of Newborns for Suspected Conditions not Found**
    Assign a code from categories P00-P04 to identify those instances when a healthy newborn is evaluated for a suspected condition that is determined after study not to be present. Do not use a code from categories P00-P04 when the patient has identified signs or symptoms of a suspected problem; in such cases, code the sign or symptom.

c. **Coding Additional Perinatal Diagnoses**

1) **Assigning codes for conditions that require treatment**

Assign codes for conditions that require treatment or further investigation, prolong the length of stay, or require resource utilization.

2) **Codes for conditions specified as having implications for future health care needs**

Assign codes for conditions that have been specified by the provider as having implications for future health care needs.

Note: This guideline should not be used for adult patients.

d. **Prematurity and Fetal Growth Retardation**

Providers utilize different criteria in determining prematurity. A code for prematurity should not be assigned unless it is documented. Assignment of codes in categories P05, Disorders of newborn related to slow fetal growth and fetal malnutrition, and P07, Disorders of newborn related to short gestation and low birth weight, not elsewhere classified, should be based on the recorded birth weight and estimated gestational age. Codes from category P05 should not be assigned with codes from category P07.

When both birth weight and gestational age are available, two codes from category P07 should be assigned, with the code for birth weight sequenced before the code for gestational age.

A code from P05 and codes from P07.2 and P07.3 may be used to specify weeks of gestation as documented by the provider in the record.

e. **Low birth weight and immaturity status**

Codes from category P07, Disorders of newborn related to short gestation and low birth weight, not elsewhere classified, are for use for a child or adult who was premature or had a low birth weight as a newborn and this is affecting the patient's current health status.

See Section I.C.21. Factors influencing health status and contact with health services, Status.

f. **Bacterial Sepsis of Newborn**

Category P36, Bacterial sepsis of newborn, includes congenital sepsis. If a perinate is documented as having sepsis without documentation of congenital or community acquired, the default is congenital and a code from category P36 should be assigned. If the P36 code includes the causal organism, an additional code from category B95, Streptococcus, Staphylococcus, and Enterococcus as the cause of diseases classified elsewhere, or B96, Other bacterial agents as the cause of diseases classified elsewhere, should not be assigned. If the P36 code does not include the causal organism, assign an additional code from category B96. If applicable, use additional codes to identify severe sepsis (R65.2-) and any associated acute organ dysfunction.

g. **Stillbirth**

Code P95, Stillbirth, is only for use in institutions that maintain separate records for stillbirths. No other code should be used with P95. Code P95 should not be used on the mother's record.

17. **Chapter 17: Congenital malformations, deformations, and chromosomal abnormalities (Q00-Q99)**

Assign an appropriate code(s) from categories Q00-Q99, Congenital malformations, deformations, and chromosomal abnormalities when a malformation/deformation or chromosomal abnormality is documented. A malformation/deformation/or chromosomal abnormality may be the principal/first-listed diagnosis on a record or a secondary diagnosis.

When a malformation/deformation/or chromosomal abnormality does not have a unique code assignment, assign additional code(s) for any manifestations that may be present.

When the code assignment specifically identifies the malformation/ deformation/or chromosomal abnormality, manifestations that are an inherent component of the anomaly should not be coded separately. Additional codes should be assigned for manifestations that are not an inherent component.

Codes from Chapter 17 may be used throughout the life of the patient. If a congenital malformation or deformity has been corrected, a personal history code should be used to identify the history of the malformation or deformity. Although present at birth, malformation/deformation/or chromosomal abnormality may not be identified until later in life. Whenever the condition is diagnosed by the physician, it is appropriate to assign a code from codes Q00-Q99.

For the birth admission, the appropriate code from category Z38, Liveborn infants, according to place of birth and type of delivery, should be sequenced as the principal diagnosis, followed by any congenital anomaly codes, Q00-Q99.

18. **Chapter 18: Symptoms, signs, and abnormal clinical and laboratory findings, not elsewhere classified (R00-R99)**
Chapter 18 includes symptoms, signs, abnormal results of clinical or other investigative procedures, and ill-defined conditions regarding which no diagnosis classifiable elsewhere is recorded. Signs and symptoms that point to a specific diagnosis have been assigned to a category in other chapters of the classification.

a. **Use of symptom codes**
Codes that describe symptoms and signs are acceptable for reporting purposes when a related definitive diagnosis has not been established (confirmed) by the provider.

b. **Use of a symptom code with a definitive diagnosis code**
Codes for signs and symptoms may be reported in addition to a related definitive diagnosis when the sign or symptom is not routinely associated with that diagnosis, such as the various signs and symptoms associated with complex syndromes. The definitive diagnosis code should be sequenced before the symptom code.

Signs or symptoms that are associated routinely with a disease process should not be assigned as additional codes, unless otherwise instructed by the classification.

c. **Combination codes that include symptoms**
ICD-10-CM contains a number of combination codes that identify both the definitive diagnosis and common symptoms of that diagnosis. When using one of these combination codes, an additional code should not be assigned for the symptom.

d. **Repeated falls**
Code R29.6, Repeated falls, is for use for encounters when a patient has recently fallen and the reason for the fall is being investigated.

Code Z91.81, History of falling, is for use when a patient has fallen in the past and is at risk for future falls. When appropriate, both codes R29.6 and Z91.81 may be assigned together.

e. *Coma* **scale**
The coma scale codes (R40.2-) can be used in conjunction with traumatic brain injury codes, acute cerebrovascular disease or sequelae of cerebrovascular disease codes. These codes are primarily for use by trauma registries, but they may be used in any setting where this information is collected. The coma scale codes should be sequenced after the diagnosis code(s).

These codes, one from each subcategory, are needed to complete the scale. The 7th character indicates when the scale was recorded. The 7th character should match for all three codes.

At a minimum, report the initial score documented on presentation at your facility. This may be a score from the emergency medicine technician (EMT) or in the emergency department. If desired, a facility may choose to capture multiple Glasgow coma scale scores.

Assign code R40.24, Glasgow coma scale, total score, when only the total score is documented in the medical record and not the individual score(s).

f. Functional quadriplegia

Functional quadriplegia (code R53.2) is the lack of ability to use one's limbs or to ambulate due to extreme debility. It is not associated with neurologic deficit or injury, and code R53.2 should not be used for cases of neurologic quadriplegia. It should only be assigned if functional quadriplegia is specifically documented in the medical record.

g. SIRS due to Non-Infectious Process

The systemic inflammatory response syndrome (SIRS) can develop as a result of certain non-infectious disease processes, such as trauma, malignant neoplasm, or pancreatitis. When SIRS is documented with a noninfectious condition, and no subsequent infection is documented, the code for the underlying condition, such as an injury, should be assigned, followed by code R65.10, Systemic inflammatory response syndrome (SIRS) of non-infectious origin without acute organ dysfunction, or code R65.11, Systemic inflammatory response syndrome (SIRS) of non-infectious origin with acute organ dysfunction. If an associated acute organ dysfunction is documented, the appropriate code(s) for the specific type of organ dysfunction(s) should be assigned in addition to code R65.11. If acute organ dysfunction is documented, but it cannot be determined if the acute organ dysfunction is associated with SIRS or due to another condition (e.g., directly due to the trauma), the provider should be queried.

h. Death NOS

Code R99, Ill-defined and unknown cause of mortality, is only for use in the very limited circumstance when a patient who has already died is brought into an emergency department or other healthcare facility and is pronounced dead upon arrival. It does not represent the discharge disposition of death.

19. Chapter 19: Injury, poisoning, and certain other consequences of external causes (S00-T88)

a. *Application of 7th Characters* in Chapter 19

Most categories in chapter 19 have **a** 7th character requirement for each applicable code. Most categories in this chapter have three **7th character values** (with the exception of fractures): A, initial encounter, D, subsequent encounter and S, sequela. **Categories for traumatic fractures have additional 7th character values.**

7th character "A", initial encounter is used while the patient is receiving active treatment for the **condition.** Examples of active treatment are: surgical treatment, emergency department encounter, and evaluation and treatment by a new physician.

7th character "D" subsequent encounter is used for encounters after the patient has received active treatment of the **condition** and is receiving routine care for the **condition** during the healing or recovery phase. Examples of subsequent care are: cast change or removal, removal of external or internal fixation device, medication adjustment, other aftercare and follow up visits following **treatment of the injury or condition.**

The aftercare Z codes should not be used for aftercare for **conditions such as** injuries **or poisonings, where 7th characters are provided to identify subsequent care. For example,** for aftercare of an injury, assign the acute injury code with the 7th character "D" (subsequent encounter).

7th character "S", sequela, is for use for complications or conditions that arise as a direct result of a **condition**, such as scar formation after a burn. The scars are sequelae of the burn. When using **7th character** "S", it is necessary to use both the injury code that precipitated the sequela and the code for the sequela itself. The "S" is added only to the injury code, not the sequela code. The **7th character** "S" identifies the injury responsible for the sequela. The specific type of sequela (e.g. scar) is sequenced first, followed by the injury code.

b. Coding of Injuries

When coding injuries, assign separate codes for each injury unless a combination code is provided, in which case the combination code is assigned. Code T07, Unspecified multiple injuries should not be assigned

in the inpatient setting unless information for a more specific code is not available. Traumatic injury codes (S00–T14.9) are not to be used for normal, healing surgical wounds or to identify complications of surgical wounds.

The code for the most serious injury, as determined by the provider and the focus of treatment, is sequenced first.

1) Superficial injuries

Superficial injuries such as abrasions or contusions are not coded when associated with more severe injuries of the same site.

2) Primary injury with damage to nerves/blood vessels

When a primary injury results in minor damage to peripheral nerves or blood vessels, the primary injury is sequenced first with additional code(s) for injuries to nerves and spinal cord (such as category S04), and/or injury to blood vessels (such as category S15). When the primary injury is to the blood vessels or nerves, that injury should be sequenced first.

c. Coding of Traumatic Fractures

The principles of multiple coding of injuries should be followed in coding fractures. Fractures of specified sites are coded individually by site in accordance with both the provisions within categories S02, S12, S22, S32, S42, S49, S52, S59, S62, S72, S79, S82, S89, S92 and the level of detail furnished by medical record content.

A fracture not indicated as open or closed should be coded to closed. A fracture not indicated whether displaced or not displaced should be coded to displaced.

More specific guidelines are as follows:

1) Initial vs. Subsequent Encounter for Fractures

Traumatic fractures are coded using the appropriate 7th character for initial encounter (A, B, C) while the patient is receiving active treatment for the fracture. Examples of active treatment are: surgical treatment, emergency department encounter, and evaluation and treatment by a new physician. The appropriate 7th character for initial encounter should also be assigned for a patient who delayed seeking treatment for the fracture or nonunion.

Fractures are coded using the appropriate 7th character for subsequent care for encounters after the patient has completed active treatment of the fracture and is receiving routine care for the fracture during the healing or recovery phase. Examples of fracture aftercare are: cast change or removal, removal of external or internal fixation device, medication adjustment, and follow-up visits following fracture treatment.

Care for complications of surgical treatment for fracture repairs during the healing or recovery phase should be coded with the appropriate complication codes.

Care of complications of fractures, such as malunion and nonunion, should be reported with the appropriate 7th character for subsequent care with nonunion (K, M, N,) or subsequent care with malunion (P, Q, R).

A code from category M80, not a traumatic fracture code, should be used for any patient with known osteoporosis who suffers a fracture, even if the patient had a minor fall or trauma, if that fall or trauma would not usually break a normal, healthy bone.

See Section I.C.13. Osteoporosis.

The aftercare Z codes should not be used for aftercare for traumatic fractures. For aftercare of a traumatic fracture, assign the acute fracture code with the appropriate 7th character.

2) Multiple fractures sequencing

Multiple fractures are sequenced in accordance with the severity of the fracture.

d. Coding of Burns and Corrosions

The ICD-10-CM makes a distinction between burns and corrosions. The burn codes are for thermal burns, except sunburns, that come from a heat source, such as a fire or hot appliance. The burn codes are also for burns resulting from electricity and radiation. Corrosions are burns due to chemicals. The guidelines are the same for burns and corrosions.

Current burns (T20-T25) are classified by depth, extent and by agent (X code). Burns are classified by depth as first degree (erythema), second degree (blistering), and third degree (full-thickness involvement). Burns of the eye and internal organs (T26-T28) are classified by site, but not by degree.

1) Sequencing of burn and related condition codes
Sequence first the code that reflects the highest degree of burn when more than one burn is present.

    a. When the reason for the admission or encounter is for treatment of external multiple burns, sequence first the code that reflects the burn of the highest degree.

    b. When a patient has both internal and external burns, the circumstances of admission govern the selection of the principal diagnosis or first-listed diagnosis.

    c. When a patient is admitted for burn injuries and other related conditions such as smoke inhalation and/or respiratory failure, the circumstances of admission govern the selection of the principal or first-listed diagnosis.

2) Burns of the same local site
Classify burns of the same local site (three-character category level, T20-T28) but of different degrees to the subcategory identifying the highest degree recorded in the diagnosis.

3) Non-healing burns
Non-healing burns are coded as acute burns.
    Necrosis of burned skin should be coded as a non-healed burn.

4) Infected Burn
For any documented infected burn site, use an additional code for the infection.

5) Assign separate codes for each burn site
When coding burns, assign separate codes for each burn site. Category T30, Burn and corrosion, body region unspecified is extremely vague and should rarely be used.

6) Burns and Corrosions Classified According to Extent of Body Surface Involved
Assign codes from category T31, Burns classified according to extent of body surface involved, or T32, Corrosions classified according to extent of body surface involved, when the site of the burn is not specified or when there is a need for additional data. It is advisable to use category T31 as additional coding when needed to provide data for evaluating burn mortality, such as that needed by burn units. It is also advisable to use category T31 as an additional code for reporting purposes when there is mention of a third-degree burn involving 20 percent or more of the body surface.

Categories T31 and T32 are based on the classic "rule of nines" in estimating body surface involved: head and neck are assigned nine percent, each arm nine percent, each leg 18 percent, the anterior trunk 18 percent, posterior trunk 18 percent, and genitalia one percent. Providers may change these percentage assignments where necessary to accommodate infants and children who have proportionately larger heads than adults, and patients who have large buttocks, thighs, or abdomen that involve burns.

7) Encounters for treatment of *sequela* of burns
Encounters for the treatment of the late effects of burns or corrosions (i.e., scars or joint contractures) should be coded with a burn or corrosion code with the 7th character "S" **for** sequela.

8) Sequelae with a late effect code and current burn
When appropriate, both a code for a current burn or corrosion with 7th character "A" or "D" and a burn or corrosion code with **7th character** "S" may be assigned on the same record (when both a current burn and sequelae of an old burn exist). Burns and corrosions do not heal at the same rate and a current healing wound may still exist with sequela of a healed burn or corrosion.

9) Use of an external cause code with burns and corrosions
An external cause code should be used with burns and corrosions to identify the source and intent of the burn, as well as the place where it occurred.

e. Adverse Effects, Poisoning , Underdosing and Toxic Effects
Codes in categories T36-T65 are combination codes that include the substance **that was taken** as well as the **intent**. No additional external cause code is required for poisonings, toxic effects, adverse effects and underdosing codes.

1) Do not code directly from the Table of Drugs
Do not code directly from the Table of Drugs and Chemicals. Always refer back to the Tabular List.

2) Use as many codes as necessary to describe
Use as many codes as necessary to describe completely all drugs, medicinal or biological substances.

3) If the same code would describe the causative agent
If the same code would describe the causative agent for more than one adverse reaction, poisoning, toxic effect or underdosing, assign the code only once.

4) If two or more drugs, medicinal or biological substances
If two or more drugs, medicinal or biological substances are reported, code each individually unless **a** combination code is listed in the Table of Drugs and Chemicals.

5) The occurrence of drug toxicity is classified in ICD-10-CM as follows:

(a) Adverse Effect
When coding an adverse effect of a drug that has been correctly prescribed and properly administered, assign the appropriate code for **the nature of the adverse effect followed by the appropriate code for the** adverse effect **of the drug (T36-T50). The code for the drug should have a 5th or 6th character "5" (for example T36.0X5-)** Examples of **the nature of an adverse effect** are tachycardia, delirium, gastrointestinal hemorrhaging, vomiting, hypokalemia, hepatitis, renal failure, or respiratory failure.

(b) Poisoning
When coding a poisoning or reaction to the improper use of a medication (e.g., overdose, wrong substance given or taken in error, wrong route of administration), **first** assign the appropriate code from categories T36-T50. **The p**oisoning codes have an associated intent **as their 5th or 6th character** (accidental, intentional self-harm, assault and undetermined. Use additional code(s) for all manifestations of poisonings.

If there is also a diagnosis of abuse or dependence **of** the substance, the abuse or dependence is **assigned** as an additional code.

Examples of poisoning include:

(i) Error was made in drug prescription Errors made in drug prescription or in the administration of the drug by provider, nurse, patient, or other person.

(ii) Overdose of a drug intentionally taken If an overdose of a drug was intentionally taken or administered and resulted in drug toxicity, it would be coded as a poisoning.

(iii) Nonprescribed drug taken with correctly prescribed and properly administered drug.
If a nonprescribed drug or medicinal agent was taken in combination with a correctly prescribed and properly administered drug, any drug toxicity or other reaction resulting from the interaction of the two drugs would be classified as a poisoning.

(iv) Interaction of drug(s) and alcohol.
When a reaction results from the interaction of a drug(s) and alcohol, this would be classified as poisoning.

See Section I.C.4. if poisoning is the result of insulin pump malfunctions.

(c) Underdosing

Underdosing refers to taking less of a medication than is prescribed by a provider or a manufacturer's instruction. For underdosing, assign the code from categories T36-T50 (fifth or sixth character "6").

Codes for underdosing should never be assigned as principal or first-listed codes. If a patient has a relapse or exacerbation of the medical condition for which the drug is prescribed because of the reduction in dose, then the medical condition itself should be coded.

Noncompliance (Z91.12-, Z91.13-) or complication of care (Y63.8-Y63.9) codes are to be used with an underdosing code to indicate intent, if known.

(d) Toxic Effects

When a harmful substance is ingested or comes in contact with a person, this is classified as a toxic effect. The toxic effect codes are in categories T51-T65.

Toxic effect codes have an associated intent: accidental, intentional self-harm, assault and undetermined.

f. Adult and child abuse, neglect and other maltreatment

Sequence first the appropriate code from categories T74.- (Adult and child abuse, neglect and other maltreatment, confirmed) or T76.- (Adult and child abuse, neglect and other maltreatment, suspected) for abuse, neglect and other maltreatment, followed by any accompanying mental health or injury code(s).

If the documentation in the medical record states abuse or neglect it is coded as confirmed (T74.-). It is coded as suspected if it is documented as suspected (T76.-).

For cases of confirmed abuse or neglect an external cause code from the assault section (X92-Y08) should be added to identify the cause of any physical injuries. A perpetrator code (Y07) should be added when the perpetrator of the abuse is known. For suspected cases of abuse or neglect, do not report external cause or perpetrator code.

If a suspected case of abuse, neglect or mistreatment is ruled out during an encounter code Z04.71, **Encounter for examination and observation following alleged physical adult abuse**, ruled out, or code Z04.72, **Encounter for examination and observation following alleged child physical abuse,** ruled out, should be used, not a code from T76.

If a suspected case of alleged rape or sexual abuse is ruled out during an encounter code Z04.41, Encounter for examination and observation following alleged physical adult abuse, ruled out, or code Z04.42, Encounter for examination and observation following alleged rape or sexual abuse, ruled out, should be used, not a code from T76.

See Section I.C.15. Abuse in a pregnant patient.

g. Complications of care

1) *General guidelines for* **complications of care**

(a) Documentation of complications of care

See Section I.B.16. for information on documentation of complications of care.

2) Pain due to medical devices

Pain associated with devices, implants or grafts left in a surgical site (for example painful hip prosthesis) is assigned to the appropriate code(s) found in Chapter 19, Injury, poisoning, and certain other consequences of external causes. Specific codes for pain due to medical devices are found in the T code section of the ICD-10-CM. Use additional code(s) from category G89 to identify acute or chronic pain due to presence of the device, implant or graft (G89.18 or G89.28).

3) Transplant complications

(a) Transplant complications other than kidney

Codes under category T86, Complications of transplanted organs and tissues, are for use for both complications and rejection of transplanted organs. A transplant complication code is only assigned if the complication affects the function of the transplanted organ. Two codes are required to fully describe a transplant complication: the appropriate code from category T86 and a secondary code that identifies the complication.

Pre-existing conditions or conditions that develop after the transplant are not coded as complications unless they affect the function of the transplanted organs.

See I.C.21. for transplant organ removal status
See I.C.2. for malignant neoplasm associated with transplanted organ.

(b) *Kidney transplant complications*

Patients who have undergone kidney transplant may still have some form of chronic kidney disease (CKD) because the kidney transplant may not fully restore kidney function. Code T86.1- should be assigned for documented complications of a kidney transplant, such as transplant failure or rejection or other transplant complication. Code T86.1- should not be assigned for post kidney transplant patients who have chronic kidney (CKD) unless a transplant complication such as transplant failure or rejection is documented. If the documentation is unclear as to whether the patient has a complication of the transplant, query the provider.

Conditions that affect the function of the transplanted kidney, other than CKD, should be assigned a code from subcategory T86.1, Complications of transplanted organ, Kidney, and a secondary code that identifies the complication.

For patients with CKD following a kidney transplant, but who do not have a complication such as failure or rejection, *see section I.C.14. Chronic kidney disease and kidney transplant status*.

4) Complication codes that include the external cause

As with certain other T codes, some of the complications of care codes have the external cause included in the code. The code includes the nature of the complication as well as the type of procedure that caused the complication. No external cause code indicating the type of procedure is necessary for these codes.

5) Complications of care codes within the body system chapters

Intraoperative and postprocedural complication codes are found within the body system chapters with codes specific to the organs and structures of that body system. These codes should be sequenced first, followed by a code(s) for the specific complication, if applicable.

20. Chapter 20: External Causes of Morbidity (V01-Y99)

Introduction: These guidelines are provided for the reporting of external causes of morbidity codes in order that there will be standardization in the process. These codes are secondary codes for use in any health care setting.

External cause codes are intended to provide data for injury research and evaluation of injury prevention strategies. These codes capture how the injury or health condition happened (cause), the intent (unintentional or accidental; or intentional, such as suicide or assault), the place where the event occurred the activity of the patient at the time of the event, and the person's status (e.g., civilian, military).

a. General External Cause Coding Guidelines

1) Used with any code in the range of A00.0-T88.9, Z00-Z99

An external cause code may be used with any code in the range of A00.0-T88.9, Z00-Z99, classification that is a health condition due to an external cause. Though they are most applicable to injuries, they are also valid for use with such things as infections or diseases due to an external source, and other health conditions, such as a heart attack that occurs during strenuous physical activity.

2) External cause code used for length of treatment

Assign the external cause code, with the appropriate 7th character (initial encounter, subsequent encounter or sequela) for each encounter for which the injury or condition is being treated.

3) Use the full range of external cause codes

Use the full range of external cause codes to completely describe the cause, the intent, the place of occurrence and if applicable, the activity of the patient at the time of the event, and the patient's status, for all injuries, and other health conditions due to an external cause.

4) Assign as many external cause codes as necessary

Assign as many external cause codes as necessary to fully explain each cause. If only one external code can be recorded, assign the code most related to the principal diagnosis.

5) The selection of the appropriate external cause code

The selection of the appropriate external cause code is guided by the Alphabetic Index of External Causes and by Inclusion and Exclusion notes in the Tabular List.

6) External cause code can never be a principal diagnosis

An external cause code can never be a principal (first-listed) diagnosis.

7) Combination external cause codes

Certain of the external cause codes are combination codes that identify sequential events that result in an injury, such as a fall which results in striking against an object. The injury may be due to either event or both. The combination external cause code used should correspond to the sequence of events regardless of which caused the most serious injury.

8) No external cause code needed in certain circumstances

No external cause code from Chapter 20 is needed if the external cause and intent are included in a code from another chapter (e.g. T36.0X1- Poisoning by penicillins, accidental (unintentional)).

b. Place of Occurrence Guideline

Codes from category Y92, Place of occurrence of the external cause, are secondary codes for use after other external cause codes to identify the location of the patient at the time of injury or other condition.

A place of occurrence code is used only once, at the initial encounter for treatment. No 7th characters are used for Y92. Only one code from Y92 should be recorded on a medical record. A place of occurrence code should be used in conjunction with an activity code, Y93.

Do not use place of occurrence code Y92.9 if the place is not stated or is not applicable.

c. Activity Code

Assign a code from category Y93, Activity code, to describe the activity of the patient at the time the injury or other health condition occurred.

An activity code is used only once, at the initial encounter for treatment. Only one code from Y93 should be recorded on a medical record. An activity code should be used in conjunction with a place of occurrence code, Y92.

The activity codes are not applicable to poisonings, **sequela**, misadventures or late effects.

Do not assign Y93.9, Unspecified activity, if the activity is not stated.

A code from category Y93 is appropriate for use with external cause and intent codes if identifying the activity provides additional information about the event.

d. Place of Occurrence, Activity, and Status Codes Used with other External Cause Code

When applicable, place of occurrence, activity, and external cause status codes are sequenced after the main external cause code(s). Regardless of the number of external cause codes assigned, there should be only one place of occurrence code, one activity code, and one external cause status code assigned to an encounter.

e. If the Reporting Format Limits the Number of External Cause Codes

If the reporting format limits the number of external cause codes that can be used in reporting clinical data, report the code for the cause/intent most related to the principal diagnosis. If the format permits capture of additional external cause codes, the cause/intent, including medical misadventures, of the additional events should be reported rather than the codes for place, activity, or external status.

f. Multiple External Cause Coding Guidelines

More than one external cause code is required to fully describe the external cause of an illness **or** injury. The assignment of external cause codes should be sequenced in the following priority:

If two or more events cause separate injuries, an external cause code should be assigned for each cause. The first-listed external cause code will be selected in the following order:

External codes for child and adult abuse take priority over all other external cause codes.

See Section I.C.19., Child and Adult abuse guidelines.

External codes for terrorism events take priority over all other external cause codes except child and adult abuse.

External cause codes for cataclysmic events take priority over all other external cause codes except child and adult abuse and terrorism.

External cause codes for transport accidents take priority over all other external cause codes except cataclysmic events, child and adult abuse and terrorism.

Activity and external cause status codes are assigned following all causal (intent) external cause codes.

The first-listed external cause code should correspond to the cause of the most serious diagnosis due to an assault, accident, or self-harm, following the order of hierarchy listed above.

g. Child and Adult Abuse Guideline

Adult and child abuse, neglect and maltreatment are classified as assault. Any of the assault codes may be used to indicate the external cause of any injury resulting from the confirmed abuse.

For confirmed cases of abuse, neglect and maltreatment, when the perpetrator is known, a code from Y07, Perpetrator of maltreatment and neglect, should accompany any other assault codes.

See Section I.C.19. Adult and child abuse, neglect and other maltreatment

h. Unknown or Undetermined Intent Guideline

If the intent (accident, self-harm, assault) of the cause of an injury or other condition is unknown or unspecified, code the intent as accidental intent. All transport accident categories assume accidental intent.

1) Use of undetermined intent

External cause codes for events of undetermined intent are only for use if the documentation in the record specifies that the intent cannot be determined.

i. *Sequelae (Late Effects) of External Cause Guidelines*

1) *Sequelae* external cause codes

Sequela are reported using the external cause code with the 7th character "S" for sequela. These codes should be used with any report of a late effect or sequela resulting from a previous injury.

2) *Sequela* external cause code with a related current injury

A **sequela** external cause code should never be used with a related current nature of injury code.

3) Use of *sequela* external cause codes for subsequent visits

Use a late effect external cause code for subsequent visits when a late effect of the initial injury is being treated. Do not use a late effect external cause code for subsequent visits for follow-up care (e.g., to assess healing, to receive rehabilitative therapy) of the injury when no late effect of the injury has been documented.

j. Terrorism Guidelines

1) Cause of injury identified by the Federal Government (FBI) as terrorism

When the cause of an injury is identified by the Federal Government (FBI) as terrorism, the first-listed external cause code should be a code from category Y38, Terrorism. The definition of terrorism employed by the FBI is found at the inclusion note at the beginning of category Y38. Use additional code for place of occurrence (Y92.-). More than one Y38 code may be assigned if the injury is the result of more than one mechanism of terrorism.

2) Cause of an injury is suspected to be the result of terrorism

When the cause of an injury is suspected to be the result of terrorism a code from category Y38 should not be assigned. Suspected cases should be classified as assault.

3) Code Y38.9, Terrorism, secondary effects

Assign code Y38.9, Terrorism, secondary effects, for conditions occurring subsequent to the terrorist event. This code should not be assigned for conditions that are due to the initial terrorist act.

It is acceptable to assign code Y38.9 with another code from Y38 if there is an injury due to the initial terrorist event and an injury that is a subsequent result of the terrorist event.

k. External cause status

A code from category Y99, External cause status, should be assigned whenever any other external cause code is assigned for an encounter, including an Activity code, except for the events noted below. Assign a code from category Y99, External cause status, to indicate the work status of the person at the time the event occurred. The status code indicates whether the event occurred during military activity, whether a non-military person was at work, whether an individual including a student or volunteer was involved in a non-work activity at the time of the causal event.

A code from Y99, External cause status, should be assigned, when applicable, with other external cause codes, such as transport accidents and falls. The external cause status codes are not applicable to poisonings, adverse effects, misadventures or late effects.

Do not assign a code from category Y99 if no other external cause codes (cause, activity) are applicable for the encounter.

An external cause status code is used only once, at the initial encounter for treatment. Only one code from Y99 should be recorded on a medical record.

Do not assign code Y99.9, Unspecified external cause status, if the status is not stated.

21. **Chapter 21: Factors influencing health status and contact with health services (Z00-Z99)**

Note: The chapter specific guidelines provide additional information about the use of Z codes for specified encounters.

a. Use of Z codes in any healthcare setting

Z codes are for use in any healthcare setting. Z codes may be used as either a first-listed (principal diagnosis code in the inpatient setting) or secondary code, depending on the circumstances of the encounter. Certain Z codes may only be used as first-listed or principal diagnosis.

b. Z Codes indicate a reason for an encounter

Z codes are not procedure codes. A corresponding procedure code must accompany a Z code to describe any procedure performed.

c. Categories of Z Codes

1) Contact/Exposure

Category Z20 indicates contact with, and suspected exposure to, communicable diseases. These codes are for patients who do not show any sign or symptom of a disease but are suspected to have been exposed to it by close personal contact with an infected individual or are in an area where a disease is epidemic.

Category Z77, indicates contact with and suspected exposures hazardous to health.

Contact/exposure codes may be used as a first-listed code to explain an encounter for testing, or, more commonly, as a secondary code to identify a potential risk.

2) Inoculations and vaccinations

Code Z23 is for encounters for inoculations and vaccinations. It indicates that a patient is being seen to receive a prophylactic inoculation against a disease. Procedure codes are required to identify the actual administration of the injection and the type(s) of immunizations given. Code Z23 may be used as a secondary code if the inoculation is given as a routine part of preventive health care, such as a well-baby visit.

3) Status

Status codes indicate that a patient is either a carrier of a disease or has the sequelae or residual of a past disease or condition. This includes such things as the presence of prosthetic or mechanical devices resulting from past treatment. A status code is informative, because the status may affect the course of treatment and its outcome. A status code is distinct from a history code. The history code indicates that the patient no longer has the condition.

A status code should not be used with a diagnosis code from one of the body system chapters, if the diagnosis code includes the information provided by the status code. For example, code Z94.1, Heart transplant status, should not be used with a code from subcategory T86.2, Complications of heart transplant. The status code does not provide additional information. The complication code indicates that the patient is a heart transplant patient.

For encounters for weaning from a mechanical ventilator, assign a code from subcategory J96.1, Chronic respiratory failure, followed by code Z99.11, Dependence on respirator [ventilator] status.

The status Z codes/categories are:

Z14   Genetic carrier

       Genetic carrier status indicates that a person carries a gene, associated with a particular disease, which may be passed to offspring who may develop that disease. The person does not have the disease and is not at risk of developing the disease.

Z15   Genetic susceptibility to disease

       Genetic susceptibility indicates that a person has a gene that increases the risk of that person developing the disease.

Codes from category Z15 should not be used as principal or first-listed codes. If the patient has the condition to which he/she is susceptible, and that condition is the reason for the encounter, the code for the current condition should be sequenced first. If the patient is being seen for follow-up after completed treatment for this condition, and the condition no longer exists, a follow-up code should be sequenced first, followed by the appropriate personal history and genetic susceptibility codes. If the purpose of the encounter is genetic counseling associated with procreative management, code Z31.5, Encounter for genetic counseling, should be assigned as the first-listed code, followed by a code from category Z15. Additional codes should be assigned for any applicable family or personal history.

Z16   <u>Resistance to antimicrobial drugs</u>

       This code indicates that a patient has **a condition that** is resistant to **antimicrobial** drug treatment. Sequence the infection code first.

Z17   Estrogen receptor status

Z18   Retained foreign body fragments

Z21   Asymptomatic HIV infection status

       This code indicates that a patient has tested positive for HIV but has manifested no signs or symptoms of the disease.

Z22   Carrier of infectious disease

       Carrier status indicates that a person harbors the specific organisms of a disease without manifest symptoms and is capable of transmitting the infection.

Z28.3   Underimmunization status

Z33.1   Pregnant state, incidental
        This code is a secondary code only for use when the pregnancy is in no way complicating the reason for visit. Otherwise, a code from the obstetric chapter is required.

Z66   Do not resuscitate
This code may be used when it is documented by the provider that a patient is on do not resuscitate status at any time during the stay.

Z67   Blood type

Z68   Body mass index (BMI)

Z74.01 Bed confinement status

Z76.82 Awaiting organ transplant status

Z78   Other specified health status
Code Z78.1, Physical restraint status, may be used when it is documented by the provider that a patient has been put in restraints during the current encounter. Please note that this code should not be reported when it is documented by the provider that a patient is temporarily restrained during a procedure.

Z79   Long-term (current) drug therapy
Codes from this category indicate a patient's continuous use of a prescribed drug (including such things as aspirin therapy) for the long-term treatment of a condition or for prophylactic use. It is not for use for patients who have addictions to drugs. This subcategory is not for use of medications for detoxification or maintenance programs to prevent withdrawal symptoms in patients with drug dependence (e.g., methadone maintenance for opiate dependence). Assign the appropriate code for the drug dependence instead.

Assign a code from Z79 if the patient is receiving a medication for an extended period as a prophylactic measure (such as for the prevention of deep vein thrombosis) or as treatment of a chronic condition (such as arthritis) or a disease requiring a lengthy course of treatment (such as cancer). Do not assign a code from category Z79 for medication being administered for a brief period of time to treat an acute illness or injury (such as a course of antibiotics to treat acute bronchitis).

Z88   Allergy status to drugs, medicaments and biological substances
        Except: Z88.9, Allergy status to unspecified drugs, medicaments and biological substances status

Z89   Acquired absence of limb

Z90   Acquired absence of organs, not elsewhere classified

Z91.0- Allergy status, other than to drugs and biological substances

Z92.82 Status post administration of tPA (rtPA) in a different facility within the last 24 hours prior to admission to a current facility
        Assign code Z92.82, Status post administration of tPA (rtPA) in a different facility within the last 24 hours prior to admission to current facility, as a secondary diagnosis when a patient is received by transfer into a facility and documentation indicates they were administered tissue plasminogen activator (tPA) within the last 24 hours prior to admission to the current facility.
        This guideline applies even if the patient is still receiving the tPA at the time they are received into the current facility.
        The appropriate code for the condition for which the tPA was administered (such as cerebrovascular disease or myocardial infarction) should be assigned first.
        Code Z92.82 is only applicable to the receiving facility record and not to the transferring facility record.

Z93   Artificial opening status

Z94   Transplanted organ and tissue status

Z95   Presence of cardiac and vascular implants and grafts

Z96   Presence of other functional implants

Z97   Presence of other devices

Z98   Other postprocedural states

Assign code Z98.85, Transplanted organ removal status, to indicate that a transplanted organ has been previously removed. This code should not be assigned for the encounter in which the transplanted organ is removed. The complication necessitating removal of the transplant organ should be assigned for that encounter.

See section I.C.19. for information on the coding of organ transplant complications.

Z99   Dependence on enabling machines and devices, not elsewhere classified

Note: Categories Z89-Z90 and Z93-Z99 are for use only if there are no complications or malfunctions of the organ or tissue replaced, the amputation site or the equipment on which the patient is dependent.

4) History (of)

There are two types of history Z codes, personal and family. Personal history codes explain a patient's past medical condition that no longer exists and is not receiving any treatment, but that has the potential for recurrence, and therefore may require continued monitoring.

Family history codes are for use when a patient has a family member(s) who has had a particular disease that causes the patient to be at higher risk of also contracting the disease.

Personal history codes may be used in conjunction with follow-up codes and family history codes may be used in conjunction with screening codes to explain the need for a test or procedure. History codes are also acceptable on any medical record regardless of the reason for visit. A history of an illness, even if no longer present, is important information that may alter the type of treatment ordered.

The history Z code categories are:

Z80   Family history of primary malignant neoplasm
Z81   Family history of mental and behavioral disorders
Z82   Family history of certain disabilities and chronic diseases (leading to disablement)
Z83   Family history of other specific disorders
Z84   Family history of other conditions
Z85   Personal history of malignant neoplasm
Z86   Personal history of certain other diseases
Z87   Personal history of other diseases and conditions
Z91.4- Personal history of psychological trauma, not elsewhere classified
Z91.5 Personal history of self-harm
Z91.8- Other specified personal risk factors, not elsewhere classified
        Exception:
        Z91.83, Wandering in diseases classified elsewhere
Z92   Personal history of medical treatment
        Except: Z92.0, Personal history of contraception
        Except: Z92.82, Status post administration of tPA (rtPA) in a different facility within the last 24 hours prior to admission to a current facility

5) Screening

Screening is the testing for disease or disease precursors in seemingly well individuals so that early detection and treatment can be provided for those who test positive for the disease (e.g., screening mammogram).

The testing of a person to rule out or confirm a suspected diagnosis because the patient has some sign or symptom is a diagnostic examination, not a screening. In these cases, the sign or symptom is used to explain the reason for the test.

A screening code may be a first-listed code if the reason for the visit is specifically the screening exam. It may also be used as an additional code if the screening is done during an office visit for other health problems. A screening code is not necessary if the screening is inherent to a routine examination, such as a pap smear done during a routine pelvic examination.

Should a condition be discovered during the screening then the code for the condition may be assigned as an additional diagnosis.

GUIDELINES (ICD-10-CM)

The Z code indicates that a screening exam is planned. A procedure code is required to confirm that the screening was performed.

The screening Z codes/categories:

Z11   Encounter for screening for infectious and parasitic diseases
Z12   Encounter for screening for malignant neoplasms
Z13   Encounter for screening for other diseases and disorders
           Except: Z13.9, Encounter for screening, unspecified
Z36   Encounter for antenatal screening for mother

6) Observation

There are two observation Z code categories. They are for use in very limited circumstances when a person is being observed for a suspected condition that is ruled out. The observation codes are not for use if an injury or illness or any signs or symptoms related to the suspected condition are present. In such cases the diagnosis/symptom code is used with the corresponding external cause code.

The observation codes are to be used as principal diagnosis only. Additional codes may be used in addition to the observation code but only if they are unrelated to the suspected condition being observed.

Codes from subcategory Z03.7 Encounter for suspected maternal and fetal conditions ruled out, may either be used as a first-listed or as an additional code assignment depending on the case. They are for use in very limited circumstances on a maternal record when an encounter is for a suspected maternal or fetal condition that is ruled out during that encounter (for example, a maternal or fetal condition may be suspected due to an abnormal test result). These codes should not be used when the condition is confirmed. In those cases, the confirmed condition should be coded. In addition, these codes are not for use if an illness or any signs or symptoms related to the suspected condition or problem are present. In such cases the diagnosis/symptom code is used.

Additional codes may be used in addition to the code from subcategory Z03.7, but only if they are unrelated to the suspected condition being evaluated.

Codes from subcategory Z03.7 may not be used for encounters for antenatal screening of mother. *See Section I.C.21. Screening.*

For encounters for suspected fetal condition that are inconclusive following testing and evaluation, assign the appropriate code from category O35, O36, O40 or O41.

The observation Z code categories:

Z03   Encounter for medical observation for suspected diseases and conditions ruled out
Z04   Encounter for examination and observation for other reasons
           Except: Z04.9, Encounter for examination and observation for unspecified reason

7) Aftercare

Aftercare visit codes cover situations when the initial treatment of a disease has been performed and the patient requires continued care during the healing or recovery phase, or for the long-term consequences of the disease. The aftercare Z code should not be used if treatment is directed at a current, acute disease. The diagnosis code is to be used in these cases.

Exceptions to this rule are codes Z51.0, Encounter for antineoplastic radiation therapy, and codes from subcategory Z51.1, Encounter for antineoplastic chemotherapy and immunotherapy. These codes are to be first-listed, followed by the diagnosis code when a patient's encounter is solely to receive radiation therapy, chemotherapy, or immunotherapy for the treatment of a neoplasm. If the reason for the encounter is more than one type of antineoplastic therapy, code Z51.0 and a code from subcategory Z51.1 may be assigned together, in which case one of these codes would be reported as a secondary diagnosis.

The aftercare Z codes should also not be used for aftercare for injuries. For aftercare of an injury, assign the acute injury code with the appropriate 7th character (for subsequent encounter).

The aftercare codes are generally first-listed to explain the specific reason for the encounter. An aftercare code may be used as an additional code when some type of aftercare is provided in addition to the reason for admission and no diagnosis code is applicable. An example of this would be the closure of a colostomy during an encounter for treatment of another condition.

Aftercare codes should be used in conjunction with other aftercare codes or diagnosis codes to provide better detail on the specifics of an aftercare encounter visit, unless otherwise directed by the classification. Should a patient receive multiple types of antineoplastic therapy during the same encounter, code Z51.0, Encounter for antineoplastic radiation therapy, and codes from subcategory Z51.1, Encounter for antineoplastic chemotherapy and immunotherapy, may be used together on a record.
The sequencing of multiple aftercare codes depends on the circumstances of the encounter.

Certain aftercare Z code categories need a secondary diagnosis code to describe the resolving condition or sequelae. For others, the condition is included in the code title.

Additional Z code aftercare category terms include fitting and adjustment, and attention to artificial openings.

Status Z codes may be used with aftercare Z codes to indicate the nature of the aftercare. For example code Z95.1, Presence of aortocoronary bypass graft, may be used with code Z48.812, Encounter for surgical aftercare following surgery on the circulatory system, to indicate the surgery for which the aftercare is being performed. A status code should not be used when the aftercare code indicates the type of status, such as using Z43.0, Encounter for attention to tracheostomy, with Z93.0, Tracheostomy status.

The aftercare Z category/codes:

Z42	Encounter for plastic and reconstructive surgery following medical procedure or healed injury
Z43	Encounter for attention to artificial openings
Z44	Encounter for fitting and adjustment of external prosthetic device
Z45	Encounter for adjustment and management of implanted device
Z46	Encounter for fitting and adjustment of other devices
Z47	Orthopedic aftercare
Z48	Encounter for other postprocedural aftercare
Z49	Encounter for care involving renal dialysis
Z51	Encounter for other aftercare

8) Follow-up

The follow-up codes are used to explain continuing surveillance following completed treatment of a disease, condition, or injury. They imply that the condition has been fully treated and no longer exists. They should not be confused with aftercare codes, or injury codes with a 7th character for subsequent encounter, that explain ongoing care of a healing condition or its sequelae. Follow-up codes may be used in conjunction with history codes to provide the full picture of the healed condition and its treatment. The follow-up code is sequenced first, followed by the history code.

A follow-up code may be used to explain multiple visits. Should a condition be found to have recurred on the follow-up visit, then the diagnosis code for the condition should be assigned in place of the follow-up code.

The follow-up Z code categories:

Z08	Encounter for follow-up examination after completed treatment for malignant neoplasm
Z09	Encounter for follow-up examination after completed treatment for conditions other than malignant neoplasm
Z39	Encounter for maternal postpartum care and examination

9) Donor

Codes in category Z52, Donors of organs and tissues, are used for living individuals who are donating blood or other body tissue. These codes are only for individuals donating for others, not for self-donations. They are not used to identify cadaveric donations.

10) Counseling

Counseling Z codes are used when a patient or family member receives assistance in the aftermath of an illness or injury, or when support is required in coping with family or social problems. They are not used in conjunction with a diagnosis code when the counseling component of care is considered integral to standard treatment.

The counseling Z codes/categories:

Z30.0-	Encounter for general counseling and advice on contraception
Z31.5	Encounter for genetic counseling
Z31.6-	Encounter for general counseling and advice on procreation
Z32.2	Encounter for childbirth instruction
Z32.3	Encounter for childcare instruction
Z69	Encounter for mental health services for victim and perpetrator of abuse
Z70	Counseling related to sexual attitude, behavior and orientation
Z71	Persons encountering health services for other counseling and medical advice, not elsewhere classified
Z76.81	Expectant mother prebirth pediatrician visit

11) Encounters for Obstetrical and Reproductive Services

See Section I.C.15. Pregnancy, Childbirth, and the Puerperium, for further instruction on the use of these codes.

Z codes for pregnancy are for use in those circumstances when none of the problems or complications included in the codes from the Obstetrics chapter exist (a routine prenatal visit or postpartum care). Codes in category Z34, Encounter for supervision of normal pregnancy, are always first listed and are not to be used with any other code from the OB chapter. **Codes in category Z3A, Weeks of gestation, may be assigned to provide additional information about the pregnancy.**

The outcome of delivery, category Z37, should be included on all maternal delivery records. It is always a secondary code. Codes in category Z37 should not be used on the newborn record.

Z codes for family planning (contraceptive) or procreative management and counseling should be included on an obstetric record either during the pregnancy or the postpartum stage, if applicable.

Z codes/categories for obstetrical and reproductive services:

Z30	Encounter for contraceptive management
Z31	Encounter for procreative management
Z32.2	Encounter for childbirth instruction
Z32.3	Encounter for childcare instruction
Z33	Pregnant state
Z34	Encounter for supervision of normal pregnancy
Z36	Encounter for antenatal screening of mother
Z3A	**Weeks of gestation**
Z37	Outcome of delivery
Z39	Encounter for maternal postpartum care and examination
Z76.81	Expectant mother prebirth pediatrician visit

12) Newborns and Infants

See Section I.C.16. Newborn (Perinatal) Guidelines, for further instruction on the use of these codes.

Newborn Z codes/categories:

Z76.1	Encounter for health supervision and care of foundling
Z00.1-	Encounter for routine child health examination
Z38	Liveborn infants according to place of birth and type of delivery

13) Routine and administrative examinations

The Z codes allow for the description of encounters for routine examinations, such as, a general check-up, or, examinations for administrative purposes, such as, a pre-employment physical. The codes are not to be used if the examination is for diagnosis of a suspected condition or for treatment purposes. In such cases the diagnosis code is used. During a routine exam, should a diagnosis or condition be discovered, it should be coded as an additional code. Pre-existing and chronic conditions and history codes may also be included as additional codes as long as the examination is for administrative purposes and not focused on any particular condition.

Some of the codes for routine health examinations distinguish between "with" and "without" abnormal findings. Code assignment depends on the information that is known at the time the encounter is being coded. For example, if no abnormal findings were found during the examination, but the encounter is being coded before test results are back, it is acceptable to assign the code for "without abnormal findings." When assigning a code for "with abnormal findings," additional code(s) should be assigned to identify the specific abnormal finding(s).

Pre-operative examination and pre-procedural laboratory examination Z codes are for use only in those situations when a patient is being cleared for a procedure or surgery and no treatment is given.

The Z codes/categories for routine and administrative examinations:

Z00   Encounter for general examination without complaint, suspected or reported diagnosis
Z01   Encounter for other special examination without complaint, suspected or reported diagnosis
Z02   Encounter for administrative examination
      Except: Z02.9, Encounter for administrative examinations, unspecified
Z32.0- Encounter for pregnancy test

14) Miscellaneous Z codes

The miscellaneous Z codes capture a number of other health care encounters that do not fall into one of the other categories. Certain of these codes identify the reason for the encounter; others are for use as additional codes that provide useful information on circumstances that may affect a patient's care and treatment.

Prophylactic Organ Removal

For encounters specifically for prophylactic removal of an organ (such as prophylactic removal of breasts due to a genetic susceptibility to cancer or a family history of cancer), the principal or first-listed code should be a code from category Z40, Encounter for prophylactic surgery, followed by the appropriate codes to identify the associated risk factor (such as genetic susceptibility or family history).

If the patient has a malignancy of one site and is having prophylactic removal at another site to prevent either a new primary malignancy or metastatic disease, a code for the malignancy should also be assigned in addition to a code from subcategory Z40.0, Encounter for prophylactic surgery for risk factors related to malignant neoplasms. A Z40.0 code should not be assigned if the patient is having organ removal for treatment of a malignancy, such as the removal of the testes for the treatment of prostate cancer.

Miscellaneous Z codes/categories:

Z28   Immunization not carried out
      Except: Z28.3, Underimmunization status
Z40   Encounter for prophylactic surgery
Z41   Encounter for procedures for purposes other than remedying health state
      Except: Z41.9, Encounter for procedure for purposes other than remedying health state, unspecified
Z53   Persons encountering health services for specific procedures and treatment, not carried out
Z55   Problems related to education and literacy
Z56   Problems related to employment and unemployment
Z57   Occupational exposure to risk factors
Z58   Problems related to physical environment
Z59   Problems related to housing and economic circumstances
Z60   Problems related to social environment
Z62   Problems related to upbringing
Z63   Other problems related to primary support group, including family circumstances

Z64	Problems related to certain psychosocial circumstances
Z65	Problems related to other psychosocial circumstances
Z72	Problems related to lifestyle
Z73	Problems related to life management difficulty
Z74	Problems related to care provider dependency
	Except: Z74.01, Bed confinement status
Z75	Problems related to medical facilities and other health care
Z76.0	Encounter for issue of repeat prescription
Z76.3	Healthy person accompanying sick person
Z76.4	Other boarder to healthcare facility
Z76.5	Malingerer [conscious simulation]
Z91.1-	Patient's noncompliance with medical treatment and regimen
Z91.83	**Wandering in diseases classified elsewhere**
Z91.89	Other specified personal risk factors, not elsewhere classified

15) Nonspecific Z codes

Certain Z codes are so non-specific, or potentially redundant with other codes in the classification, that there can be little justification for their use in the inpatient setting. Their use in the outpatient setting should be limited to those instances when there is no further documentation to permit more precise coding. Otherwise, any sign or symptom or any other reason for visit that is captured in another code should be used.

Nonspecific Z codes/categories:

Z02.9	Encounter for administrative examinations, unspecified
Z04.9	Encounter for examination and observation for unspecified reason
Z13.9	Encounter for screening, unspecified
Z41.9	Encounter for procedure for purposes other than remedying health state, unspecified
Z52.9	Donor of unspecified organ or tissue
Z86.59	Personal history of other mental and behavioral disorders
Z88.9	Allergy status to unspecified drugs, medicaments and biological substances status
Z92.0	Personal history of contraception

16) Z Codes That May Only be Principal/First-Listed Diagnosis

The following Z codes/categories may only be reported as the principal/first-listed diagnosis, except when there are multiple encounters on the same day and the medical records for the encounters are combined:

Z00	Encounter for general examination without complaint, suspected or reported diagnosis
Z01	Encounter for other special examination without complaint, suspected or reported diagnosis
Z02	Encounter for administrative examination
Z03	Encounter for medical observation for suspected diseases and conditions ruled out
Z04	Encounter for examination and observation for other reasons
Z33.2	Encounter for elective termination of pregnancy
Z31.81	Encounter for male factor infertility in female patient
Z31.82	Encounter for Rh incompatibility status
Z31.83	Encounter for assisted reproductive fertility procedure cycle
Z31.84	Encounter for fertility preservation procedure
Z34	Encounter for supervision of normal pregnancy
Z39	Encounter for maternal postpartum care and examination
Z38	Liveborn infants according to place of birth and type of delivery
Z42	Encounter for plastic and reconstructive surgery following medical procedure or healed injury
Z51.0	Encounter for antineoplastic radiation therapy
Z51.1-	Encounter for antineoplastic chemotherapy and immunotherapy
Z52	Donors of organs and tissues
	Except: Z52.9, Donor of unspecified organ or tissue
Z76.1	Encounter for health supervision and care of foundling

Z76.2   Encounter for health supervision and care of other healthy infant and child

Z99.12   Encounter for respirator [ventilator] dependence during power failure

Section II. Selection of Principal Diagnosis

The circumstances of inpatient admission always govern the selection of principal diagnosis. The principal diagnosis is defined in the Uniform Hospital Discharge Data Set (UHDDS) as "that condition established after study to be chiefly responsible for occasioning the admission of the patient to the hospital for care."

The UHDDS definitions are used by hospitals to report inpatient data elements in a standardized manner. These data elements and their definitions can be found in the July 31, 1985, Federal Register (Vol. 50, No, 147), pp. 31038-40.

Since that time the application of the UHDDS definitions has been expanded to include all nonoutpatient settings (acute care, short term, long term care and psychiatric hospitals; home health agencies; rehab facilities; nursing homes, etc).

In determining principal diagnosis, coding conventions in the ICD-10-CM, the Tabular List and Alphabetic Index take precedence over these official coding guidelines.

(See Section I.A., Conventions for the ICD-10-CM)

The importance of consistent, complete documentation in the medical record cannot be overemphasized. Without such documentation the application of all coding guidelines is a difficult, if not impossible, task.

A. Codes for symptoms, signs, and ill-defined conditions

Codes for symptoms, signs, and ill-defined conditions from Chapter 18 are not to be used as principal diagnosis when a related definitive diagnosis has been established.

B. Two or more interrelated conditions, each potentially meeting the definition for principal diagnosis.

When there are two or more interrelated conditions (such as diseases in the same ICD-10-CM chapter or manifestations characteristically associated with a certain disease) potentially meeting the definition of principal diagnosis, either condition may be sequenced first, unless the circumstances of the admission, the therapy provided, the Tabular List, or the Alphabetic Index indicate otherwise.

C. Two or more diagnoses that equally meet the definition for principal diagnosis

In the unusual instance when two or more diagnoses equally meet the criteria for principal diagnosis as determined by the circumstances of admission, diagnostic workup and/or therapy provided, and the Alphabetic Index, Tabular List, or another coding guidelines does not provide sequencing direction, any one of the diagnoses may be sequenced first.

D. Two or more comparative or contrasting conditions.

In those rare instances when two or more contrasting or comparative diagnoses are documented as "either/or" (or similar terminology), they are coded as if the diagnoses were confirmed and the diagnoses are sequenced according to the circumstances of the admission. If no further determination can be made as to which diagnosis should be principal, either diagnosis may be sequenced first.

E. A symptom(s) followed by contrasting/comparative diagnoses

When a symptom(s) is followed by contrasting/comparative diagnoses, the symptom code is sequenced first. All the contrasting/comparative diagnoses should be coded as additional diagnoses.

F. Original treatment plan not carried out

Sequence as the principal diagnosis the condition, which after study occasioned the admission to the hospital, even though treatment may not have been carried out due to unforeseen circumstances.

G. Complications of surgery and other medical care
When the admission is for treatment of a complication resulting from surgery or other medical care, the complication code is sequenced as the principal diagnosis. If the complication is classified to the T80-T88 series and the code lacks the necessary specificity in describing the complication, an additional code for the specific complication should be assigned.

H. Uncertain Diagnosis
If the diagnosis documented at the time of discharge is qualified as "probable", "suspected", "likely", "questionable", "possible", or "still to be ruled out", or other similar terms indicating uncertainty, code the condition as if it existed or was established. The bases for these guidelines are the diagnostic workup, arrangements for further workup or observation, and initial therapeutic approach that correspond most closely with the established diagnosis.

Note: This guideline is applicable only to inpatient admissions to short-term, acute, long-term care and psychiatric hospitals.

I. Admission from Observation Unit

1. Admission Following Medical Observation
When a patient is admitted to an observation unit for a medical condition, which either worsens or does not improve, and is subsequently admitted as an inpatient of the same hospital for this same medical condition, the principal diagnosis would be the medical condition which led to the hospital admission.

2. Admission Following Post-Operative Observation
When a patient is admitted to an observation unit to monitor a condition (or complication) that develops following outpatient surgery, and then is subsequently admitted as an inpatient of the same hospital, hospitals should apply the Uniform Hospital Discharge Data Set (UHDDS) definition of principal diagnosis as "that condition established after study to be chiefly responsible for occasioning the admission of the patient to the hospital for care."

J. Admission from Outpatient Surgery
When a patient receives surgery in the hospital's outpatient surgery department and is subsequently admitted for continuing inpatient care at the same hospital, the following guidelines should be followed in selecting the principal diagnosis for the inpatient admission:
- If the reason for the inpatient admission is a complication, assign the complication as the principal diagnosis.
- If no complication, or other condition, is documented as the reason for the inpatient admission, assign the reason for the outpatient surgery as the principal diagnosis.
- If the reason for the inpatient admission is another condition unrelated to the surgery, assign the unrelated condition as the principal diagnosis.

Section III. Reporting Additional Diagnoses

GENERAL RULES FOR OTHER (ADDITIONAL) DIAGNOSES
For reporting purposes the definition for "other diagnoses" is interpreted as additional conditions that affect patient care in terms of requiring:
    clinical evaluation; or
    therapeutic treatment; or
    diagnostic procedures; or
    extended length of hospital stay; or
    increased nursing care and/or monitoring.
The UHDDS item #11-b defines Other Diagnoses as "all conditions that coexist at the time of admission, that develop subsequently, or that affect the treatment received and/or the length of stay. Diagnoses that relate to an earlier episode which have no bearing on the current hospital stay are to be excluded." UHDDS definitions apply to inpatients in acute care, short-term, long term care and psychiatric hospital setting. The UHDDS definitions are used by acute care short-term hospitals to report inpatient data elements in a standardized manner.

These data elements and their definitions can be found in the July 31, 1985, Federal Register (Vol. 50, No, 147), pp. 31038-40.

Since that time the application of the UHDDS definitions has been expanded to include all nonoutpatient settings (acute care, short term, long term care and psychiatric hospitals; home health agencies; rehab facilities; nursing homes, etc). The following guidelines are to be applied in designating "other diagnoses" when neither the Alphabetic Index nor the Tabular List in ICD-10-CM provide direction. The listing of the diagnoses in the patient record is the responsibility of the attending provider.

A. Previous conditions

If the provider has included a diagnosis in the final diagnostic statement, such as the discharge summary or the face sheet, it should ordinarily be coded. Some providers include in the diagnostic statement resolved conditions or diagnoses and status-post procedures from previous admission that have no bearing on the current stay. Such conditions are not to be reported and are coded only if required by hospital policy.

However, history codes (categories Z80-Z87) may be used as secondary codes if the historical condition or family history has an impact on current care or influences treatment.

B. Abnormal findings

Abnormal findings (laboratory, x-ray, pathologic, and other diagnostic results) are not coded and reported unless the provider indicates their clinical significance. If the findings are outside the normal range and the attending provider has ordered other tests to evaluate the condition or prescribed treatment, it is appropriate to ask the provider whether the abnormal finding should be added.

Please note: This differs from the coding practices in the outpatient setting for coding encounters for diagnostic tests that have been interpreted by a provider.

C. Uncertain Diagnosis

If the diagnosis documented at the time of discharge is qualified as "probable", "suspected", "likely", "questionable", "possible", or "still to be ruled out" or other similar terms indicating uncertainty, code the condition as if it existed or was established. The bases for these guidelines are the diagnostic workup, arrangements for further workup or observation, and initial therapeutic approach that correspond most closely with the established diagnosis.

Note: This guideline is applicable only to inpatient admissions to short-term, acute, long-term care and psychiatric hospitals.

Section IV. Diagnostic Coding and Reporting Guidelines for Outpatient Services

These coding guidelines for outpatient diagnoses have been approved for use by hospitals/ providers in coding and reporting hospital-based outpatient services and provider-based office visits.

Information about the use of certain abbreviations, punctuation, symbols, and other conventions used in the ICD-10-CM Tabular List (code numbers and titles), can be found in Section IA of these guidelines, under "Conventions Used in the Tabular List." Information about the correct sequence to use in finding a code is also described in Section I.

The terms encounter and visit are often used interchangeably in describing outpatient service contacts and, therefore, appear together in these guidelines without distinguishing one from the other.

Though the conventions and general guidelines apply to all settings, coding guidelines for outpatient and provider reporting of diagnoses will vary in a number of instances from those for inpatient diagnoses, recognizing that:

The Uniform Hospital Discharge Data Set (UHDDS) definition of principal diagnosis applies only to inpatients in acute, short-term, long-term care and psychiatric hospitals.

Coding guidelines for inconclusive diagnoses (probable, suspected, rule out, etc.) were developed for inpatient reporting and do not apply to outpatients.

A. Selection of first-listed condition

In the outpatient setting, the term first-listed diagnosis is used in lieu of principal diagnosis.

In determining the first-listed diagnosis the coding conventions of ICD-10-CM, as well as the general and disease specific guidelines take precedence over the outpatient guidelines.

Diagnoses often are not established at the time of the initial encounter/ visit. It may take two or more visits before the diagnosis is confirmed.

The most critical rule involves beginning the search for the correct code assignment through the Alphabetic Index. Never begin searching initially in the Tabular List as this will lead to coding errors.

1. Outpatient Surgery

When a patient presents for outpatient surgery (same day surgery), code the reason for the surgery as the first-listed diagnosis (reason for the encounter), even if the surgery is not performed due to a contraindication.

2. Observation Stay

When a patient is admitted for observation for a medical condition, assign a code for the medical condition as the first-listed diagnosis.

When a patient presents for outpatient surgery and develops complications requiring admission to observation, code the reason for the surgery as the first reported diagnosis (reason for the encounter), followed by codes for the complications as secondary diagnoses.

B. Codes from A00.0 through T88.9, Z00-Z99

The appropriate code(s) from A00.0 through T88.9, Z00-Z99 must be used to identify diagnoses, symptoms, conditions, problems, complaints, or other reason(s) for the encounter/visit.

C. Accurate reporting of ICD-10-CM diagnosis codes

For accurate reporting of ICD-10-CM diagnosis codes, the documentation should describe the patient's condition, using terminology which includes specific diagnoses as well as symptoms, problems, or reasons for the encounter. There are ICD-10-CM codes to describe all of these.

D. Codes that describe symptoms and signs

Codes that describe symptoms and signs, as opposed to diagnoses, are acceptable for reporting purposes when a diagnosis has not been established (confirmed) by the provider. Chapter 18 of ICD-10-CM, Symptoms, Signs, and Abnormal Clinical and Laboratory Findings Not Elsewhere Classified (codes R00-R99) contain many, but not all codes for symptoms.

E. Encounters for circumstances other than a disease or injury

ICD-10-CM provides codes to deal with encounters for circumstances other than a disease or injury. The Factors Influencing Health Status and Contact with Health Services codes (Z00-Z99) are provided to deal with occasions when circumstances other than a disease or injury are recorded as diagnosis or problems.

See Section I.C.21. Factors influencing health status and contact with health services.

F. Level of Detail in Coding

1. ICD-10-CM codes with 3, 4, 5, 6 or 7 characters

ICD-10-CM is composed of codes with 3, 4, 5, 6 or 7 characters. Codes with three characters are included in ICD-10-CM as the heading of a category of codes that may be further subdivided by the use of fourth, fifth, sixth or seventh characters to provide greater specificity.

2. Use of full number of *characters* required for a code

A three-**character** code is to be used only if it is not further subdivided. A code is invalid if it has not been coded to the full number of characters required for that code, including the 7th character, if applicable.

G. ICD-10-CM code for the diagnosis, condition, problem, or other reason for encounter/visit

List first the ICD-10-CM code for the diagnosis, condition, problem, or other reason for encounter/visit shown in the medical record to be chiefly responsible for the services provided. List additional codes that describe any coexisting conditions. In some cases the first-listed diagnosis may be a symptom when a diagnosis has not been established (confirmed) by the physician.

H. Uncertain diagnosis

Do not code diagnoses documented as "probable", "suspected," "questionable," "rule out," or "working diagnosis" or other similar terms indicating uncertainty. Rather, code the condition(s) to the highest degree of certainty for that encounter/visit, such as symptoms, signs, abnormal test results, or other reason for the visit.

Please note: This differs from the coding practices used by short-term, acute care, long-term care and psychiatric hospitals.

I. Chronic diseases

Chronic diseases treated on an ongoing basis may be coded and reported as many times as the patient receives treatment and care for the condition(s)

J. Code all documented conditions that coexist

Code all documented conditions that coexist at the time of the encounter/visit, and require or affect patient care treatment or management. Do not code conditions that were previously treated and no longer exist. However, history codes (categories Z80-Z87) may be used as secondary codes if the historical condition or family history has an impact on current care or influences treatment.

K. Patients receiving diagnostic services only

For patients receiving diagnostic services only during an encounter/visit, sequence first the diagnosis, condition, problem, or other reason for encounter/visit shown in the medical record to be chiefly responsible for the outpatient services provided during the encounter/visit. Codes for other diagnoses (e.g., chronic conditions) may be sequenced as additional diagnoses.

For encounters for routine laboratory/radiology testing in the absence of any signs, symptoms, or associated diagnosis, assign Z01.89, Encounter for other specified special examinations. If routine testing is performed during the same encounter as a test to evaluate a sign, symptom, or diagnosis, it is appropriate to assign both the Z code and the code describing the reason for the non-routine test.

For outpatient encounters for diagnostic tests that have been interpreted by a physician, and the final report is available at the time of coding, code any confirmed or definitive diagnosis(es) documented in the interpretation. Do not code related signs and symptoms as additional diagnoses.

Please note: This differs from the coding practice in the hospital inpatient setting regarding abnormal findings on test results.

L. Patients receiving therapeutic services only

For patients receiving therapeutic services only during an encounter/visit, sequence first the diagnosis, condition, problem, or other reason for encounter/visit shown in the medical record to be chiefly responsible for the outpatient services provided during the encounter/visit. Codes for other diagnoses (e.g., chronic conditions) may be sequenced as additional diagnoses.

EXCEPTION The only exception to this rule is that when the primary reason for the admission/encounter is chemotherapy or radiation therapy, the appropriate Z code for the service is listed first, and the diagnosis or problem for which the service is being performed listed second.

M. Patients receiving preoperative evaluations only

For patients receiving preoperative evaluations only, sequence first a code from subcategory Z01.81, Encounter for pre-procedural examinations, to describe the pre-op consultations. Assign a code for the condition to describe the reason for the surgery as an additional diagnosis. Code also any findings related to the pre-op evaluation.

N. Ambulatory surgery

For ambulatory surgery, code the diagnosis for which the surgery was performed. If the postoperative diagnosis is known to be different from the preoperative diagnosis at the time the diagnosis is confirmed, select the postoperative diagnosis for coding, since it is the most definitive.

O. Routine outpatient prenatal visits

See Section I.C.15. Routine outpatient prenatal visits.

P. Encounters for general medical examinations with abnormal findings

The subcategories for encounters for general medical examinations, Z00.0-, provide codes for with and without abnormal findings. Should a general medical examination result in an abnormal finding, the code for general medical examination with abnormal finding should be assigned as the first-listed diagnosis. A secondary code for the abnormal finding should also be coded.

Q. Encounters for routine health screenings

See Section I.C.21. Factors influencing health status and contact with health services, Screening

Appendix I
Present on Admission Reporting Guidelines
(Effective with 2011 update)

Introduction

These guidelines are to be used as a supplement to the *ICD-10-CM Official Guidelines for Coding and Reporting* to facilitate the assignment of the Present on Admission (POA) indicator for each diagnosis and external cause of injury code reported on claim forms (UB-04 and 837 Institutional).

These guidelines are not intended to replace any guidelines in the main body of the *ICD-10-CM Official Guidelines for Coding and Reporting*. The POA guidelines are not intended to provide guidance on when a condition should be coded, but rather, how to apply the POA indicator to the final set of diagnosis codes that have been assigned in accordance with Sections I, II, and III of the official coding guidelines. Subsequent to the assignment of the ICD-10-CM codes, the POA indicator should then be assigned to those conditions that have been coded.

As stated in the Introduction to the ICD-10-CM Official Guidelines for Coding and Reporting, a joint effort between the healthcare provider and the coder is essential to achieve complete and accurate documentation, code assignment, and reporting of diagnoses and procedures. The importance of consistent, complete documentation in the medical record cannot be overemphasized. Medical record documentation from any provider involved in the care and treatment of the patient may be used to support the determination of whether a condition was present on admission or not. In the context of the official coding guidelines, the term "provider" means a physician or any qualified healthcare practitioner who is legally accountable for establishing the patient's diagnosis.

These guidelines are not a substitute for the provider's clinical judgment as to the determination of whether a condition was/was not present on admission. The provider should be queried regarding issues related to the linking of signs/symptoms, timing of test results, and the timing of findings.

General Reporting Requirements

All claims involving inpatient admissions to general acute care hospitals or other facilities that are subject to a law or regulation mandating collection of present on admission information.

Present on admission is defined as present at the time the order for inpatient admission occurs -- conditions that develop during an outpatient encounter, including emergency department, observation, or outpatient surgery, are considered as present on admission.

POA indicator is assigned to principal and secondary diagnoses (as defined in Section II of the Official Guidelines for Coding and Reporting) and the external cause of injury codes.

Issues related to inconsistent, missing, conflicting or unclear documentation must still be resolved by the provider.

If a condition would not be coded and reported based on UHDDS definitions and current official coding guidelines, then the POA indicator would not be reported.

Reporting Options

Y - Yes

N - No

U - Unknown

W - Clinically undetermined

Unreported/Not used (or "1" for Medicare usage) - (Exempt from POA reporting)

Reporting Definitions

Y = present at the time of inpatient admission

N = not present at the time of inpatient admission

U = documentation is insufficient to determine if condition is present on admission

W = provider is unable to clinically determine whether condition was present on admission or not

Timeframe for POA Identification and Documentation

There is no required timeframe as to when a provider (per the definition of "provider" used in these guidelines) must identify or document a condition to be present on admission. In some clinical situations, it may not be possible for a provider to make a definitive diagnosis (or a condition may not be recognized or reported by the patient) for a period of time after admission. In some cases it may be several days before the provider arrives at a definitive diagnosis. This does not mean that the condition was not present on admission. Determination of whether the condition was present on admission or not will be based on the applicable POA guideline as identified in this document, or on the provider's best clinical judgment.

If at the time of code assignment the documentation is unclear as to whether a condition was present on admission or not, it is appropriate to query the provider for clarification.

Assigning the POA Indicator

Condition is on the "Exempt from Reporting" list

Leave the "present on admission" field blank if the condition is on the list of ICD-10-CM codes for which this field is not applicable. This is the only circumstance in which the field may be left blank.

POA Explicitly Documented

Assign Y for any condition the provider explicitly documents as being present on admission.

Assign N for any condition the provider explicitly documents as not present at the time of admission.

Conditions diagnosed prior to inpatient admission

Assign "Y" for conditions that were diagnosed prior to admission (example: hypertension, diabetes mellitus, asthma)

Conditions diagnosed during the admission but clearly present before admission

Assign "Y" for conditions diagnosed during the admission that were clearly present but not diagnosed until after admission occurred.

Diagnoses subsequently confirmed after admission are considered present on admission if at the time of admission they are documented as suspected, possible, rule out, differential diagnosis, or constitute an underlying cause of a symptom that is present at the time of admission.

Condition develops during outpatient encounter prior to inpatient admission

Assign Y for any condition that develops during an outpatient encounter prior to a written order for inpatient admission.

Documentation does not indicate whether condition was present on admission

Assign "U" when the medical record documentation is unclear as to whether the condition was present on admission. "U" should not be routinely assigned and used only in very limited circumstances. Coders are encouraged to query the providers when the documentation is unclear.

Documentation states that it cannot be determined whether the condition was or was not present on admission

Assign "W" when the medical record documentation indicates that it cannot be clinically determined whether or not the condition was present on admission.

Chronic condition with acute exacerbation during the admission

If a single code identifies both the chronic condition and the acute exacerbation, see POA guidelines pertaining to combination codes.

If a single code only identifies the chronic condition and not the acute exacerbation (e.g., acute exacerbation of chronic leukemia), assign "Y."

Conditions documented as possible, probable, suspected, or rule out at the time of discharge

If the final diagnosis contains a possible, probable, suspected, or rule out diagnosis, and this diagnosis was based on signs, symptoms or clinical findings suspected at the time of inpatient admission, assign "Y."

If the final diagnosis contains a possible, probable, suspected, or rule out diagnosis, and this diagnosis was based on signs, symptoms or clinical findings that were not present on admission, assign "N".

Conditions documented as impending or threatened at the time of discharge

If the final diagnosis contains an impending or threatened diagnosis, and this diagnosis is based on symptoms or clinical findings that were present on admission, assign "Y".

If the final diagnosis contains an impending or threatened diagnosis, and this diagnosis is based on symptoms or clinical findings that were not present on admission, assign "N".

Acute and Chronic Conditions

Assign "Y" for acute conditions that are present at time of admission and N for acute conditions that are not present at time of admission.

Assign "Y" for chronic conditions, even though the condition may not be diagnosed until after admission.

If a single code identifies both an acute and chronic condition, see the POA guidelines for combination codes.

Combination Codes

Assign "N" if any part of the combination code was not present on admission (e.g., COPD with acute exacerbation and the exacerbation was not present on admission; gastric ulcer that does not start bleeding until after admission; asthma patient develops status asthmaticus after admission)

Assign "Y" if all parts of the combination code were present on admission (e.g., patient with acute prostatitis admitted with hematuria)

If the final diagnosis includes comparative or contrasting diagnoses, and both were present, or suspected, at the time of admission, assign "Y".

For infection codes that include the causal organism, assign "Y" if the infection (or signs of the infection) was present on admission, even though the culture results may not be known until after admission (e.g., patient is admitted with pneumonia and the provider documents pseudomonas as the causal organism a few days later).

Same Diagnosis Code for Two or More Conditions

When the same ICD-10-CM diagnosis code applies to two or more conditions during the same encounter (e.g. two separate conditions classified to the same ICD-10-CM diagnosis code):

Assign "Y" if all conditions represented by the single ICD-10-CM code were present on admission (e.g. bilateral unspecified age-related cataracts).

Assign "N" if any of the conditions represented by the single ICD-10-CM code was not present on admission (e.g. traumatic secondary and recurrent hemorrhage and seroma is assigned to a single code T79.2, but only one of the conditions was present on admission).

Obstetrical conditions

Whether or not the patient delivers during the current hospitalization does not affect assignment of the POA indicator. The determining factor for POA assignment is whether the pregnancy complication or obstetrical condition described by the code was present at the time of admission or not.

If the pregnancy complication or obstetrical condition was present on admission (e.g., patient admitted in preterm labor), assign "Y".

If the pregnancy complication or obstetrical condition was not present on admission (e.g., 2nd degree laceration during delivery, postpartum hemorrhage that occurred during current hospitalization, fetal distress develops after admission), assign "N".

If the obstetrical code includes more than one diagnosis and any of the diagnoses identified by the code were not present on admission assign "N".

(e.g., Category O11, Pre-existing hypertension with pre-eclampsia)

Perinatal conditions

Newborns are not considered to be admitted until after birth. Therefore, any condition present at birth or that developed in utero is considered present at admission and should be assigned "Y". This includes conditions that occur during delivery (e.g., injury during delivery, meconium aspiration, exposure to streptococcus B in the vaginal canal).

Congenital conditions and anomalies

Assign "Y" for congenital conditions and anomalies except for **categories** Q00-Q99**, Congenital anomalies**, which are **on the exempt list**. Congenital conditions are always considered present on admission.

External cause of injury codes

Assign "Y" for any external cause code representing an external cause of morbidity that occurred prior to inpatient admission (e.g., patient fell out of bed at home, patient fell out of bed in emergency room prior to admission)

Assign "N" for any external cause code representing an external cause of morbidity that occurred during inpatient hospitalization (e.g., patient fell out of hospital bed during hospital stay, patient experienced an adverse reaction to a medication administered after inpatient admission)

Categories and Codes
Exempt from
Diagnosis Present on Admission Requirement

Note: "Diagnosis present on admission" for these code categories are exempt because they represent circumstances regarding the healthcare encounter or factors influencing health status that do not represent a current disease or injury or are always present on admission

B90-B94, Sequelae of infectious and parasitic diseases

E64, Sequelae of malnutrition and other nutritional deficiencies

I25.2, Old myocardial infarction

I69, Sequelae of cerebrovascular disease

O09, Supervision of high risk pregnancy

O66.5, Attempted application of vacuum extractor and forceps

O80, Encounter for full-term uncomplicated delivery

O94, Sequelae of complication of pregnancy, childbirth, and the puerperium

P00, Newborn (suspected to be) affected by maternal conditions that may be unrelated to present pregnancy

Q00 - Q99, Congenital malformations, deformations and chromosomal abnormalities

S00-T88.9, Injury, poisoning and certain other consequences of external causes with 7th character representing subsequent encounter or sequela

V00.121, Fall from non-in-line roller-skates

V00.131, Fall from skateboard

V00.141, Fall from scooter (nonmotorized)

V00.311, Fall from snowboard

V00.321, Fall from snow-skis

V40-V49, Car occupant injured in transport accident

V80-V89, Other land transport accidents

V90-V94, Water transport accidents

V95-V97, Air and space transport accidents

W03, Other fall on same level due to collision with another person

W09, Fall on and from playground equipment

W15, Fall from cliff

W17.0, Fall into well

W17.1, Fall into storm drain or manhole

W18.01 Striking against sports equipment with subsequent fall

W20.8, Other cause of strike by thrown, projected or falling object

W21, Striking against or struck by sports equipment

W30, Contact with agricultural machinery

W31, Contact with other and unspecified machinery

W32-W34, Accidental handgun discharge and malfunction

W35- W40, Exposure to inanimate mechanical forces

W52, Crushed, pushed or stepped on by crowd or human stampede

W89, Exposure to man-made visible and ultraviolet light

X02, Exposure to controlled fire in building or structure

X03, Exposure to controlled fire, not in building or structure

X04, Exposure to ignition of highly flammable material

X52, Prolonged stay in weightless environment

X71-X83, Intentional self-harm

Y21, Drowning and submersion, undetermined intent

Y22, Handgun discharge, undetermined intent

Y23, Rifle, shotgun and larger firearm discharge, undetermined intent

Y24, Other and unspecified firearm discharge, undetermined intent

Y30, Falling, jumping or pushed from a high place, undetermined intent

Y35, Legal intervention

Y37, Military operations

Y36, Operations of war

Y38, Terrorism

Y92, Place of occurrence of the external cause

Y93, Activity code

Y99, External cause status

Z00, Encounter for general examination without complaint, suspected or reported diagnosis

Z01, Encounter for other special examination without complaint, suspected or reported diagnosis

Z02, Encounter for administrative examination

Z03, Encounter for medical observation for suspected diseases and conditions ruled out

Z08, Encounter for follow-up examination following completed treatment for malignant neoplasm

Z09, Encounter for follow-up examination after completed treatment for conditions other than malignant neoplasm

Z11, Encounter for screening for infectious and parasitic diseases

Z11.8, Encounter for screening for other infectious and parasitic diseases

Z12, Encounter for screening for malignant neoplasms

Z13, Encounter for screening for other diseases and disorders

Z13.4, Encounter for screening for certain developmental disorders in childhood

Z13.5, Encounter for screening for eye and ear disorders

Z13.6, Encounter for screening for cardiovascular disorders

Z13.83, Encounter for screening for respiratory disorder NEC

Z13.89, Encounter for screening for other disorder (inclusion term) (Encounter for screening for genitourinary disorders)

Z13.89, Encounter for screening for other disorder

Z14, Genetic carrier

Z15, Genetic susceptibility to disease

Z17, Estrogen receptor status

Z18, Retained foreign body fragments

Z22, Carrier of infectious disease

Z23, Encounter for immunization

Z28, Immunization not carried out and underimmunization status

Z28.3, Underimmunization status

Z30, Encounter for contraceptive management

Z31, Encounter for procreative management

Z34, Encounter for supervision of normal pregnancy

Z36, Encounter for antenatal screening of mother

Z37, Outcome of delivery

Z38, Liveborn infants according to place of birth and type of delivery

Z39, Encounter for maternal postpartum care and examination

Z41, Encounter for procedures for purposes other than remedying health state

Z42, Encounter for plastic and reconstructive surgery following medical procedure or healed injury

Z43, Encounter for attention to artificial openings

Z44, Encounter for fitting and adjustment of external prosthetic device

Z45, Encounter for adjustment and management of implanted device

Z46, Encounter for fitting and adjustment of other devices

Z47.8, Encounter for other orthopedic aftercare

Z49, Encounter for care involving renal dialysis

Z51, Encounter for other aftercare

Z51.5, Encounter for palliative care

Z51.8, Encounter for other specified aftercare

Z52, Donors of organs and tissues

Z59, Problems related to housing and economic circumstances

Z63, Other problems related to primary support group, including family circumstances

Z65, Problems related to other psychosocial circumstances

Z65.8 Other specified problems related to psychosocial circumstances

Z67.1 - Z67.9 Blood type

Z68, Body mass index (BMI)

Z72, Problems related to lifestyle

Z74.01, Bed confinement status

Z76, Persons encountering health services in other circumstances

Z77.110- Z77.128, Environmental pollution and hazards in the physical environment

Z78, Other specified health status

Z79, Long term (current) drug therapy

Z80, Family history of primary malignant neoplasm

Z81, Family history of mental and behavioral disorders

Z82, Family history of certain disabilities and chronic diseases (leading to disablement)

Z83, Family history of other specific disorders

Z84, Family history of other conditions

Z85, Personal history of primary malignant neoplasm

Z86, Personal history of certain other diseases

Z87, Personal history of other diseases and conditions

Z87.828, Personal history of other (healed) physical injury and trauma

Z87.891, Personal history of nicotine dependence

Z88, Allergy status to drugs, medicaments and biological substances

Z89, Acquired absence of limb

Z90.710, Acquired absence of both cervix and uterus

Z91.0, Allergy status, other than to drugs and biological substances

Z91.4, Personal history of psychological trauma, not elsewhere classified

Z91.5, Personal history of self-harm

Z91.8, Other specified risk factors, not elsewhere classified

Z92, Personal history of medical treatment

Z93, Artificial opening status

Z94, Transplanted organ and tissue status

Z95, Presence of cardiac and vascular implants and grafts

Z97, Presence of other devices

Z98, Other postprocedural states

Z99, Dependence on enabling machines and devices, not elsewhere classified

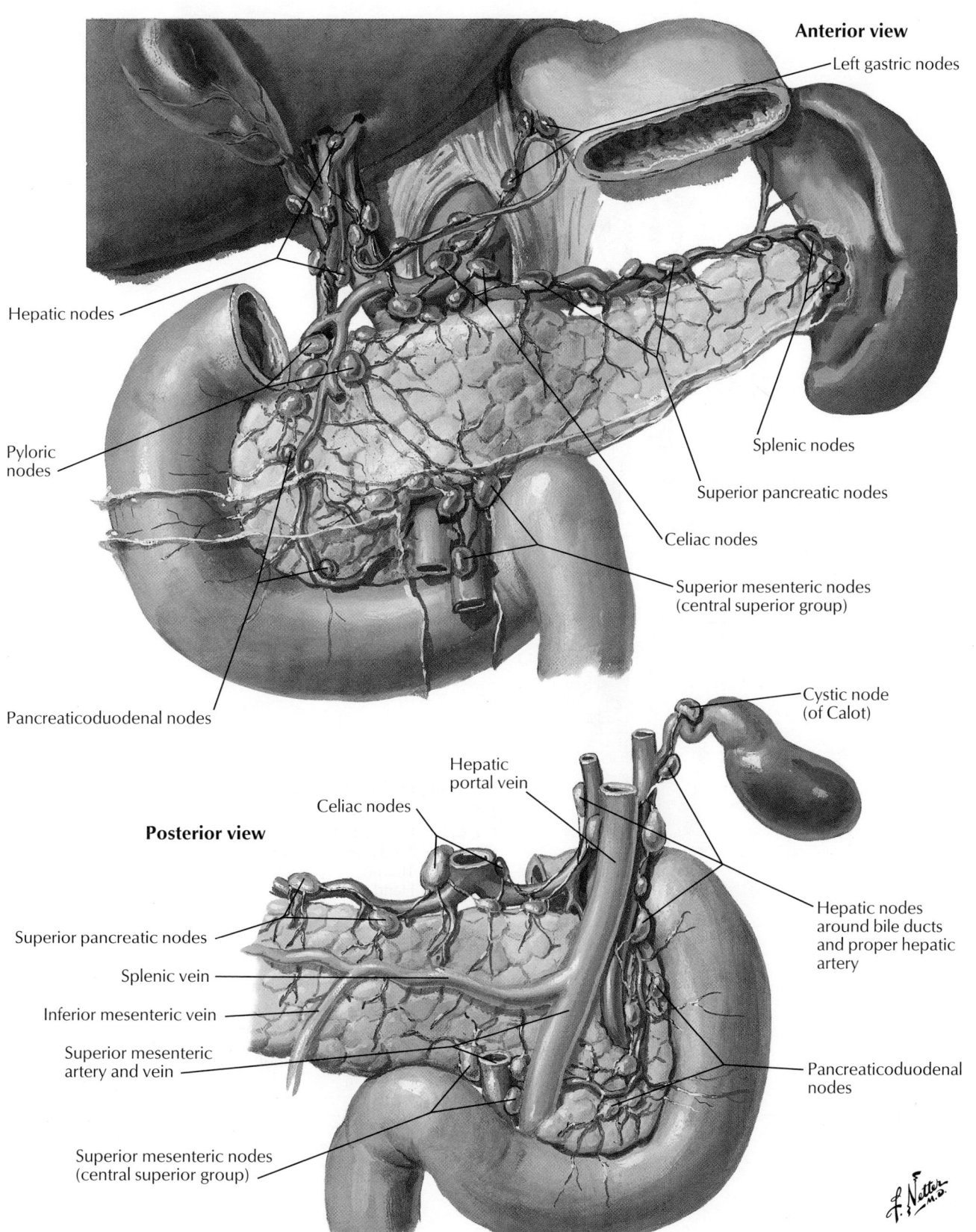

Anterior view

Left gastric nodes

Hepatic nodes

Pyloric nodes

Pancreaticoduodenal nodes

Splenic nodes

Superior pancreatic nodes

Celiac nodes

Superior mesenteric nodes (central superior group)

Posterior view

Hepatic portal vein

Celiac nodes

Cystic node (of Calot)

Hepatic nodes around bile ducts and proper hepatic artery

Superior pancreatic nodes

Splenic vein

Inferior mesenteric vein

Superior mesenteric artery and vein

Pancreaticoduodenal nodes

Superior mesenteric nodes (central superior group)

Plate 315 Lymph Vessels and Nodes of Pancreas. (Netter: Atlas of Human Anatomy, 4 ed, 2006, Saunders.)

Dermatome pattern

Levels of principal dermatomes

C5	Clavicles
C5, 6, 7	Lateral parts of upper limbs
C8; T1	Medial sides of upper limbs
C6	Thumb
C6, 7, 8	Hand
C8	Ring and little fingers
T4	Level of nipples
T10	Level of umbilicus
T12	Inguinal or groin regions
L1, 2, 3, 4	Anterior and inner surfaces of lower limbs
L4, 5; S1	Foot
L4	Medial side of great toe
L5; S1, 2	Outer and posterior sides of lower limbs
S1	Lateral margin of foot and little toe
S2, 3, 4	Perineum

Plate 164   Dermatomes. (Netter: Atlas of Human Anatomy, 4 ed, 2006, Saunders.)

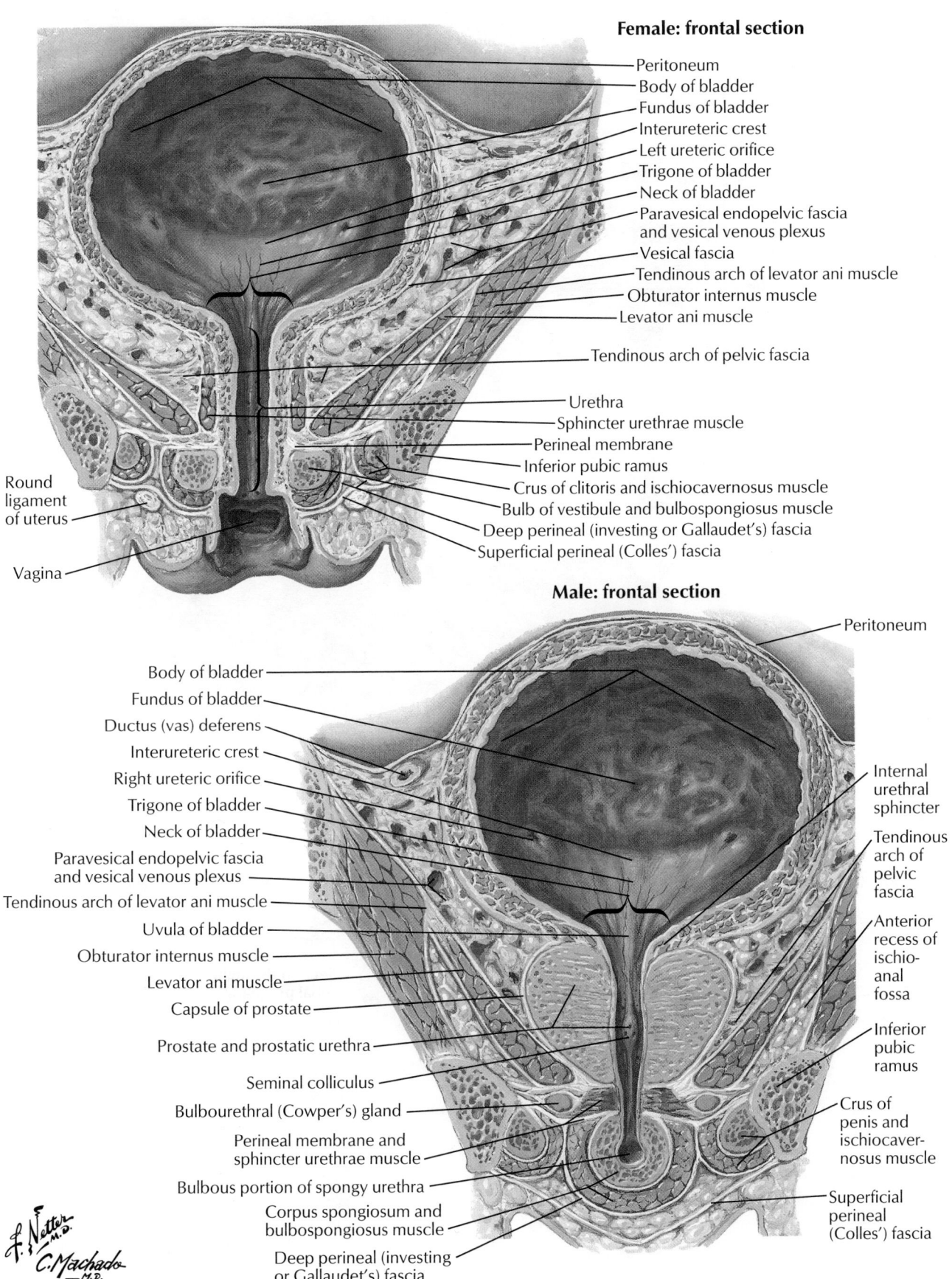

Female: frontal section

Peritoneum
Body of bladder
Fundus of bladder
Interureteric crest
Left ureteric orifice
Trigone of bladder
Neck of bladder
Paravesical endopelvic fascia and vesical venous plexus
Vesical fascia
Tendinous arch of levator ani muscle
Obturator internus muscle
Levator ani muscle

Tendinous arch of pelvic fascia

Urethra
Sphincter urethrae muscle
Perineal membrane
Inferior pubic ramus
Crus of clitoris and ischiocavernosus muscle
Bulb of vestibule and bulbospongiosus muscle
Deep perineal (investing or Gallaudet's) fascia
Superficial perineal (Colles') fascia

Round ligament of uterus

Vagina

Male: frontal section

Peritoneum

Body of bladder
Fundus of bladder
Ductus (vas) deferens
Interureteric crest
Right ureteric orifice
Trigone of bladder
Neck of bladder
Paravesical endopelvic fascia and vesical venous plexus
Tendinous arch of levator ani muscle
Uvula of bladder
Obturator internus muscle
Levator ani muscle
Capsule of prostate
Prostate and prostatic urethra
Seminal colliculus
Bulbourethral (Cowper's) gland
Perineal membrane and sphincter urethrae muscle
Bulbous portion of spongy urethra
Corpus spongiosum and bulbospongiosus muscle
Deep perineal (investing or Gallaudet's) fascia

Internal urethral sphincter
Tendinous arch of pelvic fascia
Anterior recess of ischio-anal fossa
Inferior pubic ramus
Crus of penis and ischiocavernosus muscle
Superficial perineal (Colles') fascia

Plate 366 Urinary Bladder: Female and Male. (Netter: Atlas of Human Anatomy, 4 ed, 2006, Saunders.)

Sites of ectopic implantation

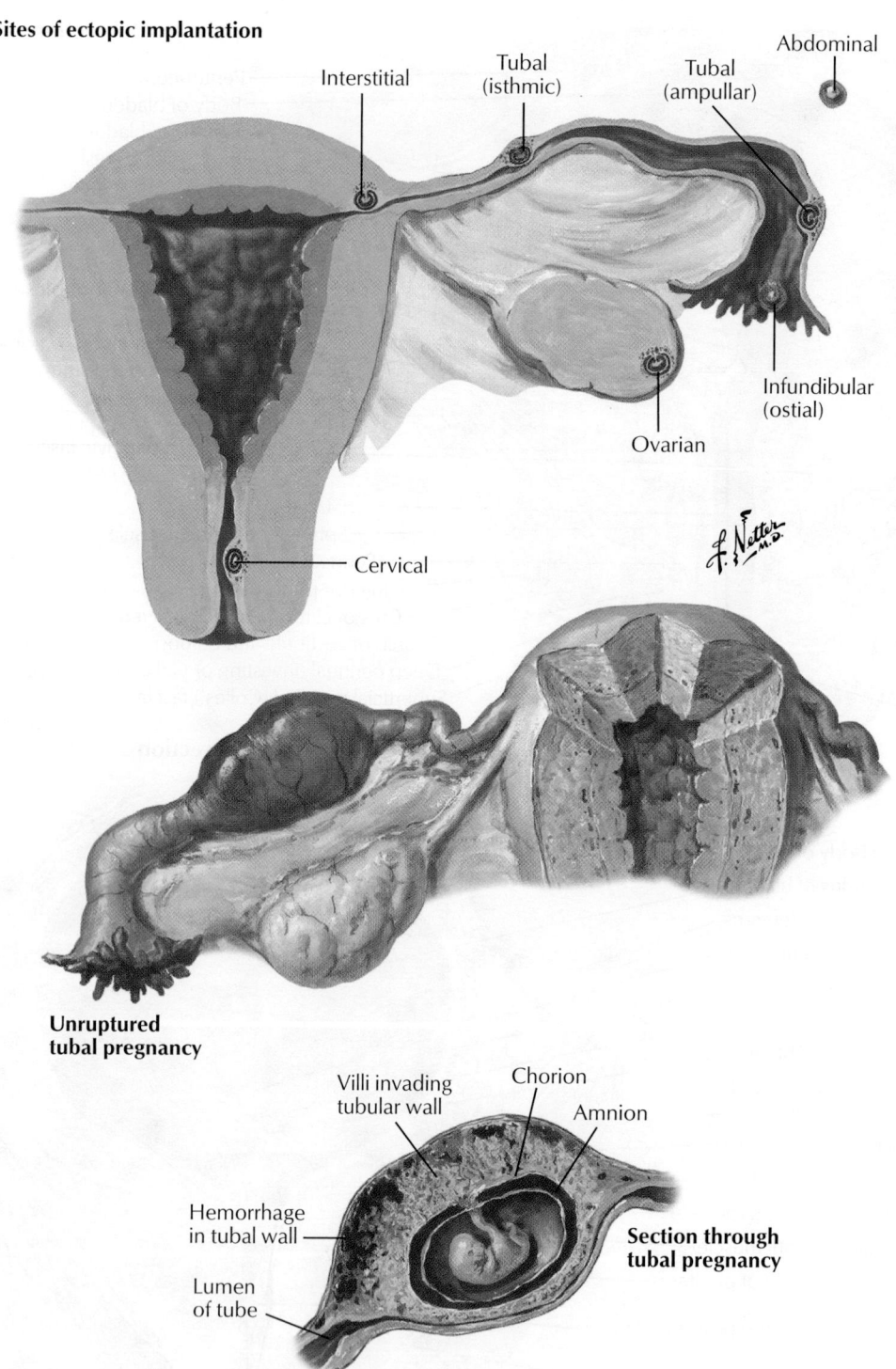

Interstitial

Tubal (isthmic)

Tubal (ampullar)

Abdominal

Infundibular (ostial)

Ovarian

Cervical

f. Netter
M.D.

Unruptured tubal pregnancy

Villi invading tubular wall

Chorion

Amnion

Hemorrhage in tubal wall

Lumen of tube

Section through tubal pregnancy

Plate 375   Ectopic Pregnancy. (Netter: Atlas of Human Anatomy, 4 ed, 2006, Saunders.)

Skin of penis

Superficial fascia
of penis (Colles' fascia)

Deep (Buck's)
fascia of penis

Testicular artery

Ductus deferens

Artery to ductus deferens

Genital branch of
genitofemoral nerve

Pampiniform (venous) plexus

Epididymis

Appendix of epididymis

Appendix of testis

Testis (covered by visceral
layer of tunica vaginalis)

Parietal layer of tunica vaginalis

Superficial
inguinal ring

External
spermatic fascia

Cremaster muscle
and fascia

Septum of scrotum
(formed by
dartos fascia)

Superficial
(dartos) fascia
of scrotum

Skin of scrotum

Superficial (dartos) fascia of scrotum

External spermatic fascia

Cremaster muscle and fascia

Internal spermatic fascia

Parietal layer of tunica vaginalis

Epididymis

Testis (covered by visceral layer of tunica vaginalis)

Skin of scrotum

Plate 387   Scrotum and Contents. (Netter: Atlas of Human Anatomy, 4 ed, 2006, Saunders.)

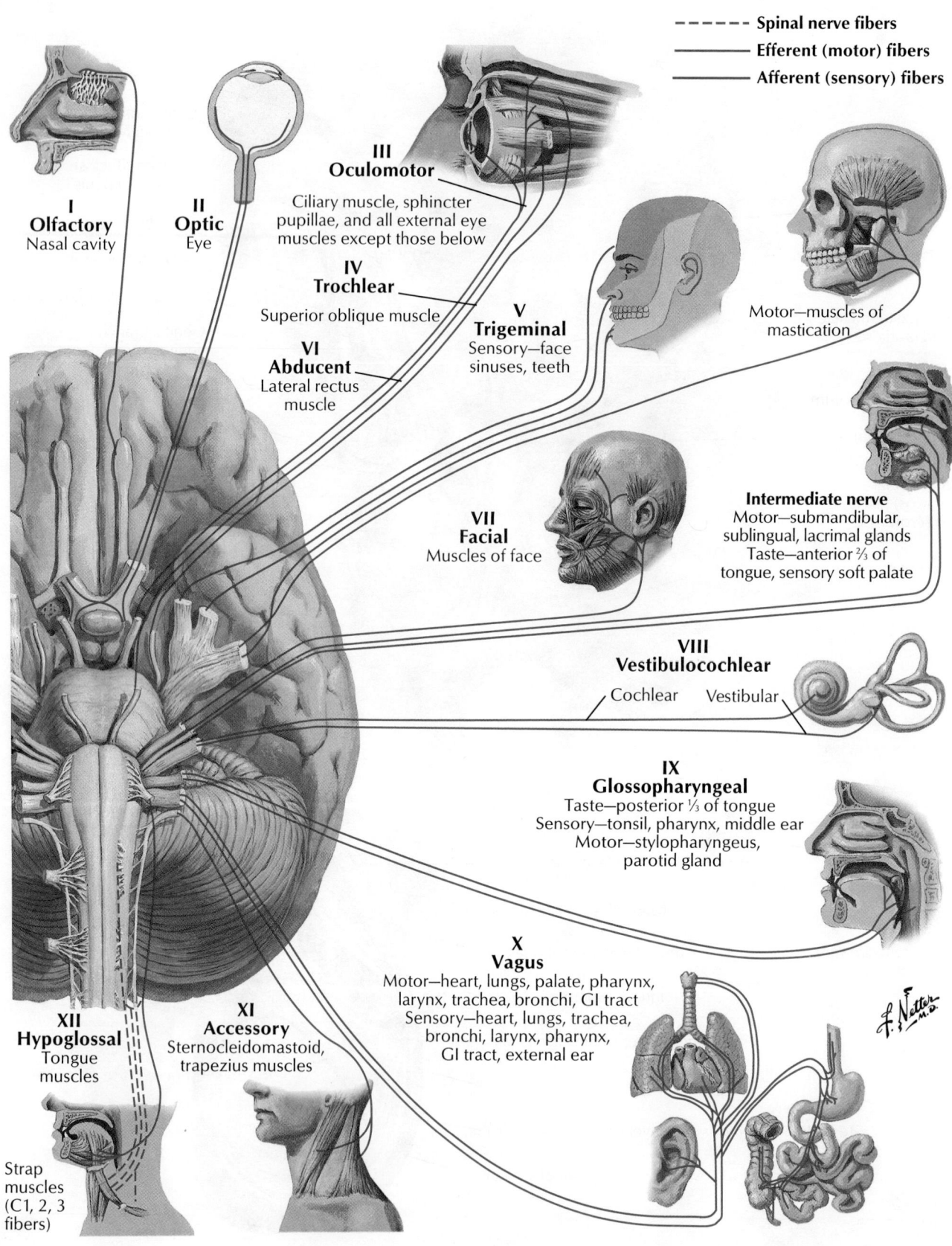

NETTER ANATOMY PLATE

- - - - - Spinal nerve fibers
———— Efferent (motor) fibers
———— Afferent (sensory) fibers

I
Olfactory
Nasal cavity

II
Optic
Eye

III
Oculomotor
Ciliary muscle, sphincter
pupillae, and all external eye
muscles except those below

IV
Trochlear
Superior oblique muscle

V
Trigeminal
Sensory—face
sinuses, teeth

VI
Abducent
Lateral rectus
muscle

Motor—muscles of
mastication

VII
Facial
Muscles of face

Intermediate nerve
Motor—submandibular,
sublingual, lacrimal glands
Taste—anterior ⅔ of
tongue, sensory soft palate

VIII
Vestibulocochlear
Cochlear   Vestibular

IX
Glossopharyngeal
Taste—posterior ⅓ of tongue
Sensory—tonsil, pharynx, middle ear
Motor—stylopharyngeus,
parotid gland

X
Vagus
Motor—heart, lungs, palate, pharynx,
larynx, trachea, bronchi, GI tract
Sensory—heart, lungs, trachea,
bronchi, larynx, pharynx,
GI tract, external ear

XII
Hypoglossal
Tongue
muscles

XI
Accessory
Sternocleidomastoid,
trapezius muscles

Strap
muscles
(C1, 2, 3
fibers)

Plate 118   Cranial Nerves (Motor and Sensory Distribution): Schema. (Netter: Atlas of Human Anatomy, 4 ed, 2006, Saunders.)

Superior view

Supratrochlear nerve
Medial rectus muscle
Superior oblique muscle
Infratrochlear nerve
Nasociliary nerve
Trochlear nerve (IV)
Common tendinous ring
Ophthalmic nerve (V₁)
Optic nerve (II)
Internal carotid artery and nerve plexus
Oculomotor nerve (III)
Trochlear nerve (IV)
Abducent nerve (VI)
Tentorium cerebelli

Medial branch } Supraorbital nerve
Lateral branch }
Levator palpebrae superioris muscle
Superior rectus muscle
Lacrimal gland
Lacrimal nerve
Lateral rectus muscle
Frontal nerve
Maxillary nerve (V₂)
Meningeal branch of maxillary nerve
Mandibular nerve (V₃)
Lesser petrosal nerve
Meningeal branch of mandibular nerve
Greater petrosal nerve
Trigeminal (semilunar) ganglion
Tentorial (meningeal) branch of ophthalmic nerve

Superior view:
levator palpebrae superioris, superior rectus, and superior oblique muscles partially cut away

Supratrochlear nerve (cut)
Supraorbital nerve branches (cut)
Infratrochlear nerve
Anterior ethmoidal nerve
Optic nerve (II)
Posterior ethmoidal nerve
Superior branch of oculomotor nerve (III) (cut)
Nasociliary nerve
Internal carotid plexus
Trochlear nerve (IV) (cut)
Oculomotor nerve (III)
Abducent nerve (VI)

Long ciliary nerves
Short ciliary nerves
Lacrimal nerve
Ciliary ganglion
Parasympathetic root of ciliary ganglion (from inferior branch of oculomotor nerve)
Sympathetic root of ciliary ganglion (from internal carotid plexus)
Sensory root of ciliary ganglion (from nasociliary nerve)
Branches to inferior and medial rectus muscles
Abducent nerve (VI)
Inferior branch of oculomotor nerve (III)
Lacrimal nerve
Frontal nerve (cut)
Ophthalmic nerve (V₁)

f. Netter m.d.

Plate 86   Nerves of Orbit. (Netter: Atlas of Human Anatomy, 4 ed, 2006, Saunders.)

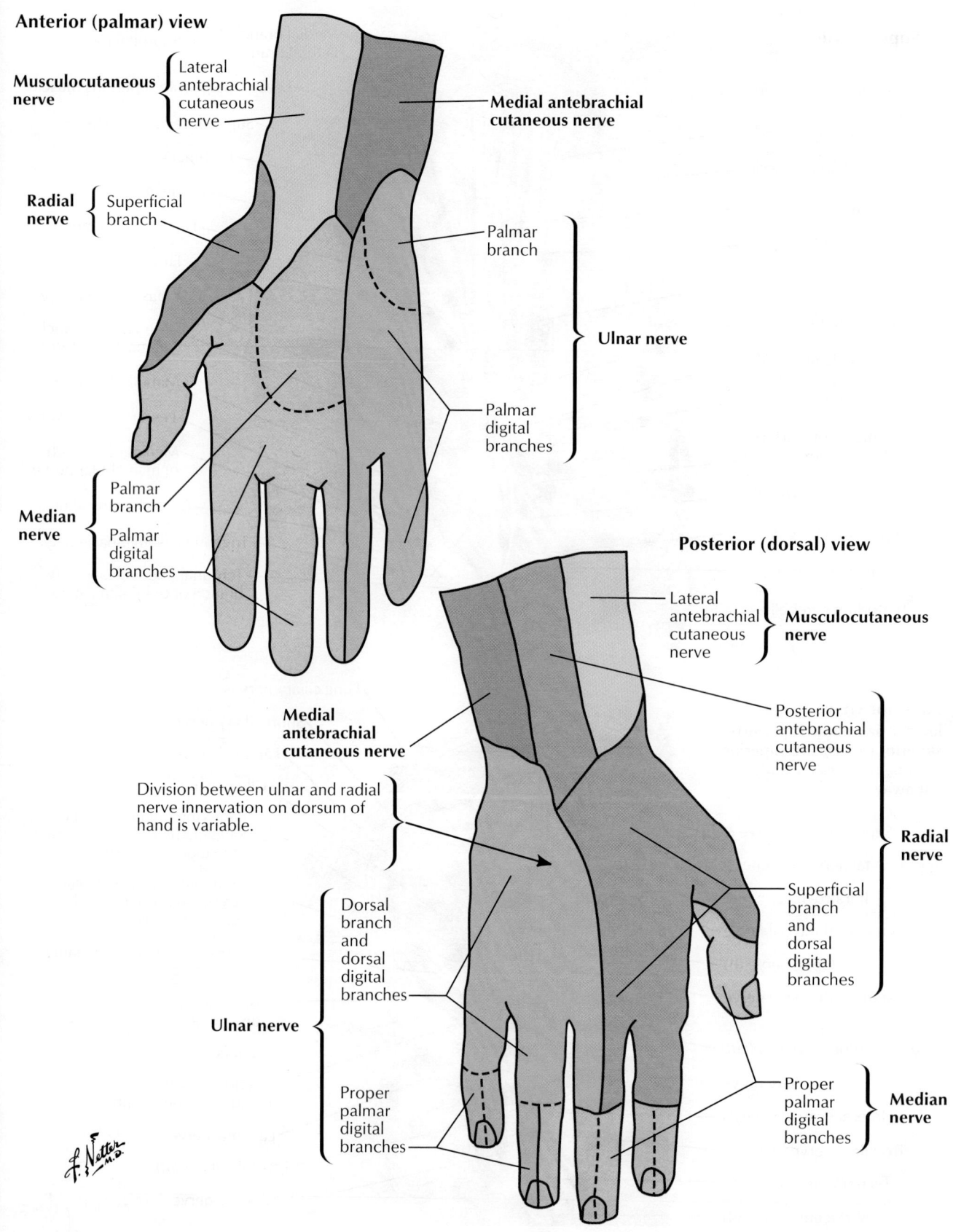

Anterior (palmar) view

Musculocutaneous nerve { Lateral antebrachial cutaneous nerve

Medial antebrachial cutaneous nerve

Radial nerve { Superficial branch

Palmar branch

Ulnar nerve

Palmar digital branches

Median nerve { Palmar branch / Palmar digital branches

Posterior (dorsal) view

Lateral antebrachial cutaneous nerve } Musculocutaneous nerve

Medial antebrachial cutaneous nerve

Posterior antebrachial cutaneous nerve

Division between ulnar and radial nerve innervation on dorsum of hand is variable.

Radial nerve

Superficial branch and dorsal digital branches

Ulnar nerve { Dorsal branch and dorsal digital branches

Proper palmar digital branches

Proper palmar digital branches } Median nerve

Plate 472 Cutaneous Innervation of Wrist and Hand. (Netter: Atlas of Human Anatomy, 4 ed, 2006, Saunders.)

Anterior view

Deltoid muscle

Coracobrachialis muscle

Biceps brachii muscle { Short head (*cut*)
Long head (*cut*)

Musculocutaneous nerve

Brachialis muscle

Biceps brachii muscle (*cut*) and tendon

Lateral antebrachial cutaneous nerve
(from musculocutaneous nerve)

Radial nerve { Deep branch
Superficial branch

Supinator muscle

Brachioradialis muscle

Radial artery

Pronator teres muscle (*partially cut*)

Median nerve

Flexor pollicis longus muscle

Flexor carpi radialis
tendon (*cut*)

Flexor retinaculum
(transverse carpal
ligament)

Superficial branch
of radial nerve

Recurrent (motor)
branch of
median nerve to
thenar muscles

Common palmar
digital branches
of median nerve

Proper palmar
digital branches
of median nerve

Intercostobrachial nerve

Medial brachial
cutaneous nerve

Radial nerve

Ulnar nerve

Medial antebrachial
cutaneous nerve

Median nerve

Brachial artery

Bicipital aponeurosis

Humeral head (*cut*) }
Ulnar head } Pronator teres muscle

Flexor carpi radialis muscle (*cut*)

Humeroulnar head } Flexor digitorum
Radial head } superficialis muscle (*cut*)

Flexor digitorum profundus muscle

Flexor carpi ulnaris muscle

Ulnar artery and nerve

Dorsal branch of ulnar nerve

Flexor digitorum superficialis tendons (*cut*)

Deep palmar branch of ulnar artery and deep branch of ulnar nerve

Superficial branch of ulnar nerve

Superficial palmar arch (*cut*)

Common palmar digital branch of ulnar nerve

Communicating branch of median nerve with ulnar nerve

Proper palmar digital branches of ulnar nerve

NETTER ANATOMY PLATE

Plate 473   Arteries and Nerves of Upper Limb. (Netter: Atlas of Human Anatomy, 4 ed, 2006, Saunders.)

Lateral cutaneous branch of subcostal nerve

Inguinal ligament (Poupart's)

Superficial circumflex iliac vein

Femoral branches of genitofemoral nerve

Lateral femoral cutaneous nerve

Saphenous opening (fossa ovalis)

Fascia lata

Anterior cutaneous branches of femoral nerve

Patellar nerve plexus

Branches of lateral sural cutaneous nerve (from common fibular [peroneal] nerve)

Deep fascia of leg (crural fascia)

Superficial fibular (peroneal) nerve
Medial dorsal cutaneous branch

Intermediate dorsal cutaneous branch

Small saphenous vein and lateral dorsal cutaneous nerve (from sural nerve)

Lateral dorsal digital nerve and vein of 5th toe

Dorsal metatarsal veins

Dorsal digital nerves and veins

Superficial epigastric vein

Ilioinguinal nerve (scrotal branch) (usually passes through superficial inguinal ring)

Genital branch of genitofemoral nerve

Femoral vein

Superficial external pudendal vein

Accessory saphenous vein

Great saphenous vein

Cutaneous branches of obturator nerve

Infrapatellar branch of saphenous nerve

Saphenous nerve (terminal branch of femoral nerve)

Great saphenous vein

Dorsal digital nerves

Dorsal venous arch

Dorsal digital nerve and vein of medial side of great toe

Dorsal digital branch of deep fibular (peroneal) nerve

Plate 544 Superficial Nerves and Veins of Lower Limb: Anterior View. (Netter: Atlas of Human Anatomy, 4 ed, 2006, Saunders.)

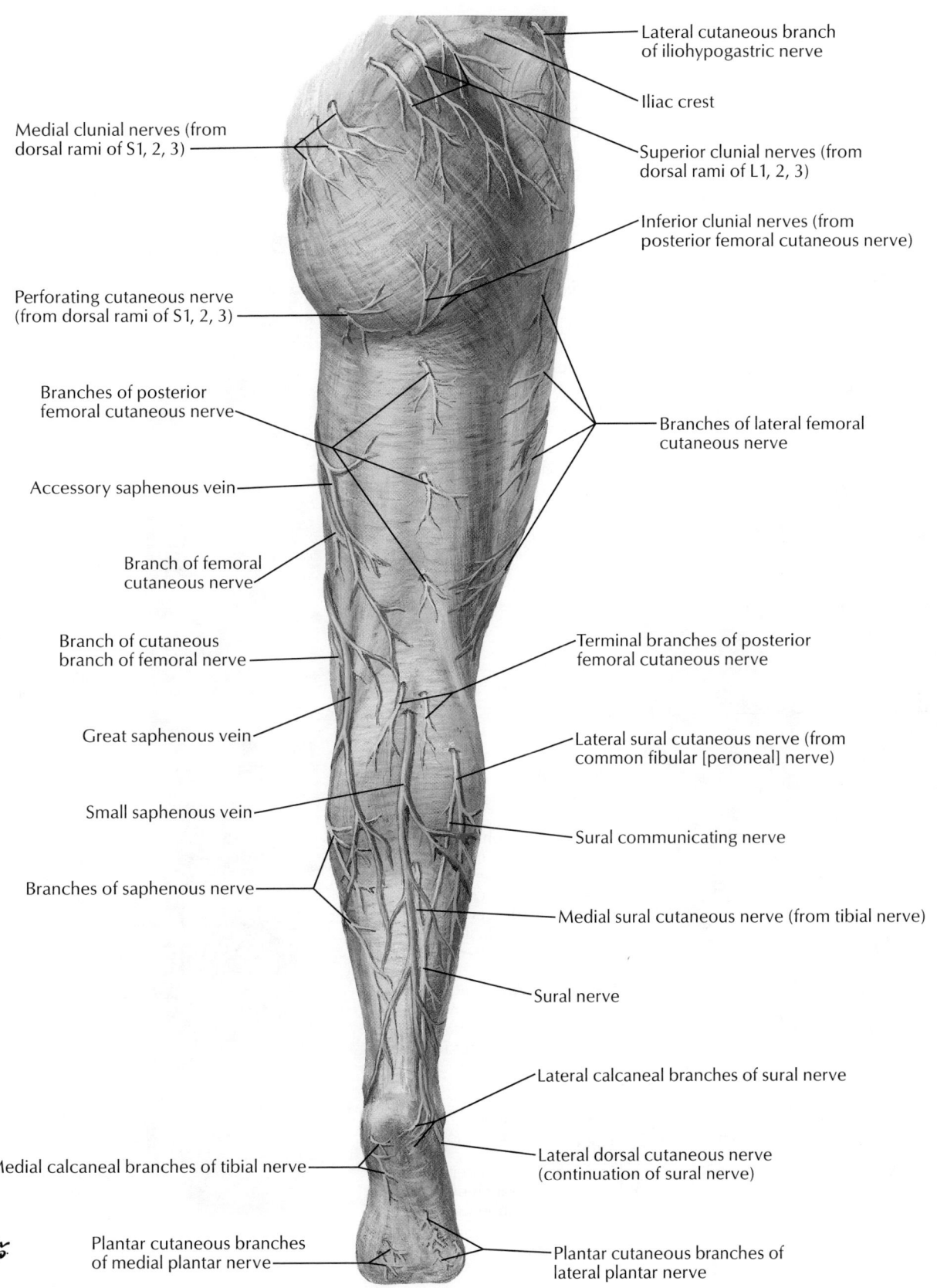

Lateral cutaneous branch of iliohypogastric nerve

Iliac crest

Medial clunial nerves (from dorsal rami of S1, 2, 3)

Superior clunial nerves (from dorsal rami of L1, 2, 3)

Inferior clunial nerves (from posterior femoral cutaneous nerve)

Perforating cutaneous nerve (from dorsal rami of S1, 2, 3)

Branches of posterior femoral cutaneous nerve

Branches of lateral femoral cutaneous nerve

Accessory saphenous vein

Branch of femoral cutaneous nerve

Branch of cutaneous branch of femoral nerve

Terminal branches of posterior femoral cutaneous nerve

Great saphenous vein

Lateral sural cutaneous nerve (from common fibular [peroneal] nerve)

Small saphenous vein

Sural communicating nerve

Branches of saphenous nerve

Medial sural cutaneous nerve (from tibial nerve)

Sural nerve

Lateral calcaneal branches of sural nerve

Medial calcaneal branches of tibial nerve

Lateral dorsal cutaneous nerve (continuation of sural nerve)

Plantar cutaneous branches of medial plantar nerve

Plantar cutaneous branches of lateral plantar nerve

Plate 545 Superficial Nerves and Veins of Lower Limb: Posterior View. (Netter: Atlas of Human Anatomy, 4 ed, 2006, Saunders.)

NETTER ANATOMY PLATE

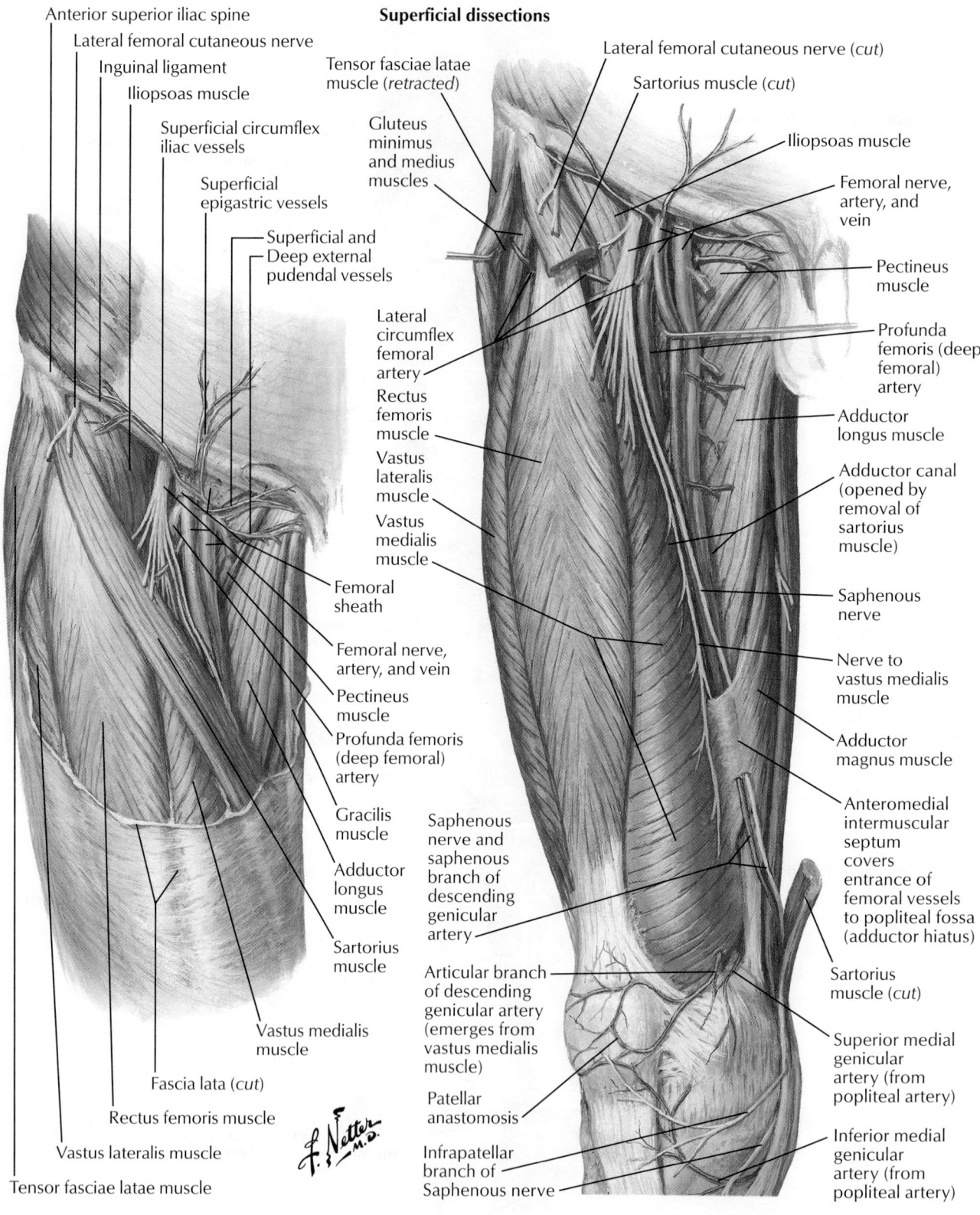

Superficial dissections

Anterior superior iliac spine

Lateral femoral cutaneous nerve

Inguinal ligament

Iliopsoas muscle

Superficial circumflex iliac vessels

Superficial epigastric vessels

Superficial and Deep external pudendal vessels

Tensor fasciae latae muscle (*retracted*)

Gluteus minimus and medius muscles

Lateral circumflex femoral artery

Rectus femoris muscle

Vastus lateralis muscle

Vastus medialis muscle

Femoral sheath

Femoral nerve, artery, and vein

Pectineus muscle

Profunda femoris (deep femoral) artery

Gracilis muscle

Adductor longus muscle

Sartorius muscle

Vastus medialis muscle

Fascia lata (*cut*)

Rectus femoris muscle

Vastus lateralis muscle

Tensor fasciae latae muscle

Lateral femoral cutaneous nerve (*cut*)

Sartorius muscle (*cut*)

Iliopsoas muscle

Femoral nerve, artery, and vein

Pectineus muscle

Profunda femoris (deep femoral) artery

Adductor longus muscle

Adductor canal (opened by removal of sartorius muscle)

Saphenous nerve

Nerve to vastus medialis muscle

Adductor magnus muscle

Anteromedial intermuscular septum covers entrance of femoral vessels to popliteal fossa (adductor hiatus)

Sartorius muscle (*cut*)

Superior medial genicular artery (from popliteal artery)

Inferior medial genicular artery (from popliteal artery)

Saphenous nerve and saphenous branch of descending genicular artery

Articular branch of descending genicular artery (emerges from vastus medialis muscle)

Patellar anastomosis

Infrapatellar branch of Saphenous nerve

f. Netter m.d.

Plate 500 Arteries and Nerves of Thigh: Anterior Views. (Netter: Atlas of Human Anatomy, 4 ed, 2006, Saunders.)

Deep dissection

Deep circumflex iliac artery

Lateral femoral cutaneous nerve

Sartorius muscle (*cut*)

Iliopsoas muscle

Tensor fasciae latae muscle (*retracted*)

Gluteus medius and minimus muscles

Femoral nerve

Rectus femoris muscle (*cut*)

Ascending, transverse and descending branches of Lateral circumflex femoral artery

Medial circumflex femoral artery

Pectineus muscle (*cut*)

Profunda femoris (deep femoral) artery

Perforating branches

Adductor longus muscle (*cut*)

Vastus lateralis muscle

Vastus intermedius muscle

Rectus femoris muscle (*cut*)

Saphenous nerve

Anteromedial intermuscular septum (*opened*)

Vastus medialis muscle

Quadriceps femoris tendon

Patella and patellar anastomosis

Medial patellar retinaculum

Patellar ligament

External iliac artery and vein

Inguinal ligament (Poupart's)

Femoral artery and vein (*cut*)

Pectineus muscle (*cut*)

Obturator canal

Obturator externus muscle

Adductor longus muscle (*cut*)

Anterior branch and Posterior branch of obturator nerve

Quadratus femoris muscle

Adductor brevis muscle

Branches of posterior branch of obturator nerve

Adductor magnus muscle

Gracilis muscle

Cutaneous branch of obturator nerve

Femoral artery and vein (*cut*)

Descending genicular artery
Articular branch
Saphenous branch

Adductor hiatus

Sartorius muscle (*cut*)

Adductor magnus tendon

Adductor tubercle on medial epicondyle of femur

Superior medial genicular artery (from popliteal artery)

Infrapatellar branch of Saphenous nerve

Inferior medial genicular artery (from popliteal artery)

Plate 501 Arteries and Nerves of Thigh: Posterior View. (Netter: Atlas of Human Anatomy, 4 ed, 2006, Saunders.)

NAP-13

NETTER ANATOMY PLATE

Deep dissection

Superior clunial nerves

Gluteus maximus muscle (cut)

Medial clunial nerves

Inferior gluteal artery and nerve

Pudendal nerve

Nerve to obturator internus (and superior gemellus)

Posterior femoral cutaneous nerve

Sacrotuberous ligament

Ischial tuberosity

Inferior clunial nerves (cut)

Adductor magnus muscle

Gracilis muscle

Sciatic nerve

Muscular branches of sciatic nerve

Semitendinosus muscle (retracted)

Semimembranosus muscle

Sciatic nerve

Articular branch

Adductor hiatus

Popliteal vein and artery

Superior medial genicular artery

Medial epicondyle of femur

Tibial nerve

Gastrocnemius muscle (medial head)

Medial sural cutaneous nerve

Small saphenous vein

Iliac crest

Gluteal aponeurosis and gluteus medius muscle (cut)

Superior gluteal artery and nerve

Gluteus minimus muscle

Tensor fasciae latae muscle

Piriformis muscle

Gluteus medius muscle (cut)

Superior gemellus muscle

Greater trochanter of femur

Obturator internus muscle

Inferior gemellus muscle

Gluteus maximus muscle (cut)

Quadratus femoris muscle

Medial circumflex femoral artery

Vastus lateralis muscle and iliotibial tract

Adductor minimus part of adductor magnus muscle

1st perforating artery (from profunda femoris artery)

Adductor magnus muscle

2nd and 3rd perforating arteries (from profunda femoris artery)

4th perforating artery (from profunda femoris artery)

Long head (retracted)
Short head } Biceps femoris muscle

Superior lateral genicular artery

Common fibular (peroneal) nerve

Plantaris muscle

Gastrocnemius muscle (lateral head)

Lateral sural cutaneous nerve

Plate 502   Arteries and Nerves of Thigh: Posterior View. (Netter: Atlas of Human Anatomy, 4 ed, 2006, Saunders.)

Horizontal section

Zonular fibers
(suspensory ligament of lens)

Scleral venous sinus
(canal of Schlemm)

Scleral spur

Ciliary body and ciliary muscle

Ciliary part of retina

Tendon of
lateral rectus
muscle

Iris

Lens

Capsule of lens

Cornea

Anterior chamber

Posterior chamber

Iridocorneal angle

Ciliary processes

Bulbar conjunctiva

Ora serrata

Tendon of
medial rectus
muscle

Optic (visual)
part of retina

Choroid

Perichoroidal space

Sclera

Fascial sheath of eyeball
(Tenon's capsule)

Episcleral space

Fovea centralis in macula (lutea)

Outer sheath of optic nerve

Subarachnoid space

Vitreous body

Hyaloid canal

Lamina cribrosa of sclera

Optic nerve (II)

Central retinal
artery and vein

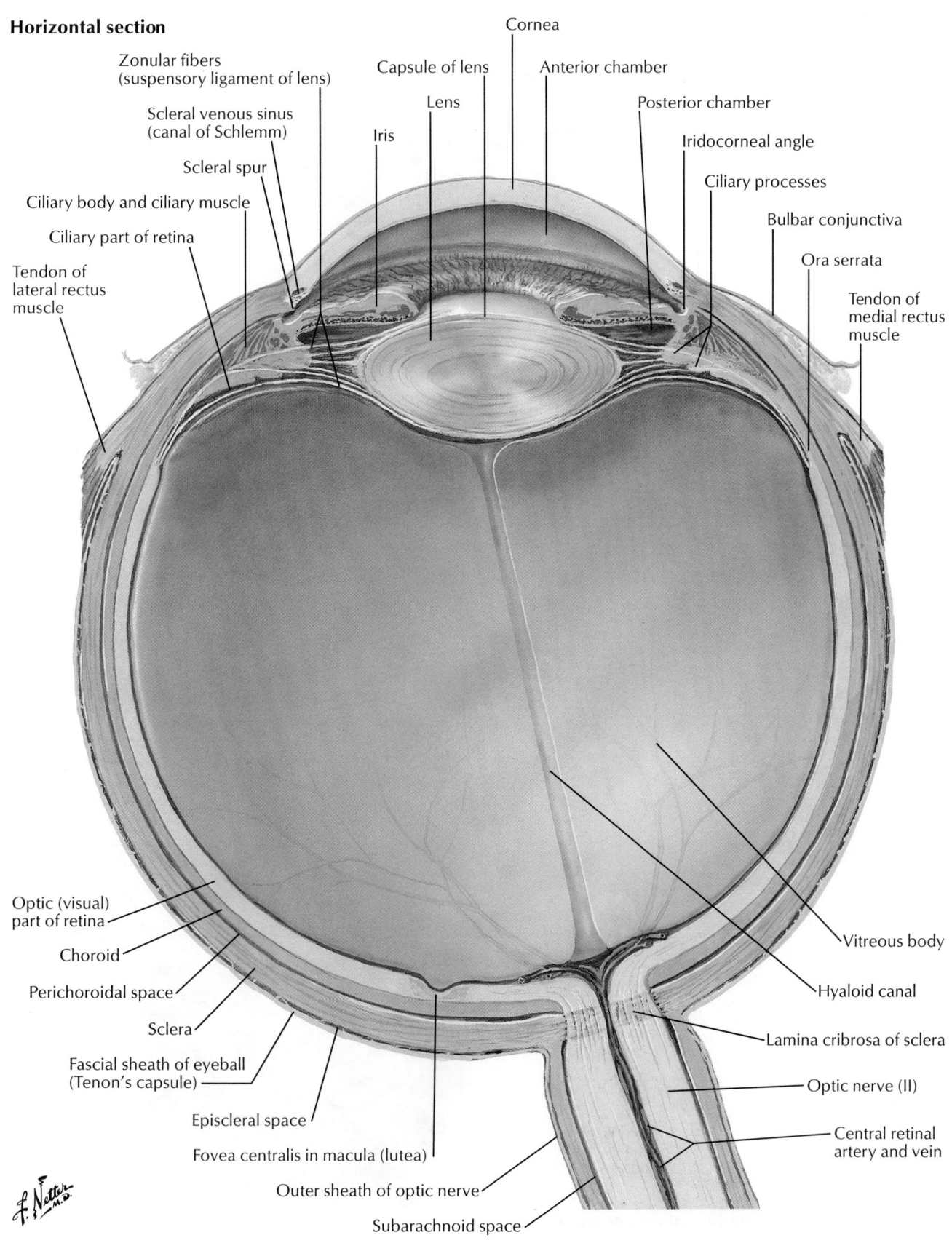

Plate 87   Eyeball. (Netter: Atlas of Human Anatomy, 4 ed, 2006, Saunders.)

NAP-15

NETTER ANATOMY PLATE

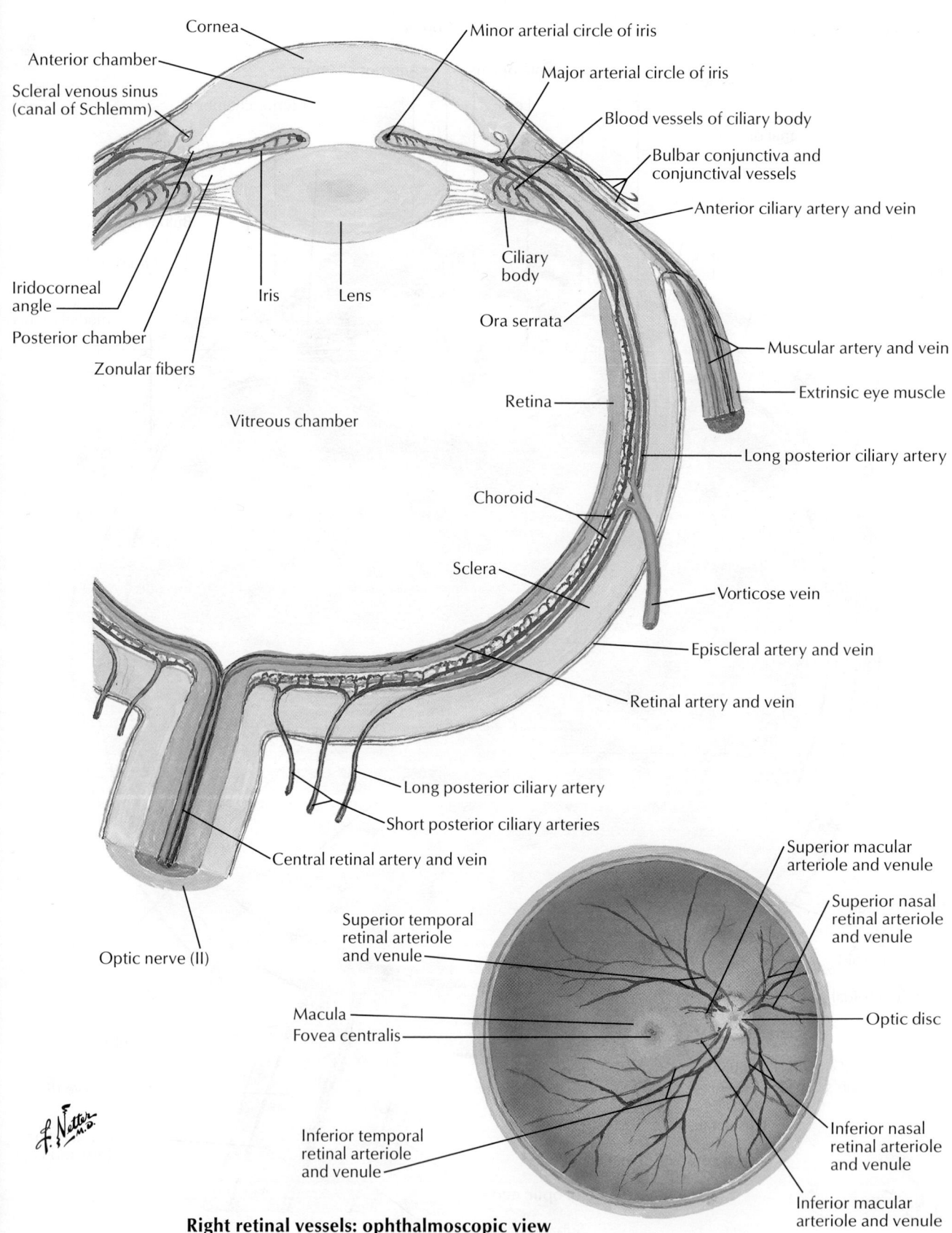

Cornea

Minor arterial circle of iris

Anterior chamber

Major arterial circle of iris

Scleral venous sinus (canal of Schlemm)

Blood vessels of ciliary body

Bulbar conjunctiva and conjunctival vessels

Anterior ciliary artery and vein

Ciliary body

Muscular artery and vein

Iridocorneal angle

Iris

Lens

Ora serrata

Extrinsic eye muscle

Posterior chamber

Long posterior ciliary artery

Zonular fibers

Retina

Vitreous chamber

Choroid

Vorticose vein

Sclera

Episcleral artery and vein

Retinal artery and vein

Long posterior ciliary artery

Short posterior ciliary arteries

Central retinal artery and vein

Optic nerve (II)

Superior macular arteriole and venule

Superior nasal retinal arteriole and venule

Superior temporal retinal arteriole and venule

Macula

Fovea centralis

Optic disc

Inferior temporal retinal arteriole and venule

Inferior nasal retinal arteriole and venule

Inferior macular arteriole and venule

Right retinal vessels: ophthalmoscopic view

Plate 90 Intrinsic Arteries and Veins of Eye. (Netter: Atlas of Human Anatomy, 4 ed, 2006, Saunders.)

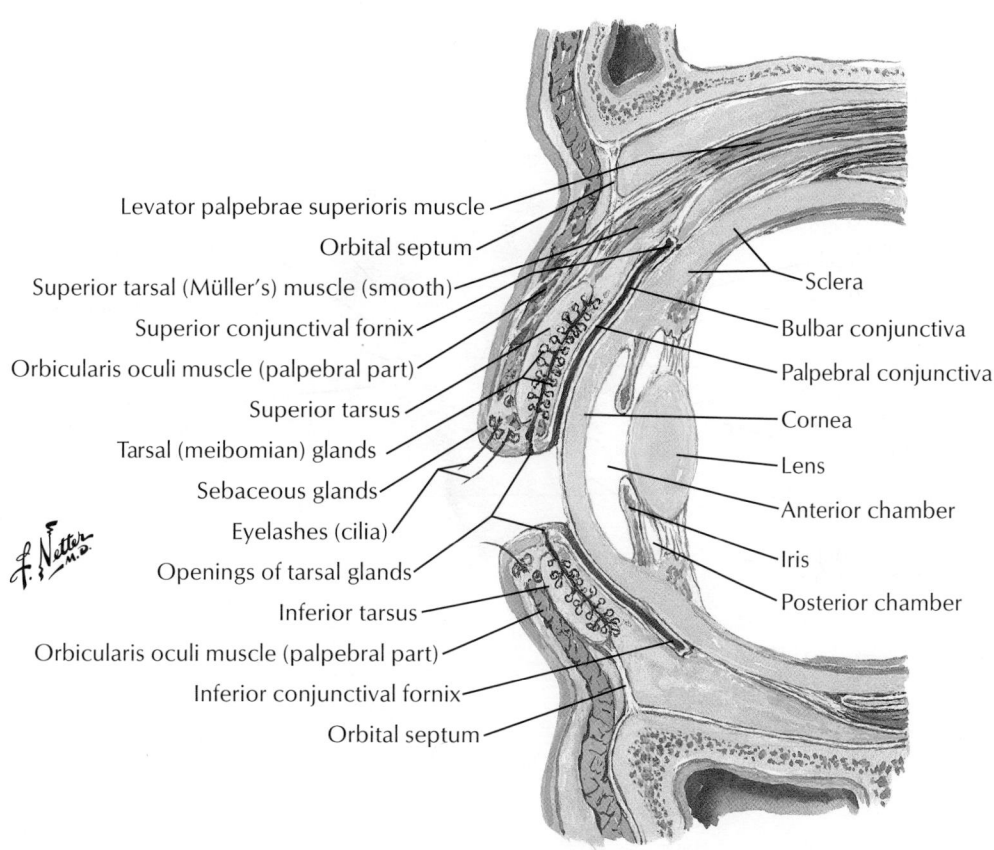

Levator palpebrae superioris muscle

Orbital septum

Superior tarsal (Müller's) muscle (smooth)

Superior conjunctival fornix

Orbicularis oculi muscle (palpebral part)

Superior tarsus

Tarsal (meibomian) glands

Sebaceous glands

Eyelashes (cilia)

Openings of tarsal glands

Inferior tarsus

Orbicularis oculi muscle (palpebral part)

Inferior conjunctival fornix

Orbital septum

Sclera

Bulbar conjunctiva

Palpebral conjunctiva

Cornea

Lens

Anterior chamber

Iris

Posterior chamber

Plate 81, Middle   Eyelids. (Netter: Atlas of Human Anatomy, 4 ed, 2006, Saunders.)

NETTER ANATOMY PLATE

Superior palpebral conjunctiva:
tarsal (meibomian) glands
shining through

Seen through { Pupil
cornea { Iris

Corneoscleral junction
(corneal limbus)

Bulbar conjunctiva
over sclera

Inferior conjunctival fornix

Inferior palpebral conjunctiva:
tarsal glands shining through

Superior lacrimal papilla and
punctum

Plica semilunaris

Lacrimal caruncle in
lacrimal lake (lacus lacrimalis)

Inferior lacrimal papilla and
punctum

Plate 81, Upper   Eyelid. (Netter: Atlas of Human Anatomy, 4 ed, 2006, Saunders.)

Orbital part of lacrimal gland

Palpebral part of lacrimal gland

Excretory ducts of lacrimal gland

Plica semilunaris

Lacrimal caruncle

Inferior lacrimal papilla and punctum

Superior lacrimal papilla and punctum

Lacrimal canaliculi

Lacrimal sac

Nasolacrimal duct

Opening of nasolacrimal duct

Frontal bone (*cut away*)

Orbital part of lacrimal gland

Palpebral part of lacrimal gland

Excretory ducts of lacrimal gland

Plica semilunaris and lacrimal lake

Lacrimal caruncle

Inferior lacrimal papilla and punctum

Opening of nasolacrimal duct

Superior lacrimal papilla and punctum

Lacrimal canaliculi

Lacrimal sac

Nasolacrimal duct

Middle nasal concha

Nasal cavity

Inferior nasal concha (*cut*)

Inferior nasal meatus

Plate 82 Lacrimal Apparatus. (Netter: Atlas of Human Anatomy, 4 ed, 2006, Saunders.)

Frontal section

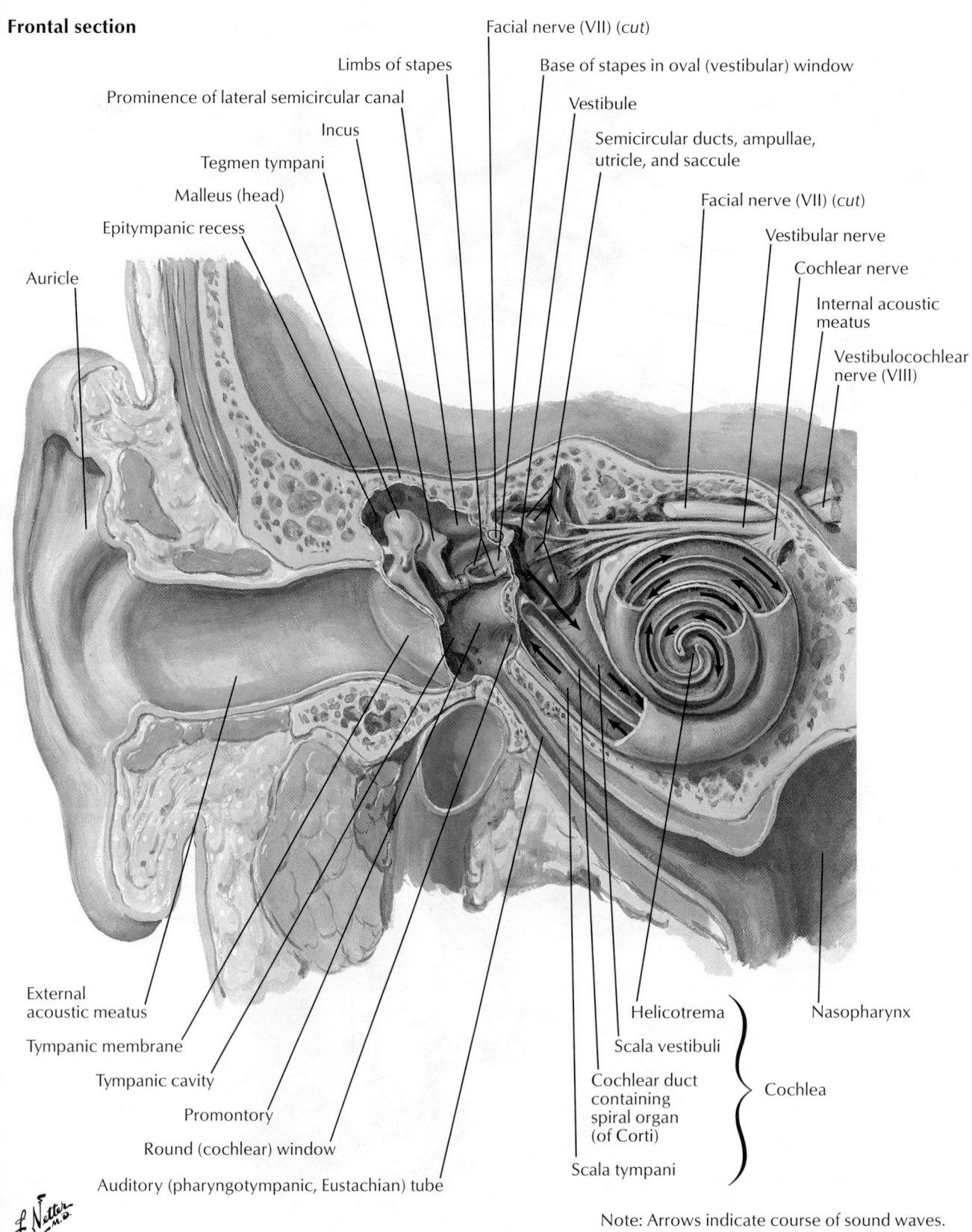

Limbs of stapes

Prominence of lateral semicircular canal

Incus

Tegmen tympani

Malleus (head)

Epitympanic recess

Auricle

Facial nerve (VII) (*cut*)

Base of stapes in oval (vestibular) window

Vestibule

Semicircular ducts, ampullae, utricle, and saccule

Facial nerve (VII) (*cut*)

Vestibular nerve

Cochlear nerve

Internal acoustic meatus

Vestibulocochlear nerve (VIII)

External acoustic meatus

Tympanic membrane

Tympanic cavity

Promontory

Round (cochlear) window

Auditory (pharyngotympanic, Eustachian) tube

Helicotrema

Scala vestibuli

Cochlear duct containing spiral organ (of Corti)

Scala tympani

Cochlea

Nasopharynx

Note: Arrows indicate course of sound waves.

NETTER ANATOMY PLATE

Plate 92 *Pathway of Sound Reception. (Netter: Atlas of Human Anatomy, 4 ed, 2006, Saunders.)*

Medial wall of tympanic cavity: lateral view

Mastoid antrum

Prominence of lateral semicircular canal

Prominence of facial canal

Geniculum (geniculate ganglion) of facial nerve

Greater petrosal nerve

Base of stapes in fossa of oval (vestibular) window

Limbs of stapes

Pyramidal eminence

Chorda tympani nerve (*cut*)

Mastoid cells

Tendon of stapedius muscle

Fossa of round (cochlear) window

Facial nerve (VII) in stylomastoid foramen

Jugular fossa

Tympanic cells

Tensor tympani muscle (*tendon cut*)

Auditory (pharyngotympanic, Eustachian) tube

Levator veli palatini muscle

Promontory with tympanic nerve (of Jacobson) and plexus under mucosa

Internal carotid artery

Plate 94 Tympanic Cavity. (Netter: Atlas of Human Anatomy, 4 ed, 2006, Saunders.)

Otoscopic view of right tympanic membrane

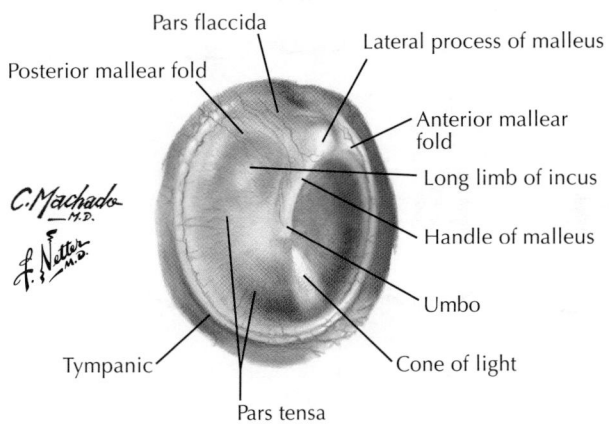

Pars flaccida

Posterior mallear fold

Lateral process of malleus

Anterior mallear fold

Long limb of incus

Handle of malleus

Umbo

Cone of light

Tympanic

Pars tensa

Plate 93 Tympanic Cavity. (Netter: Atlas of Human Anatomy, 4 ed, 2006, Saunders.)

Dissected right bony labyrinth (otic capsule): membranous labyrinth removed

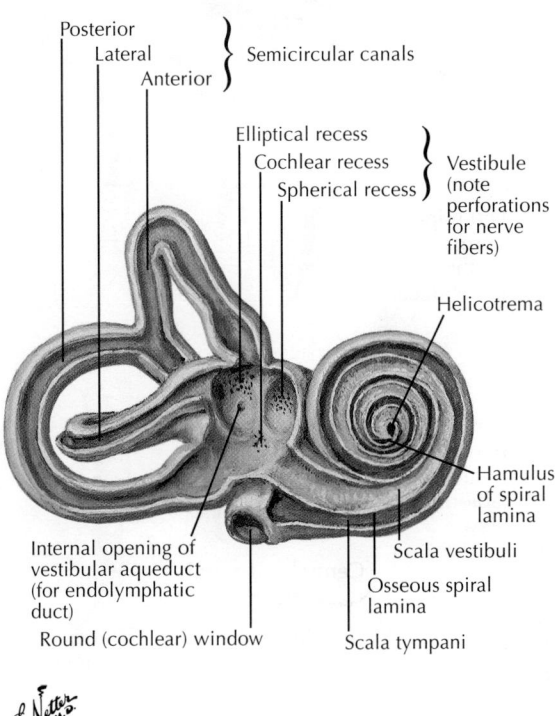

Posterior

Lateral

Anterior

Semicircular canals

Elliptical recess

Cochlear recess

Spherical recess

Vestibule (note perforations for nerve fibers)

Helicotrema

Internal opening of vestibular aqueduct (for endolymphatic duct)

Round (cochlear) window

Hamulus of spiral lamina

Scala vestibuli

Osseous spiral lamina

Scala tympani

Plate 95 Bony Membranous Labyrinth. (Netter: Atlas of Human Anatomy, 4 ed, 2006, Saunders.)

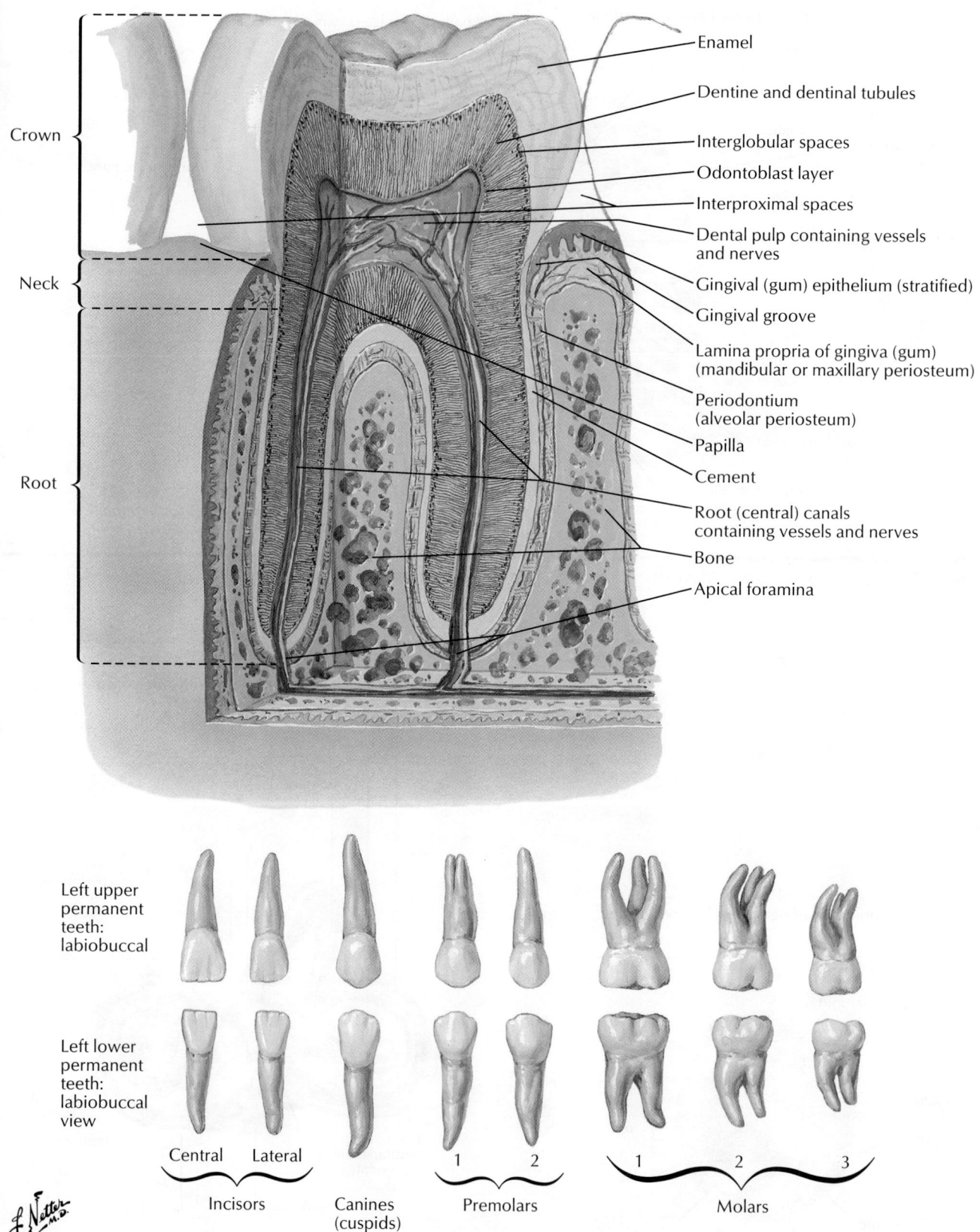

Crown

Neck

Root

Enamel

Dentine and dentinal tubules

Interglobular spaces

Odontoblast layer

Interproximal spaces

Dental pulp containing vessels and nerves

Gingival (gum) epithelium (stratified)

Gingival groove

Lamina propria of gingiva (gum) (mandibular or maxillary periosteum)

Periodontium (alveolar periosteum)

Papilla

Cement

Root (central) canals containing vessels and nerves

Bone

Apical foramina

Left upper permanent teeth: labiobuccal

Left lower permanent teeth: labiobuccal view

Central   Lateral

Incisors

Canines (cuspids)

1   2

Premolars

1   2   3

Molars

Plate 57 Teeth. (Netter: Atlas of Human Anatomy, 4 ed, 2006, Saunders.)

Tongue

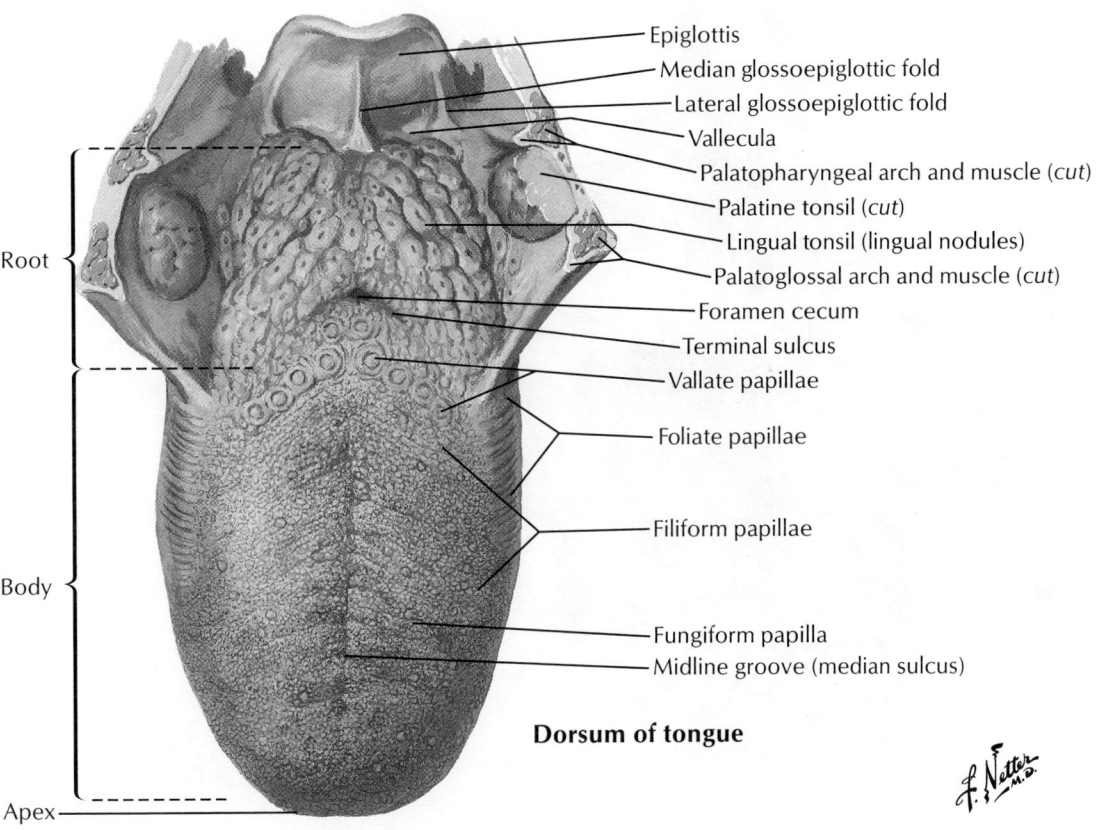

Epiglottis
Median glossoepiglottic fold
Lateral glossoepiglottic fold
Vallecula
Palatopharyngeal arch and muscle (*cut*)
Palatine tonsil (*cut*)
Lingual tonsil (lingual nodules)
Palatoglossal arch and muscle (*cut*)
Foramen cecum
Terminal sulcus
Vallate papillae
Foliate papillae
Filiform papillae
Fungiform papilla
Midline groove (median sulcus)

Root

Body

Apex

Dorsum of tongue

Plate 58   Tongue. (Netter: Atlas of Human Anatomy, 4 ed, 2006, Saunders.)

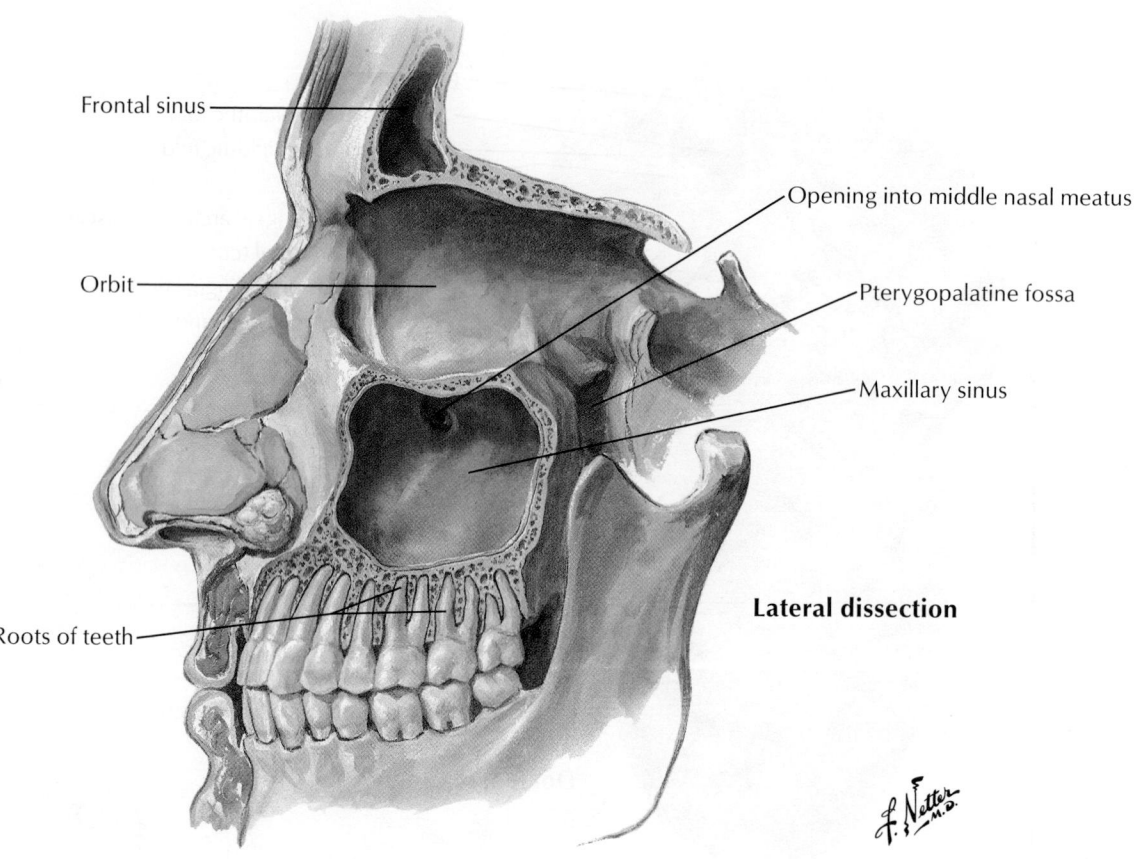

Frontal sinus

Opening into middle nasal meatus

Orbit

Pterygopalatine fossa

Maxillary sinus

Roots of teeth

Lateral dissection

Plate 49 Paranasal Sinuses. (Netter: Atlas of Human Anatomy, 4 ed, 2006, Saunders.)

Superficial temporal artery and vein and auriculotemporal nerve

Branches of facial nerve

Transverse facial artery

Accessory parotid gland

Parotid duct

Buccinator muscle (*cut*)

Masseter muscle

Lingual nerve

Submandibular ganglion

Tongue

Frenulum of tongue

Sublingual fold with openings of sublingual ducts

Sublingual caruncle with opening of submandibular duct

Sublingual gland

Submandibular duct

Sublingual artery and vein

Mylohyoid muscle (*cut*)

Digastric muscle (anterior belly)

Submandibular gland

Facial artery and vein

Hyoid bone

Parotid gland

Retromandibular vein (anterior and posterior branches)

Digastric muscle (posterior belly)

Stylohyoid muscle

External jugular vein

Sternocleidomastoid muscle

Common trunk receiving facial, anterior branch of retromandibular, and lingual veins (common facial vein)

Internal jugular vein

External carotid artery

Parotid gland: totally serous

Submandibular gland: mostly serous, partially mucous

Sublingual gland: almost completely mucous

Plate 61 Salivary Glands. (Netter: Atlas of Human Anatomy, 4 ed, 2006, Saunders.)

Coronary Arteries: Arteriographic Views

Right coronary artery: left anterior oblique view

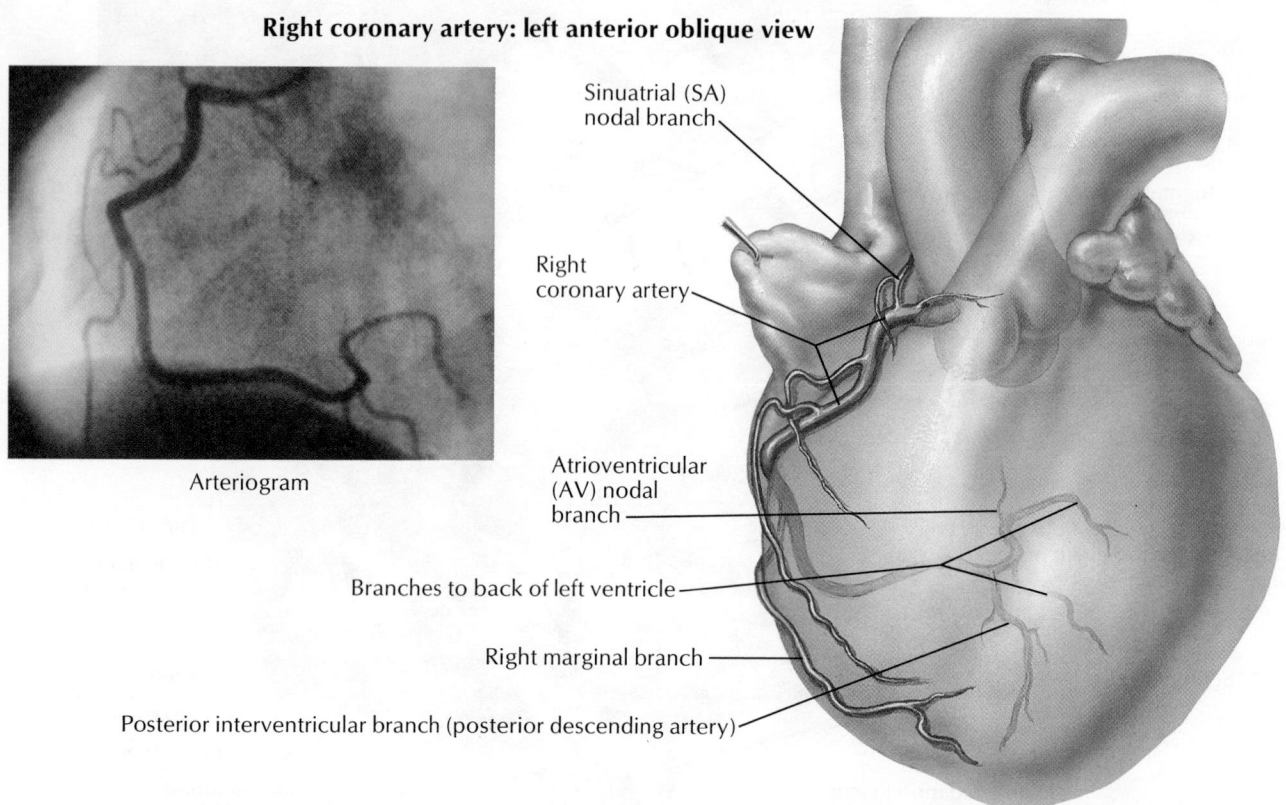

Arteriogram

Sinuatrial (SA) nodal branch

Right coronary artery

Atrioventricular (AV) nodal branch

Branches to back of left ventricle

Right marginal branch

Posterior interventricular branch (posterior descending artery)

Right coronary artery: right anterior oblique view

Sinuatrial (SA) nodal branch

Conus (arteriosus) branch

Right coronary artery

Right marginal branch

Arteriogram

Atrioventricular (AV) nodal branch

Right posterolateral branches (to back of left ventricle)

Posterior interventricular branch (posterior descending artery)

Plate 218   Coronary Arteries: Arteriographic Views. (Netter: Atlas of Human Anatomy, 4 ed, 2006, Saunders.)

Left coronary artery: left anterior oblique view

Left coronary artery

Circumflex branch

Arteriogram

Anterior interventricular branch (left anterior descending)

Diagonal branches of anterior interventricular branch

Atrioventricular branch of circumflex branch

Left (obtuse) marginal branch

Posterolateral branches

(Perforating) interventricular septal branches

Left coronary artery: right anterior oblique view

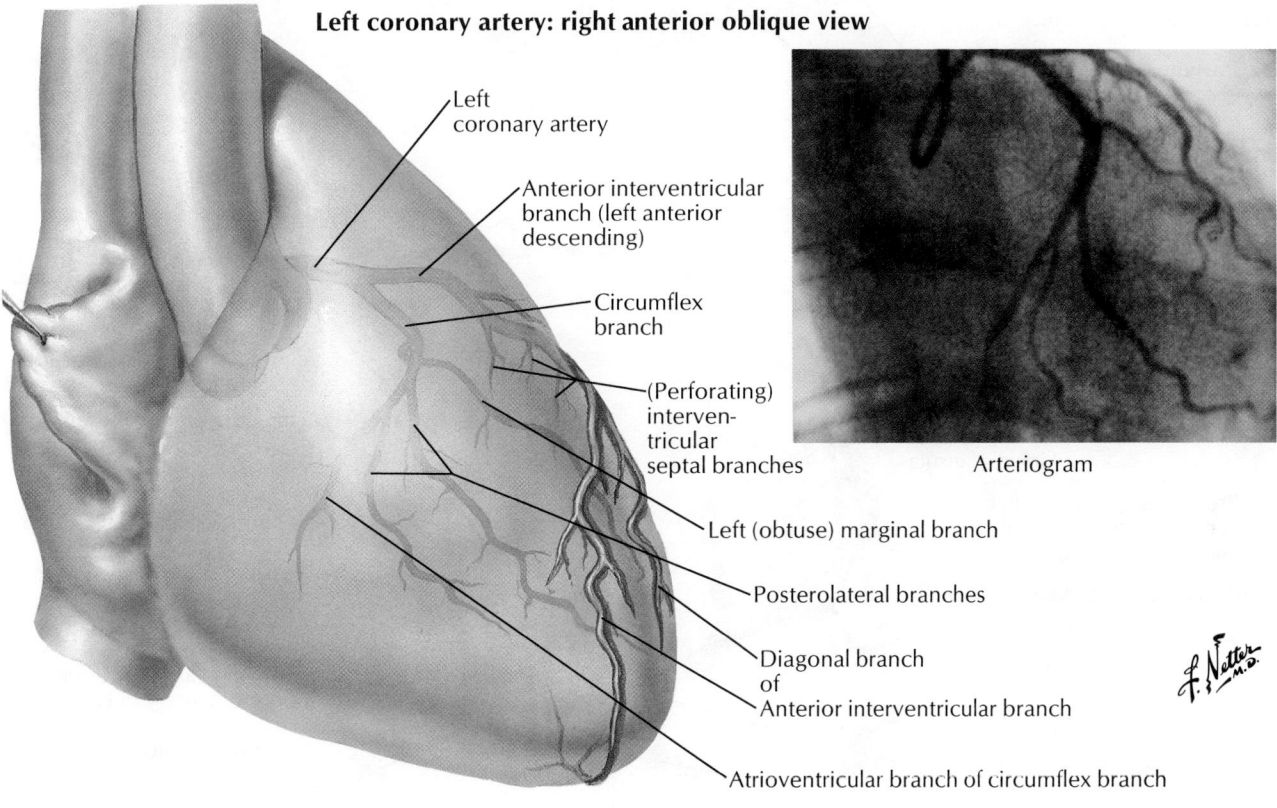

Left coronary artery

Anterior interventricular branch (left anterior descending)

Circumflex branch

(Perforating) interventricular septal branches

Arteriogram

Left (obtuse) marginal branch

Posterolateral branches

Diagonal branch of Anterior interventricular branch

Atrioventricular branch of circumflex branch

Plate 219 Coronary Arteries: Arteriographic Views. (Netter: Atlas of Human Anatomy, 4 ed, 2006, Saunders.)

Corpus callosum

Anterolateral central (lenticulostriate) arteries

Lateral frontobasal (orbitofrontal) artery

Prefrontal artery

Precentral (pre-Rolandic) and central (Rolandic) sulcal arteries

Anterior parietal (postcentral sulcal) artery

Posterior parietal artery

Branch to angular gyrus

Temporal branches (anterior, middle, and posterior)

Middle cerebral artery and branches (deep in lateral cerebral [Sylvian] sulcus)

Anterior communicating artery

Posterior communicating artery

Anterior inferior cerebellar artery (AICA)

Posterior spinal artery

Paracentral artery

Medial frontal branches

Pericallosal artery

Callosomarginal artery

Polar frontal artery

Anterior cerebral arteries

Medial frontobasal (orbitofrontal) artery

Distal medial striate artery (recurrent artery of Heubner)

Internal carotid artery

Anterior choroidal artery

Posterior cerebral artery

Superior cerebellar artery

Basilar and pontine arteries

Labyrinthine (internal acoustic) artery

Vertebral artery

Posterior inferior cerebellar artery (PICA)

Anterior spinal artery

Falx cerebri

Corpus striatum (caudate and lentiform nuclei)

Anterolateral central (lenticulostriate) arteries

Insula (island of Reil)

Limen of insula

Precentral (pre-Rolandic), central (Rolandic) sulcal, and parietal arteries

Lateral cerebral (Sylvian) sulcus

Temporal branches of middle cerebral artery

Temporal lobe

Middle cerebral artery

Internal carotid artery

Callosomarginal arteries and Pericallosal arteries (branches of anterior cerebral arteries)

Trunk of corpus callosum

Internal capsule

Septum pellucidum

Rostrum of corpus callosum

Anterior cerebral arteries

Distal medial striate artery (recurrent artery of Heubner)

Anterior communicating artery

Optic chiasm

Plate 141 Arteries of Brain: Frontal View and Section. (Netter: Atlas of Human Anatomy, 4 ed, 2006, Saunders.)

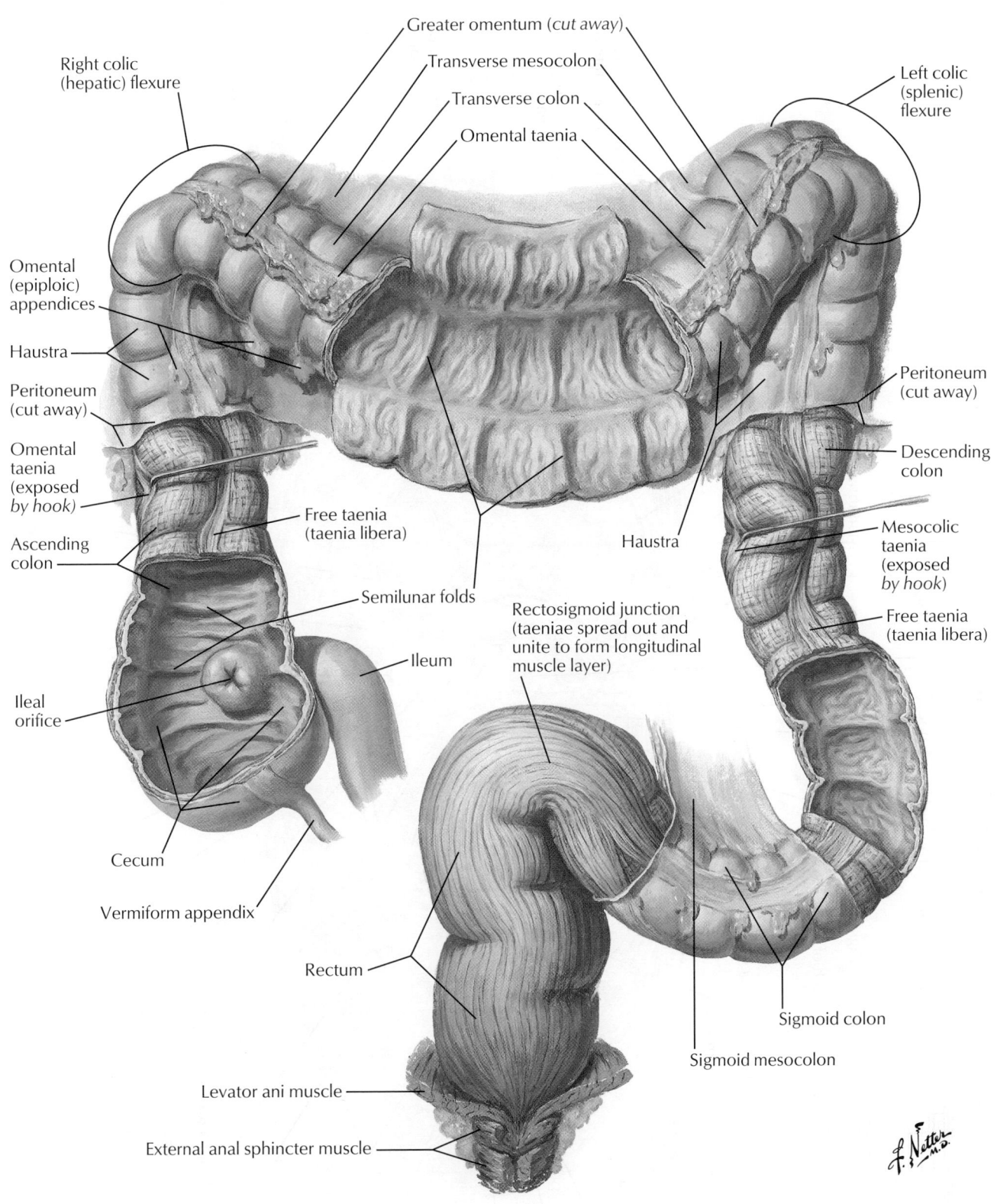

Right colic
(hepatic) flexure

Greater omentum (*cut away*)

Transverse mesocolon

Transverse colon

Omental taenia

Left colic
(splenic)
flexure

Omental
(epiploic)
appendices

Haustra

Peritoneum
(cut away)

Omental
taenia
(exposed
by hook)

Ascending
colon

Ileal
orifice

Cecum

Vermiform appendix

Free taenia
(taenia libera)

Semilunar folds

Ileum

Rectosigmoid junction
(taeniae spread out and
unite to form longitudinal
muscle layer)

Haustra

Peritoneum
(cut away)

Descending
colon

Mesocolic
taenia
(exposed
by hook)

Free taenia
(taenia libera)

Sigmoid colon

Sigmoid mesocolon

Rectum

Levator ani muscle

External anal sphincter muscle

f. Netter M.D.

Plate 284   Mucosa and Musculature of Large Intestine. (Netter: Atlas of Human Anatomy, 4 ed, 2006, Saunders.)

Transverse Section: T3–4 Intervertebral Disc, Manubrium

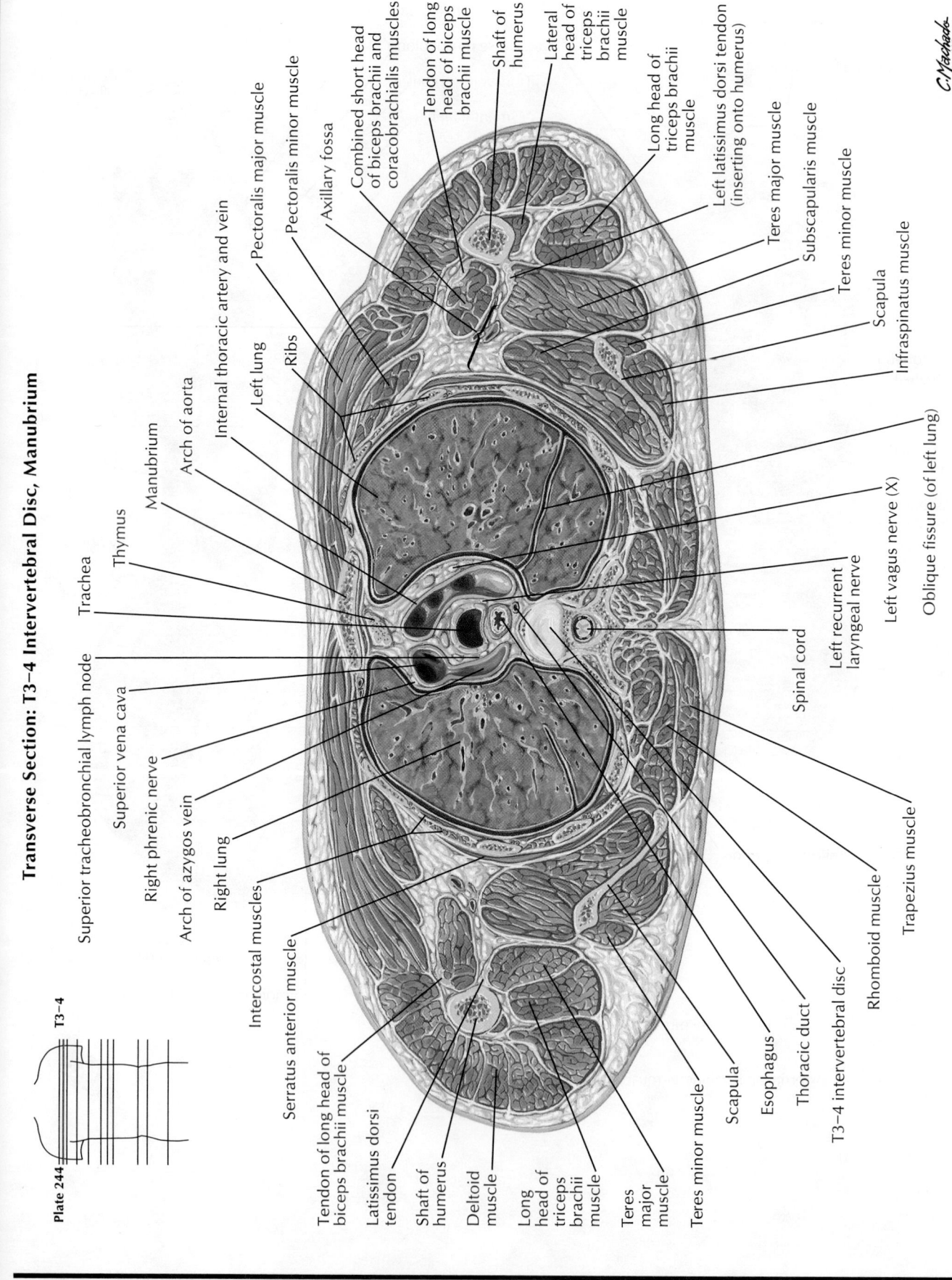

Superior tracheobronchial lymph node

Trachea

Thymus

Manubrium

Arch of aorta

Internal thoracic artery and vein

Left lung

Ribs

Axillary fossa

Pectoralis minor muscle

Pectoralis major muscle

Combined short head of biceps brachii and coracobrachialis muscles

Tendon of long head of biceps brachii muscle

Shaft of humerus

Lateral head of triceps brachii muscle

Long head of triceps brachii muscle

Left latissimus dorsi tendon (inserting onto humerus)

Teres major muscle

Subscapularis muscle

Teres minor muscle

Scapula

Infraspinatus muscle

Oblique fissure (of left lung)

Left vagus nerve (X)

Left recurrent laryngeal nerve

Spinal cord

Trapezius muscle

Rhomboid muscle

T3–4 intervertebral disc

Thoracic duct

Esophagus

Scapula

Teres minor muscle

Teres major muscle

Long head of triceps brachii muscle

Deltoid muscle

Shaft of humerus

Latissimus dorsi tendon

Tendon of long head of biceps brachii muscle

Serratus anterior muscle

Intercostal muscles

Right lung

Arch of azygos vein

Right phrenic nerve

Superior vena cava

Superior tracheobronchial lymph node

Plate 244 Cross Section of Thorax at T3-4 Disc Level. (Netter: Atlas of Human Anatomy, 4 ed, 2006, Saunders.)

Plate 244

T3–4

Right knee in extension: posterior view

Adductor tubercle on medial epicondyle of femur

Medial condyle of femur (articular surface)

Medial meniscus

Tibial collateral ligament

Medial condyle of tibia

Posterior cruciate ligament

Anterior cruciate ligament

Posterior meniscofemoral ligament

Lateral condyle of femur (articular surface)

Popliteus tendon

Fibular collateral ligament

Lateral meniscus

Head of fibula

Plate 509   Knee: Cruciate and Collateral Ligaments. (Netter: Atlas of Human Anatomy, 4 ed, 2006, Saunders.)

Paramedian (sagittal) dissection

Ureter

Uterine (fallopian) tube

Ovary

Ligament of ovary

Round ligament of uterus

Broad ligament (*cut*)

Superior pubic ramus (*cut*)

Inferior pubic ramus (*cut*)

Ischiocavernosus muscle

Body of clitoris

Labia minora

Labium majus

Rectouterine pouch (of Douglas)

Peritoneum (*cut edge*)

Vesicouterine pouch

Rectum

Ureter

Urinary bladder

Vagina

Pelvic diaphragm (levator ani muscle)

Deep transverse perineal muscle (*cut*)

External anal sphincter muscle

Median (sagittal) section

Sacral promontory

Ureter

Suspensory ligament of ovary

Uterine (fallopian) tube

Ovary

External iliac vessels

Ligament of ovary

Body of uterus

Round ligament of uterus (ligamentum teres)

Fundus of uterus

Urinary bladder

Pubic symphysis

Urethra

Sphincter urethrae

Deep transverse perineal muscle

Deep dorsal vein of clitoris

Crus of clitoris

External urethral orifice

Superficial transverse perineal muscle

Labium minus

Labium majus

Uterosacral ligament

Vesicouterine pouch

Rectouterine pouch (of Douglas)

Cervix of uterus

Posterior part of vaginal fornix

Anterior part of vaginal fornix

Rectum

Vagina

Perineal membrane

Levator ani muscle

Anal canal

External anal sphincter muscle

Anus

Vaginal orifice

Plate 360   Pelvic Viscera and Perineum: Female. (Netter: Atlas of Human Anatomy, 4 ed, 2006, Saunders.)

Alphabetic Index

A

Aarskog's syndrome Q87.1
Abandonment —see Maltreatment
Abasia (-astasia) (hysterical) F44.4
Abderhalden-Kaufmann-Lignac
    syndrome (cystinosis) E72.04
Abdomen, abdominal —see also
    condition
  acute R10.0
  angina K55.1
  muscle deficiency syndrome Q79.4
Abdominalgia —see Pain, abdominal
Abduction contracture, hip or other
    joint —see Contraction, joint
Aberrant (congenital) —see also
    Malposition, congenital
  adrenal gland Q89.1
  artery (peripheral) Q27.8
    basilar NEC Q28.1
    cerebral Q28.3
    coronary Q24.5
    digestive system Q27.8
    eye Q15.8
    lower limb Q27.8
    precerebral Q28.1
    pulmonary Q25.79
    renal Q27.2
    retina Q14.1
    specified site NEC Q27.8
    subclavian Q27.8
    upper limb Q27.8
    vertebral Q28.1
  breast Q83.8
  endocrine gland NEC Q89.2
  hepatic duct Q44.5
  pancreas Q45.3
  parathyroid gland Q89.2
  pituitary gland Q89.2
  sebaceous glands, mucous membrane,
    mouth, congenital Q38.6
  spleen Q89.09
  subclavian artery Q27.8
  thymus (gland) Q89.2
  thyroid gland Q89.2
  vein (peripheral) NEC Q27.8
    cerebral Q28.3
    digestive system Q27.8
    lower limb Q27.8
    precerebral Q28.1
    specified site NEC Q27.8
    upper limb Q27.8
Aberration
  distantial —see Disturbance, visual
  mental F99
Abetalipoproteinemia E78.6
Abiotrophy R68.89
Ablatio, ablation
  retinae —see Detachment, retina
Ablepharia, ablepharon Q10.3
Abnormal, abnormality, abnormalities —
    see also Anomaly
  acid-base balance (mixed) E87.4
  albumin R77.0
  alphafetoprotein R77.2
  alveolar ridge K08.9
  anatomical relationship Q89.9
  apertures, congenital, diaphragm Q79.1
  auditory perception H93.29-
    diplacusis —see Diplacusis
    hyperacusis —see Hyperacusis
    recruitment —see Recruitment,
      auditory

Abnormal, abnormality, abnormalities
    (Continued)
  auditory perception (Continued)
    threshold shift —see Shift, auditory
      threshold
  autosomes Q99.9
    fragile site Q95.5
  basal metabolic rate R94.8
  biosynthesis, testicular androgen
    E29.1
  bleeding time R79.1
  blood level (of)
    cobalt R79.0
    copper R79.0
    iron R79.0
    lithium R78.89
    magnesium R79.0
    mineral NEC R79.0
    zinc R79.0
  blood pressure
    elevated R03.0
    low reading (nonspecific) R03.1
  blood sugar R73.09
  blood-gas level R79.81
  bowel sounds R19.15
    absent R19.11
    hyperactive R19.12
  brain scan R94.02
  breathing R06.9
  caloric test R94.138
  cerebrospinal fluid R83.9
    cytology R83.6
    drug level R83.2
    enzyme level R83.0
    hormones R83.1
    immunology R83.4
    microbiology R83.5
    nonmedicinal level R83.3
    specified type NEC R83.8
  chemistry, blood R79.9
    C-reactive protein R79.82
    drugs —see Findings, abnormal, in
      blood
    gas level R79.81
    minerals R79.0
    pancytopenia D61.818
    PTT R79.1
    specified NEC R79.89
    toxins —see Findings, abnormal, in
      blood
  chest sounds (friction) (rales) R09.89
  chromosome, chromosomal Q99.9
    with more than three X
      chromosomes, female Q97.1
    analysis result R89.8
      bronchial washings R84.8
      cerebrospinal fluid R83.8
      cervix uteri NEC R87.89
      nasal secretions R84.8
      nipple discharge R89.8
      peritoneal fluid R85.89
      pleural fluid R84.8
      prostatic secretions R86.8
      saliva R85.89
      seminal fluid R86.8
      sputum R84.8
      synovial fluid R89.8
      throat scrapings R84.8
      vagina R87.89
      vulva R87.89
      wound secretions R89.8
    dicentric replacement Q93.2
    ring replacement Q93.2

Abnormal, abnormality, abnormalities
    (Continued)
  chromosome, chromosomal (Continued)
    sex Q99.8
      female phenotype Q97.9
        specified NEC Q97.8
      male phenotype Q98.9
        specified NEC Q98.8
      structural male Q98.6
    specified NEC Q99.8
  clinical findings NEC R68.89
  coagulation D68.9
    newborn, transient P61.6
    profile R79.1
    time R79.1
  communication —see Fistula
  conjunctiva, vascular H11.41-
  coronary artery Q24.5
  cortisol-binding globulin E27.8
  course, eustachian tube Q17.8
  creatinine clearance R94.4
  cytology
    anus R85.619
      atypical squamous cells cannot
        exclude high grade squamous
        intraepithelial lesion (ASC-H)
        R85.611
      atypical squamous cells of
        undetermined significance
        (ASC-US) R85.610
      cytologic evidence of malignancy
        R85.614
      high grade squamous intraepithelial
        lesion (HGSIL) R85.613
      human papillomavirus (HPV)
        DNA test
        high risk positive R85.81
        low risk postive R85.82
      inadequate smear R85.615
      low grade squamous intraepithelial
        lesion (LGSIL) R85.612
      satisfactory anal smear but lacking
        transformation zone R85.616
      specified NEC R85.618
      unsatisfactory smear R85.615
    female genital organs —see
      Abnormal, Papanicolaou
      (smear)
  dark adaptation curve H53.61
  dentofacial NEC —see Anomaly,
    dentofacial
  development, developmental Q89.9
    central nervous system Q07.9
  diagnostic imaging
    abdomen, abdominal region NEC R93.5
    biliary tract R93.2
    breast R92.8
    central nervous system NEC R90.89
    cerebrovascular NEC R90.89
    coronary circulation R93.1
    digestive tract NEC R93.3
    gastrointestinal (tract) R93.3
    genitourinary organs R93.8
    head R93.0
    heart R93.1
    intrathoracic organ NEC R93.8
    limbs R93.6
    liver R93.2
    lung (field) R91.8
    musculoskeletal system NEC R93.7
    retroperitoneum R93.5
    site specified NEC R93.8
    skin and subcutaneous tissue R93.8
    skull R93.0
    urinary organs R93.4

Abnormal, abnormality, abnormalities
(Continued)
direction, teeth, fully erupted M26.30
ear ossicles, acquired NEC H74.39-
  ankylosis —*see* Ankylosis, ear ossicles
  discontinuity —*see* Discontinuity,
    ossicles, ear
  partial loss —*see* Loss, ossicles, ear
    (partial)
Ebstein Q22.5
echocardiogram R93.1
echoencephalogram R90.81
echogram —*see* Abnormal, diagnostic
  imaging
electrocardiogram [ECG] [EKG]
  R94.31
electroencephalogram [EEG] R94.01
electrolyte —*see* Imbalance, electrolyte
electromyogram [EMG] R94.131
electro-oculogram [EOG] R94.110
electrophysiological intracardiac
  studies R94.39
electroretinogram [ERG] R94.111
erythrocytes
  congenital, with perinatal jaundice
    D58.9
feces (color) (contents) (mucus) R19.5
finding —*see* Findings, abnormal,
  without diagnosis
fluid
  amniotic —*see* Abnormal, specimen,
    specified
  cerebrospinal —*see* Abnormal,
    cerebrospinal fluid
  peritoneal —*see* Abnormal, specimen,
    digestive organs
  pleural —*see* Abnormal, specimen,
    respiratory organs
  synovial —*see* Abnormal, specimen,
    specified
  thorax (bronchial washings) (pleural
    fluid) —*see* Abnormal, specimen,
    respiratory organs
  vaginal —*see* Abnormal, specimen,
    female genital organs
form
  teeth K00.2
  uterus —*see* Anomaly, uterus
function studies
  auditory R94.120
  bladder R94.8
  brain R94.09
  cardiovascular R94.30
  ear R94.128
  endocrine NEC R94.7
  eye NEC R94.118
  kidney R94.4
  liver R94.5
  nervous system
    central NEC R94.09
    peripheral NEC R94.138
  pancreas R94.8
  placenta R94.8
  pulmonary R94.2
  special senses NEC R94.128
  spleen R94.8
  thyroid R94.6
  vestibular R94.121
gait —*see* Gait
  hysterical F44.4
gastrin secretion E16.4
globulin R77.1
  cortisol-binding E27.8
  thyroid-binding E07.89

Abnormal, abnormality, abnormalities
(Continued)
glomerular, minor (*see also* N00-N07
  with fourth character .0) N05.0
glucagon secretion E16.3
glucose tolerance (test) (non-fasting)
  R73.09
gravitational (G) forces or states (effect
  of) T75.81
hair (color) (shaft) L67.9
  specified NEC L67.8
hard tissue formation in pulp (dental)
  K04.3
head movement R25.0
heart
  rate R00.9
    specified NEC R00.8
  shadow R93.1
  sounds NEC R01.2
hemoglobin (disease) (*see also* Disease,
  hemoglobin) D58.2
  trait —*see* Trait, hemoglobin,
    abnormal
histology NEC R89.7
immunological findings R89.4
  in serum R76.9
    specified NEC R76.8
increase in appetite R63.2
involuntary movement —*see* Abnormal,
  movement, involuntary
jaw closure M26.51
karyotype R89.8
kidney function test R94.4
knee jerk R29.2
leukocyte (cell) (differential) NEC D72.9
liver
loss of
  height R29.890
  weight R63.4
mammogram NEC R92.8
  calcification (calculus) R92.1
  microcalcification R92.0
Mantoux test R76.11
movement (disorder) —*see also*
  Disorder, movement
  head R25.0
  involuntary R25.9
    fasciculation R25.3
    of head R25.0
    spasm R25.2
    specified type NEC R25.8
    tremor R25.1
myoglobin (Aberdeen) (Annapolis) R89.7
neonatal screening P09
oculomotor study R94.113
palmar creases Q82.8
Papanicolaou (smear)
  anus R85.619
    atypical squamous cells cannot
      exclude high grade squamous
      intraepithelial lesion (ASC-H)
      R85.611
    atypical squamous cells of
      undetermined significance
      (ASC-US) R85.610
    cytologic evidence of malignancy
      R85.614
    high grade squamous intraepithelial
      lesion (HGSIL) R85.613
    human papillomavirus (HPV)
      DNA test
      high risk positive R85.81
      low risk postive R85.82
    inadequate smear R85.615

Abnormal, abnormality, abnormalities
(Continued)
Papanicolaou *(Continued)*
  anus *(Continued)*
    low grade squamous intraepithelial
      lesion (LGSIL) R85.612
    satisfactory anal smear but lacking
      transformation zone R85.616
    specified NEC R85.618
      unsatisfactory smear R85.615
  bronchial washings R84.6
  cerebrospinal fluid R83.6
  cervix R87.619
    atypical squamous cells cannot
      exclude high grade squamous
      intraepithelial lesion (ASC-H)
      R87.611
    atypical squamous cells of
      undetermined significance
      (ASC-US) R87.610
    cytologic evidence of malignancy
      R87.614
    high grade squamous intraepithelial
      lesion (HGSIL) R87.613
    inadequate smear R87.615
    low grade squamous intraepithelial
      lesion (LGSIL) R87.612
    non-atypical endometrial cells
      R87.618
    satisfactory cervical smear but
      lacking transformation zone
      R87.616
    specified NEC R87.618
    thin preparaton R87.619
    unsatisfactory smear R87.615
  nasal secretions R84.6
  nipple discharge R89.6
  peritoneal fluid R85.69
  pleural fluid R84.6
  prostatic secretions R86.6
  saliva R85.69
  seminal fluid R86.6
  sites NEC R89.6
  sputum R84.6
  synovial fluid R89.6
  throat scrapings R84.6
  vagina R87.629
    atypical squamous cells cannot
      exclude high grade squamous
      intraepithelial lesion (ASC-H)
      R87.621
    atypical squamous cells of
      undetermined significance
      (ASC-US) R87.620
    cytologic evidence of malignancy
      R87.624
    high grade squamous intraepithelial
      lesion (HGSIL) R87.623
    inadequate smear R87.625
    low grade squamous intraepithelial
      lesion (LGSIL) R87.622
    specified NEC R87.628
    thin preparation R87.629
    unsatisfactory smear R87.625
  vulva R87.69
  wound secretions R89.6
partial thromboplastin time (PTT) R79.1
pelvis (bony) —*see* Deformity, pelvis
percussion, chest (tympany) R09.89
periods (grossly) —*see* Menstruation
phonocardiogram R94.39
plantar reflex R29.2
plasma
  protein R77.9
    specified NEC R77.8
  viscosity R70.1

Abnormal, abnormality, abnormalities *(Continued)*
pleural (folds) Q34.0
posture R29.3
product of conception O02.9
  specified type NEC O02.89
prothrombin time (PT) R79.1
pulmonary
  artery, congenital Q25.79
  function, newborn P28.89
  test results R94.2
pulsations in neck R00.2
pupillary H21.56-
  function (reaction) (reflex) —*see*
    Anomaly, pupil, function
radiological examination —*see*
  Abnormal, diagnostic imaging
red blood cell (s) (morphology)
  (volume) R71.8
reflex —*see* Reflex
renal function test R94.4
response to nerve stimulation
  R94.130
retinal correspondence H53.31
retinal function study R94.111
rhythm, heart —*see also* Arrhythmia
saliva —*see* Abnormal, specimen,
  digestive organs
scan
  kidney R94.4
  liver R93.2
  thyroid R94.6
secretion
  gastrin E16.4
  glucagon E16.3
semen, seminal fluid —*see* Abnormal,
  specimen, male genital organs
serum level (of)
  acid phosphatase R74.8
  alkaline phosphatase R74.8
  amylase R74.8
  enzymes R74.9
    specified NEC R74.8
  lipase R74.8
  triacylglycerol lipase R74.8
shape
  gravid uterus —*see* Anomaly, uterus
sinus venosus Q21.1
size, tooth, teeth K00.2
spacing, tooth, teeth, fully erupted
  M26.30
specimen
  digestive organs (peritoneal fluid)
    (saliva) R85.9
    cytology R85.69
    drug level R85.2
    enzyme level R85.0
    histology R85.7
    hormones R85.1
    immunology R85.4
    microbiology R85.5
    nonmedicinal level R85.3
    specified type NEC R85.89
  female genital organs (secretions)
    (smears) R87.9
    cytology R87.69
      cervix R87.619
        human papillomavirus (HPV)
          DNA test
          high risk positive R87.810
          low risk positive R87.820
        inadequate (unsatisfactory)
          smear R87.615
        non-atypical endometrial cells
          R87.618
        specified NEC R87.89

Abnormal, abnormality, abnormalities *(Continued)*
specimen *(Continued)*
  female genital organs *(Continued)*
    cytology *(Continued)*
      vagina R87.629
        human papillomavirus (HPV)
          DNA test
          high risk positive R87.811
          low risk positive R87.821
        inadequate (unsatisfactory)
          smear R87.625
      vulva R87.69
    drug level R87.2
    enzyme level R87.0
    histological R87.7
    hormones R87.1
    immunology R87.4
    microbiology R87.5
    nonmedicinal level R87.3
    specified type NEC R87.89
  male genital organs (prostatic
    secretions) (semen) R86.9
    cytology R86.6
    drug level R86.2
    enzyme level R86.0
    histological R86.7
    hormones R86.1
    immunology R86.4
    microbiology R86.5
    nonmedicinal level R86.3
    specified type NEC R86.8
  nipple discharge —*see* Abnormal,
    specimen, specified
  respiratory organs (bronchial
    washings) (nasal secretions)
    (pleural fluid) (sputum) R84.9
    cytology R84.6
    drug level R84.2
    enzyme level R84.0
    histology R84.7
    hormones R84.1
    immunology R84.4
    microbiology R84.5
    nonmedicinal level R84.3
    specified type NEC R84.8
  specified organ, system and tissue
    NOS R89.9
    cytology R89.6
    drug level R89.2
    enzyme level R89.0
    histology R89.7
    hormones R89.1
    immunology R89.4
    microbiology R89.5
    nonmedicinal level R89.3
    specified type NEC R89.8
  synovial fluid —*see* Abnormal,
    specimen, specified
  thorax (bronchial washings) (pleural
    fluids) —*see* Abnormal,
    specimen, respiratory organs
  vagina (secretion) (smear) R87.629
  vulva (secretion) (smear) R87.69
  wound secretion —*see* Abnormal,
    specimen, specified
spermatozoa —*see* Abnormal, specimen,
  male genital organs
sputum (amount) (color) (odor)
  R09.3
stool (color) (contents) (mucus)
  R19.5
  bloody K92.1
  guaiac positive R19.5
synchondrosis Q78.8

Abnormal, abnormality, abnormalities *(Continued)*
thermography (*see also* Abnormal,
  diagnostic imaging) R93.8
thyroid-binding globulin E07.89
tooth, teeth (form) (size) K00.2
toxicology (findings) R78.9
transport protein E88.09
tumor marker NEC R97.8
ultrasound results —*see* Abnormal,
  diagnostic imaging
umbilical cord complicating delivery
  O69.9
urination NEC R39.19
urine (constituents) R82.90
  bile R82.2
  cytological examination R82.8
  drugs R82.5
  fat R82.0
  glucose R81
  heavy metals R82.6
  hemoglobin R82.3
  histological examination R82.8
  ketones R82.4
  microbiological examination (culture)
    R82.7
  myoglobin R82.1
  positive culture R82.7
  protein —*see* Proteinuria
  specified substance NEC R82.99
    chromoabnormality NEC R82.91
  substances nonmedical R82.6
uterine hemorrhage —*see* Hemorrhage,
  uterus
vectorcardiogram R94.39
visually evoked potential (VEP)
  R94.112
white blood cells D72.9
  specified NEC D72.89
X-ray examination —*see* Abnormal,
  diagnostic imaging
Abnormity (any organ or part) —*see*
  Anomaly
Abocclusion M26.29
  hemolytic disease (newborn) P55.1
  incompatibility reaction ABO —*see*
    Complication (s), transfusion,
    incompatibility reaction, ABO
Abolition, language R48.8
Aborter, habitual or recurrent —*see* Loss
  (of), pregnancy, recurrent
Abortion (complete) (spontaneous)
  O03.9
  with retained products of conception —
    see Abortion, incomplete
  attempted (elective) (failed) O07.4
    complicated by O07.30
      afibrinogenemia O07.1
      cardiac arrest O07.36
      chemical damage of pelvic
        organ (s) O07.34
      circulatory collapse O07.31
      cystitis O07.38
      defibrination syndrome O07.1
      electrolyte imbalance O07.33
      embolism (air) (amniotic fluid)
        (blood clot) (fat) (pulmonary)
        (septic) (soap) O07.2
      endometritis O07.0
      genital tract and pelvic infection
        O07.0
      hemolysis O07.1
      hemorrhage (delayed) (excessive)
        O07.1

Abortion (Continued)
 attempted (Continued)
  complicated by (Continued)
   infection
    genital tract or pelvic O07.0
    urinary tract tract O07.38
   intravascular coagulation O07.1
   laceration of pelvic organ (s)
     O07.34
   metabolic disorder O07.33
   oliguria O07.32
   oophoritis O07.0
   parametritis O07.0
   pelvic peritonitis O07.0
   perforation of pelvic organ (s)
     O07.34
   renal failure or shutdown O07.32
   salpingitis or salpingo-oophoritis
     O07.0
   sepsis O07.37
   shock O07.31
   specified condition NEC O07.39
   tubular necrosis (renal) O07.32
   uremia O07.32
   urinary tract infection O07.38
   venous complication NEC O07.35
    embolism (air) (amniotic
      fluid) (blood clot) (fat)
      (pulmonary) (septic) (soap)
      O07.2
  complicated (by) (following) O03.80
   afibrinogenemia O03.6
   cardiac arrest O03.86
   chemical damage of pelvic organ (s)
     O03.84
   circulatory collapse O03.81
   cystitis O03.88
   defibrination syndrome O03.6
   electrolyte imbalance O03.83
   embolism (air) (amniotic fluid) (blood
     clot) (fat) (pulmonary) (septic)
     (soap) O03.7
   endometritis O03.5
   genital tract and pelvic infection
     O03.5
   hemolysis O03.6
   hemorrhage (delayed) (excessive)
     O03.6
   infection
    genital tract or pelvic O03.5
    urinary tract O03.88
   intravascular coagulation O03.6
   laceration of pelvic organ (s)
     O03.84
   metabolic disorder O03.83
   oliguria O03.82
   oophoritis O03.5
   parametritis O03.5
   pelvic peritonitis O03.5
   perforation of pelvic organ (s) O03.84
   renal failure or shutdown O03.82
   salpingitis or salpingo-oophoritis
     O03.5
   sepsis O03.87
   shock O03.81
   specified condition NEC O03.89
   tubular necrosis (renal) O03.82
   uremia O03.82
   urinary tract infection O03.88
   venous complication NEC O03.85
    embolism (air) (amniotic fluid)
      (blood clot) (fat) (pulmonary)
      (septic) (soap) O03.7
 failed —see Abortion, attempted

Abortion (Continued)
 habitual or recurrent N96
  with current abortion —see categories
    O03-O06
  without current pregnancy N96
  care in current pregnancy O26.2-
 incomplete (spontaneous) O03.4
  complicated (by) (following) O03.30
   afibrinogenemia O03.1
   cardiac arrest O03.36
   chemical damage of pelvic
     organ (s) O03.34
   circulatory collapse O03.31
   cystitis O03.38
   defibrination syndrome O03.1
   electrolyte imbalance O03.33
   embolism (air) (amniotic fluid)
     (blood clot) (fat) (pulmonary)
     (septic) (soap) O03.2
   endometritis O03.0
   genital tract and pelvic infection
     O03.0
   hemolysis O03.1
   hemorrhage (delayed) (excessive)
     O03.1
   infection
    genital tract or pelvic O03.0
    urinary tract O03.38
   intravascular coagulation O03.1
   laceration of pelvic organ (s)
     O03.34
   metabolic disorder O03.33
   oliguria O03.32
   oophoritis O03.0
   parametritis O03.0
   pelvic peritonitis O03.0
   perforation of pelvic organ (s)
     O03.34
   renal failure or shutdown O03.32
   salpingitis or salpingo-oophoritis
     O03.0
   sepsis O03.37
   shock O03.31
   specified condition NEC O03.39
   tubular necrosis (renal) O03.32
   uremia O03.32
   urinary infection O03.38
   venous complication NEC O03.35
    embolism (air) (amniotic
      fluid) (blood clot) (fat)
      (pulmonary) (septic) (soap)
      O03.2
 induced (encounter for) Z33.2
  complicated by O04.80
   afibrinogenemia O04.6
   cardiac arrest O04.86
   chemical damage of pelvic
     organ (s) O04.84
   circulatory collapse O04.81
   cystitis O04.88
   defibrination syndrome O04.6
   electrolyte imbalance O04.83
   embolism (air) (amniotic fluid)
     (blood clot) (fat) (pulmonary)
     (septic) (soap) O04.7
   endometritis O04.5
   genital tract and pelvic infection
     O04.5
   hemolysis O04.6
   hemorrhage (delayed) (excessive)
     O04.6
   infection
    genital tract or pelvic O04.5
    urinary tract O04.88

Abortion (Continued)
 induced (Continued)
  complicated by (Continued)
   intravascular coagulation O04.6
   laceration of pelvic organ (s)
     O04.84
   metabolic disorder O04.83
   oliguria O04.82
   oophoritis O04.5
   parametritis O04.5
   pelvic peritonitis O04.5
   perforation of pelvic organ (s)
     O04.84
   renal failure or shutdown O04.82
   salpingitis or salpingo-oophoritis
     O04.5
   sepsis O04.87
   shock O04.81
   specified condition NEC O04.89
   tubular necrosis (renal) O04.82
   uremia O04.82
   urinary tract infection O04.88
   venous complication NEC
     O04.85
    embolism (air) (amniotic
      fluid) (blood clot) (fat)
      (pulmonary) (septic) (soap)
      O04.7
  missed O02.1
  spontaneous —see Abortion (complete)
    (spontaneous)
  threatened O20.0
  threatened (spontaneous) O20.0
  tubal O00.1
Abortus fever A23.1
Aboulomania F60.7
Abrami's disease D59.8
Abramov-Fiedler myocarditis (acute
  isolated myocarditis) I40.1
Abrasion T14.8
 abdomen, abdominal (wall) S30.811
 alveolar process S00.512
 ankle S90.51-
 antecubital space —see Abrasion,
   elbow
 anus S30.817
 arm (upper) S40.81-
 auditory canal —see Abrasion, ear
 auricle —see Abrasion, ear
 axilla —see Abrasion, arm
 back, lower S30.810
 breast S20.11-
 brow S00.81
 buttock S30.810
 calf —see Abrasion, leg
 canthus —see Abrasion, eyelid
 cheek S00.81
  internal S00.512
 chest wall —see Abrasion, thorax
 chin S00.81
 clitoris S30.814
 cornea S05.0-
 costal region —see Abrasion, thorax
 dental K03.1
 digit (s)
   foot —see Abrasion, toe
   hand —see Abrasion, finger
 ear S00.41-
 elbow S50.31-
 epididymis S30.813
 epigastric region S30.811
 epiglottis S10.11
 esophagus (thoracic) S27.818
  cervical S10.11

Abrasion (*Continued*)
eyebrow —*see* Abrasion, eyelid
eyelid S00.21-
face S00.81
finger (s) S60.41-
  index S60.41-
  little S60.41-
  middle S60.41-
  ring S60.41-
flank S30.811
foot (except toe (s) alone) S90.81-
  toe —*see* Abrasion, toe
forearm S50.81-
  elbow only —*see* Abrasion, elbow
forehead S00.81
genital organs, external
  female S30.816
  male S30.815
groin S30.811
gum S00.512
hand S60.51-
head S00.91
  ear —*see* Abrasion, ear
  eyelid —*see* Abrasion, eyelid
  lip S00.511
  nose S00.31
  oral cavity S00.512
  scalp S00.01
  specified site NEC S00.81
heel —*see* Abrasion, foot
hip S70.21-
inguinal region S30.811
interscapular region S20.419
jaw S00.81
knee S80.21-
labium (majus) (minus) S30.814
larynx S10.11
leg (lower) S80.81-
  knee —*see* Abrasion, knee
  upper —*see* Abrasion, thigh
lip S00.511
lower back S30.810
lumbar region S30.810
malar region S00.81
mammary —*see* Abrasion, breast
mastoid region S00.81
mouth S00.512
nail
  finger —*see* Abrasion, finger
  toe —*see* Abrasion, toe
nape S10.81
nasal S00.31
neck S10.91
  specified site NEC S10.81
  throat S10.11
nose S00.31
occipital region S00.01
oral cavity S00.512
orbital region —*see* Abrasion, eyelid
palate S00.512
palm —*see* Abrasion, hand
parietal region S00.01
pelvis S30.810
penis S30.812
perineum
  female S30.814
  male S30.810
periocular area —*see* Abrasion, eyelid
phalanges
  finger —*see* Abrasion, finger
  toe —*see* Abrasion, toe
pharynx S10.11
pinna —*see* Abrasion, ear
popliteal space —*see* Abrasion, knee

Abrasion (*Continued*)
prepuce S30.812
pubic region S30.810
pudendum
  female S30.816
  male S30.815
sacral region S30.810
scalp S00.01
scapular region —*see* Abrasion, shoulder
scrotum S30.813
shin —*see* Abrasion, leg
shoulder S40.21-
skin NEC T14.8
sternal region S20.319
submaxillary region S00.81
submental region S00.81
subungual
  finger (s) —*see* Abrasion, finger
  toe (s) —*see* Abrasion, toe
supraclavicular fossa S10.81
supraorbital S00.81
temple S00.81
temporal region S00.81
testis S30.813
thigh S70.31-
thorax, thoracic (wall) S20.91
  back S20.41-
  front S20.31-
throat S10.11
thumb S60.31-
toe (s) (lesser) S90.416
  great S90.41-
tongue S00.512
tooth, teeth (dentifrice) (habitual)
  (hard tissues) (occupational)
  (ritual) (traditional) K03.1
trachea S10.11
tunica vaginalis S30.813
tympanum, tympanic membrane —*see*
  Abrasion, ear
uvula S00.512
vagina S30.814
vocal cords S10.11
vulva S30.814
wrist S60.81-
Abrism —*see* Poisoning, food, noxious, plant
Abruptio placentae O45.9-
  with
    afibrinogenemia O45.01-
    coagulation defect O45.00-
      specified NEC O45.09-
    disseminated intravascular
      coagulation O45.02-
    hypofibrinogenemia O45.01-
  specified NEC O45.8-
Abruption, placenta —*see* Abruptio
  placentae
Abscess (connective tissue) (embolic)
  (fistulous) (infective) (metastatic)
  (multiple) (pernicious) (pyogenic)
  (septic) L02.91
  with
    diverticular disease (intestine) K57.80
      with bleeding K57.81
      large intestine K57.20
        with
          bleeding K57.21
          small intestine K57.40
            with bleeding K57.41
      small intestine K57.00
        with
          bleeding K57.01
          large intestine K57.40
            with bleeding K57.41
    lymphangitis - code by site under
      Abscess

Abscess (*Continued*)
abdomen, abdominal
  cavity K65.1
  wall L02.211
abdominopelvic K65.1
accessory sinus —*see* Sinusitis
adrenal (capsule) (gland) E27.8
alveolar K04.7
  with sinus K04.6
amebic A06.4
  brain (and liver or lung abscess) A06.6
  genitourinary tract A06.82
  liver (without mention of brain or
    lung abscess) A06.4
  lung (and liver) (without mention of
    brain abscess) A06.5
  specified site NEC A06.89
  spleen A06.89
anerobic A48.0
ankle —*see* Abscess, lower limb
anorectal K61.2
antecubital space —*see* Abscess, upper
  limb
antrum (chronic) (Highmore) —*see*
  Sinusitis, maxillary
anus K61.0
apical (tooth) K04.7
  with sinus (alveolar) K04.6
appendix K35.3
areola (acute) (chronic) (nonpuerperal)
  N61
  puerperal, postpartum or
    gestational —*see* Infection,
    nipple
arm (any part) —*see* Abscess, upper
  limb
artery (wall) I77.89
atheromatous I77.2
auricle, ear —*see* Abscess, ear, external
axilla (region) L02.41-
  lymph gland or node L04.2
back (any part, except buttock) L02.212
Bartholin's gland N75.1
  with
    abortion —*see* Abortion, by type
      complicated by, sepsis
    ectopic or molar pregnancy O08.0
    following ectopic or molar pregnancy
      O08.0
Bezold's —*see* Mastoiditis, acute
bilharziasis B65.1
bladder (wall) —*see* Cystitis, specified
  type NEC
bone (subperiosteal) —*see also*
  Osteomyelitis, specified type NEC
  accessory sinus (chronic) —*see*
    Sinusitis
  chronic or old —*see* Osteomyelitis,
    chronic
  jaw (lower) (upper) M27.2
  mastoid —*see* Mastoiditis, acute,
    subperiosteal
  petrous —*see* Petrositis
  spinal (tuberculous) A18.01
    nontuberculous —*see*
      Osteomyelitis, vertebra
bowel K63.0
brain (any part) (cystic) (otogenic)
  G06.0
  amebic (with abscess of any other
    site) A06.6
  gonococcal A54.82
  pheomycotic (chromomycotic) B43.1
  tuberculous A17.81

Abscess (Continued)
  breast (acute) (chronic) (nonpuerperal)
        N61
      newborn P39.0
      puerperal, postpartum, gestational —
          see Mastitis, obstetric, purulent
  broad ligament N73.2
      acute N73.0
      chronic N73.1
  Brodie's (localized) (chronic) M86.8X-
  bronchi J98.09
  buccal cavity K12.2
  bulbourethral gland N34.0
  bursa M71.00
      ankle M71.07-
      elbow M71.02-
      foot M71.07-
      hand M71.04-
      hip M71.05-
      knee M71.06-
      multiple sites M71.09
      pharyngeal J39.1
      shoulder M71.01-
      specified site NEC M71.08
      wrist M71.03-
  buttock L02.31
  canthus —see Blepharoconjunctivitis
  cartilage —see Disorder, cartilage,
        specified type NEC
  cecum K35.3
  cerebellum, cerebellar G06.0
      sequelae G09
  cerebral (embolic) G06.0
      sequelae G09
  cervical (meaning neck) L02.11
      lymph gland or node L04.0
  cervix (stump) (uteri) —see Cervicitis
  cheek (external) L02.01
      inner K12.2
  chest J86.9
      with fistula J86.0
      wall L02.213
  chin L02.01
  choroid —see Inflammation,
        chorioretinal
  circumtonsillar J36
  cold (lung) (tuberculous) —see also
        Tuberculosis, abscess, lung
      articular —see Tuberculosis, joint
  colon (wall) K63.0
  colostomy K94.02
  conjunctiva —see Conjunctivitis, acute
  cornea H16.31-
  corpus
      cavernosum N48.21
      luteum —see Oophoritis
  Cowper's gland N34.0
  cranium G06.0
  cul-de-sac (Douglas') (posterior) —see
        Peritonitis, pelvic, female
  cutaneous —see Abscess, by site
  dental K04.7
      with sinus (alveolar) K04.6
  dentoalveolar K04.7
      with sinus K04.6
  diaphragm, diaphragmatic K65.1
  Douglas' cul-de-sac or pouch —see
        Peritonitis, pelvic, female
  Dubois A50.59
  ear (middle) —see also Otitis, media,
        suppurative
      acute —see Otitis, media,
          suppurative, acute
      external H60.0-

Abscess (Continued)
  entamebic —see Abscess, amebic
  enterostomy K94.12
  epididymis N45.4
  epidural G06.2
      brain G06.0
      spinal cord G06.1
  epiglottis J38.7
  epiploon, epiploic K65.1
  erysipelatous —see Erysipelas
  esophagus K20.8
  ethmoid (bone) (chronic) (sinus) J32.2
  external auditory canal —see Abscess,
        ear, external
  extradural G06.2
      brain G06.0
          sequelae G09
      spinal cord G06.1
  extraperitoneal K68.19
  eye —see Endophthalmitis, purulent
  eyelid H00.03-
  face (any part, except ear, eye and nose)
        L02.01
  fallopian tube —see Salpingitis
  fascia M72.8
  fauces J39.1
  fecal K63.0
  femoral (region) —see Abscess, lower limb
  filaria, filarial —see Infestation, filarial
  finger (any) —see also Abscess, hand
      nail —see Cellulitis, finger
  foot L02.61-
  forehead L02.01
  frontal sinus (chronic) J32.1
  gallbladder K81.0
  genital organ or tract
      female (external) N76.4
      male N49.9
          multiple sites N49.8
          specified NEC N49.8
  gestational mammary O91.11-
  gestational subareolar O91.11-
  gingival K05.21
  gland, glandular (lymph) (acute) —see
        Lymphadenitis, acute
  gluteal (region) L02.31
  gonorrheal —see Gonococcus
  groin L02.214
  gum K05.21
  hand L02.51-
  head NEC L02.811
      face (any part, except ear, eye and
          nose) L02.01
  heart —see Carditis
  heel —see Abscess, foot
  helminthic —see Infestation, helminth
  hepatic (cholangitic) (hematogenic)
        (lymphogenic) (pylephlebitic) K75.0
      amebic A06.4
  hip (region) —see Abscess, lower limb
  ileocecal K35.3
  ileostomy (bud) K94.12
  iliac (region) L02.214
      fossa K35.3
  infraclavicular (fossa) —see Abscess,
        upper limb
  inguinal (region) L02.214
      lymph gland or node L04.1
  intestine, intestinal NEC K63.0
      rectal K61.1
  intra-abdominal (see also Abscess,
        peritoneum) K65.1
      postoperative T81.4
          retroperitoneal K68.11

Abscess (Continued)
  intracranial G06.0
  intramammary —see Abscess, breast
  intraorbital —see Abscess, orbit
  intraperitoneal K65.1
  intrasphincteric (anus) K61.4
  intraspinal G06.1
  intratonsillar J36
  ischiorectal (fossa) K61.3
  jaw (bone) (lower) (upper) M27.2
  joint —see Arthritis, pyogenic or pyemic
      spine (tuberculous) A18.01
          nontuberculous —see
              Spondylopathy, infective
  kidney N15.1
      with calculus N20.0
          with hydronephrosis N13.6
      puerperal (postpartum) O86.21
  knee —see also Abscess, lower limb
      joint M00.9
  labium (majus) (minus) N76.4
  lacrimal
      caruncle —see Inflammation, lacrimal,
          passages, acute
      gland —see Dacryoadenitis
      passages (duct) (sac) —see
          Inflammation, lacrimal,
          passages, acute
  lacunar N34.0
  larynx J38.7
  lateral (alveolar) K04.7
      with sinus K04.6
  leg (any part) —see Abscess, lower limb
  lens H27.8
  lingual K14.0
      tonsil J36
  lip K13.0
  Littre's gland N34.0
  liver (cholangitic) (hematogenic)
        (lymphogenic) (pylephlebitic)
        (pyogenic) K75.0
      amebic (due to Entamoeba histolytica)
          (dysenteric) (tropical) A06.4
          with
              brain abscess (and liver or lung
                  abscess) A06.6
              lung abscess A06.5
  loin (region) L02.211
  lower limb L02.41-
  lumbar (tuberculous) A18.01
      nontuberculous L02.212
  lung (miliary) (putrid) J85.2
      with pneumonia J85.1
          due to specified organism (see
              Pneumonia, in (due to))
      amebic (with liver abscess) A06.5
          with
              brain abscess A06.6
              pneumonia A06.5
  lymph, lymphatic, gland or node
        (acute) —see also Lymphadenitis,
        acute
      mesentery I88.0
  malar M27.2
  mammary gland —see Abscess, breast
  marginal, anus K61.0
  mastoid —see Mastoiditis, acute
  maxilla, maxillary M27.2
      molar (tooth) K04.7
          with sinus K04.6
      premolar K04.7
      sinus (chronic) J32.0
  mediastinum J85.3
  meibomian gland —see Hordeolum
  meninges G06.2

Abscess (Continued)
mesentery, mesenteric K65.1
mesosalpinx —see Salpingitis
mons pubis L02.215
mouth (floor) K12.2
muscle —see Myositis, infective
myocardium I40.0
nabothian (follicle) —see Cervicitis
nasal J32.9
nasopharyngeal J39.1
navel L02.216
　newborn P38.9
　　with mild hemorrhage P38.1
　　without hemorrhage P38.9
neck (region) L02.11
　lymph gland or node L04.0
nephritic —see Abscess, kidney
nipple N61
　associated with
　　lactation —see Pregnancy,
　　　complicated by,
　　pregnancy —see Pregnancy,
　　　complicated by
nose (external) (fossa) (septum) J34.0
　sinus (chronic) —see Sinusitis
omentum K65.1
operative wound T81.4
orbit, orbital —see Cellulitis, orbit
otogenic G06.0
ovary, ovarian (corpus luteum) —see
　Oophoritis
oviduct —see Oophoritis
palate (soft) K12.2
　hard M27.2
palmar (space) —see Abscess, hand
pancreas (duct) —see Pancreatitis, acute
parafrenal N48.21
parametric, parametrium N73.2
　acute N73.0
　chronic N73.1
paranephric N15.1
parapancreatic —see Pancreatitis, acute
parapharyngeal J39.0
pararectal K61.1
parasinus —see Sinusitis
parauterine (see also Disease, pelvis,
　inflammatory) N73.2
paravaginal —see Vaginitis
parietal region (scalp) L02.811
parodontal K05.21
parotid (duct) (gland) K11.3
　region K12.2
pectoral (region) L02.213
pelvis, pelvic
　female —see Disease, pelvis,
　　inflammatory
　male, peritoneal K65.1
penis N48.21
　gonococcal (accessory gland)
　　(periurethral) A54.1
perianal K61.0
periapical K04.7
　with sinus (alveolar) K04.6
periappendicular K35.3
pericardial I30.1
pericecal K35.3
pericemental K05.21
pericholecystic —see Cholecystitis, acute
pericoronal K05.21
peridental K05.21
perimetric (see also Disease, pelvis,
　inflammatory) N73.2
perinephric, perinephritic —see
　Abscess, kidney

Abscess (Continued)
perineum, perineal (superficial) L02.215
　urethra N34.0
periodontal (parietal) K05.21
　apical K04.7
periosteum, periosteal —see also
　Osteomyelitis, specified type NEC
　with osteomyelitis —see also
　　Osteomyelitis, specified type
　　NEC
　　acute —see Osteomyelitis, acute
　　chronic —see Osteomyelitis, chronic
peripharyngeal J39.0
peripleuritic J86.9
　with fistula J86.0
periprostatic N41.2
perirectal K61.1
perirenal (tissue) —see Abscess, kidney
perisinuous (nose) —see Sinusitis
peritoneum, peritoneal (perforated)
　(ruptured) K65.1
　with appendicitis K35.3
　pelvic
　　female —see Peritonitis, pelvic,
　　　female
　　male K65.1
　postoperative T81.4
　puerperal, postpartum, childbirth O85
　tuberculous A18.31
peritonsillar J36
perityphlic K35.3
periureteral N28.89
periurethral N34.0
　gonococcal (accessory gland)
　　(periurethral) A54.1
periuterine (see also Disease, pelvis,
　inflammatory) N73.2
perivesical —see Cystitis, specified type
　NEC
petrous bone —see Petrositis
phagedenic NOS L02.91
　chancroid A57
pharynx, pharyngeal (lateral) J39.1
pilonidal L05.01
pituitary (gland) E23.6
pleura J86.9
　with fistula J86.0
popliteal —see Abscess, lower limb
postcecal K35.3
postlaryngeal J38.7
postnasal J34.0
postoperative (any site) T81.4
　retroperitoneal K68.11
postpharyngeal J39.0
posttonsillar J36
post-typhoid A01.09
pouch of Douglas —see Peritonitis,
　pelvic, female
premammary —see Abscess, breast
prepatellar —see Abscess, lower limb
prostate N41.2
　gonococcal (acute) (chronic) A54.22
psoas muscle K68.12
puerperal - code by site under
　Puerperal, abscess
pulmonary —see Abscess, lung
pulp, pulpal (dental) K04.0
rectovaginal septum K63.0
rectovesical —see Cystitis, specified
　type NEC
rectum K61.1
renal —see Abscess, kidney
retina —see Inflammation, chorioretinal
retrobulbar —see Abscess, orbit

Abscess (Continued)
retrocecal K65.1
retrolaryngeal J38.7
retromammary —see Abscess, breast
retroperitoneal NEC K68.19
　postprocedural K68.11
retropharyngeal J39.0
retrouterine —see Peritonitis, pelvic,
　female
retrovesical —see Cystitis, specified
　type NEC
root, tooth K04.7
　with sinus (alveolar) K04.6
round ligament (see also Disease, pelvis,
　inflammatory) N73.2
rupture (spontaneous) NOS L02.91
sacrum (tuberculous) A18.01
　nontuberculous M46.28
salivary (duct) (gland) K11.3
scalp (any part) L02.811
scapular —see Osteomyelitis, specified
　type NEC
sclera —see Scleritis
scrofulous (tuberculous) A18.2
scrotum N49.2
seminal vesicle N49.0
septal, dental K04.7
　with sinus (alveolar) K04.6
serous —see Periostitis
shoulder (region) —see Abscess, upper
　limb
sigmoid K63.0
sinus (accessory) (chronic) (nasal) —see
　also Sinusitis
　intracranial venous (any) G06.0
Skene's duct or gland N34.0
skin —see Abscess, by site
specified site NEC L02.818
spermatic cord N49.1
sphenoidal (sinus) (chronic) J32.3
spinal cord (any part) (staphylococcal)
　G06.1
　tuberculous A17.81
spine (column) (tuberculous) A18.01
　epidural G06.1
　nontuberculous —see Osteomyelitis,
　　vertebra
spleen D73.3
　amebic A06.89
stitch T81.4
subarachnoid G06.2
　brain G06.0
　spinal cord G06.1
subareolar —see Abscess, breast
subcecal K35.3
subcutaneous —see also Abscess, by site
　pheomycotic (chromomycotic) B43.2
subdiaphragmatic K65.1
subdural G06.2
　brain G06.0
　　sequelae G09
　spinal cord G06.1
subgaleal L02.811
subhepatic K65.1
sublingual K12.2
　gland K11.3
submammary —see Abscess, breast
submandibular (region) (space)
　(triangle) K12.2
　gland K11.3
submaxillary (region) L02.01
　gland K11.3
submental L02.01
　gland K11.3

Abscess *(Continued)*
subperiosteal —*see* Osteomyelitis,
    specified type NEC
subphrenic K65.1
    postoperative T81.4
suburethral N34.0
sudoriparous L75.8
supraclavicular (fossa) —*see* Abscess,
    upper limb
suprapelvic, acute N73.0
suprarenal (capsule) (gland) E27.8
sweat gland L74.8
tear duct —*see* Inflammation, lacrimal,
    passages, acute
temple L02.01
temporal region L02.01
temporosphenoidal G06.0
tendon (sheath) M65.00
    ankle M65.07-
    foot M65.07-
    forearm M65.03-
    hand M65.04-
    lower leg M65.06-
    pelvic region M65.05-
    shoulder region M65.01-
    specified site NEC M65.08
    thigh M65.05-
    upper arm M65.02-
testis N45.4
thigh —*see* Abscess, lower limb
thorax J86.9
    with fistula J86.0
throat J39.1
thumb —*see also* Abscess, hand
    nail —*see* Cellulitis, finger
thymus (gland) E32.1
thyroid (gland) E06.0
toe (any) —*see also* Abscess, foot
    nail —*see* Cellulitis, toe
tongue (staphylococcal) K14.0
tonsil (s) (lingual) J36
tonsillopharyngeal J36
tooth, teeth (root) K04.7
    with sinus (alveolar) K04.6
    supporting structures NEC
        K05.21
trachea J39.8
trunk L02.219
    abdominal wall L02.211
    back L02.212
    chest wall L02.213
    groin L02.214
    perineum L02.215
    umbilicus L02.216
tubal —*see* Salpingitis
tuberculous —*see* Tuberculosis, abscess
tubo-ovarian —*see* Salpingo-oophoritis
tunica vaginalis N49.1
umbilicus L02.216
upper
    limb L02.41-
    respiratory J39.8
urethral (gland) N34.0
urinary N34.0
uterus, uterine (wall) —*see also*
    Endometritis
    ligament (*see also* Disease, pelvis,
        inflammatory) N73.2
    neck —*see* Cervicitis
uvula K12.2
vagina (wall) —*see* Vaginitis
vaginorectal —*see* Vaginitis
vas deferens N49.1
vermiform appendix K35.3

Abscess *(Continued)*
vertebra (column) (tuberculous)
    A18.01
    nontuberculous —*see* Osteomyelitis,
        vertebra
vesical —*see* Cystitis, specified type
    NEC
vesico-uterine pouch —*see* Peritonitis,
    pelvic, female
vitreous (humor) —*see*
    Endophthalmitis, purulent
vocal cord J38.3
von Bezold's —*see* Mastoiditis, acute
vulva N76.4
vulvovaginal gland N75.1
web space —*see* Abscess, hand
wound T81.4
wrist —*see* Abscess, upper limb
Absence (of) (organ or part) (complete or
    partial)
adrenal (gland) (congenital) Q89.1
    acquired E89.6
albumin in blood E88.09
alimentary tract (congenital) Q45.8
    upper Q40.8
alveolar process (acquired) —*see*
    Anomaly, alveolar
ankle (acquired) Z89.44-
anus (congenital) Q42.3
    with fistula Q42.2
aorta (congenital) Q25.4
appendix, congenital Q42.8
arm (acquired) Z89.20-
    above elbow Z89.22-
        congenital (with hand present) —
            see Agenesis, arm, with hand
            present
        and hand —*see* Agenesis,
            forearm, and hand
    below elbow Z89.21-
        congenital (with hand present) —
            see Agenesis, arm, with hand
            present
        and hand —*see* Agenesis,
            forearm, and hand
    congenital —*see* Defect, reduction,
        upper limb
    shoulder (following explantation of
        shoulder joint prosthesis) (joint)
        (with or without presence of
        antibiotic-impregnated cement
        spacer) Z89.23-
        congenital (with hand present) —
            see Agenesis, arm, with hand
            present
artery (congenital) (peripheral) Q27.8
    brain Q28.3
    coronary Q24.5
    pulmonary Q25.79
    specified NEC Q27.8
    umbilical Q27.0
atrial septum (congenital) Q21.1
auditory canal (congenital) (external)
    Q16.1
auricle (ear), congenital Q16.0
bile, biliary duct, congenital Q44.5
bladder (acquired) Z90.6
    congenital Q64.5
bowel sounds R19.11
brain Q00.0
    part of Q04.3
breast (s) (and nipple (s)) (acquired)
    Z90.1-
    congenital Q83.8

Absence *(Continued)*
broad ligament Q50.6
bronchus (congenital) Q32.4
canaliculus lacrimalis, congenital Q10.4
cerebellum (vermis) Q04.3
cervix (acquired) (with uterus) Z90.710
    with remaining uterus Z90.712
    congenital Q51.5
chin, congenital Q18.8
cilia (congenital) Q10.3
    acquired —*see* Madarosis
clitoris (congenital) Q52.6
coccyx, congenital Q76.49
cold sense R20.8
congenital
    lumen —*see* Atresia
    organ or site NEC —*see* Agenesis
    septum —*see* Imperfect, closure
corpus callosum Q04.0
cricoid cartilage, congenital Q31.8
diaphragm (with hernia), congenital
    Q79.1
digestive organ (s) or tract, congenital
    Q45.8
    acquired NEC Z90.49
    upper Q40.8
ductus arteriosus Q28.8
duodenum (acquired) Z90.49
    congenital Q41.0
ear, congenital Q16.9
    acquired H93.8-
    auricle Q16.0
    external Q16.0
    inner Q16.5
    lobe, lobule Q17.8
    middle, except ossicles Q16.4
        ossicles Q16.3
    ossicles Q16.3
ejaculatory duct (congenital)
    Q55.4
endocrine gland (congenital) NEC
    Q89.2
    acquired E89.89
epididymis (congenital) Q55.4
    acquired Z90.79
epiglottis, congenital Q31.8
esophagus (congenital) Q39.8
    acquired (partial) Z90.49
eustachian tube (congenital) Q16.2
extremity (acquired) Z89.9
    congenital Q73.0
    knee (following explantation of knee
        joint prosthesis) (joint) (with or
        without presence of antibiotic-
        impregnated cement spacer)
        Z89.52-
    lower (above knee) Z89.619
        below knee Z89.51-
    upper —*see* Absence, arm
eye (acquired) Z90.01
    congenital Q11.1
    muscle (congenital) Q10.3
eyeball (acquired) Z90.01
eyelid (fold) (congenital) Q10.3
    acquired Z90.01
face, specified part NEC Q18.8
fallopian tube (s) (acquired) Z90.79
    congenital Q50.6
family member (causing problem in
    home) NEC (*see also*
    Disruption, family) Z63.32
femur, congenital —*see* Defect,
    reduction, lower limb,
    longitudinal, femur

Absence *(Continued)*
  fibrinogen (congenital) D68.2
    acquired D65
  finger (s) (acquired) Z89.02-
    congenital —*see* Agenesis, hand
  foot (acquired) Z89.43-
    congenital —*see* Agenesis, foot
  forearm (acquired) —*see* Absence, arm,
      below elbow
  gallbladder (acquired) Z90.49
    congenital Q44.0
  gamma globulin in blood D80.1
    hereditary D80.0
  genital organs
    acquired (female) (male) Z90.79
    female, congenital Q52.8
      external Q52.71
      internal NEC Q52.8
    male, congenital Q55.8
  genitourinary organs, congenital NEC
    female Q52.8
    male Q55.8
  globe (acquired) Z90.01
    congenital Q11.1
  glottis, congenital Q31.8
  hand and wrist (acquired) Z89.11-
    congenital —*see* Agenesis, hand
  head, part (acquired) NEC Z90.09
  heat sense R20.8
  hip (following explantation of hip joint
      prosthesis) (joint) (with or without
      presence of antibiotic-impregnated
      cement spacer) Z89.62-
  hymen (congenital) Q52.4
  ileum (acquired) Z90.49
    congenital Q41.2
  immunoglobulin, isolated NEC D80.3
    IgA D80.2
    IgG D80.3
    IgM D80.4
  incus (acquired) —*see* Loss, ossicles, ear
    congenital Q16.3
  inner ear, congenital Q16.5
  intestine (acquired) (small) Z90.49
    congenital Q41.9
      specified NEC Q41.8
    large Z90.49
      congenital Q42.9
        specified NEC Q42.8
  iris, congenital Q13.1
  jejunum (acquired) Z90.49
    congenital Q41.1
  joint
    acquired
      hip (following explantation of
          hip joint prosthesis) (with or
          without presence of antibiotic-
          impregnated cement spacer)
          Z89.62-
      knee (following explantation of
          knee joint prosthesis) (with or
          without presence of antibiotic-
          impregnated cement spacer)
          Z89.52-
      shoulder (following explantation
          of shoulder joint prosthesis)
          (with or without presence
          of antibiotic-impregnated
          cement spacer) Z89.23-
    congenital NEC Q74.8
  kidney (s) (acquired) Z90.5
    congenital Q60.2
      bilateral Q60.1
      unilateral Q60.0

Absence *(Continued)*
  knee (following explantation of knee
      joint prosthesis) (joint) (with or
      without presence of antibiotic-
      impregnated cement spacer)
      Z89.52-
  labyrinth, membranous Q16.5
  larynx (congenital) Q31.8
    acquired Z90.02
  leg (acquired) (above knee) Z89.61-
    below knee (acquired) Z89.51-
    congenital —*see* Defect, reduction,
        lower limb
  lens (acquired) —*see also* Aphakia
    congenital Q12.3
    post cataract extraction Z98.4-
  limb (acquired) —*see* Absence,
      extremity
  lip Q38.6
  liver (congenital) Q44.7
  lung (fissure) (lobe) (bilateral)
      (unilateral) (congenital) Q33.3
    acquired (any part) Z90.2
  menstruation —*see* Amenorrhea
  muscle (congenital) (pectoral) Q79.8
    ocular Q10.3
  neck, part Q18.8
  neutrophil —*see* Agranulocytosis
  nipple (s) (with breast (s)) (acquired)
      Z90.1-
    congenital Q83.2
  nose (congenital) Q30.1
    acquired Z90.09
  organ
    of Corti, congenital Q16.5
    or site, congenital NEC Q89.8
      acquired NEC Z90.89
  osseous meatus (ear) Q16.4
  ovary (acquired)
    bilateral Z90.722
    congenital
      bilateral Q50.02
      unilateral Q50.01
    unilateral Z90.721
  oviduct (acquired)
    bilateral Z90.722
    congenital Q50.6
    unilateral Z90.721
  pancreas (congenital) Q45.0
    acquired Z90.410
    complete Z90.410
    partial Z90.411
    total Z90.410
  parathyroid gland (acquired) E89.2
    congenital Q89.2
  patella, congenital Q74.1
  penis (congenital) Q55.5
    acquired Z90.79
  pericardium (congenital) Q24.8
  pituitary gland (congenital) Q89.2
    acquired E89.3
  prostate (acquired) Z90.79
    congenital Q55.4
  pulmonary valve Q22.0
  punctum lacrimale (congenital) Q10.4
  radius, congenital —*see* Defect,
      reduction, upper limb,
      longitudinal, radius
  rectum (congenital) Q42.1
    with fistula Q42.0
    acquired Z90.49
  respiratory organ NOS Q34.9
  rib (acquired) Z90.89
    congenital Q76.6

Absence *(Continued)*
  sacrum, congenital Q76.49
  salivary gland (s), congenital Q38.4
  scrotum, congenital Q55.29
  seminal vesicles (congenital) Q55.4
    acquired Z90.79
  septum
    atrial (congenital) Q21.1
    between aorta and pulmonary artery
        Q21.4
    ventricular (congenital) Q20.4
  sex chromosome
    female phenotype Q97.8
    male phenotype Q98.8
  skull bone (congenital) Q75.8
    with
      anencephaly Q00.0
      encephalocele —*see* Encephalocele
      hydrocephalus Q03.9
        with spina bifida —*see* Spina
            bifida, by site, with
            hydrocephalus
      microcephaly Q02
  spermatic cord, congenital Q55.4
  spine, congenital Q76.49
  spleen (congenital) Q89.01
    acquired Z90.81
  sternum, congenital Q76.7
  stomach (acquired) (partial) Z90.3
    congenital Q40.2
  superior vena cava, congenital Q26.8
  teeth, tooth (congenital) K00.0
    acquired (complete) K08.109
      class I K08.101
      class II K08.102
      class III K08.103
      class IV K08.104
      due to
        caries K08.139
          class I K08.131
          class II K08.132
          class III K08.133
          class IV K08.134
        periodontal disease K08.129
          class I K08.121
          class II K08.122
          class III K08.123
          class IV K08.124
      specified NEC K08.199
        class I K08.191
        class II K08.192
        class III K08.193
        class IV K08.194
      trauma K08.119
        class I K08.111
        class II K08.112
        class III K08.113
        class IV K08.114
    partial K08.409
      class I K08.401
      class II K08.402
      class III K08.403
      class IV K08.404
      due to
        caries K08.439
          class I K08.431
          class II K08.432
          class III K08.433
          class IV K08.434
        periodontal disease K08.429
          class I K08.421
          class II K08.422
          class III K08.423
          class IV K08.424

Abuse *(Continued)*
  drug NEC *(Continued)*
    hallucinogen *(Continued)*
      with *(Continued)*
        mood disorder F16.14
        other specified disorder F16.188
        perception disorder, persisting
          F16.183
        psychosis F16.159
          delusions F16.150
          hallucinations F16.151
        unspecified disorder F16.19
      hashish —*see* Abuse, drug, cannabis
      herbal or folk remedies F55.1
      hormones F55.3
      hypnotics —*see* Abuse, drug, sedative
      inhalant F18.10
        with
          anxiety disorder F18.180
          dementia, persisting F18.17
          intoxication F18.129
            with delirium F18.121
            uncomplicated F18.120
          mood disorder F18.14
          other specified disorder F18.188
          psychosis F18.159
            delusions F18.150
            hallucinations F18.151
          unspecified disorder F18.19
      laxatives F55.2
      LSD —*see* Abuse, drug, hallucinogen
      marihuana —*see* Abuse, drug,
        cannabis
      morphine type (opioids) —*see* Abuse,
        drug, opioid
      opioid F11.10
        with
          intoxication F11.129
            with
              delirium F11.121
              perceptual disturbance
                F11.122
            uncomplicated F11.120
          mood disorder F11.14
          other specified disorder
            F11.188
          psychosis F11.159
            delusions F11.150
            hallucinations F11.151
          sexual dysfunction F11.181
          sleep disorder F11.182
          unspecified disorder F11.19
      PCP (phencyclidine) (or related
        substance) —*see* Abuse, drug,
        hallucinogen
      psychoactive NEC F19.10
        with
          amnestic disorder F19.16
          anxiety disorder F19.180
          dementia F19.17
          intoxication F19.129
            with
              delirium F19.121
              perceptual disturbance
                F19.122
            uncomplicated F19.120
          mood disorder F19.14
          other specified disorder F19.188
          psychosis F19.159
            delusions F19.150
            hallucinations F19.151
          sexual dysfunction F19.181
          sleep disorder F19.182
          unspecified disorder F19.19

Abuse *(Continued)*
  drug NEC *(Continued)*
    sedative, hypnotic or anxiolytic
      F13.10
      with
        anxiety disorder F13.180
        intoxication F13.129
          with delirium F13.121
          uncomplicated F13.120
        mood disorder F13.14
        other specified disorder F13.188
        psychosis F13.159
          delusions F13.150
          hallucinations F13.151
        sexual dysfunction F13.181
        sleep disorder F13.182
        unspecified disorder F13.19
    solvent —*see* Abuse, drug, inhalant
    steroids F55.3
    stimulant NEC F15.10
      with
        anxiety disorder F15.180
        intoxication F15.129
          with
            delirium F15.121
            perceptual disturbance
              F15.122
          uncomplicated F15.120
        mood disorder F15.14
        other specified disorder F15.188
        psychosis F15.159
          delusions F15.150
          hallucinations F15.151
        sexual dysfunction F15.181
        sleep disorder F15.182
        unspecified disorder F15.19
    tranquilizers —*see* Abuse, drug,
      sedative
    vitamins F55.4
  hallucinogens —*see* Abuse, drug,
    hallucinogen
  hashish —*see* Abuse, drug, cannabis
  herbal or folk remedies F55.1
  hormones F55.3
  hypnotic —*see* Abuse, drug, sedative
  inhalant —*see* Abuse, drug, inhalant
  laxatives F55.2
  LSD —*see* Abuse, drug, hallucinogen
  marihuana —*see* Abuse, drug, cannabis
  morphine type (opioids) —*see* Abuse,
    drug, opioid
  non-psychoactive substance NEC F55.8
    antacids F55.0
    folk remedies F55.1
    herbal remedies F55.1
    hormones F55.3
    laxatives F55.2
    steroids F55.3
    vitamins F55.4
  opioids —*see* Abuse, drug, opioid
  PCP (phencyclidine) (or related
    substance) —*see* Abuse, drug,
    hallucinogen
  physical (adult) (child) —*see*
    Maltreatment
  psychoactive substance —*see* Abuse,
    drug, psychoactive NEC
  psychological (adult) (child) —*see*
    Maltreatment
  sedative —*see* Abuse, drug, sedative
  sexual —*see* Maltreatment
  solvent —*see* Abuse, drug, inhalant
  steroids F55.3
  vitamins F55.4

Acalculia R48.8
  developmental F81.2
Acanthamebiasis (with) B60.10
  conjunctiva B60.12
  keratoconjunctivitis B60.13
  meningoencephalitis B60.11
  other specified B60.19
Acanthocephaliasis B83.8
Acanthocheilonemiasis B74.4
Acanthocytosis E78.6
Acantholysis L11.9
Acanthosis (acquired) (nigricans) L83
  benign Q82.8
  congenital Q82.8
  seborrheic L82.1
    inflamed L82.0
  tongue K14.3
Acapnia E87.3
Acarbia E87.2
Acardia, acardius Q89.8
Acardiacus amorphus Q89.8
Acardiotrophia I51.4
Acariasis B88.0
  scabies B86
Acarodermatitis (urticarioides) B88.0
Acarophobia F40.218
Acatalasemia, acatalasia E80.3
Acathisia (drug induced) G25.71
Accelerated atrioventricular conduction
  I45.6
Accentuation of personality traits
  (type A) Z73.1
Accessory (congenital)
  adrenal gland Q89.1
  anus Q43.4
  appendix Q43.4
  atrioventricular conduction I45.6
  auditory ossicles Q16.3
  auricle (ear) Q17.0
  biliary duct or passage Q44.5
  bladder Q64.79
  blood vessels NEC Q27.9
    coronary Q24.5
  bone NEC Q79.8
  breast tissue, axilla Q83.1
  carpal bones Q74.0
  cecum Q43.4
  chromosome (s) NEC (nonsex)
    Q92.9
    with complex rearrangements NEC
      Q92.5
    seen only at prometaphase Q92.8
    13 —*see* Trisomy, 13
    18 —*see* Trisomy, 18
    21 —*see* Trisomy, 21
    partial Q92.9
    sex
      female phenotype Q97.8
  coronary artery Q24.5
  cusp (s), heart valve NEC Q24.8
    pulmonary Q22.3
  cystic duct Q44.5
  digit (s) Q69.9
  ear (auricle) (lobe) Q17.0
  endocrine gland NEC Q89.2
  eye muscle Q10.3
  eyelid Q10.3
  face bone (s) Q75.8
  fallopian tube (fimbria) (ostium)
    Q50.6
  finger (s) Q69.0
  foreskin N47.8
  frontonasal process Q75.8
  gallbladder Q44.1

Accessory (Continued)
  genital organ (s)
    female Q52.8
      external Q52.79
      internal NEC Q52.8
    male Q55.8
  genitourinary organs NEC Q89.8
    female Q52.8
    male Q55.8
  hallux Q69.2
  heart Q24.8
    valve NEC Q24.8
      pulmonary Q22.3
  hepatic ducts Q44.5
  hymen Q52.4
  intestine (large) (small) Q43.4
  kidney Q63.0
  lacrimal canal Q10.6
  leaflet, heart valve NEC Q24.8
  ligament, broad Q50.6
  liver Q44.7
    duct Q44.5
  lobule (ear) Q17.0
  lung (lobe) Q33.1
  muscle Q79.8
  navicular of carpus Q74.0
  nervous system, part NEC Q07.8
  nipple Q83.3
  nose Q30.8
  organ or site not listed —see Anomaly,
    by site
  ovary Q50.31
  oviduct Q50.6
  pancreas Q45.3
  parathyroid gland Q89.2
  parotid gland (and duct) Q38.4
  pituitary gland Q89.2
  preauricular appendage Q17.0
  prepuce N47.8
  renal arteries (multiple) Q27.2
  rib Q76.6
    cervical Q76.5
  roots (teeth) K00.2
  salivary gland Q38.4
  sesamoid bones Q74.8
    foot Q74.2
    hand Q74.0
  skin tags Q82.8
  spleen Q89.09
  sternum Q76.7
  submaxillary gland Q38.4
  tarsal bones Q74.2
  teeth, tooth K00.1
  tendon Q79.8
  thumb Q69.1
  thymus gland Q89.2
  thyroid gland Q89.2
  toes Q69.2
  tongue Q38.3
  tooth, teeth K00.1
  tragus Q17.0
  ureter Q62.5
  urethra Q64.79
  urinary organ or tract NEC Q64.8
  uterus Q51.2
  vagina Q52.10
  valve, heart NEC Q24.8
    pulmonary Q22.3
  vertebra Q76.49
  vocal cords Q31.8
  vulva Q52.79
Accident
  birth —see Birth, injury
  cardiac —see Infarct, myocardium
  cerebral I63.9

Accident (Continued)
  cerebrovascular (embolic) (ischemic)
      (thrombotic) I63.9
    aborted I63.9
    hemorrhagic —see Hemorrhage,
      intracranial, intracerebral
    old (without sequelae) Z86.73
      with sequelae (of) —see Sequelae,
        infarction, cerebral
  coronary —see Infarct, myocardium
  craniovascular I63.9
  vascular, brain I63.9
Accidental —see condition
Accommodation (disorder) —see also
    condition
  hysterical paralysis of F44.89
  insufficiency of H52.4
  paresis —see Paresis, of accommodation
  spasm —see Spasm, of accommodation
Accouchement —see Delivery
Accreta placenta O43.21-
Accretio cordis (nonrheumatic) I31.0
Accretions, tooth, teeth K03.6
Acculturation difficulty Z60.3
Accumulation secretion, prostate N42.89
Acephalia, acephalism, acephalus,
    acephaly Q00.0
Acephalobrachia monster Q89.8
Acephalochirus monster Q89.8
Acephalogaster Q89.8
Acephalostomus monster Q89.8
Acephalothorax Q89.8
Acerophobia F40.298
Acetonemia R79.89
  in Type 1 diabetes E10.10
    with coma E10.11
Acetonuria R82.4
Achalasia (cardia) (esophagus) K22.0
  congenital Q39.5
  pylorus Q40.0
  sphincteral NEC K59.8
Ache (s) —see Pain
Acheilia Q38.6
Achilloburisitis —see Tendinitis, Achilles
Achillodynia —see Tendinitis, Achilles
Achlorhydria, achlorhydric (neurogenic)
    K31.83
  anemia D50.8
  diarrhea K31.83
  psychogenic F45.8
  secondary to vagotomy K91.1
Achluophobia F40.228
Acholia K82.8
Acholuric jaundice (familial)
    (splenomegalic) —see also
    Spherocytosis
  acquired D59.8
Achondrogenesis Q77.0
Achondroplasia (osteosclerosis congenita)
    Q77.4
Achroma, cutis L80
Achromat (ism), achromatopsia
    (acquired) (congenital) H53.51
Achromia, congenital —see Albinism
Achromia parasitica B36.0
Achylia gastrica K31.89
  psychogenic F45.8
Acid
  burn —see Corrosion
  deficiency
    amide nicotinic E52
    ascorbic E54
    folic E53.8
    nicotinic E52
    pantothenic E53.8

Acid (Continued)
  intoxication E87.2
  peptic disease K30
  phosphatase deficiency E83.39
  stomach K30
    psychogenic F45.8
Acidemia E87.2
  argininosuccinic E72.22
  isovaleric E71.110
  metabolic (newborn) P19.9
    first noted before onset of labor P19.0
    first noted during labor P19.1
    noted at birth P19.2
  methylmalonic E71.120
  pipecolic E72.3
  propionic E71.121
Acidity, gastric (high) K30
  psychogenic F45.8
Acidocytopenia —see Agranulocytosis
Acidocytosis D72.1
Acidopenia —see Agranulocytosis
Acidosis (lactic) (respiratory) E87.2
  in Type 1 diabetes E10.10
    with coma E10.11
  kidney, tubular N25.89
  lactic E87.2
  metabolic NEC E87.2
    with respiratory acidosis E87.4
    late, of newborn P74.0
  mixed metabolic and respiratory,
    newborn P84
  newborn P84
  renal (hyperchloremic) (tubular) N25.89
  respiratory E87.2
    complicated by
      metabolic
        acidosis E87.4
        alkalosis E87.4
Aciduria
  argininosuccinic E72.22
  glutaric (type I) E72.3
    type II E71.313
    type III E71.5-
  orotic (congenital) (hereditary)
      (pyrimidine deficiency) E79.8
    anemia D53.0
Acladiosis (skin) B36.0
Aclasis, diaphyseal Q78.6
Acleistocardia Q21.1
Aclusion —see Anomaly, dentofacial,
    malocclusion
Acne L70.9
  artificialis L70.8
  atrophica L70.2
  cachecticorum (Hebra) L70.8
  conglobata L70.1
  cystic L70.0
  decalvans L66.2
  excoriée des jeunes filles L70.5
  frontalis L70.2
  indurata L70.0
  infantile L70.4
  keloid L73.0
  lupoid L70.2
  necrotic, necrotica (miliaris) L70.2
  neonatal L70.4
  nodular L70.0
  occupational L70.8
  picker's L70.5
  pustular L70.0
  rodens L70.2
  rosacea L71.9
  specified NEC L70.8
  tropica L70.3

Acne (*Continued*)
  varioliformis L70.2
  vulgaris L70.0
Acnitis (primary) A18.4
Acosta's disease T70.29
Acoustic —*see* condition
Acousticophobia F40.298
Acquired —*see also* condition
  immunodeficiency syndrome (AIDS) B20
Acrania Q00.0
Acroangiodermatitis I78.9
Acroasphyxia, chronic I73.89
Acrobystitis N47.7
Acrocephalopolysyndactyly Q87.0
Acrocephalosyndactyly Q87.0
Acrocephaly Q75.0
Acrochondrohyperplasia —*see*
  Syndrome, Marfan's
Acrocyanosis I73.8
  newborn P28.2
    meaning transient blue hands and
      feet - omit code
Acrodermatitis L30.8
  atrophicans (chronica) L90.4
  continua (Hallopeau) L40.2
  enteropathica (hereditary) E83.2
  Hallopeau's L40.2
  infantile papular L44.4
  perstans L40.2
  pustulosa continua L40.2
  recalcitrant pustular L40.2
Acrodynia —*see* Poisoning, mercury
Acromegaly, acromegalia E22.0
Acromelalgia I73.81
Acromicria, acromikria Q79.8
Acronyx L60.0
Acropachy, thyroid —*see* Thyrotoxicosis
Acroparesthesia (simple) (vasomotor)
  I73.89
Acropathy, thyroid —*see* Thyrotoxicosis
Acrophobia F40.241
Acroposthitis N47.7
Acroscleriasis, acroscleroderma,
  acrosclerosis —*see* Sclerosis,
  systemic
Acrosphacelus I96
Acrospiroma, eccrine —*see* Neoplasm,
  skin, benign
Acrostealgia —*see* Osteochondropathy
Acrotrophodynia —*see* Immersion
ACTH ectopic syndrome E24.3
Actinic —*see* condition
Actinobacillosis, actinobacillus A28.8
  mallei A24.0
  muris A25.1
Actinomyces israelii (infection) —*see*
  Actinomycosis
Actinomycetoma (foot) B47.1
Actinomycosis, actinomycotic A42.9
  with pneumonia A42.0
  abdominal A42.1
  cervicofacial A42.2
  cutaneous A42.89
  gastrointestinal A42.1
  pulmonary A42.0
  sepsis A42.7
  specified site NEC A42.89
Actinoneuritis G62.82
Action, heart
  disorder I49.9
  irregular I49.9
    psychogenic F45.8
Activated protein C resistance D68.51
Active —*see* condition

Acute —*see also* condition
  abdomen R10.0
  gallbladder —*see* Cholecystitis, acute
Acyanotic heart disease (congenital) Q24.9
Acystia Q64.5
Adair-Dighton syndrome (brittle bones
  and blue sclera, deafness) Q78.0
Adamantinoblastoma —*see*
  Ameloblastoma
Adamantinoma —*see also* Cyst, calcifying
  odontogenic
  long bones C40.90
    lower limb C40.2-
    upper limb C40.0-
  malignant C41.1
    jaw (bone) (lower) C41.1
      upper C41.0
  tibial C40.2-
Adamantoblastoma —*see* Ameloblastoma
Adams-Stokes (-Morgagni) **disease or**
  syndrome I45.9
Adaption reaction —*see* Disorder,
  adjustment
Addiction (*see also* Dependence) F19.20
  alcohol, alcoholic (ethyl) (methyl)
    (wood) (without remission) F10.20
    with remission F10.21
  drug —*see* Dependence, drug
  ethyl alcohol (without remission) F10.20
    with remission F10.21
  heroin —*see* Dependence, drug, opioid
  methyl alcohol (without remission)
    F10.20
    with remission F10.21
  methylated spirit (without remission)
    F10.20
    with remission F10.21
  morphine(-like substances) —*see*
    Dependence, drug, opioid
  nicotine —*see* Dependence, drug,
    nicotine
  opium and opioids —*see* Dependence,
    drug, opioid
  tobacco —*see* Dependence, drug,
    nicotine
Addisonian crisis E27.2
Addison's
  anemia (pernicious) D51.0
  disease (bronze) or syndrome E27.1
    tuberculous A18.7
  keloid L94.0
Addison-Biermer anemia (pernicious)
  D51.0
Addison-Schilder complex E71.528
Additional —*see also* Accessory
  chromosome (s) Q99.8
    21 —*see* Trisomy, 21
    sex —*see* Abnormal, chromosome, sex
Adduction contracture, hip or other
  joint —*see* Contraction, joint
Adenitis —*see also* Lymphadenitis
  acute, unspecified site L04.9
  axillary I88.9
    acute L04.2
    chronic or subacute I88.1
  Bartholin's gland N75.8
  bulbourethral gland —*see* Urethritis
  cervical I88.9
    acute L04.0
    chronic or subacute I88.1
  chancroid (Hemophilus ducreyi) A57
  chronic, unspecified site I88.1
  Cowper's gland —*see* Urethritis
  due to Pasteurella multocida (p. septica)
    A28.0

Adenitis (*Continued*)
  epidemic, acute B27.09
  gangrenous L04.9
  gonorrheal NEC A54.89
  groin I88.9
    acute L04.1
    chronic or subacute I88.1
  infectious (acute) (epidemic) B27.09
  inguinal I88.9
    acute L04.1
    chronic or subacute I88.1
  lymph gland or node, except mesenteric
    I88.9
    acute —*see* Lymphadenitis, acute
    chronic or subacute I88.1
  mesenteric (acute) (chronic)
    (nonspecific) (subacute) I88.0
  parotid gland (suppurative) —*see*
    Sialoadenitis
  salivary gland (any) (suppurative) —*see*
    Sialoadenitis
  scrofulous (tuberculous) A18.2
  Skene's duct or gland —*see* Urethritis
  strumous, tuberculous A18.2
  subacute, unspecified site I88.1
  sublingual gland (suppurative) —*see*
    Sialoadenitis
  submandibular gland (suppurative) —
    see Sialoadenitis
  submaxillary gland (suppurative) —*see*
    Sialoadenitis
  tuberculous —*see* Tuberculosis, lymph
    gland
  urethral gland —*see* Urethritis
  Wharton's duct (suppurative) —*see*
    Sialoadenitis
Adenoacanthoma —*see* Neoplasm,
  malignant, by site
Adenoameloblastoma —*see* Cyst,
  calcifying odontogenic
Adenocarcinoid (tumor) —*see* Neoplasm,
  malignant, by site
Adenocarcinoma —*see also* Neoplasm,
  malignant, by site
  acidophil
    specified site —*see* Neoplasm,
      malignant, by site
    unspecified site C75.1
  adrenal cortical C74.0-
  alveolar —*see* Neoplasm, lung,
    malignant
  apocrine
    breast —*see* Neoplasm, breast,
      malignant
    in situ
      breast D05.8-
      specified site NEC —*see* Neoplasm,
        skin, in situ
      unspecified site D04.9
    specified site NEC —*see* Neoplasm,
      skin, malignant
    unspecified site C44.99
  basal cell
    specified site —*see* Neoplasm, skin,
      malignant
    unspecified site C08.9
  basophil
    specified site —*see* Neoplasm,
      malignant, by site
    unspecified site C75.1
  bile duct type C22.1
    liver C22.1
    specified site NEC —*see* Neoplasm,
      malignant, by site
    unspecified site C22.1

Adenocarcinoma (*Continued*)
  bronchiolar —*see* Neoplasm, lung,
    malignant
  bronchioloalveolar —*see* Neoplasm,
    lung, malignant
  ceruminous C44.29-
  cervix, in situ (*see also* Carcinoma,
    cervix uteri, in situ) D06.9
  chromophobe
    specified site —*see* Neoplasm,
      malignant, by site
    unspecified site C75.1
  diffuse type
    specified site —*see* Neoplasm,
      malignant, by site
    unspecified site C16.9
  duct
    infiltrating
      with Paget's disease —*see*
        Neoplasm, breast,
        malignant
      specified site —*see* Neoplasm,
        malignant, by site
      unspecified site (female)
        C50.91-
        male C50.92-
    specified site —*see* Neoplasm,
      malignant, by site
    unspecified site
      female C56.9
      male C61
  eosinophil
    specified site —*see* Neoplasm,
      malignant, by site
    unspecified site C75.1
  follicular
    with papillary C73
    moderately differentiated C73
    specified site —*see* Neoplasm,
      malignant, by site
    trabecular C73
    unspecified site C73
    well differentiated C73
  Hurthle cell C73
  in
    adenomatous
      polyposis coli C18.9
  infiltrating duct
    with Paget's disease —*see* Neoplasm,
      breast, malignant
    specified site —*see* Neoplasm,
      malignant, by site
    unspecified site (female) C50.91-
      male C50.92-
  inflammatory
    specified site —*see* Neoplasm,
      malignant, by site
    unspecified site (female) C50.91-
      male C50.92-
  intestinal type
    specified site —*see* Neoplasm,
      malignant, by site
    unspecified site C16.9
  intracystic papillary
  intraductal
    breast D05.1-
    noninfiltrating
      breast D05.1-
      papillary
        with invasion
          specified site —*see* Neoplasm,
            malignant, by site
          unspecified site (female)
            C50.91-
            male C50.92-

Adenocarcinoma (*Continued*)
  intraductal (*Continued*)
    noninfiltrating (*Continued*)
      papillary (*Continued*)
        breast D05.1-
        specified site NEC —*see*
          Neoplasm, in situ, by site
        unspecified site D05.1-
      specified site NEC —*see* Neoplasm,
        in situ, by site
      unspecified site D05.1-
    papillary
      with invasion
        specified site —*see* Neoplasm,
          malignant, by site
        unspecified site (female) C50.91-
          male C50.92-
      breast D05.1-
      specified site —*see* Neoplasm, in
        situ, by site
      unspecified site D05.1-
    specified site NEC —*see* Neoplasm, in
      situ, by site
    unspecified site D05.1-
  islet cell
    with exocrine, mixed
      specified site —*see* Neoplasm,
        malignant, by site
      unspecified site C25.9
    pancreas C25.4
    specified site NEC —*see* Neoplasm,
      malignant, by site
    unspecified site C25.4
  lobular
    in situ
      breast D05.0-
      specified site NEC —*see* Neoplasm,
        in situ, by site
      unspecified site D05.0-
    specified site —*see* Neoplasm,
      malignant, by site
    unspecified site (female) C50.91-
      male C50.92-
  mucoid —*see also* Neoplasm, malignant,
    by site
    cell
      specified site —*see* Neoplasm,
        malignant, by site
      unspecified site C75.1
  nonencapsulated sclerosing C73
  papillary
    with follicular C73
    follicular variant C73
    intraductal (noninfiltrating)
      with invasion
        specified site —*see* Neoplasm,
          malignant, by site
        unspecified site (female)
          C50.91-
          male C50.92-
      breast D05.1-
      specified site NEC —*see* Neoplasm,
        in situ, by site
      unspecified site D05.1-
    serous
      specified site —*see* Neoplasm,
        malignant, by site
      unspecified site C56.9
  papillocystic
    specified site —*see* Neoplasm,
      malignant, by site
    unspecified site C56.9
  pseudomucinous
    specified site —*see* Neoplasm,
      malignant, by site
    unspecified site C56.9

Adenocarcinoma (*Continued*)
  renal cell C64-
  sebaceous —*see* Neoplasm, skin,
    malignant, by site
  serous —*see also* Neoplasm, malignant,
    by site
    papillary
      specified site —*see* Neoplasm,
        malignant, by site
      unspecified site C56.9
  sweat gland —*see* Neoplasm, skin,
    malignant
  water-clear cell C75.0
Adenocarcinoma-in-situ —*see also*
  Neoplasm, in situ, by site
  breast D05.9-
Adenofibroma
  clear cell —*see* Neoplasm, benign,
    by site
  endometrioid D27.9
    borderline malignancy D39.10
    malignant C56-
  mucinous
    specified site —*see* Neoplasm, benign,
      by site
    unspecified site D27.9
  papillary
    specified site —*see* Neoplasm, benign,
      by site
    unspecified site D27.9
  prostate —*see* Enlargement, enlarged,
    prostate
  serous
    specified site —*see* Neoplasm, benign,
      by site
    unspecified site D27.9
  specified site —*see* Neoplasm, benign,
    by site
  unspecified site D27.9
Adenofibrosis
  breast —*see* Fibroadenosis, breast
  endometrioid N80.0
Adenoiditis (chronic) J35.02
  with tonsillitis J35.03
  acute J03.90
    recurrent J03.91
    specified organism NEC J03.80
      recurrent J03.81
    staphylococcal J03.80
      recurrent J03.81
    streptococcal J03.00
      recurrent J03.01
Adenoids —*see* condition
Adenolipoma —*see* Neoplasm, benign,
  by site
Adenolipomatosis, Launois-Bensaude
  E88.89
Adenolymphoma
  specified site —*see* Neoplasm, benign,
    by site
  unspecified site D11.9
Adenoma —*see also* Neoplasm, benign,
  by site
  acidophil
    specified site —*see* Neoplasm, benign,
      by site
    unspecified site D35.2
  acidophil-basophil, mixed
    specified site —*see* Neoplasm, benign,
      by site
    unspecified site D35.2
  adrenal (cortical) D35.00
    clear cell D35.00
    compact cell D35.00
    glomerulosa cell D35.00

Adenoma *(Continued)*
  adrenal *(Continued)*
    heavily pigmented variant D35.00
    mixed cell D35.00
  alpha-cell
    pancreas D13.7
    specified site NEC —*see* Neoplasm,
      benign, by site
    unspecified site D13.7
  alveolar D14.30
  apocrine
    breast D24-
    specified site NEC —*see* Neoplasm,
      skin, benign, by site
    unspecified site D23.9
  basal cell D11.9
  basophil
    specified site —*see* Neoplasm, benign,
      by site
    unspecified site D35.2
  basophil-acidophil, mixed
    specified site —*see* Neoplasm, benign,
      by site
    unspecified site D35.2
  beta-cell
    pancreas D13.7
    specified site NEC —*see* Neoplasm,
      benign, by site
    unspecified site D13.7
  bile duct D13.4
    common D13.5
    extrahepatic D13.5
    intrahepatic D13.4
    specified site NEC —*see* Neoplasm,
      benign, by site
    unspecified site D13.4
  black D35.00
  bronchial D38.1
    cylindroid type —*see* Neoplasm,
      lung, malignant
  ceruminous D23.2-
  chief cell D35.1
  chromophobe
    specified site —*see* Neoplasm, benign,
      by site
    unspecified site D35.2
  colloid
    specified site —*see* Neoplasm, benign,
      by site
    unspecified site D34
  duct
  eccrine, papillary —*see* Neoplasm, skin,
    benign
  endocrine, multiple
    single specified site —*see* Neoplasm,
      uncertain behavior, by site
    two or more specified sites D44-
    unspecified site D44.9
  endometrioid —*see also* Neoplasm,
    benign
    borderline malignancy —*see*
      Neoplasm, uncertain behavior,
      by site
  eosinophil
    unspecified site D35.2
  fetal
    specified site —*see* Neoplasm, benign,
      by site
    unspecified site D34
  follicular
    specified site —*see* Neoplasm, benign,
      by site
    unspecified site D34
  hepatocellular D13.4
  Hurthle cell D34

Adenoma *(Continued)*
  islet cell
    pancreas D13.7
    specified site NEC —*see* Neoplasm,
      benign, by site
    unspecified site D13.7
  liver cell D13.4
  macrofollicular
    specified site —*see* Neoplasm, benign,
      by site
    unspecified site D34
  malignant, malignum —*see* Neoplasm,
    malignant, by site
  microcystic
    pancreas D13.7
    specified site NEC —*see* Neoplasm,
      benign, by site
    unspecified site D13.7
  microfollicular
    specified site —*see* Neoplasm, benign,
      by site
    unspecified site D34
  mucoid cell
    specified site —*see* Neoplasm, benign,
      by site
    unspecified site D35.2
  multiple endocrine
    single specified site —*see* Neoplasm,
      uncertain behavior, by site
    two or more specified sites D44-
    unspecified site D44.9
  nipple D24-
  papillary —*see also* Neoplasm, benign,
    by site
    eccrine —*see* Neoplasm, skin, benign,
      by site
  Pick's tubular
    specified site —*see* Neoplasm, benign,
      by site
    unspecified site
      female D27.9
      male D29.20
  pleomorphic
    carcinoma in —*see* Neoplasm,
      salivary gland, malignant
      specified site —*see* Neoplasm,
        malignant, by site
      unspecified site C08.9
  polypoid —*see also* Neoplasm,
    benign
    adenocarcinoma in —*see* Neoplasm,
      malignant, by site
    adenocarcinoma in situ —*see*
      Neoplasm, in situ, by site
  prostate —*see* Neoplasm, benign,
    prostate
  rete cell D29.20
  sebaceous —*see* Neoplasm, skin, benign
  Sertoli cell
    specified site —*see* Neoplasm, benign,
      by site
    unspecified site
      female D27.9
      male D29.20
  skin appendage —*see* Neoplasm, skin,
    benign
  sudoriferous gland —*see* Neoplasm,
    skin, benign
  sweat gland —*see* Neoplasm, skin,
    benign
  testicular
    unspecified site
      female D27.9
      male D29.20

Adenoma *(Continued)*
  tubular —*see also* Neoplasm, benign,
    by site
    adenocarcinoma in —*see* Neoplasm,
      malignant, by site
    adenocarcinoma in situ —*see*
      Neoplasm, in situ, by site
    Pick's
      specified site —*see* Neoplasm,
        benign
      unspecified site
        female D27.9
        male D29.20
  tubulovillous —*see also* Neoplasm,
    benign, by site
    adenocarcinoma in —*see* Neoplasm,
      malignant, by site
    adenocarcinoma in situ —*see*
      Neoplasm, in situ, by site
  villous —*see* Neoplasm, uncertain
    behavior, by site
    adenocarcinoma in —*see* Neoplasm,
      malignant, by site
    adenocarcinoma in situ —*see*
      Neoplasm, in situ, by site
  water-clear cell D35.1
Adenomatosis
  endocrine (multiple) E31.20
    single specified site —*see* Neoplasm,
      uncertain behavior, by site
  erosive of nipple D24-
  pluriendocrine —*see* Adenomatosis,
    endocrine
  pulmonary D38.1
    malignant —*see* Neoplasm, lung,
      malignant
    specified site —*see* Neoplasm, benign,
      by site
    unspecified site D12.6
Adenomatous
  goiter (nontoxic) E04.9
    with hyperthyroidism —*see* Hyper-
      thyroidism, with, goiter, nodular
    toxic —*see* Hyperthyroidism, with,
      goiter, nodular
Adenomyoma —*see also* Neoplasm,
  benign, by site
  prostate —*see* Enlarged, prostate
Adenomyometritis N80.0
Adenomyosis N80.0
Adenopathy (lymph gland) R59.9
  generalized R59.1
  inguinal R59.0
  localized R59.0
  mediastinal R59.0
  mesentery R59.0
  syphilitic (secondary) A51.49
  tracheobronchial R59.0
    tuberculous A15.4
      primary (progressive) A15.7
  tuberculous —*see also* Tuberculosis,
    lymph gland
    tracheobronchial A15.4
      primary (progressive) A15.7
Adenosalpingitis —*see* Salpingitis
Adenosarcoma —*see* Neoplasm,
  malignant, by site
Adenosclerosis I88.8
Adenosis (sclerosing) breast —*see*
  Fibroadenosis, breast
Adenovirus, as cause of disease
  classified elsewhere B97.0
Adentia (complete) (partial) —*see*
  Absence, teeth

Adherent —*see also* Adhesions
  labia (minora) N90.89
  pericardium (nonrheumatic) I31.0
    rheumatic I09.2
  placenta (with hemorrhage) O72.0
    without hemorrhage O73.0
  prepuce, newborn N47.0
  scar (skin) L90.5
  tendon in scar L90.5
Adhesions, adhesive (postinfective) K66.0
  with intestinal obstruction K56.5
  abdominal (wall) —*see* Adhesions,
    peritoneum
  appendix K38.8
  bile duct (common) (hepatic) K83.8
  bladder (sphincter) N32.89
  bowel —*see* Adhesions, peritoneum
  cardiac I31.0
    rheumatic I09.2
  cecum —*see* Adhesions, peritoneum
  cervicovaginal N88.1
    congenital Q52.8
    postpartal O90.89
      old N88.1
  cervix N88.1
  ciliary body NEC —*see* Adhesions, iris
  clitoris N90.89
  colon —*see* Adhesions, peritoneum
  common duct K83.8
  congenital —*see also* Anomaly, by site
    fingers —*see* Syndactylism, complex,
      fingers
    omental, anomalous Q43.3
    peritoneal Q43.3
    tongue (to gum or roof of mouth)
      Q38.3
  conjunctiva (acquired) H11.21-
    congenital Q15.8
  cystic duct K82.8
  diaphragm —*see* Adhesions,
    peritoneum
  due to foreign body —*see* Foreign body
  duodenum —*see* Adhesions,
    peritoneum
  ear
    middle H74.1-
  epididymis N50.8
  epidural —*see* Adhesions, meninges
  epiglottis J38.7
  eyelid H02.59
  female pelvis N73.6
  gallbladder K82.8
  globe H44.89
  heart I31.0
    rheumatic I09.2
  ileocecal (coil) —*see* Adhesions,
    peritoneum
  ileum —*see* Adhesions, peritoneum
  intestine —*see also* Adhesions,
    peritoneum
    with obstruction K56.5
  intra-abdominal —*see* Adhesions,
    peritoneum
  iris H21.50-
    anterior H21.51-
    goniosynechiae H21.52-
    posterior H21.54-
    to corneal graft T85.89
  joint —*see* Ankylosis
    knee M23.8X
    temporomandibular M26.61
  labium (majus) (minus), congenital Q52.5
  liver —*see* Adhesions, peritoneum
  lung J98.4

Adhesions, adhesive (Continued)
  mediastinum J98.5
  meninges (cerebral) (spinal) G96.12
    congenital Q07.8
    tuberculous (cerebral) (spinal) A17.0
  mesenteric —*see* Adhesions,
    peritoneum
  nasal (septum) (to turbinates) J34.89
  ocular muscle —*see* Strabismus,
    mechanical
  omentum —*see* Adhesions, peritoneum
  ovary N73.6
    congenital (to cecum, kidney or
      omentum) Q50.39
  paraovarian N73.6
  pelvic (peritoneal)
    female N73.6
      postprocedural N99.4
    male —*see* Adhesions, peritoneum
    postpartal (old) N73.6
    tuberculous A18.17
  penis to scrotum (congenital) Q55.8
  periappendiceal —*see also* Adhesions,
    peritoneum
  pericardium (nonrheumatic) I31.0
    focal I31.8
    rheumatic I09.2
    tuberculous A18.84
  pericholecystic K82.8
  perigastric —*see* Adhesions, peritoneum
  periovarian N73.6
  periprostatic N42.89
  perirectal —*see* Adhesions, peritoneum
  perirenal N28.89
  peritoneum, peritoneal (postinfective)
    (postprocedural) K66.0
    with obstruction (intestinal) K56.5
    congenital Q43.3
    pelvic, female N73.6
      postprocedural N99.4
    postpartal, pelvic N73.6
    to uterus N73.6
  peritubal N73.6
  periureteral N28.89
  periuterine N73.6
  perivesical N32.89
  perivesicular (seminal vesicle) N50.8
  pleura, pleuritic J94.8
    tuberculous NEC A15.6
  pleuropericardial J94.8
  postoperative (gastrointestinal tract)
    K66.0
    with obstruction K91.3
    due to foreign body accidentally
      left in wound —*see* Foreign
      body, accidentally left during a
      procedure
    pelvic peritoneal N99.4
    urethra —*see* Stricture, urethra,
      postprocedural
    vagina N99.2
  postpartal, old (vulva or perineum)
    N90.89
  preputial, prepuce N47.5
  pulmonary J98.4
  pylorus —*see* Adhesions, peritoneum
  sciatic nerve —*see* Lesion, nerve, sciatic
  seminal vesicle N50.8
  shoulder (joint) —*see* Capsulitis,
    adhesive
  sigmoid flexure —*see* Adhesions,
    peritoneum
  spermatic cord (acquired) N50.8
    congenital Q55.4

Adhesions, adhesive (Continued)
  spinal canal G96.12
  stomach —*see* Adhesions, peritoneum
  subscapular —*see* Capsulitis, adhesive
  temporomandibular M26.61
  tendinitis —*see also* Tenosynovitis,
    specified type NEC
    shoulder —*see* Capsulitis, adhesive
  testis N44.8
  tongue, congenital (to gum or roof of
    mouth) Q38.3
    acquired K14.8
  trachea J39.8
  tubo-ovarian N73.6
  tunica vaginalis N44.8
  uterus N73.6
    internal N85.6
    to abdominal wall N73.6
  vagina (chronic) N89.5
    postoperative N99.2
  vitreomacular H43.82-
  vitreous H43.89
  vulva N90.89
Adiaspiromycosis B48.8
Adie (-Holmes) pupil or syndrome —*see*
    Anomaly, pupil, function, tonic
    pupil
Adiponecrosis neonatorum P83.8
Adiposis —*see also* Obesity
  cerebralis E23.6
  dolorosa E88.2
Adiposity —*see also* Obesity
  heart —*see* Degeneration, myocardial
  localized E65
Adiposogenital dystrophy E23.6
Adjustment
  disorder —*see* Disorder, adjustment
  implanted device —*see* Encounter (for),
    adjustment (of)
  prosthesis, external —*see* Fitting
  reaction —*see* Disorder, adjustment
Administration of tPA (rtPA) in a
    different facility within the last
    24 hours prior to admission to
    current facility Z92.82
Admission (for) —*see also* Encounter
    (for)
  adjustment (of)
    artificial
      arm Z44.00-
        complete Z44.01-
        partial Z44.02-
      eye Z44.2
      leg Z44.10-
        complete Z44.11-
        partial Z44.12-
    brain neuropacemaker Z46.2
      implanted Z45.42
    breast
      implant Z45.81
      prosthesis (external) Z44.3
    colostomy belt Z46.89
    contact lenses Z46.0
    cystostomy device Z46.6
    dental prosthesis Z46.3
    device NEC
      abdominal Z46.89
      implanted Z45.89
        cardiac Z45.09
          defibrillator (with
            synchronous cardiace
            pacemaker) Z45.02
          pacemaker Z45.018
          pulse generator Z45.010

Admission (*Continued*)
adjustment (*Continued*)
device NEC (*Continued*)
implanted (*Continued*)
hearing device Z45.328
bone conduction Z45.320
cochlear Z45.321
infusion pump Z45.1
nervous system Z45.49
CSF drainage Z45.41
hearing device —*see*
Admission, adjustment,
device, implanted,
hearing device
neuropacemaker Z45.42
visual substitution Z45.31
specified NEC Z45.89
vascular access Z45.2
visual substitution Z45.31
nervous system Z46.2
implanted —*see* Admission,
adjustment, device,
implanted, nervous system
orthodontic Z46.4
prosthetic Z44.9
arm —*see* Admission,
adjustment, artificial, arm
breast Z44.3
dental Z46.3
eye Z44.2
leg —*see* Admission, adjustment,
artificial, leg
specified type NEC Z44.8
substitution
auditory Z46.2
implanted —*see* Admission,
adjustment, device,
implanted, hearing device
nervous system Z46.2
implanted —*see* Admission,
adjustment, device,
implanted, nervous
system
visual Z46.2
implanted Z45.31
urinary Z46.6
hearing aid Z46.1
implanted —*see* Admission,
adjustment, device,
implanted, hearing device
ileostomy device Z46.89
intestinal appliance or device NEC
Z46.89
neuropacemaker (brain) (peripheral
nerve) (spinal cord) Z46.2
implanted Z45.42
orthodontic device Z46.4
orthopedic (brace) (cast) (device)
(shoes) Z46.89
pacemaker
cardiac Z45.018
pulse generator Z45.010
nervous system Z46.2
implanted Z45.42
portacath (port-a-cath) Z45.2
prosthesis Z44.9
arm —*see* Admission, adjustment,
artificial, arm
breast Z44.3
dental Z46.3
eye Z44.2
leg —*see* Admission, adjustment,
artificial, leg
specified NEC Z44.8
spectacles Z46.0

Admission (*Continued*)
aftercare (*see also* Aftercare) Z51.89
postpartum
immediately after delivery Z39.0
routine follow-up Z39.2
radiation therapy (antineoplastic)
Z51.0
attention to artificial opening (of) Z43.9
artificial vagina Z43.7
colostomy Z43.3
cystostomy Z43.5
enterostomy Z43.4
gastrostomy Z43.1
ileostomy Z43.2
jejunostomy Z43.4
nephrostomy Z43.6
specified site NEC Z43.8
intestinal tract Z43.4
urinary tract Z43.6
tracheostomy Z43.0
ureterostomy Z43.6
urethrostomy Z43.6
breast augmentation or reduction
Z41.1
breast reconstruction following
mastectomy Z42.1
change of
dressing (nonsurgical) Z48.00
neuropacemaker device (brain)
(peripheral nerve) (spinal cord)
Z46.2
implanted Z45.42
surgical dressing Z48.01
circumcision, ritual or routine
(in absence of diagnosis) Z41.2
clinical research investigation (control)
(normal comparison) (participant)
Z00.6
contraceptive management Z30.9
cosmetic surgery NEC Z41.1
counseling (*see also* Counseling)
dietary Z71.3
HIV Z71.7
human immunodeficiency virus Z71.7
nonattending third party Z71.0
procreative management NEC Z31.69
delivery, full-term, uncomplicated O80
cesarean, without indication O82
dietary surveillance and counseling
Z71.3
ear piercing Z41.3
examination at health care facility (adult)
(*see also* Examination) Z00.00
with abnormal findings Z00.01
clinical research investigation
(control) (normal comparison)
(participant) Z00.6
dental Z01.20
with abnormal findings Z01.21
donor (potential) Z00.5
ear Z01.10
with abnormal findings NEC
Z01.118
eye Z01.00
with abnormal findings Z01.01
general, specified reason NEC Z00.8
hearing Z01.10
with abnormal findings NEC
Z01.118
postpartum checkup Z39.2
psychiatric (general) Z00.8
requested by authority Z04.6
vision Z01.00
with abnormal findings Z01.01

Admission (*Continued*)
fitting (of)
artificial
arm —*see* Admission, adjustment,
artificial, arm
eye Z44.2
leg —*see* Admission, adjustment,
artificial, leg
brain neuropacemaker Z46.2
implanted Z45.42
breast prosthesis (external) Z44.3
colostomy belt Z46.89
contact lenses Z46.0
cystostomy device Z46.6
dental prosthesis Z46.3
dentures Z46.3
device NEC
abdominal Z46.89
nervous system Z46.2
implanted —*see* Admission,
adjustment, device,
implanted, nervous system
orthodontic Z46.4
prosthetic Z44.9
breast Z44.3
dental Z46.3
eye Z44.2
substitution
auditory Z46.2
implanted —*see* Admission,
adjustment, device,
implanted, hearing
device
nervous system Z46.2
implanted —*see* Admission,
adjustment, device,
implanted, nervous
system
visual Z46.2
implanted Z45.31
hearing aid Z46.1
ileostomy device Z46.89
intestinal appliance or device NEC
Z46.89
neuropacemaker (brain) (peripheral
nerve) (spinal cord) Z46.2
implanted Z45.42
orthodontic device Z46.4
orthopedic device (brace) (cast)
(shoes) Z46.89
prosthesis Z44.9
arm —*see* Admission, adjustment,
artificial, arm
breast Z44.3
dental Z46.3
eye Z44.2
leg —*see* Admission, adjustment,
artificial, leg
specified type NEC Z44.8
spectacles Z46.0
follow-up examination Z09
intrauterine device management
Z30.431
initial prescription Z30.014
mental health evaluation Z00.8
requested by authority Z04.6
observation —*see* Observation
Papanicolaou smear, cervix Z12.4
for suspected malignant neoplasm
Z12.4
plastic and reconstructive surgery
following medical procedure or
healed injury NEC Z42.8
plastic surgery, cosmetic NEC Z41.1

Admission (Continued)
  postpartum observation
    immediately after delivery Z39.0
    routine follow-up Z39.2
  poststerilization (for restoration) Z31.0
    aftercare Z31.42
  procreative management Z31.9
  prophylactic (measure)
    organ removal Z40.00
      breast Z40.01
      ovary Z40.02
      specified organ NEC Z40.09
      testes Z40.09
    vaccination Z23
  psychiatric examination (general) Z00.8
    requested by authority Z04.6
  radiation therapy (antineoplastic) Z51.0
  reconstructive surgery following
    medical procedure or healed
    injury NEC Z42.8
  removal of
    cystostomy catheter Z43.5
    drains Z48.03
    dressing (nonsurgical) Z48.00
    intrauterine contraceptive device
      Z30.432
    neuropacemaker (brain) (peripheral
      nerve) (spinal cord) Z46.2
      implanted Z45.42
    staples Z48.02
    surgical dressing Z48.01
    sutures Z48.02
    ureteral stent Z46.6
  respirator [ventilator] use during power
    failure Z99.12
  restoration of organ continuity
    (poststerilization) Z31.0
    aftercare Z31.42
  sensitivity test —see also Test, skin
    allergy NEC Z01.82
    Mantoux Z11.1
  tuboplasty following previous
    sterilization Z31.0
    aftercare Z31.42
  vasoplasty following previous
    sterilization Z31.0
    aftercare Z31.42
  vision examination Z01.00
    with abnormal findings Z01.01
  waiting period for admission to other
    facility Z75.1
Adnexitis (suppurative) —see
  Salpingo-oophoritis
Adolescent X-linked adrenoleuko-
  dystrophy E71.521
Adrenal (gland) —see condition
Adrenalism, tuberculous A18.7
Adrenalitis, adrenitis E27.8
  autoimmune E27.1
  meningococcal, hemorrhagic A39.1
Adrenarche, premature E27.0
Adrenocortical syndrome —see
  Cushing's, syndrome
Adrenogenital syndrome E25.9
  acquired E25.8
  congenital E25.0
  salt loss E25.0
Adrenogenitalism, congenital E25.0
Adrenoleukodystrophy E71.529
  neonatal E71.511
  X-linked E71.529
    Addison only phenotype E71.528
    Addison-Schilder E71.528
    adolescent E71.521

Adrenoleukodystrophy (Continued)
  X-linked (Continued)
    adrenomyeloneuropathy E71.522
    childhood cerebral E71.520
    other specified E71.528
Adrenomyeloneuropathy E71.522
Adventitious bursa —see Bursopathy,
  specified type NEC
Adverse effect —see Table of drugs and
  chemicals, categories T36-T50, with
  6th character 5
Advice —see Counseling
Adynamia (episodica) (hereditary)
  (periodic) G72.3
Aeration lung imperfect, newborn —see
  Atelectasis
Aerobullosis T70.3
Aerocele —see Embolism, air
Aerodermectasia
  subcutaneous (traumatic) T79.7
Aerodontalgia T70.29
Aeroembolism T70.3
Aerogenes capsulatus infection
  A48.0
Aero-otitis media T70.0
Aerophagy, aerophagia (psychogenic)
  F45.8
Aerophobia F40.228
Aerosinusitis T70.1
Aerotitis T70.0
Affection —see Disease
Afibrinogenemia (see also Defect,
  coagulation) D68.8
  acquired D65
  congenital D68.2
  following ectopic or molar pregnancy
    O08.1
  in abortion —see Abortion, by
    type, complicated by,
    afibrinogenemia
  puerperal O72.3
African
  sleeping sickness B56.9
  tick fever A68.1
  trypanosomiasis B56.9
    gambian B56.0
    rhodesian B56.1
Aftercare (see also Care) Z51.89
  following surgery (for) (on)
    amputation Z47.81
    attention to
      drains Z48.03
      dressings (nonsurgical) Z48.00
        surgical Z48.01
      sutures Z48.02
    circulatory system Z48.812
    delayed (planned) wound closure Z48.1
    digestive system Z48.815
    explantation of joint prosthesis
      (staged procedure)
      hip Z47.32
      knee Z47.33
      shoulder Z47.31
    genitourinary system Z48.816
    joint replacement Z47.1
    neoplasm Z48.3
    nervous system Z48.811
    oral cavity Z48.814
    organ transplant
      bone marrow Z48.290
      heart Z48.21
      heart-lung Z48.280
      kidney Z48.22
      liver Z48.23

Aftercare (Continued)
  following surgery (Continued)
    organ transplant (Continued)
      lung Z48.24
      multiple organs NEC Z48.288
      specified NEC Z48.298
    orthopedic NEC Z47.89
    planned wound closure Z48.1
    removal of internal fixation device Z47.2
    respiratory system Z48.813
    scoliosis Z47.82
    sense organs Z48.810
    skin and subcutaneous tissue
      Z48.817
    specified body system
      circulatory Z48.812
      digestive Z48.815
      genitourinary Z48.816
      nervous Z48.811
      oral cavity Z48.814
      respiratory Z48.813
      sense organs Z48.810
      skin and subcutaneous tissue
        Z48.817
      teeth Z48.814
    specified NEC Z48.89
    spinal Z48.89
    teeth Z48.814
  fracture — code to fracture with
    seventh character D
  involving
    removal of
      drains Z48.03
      dressings (nonsurgical) Z48.00
      staples Z48.02
      surgical dressings Z48.01
      sutures Z48.02
    neuropacemaker (brain) (peripheral
      nerve) (spinal cord) Z46.2
      implanted Z45.42
    orthopedic NEC Z47.89
  postprocedural —see Aftercare,
    following surgery
After-cataract —see Cataract, secondary
Agalactia (primary) O92.3
  elective, secondary or therapeutic
    O92.5
Agammaglobulinemia (acquired
  (secondary)) (nonfamilial) D80.1
  with
    immunoglobulin-bearing
      B-lymphocytes D80.1
    lymphopenia D81.9
  autosomal recessive (Swiss type) D80.0
  Bruton's X-linked D80.0
  common variable (CVAgamma) D80.1
  congenital sex-linked D80.0
  hereditary D80.0
  lymphopenic D81.9
  Swiss type (autosomal recessive)
    D80.0
  X-linked (with growth hormone
    deficiency)(Bruton) D80.0
Aganglionosis (bowel) (colon) Q43.1
Age (old) —see Senility
Agenesis
  adrenal (gland) Q89.1
  alimentary tract (complete) (partial)
    NEC Q45.8
    upper Q40.8
  anus, anal (canal) Q42.3
    with fistula Q42.2
  aorta Q25.4
  appendix Q42.8

Agenesis *(Continued)*
  arm (complete) Q71.0-
    with hand present Q71.1-
  artery (peripheral) Q27.9
    brain Q28.3
    coronary Q24.5
    pulmonary Q25.79
    specified NEC Q27.8
    umbilical Q27.0
  auditory (canal) (external) Q16.1
  auricle (ear) Q16.0
  bile duct or passage Q44.5
  bladder Q64.5
  bone Q79.9
  brain Q00.0
    part of Q04.3
  breast (with nipple present) Q83.8
    with absent nipple Q83.0
  bronchus Q32.4
  canaliculus lacrimalis Q10.4
  carpus —*see* Agenesis, hand
  cartilage Q79.9
  cecum Q42.8
  cerebellum Q04.3
  cervix Q51.5
  chin Q18.8
  cilia Q10.3
  circulatory system, part NOS Q28.9
  clavicle Q74.0
  clitoris Q52.6
  coccyx Q76.49
  colon Q42.9
    specified NEC Q42.8
  corpus callosum Q04.0
  cricoid cartilage Q31.8
  diaphragm (with hernia) Q79.1
  digestive organ (s) or tract (complete)
    (partial) NEC Q45.8
    upper Q40.8
  ductus arteriosus Q28.8
  duodenum Q41.0
  ear Q16.9
    auricle Q16.0
    lobe Q17.8
  ejaculatory duct Q55.4
  endocrine (gland) NEC Q89.2
  epiglottis Q31.8
  esophagus Q39.8
  eustachian tube Q16.2
  eye Q11.1
    adnexa Q15.8
  eyelid (fold) Q10.3
  face
    bones NEC Q75.8
    specified part NEC Q18.8
  fallopian tube Q50.6
  femur —*see* Defect, reduction, lower
    limb, longitudinal, femur
  fibula —*see* Defect, reduction, lower
    limb, longitudinal, fibula
  finger (complete) (partial) —*see*
    Agenesis, hand
  foot (and toes) (complete) (partial)
    Q72.3-
  forearm (with hand present) —*see*
    Agenesis, arm, with hand present
    and hand Q71.2-
  gallbladder Q44.0
  gastric Q40.2
  genitalia, genital (organ (s))
    female Q52.8
      external Q52.71
      internal NEC Q52.8
    male Q55.8

Agenesis *(Continued)*
  glottis Q31.8
  hair Q84.0
  hand (and fingers) (complete) (partial)
    Q71.3-
  heart Q24.8
    valve NEC Q24.8
      pulmonary Q22.0
  hepatic Q44.7
  humerus —*see* Defect, reduction, upper
    limb
  hymen Q52.4
  ileum Q41.2
  incus Q16.3
  intestine (small) Q41.9
    large Q42.9
      specified NEC Q42.8
  iris (dilator fibers) Q13.1
  jaw M26.09
  jejunum Q41.1
  kidney (s) (partial) Q60.2
    bilateral Q60.1
    unilateral Q60.0
  labium (majus) (minus) Q52.71
  labyrinth, membranous Q16.5
  lacrimal apparatus Q10.4
  larynx Q31.8
  leg (complete) Q72.0-
    with foot present Q72.1-
    lower leg (with foot present) —*see*
      Agenesis, leg, with foot present
      and foot Q72.2-
  lens Q12.3
  limb (complete) Q73.0
    lower —*see* Agenesis, leg
    upper —*see* Agenesis, arm
  lip Q38.0
  liver Q44.7
  lung (fissure) (lobe) (bilateral)
    (unilateral) Q33.3
  mandible, maxilla M26.09
  metacarpus —*see* Agenesis, hand
  metatarsus —*see* Agenesis, foot
  muscle Q79.8
    eyelid Q10.3
    ocular Q15.8
  musculoskeletal system NEC Q79.8
  nail (s) Q84.3
  neck, part Q18.8
  nerve Q07.8
  nervous system, part NEC Q07.8
  nipple Q83.2
  nose Q30.1
  nuclear Q07.8
  oesophagus Q39.8
  organ
    of Corti Q16.5
    or site not listed —*see* Anomaly,
      by site
  osseous meatus (ear) Q16.1
  ovary
    bilateral Q50.02
    unilateral Q50.01
  oviduct Q50.6
  pancreas Q45.0
  parathyroid (gland) Q89.2
  parotid gland (s) Q38.4
  patella Q74.1
  pelvic girdle (complete) (partial) Q74.2
  penis Q55.5
  pericardium Q24.8
  pituitary (gland) Q89.2
  prostate Q55.4
  punctum lacrimale Q10.4

Agenesis *(Continued)*
  radioulnar —*see* Defect, reduction,
    upper limb
  radius —*see* Defect, reduction, upper
    limb, longitudinal, radius
  rectum Q42.1
    with fistula Q42.0
  renal Q60.2
    bilateral Q60.1
    unilateral Q60.0
  respiratory organ NEC Q34.8
  rib Q76.6
  roof of orbit Q75.8
  round ligament Q52.8
  sacrum Q76.49
  salivary gland Q38.4
  scapula Q74.0
  scrotum Q55.29
  seminal vesicles Q55.4
  septum
    atrial Q21.1
    between aorta and pulmonary artery
      Q21.4
    ventricular Q20.4
  shoulder girdle (complete) (partial) Q74.0
  skull (bone) Q75.8
    with
      anencephaly Q00.0
      encephalocele —*see* Encephalocele
      hydrocephalus Q03.9
        with spina bifida —*see* Spina
          bifida, by site, with
          hydrocephalus
      microcephaly Q02
  spermatic cord Q55.4
  spinal cord Q06.0
  spine Q76.49
  spleen Q89.01
  sternum Q76.7
  stomach Q40.2
  submaxillary gland (s) (congenital)
    Q38.4
  tarsus —*see* Agenesis, foot
  tendon Q79.8
  testicle Q55.0
  thymus (gland) Q89.2
  thyroid (gland) E03.1
    cartilage Q31.8
  tibia —*see* Defect, reduction, lower
    limb, longitudinal, tibia
  tibiofibular —*see* Defect, reduction,
    lower limb, specified type NEC
  toe (and foot) (complete) (partial) —*see*
    Agenesis, foot
  tongue Q38.3
  trachea (cartilage) Q32.1
  ulna —*see* Defect, reduction, upper
    limb, longitudinal, ulna
  upper limb —*see* Agenesis, arm
  ureter Q62.4
  urethra Q64.5
  urinary tract NEC Q64.8
  uterus Q51.0
  uvula Q38.5
  vagina Q52.0
  vas deferens Q55.4
  vein (s) (peripheral) Q27.9
    brain Q28.3
    great NEC Q26.8
    portal Q26.5
  vena cava (inferior) (superior) Q26.8
  vermis of cerebellum Q04.3
  vertebra Q76.49
  vulva Q52.71

Algoneurodystrophy M89.00
  ankle M89.07-
  foot M89.07-
  forearm M89.03-
  hand M89.04-
  lower leg M89.06-
  multiple sites M89.0-
  shoulder M89.01-
  specified site NEC M89.08
  thigh M89.05-
  upper arm M89.02-
Algophobia F40.298
Alienation, mental —*see* Psychosis
Alkalemia E87.3
Alkalosis E87.3
  metabolic E87.3
    with respiratory acidosis E87.4
  respiratory E87.3
Alkaptonuria E70.29
Allen-Masters syndrome N83.8
Allergy, allergic (reaction) (to) T78.40
  air-borne substance NEC (rhinitis)
      J30.89
  alveolitis (extrinsic) J67.9
    due to
      Aspergillus clavatus J67.4
      Cryptostroma corticale J67.5
      organisms (fungal, thermophilic
          actinomycete) growing in
          ventilation (air conditioning)
          systems J67.7
    specified type NEC J67.8
  anaphylactic reaction or shock T78.2
  angioneurotic edema T78.3
  animal (dander) (epidermal) (hair)
      (rhinitis) J30.81
  bee sting (anaphylactic shock) —*see*
      Toxicity, venom, arthropod, bee
  biological —*see* Allergy, drug
  colitis K52.2
  dander (animal) (rhinitis) J30.81
  dandruff (rhinitis) J30.81
  dental restorative material (existing)
      K08.55
  dermatitis —*see* Dermatitis, contact,
      allergic
  diathesis —*see* History, allergy
  drug, medicament & biological (any)
      (external) (internal) T78.40
    correct substance properly
        administered —*see* Table of
        drugs and chemicals, by drug,
        adverse effect
    wrong substance given or taken NEC
        (by accident) —*see* Table of
        drugs and chemicals, by drug,
        poisoning
  due to pollen J30.1
  dust (house) (stock) (rhinitis) J30.89
    with asthma —*see* Asthma, allergic
        extrinsic
  eczema —*see* Dermatitis, contact,
      allergic
  epidermal (animal) (rhinitis) J30.81
  feathers (rhinitis) J30.89
  food (any) (ingested) NEC T78.1
    anaphylactic shock —*see* Shock,
        anaphylactic, due to food
    dermatitis —*see* Dermatitis, due to,
        food
    dietary counseling and surveillance
        Z71.3
    in contact with skin L23.6
    rhinitis J30.5

Allergy, allergic (*Continued*)
  food NEC (*Continued*)
    status (without reaction) Z91.018
      eggs Z91.012
      milk products Z91.011
      peanuts Z91.010
      seafood Z91.013
      specified NEC Z91.018
  gastrointestinal K52.2
  grain J30.1
  grass (hay fever) (pollen) J30.1
    asthma —*see* Asthma, allergic
        extrinsic
  hair (animal) (rhinitis) J30.81
  history (of) —*see* History, allergy
  horse serum —*see* Allergy, serum
  inhalant (rhinitis) J30.89
    pollen J30.1
  kapok (rhinitis) J30.89
  medicine —*see* Allergy, drug
  milk protein K52.2
  nasal, seasonal due to pollen J30.1
  pneumonia J82
  pollen (any) (hay fever) J30.1
    asthma —*see* Asthma, allergic
        extrinsic
  primrose J30.1
  primula J30.1
  purpura D69.0
  ragweed (hay fever) (pollen) J30.1
    asthma —*see* Asthma, allergic
        extrinsic
  rose (pollen) J30.1
  seasonal NEC J30.2
  Senecio jacobae (pollen) J30.1
  serum (*see also* Reaction, serum) T80.69
    anaphylactic shock T80.59
  shock (anaphylactic) T78.2
    due to
      adverse effect of correct medicinal
          substance properly
          administered T88.6
      administration of blood and blood
          products T80.51
      immunization T80.52
      serum NEC T80.59
      vaccination T80.52
    specific NEC T78.49
  tree (any) (hay fever) (pollen) J30.1
    asthma —*see* Asthma, allergic
        extrinsic
  upper respiratory J30.9
  urticaria L50.0
  vaccine —*see* Allergy, serum
Allescheriasis B48.2
Alligator skin disease Q80.9
Allocheiria, allochiria R20.8
Almeida's disease —*see*
      Paracoccidioidomycosis
Alopecia (hereditaria) (seborrheica) L65.9
  androgenic L64.9
    drug-induced L64.0
    specified NEC L64.8
  areata L63.9
    ophiasis L63.2
    specified NEC L63.8
    totalis L63.0
    universalis L63.1
  cicatricial L66.9
    specified NEC L66.8
  circumscripta L63.9
  congenital, congenitalis Q84.0
  due to cytotoxic drugs NEC L65.8
  mucinosa L65.2

Alopecia (*Continued*)
  postinfective NEC L65.8
  postpartum L65.0
  premature L64.8
  specific (syphilitic) A51.32
  specified NEC L65.8
  syphilitic (secondary) A51.32
  totalis (capitis) L63.0
  universalis (entire body) L63.1
  X-ray L58.1
Alpers' disease G31.81
Alpine sickness T70.29
Alport syndrome Q87.81
ALTE (apparent life threatening event) in
      newborn and infant R68.13
Alteration (of), **Altered**
  awareness, transient R40.4
  mental status R41.82
  pattern of family relationships affecting
      child Z62.898
  sensation
    following
      cerebrovascular disease I69.998
        cerebral infarction I69.398
        intracerebral hemorrhage I69.198
        nontraumatic intracranial
            hemorrhage NEC I69.298
        specified disease NEC I69.898
        subarachnoid hemorrhage
            I69.098
Alternating —*see* condition
Altitude, high (effects) —*see* Effect,
      adverse, high altitude
Aluminosis (of lung) J63.0
Alveolitis
  allergic (extrinsic) —*see* Pneumonitis,
      hypersensitivity
  due to
    Aspergillus clavatus J67.4
    Cryptostroma corticale J67.6
  fibrosing (cryptogenic) (idiopathic)
      J84.112
  jaw M27.3
  sicca dolorosa M27.3
Alveolus, alveolar —*see* condition
Alymphocytosis D72.820
  thymic (with immunodeficiency) D82.1
Alymphoplasia, thymic D82.1
Alzheimer's disease or sclerosis —*see*
      Disease, Alzheimer's
Amastia (with nipple present) Q83.8
  with absent nipple Q83.0
Amathophobia F40.228
Amaurosis (acquired) (congenital) —*see*
      also Blindness
  fugax G45.3
  hysterical F44.6
  Leber's congenital H35.50
  uremic —*see* Uremia
Amaurotic idiocy (infantile) (juvenile)
      (late) E75.4
Amaxophobia F40.248
Ambiguous genitalia Q56.4
Amblyopia (congenital) (ex anopsia)
      (partial) (suppression) H53.00-
  anisometropic —*see* Amblyopia,
      refractive
  deprivation H53.01-
  hysterical F44.6
  nocturnal —*see also* Blindness, night
    vitamin A deficiency E50.5
  refractive H53.02-
  strabismic H53.03-
  tobacco H53.8

Amblyopia (Continued)
  toxic NEC H53.8
  uremic —see Uremia
Ameba, amebic (histolytica) —see also
      Amebiasis
  abscess (liver) A06.4
Amebiasis A06.9
  with abscess —see Abscess, amebic
  acute A06.0
  chronic (intestine) A06.1
    with abscess —see Abscess, amebic
  cutaneous A06.7
  cutis A06.7
  cystitis A06.81
  genitourinary tract NEC A06.82
  hepatic —see Abscess, liver, amebic
  intestine A06.0
  nondysenteric colitis A06.2
  skin A06.7
  specified site NEC A06.89
Ameboma (of intestine) A06.3
Amelia Q73.0
  lower limb —see Agenesis, leg
  upper limb —see Agenesis, arm
Ameloblastoma —see also Cyst, calcifying
      odontogenic
  long bones C40.9-
    lower limb C40.2-
    upper limb C40.0-
  malignant C41.1
    jaw (bone) (lower) C41.1
      upper C41.0
  tibial C40.2-
Amelogenesis imperfecta K00.5
  nonhereditaria (segmentalis) K00.4
Amenorrhea N91.2
  hyperhormonal E28.8
  primary N91.0
  secondary N91.1
Amentia —see Disability, intellectual
  Meynert's (nonalcoholic) F04
American
  leishmaniasis B55.2
  mountain tick fever A93.2
Ametropia —see Disorder, refraction
Amianthosis J61
Amimia R48.8
Amino-acid disorder E72.9
  anemia D53.0
Aminoacidopathy E72.9
Aminoaciduria E72.9
Amnes (t)ic syndrome (post-traumatic)
      F04
  induced by
    alcohol F10.96
      with dependence F10.26
    psychoactive NEC F19.96
      with
        abuse F19.16
        dependence F19.26
    sedative F13.96
      with dependence F13.26
Amnesia R41.3
  anterograde R41.1
  auditory R48.8
  dissociative F44.0
  hysterical F44.0
  postictal in epilepsy —see Epilepsy
  psychogenic F44.0
  retrograde R41.2
  transient global G45.4
Amnion, amniotic —see condition
Amnionitis —see Pregnancy, complicated
      by

Amok F68.8
Amoral traits F60.89
Ampulla
  lower esophagus K22.8
  phrenic K22.8
Amputation —see also Absence, by site,
      acquired
  neuroma (postoperative) (traumatic) —
      see Complications, amputation
      stump, neuroma
  stump (surgical)
    abnormal, painful, or with
        complication (late) —see
        Complications, amputation
        stump
    healed or old NOS Z89.9
  traumatic (complete) (partial)
    arm (upper) (complete) S48.91-
      at
        elbow S58.01-
          partial S58.02-
        shoulder joint (complete) S48.01-
          partial S48.02-
      between
        elbow and wrist (complete)
            S58.11-
          partial S58.12-
        shoulder and elbow (complete)
            S48.11-
          partial S48.12-
      partial S48.92-
    breast (complete) S28.21-
      partial S28.22-
    clitoris (complete) S38.211
      partial S38.212
    ear (complete) S08.11-
      partial S08.12-
    finger (complete)
        (metacarpophalangeal) S68.11-
      index S68.11-
      little S68.11-
      middle S68.11-
      partial S68.12-
        index S68.12-
        little S68.12-
        middle S68.12-
        ring S68.12-
      ring S68.11-
    thumb —see Amputation,
        traumatic, thumb
    transphalangeal (complete)
        S68.61-
      index S68.61-
      little S68.61-
      middle S68.61-
      partial S68.62-
        index S68.62-
        little S68.62-
        middle S68.62-
        ring S68.62-
      ring S68.61-
    foot (complete) S98.91-
      at ankle level S98.01-
        partial S98.02-
      midfoot S98.31-
        partial S98.32-
      partial S98.92-
    forearm (complete) S58.91-
      at elbow level (complete) S58.01-
        partial S58.02-
      between elbow and wrist
          (complete) S58.11-
        partial S58.12-
      partial S58.92-

Amputation (Continued)
  traumatic (Continued)
    genital organ (s) (external)
      female (complete) S38.211
        partial S38.212
      male
        penis (complete) S38.221
          partial S38.222
        scrotum (complete) S38.231
          partial S38.232
        testes (complete) S38.231
          partial S38.232
    hand (complete) (wrist level) S68.41-
      finger (s) alone —see Amputation,
          traumatic, finger
      partial S68.42-
      thumb alone —see Amputation,
          traumatic, thumb
      transmetacarpal (complete) S68.71-
        partial S68.72-
    head
      ear —see Amputation, traumatic,
          ear
      nose (partial) S08.812
        complete S08.811
        part S08.89
        scalp S08.0
    hip (and thigh) (complete) S78.91-
      at hip joint (complete) S78.01-
        partial S78.02-
      between hip and knee (complete)
          S78.11-
        partial S78.12-
      partial S78.92-
    labium (majus) (minus) (complete)
        S38.21-
      partial S38.21-
    leg (lower) S88.91-
      at knee level S88.01-
        partial S88.02-
      between knee and ankle S88.11-
        partial S88.12-
      partial S88.92-
    nose (partial) S08.812
      complete S08.811
    penis (complete) S38.221
      partial S38.222
    scrotum (complete) S38.231
      partial S38.232
    shoulder —see Amputation,
        traumatic, arm
      at shoulder joint —see Amputation,
          traumatic, arm, at shoulder
          joint
    testes (complete) S38.231
      partial S38.232
    thigh —see Amputation, traumatic,
        hip
    thorax, part of S28.1
      breast —see Amputation, traumatic,
          breast
    thumb (complete)
        (metacarpophalangeal) S68.01-
      partial S68.02-
      transphalangeal (complete) S68.51-
        partial S68.52-
    toe (lesser) S98.13-
      great S98.11-
        partial S98.12-
      more than one S98.21-
        partial S98.22-
      partial S98.14-
    vulva (complete) S38.211
      partial S38.212

Amputee (bilateral) (old) Z89.9
Amsterdam dwarfism Q87.1
Amusia R48.8
  developmental F80.89
Amyelencephalus, amyelencephaly
  Q00.0
Amyelia Q06.0
Amygdalitis —see Tonsillitis
Amygdalolith J35.8
Amyloid heart (disease) E85.4 [I43]
Amyloidosis (generalized) (primary) E85.9
  with lung involvement E85.4 [J99]
  familial E85.2
  genetic E85.2
  heart E85.4 [I43]
  hemodialysis-associated E85.3
  liver E85.4 [K77]
  localized E85.4
  neuropathic heredofamilial E85.1
  non-neuropathic heredofamilial E85.0
  organ limited E85.4
  Portuguese E85.1
  pulmonary E85.4 [J99]
  secondary systemic E85.3
  skin (lichen) (macular) E85.4 [L99]
  specified NEC E85.8
  subglottic E85.4 [J99]
Amylopectinosis (brancher enzyme
  deficiency) E74.03
Amylophagia —see Pica
Amyoplasia congenita Q79.8
Amyotonia M62.89
  congenita G70.2
Amyotrophia, amyotrophy, amyotrophic
  G71.8
  congenita Q79.8
  diabetic —see Diabetes, amyotrophy
  lateral sclerosis G12.21
  neuralgic G54.5
  spinal progressive G12.21
Anacidity, gastric K31.83
  psychogenic F45.8
Anaerosis of newborn P28.89
Analbuminemia E88.09
Analgesia —see Anesthesia
Analphalipoproteinemia E78.6
Anaphylactic
  purpura D69.0
  shock or reaction —see Shock,
    anaphylactic
Anaphylactoid shock or reaction —see
  Shock, anaphylactic
Anaphylactoid syndrome of pregnancy
  O88.01-
Anaphylaxis —see Shock, anaphylactic
Anaplasia cervix (see also Dysplasia,
  cervix) N87.9
Anaplasmosis, human A77.49
Anarthria R47.1
Anasarca R60.1
  cardiac —see Failure, heart, congestive
  lung J18.2
  newborn P83.2
  nutritional E43
  pulmonary J18.2
  renal N04.9
Anastomosis
  aneurysmal —see Aneurysm
  arteriovenous ruptured brain I60.8
  intestinal K63.89
    complicated NEC K91.89
      involving urinary tract N99.89
  retinal and choroidal vessels
    (congenital) Q14.8

Anatomical narrow angle H40.03-
Ancylostoma, ancylostomiasis
    (braziliense) (caninum) (ceylanicum)
    (duodenale) B76.0
  Necator americanus B76.1
Andersen's disease (glycogen storage)
  E74.09
Anderson-Fabry disease E75.21
Andes disease T70.29
Andrews' disease (bacterid) L08.89
Androblastoma
  benign
    specified site —see Neoplasm, benign,
      by site
    unspecified site
      female D27.9
      male D29.20
  malignant
    specified site —see Neoplasm,
      malignant, by site
    unspecified site
      female C56.9
      male C62.90
  specified site —see Neoplasm, uncertain
    behavior, by site
  tubular
    with lipid storage
      specified site —see Neoplasm,
        benign, by site
      unspecified site
        female D27.9
        male D29.20
    specified site —see Neoplasm, benign,
      by site
    unspecified site
      female D27.9
      male D29.20
  unspecified site
    female D39.10
    male D40.10
Androgen insensitivity syndrome
    (see also Syndrome, androgen
    insensitivity) E34.50
Androgen resistance syndrome (see also
    Syndrome, androgen insensitivity)
    E34.50
Android pelvis Q74.2
  with disproportion (fetopelvic) O33.3
    causing obstructed labor O65.3
Androphobia F40.290
Anectasis, pulmonary (newborn) —see
  Atelectasis
Anemia (essential) (general) (hemoglobin
    deficiency) (infantile) (primary)
    (profound) D64.9
  with (due to) (in)
    disorder of
      anaerobic glycolysis D55.2
      pentose phosphate pathway D55.1
    koilonychia D50.9
  achlorhydric D50.8
  achrestic D53.1
  Addison (-Biermer) (pernicious) D51.0
  agranulocytic —see Agranulocytosis
  amino-acid-deficiency D53.0
  aplastic D61.9
    congenital D61.09
    drug-induced D61.1
    due to
      drugs D61.1
      external agents NEC D61.2
      infection D61.2
      radiation D61.2
    idiopathic D61.3

Anemia (Continued)
  aplastic (Continued)
    red cell (pure) D60.9
      chronic D60.0
      congenital D61.01
      specified type NEC D60.8
      transient D60.1
    specified type NEC D61.89
    toxic D61.2
  aregenerative
    congenital D61.09
  asiderotic D50.9
  atypical (primary) D64.9
  Baghdad spring D55.0
  Balantidium coli A07.0
  Biermer's (pernicious) D51.0
  blood loss (chronic) D50.0
    acute D62
  bothriocephalus B70.0 [D63.8]
  brickmaker's B76.9 [D63.8]
  cerebral I67.89
  childhood D58.9
  chlorotic D50.8
  chronic
    blood loss D50.0
    hemolytic D58.9
      idiopathic D59.9
    simple D53.9
  chronica congenita aregenerativa
    D61.09
  combined system disease NEC D51.0
    [G32.0]
    due to dietary vitamin B12 deficiency
      D51.3 [G32.0]
  complicating pregnancy, childbirth
    or puerperium —see Pregnancy,
    complicated by (management
    affected by), anemia
  congenital P61.4
    aplastic D61.09
    due to isoimmunization NOS
      P55.9
    dyserythropoietic, dyshematopoietic
      D64.4
    following fetal blood loss P61.3
    Heinz body D58.2
    hereditary hemolytic NOS D58.9
    pernicious D51.0
    spherocytic D58.0
  Cooley's (erythroblastic) D56.1
  cytogenic D51.0
  deficiency D53.9
    2, 3 diphosphoglycurate mutase
      D55.2
    2, 3 PG D55.2
    6 phosphogluconate dehydrogenase
      D55.1
    6-PGD D55.1
    amino-acid D53.0
    combined B12 and folate D53.1
    enzyme D55.9
      drug-induced (hemolytic) D59.2
      glucose-6-phosphate
        dehydrogenase (G6PD) D55.0
      glycolytic D55.2
      nucleotide metabolism D55.3
      related to hexose monophosphate
        (HMP) shunt pathway NEC
        D55.1
    specified type NEC D55.8
    erythrocytic glutathione D55.1
    folate D52.9
      dietary D52.0
      drug-induced D52.1

Anemia *(Continued)*
  deficiency *(Continued)*
    folic acid D52.9
      dietary D52.0
      drug-induced D52.1
    G SH D55.1
    G6PD D55.0
    GGS-R D55.1
    glucose-6-phosphate dehydrogenase
        D55.0
    glutathione reductase D55.1
    glyceraldehyde phosphate
        dehydrogenase D55.2
    hexokinase D55.2
    iron D50.9
      secondary to blood loss (chronic)
          D50.0
    nutritional D53.9
      with
        poor iron absorption D50.8
        specified deficiency NEC
            D53.8
    phosphofructo-aldolase D55.2
    phosphoglycerate kinase D55.2
    PK D55.2
    protein D53.0
    pyruvate kinase D55.2
    transcobalamin II D51.2
    triose-phosphate isomerase D55.2
    vitamin B12 NOS D51.9
      dietary D51.3
      due to
        intrinsic factor deficiency D51.0
        selective vitamin B12
            malabsorption with
            proteinuria D51.1
      pernicious D51.0
      specified type NEC D51.8
  Diamond-Blackfan (congenital
      hypoplastic) D61.01
  dibothriocephalus B70.0 *[D63.8]*
  dimorphic D53.1
  diphasic D53.1
  Diphyllobothrium (Dibothriocephalus)
      B70.0 *[D63.8]*
  due to (in) (with)
    antineoplastic chemotherapy D64.81
    blood loss (chronic) D50.0
      acute D62
    chemotherapy, antineoplastic
        D64.81
    chronic disease classified elsewhere
        NEC D63.8
    chronic kidney disease D63.1
    deficiency
      amino-acid D53.0
      copper D53.8
      folate (folic acid) D52.9
        dietary D52.0
        drug-induced D52.1
      molybdenum D53.8
      protein D53.0
      zinc D53.8
    dietary vitamin B12 deficiency D51.3
    disorder of
      glutathione metabolism D55.1
      nucleotide metabolism D55.3
    drug —*see* Anemia, by type —*see also*
        Table of Drugs and Chemicals
    end stage renal disease D63.1
    enzyme disorder D55.9
    fetal blood loss P61.3
    fish tapeworm (D latum) infestation
        B70.0 *[D63.8]*

Anemia *(Continued)*
  due to *(Continued)*
    hemorrhage (chronic) D50.0
      acute D62
    impaired absorption D50.9
    loss of blood (chronic) D50.0
      acute D62
    myxedema E03.9 *[D63.8]*
    Necator americanus B76.1 *[D63.8]*
    prematurity P61.2
    selective vitamin B12 malabsorption
        with proteinuria D51.1
    transcobalamin II deficiency D51.2
  Dyke-Young type (secondary)
      (symptomatic) D59.1
  dyserythropoietic (congenital)
      D64.4
  dyshematopoietic (congenital)
      D64.4
  Egyptian B76.9 *[D63.8]*
  elliptocytosis —*see* Elliptocytosis
  enzyme-deficiency, drug-induced
      D59.2
  epidemic (*see also* Ancylostomiasis)
      B76.9 *[D63.8]*
  erythroblastic
    familial D56.1
    newborn (*see also* Disease, hemolytic)
        P55.9
    of childhood D56.1
  erythrocytic glutathione deficiency
      D55.1
  erythropoietin-resistant anemia (EPO
      resistant anemia) D63.1
  Faber's (achlorhydric anemia) D50.9
  factitious (self-induced blood letting)
      D50.0
  familial erythroblastic D56.1
  Fanconi's (congenital pancytopenia)
      D61.09
  favism D55.0
  fish tapeworm (D. latum) infestation
      B70.0 *[D63.8]*
  folate (folic acid) deficiency D52.9
  glucose-6-phosphate dehydrogenase
      (G6PD) deficiency D55.0
  glutathione-reductase deficiency D55.1
  goat's milk D52.0
  granulocytic —*see* Agranulocytosis
  Heinz body, congenital D58.2
  hemolytic D58.9
    acquired D59.9
      with hemoglobinuria NEC
          D59.6
      autoimmune NEC D59.1
      infectious D59.4
      specified type NEC D59.8
      toxic D59.4
    acute D59.9
      due to enzyme deficiency specified
          type NEC D55.8
      Lederer's D59.1
    autoimmune D59.1
      drug-induced D59.0
    chronic D58.9
      idiopathic D59.9
    cold type (secondary) (symptomatic)
        D59.1
    congenital (spherocytic) —*see*
        Spherocytosis
    due to
      cardiac conditions D59.4
      drugs (nonautoimmune) D59.2
        autoimmune D59.0

Anemia *(Continued)*
  hemolytic *(Continued)*
    due to *(Continued)*
      enzyme disorder D55.9
        drug-induced D59.2
      presence of shunt or other
          internal prosthetic device
          D59.4
    familial D58.9
    hereditary D58.9
      due to enzyme disorder
          D55.9
        specified type NEC D55.8
      specified type NEC D58.8
    idiopathic (chronic) D59.9
    mechanical D59.4
    microangiopathic D59.4
    nonautoimmune D59.4
      drug-induced D59.2
    nonspherocytic
      congenital or hereditary NEC
          D55.8
        glucose-6-phosphate
            dehydrogenase deficiency
            D55.0
        pyruvate kinase deficiency
            D55.2
        type
          I D55.1
          II D55.2
      type
        I D55.1
        II D55.2
    secondary D59.4
      autoimmune D59.1
    specified (hereditary) type NEC
        D58.8
    Stransky-Regala type (*see also*
        Hemoglobinopathy)
        D58.8
    symptomatic D59.4
      autoimmune D59.1
    toxic D59.4
    warm type (secondary)
        (symptomatic) D59.1
  hemorrhagic (chronic) D50.0
    acute D62
  Herrick's D57.1
  hexokinase deficiency D55.2
  hookworm B76.9 *[D63.8]*
  hypochromic (idiopathic) (microcytic)
      (normoblastic) D50.9
    due to blood loss (chronic) D50.0
      acute D62
    familial sex-linked D64.0
    pyridoxine-responsive D64.3
    sideroblastic, sex-linked D64.0
  hypoplasia, red blood cells D61.9
    congenital or familial D61.01
  hypoplastic (idiopathic) D61.9
    congenital or familial (of childhood)
        D61.01
  hypoproliferative (refractive) D61.9
  idiopathic D64.9
    aplastic D61.3
    hemolytic, chronic D59.9
  in (due to) (with)
    chronic kidney disease D63.1
    end stage renal disease D63.1
    failure, kidney (renal) D63.1
    neoplastic disease (*see also* Neoplasm)
        D63.0
  intertropical (*see also* Ancylostomiasis)
      D63.8

Anemia *(Continued)*
  iron deficiency D50.9
    secondary to blood loss (chronic)
      D50.0
      acute D62
    specified type NEC D50.8
  Joseph-Diamond-Blackfan (congenital
    hypoplastic) D61.01
  Lederer's (hemolytic) D59.1
  leukoerythroblastic D61.82
  macrocytic D53.9
    nutritional D52.0
    tropical D52.8
  malarial *(see also* Malaria) B54 *[D63.8]*
  malignant (progressive) D51.0
  malnutrition D53.9
  marsh *(see also* Malaria) B54 *[D63.8]*
  Mediterranean (with other
    hemoglobinopathy) D56.9
  megaloblastic D53.1
    combined B12 and folate deficiency
      D53.1
    hereditary D51.1
    nutritional D52.0
    orotic aciduria D53.0
    refractory D53.1
    specified type NEC D53.1
  megalocytic D53.1
  microcytic (hypochromic) D50.9
    due to blood loss (chronic) D50.0
      acute D62
    familial D56.8
  microdrepanocytosis D57.40
  microelliptopoikilocytic (Rietti-Greppi-
    Micheli) D56.9
  miner's B76.9 *[D63.8]*
  myelodysplastic D46.9
  myelofibrosis D75.81
  myelogenous D64.89
  myelopathic D64.89
  myelophthisic D61.82
  myeloproliferative D47.Z9
  newborn P61.4
    due to
      ABO (antibodies, isoimmunization,
        maternal/fetal
        incompatibility) P55.1
      Rh (antibodies, isoimmunization,
        maternal/fetal
        incompatibility) P55.0
    following fetal blood loss P61.3
    posthemorrhagic (fetal) P61.3
  nonspherocytic hemolytic —*see* Anemia,
    hemolytic, nonspherocytic
  normocytic (infectional) D64.9
    due to blood loss (chronic) D50.0
      acute D62
    myelophthisic D61.82
  nutritional (deficiency) D53.9
    with
      poor iron absorption D50.8
      specified deficiency NEC D53.8
    megaloblastic D52.0
  of prematurity P61.2
  orotaciduric (congenital) (hereditary)
    D53.0
  osteosclerotic D64.89
  ovalocytosis (hereditary) —*see*
    Elliptocytosis
  paludal *(see also* Malaria) B54 *[D63.8]*
  pernicious (congenital) (malignant)
    (progressive) D51.0
  pleochromic D64.89
    of sprue D52.8

Anemia *(Continued)*
  posthemorrhagic (chronic) D50.0
    acute D62
    newborn P61.3
  postoperative (postprocedural)
    due to (acute) blood loss D62
      chronic blood loss D50.0
    specified NEC D64.9
  postpartum O90.81
  pressure D64.89
  progressive D64.9
    malignant D51.0
    pernicious D51.0
  protein-deficiency D53.0
  pseudoleukemica infantum D64.89
  pure red cell D60.9
    congenital D61.01
  pyridoxine-responsive D64.3
  pyruvate kinase deficiency D55.2
  refractory D46.4
    with
      excess of blasts D46.20
        1 (RAEB 1) D46.21
        2 (RAEB 2) D46.22
        in transformation (RAEB T) —
          see Leukemia, acute
          myeloblastic
      hemochromatosis D46.1
      sideroblasts (ring) (RARS) D46.1
    without ring sideroblasts, so stated
      D46.0
    without sideroblasts without excess
      of blasts D46.0
    megaloblastic D53.1
    sideroblastic D46.1
    sideropenic D50.8
  Rietti-Greppi-Micheli D56.9
  scorbutic D53.2
  secondary to
    blood loss (chronic) D50.0
      acute D62
    hemorrhage (chronic) D50.0
      acute D62
  semiplastic D61.89
  sickle-cell —*see* Disease, sickle-cell
  sideroblastic D64.3
    hereditary D64.0
    hypochromic, sex-linked D64.0
    pyridoxine-responsive NEC D64.3
    refractory D46.1
    secondary (due to)
      disease D64.1
      drugs and toxins D64.2
    specified type NEC D64.3
  sideropenic (refractory) D50.9
    due to blood loss (chronic) D50.0
      acute D62
  simple chronic D53.9
  specified type NEC D64.89
  spherocytic (hereditary) —*see*
    Spherocytosis
  splenic D64.89
  splenomegalic D64.89
  stomatocytosis D58.8
  syphilitic (acquired) (late) A52.79
    [D63.8]
  target cell D64.89
  thalassemia D56.9
  thrombocytopenic —*see*
    Thrombocytopenia
  toxic D61.2
  tropical B76.9 *[D63.8]*
    macrocytic D52.8
  tuberculous A18.89 *[D63.8]*
  vegan D51.3

Anemia *(Continued)*
  vitamin
    B6-responsive D64.3
    B12 deficiency (dietary) pernicious
      D51.0
  von Jaksch's D64.89
  Witts' (achlorhydric anemia) D50.8
Anemophobia F40.228
Anencephalus, anencephaly Q00.0
Anergasia —*see* Psychosis, organic
Anesthesia, anesthetic R20.0
  complication or reaction NEC *(see also*
    Complications, anesthesia) T88.59
    due to
      correct substance properly
        administered —*see* Table of
        drugs and chemicals, by drug,
        adverse effect
      overdose or wrong substance
        given —*see* Table of drugs
        and chemicals, by drug,
        poisoning
  cornea H18.81-
  dissociative F44.6
  functional (hysterical) F44.6
  hyperesthetic, thalamic G89.0
  hysterical F44.6
  local skin lesion R20.0
  sexual (psychogenic) F52.1
  shock (due to) T88.2
  skin R20.0
  testicular N50.9
Anetoderma (maculosum) (of) L90.8
  Jadassohn-Pellizzari L90.2
  Schweniger-Buzzi L90.1
Aneurin deficiency E51.9
Aneurysm (anastomotic) (artery) (cirsoid)
  (diffuse) (false) (fusiform) (multiple)
  (saccular) I72.9
  abdominal (aorta) I71.4
    ruptured I71.3
    syphilitic A52.01
  aorta, aortic (nonsyphilitic) I71.9
    abdominal I71.4
      ruptured I71.3
    arch I71.2
      ruptured I71.1
    arteriosclerotic I71.9
      ruptured I71.8
    ascending I71.2
      ruptured I71.1
    congenital Q25.4
    descending I71.9
      abdominal I71.4
        ruptured I71.3
      ruptured I71.8
      thoracic I71.2
        ruptured I71.1
    ruptured I71.8
    sinus, congenital Q25.4
    syphilitic A52.01
    thoracic I71.2
      ruptured I71.1
    thoracoabdominal I71.6
      ruptured I71.5
    thorax, thoracic (arch) I71.2
      ruptured I71.1
    transverse I71.2
      ruptured I71.1
    valve (heart) *(see also* Endocarditis,
      aortic) I35.8
  arteriosclerotic I72.9
    cerebral I67.1
      ruptured —*see* Hemorrhage,
        intracranial, subarachnoid

Aneurysm (Continued)
arteriovenous (congenital) —see also
    Malformation, arteriovenous
  acquired I77.0
    brain I67.1
    coronary I25.41
    pulmonary I28.0
  brain Q28.2
    ruptured I60.8
  peripheral —see Malformation,
    arteriovenous, peripheral
  precerebral vessels Q28.0
  specified site NEC —see also
    Malformation, arteriovenous
    acquired I77.0
basal —see Aneurysm, brain
berry (congenital) (nonruptured) I67.1
  ruptured I60.7
brain I67.1
  arteriosclerotic I67.1
    ruptured —see Hemorrhage,
      intracranial, subarachnoid
  arteriovenous (congenital)
    (nonruptured) Q28.2
    acquired I67.1
      ruptured I60.8
    ruptured I60.8
  berry (congenital) (nonruptured)
    I67.1
    ruptured (see also Hemorrhage,
      intracranial, subarachnoid)
      I60.7
  congenital Q28.3
    ruptured I60.7
  meninges I67.1
    ruptured I60.8
  miliary (congenital) (nonruptured)
    I67.1
    ruptured (see also Hemorrhage,
      intracranial, subarachnoid)
      I60.7
  mycotic I33.0
  ruptured —see Hemorrhage,
    intracranial, subarachnoid
  syphilitic (hemorrhage) A52.05
cardiac (false) (see also Aneurysm, heart)
  I25.3
carotid artery (common) (external) I72.0
  internal (intracranial) I67.1
    extracranial portion I72.0
    ruptured into brain I60.0-
  syphilitic A52.09
    intracranial A52.05
cavernous sinus I67.1
  arteriovenous (congenital)
    (nonruptured) Q28.3
    ruptured I60.8
celiac I72.8
central nervous system, syphilitic
  A52.05
cerebral —see Aneurysm, brain
chest —see Aneurysm, thorax
circle of Willis I67.1
  congenital Q28.3
    ruptured I60.6
  ruptured I60.6
common iliac artery I72.3
congenital (peripheral) Q27.8
  brain Q28.3
    ruptured I60.7
  coronary Q24.5
  digestive system Q27.8
  lower limb Q27.8
  pulmonary Q25.79

Aneurysm (Continued)
congenital (Continued)
  retina Q14.1
  specified site NEC Q27.8
  upper limb Q27.8
conjunctiva —see Abnormality,
  conjunctiva, vascular
conus arteriosus —see Aneurysm, heart
coronary (arteriosclerotic) (artery)
  I25.41
  arteriovenous, congenital Q24.5
  congenital Q24.5
  ruptured —see Infarct, myocardium
  syphilitic A52.06
  vein I25.89
cylindroid (aorta) I71.9
  ruptured I71.8
  syphilitic A52.01
ductus arteriosus Q25.0
endocardial, infective (any valve) I33.0
femoral (artery) (ruptured) I72.4
gastroduodenal I72.8
gastroepiploic I72.8
heart (wall) (chronic or with a stated
  duration of over 4 weeks) I25.3
  valve —see Endocarditis
hepatic I72.8
iliac (common) (artery) (ruptured) I72.3
infective I72.9
  endocardial (any valve) I33.0
innominate (nonsyphilitic) I72.8
  syphilitic A52.09
interauricular septum —see Aneurysm,
  heart
interventricular septum —see
  Aneurysm, heart
intrathoracic (nonsyphilitic) I71.2
  ruptured I71.1
  syphilitic A52.01
lower limb I72.4
lung (pulmonary artery) I28.1
mediastinal (nonsyphilitic) I72.8
  syphilitic A52.09
miliary (congenital) I67.1
  ruptured —see Hemorrhage,
    intracerebral, subarachnoid,
    intracranial
mitral (heart) (valve) I34.8
mural —see Aneurysm, heart
mycotic I72.9
  endocardial (any valve) I33.0
  ruptured, brain —see Hemorrhage,
    intracerebral, subarachnoid
myocardium —see Aneurysm, heart
neck I72.0
pancreaticoduodenal I72.8
patent ductus arteriosus Q25.0
peripheral NEC I72.8
  congenital Q27.8
    digestive system Q27.8
    lower limb Q27.8
    specified site NEC Q27.8
    upper limb Q27.8
popliteal (artery) (ruptured) I72.4
precerebral, congenital (nonruptured)
  Q28.1
pulmonary I28.1
  arteriovenous Q25.72
    acquired I28.0
  syphilitic A52.09
  valve (heart) —see Endocarditis,
    pulmonary
racemose (peripheral) I72.9
  congenital —see Aneurysm,
    congenital

Aneurysm (Continued)
radial I72.1
Rasmussen NEC A15.0
renal (artery) I72.2
retina —see also Disorder, retina,
  microaneurysms
  congenital Q14.1
  diabetic —see Diabetes,
    microaneurysms, retinal
sinus of Valsalva Q25.4
specified NEC I72.8
spinal (cord) I72.8
  syphilitic (hemorrhage) A52.09
splenic I72.8
subclavian (artery) (ruptured) I72.8
  syphilitic A52.09
superior mesenteric I72.8
syphilitic (aorta) A52.01
  central nervous system A52.05
  congenital (late) A50.54 [I79.0]
  spine, spinal A52.09
thoracoabdominal (aorta) I71.6
  ruptured I71.5
  syphilitic A52.01
thorax, thoracic (aorta) (arch)
  (nonsyphilitic) I71.2
  ruptured I71.1
  syphilitic A52.01
traumatic (complication) (early),
  specified site —see Injury, blood
  vessel
tricuspid (heart) (valve) I07.8
ulnar I72.1
upper limb (ruptured) I72.1
valve, valvular —see Endocarditis
visceral NEC I72.8
venous (see also Varix) I86.8
  congenital Q27.8
    digestive system Q27.8
    lower limb Q27.8
    specified site NEC Q27.8
    upper limb Q27.8
ventricle —see Aneurysm, heart
Angelman syndrome Q93.5
Anger R45.4
Angiectasis, angiectopia I99.8
Angiitis I77.6
allergic granulomatous M30.1
hypersensitivity M31.0
necrotizing M31.9
  specified NEC M31.8
nervous system, granulomatous I67.7
Angina (attack) (cardiac) (chest) (heart)
  (pectoris) (syndrome) (vasomotor)
  I20.9
with
  atherosclerotic heart disease —see
    Arteriosclerosis, coronary (artery)
  documented spasm I20.1
abdominal K55.1
accelerated —see Angina, unstable
agranulocytic —see Agranulocytosis
angiospastic —see Angina, with
  documented spasm
aphthous B08.5
crescendo —see Angina, unstable
croupous J05.0
cruris I73.9
de novo effort —see Angina, unstable
diphtheritic, membranous A36.0
equivalent I20.8
exudative, chronic J37.0
following acute myocardial infarction
  I23.7

Angina (Continued)
  gangrenous diphtheritic A36.0
  intestinal K55.1
  Ludovici K12.2
  Ludwig's K12.2
  malignant diphtheritic A36.0
  membranous J05.0
    diphtheritic A36.0
    Vincent's A69.1
  mesenteric K55.1
  monocytic —see Mononucleosis,
    infectious
  of effort —see Angina, specified NEC
  phlegmonous J36
    diphtheritic A36.0
  post-infarctional I23.7
  pre-infarctional —see Angina, unstable
  Prinzmetal —see Angina, with
    documented spasm
  progressive —see Angina, unstable
  pseudomembranous A69.1
  pultaceous, diphtheritic A36.0
  spasm-induced —see Angina, with
    documented spasm
  specified NEC I20.8
  stable I20.9
  stenocardia —see Angina, specified
    NEC
  stridulous, diphtheritic A36.2
  tonsil J36
  trachealis J05.0
  unstable I20.0
  variant —see Angina, with documented
    spasm
  Vincent's A69.1
  worsening effort —see Angina, unstable
Angioblastoma —see Neoplasm,
  connective tissue, uncertain behavior
Angiocholecystitis —see Cholecystitis,
  acute
Angiocholitis (see also Cholecystitis,
  acute) K83.0
Angiodysgenesis spinalis G95.19
Angiodysplasia (cecum) (colon) K55.20
  with bleeding K55.21
  duodenum (and stomach) K31.819
    with bleeding K31.811
  stomach (and duodenum) K31.819
    with bleeding K31.811
Angioedema (allergic) (any site) (with
  urticaria) T78.3
  hereditary D84.1
Angioendothelioma —see Neoplasm,
  uncertain behavior, by site
  benign D18.00
    intra-abdominal D18.03
    intracranial D18.02
    skin D18.01
    specified site NEC D18.09
  bone —see Neoplasm, bone, malignant
  Ewing's —see Neoplasm, bone,
    malignant
Angioendotheliomatosis C85.8-
Angiofibroma —see also Neoplasm,
  benign, by site
  juvenile
    specified site —see Neoplasm, benign,
      by site
    unspecified site D10.6
Angiohemophilia (A) (B) D68.0
Angioid streaks (choroid) (macula)
  (retina) H35.33
Angiokeratoma —see Neoplasm, skin,
  benign
  corporis diffusum E75.21

Angioleiomyoma —see Neoplasm,
  connective tissue, benign
Angiolipoma —see also Lipoma
  infiltrating —see Lipoma
Angioma —see also Hemangioma, by site
  capillary I78.1
  hemorrhagicum hereditaria I78.0
  intra-abdominal D18.03
  intracranial D18.02
  malignant —see Neoplasm, connective
    tissue, malignant
  plexiform D18.00
    intra-abdominal D18.03
    intracranial D18.02
    skin D18.01
    specified site NEC D18.09
  senile I78.1
  serpiginosum L81.7
  skin D18.01
  specified site NEC D18.09
  spider I78.1
  stellate I78.1
  venous Q28.3
Angiomatosis Q82.8
  bacillary A79.89
  encephalotrigeminal Q85.8
  hemorrhagic familial I78.0
  hereditary familial I78.0
  liver K76.4
Angiomyolipoma —see Lipoma
Angiomyoliposarcoma —see Neoplasm,
  connective tissue, malignant
Angiomyoma —see Neoplasm, connective
  tissue, benign
Angiomyosarcoma —see Neoplasm,
  connective tissue, malignant
Angiomyxoma —see Neoplasm,
  connective tissue, uncertain behavior
Angioneurosis F45.8
Angioneurotic edema (allergic) (any site)
  (with urticaria) T78.3
  hereditary D84.1
Angiopathia, angiopathy I99.9
  cerebral I67.9
    amyloid E85.4 [I68.0]
  diabetic (peripheral) —see Diabetes,
    angiopathy
  peripheral I73.9
    diabetic —see Diabetes, angiopathy
    specified type NEC I73.89
  retinae syphilitica A52.05
  retinalis (juvenilis)
    diabetic —see Diabetes, retinopathy
    proliferative —see Retinopathy,
      proliferative
Angiosarcoma —see also Neoplasm,
  connective tissue, malignant
  liver C22.3
Angiosclerosis —see Arteriosclerosis
Angiospasm (peripheral) (traumatic)
  (vessel) I73.9
  brachial plexus G54.0
  cerebral G45.9
  cervical plexus G54.2
  nerve
    arm —see Mononeuropathy, upper
      limb
    axillary G54.0
    median —see Lesion, nerve,
      median
    ulnar —see Lesion, nerve, ulnar
    axillary G54.0
    leg —see Mononeuropathy, lower
      limb

Angiospasm (Continued)
  nerve (Continued)
    median —see Lesion, nerve, median
    plantar —see Lesion, nerve, plantar
    ulnar —see Lesion, nerve, ulnar
Angiospastic disease or edema I73.9
Angiostrongyliasis
  due to
    Parastrongylus
      cantonensis B83.2
      costaricensis B81.3
    intestinal B81.3
Anguillulosis —see Strongyloidiasis
Angulation
  cecum —see Obstruction, intestine
  coccyx (acquired) (see also subcategory)
    M43.8
    congenital NEC Q76.49
  femur (acquired) —see also Deformity,
    limb, specified type NEC, thigh
    congenital Q74.2
  intestine (large) (small) —see
    Obstruction, intestine
  sacrum (acquired) (see also subcategory)
    M43.8
    congenital NEC Q76.49
  sigmoid (flexure) —see Obstruction,
    intestine
  spine —see Dorsopathy, deforming,
    specified NEC
  tibia (acquired) —see also Deformity,
    limb, specified type NEC, lower
    leg
    congenital Q74.2
  ureter N13.5
    with infection N13.6
  wrist (acquired) —see also Deformity,
    limb, specified type NEC, forearm
    congenital Q74.0
Angulus infectiosus (lips) K13.0
Anhedonia R45.84
Anhidrosis L74.4
Anhydration, anhydremia E86.0
  with
    hypernatremia E87.0
    hyponatremia E87.1
Anhydremia E86.0
  with
    hypernatremia E87.0
    hyponatremia E87.1
Anidrosis L74.4
Aniridia (congenital) Q13.1
Anisakiasis (infection) (infestation) B81.0
Anisakis larvae infestation B81.0
Aniseikonia H52.32
Anisocoria (pupil) H57.02
  congenital Q13.2
Anisocytosis R71.8
Anisometropia (congenital) H52.31
Ankle —see condition
Ankyloblepharon (eyelid) (acquired) —
  see also Blepharophimosis
  filiforme (adnatum) (congenital) Q10.3
  total Q10.3
Ankyloglossia Q38.1
Ankylosis (fibrous) (osseous) (joint)
  M24.60
  ankle M24.67-
  arthrodesis status Z98.1
  cricoarytenoid (cartilage) (joint) (larynx)
    J38.7
  dental K03.5
  ear ossicles H74.31-
  elbow M24.62-

Ankylosis *(Continued)*
  foot M24.67-
  hand M24.64-
  hip M24.65-
  incostapedial joint (infectional) —*see*
      Ankylosis, ear ossicles
  jaw (temporomandibular) M26.61
  knee M24.66-
  lumbosacral (joint) M43.27
  postoperative (status) Z98.1
  produced by surgical fusion, status
      Z98.1
  sacro-iliac (joint) M43.28
  shoulder M24.61-
  spine (joint) —*see also* Fusion, spine
    spondylitic —*see* Spondylitis,
        ankylosing
  surgical Z98.1
  temporomandibular M26.61
  tooth, teeth (hard tissues) K03.5
  wrist M24.63-
Ankylostoma —*see* Ancylostoma
Ankylostomiasis —*see* Ancylostomiasis
Ankylurethria —*see* Stricture, urethra
Annular —*see also* condition
  detachment, cervix N88.8
  organ or site, congenital NEC —*see*
      Distortion
  pancreas (congenital) Q45.1
Anodontia (complete) (partial) (vera) K00.0
  acquired K08.10
Anomaly, anomalous (congenital)
      (unspecified type) Q89.9
  abdominal wall NEC Q79.59
  acoustic nerve Q07.8
  adrenal (gland) Q89.1
  Alder (-Reilly) (leukocyte granulation)
      D72.0
  alimentary tract Q45.9
    upper Q40.9
  alveolar M26.70
    hyperplasia M26.79
      mandibular M26.72
      maxillary M26.71
    hypoplasia M26.79
      mandibular M26.74
      maxillary M26.73
    ridge (process) M26.79
    specified NEC M26.79
  ankle (joint) Q74.2
  anus Q43.9
  aorta (arch) NEC Q25.4
    coarctation (preductal) (postductal)
        Q25.1
  aortic cusp or valve Q23.9
  appendix Q43.8
  apple peel syndrome Q41.1
  aqueduct of Sylvius Q03.0
    with spina bifida —*see* Spina bifida,
        with hydrocephalus
  arm Q74.0
  arteriovenous NEC
    coronary Q24.5
    gastrointestinal Q27.33
      acquired —*see* Angiodysplasia
  artery (peripheral) Q27.9
    basilar NEC Q28.1
    cerebral Q28.3
    coronary Q24.5
    digestive system Q27.8
    eye Q15.8
    great Q25.9
      specified NEC Q25.8
    lower limb Q27.8

Anomaly, anomalous *(Continued)*
  artery *(Continued)*
    peripheral Q27.9
      specified NEC Q27.8
    pulmonary NEC Q25.79
    renal Q27.2
    retina Q14.1
    specified site NEC Q27.8
    subclavian Q27.8
    umbilical Q27.0
    upper limb Q27.8
    vertebral NEC Q28.1
  aryteno-epiglottic folds Q31.8
  atrial
    bands or folds Q20.8
    septa Q21.1
  atrioventricular
    excitation I45.6
    septum Q21.0
  auditory canal Q17.8
  auricle
    ear Q17.8
      causing impairment of hearing
          Q16.9
    heart Q20.8
  Axenfeld's Q15.0
  back Q89.9
  band
    atrial Q20.8
    heart Q24.8
    ventricular Q24.8
  Bartholin's duct Q38.4
  biliary duct or passage Q44.5
  bladder Q64.70
    absence Q64.5
    diverticulum Q64.6
    exstrophy Q64.10
      cloacal Q64.12
      extroversion Q64.19
      specified type NEC Q64.19
      supravesical fissure Q64.11
    neck obstruction Q64.31
    specified type NEC Q64.79
  bone Q79.9
    arm Q74.0
    face Q75.9
    leg Q74.2
    pelvic girdle Q74.2
    shoulder girdle Q74.0
    skull Q75.9
      with
        anencephaly Q00.0
        encephalocele —*see* Encephalocele
        hydrocephalus Q03.9
          with spina bifida —*see* Spina
              bifida, by site, with
              hydrocephalus
        microcephaly Q02
  brain (multiple) Q04.9
    vessel Q28.3
  breast Q83.9
  broad ligament Q50.6
  bronchus Q32.4
  bulbus cordis Q21.9
  bursa Q79.9
  canal of Nuck Q52.4
  canthus Q10.3
  capillary Q27.9
  cardiac Q24.9
    chambers Q20.9
      specified NEC Q20.8
    septal closure Q21.9
      specified NEC Q21.8
    valve NEC Q24.8
      pulmonary Q22.3

Anomaly, anomalous *(Continued)*
  cardiovascular system Q28.8
  carpus Q74.0
  caruncle, lacrimal Q10.6
  cascade stomach Q40.2
  cauda equina Q06.3
  cecum Q43.9
  cerebral Q04.9
    vessels Q28.3
  cervix Q51.9
  Chédiak-Higashi(-Steinbrinck)
      (congenital gigantism of
      peroxidase granules) E70.330
  cheek Q18.9
  chest wall Q67.8
    bones Q76.9
  chin Q18.9
  chordae tendineae Q24.8
  choroid Q14.3
    plexus Q07.8
  chromosomes, chromosomal Q99.9
    D (1) —*see* condition, chromosome 13
    E (3) —*see* condition, chromosome 18
    G —*see* condition, chromosome 21
    sex
      female phenotype Q97.8
      gonadal dysgenesis (pure) Q99.1
      Klinefelter's Q98.4
      male phenotype Q98.9
      Turner's Q96.9
      specified NEC Q99.8
  cilia Q10.3
  circulatory system Q28.9
  clavicle Q74.0
  clitoris Q52.6
  coccyx Q76.49
  colon Q43.9
  common duct Q44.5
  communication
    coronary artery Q24.5
    left ventricle with right atrium
        Q21.0
  concha (ear) Q17.3
  connection
    portal vein Q26.5
    pulmonary venous Q26.4
      partial Q26.3
      total Q26.2
    renal artery with kidney Q27.2
  cornea (shape) Q13.4
  coronary artery or vein Q24.5
  cranium —*see* Anomaly, skull
  cricoid cartilage Q31.8
  cystic duct Q44.5
  dental
    alveolar —*see* Anomaly, alveolar
    arch relationship M26.20
      specified NEC M26.29
  dentofacial M26.9
    alveolar —*see* Anomaly, alveolar
    dental arch relationship M26.20
      specified NEC M26.29
    functional M26.50
      specified NEC M26.59
    jaw size M26.00
      macrogenia M26.05
      mandibular
        hyperplasia M26.03
        hypoplasia M26.04
      maxillary
        hyperplasia M26.01
        hypoplasia M26.02
      microgenia M26.06
      specified type NEC M26.09

Anomaly, anomalous (Continued)
  dentofacial (Continued)
    jaw-cranial base relationship
        M26.10
      asymmetry M26.12
        maxillary M26.11
      specified type NEC M26.19
    malocclusion M26.4
      dental arch relationship NEC M26.29
      jaw size —see Anomaly,
          dentofacial, jaw size
      jaw-cranial base relationship —
          see Anomaly, dentofacial,
          jaw-cranial base
          relationship
      specified type NEC M26.89
    temporomandibular joint M26.60
      adhesions M26.61
      ankylosis M26.61
      arthralgia M26.62
      articular disc M26.63
      specified type NEC M26.69
    tooth position, fully erupted
        M26.30
      specified NEC M26.39
  dermatoglyphic Q82.8
  diaphragm (apertures) NEC Q79.1
  digestive organ (s) or tract Q45.9
    lower Q43.9
    upper Q40.9
  distance, interarch (excessive)
      (inadequate) M26.25
  distribution, coronary artery Q24.5
  ductus
    arteriosus Q25.0
    botalli Q25.0
  duodenum Q43.9
  dura (brain) Q04.9
    spinal cord Q06.9
  ear (external) Q17.9
    causing impairment of hearing Q16.9
    inner Q16.5
    middle (causing impairment of
        hearing) Q16.4
      ossicles Q16.3
  Ebstein's (heart) (tricuspid valve) Q22.5
  ectodermal Q82.9
  Eisenmenger's (ventricular septal
      defect) Q21.8
  ejaculatory duct Q55.4
  elbow Q74.0
  endocrine gland NEC Q89.2
  epididymis Q55.4
  epiglottis Q31.8
  esophagus Q39.9
  eustachian tube Q17.8
  eye Q15.9
    anterior segment Q13.9
      specified NEC Q13.89
    posterior segment Q14.9
      specified NEC Q14.8
    ptosis (eyelid) Q10.0
    specified NEC Q15.8
  eyebrow Q18.8
  eyelid Q10.3
    ptosis Q10.0
  face Q18.9
    bone (s) Q75.9
  fallopian tube Q50.6
  fascia Q79.9
  femur NEC Q74.2
  fibula NEC Q74.2
  finger Q74.0
  fixation, intestine Q43.3

Anomaly, anomalous (Continued)
  flexion (joint) NOS Q74.9
    hip or thigh Q65.89
  foot NEC Q74.2
    varus (congenital) Q66.3
  foramen
    Botalli Q21.1
    ovale Q21.1
  forearm Q74.0
  forehead Q75.8
  form, teeth K00.2
  fovea centralis Q14.1
  frontal bone —see Anomaly, skull
  gallbladder (position) (shape) (size)
      Q44.1
  Gartner's duct Q52.4
  gastrointestinal tract Q45.9
  genitalia, genital organ (s) or system
    female Q52.9
      external Q52.70
      internal NOS Q52.9
    male Q55.9
      hydrocele P83.5
      specified NEC Q55.8
  genitourinary NEC
    female Q52.9
    male Q55.9
  Gerbode Q21.0
  glottis Q31.8
  granulation or granulocyte, genetic
      (constitutional) (leukocyte) D72.0
  gum Q38.6
  gyri Q07.9
  hair Q84.2
  hand Q74.0
  hard tissue formation in pulp K04.3
  head —see Anomaly, skull
  heart Q24.9
    auricle Q20.8
    bands or folds Q24.8
    fibroelastosis cordis I42.4
    obstructive NEC Q22.6
    patent ductus arteriosus (Botalli)
        Q25.0
    septum Q21.9
      auricular Q21.1
      interatrial Q21.1
      interventricular Q21.0
        with pulmonary stenosis or
            atresia, dextraposition
            of aorta and hypertrophy
            of right ventricle Q21.3
      specified NEC Q21.8
      ventricular Q21.0
        with pulmonary stenosis or
            atresia, dextraposition
            of aorta and hypertrophy
            of right ventricle Q21.3
    tetralogy of Fallot Q21.3
    valve NEC Q24.8
      aortic
        bicuspid valve Q23.1
        insufficiency Q23.1
        stenosis Q23.0
          subaortic Q24.4
      mitral
        insufficiency Q23.3
        stenosis Q23.2
      pulmonary Q22.3
        atresia Q22.0
        insufficiency Q22.2
        stenosis Q22.1
          infundibular Q24.3
          subvalvular Q24.3

Anomaly, anomalous (Continued)
  heart (Continued)
    valve NEC (Continued)
      tricuspid
        atresia Q22.4
        stenosis Q22.4
    ventricle Q20.8
  heel NEC Q74.2
  Hegglin's D72.0
  hemianencephaly Q00.0
  hemicephaly Q00.0
  hemicrania Q00.0
  hepatic duct Q44.5
  hip NEC Q74.2
  hourglass stomach Q40.2
  humerus Q74.0
  hydatid of Morgagni
    female Q50.5
    male (epididymal) Q55.4
      testicular Q55.29
  hymen Q52.4
  hypersegmentation of neutrophils,
      hereditary D72.0
  hypophyseal Q89.2
  ileocecal (coil) (valve) Q43.9
  ileum Q43.9
  ilium NEC Q74.2
  integument Q84.9
    specified NEC Q84.8
  interarch distance (excessive)
      (inadequate) M26.25
  intervertebral cartilage or disc
      Q76.49
  intestine (large) (small) Q43.9
    with anomalous adhesions, fixation
        or malrotation Q43.3
  iris Q13.2
  ischium NEC Q74.2
  jaw —see Anomaly, dentofacial
    alveolar —see Anomaly, alveolar
  jaw-cranial base relationship —see
      Anomaly, dentofacial, jaw-cranial
      base relationship
  jejunum Q43.8
  joint Q74.9
    specified NEC Q74.8
  Jordan's D72.0
  kidney (s) (calyx) (pelvis) Q63.9
    artery Q27.2
    specified NEC Q63.8
  Klippel-Feil (brevicollis) Q76.1
  knee Q74.1
  labium (majus) (minus) Q52.70
  labyrinth, membranous Q16.5
  lacrimal apparatus or duct Q10.6
  larynx, laryngeal (muscle) Q31.9
    web (bed) Q31.0
  lens Q12.9
  leucocytes, genetic D72.0
    granulation (constitutional)
        D72.0
  lid (fold) Q10.3
  ligament Q79.9
    broad Q50.6
    round Q52.8
  limb Q74.9
    lower NEC Q74.2
      reduction deformity —see Defect,
          reduction, lower limb
    upper Q74.0
  lip Q38.0
  liver Q44.7
    duct Q44.5
  lower limb NEC Q74.2

Anomaly, anomalous *(Continued)*
  lumbosacral (joint) (region) Q76.49
    kyphosis —*see* Kyphosis, congenital
    lordosis —*see* Lordosis, congenital
  lung (fissure) (lobe) Q33.9
  mandible —*see* Anomaly, dentofacial
  maxilla —*see* Anomaly, dentofacial
  May (-Hegglin) D72.0
  meatus urinarius NEC Q64.79
  meningeal bands or folds Q07.9
    constriction of Q07.8
    spinal Q06.9
  meninges Q07.9
    cerebral Q04.8
    spinal Q06.9
  meningocele Q05.9
  mesentery Q45.9
  metacarpus Q74.0
  metatarsus NEC Q74.2
  middle ear Q16.4
    ossicles Q16.3
  mitral (leaflets) (valve) Q23.9
    insufficiency Q23.3
    specified NEC Q23.8
    stenosis Q23.2
  mouth Q38.6
  Müllerian —*see also* Anomaly, by site
    uterus NEC Q51.818
  multiple NEC Q89.7
  muscle Q79.9
    eyelid Q10.3
  musculoskeletal system, except limbs
      Q79.9
  myocardium Q24.8
  nail Q84.6
  narrowness, eyelid Q10.3
  nasal sinus (wall) Q30.8
  neck (any part) Q18.9
  nerve Q07.9
    acoustic Q07.8
    optic Q07.8
  nervous system (central) Q07.9
  nipple Q83.9
  nose, nasal (bones) (cartilage) (septum)
      (sinus) Q30.9
    specified NEC Q30.8
  ocular muscle Q15.8
  omphalomesenteric duct Q43.0
  opening, pulmonary veins Q26.4
  optic
    disc Q14.2
    nerve Q07.8
  opticociliary vessels Q13.2
  orbit (eye) Q10.7
  organ Q89.9
    of Corti Q16.5
  origin
    artery
      innominate Q25.8
      pulmonary Q25.79
      renal Q27.2
      subclavian Q25.8
  osseous meatus (ear) Q16.1
  ovary Q50.39
  oviduct Q50.6
  palate (hard) (soft) NEC Q38.5
  pancreas or pancreatic duct Q45.3
  papillary muscles Q24.8
  parathyroid gland Q89.2
  paraurethral ducts Q64.79
  parotid (gland) Q38.4
  patella Q74.1
  Pelger-Huët (hereditary
      hyposegmentation) D72.0

Anomaly, anomalous *(Continued)*
  pelvic girdle NEC Q74.2
  pelvis (bony) NEC Q74.2
    rachitic E64.3
  penis (glans) Q55.69
  pericardium Q24.8
  peripheral vascular system Q27.9
  Peter's Q13.4
  pharynx Q38.8
  pigmentation L81.9
    congenital Q82.8
  pituitary (gland) Q89.2
  pleural (folds) Q34.0
  portal vein Q26.5
    connection Q26.5
  position, tooth, teeth, fully erupted
      M26.30
    specified NEC M26.39
  precerebral vessel Q28.1
  prepuce Q55.69
  prostate Q55.4
  pulmonary Q33.9
    artery NEC Q25.79
    valve Q22.3
      atresia Q22.0
      insufficiency Q22.2
      specified type NEC Q22.3
      stenosis Q22.1
        infundibular Q24.3
        subvalvular Q24.3
    venous connection Q26.4
      partial Q26.3
      total Q26.2
  pupil Q13.2
    function H57.00
      anisocoria H57.02
      Argyll Robertson pupil H57.01
      miosis H57.03
      mydriasis H57.04
      specified type NEC H57.09
      tonic pupil H57.05-
  pylorus Q40.3
  radius Q74.0
  rectum Q43.9
  reduction (extremity) (limb)
    femur (longitudinal) —*see* Defect,
      reduction, lower limb,
      longitudinal, femur
    fibula (longitudinal) —*see* Defect,
      reduction, lower limb,
      longitudinal, fibula
    lower limb —*see* Defect, reduction,
      lower limb
    radius (longitudinal) —*see* Defect,
      reduction, upper limb,
      longitudinal, radius
    tibia (longitudinal) —*see* Defect,
      reduction, lower limb,
      longitudinal, tibia
    ulna (longitudinal) —*see* Defect,
      reduction, upper limb,
      longitudinal, ulna
    upper limb —*see* Defect, reduction,
      upper limb
  refraction —*see* Disorder, refraction
  renal Q63.9
    artery Q27.2
    pelvis Q63.9
      specified NEC Q63.8
  respiratory system Q34.9
    specified NEC Q34.8
  retina Q14.1
  rib Q76.6
    cervical Q76.5

Anomaly, anomalous *(Continued)*
  Rieger's Q13.81
  rotation —*see* Malrotation
    hip or thigh Q65.89
  round ligament Q52.8
  sacroiliac (joint) NEC Q74.2
  sacrum NEC Q76.49
    kyphosis —*see* Kyphosis, congenital
    lordosis —*see* Lordosis, congenital
  saddle nose, syphilitic A50.57
  salivary duct or gland Q38.4
  scapula Q74.0
  scrotum —*see* Malformation, testis and
      scrotum
  sebaceous gland Q82.9
  seminal vesicles Q55.4
  sense organs NEC Q07.8
  sex chromosomes NEC —*see also*
      Anomaly, chromosomes
    female phenotype Q97.8
    male phenotype Q98.9
  shoulder (girdle) (joint) Q74.0
  sigmoid (flexure) Q43.9
  simian crease Q82.8
  sinus of Valsalva Q25.4
  skeleton generalized Q78.9
  skin (appendage) Q82.9
  skull Q75.9
    with
      anencephaly Q00.0
      encephalocele —*see* Encephalocele
      hydrocephalus Q03.9
        with spina bifida —*see* Spina
          bifida, by site, with
          hydrocephalus
      microcephaly Q02
  specified organ or site NEC Q89.8
  spermatic cord Q55.4
  spine, spinal NEC Q76.49
    column NEC Q76.49
      kyphosis —*see* Kyphosis,
        congenital
      lordosis —*see* Lordosis,
        congenital
    cord Q06.9
    nerve root Q07.8
  spleen Q89.09
    agenesis Q89.01
  stenonian duct Q38.4
  sternum NEC Q76.7
  stomach Q40.3
  submaxillary gland Q38.4
  tarsus NEC Q74.2
  tendon Q79.9
  testis —*see* Malformation, testis and
      scrotum
  thigh NEC Q74.2
  thorax (wall) Q67.8
    bony Q76.9
  throat Q38.8
  thumb Q74.0
  thymus gland Q89.2
  thyroid (gland) Q89.2
    cartilage Q31.8
  tibia NEC Q74.2
    saber A50.56
  toe Q74.2
  tongue Q38.3
  tooth, teeth K00.9
    eruption K00.6
    position, fully erupted M26.30
    spacing, fully erupted M26.30
  trachea (cartilage) Q32.1
  tragus Q17.9

Anomaly, anomalous (*Continued*)
tricuspid (leaflet) (valve) Q22.9
atresia or stenosis Q22.4
Ebstein's Q22.5
Uhl's (hypoplasia of myocardium, right
ventricle) Q24.8
ulna Q74.0
umbilical artery Q27.0
union
cricoid cartilage and thyroid cartilage
Q31.8
thyroid cartilage and hyoid bone Q31.8
trachea with larynx Q31.8
upper limb Q74.0
urachus Q64.4
ureter Q62.8
obstructive NEC Q62.39
cecoureterocele Q62.32
orthotopic ureterocele Q62.31
urethra Q64.70
absence Q64.5
double Q64.74
fistula to rectum Q64.73
obstructive Q64.39
stricture Q64.32
prolapse Q64.71
specified type NEC Q64.79
urinary tract Q64.9
uterus Q51.9
with only one functioning horn Q51.4
uvula Q38.5
vagina Q52.4
valleculae Q31.8
valve (heart) NEC Q24.8
coronary sinus Q24.5
inferior vena cava Q24.8
pulmonary Q22.3
sinus coronario Q24.5
venae cavae inferioris Q24.8
vas deferens Q55.4
vascular Q27.9
brain Q28.3
ring Q25.4
vein (s) (peripheral) Q27.9
brain Q28.3
cerebral Q28.3
coronary Q24.5
developmental Q28.3
great Q26.9
specified NEC Q26.8
vena cava (inferior) (superior) Q26.9
venous —*see* Anomaly, vein (s)
venous return Q26.8
ventricular
bands or folds Q24.8
septa Q21.0
vertebra Q76.49
kyphosis —*see* Kyphosis, congenital
lordosis —*see* Lordosis, congenital
vesicourethral orifice Q64.79
vessel (s) Q27.9
optic papilla Q14.2
precerebral Q28.1
vitelline duct Q43.0
vitreous body or humor Q14.0
vulva Q52.70
wrist (joint) Q74.0
Anomia R48.8
Anonychia (congenital) Q84.3
acquired L60.8
Anophthalmos, anophthalmus
(congenital) (globe) Q11.1
acquired Z90.01
Anopia, anopsia H53.46-
quadrant H53.46-

Anorchia, anorchism, anorchidism Q55.0
Anorexia R63.0
hysterical F44.89
nervosa F50.00
atypical F50.9
binge-eating type F50.2
with purging F50.02
restricting type F50.01
Anorgasmy, psychogenic (female) F52.31
male F52.32
Anosmia R43.0
hysterical F44.6
postinfectional J39.8
Anosognosia R41.89
Anosteoplasia Q78.9
Anovulatory cycle N97.0
Anoxemia R09.02
newborn P84
Anoxia (pathological) R09.02
altitude T70.29
cerebral G93.1
complicating
anesthesia (general) (local) or other
sedation T88.59
in labor and delivery O74.3
in pregnancy O29.21-
postpartum, puerperal O89.2
delivery (cesarean) (instrumental)
O75.4
during a procedure G97.81
newborn P84
resulting from a procedure G97.82
due to
drowning T75.1
high altitude T70.29
heart —*see* Insufficiency, coronary
intrauterine P84
myocardial —*see* Insufficiency, coronary
newborn P84
spinal cord G95.11
systemic (by suffocation) (low content
in atmosphere) —*see* Asphyxia,
traumatic
Anteflexion —*see* Anteversion
Antenatal
care (normal pregnancy) Z34.90
screening (encounter for) of mother Z36
Antepartum —*see* condition
Anterior —*see* condition
Antero-occlusion M26.220
Anteversion
cervix —*see* Anteversion, uterus
femur (neck), congenital Q65.89
uterus, uterine (cervix) (postinfectional)
(postpartal, old) N85.4
congenital Q51.818
in pregnancy or childbirth —*see*
Pregnancy, complicated by
Anthophobia F40.228
Anthracosilicosis J60
Anthracosis (lung) (occupational) J60
lingua K14.3
Anthrax A22.9
with pneumonia A22.1
cerebral A22.8
colitis A22.2
cutaneous A22.0
gastrointestinal A22.2
inhalation A22.1
intestinal A22.2
meningitis A22.8
pulmonary A22.1
respiratory A22.1
sepsis A22.7
specified manifestation NEC A22.8

Anthropoid pelvis Q74.2
with disproportion (fetopelvic)
O33.0
Anthropophobia F40.10
generalized F40.11
Antibodies, maternal (blood group) —
see Isoimmunization, affecting
management of pregnancy
anti-D —*see* Isoimmunization,
affecting management of
pregnancy, Rh
newborn P55.0
Antibody
anticardiolipin R76.0
with
hemorrhagic disorder D68.312
hypercoagulable state D68.61
antiphosphatidylglycerol R76.0
with
hemorrhagic disorder D68.312
hypercoagulable state D68.61
antiphosphatidylinositol R76.0
with
hemorrhagic disorder D68.312
hypercoagulable state D68.61
antiphosphatidylserine R76.0
with
hemorrhagic disorder D68.312
hypercoagulable state D68.61
antiphospholipid R76.0
with
hemorrhagic disorder D68.312
hypercoagulable state D68.61
Anticardiolipin syndrome D68.61
Anticoagulant, circulating (intrinsic)
(*see also* - Disorder, hemorrhagic)
D68.318
drug-induced (extrinsic) (*see also* -
Disorder, hemorrhagic) D68.32
Antidiuretic hormone syndrome E22.2
Antimonial cholera —*see* Poisoning,
antimony
Antiphospholipid
antibody
with hemorrhagic disorder D68.312
syndrome D68.61
Antisocial personality F60.2
Antithrombinemia —*see* Circulating
anticoagulants
Antithromboplastinemia D68.318
Antithromboplastinogenemia D68.318
Antitoxin complication or reaction —*see*
Complications, vaccination
Antlophobia F40.228
Antritis J32.0
maxilla J32.0
acute J01.00
recurrent J01.01
stomach K29.60
with bleeding K29.61
Antrum, antral —*see* condition
Anuria R34
calculus (impacted) (recurrent) (*see also*
Calculus, urinary) N20.9
following
abortion —*see* Abortion by type
complicated by, renal failure
ectopic or molar pregnancy O08.4
newborn P96.0
postprocedural N99.0
postrenal N13.8
traumatic (following crushing)
T79.5
Anus, anal —*see* condition
Anusitis K62.89

Anxiety F41.9
  depression F41.8
  episodic paroxysmal F41.0
  generalized F41.1
  hysteria F41.8
  neurosis F41.1
  panic type F41.0
  reaction F41.1
  separation, abnormal (of childhood)
    F93.0
  specified NEC F41.8
  state F41.1
Aorta, aortic —see condition
Aortectasia —see Ectasia, aorta
  with aneurysm —see Aneurysm, aorta
Aortitis (nonsyphilitic) (calcific) I77.6
  arteriosclerotic I70.0
  Doehle-Heller A52.02
  luetic A52.02
  rheumatic —see Endocarditis, acute,
    rheumatic
  specific (syphilitic) A52.02
  syphilitic A52.02
    congenital A50.54 [I79.1]
Apathetic thyroid storm —see
  Thyrotoxicosis
Apathy R45.3
Apeirophobia F40.228
Apepsia K30
  psychogenic F45.8
Aperistalsis, esophagus K22.0
Apertognathia M26.29
Apert's syndrome Q87.0
Aphagia R13.0
  psychogenic F50.9
Aphakia (acquired) (postoperative)
  H27.0-
  congenital Q12.3
Aphasia (amnestic) (global) (nominal)
    (semantic) (syntactic) R47.01
  acquired, with epilepsy (Landau-
    Kleffner syndrome) —see
    Epilepsy, specified NEC
  auditory (developmental) F80.2
  developmental (receptive type) F80.2
    expressive type F80.1
    Wernicke's F80.2
  following
    cerebrovascular disease I69.920
      cerebral infarction I69.320
      intracerebral hemorrhage I69.120
      nontraumatic intracranial
        hemorrhage NEC I69.220
      specified disease NEC I69.820
      subarachnoid hemorrhage I69.020
  primary progressive G31.01 [F02.80]
    with behavioral disturbance G31.01
      [F02.81]
  progressive isolated G31.01 [F02.80]
    with behavioral disturbance G31.01
      [F02.81]
  sensory F80.2
  syphilis, tertiary A52.19
  Wernicke's (developmental) F80.2
Aphonia (organic) R49.1
  hysterical F44.4
  psychogenic F44.4
Aphthae, aphthous —see also condition
  Bednar's K12.0
  cachectic K14.0
  epizootic B08.8
  fever B08.8
  oral (recurrent) K12.0
  stomatitis (major) (minor) K12.0
  thrush B37.0

Aphthae, aphthous (Continued)
  ulcer (oral) (recurrent) K12.0
    genital organ (s) NEC
      female N76.6
      male N50.8
    larynx J38.7
Apical —see condition
Apiphobia F40.218
Aplasia —see also Agenesis
  abdominal muscle syndrome Q79.4
  alveolar process (acquired) —see
    Anomaly, alveolar
    congenital Q38.6
  aorta (congenital) Q25.4
  axialis extracorticalis (congenita) E75.29
  bone marrow (myeloid) D61.9
    congenital D61.01
  brain Q00.0
    part of Q04.3
  bronchus Q32.4
  cementum K00.4
  cerebellum Q04.3
  cervix (congenital) Q51.5
  congenital pure red cell D61.01
  corpus callosum Q04.0
  cutis congenita Q84.8
  erythrocyte congenital D61.01
  extracortical axial E75.29
  eye Q11.1
  fovea centralis (congenital) Q14.1
  gallbladder, congenital Q44.0
  iris Q13.1
  labyrinth, membranous Q16.5
  limb (congenital) Q73.8
    lower —see Defect, reduction, lower
      limb
    upper —see Agenesis, arm
  lung, congenital (bilateral) (unilateral)
    Q33.3
  pancreas Q45.0
  parathyroid-thymic D82.1
  Pelizaeus-Merzbacher E75.29
  penis Q55.5
  prostate Q55.4
  red cell (with thymoma) D60.9
    acquired D60.9
      due to drugs D60.9
    adult D60.9
    chronic D60.0
    congenital D61.01
    constitutional D61.01
    due to drugs D60.9
    hereditary D61.01
    of infants D61.01
    primary D61.01
    pure D61.01
      due to drugs D60.9
    specified type NEC D60.8
    transient D60.1
  round ligament Q52.8
  skin Q84.8
  spermatic cord Q55.4
  spleen Q89.01
  testicle Q55.0
  thymic, with immunodeficiency D82.1
  thyroid (congenital) (with myxedema)
    E03.1
  uterus Q51.0
  ventral horn cell Q06.1
Apnea, apneic (of) (spells) R06.81
  newborn NEC P28.4
    obstructive P28.4
    sleep (central) (obstructive) (primary)
      P28.3
  prematurity P28.4

Apnea, apneic (Continued)
  sleep G47.30
    central (primary) G47.31
      in conditions classified elsewhere
        G47.37
    obstructive (adult) (pediatric) G47.33
    primary central G47.31
    specified NEC G47.39
Apneumatosis, newborn P28.0
Apocrine metaplasia (breast) —see
  Dysplasia, mammary, specified type
  NEC
Apophysitis (bone) —see also
  Osteochondropathy
  calcaneus M92.8
  juvenile M92.9
Apoplectiform convulsions (cerebral
  ischemia) I67.82
Apoplexia, apoplexy, apoplectic
  adrenal A39.1
  heart (auricle) (ventricle) —see Infarct,
    myocardium
  heat T67.0
  hemorrhagic (stroke) —see Hemorrhage,
    intracranial
  meninges, hemorrhagic —see
    Hemorrhage, intracranial,
    subarachnoid
  uremic N18.9 [I68.8]
Appearance
  bizarre R46.1
  specified NEC R46.89
  very low level of personal hygiene
    R46.0
Appendage
  epididymal (organ of Morgagni) Q55.4
  intestine (epiploic) Q43.8
  preauricular Q17.0
  testicular (organ of Morgagni) Q55.29
Appendicitis (pneumococcal) (retrocecal)
  K37
  with
    perforation or rupture K35.2
    peritoneal abscess K35.3
      with peritonitis K35.2
    peritonitis K35.2
      with perforation or rupture K35.2
      generalized K35.2
      localized K35.3
  acute (catarrhal) (fulminating)
    (gangrenous) (obstructive)
    (retrocecal) (suppurative) K35.80
    with
      perforation or rupture K35.2
      peritoneal abscess K35.3
        with peritonitis K35.2
      peritonitis K35.2
        with perforation or rupture K35.2
        generalized K35.2
        localized K35.3
    specified NEC K35.89
  amebic A06.89
  chronic (recurrent) K36
  exacerbation —see Appendicitis, acute
  gangrenous —see Appendicitis, acute
  healed (obliterative) K36
  interval K36
  neurogenic K36
  obstructive K36
  recurrent K36
  relapsing K36
  subacute (adhesive) K36
  subsiding K36
  suppurative —see Appendicitis, acute
  tuberculous A18.32

Appendicopathia oxyurica B80
Appendix, appendicular —*see also*
    condition
    epididymis Q55.4
    Morgagni
        female Q50.5
        male (epididymal) Q55.4
            testicular Q55.29
    testis Q55.29
Appetite
    depraved —*see* Pica
    excessive R63.2
    lack or loss (*see also* Anorexia) R63.0
        nonorganic origin F50.8
        psychogenic F50.8
    perverted (hysterical) —*see* Pica
Apple peel syndrome Q41.1
Apprehension state F41.1
Apprehensiveness, abnormal F41.9
Approximal wear K03.0
Apraxia (classic) (ideational) (ideokinetic)
    (ideomotor) (motor) (verbal) R48.2
    following
        cerebrovascular disease I69.990
            cerebral infarction I69.390
            intracerebral hemorrhage I69.190
            nontraumatic intracranial
                hemorrhage NEC I69.290
            specified disease NEC I69.890
            subarachnoid hemorrhage I69.090
    oculomotor, congenital H51.8
Aptyalism K11.7
Apudoma —*see* Neoplasm, uncertain
    behavior, by site
Aqueous misdirection H40.83-
Arabicum elephantiasis —*see* Infestation,
    filarial
Arachnitis —*see* Meningitis
Arachnodactyly —*see* Syndrome,
    Marfan's
Arachnoiditis (acute) (adhesive) (basal)
    (brain) (cerebrospinal) —*see*
    Meningitis
Arachnophobia F40.210
Arboencephalitis, Australian A83.4
Arborization block (heart) I45.5
ARC (AIDS-related complex) B20
Arches —*see* condition
Arcuate uterus Q51.810
Arcuatus uterus Q51.810
Arcus (cornea) senilis —*see* Degeneration,
    cornea, senile
Arc-welder's lung J63.4
Areflexia R29.2
Areola —*see* condition
Argentaffinoma —*see also* Neoplasm,
    uncertain behavior, by site
    malignant —*see* Neoplasm, malignant,
        by site
    syndrome E34.0
Argininemia E72.21
Arginosuccinic aciduria E72.22
Argyll Robertson phenomenon, pupil or
    syndrome (syphilitic) A52.19
    atypical H57.09
    nonsyphilitic H57.09
Argyria, argyriasis
    conjunctival H11.13-
    from drug or medicament —*see* Table of
        drugs and chemicals, by substance
Argyrosis, conjunctival H11.13-
Arhinencephaly Q04.1
Ariboflavinosis E53.0
Arm —*see* condition

Arnold-Chiari disease, obstruction or
    syndrome (type II) Q07.00
    with
        hydrocephalus Q07.02
            with spina bifida Q07.03
        spina bifida Q07.01
            with hydrocephalus Q07.03
    type III —*see* Encephalocele
    type IV Q04.8
Aromatic amino-acid metabolism
    disorder E70.9
    specified NEC E70.8
Arousals, confusional G47.51
Arrest, arrested
    cardiac I46.9
        complicating
            abortion —*see* Abortion, by type,
                complicated by, cardiac arrest
            anesthesia (general) (local) or
                other sedation —*see* Table of
                drugs and chemicals, by drug,
                in labor and delivery O74.2
                in pregnancy O29.11-
                postpartum, puerperal O89.1
            delivery (cesarean) (instrumental)
                O75.4
        due to
            cardiac condition I46.2
            specified condition NEC I46.8
        intraoperative I97.71-
        newborn P29.81
        postprocedural I97.12-
            obstetric procedure O75.4
    cardiorespiratory —*see* Arrest,
        cardiac
    circulatory —*see* Arrest, cardiac
    deep transverse O64.0
    development or growth
        bone —*see* Disorder, bone,
            development or growth
        child R62.50
        tracheal rings Q32.1
    epiphyseal
        complete
            femur M89.15-
            humerus M89.12-
            tibia M89.16-
            ulna M89.13-
        forearm M89.13-
            specified NEC M89.13-
            ulna —*see* Arrest, epiphyseal, by
                type, ulna
        lower leg M89.16-
            specified NEC M89.168
            tibia —*see* Arrest, epiphyseal, by
                type, tibia
        partial
            femur M89.15-
            humerus M89.12-
            tibia M89.16-
            ulna M89.13-
        specified NEC M89.18
    granulopoiesis —*see* Agranulocytosis
    growth plate —*see* Arrest, epiphyseal
    heart —*see* Arrest, cardiac
    legal, anxiety concerning Z65.3
    physeal —*see* Arrest, epiphyseal
    respiratory R09.2
        newborn P28.81
    sinus I45.5
    spermatogenesis (complete) —*see*
        Azoospermia
        incomplete —*see* Oligospermia
    transverse (deep) O64.0

Arrhenoblastoma
    benign
        specified site —*see* Neoplasm,
            benign, by site
        unspecified site
            female D27.9
            male D29.20
    malignant
        specified site —*see* Neoplasm,
            malignant, by site
        unspecified site
            female C56.9
            male C62.90
    specified site —*see* Neoplasm, uncertain
        behavior, by site
    unspecified site
        female D39.10
        male D40.10
Arrhythmia (auricle)(cardiac)
    (juvenile)(nodal) (reflex)(sinus)
    (supraventricular)(transitory)
    (ventricle) I49.9
    block I45.9
    extrasystolic I49.49
    newborn
        bradycardia P29.12
        occurring before birth P03.819
            before onset of labor P03.810
            during labor P03.811
        tachycardia P29.11
    psychogenic F45.8
    specified NEC I49.8
    vagal R55
    ventricular re-entry I47.0
Arrillaga-Ayerza syndrome (pulmonary
    sclerosis with pulmonary
    hypertension) I27.0
Arsenical pigmentation L81.8
    from drug or medicament —*see* Table of
        drugs and medicaments
Arsenism —*see* Poisoning, arsenic
Arterial —*see* condition
Arteriofibrosis —*see* Arteriosclerosis
Arteriolar sclerosis —*see* Arteriosclerosis
Arteriolith —*see* Arteriosclerosis
Arteriolitis I77.6
    necrotizing, kidney I77.5
    renal —*see* Hypertension, kidney
Arteriolosclerosis —*see* Arteriosclerosis
Arterionephrosclerosis —*see*
    Hypertension, kidney
Arteriopathy I77.9
Arteriosclerosis, arteriosclerotic
    (diffuse) (obliterans) (of) (senile)
    (with calcification) I70.90
    aorta I70.0
    arteries of extremities —*see*
        Arteriosclerosis, extremities
    brain I67.2
    bypass graft
        coronary —*see* Arteriosclerosis,
            coronary, bypass graft
        extremities —*see* Arteriosclerosis,
            extremities, bypass graft
    cardiac —*see* Disease, heart, ischemic,
        atherosclerotic
    cardiopathy —*see* Disease, heart,
        ischemic, atherosclerotic
    cardiorenal —*see* Hypertension,
        cardiorenal
    cardiovascular —*see* Disease, heart,
        ischemic, atherosclerotic
    carotid (*see also* Occlusion, artery,
        carotid) I65.2-

Arteriosclerosis, arteriosclerotic
  (Continued)
central nervous system I67.2
cerebral I67.2
cerebrovascular I67.2
coronary (artery) I25.10
  bypass graft I25.810
    with
      angina pectoris I25.709
        with documented spasm I25.701
        specified type NEC I25.708
        unstable I25.700
      ischemic chest pain I25.709
    autologous artery I25.810
      with
        angina pectoris I25.729
          with documented spasm I25.721
          specified type I25.728
          unstable I25.720
        ischemic chest pain I25.729
    autologous vein I25.810
      with
        angina pectoris I25.719
          with documented spasm I25.711
          specified type I25.718
          unstable I25.710
        ischemic chest pain I25.719
    nonautologous biological I25.810
      with
        angina pectoris I25.739
          with documented spasm I25.731
          specified type I25.738
          unstable I25.730
        ischemic chest pain I25.739
    specified type NEC I25.810
      with
        angina pectoris I25.799
          with documented spasm I25.791
          specified type I25.798
          unstable I25.790
        ischemic chest pain I25.799
  due to
    calcified coronary lesion (severely) I25.84
    lipid rich plaque I25.83
  native vessel
    with
      angina pectoris I25.119
        with documented spasm I25.111
        specified type NEC I25.118
        unstable I25.110
      ischemic chest pain I25.119
  transplanted heart I25.811
    bypass graft I25.812
      with
        angina pectoris I25.769
          with documented spasm I25.761
          specified type I25.768
          unstable I25.760
        ischemic chest pain I25.769
    native coronary artery I25.811
      with
        angina pectoris I25.759
          with documented spasm I25.751
          specified type I25.758
          unstable I25.750
        ischemic chest pain I25.759

Arteriosclerosis, arteriosclerotic
  (Continued)
extremities (native arteries) I70.209
  bypass graft I70.309
    autologous vein graft I70.409
      leg I70.409
        with
          gangrene (and intermittent claudication, rest pain and ulcer) I70.469
          intermittent claudication I70.419
          rest pain (and intermittent claudication) I70.429
      bilateral I70.403
        with
          gangrene (and intermittent claudication, rest pain and ulcer) I70.463
          intermittent claudication I70.413
          rest pain (and intermittent claudication) I70.423
        specified type NEC I70.493
      left I70.402
        with
          gangrene (and intermittent claudication, rest pain and ulcer) I70.462
          intermittent claudication I70.412
          rest pain (and intermittent claudication) I70.422
          ulceration (and intermittent claudication and rest pain) I70.449
            ankle I70.443
            calf I70.442
            foot site NEC I70.445
            heel I70.444
            lower leg NEC I70.448
            midfoot I70.444
            thigh I70.441
        specified type NEC I70.492
      right I70.401
        with
          gangrene (and intermittent claudication, rest pain and ulcer) I70.461
          intermittent claudication I70.411
          rest pain (and intermittent claudication) I70.421
          ulceration (and intermittent claudication and rest pain) I70.439
            ankle I70.433
            calf I70.432
            foot site NEC I70.435
            heel I70.434
            lower leg NEC I70.438
            midfoot I70.434
            thigh I70.431
        specified type NEC I70.491
      specified type NEC I70.499

Arteriosclerosis, arteriosclerotic
  (Continued)
extremities (Continued)
  bypass graft (Continued)
    leg (Continued)
      specified NEC I70.408
        with
          gangrene (and intermittent claudication, rest pain and ulcer) I70.468
          intermittent claudication I70.418
          rest pain (and intermittent claudication) I70.428
          ulceration (and intermittent claudication and rest pain) I70.45
        specified type NEC I70.498
    leg I70.309
      with
        gangrene (and intermittent claudication, rest pain and ulcer) I70.369
        intermittent claudication I70.319
        rest pain (and intermittent claudication) I70.329
      bilateral I70.303
        with
          gangrene (and intermittent claudication, rest pain and ulcer) I70.363
          intermittent claudication I70.313
          rest pain (and intermittent claudication) I70.323
        specified type NEC I70.393
      left I70.302
        with
          gangrene (and intermittent claudication, rest pain and ulcer) I70.362
          intermittent claudication I70.312
          rest pain (and intermittent claudication) I70.322
          ulceration (and intermittent claudication and rest pain) I70.349
            ankle I70.343
            calf I70.342
            foot site NEC I70.345
            heel I70.344
            lower leg NEC I70.348
            midfoot I70.344
            thigh I70.341
        specified type NEC I70.392
      right I70.301
        with
          gangrene (and intermittent claudication, rest pain and ulcer) I70.361
          intermittent claudication I70.311
          rest pain (and intermittent claudication) I70.321

Arteriosclerosis, arteriosclerotic
(Continued)
extremities (Continued)
bypass graft (Continued)
leg (Continued)
right (Continued)
with (Continued)
ulceration (and intermittent
claudication and rest
pain) I70.339
ankle I70.333
calf I70.332
foot site NEC I70.335
heel I70.334
lower leg NEC
I70.338
midfoot I70.334
thigh I70.331
specified type NEC
I70.391
specified type NEC I70.399
nonautologous biological graft
I70.509
leg I70.509
with
gangrene (and intermittent
claudication, rest pain
and ulcer) I70.569
intermittent claudication
I70.519
rest pain (and intermittent
claudication)
I70.529
bilateral I70.503
with
gangrene (and
intermittent
claudication, rest
pain and ulcer)
I70.563
intermittent claudication
I70.513
rest pain (and intermittent
claudication)
I70.523
specified type NEC
I70.593
left I70.502
with
gangrene (and
intermittent
claudication, rest
pain and ulcer)
I70.562
intermittent claudication
I70.512
rest pain (and intermittent
claudication)
I70.522
ulceration (and
intermittent
claudication and rest
pain) I70.549
ankle I70.543
calf I70.542
foot site NEC
I70.545
heel I70.544
lower leg NEC
I70.548
midfoot I70.544
thigh I70.541
specified type NEC
I70.592

Arteriosclerosis, arteriosclerotic
(Continued)
extremities (Continued)
bypass graft (Continued)
nonautologous biological graft
(Continued)
leg (Continued)
right I70.501
with
gangrene (and
intermittent
claudication, rest
pain and ulcer)
I70.561
intermittent claudication
I70.511
rest pain (and intermittent
claudication)
I70.521
ulceration (and
intermittent
claudication and rest
pain) I70.539
ankle I70.533
calf I70.532
foot site NEC I70.535
heel I70.534
lower leg NEC I70.538
midfoot I70.534
thigh I70.531
specified type NEC I70.591
specified type NEC I70.599
specified NEC I70.508
with
gangrene (and intermittent
claudication, rest pain
and ulcer) I70.568
intermittent claudication
I70.518
rest pain (and intermittent
claudication) I70.528
ulceration (and intermittent
claudication and rest
pain) I70.55
specified type NEC I70.598
nonbiological graft I70.609
leg I70.609
with
gangrene (and intermittent
claudication, rest pain
and ulcer) I70.669
intermittent claudication
I70.619
rest pain (and intermittent
claudication) I70.629
bilateral I70.603
with
gangrene (and
intermittent
claudication, rest
pain and ulcer)
I70.663
intermittent claudication
I70.613
rest pain (and intermittent
claudication) I70.623
specified type NEC I70.693
left I70.602
with
gangrene (and
intermittent
claudication, rest
pain and ulcer)
I70.662

Arteriosclerosis, arteriosclerotic
(Continued)
extremities (Continued)
bypass graft (Continued)
nonbiological graft (Continued)
leg (Continued)
left (Continued)
with (Continued)
intermittent claudication
I70.612
rest pain (and intermittent
claudication)
I70.622
ulceration (and
intermittent
claudication and rest
pain) I70.649
ankle I70.643
calf I70.642
foot site NEC I70.645
heel I70.644
lower leg NEC I70.648
midfoot I70.644
thigh I70.641
specified type NEC I70.692
right I70.601
with
gangrene (and
intermittent
claudication, rest
pain and ulcer)
I70.661
intermittent claudication
I70.611
rest pain (and intermittent
claudication)
I70.621
ulceration (and
intermittent
claudication and rest
pain) I70.639
ankle I70.633
calf I70.632
foot site NEC I70.635
heel I70.634
lower leg NEC I70.638
midfoot I70.634
thigh I70.631
specified type NEC I70.691
specified type NEC I70.699
specified NEC I70.608
with
gangrene (and intermittent
claudication, rest pain
and ulcer) I70.668
intermittent claudication
I70.618
rest pain (and intermittent
claudication) I70.628
ulceration (and intermittent
claudication and rest
pain) I70.65
specified type NEC I70.698
specified graft NEC I70.709
leg I70.709
with
gangrene (and intermittent
claudication, rest
pain and ulcer)
I70.769
intermittent claudication
I70.719
rest pain (and intermittent
claudication) I70.729

Arteriosclerosis, arteriosclerotic
 (Continued)
 extremities *(Continued)*
 bypass graft *(Continued)*
 specified graft NEC *(Continued)*
 leg *(Continued)*
 bilateral I70.703
 with
 gangrene (and intermittent
 claudication, rest
 pain and ulcer)
 I70.763
 intermittent claudication
 I70.713
 rest pain (and intermittent
 claudication) I70.723
 specified type NEC I70.793
 left I70.702
 with
 gangrene (and intermittent
 claudication, rest
 pain and ulcer)
 I70.762
 intermittent claudication
 I70.712
 rest pain (and intermittent
 claudication) I70.722
 ulceration (and intermittent
 claudication and rest
 pain) I70.749
 ankle I70.743
 calf I70.742
 foot site NEC I70.745
 heel I70.744
 lower leg NEC I70.748
 midfoot I70.744
 thigh I70.741
 specified type NEC I70.792
 right I70.701
 with
 gangrene (and intermittent
 claudication, rest
 pain and ulcer)
 I70.761
 intermittent claudication
 I70.711
 rest pain (and intermittent
 claudication) I70.721
 ulceration (and
 intermittent
 claudication and rest
 pain) I70.739
 ankle I70.733
 calf I70.732
 foot site NEC I70.735
 heel I70.734
 lower leg NEC I70.738
 midfoot I70.734
 thigh I70.731
 specified type NEC I70.791
 specified type NEC I70.799
 specified NEC I70.708
 with
 gangrene (and intermittent
 claudication, rest pain
 and ulcer) I70.768
 intermittent claudication
 I70.718
 rest pain (and intermittent
 claudication) I70.728
 ulceration (and intermittent
 claudication and rest
 pain) I70.75
 specified type NEC I70.798

Arteriosclerosis, arteriosclerotic
 (Continued)
 extremities *(Continued)*
 bypass graft *(Continued)*
 specified NEC I70.308
 with
 gangrene (and intermittent
 claudication, rest pain
 and ulcer) I70.368
 intermittent claudication I70.318
 rest pain (and intermittent
 claudication) I70.328
 ulceration (and intermittent
 claudication and rest
 pain) I70.35
 specified type NEC I70.398
 leg I70.209
 with
 gangrene (and intermittent
 claudication, rest pain and
 ulcer) I70.269
 intermittent claudication I70.219
 rest pain (and intermittent
 claudication) I70.229
 bilateral I70.203
 with
 gangrene (and intermittent
 claudication, rest pain
 and ulcer) I70.263
 intermittent claudication
 I70.213
 rest pain (and intermittent
 claudication) I70.223
 specified type NEC I70.293
 left I70.202
 with
 gangrene (and intermittent
 claudication, rest pain
 and ulcer) I70.262
 intermittent claudication I70.212
 rest pain (and intermittent
 claudication) I70.222
 ulceration (and intermittent
 claudication and rest
 pain) I70.249
 ankle I70.243
 calf I70.242
 foot site NEC I70.245
 heel I70.244
 lower leg NEC I70.248
 midfoot I70.244
 thigh I70.241
 specified type NEC I70.292
 right I70.201
 with
 gangrene (and intermittent
 claudication, rest pain
 and ulcer) I70.261
 intermittent claudication
 I70.211
 rest pain (and intermittent
 claudication) I70.221
 ulceration (and intermittent
 claudication and rest
 pain) I70.239
 ankle I70.233
 calf I70.232
 foot site NEC I70.235
 heel I70.234
 lower leg NEC I70.238
 midfoot I70.234
 thigh I70.231
 specified type NEC I70.291
 specified type NEC I70.299

Arteriosclerosis, arteriosclerotic
 (Continued)
 extremities *(Continued)*
 specified site NEC I70.208
 with
 gangrene (and intermittent
 claudication, rest pain and
 ulcer) I70.268
 intermittent claudication I70.218
 rest pain (and intermittent
 claudication) I70.228
 ulceration (and intermittent
 claudication and rest pain)
 I70.25
 specified type NEC I70.298
 generalized I70.91
 heart (disease) —*see* Arteriosclerosis,
 coronary (artery)
 kidney —*see* Hypertension, kidney
 medial —*see* Arteriosclerosis,
 extremities
 mesenteric (artery) K55.1
 Mönckeberg's —*see* Arteriosclerosis,
 extremities
 myocarditis I51.4
 peripheral (of extremities) —*see*
 Arteriosclerosis, extremities
 pulmonary (idiopathic) I27.0
 renal (arterioles) —*see also*
 Hypertension, kidney
 artery I70.1
 retina (vascular) I70.8 [H35.0-]
 specified artery NEC I70.8
 spinal (cord) G95.19
 vertebral (artery) I67.2
Arteriospasm I73.9
Arteriovenous —*see* condition
Arteritis I77.6
 allergic M31.0
 aorta (nonsyphilitic) I77.6
 syphilitic A52.02
 aortic arch M31.4
 brachiocephalic M31.4
 brain I67.7
 syphilitic A52.04
 cerebral I67.7
 in systemic lupus erythematosus
 M32.19
 listerial A32.89
 syphilitic A52.04
 tuberculous A18.89
 coronary (artery) I25.89
 rheumatic I01.8
 chronic I09.89
 syphilitic A52.06
 cranial (left) (right), giant cell M31.6
 deformans —*see* Arteriosclerosis
 giant cell NEC M31.6
 with polymyalgia rheumatica M31.5
 necrosing or necrotizing M31.9
 specified NEC M31.8
 nodosa M30.0
 obliterans —*see* Arteriosclerosis
 pulmonary I28.8
 rheumatic —*see* Fever, rheumatic
 senile —*see* Arteriosclerosis
 suppurative I77.2
 syphilitic (general) A52.09
 brain A52.04
 coronary A52.06
 spinal A52.09
 temporal, giant cell M31.6
 young female aortic arch syndrome
 M31.4

Artery, arterial —*see also* condition
abscess I77.89
single umbilical Q27.0
Arthralgia (allergic) —*see also* Pain, joint
in caisson disease T70.3
temporomandibular M26.62
Arthritis, arthritic (acute) (chronic)
(nonpyogenic) (subacute) M19.90
allergic —*see* Arthritis, specified form
NEC
ankylosing (crippling) (spine) —*see also*
Spondylitis, ankylosing
sites other than spine —*see* Arthritis,
specified form NEC
atrophic —*see* Osteoarthritis
spine —*see* Spondylitis, ankylosing
back —*see* Spondylopathy, inflammatory
blennorrhagic (gonococcal) A54.42
Charcot's —*see* Arthropathy,
neuropathic
diabetic —*see* Diabetes, arthropathy,
neuropathic
syringomyelic G95.0
chylous (filarial) (*see also* category M01)
B74.9
climacteric (any site) NEC —*see*
Arthritis, specified form NEC
crystal (-induced) —*see* Arthritis, in,
crystals
deformans —*see* Osteoarthritis
degenerative —*see* Osteoarthritis
due to or associated with
acromegaly E22.0
brucellosis —*see* Brucellosis
caisson disease T70.3
diabetes —*see* Diabetes, arthropathy
dracontiasis (*see also* category M01)
B72
enteritis NEC
regional —*see* Enteritis, regional
erysipelas (*see also* category M01) A46
erythema
epidemic A25.1
nodosum L52
filariasis NOS B74.9
glanders A24.0
helminthiasis (*see also* category M01)
B83.9
hemophilia D66 [M36.2]
Henoch-(Schönlein) purpura D69.0
[M36.4]
human parvovirus (*see also* category
M01) B97.6
infectious disease NEC —*see* category
M01
leprosy (*see also* category M01) (*see
also* Leprosy) A30.9
Lyme disease A69.23
mycobacteria (*see also* category M01)
A31.8
parasitic disease NEC (*see also*
category M01) B89
paratyphoid fever (*see also*
category M01) (*see also* Fever,
paratyphoid) A01.4
rat bite fever (*see also* category M01)
A25.1
regional enteritis —*see* Enteritis,
regional
respiratory disorder NOS J98.9
serum sickness (*see also* Reaction,
serum) T80.69
syringomyelia G95.0
typhoid fever A01.04

Arthritis, arthritic (Continued)
epidemic erythema A25.1
febrile —*see* Fever, rheumatic
gonococcal A54.42
gouty (acute) —*see* Gout, idiopathic
in (due to)
acromegaly (*see also* subcategory
M14.8-) E22.0
amyloidosis (*see also* subcategory
M14.8-) E85.4
bacterial disease (*see also* subcategory
M01) A49.9
Behçet's syndrome M35.2
caisson disease (*see also* subcategory
M14.8-) T70.3
coliform bacilli (Escherichia coli) —
see Arthritis, in, pyogenic
organism NEC
crystals M11.9
dicalcium phosphate —*see* Arthritis,
in, crystals, specified type NEC
hydroxyapatite M11.0-
pyrophosphate —*see* Arthritis, in,
crystals, specified type NEC
specified type NEC M11.80
ankle M11.87-
elbow M11.82-
foot joint M11.87-
hand joint M11.84-
hip M11.85-
knee M11.86-
multiple sites M11.8-
shoulder M11.81-
vertebrae M11.88
wrist M11.83-
dermatoarthritis, lipoid E78.81
dracontiasis (dracunculiasis) (*see also*
category M01) B72
endocrine disorder NEC (*see also*
subcategory M14.8-) E34.9
enteritis, infectious NEC (*see also*
category M01) A09
specified organism NEC (*see also*
category M01) A08.8
erythema
multiforme (*see also* subcategory
M14.8-) L51.9
nodosum (*see also* subcategory
M14.8-) L52
gout —*see* Gout, idiopathic
helminthiasis NEC (*see also* category
M01) B83.9
hemochromatosis (*see also*
subcategory M14.8-) E83.118
hemoglobinopathy NEC D58.2 [M36.3]
hemophilia NEC D66 [M36.2]
Hemophilus influenzae M00.8- [B96.3]
Henoch(-Schönlein) purpura D69.0
[M36.4]
hyperparathyroidism NEC (*see also*
subcategory M14.8-) E21.3
hypersensitivity reaction NEC T78.49
[M36.4]
hypogammaglobulinemia (*see also*
subcategory M14.8-) D80.1
hypothyroidism NEC (*see also*
subcategory M14.8-) E03.9
infection —*see* Arthritis, pyogenic or
pyemic
spine —*see* Spondylopathy,
infective
infectious disease NEC —*see* category
M01
leprosy (*see also* category M01) A30.9

Arthritis, arthritic (Continued)
in (Continued)
leukemia NEC C95.9- [M36.1]
lipoid dermatoarthritis E78.81
Lyme disease A69.23
Mediterranean fever, familial (*see also*
subcategory M14.8-) E85.0
Meningococcus A39.83
metabolic disorder NEC (*see also*
subcategory M14.8-) E88.9
multiple myelomatosis C90.0- [M36.1]
mumps B26.85
mycosis NEC (*see also* category M01)
B49
myelomatosis (multiple)
C90.0- [M36.1]
neurological disorder NEC G98.0
ochronosis (*see also* subcategory
M14.8-) E70.29
O'nyong-nyong (*see also* category
M01) A92.1
parasitic disease NEC (*see also*
category M01) B89
paratyphoid fever (*see also* category
M01) A01.4
Pseudomonas —*see* Arthritis,
pyogenic, bacterial NEC
psoriasis L40.50
pyogenic organism NEC —*see*
Arthritis, pyogenic, bacterial
NEC
Reiter's disease —*see* Reiter's disease
respiratory disorder NEC (*see also*
subcategory M14.8-) J98.9
reticulosis, malignant (*see also*
subcategory M14.8-) C86.0
rubella B06.82
Salmonella (arizonae) (cholerae-suis)
(enteritidis) (typhimurium)
A02.23
sarcoidosis D86.86
specified bacteria NEC —*see* Arthritis,
pyogenic, bacterial NEC
sporotrichosis B42.82
syringomyelia G95.0
thalassemia NEC D56.9 [M36.3]
tuberculosis —*see* Tuberculosis,
arthritis
typhoid fever A01.04
urethritis, Reiter's —*see* Reiter's
disease
viral disease NEC (*see also* category
M01) B34.9
infectious or infective —*see also*
Arthritis, pyogenic or pyemic
spine —*see* Spondylopathy, infective
juvenile M08.90
with systemic onset —*see* Still's
disease
ankle M08.97-
elbow M08.92-
foot joint M08.97-
hand joint M08.94-
hip M08.95-
knee M08.96-
multiple site M08.99
pauciarticular M08.40
ankle M08.47-
elbow M08.42-
foot joint M08.47-
hand joint M08.44-
hip M08.45-
knee M08.46-
shoulder M08.41-

Arthritis, arthritic (Continued)
  juvenile (Continued)
    pauciarticular (Continued)
      vertebrae M08.48
      wrist M08.43-
    psoriatic L40.54
    rheumatoid —see Arthritis,
      rheumatoid, juvenile
    shoulder M08.91-
    specified type NEC M08.80
      ankle M08.87-
      elbow M08.82-
      foot joint M08.87-
      hand joint M08.84-
      hip M08.85-
      knee M08.86-
      multiple site M08.89
      shoulder M08.81-
      specified joint NEC M08.88
      wrist M08.83-
    vertebra M08.98
    wrist M08.93-
  meningococcal A39.83
  menopausal (any site) NEC —see
    Arthritis, specified form NEC
  mutilans (psoriatic) L40.52
  mycotic NEC (see also category M01)
    B49
  neuropathic (Charcot) —see
    Arthropathy, neuropathic
    diabetic —see Diabetes, arthropathy,
      neuropathic
    nonsyphilitic NEC G98.0
    syringomyelic G95.0
  ochronotic (see also subcategory M14.8-)
    E70.29
  palindromic (any site) —see
    Rheumatism, palindromic
  pneumococcal M00.10
    ankle M00.17-
    elbow M00.12-
    foot joint —see Arthritis,
      pneumococcal, ankle
    hand joint M00.14-
    hip M00.15-
    knee M00.16-
    multiple site M00.19
    shoulder M00.11-
    vertebra M00.18
    wrist M00.13-
  postdysenteric —see Arthropathy,
    postdysenteric
  postmeningococcal A39.84
  postrheumatic, chronic —see
    Arthropathy, postrheumatic,
    chronic
  primary progressive —see also Arthritis,
    specified form NEC
    spine —see Spondylitis, ankylosing
  psoriatic L40.50
  purulent (any site except spine) —see
    Arthritis, pyogenic or pyemic
    spine —see Spondylopathy, infective
  pyogenic or pyemic (any site except
    spine) M00.9
    bacterial NEC M00.80
      ankle M00.87-
      elbow M00.82-
      foot joint —see Arthritis, pyogenic,
        bacterial NEC, ankle
      hand joint M00.84-
      hip M00.85-
      knee M00.86-
      multiple site M00.89

Arthritis, arthritic (Continued)
  pyogenic or pyemic (Continued)
    bacterial NEC (Continued)
      shoulder M00.81-
      vertebra M00.88
      wrist M00.83-
    pneumococcal —see Arthritis,
      pneumococcal
    spine —see Spondylopathy,
      infective
    staphylococcal —see Arthritis,
      staphylococcal
    streptococcal —see Arthritis,
      streptococcal NEC
    pneumococcal —see Arthritis,
      pneumococcal
  reactive —see Reiter's disease
  rheumatic —see also Arthritis,
    rheumatoid
  acute or subacute —see Fever,
    rheumatic
  rheumatoid M06.9
    with
      carditis —see Rheumatoid,
        carditis
      endocarditis —see Rheumatoid,
        carditis
      heart involvement NEC —see
        Rheumatoid, carditis
      lung involvement —see
        Rheumatoid, lung
      myocarditis —see Rheumatoid,
        carditis
      myopathy —see Rheumatoid,
        myopathy
      pericarditis —see Rheumatoid,
        carditis
      polyneuropathy —see Rheumatoid,
        polyneuropathy
      rheumatoid factor —see Arthritis,
        rheumatoid, seropositive
      splenoadenomegaly and
        leukopenia —see Felty's
        syndrome
      vasculitis —see Rheumatoid,
        vasculitis
      visceral involvement NEC —see
        Rheumatoid, arthritis,
        with involvement of organs
        NEC
    juvenile (with or without
      rheumatoid factor)
      M08.00
      ankle M08.07-
      elbow M08.02-
      foot joint M08.07-
      hand joint M08.04-
      hip M08.05-
      knee M08.06-
      multiple site M08.09
      shoulder M08.01-
      vertebra M08.08
      wrist M08.03-
      seronegative M06.00
      ankle M06.07-
      elbow M06.02-
      foot joint M06.07-
      hand joint M06.04-
      hip M06.05-
      knee M06.06-
      multiple sites M06.09
      shoulder M06.01-
      vertebra M06.08
      wrist M06.03-

Arthritis, arthritic (Continued)
  rheumatoid (Continued)
    seropositive M05.9
      without organ involvement
        M05.70
      ankle M05.77-
      elbow M05.72-
      foot joint M05.77-
      hand joint M05.74-
      hip M05.75-
      knee M05.76-
      multiple sites M05.79
      shoulder M05.71-
      vertebra —see Spondylitis,
        ankylosing
      wrist M05.73-
    specified NEC M05.80
      ankle M05.87-
      elbow M05.82-
      foot joint M05.87-
      hand joint M05.84-
      hip M05.85-
      knee M05.86-
      multiple sites M05.89
      shoulder M05.81-
      vertebra —see Spondylitis,
        ankylosing
      wrist M05.83-
    specified type NEC M06.80
      ankle M06.87-
      elbow M06.82-
      foot joint M06.87-
      hand joint M06.84-
      hip M06.85-
      knee M06.86-
      multiple site M06.89
      shoulder M06.81-
      vertebra M06.88
      wrist M06.83-
    spine —see Spondylitis, ankylosing
  rubella B06.82
  scorbutic (see also subcategory M14.8-)
    E54
  senile or senescent —see Osteoarthritis
  septic (any site except spine) —see
    Arthritis, pyogenic or pyemic
    spine —see Spondylopathy,
      infective
  serum (nontherapeutic) (therapeutic) —
    see Arthropathy, postimmunization
  specified form NEC M13.80
    ankle M13.87-
    elbow M13.82-
    foot joint M13.87-
    hand joint M13.84-
    hip M13.85-
    knee M13.86-
    multiple site M13.89
    shoulder M13.81-
    specified joint NEC M13.88
    wrist M13.83-
  spine —see also Spondylopathy,
    inflammatory
    infectious or infective NEC —see
      Spondylopathy, infective
    Marie-Strümpell —see Spondylitis,
      ankylosing
    pyogenic —see Spondylopathy,
      infective
    rheumatoid —see Spondylitis,
      ankylosing
    traumatic (old) —see Spondylopathy,
      traumatic
    tuberculous A18.01

Arthritis, arthritic *(Continued)*
staphylococcal M00.00
  ankle M00.07-
  elbow M00.02-
  foot joint —*see* Arthritis,
      staphylococcal, ankle
  hand joint M00.04-
  hip M00.05-
  knee M00.06-
  multiple site M00.09
  shoulder M00.01-
  vertebra M00.08
  wrist M00.03-
streptococcal NEC M00.20
  ankle M00.27-
  elbow M00.22-
  foot joint —*see* Arthritis,
      streptococcal, ankle
  hand joint M00.24-
  hip M00.25-
  knee M00.26-
  multiple site M00.29
  shoulder M00.21-
  vertebra M00.28
  wrist M00.23-
suppurative —*see* Arthritis, pyogenic or
    pyemic
syphilitic (late) A52.16
  congenital A50.55 *[M12.80]*
syphilitica deformans (Charcot) A52.16
temporomandibular M26.69
toxic of menopause (any site) —*see*
    Arthritis, specified form NEC
transient —*see* Arthropathy, specified
    form NEC
traumatic (chronic) —*see* Arthropathy,
    traumatic
tuberculous A18.02
  spine A18.01
uratic —*see* Gout, idiopathic
urethritica (Reiter's) —*see* Reiter's
    disease
vertebral —*see* Spondylopathy,
    inflammatory
villous (any site) —*see* Arthropathy,
    specified form NEC
Arthrocele —*see* Effusion, joint
Arthrodesis status Z98.1
Arthrodynia —*see also* Pain, joint
Arthrodysplasia Q74.9
Arthrofibrosis, joint —*see* Ankylosis
Arthrogryposis (congenital) Q68.8
  multiplex congenita Q74.3
Arthrokatadysis M24.7
Arthropathy *(see also* Arthritis) M12.9
Charcot's —*see* Arthropathy, neuropathic
  diabetic —*see* Diabetes, arthropathy,
      neuropathic
  syringomyelic G95.0
cricoarytenoid J38.7
crystal(-induced) —*see* Arthritis, in,
    crystals
diabetic NEC —*see* Diabetes,
    arthropathy
distal interphalangeal, psoriatic L40.51
enteropathic M07.60
  ankle M07.67-
  elbow M07.62-
  foot joint M07.67-
  hand joint M07.64-
  hip M07.65-
  knee M07.66-
  multiple site M07.69

Arthropathy *(Continued)*
enteropathic *(Continued)*
  shoulder M07.61-
  vertebra M07.68
  wrist M07.63-
following intestinal bypass
    M02.00
  ankle M02.07-
  elbow M02.02-
  foot joint M02.07-
  hand joint M02.04-
  hip M02.05-
  knee M02.06-
  multiple site M02.09
  shoulder M02.01-
  vertebra M02.08
  wrist M02.03-
gouty —*see also* Gout, idiopathic
  in (due to)
    Lesch-Nyhan syndrome E79.1
        [M14.8-]
    sickle-cell disorders D57- *[M14.8-]*
hemophilic NEC D66 *[M36.2]*
  in (due to)
    hyperparathyroidism NEC E21.3
        [M14.8-]
    metabolic disease NOS E88.9
        [M14.8-]
in (due to)
  acromegaly E22.0 *[M14.8-]*
  amyloidosis E85.4 *[M14.8-]*
  blood disorder NOS D75.9 *[M36.3]*
  diabetes —*see* Diabetes, arthropathy
  endocrine disease NOS E34.9
      [M14.8-]
  erythema
    multiforme L51.9 *[M14.8-]*
    nodosum L52 *[M14.8-]*
  hemochromatosis E83.118 *[M14.8-]*
  hemoglobinopathy NEC D58.2
      [M36.3]
  hemophilia NEC D66 *[M36.2]*
  Henoch-Schönlein purpura D69.0
      [M36.4]
  hyperthyroidism E05.90 *[M14.8-]*
  hypothyroidism E03.9 *[M14.8-]*
  infective endocarditis I33.0 *[M12.80]*
  leukemia NEC C95.9- *[M36.1]*
  malignant histiocytosis C96.A *[M36.1]*
  metabolic disease NOS E88.9 *[M14.8-]*
  multiple myeloma C90.0- *[M36.1]*
  neoplastic disease NOS *(see also*
      Neoplasm) D49.9 *[M36.1]*
  nutritional deficiency *(see also*
      subcategory M14.8-) E63.9
  psoriasis NOS L40.50
  sarcoidosis D86.86
  syphilis (late) A52.77
    congenital A50.55 *[M12.80]*
  thyrotoxicosis *(see also* subcategory
      M14.8-) E05.90
  ulcerative colitis K51.90 *[M07.60]*
  viral hepatitis (postinfectious) NEC
      B19.9 *[M12.80]*
  Whipple's disease *(see also*
      subcategory M14.8-) K90.81
Jaccoud —*see* Arthropathy,
    postrheumatic, chronic
juvenile —*see* Arthritis, juvenile
  psoriatic L40.54
mutilans (psoriatic) L40.52
neuropathic (Charcot) M14.60
  ankle M14.67-

Arthropathy *(Continued)*
neuropathic *(Continued)*
  diabetic —*see* Diabetes, arthropathy,
      neuropathic
  elbow M14.62-
  foot joint M14.67-
  hand joint M14.64-
  hip M14.65-
  knee M14.66-
  multiple site M14.69
  nonsyphilitic NEC G98.0
  shoulder M14.61-
  syringomyelic G95.0
  vertebra M14.68
  wrist M14.63-
osteopulmonary —*see*
    Osteoarthropathy, hypertrophic,
    specified NEC
postdysenteric M02.10
  ankle M02.17-
  elbow M02.12-
  foot joint M02.17-
  hand joint M02.14-
  hip M02.15-
  knee M02.16-
  multiple site M02.19
  shoulder M02.11-
  vertebra M02.18
  wrist M02.13-
postimmunization M02.20
  ankle M02.27-
  elbow M02.22-
  foot joint M02.27-
  hand joint M02.24-
  hip M02.25-
  knee M02.26-
  multiple site M02.29
  shoulder M02.21-
  vertebra M02.28
  wrist M02.23-
postinfectious NEC B99 *[M12.80]*
  in (due to)
    enteritis due to Yersinia
        enterocolitica A04.6 *[M12.80]*
    syphilis A52.77
    viral hepatitis NEC B19.9 *[M12.80]*
postrheumatic, chronic (Jaccoud)
    M12.00
  ankle M12.07-
  elbow M12.02-
  foot joint M12.07-
  hand joint M12.04-
  hip M12.05-
  knee M12.06-
  multiple site M12.09
  shoulder M12.01-
  specified joint NEC M12.08
  wrist M12.03-
psoriatic NEC L40.59
  interphalangeal, distal L40.51
reactive M02.9
  in (due to)
    infective endocarditis I33.0
        [M02.9]
  specified type NEC M02.80
    ankle M02.87-
    elbow M02.82-
    foot joint M02.87-
    hand joint M02.84-
    hip M02.85-
    knee M02.86-
    multiple site M02.89
    shoulder M02.81-

Arthropathy (*Continued*)
  reactive (*Continued*)
    specified type NEC (*Continued*)
      vertebra M02.88
      wrist M02.83-
    specified form NEC M12.80
      ankle M12.87-
      elbow M12.82-
      foot joint M12.87-
      hand joint M12.84-
      hip M12.85-
      knee M12.86-
      multiple site M12.89
      shoulder M12.81-
      specified joint NEC M12.88
      wrist M12.83-
    syringomyelic G95.0
    tabes dorsalis A52.16
    tabetic A52.16
    transient —*see* Arthropathy, specified
      form NEC
    traumatic M12.50
      ankle M12.57-
      elbow M12.52-
      foot joint M12.57-
      hand joint M12.54-
      hip M12.55-
      knee M12.56-
      multiple site M12.59
      shoulder M12.51-
      specified joint NEC M12.58
      wrist M12.53-
Arthropyosis —*see* Arthritis, pyogenic or
  pyemic
Arthrosis (deformans) (degenerative)
  (localized) (*see also* Osteoarthritis)
  M19.90
  spine —*see* Spondylosis
Arthus' phenomenon or reaction T78.41
  due to
    drug —*see* Table of drugs and
      chemicals, by drug
Articular —*see* condition
Articulation, reverse (teeth)
  M26.24
Artificial
  insemination complication —*see*
    Complications, artificial,
    fertilization
  opening status (functioning) (without
    complication) Z93.9
    anus (colostomy) Z93.3
    colostomy Z93.3
    cystostomy Z93.50
      appendico-vesicostomy
        Z93.52
      cutaneous Z93.51
      specified NEC Z93.59
    enterostomy Z93.4
    gastrostomy Z93.1
    ileostomy Z93.2
    intestinal tract NEC Z93.4
    jejunostomy Z93.4
    nephrostomy Z93.6
    specified site NEC Z93.8
    tracheostomy Z93.0
    ureterostomy Z93.6
    urethrostomy Z93.6
    urinary tract NEC Z93.6
    vagina Z93.8
  vagina status Z93.8
Arytenoid —*see* condition
Asbestosis (occupational) J61

ASC-H (atypical squamous cells cannot
  exclude high grade squamous
  intraepithelial lesion on cytologic
  smear)
  anus R85.611
  cervix R87.611
  vagina R87.621
ASC-US (atypical squamous cells of
  undetermined significance on
  cytologic smear)
  anus R85.610
  cervix R87.610
  vagina R87.620
Ascariasis B77.9
  with
    complications NEC B77.89
    intestinal complications B77.0
    pneumonia, pneumonitis B77.81
Ascaridosis, ascaridiasis —*see* Ascariasis
Ascaris (infection) (infestation)
  (lumbricoides) —*see* Ascariasis
Ascending —*see* condition
Aschoff's bodies —*see* Myocarditis,
  rheumatic
Ascites (abdominal) R18.8
  cardiac I50.9
  chylous (nonfilarial) I89.8
    filarial —*see* Infestation, filarial
  due to
    cirrhosis, alcoholic K70.31
    hepatitis
      alcoholic K70.11
      chronic active K71.51
      S. japonicum B65.2
  heart I50.9
  malignant R18.0
  pseudochylous R18.8
  syphilitic A52.74
  tuberculous A18.31
Aseptic —*see* condition
Asherman's syndrome N85.6
Asialia K11.7
Asiatic cholera —*see* Cholera
Asimultagnosia (simultanagnosia) R48.3
Askin's tumor —*see* Neoplasm,
  connective tissue, malignant
Asocial personality F60.2
Asomatognosia R41.4
Aspartylglucosaminuria E77.1
Asperger's disease or syndrome F84.5
Aspergilloma —*see* Aspergillosis
Aspergillosis (with pneumonia) B44.9
  bronchopulmonary, allergic B44.81
  disseminated B44.7
  generalized B44.7
  pulmonary NEC B44.1
    allergic B44.81
    invasive B44.0
    specified NEC B44.89
  tonsillar B44.2
Aspergillus (flavus) (fumigatus)
  (infection) (terreus) —*see*
  Aspergillosis
Aspermatogenesis —*see* Azoospermia
Aspermia (testis) —*see* Azoospermia
Asphyxia, asphyxiation (by) R09.01
  antenatal P84
  birth P84
  bunny bag —*see* Asphyxia, due to,
    mechanical threat to breathing,
    trapped in bed clothes
  crushing S28.0
  drowning T75.1

Asphyxia, asphyxiation (*Continued*)
  gas, fumes, or vapor —*see* Table of
    drugs and chemicals
  inhalation —*see* Inhalation
  intrauterine P84
  local I73.00
    with gangrene I73.01
  mucus —*see also* Foreign body,
    respiratory tract, causing
    asphyxia
  newborn P84
  pathological R09.01
  postnatal P84
    mechanical —*see* Asphyxia, due
      to, mechanical threat to
      breathing
  prenatal P84
  reticularis R23.1
  strangulation —*see* Asphyxia, due
    to, mechanical threat to
    breathing
  submersion T75.1
  traumatic T71.9
  due to
    crushed chest S28.0
    foreign body (in) —*see* Foreign
      body, respiratory tract,
      causing asphyxia
    low oxygen content of ambient air
      T71.20
    due to
      being trapped in
        low oxygen environment
          T71.29
        in car trunk T71.221
          circumstances
            undetermined
            T71.224
          done with intent to
            harm by
            another person
            T71.223
          self T71.222
        in refrigerator T71.231
          circumstances
            undetermined
            T71.234
          done with intent to
            harm by
            another person
            T71.233
          self T71.232
    cave-in T71.21
    mechanical threat to breathing
      (accidental) T71.191
      circumstances undetermined
        T71.194
      done with intent to harm by
        another person T71.193
      self T71.192
    hanging T71.161
      circumstances undetermined
        T71.164
      done with intent to harm by
        another person T71.163
      self T71.162
    plastic bag T71.121
      circumstances undetermined
        T71.124
      done with intent to
        harm by
        another person T71.123
      self T71.122

Asphyxia, asphyxiation (Continued)
  traumatic (Continued)
    due to (Continued)
      mechanical threat to breathing
        (Continued)
        smothering
          in furniture T71.151
            circumstances undetermined
              T71.154
            done with intent to harm by
              another person T71.153
            self T71.152
          under
            another person's body
              T71.141
              circumstances
                undetermined
                T71.144
              done with intent to harm
                T71.143
            pillow T71.111
              circumstances
                undetermined
                T71.114
              done with intent to harm
                by
                another person T71.113
                self T71.112
        trapped in bed clothes T71.131
          circumstances undetermined
            T71.134
          done with intent to harm by
            another person T71.133
            self T71.132
  vomiting, vomitus —see Foreign body,
    respiratory tract, causing
    asphyxia
Aspiration
  amniotic (clear) fluid (newborn)
    P24.10
    with
      pneumonia (pneumonitis) P24.11
      respiratory symptoms P24.11
  blood
    newborn (without respiratory
      symptoms) P24.20
      with
        pneumonia (pneumonitis)
          P24.21
        respiratory symptoms P24.21
    specified age NEC —see Foreign
      body, respiratory tract
  bronchitis J69.0
  food or foreign body (with
    asphyxiation) —see Asphyxia,
    food
  liquor (amnii) (newborn) P24.10
    with
      pneumonia (pneumonitis) P24.11
      respiratory symptoms P24.11
  meconium (newborn) (without
    respiratory symptoms) P24.00
    with
      pneumonitis (pneumonitis)
        P24.01
      respiratory symptoms P24.01
  milk (newborn) (without respiratory
    symptoms) P24.30
    with
      pneumonia (pneumonitis)
        P24.31
      respiratory symptoms P24.31
  specified age NEC —see Foreign
    body, respiratory tract

Aspiration (Continued)
  mucus —see also Foreign body, by site,
    causing asphyxia
    newborn P24.10
      with
        pneumonia (pneumonitis)
          P24.11
        respiratory symptoms P24.11
    neonatal P24.9
      specific NEC (without respiratory
        symptoms) P24.80
        with
          pneumonia (pneumonitis)
            P24.81
          respiratory symptoms P24.81
    newborn P24.9
      specific NEC (without respiratory
        symptoms) P24.80
        with
          pneumonia (pneumonitis)
            P24.81
          respiratory symptoms P24.81
  pneumonia J69.0
  pneumonitis J69.0
  syndrome of newborn —see Aspiration,
    by substance, with pneumonia
  vernix caseosa (newborn) P24.80
    with
      pneumonia (pneumonitis) P24.81
      respiratory symptoms P24.81
  vomitus —see also Foreign body,
    respiratory tract
    newborn (without respiratory
      symptoms) P24.30
      with
        pneumonia (pneumonitis)
          P24.31
        respiratory symptoms P24.31
Asplenia (congenital) Q89.01
  postsurgical Z90.81
Assam fever B55.0
Assault, sexual —see Maltreatment
Assmann's focus NEC A15.0
Astasia (-abasia) (hysterical) F44.4
Asteatosis cutis L85.3
Astereognosia, astereognosis R48.1
Asterixis R27.8
  in liver disease K71.3
Asteroid hyalitis —see Deposit,
  crystalline
Asthenia, asthenic R53.1
  cardiac (see also Failure, heart) I50.9
    psychogenic F45.8
  cardiovascular (see also Failure, heart)
    I50.9
    psychogenic F45.8
  heart (see also Failure, heart) I50.9
    psychogenic F45.8
  hysterical F44.4
  myocardial (see also Failure, heart) I50.9
    psychogenic F45.8
  nervous F48.8
  neurocirculatory F45.8
  neurotic F48.8
  psychogenic F48.8
  psychoneurotic F48.8
  psychophysiologic F48.8
  reaction (psychophysiologic) F48.8
  senile R54
Asthenopia —see also Discomfort, visual
  hysterical F44.6
  psychogenic F44.6
Asthenospermia —see Abnormal,
  specimen, male genital organs

Asthma, asthmatic (bronchial) (catarrh)
  (spasmodic) J45.909
  with
    chronic obstructive bronchitis J44.9
      with
        acute lower respiratory infection
          J44.0
        exacerbation (acute) J44.1
    chronic obstructive pulmonary
      disease J44.9
      with
        acute lower respiratory infection
          J44.0
        exacerbation (acute) J44.1
    exacerbation (acute) J45.901
    hay fever —see Asthma, allergic
      extrinsic
    rhinitis, allergic —see Asthma, allergic
      extrinsic
    status asthmaticus J45.902
  allergic extrinsic J45.909
    with
      exacerbation (acute) J45.901
      status asthmaticus J45.902
  atopic —see Asthma, allergic
    extrinsic
  cardiac —see Failure, ventricular, left
  cardiobronchial I50.1
  childhood J45.909
    with
      exacerbation (acute) J45.901
      status asthmaticus J45.902
  chronic obstructive J44.9
    with
      acute lower respiratory infection
        J44.0
      exacerbation (acute) J44.1
  collier's J60
  cough variant J45.991
  detergent J69.8
  due to
    detergent J69.8
    inhalation of fumes J68.3
  eosinophilic J82
  extrinsic, allergic —see Asthma, allergic
    extrinsic
  grinder's J62.8
  hay —see Asthma, allergic extrinsic
  heart I50.1
  idiosyncratic —see Asthma, nonallergic
  intermittent (mild) J45.20
    with
      exacerbation (acute) J45.21
      status asthmaticus J45.22
  intrinsic, nonallergic —see Asthma,
    nonallergic
  Kopp's E32.8
  late-onset J45.909
    with
      exacerbation (acute) J45.901
      status asthmaticus J45.902
  mild intermittent J45.20
    with
      exacerbation (acute) J45.21
      status asthmaticus J45.22
  mild persistent J45.30
    with
      exacerbation (acute) J45.31
      status asthmaticus J45.32
  Millar's (laryngismus stridulus) J38.5
  miner's J60
  mixed J45.909
    with
      exacerbation (acute) J45.901
      status asthmaticus J45.902

Asthma, asthmatic *(Continued)*
  moderate persistent J45.40
    with
      exacerbation (acute) J45.41
      status asthmaticus J45.42
  nervous —*see* Asthma, nonallergic
  nonallergic (intrinsic) J45.909
    with
      exacerbation (acute) J45.901
      status asthmaticus J45.902
  persistent
    mild J45.30
      with
        exacerbation (acute) J45.31
        status asthmaticus J45.32
    moderate J45.40
      with
        exacerbation (acute) J45.41
        status asthmaticus J45.42
    severe J45.50
      with
        exacerbation (acute)
          J45.51
        status asthmaticus
          J45.52
  platinum J45.998
  pneumoconiotic NEC J64
  potter's J62.8
  predominantly allergic
    J45.909
  psychogenic F54
  pulmonary eosinophilic J82
  red cedar J67.8
  Rostan's I50.1
  sandblaster's J62.8
  sequoiosis J67.8
  severe persistent J45.50
    with
      exacerbation (acute) J45.51
      status asthmaticus J45.52
  specified NEC J45.998
  stonemason's J62.8
  thymic E32.8
  tuberculous —*see* Tuberculosis,
    pulmonary
  Wichmann's (laryngismus stridulus)
    J38.5
  wood J67.8
Astigmatism (compound) (congenital)
    H52.20-
  irregular H52.21-
  regular H52.22-
Astraphobia F40.220
Astroblastoma
  specified site —*see* Neoplasm,
    malignant, by site
  unspecified site C71.9
Astrocytoma (cystic)
  anaplastic
    specified site —*see* Neoplasm,
      malignant, by site
    unspecified site C71.9
  fibrillary
    specified site —*see* Neoplasm,
      malignant, by site
    unspecified site C71.9
  fibrous
    specified site —*see* Neoplasm,
      malignant, by site
    unspecified site C71.9
  gemistocytic
    specified site —*see* Neoplasm,
      malignant, by site
    unspecified site C71.9

Astrocytoma *(Continued)*
  juvenile
    specified site —*see* Neoplasm,
      malignant, by site
    unspecified site C71.9
  pilocytic
    specified site —*see* Neoplasm,
      malignant, by site
    unspecified site C71.9
  piloid
    specified site —*see* Neoplasm,
      malignant, by site
    unspecified site C71.9
  protoplasmic
    specified site —*see* Neoplasm,
      malignant, by site
    unspecified site C71.9
  specified site NEC —*see* Neoplasm,
    malignant, by site
  subependymal D43.2
    giant cell
      specified site —*see* Neoplasm,
        uncertain behavior, by site
      unspecified site D43.2
    specified site —*see* Neoplasm,
      uncertain behavior, by site
    unspecified site D43.2
  unspecified site C71.9
Astroglioma
  specified site —*see* Neoplasm,
    malignant, by site
  unspecified site C71.9
Asymbolia R48.8
Asymmetry —*see also* Distortion
  between native and reconstructed
    breast N65.1
  face Q67.0
  jaw (lower) —*see* Anomaly, dentofacial,
    jaw-cranial base relationship,
    asymmetry
Asynergia, asynergy R27.8
  ventricular I51.89
Asystole (heart) —*see* Arrest, cardiac
At risk
  for falling Z91.81
Ataxia, ataxy, ataxic R27.0
  acute R27.8
  brain (hereditary) G11.9
  cerebellar (hereditary) G11.9
    with defective DNA repair G11.3
    alcoholic G31.2
    early-onset G11.1
    in
      alcoholism G31.2
      myxedema E03.9 *[G13.2]*
      neoplastic disease *(see also*
        Neoplasm) D49.9
        [G13.1]
      specified disease NEC G32.81
    late-onset (Marie's) G11.2
  cerebral (hereditary) G11.9
  congenital nonprogressive G11.0
  family, familial —*see* Ataxia,
    hereditary
  following
    cerebrovascular disease I69.993
      cerebral infarction I69.393
      intracerebral hemorrhage
        I69.193
      nontraumatic intracranial
        hemorrhage NEC I69.293
      specified disease NEC I69.893
      subarachnoid hemorrhage
        I69.093

Ataxia, ataxy, ataxic *(Continued)*
  Friedreich's (heredofamilial) (cerebellar)
    (spinal) G11.1
  gait R26.0
    hysterical F44.4
  general R27.8
  hereditary G11.9
    with neuropathy G60.2
    cerebellar —*see* Ataxia, cerebellar
    spastic G11.4
    specified NEC G11.8
    spinal (Friedreich's) G11.1
  heredofamilial —*see* Ataxia, hereditary
  Hunt's G11.1
  hysterical F44.4
  locomotor (progressive) (syphilitic)
    (partial) (spastic) A52.11
    diabetic —*see* Diabetes, ataxia
  Marie's (cerebellar) (heredofamilial)
    (late- onset) G11.2
  nonorganic origin F44.4
  nonprogressive, congenital G11.0
  psychogenic F44.4
  Roussy-Lévy G60.0
  Sanger-Brown's (hereditary) G11.2
  spastic hereditary G11.4
  spinal
    hereditary (Friedreich's) G11.1
    progressive (syphilitic) A52.11
  spinocerebellar, X-linked recessive
    G11.1
  telangiectasia (Louis-Bar) G11.3
Ataxia-telangiectasia (Louis-Bar)
    G11.3
Atelectasis (massive) (partial) (pressure)
    (pulmonary) J98.11
  newborn P28.10
    due to resorption P28.11
    partial P28.19
    primary P28.0
    secondary P28.19
  primary (newborn) P28.0
  tuberculous —*see* Tuberculosis,
    pulmonary
Atelocardia Q24.9
Atelomyelia Q06.1
Atheroembolism
  of
    extremities
      lower I75.02-
      upper I75.01-
    kidney I75.81
    specified NEC I75.89
Atheroma, atheromatous *(see also*
    Arteriosclerosis) I70.90
  aorta, aortic I70.0
    valve *(see also* Endocarditis, aortic)
      I35.8
  aorto-iliac I70.0
  artery —*see* Arteriosclerosis
  basilar (artery) I67.2
  carotid (artery) (common) (internal)
    I67.2
  cerebral (arteries) I67.2
  coronary (artery) I25.10
    with angina pectoris —*see* Arterio-
      sclerosis, coronary (artery)
  degeneration —*see* Arteriosclerosis
  heart, cardiac —*see* Disease, heart,
    ischemic, atherosclerotic
  mitral (valve) I34.8
  myocardium, myocardial —*see*
    Disease, heart, ischemic,
    atherosclerotic

Atheroma, atheromatous *(Continued)*
  pulmonary valve (heart) *(see also*
      Endocarditis, pulmonary) I37.8
  tricuspid (heart) (valve) I36.8
  valve, valvular —*see* Endocarditis
  vertebral (artery) I67.2
Atheromatosis —*see* Arteriosclerosis
Atherosclerosis —*see also* Arteriosclerosis
  coronary
      artery I25.10
          with angina pectoris —*see*
              Arteriosclerosis, coronary
              (artery),
          due to
              calcified coronary lesion
                  (severely) I25.84
              lipid rich plaque I25.83
      transplanted heart I25.811
          bypass graft I25.812
              with angina pectoris —*see*
                  Arteriosclerosis, coronary
                  (artery)
          native coronary artery I25.811
              with angina pectoris —*see*
                  Arteriosclerosis, coronary
                  (artery)
Athetosis (acquired) R25.8
  bilateral (congenital) G80.3
  congenital (bilateral) (double) G80.3
  double (congenital) G80.3
  unilateral R25.8
Athlete's
  foot B35.3
  heart I51.7
Athrepsia E41
Athyrea (acquired) —*see also*
      Hypothyroidism
  congenital E03.1
Atonia, atony, atonic
  bladder (sphincter) (neurogenic) N31.2
  capillary I78.8
  cecum K59.8
      psychogenic F45.8
  colon —*see* Atony, intestine
  congenital P94.2
  esophagus K22.8
  intestine K59.8
      psychogenic F45.8
  stomach K31.89
      neurotic or psychogenic F45.8
  uterus (during labor) O62.2
      with hemorrhage (postpartum)
          O72.1
      postpartum (with hemorrhage) O72.1
          without hemorrhage O75.89
Atopy —*see* History, allergy
Atransferrinemia, congenital E88.09
Atresia, atretic
  alimentary organ or tract NEC Q45.8
      upper Q40.8
  ani, anus, anal (canal) Q42.3
      with fistula Q42.2
  aorta (arch) (ring) Q25.2
  aortic (orifice) (valve) Q23.0
      arch Q25.2
      congenital with hypoplasia of
          ascending aorta and defective
          development of left ventricle
          (with mitral stenosis) Q23.4
      in hypoplastic left heart syndrome
          Q23.4
  aqueduct of Sylvius Q03.0
      with spina bifida —*see* Spina bifida,
          with hydrocephalus

Atresia, atretic *(Continued)*
  artery NEC Q27.8
      cerebral Q28.3
      coronary Q24.5
      digestive system Q27.8
      eye Q15.8
      lower limb Q27.8
      pulmonary Q25.5
      specified site NEC Q27.8
      umbilical Q27.0
      upper limb Q27.8
  auditory canal (external) Q16.1
  bile duct (common) (congenital)
          (hepatic) Q44.2
      acquired —*see* Obstruction, bile duct
  bladder (neck) Q64.39
      obstruction Q64.31
  bronchus Q32.4
  cecum Q42.8
  cervix (acquired) N88.2
      congenital Q51.828
      in pregnancy or childbirth —*see*
          Anomaly, cervix, in pregnancy
          or childbirth
          causing obstructed labor O65.5
  choana Q30.0
  colon Q42.9
      specified NEC Q42.8
  common duct Q44.2
  cricoid cartilage Q31.8
  cystic duct Q44.2
      acquired K82.8
          with obstruction K82.0
  digestive organs NEC Q45.8
  duodenum Q41.0
  ear canal Q16.1
  ejaculatory duct Q55.4
  epiglottis Q31.8
  esophagus Q39.0
      with tracheoesophageal fistula Q39.1
  eustachian tube Q17.8
  fallopian tube (congenital) Q50.6
      acquired N97.1
  follicular cyst N83.0
  foramen of
      Luschka Q03.1
          with spina bifida —*see* Spina bifida,
              with hydrocephalus
      Magendie Q03.1
          with spina bifida —*see* Spina bifida,
              with hydrocephalus
  gallbladder Q44.1
  genital organ
      external
          female Q52.79
          male Q55.8
      internal
          female Q52.8
          male Q55.8
  glottis Q31.8
  gullet Q39.0
      with tracheoesophageal fistula Q39.1
  heart valve NEC Q24.8
      pulmonary Q22.0
      tricuspid Q22.4
  hymen Q52.3
      acquired (postinfective) N89.6
  ileum Q41.2
  intestine (small) Q41.9
      large Q42.9
          specified NEC Q42.8
  iris, filtration angle Q15.0
  jejunum Q41.1

Atresia, atretic *(Continued)*
  lacrimal apparatus Q10.4
  larynx Q31.8
  meatus urinarius Q64.33
  mitral valve Q23.2
      in hypoplastic left heart syndrome
          Q23.4
  nares (anterior) (posterior) Q30.0
  nasopharynx Q34.8
  nose, nostril Q30.0
      acquired J34.89
  oesophagus Q39.0
      with tracheoesophageal fistula Q39.1
  organ or site NEC Q89.8
  osseous meatus (ear) Q16.1
  oviduct (congenital) Q50.6
      acquired N97.1
  parotid duct Q38.4
      acquired K11.8
  pulmonary (artery) Q25.5
      valve Q22.0
  pulmonic Q22.0
  pupil Q13.2
  rectum Q42.1
      with fistula Q42.0
  salivary duct Q38.4
      acquired K11.8
  sublingual duct Q38.4
      acquired K11.8
  submandibular duct Q38.4
      acquired K11.8
  submaxillary duct Q38.4
      acquired K11.8
  thyroid cartilage Q31.8
  trachea Q32.1
  tricuspid valve Q22.4
  ureter Q62.10
      pelvic junction Q62.11
      vesical orifice Q62.12
  ureteropelvic junction Q62.11
  ureterovesical orifice Q62.12
  urethra (valvular) Q64.39
      stricture Q64.32
  urinary tract NEC Q64.8
  uterus Q51.818
      acquired N85.8
  vagina (congenital) Q52.4
      acquired (postinfectional) (senile)
          N89.5
  vas deferens Q55.3
  vascular NEC Q27.8
      cerebral Q28.3
      digestive system Q27.8
      lower limb Q27.8
      specified site NEC Q27.8
      upper limb Q27.8
  vein NEC Q27.8
      digestive system Q27.8
      great Q26.8
      lower limb Q27.8
      portal Q26.5
      pulmonary Q26.3
      specified site NEC Q27.8
      upper limb Q27.8
  vena cava (inferior) (superior) Q26.8
  vesicourethral orifice Q64.31
  vulva Q52.79
      acquired N90.5
Atrichia, atrichosis —*see* Alopecia
Atrophia —*see also* Atrophy
  cutis senilis L90.8
      due to radiation L57.8
  gyrata of choroid and retina H31.23

Atrophia *(Continued)*
  senilis R54
    dermatological L90.8
      due to radiation (nonionizing)
        (solar) L57.8
  unguium L60.3
    congenita Q84.6
Atrophie blanche (en plaque) (de Milian)
  L95.0
Atrophoderma, atrophodermia (of)
  L90.9
  diffusum (idiopathic) L90.4
  maculatum L90.8
    et striatum L90.8
      due to syphilis A52.79
    syphilitic A51.39
  neuriticum L90.8
  Pasini and Pierini L90.3
  pigmentosum Q82.1
  reticulatum symmetricum faciei
    L66.4
  senile L90.8
    due to radiation (nonionizing) (solar)
      L57.8
  vermiculata (cheeks) L66.4
Atrophy, atrophic (of)
  adrenal (capsule) (gland) E27.49
    primary (autoimmune) E27.1
  alveolar process or ridge (edentulous)
    K08.20
  anal sphincter (disuse) N81.84
  appendix K38.8
  arteriosclerotic —*see* Arteriosclerosis
  bile duct (common) (hepatic) K83.8
  bladder N32.89
    neurogenic N31.8
  blanche (en plaque) (of Milian) L95.0
  bone (senile) NEC —*see also* Disorder,
    bone, specified type NEC
    due to
      tabes dorsalis (neurogenic) A52.11
  brain (cortex) (progressive) G31.9
    frontotemporal circumscribed G31.01
      [F02.80]
      with behavioral disturbance G31.01
        [F02.81]
    senile NEC G31.1
  breast N64.2
    obstetric —*see* Disorder, breast,
      specified type NEC
  buccal cavity K13.79
  cardiac —*see* Degeneration, myocardial
  cartilage (infectional) (joint) —*see*
    Disorder, cartilage, specified NEC
  cerebellar —*see* Atrophy, brain
  cerebral —*see* Atrophy, brain
  cervix (mucosa) (senile) (uteri) N88.8
    menopausal N95.8
  Charcot-Marie-Tooth G60.0
  choroid (central) (macular) (myopic)
    (retina) H31.10-
    diffuse secondary H31.12-
    gyrate H31.23
    senile H31.11-
  ciliary body —*see* Atrophy, iris
  conjunctiva (senile) H11.89
  corpus cavernosum N48.89
  cortical —*see* Atrophy, brain
  cystic duct K82.8
  Déjérine-Thomas G23.8
  disuse NEC —*see* Atrophy, muscle
  Duchenne-Aran G12.21
  ear H93.8-

Atrophy, atrophic *(Continued)*
  edentulous alveolar ridge K08.20
  endometrium (senile) N85.8
    cervix N88.8
  enteric K63.89
  epididymis N50.8
  eyeball —*see* Disorder, globe,
    degenerated condition,
    atrophy
  eyelid (senile) —*see* Disorder, eyelid,
    degenerative
  facial (skin) L90.9
  fallopian tube (senile) N83.32
    with ovary N83.33
  fascioscapulohumeral (Landouzy-
    Déjérine) G71.0
  fatty, thymus (gland) E32.8
  gallbladder K82.8
  gastric K29.40
    with bleeding K29.41
  gastrointestinal K63.89
  glandular I89.8
  globe H44.52-
  gum K06.0
  hair L67.8
  heart (brown) —*see* Degeneration,
    myocardial
  hemifacial Q67.4
    Romberg G51.8
  infantile E41
    paralysis, acute —*see* Poliomyelitis,
      paralytic
  intestine K63.89
  iris (essential) (progressive)
    H21.26-
    specified NEC H21.29
  kidney (senile) (terminal) (*see also*
    Sclerosis, renal) N26.1
    congenital or infantile Q60.5
      bilateral Q60.4
      unilateral Q60.3
    hydronephrotic —*see*
      Hydronephrosis
  lacrimal gland (primary) H04.14-
    secondary H04.15-
  Landouzy-Déjérine G71.0
  laryngitis, infective J37.0
  larynx J38.7
  Leber's optic (hereditary) H47.22
  lip K13.0
  liver (yellow) K72.90
    with coma K72.91
    acute, subacute K72.00
      with coma K72.01
    chronic K72.10
      with coma K72.11
  lung (senile) J98.4
  macular (dermatological) L90.8
    syphilitic, skin A51.39
    striated A52.79
  mandible (edentulous) K08.20
    minimal K08.21
    moderate K08.22
    severe K08.23
  maxilla K08.20
    minimal K08.24
    moderate K08.25
    severe K08.26
  muscle, muscular (diffuse) (general)
    (idiopathic) (primary) M62.50
    ankle M62.57-
    Duchenne-Aran G12.21
    foot M62.57-

Atrophy, atrophic *(Continued)*
  muscle, muscular *(Continued)*
    forearm M62.53-
    hand M62.54-
    infantile spinal G12.0
    lower leg M62.56-
    multiple sites M62.59
    myelopathic —*see* Atrophy, muscle,
      spinal
    myotonic G71.11
    neuritic G58.9
    neuropathic (peroneal) (progressive)
      G60.0
    pelvic (disuse) N81.84
    peroneal G60.0
    progressive (bulbar) G12.21
      adult G12.1
      infantile (spinal) G12.0
      spinal G12.9
        adult G12.1
        infantile G12.0
    pseudohypertrophic G71.0
    shoulder region M62.51-
    specified site NEC M62.58
    spinal G12.9
      adult form G12.1
      Aran-Duchenne G12.21
      childhood form, type II G12.1
      distal G12.1
      hereditary NEC G12.1
      infantile, type I (Werdnig-
        Hoffmann) G12.0
      juvenile form, type III (Kugelberg-
        Welander) G12.1
      progressive G12.21
      scapuloperoneal form G12.1
      specified NEC G12.8
    syphilitic A52.78
    thigh M62.55-
    upper arm M62.52-
  myocardium —*see* Degeneration,
    myocardial
  myometrium (senile) N85.8
    cervix N88.8
  myopathic NEC —*see* Atrophy, muscle
  myotonia G71.11
  nail L60.3
  nasopharynx J31.1
  nerve —*see also* Disorder, nerve
    abducens —*see* Strabismus, paralytic,
      sixth nerve
    accessory G52.8
    acoustic or auditory —*see*
      subcategory H93.3
    cranial G52.9
      eighth (auditory) —*see* subcategory
        H93.3
      eleventh (accessory) G52.8
      fifth (trigeminal) G50.8
      first (olfactory) G52.0
      fourth (trochlear) —*see* Strabismus,
        paralytic, fourth nerve
      second (optic) H47.20
      sixth (abducens) —*see* Strabismus,
        paralytic, sixth nerve
      tenth (pneumogastric) (vagus) G52.2
      third (oculomotor) —*see*
        Strabismus, paralytic, third
        nerve
      twelfth (hypoglossal) G52.3
    hypoglossal G52.3
    oculomotor —*see* Strabismus,
      paralytic, third nerve

Atrophy, atrophic (*Continued*)
nerve (*Continued*)
olfactory G52.0
optic (papillomacular bundle)
syphilitic (late) A52.15
congenital A50.44
pneumogastric G52.2
trigeminal G50.8
trochlear —*see* Strabismus, paralytic,
fourth nerve
vagus (pneumogastric) G52.2
neurogenic, bone, tabetic A52.11
nutritional E41
old age R54
olivopontocerebellar G23.8
optic (nerve) H47.20
glaucomatous H47.23-
hereditary H47.22
primary H47.21-
specified type NEC H47.29-
syphilitic (late) A52.15
congenital A50.44
orbit H05.31-
ovary (senile) N83.31
with fallopian tube N83.33
oviduct (senile) —*see* Atrophy, fallopian
tube
palsy, diffuse (progressive) G12.22
pancreas (duct) (senile) K86.8
parotid gland K11.0
pelvic muscle N81.84
penis N48.89
pharynx J39.2
pluriglandular E31.8
autoimmune E31.0
polyarthritis M15.9
prostate N42.89
pseudohypertrophic (muscle) G71.0
renal (*see also* Sclerosis, renal) N26.1
retina, retinal (postinfectional)
H35.89
rhinitis J31.0
salivary gland K11.0
scar L90.5
sclerosis, lobar (of brain) G31.09
[F02.80]
with behavioral disturbance G31.09
[F02.81]
scrotum N50.8
seminal vesicle N50.8
senile R54
due to radiation (nonionizing) (solar)
L57.8
skin (patches) (spots) L90.9
degenerative (senile) L90.8
due to radiation (nonionizing) (solar)
L57.8
senile L90.8
spermatic cord N50.8
spinal (acute) (cord) G95.89
muscular —*see* Atrophy, muscle,
spinal
paralysis G12.20
acute —*see* Poliomyelitis,
paralytic
meaning progressive muscular
atrophy G12.21
spine (column) —*see* Spondylopathy,
specified NEC
spleen (senile) D73.0
stomach K29.40
with bleeding K29.41
striate (skin) L90.6
syphilitic A52.79

Atrophy, atrophic (*Continued*)
subcutaneous L90.9
sublingual gland K11.0
submandibular gland K11.0
submaxillary gland K11.0
Sudeck's —*see* Algoneurodystrophy
suprarenal (capsule) (gland) E27.49
primary E27.1
systemic affecting central nervous
system
in
myxedema E03.9 [G13.2]
neoplastic disease (*see also*
Neoplasm) D49.9 [G13.1]
specified disease NEC G13.8
tarso-orbital fascia, congenital Q10.3
testis N50.0
thenar, partial —*see* Syndrome, carpal
tunnel
thymus (fatty) E32.8
thyroid (gland) (acquired) E03.4
with cretinism E03.1
congenital (with myxedema) E03.1
tongue (senile) K14.8
papillae K14.4
trachea J39.8
tunica vaginalis N50.8
turbinate J34.89
tympanic membrane (nonflaccid)
H73.82-
flaccid H73.81-
upper respiratory tract J39.8
uterus, uterine (senile) N85.8
cervix N88.8
due to radiation (intended effect)
N85.8
adverse effect or misadventure
N99.89
vagina (senile) N95.2
vas deferens N50.8
vascular I99.8
vertebra (senile) —*see* Spondylopathy,
specified NEC
vulva (senile) N90.5
Werdnig-Hoffmann G12.0
yellow —*see* Failure, hepatic
Attack, attacks
with alteration of consciousness (with
automatisms) —*see* Epilepsy,
localization-related, symptomatic,
with complex partial seizures
without alteration of consciousness —
see Epilepsy, localization-related,
symptomatic, with simple partial
seizures
Adams-Stokes I45.9
akinetic —*see* Epilepsy, generalized,
specified NEC
angina —*see* Angina
atonic —*see* Epilepsy, generalized,
specified NEC
benign shuddering G25.83
cataleptic —*see* Catalepsy
coronary —*see* Infarct, myocardium
cyanotic, newborn P28.2
drop NEC R55
epileptic —*see* Epilepsy
heart —*see* infarct, myocardium
hysterical F44.9
jacksonian —*see* Epilepsy, localization-
related, symptomatic, with simple
partial seizures
myocardium, myocardial —*see* Infarct,
myocardium

Attack, attacks (*Continued*)
myoclonic —*see* Epilepsy, generalized,
specified NEC
panic F41.0
psychomotor —*see* Epilepsy,
localization-related,
symptomatic, with complex
partial seizures
salaam —*see* Epilepsy, spasms
schizophreniform, brief F23
shuddering, benign G25.83
Stokes-Adams I45.9
syncope R55
transient ischemic (TIA) G45.9
specified NEC G45.8
unconsciousness R55
hysterical F44.89
vasomotor R55
vasovagal (paroxysmal) (idiopathic) R55
Attention (to)
artificial
opening (of) Z43.9
digestive tract NEC Z43.4
colon Z43.3
ilium Z43.2
stomach Z43.1
specified NEC Z43.8
trachea Z43.0
urinary tract NEC Z43.6
cystostomy Z43.5
nephrostomy Z43.6
ureterostomy Z43.6
urethrostomy Z43.6
vagina Z43.7
colostomy Z43.3
cystostomy Z43.5
deficit disorder or syndrome F98.8
with hyperactivity —*see* Disorder,
attention-deficit
hyperactivity
gastrostomy Z43.1
ileostomy Z43.2
jejunostomy Z43.4
nephrostomy Z43.6
surgical dressings Z48.01
sutures Z48.02
tracheostomy Z43.0
ureterostomy Z43.6
urethrostomy Z43.6
Attrition
gum K06.0
tooth, teeth (excessive) (hard tissues)
K03.0
Atypical, atypism —*see also* condition
cells (on cytolgocial smear)
(endocervical) (endometrial)
(glandular)
cervix R87.619
vagina R87.629
cervical N87.9
endometrium N85.9
hyperplasia N85.00
parenting situation Z62.9
Auditory —*see* condition
Aujeszky's disease B33.8
Aurantiasis, cutis E67.1
Auricle, auricular —*see also* condition
cervical Q18.2
Auriculotemporal syndrome G50.8
Austin Flint murmur (aortic
insufficiency) I35.1
Australian
Q fever A78
X disease A83.4

A

Autism, autistic (childhood) (infantile)
F84.0
  atypical F84.9
Autodigestion R68.89
Autoerythrocyte sensitization
  (syndrome) D69.2
Autographism L50.3
Autoimmune
  disease (systemic) M35.9
  inhibitors to clotting factors D68.311
  lymphoproliferative syndrome [ALPS]
    D89.82
  thyroiditis E06.3
Autointoxication R68.89
Automatism G93.89
  with temporal sclerosis G93.81
  epileptic —see Epilepsy, localization-
    related, symptomatic, with
    complex partial seizures
  paroxysmal, idiopathic —see Epilepsy,
    localization-related, symptomatic,
    with complex partial seizures
Autonomic, autonomous
  bladder (neurogenic) N31.2
  hysteria seizure F44.5
Autosensitivity, erythrocyte D69.2
Autosensitization, cutaneous L30.2
Autosome —see condition by
  chromosome involved
Autotopagnosia R48.1
Autotoxemia R68.89
Autumn —see condition
Avellis' syndrome G46.8
Aversion
  oral R63.3
    newborn P92.-
    nonorganic origin F98.2
  sexual F52.1
Aviator's
  disease or sickness —see Effect, adverse,
    high altitude
  ear T70.0

Avitaminosis (multiple) (see also
  Deficiency, vitamin) E56.9
  B E53.9
    with
      beriberi E51.11
      pellagra E52
  B2 E53.0
  B6 E53.1
  B12 E53.8
  D E55.9
    with rickets E55.0
  G E53.0
  K E56.1
  nicotinic acid E52
AVNRT (atrioventricular nodal re-entrant
  tachycardia) I47.1
AVRT (atrioventricular nodal re-entrant
  tachycardia) I47.1
Avulsion (traumatic)
  blood vessel —see Injury, blood vessel
  bone —see Fracture, by site
  cartilage —see also Dislocation, by site
    symphyseal (inner), complicating
      delivery O71.6
  external site other than limb —see
    Wound, open, by site
  eye S05.7-
  head (intracranial)
    external site NEC S08.89
    scalp S08.0
  internal organ or site —see Injury, by
    site
  joint —see also Dislocation, by site
    capsule —see Sprain, by site
  kidney S37.06-
  ligament —see Sprain, by site
  limb —see also Amputation, traumatic,
    by site
  skin and subcutaneous tissue —see
    Wound, open, by site

Avulsion (Continued)
  muscle —see Injury, muscle
  nerve (root) —see Injury, nerve
  scalp S08.0
  skin and subcutaneous tissue —see
    Wound, open, by site
  spleen S36.032
  symphyseal cartilage (inner),
    complicating delivery O71.6
  tendon —see Injury, muscle
  tooth S03.2
Awareness of heart beat R00.2
Axenfeld's
  anomaly or syndrome Q15.0
  degeneration (calcareous) Q13.4
Axilla, axillary —see also condition
  breast Q83.1
Axonotmesis —see Injury, nerve
Ayerza's disease or syndrome
  (pulmonary artery sclerosis
  with pulmonary hypertension)
  I27.0
Azoospermia (organic) N46.01
  due to
    drug therapy N46.021
    efferent duct obstruction
      N46.023
    infection N46.022
    radiation N46.024
    specified cause NEC N46.029
    systemic disease N46.025
Azotemia R79.89
  meaning uremia N19
Aztec ear Q17.3
Azygos
  continuation inferior vena cava Q26.8
  lobe (lung) Q33.1

A

B

Baastrup's disease —see Kissing spine
Babesiosis B60.0
Babington's disease (familial
hemorrhagic telangiectasia) I78.0
Babinski's syndrome A52.79
Baby
crying constantly R68.11
floppy (syndrome) P94.2
Bacillary —see condition
Bacilluria N39.0
Bacillus —see also Infection, bacillus
abortus infection A23.1
anthracis infection A22.9
coli infection (see also Escherichia coli)
B96.20
Flexner's A03.1
mallei infection A24.0
Shiga's A03.0
suipestifer infection —see Infection,
salmonella
Back —see condition
Backache (postural) M54.9
sacroiliac M53.3
specified NEC M54.89
Backflow —see Reflux
Backward reading (dyslexia) F81.0
Bacteremia R78.81
with sepsis —see Sepsis
Bactericholia —see Cholecystitis, acute
Bacterid, bacteride (pustular) L40.3
Bacterium, bacteria, bacterial
agent NEC, as cause of disease
classified elsewhere B96.89
in blood —see Bacteremia
in urine —see Bacteriuria
Bacteriuria, bacteruria N39.0
asymptomatic N39.0
Bacteroides
fragilis, as cause of disease classified
elsewhere B96.6
Bad
heart —see Disease, heart
trip
due to drug abuse —see Abuse, drug,
hallucinogen
due to drug dependence —see
Dependence, drug, hallucinogen
Baelz's disease (cheilitis glandularis
apostematosa) K13.0
Baerensprung's disease (eczema
marginatum) B35.6
Bagasse disease or pneumonitis J67.1
Bagassosis J67.1
Baker's cyst —see Cyst, Baker's
Bakwin-Krida syndrome
(craniometaphyseal dysplasia) Q78.5
Balancing side interference M26.56
Balanitis (circinata) (erosiva) (gangrenosa)
(phagedenic) (vulgaris) N48.1
amebic A06.82
candidal B37.42
due to Haemophilus ducreyi A57
gonococcal (acute) (chronic) A54.09
xerotica obliterans N48.0
Balanoposthitis N47.6
gonococcal (acute) (chronic) A54.09
ulcerative (specific) A63.8
Balanorrhagia —see Balanitis
Balantidiasis, balantidiosis A07.0
Bald tongue K14.4
Baldness —see also Alopecia
male-pattern —see Alopecia, androgenic

Balkan grippe A78
Balloon disease —see Effect, adverse,
high altitude
Balo's disease (concentric sclerosis) G37.5
Bamberger-Marie disease —see
Osteoarthropathy, hypertrophic,
specified type NEC
Bancroft's filariasis B74.0
Band (s)
adhesive —see Adhesions, peritoneum
anomalous or congenital —see also
Anomaly, by site
heart (atrial) (ventricular) Q24.8
intestine Q43.3
omentum Q43.3
cervix N88.1
constricting, congenital Q79.8
gallbladder (congenital) Q44.1
intestinal (adhesive) —see Adhesions,
peritoneum
obstructive
intestine K56.5
peritoneum K56.5
periappendiceal, congenital Q43.3
peritoneal (adhesive) —see Adhesions,
peritoneum
uterus N73.6
internal N85.6
vagina N89.5
Bandemia D72.825
Bandl's ring (contraction), complicating
delivery O62.4
Bangkok hemorrhagic fever A91
Bang's disease (brucella abortus) A23.1
Bankruptcy, anxiety concerning Z59.8
Bannister's disease T78.3
hereditary D84.1
Banti's disease or syndrome (with
cirrhosis) (with portal hypertension)
K76.6
Bar, median, prostate —see Enlargement,
enlarged, prostate
Barcoo disease or rot —see Ulcer, skin
Barlow's disease E54
Barodontalgia T70.29
Baron Münchausen syndrome —see
Disorder, factitious
Barosinusitis T70.1
Barotitis T70.0
Barotrauma T70.29
odontalgia T70.29
otitic T70.0
sinus T70.1
Barraquer (-Simons) disease or syndrome
(progressive lipodystrophy) E88.1
Barré-Guillain disease or syndrome
G61.0
Barré-Liéou syndrome (posterior cervical
sympathetic) M53.0
Barrel chest M95.4
Barrett's
disease —see Barrett's, esophagus
esophagus K22.70
with dysplasia K22.719
high grade K22.711
low grade K22.710
without dysplasia K22.70
syndrome —see Barrett's, esophagus
ulcer K22.10
with bleeding K22.11
without bleeding K22.10
Barth syndrome E78.71
Bársony (-Polgár) (-Teschendorf) syndrome
(corkscrew esophagus) K22.4

Bartholinitis (suppurating) N75.8
gonococcal (acute) (chronic) (with
abscess) A54.1
Bartonellosis A44.9
cutaneous A44.1
mucocutaneous A44.1
specified NEC A44.8
systemic A44.0
Barton's fracture S52.56-
Bartter's syndrome E26.81
Basal —see condition
Basan's (hidrotic) ectodermal dysplasia
Q82.4
Baseball finger —see Dislocation, finger
Basedow's disease (exophthalmic
goiter) —see Hyperthyroidism,
with, goiter
Basic —see condition
Basilar —see condition
Bason's (hidrotic) ectodermal dysplasia
Q82.4
Basopenia —see Agranulocytosis
Basophilia D72.824
Basophilism (cortico-adrenal) (Cushing's)
(pituitary) E24.0
Bassen-Kornzweig disease or syndrome
E78.6
Bat ear Q17.5
Bateman's
disease B08.1
purpura (senile) D69.2
Bathing cramp T75.1
Bathophobia F40.248
Batten (-Mayou) disease E75.4
retina E75.4 [H36]
Batten-Steinert syndrome G71.11
Battered —see Maltreatment
Battey Mycobacterium infection A31.0
Battle exhaustion F43.0
Battledore placenta O43.19-
Baumgarten-Cruveilhier cirrhosis,
disease or syndrome K74.69
Bauxite fibrosis (of lung) J63.1
Bayle's disease (general paresis) A52.17
Bazin's disease (primary) (tuberculous)
A18.4
Beach ear —see Swimmer's, ear
Beaded hair (congenital) Q84.1
Béal conjunctivitis or syndrome B30.2
Beard's disease (neurasthenia) F48.8
Beat (s)
atrial, premature I49.1
ectopic I49.49
elbow —see Bursitis, elbow
escaped, heart I49.49
hand —see Bursitis, hand
knee —see Bursitis, knee
premature I49.40
atrial I49.1
auricular I49.1
supraventricular I49.1
Beau's
disease or syndrome —see
Degeneration, myocardial
lines (transverse furrows on fingernails)
L60.4
Bechterev's syndrome —see Spondylitis,
ankylosing
Beck's syndrome (anterior spinal artery
occlusion) I65.8
Becker's
cardiomyopathy I42.8
disease
idiopathic mural endomyocardial
disease I42.3

Becker's *(Continued)*
  disease *(Continued)*
    myotonia congenita, recessive form
        G71.12
    dystrophy G71.0
    pigmented hairy nevus D22.5
Beckwith-Wiedemann syndrome Q87.3
Bed confinement status Z74.01
Bed sore —*see* Ulcer, pressure, by site
Bedbug bite (s) —*see* Bite (s), by site,
    superficial, insect
Bedclothes, asphyxiation or suffocation
    by —*see* Asphyxia, traumatic, due to,
    mechanical, trapped
Bednar's
  aphthae K12.0
  tumor —*see* Neoplasm, malignant, by
    site
Bedridden Z74.01
Bedsore —*see* Ulcer, pressure, by site
Bedwetting —*see* Enuresis
Bee sting (with allergic or anaphylactic
    shock) —*see* Toxicity, venom,
    arthropod, bee
Beer drinker's heart (disease) I42.6
Begbie's disease (exophthalmic goiter) —
    see Hyperthyroidism, with,
    goiter
Behavior
  antisocial
    adult Z72.811
    child or adolescent Z72.810
  disorder, disturbance —*see* Disorder,
    conduct
  disruptive —*see* Disorder, conduct
  drug seeking Z72.89
  inexplicable R46.2
  marked evasiveness R46.5
  obsessive-compulsive R46.81
  overactivity R46.3
  poor responsiveness R46.4
  self-damaging (life-style) Z72.89
  sleep-incompatible Z72.821
  slowness R46.4
  specified NEC R46.89
  strange (and inexplicable) R46.2
  suspiciousness R46.5
  type A pattern Z73.1
  undue concern or preoccupation with
    stressful events R46.6
  verbosity and circumstantial detail
    obscuring reason for contact R46.7
Behcet's disease or syndrome M35.2
Behr's disease —*see* Degeneration,
    macula
Beigel's disease or morbus (white piedra)
    B36.2
Bejel A65
Bekhterev's syndrome —*see* Spondylitis,
    ankylosing
Belching —*see* Eructation
Bell's
  mania F30.8
  palsy, paralysis G51.0
    infant or newborn P11.3
  spasm G51.3
Bence Jones albuminuria or proteinuria
    NEC R80.3
Bends T70.3
Benedikt's paralysis or syndrome G46.3
Benign (*see also* condition)
  prostatic hyperplasia —*see* Hyperplasia,
    prostate
Bennett's fracture (displaced) S62.21-
Benson's disease —*see* Deposit, crystalline

Bent
  back (hysterical) F44.4
  nose M95.0
    congenital Q67.4
Bereavement (uncomplicated) Z63.4
Bergeron's disease (hysterical chorea) F44.4
Berger's disease —*see* Nephropathy, IgA
Beriberi (dry) E51.11
  heart (disease) E51.12
  polyneuropathy E51.11
  wet E51.12
    involving circulatory system E51.11
Berlin's disease or edema (traumatic) S05.8X-
Berlock (berloque) dermatitis L56.2
Bernard-Horner syndrome G90.2
Bernard-Soulier disease or
    thrombopathia D69.1
Bernhardt (-Roth) disease —*see*
    Mononeuropathy, lower limb,
    meralgia paresthetica
Bernheim's syndrome —*see* Failure, heart,
    congestive
Bertielliasis B71.8
Berylliosis (lung) J63.2
Besnier-Boeck (-Schaumann) disease —
    see Sarcoidosis
Besnier's
  lupus pernio D86.3
  prurigo L20.0
Bestiality F65.89
Best's disease H35.50
Beta-mercaptolactate-cysteine
    disulfiduria E72.09
Betalipoproteinemia, broad or floating
    E78.2
Betting and gambling Z72.6
  pathological (compulsive) F63.0
Bezoar T18.9
  intestine T18.3
  stomach T18.2
Bezold's abscess —*see* Mastoiditis, acute
Bianchi's syndrome R48.8
Bicornate or bicornis uterus Q51.3
  in pregnancy or childbirth O34.59-
    causing obstructed labor O65.5
Bicuspid aortic valve Q23.1
Biedl-Bardet syndrome Q87.89
Bielschowsky (-Jansky) disease E75.4
Biermer's (pernicious) anemia or disease
    D51.0
Biett's disease L93.0
Bifid (congenital)
  apex, heart Q24.8
  clitoris Q52.6
  kidney Q63.8
  nose Q30.2
  patella Q74.1
  scrotum Q55.29
  toe NEC Q74.2
  tongue Q38.3
  ureter Q62.8
  uterus Q51.3
  uvula Q35.7
Biforis uterus (suprasimplex) Q51.3
Bifurcation (congenital)
  gallbladder Q44.1
  kidney pelvis Q63.8
  renal pelvis Q63.8
  rib Q76.6
  tongue, congenital Q38.3
  trachea Q32.1
  ureter Q62.8
  urethra Q64.74
  vertebra Q76.49

Big spleen syndrome D73.1
Bigeminal pulse R00.8
Bilateral —*see* condition
Bile
  duct —*see* condition
  pigments in urine R82.2
Bilharziasis —*see also* Schistosomiasis
  chyluria B65.0
  cutaneous B65.3
  galacturia B65.0
  hematochyluria B65.0
  intestinal B65.1
  lipemia B65.9
  lipuria B65.0
  oriental B65.2
  piarhemia B65.9
  pulmonary NOS B65.9 *[J99]*
    pneumonia B65.9 *[J17]*
  tropical hematuria B65.0
  vesical B65.0
Biliary —*see* condition
Bilirubin metabolism disorder E80.7
  specified NEC E80.6
Bilirubinemia, familial nonhemolytic
    E80.4
Bilirubinuria R82.2
Biliuria R82.2
Bilocular stomach K31.2
Binswanger's disease I67.3
Biparta, bipartite
  carpal scaphoid Q74.0
  patella Q74.1
  vagina Q52.10
Bird
  face Q75.8
  fancier's disease or lung J67.2
Birt-Hogg-Dube syndrome Q87.89
Birth
  complications in mother —*see* Delivery,
    complicated
  compression during NOS P15.9
  defect —*see* Anomaly
  immature (less than 37 completed
      weeks) —*see* Preterm, newborn
    extremely (less than 28 completed
        weeks) —*see* Immaturity,
        extreme
  inattention, at or after —*see*
      Maltreatment, child, neglect
  injury NOS P15.9
    basal ganglia P11.1
    brachial plexus NEC P14.3
    brain (compression) (pressure) P11.2
    central nervous system NOS P11.9
    cerebellum P11.1
    cerebral hemorrhage P10.1
    external genitalia P15.5
    eye P15.3
    face P15.4
    fracture
      bone P13.9
        specified NEC P13.8
      clavicle P13.4
      femur P13.2
      humerus P13.3
      long bone, except femur P13.3
      radius and ulna P13.3
      skull P13.0
      spine P11.5
      tibia and fibula P13.3
    intracranial P11.2
      laceration or hemorrhage P10.9
        specified NEC P10.8
    intraventricular hemorrhage P10.2

Birth (Continued)
  injury NOS (Continued)
    laceration
      brain P10.1
      by scalpel P15.8
      peripheral nerve P14.9
    liver P15.0
    meninges
      brain P11.1
      spinal cord P11.5
    nerve
      brachial plexus P14.3
      cranial NEC (except facial)
        P11.4
      facial P11.3
      peripheral P14.9
      phrenic (paralysis) P14.2
    paralysis
      facial nerve P11.3
      spinal P11.5
    penis P15.5
    rupture
      spinal cord P11.5
    scalp P12.9
    scalpel wound P15.8
    scrotum P15.5
    skull NEC P13.1
      fracture P13.0
    specified type NEC P15.8
    spinal cord P11.5
    spine P11.5
    spleen P15.1
    sternomastoid (hematoma)
      P15.2
    subarachnoid hemorrhage P10.3
    subcutaneous fat necrosis P15.6
    subdural hemorrhage P10.0
    tentorial tear P10.4
    testes P15.5
    vulva P15.5
  lack of care, at or after —*see*
    Maltreatment, child, neglect
  neglect, at or after —*see* Maltreatment,
    child, neglect
  palsy or paralysis, newborn, NOS
    (birth injury) P14.9
  premature (infant) —*see* Preterm,
    newborn
  shock, newborn P96.89
  trauma —*see* Birth, injury
  weight
    4000 grams to 4499 grams P08.1
    4500 grams or more P08.0
    low (2499 grams or less) —*see* Low,
      birthweight
      extremely (999 grams or less) —*see*
        Low, birthweight,
        extreme
Birthmark Q82.5
Bisalbuminemia E88.09
Biskra's button B55.1
Bite (s) (animal) (human)
  abdomen, abdominal
    wall S31.159
      with penetration into peritoneal
        cavity S31.659
      epigastric region S31.152
        with penetration into peritoneal
          cavity S31.652
      left
        lower quadrant S31.154
          with penetration into
            peritoneal cavity
            S31.654

Bite (s) (Continued)
  abdomen, abdominal (Continued)
    wall (Continued)
      left (Continued)
        upper quadrant S31.151
          with penetration into
            peritoneal cavity S31.651
        periumbilic region S31.155
          with penetration into peritoneal
            cavity S31.655
      right
        lower quadrant S31.153
          with penetration into
            peritoneal cavity S31.653
        upper quadrant S31.150
          with penetration into
            peritoneal cavity S31.650
      superficial NEC S30.871
        insect S30.861
    alveolar (process) —*see* Bite, oral cavity
    amphibian (venomous) —*see* Venom,
      bite, amphibian
    animal —*see also* Bite, by site
      venomous —*see* Venom
    ankle S91.05-
      superficial NEC S90.57-
      insect S90.56-
    antecubital space —*see* Bite, elbow
    anus S31.835
      superficial NEC S30.877
      insect S30.867
    arm (upper) S41.15-
      lower —*see* Bite, forearm
      superficial NEC S40.87-
      insect S40.86-
    arthropod NEC —*see* Venom, bite,
      arthropod
    auditory canal (external) (meatus) —*see*
      Bite, ear
    auricle, ear —*see* Bite, ear
    axilla —*see* Bite, arm
    back —*see also* Bite, thorax, back
      lower S31.050
        with penetration into
          retroperitoneal space S31.051
      superficial NEC S30.870
        insect S30.860
    bedbug —*see* Bite (s), by site,
      superficial, insect
    breast S21.05-
      superficial NEC S20.17-
      insect S20.16-
    brow —*see* Bite, head, specified site NEC
    buttock S31.805
      left S31.825
      right S31.815
      superficial NEC S30.870
      insect S30.860
    calf —*see* Bite, leg
    canaliculus lacrimalis —*see* Bite, eyelid
    canthus, eye —*see* Bite, eyelid
    centipede —*see* Toxicity, venom,
      arthropod, centipede
    cheek (external) S01.45-
      internal —*see* Bite, oral cavity
      superficial NEC S00.87
      insect S00.86
    chest wall —*see* Bite, thorax
    chigger B88.0
    chin —*see* Bite, head, specified site NEC
    clitoris —*see* Bite, vulva
    costal region —*see* Bite, thorax
    digit (s)
      hand —*see* Bite, finger
      toe —*see* Bite, toe

Bite (s) (Continued)
  ear (canal) (external) S01.35-
    superficial NEC S00.47-
      insect S00.46-
  elbow S51.05-
    superficial NEC S50.37-
      insect S50.36-
  epididymis —*see* Bite, testis
  epigastric region —*see* Bite, abdomen
  epiglottis —*see* Bite, neck, specified site
    NEC
  esophagus, cervical S11.25
    superficial NEC S10.17
      insect S10.16
  eyebrow —*see* Bite, eyelid
  eyelid S01.15-
    superficial NEC S00.27-
      insect S00.26-
  face NEC —*see* Bite, head, specified site
    NEC
  finger (s) S61.259
    with
      damage to nail S61.359
    index S61.258
      with
        damage to nail S61.358
      left S61.251
        with
          damage to nail S61.351
      right S61.250
        with
          damage to nail S61.350
      superficial NEC S60.478
        insect S60.46-
    little S61.25-
      with
        damage to nail S61.35-
      superficial NEC S60.47-
        insect S60.46-
    middle S61.25-
      with
        damage to nail S61.35-
      superficial NEC S60.47-
        insect S60.46-
    ring S61.25-
      with
        damage to nail S61.35-
      superficial NEC S60.47-
        insect S60.46-
    superficial NEC S60.479
      insect S60.469
    thumb —*see* Bite, thumb
  flank —*see* Bite, abdomen, wall
  flea —*see* Bite, by site, superficial, insect
  foot (except toe (s) alone) S91.35-
    superficial NEC S90.87-
      insect S90.86-
    toe —*see* Bite, toe
  forearm S51.85-
    elbow only —*see* Bite, elbow
    superficial NEC S50.87-
      insect S50.86-
  forehead —*see* Bite, head, specified site NEC
  genital organs, external
    female S31.552
      superficial NEC S30.876
        insect S30.866
      vagina and vulva —*see* Bite, vulva
    male S31.551
      penis —*see* Bite, penis
      scrotum —*see* Bite, scrotum
      superficial NEC S30.875
        insect S30.865
      testes —*see* Bite, testis

Bite (s) *(Continued)*
groin —*see* Bite, abdomen, wall
gum —*see* Bite, oral cavity
hand S61.45-
   finger —*see* Bite, finger
   superficial NEC S60.57-
      insect S60.56-
   thumb —*see* Bite, thumb
head S01.95
   cheek —*see* Bite, cheek
   ear —*see* Bite, ear
   eyelid —*see* Bite, eyelid
   lip —*see* Bite, lip
   nose —*see* Bite, nose
   oral cavity —*see* Bite, oral cavity
   scalp —*see* Bite, scalp
   specified site NEC S01.85
      superficial NEC S00.87
         insect S00.86
   superficial NEC S00.97
      insect S00.96
   temporomandibular area —*see* Bite,
      cheek
heel —*see* Bite, foot
hip S71.05-
   superficial NEC S70.27-
      insect S70.26-
hymen S31.45
hypochondrium —*see* Bite, abdomen,
   wall
hypogastric region —*see* Bite, abdomen,
   wall
inguinal region —*see* Bite, abdomen,
   wall
insect —*see* Bite, by site, superficial,
   insect
instep —*see* Bite, foot
interscapular region —*see* Bite, thorax,
   back
jaw —*see* Bite, head, specified site NEC
knee S81.05-
   superficial NEC S80.27-
      insect S80.26-
labium (majus) (minus) —*see* Bite, vulva
lacrimal duct —*see* Bite, eyelid
larynx S11.015
   superficial NEC S10.17
      insect S10.16
leg (lower) S81.85-
   ankle —*see* Bite, ankle
   foot —*see* Bite, foot
   knee —*see* Bite, knee
   superficial NEC S80.87-
      insect S80.86-
   toe —*see* Bite, toe
   upper —*see* Bite, thigh
lip S01.551
   superficial NEC S00.571
      insect S00.561
lizard (venomous) —*see* Venom, bite,
   reptile
loin —*see* Bite, abdomen, wall
lower back —*see* Bite, back, lower
lumbar region —*see* Bite, back, lower
malar region —*see* Bite, head, specified
   site NEC
mammary —*see* Bite, breast
marine animals (venomous) —*see*
   Toxicity, venom, marine animal
mastoid region —*see* Bite, head,
   specified site NEC
mouth —*see* Bite, oral cavity
nail
   finger —*see* Bite, finger
   toe —*see* Bite, toe

Bite (s) *(Continued)*
nape —*see* Bite, neck, specified site NEC
nasal (septum) (sinus) —*see* Bite, nose
nasopharynx —*see* Bite, head, specified
   site NEC
neck S11.95
   involving
      cervical esophagus —*see* Bite,
         esophagus, cervical
      larynx —*see* Bite, larynx
      pharynx —*see* Bite, pharynx
      thyroid gland S11.15
      trachea —*see* Bite, trachea
   specified site NEC S11.85
      superficial NEC S10.87
         insect S10.86
   superficial NEC S10.97
      insect S10.96
   throat S11.85
      superficial NEC S10.17
         insect S10.16
nose (septum) (sinus) S01.25
   superficial NEC S00.37
      insect S00.36
occipital region —*see* Bite, scalp
oral cavity S01.552
   superficial NEC S00.572
      insect S00.562
orbital region —*see* Bite, eyelid
palate —*see* Bite, oral cavity
palm —*see* Bite, hand
parietal region —*see* Bite, scalp
pelvis S31.050
   with penetration into retroperitoneal
      space S31.051
   superficial NEC S30.870
      insect S30.860
penis S31.25
   superficial NEC S30.872
      insect S30.862
perineum
   female —*see* Bite, vulva
   male —*see* Bite, pelvis
periocular area (with or without lacrimal
   passages) —*see* Bite, eyelid
phalanges
   finger —*see* Bite, finger
   toe —*see* Bite, toe
pharynx S11.25
   superficial NEC S10.17
      insect S10.16
pinna —*see* Bite, ear
poisonous —*see* Venom
popliteal space —*see* Bite, knee
prepuce —*see* Bite, penis
pubic region —*see* Bite, abdomen, wall
rectovaginal septum —*see* Bite, vulva
red bug B88.0
reptile NEC —*see also* Venom, bite,
   reptile
   nonvenomous —*see* Bite, by site
   snake —*see* Venom, bite, snake
sacral region —*see* Bite, back, lower
sacroiliac region —*see* Bite, back, lower
salivary gland —*see* Bite, oral cavity
scalp S01.05
   superficial NEC S00.07
      insect S00.06
scapular region —*see* Bite, shoulder
scrotum S31.35
   superficial NEC S30.873
      insect S30.863
sea-snake (venomous) —*see* Toxicity,
   venom, snake, sea snake

Bite (s) *(Continued)*
shin —*see* Bite, leg
shoulder S41.05-
   superficial NEC S40.27-
      insect S40.26-
   snake —*see also* Venom, bite, snake
   nonvenomous —*see* Bite, by site
spermatic cord —*see* Bite, testis
spider (venomous) —*see* Toxicity,
   venom, spider
   nonvenomous —*see* Bite, by site,
      superficial, insect
sternal region —*see* Bite, thorax, front
submaxillary region —*see* Bite, head,
   specified site NEC
submental region —*see* Bite, head,
   specified site NEC
subungual
   finger (s) —*see* Bite, finger
   toe —*see* Bite, toe
superficial —*see* Bite, by site, superficial
supraclavicular fossa S11.85
supraorbital —*see* Bite, head, specified
   site NEC
temple, temporal region —*see* Bite,
   head, specified site NEC
temporomandibular area —*see* Bite, cheek
testis S31.35
   superficial NEC S30.873
      insect S30.863
thigh S71.15-
   superficial NEC S70.37-
      insect S70.36-
thorax, thoracic (wall) S21.95
   back S21.25-
      with penetration into thoracic
         cavity S21.45-
   breast —*see* Bite, breast
   front S21.15-
      with penetration into thoracic
         cavity S21.35-
   superficial NEC S20.97
      back S20.47-
      front S20.37-
      insect S20.96
         back S20.46-
         front S20.36-
throat —*see* Bite, neck, throat
thumb S61.05-
   with
      damage to nail S61.15-
   superficial NEC S60.37-
      insect S60.36-
thyroid S11.15
   superficial NEC S10.87
      insect S10.86
toe (s) S91.15-
   with
      damage to nail S91.25-
   great S91.15-
      with
         damage to nail S91.25-
   lesser S91.15-
      with
         damage to nail S91.25-
   superficial NEC S90.47-
      great S90.47-
      insect S90.46-
         great S90.46-
tongue S01.552
trachea S11.025
   superficial NEC S10.17
      insect S10.16
tunica vaginalis —*see* Bite, testis

Bite (s) *(Continued)*
  tympanum, tympanic membrane —*see* Bite, ear
  umbilical region S31.155
  uvula —*see* Bite, oral cavity
  vagina —*see* Bite, vulva
  venomous —*see* Venom
  vocal cords S11.035
    superficial NEC S10.17
      insect S10.16
  vulva S31.45
    superficial NEC S30.874
      insect S30.864
  wrist S61.55-
    superficial NEC S60.87-
      insect S60.86-
Biting, cheek or lip K13.1
Biventricular failure (heart) I50.9
Björck (-Thorson) syndrome (malignant carcinoid) E34.0
Black
  death A20.9
  eye S00.1-
  hairy tongue K14.3
  heel (foot) S90.3-
  lung (disease) J60
  palm (hand) S60.22-
Blackfan-Diamond anemia or syndrome (congenital hypoplastic anemia) D61.01
Blackhead L70.0
Blackout R55
Bladder —*see* condition
Blast (air) (hydraulic) (immersion) (underwater)
  blindness S05.8X-
  injury
    abdomen or thorax —*see* Injury, by site
    ear (acoustic nerve trauma) —*see* Injury, nerve, acoustic, specified type NEC
    syndrome NEC T70.8
Blastoma —*see* Neoplasm, malignant, by site
  pulmonary —*see* Neoplasm, lung, malignant
Blastomycosis, blastomycotic B40.9
  Brazilian —*see* Paracoccidioidomycosis
  cutaneous B40.3
  disseminated B40.7
  European —*see* Cryptococcosis
  generalized B40.7
  keloidal B48.0
  North American B40.9
  primary pulmonary B40.0
  pulmonary B40.2
    acute B40.0
    chronic B40.1
  skin B40.3
  South American —*see* Paracoccidioidomycosis
  specified NEC B40.89
Bleb (s) R23.8
  emphysematous (lung) (solitary) J43.9
  endophthalmitis H59.43
  filtering (vitreous), after glaucoma surgery Z98.83
  inflamed (infected), postprocedural H59.40
    stage 1 H59.41
    stage 2 H59.42
    stage 3 H59.43

Bleb (s) *(Continued)*
  lung (ruptured) J43.9
    congenital —*see* Atelectasis
    newborn P25.8
  subpleural (emphysematous) J43.9
Blebitis, postprocedural H59.40
  stage 1 H59.41
  stage 2 H59.42
  stage 3 H59.43
Bleeder (familial) (hereditary) —*see* Hemophilia
Bleeding —*see also* Hemorrhage
  anal K62.5
  anovulatory N97.0
  atonic, following delivery O72.1
  capillary I78.8
    puerperal O72.2
  contact (postcoital) N93.0
  due to uterine subinvolution N85.3
  ear —*see* Otorrhagia
  excessive, associated with menopausal onset N92.4
  familial —*see* Defect, coagulation
  following intercourse N93.0
  gastrointestinal K92.2
  hemorrhoids —*see* Hemorrhoids
  intermenstrual (regular) N92.3
    irregular N92.1
  intraoperative —*see* Complication, intraoperative, hemorrhage
  irregular N92.6
  menopausal N92.4
  newborn, intraventricular — *see* Newborn, affected by, hemorrhage, intraventricular
  nipple N64.59
  nose R04.0
  ovulation N92.3
  postclimacteric N95.0
  postcoital N93.0
  postmenopausal N95.0
  postoperative —*see* Complication, postprocedural, hemorrhage
  preclimacteric N92.4
  puberty (excessive, with onset of menstrual periods) N92.2
  rectum, rectal K62.5
    newborn P54.2
  tendencies —*see* Defect, coagulation
  throat R04.1
  tooth socket (post-extraction) K91.840
  umbilical stump P51.9
  uterus, uterine NEC N93.9
    climacteric N92.4
    dysfunctional of functional N93.8
    menopausal N92.4
    preclimacteric or premenopausal N92.4
    unrelated to menstrual cycle N93.9
  vagina, vaginal (abnormal) N93.9
    dysfunctional or functional N93.8
    newborn P54.6
  vicarious N94.89
Blennorrhagia, blennorrhagic —*see* Gonorrhea
Blennorrhea (acute) (chronic) —*see also* Gonorrhea
  inclusion (neonatal) (newborn) P39.1
  lower genitourinary tract (gonococcal) A54.00
  neonatorum (gonococcal ophthalmia) A54.31
Blepharelosis —*see* Entropion

Blepharitis (angularis) (ciliaris) (eyelid) (marginal) (nonulcerative) H01.009
  herpes zoster B02.39
  left H01.006
    lower H01.005
    upper H01.004
  right H01.003
    lower H01.002
    upper H01.001
  squamous H01.029
    left H01.026
      lower H01.025
      upper H01.024
    right H01.023
      lower H01.022
      upper H01.021
  ulcerative H01.019
    left H01.016
      lower H01.015
      upper H01.014
    right H01.013
      lower H01.012
      upper H01.011
Blepharochalasis H02.30
  congenital Q10.0
  left H02.36
    lower H02.35
    upper H02.34
  right H02.33
    lower H02.32
    upper H02.31
Blepharoclonus H02.59
Blepharoconjunctivitis H10.50-
  angular H10.52-
  contact H10.53-
  ligneous H10.51-
Blepharophimosis (eyelid) H02.529
  congenital Q10.3
  left H02.526
    lower H02.525
    upper H02.524
  right H02.523
    lower H02.522
    upper H02.521
Blepharoptosis H02.40-
  congenital Q10.0
  mechanical H02.41-
  myogenic H02.42-
  neurogenic H02.43-
  paralytic H02.43-
Blepharopyorrhea, gonococcal A54.39
Blepharospasm G24.5
  drug induced G24.01
Blighted ovum O02.0
Blind —*see also* Blindness
  bronchus (congenital) Q32.4
  loop syndrome K90.2
    congenital Q43.8
  sac, fallopian tube (congenital) Q50.6
  spot, enlarged —*see* Defect, visual field, localized, scotoma, blind spot area
  tract or tube, congenital NEC —*see* Atresia, by site
Blindness (acquired) (congenital) (both eyes) H54.0
  blast S05.8X-
  color —*see* Deficiency, color vision
  concussion S05.8X-
  cortical H47.619
    left brain H47.612
    right brain H47.611
  day H53.11
  due to injury (current episode) S05.9-
    sequelae — code to injury with seventh character S

B

Blindness *(Continued)*
eclipse (total) —*see* Retinopathy, solar
emotional (hysterical) F44.6
face H53.16
hysterical F44.6
legal (both eyes) (USA definition) H54.8
mind R48.8
night H53.60
    abnormal dark adaptation curve
        H53.61
    acquired H53.62
    congenital H53.63
    specified type NEC H53.69
    vitamin A deficiency E50.5
one eye (other eye normal) H54.40
    left (normal vision on right) H54.42
        low vision on right H54.12
    low vision, other eye H54.10
    right (normal vision on left) H54.41
        low vision on left H54.11
psychic R48.8
river B73.01
snow —*see* Photokeratitis
sun, solar —*see* Retinopathy, solar
transient —*see* Disturbance, vision,
    subjective, loss, transient
traumatic (current episode) S05.9-
word (developmental) F81.0
    acquired R48.0
    secondary to organic lesion R48.0
Blister (nonthermal)
abdominal wall S30.821
alveolar process S00.522
ankle S90.52-
antecubital space —*see* Blister, elbow
anus S30.827
arm (upper) S40.82-
auditory canal —*see* Blister, ear
auricle —*see* Blister, ear
axilla —*see* Blister, arm
back, lower S30.820
beetle dermatitis L24.89
breast S20.12-
brow S00.82
calf —*see* Blister, leg
canthus —*see* Blister, eyelid
cheek S00.82
    internal S00.522
chest wall —*see* Blister, thorax
chin S00.82
costal region —*see* Blister, thorax
digit (s)
    foot —*see* Blister, toe
    hand —*see* Blister, finger
due to burn —*see* Burn, by site, second
    degree
ear S00.42-
elbow S50.32-
epiglottis S10.12
esophagus, cervical S10.12
eyebrow —*see* Blister, eyelid
eyelid S00.22-
face S00.82
fever B00.1
finger (s) S60.429
    index S60.42-
    little S60.42-
    middle S60.42-
    ring S60.42-
foot (except toe (s) alone) S90.82-
    toe —*see* Blister, toe
forearm S50.82-
    elbow only —*see* Blister, elbow
forehead S00.82
fracture - omit code

Blister *(Continued)*
genital organ
    female S30.826
    male S30.825
gum S00.522
hand S60.52-
head S00.92
    ear —*see* Blister, ear
    eyelid —*see* Blister, eyelid
    lip S00.521
    nose S00.32
    oral cavity S00.522
    scalp S00.02
    specified site NEC S00.82
heel —*see* Blister, foot
hip S70.22-
interscapular region S20.429
jaw S00.82
knee S80.22-
larynx S10.12
leg (lower) S80.82-
    knee —*see* Blister, knee
    upper —*see* Blister, thigh
lip S00.521
malar region S00.82
mammary —*see* Blister, breast
mastoid region S00.82
mouth S00.522
multiple, skin, nontraumatic R23.8
nail
    finger —*see* Blister, finger
    toe —*see* Blister, toe
nasal S00.32
neck S10.92
    specified site NEC S10.82
    throat S10.12
nose S00.32
occipital region S00.02
oral cavity S00.522
orbital region —*see* Blister, eyelid
palate S00.522
palm —*see* Blister, hand
parietal region S00.02
pelvis S30.820
penis S30.822
periocular area —*see* Blister, eyelid
phalanges
    finger —*see* Blister, finger
    toe —*see* Blister, toe
pharynx S10.12
pinna —*see* Blister, ear
popliteal space —*see* Blister, knee
scalp S00.02
scapular region —*see* Blister, shoulder
scrotum S30.823
shin —*see* Blister, leg
shoulder S40.22-
sternal region S20.329
submaxillary region S00.82
submental region S00.82
subungual
    finger (s) —*see* Blister, finger
    toe (s) —*see* Blister, toe
supraclavicular fossa S10.82
supraorbital S00.82
temple S00.82
temporal region S00.82
testis S30.823
thermal —*see* Burn, second degree, by
    site
thigh S70.32-
thorax, thoracic (wall) S20.92
    back S20.42-
    front S20.32-
throat S10.12

Blister *(Continued)*
thumb S60.32-
toe (s) S90.42-
    great S90.42-
tongue S00.522
trachea S10.12
tympanum, tympanic membrane —*see*
    Blister, ear
upper arm —*see* Blister, arm (upper)
uvula S00.522
vagina S30.824
vocal cords S10.12
vulva S30.824
wrist S60.82-
Bloating R14.0
Bloch-Sulzberger disease or syndrome
Q82.3
Block, blocked
alveolocapillary J84.10
arborization (heart) I45.5
arrhythmic I45.9
atrioventricular (incomplete) (partial)
    I44.30
    with atrioventricular dissociation
        I44.2
    complete I44.2
        congenital Q24.6
    congenital Q24.6
    first degree I44.0
    second degree (types I and II) I44.1
    specified NEC I44.39
    third degree I44.2
    types I and II I44.1
auriculoventricular —*see* Block,
    atrioventricular
bifascicular (cardiac) I45.2
bundle-branch (complete) (false)
    (incomplete) I45.4
    bilateral I45.2
    left I44.7
        with right bundle branch block I45.2
        hemiblock I44.60
            anterior I44.4
            posterior I44.5
        incomplete I44.7
            with right bundle branch block
                I45.2
    right I45.10
        with
            left bundle branch block I45.2
            left fascicular block I45.2
            specified NEC I45.19
        Wilson's type I45.19
cardiac I45.9
conduction I45.9
    complete I44.2
fascicular (left) I44.60
    anterior I44.4
    posterior I44.5
    right I45.0
    specified NEC I44.69
foramen Magendie (acquired) G91.1
    congenital Q03.1
        with spina bifida —*see* Spina bifida,
            by site, with hydrocephalus
heart I45.9
    bundle branch I45.4
        bilateral I45.2
    complete (atrioventricular) I44.2
    congenital Q24.6
    first degree (atrioventricular) I44.0
    second degree (atrioventricular) I44.1
    specified type NEC I45.5
    third degree (atrioventricular) I44.2
hepatic vein I82.0

Block, blocked *(Continued)*
  intraventricular (nonspecific) I45.4
    bundle branch
      bilateral I45.2
  kidney N28.9
    postcystoscopic or postprocedural
      N99.0
  Mobitz (types I and II) I44.1
  myocardial —*see* Block, heart
  nodal I45.5
  organ or site, congenital NEC —*see*
    Atresia, by site
  portal (vein) I81
  second degree (types I and II) I44.1
  sinoatrial I45.5
  sinoauricular I45.5
  third degree I44.2
  trifascicular I45.3
  tubal N97.1
  vein NOS I82.90
  Wenckebach (types I and II) I44.1
Blockage —*see* Obstruction
Blocq's disease F44.4
Blood
  constituents, abnormal R78.9
  disease D75.9
  donor —*see* Donor, blood
  dyscrasia D75.9
    with
      abortion —*see* Abortion, by type,
        complicated by, hemorrhage
      ectopic pregnancy O08.1
      molar pregnancy O08.1
    following ectopic or molar pregnancy
      O08.1
    newborn P61.9
    puerperal, postpartum O72.3
  flukes NEC —*see* Schistosomiasis
  in
    feces K92.1
      occult R19.5
    urine —*see* Hematuria
  mole O02.0
  occult in feces R19.5
  pressure
    decreased, due to shock following
      injury T79.4
    examination only Z01.30
    fluctuating I99.8
    high —*see* Hypertension
      borderline R03.0
      incidental reading, without
        diagnosis of hypertension R03.0
    low —*see also* Hypotension
      incidental reading, without
        diagnosis of hypotension R03.1
  spitting —*see* Hemoptysis
  staining cornea —*see* Pigmentation,
    cornea, stromal
  transfusion
    reaction or complication —*see*
      Complications, transfusion
  type
    A (Rh positive) Z67.10
      Rh negative Z67.11
    AB (Rh positive) Z67.30
      Rh negative Z67.31
    B (Rh positive) Z67.20
      Rh negative Z67.21
    O (Rh positive) Z67.40
      Rh negative Z67.41
    Rh (positive) Z67.90
      negative Z67.91
  vessel rupture —*see* Hemorrhage
  vomiting —*see* Hematemesis

Blood-forming organs, disease D75.9
Bloodgood's disease —*see* Mastopathy,
  cystic
Bloom (-Machacek)(-Torre) syndrome
  Q82.8
Blount's disease or osteochondrosis —*see*
  Osteochondrosis, juvenile, tibia
Blue
  baby Q24.9
  diaper syndrome E72.09
  dome cyst (breast) —*see* Cyst, breast
  dot cataract Q12.0
  nevus D22.9
  sclera Q13.5
    with fragility of bone and deafness
      Q78.0
  toe syndrome I75.02-
Blueness —*see* Cyanosis
Blues, postpartal O90.6
  baby O90.6
Blurring, visual H53.8
Blushing (abnormal) (excessive) R23.2
BMI —*see* Body, mass index
Boarder, hospital NEC Z76.4
  accompanying sick person Z76.3
  healthy infant or child Z76.2
    foundling Z76.1
Bockhart's impetigo L01.02
Bodechtel-Guttman disease (subacute
  sclerosing panencephalitis) A81.1
Boder-Sedgwick syndrome (ataxia-
  telangiectasia) G11.3
Body, bodies
  Aschoff's —*see* Myocarditis, rheumatic
  asteroid, vitreous —*see* Deposit,
    crystalline
  cytoid (retina) —*see* Occlusion, artery,
    retina
  drusen (degenerative) (macula)
    (retinal) —*see also* Degeneration,
    macula, drusen
    optic disc —*see* Drusen, optic disc
  foreign —*see* Foreign body
  loose
    joint, except knee —*see* Loose, body,
      joint
      knee M23.4-
    sheath, tendon —*see* Disorder,
      tendon, specified type NEC
  mass index (BMI)
    adult
      19 or less Z68.1
      20.0-20.9 Z68.20
      21.0-21.9 Z68.21
      22.0-22.9 Z68.22
      23.0-23.9 Z68.23
      24.0-24.9 Z68.24
      25.0-25.9 Z68.25
      26.0-26.9 Z68.26
      27.0-27.9 Z68.27
      28.0-28.9 Z68.28
      29.0-29.9 Z68.29
      30.0-30.9 Z68.30
      31.0-31.9 Z68.31
      32.0-32.9 Z68.32
      33.0-33.9 Z68.33
      34.0-34.9 Z68.34
      35.0-35.9 Z68.35
      36.0-36.9 Z68.36
      37.0-37.9 Z68.37
      38.0-38.9 Z68.38
      39.0-39.9 Z68.39
      40.0-44.9 Z68.41
      45.0-49.9 Z68.42
      50.0-59.9 Z68.43

Body, bodies *(Continued)*
  mass index *(Continued)*
    adult *(Continued)*
      60.0-69.9 Z68.44
      70 and over Z68.45
    pediatric
      5th percentile to less than 85th
        percentile for age Z68.52
      85th percentile to less than 95th
        percentile for age Z68.53
      greater than or equal to ninety-fifth
        percentile for age Z68.54
      less than fifth percentile for age
        Z68.51
  Mooser's A75.2
  rice —*see also* Loose, body, joint
    knee M23.4-
  rocking F98.4
Boeck's
  disease or sarcoid —*see* Sarcoidosis
  lupoid (miliary) D86.3
Boerhaave's syndrome (spontaneous
  esophageal rupture) K22.3
Boggy
  cervix N88.8
  uterus N85.8
Boil —*see also* Furuncle, by site
  Aleppo B55.1
  Baghdad B55.1
  Delhi B55.1
  lacrimal
    gland —*see* Dacryoadenitis
    passages (duct) (sac) —*see*
      Inflammation, lacrimal,
      passages, acute
  Natal B55.1
  orbit, orbital —*see* Abscess, orbit
  tropical B55.1
Bold hives —*see* Urticaria
Bombé, iris —*see* Membrane, pupillary
Bone —*see* condition
Bonnevie-Ullrich syndrome Q87.1
Bonnier's syndrome —*see* subcategory
  H81.8
Bonvale dam fever T73.3
Bony block of joint —*see* Ankylosis
BOOP (bronchiolitis obliterans organized
  pneumonia) J84.89
Borderline
  diabetes mellitus R73.09
  hypertension R03.0
  osteopenia M85.8-
  pelvis, with obstruction during labor
    O65.1
  personality F60.3
Borna disease A83.9
Bornholm disease B33.0
Boston exanthem A88.0
Botalli, ductus (patent) (persistent) Q25.0
Bothriocephalus latus infestation B70.0
Botulism (foodborne intoxication) A05.1
  infant A48.51
  non-foodborne A48.52
  wound A48.52
Bouba —*see* Yaws
Bouchard's nodes (with arthropathy)
  M15.2
Bouffée délirante F23
Bouillaud's disease or syndrome
  (rheumatic heart disease) I01.9
Bourneville's disease Q85.1
Boutonniere deformity (finger) —*see*
  Deformity, finger, boutonniere
Bouveret (-Hoffmann) syndrome
  (paroxysmal tachycardia) I47.9

Bovine heart —*see* Hypertrophy, cardiac
Bowel —*see* condition
Bowen's
　dermatosis (precancerous) —*see*
　　Neoplasm, skin, in situ
　disease —*see* Neoplasm, skin, in situ
　epithelioma —*see* Neoplasm, skin, in
　　situ
　type
　　epidermoid carcinoma-in-situ —*see*
　　　Neoplasm, skin, in situ
　　intraepidermal squamous cell
　　　carcinoma —*see* Neoplasm, skin,
　　　in situ
Bowing
　femur —*see also* Deformity, limb,
　　specified type NEC, thigh
　　congenital Q68.3
　fibula —*see also* Deformity, limb,
　　specified type NEC, lower leg
　　congenital Q68.4
　forearm —*see* Deformity, limb, specified
　　type NEC, forearm
　leg (s), long bones, congenital Q68.5
　radius —*see* Deformity, limb, specified
　　type NEC, forearm
　tibia —*see also* Deformity, limb,
　　specified type NEC, lower leg
　　congenital Q68.4
Bowleg (s) (acquired) M21.16-
　congenital Q68.5
　rachitic E64.3
Boyd's dysentery A03.2
Brachial —*see* condition
Brachycardia R00.1
Brachycephaly Q75.0
Bradley's disease A08.19
Bradyarrhythmia, cardiac I49.8
Bradycardia (sinoatrial) (sinus) (vagal)
　R00.1
　neonatal P29.12
　reflex G90.09
　tachycardia syndrome I49.5
Bradykinesia R25.8
Bradypnea R06.89
Bradytachycardia I49.5
Brailsford's disease or osteochondrosis
　—*see* Osteochondrosis, juvenile,
　radius
Brain —*see also* condition
　death G93.82
　syndrome —*see* Syndrome, brain
Branched-chain amino-acid disorder E71.2
Branchial —*see* condition
　cartilage, congenital Q18.2
Branchiogenic remnant (in neck) Q18.0
Brandt's syndrome (acrodermatitis
　enteropathica) E83.2
Brash (water) R12
Bravais-jacksonian epilepsy —*see*
　Epilepsy, localization-related,
　symptomatic, with simple partial
　seizures
Braxton Hicks contractions —*see* False,
　labor
Brazilian leishmaniasis B55.2
BRBPR K62.5
Break, retina (without detachment)
　H33.30-
　with retinal detachment —*see*
　　Detachment, retina
　horseshoe tear H33.31-
　multiple H33.33-
　round hole H33.32-

Breakdown
　device, graft or implant (*see also*
　　Complications, by site and type,
　　mechanical) T85.618
　arterial graft NEC —*see*
　　Complication, cardiovascular
　　device, mechanical, vascular
　breast (implant) T85.41
　catheter NEC T85.618
　　cystostomy T83.010
　　dialysis (renal) T82.41
　　　intraperitoneal T85.611
　　infusion NEC T82.514
　　　spinal (epidural) (subdural)
　　　　T85.610
　　urinary (indwelling) T83.018
　electronic (electrode) (pulse
　　generator) (stimulator)
　　bone T84.310
　　cardiac T82.119
　　　electrode T82.110
　　　pulse generator T82.111
　　　specified type NEC T82.118
　　nervous system —*see*
　　　Complication, prosthetic
　　　device, mechanical, electronic
　　　nervous system stimulator
　　urinary —*see* Complication,
　　　genitourinary, device, urinary,
　　　mechanical
　fixation, internal (orthopedic) NEC —
　　see Complication, fixation
　　device, mechanical
　gastrointestinal —*see* Complications,
　　prosthetic device, mechanical,
　　gastrointestinal device
　genital NEC T83.418
　　intrauterine contraceptive device
　　　T83.31
　　penile prosthesis T83.410
　heart NEC —*see* Complication,
　　cardiovascular device,
　　mechanical
　joint prosthesis —*see* Complications...,
　　joint prosthesis,internal,
　　mechanical, by site
　ocular NEC —*see* Complications,
　　prosthetic device, mechanical,
　　ocular device
　orthopedic NEC —*see* Complication,
　　orthopedic, device, mechanical
　specified NEC T85.618
　sutures, permanent T85.612
　　used in bone repair —*see*
　　　Complications, fixation
　　　device, internal (orthopedic),
　　　mechanical
　urinary NEC —*see also* Complication,
　　genitourinary, device, urinary,
　　mechanical
　　graft T83.21
　vascular NEC —*see* Complication,
　　cardiovascular device,
　　mechanical
　ventricular intracranial shunt T85.01
　nervous F48.8
　perineum O90.1
　respirator J95.850
　　specified NEC J95.859
　ventilator J95.850
　　specified NEC J95.859
Breast —*see also* condition
　buds E30.1
　　in newborn P96.89

Breast (*Continued*)
　dense R92.2
　nodule N63
Breath
　foul R19.6
　holder, child R06.89
　holding spell R06.89
　shortness R06.02
Breathing
　labored —*see* Hyperventilation
　mouth R06.5
　　causing malocclusion M26.5
　periodic R06.3
　　high altitude G47.32
Breathlessness R06.81
Breda's disease —*see* Yaws
Breech presentation (mother) O32.1
　causing obstructed labor O64.1
　footling O32.8
　　causing obstructed labor O64.8
　incomplete O32.8
　　causing obstructed labor O64.8
Breisky's disease N90.4
Brennemann's syndrome I88.0
Brenner
　tumor (benign) D27.9
　　borderline malignancy D39.1-
　　malignant C56
　　proliferating D39.1
Bretonneau's disease or angina
　A36.0
Breus' mole O02.0
Brevicollis Q76.49
Brickmakers' anemia B76.9
Bridge, myocardial Q24.5
Bright red blood per rectum (BRBPR)
　K62.5
Bright's disease —*see also* Nephritis
　arteriosclerotic —*see* Hypertension,
　　kidney
Brill (-Zinsser) disease (recrudescent
　typhus) A75.1
　flea-borne A75.2
　louse-borne A75.1
Brill-Symmers' disease C82.90
Brion-Kayser disease —*see* Fever,
　parathyroid
Briquet's disorder or syndrome F45.0
Brissaud's
　infantilism or dwarfism E23.0
　motor-verbal tic F95.2
Brittle
　bones disease Q78.0
　nails L60.3
　　congenital Q84.6
Broad —*see also* condition
　beta disease E78.2
　ligament laceration syndrome
　　N83.8
Broad- or floating-betalipoproteinemia
　E78.2
Brock's syndrome (atelectasis due
　to enlarged lymph nodes)
　J98.19
Brocq-Duhring disease (dermatitis
　herpetiformis) L13.0
Brodie's abscess or disease M86.8X-
Broken
　arches —*see also* Deformity, limb,
　　flat foot
　arm (meaning upper limb) —*see*
　　Fracture, arm
　back —*see* Fracture, vertebra
　bone —*see* Fracture

Broken *(Continued)*
  implant or internal device —*see*
      Complications, by site and type,
      mechanical
  leg (meaning lower limb) —*see* Fracture,
      leg
  nose S02.2
  tooth, teeth —*see* Fracture, tooth
Bromhidrosis, bromidrosis L75.0
Bromidism, bromism G92
  chronic (dependence) F13.20
  due to
    correct substance properly
      administered —*see* Table of drugs
      and chemicals, by drug, adverse
      effect
    overdose or wrong substance
      given or taken —*see* Table of
      drugs and chemicals, by drug,
      poisoning
Bromidrosiphobia F40.298
Bronchi, bronchial —*see* condition
Bronchiectasis (cylindrical) (diffuse)
  (fusiform) (localized) (saccular) J47.9
  with
    acute
      bronchitis J47.0
      lower respiratory infection J47.0
    exacerbation (acute) J47.1
  congenital Q33.4
  tuberculous NEC —*see* Tuberculosis,
    pulmonary
Bronchiolectasis —*see* Bronchiectasis
Bronchiolitis (acute) (infective) (subacute)
  J21.9
  with
    bronchospasm or obstruction J21.9
    influenza, flu or grippe —*see*
      Influenza, with, respiratory
      manifestations NEC
  chemical (chronic) J68.4
    acute J68.0
  chronic (fibrosing) (obliterative) J44.9
  due to
    external agent —*see* Bronchitis, acute,
      due to
    human metapneumovirus J21.1
    respiratory syncytial virus J21.0
    specified organism NEC J21.8
  fibrosa obliterans J44.9
  influenzal —*see* Influenza, with,
    respiratory manifestations NEC
  obliterans J42
    with organizing pneumonia (BOOP)
      J84.89
  obliterative (chronic) (subacute) J44.9
    due to chemicals, gases, fumes or
      vapors (inhalation) J68.4
    due to fumes or vapors J68.4
  respiratory, interstitial lung disease
    J84.115
Bronchitis (diffuse) (fibrinous)
  (hypostatic) (infective)
  (membranous) J40
  with
    influenza, flu or grippe —*see*
      Influenza, with, respiratory
      manifestations NEC
    obstruction (airway) (lung) J44.9
    tracheitis (15 years of age and above)
      J40
      acute or subacute J20.9
      chronic J42
      under 15 years of age J20.9

Bronchitis *(Continued)*
  acute or subacute (with bronchospasm
    or obstruction) J20.9
    with
      bronchiectasis J47.0
      chronic obstructive pulmonary
        disease J44.0
    chemical (due to gases, fumes or
      vapors) J68.0
    due to
      fumes or vapors J68.0
      Haemophilus influenzae J20.1
      Mycoplasma pneumoniae J20.0
      radiation J70.0
      specified organism NEC J20.8
      Streptococcus J20.2
      virus
        coxsackie J20.3
        echovirus J20.7
        parainfluenzae J20.4
        respiratory syncytial J20.5
        rhinovirus J20.6
    viral NEC J20.8
  allergic (acute) J45.909
    with
      exacerbation (acute) J45.901
      status asthmaticus J45.902
  arachidic T17.528
  aspiration (due to fumes or vapors) J68.0
  asthmatic J45.9
    chronic J44.9
    with
      acute lower respiratory infection
        J44.0
      exacerbation (acute) J44.1
  capillary —*see* Pneumonia, broncho
  caseous (tuberculous) A15.5
  Castellani's A69.8
  catarrhal (15 years of age and above) J40
    acute —*see* Bronchitis, acute
    chronic J41.0
    under 15 years of age J20.9
  chemical (acute) (subacute) J68.0
    chronic J68.4
    due to fumes or vapors J68.0
      chronic J68.4
  chronic J42
    with
      airways obstruction J44.9
      tracheitis (chronic) J42
    asthmatic (obstructive) J44.9
    catarrhal J41.0
    chemical (due to fumes or vapors) J68.4
    due to
      chemicals, gases, fumes or vapors
        (inhalation) J68.4
      radiation J70.1
      tobacco smoking J41.0
    emphysematous J44.9
    mucopurulent J41.1
    non-obstructive J41.0
    obliterans J44.9
    obstructive J44.9
    purulent J41.1
    simple J41.0
  croupous —*see* Bronchitis, acute
  due to gases, fumes or vapors
    (chemical) J68.0
  emphysematous (obstructive) J44.9
  exudative —*see* Bronchitis, acute
  fetid J41.1
  grippal —*see* Influenza, with,
    respiratory manifestations
    NEC

Bronchitis *(Continued)*
  in those under 15 years age —*see*
    Bronchitis, acute
    chronic —*see* Bronchitis, chronic
  influenzal —*see* Influenza, with,
    respiratory manifestations NEC
  mixed simple and mucopurulent J41.8
  moulder's J62.8
  mucopurulent (chronic) (recurrent) J41.1
    acute or subacute J20.9
    simple (mixed) J41.8
  obliterans (chronic) J44.9
  obstructive (chronic) (diffuse) J44.9
  pituitous J41.1
  pneumococcal, acute or subacute J20.2
  pseudomembranous, acute or
    subacute —*see* Bronchitis, acute
  purulent (chronic) (recurrent) J41.1
    acute or subacute —*see* Bronchitis,
      acute
  putrid J41.1
  senile (chronic) J42
  simple and mucopurulent (mixed) J41.8
  smokers' J41.0
  spirochetal NEC A69.8
  subacute —*see* Bronchitis, acute
  suppurative (chronic) J41.1
    acute or subacute —*see* Bronchitis,
      acute
  tuberculous A15.5
  under 15 years of age —*see* Bronchitis,
    acute
    chronic —*see* Bronchitis, chronic
  viral NEC, acute or subacute (*see also*
    Bronchitis, acute) J20.8
Bronchoalveolitis J18.0
Bronchoaspergillosis B44.1
Bronchocele meaning goiter E04.0
Broncholithiasis J98.09
  tuberculous NEC A15.5
Bronchomalacia J98.09
  congenital Q32.2
Bronchomycosis NOS B49 *[J99]*
  candidal B37.1
Bronchopleuropneumonia —*see*
  Pneumonia, broncho
Bronchopneumonia —*see* Pneumonia,
  broncho
Bronchopneumonitis —*see* Pneumonia,
  broncho
Bronchopulmonary —*see* condition
Bronchopulmonitis —*see* Pneumonia,
  broncho
Bronchorrhagia (*see* Hemoptysis)
Bronchorrhea J98.09
  acute J20.9
  chronic (infective) (purulent) J42
Bronchospasm (acute) J98.01
  with
    bronchiolitis, acute J21.9
    bronchitis, acute (conditions in
      J20) —*see* Bronchitis, acute
  due to external agent —*see* condition,
    respiratory, acute, due to
  exercise induced J45.990
Bronchospirochetosis A69.8
  Castellani A69.8
Bronchostenosis J98.09
Bronchus —*see* condition
Brontophobia F40.220
Bronze baby syndrome P83.8
Brooke's tumor —*see* Neoplasm, skin,
  benign
Brown enamel of teeth (hereditary) K00.5

Brown's sheath syndrome H50.61-
Brown-Séquard disease, paralysis or
   syndrome G83.81
Bruce sepsis A23.0
Brucellosis (infection) A23.9
   abortus A23.1
   canis A23.3
   dermatitis A23.9
   melitensis A23.0
   mixed A23.8
   sepsis A23.9
      melitensis A23.0
      specified NEC A23.8
   suis A23.2
Bruck-de Lange disease Q87.1
Bruck's disease —see Deformity, limb
Brugsch's syndrome Q82.8
Bruise (skin surface intact) —see also
   Contusion
   with
      open wound —see Wound, open
   internal organ —see Injury, by site
   newborn P54.5
   scalp, due to birth injury, newborn P12.3
   umbilical cord O69.5
Bruit (arterial) R09.89
   cardiac R01.1
Brush burn —see Abrasion, by site
Bruton's X-linked agammaglobulinemia
   D80.0
Bruxism
   psychogenic F45.8
   sleep related G47.63
Bubbly lung syndrome P27.0
Bubo I88.8
   blennorrhagic (gonococcal) A54.89
   chancroidal A57
   climatic A55
   due to Haemophilus ducreyi A57
   gonococcal A54.89
   indolent (nonspecific) I88.8
   inguinal (nonspecific) I88.8
      chancroidal A57
      climatic A55
      due to H. ducreyi A57
      infective I88.8
   scrofulous (tuberculous) A18.2
   soft chancre A57
   suppurating —see Lymphadenitis, acute
   syphilitic (primary) A51.0
      congenital A50.07
   tropical A55
   virulent (chancroidal) A57
Bubonic plague A20.0
Bubonocele —see Hernia, inguinal
Buccal —see condition
Buchanan's disease or osteochondrosis
   M91.0
Buchem's syndrome (hyperostosis
   corticalis) M85.2
Bucket-handle fracture or tear (semilunar
   cartilage) —see Tear, meniscus
Budd-Chiari syndrome (hepatic vein
   thrombosis) I82.0
Budgerigar fancier's disease or lung
   J67.2
Buds
   breast E30.1
      in newborn P96.89
Buerger's disease (thromboangiitis
   obliterans) I73.1
Bulbar —see condition
Bulbus cordis (left ventricle) (persistent)
   Q21.8

Bulimia (nervosa) F50.2
   atypical F50.9
   normal weight F50.9
Bulky
   stools R19.5
   uterus N85.2
Bulla (e) R23.8
   lung (emphysematous) (solitary) J43.9
      newborn P25.8
Bullet wound —see also Wound, open
   fracture - code as Fracture, by site
   internal organ —see Injury, by site
Bundle
   branch block (complete) (false)
      (incomplete) —see Block,
      bundle-branch
   of His —see condition
Bunion —see Deformity, toe, hallux
   valgus
Buphthalmia, buphthalmos (congenital)
   Q15.0
Burdwan fever B55.0
Bürger-Grütz disease or syndrome E78.3
Buried
   penis (congenital) Q55.64
      acquired N48.83
   roots K08.3
Burke's syndrome K86.8
Burkitt
   cell leukemia C91.0-
   lymphoma (malignant) C83.7-
      small noncleaved, diffuse C83.7-
      spleen C83.77
      undifferentiated C83.7-
   tumor C83.7-
   type
      acute lymphoblastic leukemia C91.0-
      undifferentiated C83.7-
Burn (electricity) (flame) (hot gas, liquid
   or hot object) (radiation) (steam)
   (thermal) T30.0
   abdomen, abdominal (muscle) (wall)
      T21.02
      first degree T21.12
      second degree T21.22
      third degree T21.32
   above elbow T22.039
      first degree T22.139
      left T22.032
         first degree T22.132
         second degree T22.232
         third degree T22.332
      right T22.031
         first degree T22.131
         second degree T22.231
         third degree T22.331
      second degree T22.239
      third degree T22.339
   acid (caustic) (external) (internal) —see
      Corrosion, by site
   alimentary tract NEC T28.2
      esophagus T28.1
      mouth T28.0
      pharynx T28.0
   alkaline (caustic) (external) (internal) —
      see Corrosion, by site
   ankle T25.019
      first degree T25.119
      left T25.012
         first degree T25.112
         second degree T25.212
         third degree T25.312
      multiple with foot —see Burn, lower,
         limb, multiple, ankle and foot

Burn (Continued)
   ankle (Continued)
      right T25.011
         first degree T25.111
         second degree T25.211
         third degree T25.311
      second degree T25.219
      third degree T25.319
   anus —see Burn, buttock
   arm (lower) (upper) —see Burn, upper,
      limb
   axilla T22.049
      first degree T22.149
      left T22.042
         first degree T22.142
         second degree T22.242
         third degree T22.342
      right T22.041
         first degree T22.141
         second degree T22.241
         third degree T22.341
      second degree T22.249
      third degree T22.349
   back (lower) T21.04
      first degree T21.14
      second degree T21.24
      third degree T21.34
      upper T21.03
         first degree T21.13
         second degree T21.23
         third degree T21.33
   blisters - code as Burn, second degree,
      by site
   breast (s) —see Burn, chest wall
   buttock (s) T21.05
      first degree T21.15
      second degree T21.25
      third degree T21.35
   calf T24.039
      first degree T24.139
      left T24.032
         first degree T24.132
         second degree T24.232
         third degree T24.332
      right T24.031
         first degree T24.131
         second degree T24.231
         third degree T24.331
      second degree T24.239
      third degree T24.339
   canthus (eye) —see Burn, eyelid
   caustic acid or alkaline —see Corrosion,
      by site
   cervix T28.3
   cheek T20.06
      first degree T20.16
      second degree T20.26
      third degree T20.36
   chemical (acids) (alkalines)
      (caustics) (external) (internal) —see
      Corrosion, by site
   chest wall T21.01
      first degree T21.11
      second degree T21.21
      third degree T21.31
   chin T20.03
      first degree T20.13
      second degree T20.23
      third degree T20.33
   colon T28.2
   conjunctiva (and cornea) —see Burn,
      cornea
   cornea (and conjunctiva) T26.1-
      chemical —see Corrosion, cornea

Burn (Continued)
corrosion (external) (internal) —see
Corrosion, by site
deep necrosis of underlying tissue -
code as Burn, third degree, by site
dorsum of hand T23.069
first degree T23.169
left T23.062
first degree T23.162
second degree T23.262
third degree T23.362
right T23.061
first degree T23.161
second degree T23.261
third degree T23.361
second degree T23.269
third degree T23.369
due to ingested chemical agent —see
Corrosion, by site
ear (auricle) (external) (canal) T20.01
first degree T20.11
second degree T20.21
third degree T20.31
elbow T22.029
first degree T22.129
left T22.022
first degree T22.122
second degree T22.222
third degree T22.322
right T22.021
first degree T22.121
second degree T22.221
third degree T22.321
second degree T22.229
third degree T22.329
epidermal loss - code as Burn, second
degree, by site
erythema, erythematous - code as Burn,
first degree, by site
esophagus T28.1
extent (percentage of body surface)
less than 10 percent T31.0
10-19 percent T31.10
with 0-9 percent third degree burns
T31.10
with 10-19 percent third degree
burns T31.11
20-29 percent T31.20
with 0-9 percent third degree burns
T31.20
with 10-19 percent third degree
burns T31.21
with 20-29 percent third degree
burns T31.22
30-39 percent T31.30
with 0-9 percent third degree burns
T31.30
with 10-19 percent third degree
burns T31.31
with 20-29 percent third degree
burns T31.32
with 30-39 percent third degree
burns T31.33
40-49 percent T31.40
with 0-9 percent third degree burns
T31.40
with 10-19 percent third degree
burns T31.41
with 20-29 percent third degree
burns T31.42
with 30-39 percent third degree
burns T31.43
with 40-49 percent third degree
burns T31.44

Burn (Continued)
extent (Continued)
50-59 percent T31.50
with 0-9 percent third degree burns
T31.50
with 10-19 percent third degree
burns T31.51
with 20-29 percent third degree
burns T31.52
with 30-39 percent third degree
burns T31.53
with 40-49 percent third degree
burns T31.54
with 50-59 percent third degree
burns T31.55
60-69 percent T31.60
with 0-9 percent third degree burns
T31.60
with 10-19 percent third degree
burns T31.61
with 20-29 percent third degree
burns T31.62
with 30-39 percent third degree
burns T31.63
with 40-49 percent third degree
burns T31.64
with 50-59 percent third degree
burns T31.65
with 60-69 percent third degree
burns T31.66
70-79 percent T31.70
with 0-9 percent third degree burns
T31.70
with 10-19 percent third degree
burns T31.71
with 20-29 percent third degree
burns T31.72
with 30-39 percent third degree
burns T31.73
with 40-49 percent third degree
burns T31.74
with 50-59 percent third degree
burns T31.75
with 60-69 percent third degree
burns T31.76
with 70-79 percent third degree
burns T31.77
80-89 percent T31.80
with 0-9 percent third degree burns
T31.80
with 10-19 percent third degree
burns T31.81
with 20-29 percent third degree
burns T31.82
with 30-39 percent third degree
burns T31.83
with 40-49 percent third degree
burns T31.84
with 50-59 percent third degree
burns T31.85
with 60-69 percent third degree
burns T31.86
with 70-79 percent third degree
burns T31.87
with 80-89 percent third degree
burns T31.88
90 percent or more T31.90
with 0-9 percent third degree burns
T31.90
with 10-19 percent third degree
burns T31.91
with 20-29 percent third degree
burns T31.92
with 30-39 percent third degree
burns T31.93

Burn (Continued)
extent (Continued)
90 percent or more (Continued)
with 40-49 percent third degree
burns T31.94
with 50-59 percent third degree
burns T31.95
with 60-69 percent third degree
burns T31.96
with 70-79 percent third degree
burns T31.97
with 80-89 percent third degree
burns T31.98
with 90 percent or more third
degree burns T31.99
extremity —see Burn, limb
eye (s) and adnexa T26.4-
with resulting rupture and destruction
of eyeball T26.2-
conjunctival sac —see Burn, cornea
cornea —see Burn, cornea
lid —see Burn, \eyelid
periocular area —see Burn eyelid
specified site NEC T26.3-
eyeball —see Burn, eye
eyelid (s) T26.0-
chemical —see Corrosion, eyelid
face —see Burn, head
finger T23.029
first degree T23.129
left T23.022
first degree T23.122
second degree T23.222
third degree T23.322
multiple sites (without thumb)
T23.039
with thumb T23.049
first degree T23.149
left T23.042
first degree T23.142
second degree T23.242
third degree T23.342
right T23.041
first degree T23.141
second degree T23.241
third degree T23.341
second degree T23.249
third degree T23.349
first degree T23.139
left T23.032
first degree T23.132
second degree T23.232
third degree T23.332
right T23.031
first degree T23.131
second degree T23.231
third degree T23.331
second degree T23.239
third degree T23.339
right T23.021
first degree T23.121
second degree T23.221
third degree T23.321
second degree T23.229
third degree T23.329
flank —see Burn, abdominal wall
foot T25.029
first degree T25.129
left T25.022
first degree T25.122
second degree T25.222
third degree T25.322
multiple with ankle —see Burn, lower,
limb, multiple, ankle and foot

Burn *(Continued)*
  foot *(Continued)*
    right T25.021
      first degree T25.121
      second degree T25.221
      third degree T25.321
    second degree T25.229
    third degree T25.329
  forearm T22.019
    first degree T22.119
    left T22.012
      first degree T22.112
      second degree T22.212
      third degree T22.312
    right T22.011
      first degree T22.111
      second degree T22.211
      third degree T22.311
    second degree T22.219
    third degree T22.319
  forehead T20.06
    first degree T20.16
    second degree T20.26
    third degree T20.36
  fourth degree - code as Burn, third
      degree, by site
  friction —*see* Burn, by site
  from swallowing caustic or corrosive
      substance NEC —*see* Corrosion,
      by site
  full thickness skin loss - code as Burn,
      third degree, by site
  gastrointestinal tract NEC T28.2
    from swallowing caustic or corrosive
        substance T28.7
  genital organs
    external
      female T21.07
        first degree T21.17
        second degree T21.27
        third degree T21.37
      male T21.06
        first degree T21.16
        second degree T21.26
        third degree T21.36
    internal T28.3
      from caustic or corrosive substance
          T28.8
  groin —*see* Burn, abdominal wall
  hand (s) T23.009
    back —*see* Burn, dorsum of hand
    finger —*see* Burn, finger
    first degree T23.109
    left T23.002
      first degree T23.102
      second degree T23.202
      third degree T23.302
    multiple sites with wrist T23.099
      first degree T23.199
      left T23.092
        first degree T23.192
        second degree T23.292
        third degree T23.392
      right T23.091
        first degree T23.191
        second degree T23.291
        third degree T23.391
      second degree T23.299
      third degree T23.399
    palm —*see* Burn, palm
    right T23.001
      first degree T23.101
      second degree T23.201
      third degree T23.301

Burn *(Continued)*
  hand (s) *(Continued)*
    second degree T23.209
    third degree T23.309
    thumb —*see* Burn, thumb
  head (and face) (and neck) T20.00
    cheek —*see* Burn, cheek
    chin —*see* Burn, chin
    ear —*see* Burn, ear
    eye (s) only —*see* Burn, eye
    first degree T20.10
    forehead —*see* Burn, forehead
    lip —*see* Burn, lip
    multiple sites T20.09
      first degree T20.19
      second degree T20.29
      third degree T20.39
    neck —*see* Burn, neck
    nose —*see* Burn, nose
    scalp —*see* Burn, scalp
    second degree T20.20
    third degree T20.30
  hip (s) —*see* Burn, lower, limb
  inhalation —*see* Burn, respiratory tract
    caustic or corrosive substance
        (fumes) —*see* Corrosion,
        respiratory tract
  internal organ (s) T28.40
    alimentary tract T28.2
      esophagus T28.1
    eardrum T28.41
    esophagus T28.1
    from caustic or corrosive substance
        (swallowing) NEC —*see*
        Corrosion, by site
    genitourinary T28.3
    mouth T28.0
    pharynx T28.0
    respiratory tract —*see* Burn,
        respiratory tract
    specified organ NEC T28.49
  interscapular region —*see* Burn, back,
      upper
  intestine (large) (small) T28.2
  knee T24.029
    first degree T24.129
    left T24.022
      first degree T24.122
      second degree T24.222
      third degree T24.322
    right T24.021
      first degree T24.121
      second degree T24.221
      third degree T24.321
    second degree T24.229
    third degree T24.329
  labium (majus) (minus) —*see* Burn,
      genital organs, external, female
  lacrimal apparatus, duct, gland or
      sac —*see* Burn, eye, specified site
      NEC
  larynx T27.0
    with lung T27.1
  leg (s) (lower) (upper) —*see* Burn,
      lower, limb
  lightning —*see* Burn, by site
  limb (s)
    lower (except ankle or foot alone) —
        see Burn, lower, limb
    upper —*see* Burn, upper limb
  lip (s) T20.02
    first degree T20.12
    second degree T20.22
    third degree T20.32

Burn *(Continued)*
  lower
    back —*see* Burn, back
    limb T24.009
      ankle —*see* Burn, ankle
      calf —*see* Burn, calf
      first degree T24.109
      foot —*see* Burn, foot
      hip —*see* Burn, thigh
      knee —*see* Burn, knee
      left T24.002
        first degree T24.102
        second degree T24.202
        third degree T24.302
      multiple sites, except ankle and
          foot T24.099
        ankle and foot T25.099
          first degree T25.199
          left T25.092
            first degree T25.192
            second degree T25.292
            third degree T25.392
          right T25.091
            first degree T25.191
            second degree T25.291
            third degree T25.391
          second degree T25.299
          third degree T25.399
        first degree T24.199
        left T24.092
          first degree T24.192
          second degree T24.292
          third degree T24.392
        right T24.091
          first degree T24.191
          second degree T24.291
          third degree T24.391
        second degree T24.299
        third degree T24.399
      right T24.001
        first degree T24.101
        second degree T24.201
        third degree T24.301
      second degree T24.209
      thigh —*see* Burn, thigh
      third degree T24.309
      toe —*see* Burn, toe
  lung (with larynx and trachea) T27.1
  mouth T28.0
  neck T20.07
    first degree T20.17
    second degree T20.27
    third degree T20.37
  nose (septum) T20.04
    first degree T20.14
    second degree T20.24
    third degree T20.34
  ocular adnexa —*see* Burn, eye
  orbit region —*see* Burn, eyelid
  palm T23.059
    first degree T23.159
    left T23.052
      first degree T23.152
      second degree T23.252
      third degree T23.352
    right T23.051
      first degree T23.151
      second degree T23.251
      third degree T23.351
    second degree T23.259
    third degree T23.359
  partial thickness - code as Burn,
      unspecified degree, by site
  pelvis —*see* Burn, trunk

Burn (*Continued*)
  penis —*see* Burn, genital organs,
    external, male
  perineum
    female —*see* Burn, genital organs,
      external, female
    male —*see* Burn, genital organs,
      external, male
  periocular area —*see* Burn, eyelid
  pharynx T28.0
  rectum T28.2
  respiratory tract T27.3
    larynx —*see* Burn, larynx
    specified part NEC T27.2
    trachea —*see* Burn, trachea
  sac, lacrimal —*see* Burn, eye, specified
    site NEC
  scalp T20.05
    first degree T20.15
    second degree T20.25
    third degree T20.35
  scapular region T22.069
    first degree T22.169
    left T22.062
      first degree T22.162
      second degree T22.262
      third degree T22.362
    right T22.061
      first degree T22.161
      second degree T22.261
      third degree T22.361
    second degree T22.269
    third degree T22.369
  sclera —*see* Burn, eye, specified site
    NEC
  scrotum —*see* Burn, genital organs,
    external, male
  shoulder T22.059
    first degree T22.159
    left T22.052
      first degree T22.152
      second degree T22.252
      third degree T22.352
    right T22.051
      first degree T22.151
      second degree T22.251
      third degree T22.351
    second degree T22.259
    third degree T22.359
  stomach T28.2
  temple —*see* Burn, head
  testis —*see* Burn, genital organs,
    external, male
  thigh T24.019
    first degree T24.119
    left T24.012
      first degree T24.112
      second degree T24.212
      third degree T24.312
    right T24.011
      first degree T24.111
      second degree T24.211
      third degree T24.311
    second degree T24.219
    third degree T24.319
  thorax (external) —*see* Burn,
    trunk
  throat (meaning pharynx)
    T28.0
  thumb (s) T23.019
    first degree T23.119
    left T23.012
      first degree T23.112
      second degree T23.212
      third degree T23.312

Burn (*Continued*)
  thumb (s) (*Continued*)
    multiple sites with fingers T23.049
      first degree T23.149
      left T23.042
        first degree T23.142
        second degree T23.242
        third degree T23.342
      right T23.041
        first degree T23.141
        second degree T23.241
        third degree T23.341
      second degree T23.249
      third degree T23.349
    right T23.011
      first degree T23.111
      second degree T23.211
      third degree T23.311
    second degree T23.219
    third degree T23.319
  toe T25.039
    first degree T25.139
    left T25.032
      first degree T25.132
      second degree T25.232
      third degree T25.332
    right T25.031
      first degree T25.131
      second degree T25.231
      third degree T25.331
    second degree T25.239
    third degree T25.339
  tongue T28.0
  tonsil (s) T28.0
  trachea T27.0
    with lung T27.1
  trunk T21.00
    abdominal wall —*see* Burn,
      abdominal wall
    anus —*see* Burn, buttock
    axilla —*see* Burn, upper limb
    back —*see* Burn, back
    breast —*see* Burn, chest wall
    buttock —*see* Burn, buttock
    chest wall —*see* Burn, chest wall
    first degree T21.10
    flank —*see* Burn, abdominal wall
    genital
      female —*see* Burn, genital organs,
        external, female
      male —*see* Burn, genital organs,
        external, male
    groin —*see* Burn, abdominal wall
    interscapular region —*see* Burn, back,
      upper
    labia —*see* Burn, genital organs,
      external, female
    lower back —*see* Burn, back
    penis —*see* Burn, genital organs,
      external, male
    perineum
      female —*see* Burn, genital organs,
        external, female
      male —*see* Burn, genital organs,
        external, male
    scapula region —*see* Burn, scapular
      region
    scrotum —*see* Burn, genital organs,
      external, male
    second degree T21.20
    specified site NEC T21.09
      first degree T21.19
      second degree T21.29
      third degree T21.39

Burn (*Continued*)
  trunk (*Continued*)
    testes —*see* Burn, genital organs,
      external, male
    third degree T21.30
    upper back —*see* Burn, back,
      upper
    vulva —*see* Burn, genital organs,
      external, female
  unspecified site with extent of
    body surface involved
    specified
    less than 10 percent T31.0
    10-19 percent (0-9 percent third
      degree) T31.10
      with 10-19 percent third degree
        T31.11
    20-29 percent (0-9 percent third
      degree) T31.20
      with
        10-19 percent third degree T31.21
        20-29 percent third degree T31.22
    30-39 percent (0-9 percent third
      degree) T31.30
      with
        10-19 percent third degree T31.31
        20-29 percent third degree T31.32
        30-39 percent third degree T31.33
    40-49 percent (0-9 percent third
      degree) T31.40
      with
        10-19 percent third degree T31.41
        20-29 percent third degree T31.42
        30-39 percent third degree T31.43
        40-49 percent third degree T31.44
    50-59 percent (0-9 percent third
      degree) T31.50
      with
        10-19 percent third degree T31.51
        20-29 percent third degree T31.52
        30-39 percent third degree T31.53
        40-49 percent third degree T31.54
        50-59 percent third degree T31.55
    60-69 percent (0-9 percent third
      degree) T31.60
      with
        10-19 percent third degree T31.61
        20-29 percent third degree T31.62
        30-39 percent third degree T31.63
        40-49 percent third degree T31.64
        50-59 percent third degree T31.65
        60-69 percent third degree T31.66
    70-79 percent (0-9 percent third
      degree) T31.70
      with
        10-19 percent third degree T31.71
        20-29 percent third degree T31.72
        30-39 percent third degree T31.73
        40-49 percent third degree T31.74
        50-59 percent third degree T31.75
        60-69 percent third degree T31.76
        70-79 percent third degree T31.77
    80-89 percent (0-9 percent third
      degree) T31.80
      with
        10-19 percent third degree T31.81
        20-29 percent third degree T31.82
        30-39 percent third degree T31.83
        40-49 percent third degree T31.84
        50-59 percent third degree T31.85
        60-69 percent third degree T31.86
        70-79 percent third degree T31.87
        80-89 percent third degree T31.88

Burn (*Continued*)
  unspecified site with extent of
    body surface involved
    specified (*Continued*)
     90 percent or more (0-9 percent third
      degree) T31.90
      with
        10-19 percent third degree T31.91
        20-29 percent third degree T31.92
        30-39 percent third degree T31.93
        40-49 percent third degree T31.94
        50-59 percent third degree T31.95
        60-69 percent third degree T31.96
        70-79 percent third degree T31.97
        80-89 percent third degree T31.98
        90-99 percent third degree T31.99
  upper limb T22.00
    above elbow —*see* Burn, above elbow
    axilla —*see* Burn, axilla
    elbow —*see* Burn, elbow
    first degree T22.10
    forearm —*see* Burn, forearm
    hand —*see* Burn, hand
    interscapular region —*see* Burn, back,
      upper
    multiple sites T22.099
      first degree T22.199
      left T22.092
        first degree T22.192
        second degree T22.292
        third degree T22.392
      right T22.091
        first degree T22.191
        second degree T22.291
        third degree T22.391
      second degree T22.299
      third degree T22.399
    scapular region —*see* Burn, scapular
      region
    second degree T22.20
    shoulder —*see* Burn, shoulder
    third degree T22.30
    wrist —*see* Burn, wrist
  uterus T28.3
  vagina T28.3
  vulva —*see* Burn, genital organs,
    external, female
  wrist T23.079
    first degree T23.179
    left T23.072
      first degree T23.172
      second degree T23.272
      third degree T23.372
    multiple sites with hand T23.099
      first degree T23.199
      left T23.092
        first degree T23.192
        second degree T23.292
        third degree T23.392
      right T23.091
        first degree T23.191
        second degree T23.291
        third degree T23.391
      second degree T23.299
      third degree T23.399
    right T23.071
      first degree T23.171
      second degree T23.271
      third degree T23.371

Burn (*Continued*)
  wrist (*Continued*)
    second degree T23.279
    third degree T23.379
Burnett's syndrome E83.52
Burning
  feet syndrome E53.9
  sensation R20.8
  tongue K14.6
Burn-out (state) Z73.0
Burns' disease or osteochondrosis —*see*
  Osteochondrosis, juvenile, ulna
Bursa —*see* condition
Bursitis M71.9
  Achilles —*see* Tendinitis, Achilles
  adhesive —*see* Bursitis, specified NEC
  ankle —*see* Enthesopathy, lower limb,
    ankle, specified type NEC
  calcaneal —*see* Enthesopathy, foot,
    specified type NEC
  collateral ligament, tibial —*see* Bursitis,
    tibial collateral
  due to use, overuse, pressure —*see also*
    Disorder, soft tissue, due to use,
    specified type NEC
  specified NEC —*see* Disorder, soft
    tissue, due to use, specified NEC
  Duplay's M75.0
  elbow NEC M70.3-
    olecranon M70.2-
  finger —*see* Disorder, soft tissue,
    due to use, specified type NEC,
    hand
  foot —*see* Enthesopathy, foot, specified
    type NEC
  gonococcal A54.49
  gouty —*see* Gout, idiopathic
  hand M70.1-
  hip NEC M70.7-
    trochanteric M70.6-
  infective NEC M71.10
    abscess —*see* Abscess, bursa
    ankle M71.17-
    elbow M71.12-
    foot M71.17-
    hand M71.14-
    hip M71.15-
    knee M71.16-
    multiple sites M71.19
    shoulder M71.11-
    specified site NEC M71.18
    wrist M71.13-
  ischial —*see* Bursitis, hip
  knee NEC M70.5-
    prepatellar M70.4-
  occupational NEC —*see also* Disorder,
    soft tissue, due to use,
  olecranon —*see* Bursitis, elbow,
    olecranon
  pharyngeal J39.1
  popliteal —*see* Bursitis, knee
  prepatellar M70.4-
  radiohumeral M77.8
  rheumatoid M06.20
    ankle M06.27-
    elbow M06.22-
    foot joint M06.27-
    hand joint M06.24-
    hip M06.25-

Bursitis (*Continued*)
  rheumatoid (*Continued*)
    knee M06.26-
    multiple site M06.29
    shoulder M06.21-
    vertebra M06.28
    wrist M06.23-
  scapulohumeral —*see* Bursitis, shoulder
  semimembranous muscle (knee) —*see*
    Bursitis, knee
  shoulder M75.5-
    adhesive —*see* Capsulitis, adhesive
  specified NEC M71.50
    ankle M71.57-
    due to use, overuse or pressure —*see*
      Disorder, soft tissue, due to, use
    elbow M71.52-
    foot M71.57-
    hand M71.54-
    hip M71.55-
    knee M71.56-
    shoulder —*see* Bursitis, shoulder
    specified site NEC M71.58
    tibial collateral M76.4-
    wrist M71.53-
  subacromial —*see* Bursitis, shoulder
  subcoracoid —*see* Bursitis, shoulder
  subdeltoid —*see* Bursitis, shoulder
  syphilitic A52.78
  Thornwaldt, Tornwaldt J39.2
  tibial collateral —*see* Bursitis, tibial
    collateral
  toe —*see* Enthesopathy, foot, specified
    type NEC
  trochanteric (area) —*see* Bursitis, hip,
    trochanteric
  wrist —*see* Bursitis, hand
Bursopathy M71.9
  specified type NEC M71.80
    ankle M71.87-
    elbow M71.82-
    foot M71.87-
    hand M71.84-
    hip M71.85-
    knee M71.86-
    multiple sites M71.89
    shoulder M71.81-
    specified site NEC M71.88
    wrist M71.83-
Burst stitches or sutures (complication of
  surgery) T81.31
  external operation wound T81.31
  internal operation wound T81.32
Buruli ulcer A31.1
Bury's disease L95.1
Buschke's
  disease B45.3
  scleredema —*see* Sclerosis, systemic
Busse-Buschke disease B45.3
Buttock —*see* condition
Button
  Biskra B55.1
  Delhi B55.1
  oriental B55.1
Buttonhole deformity (finger) —*see*
  Deformity, finger, boutonniere
Bwamba fever A92.8
Byssinosis J66.0
Bywaters' syndrome T79.5

C

Cachexia R64
  cancerous R64
  cardiac —see Disease, heart
  dehydration E86.0
    with
      hypernatremia E87.0
      hyponatremia E87.1
    due to malnutrition R64
  exophthalmic —see Hyperthyroidism
  heart —see Disease, heart
  hypophyseal E23.0
  hypopituitary E23.0
  lead —see Poisoning, lead
  malignant R64
  marsh —see Malaria
  nervous F48.8
  old age R54
  paludal —see Malaria
  pituitary E23.0
  renal N28.9
  saturnine —see Poisoning, lead
  senile R54
  Simmonds' E23.0
  splenica D73.0
  strumipriva E03.4
  tuberculous NEC —see Tuberculosis
Café au lait spots L81.3
Caffey's syndrome Q78.8
Caisson disease T70.3
Cake kidney Q63.1
Caked breast (puerperal, postpartum)
    O92.79
Calabar swelling B74.3
Calcaneal spur —see Spur, bone, calcaneal
Calcaneo-apophysitis M92.8
Calcareous —see condition
Calcicosis J62.8
Calciferol (vitamin D) deficiency E55.9
  with rickets E55.0
Calcification
  adrenal (capsule) (gland) E27.49
    tuberculous B90.8 [E35]
  aorta I70.0
  artery (annular) —see Arteriosclerosis
  auricle (ear) —see Disorder, pinna,
      specified type NEC
  basal ganglia G23.8
  bladder N32.89
    due to Schistosoma hematobium
        B65.0
  brain (cortex) —see Calcification,
      cerebral
  bronchus J98.09
  bursa M71.40
    ankle M71.47-
    elbow M71.42-
    foot M71.47-
    hand M71.44-
    hip M71.45-
    knee M71.46-
    multiple sites M71.49
    shoulder M75.3-
    specified site NEC M71.48
    wrist M71.43-
  cardiac —see Degeneration, myocardial
  cerebral (cortex) G93.89
    artery I67.2
  cervix (uteri) N88.8
  choroid plexus G93.89
  conjunctiva —see Concretion, conjunctiva
  corpora cavernosa (penis) N48.89
  cortex (brain) —see Calcification, cerebral

Calcification (Continued)
  dental pulp (nodular) K04.2
  dentinal papilla K00.4
  fallopian tube N83.8
  falx cerebri G96.19
  gallbladder K82.8
  general E83.59
  heart —see also Degeneration, myocardial
    valve —see Endocarditis
  idiopathic infantile arterial (IIAC) Q28.8
  intervertebral cartilage or disc
      (postinfective) —see Disorder, disc,
      specified NEC
  intracranial —see Calcification, cerebral
  joint —see Disorder, joint, specified type
      NEC
  kidney N28.89
    tuberculous B90.1 [N29]
  larynx (senile) J38.7
  lens —see Cataract, specified NEC
  lung (active) (postinfectional) J98.4
    tuberculous B90.9
  lymph gland or node (postinfectional)
      I89.8
    tuberculous (see also Tuberculosis,
        lymph gland) B90.8
  mammographic R92.1
  massive (paraplegic) —see Myositis,
      ossificans, in, quadriplegia
  medial —see Arteriosclerosis,
      extremities
  meninges (cerebral) (spinal) G96.19
  metastatic E83.59
  Mönckeberg's —see Arteriosclerosis,
      extremities
  muscle M61.9
    due to burns —see Myositis,
        ossificans, in, burns
    paralytic —see Myositis, ossificans, in,
        quadriplegia
    specified type NEC M61.40
      ankle M61.47-
      foot M61.47-
      forearm M61.43-
      hand M61.44-
      lower leg M61.46-
      multiple sites M61.49
      pelvic region M61.45-
      shoulder region M61.41-
      specified site NEC M61.48
      thigh M61.45-
      upper arm M61.42-
  myocardium, myocardial —see
      Degeneration, myocardial
  ovary N83.8
  pancreas K86.8
  penis N48.89
  periarticular —see Disorder, joint,
      specified type NEC
  pericardium (see also Pericarditis) I31.1
  pineal gland E34.8
  pleura J94.8
    postinfectional J94.8
    tuberculous NEC B90.9
  pulpal (dental) (nodular) K04.2
  sclera H15.89
  spleen D73.89
  subcutaneous L94.2
  suprarenal (capsule) (gland) E27.49
  tendon (sheath) —see also Tenosynovitis,
      specified type NEC
    with bursitis, synovitis or
        tenosynovitis —see Tendinitis,
        calcific

Calcification (Continued)
  trachea J39.8
  ureter N28.89
  vitreous —see Deposit, crystalline
Calcified —see Calcification
Calcinosis (interstitial) (tumoral)
    (universalis) E83.59
  with Raynaud's phenomenon,
      esophageal dysfunction,
      sclerodactyly, telangiectasia
      (CREST syndrome) M34.1
  circumscripta (skin) L94.2
  cutis L94.2
Calciphylaxis (see also Calcification, by
    site) E83.59
Calcium
  deposits —see Calcification, by site
  metabolism disorder E83.50
  salts or soaps in vitreous —see Deposit,
      crystalline
Calciuria R82.99
Calculi —see Calculus
Calculosis, intrahepatic —see Calculus,
    bile duct
Calculus, calculi, calculous
  ampulla of Vater —see Calculus, bile
      duct
  anuria (impacted) (recurrent)
      (see also Calculus, urinary)
      N20.9
  appendix K38.1
  bile duct (common) (hepatic) K80.50
    with
      calculus of gallbladder —see
          Calculus, gallbladder and bile
          duct
      cholangitis K80.30
        with
          cholecystitis —see Calculus,
              bile duct, with
              cholecystitis
          obstruction K80.31
        acute K80.32
          with
            chronic cholangitis K80.36
              with obstruction K80.37
            obstruction K80.33
        chronic K80.34
          with
            acute cholangitis K80.36
              with obstruction K80.37
            obstruction K80.35
      cholecystitis (with cholangitis)
          K80.40
        with obstruction K80.41
        acute K80.42
          with
            chronic cholecystitis K80.46
              with obstruction K80.47
            obstruction K80.43
        chronic K80.44
          with
            acute cholecystitis K80.46
              with obstruction K80.47
            obstruction K80.45
      obstruction K80.51
    biliary —see also Calculus, gallbladder
    specified NEC K80.80
      with obstruction K80.81
    bilirubin, multiple —see Calculus,
        gallbladder
  bladder (encysted) (impacted) (urinary)
      (diverticulum) N21.0
  bronchus J98.09

Calculus, calculi, calculous *(Continued)*
calyx (kidney) (renal) —*see* Calculus, kidney
cholesterol (pure) (solitary) —*see* Calculus, gallbladder
common duct (bile) —*see* Calculus, bile duct
conjunctiva —*see* Concretion, conjunctiva
cystic N21.0
duct —*see* Calculus, gallbladder
dental (subgingival) (supragingival) K03.6
diverticulum
bladder N21.0
kidney N20.0
epididymis N50.8
gallbladder K80.20
with
bile duct calculus —*see* Calculus, gallbladder and bile duct
cholecystitis K80.10
with obstruction K80.11
acute K80.00
with
chronic cholecystitis K80.12
with obstruction K80.13
obstruction K80.01
chronic K80.10
with
acute cholecystitis K80.12
with obstruction K80.13
obstruction K80.11
specified NEC K80.18
with obstruction K80.19
obstruction K80.21
gallbladder and bile duct K80.70
with
cholecystitis K80.60
with obstruction K80.61
acute K80.62
with
chronic cholecystitis K80.66
with obstruction K80.67
obstruction K80.63
chronic K80.64
with
acute cholecystitis K80.66
with obstruction K80.67
obstruction K80.65
obstruction K80.71
hepatic (duct) —*see* Calculus, bile duct
ileal conduit N21.8
intestinal (impaction) (obstruction) K56.49
kidney (impacted) (multiple) (pelvis) (recurrent) (staghorn) N20.0
with calculus, ureter N20.2
congenital Q63.8
lacrimal passages —*see* Dacryolith
liver (impacted) —*see* Calculus, bile duct
lung J98.4
mammographic R92.1
nephritic (impacted) (recurrent) —*see* Calculus, kidney
nose J34.89
pancreas (duct) K86.8
parotid duct or gland K11.5
pelvis, encysted —*see* Calculus, kidney
prostate N42.0
pulmonary J98.4
pyelitis (impacted) (recurrent) N20.0
with hydronephrosis N13.2

Calculus, calculi, calculous *(Continued)*
pyelonephritis (impacted) (recurrent) —*see* category N20
with hydronephrosis N13.2
renal (impacted) (recurrent) —*see* Calculus, kidney
salivary (duct) (gland) K11.5
seminal vesicle N50.8
staghorn —*see* Calculus, kidney
Stensen's duct K11.5
stomach K31.89
sublingual duct or gland K11.5
congenital Q38.4
submandibular duct, gland or region K11.5
submaxillary duct, gland or region K11.5
suburethral N21.8
tonsil J35.8
tooth, teeth (subgingival) (supragingival) K03.6
tunica vaginalis N50.8
ureter (impacted) (recurrent) N20.1
with calculus, kidney N20.2
with hydronephrosis N13.2
with infection N13.6
urethra (impacted) N21.1
urinary (duct) (impacted) (passage) (tract) N20.9
with hydronephrosis N13.2
with infection N13.6
in (due to)
lower N21.9
specified NEC N21.8
vagina N89.8
vesical (impacted) N21.0
Wharton's duct K11.5
xanthine E79.8 *[N22]*
Calicectasis N28.89
Caliectasis N28.89
California
disease B38.9
encephalitis A83.5
Caligo cornea —*see* Opacity, cornea, central
Callositas, callosity (infected) L84
Callus (infected) L84
bone —*see* Osteophyte
excessive, following fracture - code as Sequelae of fracture
Calorie deficiency or malnutrition *(see also* Malnutrition) E46
Calvé-Perthes disease —*see* Legg-Calve-Perthes disease
Calvé's disease —*see* Osteochondrosis, juvenile, spine
Calvities —*see* Alopecia, androgenic
Cameroon fever —*see* Malaria
Camptocormia (hysterical) F44.4
Camurati-Engelmann syndrome Q78.3
Canal —*see also* condition
atrioventricular common Q21.2
Canaliculitis (lacrimal) (acute) (subacute) H04.33-
Actinomyces A42.89
chronic H04.42-
Canavan's disease E75.29
Canceled procedure (surgical) Z53.9
because of
contraindication Z53.09
smoking Z53.01
left against medical advice (AMA) Z53.21

Canceled procedure *(Continued)*
because of *(Continued)*
patient's decision Z53.20
for reasons of belief or group pressure Z53.1
specified reason NEC Z53.29
specified reason NEC Z53.8
Cancer —*see also* Neoplasm, by site, malignant
bile duct type, liver C22.1
blood —*see* Leukemia
breast *(see also* Neoplasm, breast, malignant) C50.91-
hepatocellular C22.0
lung *(see also* Neoplasm, lung, malignant) C34.90
ovarian *(see also* Neoplasm, ovary, malignant) C56.9
unspecified site (primary) C80.1
Cancer (o)phobia F45.29
Cancerous —*see* Neoplasm, malignant, by site
Cancrum oris A69.0
Candidiasis, candidal B37.9
balanitis B37.42
bronchitis B37.1
cheilitis B37.83
congenital P37.5
cystitis B37.41
disseminated B37.7
endocarditis B37.6
enteritis B37.82
esophagitis B37.81
intertrigo B37.2
lung B37.1
meningitis B37.5
mouth B37.0
nails B37.2
neonatal P37.5
onychia B37.2
oral B37.0
osteomyelitis B37.89
otitis externa B37.84
paronychia B37.2
perionyxis B37.2
pneumonia B37.1
proctitis B37.82
pulmonary B37.1
pyelonephritis B37.49
sepsis B37.7
skin B37.2
specified site NEC B37.89
stomatitis B37.0
systemic B37.7
urethritis B37.41
urogenital site NEC B37.49
vagina B37.3
vulva B37.3
vulvovaginitis B37.3
Candidid L30.2
Candidosis —*see* Candidiasis
Candiru infection or infestation B88.8
Canities (premature) L67.1
congenital Q84.2
Canker (mouth) (sore) K12.0
rash A38.9
Cannabinosis J66.2
Canton fever A75.9
Cantrell's syndrome Q87.89
Capillariasis (intestinal) B81.1
hepatic B83.8
Capillary —*see* condition
Caplan's syndrome —*see* Rheumatoid, lung

Capsule —*see* condition
Capsulitis (joint) —*see also*
    Enthesopathy
  adhesive (shoulder) M75.0-
  hepatic K65.8
  labyrinthine —*see* Otosclerosis,
    specified NEC
  thyroid E06.9
Caput
  crepitus Q75.8
  medusae I86.8
  succedaneum P12.81
Car sickness T75.3
Carapata (disease) A68.0
Carate —*see* Pinta
Carbon lung J60
Carbuncle L02.93
  abdominal wall L02.231
  anus K61.0
  auditory canal, external —*see* Abscess,
    ear, external
  auricle ear —*see* Abscess, ear, external
  axilla L02.43-
  back (any part) L02.232
  breast N61
  buttock L02.33
  cheek (external) L02.03
  chest wall L02.233
  chin L02.03
  corpus cavernosum N48.21
  ear (any part) (external) (middle) —*see*
    Abscess, ear, external
  external auditory canal —*see* Abscess,
    ear, external
  eyelid —*see* Abscess, eyelid
  face NEC L02.03
  femoral (region) —*see* Carbuncle, lower
    limb
  finger —*see* Carbuncle, hand
  flank L02.231
  foot L02.63-
  forehead L02.03
  genital —*see* Abscess, genital
  gluteal (region) L02.33
  groin L02.234
  hand L02.53-
  head NEC L02.831
  heel —*see* Carbuncle, foot
  hip —*see* Carbuncle, lower limb
  kidney —*see* Abscess, kidney
  knee —*see* Carbuncle, lower limb
  labium (majus) (minus) N76.4
  lacrimal
    gland —*see* Dacryoadenitis
    passages (duct) (sac) —*see*
      Inflammation, lacrimal,
      passages, acute
  leg —*see* Carbuncle, lower limb
  lower limb L02.43-
  malignant A22.0
  navel L02.236
  neck L02.13
  nose (external) (septum) J34.0
  orbit, orbital —*see* Abscess, orbit
  palmar (space) —*see* Carbuncle,
    hand
  partes posteriores L02.33
  pectoral region L02.233
  penis N48.21
  perineum L02.235
  pinna —*see* Abscess, ear, external
  popliteal —*see* Carbuncle, lower limb
  scalp L02.831
  seminal vesicle N49.0

Carbuncle *(Continued)*
  shoulder —*see* Carbuncle, upper limb
  specified site NEC L02.838
  temple (region) L02.03
  thumb —*see* Carbuncle, hand
  toe —*see* Carbuncle, foot
  trunk L02.239
    abdominal wall L02.231
    back L02.232
    chest wall L02.233
    groin L02.234
    perineum L02.235
    umbilicus L02.236
  umbilicus L02.236
  upper limb L02.43-
  urethra N34.0
  vulva N76.4
Carbunculus —*see* Carbuncle
Carcinoid (tumor) —*see* Tumor,
  carcinoid
Carcinoidosis E34.0
Carcinoma (malignant) —*see also*
    Neoplasm, by site, malignant
  acidophil
    specified site —*see* Neoplasm,
      malignant, by site
    unspecified site C75.1
  acidophil-basophil, mixed
    specified site —*see* Neoplasm,
      malignant, by site
    unspecified site C75.1
  adnexal (skin) —*see* Neoplasm, skin,
    malignant
  adrenal cortical C74.0-
  alveolar —*see* Neoplasm, lung,
    malignant
    cell —*see* Neoplasm, lung, malignant
  ameloblastic C41.1
    upper jaw (bone) C41.0
  apocrine
    breast —*see* Neoplasm, breast,
      malignant
    specified site NEC —*see* Neoplasm,
      skin, malignant
    unspecified site C44.99
  basal cell (pigmented) (*see also*
    Neoplasm, skin, malignant) C44.91
    fibro-epithelial —*see* Neoplasm, skin,
      malignant
    morphea —*see* Neoplasm, skin,
      malignant
    multicentric —*see* Neoplasm, skin,
      malignant
  basaloid
  basal-squamous cell, mixed —*see*
    Neoplasm, skin, malignant
  basophil
    specified site —*see* Neoplasm,
      malignant, by site
    unspecified site C75.1
  basophil-acidophil, mixed
    specified site —*see* Neoplasm,
      malignant, by site
    urethra site C75.1
  basosquamous —*see* Neoplasm, skin,
    malignant
  bile duct
    with hepatocellular, mixed C22.0
    liver C22.1
    specified site NEC —*see* Neoplasm,
      malignant, by site
    unspecified site C22.1
  branchial or branchiogenic C10.4
  bronchial or bronchogenic —*see*
    Neoplasm, lung, malignant

Carcinoma *(Continued)*
  bronchiolar —*see* Neoplasm, lung,
    malignant
  bronchioloalveolar —*see* Neoplasm,
    lung, malignant
  C cell
    specified site —*see* Neoplasm,
      malignant, by site
    unspecified site C73
  ceruminous C44.29-
  cervix uteri
    in situ D06.9
      endocervix D06.0
      exocervix D06.1
      specified site NEC D06.7
  chorionic
    specified site —*see* Neoplasm,
      malignant, by site
    unspecified site
      female C58
      male C62.90
  chromophobe
    specified site —*see* Neoplasm,
      malignant, by site
    unspecified site C75.1
  cloacogenic
    specified site —*see* Neoplasm,
      malignant, by site
    unspecified site C21.2
  diffuse type
    specified site —*see* Neoplasm,
      malignant, by site
    unspecified site C16.9
  duct (cell)
    with Paget's disease —*see* Neoplasm,
      breast, malignant
    infiltrating
      with lobular carcinoma (in situ)
        specified site —*see* Neoplasm,
          malignant, by site
        unspecified site (female)
          C50.91-
        male C50.92-
      specified site —*see* Neoplasm,
        malignant, by site
      unspecified site (female) C50.91-
      male C50.92-
  ductal
    with lobular
      specified site —*see* Neoplasm,
        malignant, by site
      unspecified site (female) C50.91-
      male C50.92-
  ductular, infiltrating
    specified site —*see* Neoplasm,
      malignant, by site
    unspecified site (female) C50.91-
    male C50.92-
  embryonal
    liver C22.7
  endometrioid
    specified site —*see* Neoplasm,
      malignant, by site
    unspecified site
      female C56.9
      male C61
  eosinophil
    specified site —*see* Neoplasm,
      malignant, by site
    unspecified site C75.1
  epidermoid —*see also* Carcinoma,
    squamous cell
    in situ, Bowen's type —*see* Neoplasm,
      skin, in situ

Carcinoma *(Continued)*
 fibroepithelial, basal cell —*see*
  Neoplasm, skin, malignant
 follicular
  with papillary (mixed) C73
  moderately differentiated C73
  pure follicle C73
  specified site —*see* Neoplasm,
   malignant, by site
  trabecular C73
  unspecified site C73
  well differentiated C73
 generalized, with unspecified primary
  site C80.0
 glycogen-rich —*see* Neoplasm, breast,
  malignant
 granulosa cell C56-
 hepatic cell C22.0
 hepatocellular C22.0
  with bile duct, mixed C22.0
  fibrolamellar C22.0
 hepatocholangiolitic C22.0
 Hurthle cell C73
 in
  adenomatous
   polyposis coli C18.9
  pleomorphic adenoma —*see*
   Neoplasm, salivary glands,
   malignant
  situ —*see* Carcinoma-in-situ
 infiltrating
  duct
   with lobular
    specified site —*see* Neoplasm,
     malignant, by site
    unspecified site (female) C50.91-
     male C50.92-
   with Paget's disease —*see*
    Neoplasm, breast, malignant
   specified site —*see* Neoplasm,
    malignant
   unspecified site (female) C50.91-
    male C50.92-
  ductular
   specified site —*see* Neoplasm,
    malignant
   unspecified site (female) C50.91-
    male C50.92-
  lobular
   specified site —*see* Neoplasm,
    malignant
   unspecified site (female) C50.91-
    male C50.92-
 inflammatory
  specified site —*see* Neoplasm,
   malignant
  unspecified site (female) C50.91-
   male C50.92-
 intestinal type
  specified site —*see* Neoplasm,
   malignant, by site
  unspecified site C16.9
 intracystic
  noninfiltrating —*see* Neoplasm, in
   situ, by site
 intraductal (noninfiltrating)
  with Paget's disease —*see* Neoplasm,
   breast, malignant
  breast D05.1-
  papillary
   with invasion
    specified site —*see* Neoplasm,
     malignant, by site
    unspecified site (female) C50.91-
     male C50.92-

Carcinoma *(Continued)*
 intraductal *(Continued)*
  papillary *(Continued)*
   breast D05.1-
   specified site NEC —*see* Neoplasm,
    in situ, by site
   unspecified site (female) D05.1-
  specified site NEC —*see* Neoplasm, in
   situ, by site
  unspecified site (female) D05.1-
 intraepidermal —*see* Neoplasm, in situ
  squamous cell, Bowen's type —*see*
   Neoplasm, skin, in situ
 intraepithelial —*see* Neoplasm, in situ,
  by site
  squamous cell —*see* Neoplasm, in
   situ, by site
 intraosseous C41.1
  upper jaw (bone) C41.0
 islet cell
  with exocrine, mixed
   specified site —*see* Neoplasm,
    malignant, by site
   unspecified site C25.9
  pancreas C25.4
  specified site NEC —*see* Neoplasm,
   malignant, by site
  unspecified site C25.4
 juvenile, breast —*see* Neoplasm, breast,
  malignant
 large cell
  small cell
   specified site —*see* Neoplasm,
    malignant, by site
   unspecified site C34.90
 Leydig cell (testis)
  specified site —*see* Neoplasm,
   malignant, by site
  unspecified site
   female C56.9
   male C62.90
 lipid-rich (female) C50.91-
  male C50.92-
 liver cell C22.0
 liver NEC C22.7
 lobular (infiltrating)
  with intraductal
   specified site —*see* Neoplasm,
    malignant, by site
   unspecified site (female) C50.91-
    male C50.92-
  noninfiltrating
   breast D05.0-
   specified site NEC —*see* Neoplasm,
    in situ, by site
   unspecified site D05.0-
  specified site —*see* Neoplasm,
   malignant, by site
  unspecified site (female) C50.91-
   male C50.92-
 medullary
  with
   amyloid stroma
    specified site —*see* Neoplasm,
     malignant, by site
    unspecified site C73
   lymphoid stroma
    specified site —*see* Neoplasm,
     malignant, by site
    unspecified site (female) C50.91-
     male C50.92-
 Merkel cell C4A.9
  anal margin C4A.51
  anal skin C4A.51
  canthus C4A.1-

Carcinoma *(Continued)*
 Merkel cell *(Continued)*
  ear and external auricular canal C4A.2-
  external auricular canal C4A.2-
  eyelid, including canthus C4A.1-
  face C4A.30
   specified NEC C4A.39
  hip C4A.7-
  lip C4A.0
  lower limb, including hip C4A.7-
  neck C4A.4
  nodal presentation C7B.1
  nose C4A.31
  overlapping sites C4A.8
  perianal skin C4A.51
  scalp C4A.4
  secondary C7B.1
  shoulder C4A.6-
  skin of breast C4A.52
  trunk NEC C4A.59
  upper limb, including shoulder C4A.6-
  visceral metastatic C7B.1
 metastatic —*see* Neoplasm, secondary
 metatypical —*see* Neoplasm, skin,
  malignant
 morphea, basal cell —*see* Neoplasm,
  skin, malignant
 mucoid
  cell
   specified site —*see* Neoplasm,
    malignant, by site
   unspecified site C75.1
 neuroendocrine —*see also* Tumor,
  neuroendocrine
  high grade, any site C7A.1
  poorly differentiated, any site
   C7A.1
 nonencapsulated sclerosing C73
 noninfiltrating
  intracystic —*see* Neoplasm, in situ,
   by site
  intraductal
   breast D05.1-
   papillary
    breast D05.1-
    specified site NEC —*see*
     Neoplasm, in situ, by site
    unspecified site D05.1-
   specified site —*see* Neoplasm, in
    situ, by site
   unspecified site D05.1-
  lobular
   breast D05.0-
   specified site NEC —*see* Neoplasm,
    in situ, by site
   unspecified site (female) D05.0-
 oat cell
  specified site —*see* Neoplasm,
   malignant, by site
  unspecified site C34.90
 odontogenic C41.1
  upper jaw (bone) C41.0
 papillary
  with follicular (mixed) C73
  follicular variant C73
  intraductal (noninfiltrating)
   with invasion
    specified site —*see* Neoplasm,
     malignant, by site
    unspecified site (female) C50.91-
     male C50.92-
   breast D05.1-
   specified site NEC —*see* Neoplasm,
    in situ, by site
   unspecified site D05.1-

Carcinoma *(Continued)*
  papillary *(Continued)*
    serous
      specified site —*see* Neoplasm,
        malignant, by site
      surface
        specified site —*see* Neoplasm,
          malignant, by site
        unspecified site C56.9
      unspecified site C56.9
  papillocystic
    specified site —*see* Neoplasm,
      malignant, by site
    unspecified site C56.9
  parafollicular cell
    specified site —*see* Neoplasm,
      malignant, by site
    unspecified site C73
  pilomatrix —*see* Neoplasm, skin,
    malignant
  pseudomucinous
    specified site —*see* Neoplasm,
      malignant, by site
    unspecified site C56.9
  renal cell C64-
  Schmincke —*see* Neoplasm,
    nasopharynx, malignant
  Schneiderian
    specified site —*see* Neoplasm,
      malignant, by site
    unspecified site C30.0
  sebaceous —*see* Neoplasm, skin,
    malignant
  secondary —*see also* Neoplasm,
    secondary, by site
    Merkel cell C7B.1
  secretory, breast —*see* Neoplasm, breast,
    malignant
  serous
    papillary
      specified site —*see* Neoplasm,
        malignant, by site
      unspecified site C56.9
    surface, papillary
      specified site —*see* Neoplasm,
        malignant, by site
      unspecified site C56.9
  Sertoli cell
    specified site —*see* Neoplasm,
      malignant, by site
    unspecified site C62.90
      female C56.9
      male C62.90
  skin appendage —*see* Neoplasm, skin,
    malignant
  small cell
    fusiform cell
      specified site —*see* Neoplasm,
        malignant, by site
      unspecified site C34.90
    intermediate cell
      specified site —*see* Neoplasm,
        malignant, by site
      unspecified site C34.90
    large cell
      specified site —*see* Neoplasm,
        malignant, by site
      unspecified site C34.90
  solid
    with amyloid stroma
      specified site —*see* Neoplasm,
        malignant, by site
      unspecified site C73

Carcinoma *(Continued)*
  solid *(Continued)*
    microinvasive
      specified site —*see* Neoplasm,
        malignant, by site
      unspecified site C53.9
    sweat gland —*see* Neoplasm, skin,
      malignant
    theca cell C56.-
    thymic C37
    unspecified site (primary) C80.1
    water-clear cell C75.0
Carcinoma-in-situ —*see also* Neoplasm, in
  situ, by site
  breast NOS D05.9-
    specified type NEC D05.8-
  epidermoid —*see also* Neoplasm, in situ,
    by site
    with questionable stromal invasion
      cervix D06.9
      specified site NEC —*see* Neoplasm,
        in situ, by site
      unspecified site D06.9
    Bowen's type —*see* Neoplasm, skin,
      in situ
  intraductal
    breast D05.1-
    specified site NEC —*see* Neoplasm, in
      situ, by site
    unspecified site D05.1-
  lobular
    with
      infiltrating duct
        breast (female) C50.91-
          male C50.92-
        specified site NEC —*see*
          Neoplasm, malignant
        unspecified site (female) C50.91-
          male C50.92-
      intraductal
        breast D05.8-
        specified site NEC —*see*
          Neoplasm, in situ, by site
        unspecified site (female) D05.8-
    breast D05.0-
    specified site NEC —*see* Neoplasm, in
      situ, by site
    unspecified site D05.0-
  squamous cell —*see also* Neoplasm, in
    situ, by site
    with questionable stromal invasion
      cervix D06.9
      specified site NEC —*see* Neoplasm,
        in situ, by site
      unspecified site D06.9
Carcinomaphobia F45.29
Carcinomatosis C80.0
  peritonei C78.6
  unspecified site (primary) (secondary)
    C80.0
Carcinosarcoma —*see* Neoplasm,
  malignant, by site
  embryonal —*see* Neoplasm, malignant,
    by site
Cardia, cardial —*see* condition
Cardiac —*see also* condition
  death, sudden —*see* Arrest, cardiac
  pacemaker
    in situ Z95.0
    management or adjustment Z45.018
  tamponade I31.4
Cardialgia —*see* Pain, precordial
Cardiectasis —*see* Hypertrophy, cardiac
Cardiochalasia K21.9

Cardiomalacia I51.5
Cardiomegalia glycogenica diffusa
  E74.02 *[I43]*
Cardiomegaly —*see also* Hypertrophy,
  cardiac
  congenital Q24.8
  glycogen E74.02 *[I43]*
  idiopathic I51.7
Cardiomyoliposis I51.5
Cardiomyopathy (familial) (idiopathic)
  I42.9
  alcoholic I42.6
  amyloid E85.4 *[I43]*
  arteriosclerotic —*see* Disease, heart,
    ischemic, atherosclerotic
  beriberi E51.12
  cobalt-beer I42.6
  congenital I42.4
  congestive I42.0
  constrictive NOS I42.5
  dilated I42.0
  due to
    alcohol I42.6
    beriberi E51.12
    cardiac glycogenosis E74.02 *[I43]*
    drugs I42.7
    external agents NEC I42.7
    Friedreich's ataxia G11.1
    myotonia atrophica G71.11 *[I43]*
    progressive muscular dystrophy G71.0
  glycogen storage E74.02 *[I43]*
  hypertensive —*see* Hypertension, heart
  hypertrophic (nonobstructive) I42.2
    obstructive I42.1
      congenital Q24.8
  in
    Chagas' disease (chronic) B57.2
      acute B57.0
    sarcoidosis D86.85
  ischemic I25.5
  metabolic E88.9 *[I43]*
    thyrotoxic E05.90 *[I43]*
      with thyroid storm E05.91 *[I43]*
  newborn I42.8
    congenital I42.4
  nutritional E63.9 *[I43]*
    beriberi E51.12
  obscure of Africa I42.8
  peripartum O90.3
  postpartum O90.3
  restrictive NEC I42.5
  rheumatic I09.0
  secondary I42.9
  stress induced I51.81
  takotsubo I51.81
  thyrotoxic E05.90 *[I43]*
    with thyroid storm E05.91 *[I43]*
  toxic NEC I42.7
  tuberculous A18.84
  viral B33.24
Cardionephritis —*see* Hypertension,
  cardiorenal
Cardionephropathy —*see* Hypertension,
  cardiorenal
Cardionephrosis —*see* Hypertension,
  cardiorenal
Cardiopathia nigra I27.0
Cardiopathy (*see also* Disease, heart) I51.9
  idiopathic I42.9
  mucopolysaccharidosis E76.3 *[I52]*
Cardiopericarditis —*see* Pericarditis
Cardiophobia F45.29
Cardiorenal —*see* condition
Cardiorrhexis —*see* Infarct, myocardium

Cardiosclerosis —*see* Disease, heart, ischemic, atherosclerotic
Cardiosis —*see* Disease, heart
Cardiospasm (esophagus) (reflex) (stomach) K22.0
  congenital Q39.5
    with megaesophagus Q39.5
Cardiostenosis —*see* Disease, heart
Cardiosymphysis I31.0
Cardiovascular—*see* condition
Carditis (acute) (bacterial) (chronic) (subacute) I51.89
  meningococcal A39.50
  rheumatic —*see* Disease, heart, rheumatic
  rheumatoid —*see* Rheumatoid, carditis
  viral B33.20
Care (of) (for) (following)
  child (routine) Z76.2
  family member (handicapped) (sick)
    creating problem for family Z63.6
    provided away from home for holiday relief Z75.5
    unavailable, due to
      absence (person rendering care) (sufferer) Z74.2
      inability (any reason) of person rendering care Z74.2
  foundling Z76.1
  holiday relief Z75.5
  improper —*see* Maltreatment
  lack of (at or after birth) (infant) —*see* Maltreatment, child, neglect
  lactating mother Z39.1
  palliative Z51.5
  postpartum
    immediately after delivery Z39.0
    routine follow-up Z39.2
  respite Z75.5
  unavailable, due to
    absence of person rendering care Z74.2
    inability (any reason) of person rendering care Z74.2
  well-baby Z76.2
Caries
  bone NEC A18.03
  dental K02.9
    arrested (coronal) (root) K02.3
    chewing surface
      limited to enamel K02.51
      penetrating into dentin K02.52
      penetrating into pulp K02.53
    coronal surface
      chewing surface
        limited to enamel K02.51
        penetrating into dentin K02.52
        penetrating into pulp K02.53
      pit and fissure surface
        limited to enamel K02.51
        penetrating into dentin K02.52
        penetrating into pulp K02.53
      smooth surface
        limited to enamel K02.61
        penetrating into dentin K02.62
        penetrating into pulp K02.63
    pit and fissure surface
      limited to enamel K02.51
      penetrating into dentin K02.52
      penetrating into pulp K02.53
    root K02.7
    smooth surface
      limited to enamel K02.61
      penetrating into dentin K02.62
      penetrating into pulp K02.63
    external meatus —*see* Disorder, ear, external, specified type NEC

Caries *(Continued)*
  hip (tuberculous) A18.02
  initial (tooth)
    chewing surface K02.51
    pit and fissure surface K02.51
    smooth surface K02.61
  knee (tuberculous) A18.02
  labyrinth —*see* subcategory H83.8
  limb NEC (tuberculous) A18.03
  mastoid process (chronic) —*see* Mastoiditis, chronic
    tuberculous A18.03
  middle ear —*see* subcategory H74.8
  nose (tuberculous) A18.03
  orbit (tuberculous) A18.03
  ossicles, ear —*see* Abnormal, ear ossicles
  petrous bone —*see* Petrositis
  root (dental) (tooth) K02.7
  sacrum (tuberculous) A18.01
  spine, spinal (column) (tuberculous) A18.01
  syphilitic A52.77
    congenital (early) A50.02 *[M90.80]*
  tooth, teeth —*see* Caries, dental
  tuberculous A18.03
  vertebra (column) (tuberculous) A18.01
Carious teeth —*see* Caries, dental
Carneous mole O02.0
Carnitine insufficiency E71.40
Carotid body or sinus syndrome G90.01
Carotidynia G90.01
Carotinemia (dietary) E67.1
Carotinosis (cutis) (skin) E67.1
Carpal tunnel syndrome —*see* Syndrome, carpal tunnel
Carpenter's syndrome Q87.0
Carpopedal spasm —*see* Tetany
Carr-Barr-Plunkett syndrome Q97.1
Carrier (suspected) of
  amebiasis Z22.1
  bacterial disease NEC Z22.39
    diphtheria Z22.2
    intestinal infectious NEC Z22.1
      typhoid Z22.0
    meningococcal Z22.31
    sexually transmitted Z22.4
    specified NEC Z22.39
    staphylococcal (Methicillin susceptible) Z22.321
      Methicillin resistant Z22.322
    streptococcal Z22.338
      group B Z22.330
    typhoid Z22.0
  cholera Z22.1
  diphtheria Z22.2
  gastrointestinal pathogens NEC Z22.1
  genetic Z14.8
    cystic fibrosis Z14.1
    hemophilia A (asymptomatic) Z14.01
      symptomatic Z14.02
  gonorrhea Z22.4
  HAA (hepatitis Australian-antigen) Z22.59
  HB (c)(s)-AG Z22.51
  hepatitis (viral) Z22.50
    Australia-antigen (HAA) Z22.59
    B surface antigen (HBsAg) Z22.51
      with acute delta- (super)infection B17.0
    C Z22.52
    specified NEC Z22.59
  human T-cell lymphotropic virus type-1 (HTLV-1) infection Z22.6
  infectious organism Z22.9
    specified NEC Z22.8

Carrier of *(Continued)*
  meningococci Z22.31
  Salmonella typhosa Z22.0
  serum hepatitis —*see* Carrier, hepatitis
  staphylococci (Methicillin susceptible) Z22.321
    Methicillin resistant Z22.322
  streptococci Z22.338
    group B Z22.330
  syphilis Z22.4
  typhoid Z22.0
  venereal disease NEC Z22.4
Carrion's disease A44.0
Carter's relapsing fever (Asiatic) A68.1
Cartilage —*see* condition
Caruncle (inflamed)
  conjunctiva (acute) —*see* Conjunctivitis, acute
  labium (majus) (minus) N90.89
  lacrimal —*see* Inflammation, lacrimal, passages
  myrtiform N89.8
  urethral (benign) N36.2
Cascade stomach K31.2
Caseation lymphatic gland (tuberculous) A18.2
Cassidy (-Scholte) syndrome (malignant carcinoid) E34.0
Castellani's disease A69.8
Castration, traumatic, male S38.231
Casts in urine R82.99
Cat
  cry syndrome Q93.4
  ear Q17.3
  eye syndrome Q92.8
Catabolism, senile R54
Catalepsy (hysterical) F44.2
  schizophrenic F20.2
Cataplexy (idiopathic) —*see* - Narcolepsy
Cataract (cortical) (immature) (incipient) H26.9
  with
    neovascularization —*see* Cataract, complicated
  age-related —*see* Cataract, senile
  anterior
    and posterior axial embryonal Q12.0
    pyramidal Q12.0
  associated with
    galactosemia E74.21 *[H28]*
    myotonic disorders G71.19 *[H28]*
  blue Q12.0
  central Q12.0
  cerulean Q12.0
  complicated H26.20
    with
      neovascularization H26.21-
      ocular disorder H26.22-
      glaucomatous flecks H26.23-
  congenital Q12.0
  coraliform Q12.0
  coronary Q12.0
  crystalline Q12.0
  diabetic —*see* Diabetes, cataract
  drug-induced H26.3-
  due to
    ocular disorder —*see* Cataract, complicated
    radiation H26.8
  electric H26.8
  extraction status Z98.4-
  glass-blower's H26.8
  heat ray H26.8
  heterochromic —*see* Cataract, complicated

Cataract *(Continued)*
  hypermature —*see* Cataract, senile,
    morgagnian type
  in (due to)
    chronic iridocyclitis —*see* Cataract,
      complicated
      diabetes —*see* Diabetes, cataract
      endocrine disease E34.9 *[H28]*
      eye disease —*see* Cataract,
        complicated
      hypoparathyroidism E20.9 *[H28]*
      malnutrition-dehydration E46 *[H28]*
      metabolic disease E88.9 *[H28]*
      myotonic disorders G71.19 *[H28]*
      nutritional disease E63.9 *[H28]*
  infantile —*see* Cataract, presenile
  irradiational —*see* Cataract, specified
    NEC
  juvenile —*see* Cataract, presenile
  malnutrition-dehydration E46 *[H28]*
  morgagnian —*see* Cataract, senile,
    morgagnian type
  myotonic G71.19 *[H28]*
  myxedema E03.9 *[H28]*
  nuclear
  embryonal Q12.0
    sclerosis —*see* Cataract, senile, nuclear
  presenile H26.00-
    combined forms H26.06-
    cortical H26.01-
    lamellar —*see* Cataract, presenile,
      cortical
    nuclear H26.03-
    specified NEC H26.09
    subcapsular polar (anterior) H26.04-
    posterior H26.05-
      zonular —*see* Cataract, presenile,
        cortical
  secondary H26.40
    Soemmering's ring H26.41-
    specified NEC H26.49-
    to eye disease —*see* Cataract,
      complicated
  senile H25.9
    brunescens —*see* Cataract, senile,
      nuclear
    combined forms H25.81-
    coronary —*see* Cataract, senile,
      incipient
    cortical H25.01-
    hypermature —*see* Cataract, senile,
      morgagnian type
    incipient (mature) (total) H25.09-
      cortical —*see* Cataract, senile,
        cortical
      subcapsular —*see* Cataract, senile,
        subcapsular
    morgagnian type (hypermature)
      H25.2-
    nuclear (sclerosis) H25.1-
    polar subcapsular (anterior)
      (posterior) —*see* Cataract, senile,
      incipient
    punctate —*see* Cataract, senile, incipient
    specified NEC H25.89
    subcapsular polar (anterior) H25.03-
      posterior H25.04-
  snowflake —*see* Diabetes, cataract
  specified NEC H26.8
  toxic —*see* Cataract, drug-induced
  traumatic H26.10-
    localized H26.11-
    partially resolved H26.12-
    total H26.13-
  zonular (perinuclear) Q12.0

Cataracta —*see also* Cataract
  brunescens —*see* Cataract, senile,
    nuclear
  centralis pulverulenta Q12.0
  cerulea Q12.0
  complicata —*see* Cataract, complicated
  congenita Q12.0
  coralliformis Q12.0
  coronaria Q12.0
  diabetic —*see* Diabetes, cataract
  membranacea
    accreta —*see* Cataract, secondary
    congenita Q12.0
  nigra —*see* Cataract, senile, nuclear
  sunflower —*see* Cataract, complicated
Catarrh, catarrhal (acute) (febrile)
    (infectious) (inflammation) (*see also*
    condition) J00
  bronchial —*see* Bronchitis
  chest —*see* Bronchitis
  chronic J31.0
  due to congenital syphilis A50.03
  enteric —*see* Enteritis
  eustachian H68.009
  fauces —*see* Pharyngitis
  gastrointestinal —*see* Enteritis
  gingivitis K05.00
    nonplaque induced K05.01
    plaque induced K05.00
  hay —*see* Fever, hay
  intestinal —*see* Enteritis
  larynx, chronic J37.0
  liver B15.9
    with hepatic coma B15.0
  lung —*see* Bronchitis
  middle ear, chronic —*see* Otitis, media,
    nonsuppurative, chronic, serous
  mouth K12.1
  nasal (chronic) —*see* Rhinitis
  nasobronchial J31.1
  nasopharyngeal (chronic) J31.1
    acute J00
  pulmonary —*see* Bronchitis
  spring (eye) (vernal) —*see*
    Conjunctivitis, acute, atopic
  summer (hay) —*see* Fever, hay
  throat J31.2
  tubotympanal —*see also* Otitis, media,
    nonsuppurative
    chronic —*see* Otitis, media,
      nonsuppurative, chronic, serous
Catatonia (schizophrenic) F20.2
Catatonic
  disorder due to known physiologic
    condition F06.1
  schizophrenia F20.2
  stupor R40.1
Cat-scratch —*see also* Abrasion
  disease or fever A28.1
Cauda equina —*see* condition
Cauliflower ear M95.1-
Causalgia (upper limb) G56.4-
  lower limb G57.7-
Cause
  external, general effects T75.89
Caustic burn —*see* Corrosion, by site
Cavare's disease (familial periodic
    paralysis) G72.3
Cave-in, injury
  crushing (severe) —*see* Crush
  suffocation —*see* Asphyxia, traumatic,
    due to low oxygen, due to cave-in
Cavernitis (penis) N48.29
Cavernositis N48.29
Cavernous —*see* condition

Cavitation of lung —*see also* Tuberculosis,
    pulmonary
  nontuberculous J98.4
Cavities, dental —*see* Caries, dental
Cavity
  lung —*see* Cavitation of lung
  optic papilla Q14.2
  pulmonary —*see* Cavitation of lung
Cavovarus foot, congenital Q66.1
Cavus foot (congenital) Q66.7
  acquired —*see* Deformity, limb, foot,
    specified NEC
Cazenave's disease L10.2
Cecitis K52.9
  with perforation, peritonitis, or rupture
    K65.8
Cecum —*see* condition
Celiac
  artery compression syndrome I77.4
  disease K90.0
  infantilism K90.0
Cell (s), cellular —*see also* condition
  in urine R82.99
Cellulitis (diffuse) (phlegmonous) (septic)
    (suppurative) L03.90
  abdominal wall L03.311
  anaerobic A48.0
  ankle —*see* Cellulitis, lower limb
  anus K61.0
  arm —*see* Cellulitis, upper limb
  auricle (ear) —*see* Cellulitis, ear
  axilla L03.11-
  back (any part) L03.312
  broad ligament
    acute N73.0
  buttock L03.317
  cervical (meaning neck) L03.221
  cervix (uteri) —*see* Cervicitis
  cheek (external) L03.211
    internal K12.2
  chest wall L03.313
  chronic L03.90
  clostridial A48.0
  corpus cavernosum N48.22
  digit
    finger —*see* Cellulitis, finger
    toe —*see* Cellulitis, toe
  Douglas' cul-de-sac or pouch
    acute N73.0
  drainage site (following operation) T81.4
  ear (external) H60.1-
  eosinophilic (granulomatous) L98.3
  erysipelatous —*see* Erysipelas
  external auditory canal —*see* Cellulitis, ear
  eyelid —*see* Abscess, eyelid
  face NEC L03.211
  finger (intrathecal) (periosteal)
    (subcutaneous) (subcuticular)
    L03.01-
  foot —*see* Cellulitis, lower limb
  gangrenous —*see* Gangrene
  genital organ NEC
    female (external) N76.4
    male N49.9
      multiple sites N49.8
      specified NEC N49.8
  gluteal (region) L03.317
  gonococcal A54.89
  groin L03.314
  hand —*see* Cellulitis, upper limb
  head NEC L03.811
    face (any part, except ear, eye and
      nose) L03.211
  heel —*see* Cellulitis, lower limb

Cellulitis *(Continued)*
 hip —*see* Cellulitis, lower limb
 jaw (region) L03.211
 knee —*see* Cellulitis, lower limb
 labium (majus) (minus) —*see* Vulvitis
 lacrimal passages —*see* Inflammation,
   lacrimal, passages
 larynx J38.7
 leg —*see* Cellulitis, lower limb
 lip K13.0
 lower limb L03.11-
   toe —*see* Cellulitis, toe
 mouth (floor) K12.2
 multiple sites, so stated L03.90
 nasopharynx J39.1
 navel L03.316
   newborn P38.9
     with mild hemorrhage P38.1
     without hemorrhage P38.9
 neck (region) L03.221
 nose (septum) (external) J34.0
 orbit, orbital H05.01-
 palate (soft) K12.2
 pectoral (region) L03.313
 pelvis, pelvic (chronic)
   female (*see also* Disease, pelvis,
     inflammatory) N73.2
     acute N73.0
   following ectopic or molar pregnancy
     O08.0
   male K65.0
 penis N48.22
 perineal, perineum L03.315
 perirectal K61.1
 peritonsillar J36
 periurethral N34.0
 periuterine (*see also* Disease, pelvis,
   inflammatory) N73.2
   acute N73.0
 pharynx J39.1
 rectum K61.1
 retroperitoneal K68.9
 round ligament
   acute N73.0
 scalp (any part) L03.811
 scrotum N49.2
 seminal vesicle N49.0
 shoulder —*see* Cellulitis, upper limb
 specified site NEC L03.818
 submandibular (region) (space)
   (triangle) K12.2
   gland K11.3
 submaxillary (region) K12.2
   gland K11.3
 thigh —*see* Cellulitis, lower limb
 thumb (intrathecal) (periosteal)
   (subcutaneous) (subcuticular) —
   see Cellulitis, finger
 toe (intrathecal) (periosteal)
   (subcutaneous) (subcuticular)
   L03.03-
 tonsil J36
 trunk L03.319
   abdominal wall L03.311
   back (any part) L03.312
   buttock L03.317
   chest wall L03.313
   groin L03.314
   perineal, perineum L03.315
   umbilicus L03.316
 tuberculous (primary) A18.4
 umbilicus L03.316
 upper limb L03.11-
   axilla —*see* Cellulitis, axilla
   finger —*see* Cellulitis, finger
   thumb —*see* Cellulitis, finger

Cellulitis *(Continued)*
 vaccinal T88.0
 vocal cord J38.3
 vulva —*see* Vulvitis
 wrist —*see* Cellulitis, upper limb
Cementoblastoma, benign —*see* Cyst,
   calcifying odontogenic
Cementoma —*see* Cyst, calcifying
   odontogenic
Cementoperiostitis —*see* Periodontitis
Cementosis K03.4
Central auditory processing disorder
   H93.25
Central pain syndrome G89.0
Cephalematocele, cephal (o)hematocele
 newborn P52.8
   birth injury P10.8
 traumatic —*see* Hematoma, brain
Cephalematoma, cephalhematoma
   (calcified)
 newborn (birth injury) P12.0
 traumatic —*see* Hematoma, brain
Cephalgia, cephalalgia —*see also*
   Headache
 histamine G44.009
   intractable G44.001
   not intractable G44.009
 trigeminal autonomic (TAC) NEC
   G44.099
   intractable G44.091
   not intractable G44.099
Cephalic —*see* condition
Cephalitis —*see* Encephalitis
Cephalocele —*see* Encephalocele
Cephalomenia N94.89
Cephalopelvic —*see* condition
Cerclage (with cervical incompetence)
   in pregnancy —*see* Incompetence,
   cervix, in pregnancy
Cerebellitis —*see* Encephalitis
Cerebellum, cerebellar —*see* condition
Cerebral —*see* condition
Cerebritis —*see* Encephalitis
Cerebro-hepato-renal syndrome Q87.89
Cerebromalacia —*see* Softening, brain
 sequelae of cerebrovascular disease
   I69.398
Cerebroside lipidosis E75.22
Cerebrospasticity (congenital) G80.1
Cerebrospinal —*see* condition
Cerebrum —*see* condition
Ceroid-lipofuscinosis, neuronal E75.4
Cerumen (accumulation) (impacted) H61.2-
Cervical —*see also* condition
 auricle Q18.2
 dysplasia in pregnancy —*see* Abnormal,
   cervix, in pregnancy or childbirth
 erosion in pregnancy —*see* Abnormal,
   cervix, in pregnancy or childbirth
 fibrosis in pregnancy —*see* Abnormal,
   cervix, in pregnancy or childbirth
 fusion syndrome Q76.1
 rib Q76.5
 shortening (complicating pregnancy)
   O26.87-
Cervicalgia M54.2
Cervicitis (acute) (chronic) (nonvenereal)
   (senile (atrophic)) (subacute) (with
   ulceration) N72
 with
   abortion —*see* Abortion, by type
     complicated by genital tract and
     pelvic infection
   ectopic pregnancy O08.0
   molar pregnancy O08.0

Cervicitis *(Continued)*
 chlamydial A56.09
 gonococcal A54.03
 herpesviral A60.03
 puerperal (postpartum) O86.11
 syphilitic A52.76
 trichomonal A59.09
 tuberculous A18.16
Cervicocolpitis (emphysematosa) (*see also*
   Cervicitis) N72
Cervix —*see* condition
Cesarean delivery, previous, affecting
   management of pregnancy O34.21
Céstan (-Chenais) paralysis or syndrome
   G46.3
Céstan-Raymond syndrome I65.8
Cestode infestation B71.9
 specified type NEC B71.8
Cestodiasis B71.9
Chabert's disease A22.9
Chacaleh E53.8
Chafing L30.4
Chagas' (-Mazza) disease (chronic) B57.2
 with
   cardiovascular involvement NEC
     B57.2
   digestive system involvement B57.30
     megacolon B57.32
     megaesophagus B57.31
     other specified B57.39
   megacolon B57.32
   megaesophagus B57.31
   myocarditis B57.2
   nervous system involvement B57.40
     meningitis B57.41
     meningoencephalitis B57.42
     other specified B57.49
   specified organ involvement NEC
     B57.5
 acute (with) B57.1
   cardiovascular NEC B57.0
   myocarditis B57.0
Chagres fever B50.9
Chairridden Z74.09
Chalasia (cardiac sphincter) K21.9
Chalazion H00.19
 left H00.16
   lower H00.15
   upper H00.14
 right H00.13
   lower H00.12
   upper H00.11
Chalcosis —*see also* Disorder, globe,
   degenerative, chalcosis
 cornea —*see* Deposit, cornea
 crystalline lens —*see* Cataract,
   complicated
 retina H35.89
Chalicosis (pulmonum) J62.8
Chancre (any genital site) (hard)
   (hunterian) (mixed) (primary)
   (seronegative) (seropositive)
   (syphilitic) A51.0
 congenital A50.07
 conjunctiva NEC A51.2
 Ducrey's A57
 extragenital A51.2
 eyelid A51.2
 lip A51.2
 nipple A51.2
 Nisbet's A57
 of
   carate A67.0
   pinta A67.0
   yaws A66.0

Chancre *(Continued)*
  palate, soft A51.2
  phagedenic A57
  simple A57
  soft A57
    bubo A57
    palate A51.2
  urethra A51.0
  yaws A66.0
Chancroid (anus) (genital) (penis)
    (perineum) (rectum) (urethra)
    (vulva) A57
Chandler's disease (osteochondritis
      dissecans, hip) —*see* Osteochondritis,
      dissecans, hip
Change (s) (in) (of) —*see also* Removal
  arteriosclerotic —*see* Arteriosclerosis
  bone —*see also* Disorder, bone
    diabetic —*see* Diabetes, bone change
  bowel habit R19.4
  cardiorenal (vascular) —*see*
      Hypertension, cardiorenal
  cardiovascular —*see* Disease,
      cardiovascular
  circulatory I99.9
  cognitive (mild) (organic) R41.89
  color, tooth, teeth
    during formation K00.8
    posteruptive K03.7
  contraceptive device Z30.433
  corneal membrane H18.30
    Bowman's membrane fold or rupture
        H18.31-
    Descemet's membrane
        fold H18.32-
        rupture H18.33-
  coronary —*see* Disease, heart, ischemic
  degenerative, spine or vertebra —*see*
      Spondylosis
  dental pulp, regressive K04.2
  dressing (nonsurgical) Z48.00
    surgical Z48.01
  heart —*see* Disease, heart
  hip joint —*see* Derangement, joint, hip
  hyperplastic larynx J38.7
  hypertrophic
    nasal sinus J34.89
    turbinate, nasal J34.3
    upper respiratory tract J39.8
  indwelling catheter Z46.6
  inflammatory —*see also* Inflammation
    sacroiliac M46.1
  job, anxiety concerning Z56.1
  joint —*see* Derangement, joint
  life —*see* Menopause
  mental status R41.82
  minimal (glomerular) (*see also* N00-N07
    with fourth character .0) N05.0
  myocardium, myocardial —*see*
      Degeneration, myocardial - of
      life —*see* Menopause
  pacemaker Z45.018
    pulse generator Z45.010
  personality (enduring) F68.8
    due to (secondary to)
      general medical condition F07.0
      secondary (nonspecific) F60.89
  regressive, dental pulp K04.2
  renal —*see* Disease, renal
  retina H35.9
    myopic H44.2-
  sacroiliac joint M53.3
  senile (*see also* condition) R54
  sensory R20.8

Change (s) *(Continued)*
  skin R23.9
    acute, due to ultraviolet radiation
        L56.9
      specified NEC L56.8
    chronic, due to nonionizing radiation
        L57.9
      specified NEC L57.8
    cyanosis R23.0
    flushing R23.2
    pallor R23.1
    petechiae R23.3
    specified change NEC R23.8
    swelling —*see* Mass, localized
    texture R23.4
  trophic
    arm —*see* Mononeuropathy, upper
        limb
    leg —*see* Mononeuropathy, lower limb
  vascular I99.9
  vasomotor I73.9
  voice R49.9
    psychogenic F44.4
    specified NEC R49.8
Changing sleep-work schedule, affecting
    sleep G47.26
Changuinola fever A93.1
Chapping skin T69.8
Charcot-Marie-Tooth disease, paralysis
    or syndrome G60.0
Charcot's
  arthropathy —*see* Arthropathy,
      neuropathic
  cirrhosis K74.3
  disease (tabetic arthropathy) A52.16
  joint (disease) (tabetic) A52.16
    diabetic —*see* Diabetes, with,
        arthropathy
    syringomyelic G95.0
  syndrome (intermittent claudication)
      I73.9
CHARGE association Q89.8
Charley-horse (quadriceps) M62.831
  traumatic (quadriceps) S76.11-
Charlouis' disease —*see* Yaws
Cheadle's disease E54
Checking (of)
  cardiac pacemaker (battery)
      (electrode (s)) Z45.018
    pulse generator Z45.010
  intrauterine contraceptive device Z30.431
Check-up —*see* Examination
Chédiak-Higashi (-Steinbrinck)
      syndrome (congenital gigantism of
      peroxidase granules) E70.330
Cheek —*see* condition
Cheese itch B88.0
Cheese-washer's lung J67.8
Cheese-worker's lung J67.8
Cheilitis (acute) (angular) (catarrhal)
      (chronic) (exfoliative) (gangrenous)
      (glandular) (infectional)
      (suppurative) (ulcerative) (vesicular)
      K13.0
  actinic (due to sun) L56.8
    other than from sun L59.8
  candidal B37.83
Cheilodynia K13.0
Cheiloschisis —*see* Cleft, lip
Cheilosis (angular) K13.0
  with pellagra E52
  due to
    vitamin B2 (riboflavin) deficiency
        E53.0

Cheiromegaly M79.89
Cheiropompholyx L30.1
Cheloid —*see* Keloid
Chemical burn —*see* Corrosion,
    by site
Chemodectoma —*see* Paraganglioma,
    nonchromaffin
Chemosis, conjunctiva —*see* Edema,
    conjunctiva
Chemotherapy (session) (for)
  cancer Z51.11
  neoplasm Z51.11
Cherubism M27.8
Chest —*see* condition
Cheyne-Stokes breathing (respiration)
    R06.3
Chiari's
  disease or syndrome (hepatic vein
      thrombosis) I82.0
  malformation
    type I G93.5
    type II —*see* Spina bifida
  net Q24.8
Chicago disease B40.9
Chickenpox —*see* Varicella
Chiclero ulcer or sore B55.1
Chigger (infestation) B88.0
Chignon (disease) B36.8
  newborn (from vacuum extraction)
      (birth injury) P12.1
Chilaiditi's syndrome (subphrenic
    displacement, colon)
    Q43.3
Chilblain (s) (lupus) T69.1
Child
  custody dispute Z65.3
Childbirth —*see* Delivery
Childhood
  cerebral X-linked
      adrenoleukodystrophy
      E71.520
  period of rapid growth Z00.2
Chill (s) R68.83
  with fever R50.9
  without fever R68.83
  congestive in malarial regions B54
Chilomastigiasis A07.8
Chimera 46,XX/46,XY Q99.0
Chin —*see* condition
Chinese dysentery A03.9
Chionophobia F40.228
Chitral fever A93.1
Chlamydia, chlamydial A74.9
  cervicitis A56.09
  conjunctivitis A74.0
  cystitis A56.01
  endometritis A56.11
  epididymitis A56.19
  female
    pelvic inflammatory disease
        A56.11
    pelviperitonitis A56.11
  orchitis A56.19
  peritonitis A74.81
  pharyngitis A56.4
  proctitis A56.3
  psittaci (infection) A70
  salpingitis A56.11
  sexually-transmitted infection NEC
      A56.8
  specified NEC A74.89
  urethritis A56.01
  vulvovaginitis A56.02
Chlamydiosis —*see* Chlamydia

Chloasma (skin) (idiopathic) (symptomatic) L81.1
eyelid H02.719
hyperthyroid E05.90 [H02.719]
with thyroid storm E05.91 [H02.719]
left H02.716
lower H02.715
upper H02.714
right H02.713
lower H02.712
upper H02.711
Chloroma C92.3-
Chlorosis D50.9
Egyptian B76.9 [D63.8]
miner's B76.9 [D63.8]
Chlorotic anemia D50.8
Chocolate cyst (ovary) N80.1
Choked
disc or disk —see Papilledema
on food, phlegm, or vomitus NOS —see Foreign body, by site
while vomiting NOS —see Foreign body, by site
Chokes (resulting from bends) T70.3
Choking sensation R09.89
Cholangiectasis K83.8
Cholangiocarcinoma
with hepatocellular carcinoma, combined C22.0
liver C22.1
specified site NEC —see Neoplasm, malignant, by site
unspecified site C22.1
Cholangiohepatitis K83.8
due to fluke infestation B66.1
Cholangiohepatoma C22.0
Cholangiolitis (acute) (chronic) (extrahepatic) (gangrenous) (intrahepatic) K83.0
paratyphoidal —see Fever, paratyphoid
typhoidal A01.09
Cholangioma D13.4
malignant —see Cholangiocarcinoma
Cholangitis (ascending) (primary) (recurrent) (sclerosing) (secondary) (stenosing) (suppurative) K83.0
with calculus, bile duct —see Calculus, bile duct, with cholangitis
chronic nonsuppurative destructive K74.3
Cholecystectasia K82.8
Cholecystitis K81.9
with
calculus, stones in
bile duct (common) (hepatic) —see Calculus, bile duct, with cholecystitis
cystic duct —see Calculus, gallbladder, with cholecystitis
gallbladder —see Calculus, gallbladder, with cholecystitis
choledocholithiasis —see Calculus, bile duct, with cholecystitis
cholelithiasis —see Calculus, gallbladder, with cholecystitis
acute (emphysematous) (gangrenous) (suppurative) K81.0
with
calculus, stones in
cystic duct —see Calculus, gallbladder, with cholecystitis, acute

Cholecystitis (Continued)
acute (Continued)
with (Continued)
calculus, stones in (Continued)
gallbladder —see Calculus, gallbladder, with cholecystitis, acute
choledocholithiasis —see Calculus, bile duct, with cholecystitis, acute
cholelithiasis —see Calculus, gallbladder, with cholecystitis, acute
chronic cholecystitis K81.2
with gallbladder calculus K80.12
with obstruction K80.13
chronic K81.1
with acute cholecystitis K81.2
with gallbladder calculus K80.12
with obstruction K80.13
emphysematous (acute) —see Cholecystitis, acute
gangrenous —see Cholecystitis, acute
paratyphoidal, current A01.4
suppurative —see Cholecystitis, acute
typhoidal A01.09
Cholecystolithiasis —see Calculus, gallbladder
Choledochitis (suppurative) K83.0
Choledocholith —see Calculus, bile duct
Choledocholithiasis (common duct) (hepatic duct) —see Calculus, bile duct
cystic —see Calculus, gallbladder
typhoidal A01.09
Cholelithiasis (cystic duct) (gallbladder) (impacted) (multiple) —see Calculus, gallbladder
bile duct (common) (hepatic) —see Calculus, bile duct
hepatic duct —see Calculus, bile duct
specified NEC K80.80
with obstruction K80.81
Cholemia —see also Jaundice
familial (simple) (congenital) E80.4
Gilbert's E80.4
Choleperitoneum, choleperitonitis K65.3
Cholera (Asiatic) (epidemic) (malignant) A00.9
antimonial —see Poisoning, antimony
classical A00.0
due to Vibrio cholerae 01 A00.9
biovar cholerae A00.0
biovar eltor A00.1
el tor A00.1
el tor A00.1
Cholerine —see Cholera
Cholestasis NEC K83.1
with hepatocyte injury K71.0
due to total parenteral nutrition (TPN) K76.89
pure K71.0
Cholesteatoma (ear) (middle) (with reaction) H71.9-
attic H71.0-
external ear (canal) H60.4-
mastoid H71.2-
postmastoidectomy cavity (recurrent) —see Complications, postmastoidectomy, recurrent cholesteatoma
recurrent (postmastoidectomy) — see Complications, postmastoidectomy, recurrent cholesteatoma
tympanum H71.1-

Cholesteatosis, diffuse H71.3-
Cholesteremia E78.0
Cholesterin in vitreous —see Deposit, crystalline
Cholesterol
deposit
retina H35.89
vitreous —see Deposit, crystalline
elevated (high) E78.0
with elevated (high) triglycerides E78.2
screening for Z13.220
imbibition of gallbladder K82.4
Cholesterolemia (essential) (familial) (hereditary) (pure) E78.0
Cholesterolosis, cholesterosis (gallbladder) K82.4
cerebrotendinous E75.5
Cholocolic fistula K82.3
Choluria R82.2
Chondritis M94.8X9
aurical H61.03-
costal (Tietze's) M94.0
external ear H61.03-
patella, posttraumatic —see Chondromalacia, patella
pinna H61.03-
purulent M94.8X-
tuberculous NEC A18.02
intervertebral A18.01
Chondroblastoma —see also Neoplasm, bone, benign
malignant —see Neoplasm, bone, malignant
Chondrocalcinosis M11.20
ankle M11.27-
elbow M11.22-
familial M11.10
ankle M11.17-
elbow M11.12-
foot joint M11.17-
hand joint M11.14-
hip M11.15-
knee M11.16-
multiple site M11.19
shoulder M11.11-
vertebrae M11.18
wrist M11.13-
foot joint M11.27-
hand joint M11.24-
hip M11.25-
knee M11.26-
multiple site M11.29
shoulder M11.21-
specified type NEC M11.20
ankle M11.27-
elbow M11.22-
foot joint M11.27-
hand joint M11.24-
hip M11.25-
knee M11.26-
multiple site M11.29
shoulder M11.21-
vertebrae M11.28
wrist M11.23-
vertebrae M11.28
wrist M11.23-
Chondrodermatitis nodularis helicis or anthelicis —see Perichondritis, ear
Chondrodysplasia Q78.9
with hemangioma Q78.4
calcificans congenita Q77.3
fetalis Q77.4
metaphyseal (Jansen's) (McKusick's) (Schmid's) Q78.5
punctata Q77.3

Chondrodystrophy, chondrodystrophia
(familial) (fetalis) (hypoplastic)
Q78.9
calcificans congenita Q77.3
myotonic (congenital) G71.13
punctata Q77.3
Chondroectodermal dysplasia Q77.6
Chondrogenesis imperfecta Q77.4
Chondrolysis M94.35-
Chondroma —see also Neoplasm,
cartilage, benign
juxtacortical —see Neoplasm, bone,
benign
periosteal —see Neoplasm, bone,
benign
Chondromalacia (systemic) M94.20
acromioclavicular joint M94.21-
ankle M94.27-
elbow M94.22-
foot joint M94.27-
glenohumeral joint M94.21-
hand joint M94.24-
hip M94.25-
knee M94.26-
patella M22.4-
multiple sites M94.29
patella M22.4-
rib M94.28
sacroiliac joint M94.259
shoulder M94.21-
sternoclavicular joint M94.21-
vertebral joint M94.28
wrist M94.23-
Chondromatosis —see also Neoplasm,
cartilage, uncertain behavior
internal Q78.4
Chondromyxosarcoma —see Neoplasm,
cartilage, malignant
Chondro-osteodysplasia (Morquio-
Brailsford type) E76.219
Chondro-osteodystrophy E76.29
Chondro-osteoma —see Neoplasm, bone,
benign
Chondropathia tuberosa M94.0
Chondrosarcoma —see Neoplasm,
cartilage, malignant
juxtacortical —see Neoplasm, bone,
malignant
mesenchymal —see Neoplasm,
connective tissue, malignant
myxoid —see Neoplasm, cartilage,
malignant
Chordee (nonvenereal) N48.89
congenital Q54.4
gonococcal A54.09
Chorditis (fibrinous) (nodosa) (tuberosa)
J38.2
Chordoma —see Neoplasm, vertebral
(column), malignant
Chorea (chronic) (gravis)
(posthemiplegic) (senile)
(spasmodic) G25.5
with
heart involvement I02.0
active or acute (conditions in I01-)
I02.0
rheumatic I02.9
with valvular disorder I02.0
rheumatic heart disease (chronic)
(inactive)(quiescent) — code
to rheumatic heart condition
involved
drug-induced G25.4
habit F95.8

Chorea (Continued)
hereditary G10
Huntington's G10
hysterical F44.4
minor I02.9
with heart involvement I02.0
progressive G25.5
hereditary G10
rheumatic (chronic) I02.9
with heart involvement I02.0
Sydenham's I02.9
with heart involvement —see Chorea,
with rheumatic heart disease
nonrheumatic G25.5
Choreoathetosis (paroxysmal) G25.5
Chorioadenoma (destruens) D39.2
Chorioamnionitis O41.12-
Chorioangioma D26.7
Choriocarcinoma —see Neoplasm,
malignant, by site
combined with
embryonal carcinoma —see
Neoplasm, malignant, by site
other germ cell elements —see
Neoplasm, malignant, by site
teratoma —see Neoplasm,
malignant, by site
specified site —see Neoplasm,
malignant, by site
unspecified site
female C58
male C62.90
Chorioencephalitis (acute) (lymphocytic)
(serous) A87.2
Chorioepithelioma —see
Choriocarcinoma
Choriomeningitis (acute) (lymphocytic)
(serous) A87.2
Chorionepithelioma —see
Choriocarcinoma
Chorioretinitis —see also Inflammation,
chorioretinal
disseminated —see also Inflammation,
chorioretinal, disseminated
in neurosyphilis A52.19
Egyptian B76.9 [D63.8]
focal —see also Inflammation,
chorioretinal, focal
histoplasmic B39.9 [H32]
in (due to)
histoplasmosis B39.9 [H32]
syphilis (secondary) A51.43
late A52.71
toxoplasmosis (acquired) B58.01
congenital (active) P37.1 [H32]
tuberculosis A18.53
juxtapapillary, juxtapapillaris —see
Inflammation, chorioretinal, focal,
juxtapapillary
leprous A30.9 [H32]
miner's B76.9 [D63.8]
progressive myopia (degeneration)
H44.2-
syphilitic (secondary) A51.43
congenital (early) A50.01 [H32]
late A50.32
late A52.71
tuberculous A18.53
Chorioretinopathy, central serous H35.71-
Choroid —see condition
Choroideremia H31.21
Choroiditis —see Chorioretinitis
Choroidopathy —see Disorder,
choroid

Choroidoretinitis —see Chorioretinitis
Choroidoretinopathy, central serous —
see Chorioretinopathy, central serous
Christian-Weber disease M35.6
Christmas disease D67
Chromaffinoma —see also Neoplasm,
benign, by site
malignant —see Neoplasm, malignant,
by site
Chromatopsia —see Deficiency, color
vision
Chromhidrosis, chromidrosis L75.1
Chromoblastomycosis —see
Chromomycosis
Chromoconversion R82.91
Chromomycosis B43.9
brain abscess B43.1
cerebral B43.1
cutaneous B43.0
skin B43.0
specified NEC B43.8
subcutaneous abscess or cyst B43.2
Chromophytosis B36.0
Chromosome —see condition by
chromosome involved
D (1) —see condition, chromosome 13
E (3) —see condition, chromosome 18
G —see condition, chromosome 21
Chromotrichomycosis B36.8
Chronic —see condition
fracture —see Fracture, pathological
Churg-Strauss syndrome M30.1
Chyle cyst, mesentery I89.8
Chylocele (nonfilarial) I89.8
filarial (see also Infestation, filarial) B74.9
[N51]
tunica vaginalis N50.8
filarial (see also Infestation, filarial)
B74.9 [N51]
Chylomicronemia (fasting) (with
hyperprebetalipoproteinemia) E78.3
Chylopericardium I31.3
acute I30.9
Chylothorax (nonfilarial) I89.8
filarial (see also Infestation, filarial) B74.9
[J91.8]
Chylous —see condition
Chyluria (nonfilarial) R82.0
due to
bilharziasis B65.0
Brugia (malayi) B74.1
timori B74.2
schistosomiasis (bilharziasis) B65.0
Wuchereria (bancrofti) B74.0
filarial —see Infestation, filarial
Cicatricial (deformity) —see Cicatrix
Cicatrix (adherent) (contracted) (painful)
(vicious) (see also Scar) L90.5
adenoid (and tonsil) J35.8
alveolar process M26.79
anus K62.89
auricle —see Disorder, pinna, specified
type NEC
bile duct (common) (hepatic) K83.8
bladder N32.89
bone —see Disorder, bone, specified
type NEC
brain G93.89
cervix (postoperative) (postpartal) N88.1
common duct K83.8
cornea H17.9
tuberculous A18.59
duodenum (bulb), obstructive K31.5
esophagus K22.2
eyelid —see Disorder, eyelid function

Cicatrix *(Continued)*
hypopharynx J39.2
lacrimal passages —*see* Obstruction,
lacrimal
larynx J38.7
lung J98.4
middle ear —*see* subcategory H74.8
mouth K13.79
muscle M62.89
with contracture —*see* Contraction,
muscle NEC
nasopharynx J39.2
palate (soft) K13.79
penis N48.89
pharynx J39.2
prostate N42.89
rectum K62.89
retina —*see* Scar, chorioretinal
semilunar cartilage —*see* Derangement,
meniscus
seminal vesicle N50.8
skin L90.5
infected L08.89
postinfective L90.5
tuberculous B90.8
specified site NEC L90.5
throat J39.2
tongue K14.8
tonsil (and adenoid) J35.8
trachea J39.8
tuberculous NEC B90.9
urethra N36.8
uterus N85.8
vagina N89.8
postoperative N99.2
vocal cord J38.3
wrist, constricting (annular) L90.5
CIDP (chronic inflammatory
demyelinating polyneuropathy)
G61.81
CIN —*see* Neoplasia, intraepithelial, cervix
Cinchonism —*see* Deafness, ototoxic
correct substance properly
administered —*see* Table of drugs
and chemicals, by drug, adverse
effect
overdose or wrong substance given
or taken —*see* Table of drugs and
chemicals, by drug, poisoning
Circle of Willis —*see* condition
Circular —*see* condition
Circulating anticoagulants (*see also* -
Disorder, hemorrhagic) D68.318
due to drugs (*see also* - Disorder,
hemorrhagic) D68.32
following childbirth O72.3
Circulation
collateral, any site I99.8
defective (lower extremity) I99.8
congenital Q28.9
embryonic Q28.9
failure (peripheral) R57.9
newborn P29.89
fetal, persistent P29.3
heart, incomplete Q28.9
Circulatory system —*see* condition
Circulus senilis (cornea) —*see*
Degeneration, cornea, senile
Circumcision (in absence of medical
indication) (ritual) (routine) Z41.2
Circumscribed —*see* condition
Circumvallate placenta O43.11-
Cirrhosis, cirrhotic (hepatic) (liver) K74.60
alcoholic K70.30
with ascites K70.31

Cirrhosis, cirrhotic *(Continued)*
atrophic —*see* Cirrhosis, liver
Baumgarten-Cruveilhier K74.69
biliary (cholangiolitic) (cholangitic)
(hypertrophic) (obstructive)
(pericholangiolitic) K74.5
due to
Clonorchiasis B66.1
flukes B66.3
primary K74.3
secondary K74.4
cardiac (of liver) K76.1
Charcot's K74.3
cholangiolitic, cholangitic, cholostatic
(primary) K74.3
congestive K76.1
Cruveilhier-Baumgarten K74.69
cryptogenic (liver) K74.69
due to
hepatolenticular degeneration
E83.01
Wilson's disease E83.01
xanthomatosis E78.2
fatty K76.0
alcoholic K70.0
Hanot's (hypertrophic) K74.3
hepatic —*see* Cirrhosis, liver
hypertrophic K74.3
Indian childhood K74.69
kidney —*see* Sclerosis, renal
Laennec's K70.30
with ascites K70.31
alcoholic K70.30
with ascites K70.31
nonalcoholic K74.69
liver K74.60
alcoholic K70.30
with ascites K70.31
fatty K70.0
congenital P78.81
syphilitic A52.74
lung (chronic) J84.10
macronodular K74.69
alcoholic K70.30
with ascites K70.31
micronodular K74.69
alcoholic K70.30
with ascites K70.31
mixed type K74.69
monolobular K74.3
nephritis —*see* Sclerosis, renal
nutritional K74.69
alcoholic K70.30
with ascites K70.31
obstructive —*see* Cirrhosis, biliary
ovarian N83.8
pancreas (duct) K86.8
pigmentary E83.110
portal K74.69
alcoholic K70.30
with ascites K70.31
postnecrotic K74.69
alcoholic K70.30
with ascites K70.31
pulmonary J84.10
renal —*see* Sclerosis, renal
spleen D73.2
stasis K76.1
Todd's K74.3
unilobar K74.3
xanthomatous (biliary) K74.5
due to xanthomatosis (familial)
(metabolic) (primary) E78.2
Cistern, subarachnoid R93.0

Citrullinemia E72.23
Citrullinuria E72.23
Civatte's disease or poikiloderma L57.3
Clam digger's itch B65.3
Clammy skin R23.1
Clap —*see* Gonorrhea
Clarke-Hadfield syndrome (pancreatic
infantilism) K86.8
Clark's paralysis G80.9
Clastothrix L67.8
Claude Bernard-Horner syndrome G90.2
traumatic —*see* Injury, nerve, cervical
sympathetic
Claude's disease or syndrome G46.3
Claudicatio venosa intermittens I87.8
Claudication, intermittent I73.9
cerebral (artery) G45.9
spinal cord (arteriosclerotic) G95.19
syphilitic A52.09
venous (axillary) I87.8
Claustrophobia F40.240
Clavus (infected) L84
Clawfoot (congenital) Q66.89
acquired —*see* Deformity, limb,
clawfoot
Clawhand (acquired) —*see also* Deformity,
limb, clawhand
congenital Q68.1
Clawtoe (congenital) Q66.89
acquired —*see* Deformity, toe, specified
NEC
Clay eating —*see* Pica
Cleansing of artificial opening —*see*
Attention to, artificial, opening
Cleft (congenital) —*see also* Imperfect,
closure
alveolar process M26.79
branchial (cyst) (persistent) Q18.2
cricoid cartilage, posterior Q31.8
lip (unilateral) Q36.9
with cleft palate Q37.9
hard Q37.1
with soft Q37.5
soft Q37.3
with hard Q37.5
bilateral Q36.0
with cleft palate Q37.8
hard Q37.0
with soft Q37.4
soft Q37.2
with hard Q37.4
median Q36.1
nose Q30.2
palate Q35.9
with cleft lip (unilateral) Q37.9
bilateral Q37.8
hard Q35.1
with
cleft lip (unilateral) Q37.1
bilateral Q37.0
soft Q35.5
with cleft lip (unilateral) Q37.5
bilateral Q37.4
medial Q35.5
soft Q35.3
with
cleft lip (unilateral) Q37.3
bilateral Q37.2
hard Q35.5
with cleft lip (unilateral) Q37.5
bilateral Q37.4
penis Q55.69
scrotum Q55.29
thyroid cartilage Q31.8
uvula Q35.7

Cleidocranial dysostosis Q74.0
Cleptomania F63.2
Clicking hip (newborn) R29.4
Climacteric (female) —see also Menopause
    arthritis (any site) NEC —see Arthritis,
        specified form NEC
    depression (single episode) F32.8
    male (symptoms) (syndrome) NEC
        N50.8
    paranoid state F22
    polyarthritis NEC —see Arthritis,
        specified form NEC
    symptoms (female) N95.1
Clinical research investigation (clinical
    trial) (control subject) (normal
    comparison) (participant) Z00.6
Clitoris —see condition Cloaca
    (persistent) Q43.7
Clonorchiasis, clonorchis infection
    (liver) B66.1
Clonus R25.8
Closed bite M26.29
Clostridium (C.) perfringens, as cause of
    disease classified elsewhere B96.7
Closure
    congenital, nose Q30.0
    cranial sutures, premature Q75.0
    defective or imperfect NEC —see
        Imperfect, closure
    fistula, delayed —see Fistula
    foramen ovale, imperfect Q21.1
    hymen N89.6
    interauricular septum, defective Q21.1
    interventricular septum, defective Q21.0
    lacrimal duct —see also Stenosis,
        lacrimal, duct
        congenital Q10.5
    nose (congenital) Q30.0
        acquired M95.0
    of artificial opening —see Attention to,
        artificial, opening
    vagina N89.5
    valve —see Endocarditis
    vulva N90.5
Clot (blood) —see also Embolism
    artery (obstruction) (occlusion) —see
        Embolism
    bladder N32.89
    brain (intradural or extradural) —see
        Occlusion, artery, cerebral
    circulation I74.9
    heart —see also Infarct, myocardium
        not resulting in infarction I24.0
    vein —see Thrombosis
Clouded state R40.1
    epileptic —see Epilepsy, specified NEC
    paroxysmal —see Epilepsy, specified
        NEC
Cloudy antrum, antra J32.0
Clouston's (hidrotic) ectodermal
    dysplasia Q82.4
Clubbed nail pachydermoperiostosis
    M89.40 [L62]
Clubbing of finger (s) (nails) R68.3
Clubfinger R68.3
    congenital Q68.1
Clubfoot (congenital) Q66.89
    acquired —see Deformity, limb, clubfoot
    equinovarus Q66.0
    paralytic —see Deformity, limb, clubfoot
Clubhand (congenital) (radial) Q71.4-
    acquired —see Deformity, limb,
        clubhand
Clubnail R68.3
    congenital Q84.6

Clump, kidney Q63.1
Clumsiness, clumsy child syndrome F82
Cluttering F98.81
Clutton's joints A50.51 [M12.80]
Coagulation, intravascular (diffuse)
    (disseminated) —see also
        Defibrination syndrome
    complicating abortion —see Abortion,
        by type, complicated by,
        intravascular coagulation
    following ectopic or molar pregnancy
        O08.1
Coagulopathy —see also Defect,
    coagulation
    consumption D65
    intravascular D65
        newborn P60
Coalition
    calcaneo-scaphoid Q66.89
    tarsal Q66.89
Coalminer's
    elbow —see Bursitis, elbow, olecranon
    lung or pneumoconiosis J60
Coalworker's lung or pneumoconiosis J60
Coarctation
    aorta (preductal) (postductal) Q25.1
    pulmonary artery Q25.71
Coated tongue K14.3
Coats' disease (exudative retinopathy) —
    see Retinopathy, exudative
Cocainism —see Dependence, drug,
    cocaine
Coccidioidomycosis B38.9
    cutaneous B38.3
    disseminated B38.7
    generalized B38.7
    meninges B38.4
    prostate B38.81
    pulmonary B38.2
        acute B38.0
        chronic B38.1
    skin B38.3
    specified NEC B38.89
Coccidioidosis —see Coccidioidomycosis
Coccidiosis (intestinal) A07.3
Coccydynia, coccygodynia M53.3
Coccyx —see condition
Cochin-China diarrhea K90.1
Cockayne's syndrome Q87.1
Cocked up toe —see Deformity, toe,
    specified NEC
Cock's peculiar tumor L72.3
Codman's tumor —see Neoplasm, bone,
    benign
Coenurosis B71.8
Coffee-worker's lung J67.8
Cogan's syndrome H16.32-
    oculomotor apraxia H51.8
Coitus, painful (female) N94.1
    male N53.12
    psychogenic F52.6
Cold J00
    with influenza, flu, or grippe —see
        Influenza, with, respiratory
        manifestations NEC
    agglutinin disease or hemoglobinuria
        (chronic) D59.1
    bronchial —see Bronchitis
    chest —see Bronchitis
    common (head) J00
    effects of T69.9
        specified effect NEC T69.8
    excessive, effects of T69.9
        specified effect NEC T69.8
    exhaustion from T69.8

Cold (Continued)
    exposure to T69.9
        specified effect NEC T69.8
    head J00
    injury syndrome (newborn) P80.0
    on lung —see Bronchitis
    rose J30.1
    sensitivity, auto-immune D59.1
    virus J00
Coldsore B00.1
Colibacillosis A49.8
    as the cause of other disease (see also
        Escherichia coli) B96.20
    generalized A41.50
Colic (bilious) (infantile) (intestinal)
    (recurrent) (spasmodic) R10.83
    abdomen R10.83
        psychogenic F45.8
    appendix, appendicular K38.8
    bile duct —see Calculus, bile duct
    biliary —see Calculus, bile duct
    common duct —see Calculus, bile duct
    cystic duct —see Calculus, gallbladder
    Devonshire NEC —see Poisoning, lead
    gallbladder —see Calculus, gallbladder
    gallstone —see Calculus, gallbladder
        gallbladder or cystic duct —see
            Calculus, gallbladder
    hepatic (duct) —see Calculus, bile duct
    hysterical F45.8
    kidney N23
    lead NEC —see Poisoning, lead
    mucous K58.9
        with diarrhea K58.0
        psychogenic F54
    nephritic N23
    painter's NEC —see Poisoning, lead
    pancreas K86.8
    psychogenic F45.8
    renal N23
    saturnine NEC —see Poisoning, lead
    ureter N23
    urethral N36.8
        due to calculus N21.1
    uterus NEC N94.89
        menstrual —see Dysmenorrhea
    worm NOS B83.9
Colicystitis —see Cystitis
Colitis (acute) (catarrhal) (chronic)
    (noninfective) (hemorrhagic) (see also
        Enteritis) K52.9
    allergic K52.2
    amebic (acute) (see also Amebiasis) A06.0
        nondysenteric A06.2
    anthrax A22.2
    bacillary —see Infection, Shigella
    balantidial A07.0
    Clostridium difficile A04.7
    coccidial A07.3
    collagenous K52.89
    cystica superficialis K52.89
    dietary counseling and surveillance
        (for) Z71.3
    dietetic K52.2
    drug-induced K52.1
    due to radiation K52.0
    eosinophilic K52.82
    food hypersensitivity K52.2
    giardial A07.1
    granulomatous —see Enteritis, regional,
        large intestine
    infectious —see Enteritis, infectious
    ischemic K55.9
        acute (fulminant) (subacute) K55.0
        chronic K55.1

Colitis (Continued)
  ischemic (Continued)
    due to mesenteric artery insufficiency
        K55.1
    fulminant (acute) K55.0
  left sided K51.50
    with
      abscess K51.514
      complication K51.519
        specified NEC K51.518
      fistula K51.513
      obstruction K51.512
      rectal bleeding K51.511
  lymphocytic K52.89
  membranous
    psychogenic F54
  microscopic (collagenous)
      (lymphocytic) K52.89
  mucous —see Syndrome, irritable,
      bowel
    psychogenic F54
  noninfective K52.9
    specified NEC K52.89
  polyposa —see Polyps, colon,
      inflammatory
  protozoal A07.9
  pseudomembranous A04.7
  pseudomucinous —see Syndrome,
      irritable, bowel
  regional —see Enteritis, regional, large
      intestine
  segmental —see Enteritis, regional, large
      intestine
  septic —see Enteritis, infectious
  spastic K58.9
    with diarrhea K58.0
    psychogenic F54
  staphylococcal A04.8
    foodborne A05.0
  subacute ischemic K55.0
  thromboulcerative K55.0
  toxic NEC K52.1
    due to Clostridium difficile A04.7
  transmural —see Enteritis, regional,
      large intestine
  trichomonal A07.8
  tuberculous (ulcerative) A18.32
  ulcerative (chronic) K51.90
    with
      complication K51.919
        abscess K51.914
        fistula K51.913
        obstruction K51.912
        rectal bleeding K51.911
        specified complication NEC
            K51.918
    enterocolitis —see Enterocolitis,
        ulcerative
    ileocolitis —see Ileocolitis, ulcerative
    mucosal proctocolitis —see
        Proctocolitis, mucosal
    proctitis —see Proctitis, ulcerative
    pseudopolyposis —see Polyps, colon,
        inflammatory
    psychogenic F54
    rectosigmoiditis —see
        Rectosigmoiditis, ulcerative
    specified type NEC K51.80
      with
        complication K51.819
          abscess K51.814
          fistula K51.813
          obstruction K51.812
          rectal bleeding K51.811
          specified complication NEC
              K51.818

Collagenosis, collagen disease
    (nonvascular) (vascular) M35.9
  cardiovascular I42.8
  reactive perforating L87.1
  specified NEC M35.8
Collapse R55
  adrenal E27.2
  cardiorespiratory R57.0
  cardiovascular R57.0
    newborn P29.89
  circulatory (peripheral) R57.9
    during or after labor and delivery O75.1
    following ectopic or molar pregnancy
        O08.3
    newborn P29.89
  during or
    after labor and delivery O75.1
    resulting from a procedure, not
        elsewhere classified T81.10
  external ear canal —see Stenosis,
      external ear canal
  general R55
  heart —see Disease, heart
  heat T67.1
  hysterical F44.89
  labyrinth, membranous (congenital)
      Q16.5
  lung (massive) (see also Atelectasis) J98.19
    pressure due to anesthesia (general)
        (local) or other sedation T88.2
      during labor and delivery O74.1
      in pregnancy O29.02-
      postpartum, puerperal O89.09
  myocardial —see Disease, heart
  nervous F48.8
  neurocirculatory F45.8
  nose M95.0
  postoperative (cardiovascular) T81.11
  pulmonary (see also Atelectasis) J98.19
    newborn —see Atelectasis
  trachea J39.8
  tracheobronchial J98.09
  valvular —see Endocarditis
  vascular (peripheral) R57.9
    during or after labor and delivery
        O75.1
    following ectopic or molar pregnancy
        O08.3
    newborn P29.89
  vertebra M48.50-
    cervical region M48.52-
    cervicothoracic region M48.53-
    in (due to)
      metastasis —see Collapse, vertebra,
          in, specified disease NEC
      osteoporosis (see also Osteoporosis)
          M80.88
        cervical region M80.88
        cervicothoracic region M80.88
        lumbar region M80.88
        lumbosacral region M80.88
        multiple sites M80.88
        occipito-atlanto-axial region
            M80.88
        sacrococcygeal region M80.88
        thoracic region M80.88
        thoracolumbar region M80.88
      specified disease NEC M48.50-
        cervical region M48.52-
        cervicothoracic region M48.53-
        lumbar region M48.56-
        lumbosacral region M48.57-
        occipito-atlanto-axial region
            M48.51-
        sacrococcygeal region M48.58-
        thoracic region M48.54-
        thoracolumbar region M48.55-

Collapse (Continued)
  vertebra (Continued)
    lumbar region M48.56-
    lumbosacral region M48.57-
    occipito-atlanto-axial region M48.51-
    sacrococcygeal region M48.58-
    thoracic region M48.54-
    thoracolumbar region M48.55-
Collateral —see also condition
  circulation (venous) I87.8
  dilation, veins I87.8
Colles' fracture S52.53-
Collet (-Sicard) syndrome G52.7
Collier's asthma or lung J60
Collodion baby Q80.2
Colloid nodule (of thyroid) (cystic) E04.1
Coloboma (iris) Q13.0
  eyelid Q10.3
  fundus Q14.8
  lens Q12.2
  optic disc (congenital) Q14.2
    acquired H47.31-
Coloenteritis —see Enteritis
Colon —see condition
Colonization
  MRSA (Methicillin resistant
      Staphylococcus aureus) Z22.322
  MSSA (Methicillin susceptible
      Staphylococcus aureus) Z22.321
  status —see Carrier (suspected) of
Coloptosis K63.4
Color blindness —see Deficiency, color
    vision
Colostomy
  attention to Z43.3
  fitting or adjustment Z46.89
  malfunctioning K94.03
  status Z93.3
Colpitis (acute) —see Vaginitis
Colpocele N81.5
Colpocystitis —see Vaginitis
Colpospasm N94.2
Column, spinal, vertebral —see condition
Coma R40.20
  with
    motor response (none) R40.231
      abnormal R40.233
      extension R40.232
      flexion withdrawal R40.234
      localizes pain R40.235
      obeys commands R40.236
    opening of eyes (never) R40.211
      in response to
        pain R40.212
        sound R40.213
      spontaneous R40.214
    verbal response (none) R40.221
      confused conversation R40.224
      inappropriate words R40.223
      incomprehensible words R40.222
      oriented R40.225
  eclamptic —see Eclampsia
  epileptic —see Epilepsy
  Glasgow, scale score —see Glasgow
      coma scale
  hepatic —see Failure, hepatic, by type,
      with coma
  hyperglycemic (diabetic) —see Diabetes,
      coma
  hyperosmolar (diabetic) —see Diabetes,
      coma
  hypoglycemic (diabetic) —see Diabetes,
      coma, hypoglycemic
    nondiabetic E15
  in diabetes —see Diabetes, coma

Coma *(Continued)*
  insulin-induced —*see* Coma,
      hypoglycemic
  myxedematous E03.5
  newborn P91.5
  persistent vegetative state R40.3
  specified NEC, without documented
      Glasgow coma scale score, or with
      partial Glasgow coma scale score
      reported R40.244
Comatose —*see* Coma
Combat fatigue F43.0
Combined —*see* condition
Comedo, comedones (giant) L70.0
Comedocarcinoma —*see also* Neoplasm,
      breast, malignant
  noninfiltrating
      breast D05.8-
      specified site —*see* Neoplasm, in situ,
          by site
      unspecified site D05.8-
Comedomastitis —*see* Ectasia, mammary
      duct
Comminuted fracture - code as Fracture,
      closed
Common
  arterial trunk Q20.0
  atrioventricular canal Q21.2
  atrium Q21.1
  cold (head) J00
  truncus (arteriosus) Q20.0
  variable immunodeficiency —*see*
      Immunodeficiency, common
      variable
  ventricle Q20.4
Commotio, commotion (current)
  brain —*see* Injury, intracranial,
      concussion
  cerebri —*see* Injury, intracranial,
      concussion
  retinae S05.8X-
  spinal cord —*see* Injury, spinal cord, by
      region
  spinalis —*see* Injury, spinal cord, by
      region
Communication
  between
      base of aorta and pulmonary artery
          Q21.4
      left ventricle and right atrium Q20.5
      pericardial sac and pleural sac Q34.8
      pulmonary artery and pulmonary
          vein, congenital Q25.72
  congenital between uterus and
      digestive or urinary tract Q51.7
Compartment syndrome (deep)
      (posterior) (traumatic) T79.A0
  abdomen T79.A3
  lower extremity (hip, buttock, thigh,
      leg, foot, toes) T79.A2
  nontraumatic
      abdomen M79.A3
      lower extremity (hip, buttock, thigh,
          leg, foot, toes) M79.A2-
      specified site NEC M79.A9
      upper extremity (shoulder, arm,
          forearm, wrist, hand, fingers) -
          M79.A1
  specified site NEC T79.A9
  upper extremity (shoulder, arm, forearm,
      wrist, hand, fingers) T79.A1
Compensation
  failure —*see* Disease, heart
  neurosis, psychoneurosis —*see*
      Disorder, factitious

Complaint —*see also* Disease
  bowel, functional K59.9
      psychogenic F45.8
  intestine, functional K59.9
      psychogenic F45.8
  kidney —*see* Disease, renal
  miners' J60
Complete —*see* condition
Complex
  Addison-Schilder E71.528
  cardiorenal —*see* Hypertension,
      cardiorenal
  Costen's M26.69
  disseminated mycobacterium avium-
      intracellulare (DMAC) A31.2
  Eisenmenger's (ventricular septal
      defect) I27.89
  hypersexual F52.8
  jumped process, spine —*see* Dislocation,
      vertebra
  primary, tuberculous A15.7
  Schilder-Addison E71.528
  subluxation (vertebral) M99.19
      abdomen M99.19
      acromioclavicular M99.17
      cervical region M99.11
      cervicothoracic M99.11
      costochondral M99.18
      costovertebral M99.18
      head region M99.10
      hip M99.15
      lower extremity M99.16
      lumbar region M99.13
      lumbosacral M99.13
      occipitocervical M99.10
      pelvic region M99.15
      pubic M99.15
      rib cage M99.18
      sacral region M99.14
      sacrococcygeal M99.14
      sacroiliac M99.14
      specified NEC M99.19
      sternochondral M99.18
      sternoclavicular M99.17
      thoracic region M99.12
      thoracolumbar M99.12
      upper extremity M99.17
  Taussig-Bing (transposition, aorta and
      overriding pulmonary artery) Q20.1
Complication (s) (from) (of)
  accidental puncture or laceration
      during a procedure (of) —*see*
      Complications, intraoperative
      (intraprocedural), puncture or
      laceration
  amputation stump (surgical) (late) NEC
      T87.9
      dehiscence T87.81
      infection or inflammation T87.40
          lower limb T87.4-
          upper limb T87.4-
      necrosis T87.50
          lower limb T87.5-
          upper limb T87.5-
      neuroma T87.30
          lower limb T87.3-
          upper limb T87.3-
      specified type NEC T87.89
  anastomosis (and bypass) —*see also*
      Complications, prosthetic device
      or implant
      intestinal (internal) NEC K91.89
          involving urinary tract N99.89
      urinary tract (involving intestinal
          tract) N99.89

Complication (s) *(Continued)*
  anastomosis *(Continued)*
      vascular —*see* Complications,
          cardiovascular device or implant
  anesthesia, anesthetic (*see also*
      Anesthesia, complication) T88.59
      brain, postpartum, puerperal O89.2
      cardiac
          in
              labor and delivery O74.2
              pregnancy O29.19-
          postpartum, puerperal O89.1
      central nervous system
          in
              labor and delivery O74.3
              pregnancy O29.29-
          postpartum, puerperal O89.2
      difficult or failed intubation T88.4
          in pregnancy O29.6-
      failed sedation (conscious) (moderate)
          during procedure T88.52
      hyperthermia, malignant T88.3
      hypothermia T88.51
      intubation failure T88.4
      malignant hyperthermia T88.3
      pulmonary
          in
              labor and delivery O74.1
              pregnancy NEC O29.09-
          postpartum, puerperal O89.09
      shock T88.2
      spinal and epidural
          in
              labor and delivery NEC O74.6
                  headache O74.5
              pregnancy NEC O29.5X-
          postpartum, puerperal NEC O89.5
              headache O89.4
  anti-reflux device —*see* Complications,
      esophageal anti-reflux device
  aortic (bifurcation) graft —*see*
      Complications, graft, vascular
  aortocoronary (bypass) graft —*see*
      Complications, coronary artery
      (bypass) graft
  aortofemoral (bypass) graft —*see*
      Complications, extremity artery
      (bypass) graft
  arteriovenous
      fistula, surgically created T82.9
          embolism T82.818
          fibrosis T82.828
          hemorrhage T82.838
          infection or inflammation T82.7
          mechanical
              breakdown T82.510
              displacement T82.520
              leakage T82.530
              malposition T82.520
              obstruction T82.590
              perforation T82.590
              protrusion T82.590
          pain T82.848
          specified type NEC T82.898
          stenosis T82.858
          thrombosis T82.868
      shunt, surgically created T82.9
          embolism T82.818
          fibrosis T82.828
          hemorrhage T82.838
          infection or inflammation T82.7
          mechanical
              breakdown T82.511
              displacement T82.521
              leakage T82.531

Complication (s) *(Continued)*
arteriovenous *(Continued)*
  shunt, surgically created *(Continued)*
    mechanical *(Continued)*
      malposition T82.521
      obstruction T82.591
      perforation T82.591
      protrusion T82.591
    pain T82.848
    specified type NEC T82.898
    stenosis T82.858
    thrombosis T82.868
  arthroplasty —*see* Complications, joint
    prosthesis
  artificial
    fertilization or insemination N98.9
      attempted introduction (of)
        embryo in embryo transfer N98.3
        ovum following in vitro
          fertilization N98.2
      hyperstimulation of ovaries N98.1
      infection N98.0
      specified NEC N98.8
    heart T82.9
      embolism T82.817
      fibrosis T82.827
      hemorrhage T82.837
      infection or inflammation T82.7
      mechanical
        breakdown T82.512
        displacement T82.522
        leakage T82.532
        malposition T82.522
        obstruction T82.592
        perforation T82.592
        protrusion T82.592
      pain T82.847
      specified type NEC T82.897
      stenosis T82.857
      thrombosis T82.867
  opening
    cecostomy —*see* Complications,
      colostomy
    colostomy —*see* Complications,
      colostomy
    cystostomy —*see* Complications,
      cystostomy
    enterostomy —*see* Complications,
      enterostomy
    gastrostomy —*see* Complications,
      gastrostomy
    ileostomy —*see* Complications,
      enterostomy
    jejunostomy —*see* Complications,
      enterostomy
    nephrostomy —*see* Complications,
      stoma, urinary tract
    tracheostomy —*see* Complications,
      tracheostomy
    ureterostomy —*see* Complications,
      stoma, urinary tract
    urethrostomy —*see* Complications,
      stoma, urinary tract
  balloon implant or device
    gastrointestinal T85.9
      embolism T85.81
      fibrosis T85.82
      hemorrhage T85.83
      infection and inflammation T85.79
      pain T85.84
      specified type NEC T85.89
      stenosis T85.85
      thrombosis T85.86
    vascular (counterpulsation) T82.9
      embolism T82.818
      fibrosis T82.828

Complication (s) *(Continued)*
balloon implant or device *(Continued)*
  vascular *(Continued)*
    hemorrhage T82.838
    infection or inflammation T82.7
    mechanical
      breakdown T82.513
      displacement T82.523
      leakage T82.533
      malposition T82.523
      obstruction T82.593
      perforation T82.593
      protrusion T82.593
    pain T82.848
    specified type NEC T82.898
    stenosis T82.858
    thrombosis T82.868
  bariatric procedure
    gastric band procedure K95.09
      infection K95.01
    specified procedure NEC K95.89
      infection K95.81
  bile duct implant (prosthetic) T85.9
    embolism T85.81
    fibrosis T85.82
    hemorrhage T85.83
    infection and inflammation T85.79
    mechanical
      breakdown T85.510
      displacement T85.520
      malfunction T85.510
      malposition T85.520
      obstruction T85.590
      perforation T85.590
      protrusion T85.590
      specified NEC T85.590
    pain T85.84
    specified type NEC T85.89
    stenosis T85.85
    thrombosis T85.86
  bladder device (auxiliary) —*see*
    Complications, genitourinary,
    device or implant, urinary system
  bleeding (postoperative) —*see*
    Complication, postoperative,
    hemorrhage
    intraoperative —*see* Complication,
      intraoperative, hemorrhage
  blood vessel graft —*see* Complications,
    graft, vascular
  bone
    device NEC T84.9
      embolism T84.81
      fibrosis T84.82
      hemorrhage T84.83
      infection or inflammation T84.7
      mechanical
        breakdown T84.318
        displacement T84.328
        malposition T84.328
        obstruction T84.398
        perforation T84.398
        protrusion T84.398
      pain T84.84
      specified type NEC T84.89
      stenosis T84.85
      thrombosis T84.86
    graft —*see* Complications, graft, bone
    growth stimulator (electrode) —*see*
      Complications, electronic
      stimulator device, bone
    marrow transplant —*see*
      Complications, transplant,
      bone, marrow

Complication (s) *(Continued)*
brain neurostimulator (electrode) —
  see Complications, electronic
  stimulator device, brain
  breast implant (prosthetic) T85.9
    capsular contracture T85.44
    embolism T85.81
    fibrosis T85.82
    hemorrhage T85.83
    infection and inflammation T85.79
    mechanical
      breakdown T85.41
      displacement T85.42
      leakage T85.43
      malposition T85.42
      obstruction T85.49
      perforation T85.49
      protrusion T85.49
      specified NEC T85.49
    pain T85.84
    specified type NEC T85.89
    stenosis T85.85
    thrombosis T85.86
  bypass —*see also* Complications,
    prosthetic device or implant
    aortocoronary —*see* Complications,
      coronary artery (bypass) graft
    arterial —*see also* Complications,
      graft, vascular
      extremity —*see* Complications,
        extremity artery (bypass) graft
  cardiac —*see also* Disease, heart
    device, implant or graft T82.9
      embolism T82.817
      fibrosis T82.827
      hemorrhage T82.837
      infection or inflammation T82.7
      valve prosthesis T82.6
      mechanical
        breakdown T82.519
          specified device NEC T82.518
        displacement T82.529
          specified device NEC T82.528
        leakage T82.539
          specified device NEC T82.538
        malposition T82.529
          specified device NEC T82.528
        obstruction T82.599
          specified device NEC T82.598
        perforation T82.599
          specified device NEC T82.598
        protrusion T82.599
          specified device NEC T82.598
      pain T82.847
      specified type NEC T82.897
      stenosis T82.857
      thrombosis T82.867
  cardiovascular device, graft or implant
    T82.9
    aortic graft —*see* Complications,
      graft, vascular
    arteriovenous
      fistula, artificial —*see*
        Complication, arteriovenous,
        fistula, surgically created
      shunt —*see* Complication, arterio-
        venous, shunt, surgically
        created
    artificial heart —*see* Complication,
      artificial, heart
    balloon (counterpulsation) device —
      see Complication, balloon
      implant, vascular
    carotid artery graft —*see*
      Complications, graft, vascular

Complication (s) (Continued)
  cardiovascular device, graft or implant
    (Continued)
    coronary bypass graft —see
      Complication, coronary artery
      (bypass) graft
    dialysis catheter (vascular) —see
      Complication, catheter, dialysis
    electronic T82.9
     electrode T82.9
      embolism T82.817
      fibrosis T82.827
      hemorrhage T82.837
      infection T82.7
      mechanical
       breakdown T82.110
       displacement T82.120
       leakage T82.190
       obstruction T82.190
       perforation T82.190
       protrusion T82.190
       specified type NEC T82.190
      pain T82.847
      specified NEC T82.897
      stenosis T82.857
      thrombosis T82.867
     embolism T82.817
     fibrosis T82.827
     hemorrhage T82.837
     infection T82.7
     mechanical
      breakdown T82.119
      displacement T82.129
      leakage T82.199
      obstruction T82.199
      perforation T82.199
      protrusion T82.199
      specified type NEC T82.199
     pain T82.847
     pulse generator T82.9
      embolism T82.817
      fibrosis T82.827
      hemorrhage T82.837
      infection T82.7
      mechanical
       breakdown T82.111
       displacement T82.121
       leakage T82.191
       obstruction T82.191
       perforation T82.191
       protrusion T82.191
       specified type NEC T82.191
      pain T82.847
      specified NEC T82.897
      stenosis T82.857
      thrombosis T82.867
     specified condition NEC T82.897
     specified device NEC T82.9
      embolism T82.817
      fibrosis T82.827
      hemorrhage T82.837
      infection T82.7
      mechanical
       breakdown T82.118
       displacement T82.128
       leakage T82.198
       obstruction T82.198
       perforation T82.198
       protrusion T82.198
       specified type NEC T82.198
      pain T82.847
      specified NEC T82.897
      stenosis T82.857
      thrombosis T82.867
     stenosis T82.857
     thrombosis T82.867

Complication (s) (Continued)
  cardiovascular device, graft or implant
    (Continued)
    extremity artery graft —see
      Complication, extremity artery
      (bypass) graft
    femoral artery graft —see
      Complication, extremity artery
      (bypass) graft
    heart
     transplant —see Complication,
      transplant, heart
     valve —see Complication,
      prosthetic device, heart valve
     graft —see Complication, heart,
      valve, graft
    heart-lung transplant —see
      Complication, transplant, heart,
      with lung
    infection or inflammation T82.7
    umbrella device —see Complication,
      umbrella device, vascular
    vascular graft (or anastomosis) —see
      Complication, graft, vascular
  carotid artery (bypass) graft —see
    Complications, graft, vascular
  catheter (device) NEC —see also
    Complications, prosthetic device
    or implant
    cystostomy T83.9
     embolism T83.81
     fibrosis T83.82
     hemorrhage T83.83
     infection and inflammation T83.59
     mechanical
      breakdown T83.010
      displacement T83.020
      leakage T83.030
      malposition T83.020
      obstruction T83.090
      perforation T83.090
      protrusion T83.090
      specified NEC T83.090
     pain T83.84
     specified type NEC T83.89
     stenosis T83.85
     thrombosis T83.86
    dialysis (vascular) T82.9
     embolism T82.818
     fibrosis T82.828
     hemorrhage T82.838
     infection and inflammation
      T82.7
     intraperitoneal —see
      Complications, catheter,
      intraperitoneal
     mechanical
      breakdown T82.41
      displacement T82.42
      leakage T82.43
      malposition T82.42
      obstruction T82.49
      perforation T82.49
      protrusion T82.49
     pain T82.848
     specified type NEC T82.898
     stenosis T82.858
     thrombosis T82.868
    epidural infusion T85.9
     embolism T85.81
     fibrosis T85.82
     hemorrhage T85.83
     infection and inflammation
      T85.79

Complication (s) (Continued)
  catheter (device) NEC (Continued)
    epidural infusion (Continued)
     mechanical
      breakdown T85.610
      displacement T85.620
      leakage T85.630
      malfunction T85.610
      malposition T85.620
      obstruction T85.690
      perforation T85.690
      protrusion T85.690
      specified NEC T85.690
     pain T85.84
     specified type NEC T85.89
     stenosis T85.85
     thrombosis T85.86
    intraperitoneal dialysis T85.9
     embolism T85.81
     fibrosis T85.82
     hemorrhage T85.83
     infection and inflammation
      T85.71
     mechanical
      breakdown T85.611
      displacement T85.621
      leakage T85.631
      malfunction T85.611
      malposition T85.621
      obstruction T85.691
      perforation T85.691
      protrusion T85.691
      specified NEC T85.691
     pain T85.84
     specified type NEC T85.89
     stenosis T85.85
     thrombosis T85.86
    intravenous infusion T82.9
     embolism T82.818
     fibrosis T82.828
     hemorrhage T82.838
     infection or inflammation T82.7
     mechanical
      breakdown T82.514
      displacement T82.524
      leakage T82.534
      malposition T82.524
      obstruction T82.594
      perforation T82.594
      protrusion T82.594
     pain T82.848
     specified type NEC T82.898
     stenosis T82.858
     thrombosis T82.868
    subdural infusion T85.9
     embolism T85.81
     fibrosis T85.82
     hemorrhage T85.83
     infection and inflammation
      T85.79
     mechanical
      breakdown T85.610
      displacement T85.620
      leakage T85.630
      malfunction T85.610
      malposition T85.620
      obstruction T85.690
      perforation T85.690
      protrusion T85.690
      specified NEC T85.690
     pain T85.84
     specified type NEC T85.89
     stenosis T85.85
     thrombosis T85.86

Complication (s) *(Continued)*
  catheter (device) NEC *(Continued)*
    urethral, indwelling T83.9
      displacement T83.028
      embolism T83.81
      fibrosis T83.82
      hemorrhage T83.83
      infection and inflammation T83.51
      leakage T83.038
      malposition T83.028
      mechanical
        breakdown T83.018
      obstruction (mechanical) T83.098
      pain T83.84
      perforation T83.098
      protrusion T83.098
      specified type NEC T83.098
      stenosis T83.85
      thrombosis T83.86
    urinary (indwelling) —*see*
        Complications, catheter,
        urethral, indwelling
  cecostomy (stoma) —*see* Complications,
      colostomy
  cesarean delivery wound NEC O90.89
    disruption O90.0
    hematoma O90.2
    infection (following delivery) O86.0
  chemotherapy (antineoplastic) NEC
      T88.7
  chin implant (prosthetic) —*see*
      Complication, prosthetic device or
      implant, specified NEC
  circulatory system I99.8
    intraoperative I97.88
    postprocedural I97.89
      following cardiac surgery I97.19-
        postcardiotomy syndrome I97.0
      hypertension I97.3
      lymphedema after mastectomy I97.2
      postcardiotomy syndrome I97.0
      specified NEC I97.89
  colostomy (stoma) K94.00
    hemorrhage K94.01
    infection K94.02
    malfunction K94.03
    mechanical K94.03
    specified complication NEC K94.09
  contraceptive device, intrauterine —
      see Complications, intrauterine,
      contraceptive device
  cord (umbilical) —*see* Complications,
      umbilical cord
  corneal graft —*see* Complications, graft,
      cornea
  coronary artery (bypass) graft T82.9
    atherosclerosis —*see* Arteriosclerosis,
        coronary (artery)
    embolism T82.818
    fibrosis T82.828
    hemorrhage T82.838
    infection and inflammation T82.7
    mechanical
      breakdown T82.211
      displacement T82.212
      leakage T82.213
      malposition T82.212
      obstruction T82.218
      perforation T82.218
      protrusion T82.218
      specified NEC T82.218
    pain T82.848
    specified type NEC T82.897
    stenosis T82.858
    thrombosis T82.868

Complication (s) *(Continued)*
  counterpulsation device (balloon),
      intra-aortic —*see* Complications,
      balloon implant, vascular
  cystostomy (stoma) N99.518
    catheter —*see* Complications,
        catheter, cystostomy
    hemorrhage N99.510
    infection N99.511
    malfunction N99.512
    specified type NEC N99.518
  delivery *(see also* Complications,
      obstetric) O75.9
    procedure (instrumental) (manual)
        (surgical) O75.4
    specified NEC O75.89
  dialysis (peritoneal) (renal) —*see also*
      Complications, infusion
    catheter (vascular) —*see*
        Complication, catheter, dialysis
    peritoneal, intraperitoneal —*see*
        Complications, catheter,
        intraperitoneal
  dorsal column (spinal)
      neurostimulator —*see*
      Complications, electronic
      stimulator device, spinal cord
  drug NEC T88.7
  ear procedure —*see also* Disorder, ear
    intraoperative H95.88-
      hematoma —*see* Complications,
          intraoperative, hemorrhage
          (hematoma) (of), ear
      hemorrhage —*see* Complications,
          intraoperative, hemorrhage
          (hematoma) (of), ear
      laceration —*see* Complications,
          intraoperative, puncture or
          laceration..., ear
      specified NEC H95.88-
    postoperative H95.89-
      external ear canal stenosis H95.81-
      hematoma —*see* Complications,
          postprocedural, hemorrhage
          (hematoma) (of), ear
      hemorrhage —*see* Complications,
          postprocedural, hemorrhage
          (hematoma) (of), ear
      postmastoidectomy —
          see Complications,
          postmastoidectomy
      specified NEC H95.89-
  ectopic pregnancy O08.9
    damage to pelvic organs O08.6
    embolism O08.2
    genital infection O08.0
    hemorrhage (delayed) (excessive)
        O08.1
    metabolic disorder O08.5
    renal failure O08.4
    shock O08.3
    specified type NEC O08.0
    venous complication NEC O08.7
  electronic stimulator device
    bladder (urinary) —*see*
        Complications, electronic
        stimulator device, urinary
    bone T84.9
      breakdown T84.310
      displacement T84.320
      embolism T84.81
      fibrosis T84.82
      hemorrhage T84.83
      infection or inflammation T84.7
      malfunction T84.310

Complication (s) *(Continued)*
  electronic stimulator device *(Continued)*
    bone *(Continued)*
      malposition T84.320
      mechanical NEC T84.390
      obstruction T84.390
      pain T84.84
      perforation T84.390
      protrusion T84.390
      specified type NEC T84.89
      stenosis T84.85
      thrombosis T84.86
    brain T85.9
      embolism T85.81
      fibrosis T85.82
      hemorrhage T85.83
      infection and inflammation T85.79
      mechanical
        breakdown T85.110
        displacement T85.120
        leakage T85.190
        malposition T85.120
        obstruction T85.190
        perforation T85.190
        protrusion T85.190
        specified NEC T85.190
      pain T85.84
      specified type NEC T85.89
      stenosis T85.85
      thrombosis T85.86
    cardiac (defibrillator) (pacemaker) —
        see Complications,
        cardiovascular device or
        implant, electronic
    muscle T84.9
      breakdown T84.418
      displacement T84.428
      embolism T84.81
      fibrosis T84.82
      hemorrhage T84.83
      infection or inflammation T84.7
      mechanical NEC T84.498
      pain T84.84
      specified type NEC T84.89
      stenosis T84.85
      thrombosis T84.86
    nervous system T85.9
      brain —*see* Complications,
          electronic stimulator device,
          brain
      embolism T85.81
      fibrosis T85.82
      hemorrhage T85.83
      infection and inflammation T85.79
      mechanical
        breakdown T85.118
        displacement T85.128
        leakage T85.199
        malposition T85.128
        obstruction T85.199
        perforation T85.199
        protrusion T85.199
        specified NEC T85.199
      pain T85.84
      peripheral nerve —*see*
          Complications, electronic
          stimulator device, peripheral
          nerve
      specified type NEC T85.89
      spinal cord —*see* Complications,
          electronic stimulator device,
          spinal cord
      stenosis T85.85
      thrombosis T85.86

Complication (s) (Continued)
  electronic stimulator device (Continued)
    peripheral nerve T85.9
      embolism T85.81
      fibrosis T85.82
      hemorrhage T85.83
      infection and inflammation T85.79
      mechanical
        breakdown T85.111
        displacement T85.121
        leakage T85.191
        malposition T85.121
        obstruction T85.191
        perforation T85.191
        protrusion T85.191
        specified NEC T85.191
      pain T85.84
      specified type NEC T85.89
      stenosis T85.85
      thrombosis T85.86
    spinal cord T85.9
      embolism T85.81
      fibrosis T85.82
      hemorrhage T85.83
      infection and inflammation T85.79
      mechanical
        breakdown T85.112
        displacement T85.122
        leakage T85.192
        malposition T85.122
        obstruction T85.192
        perforation T85.192
        protrusion T85.192
        specified NEC T85.192
      pain T85.84
      specified type NEC T85.89
      stenosis T85.85
      thrombosis T85.86
  urinary T83.9
    embolism T83.81
    fibrosis T83.82
    hemorrhage T83.83
    infection and inflammation T83.59
    mechanical
      breakdown T83.110
      displacement T83.120
      malposition T83.120
      perforation T83.190
      protrusion T83.190
      specified NEC T83.190
    pain T83.84
    specified type NEC T83.89
    stenosis T83.85
    thrombosis T83.86
  electroshock therapy T88.9
    specified NEC T88.8
  endocrine E34.9
    postprocedural
      adrenal hypofunction E89.6
      hypoinsulinemia E89.1
      hypoparathyroidism E89.2
      hypopituitarism E89.3
      hypothyroidism E89.0
      ovarian failure E89.40
        asymptomatic E89.40
        symptomatic E89.41
      specified NEC E89.89
      testicular hypofunction E89.5
  endodontic treatment NEC M27.59
  enterostomy (stoma) K94.10
    hemorrhage K94.11
    infection K94.12
    malfunction K94.13
    mechanical K94.13
    specified complication NEC K94.19

Complication (s) (Continued)
  episiotomy, disruption O90.1
  esophageal anti-reflux device T85.9
    embolism T85.81
    fibrosis T85.82
    hemorrhage T85.83
    infection and inflammation T85.79
    mechanical
      breakdown T85.511
      displacement T85.521
      malfunction T85.511
      malposition T85.521
      obstruction T85.591
      perforation T85.591
      protrusion T85.591
      specified NEC T85.591
    pain T85.84
    specified type NEC T85.89
    stenosis T85.85
    thrombosis T85.86
  esophagostomy K94.30
    hemorrhage K94.31
    infection K94.32
    malfunction K94.33
    mechanical K94.33
    specified complication NEC K94.39
  extracorporeal circulation T80.90
  extremity artery (bypass) graft T82.9
    arteriosclerosis —see Arteriosclerosis,
        extremities, bypass graft
    embolism T82.818
    fibrosis T82.828
    hemorrhage T82.838
    infection and inflammation T82.7
    mechanical
      breakdown T82.318
        femoral artery T82.312
      displacement T82.328
        femoral artery T82.322
      leakage T82.338
        femoral artery T82.332
      malposition T82.328
        femoral artery T82.322
      obstruction T82.398
        femoral artery T82.392
      perforation T82.398
        femoral artery T82.392
      protrusion T82.398
        femoral artery T82.392
    pain T82.848
    specified type NEC T82.898
    stenosis T82.858
    thrombosis T82.868
  eye H57.9
    corneal graft —see Complications,
        graft, cornea
    implant (prosthetic) T85.9
      embolism T85.81
      fibrosis T85.82
      hemorrhage T85.83
      infection and inflammation T85.79
      mechanical
        breakdown T85.318
        displacement T85.328
        leakage T85.398
        malposition T85.328
        obstruction T85.398
        perforation T85.398
        protrusion T85.398
        specified NEC T85.398
      pain T85.84
      specified type NEC T85.89
      stenosis T85.85
      thrombosis T85.86
    intraocular lens —see Complications,
        intraocular lens

Complication (s) (Continued)
  eye (Continued)
    orbital prosthesis —see Complications,
        orbital prosthesis
  female genital N94.9
    device, implant or graft NEC —see
        Complications, genitourinary,
        device or implant, genital tract
  femoral artery (bypass) graft —see
      Complication, extremity artery
      (bypass) graft
  fixation device, internal (orthopedic)
      T84.9
    infection and inflammation
        T84.60
      arm T84.61-
        humerus T84.61-
        radius T84.61-
        ulna T84.61-
      leg T84.629
        femur T84.62-
        fibula T84.62-
        tibia T84.62-
      specified site NEC T84.69
      spine T84.63
    mechanical
      breakdown
        limb T84.119
          carpal T84.210
          femur T84.11-
          fibula T84.11-
          humerus T84.11-
          metacarpal T84.210
          metatarsal T84.213
          phalanx
            foot T84.213
            hand T84.210
          radius T84.11-
          tarsal T84.213
          tibia T84.11-
          ulna T84.11-
        specified bone NEC T84.218
        spine T84.216
      displacement
        limb T84.129
          carpal T84.220
          femur T84.12-
          fibula T84.12-
          humerus T84.12-
          metacarpal T84.220
          metatarsal T84.223
          phalanx
            foot T84.223
            hand T84.220
          radius T84.12-
          tarsal T84.223
          tibia T84.12-
          ulna T84.12-
        specified bone NEC T84.228
        spine T84.226
      malposition —see Complications,
          fixation device, internal,
          mechanical, displacement
      obstruction —see Complications,
          fixation device, internal,
          mechanical, specified
          type NEC
      perforation —see Complications,
          fixation device, internal,
          mechanical, specified
          type NEC
      protrusion —see Complications,
          fixation device, internal,
          mechanical, specified
          type NEC

Complication (s) *(Continued)*
  fixation device, internal *(Continued)*
    mechanical *(Continued)*
      specified type NEC
        limb T84.199
          carpal T84.290
          femur T84.19-
          fibula T84.19-
          humerus T84.19-
          metacarpal T84.290
          metatarsal T84.293
          phalanx
            foot T84.293
            hand T84.290
          radius T84.19-
          tarsal T84.293
          tibia T84.19-
          ulna T84.19-
        specified bone NEC T84.298
        vertebra T84.296
    specified type NEC T84.9
      embolism T84.81
      fibrosis T84.82
      hemorrhage T84.83
      pain T84.84
      specified complication NEC T84.89
      stenosis T84.85
      thrombosis T84.86
  following
    acute myocardial infarction NEC I23.8
    aneurysm (false) (of cardiac wall)
      (of heart wall) (ruptured) I23.3
    angina I23.7
    atrial
      septal defect I23.1
      thrombosis I23.6
    cardiac wall rupture I23.3
    chordae tendinae rupture I23.4
    defect
      septal
        atrial (heart) I23.1
        ventricular (heart) I23.2
    hemopericardium I23.0
    papillary muscle rupture I23.5
    rupture
      cardiac wall I23.3
        with hemopericardium I23.0
      chordae tendineae I23.4
      papillary muscle I23.5
    specified NEC I23.8
    thrombosis
      atrium I23.6
      auricular appendage I23.6
      ventricle (heart) I23.6
    ventricular
      septal defect I23.2
      thrombosis I23.6
  ectopic or molar pregnancy O08.9
    cardiac arrest O08.81
    sepsis O08.82
    specified type NEC O08.89
    urinary tract infection O08.83
  termination of pregnancy —*see*
    Abortion
  gastrointestinal K92.9
    bile duct prosthesis —*see*
      Complications, bile duct implant
    esophageal anti-reflux device —*see*
      Complications, esophageal anti-
      reflux device
    postoperative
      colostomy —*see* Complications,
        colostomy
      dumping syndrome K91.1
      enterostomy —*see* Complications,
        enterostomy

Complication (s) *(Continued)*
  gastrointestinal *(Continued)*
    postoperative *(Continued)*
      gastrostomy —*see* Complications,
        gastrostomy
      malabsorption NEC K91.2
      obstruction K91.3
      postcholecystectomy syndrome
        K91.5
      specified NEC K91.89
      vomiting after GI surgery K91.0
    prosthetic device or implant
      bile duct prosthesis —*see*
        Complications, bile duct
        implant
      esophageal anti-reflux device —*see*
        Complications, esophageal
        anti-reflux device
      specified type NEC
      embolism T85.81
        fibrosis T85.82
        hemorrhage T85.83
        mechanical
          breakdown T85.518
          displacement T85.528
          malfunction T85.518
          malposition T85.528
          obstruction T85.598
          perforation T85.598
          protrusion T85.598
          specified NEC T85.598
        pain T85.84
        specified complication NEC
          T85.89
        stenosis T85.85
        thrombosis T85.86
    gastrostomy (stoma) K94.20
      hemorrhage K94.21
      infection K94.22
      malfunction K94.23
      mechanical K94.23
      specified complication NEC K94.29
  genitourinary
    device or implant T83.9
      genital tract T83.9
        infection or inflammation T83.6
        intrauterine contraceptive
          device —*see* Complications,
          intrauterine, contraceptive
          device
        mechanical —*see* Complications,
          by device, mechanical
        mesh —*see* Complications, mesh
        penile prosthesis —*see*
          Complications, prosthetic
          device, penile
        specified type NEC T83.89
          embolism T83.81
          fibrosis T83.82
          hemorrhage T83.83
          pain T83.84
          specified complication NEC
            T83.89
          stenosis T83.85
          thrombosis T83.86
        vaginal mesh —*see*
          Complications, mesh
      urinary system T83.9
        cystostomy catheter —*see*
          Complication, catheter,
          cystostomy
        electronic stimulator —*see*
          Complications, electronic
          stimulator device, urinary

Complication (s) *(Continued)*
  genitourinary *(Continued)*
    device or implant *(Continued)*
      urinary system *(Continued)*
        indwelling urethral catheter —
          see Complications, catheter,
          urethral, indwelling
        infection or inflammation
          T83.59
          indwelling urinary catheter
          T83.51
        kidney transplant —*see*
          Complication, transplant,
          kidney
        organ graft —*see* Complication,
          graft, urinary organ
        specified type NEC T83.89
          embolism T83.81
          fibrosis T83.82
          hemorrhage T83.83
          mechanical T83.198
            breakdown T83.118
            displacement T83.128
            malfunction T83.118
            malposition T83.128
            obstruction T83.198
            perforation T83.198
            protrusion T83.198
            specified NEC T83.198
          pain T83.84
          specified complication NEC
            T83.89
          stenosis T83.85
          thrombosis T83.86
        sphincter implant —*see*
          Complications, implant,
          urinary sphincter
    postprocedural
      pelvic peritoneal adhesions N99.4
      renal failure N99.0
      specified NEC N99.89
      stoma —*see* Complications, stoma,
        urinary tract
      urethral stricture —*see* Stricture,
        urethra, postprocedural
      vaginal
        adhesions N99.2
        vault prolapse N99.3
  graft (bypass) (patch) —*see also*
    Complications, prosthetic device
    or implant
    aorta —*see* Complications, graft,
      vascular
    arterial —*see* Complication, graft,
      vascular
    bone T86.839
      failure T86.831
      infection T86.832
      mechanical T84.318
        breakdown T84.318
        displacement T84.328
        protrusion T84.398
        specified type NEC T84.398
      rejection T86.830
      specified type NEC T86.838
    carotid artery —*see* Complications,
      graft, vascular
    cornea T86.849
      failure T86.841
      infection T86.842
      mechanical T85.398
        breakdown T85.318
        displacement T85.328
        protrusion T85.398

Complication (s) *(Continued)*
  graft *(Continued)*
    cornea *(Continued)*
      mechanical *(Continued)*
        specified type NEC T85.398
      rejection T86.840
      retroprosthetic membrane T85.398
      specified type NEC T86.848
    femoral artery (bypass) —*see*
      Complication, extremity artery
      (bypass) graft
    genital organ or tract —*see*
      Complications, genitourinary,
      device or implant, genital tract
    muscle T84.9
      breakdown T84.410
      displacement T84.420
      embolism T84.81
      fibrosis T84.82
      hemorrhage T84.83
      infection and inflammation T84.7
      mechanical NEC T84.490
      pain T84.84
      specified type NEC T84.89
      stenosis T84.85
      thrombosis T84.86
    nerve —*see* Complication, prosthetic
      device or implant, specified NEC
    skin —*see* Complications, prosthetic
      device or implant, skin graft
    tendon T84.9
      breakdown T84.410
      displacement T84.420
      embolism T84.81
      fibrosis T84.82
      hemorrhage T84.83
      infection and inflammation T84.7
      mechanical NEC T84.490
      pain T84.84
      specified type NEC T84.89
      stenosis T84.85
      thrombosis T84.86
    urinary organ T83.9
      embolism T83.81
      fibrosis T83.82
      hemorrhage T83.83
      infection and inflammation T83.59
        indwelling urinary catheter T83.51
      mechanical
        breakdown T83.21
        displacement T83.22
        leakage T83.23
        malposition T83.22
        obstruction T83.29
        perforation T83.29
        protrusion T83.29
        specified NEC T83.29
      pain T83.84
      specified type NEC T83.89
      stenosis T83.85
      thrombosis T83.86
    vascular T82.9
      embolism T82.818
      femoral artery —*see* Complication,
        extremity artery (bypass) graft
      fibrosis T82.828
      hemorrhage T82.838
      mechanical
        breakdown T82.319
          aorta (bifurcation) T82.310
          carotid artery T82.311
          specified vessel NEC T82.318
        displacement T82.329
          aorta (bifurcation) T82.320
          carotid artery T82.321
          specified vessel NEC T82.328

Complication (s) *(Continued)*
  graft *(Continued)*
    vascular *(Continued)*
      mechanical *(Continued)*
        leakage T82.339
          aorta (bifurcation) T82.330
          carotid artery T82.331
          specified vessel NEC T82.338
        malposition T82.329
          aorta (bifurcation) T82.320
          carotid artery T82.321
          specified vessel NEC T82.328
        obstruction T82.399
          aorta (bifurcation) T82.390
          carotid artery T82.391
          specified vessel NEC T82.398
        perforation T82.399
          aorta (bifurcation) T82.390
          carotid artery T82.391
          specified vessel NEC T82.398
        protrusion T82.399
          aorta (bifurcation) T82.390
          carotid artery T82.391
          specified vessel NEC T82.398
      pain T82.848
      specified complication NEC T82.898
      stenosis T82.858
      thrombosis T82.868
  heart I51.9
    assist device
      infection and inflammation T82.7
    following acute myocardial
      infarction —*see* Complications,
      following, acute myocardial
      infarction
    postoperative —*see* Complications,
      circulatory system
    transplant —*see* Complication,
      transplant, heart
    and lung (s) —*see* Complications,
      transplant, heart, with lung
    valve
      graft (biological) T82.9
        embolism T82.817
        fibrosis T82.827
        hemorrhage T82.837
        infection and inflammation T82.7
        mechanical T82.228
          breakdown T82.221
          displacement T82.222
          leakage T82.223
          malposition T82.222
          obstruction T82.228
          perforation T82.228
          protrusion T82.228
        pain T82.847
        specified type NEC T82.897
        stenosis T82.857
        thrombosis T82.867
      prosthesis T82.9
        embolism T82.817
        fibrosis T82.827
        hemorrhage T82.837
        infection or inflammation T82.6
        mechanical T82.09
          breakdown T82.01
          displacement T82.02
          leakage T82.03
          malposition T82.02
          obstruction T82.09
          perforation T82.09
          protrusion T82.09
        pain T82.847
        specified type NEC T82.897
          mechanical T82.09

Complication (s) *(Continued)*
  heart *(Continued)*
    valve *(Continued)*
      prosthesis *(Continued)*
        stenosis T82.857
        thrombosis T82.867
  hematoma
    intraoperative —*see* Complication,
      intraoperative, hemorrhage
    postprocedural —*see* Complication,
      postprocedural, hemorrhage
  hemodialysis —*see* Complications,
    dialysis
  hemorrhage
    intraoperative —*see* Complication,
      intraoperative, hemorrhage
    postprocedural —*see* Complication,
      postprocedural, hemorrhage
  ileostomy (stoma) —*see* Complications,
    enterostomy
  immunization (procedure) —*see*
    Complications, vaccination
  implant —*see also* Complications, by site
    and type
    urinary sphincter T83.9
      embolism T83.81
      fibrosis T83.82
      hemorrhage T83.83
      infection and inflammation T83.59
      mechanical
        breakdown T83.111
        displacement T83.121
        leakage T83.191
        malposition T83.121
        obstruction T83.191
        perforation T83.191
        protrusion T83.191
        specified NEC T83.191
      pain T83.84
      specified type NEC T83.89
      stenosis T83.85
      thrombosis T83.86
  infusion (procedure) T80.90
    air embolism T80.0
    blood —*see* Complications,
      transfusion
    catheter —*see* Complications, catheter
    infection T80.29
    pump —*see* Complications, cardio-
      vascular, device or implant
    sepsis T80.29
    serum reaction (*see also* Reaction,
      serum) T80.69
      anaphylactic shock (*see also* Shock,
        anaphylactic) T80.59
    specified type NEC T80.89
  inhalation therapy NEC T81.81
  injection (procedure) T80.90
    drug reaction —*see* Reaction, drug
    infection T80.29
    sepsis T80.29
    serum (prophylactic) (therapeutic) —
      see Complications, vaccination
    specified type NEC T80.89
    vaccine (any) —*see* Complications,
      vaccination
  inoculation (any) —*see* Complications,
    vaccination
  insulin pump
    infection and inflammation T85.72
    mechanical
      breakdown T85.614
      displacement T85.624
      leakage T85.633

Complication (s) *(Continued)*
  insulin pump *(Continued)*
    mechanical *(Continued)*
      malposition T85.624
      obstruction T85.694
      perforation T85.694
      protrusion T85.694
      specified NEC T85.694
  intestinal pouch NEC K91.858
  intraocular lens (prosthetic) T85.9
    embolism T85.81
    fibrosis T85.82
    hemorrhage T85.83
    infection and inflammation
        T85.79
    mechanical
      breakdown T85.21
      displacement T85.22
      malposition T85.22
      obstruction T85.29
      perforation T85.29
      protrusion T85.29
      specified NEC T85.29
    pain T85.84
    specified type NEC T85.89
    stenosis T85.85
    thrombosis T85.86
  intraoperative (intraprocedural)
    cardiac arrest
      during cardiac surgery I97.710
      during other surgery I97.711
    cardiac functional disturbance NEC
      during cardiac surgery I97.790
      during other surgery I97.791
    hemorrhage (hematoma) (of)
      circulatory system organ or
          structure
        during cardiac bypass I97.411
        during cardiac catheterization
            I97.410
        during other circulatory system
            procedure I97.418
        during other procedure I97.42
      digestive system organ
        during procedure on digestive
            system K91.61
        during procedure on other organ
            K91.62
      ear
        during procedure on ear and
            mastoid process H95.21
        during procedure on other organ
            H95.22
      endocrine system organ or structure
        during procedure on endocrine
            system organ or structure
            E36.01
        during procedure on other organ
            E36.02
      eye and adnexa
        during ophthalmic procedure
            H59.11-
        during other procedure H59.12-
      genitourinary organ or structure
        during procedure on
            genitourinary organ or
            structure N99.61
        during procedure on other organ
            N99.62
      mastoid process
        during procedure on ear and
            mastoid process H95.21
        during procedure on other organ
            H95.22

Complication (s) *(Continued)*
  intraoperative *(Continued)*
    hemorrhage *(Continued)*
      musculoskeletal structure
        during musculoskeletal surgery
            M96.810
        during non-orthopedic surgery
            M96.811
        during orthopedic surgery
            M96.810
      nervous system
        during a nervous system
            procedure G97.31
        during other procedure G97.32
      respiratory system
        during other procedure J95.62
        during procedure on respiratory
            system organ or structure
            J95.61
      skin and subcutaneous tissue
        during a dermatologic procedure
            L76.01
        during a procedure on other
            organ L76.02
      spleen
        during a procedure on other
            organ D78.02
        during a procedure on the spleen
            D78.01
    puncture or laceration (accidental)
        (unintentional) (of)
      brain
        during a nervous system
            procedure G97.48
        during other procedure
            G97.49
      circulatory system organ or
          structure
        during circulatory system
            procedure I97.51
        during other procedure I97.52
      digestive system
        during procedure on digestive
            system K91.71
        during procedure on other organ
            K91.72
      ear
        during procedure on ear and
            mastoid process H95.31
        during procedure on other organ
            H95.32
      endocrine system organ or
          structure
        during procedure on endocrine
            system organ or structure
            E36.11
        during procedure on other organ
            E36.12
      eye and adnexa
        during ophthalmic procedure
            H59.21-
        during other procedure
            H59.22-
      genitourinary organ or structure
        during procedure on
            genitourinary organ or
            structure N99.71
        during procedure on other organ
            N99.72
      mastoid process
        during procedure on ear and
            mastoid process H95.31
        during procedure on other organ
            H95.32

Complication (s) *(Continued)*
  intraoperative *(Continued)*
    puncture or laceration *(Continued)*
      musculoskeletal structure
        during musculoskeletal surgery
            M96.820
        during non-orthopedic surgery
            M96.821
        during orthopedic surgery
            M96.820
      nervous system
        during a nervous system
            procedure G97.48
        during other procedure G97.49
      respiratory system
        during other procedure J95.72
        during procedure on respiratory
            system organ or structure
            J95.71
      skin and subcutaneous tissue
        during a dermatologic procedure
            L76.11
        during a procedure on other
            organ L76.12
      spleen
        during a procedure on other
            organ D78.12
        during a procedure on the spleen
            D78.11
    specified NEC
      circulatory system I97.88
      digestive system K91.81
      ear H95.88
      endocrine system E36.8
      eye and adnexa H59.88
      genitourinary system N99.81
      mastoid process H95.88
      musculoskeletal structure M96.89
      nervous system G97.81
      respiratory system J95.88
      skin and subcutaneous tissue L76.81
      spleen D78.81
  intraperitoneal catheter (dialysis)
      (infusion) —*see* Complications,
      catheter, intraperitoneal
  intrauterine
    contraceptive device
      embolism T83.81
      fibrosis T83.82
      hemorrhage T83.83
      infection and inflammation T83.6
      mechanical
        breakdown T83.31
        displacement T83.32
        malposition T83.32
        obstruction T83.39
        perforation T83.39
        protrusion T83.39
        specified NEC T83.39
      pain T83.84
      specified type NEC T83.89
      stenosis T83.85
      thrombosis T83.86
    procedure (fetal), to newborn P96.5
  jejunostomy (stoma) —*see*
      Complications, enterostomy
  joint prosthesis, internal T84.9
    breakage (fracture) T84.01-
    dislocation T84.02-
    fracture T84.01-
    infection or inflammation T84.50
    hip T84.5-
    knee T84.5-
    specified joint NEC T84.59

151

Complication (s) (*Continued*)
  joint prosthesis, internal (*Continued*)
    instability T84.02-
    malposition —*see* Complications,
      joint prosthesis, mechanical,
      displacement
    mechanical
      breakage, broken T84.01-
      dislocation T84.02-
      fracture T84.01-
      instability T84.02-
      leakage —*see* Complications,
        joint prosthesis, mechanical,
        specified NEC
      loosening T84.039
        hip T84.03-
        knee T84.03-
        specified joint NEC T84.038
      obstruction —*see* Complications,
        joint prosthesis, mechanical,
        specified NEC
      perforation —*see* Complications,
        joint prosthesis, mechanical,
        specified NEC
      periprosthetic
        fracture T84.049
          hip T84.04-
          knee T84.04-
          other specified joint T84.048
        osteolysis T84.059
          hip T84.05-
          knee T84.05-
          other specified joint T84.058
      protrusion —*see* Complications,
        joint prosthesis, mechanical,
        specified NEC
      specified complication NEC
        T84.099
        hip T84.09-
        knee T84.09-
        other specified joint T84.098
      subluxation T84.02-
      wear of articular bearing surface
        T84.069
        hip T84.06-
        knee T84.06-
        other specified joint T84.068
    specified joint NEC T84.9
      embolism T84.81
      fibrosis T84.82
      hemorrhage T84.83
      pain T84.84
      specified complication NEC
        T84.89
      stenosis T84.85
      thrombosis T84.86
    subluxation T84.02-
  kidney transplant —*see* Complications,
    transplant, kidney
  labor O75.9
    specified NEC O75.89
  liver transplant (immune or
    nonimmune) —*see* Complications,
    transplant, liver
  lumbar puncture G97.1
    cerebrospinal fluid leak G97.0
    headache or reaction G97.1
  lung transplant —*see* Complications,
    transplant, lung
    and heart —*see* Complications,
      transplant, lung, with heart
  male genital N50.9
    device, implant or graft —*see*
      Complications, genitourinary,
      device or implant, genital tract

Complication (s) (*Continued*)
  male genital (*Continued*)
    postprocedural or postoperative —*see*
      Complications, genitourinary,
      postprocedural
    specified NEC N99.89
  mastoid (process) procedure
    intraoperative H95.88-
      hematoma —*see* Complications,
        intraoperative, hemorrhage
        (hematoma) (of), mastoid
        process
      hemorrhage —*see* Complications,
        intraoperative, hemorrhage
        (hematoma) (of), mastoid
        process
      laceration —*see* Complications,
        intraoperative, puncture or
        laceration..., mastoid process
      specified NEC H95.88-
    postmastoidectomy —
      see Complications,
      postmastoidectomy
    postoperative H95.89-
      external ear canal stenosis
        H95.81-
      hematoma —*see* Complications...,
        postprocedural, hemorrhage
        (hematoma) (of), mastoid
        process
      hemorrhage —*see* Complications...,
        postprocedural, hemorrhage
        (hematoma) (of), mastoid
        process
      postmastoidectomy —
        see Complications,
        postmastoidectomy
      specified NEC H95.89-
  mastoidectomy cavity —
    see Complications,
    postmastoidectomy
  mechanical —*see* Complications, by site
    and type, mechanical
  medical procedures (*see also*
    Complication, intraoperative)
    T88.9
  metabolic E88.9
    postoperative E89.89
      specified NEC E89.89
  molar pregnancy NOS O08.9
    damage to pelvic organs O08.6
    embolism O08.2
    genital infection O08.0
    hemorrhage (delayed) (excessive)
      O08.1
    metabolic disorder O08.5
    renal failure O08.4
    shock O08.3
    specified type NEC O08.0
    venous complication NEC O08.7
  musculoskeletal system —*see also*
    Complication, intraoperative
    (intraprocedural), by site
    device, implant or graft NEC —*see*
      Complications, orthopedic,
      device or implant
    internal fixation (nail) (plate) (rod) —
      see Complications, fixation
      device, internal
    joint prosthesis —*see* Complications,
      joint prosthesis
    postoperative (postprocedural)
      M96.89
      with osteoporosis —*see*
        Osteoporosis

Complication (s) (*Continued*)
  musculoskeletal system (*Continued*)
    postoperative (*Continued*)
      fracture following insertion
        of device —*see* Fracture,
        following insertion of
        orthopedic implant, joint
        prosthesis or bone plate
      joint instability after prosthesis
        removal M96.89
      lordosis M96.4
      post radiation M96.89
        kyphosis M96.3
      postlaminectomy syndrome NEC
        M96.1
        kyphosis M96.3
      pseudarthrosis M96.0
      scoliosis M96.5
      specified complication NEC M96.89
  nephrostomy (stoma) —*see*
    Complications, stoma, urinary
    tract, external NEC
  nervous system G98.8
    central G96.9
    device, implant or graft —*see also*
      Complication, prosthetic device
      or implant, specified NEC
    electronic stimulator (electrode (s)) —
      see Complications, electronic
      stimulator device
    ventricular shunt —*see*
      Complications, ventricular
      shunt
    electronic stimulator (electrode (s)) —
      see Complications, electronic
      stimulator device
    postprocedural G97.82
      intracranial hypotension G97.2
      specified NEC G97.82
      spinal fluid leak G97.0
  newborn, due to intrauterine (fetal)
    procedure P96.5
  nonabsorbable (permanent) sutures —
    see Complication, sutures,
    permanent
  obstetric O75.9
    procedure (instrumental) (manual)
      (surgical) specified NEC O75.4
    specified NEC O75.89
    surgical wound NEC O90.89
      hematoma O90.2
      infection O86.0
  ocular lens implant —*see*
    Complications, intraocular lens
  ophthalmologic
    postprocedural bleb —*see* Blebitis
  orbital prosthesis T85.9
    embolism T85.81
    fibrosis T85.82
    hemorrhage T85.83
    infection and inflammation T85.79
    mechanical
      breakdown T85.31-
      displacement T85.32-
      malposition T85.32-
      obstruction T85.39-
      perforation T85.39-
      protrusion T85.39-
      specified NEC T85.39-
    pain T85.84
    specified type NEC T85.89
    stenosis T85.85
    thrombosis T85.86
  organ or tissue transplant (partial)
    (total) —*see* Complications,
    transplant

C

Complication (s) (Continued)
orthopedic —see also Disorder, soft
    tissue
    device or implant T84.9
      bone
        device or implant —see
          Complication, bone, device
          NEC
        graft —see Complication, graft,
          bone
      breakdown T84.418
      displacement T84.428
      electronic bone stimulator —see
        Complications, electronic
        stimulator device, bone
      embolism T84.81
      fibrosis T84.82
      fixation device —see Complication,
        fixation device, internal
      hemorrhage T84.83
      infection or inflammation T84.7
      joint prosthesis —see Complication,
        joint prosthesis, internal
      malfunction T84.418
      malposition T84.428
      mechanical NEC T84.498
      muscle graft —see Complications,
        graft, muscle
      obstruction T84.498
      pain T84.84
      perforation T84.498
      protrusion T84.498
      specified complication NEC T84.89
      stenosis T84.85
      tendon graft —see Complications,
        graft, tendon
      thrombosis T84.86
    fracture (following insertion
      of device) —see Fracture,
      following insertion of
      orthopedic implant, joint
      prosthesis or bone plate
    postprocedural M96.89
      fracture —see Fracture, following
        insertion of orthopedic
        implant, joint prosthesis or
        bone plate
      postlaminectomy syndrome NEC
        M96.1
        kyphosis M96.3
        lordosis M96.4
      postradiation
        kyphosis M96.2
        scoliosis M96.5
      pseudarthrosis post-fusion M96.0
      specified type NEC M96.89
  pacemaker (cardiac) —see
    Complications, cardiovascular
    device or implant, electronic
  pancreas transplant —see
    Complications, transplant,
    pancreas
  penile prosthesis (implant) —see
    Complications, prosthetic device,
    penile
  perfusion NEC T80.90
  perineal repair (obstetrical) NEC O90.89
    disruption O90.1
    hematoma O90.2
    infection (following delivery) O86.0
  phototherapy T88.9
    specified NEC T88.8
  postmastoidectomy NEC H95.19-
    cyst, mucosal H95.13-
    granulation H95.12-

Complication (s) (Continued)
postmastoidectomy NEC (Continued)
  inflammation, chronic H95.11-
  recurrent cholesteatoma H95.0-
postoperative —see Complications,
  postprocedural
  circulatory —see Complications,
    circulatory system
  ear —see Complications, ear
  endocrine —see Complications,
    endocrine
  eye —see Complications, eye
  lumbar puncture G97.1
    cerebrospinal fluid leak G97.0
  nervous system (central)
    (peripheral) —see
      Complications, nervous system
  respiratory system —see
    Complications, respiratory
    system
postprocedural —see also
    Complications, surgical procedure
  cardiac arrest
    following cardiac surgery I97.120
    following other surgery I97.121
  cardiac functional disturbance NEC
    following cardiac surgery I97.190
    following other surgery I97.191
  cardiac insufficiency
    following cardiac surgery I97.110
    following other surgery I97.111
  chorioretinal scars following retinal
    surgery H59.81-
  following cataract surgery
    cataract (lens) fragments H59.02-
    cystoid macular edema H59.03-
    specified NEC H59.09-
    vitreous (touch) syndrome H59.01-
  heart failure
    following cardiac surgery I97.130
    following other surgery I97.131
  hemorrhage (hematoma) (of)
    circulatory system organ or
      structure
      following a cardiac bypass I97.611
      following a cardiac
        catheterization I97.610
      following other circulatory
        system procedure I97.618
      following other procedure I97.62
    digestive system
      following procedure on digestive
        system K91.840
      following procedure on other
        organ K91.841
    ear
      following other procedure H95.42
      following procedure on ear and
        mastoid process H95.41
    endocrine system
      following endocrine system
        procedure E89.810
      following other procedure
        E89.811
    eye and adnexa
      following ophthalmic procedure
        H59.31-
      following other procedure
        H59.32-
    genitourinary organ or structure
      following procedure on
        genitourinary organ or
        structure N99.820
      following procedure on other
        organ N99.821

Complication (s) (Continued)
postprocedural (Continued)
  hemorrhage (Continued)
    mastoid process
      following other procedure H95.42
      following procedure on ear and
        mastoid process H95.41
    musculoskeletal structure
      following musculoskeletal
        surgery M96.830
      following non-orthopedic
        surgery M96.831
      following orthopedic surgery
        M96.830
    nervous system
      during a nervous system
        procedure G97.51
      during other procedure G97.52
    respiratory system
      during other procedure J95.831
      during procedure on respiratory
        system organ or structure
        J95.830
    skin and subcutaneous tissue
      following a dermatologic
        procedure L76.21
      following a procedure on other
        organ L76.22
    spleen
      following procedure on other
        organ D78.22
      following procedure on the
        spleen D78.21
  specified NEC
    circulatory system I97.89
    digestive K91.89
    ear H95.89
    endocrine E89.89
    eye and adnexa H59.89
    genitourinary N99.89
    mastoid process H95.89
    metabolic E89.89
    musculoskeletal structure
      M96.89
    nervous system G97.82
    respiratory system J95.89
    skin and subcutaneous tissue
      L76.82
    spleen D78.89
pregnancy NEC —see Pregnancy,
  complicated by
prosthetic device or implant T85.9
  bile duct —see Complications, bile
    duct implant
  breast —see Complications, breast
    implant
  cardiac and vascular NEC —see
    Complications, cardiovascular
    device or implant
  corneal transplant —see
    Complications, graft, cornea
  electronic nervous system
    stimulator —see Complications,
    electronic stimulator device
  epidural infusion catheter —see
    Complications, catheter,
    epidural
  esophageal anti-reflux device —see
    Complications, esophageal anti-
    reflux device
  genital organ or tract —see
    Complications, genitourinary,
    device or implant, genital tract
  heart valve —see Complications,
    heart, valve, prosthesis

Complication (s) *(Continued)*
  prosthetic device or implant *(Continued)*
    infection or inflammation T85.79
      intestine transplant T86.892
      liver transplant T86.43
      lung transplant T86.812
      pancreas transplant T86.892
      skin graft T86.822
    intraocular lens —*see* Complications,
        intraocular lens
    intraperitoneal (dialysis) catheter —
        see Complications, catheter,
        intraperitoneal
    joint —*see* Complications, joint
        prosthesis, internal
    mechanical NEC T85.698
      dialysis catheter (vascular) —*see
          also* Complication, catheter,
          dialysis, mechanical
        peritoneal —*see* Complication,
            catheter, intraperitoneal,
            mechanical
      gastrointestinal device T85.598
      ocular device T85.398
      subdural (infusion) catheter T85.690
      suture, permanent T85.692
        that for bone repair —*see*
            Complications, fixation
            device, internal
            (orthopedic), mechanical
      ventricular shunt
        breakdown T85.01
        displacement T85.02
        leakage T85.03
        malposition T85.02
        obstruction T85.09
        perforation T85.09
        protrusion T85.09
        specified NEC T85.09
    mesh
      erosion (to surrounding organ or
          tissue) T83.718
        vaginal (into pelvic floor
            muscles) T83.711
      exposure (into surrounding organ
          or tissue) T83.728
        vaginal (into vagina) (through
            vaginal wall) T83.721
    orbital —*see* Complications, orbital
        prosthesis
    penile T83.9
      embolism T83.81
      fibrosis T83.82
      hemorrhage T83.83
      infection and inflammation
          T83.6
      mechanical
        breakdown T83.410
        displacement T83.420
        leakage T83.490
        malposition T83.420
        obstruction T83.490
        perforation T83.490
        protrusion T83.490
        specified NEC T83.490
      pain T83.84
      specified type NEC T83.89
      stenosis T83.85
      thrombosis T83.86
    prosthetic materials NEC
      erosion (to surrounding organ or
          tissue) T83.718
        vaginal (into pelvic floor
            muscles) T83.711

Complication (s) *(Continued)*
  prosthetic device or implant *(Continued)*
    prosthetic materials NEC *(Continued)*
      exposure (into surrounding organ
          or tissue) T83.728
        vaginal (into vagina) (through
            vaginal wall) T83.721
    skin graft T86.829
      artificial skin or decellularized
          allodermis
        embolism T85.81
        fibrosis T85.82
        hemorrhage T85.83
        infection and inflammation
            T85.79
        mechanical
          breakdown T85.613
          displacement T85.623
          malfunction T85.613
          malposition T85.623
          obstruction T85.693
          perforation T85.693
          protrusion T85.693
          specified NEC T85.693
        pain T85.84
        specified type NEC T85.89
        stenosis T85.85
        thrombosis T85.86
      failure T86.821
      infection T86.822
      rejection T86.820
      specified NEC T86.828
    specified NEC T85.9
      embolism T85.81
      fibrosis T85.82
      hemorrhage T85.83
      infection and inflammation
          T85.79
      mechanical
        breakdown T85.618
        displacement T85.628
        leakage T85.638
        malfunction T85.618
        malposition T85.628
        obstruction T85.698
        perforation T85.698
        protrusion T85.698
        specified NEC T85.698
      pain T85.84
      specified type NEC T85.89
      stenosis T85.85
      thrombosis T85.86
    subdural infusion catheter —*see*
        Complications, catheter,
        subdural
    sutures —*see* Complications, sutures
    urinary organ or tract NEC —*see*
        Complications, genitourinary,
        device or implant, urinary
        system
    vascular —*see* Complications,
        cardiovascular device or
        implant
    ventricular shunt —*see*
        Complications, ventricular
        shunt (device)
  puerperium —*see* Puerperal
  puncture, spinal G97.1
    cerebrospinal fluid leak G97.0
    headache or reaction G97.1
  pyelogram N99.89
  radiation
    kyphosis M96.2
    scoliosis M96.5

Complication (s) *(Continued)*
  reattached
    extremity (infection) (rejection)
      lower T87.1X-
      upper T87.0X-
    specified body part NEC T87.2
  reconstructed breast
    asymmetry between native and
        reconstructed breast N65.1
    deformity N65.0
    disproportion between native and
        reconstructed breast N65.1
    excess tissue N65.0
    misshappen N65.0
  reimplant NEC —*see also*
      Complications, prosthetic device
      or implant
    limb (infection) (rejection) —*see*
        Complications, reattached,
        extremity
    organ (partial) (total) —*see*
        Complications, transplant
    prosthetic device NEC —*see*
        Complications, prosthetic
        device
  renal N28.9
    allograft —*see* Complications,
        transplant, kidney
    dialysis —*see* Complications, dialysis
  respirator
    mechanical J95.850
      specified NEC J95.859
  respiratory system J98.9
    device, implant or graft —*see*
        Complication, prosthetic device
        or implant, specified NEC
    lung transplant —*see* Complications,
        prosthetic device or implant,
        lung transplant
    postoperative J95.89
      air leak J95.812
      Mendelson's syndrome (chemical
          pneumonitis) J95.4
      pneumothorax J95.811
      pulmonary insufficiency (acute)
          (after nonthoracic surgery)
          J95.2
        chronic J95.3
        following thoracic surgery J95.1
      respiratory failure (acute) J95.821
        acute and chronic J95.822
      specified NEC J95.89
      subglottic stenosis J95.5
    tracheostomy complication —*see*
        Complications, tracheostomy
    therapy T81.89
  sedation during labor and delivery
      O74.9
    cardiac O74.2
    central nervous system O74.3
    pulmonary NEC O74.1
  shunt —*see also* Complications,
      prosthetic device or implant
    arteriovenous —*see* Complications,
        arteriovenous, shunt
    ventricular (communicating) —*see*
        Complications, ventricular
        shunt
  skin
    graft T86.829
      failure T86.821
      infection T86.822
      rejection T86.820
      specified type NEC T86.828

Complication (s) *(Continued)*
spinal
  anesthesia —*see* Complications,
    anesthesia, spinal
  catheter (epidural) (subdural) —*see*
    Complications, catheter
  puncture or tap G97.1
    cerebrospinal fluid leak G97.0
    headache or reaction G97.1
stent
  bile duct —*see* Complications, bile
    duct prosthesis
  urinary T83.9
    embolism T83.81
    fibrosis T83.82
    hemorrhage T83.83
    infection and inflammation
      T83.59
    mechanical
      breakdown T83.112
      displacement T83.122
      leakage T83.192
      malposition T83.122
      obstruction T83.192
      perforation T83.192
      protrusion T83.192
      specified NEC T83.192
    pain T83.84
    specified type NEC T83.89
    stenosis T83.85
    thrombosis T83.86
stoma
  digestive tract
    colostomy —*see* Complications,
      colostomy
    enterostomy —*see* Complications,
      enterostomy
    esophagostomy —*see*
      Complications,
      esophagostomy
    gastrostomy —*see* Complications,
      gastrostomy
  urinary tract N99.538
    cystostomy —*see* Complications,
      cystostomy
    external NOS N99.528
      hemorrhage N99.520
      infection N99.521
      malfunction N99.522
      specified type NEC N99.528
    hemorrhage N99.530
    infection N99.531
    malfunction N99.532
    specified type NEC N99.538
stomach banding —*see*
  Complication (s), bariatric
  procedure
stomach stapling —*see* Complication (s),
  bariatric procedure
surgical material, nonabsorbable —*see*
  Complication, suture, permanent
surgical procedure (on) T81.9
  amputation stump (late) —*see*
    Complications, amputation
    stump
  cardiac —*see* Complications,
    circulatory system
  cholesteatoma, recurrent —
    see Complications,
    postmastoidectomy, recurrent
    cholesteatoma
  circulatory (early) —*see*
    Complications, circulatory
    system

Complication (s) *(Continued)*
surgical procedure *(Continued)*
  digestive system —*see* Complications,
    gastrointestinal
  dumping syndrome
    (postgastrectomy) K91.1
  ear —*see* Complications, ear
  elephantiasis or lymphedema I97.89
    postmastectomy I97.2
  emphysema (surgical) T81.82
  endocrine —*see* Complications,
    endocrine
  eye —*see* Complications, eye
  fistula (persistent postoperative)
    T81.83
  foreign body inadvertently left
    in wound (sponge) (suture)
    (swab) —*see* Foreign body,
    accidentally left during a
    procedure
  gastrointestinal —*see* Complications,
    gastrointestinal
  genitourinary NEC N99.89
  hematoma
    intraoperative —*see* Complication,
      intraoperative, hemorrhage
    postprocedural —*see* Complication,
      postprocedural, hemorrhage
  hemorrhage
    intraoperative —*see* Complication,
      intraoperative, hemorrhage
    postprocedural —*see* Complication,
      postprocedural, hemorrhage
  hepatic failure K91.82
  hyperglycemia (postpancreatectomy)
    E89.1
  hypoinsulinemia
    (postpancreatectomy) E89.1
  hypoparathyroidism
    (postparathyroidectomy) E89.2
  hypopituitarism
    (posthypophysectomy) E89.3
  hypothyroidism (post-
    thyroidectomy) E89.0
  intestinal obstruction K91.3
  intracranial hypotension following
    ventricular shunting
    (ventriculostomy) G97.2
  lymphedema I97.89
    postmastectomy I97.2
  malabsorption (postsurgical) NEC
    K91.2
    osteoporosis —*see* Osteoporosis,
      postsurgical malabsorption
  mastoidectomy cavity NEC —
    see Complications,
    postmastoidectomy
  metabolic E89.89
    specified NEC E89.89
  musculoskeletal —*see* Complications,
    musculoskeletal system
  nervous system (central)
    (peripheral) —*see*
    Complications, nervous system
  ovarian failure E89.40
    asymptomatic E89.40
    symptomatic E89.41
  peripheral vascular —*see*
    Complications, surgical
    procedure, vascular
  postcardiotomy syndrome I97.0
  postcholecystectomy syndrome K91.5
  postcommissurotomy syndrome
    I97.0

Complication (s) *(Continued)*
surgical procedure *(Continued)*
  postgastrectomy dumping syndrome
    K91.1
  postlaminectomy syndrome NEC
    M96.1
    kyphosis M96.3
  postmastectomy lymphedema
    syndrome I97.2
  postmastoidectomy cholesteatoma —
    see Complications,
    postmastoidectomy, recurrent
    cholesteatoma
  postvagotomy syndrome K91.1
  postvalvulotomy syndrome I97.0
  pulmonary insufficiency (acute)
    J95.2
    chronic J95.3
    following thoracic surgery J95.1
  reattached body part —*see*
    Complications, reattached
  respiratory —*see* Complications,
    respiratory system
  shock (hypovolemic) T81.19
  spleen (postoperative) D78.89
    intraoperative D78.81
  stitch abscess T81.4
  subglottic stenosis (postsurgical) J95.5
  testicular hypofunction E89.5
  transplant —*see* Complications, organ
    or tissue transplant
  urinary NEC N99.89
  vaginal vault prolapse
    (posthysterectomy) N99.3
  vascular (peripheral)
    artery T81.719
      mesenteric T81.710
      renal T81.711
      specified NEC T81.718
    vein T81.72
  wound infection T81.4
suture, permanent (wire) NEC T85.9
  with repair of bone —*see* Compli-
    cations, fixation device, internal
  embolism T85.81
  fibrosis T85.82
  hemorrhage T85.83
  infection and inflammation T85.79
  mechanical
    breakdown T85.612
    displacement T85.622
    malfunction T85.612
    malposition T85.622
    obstruction T85.692
    perforation T85.692
    protrusion T85.692
    specified NEC T85.692
  pain T85.84
  specified type NEC T85.89
  stenosis T85.85
  thrombosis T85.86
tracheostomy J95.00
  granuloma J95.09
  hemorrhage J95.01
  infection J95.02
  malfunction J95.03
  mechanical J95.03
  obstruction J95.03
  specified type NEC J95.09
  tracheo-esophageal fistula J95.04
transfusion (blood) (lymphocytes)
  (plasma) T80.92
  air embolism T80.0
  circulatory overload E87.71

155

Complication (s) (Continued)
  transfusion (Continued)
    febrile nonhemolytic transfusion
      reaction R50.84
    hemochromatosis E83.111
    hemolysis T80.89
    hemolytic reaction (antigen
      unspecified) T80.919
    incompatibility reaction (antigen
      unspecified) T80.919
      ABO T80.30
        delayed serologic (DSTR) T80.39
        hemolytic transfusion reaction
          (HTR) (unspecified time
          after transfusion) T80.319
          acute (AHTR) (less than
            24 hours after transfusion)
            T80.310
          delayed (DHTR) (24 hours or
            more after transfusion)
            T80.311
        specified NEC T80.39
      acute (antigen unspecified) T80.910
      delayed (antigen unspecified)
        T80.911
      delayed serologic (DSTR) T80.89
      Non-ABO (minor antigens (Duffy)
        (Kell) (Kidd) (Lewis) (M) (N)
        (P) (S)) T80.A0
        delayed serologic (DSTR) T80.A9
        hemolytic transfusion reaction
          (HTR) (unspecified time
          after transfusion) T80.A19
          acute (AHTR) (less than
            24 hours after transfusion)
            T80.A10
          delayed (DHTR) (24 hours or
            more after transfusion)
            T80.A11
        specified NEC T80.A9
      Rh (antigens (C) (c) (D) (E) (e))
        (factor) T80.40
        delayed serologic (DSTR) T80.49
        hemolytic transfusion reaction
          (HTR) (unspecified time
          after transfusion) T80.419
          acute (AHTR) (less than
            24 hours after transfusion)
            T80.410
          delayed (DHTR) (24 hours or
            more after transfusion)
            T80.411
        specified NEC T80.49
    infection T80.29
    reaction NEC T80.89
    sepsis T80.29
    shock T80.89
  transplant T86.90
    bone T86.839
      failure T86.831
      infection T86.832
      rejection T86.830
      specified type NEC T86.838
    bone marrow T86.00
      failure T86.02
      infection T86.03
      rejection T86.01
      specified type NEC T86.09
    cornea T86.849
      failure T86.841
      infection T86.842
      rejection T86.840
      specified type NEC T86.848
    failure T86.92

Complication (s) (Continued)
  transplant (Continued)
    heart T86.20
      with lung T86.30
        cardiac allograft vasculopathy
          T86.290
        failure T86.32
        infection T86.33
        rejection T86.31
        specified type NEC T86.39
      failure T86.22
      infection T86.23
      rejection T86.21
      specified type NEC T86.298
    infection T86.93
    intestine T86.859
      failure T86.851
      infection T86.852
      rejection T86.850
      specified type NEC T86.858
    kidney T86.10
      failure T86.12
      infection T86.13
      rejection T86.11
      specified type NEC T86.19
    liver T86.40
      failure T86.42
      infection T86.43
      rejection T86.41
      specified type NEC T86.49
    lung T86.819
      with heart T86.30
        failure T86.32
        infection T86.33
        rejection T86.31
        specified type NEC T86.39
      failure T86.811
      infection T86.812
      rejection T86.810
      specified type NEC T86.818
    malignant neoplasm C80.2
    pancreas T86.899
      failure T86.891
      infection T86.892
      rejection T86.890
      specified type NEC T86.898
    peripheral blood stem cells T86.5
    post-transplant lymphoproliferative
      disorder (PTLD) D47.Z1
    rejection T86.91
    skin T86.829
      failure T86.821
      infection T86.822
      rejection T86.820
      specified type NEC T86.828
    stem cell (from peripheral blood)
      (from umbilical cord) T86.5
    umbilical cord stem cells T86.5
    specified
      tissue T86.899
        failure T86.891
        infection T86.892
        rejection T86.890
        specified type NEC T86.898
      type NEC T86.99
  trauma (early) T79.9
    specified NEC T79.8
  ultrasound therapy NEC T88.9
  umbilical cord NEC
    complicating delivery O69.9
      specified NEC O69.89
  umbrella device, vascular T82.9
    embolism T82.818
    fibrosis T82.828

Complication (s) (Continued)
  umbrella device, vascular (Continued)
    hemorrhage T82.838
    infection or inflammation T82.7
    mechanical
      breakdown T82.515
      displacement T82.525
      leakage T82.535
      malposition T82.525
      obstruction T82.595
      perforation T82.595
      protrusion T82.595
    pain T82.848
    specified type NEC T82.898
    stenosis T82.858
    thrombosis T82.868
  urethral catheter —see Complications,
    catheter, urethral, indwelling
  vaccination T88.1
    anaphylaxis NEC T80.52
    arthropathy —see Arthropathy,
      postimmunization
    cellulitis T88.0
    encephalitis or encephalomyelitis
      G04.02
    infection (general) (local) NEC T88.0
    meningitis G03.8
    myelitis G04.89
    protein sickness T80.62
    rash T88.1
    reaction (allergic) T88.1
      serum T80.62
    sepsis T88.0
    serum intoxication, sickness, rash,
      or other serum reaction NEC
      T80.62
      anaphylactic shock T80.52
    shock (allergic) (anaphylactic) T80.52
    vaccinia (generalized) (localized) T88.1
  vas deferens device or implant —see
    Complications, genitourinary,
    device or implant, genital tract
  vascular I99.9
    device or implant T82.9
      embolism T82.818
      fibrosis T82.828
      hemorrhage T82.838
      infection or inflammation T82.7
      mechanical
        breakdown T82.519
          specified device NEC T82.518
        displacement T82.529
          specified device NEC T82.528
        leakage T82.539
          specified device NEC T82.538
        malposition T82.529
          specified device NEC T82.528
        obstruction T82.599
          specified device NEC T82.598
        perforation T82.599
          specified device NEC T82.598
        protrusion T82.599
          specified device NEC T82.598
      pain T82.848
      specified type NEC T82.898
      stenosis T82.858
      thrombosis T82.868
    dialysis catheter —see Complication,
      catheter, dialysis
    following infusion, therapeutic
      injection or transfusion T80.1
    graft T82.9
      embolism T82.818
      fibrosis T82.828

Complication (s) (Continued)
  vascular (Continued)
    graft (Continued)
      hemorrhage T82.838
      mechanical
        breakdown T82.319
          aorta (bifurcation) T82.310
          carotid artery T82.311
          specified vessel NEC T82.318
        displacement T82.329
          aorta (bifurcation) T82.320
          carotid artery T82.321
          specified vessel NEC T82.328
        leakage T82.339
          aorta (bifurcation) T82.330
          carotid artery T82.331
          specified vessel NEC T82.338
        malposition T82.329
          aorta (bifurcation) T82.320
          carotid artery T82.321
          specified vessel NEC T82.328
        obstruction T82.399
          aorta (bifurcation) T82.390
          carotid artery T82.391
          specified vessel NEC T82.398
        perforation T82.399
          aorta (bifurcation) T82.390
          carotid artery T82.391
          specified vessel NEC T82.398
        protrusion T82.399
          aorta (bifurcation) T82.390
          carotid artery T82.391
          specified vessel NEC T82.398
      pain T82.848
      specified complication NEC T82.898
      stenosis T82.858
      thrombosis T82.868
    postoperative —see Complications,
      postoperative, circulatory
  vena cava device (filter) (sieve)
    (umbrella) —see Complications,
    umbrella device, vascular
  ventilation therapy NEC T81.81
  ventilator
    mechanical J95.850
      specified NEC J95.859
  ventricular (communicating) shunt
    (device) T85.9
    embolism T85.81
    fibrosis T85.82
    hemorrhage T85.83
    infection and inflammation T85.79
    mechanical
      breakdown T85.01
      displacement T85.02
      leakage T85.03
      malposition T85.02
      obstruction T85.09
      perforation T85.09
      protrusion T85.09
      specified NEC T85.09
    pain T85.84
    specified type NEC T85.89
    stenosis T85.85
    thrombosis T85.86
  wire suture, permanent (implanted) —
    see Complications, suture,
    permanent
Compressed air disease T70.3
Compression
  with injury - code by Nature of injury
  artery I77.1
    celiac, syndrome I77.4
  brachial plexus G54.0

Compression (Continued)
  brain (stem) G93.5
    due to
      contusion (diffuse) —see Injury,
        intracranial, diffuse
      focal —see Injury, intracranial,
        focal
      injury NEC —see Injury,
        intracranial, diffuse
      traumatic —see Injury, intracranial,
        diffuse
  bronchus J98.09
  cauda equina G83.4
  celiac (artery) (axis) I77.4
  cerebral —see Compression, brain
  cervical plexus G54.2
  cord
    spinal —see Compression, spinal
    umbilical —see Compression,
      umbilical cord
  cranial nerve G52.9
    eighth —see subcategory H93.3
    eleventh G52.8
    fifth G50.8
    first G52.0
    fourth —see Strabismus, paralytic,
      fourth nerve
    ninth G52.1
    second —see Disorder, nerve, optic
    seventh G52.8
    sixth —see Strabismus, paralytic,
      sixth nerve
    tenth G52.2
    third —see Strabismus, paralytic,
      third nerve
    twelfth G52.3
  diver's squeeze T70.3
  during birth (newborn) P15.9
  esophagus K22.2
  eustachian tube —see Obstruction,
    eustachian tube, cartilaginous
  facies Q67.1
  fracture —see Fracture
  heart —see Disease, heart
  intestine —see Obstruction, intestine
  laryngeal nerve, recurrent G52.2
    with paralysis of vocal cords and
      larynx J38.00
      bilateral J38.02
      unilateral J38.01
  lumbosacral plexus G54.1
  lung J98.4
  lymphatic vessel I89.0
  medulla —see Compression, brain
  nerve (see also Disorder, nerve) G58.9
    arm NEC —see Mononeuropathy,
      upper limb
    axillary G54.0
    cranial —see Compression, cranial
      nerve
    leg NEC —see Mononeuropathy,
      lower limb
    median (in carpal tunnel) —see
      Syndrome, carpal tunnel
    optic —see Disorder, nerve, optic
    plantar —see Lesion, nerve, plantar
    posterior tibial (in tarsal tunnel) —see
      Syndrome, tarsal tunnel
    root or plexus NOS (in) G54.9
      intervertebral disc disorder NEC —
        see Disorder, disc, with,
        radiculopathy
      with myelopathy —see Disorder,
        disc, with, myelopathy

Compression (Continued)
  nerve (Continued)
    root or plexus NOS (Continued)
      neoplastic disease (see also
        Neoplasm) D49.9 [G55]
      spondylosis —see Spondylosis,
        with radiculopathy
      sciatic (acute) —see Lesion, nerve,
        sciatic
      sympathetic G90.8
      traumatic —see Injury, nerve
      ulnar —see Lesion, nerve, ulnar
      upper extremity NEC —see
        Mononeuropathy, upper limb
    spinal (cord) G95.20
      by displacement of intervertebral disc
        NEC —see also Disorder, disc,
        with, myelopathy
      nerve root NOS G54.9
        due to displacement of
          intervertebral disc NEC —
          see Disorder, disc, with,
          radiculopathy
        with myelopathy —see Disorder,
          disc, with, myelopathy
      specified NEC G95.29
      spondylogenic (cervical) (lumbar,
        lumbosacral) (thoracic) —see
        Spondylosis, with myelopathy
        NEC
      anterior —see Syndrome, anterior,
        spinal artery, compression
      traumatic —see Injury, spinal cord, by
        region
    subcostal nerve (syndrome) —see
      Mononeuropathy, upper limb,
      specified NEC
    sympathetic nerve NEC G90.8
    syndrome T79.5
    trachea J39.8
    ulnar nerve (by scar tissue) —see
      Lesion, nerve, ulnar
    umbilical cord
      complicating delivery O69.2
        cord around neck O69.1
        prolapse O69.0
        specified NEC O69.2
    ureter N13.5
    vein I87.1
    vena cava (inferior) (superior) I87.1
Compulsion, compulsive
  gambling F63.0
  neurosis F42
  personality F60.5
  states F42
  swearing F42
    in Gilles de la Tourette's syndrome
      F95.2
  tics and spasms F95.9
Concato's disease (pericardial
  polyserositis) A19.9
  nontubercular I31.1
  pleural —see Pleurisy, with effusion
Concavity chest wall M95.4
Concealed penis Q55.69
Concern (normal) about sick person in
  family Z63.6
Concrescence (teeth) K00.2
Concretio cordis I31.1
  rheumatic I09.2
Concretion —see also Calculus
  appendicular K38.1
  canaliculus —see Dacryolith
  clitoris N90.89

157

Concretion (*Continued*)
  conjunctiva H11.12-
  eyelid —*see* Disorder, eyelid, specified
      type NEC
  lacrimal passages —*see* Dacryolith
  prepuce (male) N47.8
  salivary gland (any) K11.5
  seminal vesicle N50.8
  tonsil J35.8
Concussion (brain) (cerebral) (current)
      S06.0X-
  blast (air) (hydraulic) (immersion)
      (underwater)
    abdomen or thorax —*see* Injury, blast,
        by site
    ear with acoustic nerve injury —*see*
        Injury, nerve, acoustic, specified
        type NEC
  cauda equina S34.3
  conus medullaris S34.139
  ocular S05.8X-
  spinal (cord)
    cervical S14.0
    lumbar S34.01
    sacral S34.02
    thoracic S24.0
  syndrome F07.81
Condition —*see* Disease
Conditions arising in the perinatal
      period —*see* Newborn, affected by
Conduct disorder —*see* Disorder, conduct
Condyloma A63.0
  acuminatum A63.0
  gonorrheal A54.09
  latum A51.31
  syphilitic A51.31
    congenital A50.07
  venereal, syphilitic A51.31
Conflagration —*see also* Burn
  asphyxia (by inhalation of gases, fumes
      or vapors) —*see also* Table of drugs
      and chemicals T59.9-
Conflict (with) —*see also* Discord
  family Z73.9
  marital Z63.0
    involving divorce or estrangement
        Z63.5
  parent-child Z62.820
    parent-adopted child Z62.821
    parent-biological child Z62.820
    parent-foster child Z62.822
  social role NEC Z73.5
Confluent —*see* condition
Confusion, confused R41.0
  epileptic F05
  mental state (psychogenic) F44.89
  psychogenic F44.89
  reactive (from emotional stress,
      psychological trauma) F44.89
Confusional arousals G47.51
Congelation T69.9
Congenital —*see also* condition
  aortic septum Q25.4
  intrinsic factor deficiency D51.0
  malformation —*see* Anomaly
Congestion, congestive
  bladder N32.89
  bowel K63.89
  brain G93.89
  breast N64.59
  bronchial J98.09
  catarrhal J31.0
  chest R09.89
  chill, malarial —*see* Malaria

Congestion, congestive (*Continued*)
  circulatory NEC I99.8
  duodenum K31.89
  eye —*see* Hyperemia, conjunctiva
  facial, due to birth injury P15.4
  general R68.89
  glottis J37.0
  heart —*see* Failure, heart, congestive
  hepatic K76.1
  hypostatic (lung) —*see* Edema, lung
  intestine K63.89
  kidney N28.89
  labyrinth —*see* subcategory H83.8
  larynx J37.0
  liver K76.1
  lung R09.89
    active or acute —*see* Pneumonia
  malaria, malarial —*see* Malaria
  nasal R09.81
  nose R09.81
  orbit, orbital —*see also* Exophthalmos
    inflammatory (chronic) —*see*
        Inflammation, orbit
  ovary N83.8
  pancreas K86.8
  pelvic, female N94.89
  pleural J94.8
  prostate (active) N42.1
  pulmonary —*see* Congestion, lung
  renal N28.89
  retina H35.81
  seminal vesicle N50.1
  spinal cord G95.19
  spleen (chronic) D73.2
  stomach K31.89
  trachea —*see* Tracheitis
  urethra N36.8
  uterus N85.8
    with subinvolution N85.3
  venous (passive) I87.8
  viscera R68.89
Congestive —*see* Congestion
Conical
  cervix (hypertrophic elongation) N88.4
  cornea —*see* Keratoconus
  teeth K00.2
Conjoined twins Q89.4
Conjugal maladjustment Z63.0
  involving divorce or estrangement Z63.5
Conjunctiva —*see* condition
Conjunctivitis (staphylococcal)
      (streptococcal) NOS H10.9
  Acanthamoeba B60.12
  acute H10.3-
    atopic H10.1-
    chemical (*see also* Corrosion, cornea)
        H10.21-
    mucopurulent H10.02-
      follicular H10.01-
    pseudomembranous H10.22-
    serous except viral H10.23-
      viral —*see* Conjunctivitis, viral
    toxic H10.21-
  adenoviral (acute) (follicular) B30.1
  allergic (acute) —*see* Conjunctivitis,
      acute, atopic
    chronic H10.45
      vernal H10.44
  anaphylactic —*see* Conjunctivitis, acute,
      atopic
  Apollo B30.3
  atopic (acute) —*see* Conjunctivitis,
      acute, atopic
  Béal's B30.2

Conjunctivitis (*Continued*)
  blennorrhagic (gonococcal)
      (neonatorum) A54.31
  chemical (acute) (*see also* Corrosion,
      cornea) H10.21-
  chlamydial A74.0
    due to trachoma A71.1
    neonatal P39.1
  chronic (nodosa) (petrificans)
      (phlyctenular) H10.40-
    allergic H10.45
      vernal H10.44
    follicular H10.43-
    giant papillary H10.41-
    simple H10.42-
    vernal H10.44
  coxsackievirus 24 B30.3
  diphtheritic A36.86
  due to
    dust —*see* Conjunctivitis, acute,
        atopic
    filariasis B74.9
    mucocutaneous leishmaniasis B55.2
  enterovirus type 70 (hemorrhagic) B30.3
  epidemic (viral) B30.9
    hemorrhagic B30.3
  gonococcal (neonatorum) A54.31
  granular (trachomatous) A71.1
    sequelae (late effect) B94.0
  hemorrhagic (acute) (epidemic) B30.3
  herpes zoster B02.31
  in (due to)
    Acanthamoeba B60.12
    adenovirus (acute) (follicular) B30.1
    Chlamydia A74.0
    coxsackievirus 24 B30.3
    diphtheria A36.86
    enterovirus type 70 (hemorrhagic) B30.3
    filariasis B74.9
    gonococci A54.31
    herpes (simplex) virus B00.53
      zoster B02.31
    infectious disease NEC B99
    meningococci A39.89
    mucocutaneous leishmaniasis B55.2
    rosacea L71.9
    syphilis (late) A52.71
    zoster B02.31
  inclusion A74.0
  infantile P39.1
    gonococcal A54.31
  Koch-Weeks' —*see* Conjunctivitis, acute,
      mucopurulent
  light —*see* Conjunctivitis, acute, atopic
  ligneous —*see* Blepharoconjunctivitis,
      ligneous
  meningococcal A39.89
  mucopurulent —*see* Conjunctivitis,
      acute, mucopurulent
  neonatal P39.1
    gonococcal A54.31
  Newcastle B30.8
  of Béal B30.2
  parasitic
    filariasis B74.9
    mucocutaneous leishmaniasis B55.2
  Parinaud's H10.89
  petrificans H10.89
  rosacea L71.9
  specified NEC H10.89
  swimming-pool B30.1
  trachomatous A71.1
    acute A71.0
    sequelae (late effect) B94.0

Conjunctivitis *(Continued)*
   traumatic NEC H10.89
   tuberculous A18.59
   tularemic A21.1
   tularensis A21.1
   viral B30.9
     due to
       adenovirus B30.1
       enterovirus B30.3
       specified NEC B30.8
Conjunctivochalasis H11.82-
Connective tissue —*see* condition
Conn's syndrome E26.01
Conradi (-Hunermann) disease Q77.3
Consanguinity Z84.3
   counseling Z71.89
Conscious simulation (of illness) Z76.5
Consecutive —*see* condition
Consolidation lung (base) —*see*
   Pneumonia, lobar
Constipation (atonic) (neurogenic)
   (simple) (spastic) K59.00
   drug-induced —*see* Table of drugs and
     chemicals
   outlet dysfunction K59.02
   psychogenic F45.8
   slow transit K59.01
   specified NEC K59.09
Constitutional —*see also* condition
   substandard F60.7
Constitutionally substandard F60.7
Constriction —*see also* Stricture
   auditory canal —*see* Stenosis, external
     ear canal
   bronchial J98.09
   duodenum K31.5
   esophagus K22.2
   external
     abdomen, abdominal (wall) S30.841
     alveolar process S00.542
     ankle S90.54-
     antecubital space —*see* Constriction,
       external, forearm
     arm (upper) S40.84-
     auricle —*see* Constriction, external,
       ear
     axilla —*see* Constriction, external, arm
     back, lower S30.840
     breast S20.14-
     brow S00.84
     buttock S30.840
     calf —*see* Constriction, external, leg
     canthus —*see* Constriction, external,
       eyelid
     cheek S00.84
       internal S00.542
     chest wall —*see* Constriction,
       external, thorax
     chin S00.84
     clitoris S30.844
     costal region —*see* Constriction,
       external, thorax
     digit (s)
       foot —*see* Constriction, external,
         toe
       hand —*see* Constriction, external,
         finger
     ear S00.44-
     elbow S50.34-
     epididymis S30.843
     epigastric region S30.841
     esophagus, cervical S10.14
     eyebrow —*see* Constriction, external,
       eyelid

Constriction *(Continued)*
   external *(Continued)*
     eyelid S00.24-
     face S00.84
     finger (s) S60.44-
       index S60.44-
       little S60.44-
       middle S60.44-
       ring S60.44-
     flank S30.841
     foot (except toe (s) alone) S90.84-
       toe —*see* Constriction, external, toe
     forearm S50.84-
       elbow only —*see* Constriction,
         external, elbow
     forehead S00.84
     genital organs, external
       female S30.846
       male S30.845
     groin S30.841
     gum S00.542
     hand S60.54-
     head S00.94
       ear —*see* Constriction, external, ear
       eyelid —*see* Constriction, external,
         eyelid
       lip S00.541
       nose S00.34
       oral cavity S00.542
       scalp S00.04
       specified site NEC S00.84
     heel —*see* Constriction, external, foot
     hip S70.24-
     inguinal region S30.841
     interscapular region S20.449
     jaw S00.84
     knee S80.24-
     labium (majus) (minus) S30.844
     larynx S10.14
     leg (lower) S80.84-
       knee —*see* Constriction, external,
         knee
       upper —*see* Constriction, external,
         thigh
     lip S00.541
     lower back S30.840
     lumbar region S30.840
     malar region S00.84
     mammary —*see* Constriction,
       external, breast
     mastoid region S00.84
     mouth S00.542
     nail
       finger —*see* Constriction, external,
         finger
       toe —*see* Constriction, external, toe
     nasal S00.34
     neck S10.94
       specified site NEC S10.84
       throat S10.14
     nose S00.34
     occipital region S00.04
     oral cavity S00.542
     orbital region —*see* Constriction,
       external, eyelid
     palate S00.542
     palm —*see* Constriction, external,
       hand
     parietal region S00.04
     pelvis S30.840
     penis S30.842
     perineum
       female S30.844
       male S30.840

Constriction *(Continued)*
   external *(Continued)*
     periocular area —*see* Constriction,
       external, eyelid
     phalanges
       finger —*see* Constriction, external,
         finger
       toe —*see* Constriction, external, toe
     pharynx S10.14
     pinna —*see* Constriction, external, ear
     popliteal space —*see* Constriction,
       external, knee
     prepuce S30.842
     pubic region S30.840
     pudendum
       female S30.846
       male S30.845
     sacral region S30.840
     scalp S00.04
     scapular region —*see* Constriction,
       external, shoulder
     scrotum S30.843
     shin —*see* Constriction, external, leg
     shoulder S40.24-
     sternal region S20.349
     submaxillary region S00.84
     submental region S00.84
     subungual
       finger (s) —*see* Constriction,
         external, finger
       toe (s) —*see* Constriction, external,
         toe
     supraclavicular fossa S10.84
     supraorbital S00.84
     temple S00.84
     temporal region S00.84
     testis S30.843
     thigh S70.34-
     thorax, thoracic (wall) S20.94
       back S20.44-
       front S20.34-
     throat S10.14
     thumb S60.34-
     toe (s) (lesser) S90.44-
       great S90.44-
     tongue S00.542
     trachea S10.14
     tunica vaginalis S30.843
     uvula S00.542
     vagina S30.844
     vulva S30.844
     wrist S60.84-
   gallbladder —*see* Obstruction,
     gallbladder
   intestine —*see* Obstruction, intestine
   larynx J38.6
     congenital Q31.8
       specified NEC Q31.8
       subglottic Q31.1
   organ or site, congenital NEC —*see*
     Atresia, by site
   prepuce (acquired) (congenital) N47.1
   pylorus (adult hypertrophic) K31.1
     congenital or infantile Q40.0
     newborn Q40.0
   ring dystocia (uterus) O62.4
   spastic —*see also* Spasm
     ureter N13.5
   ureter N13.5
     with infection N13.6
   urethra —*see* Stricture, urethra
   visual field (peripheral) (functional) —
     see Defect, visual field
Constrictive —*see* condition

Consultation
  without complaint or sickness Z71.9
    feared complaint unfounded Z71.1
    specified reason NEC Z71.89
  medical —see Counseling, medical
  religious Z71.81
  specified reason NEC Z71.89
  spiritual Z71.81
Consumption —see Tuberculosis
Contact (with)) —see also Exposure (to
  acariasis Z20.7
  AIDS virus Z20.6
  air pollution Z77.110
  algae and algae toxins Z77.121
  algae bloom Z77.121
  anthrax Z20.810
  aromatic (hazardous) compounds NEC
    Z77.028
  aromatic amines Z77.020
  aromatic dyes NOS Z77.028
  arsenic Z77.010
  asbestos Z77.090
  bacterial disease NEC Z20.818
  benzene Z77.021
  blue-green algae bloom Z77.121
  body fluids (potentially hazardous)
    Z77.21
  brown tide Z77.121
  chemicals (chiefly nonmedicinal)
    (hazardous) NEC Z77.098
  cholera Z20.09
  chromium compounds Z77.018
  communicable disease Z20.9
    bacterial NEC Z20.818
    specified NEC Z20.89
    viral NEC Z20.828
  cyanobacteria bloom Z77.121
  dyes Z77.098
  Escherichia coli (E. coli) Z20.01
  fiberglass —see Table of drugs and
    chemicals, fiberglass
  German measles Z20.4
  gonorrhea Z20.2
  hazardous metals NEC Z77.018
  hazardous substances NEC Z77.29
  hazards in the physical environment
    NEC Z77.128
  hazards to health NEC Z77.9
  HIV Z20.6
  HTLV-III/LAV Z20.6
  human immunodeficiency virus (HIV)
    Z20.6
  infection Z20.9
    specified NEC Z20.89
  infestation (parasitic) NEC Z20.7
  intestinal infectious disease NEC
    Z20.09
    Escherichia coli (E. coli) Z20.01
  lead Z77.011
  meningococcus Z20.811
  mold (toxic) Z77.120
  nickel dust Z77.018
  noise Z77.122
  parasitic disease Z20.7
  pediculosis Z20.7
  pfiesteria piscicida Z77.121
  poliomyelitis Z20.89
  pollution
    air Z77.110
    environmental NEC Z77.118
    soil Z77.112
    water Z77.111
  polycyclic aromatic hydrocarbons
    Z77.028

Contact (Continued)
  rabies Z20.3
  radiation, naturally occurring NEC
    Z77.123
  radon Z77.123
  red tide (Florida) Z77.121
  rubella Z20.4
  sexually-transmitted disease Z20.2
  smallpox (laboratory) Z20.89
  syphilis Z20.2
  tuberculosis Z20.1
  uranium Z77.012
  varicella Z20.820
  venereal disease Z20.2
  viral disease NEC Z20.828
  viral hepatitis Z20.5
  water pollution Z77.111
Contamination, food —see Intoxication,
    foodborne
Contraception, contraceptive
  advice Z30.09
  counseling Z30.09
  device (intrauterine) (in situ) Z97.5
    causing menorrhagia T83.83
    checking Z30.431
    complications —see Complications,
      intrauterine, contraceptive
      device
    in place Z97.5
    initial prescription Z30.014
    reinsertion Z30.433
    removal Z30.432
    replacement Z30.433
  emergency (postcoital) Z30.012
  initial prescription Z30.019
    injectable Z30.013
    intrauterine device Z30.014
    pills Z30.011
    postcoital (emergency) Z30.012
    specified type NEC Z30.018
    subdermal implantable Z30.019
  maintenance Z30.40
    examination Z30.8
    injectable Z30.42
    intrauterine device Z30.431
    pills Z30.41
    specified type NEC Z30.49
    subdermal implantable Z30.49
  management Z30.9
    specified NEC Z30.8
  postcoital (emergency) Z30.012
  prescription Z30.019
    repeat Z30.40
  sterilization Z30.2
  surveillance (drug) —see Contraception,
    maintenance
Contraction (s), contracture, contracted
  Achilles tendon —see also Short, tendon,
    Achilles
    congenital Q66.89
  amputation stump (surgical) (flexion)
    (late) next proximal joint T87.89
  anus K59.8
  bile duct (common) (hepatic) K83.8
  bladder N32.89
    neck or sphincter N32.0
  bowel, cecum, colon or intestine, any
    part —see Obstruction, intestine
  Braxton Hicks —see False, labor
  breast implant, capsular T85.44
  bronchial J98.09
  burn (old) —see Cicatrix
  cervix —see Stricture, cervix
  cicatricial —see Cicatrix

Contraction (s), contracture, contracted
    (Continued)
  conjunctiva, trachomatous, active A71.1
    sequelae (late effect) B94.0
  Dupuytren's M72.0
  eyelid —see Disorder, eyelid function
  fascia (lata) (postural) M72.8
    Dupuytren's M72.0
    palmar M72.0
    plantar M72.2
  finger NEC —see also Deformity, finger
    congenital Q68.1
    joint —see Contraction, joint, hand
  flaccid —see Contraction, paralytic
  gallbladder K82.0
  heart valve —see Endocarditis
  hip —see Contraction, joint, hip
  hourglass
    bladder N32.89
      congenital Q64.79
    gallbladder K82.0
      congenital Q44.1
    stomach K31.89
      congenital Q40.2
      psychogenic F45.8
    uterus (complicating delivery) O62.4
  hysterical F44.4
  internal os —see Stricture, cervix
  joint (abduction) (acquired) (adduction)
      (flexion) (rotation) M24.50
    ankle M24.57-
    congenital NEC Q68.8
      hip Q65.89
    elbow M24.52-
    foot joint M24.57-
    hand joint M24.54-
    hip M24.55-
      congenital Q65.89
    hysterical F44.4
    knee M24.56-
    shoulder M24.51-
    wrist M24.53-
  kidney (granular) (secondary) N26.9
    congenital Q63.8
    hydronephritic —see Hydronephrosis
      Page N26.2
    pyelonephritic —see Pyelitis, chronic
      tuberculous A18.11
  ligament —see also Disorder, ligament
    congenital Q79.8
  muscle (postinfective) (postural) NEC
      M62.40
    with contracture of joint —see
      Contraction, joint
    ankle M62.47-
    congenital Q79.8
      sternocleidomastoid Q68.0
    extraocular —see Strabismus
    eye (extrinsic) —see Strabismus
    foot M62.47-
    forearm M62.43-
    hand M62.44-
    hysterical F44.4
    ischemic (Volkmann's) T79.6
    lower leg M62.46-
    multiple sites M62.49
    pelvic region M62.45-
    posttraumatic —see Strabismus,
      paralytic
    psychogenic F45.8
      conversion reaction F44.4
    shoulder region M62.41-
    specified site NEC M62.48
    thigh M62.45-
    upper arm M62.42-

Contraction (s), contracture, contracted
(Continued)
neck —see Torticollis
ocular muscle —see Strabismus
organ or site, congenital NEC —see
Atresia, by site
outlet (pelvis) —see Contraction,
pelvis
palmar fascia M72.0
paralytic
joint —see Contraction, joint
muscle —see also Contraction, muscle
NEC
ocular —see Strabismus, paralytic
pelvis (acquired) (general) M95.5
with disproportion (fetopelvic) O33.1
causing obstructed labor O65.1
inlet O33.2
mid-cavity O33.3
outlet O33.3
plantar fascia M72.2
premature
atrium I49.1
auriculoventricular I49.49
heart I49.49
junctional I49.2
supraventricular I49.1
ventricular I49.3
prostate N42.89
pylorus NEC —see also Pylorospasm
psychogenic F45.8
rectum, rectal (sphincter) K59.8
ring (Bandl's) (complicating delivery)
O62.4
scar —see Cicatrix
spine —see Dorsopathy, deforming
sternocleidomastoid (muscle),
congenital Q68.0
stomach K31.89
hourglass K31.89
congenital Q40.2
psychogenic F45.8
psychogenic F45.8
tendon (sheath) M62.40
with contracture of joint —see
Contraction, joint
Achilles —see Short, tendon, Achilles
ankle M62.47-
Achilles —see Short, tendon,
Achilles
foot M62.47-
forearm M62.43-
hand M62.44-
lower leg M62.46-
multiple sites M62.49
neck M62.48
pelvic region M62.45-
shoulder region M62.41-
specified site NEC M62.48
thigh M62.45-
thorax M62.48
trunk M62.48
upper arm M62.42-
toe —see Deformity, toe, specified NEC
ureterovesical orifice (postinfectional)
N13.5
with infection N13.6
urethra —see also Stricture, urethra
orifice N32.0
uterus N85.8
abnormal NEC O62.9
clonic (complicating delivery) O62.4
dyscoordinate (complicating
delivery) O62.4

Contraction (s), contracture, contracted
(Continued)
uterus (Continued)
hourglass (complicating delivery)
O62.4
hypertonic O62.4
hypotonic NEC O62.2
inadequate
primary O62.0
secondary O62.1
incoordinate (complicating delivery)
O62.4
poor O62.2
tetanic (complicating delivery) O62.4
vagina (outlet) N89.5
vesical N32.89
neck or urethral orifice N32.0
visual field —see Defect, visual field,
generalized
Volkmann's (ischemic) T79.6
Contusion (skin surface intact) T14.8
abdomen, abdominal (muscle) (wall)
S30.1
adnexa, eye NEC S05.8X-
adrenal gland S37.812
alveolar process S00.532
ankle S90.0-
antecubital space —see Contusion,
forearm
anus S30.3
arm (upper) S40.02-
lower (with elbow) —see Contusion,
forearm
auditory canal —see Contusion, ear
auricle —see Contusion, ear
axilla —see Contusion, arm, upper
back —see also Contusion, thorax, back
lower S30.0
bile duct S36.13
bladder S37.22
bone NEC T14.8
brain (diffuse) —see Injury, intracranial,
diffuse
focal —see Injury, intracranial, focal
brainstem S06.38-
breast S20.0-
broad ligament S37.892
brow S00.83
buttock S30.0
canthus, eye S00.1-
cauda equina S34.3
cerebellar, traumatic S06.37-
cerebral S06.33-
left side S06.32-
right side S06.31-
cheek S00.83
internal S00.532
chest (wall) —see Contusion, thorax
chin S00.83
clitoris S30.23
colon —see Injury, intestine, large,
contusion
common bile duct S36.13
conjunctiva S05.1-
with foreign body (in conjunctival
sac) —see Foreign body,
conjunctival sac
conus medullaris (spine) S34.139
cornea —see Contusion, eyeball
with foreign body —see Foreign body,
cornea
corpus cavernosum S30.21
cortex (brain) (cerebral) —see Injury,
intracranial, diffuse
focal —see Injury, intracranial, focal

Contusion (Continued)
costal region —see Contusion, thorax
cystic duct S36.13
diaphragm S27.802
duodenum S36.420
ear S00.43-
elbow S50.0-
with forearm —see Contusion, forearm
epididymis S30.22
epigastric region S30.1
epiglottis S10.0
esophagus (thoracic) S27.812
cervical S10.0
eyeball S05.1-
eyebrow S00.1-
eyelid (and periocular area) S00.1-
face NEC S00.83
fallopian tube S37.529
bilateral S37.522
unilateral S37.521
femoral triangle S30.1
finger (s) S60.00
with damage to nail (matrix) S60.10
index S60.02-
with damage to nail S60.12-
little S60.05-
with damage to nail S60.15-
middle S60.03-
with damage to nail S60.13-
ring S60.04-
with damage to nail S60.14-
thumb —see Contusion, thumb
flank S30.1
foot (except toe (s) alone) S90.3-
toe —see Contusion, toe
forearm S50.1-
elbow only —see Contusion, elbow
forehead S00.83
gallbladder S36.122
genital organs, external
female S30.202
male S30.201
globe (eye) —see Contusion, eyeball
groin S30.1
gum S00.532
hand S60.22-
finger (s) —see Contusion, finger
wrist —see Contusion, wrist
head S00.93
ear —see Contusion, ear
eyelid —see Contusion, eyelid
lip S00.531
nose S00.33
oral cavity S00.532
scalp S00.03
specified part NEC S00.83
heel —see Contusion, foot
hepatic duct S36.13
hip S70.0-
ileum S36.428
iliac region S30.1
inguinal region S30.1
interscapular region S20.229
intra-abdominal organ S36.92
colon —see Injury, intestine, large,
contusion
liver S36.112
pancreas —see Contusion, pancreas
rectum S36.62
small intestine —see Injury, intestine,
small, contusion
specified organ NEC S36.892
spleen —see Contusion, spleen
stomach S36.32

Contusion (Continued)
iris (eye) —see Contusion, eyeball
jaw S00.83
jejunum S36.428
kidney S37.01-
  major (greater than 2 cm) S37.02-
  minor (less than 2 cm) S37.01-
knee S80.0-
labium (majus) (minus) S30.23
lacrimal apparatus, gland or sac S05.8X-
larynx S10.0
leg (lower) S80.1-
  knee —see Contusion, knee
lens —see Contusion, eyeball
lip S00.531
liver S36.112
lower back S30.0
lumbar region S30.0
lung S27.329
  bilateral S27.322
  unilateral S27.321
malar region S00.83
mastoid region S00.83
membrane, brain —see Injury,
    intracranial, diffuse
  focal —see Injury, intracranial, focal
mesentery S36.892
mesosalpinx S37.529
  bilateral S37.522
  unilateral S37.521
mouth S00.532
muscle —see Contusion, by site
nail
  finger —see Contusion, finger, with
      damage to nail
  toe —see Contusion, toe, with
      damage to nail
nasal S00.33
neck S10.93
  specified site NEC S10.83
  throat S10.0
nerve —see Injury, nerve
newborn P54.5
nose S00.33
occipital
  lobe (brain) —see Injury, intracranial,
      diffuse
    focal —see Injury, intracranial, focal
  region (scalp) S00.03
orbit (region) (tissues) S05.1-
ovary S37.429
  bilateral S37.422
  unilateral S37.421
palate S00.532
pancreas S36.229
  body S36.221
  head S36.220
  tail S36.222
parietal
  lobe (brain) —see Injury, intracranial,
      diffuse
    focal —see Injury, intracranial, focal
  region (scalp) S00.03
pelvic organ S37.92
  adrenal gland S37.812
  bladder S37.22
  fallopian tube —see Contusion,
      fallopian tube
  kidney —see Contusion, kidney
  ovary —see Contusion, ovary
  prostate S37.823
  specified organ NEC S37.892
  ureter S37.12
  urethra S37.32
  uterus S37.62

Contusion (Continued)
pelvis S30.0
penis S30.21
perineum
  female S30.23
  male S30.0
periocular area S00.1-
peritoneum S36.81
periurethral tissue —see Contusion,
    urethra
pharynx S10.0
pinna —see Contusion, ear
popliteal space —see Contusion, knee
prepuce S30.21
prostate S37.822
pubic region S30.1
pudendum
  female S30.202
  male S30.201
quadriceps femoris —see Contusion,
    thigh
rectum S36.62
retroperitoneum S36.892
round ligament S37.892
sacral region S30.0
scalp S00.03
  due to birth injury P12.3
scapular region —see Contusion,
    shoulder
sclera —see Contusion, eyeball
scrotum S30.22
seminal vesicle S37.892
shoulder S40.01-
skin NEC T14.8
small intestine —see Injury, intestine,
    small, contusion
spermatic cord S30.22
spinal cord —see Injury, spinal cord, by
    region
  cauda equina S34.3
  conus medullaris S34.139
spleen S36.029
  major S36.021
  minor S36.020
sternal region S20.219
stomach S36.32
subconjunctival S05.1-
subcutaneous NEC T14.8
submaxillary region S00.83
submental region S00.83
subperiosteal NEC T14.8
subungual
  finger —see Contusion, finger, with
      damage to nail
  toe —see Contusion, toe, with
      damage to nail
supraclavicular fossa S10.83
supraorbital S00.83
suprarenal gland S37.812
temple (region) S00.83
temporal
  lobe (brain) —see Injury, intracranial,
      diffuse
    focal —see Injury, intracranial,
        focal
  region S00.83
testis S30.22
thigh S70.1-
thorax (wall) S20.20
  back S20.22-
  front S20.21-
throat S10.0
thumb S60.01-
  with damage to nail S60.11-

Contusion (Continued)
toe (s) (lesser) S90.12-
  with damage to nail S90.22-
  great S90.11-
    with damage to nail S90.21-
    specified type NEC S90.221
tongue S00.532
trachea (cervical) S10.0
  thoracic S27.52
tunica vaginalis S30.22
tympanum, tympanic membrane —see
    Contusion, ear
ureter S37.12
urethra S37.32
urinary organ NEC S37.892
uterus S37.62
uvula S00.532
vagina S30.23
vas deferens S37.892
vesical S37.22
vocal cord (s) S10.0
vulva S30.23
wrist S60.21-
Conus (congenital) (any type) Q14.8
  cornea —see Keratoconus
  medullaris syndrome G95.81
Conversion hysteria, neurosis or reaction
    F44.9
Converter, tuberculosis (test reaction)
    R76.11
Conviction (legal), anxiety concerning
    Z65.0
  with imprisonment Z65.1
Convulsions (idiopathic) (see also
    Seizure (s)) R56.9
  apoplectiform (cerebral ischemia) I67.82
  benign neonatal (familial) —see
      Epilepsy, generalized, idiopathic
  dissociative F44.5
  epileptic —see Epilepsy
  epileptiform, epileptoid —see Seizure,
      epileptiform
  ether (anesthetic) —see Table of drugs
      and chemicals, by drug
  febrile R56.00
    with status epilepticus G40.901
    complex R56.01
      with status epilepticus G40.901
    simple R56.00
  hysterical F44.5
  infantile P90
    epilepsy —see Epilepsy
  jacksonian —see Epilepsy, localization-
      related, symptomatic, with simple
      partial seizures
  myoclonic G25.3
  neonatal, benign (familial) —see
      Epilepsy, generalized, idiopathic
  newborn P90
  obstetrical (nephritic) (uremic) —see
      Eclampsia
  paretic A52.17
  post traumatic R56.1
  psychomotor —see Epilepsy,
      localization-related, symptomatic,
      with complex partial seizures
  recurrent R56.9
  reflex R25.8
  scarlatinal A38.8
  tetanus, tetanic —see Tetanus
  thymic E32.8
Convulsive —see also Convulsions
Cooley's anemia D56.1
Coolie itch B76.9

Cooper's
  disease —*see* Mastopathy, cystic
  hernia —*see* Hernia, abdomen, specified
    site NEC
Copra itch B88.0
Coprophagy F50.8
Coprophobia F40.298
Coproporphyria, hereditary E80.29
Cor
  biloculare Q20.8
  bovis, bovinum —*see* Hypertrophy,
    cardiac
  pulmonale (chronic) I27.81
    acute I26.09
  triatriatum, triatrium Q24.2
  triloculare Q20.8
    biatrium Q20.4
    biventriculare Q21.1
Corbus' disease (gangrenous balanitis)
    N48.1
Cord —*see also* condition
  around neck (tightly) (with
    compression)
    complicating delivery O69.1
  bladder G95.89
    tabetic A52.19
Cordis ectopia Q24.8
Corditis (spermatic) N49.1
Corectopia Q13.2
Cori's disease (glycogen storage)
    E74.03
Corkhandler's disease or lung J67.3
Corkscrew esophagus K22.4
Corkworker's disease or lung J67.3
Corn (infected) L84
Cornea —*see also* condition
  donor Z52.5
  plana Q13.4
Cornelia de Lange syndrome
    Q87.1
Cornu cutaneum L85.8
Cornual gestation or pregnancy
    O00.8
Coronary (artery) —*see* condition
Coronavirus, as cause of disease
    classified elsewhere B97.29
    SARS-associated B97.21
Corpora —*see also* condition
  amylacea, prostate N42.89
  cavernosa —*see* condition
Corpulence —*see* Obesity
Corpus —*see* condition
Corrected transposition Q20.5
Corrosion (injury) (acid) (caustic)
    (chemical) (lime) (external) (internal)
    T30.4
  abdomen, abdominal (muscle) (wall)
    T21.42
    first degree T21.52
    second degree T21.62
    third degree T21.72
  above elbow T22.439
    first degree T22.539
    left T22.432
      first degree T22.532
      second degree T22.632
      third degree T22.732
    right T22.431
      first degree T22.531
      second degree T22.631
      third degree T22.731
    second degree T22.639
    third degree T22.739
  alimentary tract NEC T28.7

Corrosion (Continued)
  ankle T25.419
    first degree T25.519
    left T25.412
      first degree T25.512
      second degree T25.612
      third degree T25.712
    multiple with foot —*see* Corrosion,
      lower, limb, multiple, ankle and
      foot
    right T25.411
      first degree T25.511
      second degree T25.611
      third degree T25.711
    second degree T25.619
    third degree T25.719
  anus —*see* Corrosion, buttock
  arm (s) (meaning upper limb (s)) —*see*
    Corrosion, upper limb
  axilla T22.449
    first degree T22.549
    left T22.442
      first degree T22.542
      second degree T22.642
      third degree T22.742
    right T22.441
      first degree T22.541
      second degree T22.641
      third degree T22.741
    second degree T22.649
    third degree T22.749
  back (lower) T21.44
    first degree T21.54
    second degree T21.64
    third degree T21.74
    upper T21.43
      first degree T21.53
      second degree T21.63
      third degree T21.73
  blisters - code as Corrosion, second
    degree, by site
  breast (s) —*see* Corrosion, chest wall
  buttock (s) T21.45
    first degree T21.55
    second degree T21.65
    third degree T21.75
  calf T24.439
    first degree T24.539
    left T24.432
      first degree T24.532
      second degree T24.632
      third degree T24.732
    right T24.431
      first degree T24.531
      second degree T24.631
      third degree T24.731
    second degree T24.639
    third degree T24.739
  canthus (eye) —*see* Corrosion,
    eyelid
  cervix T28.8
  cheek T20.46
    first degree T20.56
    second degree T20.66
    third degree T20.76
  chest wall T21.41
    first degree T21.51
    second degree T21.61
    third degree T21.71
  chin T20.43
    first degree T20.53
    second degree T20.63
    third degree T20.73
  colon T28.7

Corrosion (Continued)
  conjunctiva (and cornea) —*see*
    Corrosion, cornea
  cornea (and conjunctiva) T26.6-
  deep necrosis of underlying tissue - code
    as Corrosion, third degree, by site
  dorsum of hand T23.469
    first degree T23.569
    left T23.462
      first degree T23.562
      second degree T23.662
      third degree T23.762
    right T23.461
      first degree T23.561
      second degree T23.661
      third degree T23.761
    second degree T23.669
    third degree T23.769
  ear (auricle) (external) (canal) T20.41
    drum T28.91
    first degree T20.51
    second degree T20.61
    third degree T20.71
  elbow T22.429
    first degree T22.529
    left T22.422
      first degree T22.522
      second degree T22.622
      third degree T22.722
    right T22.421
      first degree T22.521
      second degree T22.621
      third degree T22.721
    second degree T22.629
    third degree T22.729
  entire body —*see* Corrosion, multiple
    body regions
  epidermal loss - code as Corrosion,
    second degree, by site
  epiglottis T27.4
  erythema, erythematous - code as
    Corrosion, first degree, by site
  esophagus T28.6
  extent (percentage of body surface)
    less than 10 percent T32.0
    10-19 percent (0-9 percent third
      degree) T32.10
      with 10-19 percent third degree
        T32.11
    20-29 percent (0-9 percent third
      degree) T32.20
      with
        10-19 percent third degree T32.21
        20-29 percent third degree T32.22
    30-39 percent (0-9 percent third
      degree) T32.30
      with
        10-19 percent third degree T32.31
        20-29 percent third degree T32.32
        30-39 percent third degree T32.33
    40-49 percent (0-9 percent third
      degree) T32.40
      with
        10-19 percent third degree T32.41
        20-29 percent third degree T32.42
        30-39 percent third degree T32.43
        40-49 percent third degree T32.44
    50-59 percent (0-9 percent third
      degree) T32.50
      with
        10-19 percent third degree T32.51
        20-29 percent third degree T32.52
        30-39 percent third degree T32.53
        40-49 percent third degree T32.54
        50-59 percent third degree T32.55

Corrosion *(Continued)*
lacrimal apparatus, duct, gland or
    sac —*see* Corrosion, eye, specified
    site NEC
larynx T27.4
    with lung T27.5
leg (s) (meaning lower limb (s)) —*see*
    Corrosion, lower limb
limb (s)
    lower —*see* Corrosion, lower, limb
    upper —*see* Corrosion, upper
    limb
lip (s) T20.42
    first degree T20.52
    second degree T20.62
    third degree T20.72
lower
    back —*see* Corrosion, back
    limb T24.409
      ankle —*see* Corrosion, ankle
      calf —*see* Corrosion, calf
      first degree T24.509
      foot —*see* Corrosion, foot
      hip —*see* Corrosion, thigh
      knee —*see* Corrosion, knee
      left T24.402
        first degree T24.502
        second degree T24.602
        third degree T24.702
      multiple sites, except ankle and
        foot T24.499
        ankle and foot T25.499
          first degree T25.599
          left T25.492
            first degree T25.592
            second degree T25.692
            third degree T25.792
          right T25.491
            first degree T25.591
            second degree T25.691
            third degree T25.791
          second degree T25.699
          third degree T25.799
      first degree T24.599
      left T24.492
        first degree T24.592
        second degree T24.692
        third degree T24.792
      right T24.491
        first degree T24.591
        second degree T24.691
        third degree T24.791
      second degree T24.699
      third degree T24.799
      right T24.401
        first degree T24.501
        second degree T24.601
        third degree T24.701
      second degree T24.609
      thigh —*see* Corrosion, thigh
      third degree T24.709
lung (with larynx and trachea)
    T27.5
mouth T28.5
neck T20.47
    first degree T20.57
    second degree T20.67
    third degree T20.77
nose (septum) T20.44
    first degree T20.54
    second degree T20.64
    third degree T20.74
ocular adnexa —*see* Corrosion, eye
orbit region —*see* Corrosion, eyelid

Corrosion *(Continued)*
palm T23.459
    first degree T23.559
    left T23.452
      first degree T23.552
      second degree T23.652
      third degree T23.752
    right T23.451
      first degree T23.551
      second degree T23.651
      third degree T23.751
    second degree T23.659
    third degree T23.759
partial thickness - code as Corrosion,
    unspecified degree, by site
pelvis —*see* Corrosion, trunk
penis —*see* Corrosion, genital organs,
    external, male
perineum
    female —*see* Corrosion, genital
      organs, external, female
    male —*see* Corrosion, genital organs,
      external, male
periocular area —*see* Corrosion, eyelid
pharynx T28.5
rectum T28.7
respiratory tract T27.7
    larynx —*see* Corrosion, larynx
    specified part NEC T27.6
    trachea —*see* Corrosion, larynx
sac, lacrimal —*see* Corrosion, eye,
    specified site NEC
scalp T20.45
    first degree T20.55
    second degree T20.65
    third degree T20.75
scapular region T22.469
    first degree T22.569
    left T22.462
      first degree T22.562
      second degree T22.662
      third degree T22.762
    right T22.461
      first degree T22.561
      second degree T22.661
      third degree T22.761
    second degree T22.669
    third degree T22.769
sclera —*see* Corrosion, eye, specified
    site NEC
scrotum —*see* Corrosion, genital organs,
    external, male
shoulder T22.459
    first degree T22.559
    left T22.452
      first degree T22.552
      second degree T22.652
      third degree T22.752
    right T22.451
      first degree T22.551
      second degree T22.651
      third degree T22.751
    second degree T22.659
    third degree T22.759
stomach T28.7
temple —*see* Corrosion, head
testis —*see* Corrosion, genital organs,
    external, male
thigh T24.419
    first degree T24.519
    left T24.412
      first degree T24.512
      second degree T24.612
      third degree T24.712

Corrosion *(Continued)*
thigh *(Continued)*
    right T24.411
      first degree T24.511
      second degree T24.611
      third degree T24.711
    second degree T24.619
    third degree T24.719
thorax (external) —*see* Corrosion,
    trunk
throat (meaning pharynx) T28.5
thumb (s) T23.419
    first degree T23.519
    left T23.412
      first degree T23.512
      second degree T23.612
      third degree T23.712
    multiple sites with fingers
      T23.449
    first degree T23.549
    left T23.442
      first degree T23.542
      second degree T23.642
      third degree T23.742
    right T23.441
      first degree T23.541
      second degree T23.641
      third degree T23.741
    second degree T23.649
    third degree T23.749
    right T23.411
      first degree T23.511
      second degree T23.611
      third degree T23.711
    second degree T23.619
    third degree T23.719
toe T25.439
    first degree T25.539
    left T25.432
      first degree T25.532
      second degree T25.632
      third degree T25.732
    right T25.431
      first degree T25.531
      second degree T25.631
      third degree T25.731
    second degree T25.639
    third degree T25.739
tongue T28.5
tonsil (s) T28.5
total body —*see* Corrosion, multiple
    body regions
trachea T27.4
    with lung T27.5
trunk T21.40
    abdominal wall —*see* Corrosion,
      abdominal wall
    anus —*see* Corrosion, buttock
    axilla —*see* Corrosion, upper limb
    back —*see* Corrosion, back
    breast —*see* Corrosion, chest wall
    buttock —*see* Corrosion, buttock
    chest wall —*see* Corrosion, chest
      wall
    first degree T21.50
    flank —*see* Corrosion, abdominal
      wall
    genital
      female —*see* Corrosion, genital
        organs, external, female
      male —*see* Corrosion, genital
        organs, external, male
    groin —*see* Corrosion, abdominal
      wall

Corrosion *(Continued)*
  trunk *(Continued)*
    interscapular region —*see* Corrosion,
      back, upper
    labia —*see* Corrosion, genital organs,
      external, female
    lower back —*see* Corrosion, back
    penis —*see* Corrosion, genital organs,
      external, male
    perineum
      female —*see* Corrosion, genital
        organs, external, female
      male —*see* Corrosion, genital
        organs, external, male
    scapular region —*see* Corrosion,
      upper limb
    scrotum —*see* Corrosion, genital
      organs, external, male
    second degree T21.60
    shoulder —*see* Corrosion, upper limb
    specified site NEC T21.49
      first degree T21.59
      second degree T21.69
      third degree T21.79
    testes —*see* Corrosion, genital organs,
      external, male
    third degree T21.70
    upper back —*see* Corrosion, back,
      upper
    vagina T28.8
    vulva —*see* Corrosion, genital organs,
      external, female
  unspecified site with extent of body
    surface involved specified
    less than 10 percent T32.0
    10-19 percent (0-9 percent third
      degree) T32.10
      with 10-19 percent third degree
        T32.11
    20-29 percent (0-9 percent third
      degree) T32.20
      with
        10-19 percent third degree T32.21
        20-29 percent third degree T32.22
    30-39 percent (0-9 percent third
      degree) T32.30
      with
        10-19 percent third degree T32.31
        20-29 percent third degree T32.32
        30-39 percent third degree T32.33
    40-49 percent (0-9 percent third
      degree) T32.40
      with
        10-19 percent third degree T32.41
        20-29 percent third degree T32.42
        30-39 percent third degree T32.43
        40-49 percent third degree T32.44
    50-59 percent (0-9 percent third
      degree) T32.50
      with
        10-19 percent third degree T32.51
        20-29 percent third degree T32.52
        30-39 percent third degree T32.53
        40-49 percent third degree T32.54
        50-59 percent third degree T32.55
    60-69 percent (0-9 percent third
      degree) T32.60
      with
        10-19 percent third degree T32.61
        20-29 percent third degree T32.62
        30-39 percent third degree T32.63
        40-49 percent third degree T32.64
        50-59 percent third degree T32.65
        60-69 percent third degree T32.66

Corrosion *(Continued)*
  unspecified site with extent of body
    surface involved specified
    (Continued)
    70-79 percent (0-9 percent third
      degree) T32.70
      with
        10-19 percent third degree T32.71
        20-29 percent third degree T32.72
        30-39 percent third degree T32.73
        40-49 percent third degree T32.74
        50-59 percent third degree T32.75
        60-69 percent third degree T32.76
        70-79 percent third degree T32.77
    80-89 percent (0-9 percent third
      degree) T32.80
      with
        10-19 percent third degree T32.81
        20-29 percent third degree T32.82
        30-39 percent third degree T32.83
        40-49 percent third degree T32.84
        50-59 percent third degree T32.85
        60-69 percent third degree T32.86
        70-79 percent third degree T32.87
        80-89 percent third degree T32.88
    90 percent or more (0-9 percent third
      degree) T32.90
      with
        10-19 percent third degree T32.91
        20-29 percent third degree T32.92
        30-39 percent third degree T32.93
        40-49 percent third degree T32.94
        50-59 percent third degree T32.95
        60-69 percent third degree T32.96
        70-79 percent third degree T32.97
        80-89 percent third degree T32.98
        90-99 percent third degree T32.99
  upper limb (axilla) (scapular region) T22.40
    above elbow —*see* Corrosion, above
      elbow
    axilla —*see* Corrosion, axilla
    elbow —*see* Corrosion, elbow
    first degree T22.50
    forearm —*see* Corrosion, forearm
    hand —*see* Corrosion, hand
    interscapular region —*see* Corrosion,
      back, upper
    multiple sites T22.499
      first degree T22.599
      left T22.492
        first degree T22.592
        second degree T22.692
        third degree T22.792
      right T22.491
        first degree T22.591
        second degree T22.691
        third degree T22.791
      second degree T22.699
      third degree T22.799
    scapular region —*see* Corrosion,
      scapular region
    second degree T22.60
    shoulder —*see* Corrosion, shoulder
    third degree T22.70
    wrist —*see* Corrosion, hand
  uterus T28.8
  vagina T28.8
  vulva —*see* Corrosion, genital organs,
    external, female
  wrist T23.479
    first degree T23.579
    left T23.472
      first degree T23.572
      second degree T23.672
      third degree T23.772

Corrosion *(Continued)*
  wrist *(Continued)*
    multiple sites with hand T23.499
      first degree T23.599
      left T23.492
        first degree T23.592
        second degree T23.692
        third degree T23.792
      right T23.491
        first degree T23.591
        second degree T23.691
        third degree T23.791
      second degree T23.699
      third degree T23.799
    right T23.471
      first degree T23.571
      second degree T23.671
      third degree T23.771
    second degree T23.679
    third degree T23.779
Corrosive burn —*see* Corrosion
Corsican fever —*see* Malaria
Cortical —*see* condition
Cortico-adrenal —*see* condition
Coryza (acute) J00
  with grippe or influenza —*see*
    Influenza, with, respiratory
    manifestations NEC
  syphilitic
    congenital (chronic) A50.05
Costen's syndrome or complex M26.69
Costiveness —*see* Constipation
Costochondritis M94.0
Cot death R99
Cotard's syndrome F22
Cotia virus B08.8
Cotton wool spots (retinal) H35.81
Cotungo's disease —*see* Sciatica
Cough (affected) (chronic) (epidemic)
  (nervous) R05
  with hemorrhage —*see* Hemoptysis
  bronchial R05
    with grippe or influenza —*see*
      Influenza, with, respiratory
      manifestations NEC
  functional F45.8
  hysterical F45.8
  laryngeal, spasmodic R05
  psychogenic F45.8
  smokers' J41.0
  tea taster's B49
Counseling (for) Z71.9
  abuse NEC
    perpetrator Z69.82
    victim Z69.81
  alcohol abuser Z71.41
    family Z71.42
  child abuse
    nonparental
      perpetrator Z69.021
      victim Z69.020
    parental
      perpetrator Z69.011
      victim Z69.010
  consanguinity Z71.89
  contraceptive Z30.09
  dietary Z71.3
  drug abuser Z71.51
    family member Z71.52
  family Z71.89
  fertility preservation (prior to cancer
    therapy) (prior to removal of
    gonads) Z31.62
  for non-attending third party Z71.0
    related to sexual behavior or
      orientation Z70.2

Counseling (Continued)
  genetic NEC Z31.5
  health (advice) (education)
      (instruction) —see Counseling,
      medical
  human immunodeficiency virus (HIV)
      Z71.7
  impotence Z70.1
  insulin pump use Z46.81
  medical (for) Z71.9
    boarding school resident Z59.3
    consanguinity Z71.89
    feared complaint and no disease
        found Z71.1
    human immunodeficiency virus
        (HIV) Z71.7
    institutional resident Z59.3
    on behalf of another Z71.0
      related to sexual behavior or
          orientation Z70.2
    person living alone Z60.2
    specified reason NEC Z71.89
  natural family planning
    procreative Z31.61
    to avoid pregnancy Z30.02
  perpetrator (of)
    abuse NEC Z69.82
    child abuse
      non-parental Z69.021
      parental Z69.011
    rape NEC Z69.82
    spousal abuse Z69.12
  procreative NEC Z31.69
    fertility preservation (prior to cancer
        therapy) (prior to removal of
        gonads) Z31.62
    using natural family planning Z31.61
  promiscuity Z70.1
  rape victim Z69.81
  religious Z71.81
  sex, sexual (related to) Z70.9
    attitude (s) Z70.0
    behavior or orientation Z70.1
    combined concerns Z70.3
    non-responsiveness Z70.1
    on behalf of third party Z70.2
    specified reason NEC Z70.8
  specified reason NEC Z71.89
  spiritual Z71.81
  spousal abuse (perpetrator) Z69.12
    victim Z69.11
  substance abuse Z71.89
    alcohol Z71.41
    drug Z71.51
    tobacco Z71.6
  tobacco use Z71.6
  use (of)
    insulin pump Z46.81
  victim (of)
    abuse Z69.81
    child abuse
      by parent Z69.010
      non-parental Z69.020
    rape NEC Z69.81
Coupled rhythm R00.8
Couvelaire syndrome or uterus
    (complicating delivery) O45.8X-
Cowperitis —see Urethritis
Cowper's gland —see condition
Cowpox B08.010
  due to vaccination T88.1
Coxa
  magna M91.4-
  plana M91.2-

Coxa (Continued)
  valga (acquired) —see also Deformity,
      limb, specified type NEC, thigh
    congenital Q65.81
    sequelae (late effect) of rickets E64.3
  vara (acquired) —see also Deformity,
      limb, specified type NEC, thigh
    congenital Q65.82
    sequelae (late effect) of rickets E64.3
Coxalgia, coxalgic (nontuberculous) —see
    also Pain, joint, hip
  tuberculous A18.02
Coxitis —see Monoarthritis, hip
Coxsackie (virus) (infection) B34.1
  as cause of disease classified elsewhere
      B97.11
  carditis B33.20
  central nervous system NEC A88.8
  endocarditis B33.21
  enteritis A08.39
  meningitis (aseptic) A87.0
  myocarditis B33.22
  pericarditis B33.23
  pharyngitis B08.5
  pleurodynia B33.0
  specific disease NEC B33.8
Crabs, meaning pubic lice B85.3
Crack baby P04.41
Cracked nipple N64.0
  associated with
    lactation O92.13
    pregnancy O92.11-
Cracked tooth K03.81
Cradle cap L21.0
Craft neurosis F48.8
Cramp (s) R25.2
  abdominal —see Pain, abdominal
  bathing T75.1
  colic R10.83
    psychogenic F45.8
  due to immersion T75.1
  fireman T67.2
  heat T67.2
  immersion T75.1
  intestinal —see Pain, abdominal
    psychogenic F45.8
  leg, sleep related G47.62
  limb (lower) (upper) NEC R25.2
    sleep related G47.62
  linotypist's F48.8
    organic G25.89
  muscle (limb) (general) R25.2
    due to immersion T75.1
    psychogenic F45.8
  occupational (hand) F48.8
    organic G25.89
  salt-depletion E87.1
  sleep related, leg G47.62
  stoker's T67.2
  swimmer's T75.1
  telegrapher's F48.8
    organic G25.89
  typist's F48.8
    organic G25.89
  uterus N94.89
    menstrual —see Dysmenorrhea
  writer's F48.8
    organic G25.89
Cranial —see condition
Craniocleidodysostosis Q74.0
Craniofenestria (skull) Q75.8
Craniolacunia (skull) Q75.8
Craniopagus Q89.4
Craniopathy, metabolic M85.2

Craniopharyngeal —see condition
Craniopharyngioma D44.4
Craniorachischisis (totalis) Q00.1
Cranioschisis Q75.8
Craniostenosis Q75.0
Craniosynostosis Q75.0
Craniotabes (cause unknown) M83.8
  neonatal P96.3
  rachitic E64.3
  syphilitic A50.56
Cranium —see condition
Craw-craw —see Onchocerciasis
Creaking joint —see Derangement, joint,
    specified type NEC
Creeping
  eruption B76.9
  palsy or paralysis G12.22
Crenated tongue K14.8
Creotoxism A05.9
Crepitus
  caput Q75.8
  joint —see Derangement, joint, specified
      type NEC
Crescent or conus choroid, congenital
    Q14.3
CREST syndrome M34.1
Cretin, cretinism (congenital) (endemic)
    (nongoitrous) (sporadic) E00.9
  pelvis
    with disproportion (fetopelvic) O33.0
      causing obstructed labor O65.0
  type
    hypothyroid E00.1
    mixed E00.2
    myxedematous E00.1
    neurological E00.0
Creutzfeldt-Jakob disease or syndrome
    (with dementia) A81.00
  familial A81.09
  iatrogenic A81.09
  specified NEC A81.09
  sporadic A81.09
  variant (vCJD) A81.01
Crib death R99
Cribriform hymen Q52.3
Cri-du-chat syndrome Q93.4
Crigler-Najjar disease or syndrome E80.5
Crime, victim of Z65.4
Crimean hemorrhagic fever A98.0
Criminalism F60.2
Crisis
  abdomen R10.0
  acute reaction F43.0
  addisonian E27.2
  adrenal (cortical) E27.2
  celiac K90.0
  Dietl's N13.8
  emotional —see also Disorder,
      adjustment
    acute reaction to stress F43.0
    specific to childhood and adolescence
        F93.8
  glaucomatocyclitic —see Glaucoma,
      secondary, inflammation
  heart —see Failure, heart
  nitritoid I95.2
    correct substance properly
        administered —see Table of
        drugs and chemicals, by drug,
        adverse effect
    overdose or wrong substance given
        or taken —see Table of drugs
        and chemicals, by drug,
        poisoning

Crisis *(Continued)*
oculogyric H51.8
psychogenic F45.8
Pel's (tabetic) A52.11
psychosexual identity F64.2
renal N28.0
sickle-cell D57.00
with
acute chest syndrome D57.01
splenic sequestration D57.02
state (acute reaction) F43.0
tabetic A52.11
thyroid —*see* Thyrotoxicosis with
thyroid storm
thyrotoxic —*see* Thyrotoxicosis with
thyroid storm
Crocq's disease (acrocyanosis) I73.89
Crohn's disease —*see* Enteritis, regional
Crooked septum, nasal J34.2
Cross syndrome E70.328
Crossbite (anterior) (posterior) M26.24
Cross-eye —*see* Strabismus, convergent
concomitant
Croup, croupous (catarrhal) (infectious)
(inflammatory) (nondiphtheritic) J05.0
bronchial J20.9
diphtheritic A36.2
false J38.5
spasmodic J38.5
diphtheritic A36.2
stridulous J38.5
diphtheritic A36.2
Crouzon's disease Q75.1
Crowding, tooth, teeth, fully erupted
M26.31
CRST syndrome M34.1
Cruchet's disease A85.8
Cruelty in children —*see also* Disorder,
conduct
Crural ulcer —*see* Ulcer, lower limb
Crush, crushed, crushing T14.8
abdomen S38.1
ankle S97.0-
arm (upper) (and shoulder) S47.-
axilla —*see* Crush, arm
back, lower S38.1
buttock S38.1
cheek S07.0
chest S28.0
cranium S07.1
ear S07.0
elbow S57.0-
extremity
lower
ankle —*see* Crush, ankle
below knee —*see* Crush, leg
foot —*see* Crush, foot
hip —*see* Crush, hip
knee —*see* Crush, knee
thigh —*see* Crush, thigh
toe —*see* Crush, toe
upper
below elbow S67.9-
elbow —*see* Crush, elbow
finger —*see* Crush, finger
forearm —*see* Crush, forearm
hand —*see* Crush, hand
thumb —*see* Crush, thumb
upper arm —*see* Crush, arm
wrist —*see* Crush, wrist
face S07.0
finger (s) S67.1-
with hand (and wrist) —*see* Crush,
hand, specified site NEC
index S67.19-

Crush, crushed, crushing *(Continued)*
finger (s) *(Continued)*
little S67.19-
middle S67.19-
ring S67.19-
thumb —*see* Crush, thumb
foot S97.8-
toe —*see* Crush, toe
forearm S57.8-
genitalia, external
female S38.002
vagina S38.03
vulva S38.03
male S38.001
penis S38.01
scrotum S38.02
testis S38.02
hand (except fingers alone) S67.2-
with wrist S67.4-
head S07.9
specified NEC S07.8
heel —*see* Crush, foot
hip S77.0-
with thigh S77.2-
internal organ (abdomen, chest, or
pelvis) NEC T14.8
knee S87.0-
labium (majus) (minus) S38.03
larynx S17.0
leg (lower) S87.8-
knee —*see* Crush, knee
lip S07.0
lower
back S38.1
leg —*see* Crush, leg
neck S17.9
nerve —*see* Injury, nerve
nose S07.0
pelvis S38.1
penis S38.01
scalp S07.8
scapular region —*see* Crush, arm
scrotum S38.02
severe, unspecified site T14.8
shoulder (and upper arm) —*see* Crush,
arm
skull S07.1
syndrome (complication of trauma)
T79.5
testis S38.02
thigh S77.1-
with hip S77.2-
throat S17.8
thumb S67.0-
with hand (and wrist) —*see* Crush,
hand, specified site NEC
toe (s) S97.10-
great S97.11-
lesser S97.12-
trachea S17.0
vagina S38.03
vulva S38.03
wrist S67.3-
with hand S67.4-
Crusta lactea L21.0
Crusts R23.4
Crutch paralysis —*see* Injury, brachial
plexus
Cruveilhier-Baumgarten cirrhosis,
disease or syndrome K74.69
Cruveilhier's atrophy or disease G12.8
Crying (constant) (continuous) (excessive)
child, adolescent, or adult R45.83
infant (baby) (newborn) R68.11

Cryofibrinogenemia D89.2
Cryoglobulinemia (essential)
(idiopathic) (mixed) (primary)
(purpura) (secondary) (vasculitis)
D89.1
with lung involvement D89.1 *[J99]*
Cryptitis (anal) (rectal) K62.89
Cryptococcosis, cryptococcus (infection)
(neoformans) B45.9
bone B45.3
cerebral B45.1
cutaneous B45.2
disseminated B45.7
generalized B45.7
meningitis B45.1
meningocerebralis B45.1
osseous B45.3
pulmonary B45.0
skin B45.2
specified NEC B45.8
Cryptopapillitis (anus) K62.89
Cryptophthalmos Q11.2
syndrome Q87.0
Cryptorchid, cryptorchism,
cryptorchidism Q53.9
bilateral Q53.20
abdominal Q53.21
perineal Q53.22
unilateral Q53.10
abdominal Q53.11
perineal Q53.12
Cryptosporidiosis A07.2
hepatobiliary B88.8
respiratory B88.8
Cryptostromosis J67.6
Crystalluria R82.99
Cubitus
congenital Q68.8
valgus (acquired) M21.0-
congenital Q68.8
sequelae (late effect) of rickets
E64.3
varus (acquired) M21.1-
congenital Q68.8
sequelae (late effect) of rickets
E64.3
Cultural deprivation or shock Z60.3
Curling esophagus K22.4
Curling's ulcer —*see* Ulcer, peptic, acute
Curschmann (-Batten) (-Steinert) **disease
or syndrome** G71.11
Curse, Ondine's —*see* Apnea, sleep
Curvature
organ or site, congenital NEC —*see*
Distortion
penis (lateral) Q55.61
Pott's (spinal) A18.01
radius, idiopathic, progressive
(congenital) Q74.0
spine (acquired) (angular) (idiopathic)
(incorrect) (postural) —*see*
Dorsopathy, deforming
congenital Q67.5
due to or associated with
Charcot-Marie-Tooth disease (*see
also* subcategory M49.8) G60.0
osteitis
deformans M88.88
fibrosa cystica (*see also*
subcategory M49.8) E21.0
tuberculosis (Pott's curvature)
A18.01
sequelae (late effect) of rickets E64.3
tuberculous A18.01

Cushingoid due to steroid therapy E24.2
correct substance properly
administered —*see* Table of drugs
and chemicals, by drug, adverse
effect
overdose or wrong substance given
or taken —*see* Table of drugs and
chemicals, by drug, poisoning
Cushing's
syndrome or disease E24.9
drug-induced E24.2
iatrogenic E24.2
pituitary-dependent E24.0
specified NEC E24.8
ulcer —*see* Ulcer, peptic, acute
Cusp, Carabelli - omit code
Cut (external) —*see also* Laceration
muscle —*see* Injury, muscle
Cutaneous —*see also* condition
hemorrhage R23.3
larva migrans B76.9
Cutis —*see also* condition
hyperelastica Q82.8
acquired L57.4
laxa (hyperelastica) —*see* Dermatolysis
marmorata R23.8
osteosis L94.2
pendula —*see* Dermatolysis
rhomboidalis nuchae L57.2
verticis gyrata Q82.8
acquired L91.8
Cyanosis R23.0
due to
patent foramen botalli Q21.1
persistent foramen ovale Q21.1
enterogenous D74.8
paroxysmal digital —*see* Raynaud's
disease
with gangrene I73.01
retina, retinal H35.89
Cyanotic heart disease I24.9
congenital Q24.9
Cycle
anovulatory N97.0
menstrual, irregular N92.6
Cyclencephaly Q04.9
Cyclical vomiting (*see also* Vomiting,
cyclical) G43.A0
psychogenic F50.8
Cyclitis (*see also* Iridocyclitis) H20.9
chronic —*see* Iridocyclitis, chronic
Fuchs' heterochromic H20.81-
granulomatous —*see* Iridocyclitis,
chronic
lens-induced —*see* Iridocyclitis,
lens-induced
posterior H30.2-
Cycloid personality F34.0
Cyclophoria H50.54
Cyclopia, cyclops Q87.0
Cyclopism Q87.0
Cyclosporiasis A07.4
Cyclothymia F34.0
Cyclothymic personality F34.0
Cyclotropia H50.41-
Cylindroma —*see also* Neoplasm,
malignant, by site
eccrine dermal —*see* Neoplasm, skin,
benign
skin —*see* Neoplasm, skin, benign
Cylindruria R82.99
Cynanche
diphtheritic A36.2
tonsillaris J36

Cynophobia F40.218
Cynorexia R63.2
Cyphosis —*see* Kyphosis
Cyprus fever —*see* Brucellosis
Cyst (colloid) (mucous) (simple) (retention)
adenoid (infected) J35.8
adrenal gland E27.8
congenital Q89.1
air, lung J98.4
allantoic Q64.4
alveolar process (jaw bone) M27.40
amnion, amniotic O41.8X-
anterior
chamber (eye) —*see* Cyst, iris
nasopalatine K09.1
antrum J34.1
anus K62.89
apical (tooth) (periodontal) K04.8
appendix K38.8
arachnoid, brain (acquired) G93.0
congenital Q04.6
arytenoid J38.7
Baker's M71.2-
ruptured M66.0
tuberculous A18.02
Bartholin's gland N75.0
bile duct (common) (hepatic) K83.5
bladder (multiple) (trigone) N32.89
blue dome (breast) —*see* Cyst, breast
bone (local) NEC M85.60
aneurysmal M85.50
ankle M85.57-
foot M85.57-
forearm M85.53-
hand M85.54-
jaw M27.49
lower leg M85.56-
multiple site M85.59
neck M85.58
rib M85.58
shoulder M85.51-
skull M85.58
specified site NEC M85.58
thigh M85.55-
toe M85.57-
upper arm M85.52-
vertebra M85.58
solitary M85.40
ankle M85.47-
fibula M85.46-
foot M85.47-
hand M85.44-
humerus M85.42-
jaw M27.49
neck M85.48
pelvis M85.45-
radius M85.43-
rib M85.48
shoulder M85.41-
skull M85.48
specified site NEC M85.48
tibia M85.46-
toe M85.47-
ulna M85.43-
vertebra M85.48
specified type NEC M85.60
ankle M85.67-
foot M85.67-
forearm M85.63-
hand M85.64-
jaw M27.40
developmental (nonodontogenic)
K09.1
odontogenic K09.0
latent M27.0

Cyst (*Continued*)
bone (local) NEC (*Continued*)
specified type NEC (*Continued*)
lower leg M85.66-
multiple site M85.69
neck M85.68
rib M85.68
shoulder M85.61-
skull M85.68
specified site NEC M85.68
thigh M85.65-
toe M85.67-
upper arm M85.62-
vertebra M85.68
brain (acquired) G93.0
congenital Q04.6
hydatid B67.99 [G94]
third ventricle (colloid), congenital
Q04.6
branchial (cleft) Q18.0
branchiogenic Q18.0
breast (benign) (blue dome)
(pedunculated) (solitary) N60.0-
involution —*see* Dysplasia,
mammary, specified type NEC
sebaceous —*see* Dysplasia, mammary,
specified type NEC
broad ligament (benign) N83.8
bronchogenic (mediastinal)
(sequestration) J98.4
congenital Q33.0
buccal K09.8
bulbourethral gland N36.8
bursa, bursal NEC M71.30
with rupture —*see* Rupture, synovium
ankle M71.37-
elbow M71.32-
foot M71.37-
hand M71.34-
hip M71.35-
multiple sites M71.39
pharyngeal J39.2
popliteal space —*see* Cyst, Baker's
shoulder M71.31-
specified site NEC M71.38
wrist M71.33-
calcifying odontogenic D16.5
upper jaw (bone) (maxilla) D16.4
canal of Nuck (female) N94.89
congenital Q52.4
canthus —*see* Cyst, conjunctiva
carcinomatous —*see* Neoplasm,
malignant, by site
cauda equina G95.89
cavum septi pellucidi —*see* Cyst, brain
celomic (pericardium) Q24.8
cerebellopontine (angle) —*see* Cyst,
brain
cerebellum —*see* Cyst, brain
cerebral —*see* Cyst, brain
cervical lateral Q18.1
cervix NEC N88.8
embryonic Q51.6
nabothian N88.8
chiasmal optic NEC —*see* Disorder,
optic, chiasm
chocolate (ovary) N80.1
choledochus, congenital Q44.4
chorion O41.8X-
choroid plexus G93.0
ciliary body —*see* Cyst, iris
clitoris N90.7
colon K63.89
common (bile) duct K83.5

Cyst (Continued)
  congenital NEC Q89.8
    adrenal gland Q89.1
    epiglottis Q31.8
    esophagus Q39.8
    fallopian tube Q50.4
    kidney Q61.00
      more than one (multiple) Q61.02
        specified as polycystic Q61.3
          adult type Q61.2
            infantile type NEC Q61.19
              collecting duct dilation
                Q61.11
      solitary Q61.01
    larynx Q31.8
    liver Q44.6
    lung Q33.0
    mediastinum Q34.1
    ovary Q50.1
    oviduct Q50.4
    periurethral (tissue) Q64.79
    prepuce Q55.69
    salivary gland (any) Q38.4
    sublingual Q38.6
    submaxillary gland Q38.6
    thymus (gland) Q89.2
    tongue Q38.3
    ureterovesical orifice Q62.8
    vulva Q52.79
  conjunctiva H11.44-
  cornea H18.89-
  corpora quadrigemina G93.0
  corpus
    albicans N83.29
    luteum (hemorrhagic) (ruptured)
      N83.1
  Cowper's gland (benign) (infected)
    N36.8
  cranial meninges G93.0
  craniobuccal pouch E23.6
  craniopharyngeal pouch E23.6
  cystic duct K82.8
  Cysticercus —see Cysticercosis
  Dandy-Walker Q03.1
    with spina bifida —see Spina bifida
  dental (root) K04.8
    developmental K09.0
    eruption K09.0
    primordial K09.0
  dentigerous (mandible) (maxilla)
    K09.0
  dermoid —see Neoplasm, benign, by
    site
    with malignant transformation C56.-
  implantation
    external area or site (skin) NEC
      L72.0
    iris —see Cyst, iris, implantation
    vagina N89.8
    vulva N90.7
  mouth K09.8
  oral soft tissue K09.8
  sacrococcygeal —see Cyst, pilonidal
  developmental K09.1
    odontogenic K09.0
    oral region (nonodontogenic) K09.1
  ovary, ovarian Q50.1
  dura (cerebral) G93.0
    spinal G96.19
  ear (external) Q18.1
  echinococcal —see Echinococcus
  embryonic
    cervix uteri Q51.6
    fallopian tube Q50.4
    vagina Q51.6

Cyst (Continued)
  endometrium, endometrial (uterus)
    N85.8
    ectopic —see Endometriosis
  enterogenous Q43.8
  epidermal, epidermoid (inclusion) (see
    also Cyst, skin) L72.0
    mouth K09.8
    oral soft tissue K09.8
  epididymis N50.3
  epiglottis J38.7
  epiphysis cerebri E34.8
  epithelial (inclusion) L72.0
  epoophoron Q50.5
  eruption K09.0
  esophagus K22.8
  ethmoid sinus J34.1
  external female genital organs NEC
    N90.7
  eye NEC H57.8
    congenital Q15.8
  eyelid (sebaceous) H02.829
    infected —see Hordeolum
    left H02.826
      lower H02.825
      upper H02.824
    right H02.823
      lower H02.822
      upper H02.821
  fallopian tube N83.8
    congenital Q50.4
  fimbrial (twisted) Q50.4
  fissural (oral region) K09.1
  follicle (graafian) (hemorrhagic) N83.0
    nabothian N88.8
  follicular (atretic) (hemorrhagic)
    (ovarian) N83.0
    dentigerous K09.0
    odontogenic K09.0
    skin L72.9
      specified NEC L72.8
  frontal sinus J34.1
  gallbladder K82.8
  ganglion —see Ganglion
  Gartner's duct Q52.4
  gingiva K09.0
  gland of Moll —see Cyst, eyelid
  globulomaxillary K09.1
  graafian follicle (hemorrhagic) N83.0
  granulosal lutein (hemorrhagic) N83.1
  hemangiomatous D18.00
    intra-abdominal D18.03
    intracranial D18.02
    skin D18.01
    specified site NEC D18.09
  hydatid (see also Echinococcus) B67.90
    brain B67.99 [G94]
    liver (see also Cyst, liver, hydatid)
      B67.8
    lung NEC B67.99 [J99]
    Morgagni
      female Q50.5
      male (epididymal) Q55.4
        testicular Q55.29
    specified site NEC B67.99
  hymen N89.8
    embryonic Q52.4
  hypopharynx J39.2
  hypophysis, hypophyseal (duct)
    (recurrent) E23.6
    cerebri E23.6
  implantation (dermoid)
    external area or site (skin) NEC L72.0
    iris —see Cyst, iris, implantation

Cyst (Continued)
  implantation (Continued)
    vagina N89.8
    vulva N90.7
  incisive canal K09.1
  inclusion (epidermal) (epithelial)
    (epidermoid) (squamous) L72.0
    not of skin - code under Cyst, by site
  intestine (large) (small) K63.89
  intracranial —see Cyst, brain
  intraligamentous —see also Disorder,
    ligament
    knee —see Derangement, knee
  intrasellar E23.6
  iris H21.309
    exudative H21.31-
    idiopathic H21.30-
    implantation H21.32-
    parasitic H21.33-
    pars plana (primary) H21.34-
      exudative H21.35-
  jaw (bone) (aneurysmal) (hemorrhagic)
    (traumatic) M27.40
    developmental (odontogenic) K09.0
    fissural K09.1
  joint NEC —see Disorder, joint, specified
    type NEC
  kidney (acquired) N28.1
    calyceal —see Hydronephrosis
    congenital Q61.00
      more than one (multiple) Q61.02
        specified as polycystic Q61.3
          adult type (autosomal dominant)
            Q61.2
          infantile type (autosomal
            recessive) NEC Q61.19
            collecting duct dilation Q61.11
    pyelogenic —see Hydronephrosis
    simple N28.1
    solitary (single) Q61.01
      acquired N28.1
  labium (majus) (minus) N90.7
    sebaceous N90.7
  lacrimal —see also Disorder, lacrimal
    system, specified NEC
    gland H04.13-
    passages or sac —see Disorder,
      lacrimal system, specified NEC
  larynx J38.7
  lateral periodontal K09.0
  lens H27.8
    congenital Q12.8
  lip (gland) K13.0
  liver (idiopathic) (simple) K76.89
    congenital Q44.6
    hydatid B67.8
      granulosus B67.0
      multilocularis B67.5
  lung J98.4
    congenital Q33.0
    giant bullous J43.9
  lutein N83.1
  lymphangiomatous D18.1
  lymphoepithelial, oral soft tissue K09.8
  macula —see Degeneration, macula, hole
  malignant —see Neoplasm, malignant,
    by site
  mammary gland —see Cyst, breast
  mandible M27.40
    dentigerous K09.0
    radicular K04.8
  maxilla M27.40
    dentigerous K09.0
    radicular K04.8
  medial, face and neck Q18.8

Cyst *(Continued)*
  median
    anterior maxillary K09.1
    palatal K09.1
  mediastinum, congenital Q34.1
  meibomian (gland) —*see* Chalazion
    infected —*see* Hordeolum
  membrane, brain G93.0
  meninges (cerebral) G93.0
    spinal G96.19
  meniscus, knee —*see* Derangement,
    knee, meniscus, cystic
  mesentery, mesenteric K66.8
    chyle I89.8
  mesonephric duct
    female Q50.5
    male Q55.4
  milk N64.89
  Morgagni (hydatid)
    female Q50.5
    male (epididymal) Q55.4
      testicular Q55.29
  mouth K09.8
  Müllerian duct Q50.4
    appendix testis Q55.29
    cervix Q51.6
    fallopian tube Q50.4
    female Q50.4
    male Q55.29
    prostatic utricle Q55.4
    vagina (embryonal) Q52.4
  multilocular (ovary) D39.10
    benign —*see* Neoplasm, benign, by
      site
  myometrium N85.8
  nabothian (follicle) (ruptured) N88.8
  nasoalveolar K09.1
  nasolabial K09.1
  nasopalatine (anterior) (duct) K09.1
  nasopharynx J39.2
  neoplastic —*see* Neoplasm, uncertain
      behavior, by site
    benign —*see* Neoplasm, benign, by
      site
  nervous system NEC G96.8
  neuroenteric (congenital) Q06.8
  nipple —*see* Cyst, breast
  nose (turbinates) J34.1
    sinus J34.1
  odontogenic, developmental K09.0
  omentum (lesser) K66.8
    congenital Q45.8
  ora serrata —*see* Cyst, retina, ora serrata
  oral
    region K09.9
      developmental (nonodontogenic)
        K09.1
      specified NEC K09.8
    soft tissue K09.9
      specified NEC K09.8
  orbit H05.81-
  ovary, ovarian (twisted) N83.20
    adherent N83.20
    chocolate N80.1
    corpus
      albicans N83.29
      luteum (hemorrhagic) N83.1
    dermoid D27.9
    developmental Q50.1
    due to failure of involution NEC
      N83.20
    endometrial N80.1
    follicular (graafian) (hemorrhagic)
      N83.0

Cyst *(Continued)*
  ovary, ovarian *(Continued)*
    hemorrhagic N83.20
    in pregnancy or childbirth O34.8-
      with obstructed labor O65.5
    multilocular D39.10
    pseudomucinous D27.9
    retention N83.29
    serous N83.20
    specified NEC N83.29
    theca lutein (hemorrhagic) N83.1
    tuberculous A18.18
  oviduct N83.8
  palate (median) (fissural) K09.1
  palatine papilla (jaw) K09.1
  pancreas, pancreatic (hemorrhagic)
      (true) K86.2
    congenital Q45.2
    false K86.3
  paralabral
    hip M24.85-
    shoulder S43.43-
  paramesonephric duct Q50.4
    female Q50.4
    male Q55.29
  paranephric N28.1
  paraphysis, cerebri, congenital Q04.6
  parasitic B89
  parathyroid (gland) E21.4
  paratubal N83.8
  paraurethral duct N36.8
  paroophoron Q50.5
  parotid gland K11.6
  parovarian Q50.5
  pelvis, female N94.89
    in pregnancy or childbirth O34.8-
      causing obstructed labor O65.5
  penis (sebaceous) N48.89
  periapical K04.8
  pericardial (congenital) Q24.8
    acquired (secondary) I31.8
  pericoronal K09.0
  periodontal K04.8
    lateral K09.0
  peripelvic (lymphatic) N28.1
  peritoneum K66.8
    chylous I89.8
  periventricular, acquired, newborn P91.1
  pharynx (wall) J39.2
  pilar L72.11
  pilonidal (infected) (rectum) L05.91
    with abscess L05.01
    malignant C44.59-
  pituitary (duct) (gland) E23.6
  placenta O43.19-
  pleura J94.8
  popliteal —*see* Cyst, Baker's
  porencephalic Q04.6
    acquired G93.0
  postanal (infected) —*see* Cyst, pilonidal
  postmastoidectomy cavity (mucosal) —
      see Complications, post-
      mastoidectomy, cyst
  preauricular Q18.1
  prepuce N47.4
    congenital Q55.69
  primordial (jaw) K09.0
  prostate N42.83
  pseudomucinous (ovary) D27.9
  pupillary, miotic H21.27-
  radicular (residual) K04.8
  radiculodental K04.8
  ranular K11.8
  Rathke's pouch E23.6
  rectum (epithelium) (mucous) K62.89

Cyst *(Continued)*
  renal —*see* Cyst, kidney
  residual (radicular) K04.8
  retention (ovary) N83.29
    salivary gland K11.6
  retina H33.19-
    ora serrata H33.11-
    parasitic H33.12-
  retroperitoneal K68.9
  sacrococcygeal (dermoid) —*see* Cyst,
      pilonidal
  salivary gland or duct (mucous
      extravasation or retention)
      K11.6
  Sampson's N80.1
  sclera H15.89
  scrotum L72.9
    sebaceous L72.3
  sebaceous (duct) (gland) L72.3
    breast —*see* Dysplasia, mammary,
      specified type NEC
    eyelid —*see* Cyst, eyelid
    genital organ NEC
      female N94.89
      male N50.8
    scrotum L72.3
  semilunar cartilage (knee) (multiple) —
      see Derangement, knee, meniscus,
      cystic
  seminal vesicle N50.8
  serous (ovary) N83.20
  sinus (accessory) (nasal) J34.1
  Skene's gland N36.8
  skin L72.9
    breast —*see* Dysplasia, mammary,
      specified type NEC
    epidermal, epidermoid L72.0
    epithelial L72.0
    eyelid —*see* Cyst, eyelid
    genital organ NEC
      female N90.7
      male N50.8
    inclusion L72.0
    scrotum L72.9
    sebaceous L72.3
    sweat gland or duct L74.8
  solitary
    bone —*see* Cyst, bone, solitary
    jaw M27.40
    kidney N28.1
  spermatic cord N50.8
  sphenoid sinus J34.1
  spinal meninges G96.19
  spleen NEC D73.4
    congenital Q89.09
    hydatid (*see also* Echinococcus) B67.99
      [D77]
  Stafne's M27.0
  subarachnoid intrasellar R93.0
  subcutaneous, pheomycotic
      (chromomycotic) B43.2
  subdural (cerebral) G93.0
    spinal cord G96.19
  sublingual gland K11.6
  submandibular gland K11.6
  submaxillary gland K11.6
  suburethral N36.8
  suprarenal gland E27.8
  suprasellar —*see* Cyst, brain
  sweat gland or duct L74.8
  synovial —*see also* Cyst, bursa
    ruptured —*see* Rupture, synovium
  tarsal —*see* Chalazion
  tendon (sheath) —*see* Disorder, tendon,
      specified type NEC

Cyst (Continued)
  testis N44.2
    tunica albuginea N44.1
  theca lutein (ovary) N83.1
  Thornwaldt's J39.2
  thymus (gland) E32.8
  thyroglossal duct (infected) (persistent) Q89.2
  thyroid (gland) E04.1
  thyrolingual duct (infected) (persistent) Q89.2
  tongue K14.8
  tonsil J35.8
  tooth —see Cyst, dental
  Tornwaldt's J39.2
  trichilemmal (proliferating) L72.12
  trichodermal L72.12
  tubal (fallopian) N83.8
    inflammatory —see Salpingitis, chronic
  tubo-ovarian N83.8
    inflammatory N70.13
  tunica
    albuginea testis N44.1
    vaginalis N50.8
  turbinate (nose) J34.1
  Tyson's gland N48.89
  urachus, congenital Q64.4
  ureter N28.89
  ureterovesical orifice N28.89
  urethra, urethral (gland) N36.8
  uterine ligament N83.8
  uterus (body) (corpus) (recurrent) N85.8
    embryonic Q51.818
      cervix Q51.6
  vagina, vaginal (implantation) (inclusion) (squamous cell) (wall) N89.8
    embryonic Q52.4
  vallecula, vallecular (epiglottis) J38.7
  vesical (orifice) N32.89
  vitreous body H43.89
  vulva (implantation) (inclusion) N90.7
    congenital Q52.79
    sebaceous gland N90.7
  vulvovaginal gland N90.7
  wolffian
    female Q50.5
    male Q55.4
Cystadenocarcinoma —see Neoplasm, malignant, by site
  bile duct C22.1
  endometrioid —see Neoplasm, malignant, by site
    specified site —see Neoplasm, malignant, by site
    unspecified site
      female C56.9
      male C61
  mucinous
    papillary
      specified site —see Neoplasm, malignant, by site
      unspecified site C56.9
    specified site —see Neoplasm, malignant, by site
    unspecified site C56.9
  papillary
    mucinous
      specified site —see Neoplasm, malignant, by site
      unspecified site C56.9

Cystadenocarcinoma (Continued)
  papillary (Continued)
    pseudomucinous
      specified site —see Neoplasm, malignant, by site
      unspecified site C56.9
    serous
      specified site —see Neoplasm, malignant, by site
      unspecified site C56.9
    specified site —see Neoplasm, malignant, by site
    unspecified site C56.9
  pseudomucinous
    papillary
      specified site —see Neoplasm, malignant, by site
      unspecified site C56.9
    specified site —see Neoplasm, malignant, by site
    unspecified site C56.9
  serous
    papillary
      specified site —see Neoplasm, malignant, by site
      unspecified site C56.9
    specified site —see Neoplasm, malignant, by site
    unspecified site C56.9
Cystadenofibroma
  clear cell —see Neoplasm, benign, by site
  endometrioid D27.9
    borderline malignancy D39.1-
    malignant C56.-
  mucinous
    specified site —see Neoplasm, benign, by site
    unspecified site D27.9
  serous
    specified site —see Neoplasm, benign, by site
    unspecified site D27.9
  specified site —see Neoplasm, benign, by site
  unspecified site D27.9
Cystadenoma —see also Neoplasm, benign, by site
  bile duct D13.4
  endometrioid —see Neoplasm, benign, by site
    borderline malignancy —see Neoplasm, uncertain behavior, by site
    malignant —see Neoplasm, malignant, by site
  mucinous
    borderline malignancy
      ovary C56.-
      specified site NEC —see Neoplasm, uncertain behavior, by site
      unspecified site C56.9
    papillary
      borderline malignancy
        ovary C56.-
        specified site NEC —see Neoplasm, uncertain behavior, by site
        unspecified site C56.9
      specified site —see Neoplasm, benign, by site
      unspecified site D27.9
    specified site —see Neoplasm, benign, by site
    unspecified site D27.9

Cystadenoma (Continued)
  papillary
    borderline malignancy
      ovary C56-
      specified site NEC —see Neoplasm, uncertain behavior, by site
      unspecified site C56.9
    lymphomatosum
      specified site —see Neoplasm, benign, by site
      unspecified site D11.9
    mucinous
      borderline malignancy
        ovary C56.-
        specified site NEC —see Neoplasm, uncertain behavior, by site
        unspecified site C56.9
      specified site —see Neoplasm, benign, by site
      unspecified site D27.9
    pseudomucinous
      borderline malignancy
        ovary C56.-
        specified site NEC —see Neoplasm, uncertain behavior, by site
        unspecified site C56.9
      specified site —see Neoplasm, benign, by site
      unspecified site D27.9
    serous
      borderline malignancy
        ovary C56.-
        specified site NEC —see Neoplasm, uncertain behavior, by site
        unspecified site C56.9
      specified site —see Neoplasm, benign, by site
      unspecified site D27.9
    specified site —see Neoplasm, benign, by site
    unspecified site D27.9
  pseudomucinous
    borderline malignancy
      ovary C56.-
      specified site NEC —see Neoplasm, uncertain behavior, by site
      unspecified site C56.9
    papillary
      borderline malignancy
        ovary C56.-
        specified site NEC —see Neoplasm, uncertain behavior, by site
        unspecified site C56.9
      specified site —see Neoplasm, benign, by site
      unspecified site D27.9
    specified site —see Neoplasm, benign, by site
    unspecified site D27.9
  serous
    borderline malignancy
      ovary C56.-
      specified site NEC —see Neoplasm, uncertain behavior, by site
      unspecified site C56.9
    papillary
      borderline malignancy
        ovary C56.-
        specified site NEC —see Neoplasm, uncertain behavior, by site
        unspecified site C56.9

Cystadenoma *(Continued)*
  serous *(Continued)*
    papillary *(Continued)*
      specified site —*see* Neoplasm,
        benign, by site
      unspecified site D27.9
    specified site —*see* Neoplasm, benign,
      by site
    unspecified site D27.9
Cystathionine synthase deficiency E72.11
Cystathioninemia E72.19
Cystathioninuria E72.19
Cystic —*see also* condition
  breast (chronic) —*see* Mastopathy, cystic
  corpora lutea (hemorrhagic) N83.1
  duct —*see* condition
  eyeball (congenital) Q11.0
  fibrosis —*see* Fibrosis, cystic
  kidney (congenital) Q61.9
    adult type Q61.2
    infantile type NEC Q61.19
      collecting duct dilatation
        Q61.11
    medullary Q61.5
  liver, congenital Q44.6
  lung disease J98.4
    congenital Q33.0
  mastitis, chronic —*see* Mastopathy,
    cystic
  medullary, kidney Q61.5
  meniscus —*see* Derangement, knee,
    meniscus, cystic
  ovary N83.20
Cysticercosis, cysticerciasis B69.9
  with
    epileptiform fits B69.0
    myositis B69.81
  brain B69.0
  central nervous system B69.0
  cerebral B69.0
  ocular B69.1
  specified NEC B69.89
Cysticercus cellulose infestation —*see*
  Cysticercosis
Cystinosis (malignant) E72.04
Cystinuria E72.01
Cystitis (exudative) (hemorrhagic)
  (septic) (suppurative) N30.90
  with
    fibrosis —*see* Cystitis, chronic,
      interstitial
    hematuria N30.91
    leukoplakia —*see* Cystitis, chronic,
      interstitial
    malakoplakia —*see* Cystitis, chronic,
      interstitial
    metaplasia —*see* Cystitis, chronic,
      interstitial
    prostatitis N41.3
  acute N30.00
    with hematuria N30.01
    of trigone N30.30
      with hematuria N30.31

Cystitis *(Continued)*
  allergic —*see* Cystitis, specified type
    NEC
  amebic A06.81
  bilharzial B65.9 *[N33]*
  blennorrhagic (gonococcal) A54.01
  bullous —*see* Cystitis, specified type
    NEC
  calculous N21.0
  chlamydial A56.01
  chronic N30.20
    with hematuria N30.21
    interstitial N30.10
      with hematuria N30.11
    of trigone N30.30
      with hematuria N30.31
    specified NEC N30.20
      with hematuria N30.21
  cystic (a) —*see* Cystitis, specified type
    NEC
  diphtheritic A36.85
  echinococcal
    granulosus B67.39
    multilocularis B67.69
  emphysematous —*see* Cystitis, specified
    type NEC
  encysted —*see* Cystitis, specified type
    NEC
  eosinophilic —*see* Cystitis, specified
    type NEC
  follicular —*see* Cystitis, of trigone
  gangrenous —*see* Cystitis, specified
    type NEC
  glandularis —*see* Cystitis, specified type
    NEC
  gonococcal A54.01
  incrusted —*see* Cystitis, specified type
    NEC
  interstitial (chronic) —*see* Cystitis,
    chronic, interstitial
  irradiation N30.40
    with hematuria N30.41
  irritation —*see* Cystitis, specified type
    NEC
  malignant —*see* Cystitis, specified type
    NEC
  of trigone N30.30
    with hematuria N30.31
  panmural —*see* Cystitis, chronic,
    interstitial
  polyposa —*see* Cystitis, specified type
    NEC
  prostatic N41.3
  puerperal (postpartum) O86.22
  radiation —*see* Cystitis, irradiation
  specified type NEC N30.80
    with hematuria N30.81
  subacute —*see* Cystitis, chronic
  submucous —*see* Cystitis, chronic,
    interstitial
  syphilitic (late) A52.76
  trichomonal A59.03
  tuberculous A18.12

Cystitis *(Continued)*
  ulcerative —*see* Cystitis, chronic,
    interstitial
Cystocele (-urethrocele)
  female N81.10
    with prolapse of uterus —*see*
      Prolapse, uterus
    lateral N81.12
    midline N81.11
    paravaginal N81.12
  in pregnancy or childbirth O34.8-
    causing obstructed labor O65.5
  male N32.89
Cystolithiasis N21.0
Cystoma —*see also* Neoplasm, benign,
  by site
  endometrial, ovary N80.1
  mucinous
    specified site —*see* Neoplasm, benign,
      by site
    unspecified site D27.9
  serous
    specified site —*see* Neoplasm, benign,
      by site
    unspecified site D27.9
  simple (ovary) N83.29
Cystoplegia N31.2
Cystoptosis N32.89
Cystopyelitis —*see* Pyelonephritis
Cystorrhagia N32.89
Cystosarcoma phyllodes D48.6-
  benign D24-
  malignant —*see* Neoplasm, breast,
    malignant
Cystostomy
  attention to Z43.5
  complication —*see* Complications,
    cystostomy
  status Z93.50
    appendico-vesicostomy Z93.52
    cutaneous Z93.51
    specified NEC Z93.59
Cystourethritis —*see* Urethritis
Cystourethrocele —*see also* Cystocele
  female N81.10
    with uterine prolapse —*see* Prolapse,
      uterus
    lateral N81.12
    midline N81.11
    paravaginal N81.12
  male N32.89
Cytomegalic inclusion disease
  congenital P35.1
Cytomegalovirus infection B25.9
Cytomycosis (reticuloendothelial) B39.4
Cytopenia D75.9
  refractory
    with multilineage dysplasia D46.A
      and ring sideroblasts
        (RCMD RS) D46.B
Czerny's disease (periodic hydrarthrosis
  of the knee) —*see* Effusion, joint,
  knee

D

Daae (-Finsen) disease (epidemic
    pleurodynia) B33.0
Dabney's grip B33.0
Da Costa's syndrome F45.8
Dacryoadenitis, dacryadenitis H04.00-
    acute H04.01-
    chronic H04.02-
Dacryocystitis H04.30-
    acute H04.32-
    chronic H04.41-
    neonatal P39.1
    phlegmonous H04.31-
    syphilitic A52.71
        congenital (early) A50.01
    trachomatous, active A71.1
        sequelae (late effect) B94.0
Dacryocystoblenorrhea —see
        Inflammation, lacrimal, passages,
        chronic
Dacryocystocele —see Disorder, lacrimal
        system, changes
Dacryolith, dacryolithiasis H04.51-
Dacryoma —see Disorder, lacrimal
        system, changes
Dacryopericystitis —see Dacryocystitis
Dacryops H04.11-
Dacryostenosis —see also Stenosis,
        lacrimal
    congenital Q10.5
Dactylitis
    bone —see Osteomyelitis
    sickle-cell D57.00
        Hb C D57.219
        Hb SS D57.00
        specified NEC D57.819
    skin L08.9
    syphilitic A52.77
    tuberculous A18.03
Dactylolysis spontanea (ainhum) L94.6
Dactylosymphysis Q70.9
    fingers —see Syndactylism, complex,
        fingers
    toes —see Syndactylism, complex, toes
Damage
    arteriosclerotic —see Arteriosclerosis
    brain (nontraumatic) G93.9
        anoxic, hypoxic G93.1
            resulting from a procedure G97.82
        child NEC G80.9
        due to birth injury P11.2
    cardiorenal (vascular) —see
        Hypertension, cardiorenal
    cerebral NEC —see Damage, brain
    coccyx, complicating delivery O71.6
    coronary —see Disease, heart, ischemic
    eye, birth injury P15.3
    liver (nontraumatic) K76.9
        alcoholic K70.9
        due to drugs —see Disease, liver, toxic
        toxic —see Disease, liver, toxic
    medication T88.7
    pelvic
        joint or ligament, during delivery
            O71.6
        organ NEC
            during delivery O71.5
            following ectopic or molar
                pregnancy O08.6
    renal —see Disease, renal
    subendocardium, subendocardial —see
        Degeneration, myocardial
    vascular I99.9

Dana-Putnam syndrome (subacute
    combined sclerosis with pernicious
    anemia) —see Degeneration,
    combined
Danbolt (-Cross) syndrome
    (acrodermatitis enteropathica) E83.2
Dandruff L21.0
Dandy-Walker syndrome Q03.1
    with spina bifida —see Spina bifida
Danlos' syndrome Q79.6
Darier (-White) disease (congenital)
    Q82.8
    meaning erythema annulare
        centrifugum L53.1
Darier-Roussy sarcoid D86.3
Darling's disease or histoplasmosis B39.4
Darwin's tubercle Q17.8
Dawson's (inclusion body) encephalitis
    A81.1
De Beurmann (-Gougerot) disease B42.1
De la Tourette's syndrome F95.2
De Lange's syndrome Q87.1
De Morgan's spots (senile angiomas) I78.1
De Quervain's
    disease (tendon sheath) M65.4
    syndrome E34.51
    thyroiditis (subacute granulomatous
        thyroiditis) E06.1
De Toni-Fanconi (-Debré) syndrome
    E72.09
    with cystinosis E72.04
Dead
    fetus, retained (mother) O36.4
        early pregnancy O02.1
    labyrinth —see subcategory H83.2
    ovum, retained O02.0
Deaf nonspeaking NEC H91.3
Deafmutism (acquired) (congenital) NEC
    H91.3
    hysterical F44.6
    syphilitic, congenital (see also
        subcategory H94.8) A50.09
Deafness (acquired) (complete)
    (hereditary) (partial) H91.9-
    with blue sclera and fragility of bone
        Q78.0
    auditory fatigue —see Deafness,
        specified type NEC
    aviation T70.0
        nerve injury —see Injury, nerve,
            acoustic, specified type NEC
    boilermaker's —see subcategory H83.3
    central —see Deafness, sensorineural
    conductive H90.2
        and sensorineural, mixed H90.8
            bilateral H90.6
        bilateral H90.0
        unilateral H90.1-
    congenital H90.5
        with blue sclera and fragility of bone
            Q78.0
    due to toxic agents —see Deafness,
        ototoxic
    emotional (hysterical) F44.6
    functional (hysterical) F44.6
    high frequency H91.9-
    hysterical F44.6
    low frequency H91.9-
    mental R48.8
    mixed conductive and sensorineural
        H90.8
        bilateral H90.6
        unilateral H90.7-
    nerve —see Deafness, sensorineural
    neural —see Deafness, sensorineural

Deafness (Continued)
    noise-induced —see also subcategory
        H83.3
        nerve injury —see Injury, nerve,
            acoustic, specified type NEC
    nonspeaking H91.3
    ototoxic —see subcategory H91.0
    perceptive —see Deafness, sensorineural
    psychogenic (hysterical) F44.6
    sensorineural H90.5
        and conductive, mixed H90.8
            bilateral H90.6
        bilateral H90.3
        unilateral H90.4-
    sensory —see Deafness, sensorineural
    specified type NEC —see subcategory
        H91.8
    sudden (idiopathic) H91.2-
    syphilitic A52.15
    transient ischemic H93.01-
    traumatic —see Injury, nerve, acoustic,
        specified type NEC
    word (developmental) H93.25
Death (cause unknown) (of) (unexplained)
    (unspecified cause) R99
    brain G93.82
    cardiac (sudden) (with successful
        resuscitation) — code to
        underlying disease
    family history of Z82.41
    personal history of Z86.74
    family member (assumed) Z63.4
Debility (chronic) (general) (nervous)
    R53.81
    congenital or neonatal NOS P96.9
    nervous R53.81
    old age R54
    senile R54
Débove's disease (splenomegaly) R16.1
Decalcification
    bone —see Osteoporosis
    teeth K03.89
Decapsulation, kidney N28.89
Decay
    dental —see Caries, dental
    senile R54
    tooth, teeth —see Caries, dental
Deciduitis (acute)
    following ectopic or molar pregnancy
        O08.0
Decline (general) —see Debility
    cognitive, age-associated R41.81
Decompensation
    cardiac (acute) (chronic) —see Disease,
        heart
    cardiovascular —see Disease,
        cardiovascular
    heart —see Disease, heart
    hepatic —see Failure, hepatic
    myocardial (acute) (chronic) —see
        Disease, heart
    respiratory J98.8
Decompression sickness T70.3
Decrease (d)
    absolute neutrophile count —see
        Neutropenia
    blood
        platelets —see Thrombocytopenia
        pressure R03.1
            due to shock following
                injury T79.4
                operation T81.19
    estrogen E28.39
        postablative E89.40
            asymptomatic E89.40
            symptomatic E89.41

Decrease (d) *(Continued)*
  fragility of erythrocytes D58.8
  function
    lipase (pancreatic) K90.3
    ovary in hypopituitarism E23.0
    parenchyma of pancreas K86.8
    pituitary (gland) (anterior) (lobe) E23.0
      posterior (lobe) E23.0
  functional activity R68.89
  glucose R73.09
  hematocrit R71.0
  hemoglobin R71.0
  leukocytes D72.819
    specified NEC D72.818
  libido R68.82
  lymphocytes D72.810
  platelets D69.6
  respiration, due to shock following
      injury T79.4
  sexual desire R68.82
  tear secretion NEC —*see* Syndrome,
      dry eye
  tolerance
    fat K90.4
    glucose R73.09
    pancreatic K90.3
    salt and water E87.8
  vision NEC H54.7
  white blood cell count D72.819
    specified NEC D72.818
Decubitus (ulcer) —*see* Ulcer, pressure,
    by site
  cervix N86
Deepening acetabulum —*see*
    Derangement, joint, specified type
    NEC, hip
Defect, defective Q89.9
  3-beta-hydroxysteroid dehydrogenase
      E25.0
  11-hydroxylase E25.0
  21-hydroxylase E25.0
  abdominal wall, congenital Q79.59
  antibody immunodeficiency D80.9
  aorticopulmonary septum Q21.4
  atrial septal (ostium secundum type)
      Q21.1
    following acute myocardial
        infarction (current
        complication) I23.1
    ostium primum type Q21.2
  atrioventricular
    canal Q21.2
    septum Q21.2
  auricular septal Q21.1
  bilirubin excretion NEC E80.6
  biosynthesis, androgen (testicular) E29.1
  bulbar septum Q21.0
  catalase E80.3
  cell membrane receptor complex (CR3)
      D71
  circulation I99.9
    congenital Q28.9
    newborn Q28.9
  coagulation (factor) *(see also* Deficiency,
      factor) D68.9
    with
      ectopic pregnancy O08.1
      molar pregnancy O08.1
    acquired D68.4
    antepartum with hemorrhage —*see*
        Hemorrhage, antepartum, with
        coagulation defect
    due to
      liver disease D68.4
      vitamin K deficiency D68.4

Defect, defective *(Continued)*
  coagulation *(Continued)*
    hereditary NEC D68.2
    intrapartum O67.0
    newborn, transient P61.6
    postpartum O72.3
    specified type NEC D68.8
  complement system D84.1
  conduction (heart) I45.9
    bone —*see* Deafness, conductive
  congenital, organ or site not listed —*see*
      Anomaly, by site
  coronary sinus Q21.1
  cushion, endocardial Q21.2
  degradation, glycoprotein E77.1
  dental bridge, crown, fillings —*see*
      Defect, dental restoration
  dental restoration K08.50
    specified NEC K08.59
  dentin (hereditary) K00.5
  Descemet's membrane, congenital
      Q13.89
  developmental —*see also* Anomaly
    cauda equina Q06.3
  diaphragm
    with elevation, eventration or
        hernia —*see* Hernia, diaphragm
    congenital Q79.1
      with hernia Q79.0
      gross (with hernia) Q79.0
  ectodermal, congenital Q82.9
  Eisenmenger's Q21.8
  enzyme
    catalase E80.3
    peroxidase E80.3
  esophagus, congenital Q39.9
  extensor retinaculum M62.89
  fibrin polymerization D68.2
  filling
    bladder R93.4
    kidney R93.4
    stomach R93.3
    ureter R93.4
  Gerbode Q21.0
  glycoprotein degradation E77.1
  Hageman (factor) D68.2
  hearing —*see* Deafness
  high grade F70
  interatrial septal Q21.1
  interauricular septal Q21.1
  interventricular septal Q21.0
    with dextroposition of aorta,
        pulmonary stenosis and
        hypertrophy of right ventricle
        Q21.3
    in tetralogy of Fallot Q21.3
  learning (specific) —*see* Disorder,
      learning
  lymphocyte function antigen-1 (LFA-1)
      D84.0
  lysosomal enzyme, post-translational
      modification E77.0
  major osseous M89.70
    ankle M89.77-
    carpus M89.74-
    clavicle M89.71-
    femur M89.75-
    fibula M89.76-
    fingers M89.74-
    foot M89.77-
    forearm M89.73-
    hand M89.74-
    humerus M89.72-
    lower leg M89.76-
    metacarpus M89.74-

Defect, defective *(Continued)*
  major osseous *(Continued)*
    metatarsus M89.77-
    multiple sites M89.79
    pelvic region M89.75-
    pelvis M89.75-
    radius M89.73-
    scapula M89.71-
    shoulder region M89.71-
    specified NEC M89.78
    tarsus M89.77-
    thigh M89.75-
    tibia M89.76-
    toes M89.77-
    ulna M89.73-
  mental —*see* Disability, intellectual
  modification, lysosomal enzymes, post-
      translational E77.0
  obstructive, congenital
    renal pelvis Q62.39
    ureter Q62.39
      atresia —*see* Atresia, ureter
      cecoureterocele Q62.32
      megaureter Q62.2
      orthotopic ureterocele Q62.31
  osseous, major M89.70
    ankle M89.77-
    carpus M89.74-
    clavicle M89.71-
    femur M89.75-
    fibula M89.76-
    fingers M89.74-
    foot M89.77-
    forearm M89.73-
    hand M89.74-
    humerus M89.72-
    lower leg M89.76-
    metacarpus M89.74-
    metatarsus M89.77-
    multiple sites M89.9
    pelvic region M89.75-
    pelvis M89.75-
    radius M89.73-
    scapula M89.71-
    shoulder region M89.71-
    specified NEC M89.78
    tarsus M89.77-
    thigh M89.75-
    tibia M89.76-
    toes M89.77-
    ulna M89.73-
  osteochondral NEC *(see also* Deformity)
      M95.8-
  ostium
    primum Q21.2
    secundum Q21.1
  peroxidase E80.3
  placental blood supply —*see*
      Insufficiency, placental
  platelets, qualitative D69.1
    constitutional D68.0
  postural NEC, spine —*see* Dorsopathy,
      deforming
  reduction
    limb Q73.8
      lower Q72.9-
        absence —*see* Agenesis, leg
          foot —*see* Agenesis, foot
        longitudinal
          femur Q72.4-
          fibula Q72.6-
          tibia Q72.5-
        specified type NEC Q72.89-
        split foot Q72.7-

Defect, defective (Continued)
 reduction (Continued)
  limb (Continued)
   specified type NEC Q73.8
   upper Q71.9-
    absence —see Agenesis, arm
    forearm —see Agenesis,
     forearm
    hand —see Agenesis, hand
    lobster-claw hand Q71.6-
    longitudinal
     radius Q71.4-
     ulna Q71.5-
    specified type NEC Q71.89-
  renal pelvis Q63.8
   obstructive Q62.39
  respiratory system, congenital Q34.9
  restoration, dental K08.50
   specified NEC K08.59
  retinal nerve bundle fibers H35.89
  septal (heart) NOS Q21.9
   acquired (atrial) (auricular)
    (ventricular) (old) I51.0
   atrial Q21.1
    concurrent with acute myocardial
     infarction —see Infarct,
     myocardium
    following acute myocardial
     infarction (current
     complication) I23.1
   ventricular (see also Defect,
    ventricular septal) Q21.0
  sinus venosus Q21.1
  speech R47.9
   developmental F80.9
   specified NEC R47.89
  Taussig-Bing (aortic transposition and
   overriding pulmonary artery)
   Q20.1
  teeth, wedge K03.1
  vascular (local) I99.9
   congenital Q27.9
  ventricular septal Q21.0
   concurrent with acute myocardial
    infarction —see Infarct,
    myocardium
   following acute myocardial infarction
    (current complication) I23.2
   in tetralogy of Fallot Q21.3
  vision NEC H54.7
  visual field H53.40
   bilateral
    heteronymous H53.47
    homonymous H53.46-
   generalized contraction H53.48-
   localized
    arcuate H53.43-
    scotoma (central area) H53.41-
     blind spot area H53.42-
    sector H53.43-
    specified type NEC H53.45-
  voice R49.9
   specified NEC R49.8
  wedge, tooth, teeth (abrasion) K03.1
Deferentitis N49.1
 gonorrheal (acute) (chronic) A54.23
Defibrination (syndrome) D65
 antepartum —see Hemorrhage,
  antepartum, with coagulation
  defect, disseminated intravascular
  coagulation
 following ectopic or molar pregnancy
  O08.1
 intrapartum O67.0

Defibrination (Continued)
 newborn P60
 postpartum O72.3
Deficiency, deficient
 3-beta hydroxysteroid dehydrogenase
  E25.0
 11-hydroxylase E25.0
 21-hydroxylase E25.0
 5-alpha reductase (with male
  pseudohermaphroditism) E29.1
 abdominal muscle syndrome Q79.4
 AC globulin (congenital) (hereditary)
  D68.2
  acquired D68.4
 accelerator globulin (Ac G) (blood) D68.2
 acid phosphatase E83.39
 activating factor (blood) D68.2
 adenosine deaminase (ADA) D81.3
 aldolase (hereditary) E74.19
 alpha-1-antitrypsin E88.01
 amino-acids E72.9
 anemia —see Anemia
 aneurin E51.9
 antibody with
  hyperimmunoglobulinemia D80.6
  near-normal immunoglobins D80.6
 antidiuretic hormone E23.2
 anti-hemophilic
  factor (A) D66
   B D67
   C D68.1
  globulin (AHG) NEC D66
 antithrombin (antithrombin III) D68.59
 ascorbic acid E54
 attention (disorder) (syndrome) F98.8
  with hyperactivity —see Disorder,
   attention-deficit hyperactivity
 autoprothrombin
  I D68.2
  II D67
  C D68.2
 beta-glucuronidase E76.29
 biotin E53.8
 biotin-dependent carboxylase D81.819
 biotinidase D81.810
 brancher enzyme (amylopectinosis)
  E74.03
 C1 esterase inhibitor (C1-INH) D84.1
 calciferol E55.9
  with
   adult osteomalacia M83.8
   rickets —see Rickets
 calcium (dietary) E58
 calorie, severe E43
  with marasmus E41
   and kwashiorkor E42
 cardiac —see Insufficiency, myocardial
 carnitine E71.40
  due to
   hemodialysis E71.43
   inborn errors of metabolism E71.42
   Valproic acid therapy E71.43
  iatrogenic E71.43
  muscle palmityltransferase E71.314
  primary E71.41
  secondary E71.448
 carotene E50.9
 central nervous system G96.8
 ceruloplasmin (Wilson) E83.01
 choline E53.8
 Christmas factor D67
 chromium E61.4
 clotting (blood) (see also Deficiency,
  coagulation factor) D68.9

Deficiency, deficient (Continued)
 clotting factor NEC (hereditary) (see also
  Deficiency, factor) D68.2
 coagulation NOS D68.9
  with
   ectopic pregnancy O08.1
   molar pregnancy O08.1
  acquired (any) D68.4
  antepartum hemorrhage —see
   Hemorrhage, antepartum, with
   coagulation defect
  clotting factor NEC (see also
   Deficiency, factor) D68.2
  due to
   hyperprothrombinemia D68.4
   liver disease D68.4
   vitamin K deficiency D68.4
  newborn, transient P61.6
  postpartum O72.3
  specified NEC D68.8
 cognitive F09
 color vision H53.50
  achromatopsia H53.51
  acquired H53.52
  deuteranomaly H53.53
  protanomaly H53.54
  specified type NEC H53.59
  tritanomaly H53.55
 combined glucocorticoid and
  mineralocorticoid E27.49
 contact factor D68.2
 copper (nutritional) E61.0
 corticoadrenal E27.40
  primary E27.1
 craniofacial axis Q75.0
 cyanocobalamin E53.8
 debrancher enzyme (limit dextrinosis)
  E74.03
 dehydrogenase
  long chain/very long chain acyl CoA
   E71.310
  medium chain acyl CoA E71.311
  short chain acyl CoA E71.312
 diet E63.9
 dihydropyrimidine dehydrogenase
  (DPD) E88.89
 disaccharidase E73.9
 edema —see Malnutrition, severe
 endocrine E34.9
 energy-supply —see Malnutrition
 enzymes, circulating NEC E88.09
 ergosterol E55.9
  with
   adult osteomalacia M83.8
   rickets —see Rickets
 essential fatty acid (EFA) E63.0
 factor —see also Deficiency, coagulation
  Hageman D68.2
  I (congenital) (hereditary) D68.2
  II (congenital) (hereditary) D68.2
  IX (congenital) (functional)
   (hereditary) (with functional
   defect) D67
  multiple (congenital) D68.8
   acquired D68.4
  V (congenital) (hereditary) D68.2
  VII (congenital) (hereditary) D68.2
  VIII (congenital) (functional)
   (hereditary) (with functional
   defect) D66
   with vascular defect D68.0
  X (congenital) (hereditary) D68.2
  XI (congenital) (hereditary) D68.1
  XII (congenital) (hereditary) D68.2
  XIII (congenital) (hereditary) D68.2

Deficiency, deficient (Continued)
femoral, proximal focal (congenital) —
see Defect, reduction, lower limb,
longitudinal, femur
fibrin-stabilizing factor (congenital)
(hereditary) D68.2
acquired D68.4
fibrinase D68.2
fibrinogen (congenital) (hereditary)
D68.2
acquired D65
folate E53.8
folic acid E53.8
foreskin N47.3
fructokinase E74.11
fructose 1,6-diphosphatase E74.19
fructose-1-phosphate aldolase E74.19
galactokinase E74.29
galactose-1-phosphate uridyl
transferase E74.29
gammaglobulin in blood D80.1
hereditary D80.0
glass factor D68.2
glucocorticoid E27.49
mineralocorticoid E27.49
glucose-6-phosphatase E74.01
glucose-6-phosphate dehydrogenase
anemia D55.0
glucuronyl transferase E80.5
glycogen synthetase E74.09
gonadotropin (isolated) E23.0
growth hormone (idiopathic) (isolated)
E23.0
Hageman factor D68.2
hemoglobin D64.9
hepatophosphorylase E74.09
homogentisate 1,2-dioxygenase E70.29
hormone
anterior pituitary (partial) NEC
E23.0
growth E23.0
growth (isolated) E23.0
pituitary E23.0
testicular E29.1
hypoxanthine-(guanine)-
phosphoribosyltransferase
(HG-PRT) (total HG-PRT) E79.1
immunity D84.9
cell-mediated D84.8
with thrombocytopenia and
eczema D82.0
combined D81.9
humoral D80.9
IgA (secretory) D80.2
IgG D80.3
IgM D80.4
immuno —see Immunodeficiency
immunoglobulin, selective
A (IgA) D80.2
G (IgG) (subclasses) D80.3
M (IgM) D80.4
inositol (B complex) E53.8
intrinsic
factor (congenital) D51.0
sphincter N36.42
with urethral hypermobility
N36.43
iodine E61.8
congenital syndrome —see Syndrome,
iodine-deficiency, congenital
iron E61.1
anemia D50.9
kalium E87.6
kappa-light chain D80.8

Deficiency, deficient (Continued)
labile factor (congenital) (hereditary)
D68.2
acquired D68.4
lacrimal fluid (acquired) —see also
Syndrome, dry eye
congenital Q10.6
lactase
congenital E73.0
secondary E73.1
Laki-Lorand factor D68.2
lecithin cholesterol acyltransferase
E78.6
lipocaic K86.8
lipoprotein (familial) (high density)
E78.6
liver phosphorylase E74.09
lysosomal alpha-1, 4 glucosidase E74.02
magnesium E61.2
major histocompatibility complex
class I D81.6
class II D81.7
manganese E61.3
menadione (vitamin K) E56.1
newborn P53
mental (familial) (hereditary) —see
Disability, intellectual
methylenetetrahydrofolate reductase
(MTHFR) E72.12
mineral NEC E61.8
mineralocorticoid E27.49
with glucocorticoid E27.49
molybdenum (nutritional) E61.5
moral F60.2
multiple nutrient elements E61.7
muscle
carnitine (palmityltransferase)
E71.314
phosphofructokinase E74.09
myoadenylate deaminase E79.2
myocardial —see Insufficiency,
myocardial
myophosphorylase E74.04
NADH diaphorase or reductase
(congenital) D74.0
NADH-methemoglobin reductase
(congenital) D74.0
natrium E87.1
niacin (amide) (-tryptophan) E52
nicotinamide E52
nicotinic acid E52
number of teeth —see Anodontia
nutrient element E61.9
multiple E61.7
specified NEC E61.8
nutrition, nutritional E63.9
sequelae —see Sequelae, nutritional
deficiency
specified NEC E63.8
ornithine transcarbamylase E72.4
ovarian E28.39
oxygen —see Anoxia
pantothenic acid E53.8
parathyroid (gland) E20.9
perineum (female) N81.89
phenylalanine hydroxylase E70.1
phosphoenolpyruvate carboxykinase
E74.4
phosphofructokinase E74.19
phosphomannomutase E74.8
phosphomannose isomerase E74.8
phosphomannosyl mutase E74.8
phosphorylase kinase, liver E74.09
pituitary hormone (isolated) E23.0

Deficiency, deficient (Continued)
plasma thromboplastin
antecedent (PTA) D68.1
component (PTC) D67
platelet NEC D69.1
constitutional D68.0
polyglandular E31.8
autoimmune E31.0
potassium (K) E87.6
prepuce N47.3
proaccelerin (congenital) (hereditary)
D68.2
acquired D68.4
proconvertin factor (congenital)
(hereditary) D68.2
acquired D68.4
protein (see also Malnutrition) E46
anemia D53.0
C D68.59
S D68.59
prothrombin (congenital) (hereditary)
D68.2
acquired D68.4
Prower factor D68.2
pseudocholinesterase E88.09
PTA (plasma thromboplastin
antecedent) D68.1
PTC (plasma thromboplastin
component) D67
purine nucleoside phosphorylase (PNP)
D81.5
pyracin (alpha) (beta) E53.1
pyridoxal E53.1
pyridoxamine E53.1
pyridoxine (derivatives) E53.1
pyruvate
carboxylase E74.4
dehydrogenase E74.4
riboflavin (vitamin B2) E53.0
salt E87.1
secretion
ovary E28.39
salivary gland (any) K11.7
urine R34
selenium (dietary) E59
serum antitrypsin, familial E88.01
short stature homeobox gene (SHOX)
with
dyschondrosteosis Q78.8
short stature (idiopathic) E34.3
Turner's syndrome Q96.9
sodium (Na) E87.1
SPCA (factor VII) D68.2
sphincter, intrinsic N36.42
with urethral hypermobility N36.43
stable factor (congenital) (hereditary)
D68.2
acquired D68.4
Stuart-Prower (factor X) D68.2
sucrase E74.39
sulfatase E75.29
sulfite oxidase E72.19
thiamin, thiaminic (chloride) E51.9
beriberi (dry) E51.11
wet E51.12
thrombokinase D68.2
newborn P53
thyroid (gland) —see Hypothyroidism
tocopherol E56.0
tooth bud K00.0
transcobalamine II (anemia) D51.2
vanadium E61.6
vascular I99.9
vasopressin E23.2

Deficiency, deficient (*Continued*)
viosterol —*see* Deficiency, calciferol
vitamin (multiple) NOS E56.9
A E50.9
with
Bitot's spot (corneal) E50.1
follicular keratosis E50.8
keratomalacia E50.4
manifestations NEC E50.8
night blindness E50.5
scar of cornea, xerophthalmic
E50.6
xeroderma E50.8
xerophthalmia E50.7
xerosis
conjunctival E50.0
and Bitot's spot E50.1
cornea E50.2
and ulceration E50.3
sequelae E64.1
B (complex) NOS E53.9
with
beriberi (dry) E51.11
wet E51.12
pellagra E52
B1 NOS E51.9
beriberi (dry) E51.11
with circulatory system
manifestations E51.11
wet E51.12
B12 E53.8
B2 (riboflavin) E53.0
B6 E53.1
C E54
sequelae E64.2
D E55.9
with
adult osteomalacia M83.8
rickets —*see* Rickets
25-hydroxylase E83.32
E E56.0
folic acid E53.8
G E53.0
group B E53.9
specified NEC E53.8
H (biotin) E53.8
K E56.1
of newborn P53
nicotinic E52
P E56.8
PP (pellagra-preventing) E52
specified NEC E56.8
thiamin E51.9
beriberi —*see* Beriberi
zinc, dietary E60
Deficit —*see also* Deficiency
attention and concentration R41.840
disorder —*see* Attention, deficit
cognitive communication R41.841
cognitive NEC R41.89
following
cerebral infarction I69.31
cerebrovascular disease I69.91
specified disease NEC I69.81
intracerebral hemorrhage I69.11
nontraumatic intracranial
hemorrhage NEC I69.21
subarachnoid hemorrhage I69.01
concentration R41.840
executive function R41.844
frontal lobe R41.844
neurologic NEC R29.818
ischemic
reversible (RIND) I63.9
prolonged (PRIND) I63.9

Deficit (*Continued*)
oxygen R09.02
prolonged reversible ischemic
neurologic (PRIND) I63.9
psychomotor R41.843
visuospatial R41.842
Deflection
radius —*see* Deformity, limb, specified
type NEC, forearm
septum (acquired) (nasal) (nose) J34.2
spine —*see* Curvature, spine
turbinate (nose) J34.2
Defluvium
capillorum —*see* Alopecia
ciliorum —*see* Madarosis
unguium L60.8
Deformity Q89.9
abdomen, congenital Q89.9
abdominal wall
acquired M95.8
congenital Q79.59
acquired (unspecified site) M95.9
adrenal gland Q89.1
alimentary tract, congenital Q45.9
upper Q40.9
ankle (joint) (acquired) —*see also*
Deformity, limb, lower leg
abduction —*see* Contraction, joint,
ankle
congenital Q68.8
contraction —*see* Contraction, joint,
ankle
specified type NEC —*see* Deformity,
limb, foot, specified NEC
anus (acquired) K62.89
congenital Q43.9
aorta (arch) (congenital) Q25.4
acquired I77.89
aortic
arch, acquired I77.89
cusp or valve (congenital) Q23.8
acquired (*see also* Endocarditis,
aortic) I35.8
arm (acquired) (upper) —*see also*
Deformity, limb, upper arm
congenital Q68.8
forearm —*see* Deformity, limb, forearm
artery (congenital) (peripheral) NOS
Q27.9
acquired I77.89
coronary (acquired) I25.9
congenital Q24.5
umbilical Q27.0
atrial septal Q21.1
auditory canal (external) (congenital) —
see also Malformation, ear, external
acquired —*see* Disorder, ear, external,
specified type NEC
auricle
ear (congenital) —*see also*
Malformation, ear, external
acquired —*see* Disorder, pinna,
deformity
back —*see* Dorsopathy, deforming
bile duct (common) (congenital)
(hepatic) Q44.5
acquired K83.8
biliary duct or passage (congenital) Q44.5
acquired K83.8
bladder (neck) (trigone) (sphincter)
(acquired) N32.89
congenital Q64.79
bone (acquired) NOS M95.9
congenital Q79.9
turbinate M95.0

Deformity (*Continued*)
brain (congenital) Q04.9
acquired G93.89
reduction Q04.3
breast (acquired) N64.89
congenital Q83.9
reconstructed N65.0
bronchus (congenital) Q32.4
acquired NEC J98.09
bursa, congenital Q79.9
canaliculi (lacrimalis) (acquired) —*see also*
Disorder, lacrimal system, changes
congenital Q10.6
canthus, acquired —*see* Disorder, eyelid,
specified type NEC
capillary (acquired) I78.8
cardiovascular system, congenital Q28.9
caruncle, lacrimal (acquired) —*see also*
Disorder, lacrimal system, changes
congenital Q10.6
cascade, stomach K31.2
cecum (congenital) Q43.9
acquired K63.89
cerebral, acquired G93.89
congenital Q04.9
cervix (uterus) (acquired) NEC N88.8
congenital Q51.9
cheek (acquired) M95.2
congenital Q18.9
chest (acquired) (wall) M95.4
congenital Q67.8
sequelae (late effect) of rickets E64.3
chin (acquired) M95.2
congenital Q18.9
choroid (congenital) Q14.3
acquired H31.8
plexus Q07.8
acquired G96.19
cicatricial —*see* Cicatrix
cilia, acquired —*see* Disorder, eyelid,
specified type NEC
clavicle (acquired) M95.8
congenital Q68.8
clitoris (congenital) Q52.6
acquired N90.89
clubfoot —*see* Clubfoot
coccyx (acquired) —*see* subcategory
M43.8
colon (congenital) Q43.9
acquired K63.89
concha (ear), congenital —*see also*
Malformation, ear, external
acquired —*see* Disorder, pinna,
deformity
cornea (acquired) H18.70
congenital Q13.4
descemetocele —*see* Descemetocele
ectasia —*see* Ectasia, cornea
specified NEC H18.79-
staphyloma —*see* Staphyloma, cornea
coronary artery (acquired) I25.9
congenital Q24.5
cranium (acquired) —*see* Deformity,
skull
cricoid cartilage (congenital) Q31.8
acquired J38.7
cystic duct (congenital) Q44.5
acquired K82.8
Dandy-Walker Q03.1
with spina bifida —*see* Spina bifida
diaphragm (congenital) Q79.1
acquired J98.6
digestive organ NOS Q45.9
ductus arteriosus Q25.0
duodenal bulb K31.89

Deformity *(Continued)*
　duodenum (congenital) Q43.9
　　acquired K31.89
　dura —*see* Deformity, meninges
　ear (acquired) —*see also* Disorder, pinna, deformity
　　congenital (external) Q17.9
　　　internal Q16.5
　　　middle Q16.4
　　　　ossicles Q16.3
　　　ossicles Q16.3
　ectodermal (congenital) NEC Q84.9
　ejaculatory duct (congenital) Q55.4
　　acquired N50.8
　elbow (joint) (acquired) —*see also* Deformity, limb, upper arm
　　congenital Q68.8
　　contraction —*see* Contraction, joint, elbow
　endocrine gland NEC Q89.2
　epididymis (congenital) Q55.4
　　acquired N50.3
　epiglottis (congenital) Q31.8
　　acquired J38.7
　esophagus (congenital) Q39.9
　　acquired K22.8
　eustachian tube (congenital) NEC Q17.8
　eye, congenital Q15.9
　eyebrow (congenital) Q18.8
　eyelid (acquired) —*see also* Disorder, eyelid, specified type NEC
　　congenital Q10.3
　face (acquired) M95.2
　　congenital Q18.9
　fallopian tube, acquired N83.8
　femur (acquired) —*see* Deformity, limb, specified type NEC, thigh
　fetal
　　with fetopelvic disproportion O33.7
　　causing obstructed labor O66.3
　finger (acquired) M20.00-
　　boutonniere M20.02-
　　congenital Q68.1
　　flexion contracture —*see* Contraction, joint, hand
　　mallet finger M20.01-
　　specified NEC M20.09-
　　swan-neck M20.03-
　flexion (joint) (acquired) (*see also* Deformity, limb, flexion) M21.20
　　congenital NOS Q74.9
　　hip Q65.89
　foot (acquired) —*see also* Deformity, limb, lower leg
　　cavovarus (congenital) Q66.1
　　congenital NOS Q66.9
　　　specified type NEC Q66.89
　　specified type NEC —*see* Deformity, limb, foot, specified NEC
　　valgus (congenital) Q66.6
　　　acquired —*see* Deformity, valgus, ankle
　　varus (congenital) NEC Q66.3
　　　acquired —*see* Deformity, varus, ankle
　forearm (acquired) —*see also* Deformity, limb, forearm
　　congenital Q68.8
　forehead (acquired) M95.2
　　congenital Q75.8
　frontal bone (acquired) M95.2
　　congenital Q75.8
　gallbladder (congenital) Q44.1
　　acquired K82.8

Deformity *(Continued)*
　gastrointestinal tract (congenital) NOS Q45.9
　　acquired K63.89
　genitalia, genital organ (s) or system NEC
　　female (congenital) Q52.9
　　　acquired N94.89
　　　external Q52.70
　　male (congenital) Q55.9
　　　acquired N50.8
　globe (eye) (congenital) Q15.8
　　acquired H44.89
　gum, acquired NEC K06.8
　hand (acquired) —*see* Deformity, limb, hand
　　congenital Q68.1
　head (acquired) M95.2
　　congenital Q75.8
　heart (congenital) Q24.9
　　septum Q21.9
　　　auricular Q21.1
　　　ventricular Q21.0
　　valve (congenital) NEC Q24.8
　　　acquired —*see* Endocarditis
　heel (acquired) —*see* Deformity, foot
　hepatic duct (congenital) Q44.5
　　acquired K83.8
　hip (joint) (acquired) —*see also* Deformity, limb, thigh
　　congenital Q65.9
　　due to (previous) juvenile osteochondrosis —*see* Coxa, plana
　　flexion —*see* Contraction, joint, hip
　hourglass —*see* Contraction, hourglass
　humerus (acquired) M21.82-
　　congenital Q74.0
　hypophyseal (congenital) Q89.2
　ileocecal (coil) (valve) (acquired) K63.89
　　congenital Q43.9
　ileum (congenital) Q43.9
　　acquired K63.89
　ilium (acquired) M95.5
　　congenital Q74.2
　integument (congenital) Q84.9
　intervertebral cartilage or disc (acquired) —*see* Disorder, disc, specified NEC
　intestine (large) (small) (congenital) NOS Q43.9
　　acquired K63.89
　intrinsic minus or plus (hand) —*see* Deformity, limb, specified type NEC, forearm
　iris (acquired) H21.89
　　congenital Q13.2
　ischium (acquired) M95.5
　　congenital Q74.2
　jaw (acquired) (congenital) M26.9
　joint (acquired) NEC M21.90
　　congenital Q68.8
　　elbow M21.92-
　　hand M21.94-
　　hip M21.95-
　　knee M21.96-
　　shoulder M21.92-
　　wrist M21.93-
　kidney (s) (calyx) (pelvis) (congenital) Q63.9
　　acquired N28.89
　　artery (congenital) Q27.2
　　　acquired I77.89
　Klippel-Feil (brevicollis) Q76.1

Deformity *(Continued)*
　knee (acquired) NEC —*see also* Deformity, limb, lower leg
　　congenital Q68.2
　labium (majus) (minus) (congenital) Q52.79
　　acquired N90.89
　lacrimal passages or duct (congenital) NEC Q10.6
　　acquired —*see* Disorder, lacrimal system, changes
　larynx (muscle) (congenital) Q31.8
　　acquired J38.7
　　web (glottic) Q31.0
　leg (upper) (acquired) NEC —*see also* Deformity, limb, thigh
　　congenital Q68.8
　　lower leg —*see* Deformity, limb, lower leg
　lens (acquired) H27.8
　　congenital Q12.9
　lid (fold) (acquired) —*see also* Disorder, eyelid, specified type NEC
　　congenital Q10.3
　ligament (acquired) —*see* Disorder, ligament
　　congenital Q79.9
　limb (acquired) M21.90
　　clawfoot M21.53-
　　clawhand M21.51-
　　clubfoot M21.54-
　　clubhand M21.52-
　　congenital, except reduction deformity Q74.9
　　flat foot M21.4-
　　flexion M21.20
　　　ankle M21.27-
　　　elbow M21.22-
　　　finger M21.24-
　　　hip M21.25-
　　　knee M21.26-
　　　shoulder M21.21-
　　　toe M21.27-
　　　wrist M21.23-
　　foot
　　　claw —*see* Deformity, limb, clawfoot
　　　club —*see* Deformity, limb, clubfoot
　　　drop M21.37-
　　　flat —*see* Deformity, limb, flat foot
　　　specified NEC M21.6X-
　　forearm M21.93-
　　hand M21.94-
　　lower leg M21.96-
　　specified type NEC M21.80
　　　forearm M21.83-
　　　lower leg M21.86-
　　　thigh M21.85-
　　　upper arm M21.82-
　　thigh M21.95-
　　unequal length M21.70
　　　short site is
　　　　femur M21.75-
　　　　fibula M21.76-
　　　　humerus M21.72-
　　　　radius M21.73-
　　　　tibia M21.76-
　　　　ulna M21.73-
　　upper arm M21.92-
　　valgus —*see* Deformity, valgus
　　varus —*see* Deformity, varus
　　wrist drop M21.33-
　lip (acquired) NEC K13.0
　　congenital Q38.0

Deformity *(Continued)*
  liver (congenital) Q44.7
    acquired K76.89
  lumbosacral (congenital) (joint) (region)
      Q76.49
    acquired —*see* subcategory M43.8
    kyphosis —*see* Kyphosis, congenital
    lordosis —*see* Lordosis, congenital
  lung (congenital) Q33.9
    acquired J98.4
  lymphatic system, congenital Q89.9
  Madelung's (radius) Q74.0
  mandible (acquired) (congenital) M26.9
  maxilla (acquired) (congenital) M26.9
  meninges or membrane (congenital)
      Q07.9
    cerebral Q04.8
      acquired G96.19
    spinal cord (congenital) G96.19
      acquired G96.19
  metacarpus (acquired) —*see* Deformity,
      limb, forearm
    congenital Q74.0
  metatarsus (acquired) —*see* Deformity,
      foot
    congenital Q66.9
  middle ear (congenital) Q16.4
    ossicles Q16.3
  mitral (leaflets) (valve) I05.8
    parachute Q23.2
    stenosis, congenital Q23.2
  mouth (acquired) K13.79
    congenital Q38.6
  multiple, congenital NEC Q89.7
  muscle (acquired) M62.89
    congenital Q79.9
      sternocleidomastoid Q68.0
  musculoskeletal system (acquired)
      M95.9
    congenital Q79.9
    specified NEC M95.8
  nail (acquired) L60.8
    congenital Q84.6
  nasal —*see* Deformity, nose
  neck (acquired) M95.3
    congenital Q18.9
      sternocleidomastoid Q68.0
  nervous system (congenital) Q07.9
  nipple (congenital) Q83.9
    acquired N64.89
  nose (acquired) (cartilage) M95.0
    bone (turbinate) M95.0
    congenital Q30.9
      bent or squashed Q67.4
    saddle M95.0
      syphilitic A50.57
    septum (acquired) J34.2
      congenital Q30.8
    sinus (wall) (congenital) Q30.8
      acquired M95.0
    syphilitic (congenital) A50.57
      late A52.73
  ocular muscle (congenital) Q10.3
    acquired —*see* Strabismus, mechanical
  opticociliary vessels (congenital) Q13.2
  orbit (eye) (acquired) H05.30
    atrophy —*see* Atrophy, orbit
    congenital Q10.7
    due to
      bone disease NEC H05.32-
      trauma or surgery H05.33-
    enlargement —*see* Enlargement, orbit
    exostosis —*see* Exostosis, orbit
  organ of Corti (congenital) Q16.5

Deformity *(Continued)*
  ovary (congenital) Q50.39
    acquired N83.8
  oviduct, acquired N83.8
  palate (congenital) Q38.5
    acquired M27.8
    cleft (congenital) —*see* Cleft, palate
  pancreas (congenital) Q45.3
    acquired K86.8
  parathyroid (gland) Q89.2
  parotid (gland) (congenital) Q38.4
    acquired K11.8
  patella (acquired) —*see* Disorder,
      patella, specified NEC
  pelvis, pelvic (acquired) (bony) M95.5
    with disproportion (fetopelvic)
        O33.0
      causing obstructed labor O65.0
    congenital Q74.2
    rachitic sequelae (late effect) E64.3
  penis (glans) (congenital) Q55.69
    acquired N48.89
  pericardium (congenital) Q24.8
    acquired —*see* Pericarditis
  pharynx (congenital) Q38.8
    acquired J39.2
  pinna, acquired —*see also* Disorder,
      pinna, deformity
    congenital Q17.9
  pituitary (congenital) Q89.2
  posture —*see* Dorsopathy, deforming
  prepuce (congenital) Q55.69
    acquired N47.8
  prostate (congenital) Q55.4
    acquired N42.89
  pupil (congenital) Q13.2
    acquired —*see* Abnormality, pupillary
  pylorus (congenital) Q40.3
    acquired K31.89
  rachitic (acquired), old or healed E64.3
  radius (acquired) —*see also* Deformity,
      limb, forearm
    congenital Q68.8
  rectum (congenital) Q43.9
    acquired K62.89
  reduction (extremity) (limb), congenital
      (*see also* condition and site) Q73.8
    brain Q04.3
    lower —*see* Defect, reduction, lower
        limb
    upper —*see* Defect, reduction, upper
        limb
  renal —*see* Deformity, kidney
  respiratory system (congenital) Q34.9
  rib (acquired) M95.4
    congenital Q76.6
    cervical Q76.5
  rotation (joint) (acquired) —*see*
      Deformity, limb, specified site NEC
    congenital Q74.9
    hip —*see* Deformity, limb, specified
        type NEC, thigh
      congenital Q65.89
  sacroiliac joint (congenital) Q74.2
    acquired —*see* subcategory M43.8
  sacrum (acquired) —*see* subcategory
      M43.8
  saddle
    back —*see* Lordosis
    nose M95.0
      syphilitic A50.57
  salivary gland or duct (congenital)
      Q38.4
    acquired K11.8

Deformity *(Continued)*
  scapula (acquired) M95.8
    congenital Q68.8
  scrotum (congenital) —*see also*
      Malformation, testis and
      scrotum
    acquired N50.8
  seminal vesicles (congenital) Q55.4
    acquired N50.8
  septum, nasal (acquired) J34.2
  shoulder (joint) (acquired) —*see*
      Deformity, limb, upper arm
    congenital Q74.0
    contraction —*see* Contraction, joint,
        shoulder
  sigmoid (flexure) (congenital) Q43.9
    acquired K63.89
  skin (congenital) Q82.9
  skull (acquired) M95.2
    congenital Q75.8
      with
        anencephaly Q00.0
        encephalocele —*see* Encephalocele
        hydrocephalus Q03.9
          with spina bifida —*see* Spina
              bifida, by site, with
              hydrocephalus
        microcephaly Q02
  soft parts, organs or tissues (of pelvis)
      in pregnancy or childbirth NEC
        O34.8-
      causing obstructed labor O65.5
  spermatic cord (congenital) Q55.4
    acquired N50.8
    torsion —*see* Torsion, spermatic cord
  spinal —*see* Dorsopathy, deforming
    column (acquired) —*see* Dorsopathy,
        deforming
    congenital Q67.5
    cord (congenital) Q06.9
      acquired G95.89
    nerve root (congenital) Q07.9
  spine (acquired) —*see also* Dorsopathy,
      deforming
    congenital Q67.5
    rachitic E64.3
    specified NEC —*see* Dorsopathy,
        deforming, specified NEC
  spleen
    acquired D73.89
    congenital Q89.09
  Sprengel's (congenital) Q74.0
  sternocleidomastoid (muscle),
      congenital Q68.0
  sternum (acquired) M95.4
    congenital NEC Q76.7
  stomach (congenital) Q40.3
    acquired K31.89
  submandibular gland (congenital)
      Q38.4
  submaxillary gland (congenital)
      Q38.4
    acquired K11.8
  talipes —*see* Talipes
  testis (congenital) —*see also*
      Malformation, testis and scrotum
    acquired N44.8
    torsion —*see* Torsion, testis
  thigh (acquired) —*see also* Deformity,
      limb, thigh
    congenital NEC Q68.8
  thorax (acquired) (wall) M95.4
    congenital Q67.8
    sequelae of rickets E64.3

Deformity (*Continued*)
- thumb (acquired) —*see also* Deformity, finger
  - congenital NEC Q68.1
- thymus (tissue) (congenital) Q89.2
- thyroid (gland) (congenital) Q89.2
  - cartilage Q31.8
    - acquired J38.7
- tibia (acquired) —*see also* Deformity, limb, specified type NEC, lower leg
  - congenital NEC Q68.8
  - saber (syphilitic) A50.56
- toe (acquired) M20.6-
  - congenital Q66.9
  - hallux rigidus M20.2-
  - hallux valgus M20.1-
  - hallux varus M20.3-
  - hammer toe M20.4-
  - specified NEC M20.5X-
- tongue (congenital) Q38.3
  - acquired K14.8
- tooth, teeth K00.2
- trachea (rings) (congenital) Q32.1
  - acquired J39.8
- transverse aortic arch (congenital) Q25.4
- tricuspid (leaflets) (valve) I07.8
  - atresia or stenosis Q22.4
  - Ebstein's Q22.5
- trunk (acquired) M95.8
  - congenital Q89.9
- ulna (acquired) —*see also* Deformity, limb, forearm
  - congenital NEC Q68.8
- urachus, congenital Q64.4
- ureter (opening) (congenital) Q62.8
  - acquired N28.89
- urethra (congenital) Q64.79
  - acquired N36.8
- urinary tract (congenital) Q64.9
  - urachus Q64.4
- uterus (congenital) Q51.9
  - acquired N85.8
- uvula (congenital) Q38.5
- vagina (acquired) N89.8
  - congenital Q52.4
- valgus NEC M21.00
  - ankle M21.07-
  - elbow M21.02-
  - hip M21.05-
  - knee M21.06-
- valve, valvular (congenital) (heart) Q24.8
  - acquired —*see* Endocarditis
- varus NEC M21.10
  - ankle M21.17-
  - elbow M21.12-
  - hip M21.15
  - knee M21.16-
  - tibia —*see* Osteochondrosis, juvenile, tibia
- vas deferens (congenital) Q55.4
  - acquired N50.8
- vein (congenital) Q27.9
  - great Q26.9
- vertebra —*see* Dorsopathy, deforming
- vertical talus (congenital) Q66.80
  - left foot Q66.82
  - right foot Q66.81
- vesicourethral orifice (acquired) N32.89
  - congenital NEC Q64.79
- vessels of optic papilla (congenital) Q14.2
- visual field (contraction) —*see* Defect, visual field
- vitreous body, acquired H43.89

Deformity (*Continued*)
- vulva (congenital) Q52.79
  - acquired N90.89
- wrist (joint) (acquired) —*see also* Deformity, limb, forearm
  - congenital Q68.8
  - contraction —*see* Contraction, joint, wrist

Degeneration, degenerative
- adrenal (capsule) (fatty) (gland) (hyaline) (infectional) E27.8
- amyloid (*see also* Amyloidosis) E85.9
- anterior cornua, spinal cord G12.29
- anterior labral S43.49-
- aorta, aortic I70.0
  - fatty I77.89
- aortic valve (heart) —*see* Endocarditis, aortic
- arteriovascular —*see* Arteriosclerosis
- artery, arterial (atheromatous) (calcareous) —*see also* Arteriosclerosis
  - cerebral, amyloid E85.4 [I68.0]
  - medial —*see* Arteriosclerosis, extremities
- articular cartilage NEC —*see* Derangement, joint, articular cartilage, by site
- atheromatous —*see* Arteriosclerosis
- basal nuclei or ganglia G23.9
  - specified NEC G23.8
- bone NEC —*see* Disorder, bone, specified type NEC
- brachial plexus G54.0
- brain (cortical) (progressive) G31.9
  - alcoholic G31.2
  - arteriosclerotic I67.2
  - childhood G31.9
    - specified NEC G31.89
  - cystic G31.89
    - congenital Q04.6
  - in
    - alcoholism G31.2
    - beriberi E51.2
    - cerebrovascular disease I67.9
    - congenital hydrocephalus Q03.9
      - with spina bifida —*see also* Spina bifida
    - Fabry-Anderson disease E75.21
    - Gaucher's disease E75.22
    - Hunter's syndrome E76.1
    - lipidosis
      - cerebral E75.4
      - generalized E75.6
    - mucopolysaccharidosis —*see* Mucopolysaccharidosis
    - myxedema E03.9 [G32.89]
    - neoplastic disease (*see also* Neoplasm) D49.6 [G32.89]
    - Niemann-Pick disease E75.249 [G32.89]
    - sphingolipidosis E75.3 [G32.89]
    - vitamin B12 deficiency E53.8 [G32.89]
  - senile NEC G31.1
- breast N64.89
- Bruch's membrane —*see* Degeneration, choroid
- capillaries (fatty) I78.8
  - amyloid E85.8 [I79.8]
- cardiac —*see also* Degeneration, myocardial
  - valve, valvular —*see* Endocarditis
- cardiorenal —*see* Hypertension, cardiorenal

Degeneration, degenerative (*Continued*)
- cardiovascular —*see also* Disease, cardiovascular
  - renal —*see* Hypertension, cardiorenal
- cerebellar NOS G31.9
  - alcoholic G31.2
  - primary (hereditary) (sporadic) G11.9
- cerebral —*see* Degeneration, brain
- cerebrovascular I67.9
  - due to hypertension I67.4
- cervical plexus G54.2
- cervix N88.8
  - due to radiation (intended effect) N88.8
    - adverse effect or misadventure N99.89
- chamber angle H21.21-
- changes, spine or vertebra —*see* Spondylosis
- chorioretinal —*see also* Degeneration, choroid
  - hereditary H31.20
- choroid (colloid) (drusen) H31.10-
  - atrophy —*see* Atrophy, choroidal
  - hereditary —*see* Dystrophy, choroidal, hereditary
- ciliary body H21.22-
- cochlear —*see* subcategory H83.8
- combined (spinal cord) (subacute) E53.8 [G32.0]
  - with anemia (pernicious) D51.0 [G32.0]
    - due to dietary vitamin B12 deficiency D51.3 [G32.0]
  - in (due to)
    - vitamin B12 deficiency E53.8 [G32.0]
    - anemia D51.9 [G32.0]
- conjunctiva H11.10
  - concretions —*see* Concretion, conjunctiva
  - deposits —*see* Deposit, conjunctiva
  - pigmentations —*see* Pigmentation, conjunctiva
  - pinguecula —*see* Pinguecula
  - xerosis —*see* Xerosis, conjunctiva
- cornea H18.40
  - calcerous H18.43
    - band keratopathy H18.42-
  - familial, hereditary —*see* Dystrophy, cornea
  - hyaline (of old scars) H18.49
  - keratomalacia —*see* Keratomalacia
  - nodular H18.45-
  - peripheral H18.46-
  - senile H18.41-
  - specified type NEC H18.49
- cortical (cerebellar) (parenchymatous) G31.89
  - alcoholic G31.2
  - diffuse, due to arteriopathy I67.2
- corticobasal G31.85
- cutis L98.8
  - amyloid E85.4 [L99]
- dental pulp K04.2
- disc disease —*see* Degeneration, intervertebral disc NEC
- dorsolateral (spinal cord) —*see* Degeneration, combined
- extrapyramidal G25.9
- eye, macular —*see also* Degeneration, macula
  - congenital or hereditary —*see* Dystrophy, retina

Degeneration, degenerative (Continued)
 facet joints —see Spondylosis
 fatty
  liver NEC K76.0
   alcoholic K70.0
 grey matter (brain) (Alpers') G31.81
 heart —see also Degeneration,
   myocardial
  amyloid E85.4 [I43]
  atheromatous —see Disease, heart,
   ischemic, atherosclerotic
  ischemic —see Disease, heart,
   ischemic
 hepatolenticular (Wilson's) E83.01
 hepatorenal K76.7
 hyaline (diffuse) (generalized)
  localized —see Degeneration, by site
 infrapatellar fat pad M79.4
 intervertebral disc NOS
  with
   myelopathy —see Disorder, disc,
    with, myelopathy
   radiculitis or radiculopathy —
    see Disorder, disc, with,
    radiculopathy
  cervical, cervicothoracic —see
    Disorder, disc, cervical,
    degeneration
   with
    myelopathy —see Disorder,
     disc, cervical, with
     myelopathy
    neuritis, radiculitis or
     radiculopathy —see
     Disorder, disc, cervical, with
     neuritis
  lumbar region M51.36
   with
    myelopathy M51.06
    neuritis, radiculitis, radiculopathy
     or sciatica M51.16
  lumbosacral region M51.37
   with
    myelopathy M51.07
    neuritis, radiculitis, radicu-
     lopathy or sciatica M51.17
  sacrococcygeal region M53.3
  thoracic region M51.34
   with
    myelopathy M51.04
    neuritis, radiculitis,
     radiculopathy M51.14
  thoracolumbar region M51.35
   with
    myelopathy M51.05
    neuritis, radiculitis,
     radiculopathy M51.15
 intestine, amyloid E85.4
 iris (pigmentary) H21.23-
 ischemic —see Ischemia
 joint disease —see Osteoarthritis
 kidney N28.89
  amyloid E85.4 [N29]
  cystic, congenital Q61.9
  fatty N28.89
  polycystic Q61.3
   adult type (autosomal dominant)
    Q61.2
   infantile type (autosomal recessive)
    NEC Q61.19
    collecting duct dilatation Q61.11
 Kuhnt-Junius (see also Degeneration,
   macula) H35.32
 lens —see Cataract

Degeneration, degenerative (Continued)
 lenticular (familial) (progressive)
   (Wilson's) (with cirrhosis of liver)
   E83.01
 liver (diffuse) NEC K76.89
  amyloid E85.4 [K77]
  cystic K76.89
   congenital Q44.6
  fatty NEC K76.0
   alcoholic K70.0
  hypertrophic K76.89
  parenchymatous, acute or subacute
    K72.00
   with coma K72.01
  pigmentary K76.89
  toxic (acute) K71.9
 lung J98.4
 lymph gland I89.8
  hyaline I89.8
 macula, macular (acquired)
   (age-related) (senile)
   H35.30
  angioid streaks H35.33
  atrophic age-related H35.31
  congenital or hereditary —see
    Dystrophy, retina
  cystoid H35.35-
  drusen H35.36-
  exudative H35.32
  hole H35.34-
  nonexudative H35.31
  puckering H35.37-
  toxic H35.38-
 membranous labyrinth, congenital
   (causing impairment of hearing)
   Q16.5
 meniscus —see Derangement, meniscus
 mitral —see Insufficiency, mitral
 Mönckeberg's —see Arteriosclerosis,
   extremities
 motor centers, senile G31.1
 multi-system G90.3
 mural —see Degeneration, myocardial
 muscle (fatty) (fibrous) (hyaline)
   (progressive) M62.89
  heart —see Degeneration, myocardial
 myelin, central nervous system G37.9
 myocardial, myocardium (fatty)
   (hyaline) (senile) I51.5
  with rheumatic fever (conditions in
    I00) I09.0
   active, acute or subacute I01.2
    with chorea I02.0
   inactive or quiescent (with chorea)
    I09.0
  hypertensive —see Hypertension, heart
  rheumatic —see Degeneration,
    myocardial, with rheumatic fever
  syphilitic A52.06
 nasal sinus (mucosa) J32.9
  frontal J32.1
  maxillary J32.0
 nerve —see Disorder, nerve
 nervous system G31.9
  alcoholic G31.2
  amyloid E85.4 [G99.8]
  autonomic G90.9
  fatty G31.89
  specified NEC G31.89
 nipple N64.89
 olivopontocerebellar (hereditary)
   (familial) G23.8
 osseous labyrinth —see subcategory
   H83.8

Degeneration, degenerative (Continued)
 ovary N83.8
  cystic N83.20
  microcystic N83.20
 pallidal pigmentary (progressive) G23.0
 pancreas K86.8
  tuberculous A18.83
 penis N48.89
 pigmentary (diffuse) (general)
  localized —see Degeneration, by site
  pallidal (progressive) G23.0
 pineal gland E34.8
 pituitary (gland) E23.6
 popliteal fat pad M79.4
 posterolateral (spinal cord) —see
   Degeneration, combined
 pulmonary valve (heart) I37.8
 pulp (tooth) K04.2
 pupillary margin H21.24-
 renal —see Degeneration, kidney
 retina H35.9
  hereditary (cerebroretinal)
    (congenital) (juvenile) (macula)
    (peripheral) (pigmentary) —see
    Dystrophy, retina
  Kuhnt-Junius (see also Degeneration,
    macula) H35.32
  macula (cystic) (exudative) (hole)
    (nonexudative) (pseudohole)
    (senile) (toxic) —see
    Degeneration, macula
  peripheral H35.40
   lattice H35.41-
   microcystoid H35.42-
   paving stone H35.43-
   secondary
    pigmentary H35.45-
    vitreoretinal H35.46-
   senile reticular H35.44-
  pigmentary (primary) —see also
    Dystrophy, retina
   secondary —see Degeneration,
    retina, peripheral, secondary
  posterior pole —see Degeneration,
    macula
 saccule, congenital (causing impairment
   of hearing) Q16.5
 senile R54
  brain G31.1
  cardiac, heart or myocardium —see
    Degeneration, myocardial
  motor centers G31.1
  vascular —see Arteriosclerosis
 sinus (cystic) —see also Sinusitis
  polypoid J33.1
 skin L98.8
  amyloid E85.4 [L99]
  colloid L98.8
 spinal (cord) G31.89
  amyloid E85.4 [G32.89]
  combined (subacute) —see
    Degeneration, combined
  dorsolateral —see Degeneration,
    combined
  familial NEC G31.89
  fatty G31.89
  funicular —see Degeneration,
    combined
  posterolateral —see Degeneration,
    combined
  subacute combined —see
    Degeneration, combined
  tuberculous A17.81
 spleen D73.0
  amyloid E85.4 [D77]

Degeneration, degenerative *(Continued)*
  stomach K31.89
  striatonigral G23.2
  suprarenal (capsule) (gland) E27.8
  synovial membrane (pulpy) —*see*
      Disorder, synovium, specified type
      NEC
  tapetoretinal —*see* Dystrophy, retina
  thymus (gland) E32.8
    fatty E32.8
  thyroid (gland) E07.89
  tricuspid (heart) (valve) I07.9
  tuberculous NEC —*see* Tuberculosis
  turbinate J34.89
  uterus (cystic) N85.8
  vascular (senile) —*see* Arteriosclerosis
    hypertensive —*see* Hypertension
  vitreoretinal, secondary —*see*
      Degeneration, retina, peripheral,
      secondary, vitreoretinal
  vitreous (body) H43.81-
  Wallerian —*see* Disorder, nerve
  Wilson's hepatolenticular E83.01
Deglutition
  paralysis R13.0
    hysterical F44.4
  pneumonia J69.0
Degos' disease I77.89
Dehiscence (of)
  amputation stump T87.81
  cesarean wound O90.0
  closure of
    cornea T81.31
    craniotomy T81.32
    fascia (muscular) (superficial) T81.32
    internal organ or tissue T81.32
    laceration (external) (internal) T81.33
    ligament T81.32
    mucosa T81.31
    muscle or muscle flap T81.32
    ribs or rib cage T81.32
    skin and subcutaneous tissue (full-
        thickness) (superficial) T81.31
    skull T81.32
    sternum (sternotomy) T81.32
    tendon T81.32
    traumatic laceration (external)
        (internal) T81.33
  episiotomy O90.1
  operation wound NEC T81.31
    external operation wound (superficial)
        T81.31
    internal operation wound (deep)
        T81.32
  perineal wound (postpartum) O90.1
  traumatic injury wound repair T81.33
  wound T81.30
    traumatic repair T81.33
Dehydration E86.0
  hypertonic E87.0
  hypotonic E87.1
  newborn P74.1
Déjérine-Roussy syndrome G93.89
Déjérine-Sottas disease or neuropathy
    (hypertrophic) G60.0
Déjérine-Thomas atrophy G23.8
Delay, delayed
  any plane in pelvis
    complicating delivery O66.9
  birth or delivery NOS O63.9
  closure, ductus arteriosus (Botalli) P29.3
  coagulation —*see* Defect, coagulation
  conduction (cardiac) (ventricular) I45.9
  delivery, second twin, triplet, etc O63.2

Delay, delayed *(Continued)*
  development R62.50
    global F88
    intellectual (specific) F81.9
    language F80.9
      due to hearing loss F80.4
    learning F81.9
    pervasive F84.9
    physiological R62.50
      specified stage NEC R62.0
    reading F81.0
    sexual E30.0
    speech F80.9
      due to hearing loss F80.4
    spelling F81.81
  gastric emptying K30
  menarche E30.0
  menstruation (cause unknown) N91.0
  milestone R62.0
  passage of meconium (newborn) P76.0
  primary respiration P28.9
  puberty (constitutional) E30.0
  separation of umbilical cord P96.82
  sexual maturation, female E30.0
  sleep phase syndrome G47.21
  union, fracture —*see* Fracture, by site
  vaccination Z28.9
Deletion (s)
  autosome Q93.9
    identified by fluorescence in situ
        hybridization (FISH) Q93.89
    identified by in situ hybridization
        (ISH) Q93.89
  chromosome
    with complex rearrangements NEC
        Q93.7
    part of NEC Q93.5
    seen only at prometaphase Q93.89
    short arm
      4 Q93.3
      5p Q93.4
      22q11.2 Q93.81
    specified NEC Q93.89
  long arm chromosome 18 or 21
      Q93.89
    with complex rearrangements NEC
        Q93.7
  microdeletions NEC Q93.88
Delhi boil or button B55.1
Delinquency (juvenile) (neurotic)
    F91.8
  group Z72.810
Delinquent immunization status
    Z28.3
Delirium, delirious (acute or subacute)
    (not alcohol or drug-induced) (with
    dementia) R41.0
  alcoholic (acute) (tremens) (withdrawal)
      F10.921
    with intoxication F10.921
    in
      abuse F10.121
      dependence F10.221
  due to (secondary to)
    alcohol
      intoxication F10.921
      in
        abuse F10.121
        dependence F10.221
      withdrawal F10.231
    amphetamine intoxication F15.921
      in
        abuse F15.121
        dependence F15.221

Delirium, delirious *(Continued)*
  due to *(Continued)*
    anxiolytic
      intoxication F13.921
        in
          abuse F13.121
          dependence F13.221
        withdrawal F13.231
    cannabis intoxication (acute) F12.921
      in
        abuse F12.121
        dependence F12.221
    cocaine intoxication (acute) F14.921
      in
        abuse F14.121
        dependence F14.221
    general medical condition F05
    hallucinogen intoxication F16.921
      in
        abuse F16.121
        dependence F16.221
    hypnotic
      intoxication F13.921
        in
          abuse F13.121
          dependence F13.221
        withdrawal F13.231
    inhalant intoxication (acute) F18.921
      in
        abuse F18.121
        dependence F18.221
    multiple etiologies F05
    opioid intoxication (acute) F11.921
      in
        abuse F11.121
        dependence F11.221
    phencyclidine intoxication (acute)
        F16.921
      in
        abuse F16.121
        dependence F16.221
    psychoactive substance NEC
        intoxication (acute) F19.921
      in
        abuse F19.121
        dependence F19.221
    sedative
      intoxication F13.921
        in
          abuse F13.121
          dependence F13.221
        withdrawal F13.231
    unknown etiology F05
  exhaustion F43.0
  hysterical F44.89
  postprocedural (postoperative) F05
  puerperal F05
  thyroid —*see* Thyrotoxicosis with
      thyroid storm
  traumatic —*see* Injury, intracranial
  tremens (alcohol-induced) F10.231
    sedative-induced F13.231
Delivery (childbirth) (labor)
  arrested active phase O62.1
  cesarean (for)
    without indication O82
    abnormal
      pelvis (bony) (deformity) (major)
          NEC with disproportion
          (fetopelvic) O33.0
        with obstructed labor O65.0
      presentation or position O32.9
    abruptio placentae (*see also* Abruptio
        placentae) O45.9-
    acromion presentation O32.2

Delivery *(Continued)*
  cesarean *(Continued)*
    atony, uterus O62.2
    breech presentation O32.1
      incomplete O32.8
    brow presentation O32.3
    cephalopelvic disproportion O33.9
    cerclage O34.3-
    chin presentation O32.3
    cicatrix of cervix O34.4-
    contracted pelvis (general)
      inlet O33.2
      outlet O33.3
    cord presentation or prolapse
      O69.0
    cystocele O34.8-
    deformity (acquired) (congenital)
      pelvic organs or tissues NEC
        O34.8-
      pelvis (bony) NEC O33.0
    disproportion NOS O33.9
    eclampsia —*see* Eclampsia
    face presentation O32.3
    failed
      forceps O66.5
      induction of labor O61.9
        instrumental O61.1
        mechanical O61.1
        medical O61.0
        specified NEC O61.8
        surgical O61.1
      trial of labor NOS O66.40
        following previous cesarean
          delivery O66.41
      vacuum extraction O66.5
      ventouse O66.5
    fetal-maternal hemorrhage O43.01-
    hemorrhage (intrapartum) O67.9
      with coagulation defect O67.0
      specified cause NEC O67.8
    high head at term O32.4
    hydrocephalic fetus O33.6
    incarceration of uterus O34.51-
    incoordinate uterine action O62.4
    increased size, fetus O33.5
    inertia, uterus O62.2
      primary O62.0
      secondary O62.1
    lateroversion, uterus O34.59-
    mal lie O32.9
    malposition
      fetus O32.9
      pelvic organs or tissues NEC O34.8-
      uterus NEC O34.59-
    malpresentation NOS O32.9
    oblique presentation O32.2
    occurring after 37 completed weeks
      of gestation but before 39
      completed weeks gestation due
      to (spontaneous) onset of labor
      O75.82
    oversize fetus O33.5
    pelvic tumor NEC O34.8-
    placenta previa O44.1-
      without hemorrhage O44.0-
    placental insufficiency O36.51-
    planned, occurring after 37
      completed weeks of gestation
      but before 39 completed weeks
      gestation due to (spontaneous)
      onset of labor O75.82
    polyp, cervix O34.4-
      causing obstructed labor O65.5
    poor dilatation, cervix O62.0

Delivery *(Continued)*
  cesarean *(Continued)*
    pre-eclampsia O14.9-
      mild O14.0-
      moderate O14.0-
      severe
        with hemolysis, elevated liver
          enzymes and low platelet
          count (HELLP) O14.2-
    previous
      cesarean delivery O34.21
      surgery (to)
        cervix O34.4-
        gynecological NEC O34.8-
        rectum O34.7-
        uterus O34.29
        vagina O34.6-
    prolapse
      arm or hand O32.2
      uterus O34.52-
    prolonged labor NOS O63.9
    rectocele O34.8-
    retroversion
      uterus O34.53-
    rigid
      cervix O34.4-
      pelvic floor O34.8-
      perineum O34.7-
      vagina O34.6-
      vulva O34.7-
    sacculation, pregnant uterus O34.59-
    scar (s)
      cervix O34.4-
      cesarean delivery O34.21
      uterus O34.29
    Shirodkar suture in situ O34.3-
    shoulder presentation O32.2
    stenosis or stricture, cervix O34.4-
    streptococcus B carrier state O99.824
    transverse presentation or lie O32.2
    tumor, pelvic organs or tissues NEC
      O34.8-
      cervix O34.4-
    umbilical cord presentation or
      prolapse O69.0
  completely normal case O80
  complicated O75.9
    by
      abnormal, abnormality (of)
        forces of labor O62.9
          specified type NEC O62.8
        glucose O99.814
        uterine contractions NOS O62.9
      abruptio placentae (*see also*
        Abruptio placentae) O45.9-
      abuse
        physical O9A.32
        psychological O9A.52
        sexual O9A.42
      adherent placenta O72.0
        without hemorrhage O73.0
      alcohol use O99.314
      anemia (pre-existing) O99.02
      anesthetic death O74.8
      annular detachment of cervix O71.3
      atony, uterus O62.2
      attempted vacuum extraction and
        forceps O66.5
      Bandl's ring O62.4
      bariatric surgery status O99.844
      biliary tract disorder O26.62
      bleeding —*see* Delivery,
        complicated by, hemorrhage
      blood disorder NEC O99.12

Delivery *(Continued)*
  complicated *(Continued)*
    by *(Continued)*
      cervical dystocia (hypotonic) O62.2
        primary O62.0
        secondary O62.1
      circulatory system disorder O99.42
      compression of cord (umbilical)
        NEC O69.2
      condition NEC O99.89
      contraction, contracted ring O62.4
      cord (umbilical)
        around neck
          with compression O69.1
          without compression O69.81
        bruising O69.5
        complication O69.9
          specified NEC O69.89
        compression NEC O69.2
        entanglement O69.2
          without compression O69.82
        hematoma O69.5
        presentation O69.0
        prolapse O69.0
        short O69.3
        thrombosis (vessels) O69.5
        vascular lesion O69.5
      Couvelaire uterus O45.8X-
      damage to (injury to) NEC
        perineum O71.82
        periurethral tissue O71.82
        vulva O71.82
      delay following rupture of
        membranes (spontaneous) —
        see Pregnancy, complicated
        by, premature rupture of
        membranes
      depressed fetal heart tones O76
      diabetes O24.92
        gestational O24.429
          diet controlled O24.420
          insulin controlled O24.424
        pre-existing O24.32
          specified NEC O24.82
          type 1 O24.02
          type 2 O24.12
      diastasis recti (abdominis) O71.89
      dilatation
        bladder O66.8
        cervix incomplete, poor or slow
          O62.0
      disease NEC O99.89
      disruptio uteri —*see* Delivery,
        complicated by, rupture, uterus
      drug use O99.324
      dysfunction, uterus NOS O62.9
        hypertonic O62.4
        hypotonic O62.2
          primary O62.0
          secondary O62.1
        incoordinate O62.4
      eclampsia O15.1
      embolism (pulmonary) —*see*
        Embolism, obstetric
      endocrine, nutritional or metabolic
        disease NEC O99.284
      failed
        attempted vaginal birth after
          previous cesarean delivery
          O66.41
        induction of labor O61.9
          instrumental O61.1
          mechanical O61.1
          medical O61.0

Delivery *(Continued)*
 complicated *(Continued)*
  by *(Continued)*
   failed *(Continued)*
    induction of labor *(Continued)*
     specified NEC O61.8
     surgical O61.1
    trial of labor O66.40
   female genital mutilation O65.5
   fetal
    abnormal acid-base balance O68
    acidemia O68
    acidosis O68
    alkalosis O68
    death, early O02.1
    deformity O66.3
    heart rate or rhythm (abnormal) (non-reassuring) O76
    hypoxia O77.8
    stress O77.9
     due to drug administration O77.1
     electrocardiographic evidence of O77.8
     specified NEC O77.8
     ultrasound evidence of O77.8
   fever during labor O75.2
   gastric banding status O99.844
   gastric bypass status O99.844
   gastrointestinal disease NEC O99.62
   gestational diabetes O24.429
    diet controlled O24.420
    insulin (and diet) controlled O24.424
   gonorrhea O98.22
   hematoma O71.7
    ischial spine O71.7
    pelvic O71.7
    vagina O71.7
    vulva or perineum O71.7
   hemorrhage (uterine) O67.9
    associated with
     afibrinogenemia O67.0
     coagulation defect O67.0
     hyperfibrinolysis O67.0
     hypofibrinogenemia O67.0
    due to
     low-lying placenta O44.1-
     placenta previa O44.1-
     premature separation of placenta (normally implanted) *(see also* Abruptio placentae) O45.9-
     retained placenta O72.0
     uterine leiomyoma O67.8
    placenta NEC O67.8
    postpartum NEC (atonic) (immediate) O72.1
     with retained or trapped placenta O72.0
     delayed O72.2
     secondary O72.2
     third stage O72.0
   hourglass contraction, uterus O62.4
   hypertension, hypertensive (pre-existing) *—see* Hypertension, complicated by, childbirth (labor)
   hypotension O26.5-
   incomplete dilatation (cervix) O62.0
   incoordinate uterus contractions O62.4

Delivery *(Continued)*
 complicated *(Continued)*
  by *(Continued)*
   inertia, uterus O62.2
    during latent phase of labor O62.0
    primary O62.0
    secondary O62.1
   infection (maternal) O98.92
    carrier state NEC O99.834
    gonorrhea O98.22
    human immunodeficiency virus (HIV) O98.72
    sexually transmitted NEC O98.32
    specified NEC O98.82
    syphilis O98.12
    tuberculosis O98.02
    viral hepatitis O98.42
    viral NEC O98.52
   injury (to mother) *(see also* Delivery, complicated, by, damage to) O71.9
    nonobstetric O9A.22
     caused by abuse *—see* Delivery, complicated by, abuse
   intrauterine fetal death, early O02.1
   inversion, uterus O71.2
   laceration (perineal) O70.9
    anus (sphincter) O70.4
     with third degree laceration O70.2
      with mucosa O70.3
     without third degree laceration O70.4
    bladder (urinary) O71.5
    bowel O71.5
    cervix (uteri) O71.3
    fourchette O70.0
    hymen O70.0
    labia O70.0
    pelvic
     floor O70.1
     organ NEC O71.5
    perineum, perineal O70.9
     first degree O70.0
     fourth degree O70.3
     muscles O70.1
     second degree O70.1
     skin O70.0
     slight O70.0
     third degree O70.2
    peritoneum (pelvic) O71.5
    rectovaginal (septum) (without perineal laceration) O71.4
     with perineum O70.2
      with anal or rectal mucosa O70.3
    specified NEC O71.89
    sphincter ani *—see* Delivery, complicated, by, laceration, anus (sphincter)
    urethra O71.5
    uterus O71.81
     before labor O71.81
    vagina, vaginal (deep) (high) (without perineal laceration) O71.4
     with perineum O70.0
      muscles, with perineum O70.1
    vulva O70.0
   liver disorder O26.62
   malignancy O9A.12
   malnutrition O25.2

Delivery *(Continued)*
 complicated *(Continued)*
  by *(Continued)*
   malposition, malpresentation
    without obstruction O32.9 *—see also* Delivery, complicated by, obstruction
     breech O32.1
     compound O32.6
     face (brow) (chin) O32.3
     footling O38.8
     high head O32.4
     oblique O32.2
     specified NEC O32.8
     transverse O32.2
     unstable lie O32.0
    placenta (with hemorrhage) O44.1-
     without hemorrhage O44.0-
    uterus or cervix O65.5
   meconium in amniotic fluid O77.0
   mental disorder NEC O99.344
   metrorrhexis *—see* Delivery, complicated by, rupture, uterus
   nervous system disorder O99.354
   obesity (pre-existing) O99.214
   obesity surgery status O99.844
   obstetric trauma O71.9
    specified NEC O71.89
   obstructed labor
    due to
     breech (complete) (frank) presentation O64.1
      incomplete O64.8
     brow presentation O64.3
     buttock presentation O64.1
     chin presentation O64.2
     compound presentation O64.5
     contracted pelvis O65.1
     deep transverse arrest O64.0
     deformed pelvis O65.0
     dystocia (fetal) O66.9
      due to
       conjoined twins O66.3
       fetal
        abnormality NEC O66.3
        ascites O66.3
        hydrops O66.3
        meningomyelocele O66.3
        sacral teratoma O66.3
        tumor O66.3
       hydrocephalic fetus O66.3
      shoulder O66.0
     face presentation O64.2
     fetopelvic disproportion O65.4
     footling presentation O64.8
     impacted shoulders O66.0
     incomplete rotation of fetal head O64.0
     large fetus O66.2
     locked twins O66.1
     malposition O64.9
      specified NEC O64.8
     malpresentation O64.9
      specified NEC O64.8
     multiple fetuses NEC O66.6
     pelvic
      abnormality (maternal) O65.9
       organ O65.5
       specified NEC O65.8
      contraction
       inlet O65.2
       mid-cavity O65.3
       outlet O65.3

Delivery *(Continued)*
  complicated *(Continued)*
    by *(Continued)*
      obstructed labor *(Continued)*
        due to *(Continued)*
          persistent (position)
            occipitoiliac O64.0
            occipitoposterior O64.0
            occipitosacral O64.0
            occipitotransverse O64.0
          prolapsed arm O64.4
          shoulder presentation O64.4
        specified NEC O66.8
      pathological retraction ring, uterus
          O62.4
      penetration, pregnant uterus by
          instrument O71.1
      perforation —*see* Delivery,
          complicated by, laceration
      placenta, placental
        ablatio (*see also* Abruptio
            placentae) O45.9-
        abnormality O43.9-
          specified NEC O43.89-
        abruptio (*see also* Abruptio
            placentae) O45.9-
        accreta O43.21-
        adherent (with hemorrhage) O72.0
          without hemorrhage O73.0
        detachment (premature) (*see also*
            Abruptio placentae) O45.9-
        disorder O43.9-
          specified NEC O43.89-
        hemorrhage NEC O67.8
        increta - O43.22
        low (implantation) O44.1-
          without hemorrhage O44.0-
        malformation O43.10-
        malposition O44.1-
          without hemorrhage O44.0-
        percreta - O43.23
        previa (central) (lateral) (low)
            (marginal) (partial) (total)
            O44.1-
          without hemorrhage O44.0-
        retained (with hemorrhage) O72.0
          without hemorrhage O73.0
        separation (premature) O45.9-
          specified NEC O45.8X-
        vicious insertion O44.1-
      precipitate labor O62.3
      premature rupture, membranes (*see
          also* Pregnancy, complicated
          by, premature rupture of
          membranes) O42.90
      prolapse
        arm or hand O32.2
        cord (umbilical) O69.0
        foot or leg O32.8
        uterus O34.52-
      prolonged labor O63.9
        first stage O63.0
        second stage O63.1
      protozoal disease (maternal) O98.62
      respiratory disease NEC O99.52
      retained membranes or portions of
          placenta O72.2
        without hemorrhage O73.1
      retarded birth O63.9
      retention of secundines (with
          hemorrhage) O72.0
        without hemorrhage O73.0
        partial O72.2
          without hemorrhage O73.1

Delivery *(Continued)*
  complicated *(Continued)*
    by *(Continued)*
      rupture
        bladder (urinary) O71.5
        cervix O71.3
        pelvic organ NEC O71.5
        urethra O71.5
        uterus (during or after labor)
            O71.1
          before labor O71.0-
      separation, pubic bone (symphysis
          pubis) O71.6
      shock O75.1
      shoulder presentation O64.4
      skin disorder NEC O99.72
      spasm, cervix O62.4
      stenosis or stricture, cervix O65.5
      streptococcus B carrier state O99.824
      subluxation of symphysis (pubis)
          O26.72
      syphilis (maternal) O98.12
      tear —*see* Delivery, complicated by,
          laceration
      tetanic uterus O62.4
      trauma (obstetrical) (*see also*
          Delivery, complicated, by,
          damage to) O71.9
        non-obstetric O9A.22
        periurethral O71.82
        specified NEC O71.89
      tuberculosis (maternal) O98.02
      tumor, pelvic organs or tissues
          NEC O65.5
      umbilical cord around neck
        with compression O69.1
        without compression O69.81
      uterine inertia O62.2
        during latent phase of labor O62.0
        primary O62.0
        secondary O62.1
      vasa previa O69.4
      velamentous insertion of cord
          O43.12-
    specified complication NEC O75.89
  delayed NOS O63.9
    following rupture of membranes
        artificial O75.5
    second twin, triplet, etc. O63.2
  forceps, low following failed vacuum
      extraction O66.5
  missed (at or near term) O36.4
  normal O80
  obstructed —*see* Delivery, complicated
      by, obstruction
  precipitate O62.3
  preterm (*see also* Pregnancy,
      complicated by, preterm labor)
      O60.10
  spontaneous O80
  term pregnancy NOS O80
  uncomplicated O80
  vaginal, following previous cesarean
      delivery O34.21
Delusions (paranoid) —*see* Disorder,
    delusional
Dementia (degenerative (primary)) (old
    age) (persisting) F03.90
  with
    aggressive behavior F03.91
    behavioral disturbance F03.91
    combative behavior F03.91
    Lewy bodies G31.83 [F02.80]
      with behavioral disturbance G31.83
          [F02.81]

Dementia *(Continued)*
  with *(Continued)*
    Parkinson's disease G20 [F02.80]
      with behavioral disturbance G20
          [F02.81]
    Parkinsonism G31.83 [F02.80]
      with behavioral disturbance G31.83
          [F02.81]
    violent behavior F03.91
  alcoholic F10.97
    with dependence F10.27
  Alzheimer's type —*see* Disease,
      Alzheimer's
  arteriosclerotic —*see* Dementia,
      vascular
  atypical, Alzheimer's type —*see*
      Disease, Alzheimer's, specified
      NEC
  congenital —*see* Disability,
      intellectual
  frontal (lobe) G31.09 [F02.80]
    with behavioral disturbance G31.09
        [F02.81]
  frontotemporal G31.09 [F02.80]
    with behavioral disturbance G31.09
        [F02.81]
    specified NEC G31.09 [F02.80]
      with behavioral disturbance G31.09
          [F02.81]
  in (due to)
    alcohol F10.97
      with dependence F10.27
    Alzheimer's disease —*see* Disease,
        Alzheimer's
    arteriosclerotic brain disease —*see*
        Dementia, vascular
    cerebral lipidoses E75.- [F02.80]
      with behavioral disturbance
          E75.- [F02.81]
    Creutzfeldt-Jakob disease) (*see also*
        Creutzfeldt-Jakob disease or
        syndrome (with dementia)
        A81.00
    epilepsy G40.- [F02.80]
      with behavioral disturbance
          G40.- [F02.81]
    hepatolenticular degeneration E83.01
        [F02.80]
      with behavioral disturbance E83.01
          [F02.81]
    human immunodeficiency virus
        (HIV) disease B20 [F02.80]
      with behavioral disturbance B20
          [F02.81]
    Huntington's disease or chorea
        G10
    hypercalcemia E83.52 [F02.80]
      with behavioral disturbance E83.52
          [F02.81]
    hypothyroidism, acquired E03.9
        [F02.80]
      with behavioral disturbance E03.9
          [F02.81]
    due to iodine deficiency E01.8
        [F02.80]
      with behavioral disturbance
          E01.8 [F02.81]
    inhalants F18.97
      with dependence F18.27
    multiple
      etiologies F03
    sclerosis G35 [F02.80]
      with behavioral disturbance G35
          [F02.81]

Dementia *(Continued)*
in *(Continued)*
neurosyphilis A52.17 *[F02.80]*
with behavioral disturbance A52.17
[F02.81]
juvenile A50.49 *[F02.80]*
with behavioral disturbance
A50.49 *[F02.81]*
niacin deficiency E52 *[F02.80]*
with behavioral disturbance E52
[F02.81]
paralysis agitans G20 *[F02.80]*
with behavioral disturbance G20
[F02.81]
Parkinson's disease G20 *[F02.80]*
pellagra E52 *[F02.80]*
with behavioral disturbance E52
[F02.81]
Pick's G31.01 *[F02.80]*
with behavioral disturbance G31.01
[F02.81]
polyarteritis nodosa M30.0 *[F02.80]*
with behavioral disturbance M30.0
[F02.81]
psychoactive drug F19.97
with dependence F19.27
inhalants F18.97
with dependence F18.27
sedatives, hypnotics or anxiolytics
F13.97
with dependence F13.27
sedatives, hypnotics or anxiolytics
F13.97
with dependence F13.27
systemic lupus erythematosus
M32.- *[F02.80]*
with behavioral disturbance
M32.- *[F02.81]*
trypanosomiasis
African B56.9 *[F02.80]*
with behavioral disturbance
B56.9 *[F02.81]*
unknown etiology F03
vitamin B12 deficiency E53.8 *[F02.80]*
with behavioral disturbance E53.8
[F02.81]
volatile solvents F18.97
with dependence F18.27
infantile, infantilis F84.3
Lewy body G31.83 *[F02.80]*
with behavioral disturbance G31.83
[F02.81]
multi-infarct —*see* Dementia, vascular
paralytica, paralytic (syphilitic) A52.17
[F02.80]
with behavioral disturbance A52.17
[F02.81]
juvenilis A50.45
paretic A52.17
praecox —*see* Schizophrenia
presenile F03
Alzheimer's type —*see* Disease,
Alzheimer's, early onset
primary degenerative F03
progressive, syphilitic A52.17
senile F03
with acute confusional state F05
Alzheimer's type —*see* Disease,
Alzheimer's, late onset
depressed or paranoid type F03
vascular (acute onset) (mixed)
(multi-infarct) (subcortical)
F01.50
with behavioral disturbance
F01.51

Demineralization, bone —*see*
Osteoporosis
Demodex folliculorum (infestation)
B88.0
Demophobia F40.248
Demoralization R45.3
Demyelination, demyelinization
central nervous system G37.9
specified NEC G37.8
corpus callosum (central) G37.1
disseminated, acute G36.9
specified NEC G36.8
global G35
in optic neuritis G36.0
Dengue (classical) (fever) A90
hemorrhagic A91
sandfly A93.1
Dennie-Marfan syphilitic syndrome
A50.45
Dens evaginatus, in dente or invaginatus
K00.2
Dense breasts R92.2
Density
increased, bone (disseminated)
(generalized) (spotted) —*see*
Disorder, bone, density and
structure, specified type NEC
lung (nodular) J98.4
Dental —*see also* condition
examination Z01.20
with abnormal findings Z01.21
restoration
aesthetically inadequate or
displeasing K08.56
defective K08.50
specified NEC K08.59
failure of marginal integrity K08.51
failure of periodontal anatomical
integrity K08.54
Dentia praecox K00.6
Denticles (pulp) K04.2
Dentigerous cyst K09.0
Dentin
irregular (in pulp) K04.3
opalescent K00.5
secondary (in pulp) K04.3
sensitive K03.89
Dentinogenesis imperfecta K00.5
Dentinoma —*see* Cyst, calcifying
odontogenic
Dentition (syndrome) K00.7
delayed K00.6
difficult K00.7
precocious K00.6
premature K00.6
retarded K00.6
Dependence (on) (syndrome) F19.20
with remission F19.21
alcohol (ethyl) (methyl) (without
remission) F10.20
with
amnestic disorder, persisting F10.26
anxiety disorder F10.280
dementia, persisting F10.27
intoxication F10.229
with delirium F10.221
uncomplicated F10.220
mood disorder F10.24
psychotic disorder F10.259
with
delusions F10.250
hallucinations F10.251
remission F10.21
sexual dysfunction F10.281

Dependence *(Continued)*
alcohol *(Continued)*
with *(Continued)*
sleep disorder F10.282
specified disorder NEC F10.288
withdrawal F10.239
with
delirium F10.231
perceptual disturbance
F10.232
uncomplicated F10.230
counseling and surveillance Z71.41
amobarbital —*see* Dependence, drug,
sedative
amphetamine (s) (type) —*see*
Dependence, drug, stimulant NEC
amytal (sodium) —*see* Dependence,
drug, sedative
analgesic NEC F55.8
anesthetic (agent) (gas) (general) (local)
NEC —*see* Dependence, drug,
psychoactive NEC
anxiolytic NEC —*see* Dependence,
drug, sedative
barbital (s) —*see* Dependence, drug,
sedative
barbiturate (s) (compounds) (drugs
classifiable to T42) —*see*
Dependence, drug, sedative
benzedrine —*see* Dependence, drug,
stimulant NEC
bhang —*see* Dependence, drug,
cannabis
bromide (s) NEC —*see* Dependence,
drug, sedative
caffeine —*see* Dependence, drug,
stimulant NEC
cannabis (sativa) (indica) (resin)
(derivatives) (type) —*see*
Dependence, drug, cannabis
chloral (betaine) (hydrate) —*see*
Dependence, drug, sedative
chlordiazepoxide —*see* Dependence,
drug, sedative
coca (leaf) (derivatives) —*see*
Dependence, drug, cocaine
cocaine —*see* Dependence, drug,
cocaine
codeine —*see* Dependence, drug,
opioid
combinations of drugs F19.20
dagga —*see* Dependence, drug,
cannabis
demerol —*see* Dependence, drug,
opioid
dexamphetamine —*see* Dependence,
drug, stimulant NEC
dexedrine —*see* Dependence, drug,
stimulant NEC
dextromethorphan —*see* Dependence,
drug, opioid
dextromoramide —*see* Dependence,
drug, opioid
dextro-nor-pseudo-ephedrine —*see*
Dependence, drug, stimulant
NEC
dextrorphan —*see* Dependence, drug,
opioid
diazepam —*see* Dependence, drug,
sedative
dilaudid —*see* Dependence, drug,
opioid
D-lysergic acid diethylamide —*see*
Dependence, drug, hallucinogen

Dependence *(Continued)*
  drug NEC F19.20
    with sleep disorder F19.282
    cannabis F12.20
      with
        anxiety disorder F12.280
        intoxication F12.229
          with
            delirium F12.221
            perceptual disturbance
              F12.222
          uncomplicated F12.220
        other specified disorder F12.288
        psychosis F12.259
          delusions F12.250
          hallucinations F12.251
        unspecified disorder F12.29
      in remission F12.21
    cocaine F14.20
      with
        anxiety disorder F14.280
        intoxication F14.229
          with
            delirium F14.221
            perceptual disturbance
              F14.222
          uncomplicated F14.220
        mood disorder F14.24
        other specified disorder
          F14.288
        psychosis F14.259
          delusions F14.250
          hallucinations F14.251
        sexual dysfunction F14.281
        sleep disorder F14.282
        unspecified disorder F14.29
        withdrawal F14.23
      in remission F14.21
      withdrawal symptoms in newborn
        P96.1
    counseling and surveillance Z71.51
    hallucinogen F16.20
      with
        anxiety disorder F16.280
        flashbacks F16.283
        intoxication F16.229
          with delirium F16.221
          uncomplicated F16.220
        mood disorder F16.24
        other specified disorder
          F16.288
        perception disorder, persisting
          F16.283
        psychosis F16.259
          delusions F16.250
          hallucinations F16.251
        unspecified disorder F16.29
      in remission F16.21
    in remission F19.21
    inhalant F18.20
      with
        anxiety disorder F18.280
        dementia, persisting F18.27
        intoxication F18.229
          with delirium F18.221
          uncomplicated F18.220
        mood disorder F18.24
        other specified disorder
          F18.288
        psychosis F18.259
          delusions F18.250
          hallucinations F18.251
        unspecified disorder F18.29
      in remission F18.21

Dependence *(Continued)*
  drug NEC *(Continued)*
    nicotine F17.200
      with disorder F17.209
        remission F17.201
        specified disorder NEC F17.208
        withdrawal F17.203
      chewing tobacco F17.220
        with disorder F17.229
          remission F17.221
          specified disorder NEC F17.228
          withdrawal F17.223
      cigarettes F17.210
        with disorder F17.219
          remission F17.211
          specified disorder NEC
            F17.218
          withdrawal F17.213
      specified product NEC F17.290
        with disorder F17.299
          remission F17.291
          specified disorder NEC F17.298
          withdrawal F17.293
    opioid F11.20
      with
        intoxication F11.229
          with
            delirium F11.221
            perceptual disturbance
              F11.222
          uncomplicated F11.220
        mood disorder F11.24
        other specified disorder F11.288
        psychosis F11.259
          delusions F11.250
          hallucinations F11.251
        sexual dysfunction F11.281
        sleep disorder F11.282
        unspecified disorder F11.29
        withdrawal F11.23
      in remission F11.21
    psychoactive NEC F19.20
      with
        amnestic disorder F19.26
        anxiety disorder F19.280
        dementia F19.27
        intoxication F19.229
          with
            delirium F19.221
            perceptual disturbance
              F19.222
          uncomplicated F19.220
        mood disorder F19.24
        other specified disorder F19.288
        psychosis F19.259
          delusions F19.250
          hallucinations F19.251
        sexual dysfunction F19.281
        sleep disorder F19.282
        unspecified disorder F19.29
        withdrawal F19.239
          with
            delirium F19.231
            perceptual disturbance
              F19.232
          uncomplicated F19.230
    sedative, hypnotic or anxiolytic F13.20
      with
        amnestic disorder F13.26
        anxiety disorder F13.280
        dementia, persisting F13.27
        intoxication F13.229
          with delirium F13.221
          uncomplicated F13.220

Dependence *(Continued)*
  drug NEC *(Continued)*
    sedative, hypnotic or anxiolytic
      (Continued)
      with *(Continued)*
        mood disorder F13.24
        other specified disorder F13.288
        psychosis F13.259
          delusions F13.250
          hallucinations F13.251
        sexual dysfunction F13.281
        sleep disorder F13.282
        unspecified disorder F13.29
        withdrawal F13.239
          with
            delirium F13.231
            perceptual disturbance
              F13.232
          uncomplicated F13.230
      in remission F13.21
    stimulant NEC F15.20
      with
        anxiety disorder F15.280
        intoxication F15.229
          with
            delirium F15.221
            perceptual disturbance
              F15.222
          uncomplicated F15.220
        mood disorder F15.24
        other specified disorder F15.288
        psychosis F15.259
          delusions F15.250
          hallucinations F15.251
        sexual dysfunction F15.281
        sleep disorder F15.282
        unspecified disorder F15.29
        withdrawal F15.23
      in remission F15.21
    ethyl
      alcohol (without remission) F10.20
        with remission F10.21
      bromide —*see* Dependence, drug,
        sedative
      carbamate F19.20
      chloride F19.20
      morphine —*see* Dependence, drug,
        opioid
    ganja —*see* Dependence, drug, cannabis
    glue (airplane) (sniffing) —*see*
      Dependence, drug, inhalant
    glutethimide —*see* Dependence, drug,
      sedative
    hallucinogenics —*see* Dependence,
      drug, hallucinogen
    hashish —*see* Dependence, drug,
      cannabis
    hemp —*see* Dependence, drug, cannabis
    heroin (salt) (any) —*see* Dependence,
      drug, opioid
    hypnotic NEC —*see* Dependence, drug,
      sedative
    Indian hemp —*see* Dependence, drug,
      cannabis
    inhalants —*see* Dependence, drug,
      inhalant
    khat —*see* Dependence, drug, stimulant
      NEC
    laudanum —*see* Dependence, drug,
      opioid
    LSD (-25) (derivatives) —*see*
      Dependence, drug, hallucinogen
    luminal —*see* Dependence, drug,
      sedative

Dependence (*Continued*)

lysergic acid —*see* Dependence, drug, hallucinogen

maconha —*see* Dependence, drug, cannabis

marihuana —*see* Dependence, drug, cannabis

meprobamate —*see* Dependence, drug, sedative

mescaline —*see* Dependence, drug, hallucinogen

methadone —*see* Dependence, drug, opioid

methamphetamine (s) —*see* Dependence, drug, stimulant NEC

methaqualone —*see* Dependence, drug, sedative

methyl
  alcohol (without remission) F10.20
    with remission F10.21
  bromide —*see* Dependence, drug, sedative
  morphine —*see* Dependence, drug, opioid
  phenidate —*see* Dependence, drug, stimulant NEC
  sulfonal —*see* Dependence, drug, sedative

morphine (sulfate) (sulfite) (type) —*see* Dependence, drug, opioid

narcotic (drug) NEC —*see* Dependence, drug, opioid

nembutal —*see* Dependence, drug, sedative

neraval —*see* Dependence, drug, sedative

neravan —*see* Dependence, drug, sedative

neurobarb —*see* Dependence, drug, sedative

nicotine —*see* Dependence, drug, nicotine

nitrous oxide F19.20

nonbarbiturate sedatives and tranquilizers with similar effect — *see* Dependence, drug, sedative

on
  aspirator Z99.0
  care provider (because of) Z74.9
    impaired mobility Z74.09
    need for
      assistance with personal care Z74.1
      continuous supervision Z74.3
      no other household member able to render care Z74.2
      specified reason NEC Z74.8
  machine Z99.89
    enabling NEC Z99.89
    specified type NEC Z99.89
  renal dialysis (hemodialysis) (peritoneal) Z99.2
  respirator Z99.11
  ventilator Z99.11
  wheelchair Z99.3

opiate —*see* Dependence, drug, opioid

opioids —*see* Dependence, drug, opioid

opium (alkaloids) (derivatives) (tincture) —*see* Dependence, drug, opioid

oxygen (long-term) (supplemental) Z99.81

Dependence (*Continued*)

paraldehyde —*see* Dependence, drug, sedative

paregoric —*see* Dependence, drug, opioid

PCP (phencyclidine) (*see also* Abuse, drug, hallucinogen) F16.20

pentobarbital —*see* Dependence, drug, sedative

pentobarbitone (sodium) —*see* Dependence, drug, sedative

pentothal —*see* Dependence, drug, sedative

peyote —*see* Dependence, drug, hallucinogen

phencyclidine (PCP) (and related substances) (*see also* Abuse, drug, hallucinogen) F16.20

phenmetrazine —*see* Dependence, drug, stimulant NEC

phenobarbital —*see* Dependence, drug, sedative

polysubstance F19.20

psilocibin, psilocin, psilocyn, psilocyline —*see* Dependence, drug, hallucinogen

psychostimulant NEC —*see* Dependence, drug, stimulant NEC

secobarbital —*see* Dependence, drug, sedative

seconal —*see* Dependence, drug, sedative

sedative NEC —*see* Dependence, drug, sedative

specified drug NEC —*see* Dependence, drug

stimulant NEC —*see* Dependence, drug, stimulant NEC

substance NEC —*see* Dependence, drug

supplemental oxygen Z99.81

tobacco —*see* Dependence, drug, nicotine
  counseling and surveillance Z71.6

tranquilizer NEC —*see* Dependence, drug, sedative

vitamin B6 E53.1

volatile solvents —*see* Dependence, drug, inhalant

Dependency
care-provider Z74.9
passive F60.7
reactions (persistent) F60.7

Depersonalization (in neurotic state) (neurotic) (syndrome) F48.1

Depletion
extracellular fluid E86.9
plasma E86.1
potassium E87.6
  nephropathy N25.89
salt or sodium E87.1
  causing heat exhaustion or prostration T67.4
  nephropathy N28.9
volume NOS E86.9

Deployment (current) (military) status Z56.82
in theater or in support of military war, peacekeeping and humanitarian operations Z56.82
personal history of Z91.82
  military war, peacekeeping and humanitarian deployment (current or past conflict) Z91.82
returned from Z91.82

Depolarization, premature I49.40
atrial I49.1
junctional I49.2
specified NEC I49.49
ventricular I49.3

Deposit
bone in Boeck's sarcoid D86.89
calcareous, calcium —*see* Calcification
cholesterol
  retina H35.89
  vitreous (body) (humor) —*see* Deposit, crystalline
conjunctiva H11.11-
cornea H18.00-
  argentous H18.02-
  due to metabolic disorder H18.03-
  Kayser-Fleischer ring H18.04-
  pigmentation —*see* Pigmentation, cornea
crystalline, vitreous (body) (humor) H43.2-
hemosiderin in old scars of cornea —*see* Pigmentation, cornea, stromal
metallic in lens —*see* Cataract, specified NEC
skin R23.8
tooth, teeth (betel) (black) (green) (materia alba) (orange) (tobacco) K03.6
urate, kidney —*see* Calculus, kidney

Depraved appetite —*see* Pica

Depressed
HDL cholesterol E78.6

Depression (acute) (mental) F32.9
agitated (single episode) F32.2
anaclitic —*see* Disorder, adjustment
anxiety F41.8
  persistent F34.1
arches —*see also* Deformity, limb, flat foot
atypical (single episode) F32.8
basal metabolic rate R94.8
bone marrow D75.89
central nervous system R09.2
cerebral R29.818
  newborn P91.4
cerebrovascular I67.9
chest wall M95.4
climacteric (single episode) F32.8
endogenous (without psychotic symptoms) F33.2
  with psychotic symptoms F33.3
functional activity R68.89
hysterical F44.89
involutional (single episode) F32.8
major F32.9
  with psychotic symptoms F32.3
  recurrent —*see* Disorder, depressive, recurrent
manic-depressive —*see* Disorder, depressive, recurrent
masked (single episode) F32.8
medullary G93.89
menopausal (single episode) F32.8
metatarsus —*see* Depression, arches
monopolar F33.9
nervous F34.1
neurotic F34.1
nose M95.0
postnatal F53
postpartum F53
post-psychotic of schizophrenia F32.8
post-schizophrenic F32.8

Depression (Continued)
  psychogenic (reactive) (single episode) F32.9
  psychoneurotic F34.1
  psychotic (single episode) F32.3
    recurrent F33.3
  reactive (psychogenic) (single episode) F32.9
    psychotic (single episode) F32.3
  recurrent —see Disorder, depressive, recurrent
  respiratory center G93.89
  seasonal —see Disorder, depressive, recurrent
  senile F03
  severe, single episode F32.2
  situational F43.21
  skull Q67.4
  specified NEC (single episode) F32.8
  sternum M95.4
  visual field —see Defect, visual field
  vital (recurrent) (without psychotic symptoms) F33.2
    with psychotic symptoms F33.3
    single episode F32.2
Deprivation
  cultural Z60.3
  effects NOS T73.9
    specified NEC T73.8
  emotional NEC Z65.8
    affecting infant or child —see Maltreatment, child, psychological
  food T73.0
  protein —see Malnutrition
  sleep Z72.820
  social Z60.4
    affecting infant or child —see Maltreatment, child, psychological
  specified NEC T73.8
  vitamins —see Deficiency, vitamin
  water T73.1
Derangement
  ankle (internal) —see Derangement, joint, ankle
  cartilage (articular) NEC —see Derangement, joint, articular cartilage, by site
    recurrent —see Dislocation, recurrent
  cruciate ligament, anterior, current injury —see Sprain, knee, cruciate, anterior
  elbow (internal) —see Derangement, joint, elbow
  hip (joint) (internal) (old) —see Derangement, joint, hip
  joint (internal) M24.9
    ankylosis —see Ankylosis
    articular cartilage M24.10
      ankle M24.17-
      elbow M24.12-
      foot M24.17-
      hand M24.14-
      hip M24.15-
      knee NEC M23.9-
      loose body —see Loose, body
      shoulder M24.11-
      wrist M24.13-
    contracture —see Contraction, joint
    current injury —see also Dislocation
      knee, meniscus or cartilage —see Tear, meniscus

Derangement (Continued)
  joint (Continued)
    dislocation
      pathological —see Dislocation, pathological
      recurrent —see Dislocation, recurrent
      knee —see Derangement, knee
      ligament —see Disorder, ligament
      loose body —see Loose, body
      recurrent —see Dislocation, recurrent
      specified type NEC M24.80
        ankle M24.87-
        elbow M24.82-
        foot joint M24.87-
        hand joint M24.84-
        hip M24.85-
        shoulder M24.81-
        wrist M24.83-
      temporomandibular M26.69
    knee (recurrent) M23.9-
      ligament disruption, spontaneous M23.60-
        anterior cruciate M23.61-
        capsular M23.67-
        instability, chronic M23.5-
        lateral collateral M23.64-
        medial collateral M23.63-
        posterior cruciate M23.62-
      loose body M23.4-
      meniscus M23.30-
        cystic M23.00-
          lateral M23.02-
            anterior horn M23.04-
            posterior horn M23.05-
            specified NEC M23.06-
          medial M23.00-
            anterior horn M23.01-
            posterior horn M23.02-
            specified NEC M23.03-
        degenerate —see Derangement, knee, meniscus, specified NEC
        detached —see Derangement, knee, meniscus, specified NEC
        due to old tear or injury M23.20-
          lateral M23.20-
            anterior horn M23.24-
            posterior horn M23.25-
            specified NEC M23.26-
          medial M23.20-
            anterior horn M23.21-
            posterior horn M23.22-
            specified NEC M23.23-
        retained —see Derangement, knee, meniscus, specified NEC
        specified NEC M23.30-
          lateral M23.30-
            anterior horn M23.34-
            posterior horn M23.35-
            specified NEC M23.36-
          medial M23.30-
            anterior horn M23.31-
            posterior horn M23.32-
            specified NEC M23.33-
      old M23.8X-
      specified NEC —see subcategory M23.8
    low back NEC —see Dorsopathy, specified NEC
    meniscus —see Derangement, knee, meniscus
    mental —see Psychosis
    patella, specified NEC —see Disorder, patella, derangement NEC

Derangement (Continued)
  semilunar cartilage (knee) —see Derangement, knee, meniscus, specified NEC
  shoulder (internal) —see Derangement, joint, shoulder
Dercum's disease E88.2
Derealization (neurotic) F48.1
Dermal —see condition
Dermaphytid —see Dermatophytosis
Dermatitis (eczematous) L30.9
  ab igne L59.0
  acarine B88.0
  actinic (due to sun) L57.8
    other than from sun L59.8
  allergic —see Dermatitis, contact, allergic
  ambustionis, due to burn or scald —see Burn
  amebic A06.7
  ammonia L22
  arsenical (ingested) L27.8
  artefacta L98.1
    psychogenic F54
  atopic L20.9
    psychogenic F54
    specified NEC L20.89
  autoimmune progesterone L30.8
  berlock, berloque L56.2
  blastomycotic B40.3
  blister beetle L24.89
  bullous, bullosa L13.9
    mucosynechial, atrophic L12.1
    seasonal L30.8
    specified NEC L13.8
  calorica L59.0
    due to burn or scald —see Burn
  caterpillar L24.89
  cercarial B65.3
  combustionis L59.0
    due to burn or scald —see Burn
  congelationis T69.1
  contact (occupational) L25.9
    allergic L23.9
      due to
        adhesives L23.1
        cement L23.5
        chemical products NEC L23.5
        chromium L23.0
        cosmetics L23.2
        dander (cat) (dog) L23.81
        drugs in contact with skin L23.3
        dyes L23.4
        food in contact with skin L23.6
        hair (cat) (dog) L23.81
        insecticide L23.5
        metals L23.0
        nickel L23.0
        plants, non-food L23.7
        plastic L23.5
        rubber L23.5
        specified agent NEC L23.89
    due to
      chemical products NEC L25.3
      cosmetics L25.0
      dander (cat) (dog) L23.81
      drugs in contact with skin L25.1
      dyes L25.2
      food in contact with skin L25.4
      hair (cat) (dog) L23.81
      plants, non-food L25.5
      specified agent NEC L25.8

Dermatitis *(Continued)*
  contact *(Continued)*
    irritant L24.9
      due to
        chemical products NEC L24.5
        cosmetics L24.3
        detergents L24.0
        drugs in contact with skin
          L24.4
        food in contact with skin L24.6
        oils and greases L24.1
        plants, non-food L24.7
        solvents L24.2
        specified agent NEC L24.89
  contusiformis L52
  diabetic —*see* E08-E13 with .620
  diaper L22
  diphtheritica A36.3
  dry skin L85.3
  due to
    acetone (contact) (irritant) L24.2
    acids (contact) (irritant) L24.5
    adhesive (s) (allergic) (contact)
      (plaster) L23.1
      irritant L24.5
    alcohol (irritant) (skin contact)
      (substances in T51.00-T51.93)
      L24.2
      taken internally L27.8
    alkalis (contact) (irritant) L24.5
    arsenic (ingested) L27.8
    carbon disulfide (contact) (irritant)
      L24.2
    caustics (contact) (irritant) L24.5
    cement (contact) L24.5
    cereal (ingested) L27.2
    chemical (s) NEC L24.5
      taken internally L27.8
    chlorocompounds L24.2
    chromium (contact) (irritant) L24.81
    coffee (ingested) L27.2
    cold weather L30.8
    cosmetics (contact) L25.0
      allergic L23.2
      irritant L24.3
    cyclohexanes L24.2
    dander (cat) (dog) L23.81
    Demodex species B88.0
    Dermanyssus gallinae B88.0
    detergents (contact) (irritant) L24.0
    dichromate L24.81
    drugs and medicaments (generalized)
      (internal use) L27.0
      external —*see* Dermatitis, due to,
        drugs, in contact with skin
      in contact with skin L25.1
        allergic L23.3
        irritant L24.4
      localized skin eruption L27.1
      specified substance —*see* Table of
        drugs and chemicals
    dyes (contact) L25.2
      allergic L23.4
      irritant L24.89
    epidermophytosis —*see*
      Dermatophytosis
    esters L24.2
    external irritant NEC L24.9
    fish (ingested) L27.2
    flour (ingested) L27.2
    food (ingested) L27.2
      in contact with skin L25.4
    fruit (ingested) L27.2
    furs (allergic) (contact) L23.81

Dermatitis *(Continued)*
  due to *(Continued)*
    glues —*see* Dermatitis, due to,
      adhesives
    glycols L24.2
    greases NEC (contact) (irritant) L24.1
    hair (cat) (dog) L23.81
    hot
      objects and materials —*see* Burn
      weather or places L59.0
    hydrocarbons L24.2
    infrared rays L59.8
    ingestion, ingested substance L27.9
      chemical NEC L27.8
      drugs and medicaments —*see*
        Dermatitis, due to, drugs
      food L27.2
      specified NEC L27.8
    insecticide in contact with skin L24.5
    internal agent L27.9
      drugs and medicaments
        (generalized) —*see* Dermatitis,
        due to, drugs
      food L27.2
    irradiation —*see* Dermatitis, due to,
      radioactive substance
    ketones L24.2
    lacquer tree (allergic) (contact) L23.7
    light (sun) NEC L57.8
      acute L56.8
      other L59.8
    Liponyssoides sanguineus B88.0
    low temperature L30.8
    meat (ingested) L27.2
    metals, metal salts (contact) (irritant)
      L24.81
    milk (ingested) L27.2
    nickel (contact) (irritant) L24.81
    nylon (contact) (irritant) L24.5
    oils NEC (contact) (irritant) L24.1
    paint solvent (contact) (irritant) L24.2
    petroleum products (contact)
      (irritant) (substances in T52)
      L24.2
    plants NEC (contact) L25.5
      allergic L23.7
      irritant L24.7
    plasters (adhesive) (any) (allergic)
      (contact) L23.1
      irritant L24.5
    plastic (contact) L24.5
    preservatives (contact) —*see*
      Dermatitis, due to, chemical, in
      contact with skin
    primrose (allergic) (contact) L23.7
    primula (allergic) (contact) L23.7
    radiation L59.8
      nonionizing (chronic exposure)
        L57.8
      sun NEC L57.8
        acute L56.8
    radioactive substance L58.9
      acute L58.0
      chronic L58.1
    radium L58.9
      acute L58.0
      chronic L58.1
    ragweed (allergic) (contact) L23.7
    Rhus (allergic) (contact) (diversiloba)
      (radicans) (toxicodendron)
      (venenata) (verniciflua) L23.7
    rubber (contact) L24.5
    Senecio jacobaea (allergic) (contact)
      L23.7

Dermatitis *(Continued)*
  due to *(Continued)*
    solvents (contact) (irritant) (substances
      in T52.00-T53.93) L24.2
    specified agent NEC (contact) L25.8
      allergic L23.89
      irritant L24.89
    sunshine NEC L57.8
      acute L56.8
    tetrachlorethylene (contact) (irritant)
      L24.2
    toluene (contact) (irritant) L24.2
    turpentine (contact) L24.2
    ultraviolet rays (sun NEC) (chronic
      exposure) L57.8
      acute L56.8
    vaccine or vaccination L27.0
      specified substance —*see* Table of
        drugs and chemicals
    varicose veins —*see* Varix, leg, with,
      inflammation
    X-rays L58.9
      acute L58.0
      chronic L58.1
  dyshydrotic L30.1
  dysmenorrheica N94.6
  escharotica —*see* Burn
  exfoliative, exfoliativa (generalized) L26
    neonatorum L00
  eyelid —*see also* Dermatosis, eyelid
    allergic H01.119
      left H01.116
        lower H01.115
        upper H01.114
      right H01.113
        lower H01.112
        upper H01.111
    contact —*see* Dermatitis, eyelid,
      allergic
    due to
      Demodex species B88.0
      herpes (zoster) B02.39
        simplex B00.59
    eczematous H01.139
      left H01.136
        lower H01.135
        upper H01.134
      right H01.133
        lower H01.132
        upper H01.131
  facta, factitia, factitial L98.1
    psychogenic F54
  flexural NEC L20.82
  friction L30.4
  fungus B36.9
    specified type NEC B36.8
  gangrenosa, gangrenous infantum
    L08.0
  harvest mite B88.0
  heat L59.0
  herpesviral, vesicular (ear) (lip) B00.1
  herpetiformis (bullous) (erythematous)
    (pustular) (vesicular) L13.0
    juvenile L12.2
    senile L12.0
  hiemalis L30.8
  hypostatic, hypostatica —*see* Varix, leg,
    with, inflammation
  infectious eczematoid L30.3
  infective L30.3
  irritant —*see* Dermatitis, contact, irritant
  Jacquet's (diaper dermatitis) L22
  Leptus B88.0
  lichenified NEC L28.0

Dermatitis (Continued)
  medicamentosa (generalized) (internal
      use) —see Dermatitis, due to drugs
  mite B88.0
  multiformis L13.0
      juvenile L12.2
  napkin L22
  neurotica L13.0
  nummular L30.0
  papillaris capillitii L73.0
  pellagrous E52
  perioral L71.0
  photocontact L56.2
  polymorpha dolorosa L13.0
  pruriginosa L13.0
  pruritic NEC L30.8
  psychogenic F54
  purulent L08.0
  pustular
      contagious B08.02
      subcorneal L13.1
  pyococcal L08.0
  pyogenica L08.0
  repens L40.2
  Ritter's (exfoliativa) L00
  Schamberg's L81.7
  schistosome B65.3
  seasonal bullous L30.8
  seborrheic L21.9
      infantile L21.1
      specified NEC L21.8
  sensitization NOS L23.9
  septic L08.0
  solare L57.8
  specified NEC L30.8
  stasis I87.2
      with varicose ulcer —see Varix, leg,
          with ulcer, with inflammation
      due to postthrombotic syndrome —
          see Syndrome, postthrombotic
  suppurative L08.0
  traumatic NEC L30.4
  trophoneurotica L13.0
  ultraviolet (sun) (chronic exposure)
      L57.8
      acute L56.8
  varicose —see Varix, leg, with,
      inflammation
  vegetans L10.1
  verrucosa B43.0
  vesicular, herpesviral B00.1
Dermatoarthritis, lipoid E78.81
Dermatochalasis, eyelid H02.839
  left H02.836
      lower H02.835
      upper H02.834
  right H02.833
      lower H02.832
      upper H02.831
Dermatofibroma (lenticulare) —see
    Neoplasm, skin, benign
  protuberans —see Neoplasm, skin,
      uncertain behavior
Dermatofibrosarcoma (pigmented)
    (protuberans) —see Neoplasm, skin,
    malignant
Dermatographia L50.3
Dermatolysis (exfoliativa) (congenital)
    Q82.8
  acquired L57.4
  eyelids —see Blepharochalasis
  palpebrarum —see Blepharochalasis
  senile L57.4
Dermatomegaly NEC Q82.8

Dermatomucosomyositis M33.10
  with
      myopathy M33.12
      respiratory involvement M33.11
      specified organ involvement NEC
          M33.19
Dermatomycosis B36.9
  furfuracea B36.0
  specified type NEC B36.8
Dermatomyositis (acute) (chronic) —see
    also Dermatopolymyositis
  in (due to) neoplastic disease (see also
      Neoplasm) D49.9 [M36.0]
Dermatoneuritis of children —see
    Poisoning, mercury
Dermatophilosis A48.8
Dermatophytid L30.2
Dermatophytide —see Dermatophytosis
Dermatophytosis (epidermophyton)
    (infection) (Microsporum) (tinea)
    (Trichophyton) B35.9
  beard B35.0
  body B35.4
  capitis B35.0
  corporis B35.4
  deep-seated B35.8
  disseminated B35.8
  foot B35.3
  granulomatous B35.8
  groin B35.6
  hand B35.2
  nail B35.1
  perianal (area) B35.6
  scalp B35.0
  specified NEC B35.8
Dermatopolymyositis M33.90
  with
      myopathy M33.92
      respiratory involvement M33.91
      specified organ involvement NEC
          M33.99
  in neoplastic disease (see also Neoplasm)
      D49.9 [M36.0]
  juvenile M33.00
      with
          myopathy M33.02
          respiratory involvement M33.01
          specified organ involvement NEC
              M33.09
  specified NEC M33.10
      myopathy M33.12
      respiratory involvement M33.11
      specified organ involvement NEC
          M33.19
Dermatopolyneuritis —see Poisoning,
    mercury
Dermatorrhexis Q79.6
  acquired L57.4
Dermatosclerosis —see also Scleroderma
  localized L94.0
Dermatosis L98.9
  Andrews' L08.89
  Bowen's —see Neoplasm, skin, in situ
  bullous L13.9
      specified NEC L13.8
  exfoliativa L26
  eyelid (noninfectious)
      dermatitis —see Dermatitis, eyelid
      discoid lupus erythematosus —see
          Lupus, erythematosus, eyelid
      xeroderma —see Xeroderma,
          acquired, eyelid
  factitial L98.1
  febrile neutrophilic L98.2

Dermatosis (Continued)
  gonococcal A54.89
  herpetiformis L13.0
      juvenile L12.2
  linear IgA L13.8
  menstrual NEC L98.8
  neutrophilic, febrile L98.2
  occupational —see Dermatitis, contact
  papulosa nigra L82.1
  pigmentary L81.9
      progressive L81.7
      Schamberg's L81.7
  psychogenic F54
  purpuric, pigmented L81.7
  pustular, subcorneal L13.1
  transient acantholytic L11.1
Dermographia, dermographism L50.3
Dermoid (cyst) —see also Neoplasm,
    benign, by site
  with malignant transformation C56-
  due to radiation (nonionizing) L57.8
Dermopathy
  infiltrative with thyrotoxicosis —see
      Thyrotoxicosis
  nephrogenic fibrosing L90.8
Dermophytosis —see Dermatophytosis
Descemetocele H18.73-
Descemet's membrane —see condition
Descending —see condition
Descensus uteri —see Prolapse, uterus
Desert
  rheumatism B38.0
  sore —see Ulcer, skin
Desertion (newborn) —see Maltreatment
Desmoid (extra-abdominal) (tumor) —
    see Neoplasm, connective tissue,
    uncertain behavior
  abdominal D48.1
Despondency F32.9
Desquamation, skin R23.4
Destruction, destructive —see also
    Damage
  articular facet —see also Derangement,
      joint, specified type NEC
      knee M23.8X-
      vertebra —see Spondylosis
  bone —see also Disorder, bone, specified
      type NEC
      syphilitic A52.77
  joint —see also Derangement, joint,
      specified type NEC
      sacroiliac M53.3
  rectal sphincter K62.89
  septum (nasal) J34.89
  tuberculous NEC —see Tuberculosis
  tympanum, tympanic membrane
      (nontraumatic) —see Disorder,
      tympanic membrane, specified
      NEC
  vertebral disc —see Degeneration,
      intervertebral disc
Destructiveness —see also Disorder,
    conduct
  adjustment reaction —see Disorder,
      adjustment
Desultory labor O62.2
Detachment
  cartilage —see Sprain
  cervix, annular N88.8
      complicating delivery O71.3
  choroid (old) (postinfectional) (simple)
      (spontaneous) H31.40-
      hemorrhagic H31.41-
      serous H31.42-

Detachment *(Continued)*
ligament —*see* Sprain
meniscus (knee) —*see also*
  Derangement, knee, meniscus,
  specified NEC
  current injury —*see* Tear, meniscus
  due to old tear or injury —*see*
    Derangement, knee, meniscus,
    due to old tear
retina (without retinal break) (serous)
  H33.2-
  with retinal:
    break H33.00-
      giant H33.03-
      multiple H33.02-
      single H33.01-
    dialysis H33.04-
  pigment epithelium —*see*
    Degeneration, retina, separation
    of layers, pigment epithelium
    detachment
  rhegmatogenous —*see* Detachment,
    retina, with retinal, break
  specified NEC H33.8
  total H33.05-
  traction H33.4-
vitreous (body) H43.81
Detergent asthma J69.8
Deterioration
epileptic F06.8
general physical R53.81
heart, cardiac —*see* Degeneration,
  myocardial
mental —*see* Psychosis
myocardial, myocardium —*see*
  Degeneration, myocardial
senile (simple) R54
Deuteranomaly (anomalous trichromat)
  H53.53
Deuteranopia (complete) (incomplete)
  H53.53
Development
abnormal, bone Q79.9
arrested R62.50
  bone —*see* Arrest, development or
    growth, bone
  child R62.50
  due to malnutrition E45
defective, congenital —*see also*
  Anomaly, by site
  cauda equina Q06.3
  left ventricle Q24.8
    in hypoplastic left heart syndrome
      Q23.4
  valve Q24.8
  pulmonary Q22.3
delayed (*see also* Delay, development)
  R62.50
  arithmetical skills F81.2
  language (skills) (expressive)
    F80.1
  learning skill F81.9
  mixed skills F88
  motor coordination F82
  reading F81.0
  specified learning skill NEC
    F81.89
  speech F80.9
  spelling F81.81
  written expression F81.81
imperfect, congenital —*see also*
  Anomaly, by site
  heart Q24.9
  lungs Q33.6

Development *(Continued)*
incomplete
  bronchial tree Q32.4
  organ or site not listed —*see*
    Hypoplasia, by site
  respiratory system Q34.9
sexual, precocious NEC E30.1
tardy, mental (*see also* Disability,
  intellectual) F79
Developmental —*see* condition
testing, child —*see* Examination, child
Devergie's disease (pityriasis rubra
  pilaris) L44.0
Deviation (in)
conjugate palsy (eye) (spastic) H51.0
esophagus (acquired) K22.8
eye, skew H51.8
midline (jaw) (teeth) (dental arch) M26.29
  specified site NEC —*see* Malposition
nasal septum J34.2
  congenital Q67.4
opening and closing of the mandible
  M26.53
organ or site, congenital NEC —*see*
  Malposition, congenital
septum (nasal) (acquired) J34.2
  congenital Q67.4
sexual F65.9
  bestiality F65.89
  erotomania F52.8
  exhibitionism F65.2
  fetishism, fetishistic F65.0
    transvestism F65.1
  frotteurism F65.81
  masochism F65.51
  multiple F65.89
  necrophilia F65.89
  nymphomania F52.8
  pederosis F65.4
  pedophilia F65.4
  sadism, sadomasochism F65.52
  satyriasis F52.8
  specified type NEC F65.89
  transvestism F64.1
  voyeurism F65.3
teeth, midline M26.29
trachea J39.8
ureter, congenital Q62.61
Device
cerebral ventricle (communicating) in
  situ Z98.2
contraceptive —*see* Contraceptive,
  device
drainage, cerebrospinal fluid, in situ
  Z98.2
Devic's disease G36.0
Devil's
grip B33.0
pinches (purpura simplex) D69.2
Devitalized tooth K04.99
Devonshire colic —*see* Poisoning, lead
Dextraposition, aorta Q20.3
  in tetralogy of Fallot Q21.3
Dextrinosis, limit (debrancher enzyme
  deficiency) E74.03
Dextrocardia (true) Q24.0
  with
    complete transposition of viscera
      Q89.3
    situs inversus Q89.3
Dextrotransposition, aorta Q20.3
d-glycericacidemia E72.59
Dhat syndrome F48.8
Dhobi itch B35.6

Di George's syndrome D82.1
Di Guglielmo's disease C94.0-
Diabetes, diabetic (mellitus) (sugar) E11.9
  with
    amyotrophy E11.44
    arthropathy NEC E11.618
    autonomic (poly)neuropathy E11.43
    cataract E11.36
    Charcot's joints E11.610
    chronic kidney disease E11.22
    circulatory complication NEC
      E11.59
    complication E11.8
      specified NEC E11.69
    dermatitis E11.620
    foot ulcer E11.621
    gangrene E11.52
    gastroparesis E11.43
    glomerulonephrosis, intracapillary
      E11.21
    glomerulosclerosis, intercapillary
      E11.21
    hyperglycemia E11.65
    hyperosmolarity E11.00
      with coma E11.01
    hypoglycemia E11.649
      with coma E11.641
    kidney complications NEC E11.29
    Kimmelstiel-Wilson disease E11.21
    loss of protective sensation (LOPS) —
      see Diabetes, by type, with
      neuropathy
    mononeuropathy E11.41
    myasthenia E11.44
    necrobiosis lipoidica E11.620
    nephropathy E11.21
    neuralgia E11.42
    neurologic complication NEC E11.49
    neuropathic arthropathy E11.610
    neuropathy E11.40
    ophthalmic complication NEC E11.39
    oral complication NEC E11.638
    periodontal disease E11.630
    peripheral angiopathy E11.51
      with gangrene E11.52
    polyneuropathy E11.42
    renal complication NEC E11.29
    renal tubular degeneration E11.29
    retinopathy E11.319
      with macular edema E11.311
      nonproliferative E11.329
        with macular edema E11.321
        mild E11.329
          with macular edema E11.321
        moderate E11.339
          with macular edema E11.331
        severe E11.349
          with macular edema E11.341
      proliferative E11.359
        with macular edema E11.351
    skin complication NEC E11.628
    skin ulcer NEC E11.622
  bronzed E83.110
  complicating pregnancy —*see*
    Pregnancy, complicated by,
    diabetes
  dietary counseling and surveillance
    Z71.3
  due to drug or chemical E09.9
    with
      amyotrophy E09.44
      arthropathy NEC E09.618
      autonomic (poly)neuropathy
        E09.43

Diabetes, diabetic *(Continued)*
  due to drug or chemical *(Continued)*
    with *(Continued)*
      cataract E09.36
      Charcot's joints E09.610
      chronic kidney disease E09.22
      circulatory complication NEC E09.59
      complication E09.8
        specified NEC E09.69
      dermatitis E09.620
      foot ulcer E09.621
      gangrene E09.52
      gastroparesis E09.43
      glomerulonephrosis, intracapillary E09.21
      glomerulosclerosis, intercapillary E09.21
      hyperglycemia E09.65
      hyperosmolarity E09.00
        with coma E09.01
      hypoglycemia E09.649
        with coma E09.641
      ketoacidosis E09.10
        with coma E09.11
      kidney complications NEC E09.29
      Kimmelsteil-Wilson disease E09.21
      mononeuropathy E09.41
      myasthenia E09.44
      necrobiosis lipoidica E09.620
      nephropathy E09.21
      neuralgia E09.42
      neurologic complication NEC E09.49
      neuropathic arthropathy E09.610
      neuropathy E09.40
      ophthalmic complication NEC E09.39
      oral complication NEC E09.638
      periodontal disease E09.630
      peripheral angiopathy E09.51
        with gangrene E09.52
      polyneuropathy E09.42
      renal complication NEC E09.29
      renal tubular degeneration E09.29
      retinopathy E09.319
        with macular edema E09.311
        nonproliferative E09.329
          with macular edema E09.321
          mild E09.329
            with macular edema E09.321
          moderate E09.339
            with macular edema E09.331
          severe E09.349
            with macular edema E09.341
        proliferative E09.359
          with macular edema E09.351
      skin complication NEC E09.628
      skin ulcer NEC E09.622
  due to underlying condition E08.9
    with
      amyotrophy E08.44
      arthropathy NEC E08.618
      autonomic (poly)neuropathy E08.43
      cataract E08.36
      Charcot's joints E08.610
      chronic kidney disease E08.22
      circulatory complication NEC E08.59
      complication E08.8
        specified NEC E08.69
      dermatitis E08.620
      foot ulcer E08.621

Diabetes, diabetic *(Continued)*
  due to underlying condition *(Continued)*
    with *(Continued)*
      gangrene E08.52
      gastroparesis E08.43
      glomerulonephrosis, intracapillary E08.21
      glomerulosclerosis, intercapillary E08.21
      hyperglycemia E08.69
      hyperosmolarity E08.00
        with coma E08.01
      hypoglycemia E08.649
        with coma E08.641
      ketoacidosis E08.10
        with coma E08.11
      kidney complications NEC E08.29
      Kimmelsteil-WIlson disease E08.21
      mononeuropathy E08.41
      myasthenia E08.44
      necrobiosis lipoidica E08.620
      nephropathy E08.21
      neuralgia E08.42
      neurologic complication NEC E08.49
      neuropathic arthropathy E08.610
      neuropathy E08.40
      ophthalmic complication NEC E08.39
      oral complication NEC E08.638
      periodontal disease E08.630
      peripheral angiopathy E08.51
        with gangrene E08.52
      polyneuropathy E08.42
      renal complication NEC E08.29
      renal tubular degeneration E08.29
      retinopathy E08.319
        with macular edema E08.311
        nonproliferative E08.329
          with macular edema E08.321
          mild E08.329
            with macular edema E08.321
          moderate E08.339
            with macular edema E08.331
          severe E08.349
            with macular edema E08.341
        proliferative E08.359
          with macular edema E08.351
      skin complication NEC E08.628
      skin ulcer NEC E08.622
  gestational (in pregnancy) O24.419
    affecting newborn P70.0
    diet-controlled O24.410
    in childbirth O24.429
      diet-controlled O24.420
      insulin (and diet) controlled O24.424
    insulin (and diet) controlled O24.414
    puerperal O24.439
      diet-controlled O24.430
      insulin (and diet) controlled O24.434
  hepatogenous E13.9
  inadequately controlled — code to Diabetes, by type, with hyperglycemia
  insipidus E23.2
    nephrogenic N25.1
    pituitary E23.2
    vasopressin resistant N25.1
  insulin dependent — code to type of diabetes
  juvenile-onset —*see* Diabetes, type 1
  ketosis-prone —*see* Diabetes, type 1
  latent R73.09
  neonatal (transient) P70.2

Diabetes, diabetic *(Continued)*
  non-insulin dependent — code to type of diabetes
  out of control — code to Diabetes, by type, with hyperglycemia
  phosphate E83.39
  poorly controlled — code to Diabetes, by type, with hyperglycemia
  postpancreatectomy —*see* Diabetes, specified type NEC
  postprocedural —*see* Diabetes, specified type NEC
  secondary diabetes mellitus NEC —*see* Diabetes, specified type NEC
  specified type NEC E13.9
    with
      amyotrophy E13.44
      arthropathy NEC E13.618
      autonomic (poly)neuropathy E13.43
      cataract E13.36
      Charcot's joints E13.610
      chronic kidney disease E13.22
      circulatory complication NEC E13.59
      complication E13.8
        specified NEC E13.69
      dermatitis E13.620
      foot ulcer E13.621
      gangrene E13.52
      gastroparesis E13.43
      glomerulonephrosis, intracapillary E13.21
      glomerulosclerosis, intercapillary E13.21
      hyperglycemia E13.65
      hyperosmolarity E13.00
        with coma E13.01
      hypoglycemia E13.649
        with coma E13.641
      ketoacidosis E13.10
        with coma E13.11
      kidney complications NEC E13.29
      Kimmelsteil-Wilson disease E13.21
      mononeuropathy E13.41
      myasthenia E13.44
      necrobiosis lipoidica E13.620
      nephropathy E13.21
      neuralgia E13.42
      neurologic complication NEC E13.49
      neuropathic arthropathy E13.610
      neuropathy E13.40
      ophthalmic complication NEC E13.39
      oral complication NEC E13.638
      periodontal disease E13.630
      peripheral angiopathy E13.51
        with gangrene E13.52
      polyneuropathy E13.42
      renal complication NEC E13.29
      renal tubular degeneration E13.29
      retinopathy E13.319
        with macular edema E13.311
        nonproliferative E13.329
          with macular edema E13.321
          mild E13.329
            with macular edema E13.321
          moderate E13.339
            with macular edema E13.331
          severe E13.349
            with macular edema E13.341
        proliferative E13.359
          with macular edema E13.351
      skin complication NEC E13.628
      skin ulcer NEC E13.622
  steroid-induced —*see* Diabetes, due to, drug or chemical

Diabetes, diabetic *(Continued)*
  type 1 E10.9
    with
      amyotrophy E10.44
      arthropathy NEC E10.618
      autonomic (poly)neuropathy
        E10.43
      cataract E10.36
      Charcot's joints E10.610
      chronic kidney disease E10.22
      circulatory complication NEC
        E10.59
      complication E10.8
        specified NEC E10.69
      dermatitis E10.620
      foot ulcer E10.621
      gangrene E10.52
      gastroparesis E10.43
      glomerulonephrosis, intracapillary
        E10.21
      glomerulosclerosis, intercapillary
        E10.21
      hyperglycemia E10.65
      hypoglycemia E10.649
        with coma E10.641
      ketoacidosis E10.10
        with coma E10.11
      kidney complications NEC E10.29
      Kimmelsteil-Wilson disease E10.21
      mononeuropathy E10.41
      myasthenia E10.44
      necrobiosis lipoidica E10.620
      nephropathy E10.21
      neuralgia E10.42
      neurologic complication NEC
        E10.49
      neuropathic arthropathy E10.610
      neuropathy E10.40
      ophthalmic complication NEC
        E10.39
      oral complication NEC E10.638
      periodontal disease E10.630
      peripheral angiopathy E10.51
        with gangrene E10.52
      polyneuropathy E10.42
      renal complication NEC E10.29
      renal tubular degeneration E10.29
      retinopathy E10.319
        with macular edema E10.311
        nonproliferative E10.329
          with macular edema E10.321
          mild E10.329
            with macular edema E10.321
          moderate E10.339
            with macular edema E10.331
          severe E10.349
            with macular edema E10.341
        proliferative E10.359
          with macular edema E10.351
      skin complication NEC E10.628
      skin ulcer NEC E10.622
  type 2 E11.9
    with
      amyotrophy E11.44
      arthropathy NEC E11.618
      autonomic (poly)neuropathy E11.43
      cataract E11.36
      Charcot's joints E11.610
      chronic kidney disease E11.22
      circulatory complication NEC
        E11.59
      complication E11.8
        specified NEC E11.69
      dermatitis E11.620

Diabetes, diabetic *(Continued)*
  type 2 *(Continued)*
    with *(Continued)*
      foot ulcer E11.621
      gangrene E11.52
      gastroparesis E11.43
      glomerulonephrosis, intracapillary
        E11.21
      glomerulosclerosis, intercapillary
        E11.21
      hyperglycemia E11.65
      hyperosmolarity E11.00
        with coma E11.01
      hypoglycemia E11.649
        with coma E11.641
      kidney complications NEC E11.29
      Kimmelsteil-Wilson disease E11.21
      mononeuropathy E11.41
      myasthenia E11.44
      necrobiosis lipoidica E11.620
      nephropathy E11.21
      neuralgia E11.42
      neurologic complication NEC
        E11.49
      neuropathic arthropathy E11.610
      neuropathy E11.40
      ophthalmic complication NEC
        E11.39
      oral complication NEC E11.638
      periodontal disease E11.630
      peripheral angiopathy E11.51
        with gangrene E11.52
      polyneuropathy E11.42
      renal complication NEC E11.29
      renal tubular degeneration E11.29
      retinopathy E11.319
        with macular edema E11.311
        nonproliferative E11.329
          with macular edema E11.321
          mild E11.329
            with macular edema E11.321
          moderate E11.339
            with macular edema E11.331
          severe E11.349
            with macular edema E11.341
        proliferative E11.359
          with macular edema E11.351
      skin complication NEC E11.628
      skin ulcer NEC E11.622
Diacyclothrombopathia D69.1
Diagnosis deferred R69
Dialysis (intermittent) (treatment)
  noncompliance (with) Z91.15
  renal (hemodialysis) (peritoneal), status
    Z99.2
  retina, retinal —*see* Detachment, retina,
    with retinal, dialysis
Diamond-Blackfan anemia (congenital
  hypoplastic) D61.01
Diamond-Gardener syndrome
  (autoerythrocyte sensitization)
  D69.2
Diaper rash L22
Diaphoresis (excessive) R61
Diaphragm —*see* condition
Diaphragmalgia R07.1
Diaphragmatitis, diaphragmitis J98.6
Diaphysial aclasis Q78.6
Diaphysitis —*see* Osteomyelitis, specified
  type NEC
Diarrhea, diarrheal (disease) (infantile)
  (inflammatory) R19.7
  achlorhydric K31.83
  allergic K52.2

Diarrhea, diarrheal *(Continued)*
  amebic (*see also* Amebiasis) A06.0
    with abscess —*see* Abscess, amebic
    acute A06.0
    chronic A06.1
    nondysenteric A06.2
  bacillary —*see* Dysentery, bacillary
  balantidial A07.0
  cachectic NEC K52.89
  Chilomastix A07.8
  choleriformis A00.1
  chronic (noninfectious) K52.9
  coccidial A07.3
  Cochin-China K90.1
    strongyloidiasis B78.0
  Dientamoeba A07.8
  dietetic K52.2
  drug-induced K52.1
  due to
    bacteria A04.9
      specified NEC A04.8
    Campylobacter A04.5
    Capillaria philippinensis B81.1
    Clostridium difficile A04.7
    Clostridium perfringens (C) (F) A04.8
    Cryptosporidium A07.2
    drugs K52.1
    Escherichia coli A04.4
      enteroaggregative A04.4
      enterohemorrhagic A04.3
      enteroinvasive A04.2
      enteropathogenic A04.0
      enterotoxigenic A04.1
      specified NEC A04.4
    food hypersensitivity K52.2
    Necator americanus B76.1
    S. japonicum B65.2
    specified organism NEC A08.8
      bacterial A04.8
      viral A08.39
    Staphylococcus A04.8
    Trichuris trichiuria B79
    virus —*see* Enteritis, viral
    Yersinia enterocolitica A04.6
  dysenteric A09
  endemic A09
  epidemic A09
  flagellate A07.9
  Flexner's (ulcerative) A03.1
  functional K59.1
    following gastrointestinal surgery
      K91.89
    psychogenic F45.8
  Giardia lamblia A07.1
  giardial A07.1
  hill K90.1
  infectious A09
  malarial —*see* Malaria
  mite B88.0
  mycotic NEC B49
  neonatal (noninfectious) P78.3
  nervous F45.8
  neurogenic K59.1
  noninfectious K52.9
  postgastrectomy K91.1
  postvagotomy K91.1
  protozoal A07.9
    specified NEC A07.8
  psychogenic F45.8
  specified
    bacterium NEC A04.8
    virus NEC A08.39
  strongyloidiasis B78.0
  toxic K52.1

Diarrhea, diarrheal (Continued)
  trichomonal A07.8
  tropical K90.1
  tuberculous A18.32
  viral —see Enteritis, viral
Diastasis
  cranial bones M84.88
    congenital NEC Q75.8
  joint (traumatic) —see Dislocation
  muscle M62.00
    ankle M62.07-
    congenital Q79.8
    foot M62.07-
    forearm M62.03-
    hand M62.04-
    lower leg M62.06-
    pelvic region M62.05-
    shoulder region M62.01-
    specified site NEC M62.08
    thigh M62.05-
    upper arm M62.02-
  recti (abdomen)
    complicating delivery O71.89
    congenital Q79.59
Diastema, tooth, teeth, fully erupted
    M26.32
Diastematomyelia Q06.2
Diataxia, cerebral G80.4
Diathesis
  allergic —see History, allergy
  bleeding (familial) D69.9
  cystine (familial) E72.00
  gouty —see Gout
  hemorrhagic (familial) D69.9
    newborn NEC P53
  spasmophilic R29.0
Diaz's disease or osteochondrosis
    (juvenile) (talus) —see
    Osteochondrosis, juvenile, tarsus
Dibothriocephalus, dibothriocephaliasis
    (latus) (infection) (infestation) B70.0
    larval B70.1
Dicephalus, dicephaly Q89.4
Dichotomy, teeth K00.2
Dichromat, dichromatopsia (congenital) —
    see Deficiency, color vision
Dichuchwa A65
Dicroceliasis B66.2
Didelphia, didelphys —see Double uterus
Didymytis N45.1
  with orchitis N45.3
Dietary
  inadequacy or deficiency E63.9
  surveillance and counseling Z71.3
Dietl's crisis N13.8
Dieulafoy lesion (hemorrhagic)
  duodenum K31.82
  esophagus K22.8
  intestine (colon) K63.81
  stomach K31.82
Difficult, difficulty (in)
  acculturation Z60.3
  feeding R63.3
    newborn P92.9
      breast P92.5
      specified NEC P92.8
    nonorganic (infant or child) F98.29
  intubation, in anesthesia T88.4
  mechanical, gastroduodenal stoma
      K91.89
    causing obstruction K91.3
  reading (developmental) F81.0
    secondary to emotional disorders
        F93.9

Difficult, difficulty (in) (Continued)
  spelling (specific) F81.81
    with reading disorder F81.89
    due to inadequate teaching Z55.8
  swallowing —see Dysphagia
  walking R26.2
  work
    conditions NEC Z56.5
    schedule Z56.3
Diffuse —see condition
DiGeorge's syndrome (thymic
    hypoplasia) D82.1
Digestive —see condition
Dihydropyrimidine dehydrogenase
    disease (DPD) E88.89
Diktyoma —see Neoplasm, malignant,
    by site
Dilaceration, tooth K00.4
Dilatation
  anus K59.8
    venule —see Hemorrhoids
  aorta (focal) (general) —see Ectasia,
    aorta
    with aneurysm —see Aneurysm,
      aorta
  artery —see Aneurysm
  bladder (sphincter) N32.89
    congenital Q64.79
  blood vessel I99.8
  bronchial J47.9
    with
      exacerbation (acute) J47.1
      lower respiratory infection J47.0
  calyx (due to obstruction) —see
      Hydronephrosis
  capillaries I78.8
  cardiac (acute) (chronic) —see also
      Hypertrophy, cardiac
    congenital Q24.8
      valve NEC Q24.8
        pulmonary Q22.3
      valve —see Endocarditis
  cavum septi pellucidi Q06.8
  cervix (uteri) —see also Incompetency,
      cervix
    incomplete, poor, slow complicating
        delivery O62.0
  colon K59.3
    congenital Q43.1
    psychogenic F45.8
  common duct (acquired) K83.8
    congenital Q44.5
  cystic duct (acquired) K82.8
    congenital Q44.5
  duct, mammary —see Ectasia,
      mammary duct
  duodenum K59.8
  esophagus K22.8
    congenital Q39.5
    due to achalasia K22.0
  eustachian tube, congenital Q17.8
  gallbladder K82.8
  gastric —see Dilatation, stomach
  heart (acute) (chronic) —see also
      Hypertrophy, cardiac
    congenital Q24.8
      valve —see Endocarditis
  ileum K59.8
    psychogenic F45.8
  jejunum K59.8
    psychogenic F45.8
  kidney (calyx) (collecting structures)
      (cystic) (parenchyma) (pelvis)
      (idiopathic) N28.89

Dilatation (Continued)
  lacrimal passages or duct —see
      Disorder, lacrimal system, changes
  lymphatic vessel I89.0
  mammary duct —see Ectasia, mammary
      duct
  Meckel's diverticulum (congenital)
      Q43.0
    malignant —see Table of Neoplasms,
        small intestine, malignant
  myocardium (acute) (chronic) —see
      Hypertrophy, cardiac organ or site,
      congenital NEC —see Distortion
  pancreatic duct K86.8
  pericardium —see Pericarditis
  pharynx J39.2
  prostate N42.89
  pulmonary
    artery (idiopathic) I28.8
    valve, congenital Q22.3
  pupil H57.04
  rectum K59.3
  saccule, congenital Q16.5
  salivary gland (duct) K11.8
  sphincter ani K62.89
  stomach K31.89
    acute K31.0
    psychogenic F45.8
  submaxillary duct K11.8
  trachea, congenital Q32.1
  ureter (idiopathic) N28.82
    congenital Q62.2
    due to obstruction N13.4
  urethra (acquired) N36.8
  vasomotor I73.9
  vein I86.8
  ventricular, ventricle (acute)
      (chronic) —see also Hypertrophy,
      cardiac
    cerebral, congenital Q04.8
  venule NEC I86.8
  vesical orifice N32.89
Dilated, dilation —see Dilatation
Diminished, diminution
  hearing (acuity) —see Deafness
  sense or sensation (cold) (heat) (tactile)
      (vibratory) R20.8
  vision NEC H54.7
  vital capacity R94.2
Diminuta taenia B71.0
Dimitri-Sturge-Weber disease Q85.8
Dimple
  parasacral, pilonidal or postanal —see
      Cyst, pilonidal
Dioctophyme renalis (infection)
    (infestation) B83.8
Dipetalonemiasis B74.4
Diphallus Q55.69
Diphtheria, diphtheritic (gangrenous)
    (hemorrhagic) A36.9
  carrier (suspected) Z22.2
  cutaneous A36.3
  faucial A36.0
  infection of wound A36.3
  laryngeal A36.2
  myocarditis A36.81
  nasal, anterior A36.89
  nasopharyngeal A36.1
  neurological complication A36.89
  pharyngeal A36.0
  specified site NEC A36.89
  tonsillar A36.0
Diphyllobothriasis (intestine) B70.0
  larval B70.1
Diplacusis H93.22-

Diplegia (upper limbs) G83.0
  congenital (cerebral) G80.8
  facial G51.0
  lower limbs G82.20
  spastic G80.1
Diplococcus, diplococcal —*see* condition
Diplopia H53.2
Dipsomania F10.20
  with
    psychosis —*see* Psychosis, alcoholic
    remission F10.21
Dipylidiasis B71.1
Direction, teeth, abnormal, fully erupted
  M26.30
Dirofilariasis B74.8
Dirt-eating child F98.3
Disability, disabilities
  heart —*see* Disease, heart
  intellectual F79
    with
      autistic features F84.9
    mild (I.Q. 50-69) F70
    moderate (I.Q. 35-49) F71
    profound (I.Q. under 20) F73
    severe (I.Q. 20-34) F72
    specified level NEC F78
  knowledge acquisition F81.9
  learning F81.9
  limiting activities Z73.6
  spelling, specific F81.81
Disappearance of family member Z63.4
Disarticulation —*see* Amputation
  meaning traumatic amputation —*see*
    Amputation, traumatic
Discharge (from)
  abnormal finding in —*see* Abnormal,
    specimen
  breast (female) (male) N64.52
  diencephalic autonomic idiopathic —*see*
    Epilepsy, specified NEC
  ear —*see also* Otorrhea
    blood —*see* Otorrhagia
  excessive urine R35.8
  nipple N64.52
  penile R36.9
  postnasal R09.82
  prison, anxiety concerning Z65.2
  urethral R36.9
    without blood R36.0
    hematospermia R36.1
  vaginal N89.8
Discitis, diskitis M46.40
  cervical region M46.42
  cervicothoracic region M46.43
  lumbar region M46.46
  lumbosacral region M46.47
  multiple sites M46.49
  occipito-atlanto-axial region M46.41
  pyogenic —*see* Infection, intervertebral
    disc, pyogenic
  sacrococcygeal region M46.48
  thoracic region M46.44
  thoracolumbar region M46.45
Discoid
  meniscus (congenital) Q68.6
  semilunar cartilage (congenital) —*see*
    Derangement, knee, meniscus,
    specified NEC
Discoloration
  nails L60.8
  teeth (posteruptive) K03.7
    during formation K00.8
Discomfort
  chest R07.89
  visual H53.14-

Discontinuity, ossicles, ear H74.2-
Discord (with)
  boss Z56.4
  classmates Z55.4
  counselor Z64.4
  employer Z56.4
  family Z63.8
  fellow employees Z56.4
  in-laws Z63.1
  landlord Z59.2
  lodgers Z59.2
  neighbors Z59.2
  probation officer Z64.4
  social worker Z64.4
  teachers Z55.4
  workmates Z56.4
Discordant connection
  atrioventricular (congenital) Q20.5
  ventriculoarterial Q20.3
Discrepancy
  centric occlusion maximum
    intercuspation M26.55
  leg length (acquired) —*see* Deformity,
    limb, unequal length
    congenital —*see* Defect, reduction,
      lower limb
  uterine size date O26.84-
Discrimination
  ethnic Z60.5
  political Z60.5
  racial Z60.5
  religious Z60.5
  sex Z60.5
Disease, diseased —*see also* Syndrome
  absorbent system I87.8
  acid-peptic K30
  Acosta's T70.29
  Adams-Stokes (-Morgagni) (syncope
    with heart block) I45.9
  Addison's anemia (pernicious) D51.0
  adenoids (and tonsils) J35.9
  adrenal (capsule) (cortex) (gland)
    (medullary) E27.9
    hyperfunction E27.0
    specified NEC E27.8
  ainhum L94.6
  airway
    obstructive, chronic J44.9
      due to
        cotton dust J66.0
        specific organic dusts NEC J66.8
    reactive —*see* Asthma
  akamushi (scrub typhus) A75.3
  Albers-Schönberg (marble bones)
    Q78.2
  Albert's —*see* Tendinitis, Achilles
  alimentary canal K63.9
  alligator-skin Q80.9
    acquired L85.0
  alpha heavy chain C88.3
  alpine T70.29
  altitude T70.20
  alveolar ridge
    edentulous K06.9
      specified NEC K06.8
  alveoli, teeth K08.9
  Alzheimer's G30.9 [F02.80]
    with behavioral disturbance G30.9
      [F02.81]
    early onset G30.0 [F02.80]
      with behavioral disturbance G30.0
        [F02.81]
    late onset G30.1 [F02.80]
      with behavioral disturbance G30.1
        [F02.81]

Disease, diseased (*Continued*)
  Alzheimer's (*Continued*)
    specified NEC G30.8 [F02.80]
      with behavioral disturbance G30.8
        [F02.81]
  amyloid —*see* Amyloidosis
  Andersen's (glycogenosis IV) E74.09
  Andes T70.29
  Andrews' (bacterid) L08.89
  angiospastic I73.9
    cerebral G45.9
    vein I87.8
  anterior
    chamber H21.9
    horn cell G12.29
  antiglomerular basement membrane
    (anti-GBM) antibody M31.0
    tubulo-interstitial nephritis N12
  antral —*see* Sinusitis, maxillary
  anus K62.9
    specified NEC K62.89
  aorta (nonsyphilitic) I77.9
    syphilitic NEC A52.02
  aortic (heart) (valve) I35.9
    rheumatic I06.9
  Apollo B30.3
  aponeuroses —*see* Enthesopathy
  appendix K38.9
    specified NEC K38.8
  aqueous (chamber) H21.9
  Arnold-Chiari —*see* Arnold-Chiari
    disease
  arterial I77.9
    occlusive —*see* Occlusion, by site
    due to stricture or stenosis I77.1
  arteriocardiorenal —*see* Hypertension,
    cardiorenal
  arteriolar (generalized) (obliterative)
    I77.9
  arteriorenal —*see* Hypertension,
    kidney
  arteriosclerotic —*see also*
    Arteriosclerosis
    cardiovascular —*see* Disease, heart,
      ischemic, atherosclerotic
    coronary (artery) —*see* Disease, heart,
      ischemic, atherosclerotic
    heart —*see* Disease, heart, ischemic,
      atherosclerotic
  artery I77.9
    cerebral I67.9
    coronary I25.10
      with angina pectoris —*see*
        Arteriosclerosis, coronary
        (artery),
  arthropod-borne NOS (viral) A94
    specified type NEC A93.8
  atticoantral, chronic H66.20
    left H66.22
      with right H66.23
    right H66.21
      with left H66.23
  auditory canal —*see* Disorder, ear,
    external
  auricle, ear NEC —*see* Disorder, pinna
  Australian X A83.4
  autoimmune (systemic) NOS M35.9
    hemolytic (cold type) (warm type)
      D59.1
      drug-induced D59.0
    thyroid E06.3
  aviator's —*see* Effect, adverse, high
    altitude
  Ayala's Q78.5

Disease, diseased *(Continued)*
Ayerza's (pulmonary artery sclerosis with pulmonary hypertension) I27.0
Babington's (familial hemorrhagic telangiectasia) I78.0
bacterial A49.9
  specified NEC A48.8
  zoonotic A28.9
    specified type NEC A28.8
Baelz's (cheilitis glandularis apostematosa) K13.0
bagasse J67.1
balloon —*see* Effect, adverse, high altitude
Bang's (brucella abortus) A23.1
Bannister's T78.3
barometer makers' —*see* Poisoning, mercury
Barraquer (-Simons') (progressive lipodystrophy) E88.1
Barrett's —*see* Barrett's, esophagus
Bartholin's gland N75.9
basal ganglia G25.9
  degenerative G23.9
    specified NEC G23.8
  specified NEC G25.89
Basedow's (exophthalmic goiter) —*see* Hyperthyroidism, with, goiter (diffuse)
Bateman's B08.1
Batten-Steinert G71.11
Battey A31.0
Beard's (neurasthenia) F48.8
Becker
  idiopathic mural endomyocardial I42.3
  myotonia congenita G71.12
Begbie's (exophthalmic goiter) —*see* Hyperthyroidism, with, goiter (diffuse)
behavioral, organic F07.9
Beigel's (white piedra) B36.2
Benson's —*see* Deposit, crystalline
Bernard-Soulier (thrombopathy) D69.1
Bernhardt (-Roth) —*see* Mononeuropathy, lower limb, meralgia paresthetica
Biermer's (pernicious anemia) D51.0
bile duct (common) (hepatic) K83.9
  with calculus, stones —*see* Calculus, bile duct
  specified NEC K83.8
biliary (tract) K83.9
  specified NEC K83.8
Billroth's —*see* Spina bifida
bird fancier's J67.2
black lung J60
bladder N32.9
  in (due to)
    schistosomiasis (bilharziasis) B65.0 [N33]
  specified NEC N32.89
bleeder's D66
blood D75.9
  forming organs D75.9
  vessel I99.9
Bloodgood's —*see* Mastopathy, cystic
Bodechtel-Guttmann (subacute sclerosing panencephalitis) A81.1
bone —*see also* Disorder, bone
  aluminum M83.4
  fibrocystic NEC
    jaw M27.49

Disease, diseased *(Continued)*
bone-marrow D75.9
Borna A83.9
Bornholm (epidemic pleurodynia) B33.0
Bouchard's (myopathic dilatation of the stomach) K31.0
Bouillaud's (rheumatic heart disease) I01.9
Bourneville (-Brissaud) (tuberous sclerosis) Q85.1
Bouveret (-Hoffmann) (paroxysmal tachycardia) I47.9
bowel K63.9
  functional K59.9
    psychogenic F45.8
brain G93.9
  arterial, artery I67.9
  arteriosclerotic I67.2
  congenital Q04.9
  degenerative —*see* Degeneration, brain
  inflammatory —*see* Encephalitis
  organic G93.9
    arteriosclerotic I67.2
  parasitic NEC B71.9 [G94]
  senile NEC G31.1
  specified NEC G93.89
breast (*see also* Disorder, breast) N64.9
  cystic (chronic) —*see* Mastopathy, cystic
  fibrocystic —*see* Mastopathy, cystic
  Paget's
    female, unspecified side C50.91-
    male, unspecified side C50.92-
  specified NEC N64.89
Breda's —*see* Yaws
Bretonneau's (diphtheritic malignant angina) A36.0
Bright's —*see* Nephritis
  arteriosclerotic —*see* Hypertension, kidney
Brill's (recrudescent typhus) A75.1
Brill-Zinsser (recrudescent typhus) A75.1
Brion-Kayser —*see* Fever, paratyphoid
broad
  beta E78.2
  ligament (noninflammatory) N83.9
    inflammatory —*see* Disease, pelvis, inflammatory
    specified NEC N83.8
Brocq-Duhring (dermatitis herpetiformis) L13.0
Brocq's
  meaning
    dermatitis herpetiformis L13.0
    prurigo L28.2
bronchopulmonary J98.4
bronchus NEC J98.09
bronze Addison's E27.1
  tuberculous A18.7
budgerigar fancier's J67.2
Buerger's (thromboangiitis obliterans) I73.1
bullous L13.9
  chronic of childhood L12.2
  specified NEC L13.8
Bürger-Grütz (essential familial hyperlipemia) E78.3
bursa —*see* Bursopathy
caisson T70.3
California —*see* Coccidioidomycosis
capillaries I78.9
  specified NEC I78.8

Disease, diseased *(Continued)*
Carapata A68.0
cardiac —*see* Disease, heart
cardiopulmonary, chronic I27.9
cardiorenal (hepatic) (hypertensive) (vascular) —*see* Hypertension, cardiorenal
cardiovascular (atherosclerotic) I25.10
  with angina pectoris —*see* Arteriosclerosis, coronary (artery),
  congenital Q28.9
  hypertensive —*see* Hypertension, heart
  newborn P29.9
    specified NEC P29.89
  renal (hypertensive) —*see* Hypertension, cardiorenal
  syphilitic (asymptomatic) A52.00
cartilage —*see* Disorder, cartilage
Castellani's A69.8
cat-scratch A28.1
Cavare's (familial periodic paralysis) G72.3
cecum K63.9
celiac (adult) (infantile) K90.0
cellular tissue L98.9
central core G71.2
cerebellar, cerebellum —*see* Disease, brain
cerebral —*see also* Disease, brain
  degenerative —*see* Degeneration, brain
cerebrospinal G96.9
cerebrovascular I67.9
  acute I67.89
    embolic I63.4-
    thrombotic I63.3-
  arteriosclerotic I67.2
  specified NEC I67.89
cervix (uteri) (noninflammatory) N88.9
  inflammatory —*see* Cervicitis
  specified NEC N88.8
Chabert's A22.9
Chandler's (osteochondritis dissecans, hip) —*see* Osteochondritis, dissecans, hip
Charlouis —*see* Yaws
Chédiak-Steinbrinck (-Higashi) (congenital gigantism of peroxidase granules) E70.330
chest J98.9
Chiari's (hepatic vein thrombosis) I82.0
Chicago B40.9
Chignon B36.8
chigo, chigoe B88.1
childhood granulomatous D71
Chinese liver fluke B66.1
chlamydial A74.9
  specified NEC A74.89
cholecystic K82.9
choroid H31.9
  specified NEC H31.8
Christmas D67
chronic bullous of childhood L12.2
chylomicron retention E78.3
ciliary body H21.9
  specified NEC H21.89
circulatory (system) NEC I99.8
  newborn P29.9
  syphilitic A52.00
    congenital A50.54
coagulation factor deficiency (congenital) —*see* Defect, coagulation

Disease, diseased *(Continued)*
coccidioidal —*see* Coccidioidomycosis
cold
  agglutinin or hemoglobinuria D59.1
    paroxysmal D59.6
  hemagglutinin (chronic) D59.1
collagen NOS (nonvascular) (vascular)
  M35.9
  specified NEC M35.8
colon K63.9
  functional K59.9
    congenital Q43.2
  ischemic K55.0
combined system —*see* Degeneration,
  combined
compressed air T70.3
Concato's (pericardial polyserositis)
  A19.9
  nontubercular I31.1
  pleural —*see* Pleurisy, with effusion
conjunctiva H11.9
  chlamydial A74.0
  specified NEC H11.89
  viral B30.9
    specified NEC B30.8
connective tissue, systemic (diffuse)
  M35.9
  in (due to)
    hypogammaglobulinemia D80.1
      [M36.8]
    ochronosis E70.29 [M36.8]
  specified NEC M35.8
Conor and Bruch's (boutonneuse fever)
  A77.1
Cooper's —*see* Mastopathy, cystic
Cori's (glycogenosis III) E74.03
corkhandler's or corkworker's J67.3
cornea H18.9
  specified NEC H18.89-
coronary (artery) —*see* Disease, heart,
  ischemic, atherosclerotic
  congenital Q24.5
  ostial, syphilitic (aortic) (mitral)
    (pulmonary) A52.03
corpus cavernosum N48.9
  specified NEC N48.89
Cotugno's —*see* Sciatica
coxsackie (virus) NEC B34.1
cranial nerve NOS G52.9
Creutzfeldt-Jakob —*see* Creutzfeldt-
  Jakob disease or syndrome
Crocq's (acrocyanosis) I73.89
Crohn's —*see* Enteritis, regional
Curschmann G71.11
cystic
  breast (chronic) —*see* Mastopathy,
    cystic
  kidney, congenital Q61.9
  liver, congenital Q44.6
  lung J98.4
    congenital Q33.0
cytomegalic inclusion (generalized)
  B25.9
  with pneumonia B25.0
  congenital P35.1
cytomegaloviral B25.9
  specified NEC B25.8
Czerny's (periodic hydrarthrosis of the
  knee) —*see* Effusion, joint, knee
Daae (-Finsen) (epidemic pleurodynia)
  B33.0
Darling's —*see* Histoplasmosis capsulati
Débove's (splenomegaly) R16.1
deer fly —*see* Tularemia
Degos' I77.8

Disease, diseased *(Continued)*
demyelinating, demyelinizating
  (nervous system) G37.9
  multiple sclerosis G35
  specified NEC G37.8
dense deposit *(see also* N00-N07 with
  fourth character .6) N05.6
deposition, hydroxyapatite —*see*
  Disease, hydroxyapatite
  deposition
de Quervain's (tendon sheath) M65.4
  thyroid (subacute granulomatous
    thyroiditis) E06.1
Devergie's (pityriasis rubra pilaris) L44.0
Devic's G36.0
diaphorase deficiency D74.0
diaphragm J98.6
diarrheal, infectious NEC A09
digestive system K92.9
  specified NEC K92.89
disc, degenerative —*see* Degeneration,
  intervertebral disc
discogenic —*see also* Displacement,
  intervertebral disc NEC
  with myelopathy —*see* Disorder, disc,
    with, myelopathy
diverticular —*see* Diverticula
Dubois (thymus) A50.59 *[E35]*
Duchenne-Griesinger G71.0
Duchenne's
  muscular dystrophy G71.0
  pseudohypertrophy, muscles G71.0
ductless glands E34.9
Duhring's (dermatitis herpetiformis)
  L13.0
duodenum K31.9
  specified NEC K31.89
Dupré's (meningism) R29.1
Dupuytren's (muscle contracture) M72.0
Durand-Nicholas-Favre (climatic bubo)
  A55
Duroziez's (congenital mitral stenosis)
  Q23.2
ear —*see* Disorder, ear
Eberth's —*see* Fever, typhoid
Ebola (virus) A98.4
Ebstein's heart Q22.5
Echinococcus —*see* Echinococcus
echovirus NEC B34.1
Eddowes' (brittle bones and blue sclera)
  Q78.0
edentulous (alveolar) ridge K06.9
  specified NEC K06.8
Edsall's T67.2
Eichstedt's (pityriasis versicolor) B36.0
Ellis-van Creveld (chondroectodermal
  dysplasia) Q77.6
end stage renal (ESRD) N18.6
  due to hypertension I12.0
endocrine glands or system NEC E34.9
endomyocardial (eosinophilic) I42.3
English (rickets) E55.0
enteroviral, enterovirus NEC B34.1
  central nervous system NEC A88.8
epidemic B99.9
  specified NEC B99.8
epididymis N50.9
Erb (-Landouzy) G71.0
Erdheim-Chester (ECD) E88.89
esophagus K22.9
  functional K22.4
  psychogenic F45.8
  specified NEC K22.8
Eulenburg's (congenital paramyotonia)
  G71.19

Disease, diseased *(Continued)*
eustachian tube —*see* Disorder,
  eustachian tube
external
  auditory canal —*see* Disorder, ear,
    external
  ear —*see* Disorder, ear, external
extrapyramidal G25.9
  specified NEC G25.89
eye H57.9
  anterior chamber H21.9
  inflammatory NEC H57.8
  muscle (external) —*see* Strabismus
  specified NEC H57.8
  syphilitic —*see* Oculopathy, syphilitic
eyeball H44.9
  specified NEC H44.89
eyelid —*see* Disorder, eyelid
  specified NEC —*see* Disorder, eyelid,
    specified type NEC
eyeworm of Africa B74.3
facial nerve (seventh) G51.9
  newborn (birth injury) P11.3
Fahr (of brain) G23.8
Fahr Volhard (of kidney) I12.-
fallopian tube (noninflammatory) N83.9
  inflammatory —*see*
    Salpingo-oophoritis
  specified NEC N83.8
familial periodic paralysis G72.3
Fanconi's (congenital pancytopenia)
  D61.09
fascia NEC —*see also* Disorder, muscle
  inflammatory —*see* Myositis
  specified NEC M62.89
Fauchard's (periodontitis) —*see*
  Periodontitis
Favre-Durand-Nicolas (climatic bubo)
  A55
Fede's K14.0
Feer's —*see* Poisoning, mercury
female pelvic inflammatory *(see also*
  Disease, pelvis, inflammatory)
  N73.9
  syphilitic (secondary) A51.42
  tuberculous A18.17
Fernels' (aortic aneurysm) I71.9
fibrocaseous of lung —*see* Tuberculosis,
  pulmonary
fibrocystic —*see* Fibrocystic disease
Fiedler's (leptospiral jaundice) A27.0
fifth B08.3
file-cutter's —*see* Poisoning, lead
fish-skin Q80.9
  acquired L85.0
Flajani (-Basedow) (exophthalmic
  goiter) —*see* Hyperthyroidism,
  with, goiter (diffuse)
flax-dresser's J66.1
fluke —*see* Infestation, fluke
foot and mouth B08.8
foot process N04.9
Forbes' (glycogenosis III) E74.03
Fordyce-Fox (apocrine miliaria) L75.2
Fordyce's (ectopic sebaceous glands)
  (mouth) Q38.6
Forestier's (rhizomelic
  pseudopolyarthritis) M35.3
  meaning ankylosing hyperostosis —
    see Hyperostosis, ankylosing
Fothergill's
  neuralgia —*see* Neuralgia, trigeminal
  scarlatina anginosa A38.9
Fournier (gangrene) N49.3
  female N76.89

Disease, diseased (Continued)
  fourth B08.8
  Fox (-Fordyce) (apocrine miliaria)
      L75.2
  Francis' —see Tularemia
  Franklin C88.2
  Frei's (climatic bubo) A55
  Friedreich's
      combined systemic or ataxia G11.1
      myoclonia G25.3
  frontal sinus —see Sinusitis, frontal
  fungus NEC B49
  Gaisböck's (polycythemia hypertonica)
      D75.1
  gallbladder K82.9
      calculus —see Calculus, gallbladder
      cholecystitis —see Cholecystitis
      cholesterolosis K82.4
      fistula —see Fistula, gallbladder
      hydrops K82.1
      obstruction —see Obstruction,
          gallbladder
      perforation K82.2
      specified NEC K82.8
  gamma heavy chain C88.2
  Gamna's (siderotic splenomegaly) D73.2
  Gamstorp's (adynamia episodica
      hereditaria) G72.3
  Gandy-Nanta (siderotic splenomegaly)
      D73.2
  ganister J62.8
  gastric —see Disease, stomach
  gastroesophageal reflux (GERD) K21.9
      with esophagitis K21.0
  gastrointestinal (tract) K92.9
      amyloid E85.4
      functional K59.9
          psychogenic F45.8
      specified NEC K92.89
  Gee (-Herter) (-Heubner) (-Thaysen)
      (nontropical sprue) K90.0
  genital organs
      female N94.9
      male N50.9
  Gerhardt's (erythromelalgia) I73.81
  Gibert's (pityriasis rosea) L42
  Gierke's (glycogenosis I) E74.01
  Gilles de la Tourette's (motor-verbal tic)
      F95.2
  gingiva K06.9
      specified NEC K06.8
  gland (lymph) I89.9
  Glanzmann's (hereditary hemorrhagic
      thrombasthenia) D69.1
  glass-blower's (cataract) —see Cataract,
      specified NEC
  salivary gland hypertrophy K11.1
  Glisson's —see Rickets
  globe H44.9
      specified NEC H44.89
  glomerular —see also
          Glomerulonephritis
      with edema —see Nephrosis
      acute —see Nephritis, acute
      chronic —see Nephritis, chronic
      minimal change N05.0
      rapidly progressive N01.9
  glycogen storage E74.00
      Andersen's E74.09
      Cori's E74.03
      Forbes' E74.03
      generalized E74.00
      glucose-6-phosphatase deficiency
          E74.01

Disease, diseased (Continued)
  glycogen storage (Continued)
      heart E74.02 [I43]
      hepatorenal E74.09
      Hers' E74.09
      liver and kidney E74.09
      McArdle's E74.04
      muscle phosphofructokinase E74.09
      myocardium E74.02 [I43]
      Pompe's E74.02
      Tauri's E74.09
      type 0 E74.09
      type I E74.01
      type II E74.02
      type III E74.03
      type IV E74.09
      type V E74.04
      type VI-XI E74.09
      Von Gierke's E74.01
  Goldstein's (familial hemorrhagic
      telangiectasia) I78.0
  gonococcal NOS A54.9
  graft-versus-host (GVH) D89.813
      acute D89.810
      acute on chronic D89.812
      chronic D89.811
  grainhandler's J67.8
  granulomatous (childhood) (chronic)
      D71
  Graves' (exophthalmic goiter) —see
      Hyperthyroidism, with, goiter
      (diffuse)
  Griesinger's —see Ancylostomiasis
  Grisel's M43.6
  Gruby's (tinea tonsurans) B35.0
  Guillain-Barr, G61.0
  Guinon's (motor-verbal tic) F95.2
  gum K06.9
  gynecological N94.9
  H (Hartnup's) E72.02
  Haff —see Poisoning, mercury
  Hageman (congenital factor XII
      deficiency) D68.2
  hair (color) (shaft) L67.9
      follicles L73.9
          specified NEC L73.8
  Hamman's (spontaneous mediastinal
      emphysema) J98.2
  hand, foot and mouth B08.4
  Hansen's —see Leprosy
  Hantavirus, with pulmonary
      manifestations B33.4
      with renal manifestations A98.5
  Harada's H30.81-
  Hartnup (pellagra-cerebellar ataxia-
      renal aminoaciduria) E72.02
  Hart's (pellagra-cerebellar ataxia-renal
      aminoaciduria) E72.02
  Hashimoto's (struma lymphomatosa)
      E06.3
  Hb —see Disease, hemoglobin
  heart (organic) I51.9
      with
          pulmonary edema (acute) (see also
              Failure, ventricular, left) I50.1
          rheumatic fever (conditions in I00)
              active I01.9
                  with chorea I02.0
                  specified NEC I01.8
              inactive or quiescent (with
                  chorea) I09.9
                  specified NEC I09.89
      amyloid E85.4 [I43]
      aortic (valve) I35.9

Disease, diseased (Continued)
  heart (Continued)
      arteriosclerotic or sclerotic (senile) —
          see Disease, heart, ischemic,
          atherosclerotic
      artery, arterial —see Disease, heart,
          ischemic, atherosclerotic
      beer drinkers' I42.6
      beriberi (wet) E51.12
      black I27.0
      congenital Q24.9
          cyanotic Q24.9
          specified NEC Q24.8
      coronary —see Disease, heart,
          ischemic
      cryptogenic I51.9
      fibroid —see Myocarditis
      functional I51.89
          psychogenic F45.8
      glycogen storage E74.02 [I43]
      gonococcal A54.83
      hypertensive —see Hypertension,
          heart
      hyperthyroid (see also
          Hyperthyroidism) E05.90 [I43]
          with thyroid storm E05.91 [I43]
      ischemic (chronic or with a stated
          duration of over 4 weeks) I25.9
          atherosclerotic (of) I25.10
              with angina pectoris —see
                  Arteriosclerosis, coronary
                  (artery)
              coronary artery bypass graft —
                  see Arteriosclerosis,
                  coronary (artery),
          cardiomyopathy I25.5
          diagnosed on ECG or other special
              investigation, but currently
              presenting no symptoms I25.6
          silent I25.6
          specified form NEC I25.89
      kyphoscoliotic I27.1
      meningococcal A39.50
          endocarditis A39.51
          myocarditis A39.52
          pericarditis A39.53
      mitral I05.9
          specified NEC I05.8
      muscular —see Degeneration,
          myocardial
      psychogenic (functional) F45.8
      pulmonary (chronic) I27.9
          in schistosomiasis B65.9 [I52]
          specified NEC I27.89
      rheumatic (chronic) (inactive) (old)
          (quiescent) (with chorea) I09.9
          active or acute I01.9
              with chorea (acute) (rheumatic)
                  (Sydenham's) I02.0
          specified NEC I09.89
      senile —see Myocarditis
      syphilitic A52.06
          aortic A52.03
              aneurysm A52.01
          congenital A50.54 [I52]
      thyrotoxic (see also Thyrotoxicosis)
          E05.90 [I43]
          with thyroid storm E05.91 [I43]
      valve, valvular (obstructive)
          (regurgitant) —see also
          Endocarditis
          congenital NEC Q24.8
              pulmonary Q22.3
      vascular —see Disease, cardiovascular

Disease, diseased *(Continued)*
heavy chain NEC C88.2
  alpha C88.3
  gamma C88.2
  mu C88.2
Hebra's
  pityriasis
    maculata et circinata L42
    rubra pilaris L44.0
  prurigo L28.2
hematopoietic organs D75.9
hemoglobin or Hb
  abnormal (mixed) NEC D58.2
    with thalassemia D56.9
  AS genotype D57.3
  Bart's D56.0
  C (Hb-C) D58.2
    with other abnormal hemoglobin
      NEC D58.2
    elliptocytosis D58.1
    Hb-S D57.2-
    sickle-cell D57.2-
    thalassemia D56.8
  Constant Spring D58.2
  D (Hb-D) D58.2
  E (Hb-E) D58.2
  E-beta thalassemia D56.5
  elliptocytosis D58.1
  H (Hb-H) (thalassemia) D56.0
    with other abnormal hemoglobin
      NEC D56.9
    Constant Spring D56.0
  I thalassemia D56.9
  M D74.0
  S or SS D57.1
  SC D57.2-
  SD D57.8-
  SE D57.8-
  spherocytosis D58.0
  unstable, hemolytic D58.2
hemolytic (newborn) P55.9
  autoimmune (cold type) (warm type)
    D59.1
  drug-induced D59.0
  due to or with
    incompatibility
      ABO (blood group) P55.1
      blood (group) (Duffy) (K(ell))
        (Kidd) (Lewis) (M) (S) NEC
        P55.8
      Rh (blood group) (factor) P55.0
      Rh negative mother P55.0
  specified type NEC P55.8
  unstable hemoglobin D58.2
hemorrhagic D69.9
  newborn P53
Henoch (-Schönlein) (purpura nervosa)
  D69.0
hepatic —*see* Disease, liver
hepatolenticular E83.01
heredodegenerative NEC
  spinal cord G95.89
herpesviral, disseminated B00.7
Hers' (glycogenosis VI) E74.09
Herter (-Gee) (-Heubner) (nontropical
  sprue) K90.0
Heubner-Herter (nontropical sprue)
  K90.0
high fetal gene or hemoglobin
  thalassemia D56.9
Hildenbrand's —*see* Typhus
hip (joint) M25.9
  congenital Q65.89
  suppurative M00.9
  tuberculous A18.02

Disease, diseased *(Continued)*
His (-Werner) (trench fever) A79.0
Hodgson's I71.2
  ruptured I71.1
Holla —*see* Spherocytosis
hookworm B76.9
  specified NEC B76.8
host-versus-graft D89.813
  acute D89.810
  acute on chronic D89.812
  chronic D89.811
human immunodeficiency virus (HIV)
  B20
Huntington's G10
Hutchinson's (cheiropompholyx) —*see*
  Hutchinson's disease
hyaline (diffuse) (generalized)
  membrane (lung) (newborn)
    P22.0
    adult J80
hydatid —*see* Echinococcus
hydroxyapatite deposition M11.00
  ankle M11.07-
  elbow M11.02-
  foot joint M11.07-
  hand joint M11.04-
  hip M11.05-
  knee M11.06-
  multiple site M11.09
  shoulder M11.01-
  vertebra M11.08
  wrist M11.03-
hyperkinetic —*see* Hyperkinesia
hypertensive —*see* Hypertension
hypophysis E23.7
Iceland G93.3
I-cell E77.0
immune D89.9
immunoproliferative (malignant)
  C88.9
  small intestinal C88.3
  specified NEC C88.8
inclusion B25.9
  salivary gland B25.9
infectious, infective B99.9
  congenital P37.9
    specified NEC P37.8
    viral
  specified NEC B99.8
inflammatory
  penis N48.29
    abscess N48.21
    cellulitis N48.22
  prepuce N47.7
    balanoposthitis N47.6
  tubo-ovarian —*see*
    Salpingo-oophoritis
intervertebral disc —*see also* Disorder,
  disc
  with myelopathy —*see* Disorder,
    disc, with, myelopathy
  cervical, cervicothoracic —*see*
    Disorder, disc, cervical
    with
      myelopathy —*see* Disorder,
        disc, cervical, with
        myelopathy
      neuritis, radiculitis or
        radiculopathy —*see*
        Disorder, disc, cervical,
        with neuritis
    specified NEC —*see* Disorder,
      disc, cervical, specified type
      NEC

Disease, diseased *(Continued)*
intervertebral disc *(Continued)*
  lumbar (with)
    myelopathy M51.06
    neuritis, radiculitis, radiculopathy
      or sciatica M51.16
    specified NEC M51.86
  lumbosacral (with)
    myelopathy M51.07
    neuritis, radiculitis, radiculopathy
      or sciatica M51.17
    specified NEC M51.87
  specified NEC —*see* Disorder, disc,
    specified NEC
  thoracic (with)
    myelopathy M51.04
    neuritis, radiculitis or
      radiculopathy M51.14
    specified NEC M51.84
  thoracolumbar (with)
    myelopathy M51.05
    neuritis, radiculitis or
      radiculopathy M51.15
    specified NEC M51.85
intestine K63.9
  functional K59.9
    psychogenic F45.8
    specified NEC K59.8
  organic K63.9
  protozoal A07.9
  specified NEC K63.89
iris H21.9
  specified NEC H21.89
iron metabolism or storage
  E83.10
island (scrub typhus) A75.3
itai-itai —*see* Poisoning, cadmium
Jakob-Creutzfeldt —*see* Creutzfeldt-
  Jakob disease or syndrome
jaw M27.9
  fibrocystic M27.49
  specified NEC M27.8
jigger B88.1
joint —*see also* Disorder, joint
  Charcot's —*see* Arthropathy,
    neuropathic (Charcot)
  degenerative —*see* Osteoarthritis
    multiple M15.9
    spine —*see* Spondylosis
  hypertrophic —*see* Osteoarthritis
  sacroiliac M53.3
  specified NEC —*see* Disorder, joint,
    specified type NEC
  spine NEC —*see* Dorsopathy
  suppurative —*see* Arthritis, pyogenic
    or pyemic
Jourdain's (acute gingivitis) K05.00
  nonplaque induced K05.01
  plaque induced K05.00
Kaschin-Beck (endemic polyarthritis)
  M12.10
  ankle M12.17-
  elbow M12.12-
  foot joint M12.17-
  hand joint M12.14-
  hip M12.15-
  knee M12.16-
  multiple site M12.19
  shoulder M12.11-
  vertebra M12.18
  wrist M12.13-
Katayama B65.2
Kedani (scrub typhus) A75.3
Keshan E59

Disease, diseased (Continued)
kidney (functional) (pelvis) N28.9
  chronic N18.9
    hypertensive —see Hypertension,
      kidney
    stage 1 N18.1
    stage 2 (mild) N18.2
    stage 3 (moderate) N18.3
    stage 4 (severe) N18.4
    stage 5 N18.5
  complicating pregnancy —see
    Pregnancy, complicated by, renal
    disease
  cystic (congenital) Q61.9
  fibrocystic (congenital) Q61.8
  hypertensive —see Hypertension,
    kidney
  in (due to)
    schistosomiasis (bilharziasis) B65.9
      [N29]
  multicystic Q61.4
  polycystic Q61.3
    adult type Q61.2
    childhood type NEC Q61.19
      collecting duct dilatation Q61.11
  Kimmelstiel (-Wilson) (intercapillary
    polycystic (congenital)
    glomerulosclerosis) —see E08-E13
    with .21
Kinnier Wilson's (hepatolenticular
  degeneration) E83.01
kissing —see Mononucleosis, infectious
Klebs' (see also Glomerulonephritis) N05.-
Klippel-Feil (brevicollis) Q76.1
Köhler-Pellegrini-Stieda (calcification,
  knee joint) —see Bursitis, tibial
  collateral
Kok Q89.8
König's (osteochondritis dissecans) —
  see Osteochondritis, dissecans
Korsakoff's (nonalcoholic) F04
  alcoholic F10.96
    with dependence F10.26
Kostmann's (infantile genetic
  agranulocytosis) D70.0
kuru A81.81
Kyasanur Forest A98.2
labyrinth, ear —see Disorder, ear, inner
lacrimal system —see Disorder, lacrimal
  system
Lafora's —see Epilepsy, generalized,
  idiopathic
Lancereaux-Mathieu (leptospiral
  jaundice) A27.0
Landry's G61.0
Larrey-Weil (leptospiral jaundice)
  A27.0
larynx J38.7
legionnaires' A48.1
  nonpneumonic A48.2
Lenegre's I44.2
lens H27.9
  specified NEC H27.8
Lev's (acquired complete heart block)
  I44.2
Lewy body (dementia) G31.83 [F02.80]
  with behavioral disturbance G31.83
    [F02.81]
Lichtheim's (subacute combined sclerosis
  with pernicious anemia) D51.0
Lightwood's (renal tubular acidosis)
  N25.89
Lignac's (cystinosis) E72.04
lip K13.0

Disease, diseased (Continued)
lipid-storage E75.6
  specified NEC E75.5
Lipschütz's N76.6
liver (chronic) (organic) K76.9
  alcoholic (chronic) K70.9
    acute —see Disease, liver, alcoholic,
      hepatitis
    cirrhosis K70.30
      with ascites K70.31
    failure K70.40
      with coma K70.41
    fatty liver K70.0
    fibrosis K70.2
    hepatitis K70.10
      with ascites K70.11
    sclerosis K70.2
  cystic, congenital Q44.6
  drug-induced (idiosyncratic) (toxic)
    (predictable) (unpredictable) —
    see Disease, liver, toxic
  end stage K72.90
    due to hepatitis —see Hepatitis
  fatty, nonalcoholic (NAFLD) K76.0
    alcoholic K70.0
  fibrocystic (congenital) Q44.6
  fluke
    Chinese B66.1
    oriental B66.1
    sheep B66.3
  glycogen storage E74.09 [K77]
  in (due to)
    schistosomiasis (bilharziasis) B65.9
      [K77]
  inflammatory K75.9
    alcoholic K70.1
    specified NEC K75.89
  polycystic (congenital) Q44.6
  toxic K71.9
    with
      cholestasis K71.0
      cirrhosis (liver) K71.7
      fibrosis (liver) K71.7
      focal nodular hyperplasia K71.8
      hepatic granuloma K71.8
      hepatic necrosis K71.10
        with coma K71.11
      hepatitis NEC K71.6
        acute K71.2
        chronic
          active K71.50
            with ascites K71.51
          lobular K71.4
          persistent K71.3
        lupoid K71.50
          with ascites K71.51
      peliosis hepatis K71.8
      veno-occlusive disease (VOD) of
        liver K71.8
  veno-occlusive K76.5
Lobo's (keloid blastomycosis) B48.0
Lobstein's (brittle bones and blue
  sclera) Q78.0
Ludwig's (submaxillary cellulitis)
  K12.2
lumbosacral region M53.87
lung J98.4
  black J60
  congenital Q33.9
  cystic J98.4
    congenital Q33.0
  fibroid (chronic) —see Fibrosis, lung
  fluke B66.4
    oriental B66.4

Disease, diseased (Continued)
lung (Continued)
  in
    amyloidosis E85.4 [J99]
    sarcoidosis D86.0
    Sjögren's syndrome M35.02
    systemic
      lupus erythematosus M32.13
      sclerosis M34.81
  interstitial J84.9
    of childhood, specified NEC
      J84.848
    respiratory bronchiolitis J84.115
    specified NEC J84.89
  obstructive (chronic) J44.9
    with
      acute
        bronchitis J44.0
        exacerbation NEC J44.1
        lower respiratory infection J44.0
      alveolitis, allergic J67.9
      asthma J44.9
      bronchiectasis J47.9
        with
          exacerbation (acute) J47.1
          lower respiratory infection
            J47.0
      bronchitis J44.9
        with
          exacerbation (acute) J44.1
          lower respiratory infection
            J44.0
      emphysema J44.9
      hypersensitivity pneumonitis J67.9
    decompensated J44.1
      with
        exacerbation (acute) J44.1
  polycystic J98.4
    congenital Q33.0
  rheumatoid (diffuse) (interstitial) —
    see Rheumatoid, lung
Lutembacher's (atrial septal defect with
  mitral stenosis) Q21.1
Lyme A69.20
lymphatic (gland) (system) (channel)
  (vessel) I89.9
lymphoproliferative D47.9
  specified NEC D47.Z9
  T-gamma D47.Z9
  X-linked D82.3
Magitot's M27.2
malarial —see Malaria
malignant —see also Neoplasm,
  malignant, by site
Manson's B65.1
maple bark J67.6
maple-syrup-urine E71.0
Marburg (virus) A98.3
Marion's (bladder neck obstruction)
  N32.0
Marsh's (exophthalmic goiter) —see
  Hyperthyroidism, with, goiter
  (diffuse)
mastoid (process) —see Disorder, ear,
  middle
Mathieu's (leptospiral jaundice) A27.0
Maxcy's A75.2
McArdle (-Schmid-Pearson)
  (glycogenosis V) E74.04
mediastinum J98.5
medullary center (idiopathic)
  (respiratory) G93.89
Meige's (chronic hereditary edema)
  Q82.0

Disease, diseased *(Continued)*
  meningococcal —*see* Infection,
     meningococcal
  mental F99
    organic F09
  mesenchymal M35.9
  mesenteric embolic K55.0
  metabolic, metabolism E88.9
    bilirubin E80.7
  metal-polisher's J62.8
  metastatic (*see also* Neoplasm,
    secondary, by site) C79.9
  microvascular — code to condition
  microvillus
    atrophy Q43.8
    inclusion (MVD) Q43.8
  middle ear —*see* Disorder, ear, middle
  Mikulicz' (dryness of mouth, absent or
    decreased lacrimation) K11.8
  Milroy's (chronic hereditary edema)
    Q82.0
  Minamata —*see* Poisoning, mercury
  minicore G71.2
  Minor's G95.19
  Minot's (hemorrhagic disease,
    newborn) P53
  Minot-von Willebrand-Jürgens
    (angiohemophilia) D68.0
  Mitchell's (erythromelalgia) I73.81
  mitral (valve) I05.9
    nonrheumatic I34.9
  mixed connective tissue M35.1
  moldy hay J67.0
  Monge's T70.29
  Morgagni-Adams-Stokes (syncope with
    heart block) I45.9
  Morgagni's (syndrome) (hyperostosis
    frontalis interna) M85.2
  Morton's (with metatarsalgia) —*see*
    Lesion, nerve, plantar
  Morvan's G60.8
  motor neuron (bulbar) (familial) (mixed
    type) (spinal) G12.20
    amyotrophic lateral sclerosis
      G12.21
    progressive bulbar palsy G12.22
    specified NEC G12.29
  moyamoya I67.5
  mu heavy chain disease C88.2
  multicore G71.2
  muscle —*see also* Disorder, muscle
    inflammatory —*see* Myositis
    ocular (external) —*see* Strabismus
  musculoskeletal system, soft tissue —
    see also Disorder, soft tissue
    specified NEC —*see* Disorder, soft
      tissue, specified type NEC
  mushroom workers' J67.5
  mycotic B49
  myelodysplastic, not classified C94.6
  myeloproliferative, not classified
    C94.6
    chronic D47.1
  myocardium, myocardial (*see also*
    Degeneration, myocardial) I51.5
    primary (idiopathic) I42.9
  myoneural G70.9
  Naegeli's D69.1
  nails L60.9
    specified NEC L60.8
  Nairobi (sheep virus) A93.8
  nasal J34.9
  nemaline body G71.2
  nerve —*see* Disorder, nerve

Disease, diseased *(Continued)*
  nervous system G98.8
    autonomic G90.9
    central G96.9
      specified NEC G96.8
    congenital Q07.9
    parasympathetic G90.9
    specified NEC G98.8
    sympathetic G90.9
    vegetative G90.9
  neuromuscular system G70.9
  Newcastle B30.8
  Nicolas (-Durand)-Favre (climatic bubo)
    A55
  nipple N64.9
    Paget's C50.01-
      female C50.01-
      male C50.02-
  Nishimoto (-Takeuchi) I67.5
  nonarthropod-borne NOS (viral) B34.9
    enterovirus NEC B34.1
  nonautoimmune hemolytic D59.4
    drug-induced D59.2
  Nonne-Milroy-Meige (chronic
    hereditary edema) Q82.0
  nose J34.9
  nucleus pulposus —*see* Disorder, disc
  nutritional E63.9
  oast-house-urine E72.19
    ocular
      herpesviral B00.50
      zoster B02.30
  obliterative vascular I77.1
  Ohara's —*see* Tularemia
  Opitz's (congestive splenomegaly) D73.2
  Oppenheim-Urbach (necrobiosis
    lipoidica diabeticorum) —*see*
    E08-E13 with .620
  optic nerve NEC —*see* Disorder, nerve,
    optic orbit —*see* Disorder, orbit
  Oriental liver fluke B66.1
  Oriental lung fluke B66.4
  Ormond's N13.5
  Oropouche virus A93.0
  Osler-Rendu (familial hemorrhagic
    telangiectasia) I78.0
  osteofibrocystic E21.0
  Otto's M24.7
  outer ear —*see* Disorder, ear, external
  ovary (noninflammatory) N83.9
    cystic N83.20
    inflammatory —*see*
      Salpingo-oophoritis
    polycystic E28.2
    specified NEC N83.8
  Owren's (congenital) —*see* Defect,
    coagulation
  pancreas K86.9
    cystic K86.2
    fibrocystic E84.9
    specified NEC K86.8
  panvalvular I08.9
    specified NEC I08.8
  parametrium (noninflammatory) N83.9
  parasitic B89
    cerebral NEC B71.9 *[G94]*
    intestinal NOS B82.9
    mouth B37.0
    skin NOS B88.9
    specified type —*see* Infestation
    tongue B37.0
  parathyroid (gland) E21.5
    specified NEC E21.4
  Parkinson's G20

Disease, diseased *(Continued)*
  parodontal K05.6
  Parrot's (syphilitic osteochondritis)
    A50.02
  Parry's (exophthalmic goiter) —*see*
    Hyperthyroidism, with, goiter
    (diffuse)
  Parson's (exophthalmic goiter) —*see*
    Hyperthyroidism, with, goiter
    (diffuse)
  Paxton's (white piedra) B36.2
  pearl-worker's —*see* Osteomyelitis,
    specified type NEC
  Pellegrini-Stieda (calcification, knee
    joint) —*see* Bursitis, tibial collateral
  pelvis, pelvic
    female NOS N94.9
      specified NEC N94.89
    gonococcal (acute) (chronic) A54.24
    inflammatory (female) N73.9
      acute N73.0
      chronic N73.1
      specified NEC N73.8
      syphilitic (secondary) A51.42
        late A52.76
      tuberculous A18.17
    organ, female N94.9
    peritoneum, female NEC N94.89
  penis N48.9
    inflammatory N48.29
      abscess N48.21
      cellulitis N48.22
    specified NEC N48.89
  periapical tissues NOS K04.90
  periodontal K05.6
    specified NEC K05.5
  periosteum —*see* Disorder, bone,
    specified type NEC
  peripheral
    arterial I73.9
    autonomic nervous system G90.9
    nerves —*see* Polyneuropathy
    vascular NOS I73.9
  peritoneum K66.9
    pelvic, female NEC N94.89
    specified NEC K66.8
  persistent mucosal (middle ear)
    H66.20
    left H66.22
      with right H66.23
    right H66.21
      with left H66.23
  Petit's —*see* Hernia, abdomen, specified
    site NEC
  pharynx J39.2
    specified NEC J39.2
  Phocas' —*see* Mastopathy, cystic
  photochromogenic (acid-fast bacilli)
    (pulmonary) A31.0
    nonpulmonary A31.9
  Pick's G31.01 *[F02.80]*
    with behavioral disturbance G31.01
      [F02.81]
  pigeon fancier's J67.2
  pineal gland E34.8
  pink —*see* Poisoning, mercury
  Pinkus' (lichen nitidus) L44.1
  pinworm B80
  Piry virus A93.8
  pituitary (gland) E23.7
  pituitary-snuff-taker's J67.8
  pleura (cavity) J94.9
    specified NEC J94.8
  pneumatic drill (hammer) T75.21

Disease, diseased *(Continued)*
Pollitzer's (hidradenitis suppurativa)
   L73.2
polycystic
   kidney or renal Q61.3
      adult type Q61.2
      childhood type NEC Q61.19
         collecting duct dilatation Q61.11
   liver or hepatic Q44.6
   lung or pulmonary J98.4
      congenital Q33.0
   ovary, ovaries E28.2
   spleen Q89.09
polyethylene T84.05-
Pompe's (glycogenosis II) E74.02
Posadas-Wernicke B38.9
Potain's (pulmonary edema) —*see*
   Edema, lung
prepuce N47.8
   inflammatory N47.7
      balanoposthitis N47.6
Pringle's (tuberous sclerosis) Q85.1
prion, central nervous system A81.9
   specified NEC A81.89
prostate N42.9
   specified NEC N42.89
protozoal B64
   acanthamebiasis —*see*
      Acanthamebiasis
   African trypanosomiasis —*see*
      African trypanosomiasis
   babesiosis B60.0
   Chagas disease —*see* Chagas disease
   intestine, intestinal A07.9
   leishmaniasis —*see* Leishmaniasis
   malaria —*see* Malaria
   naegleriasis B60.2
   pneumocystosis B59
   specified organism NEC B60.8
   toxoplasmosis —*see* Toxoplasmosis
pseudo-Hurler's E77.0
psychiatric F99
psychotic —*see* Psychosis
Puente's (simple glandular cheilitis)
   K13.0
puerperal *(see also* Puerperal) O90.89
pulmonary —*see also* Disease, lung
   artery I28.9
   chronic obstructive J44.9
      with
         acute bronchitis J44.0
         exacerbation (acute) J44.1
         lower respiratory infection
            (acute) J44.0
      decompensated J44.1
        with
           exacerbation (acute) J44.1
   heart I27.9
      specified NEC I27.89
   hypertensive (vascular) I27.0
   valve I37.9
      rheumatic I09.89
pulp (dental) NOS K04.90
pulseless M31.4
Putnam's (subacute combined sclerosis
   with pernicious anemia) D51.0
Pyle (-Cohn) (craniometaphyseal
   dysplasia) Q78.5
ragpicker's or ragsorter's A22.1
Raynaud's —*see* Raynaud's disease
reactive airway —*see* Asthma
Reclus' (cystic) —*see* Mastopathy, cystic
rectum K62.9
   specified NEC K62.89

Disease, diseased *(Continued)*
Refsum's (heredopathia atactica
   polyneuritiformis) G60.1
renal (functional) (pelvis) *(see also*
   Disease, kidney) N28.9
   with
      edema —*see* Nephrosis
      glomerular lesion —*see*
         Glomerulonephritis
         with edema —*see* Nephrosis
      interstitial nephritis N12
   acute N28.9
   chronic *(see also* Disease, kidney,
      chronic) N18.9
   cystic, congenital Q61.9
   diabetic —*see* E08-E13 with .22
   end-stage (failure) N18.6
      due to hypertension I12.0
   fibrocystic (congenital) Q61.8
   hypertensive —*see* Hypertension,
      kidney
   lupus M32.14
   phosphate-losing (tubular) N25.0
   polycystic (congenital) Q61.3
      adult type Q61.2
      childhood type NEC Q61.19
         collecting duct dilatation Q61.11
   rapidly progressive N01.9
   subacute N01.9
Rendu-Osler-Weber (familial
   hemorrhagic telangiectasia) I78.0
renovascular (arteriosclerotic) —*see*
   Hypertension, kidney
respiratory (tract) J98.9
   acute or subacute NOS J06.9
      due to
         chemicals, gases, fumes or
            vapors (inhalation) J68.3
         external agent J70.9
            specified NEC J70.8
         radiation J70.0
         smoke inhalation J70.5
      noninfectious J39.8
   chronic NOS J98.9
      due to
         chemicals, gases, fumes or
            vapors J68.4
         external agent J70.9
            specified NEC J70.8
         radiation J70.1
      newborn P27.9
         specified NEC P27.8
   due to
      chemicals, gases, fumes or vapors
         J68.9
         acute or subacute NEC J68.3
         chronic J68.4
      external agent J70.9
         specified NEC J70.8
   newborn P28.9
      specified type NEC P28.89
   upper J39.9
      acute or subacute J06.9
      noninfectious NEC J39.8
      specified NEC J39.8
      streptococcal J06.9
retina, retinal H35.9
   Batten's or Batten-Mayou E75.4 [H36]
   specified NEC H35.89
rheumatoid —*see* Arthritis, rheumatoid
rickettsial NOS A79.9
   specified type NEC A79.89
Riga (-Fede) (cachectic aphthae) K14.0
Riggs' (compound periodontitis) —*see*
   Periodontitis

Disease, diseased *(Continued)*
Ritter's L00
Rivalta's (cervicofacial actinomycosis)
   A42.2
Robles' (onchocerciasis) B73.01
Roger's (congenital interventricular
   septal defect) Q21.0
Rosenthal's (factor XI deficiency)
   D68.1
Ross River B33.1
Rossbach's (hyperchlorhydria) K30
Rotes Quérol —*see* Hyperostosis,
   ankylosing
Roth (-Bernhardt) —*see*
   Mononeuropathy, lower limb,
   meralgia paresthetica
Runeberg's (progressive pernicious
   anemia) D51.0
sacroiliac NEC M53.3
salivary gland or duct K11.9
   inclusion B25.9
   specified NEC K11.8
   virus B25.9
sandworm B76.9
Schimmelbusch's —*see* Mastopathy,
   cystic
Schmorl's —*see* Schmorl's disease or
   nodes
Schönlein (-Henoch) (purpura
   rheumatica) D69.0
Schottmüller's —*see* Fever, paratyphoid
Schultz's (agranulocytosis) —*see*
   Agranulocytosis
Schwalbe-Ziehen-Oppenheim G24.1
Schwartz-Jampel G71.13
sclera H15.9
   specified NEC H15.89
scrofulous (tuberculous) A18.2
scrotum N50.9
sebaceous glands L73.9
semilunar cartilage, cystic —*see also*
   Derangement, knee, meniscus,
   cystic
seminal vesicle N50.9
serum NEC *(see also* Reaction, serum)
   T80.69
sexually transmitted A64
   anogenital
      herpesviral infection —*see* Herpes,
         anogenital
      warts A63.0
   chancroid A57
   chlamydial infection —*see* Chlamydia
   gonorrhea —*see* Gonorrhea
   granuloma inguinale A58
   specified organism NEC A63.8
   syphilis —*see* Syphilis
   trichomoniasis —*see* Trichmoniasis
Sézary C84.1-
shimamushi (scrub typhus) A75.3
shipyard B30.0
sickle-cell D57.1
   with crisis (vasoocclusive pain) D57.00
      with
         acute chest syndrome D57.01
         splenic sequestration D57.02
   elliptocytosis D57.8-
   Hb-C D57.20
      with crisis (vasoocclusive pain)
         D57.219
         with
           acute chest syndrome D57.211
           splenic sequestration D57.212
      without crisis D57.20

Disease, diseased *(Continued)*
sickle-cell *(Continued)*
Hb-SD D57.80
with crisis D57.819
with
acute chest syndrome D57.811
splenic sequestration D57.812
Hb-SE D57.80
with crisis D57.819
with
acute chest syndrome D57.811
splenic sequestration D57.812
specified NEC D57.80
with crisis D57.819
with
acute chest syndrome D57.811
splenic sequestration D57.812
spherocytosis D57.80
with crisis D57.819
with
acute chest syndrome D57.811
splenic sequestration D57.812
thalassemia D57.40
with crisis (vasoocclusive pain)
D57.419
with
acute chest syndrome D57.411
splenic sequestration D57.412
without crisis D57.40
silo-filler's J68.8
bronchitis J68.0
pneumonitis J68.0
pulmonary edema J68.1
simian B B00.4
Simons' (progressive lipodystrophy)
E88.1
sin nombre virus B33.4
sinus —*see* Sinusitis
Sirkari's B55.0
sixth B08.20
due to human herpesvirus 6 B08.21
due to human herpesvirus 7 B08.22
skin L98.9
due to metabolic disorder NEC E88.9
[L99]
specified NEC L98.8
slim (HIV) B20
small vessel I73.9
Sneddon-Wilkinson (subcorneal
pustular dermatosis) L13.1
South African creeping B88.0
spinal (cord) G95.9
congenital Q06.9
specified NEC G95.89
spine —*see also* Spondylopathy
joint —*see* Dorsopathy
tuberculous A18.01
spinocerebellar (hereditary) G11.9
specified NEC G11.8
spleen D73.9
amyloid E85.4 *[D77]*
organic D73.9
polycystic Q89.09
postinfectional D73.89
sponge-diver's —*see* Toxicity, venom,
marine animal, sea anemone
Startle Q89.8
Steinert's G71.11
Sticker's (erythema infectiosum) B08.3
Stieda's (calcification, knee joint) —*see*
Bursitis, tibial collateral
Stokes' (exophthalmic goiter) —*see*
Hyperthyroidism, with, goiter
(diffuse)

Disease, diseased *(Continued)*
Stokes-Adams (syncope with heart
block) I45.9
stomach K31.9
functional, psychogenic F45.8
specified NEC K31.89
stonemason's J62.8
storage
glycogen —*see* Disease, glycogen
storage
mucopolysaccharide —*see*
Mucopolysaccharidosis
striatopallidal system NEC G25.89
Stuart-Prower (congenital factor X
deficiency) D68.2
Stuart's (congenital factor X deficiency)
D68.2
subcutaneous tissue —*see* Disease, skin
supporting structures of teeth K08.9
specified NEC K08.8
suprarenal (capsule) (gland) E27.9
hyperfunction E27.0
specified NEC E27.8
sweat glands L74.9
specified NEC L74.8
Sweeley-Klionsky E75.21
Swift (-Feer) —*see* Poisoning, mercury
swimming-pool granuloma A31.1
Sylvest's (epidemic pleurodynia) B33.0
sympathetic nervous system G90.9
synovium —*see* Disorder, synovium
syphilitic —*see* Syphilis
systemic tissue mast cell C96.2
tanapox (virus) B08.71
Tangier E78.6
Tarral-Besnier (pityriasis rubra pilaris)
L44.0
Tauri's E74.09
tear duct —*see* Disorder, lacrimal system
tendon, tendinous —*see also* Disorder,
tendon
nodular —*see* Trigger finger
terminal vessel I73.9
testis N50.9
thalassemia Hb-S —*see* Disease, sickle-
cell, thalassemia
Thaysen-Gee (nontropical sprue) K90.0
Thomsen G71.12
throat J39.2
septic J02.0
thromboembolic —*see* Embolism
thymus (gland) E32.9
specified NEC E32.8
thyroid (gland) E07.9
heart (*see also* Hyperthyroidism)
E05.90 *[I43]*
with thyroid storm E05.91 *[I43]*
specified NEC E07.89
Tietze's M94.0
tongue K14.9
specified NEC K14.8
tonsils, tonsillar (and adenoids) J35.9
tooth, teeth K08.9
hard tissues K03.9
specified NEC K03.89
pulp NEC K04.99
specified NEC K08.8
Tourette's F95.2
trachea NEC J39.8
tricuspid I07.9
nonrheumatic I36.9
triglyceride-storage E75.5
trophoblastic —*see* Mole, hydatidiform
tsutsugamushi A75.3

Disease, diseased *(Continued)*
tube (fallopian) (noninflammatory) N83.9
inflammatory —*see* Salpingitis
specified NEC N83.8
tuberculous NEC —*see* Tuberculosis
tubo-ovarian (noninflammatory) N83.9
inflammatory —*see*
Salpingo-oophoritis
specified NEC N83.8
tubotympanic, chronic —*see* Otitis,
media, suppurative, chronic,
tubotympanic
tubulo-interstitial N15.9
specified NEC N15.8
tympanum —*see* Disorder, tympanic
membrane
Uhl's Q24.8
Underwood's (sclerema neonatorum)
P83.0
Unverricht (-Lundborg) —*see* Epilepsy,
generalized, idiopathic
Urbach-Oppenheim (necrobiosis
lipoidica diabeticorum) —*see*
E08-E13 with .620
ureter N28.9
in (due to)
schistosomiasis (bilharziasis) B65.0
[N29]
urethra N36.9
specified NEC N36.8
urinary (tract) N39.9
bladder N32.9
specified NEC N32.89
specified NEC N39.8
uterus (noninflammatory) N85.9
infective —*see* Endometritis
inflammatory —*see* Endometritis
specified NEC N85.8
uveal tract (anterior) H21.9
posterior H31.9
vagabond's B85.1
vagina, vaginal (noninflammatory) N89.9
inflammatory NEC N76.89
specified NEC N89.8
valve, valvular I38
multiple I08.9
specified NEC I08.8
van Creveld-von Gierke
(glycogenosis I) E74.01
vas deferens N50.9
vascular I99.9
arteriosclerotic —*see* Arteriosclerosis
ciliary body NEC —*see* Disorder, iris,
vascular
hypertensive —*see* Hypertension
iris NEC —*see* Disorder, iris, vascular
obliterative I77.1
peripheral I73.9
occlusive I99.8
peripheral (occlusive) I73.9
in diabetes mellitus —*see* E08-E13
with .51
vasomotor I73.9
vasospastic I73.9
vein I87.9
venereal (*see also* Disease, sexually
transmitted) A64
chlamydial NEC A56.8
anus A56.3
genitourinary NOS A56.2
pharynx A56.4
rectum A56.3
fifth A55
sixth A55
specified nature or type NEC A63.8

Disease, diseased *(Continued)*
 vertebra, vertebral —*see also*
  Spondylopathy
 disc —*see* Disorder, disc
 vibration —*see* Vibration, adverse
  effects
 viral, virus (*see also* Disease, by type of
  virus) B34.9
  arbovirus NOS A94
  arthropod-borne NOS A94
  congenital P35.9
   specified NEC P35.8
  Hanta (with renal manifestations)
   (Dobrava) (Puumala) (Seoul)
   A98.5
   with pulmonary manifestations
    (Andes) (Bayou) (Bermejo)
    (Black Creek Canal) (Choclo)
    (Juquitiba) (Laguna negra)
    (Lechiguanas) (New York)
    (Oran) (Sin nombre) B33.4
  Hantaan (Korean hemorrhagic fever)
   A98.5
  human immunodeficiency (HIV) B20
  Kunjin A83.4
  nonarthropod-borne NOS B34.9
  Powassan A84.8
  Rocio (encephalitis) A83.6
  Sin nombre (Hantavirus) (cardio)-
   pulmonary syndrome B33.4
  Tahyna B33.8
  vesicular stomatitis A93.8
 vitreous H43.9
  specified NEC H43.89
 vocal cord J38.3
 Volkmann's, acquired T79.6
 von Eulenburg's (congenital
  paramyotonia) G71.19
 von Gierke's (glycogenosis I) E74.01
 von Graefe's —*see* Strabismus,
  paralytic, ophthalmoplegia,
  progressive
 von Willebrand (-Jürgens)
  (angiohemophilia) D68.0
 Vrolik's (osteogenesis imperfecta) Q78.0
 vulva (noninflammatory) N90.9
  inflammatory NEC N76.89
  specified NEC N90.89
 Wallgren's (obstruction of splenic vein
  with collateral circulation) I87.8
 Wassilieff's (leptospiral jaundice) A27.0
 wasting NEC R64
  due to malnutrition E41
 Waterhouse-Friderichsen A39.1
 Wegner's (syphilitic osteochondritis)
  A50.02
 Weil's (leptospiral jaundice of lung)
  A27.0
 Weir Mitchell's (erythromelalgia) I73.81
 Werdnig-Hoffmann G12.0
 Wermer's E31.21
 Werner-His (trench fever) A79.0
 Werner-Schultz (neutropenic
  splenomegaly) D73.81
 Wernicke-Posadas B38.9
 whipworm B79
 white blood cells D72.9
  specified NEC D72.89
 white matter R90.82
 white-spot, meaning lichen sclerosus et
  atrophicus L90.0
  penis N48.0
  vulva N90.4
 Wilkie's K55.1

Disease, diseased *(Continued)*
 Wilkinson-Sneddon (subcorneal
  pustular dermatosis) L13.1
 Willis' —*see* Diabetes
 Wilson's (hepatolenticular
  degeneration) E83.01
 woolsorter's A22.1
 yaba monkey tumor B08.72
 yaba pox (virus) B08.72
 zoonotic, bacterial A28.9
  specified type NEC A28.8
Disfigurement (due to scar) L90.5
Disgerminoma —*see* Dysgerminoma
DISH (diffuse idiopathic skeletal
  hyperostosis) —*see* Hyperostosis,
  ankylosing
Disinsertion, retina —*see* Detachment,
  retina
Dislocatable hip, congenital Q65.6
Dislocation (articular)
 with fracture —*see* Fracture
 acromioclavicular (joint) S43.10-
  with displacement
   100%-200% S43.12-
   more than 200% S43.13-
  inferior S43.14-
  posterior S43.15-
 ankle S93.0-
 astragalus —*see* Dislocation, ankle
 atlantoaxial S13.121
 atlantooccipital S13.111
 atloidooccipital S13.111
 breast bone S23.29
 capsule, joint code by site under
  Dislocation
 carpal (bone) —*see* Dislocation, wrist
 carpometacarpal (joint) NEC S63.05-
  thumb S63.04-
 cartilage (joint) - code by site under
  Dislocation
 cervical spine (vertebra) —*see*
  Dislocation, vertebra, cervical
 chronic —*see* Dislocation, recurrent
 clavicle —*see* Dislocation,
  acromioclavicular joint
 coccyx S33.2
 congenital NEC Q68.8
 coracoid —*see* Dislocation, shoulder
 costal cartilage S23.29
 costochondral S23.29
 cricoarytenoid articulation S13.29
 cricothyroid articulation S13.29
 dorsal vertebra —*see* Dislocation,
  vertebra, thoracic
 ear ossicle —*see* Discontinuity, ossicles,
  ear
 elbow S53.10-
  congenital Q68.8
  pathological —*see* Dislocation,
   pathological NEC, elbow
  radial head alone —*see* Dislocation,
   radial head
  recurrent —*see* Dislocation, recurrent,
   elbow
  traumatic S53.10-
   anterior S53.11-
   lateral S53.14-
   medial S53.13-
   posterior S53.12-
   specified type NEC S53.19-
 eye, nontraumatic —*see* Luxation,
  globe
 eyeball, nontraumatic —*see* Luxation,
  globe

Dislocation *(Continued)*
 femur
  distal end —*see* Dislocation, knee
  proximal end —*see* Dislocation, hip
 fibula
  distal end —*see* Dislocation, ankle
  proximal end —*see* Dislocation,
   knee
 finger S63.25-
  index S63.25-
  interphalangeal S63.27-
   distal S63.29-
    index S63.29-
    little S63.29-
    middle S63.29-
    ring S63.29-
   index S63.27-
   little S63.27-
   middle S63.27-
   proximal S63.28-
    index S63.28-
    little S63.28-
    middle S63.28-
    ring S63.28-
   ring S63.27-
  little S63.25-
  metacarpophalangeal S63.26-
   index S63.26-
   little S63.26-
   middle S63.26-
   ring S63.26-
  middle S63.25-
  recurrent —*see* Dislocation, recurrent,
   finger
  ring S63.25-
  thumb —*see* Dislocation, thumb
 foot S93.30-
  recurrent —*see* Dislocation, recurrent,
   foot
  specified site NEC S93.33-
  tarsal joint S93.31-
  tarsometatarsal joint S93.32-
  toe —*see* Dislocation, toe
 fracture —*see* Fracture
 glenohumeral (joint) —*see* Dislocation,
  shoulder
 glenoid —*see* Dislocation, shoulder
 habitual —*see* Dislocation, recurrent
 hip S73.00-
  anterior S73.03-
   obturator S73.02-
  central S73.04-
  congenital (total) Q65.2
   bilateral Q65.1
   partial Q65.5
    bilateral Q65.4
    unilateral Q65.3-
   unilateral Q65.0-
  developmental M24.85-
  pathological —*see* Dislocation,
   pathological NEC, hip
  posterior S73.01-
  recurrent —*see* Dislocation, recurrent,
   hip
 humerus, proximal end —*see*
  Dislocation, shoulder
 incomplete —*see* Subluxation, by site
 incus —*see* Discontinuity, ossicles, ear
 infracoracoid —*see* Dislocation,
  shoulder
 innominate (pubic junction) (sacral
  junction) S33.39
  acetabulum —*see* Dislocation,
   hip

Dislocation (Continued)
  tibia
    distal end —see Dislocation, ankle
    proximal end —see Dislocation, knee
  tibiofibular (joint)
    distal —see Dislocation, ankle
    superior —see Dislocation, knee
  toe (s) S93.106
    great S93.10-
      interphalangeal joint S93.11-
      metatarsophalangeal joint
        S93.12-
    interphalangeal joint S93.119
    lesser S93.106
      interphalangeal joint S93.11-
      metatarsophalangeal joint
        S93.12-
    metatarsophalangeal joint S93.12-
  tooth S03.2
  trachea S23.29
  ulna
    distal end S63.07-
    proximal end —see Dislocation, elbow
  ulnohumeral (joint) —see Dislocation,
      elbow
  vertebra (articular process) (body)
      (traumatic)
    cervical S13.101
      atlantoaxial joint S13.121
      atlantooccipital joint S13.111
      atloidooccipital joint S13.111
      joint between
        C0 and C1 S13.111
        C1 and C2 S13.121
        C2 and C3 S13.131
        C3 and C4 S13.141
        C4 and C5 S13.151
        C5 and C6 S13.161
        C6 and C7 S13.171
        C7 and T1 S13.181
      occipitoatloid joint S13.111
    congenital Q76.49
    lumbar S33.101
      joint between
        L1 and L2 S33.111
        L2 and L3 S33.121
        L3 and L4 S33.131
        L4 and L5 S33.141
    nontraumatic —see Displacement,
        intervertebral disc
    partial —see Subluxation, by site
    recurrent NEC —see subcategory
        M43.5
    thoracic S23.101
      joint between
        T1 and T2 S23.111
        T2 and T3 S23.121
        T3 and T4 S23.123
        T4 and T5 S23.131
        T5 and T6 S23.133
        T6 and T7 S23.141
        T7 and T8 S23.143
        T8 and T9 S23.151
        T9 and T10 S23.153
        T10 and T11 S23.161
        T11 and T12 S23.163
        T12 and L1 S23.171
  wrist (carpal bone) S63.006
    carpometacarpal joint —see
        Dislocation, carpometacarpal
        (joint)
    distal radioulnar joint —see
        Dislocation, radioulnar (joint),
        distal

Dislocation (Continued)
  wrist (Continued)
    metacarpal bone, proximal —see
        Dislocation, metacarpal (bone),
        proximal end
    midcarpal —see Dislocation,
        midcarpal (joint)
    radiocarpal joint —see Dislocation,
        radiocarpal (joint)
    recurrent —see Dislocation, recurrent,
        wrist
    specified site NEC S63.09-
    ulna —see Dislocation, ulna, distal
        end
  xiphoid cartilage S23.29
Disorder (of) —see also Disease
  acantholytic L11.9
    specified NEC L11.8
  acute
    psychotic —see Psychosis, acute
    stress F43.0
  adjustment (grief) F43.20
    with
      anxiety F43.22
        with depressed mood F43.23
      conduct disturbance F43.24
        with emotional disturbance F43.25
      depressed mood F43.21
        with anxiety F43.23
      other specified symptom F43.29
  adrenal (capsule) (gland) (medullary)
      E27.9
    specified NEC E27.8
  adrenogenital E25.9
    drug-induced E25.8
    iatrogenic E25.8
    idiopathic E25.8
  adult personality (and behavior) F69
    specified NEC F68.8
  affective (mood) —see Disorder, mood
  aggressive, unsocialized F91.1
  alcohol-related F10.99
    with
      amnestic disorder, persisting F10.96
      anxiety disorder F10.980
      dementia, persisting F10.97
      intoxication F10.929
        with delirium F10.921
        uncomplicated F10.920
      mood disorder F10.94
      other specified F10.988
      psychotic disorder F10.959
        with
          delusions F10.950
          hallucinations F10.951
      sexual dysfunction F10.981
      sleep disorder F10.982
  allergic —see Allergy
  alveolar NEC J84.09
  amino-acid
    cystathioninuria E72.19
    cystinosis E72.04
    cystinuria E72.01
    glycinuria E72.09
    homocystinuria E72.11
    metabolism —see Disturbance,
        metabolism, amino-acid
    specified NEC E72.8
    neonatal, transitory P74.8
    renal transport NEC E72.09
    transport NEC E72.09
  amnesic, amnestic
    alcohol-induced F10.96
      with dependence F10.26

Disorder (Continued)
  amnesic, amnestic (Continued)
    due to (secondary to) general medical
        condition F04
    psychoactive NEC-induced F19.96
      with
        abuse F19.16
        dependence F19.26
    sedative, hypnotic or anxiolytic-
        induced F13.96
      with dependence F13.26
  anaerobic glycolysis with anemia
      D55.2
  anxiety F41.9
    due to (secondary to)
      alcohol F10.980
      amphetamine F15.980
        in
          abuse F15.180
          dependence F15.280
      anxiolytic F13.980
        in
          abuse F13.180
          dependence F13.280
      caffeine F15.980
        in
          abuse F15.180
          dependence F15.280
      cannabis F12.980
        in
          abuse F12.180
          dependence F12.280
      cocaine F14.980
        in
          abuse F14.180
          dependence F14.180
      general medical condition F06.4
      hallucinogen F16.980
        in
          abuse F16.180
          dependence F16.280
      hypnotic F13.980
        in
          abuse F13.180
          dependence F13.280
      inhalant F18.980
        in
          abuse F18.180
          dependence F18.280
      phencyclidine F16.980
        in
          abuse F16.180
          dependence F16.280
      psychoactive substance NEC
          F19.980
        in
          abuse F19.180
          dependence F19.280
      sedative F13.980
        in
          abuse F13.180
          dependence F13.280
      volatile solvents F18.980
        in
          abuse F18.180
          dependence F18.280
    generalized F41.1
    mixed
      with depression (mild) F41.8
      specified NEC F41.3
    organic F06.4
    phobic F40.9
      of childhood F40.8
    specified NEC F41.8

Disorder *(Continued)*
  aortic valve —*see* Endocarditis, aortic
  aromatic amino-acid metabolism
    E70.9
    specified NEC E70.8
  arteriole NEC I77.89
  artery NEC I77.89
  articulation —*see* Disorder, joint
  attachment (childhood)
    disinhibited F94.2
    reactive F94.1
  attention-deficit hyperactivity
    (adolescent) (adult) (child) F90.9
    combined type F90.2
    hyperactive type F90.1
    inattentive type F90.0
    specified type NEC F90.8
  attention-deficit without hyperactivity
    (adolescent) (adult) (child) F90.0
  auditory processing (central) H93.25
  autistic F84.0
  autonomic nervous system G90.9
    specified NEC G90.8
  avoidant, child or adolescent F40.10
  balance
    acid-base E87.8
      mixed E87.4
    electrolyte E87.8
    fluid NEC E87.8
  behavioral (disruptive) —*see* Disorder,
    conduct
  beta-amino-acid metabolism E72.8
  bile acid and cholesterol metabolism
    E78.70
    Barth syndrome E78.71
    other specified E78.79
    Smith-Lemli-Opitz syndrome
      E78.72
  bilirubin excretion E80.6
  binocular
    movement H51.9
      convergence
        excess H51.12
        insufficiency H51.11
      internuclear ophthalmoplegia —
        see Ophthalmoplegia,
        internuclear
      palsy of conjugate gaze H51.0
      specified type NEC H51.8
    vision NEC —*see* Disorder, vision,
      binocular
  bipolar (I) F31.9
    current episode
      depressed F31.9
        with psychotic features F31.5
        without psychotic features
          F31.30
          mild F31.31
          moderate F31.32
          severe (without psychotic
            features) F31.4
            with psychotic features
              F31.5
      hypomanic F31.0
      manic F31.9
        with psychotic features F31.2
        without psychotic features
          F31.10
          mild F31.11
          moderate F31.12
          severe (without psychotic
            features) F31.13
            with psychotic features
              F31.2

Disorder *(Continued)*
  bipolar *(Continued)*
    current episode *(Continued)*
      mixed F31.60
        mild F31.61
        moderate F31.62
        severe (without psychotic
          features) F31.63
          with psychotic features F31.64
        severe depression (without
          psychotic features) F31.4
          with psychotic features F31.5
      II F31.81
      in remission (currently) F31.70
      in full remission
        most recent episode
          depressed F31.76
          hypomanic F31.72
          manic F31.74
          mixed F31.78
      in partial remission
        most recent episode
          depressed F31.75
          hypomanic F31.71
          manic F31.73
          mixed F31.77
    organic F06.30
    single manic episode F30.9
      mild F30.11
      moderate F30.12
      severe (without psychotic
        symptoms) F30.13
        with psychotic symptoms F30.2
    specified NEC F31.89
  bladder N32.9
    functional NEC N31.9
    in schistosomiasis B65.0 *[N33]*
    specified NEC N32.89
  bleeding D68.9
  blood D75.9
    in congenital early syphilis A50.09
      [D77]
  body dysmorphic F45.22
  bone M89.9
    continuity M84.9
      specified type NEC M84.80
        ankle M84.87-
        fibula M84.86-
        foot M84.87-
        hand M84.84-
        humerus M84.82-
        neck M84.88
        pelvis M84.859
        radius M84.83-
        rib M84.88
        shoulder M84.81-
        skull M84.88
        thigh M84.85-
        tibia M84.86-
        ulna M84.83-
        vertebra M84.88
    density and structure M85.9
      cyst —*see also* Cyst, bone, specified
        type NEC
        aneurysmal —*see* Cyst, bone,
          aneurysmal
        solitary —*see* Cyst, bone, solitary
      diffuse idiopathic skeletal
        hyperostosis —*see*
        Hyperostosis, ankylosing
      fibrous dysplasia (monostotic) —
        see Dysplasia, fibrous, bone
      fluorosis —*see* Fluorosis, skeletal
      hyperostosis of skull M85.2

Disorder *(Continued)*
  bone *(Continued)*
    density and structure *(Continued)*
      osteitis condensans —*see* Osteitis,
        condensans
      specified type NEC M85.8-
        ankle M85.87-
        foot M85.87-
        forearm M85.83-
        hand M85.84-
        lower leg M85.86-
        multiple sites M85.89
        neck M85.88
        rib M85.88
        shoulder M85.81-
        skull M85.88
        thigh M85.85-
        upper arm M85.82-
        vertebra M85.88
    development and growth NEC
      M89.20
      carpus M89.24-
      clavicle M89.21-
      femur M89.25-
      fibula M89.26-
      finger M89.24-
      humerus M89.22-
      ilium M89.259
      ischium M89.259
      metacarpus M89.24-
      metatarsus M89.27-
      multiple sites M89.29
      neck M89.28
      radius M89.23-
      rib M89.28
      scapula M89.21-
      skull M89.28
      tarsus M89.27-
      tibia M89.26-
      toe M89.27-
      ulna M89.23-
      vertebra M89.28
    specified type NEC M89.8X-
  brachial plexus G54.0
  branched-chain amino-acid metabolism
    E71.2
    specified NEC E71.19
  breast N64.9
    agalactia —*see* Agalactia
    associated with
      lactation O92.70
        specified NEC O92.79
      pregnancy O92.20
        specified NEC O92.29
      puerperium O92.20
        specified NEC O92.29
    cracked nipple —*see* Cracked nipple
    galactorrhea —*see* Galactorrhea
    hypogalactia O92.4
    lactation disorder NEC O92.79
    mastitis —*see* Mastitis
    nipple infection —*see* Infection,
      nipple
    retracted nipple —*see* Retraction,
      nipple
    specified type NEC N64.89
  Briquet's F45.0
  bullous, in diseases classified elsewhere
    L14
  cannabis use
    due to drug abuse —*see* Abuse, drug,
      cannabis
    due to drug dependence —*see*
      Dependend, drug, cannabis

Disorder *(Continued)*
  carbohydrate
    absorption, intestinal NEC E74.39
    metabolism (congenital) E74.9
      specified NEC E74.8
  cardiac, functional I51.89
  carnitine metabolism E71.40
  cartilage M94.9
    articular NEC —*see* Derangement,
      joint, articular cartilage
    chondrocalcinosis —*see*
      Chondrocalcinosis
    specified type NEC M94.8X-
      articular —*see* Derangement, joint,
        articular cartilage
      multiple sites M94.8X0
  catatonic
    due to (secondary to) known
      physiological condition F06.1
    organic F06.1
  central auditory processing H93.25
  cervical
    region NEC M53.82
    root (nerve) NEC G54.2
  character NOS F60.9
  childhood disintegrative NEC F84.3
  cholesterol and bile acid metabolism
    E78.70
    Barth syndrome E78.71
    other specified E78.79
    Smith-Lemli-Opitz syndrome E78.72
  choroid H31.9
    atrophy —*see* Atrophy, choroid
    degeneration —*see* Degeneration,
      choroid
    detachment —*see* Detachment,
      choroid
    dystrophy —*see* Dystrophy, choroid
    hemorrhage —*see* Hemorrhage,
      choroid
    rupture —*see* Rupture, choroid
    scar —*see* Scar, chorioretinal
    solar retinopathy —*see* Retinopathy,
      solar
    specified type NEC H31.8
  ciliary body —*see* Disorder, iris
    degeneration —*see* Degeneration,
      ciliary body
  coagulation (factor) (*see also* Defect,
    coagulation) D68.9
    newborn, transient P61.6
  coccyx NEC M53.3
  cognitive F09
    due to (secondary to) general medical
      condition F09
    persisting R41.89
      due to
        alcohol F10.97
          with dependence F10.27
        anxiolytics F13.97
          with dependence F13.27
        hypnotics F13.97
          with dependence F13.27
        sedatives F13.97
          with dependence F13.27
        specified substance NEC F19.97
          with
            abuse F19.17
            dependence F19.27
  communication F80.9
  conduct (childhood) F91.9
    adjustment reaction —*see* Disorder,
      adjustment
    adolescent onset type F91.2

Disorder *(Continued)*
  conduct *(Continued)*
    childhood onset type F91.1
    compulsive F63.9
    confined to family context F91.0
    depressive F91.8
    group type F91.2
    hyperkinetic —*see* Disorder,
      attention-deficit hyperactivity
    oppositional defiance F91.3
    socialized F91.2
    solitary aggressive type F91.1
    specified NEC F91.8
    unsocialized (aggressive) F91.1
  conduction, heart I45.9
  congenital glycosylation (CDG)
    E74.8
  conjunctiva H11.9
    infection —*see* Conjunctivitis
  connective tissue, localized L94.9
    specified NEC L94.8
  conversion —*see* Disorder, dissociative
  convulsive (secondary) —*see*
    Convulsions
  cornea H18.9
    deformity —*see* Deformity, cornea
    degeneration —*see* Degeneration,
      cornea
    deposits —*see* Deposit, cornea
    due to contact lens H18.82-
      specified as edema —*see* Edema,
        cornea
    edema —*see* Edema, cornea
    keratitis —*see* Keratitis
    keratoconjunctivitis —*see*
      Keratoconjunctivitis
    membrane change —*see* Change,
      corneal membrane
    neovascularization —*see*
      Neovascularization, cornea
    scar —*see* Opacity, cornea
    specified type NEC H18.89-
    ulcer —*see* Ulcer, cornea
  corpus cavernosum N48.9
  cranial nerve —*see* Disorder, nerve,
    cranial
  cyclothymic F34.0
  defiant oppositional F91.3
  delusional (persistent) (systematized)
    F22
    induced F24
  depersonalization F48.1
  depressive F32.9
    major F32.9
      with psychotic symptoms F32.3
      in remission (full) F32.5
        partial F32.4
      recurrent F33.9
      single episode F32.9
        mild F32.0
        moderate F32.1
        severe (without psychotic
          symptoms) F32.2
          with psychotic symptoms
            F32.3
    organic F06.31
    recurrent F33.9
      current episode
        mild F33.0
        moderate F33.1
        severe (without psychotic
          symptoms) F33.2
          with psychotic symptoms
            F33.3

Disorder *(Continued)*
  depressive *(Continued)*
    recurrent *(Continued)*
      in remission F33.40
        full F33.42
        partial F33.41
      specified NEC F33.8
    single episode —*see* Episode,
      depressive
  developmental F89
    arithmetical skills F81.2
    coordination (motor) F82
    expressive writing F81.81
    language F80.9
      expressive F80.1
      mixed receptive and expressive
        F80.2
      receptive type F80.2
      specified NEC F80.89
    learning F81.9
      arithmetical F81.2
      reading F81.0
    mixed F88
    motor coordination or function F82
    pervasive F84.9
      specified NEC F84.8
    phonological F80.0
    reading F81.0
    scholastic skills —*see also* Disorder,
      learning
      mixed F81.89
    specified NEC F88
    speech F80.9
      articulation F80.0
      specified NEC F80.89
    written expression F81.81
  diaphragm J98.6
  digestive (system) K92.9
    newborn P78.9
      specified NEC P78.89
    postprocedural —*see* Complication,
      gastrointestinal
    psychogenic F45.8
  disc (intervertebral) M51.9
    with
      myelopathy
        cervical region M50.00
        cervicothoracic region M50.03
        lumbar region M51.06
        lumbosacral region M51.07
        mid-cervical region M50.02
        occipito-atlanto-axial region
          M50.01
        sacrococcygeal region M53.3
        thoracic region M51.04
        thoracolumbar region M51.05
      radiculopathy
        cervical region M50.10
        cervicothoracic region M50.13
        lumbar region M51.16
        lumbosacral region M51.17
        mid-cervical region M50.12
        occipito-atlanto-axial region
          M50.11
        sacrococcygeal region M53.3
        thoracic region M51.14
        thoracolumbar region M51.15
    cervical M50.90
      with
        myelopathy M50.00
          cervicothoracic region M50.03
          mid-cervical region M50.02
          occipito-atlanto-axial region
            M50.01

Disorder *(Continued)*
 disc *(Continued)*
  cervical *(Continued)*
   with *(Continued)*
    neuritis, radiculitis or
     radiculopathy M50.10
      cervicothoracic region M50.13
      mid-cervical region M50.12
      occipito-atlanto-axial region
       M50.11
    cervicothoracic region M50.93
   degeneration M50.30
    cervicothoracic region M50.33
    mid-cervical region M50.32
    occipito-atlanto-axial region
     M50.31
   displacement M50.20
    cervicothoracic region M50.23
    mid-cervical region M50.22
    occipito-atlanto-axial region
     M50.21
   mid-cervical region M50.92
   occipito-atlanto-axial region
    M50.91
   specified type NEC M50.80
    cervicothoracic region M50.83
    mid-cervical region M50.82
    occipito-atlanto-axial region
     M50.81
  specified NEC
   lumbar region M51.86
   lumbosacral region M51.87
   sacrococcygeal region M53.3
   thoracic region M51.84
   thoracolumbar region M51.85
 disinhibited attachment (childhood)
  F94.2
 disintegrative, childhood NEC F84.3
 disruptive behavior F98.9
 dissocial personality F60.2
 dissociative F44.9
  affecting
   motor function F44.4
    and sensation F44.7
   sensation F44.6
    and motor function F44.7
  brief reactive F43.0
  due to (secondary to) general medical
   condition F06.8
  mixed F44.7
  organic F06.8
  other specified NEC F44.89
 double heterozygous sickling —*see*
  Disease, sickle-cell
 dream anxiety F51.5
 drug induced hemorrhagic D68.32
 drug related F19.99
  abuse —*see* Abuse, drug
  dependence —*see* Dependence, drug
 dysmorphic body F45.1
 dysthymic F34.1
 ear H93.9-
  bleeding —*see* Otorrhagia
  deafness —*see* Deafness
  degenerative H93.09-
  discharge —*see* Otorrhea
  external H61.9-
   auditory canal stenosis —*see*
    Stenosis, external ear canal
   exostosis —*see* Exostosis, external
    ear canal
   impacted cerumen —*see* Impaction,
    cerumen
   otitis —*see* Otitis, externa

Disorder *(Continued)*
 ear *(Continued)*
  external *(Continued)*
   perichondritis —*see* Perichondritis,
    ear
   pinna —*see* Disorder, pinna
   specified type NEC H61.89-
  inner H83.9-
   vestibular dysfunction —*see*
    Disorder, vestibular function
  middle H74.9-
   adhesive H74.1-
   ossicle —*see* Abnormal, ear ossicles
   polyp —*see* Polyp, ear (middle)
   specified NEC, in diseases
    classified elsewhere H75.8-
   postprocedural —*see* Complications,
    ear, procedure
   specified NEC, in diseases classified
    elsewhere H94.8-
  eating (adult) (psychogenic) F50.9
   anorexia —*see* Anorexia
   bulimia F50.2
   child F98.29
    pica F98.3
    rumination disorder F98.21
   pica F50.8
    childhood F98.3
  electrolyte (balance) NEC E87.8
   with
    abortion —*see* Abortion by type
     complicated by specified
     condition NEC
    ectopic pregnancy O08.5
    molar pregnancy O08.5
   acidosis (metabolic) (respiratory) E87.2
   alkalosis (metabolic) (respiratory)
    E87.3
  elimination, transepidermal L87.9
   specified NEC L87.8
  emotional (persistent) F34.9
   of childhood F93.9
    specified NEC F93.8
  endocrine E34.9
   postprocedural E89.89
   specified NEC E89.89
  erectile (male) (organic) (*see also*
   Dysfunction, sexual, male,
   erectile) N52.9
   nonorganic F52.21
  erythematous —*see* Erythema
  esophagus K22.9
   functional K22.4
   psychogenic F45.8
  eustachian tube H69.9-
   infection —*see* Salpingitis, eustachian
   obstruction —*see* Obstruction,
    eustachian tube
   patulous —*see* Patulous, eustachian
    tube
   specified NEC H69.8-
  extrapyramidal G25.9
   specified type NEC G25.89
  eye H57.9
   postprocedural —*see* Complication,
    postprocedural, eye
  eyelid H02.9
   cyst —*see* Cyst, eyelid
   degenerative H02.70
    chloasma —*see* Chloasma, eyelid
    madarosis —*see* Madarosis
    specified type NEC H02.79
    vitiligo —*see* Vitiligo, eyelid
    xanthelasma —*see* Xanthelasma

Disorder *(Continued)*
 eyelid *(Continued)*
  dermatochalasis —*see*
   Dermato-chalasis
  edema —*see* Edema, eyelid
  elephantiasis —*see* Elephantiasis,
   eyelid
  foreign body, retained —*see* Foreign
   body, retained, eyelid
  function H02.59
   abnormal innervation syndrome —
    see Syndrome, abnormal
    innervation
   blepharochalasis —*see*
    Blepharochalasis
   blepharoclonus —*see*
    Blepharoclonus
   blepharophimosis —*see*
    Blepharophimosis
   blepharoptosis —*see* Blepharoptosis
   lagophthalmos —*see*
    Lagophthalmos
   lid retraction —*see* Retraction, lid
   hypertrichosis —*see* Hypertrichosis,
    eyelid
   specified type NEC H02.89
  vascular H02.879
   left H02.876
    lower H02.875
    upper H02.874
   right H02.873
    lower H02.872
    upper H02.871
 factitious F68.10
  with predominantly
   physical symptoms F68.12
    with psychological symptoms
     F68.13
   psychological symptoms F68.11
    with physical symptoms F68.13
 factor, coagulation —*see* Defect,
  coagulation
 fatty acid
  metabolism E71.30
   specified NEC E71.39
  oxidation
   LCAD E71.310
   MCAD E71.311
   SCAD E71.312
   specified deficiency NEC E71.318
 feeding (infant or child) (*see also*
  Disorder, eating) R63.3-
 feigned (with obvious motivation) Z76.5
  without obvious motivation —*see*
   Disorder, factitious
 female
  hypoactive sexual desire F52.0
  orgasmic F52.31
  sexual arousal F52.22
 fibroblastic M72.9
  specified NEC M72.8
 fluency
  adult onset F98.5
  childhood onset F80.81
  following
   cerebral infarction I69.323
   cerebrovascular disease I69.923
    specified disease NEC I69.823
   intracerebral hemorrhage I69.123
   nontraumatic intracranial
    hemorrhage NEC I69.223
   subarachnoid hemorrhage I69.023
  in conditions classified elsewhere
   R47.82
 fluid balance E87.8

Disorder (*Continued*)
follicular (skin) L73.9
  specified NEC L73.8
fructose metabolism E74.10
  essential fructosuria E74.11
  fructokinase deficiency E74.11
  fructose-1, 6-diphosphatase
    deficiency E74.19
  hereditary fructose intolerance E74.12
  other specified E74.19
functional polymorphonuclear
  neutrophils D71
gallbladder, biliary tract and pancreas in
  diseases classified elsewhere K87
gamma-glutamyl cycle E72.8
gastric (functional) K31.9
  motility K30
  psychogenic F45.8
  secretion K30
gastrointestinal (functional) NOS K92.9
  newborn P78.9
  psychogenic F45.8
gender-identity or -role F64.9
  childhood F64.2
  effect on relationship F66
  of adolescence or adulthood
    (nontranssexual) F64.1
  specified NEC F64.8
  uncertainty F66
genitourinary system
  female N94.9
  male N50.9
  psychogenic F45.8
globe H44.9
  degenerated condition H44.50
    absolute glaucoma H44.51-
    atrophy H44.52-
    leucocoria H44.53-
  degenerative H44.30
    chalcosis H44.31-
    myopia H44.2-
    siderosis H44.32-
    specified type NEC H44.39-
  endophthalmitis —*see*
    Endophthalmitis
  foreign body, retained —*see* Foreign
    body, intraocular, old, retained
  hemophthalmos —*see*
    Hemophthalmos
  hypotony H44.40
    due to
      ocular fistula H44.42-
      specified disorder NEC H44.43-
    flat anterior chamber H44.41-
    primary H44.44-
  luxation —*see* Luxation, globe
  specified NEC H44.89
glomerular (in) N05.9
  amyloidosis E85.4 [N08]
  cryoglobulinemia D89.1 [N08]
  disseminated intravascular
    coagulation D65 [N08]
  Fabry's disease E75.21 [N08]
  familial lecithin cholesterol
    acyltransferase deficiency E78.6
    [N08]
  Goodpasture's syndrome M31.0
  hemolytic-uremic syndrome D59.3
  Henoch (-Schönlein) purpura D69.0
    [N08]
  malariae malaria B52.0
  microscopic polyangiitis M31.7 [N08]
  multiple myeloma C90.0- [N08]
  mumps B26.83

Disorder (*Continued*)
 glomerular (in) (*Continued*)
  schistosomiasis B65.9 [N08]
  sepsis NEC A41.- [N08]
    streptococcal A40.- [N08]
  sickle-cell disorders D57.- [N08]
  strongyloidiasis B78.9 [N08]
  subacute bacterial endocarditis
    I33.0 [N08]
  syphilis A52.75
  systemic lupus erythematosus M32.14
  thrombotic thrombocytopenic
    purpura M31.1 [N08]
  Waldenström macroglobulinemia
    C88.0 [N08]
  Wegener's granulomatosis M31.31
 gluconeogenesis E74.4
 glucosaminoglycan metabolism —
    see Disorder, metabolism,
    glucosaminoglycan
 glycine metabolism E72.50
  d-glycericacidemia E72.59
  hyperhydroxyprolinemia E72.59
  hyperoxaluria E72.53
  hyperprolinemia E72.59
  non-ketotic hyperglycinemia E72.51
  oxalosis E72.53
  oxaluria E72.53
  sarcosinemia E72.59
  trimethylaminuria E72.52
 glycoprotein metabolism E77.9
  specified NEC E77.8
 habit (and impulse) F63.9
  involving sexual behavior NEC
    F65.9
  specified NEC F63.89
 heart action I49.9
 hematological D75.9
  newborn (transient) P61.9
    specified NEC P61.8
 hematopoietic organs D75.9
 hemorrhagic NEC D69.9
  drug-induced D68.32
  due to
    extrinsic circulating anticoagulants
      D68.32
    increase in
      anti-IIa D68.32
      anti-Xa D68.32
    intrinsic
      circulating anticoagulants
        D68.318
      increase in
        antithrombin D68.318
        anti-VIIIa D68.318
        anti-IXa D68.318
        anti-XIa D68.318
  following childbirth O72.3
 hemostasis —*see* Defect, coagulation
 histidine metabolism E70.40
  histidinemia E70.41
  other specified E70.49
 hyperkinetic —*see* Disorder, attention-
    deficit hyperactivity
 hyperleucine-isoleucinemia E71.19
 hypervalinemia E71.19
 hypoactive sexual desire F52.0
 hypochondriacal F45.20
  body dysmorphic F45.22
  neurosis F45.21
  other specified F45.29
 identity
  dissociative F44.81
  of childhood F93.8

Disorder (*Continued*)
immune mechanism (immunity) D89.9
  specified type NEC D89.89
impaired renal tubular function N25.9
  specified NEC N25.89
impulse (control) F63.9
inflammatory
  penis N48.29
    abscess N48.21
    cellulitis N48.22
integument, newborn P83.9
  specified NEC P83.8
intermittent explosive F63.81
internal secretion pancreas —*see*
    Increased, secretion, pancreas,
    endocrine
intestine, intestinal
  carbohydrate absorption NEC E74.39
    postoperative K91.2
  functional NEC K59.9
    postoperative K91.89
  psychogenic F45.8
  vascular K55.9
    chronic K55.1
    specified NEC K55.8
intraoperative (intraprocedural) —*see*
    Complications, intraoperative
involuntary emotional expression
  (IEED) F07.89
iris H21.9
  adhesions —*see* Adhesions, iris
  atrophy —*see* Atrophy, iris
  chamber angle recession —*see*
    Recession, chamber angle
  cyst —*see* Cyst, iris
  degeneration —*see* Degeneration, iris
  in diseases classified elsewhere H22
  iridodialysis —*see* Iridodialysis
  iridoschisis —*see* Iridoschisis
  miotic pupillary cyst —*see* Cyst,
    pupillary
  pupillary
    abnormality —*see* Abnormality,
      pupillary
    membrane —*see* Membrane,
      pupillary
  specified type NEC H21.89
  vascular NEC H21.1X-
iron metabolism E83.10
  specified NEC E83.19
isovaleric acidemia E71.110
jaw, developmental M27.0
  temporomandibular —*see* Anomaly,
    dentofacial, temporomandibular
    joint
joint M25.9
  derangement —*see* Derangement,
    joint
  effusion —*see* Effusion, joint
  fistula —*see* Fistula, joint
  hemarthrosis —*see* Hemarthrosis
  instability —*see* Instability, joint
  osteophyte —*see* Osteophyte
  pain —*see* Pain, joint
  psychogenic F45.8
  specified type NEC M25.80
    ankle M25.87-
    elbow M25.82-
    foot joint M25.87-
    hand joint M25.84-
    hip M25.85-
    knee M25.86-
    shoulder M25.81-
    wrist M25.83-
  stiffness —*see* Stiffness, joint

Disorder *(Continued)*
  ketone metabolism E71.32
  kidney N28.9
    functional (tubular) N25.9
    in
      schistosomiasis B65.9 *[N29]*
    tubular function N25.9
      specified NEC N25.89
  lacrimal system H04.9
    changes H04.69
    fistula —*see* Fistula, lacrimal
    gland H04.19
      atrophy —*see* Atrophy, lacrimal
        gland
      cyst —*see* Cyst, lacrimal, gland
      dacryops —*see* Dacryops
      dislocation —*see* Dislocation,
        lacrimal gland
      dry eye syndrome —*see* Syndrome,
        dry eye
      infection —*see* Dacryoadenitis
      granuloma —*see* Granuloma, lacrimal
      inflammation —*see* Inflammation,
        lacrimal
      obstruction —*see* Obstruction,
        lacrimal
      specified NEC H04.89
  lactation NEC O92.79
  language (developmental) F80.9
    expressive F80.1
    mixed receptive and expressive
      F80.2
    receptive F80.2
  late luteal phase dysphoric N94.89
  learning (specific) F81.9
    acalculia R48.8
    alexia R48.0
    mathematics F81.2
    reading F81.0
    specified NEC F81.89
    spelling F81.81
    written expression F81.81
  lens H27.9
    aphakia —*see* Aphakia
    cataract —*see* Cataract
    dislocation —*see* Dislocation, lens
    specified type NEC H27.8
  ligament M24.20
    ankle M24.27-
    attachment, spine —*see* Enthesopathy,
      spinal
    elbow M24.22-
    foot joint M24.27-
    hand joint M24.24-
    hip M24.25-
    knee —*see* Derangement, knee,
      specified NEC
    shoulder M24.21-
    vertebra M24.28
    wrist M24.23-
  ligamentous attachments —*see also*
      Enthesopathy
    spine —*see* Enthesopathy, spinal
  lipid
    metabolism, congenital E78.9
    storage E75.6
      specified NEC E75.5
  lipoprotein
    deficiency (familial) E78.6
    metabolism E78.9
      specified NEC E78.89
  liver K76.9
    malarial B54 *[K77]*
  low back —*see also* Dorsopathy,
      specified NEC

Disorder *(Continued)*
  lumbosacral
    plexus G54.1
    root (nerve) NEC G54.4
  lung, interstitial, drug-induced J70.4
    acute J70.2
    chronic J70.3
  lymphoproliferative, post-transplant
      (PTLD) D47.Z1
  lysine and hydroxylysine metabolism
      E72.3
  male
    erectile (organic) (*see also* Dysfunction,
      sexual, male, erectile) N52.9
      nonorganic F52.21
    hypoactive sexual desire F52.0
    orgasmic F52.32
  manic F30.9
    organic F06.33
  mastoid —*see also* Disorder, ear, middle
    postprocedural —*see* Complications,
      ear, procedure
  meniscus —*see* Derangement, knee,
      meniscus
  menopausal N95.9
    specified NEC N95.8
  menstrual N92.6
    psychogenic F45.8
    specified NEC N92.5
  mental (or behavioral) (nonpsychotic)
      F99
    due to (secondary to)
      amphetamine
        due to drug abuse —*see* Abuse,
          drug, stimulant
        due to drug dependence —*see*
          Dependence, drug, stimulant
      brain disease, damage and
        dysfunction F09
      caffeine use
        due to drug abuse —*see* Abuse,
          drug, stimulant
        due to drug dependence —
          see Dependence, drug,
          stimulant
      cannabis use
        due to drug abuse —*see* Abuse,
          drug, cannabis
        due to drug dependence —
          see Dependence, drug,
          cannabis
      general medical condition F09
      sedative or hypnotic use
        due to drug abuse —*see* Abuse,
          drug, sedative
        due to drug dependence —*see*
          Dependence, drug, sedative
      tobacco (nicotine) use —*see*
        Dependence, drug, nicotine
    following organic brain damage F07.9
      frontal lobe syndrome F07.0
      personality change F07.0
      postconcussional syndrome F07.81
      specified NEC F07.89
    infancy, childhood or adolescence
      F98.9
    neurotic —*see* Neurosis
    organic or symptomatic F09
    presenile, psychotic F03
    problem NEC
    psychoneurotic —*see* Neurosis
    psychotic —*see* Psychosis
    puerperal F53
    senile, psychotic NEC F03

Disorder *(Continued)*
  metabolic, amino acid, transitory,
      newborn P74.8
  metabolism NOS E88.9
    amino-acid E72.9
      aromatic E70.9
        albinism —*see* Albinism
        histidine E70.40
          histidinemia E70.41
          other specified E70.49
        hyperphenylalaninemia E70.1
          classical phenylketonuria E70.0
        other specified E70.8
        tryptophan E70.5
        tyrosine E70.20
          hypertyrosinemia E70.21
          other specified E70.29
      branched chain E71.2
        3-methylglutaconic aciduria
          E71.111
        hyperleucine-isoleucinemia
          E71.19
        hypervalinemia E71.19
        isovaleric acidemia E71.110
        maple syrup urine disease E71.0
        methylmalonic acidemia E71.120
        organic aciduria NEC E71.118
        other specified E71.19
        proprionate NEC E71.128
        proprionic acidemia E71.121
      glycine E72.50
        d-glycericacidemia E72.59
        hyperhydroxyprolinemia E72.59
        hyperoxaluria E72.53
        hyperprolinemia E72.59
        non-ketotic hyperglycinemia
          E72.51
        other specified E72.59
        sarcosinemia E72.59
        trimethylaminuria E72.52
      hydroxylysine E72.3
      lysine E72.3
      ornithine E72.4
      other specified E72.8
        beta-amino acid E72.8
        gamma-glutamyl cycle E72.8
      straight-chain E72.8
      sulfur-bearing E72.10
        homocystinuria E72.11
        methylenetetrahydrofolate
          reductase deficiency E72.12
        other specified E72.19
    bile acid and cholesterol metabolism
      E78.70
    bilirubin E80.7
      specified NEC E80.6
    calcium E83.50
      hypercalcemia E83.52
      hypocalcemia E83.51
      other specified E83.59
    carbohydrate E74.9
      specified NEC E74.8
    cholesterol and bile acid metabolism
      E78.70
    congenital E88.9
    copper E83.00
      specified type NEC E83.09
      Wilson's disease E83.01
    cystinuria E72.01
    fructose E74.10
    galactose E74.20
    glucosaminoglycan E76.9
      mucopolysaccharidosis —*see*
        Mucopolysaccharidosis
      specified NEC E76.8

Disorder *(Continued)*
  metabolism *(Continued)*
    glutamine E72.8
    glycine E72.50
    glycogen storage (hepatorenal) E74.09
    glycoprotein E77.9
      specified NEC E77.8
    glycosaminoglycan E76.9
      specified NEC E76.8
    in labor and delivery O75.89
    iron E83.10
    isoleucine E71.19
    leucine E71.19
    lipoid E78.9
    lipoprotein E78.9
      specified NEC E78.89
    magnesium E83.40
      hypermagnesemia E83.41
      hypomagnesemia E83.42
      other specified E83.49
    mineral E83.9
      specified NEC E83.89
    mitochondrial E88.40
      MELAS syndrome E88.41
      MERRF syndrome (myoclonic
        epilepsy associated with
        ragged-red fibers) E88.42
      other specified E88.49
    ornithine E72.4
    phosphatases E83.30
    phosphorus E83.30
      acid phosphatase deficiency E83.39
      hypophosphatasia E83.39
      hypophosphatemia E83.39
        familial E83.31
      other specified E83.39
      pseudovitamin D deficiency E83.32
    plasma protein NEC E88.09
    porphyrin —*see* Porphyria
    postprocedural E89.89
      specified NEC E89.89
    purine E79.9
      specified NEC E79.8
    pyrimidine E79.9
      specified NEC E79.8
    pyruvate E74.4
    serine E72.8
    sodium E87.8
    specified NEC E88.89
    threonine E72.8
    valine E71.19
    zinc E83.2
  methylmalonic acidemia E71.120
  micturition NEC R39.19
    feeling of incomplete emptying
      R39.14
    hesitancy R39.11
    poor stream R39.12
    psychogenic F45.8
    split stream R39.13
    straining R39.16
    urgency R39.15
  mitochondrial metabolism E88.40
  mitral (valve) —*see* Endocarditis,
    mitral
  mixed
    anxiety and depressive F41.8
    of scholastic skills (developmental)
      F81.89
    receptive expressive language F80.2
  mood F39
    bipolar —*see* Disorder, bipolar
    depressive —*see* Disorder,
      depressive

Disorder *(Continued)*
  mood *(Continued)*
    due to (secondary to)
      alcohol F10.94
      amphetamine F15.94
        in
          abuse F15.14
          dependence F15.24
      anxiolytic F13.94
        in
          abuse F13.14
          dependence F13.24
      cocaine F14.94
        in
          abuse F14.14
          dependence F14.24
      general medical condition F06.30
      hallucinogen F16.94
        in
          abuse F16.14
          dependence F16.24
      hypnotic F13.94
        in
          abuse F13.14
          dependence F13.24
      inhalant F18.94
        in
          abuse F18.14
          dependence F18.24
      opioid F11.94
        in
          abuse F11.14
          dependence F11.24
      phencyclidine (PCP) F16.94
        in
          abuse F16.14
          dependence F16.24
      physiological condition F06.30
        with
          depressive features F06.31
          major depressive-like episode
            F06.32
          manic features F06.33
          mixed features F06.34
      psychoactive substance NEC F19.94
        in
          abuse F19.14
          dependence F19.24
      sedative F13.94
        in
          abuse F13.14
          dependence F13.24
      volatile solvents F18.94
        in
          abuse F18.14
          dependence F18.24
    manic episode F30.9
      with psychotic symptoms F30.2
      without psychotic symptoms
        F30.10
        mild F30.11
        moderate F30.12
        severe F30.13
      in remission (full) F30.4
        partial F30.3
      specified type NEC F30.8
    organic F06.30
      right hemisphere F07.89
    persistent F34.9
      cyclothymia F34.0
      dysthymia F34.1
      specified type NEC F34.8
    recurrent F39
    right hemisphere organic F07.89

Disorder *(Continued)*
  movement G25.9
    drug-induced G25.70
      akathisia G25.71
      specified NEC G25.79
    hysterical F44.4
    periodic limb G47.61
      sleep related G47.61
    sleep related NEC G47.69
    specified NEC G25.89
    stereotyped F98.4
    treatment-induced G25.9
  multiple personality F44.81
  muscle M62.9
    attachment, spine —*see* Enthesopathy,
      spinal
    in trichinellosis —*see* Trichinellosis,
      with muscle disorder
    psychogenic F45.8
    specified type NEC M62.89
    tone, newborn P94.9
      specified NEC P94.8
  muscular
    attachments —*see also* Enthesopathy
      spine —*see* Enthesopathy, spinal
    urethra N36.44
  musculoskeletal system, soft tissue —
    see Disorder, soft tissue
    postprocedural M96.89
    psychogenic F45.8
  myoneural G70.9
    due to lead G70.1
    specified NEC G70.89
    toxic G70.1
  myotonic NEC G71.19
  nail, in diseases classified elsewhere L62
  neck region NEC —*see* Dorsopathy,
    specified NEC
  nerve G58.9
    abducent NEC —*see* Strabismus,
      paralytic, sixth nerve
    accessory G52.8
    acoustic —*see* subcategory H93.3
    auditory —*see* subcategory H93.3
    auriculotemporal G50.8
    axillary G54.0
    cerebral —*see* Disorder, nerve, cranial
    cranial G52.9
      eighth —*see* subcategory H93.3
      eleventh G52.8
      fifth G50.9
      first G52.0
      fourth NEC —*see* Strabismus,
        paralytic, fourth nerve
      multiple G52.7
      ninth G52.1
      second NEC —*see* Disorder, nerve,
        optic
      seventh NEC G51.8
      sixth NEC —*see* Strabismus,
        paralytic, sixth nerve
      specified NEC G52.8
      tenth G52.2
      third NEC —*see* Strabismus,
        paralytic, third nerve
      twelfth G52.3
    entrapment —*see* Neuropathy,
      entrapment
    facial G51.9
      specified NEC G51.8
    femoral —*see* Lesion, nerve, femoral
    glossopharyngeal NEC G52.1
    hypoglossal G52.3
    intercostal G58.0

Disorder *(Continued)*
 nerve *(Continued)*
  lateral
   cutaneous of thigh —*see*
     Mononeuropathy, lower limb,
     meralgia paresthetica
   popliteal —*see* Lesion, nerve,
     popliteal
  lower limb —*see* Mononeuropathy,
    lower limb
  medial popliteal —*see* Lesion, nerve,
    popliteal, medial
  median NEC —*see* Lesion, nerve,
    median
  multiple G58.7
  oculomotor NEC —*see* Strabismus,
    paralytic, third nerve
  olfactory G52.0
  optic NEC H47.09-
   hemorrhage into sheath —*see*
     Hemorrhage, optic nerve
   ischemic H47.01-
  peroneal —*see* Lesion, nerve,
    popliteal
  phrenic G58.8
  plantar —*see* Lesion, nerve, plantar
  pneumogastric G52.2
  posterior tibial —*see* Syndrome, tarsal
    tunnel
  radial —*see* Lesion, nerve, radial
  recurrent laryngeal G52.2
  root G54.9
   cervical G54.2
   lumbosacral G54.1
   specified NEC G54.8
   thoracic G54.3
  sciatic NEC —*see* Lesion, nerve,
    sciatic
  specified NEC G58.8
   lower limb —*see* Mononeuropathy,
     lower limb, specified NEC
   upper limb —*see* Mononeuropathy,
     upper limb, specified NEC
  sympathetic G90.9
  tibial —*see* Lesion, nerve, popliteal,
    medial
  trigeminal G50.9
   specified NEC G50.8
  trochlear NEC —*see* Strabismus,
    paralytic, fourth nerve
  ulnar —*see* Lesion, nerve, ulnar
  upper limb —*see* Mononeuropathy,
    upper limb
  vagus G52.2
 nervous system G98.8
  autonomic (peripheral) G90.9
   specified NEC G90.8
  central G96.9
   specified NEC G96.8
  parasympathetic G90.9
  specified NEC G98.8
  sympathetic G90.9
  vegetative G90.9
 neurohypophysis NEC E23.3
 neurological NEC R29.818
 neuromuscular G70.9
  hereditary NEC G71.9
  specified NEC G70.89
  toxic G70.1
 neurotic F48.9
  specified NEC F48.8
 neutrophil, polymorphonuclear D71
 nicotine use —*see* Dependence, drug,
   nicotine

Disorder *(Continued)*
 nightmare F51.5
 nose J34.9
  specified NEC J34.89
 obsessive-compulsive F42
 odontogenesis NOS K00.9
 oesophagus —*see* Disorder, esophagus
 opioid use
  due to drug abuse —*see* Abuse, drug,
    opioid
  due to drug dependence —*see*
    Dependence, drug, opioid
 oppositional defiant F91.3
 optic
  chiasm H47.49
   due to
    inflammatory disorder H47.41
    neoplasm H47.42
    vascular disorder H47.43
  disc H47.39-
   coloboma —*see* Coloboma, optic
     disc
   drusen —*see* Drusen, optic disc
   pseudopapilledema —*see*
     Pseudopapilledema
  radiations —*see* Disorder, visual,
    pathway
  tracts —*see* Disorder, visual, pathway
 orbit H05.9
  cyst —*see* Cyst, orbit
  deformity —*see* Deformity, orbit
  edema —*see* Edema, orbit
  enophthalmos —*see* Enophthalmos
  exophthalmos —*see* Exophthalmos
  hemorrhage —*see* Hemorrhage, orbit
  inflammation —*see* Inflammation,
    orbit
  myopathy —*see* Myopathy,
    extraocular muscles
  retained foreign body —*see* Foreign
    body, orbit, old
  specified type NEC H05.89
 organic
  anxiety F06.4
  catatonic F06.1
  delusional F06.2
  dissociative F06.8
  emotionally labile (asthenic) F06.8
  mood (affective) F06.30
  schizophrenia-like F06.2
 orgasmic (female) F52.31
  male F52.32
 ornithine metabolism E72.4
 overanxious F41.1
  of childhood F93.8
 pain
  with related psychological factors
    F45.42
  exclusively related to psychological
    factors F45.41
 pancreatic internal secretion E16.9
  specified NEC E16.8
 panic F41.0
  with agoraphobia F40.01
 papulosquamous L44.9
  in diseases classified elsewhere L45
  specified NEC L44.8
 paranoid F22
  induced F24
  shared F24
 parathyroid (gland) E21.5
  specified NEC E21.4
 parietoalveolar NEC J84.09
 paroxysmal, mixed R56.9

Disorder *(Continued)*
 patella M22.9-
  chondromalacia —*see*
    Chondromalacia, patella
  derangement NEC M22.3X-
  recurrent
   dislocation —*see* Dislocation,
     patella, recurrent
   subluxation —*see* Dislocation,
     patella, recurrent, incomplete
  specified NEC M22.8X-
 patellofemoral M22.2X-
 pentose phosphate pathway with
   anemia D55.1
 perception, due to hallucinogens
   F16.983
  in
   abuse F16.183
   dependence F16.283
 peripheral nervous system NEC G64
 peroxisomal E71.50
  biogenesis
   neonatal adrenoleukodystrophy
     E71.511
   specified disorder NEC E71.518
   Zellweger syndrome E71.510
  rhizomelic chondrodysplasia
    punctata E71.540
  specified form NEC E71.548
   group 1 E71.518
   group 2 E71.53
   group 3 E71.542
  X-linked adrenoleukodystrophy
    E71.529
   adolescent E71.521
   adrenomyeloneuropathy E71.522
   childhood E71.520
   specified form NEC E71.528
  Zellweger-like syndrome E71.541
 persistent
  (somatoform) pain F45.41
  affective (mood) F34.9
 personality *(see also* Personality) F60.9
  affective F34.9
  aggressive F60.3
  amoral F60.2
  anankastic F60.5
  antisocial F60.2
  anxious F60.6
  asocial F60.2
  asthenic F60.7
  avoidant F60.6
  borderline F60.3
  change (secondary) due to general
    medical condition F07.0
  compulsive F60.5
  cyclothymic F34.0
  dependent (passive) F60.7
  depressive F34.1
  dissocial F60.2
  emotional instability F60.3
  expansive paranoid F60.0
  explosive F60.3
  following organic brain damage F07.9
  histrionic F60.4
  hyperthymic F34.0
  hypothymic F34.1
  hysterical F60.4
  immature F60.89
  inadequate F60.7
  labile F60.3
  mixed (nonspecific) F60.89
  moral deficiency F60.2
  narcissistic F60.81

Disorder *(Continued)*
  personality *(Continued)*
    negativistic F60.89
    obsessional F60.5
    obsessive (-compulsive) F60.5
    organic F07.9
    overconscientious F60.5
    paranoid F60.0
    passive (-dependent) F60.7
    passive-aggressive F60.89
    pathological NEC F60.9
    pseudosocial F60.2
    psychopathic F60.2
    schizoid F60.1
    schizotypal F21
    self-defeating F60.7
    specified NEC F60.89
    type A F60.5
    unstable (emotional) F60.3
  pervasive, developmental F84.9
  phobic anxiety, childhood F40.8
  phosphate-losing tubular N25.0
  pigmentation L81.9
    choroid, congenital Q14.3
    diminished melanin formation L81.6
    iron L81.8
    specified NEC L81.8
  pinna (noninfective) H61.10-
    deformity, acquired H61.11-
    hematoma H61.12-
    perichondritis —*see* Perichondritis, ear
    specified type NEC H61.19-
  pituitary gland E23.7
    iatrogenic (postprocedural) E89.3
    specified NEC E23.6
  platelets D69.1
  plexus G54.9
    specified NEC G54.8
  polymorphonuclear neutrophils D71
  porphyrin metabolism —*see* Porphyria
  postconcussional F07.81
  posthallucinogen perception F16.983
    in
      abuse F16.183
      dependence F16.283
  postmenopausal N95.9
    specified NEC N95.8
  postprocedural (postoperative) —*see* Complications, postprocedural
  post-transplant lymphoproliferative D47.z1
  post-traumatic stress (PTSD) F43.10
    acute F43.11
    chronic F43.12
  premenstrual dysphoric (PMDD) N94.3
  prepuce N47.8
  propionic acidemia E71.121
  prostate N42.9
    specified NEC N42.89
  psychogenic NOS *(see also* condition) F45.9
    anxiety F41.8
    appetite F50.9
    asthenic F48.8
    cardiovascular (system) F45.8
    compulsive F42
    cutaneous F54
    depressive F32.9
    digestive (system) F45.8
    dysmenorrheic F45.8
    dyspneic F45.8
    endocrine (system) F54
    eye NEC F45.8
    feeding —*see* Disorder, eating

Disorder *(Continued)*
  psychogenic NOS *(Continued)*
    functional NEC F45.8
    gastric F45.8
    gastrointestinal (system) F45.8
    genitourinary (system) F45.8
    heart (function) (rhythm) F45.8
    hyperventilatory F45.8
    hypochondriacal —*see* Disorder, hypochondriacal
    intestinal F45.8
    joint F45.8
    learning F81.9
    limb F45.8
    lymphatic (system) F45.8
    menstrual F45.8
    micturition F45.8
    monoplegic NEC F44.4
    motor F44.4
    muscle F45.8
    musculoskeletal F45.8
    neurocirculatory F45.8
    obsessive F42
    occupational F48.8
    organ or part of body NEC F45.8
    paralytic NEC F44.4
    phobic F40.9
    physical NEC F45.8
    rectal F45.8
    respiratory (system) F45.8
    rheumatic F45.8
    sexual (function) F52.9
    skin (allergic) (eczematous) F54
    sleep F51.9
    specified part of body NEC F45.8
    stomach F45.8
  psychological F99
    associated with
      disease classified elsewhere F54
      sexual
        development F66
        relationship F66
      uncertainty about gender identity F66
  psychomotor NEC F44.4
    hysterical F44.4
  psychoneurotic —*see also* Neurosis
    mixed NEC F48.8
  psychophysiologic —*see* Disorder, somatoform
  psychosexual F65.9
    development F66
    identity of childhood F64.2
  psychosomatic NOS —*see* Disorder, somatoform
    multiple F45.0
    undifferentiated F45.1
  psychotic —*see* Psychosis
    transient (acute) F23
  puberty E30.9
    specified NEC E30.8
  pulmonary (valve) —*see* Endocarditis, pulmonary
  purine metabolism E79.9
  pyrimidine metabolism E79.9
  pyruvate metabolism E74.4
  reactive attachment (childhood) F94.1
  reading R48.0
    developmental (specific) F81.0
  receptive language F80.2
  receptor, hormonal, peripheral *(see also* Syndrome, androgen insensitivity) E34.50
  recurrent brief depressive F33.8

Disorder *(Continued)*
  reflex R29.2
  refraction H52.7
    aniseikonia H52.32
    anisometropia H52.31
    astigmatism —*see* Astigmatism
    hypermetropia —*see* Hypermetropia
    myopia —*see* Myopia
    presbyopia H52.4
    specified NEC H52.6
  relationship F68.8
    due to sexual orientation F66
  REM sleep behavior G47.52
  renal function, impaired (tubular) N25.9
  resonance R49.9
    specified NEC R49.8
  respiratory function, impaired —*see also* Failure, respiration
    postprocedural —*see* Complication, postoperative, respiratory system
    psychogenic F45.8
  retina H35.9
    angioid streaks H35.33
    changes in vascular appearance H35.01-
    degeneration —*see* Degeneration, retina
    dystrophy (hereditary) —*see* Dystrophy, retina
    edema H35.81
    hemorrhage —*see* Hemorrhage, retina
    ischemia H35.82
    macular degeneration —*see* Degeneration, macula
    microaneurysms H35.04-
    microvascular abnormality NEC H35.09
    neovascularization —*see* Neovascularization, retina
    retinopathy —*see* Retinopathy
    separation of layers H35.70
      central serous chorioretinopathy H35.71-
      pigment epithelium detachment (serous) H35.72-
      hemorrhagic H35.73-
    specified type NEC H35.89
    telangiectasis —*see* Telangiectasis, retina
    vasculitis —*see* Vasculitis, retina
  retroperitoneal K68.9
  right hemisphere organic affective F07.89
  rumination (infant or child) F98.21
  sacrum, sacrococcygeal NEC M53.3
  schizoaffective F25.9
    bipolar type F25.0
    depressive type F25.1
    manic type F25.0
    mixed type F25.0
    specified NEC F25.8
  schizoid of childhood F84.5
  schizophreniform F20.81
    brief F23
  schizotypal (personality) F21
  secretion, thyrocalcitonin E07.0
  seizure *(see also* Epilepsy) G40.909
    intractable G40.919
      with status epilepticus G40.911
  semantic pragmatic F80.89
    with autism F84.0
  sense of smell R43.1
    psychogenic F45.8
  separation anxiety, of childhood F93.0

Disorder (Continued)
  stress F43.9
    post-traumatic F43.10
      acute F43.11
      chronic F43.12
  sulfur-bearing amino-acid metabolism
      E72.10
  sweat gland (eccrine) L74.9
    apocrine L75.9
      specified NEC L75.8
    specified NEC L74.8
  synovium M67.90
    acromioclavicular M67.91-
    ankle M67.97-
    elbow M67.92-
    foot M67.97-
    forearm M67.93-
    hand M67.94-
    hip M67.95-
    knee M67.96-
    multiple sites M67.99
    rupture —see Rupture, synovium
    shoulder M67.91-
    specified type NEC M67.80
      acromioclavicular M67.81-
      ankle M67.87-
      elbow M67.82-
      foot M67.87-
      hand M67.84-
      hip M67.85-
      knee M67.86-
      multiple sites M67.89
      wrist M67.83-
    synovitis —see Synovitis
    upper arm M67.92-
    wrist M67.93-
  temperature regulation, newborn P81.9
    specified NEC P81.8
  temporomandibular joint —see
      Anomaly, dentofacial,
      temporomandibular joint
  tendon M67.90
    acromioclavicular M67.91-
    ankle M67.97-
    contracture —see Contracture,
      tendon
    elbow M67.92-
    foot M67.97-
    forearm M67.93-
    hand M67.94-
    hip M67.95-
    knee M67.96-
    multiple sites M67.99
    rupture —see Rupture, tendon
    shoulder M67.91-
    specified type NEC M67.80
      acromioclavicular M67.81-
      ankle M67.87-
      elbow M67.82-
      foot M67.87-
      hand M67.84-
      hip M67.85-
      knee M67.86-
      multiple sites M67.89
      trunk M67.88
      wrist M67.83-
    synovitis —see Synovitis
    tendinitis —see Tendinitis
    tenosynovitis —see Tenosynovitis
    trunk M67.98
    upper arm M67.92-
    wrist M67.93-
  thoracic root (nerve) NEC G54.3
  thyrocalcitonin hypersecretion E07.0

Disorder (Continued)
  thyroid (gland) E07.9
    function NEC, neonatal, transitory
      P72.2
    iodine-deficiency related E01.8
    specified NEC E07.89
  tic —see Tic
  tooth K08.9
    development K00.9
      specified NEC K00.8
    eruption K00.6
  Tourette's F95.2
  trance and possession F44.89
  tricuspid (valve) —see Endocarditis,
      tricuspid
  tryptophan metabolism E70.5
  tubular, phosphate-losing N25.0
  tubulo-interstitial (in)
    brucellosis A23.9 [N16]
    cystinosis E72.04
    diphtheria A36.84
    glycogen storage disease E74.00 [N16]
    leukemia NEC C95.9- [N16]
    lymphoma NEC C85.9- [N16]
    mixed cryoglobulinemia D89.1
      [N16]
    multiple myeloma C90.0- [N16]
    Salmonella infection A02.25
    sarcoidosis D86.84
    sepsis A41.9 [N16]
      streptococcal A40.9 [N16]
    systemic lupus erythematosus
      M32.15
    toxoplasmosis B58.83
    transplant rejection T86.91 [N16]
    Wilson's disease E83.01 [N16]
  tubulo-renal function, impaired N25.9
    specified NEC N25.89
  tympanic membrane H73.9-
    atrophy —see Atrophy, tympanic
      membrane
    infection —see Myringitis
    perforation —see Perforation,
      tympanum
    specified NEC H73.89-
  unsocialized aggressive F91.1
  urea cycle metabolism E72.20
    argininemia E72.21
    arginosuccinic aciduria E72.22
    citrullinemia E72.23
    ornithine transcarbamylase
      deficiency E72.4
    other specified E72.29
  ureter (in) N28.9
    schistosomiasis B65.0 [N29]
    tuberculosis A18.11
  urethra N36.9
    specified NEC N36.8
  urinary system N39.9
    specified NEC N39.8
  valve, heart
    aortic —see Endocarditis, aortic
    mitral —see Endocarditis, mitral
    pulmonary —see Endocarditis,
      pulmonary
    rheumatic
      aortic —see Endocarditis, aortic,
        rheumatic
      mitral —see Endocarditis, mitral
      pulmonary —see Endocarditis,
        pulmonary, rheumatic
      tricuspid —see Endocarditis,
        tricuspid
    tricuspid —see Endocarditis, tricuspid

Disorder (Continued)
  vestibular function H81.9-
    specified NEC —see subcategory
      H81.8
    in diseases classified elsewhere
      H82.-
  vertigo —see Vertigo
  vision, binocular H53.30
    abnormal retinal correspondence
      H53.31
    diplopia H53.2
    fusion with defective stereopsis H53.32
    simultaneous perception H53.33
    suppression H53.34
  visual
    cortex
      blindness H47.619
        left brain H47.612
        right brain H47.611
      due to
        inflammatory disorder H47.629
          left brain H47.622
          right brain H47.621
        neoplasm H47.639
          left brain H47.632
          right brain H47.631
        vascular disorder H47.649
          left brain H47.642
          right brain H47.641
    pathway H47.9
      due to
        inflammatory disorder H47.51-
        neoplasm H47.52-
        vascular disorder H47.53-
      optic chiasm —see Disorder, optic,
        chiasm
  vitreous body H43.9
    crystalline deposits —see Deposit,
      crystalline
    degeneration —see Degeneration,
      vitreous
    hemorrhage —see Hemorrhage,
      vitreous
    opacities —see Opacity, vitreous
    prolapse —see Prolapse, vitreous
    specified type NEC H43.89
  voice R49.9
    specified type NEC R49.8
  volatile solvent use
    due to drug abuse —see Abuse, drug,
      inhalant
    due to drug dependence —see
      Dependence, drug, inhalant
  white blood cells D72.9
    specified NEC D72.89
  withdrawing, child or adolescent F40.10
Disorientation R41.0
Displacement, displaced
  acquired traumatic of bone, cartilage,
      joint, tendon NEC —see
      Dislocation
  adrenal gland (congenital) Q89.1
  appendix, retrocecal (congenital) Q43.8
  auricle (congenital) Q17.4
  bladder (acquired) N32.89
    congenital Q64.19
  brachial plexus (congenital) Q07.8
  brain stem, caudal (congenital) Q04.8
  canaliculus (lacrimalis), congenital
      Q10.6
  cardia through esophageal hiatus
      (congenital) Q40.1
  cerebellum, caudal (congenital) Q04.8
  cervix —see Malposition, uterus

Displacement, displaced (Continued)
colon (congenital) Q43.3
device, implant or graft (see also
    Complications, by site and type,
    mechanical) T85.628
    arterial graft NEC —see
        Complication, cardiovascular
        device, mechanical, vascular
    breast (implant) T85.42
    catheter NEC T85.628
        dialysis (renal) T82.42
            intraperitoneal T85.621
        infusion NEC T82.524
            spinal (epidural) (subdural)
                T85.620
        urinary (indwelling) T83.028
            cystostomy T83.020
    electronic (electrode) (pulse
        generator) (stimulator) —see
        Complication, electronic
        stimulator
    fixation, internal (orthopedic) NEC —
        see Complication, fixation
        device, mechanical
    gastrointestinal —see Complications,
        prosthetic device, mechanical,
        gastrointestinal device
    genital NEC T83.428
        intrauterine contraceptive device
            T83.32
        penile prosthesis T83.420
    heart NEC —see Complication,
        cardiovascular device,
        mechanical
    joint prosthesis —see Complications,
        joint prosthesis, mechanical
    ocular —see Complications, prosthetic
        device, mechanical, ocular
        device
    orthopedic NEC —see Complication,
        orthopedic, device or graft,
        mechanical
    specified NEC T85.628
    urinary NEC —see also Complication,
        genitourinary, device, urinary,
        mechanical
        graft T83.22
    vascular NEC —see Complication,
        cardiovascular device,
        mechanical
    ventricular intracranial shunt
        T85.02
electronic stimulator
    bone T84.320
    cardiac —see Complications, cardiac
        device, electronic
    nervous system —see Complication,
        prosthetic device, mechanical,
        electronic nervous system
        stimulator
    urinary —see Complications,
        electronic stimulator, urinary
esophageal mucosa into cardia of
    stomach, congenital Q39.8
esophagus (acquired) K22.8
    congenital Q39.8
eyeball (acquired) (lateral) (old) —see
    Displacement, globe
    congenital Q15.8
    current —see Avulsion, eye
fallopian tube (acquired) N83.4
    congenital Q50.6
    opening (congenital) Q50.6
gallbladder (congenital) Q44.1

Displacement, displaced (Continued)
gastric mucosa (congenital) Q40.2
globe (acquired) (old) (lateral) H05.21-
    current —see Avulsion, eye
heart (congenital) Q24.8
    acquired I51.89
hymen (upward) (congenital) Q52.4
intervertebral disc NEC
    with myelopathy —see Disorder, disc,
        with, myelopathy
    cervical, cervicothoracic (with)
        M50.20
        myelopathy —see Disorder, disc,
            cervical, with myelopathy
        neuritis, radiculitis or
            radiculopathy —see Disorder,
            disc, cervical, with neuritis
    due to trauma —see Dislocation,
        vertebra
    lumbar region M51.26
        with
            myelopathy M51.06
            neuritis, radiculitis, radiculopathy
                or sciatica M51.16
    lumbosacral region M51.27
        with
            myelopathy M51.07
            neuritis, radiculitis, radiculopathy
                or sciatica M51.17
    sacrococcygeal region M53.3
    thoracic region M51.24
        with
            myelopathy M51.04
            neuritis, radiculitis,
                radiculopathy M51.14
    thoracolumbar region M51.25
        with
            myelopathy M51.05
            neuritis, radiculitis,
                radiculopathy M51.15
intrauterine device T83.32
kidney (acquired) N28.83
    congenital Q63.2
lachrymal, lacrimal apparatus or duct
    (congenital) Q10.6
lens, congenital Q12.1
macula (congenital) Q14.1
Meckel's diverticulum Q43.0
    malignant —see Table of Neoplasms,
        small intestine, malignant
nail (congenital) Q84.6
    acquired L60.8
oesophagus (acquired) —see
    Displacement, esophagus
opening of Wharton's duct in mouth
    Q38.4
organ or site, congenital NEC —see
    Malposition, congenital
ovary (acquired) N83.4
    congenital Q50.39
    free in peritoneal cavity (congenital)
        Q50.39
    into hernial sac N83.4
oviduct (acquired) N83.4
    congenital Q50.6
parathyroid (gland) E21.4
parotid gland (congenital) Q38.4
punctum lacrimale (congenital) Q10.6
sacro-iliac (joint) (congenital) Q74.2
    current injury S33.2
    old —see subcategory M53.2
salivary gland (any) (congenital) Q38.4
spleen (congenital) Q89.09
stomach, congenital Q40.2

Displacement, displaced (Continued)
sublingual duct Q38.4
tongue (downward) (congenital)
    Q38.3
tooth, teeth, fully erupted M26.30
    horizontal M26.33
    vertical M26.34
trachea (congenital) Q32.1
ureter or ureteric opening or orifice
    (congenital) Q62.62
uterine opening of oviducts or fallopian
    tubes Q50.6
uterus, uterine —see Malposition,
    uterus
ventricular septum Q21.0
    with rudimentary ventricle Q20.4
Disproportion
between native and reconstructed
    breast N65.1
fiber-type G71.2
Disruptio uteri —see Rupture, uterus
Disruption (of)
ciliary body NEC H21.89
closure of
    cornea T81.31
    craniotomy T81.32
    fascia (muscular) (superficial)
        T81.32
    internal organ or tissue T81.32
    laceration (external) (internal)
        T81.33
    ligament T81.32
    mucosa T81.31
    muscle or muscle flap T81.32
    ribs or rib cage T81.32
    skin and subcutaneous tissue (full-
        thickness) (superficial) T81.31
    skull T81.32
    sternum (sternotomy) T81.32
    tendon T81.32
    traumatic laceration (external)
        (internal) T81.33
family Z63.8
    due to
        absence of family member due to
            military deployment Z63.31
        absence of family member NEC
            Z63.32
        alcoholism and drug addiction in
            family Z63.72
        bereavement Z63.4
        death (assumed) or disappearance
            of family member Z63.4
        divorce or separation Z63.5
        drug addiction in family Z63.72
        return of family member from
            military deployment (current
            or past conflict) Z63.71
        stressful life events NEC Z63.79
iris NEC H21.89
ligament (s) —see also Sprain
    knee
        current injury —see Dislocation,
            knee
        old (chronic) —see Derangement,
            knee, instability
        spontaneous NEC —see
            Derangement, knee,
            disruption ligament
ossicular chain —see Discontinuity,
    ossicles, ear
pelvic ring (stable) S32.810
    unstable S32.811
traumatic injury wound repair T81.33

Disruption *(Continued)*
  wound T81.30
    episiotomy O90.1
    operation T81.31
      cesarean O90.0
      external operation wound
        (superficial) T81.31
      internal operation wound (deep)
        T81.32
    perineal (obstetric) O90.1
  traumatic injury repair T81.33
Dissatisfaction with
  employment Z56.9
  school environment Z55.4
Dissecting —*see* condition
Dissection
  aorta I71.00
    abdominal I71.02
    thoracic I71.01
    thoracoabdominal I71.03
  artery
    carotid I77.71
    cerebral (nonruptured) I67.0
      ruptured —*see* Hemorrhage,
        intracranial, subarachnoid
    coronary I25.42
    iliac I77.72
    renal I77.73
    specified NEC I77.79
    vertebral I77.74
  traumatic —*see* Wound, open, by site
  vascular I99.8
  wound —*see* Wound, open
Disseminated —*see* condition
Dissociation
  auriculoventricular or atrioventricular
    (AV) (any degree) (isorhythmic)
    I45.89
    with heart block I44.2
  interference I45.89
Dissociative reaction, state F44.9
Dissolution, vertebra —*see* Osteoporosis
Distension, distention
  abdomen R14.0
  bladder N32.89
  cecum K63.89
  colon K63.89
  gallbladder K82.8
  intestine K63.89
  kidney N28.89
  liver K76.89
  seminal vesicle N50.8
  stomach K31.89
    acute K31.0
    psychogenic F45.8
  ureter —*see* Dilatation, ureter
  uterus N85.8
Distoma hepaticum infestation B66.3
Distomiasis B66.9
  bile passages B66.3
  hemic B65.9
  hepatic B66.3
    due to Clonorchis sinensis B66.1
  intestinal B66.5
  liver B66.3
    due to Clonorchis sinensis B66.1
  lung B66.4
  pulmonary B66.4
Distomolar (fourth molar) K00.1
Disto-occlusion (Division I) (Division II)
  M26.212
Distortion (s) (congenital)
  adrenal (gland) Q89.1
  arm NEC Q68.8

Distortion (s) *(Continued)*
  bile duct or passage Q44.5
  bladder Q64.79
  brain Q04.9
  cervix (uteri) Q51.9
  chest (wall) Q67.8
    bones Q76.8
  clavicle Q74.0
  clitoris Q52.6
  coccyx Q76.49
  common duct Q44.5
  coronary Q24.5
  cystic duct Q44.5
  ear (auricle) (external) Q17.3
    inner Q16.5
    middle Q16.4
      ossicles Q16.3
  endocrine NEC Q89.2
  eustachian tube Q17.8
  eye (adnexa) Q15.8
  face bone (s) NEC Q75.8
  fallopian tube Q50.6
  femur NEC Q68.8
  fibula NEC Q68.8
  finger (s) Q68.1
  foot Q66.9
  genitalia, genital organ (s)
    female Q52.8
      external Q52.79
      internal NEC Q52.8
  gyri Q04.8
  hand bone (s) Q68.1
  heart (auricle) (ventricle) Q24.8
    valve (cusp) Q24.8
  hepatic duct Q44.5
  humerus NEC Q68.8
  hymen Q52.4
  intrafamilial communications
    Z63.8
  jaw NEC M26.89
  labium (majus) (minus) Q52.79
  leg NEC Q68.8
  lens Q12.8
  liver Q44.7
  lumbar spine Q76.49
    with disproportion O33.8
      causing obstructed labor O65.0
  lumbosacral (joint) (region) Q76.49
    kyphosis —*see* Kyphosis, congenital
    lordosis —*see* Lordosis, congenital
  nerve Q07.8
  nose Q30.8
  organ
    of Corti Q16.5
    or site not listed —*see* Anomaly, by
      site ossicles, ear Q16.3
  oviduct Q50.6
  pancreas Q45.3
  parathyroid (gland) Q89.2
  pituitary (gland) Q89.2
  radius NEC Q68.8
  sacroiliac joint Q74.2
  sacrum Q76.49
  scapula Q74.0
  shoulder girdle Q74.0
  skull bone (s) NEC Q75.8
    with
      anencephalus Q00.0
      encephalocele —*see* Encephalocele
      hydrocephalus Q03.9
        with spina bifida —*see* Spina
          bifida, with hydrocephalus
      microcephaly Q02
  spinal cord Q06.8

Distortion (s) *(Continued)*
  spine Q76.49
    kyphosis —*see* Kyphosis, congenital
    lordosis —*see* Lordosis, congenital
  spleen Q89.09
  sternum NEC Q76.7
  thorax (wall) Q67.8
    bony Q76.8
  thymus (gland) Q89.2
  thyroid (gland) Q89.2
  tibia NEC Q68.8
  toe (s) Q66.9
  tongue Q38.3
  trachea (cartilage) Q32.1
  ulna NEC Q68.8
  ureter Q62.8
  urethra Q64.79
    causing obstruction Q64.39
  uterus Q51.9
  vagina Q52.4
  vertebra Q76.49
    kyphosis —*see* Kyphosis, congenital
    lordosis —*see* Lordosis, congenital
  visual —*see also* Disturbance, vision
    shape and size H53.15
  vulva Q52.79
  wrist (bones) (joint) Q68.8
Distress
  abdomen —*see* Pain, abdominal
  acute respiratory (adult) (child) J80
  epigastric R10.13
  fetal P84
    complicating pregnancy —*see* Stress,
      fetal
  gastrointestinal (functional) K30
    psychogenic F45.8
  intestinal (functional) NOS K59.9
    psychogenic F45.8
  maternal, during labor and delivery
    O75.0
  respiratory R06.00
    adult J80
    child J80
    newborn P22.9
      specified NEC P22.8
    orthopnea R06.01
    psychogenic F45.8
    shortness of breath R06.02
    specified type NEC R06.09
Distribution vessel, atypical Q27.9
  coronary artery Q24.5
  precerebral Q28.1
Districhiasis L68.8
Disturbance (s) —*see also* Disease
  absorption K90.9
    calcium E58
    carbohydrate K90.4
    fat K90.4
      pancreatic K90.3
    protein K90.4
    starch K90.4
    vitamin —*see* Deficiency, vitamin
  acid-base equilibrium E87.8
    mixed E87.4
  activity and attention (with
    hyperkinesis) —*see* Disorder,
    attention-deficit hyperactivity
  amino acid transport E72.00
  assimilation, food K90.9
  auditory nerve, except deafness —*see*
    subcategory H93.3
  behavior —*see* Disorder, conduct
  blood clotting (mechanism) (*see also*
    Defect, coagulation) D68.9

Disturbance (s) (Continued)
cerebral
  nerve —see Disorder, nerve, cranial
  status, newborn P91.9
    specified NEC P91.8
circulatory I99.9
conduct (see also Disorder, conduct)
    F91.9
  adjustment reaction —see Disorder,
    adjustment
  compulsive F63.9
  disruptive F91.9
  hyperkinetic —see Disorder,
    attention-deficit hyperactivity
  socialized F91.2
  specified NEC F91.8
  unsocialized F91.1
coordination R27.8
cranial nerve —see Disorder, nerve,
    cranial
deep sensibility —see Disturbance,
    sensation
digestive K30
  psychogenic F45.8
electrolyte —see also Imbalance,
    electrolyte
  newborn, transitory P74.4
    hyperammonemia P74.6
    potassium balance P74.3
    sodium balance P74.2
    specified type NEC P74.4
emotions specific to childhood and
    adolescence F93.9
  with
    anxiety and fearfulness NEC F93.8
    elective mutism F94.0
    oppositional disorder F91.3
    sensitivity (withdrawal) F40.10
    shyness F40.10
    social withdrawal F40.10
  involving relationship problems
    F93.8
  mixed F93.8
  specified NEC F93.8
endocrine (gland) E34.9
  neonatal, transitory P72.9
    specified NEC P72.8
equilibrium R42
fructose metabolism E74.10
gait —see Gait
  hysterical F44.4
  psychogenic F44.4
gastrointestinal (functional) K30
  psychogenic F45.8
habit, child F98.9
hearing, except deafness and tinnitus —
    see Abnormal, auditory perception
heart, functional (conditions in I44-I50)
  due to presence of (cardiac)
    prosthesis I97.19-
  postoperative I97.89
    cardiac surgery I97.19-
hormones E34.9
innervation uterus (parasympathetic)
    (sympathetic) N85.8
keratinization NEC
  gingiva K05.10
    nonplaque induced K05.11
    plaque induced K05.10
  lip K13.0
  oral (mucosa) (soft tissue) K13.29
  tongue K13.29
learning (specific) —see Disorder,
    learning

Disturbance (s) (Continued)
memory —see Amnesia
  mild, following organic brain damage
    F06.8
mental F99
  associated with diseases classified
    elsewhere F54
metabolism E88.9
  with
    abortion —see Abortion, by
      type with other specified
      complication
    ectopic pregnancy O08.5
    molar pregnancy O08.5
  amino-acid E72.9
    aromatic E70.9
    branched-chain E71.2
    straight-chain E72.8
    sulfur-bearing E72.10
  ammonia E72.20
  arginine E72.21
  arginosuccinic acid E72.22
  carbohydrate E74.9
  cholesterol E78.9
  citrulline E72.23
  cystathionine E72.19
  general E88.9
  glutamine E72.8
  histidine E70.40
  homocystine E72.19
  hydroxylysine E72.3
  in labor or delivery O75.89
  iron E83.10
  lipoid E78.9
  lysine E72.3
  methionine E72.19
  neonatal, transitory P74.9
    calcium and magnesium P71.9
      specified type NEC P71.8
    carbohydrate metabolism P70.9
      specified type NEC P70.8
    specified NEC P74.8
  ornithine E72.4
  phosphate E83.39
  sodium NEC E87.8
  threonine E72.8
  tryptophan E70.5
  tyrosine E70.20
  urea cycle E72.20
motor R29.2
nervous, functional R45.0
neuromuscular mechanism (eye), due
    to syphilis A52.15
nutritional E63.9
  nail L60.3
ocular motion H51.9
  psychogenic F45.8
oculogyric H51.8
  psychogenic F45.8
oculomotor H51.9
  psychogenic F45.8
olfactory nerve R43.1
optic nerve NEC —see Disorder, nerve,
    optic
oral epithelium, including tongue NEC
    K13.29
perceptual due to
  alcohol withdrawal F10.232
  amphetamine intoxication
    F15.922
    in
      abuse F15.122
      dependence F15.222
  anxiolytic withdrawal F13.232

Disturbance (s) (Continued)
perceptual due to (Continued)
  cannabis intoxication (acute) F12.922
    in
      abuse F12.122
      dependence F12.222
  cocaine intoxication (acute) F14.922
    in
      abuse F14.122
      dependence F14.222
  hypnotic withdrawal F13.232
  opioid intoxication (acute) F11.922
    in
      abuse F11.122
      dependence F11.222
  phencyclidine intoxication (acute)
    F19.922
    in
      abuse F19.122
      dependence F19.222
  sedative withdrawal F13.232
personality (pattern) (trait) (see also
    Disorder, personality) F60.9
  following organic brain damage
    F07.9
polyglandular E31.9
  specified NEC E31.8
potassium balance, newborn P74.3
psychogenic F45.9
psychomotor F44.4
psychophysical visual H53.16
pupillary —see Anomaly, pupil,
    function
reflex R29.2
rhythm, heart I49.9
salivary secretion K11.7
sensation (cold) (heat) (localization)
    (tactile discrimination) (texture)
    (vibratory) NEC R20.9
  hysterical F44.6
  skin R20.9
    anesthesia R20.0
    hyperesthesia R20.3
    hypoesthesia R20.1
    paresthesia R20.2
    specified type NEC R20.8
  smell R43.9
    and taste (mixed) R43.8
    anosmia R43.0
    parosmia R43.1
    specified NEC R43.8
  taste R43.9
    and smell (mixed) R43.8
    parageusia R43.2
    specified NEC R43.8
sensory —see Disturbance, sensation
situational (transient) —see also
    Disorder, adjustment
  acute F43.0
sleep G47.9
  nonorganic origin F51.9
smell —see Disturbance, sensation, smell
sociopathic F60.2
sodium balance, newborn P74.2
speech R47.9
  developmental F80.9
  specified NEC R47.89
stomach (functional) K31.9
sympathetic (nerve) G90.9
taste —see Disturbance, sensation, taste
temperature
  regulation, newborn P81.9
    specified NEC P81.8
  sense R20.8
    hysterical F44.6

221

Disturbance (s) (*Continued*)
tooth
eruption K00.6
formation K00.4
structure, hereditary NEC K00.5
touch —*see* Disturbance, sensation
vascular I99.9
arteriosclerotic —*see* Arteriosclerosis
vasomotor I73.9
vasospastic I73.9
vision, visual H53.9
following
cerebral infarction I69.398
cerebrovascular disease I69.998
intracerebral hemorrhage
I69.198
nontraumatic intracranial
hemorrhage NEC I69.298
specified disease NEC I69.898
subarachnoid hemorrhage
I69.098
specified NEC I69.898
psychophysical H53.16
specified NEC H53.8
subjective H53.10
day blindness H53.11
discomfort H53.14-
distortions of shape and size
H53.15
loss
sudden H53.13-
transient H53.12-
specified type NEC H53.19
voice R49.9
psychogenic F44.4
specified NEC R49.8
Diuresis R35.8
Diver's palsy, paralysis or squeeze
T70.3
Diverticulitis (acute) K57.92
bladder —*see* Cystitis
ileum —*see* Diverticulitis, intestine,
small
intestine K57.92
with
abscess, perforation or peritonitis
K57.80
with bleeding K57.81
bleeding K57.93
congenital Q43.8
large K57.32
with
abscess, perforation or peritonitis
K57.20
with bleeding K57.21
bleeding K57.33
small intestine K57.52
with
abscess, perforation or
peritonitis K57.40
with bleeding K57.41
bleeding K57.53
small K57.12
with
abscess, perforation or peritonitis
K57.00
with bleeding K57.01
bleeding K57.13
large intestine K57.52
with
abscess, perforation or
peritonitis K57.40
with bleeding K57.41
bleeding K57.53

Diverticulosis K57.90
with bleeding K57.91
large intestine K57.30
with
bleeding K57.31
small intestine K57.50
with bleeding K57.51
small intestine K57.10
with
bleeding K57.11
large intestine K57.50
with bleeding K57.51
Diverticulum, diverticula (multiple)
K57.90
appendix (noninflammatory) K38.2
bladder (sphincter) N32.3
congenital Q64.6
bronchus (congenital) Q32.4
acquired J98.09
calyx, calyceal (kidney) N28.89
cardia (stomach) K31.4
cecum —*see* Diverticulosis, intestine,
large
congenital Q43.8
colon —*see* Diverticulosis, intestine, large
congenital Q43.8
duodenum —*see* Diverticulosis,
intestine, small
congenital Q43.8
epiphrenic (esophagus) K22.5
esophagus (congenital) Q39.6
acquired (epiphrenic) (pulsion)
(traction) K22.5
eustachian tube —*see* Disorder,
eustachian tube, specified NEC
fallopian tube N83.8
gastric K31.4
heart (congenital) Q24.8
ileum —*see* Diverticulosis, intestine,
small
jejunum —*see* Diverticulosis, intestine,
small
kidney (pelvis) (calyces) N28.89
with calculus —*see* Calculus, kidney
Meckel's (displaced) (hypertrophic)
Q43.0
malignant —*see* Table of Neoplasms,
small intestine, malignant
midthoracic K22.5
organ or site, congenital NEC —*see*
Distortion
pericardium (congenital) (cyst) Q24.8
acquired I31.8
pharyngoesophageal (congenital) Q39.6
acquired K22.5
pharynx (congenital) Q38.7
rectosigmoid —*see* Diverticulosis,
intestine, large
congenital Q43.8
rectum —*see* Diverticulosis, intestine,
large
Rokitansky's K22.5
seminal vesicle N50.8
sigmoid —*see* Diverticulosis, intestine,
large
congenital Q43.8
stomach (acquired) K31.4
congenital Q40.2
trachea (acquired) J39.8
ureter (acquired) N28.89
congenital Q62.8
ureterovesical orifice N28.89
urethra (acquired) N36.1
congenital Q64.79

Diverticulum, diverticula (*Continued*)
ventricle, left (congenital) Q24.8
vesical N32.3
congenital Q64.6
Zenker's (esophagus) K22.5
Division
cervix uteri (acquired) N88.8
glans penis Q55.69
labia minora (congenital) Q52.79
ligament (partial or complete)
(current) —*see also* Sprain
with open wound —*see* Wound, open
muscle (partial or complete)
(current) —*see also* Injury, muscle
with open wound —*see* Wound, open
nerve (traumatic) —*see* Injury, nerve
spinal cord —*see* Injury, spinal cord, by
region
vein I87.8
Divorce, causing family disruption
Z63.5
Dix-Hallpike neurolabyrinthitis —*see*
Neuronitis, vestibular
Dizziness R42
hysterical F44.89
psychogenic F45.8
DMAC (disseminated mycobacterium
avium-intracellulare complex)
A31.2
DNR (do not resuscitate) Z66
Doan-Wiseman syndrome (primary
splenic neutropenia) —*see*
Agranulocytosis
Doehle-Heller aortitis A52.02
Dog bite —*see* Bite
Dohle body panmyelopathic syndrome
D72.0
Dolichocephaly Q67.2
Dolichocolon Q43.8
Dolichostenomelia —*see* Syndrome,
Marfan's
Donohue's syndrome E34.8
Donor (organ or tissue) Z52.9
blood (whole) Z52.000
autologous Z52.010
specified component (lymphocytes)
(platelets) NEC Z52.008
autologous Z52.018
specified donor NEC Z52.098
specified donor NEC Z52.090
stem cells Z52.001
autologous Z52.011
specified donor NEC Z52.091
bone Z52.20
autologous Z52.21
marrow Z52.3
specified type NEC Z52.29
cornea Z52.5
egg (Oocyte) Z52.819
age 35 and over Z52.812
anonymous recipient Z52.812
designated recipient Z52.813
under age 35 Z52.810
anonymous recipient Z52.810
designated recipient Z52.811
kidney Z52.4
liver Z52.6
lung Z52.89
lymphocyte —*see* Donor, blood,
specified components NEC
Oocyte —*see* Donor, egg
platelets Z52.008
potential, examination of Z00.5
semen Z52.89

Donor *(Continued)*
skin Z52.10
autologous Z52.11
specified type NEC Z52.19
specified organ or tissue NEC Z52.89
sperm Z52.89
Donovanosis A58
Dorsalgia M54.9
psychogenic F45.41
specified NEC M54.89
Dorsopathy M53.9
deforming M43.9
specified NEC —*see* subcategory
M43.8
specified NEC M53.80
cervical region M53.82
cervicothoracic region M53.83
lumbar region M53.86
lumbosacral region M53.87
occipito-atlanto-axial region M53.81
sacrococcygeal region M53.88
thoracic region M53.84
thoracolumbar region M53.85
Double
albumin E88.09
aortic arch Q25.4
auditory canal Q17.8
auricle (heart) Q20.8
bladder Q64.79
cervix Q51.820
with doubling of uterus (and vagina)
Q51.10
with obstruction Q51.11
inlet ventricle Q20.4
kidney with double pelvis (renal) Q63.0
meatus urinarius Q64.75
monster Q89.4
outlet
left ventricle Q20.2
right ventricle Q20.1
pelvis (renal) with double ureter Q62.5
tongue Q38.3
ureter (one or both sides) Q62.5
with double pelvis (renal) Q62.5
urethra Q64.74
urinary meatus Q64.75
uterus Q51.2
with
doubling of cervix (and vagina)
Q51.10
with obstruction Q51.11
in pregnancy or childbirth O34.59-
causing obstructed labor O65.5
vagina Q52.10
with doubling of uterus (and cervix)
Q51.10
with obstruction Q51.11
vision H53.2
vulva Q52.79
Douglas' pouch, cul-de-sac —*see*
condition
Down syndrome Q90.9
meiotic nondisjunction Q90.0
mitotic nondisjunction Q90.1
mosaicism Q90.1
translocation Q90.2
**DPD (dihydropyrimidine dehydrogenase
deficiency)** E88.89
Dracontiasis B72
Dracunculiasis, dracunculosis B72
Dream state, hysterical F44.89
Drepanocytic anemia —*see* Disease,
sickle-cell
Dresbach's syndrome (elliptocytosis) D58.1

Dreschlera (hawaiiensis) (infection) B43.8
Dressler's syndrome I24.1
Drift, ulnar —*see* Deformity, limb,
specified type NEC, forearm
Drinking (alcohol)
excessive, to excess NEC (without
dependence) F10.10
habitual (continual) (without
remission) F10.20
with remission F10.21
Drip, postnasal (chronic) R09.82
due to
allergic rhinitis —*see* Rhinitis, allergic
common cold J00
gastroesophageal reflux —*see* Reflux,
gastroesophageal
nasopharyngitis —*see*
Nasopharyngitis
other known condition — code to
condition
sinusitis —*see* Sinusitis
Droop
facial R29.810
cerebrovascular disease I69.992
cerebral infarction I69.392
intracerebral hemorrhage I69.192
nontraumatic intracranial
hemorrhage NEC I69.292
specified disease NEC I69.892
subarachnoid hemorrhage I69.092
Drop (in)
attack NEC R55
finger —*see* Deformity, finger
foot —*see* Deformity, limb, foot, drop
hematocrit (precipitous) R71.0
hemoglobin R71.0
toe —*see* Deformity, toe, specified NEC
wrist —*see* Deformity, limb, wrist drop
Dropped heart beats I45.9
Dropsy, dropsical —*see also* Hydrops
abdomen R18.8
brain —*see* Hydrocephalus
cardiac, heart —*see* Failure, heart,
congestive
gangrenous —*see* Gangrene
heart —*see* Failure, heart, congestive
kidney —*see* Nephrosis
lung —*see* Edema, lung
newborn due to isoimmunization P56.0
pericardium —*see* Pericarditis
Drowned, drowning (near) T75.1
Drowsiness R40.0
Drug
abuse counseling and surveillance Z71.51
addiction —*see* Dependence
dependence —*see* Dependence
habit —*see* Dependence
harmful use —*see* Abuse, drug
induced fever R50.2
overdose —*see* Table of drugs and
chemicals, by drug, poisoning
poisoning —*see* Table of drugs and
chemicals, by drug, poisoning
resistant organism infection (*see also*
Resistant, organism, to, drug)
Z16.30
therapy
long term (current) (prophylactic) —
see Therapy, drug long-term
(current) (prophylactic)
short term - omit code
wrong substance given or taken in
error —*see* Table of drugs and
chemicals, by drug, poisoning

Drunkenness (without dependence)
F10.129
acute in alcoholism F10.229
chronic (without remission) F10.20
with remission F10.21
pathological (without dependence)
F10.129
with dependence F10.229
sleep F51.9
Drusen
macula (degenerative) (retina) —*see*
Degeneration, macula, drusen
optic disc H47.32-
Dry, dryness —*see also* condition
larynx J38.7
mouth R68.2
due to dehydration E86.0
nose J34.89
socket (teeth) M27.3
throat J39.2
DSAP L56.5
Duane's syndrome H50.81-
Dubin-Johnson disease or syndrome E80.6
Dubois' disease (thymus gland) A50.59
[E35]
Dubowitz' syndrome Q87.1
Duchenne-Aran muscular atrophy G12.21
Duchenne-Griesinger disease G71.0
Duchenne's
disease or syndrome
motor neuron disease G12.22
muscular dystrophy G71.0
locomotor ataxia (syphilitic) A52.11
paralysis
birth injury P14.0
due to or associated with
motor neuron disease G12.22
muscular dystrophy G71.0
Ducrey's chancre A57
Duct, ductus —*see* condition
**Duhring's disease (dermatitis
herpetiformis)** L13.0
Dullness, cardiac (decreased) (increased)
R01.2
Dumb ague —*see* Malaria
Dumbness —*see* Aphasia
Dumdum fever B55.0
Dumping syndrome (postgastrectomy)
K91.1
Duodenitis (nonspecific) (peptic) K29.80
with bleeding K29.81
Duodenocholangitis —*see* Cholangitis
Duodenum, duodenal —*see* condition
Duplay's bursitis or periarthritis —*see*
Tendinitis, calcific, shoulder
Duplication, duplex —*see also* Accessory
alimentary tract Q45.8
anus Q43.4
appendix (and cecum) Q43.4
biliary duct (any) Q44.5
bladder Q64.79
cecum (and appendix) Q43.4
cervix Q51.820
chromosome NEC
with complex rearrangements NEC
Q92.5
seen only at prometaphase Q92.8
cystic duct Q44.5
digestive organs Q45.8
esophagus Q39.8
frontonasal process Q75.8
intestine (large) (small) Q43.4
kidney Q63.0
liver Q44.7

Duplication, duplex (*Continued*)
oesophagus Q39.8
pancreas Q45.3
penis Q55.69
respiratory organs NEC Q34.8
salivary duct Q38.4
spinal cord (incomplete) Q06.2
stomach Q40.2
Dupré's disease (meningism) R29.1
Dupuytren's contraction or disease M72.0
Durand-Nicolas-Favre disease A55
Durotomy (inadvertent) (incidental) G97.41
Duroziez's disease (congenital mitral
stenosis) Q23.2
Dutton's relapsing fever (West African)
A68.1
Dwarfism E34.3
achondroplastic Q77.4
congenital E34.3
constitutional E34.3
hypochondroplastic Q77.4
hypophyseal E23.0
infantile E34.3
Laron-type E34.3
Lorain (-Levi) type E23.0
metatropic Q77.8
nephrotic-glycosuric (with
hypophosphatemic rickets) E72.09
nutritional E45
pancreatic K86.8
pituitary E23.0
renal N25.0
thanatophoric Q77.1
Dyke-Young anemia (secondary)
(symptomatic) D59.1
Dysacusis —*see* Abnormal, auditory
perception
Dysadrenocortism E27.9
hyperfunction E27.0
Dysarthria R47.1
following
cerebral infarction I69.322
cerebrovascular disease I69.922
specified disease NEC I69.822
intracerebral hemorrhage I69.122
nontraumatic intracranial
hemorrhage NEC I69.222
subarachnoid hemorrhage I69.022
Dysautonomia (familial) G90.1
Dysbarism T70.3
Dysbasia R26.2
angiosclerotica intermittens I73.9
hysterical F44.4
lordotica (progressiva) G24.1
nonorganic origin F44.4
psychogenic F44.4
Dysbetalipoproteinemia (familial) E78.2
Dyscalculia R48.8
developmental F81.2
Dyschezia K59.00
Dyschondroplasia (with hemangiomata)
Q78.4
Dyschromia (skin) L81.9
Dyscollagenosis M35.9
Dyscranio-pygo-phalangy Q87.0
Dyscrasia
blood (with) D75.9
antepartum hemorrhage —*see*
Hemorrhage, antepartum, with
coagulation defect
intrapartum hemorrhage O67.0
newborn P61.9
specified type NEC P61.8
puerperal, postpartum O72.3
polyglandular, pluriglandular E31.9

Dysendocrinism E34.9
Dysentery, dysenteric (catarrhal)
(diarrhea) (epidemic) (hemorrhagic)
(infectious) (sporadic) (tropical)
A09
abscess, liver A06.4
amebic (*see also* Amebiasis) A06.0
with abscess —*see* Abscess, amebic
acute A06.0
chronic A06.1
arthritis (*see also* category M01) A09
bacillary (*see also* category M01)
A03.9
bacillary A03.9
arthritis (*see also* category M01)
A03.9
Boyd A03.2
Flexner A03.1
Schmitz (-Stutzer) A03.0
Shiga (-Kruse) A03.0
Shigella A03.9
boydii A03.2
dysenteriae A03.0
flexneri A03.1
group A A03.0
group B A03.1
group C A03.2
group D A03.3
sonnei A03.3
specified type NEC A03.8
Sonne A03.3
specified type NEC A03.8
balantidial A07.0
Balantidium coli A07.0
Boyd's A03.2
candidal B37.82
Chilomastix A07.8
Chinese A03.9
coccidial A07.3
Dientamoeba (fragilis) A07.8
Embadomonas A07.8
Entamoeba, entambic —*see* Dysentery,
amebic
Flexner-Boyd A03.2
Flexner's A03.1
Giardia lamblia A07.1
Hiss-Russell A03.1
Lamblia A07.1
leishmanial B55.0
malarial —*see* Malaria
metazoal B82.0
monilial B37.82
protozoal A07.9
Salmonella A02.0
schistosomal B65.1
Schmitz (-Stutzer) A03.0
Shiga (-Kruse) A03.0
Shigella NOS —*see* Dysentery,
bacillary
Sonne A03.3
strongyloidiasis B78.0
trichomonal A07.8
viral (*see also* Enteritis, viral) A08.4
Dysequilibrium R42
Dysesthesia R20.8
hysterical F44.6
Dysfibrinogenemia (congenital)
D68.2
Dysfunction
adrenal E27.9
hyperfunction E27.0
autonomic
due to alcohol G31.2
somatoform F45.8

Dysfunction (*Continued*)
bladder N31.9
neurogenic NOS —*see* Dysfunction,
bladder, neuromuscular
neuromuscular NOS N31.9
atonic (motor) (sensory)
N31.2
autonomous N31.2
flaccid N31.2
nonreflex N31.2
reflex N31.1
specified NEC N31.8
uninhibited N31.0
bleeding, uterus N93.8
cerebral G93.89
colon K59.9
psychogenic F45.8
colostomy K94.03
cystic duct K82.8
cystostomy (stoma) —*see*
Complications, cystostomy
ejaculatory N53.19
anejaculatory orgasm N53.13
painful N53.12
premature F52.4
retarded N53.11
endocrine NOS E34.9
endometrium N85.8
enterostomy K94.13
gallbladder K82.8
gastrostomy (stoma) K94.23
gland, glandular NOS E34.9
heart I51.89
hemoglobin D75.89
hepatic K76.89
hypophysis E23.7
hypothalamic NEC E23.3
ileostomy (stoma) K94.13
jejunostomy (stoma) K94.13
kidney —*see* Disease, renal
labyrinthine —*see* subcategory
H83.2
left ventricular, following sudden
emotional stress I51.81
liver K76.89
male —*see* Dysfunction, sexual,
male
orgasmic (female) F52.31
male F52.32
ovary E28.9
specified NEC E28.8
papillary muscle I51.89
parathyroid E21.4
physiological NEC R68.89
psychogenic F59
pineal gland E34.8
pituitary (gland) E23.3
platelets D69.1
polyglandular E31.9
specified NEC E31.8
psychophysiologic F59
psychosexual F52.9
with
dyspareunia F52.6
premature ejaculation F52.4
vaginismus F52.5
pylorus K31.9
rectum K59.9
psychogenic F45.8
reflex (sympathetic) —*see* Syndrome,
pain, complex regional I
segmental —*see* Dysfunction,
somatic
senile R54

Dysfunction *(Continued)*
 sexual (due to) R37
  alcohol F10.981
  amphetamine F15.981
   in
    abuse F15.181
    dependence F15.281
  anxiolytic F13.981
   in
    abuse F13.181
    dependence F13.281
  cocaine F14.981
   in
    abuse F14.181
    dependence F14.281
  excessive sexual drive F52.8
  failure of genital response (male)
    F52.21
   female F52.22
  female N94.9
   aversion F52.1
   dyspareunia N94.1
    psychogenic F52.6
   frigidity F52.22
   nymphomania F52.8
   orgasmic F52.31
   psychogenic F52.9
    aversion F52.1
    dyspareunia F52.6
    frigidity F52.22
    nymphomania F52.8
    orgasmic F52.31
    vaginismus F52.5
   vaginismus N94.2
    psychogenic F52.5
  hypnotic F13.981
   in
    abuse F13.181
    dependence F13.281
  inhibited orgasm (female) F52.31
   male F52.32
  lack
   of sexual enjoyment F52.1
   or loss of sexual desire F52.0
  male N53.9
   anejaculatory orgasm N53.13
   ejaculatory N53.19
    painful N53.12
    premature F52.4
    retarded N53.11
   erectile N52.9
    drug induced N52.2
    due to
     disease classified elsewhere
       N52.1
     drug N52.2
     postoperative (postprocedural)
       N52.39
     following
       prostatectomy N52.34
        radical N52.31
       radical cystectomy
         N52.32
       urethral surgery N52.33
    psychogenic F52.21
    specified cause NEC N52.8
    vasculogenic
     arterial insufficiency N52.01
      with corporo-venous
        occlusive N52.03
     corporo-venous occlusive
       N52.02
      with arterial insufficiency
        N52.03

Dysfunction *(Continued)*
 sexual *(Continued)*
  male *(Continued)*
   impotence —*see* Dysfunction,
      sexual, male, erectile
   psychogenic F52.9
    aversion F52.1
    erectile F52.21
    orgasmic F52.32
    premature ejaculation F52.4
    satyriasis F52.8
    specified type NEC F52.8
   specified type NEC N53.8
  nonorganic F52.9
   specified NEC F52.8
  opioid F11.981
   in
    abuse F11.181
    dependence F11.281
  orgasmic dysfunction (female)
    F52.31
   male F52.32
  premature ejaculation F52.4
  psychoactive substances NEC
    F19.981
   in
    abuse F19.181
    dependence F19.281
  psychogenic F52.9
  sedative F13.981
   in
    abuse F13.181
    dependence F13.281
  sexual aversion F52.1
  vaginismus (nonorganic)
    (psychogenic) F52.5
 sinoatrial node I49.5
 somatic M99.09
  abdomen M99.09
  acromioclavicular M99.07
  cervical region M99.01
  cervicothoracic M99.01
  costochondral M99.08
  costovertebral M99.08
  head region M99.00
  hip M99.05
  lower extremity M99.06
  lumbar region M99.03
  lumbosacral M99.03
  occipitocervical M99.00
  pelvic region M99.05
  pubic M99.05
  rib cage M99.08
  sacral region M99.04
  sacrococcygeal M99.04
  sacroiliac M99.04
  specified NEC M99.09
  sternochondral M99.08
  sternoclavicular M99.07
  thoracic region M99.02
  thoracolumbar M99.02
  upper extremity M99.07
 somatoform autonomic F45.8
 stomach K31.89
  psychogenic F45.8
 suprarenal E27.9
  hyperfunction E27.0
 symbolic R48.9
  specified type NEC R48.8
 temporomandibular (joint) M26.69
  joint-pain syndrome M26.62
 testicular (endocrine) E29.9
  specified NEC E29.8
 thymus E32.9

Dysfunction *(Continued)*
 thyroid E07.9
 ureterostomy (stoma) —*see*
    Complications, stoma, urinary
    tract
 urethrostomy (stoma) —*see*
    Complications, stoma, urinary
    tract
 uterus, complicating delivery O62.9
  hypertonic O62.4
  hypotonic O62.2
   primary O62.0
   secondary O62.1
 ventricular I51.9
  with congestive heart failure I50.9-
  left, reversible, following sudden
    emotional stress I51.81
Dysgenesis
 gonadal (due to chromosomal anomaly)
    Q96.9
  pure Q99.1
 renal Q60.5
  bilateral Q60.4
  unilateral Q60.3
 reticular D72.0
 tidal platelet D69.3
Dysgerminoma
 specified site —*see* Neoplasm,
    malignant, by site
 unspecified site
  female C56.9
  male C62.90
Dysgeusia R43.2
Dysgraphia R27.8
Dyshidrosis, dysidrosis L30.1
Dyskaryotic cervical smear R87.619
Dyskeratosis L85.8
 cervix —*see* Dysplasia, cervix
 congenital Q82.8
 uterus NEC N85.8
Dyskinesia G24.9
 biliary (cystic duct or gallbladder)
    K82.8
 drug induced
  orofacial G24.01
 esophagus K22.4
 hysterical F44.4
 intestinal K59.8
 nonorganic origin F44.4
 orofacial (idiopathic) G24.4
  drug induced G24.01
 psychogenic F44.4
 subacute, drug induced G24.01
 tardive G24.01
  neuroleptic induced G24.01
 trachea J39.8
 tracheobronchial J98.09
Dyslalia (developmental) F80.0
Dyslexia R48.0
 developmental F81.0
Dyslipidemia E78.5
 depressed HDL cholesterol E78.6
 elevated fasting triglycerides E78.1
Dysmaturity —*see also* Light for dates
 pulmonary (newborn) (Wilson-Mikity)
    P27.0
Dysmenorrhea (essential) (exfoliative)
    N94.6
 congestive (syndrome) N94.6
 primary N94.4
 psychogenic F45.8
 secondary N94.5
Dysmetabolic syndrome X E88.81
Dysmetria R27.8

Dystocia O66.9
affecting newborn P03.1
cervical (hypotonic) O62.2
affecting newborn P03.6
primary O62.0
secondary O62.1
contraction ring O62.4
fetal O66.9
abnormality NEC O66.3
conjoined twins O66.3
oversize O66.2
maternal O66.9
positional O64.9
shoulder (girdle) O66.0
causing obstructed labor O66.0
uterine NEC O62.4
Dystonia G24.9
deformans progressiva G24.1
drug induced NEC G24.09
acute G24.02
specified NEC G24.09
familial G24.1
idiopathic G24.1
familial G24.1
nonfamilial G24.2
orofacial G24.4
lenticularis G24.8
musculorum deformans G24.1
neuroleptic induced (acute)
G24.02
orofacial (idiopathic) G24.4
oromandibular G24.4
due to drug G24.01
specified NEC G24.8
torsion (familial) (idiopathic) G24.1
acquired G24.8
genetic G24.1
symptomatic (nonfamilial) G24.2
Dystonic movements R25.8
Dystrophy, dystrophia
adiposogenital E23.6
Becker's type G71.0
cervical sympathetic G90.2

Dystrophy, dystrophia (Continued)
choroid (hereditary) H31.20
central areolar H31.22
choroideremia H31.21
gyrate atrophy H31.23
specified type NEC H31.29
cornea (hereditary) H18.50
endothelial H18.51
epithelial H18.52
granular H18.53
lattice H18.54
macular H18.55
specified type NEC H18.59
Duchenne's type G71.0
due to malnutrition E45
Erb's G71.0
Fuchs' H18.51
Gower's muscular G71.0
hair L67.8
infantile neuraxonal G31.89
Landouzy-Déjérine G71.0
Leyden-Möbius G71.0
muscular G71.0
benign (Becker type) G71.0
congenital (hereditary) (progressive)
(with specific morphological
abnormalities of the muscle
fiber) G71.0
myotonic G71.11
distal G71.0
Duchenne type G71.0
Emery-Dreifuss G71.0
Erb type G71.0
facioscapulohumeral G71.0
Gower's G71.0
hereditary (progressive) G71.0
Landouzy-Déjérine type G71.0
limb-girdle G71.0
myotonic G71.11
progressive (hereditary) G71.0
Charcot-Marie (-Tooth) type G60.0
pseudohypertrophic (infantile) G71.0
severe (Duchenne type) G71.0

Dystrophy, dystrophia (Continued)
myocardium, myocardial —see
Degeneration, myocardial
myotonic, myotonica G71.11
nail L60.3
congenital Q84.6
nutritional E45
ocular G71.0
oculocerebrorenal E72.03
oculopharyngeal G71.0
ovarian N83.8
polyglandular E31.8
reflex (neuromuscular) (sympathetic) —
see Syndrome, pain, complex
regional I
retinal (hereditary) H35.50
in
lipid storage disorders E75.6
[H36]
systemic lipidoses E75.6 [H36]
involving
pigment epithelium H35.54
sensory area H35.53
pigmentary H35.52
vitreoretinal H35.51
Salzmann's nodular —see Degeneration,
cornea, nodular
scapuloperoneal G71.0
skin NEC L98.8
sympathetic (reflex) —see Syndrome,
pain, complex regional I
cervical G90.2
tapetoretinal H35.54
thoracic, asphyxiating Q77.2
unguium L60.3
congenital Q84.6
vitreoretinal H35.51
vulva N90.4
yellow (liver) —see Failure, hepatic
Dysuria R30.0
psychogenic F45.8

E

Eales' disease H35.06-
Ear —*see also* condition
  piercing Z41.3
  tropical B36.8
  wax (impacted) H61.20
    left H61.22
      with right H61.23
    right H61.21
      with left H61.23
Earache —*see* subcategory H92.0
Early satiety R68.81
Eaton-Lambert syndrome—*see*
    Syndrome, Lambert-Eaton
Eberth's disease (typhoid fever) A01.00
Ebola virus disease A98.4
Ebstein's anomaly or syndrome (heart)
    Q22.5
Eccentro-osteochondrodysplasia E76.29
Ecchondroma —*see* Neoplasm, bone,
    benign
Ecchondrosis D48.0
Ecchymosis R58
  conjunctiva —*see* Hemorrhage,
    conjunctiva
  eye (traumatic) —*see* Contusion,
    eyeball
  eyelid (traumatic) —*see* Contusion,
    eyelid
  newborn P54.5
  spontaneous R23.3
  traumatic —*see* Contusion
Echinococciasis —*see* Echinococcus
Echinococcosis —*see* Echinococcus
Echinococcus (infection) B67.90
  granulosus B67.4
    bone B67.2
    liver B67.0
    lung B67.1
    multiple sites B67.32
    specified site NEC B67.39
    thyroid B67.31 [E35]
  liver NOS B67.8
    granulosus B67.0
    multilocularis B67.5
  lung NEC B67.99
    granulosus B67.1
    multilocularis B67.69
  multilocularis B67.7
    liver B67.5
    multiple sites B67.61
    specified site NEC B67.69
  specified site NEC B67.99
    granulosus B67.39
    multilocularis B67.69
  thyroid NEC B67.99
    granulosus B67.31 [E35]
    multilocularis B67.69 [E35]
Echinorhynchiasis B83.8
Echinostomiasis B66.8
Echolalia R48.8
Echovirus, as cause of disease classified
    elsewhere B97.12
Eclampsia, eclamptic (coma)
    (convulsions) (delirium) (with
    hypertension) NEC O15.9
  during labor and delivery O15.1
  postpartum O15.2
  pregnancy O15.0-
  puerperal O15.2
Economic circumstances affecting care
    Z59.9
Economo's disease A85.8

Ectasia, ectasis
  annuloaortic I35.8
  aorta I77.819
    with aneurysm —*see* Aneurysm, aorta
    abdominal I77.811
    thoracic I77.810
    thoracoabdominal I77.812
  breast —*see* Ectasia, mammary duct
  capillary I78.8
  cornea H18.71-
  gastric antral vascular (GAVE) K31.819
    with hemorrhage K31.811
    without hemorrhage K31.819
  mammary duct N60.4-
  salivary gland (duct) K11.8
  sclera —*see* Sclerectasia
Ecthyma L08.0
  contagiosum B08.02
  gangrenosum L08.0
  infectiosum B08.02
Ectocardia Q24.8
Ectodermal dysplasia (anhidrotic) Q82.4
Ectodermosis erosiva pluriorificialis L51.1
Ectopic, ectopia (congenital)
  abdominal viscera Q45.8
    due to defect in anterior abdominal
      wall Q79.59
  ACTH syndrome E24.3
  adrenal gland Q89.1
  anus Q43.5
  atrial beats I49.1
  beats I49.49
    atrial I49.1
    ventricular I49.3
  bladder Q64.10
  bone and cartilage in lung Q33.5
  brain Q04.8
  breast tissue Q83.8
  cardiac Q24.8
  cerebral Q04.8
  cordis Q24.8
  endometrium —*see* Endometriosis
  gastric mucosa Q40.2
  gestation —*see* Pregnancy, by site
  heart Q24.8
  hormone secretion NEC E34.2
  kidney (crossed) (pelvis) Q63.2
  lens, lentis Q12.1
  mole —*see* Pregnancy, by site
  organ or site NEC —*see* Malposition,
    congenital
  pancreas Q45.3
  pregnancy —*see* Pregnancy, ectopic
  pupil —*see* Abnormality, pupillary
  renal Q63.2
  sebaceous glands of mouth Q38.6
  spleen Q89.09
  testis Q53.00
    bilateral Q53.02
    unilateral Q53.01
  thyroid Q89.2
  tissue in lung Q33.5
  ureter Q62.63
  ventricular beats I49.3
  vesicae Q64.10
Ectromelia Q73.8
  lower limb —*see* Defect, reduction,
    limb, lower, specified type NEC
  upper limb —*see* Defect, reduction,
    limb, upper, specified type NEC
Ectropion H02.109
  cervix N86
    with cervicitis N72
  congenital Q10.1

Ectropion (*Continued*)
  eyelid (paralytic) H02.109
    cicatricial H02.119
      left H02.116
        lower H02.115
        upper H02.114
      right H02.113
        lower H02.112
        upper H02.111
    congenital Q10.1
      left H02.106
        lower H02.105
        upper H02.104
    mechanical H02.129
      left H02.126
        lower H02.125
        upper H02.124
      right H02.123
        lower H02.122
        upper H02.121
    right H02.103
      lower H02.102
      upper H02.101
    senile H02.139
      left H02.136
        lower H02.135
        upper H02.134
      right H02.133
        lower H02.132
        upper H02.131
    spastic H02.149
      left H02.146
        lower H02.145
        upper H02.144
      right H02.143
        lower H02.142
        upper H02.141
  iris H21.89
  lip (acquired) K13.0
    congenital Q38.0
  urethra N36.8
  uvea H21.89
Eczema (acute) (chronic) (erythematous)
    (fissum) (rubrum) (squamous) (*see
    also* Dermatitis) L30.9
  contact —*see* Dermatitis, contact
  dyshydrotic L30.1
  external ear —*see* Otitis, externa, acute,
    eczematoid
  flexural L20.82
  herpeticum B00.0
  hypertrophicum L28.0
  hypostatic —*see* Varix, leg, with,
    inflammation
  impetiginous L01.1
  infantile (due to any substance) L20.83
    intertriginous L21.1
    seborrheic L21.1
  intertriginous NEC L30.4
    infantile L21.1
  intrinsic (allergic) L20.84
  lichenified NEC L28.0
  marginatum (hebrae) B35.6
  pustular L30.3
  stasis —*see* Varix, leg, with, inflammation
  vaccination, vaccinatum T88.1
  varicose —*see* Varix, leg, with,
    inflammation
Eczematid L30.2
Eddowes (-Spurway) syndrome Q78.0
Edema, edematous (infectious) (pitting)
    (toxic) R60.9
  with nephritis —*see* Nephrosis
  allergic T78.3

Edema, edematous (*Continued*)
amputation stump (surgical) (sequelae (late effect)) T87.89
angioneurotic (allergic) (any site) (with urticaria) T78.3
  hereditary D84.1
angiospastic I73.9
Berlin's (traumatic) S05.8X-
brain (cytotoxic) (vasogenic) G93.6
  due to birth injury P11.0
  newborn (anoxia or hypoxia) P52.4
    birth injury P11.0
  traumatic —*see* Injury, intracranial, cerebral edema
cardiac —*see* Failure, heart, congestive
cardiovascular —*see* Failure, heart, congestive
cerebral —*see* Edema, brain
cerebrospinal —*see* Edema, brain
cervix (uteri) (acute) N88.8
  puerperal, postpartum O90.89
chronic hereditary Q82.0
circumscribed, acute T78.3
  hereditary D84.1
conjunctiva H11.42-
cornea H18.2-
  idiopathic H18.22-
  secondary H18.23-
  due to contact lens H18.21-
due to
  lymphatic obstruction I89.0
  salt retention E87.0
epiglottis —*see* Edema, glottis
essential, acute T78.3
  hereditary D84.1
extremities, lower —*see* Edema, legs
eyelid NEC H02.849
  left H02.846
    lower H02.845
    upper H02.844
  right H02.843
    lower H02.842
    upper H02.841
familial, hereditary Q82.0
famine —*see* Malnutrition, severe
generalized R60.1
glottis, glottic, glottidis (obstructive) (passive) J38.4
  allergic T78.3
  hereditary D84.1
heart —*see* Failure, heart, congestive
heat T67.7
hereditary Q82.0
inanition —*see* Malnutrition, severe
intracranial G93.6
iris H21.89
joint —*see* Effusion, joint
larynx —*see* Edema, glottis
legs R60.0
  due to venous obstruction I87.1
  hereditary Q82.0
localized R60.0
  due to venous obstruction I87.1
lower limbs —*see* Edema, legs
lung J81.1
  with heart condition or failure —*see* Failure, ventricular, left
  acute J81.0
  chemical (acute) J68.1
    chronic J68.1
  chronic J81.1
    due to
      chemicals, gases, fumes or vapors (inhalation) J68.1

Edema, edematous (*Continued*)
lung (*Continued*)
  chronic (*Continued*)
    due to (*Continued*)
      external agent J70.9
        specified NEC J70.8
      radiation J70.1
    due to
      chemicals, fumes or vapors (inhalation) J68.1
      external agent J70.9
        specified NEC J70.8
      high altitude T70.29
      near drowning T75.1
      radiation J70.0
    meaning failure, left ventricle I50.1
lymphatic I89.0
  due to mastectomy I97.2
macula H35.81
  cystoid, following cataract surgery —*see* Complications, postprocedural, following cataract surgery
  diabetic —*see* Diabetes, macular edema
malignant —*see* Gangrene, gas
Milroy's Q82.0
nasopharynx J39.2
newborn P83.30
  hydrops fetalis —*see* Hydrops, fetalis
  specified NEC P83.39
nutritional —*see also* Malnutrition, severe
  with dyspigmentation, skin and hair E40
optic disc or nerve —*see* Papilledema
orbit H05.22-
pancreas K86.8
papilla, optic —*see* Papilledema
penis N48.89
periodic T78.3
  hereditary D84.1
pharynx J39.2
pulmonary —*see* Edema, lung
Quincke's T78.3
  hereditary D84.1
renal —*see* Nephrosis
retina H35.81
  diabetic —*see* Diabetes, macular edema
salt E87.0
scrotum N50.8
seminal vesicle N50.8
spermatic cord N50.8
spinal (cord) (vascular) (nontraumatic) G95.19
starvation —*see* Malnutrition, severe
stasis —*see* Hypertension, venous, (chronic)
subglottic —*see* Edema, glottis
supraglottic —*see* Edema, glottis
testis N44.8
tunica vaginalis N50.8
vas deferens N50.8
vulva (acute) N90.89
Edentulism —*see* Absence, teeth, acquired
Edsall's disease T67.2
Educational handicap Z55.9
  specified NEC Z55.8
Edward's syndrome —*see* Trisomy, 18
Effect, adverse
abnormal gravitational (G) forces or states T75.81
abuse —*see* Maltreatment

Effect, adverse (*Continued*)
air pressure T70.9
  specified NEC T70.8
altitude (high) —*see* Effect, adverse, high altitude
anesthesia (*see also* Anesthesia) T88.59
  in labor and delivery O74.9
  in pregnancy NEC O29.3-
  local, toxic
    in labor and delivery O74.4-
    postpartum, puerperal O89.3
  postpartum, puerperal O89.9
  specified NEC T88.59
    in labor and delivery O74.8
    postpartum, puerperal O89.8
  spinal and epidural T88.59
    headache T88.59
      in labor and delivery O74.5
      postpartum, puerperal O89.4
    specified NEC
      in labor and delivery O74.6
      postpartum, puerperal O89.5
antitoxin —*see* Complications, vaccination
atmospheric pressure T70.9
  due to explosion T70.8
  high T70.3
  low —*see* Effect, adverse, high altitude
  specified effect NEC T70.8
biological, correct substance properly administered —*see* Effect, adverse, drug
blood (derivatives) (serum) (transfusion) —*see* Complications, transfusion
chemical substance —*see* Table of drugs and chemicals
cold (temperature) (weather) T69.9
  chilblains T69.1
  frostbite —*see* Frostbite
  specified effect NEC T69.8
drugs and medicaments T88.7
  specified drug —*see* Table of drugs and chemicals, by drug, adverse effect
  specified effect — code to condition
electric current, electricity (shock) T75.4
  burn —*see* Burn
exertion (excessive) T73.3
exposure —*see* Exposure
external cause NEC T75.89
foodstuffs T78.1
  allergic reaction —*see* Allergy, food
    causing anaphylaxis —*see* Shock, anaphylactic, due to food
  noxious —*see* Poisoning, food, noxious
gases, fumes, or vapors T59.9-
  specified agent —*see* Table of drugs and chemicals
glue (airplane) sniffing
  due to drug abuse —*see* Abuse, drug, inhalant
  due to drug dependence —*see* Dependence, drug, inhalant
heat —*see* Heat
high altitude NEC T70.29
  anoxia T70.29
  on
    ears T70.0
    sinuses T70.1
  polycythemia D75.1
high pressure fluids T70.4
hot weather —*see* Heat

Effect, adverse *(Continued)*
  hunger T73.0
  immersion, foot —*see* Immersion
  immunization —*see* Complications,
    vaccination
  immunological agents —*see*
    Complications, vaccination
  infrared (radiation) (rays) NOS T66
    dermatitis or eczema L59.8
  infusion —*see* Complications, infusion
  lack of care of infants —*see*
    Maltreatment, child
  lightning —*see* Lightning
  medical care T88.9
    specified NEC T88.8
  medicinal substance, correct, properly
    administered —*see* Effect, adverse,
    drug
  motion T75.3
  noise, on inner ear —*see* subcategory
    H83.3
  overheated places —*see* Heat
  psychosocial, of work environment
    Z56.5
  radiation (diagnostic) (infrared) (natural
    source) (therapeutic) (ultraviolet)
    (X-ray) NOS T66
    dermatitis or eczema —*see*
      Dermatitis, due to, radiation
    fibrosis of lung J70.1
    pneumonitis J70.0
    pulmonary manifestations
      acute J70.0
      chronic J70.1
    skin L59.9
  radioactive substance NOS
    dermatitis or eczema —*see*
      Radiodermatitis
  reduced temperature T69.9
    immersion foot or hand —*see*
      Immersion
    specified effect NEC T69.8
  serum NEC (*see also* Reaction, serum)
    T80.69
  specified NEC T78.8
    external cause NEC T75.89
  strangulation —*see* Asphyxia, traumatic
  submersion T75.1
  thirst T73.1
  toxic —*see* Toxicity
  transfusion —*see* Complications,
    transfusion
  ultraviolet (radiation) (rays) NOS T66
    burn —*see* Burn
    dermatitis or eczema —*see* Dermatitis,
      due to, ultraviolet rays
      acute L56.8
  vaccine (any) —*see* Complications,
    vaccination
  vibration —*see* Vibration, adverse
    effects
  water pressure NEC T70.9
    specified NEC T70.8
  weightlessness T75.82
  whole blood —*see* Complications,
    transfusion
  work environment Z56.5
Effect (s) (of) (from) —*see* Effect, adverse
  NEC
Effects, late —*see* Sequelae
Effluvium
  anagen L65.1
  telogen L65.0
Effort syndrome (psychogenic) F45.8

Effusion
  amniotic fluid —*see* Pregnancy,
    complicated by, prematue rupture
    of membranes
  brain (serous) G93.6
  bronchial —*see* Bronchitis
  cerebral G93.6
  cerebrospinal —*see also* Meningitis
    vessel G93.6
  chest —*see* Effusion, pleura
  chylous, chyliform (pleura) J94.0
  intracranial G93.6
  joint M25.40
    ankle M25.47-
    elbow M25.42-
    foot joint M25.47-
    hand joint M25.44-
    hip M25.45-
    knee M25.46-
    shoulder M25.41-
    specified joint NEC M25.48
    wrist M25.43-
  malignant pleural J91.0
  meninges —*see* Meningitis
  pericardium, pericardial
    (noninflammatory) I31.3
    acute —*see* Pericarditis, acute
  peritoneal (chronic) R18.8
  pleura, pleurisy, pleuritic,
    pleuropericardial J90
    chylous, chyliform J94.0
    due to systemic lupus erythematosis
      M32.13
    influenzal —*see* Influenza, with,
      respiratory manifestations NEC
    malignant J91.0
    newborn P28.89
    tuberculous NEC A15.6
      primary (progressive) A15.7
  spinal —*see* Meningitis
  thorax, thoracic —*see* Effusion, pleura
Egg shell nails L60.3
  congenital Q84.6
Egyptian splenomegaly B65.1
Ehlers-Danlos syndrome Q79.6
Ehrlichiosis A77.40
  due to
    E. chafeensis A77.41
    E. sennetsu A79.81
    specified organism NEC A77.49
Eichstedt's disease B36.0
Eisenmenger's
  complex or syndrome I27.89
  defect Q21.8
Ejaculation
  painful N53.12
  premature F52.4
  retarded N53.11
  retrograde N53.14
  semen, painful N53.12
    psychogenic F52.6
Ekbom's syndrome (restless legs) G25.81
Ekman's syndrome (brittle bones and
  blue sclera) Q78.0
Elastic skin Q82.8
  acquired L57.4
Elastofibroma —*see* Neoplasm, connective
  tissue, benign
Elastoma (juvenile) Q82.8
  Miescher's L87.2
Elastomyofibrosis I42.4
Elastosis
  actinic, solar L57.8
  atrophicans (senile) L57.4

Elastosis *(Continued)*
  perforans serpiginosa L87.2
  senilis L57.4
Elbow —*see* condition
Electric current, electricity, effects
  (concussion) (fatal) (nonfatal) (shock)
    T75.4
  burn —*see* Burn
Electric feet syndrome E53.8
Electrocution T75.4
  from electroshock gun (taser) T75.4
Electrolyte imbalance E87.8
  with
    abortion —*see* Abortion by type,
      complicated by, electrolyte
      imbalance
    ectopic pregnancy O08.5
    molar pregnancy O08.5
Elephantiasis (nonfilarial) I89.0
  arabicum —*see* Infestation, filarial
  bancroftian B74.0
  congenital (any site) (hereditary) Q82.0
  due to
    Brugia (malayi) B74.1
      timori B74.2
    mastectomy I97.2
    Wuchereria (bancrofti) B74.0
  eyelid H02.859
    left H02.856
      lower H02.855
      upper H02.854
    right H02.853
      lower H02.852
      upper H02.851
  filarial, filariensis —*see* Infestation,
    filarial
  glandular I89.0
  graecorum A30.9
  lymphangiectatic I89.0
  lymphatic vessel I89.0
    due to mastectomy I97.2
  scrotum (nonfilarial) I89.0
  streptococcal I89.0
  surgical I97.89
    postmastectomy I97.2
  telangiectodes I89.0
  vulva (nonfilarial) N90.89
Elevated, elevation
  antibody titer R76.0
  basal metabolic rate R94.8
  blood pressure —*see also* Hypertension
    reading (incidental) (isolated)
      (nonspecific), no diagnosis of
      hypertension R03.0
  blood sugar R73.9
  body temperature (of unknown origin)
    R50.9
  C-reactive protein (CRP) R79.82
  cancer antigen 125 [CA 125] R97.1
  carcinoembryonic antigen [CEA] R97.0
  cholesterol E78.0
    with high triglycerides E78.2
  conjugate, eye H51.0
  diaphragm, congenital Q79.1
  erythrocyte sedimentation rate R70.0
  fasting glucose R73.01
  fasting triglycerides E78.1
  finding on laboratory examination —*see*
    Findings, abnormal, inconclusive,
    without diagnosis, by type of exam
  GFR (glomerular filtration rate) —*see*
    Findings, abnormal, inconclusive,
    without diagnosis, by type of exam
  glucose tolerance (oral) R73.02
  immunoglobulin level R76.8

Elevated, elevation *(Continued)*
  indoleacetic acid R82.5
  lactic acid dehydrogenase (LDH) level
      R74.0
  leukocytes D72.829
  lipoprotein a level E78.8
  liver function
    study R94.5
    test R79.89
      alkaline phosphatase R74.8
      aminotransferase R74.0
      bilirubin R17
      hepatic enzyme R74.8
      lactate dehydrogenase R74.0
  lymphocytes D72.820
  prostate specific antigen [PSA] R97.2
  Rh titer —*see* Complication (s),
      transfusion, incompatibility
      reaction, Rh (factor)
  scapula, congenital Q74.0
  sedimentation rate R70.0
  SGOT R74.0
  SGPT R74.0
  transaminase level R74.0
  triglycerides E78.1
    with high cholesterol E78.2
  tumor associated antigens [TAA] NEC
      R97.8
  tumor specific antigens [TSA] NEC R97.8
  urine level of
      17-ketosteroids R82.5
      catecholamine R82.5
      indoleacetic acid R82.5
      steroids R82.5
      vanillylmandelic acid (VMA) R82.5
  venous pressure I87.8
  white blood cell count D72.829
    specified NEC D72.828
Elliptocytosis (congenital) (hereditary)
      D58.1
  Hb C (disease) D58.1
  hemoglobin disease D58.1
  sickle-cell (disease) D57.8-
    trait D57.3
Ellison-Zollinger syndrome E16.4
Ellis-van Creveld syndrome
      (chondroectodermal dysplasia)
      Q77.6
Elongated, elongation (congenital) —*see*
      also Distortion
  bone Q79.9
  cervix (uteri) Q51.828
    acquired N88.4
      hypertrophic N88.4
  colon Q43.8
  common bile duct Q44.5
  cystic duct Q44.5
  frenulum, penis Q55.69
  labia minora (acquired) N90.6
  ligamentum patellae Q74.1
  petiolus (epiglottidis) Q31.8
  tooth, teeth K00.2
  uvula Q38.6
Eltor cholera A00.1
Emaciation (due to malnutrition) E41
Embadomoniasis A07.8
Embedded tooth, teeth K01.0
  root only K08.3
Embolic —*see* condition
Embolism (multiple) (paradoxical) I74.9
  air (any site) (traumatic) T79.0
    following
      abortion —*see* Abortion by type
          complicated by embolism
      ectopic pregnancy O08.2

Embolism *(Continued)*
  air *(Continued)*
    following *(Continued)*
      infusion, therapeutic injection or
          transfusion T80.0
      molar pregnancy O08.2
      procedure NEC
        artery T81.719
          mesenteric T81.710
          renal T81.711
          specified NEC T81.718
        vein T81.72
    in pregnancy, childbirth or
        puerperium —*see* Embolism,
        obstetric
  amniotic fluid (pulmonary) —*see also*
      Embolism, obstetric
    following
      abortion —*see* Abortion by type
          complicated by embolism
      ectopic pregnancy O08.2
      molar pregnancy O08.2
  aorta, aortic I74.10
    abdominal I74.09
      saddle I74.01
    bifurcation I74.09
    saddle I74.01
    thoracic I74.11
  artery I74.9
    auditory, internal I65.8
    basilar —*see* Occlusion, artery, basilar
    carotid (common) (internal) —*see*
        Occlusion, artery, carotid
    cerebellar (anterior inferior) (posterior
        inferior) (superior) I66.3
    cerebral —*see* Occlusion, artery,
        cerebral
    choroidal (anterior) I66.8
    communicating posterior I66.8
    coronary —*see also* Infarct,
        myocardium
      not resulting in infarction I24.0
    extremity I74.4
      lower I74.3
      upper I74.2
    hypophyseal I66.8
    iliac I74.5
    limb I74.4
      lower I74.3
      upper I74.2
    mesenteric (with gangrene) K55.0
    ophthalmic —*see* Occlusion, artery,
        retina
    peripheral I74.4
    pontine I66.8
    precerebral —*see* Occlusion, artery,
        precerebral
    pulmonary —*see* Embolism,
        pulmonary
    renal N28.0
    retinal —*see* Occlusion, artery, retina
    septic I76
    specified NEC I74.8
    vertebral —*see* Occlusion, artery,
        vertebral
  basilar (artery) I65.1
  blood clot
    following
      abortion —*see* Abortion by type
          complicated by embolism
      ectopic or molar pregnancy O08.2
    in pregnancy, childbirth or
        puerperium —*see* Embolism,
        obstetric

Embolism *(Continued)*
  brain —*see also* Occlusion, artery, cerebral
    following
      abortion —*see* Abortion by type
          complicated by embolism
      ectopic or molar pregnancy O08.2
    puerperal, postpartum, childbirth —
        see Embolism, obstetric
  capillary I78.8
  cardiac —*see also* Infarct, myocardium
    not resulting in infarction I24.0
  carotid (artery) (common) (internal) —
      see Occlusion, artery, carotid
  cavernous sinus (venous) —*see*
      Embolism, intracranial venous
      sinus
  cerebral —*see* Occlusion, artery, cerebral
  cholesterol —*see* Atheroembolism
  coronary (artery or vein) (systemic) —
      see Occlusion, coronary
  due to device, implant or graft —*see also*
      Complications, by site and type,
      specified NEC
    arterial graft NEC T82.818
    breast (implant) T85.81
    catheter NEC T85.81
      dialysis (renal) T82.818
        intraperitoneal T85.81
      infusion NEC T82.818
        spinal (epidural) (subdural)
            T85.81
      urinary (indwelling) T83.81
    electronic (electrode) (pulse
        generator) (stimulator)
      bone T84.81
      cardiac T82.817
      nervous system (brain) (peripheral
          nerve) (spinal) T85.81
      urinary T83.81
    fixation, internal (orthopedic) NEC
        T84.81
    gastrointestinal (bile duct)
        (esophagus) T85.81
    genital NEC T83.81
    heart (graft) (valve) T82.817
    joint prosthesis T84.81
    ocular (corneal graft) (orbital
        implant) T85.81
    orthopedic (bone graft) NEC T86.838
    specified NEC T85.81
    urinary (graft) NEC T83.81
    vascular NEC T82.818
    ventricular intracranial shunt T85.81
  extremities
    lower —*see* Embolism, vein, lower
        extremity
      arterial I74.3
    upper I74.2
  eye H34.9
  fat (cerebral) (pulmonary) (systemic)
      T79.1
    complicating delivery —*see*
        Embolism, obstetric
    following
      abortion —*see* Abortion by type
          complicated by embolism
      ectopic or molar pregnancy O08.2
  following
    abortion —*see* Abortion by type
        complicated by embolism
    ectopic or molar pregnancy O08.2
    infusion, therapeutic injection or
        transfusion
      air T80.0

Embolism *(Continued)*
  heart (fatty) —*see also* Infarct,
      myocardium
    not resulting in infarction I24.0
  hepatic (vein) I82.0
  in pregnancy, childbirth or
      puerperium —*see* Embolism,
      obstetric
  intestine (artery) (vein) (with gangrene)
      K55.0
  intracranial —*see also* Occlusion, artery,
      cerebral
    venous sinus (any) G08
      nonpyogenic I67.6
  intraspinal venous sinuses or veins G08
    nonpyogenic G95.19
  kidney (artery) N28.0
  lateral sinus (venous) —*see* Embolism,
      intracranial, venous sinus
  leg —*see* Embolism, vein, lower
      extremity
    arterial I74.3
  longitudinal sinus (venous) —*see*
      Embolism, intracranial, venous
      sinus
  lung (massive) —*see* Embolism,
      pulmonary
  meninges I66.8
  mesenteric (artery) (vein) (with
      gangrene) K55.0
  obstetric (in) (pulmonary)
    childbirth O88.82
      air O88.02
      amniotic fluid O88.12
      blood clot O88.22
      fat O88.82
      pyemic O88.32
      septic O88.32
      specified type NEC O88.82
    pregnancy O88.81-
      air O88.01-
      amniotic fluid O88.11-
      blood clot O88.21-
      fat O88.81-
      pyemic O88.31-
      septic O88.31-
      specified type NEC O88.81-
    puerperal O88.83
      air O88.03
      amniotic fluid O88.13
      blood clot O88.23
      fat O88.83
      pyemic O88.33
      septic O88.33
      specified type NEC O88.83
  ophthalmic —*see* Occlusion, artery,
      retina
  penis N48.81
  peripheral artery NOS I74.4
  pituitary E23.6
  popliteal (artery) I74.3
  portal (vein) I81
  postoperative, postprocedural
    artery T81.719
      mesenteric T81.710
      renal T81.711
      specified NEC T81.718
    vein T81.72
  precerebral artery —*see* Occlusion,
      artery, precerebral
  puerperal —*see* Embolism, obstetric
  pulmonary (acute) (artery) (vein)
      I26.99
    with acute cor pulmonale I26.09
    chronic I27.82

Embolism *(Continued)*
  pulmonary *(Continued)*
    following
      abortion —*see* Abortion by type
          complicated by embolism
      ectopic or molar pregnancy O08.2
    healed or old Z86.711
    in pregnancy, childbirth or
        puerperium —*see* Embolism,
        obstetric
    personal history of Z86.711
    saddle I26.92
      with acute cor pulmonale I26.02
    septic I26.90
      with acute cor pulmonale I26.01
  pyemic (multiple) I76
    following
      abortion —*see* Abortion by type
          complicated by embolism
      ectopic or molar pregnancy O08.2
    Hemophilus influenzae A41.3
    pneumococcal A40.3
      with pneumonia J13
    puerperal, postpartum, childbirth
        (any organism) —*see* Embolism,
        obstetric
    specified organism NEC A41.89
    staphylococcal A41.2
    streptococcal A40.9
  renal (artery) N28.0
    vein I82.3
  retina, retinal —*see* Occlusion, artery,
      retina
  saddle
    abdominal aorta I74.01
    pulmonary artery I26.92
      with acute cor pulmonale I26.02
  septic (arterial) I76
    complicating abortion —*see* Abortion,
        by type, complicated by, embolism
  sinus —*see* Embolism, intracranial,
      venous sinus
  soap complicating abortion —*see*
      Abortion, by type, complicated by,
      embolism
  spinal cord G95.19
    pyogenic origin G06.1
  spleen, splenic (artery) I74.8
  upper extremity I74.2
  vein (acute) I82.90
    antecubital I82.61-
      chronic I82.71-
    axillary I82.A1-
      chronic I82.A2-
    basilic I82.61-
      chronic I82.71-
    brachial I82.62-
      chronic I82.72-
    brachiocephalic (innominate) I82.290
      chronic I82.291
    cephalic I82.61-
      chronic I82.71-
    chronic I82.91
    deep (DVT) I82.40-
      calf I82.4Z-
        chronic I82.5Z-
      lower leg I82.4Z-
        chronic I82.5Z-
      thigh I82.4Y-
        chronic I82.5Y-
      upper leg I82.4Y
        chronic I82.5y--
    femoral I82.41-
      chronic I82.51-

Embolism *(Continued)*
  vein *(Continued)*
    iliac (iliofemoral) I82.42-
      chronic I82.52-
    innominate I82.290
      chronic I82.291
    internal jugular I82.C1-
      chronic I82.C2-
    lower extremity
      deep I82.40-
        chronic I82.50-
          specified NEC I82.49-
            chronic NEC I82.59-
      distal
        deep I82.4Z-
      proximal
        deep I82.4Y-
          chronic I82.5Y-
      superficial I82.81-
    popliteal I82.43-
      chronic I82.53-
    radial I82.62-
      chronic I82.72-
    renal I82.3
    saphenous (greater) (lesser) I82.81-
    specified NEC I82.890
      chronic NEC I82.891
    subclavian I82.B1-
      chronic I82.B2-
    thoracic NEC I82.290
      chronic I82.291
    tibial I82.44-
      chronic I82.54-
    ulnar I82.62-
      chronic I82.72-
    upper extremity I82.60-
      chronic I82.70-
      deep I82.62-
        chronic I82.72-
      superficial I82.61-
        chronic I82.71-
    vena cava
      inferior (acute) I82.220
        chronic I82.221
      superior (acute) I82.210
        chronic I82.211
    venous sinus G08
    vessels of brain —*see* Occlusion, artery,
        cerebral
Embolus —*see* Embolism
Embryoma —*see also* Neoplasm, uncertain
    behavior, by site
  benign —*see* Neoplasm, benign, by site
  kidney C64.-
  liver C22.0
  malignant —*see also* Neoplasm,
      malignant, by site
    kidney C64.-
    liver C22.0
    testis C62.9-
      descended (scrotal) C62.1-
      undescended C62.0-
  testis C62.9-
    descended (scrotal) C62.1-
    undescended C62.0-
Embryonic
  circulation Q28.9
  heart Q28.9
  vas deferens Q55.4
Embryopathia NOS Q89.9
Embryotoxon Q13.4
Emesis —*see* Vomiting
Emotional lability R45.86
Emotionality, pathological F60.3

Emotogenic disease —*see* Disorder, psychogenic
Emphysema (atrophic) (bullous) (chronic) (interlobular) (lung) (obstructive) (pulmonary) (senile) (vesicular) J43.9
  cellular tissue (traumatic) T79.7
    surgical T81.82
  centrilobular J43.2
  compensatory J98.3
  congenital (interstitial) P25.0
  conjunctiva H11.89
  connective tissue (traumatic) T79.7
    surgical T81.82
  due to chemicals, gases, fumes or vapors J68.4
  eyelid (s) —*see* Disorder, eyelid, specified type NEC
    surgical T81.82
    traumatic T79.7
  interstitial J98.2
    congenital P25.0
    perinatal period P25.0
  laminated tissue T79.7
    surgical T81.82
  mediastinal J98.2
    newborn P25.2
  orbit, orbital —*see* Disorder, orbit, specified type NEC
  panacinar J43.1
  panlobular J43.1
  specified NEC J43.8
  subcutaneous (traumatic) T79.7
    nontraumatic J98.2
    postprocedural T81.82
    surgical T81.82
  surgical T81.82
  thymus (gland) (congenital) E32.8
  traumatic (subcutaneous) T79.7
  unilateral J43.0
Empty nest syndrome Z60.0
Empyema (acute) (chest) (double) (pleura) (supradiaphragmatic) (thorax) J86.9
  with fistula J86.0
  accessory sinus (chronic) —*see* Sinusitis
  antrum (chronic) —*see* Sinusitis, maxillary
  brain (any part) —*see* Abscess, brain
  ethmoidal (chronic) (sinus) —*see* Sinusitis, ethmoidal
  extradural —*see* Abscess, extradural
  frontal (chronic) (sinus) —*see* Sinusitis, frontal
  gallbladder K81.0
  mastoid (process) (acute) —*see* Mastoiditis, acute
  maxilla, maxillary M27.2
    sinus (chronic) —*see* Sinusitis, maxillary
  nasal sinus (chronic) —*see* Sinusitis
  sinus (accessory) (chronic) (nasal) —*see* Sinusitis
  sphenoidal (sinus) (chronic) —*see* Sinusitis, sphenoidal
  subarachnoid —*see* Abscess, extradural
  subdural —*see* Abscess, subdural
  tuberculous A15.6
  ureter —*see* Ureteritis
  ventricular —*see* Abscess, brain
En coup de sabre lesion L94.1
Enamel pearls K00.2
Enameloma K00.2
Enanthema, viral B09

Encephalitis (chronic) (hemorrhagic) (idiopathic) (nonepidemic) (spurious) (subacute) G04.90
  acute (*see also* Encephalitis, viral) A86
    disseminated G04.00
      infectious G04.01
      noninfectious G04.81
      postimmunization (postvaccination) G04.02
      postinfectious G04.01
    inclusion body A85.8
    necrotizing hemorrhagic G04.30
      postimmunization G04.32
      postinfectious G04.31
      specified NEC G04.39
  arboviral, arbovirus NEC A85.2
  arthropod-borne NEC (viral) A85.2
  Australian A83.4
  California (virus) A83.5
  Central European (tick-borne) A84.1
  Czechoslovakian A84.1
  Dawson's (inclusion body) A81.1
  diffuse sclerosing A81.1
  disseminated, acute G04.00
  due to
    cat scratch disease A28.1
    human immunodeficiency virus [HIV] disease B20 *[G05]*
    malaria —*see* Malaria
    rickettsiosis —*see* Rickettsiosis
    smallpox inoculation G04.02
    typhus —*see* Typhus
  Eastern equine A83.2
  endemic (viral) A86
  epidemic NEC (viral) A86
  equine (acute) (infectious) (viral) A83.9
    Eastern A83.2
    Venezuelan A92.2
    Western A83.1
  Far Eastern (tick-borne) A84.0
  following vaccination or other immunization procedure G04.02
  herpes zoster B02.0
  herpesviral B00.4
    due to herpesvirus 6 B10.01
    due to herpesvirus 7 B10.09
    specified NEC B10.09
  Ilheus (virus) A83.8
  in (due to)
    actinomycosis A42.82
    adenovirus A85.1
    African trypanosomiasis B56.9 *[G05.3]*
    Chagas' disease (chronic) B57.42
    cytomegalovirus B25.8
    enterovirus A85.0
    herpes (simplex) virus B00.4
      due to herpesvirus 6 B10.01
      due to herpesvirus 7 B10.09
      specified NEC B10.09
    infectious disease NEC B99 *[G05.3]*
    influenza —*see* Influenza, with, encephalopathy
    listeriosis A32.12
    measles B05.0
    mumps B26.2
    naegleriasis B60.2
    parasitic disease NEC B89 *[G05.3]*
    poliovirus A80.9 *[G05.3]*
    rubella B06.01
    syphilis
      congenital A50.42
      late A52.14
    systemic lupus erythematosus M32.19

Encephalitis (*Continued*)
  in (*Continued*)
    toxoplasmosis (acquired) B58.2
      congenital P37.1
    tuberculosis A17.82
    zoster B02.0
  inclusion body A81.1
  infectious (acute) (virus) NEC A86
  Japanese (B type) A83.0
  La Crosse A83.5
  lead —*see* Poisoning, lead
  lethargica (acute) (infectious) A85.8
  louping ill A84.8
  lupus erythematosus, systemic M32.19
  lymphatica A87.2
  Mengo A85.8
  meningococcal A39.81
  Murray Valley A83.4
  otitic NEC H66.40 *[G05.3]*
  parasitic NOS B71.9
  periaxial G37.0
  periaxialis (concentrica) (diffuse) G37.5
  postchickenpox B01.11
  postexanthematous NEC B09
  postimmunization G04.02
  postinfectious NEC G04.01
  postmeasles B05.0
  postvaccinal G04.02
  postvaricella B01.11
  postviral NEC A86
  Powassan A84.8
  Rasmussen G04.81
  Rio Bravo A85.8
  Russian
    autumnal A83.0
    spring-summer (taiga) A84.0
  saturnine —*see* Poisoning, lead
  specified NEC G04.81
  St. Louis A83.3
  subacute sclerosing A81.1
  summer A83.0
  suppurative G04.81
  tick-borne A84.9
  Torula, torular (cryptococcal) B45.1
  toxic NEC G92
  trichinosis B75 *[G05.3]*
  type
    B A83.0
    C A83.3
  van Bogaert's A81.1
  Venezuelan equine A92.2
  Vienna A85.8
  viral, virus A86
    arthropod-borne NEC A85.2
    mosquito-borne A83.9
      Australian X disease A83.4
      California virus A83.5
      Eastern equine A83.2
      Japanese (B type) A83.0
      Murray Valley A83.4
      specified NEC A83.8
      St. Louis A83.3
      type B A83.0
      type C A83.3
      Western equine A83.1
    tick-borne A84.9
      biundulant A84.1
      central European A84.1
      Czechoslovakian A84.1
      diphasic meningoencephalitis A84.1

Encephalitis (Continued)
  viral, virus (Continued)
    arthropod-borne NEC (Continued)
      tick-borne (Continued)
        Far Eastern A84.0
        Russian spring-summer (taiga) A84.0
        specified NEC A84.8
      specified type NEC A85.8
      Western equine A83.1
Encephalocele Q01.9
  frontal Q01.0
  nasofrontal Q01.1
  occipital Q01.2
  specified NEC Q01.8
Encephalocystocele —see Encephalocele
Encephaloduroarteriomyosynangiosis (EDAMS) I67.5
Encephalomalacia (brain) (cerebellar) (cerebral) —see Softening, brain
Encephalomeningitis —see Meningoencephalitis
Encephalomeningocele —see Encephalocele
Encephalomeningomyelitis —see Meningoencephalitis
Encephalomyelitis (see also Encephalitis) G04.90
  acute disseminated G04.00
    infectious G04.01
    noninfectious G04.81
    postinfectious G04.01
    postimmunization G04.02
  acute necrotizing hemorrhagic G04.30
    postimmunization G04.32
    postinfectious G04.31
    specified NEC G04.39
  benign myalgic G93.3
  equine A83.9
    Eastern A83.2
    Venezuelan A92.2
    Western A83.1
  in diseases classified elsewhere G05.3
  myalgic, benign G93.3
  postchickenpox B01.11
  postinfectious NEC G04.01
  postmeasles B05.0
  postvaccinal G04.02
  postvaricella B01.11
  rubella B06.01
  specified NEC G04.81
  Venezuelan equine A92.2
Encephalomyelocele —see Encephalocele
Encephalomyelomeningitis —see Meningoencephalitis
Encephalomyelopathy G96.9
Encephalomyeloradiculitis (acute) G61.0
Encephalomyeloradiculoneuritis (acute) (Guillain-Barré) G61.0
Encephalomyeloradiculopathy G96.9
Encephalopathia hyperbilirubinemica, newborn P57.9
  due to isoimmunization (conditions in P55) P57.0
Encephalopathy (acute) G93.40
  acute necrotizing hemorrhagic G04.30
    postimmunization G04.32
    postinfectious G04.31
    specified NEC G04.39
  alcoholic G31.2
  anoxic —see Damage, brain, anoxic
  arteriosclerotic I67.2
  centrolobar progressive (Schilder) G37.0
  congenital Q07.9

Encephalopathy (Continued)
  degenerative, in specified disease NEC G32.89
  due to
    drugs (see also Table of Drugs and Chemicals) G92
  demyelinating callosal G37.1
  hepatic —see Failure, hepatic
  hyperbilirubinemic, newborn P57.9
    due to isoimmunization (conditions in P55) P57.0
  hypertensive I67.4
  hypoglycemic E16.2
  hypoxic —see Damage, brain, anoxic
  hypoxic ischemic P91.60
    mild P91.61
    moderate P91.62
    severe P91.63
  in (due to) (with)
    birth injury P11.1
    hyperinsulinism E16.1 [G94]
    influenza —see Influenza, with, encephalopathy
    lack of vitamin (see also Deficiency, vitamin) E56.9 [G32.89]
    neoplastic disease (see also Neoplasm) D49.9 [G13.1]
    serum (see also Reaction, serum) T80.69
    syphilis A52.17
    trauma (postconcussional) F07.81
      current injury —see Injury, intracranial
    vaccination G04.02
  lead —see Poisoning, lead
  metabolic G93.41
    drug induced G92
    toxic G92
  myoclonic, early, symptomatic —see Epilepsy, generalized, specified NEC
  necrotizing, subacute (Leigh) G31.82
  pellagrous E52 [G32.89]
  portosystemic —see Failure, hepatic
  postcontusional F07.81
    current injury —see Injury, intracranial, diffuse
  posthypoglycemic (coma) E16.1 [G94]
  postradiation G93.89
  saturnine —see Poisoning, lead
  septic G93.41
  specified NEC G93.49
  spongiform, subacute (viral) A81.09
  toxic G92
    metabolic G92
  traumatic (postconcussional) F07.81
    current injury —see Injury, intracranial
  vitamin B deficiency NEC E53.9 [G32.89]
    vitamin B1 E51.2
  Wernicke's E51.2
Encephalorrhagia —see Hemorrhage, intracranial, intracerebral
Encephalosis, posttraumatic F07.81
Enchondroma —see also Neoplasm, bone, benign
Enchondromatosis (cartilaginous) (multiple) Q78.4
Encopresis R15.9
  functional F98.1
  nonorganic origin F98.1
  psychogenic F98.1

Encounter (with health service) (for) Z76.89
  adjustment and management (of)
    breast implant Z45.81
    implanted device NEC Z45.89
    myringotomy device (stent) (tube) Z45.82
  administrative purpose only Z02.9
    examination for
      adoption Z02.82
      armed forces Z02.3
      disability determination Z02.71
      driving license Z02.4
      employment Z02.1
      insurance Z02.6
      medical certificate NEC Z02.79
      paternity testing Z02.81
      residential institution admission Z02.2
      school admission Z02.0
      sports Z02.5
    specified reason NEC Z02.89
  aftercare —see Aftercare
  antenatal screening Z36
  assisted reproductive fertility procedure cycle Z31.83
  blood typing Z01.83
    Rh typing Z01.83
  breast augmentation or reduction Z41.1
  breast implant exchange (different material) (different size) Z45.81
  breast reconstruction following mastectomy Z42.1
  check-up —see Examination
  chemotherapy for neoplasm Z51.11
  colonoscopy, screening Z12.11
  counseling —see Counseling
  delivery, full-term, uncomplicated O80
    cesarean, without indication O82
  ear piercing Z41.3
  examination —see Examination
  expectant parent (s) (adoptive) pre-birth pediatrician visit Z76.81
  fertility preservation procedure (prior to cancer therapy) (prior to removal of gonads) Z31.84
  fitting (of) —see Fitting (and adjustment) (of)
  genetic
    counseling Z31.5
    testing —see Test, genetic
  hearing conservation and treatment Z01.12
  immunotherapy for neoplasm Z51.12
  in vitro fertilization cycle Z31.83
  instruction (in)
    child care (postpartal) (prenatal) Z32.3
    childbirth Z32.2
    natural family planning
      procreative Z31.61
      to avoid pregnancy Z30.02
  insulin pump titration Z46.81
  joint prosthesis insertion following prior explantation of joint prosthesis (staged procedure)
    hip Z47.32
    knee Z47.33
    shoulder Z47.31
  laboratory (as part of a general medical examination) Z00.00
    with abnormal findings Z00.01

Encounter (*Continued*)
mental health services (for)
  abuse NEC
    perpetrator Z69.82
    victim Z69.81
  child abuse
    nonparental
      perpetrator Z69.021
      victim Z69.020
    parental
      perpetrator Z69.011
      victim Z69.010
  spousal or partner abuse
    perpetrator Z69.12
    victim Z69.11
observation (for) (ruled out)
  exposure to (suspected)
    anthrax Z03.810
    biological agent NEC Z03.818
  pediatrician visit, by expectant
    parent (s) (adoptive) Z76.81
  plastic and reconstructive surgery
    following medical procedure or
    healed injury NEC Z42.8
  pregnancy
    supervision of —*see* Pregnancy,
      supervision of
  test Z32.00
    result negative Z32.02
    result positive Z32.01
radiation therapy (antineoplastic)
  Z51.0
radiological (as part of a general medical
  examination) Z00.00
  with abnormal findings Z00.01
reconstructive surgery following
  medical procedure or healed
  injury NEC Z42.8
removal (of) —*see also* Removal
  artificial
    arm Z44.00-
      complete Z44.01-
      partial Z44.02-
    eye Z44.2-
    leg Z44.10-
      complete Z44.11-
      partial Z44.12-
  breast implant Z45.81
    tissue expander (without
      synchronous insertion of
      permanent implant) Z45.81
  device Z46.9
    specified NEC Z46.89
  external
    fixation device — code to fracture
      with seventh character D
    prosthesis, prosthetic device
      Z44.9
      breast Z44.3-
      specified NEC Z44.8
  implanted device NEC Z45.89
  insulin pump Z46.81
  internal fixation device Z47.2
  myringotomy device (stent) (tube)
    Z45.82
  nervous system device NEC Z46.2
    brain neuropacemaker Z46.2
    visual substitution device Z46.2
      implanted Z45.31
  non-vascular catheter Z46.82
  orthodontic device Z46.4
  stent
    ureteral Z46.6
  urinary device Z46.6

Encounter (*Continued*)
repeat cervical smear to confirm findings
  of recent normal smear following
  initial abnormal smear Z01.42
respirator [ventilator] use during power
  failure (Z99.12)
Rh typing Z01.83
screening —*see* Screening
specified NEC Z76.89
sterilization Z30.2
suspected condition, ruled out
  amniotic cavity and membrane Z03.71
  cervical shortening Z03.75
  fetal anomaly Z03.73
  fetal growth Z03.74
  maternal and fetal conditions NEC
    Z03.79
  oligohydramnios Z03.71
  placental problem Z03.72
  polyhydramnios Z03.71
suspected exposure (to), ruled out
  anthrax Z03.810
  biological agents NEC Z03.818
termination of pregnancy, elective Z33.2
testing —*see* Test
therapeutic drug level monitoring Z51.81
titration, insulin pump Z46.81
to determine fetal viability of
  pregnancy O36.80
training
  insulin pump Z46.81
X-ray of chest (as part of a general
  medical examination Z00.00)
  with abnormal findings Z00.01
Encystment —*see* Cyst
Endarteritis (bacterial, subacute)
  (infective) I77.6
  brain I67.7
  cerebral or cerebrospinal I67.7
  deformans —*see* Arteriosclerosis
  embolic —*see* Embolism
  obliterans —*see also* Arteriosclerosis
    pulmonary I28.8
  pulmonary I28.8
  retina —*see* Vasculitis, retina
  senile —*see* Arteriosclerosis
  syphilitic A52.09
    brain or cerebral A52.04
    congenital A50.54 [I79.8]
  tuberculous A18.89
Endemic —*see* condition
Endocarditis (chronic) (marantic)
  (nonbacterial) (thrombotic)
  (valvular) I38
  with rheumatic fever (conditions in I00)
    active —*see* Endocarditis, acute,
      rheumatic
    inactive or quiescent (with chorea)
      I09.1
  acute or subacute I33.9
    infective I33.0
    rheumatic (aortic) (mitral)
      (pulmonary) (tricuspid) I01.1
      with chorea (acute) (rheumatic)
        (Sydenham's) I02.0
  aortic (heart) (nonrheumatic) (valve)
    I35.8
    with
      mitral disease I08.0
        with tricuspid (valve) disease
          I08.3
        active or acute I01.1
          with chorea (acute) (rheumatic)
            (Sydenham's) I02.0

Endocarditis (*Continued*)
aortic (*Continued*)
  with (*Continued*)
    rheumatic fever (conditions in I00)
      active —*see* Endocarditis, acute,
        rheumatic
      inactive or quiescent (with
        chorea) I06.9
    tricuspid (valve) disease I08.2
      with mitral (valve) disease I08.3
  acute or subacute I33.9
  arteriosclerotic I35.8
  rheumatic I06.9
    with mitral disease I08.0
      with tricuspid (valve) disease
        I08.3
      active or acute I01.1
        with chorea (acute) (rheumatic)
          (Sydenham's) I02.0
    active or acute I01.1
      with chorea (acute) (rheumatic)
        (Sydenham's) I02.0
    specified NEC I06.8
  specified cause NEC I35.8
  syphilitic A52.03
arteriosclerotic I38
atypical verrucous (Libman-Sacks)
  M32.11
bacterial (acute) (any valve) (subacute)
  I33.0
candidal B37.6
congenital Q24.8
constrictive I33.0
Coxiella burnetii A78 [I39]
Coxsackie B33.21
due to
  prosthetic cardiac valve T82.6
  Q fever A78 [I39]
  Serratia marcescens I33.0
  typhoid (fever) A01.02
gonococcal A54.83
infectious or infective (acute) (any
  valve) (subacute) I33.0
lenta (acute) (any valve) (subacute) I33.0
Libman-Sacks M32.11
listerial A32.82
Löffler's I42.3
malignant (acute) (any valve)
  (subacute) I33.0
meningococcal A39.51
mitral (chronic) (double) (fibroid)
  (heart) (inactive) (valve) (with
  chorea) I05.9
  with
    aortic (valve) disease I08.0
      with tricuspid (valve) disease
        I08.3
      active or acute I01.1
        with chorea (acute) (rheumatic)
          (Sydenham's) I02.0
    rheumatic fever (conditions in I00)
      active —*see* Endocarditis, acute,
        rheumatic
      inactive or quiescent (with
        chorea) I05.9
    tricuspid (valve) disease I08.1
      with aortic (valve) disease I08.3
  active or acute I01.1
    with chorea (acute) (rheumatic)
      (Sydenham's) I02.0
  bacterial I33.0
  arteriosclerotic I34.8
  nonrheumatic I34.8
    acute or subacute I33.9
  specified NEC I05.8

Endocarditis (Continued)
 monilial B37.6
 multiple valves I08.9
  specified disorders I08.8
 mycotic (acute) (any valve) (subacute)
  I33.0
 pneumococcal (acute) (any valve)
  (subacute) I33.0
 pulmonary (chronic) (heart) (valve) I37.8
  with rheumatic fever (conditions in
   I00)
    active —see Endocarditis, acute,
     rheumatic
    inactive or quiescent (with chorea)
     I09.89
      with aortic, mitral or tricuspid
       disease I08.8
  acute or subacute I33.9
   rheumatic I01.1
    with chorea (acute) (rheumatic)
     (Sydenham's) I02.0
  arteriosclerotic I37.8
  congenital Q22.2
  rheumatic (chronic) (inactive) (with
   chorea) I09.89
    active or acute I01.1
     with chorea (acute) (rheumatic)
      (Sydenham's) I02.0
  syphilitic A52.03
 purulent (acute) (any valve) (subacute)
  I33.0
 Q fever A78 [I39]
 rheumatic (chronic) (inactive) (with
  chorea) I09.1
   active or acute (aortic) (mitral)
    (pulmonary) (tricuspid) I01.1
    with chorea (acute) (rheumatic)
     (Sydenham's) I02.0
 rheumatoid —see Rheumatoid, carditis
 septic (acute) (any valve) (subacute) I33.0
 streptococcal (acute) (any valve)
  (subacute) I33.0
 subacute —see Endocarditis, acute
 suppurative (acute) (any valve)
  (subacute) I33.0
 syphilitic A52.03
 toxic I33.9
 tricuspid (chronic) (heart) (inactive)
  (rheumatic) (valve) (with chorea)
  I07.9
  with
   aortic (valve) disease I08.2
    mitral (valve) disease I08.3
   mitral (valve) disease I08.1
    aortic (valve) disease I08.3
   rheumatic fever (conditions in I00)
    active —see Endocarditis, acute,
     rheumatic
    inactive or quiescent (with
     chorea) I07.8
   active or acute I01.1
    with chorea (acute) (rheumatic)
     (Sydenham's) I02.0
  arteriosclerotic I36.8
  nonrheumatic I36.8
   acute or subacute I33.9
  specified cause, except rheumatic I36.8
 tuberculous —see Tuberculosis,
  endocarditis
 typhoid A01.02
 ulcerative (acute) (any valve) (subacute)
  I33.0
 vegetative (acute) (any valve)
  (subacute) I33.0

Endocarditis (Continued)
 verrucous (atypical) (nonbacterial)
  (nonrheumatic) M32.11
Endocardium, endocardial —see also
  condition
 cushion defect Q21.2
Endocervicitis —see also Cervicitis
 due to intrauterine (contraceptive)
  device T83.6
 hyperplastic N72
Endocrine —see condition
Endocrinopathy, pluriglandular E31.9
Endodontic
 overfill M27.52
 underfill M27.53
Endodontitis K04.0
Endomastoiditis —see Mastoiditis
Endometrioma N80.9
Endometriosis N80.9
 appendix N80.5
 bladder N80.8
 bowel N80.5
 broad ligament N80.3
 cervix N80.0
 colon N80.5
 cul-de-sac (Douglas') N80.3
 exocervix N80.0
 fallopian tube N80.2
 female genital organ NEC N80.8
 gallbladder N80.8
 in scar of skin N80.6
 internal N80.0
 intestine N80.5
 lung N80.8
 myometrium N80.0
 ovary N80.1
 parametrium N80.3
 pelvic peritoneum N80.3
 peritoneal (pelvic) N80.3
 rectovaginal septum N80.4
 rectum N80.5
 round ligament N80.3
 skin (scar) N80.6
 specified site NEC N80.8
 stromal D39.0
 umbilicus N80.8
 uterus (internal) N80.0
 vagina N80.4
 vulva N80.8
Endometritis (decidual) (nonspecific)
  (purulent) (senile (atrophic)
  (suppurative) N71.9
 with ectopic pregnancy O08.0
 acute N71.0
 blenorrhagic (gonococcal) (acute)
  (chronic) A54.24
 cervix, cervical (with erosion or
  ectropion) —see also Cervicitis
  hyperplastic N72
 chlamydial A56.11
 chronic N71.1
 following
  abortion —see Abortion by type
   complicated by genital infection
  ectopic or molar pregnancy O08.0
 gonococcal, gonorrheal (acute) (chronic)
  A54.24
 hyperplastic (see also Hyperplasia,
  endometrial) N85.00
  cervix N72
 puerperal, postpartum, childbirth O86.12
 subacute N71.0
 tuberculous A18.17
Endometrium —see condition

Endomyocardiopathy, South African I42.3
Endomyocarditis —see Endocarditis
Endomyofibrosis I42.3
Endomyometritis —see Endometritis
Endopericarditis —see Endocarditis
Endoperineuritis —see Disorder, nerve
Endophlebitis —see Phlebitis
Endophthalmia —see Endophthalmitis,
  purulent
Endophthalmitis (acute) (infective)
  (metastatic) (subacute) H44.009
 bleb associated H59.4 —see also
   Bleb, inflammed (infected),
   postprocedural
 gonorrheal A54.39
 in (due to)
  cysticercosis B69.1
  onchocerciasis B73.01
  toxocariasis B83.0
 panuveitis —see Panuveitis
 parasitic H44.12-
 purulent H44.00-
  panophthalmitis —see
   Panophthalmitis
  vitreous abscess H44.02-
 specified NEC H44.19
 sympathetic —see Uveitis, sympathetic
Endosalpingioma D28.2
Endosalpingiosis N94.89
Endosteitis —see Osteomyelitis
Endothelioma, bone —see Neoplasm,
  bone, malignant
Endotheliosis (hemorrhagic infectional)
  D69.8
Endotoxemia — code to condition
Endotrachelitis —see Cervicitis
Engelmann (-Camurati) syndrome Q78.3
English disease —see Rickets
Engman's disease L30.3
Engorgement
 breast N64.59
  newborn P83.4
  puerperal, postpartum O92.79
 lung (passive) —see Edema, lung
 pulmonary (passive) —see Edema, lung
 stomach K31.89
 venous, retina —see Occlusion, retina,
  vein, engorgement
Enlargement, enlarged —see also
  Hypertrophy
 adenoids J35.2
  with tonsils J35.3
 alveolar ridge K08.8
  congenital —see Anomaly, alveolar
 apertures of diaphragm (congenital) Q79.1
 gingival K06.1
 heart, cardiac —see Hypertrophy,
  cardiac
 lacrimal gland, chronic H04.03-
 liver —see Hypertrophy, liver
 lymph gland or node R59.9
  generalized R59.1
  localized R59.0
 orbit H05.34-
 organ or site, congenital NEC —see
  Anomaly, by site
 parathyroid (gland) E21.0
 pituitary fossa R93.0
 prostate N40.0
  with lower urinary tract symptoms
   (LUTS) N40.1
  without lower urinary tract
   symptoms (LUTS) N40.0
 sella turcica R93.0

Enlargement, enlarged *(Continued)*
  spleen —*see* Splenomegaly
  thymus (gland) (congenital) E32.0
  thyroid (gland) —*see* Goiter
  tongue K14.8
  tonsils J35.1
    with adenoids J35.3
  uterus N85.2
Enophthalmos H05.40-
  due to
    orbital tissue atrophy H05.41-
    trauma or surgery H05.42-
Enostosis M27.8
Entamebic, entamebiasis —*see* Amebiasis
Entanglement
  umbilical cord (s) O69.2
    with compression O69.2
      without compression O69.82
    around neck (with compression) O69.1
      without compression O69.81
    of twins in monoamniotic sac O69.2
Enteralgia —*see* Pain, abdominal
Enteric —*see* condition
Enteritis (acute) (diarrheal) (hemorrhagic) (noninfective) (septic) K52.9
  adenovirus A08.2
  aertrycke infection A02.0
  allergic K52.2
  amebic (acute) A06.0
    with abscess —*see* Abscess, amebic
    chronic A06.1
      with abscess —*see* Abscess, amebic
      nondysenteric A06.2
    nondysenteric A06.2
  astrovirus A08.32
  bacillary NOS A03.9
  bacterial A04.9
    specified NEC A04.8
  calicivirus A08.31
  candidal B37.82
  Chilomastix A07.8
  choleriformis A00.1
  chronic (noninfectious) K52.9
    ulcerative —*see* Colitis, ulcerative
  cicatrizing (chronic) —*see* Enteritis, regional, small intestine
  Clostridium
    botulinum (food poisoning) A05.1
    difficile A04.7
  coccidial A07.3
  coxsackie virus A08.39
  dietetic K52.2
  drug-induced K52.1
  due to
    astrovirus A08.32
    calicivirus A08.31
    coxsackie virus A08.39
    drugs K52.1
    echovirus A08.39
    enterovirus NEC A08.39
    food hypersensitivity K52.2
    infectious organism (bacterial) (viral) —*see* Enteritis, infectious
    torovirus A08.39
    Yersinia enterocolitica A04.6
  echovirus A08.39
  eltor A00.1
  enterovirus NEC A08.39
  eosinophilic K52.81
  epidemic (infectious) A09
  fulminant K55.0
  gangrenous —*see* Enteritis, infectious
  giardial A07.1

Enteritis *(Continued)*
  infectious NOS A09
    due to
      adenovirus A08.2
      Aerobacter aerogenes A04.8
      Arizona (bacillus) A02.0
      bacteria NOS A04.9
        specified NEC A04.8
      Campylobacter A04.5
      Clostridium difficile A04.7
      Clostridium perfringens A04.8
      Enterobacter aerogenes A04.8
      enterovirus A08.39
      Escherichia coli A04.4
        enteroaggregative A04.4
        enterohemorrhagic A04.3
        enteroinvasive A04.2
        enteropathogenic A04.0
        enterotoxigenic A04.1
        specified NEC A04.4
      specified
        bacteria NEC A04.8
        virus NEC A08.39
      Staphylococcus A04.8
      virus NEC A08.4
        specified type NEC A08.39
      Yersinia enterocolitica A04.6
    specified organism NEC A08.8
  influenzal —*see* Influenza, with, digestive manifestations
  ischemic K55.9
    acute K55.0
    chronic K55.1
  microsporidial A07.8
  mucomembranous, myxomembranous —*see* Syndrome, irritable bowel
  mucous —*see* Syndrome, irritable bowel
  necroticans A05.2
  necrotizing of newborn —*see* Enterocolitis, necrotizing, in newborn
  neurogenic —*see* Syndrome, irritable bowel
  newborn necrotizing —*see* Enterocolitis, necrotizing, in newborn
  noninfectious K52.9
  norovirus A08.11
  parasitic NEC B82.9
  paratyphoid (fever) —*see* Fever, paratyphoid
  protozoal A07.9
    specified NEC A07.8
  radiation K52.0
  regional (of) K50.90
    with
      complication K50.919
        abscess K50.914
        fistula K50.913
        intestinal obstruction K50.912
        rectal bleeding K50.911
        specified complication NEC K50.918
    colon —*see* Enteritis, regional, large intestine
    duodenum —*see* Enteritis, regional, small intestine
    ileum —*see* Enteritis, regional, small intestine
    jejunum —*see* Enteritis, regional, small intestine
    large bowel —*see* Enteritis, regional, large intestine

Enteritis *(Continued)*
  regional *(Continued)*
    large intestine (colon) (rectum) K50.10
      with
        complication K50.119
          abscess K50.114
          fistula K50.113
          intestinal obstruction K50.112
          rectal bleeding K50.111
          small intestine (duodenum) (ileum) (jejunum) involvement K50.80
          with
            complication K50.819
              abscess K50.814
              fistula K50.813
              intestinal obstruction K50.812
              rectal bleeding K50.811
              specified complication NEC K50.818
        specified complication NEC K50.118
    rectum —*see* Enteritis, regional, large intestine
    small intestine (duodenum) (ileum) (jejunum) K50.00
      with
        complication K50.019
          abscess K50.014
          fistula K50.013
          intestinal obstruction K50.012
          large intestine (colon) (rectum) involvement K50.80
          with
            complication K50.819
              abscess K50.814
              fistula K50.813
              intestinal obstruction K50.812
              rectal bleeding K50.811
              specified complication NEC K50.818
        rectal bleeding K50.011
        specified complication NEC K50.018
  rotaviral A08.0
  Salmonella, salmonellosis (arizonae) (cholerae-suis) (enteritidis) (typhimurium) A02.0
  segmental —*see* Enteritis, regional
  septic A09
  Shigella —*see* Infection, Shigella
  small round structured NEC A08.19
  spasmodic, spastic —*see* Syndrome, irritable bowel
  staphylococcal A04.8
    due to food A05.0
  torovirus A08.39
  toxic NEC K52.1
    due to Clostridium difficile A04.7
  trichomonal A07.8
  tuberculous A18.32
  typhosa A01.00
  ulcerative (chronic) —*see* Colitis, ulcerative
  viral A08.4
    adenovirus A08.2
    enterovirus A08.39
    Rotavirus A08.0
    small round structured NEC A08.19
    specified NEC A08.39
    virus specified NEC A08.39

Enterobiasis B80
Enterobius vermicularis (infection) (infestation) B80
Enterocele —see also Hernia, abdomen
    pelvic, pelvis (acquired) (congenital) N81.5
    vagina, vaginal (acquired) (congenital) NEC N81.5
Enterocolitis (see also Enteritis) K52.9
    due to Clostridium difficile A04.7
    fulminant ischemic K55.0
    granulomatous —see Enteritis, regional
    hemorrhagic (acute) K55.0
        chronic K55.1
    infectious NEC A09
    ischemic K55.9
    necrotizing
        due to Clostridium difficile A04.7
        in newborn P77.9
            stage 1 (without pneumatosis, without perforation) P77.1
            stage 2 (with pneumatosis, without perforation) P77.2
            stage 3 (with pneumatosis, with perforation) P77.3
    noninfectious K52.9
        newborn —see Enterocolitis, necrotizing, in newborn
    pseudomembranous (newborn) A04.7
    radiation K52.0
        newborn —see Enterocolitis, necrotizing, in newborn
    ulcerative (chronic) —see Pancolitis, ulcerative (chronic)
Enterogastritis —see Enteritis
Enteropathy K63.9
    gluten-sensitive K90.0
    hemorrhagic, terminal K55.0
    protein-losing K90.4
Enteroperitonitis —see Peritonitis
Enteroptosis K63.4
Enterorrhagia K92.2
Enterospasm —see also Syndrome, irritable, bowel
    psychogenic F45.8
Enterostenosis (see also Obstruction, intestine) K56.69
Enterostomy
    complication —see Complication, enterostomy
    status Z93.4
Enterovirus, as cause of disease classified elsewhere B97.10
    coxsackievirus B97.11
    echovirus B97.12
    other specified B97.19
Enthesopathy (peripheral) M77.9
    Achilles tendinitis —see Tendinitis, Achilles
    ankle and tarsus M77.9
        specified type NEC —see Enthesopathy, foot, specified type NEC
    anterior tibial syndrome M76.81-
    calcaneal spur —see Spur, bone, calcaneal
    elbow region M77.8
        lateral epicondylitis —see Epicondylitis, lateral
        medial epicondylitis —see Epicondylitis, medial
    foot NEC M77.9
        metatarsalgia —see Metatarsalgia
        specified type NEC M77.5-
    forearm M77.9

Enthesopathy (Continued)
    gluteal tendinitis —see Tendinitis, gluteal
    hand M77.9
    hip —see Enthesopathy, lower limb, specified type NEC
    iliac crest spur —see Spur, bone, iliac crest
    iliotibial band syndrome —see Syndrome, iliotibial band
    knee —see Enthesopathy, lower limb, lower leg, specified type NEC
    lateral epicondylitis —see Epicondylitis, lateral
    lower limb (excluding foot) M76.9
        Achilles tendinitis —see Tendinitis, Achilles
        anterior tibial syndrome M76.81-
        gluteal tendinitis —see Tendinitis, gluteal
        iliac crest spur —see Spur, bone, iliac crest
        iliotibial band syndrome —see Syndrome, iliotibial band
        patellar tendinitis —see Tendinitis, patellar
        pelvic region —see Enthesopathy, lower limb, specified type NEC
        peroneal tendinitis —see Tendinitis, peroneal
        posterior tibial syndrome M76.82-
        psoas tendinitis —see Tendinitis, psoas
        shoulder M77.9
        specified type NEC M76.89-
        tibial collateral bursitis —see Bursitis, tibial collateral
    medial epicondylitis —see Epicondylitis, medial
    multiple sites M77.9
    patellar tendinitis —see Tendinitis, patellar
    pelvis M77.9
    periarthritis of wrist —see Periarthritis, wrist
    peroneal tendinitis —see Tendinitis, peroneal
    posterior tibial syndrome M76.82-
    psoas tendinitis —see Tendinitis, psoas
    shoulder region —see Lesion, shoulder
    specified site NEC M77.9
    specified type NEC M77.8
    spinal M46.00
        cervical region M46.02
        cervicothoracic region M46.03
        lumbar region M46.06
        lumbosacral region M46.07
        multiple sites M46.09
        occipito-atlanto-axial region M46.01
        sacrococcygeal region M46.08
        thoracic region M46.04
        thoracolumbar region M46.05
        tibial collateral bursitis —see Bursitis, tibial collateral
    upper arm M77.9
    wrist and carpus NEC M77.8
        calcaneal spur —see Spur, bone, calcaneal
        periarthritis of wrist —see Periarthritis, wrist
Entomophobia F40.218
Entomophthoromycosis B46.8
Entrance, air into vein —see Embolism, air

Entrapment, nerve —see Neuropathy, entrapment
Entropion (eyelid) (paralytic) H02.009
    cicatricial H02.019
        left H02.016
            lower H02.015
            upper H02.014
        right H02.013
            lower H02.012
            upper H02.011
    congenital Q10.2
    left H02.006
        lower H02.005
        upper H02.004
    mechanical H02.029
        left H02.026
            lower H02.025
            upper H02.024
        right H02.023
            lower H02.022
            upper H02.021
    right H02.003
        lower H02.002
        upper H02.001
    senile H02.039
        left H02.036
            lower H02.035
            upper H02.034
        right H02.033
            lower H02.032
            upper H02.031
    spastic H02.049
        left H02.046
            lower H02.045
            upper H02.044
        right H02.043
            lower H02.042
            upper H02.041
Enucleated eye (traumatic, current) S05.7-
Enuresis R32
    functional F98.0
    habit disturbance F98.0
    nocturnal N39.44
        psychogenic F98.0
    nonorganic origin F98.0
    psychogenic F98.0
Eosinopenia —see Agranulocytosis
Eosinophilia (allergic) (hereditary) (idiopathic) (secondary) D72.1
    with
        angiolymphoid hyperplasia (ALHE) D18.01
    infiltrative J82
    Löffler's J82
    peritoneal —see Peritonitis, eosinophilic
    pulmonary NEC J82
    tropical (pulmonary) J82
Eosinophilia-myalgia syndrome M35.8
Ependymitis (acute) (cerebral) (chronic) (granular) —see Encephalomyelitis
Ependymoblastoma
    specified site —see Neoplasm, malignant, by site
    unspecified site C71.9
Ependymoma (epithelial) (malignant)
    anaplastic
        specified site —see Neoplasm, malignant, by site
        unspecified site C71.9
    benign
        specified site —see Neoplasm, benign, by site
        unspecified site D33.2

Ependymoma (Continued)
  myxopapillary D43.2
    specified site —see Neoplasm,
      uncertain behavior, by site
    unspecified site D43.2
  papillary D43.2
    specified site —see Neoplasm,
      uncertain behavior, by site
    unspecified site D43.2
  specified site —see Neoplasm,
    malignant, by site
  unspecified site C71.9
Ependymopathy G93.89
Ephelis, ephelides L81.2
Epiblepharon (congenital) Q10.3
Epicanthus, epicanthic fold (eyelid)
  (congenital) Q10.3
Epicondylitis (elbow)
  lateral M77.1-
  medial M77.0-
Epicystitis —see Cystitis
Epidemic —see condition
Epidermidalization, cervix —see
  Dysplasia, cervix
Epidermis, epidermal —see condition
Epidermodysplasia verruciformis B07.8
Epidermolysis
  bullosa (congenital) Q81.9
    acquired L12.30
      drug-induced L12.31
      specified cause NEC L12.35
    dystrophica Q81.2
    letalis Q81.1
    simplex Q81.0
    specified NEC Q81.8
  necroticans combustiformis L51.2
    due to drug —see Table of drugs and
      chemicals, by drug
Epidermophytid —see Dermatophytosis
Epidermophytosis (infected) —see
  Dermatophytosis
Epididymis —see condition
Epididymitis (acute) (nonvenereal)
  (recurrent) (residual) N45.1
  with orchitis N45.3
  blennorrhagic (gonococcal) A54.23
  caseous (tuberculous) A18.15
  chlamydial A56.19
  filarial B74.9
  gonococcal A54.23
  syphilitic A52.76
  tuberculous A18.15
Epididymo-orchitis (see also Epididymitis)
  N45.3
Epidural —see condition
Epigastrium, epigastric —see condition
Epigastrocele —see Hernia, ventral
Epiglottis —see condition
Epiglottitis, epiglottiditis (acute) J05.10
  with obstruction J05.11
  chronic J37.0
Epignathus Q89.4
Epilepsia partialis continua (see also
  Kozhevnikof's epilepsy) G40.1-
Epilepsy, epileptic, epilepsia (attack)
  (cerebral) (convulsion) (fit) (seizure)
  G40.909

Note: the following terms are to be
considered equivalent to intractable:
pharmacoresistant (pharmacologically
resistant), treatment resistant,
refractory (medically) and poorly
controlled

Epilepsy, epileptic, epilepsia (Continued)
  with
    complex partial seizures —see
      Epilepsy, localization-related,
      symptomatic, with complex
      partial seizures
    grand mal seizures on awakening —
      see Epilepsy, generalized,
      specified NEC
    myoclonic absences —see Epilepsy,
      generalized, specified NEC
    myoclonic-astatic seizures —see
      Epilepsy, generalized, specified
      NEC
    simple partial seizures —see
      Epilepsy, localization-related,
      symptomatic, with simple
      partial seizures
  akinetic —see Epilepsy, generalized,
    specified NEC
  benign childhood with centrotemporal
    EEG spikes —see Epilepsy,
    localization-related, idiopathic
  benign myoclonic in infancy G40.80-
  Bravais-jacksonian —see Epilepsy,
    localization-related, symptomatic,
    with simple partial seizures
  childhood with occipital EEG
    paroxysms —see Epilepsy,
    localization-related, idiopathic
  childhood absence G40.A09
    intractable G40.A19
      with status epilepticus G40.A11
      without status epilepticus G40.A19
    not intractable G40.A09
      with status epilepticus G40.A01
      without status epilepticus G40.A09
  climacteric —see Epilepsy, specified
    NEC
  cysticercosis B69.0
  deterioration (mental) F06.8
  due to syphilis A52.19
  focal —see Epilepsy, localization-related,
    symptomatic, with simple partial
    seizures
  generalized
    idiopathic G40.309
      intractable G40.319
        with status epilepticus G40.311
        without status epilepticus
          G40.319
      not intractable G40.309
        with status epilepticus G40.301
        without status epilepticus
          G40.309
    specified NEC G40.409
      intractable G40.419
        with status epilepticus G40.411
        without status epilepticus
          G40.419
      not intractable G40.409
        with status epilepticus G40.401
        without status epilepticus
          G40.409
  impulsive petit mal —see Epilepsy,
    juvenile myoclonic
  intractable G40.919
    with status epilepticus G40.911
    without status epilepticus G40.919
  juvenile absence G40.A09
    intractable G40.A19
      with status epilepticus G40.A11
      without status epilepticus
        G40.A19

Epilepsy, epileptic, epilepsia (Continued)
  juvenile absence (Continued)
    not intractable G40.A09
      with status epilepticus G40.A01
      without status epilepticus G40.A09
    juvenile myoclonic G40.B11
      intractable G40.B19
        with status epilepticus G40.B11
        without status epilepticus G40.B19
      not intractable G40.B09
        with status epilepticus G40.B01
        without status epilepticus G40.B09
  localization-related (focal) (partial)
    idiopathic G40.009
      with seizures of localized onset
        G40.009
        intractable G40.019
          with status epilepticus G40.011
          without status epilepticus
            G40.019
        not intractable G40.009
          with status epilepticus G40.001
          without status epilepticus
            G40.009
    symptomatic
      with complex partial seizures
        G40.209
        intractable G40.219
          with status epilepticus G40.211
          without status epilepticus
            G40.219
        not intractable G40.209
          with status epilepticus G40.201
          without status epilepticus
            G40.209
      with simple partial seizures G40.109
        intractable G40.119
          with status epilepticus G40.111
          without status epilepticus
            G40.119
        not intractable G40.109
          with status epilepticus G40.101
          without status epilepticus
            G40.109
  myoclonus, myoclonic (progressive) —
    see Epilepsy, generalized, specified
    NEC
  not intractable G40.909
    with status epilepticus G40.901
    without status epilepticus G40.909
  on awakening —see Epilepsy,
    generalized, specified NEC
  parasitic NOS B71.9 [G94]
  partialis continua (see also
    Kozhevnikof's epilepsy) G40.1-
  peripheral —see Epilepsy, specified
    NEC
  procursiva —see Epilepsy, localization-
    related, symptomatic, with simple
    partial seizures
  progressive (familial) myoclonic —see
    Epilepsy, generalized, idiopathic
  reflex —see Epilepsy, specified NEC
  related to
    alcohol G40.509
      not intractable G40.509
        with status epilepticus G40.501
        without status epliepticus
          G40.509
    drugs G40.509
      not intractable G40.509
        with status epilepticus G40.501
        without status epliepticus
          G40.509

Erb (-Duchenne) **paralysis** (birth injury) (newborn) P14.0
Erb's
  disease G71.0
  palsy, paralysis (brachial) (birth) (newborn) P14.0
    spinal (spastic) syphilitic A52.17
  pseudohypertrophic muscular dystrophy G71.0
Erb-Goldflam disease or syndrome G70.00
  with exacerbation (acute) G70.01
  in crisis G70.01
Erdheim's syndrome (acromegalic macrospondylitis) E22.0
Erection, painful (persistent) —*see* Priapism
Ergosterol deficiency (vitamin D) E55.9
  with
    adult osteomalacia M83.8
    rickets —*see* Rickets
Ergotism —*see also* Poisoning, food, noxious, plant
  from ergot used as drug (migraine therapy) —*see* Table of Drugs and Chemicals
Erosio interdigitalis blastomycetica B37.2
Erosion
  artery I77.2
    without rupture I77.89
  bone —*see* Disorder, bone, density and structure, specified NEC
  bronchus J98.09
  cartilage (joint) —*see* Disorder, cartilage, specified type NEC
  cervix (uteri) (acquired) (chronic) (congenital) N86
    with cervicitis N72
  cornea (nontraumatic) —*see* Ulcer, cornea
    recurrent H18.83-
    traumatic —*see* Abrasion, cornea
  dental (idiopathic) (occupational) (due to diet, drugs or vomiting) K03.2
  duodenum, postpyloric —*see* Ulcer, duodenum
  esophagus K22.10
    with bleeding K22.11
  gastric —*see* Ulcer, stomach
  gastrojejunal —*see* Ulcer, gastrojejunal
  implanted mesh —*see* Complications, mesh
  intestine K63.3
  lymphatic vessel I89.8
  pylorus, pyloric (ulcer) —*see* Ulcer, stomach
  spine, aneurysmal A52.09
  stomach —*see* Ulcer, stomach
  teeth (idiopathic) (occupational) (due to diet, drugs or vomiting) K03.2
  urethra N36.8
  uterus N85.8
Erotomania F52.8
Error
  metabolism, inborn —*see* Disorder, metabolism
  refractive —*see* Disorder, refraction
Eructation R14.2
  nervous or psychogenic F45.8

Eruption
  creeping B76.9
  drug (generalized) (taken internally) L27.0
    fixed L27.1
    in contact with skin —*see* Dermatitis, due to drugs
    localized L27.1
  Hutchinson, summer L56.4
  Kaposi's varicelliform B00.0
  napkin L22
  polymorphous light (sun) L56.4
  recalcitrant pustular L13.8
  ringed R23.8
  skin (nonspecific) R21
    creeping (meaning hookworm) B76.9
    due to inoculation/vaccination (generalized) (*see also* Dermatitis, due to, vaccine) L27.0
      localized L27.1
    erysipeloid A26.0
    feigned L98.1
    Kaposi's varicelliform B00.0
    lichenoid L28.0
    meaning dermatitis —*see* Dermatitis
    toxic NEC L53.0
  tooth, teeth, abnormal (incomplete) (late) (premature) (sequence) K00.6
  vesicular R23.8
Erysipelas (gangrenous) (infantile) (newborn) (phlegmonous) (suppurative) A46
  external ear A46 [H62.40]
  puerperal, postpartum O86.89
Erysipeloid A26.9
  cutaneous (Rosenbach's) A26.0
  disseminated A26.8
  sepsis A26.7
  specified NEC A26.8
Erythema, erythematous (infectional) (inflammation) L53.9
  ab igne L59.0
  annulare (centrifugum) (rheumaticum) L53.1
  arthriticum epidemicum A25.1
  brucellum —*see* Brucellosis
  chronic figurate NEC L53.3
  chronicum migrans (Borrelia burgdorferi) A69.20
  diaper L22
  due to
    chemical NEC L53.0
      in contact with skin L24.5
    drug (internal use) —*see* Dermatitis, due to, drugs
  elevatum diutinum L95.1
  endemic E52
  epidemic, arthritic A25.1
  figuratum perstans L53.3
  gluteal L22
  heat - code by site under Burn, first degree
  ichthyosiforme congenitum bullous Q80.3
  in diseases classified elsewhere L54
  induratum (nontuberculous) L52
    tuberculous A18.4
  infectiosum B08.3
  intertrigo L30.4
  iris L51.9
  marginatum L53.2
    in (due to) acute rheumatic fever I00

Erythema, erythematous (*Continued*)
  medicamentosum —*see* Dermatitis, due to, drugs
  migrans A26.0
    chronicum A69.20
    tongue K14.1
  multiforme (major) (minor) L51.9
    bullous, bullosum L51.1
    conjunctiva L51.1
    nonbullous L51.0
    pemphigoides L12.0
    specified NEC L51.8
  napkin L22
  neonatorum P83.8
    toxic P83.1
  nodosum L52
    tuberculous A18.4
  palmar L53.8
  pernio T69.1
  rash, newborn P83.8
  scarlatiniform (recurrent) (exfoliative) L53.8
  solare L55.0
  specified NEC L53.8
  toxic, toxicum NEC L53.0
    newborn P83.1
  tuberculous (primary) A18.4
Erythematous, erythematosus —*see* condition
Erythermalgia (primary) I73.81
Erythralgia I73.81
Erythrasma L08.1
Erythredema (polyneuropathy) —*see* Poisoning, mercury
Erythremia (acute) C94.0-
  chronic D45
  secondary D75.1
Erythroblastopenia (*see also* Aplasia, red cell) D60.9
  congenital D61.01
Erythroblastophthisis D61.09
Erythroblastosis (fetalis) (newborn) P55.9
  due to
    ABO (antibodies) (incompatibility) (isoimmunization) P55.1
    Rh (antibodies) (incompatibility) (isoimmunization) P55.0
Erythrocyanosis (crurum) I73.89
Erythrocythemia —*see* Erythremia
Erythrocytosis (megalosplenic) (secondary) D75.1
  familial D75.0
  oval, hereditary —*see* Elliptocytosis
  secondary D75.1
  stress D75.1
Erythroderma (secondary) (*see also* Erythema) L53.9
  bullous ichthyosiform, congenital Q80.3
  desquamativum L21.1
  ichthyosiform, congenital (bullous) Q80.3
  neonatorum P83.8
  psoriaticum L40.8
Erythrodysesthesia, palmar plantar (PPE) L27.1
Erythrogenesis imperfecta D61.09
Erythroleukemia C94.0-
Erythromelalgia I73.81
Erythrophagocytosis D75.89
Erythrophobia F40.298
Erythroplakia, oral epithelium, and tongue K13.29

Erythroplasia (Queyrat) D07.4
    specified site —*see* Neoplasm, skin, in
        situ
    unspecified site D07.4
Escherichia coli (E. coli), as cause of
        disease classified elsewhere B96.20
    non-O157 Shiga toxin-producing (with
        known O group) B96.22
    non-Shiga toxin-producing B96.29
    O157 with confirmation of Shiga toxin
        when H antigen is unknown, or is
        not H7 B96.21
    O157:H- (nonmotile) with confirmation
        of Shiga toxin B96.21
    O157:H7 with or without confirmation
        of Shiga toxin-production B96.21
    Shiga toxin-producing (with
        unspecified O group) (STEC)
        B96.23
        O157 B96.21
        O157:H7 with or without
            confirmation of Shiga toxin-
            production B96.21
        specified NEC B96.22
    specified NEC B96.29
Esophagismus K22.4
Esophagitis (acute) (alkaline) (chemical)
        (chronic) (infectional) (necrotic)
        (peptic) (postoperative) K20.9
    candidal B37.81
    due to gastrointestinal reflux disease
        K21.0
    eosinophilic K20.0
    reflux K21.0
    specified NEC K20.8
    tuberculous A18.83
    ulcerative K22.10
        with bleeding K22.11
Esophagocele K22.5
Esophagomalacia K22.8
Esophagospasm K22.4
Esophagostenosis K22.2
Esophagostomiasis B81.8
Esophagotracheal —*see* condition
Esophagus —*see* condition
Esophoria H50.51
    convergence, excess H51.12
    divergence, insufficiency H51.8
Esotropia —*see* Strabismus, convergent
        concomitant
Espundia B55.2
Essential —*see* condition
Esthesioneuroblastoma C30.0
Esthesioneurocytoma C30.0
Esthesioneuroepithelioma C30.0
Esthiomene A55
Estivo-autumnal malaria (fever) B50.9
Estrangement (marital) Z63.5
    parent-child NEC Z62.890
Estriasis —*see* Myiasis
Ethanolism —*see* Alcoholism
Etherism —*see* Dependence, drug,
        inhalant
Ethmoid, ethmoidal —*see* condition
Ethmoiditis (chronic) (nonpurulent)
        (purulent) —*see also* Sinusitis,
        ethmoidal
    influenzal —*see* Influenza, with,
        respiratory manifestations NEC
    Woakes' J33.1
Ethylism —*see* Alcoholism
Eulenburg's disease (congenital
        paramyotonia) G71.19
Eumycetoma B47.0

Eunuchoidism E29.1
    hypogonadotropic E23.0
European blastomycosis —*see*
        Cryptococcosis
Eustachian —*see* condition
Evaluation (for) (of)
    development state
        adolescent Z00.3
        period of
            delayed growth in childhood Z00.70
                with abnormal findings Z00.71
            rapid growth in childhood Z00.2
        puberty Z00.3
    growth and developmental state
        (period of rapid growth) Z00.2
        delayed growth Z00.70
            with abnormal findings Z00.71
    mental health (status) Z00.8
        requested by authority Z04.6
    period of
        delayed growth in childhood Z00.70
            with abnormal findings Z00.71
        rapid growth in childhood Z00.2
    suspected condition —*see* Observation
Evans syndrome D69.41
Event, apparent life threatening in
        newborn and infant (ALTE) R68.13
Eventration —*see also* Hernia, ventral
    colon into chest —*see* Hernia,
        diaphragm
    diaphragm (congenital) Q79.1
Eversion
    bladder N32.89
    cervix (uteri) N86
        with cervicitis N72
    foot NEC —*see also* Deformity, valgus,
        ankle
        congenital Q66.6
    punctum lacrimale (postinfectional)
        (senile) H04.52-
    ureter (meatus) N28.89
    urethra (meatus) N36.8
    uterus N81.4
Evidence
    cytologic
        of malignancy on anal smear R85.614
        of malignancy on cervical smear
            R87.614
        of malignancy on vaginal smear
            R87.624
Evisceration
    birth injury P15.8
    traumatic NEC
        eye —*see* Enucleated eye
Evulsion —*see* Avulsion
Ewing's sarcoma or tumor —*see*
        Neoplasm, bone, malignant
Examination (for) (following) (general)
        (of) (routine) Z00.00
    with abnormal findings Z00.01
    abuse, physical (alleged), ruled out
        adult Z04.71
        child Z04.72
    adolescent (development state) Z00.3
    alleged rape or sexual assault (victim),
        ruled out
        adult Z04.41
        child Z04.42
    allergy Z01.82
    annual (adult) (periodic) (physical)
        Z00.00
        with abnormal findings Z00.01
    gynecological Z01.419
        with abnormal findings Z01.411

Examination (*Continued*)
    antibody response Z01.84
        blood —*see* Examination, laboratory
    blood pressure Z01.30
        with abnormal findings Z01.31
    cancer staging —*see* Neoplasm,
        malignant, by site
    cervical Papanicolaou smear Z12.4
        as part of routine gynecological
            examination Z01.419
            with abnormal findings Z01.411
    child (over 28 days old) Z00.129
        with abnormal findings Z00.121
        under 28 days old —*see* Newborn,
            examination
    clinical research control or normal
        comparison (control) (participant)
        Z00.6
    contraceptive (drug) maintenance
        (routine) Z30.8
        device (intrauterine) Z30.431
    dental Z01.20
        with abnormal findings Z01.21
    developmental —*see* Examination, child
    donor (potential) Z00.5
    ear Z01.10
        with abnormal findings NEC Z01.118
    eye Z01.00
        with abnormal findings Z01.01
    following
        accident NEC Z04.3
            transport Z04.1
            work Z04.2
        assault, alleged, ruled out
            adult Z04.71
            child Z04.72
        motor vehicle accident Z04.1
        treatment (for) Z09
            combined NEC Z09
                fracture Z09
                malignant neoplasm Z08
            malignant neoplasm Z08
            mental disorder Z09
            specified condition NEC Z09
    follow-up (routine) (following) Z09
        chemotherapy NEC Z09
            malignant neoplasm Z08
        fracture Z09
        malignant neoplasm Z08
        postpartum Z39.2
        psychotherapy Z09
        radiotherapy NEC Z09
            malignant neoplasm Z08
        surgery NEC Z09
            malignant neoplasm Z08
    gynecological Z01.419
        with abnormal findings Z01.411
        for contraceptive maintenance Z30.8
    health —*see* Examination, medical
    hearing Z01.10
        with abnormal findings NEC
            Z01.118
        following failed hearing screening
            Z01.110
    immunity status testing Z01.84
    laboratory (as part of a general medical
        examination) Z00.00
        with abnormal findings Z00.01
        preprocedural Z01.812
    lactating mother Z39.1
    medical (adult) (for) (of) Z00.00
        with abnormal findings Z00.01
        administrative purpose only Z02.9
            specified NEC Z02.89

Examination *(Continued)*
  medical *(Continued)*
    admission to
      armed forces Z02.3
      old age home Z02.2
      prison Z02.89
      residential institution Z02.2
      school Z02.0
        following illness or medical
          treatment Z02.0
      summer camp Z02.89
    adoption Z02.82
    blood alcohol or drug level Z02.83
    camp (summer) Z02.89
    clinical research, normal subject
      (control) (participant) Z00.6
    control subject in clinical research
      (normal comparison)
      (participant) Z00.6
    donor (potential) Z00.5
    driving license Z02.4
    general (adult) Z00.00
      with abnormal findings Z00.01
    immigration Z02.89
    insurance purposes Z02.6
    marriage Z02.89
    medicolegal reasons NEC Z04.8
    naturalization Z02.89
    participation in sport Z02.5
    paternity testing Z02.81
    population survey Z00.8
    pre-employment Z02.1
    pre-operative —see Examination,
      pre-procedural
    pre-procedural
      cardiovascular Z01.810
      respiratory Z01.811
      specified NEC Z01.818
    preschool children
      for admission to school Z02.0
    prisoners
      for entrance into prison
        Z02.89
    recruitment for armed forces
      Z02.3
    specified NEC Z00.8
    sport competition Z02.5
  medicolegal reason NEC Z04.8
  newborn —see Newborn, examination
  pelvic (annual) (periodic) Z01.419
    with abnormal findings Z01.411
  period of rapid growth in childhood
    Z00.2
  periodic (adult) (annual) (routine)
    Z00.00
    with abnormal findings Z00.01
  physical (adult) (see also Examination,
    medical) Z00.00
    sports Z02.5
  postpartum
    immediately after delivery
      Z39.0
    routine follow-up Z39.2
  pre-chemotherapy (antineoplastic)
    Z01.818
  prenatal (normal pregnancy) (see also
    Pregnancy, normal) Z34.9-
  pre-procedural (pre-operative)
    cardiovascular Z01.810
    laboratory Z01.812
    respiratory Z01.811
    specified NEC Z01.818
  prior to chemotherapy (antineoplastic)
    Z01.818

Examination *(Continued)*
  psychiatric NEC Z00.8
    follow-up not needing further care
      Z09
    requested by authority Z04.6
  radiological (as part of a general
    medical examination) Z00.00
    with abnormal findings Z00.01
  repeat cervical smear to confirm
    findings of recent normal smear
    following initial abnormal smear
    Z01.42
  skin (hypersensitivity) Z01.82
  special (see also Examination, by type)
    Z01.89
    specified type NEC Z01.89
  specified type or reason NEC Z04.8
  teeth Z01.20
    with abnormal findings Z01.21
  urine —see Examination, laboratory
  vision Z01.00
    with abnormal findings Z01.01
Exanthem, exanthema —see also Rash
  with enteroviral vesicular stomatitis
    B08.4
  Boston A88.0
  epidemic with meningitis A88.0
    [G02]
  subitum B08.20
    due to human herpesvirus 6
      B08.21
    due to human herpesvirus 7
      B08.22
  viral, virus B09
    specified type NEC B08.8
Excess, excessive, excessively
  alcohol level in blood R78.0
  androgen (ovarian) E28.1
  attrition, tooth, teeth K03.0
  carotene, carotin (dietary) E67.1
  cold, effects of T69.9
    specified effect NEC T69.8
  convergence H51.12
  crying
    in child, adolescent, or adult
      R45.83
    in infant R68.11
  development, breast N62
  divergence H51.8
  drinking (alcohol) NEC (without
    dependence) F10.10
    habitual (continual) (without
      remission) F10.20
  eating R63.2
  estrogen E28.0
  fat —see also Obesity
    in heart —see Degeneration,
      myocardial
    localized E65
  foreskin N47.8
  gas R14.0
  glucagon E16.3
  heat —see Heat
  intermaxillary vertical dimension of
    fully erupted teeth M26.37
  interocclusal distance of fully erupted
    teeth M26.37
  kalium E87.5
  large
    colon K59.3
      congenital Q43.8
      infant P08.0
    organ or site, congenital NEC —see
      Anomaly, by site

Excess, excessive, excessively *(Continued)*
  long
    organ or site, congenital NEC —see
      Anomaly, by site
  menstruation (with regular cycle)
    N92.0
    with irregular cycle N92.1
  napping Z72.821
  natrium E87.0
  number of teeth K00.1
  nutrient (dietary) NEC R63.2
  potassium (K) E87.5
  salivation K11.7
  secretion —see also Hypersecretion
    milk O92.6
    sputum R09.3
    sweat R61
  sexual drive F52.8
  short
    organ or site, congenital NEC —see
      Anomaly, by site
    umbilical cord in labor or delivery
      O69.3
  skin, eyelid (acquired) —see
    Blepharochalasis
    congenital Q10.3
  sodium (Na) E87.0
  spacing of fully erupted teeth
    M26.32
  sputum R09.3
  sweating R61
  thirst R63.1
    due to deprivation of water
      T73.1
  tuberosity of jaw M26.07
  vitamin
    A (dietary) E67.0
      administered as drug (prolonged
        intake) —see Table of drugs
        and chemicals, vitamins,
        adverse effect
      overdose or wrong substance given
        or taken —see Table of drugs
        and chemicals, vitamins,
        poisoning
    D (dietary) E67.3
      administered as drug (prolonged
        intake) —see Table of drugs
        and chemicals, vitamins,
        adverse effect
      overdose or wrong substance given
        or taken —see Table of drugs
        and chemicals, vitamins,
        poisoning
  weight
    gain R63.5
    loss R63.4
Excitability, abnormal, under minor
  stress (personality disorder) F60.3
Excitation
  anomalous atrioventricular I45.6
  psychogenic F30.8
  reactive (from emotional stress,
    psychological trauma) F30.8
Excitement
  hypomanic F30.8
  manic F30.9
  mental, reactive (from emotional stress,
    psychological trauma) F30.8
  state, reactive (from emotional stress,
    psychological trauma) F30.8
Excoriation (traumatic) —see also
  Abrasion
  neurotic L98.1

Exfoliation
  due to erythematous conditions
      according to extent of body
      surface involved L49.0
    10-19 percent of body surface L49.1
    20-29 percent of body surface L49.2
    30-39 percent of body surface L49.3
    40-49 percent of body surface L49.4
    50-59 percent of body surface L49.5
    60-69 percent of body surface L49.6
    70-79 percent of body surface L49.7
    80-89 percent of body surface L49.8
    90-99 percent of body surface L49.9
    less than 10 percent of body surface
      L49.0
  teeth, due to systemic causes K08.0
Exfoliative —see condition
Exhaustion, exhaustive (physical NEC)
    R53.83
  battle F43.0
  cardiac —see Failure, heart
  delirium F43.0
  due to
    cold T69.8
    excessive exertion T73.3
    exposure T73.2
    neurasthenia F48.8
  heart —see Failure, heart
  heat (see also Heat, exhaustion) T67.5
    due to
      salt depletion T67.4
      water depletion T67.3
  maternal, complicating delivery O75.81
  mental F48.8
  myocardium, myocardial —see Failure,
    heart
  nervous F48.8
  old age R54
  psychogenic F48.8
  psychosis F43.0
  senile R54
  vital NEC Z73.0
Exhibitionism F65.2
Exocervicitis —see Cervicitis
Exomphalos Q79.2
  meaning hernia —see Hernia,
    umbilicus
Exophoria H50.52
  convergence, insufficiency H51.11
  divergence, excess H51.8
Exophthalmos H05.2-
  congenital Q15.8
  constant NEC H05.24-
  displacement, globe —see
    Displacement, globe
  due to thyrotoxicosis
    (hyperthyroidism) —see
    Hyperthyroidism, with, goiter
    (diffuse)
  dysthyroid —see Hyperthyroidism,
    with, goiter (diffuse)
  goiter —see Hyperthyroidism, with,
    goiter (diffuse)
  intermittent NEC H05.25-
  malignant —see Hyperthyroidism, with,
    goiter (diffuse)
  orbital
    edema —see Edema, orbit
    hemorrhage —see Hemorrhage,
      orbit
  pulsating NEC H05.26-
  thyrotoxic, thyrotropic —see
    Hyperthyroidism, with, goiter
    (diffuse)

Exostosis —see also Disorder, bone
  cartilaginous —see Neoplasm, bone,
    benign
  congenital (multiple) Q78.6
  external ear canal H61.81-
  gonococcal A54.49
  jaw (bone) M27.8
  multiple, congenital Q78.6
  orbit H05.35-
  osteocartilaginous —see Neoplasm,
    bone, benign
  syphilitic A52.77
Exotropia —see Strabismus, divergent
    concomitant
Explanation of
  investigation finding Z71.2
  medication Z71.89
Exposure (to) (see also Contact, with) T75.89
  acariasis Z20.7
  AIDS virus Z20.6
  air pollution Z77.110
  algae and algae toxins Z77.121
  algae bloom Z77.121
  anthrax Z20.810
  aromatic amines Z77.020
  aromatic (hazardous) compounds NEC
    Z77.028
  aromatic dyes NOS Z77.028
  arsenic Z77.010
  asbestos Z77.090
  bacterial disease NEC Z20.818
  benzene Z77.021
  blue-green algae bloom Z77.121
  body fluids (potentially hazardous)
    Z77.21
  brown tide Z77.121
  chemicals (chiefly nonmedicinal)
    (hazardous) NEC Z77.098
  cholera Z20.09
  chromium compounds Z77.018
  cold, effects of T69.9
    specified effect NEC T69.8
  communicable disease Z20.9
    bacterial NEC Z20.818
    specified NEC Z20.89
    viral NEC Z20.828
  cyanobacteria bloom Z77.121
  disaster Z65.5
  discrimination Z60.5
  dyes Z77.098
  effects of T73.9
  environmental tobacco smoke (acute)
    (chronic) Z77.22
  Escherichia coli (E. coli) Z20.01
  exhaustion due to T73.3
  fiberglass —see Table of drugs and
    chemicals, fiberglass
  German measles Z20.4
  gonorrhea Z20.2
  hazardous metals NEC Z77.018
  hazardous substances NEC Z77.29
  hazards in the physical environment
    NEC Z77.128
  hazards to health NEC Z77.9
  human immunodeficiency virus (HIV)
    Z20.6
  human T-lymphotropic virus type-1
    (HTLV-1) Z20.89
  implanted
    mesh —see Complications, mesh
    prosthetic materials NEC —see
      Complications, prosthetic
      materials NEC
  infestation (parasitic) NEC Z20.7

Exposure (Continued)
  intestinal infectious disease NEC Z20.09
    Escherichia coli (E. coli) Z20.01
  lead Z77.011
  meningococcus Z20.811
  mold (toxic) Z77.120
  nickel dust Z77.018
  noise Z77.122
  occupational
    air contaminants NEC Z57.39
    dust Z57.2
    environmental tobacco smoke Z57.31
    extreme temperature Z57.6
    noise Z57.0
    radiation Z57.1
    risk factors Z57.9
      specified NEC Z57.8
    toxic agents (gases) (liquids) (solids)
      (vapors) in agriculture Z57.4
    toxic agents (gases) (liquids) (solids)
      (vapors) in industry NEC Z57.5
    vibration Z57.7
  parasitic disease NEC Z20.7
  pediculosis Z20.7
  persecution Z60.5
  pfiesteria piscicida Z77.121
  poliomyelitis Z20.89
  pollution
    air Z77.110
    environmental NEC Z77.118
    soil Z77.112
    water Z77.111
  polycyclic aromatic hydrocarbons
    Z77.028
  prenatal (drugs) (toxic chemicals) —see
    Newborn, affected by (suspected
    to be), noxious substances
    transmitted via placenta or breast
    milk
  rabies Z20.3
  radiation, naturally occurring NEC
    Z77.123
  radon Z77.123
  red tide (Florida) Z77.121
  rubella Z20.4
  second hand tobacco smoke (acute)
    (chronic) Z77.22
    in the perinatal period P96.81
  sexually-transmitted disease Z20.2
  smallpox (laboratory) Z20.89
  syphilis Z20.2
  terrorism Z65.4
  torture Z65.4
  tuberculosis Z20.1
  uranium Z77.012
  varicella Z20.820
  venereal disease Z20.2
  viral disease NEC Z20.828
  war Z65.5
  water pollution Z77.111
Exsanguination —see Hemorrhage
Exstrophy
  abdominal contents Q45.8
  bladder Q64.10
    cloacal Q64.12
    specified type NEC Q64.19
    supravesical fissure Q64.11
Extensive —see condition
Extra —see also Accessory
  marker chromosomes (normal
    individual) Q92.61
    in abnormal individual Q92.62
  rib Q76.6
    cervical Q76.5

Extrasystoles (supraventricular) I49.49
    atrial I49.1
    auricular I49.1
    junctional I49.2
    ventricular I49.3
Extrauterine gestation or pregnancy —*see* Pregnancy, by site
Extravasation
    blood R58
    chyle into mesentery I89.8
    pelvicalyceal N13.8
    pyelosinus N13.8
    urine (from ureter) R39.0

Extravasation *(Continued)*
    vesicant agent
        antineoplastic chemotherapy T80.810
        other agent NEC T80.818
Extremity —*see* condition, limb
Extrophy —*see* Exstrophy
Extroversion
    bladder Q64.19
    uterus N81.4
        complicating delivery O71.2
        postpartal (old) N81.4
Extruded tooth (teeth) M26.34
Extrusion
    breast implant (prosthetic) T85.42
    eye implant (globe) (ball) T85.328

Extrusion *(Continued)*
    intervertebral disc —*see* Displacement, intervertebral disc
    ocular lens implant (prosthetic) —*see* Complications, intraocular lens
    vitreous —*see* Prolapse, vitreous
Exudate
    pleural —*see* Effusion, pleura
    retina H35.89
Exudative —*see* condition
Eye, eyeball, eyelid —*see* condition
Eyestrain —*see* Disturbance, vision, subjective
Eyeworm disease of Africa B74.3

F

Faber's syndrome (achlorhydric anemia) D50.9
Fabry (-Anderson) disease E75.21
Faciocephalalgia, autonomic (*see also* Neuropathy, peripheral, autonomic) G90.09
Factor (s)
  psychic, associated with diseases classified elsewhere F54
  psychological
    affecting physical conditions F54
    or behavioral
      affecting general medical condition F54
      associated with disorders or diseases classified elsewhere F54
Fahr disease (of brain) G23.8
Fahr Volhard disease (of kidney) I12.-
Failure, failed
  abortion —*see* Abortion, attempted
  aortic (valve) I35.8
    rheumatic I06.8
  attempted abortion —*see* Abortion, attempted
  biventricular I50.9
  bone marrow —*see* Anemia, aplastic
  cardiac —*see* Failure, heart
  cardiorenal (chronic) I50.9
    hypertensive I13.2
  cardiorespiratory (*see also* Failure, heart) R09.2
  cardiovascular (chronic) —*see* Failure, heart
  cerebrovascular I67.9
  cervical dilatation in labor O62.0
  circulation, circulatory (peripheral) R57.9
    newborn P29.89
  compensation —*see* Disease, heart
  compliance with medical treatment or regimen —*see* Noncompliance
  congestive —*see* Failure, heart, congestive
  dental implant (endosseous) M27.69
    due to
      failure of dental prosthesis M27.63
      lack of attached gingiva M27.62
      occlusal trauma (poor prosthetic design) M27.62
      parafunctional habits M27.62
      periodontal infection (peri-implantitis) M27.62
      poor oral hygiene M27.62
    osseointegration M27.61
      due to
        complications of systemic disease M27.61
        poor bone quality M27.61
      iatrogenic M27.61
    post-osseointegration
      biological M27.62
      due to complications of systemic disease M27.62
      iatrogenic M27.62
      mechanical M27.63
    pre-integration M27.61
    pre-osseointegration M27.61
    specified NEC M27.69
  descent of head (at term) of pregnancy (mother) O32.4
  endosseous dental implant —*see* Failure, dental implant

Failure, failed (*Continued*)
  engagement of head (term of pregnancy) (mother) O32.4
  erection (penile) (*see also* Dysfunction, sexual, male, erectile) N52.9
    nonorgqanic F52.21
  examination (s), anxiety concerning Z55.2
  expansion terminal respiratory units (newborn) (primary) P28.0
  forceps NOS (with subsequent cesarean delivery) O66.5
  gain weight (child over 28 days old) R62.51
    adult R62.7
    newborn P92.6
  genital response (male) F52.21
    female F52.22
  heart (acute) (senile) (sudden) I50.9
    with
      acute pulmonary edema —*see* Failure, ventricular, left
      decompensation —*see* Failure, heart, congestive
      dilatation —*see* Disease, heart
    arteriosclerotic I70.90
    biventricular I50.9
    combined left-right sided I50.9
    compensated I50.9
    complicating
      anesthesia (general) (local) or other sedation
        in labor and delivery O74.2
        in pregnancy O29.12-
        postpartum, puerperal O89.1
      delivery (cesarean) (instrumental) O75.4
    congestive (compensated) (decompensated) I50.9
      with rheumatic fever (conditions in I00)
        active I01.8
        inactive or quiescent (with chorea) I09.81
      newborn P29.0
      rheumatic (chronic) (inactive) (with chorea) I09.81
        active or acute I01.8
        with chorea I02.0
    decompensated I50.9
    degenerative —*see* Degeneration, myocardial
    diastolic (congestive) I50.30
      acute (congestive) I50.31
        and (on) chronic (congestive) I50.33
      chronic (congestive) I50.32
        and (on) acute (congestive) I50.33
      combined with systolic (congestive) I50.40
      acute (congestive) I50.41
        and (on) chronic (congestive) I50.43
      chronic (congestive) I50.42
        and (on) acute (congestive) I50.43
    due to presence of cardiac prosthesis I97.13-
    following cardiac surgery I97.13-
    high output NOS I50.9
    hypertensive —*see* Hypertension, heart
    left (ventricular) —*see* Failure, ventricular, left

Failure, failed (*Continued*)
  heart (*Continued*)
    low output (syndrome) NOS I50.9
    newborn P29.0
    organic —*see* Disease, heart
    peripartum O90.3
    postprocedural I97.13-
    rheumatic (chronic) (inactive) I09.9
    right (ventricular) (secondary to left heart failure) —*see* Failure, heart, congestive
    systolic (congestive) I50.20
      acute (congestive) I50.21
        and (on) chronic (congestive) I50.23
      chronic (congestive) I50.22
        and (on) acute (congestive) I50.23
      combined with diastolic (congestive) I50.40
      acute (congestive) I50.41
        and (on) chronic (congestive) I50.43
      chronic (congestive) I50.42
        and (on) acute (congestive) I50.43
    thyrotoxic (*see also* Thyrotoxicosis) E05.90 [I43]
      with thyroid storm E05.91 [I43]
    valvular —*see* Endocarditis
  hepatic K72.90
    with coma K72.91
    acute or subacute K72.00
      with coma K72.01
      due to drugs K71.10
        with coma K71.11
    alcoholic (acute) (chronic) (subacute) K70.40
      with coma K70.41
    chronic K72.10
      with coma K72.11
      due to drugs (acute) (subacute) (chronic) K71.10
        with coma K71.11
    due to drugs (acute) (subacute) (chronic) K71.10
      with coma K71.11
    postprocedural K91.82
  hepatorenal K76.7
  induction (of labor) O61.9
    abortion —*see* Abortion, attempted
    by
      oxytocic drugs O61.0
      prostaglandins O61.0
    instrumental O61.1
    mechanical O61.1
    medical O61.0
    specified NEC O61.8
    surgical O61.1
  intubation during anesthesia T88.4
    in pregnancy O29.6-
    labor and delivery O74.7
    postpartum, puerperal O89.6
  involution, thymus (gland) E32.0
  kidney (*see also* Disease, kidney, chronic) N19
    acute (*see also* Failure, renal, acute) N17.9
  lactation (complete) O92.3
    partial O92.4
  Leydig's cell, adult E29.1
  liver —*see* Failure, hepatic
  menstruation at puberty N91.0
  mitral I05.8

Failure, failed *(Continued)*
  myocardial, myocardium *(see also Failure, heart)* I50.9
    chronic *(see also Failure, heart, congestive)* I50.9
    congestive *(see also Failure, heart, congestive)* I50.9
  orgasm (female) (psychogenic) F52.31
    male F52.32
  ovarian (primary) E28.39
    iatrogenic E89.40
      asymptomatic E89.40
      symptomatic E89.41
    postprocedural (postablative) (postirradiation) (postsurgical) E89.40
      asymptomatic E89.40
      symptomatic E89.41
  ovulation causing infertility N97.0
  polyglandular, autoimmune E31.0
  prosthetic joint implant —*see* Complications, joint prosthesis, mechanical, breakdown, by site
  renal N19
    with
      tubular necrosis (acute) N17.0
    acute N17.9
      with
        cortical necrosis N17.1
        medullary necrosis N17.2
        tubular necrosis N17.0
      specified NEC N17.8
    chronic N18.9
      hypertensive —*see* Hypertension, kidney
    congenital P96.0
    end stage (chronic) N18.6
      due to hypertension I12.0
    following
      abortion —*see* Abortion by type complicated by specified condition NEC
      crushing T79.5
      ectopic or molar pregnancy O08.4
      labor and delivery (acute) O90.4
    hypertensive —*see* Hypertension, kidney
    postprocedural N99.0
  respiration, respiratory J96.9
    with
      hypercapnia J96.92
      hypoxia J96.91
    acute J96.00
      with
        hypercapnia J96.02
        hypoxia J96.01
    acute and (on) chronic J96.20
      with
        hypercapnia J96.22
        hypoxia J96.21
    center G93.89
    chronic J96.10
      with
        hypercapnia J96.12
        hypoxia J96.11
    newborn P28.5
    postprocedural (acute) J95.821
      acute and chronic J95.822
  rotation
    cecum Q43.3
    colon Q43.3
    intestine Q43.3
    kidney Q63.2
  sedation (conscious) (moderate) during procedure T88.52
    history of Z92.83

Failure, failed *(Continued)*
  segmentation —*see also* Fusion
    fingers —*see* Syndactylism, complex, fingers
    vertebra Q76.49
      with scoliosis Q76.3
  seminiferous tubule, adult E29.1
  senile (general) R54
  sexual arousal (male) F52.21
    female F52.22
  testicular endocrine function E29.1
  to thrive (child over 28 days old) R62.51
    adult R62.7
    newborn P92.6
  transplant T86.92
    bone T86.831
      marrow T86.02
    cornea T86.841
    heart T86.22
      with lung (s) T86.32
    intestine T86.851
    kidney T86.12
    liver T86.42
    lung (s) T86.811
      with heart T86.32
    pancreas T86.891
    skin (allograft) (autograft) T86.821
    specified organ or tissue NEC T86.891
    stem cell (peripheral blood) (umbilical cord) T86.5
  trial of labor (with subsequent cesarean delivery) O66.40
    following previous cesarean delivery O66.41
  tubal ligation N99.89
  urinary —*see* Disease, kidney, chronic
  vacuum extraction NOS (with subsequent cesarean delivery) O66.5
  vasectomy N99.89
  ventouse NOS (with subsequent cesarean delivery) O66.5
  ventricular *(see also Failure, heart)* I50.9
    left I50.1
      with rheumatic fever (conditions in I00)
        active I01.8
          with chorea I02.0
        inactive or quiescent (with chorea) I09.81
      rheumatic (chronic) (inactive) (with chorea) I09.81
        active or acute I01.8
          with chorea I02.0
    right *(see also Failure, heart, congestive)* I50.9
  vital centers, newborn P91.8
Fainting (fit) R55
Fallen arches —*see* Deformity, limb, flat foot
Falling, falls (repeated) R29.6
  any organ or part —*see* Prolapse
Fallopian
  insufflation Z31.41
  tube —*see* condition
Fallot's
  pentalogy Q21.8
  tetrad or tetralogy Q21.3
  triad or trilogy Q22.3
False —*see also* condition
  croup J38.5
  joint —*see* Nonunion, fracture
  labor (pains) O47.9
    at or after 37 completed weeks of gestation O47.1
    before 37 completed weeks of gestation O47.0-

False *(Continued)*
  passage, urethra (prostatic) N36.5
  pregnancy F45.8
Family, familial —*see also* condition
  disruption Z63.8
    involving divorce or separation Z63.5
  Li-Fraumeni (syndrome) Z15.01
  planning advice Z30.09
  problem Z63.9
    specified NEC Z63.8
  retinoblastoma C69.2-
Famine (effects of) T73.0
  edema —*see* Malnutrition, severe
Fanconi (-de Toni)(-Debré) syndrome E72.09
  with cystinosis E72.04
Fanconi's anemia (congenital pancytopenia) D61.09
Farber's disease or syndrome E75.29
Farcy A24.0
Farmer's
  lung J67.0
  skin L57.8
Farsightedness —*see* Hypermetropia
Fascia —*see* condition
Fasciculation R25.3
Fasciitis M72.9
  diffuse (eosinophilic) M35.4
  infective M72.8
    necrotizing M72.6
  necrotizing M72.6
  nodular M72.4
  perirenal (with ureteral obstruction) N13.5
    with infection N13.6
  plantar M72.2
  specified NEC M72.8
  traumatic (old) M72.8
    current - code by site under Sprain
Fascioliasis B66.3
Fasciolopsis, fasciolopsiasis (intestinal) B66.5
Fascioscapulohumeral myopathy G71.0
Fast pulse R00.0
Fat
  embolism —*see* Embolism, fat
  excessive —*see also* Obesity
    in heart —*see* Degeneration, myocardial
  in stool R19.5
  localized (pad) E65
    heart —*see* Degeneration, myocardial
    knee M79.4
    retropatellar M79.4
  necrosis
    breast N64.1
    mesentery K65.4
    omentum K65.4
  pad E65
    knee M79.4
Fatigue R53.83
  auditory deafness —*see* Deafness
  chronic R53.82
  combat F43.0
  general R53.83
    psychogenic F48.8
  heat (transient) T67.6
  muscle M62.89
  myocardium —*see* Failure, heart
  neoplasm-related R53.0
  nervous, neurosis F48.8
  operational F48.8
  psychogenic (general) F48.8
  senile R54
  voice R49.8

Fatness —*see* Obesity
Fatty —*see also* condition
　apron E65
　degeneration —*see* Degeneration, fatty
　heart (enlarged) —*see* Degeneration,
　　myocardial
　liver NEC K76.0
　　alcoholic K70.0
　　nonalcoholic K76.0
　necrosis —*see* Degeneration, fatty
Fauces —*see* condition
Fauchard's disease (periodontitis) —*see*
　Periodontitis
Faucitis J02.9
Favism (anemia) D55.0
Favus —*see* Dermatophytosis
Fazio-Londe disease or syndrome G12.1
Fear complex or reaction F40.9
Fear of —*see* Phobia
Feared complaint unfounded Z71.1
Febris, febrile —*see also* Fever
　flava (*see also* Fever, yellow) A95.9
　melitensis A23.0
　pestis —*see* Plague
　recurrens —*see* Fever, relapsing
　rubra A38.9
Fecal
　incontinence R15.9
　smearing R15.1
　soiling R15.1
　urgency R15.2
Fecalith (impaction) K56.41
　appendix K38.1
　congenital P76.8
Fede's disease K14.0
Feeble rapid pulse due to shock
　following injury T79.4
Feeble-minded F70
Feeding
　difficulties R63.3
　problem R63.3
　　newborn P92.9
　　　specified NEC P92.8
　　nonorganic (adult) —*see* Disorder,
　　　eating
Feeling (of)
　foreign body in throat R09.89
Feer's disease —*see* Poisoning, mercury
Feet —*see* condition
Feigned illness Z76.5
Feil-Klippel syndrome (brevicollis) Q76.1
Feinmesser's (hidrotic) ectodermal
　dysplasia Q82.4
Felinophobia F40.218
Felon —*see also* Cellulitis, digit
　with lymphangitis —*see* Lymphangitis,
　　acute, digit
Felty's syndrome M05.00
　ankle M05.07-
　elbow M05.02-
　foot joint M05.07-
　hand joint M05.04-
　hip M05.05-
　knee M05.06-
　multiple site M05.09
　shoulder M05.01-
　vertebra —*see* Spondylitis, ankylosing
　wrist M05.03-
Female gential cutting status —*see*
　Female genital mutilation status
　(FGM)
Female genital mutilation status (FGM)
　N90.810
　specified NEC N90.818
　type I (clitorectomy status) N90.811

Female genital mutilation status
　(*Continued*)
　type II (clitorectomy with excision of
　　labia minora status) N90.812
　type III (infibulation status) N90.813
　type IV N90.818
Femur, femoral —*see* condition
Fenestration, fenestrated —*see also*
　Imperfect, closure
　aortico-pulmonary Q21.4
　cusps, heart valve NEC Q24.8
　　pulmonary Q22.3
　pulmonic cusps Q22.3
Fernell's disease (aortic aneurysm) I71.9
Fertile eunuch syndrome E23.0
Fetid
　breath R19.6
　sweat L75.0
Fetishism F65.0
　transvestic F65.1
Fetus, fetal —*see also* condition
　alcohol syndrome (dysmorphic) Q86.0
　compressus O31.0-
　hydantoin syndrome Q86.1
　lung tissue P28.0
　papyraceous O31.0-
Fever (inanition) (of unknown origin)
　　(persistent) (with chills) (with rigor)
　　R50.9
　abortus A23.1
　Aden (dengue) A90
　African tick-borne A68.1
　American
　　mountain (tick) A93.2
　　spotted A77.0
　aphthous B08.8
　arbovirus, arboviral A94
　　hemorrhagic A94
　　specified NEC A93.8
　Argentinian hemorrhagic A96.0
　Assam B55.0
　Australian Q A78
　Bangkok hemorrhagic A91
　Barmah forest A92.8
　Bartonella A44.0
　bilious, hemoglobinuric B50.8
　blackwater B50.8
　blister B00.1
　Bolivian hemorrhagic A96.1
　Bonvale dam T73.3
　boutonneuse A77.1
　brain —*see* Encephalitis
　Brazilian purpuric A48.4
　breakbone A90
　Bullis A77.0
　Bunyamwera A92.8
　Burdwan B55.0
　Bwamba A92.8
　Cameroon —*see* Malaria
　Canton A75.9
　catarrhal (acute) J00
　　chronic J31.0
　cat-scratch A28.1
　Central Asian hemorrhagic A98.0
　cerebral —*see* Encephalitis
　cerebrospinal meningococcal A39.0
　Chagres B50.9
　Chandipura A92.8
　Changuinola A93.1
　Charcot's (biliary) (hepatic)
　　(intermittent) —*see* Calculus,
　　bile duct
　Chikungunya (viral) (hemorrhagic) A92.0
　Chitral A93.1
　Colombo —*see* Fever, paratyphoid

Fever (*Continued*)
　Colorado tick (virus) A93.2
　congestive (remittent) —*see* Malaria
　Congo virus A98.0
　continued malarial B50.9
　Corsican —*see* Malaria
　Crimean-Congo hemorrhagic A98.0
　Cyprus —*see* Brucellosis
　dandy A90
　deer fly —*see* Tularemia
　dengue (virus) A90
　　hemorrhagic A91
　　sandfly A93.1
　desert B38.0
　drug induced R50.2
　due to conditions classified elsewhere
　　R50.81
　due to heat T67.0
　enteric A01.00
　enteroviral exanthematous (Boston
　　exanthem) A88.0
　ephemeral (of unknown origin) R50.9
　epidemic hemorrhagic A98.5
　erysipelatous —*see* Erysipelas
　estivo-autumnal (malarial) B50.9
　famine A75.0
　five day A79.0
　following delivery O86.4
　Fort Bragg A27.89
　gastroenteric A01.00
　gastromalarial —*see* Malaria
　Gibraltar —*see* Brucellosis
　glandular —*see* Mononucleosis,
　　infectious
　Guama (viral) A92.8
　Haverhill A25.1
　hay (allergic) J30.1
　　with asthma (bronchial) J45.909
　　　with
　　　　exacerbation (acute) J45.901
　　　　status asthmaticus J45.902
　　　due to
　　　　allergen other than pollen J30.89
　　　　pollen, any plant or tree J30.1
　heat (effects) T67.0
　hematuric, bilious B50.8
　hemoglobinuric (malarial) (bilious) B50.8
　hemorrhagic (arthropod-borne) NOS A94
　　with renal syndrome A98.5
　　arenaviral A96.9
　　　specified NEC A96.8
　　Argentinian A96.0
　　Bangkok A91
　　Bolivian A96.1
　　Central Asian A98.0
　　Chikungunya A92.0
　　Crimean-Congo A98.0
　　dengue (virus) A91
　　epidemic A98.5
　　Junin (virus) A96.0
　　Korean A98.5
　　Kyasanur forest A98.2
　　Machupo (virus) A96.1
　　mite-borne A93.8
　　mosquito-borne A92.8
　　Omsk A98.1
　　Philippine A91
　　Russian A98.5
　　Singapore A91
　　Southeast Asia A91
　　Thailand A91
　　tick-borne NEC A93.8
　　viral A99
　　　specified NEC A98.8

Fever *(Continued)*
  hepatic —*see* Cholecystitis
  herpetic —*see* Herpes
  icterohemorrhagic A27.0
  Indiana A93.8
  infective B99.9
    specified NEC B99.8
  intermittent (bilious) —*see also* Malaria
    of unknown origin R50.9
    pernicious B50.9
  iodide R50.2
  Japanese river A75.3
  jungle —*see also* Malaria
    yellow A95.0
  Junin (virus) hemorrhagic A96.0
  Katayama B65.2
  kedani A75.3
  Kenya (tick) A77.1
  Kew Garden A79.1
  Korean hemorrhagic A98.5
  Lassa A96.2
  Lone Star A77.0
  Machupo (virus) hemorrhagic A96.1
  malaria, malarial —*see* Malaria
  Malta A23.9
  Marseilles A77.1
  marsh —*see* Malaria
  Mayaro (viral) A92.8
  Mediterranean (*see also* Brucellosis) A23.9
    familial E85.0
    tick A77.1
  meningeal —*see* Meningitis
  Meuse A79.0
  Mexican A75.2
  mianeh A68.1
  miasmatic —*see* Malaria
  mosquito-borne (viral) A92.9
    hemorrhagic A92.8
  mountain —*see also* Brucellosis
    meaning Rocky Mountain spotted
      fever A77.0
    tick (American) (Colorado) (viral)
      A93.2
  Mucambo (viral) A92.8
  mud A27.9
  Neapolitan —*see* Brucellosis
  neutropenic D70.9
  newborn P81.9
    environmental P81.0
  Nine-Mile A78
  non-exanthematous tick A93.2
  North Asian tick-borne A77.2
  Omsk hemorrhagic A98.1
  O'nyong-nyong (viral) A92.1
  Oropouche (viral) A93.0
  Oroya A44.0
  paludal —*see* Malaria
  Panama (malarial) B50.9
  Pappataci A93.1
  paratyphoid A01.4
    A A01.1
    B A01.2
    C A01.3
  parrot A70
  periodic (Mediterranean) E85.0
  persistent (of unknown origin) R50.9
  petechial A39.0
  pharyngoconjunctival B30.2
  Philippine hemorrhagic A91
  phlebotomus A93.1
  Piry (virus) A93.8
  Pixuna (viral) A92.8
  Plasmodium ovale B53.0
  polioviral (nonparalytic) A80.4

Fever *(Continued)*
  Pontiac A48.2
  postimmunization R50.83
  postoperative R50.82
    due to infection T81.4
  posttransfusion R50.84
  postvaccination R50.83
  presenting with conditions classified
    elsewhere R50.81
  pretibial A27.89
  puerperal O86.4
  Q A78
  quadrilateral A78
  quartan (malaria) B52.9
  Queensland (coastal) (tick) A77.3
  quintan A79.0
  rabbit —*see* Tularemia
  rat-bite A25.9
    due to
      Spirillum A25.0
      Streptobacillus moniliformis A25.1
  recurrent —*see* Fever, relapsing
  relapsing (Borrelia) A68.9
    Carter's (Asiatic) A68.1
    Dutton's (West African) A68.1
    Koch's A68.9
    louse-borne A68.0
    Novy's
      louse-borne A68.0
      tick-borne A68.1
    Obermeyer's (European) A68.0
    tick-borne A68.1
  remittent (bilious) (congestive)
    (gastric) —*see* Malaria
  rheumatic (active) (acute) (chronic)
    (subacute) I00
    with central nervous system
      involvement I02.9
    active with heart involvement (*see*
      category) I01
    inactive or quiescent with
      cardiac hypertrophy I09.89
      carditis I09.9
      endocarditis I09.1
        aortic (valve) I06.9
          with mitral (valve) disease I08.0
        mitral (valve) I05.9
          with aortic (valve) disease I08.0
        pulmonary (valve) I09.89
        tricuspid (valve) I07.8
      heart disease NEC I09.89
      heart failure (congestive)
        (conditions in I50.9) I09.81
      left ventricular failure (conditions
        in I50.1) I09.81
      myocarditis, myocardial
        degeneration (conditions
        in I51.4) I09.0
      pancarditis I09.9
      pericarditis I09.2
  Rift Valley (viral) A92.4
  Rocky Mountain spotted A77.0
  rose J30.1
  Ross River B33.1
  Russian hemorrhagic A98.5
  San Joaquin (Valley) B38.0
  sandfly A93.1
  Sao Paulo A77.0
  scarlet A38.9
  seven day (leptospirosis) (autumnal)
    (Japanese) A27.89
    dengue A90
  shin-bone A79.0
  Singapore hemorrhagic A91

Fever *(Continued)*
  solar A90
  Songo A98.5
  sore B00.1
  South African tick-bite A68.1
  Southeast Asia hemorrhagic A91
  spinal —*see* Meningitis
  spirillary A25.0
  splenic —*see* Anthrax
  spotted A77.9
    American A77.0
    Brazilian A77.0
    cerebrospinal meningitis A39.0
    Colombian A77.0
    due to Rickettsia
      australis A77.3
      conorii A77.1
      rickettsii A77.0
      sibirica A77.2
      specified type NEC A77.8
    Ehrlichiosis A77.40
      due to
        E. chafeensis A77.41
        specified organism NEC
          A77.49
    Rocky Mountain A77.0
  steroid R50.2
  streptobacillary A25.1
  subtertian B50.9
  Sumatran mite A75.3
  sun A90
  swamp A27.9
  swine A02.8
  sylvatic, yellow A95.0
  Tahyna B33.8
  tertian —*see* Malaria, tertian
  Thailand hemorrhagic A91
  thermic T67.0
  three-day A93.1
  tick
    American mountain A93.2
    Colorado A93.2
    Kemerovo A93.8
    Mediterranean A77.1
    mountain A93.2
    nonexanthematous A93.2
    Quaranfil A93.8
  tick-bite NEC A93.8
  tick-borne (hemorrhagic) NEC
    A93.8
  trench A79.0
  tsutsugamushi A75.3
  typhogastric A01.00
  typhoid (abortive) (hemorrhagic)
    (intermittent) (malignant)
    A01.00
    complicated by
      arthritis A01.04
      heart involvement A01.02
      meningitis A01.01
      osteomyelitis A01.05
      pneumonia A01.03
      specified NEC A01.09
  typhomalarial —*see* Malaria
  typhus —*see* Typhus (fever)
  undulant —*see* Brucellosis
  unknown origin R50.9
  uveoparotid D86.89
  valley B38.0
  Venezuelan equine A92.2
  vesicular stomatitis A93.8
  viral hemorrhagic —*see* Fever,
    hemorrhagic, by type of virus
  Volhynian A79.0
  Wesselsbron (viral) A92.8

Fever *(Continued)*
West
  African B50.8
  Nile (viral) A92.30
    with
      complications NEC A92.39
      cranial nerve disorders A92.32
      encephalitis A92.31
      encephalomyelitis A92.31
      neurologic manifestation NEC
        A92.32
      optic neuritis A92.32
      polyradiculitis A92.32
  Whitmore's —*see* Melioidosis
  Wolhynian A79.0
  worm B83.9
  yellow A95.9
    jungle A95.0
    sylvatic A95.0
    urban A95.1
  Zika (viral) A92.8
Fibrillation
  atrial or auricular (established) I48.91
    chronic I48.2
    paroxysmal I48.0
    permanent I48.2
    persistent I48.1
  cardiac I49.8
  heart I49.8
  muscular M62.89
  ventricular I49.01
Fibrin
  ball or bodies, pleural (sac) J94.1
  chamber, anterior (eye) (gelatinous
    exudate) —*see* Iridocyclitis, acute
Fibrinogenolysis —*see* Fibrinolysis
Fibrinogenopenia D68.8
  acquired D65
  congenital D68.2
Fibrinolysis (hemorrhagic) (acquired) D65
  antepartum hemorrhage —*see*
    Hemorrhage, antepartum, with
    coagulation defect
  following
    abortion —*see* Abortion by type
      complicated by hemorrhage
    ectopic or molar pregnancy O08.1
  intrapartum O67.0
  newborn, transient P60
  postpartum O72.3
Fibrinopenia (hereditary) D68.2
  acquired D68.4
Fibrinopurulent —*see* condition
Fibrinous —*see* condition
Fibroadenoma
  cellular intracanalicular D24-
  giant D24-
  intracanalicular
    cellular D24-
    giant D24-
    specified site —*see* Neoplasm, benign,
      by site
    unspecified site D24-
  juvenile D24-
  pericanalicular
    specified site —*see* Neoplasm, benign,
      by site
    unspecified site D24-
  phyllodes D24-
  prostate D29.1
  specified site NEC —*see* Neoplasm,
    benign, by site
  unspecified site D24-
Fibroadenosis, breast (chronic) (cystic)
  (diffuse) (periodic) (segmental) N60.2-

Fibroangioma —*see also* Neoplasm,
  benign, by site
  juvenile
    specified site —*see* Neoplasm, benign,
      by site
    unspecified site D10.6
Fibrochondrosarcoma —*see* Neoplasm,
  cartilage, malignant
Fibrocystic
  disease —*see also* Fibrosis, cystic
    breast —*see* Mastopathy, cystic
    jaw M27.49
    kidney (congenital) Q61.8
    liver Q44.6
    pancreas E84.9
  kidney (congenital) Q61.8
Fibrodysplasia ossificans progressiva —
  see Myositis, ossificans, progressiva
Fibroelastosis (cordis) (endocardial)
  (endomyocardial) I42.4
Fibroid (tumor) —*see also* Neoplasm,
  connective tissue, benign
  disease, lung (chronic) —*see* Fibrosis,
    lung
  heart (disease) —*see* Myocarditis
  in pregnancy or childbirth O34.1-
    causing obstructed labor O65.5
  induration, lung (chronic) —*see*
    Fibrosis, lung
  lung —*see* Fibrosis, lung
  pneumonia (chronic) —*see* Fibrosis,
    lung
  uterus D25.9
Fibrolipoma —*see* Lipoma
Fibroliposarcoma —*see* Neoplasm,
  connective tissue, malignant
Fibroma —*see also* Neoplasm, connective
  tissue, benign
  ameloblastic —*see* Cyst, calcifying
    odontogenic
  bone (nonossifying) —*see* Disorder,
    bone, specified type NEC
    ossifying —*see* Neoplasm, bone,
      benign
  cementifying —*see* Neoplasm, bone,
    benign
  chondromyxoid —*see* Neoplasm, bone,
    benign
  desmoplastic —*see* Neoplasm,
    connective tissue, uncertain
    behavior
  durum —*see* Neoplasm, connective
    tissue, benign
  fascial —*see* Neoplasm, connective
    tissue, benign
  invasive —*see* Neoplasm, connective
    tissue, uncertain behavior
  molle —*see* Lipoma
  myxoid —*see* Neoplasm, connective
    tissue, benign
  nasopharynx, nasopharyngeal
    (juvenile) D10.6
  nonosteogenic (nonossifying) —*see*
    Dysplasia, fibrous
  odontogenic (central) —*see* Cyst,
    calcifying odontogenic
  ossifying —*see* Neoplasm, bone, benign
  periosteal —*see* Neoplasm, bone, benign
  soft —*see* Lipoma
Fibromatosis M72.9
  abdominal —*see* Neoplasm, connective
    tissue, uncertain behavior
  aggressive —*see* Neoplasm, connective
    tissue, uncertain behavior

Fibromatosis *(Continued)*
  congenital generalized —*see* Neoplasm,
    connective tissue, uncertain
    behavior
  Dupuytren's M72.0
  gingival K06.1
  palmar (fascial) M72.0
  plantar (fascial) M72.2
  pseudosarcomatous (proliferative)
    (subcutaneous) M72.4
  retroperitoneal D48.3
  specified NEC M72.8
Fibromyalgia M79.7
Fibromyoma —*see also* Neoplasm,
  connective tissue, benign
  uterus (corpus) —*see also* Leiomyoma,
    uterus
  in pregnancy or childbirth —*see*
    Fibroid, in pregnancy or
    childbirth
  causing obstructed labor O65.5
Fibromyositis M79.7
Fibromyxolipoma D17.9
Fibromyxoma —*see* Neoplasm, connective
  tissue, benign
Fibromyxosarcoma —*see* Neoplasm,
  connective tissue, malignant
Fibro-odontoma, ameloblastic —*see* Cyst,
  calcifying odontogenic
Fibro-osteoma —*see* Neoplasm, bone,
  benign
Fibroplasia, retrolental H35.17
Fibropurulent —*see* condition
Fibrosarcoma —*see also* Neoplasm,
  connective tissue, malignant
  ameloblastic C41.1
    upper jaw (bone) C41.0
  congenital —*see* Neoplasm, connective
    tissue, malignant
  fascial —*see* Neoplasm, connective
    tissue, malignant
  infantile —*see* Neoplasm, connective
    tissue, malignant
  odontogenic C41.1
    upper jaw (bone) C41.0
  periosteal —*see* Neoplasm, bone,
    malignant
Fibrosclerosis
  breast N60.3-
  multifocal M35.5
  penis (corpora cavernosa)
    N48.6
Fibrosis, fibrotic
  adrenal (gland) E27.8
  amnion O41.8X-
  anal papillae K62.89
  arteriocapillary —*see* Arteriosclerosis
  bladder N32.89
    interstitial —*see* Cystitis, chronic,
      interstitial
    localized submucosal —*see* Cystitis,
      chronic, interstitial
    panmural —*see* Cystitis, chronic,
      interstitial
  breast —*see* Fibrosclerosis, breast
  capillary (*see also* Arteriosclerosis)
    I70.90
    lung (chronic) —*see* Fibrosis,
      lung
  cardiac —*see* Myocarditis
  cervix N88.8
  chorion O41.8X-
  corpus cavernosum (sclerosing)
    N48.6

Fibrosis, fibrotic (Continued)
cystic (of pancreas) E84.9
  with
    distal intestinal obstruction
        syndrome E84.19
    fecal impaction E84.19
    intestinal manifestations NEC E84.19
    pulmonary manifestations E84.0
    specified manifestations NEC E84.8
  due to device, implant or graft (see also
      Complications, by site and type,
      specified NEC) T85.82
    arterial graft NEC T82.828
    breast (implant) T85.82
    catheter NEC T85.82
      dialysis (renal) T82.828
        intraperitoneal T85.82
      infusion NEC T82.828
        spinal (epidural) (subdural)
            T85.82
      urinary (indwelling) T83.82
    electronic (electrode) (pulse
        generator) (stimulator)
      bone T84.82
      cardiac T82.827
      nervous system (brain) (peripheral
          nerve) (spinal) T85.82
      urinary T83.82
    fixation, internal (orthopedic) NEC
        T84.82
    gastrointestinal (bile duct)
        (esophagus) T85.82
    genital NEC T83.82
    heart NEC T82.827
    joint prosthesis T84.82
    ocular (corneal graft) (orbital
        implant) NEC T85.82
    orthopedic NEC T84.82
    specified NEC T85.82
    urinary NEC T83.82
    vascular NEC T82.828
    ventricular intracranial shunt T85.82
  ejaculatory duct N50.8
  endocardium —see Endocarditis
  endomyocardial (tropical) I42.3
  epididymis N50.8
  eye muscle —see Strabismus,
      mechanical
  heart —see Myocarditis
  hepatic —see Fibrosis, liver
  hepatolienal (portal hypertension)
      K76.6
  hepatosplenic (portal hypertension)
      K76.6
  infrapatellar fat pad M79.4
  intrascrotal N50.8
  kidney N26.9
  liver K74.0
    with sclerosis K74.2
    alcoholic K70.2
  lung (atrophic) (chronic) (confluent)
      (massive) (perialveolar)
      (peribronchial) J84.10
    with
      anthracosilicosis J60
      anthracosis J60
      asbestosis J61
      bagassosis J67.1
      bauxite J63.1
      berylliosis J63.2
      byssinosis J66.0
      calcicosis J62.8
      chalicosis J62.8
      dust reticulation J64

Fibrosis, fibrotic (Continued)
  lung (Continued)
    with (Continued)
      farmer's lung J67.0
      ganister disease J62.8
      graphite J63.3
      pneumoconiosis NOS J64
      siderosis J63.4
      silicosis J62.8
    capillary J84.10
    congenital P27.8
    diffuse (idiopathic) J84.10
      chemicals, gases, fumes or vapors
          (inhalation) J68.4
      interstitial J84.10
        acute J84.114
      talc J62.0
    following radiation J70.1
    idiopathic J84.112
    postinflammatory J84.10
    silicotic J62.8
    tuberculous —see Tuberculosis,
        pulmonary
  lymphatic gland I89.8
  median bar —see Hyperplasia,
      prostate
  mediastinum (idiopathic) J98.5
  meninges G96.19
  myocardium, myocardial —see
      Myocarditis
  ovary N83.8
  oviduct N83.8
  pancreas K86.8
  penis NEC N48.6
  pericardium I31.0
  perineum, in pregnancy or childbirth
      O34.7-
    causing obstructed labor
        O65.5
  pleura J94.1
  popliteal fat pad M79.4
  prostate (chronic) —see Hyperplasia,
      prostate
  pulmonary (see also Fibrosis, lung)
      J84.10
    congenital P27.8
    idiopathic J84.112
  rectal sphincter K62.89
  retroperitoneal, idiopathic (with
      ureteral obstruction) N13.5
    with infection N13.6
  sclerosing mesenteric (idiopathic)
      K65.4
  scrotum N50.8
  seminal vesicle N50.8
  senile R54
  skin L90.5
  spermatic cord N50.8
  spleen D73.89
    in schistosomiasis (bilharziasis) B65.9
        [D77]
  subepidermal nodular —see Neoplasm,
      skin, benign
  submucous (oral) (tongue) K13.5
  testis N44.8
    chronic, due to syphilis A52.76
  thymus (gland) E32.8
  tongue, submucous K13.5
  tunica vaginalis N50.8
  uterus (non-neoplastic) N85.8
  vagina N89.8
  valve, heart —see Endocarditis
  vas deferens N50.8
  vein I87.8

Fibrositis (periarticular) M79.7
  nodular, chronic (Jaccoud's)
      (rheumatoid) —see Arthropathy,
      postrheumatic, chronic
      Fibrothorax J94.1
Fibrotic —see Fibrosis
Fibrous —see condition
Fibroxanthoma —see also Neoplasm,
    connective tissue, benign
  atypical —see Neoplasm, connective
      tissue, uncertain behavior
  malignant —see Neoplasm, connective
      tissue, malignant
Fibroxanthosarcoma —see Neoplasm,
    connective tissue, malignant
Fiedler's
  disease (icterohemorrhagic
      leptospirosis) A27.0
  myocarditis (acute) I40.1
Fifth disease B08.3
  venereal A55
Filaria, filarial, filariasis —see Infestation,
    filarial
Filatov's disease —see Mononucleosis,
    infectious
File-cutter's disease —see Poisoning,
    lead
Filling defect
  biliary tract R93.2
  bladder R93.4
  duodenum R93.3
  gallbladder R93.2
  gastrointestinal tract R93.3
  intestine R93.3
  kidney R93.4
  stomach R93.3
  ureter R93.4
Fimbrial cyst Q50.4
Financial problem affecting care NOS
    Z59.9
  bankruptcy Z59.8
  foreclosure on loan Z59.8
Findings, abnormal, inconclusive,
    without diagnosis —see also
    Abnormal
  17-ketosteroids, elevated R82.5
  acetonuria R82.4
  alcohol in blood R78.0
  anisocytosis R71.8
  antenatal screening of mother O28.9
    biochemical O28.1
    chromosomal O28.5
    cytological O28.2
    genetic O28.5
    hematological O28.0
    radiological O28.4
    specified NEC O28.8
    ultrasonic O28.3
  antibody titer, elevated R76.0
  anticardiolipin antibody R76.0
  antiphosphatidylglycerol antibody
      R76.0
  antiphosphatidylinositol antibody
      R76.0
  antiphosphatidylserine antibody R76.0
  antiphospholipid antibody R76.0
  bacteriuria N39.0
  bicarbonate E87.8
  bile in urine R82.2
  blood sugar R73.09
    high R73.9
    low (transient) E16.2
  body fluid or substance, specified NEC
      R88.8

Findings, abnormal, inconclusive,
   without diagnosis (Continued)
casts, urine R82.99
catecholamines R82.5
cells, urine R82.99
chloride E87.8
cholesterol E78.9
   high E78.0
      with high triglycerides E78.2
chyluria R82.0
cloudy
   dialysis effluent R88.0
   urine R82.90
creatinine clearance R94.4
crystals, urine R82.99
culture
   blood R78.81
   positive —see Positive, culture
echocardiogram R93.1
electrolyte level, urinary R82.99
function study NEC R94.8
   bladder R94.8
   endocrine NEC R94.7
      thyroid R94.6
   kidney R94.4
   liver R94.5
   pancreas R94.8
   placenta R94.8
   pulmonary R94.2
   spleen R94.8
gallbladder, nonvisualization R93.2
glucose (tolerance test) (non-fasting)
   R73.09
glycosuria R81
heart
   shadow R93.1
   sounds R01.2
hematinuria R82.3
hematocrit drop (precipitous) R71.0
hemoglobinuria R82.3
human papillomavirus (HPV) DNA test
   positive
   cervix
      high risk R87.810
      low risk R87.820
   vagina
      high risk R87.811
      low risk R87.821
in blood (of substance not normally
   found in blood) R78.9
   addictive drug NEC R78.4
   alcohol (excessive level) R78.0
   cocaine R78.2
   hallucinogen R78.3
   heavy metals (abnormal level) R78.79
   lead R78.71
   lithium (abnormal level) R78.89
   opiate drug R78.1
   psychotropic drug R78.5
   specified substance NEC R78.89
   steroid agent R78.6
indoleacetic acid, elevated R82.5
ketonuria R82.4
lactic acid dehydrogenase (LDH) R74.0
liver function test R79.89
mammogram NEC R92.8
   calcification (calculus) R92.1
   inconclusive result (due to dense
      breasts) R92.2
   microcalcification R92.0
mediastinal shift R93.8
melanin, urine R82.99
myoglobinuria R82.1
neonatal screening P09

Findings, abnormal, inconclusive,
   without diagnosis (Continued)
nonvisualization of gallbladder
   R93.2
odor of urine NOS R82.90
Papanicolaou cervix R87.619
   non-atypical endometrial cells
      R87.618
pneumoencephalogram R93.0
poikilocytosis R71.8
potassium (deficiency) E87.6
   excess E87.5
PPD R76.11
radiologic (X-ray) R93.8
   abdomen R93.5
   biliary tract R93.2
   breast R92.8
   gastrointestinal tract R93.3
   genitourinary organs R93.8
   head R93.0
   inconclusive due to excess body fat of
      patient R93.9
   intrathoracic organs NEC R93.1
   placenta R93.8
   retroperitoneum R93.5
   skin R93.8
   skull R93.0
   subcutaneous tissue R93.8
red blood cell (count) (morphology)
   (sickling) (volume) R71.8
scan NEC R94.8
   bladder R94.8
   bone R94.8
   kidney R94.4
   liver R93.2
   lung R94.2
   pancreas R94.8
   placental R94.8
   spleen R94.8
   thyroid R94.6
sedimentation rate, elevated R70.0
SGOT R74.0
SGPT R74.0
sodium (deficiency) E87.1
   excess E87.0
specified body fluid NEC R88.8
stress test R94.39
thyroid (function) (metabolic rate)
   (scan) (uptake) R94.6
transaminase (level) R74.0
triglycerides E78.9
   high E78.1
      with high cholesterol E78.2
tuberculin skin test (without active
   tuberculosis) R76.11
urine R82.90
   acetone R82.4
   bacteria N39.0
   bile R82.2
   casts or cells R82.99
   chyle R82.0
   culture positive R82.7
   glucose R81
   hemoglobin R82.3
   ketone R82.4
   sugar R81
vanillylmandelic acid (VMA), elevated
   R82.5
vectorcardiogram (VCG) R94.39
ventriculogram R93.0
white blood cell (count) (differential)
   (morphology) D72.9
xerography R92.8
Finger —see condition
Fire, Saint Anthony's —see Erysipelas

Fire-setting
   pathological (compulsive) F63.1
Fish hook stomach K31.89
Fishmeal-worker's lung J67.8
Fissure, fissured
   anus, anal K60.2
      acute K60.0
      chronic K60.1
      congenital Q43.8
   ear, lobule, congenital Q17.8
   epiglottis (congenital) Q31.8
   larynx J38.7
      congenital Q31.8
   lip K13.0
      congenital —see Cleft, lip
   nipple N64.0
      associated with
         lactation O92.13
         pregnancy O92.11-
         puerperium O92.12
   nose Q30.2
   palate (congenital) —see Cleft, palate
   skin R23.4
   spine (congenital) —see also Spina bifida
      with hydrocephalus —see
         Spina bifida, by site, with
         hydrocephalus
   tongue (acquired) K14.5
      congenital Q38.3
Fistula (cutaneous) L98.8
   abdomen (wall) K63.2
      bladder N32.2
      intestine NEC K63.2
      ureter N28.89
      uterus N82.5
   abdominorectal K63.2
   abdominosigmoidal K63.2
   abdominothoracic J86.0
   abdominouterine N82.5
      congenital Q51.7
   abdominovesical N32.2
   accessory sinuses —see Sinusitis
   actinomycotic —see Actinomycosis
   alveolar antrum —see Sinusitis,
      maxillary
   alveolar process K04.6
   anorectal K60.5
   antrobuccal —see Sinusitis, maxillary
   antrum —see Sinusitis, maxillary
   anus, anal (recurrent) (infectional) K60.3
      congenital Q43.6
         with absence, atresia and stenosis
            Q42.2
      tuberculous A18.32
   aorta-duodenal I77.2
   appendix, appendicular K38.3
   arteriovenous (acquired) (nonruptured)
      I77.0
      brain I67.1
         congenital Q28.2
            ruptured I60.8
         ruptured I60.8
      cerebral —see Fistula, arteriovenous,
         brain
      congenital (peripheral) —see also
         Malformation, arteriovenous
        brain Q28.2
           ruptured I60.8
        coronary Q24.5
        pulmonary Q25.72
      coronary I25.41
        congenital Q24.5
      pulmonary I28.0
        congenital Q25.72

Fistula *(Continued)*
    arteriovenous *(Continued)*
        surgically created (for dialysis) Z99.2
            complication —*see* Complication,
                arteriovenous, fistula,
                surgically created
            traumatic —*see* Injury, blood vessel
    artery I77.2
    aural (mastoid) —*see* Mastoiditis,
        chronic
    auricle —*see also* Disorder, pinna,
        specified type NEC
        congenital Q18.1
    Bartholin's gland N82.8
    bile duct (common) (hepatic) K83.3
        with calculus, stones —*see* Calculus,
            bile duct
    biliary (tract) —*see* Fistula, bile duct
    bladder (sphincter) NEC *(see also*
        Fistula, vesico-) N32.2
        into seminal vesicle N32.2
    bone —*see also* Disorder, bone, specified
        type NEC
        with osteomyelitis, chronic —*see*
            Osteomyelitis, chronic, with
            draining sinus
    brain G93.89
        arteriovenous (acquired) I67.1
            congenital Q28.2
    branchial (cleft) Q18.0
    branchiogenous Q18.0
    breast N61
        puerperal, postpartum or gestational,
            due to mastitis (purulent) —*see*
            Mastitis, obstetric, purulent
    bronchial J86.0
    bronchocutaneous, bronchomediastinal,
        bronchopleural,
        bronchopleuromediastinal
        (infective) J86.0
        tuberculous NEC A15.5
    bronchoesophageal J86.0
        congenital Q39.2
            with atresia of esophagus Q39.1
    bronchovisceral J86.0
    buccal cavity (infective) K12.2
    cecosigmoidal K63.2
    cecum K63.2
    cerebrospinal (fluid) G96.0
    cervical, lateral Q18.1
    cervicoaural Q18.1
    cervicosigmoidal N82.4
    cervicovesical N82.1
    cervix N82.8
    chest (wall) J86.0
    cholecystenteric —*see* Fistula,
        gallbladder
    cholecystocolic —*see* Fistula,
        gallbladder
    cholecystocolonic —*see* Fistula,
        gallbladder
    cholecystoduodenal —*see* Fistula,
        gallbladder
    cholecystogastric —*see* Fistula,
        gallbladder
    cholecystointestinal —*see* Fistula,
        gallbladder
    choledochoduodenal —*see* Fistula, bile
        duct
    cholocolic K82.3
    coccyx —*see* Sinus, pilonidal
    colon K63.2
    colostomy K94.09
    common duct —*see* Fistula, bile duct

Fistula *(Continued)*
    congenital, site not listed —*see*
        Anomaly, by site
    coronary, arteriovenous I25.41
        congenital Q24.5
    costal region J86.0
    cul-de-sac, Douglas' N82.8
    cystic duct —*see also* Fistula, gallbladder
        congenital Q44.5
    dental K04.6
    diaphragm J86.0
    duodenum K31.6
    ear (external) (canal) —*see* Disorder, ear,
        external, specified type NEC
    enterocolic K63.2
    enterocutaneous K63.2
    enterouterine N82.4
        congenital Q51.7
    enterovaginal N82.4
        congenital Q52.2
        large intestine N82.3
        small intestine N82.2
    enterovesical N32.1
    epididymis N50.8
        tuberculous A18.15
    esophagobronchial J86.0
        congenital Q39.2
            with atresia of esophagus Q39.1
    esophagocutaneous K22.8
    esophagopleural-cutaneous J86.0
    esophagotracheal J86.0
        congenital Q39.2
            with atresia of esophagus Q39.1
    esophagus K22.8
        congenital Q39.2
            with atresia of esophagus Q39.1
    ethmoid —*see* Sinusitis, ethmoidal
    eyeball (cornea) (sclera) —*see* Disorder,
        globe, hypotony
    eyelid H01.8
    fallopian tube, external N82.5
    fecal K63.2
        congenital Q43.6
    from periapical abscess K04.6
    frontal sinus —*see* Sinusitis, frontal
    gallbladder K82.3
        with calculus, cholelithiasis, stones —
            see Calculus, gallbladder
    gastric K31.6
    gastrocolic K31.6
        congenital Q40.2
        tuberculous A18.32
    gastroenterocolic K31.6
    gastroesophageal K31.6
    gastrojejunal K31.6
    gastrojejunocolic K31.6
    genital tract (female) N82.9
        specified NEC N82.8
        to intestine NEC N82.4
        to skin N82.5
    hepatic artery-portal vein, congenital
        Q26.6
    hepatopleural J86.0
    hepatopulmonary J86.0
    ileorectal or ileosigmoidal K63.2
    ileovaginal N82.2
    ileovesical N32.1
    ileum K63.2
    in ano K60.3
        tuberculous A18.32
    inner ear (labyrinth) —*see* subcategory
        H83.1
    intestine NEC K63.2
    intestinocolonic (abdominal) K63.2

Fistula *(Continued)*
    intestinoureteral N28.89
    intestinouterine N82.4
    intestinovaginal N82.4
        large intestine N82.3
        small intestine N82.2
    intestinovesical N32.1
    ischiorectal (fossa) K61.3
    jejunum K63.2
    joint M25.10
        ankle M25.17-
        elbow M25.12-
        foot joint M25.17-
        hand joint M25.14-
        hip M25.15-
        knee M25.16-
        shoulder M25.11-
        specified joint NEC M25.18
        tuberculous —*see* Tuberculosis, joint
        wrist M25.13-
    kidney N28.89
    labium (majus) (minus) N82.8
    labyrinth —*see* subcategory H83.1
    lacrimal (gland) (sac) H04.61-
    lacrimonasal duct —*see* Fistula, lacrimal
    laryngotracheal, congenital Q34.8
    larynx J38.7
    lip K13.0
        congenital Q38.0
    lumbar, tuberculous A18.01
    lung J86.0
    lymphatic I89.8
    mammary (gland) N61
    mastoid (process) (region) —*see*
        Mastoiditis, chronic
    maxillary J32.0
    medial, face and neck Q18.8
    mediastinal J86.0
    mediastinobronchial J86.0
    mediastinocutaneous J86.0
    middle ear —*see* subcategory H74.8
    mouth K12.2
    nasal J34.89
        sinus —*see* Sinusitis
    nasopharynx J39.2
    nipple N64.0
    nose J34.89
    oral (cutaneous) K12.2
        maxillary J32.0
        nasal (with cleft palate) —*see* Cleft,
            palate
    orbit, orbital —*see* Disorder, orbit,
        specified type NEC
    oroantral J32.0
    oviduct, external N82.5
    palate (hard) M27.8
    pancreatic K86.8
    pancreaticoduodenal K86.8
    parotid (gland) K11.4
        region K12.2
    penis N48.89
    perianal K60.3
    pericardium (pleura) (sac) —*see*
        Pericarditis
    pericecal K63.2
    perineorectal K60.4
    perineosigmoidal K63.2
    perineum, perineal (with urethral
        involvement) NEC N36.0
        tuberculous A18.13
        ureter N28.89
    perirectal K60.4
        tuberculous A18.32
    peritoneum K65.9

Fistula *(Continued)*
  pharyngoesophageal J39.2
  pharynx J39.2
    branchial cleft (congenital)
      Q18.0
  pilonidal (infected) (rectum) —*see*
      Sinus, pilonidal
  pleura, pleural, pleurocutaneous,
      pleuroperitoneal J86.0
    tuberculous NEC A15.6
  pleuropericardial I31.8
  portal vein-hepatic artery, congenital
      Q26.6
  postauricular H70.81-
  postoperative, persistent T81.83
    specified site —*see* Fistula, by site
  preauricular (congenital) Q18.1
  prostate N42.89
  pulmonary J86.0
    arteriovenous I28.0
      congenital Q25.72
    tuberculous —*see* Tuberculosis,
      pulmonary
  pulmonoperitoneal J86.0
  rectolabial N82.4
  rectosigmoid (intercommunicating)
      K63.2
  rectoureteral N28.89
  rectourethral N36.0
    congenital Q64.73
  rectouterine N82.4
    congenital Q51.7
  rectovaginal N82.3
    congenital Q52.2
    tuberculous A18.18
  rectovesical N32.1
    congenital Q64.79
  rectovesicovaginal N82.3
  rectovulval N82.4
    congenital Q52.79
  rectum (to skin) K60.4
    congenital Q43.6
      with absence, atresia and stenosis
        Q42.0
    tuberculous A18.32
  renal N28.89
  retroauricular —*see* Fistula,
      postauricular
  salivary duct or gland (any) K11.4
    congenital Q38.4
  scrotum (urinary) N50.8
    tuberculous A18.15
  semicircular canals —*see* subcategory
      H83.1
  sigmoid K63.2
    to bladder N32.1
  sinus —*see* Sinusitis
  skin L98.8
    to genital tract (female) N82.5
  splenocolic D73.89
  stercoral K63.2
  stomach K31.6
  sublingual gland K11.4
  submandibular gland K11.4
  submaxillary (gland) K11.4
    region K12.2
  thoracic J86.0
    duct I89.8
  thoracoabdominal J86.0
  thoracogastric J86.0
  thoracointestinal J86.0
  thorax J86.0
  thyroglossal duct Q89.2
  thyroid E07.89

Fistula *(Continued)*
  trachea, congenital (external) (internal)
      Q32.1
  tracheoesophageal J86.0
    congenital Q39.2
      with atresia of esophagus Q39.1
    following tracheostomy J95.04
  traumatic arteriovenous —*see* Injury,
      blood vessel, by site
  tuberculous - code by site under
      Tuberculosis
  typhoid A01.09
  umbilicourinary Q64.8
  urachus, congenital Q64.4
  ureter (persistent) N28.89
  ureteroabdominal N28.89
  ureterorectal N28.89
  ureterosigmoido-abdominal N28.89
  ureterovaginal N82.1
  ureterovesical N32.2
  urethra N36.0
    congenital Q64.79
    tuberculous A18.13
  urethroperineal N36.0
  urethroperineovesical N32.2
  urethrorectal N36.0
    congenital Q64.73
  urethroscrotal N50.8
  urethrovaginal N82.1
  urethrovesical N32.2
  urinary (tract) (persistent) (recurrent)
      N36.0
  uteroabdominal N82.5
    congenital Q51.7
  uteroenteric, uterointestinal N82.4
    congenital Q51.7
  uterorectal N82.4
    congenital Q51.7
  uteroureteric N82.1
  uterourethral Q51.7
  uterovaginal N82.8
  uterovesical N82.1
    congenital Q51.7
  uterus N82.8
  vagina (postpartal) (wall) N82.8
  vaginocutaneous (postpartal)
      N82.5
  vaginointestinal NEC N82.4
    large intestine N82.3
    small intestine N82.2
  vaginoperineal N82.5
  vasocutaneous, congenital Q55.7
  vesical NEC N32.2
  vesicoabdominal N32.2
  vesicocervicovaginal N82.1
  vesicocolic N32.1
  vesicocutaneous N32.2
  vesicoenteric N32.1
  vesicointestinal N32.1
  vesicometrorectal N82.4
  vesicoperineal N32.2
  vesicorectal N32.1
    congenital Q64.79
  vesicosigmoidal N32.1
  vesicosigmoidovaginal N82.3
  vesicoureteral N32.2
  vesicoureterovaginal N82.1
  vesicourethral N32.2
  vesicourethrorectal N32.1
  vesicouterine N82.1
    congenital Q51.7
  vesicovaginal N82.0
  vulvorectal N82.4
    congenital Q52.79

Fit R56.9
  epileptic —*see* Epilepsy
  fainting R55
  hysterical F44.5
  newborn P90
Fitting (and adjustment) (of)
  artificial
    arm —*see* Admission, adjustment,
        artificial, arm
    breast Z44.3
    eye Z44.2
    leg —*see* Admission, adjustment,
        artificial, leg
  automatic implantable cardiac
      defibrillator (with synchronous
      cardiac pacemaker) Z45.02
  brain neuropacemaker Z46.2
    implanted Z45.42
  cardiac defibrillator —*see* Fitting
      (and adjustment) (of), automatic
      implantable cardiac defibrillator
  catheter, non-vascular Z46.82
  colostomy belt Z46.89
  contact lenses Z46.0
  cystostomy device Z46.6
  defibrillator, cardiac —*see* Fitting
      (and adjustment) (of), automatic
      implantable cardiac defibrillator
  dentures Z46.3
  device NOS Z46.9
    abdominal Z46.89
    gastrointestinal NEC Z46.59
    implanted NEC Z45.89
    nervous system Z46.2
      implanted —*see* Admission,
          adjustment, device,
          implanted, nervous system
    orthodontic Z46.4
    orthoptic Z46.0
    orthotic Z46.89
    prosthetic (external) Z44.9
      breast Z44.3
      dental Z46.3
      eye Z44.2
      specified NEC Z44.8
    specified NEC Z46.89
    substitution
      auditory Z46.2
        implanted —*see* Admission,
            adjustment, device,
            implanted, hearing device
      nervous system Z46.2
        implanted —*see* Admission,
            adjustment, device,
            implanted, nervous system
      visual Z46.2
        implanted Z45.31
      urinary Z46.6
  gastric lap band Z46.51
  gastrointestinal appliance NEC
      Z46.59
  glasses (reading) Z46.0
  hearing aid Z46.1
  ileostomy device Z46.89
  insulin pump Z46.81
  intestinal appliance NEC Z46.89
  myringotomy device (stent) (tube)
      Z45.82
  neuropacemaker Z46.2
    implanted Z45.42
  non-vascular catheter Z46.82
  orthodontic device Z46.4
  orthopedic device (brace) (cast) (corset)
      (shoes) Z46.89

Fitting (Continued)
  pacemaker (cardiac) Z45.018
    nervous system (brain) (peripheral
      nerve) (spinal cord) Z46.2
      implanted Z45.42
    pulse generator Z45.010
  portacath (port-a-cath) Z45.2
  prosthesis (external) Z44.9
    arm —see Admission, adjustment,
      artificial, arm
    breast Z44.3
    dental Z46.3
    eye Z44.2
    leg —see Admission, adjustment,
      artificial, leg
    specified NEC Z44.8
  spectacles Z46.0
  wheelchair Z46.89
Fitzhugh-Curtis syndrome
  due to
    Chlamydia trachomatis A74.81
    Neisseria gonorrhorea (gonococcal
      peritonitis) A54.85
Fitz's syndrome (acute hemorrhagic
  pancreatitis) K85.8
Fixation
  joint —see Ankylosis
  larynx J38.7
  stapes —see Ankylosis, ear ossicles
    deafness —see Deafness, conductive
  uterus (acquired) —see Malposition,
    uterus
  vocal cord J38.3
Flabby ridge K06.8
Flaccid —see also condition
  palate, congenital Q38.5
Flail
  chest S22.5-
    newborn (birth injury) P13.8
  joint (paralytic) M25.20
    ankle M25.27-
    elbow M25.22-
    foot joint M25.27-
    hand joint M25.24-
    hip M25.25-
    knee M25.26-
    shoulder M25.21-
    specified joint NEC M25.28
    wrist M25.23-
Flajani's disease —see Hyperthyroidism,
  with, goiter (diffuse)
Flap, liver K71.3
Flashbacks (residual to hallucinogen use)
  F16.283
Flat
  chamber (eye) —see Disorder, globe,
    hypotony, flat anterior chamber
  chest, congenital Q67.8
  foot (acquired) (fixed type) (painful)
    (postural) —see also Deformity,
    limb, flat foot
    congenital (rigid) (spastic (everted))
      Q66.5-
    rachitic sequelae (late effect)
      E64.3
  organ or site, congenital NEC —see
    Anomaly, by site
  pelvis M95.5
    with disproportion (fetopelvic)
      O33.0
      causing obstructed labor
        O65.0
    congenital Q74.2
Flatau-Schilder disease G37.0

Flatback syndrome M40.30
  lumbar region M40.36
  lumbosacral region M40.37
  thoracolumbar region M40.35
Flattening
  head, femur M89.8X5
  hip —see Coxa, plana
  lip (congenital) Q18.8
  nose (congenital) Q67.4
    acquired M95.0
Flatulence R14.3
  psychogenic F45.8
Flatus R14.3
  vaginalis N89.8
Flax-dresser's disease J66.1
Flea bite —see Injury, bite, by site,
  superficial, insect
Flecks, glaucomatous (subcapsular) —see
  Cataract, complicated
Fleischer (-Kayser) ring (cornea)
  H18.04-
Fleshy mole O02.0
Flexibilitas cerea —see Catalepsy
Flexion
  amputation stump (surgical) T87.89
  cervix —see Malposition, uterus
  contracture, joint —see Contraction,
    joint
  deformity, joint (see also Deformity,
    limb, flexion) M21.20
    hip, congenital Q65.89
  uterus —see also Malposition,
    uterus
    lateral —see Lateroversion,
      uterus
Flexner-Boyd dysentery A03.2
Flexner's dysentery A03.1
Flexure —see Flexion
Flint murmur (aortic insufficiency)
  I35.1
Floater, vitreous —see Opacity,
  vitreous
Floating
  cartilage (joint) —see also Loose, body,
    joint
    knee —see Derangement, knee, loose
      body
  gallbladder, congenital Q44.1
  kidney N28.89
    congenital Q63.8
  spleen D73.89
Flooding N92.0
Floor —see condition
Floppy
  baby syndrome (nonspecific)
    P94.2
  iris syndrome (intraoperative)
    (IFIS) H21.81
  nonrheumatic mitral valve syndrome
    I34.1
Flu —see also Influenza
  avian (see also Influenza, due to,
    identified novel influenza
    A virus) J09.X2
  bird (see also Influenza, due to,
    identified novel influenza
    A virus) J09.X2
  intestinal NEC A08.4
  swine (viruses that normally cause
    infections in pigs) (see also
    Influenza, due to, identified
    novel influenza A virus)
    J09.X2
Fluctuating blood pressure I99.8

Fluid
  abdomen R18.8
  chest J94.8
  heart —see Failure, heart, congestive
  joint —see Effusion, joint
  loss (acute) E86.9
    with
      hypernatremia E87.0
      hyponatremia E87.1
  lung —see Edema, lung
  overload E87.70
    specified NEC E87.79
  peritoneal cavity R18.8
  pleural cavity J94.8
  retention R60.9
Flukes NEC —see also Infestation,
  fluke
  blood NEC —see Schistosomiasis
  liver B66.3
Fluor (vaginalis) N89.8
  trichomonal or due to Trichomonas
    (vaginalis) A59.00
Fluorosis
  dental K00.3
  skeletal M85.10
    ankle M85.17-
    foot M85.17-
    forearm M85.13-
    hand M85.14-
    lower leg M85.16-
    multiple site M85.19
    neck M85.18
    rib M85.18
    shoulder M85.11-
    skull M85.18
    specified site NEC M85.18
    thigh M85.15-
    toe M85.17-
    upper arm M85.12-
    vertebra M85.18
Flush syndrome E34.0
Flushing R23.2
  menopausal N95.1
Flutter
  atrial or auricular I48.92
    atypical I48.4
    type I I48.3
    type II I48.4
    typical I48.3
  heart I49.8
    atrial or auricular I48.92
      atypical I48.4
      type I I48.3
      type II I48.4
      typical I48.3
    ventricular I49.02
  ventricular I49.02
FNHTR (febrile nonhemolytic transfusion
  reaction) R50.84
Fochier's abscess - code by site under
  Abscess
Focus, Assmann's —see Tuberculosis,
  pulmonary
Fogo selvagem L10.3
Foix-Alajouanine syndrome
  G95.19
Fold, folds (anomalous) —see also
  Anomaly, by site
  Descemet's membrane —see Change,
    corneal membrane, Descemet's,
    fold
  epicanthic Q10.3
  heart Q24.8
Folie à deux F24

Follicle
- cervix (nabothian) (ruptured) N88.8
- graafian, ruptured, with hemorrhage N83.0
- nabothian N88.8

Follicular —*see* condition

Folliculitis (superficial) L73.9
- abscedens et suffodiens L66.3
- cyst N83.0
- decalvans L66.2
- deep —*see* Furuncle, by site
- gonococcal (acute) (chronic) A54.01
- keloid, keloidalis L73.0
- pustular L01.02
- ulerythematosa reticulata L66.4

Folliculome lipidique
- specified site —*see* Neoplasm, benign, by site
- unspecified site
  - female D27.9
  - male D29.20

Følling's disease E70.0

Follow-up —*see* Examination, follow-up

Fong's syndrome (hereditary osteo-onychodysplasia) Q78.5

Food
- allergy L27.2
- asphyxia (from aspiration or inhalation) —*see* Foreign body, by site
- choked on —*see* Foreign body, by site
- deprivation T73.0
  - specified kind of food NEC E63.8
- intoxication —*see* Poisoning, food
- lack of T73.0
- poisoning —*see* Poisoning, food
- rejection NEC —*see* Disorder, eating
- strangulation or suffocation —*see* Foreign body, by site
- toxemia —*see* Poisoning, food

Foot —*see* condition

Foramen ovale (nonclosure) (patent) (persistent) Q21.1

Forbes' glycogen storage disease E74.03

Fordyce-Fox disease L75.2

Fordyce's disease (mouth) Q38.6

Forearm —*see* condition

Foreign body
- with
  - laceration —*see* Laceration, by site, with foreign body
  - puncture wound —*see* Puncture, by site, with foreign body
- accidentally left following a procedure T81.509
  - aspiration T81.506
    - resulting in
      - adhesions T81.516
      - obstruction T81.526
      - perforation T81.536
      - specified complication NEC T81.596
  - cardiac catheterization T81.505
    - resulting in
      - acute reaction T81.60
        - aseptic peritonitis T81.61
        - specified NEC T81.69
      - adhesions T81.515
      - obstruction T81.525
      - perforation T81.535
      - specified complication NEC T81.595

Foreign body (*Continued*)
- accidentally left following a procedure (*Continued*)
  - causing
    - acute reaction T81.60
      - aseptic peritonitis T81.61
      - specified complication NEC T81.69
    - adhesions T81.519
    - aseptic peritonitis T81.61
    - obstruction T81.529
    - perforation T81.539
    - specified complication NEC T81.599
  - endoscopy T81.504
    - resulting in
      - adhesions T81.514
      - obstruction T81.524
      - perforation T81.534
      - specified complication NEC T81.594
  - immunization T81.503
    - resulting in
      - adhesions T81.513
      - obstruction T81.523
      - perforation T81.533
      - specified complication NEC T81.593
  - infusion T81.501
    - resulting in
      - adhesions T81.511
      - obstruction T81.521
      - perforation T81.531
      - specified complication NEC T81.591
  - injection T81.503
    - resulting in
      - adhesions T81.513
      - obstruction T81.523
      - perforation T81.533
      - specified complication NEC T81.593
  - kidney dialysis T81.502
    - resulting in
      - adhesions T81.512
      - obstruction T81.522
      - perforation T81.532
      - specified complication NEC T81.592
  - packing removal T81.507
    - resulting in
      - acute reaction T81.60
        - aseptic peritonitis T81.61
        - specified NEC T81.69
      - adhesions T81.517
      - obstruction T81.527
      - perforation T81.537
      - specified complication NEC T81.597
  - puncture T81.506
    - resulting in
      - adhesions T81.516
      - obstruction T81.526
      - perforation T81.536
      - specified complication NEC T81.596
  - specified procedure NEC T81.508
    - resulting in
      - acute reaction T81.60
        - aseptic peritonitis T81.61
        - specified NEC T81.69
      - adhesions T81.518
      - obstruction T81.528
      - perforation T81.538
      - specified complication NEC T81.598

Foreign body (*Continued*)
- accidentally left following a procedure (*Continued*)
  - surgical operation T81.500
    - resulting in
      - acute reaction T81.60
        - aseptic peritonitis T81.61
        - specified NEC T81.69
      - adhesions T81.510
      - obstruction T81.520
      - perforation T81.530
      - specified complication NEC T81.590
  - transfusion T81.501
    - resulting in
      - adhesions T81.511
      - obstruction T81.521
      - perforation T81.531
      - specified complication NEC T81.591
- alimentary tract T18.9
  - anus T18.5
  - colon T18.4
  - esophagus —*see* Foreign body, esophagus
  - mouth T18.0
  - multiple sites T18.8
  - rectosigmoid (junction) T18.5
  - rectum T18.5
  - small intestine T18.3
  - specified site NEC T18.8
  - stomach T18.2
- anterior chamber (eye) S05.5-
- auditory canal —*see* Foreign body, entering through orifice, ear
- bronchus T17.508
  - causing
    - asphyxiation T17.500
      - food (bone) (seed) T17.520
      - gastric contents (vomitus) T17.510
      - specified type NEC T17.590
    - injury NEC T17.508
      - food (bone) (seed) T17.528
      - gastric contents (vomitus) T17.518
      - specified type NEC T17.598
- canthus —*see* Foreign body, conjunctival sac
- ciliary body (eye) S05.5-
- conjunctival sac T15.1-
- cornea T15.0-
- entering through orifice
  - accessory sinus T17.0
  - alimentary canal T18.9
    - multiple parts T18.8
    - specified part NEC T18.8
  - alveolar process T18.0
  - antrum (Highmore's) T17.0
  - anus T18.5
  - appendix T18.4
  - auditory canal —*see* Foreign body, entering through orifice, ear
  - auricle —*see* Foreign body, entering through orifice, ear
  - bladder T19.1
  - bronchioles —*see* Foreign body, respiratory tract, specified site NEC
  - bronchus (main) —*see* Foreign body, bronchus
  - buccal cavity T18.0
  - canthus (inner) —*see* Foreign body, conjunctival sac
  - cecum T18.4

Foreign body (*Continued*)
  entering through orifice (*Continued*)
    cervix (canal) (uteri) T19.3
    colon T18.4
    conjunctival sac —*see* Foreign body, conjunctival sac
    cornea —*see* Foreign body, cornea
    digestive organ or tract NOS T18.9
      multiple parts T18.8
      specified part NEC T18.8
    duodenum T18.3
    ear (external) T16.-
    esophagus —*see* Foreign body, esophagus
    eye (external) NOS T15.9-
      conjunctival sac —*see* Foreign body, conjunctival sac
      cornea —*see* Foreign body, cornea
      specified part NEC T15.8-
    eyeball —*see also* Foreign body, entering through orifice, eye, specified part NEC
      with penetrating wound —*see* Puncture, eyeball
    eyelid —*see also* Foreign body, conjunctival sac
      with
        laceration —*see* Laceration, eyelid, with foreign body
        puncture —*see* Puncture, eyelid, with foreign body
        superficial injury —*see* Foreign body, superficial, eyelid
    gastrointestinal tract T18.9
      multiple parts T18.8
      specified part NEC T18.8
    genitourinary tract T19.9
      multiple parts T19.8
      specified part NEC T19.8
    globe —*see* Foreign body, entering through orifice, eyeball
    gum T18.0
    Highmore's antrum T17.0
    hypopharynx —*see* Foreign body, pharynx
    ileum T18.3
    intestine (small) T18.3
      large T18.4
    lacrimal apparatus (punctum) —*see* Foreign body, entering through orifice, eye, specified part NEC
    large intestine T18.4
    larynx —*see* Foreign body, larynx
    lung —*see* Foreign body, respiratory tract, specified site NEC
    maxillary sinus T17.0
    mouth T18.0
    nasal sinus T17.0
    nasopharynx —*see* Foreign body, pharynx
    nose (passage) T17.1
    nostril T17.1
    oral cavity T18.0
    palate T18.0
    penis T19.4
    pharynx —*see* Foreign body, pharynx
    piriform sinus —*see* Foreign body, pharynx
    rectosigmoid (junction) T18.5
    rectum T18.5
    respiratory tract —*see* Foreign body, respiratory tract

Foreign body (*Continued*)
  entering through orifice (*Continued*)
    sinus (accessory) (frontal) (maxillary) (nasal) T17.0
      piriform —*see* Foreign body, pharynx
    small intestine T18.3
    stomach T18.2
    suffocation by —*see* Foreign body, by site
    tear ducts or glands —*see* Foreign body, entering through orifice, eye, specified part NEC
    throat —*see* Foreign body, pharynx
    tongue T18.0
    tonsil, tonsillar (fossa) —*see* Foreign body, pharynx
    trachea —*see* Foreign body, trachea
    ureter T19.8
    urethra T19.0
    uterus (any part) T19.3
    vagina T19.2
    vulva T19.2
  esophagus T18.108
    causing
      injury NEC T18.108
        food (bone) (seed) T18.128
        gastric contents (vomitus) T18.118
        specified type NEC T18.198
      tracheal compression T18.100
        food (bone) (seed) T18.120
        gastric contents (vomitus) T18.110
        specified type NEC T18.190
  felling of, in throat R09.89
  fragment —*see* Retained, foreign body fragments (type of)
  genitourinary tract T19.9
    bladder T19.1
    multiple parts T19.8
    penis T19.4
    specified site NEC T19.8
    urethra T19.0
    uterus T19.3
      IUD Z97.5
    vagina T19.2
      contraceptive device Z97.5
    vulva T19.2
  granuloma (old) (soft tissue) —*see also* Granuloma, foreign body
    skin L92.3
  in
    laceration —*see* Laceration, by site, with foreign body
    puncture wound —*see* Puncture, by site, with foreign body
    soft tissue (residual) M79.5
  inadvertently left in operation wound —*see* Foreign body, accidentally left during a procedure
  ingestion, ingested NOS T18.9
  inhalation or inspiration —*see* Foreign body, by site
  internal organ, not entering through a natural orifice - code as specific injury with foreign body
  intraocular S05.5-
    old, retained (nonmagnetic) H44.70-
      anterior chamber H44.71-
      ciliary body H44.72-
      iris H44.72-
      lens H44.73-

Foreign body (*Continued*)
  intraocular (*Continued*)
    old, retained (*Continued*)
      magnetic H44.60-
        anterior chamber H44.61-
        ciliary body H44.62-
        iris H44.62-
        lens H44.63-
        posterior wall H44.64-
        specified site NEC H44.69-
        vitreous body H44.65-
      posterior wall H44.74-
      specified site NEC H44.79-
      vitreous body H44.75-
    iris —*see* Foreign body, intraocular
    lacrimal punctum —*see* Foreign body, entering through orifice, eye, specified part NEC
  larynx T17.308
    causing
      asphyxiation T17.300
        food (bone) (seed) T17.320
        gastric contents (vomitus) T17.310
        specified type NEC T17.390
      injury NEC T17.308
        food (bone) (seed) T17.328
        gastric contents (vomitus) T17.318
        specified type NEC T17.398
  lens —*see* Foreign body, intraocular
  ocular muscle S05.4-
    old, retained —*see* Foreign body, orbit, old
  old or residual
    soft tissue (residual) M79.5
  operation wound, left accidentally —*see* Foreign body, accidentally left during a procedure
  orbit S05.4-
    old, retained H05.5-
  pharynx T17.208
    causing
      asphyxiation T17.200
        food (bone) (seed) T17.220
        gastric contents (vomitus) T17.210
        specified type NEC T17.290
      injury NEC T17.208
        food (bone) (seed) T17.228
        gastric contents (vomitus) T17.218
        specified type NEC T17.298
  respiratory tract T17.908
    bronchioles —*see* Foreign body, respiratory tract, specified site NEC
    bronchus —*see* Foreign body, bronchus
    causing
      asphyxiation T17.900
        food (bone) (seed) T17.920
        gastric contents (vomitus) T17.910
        specified type NEC T17.990
      injury NEC T17.908
        food (bone) (seed) T17.928
        gastric contents (vomitus) T17.918
        specified type NEC T17.998
    larynx —*see* Foreign body, larynx
    lung —*see* Foreign body, respiratory tract, specified site NEC
    multiple parts —*see* Foreign body, respiratory tract, specified site NEC

Foreign body (Continued)
  respiratory tract (Continued)
    nasal sinus T17.0
    nasopharynx —see Foreign body,
      pharynx
    nose T17.1
    nostril T17.1
    pharynx —see Foreign body,
      pharynx
    specified site NEC T17.808
      causing
        asphyxiation T17.800
          food (bone) (seed) T17.820
          gastric contents (vomitus)
            T17.810
          specified type NEC T17.890
        injury NEC T17.808
          food (bone) (seed) T17.828
          gastric contents (vomitus)
            T17.818
          specified type NEC T17.898
    throat —see Foreign body, pharynx
    trachea —see Foreign body, trachea
  retained (old) (nonmagnetic) (in)
    anterior chamber (eye) —see Foreign
      body, intraocular, old, retained,
      anterior chamber
      magnetic —see Foreign body,
        intraocular, old, retained,
        magnetic, anterior chamber
    ciliary body —see Foreign body,
      intraocular, old, retained, ciliary
      body
      magnetic —see Foreign body,
        intraocular, old, retained,
        magnetic, ciliary body
    eyelid H02.819
      left H02.816
        lower H02.815
        upper H02.814
      right H02.813
        lower H02.812
        upper H02.811
    fragments —see Retained, foreign
      body fragments (type of)
    globe —see Foreign body, intraocular,
      old, retained
      magnetic —see Foreign body,
        intraocular, old, retained,
        magnetic
    intraocular —see Foreign body,
      intraocular, old, retained
      magnetic —see Foreign body,
        intraocular, old, retained,
        magnetic
    iris —see Foreign body, intraocular,
      old, retained, iris
      magnetic —see Foreign body,
        intraocular, old, retained,
        magnetic, iris
    lens —see Foreign body, intraocular,
      old, retained, lens
      magnetic —see Foreign body,
        intraocular, old, retained,
        magnetic, lens
    muscle —see Foreign body, retained,
      soft tissue
    orbit —see Foreign body, orbit, old
    posterior wall of globe —see Foreign
      body, intraocular, old, retained,
      posterior wall
      magnetic —see Foreign body,
        intraocular, old, retained,
        magnetic, posterior wall

Foreign body (Continued)
  retained (Continued)
    retrobulbar —see Foreign body, orbit,
      old, retrobulbar
    soft tissue M79.5
    vitreous —see Foreign body,
      intraocular, old, retained,
      vitreous body
      magnetic —see Foreign body,
        intraocular, old, retained,
        magnetic, vitreous body
  retina S05.5-
  superficial, without open wound
    abdomen, abdominal (wall) S30.851
    alveolar process S00.552
    ankle S90.55-
    antecubital space —see Foreign body,
      superficial, forearm
    anus S30.857
    arm (upper) S40.85-
    auditory canal —see Foreign body,
      superficial, ear
    auricle —see Foreign body,
      superficial, ear
    axilla —see Foreign body, superficial,
      arm
    back, lower S30.850
    breast S20.15-
    brow S00.85
    buttock S30.850
    calf —see Foreign body, superficial,
      leg
    canthus —see Foreign body,
      superficial, eyelid
    cheek S00.85
      internal S00.552
    chest wall —see Foreign body,
      superficial, thorax
    chin S00.85
    clitoris S30.854
    costal region —see Foreign body,
      superficial, thorax
    digit (s)
      foot —see Foreign body, superficial,
        toe
      hand —see Foreign body,
        superficial, finger
    ear S00.45-
    elbow S50.35-
    epididymis S30.853
    epigastric region S30.851
    epiglottis S10.15
    esophagus, cervical S10.15
    eyebrow —see Foreign body,
      superficial, eyelid
    eyelid S00.25-
    face S00.85
    finger (s) S60.459
      index S60.45-
      little S60.45-
      middle S60.45-
      ring S60.45-
    flank S30.851
    foot (except toe (s) alone) S90.85-
      toe —see Foreign body, superficial,
        toe
    forearm S50.85-
      elbow only —see Foreign body,
        superficial, elbow
    forehead S00.85
    genital organs, external
      female S30.856
      male S30.855
    groin S30.851

Foreign body (Continued)
  superficial, without open wound
    (Continued)
    gum S00.552
    hand S60.55-
    head S00.95
      ear —see Foreign body, superficial,
        ear
      eyelid —see Foreign body,
        superficial, eyelid
      lip S00.551
      nose S00.35
      oral cavity S00.552
      scalp S00.05
      specified site NEC S00.85
    heel —see Foreign body, superficial,
      foot
    hip S70.25-
    inguinal region S30.851
    interscapular region S20.459
    jaw S00.85
    knee S80.25-
    labium (majus) (minus) S30.854
    larynx S10.15
    leg (lower) S80.85-
      knee —see Foreign body,
        superficial, knee
      upper —see Foreign body,
        superficial, thigh
    lip S00.551
    lower back S30.850
    lumbar region S30.850
    malar region S00.85
    mammary —see Foreign body,
      superficial, breast
    mastoid region S00.85
    mouth S00.552
    nail
      finger —see Foreign body,
        superficial, finger
      toe —see Foreign body, superficial,
        toe
    nape S10.85
    nasal S00.35
    neck S10.95
      specified site NEC S10.85
      throat S10.15
    nose S00.35
    occipital region S00.05
    oral cavity S00.552
    orbital region —see Foreign body,
      superficial, eyelid
    palate S00.552
    palm —see Foreign body, superficial,
      hand
    parietal region S00.05
    pelvis S30.850
    penis S30.852
    perineum
      female S30.854
      male S30.850
    periocular area —see Foreign body,
      superficial, eyelid
    phalanges
      finger —see Foreign body,
        superficial, finger
      toe —see Foreign body, superficial,
        toe
    pharynx S10.15
    pinna —see Foreign body, superficial,
      ear
    popliteal space —see Foreign body,
      superficial, knee
    prepuce S30.852
    pubic region S30.850

Foreign body (Continued)
  superficial, without open wound
      (Continued)
    pudendum
      female S30.856
      male S30.855
    sacral region S30.850
    scalp S00.05
    scapular region —see Foreign body,
        superficial, shoulder
    scrotum S30.853
    shin —see Foreign body, superficial,
        leg
    shoulder S40.25-
    sternal region S20.359
    submaxillary region S00.85
    submental region S00.85
    subungual
      finger (s) —see Foreign body,
          superficial, finger
      toe (s) —see Foreign body,
          superficial, toe
    supraclavicular fossa S10.85
    supraorbital S00.85
    temple S00.85
    temporal region S00.85
    testis S30.853
    thigh S70.35-
    thorax, thoracic (wall) S20.95
      back S20.45-
      front S20.35-
    throat S10.15
    thumb S60.35-
    toe (s) (lesser) S90.456
      great S90.45-
    tongue S00.552
    trachea S10.15
    tunica vaginalis S30.853
    tympanum, tympanic membrane —
        see Foreign body, superficial, ear
    uvula S00.552
    vagina S30.854
    vocal cords S10.15
    vulva S30.854
    wrist S60.85-
  swallowed T18.9
  trachea T17.408
    causing
      asphyxiation T17.400
        food (bone) (seed) T17.420
        gastric contents (vomitus)
            T17.410
        specified type NEC T17.490
      injury NEC T17.408
        food (bone) (seed) T17.428
        gastric contents (vomitus)
            T17.418
        specified type NEC T17.498
  type of fragment —see Retained, foreign
      body fragments (type of)
  vitreous (humor) S05.5-
Forestier's disease (rhizomelic
    pseudopolyarthritis) M35.3 -
  meaning ankylosing hyperostosis —
      see Hyperostosis, ankylosing
Formation
  hyalin in cornea —see Degeneration,
      cornea
  sequestrum in bone (due to infection) —
      see Osteomyelitis, chronic
  valve
    colon, congenital Q43.8
    ureter (congenital) Q62.39
Formication R20.2
Fort Bragg fever A27.89

Fossa —see also condition
  pyriform —see condition
Foster-Kennedy syndrome H47.14-
Fothergill's
  disease (trigeminal neuralgia) —see also
      Neuralgia, trigeminal
  scarlatina anginosa A38.9
Foul breath R19.6
Foundling Z76.1
Fournier disease or gangrene
    N49.3
  female N76.89
Fourth
  cranial nerve —see condition
  molar K00.1
Foville's (peduncular) disease or
    syndrome G46.3
Fox (-Fordyce) disease (apocrine miliaria)
    L75.2
Fracture, burst —see Fracture, traumatic,
    by site
Fracture, chronic —see Fracture,
    pathological
Fracture, insufficiency —see Fracture,
    pathologic, by site
Fracture, pathological (pathologic) (see also
    Fracture, traumatic) M84.40
  ankle M84.47-
  carpus M84.44-
  clavicle M84.41-
  dental implant M27.63
  dental restorative material K08.539
    with loss of material K08.531
    without loss of material K08.530
  due to
    neoplastic disease NEC (see also
        Neoplasm) M84.50
      ankle M84.57-
      carpus M84.54-
      clavicle M84.51-
      femur M84.55-
      fibula M84.56-
      finger M84.54-
      hip M84.559
      humerus M84.52-
      ilium M84.550
      ischium M84.550
      metacarpus M84.54-
      metatarsus M84.57-
      neck M84.58
      pelvis M84.550
      radius M84.53-
      rib M84.58
      scapula M84.51-
      skull M84.58
      tarsus M84.57-
      tibia M84.56-
      toe M84.57-
      ulna M84.53-
      vertebra M84.58
    osteoporosis M80.80
      disuse —see Osteoporosis, specified
          type NEC, with pathological
          fracture
      drug-induced —see Osteoporosis,
          drug induced, with
          pathological fracture
      idiopathic —see Osteoporosis,
          specified type NEC, with
          pathological fracture
      postmenopausal —
          see Osteoporosis,
          postmenopausal, with
          pathological fracture

Fracture, pathological (Continued)
  due to (Continued)
    osteoporosis (Continued)
      postoophorectomy —see Osteo-
          porosis, postoophorectomy,
          with pathological fracture
      postsurgical malabsorption —see
          Osteoporosis, specified type
          NEC, with pathological
          fracture
      specified cause NEC —see
          Osteoporosis, specified type
          NEC, with pathological
          fracture
  specified disease NEC M84.60
    ankle M84.67-
    carpus M84.64-
    clavicle M84.61-
    femur M84.65-
    fibula M84.66-
    finger M84.64-
    hip M84.65-
    humerus M84.62-
    ilium M84.650
    ischium M84.650
    metacarpus M84.64-
    metatarsus M84.67-
    neck M84.68
    radius M84.63-
    rib M84.68
    scapula M84.61-
    skull M84.68
    tarsus M84.67-
    tibia M84.66-
    toe M84.67-
    ulna M84.63-
    vertebra M84.68
  femur M84.45-
  fibula M84.46-
  finger M84.44-
  hip M84.459
  humerus M84.42-
  ilium M84.454
  ischium M84.454
  joint prosthesis —see Complications,
      joint prosthesis, mechanical,
      breakdown, by site
  periprosthetic —see Complications,
      joint prosthesis, mechanical,
      periprosthesis, fracture, by site
  metacarpus M84.44-
  metatarsus M84.47-
  neck M84.48
  pelvis M84.454
  radius M84.43-
  restorative material (dental) K08.539
    with loss of material K08.531
    without loss of material K08.530
  rib M84.48
  scapula M84.41-
  skull M84.48
  tarsus M84.47-
  tibia M84.46-
  toe M84.47-
  ulna M84.43-
  vertebra M84.48
Fracture, traumatic (abduction)
    (adduction) (separation) (see also
    Fracture, pathological) T14.8
  acetabulum S32.40-
    column
      anterior (displaced) (iliopubic)
          S32.43-
        nondisplaced S32.436

Fracture, traumatic *(Continued)*
  acetabulum *(Continued)*
    column *(Continued)*
      posterior (displaced) (ilioischial)
        S32.443
        nondisplaced S32.44-
    dome (displaced) S32.48-
      nondisplaced S32.48
    specified NEC S32.49-
    transverse (displaced) S32.45-
      with associated posterior wall
        fracture (displaced) S32.46-
        nondisplaced S32.46-
      nondisplaced S32.45-
    wall
      anterior (displaced) S32.41-
        nondisplaced S32.41-
      medial (displaced) S32.47-
        nondisplaced S32.47-
      posterior (displaced) S32.42-
        with associated transverse
          fracture (displaced)
          S32.46-
          nondisplaced S32.46-
        nondisplaced S32.42-
  acromion —*see* Fracture, scapula,
    acromial process
  ankle S82.899
    bimalleolar (displaced) S82.84-
      nondisplaced S82.84-
    lateral malleolus only (displaced)
      S82.6-
      nondisplaced S82.6-
    medial malleolus (displaced)
      S82.5-
      associated with Maisonneuve's
        fracture —*see* Fracture,
        Maisonneuve's
      nondisplaced S82.5-
    talus —*see* Fracture, tarsal, talus
    trimalleolar (displaced) S82.85-
      nondisplaced S82.85-
  arm (upper) —*see also* Fracture,
    humerus, shaft
    humerus —*see* Fracture, humerus
    radius —*see* Fracture, radius
    ulna —*see* Fracture, ulna
  astragalus —*see* Fracture, tarsal, talus
  atlas —*see* Fracture, neck, cervical
    vertebra, first
  axis —*see* Fracture, neck, cervical
    vertebra, second
  back —*see* Fracture, vertebra
  Barton's —*see* Barton's fracture
  base of skull —*see* Fracture, skull, base
  basicervical (basal) (femoral) S72.0
  Bennett's —*see* Bennett's fracture
  bimalleolar —*see* Fracture, ankle,
    bimalleolar
  blow-out S02.3
  bone NEC T14.8
    birth injury P13.9
    following insertion of orthopedic
      implant, joint prosthesis or
      bone plate —*see* Fracture,
      following insertion of
      orthopedic implant, joint
      prosthesis or
      bone plate
    in (due to) neoplastic disease NEC —
      see Fracture, pathological, due
      to, neoplastic disease
    pathological (cause unknown) —*see*
      Fracture, pathological

Fracture, traumatic *(Continued)*
  breast bone —*see* Fracture, sternum
  bucket handle (semilunar cartilage) —
    see Tear, meniscus
  burst —*see* Fracture, traumatic, by site
  calcaneus —*see* Fracture, tarsal,
    calcaneus
  carpal bone (s) S62.10-
    capitate (displaced) S62.13-
      nondisplaced S62.13-
    cuneiform —*see* Fracture, carpal
      bone, triquetrum
    hamate (body) (displaced) S62.143
      hook process (displaced) S62.15-
        nondisplaced S62.15-
      nondisplaced S62.14-
    larger multangular —*see* Fracture,
      carpal bones, trapezium
    lunate (displaced) S62.12-
      nondisplaced S62.12-
    navicular S62.00-
      distal pole (displaced) S62.01-
        nondisplaced S62.01-
      middle third (displaced) S62.02-
        nondisplaced S62.02-
      proximal third (displaced) S62.03-
        nondisplaced S62.03-
      volar tuberosity —*see* Fracture,
        carpal bones, navicular, distal
        pole
    os magnum —*see* Fracture, carpal
      bones, capitate
    pisiform (displaced) S62.16-
      nondisplaced S62.16-
    semilunar —*see* Fracture, carpal
      bones, lunate
    smaller multangular —*see* Fracture,
      carpal bones, trapezoid
    trapezium (displaced) S62.17-
      nondisplaced S62.17-
    trapezoid (displaced) S62.18-
      nondisplaced S62.18-
    triquetrum (displaced) S62.11-
      nondisplaced S62.11-
    unciform —*see* Fracture, carpal bones,
      hamate
  cervical —*see* Fracture, vertebra,
    cervical
  clavicle S42.00-
    acromial end (displaced) S42.03-
      nondisplaced S42.03-
    birth injury P13.4
    lateral end —*see* Fracture, clavicle,
      acromial end
    shaft (displaced) S42.02-
      nondisplaced S42.02-
    sternal end (anterior) (displaced)
      S42.01-
      nondisplaced S42.01-
      posterior S42.01-
  coccyx S32.2
  collapsed —*see* Collapse, vertebra
  collar bone —*see* Fracture, clavicle
  Colles' —*see* Colles' fracture
  compression, not due to trauma —*see*
    Collapse, vertebra
  coronoid process —*see* Fracture, ulna,
    upper end, coronoid process
  corpus cavernosum penis S39.840
  costochondral cartilage S23.41
  costochondral, costosternal junction —
    see Fracture, rib
  cranium —*see* Fracture, skull
  cricoid cartilage S12.8

Fracture, traumatic *(Continued)*
  cuboid (ankle) —*see* Fracture, tarsal,
    cuboid
  cuneiform
    foot —*see* Fracture, tarsal, cuneiform
    wrist —*see* Fracture, carpal,
      triquetrum
  delayed union —*see* Delay, union,
    fracture
  dental restorative material K08.539
    with loss of material K08.531
    without loss of material K08.530
  due to
    birth injury —*see* Birth, injury,
      fracture
    osteoporosis —*see* Osteoporosis, with
      fracture
  Dupuytren's —*see* Fracture, ankle,
    lateral malleolus
  elbow S42.40-
  ethmoid (bone) (sinus) —*see* Fracture,
    skull, base
  face bone S02.92
  fatigue —*see also* Fracture, stress
    vertebra M48.40
      cervical region M48.42
      cervicothoracic region M48.43
      lumbar region M48.46
      lumbosacral region M48.47
      occipito-atlanto-axial region
        M48.41
      sacrococcygeal region M48.48
      thoracic region M48.44
      thoracolumbar region M48.45
  femur, femoral S72.9-
    basicervical (basal) S72.0
    birth injury P13.2
    capital epiphyseal S79.01-
    condyles, epicondyles —*see* Fracture,
      femur, lower end
    distal end —*see* Fracture, femur,
      lower end
    epiphysis
      head —*see* Fracture, femur, upper
        end, epiphysis
      lower —*see* Fracture, femur, lower
        end, epiphysis
      upper —*see* Fracture, femur, upper
        end, epiphysis
    following insertion of implant,
      prosthesis or plate M96.66-
    head —*see* Fracture, femur, upper
      end, head
    intertrochanteric —*see* Fracture,
      femur, trochanteric
    intratrochanteric —*see* Fracture,
      femur, trochanteric
    lower end S72.40-
      condyle (displaced) S72.41-
        lateral (displaced) S72.42-
          nondisplaced S72.42-
        medial (displaced) S72.43-
          nondisplaced S72.43-
        nondisplaced S72.41-
      epiphysis (displaced) S72.44-
        nondisplaced S72.44-
      physeal S79.10-
        Salter-Harris
          Type I S79.11-
          Type II S79.12-
          Type III S79.13-
          Type IV S79.14-
        specified NEC S79.19-
      specified NEC S72.49-

Fracture, traumatic *(Continued)*
  femur, femoral *(Continued)*
    lower end *(Continued)*
      supracondylar (displaced) S72.45-
        with intracondylar extension
          (displaced) S72.46-
          nondisplaced S72.46-
        nondisplaced S72.45-
      torus S72.47-
    neck —*see* Fracture, femur, upper
      end, neck
    pertrochanteric —*see* Fracture, femur,
      trochanteric
    shaft (lower third) (middle third)
      (upper third) S72.30-
      comminuted (displaced) S72.35-
        nondisplaced S72.35-
      oblique (displaced) S72.33-
        nondisplaced S72.33-
      segmental (displaced) S72.36-
        nondisplaced S72.36-
      specified NEC S72.39-
      spiral (displaced) S72.34-
        nondisplaced S72.34-
      transverse (displaced) S72.32-
        nondisplaced S72.32-
    specified site NEC —*see* subcategory
      S72.8
    subcapital (displaced) S72.01-
    subtrochanteric (region) (section)
      (displaced) S72.2-
      nondisplaced S72.2-
    transcervical —*see* Fracture, femur,
      upper end, neck
    transtrochanteric —*see* Fracture,
      femur, trochanteric
    trochanteric S72.10-
      apophyseal (displaced) S72.14-
        nondisplaced S72.14-
      greater trochanter (displaced)
        S72.11-
        nondisplaced S72.11-
      intertrochanteric (displaced) S72.13-
        nondisplaced S72.13-
      lesser trochanter (displaced)
        S72.12-
        nondisplaced S72.12-
    upper end S72.00-
      apophyseal (displaced) S72.13-
        nondisplaced S72.13-
      cervicotrochanteric —*see* Fracture,
        femur, upper end, neck, base
      epiphysis (displaced) S72.02-
        nondisplaced S72.02-
      head S72.05-
        articular (displaced) S72.06-
          nondisplaced S72.06-
        specified NEC S72.09-
      intertrochanteric (displaced)
        S72.14-
        nondisplaced S72.14-
      intracapsular S72.01-
      midcervical (displaced) S72.03-
        nondisplaced S72.03-
      neck S72.00-
        base (displaced) S72.04-
          nondisplaced S72.04-
        specified NEC S72.09-
      pertrochanteric —*see* Fracture,
        femur, upper end, trochanteric
      physeal S79.00-
        Salter-Harris type I S79.01-
        specified NEC S79.09-
      subcapital (displaced) S72.01-

Fracture, traumatic *(Continued)*
  femur, femoral *(Continued)*
    upper end *(Continued)*
      subtrochanteric (displaced) S72.2-
        nondisplaced S72.2-
      transcervical —*see* Fracture, femur,
        upper end, midcervical
      trochanteric S72.10-
        greater (displaced) S72.11-
          nondisplaced S72.11-
        lesser (displaced) S72.12-
          nondisplaced S72.12-
  fibula (shaft) (styloid) S82.40-
    comminuted (displaced) S82.45-
      nondisplaced S82.45-
    following insertion of implant,
      prosthesis or plate M96.67-
    involving ankle or malleolus —
      see Fracture, fibula, lateral
      malleolus
    lateral malleolus (displaced) S82.6-
      nondisplaced S82.6-
    lower end
      physeal S89.30-
        Salter-Harris
          Type I S89.31-
          Type II S89.32-
        specified NEC S89.39-
      specified NEC S82.83-
      torus S82.82-
    oblique (displaced) S82.43-
      nondisplaced S82.43-
    segmental (displaced) S82.46-
      nondisplaced S82.46-
    specified NEC S82.49-
    spiral (displaced) S82.44-
      nondisplaced S82.44-
    transverse (displaced) S82.42-
      nondisplaced S82.42-
    upper end
      physeal S89.20-
        Salter-Harris
          Type I S89.21-
          Type II S89.22-
        specified NEC S89.29-
      specified NEC S82.83-
      torus S82.81-
  finger (except thumb) S62.60-
    distal phalanx (displaced) S62.63-
      nondisplaced S62.66-
    index S62.60-
      distal phalanx (displaced) S62.63-
        nondisplaced S62.66-
      medial phalanx (displaced) S62.62-
        nondisplaced S62.65-
      proximal phalanx (displaced) S62.61-
        nondisplaced S62.64-
    little S62.60-
      distal phalanx (displaced) S62.63-
        nondisplaced S62.66-
      medial phalanx (displaced) S62.62-
        nondisplaced S62.65-
      proximal phalanx (displaced) S62.61-
        nondisplaced S62.64-
    medial phalanx (displaced) S62.62-
      nondisplaced S62.65-
    middle S62.60-
      distal phalanx (displaced) S62.63-
        nondisplaced S62.66-
      medial phalanx (displaced) S62.62-
        nondisplaced S62.65-
      proximal phalanx (displaced)
        S62.61-
        nondisplaced S62.64-

Fracture, traumatic *(Continued)*
  finger *(Continued)*
    proximal phalanx (displaced) S62.61-
      nondisplaced S62.64-
    ring S62.60-
      distal phalanx (displaced) S62.63-
        nondisplaced S62.66-
      medial phalanx (displaced) S62.62-
        nondisplaced S62.65-
      proximal phalanx (displaced)
        S62.61-
        nondisplaced S62.64-
    thumb —*see* Fracture, thumb
  following insertion (intraoperative)
    (postoperative) of orthopedic
    implant, joint prosthesis or bone
    plate M96.69
    femur M96.66-
    fibula M96.67-
    humerus M96.62-
    pelvis M96.65
    radius M96.63-
    specified bone NEC M96.69
    tibia M96.67-
    ulna M96.63-
  foot S92.90-
    astragalus —*see* Fracture, tarsal,
      talus
    calcaneus —*see* Fracture, tarsal,
      calcaneus
    cuboid —*see* Fracture, tarsal, cuboid
    cuneiform —*see* Fracture, tarsal,
      cuneiform
    metatarsal —*see* Fracture, metatarsal
    navicular —*see* Fracture, tarsal,
      navicular
    talus —*see* Fracture, tarsal, talus
    tarsal —*see* Fracture, tarsal
    toe —*see* Fracture, toe
  forearm S52.9-
    radius —*see* Fracture, radius
    ulna —*see* Fracture, ulna
  fossa (anterior) (middle) (posterior)
    S02.19
  frontal (bone) (skull) S02.0
    sinus S02.19
  glenoid (cavity) (scapula) —*see*
    Fracture, scapula, glenoid cavity
  greenstick —*see* Fracture, by site
  hallux —*see* Fracture, toe, great
  hand S62.9-
    carpal —*see* Fracture, carpal bone
    finger (except thumb) —*see* Fracture,
      finger
    metacarpal —*see* Fracture, metacarpal
    navicular (scaphoid) (hand) —*see*
      Fracture, carpal bone, navicular
    thumb —*see* Fracture, thumb
  healed or old
    with complications - code by Nature
      of the complication
  heel bone —*see* Fracture, tarsal,
    calcaneus
  Hill-Sachs S42.29-
  hip —*see* Fracture, femur, neck
  humerus S42.30-
    anatomical neck —*see* Fracture,
      humerus, upper end
    articular process —*see* Fracture,
      humerus, lower end
    capitellum —*see* Fracture, humerus,
      lower end, condyle, lateral
    distal end —*see* Fracture, humerus,
      lower end

Fracture, traumatic *(Continued)*
  humerus *(Continued)*
    epiphysis
      lower —*see* Fracture, humerus, lower end, physeal
      upper —*see* Fracture, humerus, upper end, physeal
    external condyle —*see* Fracture, humerus, lower end, condyle, lateral
    following insertion of implant, prosthesis or plate M96.62-
    great tuberosity —*see* Fracture, humerus, upper end, greater tuberosity
    intercondylar —*see* Fracture, humerus, lower end
    internal epicondyle —*see* Fracture, humerus, lower end, epicondyle, medial
    lesser tuberosity —*see* Fracture, humerus, upper end, lesser tuberosity
    lower end S42.40-
      condyle
        lateral (displaced) S42.45-
          nondisplaced S42.45-
        medial (displaced) S42.46-
          nondisplaced S42.46-
      epicondyle
        lateral (displaced) S42.43-
          nondisplaced S42.43-
        medial (displaced) S42.44-
          incarcerated S42.44-
          nondisplaced S42.44-
      physeal S49.10-
        Salter-Harris
          Type I S49.11-
          Type II S49.12-
          Type III S49.13-
          Type IV S49.14-
          specified NEC S49.19-
      specified NEC (displaced) S42.49-
        nondisplaced S42.49-
      supracondylar (simple) (displaced) S42.41-
        comminuted (displaced) S42.42-
          nondisplaced S42.42-
        nondisplaced S42.41-
      torus S42.48-
      transcondylar (displaced) S42.47-
        nondisplaced S42.47-
    proximal end —*see* Fracture, humerus, upper end
    shaft S42.30-
      comminuted (displaced) S42.35-
        nondisplaced S42.35-
      greenstick S42.31-
      oblique (displaced) S42.33-
        nondisplaced S42.33-
      segmental (displaced) S42.36-
        nondisplaced S42.36-
      specified NEC S42.39-
      spiral (displaced) S42.34-
        nondisplaced S42.34-
      transverse (displaced) S42.32-
        nondisplaced S42.32-
    supracondylar —*see* Fracture, humerus, lower end
    surgical neck —*see* Fracture, humerus, upper end, surgical neck
    trochlea —*see* Fracture, humerus, lower end, condyle, medial

Fracture, traumatic *(Continued)*
  humerus *(Continued)*
    tuberosity —*see* Fracture, humerus, upper end
    upper end S42.20-
      anatomical neck —*see* Fracture, humerus, upper end, specified NEC
      articular head —*see* Fracture, humerus, upper end, specified NEC
      epiphysis —*see* Fracture, humerus, upper end, physeal
      greater tuberosity (displaced) S42.25-
        nondisplaced S42.25-
      lesser tuberosity (displaced) S42.26-
        nondisplaced S42.26-
      physeal S49.00-
        Salter-Harris
          Type I S49.01-
          Type II S49.02-
          Type III S49.03-
          Type IV S49.04-
          specified NEC S49.09-
      specified NEC (displaced) S42.29-
        nondisplaced S42.29-
      surgical neck (displaced) S42.21-
        four-part S42.24-
        nondisplaced S42.21-
        three-part S42.23-
        two-part (displaced) S42.22-
          nondisplaced S42.22-
      torus S42.27-
      transepiphyseal —*see* Fracture, humerus, upper end, physeal
  hyoid bone S12.8
  ilium S32.30-
    with disruption of pelvic ring —*see* Disruption, pelvic ring
    avulsion (displaced) S32.31-
      nondisplaced S32.31-
    specified NEC S32.39-
  impaction, impacted - code as Fracture, by site
  innominate bone —*see* Fracture, ilium
  instep —*see* Fracture, foot
  ischium S32.60-
    with disruption of pelvic ring —*see* Disruption, pelvic ring
    avulsion (displaced) S32.61-
      nondisplaced S32.61-
    specified NEC S32.69-
  jaw (bone) (lower) —*see* Fracture, mandible
    upper —*see* Fracture, maxilla
  joint prosthesis —*see* Complications, joint prosthesis, mechanical, breakdown, by site
    periprosthetic —*see* Complications, joint prosthesis, mechanical, periprosthesis, fracture, by site
  knee cap —*see* Fracture, patella
  larynx S12.8
  late effects —*see* Sequelae, fracture
  leg (lower) S82.9-
    ankle —*see* Fracture, ankle
    femur —*see* Fracture, femur
    fibula —*see* Fracture, fibula
    malleolus —*see* Fracture, ankle
    patella —*see* Fracture, patella
    specified site NEC S82.89-
    tibia —*see* Fracture, tibia

Fracture, traumatic *(Continued)*
  lumbar spine —*see* Fracture, vertebra, lumbar
  lumbosacral spine S32.9
  Maisonneuve's (displaced) S82.86-
    nondisplaced S82.86-
  malar bone (*see also* Fracture, maxilla) S02.400
  malleolus —*see* Fracture, ankle
  malunion —*see* Fracture, by site
  mandible (lower jawbone) S02.609
    alveolus S02.67
    angle (of jaw) S02.65
    body, unspecified S02.600
    condylar process S02.61
    coronoid process S02.63
    ramus, unspecified S02.64
    specified site NEC S02.69
    subcondylar process S02.62
    symphysis S02.66
  manubrium (sterni) S22.21
    dissociation from sternum S22.23
  march —*see* Fracture, traumatic, stress, by site
  maxilla, maxillary (bone) (sinus) (superior) (upper jaw) S02.401
    alveolus S02.42
    inferior —*see* Fracture, mandible
    LeFort I S02.411
    LeFort II S02.412
    LeFort III S02.413
  metacarpal S62.309
    base (displaced) S62.319
      nondisplaced S62.349
    fifth S62.30-
      base (displaced) S62.31-
        nondisplaced S62.34-
      neck (displaced) S62.33-
        nondisplaced S62.36-
      shaft (displaced) S62.32-
        nondisplaced S62.35-
      specified NEC S62.398
    first S62.20-
      base NEC (displaced) S62.23-
        nondisplaced S62.23-
      Bennett's —*see* Bennett's fracture
      neck (displaced) S62.25-
        nondisplaced S62.25-
      shaft (displaced) S62.24-
        nondisplaced S62.24-
      specified NEC S62.29-
    fourth S62.30-
      base (displaced) S62.31-
        nondisplaced S62.34-
      neck (displaced) S62.33-
        nondisplaced S62.36-
      shaft (displaced) S62.32-
        nondisplaced S62.35-
      specified NEC S62.39-
    neck (displaced) S62.33-
      nondisplaced S62.36-
    Rolando's —*see* Rolando's fracture
    second S62.30-
      base (displaced) S62.31-
        nondisplaced S62.34-
      neck (displaced) S62.33-
        nondisplaced S62.36-
      shaft (displaced) S62.32-
        nondisplaced S62.35-
      specified NEC S62.39-
    shaft (displaced) S62.32-
      nondisplaced S62.35-
    specified NEC S62.399

Fracture, traumatic (Continued)
  metacarpal (Continued)
    third S62.30-
      base (displaced) S62.31-
        nondisplaced S62.34-
      neck (displaced) S62.33-
        nondisplaced S62.36-
      shaft (displaced) S62.32-
        nondisplaced S62.35-
      specified NEC S62.39-
    metastatic —see Fracture, pathological,
        due to, neoplastic disease —see also
        Neoplasm
  metatarsal bone S92.30-
    fifth (displaced) S92.35-
      nondisplaced S92.35-
    first (displaced) S92.31-
      nondisplaced S92.31-
    fourth (displaced) S92.34-
      nondisplaced S92.34-
    second (displaced) S92.32-
      nondisplaced S92.32-
    third (displaced) S92.33-
      nondisplaced S92.33-
  Monteggia's —see Monteggia's fracture
  multiple
    hand (and wrist) NEC —see Fracture,
        by site
    ribs —see Fracture, rib, multiple
  nasal (bone (s)) S02.2
  navicular (scaphoid) (foot) —see also
      Fracture, tarsal, navicular
    hand —see Fracture, carpal, navicular
  neck S12.9
    cervical vertebra S12.9
      fifth (displaced) S12.400
        nondisplaced S12.401
        specified type NEC (displaced)
            S12.490
          nondisplaced S12.491
      first (displaced) S12.000
        burst (stable) S12.01
          unstable S12.02
        lateral mass (displaced)
            S12.040
          nondisplaced S12.041
        nondisplaced S12.001
        posterior arch (displaced)
            S12.030
          nondisplaced S12.031
        specified type NEC (displaced)
            S12.090
          nondisplaced S12.091
      fourth (displaced) S12.300
        nondisplaced S12.301
        specified type NEC (displaced)
            S12.390
          nondisplaced S12.391
      second (displaced) S12.100
        dens (anterior) (displaced)
            (type II) S12.110
          nondisplaced S12.112
          posterior S12.111
        specified type NEC (displaced)
            S12.120
          nondisplaced S12.121
        nondisplaced S12.101
        specified type NEC (displaced)
            S12.190
          nondisplaced S12.191
      seventh (displaced) S12.600
        nondisplaced S12.601
        specified type NEC (displaced)
            S12.690
          displaced S12.691

Fracture, traumatic (Continued)
  neck (Continued)
    cervical vertebra (Continued)
      sixth (displaced) S12.500
        nondisplaced S12.501
        specified type NEC (displaced)
            S12.590
          displaced S12.591
      third (displaced) S12.200
        nondisplaced S12.201
        specified type NEC (displaced)
            S12.290
          displaced S12.291
    hyoid bone S12.8
    larynx S12.8
    specified site NEC S12.8
    thyroid cartilage S12.8
    trachea S12.8
  neoplastic NEC —see Fracture,
      pathological, due to, neoplastic
      disease
  neural arch —see Fracture, vertebra
  newborn —see Birth, injury, fracture
  nontraumatic —see Fracture,
      pathological
  nonunion —see Nonunion, fracture
  nose, nasal (bone) (septum) S02.2
  occiput —see Fracture, skull, base,
      occiput
  odontoid process —see Fracture, neck,
      cervical vertebra, second
  olecranon (process) (ulna) —see
      Fracture, ulna, upper end,
      olecranon process
  orbit, orbital (bone) (region) S02.8
    floor (blow-out) S02.3
    roof S02.19
  os
    calcis —see Fracture, tarsal,
        calcaneus
    magnum —see Fracture, carpal,
        capitate
    pubis —see Fracture, pubis
  palate S02.8
  parietal bone (skull) S02.0
  patella S82.00-
    comminuted (displaced) S82.04-
      nondisplaced S82.04-
    longitudinal (displaced) S82.02-
      nondisplaced S82.02-
    osteochondral (displaced) S82.01-
      nondisplaced S82.01-
    specified NEC S82.09-
    transverse (displaced) S82.03-
      nondisplaced S82.03-
  pedicle (of vertebral arch) —see
      Fracture, vertebra
  pelvis, pelvic (bone) S32.9
    acetabulum —see Fracture,
        acetabulum
    circle —see Disruption, pelvic ring
    following insertion of implant,
        prosthesis or plate M96.65
    ilium —see Fracture, ilium
    ischium —see Fracture, ischium
    multiple
      with disruption of pelvic ring
          (circle) —see Disruption,
          pelvic ring
      without disruption of pelvic ring
          (circle) S32.82
    pubis —see Fracture, pubis
    sacrum —see Fracture, sacrum
    specified site NEC S32.89

Fracture, traumatic (Continued)
  phalanx
    foot —see Fracture, toe
    hand —see Fracture, finger
  pisiform —see Fracture, carpal,
      pisiform
  pond —see Fracture, skull
  prosthetic device, internal —see
      Complications, prosthetic device,
      by site, mechanical
  pubis S32.50-
    with disruption of pelvic ring —see
        Disruption, pelvic ring
    specified site NEC S32.59-
    superior rim S32.59-
  radius S52.9-
    distal end —see Fracture, radius,
        lower end
    following insertion of implant,
        prosthesis or plate M96.63-
    head —see Fracture, radius, upper
        end, head
    lower end S52.50-
      Barton's —see Barton's fracture
      Colles' —see Colles' fracture
      extraarticular NEC S52.55-
      intraarticular NEC S52.57-
      physeal S59.20-
        Salter-Harris
          Type I S59.21-
          Type II S59.22-
          Type III S59.23-
          Type IV S59.24-
        specified NEC S59.29-
      Smith's —see Smith's fracture
      specified NEC S52.59-
      styloid process (displaced)
          S52.51-
        nondisplaced S52.51-
      torus S52.52-
    neck —see Fracture, radius, upper
        end
    proximal end —see Fracture, radius,
        upper end
    shaft S52.30-
      bent bone S52.38-
      comminuted (displaced) S52.35-
        nondisplaced S52.35-
      Galeazzi's —see Galeazzi's
          fracture
      greenstick S52.31-
      oblique (displaced) S52.33-
        nondisplaced S52.33-
      segmental (displaced) S52.36-
        nondisplaced S52.36-
      specified NEC S52.39-
      spiral (displaced) S52.34-
        nondisplaced S52.34-
      transverse (displaced) S52.32-
        nondisplaced S52.32-
    upper end S52.10-
      head (displaced) S52.12-
        nondisplaced S52.12-
      neck (displaced) S52.13-
        nondisplaced S52.13-
      physeal S59.10-
        Salter-Harris
          Type I S59.11-
          Type II S59.12-
          Type III S59.13-
          Type IV S59.14-
        specified NEC S59.19-
      specified NEC S52.18-
      torus S52.11-

Fracture, traumatic (Continued)
  ramus
    inferior or superior, pubis —see
        Fracture, pubis
    mandible —see Fracture, mandible
  restorative material (dental) K08.539
    with loss of material K08.531
    without loss of material K08.530
  rib S22.3-
    with flail chest —see Flail, chest
    multiple S22.4-
      with flail chest —see Flail, chest
  root, tooth —see Fracture, tooth
  sacrum S32.10
    specified NEC S32.19
    Type
      1 S32.14
      2 S32.15
      3 S32.16
      4 S32.17
    Zone
      I S32.119
        displaced (minimally) S32.111
          severely S32.112
        nondisplaced S32.110
      II S32.129
        displaced (minimally) S32.121
          severely S32.122
        nondisplaced S32.120
      III S32.139
        displaced (minimally) S32.131
          severely S32.132
        nondisplaced S32.130
  scaphoid (hand) —see also Fracture,
      carpal, navicular
    foot —see Fracture, tarsal, navicular
  scapula S42.10-
    acromial process (displaced) S42.12-
      nondisplaced S42.12-
    body (displaced) S42.11-
      nondisplaced S42.11-
    coracoid process (displaced) S42.13-
      nondisplaced S42.13-
    glenoid cavity (displaced) S42.14-
      nondisplaced S42.14-
    neck (displaced) S42.15-
      nondisplaced S42.15-
    specified NEC S42.19-
  semilunar bone, wrist —see Fracture,
      carpal, lunate
  sequelae —see Sequelae, fracture
  sesamoid bone
    hand —see Fracture, carpal
    other - code by site under Fracture
  shepherd's —see Fracture, tarsal, talus
  shoulder (girdle) S42.9-
    blade —see Fracture, scapula
  sinus (ethmoid) (frontal) S02.19
  skull S02.91
    base S02.10
      occiput S02.119
        condyle S02.113
          type I S02.110
          type II S02.111
          type III S02.112
          specified NEC S02.118
        specified NEC S02.19
    birth injury P13.0
    frontal bone S02.0
    parietal bone S02.0
    specified site NEC S02.8
    temporal bone S02.19
    vault S02.0
  Smith's —see Smith's fracture

Fracture, traumatic (Continued)
  sphenoid (bone) (sinus) S02.19
  spine —see Fracture, vertebra
  spinous process —see Fracture, vertebra
  spontaneous (cause unknown) —see
      Fracture, pathological
  stave (of thumb) —see Fracture,
      metacarpal, first
  sternum S22.20
    with flail chest —see Flail, chest
    body S22.22
    manubrium S22.21
    xiphoid (process) S22.24
  stress M84.30
    ankle M84.37-
    carpus M84.34-
    clavicle M84.31-
    femoral neck M84.359
    femur M84.35-
    fibula M84.36-
    finger M84.34-
    hip M84.359
    humerus M84.32-
    ilium M84.350
    ischium M84.350
    metacarpus M84.34-
    metatarsus M84.37-
    neck —see Fracture, fatigue, vertebra
    pelvis M84.350
    radius M84.33-
    rib M84.38
    scapula M84.31-
    skull M84.38
    tarsus M84.37-
    tibia M84.36-
    toe M84.37-
    ulna M84.33-
    vertebra —see Fracture, fatigue,
        vertebra
  supracondylar, elbow —see
      Fracture, humerus, lower end,
      supracondylar
  symphysis pubis —see Fracture, pubis
  talus (ankle bone) —see Fracture, tarsal,
      talus
  tarsal bone (s) S92.20-
    astragalus —see Fracture, tarsal,
        talus
    calcaneus S92.00-
      anterior process (displaced)
          S92.02-
        nondisplaced S92.02-
      body (displaced) S92.01-
        nondisplaced S92.01-
      extraarticular NEC (displaced)
          S92.05-
        nondisplaced S92.05-
      intraarticular (displaced) S92.06-
        nondisplaced S92.06-
      tuberosity (displaced) S92.04-
        avulsion (displaced) S92.03-
          nondisplaced S92.03-
        nondisplaced S92.04-
    cuboid (displaced) S92.21-
      nondisplaced S92.21-
    cuneiform
      intermediate (displaced) S92.23-
        nondisplaced S92.23-
      lateral (displaced) S92.22-
        nondisplaced S92.22-
      medial (displaced) S92.24-
        nondisplaced S92.24-
    navicular (displaced) S92.25-
      nondisplaced S92.25-

Fracture, traumatic (Continued)
  tarsal bone (s) (Continued)
    scaphoid —see Fracture, tarsal,
        navicular
    talus S92.10-
      avulsion (displaced) S92.15-
        nondisplaced S92.15-
      body (displaced) S92.12-
        nondisplaced S92.12-
      dome (displaced) S92.14-
        nondisplaced S92.14-
      head (displaced) S92.12-
        nondisplaced S92.12-
      lateral process (displaced) S92.14-
        nondisplaced S92.14-
      neck (displaced) S92.11-
        nondisplaced S92.11-
      posterior process (displaced) S92.13-
        nondisplaced S92.13-
      specified NEC S92.19-
  temporal bone (styloid) S02.19
  thorax (bony) S22.9
    with flail chest —see Flail, chest
    rib S22.3-
      multiple S22.4-
        with flail chest —see Flail, chest
    sternum S22.20
      body S22.22
      manubrium S22.21
      xiphoid process S22.24
    vertebra (displaced) S22.009
      burst (stable) S22.001
        unstable S22.002
      eighth S22.069
        burst (stable) S22.061
          unstable S22.062
        specified type NEC S22.068
        wedge compression S22.060
      eleventh S22.089
        burst (stable) S22.081
          unstable S22.082
        specified type NEC S22.088
        wedge compression S22.080
      fifth S22.059
        burst (stable) S22.051
          unstable S22.052
        specified type NEC S22.058
        wedge compression S22.050
      first S22.019
        burst (stable) S22.011
          unstable S22.012
        specified type NEC S22.018
        wedge compression S22.010
      fourth S22.049
        burst (stable) S22.041
          unstable S22.042
        specified type NEC S22.048
        wedge compression S22.040
      ninth S22.079
        burst (stable) S22.071
          unstable S22.072
        specified type NEC S22.078
        wedge compression S22.070
      nondisplaced S22.001
      second S22.029
        burst (stable) S22.021
          unstable S22.022
        specified type NEC S22.028
        wedge compression S22.020
      seventh S22.069
        burst (stable) S22.061
          unstable S22.062
        specified type NEC S22.068
        wedge compression S22.060

Fracture, traumatic *(Continued)*
  thorax *(Continued)*
    vertebra *(Continued)*
      sixth S22.059
        burst (stable) S22.051
          unstable S22.052
        specified type NEC S22.058
        wedge compression S22.050
      specified type NEC S22.008
      tenth S22.079
        burst (stable) S22.071
          unstable S22.072
        specified type NEC S22.078
        wedge compression S22.070
      third S22.039
        burst (stable) S22.031
          unstable S22.032
        specified type NEC S22.038
        wedge compression S22.030
      twelfth S22.089
        burst (stable) S22.081
          unstable S22.082
        specified type NEC S22.088
        wedge compression S22.080
      wedge compression S22.000
  thumb S62.50-
    distal phalanx (displaced) S62.52-
      nondisplaced S62.52-
    proximal phalanx (displaced) S62.51-
      nondisplaced S62.51-
  thyroid cartilage S12.8
  tibia (shaft) S82.20-
    comminuted (displaced) S82.25-
      nondisplaced S82.25-
    condyles —*see* Fracture, tibia, upper
      end
    distal end —*see* Fracture, tibia, lower
      end
    epiphysis
      lower —*see* Fracture, tibia, lower
        end
      upper —*see* Fracture, tibia, upper
        end
    following insertion of implant,
      prosthesis or plate M96.67-
    head (involving knee joint) —*see*
      Fracture, tibia, upper end
    intercondyloid eminence —*see*
      Fracture, tibia, upper end
    involving ankle or malleolus —*see*
      Fracture, ankle, medial malleolus
    lower end S82.30-
      physeal S89.10-
        Salter-Harris
          Type I S89.11-
          Type II S89.12-
          Type III S89.13-
          Type IV S89.14-
        specified NEC S89.19-
      pilon (displaced) S82.87-
        nondisplaced S82.87-
      specified NEC S82.39-
      torus S82.31-
    malleolus —*see* Fracture, ankle,
      medial malleolus
    oblique (displaced) S82.23-
      nondisplaced S82.23-
    pilon —*see* Fracture, tibia, lower end,
      pilon
    proximal end —*see* Fracture, tibia,
      upper end
    segmental (displaced) S82.26-
      nondisplaced S82.26-
    specified NEC S82.29-

Fracture, traumatic *(Continued)*
  tibia *(Continued)*
    spine —*see* Fracture, upper end, spine
    spiral (displaced) S82.24-
      nondisplaced S82.24-
    transverse (displaced) S82.22-
      nondisplaced S82.22-
    tuberosity —*see* Fracture, tibia, upper
      end, tuberosity
    upper end S82.10-
      bicondylar (displaced) S82.14-
        nondisplaced S82.14-
      lateral condyle (displaced) S82.12-
        nondisplaced S82.12-
      medial condyle (displaced) S82.13-
        nondisplaced S82.13-
      physeal S89.00-
        Salter-Harris
          Type I S89.01-
          Type II S89.02-
          Type III S89.03-
          Type IV S89.04-
        specified NEC S89.09-
      plateau —*see* Fracture, tibia, upper
        end, bicondylar
      specified NEC S82.19-
      spine (displaced) S82.11-
        nondisplaced S82.11-
      torus S82.16-
      tuberosity (displaced) S82.15-
        nondisplaced S82.15-
  toe S92.91-
    great (displaced) S92.40-
      distal phalanx (displaced) S92.42-
        nondisplaced S92.42-
      nondisplaced S92.40-
      proximal phalanx (displaced)
        S92.41-
        nondisplaced S92.41-
      specified NEC S92.49-
    lesser (displaced) S92.50-
      distal phalanx (displaced) S92.53-
        nondisplaced S92.53-
      medial phalanx (displaced) S92.52-
        nondisplaced S92.52-
      nondisplaced S92.50-
      proximal phalanx (displaced)
        S92.51-
        nondisplaced S92.51-
      specified NEC S92.59-
  tooth (root) S02.5
  trachea (cartilage) S12.8
  transverse process —*see* Fracture,
    vertebra
  trapezium or trapezoid bone —*see*
    Fracture, carpal
  trimalleolar —*see* Fracture, ankle,
    trimalleolar
  triquetrum (cuneiform of carpus) —*see*
    Fracture, carpal, triquetrum
  trochanter —*see* Fracture, femur,
    trochanteric
  tuberosity (external) - code by site
    under Fracture
  ulna (shaft) S52.20-
    bent bone S52.28-
    coronoid process —*see* Fracture,
      ulna, upper end, coronoid
      process
    distal end —*see* Fracture, ulna, lower
      end
    following insertion of implant,
      prosthesis or plate M96.63-
    head S52.00-

Fracture, traumatic *(Continued)*
  ulna *(Continued)*
    lower end S52.60-
      physeal S59.00-
        Salter-Harris
          Type I S59.01-
          Type II S59.02-
          Type III S59.03-
          Type IV S59.04-
        specified NEC S59.09-
      specified NEC S52.69-
      styloid process (displaced) S52.61-
        nondisplaced S52.61-
      torus S52.62-
    proximal end —*see* Fracture, ulna,
      upper end
    shaft S52.20-
      comminuted (displaced) S52.25-
        nondisplaced S52.25-
      greenstick S52.21-
      Monteggia's —*see* Monteggia's
        fracture
      oblique (displaced) S52.23-
        nondisplaced S52.23-
      segmental (displaced) S52.26-
        nondisplaced S52.26-
      specified NEC S52.29-
      spiral (displaced) S52.24-
        nondisplaced S52.24-
      transverse (displaced) S52.22-
        nondisplaced S52.22-
    upper end S52.00-
      coronoid process (displaced)
        S52.04-
        nondisplaced S52.04-
      olecranon process (displaced)
        S52.02-
        with intraarticular extension
          S52.03-
        with intraarticular extension
          S52.03-
        nondisplaced S52.02-
        with intraarticular extension
          S52.03-
      specified NEC S52.09-
      torus S52.01-
  unciform —*see* Fracture, carpal, hamate
  vault of skull S02.0
  vertebra, vertebral (arch) (body)
    (column) (neural arch) (pedicle)
    (spinous process) (transverse
    process)
    atlas —*see* Fracture, neck, cervical
      vertebra, first
    axis —*see* Fracture, neck, cervical
      vertebra, second
    cervical (teardrop) S12.9
      axis —*see* Fracture, neck, cervical
        vertebra, second
      first (atlas) —*see* Fracture, neck,
        cervical vertebra, first
      second (axis) —*see* Fracture, neck,
        cervical vertebra, second
    chronic M84.48
    coccyx S32.2
    dorsal —*see* Fracture, thorax, vertebra
    lumbar S32.009
      burst (stable) S32.001
        unstable S32.002
      fifth S32.059
        burst (stable) S32.051
          unstable S32.052
        specified type NEC S32.058
        wedge compression S32.050

Fracture, traumatic *(Continued)*
vertebra, vertebral *(Continued)*
lumbar *(Continued)*
first S32.019
burst (stable) S32.011
unstable S32.012
specified type NEC S32.018
wedge compression S32.010
fourth S32.049
burst (stable) S32.041
unstable S32.042
specified type NEC S32.048
wedge compression S32.040
second S32.029
burst (stable) S32.021
unstable S32.022
specified type NEC S32.028
wedge compression S32.020
specified type NEC S32.008
third S32.039
burst (stable) S32.031
unstable S32.032
specified type NEC S32.038
wedge compression S32.030
wedge compression S32.000
metastatic —*see* Collapse, vertebra,
in, specified disease NEC —*see*
also Neoplasm
newborn (birth injury) P11.5
sacrum S32.10
specified NEC S32.19
Type
1 S32.14
2 S32.15
3 S32.16
4 S32.17
Zone
I S32.119
displaced (minimally) S32.111
severely S32.112
nondisplaced S32.110
II S32.129
displaced (minimally) S32.121
severely S32.122
nondisplaced S32.120
III S32.139
displaced (minimally) S32.131
severely S32.132
nondisplaced S32.130
thoracic —*see* Fracture, thorax,
vertebra
vertex S02.0
vomer (bone) S02.2
wrist S62.10-
carpal —*see* Fracture, carpal bone
navicular (scaphoid) (hand) —*see*
Fracture, carpal, navicular
xiphisternum, xiphoid (process) S22.24
zygoma S02.442
Fragile, fragility
autosomal site Q95.5
bone, congenital (with blue sclera)
Q78.0
capillary (hereditary) D69.8
hair L67.8
nails L60.3
non-sex chromosome site Q95.5
X chromosome Q99.2
Fragilitas
crinium L67.8
ossium (with blue sclerae) (hereditary)
Q78.0
unguium L60.3
congenital Q84.6

Fragments, cataract (lens), following
cataract surgery H59.02-
retained foreign body —*see* Retained,
foreign body fragments (type of)
Frailty (frail) R54
mental R41.81
Frambesia, frambesial (tropica) —*see also*
Yaws
initial lesion or ulcer A66.0
primary A66.0
Frambeside
gummatous A66.4
of early yaws A66.2
Frambesioma A66.1
Franceschetti-Klein (-Wildervanck)
disease or syndrome Q75.4
Francis' disease —*see* Tularemia
Franklin disease C88.2
Frank's essential thrombocytopenia D69.3
Fraser's syndrome Q87.0
Freckle (s) L81.2
malignant melanoma in —*see*
Melanoma
melanotic (Hutchinson's) —*see*
Melanoma, in situ
retinal D49.81
Frederickson's hyperlipoproteinemia,
type
I and V E78.3
IIA E78.0
IIB and III E78.2
IV E78.1
Freeman Sheldon syndrome Q87.0
Freezing —*see also* Effect, adverse, cold
T69.9
Freiberg's disease (infraction
of metatarsal head or
osteochondrosis) —*see*
Osteochondrosis, juvenile,
metatarsus
Frei's disease A55
Fremitus, friction, cardiac R01.2
Frenum, frenulum
external os Q51.828
tongue (shortening) (congenital) Q38.1
Frequency micturition (nocturnal) R35.0
psychogenic F45.8
Frey's syndrome
auriculotemporal G50.8
hyperhidrosis L74.52
Friction
burn —*see* Burn, by site
fremitus, cardiac R01.2
precordial R01.2
sounds, chest R09.89
Friderichsen-Waterhouse syndrome or
disease A39.1
Friedländer's B (bacillus) NEC (*see also*
condition) A49.8
Friedreich's
ataxia G11.1
combined systemic disease G11.1
facial hemihypertrophy Q67.4
sclerosis (cerebellum) (spinal cord)
G11.1
Frigidity F52.22
Fröhlich's syndrome E23.6
Frontal —*see also* condition
lobe syndrome F07.0
Frostbite (superficial) T33.90
with
partial thickness skin loss —*see*
Frostbite (superficial), by site
tissue necrosis T34.90

Frostbite *(Continued)*
abdominal wall T33.3
with tissue necrosis T34.3
ankle T33.81-
with tissue necrosis T34.81-
arm T33.4-
with tissue necrosis T34.4-
finger (s) —*see* Frostbite, finger
hand —*see* Frostbite, hand
wrist —*see* Frostbite, wrist
ear T33.01-
with tissue necrosis T34.01-
face T33.09
with tissue necrosis T34.09
finger T33.53-
with tissue necrosis T34.53-
foot T33.82-
with tissue necrosis T34.82-
hand T33.52-
with tissue necrosis T34.52-
head T33.09
with tissue necrosis T34.09
ear —*see* Frostbite, ear
nose —*see* Frostbite, nose
hip (and thigh) T33.6-
with tissue necrosis T34.6-
knee T33.7-
with tissue necrosis T34.7-
leg T33.9-
with tissue necrosis T34.9-
ankle —*see* Frostbite, ankle
foot —*see* Frostbite, foot
knee —*see* Frostbite, knee
lower T33.7-
with tissue necrosis T34.7-
thigh —*see* Frostbite, hip
toe —*see* Frostbite, toe
limb
lower T33.99
with tissue necrosis T34.99
upper —*see* Frostbite, arm
neck T33.1
with tissue necrosis T34.1
nose T33.02
with tissue necrosis T34.02
pelvis T33.3
with tissue necrosis T34.3
specified site NEC T33.99
with tissue necrosis T34.99
thigh —*see* Frostbite, hip
thorax T33.2
with tissue necrosis T34.2
toes T33.83-
with tissue necrosis T34.83-
trunk T33.99
with tissue necrosis T34.99
wrist T33.51-
with tissue necrosis T34.51-
Frotteurism F65.81
Frozen (*see also* Effect, adverse, cold) T69.9
pelvis (female) N94.89
male K66.8
shoulder —*see* Capsulitis, adhesive
Fructokinase deficiency E74.11
Fructose 1,6 diphosphatase deficiency
E74.19
Fructosemia (benign) (essential) E74.12
Fructosuria (benign) (essential) E74.11
Fuchs'
black spot (myopic) H44.2-
dystrophy (corneal endothelium)
H18.51
heterochromic cyclitis —*see* Cyclitis,
Fuchs' heterochromic

Fucosidosis E77.1
Fugue R68.89
  dissociative F44.1
  hysterical (dissociative) F44.1
  postictal in epilepsy —see Epilepsy
  reaction to exceptional stress (transient)
    F43.0
Fulminant, fulminating —see condition
Functional —see also condition
  bleeding (uterus) N93.8
Functioning, intellectual, borderline
    R41.83
Fundus —see condition
Fungemia NOS B49
Fungus, fungous
  cerebral G93.89
  disease NOS B49
  infection —see Infection, fungus
Funiculitis (acute) (chronic) (endemic)
    N49.1
  gonococcal (acute) (chronic) A54.23
  tuberculous A18.15
Funnel
  breast (acquired) M95.4
    congenital Q67.6
    sequelae (late effect) of rickets E64.3
  chest (acquired) M95.4
    congenital Q67.6
    sequelae (late effect) of rickets E64.3
  pelvis (acquired) M95.5
    with disproportion (fetopelvic) O33.3
      causing obstructed labor O65.3
    congenital Q74.2
FUO (fever of unknown origin) R50.9
Furfur L21.0
  microsporon B36.0
Furrier's lung J67.8
Furrowed K14.5
  nail (s) (transverse) L60.4
    congenital Q84.6
  tongue K14.5
    congenital Q38.3
Furuncle L02.92
  abdominal wall L02.221
  ankle —see Furuncle, lower limb
  antecubital space —see Furuncle, upper
    limb
  anus K61.0
  arm —see Furuncle, upper limb
  auditory canal, external —see Abscess,
    ear, external
  auricle (ear) —see Abscess, ear, external
  axilla (region) L02.42-
  back (any part) L02.222
  breast N61
  buttock L02.32
  cheek (external) L02.02
  chest wall L02.223
  chin L02.02
  corpus cavernosum N48.21
  ear, external —see Abscess, ear, external
  external auditory canal —see Abscess,
    ear, external
  eyelid —see Abscess, eyelid

Furuncle (Continued)
  face L02.02
  femoral (region) —see Furuncle, lower
    limb
  finger —see Furuncle, hand
  flank L02.221
  foot L02.62-
  forehead L02.02
  gluteal (region) L02.32
  groin L02.224
  hand L02.52-
  head L02.821
    face L02.02
  hip —see Furuncle, lower limb
  kidney —see Abscess, kidney
  knee —see Furuncle, lower limb
  labium (majus) (minus) N76.4
  lacrimal
    gland —see Dacryoadenitis
    passages (duct) (sac) —see
      Inflammation, lacrimal,
      passages, acute
  leg (any part) —see Furuncle,
    lower limb
  lower limb L02.42-
  malignant A22.0
  mouth K12.2
  navel L02.226
  neck L02.12
  nose J34.0
  orbit, orbital —see Abscess, orbit
  palmar (space) —see Furuncle, hand
  partes posteriores L02.32
  pectoral region L02.223
  penis N48.21
  perineum L02.225
  pinna —see Abscess, ear, external
  popliteal —see Furuncle, lower limb
  prepatellar —see Furuncle, lower limb
  scalp L02.821
  seminal vesicle N49.0
  shoulder —see Furuncle, upper limb
  specified site NEC L02.828
  submandibular K12.2
  temple (region) L02.02
  thumb —see Furuncle, hand
  toe —see Furuncle, foot
  trunk L02.229
    abdominal wall L02.221
    back L02.222
    chest wall L02.223
    groin L02.224
    perineum L02.225
    umbilicus L02.226
  umbilicus L02.226
  upper limb L02.42-
  vulva N76.4
Furunculosis —see Furuncle
Fused —see Fusion, fused
Fusion, fused (congenital)
  astragaloscaphoid Q74.2
  atria Q21.1
  auditory canal Q16.1
  auricles, heart Q21.1

Fusion, fused (Continued)
  binocular with defective stereopsis
    H53.32
  bone Q79.8
  cervical spine M43.22
  choanal Q30.0
  commissure, mitral valve Q23.2
  cusps, heart valve NEC Q24.8
    mitral Q23.2
    pulmonary Q22.1
    tricuspid Q22.4
  ear ossicles Q16.3
  fingers - Q70.0
  hymen Q52.3
  joint (acquired) —see also Ankylosis
    congenital Q74.8
  kidneys (incomplete) Q63.1
  labium (majus) (minus) Q52.5
  larynx and trachea Q34.8
  limb, congenital Q74.8
    lower Q74.2
    upper Q74.0
  lobes, lung Q33.8
  lumbosacral (acquired) M43.27
    arthrodesis status Z98.1
    congenital Q76.49
    postprocedural status Z98.1
  nares, nose, nasal, nostril (s) Q30.0
  organ or site not listed —see Anomaly,
    by site
  ossicles Q79.9
    auditory Q16.3
  pulmonic cusps Q22.1
  ribs Q76.6
  sacroiliac (joint) (acquired) M43.28
    arthrodesis status Z98.1
    congenital Q74.2
    postprocedural status Z98.1
  spine (acquired) NEC M43.20
    arthrodesis status Z98.1
    cervical region M43.22
    cervicothoracic region M43.23
    congenital Q76.49
    lumbar M43.26
    lumbosacral region M43.27
    occipito-atlanto-axial region M43.21
    postoperative status Z98.1
    sacrococcygeal region M43.28
    thoracic region M43.24
    thoracolumbar region M43.25
  sublingual duct with submaxillary duct
    at opening in mouth Q38.4
  testes Q55.1
  toes Q70.2
  tooth, teeth K00.2
  trachea and esophagus Q39.8
  twins Q89.4
  vagina Q52.4
  ventricles, heart Q21.0
  vertebra (arch) —see Fusion, spine
  vulva Q52.5
Fusospirillosis (mouth) (tongue)
    (tonsil) A69.1
Fussy baby R68.12

G

Gain in weight (abnormal) (excessive) —
  see also Weight, gain
Gaisböck's disease (polycythemia
  hypertonica) D75.1
Gait abnormality R26.9
  ataxic R26.0
  falling R29.6
  hysterical (ataxic) (staggering) F44.4
  paralytic R26.1
  spastic R26.1
  specified type NEC R26.89
  staggering R26.0
  unsteadiness R26.81
  walking difficulty NEC R26.2
Galactocele (breast) N64.89
  puerperal, postpartum O92.79
Galactokinase deficiency E74.29
Galactophoritis N61
  gestational, puerperal, postpartum
    O91.2-
Galactorrhea O92.6
  not associated with childbirth N64.3
Galactosemia (classic) (congenital)
  E74.21
Galactosuria E74.29
Galacturia R82.0
  schistosomiasis (bilharziasis) B65.0
Galeazzi's fracture S52.37-
Galen's vein —*see* condition
Galeophobia F40.218
Gall duct —*see* condition
Gallbladder —*see also* condition
  acute K81.0
Gallop rhythm R00.8
Gallstone (colic) (cystic duct) (gallbladder)
  (impacted) (multiple) —*see also*
  Calculus, gallbladder
  with
    cholecystitis —*see* Calculus,
      gallbladder, with cholecystitis
    bile duct (common) (hepatic) —*see*
      Calculus, bile duct
    causing intestinal obstruction K56.3
    specified NEC K80.80
      with obstruction K80.81
Gambling Z72.6
  pathological (compulsive) F63.0
Gammopathy (of undetermined
  significance [MGUS]) D47.2
  associated with lymphoplasmacytic
    dyscrasia D47.2
  monoclonal D47.2
  polyclonal D89.0
Gamna's disease (siderotic splenomegaly)
  D73.1
Gamophobia F40.298
Gampsodactylia (congenital) Q66.7
Gamstorp's disease (adynamia episodica
  hereditaria) G72.3
Gandy-Nanta disease (siderotic
  splenomegaly) D73.1
Gang
  membership offenses Z72.810
Gangliocytoma D36.10
Ganglioglioma —*see* Neoplasm,
  uncertain behavior, by site
Ganglion (compound) (diffuse) (joint)
  (tendon (sheath)) M67.40
  ankle M67.47-
  foot M67.47-
  forearm M67.43-
  hand M67.44-

Ganglion (*Continued*)
  lower leg M67.46-
  multiple sites M67.49
  of yaws (early) (late) A66.6
  pelvic region M67.45-
  periosteal —*see* Periostitis
  shoulder region M67.41-
  specified site NEC M67.48
  thigh region M67.45-
  tuberculous A18.09
  upper arm M67.42-
  wrist M67.43-
Ganglioneuroblastoma —*see* Neoplasm,
  nerve, malignant
Ganglioneuroma D36.10
  malignant —*see* Neoplasm, nerve,
    malignant
Ganglioneuromatosis D36.10
Ganglionitis
  fifth nerve —*see* Neuralgia, trigeminal
  gasserian (postherpetic) (postzoster)
    B02.21
  geniculate G51.1
    newborn (birth injury) P11.3
    postherpetic, postzoster B02.21
  herpes zoster B02.21
  postherpetic geniculate B02.21
Gangliosidosis E75.10
  GM1 E75.19
  GM2 E75.00
    other specified E75.09
    Sandhoff disease E75.01
    Tay-Sachs disease E75.02
  GM3 E75.19
  mucolipidosis IV E75.11
Gangosa A66.5
Gangrene, gangrenous (connective
  tissue) (dropsical) (dry) (moist) (skin)
  (ulcer) (*see also* Necrosis) I96
  with diabetes (mellitus) —*see* Diabetes,
    gangrene
  abdomen (wall) I96
  alveolar M27.3
  appendix K35.3
    with
      perforation or rupture K35.2
      peritoneal abscess K35.3
      peritonitis, localized K35.3
        with perforation or rupture K35.2
        generalized K35.2
  arteriosclerotic (general) (senile) —*see*
    Arteriosclerosis, extremities, with,
    gangrene
  auricle I96
  Bacillus welchii A48.0
  bladder (infectious) —*see* Cystitis,
    specified type NEC
  bowel, cecum, or colon —*see* Gangrene,
    intestine
  Clostridium perfringens or welchii
    A48.0
  cornea H18.89-
  corpora cavernosa N48.29
    noninfective N48.89
  cutaneous, spreading I96
  decubital —*see* Ulcer, pressure, by site
  diabetic (any site) —*see* Diabetes,
    gangrene
  emphysematous —*see* Gangrene, gas
  epidemic —*see* Poisoning, food,
    noxious, plant
  epididymis (infectional) N45.1
  erysipelas —*see* Erysipelas
  extremity (lower) (upper) I96

Gangrene, gangrenous (*Continued*)
  Fournier N49.3
    female N76.89
  fusospirochetal A69.0
  gallbladder —*see* Cholecystitis, acute
  gas (bacillus) A48.0
    following
      abortion —*see* Abortion by type
        complicated by infection
      ectopic or molar pregnancy O08.0
  glossitis K14.0
  hernia —*see* Hernia, by site, with
    gangrene
  intestine, intestinal (hemorrhagic)
    (massive) K55.0
    with
      mesenteric embolism K55.0
      obstruction —*see* Obstruction,
        intestine
  laryngitis J04.0
  limb (lower) (upper) I96
  lung J85.0
    spirochetal A69.8
  lymphangitis I89.1
  Meleney's (synergistic) —*see* Ulcer, skin
  mesentery K55.0
    with
      embolism K55.0
      intestinal obstruction —*see*
        Obstruction, intestine
  mouth A69.0
  ovary —*see* Oophoritis
  pancreas K85.9
  penis N48.29
    noninfective N48.89
  perineum I96
  pharynx —*see also* Pharyngitis
    Vincent's A69.1
  presenile I73.1
  progressive synergistic —*see* Ulcer, skin
  pulmonary J85.0
  pulpal (dental) K04.1
  quinsy J36
  Raynaud's (symmetric gangrene) I73.01
  retropharyngeal J39.2
  scrotum N49.3
    noninfective N50.8
  senile (atherosclerotic) —*see*
    Arteriosclerosis, extremities,
    with, gangrene
  spermatic cord N49.1
    noninfective N50.8
  spine I96
  spirochetal NEC A69.8
  spreading cutaneous I96
  stomatitis A69.0
  symmetrical I73.01
  testis (infectional) N45.2
    noninfective N44.8
  throat —*see also* Pharyngitis
    diphtheritic A36.0
    Vincent's A69.1
  thyroid (gland) E07.89
  tooth (pulp) K04.1
  tuberculous NEC —*see* Tuberculosis
  tunica vaginalis N49.1
    noninfective N50.8
  umbilicus I96
  uterus —*see* Endometritis
  uvulitis K12.2
  vas deferens N49.1
    noninfective N50.8
  vulva N76.89
Ganister disease J62.8
Ganser's syndrome (hysterical) F44.89

Gardner-Diamond syndrome
  (autoerythrocyte sensitization) D69.2
Gargoylism E76.01
Garré's disease, osteitis (sclerosing),
  osteomyelitis —see Osteomyelitis,
  specified type NEC
Garrod's pad, knuckle M72.1
Gartner's duct
  cyst Q52.4
  persistent Q50.6
Gas R14.3
  asphyxiation, inhalation, poisoning,
    suffocation NEC —see Table of
    drugs and chemicals
  excessive R14.0
  gangrene A48.0
    following
      abortion —see Abortion by type
        complicated by infection
      ectopic or molar pregnancy O08.0
  on stomach R14.0
  pains R14.1
Gastralgia —see also Pain, abdominal
Gastrectasis K31.0
  psychogenic F45.8
Gastric —see condition
Gastrinoma
  malignant
    pancreas C25.4
    specified site NEC —see Neoplasm,
      malignant, by site
    unspecified site C25.4
  specified site —see Neoplasm, uncertain
    behavior
  unspecified site D37.9
Gastritis (simple) K29.70
  with bleeding K29.71
  acute (erosive) K29.00
    with bleeding K29.01
  alcoholic K29.20
    with bleeding K29.21
  allergic K29.60
    with bleeding K29.61
  atrophic (chronic) K29.40
    with bleeding K29.41
  chronic (antral) (fundal) K29.50
    with bleeding K29.51
    atrophic K29.40
      with bleeding K29.41
    superficial K29.30
      with bleeding K29.31
  dietary counseling and surveillance
    Z71.3
  due to diet deficiency E63.9
  eosinophilic K52.81
  giant hypertrophic K29.60
    with bleeding K29.61
  granulomatous K29.60
    with bleeding K29.61
  hypertrophic (mucosa) K29.60
    with bleeding K29.61
  nervous F54
  spastic K29.60
    with bleeding K29.61
  specified NEC K29.60
    with bleeding K29.61
  superficial chronic K29.30
    with bleeding K29.31
  tuberculous A18.83
  viral NEC A08.4
Gastrocarcinoma —see Neoplasm,
  malignant, stomach
Gastrocolic —see condition
Gastrodisciasis, gastrodiscoidiasis B66.8

Gastroduodenitis K29.90
  with bleeding K29.91
  virus, viral A08.4
    specified type NEC A08.39
Gastrodynia —see Pain, abdominal
Gastroenteritis (acute) (chronic)
  (noninfectious) (see also Enteritis) K52.9
  allergic K52.2
  dietetic K52.2
  drug-induced K52.1
  due to
    Cryptosporidium A07.2
    drugs K52.1
    food poisoning —see Intoxication,
      foodborne
    radiation K52.0
  eosinophilic K52.81
  epidemic (infectious) A09
  food hypersensitivity K52.2
  infectious —see Enteritis, infectious
  influenzal —see Influenza, with
    gastroenteritis
  noninfectious K52.9
    specified NEC K52.89
  rotaviral A08.0
  Salmonella A02.0
  toxic K52.1
  viral NEC A08.4
    acute infectious A08.39
      type Norwalk A08.11
    infantile (acute) A08.39
    Norwalk agent A08.11
    rotaviral A08.0
    severe of infants A08.39
    specified type NEC A08.39
Gastroenteropathy (see also
  Gastroenteritis) K52.9
  acute, due to Norovirus A08.11
  acute, due to Norwalk agent A08.11
  infectious A09
Gastroenteroptosis K63.4
  Gastroesophageal laceration
    hemorrhage syndrome K22.6
Gastrointestinal —see condition
Gastrojejunal —see condition
Gastrojejunitis (see also Enteritis) K52.9
Gastrojejunocolic —see condition
Gastroliths K31.89
Gastromalacia K31.89
Gastroparalysis K31.84
  diabetic —see Diabetes, gastroparalysis
Gastroparesis K31.84
  diabetic —see Diabetes, by type, with
    gastroparesis
Gastropathy K31.9
  congestive portal K31.89
  erythematous K29.70
  exudative K90.89
  portal hypertensive K31.89
Gastroptosis K31.89
Gastrorrhagia K92.2
  psychogenic F45.8
Gastroschisis (congenital) Q79.3
Gastrospasm (neurogenic) (reflex) K31.89
  neurotic F45.8
  psychogenic F45.8
Gastrostaxis —see Gastritis, with bleeding
Gastrostenosis K31.89
Gastrostomy
  attention to Z43.1
  status Z93.1
Gastrosuccorrhea (continuous)
  (intermittent) K31.89
  neurotic F45.8
  psychogenic F45.8

Gatophobia F40.218
Gaucher's disease or splenomegaly
  (adult) (infantile) E75.22
Gee (-Herter)(-Thaysen) **disease**
  (nontropical sprue) K90.0
Gélineau's syndrome G47.419
  with cataplexy G47.411
Gemination, tooth, teeth K00.2
Gemistocytoma
  specified site —see Neoplasm,
    malignant, by site
  unspecified site C71.9
General, generalized —see condition
Genetic
  carrier (status)
    cystic fibrosis Z14.1
    hemophilia A (asymptomatic) Z14.01
      symptomatic Z14.02
    specified NEC Z14.8
  susceptibility to disease NEC Z15.89
    malignant neoplasm Z15.09
      breast Z15.01
      endometrium Z15.04
      ovary Z15.02
      prostate Z15.03
      specified NEC Z15.09
    multiple endocrine neoplasia Z15.81
Genital —see condition
Genito-anorectal syndrome A55
Genitourinary system —see condition
Genu
  congenital Q74.1
  extrorsum (acquired) —see also
    Deformity, varus, knee
    congenital Q74.1
    sequelae (late effect) of rickets E64.3
  introrsum (acquired) —see also
    Deformity, valgus, knee
    congenital Q74.1
    sequelae (late effect) of rickets E64.3
  rachitic (old) E64.3
  recurvatum (acquired) —see also
    Deformity, limb, specified type
    NEC, lower leg
    congenital Q68.2
    sequelae (late effect) of rickets E64.3
  valgum (acquired) (knock-knee) M21.06-
    congenital Q74.1
    sequelae (late effect) of rickets E64.3
  varum (acquired) (bowleg) M21.16-
    congenital Q74.1
    sequelae (late effect) of rickets E64.3
Geographic tongue K14.1
Geophagia —see Pica
Geotrichosis B48.3
  stomatitis B48.3
Gephyrophobia F40.242
Gerbode defect Q21.0
GERD (gastroesophageal reflux disease)
  K21.9
Gerhardt's
  disease (erythromelalgia) I73.81
  syndrome (vocal cord paralysis) J38.00
    bilateral J38.02
    unilateral J38.01
German measles —see also Rubella
  exposure to Z20.4
Germinoblastoma (diffuse) C85.9-
  follicular C82.9-
Germinoma —see Neoplasm, malignant,
  by site
Gerontoxon —see Degeneration, cornea,
  senile
Gerstmann-Sträussler-Scheinker
  syndrome (GSS) A81.82

Gerstmann's syndrome R48.8
  developmental F81.2
Gestation (period) —see also Pregnancy
  ectopic —see Pregnancy, by site
  multiple O30.9-
    greater than quadruplets —see
        Pregnancy, multiple (gestation),
        specified NEC
    specified NEC —see Pregnancy,
        multiple (gestation), specified
        NEC
Gestational
  mammary abscess O91.11-
  purulent mastitis O91.11-
  subareolar abscess O91.11-
Ghon tubercle, primary infection
    A15.7
Ghost
  teeth K00.4
  vessels (cornea) H16.41-
Ghoul hand A66.3
Gianotti-Crosti disease L44.4
Giant
  cell
    epulis K06.8
    peripheral granuloma K06.8
  esophagus, congenital Q39.5
  kidney, congenital Q63.3
  oesophagus, congenital Q39.5
  urticaria T78.3
    hereditary D84.1
Giardiasis A07.1
Gibert's disease or pityriasis L42
Giddiness R42
  hysterical F44.89
  psychogenic F45.8
Gierke's disease (glycogenosis I) E74.01
Gigantism (cerebral) (hypophyseal)
    (pituitary) E22.0
  constitutional E34.4
Gilbert's disease or syndrome E80.4
Gilchrist's disease B40.9
Gilford-Hutchinson disease E34.8
Gilles de la Tourette's disease
    or syndrome (motor-verbal tic) F95.2
Gingivitis K05.10
  acute (catarrhal) K05.00
    necrotizing A69.1
    nonplaque induced K05.01
    plaque induced K05.00
  chronic (desquamative) (hyperplastic)
      (simple marginal) (ulcerative)
      K05.10
    nonplaque induced K05.11
    plaque induced K05.10
  expulsiva —see Periodontitis
  necrotizing ulcerative (acute) A69.1
  pellagrous E52
    acute necrotizing A69.1
  Vincent's A69.1
Gingivoglossitis K14.0
Gingivopericementitis —see Periodontitis
Gingivosis —see Gingivitis, chronic
Gingivostomatitis K05.10
  herpesviral B00.2
  necrotizing ulcerative (acute) A69.1
Gland, glandular —see condition
Glanders A24.0
Glanzmann (-Naegeli) disease or
    thrombasthenia D69.1
Glasgow coma scale
  total score
    3-8 R40.243
    9-12 R40.242
    13-15 R40.241

Glass-blower's disease (cataract) —see
    Cataract, specified NEC
Glaucoma H40.9
  with
    increased episcleral venous pressure
        H40.81-
    pseudoexfoliation of lens —see
        Glaucoma, open angle, primary,
        capsular
  absolute H44.51-
  angle-closure (primary) H40.20-
    acute (attack) (crisis) H40.21-
    chronic H40.22-
    intermittent H40.23-
    residual stage H40.24-
  borderline H40.00-
  capsular (with pseudoexfoliation of
      lens) —see Glaucoma, open angle,
      primary, capsular
  childhood Q15.0
  closed angle —see Glaucoma,
      angle-closure
  congenital Q15.0
  corticosteroid-induced —see Glaucoma,
      secondary, drugs
  hypersecretion H40.82-
  in (due to)
    amyloidosis E85.4 [H42]
    aniridia Q13.1 [H42]
    concussion of globe —see Glaucoma,
        secondary, trauma
    dislocation of lens —see Glaucoma,
        secondary
    disorder of lens NEC —see Glaucoma,
        secondary
    drugs —see Glaucoma, secondary,
        drugs
    endocrine disease NOS E34.9
        [H42]
    eye
      inflammation —see Glaucoma,
          secondary, inflammation
      trauma —see Glaucoma, secondary,
          trauma
    hypermature cataract —see
        Glaucoma, secondary
    iridocyclitis —see Glaucoma,
        secondary, inflammation
    lens disorder —see Glaucoma,
        secondary, Lowe's syndrome
        E72.03 [H42]
    metabolic disease NOS E88.9
        [H42]
    ocular disorders NEC —see
        Glaucoma, secondary
    onchocerciasis B73.02
    pupillary block —see Glaucoma,
        secondary
    retinal vein occlusion —see
        Glaucoma, secondary
    Rieger's anomaly Q13.81 [H42]
    rubeosis of iris —see Glaucoma,
        secondary
    tumor of globe —see Glaucoma,
        secondary
  infantile Q15.0
  low tension —see Glaucoma, open
      angle, primary, low-tension
  malignant H40.83-
  narrow angle —see Glaucoma,
      angle-closure
  newborn Q15.0
  noncongestive (chronic) —see
      Glaucoma, open angle

Glaucoma (Continued)
  nonobstructive —see Glaucoma, open
      angle
  obstructive —see also Glaucoma,
      angle-closure
    due to lens changes —see Glaucoma,
        secondary
  open angle H40.10-
    primary H40.11-
      capsular (with pseudoexfoliation of
          lens) H40.14-
      low-tension H40.12-
      pigmentary H40.13-
      residual stage H40.15-
  phacolytic —see Glaucoma,
      secondary
  pigmentary —see Glaucoma,
      open angle, primary, pigmentary
  postinfectious —see Glaucoma,
      secondary, inflammation
  secondary (to) H40.5-
    drugs H40.6-
    inflammation H40.4-
    trauma H40.3-
  simple (chronic) H40.11
  simplex H40.11
  specified type NEC H40.89
  suspect H40.00-
  syphilitic A52.71
  traumatic —see also Glaucoma,
      secondary, trauma
    newborn (birth injury) P15.3
  tuberculous A18.59
Glaucomatous flecks (subcapsular) —see
    Cataract, complicated
Glazed tongue K14.4
Gleet (gonococcal) A54.01
Glénard's disease K63.4
Glioblastoma (multiforme)
  with sarcomatous component
    specified site —see Neoplasm,
        malignant, by site
    unspecified site C71.9
  giant cell
    specified site —see Neoplasm,
        malignant, by site
    unspecified site C71.9
  specified site —see Neoplasm,
      malignant, by site
  unspecified site C71.9
Glioma (malignant)
  astrocytic
    specified site —see Neoplasm,
        malignant, by site
    unspecified site C71.9
  mixed
    specified site —see Neoplasm,
        malignant, by site
    unspecified site C71.9
  nose Q30.8
  specified site NEC —see Neoplasm,
      malignant, by site
  subependymal D43.2
    specified site —see Neoplasm,
        uncertain behavior, by site
    unspecified site D43.2
  unspecified site C71.9
Gliomatosis cerebri C71.0
Glioneuroma —see Neoplasm, uncertain
    behavior, by site
Gliosarcoma
  specified site —see Neoplasm,
      malignant, by site
  unspecified site C71.9

Gliosis (cerebral) G93.89
  spinal G95.89
Glisson's disease —see Rickets
Globinuria R82.3
Globus (hystericus) F45.8
Glomangioma D18.00
  intra-abdominal D18.03
  intracranial D18.02
  skin D18.01
  specified site NEC D18.09
Glomangiomyoma D18.00
  intra-abdominal D18.03
  intracranial D18.02
  skin D18.01
  specified site NEC D18.09
Glomangiosarcoma —see Neoplasm,
    connective tissue, malignant
Glomerular
  disease in syphilis A52.75
  nephritis —see Glomerulonephritis
Glomerulitis —see Glomerulonephritis
Glomerulonephritis (see also Nephritis)
    N05.9
  with
    edema —see Nephrosis
    minimal change N05.0
    minor glomerular abnormality N05.0
  acute N00.9
  chronic N03.9
  crescentic (diffuse) NEC (see also
      N00-N07 with fourth character .7)
      N05.7
  dense deposit (see also N00-N07 with
      fourth character .6) N05.6
  diffuse
    crescentic (see also N00-N07 with
        fourth character .7) N05.7
    endocapillary proliferative (see also
        N00N07 with fourth character
        .4) N05.4
    membranous (see also N00-N07 with
        fourth character .2) N05.2
    mesangial proliferative (see also N00N07
        with fourth character .3) N05.3
    mesangiocapillary (see also N00-N07
        with fourth character .5) N05.5
    sclerosing N05.8
  endocapillary proliferative (diffuse)
      NEC (see also N00-N07 with fourth
      character .4) N05.4
  extracapillary NEC (see also N00-N07
      with fourth character .7) N05.7
  focal (and segmental) (see also N00-N07
      with fourth character .1) N05.1
  hypocomplementemic —see
      Glomerulonephritis,
      membranoproliferative
  IgA —see Nephropathy, IgA
  immune complex (circulating) NEC N05.8
  in (due to)
    amyloidosis E85.4 [N08]
    bilharziasis B65.9 [N08]
    cryoglobulinemia D89.1 [N08]
    defibrination syndrome D65 [N08]
    diabetes mellitus —see Diabetes,
        glomerulosclerosis
    disseminated intravascular
        coagulation D65 [N08]
    Fabry (-Anderson) disease E75.21
        [N08]
    Goodpasture's syndrome M31.0
    hemolytic-uremic syndrome D59.3
    Henoch (-Schönlein) purpura D69.0
        [N08]

Glomerulonephritis (Continued)
  in (due to) (Continued)
    lecithin cholesterol acyltransferase
        deficiency E78.6 [N08]
    microscopic polyangiitis M31.7 [N08]
    multiple myeloma C90.0- [N08]
    Plasmodium malariae B52.0
    schistosomiasis B65.9 [N08]
    sepsis A41.9- [N08]
      streptococcal A40- [N08]
    sickle-cell disorders D57.- [N08]
    strongyloidiasis B78.9 [N08]
    subacute bacterial endocarditis I33.0
        [N08]
    syphilis (late) congenital A50.59
        [N08]
    systemic lupus erythematosus
        M32.14
    thrombotic thrombocytopenic
        purpura M31.1 [N08]
    typhoid fever A01.09
    Waldenström macroglobulinemia
        C88.0 [N08]
    Wegener's granulomatosis M31.31
  latent or quiescent N03.9
  lobular, lobulonodular —see
      Glomerulonephritis,
      membranoproliferative
  membranoproliferative (diffuse) (type 1
      or 3) (see also N00-N07 with fourth
      character .5) N05.5
    dense deposit (type 2) NEC (see
        also N00-N07 with fourth
        character .6) N05.6
  membranous (diffuse) NEC (see also
      N00-N07 with fourth character .2)
      N05.2
  mesangial
    IgA/IgG —see Nephropathy, IgA
    proliferative (diffuse) NEC (see
        also N00-N07 with fourth
        character .3) N05.3
  mesangiocapillary (diffuse) NEC (see also
      N00-N07 with fourth character .5)
      N05.5
  necrotic, necrotizing NEC (see also
      N00-N07 with fourth character .8)
      N05.8
  nodular —see Glomerulonephritis,
      membranoproliferative
  poststreptococcal NEC N05.9
    acute N00.9
    chronic N03.9
    rapidly progressive N01.9
  proliferative NEC (see also N00-N07
      with fourth character .8) N05.8
    diffuse (lupus) M32.14
  rapidly progressive N01.9
  sclerosing, diffuse N05.8
  specified pathology NEC (see also
      N00-N07 with fourth character .8)
      N05.8
  subacute N01.9
Glomerulopathy —see
    Glomerulonephritis
Glomerulosclerosis —see also Sclerosis,
    renal
  intercapillary (nodular) (with
      diabetes) —see Diabetes,
      glomerulosclerosis
  intracapillary —see Diabetes,
      glomerulosclerosis
Glossagra K14.6
Glossalgia K14.6

Glossitis (chronic superficial)
    (gangrenous) (Moeller's) K14.0
  areata exfoliativa K14.1
  atrophic K14.4
  benign migratory K14.1
  cortical superficial, sclerotic K14.0
  Hunter's D51.0
  interstitial, sclerous K14.0
  median rhomboid K14.2
  pellagrous E52
  superficial, chronic K14.0
Glossocele K14.8
Glossodynia K14.6
  exfoliativa K14.4
Glossoncus K14.8
Glossopathy K14.9
Glossophytia K14.3
Glossoplegia K14.8
Glossoptosis K14.8
Glossopyrosis K14.6
Glossotrichia K14.3
Glossy skin L90.8
Glottis —see condition
Glottitis (see also Laryngitis) J04.0
Glucagonoma
  pancreas
    benign D13.7
    malignant C25.4
    uncertain behavior D37.8
  specified site NEC
    benign —see Neoplasm, benign, by
        site
    malignant —see Neoplasm,
        malignant, by site
    uncertain behavior —see Neoplasm,
        uncertain behavior, by site
  unspecified site
    benign D13.7
    malignant C25.4
    uncertain behavior D37.8
Glucoglycinuria E72.51
Glucose-galactose malabsorption
    E74.39
Glue
  ear —see Otitis, media, nonsuppurative,
      chronic, mucoid
  sniffing (airplane) —see Abuse, drug,
      inhalant
    dependence —see Dependence, drug,
        inhalant
Glutaric aciduria E72.3
Glycinemia E72.51
Glycinuria (renal) (with ketosis) E72.09
Glycogen
  infiltration —see Disease, glycogen
      storage
  storage disease —see Disease, glycogen
      storage
Glycogenosis (diffuse) (generalized) —see
    also Disease, glycogen storage
  cardiac E74.02 [I43]
  diabetic, secondary —see Diabetes,
      glycogenosis, secondary
  pulmonary interstitial J84.842
Glycopenia E16.2
Glycosuria R81
  renal E74.8
Gnathostoma spinigerum (infection)
    (infestation), gnathostomiasis
    (wandering swelling) B83.1
Goiter (plunging) (substernal) E04.9
  with
    hyperthyroidism (recurrent) —see
        Hyperthyroidism, with, goiter

Goiter *(Continued)*
with *(Continued)*
thyrotoxicosis —*see*
Hyperthyroidism, with, goiter
adenomatous —*see* Goiter, nodular
cancerous C73
congenital (nontoxic) E03.0
diffuse E03.0
parenchymatous E03.0
transitory, with normal functioning
P72.0
cystic E04.2
due to iodine-deficiency E01.1
due to
enzyme defect in synthesis of thyroid
hormone E07.1
iodine-deficiency (endemic) E01.2
dyshormonogenetic (familial) E07.1
endemic (iodine-deficiency) E01.2
diffuse E01.0
multinodular E01.1
exophthalmic —*see* Hyperthyroidism,
with, goiter
iodine-deficiency (endemic) E01.2
diffuse E01.0
multinodular E01.1
nodular E01.1
lingual Q89.2
lymphadenoid E06.3
malignant C73
multinodular (cystic) (nontoxic) E04.2
toxic or with hyperthyroidism E05.20
with thyroid storm E05.21
neonatal NEC P72.0
nodular (nontoxic) (due to) E04.9
with
hyperthyroidism E05.20
with thyroid storm E05.21
thyrotoxicosis E05.20
with thyroid storm E05.21
endemic E01.1
iodine-deficiency E01.1
sporadic E04.9
toxic E05.20
with thyroid storm E05.21
nontoxic E04.9
diffuse (colloid) E04.0
multinodular E04.2
simple E04.0
specified NEC E04.8
uninodular E04.1
simple E04.0
toxic —*see* Hyperthyroidism, with, goiter
uninodular (nontoxic) E04.1
toxic or with hyperthyroidism E05.10
with thyroid storm E05.11
Goiter-deafness syndrome E07.1
Goldberg syndrome Q89.8
Goldberg-Maxwell syndrome E34.51
Goldblatt's hypertension or kidney I70.1
Goldenhar (-Gorlin) syndrome Q87.0
Goldflam-Erb disease or syndrome
G70.00
with exacerbation (acute) G70.01
in crisis G70.01
Goldscheider's disease Q81.8
Goldstein's disease (familial hemorrhagic
telangiectasia) I78.0
Golfer's elbow —*see* Epicondylitis, medial
Gonadoblastoma
specified site —*see* Neoplasm, uncertain
behavior, by site
unspecified site
female D39.10
male D40.10

Gonecystitis —*see* Vesiculitis
Gongylonemiasis B83.8
Goniosynechiae —*see* Adhesions, iris,
goniosynechiae
Gonococcemia A54.86
Gonococcus, gonococcal (disease)
(infection) (*see also* condition)
A54.9
anus A54.6
bursa, bursitis A54.49
conjunctiva, conjunctivitis
(neonatorum) A54.31
endocardium A54.83
eye A54.30
conjunctivitis A54.31
iridocyclitis A54.32
keratitis A54.33
newborn A54.31
other specified A54.39
fallopian tubes (acute) (chronic)
A54.24
genitourinary (organ) (system) (tract)
(acute)
lower A54.00
with abscess (accessory gland)
(periurethral) A54.1
upper (*see also* condition) A54.29
heart A54.83
iridocyclitis A54.32
joint A54.42
lymphatic (gland) (node) A54.89
meninges, meningitis A54.81
musculoskeletal A54.40
arthritis A54.42
osteomyelitis A54.43
other specified A54.49
spondylopathy A54.41
pelviperitonitis A54.24
pelvis (acute) (chronic) A54.24
pharynx A54.5
proctitis A54.6
pyosalpinx (acute) (chronic) A54.24
rectum A54.6
skin A54.89
specified site NEC A54.89
tendon sheath A54.49
throat A54.5
urethra (acute) (chronic) A54.01
with abscess (accessory gland)
(periurethral) A54.1
vulva (acute) (chronic) A54.02
Gonocytoma
specified site —*see* Neoplasm, uncertain
behavior, by site
unspecified site
female D39.10
male D40.10
Gonorrhea (acute) (chronic) A54.9
Bartholin's gland (acute) (chronic)
(purulent) A54.02
with abscess (accessory gland)
(periurethral) A54.1
bladder A54.01
cervix A54.03
conjunctiva, conjunctivitis
(neonatorum) A54.31
contact Z20.2
Cowper's gland (with abscess) A54.1
exposure to Z20.2
fallopian tube (acute) (chronic) A54.24
kidney (acute) (chronic) A54.21
lower genitourinary tract A54.00
with abscess (accessory gland)
(periurethral) A54.1
ovary (acute) (chronic) A54.24

Gonorrhea *(Continued)*
pelvis (acute) (chronic) A54.24
female pelvic inflammatory disease
A54.24
penis A54.09
prostate (acute) (chronic) A54.22
seminal vesicle (acute) (chronic) A54.23
specified site not listed (*see also*
Gonococcus) A54.89
spermatic cord (acute) (chronic) A54.23
urethra A54.01
with abscess (accessory gland)
(periurethral) A54.1
vagina A54.02
vas deferens (acute) (chronic) A54.23
vulva A54.02
Goodall's disease A08.19
Goodpasture's syndrome M31.0
Gopalan's syndrome (burning feet) E53.0
Gorlin-Chaudry-Moss syndrome Q87.0
Gottron's papules L94.4
Gougerot's syndrome (trisymptomatic)
L81.7
Gougerot-Blum syndrome (pigmented
purpuric lichenoid dermatitis) L81.7
Gougerot-Carteaud disease or
syndrome (confluent reticulate
papillomatosis) L83
Gouley's syndrome (constrictive
pericarditis) I31.1
Goundou A66.6
Gout, chronic (*see also* Gout, gouty)
M1A.9-
drug-induced M1A.20
ankle M1A.27-
elbow M1A.22-
foot joint M1A.27-
hand joint M1A.24-
hip M1A.25-
knee M1A.26-
multiple site M1A.29-
shoulder M1A.21-
vertebrae M1A.28
wrist M1A.23-
idiopathic M1A.00
ankle M1A.07-
elbow M1A.02-
foot joint M1A.07-
hand joint M1A.04-
hip M1A.05-
knee M1A.06-
multiple site M1A.09
shoulder M1A.01-
vertebrae M1A.08
wrist M1A.03-
in (due to) renal impairment M1A.30
ankle M1A.37-
elbow M1A.32-
foot joint M1A.37-
hand joint M1A.34-
hip M1A.35-
knee M1A.36-
multiple site M1A.39
shoulder M1A.31-
vertebrae M1A.38
wrist M1A.33-
lead-induced M1A.10
ankle M1A.17-
elbow M1A.12-
foot joint M1A.17-
hand joint M1A.14-
hip M1A.15-
knee M1A.16-
multiple site M1A.19
shoulder M1A.11-

Gout, chronic (Continued)
  lead-induced (Continued)
    vertebrae M1A.18
    wrist M1A.13-
  primary —see Gout, chronic, idiopathic
  saturnine —see Gout, chronic,
      lead-induced
  secondary NEC M1A.40
    ankle M1A.47-
    elbow M1A.42-
    foot joint M1A.47-
    hand joint M1A.44-
    hip M1A.45-
    knee M1A.46-
    multiple site M1A.49
    shoulder M1A.41-
    vertebrae M1A.48
    wrist M1A.43-
  syphilitic (see also subcategory M14.8-)
      A52.77
  tophi —see Gout by type
Gout, gouty (acute) (attack) (flare) (see also
      Gout, chronic) M10.9-
  drug-induced M10.20
    ankle M10.27-
    elbow M10.22-
    foot joint M10.27-
    hand joint M10.24-
    hip M10.25-
    knee M10.26-
    multiple site M10.29
    shoulder M10.21-
    vertebrae M10.28
    wrist M10.23-
  idiopathic M10.00
    ankle M10.07-
    elbow M10.02-
    foot joint M10.07-
    hand joint M10.04-
    hip M10.05-
    knee M10.06-
    multiple site M10.09
    shoulder M10.01-
    vertebrae M10.08
    wrist M10.03-
  in (due to) renal impairment M10.30
    ankle M10.37-
    elbow M10.32-
    foot joint M10.37-
    hand joint M10.34-
    hip M10.35-
    knee M10.36-
    multiple site M10.39
    shoulder M10.31-
    vertebrae M10.38
    wrist M10.33-
  lead-induced M10.10
    ankle M10.17-
    elbow M10.12-
    foot joint M10.17-
    hand joint M10.14-
    hip M10.15-
    knee M10.16-
    multiple site M10.19
    shoulder M10.11-
    vertebrae M10.18
    wrist M10.13-
  primary —see Gout, idiopathic
  saturnine —see Gout, lead-induced
  secondary NEC M10.40
    ankle M10.47-
    elbow M10.42-
    foot joint M10.47-
    hand joint M10.44-

Gout, gouty (Continued)
  secondary NEC (Continued)
    hip M10.45-
    knee M10.46-
    multiple site M10.49
    shoulder M10.41-
    vertebrae M10.48
    wrist M10.43-
  syphilitic (see also subcategory M14.8-)
      A52.77
  tophi NEC —see Gout by type
Gower's
  muscular dystrophy G71.0
  syndrome (vasovagal attack) R55
Gradenigo's syndrome —see Otitis,
    media, suppurative, acute
Graefe's disease —see Strabismus,
    paralytic, ophthalmoplegia,
    progressive
Graft-versus-host disease D89.813
  acute D89.810
  acute on chronic D89.812
  chronic D89.811
Grain mite (itch) B88.0
Grainhandler's disease or lung J67.8
Grand mal —see Epilepsy, generalized,
    specified NEC
Grand multipara status only (not
    pregnant) Z64.1
  pregnant —see Pregnancy, complicated
    by, grand multiparity
Granite worker's lung J62.8
Granular —see also condition
  inflammation, pharynx J31.2
  kidney (contracting) —see Sclerosis,
    renal
  liver K74.69
Granulation tissue (abnormal) (excessive)
    L92.9
  postmastoidectomy cavity —
    see Complications,
    postmastoidectomy, granulation
Granulocytopenia (primary)
    (malignant) —see Agranulocytosis
Granuloma L92.9
  abdomen K66.8
    from residual foreign body L92.3
    pyogenicum L98.0
  actinic L57.5
  annulare (perforating) L92.0
  apical K04.5
  aural —see Otitis, externa, specified
    NEC
  beryllium (skin) L92.3
  bone
    eosinophilic C96.6
    from residual foreign body —see
      Osteomyelitis, specified type
      NEC
    lung C96.6
  brain (any site) G06.0
    schistosomiasis B65.9 [G07]
  canaliculus lacrimalis —see Granuloma,
    lacrimal
  candidal (cutaneous) B37.2
  cerebral (any site) G06.0
  coccidioidal (primary) (progressive)
      B38.7
    lung B38.1
    meninges B38.4
  colon K63.89
  conjunctiva H11.22-
  dental K04.5
  ear, middle —see Cholesteatoma

Granuloma (Continued)
  eosinophilic C96.6
    bone C96.6
    lung C96.6
    oral mucosa K13.4
    skin L92.2
  eyelid H01.8
  facial (e) L92.2
  foreign body (in soft tissue) NEC
      M60.20
    ankle M60.27-
    foot M60.27-
    forearm M60.23-
    hand M60.24-
    in operation wound —see Foreign
      body, accidentally left during a
      procedure
    lower leg M60.26-
    pelvic region M60.25-
    shoulder region M60.21-
    skin L92.3
    specified site NEC M60.28
    subcutaneous tissue L92.3
    thigh M60.25-
    upper arm M60.22-
  gangraenescens M31.2
  genito-inguinale A58
  giant cell (central) (reparative) (jaw)
      M27.1
    gingiva (peripheral) K06.8
  gland (lymph) I88.8
  hepatic NEC K75.3
    in (due to)
      berylliosis J63.2 [K77]
      sarcoidosis D86.89
  Hodgkin C81.9
  ileum K63.89
  infectious B99.9
    specified NEC B99.8
  inguinale (Donovan) (venereal) A58
  intestine NEC K63.89
  intracranial (any site) G06.0
  intraspinal (any part) G06.1
  iridocyclitis —see Iridocyclitis, chronic
  jaw (bone) (central) M27.1
    reparative giant cell M27.1
  kidney (see also Infection, kidney)
      N15.8
  lacrimal H04.81-
  larynx J38.7
  lethal midline (faciale (e)) M31.2
  liver NEC —see Granuloma, hepatic
  lung (infectious) —see also Fibrosis,
      lung
    coccidioidal B38.1
    eosinophilic C96.6
  Majocchi's B35.8
  malignant (facial (e)) M31.2
  mandible (central) M27.1
  midline (lethal) M31.2
  monilial (cutaneous) B37.2
  nasal sinus —see Sinusitis
  operation wound T81.89
    foreign body —see Foreign body,
      accidentally left during a
      procedure
    stitch T81.89
    talc —see Foreign body, accidentally
      left during a procedure
  oral mucosa K13.4
  orbit, orbital H05.11-
  paracoccidioidal B41.8
  penis, venereal A58
  periapical K04.5

273

Granuloma *(Continued)*
  peritoneum K66.8
    due to ova of helminths NOS *(see also*
      Helminthiasis) B83.9 *[K67]*
  postmastoidectomy cavity —
    see Complications,
    postmastoidectomy, recurrent
    cholesteatoma
  prostate N42.89
  pudendi (ulcerating) A58
  pulp, internal (tooth) K03.3
  pyogenic, pyogenicum (of) (skin) L98.0
    gingiva K06.8
    maxillary alveolar ridge K04.5
    oral mucosa K13.4
  rectum K62.89
  reticulohistiocytic D76.3
  rubrum nasi L74.8
  Schistosoma —*see* Schistosomiasis
  septic (skin) L98.0
  silica (skin) L92.3
  sinus (accessory) (infective) (nasal) —
    see Sinusitis
  skin L92.9
    from residual foreign body L92.3
    pyogenicum L98.0
  spine
    syphilitic (epidural) A52.19
    tuberculous A18.01
  stitch (postoperative) T81.89
  suppurative (skin) L98.0
  swimming pool A31.1
  talc —*see also* Granuloma, foreign body
    in operation wound —*see* Foreign
      body, accidentally left during a
      procedure
  telangiectaticum (skin) L98.0
  tracheostomy J95.09
  trichophyticum B35.8
  tropicum A66.4
  umbilicus L92.9
  urethra N36.8
  uveitis —*see* Iridocyclitis, chronic
  vagina A58
  venereum A58
  vocal cord J38.3
Granulomatosis L92.9
  lymphoid C83.8-
  miliary (listerial) A32.89
  necrotizing, respiratory M31.30
  progressive septic D71
  specified NEC L92.8
  Wegener's M31.30
    with renal involvement M31.31
Granulomatous tissue (abnormal)
  (excessive) L92.9
Granulosis rubra nasi L74.8
Graphite fibrosis (of lung) J63.3
Graphospasm F48.8
  organic G25.89

Grating scapula M89.8X1
Gravel (urinary) —*see* Calculus, urinary
Graves' disease —*see* Hyperthyroidism,
  with, goiter
Gravis —*see* condition
Grawitz tumor C64.-
Gray syndrome (newborn) P93.0
Grayness, hair (premature) L67.1
  congenital Q84.2
Green sickness D50.8
Greenfield's disease
  meaning
    concentric sclerosis (encephalitis
      periaxialis concentrica) G37.5
    metachromatic leukodystrophy E75.25
Greenstick fracture - code as Fracture,
  by site
Grey syndrome (newborn) P93.0
Grief F43.21
  prolonged F43.29
  reaction *(see also* Disorder, adjustment)
    F43.20
Griesinger's disease B76.9
Grinder's lung or pneumoconiosis J62.8
Grinding, teeth
  psychogenic F45.8
  sleep related G47.63
Grip
  Dabney's B33.0
  devil's B33.0
Grippe, grippal —*see also* Influenza
  Balkan A78
  summer, of Italy A93.1
Grisel's disease M43.6
Groin —*see* condition
Grooved tongue K14.5
Ground itch B76.9
Grover's disease or syndrome L11.1
Growing pains, children R29.898
Growth (fungoid) (neoplastic) (new) —*see*
  also Neoplasm
  adenoid (vegetative) J35.8
  benign —*see* Neoplasm, benign, by site
  malignant —*see* Neoplasm, malignant,
    by site
  rapid, childhood Z00.2
  secondary —*see* Neoplasm, secondary,
    by site
Gruby's disease B35.0
Gubler-Millard paralysis or syndrome
  G46.3
Guerin-Stern syndrome Q74.3
Guidance, insufficient anterior (occlusal)
  M26.54
Guillain-Barré disease or syndrome G61.0
  sequelae G65.0
Guinea worms (infection) (infestation) B72
Guinon's disease (motor-verbal tic) F95.2
Gull's disease E03.4
Gum —*see* condition

Gumboil K04.7
  with sinus K04.6
Gumma (syphilitic) A52.79
  artery A52.09
    cerebral A52.04
  bone A52.77
    of yaws (late) A66.6
  brain A52.19
  cauda equina A52.19
  central nervous system A52.3
  ciliary body A52.71
  congenital A50.59
  eyelid A52.71
  heart A52.06
  intracranial A52.19
  iris A52.71
  kidney A52.75
  larynx A52.73
  leptomeninges A52.19
  liver A52.74
  meninges A52.19
  myocardium A52.06
  nasopharynx A52.73
  neurosyphilitic A52.3
  nose A52.73
  orbit A52.71
  palate (soft) A52.79
  penis A52.76
  pericardium A52.06
  pharynx A52.73
  pituitary A52.79
  scrofulous (tuberculous) A18.4
  skin A52.79
  specified site NEC A52.79
  spinal cord A52.19
  tongue A52.79
  tonsil A52.73
  trachea A52.73
  tuberculous A18.4
  ulcerative due to yaws A66.4
  ureter A52.75
  yaws A66.4
    bone A66.6
Gunn's syndrome Q07.8
Gunshot wound —*see also* Wound, open
  fracture - code as Fracture, by site
  internal organs —*see* Injury, by site
Gynandrism Q56.0
Gynandroblastoma
  specified site —*see* Neoplasm, uncertain
    behavior, by site
  unspecified site
    female D39.10
    male D40.10
Gynecological examination (periodic)
  (routine) Z01.419
  with abnormal findings Z01.411
Gynecomastia N62
Gynephobia F40.291
Gyrate scalp Q82.8

H

H (Hartnup's) disease E72.02
Haas' disease or osteochondrosis
  (juvenile) (head of humerus) —see
  Osteochondrosis, juvenile, humerus
Habit, habituation
  bad sleep Z72.821
  chorea F95.8
  disturbance, child F98.9
  drug —see Dependence, drug
  irregular sleep Z72.821
  laxative F55.2
  spasm —see Tic
  tic —see Tic
Haemophilus (H.) influenzae, as cause of
  disease classified elsewhere B96.3
Haff disease —see Poisoning, mercury
Hageman's factor defect, deficiency or
  disease D68.2
Haglund's disease or osteochondrosis
  (juvenile) (os tibiale externum) —see
  Osteochondrosis, juvenile, tarsus
Hailey-Hailey disease Q82.8
Hair —see also condition
  plucking F63.3
    in stereotyped movement disorder
      F98.4
  tourniquet syndrome —see also
      Constriction, external, by site
    finger S60.44-
    penis S30.842
    thumb S60.34-
    toe S90.44-
Hairball in stomach T18.2
Hair-pulling, pathological (compulsive)
  F63.3
Hairy black tongue K14.3
Half vertebra Q76.49
Halitosis R19.6
Hallerman-Streiff syndrome Q87.0
Hallervorden-Spatz disease G23.0
Hallopeau's acrodermatitis or disease
  L40.2
Hallucination R44.3
  auditory R44.0
  gustatory R44.2
  olfactory R44.2
  specified NEC R44.2
  tactile R44.2
  visual R44.1
Hallucinosis (chronic) F28
  alcoholic (acute) F10.951
    in
      abuse F10.151
      dependence F10.251
  drug-induced F19.951
    cannabis F12.951
    cocaine F14.951
    hallucinogen F16.151
    in
      abuse F19.151
        cannabis F12.151
        cocaine F14.151
        hallucinogen F16.151
        inhalant F18.151
        opioid F11.151
        sedative, anxiolytic or hypnotic
          F13.151
        stimulant NEC F15.151
      dependence F19.251
        cannabis F12.251
        cocaine F14.251
        hallucinogen F16.251

Hallucinosis (Continued)
  drug-induced (Continued)
    in (Continued)
      dependence (Continued)
        inhalant F18.251
        opioid F11.251
        sedative, anxiolytic or hypnotic
          F13.251
        stimulant NEC F15.251
    inhalant F18.951
    opioid F11.951
    sedative, anxiolytic or hypnotic F13.951
    stimulant NEC F15.951
  organic F06.0
Hallux
  deformity (acquired) NEC M20.5X-
  limitus M20.5X-
  malleus (acquired) NEC M20.3-
  rigidus (acquired) M20.2-
    congenital Q74.2
    sequelae (late effect) of rickets E64.3
  valgus (acquired) M20.1-
    congenital Q66.6
  varus (acquired) M20.3-
    congenital Q66.3
Halo, visual H53.19
Hamartoma, hamartoblastoma Q85.9
  epithelial (gingival), odontogenic,
    central or peripheral —see Cyst,
    calcifying odontogenic
Hamartosis Q85.9
Hamman-Rich syndrome J84.114
Hammer toe (acquired) NEC —see also
    Deformity, toe, hammer toe
  congenital Q66.89
  sequelae (late effect) of rickets E64.3
Hand —see condition
Hand-foot syndrome L27.1
Handicap, handicapped
  educational Z55.9
    specified NEC Z55.8
Hand-Schüller-Christian disease or
  syndrome C96.5
Hanging (asphyxia) (strangulation)
  (suffocation) —see Asphyxia,
  traumatic, due to mechanical threat
Hangnail —see also Cellulitis, digit
  with lymphangitis —see Lymphangitis,
    acute, digit
Hangover (alcohol) F10.129
Hanhart's syndrome Q87.0
Hanot-Chauffard (-Troisier) syndrome
  E83.19
Hanot's cirrhosis or disease K74.3
Hansen's disease —see Leprosy
Hantaan virus disease (Korean
  hemorrhagic fever) A98.5
Hantavirus disease (with renal
  manifestations) (Dobrava) (Puumala)
  (Seoul) A98.5
  with pulmonary manifestations (Andes)
    (Bayou) (Bermejo) (Black Creek
    Canal) (Choclo) (Juquitiba) (Laguna
    negra) (Lechiguanas) (New York)
    (Oran) (Sin nombre) B33.4
Happy puppet syndrome Q93.5
Harada's disease or syndrome H30.81-
Hardening
  artery —see Arteriosclerosis
  brain G93.89
Harelip (complete) (incomplete) —see
  Cleft, lip
Harlequin (newborn) Q80.4
Harley's disease D59.6

Harmful use (of)
  alcohol F10.10
  anxiolytics —see Abuse, drug, sedative
  cannabinoids —see Abuse, drug, cannabis
  cocaine —see Abuse, drug, cocaine
  drug —see Abuse, drug
  hallucinogens —see Abuse, drug,
    hallucinogen
  hypnotics —see Abuse, drug, sedative -
    opioids —see Abuse, drug, opioid
  PCP (phencyclidine) —see Abuse, drug,
    hallucinogen
  sedatives —see Abuse, drug, sedative
  stimulants NEC —see Abuse, drug,
    stimulant
Harris' lines —see Arrest, epiphyseal
Hartnup's disease E72.02
Harvester's lung J67.0
Harvesting ovum for in vitro
  fertilization Z31.83
Hashimoto's disease or thyroiditis E06.3
Hashitoxicosis (transient) E06.3
Hassal-Henle bodies or warts (cornea)
  H18.49
Haut mal —see Epilepsy, generalized,
  specified NEC
Haverhill fever A25.1
Hay fever (see also Fever, hay) J30.1
Hayem-Widal syndrome D59.8
Haygarth's nodes M15.8
Haymaker's lung J67.0
Hb (abnormal)
  Bart's disease D56.0
  disease —see Disease, hemoglobin
  trait —see Trait
Head —see condition
Headache R51
  allergic NEC G44.89
  associated with sexual activity G44.82
  chronic daily R51
  cluster G44.009
    chronic G44.029
      intractable G44.021
      not intractable G44.029
    episodic G44.019
      intractable G44.011
      not intractable G44.019
    intractable G44.001
    not intractable G44.009
  cough (primary) G44.83
  daily chronic R51
  drug-induced NEC G44.40
    intractable G44.41
    not intractable G44.40
  exertional (primary) G44.84
  histamine G44.009
    intractable G44.001
    not intractable G44.009
  hypnic G44.81
  lumbar puncture G97.1
  medication overuse G44.40
    intractable G44.41
    not intractable G44.40
  menstrual —see Migraine, menstrual
  migraine (type) (see also Migraine)
    G43.909
  nasal septum R51
  neuralgiform, short lasting unilateral,
    with conjunctival injection and
    tearing (SUNCT) G44.059
    intractable G44.051
    not intractable G44.059
  new daily persistent (NDPH) G44.52
  orgasmic G44.82

Headache *(Continued)*
  periodic syndromes in adults and
      children G43.C0
    with refractory migraine G43.C1
      intractable G43.C1
      not intractable G43.C0
    without refractory migraine G43.C0
  postspinal puncture G97.1
  post-traumatic G44.309
    acute G44.319
      intractable G44.311
      not intractable G44.319
    chronic G44.329
      intractable G44.321
      not intractable G44.329
    intractable G44.301
    not intractable G44.309
  pre-menstrual —*see* Migraine,
      menstrual
  preorgasmic G44.82
  primary
    cough G44.83
    exertional G44.84
    stabbing G44.85
    thunderclap G44.53
  rebound G44.40
    intractable G44.41
    not intractable G44.40
  short lasting unilateral neuralgiform,
      with conjunctival injection and
      tearing (SUNCT) G44.059
    intractable G44.051
    not intractable G44.059
  specified syndrome NEC G44.89
  spinal and epidural anesthesia -
      induced T88.59
    in labor and delivery O74.5
    in pregnancy O29.4-
    postpartum, puerperal O89.4
  spinal fluid loss (from puncture) G97.1
  stabbing (primary) G44.85
  tension (-type) G44.209
    chronic G44.229
      intractable G44.221
      not intractable G44.229
    episodic G44.219
      intractable G44.211
      not intractable G44.219
    intractable G44.201
    not intractable G44.209
  thunderclap (primary) G44.53
  vascular NEC G44.10
    intractable G44.11
    not intractable G44.10
Healthy
  infant
    accompanying sick mother Z76.3
    receiving care Z76.2
  person accompanying sick person
    Z76.3
Hearing examination Z01.10
  with abnormal findings NEC Z01.118
  following failed hearing screening
    Z01.110
  for hearing conservation and treatment
    Z01.12
Heart —*see* condition
Heart beat
  abnormality R00.9
    specified NEC R00.8
  awareness R00.2
  rapid R00.0
  slow R00.1
Heartburn R12
  psychogenic F45.8

Heat (effects) T67.9
  apoplexy T67.0
  burn (*see also* Burn) L55.9
  collapse T67.1
  cramps T67.2
  dermatitis or eczema L59.0
  edema T67.7
  erythema - code by site under Burn,
    first degree
  excessive T67.9
    specified effect NEC T67.8
  exhaustion T67.5
    anhydrotic T67.3
    due to
      salt (and water) depletion T67.4
      water depletion T67.3
        with salt depletion T67.4
  fatigue (transient) T67.6
  fever T67.0
  hyperpyrexia T67.0
  prickly L74.0
  prostration —*see* Heat, exhaustion
  pyrexia T67.0
  rash L74.0
  specified effect NEC T67.8
  stroke T67.0
  sunburn —*see* Sunburn
  syncope T67.1
Heavy-for-dates NEC (infant) (4000g to
    4499g) P08.1
  exceptionally (4500g or more) P08.0
Hebephrenia, hebephrenic
    (schizophrenia) F20.1
Heberden's disease or nodes (with
    arthropathy) M15.1
Hebra's
  pityriasis L26
  prurigo L28.2
Heel —*see* condition
Heerfordt's disease D86.89
Hegglin's anomaly or syndrome D72.0
Heilmeyer-Schoner disease D45
Heine-Medin disease A80.9
Heinz body anemia, congenital D58.2
Heliophobia F40.228
Heller's disease or syndrome F84.3
HELLP syndrome (hemolysis, elevated
    liver enzymes and low platelet
    count) O14.2-
Helminthiasis —*see also* Infestation,
  helminth
  Ancylostoma B76.0
  intestinal B82.0
    mixed types (types classifiable to
      more than one of the titles
      B65.0-B81.3 and B81.8) B81.4
    specified type NEC B81.8
  mixed types (intestinal) (types
      classifiable to more than one of the
      titles B65.0-B81.3 and B81.8) B81.4
  Necator (americanus) B76.1
  specified type NEC B83.8
Heloma L84
Hemangioblastoma —*see* Neoplasm,
  connective tissue, uncertain behavior
  malignant —*see* Neoplasm, connective
    tissue, malignant
Hemangioendothelioma —*see also*
    Neoplasm, uncertain behavior,
    by site
  benign D18.00
    intra-abdominal D18.03
    intracranial D18.02
    skin D18.01
    specified site NEC D18.09

Hemangioendothelioma *(Continued)*
  bone (diffuse) —*see* Neoplasm, bone,
    malignant
  epithelioid —*see also* Neoplasm,
    uncertain behavior, by site
    malignant —*see* Neoplasm,
      malignant, by site
  malignant —*see* Neoplasm, connective
    tissue, malignant
Hemangiofibroma —*see* Neoplasm,
  benign, by site
Hemangiolipoma —*see* Lipoma
Hemangioma D18.00
  arteriovenous D18.00
    intra-abdominal D18.03
    intracranial D18.02
    skin D18.01
    specified site NEC D18.09
  capillary D18.00
    intra-abdominal D18.03
    intracranial D18.02
    skin D18.01
    specified site NEC D18.09
  cavernous D18.00
    intra-abdominal D18.03
    intracranial D18.02
    skin D18.01
    specified site NEC D18.09
  epithelioid D18.00
    intra-abdominal D18.03
    intracranial D18.02
    skin D18.01
    specified site NEC D18.09
  histiocytoid D18.00
    intra-abdominal D18.03
    intracranial D18.02
    skin D18.01
    specified site NEC D18.09
  infantile D18.00
    intra-abdominal D18.03
    intracranial D18.02
    skin D18.01
    specified site NEC D18.09
  intra-abdominal D18.03
  intracranial D18.02
  intramuscular D18.00
    intra-abdominal D18.03
    intracranial D18.02
    skin D18.01
    specified site NEC D18.09
  juvenile D18.00
  malignant —*see* Neoplasm, connective
    tissue, malignant
  plexiform D18.00
    intra-abdominal D18.03
    intracranial D18.02
    skin D18.01
    specified site NEC D18.09
  racemose D18.00
    intra-abdominal D18.03
    intracranial D18.02
    skin D18.01
    specified site NEC D18.09
  sclerosing —*see* Neoplasm, skin, benign
  simplex D18.00
    intra-abdominal D18.03
    intracranial D18.02
    skin D18.01
    specified site NEC D18.09
  skin D18.01
  specified site NEC D18.09
  venous D18.00
    intra-abdominal D18.03
    intracranial D18.02

Hemangioma (*Continued*)
  venous (*Continued*)
    skin D18.01
    specified site NEC D18.09
  verrucous keratotic D18.00
    intra-abdominal D18.03
    intracranial D18.02
    skin D18.01
    specified site NEC D18.09
Hemangiomatosis (systemic) I78.8
  involving single site —*see* Hemangioma
Hemangiopericytoma —*see also*
    Neoplasm, connective tissue,
    uncertain behavior
  benign —*see* Neoplasm, connective
    tissue, benign
  malignant —*see* Neoplasm, connective
    tissue, malignant
Hemangiosarcoma —*see* Neoplasm,
    connective tissue, malignant
Hemarthrosis (nontraumatic) M25.00
  ankle M25.07-
  elbow M25.02-
  foot joint M25.07-
  hand joint M25.04-
  hip M25.05-
  in hemophilic arthropathy —*see*
    Arthropathy, hemophilic
  knee M25.06-
  shoulder M25.01-
  specified joint NEC M25.08
  traumatic —*see* Sprain, by site
  wrist M25.03-
Hematemesis K92.0
  with ulcer - code by site under Ulcer,
    with hemorrhage K27.4
  newborn, neonatal P54.0
    due to swallowed maternal blood
      P78.2
Hematidrosis L74.8
Hematinuria —*see also* Hemoglobinuria
  malarial B50.8
Hematobilia K83.8
Hematocele
  female NEC N94.89
    with ectopic pregnancy O00.9
    ovary N83.8
  male N50.1
Hematochezia (*see also* Melena) K92.1
Hematochyluria —*see also* Infestation,
    filarial
  schistosomiasis (bilharziasis) B65.0
Hematocolpos (with hematometra or
    hematosalpinx) N89.7
Hematocornea —*see* Pigmentation,
    cornea, stromal
Hematogenous —*see* condition
Hematoma (traumatic) (skin surface
    intact) —*see also* Contusion
  with
    injury of internal organs —*see* Injury,
      by site
    open wound —*see* Wound, open
  amputation stump (surgical) (late) T87.89
  aorta, dissecting I71.00
    abdominal I71.02
    thoracic I71.01
    thoracoabdominal I71.03
  aortic intramural —*see* Dissection, aorta
  arterial (complicating trauma) —*see*
      Injury, blood vessel, by site
  auricle —*see* Contusion, ear
    nontraumatic —*see* Disorder, pinna,
      hematoma

Hematoma (*Continued*)
  birth injury NEC P15.8
  brain (traumatic)
    with
      cerebral laceration or contusion
        (diffuse) —*see* Injury,
        intracranial, diffuse
      focal —*see* Injury, intracranial,
        focal
    cerebellar, traumatic S06.37-
    intracerebral, traumatic —*see* Injury,
      intracranial, intracerebral
      hemorrhage
    newborn NEC P52.4
      birth injury P10.1
    nontraumatic —*see* Hemorrhage,
      intracranial
    subarachnoid, arachnoid, traumatic —
      see Injury, intracranial,
      subarachnoid hemorrhage
    subdural, traumatic —*see* Injury,
      intracranial, subdural
      hemorrhage
  breast (nontraumatic) N64.89
  broad ligament (nontraumatic) N83.7
    traumatic S37.892
  cerebellar, traumatic S06.37-
  cerebral —*see* Hematoma, brain
  cerebrum S06.36-
    left S06.35-
    right S06.34-
  cesarean delivery wound O90.2
  complicating delivery (perineal)
    (pelvic) (vagina) (vulva) O71.7
  corpus cavernosum (nontraumatic)
    N48.89
  epididymis (nontraumatic) N50.1
  epidural (traumatic) —*see* Injury,
    intracranial, epidural hemorrhage
    spinal —*see* Injury, spinal cord, by
      region
  episiotomy O90.2
  face, birth injury P15.4
  genital organ NEC (nontraumatic)
    female (nonobstetric) N94.89
      traumatic S30.202
    male N50.1
      traumatic S30.201
  internal organs —*see* Injury, by site
  intracerebral, traumatic —*see* Injury,
    intracranial, intracerebral
    hemorrhage
  intraoperative —*see* Complications,
    intraoperative, hemorrhage
  labia (nontraumatic) (nonobstetric) N90.8
  liver (subcapsular) (nontraumatic) K76.89
    birth injury P15.0
  mediastinum —*see* Injury, intrathoracic
  mesosalpinx (nontraumatic) N83.7
    traumatic S37.529
      bilateral S37.522
      unilateral S37.521
  muscle - code by site under Contusion
  nontraumatic
    muscle M79.81
    soft tissue M79.81
  obstetrical surgical wound O90.2
  orbit, orbital (nontraumatic) —*see also*
    Hemorrhage, orbit
    traumatic —*see* Contusion, orbit
  pelvis (female) (nontraumatic)
    (nonobstetric) N94.89
    obstetric O71.7
    traumatic —*see* Injury, by site

Hematoma (*Continued*)
  penis (nontraumatic) N48.89
    birth injury P15.5
  perianal (nontraumatic) K64.5
  perineal S30.23
    complicating delivery O71.7
  perirenal —*see* Injury, kidney
  pinna —*see* Contusion, ear
    nontraumatic —*see* Disorder, pinna,
      hematoma
  placenta O43.89-
  postoperative (postprocedural) —*see*
    Complication, postprocedural,
    hemorrhage
  retroperitoneal (nontraumatic) K66.1
    traumatic S36.892
  scrotum, superficial S30.22
    birth injury P15.5
  seminal vesicle (nontraumatic) N50.1
    traumatic S37.892
  spermatic cord (traumatic) S37.892
    nontraumatic N50.1
  spinal (cord) (meninges) —*see also*
    Injury, spinal cord, by region
    newborn (birth injury) P11.5
  spleen D73.5
    intraoperative —*see* Complications,
      intraoperative, hemorrhage,
      spleen
    postprocedural (postoperative) —*see*
      Complications, postprocedural,
      hemorrhage, spleen
  sternocleidomastoid, birth injury P15.2
  sternomastoid, birth injury P15.2
  subarachnoid (traumatic) —*see* Injury,
    intracranial, subarachnoid
    hemorrhage
    newborn (nontraumatic) P52.5
      due to birth injury P10.3
    nontraumatic —*see* Hemorrhage,
      intracranial, subarachnoid
  subdural (traumatic) —*see* Injury,
    intracranial, subdural hemorrhage
    newborn (localized) P52.8
      birth injury P10.0
    nontraumatic —*see* Hemorrhage,
      intracranial, subdural
  superficial, newborn P54.5
  testis (nontraumatic) N50.1
    birth injury P15.5
  tunica vaginalis (nontraumatic) N50.1
  umbilical cord, complicating delivery
    O69.5
  uterine ligament (broad) (nontraumatic)
    N83.7
    traumatic S37.62
  vagina (ruptured) (nontraumatic) N89.8
    complicating delivery O71.7
  vas deferens (nontraumatic) N50.1
    traumatic S37.892
  vitreous —*see* Hemorrhage, vitreous
  vulva (nontraumatic) (nonobstetric)
    N90.89
    complicating delivery O71.7
    newborn (birth injury) P15.5
Hematometra N85.7
  with hematocolpos N89.7
Hematomyelia (central) G95.19
  newborn (birth injury) P11.5
  traumatic T14.8
Hematomyelitis G04.90
Hematoperitoneum —*see*
    Hemoperitoneum
Hematophobia F40.230

Hematopneumothorax (see Hemothorax)
Hematopoiesis, cyclic D70.4
Hematoporphyria —see Porphyria
Hematorachis, hematorrhachis G95.19
  newborn (birth injury) P11.5
Hematosalpinx N83.6
  with
    hematocolpos N89.7
    hematometra N85.7
      with hematocolpos N89.7
  infectional —see Salpingitis
Hematospermia R36.1
Hematothorax (see Hemothorax)
Hematuria R31.9
  benign (familial) (of childhood) —see
    also Hematuria, idiopathic
    essential microscopic R31.1
  due to sulphonamide, sulfonamide —
    see Table of drugs and chemicals,
    by drug
  endemic (see also Schistosomiasis)
    B65.0
  gross R31.0
  idiopathic N02.9
    with glomerular lesion
      crescentic (diffuse)
        glomerulonephritis N02.7
      dense deposit disease N02.6
      endocapillary proliferative
        glomerulonephritis N02.4
      focal and segmental hyalinosis or
        sclerosis N02.1
      membranoproliferative (diffuse)
        N02.5
      membranous (diffuse) N02.2
      mesangial proliferative (diffuse)
        N02.3
      mesangiocapillary (diffuse) N02.5
      minor abnormality N02.0
      proliferative NEC N02.8
      specified pathology NEC N02.8
  intermittent —see Hematuria, idiopathic
  malarial B50.8
  microscopic NEC R31.2
    benign essential R31.1
  paroxysmal —see also Hematuria,
    idiopathic
    nocturnal D59.5
  persistent —see Hematuria, idiopathic
  recurrent —see Hematuria, idiopathic
  tropical (see also Schistosomiasis) B65.0
  tuberculous A18.13
Hemeralopia (day blindness) H53.11
  vitamin A deficiency E50.5
Hemi-akinesia R41.4
Hemianalgesia R20.0
Hemianencephaly Q00.0
Hemianesthesia R20.0
Hemianopia, hemianopsia
  (heteronymous) H53.47
  homonymous H53.46-
  syphilitic A52.71
Hemiathetosis R25.8
Hemiatrophy R68.89
  cerebellar G31.9
  face, facial, progressive (Romberg)
    G51.8
  tongue K14.8
Hemiballism (us) G25.5
Hemicardia Q24.8
Hemicephalus, hemicephaly Q00.0
Hemichorea G25.5
Hemicolitis, left —see Colitis, left
  sided

Hemicrania
  congenital malformation Q00.0
  continua G44.51
  meaning migraine (see also Migraine)
    G43.909
  paroxysmal G44.039
    chronic G44.049
      intractable G44.041
      not intractable G44.049
    episodic G44.039
      intractable G44.031
      not intractable G44.039
    intractable G44.031
    not intractable G44.039
Hemidystrophy —see Hemiatrophy
Hemiectromelia Q73.8
Hemihypalgesia R20.8
Hemihypesthesia R20.1
Hemi-inattention R41.4
Hemimelia Q73.8
  lower limb —see Defect, reduction,
    lower limb, specified type NEC
  upper limb —see Defect, reduction,
    upper limb, specified type NEC
Hemiparalysis —see Hemiplegia
Hemiparesis —see Hemiplegia
Hemiparesthesia R20.2
Hemiparkinsonism G20
Hemiplegia G81.9-
  alternans facialis G83.89
  ascending NEC G81.90
    spinal G95.89
  congenital (cerebral) G80.8
    spastic G80.2
  embolic (current episode) I63.4-
  flaccid G81.0-
    following
      cerebrovascular disease I69.959
        cerebral infarction I69.35-
        intracerebral hemorrhage I69.15-
        nontraumatic intracranial
          hemorrhage NEC I69.25-
        specified disease NEC I69.85-
        stroke NOS I69.35-
        subarachnoid hemorrhage
          I69.05-
  hysterical F44.4
  newborn NEC P91.8
    birth injury P11.9
  spastic G81.1-
    congenital G80.2
  thrombotic (current episode) I63.3
Hemisection, spinal cord —see Injury,
  spinal cord, by region
Hemispasm (facial) R25.2
Hemisporosis B48.8
Hemitremor R25.1
Hemivertebra Q76.49
  failure of segmentation with scoliosis
    Q76.3
  fusion with scoliosis Q76.3
Hemochromatosis E83.119
  with refractory anemia D46.1
  due to repeated red blood cell
    transfusion E83.111
  hereditary (primary) E83.110
  primary E83.110
  specified NEC E83.118
Hemoglobin —see also condition
  abnormal (disease) —see Disease,
    hemoglobin
  AS genotype D57.3
  Constant Spring D58.2
  E-beta thalassemia D56.5

Hemoglobin (Continued)
  fetal, hereditary persistence (HPFH)
    D56.4
  H Constant Spring D56.0
  low NOS D64.9
  S (Hb S), heterozygous D57.3
Hemoglobinemia D59.9
  due to blood transfusion T80.89
  paroxysmal D59.6
    nocturnal D59.5
Hemoglobinopathy (mixed) D58.2
  with thalassemia D56.8
  sickle-cell D57.1
    with thalassemia D57.40
      with crisis (vasoocclusive pain)
        D57.419
        with
          acute chest syndrome D57.411
          splenic sequestration D57.412
      without crisis D57.40
Hemoglobinuria R82.3
  with anemia, hemolytic, acquired
    (chronic) NEC D59.6
  cold (agglutinin) (paroxysmal) (with
    Raynaud's syndrome) D59.6
  due to exertion or hemolysis NEC D59.6
  intermittent D59.6
  malarial B50.8
  march D59.6
  nocturnal (paroxysmal) D59.5
  paroxysmal (cold) D59.6
    nocturnal D59.5
Hemolymphangioma D18.1
Hemolysis
  intravascular
    with
      abortion —see Abortion, by type,
        complicated by, hemorrhage
      ectopic or molar pregnancy O08.1
      hemorrhage
        antepartum —see Hemorrhage,
          antepartum, with
          coagulation defect
        intrapartum (see also
          Hemorrhage, complicating,
          delivery) O67.0
    postpartum O72.3
  neonatal (excessive) P58.9
    specified NEC P58.8
Hemolytic —see condition
Hemopericardium I31.2
  following acute myocardial infarction
    (current complication) I23.0
  newborn P54.8
  traumatic —see Injury, heart, with
    hemopericardium
Hemoperitoneum K66.1
  infectional K65.9
  traumatic S36.899
    with open wound —see Wound,
      open, with penetration into
      peritoneal cavity
Hemophilia (classical) (familial)
  (hereditary) D66
  A D66
  B D67
  C D68.1
  acquired D68.311
  autoimmune D68.311
  calcipriva (see also Defect, coagulation)
    D68.4
  nonfamilial (see also Defect, coagulation)
    D68.4
  secondary D68.311
  vascular D68.0

Hemophthalmos H44.81-
Hemopneumothorax —see also
   Hemothorax
   traumatic S27.2
Hemoptysis R04.2
   newborn P26.9
   tuberculous —see Tuberculosis,
      pulmonary
Hemorrhage, hemorrhagic (concealed)
   R58
   abdomen R58
   accidental antepartum —see
      Hemorrhage, antepartum
   acute idiopathic pulmonary, in infants
      R04.81
   adenoid J35.8
   adrenal (capsule) (gland) E27.49
      medulla E27.8
      newborn P54.4
   after delivery —see Hemorrhage,
      postpartum
   alveolar
      lung, newborn P26.8
      process K08.8
   alveolus K08.8
   amputation stump (surgical) T87.89
   anemia (chronic) D50.0
      acute D62
   antepartum (with) O46.90
      with coagulation defect O46.00-
        afibrinogenemia O46.01-
        disseminated intravascular
          coagulation O46.02-
        hypofibrinogenemia O46.01-
        specified defect NEC O46.09-
      before 20 weeks gestation O20.9
        specified type NEC O20.8
        threatened abortion O20.0
      due to
        abruptio placenta (see also Abruptio
          placentae) O45.9-
        leiomyoma, uterus —see
          Hemorrhage, antepartum,
          specified cause NEC
        placenta previa O44.1-
      specified cause NEC —see
        subcategory O46.8X-
   anus (sphincter) K62.5
   apoplexy (stroke) —see Hemorrhage,
      intracranial, intracerebral
   arachnoid —see Hemorrhage,
      intracranial, subarachnoid
   artery R58
      brain —see Hemorrhage, intracranial,
        intracerebral
   basilar (ganglion) I61.0
   bladder N32.89
   bowel K92.2
      newborn P54.3
   brain (miliary) (nontraumatic) —see
      Hemorrhage, intracranial,
      intracerebral
      due to
        birth injury P10.1
        syphilis A52.05
      epidural or extradural (traumatic) —
        see Injury, intracranial, epidural
        hemorrhage
      newborn P52.4
        birth injury P10.1
      subarachnoid —see Hemorrhage,
        intracranial, subarachnoid
      subdural —see Hemorrhage,
        intracranial, subdural

Hemorrhage, hemorrhagic (Continued)
   brainstem (nontraumatic) I61.3
      traumatic S06.38-
   breast N64.59
   bronchial tube —see Hemorrhage, lung
   bronchopulmonary —see Hemorrhage,
      lung
   bronchus —see Hemorrhage, lung
   bulbar I61.5
   capillary I78.8
      primary D69.8
   cecum K92.2
   cerebellar, cerebellum (nontraumatic)
      I61.4
      newborn P52.6
      traumatic S06.37-
   cerebral, cerebrum —see also
      Hemorrhage, intracranial,
      intracerebral
      lobe I61.1
      newborn (anoxic) P52.4
        birth injury P10.1
   cerebromeningeal I61.8
   cerebrospinal —see Hemorrhage,
      intracranial, intracerebral
   cervix (uteri) (stump) NEC N88.8
   chamber, anterior (eye) —see Hyphema
   childbirth —see Hemorrhage,
      complicating, delivery
   choroid H31.30-
      expulsive H31.31-
   ciliary body —see Hyphema
   cochlea —see subcategory H83.8
   colon K92.2
   complicating
      abortion —see Abortion, by type,
        complicated by, hemorrhage
      delivery O67.9
        associated with coagulation defect
          (afibrinogenemia) (DIC)
          (hyperfibrinolysis) O67.0
        specified cause NEC O67.8
        surgical procedure —see Hemorrhage,
          intraoperative
   conjunctiva H11.3-
   newborn P54.8
   cord, newborn (stump) P51.9
   corpus luteum (ruptured) cyst N83.1
   cortical (brain) I61.1
   cranial —see Hemorrhage, intracranial
   cutaneous R23.3
      due to autosensitivity, erythrocyte
        D69.2
      newborn P54.5
   delayed
      following ectopic or molar pregnancy
        O08.1
      postpartum O72.2
   diathesis (familial) D69.9
   disease D69.9
      newborn P53
      specified type NEC D69.8
   due to or associated with
      afibrinogenemia or other coagulation
        defect (conditions in categories
        D65-D69)
        antepartum —see Hemorrhage,
          antepartum, with coagulation
          defect
        intrapartum O67.0
      dental implant M27.61
      device, implant or graft (see also
        Complications, by site and type,
        specified NEC) T85.83

Hemorrhage, hemorrhagic (Continued)
   due to or associated with (Continued)
      device, implant or graft (Continued)
        arterial graft NEC T82.838
        breast T85.83
        catheter NEC T85.83
          dialysis (renal) T82.838
            intraperitoneal T85.83
          infusion NEC T82.838
            spinal (epidural) (subdural)
              T85.83
          urinary (indwelling) T83.83
        electronic (electrode) (pulse
          generator) (stimulator)
        bone T84.83
        cardiac T82.837
        nervous system (brain)
          (peripheral nerve)
          (spinal) T85.83
        urinary T83.83
      fixation, internal (orthopedic) NEC
        T84.83
      gastrointestinal (bile duct)
        (esophagus) T85.83
      genital NEC T83.83
      heart NEC T82.837
      joint prosthesis T84.83
      ocular (corneal graft) (orbital
        implant) NEC T85.83
      orthopedic NEC T84.83
        bone graft T86.838
      specified NEC T85.83
      urinary NEC T83.83
      vascular NEC T82.838
      ventricular intracranial shunt T85.83
   duodenum, duodenal K92.2
      ulcer —see Ulcer, duodenum, with
        hemorrhage
   dura mater —see Hemorrhage,
      intracranial, subdural
   endotracheal —see Hemorrhage, lung
   epicranial subaponeurotic (massive),
      birth injury P12.2
   epidural (traumatic) —see also Injury,
      intracranial, epidural hemorrhage
      nontraumatic I62.1
   esophagus K22.8
      varix I85.01
        secondary I85.11
   excessive, following ectopic gestation
      (subsequent episode) O08.1
   extradural (traumatic) —see Injury,
      intracranial, epidural hemorrhage
      birth injury P10.8
      newborn (anoxic) (nontraumatic) P52.8
      nontraumatic I62.1
   eye NEC H57.8
      fundus —see Hemorrhage, retina
      lid —see Disorder, eyelid, specified
        type NEC
   fallopian tube N83.6
   fibrinogenolysis —see Fibrinolysis
   fibrinolytic (acquired) —see Fibrinolysis
   from
      ear (nontraumatic) —see Otorrhagia
      tracheostomy stoma J95.01
   fundus, eye —see Hemorrhage, retina
   funis —see Hemorrhage, umbilicus,
      cord
   gastric —see Hemorrhage, stomach
   gastroenteric K92.2
      newborn P54.3
   gastrointestinal (tract) K92.2
      newborn P54.3

Hemorrhage, hemorrhagic *(Continued)*
  genital organ, male N50.1
  genitourinary (tract) NOS R31.9
  gingiva K06.8
  globe (eye) —*see* Hemophthalmos
  graafian follicle cyst (ruptured) N83.0
  gum K06.8
  heart I51.89
  hypopharyngeal (throat) R04.1
  intermenstrual (regular) N92.3
    irregular N92.1
  internal (organs) NEC R58
    capsule I61.0
    ear —*see* subcategory H83.8
    newborn P54.8
  intestine K92.2
    newborn P54.3
  intra-abdominal R58
  intra-alveolar (lung), newborn P26.8
  intracerebral (nontraumatic) —*see*
      Hemorrhage, intracranial,
      intracerebral
  intracranial (nontraumatic) I62.9
    birth injury P10.9
    epidural, nontraumatic I62.1
    extradural, nontraumatic I62.1
    intracerebral (nontraumatic) (in) I61.9
      brain stem I61.3
      cerebellum I61.4
      hemisphere I61.2
        cortical (superficial) I61.1
        subcortical (deep) I61.0
      intraoperative
        during a nervous system
            procedure G97.31
        during other procedure G97.32
      intraventricular I61.5
      multiple localized I61.6
      newborn P52.4
        birth injury P10.1
      postprocedural
        during a nervous system
            procedure G97.51
        during other procedure G97.52
      specified NEC I61.8
      superficial I61.1
      traumatic (diffuse) —*see* Injury,
          intracranial, diffuse
        focal —*see* Injury, intracranial,
            focal
      newborn P52.9
        specified NEC P52.8
    subarachnoid (nontraumatic) (from)
        I60.9
      intracranial (cerebral) artery I60.7
        anterior communicating I60.2-
        basilar I60.4
        carotid siphon and bifurcation
            I60.0-
        communicating I60.7
          anterior I60.2-
          posterior I60.3-
        middle cerebral I60.1-
        posterior communicating I60.3-
        specified artery NEC I60.6
        vertebral I60.5-
      newborn P52.5
        birth injury P10.3
      specified NEC I60.8
      traumatic S06.6X-
    subdural (nontraumatic) I62.00
      acute I62.01
      birth injury P10.0
      chronic I62.03

Hemorrhage, hemorrhagic *(Continued)*
  intracranial *(Continued)*
    subdural *(Continued)*
      newborn (anoxic) (hypoxic)
          P52.8
        birth injury P10.0
      spinal G95.19
      subacute I62.02
      traumatic —*see* Injury, intracranial,
          subdural hemorrhage
    traumatic —*see* Injury, intracranial,
        focal brain injury
  intramedullary NEC G95.19
  intraocular —*see* Hemophthalmos
  intraoperative, intraprocedural —*see*
      Complication, hemorrhage
      (hematoma), intraoperative
      (intraprocedural), by site
  intrapartum —*see* Hemorrhage,
      complicating, delivery
  intrapelvic
    female N94.89
    male K66.1
  intraperitoneal K66.1
  intrapontine I61.3
  intraprocedural —*see* Complication,
      hemorrhage (hematoma),
      intraoperative (intraprocedural),
      by site
  intrauterine N85.7
    complicating delivery (*see also*
        Hemorrhage, complicating,
        delivery) O67.9
    postpartum —*see* Hemorrhage,
        postpartum
  intraventricular I61.5
    newborn (nontraumatic) (*see
        also* Newborn, affected by,
        hemorrhage) P52.3
    due to birth injury P10.2
    grade
      1 P52.0
      2 P52.1
      3 P52.21
      4 P52.22
  intravesical N32.89
  iris (postinfectional) (postinflammatory)
      (toxic) —*see* Hyphema
  joint (nontraumatic) —*see* Hemarthrosis
  kidney N28.89
  knee (joint) (nontraumatic) —*see*
      Hemarthrosis, knee
  labyrinth —*see* subcategory H83.8
  lenticular striate artery I61.0
  ligature, vessel —*see* Hemorrhage,
      postoperative
  liver K76.89
  lung R04.89
    newborn P26.9
      massive P26.1
      specified NEC P26.8
    tuberculous —*see* Tuberculosis,
        pulmonary
  massive umbilical, newborn P51.0
  mediastinum —*see* Hemorrhage, lung
  medulla I61.3
  membrane (brain) I60.8
    spinal cord —*see* Hemorrhage, spinal
        cord
  meninges, meningeal (brain) (middle)
      I60.8
    spinal cord —*see* Hemorrhage, spinal
        cord
  mesentery K66.1

Hemorrhage, hemorrhagic *(Continued)*
  metritis —*see* Endometritis
  mouth K13.79
  mucous membrane NEC R58
    newborn P54.8
  muscle M62.89
  nail (subungual) L60.8
  nasal turbinate R04.0
    newborn P54.8
  navel, newborn P51.9
  newborn P54.9
    specified NEC P54.8
  nipple N64.59
  nose R04.0
    newborn P54.8
  omentum K66.1
  optic nerve (sheath) H47.02-
  orbit, orbital H05.23-
  ovary NEC N83.8
  oviduct N83.6
  pancreas K86.8
  parathyroid (gland) (spontaneous)
      E21.4
  parturition —*see* Hemorrhage,
      complicating, delivery
  penis N48.89
  pericardium, pericarditis I31.2
  peritoneum, peritoneal K66.1
  peritonsillar tissue J35.8
    due to infection J36
  petechial R23.3
    due to autosensitivity, erythrocyte
        D69.2
  pituitary (gland) E23.6
  pleura —*see* Hemorrhage, lung
  polioencephalitis, superior E51.2
  polymyositis —*see* Polymyositis
  pons, pontine I61.3
  posterior fossa (nontraumatic) I61.8
    newborn P52.6
  postmenopausal N95.0
  postnasal R04.0
  postoperative —*see* Complications,
      postprocedural, hemorrhage, by
      site
  postpartum NEC (following delivery
      of placenta) O72.1
    delayed or secondary O72.2
    retained placenta O72.0
    third stage O72.0
  pregnancy —*see* Hemorrhage,
      antepartum
  preretinal —*see* Hemorrhage, retina
  prostate N42.1
  puerperal —*see* Hemorrhage,
      postpartum
    delayed or secondary O72.2
  pulmonary R04.89
    newborn P26.9
      massive P26.1
      specified NEC P26.8
    tuberculous —*see* Tuberculosis,
        pulmonary
  purpura (primary) D69.3
  rectum (sphincter) K62.5
    newborn P54.2
  recurring, following initial hemorrhage
      at time of injury T79.2
  renal N28.89
  respiratory passage or tract R04.9
    specified NEC R04.89
  retina, retinal (vessels) H35.6-
    diabetic —*see* Diabetes, retinal,
        hemorrhage

Hemorrhage, hemorrhagic (*Continued*)
retroperitoneal R58
scalp R58
scrotum N50.1
secondary (nontraumatic) R58
  following initial hemorrhage at time
    of injury T79.2
seminal vesicle N50.1
skin R23.3
  newborn P54.5
slipped umbilical ligature P51.8
spermatic cord N50.1
spinal (cord) G95.19
  newborn (birth injury) P11.5
spleen D73.5
  intraoperative —*see* Complications,
    intraoperative, hemorrhage,
    spleen
  postprocedural —*see* Complications,
    postprocedural, hemorrhage,
    spleen
stomach K92.2
  newborn P54.3
  ulcer —*see* Ulcer, stomach, with
    hemorrhage
subarachnoid (nontraumatic) —*see*
  Hemorrhage, intracranial,
  subarachnoid
subconjunctival —*see also* Hemorrhage,
  conjunctiva
  birth injury P15.3
subcortical (brain) I61.0
subcutaneous R23.3
subdiaphragmatic R58
subdural (acute) (nontraumatic) —
  see Hemorrhage, intracranial,
  subdural
subependymal
  newborn P52.0
    with intraventricular extension
      P52.1
      and intracerebral extension
        P52.22
subhyaloid —*see* Hemorrhage, retina
subperiosteal —*see* Disorder, bone,
  specified type NEC
subretinal —*see* Hemorrhage, retina
subtentorial —*see* Hemorrhage,
  intracranial, subdural
subungual L60.8
suprarenal (capsule) (gland) E27.49
  newborn P54.4
tentorium (traumatic) NEC —*see*
  Hemorrhage, brain
  newborn (birth injury) P10.4
testis N50.1
third stage (postpartum) O72.0
thorax —*see* Hemorrhage, lung
throat R04.1
thymus (gland) E32.8
thyroid (cyst) (gland) E07.89
tongue K14.8
tonsil J35.8
trachea —*see* Hemorrhage, lung
tracheobronchial R04.89
  newborn P26.0
traumatic — code to specific injury
  cerebellar —*see* Hemorrhage, brain
  intracranial —*see* Hemorrhage,
    brain
  recurring or secondary (following
    initial hemorrhage at time of
    injury) T79.2

Hemorrhage, hemorrhagic (*Continued*)
tuberculous NEC (*see also* Tuberculosis,
  pulmonary) A15.0
tunica vaginalis N50.1
ulcer - code by site under Ulcer, with
  hemorrhage K27.4
umbilicus, umbilical
  cord
    after birth, newborn P51.9
    complicating delivery O69.5
  newborn P51.9
    massive P51.0
    slipped ligature P51.8
  stump P51.9
urethra (idiopathic) N36.8
uterus, uterine (abnormal) N93.9
  climacteric N92.4
  complicating delivery —*see*
    Hemorrhage, complicating,
    delivery
  dysfunctional or functional N93.8
  intermenstrual (regular) N92.3
    irregular N92.1
  postmenopausal N95.0
  postpartum —*see* Hemorrhage,
    postpartum
  preclimacteric or premenopausal
    N92.4
  prepubertal N93.8
  pubertal N92.2
vagina (abnormal) N93.9
  newborn P54.6
vas deferens N50.1
vasa previa O69.4
ventricular I61.5
vesical N32.89
viscera NEC R58
  newborn P54.8
vitreous (humor) (intraocular) H43.1-
vulva N90.89

Hemorrhoids (bleeding) (without
  mention of degree) K64.9
1st degree (grade/stage I) (without
  prolapse outside of anal canal)
  K64.0
2nd degree (grade/stage II) (that
  prolapse with straining but retract
  spontaneously) K64.1
3rd degree (grade/stage III) (that
  prolapse with straining and
  require manual replacement back
  inside anal canal) K64.2
4th degree (grade/stage IV) (with
  prolapsed tissue that cannot be
  manually replaced) K64.3
complicating
  pregnancy O22.4
  puerperium O87.2
external K64.4
  with
    thrombosis K64.5
internal (without mention of degree)
  K64.8
prolapsed K64.8
skin tags
  anus K64.4
  residual K64.4
specified NEC K64.8
strangulated (*see also* Hemorrhoids, by
  degree) K64.8
thrombosed (*see also* Hemorrhoids, by
  degree) K64.5
ulcerated (*see also* Hemorrhoids, by
  degree) K64.8

Hemosalpinx N83.6
with
  hematocolpos N89.7
  hematometra N85.7
    with hematocolpos N89.7
Hemosiderosis (dietary) E83.19
  pulmonary, idiopathic E83.1 *[J84.03]*
  transfusion T80.89
Hemothorax (bacterial) (nontuberculous)
  J94.2
  newborn P54.8
  traumatic S27.1
    with pneumothorax S27.2
  tuberculous NEC A15.6
Henoch (-Schönlein) **disease or syndrome**
  (purpura) D69.0
Henpue, henpuye A66.6
Hepar lobatum (syphilitic) A52.74
Hepatalgia K76.89
Hepatitis K75.9
  acute B17.9
    with coma K72.01
    with hepatic failure —*see* Failure,
      hepatic
    alcoholic —*see* Hepatitis, alcoholic
    infectious B15.9
      with hepatic coma B15.0
    viral B17.9
  alcoholic (acute) (chronic) K70.10
    with ascites K70.11
  amebic —*see* Abscess, liver, amebic
  anicteric (viral) —*see* Hepatitis,
    viral
  antigen-associated (HAA) —*see*
    Hepatitis, B
  Australia-antigen (positive) —*see*
    Hepatitis, B
  autoimmune K75.4
  B B19.10
    with hepatic coma B19.11
    acute B16.9
      with
        delta-agent (coinfection)
          (without hepatic coma)
          B16.1
          with hepatic coma B16.0
        hepatic coma (without delta-
          agent coinfection) B16.2
    chronic B18.1
      with delta-agent B18.0
  bacterial NEC K75.89
  C (viral) B19.20
    with hepatic coma B19.21
    acute B17.10
      with hepatic coma B17.11
    chronic B18.2
  catarrhal (acute) B15.9
    with hepatic coma B15.0
  cholangiolitic K75.89
  cholestatic K75.89
  chronic K73.9
    active NEC K73.2
    lobular NEC K73.1
    persistent NEC K73.0
    specified NEC K73.8
  cytomegaloviral B25.1
  due to ethanol (acute) (chronic) —*see*
    Hepatitis, alcoholic
  epidemic B15.9
    with hepatic coma B15.0
  fulminant NEC (viral) —*see* Hepatitis,
    viral
  granulomatous NEC K75.3
  herpesviral B00.81

Hepatitis *(Continued)*
history of
  B Z86.19
  C Z86.19
homologous serum —*see* Hepatitis,
  viral, type B
in (due to)
  mumps B26.81
  toxoplasmosis (acquired) B58.1
    congenital (active) P37.1 *[K77]*
infectious, infective (acute) (chronic)
  (subacute) B15.9
  with hepatic coma B15.0
inoculation —*see* Hepatitis, viral,
  type B
interstitial (chronic) K74.69
lupoid NEC K75.2
malignant NEC (with hepatic failure)
  K72.90
  with coma K72.91
neonatal giant cell P59.29
neonatal (idiopathic) (toxic) P59.29
newborn P59.29
postimmunization —*see* Hepatitis, viral,
  type B
post-transfusion —*see* Hepatitis, viral,
  type B
reactive, nonspecific K75.2
serum —*see* Hepatitis, viral, type B
specified type NEC
  with hepatic failure —*see* Failure,
    hepatic
syphilitic (late) A52.74
  congenital (early) A50.08 *[K77]*
    late A50.59 *[K77]*
  secondary A51.45
toxic *(see also* Disease, liver, toxic) K71.6
tuberculous A18.83
viral, virus B19.9
  with hepatic coma B19.0
  acute B17.9
  chronic B18.9
    specified NEC B18.8
    type
      B B18.1
        with delta-agent B18.0
      C B18.2
  congenital P35.3
  coxsackie B33.8 *[K77]*
  cytomegalic inclusion B25.1
  in remission, any type — code to
    Hepatitis, chronic, by type
  non-A, non-B B17.8
  specified type NEC (with or without
    coma) B17.8
  type
    A B15.9
      with hepatic coma B15.0
    B B19.10
      with hepatic coma B19.11
      acute B16.9
        with
          delta-agent (coinfection)
            (without hepatic coma)
            B16.1
            with hepatic coma B16.0
          hepatic coma (without delta-
            agent coinfection) B16.2
      chronic B18.1
        with delta-agent B18.0
    C B19.20
      with hepatic coma B19.21
      acute B17.10
        with hepatic coma B17.11
      chronic B18.2

Hepatitis *(Continued)*
viral, virus *(Continued)*
  type *(Continued)*
    E B17.2
    non-A, non-B B17.8
Hepatization lung (acute) —*see*
  Pneumonia, lobar
Hepatoblastoma C22.2
Hepatocarcinoma C22.0
Hepatocholangiocarcinoma C22.0
Hepatocholangioma, benign D13.4
Hepatocholangitis K75.89
Hepatolenticular degeneration E83.01
Hepatoma (malignant) C22.0
  benign D13.4
  embryonal C22.0
Hepatomegaly —*see also* Hypertrophy,
  liver
  with splenomegaly R16.2
  congenital Q44.7
  in mononucleosis
    gammaherpesviral B27.09
    infectious specified NEC B27.89
Hepatoptosis K76.89
Hepatorenal syndrome following labor
  and delivery O90.4
Hepatosis K76.89
Hepatosplenomegaly R16.2
  hyperlipemic (Bürger-Grütz type) E78.3
    [K77]
Hereditary —*see* condition
Heredodegeneration, macular —*see*
  Dystrophy, retina
Heredopathia atactica polyneuritiformis
  G60.1
Heredosyphilis —*see* Syphilis, congenital
Herlitz' syndrome Q81.1
Hermansky-Pudlak syndrome E70.331
Hermaphrodite, hermaphroditism (true)
  Q56.0
  46,XX with streak gonads Q99.1
  46,XX/46,XY Q99.0
  46,XY with streak gonads Q99.1
  chimera 46,XX/46,XY Q99.0
Hernia, hernial (acquired) (recurrent) K46.9
  with
    gangrene —*see* Hernia, by site, with,
      gangrene
    incarceration —*see* Hernia, by site,
      with, obstruction
    irreducible —*see* Hernia, by site, with,
      obstruction
    obstruction —*see* Hernia, by site,
      with, obstruction
    strangulation —*see* Hernia, by site,
      with, obstruction
  abdomen, abdominal K46.9
    with
      gangrene (and obstruction) K46.1
      obstruction K46.0
    femoral —*see* Hernia, femoral
    incisional —*see* Hernia, incisional
    inguinal —*see* Hernia, inguinal
    specified site NEC K45.8
      with
        gangrene (and obstruction) K45.1
        obstruction K45.0
    umbilical —*see* Hernia, umbilical
    wall —*see* Hernia, ventral
  appendix —*see* Hernia, abdomen
  bladder (mucosa) (sphincter)
    congenital (female) (male) Q79.51
    female —*see* Cystocele
    male N32.89

Hernia, hernial *(Continued)*
brain, congenital —*see* Encephalocele
cartilage, vertebra —*see* Displacement,
  intervertebral disc
cerebral, congenital —*see also*
  Encephalocele
  endaural Q01.8
ciliary body (traumatic) S05.2-
colon —*see* Hernia, abdomen
Cooper's —*see* Hernia, abdomen,
  specified site NEC
crural —*see* Hernia, femoral
diaphragm, diaphragmatic K44.9
  with
    gangrene (and obstruction) K44.1
    obstruction K44.0
  congenital Q79.0
direct (inguinal) —*see* Hernia, inguinal
diverticulum, intestine —*see* Hernia,
  abdomen
double (inguinal) —*see* Hernia,
  inguinal, bilateral
due to adhesions (with obstruction)
  K56.5
epigastric *(see also* Hernia, ventral) K43.9
esophageal hiatus —*see* Hernia, hiatal
external (inguinal) —*see* Hernia,
  inguinal
fallopian tube N83.4
fascia M62.89
femoral K41.90
  with
    gangrene (and obstruction) K41.40
      not specified as recurrent K41.40
      recurrent K41.41
    obstruction K41.30
      not specified as recurrent K41.30
      recurrent K41.31
  bilateral K41.20
    with
      gangrene (and obstruction)
        K41.10
        not specified as recurrent
          K41.10
        recurrent K41.11
      obstruction K41.00
        not specified as recurrent
          K41.00
        recurrent K41.01
    not specified as recurrent K41.20
    recurrent K41.21
  not specified as recurrent K41.90
  recurrent K41.91
  unilateral K41.90
    with
      gangrene (and obstruction)
        K41.40
        not specified as recurrent
          K41.40
        recurrent K41.41
      obstruction K41.30
        not specified as recurrent
          K41.30
        recurrent K41.31
    not specified as recurrent K41.90
    recurrent K41.91
foramen magnum G93.5
  congenital Q01.8
funicular (umbilical) —*see also* Hernia,
  umbilicus
  spermatic (cord) —*see* Hernia,
    inguinal
gastrointestinal tract —*see* Hernia,
  abdomen

Hernia, hernial *(Continued)*
Hesselbach's —*see* Hernia, femoral, specified site NEC
hiatal (esophageal) (sliding) K44.9
  with
    gangrene (and obstruction) K44.1
    obstruction K44.0
  congenital Q40.1
hypogastric —*see* Hernia, ventral
incarcerated —*see also* Hernia, by site, with obstruction
  with gangrene —*see* Hernia, by site, with gangrene
incisional K43.92
  with
    gangrene (and obstruction) K43.1
    obstruction K43.0
indirect (inguinal) —*see* Hernia, inguinal
inguinal (direct) (external) (funicular) (indirect) (internal) (oblique) (scrotal) (sliding) K40.90
  with
    gangrene (and obstruction) K40.40
      not specified as recurrent K40.40
      recurrent K40.41
    obstruction K40.30
      not specified as recurrent K40.30
      recurrent K40.31
  bilateral K40.20
    with
      gangrene (and obstruction) K40.10
        not specified as recurrent K40.10
        recurrent K40.11
      obstruction K40.00
        not specified as recurrent K40.00
        recurrent K40.01
    not specified as recurrent K40.20
    recurrent K40.21
  not specified as recurrent K40.90
  recurrent K40.91
  unilateral K40.90
    with
      gangrene (and obstruction) K40.40
        not specified as recurrent K40.40
        recurrent K40.41
      obstruction K40.30
        not specified as recurrent K40.30
        recurrent K40.31
    not specified as recurrent K40.90
    recurrent K40.91
internal —*see also* Hernia, abdomen
  inguinal —*see* Hernia, inguinal
interstitial —*see* Hernia, abdomen
intervertebral cartilage or disc —*see* Displacement, intervertebral disc
intestine, intestinal —*see* Hernia, by site
intra-abdominal —*see* Hernia, abdomen
iris (traumatic) S05.2-
irreducible —*see also* Hernia, by site, with obstruction
  with gangrene —*see* Hernia, by site, with gangrene
ischiatic —*see* Hernia, abdomen, specified site NEC
ischiorectal —*see* Hernia, abdomen, specified site NEC
lens (traumatic) S05.2-

Hernia, hernial *(Continued)*
linea (alba) (semilunaris) —*see* Hernia, ventral
Littre's —*see* Hernia, abdomen
lumbar —*see* Hernia, abdomen, specified site NEC
lung (subcutaneous) J98.4
mediastinum J98.5
mesenteric (internal) —*see* Hernia, abdomen
midline —*see* Hernia, ventral
muscle (sheath) M62.89
nucleus pulposus —*see* Displacement, intervertebral disc
oblique (inguinal) —*see* Hernia, inguinal
obstructive —*see also* Hernia, by site, with obstruction
  with gangrene —*see* Hernia, by site, with gangrene
obturator —*see* Hernia, abdomen, specified site NEC
omental —*see* Hernia, abdomen
ovary N83.4
oviduct N83.4
paraesophageal —*see also* Hernia, diaphragm
  congenital Q40.1
parastomal K43.5
  with
    gangrene (and obstruction) K43.4
    obstruction K43.3
paraumbilical —*see* Hernia, umbilicus
perineal —*see* Hernia, abdomen, specified site NEC
Petit's —*see* Hernia, abdomen, specified site NEC
postoperative —*see* Hernia, incisional
pregnant uterus —*see* Abnormal, uterus in pregnancy or childbirth
prevesical N32.89
properitoneal —*see* Hernia, abdomen, specified site NEC
pudendal —*see* Hernia, abdomen, specified site NEC
rectovaginal N81.6
retroperitoneal —*see* Hernia, abdomen, specified site NEC
Richter's —*see* Hernia, abdomen, with obstruction
Rieux's, Riex's —*see* Hernia, abdomen, specified site NEC
sac condition (adhesion) (dropsy) (inflammation) (laceration) (suppuration) - code by site under Hernia
sciatic —*see* Hernia, abdomen, specified site NEC
scrotum, scrotal —*see* Hernia, inguinal
sliding (inguinal) —*see also* Hernia, inguinal
  hiatus —*see* Hernia, hiatal
spigelian —*see* Hernia, ventral
spinal —*see* Spina bifida
strangulated —*see also* Hernia, by site, with obstruction
  with gangrene —*see* Hernia, by site, with gangrene
subxiphoid —*see* Hernia, ventral
supra-umbilicus —*see* Hernia, ventral
tendon —*see* Disorder, tendon, specified type NEC
Treitz's (fossa) —*see* Hernia, abdomen, specified site NEC

Hernia, hernial *(Continued)*
tunica vaginalis Q55.29
umbilicus, umbilical K42.9
  with
    gangrene (and obstruction) K42.1
    obstruction K42.0
ureter N28.89
urethra, congenital Q64.79
urinary meatus, congenital Q64.79
uterus N81.4
  pregnant —*see* Abnormal, uterus in pregnancy or childbirth
vaginal (anterior) (wall) —*see* Cystocele
Velpeau's —*see* Hernia, femoral
ventral K43.90
  with
    gangrene (and obstruction) K43.7
    obstruction K43.6
  incisional K43.2
    with
      gangrene (and obstruction) K43.1
      obstruction K43.0
    recurrent —*see* Hernia, incisional
  specified NEC K43.9
    with
      gangrene (and obstruction) K43.7
      obstruction K43.6
vesical
  congenital (female) (male) Q79.51
  female —*see* Cystocele
  male N32.89
vitreous (into wound) S05.2-
  into anterior chamber —*see* Prolapse, vitreous
Herniation —*see also* Hernia
brain (stem) G93.5
cerebral G93.5
mediastinum J98.5
nucleus pulposus —*see* Displacement, intervertebral disc
Herpangina B08.5
Herpes, herpesvirus, herpetic B00.9
anogenital A60.9
  perianal skin A60.1
  rectum A60.1
  urogenital tract A60.00
    cervix A60.03
    male genital organ NEC A60.02
    penis A60.01
    specified site NEC A60.09
    vagina A60.04
    vulva A60.04
blepharitis (zoster) B02.39
  simplex B00.59
circinatus B35.4
  bullosus L12.0
conjunctivitis (simplex) B00.53
  zoster B02.31
cornea B02.33
encephalitis B00.4
  due to herpesvirus 6 B10.01
  due to herpesvirus 7 B10.09
  specified NEC B10.09
eye (zoster) B02.30
  simplex B00.50
eyelid (zoster) B02.39
  simplex B00.59
facialis B00.1
febrilis B00.1
geniculate ganglionitis B02.21
genital, genitalis A60.00
  female A60.09
  male A60.02

Herpes, herpesvirus, herpetic (Continued)
gestational, gestationis O26.4-
gingivostomatitis B00.2
human B00.9
  1 —see Herpes, simplex
  2 —see Herpes, simplex
  3 —see Varicella
  4 —see Mononucleosis, Epstein-Barr
    (virus)
  5 —see Disease, cytomegalic inclusion
    (generalized)
  6
    encephalitis B10.01
    specified NEC B10.81
  7
    encephalitis B10.09
    specified NEC B10.82
  8 B10.89
infection NEC B10.89
  Kaposi's sarcoma associated B10.89
iridocyclitis (simplex) B00.51
  zoster B02.32
iris (vesicular erythema multiforme)
  L51.9
iritis (simplex) B00.51
Kaposi's sarcoma associated B10.89
keratitis (simplex) (dendritic)
  (disciform) (interstitial) B00.52
  zoster (interstitial) B02.33
keratoconjunctivitis (simplex) B00.52
  zoster B02.33
labialis B00.1
lip B00.1
meningitis (simplex) B00.3
  zoster B02.1
ophthalmicus (zoster) NEC B02.30
  simplex B00.50
penis A60.01
perianal skin A60.1
pharyngitis, pharyngotonsillitis B00.2
rectum A60.1
scrotum A60.02
sepsis B00.7
simplex B00.9
  complicated NEC B00.89
  congenital P35.2
  conjunctivitis B00.53
  external ear B00.1
  eyelid B00.59
  hepatitis B00.81
  keratitis (interstitial) B00.52
  myelitis B00.82
  specified complication NEC B00.89
  visceral B00.89
stomatitis B00.2
tonsurans B35.0
visceral B00.89
vulva A60.04
whitlow B00.89
zoster (see also condition) B02.9
  auricularis B02.21
  complicated NEC B02.8
  conjunctivitis B02.31
  disseminated B02.7
  encephalitis B02.0
  eye(lid) B02.39
  geniculate ganglionitis B02.21
  keratitis (interstitial) B02.33
  meningitis B02.1
  myelitis B02.24
  neuritis, neuralgia B02.29
  ophthalmicus NEC B02.30
  oticus B02.21
  polyneuropathy B02.23
  specified complication NEC B02.8
  trigeminal neuralgia B02.22

Herpesvirus (human) —see Herpes
Herpetophobia F40.218
Herrick's anemia —see Disease, sickle-
  cell
Hers' disease E74.09
Herter-Gee syndrome K90.0
Herxheimer's reaction R68.89
Hesitancy
  of micturition R39.11
  urinary R39.11
Hesselbach's hernia —see Hernia,
  femoral, specified site NEC
Heterochromia (congenital) Q13.2
  cataract —see Cataract, complicated
  cyclitis (Fuchs) —see Cyclitis, Fuchs'
    heterochromic
  hair L67.1
  iritis —see Cyclitis, Fuchs'
    heterochromic
  retained metallic foreign body
    (nonmagnetic) —see Foreign body,
    intraocular, old, retained
    magnetic —see Foreign body,
      intraocular, old, retained,
      magnetic
  uveitis —see Cyclitis, Fuchs'
    heterochromic
Heterophoria —see Strabismus,
  heterophoria
Heterophyes, heterophyiasis (small
  intestine) B66.8
Heterotopia, heterotopic —see also
  Malposition, congenital
  cerebralis Q04.8
Heterotropia —see Strabismus
Heubner-Herter disease K90.0
Hexadactylism Q69.9
HGSIL (cytology finding) (high grade
  squamous intraepithelial lesion
  on cytologic smear) (Pap smear
  finding)
  anus R85.613
  cervix R87.613
    biopsy (histology) finding — code to
      CIN II or CIN III
  vagina R87.623
    biopsy (histology) finding — code to
      VAIN II or VAIN III
Hibernoma —see Lipoma
Hiccup, hiccough R06.6
  epidemic B33.0
  psychogenic F45.8
Hidden penis (congenital) Q55.64
  acquired N48.83
Hidradenitis (axillaris) (suppurative)
  L73.2
Hidradenoma (nodular) —see also
  Neoplasm, skin, benign
  clear cell —see Neoplasm, skin, benign
  papillary —see Neoplasm, skin, benign
Hidrocystoma —see Neoplasm, skin,
  benign
High
  altitude effects T70.20
    anoxia T70.29
    on
      ears T70.0
      sinuses T70.1
    polycythemia D75.1
  arch
    foot Q66.7
    palate, congenital Q38.5
  arterial tension —see Hypertension
  basal metabolic rate R94.8

High (Continued)
  blood pressure —see also Hypertension
    borderline R03.0
    reading (incidental) (isolated)
      (nonspecific), without diagnosis
      of hypertension R03.0
  cholesterol E78.0
    with high triglycerides E78.2
  diaphragm (congenital) Q79.1
  expressed emotional level within family
    Z63.8
  head at term O32.4
  palate, congenital Q38.5
  risk
    infant NEC Z76.2
    sexual behavior (heterosexual) Z72.51
      bisexual Z72.53
      homosexual Z72.52
  temperature (of unknown origin) R50.9
  thoracic rib Q76.6
  triglycerides E78.1
    with high cholesterol E78.2
Hildenbrand's disease A75.0
Hilum —see condition Hip —see
  condition
Hippel's disease Q85.8
Hippophobia F40.218
Hippus H57.09
Hirschsprung's disease or megacolon
  Q43.1
Hirsutism, hirsuties L68.0
Hirudiniasis
  external B88.3
  internal B83.4
Hiss-Russell dysentery A03.1
Histidinemia, histidinuria E70.41
Histiocytoma —see also Neoplasm, skin,
  benign
  fibrous —see also Neoplasm, skin,
    benign
    atypical —see Neoplasm, connective
      tissue, uncertain behavior
    malignant —see Neoplasm,
      connective tissue, malignant
Histiocytosis D76.3
  acute differentiated progressive C96.0
  Langerhans' cell NEC C96.6
    multifocal X
      multisystemic (disseminated)
        C96.0
      unisystemic C96.5
    pulmonary, adult (adult PLCH) J84.82
    unifocal (X) C96.6
  lipid, lipoid D76.3
    essential E75.29
  malignant C96.A
  mononuclear phagocytes NEC D76.1
    Langerhans' cells C96.6
  non-Langerhans cell D76.3
  polyostotic sclerosing D76.3
  sinus, with massive lymphadenopathy
    D76.3
  syndrome NEC D76.3
  X NEC C96.6
    acute (progressive) C96.0
    chronic C96.6
    multifocal C96.5
    multisystemic C96.0
    unifocal C96.6
Histoplasmosis B39.9
  with pneumonia NEC B39.2 [J17]
  African B39.5
  American —see Histoplasmosis,
    capsulati

Histoplasmosis *(Continued)*
  capsulati B39.4
    disseminated B39.3
    generalized B39.3
    pulmonary B39.2
      acute B39.0
      chronic B39.1
  Darling's B39.4
  duboisii B39.5
  lung NEC B39.2
History
  family (of) —*see also* History, personal
        (of)
    alcohol abuse Z81.1
    allergy NEC Z84.89
    anemia Z83.2
    arthritis Z82.61
    asthma Z82.5
    blindness Z82.1
    cardiac death (sudden) Z82.41
    carrier of genetic disease Z84.81
    chromosomal anomaly Z82.79
    chronic
      disabling disease NEC Z82.8
      lower respiratory disease
          Z82.5
    colonic polyps Z83.71
    congenital malformations and
        deformations Z82.79
      polycystic kidney Z82.71
    consanguinity Z84.3
    deafness Z82.2
    diabetes mellitus Z83.3
    disability NEC Z82.8
    disease or disorder (of)
      allergic NEC Z84.89
      behavioral NEC Z81.8
      blood and blood-forming organs
          Z83.2
      cardiovascular NEC Z82.49
      chronic disabling NEC Z82.8
      digestive Z83.79
      ear NEC Z83.52
      endocrine NEC Z83.49
      eye NEC Z83.518
        glaucoma Z83.511
      genitourinary NEC Z84.2
      glaucoma Z83.511
      hematological Z83.2
      immune mechanism Z83.2
      infectious NEC Z83.1
      ischemic heart Z82.49
      kidney Z84.1
      mental NEC Z81.8
      metabolic Z83.49
      musculoskeletal NEC Z82.69
      neurological NEC Z82.0
      nutritional Z83.49
      parasitic NEC Z83.1
      psychiatric NEC Z81.8
      respiratory NEC Z83.6
      skin and subcutaneous tissue NEC
          Z84.0
      specified NEC Z84.89
    drug abuse NEC Z81.3
    epilepsy Z82.0
    genetic disease carrier Z84.81
    glaucoma Z83.511
    hearing loss Z82.2
    human immunodeficiency virus
        (HIV) infection Z83.0
    Huntington's chorea Z82.0
    intellectual disability Z81.0
    leukemia Z80.6

History *(Continued)*
  family *(Continued)*
    malignant neoplasm (of) NOS
        Z80.9
      bladder Z80.52
      breast Z80.3
      bronchus Z80.1
      digestive organ Z80.0
      gastrointestinal tract Z80.0
      genital organ Z80.49
        ovary Z80.41
        prostate Z80.42
        specified organ NEC Z80.49
        testis Z80.43
      hematopoietic NEC Z80.7
      intrathoracic organ NEC Z80.2
      kidney Z80.51
      lung Z80.1
      lymphatic NEC Z80.7
      ovary Z80.41
      prostate Z80.42
      respiratory organ NEC Z80.2
      specified site NEC Z80.8
      testis Z80.43
      trachea Z80.1
      urinary organ or tract Z80.59
        bladder Z80.52
        kidney Z80.51
    mental
      disorder NEC Z81.8
    multiple endocrine neoplasia (MEN)
          syndrome Z83.41
    osteoporosis Z82.62
    polycystic kidney Z82.71
    polyps (colon) Z83.71
    psychiatric disorder Z81.8
    psychoactive substance abuse NEC
        Z81.3
    respiratory condition NEC Z83.6
      asthma and other lower
          respiratory conditions
          Z82.5
    self-harmful behavior Z81.8
    skin condition Z84.0
    specified condition NEC Z84.89
    stroke (cerebrovascular) Z82.3
    substance abuse NEC Z81.4
      alcohol Z81.1
      drug NEC Z81.3
      psychoactive NEC Z81.3
      tobacco Z81.2
    sudden cardiac death Z82.41
    tobacco abuse Z81.2
    violence, violent behavior Z81.8
    visual loss Z82.1
  personal (of) —*see also* History, family
        (of)
    abuse
      adult Z91.419
        physical and sexual Z91.410
        psychological Z91.411
      childhood Z62.819
        physical Z62.810
        psychological Z62.811
        sexual Z62.810
    alcohol dependence F10.21
    allergy (to) Z88.9
      analgesic agent NEC Z88.6
      anesthetic Z88.4
      antibiotic agent NEC Z88.1
      anti-infective agent NEC Z88.3
      contrast media Z91.041
      drugs, medicaments and biological
          substances Z88.9
        specified NEC Z88.8

History *(Continued)*
  personal *(Continued)*
    allergy *(Continued)*
      food Z91.018
        additives Z91.02
        eggs Z91.012
        milk products Z91.011
        peanuts Z91.010
        seafood Z91.013
        specified food NEC Z91.018
      insect Z91.038
        bee Z91.030
      latex Z91.040
      medicinal agents Z88.9
        specified NEC Z88.8
      narcotic agent NEC Z88.5
      nonmedicinal agents Z91.048
      penicillin Z88.0
      serum Z88.7
      specified NEC Z91.09
      sulfonamides Z88.2
      vaccine Z88.7
    anaphylactic shock Z87.892
    anaphylaxis Z87.892
    blood and blood-forming organs
        Z86.2
    circulatory system Z86.79
      specified condition NEC Z86.79
    connective tissue NEC Z87.39
    digestive system Z87.19
      colonic polyp Z86.010
      peptic ulcer disease Z87.11
      specified condition NEC Z87.19
    ear Z86.69
    endocrine Z86.39
      diabetic foot ulcer Z86.31
      gestational diabetes Z86.32
      specified type NEC Z86.39
    eye Z86.69
    genital (track) system NEC
      female Z87.42
      male Z87.438
    hematological Z86.2
    Hodgkin Z85.71
    immune mechanism Z86.2
    infectious Z86.19
      malaria Z86.13
      Methicillin resistant
          Staphylococcus aureus
          (MRSA) Z86.14
      poliomyelitis Z86.12
      specified NEC Z86.19
      tuberculosis Z86.11
    mental NEC Z86.59
    metabolic Z86.39
      diabetic foot ulcer Z86.31
      gestational diabetes Z86.32
      specified type NEC Z86.39
    musculoskeletal NEC Z87.39
    nervous system Z86.69
    nutritional Z86.39
    parasitic Z86.19
    respiratory system NEC Z87.09
    sense organs Z86.69
    skin Z87.2
    specified site or type NEC Z87.898
    subcutaneous tissue Z87.2
    trophoblastic Z87.59
    urinary system NEC Z87.448
  behavioral disorders Z86.59
  benign carcinoid tumor Z86.012
  benign neoplasm Z86.018
    brain Z86.011
    carcinoid Z86.012
    colonic polyps Z86.010

History *(Continued)*
  personal *(Continued)*
    brain injury (traumatic) Z87.820
    breast implant removal Z98.86
    calculi, renal Z87.442
    cancer —*see* History, personal (of),
      malignant neoplasm (of)
    cardiac arrest (death), successfully
      resuscitated Z86.74
    cerebral infarction without residual
      deficit Z86.73
    cervical dysplasia Z87.410
    chemotherapy for neoplastic
      condition Z92.21
    childhood abuse —*see* History,
      personal (of), abuse
    cleft lip (corrected) Z87.730
    cleft palate (corrected) Z87.730
    collapsed vertebra (healed) Z87.311
      due to osteoporosis Z87.310
    combat and operational stress
      reaction Z86.51
    congenital malformation (corrected)
      Z87.798
      circulatory system (corrected)
        Z87.74
      digestive system (corrected) NEC
        Z87.738
      ear (corrected) Z87.720
      eye (corrected) Z87.721
      face and neck (corrected) Z87.790
      genitourinary system (corrected)
        NEC Z87.718
      heart (corrected) Z87.74
      integument (corrected) Z87.76
      limb (s) (corrected) Z87.76
      musculoskeletal system (corrected)
        Z87.76
      neck (corrected) Z87.790
      nervous system (corrected) NEC
        Z87.728
      respiratory system (corrected)
        Z87.75
      sense organs (corrected) NEC
        Z87.728
      specified NEC Z87.798
    contraception Z92.0
    deployment (military) Z91.82
    diabetic foot ulcer Z86.31
    disease or disorder (of) Z87.898
    drug dependence —*see* Dependence,
      drug, by type, in remission
    drug therapy
      antineoplastic chemotherapy Z92.21
      estrogen Z92.23
      immunosupression Z92.25
      inhaled steroids Z92.240
      monoclonal drug Z92.22
      specified NEC Z92.29
      steroid Z92.241
      systemic steroids Z92.241
    dysplasia
      cervical Z87.410
      prostatic Z87.430
      vaginal Z87.411
      vulvar Z87.412
    embolism (venous) Z86.718
      pulmonary Z86.711
    encephalitis Z86.61
    estrogen therapy Z92.23
    extracorporeal membrane
      oxygenation (ECMO) Z92.81
    failed conscious sedation Z92.83
    failed moderate sedation Z92.83
    fall, falling Z91.81

History *(Continued)*
  personal *(Continued)*
    fracture (healed)
      fatigue Z87.312
      fragility Z87.310
      osteoporosis Z87.310
      pathological NEC Z87.311
      stress Z87.312
      traumatic Z87.81
    gestational diabetes Z86.32
    hepatitis
      B Z86.19
      C Z86.19
    Hodgkin disease Z85.71
    hyperthermia, malignant Z88.4
    hypospadias (corrected) Z87.710
    hysterectomy Z90.710
    immunosupression therapy Z92.25
    in situ neoplasm
      breast Z86.000
      cervix uteri Z86.001
      specified NEC Z86.008
    infection NEC Z86.19
      central nervous system Z86.61
      Methicillin resistant
        Staphylococcus aureus
        (MRSA) Z86.14
      urinary (tract) Z87.41
    injury NEC Z87.828
    in utero procedure during pregnancy
      Z98.870
    in utero procedure while a fetus
      Z98.871
    irradiation Z92.3
    kidney stones Z87.442
    leukemia Z85.6
    lymphoma (non-Hodgkin) Z85.72
    malignant melanoma (skin) Z85.820
    malignant neoplasm (of) Z85.9
      accessory sinuses Z85.22
      anus NEC Z85.048
        carcinoid Z85.040
      bladder Z85.51
      bone Z85.830
      brain Z85.841
      breast Z85.3
      bronchus NEC Z85.118
        carcinoid Z85.110
      carcinoid —*see* History, personal
        (of), malignant neoplasm, by
        site, carcinioid
      cervix Z85.41
      colon NEC Z85.038
        carcinoid Z85.030
      digestive organ Z85.00
        specified NEC Z85.09
      endocrine gland NEC Z85.858
      epididymis Z85.48
      esophagus Z85.01
      eye Z85.840
      gastrointestinal tract —*see* History,
        malignant neoplasm,
        digestive organ
      genital organ
        female Z85.40
          specified NEC Z85.44
        male Z85.45
          specified NEC Z85.49
      hematopoietic NEC Z85.79
      intrathoracic organ Z85.20-
      kidney NEC Z85.528
        carcinoid Z85.520
      large intestine NEC Z85.038
        carcinoid Z85.030

History *(Continued)*
  personal *(Continued)*
    malignant neoplasm *(Continued)*
      larynx Z85.21
      liver Z85.05
      lung NEC Z85.118
        carcinoid Z85.110
      mediastinum Z85.29
      Merkel cell Z85.821
      middle ear Z85.22
      nasal cavities Z85.22
      nervous system NEC Z85.848
      oral cavity Z85.819
        specified site NEC Z85.818
      ovary Z85.43
      pancreas Z85.07
      pelvis Z85.53
      pharynx Z85.819
        specified site NEC Z85.818
      pleura Z85.29
      prostate Z85.46
      rectosigmoid junction NEC Z85.048
        carcinoid Z85.040
      rectum NEC Z85.048
        carcinoid Z85.040
      respiratory organ Z85.20
      sinuses, accessory Z85.22
      skin NEC Z85.828
        melanoma Z85.820
        Merkel cell Z85.821
      small intestine NEC Z85.068
        carcinoid Z85.060
      soft tissue Z85.831
      specified site NEC Z85.89
      stomach NEC Z85.028
        carcinoid Z85.020
      testis Z85.47
      thymus NEC Z85.238
        carcinoid Z85.230
      thyroid Z85.850
      tongue Z85.810
      trachea Z85.12
      urinary organ or tract Z85.50
        specified NEC Z85.59
      uterus Z85.42
    maltreatment Z91.89
    medical treatment NEC Z92.89
    melanoma (malignant) (skin) Z85.820
    meningitis Z86.61
    mental disorder Z86.59
    Merkel cell carcinoma (skin) Z85.821
    Methicillin resistant Staphylococcus
      aureus (MRSA) Z86.14
    military deployment Z91.82
    military war, peacekeeping and
      humanitarian deployment
      (current or past conflict) Z91.82
    myocardial infarction (old) I25.2
    neglect (in)
      adult Z91.412
      childhood Z62.812
    neoplasm
      benign Z86.018
        brain Z86.011
        colon polyp Z86.010
      in situ
        breast Z86.000
        cervix uteri Z86.001
        specified NEC Z86.008
      malignant —*see* History of,
        malignant neoplasm
      uncertain behavior Z86.03
    nephrotic syndrome Z87.441
    nicotine dependence Z87.891

History (Continued)
  personal (Continued)
    noncompliance with medical
        treatment or regimen —see
        Noncompliance
    nutritional deficiency Z86.39
    obstetric complications Z87.59
        childbirth Z87.59
        pregnancy Z87.59
        pre-term labor Z87.51
        puerperium Z87.59
    osteoporosis fractures Z87.31
    parasuicide (attempt) Z91.5
    physical trauma NEC Z87.828
        self-harm or suicide attempt Z91.5
    pneumonia (recurrent) Z87.01
    poisoning NEC Z91.89
        self-harm or suicide attempt Z91.5
    poor personal hygiene Z91.89
    preterm labor Z87.51
    procedure during pregnancy Z98.870
    procedure while a fetus Z98.871
    prolonged reversible ischemic
        neurologic deficit (PRIND)
        Z86.73
    prostatic dysplasia Z87.430
    psychiatric disorder NEC Z87.89
    psychological
        abuse
            adult Z91.411
            child Z62.811
        trauma, specified NEC Z91.49
    radiation therapy Z92.3
    removal
        implant
            breast Z98.86
    renal calculi Z87.442
    respiratory condition NEC Z87.09
    retained foreign body fully removed
        Z87.821
    risk factors NEC Z91.89
    self-harm Z91.5
    self-poisoning attempt Z91.5
    sex reassignment Z87.890
    sleep-wake cycle problem Z72.821
    specified NEC Z87.898
    steroid therapy (systemic) Z92.241
        inhaled Z92.240
    stroke without residual deficits
        Z86.73
    substance abuse NEC F10 - with fifth
        character 1 F19
    sudden cardiac arrest Z86.74
    sudden cardiac death successfully
        resuscitated Z86.74
    suicide attempt Z91.5
    surgery NEC Z98.89
        sex reassignment Z87.890
        transplant —see Transplant
    thrombophlebitis Z86.72
    thrombosis (venous) Z86.718
        pulmonary Z86.711
    tobacco dependence Z87.891
    transient ischemic attack (TIA)
        without residual deficits Z86.73
    trauma (physical) NEC Z87.828
        psychological NEC Z91.49
        self-harm Z91.5
    traumatic brain injury Z87.820
    unhealthy sleep-wake cycle Z72.821
    urinary (recurrent) (tract) infection (s)
        Z87.440
    urinary calculi Z87.43
    vaginal dysplasia Z87.411

History (Continued)
  personal (Continued)
    venous thrombosis or embolism
        Z86.718
        pulmonary Z86.711
    vulvar dysplasia Z87.412
His-Werner disease A79.0
HIV (see also Human, immunodeficiency
    virus) B20
    laboratory evidence (nonconclusive)
        R75
    nonconclusive test (in infants) R75
    positive, seropositive Z21
Hives (bold) —see Urticaria
Hoarseness R49.0
Hobo Z59.0
Hodgkin disease —see Lymphoma,
    Hodgkin
Hodgson's disease I71.2
    ruptured I71.1
Hoffa-Kastert disease E88.89
Hoffa's disease E88.89
Hoffmann-Bouveret syndrome I47.9
Hoffmann's syndrome E03.9 [G73.7]
Hole (round)
    macula H35.34-
    retina (without detachment) —see
        Break, retina, round hole
        with detachment —see Detachment,
            retina, with retinal, break
Holiday relief care Z75.5
Hollenhorst's plaque —see Occlusion,
    artery, retina
Hollow foot (congenital) Q66.7
    acquired —see Deformity, limb, foot,
        specified NEC
Holoprosencephaly Q04.2
Holt-Oram syndrome Q87.2
Homelessness Z59.0
Homesickness —see Disorder, adjustment
Homocystinemia, homocystinuria
    E72.11
Homogentisate 1,2-dioxygenase
    deficiency E70.29
Homologous serum hepatitis
        (prophylactic) (therapeutic) —see
        Hepatitis, viral, type B
Honeycomb lung J98.4
    congenital Q33.0
Hooded
    clitoris Q52.6
    penis Q55.69
Hookworm (anemia) (disease) (infection)
        (infestation) B76.9
    specified NEC B76.8
Hordeolum (eyelid) (externum)
        (recurrent) H00.019
    internum H00.029
        left H00.026
            lower H00.025
            upper H00.024
        right H00.023
            lower H00.022
            upper H00.021
    left H00.016
        lower H00.015
        upper H00.014
    right H00.013
        lower H00.012
        upper H00.011
Horn
    cutaneous L85.8
    nail L60.2
        congenital Q84.6

Horner (-Claude Bernard) syndrome
    G90.2
    traumatic —see Injury, nerve, cervical
        sympathetic
Horseshoe kidney (congenital) Q63.1
Horton's headache or neuralgia
    G44.099
    intractable G44.091
    not intractable G44.099
Hospital hopper syndrome —see
    Disorder, factitious
Hospitalism in children —see Disorder,
    adjustment
Hostility R45.5
    towards child Z62.3
Hot flashes
    menopausal N95.1
Hourglass (contracture) —see also
        Contraction, hourglass
    stomach K31.89
        congenital Q40.2
        stricture K31.2
Household, housing circumstance
        affecting care Z59.9
    specified NEC Z59.8
Housemaid's knee —see Bursitis,
    prepatellar
Hudson (-Stähli) line (cornea) —see
    Pigmentation, cornea, anterior
Human
    bite (open wound) —see also Bite
        intact skin surface —see Bite,
            superficial
    herpesvirus —see Herpes
    immunodeficiency virus (HIV) disease
        (infection) B20
        asymptomatic status Z21
        contact Z20.6
        counseling Z71.7
        dementia B20 [F02.80]
            with behavioral disturbance B20
                [F02.81]
        exposure to Z20.6
        laboratory evidence R75
        type-2 (HIV 2) as cause of disease
            classified elsewhere B97.35
    papillomavirus (HPV)
        DNA test positive
            high risk
                cervix R87.810
                vagina R87.811
            low risk
                cervix R87.820
                vagina R87.821
        screening for Z11.51
    T-cell lymphotropic virus
        type-1 (HTLV-I) infection B33.3
            as cause of disease classified
                elsewhere B97.33
            carrier Z22.6
        type-2 (HTLV-II) as cause of disease
            classified elsewhere B97.34
Humidifier lung or pneumonitis J67.7
Humiliation (experience) in childhood
    Z62.898
Humpback (acquired) —see Kyphosis
Hunchback (acquired) —see Kyphosis
Hunger T73.0
    air, psychogenic F45.8
Hungry bone syndrome E83.81
Hunner's ulcer —see Cystitis, chronic,
    interstitial
Hunter's
    glossitis D51.0
    syndrome E76.1

Huntington's disease or chorea G10
  with dementia G10 [F02.80]
    with behavioral disturbance G10
      [F02.81]
Hunt's
  disease or syndrome (herpetic
    geniculate ganglionitis) B02.21
  dyssynergia cerebellaris myoclonica
    G11.1
  neuralgia B02.21
Hurler (-Scheie) disease or syndrome
  E76.02
Hurst's disease G36.1
Hurthle cell
  adenocarcinoma C73
  adenoma D34
  carcinoma C73
  tumor D34
Hutchinson-Boeck disease or
  syndrome —see Sarcoidosis
Hutchinson-Gilford disease or syndrome
  E34.8
Hutchinson's
  disease, meaning
    angioma serpiginosum L81.7
    pompholyx (cheiropompholyx) L30.1
    prurigo estivalis L56.4
    summer eruption or summer prurigo
      L56.4
  melanotic freckle —see Melanoma, in
    situ
    malignant melanoma in —see
      Melanoma
  teeth or incisors (congenital syphilis)
    A50.52
  triad (congenital syphilis) A50.53
Hyalin plaque, sclera, senile H15.89
Hyaline membrane (disease) (lung)
  (pulmonary) (newborn) P22.0
Hyalinosis
  cutis (et mucosae) E78.89
  focal and segmental (glomerular)
    (see also N00-N07 with fourth
    character .1) N05.1
Hyalitis, hyalosis, asteroid —see also
  Deposit, crystalline
  syphilitic (late) A52.71
Hydatid
  cyst or tumor —see Echinococcus
  mole —see Hydatidiform mole
  Morgagni
    female Q50.5
    male (epididymal) Q55.4
    testicular Q55.29
Hydatidiform mole (benign)
  (complicating pregnancy) (delivered)
  (undelivered) O01.9
  classical O01.0
  complete O01.0
  incomplete O01.1
  invasive D39.2
  malignant D39.2
  partial O01.1
Hydatidosis —see Echinococcus
Hydradenitis (axillaris) (suppurative)
  L73.2
Hydradenoma —see Hidradenoma
Hydramnios O40.-
Hydrancephaly, hydranencephaly
  Q04.3
  with spina bifida —see Spina bifida,
    with hydrocephalus
Hydrargyrism NEC —see Poisoning,
  mercury

Hydrarthrosis —see also Effusion, joint
  gonococcal A54.42
  intermittent M12.40
    ankle M12.47-
    elbow M12.42-
    foot joint M12.47-
    hand joint M12.44-
    hip M12.45-
    knee M12.46-
    multiple site M12.49
    shoulder M12.41-
    specified joint NEC M12.48
    wrist M12.43-
  of yaws (early) (late) (see also
    subcategory M14.8-) A66.6
  syphilitic (late) A52.77
    congenital A50.55 [M12.80]
Hydremia D64.89
Hydrencephalocele (congenital) —see
  Encephalocele
Hydrencephalomeningocele
  (congenital) —see Encephalocele
Hydroa R23.8
  aestivale L56.4
  vacciniforme L56.4
Hydroadenitis (axillaris) (suppurative)
  L73.2
Hydrocalycosis —see Hydronephrosis
Hydrocele (spermatic cord) (testis) (tunica
  vaginalis) N43.3
  canal of Nuck N94.89
  communicating N43.2
    congenital P83.5
  congenital P83.5
  encysted N43.0
  female NEC N94.89
  infected N43.1
  newborn P83.5
  round ligament N94.89
  specified NEC N43.2
  spinalis —see Spina bifida
  vulva N90.89
Hydrocephalus (acquired) (external)
  (internal) (malignant) (recurrent)
  G91.9
  aqueduct Sylvius stricture Q03.0
  causing disproportion O33.6
    with obstructed labor O66.3
  communicating G91.0
  congenital (external) (internal) Q03.9
    with spina bifida Q05.4
      cervical Q05.0
      dorsal Q05.1
      lumbar Q05.2
      lumbosacral Q05.2
      sacral Q05.3
      thoracic Q05.1
      thoracolumbar Q05.1
    specified NEC Q03.8
  due to toxoplasmosis (congenital) P37.1
  foramen Magendie block (acquired)
    G91.1
    congenital (see also Hydrocephalus,
      congenital) Q03.1
  in (due to)
    infectious disease NEC B89 [G91.4]
    neoplastic disease NEC (see also
      Neoplasm) G91.4
    parasitic disease B89 [G91.4]
  newborn Q03.9
    with spina bifida —see Spina bifida,
      with hydrocephalus
  noncommunicating G91.1
  normal pressure G91.2
    secondary G91.0

Hydrocephalus (Continued)
  obstructive G91.1
  otitic G93.2
  post-traumatic NEC G91.3
  secondary G91.4
    post-traumatic G91.3
  specified NEC G91.8
  syphilitic, congenital A50.49
Hydrocolpos (congenital) N89.8
Hydrocystoma —see Neoplasm, skin,
  benign
Hydroencephalocele (congenital) —see
  Encephalocele
Hydroencephalomeningocele
  (congenital) —see Encephalocele
Hydrohematopneumothorax —see
  Hemothorax
Hydromeningitis —see Meningitis
Hydromeningocele (spinal) —see also
  Spina bifida
  cranial —see Encephalocele
Hydrometra N85.8
Hydrometrocolpos N89.8
Hydromicrocephaly Q02
Hydromphalos (since birth) Q45.8
Hydromyelia Q06.4
Hydromyelocele —see Spina bifida
Hydronephrosis (atrophic) (early)
  (functionless) (intermittent)
  (primary) (secondary) NEC
  N13.30
  with
    infection N13.6
    obstruction (by) (of)
      renal calculus N13.2
        with infection N13.6
      ureteral NEC N13.1
        with infection N13.6
        calculus N13.2
          with infection N13.6
      ureteropelvic junction (congenital)
        Q62.0
        with infection N13.6
    ureteral stricture NEC N13.1
      with infection N13.6
  congenital Q62.0
  specified type NEC N13.39
  tuberculous A18.11
Hydropericarditis —see Pericarditis
Hydropericardium —see Pericarditis
Hydroperitoneum R18.8
Hydrophobia —see Rabies
Hydrophthalmos Q15.0
Hydropneumohemothorax —see
  Hemothorax
Hydropneumopericarditis —see
  Pericarditis
Hydropneumopericardium —see
  Pericarditis
Hydropneumothorax J94.8
  traumatic —see Injury, intrathoracic,
    lung
  tuberculous NEC A15.6
Hydrops R60.9
  abdominis R18.8
  articulorum intermittens —see
    Hydrarthrosis, intermittent
  cardiac —see Failure, heart,
    congestive
  causing obstructed labor (mother)
    O66.3
  endolymphatic H81.0-
  fetal —see Pregnancy, complicated by,
    hydrops, fetalis

Hydrops *(Continued)*
fetalis P83.2
due to
ABO isoimmunization P56.0
alpha thalassemia D56.0
hemolytic disease P56.90
specified NEC P56.99
isoimmunization (ABO) (Rh) P56.0
other specified nonhemolytic
disease NEC P83.2
Rh incompatibility P56.0
during pregnancy —*see* Pregnancy,
complicated by, hydrops, fetalis
gallbladder K82.1
joint —*see* Effusion, joint
labyrinth H81.0
newborn (idiopathic) P83.2
due to
ABO isoimmunization P56.0
alpha thalassemia D56.0
hemolytic disease P56.90
specified NEC P56.99
isoimmunization (ABO) (Rh)
P56.0
Rh incompatibility P56.0
nutritional —*see* Malnutrition, severe
pericardium —*see* Pericarditis
pleura —*see* Hydrothorax
spermatic cord —*see* Hydrocele
Hydropyonephrosis N13.6
Hydrorachis Q06.4
Hydrorrhea (nasal) J34.89
pregnancy —*see* Rupture, membranes,
premature
Hydrosadenitis (axillaris) (suppurative)
L73.2
Hydrosalpinx (fallopian tube)
(follicularis) N70.11
Hydrothorax (double) (pleura) J94.8
chylous (nonfilarial) I89.8
filarial (*see also* Infestation, filarial)
B74.9 [J91.8]
traumatic —*see* Injury, intrathoracic
tuberculous NEC (non primary) A15.6
Hydroureter (*see also* Hydronephrosis)
N13.4
with infection N13.6
congenital Q62.39
Hydroureteronephrosis —*see*
Hydronephrosis
Hydrourethra N36.8
Hydroxykynureninuria E70.8
Hydroxylysinemia E72.3
Hydroxyprolinemia E72.59
Hygiene, sleep
abuse Z72.821
inadequate Z72.821
poor Z72.821
Hygroma (congenital) (cystic) D18.1
praepatellare, prepatellar —*see* Bursitis,
prepatellar
Hymen —*see* condition
Hymenolepis, hymenolepiasis
(diminuta) (infection) (infestation)
(nana) B71.0
Hypalgesia R20.8
Hyperacidity (gastric) K31.89
psychogenic F45.8
Hyperactive, hyperactivity F90.9
basal cell, uterine cervix —*see*
Dysplasia, cervix
bowel sounds R19.12
cervix epithelial (basal) —*see* Dysplasia,
cervix

Hyperactive, hyperactivity *(Continued)*
child F90.9
attention deficit —*see* Disorder,
attention-deficit hyperactivity
detrusor muscle N32.81
gastrointestinal K31.89
psychogenic F45.8
nasal mucous membrane J34.3
stomach K31.89
thyroid (gland) —*see* Hyperthyroidism
Hyperacusis H93.23-
Hyperadrenalism E27.5
Hyperadrenocorticism E24.9
congenital E25.0
iatrogenic E24.2
correct substance properly
administered —*see* Table of drugs
and chemicals, by drug, adverse
effect
overdose or wrong substance given
or taken —*see* Table of drugs and
chemicals, by drug, poisoning
not associated with Cushing's
syndrome E27.0
pituitary-dependent E24.0
Hyperaldosteronism E26.9
familial (type I) E26.02
glucocorticoid-remediable E26.02
primary (due to (bilateral) adrenal
hyperplasia) E26.09
primary NEC E26.09
secondary E26.1
specified NEC E26.89
Hyperalgesia R20.8
Hyperalimentation R63.2
carotene, carotin E67.1
specified NEC E67.8
vitamin
A E67.0
D E67.3
Hyperaminoaciduria
arginine E72.21
cystine E72.01
lysine E72.3
ornithine E72.4
Hyperammonemia (congenital) E72.20
Hyperazotemia —*see* Uremia
Hyperbetalipoproteinemia (familial) E78.0
with prebetalipoproteinemia E78.2
Hyperbilirubinemia
constitutional E80.6
familial conjugated E80.6
neonatal (transient) —*see* Jaundice,
newborn
Hypercalcemia, hypocalciuric, familial
E83.52
Hypercalciuria, idiopathic E83.52
Hypercapnia R06.89
newborn P84
Hypercarotenemia, hypercarotinemia
(dietary) E67.1
Hypercementosis K03.4
Hyperchloremia E87.8
Hyperchlorhydria K31.89
neurotic F45.8
psychogenic F45.8
Hypercholesterinemia —*see*
Hypercholesterolemia
Hypercholesterolemia (essential) (familial)
(hereditary) (primary) (pure) E78.0
with hyperglyceridemia, endogenous
E78.2
dietary counseling and surveillance
Z71.3

Hyperchylia gastrica, psychogenic F45.8
Hyperchylomicronemia (familial)
(primary) E78.3
with hyperbetalipoproteinemia E78.3
Hypercoagulable (state) D68.59
activated protein C resistance D68.51
antithrombin (III) deficiency D68.59
factor V Leiden mutation D68.51
primary NEC D68.59
protein C deficiency D68.59
protein S deficiency D68.59
prothrombin gene mutation D68.52
secondary D68.69
specified NEC D68.69
Hypercoagulation (state) D68.59
Hypercorticalism, pituitary-dependent
E24.0
Hypercorticosolism —*see* Cushing's,
syndrome
Hypercorticosteronism E24.2
correct substance properly
administered —*see* Table of drugs
and chemicals, by drug, adverse
effect
overdose or wrong substance given
or taken —*see* Table of drugs and
chemicals, by drug, poisoning
Hypercortisonism E24.2
correct substance properly
administered —*see* Table of
drugs and chemicals, by drug,
adverse effect
overdose or wrong substance given
or taken —*see* Table of drugs and
chemicals, by drug, poisoning
Hyperekplexia Q89.8
Hyperelectrolytemia E87.8
Hyperemesis R11.10
with nausea R11.2
gravidarum (mild) O21.0
with
carbohydrate depletion O21.1
dehydration O21.1
electrolyte imbalance O21.1
metabolic disturbance O21.1
severe (with metabolic disturbance)
O21.1
projectile R11.12
psychogenic F45.8
Hyperemia (acute) (passive) R68.89
anal mucosa K62.89
bladder N32.89
cerebral I67.89
conjunctiva H11.43-
ear internal, acute —*see* subcategory
H83.0
enteric K59.8
eye —*see* Hyperemia, conjunctiva
eyelid (active) (passive) —*see* Disorder,
eyelid, specified type NEC
intestine K59.8
iris —*see* Disorder, iris, vascular
kidney N28.89
labyrinth —*see* subcategory H83.0
liver (active) K76.89
lung (passive) —*see* Edema, lung
pulmonary (passive) —*see* Edema, lung
renal N28.89
retina H35.89
stomach K31.89
Hyperesthesia (body surface) R20.3
larynx (reflex) J38.7
hysterical F44.89
pharynx (reflex) J39.2
hysterical F44.89

Hyperestrogenism (drug-induced)
(iatrogenic) E28.0
Hyperexplexia Q89.8
Hyperfibrinolysis —*see* Fibrinolysis
Hyperfructosemia E74.19
Hyperfunction
adrenal cortex, not associated with
Cushing's syndrome E27.0
medulla E27.5
adrenomedullary E27.5
virilism E25.9
congenital E25.0
ovarian E28.8
pancreas K86.8
parathyroid (gland) E21.3
pituitary (gland) (anterior) E22.9
specified NEC E22.8
polyglandular E31.1
testicular E29.0
Hypergammaglobulinemia D89.2
polyclonal D89.0
Waldenström D89.0
Hypergastrinemia E16.4
Hyperglobulinemia R77.1
Hyperglycemia, hyperglycemic
(transient) R73.9
coma —*see* Diabetes, by type, with coma
postpancreatectomy E89.1
Hyperglyceridemia (endogenous)
(essential) (familial) (hereditary)
(pure) E78.1
mixed E78.3
Hyperglycinemia (non-ketotic) E72.51
Hypergonadism
ovarian E28.8
testicular (primary) (infantile) E29.0
Hyperheparinemia D68.32
Hyperhidrosis, hyperidrosis R61
focal
primary L74.519
axilla L74.510
face L74.511
palms L74.512
soles L74.513
secondary L74.52
generalized R61
localized
primary L74.519
axilla L74.510
face L74.511
palms L74.512
soles L74.513
secondary L74.52
psychogenic F45.8
secondary R61
focal L74.52
Hyperhistidinemia E70.41
Hyperhomocysteinemia E72.11
Hyperhydroxyprolinemia E72.59
Hyperinsulinism (functional) E16.1
with
coma (hypoglycemic) E15
encephalopathy E16.1 *[G94]*
ectopic E16.1
therapeutic misadventure (from
administration of insulin) —*see*
subcategory T38.3
Hyperkalemia E87.5
Hyperkeratosis (*see also* Keratosis) L85.9
cervix N88.0
due to yaws (early) (late) (palmar or
plantar) A66.3
follicularis Q82.8
penetrans (in cutem) L87.0

Hyperkeratosis (*Continued*)
palmoplantaris climacterica L85.1
pinta A67.1
senile (with pruritus) L57.0
universalis congenita Q80.8
vocal cord J38.3
vulva N90.4
Hyperkinesia, hyperkinetic (disease)
(reaction) (syndrome) (childhood)
(adolescence) —*see also* Disorder,
attention-deficit hyperactivity
heart I51.89
Hyperleucine-isoleucinemia E71.19
Hyperlipemia, hyperlipidemia E78.5
combined E78.2
familial E78.4
group
A E78.0
B E78.1
C E78.2
D E78.3
mixed E78.2
specified NEC E78.4
Hyperlipidosis E75.6
hereditary NEC E75.5
Hyperlipoproteinemia E78.5
Fredrickson's type
I E78.3
IIa E78.0
IIb E78.2
III E78.2
IV E78.1
V E78.3
low-density-lipoprotein-type (LDL) E78.0
very-low-density-lipoprotein-type
(VLDL) E78.1
Hyperlucent lung, unilateral J43.0
Hyperlysinemia E72.3
Hypermagnesemia E83.41
neonatal P71.8
Hypermenorrhea N92.0
Hypermethioninemia E72.19
Hypermetropia (congenital) H52.0-
Hypermobility, hypermotility
cecum —*see* Syndrome, irritable bowel
coccyx —*see* subcategory M53.2
colon —*see* Syndrome, irritable bowel
psychogenic F45.8
ileum K58.9
intestine (*see also* Syndrome, irritable
bowel) K58.9
psychogenic F45.8
meniscus (knee) —*see* Derangement,
knee, meniscus
scapula —*see* Instability, joint, shoulder
stomach K31.89
psychogenic F45.8
syndrome M35.7
urethra N36.41
with intrinsic sphincter deficiency
N36.43
Hypernasality R49.21
Hypernatremia E87.0
Hypernephroma C64.-
Hyperopia —*see* Hypermetropia
Hyperorexia nervosa F50.2
Hyperornithinemia E72.4
Hyperosmia R43.1
Hyperosmolality E87.0
Hyperostosis (monomelic) —*see also*
Disorder, bone, density and
structure, specified NEC
ankylosing (spine) M48.10
cervical region M48.12
cervicothoracic region M48.13

Hyperostosis (*Continued*)
ankylosing (*Continued*)
lumbar region M48.16
lumbosacral region M48.17
multiple sites M48.19
occipito-atlanto-axial region M48.11
sacrococcygeal region M48.18
thoracic region M48.14
thoracolumbar region M48.15
cortical (skull) M85.2
infantile M89.8X-
frontal, internal of skull M85.2
interna frontalis M85.2
skeletal, diffuse idiopathic —*see*
Hyperostosis, ankylosing
skull M85.2
congenital Q75.8
vertebral, ankylosing —*see*
Hyperostosis, ankylosing
Hyperovarism E28.8
Hyperoxaluria (primary) E72.53
Hyperparathyroidism E21.3
primary E21.0
secondary (renal) N25.81
non-renal E21.1
specified NEC E21.2
tertiary E21.2
Hyperpathia R20.8
Hyperperistalsis R19.2
psychogenic F45.8
Hyperpermeability, capillary I78.8
Hyperphagia R63.2
Hyperphenylalaninemia NEC E70.1
Hyperphoria (alternating) H50.53
Hyperphosphatemia E83.39
Hyperpiesis, hyperpiesia —*see*
Hypertension
Hyperpigmentation —*see also*
Pigmentation
melanin NEC L81.4
postinflammatory L81.0
Hyperpinealism E34.8
Hyperpituitarism E22.9
Hyperplasia, hyperplastic
adenoids J35.2
adrenal (capsule) (cortex) (gland) E27.8
with
sexual precocity (male) E25.9
congenital E25.0
virilism, adrenal E25.9
congenital E25.0
virilization (female) E25.9
congenital E25.0
congenital E25.0
salt-losing E25.0
adrenomedullary E27.5
angiolymphoid, eosinophilia (ALHE)
D18.01
appendix (lymphoid) K38.0
artery, fibromuscular I77.3
bone —*see also* Hypertrophy, bone
marrow D75.89
breast —*see also* Hypertrophy, breast
ductal (atypical) N60.9-
C-cell, thyroid E07.0
cementation (tooth) (teeth) K03.4
cervical gland R59.0
cervix (uteri) (basal cell) (endometrium)
(polypoid) —*see also* Dysplasia,
cervix
congenital Q51.828
clitoris, congenital Q52.6
denture K06.2
endocervicitis N72

Hyperplasia, hyperplastic (Continued)
endometrium, endometrial
(adenomatous) (benign) (cystic)
(glandular) (glandular-cystic)
(polypoid) N85.00
with atypia N85.02
cervix —see Dysplasia, cervix
complex (without atypia) N85.01
simple (without atypia) N85.01
epithelial L85.9
focal, oral, including tongue K13.29
nipple N62
skin L85.9
tongue K13.29
vaginal wall N89.3
erythroid D75.89
fibromuscular of artery (carotid) (renal)
I77.3
genital
female NEC N94.89
male N50.8
gingiva K06.1
glandularis cystica uteri (interstitialis)
(see also Hyperplasia, endometrial)
N85.00
gum K06.1
hymen, congenital Q52.4
irritative, edentulous (alveolar) K06.2
jaw M26.09
alveolar M26.79
lower M26.03
alveolar M26.72
upper M26.01
alveolar M26.71
kidney (congenital) Q63.3
labia N90.6
epithelial N90.3
liver (congenital) Q44.7
nodular, focal K76.89
lymph gland or node R59.9
mandible, mandibular M26.03
alveolar M26.72
unilateral condylar M27.8
maxilla, maxillary M26.01
alveolar M26.71
myometrium, myometrial N85.2
neuroendocrine cell, of infancy J84.841
nose
lymphoid J34.89
polypoid J33.9
oral mucosa (irritative) K13.6
organ or site, congenital NEC —see
Anomaly, by site
ovary N83.8
palate, papillary (irritative) K13.6
pancreatic islet cells E16.9
alpha E16.8
with excess
gastrin E16.4
glucagon E16.3
beta E16.1
parathyroid (gland) E21.0
pharynx (lymphoid) J39.2
prostate (adenofibromatous) (nodular)
N40.0
with lower urinary tract symptoms
(LUTS) N40.1
without lower urinary tract
symptoms (LUTS) N40.0
renal artery I77.89
reticulo-endothelial (cell) D75.89
salivary gland (any) K11.1
Schimmelbusch's —see Mastopathy,
cystic

Hyperplasia, hyperplastic (Continued)
suprarenal capsule (gland) E27.8
thymus (gland) (persistent) E32.0
thyroid (gland) —see Goiter
tonsils (faucial) (infective)
(lingual) (lymphoid)
J35.1
with adenoids J35.3
unilateral condylar M27.8
uterus, uterine N85.2
endometrium (glandular) (see also
Hyperplasia, endometrial)
N85.00
vulva N90.6
epithelial N90.3
Hyperpnea —see Hyperventilation
Hyperpotassemia E87.5
Hyperprebetalipoproteinemia (familial)
E78.1
Hyperprolactinemia E22.1
Hyperprolinemia (type I) (type II)
E72.59
Hyperproteinemia E88.09
Hyperprothrombinemia, causing
coagulation factor deficiency
D68.4
Hyperpyrexia R50.9
heat (effects) T67.0
malignant, due to anesthetic T88.3
rheumatic —see Fever, rheumatic
unknown origin R50.9
Hyper-reflexia R29.2
Hypersalivation K11.7
Hypersecretion
ACTH (not associated with
Cushing's syndrome)
E27.0
pituitary E24.0
adrenaline E27.5
adrenomedullary E27.5
androgen (testicular) E29.0
ovarian (drug-induced) (iatrogenic)
E28.1
calcitonin E07.0
catecholamine E27.5
corticoadrenal E24.9
cortisol E24.9
epinephrine E27.5
estrogen E28.0
gastric K31.89
psychogenic F45.8
gastrin E16.4
glucagon E16.3
hormone (s)
ACTH (not associated with
Cushing's syndrome)
E27.0
pituitary E24.0
antidiuretic E22.2
growth E22.0
intestinal NEC E34.1
ovarian androgen E28.1
pituitary E22.9
testicular E29.0
thyroid stimulating E05.80
with thyroid storm E05.81
insulin —see Hyperinsulinism
lacrimal glands —see Epiphora
medulloadrenal E27.5
milk O92.6
ovarian androgens E28.1
salivary gland (any) K11.7
thyrocalcitonin E07.0
upper respiratory J39.8

Hypersegmentation, leukocytic,
hereditary D72.0
Hypersensitive, hypersensitiveness,
hypersensitivity —see also
Allergy
carotid sinus G90.01
colon —see Irritable, colon
drug T88.7
gastrointestinal K52.2
psychogenic F45.8
labyrinth —see subcategory H83.2
pain R20.8
pneumonitis —see Pneumonitis,
allergic
reaction T78.40
upper respiratory tract NEC
J39.3
Hypersomnia (organic) G47.10
due to
alcohol
abuse F10.182
dependence F10.282
use F10.982
amphetamines
abuse F15.182
dependence F15.282
use F15.982
caffeine
abuse F15.182
dependence F15.282
use F15.982
cocaine
abuse F14.182
dependence F14.282
use F14.982
drug NEC
abuse F19.182
dependence F19.282
use F19.982
medical condition G47.14
mental disorder F51.13
opioid
abuse F11.182
dependence F11.282
use F11.982
psychoactive substance NEC
abuse F19.182
dependence F19.282
use F19.982
sedative, hypnotic, or anxiolytic
abuse F13.182
dependence F13.282
use F13.982
stimulant NEC
abuse F15.182
dependence F15.282
use F15.982
idiopathic G47.11
with long sleep time G47.11
without long sleep time G47.12
menstrual related G47.13
nonorganic origin F51.11
specified NEC F51.19
not due to a substance or known
physiological condition F51.11
specified NEC F51.19
primary F51.11
recurrent G47.13
specified NEC G47.19
Hypersplenia, hypersplenism D73.1
Hyperstimulation, ovaries (associated
with induced ovulation) N98.1
Hypersusceptibility —see Allergy
Hypertelorism (ocular) (orbital) Q75.2

Hypertension, hypertensive (accelerated) (benign) (essential) (idiopathic) (malignant) (systemic) I10
with
  heart involvement (conditions in I51.4-I51.9 due to hypertension) —see Hypertension, heart
  kidney involvement —see Hypertension, kidney
benign, intracranial G93.2
borderline R03.0
cardiorenal (disease) I13.10
  with heart failure I13.0
    with stage 1 through stage 4 chronic kidney disease I13.0
    with stage 5 or end stage renal disease I13.2
  without heart failure I13.10
    with stage 1 through stage 4 chronic kidney disease I13.10
    with stage 5 or end stage renal disease I13.11
cardiovascular
  disease (arteriosclerotic) (sclerotic) —see Hypertension, heart
  renal (disease) —see Hypertension, cardiorenal
chronic venous —see Hypertension, venous (chronic)
complicating
  childbirth (labor) O10.92
    with
      heart disease O10.12
        with renal disease O10.32
      renal disease O10.22
        with heart disease O10.32
      essential O10.02
      secondary O10.42
  pregnancy O16.-
    with edema (see also Pre-eclampsia) O14.9-
    gestational (pregnancy induced) (transient) (without proteinuria) O13.-
      with proteinuria O14.9-
        mild pre-eclampsia O14.0-
        moderate pre-eclampsia O14.0-
        severe pre-eclampsia O14.1-
          with hemolysis, elevated liver enzymes and low platelet count (HELLP) O14.2-
    pre-existing O10.91-
      with
        heart disease O10.11-
          with renal disease O10.31-
        pre-eclampsia O11.-
        renal disease O10.21-
          with heart disease O10.31-
        essential O10.01-
        secondary O10.41-
  puerperium O10.93
    with
      heart disease O10.13
        with renal disease O10.33
      renal disease O10.23
        with heart disease O10.33
      essential O10.03
      secondary O10.43
due to
  endocrine disorders I15.2
  pheochromocytoma I15.2

Hypertension, hypertensive (Continued)
due to (Continued)
  renal disorders NEC I15.1
    arterial I15.0
  renovascular disorders I15.0
  specified disease NEC I15.8
encephalopathy I67.4
gestational (without significant proteinuria) (pregnancy-induced) (transient) O13.-
  with significant proteinuria —see Pre-eclampsia
Goldblatt's I70.1
heart (disease) (conditions in I51.4-I51.9 due to hypertension) I11.9
  with
    heart failure (congestive) I11.0
    kidney disease (chronic) —see Hypertension, cardiorenal
intracranial (benign) G93.2
kidney I12.9
  with
    heart disease —see Hypertension, cardiorenal
    stage 1 through stage 4 chronic kidney disease I12.9
    stage 5 chronic kidney disease (CKD) or end stage renal disease (ESRD) I12.0
lesser circulation I27.0
newborn P29.2
  pulmonary (persistent) P29.3
ocular H40.05-
pancreatic duct — code to underlying condition
  with chronic pancreatitis K86.1
portal (due to chronic liver disease) (idiopathic) K76.6
  gastropathy K31.89
  in (due to) schistosomiasis (bilharziasis) B65.9 [K77]
postoperative I97.3
psychogenic F45.8
pulmonary (artery) (secondary) NEC I27.2
  with
    cor pulmonale (chronic) I27.2
      acute I26.09
    right heart ventricular strain/ failure I27.2
      acute I26.09
  of newborn (persistent) P29.3
  primary (idiopathic) I27.0
renal —see Hypertension, kidney
renovascular I15.0
secondary NEC I15.9
  due to
    endocrine disorders I15.2
    pheochromocytoma I15.2
    renal disorders NEC I15.1
      arterial I15.0
    renovascular disorders I15.0
  specified NEC I15.8
venous (chronic)
  due to
    deep vein thrombosis —see Syndrome, postthrombotic
  idiopathic I87.309
    with
      inflammation I87.32-
        with ulcer I87.33-
      specified complication NEC I87.39-
      ulcer I87.31-
        with inflammation I87.33-
    asymptomatic I87.30-

Hypertensive urgency —see Hypertension
Hyperthecosis ovary E28.8
Hyperthermia (of unknown origin) —see also Hyperpyrexia
  malignant, due to anesthesia T88.3
  newborn P81.9
    environmental P81.0
Hyperthyroid (recurrent) —see Hyperthyroidism
Hyperthyroidism (latent) (pre-adult) (recurrent) E05.90
  with
    goiter (diffuse) E05.00
      with thyroid storm E05.01
      nodular (multinodular) E05.20
        with thyroid storm E05.21
        uninodular E05.10
          with thyroid storm E05.11
    storm E05.91
  due to ectopic thyroid tissue E05.30
    with thyroid storm E05.31
  neonatal, transitory P72.1
  specified NEC E05.80
    with thyroid storm E05.81
Hypertony, hypertonia, hypertonicity
  bladder N31.8
  congenital P94.1
  stomach K31.89
    psychogenic F45.8
  uterus, uterine (contractions) (complicating delivery) O62.4
Hypertrichosis L68.9
  congenital Q84.2
  eyelid H02.869
    left H02.866
      lower H02.865
      upper H02.864
    right H02.863
      lower H02.862
      upper H02.861
  lanuginosa Q84.2
    acquired L68.1
  localized L68.2
  specified NEC L68.8
Hypertriglyceridemia, essential E78.1
Hypertrophy, hypertrophic
  adenofibromatous, prostate —see Enlargement, enlarged, prostate
  adenoids (infective) J35.2
    with tonsils J35.3
  adrenal cortex E27.8
  alveolar process or ridge —see Anomaly, alveolar
  anal papillae K62.89
  artery I77.89
    congenital NEC Q27.8
      digestive system Q27.8
      lower limb Q27.8
      specified site NEC Q27.8
      upper limb Q27.8
  auricular —see Hypertrophy, cardiac
  Bartholin's gland N75.8
  bile duct (common) (hepatic) K83.8
  bladder (sphincter) (trigone) N32.89
  bone M89.30
    carpus M89.34-
    clavicle M89.31-
    femur M89.35-
    fibula M89.36-
    finger M89.34-
    humerus M89.32-
    ilium M89.359
    ischium M89.359
    metacarpus M89.34-

Hypertrophy, hypertrophic (*Continued*)
  bone (*Continued*)
    metatarsus M89.37-
    multiple sites M89.39
    neck M89.38
    radius M89.33-
    rib M89.38
    scapula M89.31-
    skull M89.38
    tarsus M89.37-
    tibia M89.36-
    toe M89.37-
    ulna M89.33-
    vertebra M89.38
  brain G93.89
  breast N62
    cystic —*see* Mastopathy, cystic
    newborn P83.4
    pubertal, massive N62
    puerperal, postpartum —*see* Disorder,
      breast, specified type NEC
    senile (parenchymatous) N62
  cardiac (chronic) (idiopathic) I51.7
    with rheumatic fever (conditions in I00)
      active I01.8
      inactive or quiescent (with chorea)
        I09.89
    congenital NEC Q24.8
    fatty —*see* Degeneration, myocardial
    hypertensive —*see* Hypertension,
      heart
    rheumatic (with chorea) I09.89
      active or acute I01.8
      with chorea I02.0
    valve —*see* Endocarditis
  cartilage —*see* Disorder, cartilage,
    specified type NEC
  cecum —*see* Megacolon
  cervix (uteri) N88.8
    congenital Q51.828
    elongation N88.4
  clitoris (cirrhotic) N90.89
    congenital Q52.6
  colon —*see also* Megacolon
    congenital Q43.2
  conjunctiva, lymphoid H11.89
  corpora cavernosa N48.89
  cystic duct K82.8
  duodenum K31.89
  endometrium (glandular) (*see also*
    Hyperplasia, endometrial) N85.00
    cervix N88.8
  epididymis N50.8
  esophageal hiatus (congenital) Q79.1
    with hernia —*see* Hernia, hiatal
  eyelid —*see* Disorder, eyelid, specified
    type NEC
  fat pad E65
    knee (infrapatellar) (popliteal)
      (prepatellar) (retropatellar)
      M79.4
  foot (congenital) Q74.2
  frenulum, frenum (tongue) K14.8
    lip K13.0
  gallbladder K82.8
  gastric mucosa K29.60
    with bleeding K29.61
  gland, glandular R59.9
    generalized R59.1
    localized R59.0
  gum (mucous membrane) K06.1
  heart (idiopathic) —*see also*
    Hypertrophy, cardiac
    valve (*see also* Endocarditis) I38

Hypertrophy, hypertrophic (*Continued*)
  hemifacial Q67.4
  hepatic —*see* Hypertrophy, liver
  hiatus (esophageal) Q79.1
  hilus gland R59.0
  hymen, congenital Q52.4
  ileum K63.89
  intestine NEC K63.89
  jejunum K63.89
  kidney (compensatory) N28.81
    congenital Q63.3
  labium (majus) (minus) N90.6
  ligament —*see* Disorder, ligament
  lingual tonsil (infective) J35.1
    with adenoids J35.3
  lip K13.0
    congenital Q18.6
  liver R16.0
    acute K76.89
    cirrhotic —*see* Cirrhosis, liver
    congenital Q44.7
    fatty —*see* Fatty, liver
  lymph, lymphatic gland R59.9
    generalized R59.1
    localized R59.0
    tuberculous —*see* Tuberculosis,
      lymph gland
  mammary gland —*see* Hypertrophy,
    breast
  Meckel's diverticulum (congenital) Q43.0
    malignant —*see* Table of Neoplasms,
      small intestine, malignant
  median bar —*see* Hyperplasia, prostate
  meibomian gland —*see* Chalazion
  meniscus, knee, congenital Q74.1
  metatarsal head —*see* Hypertrophy,
    bone, metatarsus
  metatarsus —*see* Hypertrophy, bone,
    metatarsus
  mucous membrane
    alveolar ridge K06.2
    gum K06.1
    nose (turbinate) J34.3
  muscle M62.89
  muscular coat, artery I77.89
  myocardium —*see also* Hypertrophy,
    cardiac
    idiopathic I42.2
  myometrium N85.2
  nail L60.2
    congenital Q84.5
  nasal J34.89
    alae J34.89
    bone J34.89
    cartilage J34.89
    mucous membrane (septum) J34.3
    sinus J34.89
    turbinate J34.3
  nasopharynx, lymphoid (infectional)
    (tissue) (wall) J35.2
  nipple N62
  organ or site, congenital NEC —*see*
    Anomaly, by site - ovary N83.8
  palate (hard) M27.8
    soft K13.79
  pancreas, congenital Q45.3
  parathyroid (gland) E21.0
  parotid gland K11.1
  penis N48.89
  pharyngeal tonsil J35.2
  pharynx J39.2
    lymphoid (infectional) (tissue) (wall)
      J35.2
  pituitary (anterior) (fossa) (gland) E23.6

Hypertrophy, hypertrophic (*Continued*)
  prepuce (congenital) N47.8
    female N90.89
  prostate —*see* Enlargement, enlarged,
    prostate
    congenital Q55.4
  pseudomuscular G71.0
  pylorus (adult) (muscle) (sphincter)
    K31.1
    congenital or infantile Q40.0
  rectal, rectum (sphincter) K62.89
  rhinitis (turbinate) J31.0
  salivary gland (any) K11.1
    congenital Q38.4
  scaphoid (tarsal) —*see* Hypertrophy,
    bone, tarsus
  scar L91.0
  scrotum N50.8
  seminal vesicle N50.8
  sigmoid —*see* Megacolon
  skin L91.9
    specified NEC L91.8
  spermatic cord N50.8
  spleen —*see* Splenomegaly
  spondylitis —*see* Spondylosis
  stomach K31.89
  sublingual gland K11.1
  submandibular gland K11.1
  suprarenal cortex (gland) E27.8
  synovial NEC M67.20
    acromioclavicular M67.21-
    ankle M67.27-
    elbow M67.22-
    foot M67.27-
    hand M67.24-
    hip M67.25-
    knee M67.26-
    multiple sites M67.29
    specified site NEC M67.28
    wrist M67.23-
  tendon —*see* Disorder, tendon, specified
    type NEC
  testis N44.8
    congenital Q55.29
  thymic, thymus (gland) (congenital)
    E32.0
  thyroid (gland) —*see* Goiter
  toe (congenital) Q74.2
    acquired —*see also* Deformity, toe,
      specified NEC
  tongue K14.8
    congenital Q38.2
    papillae (foliate) K14.3
  tonsils (faucial) (infective) (lingual)
    (lymphoid) J35.1
    with adenoids J35.3
  tunica vaginalis N50.8
  ureter N28.89
  urethra N36.8
  uterus N85.2
    neck (with elongation) N88.4
    puerperal O90.89
  uvula K13.79
  vagina N89.8
  vas deferens N50.8
  vein I87.8
  ventricle, ventricular (heart) —*see also*
    Hypertrophy, cardiac
    congenital Q24.8
    in tetralogy of Fallot Q21.3
  verumontanum N36.8
  vocal cord J38.3
  vulva N90.6
    stasis (nonfilarial) N90.6

Hypertropia H50.2-
Hypertyrosinemia E70.21
Hyperuricemia (asymptomatic) E79.0
Hypervalinemia E71.19
Hyperventilation (tetany) R06.4
  hysterical F45.8
  psychogenic F45.8
  syndrome F45.8
Hypervitaminosis (dietary) NEC E67.8
  A E67.0
    administered as drug (prolonged
        intake) —see Table of drugs and
        chemicals, vitamins, adverse
        effect
    overdose or wrong substance given
        or taken —see Table of drugs and
        chemicals, vitamins, poisoning
  B6 E67.2
  D E67.3
    administered as drug (prolonged
        intake) —see Table of drugs and
        chemicals, vitamins, adverse
        effect
    overdose or wrong substance given
        or taken —see Table of drugs
        and chemicals, vitamins,
        poisoning
  K E67.8
    administered as drug (prolonged
        intake) —see Table of drugs and
        chemicals, vitamins, adverse
        effect
    overdose or wrong substance given
        or taken —see Table of drugs
        and chemicals, vitamins,
        poisoning
Hypervolemia E87.70
  specified NEC E87.79
Hypesthesia R20.1
  cornea —see Anesthesia, cornea
Hyphema H21.0-
  traumatic S05.1-
Hypoacidity, gastric K31.89
  psychogenic F45.8
Hypoadrenalism, hypoadrenia E27.40
  primary E27.1
  tuberculous A18.7
Hypoadrenocorticism E27.40
  pituitary E23.0
  primary E27.1
Hypoalbuminemia E88.09
Hypoaldosteronism E27.40
Hypoalphalipoproteinemia E78.6
Hypobarism T70.29
Hypobaropathy T70.29
Hypobetalipoproteinemia (familial) E78.6
Hypocalcemia E83.51
  dietary E58
  neonatal P71.1
    due to cow's milk P71.0
  phosphate-loading (newborn) P71.1
Hypochloremia E87.8
Hypochlorhydria K31.89
  neurotic F45.8
  psychogenic F45.8
Hypochondria, hypochondriac,
    hypochondriasis (reaction) F45.21
  sleep F51.03
Hypochondrogenesis Q77.0
Hypochondroplasia Q77.4
Hypochromasia, blood cells D50.8
Hypodontia —see Anodontia
Hypoeosinophilia D72.89
Hypoesthesia R20.1

Hypofibrinogenemia D68.8
  acquired D65
  congenital (hereditary) D68.2
Hypofunction
  adrenocortical E27.40
    drug-induced E27.3
    postprocedural E89.6
    primary E27.1
  adrenomedullary, postprocedural E89.6
  cerebral R29.818
  corticoadrenal NEC E27.40
  intestinal K59.8
  labyrinth —see subcategory H83.2
  ovary E28.39
  pituitary (gland) (anterior) E23.0
  testicular E29.1
    postprocedural (postsurgical)
        (postirradiation) (iatrogenic)
        E89.5
Hypogalactia O92.4
Hypogammaglobulinemia (see also
    Agammaglobulinemia) D80.1
  hereditary D80.0
  nonfamilial D80.1
  transient, of infancy D80.7
Hypogenitalism (congenital) —see
    Hypogonadism
Hypoglossia Q38.3
Hypoglycemia (spontaneous) E16.2
  coma E15
    diabetic —see Diabetes, coma
  diabetic —see Diabetes, hypoglycemia
  dietary counseling and surveillance Z71.3
  drug-induced E16.0
    with coma (nondiabetic) E15
  due to insulin E16.0
    with coma (nondiabetic) E15
    therapeutic misadventure —see
        subcategory T38.3
  functional, nonhyperinsulinemic E16.1
  iatrogenic E16.0
    with coma (nondiabetic) E15
  in infant of diabetic mother P70.1
    gestational diabetes P70.0
  infantile E16.1
  leucine-induced E71.19
  neonatal (transitory) P70.4
    iatrogenic P70.3
  reactive (not drug-induced) E16.1
  transitory neonatal P70.4
Hypogonadism
  female E28.39
  hypogonadotropic E23.0
  male E29.1
  ovarian (primary) E28.39
  pituitary E23.0
  testicular (primary) E29.1
Hypohidrosis, hypoidrosis L74.4
Hypoinsulinemia, postprocedural E89.1
Hypokalemia E87.6
Hypoleukocytosis —see Agranulocytosis
Hypolipoproteinemia (alpha) (beta) E78.6
Hypomagnesemia E83.42
  neonatal P71.2
Hypomania, hypomanic reaction F30.8
Hypomenorrhea —see Oligomenorrhea
Hypometabolism R63.8
Hypomotility
  gastrointestinal (tract) K31.89
    psychogenic F45.8
  intestine K59.8
    psychogenic F45.8
  stomach K31.89
    psychogenic F45.8

Hyponasality R49.22
Hyponatremia E87.1
Hypo-osmolality E87.1
Hypo-ovarianism, hypo-ovarism E28.39
Hypoparathyroidism E20.9
  familial E20.8
  idiopathic E20.0
  neonatal, transitory P71.4
  postprocedural E89.2
  specified NEC E20.8
Hypoperfusion (in)
  newborn P96.89
Hypopharyngitis —see
    Laryngopharyngitis
Hypophoria H50.53
Hypophosphatemia, hypophosphatasia
    (acquired) (congenital) (renal) E83.39
  familial E83.31
Hypophyseal, hypophysis —see also
    condition
  dwarfism E23.0
  gigantism E22.0
Hypopiesis —see Hypotension
Hypopinealism E34.8
Hypopituitarism (juvenile) E23.0
  drug-induced E23.1
  due to
    hypophysectomy E89.3
    radiotherapy E89.3
  iatrogenic NEC E23.1
  postirradiation E89.3
  postpartum E23.0
  postprocedural E89.3
Hypoplasia, hypoplastic
  adrenal (gland), congenital Q89.1
  alimentary tract, congenital Q45.8
    upper Q40.8
  anus, anal (canal) Q42.3
    with fistula Q42.2
  aorta, aortic Q25.4
    ascending, in hypoplastic left heart
        syndrome Q23.4
    valve Q23.1
      in hypoplastic left heart syndrome
          Q23.4
  areola, congenital Q83.8
  arm (congenital) —see Defect,
      reduction, upper limb
  artery (peripheral) Q27.8
    brain (congenital) Q28.3
    coronary Q24.5
    digestive system Q27.8
    lower limb Q27.8
    pulmonary Q25.79
      functional, unilateral J43.0
    retinal (congenital) Q14.1
    specified site NEC Q27.8
    umbilical Q27.0
    upper limb Q27.8
  auditory canal Q17.8
    causing impairment of hearing
        Q16.9
  biliary duct or passage Q44.5
  bone NOS Q79.9
    face Q75.8
    marrow D61.9
      megakaryocytic D69.49
    skull —see Hypoplasia, skull
  brain Q02
    gyri Q04.3
    part of Q04.3
  breast (areola) N64.82
  bronchus Q32.4
  cardiac Q24.8

Hypoplasia, hypoplastic *(Continued)*
carpus —*see* Defect, reduction, upper
    limb, specified type NEC
cartilage hair Q78.5
cecum Q42.8
cementum K00.4
cephalic Q02
cerebellum Q04.3
cervix (uteri), congenital Q51.821
clavicle (congenital) Q74.0
coccyx Q76.49
colon Q42.9
    specified NEC Q42.8
corpus callosum Q04.0
cricoid cartilage Q31.2
digestive organ (s) or tract NEC
    Q45.8
    upper (congenital) Q40.8
ear (auricle) (lobe) Q17.2
    middle Q16.4
enamel of teeth (neonatal) (postnatal)
    (prenatal) K00.4
endocrine (gland) NEC Q89.2
endometrium N85.8
epididymis (congenital) Q55.4
epiglottis Q31.2
erythroid, congenital D61.01
esophagus (congenital) Q39.8
eustachian tube Q17.8
eye Q11.2
eyelid (congenital) Q10.3
face Q18.8
    bone (s) Q75.8
femur (congenital) —*see* Defect,
    reduction, lower limb, specified
    type NEC
fibula (congenital) —*see* Defect,
    reduction, lower limb, specified
    type NEC
finger (congenital) —*see* Defect,
    reduction, upper limb, specified
    type NEC
focal dermal Q82.8
foot —*see* Defect, reduction, lower limb,
    specified type NEC
gallbladder Q44.0
genitalia, genital organ (s)
    female, congenital Q52.8
        external Q52.79
        internal NEC Q52.8
    in adiposogenital dystrophy E23.6
glottis Q31.2
hair Q84.2
hand (congenital) —*see* Defect,
    reduction, upper limb, specified
    type NEC
heart Q24.8
humerus (congenital) —*see* Defect,
    reduction, upper limb, specified
    type NEC
intestine (small) Q41.9
    large Q42.9
        specified NEC Q42.8
jaw M26.09
    alveolar M26.79
    lower M26.04
        alveolar M26.74
    upper M26.02
        alveolar M26.73
kidney (s) Q60.5
    bilateral Q60.4
    unilateral Q60.3
labium (majus) (minus), congenital
    Q52.79

Hypoplasia, hypoplastic *(Continued)*
larynx Q31.2
left heart syndrome Q23.4
leg (congenital) —*see* Defect, reduction,
    lower limb
limb Q73.8
    lower (congenital) —*see* Defect,
        reduction, lower limb
    upper (congenital) —*see* Defect,
        reduction, upper limb
liver Q44.7
lung (lobe) (not associated with short
    gestation) Q33.6
    associated with immaturity, low birth
        weight, prematurity, or short
        gestation P28.0
mammary (areola), congenital
    Q83.8
mandible, mandibular M26.04
    alveolar M26.74
    unilateral condylar M27.8
maxillary M26.02
    alveolar M26.73
medullary D61.9
megakaryocytic D69.49
metacarpus —*see* Defect, reduction,
    upper limb, specified type NEC
metatarsus —*see* Defect, reduction,
    lower limb, specified type NEC
muscle Q79.8
nail (s) Q84.6
nose, nasal Q30.1
optic nerve H47.03-
osseous meatus (ear) Q17.8
ovary, congenital Q50.39
pancreas Q45.0
parathyroid (gland) Q89.2
parotid gland Q38.4
patella Q74.1
pelvis, pelvic girdle Q74.2
penis (congenital) Q55.62
peripheral vascular system Q27.8
    digestive system Q27.8
    lower limb Q27.8
    specified site NEC Q27.8
    upper limb Q27.8
pituitary (gland) (congenital) Q89.2
pulmonary (not associated with short
    gestation) Q33.6
    artery, functional J43.0
    associated with short gestation P28.0
radioulnar —*see* Defect, reduction,
    upper limb, specified type NEC
radius —*see* Defect, reduction, upper
    limb
rectum Q42.1
    with fistula Q42.0
respiratory system NEC Q34.8
rib Q76.6
right heart syndrome Q22.6
sacrum Q76.49
scapula Q74.0
scrotum Q55.1
shoulder girdle Q74.0
skin Q82.8
skull (bone) Q75.8
    with
        anencephaly Q00.0
        encephalocele —*see* Encephalocele
        hydrocephalus Q03.9
            with spina bifida —*see* Spina
                bifida, by site, with
                hydrocephalus
        microcephaly Q02

Hypoplasia, hypoplastic *(Continued)*
spinal (cord) (ventral horn cell) Q06.1
spine Q76.49
sternum Q76.7
tarsus —*see* Defect, reduction, lower
    limb, specified type NEC
testis Q55.1
thymic, with immunodeficiency D82.1
thymus (gland) Q89.2
    with immunodeficiency D82.1
thyroid (gland) E03.1
    cartilage Q31.2
tibiofibular (congenital) —*see* Defect,
    reduction, lower limb, specified
    type NEC
toe —*see* Defect, reduction, lower limb,
    specified type NEC
tongue Q38.3
Turner's K00.4
ulna (congenital) —*see* Defect,
    reduction, upper limb
umbilical artery Q27.0
unilateral condylar M27.8
ureter Q62.8
uterus, congenital Q51.811
vagina Q52.4
vascular NEC peripheral Q27.8
    brain Q28.3
    digestive system Q27.8
    lower limb Q27.8
    specified site NEC Q27.8
    upper limb Q27.8
vein (s) (peripheral) Q27.8
    brain Q28.3
    digestive system Q27.8
    great Q26.8
    lower limb Q27.8
    specified site NEC Q27.8
    upper limb Q27.8
vena cava (inferior) (superior) Q26.8
vertebra Q76.49
vulva, congenital Q52.79
zonule (ciliary) Q12.8
Hypopotassemia E87.6
Hypoproconvertinemia, congenital
    (hereditary) D68.2
Hypoproteinemia E77.8
Hypoprothrombinemia (congenital)
    (hereditary) (idiopathic) D68.2
    acquired D68.4
    newborn, transient P61.6
Hypoptyalism K11.7
Hypopyon (eye) (anterior chamber) —*see*
    Iridocyclitis, acute, hypopyon
Hypopyrexia R68.0
Hyporeflexia R29.2
Hyposecretion
    ACTH E23.0
    antidiuretic hormone E23.2
    ovary E28.39
    salivary gland (any) K11.7
    vasopressin E23.2
Hyposegmentation, leukocytic,
    hereditary D72.0
Hyposiderinemia D50.9
Hypospadias Q54.9
    balanic Q54.0
    coronal Q54.0
    glandular Q54.0
    penile Q54.1
    penoscrotal Q54.2
    perineal Q54.3
    specified NEC Q54.8
Hypospermatogenesis —*see* Oligospermia

Hyposplenism D73.0
Hypostasis pulmonary, passive —*see* Edema, lung
Hypostatic —*see* condition
Hyposthenuria N28.89
Hypotension (arterial) (constitutional) I95.9
  chronic I95.89
  drug-induced I95.2
  due to (of) hemodialysis I95.3
  iatrogenic I95.89
  idiopathic (permanent) I95.0
  intracranial, following ventricular shunting (ventriculostomy) G97.2
  intra-dialytic I95.3
  maternal, syndrome (following labor and delivery) O26.5-
  neurogenic, orthostatic G90.3
  orthostatic (chronic) I95.1
    due to drugs I95.2
    neurogenic G90.3
  postoperative I95.81
  postural I95.1
  specified NEC I95.89
Hypothermia (accidental) T68
  due to anesthesia, anesthetic T88.51
  low environmental temperature T68
  neonatal P80.9
    environmental (mild) NEC P80.8
    mild P80.8
    severe (chronic) (cold injury syndrome) P80.0
    specified NEC P80.8
  not associated with low environmental temperature R68.0

Hypothyroidism (acquired) E03.9
  congenital (without goiter) E03.1
    with goiter (diffuse) E03.0
  due to
    exogenous substance NEC E03.2
    iodine-deficiency, acquired E01.8
      subclinical E02
    irradiation therapy E89.0
    medicament NEC E03.2
    P-aminosalicylic acid (PAS) E03.2
    phenylbutazone E03.2
    resorcinol E03.2
    sulfonamide E03.2
    surgery E89.0
    thiourea group drugs E03.2
  iatrogenic NEC E03.2
  iodine-deficiency (acquired) E01.8
  congenital —*see* Syndrome, iodine-deficiency, congenital
    subclinical E02
  neonatal, transitory P72.2
  postinfectious E03.3
  postirradiation E89.0
  postprocedural E89.0
  postsurgical E89.0
  specified NEC E03.8
  subclinical, iodine-deficiency related E02
Hypotonia, hypotonicity, hypotony
  bladder N31.2
  congenital (benign) P94.2
  eye —*see* Disorder, globe, hypotony
Hypotrichosis —*see* Alopecia
Hypotropia H50.2-

Hypoventilation R06.89
  congenital central alveolar G47.35
  sleep related
    idiopathic nonobstructive alveolar G47.34
    in conditions classified elsewhere G47.36
Hypovitaminosis —*see* Deficiency, vitamin
Hypovolemia E86.1
  surgical shock T81.19
  traumatic (shock) T79.4
Hypoxemia R09.02
  newborn P84
  sleep related, in conditions classified elsewhere G47.36
Hypoxia (*see also* Anoxia) R09.02
  cerebral, during a procedure NEC G97.81
    postprocedural NEC G97.82
  intrauterine P84
  myocardial —*see* Insufficiency, coronary
  newborn P84
  sleep-related G47.34
Hypsarhythmia —*see* Epilepsy, generalized, specified NEC
Hysteralgia, pregnant uterus O26.89-
Hysteria, hysterical (conversion) (dissociative state) F44.9
  anxiety F41.8
  convulsions F44.5
  psychosis, acute F44.9
Hysteroepilepsy F44.5

I

Ichthyoparasitism due to Vandellia cirrhosa B88.8
Ichthyosis (congenital) Q80.9
  acquired L85.0
  fetalis Q80.4
  hystrix Q80.8
  lamellar Q80.2
  lingual K13.29
  palmaris and plantaris Q82.8
  simplex Q80.0
  vera Q80.8
  vulgaris Q80.0
  X-linked Q80.1
Ichthyotoxism —see Poisoning, fish
  bacterial —see Intoxication, foodborne
Icteroanemia, hemolytic (acquired) D59.9
  congenital —see Spherocytosis
Icterus —see also Jaundice
  conjunctiva R17
  gravis, newborn P55.0
  hematogenous (acquired) D59.9
  hemolytic (acquired) D59.9
    congenital —see Spherocytosis
  hemorrhagic (acute) (leptospiral) (spirochetal) A27.0
    newborn P53
  infectious B15.9
    with hepatic coma B15.0
    leptospiral A27.0
    spirochetal A27.0
  neonatorum —see Jaundice, newborn
  newborn P59.9
  spirochetal A27.0
Ictus solaris, solis T67.0
Id reaction (due to bacteria) L30.2
Ideation
  homicidal R45.850
  suicidal R45.851
Identity disorder (child) F64.9
  gender role F64.2
  psychosexual F64.2
Idioglossia F80.0
Idiopathic —see condition
Idiot, idiocy (congenital) F73
  amaurotic (Bielschowsky(-Jansky)) (family) (infantile (late)) (juvenile (late)) (Vogt-Spielmeyer) E75.4
  microcephalic Q02
IgE asthma J45.909
IIAC (idiopathic infantile arterial calcification) Q28.8
Ileitis (chronic) (noninfectious) (see also Enteritis) K52.9
  backwash —see Pancolitis, ulcerative (chronic)
  infectious A09
  regional (ulcerative) —see Enteritis, regional, small intestine
  segmental —see Enteritis, regional
  terminal (ulcerative) —see Enteritis, regional, small intestine
Ileocolitis (see also Enteritis) K52.9
  infectious A09
  regional —see Enteritis, regional
Ileostomy
  attention to Z43.2
  malfunctioning K94.13
  status Z93.2
    with complication —see Complications, enterostomy
Ileotyphus —see Typhoid
Ileum —see condition

Ileus (bowel) (colon) (inhibitory) (intestine) K56.7
  adynamic K56.0
  due to gallstone (in intestine) K56.3
  duodenal (chronic) K31.5
  gallstone K56.3
  mechanical NEC K56.69
  meconium P76.0
    in cystic fibrosis E84.11
    meaning meconium plug (without cystic fibrosis) P76.0
  myxedema K59.8
  neurogenic K56.0
    Hirschsprung's disease or megacolon Q43.1
  newborn
    due to meconium P76.0
      in cystic fibrosis E84.11
      meaning meconium plug (without cystic fibrosis) P76.0
    transitory P76.1
  obstructive K56.69
  paralytic K56.0
Iliac —see condition
Iliotibial band syndrome M76.3-
Illiteracy Z55.0
Illness (see also Disease) R69
  manic-depressive —see Disorder, bipolar
Imbalance R26.89
  autonomic G90.8
  constituents of food intake E63.1
  electrolyte E87.8
    with
      abortion —see Abortion by type, complicated by, electrolyte imbalance
      molar pregnancy O08.5
    due to hyperemesis gravidarum O21.1
    following ectopic or molar pregnancy O08.5
    neonatal, transitory NEC P74.4
      potassium P74.3
      sodium P74.2
  endocrine E34.9
  eye muscle NOS H50.9
  hormone E34.9
  hysterical F44.4
  labyrinth —see subcategory H83.2
  posture R29.3
  protein-energy —see Malnutrition
  sympathetic G90.8
Imbecile, imbecility (I.Q. 35-49) F71
Imbedding, intrauterine device T83.39
Imbibition, cholesterol (gallbladder) K82.4
Imbrication, teeth, fully erupted M26.30
Imerslund (-Gräsbeck) syndrome D51.1
Immature —see also Immaturity
  birth (less than 37 completed weeks) —see Preterm, newborn
  extremely (less than 28 completed weeks) —see Immaturity, extreme
  personality F60.89
Immaturity (less than 37 completed weeks) —see also Preterm, newborn
  extreme of newborn (less than 28 completed weeks of gestation) (less than 196 completed days of gestation) (unspecified weeks of gestation) P07.20
    gestational age
      23 completed weeks (23 weeks, 0 days through 23 weeks, 6 days) P07.22

Immaturity (Continued)
  extreme of newborn (Continued)
    gestational age (Continued)
      24 completed weeks (24 weeks, 0 days through 24 weeks, 6 days) P07.23
      25 completed weeks (25 weeks, 0 days through 25 weeks, 6 days) P07.24
      26 completed weeks (26 weeks, 0 days through 26 weeks, 6 days) P07.25
      27 completed weeks (27 weeks, 0 days through 27 weeks, 6 days) P07.26
      less than 23 completed weeks P07.21
  fetus or infant light-for-dates —see Light-for-dates
  lung, newborn P28.0
  organ or site NEC —see Hypoplasia
  pulmonary, newborn P28.0
  reaction F60.89
  sexual (female) (male), after puberty E30.0
Immersion T75.1
  foot T69.02-
  hand T69.01-
Immobile, immobility
  complete, due to severe physical disability or frailty R53.2
  intestine K59.8
  syndrome (paraplegic) M62.3
Immune reconstitution (inflammatory) syndrome [IRIS] D89.3
Immunization —see also Vaccination
  ABO —see Incompatibility, ABO
    in newborn P55.1
  complication —see Complications, vaccination
  encounter for Z23
  not done (not carried out) Z28.9
    because (of)
      acute illness of patient Z28.01
      allergy to vaccine (or component) Z28.04
      caregiver refusal Z28.82
      chronic illness of patient Z28.02
      contraindication NEC Z28.09
      group pressure Z28.1
      guardian refusal Z28.82
      immune compromised state of patient Z28.03
      parent refusal Z28.82
      patient's belief Z28.1
      patient had disease being vaccinated against Z28.81
      patient refusal Z28.21
      religious beliefs of patient Z28.1
      specified reason NEC Z28.89
        of patient Z28.29
      unspecified patient reason Z28.20
  Rh factor
    affecting management of pregnancy NEC O36.09-
    anti-D antibody O36.01-
    from transfusion —see Complication (s), transfusion, incompatibility reaction, Rh (factor)
Immunocytoma C83.0-

Immunodeficiency D84.9
  with
    adenosine-deaminase deficiency D81.3
    antibody defects D80.9
      specified type NEC D80.8
    hyperimmunoglobulinemia D80.6
    increased immunoglobulin M (IgM)
        D80.5
    major defect D82.9
      specified type NEC D82.8
    partial albinism D82.8
    short-limbed stature D82.2
    thrombocytopenia and eczema D82.0
  antibody with
    hyperimmunoglobulinemia D80.6
    near-normal immunoglobulins D80.6
  autosomal recessive, Swiss type D80.0
  combined D81.9
    biotin-dependent carboxylase D81.819
      biotinidase D81.810
      holocarboxylase synthetase D81.818
      specified type NEC D81.818
    severe (SCID) D81.9
      with
        low or normal B-cell numbers
            D81.2
        low T- and B-cell numbers D81.1
        reticular dysgenesis D81.0
    specified type NEC D81.89
  common variable D83.9
    with
      abnormalities of B-cell numbers
          and function D83.0
      autoantibodies to B- or T-cells D83.2
      immunoregulatory T-cell disorders
          D83.1
    specified type NEC D83.8
  following hereditary defective response
      to Epstein-Barr virus (EBV) D82.3
  selective, immunoglobulin
    A (IgA) D80.2
    G (IgG) (subclasses) D80.3
    M (IgM) D80.4
  severe combined (SCID) D81.9
  specified type NEC D84.8
  X-linked, with increased IgM D80.5
Immunotherapy (encounter for)
  antineoplastic Z51.12
Impaction, impacted
  bowel, colon, rectum (see also Impaction,
      fecal) K56.49
    by gallstone K56.3
  calculus —see Calculus
  cerumen (ear) (external) H61.2-
  cuspid —see Impaction, tooth
  dental (same or adjacent tooth) K01.1
  fecal, feces K56.41
  fracture —see Fracture, by site
  gallbladder —see Calculus, gallbladder
  gallstone (s) —see Calculus, gallbladder
    bile duct (common) (hepatic) —see
        Calculus, bile duct
    cystic duct —see Calculus,
        gallbladder
    in intestine, with obstruction (any
        part) K56.3
  intestine (calculous) NEC (see also
      Impaction, fecal) K56.49
    gallstone, with ileus K56.3
  intrauterine device (IUD) T83.39
  molar —see Impaction, tooth
  shoulder, causing obstructed labor O66.0
  tooth, teeth K01.1
  turbinate J34.89

Impaired, impairment (function)
  auditory discrimination —see
      Abnormal, auditory perception
  cognitive, mild, so stated G31.84
  dual sensory Z73.82
  fasting glucose R73.01
  glucose tolerance (oral) R73.02
  hearing —see Deafness
  heart —see Disease, heart
  kidney N28.9
    disorder resulting from N25.9
      specified NEC N25.89
  liver K72.90
    with coma K72.91
  mastication K08.8
  mild cognitive, so stated G31.84
  mobility
    ear ossicles —see Ankylosis, ear
        ossicles
    requiring care provider Z74.09
  myocardium, myocardial —see
      Insufficiency, myocardial
  rectal sphincter R19.8
  renal (acute) (chronic) N28.9
    disorder resulting from N25.9
      specified NEC N25.89
  vision NEC H54.7
    both eyes H54.3
Impediment, speech R47.9
  psychogenic (childhood) F98.8
  slurring R47.81
  specified NEC R47.89
Impending
  coronary syndrome I20.0
  delirium tremens F10.239
  myocardial infarction I20.0
Imperception auditory (acquired) —see
    also Deafness
  congenital H93.25
Imperfect
  aeration, lung (newborn) NEC —see
      Atelectasis
  closure (congenital)
    alimentary tract NEC Q45.8
      lower Q43.8
      upper Q40.8
    atrioventricular ostium Q21.2
    atrium (secundum) Q21.1
    branchial cleft or sinus Q18.0
    choroid Q14.3
    cricoid cartilage Q31.8
    cusps, heart valve NEC Q24.8
      pulmonary Q22.3
    ductus
      arteriosus Q25.0
      Botalli Q25.0
    ear drum (causing impairment of
        hearing) Q16.4
    esophagus with communication to
        bronchus or trachea Q39.1
    eyelid Q10.3
    foramen
      botalli Q21.1
      ovale Q21.1
    genitalia, genital organ (s) or system
      female Q52.8
        external Q52.79
        internal NEC Q52.8
      male Q55.8
    glottis Q31.8
    interatrial ostium or septum Q21.1
    interauricular ostium or septum Q21.1
    interventricular ostium or septum
        Q21.0

Imperfect (Continued)
  closure (Continued)
    larynx Q31.8
    lip —see Cleft, lip
    nasal septum Q30.3
    nose Q30.2
    omphalomesenteric duct Q43.0
    optic nerve entry Q14.2
    organ or site not listed —see
        Anomaly, by site
    ostium
      interatrial Q21.1
      interauricular Q21.1
      interventricular Q21.0
    palate —see Cleft, palate
    preauricular sinus Q18.1
    retina Q14.1
    roof of orbit Q75.8
    sclera Q13.5
    septum
      aorticopulmonary Q21.4
      atrial (secundum) Q21.1
      between aorta and pulmonary
          artery Q21.4
      heart Q21.9
      interatrial (secundum) Q21.1
      interauricular (secundum) Q21.1
      interventricular Q21.0
        in tetralogy of Fallot Q21.3
      nasal Q30.3
      ventricular Q21.0
        with pulmonary stenosis or
            atresia, dextraposition of
            aorta, and hypertrophy of
            right ventricle Q21.3
        in tetralogy of Fallot Q21.3
    skull Q75.0
      with
        anencephaly Q00.0
        encephalocele —see
            Encephalocele
        hydrocephalus Q03.9
          with spina bifida —see Spina
              bifida, by site, with
              hydrocephalus
        microcephaly Q02
    spine (with meningocele) —see Spina
        bifida
    trachea Q32.1
    tympanic membrane (causing
        impairment of hearing) Q16.4
    uterus Q51.818
    vitelline duct Q43.0
  erection —see Dysfunction, sexual,
      male, erectile
  fusion —see Imperfect, closure
  inflation, lung (newborn) —see
      Atelectasis
  posture R29.3
  rotation, intestine Q43.3
  septum, ventricular Q21.0
Imperfectly descended testis —see
    Cryptorchid
Imperforate (congenital) —see also Atresia
  anus Q42.3
    with fistula Q42.2
  cervix (uteri) Q51.828
  esophagus Q39.0
    with tracheoesophageal fistula Q39.1
  hymen Q52.3
  jejunum Q41.1
  pharynx Q38.8
  rectum Q42.1
    with fistula Q42.0

Imperforate (Continued)
  urethra Q64.39
  vagina Q52.4
Impervious (congenital) —see also
    Atresia
  anus Q42.3
    with fistula Q42.2
  bile duct Q44.2
  esophagus Q39.0
    with tracheoesophageal fistula
      Q39.1
  intestine (small) Q41.9
    large Q42.9
      specified NEC Q42.8
  rectum Q42.1
    with fistula Q42.0
  ureter —see Atresia, ureter
  urethra Q64.39
Impetiginization of dermatoses L01.1
Impetigo (any organism) (any site)
      (circinate) (contagiosa) (simplex)
      (vulgaris) L01.00
  Bockhart's L01.02
  bullous, bullosa L01.03
  external ear L01.00 [H62.40]
  follicularis L01.02
  furfuracea L30.5
  herpetiformis L40.1
    nonobstetrical L40.1
  neonatorum L01.03
  nonbullous L01.01
  specified type NEC L01.09
  ulcerative L01.09
Impingement (on teeth)
  soft tissue
    anterior M26.81
    posterior M26.82
Implant, endometrial N80.9
Implantation
  anomalous —see Anomaly, by site
    ureter Q62.63
  cyst
    external area or site (skin) NEC
      L72.0
    iris —see Cyst, iris, implantation
    vagina N89.8
    vulva N90.7
  dermoid (cyst) —see Implantation,
      cyst
Impotence (sexual) N52.9
  counseling Z70.1
  organic origin (see also Dysfunction,
      sexual, male, erectile) N52.9
  psychogenic F52.21
Impression, basilar Q75.8
Imprisonment, anxiety concerning Z65.1
Improper care (child) (newborn) —see
    Maltreatment
Improperly tied umbilical cord (causing
    hemorrhage) P51.8
Impulsiveness (impulsive) R45.87
Inability to swallow —see Aphagia
Inaccessible, inaccessibility
  health care NEC Z75.3
    due to
      waiting period Z75.2
        for admission to facility
          elsewhere Z75.1
    other helping agencies Z75.4
Inactive —see condition
Inadequate, inadequacy
  aesthetics of dental restoration K08.56
  biologic, constitutional, functional, or
    social F60.7

Inadequate, inadequacy (Continued)
  development
    child R62.50
    genitalia
      after puberty NEC E30.0
      congenital
        female Q52.8
          external Q52.79
          internal Q52.8
        male Q55.8
    lungs Q33.6
      associated with short gestation P28.0
    organ or site not listed —see
        Anomaly, by site
  diet (causing nutritional deficiency)
      E63.9
  eating habits Z72.4
  environment, household Z59.1
  family support Z63.8
  food (supply) NEC Z59.4
    hunger effects T73.0
  functional F60.7
  household care, due to
    family member
      handicapped or ill Z74.2
      on vacation Z75.0
      temporarily away from home Z74.2
    technical defects in home Z59.1
    temporary absence from home of
        person rendering care Z74.2
  housing (heating) (space) Z59.1
  income (financial) Z59.6
  intrafamilial communication Z63.8
  material resources Z59.9
  mental —see Disability, intellectual
  parental supervision or control of child
      Z62.0
  personality F60.7
  pulmonary
    function R06.89
      newborn P28.5
    ventilation, newborn P28.5
  sample of cytologic smear
    anus R85.615
    cervix R87.615
    vagina R87.625
  social F60.7
    insurance Z59.7
    skills NEC Z73.4
  supervision of child by parent Z62.0
  teaching affecting education Z55.8
  welfare support Z59.7
Inanition R64
  with edema —see Malnutrition, severe
  due to
    deprivation of food T73.0
    malnutrition —see Malnutrition
  fever R50.9
Inappropriate
  change in quantitative human chorionic
      gonadotropin (hCG) in early
      pregnancy O02.81
  diet or eating habits Z72.4
  level of quantitative human chorionic
      gonadotropin (hCG) for
      gestational age in early pregnancy
      O02.81
  secretion
    antidiuretic hormone (ADH)
      (excessive) E22.2
      deficiency E23.2
    pituitary (posterior) E22.2
Inattention at or after birth —see
    Neglect

Incarceration, incarcerated
  enterocele K46.0
    gangrenous K46.1
  epiplocele K46.0
    gangrenous K46.1
  exophthalmos K42.0
    gangrenous K42.1
  hernia —see also Hernia, by site, with
      obstruction
    with gangrene —see Hernia, by site,
        with gangrene
  iris, in wound —see Injury, eye,
      laceration, with prolapse
  lens, in wound —see Injury, eye,
      laceration, with prolapse
  omphalocele K42.0
  prison, anxiety concerning Z65.1
  rupture —see Hernia, by site
  sarcoepiplocele K46.0
    gangrenous K46.1
  sarcoepiplomphalocele K42.0
    with gangrene K42.1
  uterus N85.8
    gravid O34.51-
      causing obstructed labor
        O65.5
Incised wound
  external —see Laceration
  internal organs —see Injury, by site
Incision, incisional
  hernia K43.2
    with
      gangrene (and obstruction) K43.1
      obstruction K43.0
    surgical, complication —see
        Complications, surgical procedure
  traumatic
    external —see Laceration
    internal organs —see Injury, by site
Inclusion
  azurophilic leukocytic D72.0
  blennorrhea (neonatal) (newborn) P39.1
  gallbladder in liver (congenital) Q44.1
Incompatibility
  ABO
    affecting management of pregnancy
        O36.11-
      anti-A sensitization O36.11-
      anti-B sensitization O36.19-
      specified NEC O36.19-
    infusion or transfusion reaction —see
        Complication (s), transfusion,
        incompatibility reaction, ABO
    newborn P55.1
  blood (group) (Duffy) (K(ell)) (Kidd)
      (Lewis) (M) (S) NEC
    affecting management of pregnancy
        O36.11-
      anti-A sensitization O36.11-
      anti-B sensitization O36.19-
    infusion or transfusion reaction
        T80.89
    newborn P55.8
  divorce or estrangement Z63.5
  Rh (blood group) (factor) Z31.82
    affecting management of pregnancy
        NEC O36.09-
      anti-D antibody O36.01-
    infusion or transfusion reaction —see
        Complication (s), transfusion,
        incompatibility reaction, Rh
        (factor)
    newborn P55.0
  rhesus —see Incompatibility, Rh

Incompetency, incompetent,
    incompetence
  annular
    aortic (valve) —see Insufficiency, aortic
    mitral (valve) I34.0
    pulmonary valve (heart) I37.1
  aortic (valve) —see Insufficiency, aortic
  cardiac valve —see Endocarditis
  cervix, cervical (os) N88.3
    in pregnancy O34.3-
  chronotropic I45.89
    with
      autonomic dysfunction G90.8
      ischemic heart disease I25.89
      left ventricular dysfunction I51.89
      sinus node dysfunction I49.8
  esophagogastric (junction) (sphincter)
    K22.0
  mitral (valve) —see Insufficiency, mitral
  pelvic fundus N81.89
  pubocervical tissue N81.82
  pulmonary valve (heart) I37.1
    congenital Q22.3
  rectovaginal tissue N81.83
  tricuspid (annular) (valve) —see
    Insufficiency, tricuspid
  valvular —see Endocarditis
    congenital Q24.8
  vein, venous (saphenous) (varicose) —
    see Varix, leg
Incomplete —see also condition
  bladder, emptying R33.9
  defecation R15.0
  expansion lungs (newborn) NEC —see
    Atelectasis
  rotation, intestine Q43.3
Inconclusive
  diagnostic imaging due to excess body
    fat of patient R93.9
  findings on diagnostic imaging of
    breast NEC R92.8
  mammogram (due to dense breasts)
    R92.2
Incontinence R32
  anal sphincter R15.9
  feces R15.9
    nonorganic origin F98.1
  overflow N39.490
  psychogenic F45.8
  rectal R15.9
  reflex N39.498
  stress (female) (male) N39.3
    and urge N39.46
  urethral sphincter R32
  urge N39.41
    and stress (female) (male) N39.46
  urine (urinary) R32
    continuous N39.45
    due to cognitive impairment, or
      severe physical disability or
      immobility R39.81
    functional R39.81
    mixed (stress and urge) N39.46
    nocturnal N39.44
    nonorganic origin F98.0
    overflow N39.490
    post dribbling N39.43
    reflex N39.498
    specified NEC N39.498
    stress (female) (male) N39.3
      and urge N39.46
    total N39.498
    unaware N39.42
    urge N39.41
      and stress (female) (male) N39.46

Incontinentia pigmenti Q82.3
Incoordinate, incoordination
  esophageal-pharyngeal (newborn) —see
    Dysphagia
  muscular R27.8
  uterus (action) (contractions)
    (complicating delivery) O62.4
Increase, increased
  abnormal, in development R63.8
  androgens (ovarian) E28.1
  anticoagulants (antithrombin)
    (anti-VIIIa) (anti-IXa) (anti-Xa)
    (anti-XIa) —see Circulating
    anticoagulants)
  cold sense R20.8
  estrogen E28.0
  function
    adrenal
      cortex —see Cushing's, syndrome
      medulla E27.5
    pituitary (gland) (anterior) (lobe) E22.9
      posterior E22.2
  heat sense R20.8
  intracranial pressure (benign) G93.2
  permeability, capillaries I78.8
  pressure, intracranial G93.2
  secretion
    gastrin E16.4
    glucagon E16.3
    pancreas, endocrine E16.9
      growth hormone-releasing
        hormone E16.8
      pancreatic polypeptide E16.8
      somatostatin E16.8
      vasoactive-intestinal polypeptide
        E16.8
  sphericity, lens Q12.4
  splenic activity D73.1
  venous pressure I87.8
    portal K76.6
Increta placenta O43.22-
Incrustation, cornea, foreign body (lead)
  (zinc) —see Foreign body, cornea
Incyclophoria H50.54
Incyclotropia —see Cyclotropia
Indeterminate sex Q56.4
India rubber skin Q82.8
Indigestion (acid) (bilious) (functional)
  K30
  catarrhal K31.89
  due to decomposed food NOS A05.9
  nervous F45.8
  psychogenic F45.8
Indirect —see condition
Induratio penis plastica N48.6
Induration, indurated
  brain G93.89
  breast (fibrous) N64.51
    puerperal, postpartum O92.29
  broad ligament N83.8
  chancre
    anus A51.1
    congenital A50.07
    extragenital NEC A51.2
  corpora cavernosa (penis) (plastic)
    N48.6
  liver (chronic) K76.89
  lung (black) (chronic) (fibroid) (see also
    Fibrosis, lung) J84.10
    essential brown J84.03
  penile (plastic) N48.6
  phlebitic —see Phlebitis
  skin R23.4
Inebriety (without dependence) —see
  Alcohol, intoxication

Inefficiency, kidney N28.9
Inelasticity, skin R23.4
Inequality, leg (length) (acquired) —see
  also Deformity, limb, unequal length
  congenital —see Defect, reduction,
    lower limb
  lower leg —see Deformity, limb,
    unequal length
Inertia
  bladder (neurogenic) N31.2
  stomach K31.89
    psychogenic F45.8
  uterus, uterine during labor O62.2
    during latent phase of labor O62.0
    primary O62.0
    secondary O62.1
  vesical (neurogenic) N31.2
Infancy, infantile, infantilism —see also
  condition
  celiac K90.0
  genitalia, genitals (after puberty) E30.0
  Herter's (nontropical sprue) K90.0
  intestinal K90.0
  Lorain E23.0
  pancreatic K86.8
  pelvis M95.5
    with disproportion (fetopelvic)
      O33.1
      causing obstructed labor O65.1
  pituitary E23.0
  renal N25.0
  uterus —see Infantile, genitalia
Infant (s) —see also Infancy
  excessive crying R68.11
  irritable child R68.12
  lack of care —see Neglect
  liveborn (singleton) Z38.2
    born in hospital Z38.00
      by cesarean Z38.01
    born outside hospital Z38.1
    multiple NEC Z38.8
      born in hospital Z38.68
        by cesarean Z38.69
      born outside hospital Z38.7
    quadruplet Z38.8
      born in hospital Z38.63
        by cesarean Z38.64
      born outside hospital Z38.7
    quintuplet Z38.8
      born in hospital Z38.65
        by cesarean Z38.66
      born outside hospital Z38.7
    triplet Z38.8
      born in hospital Z38.61
        by cesarean Z38.62
      born outside hospital Z38.7
    twin Z38.5
      born in hospital Z38.30
        by cesarean Z38.31
      born outside hospital Z38.4
  of diabetic mother (syndrome of)
    P70.1
    gestational diabetes P70.0
Infantile —see also condition
  genitalia, genitals E30.0
  os, uterine E30.0
  penis E30.0
  testis E29.1
  uterus E30.0
Infantilism —see Infancy
Infarct, infarction
  adrenal (capsule) (gland) E27.49
  appendices epiploicae K55.0
  bowel K55.0

Infarct, infarction (Continued)
brain (stem) —see Infarct, cerebral
breast N64.89
brewer's (kidney) N28.0
cardiac —see Infarct, myocardium
cerebellar —see Infarct, cerebral
cerebral (see also Occlusion, artery
  cerebral or precerebral, with
  infarction) I63.9
  aborted I63.9
  cortical I63.9
  due to
    cerebral venous thrombosis,
      nonpyogenic I63.6
    embolism
      cerebral arteries I63.4-
      precerebral arteries I63.1-
    occlusion NEC
      cerebral arteries I63.5-
      precerebral arteries I63.2-
    stenosis NEC
      cerebral arteries I63.5-
      precerebral arteries I63.2-
    thrombosis
      cerebral artery I63.3-
      precerebral artery I63.0-
  intraoperative
    during cardiac surgery
      I97.810
    during other surgery I97.811
  postprocedural
    following cardiac surgery
      I97.820
    following other surgery
      I97.821
  specified NEC I63.8
colon (acute) (agnogenic) (embolic)
  (hemorrhagic) (nonocclusive)
  (nonthrombotic) (occlusive)
  (segmental) (thrombotic) (with
  gangrene) K55.0
coronary artery —see Infarct,
  myocardium
embolic —see Embolism
fallopian tube N83.8
gallbladder K82.8
heart —see Infarct, myocardium
hepatic K76.3
hypophysis (anterior lobe) E23.6
impending (myocardium) I20.0
intestine (acute) (agnogenic) (embolic)
  (hemorrhagic) (nonocclusive)
  (nonthrombotic) (occlusive)
  (thrombotic) (with gangrene)
  K55.0
kidney N28.0
liver K76.3
lung (embolic) (thrombotic) —see
  Embolism, pulmonary
lymph node I89.8
mesentery, mesenteric (embolic)
  (thrombotic) (with gangrene)
  K55.0
muscle (ischemic) M62.20
  ankle M62.27-
  foot M62.27-
  forearm M62.23-
  hand M62.24-
  lower leg M62.26-
  pelvic region M62.25-
  shoulder region M62.21-
  specified site NEC M62.28
  thigh M62.25-
  upper arm M62.22-

Infarct, infarction (Continued)
myocardium, myocardial (acute) (with
  stated duration of 4 weeks or less)
  I21.3
  diagnosed on ECG, but presenting no
    symptoms I25.2
  healed or old I25.2
  intraoperative
    during cardiac surgery I97.790
    during other surgery I97.791
  non-Q wave I21.4
  non-ST elevation (NSTEMI) I21.4
    subsequent I22.2
  nontransmural I21.4
  past (diagnosed on ECG or other
    investigation, but currently
    presenting no symptoms) I25.2
  postprocedural
    following cardiac surgery I97.190
    following other surgery I97.191
  Q wave (see also, Infarct,
    myocardium, by site) I21.3
  ST elevation (STEMI) I21.3
    anterior (anteroapical)
      (anterolateral) (anteroseptal)
      (Q wave) (wall) I21.09
      subsequent I22.0
    inferior (diaphragmatic)
      (inferolateral) (inferoposterior)
      (wall) NEC I21.19
      subsequent I22.1
    inferoposterior transmural (Q
      wave) I21.11
    involving
      coronary artery of anterior wall
        NEC I21.09
      coronary artery of inferior wall
        NEC I21.19
      diagonal coronary artery I21.02
      left anterior descending coronary
        artery I21.02
      left circumflex coronary artery
        I21.21
      left main coronary artery I21.01
      oblique marginal coronary artery
        I21.21
      right coronary artery I21.11
    lateral (apical-lateral) (basal-lateral)
      (high) I21.29
      subsequent I22.8
    posterior (posterobasal)
      (posterolateral)
      (posteroseptal) (true) I21.29
      subsequent I22.8
    septal I21.29
      subsequent I22.8
    specified NEC I21.29
      subsequent I22.8
    subsequent I22.9
  subsequent (recurrent) (reinfarction)
    I22.9
    anterior (anteroapical)
      (anterolateral) (anteroseptal)
      (wall) I22.0
    diaphragmatic (wall) I22.1
    inferior (diaphragmatic)
      (inferolateral)
      (inferoposterior) (wall) I22.1
    lateral (apical-lateral) (basal-lateral)
      (high) I22.8
    non-ST elevation (NSTEMI) I22.2
    posterior (posterobasal)
      (posterolateral)
      (posteroseptal) (true) I22.8

Infarct, infarction (Continued)
myocardium, myocardial (Continued)
  subsequent (Continued)
    septal I22.8
    specified NEC I22.8
    ST elevation I22.9
      anterior (anteroapical)
        (anterolateral)
        (anteroseptal) (wall) I22.0
      inferior (diaphragmatic)
        (inferolateral)
        (inferoposterior) (wall) I22.1
      specified NEC I22.8
    subendocardial I22.2
    transmural I22.9
      anterior (anteroapical)
        (anterolateral)
        (anteroseptal) (wall) I22.0
      diaphragmatic (wall) I22.1
      inferior (diaphragmatic)
        (inferolateral)
        (inferoposterior) (wall) I22.1
      lateral (apical-lateral) (basal-
        lateral) (high) I22.8
      posterior (posterobasal)
        (posterolateral)
        (posteroseptal) (true) I22.8
      specified NEC I22.8
  syphilitic A52.06
  transmural I21.3
    anterior (anteroapical)
      (anterolateral) (anteroseptal)
      (Q wave) (wall) NEC I21.09
    inferior (diaphragmatic)
      (inferolateral)
      (inferoposterior) (Q wave)
      (wall) NEC I21.19
    inferoposterior (Q wave) I21.11
    lateral (apical-lateral) (basal-lateral)
      (high) NEC I21.29
    posterior (posterobasal)
      (posterolateral) (posteroseptal)
      (true) NEC I21.29
    septal NEC I21.29
    specified NEC I21.29
  nontransmural I21.4
  omentum K55.0
  ovary N83.8
  pancreas
  papillary muscle —see Infarct,
    myocardium
  parathyroid gland E21.4
  pituitary (gland) E23.6
  placenta O43.81-
  prostate N42.89
  pulmonary (artery) (vein)
    (hemorrhagic) —see Embolism,
    pulmonary
  renal (embolic) (thrombotic) N28.0
  retina, retinal (artery) —see Occlusion,
    artery, retina
  spinal (cord) (acute) (embolic)
    (nonembolic) G95.11
  spleen D73.5
    embolic or thrombotic I74.8
  subendocardial (acute) (nontransmural)
    I21.4
  suprarenal (capsule) (gland) E27.49
  testis N50.1
  thrombotic —see also Thrombosis
    artery, arterial —see Embolism
  thyroid (gland) E07.89
  ventricle (heart) —see Infarct,
    myocardium

Infecting —see condition
Infection, infected, infective
    (opportunistic) B99.9
    with
        drug resistant organism —see
            Resistance (to), drug —see also
            specific organism
        lymphangitis —see Lymphangitis
        organ dysfunction (acute) R65.20
            with septic shock R65.21
    abscess (skin) - code by site under
        Abscess
    Absidia —see Mucormycosis
    Acanthamoeba —see Acanthamebiasis
    Acanthocheilonema (perstans)
        (streptocerca) B74.4
    accessory sinus (chronic) —see Sinusitis
    achorion —see Dermatophytosis
    Acremonium falciforme B47.0
    acromioclavicular M00.9
    Actinobacillus (actinomycetem-
        comitans) A28.8
        mallei A24.0
        muris A25.1
    Actinomadura B47.1
    Actinomyces (israelii) (see also
        Actinomycosis) A42.9
    Actinomycetales —see Actinomycosis
    actinomycotic NOS —see Actinomycosis
    adenoid (and tonsil) J03.90
        chronic J35.02
    adenovirus NEC
        as cause of disease classified
            elsewhere B97.0
        unspecified nature or site B34.0
    aerogenes capsulatus A48.0
    aertrycke —see Infection, salmonella
    alimentary canal NOS —see Enteritis,
        infectious
    Allescheria boydii B48.2
    Alternaria B48.8
    alveolus, alveolar (process) K04.7
    Ameba, amebic (histolytica) —see
        Amebiasis
    amniotic fluid, sac or cavity O41.10-
        chorioamnionitis O41.12-
        placentitis O41.14-
    amputation stump (surgical) —see
        Complication, amputation stump,
        infection
    Ancylostoma (duodenalis) B76.0
    Anisakiasis, Anisakis larvae B81.0
    anthrax —see Anthrax
    antrum (chronic) —see Sinusitis, maxillary
    anus, anal (papillae) (sphincter) K62.89
    arbovirus (arbor virus) A94
        specified type NEC A93.8
    artificial insemination N98.0
    Ascaris lumbricoides —see Ascariasis
    Ascomycetes B47.0
    Aspergillus (flavus) (fumigatus)
        (terreus) —see Aspergillosis
    atypical
        acid-fast (bacilli) —see
            Mycobacterium, atypical
        mycobacteria —see Mycobacterium,
            atypical
        virus A81.9
            specified type NEC A81.89
    auditory meatus (external) —see Otitis,
        externa, infective
    auricle (ear) —see Otitis, externa,
        infective
    axillary gland (lymph) L04.2

Infection, infected, infective (Continued)
    Bacillus A49.9
        abortus A23.1
        anthracis —see Anthrax
        Ducrey's (any location) A57
        Flexner's A03.1
        Friedländer's NEC A49.8
        gas (gangrene) A48.0
        mallei A24.0
        melitensis A23.0
        paratyphoid, paratyphosus
            A01.4
            A A01.1
            B A01.2
            C A01.3
        Shiga (-Kruse) A03.0
        suipestifer —see Infection,
            salmonella
        swimming pool A31.1
        typhosa A01.00
        welchii —see Gangrene, gas
    bacterial NOS A49.9
        as cause of disease classified
            elsewhere B96.89
            Bacteroides fragilis [B. fragilis]
                B96.6
            Clostridium perfringens
                [C. perfringens] B96.7
            Enterobacter sakazakii
                B96.89
            Enterococcus B95.2
            Escherichia coli [E. coli] (see also
                Escherichia coli) B96.20
            Helicobacter pylori [H.pylori]
                B96.81
            Hemophilus influenzae
                [H. influenzae] B96.3
            Klebsiella pneumoniae
                [K. pneumoniae] B96.1
            Mycoplasma pneumoniae
                [M. pneumoniae] B96.0
            Proteus (mirabilis) (morganii)
                B96.4
            Pseudomonas (aeruginosa)
                (mallei) (pseudomallei)
                B96.5
            Staphylococcus B95.8
                aureus (methicillin susceptible)
                    (MSSA) B95.61
                    methicillin resistant (MRSA)
                        B95.62
                specified NEC B95.7
            Streptococcus B95.5
                group A B95.0
                group B B95.1
                pneumoniae B95.3
                specified NEC B95.4
                Vibrio vulnificus B96.82
        specified NEC A48.8
    Bacterium
        paratyphosum A01.4
            A A01.1
            B A01.2
            C A01.3
        typhosum A01.00
    Bacteroides NEC A49.8
        fragilis, as cause of disease classified
            elsewhere B96.6
    Balantidium coli A07.0
    Bartholin's gland N75.8
    Basidiobolus B46.8
    bile duct (common) (hepatic) —see
        Cholangitis
    bladder —see Cystitis

Infection, infected, infective (Continued)
    Blastomyces, blastomycotic —see also
        Blastomycosis
        brasiliensis —see
            Paracoccidioidomycosis
        dermatitidis —see Blastomycosis
        European —see Cryptococcosis
        Loboi B48.0
        North American B40.9
        South American —see
            Paracoccidioidomycosis
    bleb, postprocedure —see Blebitis
    bone —see Osteomyelitis
    Bordetella —see Whooping cough
    Borrelia bergdorfi A69.20
    brain (see also Encephalitis)
        G04.90
        membranes —see Meningitis
        septic G06.0
            meninges —see Meningitis,
                bacterial
    branchial cyst Q18.0
    breast —see Mastitis
    bronchus —see Bronchitis
    Brucella A23.9
        abortus A23.1
        canis A23.3
        melitensis A23.0
        mixed A23.8
        specified NEC A23.8
        suis A23.2
    Brugia (malayi) B74.1
        timori B74.2
    bursa —see Bursitis, infective
    buttocks (skin) L08.9
    Campylobacter, intestinal A04.5
        as cause of disease classified
            elsewhere B96.81
    Candida (albicans) (tropicalis) —see
        Candidiasis
    candiru B88.8
    Capillaria (intestinal) B81.1
        hepatica B83.8
        philippinensis B81.1
    cartilage —see Disorder, cartilage,
        specified type NEC
    cat liver fluke B66.0
    catheter-related bloodstream (CRBSI)
        T80.211
    cellulitis - code by site under Cellulitis
    central line-associated T80.219
        bloodstream (CLABSI) T80.211
        specified NEC T80.218
    Cephalosporium falciforme
        B47.0
    cerebrospinal —see Meningitis
    cervical gland (lymph) L04.0
    cervix —see Cervicitis
    cesarean delivery wound (puerperal)
        O86.0
    cestodes —see Infestation, cestodes
    chest J22
    Chilomastix (intestinal) A07.8
    Chlamydia, chlamydial A74.9
        anus A56.3
        genitourinary tract A56.2
            lower A56.00
            specified NEC A56.19
        lymphogranuloma A55
        pharynx A56.4
        psittaci A70
        rectum A56.3
        sexually transmitted NEC A56.8
    cholera —see Cholera

Infection, infected, infective (*Continued*)
  Cladosporium
    bantianum (brain abscess) B43.1
    carrionii B43.0
    castellanii B36.1
    trichoides (brain abscess) B43.1
    werneckii B36.1
  Clonorchis (sinensis) (liver) B66.1
  Clostridium NEC
    bifermentans A48.0
    botulinum (food poisoning) A05.1
      infant A48.51
      wound A48.52
    difficile
      as cause of disease classified
          elsewhere B96.89
      foodborne (disease) A04.7
      gas gangrene A48.0
      necrotizing enterocolitis A04.7
      sepsis A41.4
    gas-forming NEC A48.0
    histolyticum A48.0
    novyi, causing gas gangrene A48.0
    oedematiens A48.0
    perfringens
      as cause of disease classified
          elsewhere B96.7
      due to food A05.2
      foodborne (disease) A05.2
      gas gangrene A48.0
      sepsis A41.4
    septicum, causing gas gangrene A48.0
    sordellii, causing gas gangrene A48.0
    welchii
      as cause of disease classified
          elsewhere B96.7
      foodborne (disease) A05.2
      gas gangrene A48.0
      necrotizing enteritis A05.2
      sepsis A41.4
  Coccidioides (immitis) —*see*
      Coccidioidomycosis
  colon —*see* Enteritis, infectious
  colostomy K94.02
  common duct —*see* Cholangitis
  congenital P39.9
    Candida (albicans) P37.5
    cytomegalovirus P35.1
    hepatitis, viral P35.3
    herpes simplex P35.2
    infectious or parasitic disease P37.9
      specified NEC P37.8
    listeriosis (disseminated) P37.2
    malaria NEC P37.4
      falciparum P37.3
    Plasmodium falciparum P37.3
    poliomyelitis P35.8
    rubella P35.0
    skin P39.4
    toxoplasmosis (acute) (subacute)
        (chronic) P37.1
    tuberculosis P37.0
    urinary (tract) P39.3
    vaccinia P35.8
    virus P35.9
      specified type NEC P35.8
  Conidiobolus B46.8
  coronavirus NEC B34.2
    as cause of disease classified
        elsewhere B97.29
    severe acute respiratory syndrome
        (SARS associated) B97.21
  corpus luteum —*see*
      Salpingo-oophoritis

Infection, infected, infective (*Continued*)
  Corynebacterium diphtheriae —*see*
      Diphtheria
  cotia virus B08.8
  Coxiella burnetii A78
  coxsackie —*see* Coxsackie
  Cryptococcus neoformans —*see*
      Cryptococcosis
  Cryptosporidium A07.2
  Cunninghamella —*see* Mucormycosis
  cyst —*see* Cyst
  cystic duct (*see also* Cholecystitis) K81.9
  Cysticercus cellulosae —*see*
      Cysticercosis
  cytomegalovirus, cytomegaloviral B25.9
    congenital P35.1
    maternal, maternal care for (suspected)
        damage to fetus O35.3
    mononucleosis B27.10
      with
        complication NEC B27.19
        meningitis B27.12
        polyneuropathy B27.11
  delta-agent (acute), in hepatitis B carrier
      B17.0
  dental (pulpal origin) K04.7
  Deuteromycetes B47.0
  Dicrocoelium dendriticum B66.2
  Dipetalonema (perstans) (streptocerca)
      B74.4
  diphtherial —*see* Diphtheria
  Diphyllobothrium (adult) (latum)
      (pacificum) B70.0
    larval B70.1
  Diplogonoporus (grandis) B71.8
  Dipylidium caninum B67.4
  Dirofilaria B74.8
  Dracunculus medinensis B72
  Drechslera (hawaiiensis) B43.8
  Ducrey Haemophilus (any location)
      A57
  due to or resulting from
    artificial insemination N98.0
    central venous catheter T80.219
      bloodstream T80.211
      exit or insertion site T80.212
      localized T80.212
      port or reservoir T80.212
      specified NEC T80.218
      tunnel T80.212
    device, implant or graft (*see also*
        Complications, by site and
        type, infection or inflammation)
        T85.79
      arterial graft NEC T82.7
      breast (implant) T85.79
      catheter NEC T85.79
        dialysis (renal) T82.7
          intraperitoneal T85.71
        infusion NEC T82.7
          spinal (epidural) (subdural)
              T85.79
        urinary (indwelling) T83.51
      electronic (electrode) (pulse
          generator) (stimulator)
        bone T84.7
        cardiac T82.7
        nervous system (brain)
            (peripheral nerve) (spinal)
            T85.79
        urinary T83.59
      fixation, internal (orthopedic)
          NEC —*see* Complication,
          fixation device, infection

Infection, infected, infective (*Continued*)
  due to or resulting from (*Continued*)
    device, implant or graft (*Continued*)
      gastrointestinal (bile duct)
          (esophagus) T85.79
      genital NEC T83.6
      heart NEC T82.7
        valve (prosthesis) T82.6
        graft T82.7
      joint prosthesis —*see* Complication,
          joint prosthesis, infection
      ocular (corneal graft) (orbital
          implant) NEC T85.79
      orthopedic NEC T84.7
      specified NEC T85.79
      urinary NEC T83.59
      vascular NEC T82.7
      ventricular intracranial shunt T85.79
    Hickman catheter T80.219
      bloodstream T80.211
      localized T80.212
      specified NEC T80.218
    immunization or vaccination T88.0
    infusion, injection or transfusion
        NEC T80.29
    injury NEC - code by site under
        Wound, open
    peripherally inserted central catheter
        (PICC) T80.219
      bloodstream T80.211
      localized T80.212
      specified NEC T80.218
    portacath (port-a-cath) T80.219
      bloodstream T80.211
      localized T80.212
      specified NEC T80.218
    surgery T81.4
    triple lumen catheter T80.219
      bloodstream T80.211
      localized T80.212
      specified NEC T80.218
    umbilical venous catheter T80.219
      bloodstream T80.211
      localized T80.212
      specified NEC T80.218
  during labor NEC O75.3
  ear (middle) —*see also* Otitis media
    external —*see* Otitis, externa,
        infective
    inner —*see* subcategory H83.0
  Eberthella typhosa A01.00
  Echinococcus —*see* Echinococcus
  echovirus
    as cause of disease classified
        elsewhere B97.12
    unspecified nature or site B34.1
  endocardium I33.0
  endocervix —*see* Cervicitis
  Entamoeba —*see* Amebiasis
  enteric —*see* Enteritis, infectious
  Enterobacter sakazakii B96.89
  Enterobius vermicularis B80
  enterostomy K94.12
  enterovirus B34.1
    as cause of disease classified
        elsewhere B97.10
      coxsackievirus B97.11
      echovirus B97.12
      specified NEC B97.19
  Entomophthora B46.8
  Epidermophyton —*see*
      Dermatophytosis
  epididymis —*see* Epididymitis
  episiotomy (puerperal) O86.0

Infection, infected, infective (Continued)
  Erysipelothrix (insidiosa)
      (rhusiopathiae) —see Erysipeloid
  erythema infectiosum B08.3
  Escherichia (E.) coli NEC A49.8
    as cause of disease classified
        elsewhere (see also Escherichia
        coli) B96.20
    congenital P39.8
      sepsis P36.4
    generalized A41.51
    intestinal —see Enteritis, infectious,
        due to, Escherichia coli
  ethmoidal (chronic) (sinus) —see
      Sinusitis, ethmoidal
  eustachian tube (ear) —see Salpingitis,
      eustachian
  external auditory canal (meatus)
      NEC —see Otitis, externa, infective
  eye (purulent) —see Endophthalmitis,
      purulent
  eyelid —see Inflammation, eyelid
  fallopian tube —see Salpingo-oophoritis
  Fasciola (gigantica) (hepatica) (indica)
      B66.3
  Fasciolopsis (buski) B66.5
  filarial —see Infestation, filarial
  finger (skin) L08.9
    nail L03.01-
      fungus B35.1
  fish tapeworm B70.0
    larval B70.1
  flagellate, intestinal A07.9
  fluke —see Infestation, fluke
  focal
    teeth (pulpal origin) K04.7
    tonsils J35.01
  Fonsecaea (compactum) (pedrosoi)
      B43.0
  food —see Intoxication, foodborne
  foot (skin) L08.9
    dermatophytic fungus B35.3
  Francisella tularensis —see Tularemia
  frontal (sinus) (chronic) —see Sinusitis,
      frontal
  fungus NOS B49
    beard B35.0
    dermatophytic —see
        Dermatophytosis
    foot B35.3
    groin B35.6
    hand B35.2
    nail B35.1
    pathogenic to compromised host only
        B48.8
    perianal (area) B35.6
    scalp B35.0
    skin B36.9
      foot B35.3
      hand B35.2
      toenails B35.1
  Fusarium B48.8
  gallbladder —see Cholecystitis
  gas bacillus —see Gangrene, gas
  gastrointestinal —see Enteritis, infectious
  generalized NEC —see Sepsis
  genital organ or tract
    female —see Disease, pelvis,
        inflammatory
    male N49.9
      multiple sites N49.8
      specified NEC N49.8
  Ghon tubercle, primary A15.7
  Giardia lamblia A07.1

Infection, infected, infective (Continued)
  gingiva (chronic) K05.10
    acute K05.00
      nonplaque induced K05.01
      plaque induced K05.00
    nonplaque induced K05.11
    plaque induced K05.10
  glanders A24.0
  glenosporopsis B48.0
  Gnathostoma (spinigerum) B83.1
  Gongylonema B83.8
  gonococcal —see Gonococcus
  gram-negative bacilli NOS A49.9
  guinea worm B72
  gum (chronic) K05.10
    acute K05.00
      nonplaque induced K05.01
      plaque induced K05.00
    nonplaque induced K05.11
    plaque induced K05.10
  Haemophilus —see Infection,
      Hemophilus
  heart —see Carditis
  Helicobacter pylori A04.5
    as cause of disease classified
        elsewhere B96.81
  helminths B83.9
    intestinal B82.0
      mixed (types classifiable to
          more than one of the titles
          B65.0-B81.3 and B81.8) B81.4
      specified type NEC B81.8
    specified type NEC B83.8
  Hemophilus
    aegyptius, systemic A48.4
    ducrey (any location) A57
    generalized A41.3
    influenzae NEC A49.2
      as cause of disease classified
          elsewhere B96.3
  herpes (simplex) —see also Herpes
    congenital P35.2
    disseminated B00.7
    zoster B02.9
  herpesvirus, herpesviral —see Herpes
  Heterophyes (heterophyes) B66.8
  hip (joint) NEC M00.9
    due to internal joint prosthesis
      left T84.52
      right T84.51
    skin NEC L08.9
  Histoplasma —see Histoplasmosis
    American B39.4
    capsulatum B39.4
  hookworm B76.9
  human
    papilloma virus A63.0
    T-cell lymphotropic virus type-1
        (HTLV-1) B33.3
  hydrocele N43.0
  Hymenolepis B71.0
  hypopharynx —see Pharyngitis
  inguinal (lymph) glands L04.1
    due to soft chancre A57
  intervertebral disc, pyogenic M46.30
    cervical region M46.32
    cervicothoracic region M46.33
    lumbar region M46.36
    lumbosacral region M46.37
    multiple sites M46.39
    occipito-atlanto-axial region M46.31
    sacrococcygeal region M46.38
    thoracic region M46.34
    thoracolumbar region M46.35

Infection, infected, infective (Continued)
  intestine, intestinal —see Enteritis,
      infectious
    specified NEC A08.8
  intra-amniotic affecting newborn NEC
      P39.2
  Isospora belli or hominis A07.3
  Japanese B encephalitis A83.0
  jaw (bone) (lower) (upper) M27.2
  joint NEC M00.9
    due to internal joint prosthesis T84.50
  kidney (cortex) (hematogenous) N15.9
    with calculus N20.0
      with hydronephrosis N13.6
    following ectopic gestation O08.89
    pelvis and ureter (cystic) N28.85
    puerperal (postpartum) O86.21
    specified NEC N15.8
  Klebsiella (K.) pneumoniae NEC A49.8
    as cause of disease classified
        elsewhere B96.1
  knee (joint) NEC M00.9
    due to internal joint prosthesis
      left T84.54
      right T84.53
    joint M00.9
    skin L08.9
  Koch's —see Tuberculosis
  labia (majora) (minora) (acute) —see
      Vulvitis
  lacrimal
    gland —see Dacryoadenitis
    passages (duct) (sac) —see
        Inflammation, lacrimal, passages
  lancet fluke B66.2
  larynx NEC J38.7
  leg (skin) NOS L08.9
  Legionella pneumophila A48.1
    nonpneumonic A48.2
  Leishmania —see also Leishmaniasis
    aethiopica B55.1
    braziliensis B55.2
    chagasi B55.0
    donovani B55.0
    infantum B55.0
    major B55.1
    mexicana B55.1
    tropica B55.1
  lentivirus, as cause of disease classified
      elsewhere B97.31
  Leptosphaeria senegalensis B47.0
  Leptospira interrogans A27.9
    autumnalis A27.89
    canicola A27.89
    hebdomadis A27.89
    icterohaemorrhagiae A27.0
    pomona A27.89
    specified type NEC A27.89
  leptospirochetal NEC —see
      Leptospirosis
  Listeria monocytogenes —see also
      Listeriosis
    congenital P37.2
  Loa loa B74.3
    with conjunctival infestation B74.3
    eyelid B74.3
  Loboa loboi B48.0
  local, skin (staphylococcal)
      (streptococcal) L08.9
    abscess - code by site under Abscess
    cellulitis - code by site under
        Cellulitis
    specified NEC L08.89
    ulcer —see Ulcer, skin

Infection, infected, infective (*Continued*)
Loefflerella mallei A24.0
lung (*see also* Pneumonia) J18.9
  atypical Mycobacterium A31.0
  spirochetal A69.8
  tuberculous —*see* Tuberculosis, pulmonary
  virus —*see* Pneumonia, viral
lymph gland —*see also* Lymphadenitis, acute
  mesenteric I88.0
lymphoid tissue, base of tongue or posterior pharynx, NEC (chronic) J35.03
Madurella (grisea) (mycetomii) B47.0
major
  following ectopic or molar pregnancy O08.0
  puerperal, postpartum, childbirth O85
Malassezia furfur B36.0
Malleomyces
  mallei A24.0
  pseudomallei (whitmori) —*see* Melioidosis
mammary gland N61
Mansonella (ozzardi) (perstans) (streptocerca) B74.4
mastoid —*see* Mastoiditis
maxilla, maxillary M27.2
  sinus (chronic) —*see* Sinusitis, maxillary
mediastinum J98.5
Medina (worm) B72
meibomian cyst or gland —*see* Hordeolum
meninges —*see* Meningitis, bacterial
meningococcal (*see also* condition) A39.9
  adrenals A39.1
  brain A39.81
  cerebrospinal A39.0
  conjunctiva A39.89
  endocardium A39.51
  heart A39.50
    endocardium A39.51
    myocardium A39.52
    pericardium A39.53
  joint A39.83
  meninges A39.0
  meningococcemia A39.4
    acute A39.2
    chronic A39.3
  myocardium A39.52
  pericardium A39.53
  retrobulbar neuritis A39.82
  specified site NEC A39.89
mesenteric lymph nodes or glands NEC I88.0
Metagonimus B66.8
metatarsophalangeal M00.9
methicillin
  resistant Staphylococcus aureus (MRSA) A49.02
  susceptible Staphylococcus aureus (MSSA) A49.01
Microsporum, microsporic —*see* Dermatophytosis
mixed flora (bacterial) NEC A49.8
Monilia —*see* Candidiasis
Monosporium apiospermum B48.2
mouth, parasitic B37.0

Infection, infected, infective (*Continued*)
Mucor —*see* Mucormycosis
muscle NEC —*see* Myositis, infective
mycelium NOS B49
mycetoma B47.9
  actinomycotic NEC B47.1
  mycotic NEC B47.0
Mycobacterium, mycobacterial —*see* Mycobacterium
Mycoplasma NEC A49.3
  pneumoniae, as cause of disease classified elsewhere B96.0
mycotic NOS B49
  pathogenic to compromised host only B48.8
  skin NOS B36.9
myocardium NEC I40.0
nail (chronic)
  with lymphangitis —*see* Lymphangitis, acute, digit
  finger L03.01-
    fungus B35.1
  ingrowing L60.0
  toe L03.03-
    fungus B35.1
nasal sinus (chronic) —*see* Sinusitis
nasopharynx —*see* Nasopharyngitis
navel L08.82
Necator americanus B76.1
Neisseria —*see* Gonococcus
Neotestudina rosatii B47.0
newborn P39.9
  intra-amniotic NEC P39.2
  skin P39.4
  specified type NEC P39.8
nipple N61
  associated with
    lactation O91.03
    pregnancy O91.01-
    puerperium O91.02
Nocardia —*see* Nocardiosis
obstetrical surgical wound (puerperal) O86.0
Oesophagostomum (apiostomum) B81.8
Oestrus ovis —*see* Myiasis
Oidium albicans B37.9
Onchocerca (volvulus) —*see* Onchocerciasis - oncovirus, as cause of disease classified elsewhere B97.32
operation wound T81.4
Opisthorchis (felineus) (viverrini) B66.0
orbit, orbital —*see* Inflammation, orbit
orthopoxvirus NEC B08.09
ovary —*see* Salpingo-oophoritis
Oxyuris vermicularis B80
pancreas (acute) K85.9
  abscess —*see* Pancreatitis, acute
  specified NEC K85.8
papillomavirus, as cause of disease classified elsewhere B97.7
papovavirus NEC B34.4
Paracoccidioides brasiliensis —*see* Paracoccidioidomycosis
Paragonimus (westermani) B66.4
parainfluenza virus B34.8
parameningococcus NOS A39.9
parapoxvirus B08.60
  specified NEC B08.69
parasitic B89

Infection, infected, infective (*Continued*)
Parastrongylus
  cantonensis B83.2
  costaricensis B81.3
paratyphoid A01.4
  Type A A01.1
  Type B A01.2
  Type C A01.3
paraurethral ducts N34.2
parotid gland —*see* Sialoadenitis
parvovirus NEC B34.3
  as cause of disease classified elsewhere B97.6
Pasteurella NEC A28.0
  multocida A28.0
  pestis —*see* Plague
  pseudotuberculosis A28.0
  septica (cat bite) (dog bite) A28.0
  tularensis —*see* Tularemia
pelvic, female —*see* Disease, pelvis, inflammatory
Penicillium (marneffei) B48.4
penis (glans) (retention) NEC N48.29
periapical K04.5
peridental, periodontal K05.20
  generalized K05.22
  localized K05.21
perinatal period P39.9
  specified type NEC P39.8
perineal repair (puerperal) O86.0
periorbital —*see* Inflammation, orbit
perirectal K62.89
perirenal —*see* Infection, kidney
peritoneal —*see* Peritonitis
periureteral N28.89
Petriellidium boydii B48.2
pharynx —*see also* Pharyngitis
  coxsackievirus B08.5
  posterior, lymphoid (chronic) J35.03
Phialophora
  gougerotii (subcutaneous abscess or cyst) B43.2
  jeanselmei (subcutaneous abscess or cyst) B43.2
  verrucosa (skin) B43.0
Piedraia hortae B36.3
pinta A67.9
  intermediate A67.1
  late A67.2
  mixed A67.3
  primary A67.0
pinworm B80
pityrosporum furfur B36.0
pleuro-pneumonia-like organism (PPLO) NEC A49.3
  as cause of disease classified elsewhere B96.0
pneumococcus, pneumococcal NEC A49.1
  as cause of disease classified elsewhere B95.3
  generalized (purulent) A40.3
  with pneumonia J13
Pneumocystis carinii (pneumonia) B59
Pneumocystis jiroveci (pneumonia) B59
port or reservoir T80.212
postoperative T81.4
postoperative wound T81.4
postprocedural T81.4
postvaccinal T88.0
prepuce NEC N47.7
  with penile inflammation N47.6
prion —*see* Disease, prion, central nervous system

Infection, infected, infective (*Continued*)
prostate (capsule) —*see* Prostatitis
Proteus (mirabilis) (morganii) (vulgaris)
   NEC A49.8
   as cause of disease classified
      elsewhere B96.4
protozoal NEC B64
   intestinal A07.9
     specified NEC A07.8
   specified NEC B60.8
Pseudoallescheria boydii B48.2
Pseudomonas NEC A49.8
   as cause of disease classified
      elsewhere B96.5
   mallei A24.0
   pneumonia J15.1
   pseudomallei —*see* Melioidosis
puerperal O86.4
   genitourinary tract NEC O86.89
   major or generalized O85
   minor O86.4
   specified NEC O86.89
pulmonary —*see* Infection, lung
purulent —*see* Abscess
Pyrenochaeta romeroi B47.0
Q fever A78
rectum (sphincter) K62.89
renal —*see also* Infection, kidney
   pelvis and ureter (cystic) N28.85
reovirus, as cause of disease classified
   elsewhere B97.5
respiratory (tract) NEC J98.8
   acute J22
   chronic J98.8
   influenzal (upper) (acute) —*see*
     Influenza, with, respiratory
     manifestations NEC
   lower (acute) J22
     chronic —*see* Bronchitis, chronic
   rhinovirus J00
   syncytial virus, as cause of disease
     classified elsewhere B97.4
   upper (acute) NOS J06.9
     chronic J39.8
     streptococcal J06.9
     viral NOS J06.9
resulting from
   presence of internal prosthesis,
     implant, graft —*see*
     Complications, by site and type,
     infection
retortamoniasis A07.8
retroperitoneal NEC K68.9
retrovirus B33.3
   as cause of disease classified
     elsewhere B97.30
   human
     immunodeficiency, type 2
      (HIV 2) B97.35
     T-cell lymphotropic
      type I (HTLV-I) B97.33
      type II (HTLV-II) B97.34
   lentivirus B97.31
   oncovirus B97.32
   specified NEC B97.39
Rhinosporidium (seeberi) B48.1
rhinovirus
   as cause of disease classified
     elsewhere B97.89
   unspecified nature or site B34.8
Rhizopus —*see* Mucormycosis
rickettsial NOS A79.9
roundworm (large) NEC B82.0
   Ascariasis (*see also* Ascariasis) B77.9

Infection, infected, infective (*Continued*)
rubella —*see* Rubella
Saccharomyces —*see* Candidiasis
salivary duct or gland (any) —*see*
   Sialoadenitis
Salmonella (aertrycke) (arizonae)
   (callinarum) (cholerae-suis)
   (enteritidis) (suipestifer)
   (typhimurium) A02.9
   with
     (gastro) enteritis A02.0
     sepsis A02.1
     specified manifestation NEC
      A02.8
   due to food (poisoning) A02.9
   hirschfeldii A01.3
   localized A02.20
     arthritis A02.23
     meningitis A02.21
     osteomyelitis A02.24
     pneumonia A02.22
     pyelonephritis A02.25
     specified NEC A02.29
   paratyphi A01.4
     A A01.1
     B A01.2
     C A01.3
   schottmuelleri A01.2
   typhi, typhosa —*see* Typhoid
Sarcocystis A07.8
scabies B86
Schistosoma —*see* Infestation,
   Schistosoma
scrotum (acute) NEC N49.2
seminal vesicle —*see* Vesiculitis
septic
   localized, skin —*see* Abscess
sheep liver fluke B66.3
Shigella A03.9
   boydii A03.2
   dysenteriae A03.0
   flexneri A03.1
   group
     A A03.0
     B A03.1
     C A03.2
     D A03.3
   Schmitz (-Stutzer) A03.0
   schmitzii A03.0
   shigae A03.0
   sonnei A03.3
   specified NEC A03.8
shoulder (joint) NEC M00.9
   due to internal joint prosthesis
     T84.59
   skin NEC L08.9
sinus (accessory) (chronic) (nasal) —*see*
   also Sinusitis
   pilonidal —*see* Sinus, pilonidal
   skin NEC L08.89
Skene's duct or gland —*see* Urethritis
skin (local) (staphylococcal)
   (streptococcal) L08.9
   abscess - code by site under Abscess
   cellulitis - code by site under
     Cellulitis
   due to fungus B36.9
     specified type NEC B36.8
   mycotic B36.9
     specified type NEC B36.8
   newborn P39.4
   ulcer —*see* Ulcer, skin
slow virus A81.9
   specified NEC A81.89
Sparganum (mansoni) (proliferum)
   (baxteri) B70.1

Infection, infected, infective (*Continued*)
specific —*see also* Syphilis
   to perinatal period —*see* Infection,
     congenital
specified NEC B99.8
spermatic cord NEC N49.1
sphenoidal (sinus) —*see* Sinusitis,
   sphenoidal
spinal cord NOS (*see also* Myelitis) G04.91
   abscess G06.1
   meninges —*see* Meningitis
   streptococcal G04.89
Spirillum A25.0
spirochetal NOS A69.9
   lung A69.8
   specified NEC A69.8
Spirometra larvae B70.1
spleen D73.89
Sporotrichum, Sporothrix (schenckii) —
   see Sporotrichosis
staphylococcal, unspecified site
   aureus (methicillin susceptible)
     (MSSA) A49.01
     methicillin resistant (MRSA)
      A49.02
   as cause of disease classified
     elsewhere B95.8
     aureus (methicillin susceptible)
      (MSSA) B95.61
      methicillin resistant (MRSA)
       B95.62
     specified NEC B95.7
   food poisoning A05.0
   generalized (purulent) A41.2
   pneumonia —*see* Pneumonia,
     staphylococcal
Stellantchasmus falcatus B66.8
streptobacillus moniliformis A25.1
streptococcal NEC A49.1
   as cause of disease classified
     elsewhere B95.5
   B genitourinary complicating
     childbirth O98.82
     pregnancy O98.81-
     puerperium O98.83
   congenital
     sepsis P36.10
      group B P36.0
      specified NEC P36.19
   generalized (purulent) A40.9
Streptomyces B47.1
Strongyloides (stercoralis) —*see*
   Strongyloidiasis
stump (amputation) (surgical) —*see*
   Complication, amputation stump,
   infection
subcutaneous tissue, local L08.9
suipestifer —*see* Infection, salmonella
swimming pool bacillus A31.1
Taenia —*see* Infestation, Taenia
Taeniarhynchus saginatus B68.1
tapeworm —*see* Infestation, tapeworm
tendon (sheath) —*see* Tenosynovitis,
   infective NEC
Ternidens diminutus B81.8
testis —*see* Orchitis
threadworm B80
throat —*see* Pharyngitis
thyroglossal duct K14.8
toe (skin) L08.9
   cellulitis L03.03-
     fungus B35.1
   nail L03.03-
     fungus B35.1
tongue NEC K14.0
   parasitic B37.0

Infection, infected, infective *(Continued)*
  tonsil (and adenoid) (faucial) (lingual)
      (pharyngeal) —*see* Tonsillitis
  tooth, teeth K04.7
    periapical K04.7
    peridental, periodontal K05.20
      generalized K05.22
      localized K05.21
    pulp K04.0
    socket M27.3
  TORCH —*see* Infection, congenital
      without active infection P00.2
  Torula histolytica —*see* Cryptococcosis
  Toxocara (canis) (cati) (felis) B83.0
  Toxoplasma gondii —*see* Toxoplasma
  trachea, chronic J42
  trematode NEC —*see* Infestation, fluke
  trench fever A79.0
  Treponema pallidum —*see* Syphilis
  Trichinella (spiralis) B75
  Trichomonas A59.9
    cervix A59.09
    intestine A07.8
    prostate A59.02
    specified site NEC A59.8
    urethra A59.03
    urogenitalis A59.00
    vagina A59.01
    vulva A59.01
  Trichophyton, trichophytic —*see*
      Dermatophytosis
  Trichosporon (beigelii) cutaneum B36.2
  Trichostrongylus B81.2
  Trichuris (trichiura) B79
  Trombicula (irritans) B88.0
  Trypanosoma
    brucei
      gambiense B56.0
      rhodesiense B56.1
    cruzi —*see* Chagas' disease
  tubal —*see* Salpingo-oophoritis
  tuberculous NEC —*see* Tuberculosis
  tubo-ovarian —*see* Salpingo-oophoritis
  tunica vaginalis N49.1
  tunnel T80.212
  tympanic membrane NEC —*see*
      Myringitis
  typhoid (abortive) (ambulant)
      (bacillus) —*see* Typhoid
  typhus A75.9
    flea-borne A75.2
    mite-borne A75.3
    recrudescent A75.1
    tick-borne A77.9
      African A77.1
      North Asian A77.2
  umbilicus L08.82
  ureter N28.86
  urethra —*see* Urethritis
  urinary (tract) N39.0
    bladder —*see* Cystitis
    complicating
      pregnancy O23.4-
        specified type NEC O23.3-
    kidney —*see* Infection, kidney
    newborn P39.3
    puerperal (postpartum) O86.20
    tuberculous A18.13
    urethra —*see* Urethritis
  uterus, uterine —*see* Endometritis
  vaccination T88.0
  vaccinia not from vaccination B08.011
  vagina (acute) —*see* Vaginitis
  varicella B01.9
  varicose veins —*see* Varix

Infection, infected, infective *(Continued)*
  vas deferens NEC N49.1
  vesical —*see* Cystitis
  Vibrio
    cholerae A00.0
      El Tor A00.1
    parahaemolyticus (food poisoning)
        A05.3
    vulnificus
      as cause of disease classified
          elsewhere B96.82
      foodborne intoxication A05.5
  Vincent's (gum) (mouth) (tonsil) A69.1
  virus, viral NOS B34.9
    adenovirus
      as cause of disease classified
          elsewhere B97.0
      unspecified nature or site
          B34.0
    arborvirus, arbovirus arthropod-
        borne A94
    as cause of disease classified
        elsewhere B97.89
      adenovirus B97.0
      coronavirus B97.29
        SARS-associated B97.21
      coxsackievirus B97.11
      echovirus B97.12
      enterovirus B97.10
        coxsackievirus B97.11
        echovirus B97.12
        specified NEC B97.19
      human
        immunodeficiency, type 2
            (HIV 2) B97.35
        metapneumovirus B97.81
        T-cell lymphotropic,
            type I (HTLV-I) B97.33
            type II (HTLV-II) B97.34
      papillomavirus B97.7
      parvovirus B97.6
      reovirus B97.5
      respiratory syncytial B97.4
      retrovirus B97.30
        human
          immunodeficiency, type 2
              (HIV 2) B97.35
          T-cell lymphotropic,
              type I (HTLV-I) B97.33
              type II (HTLV-II)
              B97.34
        lentivirus B97.31
        oncovirus B97.32
        specified NEC B97.39
      specified NEC B97.89
    central nervous system A89
    atypical A81.9
      specified NEC A81.89
    enterovirus NEC A88.8
      meningitis A87.0
    slow virus A81.9
      specified NEC A81.89
    specified NEC A88.8
    chest J98.8
    cotia B08.8
    coxsackie (*see also* Infection,
        coxsackie) B34.1
      as cause of disease classified
          elsewhere B97.11
    ECHO
      as cause of disease classified
          elsewhere B97.12
      unspecified nature or site B34.1
    encephalitis, tick-borne A84.9

Infection, infected, infective *(Continued)*
  virus, viral NOS *(Continued)*
    enterovirus, as cause of disease
        classified elsewhere B97.10
      coxsackievirus B97.11
      echovirus B97.12
      specified NEC B97.19
    exanthem NOS B09
    human metapneumovirus as cause
        of disease classified elsewhere
        B97.81
    human papilloma as cause of
        disease classified elsewhere
        B97.7
    intestine —*see* Enteritis, viral
    respiratory syncytial
      as cause of disease classified
          elsewhere B97.4
      bronchopneumonia J12.1
      common cold syndrome J00
      nasopharyngitis (acute) J00
    rhinovirus
      as cause of disease classified
          elsewhere B97.89
      unspecified nature or site
          B34.8
    slow A81.9
      specified NEC A81.89
    specified type NEC B33.8
      as cause of disease classified
          elsewhere B97.89
      unspecified nature or site B34.8
    unspecified nature or site B34.9
    West Nile —*see* Virus, West Nile
    vulva (acute) —*see* Vulvitis
  West Nile —*see* Virus, West Nile
  whipworm B79
  worms B83.9
    specified type NEC B83.8
  Wuchereria (bancrofti) B74.0
    malayi B74.1
  yatapoxvirus B08.70
    specified NEC B08.79
  yeast (*see also* Candidiasis) B37.9
  yellow fever —*see* Fever, yellow
  Yersinia
    enterocolitica (intestinal) A04.6
    pestis —*see* Plague
    pseudotuberculosis A28.2
  Zeis' gland —*see* Hordeolum
  zoonotic bacterial NOS A28.9
  Zopfia senegalensis B47.0
Infective, infectious —*see* condition
Infertility
  female N97.9
    age-related N97.8
    associated with
      anovulation N97.0
      cervical (mucus) disease or
          anomaly N88.3
      congenital anomaly
        cervix N88.3
        fallopian tube N97.1
        uterus N97.2
        vagina N97.8
      dysmucorrhea N88.3
      fallopian tube disease or anomaly
          N97.1
      pituitary-hypothalamic origin
          E23.0
      specified origin NEC N97.8
      Stein-Leventhal syndrome E28.2
      uterine disease or anomaly N97.2
      vaginal disease or anomaly N97.8

Infertility (Continued)
female (Continued)
due to
cervical anomaly N88.3
fallopian tube anomaly N97.1
ovarian failure E28.39
Stein-Leventhal syndrome E28.2
uterine anomaly N97.2
vaginal anomaly N97.8
nonimplantation N97.2
origin
cervical N88.3
tubal (block) (occlusion) (stenosis)
N97.1
uterine N97.2
vaginal N97.8
male N46.9
azoospermia N46.01
extratesticular cause N46.029
drug therapy N46.021
efferent duct obstruction N46.023
infection N46.022
radiation N46.024
specified cause NEC N46.029
systemic disease N46.025
oligospermia N46.11
extratesticular cause N46.129
drug therapy N46.121
efferent duct obstruction N46.123
infection N46.122
radiation N46.124
specified cause NEC N46.129
systemic disease N46.125
specified type NEC N46.8
Infestation B88.9
Acanthocheilonema (perstans)
(streptocerca) B74.4
Acariasis B88.0
demodex folliculorum B88.0
sarcoptes scabiei B86
trombiculae B88.0
Agamofilaria streptocerca B74.4
Ancylostoma, ankylostoma (braziliense)
(caninum) (ceylanicum)
(duodenale) B76.0
americanum B76.1
new world B76.1
Anisakis larvae, anisakiasis B81.0
arthropod NEC B88.2
Ascaris lumbricoides —see Ascariasis
Balantidium coli A07.0
beef tapeworm B68.1
Bothriocephalus (latus) B70.0
larval B70.1
broad tapeworm B70.0
larval B70.1
Brugia (malayi) B74.1
timori B74.2
candiru B88.8
Capillaria
hepatica B83.8
philippinensis B81.1
cat liver fluke B66.0
cestodes B71.9
diphyllobothrium —see Infestation,
diphyllobothrium
dipylidiasis B71.1
hymenolepiasis B71.0
specified type NEC B71.8
chigger B88.0
chigo, chigoe B88.1
Clonorchis (sinensis) (liver) B66.1
coccidial A07.3
crab-lice B85.3

Infestation (Continued)
Cysticercus cellulosae —see
Cysticercosis
Demodex (folliculorum) B88.0
Dermanyssus gallinae B88.0
Dermatobia (hominis) —see Myiasis
Dibothriocephalus (latus) B70.0
larval B70.1
Dicrocoelium dendriticum B66.2
Diphyllobothrium (adult) (latum)
(intestinal) (pacificum) B70.0
larval B70.1
Diplogonoporus (grandis) B71.8
Dipylidium caninum B67.4
Distoma hepaticum B66.3
dog tapeworm B67.4
Dracunculus medinensis B72
dragon worm B72
dwarf tapeworm B71.0
Echinococcus —see Echinococcus
Echinostomum ilocanum B66.8
Entamoeba (histolytica) —see Infection,
Ameba
Enterobius vermicularis B80
eyelid
in (due to)
leishmaniasis B55.1
loiasis B74.3
onchocerciasis B73.09
phthiriasis B85.3
parasitic NOS B89
eyeworm B74.3
Fasciola (gigantica) (hepatica) (indica)
B66.3
Fasciolopsis (buski) (intestine) B66.5
filarial B74.9
bancroftian B74.0
conjunctiva B74.9
due to
Acanthocheilonema (perstans)
(streptocerca) B74.4
Brugia (malayi) B74.1
timori B74.2
Dracunculus medinensis B72
guinea worm B72
loa loa B74.3
Mansonella (ozzardi) (perstans)
(streptocerca) B74.4
Onchocerca volvulus B73.00
eye B73.00
eyelid B73.09
Wuchereria (bancrofti) B74.0
Malayan B74.1
ozzardi B74.4
specified type NEC B74.8
fish tapeworm B70.0
larval B70.1
fluke B66.9
blood NOS —see Schistosomiasis
cat liver B66.0
intestinal B66.5
lancet B66.2
liver (sheep) B66.3
cat B66.0
Chinese B66.1
due to clonorchiasis B66.1
oriental B66.1
lung (oriental) B66.4
sheep liver B66.3
specified type NEC B66.8
fly larvae —see Myiasis
Gasterophilus (intestinalis) —see
Myiasis
Gastrodiscoides hominis B66.8

Infestation (Continued)
Giardia lamblia A07.1
Gnathostoma (spinigerum) B83.1
Gongylonema B83.8
guinea worm B72
helminth B83.9
angiostrongyliasis B83.2
intestinal B81.3
gnathostomiasis B83.1
hirudiniasis, internal B83.4
intestinal B82.0
angiostrongyliasis B81.3
anisakiasis B81.0
ascariasis —see Ascariasis
capillariasis B81.1
cysticercosis —see Cysticercosis
diphyllobothriasis —see Infestation,
diphyllobothriasis
dracunculiasis B72
echinococcus —see Echinococcosis
enterobiasis B80
filariasis —see Infestation, filarial
fluke —see Infestation, fluke
hookworm —see Infestation,
hookworm
mixed (types classifiable to
more than one of the titles
B65.0-B81.3 and B81.8) B81.4
onchocerciasis —see Onchocerciasis
schistosomiasis —see Infestation,
schistosoma
specified
cestode NEC —see Infestation,
cestode
type NEC B81.8
strongyloidiasis —see
Strongyloidiasis
taenia —see Infestation, taenia
trichinellosis B75
trichostrongyliasis B81.2
trichuriasis B79
specified type NEC B83.8
syngamiasis B83.3
visceral larva migrans B83.0
Heterophyes (heterophyes) B66.8
hookworm B76.9
ancylostomiasis B76.0
necatoriasis B76.1
specified type NEC B76.8
Hymenolepis (diminuta) (nana)
B71.0
intestinal NEC B82.9
leeches (aquatic) (land) —see
Hirudiniasis
Leishmania —see Leishmaniasis
lice, louse —see Infestation, Pediculus
Linguatula B88.8
Liponyssoides sanguineus B88.0
Loa loa B74.3
conjunctival B74.3
eyelid B74.3
louse —see Infestation, Pediculus
maggots —see Myiasis
Mansonella (ozzardi) (perstans)
(streptocerca) B74.4
Medina (worm) B72
Metagonimus (yokogawai) B66.8
microfilaria streptocerca —see
Onchocerciasis
eye B73.00
eyelid B73.09
mites B88.9
scabic B86
Monilia (albicans) —see Candidiasis

Infestation *(Continued)*
  mouth B37.0
  Necator americanus B76.1
  nematode NEC (intestinal) B82.0
    Ancylostoma B76.0
    conjunctiva NEC B83.9
    Enterobius vermicularis B80
    Gnathostoma spinigerum B83.1
    physaloptera B80
    specified NEC B81.8
    trichostrongylus B81.2
    trichuris (trichuria) B79
  Oesophagostomum (apiostomum) B81.8
  Oestrus ovis (*see also* Myiasis) B87.9
  Onchocerca (volvulus) —*see*
      Onchocerciasis
  Opisthorchis (felineus) (viverrini) B66.0
  orbit, parasitic NOS B89
  Oxyuris vermicularis B80
  Paragonimus (westermani) B66.4
  parasite, parasitic B89
    eyelid B89
    intestinal NOS B82.9
    mouth B37.0
    skin B88.9
    tongue B37.0
  Parastrongylus
    cantonensis B83.2
    costaricensis B81.3
  Pediculus B85.2
    body B85.1
    capitis (humanus) (any site) B85.0
    corporis (humanus) (any site) B85.1
    head B85.0
    mixed (classifiable to more than one
        of the titles B85.0-B85.3) B85.4
    pubis (any site) B85.3
  Pentastoma B88.8
  Phthirus (pubis) (any site) B85.3
    with any infestation classifiable to
        B85.0-B85.2 B85.4
  pinworm B80
  pork tapeworm (adult) B68.0
  protozoal NEC B64
    intestinal A07.9
      specified NEC A07.8
    specified NEC B60.8
  pubic, louse B85.3
  rat tapeworm B71.0
  red bug B88.0
  roundworm (large) NEC B82.0
    Ascariasis (*see also* Ascariasis) B77.9
  sandflea B88.1
  Sarcoptes scabiei B86
  scabies B86
  Schistosoma B65.9
    bovis B65.8
    cercariae B65.3
    haematobium B65.0
    intercalatum B65.8
    japonicum B65.2
    mansoni B65.1
    mattheei B65.8
    mekongi B65.8
    specified type NEC B65.8
    spindale B65.8
  screw worms —*see* Myiasis
  skin NOS B88.9
  Sparganum (mansoni) (proliferum)
      (baxteri) B70.1
    larval B70.1
  specified type NEC B88.8
  Spirometra larvae B70.1
  Stellantchasmus falcatus B66.8

Infestation *(Continued)*
  Strongyloides stercoralis —*see*
      Strongyloidiasis
  Taenia B68.9
    diminuta B71.0
    echinococcus —*see* Echinococcus
    mediocanellata B68.1
    nana B71.0
    saginata B68.1
    solium (intestinal form) B68.0
      larval form —*see* Cysticercosis
  Taeniarhynchus saginatus B68.1
  tapeworm B71.9
    beef B68.1
    broad B70.0
      larval B70.1
    dog B67.4
    dwarf B71.0
    fish B70.0
      larval B70.1
    pork B68.0
    rat B71.0
  Ternidens diminutus B81.8
  Tetranychus molestissimus B88.0
  threadworm B80
  tongue B37.0
  Toxocara (canis) (cati) (felis) B83.0
  trematode (s) NEC —*see* Infestation,
      fluke
  Trichinella (spiralis) B75
  Trichocephalus B79
  Trichomonas —*see* Trichomoniasis
  Trichostrongylus B81.2
  Trichuris (trichiura) B79
  Trombicula (irritans) B88.0
  Tunga penetrans B88.1
  Uncinaria americana B76.1
  Vandellia cirrhosa B88.8
  whipworm B79
  worms B83.9
    intestinal B82.0
  Wuchereria (bancrofti) B74.0
Infiltrate, infiltration
  amyloid (generalized) (localized) —*see*
      Amyloidosis
  calcareous NEC R89.7
    localized —*see* Degeneration, by site
  calcium salt R89.7
  cardiac
    fatty —*see* Degeneration, myocardial
    glycogenic E74.02 *[I43]*
  corneal —*see* Edema, cornea
  eyelid —*see* Inflammation, eyelid
  glycogen, glycogenic —*see* Disease,
      glycogen storage
  heart, cardiac
    fatty —*see* Degeneration, myocardial
    glycogenic E74.02 *[I43]*
  inflammatory in vitreous H43.89
  kidney N28.89
  leukemic —*see* Leukemia
  liver K76.89
    fatty —*see* Fatty, liver NEC
    glycogen (*see also* Disease, glycogen
        storage) E74.03 *[K77]*
  lung R91.8
    eosinophilic J82
  lymphatic (*see also* Leukemia,
      lymphatic) C91.9-
    gland I88.9
  muscle, fatty M62.89
  myocardium, myocardial
    fatty —*see* Degeneration, myocardial
    glycogenic E74.02 *[I43]*

Infiltrate, infiltration *(Continued)*
  on chest x-ray R91.8
  pulmonary R91.8
    with eosinophilia J82
  skin (lymphocytic) L98.6
  thymus (gland) (fatty) E32.8
  urine R39.0
  vesicant agent
    antineoplastic chemotherapy
        T80.810
    other agent NEC T80.818
  vitreous body H43.89
Infirmity R68.89
  senile R54
Inflammation, inflamed, inflammatory
    (with exudation)
  abducent (nerve) —*see* Strabismus,
      paralytic, sixth nerve
  accessory sinus (chronic) —*see*
      Sinusitis
  adrenal (gland) E27.8
  alveoli, teeth M27.3
    scorbutic E54
  anal canal, anus K62.89
  antrum (chronic) —*see* Sinusitis,
      maxillary
  appendix —*see* Appendicitis
  arachnoid —*see* Meningitis
  areola N61
    puerperal, postpartum or
        gestational —*see* Infection, nipple
  areolar tissue NOS L08.9
  artery —*see* Arteritis
  auditory meatus (external) —*see* Otitis,
      externa
  Bartholin's gland N75.8
  bile duct (common) (hepatic) or
      passage —*see* Cholangitis
  bladder —*see* Cystitis
  bone —*see* Osteomyelitis
  brain —*see also* Encephalitis
    membrane —*see* Meningitis
  breast N61
    puerperal, postpartum, gestational —
        see Mastitis, obstetric
  broad ligament —*see* Disease, pelvis,
      inflammatory
  bronchi —*see* Bronchitis
  catarrhal J00
  cecum —*see* Appendicitis
  cerebral —*see also* Encephalitis
    membrane —*see* Meningitis
  cerebrospinal
    meningococcal A39.0
  cervix (uteri) —*see* Cervicitis
  chest J98.8
  chorioretinal H30.9-
    cyclitis —*see* Cyclitis
    disseminated H30.10-
      generalized H30.13-
      peripheral H30.12-
      posterior pole H30.11-
    epitheliopathy —*see* Epitheliopathy
    focal H30.00-
      juxtapapillary H30.01-
      macular H30.04-
      paramacular —*see* Inflammation,
          chorioretinal, focal,
          macular
      peripheral H30.03-
      posterior pole H30.02-
    specified type NEC H30.89-
  choroid —*see* Inflammation,
      chorioretinal

Inflammation, inflamed, inflammatory
(Continued)
chronic, postmastoidectomy
cavity —see Complications,
postmastoidectomy,
inflammation
colon —see Enteritis
connective tissue (diffuse) NEC —see
Disorder, soft tissue, specified type
NEC
cornea —see Keratitis
corpora cavernosa N48.29
cranial nerve —see Disorder, nerve,
cranial
Douglas' cul-de-sac or pouch (chronic)
N73.0
due to device, implant or graft —see also
Complications, by site and type,
infection or inflammation
arterial graft T82.7
breast (implant) T85.79
catheter T85.79
dialysis (renal) T82.7
intraperitoneal T85.71
infusion T82.7
spinal (epidural) (subdural)
T85.79
urinary (indwelling) T83.51
electronic (electrode) (pulse
generator) (stimulator)
bone T84.7
cardiac T82.7
nervous system (brain) (peripheral
nerve) (spinal) T85.79
urinary T83.59
fixation, internal (orthopedic) NEC —
see Complication, fixation
device, infection
gastrointestinal (bile duct)
(esophagus) T85.79
genital NEC T83.6
heart NEC T82.7
valve (prosthesis) T82.6
graft T82.7
joint prosthesis —see Complication,
joint prosthesis, infection
ocular (corneal graft) (orbital
implant) NEC T85.79
orthopedic NEC T84.7
specified NEC T85.79
urinary NEC T83.59
vascular NEC T82.7
ventricular intracranial shunt T85.79
duodenum K29.80
with bleeding K29.81
dura mater —see Meningitis
ear (middle) —see also Otitis, media
external —see Otitis, externa
inner —see subcategory H83.0
epididymis —see Epididymitis
esophagus K20.9
ethmoidal (sinus) (chronic) —see
Sinusitis, ethmoidal
eustachian tube (catarrhal) —see
Salpingitis, eustachian
eyelid H01.9
abscess —see Abscess, eyelid
blepharitis —see Blepharitis
chalazion —see Chalazion
dermatosis (noninfectious) —see
Dermatosis, eyelid
hordeolum —see Hordeolum
specified NEC H01.8
fallopian tube —see Salpingo-oophoritis

Inflammation, inflamed, inflammatory
(Continued)
fascia —see Myositis
follicular, pharynx J31.2
frontal (sinus) (chronic) —see Sinusitis,
frontal
gallbladder —see Cholecystitis
gastric —see Gastritis
gastrointestinal —see Enteritis
genital organ (internal) (diffuse)
female —see Disease, pelvis,
inflammatory
male N49.9
multiple sites N49.8
specified NEC N49.8
gland (lymph) —see Lymphadenitis
glottis —see Laryngitis
granular, pharynx J31.2
gum K05.10
nonplaque induced K05.11
plaque induced K05.10
heart —see Carditis
hepatic duct —see Cholangitis
ileoanal (internal) pouch K91.850
ileum —see also Enteritis
regional or terminal —see Enteritis,
regional
intestinal pouch K91.850
intestine (any part) —see Enteritis
jaw (acute) (bone) (chronic) (lower)
(suppurative) (upper) M27.2
joint NEC —see Arthritis
sacroiliac M46.1
kidney —see Nephritis
knee (joint) M13.169
tuberculous A18.02
labium (majus) (minus) —see Vulvitis
lacrimal
gland —see Dacryoadenitis
passages (duct) (sac) —see also
Dacryocystitis
canaliculitis —see Canaliculitis,
lacrimal
larynx —see Laryngitis
leg NOS L08.9
lip K13.0
liver (capsule) —see also Hepatitis
chronic K73.9
suppurative K75.0
lung (acute) —see also Pneumonia
chronic J98.4
lymph gland or node —see
Lymphadenitis
lymphatic vessel —see Lymphangitis
maxilla, maxillary M27.2
sinus (chronic) —see Sinusitis,
maxillary
membranes of brain or spinal cord —see
Meningitis
meninges —see Meningitis
mouth K12.1
muscle —see Myositis
myocardium —see Myocarditis
nasal sinus (chronic) —see Sinusitis
nasopharynx —see Nasopharyngitis
navel L08.82
nerve NEC —see Neuralgia
nipple N61
puerperal, postpartum or
gestational —see Infection,
nipple
nose —see Rhinitis
oculomotor (nerve) —see Strabismus,
paralytic, third nerve
optic nerve —see Neuritis, optic

Inflammation, inflamed, inflammatory
(Continued)
orbit (chronic) H05.10
acute H05.00
abscess —see Abscess, orbit
cellulitis —see Cellulitis, orbit
osteomyelitis —see Osteomyelitis,
orbit
periostitis —see Periostitis, orbital
tenonitis —see Tenonitis, eye
granuloma —see Granuloma, orbit
myositis —see Myositis, orbital
ovary —see Salpingo-oophoritis
oviduct —see Salpingo-oophoritis
pancreas (acute) —see Pancreatitis
parametrium N73.0
parotid region L08.9
pelvis, female —see Disease, pelvis,
inflammatory
penis (corpora cavernosa) N48.29
perianal K62.89
pericardium —see Pericarditis
perineum (female) (male) L08.9
perirectal K62.89
peritoneum —see Peritonitis
periuterine —see Disease, pelvis,
inflammatory
perivesical —see Cystitis
petrous bone (acute) (chronic) —see
Petrositis
pharynx (acute) —see Pharyngitis
pia mater —see Meningitis
pleura —see Pleurisy
polyp, colon (see also Polyp, colon,
inflammatory) K51.40
prostate —see also Prostatitis
specified type NEC N41.8
rectosigmoid —see Rectosigmoiditis
rectum (see also Proctitis) K62.89
respiratory, upper (see also Infection,
respiratory, upper) J06.9
acute, due to radiation J70.0
chronic, due to external agent —see
condition, respiratory, chronic,
due to
due to
chemicals, gases, fumes or vapors
(inhalation) J68.2
radiation J70.1
retina —see Chorioretinitis
retrocecal —see Appendicitis
retroperitoneal —see Peritonitis
salivary duct or gland (any)
(suppurative) —see Sialoadenitis
scorbutic, alveoli, teeth E54
scrotum N49.2
seminal vesicle —see Vesiculitis
sigmoid —see Enteritis
sinus —see Sinusitis
Skene's duct or gland —see Urethritis
skin L08.9
spermatic cord N49.1
sphenoidal (sinus) —see Sinusitis,
sphenoidal
spinal
cord —see Encephalitis
membrane —see Meningitis
nerve —see Disorder, nerve
spine —see Spondylopathy,
inflammatory
spleen (capsule) D73.89
stomach —see Gastritis
subcutaneous tissue L08.9
suprarenal (gland) E27.8
synovial —see Tenosynovitis

Inflammation, inflamed, inflammatory
(Continued)
  tendon (sheath) NEC —*see*
      Tenosynovitis
  testis —*see* Orchitis
  throat (acute) —*see* Pharyngitis
  thymus (gland) E32.8
  thyroid (gland) —*see* Thyroiditis
  tongue K14.0
  tonsil —*see* Tonsillitis
  trachea —*see* Tracheitis
  trochlear (nerve) —*see* Strabismus,
      paralytic, fourth nerve
  tubal —*see* Salpingo-oophoritis
  tuberculous NEC —*see* Tuberculosis
  tubo-ovarian —*see* Salpingo-oophoritis
  tunica vaginalis N49.1
  tympanic membrane —*see* Tympanitis
  umbilicus, umbilical L08.82
  uterine ligament —*see* Disease, pelvis,
      inflammatory
  uterus (catarrhal) —*see* Endometritis
  uveal tract (anterior) NOS —*see also*
      Iridocyclitis
    posterior —*see* Chorioretinitis
  vagina —*see* Vaginitis
  vas deferens N49.1
  vein —*see also* Phlebitis
    intracranial or intraspinal (septic)
        G08
    thrombotic I80.9
      leg —*see* Phlebitis, leg
      lower extremity —*see* Phlebitis, leg
  vocal cord J38.3
  vulva —*see* Vulvitis
  Wharton's duct (suppurative) —*see*
      Sialoadenitis
Inflation, lung, imperfect (newborn) —*see*
    Atelectasis
Influenza (bronchial) (epidemic)
    (respiratory (upper)) (unidentified
    influenza virus) J11.1
  with
    digestive manifestations J11.2
    encephalopathy J11.81
    enteritis J11.2
    gastroenteritis J11.2
    gastrointestinal manifestations J11.2
    laryngitis J11.1
    myocarditis J11.82
    otitis media J11.83
    pharyngitis J11.1
    pneumonia J11.00
      specified type J11.08
    respiratory manifestations NEC J11.1
    specified manifestation NEC J11.89
  A/H5N1 —*see also* Influenza, due to,
      identified novel influenza A virus
      J09.X2
  avian —*see also* Influenza, due to,
      identified novel influenza A virus
      J09.X2
  bird (*see also* Influenza, due to,
      identified novel influenza A virus)
      J09.X2
  novel (2009) H1N1 influenza (*see also*
      Influenza, due to, identified
      influenza virus NEC) J10.1
  novel influenza A/H1N1 (*see also*
      Influenza, due to, identified
      influenza virus NEC) J10.1
  due to
    avian (*see also* Influenza, due to,
        identified novel influenza A
        virus) J09.X2

Influenza *(Continued)*
  due to *(Continued)*
    identified influenza virus NEC J10.1
      with
        digestive manifestations J10.2
        encephalopathy J10.81
        enteritis J10.2
        gastroenteritis J10.2
        gastrointestinal manifestations
            J10.2
        laryngitis J10.1
        myocarditis J10.82
        otitis media J10.83
        pharyngitis J10.1
        pneumonia (unspecified type)
            J10.00
          with same identified influenza
              virus J10.01
          specified type NEC J10.08
        respiratory manifestations NEC
            J10.1
        specified manifestation NEC
            J10.89
    identified novel influenza A virus
        J09.X2
      with
        digestive manifestations J09.X3
        encephalopathy J09.X9
        enteritis J09.X3
        gastroenteritis J09.X3
        gastrointestinal manifestations
            J09.X3
        laryngitis J09.X2
        myocarditis J09.X9
        otitis media J09.X9
        pharyngitis J09.X2
        pneumonia J09.X1
        respiratory manifestations NEC
            J09.X2
        specified manifestation NEC
            J09.X9
        upper respiratory symptoms
            J09.X2
    of other animal origin, not bird or swine
        (*see also* Influenza, due to, identified
        novel influenza A virus) J09.X2
    swine (viruses that normally cause
        infections in pigs) (*see also*
        Influenza, due to, identified novel
        influenza A virus) J09.X2
Influenza-like disease —*see* Influenza
Influenzal —*see* Influenza
Infraction, Freiberg's (metatarsal head) —
    see Osteochondrosis, juvenile,
    metatarsus
Infraeruption of tooth (teeth) M26.34
**Infusion complication, misadventure,
    or reaction** —*see* Complications,
    infusion
Ingestion
  chemical —*see* Table of drugs and
      chemicals, by substance, poisoning
  drug or medicament
    correct substance properly
        administered —*see* Table
        of drugs and chemicals,
        by drug, adverse effect
    overdose or wrong substance
        given or taken —*see* Table of
        drugs and chemicals, by drug,
        poisoning
  foreign body —*see* Foreign body,
      alimentary tract
  tularemia A21.3

Ingrowing
  hair (beard) L73.1
  nail (finger) (toe) L60.0
Inguinal —*see also* condition
  testicle Q53.9
    bilateral Q53.21
    unilateral Q53.11
Inhalation
  anthrax A22.1
  flame T27.3
  food or foreign body —*see* Foreign
      body, by site
  gases, fumes, or vapors NEC T59.9-
    specified agent —*see* Table of drugs
        and chemicals, by substance
  liquid or vomitus —*see* Asphyxia
  meconium (newborn) P24.00
    with
      with respiratory symptoms P24.01
      pneumonia (pneumonitis) P24.01
  mucus —*see* Asphyxia, mucus
  oil or gasoline (causing suffocation) —
      see Foreign body, by site
  smoke J70.5
    due to chemicals, gases, fumes and
        vapors J68.9
  steam —*see* Toxicity, vapors
  stomach contents or secretions —*see*
      Foreign body, by site
    due to anesthesia (general) (local) or
        other sedation T88.59
      in labor and delivery O74.0
      in pregnancy O29.01-
      postpartum, puerperal O89.01
Inhibition, orgasm
  female F52.31
  male F52.32
Inhibitor, systemic lupus erythematosus
    (presence of) D68.62
Iniencephalus, iniencephaly Q00.2
Injection, traumatic jet (air) (industrial)
    (water) (paint or dye) T70.4
Injury (*see also* specified injury type) T14.90
  abdomen, abdominal S39.91
    blood vessel —*see* Injury, blood
        vessel, abdomen
    cavity —*see* Injury, intra-abdominal
    contusion S30.1
    internal —*see* Injury, intra-abdominal
    intra-abdominal organ —*see* Injury,
        intra-abdominal
    nerve —*see* Injury, nerve, abdomen
    open —*see* Wound, open, abdomen
    specified NEC S39.81
    superficial —*see* Injury, superficial,
        abdomen
  Achilles tendon S86.00-
    laceration S86.02-
    specified type NEC S86.09-
    strain S86.01-
  acoustic, resulting in deafness —*see*
      Injury, nerve, acoustic
  adrenal (gland) S37.819
    contusion S37.812
    laceration S37.813
    specified type NEC S37.818
  alveolar (process) S09.93
  ankle S99.91-
    contusion —*see* Contusion, ankle
    dislocation —*see* Dislocation, ankle
    fracture —*see* Fracture, ankle
    nerve —*see* Injury, nerve, ankle
    open —*see* Wound, open, ankle
    specified type NEC S99.81-
    sprain —*see* Sprain, ankle

Injury (Continued)
  ankle (Continued)
    superficial —see Injury, superficial, ankle
  anterior chamber, eye —see Injury, eye, specified site NEC
  anus —see Injury, abdomen
  aorta (thoracic) S25.00
    abdominal S35.00
      laceration (minor) (superficial) S35.01
      major S35.02
      specified type NEC S35.09
    laceration (minor) (superficial) S25.01
      major S25.02
    specified type NEC S25.09
  arm (upper) S49.9-
    blood vessel —see Injury, blood vessel, arm
    contusion —see Contusion, arm, upper
    fracture —see Fracture, humerus
    lower —see Injury, forearm
    muscle —see Injury, muscle, shoulder
    nerve —see Injury, nerve, arm
    open —see Wound, open, arm
    specified type NEC S49.8-
    superficial —see Injury, superficial, arm
  artery (complicating trauma) —see also Injury, blood vessel, by site
    cerebral or meningeal —see Injury, intracranial
  auditory canal (external) (meatus) S09.91
  auricle, auris, ear S09.91
  axilla —see Injury, shoulder
  back —see Injury, back, lower
  bile duct —see Injury, gallbladder
  birth —see also Birth, injury P15.9
  bladder (sphincter) S37.20
    at delivery O71.5
    contusion S37.22
    laceration S37.23
    obstetrical trauma O71.5
    specified type NEC S37.29
  blast (air) (hydraulic) (immersion) (underwater) NEC T14.8
    acoustic nerve trauma —see Injury, nerve, acoustic
    bladder —see Injury, bladder, blast injury
    brain —see Concussion
    colon —see Injury, intestine, large, blast injury
    ear (primary) S09.31-
      secondary S09.39-
    generalized T70.8
    lung —see Injury, intrathoracic, lung, blast injury
    multiple body organs T70.8
    peritoneum S36.81
    rectum S36.61
    retroperitoneum S36.898
    small intestine S36.419
      duodenum S36.410
      specified site NEC S36.418
    specified
      intra-abdominal organ NEC S36.898
      pelvic organ NEC S37.899
  blood vessel NEC T14.8
    abdomen S35.90
      aorta —see Injury, aorta, abdominal
      celiac artery —see Injury, blood vessel, celiac artery

Injury (Continued)
  blood vessel NEC (Continued)
    abdomen (Continued)
      iliac vessel —see Injury, blood vessel, iliac
      laceration S35.91
      mesenteric vessel —see Injury, mesenteric
      portal vein —see Injury, blood vessel, portal vein
      renal vessel —see Injury, blood vessel, renal
      specified T14.8
        site NEC —see subcategory S35.8
        type NEC S35.99
      splenic vessel —see Injury, blood vessel, splenic
      vena cava —see Injury, vena cava, inferior
    ankle —see Injury, blood vessel, foot
    aorta (abdominal) (thoracic) —see Injury, aorta
    arm (upper) NEC S45.90-
      forearm —see Injury, blood vessel, forearm
      laceration S45.91-
      specified
        site NEC S45.80-
          laceration S45.81-
          specified type NEC S45.89-
        type NEC S45.99-
      superficial vein S45.30-
        laceration S45.31-
        specified type NEC S45.39-
    axillary
      artery S45.00-
        laceration S45.01-
        specified type NEC S45.09-
      vein S45.20-
        laceration S45.21-
        specified type NEC S45.29-
    azygos vein —see Injury, blood vessel, thoracic, specified site NEC
    brachial
      artery S45.10-
        laceration S45.11-
        specified type NEC S45.19-
      vein S45.20-
        laceration S45.219
        specified type NEC S45.29-
    carotid artery (common) (external) (internal, extracranial) S15.00-
      internal, intracranial S06.8-
      laceration (minor) (superficial) S15.01-
        major S15.02-
      specified type NEC S15.09-
    celiac artery S35.219
      branch S35.299
        laceration (minor) (superficial) S35.291
          major S35.292
        specified NEC S35.298
      laceration (minor) (superficial) S35.211
        major S35.212
      specified type NEC S35.218
    cerebral —see Injury, intracranial
    deep plantar —see Injury, nerve, medial plantar
    digital (hand) —see Injury, blood vessel, finger

Injury (Continued)
  blood vessel NEC (Continued)
    dorsal
      artery (foot) S95.00-
        laceration S95.01-
        specified type NEC S95.09-
      vein (foot) S95.20-
        laceration S95.21-
        specified type NEC S95.29-
    due to accidental laceration during procedure —see Laceration, accidental complicating surgery
    extremity —see Injury, blood vessel, limb
    femoral
      artery (common) (superficial) S75.00-
        laceration (minor) (superficial) S75.01-
          major S75.02-
        specified type NEC S75.09-
      vein (hip level) (thigh level) S75.10-
        laceration (minor) (superficial) S75.11-
          major S75.12-
        specified type NEC S75.19-
    finger S65.50-
      index S65.50-
        laceration S65.51-
        specified type NEC S65.59-
      laceration S65.51-
      little S65.50-
        laceration S65.51-
        specified type NEC S65.59-
      middle S65.50-
        laceration S65.51-
        specified type NEC S65.59-
      specified type NEC S65.59-
      thumb —see Injury, blood vessel, thumb
    foot S95.90-
      dorsal
        artery —see Injury, blood vessel, dorsal, artery
        vein —see Injury, blood vessel, dorsal, vein
      laceration S95.91-
      plantar artery —see Injury, blood vessel, plantar artery
      specified
        site NEC S95.80-
          laceration S95.81-
          specified type NEC S95.89-
        specified type NEC S95.99-
    forearm S55.90-
      laceration S55.91-
      radial artery —see Injury, blood vessel, radial artery
      specified
        site NEC S55.80-
          laceration S55.81-
          specified type NEC S55.89-
        type NEC S55.99-
      ulnar artery —see Injury, blood vessel, ulnar artery
      vein S55.20-
        laceration S55.21-
        specified type NEC S55.29-
    gastric
      artery —see Injury, mesenteric, artery, branch
      vein —see Injury, blood vessel, abdomen
    gastroduodenal artery —see Injury, mesenteric, artery, branch

Injury *(Continued)*
blood vessel NEC *(Continued)*
greater saphenous vein (lower leg
level) S85.30-
hip (and thigh) level S75.20-
laceration (minor) (superficial)
S75.21-
major S75.22-
specified type NEC S75.29-
laceration S85.31-
specified type NEC S85.39-
hand (level) S65.90-
finger —*see* Injury, blood vessel,
finger
laceration S65.91-
palmar arch —*see* Injury, blood
vessel, palmar arch
radial artery —*see* Injury, blood
vessel, radial artery, hand
specified
site NEC S65.80-
laceration S65.81-
specified type NEC S65.89-
type NEC S65.99-
thumb —*see* Injury, blood vessel,
thumb
ulnar artery —*see* Injury, blood
vessel, ulnar artery, hand
head S09.0
intracranial —*see* Injury,
intracranial
multiple S09.0
hepatic
artery —*see* Injury, mesenteric,
artery
vein —*see* Injury, vena cava,
inferior
hip S75.90-
femoral artery —*see* Injury, blood
vessel, femoral, artery
femoral vein —*see* Injury, blood
vessel, femoral, vein
greater saphenous vein —*see*
Injury, blood vessel, greater
saphenous, hip level
laceration S75.91-
specified
site NEC S75.80-
laceration S75.81-
specified type NEC
S75.89-
type NEC S75.99-
hypogastric (artery) (vein) —*see*
Injury, blood vessel, iliac
iliac S35.5-
artery S35.51-
specified vessel NEC S35.5-
uterine vessel —*see* Injury, blood
vessel, uterine
vein S35.51-
innominate —*see* Injury, blood vessel,
thoracic, innominate
intercostal (artery) (vein) —*see*
Injury, blood vessel, thoracic,
intercostal
jugular vein (external) S15.20-
internal S15.30-
laceration (minor) (superficial)
S15.31-
major S15.32-
specified type NEC S15.39-
laceration (minor) (superficial)
S15.21-
major S15.22-
specified type NEC S15.29-

Injury *(Continued)*
blood vessel NEC *(Continued)*
leg (level) (lower) S85.90-
greater saphenous —*see* Injury,
blood vessel, greater
saphenous
laceration S85.91-
lesser saphenous —*see* Injury,
blood vessel, lesser saphenous
peroneal artery —*see* Injury, blood
vessel, peroneal artery
popliteal
artery —*see* Injury, blood vessel,
popliteal, artery
vein —*see* Injury, blood vessel,
popliteal, vein
specified
site NEC S85.80-
laceration S85.81-
specified type NEC S85.89-
type NEC S85.99-
thigh —*see* Injury, blood vessel,
hip
tibial artery —*see* Injury, blood
vessel, tibial artery
lesser saphenous vein (lower leg
level) S85.40-
laceration S85.41-
specified type NEC S85.49-
limb
lower —*see* Injury, blood vessel,
leg
upper —*see* Injury, blood vessel,
arm
lower back —*see* Injury, blood vessel,
abdomen
specified NEC —*see* Injury, blood
vessel, abdomen, specified,
site NEC
mammary (artery) (vein) —*see* Injury,
blood vessel, thoracic, specified
site NEC
mesenteric (inferior) (superior)
artery —*see* Injury, mesenteric,
artery
vein —*see* Injury, blood vessel,
portal vein
neck S15.9
specified site NEC S15.8
ovarian (artery) (vein) —*see*
subcategory S35.8
palmar arch (superficial) S65.20-
deep S65.30-
laceration S65.31-
specified type NEC S65.39-
laceration S65.21-
specified type NEC S65.29-
pelvis —*see* Injury, blood vessel,
abdomen
specified NEC —*see* Injury, blood
vessel, abdomen, specified,
site NEC
peroneal artery S85.20-
laceration S85.21-
specified type NEC S85.29-
plantar artery (deep) (foot) S95.10-
laceration S95.11-
specified type NEC S95.19-
popliteal
artery S85.00-
laceration S85.01-
specified type NEC S85.09-
vein S85.50-
laceration S85.51-
specified type NEC S85.59-

Injury *(Continued)*
blood vessel NEC *(Continued)*
portal vein S35.319
laceration S35.311
specified type NEC S35.318
precerebral —*see* Injury, blood vessel,
neck
pulmonary (artery) (vein) —*see*
Injury, blood vessel, thoracic,
pulmonary
radial artery (forearm level) S55.10-
hand and wrist (level) S65.10-
laceration S65.11-
specified type NEC S65.19-
laceration S55.11-
specified type NEC S55.19-
renal
artery S35.40-
laceration S35.41-
specified NEC S35.49-
vein S35.40-
laceration S35.41-
specified NEC S35.49-
saphenous vein (greater) (lower leg
level) —*see* Injury, blood vessel,
greater saphenous
hip and thigh level —*see* Injury,
blood vessel, greater
saphenous, hip level
lesser —*see* Injury, blood vessel,
lesser saphenous
shoulder
specified NEC —*see* Injury,
blood vessel, arm, specified
site NEC
superficial vein —*see* Injury,
blood vessel, arm, superficial
vein
specified NEC
splenic
artery —*see* Injury, blood vessel,
celiac artery, branch
vein S35.329
laceration S35.321
specified NEC S35.328
subclavian —*see* Injury, blood vessel,
thoracic, innominate
thigh —*see* Injury, blood vessel, hip
thoracic S25.90
aorta S25.00
laceration (minor) (superficial)
S25.01
major S25.02
specified type NEC S25.09
azygos vein —*see* Injury, blood
vessel, thoracic, specified, site
NEC
innominate
artery S25.10-
laceration (minor) (superficial)
S25.11-
major S25.12-
specified type NEC S25.19-
vein S25.30-
laceration (minor) (superficial)
S25.31-
major S25.32-
specified type NEC S25.39-
intercostal S25.50-
laceration S25.51-
specified type NEC S25.59-
laceration S25.91
mammary vessel —*see* Injury,
blood vessel, thoracic,
specified, site NEC

Injury *(Continued)*
  blood vessel NEC *(Continued)*
    thoracic *(Continued)*
      pulmonary S25.40-
        laceration (minor) (superficial)
          S25.41-
          major S25.42-
        specified type NEC S25.49-
      specified
        site NEC S25.80-
          laceration S25.81-
            specified type NEC S25.89-
        type NEC S25.99
      subclavian —*see* Injury, blood
          vessel, thoracic, innominate
      vena cava (superior) S25.20
        laceration (minor) (superficial)
          S25.21
          major S25.22
        specified type NEC S25.29
    thumb S65.40-
      laceration S65.41-
      specified type NEC S65.49-
    tibial artery S85.10-
      anterior S85.13-
        laceration S85.14-
        specified injury NEC S85.15-
      laceration S85.11-
      posterior S85.16-
        laceration S85.17-
        specified injury NEC S85.18-
      specified injury NEC S85.12-
    ulnar artery (forearm level)
          S55.00-
      hand and wrist (level) S65.00-
        laceration S65.01-
        specified type NEC S65.09-
      laceration S55.01-
      specified type NEC S55.09-
    upper arm (level) —*see* Injury, blood
        vessel, arm
    superficial vein —*see* Injury, blood
        vessel, arm, superficial vein
    uterine S35.5-
      artery S35.53-
      vein S35.53-
    vena cava —*see* Injury, vena cava
    vertebral artery S15.10-
      laceration (minor) (superficial)
          S15.11-
      major S15.12-
      specified type NEC S15.19-
    wrist (level) —*see* Injury, blood vessel,
        hand
  brachial plexus S14.3
    newborn P14.3
  brain (traumatic) S06.9-
    diffuse (axonal) S06.2X-
    focal S06.30-
    traumatic —*see* category S06
  brainstem S06.38-
  breast NOS S29.9
  broad ligament —*see* Injury, pelvic
      organ, specified site NEC
  bronchus, bronchi —*see* Injury,
      intrathoracic, bronchus
  brow S09.90
  buttock S39.92
  canthus, eye S05.90
  cardiac plexus —*see* Injury, nerve,
      thorax, sympathetic
  cauda equina S34.3
  cavernous sinus —*see* Injury,
      intracranial

Injury *(Continued)*
  cecum —*see* Injury, colon
  celiac ganglion or plexus —*see* Injury,
      nerve, lumbosacral, sympathetic
  cerebellum —*see* Injury, intracranial
  cerebral —*see* Injury, intracranial
  cervix (uteri) —*see* Injury, uterus
  cheek (wall) S09.93
  chest —*see* Injury, thorax
  childbirth (newborn) —*see also* Birth,
      injury
    maternal NEC O71.9
  chin S09.93
  choroid (eye) —*see* Injury, eye, specified
      site NEC
  clitoris S39.94
  coccyx —*see also* Injury, back, lower
    complicating delivery O71.6
  colon —*see* Injury, intestine, large
  common bile duct —*see* Injury, liver
  conjunctiva (superficial) —*see* Injury,
      eye, conjunctiva
  conus medullaris —*see* Injury, spinal,
      sacral
  cord
    spermatic (pelvic region) S37.898
      scrotal region S39.848
    spinal —*see* Injury, spinal cord, by
        region
  cornea —*see* Injury, eye, specified site
      NEC
    abrasion —*see* Injury, eye, cornea,
        abrasion
  cortex (cerebral) —*see also* Injury,
      intracranial
    visual —*see* Injury, nerve, optic
  costal region NEC S29.9
  costochondral NEC S29.9
  cranial
    cavity —*see* Injury, intracranial
    nerve —*see* Injury, nerve, cranial
  crushing —*see* Crush
  cutaneous sensory nerve
  cystic duct —*see* Injury, liver
  deep tissue —*see* Contusion, by site
    meaning pressure ulcer —*see* Ulcer,
        pressure, unstageable, by site
  delivery (newborn) P15.9
    maternal NEC O71.9
  Descemet's membrane —*see* Injury,
      eyeball, penetrating
  diaphragm —*see* Injury, intrathoracic,
      diaphragm
  duodenum —*see* Injury, intestine, small,
      duodenum
  ear (auricle) (external) (canal) S09.91
    abrasion —*see* Abrasion, ear
    bite —*see* Bite, ear
    blister —*see* Blister, ear
    bruise —*see* Contusion, ear
    contusion —*see* Contusion, ear
    external constriction —*see*
        Constriction, external, ear
    hematoma —*see* Hematoma, ear
    inner —*see* Injury, ear, middle
    laceration —*see* Laceration, ear
    middle S09.30-
      blast —*see* Injury, blast, ear
      specified NEC S09.39-
      puncture —*see* Puncture, ear
    superficial —*see* Injury, superficial, ear
  eighth cranial nerve (acoustic or
      auditory) —*see* Injury, nerve,
      acoustic

Injury *(Continued)*
  elbow S59.90-
    contusion —*see* Contusion, elbow
    dislocation —*see* Dislocation, elbow
    fracture —*see* Fracture, ulna, upper
        end
    open —*see* Wound, open, elbow
    specified NEC S59.80-
    sprain —*see* Sprain, elbow
    superficial —*see* Injury, superficial,
        elbow
  eleventh cranial nerve (accessory) —*see*
      Injury, nerve, accessory
  epididymis S39.94
  epigastric region S39.91
  epiglottis NEC S19.89
  esophageal plexus —*see* Injury, nerve,
      thorax, sympathetic
  esophagus (thoracic part) —*see also*
      Injury, intrathoracic, esophagus
    cervical NEC S19.85
  eustachian tube S09.91
  eye S05.9-
    avulsion S05.7-
    ball —*see* Injury, eyeball
    conjunctiva S05.0-
    cornea
      abrasion S05.0-
      laceration S05.3-
        with prolapse S05.2-
    lacrimal apparatus S05.8X-
    orbit penetration S05.4-
    specified site NEC S05.8X-
  eyeball S05.8X-
    contusion S05.1-
    penetrating S05.6-
      with
        foreign body S05.5-
        prolapse or loss of intraocular
            tissue S05.2-
        without prolapse or loss of
            intraocular tissue S05.3-
    specified type NEC S05.8-
  eyebrow S09.93
  eyelid S09.93
    abrasion —*see* Abrasion, eyelid
    contusion —*see* Contusion, eyelid
    open —*see* Wound, open, eyelid
  face S09.93
  fallopian tube S37.509
    bilateral S37.502
      blast injury S37.512
      contusion S37.522
      laceration S37.532
      specified type NEC S37.592
    blast injury (primary) S37.519
      bilateral S37.512
      secondary —*see* Injury, fallopian
          tube, specified type NEC
      unilateral S37.511
    contusion S37.529
      bilateral S37.522
      unilateral S37.521
    laceration S37.539
      bilateral S37.532
      unilateral S37.531
    specified type NEC S37.599
      bilateral S37.592
      unilateral S37.591
    unilateral S37.501
      blast injury S37.511
      contusion S37.521
      laceration S37.531
      specified type NEC S37.591

Injury (Continued)

fascia —see Injury, muscle

fifth cranial nerve (trigeminal) —see
Injury, nerve, trigeminal

finger (nail) S69.9-
blood vessel —see Injury, blood
vessel, finger
contusion —see Contusion, finger
dislocation —see Dislocation, finger
fracture —see Fracture, finger
muscle —see Injury, muscle, finger
nerve —see Injury, nerve, digital,
finger
open —see Wound, open, finger
specified NEC S69.8-
sprain —see Sprain, finger
superficial —see Injury, superficial,
finger

first cranial nerve (olfactory) —see
Injury, nerve, olfactory

flank —see Injury, abdomen

foot S99.92-
blood vessel —see Injury, blood
vessel, foot
contusion —see Contusion, foot
dislocation —see Dislocation, foot
fracture —see Fracture, foot
muscle —see Injury, muscle, foot
open —see Wound, open, foot
specified type NEC S99.82-
sprain —see Sprain, foot
superficial —see Injury, superficial,
foot

forceps NOS P15.9

forearm S59.91-
blood vessel —see Injury, blood
vessel, forearm
contusion —see Contusion, forearm
fracture —see Fracture, forearm
muscle —see Injury, muscle, forearm
nerve —see Injury, nerve, forearm
open —see Wound, open, forearm
specified NEC S59.81-
superficial —see Injury, superficial,
forearm

forehead S09.90

fourth cranial nerve (trochlear) —see
Injury, nerve, trochlear

gallbladder S36.129
contusion S36.122
laceration S36.123
specified NEC S36.128

ganglion
celiac, coeliac —see Injury, nerve,
lumbosacral, sympathetic
gasserian —see Injury, nerve,
trigeminal
stellate —see Injury, nerve, thorax,
sympathetic
thoracic sympathetic —see Injury,
nerve, thorax, sympathetic

gasserian ganglion —see Injury, nerve,
trigeminal

gastric artery —see Injury, blood vessel,
celiac artery, branch

gastroduodenal artery —see Injury,
blood vessel, celiac artery, branch

gastrointestinal tract —see Injury,
intra-abdominal
with open wound into abdominal
cavity —see Wound, open, with
penetration into peritoneal
cavity
colon —see Injury, intestine, large

Injury (Continued)

gastrointestinal tract (Continued)
rectum —see Injury, intestine, large,
rectum
with open wound into abdominal
cavity S36.61
small intestine —see Injury, intestine,
small
specified site NEC —see Injury, intra-
abdominal, specified, site NEC
stomach —see Injury, stomach

genital organ (s)
external S39.94
specified NEC S39.848
internal S37.90
fallopian tube —see Injury,
fallopian tube
ovary —see Injury, ovary
prostate —see Injury, prostate
seminal vesicle —see Injury, pelvis,
organ, specified site NEC
uterus —see Injury, uterus
vas deferens —see Injury, pelvis,
organ, specified site NEC
obstetrical trauma O71.9

gland
lacrimal laceration —see Injury, eye,
specified site NEC
salivary S09.90
thyroid NEC S19.84

globe (eye) S05.90
specified NEC S05.8X-

groin —see Injury, abdomen

gum S09.90

hand S69.9-
blood vessel —see Injury, blood
vessel, hand
contusion —see Contusion, hand
fracture —see Fracture, hand
muscle —see Injury, muscle, hand
nerve —see Injury, nerve, hand
open —see Wound, open, hand
specified NEC S69.8-
sprain —see Sprain, hand
superficial —see Injury, superficial,
hand

head S09.90
with loss of consciousness S06.9-
specified NEC S09.8-

heart S26.90
with hemopericardium S26.00
contusion S26.01
laceration (mild) S26.020
major S26.022
moderate S26.021
specified type NEC S26.09
without hemopericardium S26.10
contusion S26.11
laceration S26.12
specified type NEC S26.19
contusion S26.91
laceration S26.92
specified type NEC S26.99

heel —see Injury, foot

hepatic
artery —see Injury, blood vessel,
celiac artery, branch
duct —see Injury, liver
vein —see Injury, vena cava,
inferior

hip S79.91-
blood vessel —see Injury, blood
vessel, hip
contusion —see Contusion, hip

Injury (Continued)

hip (Continued)
dislocation —see Dislocation, hip
fracture —see Fracture, femur, neck
muscle —see Injury, muscle, hip
nerve —see Injury, nerve, hip
open —see Wound, open, hip
specified NEC S79.81-
sprain —see Sprain, hip
superficial —see Injury, superficial,
hip

hymen S39.94

hypogastric
blood vessel —see Injury, blood
vessel, iliac
plexus —see Injury, nerve,
lumbosacral, sympathetic

ileum —see Injury, intestine, small

iliac region S39.91

instrumental (during surgery) —
see Laceration, accidental
complicating surgery
birth injury —see Birth, injury
nonsurgical —see Injury, by site

obstetrical O71.9
bladder O71.5
cervix O71.3
high vaginal O71.4
perineal NOS O70.9
urethra O71.5
uterus O71.5
with rupture or perforation
O71.1

internal T14.8
aorta —see Injury, aorta
bladder (sphincter) —see Injury,
bladder
with
ectopic or molar pregnancy
O08.6
following ectopic or molar
pregnancy O08.6
obstetrical trauma O71.5
bronchus, bronchi —see Injury,
intrathoracic, bronchus
cecum —see Injury, intestine, large
cervix (uteri) —see also Injury, uterus
with ectopic or molar pregnancy
O08.6
following ectopic or molar
pregnancy O08.6
obstetrical trauma O71.3
chest —see Injury, intrathoracic
gastrointestinal tract —see Injury,
intra-abdominal
heart —see Injury, heart
intestine NEC —see Injury, intestine
intrauterine —see Injury, uterus
mesentery —see Injury, intra-
abdominal, specified, site NEC
pelvis, pelvic (organ) S37.90
following ectopic or molar
pregnancy (subsequent
episode) O08.6
obstetrical trauma NEC O71.5
rupture or perforation O71.1
specified NEC S39.83
rectum —see Injury, intestine, large,
rectum
stomach —see Injury, stomach
ureter —see Injury, ureter
urethra (sphincter) following ectopic
or molar pregnancy O08.6
uterus —see Injury, uterus

Injury *(Continued)*
  interscapular area —*see* Injury, thorax
  intestine
    large S36.509
      ascending (right) S36.500
        blast injury (primary)
          S36.510
          secondary S36.590
        contusion S36.520
        laceration S36.530
        specified type NEC S36.590
      blast injury (primary) S36.519
        ascending (right) S36.510
        descending (left) S36.512
        rectum S36.61
        sigmoid S36.513
        specified site NEC S36.518
        transverse S36.511
      contusion S36.529
        ascending (right) S36.520
        descending (left) S36.522
        rectum S36.62
        sigmoid S36.523
        specified site NEC S36.528
        transverse S36.521
      descending (left) S36.502
        blast injury (primary)
          S36.512
          secondary S36.592
        contusion S36.522
        laceration S36.532
        specified type NEC S36.592
      laceration S36.539
        ascending (right) S36.530
        descending (left) S36.532
        rectum S36.63
        sigmoid S36.533
        specified site NEC S36.538
        transverse S36.531
      rectum S36.60
        blast injury (primary) S36.61
          secondary S36.69
        contusion S36.62
        laceration S36.63
        specified type NEC S36.69
      sigmoid S36.503
        blast injury (primary) S36.513
          secondary S36.593
        contusion S36.523
        laceration S36.533
        specified type NEC S36.593
      specified
        site NEC S36.508
          blast injury (primary)
            S36.518
            secondary S36.598
          contusion S36.528
          laceration S36.538
          specified type NEC S36.598
        type NEC S36.599
          ascending (right) S36.590
          descending (left) S36.592
          rectum S36.69
          sigmoid S36.593
          specified site NEC S36.598
          transverse S36.591
      transverse S36.501
        blast injury (primary)
          S36.511
          secondary S36.591
        contusion S36.521
        laceration S36.531
        specified type NEC
          S36.591

Injury *(Continued)*
  intestine *(Continued)*
    small S36.409
      blast injury (primary) S36.419
        duodenum S36.410
        secondary S36.499
          duodenum S36.490
          specified site NEC S36.498
        specified site NEC S36.418
      contusion S36.429
        duodenum S36.420
        specified site NEC S36.428
      duodenum S36.400
        blast injury (primary) S36.410
          secondary S36.490
        contusion S36.420
        laceration S36.430
        specified NEC S36.490
      laceration S36.439
        duodenum S36.430
        specified site NEC S36.438
      specified
        site NEC S36.408
        type NEC S36.499
          duodenum S36.490
          specified site NEC S36.498
  intra-abdominal S36.90
    adrenal gland —*see* Injury, adrenal
      gland
    bladder —*see* Injury, bladder
    colon —*see* Injury, intestine, large
    contusion S36.92
    fallopian tube —*see* Injury, fallopian
      tube
    gallbladder —*see* Injury, gallbladder
    intestine —*see* Injury, intestine
    kidney —*see* Injury, kidney
    laceration S36.93
    liver —*see* Injury, liver
    ovary —*see* Injury, ovary
    pancreas —*see* Injury, pancreas
    pelvic NOS S37.90
    peritoneum —*see* Injury, intra-
      abdominal, specified, site NEC
    prostate —*see* Injury, prostate
    rectum —*see* Injury, intestine, large,
      rectum
    retroperitoneum —*see* Injury, intra-
      abdominal, specified,
      site NEC
    seminal vesicle —*see* Injury, pelvis,
      organ, specified
      site NEC
    small intestine —*see* Injury, intestine,
      small
    specified
      pelvic S37.90
        specified
          site NEC S37.899
            specified type NEC
              S37.898
            type NEC S37.99
      site NEC S36.899
        contusion S36.892
        laceration S36.893
        specified type NEC S36.898
      type NEC S36.99
    spleen —*see* Injury, spleen
    stomach —*see* Injury, stomach
    ureter —*see* Injury, ureter
    urethra —*see* Injury, urethra
    uterus —*see* Injury, uterus
    vas deferens —*see* Injury, pelvis,
      organ, specified site NEC

Injury *(Continued)*
  intracranial (traumatic) S06.9-
    cerebellar hemorrhage, traumatic —
      see Injury, intracranial, focal
    cerebral edema, traumatic S06.1X-
      diffuse S06.1X-
      focal S06.1X-
    diffuse (axonal) S06.2X-
    epidural hemorrhage (traumatic)
      S06.4X-
    focal brain injury S06.30-
      contusion —*see* Contusion,
        cerebral
      laceration —*see* Laceration,
        cerebral
    intracerebral hemorrhage, traumatic
      S06.36-
      left side S06.35-
      right side S06.34-
    subarachnoid hemorrhage, traumatic
      S06.6X-
    subdural hemorrhage, traumatic
      S06.5X-
  intraocular —*see* Injury, eyeball,
    penetrating
  intrathoracic S27.9
    bronchus S27.409
      bilateral S27.402
      blast injury (primary) S27.419
        bilateral S27.412
        secondary —*see* Injury,
          intrathoracic, bronchus,
          specified type NEC
        unilateral S27.411
      contusion S27.429
        bilateral S27.422
        unilateral S27.421
      laceration S27.439
        bilateral S27.432
        unilateral S27.431
      specified type NEC S27.499
        bilateral S27.492
        unilateral S27.491
      unilateral S27.401
    diaphragm S27.809
      contusion S27.802
      laceration S27.803
      specified type NEC S27.808
    esophagus (thoracic) S27.819
      contusion S27.812
      laceration S27.813
      specified type NEC S27.818
    heart —*see* Injury, heart
    hemopneumothorax S27.2
    hemothorax S27.1
    lung S27.309
      aspiration J69.0
      bilateral S27.302
      blast injury (primary) S27.319
        bilateral S27.312
        secondary —*see* Injury,
          intrathoracic, lung,
          specified type NEC
        unilateral S27.311
      contusion S27.329
        bilateral S27.322
        unilateral S27.321
      laceration S27.339
        bilateral S27.332
        unilateral S27.331
      specified type NEC S27.399
        bilateral S27.392
        unilateral S27.391
      unilateral S27.301

Injury *(Continued)*
  muscle *(Continued)*
    finger *(Continued)*
      little *(Continued)*
        extensor *(Continued)*
          laceration S56.42-
          specified type NEC S56.49-
          strain S56.41-
        flexor (forearm level)
          hand level S66.10-
            laceration S66.12-
            specified type NEC S66.19-
            strain S66.11-
          laceration S56.12-
          specified type NEC S56.19-
          strain S56.11-
        intrinsic S66.50-
          laceration S66.52-
          specified type NEC S66.59-
          strain S66.51-
      middle
        extensor (forearm level)
          hand level S66.30-
            laceration S66.32-
            specified type NEC S66.39-
            strain S66.31-
          laceration S56.42-
          specified type NEC S56.49-
          strain S56.41-
        flexor (forearm level)
          hand level S66.10-
            laceration S66.12-
            specified type NEC S66.19-
            strain S66.11-
          laceration S56.12-
          specified type NEC S56.19-
          strain S56.11-
        intrinsic S66.50-
          laceration S66.52-
          specified type NEC S66.59-
          strain S66.51-
      ring
        extensor (forearm level)
          hand level S66.30-
            laceration S66.32-
            specified type NEC S66.39-
            strain S66.31-
          laceration S56.42-
          specified type NEC S56.49-
          strain S56.41-
        flexor (forearm level)
          hand level S66.10-
            laceration S66.12-
            specified type NEC
              S66.19-
            strain S66.11-
          laceration S56.12-
          specified type NEC S56.19-
          strain S56.11-
        intrinsic S66.50-
          laceration S66.52-
          specified type NEC S66.59-
          strain S66.51-
    flexor
      finger (s) (other than thumb) —
        see Injury, muscle, finger
      forearm level, specified NEC —
        see Injury, muscle, forearm,
        flexor
      thumb —*see* Injury, muscle, thumb,
        flexor
      toe (long) (ankle level) (foot
        level) —*see* Injury, muscle, toe,
        flexor

Injury *(Continued)*
  muscle *(Continued)*
    foot S96.90-
      intrinsic S96.20-
        laceration S96.22-
        specified type NEC S96.29-
        strain S96.21-
      laceration S96.92-
      long extensor, toe —*see* Injury,
        muscle, toe, extensor
      long flexor, toe —*see* Injury, muscle,
        toe, flexor
      specified
        site NEC S96.80-
          laceration S96.82-
          specified type NEC S96.89-
          strain S96.81-
        type NEC S96.99-
      strain S96.91-
    forearm (level) S56.90-
      extensor S56.50-
        laceration S56.52-
        specified type NEC S56.59-
        strain S56.51-
      flexor S56.20-
        laceration S56.22-
        specified type NEC S56.29-
        strain S56.21-
      laceration S56.92-
      specified S56.99-
        site NEC S56.80-
          laceration S56.82-
          strain S56.81-
        type NEC S56.89-
      strain S56.91-
    hand (level) S66.90-
      laceration S66.92-
      specified
        site NEC S66.80-
          laceration S66.82-
          specified type NEC S66.89-
          strain S66.81-
        type NEC S66.99-
      strain S66.91-
    head S09.10
      laceration S09.12
      specified type NEC S09.19
      strain S09.11
    hip NEC S76.00-
      laceration S76.02-
      specified type NEC S76.09-
      strain S76.01-
    intrinsic
      ankle and foot level —*see* Injury,
        muscle, foot, intrinsic
      finger (other than thumb) —*see*
        Injury, muscle, finger by site,
        intrinsic
      foot (level) —*see* Injury, muscle,
        foot, intrinsic
      thumb —*see* Injury, muscle, thumb,
        intrinsic
    leg (level) (lower) S86.90-
      Achilles tendon —*see* Injury,
        Achilles tendon
      anterior muscle group —*see* Injury,
        muscle, anterior muscle group
      laceration S86.92-
      peroneal muscle group —*see* Injury,
        muscle, peroneal muscle
        group
      posterior muscle group —*see*
        Injury, muscle, posterior
        muscle group, leg level

Injury *(Continued)*
  muscle *(Continued)*
    leg *(Continued)*
      specified
        site NEC S86.80-
          laceration S86.82-
          specified type NEC S86.89-
          strain S86.81-
        type NEC S86.99-
      strain S86.91-
    long
      extensor toe, at ankle and foot
        level —*see* Injury, muscle, toe,
        extensor
      flexor, toe, at ankle and foot
        level —*see* Injury, muscle, toe,
        flexor
      head, biceps —*see* Injury, muscle,
        biceps, long head
    lower back S39.002
      laceration S39.022
      specified type NEC S39.092
      strain S39.012
    neck (level) S16.9
      laceration S16.2
      specified type NEC S16.8
      strain S16.1
    pelvis S39.003
      laceration S39.023
      specified type NEC S39.093
      strain S39.013
    peroneal muscle group, at leg level
      (lower) S86.30-
      laceration S86.32-
      specified type NEC S86.39-
      strain S86.31-
    posterior muscle (group)
      leg level (lower) S86.10-
        laceration S86.12-
        specified type NEC S86.19-
        strain S86.11-
      thigh level S76.30-
        laceration S76.32-
        specified type NEC S76.39-
        strain S76.31-
    quadriceps (thigh) S76.10-
      laceration S76.12-
      specified type NEC S76.19-
      strain S76.11-
    shoulder S46.90-
      laceration S46.92-
      rotator cuff —*see* Injury, rotator cuff
      specified site NEC S46.80-
        laceration S46.82-
        specified type NEC S46.89-
        strain S46.81-
      specified type NEC S46.99-
      strain S46.91-
    thigh NEC (level) S76.90-
      adductor —*see* Injury, muscle,
        adductor, thigh
      laceration S76.92-
      posterior muscle (group) —*see*
        Injury, muscle, posterior
        muscle, thigh level
      quadriceps —*see* Injury, muscle,
        quadriceps
      specified
        site NEC S76.80-
          laceration S76.82-
          specified type NEC S76.89-
          strain S76.81-
        type NEC S76.99-
      strain S76.91-

Injury *(Continued)*
  muscle *(Continued)*
    thorax (level) S29.009
      back wall S29.002
      front wall S29.001
      laceration S29.029
        back wall S29.022
        front wall S29.021
      specified type NEC S29.099
        back wall S29.092
        front wall S29.091
      strain S29.019
        back wall S29.012
        front wall S29.011
    thumb
      abductor (forearm level) S56.30-
        laceration S56.32-
        specified type NEC S56.39-
        strain S56.31-
      extensor (forearm level) S56.30-
        hand level S66.20-
          laceration S66.22-
          specified type NEC S66.29-
          strain S66.21-
        laceration S56.32-
        specified type NEC S56.39-
        strain S56.31-
      flexor (forearm level) S56.00-
        hand level S66.00-
          laceration S66.02-
          specified type NEC S66.09-
          strain S66.01-
        laceration S56.02-
        specified type NEC S56.09-
        strain S56.01-
        wrist level —*see* Injury, muscle,
          thumb, flexor, hand level
      intrinsic S66.40-
        laceration S66.42-
        specified type NEC S66.49-
        strain S66.41-
    toe —*see also* Injury, muscle, foot
      extensor, long S96.10-
        laceration S96.12-
        specified type NEC S96.19-
        strain S96.11-
      flexor, long S96.00-
        laceration S96.02-
        specified type NEC S96.09-
        strain S96.01-
    triceps S46.30-
      laceration S46.32-
      specified type NEC S46.39-
      strain S46.31-
    wrist (and hand) level —*see* Injury,
      muscle, hand
  musculocutaneous nerve —*see* Injury,
    nerve, musculocutaneous
  myocardium —*see* Injury, heart
  nape —*see* Injury, neck
  nasal (septum) (sinus) S09.92
  nasopharynx S09.92
  neck S19.9
    specified NEC S19.80
      specified site NEC S19.89
  nerve NEC T14.8
    abdomen S34.9
      peripheral S34.6
      specified site NEC S34.8
    abducens S04.4-
      contusion S04.4-
      laceration S04.4-
      specified type NEC S04.4-
    abducent —*see* Injury, nerve,
      abducens

Injury *(Continued)*
  nerve NEC *(Continued)*
    accessory S04.7-
      contusion S04.7-
      laceration S04.7-
      specified type NEC S04.7-
    acoustic S04.6-
      contusion S04.6-
      laceration S04.6-
      specified type NEC S04.6-
    ankle S94.9-
      cutaneous sensory S94.3-
      specified site NEC —*see*
        subcategory S94.8
    anterior crural, femoral —*see* Injury,
      nerve, femoral
    arm (upper) S44.9-
      axillary —*see* Injury, nerve, axillary
      cutaneous —*see* Injury, nerve,
        cutaneous, arm
      median —*see* Injury, nerve, median,
        upper arm
      musculocutaneous —*see* Injury,
        nerve, musculocutaneous
      radial —*see* Injury, nerve, radial,
        upper arm
      specified site NEC —*see*
        subcategory S44.8
      ulnar —*see* Injury, nerve, ulnar, arm
    auditory —*see* Injury, nerve, acoustic
    axillary S44.3-
    brachial plexus —*see* Injury, brachial
      plexus
    cervical sympathetic S14.5
    cranial S04.9
      contusion S04.9
      eighth (acoustic or auditory) —*see*
        Injury, nerve, acoustic
      eleventh (accessory) —*see* Injury,
        nerve, accessory
      fifth (trigeminal) —*see* Injury,
        nerve, trigeminal
      first (olfactory) —*see* Injury, nerve,
        olfactory
      fourth (trochlear) —*see* Injury,
        nerve, trochlear
      laceration S04.9
      ninth (glossopharyngeal) —*see*
        Injury, nerve, glossopharyngeal
      second (optic) —*see* Injury, nerve,
        optic
      seventh (facial) —*see* Injury, nerve,
        facial
      sixth (abducent) —*see* Injury, nerve,
        abducens
      specified
        nerve NEC S04.89-
          contusion S04.89-
          laceration S04.89-
          specified type NEC S04.89-
        type NEC S04.9
      tenth (pneumogastric or vagus) —
        see Injury, nerve, vagus
      third (oculomotor) —*see* Injury,
        nerve, oculomotor
      twelfth (hypoglossal) —*see* Injury,
        nerve, hypoglossal
    cutaneous sensory
      ankle (level) S94.3-
      arm (upper) (level) S44.5-
      foot (level) —*see* Injury, nerve,
        cutaneous sensory, ankle
      forearm (level) S54.3-
      hip (level) S74.2-

Injury *(Continued)*
  nerve NEC *(Continued)*
    cutaneous sensory *(Continued)*
      leg (lower level) S84.2-
      shoulder (level) —*see* Injury, nerve,
        cutaneous sensory, arm
      thigh (level) —*see* Injury, nerve,
        cutaneous sensory, hip
    deep peroneal —*see* Injury, nerve,
      peroneal, foot
    digital
      finger S64.4-
        index S64.49-
        little S64.49-
        middle S64.49-
        ring S64.49-
        thumb S64.3-
      toe —*see* Injury, nerve, ankle,
        specified site NEC
    eighth cranial (acoustic or
      auditory) —*see* Injury, nerve,
      acoustic
    eleventh cranial (accessory) —*see*
      Injury, nerve, accessory
    facial S04.5-
      contusion S04.5-
      laceration S04.5-
      newborn P11.3
      specified type NEC S04.5-
    femoral (hip level) (thigh level) S74.1-
    fifth cranial (trigeminal) —*see* Injury,
      nerve, trigeminal
    finger (digital) —*see* Injury, nerve,
      digital, finger
    first cranial (olfactory) —*see* Injury,
      nerve, olfactory
    foot S94.9-
      cutaneous sensory S94.3-
      deep peroneal S94.2-
      lateral plantar S94.0-
      medial plantar S94.1-
      specified site NEC —*see*
        subcategory S94.8
    forearm (level) S54.9-
      cutaneous sensory —*see* Injury,
        nerve, cutaneous sensory,
        forearm
      median —*see* Injury, nerve, median
      radial —*see* Injury, nerve, radial
      specified site NEC —*see*
        subcategory S54.8
      ulnar —*see* Injury, nerve, ulnar
    fourth cranial (trochlear) —*see* Injury,
      nerve, trochlear
    glossopharyngeal S04.89-
      specified type NEC S04.89-
    hand S64.9-
      median —*see* Injury, nerve, median,
        hand
      radial —*see* Injury, nerve, radial,
        hand
      specified NEC —*see* subcategory
        S64.8
      ulnar —*see* Injury, nerve, ulnar,
        hand
    hip (level) S74.9-
      cutaneous sensory —*see* Injury,
        nerve, cutaneous sensory, hip
      femoral —*see* Injury, nerve, femoral
      sciatic —*see* Injury, nerve, sciatic
      specified site NEC —*see*
        subcategory S74.8
    hypoglossal S04.89-
      specified type NEC S04.89-

Injury *(Continued)*
  nerve NEC *(Continued)*
    lateral plantar S94.0-
    leg (lower) S84.9-
      cutaneous sensory —*see* Injury,
        nerve, cutaneous sensory, leg
      peroneal —*see* Injury, nerve,
        peroneal
      specified site NEC —*see*
        subcategory S84.8
      tibial —*see* Injury, nerve, tibial
      upper —*see* Injury, nerve, thigh
    lower
      back —*see* Injury, nerve, abdomen,
        specified site NEC
        peripheral —*see* Injury, nerve,
          abdomen, peripheral
      limb —*see* Injury, nerve, leg
    lumbar plexus —*see* Injury, nerve,
      lumbosacral, sympathetic
    lumbar spinal —*see* Injury, nerve,
      spinal, lumbar
    lumbosacral
      plexus —*see* Injury, nerve,
        lumbosacral, sympathetic
      sympathetic S34.5
    medial plantar S94.1-
    median (forearm level) S54.1-
      hand (level) S64.1-
      upper arm (level) S44.1-
      wrist (level) —*see* Injury, nerve,
        median, hand
    musculocutaneous S44.4-
    musculospiral (upper arm level) —*see*
      Injury, nerve, radial, upper arm
    neck S14.9
      peripheral S14.4
      specified site NEC S14.8
      sympathetic S14.5
    ninth cranial (glossopharyngeal) —*see*
      Injury, nerve, glossopharyngeal
    oculomotor S04.1-
      contusion S04.1-
      laceration S04.1-
      specified type NEC S04.1-
    olfactory S04.81-
      specified type NEC S04.81-
    optic S04.01-
      contusion S04.01-
      laceration S04.01-
      specified type NEC S04.01-
    pelvic girdle —*see* Injury, nerve,
      hip
    pelvis —*see* Injury, nerve, abdomen,
      specified site NEC
      peripheral —*see* Injury, nerve,
        abdomen, peripheral
    peripheral NEC T14.8
      abdomen —*see* Injury, nerve,
        abdomen, peripheral
      lower back —*see* Injury, nerve,
        abdomen, peripheral
      neck —*see* Injury, nerve, neck,
        peripheral
      pelvis —*see* Injury, nerve,
        abdomen, peripheral
      specified NEC T14.8
    peroneal (lower leg level) S84.1-
      foot S94.2-
    plexus
      brachial —*see* Injury, brachial
        plexus
      celiac, coeliac —*see* Injury, nerve,
        lumbosacral, sympathetic

Injury *(Continued)*
  nerve NEC *(Continued)*
    plexus *(Continued)*
      mesenteric, inferior —*see*
        Injury, nerve, lumbosacral,
        sympathetic
      sacral —*see* Injury, lumbosacral
        plexus
      spinal
        brachial —*see* Injury, brachial
          plexus
        lumbosacral —*see* Injury,
          lumbosacral plexus
      pneumogastric —*see* Injury, nerve,
        vagus
    radial (forearm level) S54.2-
      hand (level) S64.2-
      upper arm (level) S44.2-
      wrist (level) —*see* Injury, nerve,
        radial, hand
    root —*see* Injury, nerve, spinal, root
    sacral plexus —*see* Injury,
      lumbosacral plexus
    sacral spinal —*see* Injury, nerve,
      spinal, sacral
    sciatic (hip level) (thigh level) S74.0-
    second cranial (optic) —*see* Injury,
      nerve, optic
    seventh cranial (facial) —*see* Injury,
      nerve, facial
    shoulder —*see* Injury, nerve, arm
    sixth cranial (abducent) —*see* Injury,
      nerve, abducens
    spinal
      plexus —*see* Injury, nerve, plexus,
        spinal
      root
        cervical S14.2
        dorsal S24.2
        lumbar S34.21
        sacral S34.22
        thoracic —*see* Injury, nerve,
          spinal, root, dorsal
    splanchnic —*see* Injury, nerve,
      lumbosacral, sympathetic
    sympathetic NEC —*see* Injury, nerve,
      lumbosacral, sympathetic
      cervical —*see* Injury, nerve, cervical
        sympathetic
    tenth cranial (pneumogastric or
      vagus) —*see* Injury, nerve,
      vagus
    thigh (level) —*see* Injury, nerve, hip
      cutaneous sensory —*see* Injury,
        nerve, cutaneous sensory, hip
      femoral —*see* Injury, nerve, femoral
      sciatic —*see* Injury, nerve, sciatic
      specified NEC —*see* Injury, nerve,
        hip
    third cranial (oculomotor) —*see*
      Injury, nerve, oculomotor
    thorax S24.9
      peripheral S24.3
      specified site NEC S24.8
      sympathetic S24.4
    thumb, digital —*see* Injury, nerve,
      digital, thumb
    tibial (lower leg level) (posterior)
      S84.0-
    toe —*see* Injury, nerve, ankle
    trigeminal S04.3-
      contusion S04.3-
      laceration S04.3-
      specified type NEC S04.3-

Injury *(Continued)*
  nerve NEC *(Continued)*
    trochlear S04.2-
      contusion S04.2-
      laceration S04.2-
      specified type NEC S04.2-
    twelfth cranial (hypoglossal) —*see*
      Injury, nerve, hypoglossal
    ulnar (forearm level) S54.0-
      arm (upper) (level) S44.0-
      hand (level) S64.0-
      wrist (level) —*see* Injury, nerve,
        ulnar, hand
    vagus S04.89-
      specified type NEC S04.89-
      wrist (level) —*see* Injury, nerve,
        hand
    ninth cranial nerve
      (glossopharyngeal) —*see* Injury,
      nerve, glossopharyngeal
    nose (septum) S09.92
    obstetrical O71.9
      specified NEC O71.89
    occipital (region) (scalp) S09.90
      lobe —*see* Injury, intracranial
    optic chiasm S04.02
    optic radiation S04.03-
    optic tract and pathways S04.03-
    orbit, orbital (region) —*see* Injury, eye
      penetrating (with foreign body) —*see*
        Injury, eye, orbit, penetrating
      specified NEC —*see* Injury, eye,
        specified site NEC
    ovary, ovarian S37.409
      bilateral S37.402
        contusion S37.422
        laceration S37.432
        specified type NEC S37.492
      blood vessel —*see* Injury, blood
        vessel, ovarian
      contusion S37.429
        bilateral S37.422
        unilateral S37.421
      laceration S37.439
        bilateral S37.432
        unilateral S37.431
      specified type NEC S37.499
        bilateral S37.492
        unilateral S37.491
      unilateral S37.401
        contusion S37.421
        laceration S37.431
        specified type NEC S37.491
    palate (hard) (soft) S09.93
    pancreas S36.209
      body S36.201
        contusion S36.221
        laceration S36.231
          major S36.261
          minor S36.241
          moderate S36.251
        specified type NEC S36.291
      contusion S36.229
      head S36.200
        contusion S36.220
        laceration S36.230
          major S36.260
          minor S36.240
          moderate S36.250
        specified type NEC S36.290
      laceration S36.239
        major S36.269
        minor S36.249
        moderate S36.259

Injury *(Continued)*
  pancreas *(Continued)*
    specified type NEC S36.299
    tail S36.202
      contusion S36.222
      laceration S36.232
        major S36.262
        minor S36.242
        moderate S36.252
      specified type NEC S36.292
  parietal (region) (scalp) S09.90
    lobe —*see* Injury, intracranial
  patellar ligament (tendon) S76.10-
    laceration S76.12-
    specified NEC S76.19-
    strain S76.11-
  pelvis, pelvic (floor) S39.93
    complicating delivery O70.1
    joint or ligament, complicating
        delivery O71.6
    organ S37.90
      with ectopic or molar pregnancy
          O08.6
      complication of abortion —*see*
          Abortion
      contusion S37.92
      following ectopic or molar
          pregnancy O08.6
      laceration S37.93
      obstetrical trauma NEC O71.5
      specified
        site NEC S37.899
          contusion S37.892
          laceration S37.893
          specified type NEC S37.898
        type NEC S37.99
    specified NEC S39.83
  penis S39.94
  perineum S39.94
  peritoneum —*see* Injury, intra-
      abdominal, specified site NEC
  periurethral tissue —*see* Injury, urethra
    complicating delivery O71.82
  phalanges
    foot —*see* Injury, foot
    hand —*see* Injury, hand
  pharynx NEC S19.85
  pleura —*see* Injury, intrathoracic, pleura
  plexus
    brachial —*see* Injury, brachial plexus
    cardiac —*see* Injury, nerve, thorax,
        sympathetic
    celiac, coeliac —*see* Injury, nerve,
        lumbosacral, sympathetic
    esophageal —*see* Injury, nerve,
        thorax, sympathetic
    hypogastric —*see* Injury, nerve,
        lumbosacral, sympathetic
    lumbar, lumbosacral —*see* Injury,
        lumbosacral plexus
    mesenteric —*see* Injury, nerve,
        lumbosacral, sympathetic
    pulmonary —*see* Injury, nerve,
        thorax, sympathetic
  postcardiac surgery (syndrome) I97.0
  prepuce S39.94
  prostate S37.829
    contusion S37.822
    laceration S37.823
    specified type NEC S37.828
  pubic region S39.94
  pudendum S39.94
  pulmonary plexus —*see* Injury, nerve,
      thorax, sympathetic

Injury *(Continued)*
  rectovaginal septum NEC S39.83
  rectum —*see* Injury, intestine, large,
      rectum
  retina —*see* Injury, eye, specified site
      NEC
    penetrating —*see* Injury, eyeball,
        penetrating
  retroperitoneal —*see* Injury, intra-
      abdominal, specified site NEC
  rotator cuff (muscle (s)) (tendon (s))
      S46.00-
    laceration S46.02-
    specified type NEC S46.09-
    strain S46.01-
  round ligament —*see* Injury, pelvic
      organ, specified site NEC
  sacral plexus —*see* Injury, lumbosacral
      plexus
  salivary duct or gland S09.93
  scalp S09.90
    newborn (birth injury) P12.9
      due to monitoring (electrode)
          (sampling incision) P12.4
      specified NEC P12.89
        caput succedaneum P12.81
  scapular region —*see* Injury, shoulder
  sclera —*see* Injury, eye, specified site
      NEC
    penetrating —*see* Injury, eyeball,
        penetrating
  scrotum S39.94
  second cranial nerve (optic) —*see* Injury,
      nerve, optic
  seminal vesicle —*see* Injury, pelvic
      organ, specified site NEC
  seventh cranial nerve (facial) —*see*
      Injury, nerve, facial
  shoulder S49.9-
    blood vessel —*see* Injury, blood
        vessel, arm
    contusion —*see* Contusion, shoulder
    dislocation —*see* Dislocation,
        shoulder
    fracture —*see* Fracture, shoulder
    muscle —*see* Injury, muscle,
        shoulder
    nerve —*see* Injury, nerve, shoulder
    open —*see* Wound, open, shoulder
    specified type NEC S49.8-
    sprain —*see* Sprain, shoulder girdle
    superficial —*see* Injury, superficial,
        shoulder
  sinus
    cavernous —*see* Injury, intracranial
    nasal S09.92
  sixth cranial nerve (abducent) —*see*
      Injury, nerve, abducens
  skeleton, birth injury P13.9
    specified part NEC P13.8
  skin NEC T14.8
    surface intact —*see* Injury, superficial
  skull NEC S09.90
  specified NEC T14.8
  spermatic cord (pelvic region) S37.898
    scrotal region S39.848
  spinal (cord)
    cervical (neck) S14.109
      anterior cord syndrome S14.139
        C1 level S14.131
        C2 level S14.132
        C3 level S14.133
        C4 level S14.134
        C5 level S14.135

Injury *(Continued)*
  spinal *(Continued)*
    cervical *(Continued)*
      anterior cord syndrome
          (Continued)
        C6 level S14.136
        C7 level S14.137
        C8 level S14.138
      Brown-Séquard syndrome
          S14.149
        C1 level S14.141
        C2 level S14.142
        C3 level S14.143
        C4 level S14.144
        C5 level S14.145
        C6 level S14.146
        C7 level S14.147
        C8 level S14.148
      C1 level S14.101
      C2 level S14.102
      C3 level S14.103
      C4 level S14.104
      C5 level S14.105
      C6 level S14.106
      C7 level S14.107
      C8 level S14.108
      central cord syndrome S14.129
        C1 level S14.121
        C2 level S14.122
        C3 level S14.123
        C4 level S14.124
        C5 level S14.125
        C6 level S14.126
        C7 level S14.127
        C8 level S14.128
      complete lesion S14.119
        C1 level S14.111
        C2 level S14.112
        C3 level S14.113
        C4 level S14.114
        C5 level S14.115
        C6 level S14.116
        C7 level S14.117
        C8 level S14.118
      concussion S14.0
      edema S14.0
      incomplete lesion specified NEC
          S14.159
        C1 level S14.151
        C2 level S14.152
        C3 level S14.153
        C4 level S14.154
        C5 level S14.155
        C6 level S14.156
        C7 level S14.157
        C8 level S14.158
      posterior cord syndrome S14.159
        C1 level S14.151
        C2 level S14.152
        C3 level S14.153
        C4 level S14.154
        C5 level S14.155
        C6 level S14.156
        C7 level S14.157
        C8 level S14.158
    dorsal —*see* Injury, spinal, thoracic
    lumbar S34.109
      complete lesion S34.119
        L1 level S34.111
        L2 level S34.112
        L3 level S34.113
        L4 level S34.114
        L5 level S34.115
      concussion S34.01

321

Injury *(Continued)*
  spinal *(Continued)*
    lumbar *(Continued)*
      edema S34.01
      incomplete lesion S34.129
        L1 level S34.121
        L2 level S34.122
        L3 level S34.123
        L4 level S34.124
        L5 level S34.125
        L1 level S34.101
        L2 level S34.102
        L3 level S34.103
        L4 level S34.104
        L5 level S34.105
    nerve root NEC
      cervical —*see* Injury, nerve, spinal,
        root, cervical
      dorsal —*see* Injury, nerve, spinal,
        root, dorsal
      lumbar S34.21
      sacral S34.22
      thoracic —*see* Injury, nerve, spinal,
        root, dorsal
    plexus
      brachial —*see* Injury, brachial
        plexus
      lumbosacral —*see* Injury,
        lumbosacral plexus
    sacral S34.139
      complete lesion S34.131
      incomplete lesion S34.132
    thoracic S24.109
      anterior cord syndrome
        S24.139
        T1 level S24.131
        T2-T6 level S24.132
        T7-T10 level S24.133
        T11-T12 level S24.134
      Brown-Séquard syndrome
        S24.149
        T1 level S24.141
        T2-T6 level S24.142
        T7-T10 level S24.143
        T11-T12 level S24.144
      complete lesion S24.119
        T1 level S24.111
        T2-T6 level S24.112
        T7-T10 level S24.113
        T11-T12 level S24.114
      concussion S24.0
      edema S24.0
      incomplete lesion specified NEC
        S24.159
        T1 level S24.151
        T2-T6 level S24.152
        T7-T10 level S24.153
        T11-T12 level S24.154
      posterior cord syndrome
        S24.159
        T1 level S24.151
        T2-T6 level S24.152
        T7-T10 level S24.153
        T11-T12 level S24.154
        T1 level S24.101
        T2-T6 level S24.102
        T7-T10 level S24.103
        T11-T12 level S24.104
  splanchnic nerve —*see* Injury, nerve,
    lumbosacral, sympathetic
  spleen S36.00
    contusion S36.029
      major S36.021
      minor S36.020

Injury *(Continued)*
  spleen *(Continued)*
    laceration S36.039
      major (massive) (stellate) S36.032
      moderate S36.031
      superficial (capsular) (minor)
        S36.030
    specified type NEC S36.09
  splenic artery —*see* Injury, blood vessel,
    celiac artery, branch
  stellate ganglion —*see* Injury, nerve,
    thorax, sympathetic
  sternal region S29.9
  stomach S36.30
    contusion S36.32
    laceration S36.33
    specified type NEC S36.39
  subconjunctival —*see* Injury, eye,
    conjunctiva
  subcutaneous NEC T14.8
  submaxillary region S09.93
  submental region S09.93
  subungual
    fingers —*see* Injury, hand
    toes —*see* Injury, foot
  superficial NEC T14.8
    abdomen, abdominal (wall) S30.92
      abrasion S30.811
      bite S30.871
        insect S30.861
      contusion S30.1
      external constriction S30.841
      foreign body S30.851
    abrasion —*see* Abrasion, by site
    adnexa, eye NEC —*see* Injury, eye,
      specified site NEC
    alveolar process —*see* Injury,
      superficial, oral cavity
    ankle S90.91-
      abrasion —*see* Abrasion, ankle
      bite —*see* Bite, ankle
      blister —*see* Blister, ankle
      contusion —*see* Contusion, ankle
      external constriction —*see*
        Constriction, external, ankle
      foreign body —*see* Foreign body,
        superficial, ankle
    anus S30.98
    arm (upper) S40.92-
      abrasion —*see* Abrasion, arm
      bite —*see* Bite, superficial, arm
      blister —*see* Blister, arm (upper)
      contusion —*see* Contusion, arm
      external constriction —*see*
        Constriction, external, arm
      foreign body —*see* Foreign body,
        superficial, arm
    auditory canal (external) (meatus) —
      see Injury, superficial, ear
    auricle —*see* Injury, superficial, ear
    axilla —*see* Injury, superficial, arm
    back —*see also* Injury, superficial,
      thorax, back
      lower S30.91
        abrasion S30.810
        contusion S30.0
        external constriction S30.840
        superficial
          bite NEC S30.870
            insect S30.860
          foreign body S30.850
    bite NEC —*see* Bite, superficial NEC,
      by site
    blister —*see* Blister, by site

Injury *(Continued)*
  superficial NEC *(Continued)*
    breast S20.10-
      abrasion —*see* Abrasion, breast
      bite —*see* Bite, superficial, breast
      contusion —*see* Contusion, breast
      external constriction —*see*
        Constriction, external,
        breast
      foreign body —*see* Foreign body,
        superficial, breast
    brow —*see* Injury, superficial, head,
      specified NEC
    buttock S30.91
    calf —*see* Injury, superficial, leg
    canthus, eye —*see* Injury, superficial,
      periocular area
    cheek (external) —*see* Injury,
      superficial, head, specified
      NEC
      internal —*see* Injury, superficial,
        oral cavity
    chest wall —*see* Injury, superficial,
      thorax
    chin —*see* Injury, superficial, head
      NEC
    clitoris S30.95
    conjunctiva —*see* Injury, eye,
      conjunctiva
      with foreign body (in conjunctival
        sac) —*see* Foreign body,
        conjunctival sac
    contusion —*see* Contusion, by site
    costal region —*see* Injury, superficial,
      thorax
    digit (s)
      hand —*see* Injury, superficial,
        finger
    ear (auricle) (canal) (external)
      S00.40-
      abrasion —*see* Abrasion, ear
      bite —*see* Bite, superficial, ear
      contusion —*see* Contusion, ear
      external constriction —*see*
        Constriction, external, ear
      foreign body —*see* Foreign body,
        superficial, ear
    elbow S50.90-
      abrasion —*see* Abrasion, elbow
      bite —*see* Bite, superficial, elbow
      blister —*see* Blister, elbow
      contusion —*see* Contusion, elbow
      external constriction —*see*
        Constriction, external, elbow
      foreign body —*see* Foreign body,
        superficial, elbow
    epididymis S30.94
    epigastric region S30.92
    epiglottis —*see* Injury, superficial,
      throat
    esophagus
      cervical —*see* Injury, superficial,
        throat
    external constriction —*see*
      Constriction, external, by site
    extremity NEC T14.8
    eyeball NEC —*see* Injury, eye,
      specified site NEC
    eyebrow —*see* Injury, superficial,
      periocular area
    eyelid S00.20-
      abrasion —*see* Abrasion, eyelid
      bite —*see* Bite, superficial, eyelid
      contusion —*see* Contusion, eyelid

Injury (Continued)
   superficial NEC (Continued)
      eyelid (Continued)
         external constriction —see
            Constriction, external, eyelid
         foreign body —see Foreign body,
            superficial, eyelid
      face NEC —see Injury, superficial,
         head, specified NEC
      finger (s) S60.949
         abrasion —see Abrasion, finger
         bite —see Bite, superficial, finger
         blister —see Blister, finger
         contusion —see Contusion, finger
         external constriction —see
            Constriction, external, finger
         foreign body —see Foreign body,
            superficial, finger
         index S60.94-
         insect bite —see Bite, by site,
            superficial, insect
         little S60.94-
         middle S60.94-
         ring S60.94-
      flank S30.92
      foot S90.92-
         abrasion —see Abrasion, foot
         bite —see Bite, foot
         blister —see Blister, foot
         contusion —see Contusion, foot
         external constriction —see
            Constriction, external, foot
         foreign body —see Foreign body,
            superficial, foot
      forearm S50.91-
         abrasion —see Abrasion, forearm
         bite —see Bite, forearm, superficial
         blister —see Blister, forearm
         contusion —see Contusion, forearm
         elbow only —see Injury, superficial,
            elbow
         external constriction —see
            Constriction, external,
            forearm
         foreign body —see Foreign body,
            superficial, forearm
      forehead —see Injury, superficial,
         head NEC
      foreign body —see Foreign body,
         superficial
      genital organs, external
         female S30.97
         male S30.96
      globe (eye) —see Injury, eye, specified
         site NEC
      groin S30.92
      gum —see Injury, superficial, oral
         cavity
      hand S60.92-
         abrasion —see Abrasion, hand
         bite —see Bite, superficial, hand
         contusion —see Contusion, hand
         external constriction —see
            Constriction, external, hand
         foreign body —see Foreign body,
            superficial, hand
      head S00.90
         ear —see Injury, superficial, ear
         eyelid —see Injury, superficial,
            eyelid
         nose S00.30
         oral cavity S00.502
         scalp S00.00
         specified site NEC S00.80

Injury (Continued)
   superficial NEC (Continued)
      heel —see Injury, superficial, foot
      hip S70.91-
         abrasion —see Abrasion, hip
         bite —see Bite, superficial, hip
         blister —see Blister, hip
         contusion —see Contusion, hip
         external constriction —see
            Constriction, external, hip
         foreign body —see Foreign body,
            superficial, hip
      iliac region —see Injury, superficial,
         abdomen
      inguinal region —see Injury,
         superficial, abdomen
      insect bite —see Bite, by site,
         superficial, insect
      interscapular region —see Injury,
         superficial, thorax, back
      jaw —see Injury, superficial, head,
         specified NEC
      knee S80.91-
         abrasion —see Abrasion, knee
         bite —see Bite, superficial, knee
         blister —see Blister, knee
         contusion —see Contusion, knee
         external constriction —see
            Constriction, external,
            knee
         foreign body —see Foreign body,
            superficial, knee
      labium (majus) (minus) S30.95
      lacrimal (apparatus) (gland) (sac) —
         see Injury, eye, specified site
         NEC
      larynx —see Injury, superficial, throat
      leg (lower) S80.92-
         abrasion —see Abrasion, leg
         bite —see Bite, superficial, leg
         contusion —see Contusion, leg
         external constriction —see
            Constriction, external, leg
         foreign body —see Foreign body,
            superficial, leg
         knee —see Injury, superficial,
            knee
      limb NEC T14.8
      lip S00.501
      lower back S30.91
      lumbar region S30.91
      malar region —see Injury, superficial,
         head, specified NEC
      mammary —see Injury, superficial,
         breast
      mastoid region —see Injury,
         superficial, head, specified NEC
      mouth —see Injury, superficial, oral
         cavity
      muscle NEC T14.8
      nail NEC T14.8
         finger —see Injury, superficial,
            finger
         toe —see Injury, superficial, toe
      nasal (septum) —see Injury,
         superficial, nose
      neck S10.90
         specified site NEC S10.80
      nose (septum) S00.30
      occipital region —see Injury,
         superficial, scalp
      oral cavity S00.502
      orbital region —see Injury, superficial,
         periocular area

Injury (Continued)
   superficial NEC (Continued)
      palate —see Injury, superficial, oral
         cavity
      palm —see Injury, superficial, hand
      parietal region —see Injury,
         superficial, scalp
      pelvis S30.91
         girdle —see Injury, superficial, hip
      penis S30.93
      perineum
         female S30.95
         male S30.91
      periocular area S00.20-
         abrasion —see Abrasion, eyelid
         bite —see Bite, superficial, eyelid
         contusion —see Contusion, eyelid
         external constriction —see
            Constriction, external, eyelid
         foreign body —see Foreign body,
            superficial, eyelid
      phalanges
         finger —see Injury, superficial,
            finger
         toe —see Injury, superficial, toe
      pharynx —see Injury, superficial,
         throat
      pinna —see Injury, superficial, ear
      popliteal space —see Injury,
         superficial, knee
      prepuce S30.93
      pubic region S30.91
      pudendum
         female S30.97
         male S30.96
      sacral region S30.91
      scalp S00.00
      scapular region —see Injury,
         superficial, shoulder
      sclera —see Injury, eye, specified site
         NEC
      scrotum S30.94
      shin —see Injury, superficial, leg
      shoulder S40.91-
         abrasion —see Abrasion, shoulder
         bite —see Bite, superficial, shoulder
         blister —see Blister, shoulder
         contusion —see Contusion,
            shoulder
         external constriction —see
            Constriction, external,
            shoulder
         foreign body —see Foreign body,
            superficial, shoulder
      skin NEC T14.8
      sternal region —see Injury, superficial,
         thorax, front
      subconjunctival —see Injury, eye,
         specified site NEC
      subcutaneous NEC T14.8
      submaxillary region —see Injury,
         superficial, head, specified NEC
      submental region —see Injury,
         superficial, head, specified NEC
      subungual
         finger (s) —see Injury, superficial,
            finger
         toe (s) —see Injury, superficial, toe
      supraclavicular fossa —see Injury,
         superficial, neck
      supraorbital —see Injury, superficial,
         head, specified NEC
      temple —see Injury, superficial, head,
         specified NEC

Injury *(Continued)*
  superficial NEC *(Continued)*
    temporal region —*see* Injury,
      superficial, head, specified NEC
    testis S30.94
    thigh S70.92-
      abrasion —*see* Abrasion, thigh
      bite —*see* Bite, superficial, thigh
      blister —*see* Blister, thigh
      contusion —*see* Contusion, thigh
      external constriction —*see*
        Constriction, external, thigh
      foreign body —*see* Foreign body,
        superficial, thigh
    thorax, thoracic (wall) S20.90
      abrasion —*see* Abrasion, thorax
      back S20.40-
      bite —*see* Bite, thorax, superficial
      blister —*see* Blister, thorax
      contusion —*see* Contusion, thorax
      external constriction —*see*
        Constriction, external, thorax
      foreign body —*see* Foreign body,
        superficial, thorax
      front S20.30-
    throat S10.10
      abrasion S10.11
      bite S10.17
        insect S10.16
      blister S10.12
      contusion S10.0
      external constriction S10.14
      foreign body S10.15
    thumb S60.93-
      abrasion —*see* Abrasion, thumb
      bite —*see* Bite, superficial, thumb
      blister —*see* Blister, thumb
      contusion —*see* Contusion, thumb
      external constriction —*see*
        Constriction, external, thumb
      foreign body —*see* Foreign body,
        superficial, thumb
      insect bite —*see* Bite, by site,
        superficial, insect
        specified type NEC S60.392
        specified type NEC S60.391
      specified type NEC S60.399
    toe (s) S90.93-
      abrasion —*see* Abrasion, toe
      bite —*see* Bite, toe
      blister —*see* Blister, toe
      contusion —*see* Contusion, toe
      external constriction —*see*
        Constriction, external, toe
      foreign body —*see* Foreign body,
        superficial, toe
      great S90.93-
    tongue —*see* Injury, superficial, oral
      cavity
    tooth, teeth —*see* Injury, superficial,
      oral cavity
    trachea S10.10
    tunica vaginalis S30.94
    tympanum, tympanic membrane —
      see Injury, superficial, ear
    uvula —*see* Injury, superficial, oral
      cavity
    vagina S30.95
    vocal cords —*see* Injury, superficial,
      throat
    vulva S30.95
    wrist S60.91-
  supraclavicular region —*see* Injury,
    neck
  supraorbital S09.93

Injury *(Continued)*
  suprarenal gland (multiple) —*see* Injury,
    adrenal
  surgical complication (external or
    internal site) —*see* Laceration,
    accidental complicating
    surgery
  temple S09.90
  temporal region S09.90
  tendon —*see also* Injury, muscle,
    by site
    abdomen —*see* Injury, muscle,
      abdomen
    Achilles —*see* Injury, Achilles
      tendon
    lower back —*see* Injury, muscle,
      lower back
    pelvic organs —*see* Injury, muscle,
      pelvis
  tenth cranial nerve (pneumogastric
    or vagus) —*see* Injury, nerve,
    vagus
  testis S39.94
  thigh S79.92-
    blood vessel —*see* Injury, blood
      vessel, hip
    contusion —*see* Contusion, thigh
    fracture —*see* Fracture, femur
    muscle —*see* Injury, muscle, thigh
    nerve —*see* Injury, nerve, thigh
    open —*see* Wound, open, thigh
    specified NEC S79.82-
    superficial —*see* Injury, superficial,
      thigh
  third cranial nerve (oculomotor) —*see*
    Injury, nerve, oculomotor
  thorax, thoracic S29.9
    blood vessel —*see* Injury, blood
      vessel, thorax
    cavity —*see* Injury, intrathoracic
    dislocation —*see* Dislocation, thorax
    external (wall) S29.9
      contusion —*see* Contusion,
        thorax
      nerve —*see* Injury, nerve, thorax
      open —*see* Wound, open, thorax
      specified NEC S29.8
      sprain —*see* Sprain, thorax
      superficial —*see* Injury, superficial,
        thorax
    fracture —*see* Fracture, thorax
    internal —*see* Injury, intrathoracic
    intrathoracic organ —*see* Injury,
      intrathoracic
    sympathetic ganglion —*see* Injury,
      nerve, thorax, sympathetic
  throat (*see also* Injury, neck) S19.9
  thumb S69.9-
    blood vessel —*see* Injury, blood
      vessel, thumb
    contusion —*see* Contusion, thumb
    dislocation —*see* Dislocation, thumb
    fracture —*see* Fracture, thumb
    muscle —*see* Injury, muscle, thumb
    nerve —*see* Injury, nerve, digital,
      thumb
    open —*see* Wound, open, thumb
    specified NEC S69.8-
    sprain —*see* Sprain, thumb
    superficial —*see* Injury, superficial,
      thumb
  thymus (gland) —*see* Injury,
    intrathoracic, specified organ NEC
  thyroid (gland) NEC S19.84

Injury *(Continued)*
  toe S99.92-
    contusion —*see* Contusion, toe
    dislocation —*see* Dislocation, toe
    fracture —*see* Fracture, toe
    muscle —*see* Injury, muscle, toe
    open —*see* Wound, open, toe
    specified type NEC S99.82-
    sprain —*see* Sprain, toe
    superficial —*see* Injury, superficial,
      toe
  tongue S09.93
  tonsil S09.93
  tooth S09.93
  trachea (cervical) NEC S19.82
    thoracic —*see* Injury, intrathoracic,
      trachea, thoracic
  transfusion-related acute lung (TRALI)
    J95.84
  tunica vaginalis S39.94
  twelfth cranial nerve (hypoglossal) —
    see Injury, nerve, hypoglossal
  ureter S37.10
    contusion S37.12
    laceration S37.13
    specified type NEC S37.19
  urethra (sphincter) S37.30
    at delivery O71.5
    contusion S37.32
    laceration S37.33
    specified type NEC S37.38
  urinary organ S37.899
    contusion S37.92
    laceration S37.93
    specified
      site NEC S37.899
        contusion S37.892
        laceration S37.893
        specified type NEC S37.898
      type NEC S37.99
  uterus, uterine S37.60
    with ectopic or molar pregnancy
      O08.6
    blood vessel —*see* Injury, blood
      vessel, iliac
    contusion S37.62
    laceration S37.63
      cervix at delivery O71.3
    rupture associated with obstetrics —
      see Rupture, uterus
    specified type NEC S37.69
  uvula S09.93
  vagina S39.93
    abrasion S30.814
    bite S31.45
      insect S30.864
      superficial NEC S30.874
    contusion S30.23
    crush S38.03
    during delivery —*see* Laceration,
      vagina, during delivery
    external constriction S30.844
    insect bite S30.864
    laceration S31.41
      with foreign body S31.42
    open wound S31.40
    puncture S31.43
      with foreign body S31.44
    superficial S30.95
      foreign body S30.854
  vas deferens —*see* Injury, pelvic organ,
    specified site NEC
  vascular NEC T14.8
  vein —*see* Injury, blood vessel

Injury (*Continued*)
vena cava (superior) S25.20
  inferior S35.10
    laceration (minor) (superficial)
      S35.11
      major S35.12
    specified type NEC S35.19
  laceration (minor) (superficial) S25.21
    major S25.22
  specified type NEC S25.29
vesical (sphincter) —*see* Injury, bladder
visual cortex S04.04-
vitreous (humor) S05.90
  specified NEC S05.8X-
vocal cord NEC S19.83
vulva S39.94
  abrasion S30.814
  bite S31.45
    insect S30.864
    superficial NEC S30.874
  contusion S30.23
  crush S38.03
  during delivery —*see* Laceration,
    perineum, female, during
    delivery
  external constriction S30.844
  insect bite S30.864
  laceration S31.41
    with foreign body S31.42
  open wound S31.40
  puncture S31.43
    with foreign body S31.44
  superficial S30.95
    foreign body S30.854
whiplash (cervical spine) S13.4
wrist S69.9-
  blood vessel —*see* Injury, blood
    vessel, hand
  contusion —*see* Contusion, wrist
  dislocation —*see* Dislocation, wrist
  fracture —*see* Fracture, wrist
  muscle —*see* Injury, muscle, hand
  nerve —*see* Injury, nerve, hand
  open —*see* Wound, open, wrist
  specified NEC S69.8-
  sprain —*see* Sprain, wrist
  superficial —*see* Injury, superficial,
    wrist
Inoculation —*see also* Vaccination
complication or reaction —*see*
  Complications, vaccination
Insanity, insane —*see also* Psychosis
adolescent —*see* Schizophrenia
confusional F28
  acute or subacute F05
delusional F22
senile F03
Insect
bite —*see* Bite, by site, superficial, insect
venomous, poisoning NEC (by) —*see*
  Venom, arthropod
Insensitivity
adrenocorticotropin hormone (ACTH)
  E27.49
androgen E34.50
  complete E34.51
  partial E34.52
Insertion
cord (umbilical) lateral or velamentous
  O43.12-
intrauterine contraceptive device
  (encounter for) —*see* Intrauterine
  contraceptive device
Insolation (sunstroke) T67.0

Insomnia (organic) G47.00
without objective findings F51.02
  adjustment F51.02
  adjustment disorder F51.02
behavioral, of childhood Z73.819
  combined type Z73.812
  limit setting type Z73.811
  sleep-onset association type
    Z73.810
childhood Z73.819
chronic F51.04
  somatized tension F51.04
conditioned F51.04
due to
  alcohol
    abuse F10.182
    dependence F10.282
    use F10.982
  amphetamines
    abuse F15.182
    dependence F15.282
    use F15.982
  anxiety disorder F51.05
  caffeine
    abuse F15.182
    dependence F15.282
    use F15.982
  cocaine
    abuse F14.182
    dependence F14.282
    use F14.982
  depression F51.05
  drug NEC
    abuse F19.182
    dependence F19.282
    use F19.982
  medical condition G47.01
  mental disorder NEC F51.05
  opioid
    abuse F11.182
    dependence F11.282
    use F11.982
  psychoactive substance NEC
    abuse F19.182
    dependence F19.282
    use F19.982
  sedative, hypnotic, or anxiolytic
    abuse F13.182
    dependence F13.282
    use F13.982
  stimulant NEC
    abuse F15.182
    dependence F15.282
    use F15.982
fatal familial (FFI) A81.83
idiopathic F51.01
learned F51.3
nonorganic origin F51.01
not due to a substance or known
  physiological condition F51.01
  specified NEC F51.09
paradoxical F51.03
primary F51.01
psychiatric F51.05
psychophysiologic F51.04
related to psychopathology F51.05
short-term F51.02
specified NEC G47.09
stress-related F51.02
transient F51.02
Inspiration
food or foreign body —*see* Foreign
  body, by site
mucus —*see* Asphyxia, mucus

Inspissated bile syndrome (newborn)
  P59.1
Instability
emotional (excessive) F60.3
joint (post-traumatic) M25.30
  ankle M25.37-
  due to old ligament injury —*see*
    Disorder, ligament
  elbow M25.32-
  flail —*see* Flail, joint
  foot M25.37-
  hand M25.34-
  hip M25.35-
  knee M25.36-
  lumbosacral —*see* subcategory M53.2
  prosthesis —*see* Complications,
    joint prosthesis, mechanical,
    displacement, by site
  sacroiliac —*see* subcategory M53.2
  secondary to
    old ligament injury —*see* Disorder,
      ligament
    removal of joint prosthesis M96.89
  shoulder (region) M25.31-
  spine —*see* subcategory M53.2
  wrist M25.33-
knee (chronic) M23.5-
lumbosacral —*see* subcategory M53.2
nervous F48.8
personality (emotional) F60.3
spine —*see* Instability, joint, spine
vasomotor R55
Institutional syndrome (childhood) F94.2
Institutionalization, affecting child Z62.22
disinhibited attachment F94.2
Insufficiency, insufficient
accommodation, old age H52.4
adrenal (gland) E27.40
  primary E27.1
adrenocortical E27.40
  drug-induced E27.3
  iatrogenic E27.3
  primary E27.1
anterior (occlusal) guidance M26.54
anus K62.89
aortic (valve) I35.1
  with
    mitral (valve) disease I08.0
      with tricuspid (valve) disease I08.3
    stenosis I35.2
    tricuspid (valve) disease I08.2
      with mitral (valve) disease I08.3
  congenital Q23.1
  rheumatic I06.1
    with
      mitral (valve) disease I08.0
        with tricuspid (valve) disease
          I08.3
      stenosis I06.2
        with mitral (valve) disease
          I08.0
          with tricuspid (valve)
            disease I08.3
      tricuspid (valve) disease I08.2
        with mitral (valve) disease
          I08.3
  specified cause NEC I35.1
  syphilitic A52.03
arterial I77.1
  basilar G45.0
  carotid (hemispheric) G45.1
  cerebral I67.81
  coronary (acute or subacute) I24.8
  mesenteric K55.1

Insufficiency, insufficient (Continued)
arterial (Continued)
  peripheral I73.9
  precerebral (multiple) (bilateral)
    G45.2
  vertebral G45.0
arteriovenous I99.8
biliary K83.8
cardiac —see also Insufficiency,
  myocardial
  due to presence of (cardiac)
    prosthesis I97.11-
  postprocedural I97.11-
cardiorenal, hypertensive I13.2
cardiovascular —see Disease,
  cardiovascular
cerebrovascular (acute) I67.81
  with transient focal neurological
    signs and symptoms G45.8
circulatory NEC I99.8
  newborn P29.89
convergence H51.11
coronary (acute or subacute) I24.8
  chronic or with a stated duration of
    over 4 weeks I25.89
corticoadrenal E27.40
  primary E27.1
dietary E63.9
divergence H51.8
food T73.0
gastroesophageal K22.8
gonadal
  ovary E28.39
  testis E29.1
heart —see also Insufficiency,
  myocardial
  newborn P29.0
  valve —see Endocarditis
hepatic —see Failure, hepatic
idiopathic autonomic G90.09
interocclusal distance of fully erupted
  teeth (ridge) M26.36
kidney N28.9
  acute N28.9
  chronic N18.9
lacrimal (secretion) H04.12-
  passages —see Stenosis, lacrimal
liver —see Failure, hepatic
lung —see Insufficiency, pulmonary
mental (congenital) —see Disability,
  intellectual
mesenteric K55.1
mitral (valve) I34.0
  with
    aortic valve disease I08.0
      with tricuspid (valve) disease
        I08.3
    obstruction or stenosis I05.2
      with aortic valve disease I08.0
    tricuspid (valve) disease I08.1
      with aortic (valve) disease I08.3
  congenital Q23.3
  rheumatic I05.1
    with
      aortic valve disease I08.0
        with tricuspid (valve) disease
          I08.3
      obstruction or stenosis I05.2
        with aortic valve disease I08.0
          with tricuspid (valve)
            disease I08.3
        tricuspid (valve) disease I08.1
          with aortic (valve) disease
            I08.3

Insufficiency, insufficient (Continued)
mitral (Continued)
  rheumatic (Continued)
    active or acute I01.1
      with chorea, rheumatic
        (Sydenham's) I02.0
    specified cause, except rheumatic
      I34.0
muscle —see also Disease, muscle
  heart —see Insufficiency, myocardial
ocular NEC H50.9
myocardial, myocardium (with
  arteriosclerosis) I50.9
  with
    rheumatic fever (conditions in
      I00) I09.0
    active, acute or subacute I01.2
      with chorea I02.0
    inactive or quiescent (with
      chorea) I09.0
  congenital Q24.8
  hypertensive —see Hypertension, heart
  newborn P29.0
  rheumatic I09.0
    active, acute, or subacute I01.2
  syphilitic A52.06
nourishment T73.0
pancreatic K86.8
parathyroid (gland) E20.9
peripheral vascular (arterial) I73.9
pituitary E23.0
placental (mother) O36.51-
platelets D69.6
prenatal care affecting management of
  pregnancy O09.3-
progressive pluriglandular E31.0
pulmonary J98.4
  acute, following surgery
    (nonthoracic) J95.2
    thoracic J95.1
  chronic, following surgery J95.3
  following
    shock J80
    trauma J80
  newborn P28.5
  valve I37.1
    with stenosis I37.2
    congenital Q22.2
    rheumatic I09.89
      with aortic, mitral or tricuspid
        (valve) disease I08.8
pyloric K31.89
renal (acute) N28.9
  chronic N18.9
respiratory R06.89
  newborn P28.5
rotation —see Malrotation
sleep syndrome F51.12
social insurance Z59.7
suprarenal E27.40
  primary E27.1
tarso-orbital fascia, congenital Q10.3
testis E29.1
thyroid (gland) (acquired) E03.9
  congenital E03.1
tricuspid (valve) (rheumatic) I07.1
  with
    aortic (valve) disease I08.2
      with mitral (valve) disease I08.3
    mitral (valve) disease I08.1
      with aortic (valve) disease I08.3
    obstruction or stenosis I07.2
      with aortic (valve) disease I08.2
        with mitral (valve) disease I08.3

Insufficiency, insufficient (Continued)
tricuspid (Continued)
  congenital Q22.8
  nonrheumatic I36.1
    with stenosis I36.2
urethral sphincter R32
valve, valvular (heart) —see
  Endocarditis
  congenital Q24.8
vascular I99.8
  intestine K55.9
    acute K55.0
  mesenteric K55.1
  peripheral I73.9
  renal —see Hypertension, kidney
velopharyngeal
  acquired K13.79
  congenital Q38.8
venous (chronic) (peripheral) I87.2
ventricular —see Insufficiency,
  myocardial
welfare support Z59.7
Insufflation, fallopian Z31.41
Insular —see condition
Insulinoma
pancreas
  benign D13.7
  malignant C25.4
  uncertain behavior D37.8
specified site
  benign —see Neoplasm, by site,
    benign
  malignant —see Neoplasm, by site,
    malignant
  uncertain behavior —see Neoplasm,
    by site, uncertain behavior
unspecified site
  benign D13.7
  malignant C25.4
  uncertain behavior D37.8
Insuloma —see Insulinoma
Interference
balancing side M26.56
non-working side M26.56
Intermenstrual —see condition
Intermittent —see condition
Internal —see condition
Interrogation
cardiac defibrillator (automatic)
  (implantable) Z45.02
cardiac pacemaker Z45.018
cardiac (event) (loop) recorder Z45.09
infusion pump (implanted) (intrathecal)
  Z45.1
neurostimulator Z46.2
Interruption
phase-shift, sleep cycle —see Disorder,
  sleep, circadian rhythm
sleep phase-shift, or 24 hour sleep-
  wake cycle —see Disorder, sleep,
  circadian rhythm
Interstitial —see condition
Intertrigo L30.4
labialis K13.0
Intervertebral disc —see condition
Intestine, intestinal —see condition
Intolerance
carbohydrate K90.4
disaccharide, hereditary E73.0
fat NEC K90.4
  pancreatic K90.3
food K90.4
  dietary counseling and surveillance
    Z71.3

Intolerance *(Continued)*
  fructose E74.10
    hereditary E74.12
  glucose(-galactose) E74.39
  gluten K90.0
  lactose E73.9
    specified NEC E73.8
  lysine E72.3
  milk NEC K90.4
    lactose E73.9
  protein K90.4
  starch NEC K90.4
  sucrose (-isomaltose) E74.31
Intoxicated NEC (without dependence) —
  see Alcohol, intoxication
Intoxication
  acid E87.2
  alcoholic (acute) (without
    dependence) —*see* Alcohol,
    intoxication
  alimentary canal K52.1
  amphetamine (without dependence) —
    see Abuse, drug, stimulant, with
    intoxication
    with dependence —*see* Dependence,
      drug, stimulant,
      with intoxication
  anxiolytic (acute) (without
    dependence) —*see* Abuse, drug,
    sedative, with intoxication
    with dependence —*see* Dependence,
      drug, sedative, with intoxication
  caffeine (acute) (without
    dependence) —*see* Abuse, drug,
    stimulant, with intoxication
    with dependence —*see* Dependence,
      drug, stimulant, with intoxication
  cannabinoids (acute) (without
    dependence) —*see* Abuse, drug,
    cannabis, with intoxication
    with dependence —*see* Dependence,
      drug, cannabis, with intoxication
  chemical —*see* Table of drugs and
    chemicals
    via placenta or breast milk —*see* -
      Absorption, chemical, through
      placenta
  cocaine (acute) (without
    dependence) —*see* Abuse, drug,
    cocaine, with intoxication
    with dependence —*see* Dependence,
      drug, cocaine, with intoxication
  drug
    acute (without dependence) —*see*
      Abuse, drug, by type with
      intoxication
      with dependence —*see* Dependence,
        drug, by type with
        intoxication
    addictive
      via placenta or breast milk —*see*
        Absorption, drug, addictive,
        through placenta
    newborn P93.8
      gray baby syndrome P93.0
    overdose or wrong substance
      given or taken —*see* Table of
      drugs and chemicals, by drug,
      poisoning
  enteric K52.1
  foodborne A05.9
    bacterial A05.9
    classical (Clostridium botulinum)
      A05.1

Intoxication *(Continued)*
  foodborne *(Continued)*
    due to
      Bacillus cereus A05.4
      bacterium A05.9
        specified NEC A05.8
      Clostridium
        botulinum A05.1
        perfringens A05.2
        welchii A05.2
      Salmonella A02.9
        with
          (gastro) enteritis A02.0
          localized infection (s) A02.20
            arthritis A02.23
            meningitis A02.21
            osteomyelitis A02.24
            pneumonia A02.22
            pyelonephritis A02.25
            specified NEC A02.29
          sepsis A02.1
          specified manifestation NEC
            A02.8
      Staphylococcus A05.0
      Vibrio
        parahaemolyticus A05.3
        vulnificus A05.5
    enterotoxin, staphylococcal A05.0
    noxious —*see* Poisoning, food, noxious
  gastrointestinal K52.1
  hallucinogenic (without dependence) —
    see Abuse, drug, hallucinogen,
    with intoxication
    with dependence —*see* Dependence,
      drug, hallucinogen, with
      intoxication
  hypnotic (acute) (without
    dependence) —*see* Abuse, drug,
    sedative, with intoxication
    with dependence —*see* Dependence,
      drug, sedative, with intoxication
  inhalant (acute) (without
    dependence) —*see* Abuse, drug,
    inhalant, with intoxication
    with dependence —*see* Dependence,
      drug, inhalant, with intoxication
  meaning
    inebriation —*see* category F10
    poisoning —*see* Table of drugs and
      chemicals
  methyl alcohol (acute) (without
    dependence) —*see* Alcohol,
    intoxication
  opioid (acute) (without dependence) —
    see Abuse, drug, opioid, with
    intoxication
    with dependence —*see* Dependence,
      drug, opioid, with intoxication
  pathologic NEC (without dependence) —
    see Alcohol, intoxication
  phencyclidine (without dependence) —
    see Abuse, drug, psychoactive
    NEC, with intoxication
    with dependence —*see* Dependence,
      drug, psychoactive NEC, with
      intoxication
  potassium (K) E87.5
  psychoactive substance NEC (without
    dependence) —*see* Abuse,
    drug, psychoactive NEC, with
    intoxication
    with dependence —*see* Dependence,
      drug, psychoactive NEC, with
      intoxication

Intoxication *(Continued)*
  sedative (acute) (without
    dependence) —*see* Abuse, drug,
    sedative, with intoxication
    with dependence —*see* Dependence,
      drug, sedative, with
      intoxication
  serum (*see also* Reaction, serum) T80.69
  uremic —*see* Uremia
  volatile solvents (acute) (without
    dependence) —*see* Abuse, drug,
    inhalant, with intoxication
    with dependence —*see* Dependence,
      drug, inhalant, with intoxication
  water E87.79
Intracranial —*see* condition
Intrahepatic gallbladder Q44.1
Intraligamentous —*see* condition
Intrathoracic —*see also* condition
  kidney Q63.2
Intrauterine contraceptive device
  checking Z30.431
  in situ Z97.5
  insertion Z30.430
    immediately following removal
      Z30.433
  management Z30.431
  reinsertion Z30.433
  removal Z30.432
  replacement Z30.433
  retention in pregnancy O26.3-
Intraventricular —*see* condition
Intrinsic deformity —*see* Deformity
Intubation, difficult or failed T88.4
Intumescence, lens (eye) (cataract) —*see*
  Cataract
Intussusception (bowel) (colon) (enteric)
  (ileocecal) (ileocolic) (intestine)
  (rectum) K56.1
  appendix K38.8
  congenital Q43.8
  ureter (with obstruction) N13.5
Invagination (bowel, colon, intestine or
  rectum) K56.1
Inversion
  albumin-globulin (A-G) ratio E88.09
  bladder N32.89
  cecum —*see* Intussusception
  cervix N88.8
  chromosome in normal individual Q95.1
  circadian rhythm —*see* Disorder, sleep,
    circadian rhythm
  nipple N64.59
    congenital Q83.8
    gestational —*see* Retraction, nipple
    puerperal, postpartum —*see*
      Retraction, nipple
  nyctohemeral rhythm —*see* Disorder,
    sleep, circadian rhythm
  optic papilla Q14.2
  organ or site, congenital NEC —*see*
    Anomaly, by site
  sleep rhythm —*see* Disorder, sleep,
    circadian rhythm
  testis (congenital) Q55.29
  uterus (chronic) (postinfectional)
    (postpartal, old) N85.5
    postpartum O71.2
  vagina (posthysterectomy) N99.3
  ventricular Q20.5
Investigation (*see also* Examination) Z04.9
  clinical research subject (control)
    (normal comparison) (participant)
    Z00.6

Involuntary movement, abnormal
R25.9
Involution, involutional —see also
    condition
    breast, cystic —see Dysplasia,
        mammary, specified type NEC
    depression (single episode) F32.8
        recurrent episode F33.9
    melancholia (recurrent episode) (single
        episode) F32.8
    ovary, senile —see Atrophy, ovary
    thymus failure E32.8
I.Q.
    under 20 F73
    20-34 F72
    35-49 F71
    50-69 F70
IRDS (type I) P22.0
    type II P22.1
Irideremia Q13.1
Iridis rubeosis —see Disorder, iris,
    vascular
Iridochoroiditis (panuveitis) —see
    Panuveitis
Iridocyclitis H20.9-
    acute H20.0-
        hypopyon H20.05-
        primary H20.01-
        recurrent H20.02-
        secondary (noninfectious) H20.04-
            infectious H20.03-
    chronic H20.1-
    due to allergy —see Iridocyclitis, acute,
        secondary
    endogenous —see Iridocyclitis, acute,
        primary
    Fuchs' —see Cyclitis, Fuchs'
        heterochromic
    gonococcal A54.32
    granulomatous —see Iridocyclitis,
        chronic
    herpes, herpetic (simplex) B00.51
        zoster B02.32
    hypopyon —see Iridocyclitis, acute,
        hypopyon
    in (due to)
        ankylosing spondylitis M45.9
        gonococcal infection A54.32
        herpes (simplex) virus B00.51
            zoster B02.32
        infectious disease NOS B99
        parasitic disease NOS B89 [H22]
        sarcoidosis D86.83
        syphilis A51.43
        tuberculosis A18.54
        zoster B02.32
    lens-induced H20.2-
    nongranulomatous —see Iridocyclitis,
        acute
    recurrent —see Iridocyclitis, acute,
        recurrent
    rheumatic —see Iridocyclitis, chronic
    subacute —see Iridocyclitis, acute
    sympathetic —see Uveitis, sympathetic
    syphilitic (secondary) A51.43
    tuberculous (chronic) A18.54
    Vogt-Koyanagi H20.82-
Iridocyclochoroiditis (panuveitis) —see
    Panuveitis
Iridodialysis H21.53-
Iridodonesis H21.89
Iridoplegia (complete) (partial) (reflex)
    H57.09
Iridoschisis H21.25-

Iris —see also condition
    bombé —see Membrane, pupillary
Iritis —see also Iridocyclitis
    chronic —see Iridocyclitis, chronic
    diabetic —see E08-E13 with .39
    due to
        herpes simplex B00.51
        leprosy A30.9 [H22]
    gonococcal A54.32
    gouty M10.9
    granulomatous —see Iridocyclitis,
        chronic
    lens induced —see Iridocyclitis,
        lens-induced
    papulosa (syphilitic) A52.71
    rheumatic —see Iridocyclitis, chronic
    syphilitic (secondary) A51.43
        congenital (early) A50.01
        late A52.71
    tuberculous A18.54
Iron —see condition
Iron-miner's lung J63.4
Irradiated enamel (tooth, teeth)
    K03.89
Irradiation effects, adverse T66
Irreducible, irreducibility —see
    condition
Irregular, irregularity
    action, heart I49.9
    alveolar process K08.8
    bleeding N92.6
    breathing R06.89
    contour of cornea (acquired) —see
        Deformity, cornea
        congenital Q13.4
    contour, reconstructed breast N65.0
    dentin (in pulp) K04.3
    eye movements H55.89
        nystagmus —see Nystagmus
        saccadic H55.81
    labor O62.2
    menstruation (cause unknown)
        N92.6
    periods N92.6
    prostate N42.9
    pupil —see Abnormality, pupillary
    reconstructed breast N65.0
    respiratory R06.89
    septum (nasal) J34.2
    shape, organ or site, congenital NEC —
        see Distortion
    sleep-wake pattern (rhythm) G47.23
Irritable, irritability R45.4
    bladder N32.89
    bowel (syndrome) K58.9
        with diarrhea K58.0
        psychogenic F45.8
    bronchial —see Bronchitis
    cerebral, in newborn P91.3
    colon K58.9
        with diarrhea K58.0
        psychogenic F45.8
    duodenum K59.8
    heart (psychogenic) F45.8
    hip —see Derangement, joint, specified
        type NEC, hip
    ileum K59.8
    infant R68.12
    jejunum K59.8
    rectum K59.8
    stomach K31.89
        psychogenic F45.8
    sympathetic G90.8
    urethra N36.8

Irritation
    anus K62.89
    axillary nerve G54.0
    bladder N32.89
    brachial plexus G54.0
    bronchial —see Bronchitis
    cervical plexus G54.2
    cervix —see Cervicitis
    choroid, sympathetic —see
        Endophthalmitis
    cranial nerve —see Disorder, nerve,
        cranial
    gastric K31.89
        psychogenic F45.8
    globe, sympathetic —see Uveitis,
        sympathetic
    labyrinth —see subcategory H83.2
    lumbosacral plexus G54.1
    meninges (traumatic) —see Injury,
        intracranial
        nontraumatic —see Meningismus
    nerve —see Disorder, nerve
    nervous R45.0
    penis N48.89
    perineum NEC L29.3
    peripheral autonomic nervous system
        G90.8
    peritoneum —see Peritonitis
    pharynx J39.2
    plantar nerve —see Lesion, nerve,
        plantar
    spinal (cord) (traumatic) —see also
        Injury, spinal cord, by region
        nerve G58.9
        root NEC —see Radiculopathy
        nontraumatic —see Myelopathy
    stomach K31.89
        psychogenic F45.8
    sympathetic nerve NEC G90.8
    ulnar nerve —see Lesion, nerve, ulnar
    vagina N89.8
Ischemia, ischemic I99.8
    bowel (transient)
        acute K55.0
        chronic K55.1
        due to mesenteric artery insufficiency
            K55.1
    brain —see Ischemia, cerebral
    cardiac (see Disease, heart, ischemic)
    cardiomyopathy I25.5
    cerebral (chronic) (generalized) I67.82
        arteriosclerotic I67.2
        intermittent G45.9
        newborn P91.0
        recurrent focal G45.8
        transient G45.9
    colon chronic (due to mesenteric artery
        insufficiency) K55.1
    coronary —see Disease, heart,
        ischemic
    demand (coronary) (see also Angina)
        I24.8
    heart (chronic or with a stated duration
        of over 4 weeks) I25.9
        acute or with a stated duration of
            4 weeks or less I24.9
        subacute I24.9
    infarction, muscle —see Infarct, muscle
    intestine (large) (small) (transient) K55.9
        acute K55.0
        chronic K55.1
        due to mesenteric artery
            insufficiency K55.1
    kidney N28.0

Ischemia, ischemic *(Continued)*
  mesenteric, acute K55.0
  muscle, traumatic T79.6
  myocardium, myocardial (chronic or
      with a stated duration of over
      4 weeks) I25.9
    acute, without myocardial infarction
        I24.0
    silent (asymptomatic) I25.6
    transient of newborn P29.4
  renal N28.0
  retina, retinal —*see* Occlusion, artery,
      retina
  small bowel
    acute K55.0
    chronic K55.1
    due to mesenteric artery
        insufficiency K55.1
  spinal cord G95.11
  subendocardial —*see* Insufficiency,
      coronary
  supply (coronary) (*see also* Angina) I25.9
    due to vasospasm I20.1
Ischial spine —*see* condition
Ischialgia —*see* Sciatica
Ischiopagus Q89.4
Ischium, ischial —*see* condition
Ischuria R34
Iselin's disease or osteochondrosis —*see*
      Osteochondrosis, juvenile, metatarsus
Islands of
  parotid tissue in
    lymph nodes Q38.6
    neck structures Q38.6
  submaxillary glands in
    fascia Q38.6
    lymph nodes Q38.6
    neck muscles Q38.6

Islet cell tumor, pancreas D13.7
Isoimmunization NEC —*see also*
      Incompatibility
  affecting management of pregnancy
      (ABO) (with hydrops fetalis)
      O36.11-
    anti-A sensitization O36.11-
    anti-B sensitization O36.19-
    anti-c sensitization O36.09-
    anti-C sensitization O36.09-
    anti-e sensitization O36.09-
    anti-E sensitization O36.09-
    Rh NEC O36.09-
      anti-D antibody O36.01-
    specified NEC O36.19-
  newborn P55.9
    with
      hydrops fetalis P56.0
      kernicterus P57.0
    ABO (blood groups) P55.1
    Rhesus (Rh) factor P55.0
    specified type NEC P55.8
Isolation, isolated
  dwelling Z59.8
  family Z63.79
  social Z60.4
Isoleucinosis E71.19
Isomerism atrial appendages (with
      asplenia or polysplenia) Q20.6
Isosporiasis, isosporosis A07.3
Isovaleric acidemia E71.110
Issue of
  medical certificate Z02.79
    for disability determination Z02.71
  repeat prescription (appliance)
      (glasses) (medicinal substance,
      medicament, medicine) Z76.0
    contraception —*see* Contraception

Itch, itching —*see also* Pruritus
  baker's L23.6
  barber's B35.0
  bricklayer's L24.5
  cheese B88.0
  clam digger's B65.3
  coolie B76.9
  copra B88.0
  dew B76.9
  dhobi B35.6
  filarial —*see* Infestation, filarial
  grain B88.0
  grocer's B88.0
  ground B76.9
  harvest B88.0
  jock B35.6
  Malabar B35.5
    beard B35.0
    foot B35.3
    scalp B35.0
  meaning scabies B86
  Norwegian B86
  perianal L29.0
  poultrymen's B88.0
  sarcoptic B86
  scabies B86
  scrub B88.0
  straw B88.0
  swimmer's B65.3
  water B76.9
  winter L29.8
Ivemark's syndrome (asplenia with
      congenital heart disease)
      Q89.01
Ivory bones Q78.2
Ixodiasis NEC B88.8

J

Jaccoud's syndrome —*see* Arthropathy, postrheumatic, chronic

Jackson's
 membrane Q43.3
 paralysis or syndrome G83.89
 veil Q43.3

Jacquet's dermatitis (diaper dermatitis) L22

Jadassohn-Pellizari's disease or anetoderma L90.2

Jadassohn's
 blue nevus —*see* Nevus
 intraepidermal epithelioma —*see* Neoplasm, skin, benign

Jaffe-Lichtenstein (-Uehlinger)
 syndrome —*see* Dysplasia, fibrous, bone NEC

Jakob-Creutzfeldt disease or syndrome —*see* Creutzfeldt-Jakob disease or syndrome

Jaksch-Luzet disease D64.89

Jamaican
 neuropathy G92
 paraplegic tropical ataxic-spastic syndrome G92

Janet's disease F48.8

Janiceps Q89.4

Jansky-Bielschowsky amaurotic idiocy E75.4

Japanese
 B-type encephalitis A83.0
 river fever A75.3

Jaundice (yellow) R17
 acholuric (familial) (splenomegalic) — *see also* Spherocytosis
  acquired D59.8
 breast-milk (inhibitor) P59.3
 catarrhal (acute) B15.9
  with hepatic coma B15.0
 cholestatic (benign) R17
 due to or associated with
  delayed conjugation P59.8
   associated with (due to) preterm delivery P59.0
  preterm delivery P59.0
 epidemic (catarrhal) B15.9
  with hepatic coma B15.0
  leptospiral A27.0
  spirochetal A27.0
 familial nonhemolytic (congenital) (Gilbert) E80.4
  Crigler-Najjar E80.5
 febrile (acute) B15.9
  with hepatic coma B15.0
  leptospiral A27.0
  spirochetal A27.0
 hematogenous D59.9
 hemolytic (acquired) D59.9
  congenital —*see* Spherocytosis
 hemorrhagic (acute) (leptospiral) (spirochetal) A27.0

Jaundice (Continued)
 infectious (acute) (subacute) B15.9
  with hepatic coma B15.0
  leptospiral A27.0
  spirochetal A27.0
 leptospiral (hemorrhagic) A27.0
 malignant (without coma) K72.90
  with coma K72.91
 neonatal —*see* Jaundice, newborn
 newborn P59.9
  due to or associated with
   ABO
    antibodies P55.1
    incompatibility, maternal/fetal P55.1
    isoimmunization P55.1
   absence or deficiency of enzyme system for bilirubin conjugation (congenital) P59.8
   bleeding P58.1
   breast milk inhibitors to conjugation P59.3
    associated with preterm delivery P59.0
   bruising P58.0
   Crigler-Najjar syndrome E80.5
   delayed conjugation P59.8
    associated with preterm delivery P59.0
   drugs or toxins
    given to newborn P58.42
    transmitted from mother P58.41
   excessive hemolysis P58.9
    due to
     bleeding P58.1
     bruising P58.0
     drugs or toxins
      given to newborn P58.42
      transmitted from mother P58.41
     infection P58.2
     polycythemia P58.3
     swallowed maternal blood P58.5
    specified type NEC P58.8
   galactosemia E74.21
   Gilbert syndrome E80.4
   hemolytic disease P55.9
    ABO isoimmunization P55.1
    Rh isoimmunization P55.0
    specified NEC P55.8
   hepatocellular damage P59.20
    specified NEC P59.29
   hereditary hemolytic anemia P58.8
   hypothyroidism, congenital E03.1
   incompatibility, maternal/fetal NOS P55.9
   infection P58.2
   inspissated bile syndrome P59.1
   isoimmunization NOS P55.9

Jaundice (Continued)
 newborn (Continued)
  due to or associated with (Continued)
   mucoviscidosis E84.9
   polycythemia P58.3
   preterm delivery P59.0
   Rh
    antibodies P55.0
    incompatibility, maternal/fetal P55.0
    isoimmunization P55.0
   specified cause NEC P59.8
   swallowed maternal blood P58.5
   spherocytosis (congenital) D58.0
  nonhemolytic congenital familial (Gilbert) E80.4
  nuclear, newborn (*see also* Kernicterus of newborn) P57.9
  obstructive (*see also* Obstruction, bile duct) K83.1
  post-immunization —*see* Hepatitis, viral, type, B
  post-transfusion —*see* Hepatitis, viral, type, B
  regurgitation (*see also* Obstruction, bile duct) K83.1
  serum (homologous) (prophylactic) (therapeutic) —*see* Hepatitis, viral, type, B
  spirochetal (hemorrhagic) A27.0
  symptomatic R17
   newborn P59.9

Jaw —*see* condition

Jaw-winking phenomenon or syndrome Q07.8

Jealousy
 alcoholic F10.988
 childhood F93.8
 sibling F93.8

Jejunitis —*see* Enteritis

Jejunostomy status Z93.4

Jejunum, jejunal —*see* condition

Jensen's disease —*see* Inflammation, chorioretinal, focal, juxtapapillary

Jerks, myoclonic G25.3

Jervell-Lange-Nielsen syndrome I45.81

Jeune's disease Q77.2

Jigger disease B88.1

Job's syndrome (chronic granulomatous disease) D71

Joint —*see also* condition
 mice —*see* Loose, body, joint
  knee M23.4-

Jordan's anomaly or syndrome D72.0

Joseph-Diamond-Blackfan anemia (congenital hypoplastic) D61.01

Jungle yellow fever A95.0

Jüngling's disease —*see* Sarcoidosis

Juvenile —*see* condition

K

Kahler's disease C90.0-
Kakke E51.11
Kala-azar B55.0
Kallmann's syndrome E23.0
Kanner's syndrome (autism) —see
        Psychosis, childhood
Kaposi's
    dermatosis (xeroderma pigmentosum)
        Q82.1
    lichen ruber L44.0
        acuminatus L44.0
    sarcoma
        colon C46.4
        connective tissue C46.1
        gastrointestinal organ C46.4
        lung C46.5-
        lymph node (multiple) C46.3
        palate (hard) (soft) C46.2
        rectum C46.4
        skin (multiple sites) C46.0
        specified site NEC C46.7
        stomach C46.4
        unspecified site C46.9
    varicelliform eruption B00.0
        vaccinia T88.1
Kartagener's syndrome or triad
        (sinusitis, bronchiectasis, situs
        inversus) Q89.3
Karyotype
    with abnormality except iso (Xq)
        Q96.2
    45,X Q96.0
    46,X
        iso (Xq) Q96.1
    46,XX Q98.3
        with streak gonads Q50.32
        hermaphrodite (true) Q99.1
        male Q98.3
    46,XY
        with streak gonads Q56.1
        female Q97.3
        hermaphrodite (true) Q99.1
    47,XXX Q97.0
    47,XXY Q98.0
    47,XYY Q98.5
Kaschin-Beck disease —see Disease,
        Kaschin-Beck
Katayama's disease or fever B65.2
Kawasaki's syndrome M30.3
Kayser-Fleischer ring (cornea)
        (pseudosclerosis) H18.04-
Kaznelson's syndrome (congenital
        hypoplastic anemia) D61.01
Kearns-Sayre syndrome H49.81-
Kedani fever A75.3
Kelis L91.0
Kelly (-Patterson) syndrome (sideropenic
        dysphagia) D50.1
Keloid, cheloid L91.0
    acne L73.0
    Addison's L94.0
    cornea —see Opacity, cornea
    Hawkin's L91.0
    scar L91.0
Keloma L91.0
Kenya fever A77.1
Keratectasia —see also Ectasia, cornea
    congenital Q13.4
Keratinization of alveolar ridge
        mucosa
    excessive K13.23
    minimal K13.22

Keratinized residual ridge mucosa
    excessive K13.23
    minimal K13.22
Keratitis (nodular) (nonulcerative)
        (simple) (zonular) H16.9
    with ulceration (central) (marginal)
        (perforated) (ring) —see Ulcer,
        cornea
    actinic —see Photokeratitis
    arborescens (herpes simplex) B00.52
    areolar H16.11-
    bullosa H16.8
    deep H16.309
        specified type NEC H16.399
    dendritic (a) (herpes simplex) B00.52
    disciform (is) (herpes simplex) B00.52
        varicella B01.81
    filamentary H16.12-
    gonococcal (congenital or prenatal)
        A54.33
    herpes, herpetic (simplex) B00.52
        zoster B02.33
    in (due to)
        acanthamebiasis B60.13
        adenovirus B30.0
        exanthema (see also Exanthem) B09
        herpes (simplex) virus B00.52
        measles B05.81
        syphilis A50.31
        tuberculosis A18.52
        zoster B02.33
    interstitial (nonsyphilitic) H16.30-
        diffuse H16.32-
        herpes, herpetic (simplex) B00.52
            zoster B02.33
        sclerosing H16.33-
        specified type NEC H16.39-
        syphilitic (congenital) (late) A50.31
        tuberculous A18.52
    macular H16.11-
    nummular H16.11-
    oyster shuckers' H16.8
    parenchymatous —see Keratitis,
        interstitial
    petrificans H16.8
    postmeasles B05.81
    punctata
        leprosa A30.9 [H16.14-]
        syphilitic (profunda) A50.31
    punctate H16.14-
    purulent H16.8
    rosacea L71.8
    sclerosing H16.33-
    specified type NEC H16.8
    stellate H16.11-
    striate H16.11-
    superficial H16.10-
        with conjunctivitis —see
            Keratoconjunctivitis
        due to light —see Photokeratitis
    suppurative H16.8
    syphilitic (congenital) (prenatal) A50.31
    trachomatous A71.1
        sequelae B94.0
    tuberculous A18.52
    vesicular H16.8
    xerotic (see also Keratomalacia) H16.8
        vitamin A deficiency E50.4
Keratoacanthoma L85.8
Keratocele —see Descemetocele
Keratoconjunctivitis H16.20-
    Acanthamoeba B60.13
    adenoviral B30.0
    epidemic B30.0

Keratoconjunctivitis (Continued)
    exposure H16.21-
    herpes, herpetic (simplex) B00.52
        zoster B02.33
    in exanthema (see also Exanthem) B09
    infectious B30.0
    lagophthalmic —see
            Keratoconjunctivitis, specified type
            NEC
    neurotrophic H16.23-
    phlyctenular H16.25-
    postmeasles B05.81
    shipyard B30.0
    sicca (Sjogren's) M35.0-
        not Sjogren's H16.22-
    specified type NEC H16.29-
    tuberculous (phlyctenular) A18.52
    vernal H16.26-
Keratoconus H18.60-
    congenital Q13.4
    stable H18.61-
    unstable H18.62-
Keratocyst (dental) (odontogenic) —see
        Cyst, calcifying odontogenic
Keratoderma, keratodermia (congenital)
        (palmaris et plantaris) (symmetrical)
        Q82.8
    acquired L85.1
        in diseases classified elsewhere L86
    climactericum L85.1
    gonococcal A54.89
    gonorrheal A54.89
    punctata L85.2
    Reiter's —see Reiter's disease
Keratodermatocele —see Descemetocele
Keratoglobus H18.79
    congenital Q15.8
        with glaucoma Q15.0
Keratohemia —see Pigmentation, cornea,
        stromal
Keratoiritis —see also Iridocyclitis
    syphilitic A50.39
    tuberculous A18.54
Keratoma L57.0
    palmaris and plantaris hereditarium
        Q82.8
    senile L57.0
Keratomalacia H18.44-
    vitamin A deficiency E50.4
Keratomegaly Q13.4
Keratomycosis B49
    nigrans, nigricans (palmaris) B36.1
Keratopathy H18.9
    band H18.42-
    bullous H18.1-
    bullous (aphakic), following cataract
        surgery H59.01-
Keratoscleritis, tuberculous A18.52
Keratosis L57.0
    actinic L57.0
    arsenical L85.8
    congenital, specified NEC Q80.8
    female genital NEC N94.89
    follicularis Q82.8
        acquired L11.0
        congenita Q82.8
        et parafollicularis in cutem penetrans
            L87.0
        spinulosa (decalvans) Q82.8
        vitamin A deficiency E50.8
    gonococcal A54.89
    male genital (external) N50.8
    nigricans L83
    obturans, external ear (canal) —see
            Cholesteatoma, external ear

Keratosis *(Continued)*
  palmaris et plantaris (inherited)
      (symmetrical) Q82.8
    acquired L85.1
  penile N48.89
  pharynx J39.2
  pilaris, acquired L85.8
  punctata (palmaris et plantaris) L85.2
  scrotal N50.8
  seborrheic L82.1
    inflamed L82.0
  senile L57.0
  solar L57.0
  tonsillaris J35.8
  vagina N89.4
  vegetans Q82.8
  vitamin A deficiency E50.8
  vocal cord J38.3
Kerato-uveitis —*see* Iridocyclitis
Kerion (celsi) B35.0
Kernicterus of newborn (not due to
    isoimmunization) P57.9
  due to isoimmunization (conditions in
      P55.0-P55.9) P57.0
  specified type NEC P57.8
Kerunoparalysis T75.09
Keshan disease E59
Ketoacidosis E87.2
  diabetic —*see* Diabetes, by type, with
    ketoacidosis
Ketonuria R82.4
Ketosis NEC E88.89
  diabetic —*see* Diabetes, by type, with
    ketoacidosis
Kew Garden fever A79.1
Kidney —*see* condition
Kienböck's disease —*see also*
    Osteochondrosis, juvenile, hand,
    carpal lunate
  adult M93.1
Kimmelstiel (-Wilson) disease —*see*
    Diabetes, Kimmelstiel (-Wilson)
    disease
Kink, kinking
  artery I77.1
  hair (acquired) L67.8
  ileum or intestine —*see* Obstruction,
    intestine
  Lane's —*see* Obstruction, intestine
  organ or site, congenital NEC —*see*
    Anomaly, by site
  ureter (pelvic junction) N13.5
    with
        hydronephrosis N13.1
          with infection N13.6
        pyelonephritis (chronic) N11.1
    congenital Q62.39
  vein (s) I87.8
    caval I87.1
    peripheral I87.1
Kinnier Wilson's disease (hepatolenticular
    degeneration) E83.01
Kissing spine M48.20
  cervical region M48.22
  cervicothoracic region M48.23
  lumbar region M48.26
  lumbosacral region M48.27
  occipito-atlanto-axial region M48.21
  thoracic region M48.24
  thoracolumbar region M48.25
Klatskin's tumor C22.1
Klauder's disease A26.8
Klebs' disease *(see also*
    Glomerulonephritis) N05.-

Klebsiella (K.) pneumoniae, as cause of
    disease classified elsewhere B96.1
Klein (e)-Levin syndrome G47.13
Kleptomania F63.2
Klinefelter's syndrome Q98.4
  karyotype 47,XXY Q98.0
  male with more than two X
    chromosomes Q98.1
Klippel-Feil deficiency, disease, or
    syndrome (brevicollis) Q76.1
Klippel's disease I67.2
Klippel-Trenaunay (-Weber) syndrome
    Q87.2
Klumpke (-Déjerine) palsy, paralysis
    (birth) (newborn) P14.1
Knee —*see* condition
Knock knee (acquired) M21.06-
  congenital Q74.1
Knot (s)
  intestinal, syndrome (volvulus) K56.2
  surfer S89.8-
  umbilical cord (true) O69.2
Knotting (of)
  hair L67.8
  intestine K56.2
Knuckle pad (Garrod's) **M72.1**
Koch's
  infection —*see* Tuberculosis
  relapsing fever A68.9
Koch-Weeks' conjunctivitis —*see*
    Conjunctivitis, acute, mucopurulent
Köebner's syndrome Q81.8
Köenig's disease (osteochondritis
    dissecans) —*see* Osteochondritis,
    dissecans
Köhler-Pellegrini-Steida disease or
    syndrome (calcification, knee
    joint) —*see* Bursitis, tibial collateral
Köhler's disease
  patellar —*see* Osteochondrosis, juvenile,
    patella
  tarsal navicular —*see* Osteochondrosis,
    juvenile, tarsus
Koilonychia L60.3
  congenital Q84.6
Kojevnikov's, epilepsy —*see*
    Kozhevnikof's epilepsy
Koplik's spots B05.9
Kopp's asthma E32.8
Korsakoff's (Wernicke) disease,
    psychosis or syndrome (alcoholic)
    F10.96
  with dependence F10.26
  drug-induced
    due to drug abuse —*see* Abuse, drug,
        by type, with amnestic disorder
    due to drug dependence —*see*
        Dependence, drug, by type, with
        amnestic disorder
  nonalcoholic F04
Korsakov's disease, psychosis or
    syndrome —*see* Korsakoff's disease
Korsakow's disease, psychosis or
    syndrome —*see* Korsakoff's disease
Kostmann's disease or syndrome
    (infantile genetic agranulocytosis) —
    see Agranulocytosis
Kozhevnikof's epilepsy G40.109
  intractable G40.119
    with status epilepticus G40.111
    without status epilepticus G40.119
  not intractable G40.109
    with status epilepticus G40.101
    without status epilepticus G40.109

Krabbe's
  disease E75.23
  syndrome, congenital muscle
    hypoplasia Q79.8
Kraepelin-Morel disease —*see*
    Schizophrenia
Kraft-Weber-Dimitri disease Q85.8
Kraurosis
  ani K62.89
  penis N48.0
  vagina N89.8
  vulva N90.4
Kreotoxism A05.9
Krukenberg's
  spindle —*see* Pigmentation, cornea,
    posterior
  tumor C79.6-
Kufs' disease E75.4
Kugelberg-Welander disease G12.1
Kuhnt-Junius degeneration (*see also*
    Degeneration, macula) H35.32
Kümmell's disease or spondylitis —*see*
    Spondylopathy, traumatic
Kupffer cell sarcoma C22.3
Kuru A81.81
Kussmaul's
  disease M30.0
  respiration E87.2
    in diabetic acidosis —*see* Diabetes,
        by type, with ketoacidosis
Kwashiorkor E40
  marasmic, marasmus type E42
Kyasanur Forest disease A98.2
Kyphoscoliosis, kyphoscoliotic
    (acquired) (*see also* Scoliosis)
    M41.9
  congenital Q67.5
  heart (disease) I27.1
  sequelae of rickets E64.3
  tuberculous A18.01
Kyphosis, kyphotic (acquired) M40.209
  cervical region M40.202
  cervicothoracic region M40.203
  congenital Q76.419
    cervical region Q76.412
    cervicothoracic region Q76.413
    occipito-atlanto-axial region
        Q76.411
    thoracic region Q76.414
    thoracolumbar region Q76.415
  Morquio-Brailsford type (spinal) (*see
      also* subcategory M49.8) E76.219
  postlaminectomy M96.3
  postradiation therapy M96.2
  postural (adolescent) M40.00
    cervicothoracic region M40.03
    thoracic region M40.04
    thoracolumbar region M40.05
  secondary NEC M40.10
    cervical region M40.12
    cervicothoracic region M40.13
    thoracic region M40.14
    thoracolumbar region M40.15
  sequelae of rickets E64.3
  specified type NEC M40.299
    cervical region M40.292
    cervicothoracic region M40.293
    thoracic region M40.294
    thoracolumbar region M40.295
  syphilitic, congenital A50.56
    thoracic region M40.204
    thoracolumbar region M40.205
  tuberculous A18.01
Kyrle disease L87.0

L

Labia, labium —*see* condition
Labile
  blood pressure R09.89
  vasomotor system I73.9
Labioglossal paralysis G12.29
Labium leporinum —*see* Cleft, lip
Labor —*see* Delivery
Labored breathing —*see* Hyperventilation
Labyrinthitis (circumscribed) (destructive)
    (diffuse) (inner ear) (latent) (purulent)
    (suppurative) (*see also* subcategory)
    H83.0
  syphilitic A52.79
Laceration
  with abortion —*see* Abortion, by type,
    complicated by laceration of pelvic
    organs
  abdomen, abdominal
    wall S31.119
      with
        foreign body S31.129
        penetration into peritoneal cavity
          S31.619
          with foreign body S31.629
      epigastric region S31.112
        with
          foreign body S31.122
          penetration into peritoneal
            cavity S31.612
            with foreign body S31.622
      left
        lower quadrant S31.114
          with
            foreign body S31.124
            penetration into peritoneal
              cavity S31.614
              with foreign body
                S31.624
        upper quadrant S31.111
          with
            foreign body S31.121
            penetration into peritoneal
              cavity S31.611
              with foreign body
                S31.621
      periumbilic region S31.115
        with
          foreign body S31.125
          penetration into peritoneal
            cavity S31.615
            with foreign body
              S31.625
      right
        lower quadrant S31.113
          with
            foreign body S31.123
            penetration into peritoneal
              cavity S31.613
              with foreign body
                S31.623
        upper quadrant S31.110
          with
            foreign body S31.120
            penetration into peritoneal
              cavity S31.610
              with foreign body
                S31.620
  accidental, complicating surgery —*see*
    Complications, surgical, accidental
    puncture or laceration
  Achilles tendon S86.02-
  adrenal gland S37.813

Laceration (*Continued*)
  alveolar (process) —*see* Laceration,
    oral cavity
  ankle S91.01-
    with
      foreign body S91.02-
  antecubital space —*see* Laceration,
    elbow
  anus (sphincter) S31.831
    with
      ectopic or molar pregnancy
        O08.6
      foreign body S31.832
    complicating delivery —*see* Delivery,
      complicated, by, laceration,
      anus (sphincter)
    following ectopic or molar pregnancy
      O08.6
    nontraumatic, nonpuerperal —*see*
      Fissure, anus
  arm (upper) S41.11-
    with foreign body S41.12-
    lower —*see* Laceration, forearm
  auditory canal (external) (meatus) —*see*
    Laceration, ear
  auricle, ear —*see* Laceration, ear
  axilla —*see* Laceration, arm
  back —*see also* Laceration, thorax, back
    lower S31.010
      with
        foreign body S31.020
          with penetration into
            retroperitoneal space
            S31.021
        penetration into retroperitoneal
          space S31.011
  bile duct S36.13
  bladder S37.23
    with ectopic or molar pregnancy O08.6
    following ectopic or molar pregnancy
      O08.6
    obstetrical trauma O71.5
  blood vessel —*see* Injury, blood vessel
  bowel —*see also* Laceration, intestine
    with ectopic or molar pregnancy O08.6
    complicating abortion —*see* Abortion,
      by type, complicated by,
      specified condition NEC
    following ectopic or molar pregnancy
      O08.6
    obstetrical trauma O71.5
  brain (any part) (cortex) (diffuse)
      (membrane) —*see also* Injury,
      intracranial, diffuse
    during birth P10.8
      with hemorrhage P10.1
    focal —*see* Injury, intracranial, focal
      brain injury
  brainstem S06.38-
  breast S21.01-
    with foreign body S21.02-
  broad ligament S37.893
    with ectopic or molar pregnancy O08.6
    following ectopic or molar pregnancy
      O08.6
    laceration syndrome N83.8
    obstetrical trauma O71.6
    syndrome (laceration) N83.8
  buttock S31.801
    with foreign body S31.802
    left S31.821
      with foreign body S31.822
    right S31.811
      with foreign body S31.812

Laceration (*Continued*)
  calf —*see* Laceration, leg
  canaliculus lacrimalis —*see* Laceration,
    eyelid
  canthus, eye —*see* Laceration, eyelid
  capsule, joint —*see* Sprain
  causing eversion of cervix uteri (old)
    N86
  central (perineal), complicating delivery
    O70.9
  cerebellum, traumatic S06.37-
  cerebral S06.33-
    during birth P10.8
      with hemorrhage P10.1
    left side S06.32-
    right side S06.31-
  cervix (uteri)
    with ectopic or molar pregnancy
      O08.6
    following ectopic or molar pregnancy
      O08.6
    nonpuerperal, nontraumatic
      N88.1
    obstetrical trauma (current)
      O71.3
    old (postpartal) N88.1
    traumatic S37.63
  cheek (external) S01.41-
    with foreign body S01.42-
    internal —*see* Laceration, oral
      cavity
  chest wall —*see* Laceration, thorax
  chin —*see* Laceration, head, specified
    site NEC
  chordae tendinae NEC I51.1
    concurrent with acute myocardial
      infarction —*see* Infarct,
      myocardium
    following acute myocardial infarc-
      tion (current complication)
      I23.4
  clitoris —*see* Laceration, vulva
  colon —*see* Laceration, intestine, large,
    colon
  common bile duct S36.13
  cortex (cerebral) —*see* Injury,
    intracranial, diffuse
  costal region —*see* Laceration, thorax
  cystic duct S36.13
  diaphragm S27.803
  digit (s)
    foot —*see* Laceration, toe
    hand —*see* Laceration, finger
  duodenum S36.430
  ear (canal) (external) S01.31-
    with foreign body S01.32-
    drum S09.2-
  elbow S51.01-
    with
      foreign body S51.02-
  epididymis —*see* Laceration, testis
  epigastric region —*see* Laceration,
    abdomen, wall, epigastric
    region
  esophagus K22.8
    traumatic
      cervical S11.21
        with foreign body S11.22
      thoracic S27.813
  eye (ball) S05.3-
    with prolapse or loss of intraocular
      tissue S05.2-
    penetrating S05.6-
  eyebrow —*see* Laceration, eyelid

Laceration (Continued)
eyelid S01.11-
  with foreign body S01.12-
face NEC —see Laceration, head,
    specified site NEC
fallopian tube S37.539
  bilateral S37.532
  unilateral S37.531
finger (s) S61.219
  with
    damage to nail S61.319
      with
        foreign body S61.329
    foreign body S61.229
  index S61.218
    with
      damage to nail S61.318
        with
          foreign body S61.328
      foreign body S61.228
    left S61.211
      with
        damage to nail S61.311
          with
            foreign body S61.321
        foreign body S61.221
    right S61.210
      with
        damage to nail S61.310
          with
            foreign body S61.320
        foreign body S61.220
  little S61.218
    with
      damage to nail S61.318
        with
          foreign body S61.328
      foreign body S61.228
    left S61.217
      with
        damage to nail S61.317
          with
            foreign body S61.327
        foreign body S61.227
    right S61.216
      with
        damage to nail S61.316
          with
            foreign body S61.326
        foreign body S61.226
  middle S61.218
    with
      damage to nail S61.318
        with
          foreign body S61.328
      foreign body S61.228
    left S61.213
      with
        damage to nail S61.313
          with
            foreign body S61.323
        foreign body S61.223
    right S61.212
      with
        damage to nail S61.312
          with
            foreign body S61.322
        foreign body S61.222
  ring S61.218
    with
      damage to nail S61.318
        with
          foreign body S61.328
      foreign body S61.228

Laceration (Continued)
finger (s) (Continued)
  ring (Continued)
    left S61.215
      with
        damage to nail S61.315
          with
            foreign body S61.325
        foreign body S61.225
    right S61.214
      with
        damage to nail S61.314
          with
            foreign body S61.324
        foreign body S61.224
flank S31.119
  with foreign body S31.129
foot (except toe (s) alone) S91.319
  with foreign body S91.329
  left S91.312
    with foreign body S91.322
  right S91.311
    with foreign body S91.321
  toe —see Laceration, toe
forearm S51.819
  with
    foreign body S51.829
  elbow only —see Laceration, elbow
  left S51.812
    with
      foreign body S51.822
  right S51.811
    with
      foreign body S51.821
forehead S01.81
  with foreign body S01.82
fourchette O70.0
  with ectopic or molar pregnancy
    O08.6
  complicating delivery O70.0
  following ectopic or molar pregnancy
    O08.6
gallbladder S36.123
genital organs, external
  female S31.512
    with foreign body S31.522
    vagina —see Laceration, vagina
    vulva —see Laceration, vulva
  male S31.511
    with foreign body S31.521
    penis —see Laceration, penis
    scrotum —see Laceration, scrotum
    testis —see Laceration, testis
groin —see Laceration, abdomen,
    wall
gum —see Laceration, oral cavity
hand S61.419
  with
    foreign body S61.429
  finger —see Laceration, finger
  left S61.412
    with
      foreign body S61.422
  right S61.411
    with
      foreign body S61.421
  thumb —see Laceration, thumb
head S01.91
  with foreign body S01.92
  cheek —see Laceration, cheek
  ear —see Laceration, ear
  eyelid —see Laceration, eyelid
  lip —see Laceration, lip
  nose —see Laceration, nose

Laceration (Continued)
head (Continued)
  oral cavity —see Laceration, oral cavity
  scalp S01.01
    with foreign body S01.02
    specified site NEC S01.81
      with foreign body S01.82
    temporomandibular area —see
      Laceration, cheek
  heart —see Injury, heart, laceration
  heel —see Laceration, foot
  hepatic duct S36.13
  hip S71.019
    with foreign body S71.029
    left S71.012
      with foreign body S71.022
    right S71.011
      with foreign body S71.021
  hymen —see Laceration, vagina
  hypochondrium —see Laceration,
    abdomen, wall
  hypogastric region —see Laceration,
    abdomen, wall
  ileum S36.438
  inguinal region —see Laceration,
    abdomen, wall
  instep —see Laceration, foot
  internal organ —see Injury, by site
  interscapular region —see Laceration,
    thorax, back
  intestine
    large
      colon S36.539
        ascending S36.530
        descending S36.532
        sigmoid S36.533
        specified site NEC S36.538
      rectum S36.63
      transverse S36.531
    small S36.439
      duodenum S36.430
      specified site NEC S36.438
  intra-abdominal organ S36.93
    intestine —see Laceration, intestine
    liver —see Laceration, liver
    pancreas —see Laceration,
      pancreas
    peritoneum S36.81
    specified site NEC S36.893
    spleen —see Laceration, spleen
    stomach —see Laceration, stomach
  intracranial NEC —see also Injury,
    intracranial, diffuse
    birth injury P10.9
  jaw —see Laceration, head, specified
    site NEC
  jejunum S36.438
  joint capsule —see Sprain, by site
  kidney S37.03-
    major (greater than 3 cm) (massive)
      (stellate) S37.06-
    minor (less than 1 cm) S37.04-
    moderate (1 to 3 cm) S37.05-
    multiple S37.06-
  knee S81.01-
    with foreign body S81.02-
  labium (majus) (minus) —see
    Laceration, vulva
  lacrimal duct —see Laceration,
    eyelid
  large intestine —see Laceration,
    intestine, large
  larynx S11.011
    with foreign body S11.012

Laceration (Continued)
leg (lower) S81.819
with foreign body S81.829
foot —see Laceration, foot
knee —see Laceration, knee
left S81.812
with foreign body S81.822
right S81.811
with foreign body S81.821
upper —see Laceration, thigh
ligament —see Sprain
lip S01.511
with foreign body S01.521
liver S36.113
major (stellate) S36.116
minor S36.114
moderate S36.115
loin —see Laceration, abdomen, wall
lower back —see Laceration, back, lower
lumbar region —see Laceration, back, lower
lung S27.339
bilateral S27.332
unilateral S27.331
malar region —see Laceration, head, specified site NEC
mammary —see Laceration, breast
mastoid region —see Laceration, head, specified site NEC
meninges —see Injury, intracranial, diffuse
meniscus —see Tear, meniscus
mesentery S36.893
mesosalpinx S37.539
bilateral S37.532
unilateral S37.531
mouth —see Laceration, oral cavity
muscle —see Injury, muscle, by site, laceration
nail
finger —see Laceration, finger, with damage to nail
toe —see Laceration, toe, with damage to nail
nasal (septum) (sinus) —see Laceration, nose
nasopharynx —see Laceration, head, specified site NEC
neck S11.91
with foreign body S11.92
involving
cervical esophagus S11.21
with foreign body S11.22
larynx —see Laceration, larynx
pharynx —see Laceration, pharynx
thyroid gland —see Laceration, thyroid gland
trachea —see Laceration, trachea
specified site NEC S11.81
with foreign body S11.82
nerve —see Injury, nerve
nose (septum) (sinus) S01.21
with foreign body S01.22
ocular NOS S05.3-
adnexa NOS S01.11-
oral cavity S01.512
with foreign body S01.522
orbit (eye) —see Wound, open, ocular, orbit
ovary S37.439
bilateral S37.432
unilateral S37.431
palate —see Laceration, oral cavity
palm —see Laceration, hand

Laceration (Continued)
pancreas S36.239
body S36.231
major S36.261
minor S36.241
moderate S36.251
head S36.230
major S36.260
minor S36.240
moderate S36.250
major S36.269
minor S36.249
moderate S36.259
tail S36.232
major S36.262
minor S36.242
moderate S36.252
pelvic S31.010
with
foreign body S31.020
penetration into retroperitoneal cavity S31.021
penetration into retroperitoneal cavity S31.011
floor —see also Laceration, back, lower
with ectopic or molar pregnancy O08.6
complicating delivery O70.1
following ectopic or molar pregnancy O08.6
old (postpartal) N81.89
organ S37.93
with ectopic or molar pregnancy O08.6
adrenal gland S37.813
bladder S37.23
fallopian tube —see Laceration, fallopian tube
following ectopic or molar pregnancy O08.6
kidney —see Laceration, kidney
obstetrical trauma O71.5
ovary —see Laceration, ovary
prostate S37.823
specified site NEC S37.893
ureter S37.13
urethra S37.33
uterus S37.63
penis S31.21
with foreign body S31.22
perineum
female S31.41
with
ectopic or molar pregnancy O08.6
foreign body S31.42
during delivery O70.9
first degree O70.0
fourth degree O70.3
second degree O70.1
third degree O70.2
old (postpartal) N81.89
postpartal N81.89
secondary (postpartal) O90.1
male S31.119
with foreign body S31.129
periocular area (with or without lacrimal passages) —see Laceration, eyelid
peritoneum S36.893
periumbilic region —see Laceration, abdomen, wall, periumbilic
periurethral tissue —see Laceration, urethra
phalanges
finger —see Laceration, finger

Laceration (Continued)
phalanges (Continued)
toe —see Laceration, toe
pharynx S11.21
with foreign body S11.22
pinna —see Laceration, ear
popliteal space —see Laceration, knee
prepuce —see Laceration, penis
prostate S37.823
pubic region S31.119
with foreign body S31.129
pudendum —see Laceration, genital organs, external
rectovaginal septum —see Laceration, vagina
rectum S36.63
retroperitoneum S36.893
round ligament S37.893
sacral region —see Laceration, back, lower
sacroiliac region —see Laceration, back, lower
salivary gland —see Laceration, oral cavity
scalp S01.01
with foreign body S01.02
scapular region —see Laceration, shoulder
scrotum S31.31
with foreign body S31.32
seminal vesicle S37.893
shin —see Laceration, leg
shoulder S41.019
with foreign body S41.029
left S41.012
with foreign body S41.022
right S41.011
with foreign body S41.021
small intestine —see Laceration, intestine, small
spermatic cord —see Laceration, testis
spinal cord (meninges) —see also Injury, spinal cord, by region
due to injury at birth P11.5
newborn (birth injury) P11.5
spleen S36.039
major (massive) (stellate) S36.032
moderate S36.031
superficial (minor) S36.030
sternal region —see Laceration, thorax, front
stomach S36.33
submaxillary region —see Laceration, head, specified site NEC
submental region —see Laceration, head, specified site NEC
subungual
finger (s) —see Laceration, finger, with damage to nail
toe (s) —see Laceration, toe, with damage to nail
suprarenal gland —see Laceration, adrenal gland
temple, temporal region —see Laceration, head, specified site NEC
temporomandibular area —see Laceration, cheek
tendon —see Injury, muscle, by site, laceration
Achilles S86.02-
tentorium cerebelli —see Injury, intracranial, diffuse
testis S31.31
with foreign body S31.32

Laceration *(Continued)*
    thigh S71.11-
        with foreign body S71.12-
    thorax, thoracic (wall) S21.91
        with foreign body S21.92
        back S21.22-
            with penetration into thoracic
                cavity S21.42-
        front S21.12-
            with penetration into thoracic
                cavity S21.32-
        back S21.21-
            with
                foreign body S21.22-
                    with penetration into thoracic
                        cavity S21.42-
                penetration into thoracic cavity
                    S21.41-
        breast —*see* Laceration, breast
        front S21.11-
            with
                foreign body S21.12-
                    with penetration into thoracic
                        cavity S21.32-
                penetration into thoracic cavity
                    S21.31-
    thumb S61.019
        with
            damage to nail S61.119
                with
                    foreign body S61.129
            foreign body S61.029
        left S61.012
            with
                damage to nail S61.112
                    with
                        foreign body S61.122
                foreign body S61.022
        right S61.011
            with
                damage to nail S61.111
                    with
                        foreign body S61.121
                foreign body S61.021
    thyroid gland S11.11
        with foreign body S11.12
    toe (s) S91.119
        with
            damage to nail S91.219
                with
                    foreign body S91.229
            foreign body S91.129
        great S91.113
            with
                damage to nail S91.213
                    with
                        foreign body S91.223
                foreign body S91.123
            left S91.112
                with
                    damage to nail S91.212
                        with
                            foreign body S91.222
                    foreign body S91.122
            right S91.111
                with
                    damage to nail S91.211
                        with
                            foreign body S91.221
                    foreign body S91.121
        lesser S91.116
            with
                damage to nail S91.216
                    with
                        foreign body S91.226
                foreign body S91.126

Laceration *(Continued)*
    toe (s) *(Continued)*
        lesser *(Continued)*
            left S91.115
                with
                    damage to nail S91.215
                        with
                            foreign body S91.225
                    foreign body S91.125
            right S91.114
                with
                    damage to nail S91.214
                        with
                            foreign body S91.224
                    foreign body S91.124
    tongue —*see* Laceration, oral cavity
    trachea S11.021
        with foreign body S11.022
    tunica vaginalis —*see* Laceration, testis
    tympanum, tympanic membrane —*see*
        Laceration, ear, drum
    umbilical region S31.115
        with foreign body S31.125
    ureter S37.13
    urethra S37.33
        with or following ectopic or molar
            pregnancy O08.6
        obstetrical trauma O71.5
    urinary organ NEC S37.893
    uterus S37.63
        with ectopic or molar pregnancy O08.6
        following ectopic or molar pregnancy
            O08.6
        nonpuerperal, nontraumatic N85.8
        obstetrical trauma NEC O71.81
        old (postpartal) N85.8
    uvula —*see* Laceration, oral cavity
    vagina S31.41
        with
            ectopic or molar pregnancy O08.6
            foreign body S31.42
        during delivery O71.4
            with perineal laceration —*see*
                Laceration, perineum, female,
                during delivery
        following ectopic or molar pregnancy
            O08.6
        nonpuerperal, nontraumatic N89.8
        old (postpartal) N89.8
    vas deferens S37.893
    vesical —*see* Laceration, bladder
    vocal cords S11.031
        with foreign body S11.032
    vulva S31.41
        with
            ectopic or molar pregnancy O08.6
            foreign body S31.42
        complicating delivery O70.0
        following ectopic or molar pregnancy
            O08.6
        nonpuerperal, nontraumatic N90.89
        old (postpartal) N90.89
    wrist S61.519
        with
            foreign body S61.529
        left S61.512
            with
                foreign body S61.522
        right S61.511
            with
                foreign body S61.521
Lack of
    achievement in school Z55.3
    adequate
        food Z59.4

Lack of *(Continued)*
    adequate *(Continued)*
        intermaxillary vertical dimension of
            fully erupted teeth M26.36
        sleep Z72.820
    appetite (*see* Anorexia) R63.0
    awareness R41.9
    care
        in home Z74.2
        of infant (at or after birth) T76.02
            confirmed T74.02
    cognitive functions R41.9
    coordination R27.9
        ataxia R27.0
        specified type NEC R27.8
    development (physiological) R62.50
        failure to thrive (child over 28 days
            old) R62.51
            adult R62.7
            newborn P92.6
        short stature R62.52
        specified type NEC R62.59
    energy R53.83
    financial resources Z59.6
    food T73.0
    growth R62.52
    heating Z59.1
    housing (permanent) (temporary) Z59.0
        adequate Z59.1
    learning experiences in childhood
        Z62.898
    leisure time (affecting life-style) Z73.2
    material resources Z59.9
    memory —*see also* Amnesia
        mild, following organic brain damage
            F06.8
    ovulation N97.0
    parental supervision or control of child
        Z62.0
    person able to render necessary care
        Z74.2
    physical exercise Z72.3
    play experience in childhood Z62.898
    posterior occlusal support M26.57
    relaxation (affecting life-style) Z73.2
    sexual
        desire F52.0
        enjoyment F52.1
    shelter Z59.0
    sleep (adequate) Z72.820
    supervision of child by parent Z62.0
    support, posterior occlusal M26.57
    water T73.1
Lacrimal —*see* condition
Lacrimation, abnormal —*see* Epiphora
Lacrimonasal duct —*see* condition
Lactation, lactating (breast) (puerperal,
    postpartum)
    associated
        cracked nipple O92.13
        retracted nipple O92.03
    defective O92.4
    disorder NEC O92.79
    excessive O92.6
    failed (complete) O92.3
        partial O92.4
    mastitis NEC —*see* Mastitis, obstetric
    mother (care and/or examination) Z39.1
    nonpuerperal N64.3
Lacticemia, excessive E87.2
Lacunar skull Q75.8
Laennec's cirrhosis K74.69
    alcoholic K70.30
        with ascites K70.31

Lafora's disease —*see* Epilepsy,
   generalized, idiopathic
Lag, lid (nervous) —*see* Retraction, lid
Lagophthalmos (eyelid) (nervous) H02.209
   cicatricial H02.219
      left H02.216
         lower H02.215
         upper H02.214
      right H02.213
         lower H02.212
         upper H02.211
   keratoconjunctivitis —*see*
      Keratoconjunctivitis
   left H02.206
      lower H02.205
      upper H02.204
   mechanical H02.229
      left H02.226
         lower H02.225
         upper H02.224
      right H02.223
         lower H02.222
         upper H02.221
   paralytic H02.239
      left H02.236
         lower H02.235
         upper H02.234
      right H02.233
         lower H02.232
         upper H02.231
   right H02.203
      lower H02.202
      upper H02.201
Laki-Lorand factor deficiency —*see*
   Defect, coagulation, specified type
   NEC
Lalling F80.0
Lambert-Eaton syndrome —*see*
   Syndrome, Lambert-Eaton
Lambliasis, lambliosis A07.1
Landau-Kleffner syndrome —*see*
   Epilepsy, specified NEC
Landouzy-Déjérine dystrophy or
   facioscapulohumeral atrophy
   G71.0
Landouzy's disease (icterohemorrhagic
   leptospirosis) A27.0
Landry-Guillain-Barré, syndrome or
   paralysis G61.0
Landry's disease or paralysis G61.0
Lane's
   band Q43.3
   kink —*see* Obstruction, intestine
   syndrome K90.2
Langdon Down's syndrome —*see*
   Trisomy, 21
Lapsed immunization schedule status
   Z28.3
Large
   baby (regardless of gestational age)
      (4000g to 4499g) P08.1
   ear, congenital Q17.1
   physiological cup Q14.2
   stature R68.89
Large-for-dates NEC (infant) (4000g to
   4499g) P08.1
   affecting management of pregnancy
      O36.6-
   exceptionally (4500g or more) P08.0
Larsen-Johansson disease
   orosteochondrosis —*see*
      Osteochondrosis, juvenile, patella
Larsen's syndrome (flattened facies and
   multiple congenital dislocations) Q74.8

Larva migrans
   cutaneous B76.9
      Ancylostoma B76.0
   visceral B83.0
Laryngeal —*see* condition
Laryngismus (stridulus) J38.5
   congenital P28.89
   diphtheritic A36.2
Laryngitis (acute) (edematous) (fibrinous)
   (infective) (infiltrative) (malignant)
   (membranous) (phlegmonous)
   (pneumococcal) (pseudomembranous)
   (septic) (subglottic) (suppurative)
   (ulcerative) J04.0
   with
      influenza, flu, or grippe —*see*
         Influenza, with, laryngitis
      tracheitis (acute) —*see*
         Laryngotracheitis
   atrophic J37.0
   catarrhal J37.0
   chronic J37.0
      with tracheitis (chronic) J37.1
   diphtheritic A36.2
   due to external agent —*see*
      Inflammation, respiratory, upper,
      due to
   Hemophilus influenzae J04.0
   H. influenzae J04.0
   hypertrophic J37.0
   influenzal —*see* Influenza, with,
      respiratory manifestations NEC
   obstructive J05.0
   sicca J37.0
   spasmodic J05.0
      acute J04.0
   streptococcal J04.0
   stridulous J05.0
   syphilitic (late) A52.73
      congenital A50.59 *[J99]*
      early A50.03 *[J99]*
   tuberculous A15.5
   Vincent's A69.1
Laryngocele (congenital) (ventricular)
   Q31.3
Laryngofissure J38.7
   congenital Q31.8
Laryngomalacia (congenital) Q31.5
Laryngopharyngitis (acute) J06.0
   chronic J37.0
   due to external agent —*see*
      Inflammation, respiratory, upper,
      due to
Laryngoplegia J38.00
   bilateral J38.02
   unilateral J38.01
Laryngoptosis J38.7
Laryngospasm J38.5
Laryngostenosis J38.6
Laryngotracheitis (acute) (Infectional)
   (infective) (viral) J04.2
   atrophic J37.1
   catarrhal J37.1
   chronic J37.1
   diphtheritic A36.2
   due to external agent —*see*
      Inflammation, respiratory, upper,
      due to
   Hemophilus influenzae J04.2
   hypertrophic J37.1
   influenzal —*see* Influenza, with,
      respiratory manifestations NEC
   pachydermic J38.7
   sicca J37.1

Laryngotracheitis *(Continued)*
   spasmodic J38.5
      acute J05.0
   streptococcal J04.2
   stridulous J38.5
   syphilitic (late) A52.73
      congenital A50.59 *[J99]*
      early A50.03 *[J99]*
   tuberculous A15.5
   Vincent's A69.1
Laryngotracheobronchitis —*see*
   Bronchitis
Larynx, laryngeal —*see* condition
Lassa fever A96.2
Lassitude —*see* Weakness
Late
   talker R62.0
   walker R62.0
Late effect (s) —*see* Sequelae
Latent —*see* condition
Laterocession —*see* Lateroversion
Lateroflexion —*see* Lateroversion
Lateroversion
   cervix —*see* Lateroversion, uterus
   uterus, uterine (cervix) (postinfectional)
      (postpartal, old) N85.4
   congenital Q51.818
   in pregnancy or childbirth O34.59-
Lathyrism —*see* Poisoning, food, noxious,
   plant
Launois' syndrome (pituitary gigantism)
   E22.0
Launois-Bensaude adenolipomatosis
   E88.89
Laurence-Moon (-Bardet)-Biedl
   syndrome Q87.89
Lax, laxity —*see also* Relaxation
   ligament (ous) —*see also* Disorder,
      ligament
   familial M35.7
   knee —*see* Derangement, knee
   skin (acquired) L57.4
      congenital Q82.8
Laxative habit F55.2
Lazy leukocyte syndrome D70.8
Lead miner's lung J63.6
Leak, leakage
   air NEC J93.82
      postprocedural J95.812
   amniotic fluid —*see* Rupture,
      membranes, premature
   blood (microscopic), fetal, into maternal
      circulation affecting management
      of pregnancy —*see* Pregnancy,
      complicated by
   cerebrospinal fluid G96.0
      from spinal (lumbar) puncture G97.0
   device, implant or graft —*see also*
      Complications, by site and type,
      mechanical
      arterial graft NEC —*see*
         Complication, cardiovascular
         device, mechanical, vascular
      breast (implant) T85.43
      catheter NEC T85.638
         dialysis (renal) T82.43
            intraperitoneal T85.631
         infusion NEC T82.534
            spinal (epidural) (subdural) T85.630
         urinary, indwelling T83.038
            cystostomy T83.030
      gastrointestinal —*see* Complications,
         prosthetic device, mechanical,
         gastrointestinal device

Leak, leakage (*Continued*)
  device, implant or graft (*Continued*)
    genital NEC T83.498
      penile prosthesis T83.490
    heart NEC —*see* Complication,
      cardiovascular device,
      mechanical
    joint prosthesis —*see* Complications,
      joint prosthesis, mechanical,
      specified NEC, by site
    ocular NEC —*see* Complications,
      prosthetic device, mechanical,
      ocular device
    orthopedic NEC —*see* Complication,
      orthopedic, device, mechanical
    persistent air J93.82
    specified NEC T85.638
    urinary NEC —*see also* Complication,
      genitourinary, device, urinary,
      mechanical
      graft T83.23
    vascular NEC —*see* Complication,
      cardiovascular device,
      mechanical
    ventricular intracranial shunt T85.03
  urine —*see* Incontinence
Leaky heart —*see* Endocarditis
Learning defect (specific) F81.9
Leather bottle stomach C16.9
Leber's
  congenital amaurosis H35.50
  optic atrophy (hereditary) H47.22
Lederer's anemia D59.1
Leeches (external) —*see* Hirudiniasis
Leg —*see* condition
Legg (-Calvé)**-Perthes disease, syndrome**
  or osteochondrosis M91.1-
Legionellosis A48.1
  nonpneumonic A48.2
Legionnaires'
  disease A48.1
    nonpneumonic A48.2
  pneumonia A48.1
Leigh's disease G31.82
Leiner's disease L21.1
Leiofibromyoma —*see* Leiomyoma
Leiomyoblastoma —*see* Neoplasm,
  connective tissue, benign
Leiomyofibroma —*see also* Neoplasm,
  connective tissue, benign
  uterus (cervix) (corpus) D25.9
Leiomyoma —*see also* Neoplasm,
  connective tissue, benign
  bizarre —*see* Neoplasm, connective
    tissue, benign
  cellular —*see* Neoplasm, connective
    tissue, benign
  epithelioid —*see* Neoplasm, connective
    tissue, benign
  uterus (cervix) (corpus) D25.9
    intramural D25.1
    submucous D25.0
    subserosal D25.2
  vascular —*see* Neoplasm, connective
    tissue, benign
Leiomyoma, leiomyomatosis
  (intravascular) —*see* Neoplasm,
  connective tissue, uncertain behavior
Leiomyosarcoma —*see also* Neoplasm,
  connective tissue, malignant
  epithelioid —*see* Neoplasm, connective
    tissue, malignant
  myxoid —*see* Neoplasm, connective
    tissue, malignant

Leishmaniasis B55.9
  American (mucocutaneous) B55.2
    cutaneous B55.1
  Asian Desert B55.1
  Brazilian B55.2
  cutaneous (any type) B55.1
  dermal —*see also* Leishmaniasis,
    cutaneous
    post-kala-azar B55.0
  eyelid B55.1
  infantile B55.0
  Mediterranean B55.0
  mucocutaneous (American) (New
    World) B55.2
  naso-oral B55.2
  nasopharyngeal B55.2
  old world B55.1
  tegumentaria diffusa B55.1
  visceral B55.0
Leishmanoid, dermal —*see also*
  Leishmaniasis, cutaneous
  post-kala-azar B55.0
Lenegre's disease I44.2
Lengthening, leg —*see* Deformity, limb,
  unequal length
Lennert's lymphoma —*see* Lymphoma,
  Lennert's
Lennox-Gastaut syndrome G40.812
  intractable G40.814
    with status epilepticus G40.813
    without status epilepticus G40.814
  not intractable G40.812
    with status epilepticus G40.811
    without status epilepticus G40.812
Lens —*see* condition
Lenticonus (anterior) (posterior)
  (congenital) Q12.8
Lenticular degeneration, progressive
  E83.01
Lentiglobus (posterior) (congenital) Q12.8
Lentigo (congenital) L81.4
  maligna —*see also* Melanoma, in situ
    melanoma —*see* Melanoma
Lentivirus, as cause of disease classified
  elsewhere B97.31
Leontiasis
  ossium M85.2
  syphilitic (late) A52.78
    congenital A50.59
Lepothrix A48.8
Lepra —*see* Leprosy
Leprechaunism E34.8
Leprosy A30.-
  with muscle disorder A30.9 [*M63.80*]
    ankle A30.9 [*M63.87-*]
    foot A30.9 [*M63.87-*]
    forearm A30.9 [*M63.83-*]
    hand A30.9 [*M63.84-*]
    lower leg A30.9 [*M63.86-*]
    multiple sites A30.9 [*M63.89*]
    pelvic region A30.9 [*M63.85-*]
    shoulder region A30.9 [*M63.81-*]
    specified site NEC A30.9 [*M63.88*]
    thigh A30.9 [*M63.85-*]
    upper arm A30.9 [*M63.82-*]
  anesthetic A30.9
  BB A30.3
  BL A30.4
  borderline (infiltrated) (neuritic) A30.3
    lepromatous A30.4
    tuberculoid A30.2
  BT A30.2
  dimorphous (infiltrated) (neuritic) A30.3
  I A30.0

Leprosy (*Continued*)
  indeterminate (macular) (neuritic) A30.0
  lepromatous (diffuse) (infiltrated)
    (macular) (neuritic) (nodular) A30.5
  LL A30.5
  macular (early) (neuritic) (simple) A30.9
  maculoanesthetic A30.9
  mixed A30.3
  neural A30.9
  nodular A30.5
  primary neuritic A30.3
  specified type NEC A30.8
  TT A30.1
  tuberculoid (major) (minor) A30.1
Leptocytosis, hereditary D56.9
Leptomeningitis (chronic)
  (circumscribed) (hemorrhagic)
  (nonsuppurative) —*see* Meningitis
Leptomeningopathy G96.19
Leptospiral —*see* condition
Leptospirochetal —*see* condition
Leptospirosis A27.9
  canicola A27.89
  due to Leptospira interrogans serovar
    icterohaemorrhagiae A27.0
  icterohemorrhagica A27.0
  pomona A27.89
  Weil's disease A27.0
Leptus dermatitis B88.0
Leriche's syndrome (aortic bifurcation
  occlusion) I74.09
Leri's pleonosteosis Q78.8
Leri-Weill syndrome Q77.8
Lermoyez' syndrome —*see* Vertigo,
  peripheral NEC
Lesch-Nyhan syndrome E79.1
Leser-Trélat disease L82.1
  inflamed L82.0
Lesion (s) (nontraumatic)
  abducens nerve —*see* Strabismus,
    paralytic, sixth nerve
  alveolar process K08.9
  angiocentric immunoproliferative D47.Z9
  anorectal K62.9
  aortic (valve) I35.9
  auditory nerve —*see* subcategory H93.3
  basal ganglion G25.9
  bile duct —*see* Disease, bile duct
  biomechanical M99.9
    specified type NEC M99.89
      abdomen M99.89
      acromioclavicular M99.87
      cervical region M99.81
      cervicothoracic M99.81
      costochondral M99.88
      costovertebral M99.88
      head region M99.80
      hip M99.85
      lower extremity M99.86
      lumbar region M99.83
      lumbosacral M99.83
      occipitocervical M99.80
      pelvic region M99.85
      pubic M99.85
      rib cage M99.88
      sacral region M99.84
      sacrococcygeal M99.84
      sacroiliac M99.84
      specified NEC M99.89
      sternochondral M99.88
      sternoclavicular M99.87
      thoracic region M99.82
      thoracolumbar M99.82
      upper extremity M99.87

Lesion (Continued)
  bladder N32.9
  bone —see Disorder, bone
  brachial plexus G54.0
  brain G93.9
    congenital Q04.9
    vascular I67.9
      degenerative I67.9
      hypertensive I67.4
  buccal cavity K13.79
  calcified —see Calcification
  canthus —see Disorder, eyelid
  carate —see Pinta, lesions
  cardia K22.9
  cardiac (see also Disease, heart) I51.9
    congenital Q24.9
    valvular —see Endocarditis
  cauda equina G83.4
  cecum K63.9
  cerebral —see Lesion, brain
  cerebrovascular I67.9
    degenerative I67.9
    hypertensive I67.4
  cervical (nerve) root NEC G54.2
  chiasmal —see Disorder, optic, chiasm
  chorda tympani G51.8
  coin, lung R91.1
  colon K63.9
  congenital —see Anomaly, by site
  conjunctiva H11.9
  conus medullaris —see Injury, conus
      medullaris
  coronary artery —see Ischemia, heart
  cranial nerve G52.9
    eighth —see Disorder, ear
    eleventh G52.9
    fifth G50.9
    first G52.0
    fourth —see Strabismus, paralytic,
        fourth nerve
    seventh G51.9
    sixth —see Strabismus, paralytic,
        sixth nerve
    tenth G52.2
    twelfth G52.3
  cystic —see Cyst
  degenerative —see Degeneration
  duodenum K31.9
  edentulous (alveolar) ridge, associated
      with trauma, due to traumatic
      occlusion K06.2
  en coup de sabre L94.1
  eyelid —see Disorder, eyelid
  gasserian ganglion G50.8
  gastric K31.9
  gastroduodenal K31.9
  gastrointestinal K63.9
  gingiva, associated with trauma K06.2
  glomerular
    focal and segmental (see also N00-N07
        with fourth character .1) N05.1
    minimal change (see also N00-N07
        with fourth character .0) N05.0
  heart (organic) —see Disease, heart
  hyperchromic, due to pinta (carate)
      A67.1
  hyperkeratotic —see Hyperkeratosis
  hypothalamic E23.7
  ileocecal K63.9
  ileum K63.9
  iliohypogastric nerve G57.8-
  inflammatory —see Inflammation
  intestine K63.9
  intracerebral —see Lesion, brain

Lesion (Continued)
  intrachiasmal (optic) —see Disorder,
      optic, chiasm
  intracranial, space-occupying R90.0
  joint —see Disorder, joint
    sacroiliac (old) M53.3
  keratotic —see Keratosis
  kidney —see Disease, renal
  laryngeal nerve (recurrent) G52.2
  lip K13.0
  liver K76.9
  lumbosacral
    plexus G54.1
    root (nerve) NEC G54.4
  lung (coin) R91.2
  maxillary sinus J32.0
  mitral I05.9
  Morel-Lavallée —see Hematoma, by site
  motor cortex NEC G93.89
  mouth K13.79
  nerve G58.9
    femoral G57.2-
    median G56.1-
      carpal tunnel syndrome —see
          Syndrome, carpal tunnel
    plantar G57.6-
    popliteal (lateral) G57.3-
    medial G57.4-
    radial G56.3-
    sciatic G57.0-
    spinal —see Injury, nerve, spinal
    ulnar G56.2-
  nervous system, congenital Q07.9
  nonallopathic —see Lesion,
      biomechanical
  nose (internal) J34.89
  obstructive —see Obstruction
  obturator nerve G57.8-
  oral mucosa K13.70
  organ or site NEC —see Disease, by site
  osteolytic —see Osteolysis
  peptic K27.9
  periodontal, due to traumatic occlusion
      K05.5
  pharynx J39.2
  pigment, pigmented (skin) L81.9
  pinta —see Pinta, lesions
  polypoid —see Polyp
  prechiasmal (optic) —see Disorder,
      optic, chiasm
  primary (see also Syphilis, primary) A51.0
    carate A67.0
    pinta A67.0
    yaws A66.0
  pulmonary J98.4
    valve I37.9
  pylorus K31.9
  rectosigmoid K63.9
  retina, retinal H35.9
  sacroiliac (joint) (old) M53.3
  salivary gland K11.9
    benign lymphoepithelial K11.8
  saphenous nerve G57.8-
  sciatic nerve G57.0-
  secondary —see Syphilis, secondary
  shoulder (region) M75.9-
    specified NEC M75.8-
  sigmoid K63.9
  sinus (accessory) (nasal) J34.89
  skin L98.9
    suppurative L08.0
  SLAP S43.43-
  spinal cord G95.9
    congenital Q06.9

Lesion (Continued)
  spleen D73.89
  stomach K31.9
  superior glenoid labrum S43.43-
  syphilitic —see Syphilis
  tertiary —see Syphilis, tertiary
  thoracic root (nerve) NEC G54.3
  tonsillar fossa J35.9
  tooth, teeth K08.9
    white spot
      chewing surface K02.51
      pit and fissure surface K02.51
      smooth surface K02.61
  traumatic —see specific type of injury
      by site
  tricuspid (valve) I07.9
    nonrheumatic I36.9
  trigeminal nerve G50.9
  ulcerated or ulcerative —see Ulcer, skin
  uterus N85.9
  vagus nerve G52.2
  valvular —see Endocarditis
  vascular I99.9
    affecting central nervous system I67.9
    following trauma NEC T14.8
    umbilical cord, complicating delivery
        O69.5
  warty —see Verruca
  white spot (tooth)
    chewing surface K02.51
    pit and fissure surface K02.51
    smooth surface K02.61
Lethargic —see condition
Lethargy R53.83
Letterer-Siwe's disease C96.0
Leuc (o) —see Leuk (o)
Leukemia, leukemic C95.9-
  acute basophilic C94.8-
  acute bilineal C95.0-
  acute erythroid C94.0-
  acute lymphoblastic C91.0-
  acute megakaryoblastic C94.2-
  acute megakaryocytic C94.2-
  acute mixed lineage C95.0-
  acute monoblastic (monoblastic/
      monocytic) C93.0-
  acute monocytic (monoblastic/
      monocytic) C93.0-
  acute myeloblastic (minimal
      differentiation) (with maturation)
      C92.0-
  acute myeloid
    with
      11q23-abnormality C92.6-
      dysplasia of remaining
          hematopoesis and/or
          myelodysplastic disease
          in its history C92.A-
      multilineage dysplasia C92.A-
      variation of MLL-gene C92.6-
    M6 (a)(b) C94.0-
    M7 C94.2-
  acute myelomonocytic C92.5-
  acute promyelocytic C92.4-
  adult T-cell (HTLV-1-associated)
      (acute variant) (chronic variant)
      (lymphomatoid variant)
      (smouldering variant) C91.5-
  aggressive NK-cell C94.8-
  AML (1/ETO) (M0) (M1) (M2) (without
      a FAB classification) C92.0-
  AML M3 C92.4-
  AML M4 (Eo with inv(16) or t(16;16))
      C92.5-

Leukemia, leukemic (Continued)
AML M5 C93.0-
AML M5a C93.0-
AML M5b C93.0-
AML Me with t (15;17) and variants
C92.4-
atypical chronic myeloid, BCR/ABL-
negative C92.2-
biphenotypic acute C95.0-
blast cell C95.0-
Burkitt-type, mature B-cell C91.A-
chronic lymphocytic, of B-cell type C91.1-
chronic monocytic C93.1-
chronic myelogenous (Philadelphia
chromosome (Ph1) positive)
(t(9;22)) (q34;q11) (with crisis of
blast cells) C92.1-
chronic myeloid, BCR/ABL-positive
C92.1-
atypical, BCR/ABL-negative C92.2-
chronic myelomonocytic C93.1-
chronic neutrophilic D47.1
CMML (-1) (-2) (with eosinophilia) C93.1-
granulocytic (see also Category C92)
C92.9-
hairy-cell C91.4-
juvenile myelomonocytic C93.3-
lymphoid C91.9-
specified NEC C91.Z-
mast cell C94.3-
mature B-cell, Burkitt-type C91.A-
monocytic (subacute) C93.9-
specified NEC C93.Z-
myelogenous (see also Category C92)
C92.9-
myeloid C92.9-
specified NEC C92.Z-
plasma cell C90.1-
plasmacytic C90.1-
prolymphocytic
of B-cell type C91.3-
of T-cell type C91.6-
specified NEC C94.8-
stem cell, of unclear lineage C95.0-
subacute lymphocytic C91.9-
T-cell large granular lymphocytic C91.Z-
unspecified cell type C95.9-
acute C95.0-
chronic C95.1-
Leukemoid reaction (see also Reaction,
leukemoid) D72.823
Leukoaraiosis (hypertensive) I67.81
Leukoariosis —see Leukoaraiosis
Leukocoria —see Disorder, globe,
degenerated condition, leucocoria
Leukocytopenia D72.819
Leukocytosis D72.829
eosinophilic D72.1
Leukoderma, leukodermia NEC L81.5
syphilitic A51.39
late A52.79
Leukodystrophy E75.29
Leukoedema, oral epithelium K13.29
Leukoencephalitis G04.81
acute (subacute) hemorrhagic G36.1
postimmunization or postvaccinal
G04.02
postinfectious G04.01
subacute sclerosing A81.1
van Bogaert's (sclerosing) A81.1
Leukoencephalopathy (see also
Encephalopathy) G93.49
Binswanger's I67.3
heroin vapor G92
metachromatic E75.25

Leukoencephalopathy (Continued)
multifocal (progressive) A81.2
postimmunization and postvaccinal
G04.02
progressive multifocal A81.2
reversible, posterior G93.6
van Bogaert's (sclerosing) A81.1
vascular, progressive I67.3
Leukoerythroblastosis D75.9
Leukokeratosis —see also Leukoplakia
mouth K13.21
nicotina palati K13.24
oral mucosa K13.21
tongue K13.21
vocal cord J38.3
Leukokraurosis vulva (e) N90.4
Leukoma (cornea) —see also Opacity,
cornea
adherent H17.0-
interfering with central vision —see
Opacity, cornea, central
Leukomalacia, cerebral, newborn P91.2
periventricular P91.2
Leukomelanopathy, hereditary D72.0
Leukonychia (punctata) (striata) L60.8
congenital Q84.4
Leukopathia unguium L60.8
congenital Q84.4
Leukopenia D72.819
basophilic D72.818
chemotherapy (cancer) induced D70.1
congenital D70.0
cyclic D70.0
drug induced NEC D70.2
due to cytoreductive cancer
chemotherapy D70.1
eosinophilic D72.818
familial D70.0
infantile genetic D70.0
malignant D70.9
periodic D70.0
transitory neonatal P61.5
Leukopenic —see condition
Leukoplakia
anus K62.89
bladder (postinfectional) N32.89
buccal K13.21
cervix (uteri) N88.0
esophagus K22.8
gingiva K13.21
hairy (oral mucosa) (tongue) K13.3
kidney (pelvis) N28.89
larynx J38.7
lip K13.21
mouth K13.21
oral epithelium, including tongue
(mucosa) K13.21
palate K13.21
pelvis (kidney) N28.89
penis (infectional) N48.0
rectum K62.89
syphilitic (late) A52.79
tongue K13.21
ureter (postinfectional) N28.89
urethra (postinfectional) N36.8
uterus N85.8
vagina N89.4
vocal cord J38.3
vulva N90.4
Leukorrhea N89.8
due to Trichomonas (vaginalis) A59.00
trichomonal A59.00
Leukosarcoma C85.9
Levocardia (isolated) Q24.1
with situs inversus Q89.3

Levotransposition Q20.5
Lev's disease or syndrome (acquired
complete heart block) I44.2
Levulosuria —see Fructosuria
Levurid L30.2
Lewy body (ies) (dementia) (disease)
G31.83
Leyden-Moebius dystrophy G71.0
Leydig cell
carcinoma
specified site —see Neoplasm,
malignant, by site
unspecified site
female C56.9-
male C62.9-
tumor
benign
specified site —see Neoplasm,
benign, by site
unspecified site
female D27.-
male D29.2-
malignant
specified site —see Neoplasm,
malignant, by site
unspecified site
female C56.-
male C62.9-
specified site —see Neoplasm,
uncertain behavior, by site
unspecified site
female D39.1-
male D40.1-
Leydig-Sertoli cell tumor
specified site —see Neoplasm, benign,
by site
unspecified site
female D27.-
male D29.2-
LGSIL (Low grade squamous
intraepithelial lesion on cytologic
smear of)
anus R85.612
cervix R87.612
vagina R87.622
Liar, pathologic F60.2
Libido
decreased R68.82
Libman-Sacks disease M32.11
Lice (infestation) B85.2
body (Pediculus corporis) B85.1
crab B85.3
head (Pediculus capitis) B85.0
mixed (classifiable to more than one of
the titles B85.0-B85.3) B85.4
pubic (Phthirus pubis) B85.3
Lichen L28.0
albus L90.0
penis N48.0
vulva N90.4
amyloidosis E85.4 [L99]
atrophicus L90.0
penis N48.0
vulva N90.4
congenital Q82.8
myxedematosus L98.5
nitidus L44.1
pilaris Q82.8
acquired L85.8
planopilaris L66.1
planus (chronicus) L43.9
annularis L43.8
bullous L43.1
follicular L66.1

Lichen *(Continued)*
　planus *(Continued)*
　　hypertrophic L43.0
　　moniliformis L44.3
　　of Wilson L43.9
　　specified NEC L43.8
　　subacute (active) L43.3
　　tropicus L43.3
　ruber
　　acuminatus L44.0
　　moniliformis L44.3
　　planus L43.9
　sclerosus (et atrophicus) L90.0
　　penis N48.0
　　vulva N90.4
　scrofulosus (primary) (tuberculous)
　　A18.4
　simplex (chronicus) (circumscriptus)
　　L28.0
　striatus L44.2
　urticatus L28.2
Lichenification L28.0
Lichenoides tuberculosis (primary) A18.4
Lichtheim's disease or syndrome —*see*
　Degeneration, combined
Lien migrans D73.89
Ligament —*see* condition
Light
　for gestational age —*see* Light for dates
　headedness R42
Light-for-dates (infant) P05.00
　with weight of
　　499 grams or less P05.01
　　500-749 grams P05.02
　　750-999 grams P05.03
　　1000-1249 grams P05.04
　　1250-1499 grams P05.05
　　1500-1749 grams P05.06
　　1750-1999 grams P05.07
　　2000-2499 grams P05.08
　affecting management of pregnancy
　　O36.59-
　and small-for-dates —*see* Small for
　　dates
Lightning (effects) (stroke) (struck by) T75.00
　burn —*see* Burn
　foot E53.8
　shock T75.01
　specified effect NEC T75.09
Lightwood-Albright syndrome N25.89
Lightwood's disease or syndrome (renal
　tubular acidosis) N25.89
Lignac (-de Toni) (-Fanconi) (-Debré)
　disease or syndrome E72.09
　with cystinosis E72.04
Ligneous thyroiditis E06.5
Likoff's syndrome I20.8
Limb —*see* condition
Limbic epilepsy personality syndrome F07.0
Limitation, limited
　activities due to disability Z73.6
　cardiac reserve —*see* Disease, heart
　eye muscle duction, traumatic —*see*
　　Strabismus, mechanical
　mandibular range of motion M26.52
Lindau (-von Hippel) disease Q85.8
Line (s)
　Beau's L60.4
　Harris' —*see* Arrest, epiphyseal
　Hudson's (cornea) —*see* Pigmentation,
　　cornea, anterior
　Stähli's (cornea) —*see* Pigmentation,
　　cornea, anterior
Linea corneae senilis —*see* Change,
　cornea, senile

Lingua
　geographica K14.1
　nigra (villosa) K14.3
　plicata K14.5
　tylosis K13.29
Lingual —*see* condition
Linguatulosis B88.8
Linitis (gastric) plastica C16.9
Lip —*see* condition
Lipedema —*see* Edema
Lipemia —*see also* Hyperlipidemia
　retina, retinalis E78.3
Lipidosis E75.6
　cerebral (infantile) (juvenile) (late) E75.4
　cerebroretinal E75.4
　cerebroside E75.22
　cholesterol (cerebral) E75.5
　glycolipid E75.21
　hepatosplenomegalic E78.3
　sphingomyelin —*see* Niemann-Pick
　　disease or syndrome
　sulfatide E75.29
Lipoadenoma —*see* Neoplasm, benign,
　by site
Lipoblastoma —*see* Lipoma
Lipoblastomatosis —*see* Lipoma
Lipochondrodystrophy E76.01
Lipochrome histiocytosis (familial) D71
Lipodermatosclerosis —*see* Varix, leg,
　with, inflammation
　ulcerated —*see* Varix, leg, with, ulcer,
　　with inflammation by site
Lipodystrophia progressiva E88.1
Lipodystrophy (progressive) E88.1
　insulin E88.1
　intestinal K90.81
　mesenteric K65.4
Lipofibroma —*see* Lipoma
Lipofuscinosis, neuronal (with
　ceroidosis) E75.4
Lipogranuloma, sclerosing L92.8
Lipogranulomatosis E78.89
Lipoid —*see also* condition
　histiocytosis D76.3
　　essential E75.29
　nephrosis N04.9
　proteinosis of Urbach E78.89
Lipoidemia —*see* Hyperlipidemia
Lipoidosis —*see* Lipidosis
Lipoma D17.9
　fetal D17.9
　　fat cell D17.9
　infiltrating D17.9
　intramuscular D17.9
　pleomorphic D17.9
　site classification
　　arms (skin) (subcutaneous) D17.2-
　　connective tissue D17.30
　　　intra-abdominal D17.5
　　　intrathoracic D17.4
　　　peritoneum D17.79
　　　retroperitoneum D17.79
　　　specified site NEC D17.39
　　　spermatic cord D17.6
　　face (skin) (subcutaneous) D17.0
　　genitourinary organ NEC D17.72
　　head (skin) (subcutaneous) D17.0
　　intra-abdominal D17.5
　　intrathoracic D17.4
　　kidney D17.71
　　legs (skin) (subcutaneous) D17.2-
　　neck (skin) (subcutaneous) D17.0
　　peritoneum D17.79
　　retroperitoneum D17.79

Lipoma *(Continued)*
　site classification *(Continued)*
　　skin D17.30
　　　specified site NEC D17.39
　　specified site NEC D17.79
　　spermatic cord D17.6
　　subcutaneous D17.30
　　　specified site NEC D17.39
　　trunk (skin) (subcutaneous)
　　　D17.1
　　unspecified D17.9
　spindle cell D17.9
Lipomatosis E88.2
　dolorosa (Dercum) E88.2
　fetal —*see* Lipoma
　Launois-Bensaude E88.89
Lipomyoma —*see* Lipoma
Lipomyxoma —*see* Lipoma
Lipomyxosarcoma —*see* Neoplasm,
　connective tissue, malignant
Lipoprotein metabolism disorder
　E78.9
Lipoproteinemia E78.5
　broad-beta E78.2
　floating-beta E78.2
　hyper-pre-beta E78.1
Liposarcoma —*see also* Neoplasm,
　connective tissue, malignant
　dedifferentiated —*see* Neoplasm,
　　connective tissue, malignant
　differentiated type —*see* Neoplasm,
　　connective tissue, malignant
　embryonal —*see* Neoplasm, connective
　　tissue, malignant
　mixed type —*see* Neoplasm, connective
　　tissue, malignant
　myxoid —*see* Neoplasm, connective
　　tissue, malignant
　pleomorphic —*see* Neoplasm,
　　connective tissue, malignant
　round cell —*see* Neoplasm, connective
　　tissue, malignant
　well differentiated type —*see*
　　Neoplasm, connective tissue,
　　malignant
Liposynovitis prepatellaris E88.89
Lipping, cervix N86
Lipschütz disease or ulcer N76.6
Lipuria R82.0
　schistosomiasis (bilharziasis) B65.0
Lisping F80.0
Lissauer's paralysis A52.17
Lissencephalia, lissencephaly Q04.3
Listeriosis, listerellosis A32.9
　congenital (disseminated) P37.2
　cutaneous A32.0
　neonatal, newborn (disseminated) P37.2
　oculoglandular A32.81
　specified NEC A32.89
Lithemia E79.0
Lithiasis —*see* Calculus
Lithosis J62.8
Lithuria R82.99
Litigation, anxiety concerning Z65.3
Little leaguer's elbow —*see* Epicondylitis,
　medial
Little's disease G80.9
Littre's
　gland —*see* condition
　hernia —*see* Hernia, abdomen
Littritis —*see* Urethritis
Livedo (annularis) (racemosa) (reticularis)
　R23.1
Liver —*see* condition

341

Living alone (problems with) Z60.2
  with handicapped person Z74.2
Lloyd's syndrome —see Adenomatosis,
    endocrine
Loa loa, loaiasis, loasis B74.3
Lobar —see condition
Lobomycosis B48.0
Lobo's disease B48.0
Lobotomy syndrome F07.0
Lobstein (-Ekman) disease or syndrome
    Q78.0
Lobster-claw hand Q71.6-
Lobulation (congenital) —see also
    Anomaly, by site
  kidney, Q63.1
  liver, abnormal Q44.7
  spleen Q89.09
Lobule, lobular —see condition
Local, localized —see condition
Locked twins causing obstructed labor
    O66.1
Locked-in state G83.5
Locking
  joint —see Derangement, joint, specified
      type NEC
    knee —see Derangement, knee
Lockjaw —see Tetanus
Löffler's
  endocarditis I42.3
  eosinophilia J82
  pneumonia J82
  syndrome (eosinophilic pneumonitis)
      J82
Loiasis (with conjunctival infestation)
    (eyelid) B74.3
Lone Star fever A77.0
Long
  labor O63.9
    first stage O63.0
    second stage O63.1
  QT syndrome I45.81
Long-term (current) (prophylactic) drug
    therapy (use of)
  agents affecting estrogen receptors and
      estrogen levels NEC Z79.818
  anastrozole (Arimidex) Z79.811
  antibiotics Z79.2
    short-term use - omit code
  anticoagulants Z79.01
  anti-inflammatory, non-steroidal
      (NSAID) Z79.1
  antiplatelet Z79.02
  antithrombotics Z79.02
  aromatase inhibitors Z79.811
  aspirin Z79.82
  birth control pill or patch Z79.3
  bisphosphonates Z79.83
  contraceptive, oral Z79.3
  drug, specified NEC Z79.899
  estrogen receptor downregulators Z79.818
  Evista Z79.810
  exemestane (Aromasin) Z79.811
  Fareston Z79.810
  fulvestrant (Faslodex) Z79.818
  gonadotropin-releasing hormone
      (GnRH) agonist Z79.818
  goserelin acetate (Zoladex) Z79.818
  hormone replacement
      (postmenopausal) Z79.890
  insulin Z79.4
  letrozole (Femara) Z79.811
  leuprolide acetate (leuprorelin)
      (Lupron) Z79.818
  megestrol acetate (Megace) Z79.818

Long-term (Continued)
  methadone for pain management Z79.891
  Nolvadex Z79.810
  non-steroidal anti-inflammatories
      (NSAID) Z79.1
  opiate analgesic Z79.891
  oral contraceptive Z79.3
  raloxifene (Evista) Z79.810
  selective estrogen receptor modulators
      (SERMs) Z79.810
  steroids
    inhaled Z79.51
    systemic Z79.52
  tamoxifen (Nolvadex) Z79.810
  toremifene (Fareston) Z79.810
Longitudinal stripes or grooves, nails
    L60.8
  congenital Q84.6
Loop
  intestine —see Volvulus
  vascular on papilla (optic) Q14.2
Loose —see also condition
  body
    joint M24.00
      ankle M24.07-
      elbow M24.02-
      hand M24.04-
      hip M24.05-
      knee M23.4-
      shoulder (region) M24.01-
      specified site NEC M24.08
      toe M24.07-
      vertebra M24.08
      wrist M24.03-
    knee M23.4-
    sheath, tendon —see Disorder,
        tendon, specified type NEC
  cartilage —see Loose, body, joint
  tooth, teeth K08.8
Loosening
  aseptic
    joint prosthesis —see Complications,
        joint prosthesis, mechanical,
        loosening, by site
    epiphysis —see Osteochondropathy
  mechanical
    joint prosthesis —see Complications,
        joint prosthesis, mechanical,
        loosening, by site
Looser-Milkman (-Debray) syndrome
    M83.8
Lop ear (deformity) Q17.3
Lorain (-Levi) short stature syndrome
    E23.0
Lordosis M40.50
  acquired —see Lordosis, specified type
      NEC
  congenital Q76.429
    lumbar region Q76.426
    lumbosacral region Q76.427
    sacral region Q76.428
    sacrococcygeal region Q76.428
    thoracolumbar region Q76.425
  lumbar region M40.56
  lumbosacral region M40.57
  postsurgical M96.4
  postural —see Lordosis, specified type
      NEC
  rachitic (late effect) (sequelae) E64.3
  sequelae of rickets E64.3
  specified type NEC M40.40
    lumbar region M40.46
    lumbosacral region M40.47
    thoracolumbar region M40.45

Lordosis (Continued)
  thoracolumbar region M40.55
  tuberculous A18.01
Loss (of)
  appetite (see Anorexia) R63.0
    hysterical F50.8
    nonorganic origin F50.8
    psychogenic F50.8
  blood —see Hemorrhage
  consciousness, transient R55
    traumatic —see Injury,
        intracranial
  control, sphincter, rectum R15.9
    nonorganic origin F98.1
  elasticity, skin R23.4
  family (member) in childhood
      Z62.898
  fluid (acute) E86.9
    with
      hypernatremia E87.0
      hyponatremia E87.1
  function of labyrinth —see subcategory
      H83.2
  hair, nonscarring —see Alopecia
  hearing —see also Deafness
    central NOS H90.5
    neural NOS H90.5
    perceptive NOS H90.5
    sensorineural NOS H90.5
    sensory NOS H90.5
  height R29.890
  limb or member, traumatic, current —
      see Amputation, traumatic
  love relationship in childhood
      Z62.898
  memory —see also Amnesia
    mild, following organic brain damage
        F06.8
  mind —see Psychosis
  occlusal vertical dimension of fully
      erupted teeth M26.37
  organ or part —see Absence, by site,
      acquired
  ossicles, ear (partial) H74.32-
  parent in childhood Z63.4
  pregnancy, recurrent N96
    without current pregnancy N96
    care in current pregnancy
        O26.2-
  recurrent pregnancy —see Loss,
      pregnancy, recurrent
  self-esteem, in childhood Z62.898
  sense of
    smell —see Disturbance, sensation,
        smell
    taste —see Disturbance, sensation,
        taste
    touch R20.8
  sensory R44.9
    dissociative F44.6
  sexual desire F52.0
  sight (acquired) (complete)
      (congenital) —see Blindness
  substance of
    bone —see Disorder, bone,
        density and structure,
        specified NEC
    cartilage —see Disorder, cartilage,
        specified type NEC
      auricle (ear) —see Disorder, pinna,
          specified type NEC
    vitreous (humor) H15.89
  tooth, teeth —see Absence, teeth,
      acquired

Loss (of) *(Continued)*
vision, visual H54.7
both eyes H54.3
one eye H54.60
left (normal vision on right) H54.62
right (normal vision on left) H54.61
specified as blindness —*see* Blindness
subjective
sudden H53.13-
transient H53.12-
vitreous —*see* Prolapse, vitreous
voice —*see* Aphonia
weight (abnormal) (cause unknown) R63.4
Louis-Bar syndrome (ataxia-telangiectasia) G11.3
Louping ill (encephalitis) A84.8
Louse, lousiness —*see* Lice
Low
achiever, school Z55.3
back syndrome M54.5
basal metabolic rate R94.8
birthweight (2499 grams or less) P07.10
with weight of
1000-1249 grams P07.14
1250-1499 grams P07.15
1500-1749 grams P07.16
1750-1999 grams P07.17
2000-2499 grams P07.18
extreme (999 grams or less) P07.00
with weight of
499 grams or less P07.01
500-749 grams P07.02
750-999 grams P07.03
for gestational age —*see* Light for dates
blood pressure —*see also* Hypotension
reading (incidental) (isolated) (nonspecific) R03.1
cardiac reserve —*see* Disease, heart
function —*see also* Hypofunction
kidney N28.9
hematocrit D64.9
hemoglobin D64.9
income Z59.6
level of literacy Z55.0
lying
kidney N28.89
organ or site, congenital —*see* Malposition, congenital
output syndrome (cardiac) —*see* Failure, heart
platelets (blood) —*see* Thrombocytopenia
reserve, kidney N28.89
salt syndrome E87.1
self esteem R45.81
set ears Q17.4
vision H54.2
one eye (other eye normal) H54.50
left (normal vision on right) H54.52
other eye blind —*see* Blindness
right (normal vision on left) H54.51
Low-density-lipoprotein-type (LDL) hyperlipoproteinemia E78.0
Lowe's syndrome E72.03
Lown-Ganong-Levine syndrome I45.6
LSD reaction (acute) (without dependence) F16.90
with dependence F16.20
L-shaped kidney Q63.8
Ludwig's angina or disease K12.2
Lues (venerea), luetic —*see* Syphilis
Luetscher's syndrome (dehydration) E86.0

Lumbago, lumbalgia M54.5
with sciatica M54.4-
due to intervertebral disc disorder M51.17
due to displacement, intervertebral disc M51.27
with sciatica M51.17
Lumbar —*see* condition
Lumbarization, vertebra, congenital Q76.49
Lumbermen's itch B88.0
Lump —*see* Mass
Lunacy —*see* Psychosis
Lung —*see* condition
Lupoid (miliary) of Boeck D86.3
Lupus
anticoagulant D68.62
with
hemorrhagic disorder D68.312
hypercoagulable state D68.62
finding without diagnosis R76.0
discoid (local) L93.0
erythematosus (discoid) (local) L93.0
disseminated —*see* Lupus, erythematosus, systemic
eyelid H01.129
left H01.126
lower H01.125
upper H01.124
right H01.123
lower H01.122
upper H01.121
profundus L93.2
specified NEC L93.2
subacute cutaneous L93.1
systemic M32.9
with organ or system involvement M32.10
endocarditis M32.11
lung M32.13
pericarditis M32.12
renal (glomerular) M32.14
tubulo-interstitial M32.15
specified organ or system NEC M32.19
drug-induced M32.0
inhibitor (presence of) D68.62
with
hemorrhagic disorder D68.312
hypercoagulable state D68.62
finding without diagnosis R76.0
specified NEC M32.8
exedens A18.4
hydralazine M32.0
correct substance properly administered —*see* Table of drugs and chemicals, by drug, adverse effect
overdose or wrong substance given or taken —*see* Table of drugs and chemicals, by drug, poisoning
nephritis (chronic) M32.14
nontuberculous, not disseminated L93.0
panniculitis L93.2
pernio (Besnier) D86.3
systemic —*see* Lupus, erythematosus, systemic
tuberculous A18.4
eyelid A18.4
vulgaris A18.4
eyelid A18.4

Luteinoma D27.-
Lutembacher's disease or syndrome (atrial septal defect with mitral stenosis) Q21.1
Luteoma D27.-
Lutz (-Splendore-de Almeida) disease — *see* Paracoccidioidomycosis
Luxation —*see also* Dislocation
eyeball (nontraumatic) —*see* Luxation, globe
birth injury P15.3
globe, nontraumatic H44.82-
lacrimal gland —*see* Dislocation, lacrimal gland
lens (old) (partial) (spontaneous)
congenital Q12.1
syphilitic A50.39
Lycanthropy F22
Lyell's syndrome L51.2
due to drug L51.2
correct substance properly administered —*see* Table of drugs and chemicals, by drug, adverse effect
overdose or wrong substance given or taken —*see* Table of drugs and chemicals, by drug, poisoning
Lyme disease A69.20
Lymph
gland or node —*see* condition
scrotum —*see* Infestation, filarial
Lymphadenitis I88.9
with ectopic or molar pregnancy O08.0
acute L04.9
axilla L04.2
face L04.0
head L04.0
hip L04.3
limb
lower L04.3
upper L04.2
neck L04.0
shoulder L04.2
specified site NEC L04.8
trunk L04.1
anthracosis (occupational) J60
any site, except mesenteric I88.9
chronic I88.1
subacute I88.1
breast
gestational —*see* Mastitis, obstetric
puerperal, postpartum (nonpurulent) O91.22
chancroidal (congenital) A57
chronic I88.1
mesenteric I88.0
due to
Brugia (malayi) B74.1
timori B74.2
chlamydial lymphogranuloma A55
diphtheria (toxin) A36.89
lymphogranuloma venereum A55
Wuchereria bancrofti B74.0
following ectopic or molar pregnancy O08.0
gonorrheal A54.89
infective —*see* Lymphadenitis, acute
mesenteric (acute) (chronic) (nonspecific) (subacute) I88.0
due to Salmonella typhi A01.09
tuberculous A18.39
mycobacterial A31.8
purulent —*see* Lymphadenitis, acute

343

Lymphadenitis (Continued)
  pyogenic —see Lymphadenitis, acute
  regional, nonbacterial I88.8
  septic —see Lymphadenitis, acute
  subacute, unspecified site I88.1
  suppurative —see Lymphadenitis,
    acute
  syphilitic (early) (secondary) A51.49
    late A52.79
  tuberculous —see Tuberculosis, lymph
    gland
  venereal (chlamydial) A55
Lymphadenoid goiter E06.3
Lymphadenopathy (generalized) R59.1
  angioimmunoblastic, with
    dysproteinemia (AILD) C86.5
  due to toxoplasmosis (acquired)
    B58.89
    congenital (acute) (subacute)
      (chronic) P37.1
  localized R59.0
  syphilitic (early) (secondary) A51.49
Lymphadenosis R59.1
Lymphangiectasis I89.0
  conjunctiva H11.89
  postinfectional I89.0
  scrotum I89.0
Lymphangiectatic elephantiasis,
  nonfilarial I89.0
Lymphangioendothelioma D18.1
  malignant —see Neoplasm, connective
    tissue, malignant
Lymphangioleiomyomatosis J84.81
Lymphangioma D18.1
  capillary D18.1
  cavernous D18.1
  cystic D18.1
  malignant —see Neoplasm, connective
    tissue, malignant
Lymphangiomyoma D18.1
Lymphangiomyomatosis J84.81
Lymphangiosarcoma —see Neoplasm,
  connective tissue, malignant
Lymphangitis I89.1
  with
    abscess - code by site under Abscess
    cellulitis - code by site under Cellulitis
    ectopic or molar pregnancy O08.0
  acute L03.91
    abdominal wall L03.321
    ankle —see Lymphangitis, acute,
      lower limb
    arm —see Lymphangitis, acute, upper
      limb
    auricle (ear) —see Lymphangitis,
      acute, ear
    axilla L03.12-
    back (any part) L03.322
    buttock L03.327
    cervical (meaning neck) L03.222
    cheek (external) L03.212
    chest wall L03.323
    digit
      finger —see Lymphangitis, acute,
        finger
      toe —see Lymphangitis, acute, toe
    ear (external) H60.1-
    external auditory canal —see
      Lymphangitis, acute, ear
    eyelid —see Abscess, eyelid
    face NEC L03.212
    finger (intrathecal) (periosteal)
      (subcutaneous) (subcuticular)
      L03.02-

Lymphangitis (Continued)
  acute (Continued)
    foot —see Lymphangitis, acute, lower
      limb
    gluteal (region) L03.327
    groin L03.324
    hand —see Lymphangitis, acute,
      upper limb
    head NEC L03.891
      face (any part, except ear, eye and
        nose) L03.212
    heel —see Lymphangitis, acute, lower
      limb
    hip —see Lymphangitis, acute, lower
      limb
    jaw (region) L03.212
    knee —see Lymphangitis, acute,
      lower limb
    leg —see Lymphangitis, acute, lower
      limb
    lower limb L03.12-
      toe —see Lymphangitis, acute, toe
    navel L03.326
    neck (region) L03.222
    orbit, orbital —see Cellulitis, orbit
    pectoral (region) L03.323
    perineal, perineum L03.325
    scalp (any part) L03.891
    shoulder —see Lymphangitis, acute,
      upper limb
    specified site NEC L03.898
    thigh —see Lymphangitis, acute,
      lower limb
    thumb (intrathecal) (periosteal)
      (subcutaneous) (subcuticular) —
      see Lymphangitis, acute, finger
    toe (intrathecal) (periosteal)
      (subcutaneous) (subcuticular)
      L03.04-
    trunk L03.329
      abdominal wall L03.321
      back (any part) L03.322
      buttock L03.327
      chest wall L03.323
      groin L03.324
      perineal, perineum L03.325
      umbilicus L03.326
    umbilicus L03.326
    upper limb L03.12-
      axilla —see Lymphangitis, acute,
        axilla
      finger —see Lymphangitis, acute,
        finger
      thumb —see Lymphangitis, acute,
        finger
      wrist —see Lymphangitis, acute,
        upper limb
  breast
    gestational —see Mastitis, obstetric
  chancroidal A57
  chronic (any site) I89.1
  due to
    Brugia (malayi) B74.1
      timori B74.2
    Wuchereria bancrofti B74.0
  following ectopic or molar pregnancy
    O08.89
  penis
    acute N48.29
    gonococcal (acute) (chronic) A54.09
  puerperal, postpartum, childbirth O86.89
  strumous, tuberculous A18.2
  subacute (any site) I89.1
  tuberculous —see Tuberculosis, lymph
    gland

Lymphatic (vessel) —see condition
Lymphatism E32.8
Lymphectasia I89.0
Lymphedema (acquired) —see also
  Elephantiasis
  congenital Q82.0
  hereditary (chronic) (idiopathic) Q82.0
  postmastectomy I97.2
  praecox I89.0
  secondary I89.0
  surgical NEC I97.89
    postmastectomy (syndrome) I97.2
Lymphoblastic —see condition
Lymphoblastoma (diffuse) —see
    Lymphoma, lymphoblastic (diffuse)
  giant follicular —see Lymphoma,
    lymphoblastic (diffuse)
  macrofollicular —see Lymphoma,
    lymphoblastic (diffuse)
Lymphocele I89.8
Lymphocytic
  chorioencephalitis (acute) (serous)
    A87.2
  choriomeningitis (acute) (serous)
    A87.2
  meningoencephalitis A87.2
Lymphocytoma, benign cutis L98.8
Lymphocytopenia D72.810
Lymphocytosis (symptomatic) D72.820
  infectious (acute) B33.8
Lymphoepithelioma —see Neoplasm,
  malignant, by site
Lymphogranuloma (malignant) —see also
    Lymphoma, Hodgkin
  chlamydial A55
  inguinale A55
  venereum (any site) (chlamydial) (with
    stricture of rectum) A55
Lymphogranulomatosis (malignant) —see
    also Lymphoma, Hodgkin
  benign (Boeck's sarcoid) (Schaumann's)
    D86.1
Lymphohistiocytosis, hemophagocytic
  (familial) D76.1
Lymphoid —see condition
Lymphoma (of) (malignant) C85.90
  adult T-cell (HTLV-1-associated)
    (acute variant) (chronic variant)
    (lymphomatoid variant)
    (smouldering variant) C91.5-
  anaplastic large cell
    ALK-negative C84.7-
    ALK-positive C84.6-
    CD30-positive C84.6-
    primary cutaneous C86.6
  angioimmunoblastic T-cell C86.5
  BALT C88.4
  B-cell C85.1-
  B-precursor C83.5-
  blastic NK-cell C86.4
  bronchial-associated lymphoid tissue
    [BALT-lymphoma] C88.4
  Burkitt (atypical) C83.7-
  Burkitt-like C83.7-
  centrocytic C83.1-
  cutaneous follicle center C82.6-
  cutaneous T-cell C84.A-
  diffuse follicle center C82.5-
  diffuse large cell C83.3-
    anaplastic C83.3-
    B-cell C83.3-
    CD30-positive C83.3-
    centroblastic C83.3-
    immunoblastic C83.3-

Lymphoma *(Continued)*
  diffuse large cell *(Continued)*
    plasmablastic C83.3-
    subtype not specified C83.3-
    T-cell rich C83.3-
  enteropathy-type (associated)
      (intestinal) T-cell C86.2
  extranodal marginal zone B-cell
      lymphoma of mucosa-associated
      lymphoid tissue [MALT-
      lymphoma] C88.4
  extranodal NK/T-cell, nasal type C86.0
  follicular C82.9-
    grade
      I C82.0-
      II C82.1-
      III C82.2-
      IIIa C82.3-
      IIIb C82.4-
    specified NEC C82.8-
  hepatosplenic T-cell (alpha-beta)
      (gamma-delta) C86.1
  histiocytic C85.9-
    true C96.A
  Hodgkin C81.9
    classical C81.7-
      lymphocyte-rich C81.4-
      lymphocytic depletion C81.3-
      mixed cellularity C81.2-
      nodular sclerosis C81.1-
      specified NEC C81.7-
    lymphocyte-rich classical C81.4-
    lymphocyte depleted classical C81.3-

Lymphoma *(Continued)*
  Hodgkin *(Continued)*
    mixed cellularity classical C81.2-
    nodular
      lymphocyte predominant C81.0-
      sclerosis classical C81.1-
  intravascular large B-cell C83.8-
  Lennert's C84.4-
  lymphoblastic (diffuse) C83.5-
  lymphoblastic B-cell C83.5-
  lymphoblastic T-cell C83.5-
  lymphoepithelioid C84.4-
  lymphoplasmacytic C83.0-
    with IgM-production C88.0
  MALT C88.4
  mantle cell C83.1-
  mature T-cell NEC C84.4-
  mature T/NK-cell C84.9-
    specified NEC C84.Z-
  mediastinal (thymic) large B-cell C85.2-
  Mediterranean C88.3
  mucosa-associated lymphoid tissue
      [MALT-lymphoma] C88.4
  NK/T cell C84.9-
  nodal marginal zone C83.0-
  non-follicular (diffuse) C83.9-
    specified NEC C83.8-
  non-Hodgkin *(see also* Lymphoma, by
      type) C85.9-
    specified NEC C85.8-
  non-leukemic variant of B-CLL
      C83.0-
  peripheral T-cell, not classified C84.4-

Lymphoma *(Continued)*
  primary cutaneous
    anaplastic large cell C86.6
    CD30-positive large T-cell C86.6
  primary effusion B-cell C83.8-
  SALT C88.4
  skin-associated lymphoid tissue
      [SALT-lymphoma] C88.4
  small cell B-cell C83.0-
  splenic marginal zone C83.0-
  subcutaneous panniculitis-like T-cell
      C86.3
  T-precursor C83.5-
  true histiocytic C96.A
Lymphomatosis —*see* Lymphoma
Lymphopathia venereum, veneris
    A55
Lymphopenia D72.810
Lymphoplasmacytic leukemia —*see*
    Leukemia, chronic lymphocytic,
    B-cell type
Lymphoproliferation, X-linked disease
    D82.3
Lymphoreticulosis, benign (of
    inoculation) A28.1
Lymphorrhea I89.8
Lymphosarcoma (diffuse) *(see also*
    Lymphoma) C85.9-
Lymphostasis I89.8
Lypemania —*see* Melancholia
Lysine and hydroxylysine metabolism
    disorder E72.3
Lyssa —*see* Rabies

M

Macacus ear Q17.3
Maceration, wet feet, tropical (syndrome)
    T69.02-
MacLeod's syndrome J43.0
Macrocephalia, macrocephaly Q75.3
Macrocheilia, macrochilia (congenital)
    Q18.6
Macrocolon (see also Megacolon) Q43.1
Macrocornea Q15.8
    with glaucoma Q15.0
Macrocytic —see condition
Macrocytosis D75.89
Macrodactylia, macrodactylism (fingers)
    (thumbs) Q74.0
    toes Q74.2
Macrodontia K00.2
Macrogenia M26.05
Macrogenitosomia (adrenal) (male)
    (praecox) E25.9
    congenital E25.0
Macroglobulinemia (idiopathic)
    (primary) C88.0
    monoclonal (essential) D47.2
    Waldenström C88.0
Macroglossia (congenital) Q38.2
    acquired K14.8
Macrognathia, macrognathism (congenital)
    (mandibular) (maxillary) M26.09
Macrogyria (congenital) Q04.8
Macrohydrocephalus —see Hydrocephalus
Macromastia —see Hypertrophy, breast
Macrophthalmos Q11.3
    in congenital glaucoma Q15.0
Macropsia H53.15
Macrosigmoid K59.3
    congenital Q43.2
Macrospondylitis, acromegalic E22.0
Macrostomia (congenital) Q18.4
Macrotia (external ear) (congenital) Q17.1
Macula
    cornea, corneal —see Opacity, cornea
    degeneration (atrophic) (exudative)
        (senile) —see also Degeneration,
        macula
    hereditary —see Dystrophy, retina
Maculae ceruleae — B85.1
Maculopathy, toxic —see Degeneration,
    macula, toxic
Madarosis (eyelid) H02.729
    left H02.726
        lower H02.725
        upper H02.724
    right H02.723
        lower H02.722
        upper H02.721
Madelung's
    deformity (radius) Q74.0
    disease
        radial deformity Q74.0
        symmetrical lipomas, neck E88.89
Madness —see Psychosis
Madura
    foot B47.9
        actinomycotic B47.1
        mycotic B47.0
Maduromycosis B47.0
Maffucci's syndrome Q78.4
Magnesium metabolism disorder —see
    Disorder, metabolism, magnesium
Main en griffe (acquired) —see also
    Deformity, limb, clawhand
    congenital Q74.0

Maintenance (encounter for)
    antineoplastic chemotherapy Z51.11
    antineoplastic radiation therapy
        Z51.0
    methadone F11.20
Majocchi's
    disease L81.7
    granuloma B35.8
Major —see condition
Malabar itch (any site) B35.5
Malabsorption K90.9
    calcium K90.89
    carbohydrate K90.4
    disaccharide E73.9
    fat K90.4
    galactose E74.20
    glucose(-galactose) E74.39
    intestinal K90.9
        specified NEC K90.89
    isomaltose E74.31
    lactose E73.9
    methionine E72.19
    monosaccharide E74.39
    postgastrectomy K91.2
    postsurgical K91.2
    protein K90.4
    starch K90.4
    sucrose E74.39
    syndrome K90.9
        postsurgical K91.2
Malacia, bone (adult) M83.9
    juvenile —see Rickets
Malacoplakia
    bladder N32.89
    pelvis (kidney) N28.89
    ureter N28.89
    urethra N36.8
Malacosteon, juvenile —see Rickets
Maladaptation —see Maladjustment
Maladie de Roger Q21.0
Maladjustment
    conjugal Z63.0
        involving divorce or estrangement
            Z63.5
    educational Z55.4
    family Z63.9
    marital Z63.0
        involving divorce or estrangement
            Z63.5
    occupational NEC Z56.89
    simple, adult —see Disorder,
        adjustment
    situational —see Disorder, adjustment
    social Z60.9
        due to
            acculturation difficulty Z60.3
            discrimination and persecution
                (perceived) Z60.5
            exclusion and isolation Z60.4
            life-cycle (phase of life) transition
                Z60.0
            rejection Z60.4
            specified reason NEC Z60.8
Malaise R53.81
Malakoplakia —see Malacoplakia
Malaria, malarial (fever) B54
    with
        blackwater fever B50.8
            hemoglobinuric (bilious) B50.8
        hemoglobinuria B50.8
    accidentally induced (therapeutically) -
        code by type under Malaria
    algid B50.9
    cerebral B50.0 [G94]

Malaria, malarial (Continued)
    clinically diagnosed (without
        parasitological confirmation) B54
    congenital NEC P37.4
        falciparum P37.3
    congestion, congestive B54
    continued (fever) B50.9
    estivo-autumnal B50.9
    falciparum B50.9
        with complications NEC B50.8
            cerebral B50.0 [G94]
            severe B50.8
    hemorrhagic B54
    malariae B52.9
        with
            complications NEC B52.8
            glomerular disorder B52.0
    malignant (tertian) —see Malaria,
        falciparum
    mixed infections — code to first listed
        type in B50-B53
    ovale B53.0
    parasitologically confirmed NEC
        B53.8
    pernicious, acute —see Malaria,
        falciparum
    Plasmodium (P.)
        falciparum NEC —see Malaria,
            falciparum
        malariae NEC B52.9
            with Plasmodium
                falciparum (and or vivax) —see
                    Malaria, falciparum
                vivax —see also Malaria, vivax
                    and falciparum —see Malaria,
                        falciparum
        ovale B53.0
            with Plasmodium malariae —see
                also Malaria, malariae
                and vivax —see also Malaria,
                    vivax
                and falciparum —see also Malaria,
                    falciparum
        simian B53.1
            with Plasmodium malariae —see
                also Malaria, malariae
                and vivax —see also Malaria,
                    vivax
                and falciparum —see Malaria,
                    falciparum
        vivax NEC B51.9
            with Plasmodium falciparum —see
                Malaria, falciparum
    quartan —see Malaria, malariae
    quotidian —see Malaria, falciparum
    recurrent B54
    remittent B54
    specified type NEC (parasitologically
        confirmed) B53.8
    spleen B54
    subtertian (fever) —see Malaria,
        falciparum
    tertian (benign) —see also Malaria, vivax
        malignant B50.9
    tropical B50.9
    typhoid B54
    vivax B51.9
        with
            complications NEC B51.8
            ruptured spleen B51.0
Malassez's disease (cystic) N50.8
Malassimilation K90.9
Mal de los pintos —see Pinta
Mal de mer T75.3

Maldescent, testis Q53.9
  bilateral Q53.20
    abdominal Q53.21
    perineal Q53.22
  unilateral Q53.10
    abdominal Q53.11
    perineal Q53.12
Maldevelopment —see also Anomaly
  brain Q07.9
  colon Q43.9
  hip Q74.2
    congenital dislocation Q65.2
      bilateral Q65.1
      unilateral Q65.0-
  mastoid process Q75.8
  middle ear Q16.4
    except ossicles Q16.4
    ossicles Q16.3
  ossicles Q16.3
  spine Q76.49
  toe Q74.2
Male type pelvis Q74.2
  with disproportion (fetopelvic)
      O33.3
    causing obstructed labor O65.3
Malformation (congenital) —see also
      Anomaly
  adrenal gland Q89.1
  affecting multiple systems with
      skeletal changes NEC Q87.5
  alimentary tract Q45.9
    specified type NEC Q45.8
    upper Q40.9
      specified type NEC Q40.8
  aorta Q25.9
    atresia Q25.2
    coarctation (preductal) (postductal)
        Q25.1
    patent ductus arteriosus Q25.0
    specified type NEC Q25.4
    stenosis (supravalvular) Q25.3
  aortic valve Q23.9
    specified NEC Q23.8
  arteriovenous, aneurysmatic
      (congenital) Q27.30
    brain Q28.2
    cerebral Q28.2
    peripheral Q27.30
      digestive system Q27.33
      lower limb Q27.32
      other specified site Q27.39
      renal vessel Q27.34
      upper limb Q27.31
    precerebral vessels (nonruptured)
        Q28.0
  auricle
    ear (congenital) Q17.3
      acquired H61.119
        left H61.112
          with right H61.113
        right H61.111
          with left H61.113
  bile duct Q44.5
  bladder Q64.79
    aplasia Q64.5
    diverticulum Q64.6
    exstrophy —see Exstrophy,
        bladder
    neck obstruction Q64.31
  bone Q79.9
    face Q75.9
      specified type NEC Q75.8
    skull Q75.9
      specified type NEC Q75.8

Malformation (Continued)
  brain (multiple) Q04.9
    arteriovenous Q28.2
    specified type NEC Q04.8
  branchial cleft Q18.2
  breast Q83.9
    specified type NEC Q83.8
  broad ligament Q50.6
  bronchus Q32.4
  bursa Q79.9
  cardiac
    chambers Q20.9
      specified type NEC Q20.8
    septum Q21.9
      specified type NEC Q21.8
  cerebral Q04.9
    vessels Q28.3
  cervix uteri Q51.9
    specified type NEC Q51.828
  Chiari
    Type I G93.5
    Type II Q07.01
  choroid (congenital) Q14.3
    plexus Q07.8
  circulatory system Q28.9
  cochlea Q16.5
  cornea Q13.4
  coronary vessels Q24.5
  corpus callosum (congenital) Q04.0
  diaphragm Q79.1
  digestive system NEC, specified type
      NEC Q45.8
  dura Q07.9
    brain Q04.9
    spinal Q06.9
  ear Q17.9
    causing impairment of hearing
        Q16.9
    external Q17.9
      accessory auricle Q17.0
      causing impairment of hearing
          Q16.9
      absence of
        auditory canal Q16.1
        auricle Q16.0
      macrotia Q17.1
      microtia Q17.2
      misplacement Q17.4
      misshapen NEC Q17.3
      prominence Q17.5
      specified type NEC Q17.8
    inner Q16.5
    middle Q16.4
      absence of eustachian tube
          Q16.2
      ossicles (fusion) Q16.3
      ossicles Q16.3
      specified type NEC Q17.8
  epididymis Q55.4
  esophagus Q39.9
    specified type NEC Q39.8
  eye Q15.9
    lid Q10.3
    specified NEC Q15.8
  fallopian tube Q50.6
  genital organ —see Anomaly,
      genitalia
  great
    artery Q25.9
      aorta —see Malformation, aorta
      pulmonary artery —see
          Malformation, pulmonary,
          artery
      specified type NEC Q25.8

Malformation (Continued)
  great (Continued)
    vein Q26.9
      anomalous
        portal venous connection Q26.5
        pulmonary venous connection
            Q26.4
        partial Q26.3
        total Q26.2
      persistent left superior vena cava
          Q26.1
      portal vein-hepatic artery fistula
          Q26.6
      specified type NEC Q26.8
      vena cava stenosis, congenital
          Q26.0
  gum Q38.6
  hair Q84.2
  heart Q24.9
    specified type NEC Q24.8
  integument Q84.9
    specified type NEC Q84.8
  internal ear Q16.5
  intestine Q43.9
    specified type NEC Q43.8
  iris Q13.2
  joint Q74.9
    ankle Q74.2
    lumbosacral Q76.49
    sacroiliac Q74.2
    specified type NEC Q74.8
  kidney Q63.9
    accessory Q63.0
    giant Q63.3
    horseshoe Q63.1
    hydronephrosis Q62.0
    malposition Q63.2
    specified type NEC Q63.8
  lacrimal apparatus Q10.6
  lingual Q38.3
  lip Q38.0
  liver Q44.7
  lung Q33.9
  meninges or membrane (congenital)
      Q07.9
    cerebral Q04.8
    spinal (cord) Q06.9
  middle ear Q16.4
    ossicles Q16.3
  mitral valve Q23.9
    specified NEC Q23.8
  Mondini's (congenital) (malformation,
      cochlea) Q16.5
  mouth (congenital) Q38.6
  multiple types NEC Q89.7
  musculoskeletal system Q79.9
  myocardium Q24.8
  nail Q84.6
  nervous system (central) Q07.9
  nose Q30.9
    specified type NEC Q30.8
  optic disc Q14.2
  orbit Q10.7
  ovary Q50.39
  palate Q38.5
  parathyroid gland Q89.2
  pelvic organs or tissues NEC
    in pregnancy or childbirth O34.8-
      causing obstructed labor O65.5
  penis Q55.69
    aplasia Q55.5
    curvature (lateral) Q55.61
    hypoplasia Q55.62
  pericardium Q24.8

Malformation *(Continued)*
peripheral vascular system
Q27.9
specified type NEC Q27.8
pharynx Q38.8
precerebral vessels Q28.1
prostate Q55.4
pulmonary
arteriovenous Q25.72
artery Q25.9
atresia Q25.5
specified type NEC Q25.79
stenosis Q25.6
valve Q22.3
renal artery Q27.2
respiratory system Q34.9
retina Q14.1
scrotum —*see* Malformation, testis
and scrotum
seminal vesicles Q55.4
sense organs NEC Q07.9
skin Q82.9
specified NEC Q89.8
spinal
cord Q06.9
nerve root Q07.8
spine Q76.49
kyphosis —*see* Kyphosis, congenital
lordosis —*see* Lordosis, congenital
spleen Q89.09
stomach Q40.3
specified type NEC Q40.2
teeth, tooth K00.9
tendon Q79.9
testis and scrotum Q55.20
aplasia Q55.0
hypoplasia Q55.1
polyorchism Q55.21
retractile testis Q55.22
scrotal transposition Q55.23
specified NEC Q55.29
thorax, bony Q76.9
throat Q38.8
thyroid gland Q89.2
tongue (congenital) Q38.3
hypertrophy Q38.2
tie Q38.1
trachea Q32.1
tricuspid valve Q22.9
specified type NEC Q22.8
umbilical cord NEC (complicating
delivery) O69.89
umbilicus Q89.9
ureter Q62.8
agenesis Q62.4
duplication Q62.5
malposition —*see* Malposition,
congenital, ureter
obstructive defect —*see* Defect,
obstructive, ureter
vesico-uretero-renal reflux Q62.7
urethra Q64.79
aplasia Q64.5
duplication Q64.74
posterior valves Q64.2
prolapse Q64.71
stricture Q64.32
urinary system Q64.9
uterus Q51.9
specified type NEC Q51.818
vagina Q52.4
vascular system, peripheral Q27.9
vas deferens Q55.4
atresia Q55.3

Malformation *(Continued)*
venous —*see* Anomaly, vein (s)
vulva Q52.70
Malfunction —*see also* Dysfunction
cardiac electronic device T82.119
electrode T82.110
pulse generator T82.111
specified type NEC T82.118
catheter device NEC T85.618
cystostomy T83.010
dialysis (renal) (vascular) T82.41
intraperitoneal T85.611
infusion NEC T82.514
spinal (epidural) (subdural)
T85.610
urinary, indwelling T83.018
colostomy K94.03
valve K94.03
cystostomy (stoma) N99.512
catheter T83.010
enteric stoma K94.13
enterostomy K94.13
esophagostomy K94.33
gastroenteric K31.89
gastrostomy K94.23
ileostomy K94.13
valve K94.13
jejunostomy K94.13
pacemaker —*see* Malfunction, cardiac
electronic device
prosthetic device, internal —*see*
Complications, prosthetic device,
by site, mechanical
tracheostomy J95.03
urinary device NEC —*see* Complication,
genitourinary, device, urinary,
mechanical
valve
colostomy K94.03
heart T82.09
ileostomy K94.13
vascular graft or shunt NEC —*see*
Complication, cardiovascular
device, mechanical, vascular
ventricular (communicating shunt)
T85.01
Malherbe's tumor —*see* Neoplasm, skin,
benign
Malibu disease L98.8-
Malignancy —*see also* Neoplasm,
malignant, by site
unspecified site (primary) C80.1
Malignant —*see* condition
Malingerer, malingering Z76.5
Mallet finger (acquired) —*see* Deformity,
finger, mallet finger
congenital Q74.0
sequelae of rickets E64.3
Malleus A24.0
Mallory's bodies R89.7
Mallory-Weiss syndrome K22.6
Malnutrition E46
degree
first E44.1
mild (protein) E44.1
moderate (protein) E44.0
second E44.0
severe (protein-energy) E43
intermediate form E42
with
kwashiorkor (and marasmus)
E42
marasmus E41
third E43

Malnutrition *(Continued)*
following gastrointestinal surgery K91.2
intrauterine
light-for-dates —*see* Light for dates
small-for-dates —*see* Small for dates
lack of care, or neglect (child) (infant)
T76.02
confirmed T74.02
malignant E40
protein E46
calorie E46
mild E44.1
moderate E44.0
severe E43
intermediate form E42
with
kwashiorkor (and
marasmus) E42
marasmus E41
energy E46
mild E44.1
moderate E44.0
severe E43
intermediate form E42
with
kwashiorkor (and
marasmus) E42
marasmus E41
severe (protein-energy) E43
with
kwashiorkor (and marasmus) E42
marasmus E41
Malocclusion (teeth) M26.4
Angle's M26.219
class I M26.211
class II M26.212
class III M26.213
due to
abnormal swallowing M26.59
mouth breathing M26.59
tongue, lip or finger habits M26.59
temporomandibular (joint) M26.69
Malposition
cervix —*see* Malposition, uterus
congenital
adrenal (gland) Q89.1
alimentary tract Q45.8
lower Q43.8
upper Q40.8
aorta Q25.4
appendix Q43.8
arterial trunk Q20.0
artery (peripheral) Q27.8
coronary Q24.5
digestive system Q27.8
lower limb Q27.8
pulmonary Q25.79
specified site NEC Q27.8
upper limb Q27.8
auditory canal Q17.8
causing impairment of hearing
Q16.9
auricle (ear) Q17.4
causing impairment of hearing
Q16.9
cervical Q18.2
biliary duct or passage Q44.5
bladder (mucosa) —*see* Exstrophy,
bladder
brachial plexus Q07.8
brain tissue Q04.8
breast Q83.8
bronchus Q32.4
cecum Q43.8

Malposition *(Continued)*
  congenital *(Continued)*
    clavicle Q74.0
    colon Q43.8
    digestive organ or tract NEC Q45.8
      lower Q43.8
      upper Q40.8
    ear (auricle) (external) Q17.4
      ossicles Q16.3
    endocrine (gland) NEC Q89.2
    epiglottis Q31.8
    eustachian tube Q17.8
    eye Q15.8
    facial features Q18.8
    fallopian tube Q50.6
    finger (s) Q68.1
      supernumerary Q69.0
    foot Q66.9
    gallbladder Q44.1
    gastrointestinal tract Q45.8
    genitalia, genital organ (s) or tract
      female Q52.8
        external Q52.79
        internal NEC Q52.8
      male Q55.8
    glottis Q31.8
    hand Q68.1
    heart Q24.8
      dextrocardia Q24.0
        with complete transposition of
          viscera Q89.3
    hepatic duct Q44.5
    hip (joint) Q65.89
    intestine (large) (small) Q43.8
      with anomalous adhesions, fixation
        or malrotation Q43.3
    joint NEC Q68.8
    kidney Q63.2
    larynx Q31.8
    limb Q68.8
      lower Q68.8
      upper Q68.8
    liver Q44.7
    lung (lobe) Q33.8
    nail (s) Q84.6
    nerve Q07.8
    nervous system NEC Q07.8
    nose, nasal (septum) Q30.8
    organ or site not listed —*see*
      Anomaly, by site
    ovary Q50.39
    pancreas Q45.3
    parathyroid (gland) Q89.2
    patella Q74.1
    peripheral vascular system Q27.8
    pituitary (gland) Q89.2
    respiratory organ or system NEC
      Q34.8
    rib (cage) Q76.6
      supernumerary in cervical region
        Q76.5
    scapula Q74.0
    shoulder Q74.0
    spinal cord Q06.8
    spleen Q89.09
    sternum NEC Q76.7
    stomach Q40.2
    symphysis pubis Q74.2
    thymus (gland) Q89.2
    thyroid (gland) (tissue) Q89.2
      cartilage Q31.8
    toe (s) Q66.9
      supernumerary Q69.2
    tongue Q38.3

Malposition *(Continued)*
  congenital *(Continued)*
    trachea Q32.1
    ureter Q62.60
      deviation Q62.61
      displacement Q62.62
      ectopia Q62.63
      specified type NEC Q62.69
    uterus Q51.818
    vein (s) (peripheral) Q27.8
      great Q26.8
    vena cava (inferior) (superior) Q26.8
  device, implant or graft (*see also*
    Complications, by site and type,
    mechanical) T85.628
    arterial graft NEC —*see*
      Complication, cardiovascular
      device, mechanical, vascular
    breast (implant) T85.42
    catheter NEC T85.628
      cystostomy T83.020
      dialysis (renal) T82.42
        intraperitoneal T85.621
      infusion NEC T82.524
        spinal (epidural) (subdural)
          T85.620
      urinary, indwelling T83.028
    electronic (electrode) (pulse
      generator) (stimulator)
    bone T84.320
    cardiac T82.129
      electrode T82.120
      pulse generator T82.121
      specified type NEC T82.128
    nervous system —*see*
      Complication, prosthetic
      device, mechanical, electronic
      nervous system stimulator
    urinary —*see* Complication,
      genitourinary, device, urinary,
      mechanical
    fixation, internal (orthopedic) NEC —
      see Complication, fixation
      device, mechanical
    gastrointestinal —*see* Complications,
      prosthetic device, mechanical,
      gastrointestinal device
    genital NEC T83.428
      intrauterine contraceptive device
        T83.32
      penile prosthesis T83.420
    heart NEC —*see* Complication,
      cardiovascular device,
      mechanical
    joint prosthesis —*see* Complication,
      joint prosthesis, mechanical
    ocular NEC —*see* Complications,
      prosthetic device, mechanical,
      ocular device
    orthopedic NEC —*see* Complication,
      orthopedic, device, mechanical
    specified NEC T85.628
    urinary NEC —*see also* Complication,
      genitourinary, device, urinary,
      mechanical
      graft T83.22
    vascular NEC —*see* Complication,
      cardiovascular device,
      mechanical
    ventricular intracranial shunt T85.02
  fetus —*see* Pregnancy, complicated
    by (management affected by),
    presentation, fetal
  gallbladder K82.8

Malposition *(Continued)*
  gastrointestinal tract, congenital
    Q45.8
  heart, congenital NEC Q24.8
  joint prosthesis —*see* Complications,
    joint prosthesis, mechanical,
    displacement, by site
  stomach K31.89
    congenital Q40.2
  tooth, teeth, fully erupted M26.30
  uterus (acute) (acquired) (adherent)
    (asymptomatic) (postinfectional)
    (postpartal, old) N85.4
    anteflexion or anteversion N85.4
      congenital Q51.818
    flexion N85.4
      lateral —*see* Lateroversion,
        uterus
    inversion N85.5
    lateral (flexion) (version) —*see*
      Lateroversion, uterus
      in pregnancy or childbirth —*see*
        subcategory O34.5
    retroflexion or retroversion —*see*
      Retroversion, uterus
Malposture R29.3
Malrotation
  cecum Q43.3
  colon Q43.3
  intestine Q43.3
  kidney Q63.2
Malta fever —*see* Brucellosis
Maltreatment
  adult
    abandonment
      confirmed T74.01
      suspected T76.01
    confirmed T74.91
    history of Z91.419
    neglect
      confirmed T74.01
      suspected T76.01
    physical abuse
      confirmed T74.11
      suspected T76.11
    psychological abuse
      confirmed T74.31
      history of Z91.411
      suspected T76.31
    sexual abuse
      confirmed T74.21
      suspected T76.21
    suspected T76.91
  child
    abandonment
      confirmed T74.02
      suspected T76.02
    confirmed T74.92
    history of —*see* History, personal (of),
      abuse
    neglect
      confirmed T74.02
      history of —*see* History, personal
        (of), abuse
      suspected T76.02
    physical abuse
      confirmed T74.12
      history of —*see* History, personal
        (of), abuse
      suspected T76.12
    psychological abuse
      confirmed T74.32
      history of —*see* History, personal
        (of), abuse
      suspected T76.32

Maltreatment (Continued)
  child (Continued)
    sexual abuse
      confirmed T74.22
      history of —see History, personal
        (of), abuse
      suspected T76.22
    suspected T76.92
    personal history of Z91.89
Maltworker's lung J67.4
Malunion, fracture —see Fracture,
  by site
Mammillitis N61
  puerperal, postpartum O91.02
Mammitis —see Mastitis
Mammogram (examination) Z12.39
  routine Z12.31
Mammoplasia N62
Management (of)
  bone conduction hearing device
    (implanted) Z45.320
  cardiac pacemaker NEC Z45.018
  cerebrospinal fluid drainage device
    Z45.41
  cochlear device (implanted) Z45.321
  contraceptive Z30.9
    specified NEC Z30.8
  implanted device Z45.9
    specified NEC Z45.89
  infusion pump Z45.1
  procreative Z31.9
    male factor infertility in female Z31.81
    specified NEC Z31.89
  prosthesis (external) (see also Fitting) Z44.9
    implanted Z45.9
      specified NEC Z45.89
  renal dialysis catheter Z49.01
  vascular access device Z45.2
Mangled —see specified injury by site
Mania (monopolar) —see also Disorder,
  mood, manic episode
  with psychotic symptoms F30.2
  without psychotic symptoms F30.10
    mild F30.11
    moderate F30.12
    severe F30.13
  Bell's F30.8
  chronic (recurrent) F31.89
  hysterical F44.89
  puerperal F30.8
  recurrent F31.89
Manic-depressive insanity, psychosis, or
  syndrome —see Disorder, bipolar
Mannosidosis E77.1
Mansonelliasis, mansonellosis B74.4
Manson's
  disease B65.1
  schistosomiasis B65.1
Manual —see condition
Maple-bark-stripper's lung (disease)
  J67.6
Maple-syrup-urine disease E71.0
Marable's syndrome (celiac artery
  compression) I77.4
Marasmus E41
  due to malnutrition E41
  intestinal E41
  nutritional E41
  senile R54
  tuberculous NEC —see Tuberculosis
Marble
  bones Q78.2
  skin R23.8
Marburg virus disease A98.3

March
  fracture —see Fracture, traumatic,
    stress, by site
  hemoglobinuria D59.6
Marchesani (-Weill) syndrome Q87.0
Marchiafava (-Bignami) syndrome or
  disease G37.1
Marchiafava-Micheli syndrome D59.5
Marcus Gunn's syndrome Q07.8
Marfan's syndrome —see Syndrome,
  Marfan's
Marie-Bamberger disease —see
  Osteoarthropathy, hypertrophic,
  specified NEC
Marie-Charcot-Tooth neuropathic
  muscular atrophy G60.0
Marie's
  cerebellar ataxia (late-onset) G11.2
  disease or syndrome (acromegaly) E22.0
Marie-Strümpell arthritis, disease
  or spondylitis —see Spondylitis,
  ankylosing
Marion's disease (bladder neck
  obstruction) N32.0
Marital conflict Z63.0
Mark
  port wine Q82.5
  raspberry Q82.5
  strawberry Q82.5
  stretch L90.6
  tattoo L81.8
Marker heterochromatin —see Extra,
  marker chromosomes
Maroteaux-Lamy syndrome (mild)
  (severe) E76.29
Marrow (bone)
  arrest D61.9
  poor function D75.89
Marseilles fever A77.1
Marsh fever —see Malaria
Marshall's (hidrotic) **ectodermal**
  dysplasia Q82.4
Marsh's disease (exophthalmic goiter)
  E05.00
  with storm E05.01
Masculinization (female) **with adrenal**
  hyperplasia E25.9
  congenital E25.0
Masculinovoblastoma D27.-
Masochism (sexual) F65.51
Mason's lung J62.8
Mass
  abdominal R19.00
    epigastric R19.06
    generalized R19.07
    left lower quadrant R19.04
    left upper quadrant R19.02
    periumbilic R19.05
    right lower quadrant R19.03
    right upper quadrant R19.01
    specified site NEC R19.09
  breast N63
  chest R22.2
  cystic —see Cyst
  ear H93.8-
  head R22.0
  intra-abdominal (diffuse)
    (generalized) —see Mass,
    abdominal
  kidney N28.89
  liver R16.0
  localized (skin) R22.9
    chest R22.2
    head R22.0

Mass (Continued)
  localized (Continued)
    limb
      lower R22.4-
      upper R22.3-
    neck R22.1
    trunk R22.2
  lung R91.8
  malignant —see Neoplasm, malignant,
    by site
  neck R22.1
  pelvic (diffuse) (generalized) —see
    Mass, abdominal
  specified organ NEC —see Disease, by
    site
  splenic R16.1
  substernal thyroid —see Goiter
  superficial (localized) R22.9
  umbilical (diffuse) (generalized)
    R19.09
Massive —see condition
Mast cell
  disease, systemic tissue D47.0
  leukemia C94.3-
  sarcoma C96.2
  tumor D47.0
    malignant C96.2
Mastalgia N64.4
Masters-Allen syndrome N83.8
Mastitis (acute) (diffuse) (nonpuerperal)
  (subacute) N61
  chronic (cystic) —see Mastopathy,
    cystic
  cystic (Schimmelbusch's type) —see
    Mastopathy, cystic
  fibrocystic —see Mastopathy, cystic
  infective N61
    newborn P39.0
  interstitial, gestational or puerperal —
    see Mastitis, obstetric
  neonatal (noninfective) P83.4
    infective P39.0
  obstetric (interstitial) (nonpurulent)
    associated with
      lactation O91.23
      pregnancy O91.21-
      puerperium O91.22
    purulent
      associated with
        lactation O91.13
        pregnancy O91.11-
        puerperium O91.12
  periductal —see Ectasia, mammary duct
  phlegmonous —see Mastopathy, cystic
  plasma cell —see Ectasia, mammary
    duct
Mastocytoma D47.0
  malignant C96.2
Mastocytosis Q82.2
  aggressive systemic C96.2
  indolent systemic D47.0
  malignant C96.2
  systemic, associated with clonal
    hematopoetic non-mast-cell
    disease (SM-AHNMD) D47.0
Mastodynia N64.4
Mastoid —see condition
Mastoidalgia —see subcategory H92.0
Mastoiditis (coalescent) (hemorrhagic)
  (suppurative) H70.9-
  acute, subacute H70.00-
    complicated NEC H70.09-
    subperiosteal H70.01-
  chronic (necrotic) (recurrent) H70.1-

Mastoiditis (Continued)
  in (due to)
    infectious disease NEC B99 [H75.0-]
    parasitic disease NEC B89 [H75.0-]
    tuberculosis A18.03
  petrositis —see Petrositis
  postauricular fistula —see Fistula, postauricular
  specified NEC H70.89-
  tuberculous A18.03
Mastopathy, mastopathia N64.9
  chronica cystica —see Mastopathy, cystic
  cystic (chronic) (diffuse) N60.1
    with epithelial proliferation N60.3-
  diffuse cystic —see Mastopathy, cystic
  estrogenic, oestrogenica N64.89
  ovarian origin N64.89
Mastoplasia, mastoplastia N62
Masturbation (excessive) F98.8
Maternal care (for) —see Pregnancy (complicated by) (management affected by)
Matheiu's disease (leptospiral jaundice) A27.0
Mauclaire's disease or osteochondrosis —see Osteochondrosis, juvenile, hand, metacarpal
Maxcy's disease A75.2
Maxilla, maxillary —see condition
May (-Hegglin) anomaly or syndrome D72.0
McArdle (-Schmid)(-Pearson) disease (glycogen storage) E74.04
McCune-Albright syndrome Q78.1
McQuarrie's syndrome (idiopathic familial hypoglycemia) E16.2
Meadow's syndrome Q86.1
Measles (black) (hemorrhagic) (suppressed) B05.9
  with
    complications NEC B05.89
    encephalitis B05.0
    intestinal complications B05.4
    keratitis (keratoconjunctivitis) B05.81
    meningitis B05.1
    otitis media B05.3
    pneumonia B05.2
  French —see Rubella
  German —see Rubella
  Liberty —see Rubella
Meatitis, urethral —see Urethritis
Meatus, meatal —see condition
Meat-wrappers' asthma J68.9
Meckel-Gruber syndrome Q61.9
Meckel's diverticulitis, diverticulum (displaced) (hypertrophic) Q43.0
Meconium
  ileus, newborn P76.0
    in cystic fibrosis E84.11
    meaning meconium plug (without cystic fibrosis) P76.0
  obstruction, newborn P76.0
    due to fecaliths P76.0
    in mucoviscidosis E84.11
  peritonitis P78.0
  plug syndrome (newborn) NEC P76.0
Median —see also condition
  arcuate ligament syndrome I77.4
  bar (prostate) (vesical orifice) —see Hyperplasia, prostate
  rhomboid glossitis K14.2

Mediastinal shift R93.8
Mediastinitis (acute) (chronic) J98.5
  syphilitic A52.73
  tuberculous A15.8
Mediastinopericarditis —see also Pericarditis
  acute I30.9
  adhesive I31.0
  chronic I31.8
    rheumatic I09.2
Mediastinum, mediastinal —see condition
Medical services provided for —see Health, services provided because (of)
Medicine poisoning —see Table of drugs and chemicals, by drug, poisoning
Mediterranean
  fever —see Brucellosis
    familial E85.0
    tick A77.1
  kala-azar B55.0
  leishmaniasis B55.0
  tick fever A77.1
Medulla —see condition
Medullary cystic kidney Q61.5
Medullated fibers
  optic (nerve) Q14.8
  retina Q14.1
Medulloblastoma
  desmoplastic C71.6
  specified site —see Neoplasm, malignant, by site
  unspecified site C71.6
Medulloepithelioma —see also Neoplasm, malignant, by site
  teratoid —see Neoplasm, malignant, by site
Medullomyoblastoma
  specified site —see Neoplasm, malignant, by site
  unspecified site C71.6
Meekeren-Ehlers-Danlos syndrome Q79.6
Megacolon (acquired) (functional) (not Hirschsprung's disease) (in) K59.3
  Chagas' disease B57.32
  congenital, congenitum (aganglionic) Q43.1
  Hirschsprung's (disease) Q43.1
  toxic NEC K59.3
    due to Clostridium difficile A04.7
Megaesophagus (functional) K22.0
  congenital Q39.5
  in (due to) Chagas' disease B57.31
Megalencephaly Q04.5
Megalerythema (epidemic) B08.3
Megaloappendix Q43.8
Megalocephalus, megalocephaly NEC Q75.3
Megalocornea Q15.8
  with glaucoma Q15.0
Megalocytic anemia D53.1
Megalodactylia (fingers) (thumbs) (congenital) Q74.0
  toes Q74.2
Megaloduodenum Q43.8
Megaloesophagus (functional) K22.0
  congenital Q39.5
Megalogastria (acquired) K31.89
  congenital Q40.2
Megalophthalmos Q11.3
Megalopsia H53.15
Megalosplenia —see Splenomegaly
Megaloureter N28.82
  congenital Q62.2
Megarectum K62.89

Megasigmoid K59.3
  congenital Q43.2
Megaureter N28.82
  congenital Q62.2
Megavitamin-B6 syndrome E67.2
Megrim —see Migraine
Meibomian
  cyst, infected —see Hordeolum
  gland —see condition
  sty, stye —see Hordeolum
Meibomitis —see Hordeolum
Meige-Milroy disease (chronic hereditary edema) Q82.0
Meige's syndrome Q82.0
Melalgia, nutritional E53.8
Melancholia F32.9
  climacteric (single episode) F32.8
    recurrent episode F33.9
  hypochondriac F45.29
  intermittent (single episode) F32.8
    recurrent episode F33.9
  involutional (single episode) F32.8
    recurrent episode F33.9
  menopausal (single episode) F32.8
    recurrent episode F33.9
  puerperal F32.8
  reactive (emotional stress or trauma) F32.3
  recurrent F33.9
  senile F03
  stuporous (single episode) F32.8
    recurrent episode F33.9
Melanemia R79.89
Melanoameloblastoma —see Neoplasm, bone, benign
Melanoblastoma —see Melanoma
Melanocarcinoma —see Melanoma
Melanocytoma, eyeball D31.4-
Melanocytosis, neurocutaneous Q82.8
Melanoderma, melanodermia L81.4
Melanodontia, infantile K03.89
Melanodontoclasia K03.89
Melanoepithelioma —see Melanoma
Melanoma (malignant) C43.9
  acral lentiginous, malignant —see Melanoma, skin, by site
  amelanotic —see Melanoma, skin, by site
  balloon cell —see Melanoma, skin, by site
  benign —see Nevus
  desmoplastic, malignant —see Melanoma, skin, by site
  epithelioid cell —see Melanoma, skin, by site
    with spindle cell, mixed —see Melanoma, skin, by site
  in
    giant pigmented nevus —see Melanoma, skin, by site
    Hutchinson's melanotic freckle —see Melanoma, skin, by site
    junctional nevus —see Melanoma, skin, by site
    precancerous melanosis —see Melanoma, skin, by site
  in situ D03.9
    abdominal wall D03.59
    ala nasi D03.39
    ankle D03.7-
    anus, anal (margin) (skin) D03.51
    arm D03.6-
    auditory canal D03.2-
    auricle (ear) D03.2-

M

Melanoma (Continued)
  in situ (Continued)
    auricular canal (external) D03.2-
    axilla, axillary fold D03.59
    back D03.59
    breast D03.52
    brow D03.39
    buttock D03.59
    canthus (eye) D03.1-
    cheek (external) D03.39
    chest wall D03.59
    chin D03.39
    choroid D03.8
    conjunctiva D03.8
    ear (external) D03.2-
    external meatus (ear) D03.2-
    eye D03.8
    eyebrow D03.39
    eyelid (lower) (upper) D03.1-
    face D03.30
      specified NEC D03.39
    female genital organ (external) NEC
      D03.8
    finger D03.6-
    flank D03.59
    foot D03.7-
    forearm D03.6-
    forehead D03.39
    foreskin D03.8
    gluteal region D03.59
    groin D03.59
    hand D03.6-
    heel D03.7-
    helix D03.2-
    hip D03.7-
    interscapular region D03.59
    iris D03.8
    jaw D03.39
    knee D03.7-
    labium (majus) (minus) D03.8
    lacrimal gland D03.8
    leg D03.7-
    lip (lower) (upper) D03.0
    lower limb NEC D03.7-
    male genital organ (external) NEC
      D03.8
    nail D03.9
      finger D03.6-
      toe D03.7-
    neck D03.4
    nose (external) D03.39
    orbit D03.8
    penis D03.8
    perianal skin D03.51
    perineum D03.51
    pinna D03.2-
    popliteal fossa or space D03.7-
    prepuce D03.8
    pudendum D03.8
    retina D03.8
    retrobulbar D03.8
    scalp D03.4
    scrotum D03.8
    shoulder D03.6-
    specified site NEC D03.8
    submammary fold D03.52
    temple D03.39
    thigh D03.7-
    toe D03.7-
    trunk NEC D03.59
    umbilicus D03.59
    upper limb NEC D03.6-
    vulva D03.8
  juvenile —see Nevus

Melanoma (Continued)
  malignant, of soft parts except skin —
      see Neoplasm, connective tissue,
      malignant
  metastatic
    breast C79.81
    genital organ C79.82
    specified site NEC C79.89
  neurotropic, malignant —see
      Melanoma, skin, by site
  nodular —see Melanoma, skin, by site
  regressing, malignant —see Melanoma,
      skin, by site
  skin C43.9
    abdominal wall C43.59
    ala nasi C43.31
    ankle C43.7-
    anus, anal (skin) C43.51
    arm C43.6-
    auditory canal (external) C43.2-
    auricle (ear) C43.2-
    auricular canal (external) C43.2-
    axilla, axillary fold C43.59
    back C43.59
    breast (female) (male) C43.52
    brow C43.39
    buttock C43.59
    canthus (eye) C43.1-
    cheek (external) C43.39
    chest wall C43.59
    chin C43.39
    ear (external) C43.2-
    elbow C43.6-
    external meatus (ear) C43.2-
    eyebrow C43.39
    eyelid (lower) (upper) C43.1-
    face C43.30
      specified NEC C43.39
    female genital organ (external) NEC
      C51.9
    finger C43.6-
    flank C43.59
    foot C43.7-
    forearm C43.6-
    forehead C43.39
    foreskin C60.0
    glabella C43.39
    gluteal region C43.59
    groin C43.59
    hand C43.6-
    heel C43.7-
    helix C43.2-
    hip C43.7-
    interscapular region C43.59
    jaw (external) C43.39
    knee C43.7-
    labium C51.9
      majus C51.0
      minus C51.1
    leg C43.7-
    lip (lower) (upper) C43.0
    lower limb NEC C43.7-
    male genital organ (external) NEC
      C63.9
    nail
      finger C43.6-
      toe C43.7-
    nasolabial groove C43.39
    nates C43.59
    neck C43.4
    nose (external) C43.31
    overlapping site C43.8
    palpebra C43.1-
    penis C60.9

Melanoma (Continued)
  skin (Continued)
    perianal skin C43.51
    perineum C43.51
    pinna C43.2-
    popliteal fossa or space C43.7-
    prepuce C60.0
    pudendum C51.9
    scalp C43.4
    scrotum C63.2
    shoulder C43.6-
    skin NEC C43.9
    submammary fold C43.52
    temple C43.39
    thigh C43.7-
    toe C43.7-
    trunk NEC C43.59
    umbilicus C43.59
    upper limb NEC C43.6-
    vulva C51.9
      overlapping sites C51.8
    spindle cell
      with epithelioid, mixed —see
        Melanoma, skin, by site
      type A C69.4-
      type B C69.4-
    superficial spreading —see Melanoma,
      skin, by site
Melanosarcoma —see also Melanoma
  epithelioid cell —see Melanoma
Melanosis L81.4
  addisonian E27.1
    tuberculous A18.7
  adrenal E27.1
  colon K63.89
  conjunctiva —see Pigmentation,
    conjunctiva
    congenital Q13.89
  cornea (presenile) (senile) —see also
      Pigmentation, cornea
    congenital Q13.4
  eye NEC H57.8
    congenital Q15.8
  lenticularis progressiva Q82.1
  liver K76.89
  precancerous —see also Melanoma,
    in situ
    malignant melanoma in —see
      Melanoma
  Riehl's L81.4
  sclera H15.89
    congenital Q13.89
  suprarenal E27.1
  tar L81.4
  toxic L81.4
Melanuria R82.99
MELAS syndrome E88.41
Melasma L81.1
  adrenal (gland) E27.1
  suprarenal (gland) E27.1
Melena K92.1
  with ulcer - code by site under
    Ulcer, with hemorrhage
    K27.4
  due to swallowed maternal blood
    P78.2
  newborn, neonatal P54.1
    due to swallowed maternal blood
      P78.2
Meleney's
  gangrene (cutaneous) —see Ulcer,
    skin
  ulcer (chronic undermining) —see Ulcer,
    skin

Melioidosis A24.9
  acute A24.1
  chronic A24.2
  fulminating A24.1
  pneumonia A24.1
  pulmonary (chronic) A24.2
    acute A24.1
    subacute A24.2
  sepsis A24.1
  specified NEC A24.3
  subacute A24.2
Melitensis, febris A23.0
Melkersson (-Rosenthal) syndrome G51.2
Mellitus, diabetes —see Diabetes
Melorheostosis (bone) —see Disorder, bone, density and structure, specified NEC
Meloschisis Q18.4
Melotia Q17.4
Membrana
  capsularis lentis posterior Q13.89
  epipapillaris Q14.2
Membranacea placenta O43.19-
Membranaceous uterus N85.8
Membrane (s), membranous —see also condition
  cyclitic —see Membrane, pupillary
  folds, congenital —see Web
  Jackson's Q43.3
  over face of newborn P28.9
  premature rupture —see Rupture, membranes, premature
  pupillary H21.4-
    persistent Q13.89
  retained (with hemorrhage) (complicating delivery) O72.2
    without hemorrhage O73.1
  secondary cataract —see Cataract, secondary
  unruptured (causing asphyxia) —see Asphyxia, newborn
  vitreous —see Opacity, vitreous, membranes and strands
Membranitis —see Chorioamnionitis
Memory disturbance, lack or loss —see also Amnesia
  mild, following organic brain damage F06.8
Menadione deficiency E56.1
Menarche
  delayed E30.0
  precocious E30.1
Mendacity, pathologic F60.2
Mendelson's syndrome (due to anesthesia) J95.4
  in labor and delivery O74.0
  in pregnancy O29.01-
  obstetric O74.0
  postpartum, puerperal O89.01
Ménétrier's disease or syndrome K29.60
  with bleeding K29.61
Ménière's disease, syndrome or vertigo H81.0-
Meninges, meningeal —see condition
Meningioma —see also Neoplasm, meninges, benign
  angioblastic —see Neoplasm, meninges, benign
  angiomatous —see Neoplasm, meninges, benign
  endotheliomatous —see Neoplasm, meninges, benign

Meningioma (Continued)
  fibroblastic —see Neoplasm, meninges, benign
  fibrous —see Neoplasm, meninges, benign
  hemangioblastic —see Neoplasm, meninges, benign
  hemangiopericytic —see Neoplasm, meninges, benign
  malignant —see Neoplasm, meninges, malignant
  meningiothelial —see Neoplasm, meninges, benign
  meningotheliomatous —see Neoplasm, meninges, benign
  mixed —see Neoplasm, meninges, benign
  multiple —see Neoplasm, meninges, uncertain behavior
  papillary —see Neoplasm, meninges, uncertain behavior
  psammomatous —see Neoplasm, meninges, benign
  syncytial —see Neoplasm, meninges, benign
  transitional —see Neoplasm, meninges, benign
Meningiomatosis (diffuse) —see Neoplasm, meninges, uncertain behavior
Meningism —see Meningismus
Meningismus (infectional) (pneumococcal) R29.1
  due to serum or vaccine R29.1
  influenzal —see Influenza, with, manifestations NEC
Meningitis (basal) (basic) (brain) (cerebral) (cervical) (congestive) (diffuse) (hemorrhagic) infantile (membranous) (metastatic) (nonspecific) (pontine) (progressive) (simple) (spinal) (subacute) (sympathetic) (toxic) G03.9
  abacterial G03.0
  actinomycotic A42.81
  adenoviral A87.1
  arbovirus A87.8
  aseptic (acute) G03.0
  bacterial G00.9
    Escherichia coli (E. coli) G00.8
    Friedländer (bacillus) G00.8
    gram-negative G00.9
    H. influenzae G00.0
    Klebsiella G00.8
    pneumococcal G00.1
    specified organism NEC G00.8
    staphylococcal G00.3
    streptococcal (acute) G00.2
  benign recurrent (Mollaret) G03.2
  candidal B37.5
  caseous (tuberculous) A17.0
  cerebrospinal A39.0
  chronic NEC G03.1
  clear cerebrospinal fluid NEC G03.0
  coxsackievirus A87.0
  cryptococcal B45.1
  diplococcal (gram positive) A39.0
  echovirus A87.0
  enteroviral A87.0
  eosinophilic B83.2
  epidemic NEC A39.0
  Escherichia coli (E. coli) G00.8
  fibrinopurulent G00.9
    specified organism NEC G00.8

Meningitis (Continued)
  Friedländer (bacillus) G00.8
  gonococcal A54.81
  gram-negative cocci G00.9
  gram-positive cocci G00.9
  Haemophilus (influenzae) G00.0
  H. influenzae G00.0
  in (due to)
    adenovirus A87.1
    African trypanosomiasis B56.9 [G02]
    anthrax A22.8
    bacterial disease NEC A48.8 [G01]
    Chagas' disease (chronic) B57.41
    chickenpox B01.0
    coccidioidomycosis B38.4
    Diplococcus pneumoniae G00.1
    enterovirus A87.0
    herpes (simplex) virus B00.3
      zoster B02.1
    infectious mononucleosis B27.92
    leptospirosis A27.81
    Listeria monocytogenes A32.11
    Lyme disease A69.21
    measles B05.1
    mumps (virus) B26.1
    neurosyphilis (late) A52.13
    parasitic disease NEC B89 [G02]
    poliovirus A80.9 [G02]
    preventive immunization, inoculation or vaccination G03.8
    rubella B06.02
    Salmonella infection A02.21
    specified cause NEC G03.8
    typhoid fever A01.01
    varicella B01.0
    viral disease NEC A87.8
    whooping cough A37.90
    zoster B02.1
  infectious G00.9
  influenzal (H. influenzae) G00.0
  Klebsiella G00.8
  leptospiral (aseptic) A27.81
  lymphocytic (acute) (benign) (serous) A87.2
  meningococcal A39.0
  Mima polymorpha G00.8
  Mollaret (benign recurrent) G03.2
  monilial B37.5
  mycotic NEC B49 [G02]
  Neisseria A39.0
  nonbacterial G03.0
  nonpyogenic NEC G03.0
  ossificans G96.19
  pneumococcal G00.1
  poliovirus A80.9 [G02]
  postmeasles B05.1
  purulent G00.9
    specified organism NEC G00.8
  pyogenic G00.9
    specified organism NEC G00.8
  Salmonella (arizonae) (Cholerae-Suis) (enteritidis) (typhimurium) A02.21
  septic G00.9
    specified organism NEC G00.8
  serosa circumscripta NEC G03.0
  serous NEC G93.2
  specified organism NEC G00.8
  sporotrichosis B42.81
  staphylococcal G00.3
  sterile G03.0
  streptococcal (acute) G00.2
  suppurative G00.9
    specified organism NEC G00.8

Meningitis *(Continued)*
  syphilitic (late) (tertiary) A52.13
    acute A51.41
    congenital A50.41
    secondary A51.41
  Torula histolytica (cryptococcal) B45.1
  traumatic (complication of injury) T79.8
  tuberculous A17.0
  typhoid A01.01
  viral NEC A87.9
  Yersinia pestis A20.3
Meningocele (spinal) *—see also* Spina
    bifida
  with hydrocephalus *—see* Spina bifida,
    by site, with hydrocephalus
  acquired (traumatic) G96.19
  cerebral *—see* Encephalocele
Meningocerebritis *—see*
    Meningoencephalitis
Meningococcemia A39.4
  acute A39.2
  chronic A39.3
Meningococcus, meningococcal *(see also*
    condition) A39.9
  adrenalitis, hemorrhagic A39.1
  carrier (suspected) of Z22.31
  meningitis (cerebrospinal) A39.0
Meningoencephalitis *(see also*
    Encephalitis) G04.90
  acute NEC *(see also* Encephalitis, viral)
    A86
  bacterial NEC G04.2
  California A83.5
  diphasic A84.1
  eosinophilic B83.2
  epidemic A39.81
  herpesviral, herpetic B00.4
    due to herpesvirus 6 B10.01
    due to herpesvirus 7 B10.09
    specified NEC B10.09
  in (due to)
    blastomycosis NEC B40.81
    diseases classified elsewhere G05.3
    free-living amebae B60.2
    Hemophilus influenzae
        (H. influenzae) G04.2
    herpes B00.4
      due to herpesvirus 6 B10.01
      due to herpesvirus 7 B10.09
      specified NEC B10.09
    H. influenzae G00.0
    Lyme disease A69.22
    mercury *—see* subcategory T56.1
    mumps B26.2
    Naegleria (amebae) (organisms)
        (fowleri) B60.2
    Parastrongylus cantonensis B83.2
    toxoplasmosis (acquired) B58.2
      congenital P37.1
  infectious (acute) (viral) A86
  influenzal (H. influenzae) G04.2
  Listeria monocytogenes A32.12
  lymphocytic (serous) A87.2
  mumps B26.2
  parasitic NEC [G05.3 B89
  pneumococcal G00.1
  primary amebic B60.2
  specific (syphilitic) A52.14
  specified organism NEC G04.81
  staphylococcal G04.2
  streptococcal G04.2
  syphilitic A52.14
  toxic NEC G92
    due to mercury *—see* subcategory T56.1

Meningoencephalitis *(Continued)*
  tuberculous A17.82
  virus NEC A86
Meningoencephalocele *—see also*
    Encephalocele
  syphilitic A52.19
    congenital A50.49
Meningoencephalomyelitis *—see also*
    Meningoencephalitis
  acute NEC (viral) A86
    disseminated G04.00
      postimmunization or
          postvaccination G04.02
      postinfectious G04.01
    due to
      actinomycosis A42.82
      Torula B45.1
      Toxoplasma or toxoplasmosis
          (acquired) B58.2
        congenital P37.1
    postimmunization or postvaccination
      G04.02
Meningoencephalomyelopathy G96.9
Meningoencephalopathy G96.9
Meningomyelitis *—see also*
    Meningoencephalitis
  bacterial NEC G04.2
  blastomycotic NEC B40.81
  cryptococcal B45.1
  in diseases classified elsewhere G05.4
  meningococcal A39.81
  syphilitic A52.14
  tuberculous A17.82
Meningomyelocele *—see also* Spina bifida
  syphilitic A52.19
Meningomyeloneuritis *—see*
    Meningoencephalitis
Meningoradiculitis *—see* Meningitis
Meningovascular *—see* condition
Menkes' disease or syndrome E83.09
  meaning maple-syrup-urine disease
    E71.0
Menometrorrhagia N92.1
Menopause, menopausal (asymptomatic)
    (state) Z78.0
  arthritis (any site) NEC *—see* Arthritis,
    specified form NEC
  bleeding N92.4
  depression (single episode) F32.8
    agitated (single episode) F32.2
      recurrent episode F33.9
    psychotic (single episode) F32.8
      recurrent episode F33.9
    recurrent episode F33.9
  melancholia (single episode) F32.8
    recurrent episode F33.9
  paranoid state F22
  premature E28.319
    asymptomatic E28.319
      postirradiation E89.40
      postsurgical E89.40
    symptomatic E28.310
      postirradiation E89.41
      postsurgical E89.41
  psychosis NEC F28
  symptomatic N95.1
  toxic polyarthritis NEC *—see* Arthritis,
    specified form NEC
Menorrhagia (primary) N92.0
  climacteric N92.4
    menopausal N92.4
  menopausal N92.4
  postclimacteric N95.0
  postmenopausal N95.0

Menorrhagia *(Continued)*
  preclimacteric or premenopausal
    N92.4
  pubertal (menses retained) N92.2
Menostaxis N92.0
Menses, retention N94.89
Menstrual *—see* Menstruation
Menstruation
  absent *—see* Amenorrhea
  anovulatory N97.0
  cycle, irregular N92.6
  delayed N91.0
  disorder N93.9
    psychogenic F45.8
  during pregnancy O20.8
  excessive (with regular cycle) N92.0
    with irregular cycle N92.1
    at puberty N92.2
  frequent N92.0
  infrequent *—see* Oligomenorrhea
  irregular N92.6
    specified NEC N92.5
  latent N92.5
  membranous N92.5
  painful *(see also* Dysmenorrhea) N94.6
    primary N94.4
    psychogenic F45.8
    secondary N94.5
  passage of clots N92.0
  precocious E30.1
  protracted N92.5
  rare *—see* Oligomenorrhea
  retained N94.89
  retrograde N92.5
  scanty *—see* Oligomenorrhea
  suppression N94.89
  vicarious (nasal) N94.89
Mental *—see also* condition
  deficiency *—see* Disability, intellectual
  deterioration *—see* Psychosis
  disorder *—see* Disorder, mental
  exhaustion F48.8
  insufficiency (congenital) *—see*
    Disability, intellectual
  observation without need for further
    medical care Z03.89
  retardation *—see* Disability, intellectual
  subnormality *—see* Disability,
    intellectual
  upset *—see* Disorder, mental
Meralgia paresthetica G57.1-
Mercurial *—see* condition
Mercurialism *—see* subcategory T56.1
MERRF syndrome (myoclonic epilepsy
    associated with ragged-red fiber)
    E88.42
Merkel cell tumor *—see* Carcinoma,
    Merkel cell
Merocele *—see* Hernia, femoral
Meromelia
  lower limb *—see* Defect, reduction,
    lower limb
    intercalary
      femur *—see* Defect, reduction,
          lower limb, specified type
          NEC
        tibiofibular (complete)
            (incomplete) *—see* Defect,
            reduction, lower limb
  upper limb *—see* Defect, reduction,
    upper limb
    intercalary, humeral, radioulnar *—see*
      Agenesis, arm, with hand
      present

Merzbacher-Pelizaeus disease E75.29
Mesaortitis —see Aortitis
Mesarteritis —see Arteritis
Mesencephalitis —see Encephalitis
Mesenchymoma —see also Neoplasm,
    connective tissue, uncertain behavior
  benign —see Neoplasm, connective
      tissue, benign
  malignant —see Neoplasm, connective
      tissue, malignant
Mesenteritis
  retractile K65.4
  sclerosing K65.4
Mesentery, mesenteric —see condition
Mesiodens, mesiodentes K00.1
Mesio-occlusion M26.213
Mesocolon —see condition
Mesonephroma (malignant) —see
    Neoplasm, malignant, by site
  benign —see Neoplasm, benign, by site
Mesophlebitis —see Phlebitis
Mesostromal dysgenesis Q13.89
Mesothelioma (malignant) C45.9
  benign
    mesentery D19.1
    mesocolon D19.1
    omentum D19.1
    peritoneum D19.1
    pleura D19.0
    specified site NEC D19.7
    unspecified site D19.9
  biphasic C45.9
    benign
      mesentery D19.1
      mesocolon D19.1
      omentum D19.1
      peritoneum D19.1
      pleura D19.0
      specified site NEC D19.7
      unspecified site D19.9
  cystic D48.4
  epithelioid C45.9
    benign
      mesentery D19.1
      mesocolon D19.1
      omentum D19.1
      peritoneum D19.1
      pleura D19.0
      specified site NEC D19.7
      unspecified site D19.9
  fibrous C45.9
    benign
      mesentery D19.1
      mesocolon D19.1
      omentum D19.1
      peritoneum D19.1
      pleura D19.0
      specified site NEC D19.7
      unspecified site D19.9
  site classification
    liver C45.7
    lung C45.7
    mediastinum C45.7
    mesentery C45.1
    mesocolon C45.1
    omentum C45.1
    pericardium C45.2
    peritoneum C45.1
    pleura C45.0
      parietal C45.0
    retroperitoneum C45.7
    specified site NEC C45.7
    unspecified C45.9
Metabolic syndrome E88.81

Metagonimiasis B66.8
Metagonimus infestation (intestine)
    B66.8
Metal
  pigmentation L81.8
  polisher's disease J62.8
Metamorphopsia H53.15
Metaplasia
  apocrine (breast) —see Dysplasia,
      mammary, specified type NEC
  cervix (squamous) —see Dysplasia,
      cervix
  endometrium (squamous) (uterus)
      N85.8
  esophagus
  kidney (pelvis) (squamous) N28.89
  myelogenous D73.1
  myeloid (agnogenic) (megakaryocytic)
      D73.1
  spleen D73.1
  squamous cell, bladder N32.89
Metastasis, metastatic
  abscess —see Abscess
  calcification E83.59
  cancer
    from specified site —see Neoplasm,
        malignant, by site
    to specified site —see Neoplasm,
        secondary, by site
  deposits (in) —see Neoplasm,
      secondary, by site
  disease (see also Neoplasm, secondary,
      by site) C79.9
  spread (to) —see Neoplasm, secondary,
      by site
Metastrongyliasis B83.8
Metatarsalgia M77.4-
  anterior G57.6-
  Morton's G57.6-
Metatarsus, metatarsal —see also
    condition
  valgus (abductus), congenital Q66.6
  varus (adductus) (congenital) Q66.2
Methadone use F11.20
Methemoglobinemia D74.9
  acquired (with sulfhemoglobinemia)
      D74.8
  congenital D74.0
  enzymatic (congenital) D74.0
  Hb M disease D74.0
  hereditary D74.0
  toxic D74.8
Methemoglobinuria —see
    Hemoglobinuria
Methioninemia E72.19
Methylmalonic acidemia E71.120
Metritis (catarrhal) (hemorrhagic) (septic)
    (suppurative) —see also Endometritis
  cervical —see Cervicitis
Metropathia hemorrhagica N93.8
Metroperitonitis —see Peritonitis, pelvic,
    female
Metrorrhagia N92.1
  climacteric N92.4
  menopausal N92.4
  postpartum NEC (atonic) (following
      delivery of placenta) O72.1
    delayed or secondary O72.2
  preclimacteric or premenopausal N92.4
  psychogenic F45.8
Metrorrhexis —see Rupture, uterus
Metrosalpingitis N70.91
Metrostaxis N93.8
Metrovaginitis —see Endometritis

Meyer-Schwickerath and Weyers
    syndrome Q87.0
Meynert's amentia (nonalcoholic) F04
  alcoholic F10.96
    with dependence F10.26
Mibelli's disease (porokeratosis) Q82.8
Mice, joint —see Loose, body, joint
    knee M23.4
Micrencephalon, micrencephaly Q02
Microalbuminuria R80.9
Microaneurysm, retinal —see also
    Disorder, retina, microaneurysms
  diabetic —see E08-E13 with .31
Microangiopathy (peripheral) I73.9
  thrombotic M31.1
Microcalcifications, breast R92.0
Microcephalus, microcephalic,
    microcephaly Q02
  due to toxoplasmosis (congenital) P37.1
Microcheilia Q18.7
Microcolon (congenital) Q43.8
Microcornea (congenital) Q13.4
Microcytic —see condition D57.40
Microdeletions NEC Q93.88
Microdontia K00.2
Microdrepanocytosis D57.40
  with sickle-cell crisis D57.41
Microembolism
  atherothrombotic —see Atheroembolism
  retinal —see Occlusion, artery, retina
Microencephalon Q02
Microfilaria streptocerca infestation —see
    Onchocerciasis
Microgastria (congenital) Q40.2
Microgenia M26.06
Microgenitalia, congenital
  female Q52.8
  male Q55.8
Microglioma —see Lymphoma, non-
    Hodgkin, specified NEC
Microglossia (congenital) Q38.3
Micrognathia, micrognathism (congenital)
    (mandibular) (maxillary) M26.09
Microgyria (congenital) Q04.3
Microinfarct of heart —see Insufficiency,
    coronary
Microlentia (congenital) Q12.8
Microlithiasis, alveolar, pulmonary
    J84.02
Micromastia N64.82
Micromyelia (congenital) Q06.8
Micropenis Q55.62
Microphakia (congenital) Q12.8
Microphthalmos, microphthalmia
    (congenital) Q11.2
  due to toxoplasmosis P37.1
Micropsia H53.15
Microscopic polyangiitis (polyarteritis)
    M31.7
Microsporidiosis B60.8
  intestinal A07.8
Microsporon furfur infestation B36.0
Microsporosis —see also Dermatophytosis
    nigra B36.1
Microstomia (congenital) Q18.5
Microtia (congenital) (external ear) Q17.2
Microtropia H50.40
Microvillus inclusion disease (MVD)
    (MVID) Q43.8
Micturition
  disorder NEC R39.19
    psychogenic F45.8
  frequency R35.0
    psychogenic F45.8

Micturition (*Continued*)
  hesitancy R39.11
  incomplete emptying R39.14
  nocturnal R35.1
  painful R30.9
    dysuria R30.0
    psychogenic F45.8
    tenesmus R30.1
  poor stream R39.12
  split stream R39.13
  straining R39.16
  urgency R39.15
Mid plane —*see* condition
Middle
  ear —*see* condition
  lobe (right) syndrome J98.19
Miescher's elastoma L87.2
Mietens' syndrome Q87.2
Migraine (idiopathic) G43.909
  with refractory migraine G43.919
    with status migrainosus G43.911
    without status migrainosus
      G43.919
  with aura (acute-onset) (prolonged)
    (typical) (without headache)
    G43.109
    with refractory migraine G43.119
      with status migrainosus G43.111
      without status migrainosus
        G43.119
    intractable G43.119
      with status migrainosus G43.111
      without status migrainosus
        G43.119
    not intractable G43.109
      with status migrainosus G43.101
      without status migrainosus
        G43.109
  persistent G43.509
    with cerebral infarction G43.609
      with refractory migraine
        G43.619
        with status migrainosus
          G43.611
        without status migrainosus
          G43.619
      intractable G43.619
        with status migrainosus
          G43.611
        without status migrainosus
          G43.619
      not intractable G43.609
        with status migrainosus
          G43.601
        without status migrainosus
          G43.609
      without refractory migraine
        G43.609
        with status migrainosus
          G43.601
        without status migrainosus
          G43.609
    without cerebral infarction
      G43.509
      with refractory migraine G43.519
        with status migrainosus
          G43.511
        without status migrainosus
          G43.519
      intractable G43.519
        with status migrainosus
          G43.511
        without status migrainosus
          G43.519

Migraine (*Continued*)
  with aura (*Continued*)
    persistent (*Continued*)
      without cerebral infarction
      (*Continued*)
        not intractable G43.509
          with status migrainosus
            G43.501
          without status migrainosus
            G43.509
        without refractory migraine
          G43.509
          with status migrainosus
            G43.501
          without status migrainosus
            G43.509
    without mention of refractory
      migraine G43.109
      with status migrainosus G43.101
      without status migrainosus
        G43.109
  abdominal G43.D0
    with refractory migraine G43.D1
    intractable G43.D1
    not intractable G43.D0
    without refractory migraine G43.D0
  basilar —*see* Migraine, with aura
  classical —*see* Migraine, with aura
  common —*see* Migraine, without aura
  complicated G43.109
  equivalents —*see* Migraine, with aura
  familiar —*see* Migraine, hemiplegic
  hemiplegic G43.409
    with refractory migraine G43.419
      with status migrainosus G43.411
      without status migrainosus G43.419
    intractable G43.419
      with status migrainosus G43.411
      without status migrainosus G43.419
    not intractable G43.409
      with status migrainosus G43.401
      without status migrainosus G43.409
    without refractory migraine G43.409
      with status migrainosus G43.401
      without status migrainosus G43.409
  intractable G43.919
    with status migrainosus G43.911
    without status migrainosus G43.919
  menstrual G43.829
    with refractory migraine G43.839
      with status migrainosus G43.831
      without status migrainosus G43.839
    intractable G43.839
      with status migrainosus G43.831
      without status migrainosus G43.839
    not intractable G43.829
      with status migrainosus G43.821
      without status migrainosus G43.829
    without refractory migraine G43.829
      with status migrainosus G43.821
      without status migrainosus G43.829
  menstrually related —*see* Migraine,
    menstrual
  not intractable G43.909
    with status migrainosus G43.901
    without status migrainosus G43.919
  ophthalmoplegic G43.B0
    with refractory migraine G43.B1
    intractable G43.B1
    not intractable G43.B0
    without refractory migraine G43.B0
  persistent aura (with, without) cerebral
    infarction —*see* Migraine, with
    aura, persistent

Migraine (*Continued*)
  preceded or accompanied by transient
    focal neurological phenomena —
    see Migraine, with aura
  pre-menstrual —*see* Migraine,
    menstrual
  pure menstrual —*see* Migraine,
    menstrual
  retinal —*see* Migraine, with aura
  specified NEC G43.809
    intractable G43.819
      with status migrainosus
        G43.811
      without status migrainosus
        G43.819
    not intractable G43.809
      with status migrainosus
        G43.801
      without status migrainosus
        G43.809
  sporadic —*see* Migraine, hemiplegic
  transformed —*see* Migraine, without
    aura, chronic
  triggered seizures —*see* Migraine, with
    aura
  without aura G43.009
    with refractory migraine G43.019
      with status migrainosus G43.011
      without status migrainosus
        G43.019
    chronic G43.709
      with refractory migraine G43.719
        with status migrainosus
          G43.711
        without status migrainosus
          G43.719
      intractable
        with status migrainosus G43.711
        without status migrainosus
          G43.719
      not intractable
        with status migrainosus G43.701
        without status migrainosus
          G43.709
      without refractory migraine
        G43.709
        with status migrainosus
          G43.701
        without status migrainosus
          G43.709
    intractable
      with status migrainosus G43.011
      without status migrainosus
        G43.019
    not intractable
      with status migrainosus G43.001
      without status migrainosus
        G43.009
    without mention of refractory
      migraine G43.009
      with status migrainosus G43.001
      without status migrainosus
        G43.009
  without refractory migraine G43.909
    with status migrainosus G43.901
    without status migrainosus G43.919
Migrant, social Z59.0
Migration, anxiety concerning Z60.3
Migratory, migrating —*see also* condition
  person Z59.0
  testis Q55.29
Mikity-Wilson disease or syndrome
  P27.0
Mikulicz' disease or syndrome K11.8

Miliaria L74.3
  alba L74.1
  apocrine L75.2
  crystallina L74.1
  profunda L74.2
  rubra L74.0
  tropicalis L74.2
Miliary —*see* condition
Milium L72.0
  colloid L57.8
Milk
  crust L21.0
  excessive secretion O92.6
  poisoning —*see* Poisoning, food, noxious
  retention O92.79
  sickness —*see* Poisoning, food, noxious
  spots I31.0
Milk-alkali disease or syndrome E83.52
Milk-leg (deep vessels) (nonpuerperal) —
  see Embolism, vein, lower extremity
  complicating pregnancy O22.3-
  puerperal, postpartum, childbirth O87.1
Milkman's disease or syndrome M83.8
Milky urine —*see* Chyluria
Millard-Gubler (-Foville) paralysis or
  syndrome G46.3
Millar's asthma J38.5
Miller-Fisher syndrome G61.0
Mills' disease —*see* Hemiplegia
Millstone maker's pneumoconiosis J62.8
Milroy's disease (chronic hereditary
  edema) Q82.0
Minamata disease T26.1
Miners' asthma or lung J60
Minkowski-Chauffard syndrome —*see*
  Spherocytosis
Minor —*see* condition
Minor's disease (hematomyelia) G95.19
Minot's disease (hemorrhagic disease),
  newborn P53
Minot-von Willebrand-Jurgens disease or
  syndrome (angiohemophilia) D68.0
Minus (and plus) hand (intrinsic) —*see*
  Deformity, limb, specified type NEC,
  forearm
Miosis (pupil) H57.03
Mirizzi's syndrome (hepatic duct
  stenosis) K83.1
Mirror writing F81.0
Misadventure (of) (prophylactic)
  (therapeutic) (*see also* Complications)
  T88.9
  administration of insulin (by
    accident) —*see* subcategory T38.3
  infusion —*see* Complications, infusion
  local applications (of fomentations,
    plasters, etc.) T88.9
    burn or scald —*see* Burn
    specified NEC T88.8
  medical care (early) (late) T88.9
    adverse effect of drugs or
      chemicals —*see* Table of drugs
      and chemicals
  medical care (early) (late)
    burn or scald —*see* Burn
    specified NEC T88.8
  specified NEC T88.8
  surgical procedure (early) (late) —*see*
    Complications, surgical procedure
  transfusion —*see* Complications,
    transfusion
  vaccination or other immunological
    procedure —*see* Complications,
    vaccination

Miscarriage O03.9
Misdirection, aqueous H40.83-
Misperception, sleep state F51.02
Misplaced, misplacement
  ear Q17.4
  kidney (acquired) N28.89
    congenital Q63.2
  organ or site, congenital NEC —*see*
    Malposition, congenital
Missed
  abortion O02.1
  delivery O36.4
Missing —*see* Absence
Misuse of drugs F19.99
Mitchell's disease (erythromelalgia)
  I73.81
Mite (s) (infestation) B88.9
  diarrhea B88.0
  grain (itch) B88.0
  hair follicle (itch) B88.0
  in sputum B88.0
Mitral —*see* condition
Mittelschmerz N94.0
Mixed —*see* condition
MNGIE (Mitochondrial
  Neurogastrointestinal
  Encephalopathy) syndrome E88.49
Mobile, mobility
  cecum Q43.3
  excessive —*see* Hypermobility
  gallbladder, congenital Q44.1
  kidney N28.89
  organ or site, congenital NEC —*see*
    Malposition, congenital
Mobitz heart block (atrioventricular)
  I44.1
Moebius, Möbius
  disease (ophthalmoplegic migraine) —
    see Migraine, ophthalmoplegic
  syndrome Q87.0
    congenital oculofacial paralysis (with
      other anomalies) Q87.0
    ophthalmoplegic migraine —*see*
      Migraine, ophthalmoplegic
Moeller's glossitis K14.0
Mohr's syndrome (Types I and II) Q87.0
Mola destruens D39.2
Molar pregnancy O02.0
Molarization of premolars K00.2
Molding, head (during birth) - omit code
Mole (pigmented) —*see also* Nevus
  blood O02.0
  Breus' O02.0
  cancerous —*see* Melanoma
  carneous O02.0
  destructive D39.2
  fleshy O02.0
  hydatid, hydatidiform (benign)
    (complicating pregnancy)
    (delivered) (undelivered) O01.9
    classical O01.0
    complete O01.0
    incomplete O01.1
    invasive D39.2
    malignant D39.2
    partial O01.1
  intrauterine O02.0
  invasive (hydatidiform) D39.2
  malignant
    meaning
      malignant hydatidiform mole
      D39.2
      melanoma —*see* Melanoma
  nonhydatidiform O02.0

Mole *(Continued)*
  nonpigmented —*see* Nevus
  pregnancy NEC O02.0
  skin —*see* Nevus
  tubal O00.1
  vesicular —*see* Mole, hydatidiform
Molimen, molimina (menstrual) N94.3
Molluscum contagiosum (epitheliale)
  B08.1
Mönckeberg's arteriosclerosis, disease,
  or sclerosis —*see* Arteriosclerosis,
  extremities
Mondini's malformation (cochlea) Q16.5
Mondor's disease I80.8
Monge's disease T70.29
Monilethrix (congenital) Q84.1
Moniliasis (*see also* Candidiasis) B37.9
  neonatal P37.5
Monitoring (encounter for)
  therapeutic drug level Z51.81
Monkey malaria B53.1
Monkeypox B04
Monoarthritis M13.10
  ankle M13.17-
  elbow M13.12-
  foot joint M13.17-
  hand joint M13.14-
  hip M13.15-
  knee M13.16-
  shoulder M13.11-
  wrist M13.13-
Monoblastic —*see* condition
Monochromat (ism), monochromatopsia
  (acquired) (congenital) H53.51
Monocytic —*see* condition
Monocytopenia D72.818
Monocytosis (symptomatic) D72.821
Monomania —*see* Psychosis
Mononeuritis G58.9
  cranial nerve —*see* Disorder, nerve,
    cranial
  femoral nerve G57.2-
  lateral
    cutaneous nerve of thigh G57.1-
    popliteal nerve G57.3-
  lower limb G57.9-
    specified nerve NEC G57.8-
  medial popliteal nerve G57.4-
  median nerve G56.1-
  multiplex G58.7
  plantar nerve G57.6-
  posterior tibial nerve G57.5-
  radial nerve G56.3-
  sciatic nerve G57.0-
  specified NEC G58.8
  tibial nerve G57.4-
  ulnar nerve G56.2-
  upper limb G56.9-
    specified nerve NEC G56.8-
  vestibular —*see* subcategory H93.3
Mononeuropathy G58.9
  carpal tunnel syndrome —*see*
    Syndrome, carpal tunnel
  diabetic NEC —*see* E08-E13 with .41
  femoral nerve —*see* Lesion, nerve,
    femoral
  ilioinguinal nerve G57.8-
  intercostal G58.0
  lower limb G57.9-
    causalgia —*see* Causalgia, lower
      limb
    femoral nerve —*see* Lesion, nerve,
      femoral
    meralgia paresthetica G57.1-

M

Mononeuropathy *(Continued)*
  lower limb *(Continued)*
    plantar nerve —*see* Lesion, nerve, plantar
    popliteal nerve —*see* Lesion, nerve, popliteal
    sciatic nerve —*see* Lesion, nerve, sciatic
    specified NEC G57.8-
    tarsal tunnel syndrome —*see* Syndrome, tarsal tunnel
   median nerve —*see* Lesion, nerve, median
   multiplex G58.7
   obturator nerve G57.8-
   popliteal nerve —*see* Lesion, nerve, popliteal
   radial nerve —*see* Lesion, nerve, radial
   saphenous nerve G57.8-
   specified NEC G58.8
   tarsal tunnel syndrome —*see* Syndrome, tarsal tunnel
   tuberculous A17.83
   ulnar nerve —*see* Lesion, nerve, ulnar
  upper limb G56.9-
    carpal tunnel syndrome —*see* Syndrome, carpal tunnel
    causalgia —*see* Causalgia
    median nerve —*see* Lesion, nerve, median
    radial nerve —*see* Lesion, nerve, radial
    specified site NEC G56.8-
    ulnar nerve —*see* Lesion, nerve, ulnar
Mononucleosis, infectious B27.90
  with
   complication NEC B27.99
   meningitis B27.92
   polyneuropathy B27.91
  cytomegaloviral B27.10
   with
    complication NEC B27.19
    meningitis B27.12
    polyneuropathy B27.11
  Epstein-Barr (virus) B27.00
   with
    complication NEC B27.09
    meningitis B27.02
    polyneuropathy B27.01
  gammaherpesviral B27.00
   with
    complication NEC B27.09
    meningitis B27.02
    polyneuropathy B27.01
  specified NEC B27.80
   with
    complication NEC B27.89
    meningitis B27.82
    polyneuropathy B27.81
Monoplegia G83.3-
  congenital (cerebral) G80.8
   spastic G80.1
  embolic (current episode) I63.4
  following
   cerebrovascular disease
    cerebral infarction
     lower limb I69.34-
     upper limb I69.33-
    intracerebral hemorrhage
     lower limb I69.14-
     upper limb I69.13-
     lower limb I69.94-

Monoplegia *(Continued)*
  following *(Continued)*
   cerebrovascular disease *(Continued)*
    nontraumatic intracranial hemorrhage NEC
     lower limb I69.24-
     upper limb I69.23-
    specified disease NEC
     lower limb I69.84-
     upper limb I69.83-
    stroke NOS
     lower limb I69.34-
     upper limb I69.33-
    subarachnoid hemorrhage
     lower limb I69.04-
     upper limb I69.03-
    upper limb I69.93-
  hysterical (transient) F44.4
  lower limb G83.1-
  psychogenic (conversion reaction) F44.4
  thrombotic (current episode) I63.3
  transient R29.818
  upper limb G83.2-
Monorchism, monorchidism Q55.0
Monosomy *(see also* Deletion, chromosome) Q93.9
  specified NEC Q93.89
  whole chromosome
   meiotic nondisjunction Q93.0
   mitotic nondisjunction Q93.1
   mosaicism Q93.1
  X Q96.9
Monster, monstrosity (single) Q89.7
  acephalic Q00.0
  twin Q89.4
Monteggia's fracture (-dislocation) S52.27-
Mooren's ulcer (cornea) —*see* Ulcer, cornea, Mooren's
Moore's syndrome —*see* Epilepsy, specified NEC
Mooser-Neill reaction A75.2
Mooser's bodies A75.2
Morbidity not stated or unknown R69
Morbilli —*see* Measles
Morbus —*see also* Disease
  angelicus, anglorum E55.0
  Beigel B36.2
  caducus —*see* Epilepsy
  celiacus K90.0
  comitialis —*see* Epilepsy
  cordis *(see also* Disease, heart) I51.9
   valvulorum —*see* Endocarditis
  coxae senilis M16.9
   tuberculous A18.02
  hemorrhagicus neonatorum P53
  maculosus neonatorum P54.5
Morel (-Stewart)(-Morgagni) **syndrome** M85.2
Morel-Kraepelin disease —*see* Schizophrenia
Morel-Moore syndrome M85.2
Morgagni's
  cyst, organ, hydatid, or appendage
   female Q50.5
   male (epididymal) Q55.4
    testicular Q55.29
  syndrome M85.2
Morgagni-Stewart-Morel syndrome M85.2
Morgagni-Stokes-Adams syndrome I45.9
Morgagni-Turner (-Albright) **syndrome** Q96.9

Moria F07.0
Moron (I.Q. 50-69) F70
Morphea L94.0
Morphinism (without remission) F11.20
  with remission F11.21
Morphinomania (without remission) F11.20
  with remission F11.21
Morquio (-Ullrich)(-Brailsford) **disease or syndrome** —*see* Mucopolysaccharidosis
Mortification (dry) (moist) —*see* Gangrene
Morton's metatarsalgia (neuralgia) (neuroma) (syndrome) G57.6
Morvan's disease or syndrome G60.8
Mosaicism, mosaic (autosomal) (chromosomal)
  45,X/46,XX Q96.3
  45,X/other cell lines NEC with abnormal sex chromosome Q96.4
  sex chromosome
   female Q97.8
   lines with various numbers of X chromosomes Q97.2
   male Q98.7
   XY Q96.3
Moschowitz' disease M31.1
Mother yaw A66.0
Motion sickness (from travel, any vehicle) (from roundabouts or swings) T75.3
Mottled, mottling, teeth (enamel) (endemic) (nonendemic) K00.3
Mounier-Kuhn syndrome Q32.4
  with bronchiectasis J47.9
   exacerbation (acute) J47.1
   lower respiratory infection J47.0
  acquired J98.09
   with bronchiectasis J47.9
    with
     exacerbation (acute) J47.1
     lower respiratory infection J47.0
Mountain
  sickness T70.29
   with polycythemia , acquired (acute) D75.1
  tick fever A93.2
Mouse, joint —*see* Loose, body, joint
  knee M23.4-
Mouth —*see* condition
Movable
  coccyx —*see* subcategory M53.2
  kidney N28.89
   congenital Q63.8
  spleen D73.89
Movements, dystonic R25.8
Moyamoya disease I67.5
MRSA (Methicillin resistant Staphylococcus aureus)
  infection A49.02
   as the cause of diseases classified elsewhere B95.62
  sepsis A41.02
MSSA (Methicillin susceptible Staphylococcus aureus)
  infection A49.01
   as the cause of diseases classified elsewhere B95.61
  sepsis A41.01
Mucha-Habermann disease L41.0
Mucinosis (cutaneous) (focal) (papular) (skin) L98.5
  oral K13.79

Mucocele
  appendix K38.8
  buccal cavity K13.79
  gallbladder K82.1
  lacrimal sac, chronic H04.43-
  nasal sinus J34.1
  nose J34.1
  salivary gland (any) K11.6
  sinus (accessory) (nasal) J34.1
  turbinate (bone) (middle) (nasal)
    J34.1
  uterus N85.8
Mucolipidosis
  I E77.1
  II, III E77.0
  IV E75.11
Mucopolysaccharidosis E76.3
  beta-gluduronidase deficiency
    E76.29
  cardiopathy E76.3 [I52]
  Hunter's syndrome E76.1
  Hurler's syndrome E76.01
  Hurler-Scheie syndrome E76.02
  Maroteaux-Lamy syndrome E76.29
  Morquio syndrome E76.219
    A E76.210
    B E76.211
    classic E76.210
  Sanfilippo syndrome E76.22
  Scheie's syndrome E76.03
  specified NEC E76.29
  type
    I
      Hurler's syndrome E76.01
      Hurler-Scheie syndrome E76.02
      Scheie's syndrome E76.03
    II E76.1
    III E76.22
    IV E76.219
    IVA E76.210
    IVB E76.211
    VI E76.29
    VII E76.29
Mucormycosis B46.5
  cutaneous B46.3
  disseminated B46.4
  gastrointestinal B46.2
  generalized B46.4
  pulmonary B46.0
  rhinocerebral B46.1
  skin B46.3
  subcutaneous B46.3
Mucositis (ulcerative) K12.30
  due to drugs NEC K12.32
  gastrointestinal K92.81
  mouth (oral) (oropharyngeal) K12.30
    due to antineoplastic therapy
      K12.31
    due to drugs NEC K12.32
    due to radiation K12.33
    specified NEC K12.39
    viral K12.39
  nasal J34.81
  oral cavity —see Mucositis, mouth
  oral soft tissues —see Mucositis,
    mouth
  vagina and vulva N76.81
Mucositis necroticans agranulocytica —
  see Agranulocytosis
Mucous —see also condition
  patches (syphilitic) A51.39
    congenital A50.07
Mucoviscidosis E84.9
  with meconium obstruction E84.11

Mucus
  asphyxia or suffocation —see Asphyxia,
    mucus
  in stool R19.5
  plug —see Asphyxia, mucus
Muguet B37.0
Mulberry molars (congenital syphilis)
  A50.52
Müllerian mixed tumor
  specified site —see Neoplasm,
    malignant, by site
  unspecified site C54.9
Multicystic kidney (development)
  Q61.4
Multiparity (grand) Z64.1
  affecting management of pregnancy,
    labor and delivery (supervision
    only) O09.4-
  requiring contraceptive management —
    see Contraception
Multipartita placenta O43.19-
Multiple, multiplex —see also condition
  digits (congenital) Q69.9
  endocrine neoplasia —see Neoplasia,
    endocrine, multiple [MEN}
  personality F44.81
Mumps B26.9
  arthritis B26.85
  complication NEC B26.89
  encephalitis B26.2
  hepatitis B26.81
  meningitis (aseptic) B26.1
  meningoencephalitis B26.2
  myocarditis B26.82
  oophoritis B26.89
  orchitis B26.0
  pancreatitis B26.3
  polyneuropathy B26.84
Mumu (see also Infestation, filarial) B74.9
  [N51]
Münchhausen's syndrome —see Disorder,
  factitious
Münchmeyer's syndrome —see Myositis,
  ossificans, progressiva
Mural —see condition
Murmur (cardiac) (heart) (organic)
    R01.1
  abdominal R19.15
  aortic (valve) —see Endocarditis,
    aortic
  benign R01.0
  diastolic —see Endocarditis
  Flint I35.1
  functional R01.0
  Graham Steell I37.1
  innocent R01.0
  mitral (valve) —see Insufficiency, mitral
  nonorganic R01.0
  presystolic, mitral —see Insufficiency,
    mitral
  pulmonic (valve) I37.8
  systolic (valvular) —see Endocarditis
  tricuspid (valve) I07.9
  valvular —see Endocarditis
Murri's disease (intermittent
  hemoglobinuria) D59.6
Muscle, muscular —see also condition
  carnitine (palmityltransferase)
    deficiency E71.314
Musculoneuralgia —see Neuralgia
Mushroom-workers' (pickers') disease or
  lung J67.5
Mushrooming hip —see Derangement,
  joint, specified NEC, hip

Mutation (s)
  factor V Leiden D68.51
  surfactant, of lung J84.83
  prothrombin gene D68.52
Mutism —see also Aphasia
  deaf (acquired) (congenital) NEC
    H91.3
  elective (adjustment reaction)
    (childhood) F94.0
  hysterical F44.4
  selective (childhood) F94.0
MVD (microvillus inclusion disease)
  Q43.8
MVID (microvillus inclusion disease)
  Q43.8
Myalgia M79.1
  epidemic (cervical) B33.0
  traumatic NEC T14.8
Myasthenia G70.9
  congenital G70.2
  cordis —see Failure, heart
  developmental G70.2
  gravis G70.00
    with exacerbation (acute) G70.01
    in crisis G70.01
    neonatal, transient P94.0
    pseudoparalytica G70.00
      with exacerbation (acute) G70.01
      in crisis G70.01
  stomach, psychogenic F45.8
  syndrome
    in
      diabetes mellitus —see E08-E13
        with .44
      neoplastic disease (see also
        Neoplasm) D49.9 [G73.3]
      pernicious anemia D51.0 [G73.3]
      thyrotoxicosis E05.90 [G73.3]
        with thyroid storm E05.91
          [G73.3]
Myasthenic M62.81
Mycelium infection B49
Mycetismus —see Poisoning, food,
  noxious, mushroom
Mycetoma B47.9
  actinomycotic B47.1
  bone (mycotic) B47.9 [M90.80]
  eumycotic B47.0
  foot B47.9
    actinomycotic B47.1
    mycotic B47.0
  madurae NEC B47.9
    mycotic B47.0
  maduromycotic B47.0
  mycotic B47.0
  nocardial B47.1
Mycobacteriosis —see Mycobacterium
Mycobacterium, mycobacterial
    (infection) A31.9
  anonymous A31.9
  atypical A31.9
    cutaneous A31.1
    pulmonary A31.0
      tuberculous —see Tuberculosis,
        pulmonary
    specified site NEC A31.8
  avium (intracellulare complex) A31.0
  balnei A31.1
  Battey A31.0
  chelonei A31.8
  cutaneous A31.1
  extrapulmonary systemic A31.8
  fortuitum A31.8
  intracellulare (Battey bacillus) A31.0

Mycobacterium, mycobacterial
    (Continued)
    kakaferifu A31.8
    kansasii (yellow bacillus) A31.0
    kasongo A31.8
    leprae *(see also* Leprosy) A30.9
    luciflavum A31.1
    marinum (M. balnei) A31.1
    nonspecific —*see* Mycobacterium,
        atypical
    pulmonary (atypical) A31.0
        tuberculous —*see* Tuberculosis,
            pulmonary
    scrofulaceum A31.8
    simiae A31.8
    systemic, extrapulmonary A31.8
    szulgai A31.8
    terrae A31.8
    triviale A31.8
    tuberculosis (human, bovine) —*see*
        Tuberculosis
    ulcerans A31.1
    xenopi A31.8
Mycoplasma (M.) pneumoniae, as cause
        of disease classified elsewhere
        B96.0
Mycosis, mycotic B49
    cutaneous NEC B36.9
    ear B36.8
    fungoides (extranodal) (solid organ)
        C84.0-
    mouth B37.0
    nails B35.1
    opportunistic B48.8
    skin NEC B36.9
    specified NEC B48.8
    stomatitis B37.0
    vagina, vaginitis (candidal) B37.3
Mydriasis (pupil) H57.04
Myelatelia Q06.1
Myelinolysis, pontine, central G37.2
Myelitis (acute) (ascending) (childhood)
        (chronic) (descending) (diffuse)
        (disseminated) (idiopathic) (pressure)
        (progressive) (spinal cord) (subacute)
        (see also Encephalitis) G04.91
    herpes simplex B00.82
    herpes zoster B02.24
    in diseases classified elsewhere
        G05.4
    necrotizing, subacute G37.4
    optic neuritis in G36.0
    postchickenpox B01.12
    postherpetic B02.24
    postimmunization G04.89
    postinfectious NEC G04.89
    postvaccinal G04.89
    specified NEC G04.89
    syphilitic (transverse) A52.14
    toxic G92
    transverse (in demyelinating diseases
        of central nervous system) G37.3
    tuberculous A17.82
    varicella B01.12
Myeloblastic —*see* condition
Myeloblastoma
    granular cell —*see also* Neoplasm,
        connective tissue
    malignant —*see* Neoplasm,
        connective tissue, malignant
    tongue D10.1
Myelocele —*see* Spina bifida
Myelocystocele —*see* Spina bifida
Myelocytic —*see* condition

Myelodysplasia D46.9
    specified NEC D46.Z
    spinal cord (congenital) Q06.1
Myelodysplastic syndrome D46.9
    with
        5q deletion D46.C
        isolated del (5q) chromosomal
            abnormality C46.C
    specified NEC D46.Z
Myeloencephalitis —*see* Encephalitis
Myelofibrosis D75.81
    with myeloid metaplasia D47.4
    acute C94.4-
    idiopathic (chronic) D47.4
    primary D47.1
    secondary D75.81
        in myeloproliferative disease D47.4
Myelogenous —*see* condition
Myeloid —*see* condition
Myelokathexis D70.9
Myeloleukodystrophy E75.29
Myelolipoma —*see* Lipoma
Myeloma (multiple) C90.0-
    monostotic C90.3
        plasma cell C90.0-
    plasma cell C90.0-
    solitary *(see also* Plasmacytoma, solitary)
        C90.3-
Myelomalacia G95.89
Myelomatosis C90.0-
Myelomeningitis —*see*
        Meningoencephalitis
Myelomeningocele (spinal cord) —*see*
        Spina bifida
Myelo-osteo-musculodysplasia
        hereditaria Q79.8
Myelopathic
    anemia D64.89
    muscle atrophy —*see* Atrophy, muscle,
        spinal
    pain syndrome G89.0
Myelopathy (spinal cord) G95.9
    drug-induced G95.89
    in (due to)
        degeneration or displacement,
            intervertebral disc NEC —*see*
            Disorder, disc, with,
            myelopathy
        infection —*see* Encephalitis
        intervertebral disc disorder —*see also*
            Disorder, disc, with, myelopathy
        mercury —*see* subcategory T56.1
        neoplastic disease *(see also* Neoplasm)
            D49.9 *[G99.2]*
        pernicious anemia D51.0 *[G99.2]*
        spondylosis —*see* Spondylosis, with
            myelopathy NEC
    necrotic (subacute) (vascular) G95.19
    radiation-induced G95.89
    spondylogenic NEC —*see* Spondylosis,
        with myelopathy NEC
    toxic G95.89
    transverse, acute G37.3
    vascular G95.19
    vitamin B12 E53.8 *[G32.0]*
Myelophthisis D61.82
Myeloradiculitis G04.91
Myeloradiculodysplasia (spinal) Q06.1
Myelosarcoma C92.3-
Myelosclerosis D75.89
    with myeloid metaplasia D47.4
    disseminated, of nervous system G35
    megakaryocytic D47.4
        with myeloid metaplasia D47.4

Myelosis
    acute C92.0-
    aleukemic C92.9-
    chronic D47.1
    erythremic (acute) C94.0-
    megakaryocytic C94.2-
    nonleukemic D72.828
    subacute C92.9-
Myiasis (cavernous) B87.9
    aural B87.4
    creeping B87.0
    cutaneous B87.0
    dermal B87.0
    ear (external) (middle) B87.4
    eye B87.2
    genitourinary B87.81
    intestinal B87.82
    laryngeal B87.3
    nasopharyngeal B87.3
    ocular B87.2
    orbit B87.2
    skin B87.0
    specified site NEC B87.89
    traumatic B87.1
    wound B87.1
Myoadenoma, prostate —*see*
        Hyperplasia, prostate
Myoblastoma
    granular cell —*see also* Neoplasm,
        connective tissue, benign
    malignant —*see* Neoplasm,
        connective tissue, malignant
    tongue D10.1
Myocardial —*see* condition
Myocardiopathy (congestive)
        (constrictive) (familial) (hypertrophic
        nonobstructive) (idiopathic)
        (infiltrative) (obstructive) (primary)
        (restrictive) (sporadic) *(see also*
        Cardiomyopathy) I42.9
    alcoholic I42.6
    cobalt-beer I42.6
    glycogen storage E74.02 *[I43]*
    hypertrophic obstructive I42.1
    in (due to)
        beriberi E51.12
        cardiac glycogenosis E74.02 *[I43]*
        Friedreich's ataxia G11.1 *[I43]*
        myotonia atrophica G71.19 *[I43]*
        progressive muscular dystrophy
            G71.0 *[I43]*
    obscure (African) I42.8
    secondary I42.9
    thyrotoxic E05.90 *[I43]*
        with storm E05.91 *[I43]*
    toxic NEC I42.7
Myocarditis (with arteriosclerosis)
        (chronic)(fibroid) (interstitial) (old)
        (progressive) (senile) I51.4
    with
        rheumatic fever (conditions in I00)
            I09.0
            active —*see* Myocarditis, acute,
                rheumatic
            inactive or quiescent (with chorea)
                I09.0
    active I40.9
        rheumatic I01.2
            with chorea (acute) (rheumatic)
                (Sydenham's) I02.0
    acute or subacute (interstitial) I40.9
        due to
            streptococcus (beta-hemolytic)
                I01.2

M

Myocarditis (Continued)
  acute or subacute (Continued)
    idiopathic I40.1
    rheumatic I01.2
      with chorea (acute) (rheumatic)
        (Sydenham's) I02.0
    specified NEC I40.8
  aseptic of newborn B33.22
  bacterial (acute) I40.0
  Coxsackie (virus) B33.22
  diphtheritic A36.81
  eosinophilic I40.1
  epidemic of newborn (Coxsackie)
    B33.22
  Fiedler's (acute) (isolated) I40.1
  giant cell (acute) (subacute) I40.1
  gonococcal A54.83
  granulomatous (idiopathic) (isolated)
    (nonspecific) I40.1
  hypertensive —see Hypertension, heart
  idiopathic (granulomatous) I40.1
  in (due to)
    diphtheria A36.81
    epidemic louse-borne typhus A75.0
      [I41]
    Lyme disease A69.29
    sarcoidosis D86.85
    scarlet fever A38.1
    toxoplasmosis (acquired) B58.81
    typhoid A01.02
    typhus NEC A75.9 [I41]
  infective I40.0
  influenzal —see Influenza, with,
    myocarditis
  isolated (acute) I40.1
  meningococcal A39.52
  mumps B26.82
  nonrheumatic, active I40.9
  parenchymatous I40.9
  pneumococcal I40.0
  rheumatic (chronic) (inactive) (with
    chorea) I09.0
    active or acute I01.2
      with chorea (acute) (rheumatic)
        (Sydenham's) I02.0
  rheumatoid —see Rheumatoid, carditis
  septic I40.0
  staphylococcal I40.0
  suppurative I40.0
  syphilitic (chronic) A52.06
  toxic I40.8
    rheumatic —see Myocarditis, acute,
      rheumatic
  tuberculous A18.84
  typhoid A01.02
  valvular —see Endocarditis
  virus, viral I40.0
    of newborn (Coxsackie) B33.22
Myocardium, myocardial —see condition
Myocardosis —see Cardiomyopathy
Myoclonus, myoclonic, myoclonia
    (familial) (essential) (multifocal)
    (simplex) G25.3
  drug-induced G25.3
  epilepsy (see also Epilepsy, generalized,
    specified NEC) G40.4-
    familial (progressive) G25.3
  epileptica G40.409
    with status epilepticus G40.401
  facial G51.3
  familial progressive G25.3
  Friedreich's G25.3
  jerks G25.3
  massive G25.3

Myoclonus, myoclonic, myoclonia
    (Continued)
  palatal G25.3
  pharyngeal G25.3
Myocytolysis I51.5
Myodiastasis —see Diastasis, muscle
Myoendocarditis —see Endocarditis
Myoepithelioma —see Neoplasm, benign,
    by site
Myofasciitis (acute) —see Myositis
Myofibroma —see also Neoplasm,
    connective tissue, benign
  uterus (cervix) (corpus) —see
    Leiomyoma
Myofibromatosis D48.1
  infantile Q89.8
Myofibrosis M62.89
  heart —see Myocarditis
  scapulohumeral —see Lesion, shoulder,
    specified NEC
Myofibrositis M79.7
  scapulohumeral —see Lesion, shoulder,
    specified NEC
Myoglobulinuria, myoglobinuria
    (primary) R82.1
Myokymia, facial G51.4
Myolipoma —see Lipoma
Myoma —see also Neoplasm, connective
    tissue, benign
  malignant —see Neoplasm, connective
    tissue, malignant
  prostate D29.1
  uterus (cervix) (corpus) —see
    Leiomyoma
Myomalacia M62.89
Myometritis —see Endometritis
Myometrium —see condition
Myonecrosis, clostridial A48.0
Myopathy G72.9
  acute
    necrotizing G72.81
      quadriplegic G72.81
  alcoholic G72.1
  benign congenital G71.2
  central core G71.2
  centronuclear G71.2
  congenital (benign) G71.2
  critical illness G72.81
  distal G71.0
  drug-induced G72.0
  endocrine NEC E34.9 [G73.7]
  extraocular muscles H05.82-
  facioscapulohumeral G71.0
  hereditary G71.9
    specified NEC G71.8
  immune NEC G72.49
  in (due to)
    Addison's disease E27.1 [G73.7]
    alcohol G72.1
    amyloidosis E85.0 [G73.7]
    cretinism E00.9 [G73.7]
    Cushing's syndrome E24.9 [G73.7]
    drugs G72.0
    endocrine disease NEC E34.9 [G73.7]
    giant cell arteritis M31.6 [G73.7]
    glycogen storage disease E74.00
      [G73.7]
    hyperadrenocorticism E24.9 [G73.7]
    hyperparathyroidism NEC E21.3
      [G73.7]
    hypoparathyroidism E20.9 [G73.7]
    hypopituitarism E23.0 [G73.7]
    hypothyroidism E03.9 [G73.7]
    infectious disease NEC B99 [G73.7]

Myopathy (Continued)
  in (Continued)
    lipid storage disease E75.6 [G73.7]
    metabolic disease NEC E88.9 [G73.7]
    myxedema E03.9 [G73.7]
    parasitic disease NEC B89 [G73.7]
    polyarteritis nodosa M30.0 [G73.7]
    rheumatoid arthritis —see
      Rheumatoid, myopathy
    sarcoidosis D86.87
    scleroderma M34.82
    sicca syndrome M35.03
    Sjögren's syndrome M35.03
    systemic lupus erythematosus
      M32.19
    thyrotoxicosis (hyperthyroidism)
      E05.90 [G73.7]
      with thyroid storm E05.91 [G73.7]
    toxic agent NEC G72.2
  inflammatory NEC G72.49
  intensive care (ICU) G72.81
  limb-girdle G71.0
  mitochondrial NEC G71.3
  myotubular G71.2
  mytonic, proximal (PROMM) G71.11
  nemaline G71.2
  ocular G71.0
  oculopharyngeal G71.0
  of critical illness G72.81
  primary G71.9
    specified NEC G71.8
  progressive NEC G72.89
  proximal myotonic (PROMM)
    G71.11
  rod G71.2
  scapulohumeral G71.0
  specified NEC G72.89
  toxic G72.2
Myopericarditis —see also Pericarditis
  chronic rheumatic I09.2
Myopia (axial) (congenital) H52.1-
  degenerative (malignant) H44.2-
  malignant H44.2-
  pernicious H44.2-
  progressive high (degenerative)
    H44.2-
Myosarcoma —see Neoplasm, connective
    tissue, malignant
Myosis (pupil) H57.03
  stromal (endolymphatic) D39.0
Myositis M60.9
  clostridial A48.0
  due to posture —see Myositis, specified
    type NEC
  epidemic B33.0
  fibrosa or fibrous (chronic), Volkmann's
    T79.6
  foreign body granuloma —see
    Granuloma, foreign body
  in (due to)
    bilharziasis B65.9 [M63.8-]
    cysticercosis B69.81
    leprosy A30.9 [M63.8-]
    mycosis B49 [M63.8-]
    sarcoidosis D86.87
    schistosomiasis B65.9 [M63.8-]
    syphilis
      late A52.78
      secondary A51.49
    toxoplasmosis (acquired)
      B58.82
    trichinellosis B75 [M63.8-]
    tuberculosis A18.09
  inclusion body [IBM] G72.41

Myositis *(Continued)*
  infective M60.009
    arm M60.002
      left M60.001
      right M60.000
    leg M60.005
      left M60.004
      right M60.003
    lower limb M60.005
      ankle M60.07-
      foot M60.07-
      lower leg M60.06-
      thigh M60.05-
      toe M60.07-
    multiple sites M60.09
    specified site NEC M60.08
    upper limb M60.002
      finger M60.04-
      forearm M60.03-
      hand M60.04-
      shoulder region M60.01-
      upper arm M60.02-
  interstitial M60.10
    ankle M60.17-
    foot M60.17-
    forearm M60.13-
    hand M60.14-
    lower leg M60.16-
    multiple sites M60.19
    shoulder region M60.11-
    specified site NEC M60.18
    thigh M60.15-
    upper arm M60.12-
  mycotic B49 [M63.8-]
  ossificans or ossifying (circumscripta) —
    see also Ossification, muscle,
    specified NEC
    in (due to)
      burns M61.30
        ankle M61.37-
        foot M61.37-
        forearm M61.33-
        hand M61.34-
        lower leg M61.36-
        multiple sites M61.39
        pelvic region M61.35-
        shoulder region M61.31-
        specified site NEC M61.38
        thigh M61.35-
        upper arm M61.32-
      quadriplegia or paraplegia M61.20
        ankle M61.27-
        foot M61.27-
        forearm M61.23-
        hand M61.24-

Myositis *(Continued)*
  ossificans or ossifying *(Continued)*
    in *(Continued)*
      quadriplegia or paraplegia
        (Continued)
        lower leg M61.26-
        multiple sites M61.29
        pelvic region M61.25-
        shoulder region M61.21-
        specified site NEC M61.28
        thigh M61.25-
        upper arm M61.22-
    progressiva M61.10
      ankle M61.17-
      finger M61.14-
      foot M61.17-
      forearm M61.13-
      hand M61.14-
      lower leg M61.16-
      multiple sites M61.19
      pelvic region M61.15-
      shoulder region M61.11-
      specified site NEC M61.18
      thigh M61.15-
      toe M61.17-
      upper arm M61.12-
    traumatica M61.00
      ankle M61.07-
      foot M61.07-
      forearm M61.03-
      hand M61.04-
      lower leg M61.06-
      multiple sites M61.09
      pelvic region M61.05-
      shoulder region M61.01-
      specified site NEC M61.08
      thigh M61.05-
      upper arm M61.02-
  purulent —*see* Myositis, infective
  specified type NEC M60.80
    ankle M60.87-
    foot M60.87-
    forearm M60.83-
    hand M60.84-
    lower leg M60.86-
    multiple sites M60.89
    pelvic region M60.85-
    shoulder region M60.81-
    specified site NEC M60.88
    thigh M60.85-
    upper arm M60.82-
  suppurative —*see* Myositis, infective
  traumatic (old) —*see* Myositis, specified
    type NEC
Myospasia impulsiva F95.2

Myotonia (acquisita) (intermittens)
  M62.89
  atrophica G71.11
  chondrodystrophic G71.13
  congenita (acetazolamide responsive)
    (dominant) (recessive) G71.12
  drug-induced G71.14
  dystrophica G71.11
  fluctuans G71.19
  levior G71.12
  permanens G71.19
  symptomatic G71.19
Myotonic pupil —*see* Anomaly, pupil,
  function, tonic pupil
Myriapodiasis B88.2
Myringitis H73.2-
  with otitis media —*see* Otitis, media
  acute H73.00-
    bullous H73.01-
    specified NEC H73.09-
  bullous —*see* Myringitis, acute, bullous
  chronic H73.1-
Mysophobia F40.228
Mytilotoxism —*see* Poisoning, fish
Myxadenitis labialis K13.0
Myxedema (adult) (idiocy) (infantile)
  (juvenile) (*see also* Hypothyroidism)
  E03.9
  circumscribed E05.90
    with storm E05.91
  coma E03.5
  congenital E00.1
  cutis L98.5
  localized (pretibial) E05.90
    with storm E05.91
  papular L98.5
Myxochondrosarcoma —*see* Neoplasm,
  cartilage, malignant
Myxofibroma —*see* Neoplasm, connective
  tissue, benign
  odontogenic —*see* Cyst, calcifying
    odontogenic
Myxofibrosarcoma —*see* Neoplasm,
  connective tissue, malignant
Myxolipoma D17.9
Myxoliposarcoma —*see* Neoplasm,
  connective tissue, malignant
Myxoma —*see also* Neoplasm, connective
  tissue, benign
  nerve sheath —*see* Neoplasm, nerve,
    benign
  odontogenic —*see* Cyst, calcifying
    odontogenic
Myxosarcoma —*see* Neoplasm, connective
  tissue, malignant

N

Naegeli's
  disease Q82.8
  leukemia, monocytic C93.1-
Naegleriasis (with meningoencephalitis)
  B60.2
Naffziger's syndrome G54.0
Naga sore —see Ulcer, skin
Nägele's pelvis M95.5
  with disproportion (fetopelvic) O33.0
    causing obstructed labor O65.0
Nail —see also condition
  biting F98.8
  patella syndrome Q87.2
Nanism, nanosomia —see Dwarfism
Nanophyetiasis B66.8
Nanukayami A27.89
Napkin rash L22
Narcolepsy G47.419
  with cataplexy G47.411
  in conditions classified elsewhere
    G47.429
    with cataplexy G47.421
Narcosis R06.89
Narcotism —see Dependence
NARP (Neuropathy, Ataxia and Retinitis
    pigmentosa) syndrome E88.49
Narrow
  anterior chamber angle H40.03-
  pelvis —see Contraction, pelvis
Narrowing —see also Stenosis
  artery I77.1
    auditory, internal I65.8
    basilar —see Occlusion, artery,
      basilar
    carotid —see Occlusion, artery,
      carotid
    cerebellar —see Occlusion, artery,
      cerebellar
    cerebral —see Occlusion artery,
      cerebral
    choroidal —see Occlusion, artery,
      cerebral, specified NEC
    communicating posterior —see
      Occlusion, artery, cerebral,
      specified NEC
    coronary —see also Disease, heart,
      ischemic, atherosclerotic
      congenital Q24.5
      syphilitic A50.54 [I52]
      due to syphilis NEC A52.06
    hypophyseal —see Occlusion, artery,
      cerebral, specified NEC
    pontine —see Occlusion, artery,
      cerebral, specified NEC
    precerebral —see Occlusion, artery,
      precerebral
    vertebral —see Occlusion, artery,
      vertebral
  auditory canal (external) —see Stenosis,
    external ear canal
  eustachian tube —see Obstruction,
    eustachian tube
  eyelid —see Disorder, eyelid function
  larynx J38.6
  mesenteric artery K55.0
  palate M26.89
  palpebral fissure —see Disorder, eyelid
    function
  ureter N13.5
    with infection N13.6
  urethra —see Stricture, urethra
Narrowness, abnormal, eyelid Q10.3

Nasal —see condition
Nasolachrymal, nasolacrimal —see
  condition
Nasopharyngeal —see also condition
  pituitary gland Q89.2
  torticollis M43.6
Nasopharyngitis (acute) (infective)
  (streptococcal) (subacute) J00
  chronic (suppurative) (ulcerative) J31.1
Nasopharynx, nasopharyngeal —see
  condition
Natal tooth, teeth K00.6
Nausea (without vomiting) R11.0
  with vomiting R11.2
    gravidarum —see Hyperemesis,
      gravidarum
    marina T75.3
    navalis T75.3
Navel —see condition
Neapolitan fever —see Brucellosis
Near drowning T75.1
Nearsightedness —see Myopia
Near-syncope R55
Nebula, cornea —see Opacity, cornea
Necator americanus infestation
  B76.1
Necatoriasis B76.1
Neck —see condition
Necrobiosis R68.89
  lipoidica NEC L92.1
    with diabetes —see E08-E13 with .620
Necrolysis, toxic epidermal L51.2
  due to drug
    correct substance properly
      administered —see Table of
        drugs and chemicals, by drug,
        adverse effect
    overdose or wrong substance
      given or taken —see Table of
        drugs and chemicals, by drug,
        poisoning
Necrophilia F65.89
Necrosis, necrotic (ischemic) —see also
    Gangrene
  adrenal (capsule) (gland) E27.49
  amputation stump (surgical) (late)
    T87.50
    arm T87.5-
    leg T87.5-
  antrum J32.0
  aorta (hyaline) —see also Aneurysm,
    aorta
    cystic medial —see Dissection, aorta
  artery I77.5
  bladder (aseptic) (sphincter) N32.89
  bone (see also Osteonecrosis) M87.9
    aseptic or avascular —see
      Osteonecrosis
    idiopathic M87.00
    ethmoid J32.2
    jaw M27.2
    tuberculous —see Tuberculosis, bone
  brain I67.89
  breast (aseptic) (fat) (segmental) N64.1
  bronchus J98.09
  central nervous system NEC I67.89
  cerebellar I67.89
  cerebral I67.89
  colon K55.0
  cornea H18.40
  cortical (acute) (renal) N17.1
  cystic medial (aorta) —see Dissection,
    aorta
  dental pulp K04.1

Necrosis, necrotic (Continued)
  esophagus K22.8
  ethmoid (bone) J32.2
  eyelid —see Disorder, eyelid,
    degenerative
  fat, fatty (generalized) —see also
      Disorder, soft tissue, specified type
      NEC
    abdominal wall K65.4
    breast (aseptic) (segmental) N64.1
    localized —see Degeneration, by site,
      fatty
    mesentery K65.4
    omentum K65.4
    pancreas K86.8
    peritoneum K65.4
    skin (subcutaneous), newborn P83.0
    subcutaneous, due to birth injury
      P15.6
  gallbladder —see Cholecystitis, acute
  heart —see Infarct, myocardium
  hip, aseptic or avascular —see
    Osteonecrosis, by type, femur
  intestine (acute) (hemorrhagic)
    (massive) K55.0
  jaw M27.2
  kidney (bilateral) N28.0
    acute N17.9
    cortical (acute) (bilateral) N17.1
      with ectopic or molar pregnancy
        O08.4
    medullary (bilateral) (in acute renal
      failure) (papillary) N17.2
    papillary (bilateral) (in acute renal
      failure) N17.2
    tubular N17.0
      with ectopic or molar pregnancy
        O08.4
      complicating
        abortion —see Abortion, by type,
          complicated by, tubular
          necrosis
        ectopic or molar pregnancy
          O08.4
        pregnancy —see Pregnancy,
          complicated by, diseases
          of, specified type or system
          NEC
      following ectopic or molar
        pregnancy O08.4
      traumatic T79.5
  larynx J38.7
  liver (with hepatic failure) (cell) —see
    Failure, hepatic
    hemorrhagic, central K76.2
  lung J85.0
  lymphatic gland —see Lymphadenitis,
    acute
  mammary gland (fat) (segmental) N64.1
  mastoid (chronic) —see Mastoiditis,
    chronic
  medullary (acute) (renal) N17.2
  mesentery K55.0
    fat K65.4
  mitral valve —see Insufficiency, mitral
  myocardium, myocardial —see Infarct,
    myocardium
  nose J34.0
  omentum (with mesenteric infarction)
    K55.0
    fat K65.4
  orbit, orbital —see Osteomyelitis, orbit
  ossicles, ear —see Abnormal, ear
    ossicles

Necrosis, necrotic (*Continued*)
  ovary N70.92
  pancreas (aseptic) (duct) (fat) K86.8
    acute (infective) —*see* Pancreatitis,
      acute
    infective —*see* Pancreatitis, acute
  papillary (acute) (renal) N17.2
  perineum N90.89
  peritoneum (with mesenteric infarction)
      K55.0
    fat K65.4
  pharynx J02.9
    in granulocytopenia —*see*
      Neutropenia
    Vincent's A69.1
  phosphorus —*see* subcategory T54.2
  pituitary (gland) (postpartum)
      (Sheehan) E23.0
  pressure —*see* Ulcer, pressure, by site
  pulmonary J85.0
  pulp (dental) K04.1
  radiation —*see* Necrosis, by site
  radium —*see* Necrosis, by site
  renal —*see* Necrosis, kidney
  sclera H15.89
  scrotum N50.8
  skin or subcutaneous tissue NEC I96
  spine, spinal (column) —*see also*
      Osteonecrosis, by type, vertebra
    cord G95.19
  spleen D73.5
  stomach K31.89
  stomatitis (ulcerative) A69.0
  subcutaneous fat, newborn P83.8
  subendocardial (acute) I21.4
    chronic I25.89
  suprarenal (capsule) (gland) E27.49
  testis N50.8
  thymus (gland) E32.8
  tonsil J35.8
  trachea J39.8
  tuberculous NEC —*see* Tuberculosis
  tubular (acute) (anoxic) (renal) (toxic)
      N17.0
    postprocedural N99.0
  vagina N89.8
  vertebra —*see also* Osteonecrosis, by
      type, vertebra
    tuberculous A18.01
  vulva N90.89
  X-ray —*see* Necrosis, by site
Necrospermia —*see* Infertility, male
Need (for)
  care provider because (of)
    assistance with personal care
      Z74.1
    continuous supervision required
      Z74.3
    impaired mobility Z74.09
    no other household member able to
      render care Z74.2
    specified reason NEC Z74.8
  immunization —*see* Vaccination
  vaccination —*see* Vaccination
Neglect
  adult
    confirmed T74.01
    history of Z91.412
    suspected T76.01
  child (childhood)
    confirmed T74.02
    history of Z62.812
    suspected T76.02
  emotional, in childhood Z62.898

Neglect (*Continued*)
  hemispatial R41.4
  left-sided R41.4
  sensory R41.4
  visuospatial R41.4
Neisserian infection NEC —*see*
    Gonococcus
Nelaton's syndrome G60.8
Nelson's syndrome E24.1
Nematodiasis (intestinal) B82.0
  Ancylostoma B76.0
Neonatal —*see also* Newborn
  acne L70.4
  bradycardia P29.12
  screening, abnormal findings on P09
  tachycardia P29.11
  tooth, teeth K00.6
Neonatorum —*see* condition
Neoplasia
  endocrine, multiple (MEN) E31.20
    type I E31.21
    type IIA E31.22
    type IIB E31.23
  intraepithelial (histologically confirmed)
    anal (AIN) (histologically confirmed)
      K62.82
      grade I K62.82
      grade II K62.82
      severe D01.3
    cervical glandular (histologically
      confirmed) D06.9
    cervix (uteri) (CIN) (histologically
      confirmed) N87.9
      glandular D06.9
      grade I N87.0
      grade II N87.1
      grade III (severe dysplasia) —*see
        also* Carcinoma, cervix uteri,
        in situ D06.9
    prostate (histologically confirmed)
      (PIN I) (PIN II) N42.3
      grade I N42.3
      grade II N42.3
      severe D07.5
    vagina (histologically confirmed)
      (VAIN) N89.3
      grade I N89.0
      grade II N89.1
      grade III (severe dysplasia) D07.2
    vulva (histologically confirmed)
      (VIN) N90.3
      grade I N90.0
      grade II N90.1
      grade III (severe dysplasia) D07.1
Neoplasm, neoplastic —*see also* Table of
    Neoplasms
  lipomatous, benign —*see* Lipoma
Neovascularization
  ciliary body —*see* Disorder, iris, vascular
  cornea H16.40-
    deep H16.44-
    ghost vessels —*see* Ghost, vessels
    localized H16.43-
    pannus —*see* Pannus
  iris —*see* Disorder, iris, vascular
  retina H35.05-
Nephralgia N23
Nephritis, nephritic (albuminuric)
    (azotemic) (congenital) (disseminated)
    (epithelial) (familial) (focal)
    (granulomatous) (hemorrhagic)
    (infantile) (nonsuppurative, excretory)
    (uremic) N05.9
  with
    dense deposit disease N05.6

Nephritis, nephritic (*Continued*)
  with (*Continued*)
    diffuse
      crescentic glomerulonephritis N05.7
      endocapillary proliferative
        glomerulonephritis N05.4
      membranous glomerulonephritis
        N05.2
      mesangial proliferative
        glomerulonephritis N05.3
      mesangiocapillary
        glomerulonephritis N05.5
    edema —*see* Nephrosis
    focal and segmental glomerular
      lesions N05.1
    foot process disease N04.9
    glomerular lesion
      diffuse sclerosing N05.8
      hypocomplementemic —
        see Nephritis,
        membranoproliferative
      IgA —*see* Nephropathy, IgA
      lobular, lobulonodular —
        see Nephritis,
        membranoproliferative
      nodular —*see* Nephritis,
        membranoproliferative
    lesion of
      glomerulonephritis, proliferative
        N05.8
      renal necrosis N05.9
    minor glomerular abnormality
      N05.0
    specified morphological changes
      NEC N05.8
  acute N00.9
    with
      dense deposit disease N00.6
      diffuse
        crescentic glomerulonephritis
          N00.7
        endocapillary proliferative
          glomerulonephritis N00.4
        membranous glomerulonephritis
          N00.2
        mesangial proliferative
          glomerulonephritis N00.3
        mesangiocapillary
          glomerulonephritis N00.5
      focal and segmental glomerular
        lesions N00.1
      minor glomerular abnormality
        N00.0
      specified morphological changes
        NEC N00.8
  amyloid E85.4 [N08]
  antiglomerular basement membrane
      (anti-GBM) antibody NEC
    in Goodpasture's syndrome M31.0
  antitubular basement membrane
      (tubulo-interstitial) NEC N12
  toxic —*see* Nephropathy, toxic
  arteriolar —*see* Hypertension, kidney
  arteriosclerotic —*see* Hypertension,
      kidney
  ascending —*see* Nephritis,
      tubulo-interstitial
  atrophic N03.9
  Balkan (endemic) N15.0
  calculous, calculus —*see* Calculus,
      kidney
  cardiac —*see* Hypertension, kidney
  cardiovascular —*see* Hypertension,
      kidney

Nephritis, nephritic (Continued)
chronic N03.9
  with
    dense deposit disease N03.6
    diffuse
      crescentic glomerulonephritis
        N03.7
      endocapillary proliferative
        glomerulonephritis N03.4
      membranous glomerulonephritis
        N03.2
      mesangial proliferative
        glomerulonephritis N03.3
      mesangiocapillary
        glomerulonephritis N03.5
    focal and segmental glomerular
      lesions N03.1
    minor glomerular abnormality
      N03.0
    specified morphological changes
      NEC N03.8
arteriosclerotic —see Hypertension,
  kidney
cirrhotic N26.9
complicating pregnancy O26.83-
croupous N00.9
degenerative —see Nephrosis
diffuse sclerosing N05.8
due to
  diabetes mellitus —see E08-E13 with
    .21
  subacute bacterial endocarditis
    I33.0
  systemic lupus erythematosus
    (chronic) M32.14
  typhoid fever A01.09
gonococcal (acute) (chronic) A54.21
hypocomplementemic —see Nephritis,
  membranoproliferative
IgA —see Nephropathy, IgA
immune complex (circulating) NEC
  N05.8
infective —see Nephritis,
  tubulo-interstitial
interstitial —see Nephritis,
  tubulo-interstitial
lead N14.3
membranoproliferative (diffuse) (type 1
  or 3) (see also N00-N07 with fourth
  character .5) N05.5
  type 2 (see also N00-N07 with fourth
    character .6) N05.6
minimal change N05.0
necrotic, necrotizing NEC (see also
  N00-N07 with fourth character .8)
  N05.8
nephrotic —see Nephrosis
nodular —see Nephritis,
  membranoproliferative
polycystic Q61.3
  adult type Q61.2
  autosomal
    dominant Q61.2
    recessive NEC Q61.19
  childhood type NEC Q61.19
  infantile type NEC Q61.19
poststreptococcal N05.9
  acute N00.9
  chronic N03.9
  rapidly progressive N01.9
proliferative NEC (see also N00-N07
  with fourth character .8) N05.8
purulent —see Nephritis,
  tubulo-interstitial

Nephritis, nephritic (Continued)
rapidly progressive N01.9
  with
    dense deposit disease N01.6
    diffuse
      crescentic glomerulonephritis
        N01.7
      endocapillary proliferative
        glomerulonephritis N01.4
      membranous glomerulonephritis
        N01.2
      mesangial proliferative
        glomerulonephritis N01.3
      mesangiocapillary
        glomerulonephritis N01.5
    focal and segmental glomerular
      lesions N01.1
    minor glomerular abnormality
      N01.0
    specified morphological changes
      NEC N01.8
salt losing or wasting NEC N28.89
saturnine N14.3
sclerosing, diffuse N05.8
septic —see Nephritis, tubulo-interstitial
specified pathology NEC (see also
  N00-N07 with fourth character .8)
  N05.8
subacute N01.9
suppurative —see Nephritis,
  tubulo-interstitial
syphilitic (late) A52.75
  congenital A50.59 [N08]
  early (secondary) A51.44
toxic —see Nephropathy, toxic
tubal, tubular —see Nephritis,
  tubulo-interstitial
tuberculous A18.11
tubulo-interstitial (in) N12
  acute (infectious) N10
  chronic (infectious) N11.9
    nonobstructive N11.8
      reflux-associated N11.0
    obstructive N11.1
    specified NEC N11.8
  due to
    brucellosis A23.9 [N16]
    cryoglobulinemia D89.1 [N16]
    glycogen storage disease E74.00
      [N16]
    Sjögren's syndrome M35.04
  vascular —see Hypertension, kidney
  war N00.9
Nephroblastoma (epithelial)
  (mesenchymal) C64-
Nephrocalcinosis E83.59 [N29]
Nephrocystitis, pustular —see Nephritis,
  tubulo-interstitial
Nephrolithiasis (congenital) (pelvis)
  (recurrent) —see also Calculus,
  kidney
Nephroma C64-
  mesoblastic D41.0-
Nephronephritis —see Nephrosis
Nephronophthisis Q61.5
Nephropathia epidemica A98.5
Nephropathy (see also Nephritis) N28.9
  with
    edema —see Nephrosis
    glomerular lesion —see
      Glomerulonephritis
  amyloid, hereditary E85.0
  analgesic N14.0
    with medullary necrosis, acute N17.2

Nephropathy (Continued)
Balkan (endemic) N15.0
chemical —see Nephropathy, toxic
diabetic —see E08-E13 with .21
drug-induced N14.2
  specified NEC N14.1
focal and segmental hyalinosis or
  sclerosis N02.1
heavy metal-induced N14.3
hereditary NEC N07.9
  with
    dense deposit disease N07.6
    diffuse
      crescentic glomerulonephritis
        N07.7
      endocapillary proliferative
        glomerulonephritis N07.4
      membranous glomerulonephritis
        N07.2
      mesangial proliferative
        glomerulonephritis N07.3
      mesangiocapillary
        glomerulonephritis N07.5
    focal and segmental glomerular
      lesions N07.1
    minor glomerular abnormality N07.0
    specified morphological changes
      NEC N07.8
hypercalcemic N25.89
hypertensive —see Hypertension,
  kidney
hypokalemic (vacuolar) N25.89
IgA N02.8
  with glomerular lesion N02.9
    focal and segmental hyalinosis or
      sclerosis N02.1
    membranoproliferative (diffuse)
      N02.5
    membranous (diffuse) N02.2
    mesangial proliferative (diffuse)
      N02.3
    mesangiocapillary (diffuse)
      N02.5
    proliferative NEC N02.8
    specified pathology NEC N02.8
lead N14.3
membranoproliferative (diffuse)
  N02.5
membranous (diffuse) N02.2
mesangial (IgA/IgG) —see
  Nephropathy, IgA
  proliferative (diffuse) N02.3
mesangiocapillary (diffuse) N02.5
obstructive N13.8
phenacetin N17.2
phosphate-losing N25.0
potassium depletion N25.89
pregnancy-related O26.83-
proliferative NEC (see also N00-N07
  with fourth character .8) N05.8
protein-losing N25.89
saturnine N14.3
sickle-cell D57.- [N08]
toxic NEC N14.4
  due to
    drugs N14.2
      analgesic N14.0
      specified NEC N14.1
    heavy metals N14.3
vasomotor N17.0
water-losing N25.89
Nephroptosis N28.83
Nephropyosis —see Abscess, kidney
Nephrorrhagia N28.89

Nephrosclerosis (arteriolar)
(arteriosclerotic) (chronic)
(hyaline) —see also Hypertension,
kidney
hyperplastic —see Hypertension,
kidney
senile N26.9
Nephrosis, nephrotic (Epstein's)
(syndrome) (congenital) N04.9
with
foot process disease N04.9
glomerular lesion N04.1
hypocomplementemic N04.5
acute N04.9
anoxic —see Nephrosis, tubular
chemical —see Nephrosis, tubular
cholemic K76.7
diabetic —see E08-E13 with .21
Finnish type (congenital) Q89.8
hemoglobin N10
hemoglobinuric —see Nephrosis,
tubular
in
amyloidosis E85.4 [N08]
diabetes mellitus —see E08-E13 with
.21
epidemic hemorrhagic fever A98.5
malaria (malariae) B52.0
ischemic —see Nephrosis, tubular
lipoid N04.9
lower nephron —see Nephrosis,
tubular
malarial (malariae) B52.0
minimal change N04.0
myoglobin N10
necrotizing —see Nephrosis, tubular
osmotic (sucrose) N25.89
radiation N04.9
syphilitic (late) A52.75
toxic —see Nephrosis, tubular
tubular (acute) N17.0
postprocedural N99.0
radiation N04.9
Nephrosonephritis, hemorrhagic
(endemic) A98.5
Nephrostomy
attention to Z43.6
status Z93.6
Nerve —see also condition
injury —see Injury, nerve, by body
site
Nerves R45.0
Nervous (see also condition) R45.0
heart F45.8
stomach F45.8
tension R45.0
Nervousness R45.0
Nesidioblastoma
pancreas D13.7
specified site NEC —see Neoplasm,
benign, by site
unspecified site D13.7
Nettleship's syndrome Q82.2
Neumann's disease or syndrome
L10.1
Neuralgia, neuralgic (acute) M79.2
accessory (nerve) G52.8
acoustic (nerve) —see subcategory
H93.3
auditory (nerve) —see subcategory
H93.3
ciliary G44.009
intractable G44.001
not intractable G44.009

Neuralgia, neuralgic (Continued)
cranial
nerve —see also Disorder, nerve,
cranial
fifth or trigeminal —see Neuralgia,
trigeminal
postherpetic, postzoster B02.29
ear —see subcategory H92.0
facialis vera G51.1
Fothergill's —see Neuralgia, trigeminal
glossopharyngeal (nerve) G52.1
Horton's G44.099
intractable G44.091
not intractable G44.099
Hunt's B02.21
hypoglossal (nerve) G52.3
infraorbital —see Neuralgia, trigeminal
malarial —see Malaria
migrainous G44.009
intractable G44.001
not intractable G44.009
Morton's G57.6-
nerve, cranial —see Disorder, nerve,
cranial
nose G52.0
occipital M54.81
olfactory G52.0
penis N48.9
perineum R10.2
postherpetic NEC B02.29
trigeminal B02.22
pubic region R10.2
scrotum R10.2
Sluder's G44.89
specified nerve NEC G58.8
spermatic cord R10.2
sphenopalatine (ganglion) G90.09
trifacial —see Neuralgia, trigeminal
trigeminal G50.0
postherpetic, postzoster B02.22
vagus (nerve) G52.2
writer's F48.8
organic G25.89
Neurapraxia —see Injury, nerve
Neurasthenia F48.8
cardiac F45.8
gastric F45.8
heart F45.8
Neurilemmoma —see also Neoplasm,
nerve, benign
acoustic (nerve) D33.3
malignant —see also Neoplasm, nerve,
malignant
acoustic (nerve) C72.4
Neurilemmosarcoma —see Neoplasm,
nerve, malignant
Neurinoma —see Neoplasm, nerve,
benign
Neurinomatosis —see Neoplasm, nerve,
uncertain behavior
Neuritis (rheumatoid) M79.2
abducens (nerve) —see Strabismus,
paralytic, sixth nerve
accessory (nerve) G52.8
acoustic (nerve) (see also subcategory)
H93.3
in (due to)
infectious disease NEC B99
[H94.0-]
parasitic disease NEC B89 [H94.0-]
syphilitic A52.15
alcoholic G62.1
with psychosis —see Psychosis,
alcoholic

Neuritis (Continued)
amyloid, any site E85.4 [G63]
auditory (nerve) —see subcategory
H93.3
brachial —see Radiculopathy
due to displacement, intervertebral
disc —see Disorder, disc,
cervical, with neuritis
cranial nerve
due to Lyme disease A69.22
eighth or acoustic or auditory —see
subcategory H93.3
eleventh or accessory G52.8
fifth or trigeminal G51.0
first or olfactory G52.0
fourth or trochlear —see Strabismus,
paralytic, fourth nerve
second or optic —see Neuritis,
optic
seventh or facial G51.8
newborn (birth injury) P11.3
sixth or abducent —see Strabismus,
paralytic, sixth nerve
tenth or vagus G52.2
third or oculomotor —see Strabismus,
paralytic, third nerve
twelfth or hypoglossal G52.3
Déjérine-Sottas G60.0
diabetic (mononeuropathy) —see
E08-E13 with .41
polyneuropathy —see E08-E13 with .42
due to
beriberi E51.11
displacement, prolapse or rupture,
intervertebral disc —see
Disorder, disc, with,
radiculopathy
herniation, nucleus pulposus M51.9
[G55]
endemic E51.11
facial G51.8
newborn (birth injury) P11.3
general —see Polyneuropathy
geniculate ganglion G51.1
due to herpes (zoster) B02.21
gouty M10.00 [G63]
hypoglossal (nerve) G52.3
ilioinguinal (nerve) G57.9-
infectious (multiple) NEC G61.0
interstitial hypertrophic progressive
G60.0
lumbar M54.16
lumbosacral M54.17
multiple —see also Polyneuropathy
endemic E51.11
infective, acute G61.0
multiplex endemica E51.11
nerve root —see Radiculopathy
oculomotor (nerve) —see Strabismus,
paralytic, third nerve
olfactory nerve G52.0
optic (nerve) (hereditary) (sympathetic)
H46.9
with demyelination G36.0
in myelitis G36.0
nutritional H46.2
papillitis —see Papillitis, optic
retrobulbar H46.1-
specified type NEC H46.8
toxic H46.3
peripheral (nerve) G62.9
multiple —see Polyneuropathy
single —see Mononeuritis
pneumogastric (nerve) G52.2

Neuritis (Continued)
  postherpetic, postzoster B02.29
  progressive hypertrophic interstitial
      G60.0
  retrobulbar —see also Neuritis, optic,
      retrobulbar
    in (due to)
      late syphilis A52.15
      meningococcal infection A39.82
      meningococcal A39.82
      syphilitic A52.15
  sciatic (nerve) —see also Sciatica
    due to displacement of intervertebral
        disc —see Disorder, disc, with,
        radiculopathy
  serum (see also Reaction, serum) T80.69
  shoulder-girdle G54.5
  specified nerve NEC G58.8
  spinal (nerve) root —see Radiculopathy
  syphilitic A52.15
  thenar (median) G56.1-
  thoracic M54.14
  toxic NEC G62.2
  trochlear (nerve) —see Strabismus,
      paralytic, fourth nerve
  vagus (nerve) G52.2
Neuroastrocytoma —see Neoplasm,
    uncertain behavior, by site
Neuroavitaminosis E56.9 [G99.8]
Neuroblastoma
  olfactory C30.0
  specified site —see Neoplasm,
      malignant, by site
  unspecified site C74.90
Neurochorioretinitis —see Chorioretinitis
Neurocirculatory asthenia F45.8
Neurocysticercosis B69.0
Neurocytoma —see Neoplasm, benign,
    by site
Neurodermatitis (circumscribed)
    (circumscripta) (local) L28.0
  atopic L20.81
  diffuse (Brocq) L20.81
  disseminated L20.81
Neuroencephalomyelopathy, optic G36.0
Neuroepithelioma —see also Neoplasm,
    malignant, by site
  olfactory C30.0
Neurofibroma —see also Neoplasm, nerve,
    benign
  melanotic —see Neoplasm, nerve, benign
  multiple —see Neurofibromatosis
  plexiform —see Neoplasm, nerve,
      benign
Neurofibromatosis (multiple)
    (nonmalignant) Q85.00
  acoustic Q85.02
  malignant —see Neoplasm, nerve,
      malignant
  specified NEC Q85.09
  type 1 (von Recklinghausen) Q85.01
  type 2 Q85.02
Neurofibrosarcoma —see Neoplasm,
    nerve, malignant
Neurogenic —see also condition
  bladder (see also Dysfunction, bladder,
      neuromuscular) N31.9
    cauda equina syndrome G83.4
  bowel NEC K59.2
  heart F45.8
Neuroglioma —see Neoplasm, uncertain
    behavior, by site
Neurolabyrinthitis (of Dix and
    Hallpike) —see Neuronitis, vestibular

Neurolathyrism —see Poisoning, food,
    noxious, plant
Neuroleprosy A30.9
Neuroma —see also Neoplasm, nerve,
    benign
  acoustic (nerve) D33.3
  amputation (stump) (traumatic)
      (surgical complication) (late)
      T87.3-
    arm T87.3-
    leg T87.3-
  digital (toe) G57.6-
  interdigital (toe) G58.8
    lower limb G57.8-
    upper limb G56.8-
  intermetatarsal G57.8-
  Morton's G57.6-
  nonneoplastic
    arm G56.9-
    leg G57.9-
    lower extremity G57.9-
    upper extremity G56.9-
  optic (nerve) D33.3
  plantar G57.6-
  plexiform —see Neoplasm, nerve,
      benign
  surgical (nonneoplastic)
    arm G56.9-
    leg G57.9-
    lower extremity G57.9-
    upper extremity G56.9-
Neuromyalgia —see Neuralgia
Neuromyasthenia (epidemic)
    (postinfectious) G93.3
Neuromyelitis G36.9
  ascending G61.0
  optica G36.0
Neuromyopathy G70.9
  paraneoplastic D49.9 [G13.0]
Neuromyotonia (Isaacs) G71.19
Neuronevus —see Nevus
Neuronitis G58.9
  ascending (acute) G57.2-
  vestibular H81.2-
Neuroparalytic —see condition
Neuropathy, neuropathic G62.9
  acute motor G62.81
  alcoholic G62.1
    with psychosis —see Psychosis,
        alcoholic
  arm G56.9-
  autonomic, peripheral —see
      Neuropathy, peripheral,
      autonomic
  axillary G56.9-
  bladder N31.9
    atonic (motor) (sensory) N31.2
    autonomous N31.2
    flaccid N31.2
    nonreflex N31.2
    reflex N31.1
    uninhibited N31.0
  brachial plexus G54.0
  cervical plexus G54.2
  chronic
    progressive segmentally
        demyelinating G62.89
    relapsing demyelinating G62.89
  Déjérine-Sottas G60.0
  diabetic —see E08-E13 with .40
    mononeuropathy —see E08-E13 with
        .41
    polyneuropathy —see E08-E13 with
        .42

Neuropathy, neuropathic (Continued)
  entrapment G58.9
    iliohypogastric nerve G57.8-
    ilioinguinal nerve G57.8-
    lateral cutaneous nerve of thigh G57.1-
    median nerve G56.0-
    obturator nerve G57.8-
    peroneal nerve G57.3-
    posterior tibial nerve G57.5-
    saphenous nerve G57.8-
    ulnar nerve G56.2-
  facial nerve G51.9
  hereditary G60.9
    motor and sensory (types I-IV) G60.0
    sensory G60.8
    specified NEC G60.8
  hypertrophic G60.0
    Charcot-Marie-Tooth G60.0
    Déjérine-Sottas G60.0
    interstitial progressive G60.0
    of infancy G60.0
    Refsum G60.1
  idiopathic G60.9
    progressive G60.3
    specified NEC G60.8
  in association with hereditary ataxia
      G60.2
  intercostal G58.0
  ischemic —see Disorder, nerve
  Jamaica (ginger) G62.2
  leg NEC G57.9-
  lower extremity G57.9-
  lumbar plexus G54.1
  median nerve G56.1-
  motor and sensory —see also
      Polyneuropathy
    hereditary (types I-IV) G60.0
  multiple (acute) (chronic) —see
      Polyneuropathy
  optic (nerve) —see also Neuritis, optic
    ischemic H47.01-
  paraneoplastic (sensorial) (Denny
      Brown) D49.9 [G13.0]
  peripheral (nerve) (see also
      Polyneuropathy) G62.9
    autonomic G90.9
      idiopathic G90.09
      in (due to)
        amyloidosis E85.4 [G99.0]
        diabetes mellitus —see E08-E13
            with .43
        endocrine disease NEC E34.9
            [G99.0]
        gout M10.00 [G99.0]
        hyperthyroidism E05.90
            [G99.0]
          with thyroid storm E05.91
              [G99.0]
        metabolic disease NEC E88.9
            [G99.0]
    idiopathic G60.9
      progressive G60.3
    in (due to)
      antitetanus serum G62.0
      arsenic G62.2
      drugs NEC G62.0
      lead G62.2
      organophosphate compounds G62.2
      toxic agent NEC G62.2
  plantar nerves G57.6-
  progressive
    hypertrophic interstitial G60.0
    inflammatory G62.81
  radicular NEC —see Radiculopathy

Neuropathy, neuropathic *(Continued)*
  sacral plexus G54.1
  sciatic G57.0-
  serum G61.1
  toxic NEC G62.2
  trigeminal sensory G50.8
  ulnar nerve G56.2-
  uremic N18.9 *[G63]*
  vitamin B12 E53.8 *[G63]*
    with anemia (pernicious) D51.0 *[G63]*
      due to dietary deficiency D51.3
        [G63]
Neurophthisis —*see also* Disorder, nerve
  peripheral, diabetic —*see* E08-E13 with
    .42
Neuroretinitis —*see* Chorioretinitis
Neuroretinopathy, hereditary optic
  H47.22
Neurosarcoma —*see* Neoplasm, nerve,
  malignant
Neurosclerosis —*see* Disorder, nerve
Neurosis, neurotic F48.9
  anankastic F42
  anxiety (state) F41.1
    panic type F41.0
  asthenic F48.8
  bladder F45.8
  cardiac (reflex) F45.8
  cardiovascular F45.8
  character F60.9
  colon F45.8
  compensation F68.1
  compulsive, compulsion F42
  conversion F44.9
  craft F48.8
  cutaneous F45.8
  depersonalization F48.1
  depressive (reaction) (type) F34.1
  environmental F48.8
  excoriation L98.1
  fatigue F48.8
  functional —*see* Disorder, somatoform
  gastric F45.8
  gastrointestinal F45.8
  heart F45.8
  hypochondriacal F45.21
  hysterical F44.9
  incoordination F45.8
    larynx F45.8
    vocal cord F45.8
  intestine F45.8
  larynx (sensory) F45.8
    hysterical F44.4
  mixed NEC F48.8
  musculoskeletal F45.8
  obsessional F42
  obsessive-compulsive F42
  occupational F48.8
  ocular NEC F45.8
  organ —*see* Disorder, somatoform
  pharynx F45.8
  phobic F40.9
  posttraumatic (situational) F43.10
    acute F43.11
    chronic F43.12
  psychasthenic (type) F48.8
  railroad F48.8
  rectum F45.8
  respiratory F45.8
  rumination F45.8
  sexual F65.9
  situational F48.8
  social F40.10
    generalized F40.11

Neurosis, neurotic *(Continued)*
  specified type NEC F48.8
  state F48.9
    with depersonalization episode
      F48.1
  stomach F45.8
  traumatic F43.10
    acute F43.11
    chronic F43.12
  vasomotor F45.8
  visceral F45.8
  war F48.8
Neurospongioblastosis diffusa Q85.1
Neurosyphilis (arrested) (early) (gumma)
  (late) (latent) (recurrent) (relapse)
  A52.3
  with ataxia (cerebellar) (locomotor)
    (spastic) (spinal) A52.19
  aneurysm (cerebral) A52.05
  arachnoid (adhesive) A52.13
  arteritis (any artery) (cerebral) A52.04
  asymptomatic A52.2
  congenital A50.40
  dura (mater) A52.13
  general paresis A52.17
  hemorrhagic A52.05
  juvenile (asymptomatic) (meningeal)
    A50.40
  leptomeninges (aseptic) A52.13
  meningeal, meninges (adhesive) A52.13
  meningitis A52.13
  meningovascular (diffuse) A52.13
  optic atrophy A52.15
  parenchymatous (degenerative) A52.19
  paresis, paretic A52.17
    juvenile A50.45
  remission in (sustained) A52.3
  serological (without symptoms) A52.2
  specified nature or site NEC A52.19
  tabes, tabetic (dorsalis) A52.11
    juvenile A50.45
  taboparesis A52.17
    juvenile A50.45
  thrombosis (cerebral) A52.05
  vascular (cerebral) NEC A52.05
Neurothekeoma —*see* Neoplasm, nerve,
  benign
Neurotic —*see* Neurosis
Neurotoxemia —*see* Toxemia
Neutroclusion M26.211
Neutropenia, neutropenic (chronic)
  (genetic) (idiopathic) (immune)
  (infantile) (malignant) (pernicious)
  (splenic) D70.9
  congenital (primary) D70.0
  cyclic D70.4
  cytoreductive cancer chemotherapy
    sequela D70.1
  drug-induced D70.2
    due to cytoreductive cancer
      chemotherapy D70.1
  due to infection D70.3
  fever D70.9
  neonatal, transitory (isoimmune)
    (maternal transfer) P61.5
  periodic D70.4
  secondary (cyclic) (periodic) (splenic)
    D70.4
    drug-induced D70.2
      due to cytoreductive cancer
        chemotherapy D70.1
  toxic D70.8
Neutrophilia, hereditary giant D72.0
Nevocarcinoma —*see* Melanoma

Nevus D22.9
  achromic —*see* Neoplasm, skin, benign
  amelanotic —*see* Neoplasm, skin,
    benign
  angiomatous D18.00
    intra-abdominal D18.03
    intracranial D18.02
    skin D18.01
    specified site NEC D18.09
  araneus I78.1
  balloon cell —*see* Neoplasm, skin,
    benign
  bathing trunk D48.5
  blue —*see* Neoplasm, skin, benign
    cellular —*see* Neoplasm, skin, benign
    giant —*see* Neoplasm, skin, benign
    Jadassohn's —*see* Neoplasm, skin,
      benign
    malignant —*see* Melanoma
  capillary D18.00
    intra-abdominal D18.03
    intracranial D18.02
    skin D18.01
    specified site NEC D18.09
  cavernous D18.00
    intra-abdominal D18.03
    intracranial D18.02
    skin D18.01
    specified site NEC D18.09
  cellular —*see* Neoplasm, skin, benign
    blue —*see* Neoplasm, skin, benign
  choroid D31.3-
  comedonicus Q82.5
  conjunctiva D31.0-
  dermal —*see* Neoplasm, skin, benign
    with epidermal nevus —*see*
      Neoplasm, skin, benign
  dysplastic —*see* Neoplasm, skin, benign
  eye D31.9-
  flammeus Q82.5
  hemangiomatous D18.00
    intra-abdominal D18.03
    intracranial D18.02
    skin D18.01
    specified site NEC D18.09
  iris D31.4-
  lacrimal gland D31.5-
  lymphatic D18.1
  magnocellular
    specified site —*see* Neoplasm, benign,
      by site
    unspecified site D31.40
  malignant —*see* Melanoma
  meaning hemangioma D18.00
    intra-abdominal D18.03
    intracranial D18.02
    skin D18.01
    specified site NEC D18.09
  mouth (mucosa) D10.30
    specified site NEC D10.39
    white sponge Q38.6
  multiplex Q85.1
  non-neoplastic I78.1
  oral mucosa D10.30
    specified site NEC D10.39
    white sponge Q38.6
  orbit D31.6-
  pigmented
    giant (*see also* Neoplasm, skin,
      uncertain behavior) D48.5
    malignant melanoma in —*see*
      Melanoma
  portwine Q82.5
  retina D31.2-

Nevus *(Continued)*
retrobulbar D31.6-
sanguineous Q82.5
senile I78.1
skin D22.9
    abdominal wall D22.5
    ala nasi D22.39
    ankle D22.7-
    anus, anal D22.5
    arm D22.6-
    auditory canal (external) D22.2-
    auricle (ear) D22.2-
    auricular canal (external) D22.2-
    axilla, axillary fold D22.5
    back D22.5
    breast D22.5
    brow D22.39
    buttock D22.5
    canthus (eye) D22.1-
    cheek (external) D22.39
    chest wall D22.5
    chin D22.39
    ear (external) D22.2-
    external meatus (ear) D22.2-
    eyebrow D22.39
    eyelid (lower) (upper) D22.1-
    face D22.30
        specified NEC D22.39
    female genital organ (external) NEC
        D28.0
    finger D22.6-
    flank D22.5
    foot D22.7-
    forearm D22.6-
    forehead D22.39
    foreskin D29.0
    genital organ (external) NEC
        female D28.0
        male D29.9
    gluteal region D22.5
    groin D22.5
    hand D22.6-
    heel D22.7-
    helix D22.2-
    hip D22.7-
    interscapular region D22.5
    jaw D22.39
    knee D22.7-
    labium (majus) (minus) D28.0
    leg D22.7-
    lip (lower) (upper) D22.0
    lower limb D22.7-
    male genital organ (external) D29.9
    nail D22.9
        finger D22.6-
        toe D22.7-
    nasolabial groove D22.39
    nates D22.5
    neck D22.4
    nose (external) D22.39
    palpebra D22.1-
    penis D29.0
    perianal skin D22.5
    perineum D22.5
    pinna D22.2-
    popliteal fossa or space D22.7-
    prepuce D29.0
    pudendum D28.0
    scalp D22.4
    scrotum D29.4
    shoulder D22.6-
    submammary fold D22.5
    temple D22.39
    thigh D22.7-

Nevus *(Continued)*
skin *(Continued)*
    toe D22.7-
    trunk NEC D22.5
    umbilicus D22.5
    upper limb D22.6-
    vulva D28.0
specified site NEC —*see* Neoplasm,
    benign, by site
spider I78.1
stellar I78.1
strawberry Q82.5
Sutton's —*see* Neoplasm, skin, benign
unius lateris Q82.5
Unna's Q82.5
vascular Q82.5
verrucous Q82.5
Newborn (infant) (liveborn) (singleton)
    Z38.2
abstinence syndrome P96.1
acne L70.4
affected by (suspected to be)
    abnormalities of membranes P02.9
        specified NEC P02.8
    abruptio placenta P02.1
    amino-acid metabolic disorder,
        transitory P74.8
    amniocentesis (while in utero)
        P00.6
    amnionitis P02.7
    apparent life threatening event
        (ALTE) R68.13
    bleeding (into)
        cerebral cortex P52.22
        germinal matrix P52.0
        ventricles P52.1
    breech delivery P03.0
    cardiac arrest P29.81
    cardiomyopathy I42.8
        congenital I42.4
    cerebral ischemia P91.0
    Cesarean delivery P03.4
    chemotherapy agents P04.1
    chorioamnionitis P02.7
    cocaine (crack) P04.41
    complications of labor and delivery
        P03.9
        specified NEC P03.89
    compression of umbilical cord NEC
        P02.5
    contracted pelvis P03.1
    delivery P03.9
        Cesarean P03.4
        forceps P03.2
        vacuum extractor P03.3
    entanglement (knot) in umbilical cord
        P02.5
    environmental chemicals P04.6
    fetal (intrauterine)
        growth retardation P05.9
        malnutrition not light or small for
            gestational age P05.2
    forceps delivery P03.2
    heart rate abnormalities
        bradycardia P29.12
        intrauterine P03.819
            before onset of labor P03.810
            during labor P03.811
        tachycardia P29.11
    hemorrhage (antepartum) P02.1
        cerebellar (nontraumatic) P52.6
        intracerebral (nontraumatic) P52.4
        intracranial (nontraumatic) P52.9
            specified NEC P52.8

Newborn *(Continued)*
affected by *(Continued)*
    hemorrhage *(Continued)*
        intraventricular (nontraumatic)
            P52.3
            grade 1 P52.0
            grade 2 P52.1
            grade 3 P52.21
            grade 4 P52.22
        posterior fossa (nontraumatic) P52.6
        subarachnoid (nontraumatic) P52.5
        subependymal P52.0
            with intracerebral extension
                P52.22
            with intraventricular extension
                P52.1
                with enlargment of ventricles
                    P52.21
            without intraventricular
                extension P52.0
    hypoxic ischemic encephalopathy
        [HIE] P91.60
        mild P91.61
        moderate P91.62
        severe P91.63
    induction of labor P03.89
    intestinal perforation P78.0
    intrauterine (fetal) blood loss P50.9
        due to (from)
            cut end of co-twin cord P50.5
            hemorrhage into
                co-twin P50.3
                maternal circulation P50.4
            placenta P50.2
            ruptured cord blood P50.1
            vasa previa P50.0
        specified NEC P50.8
    intrauterine (fetal) hemorrhage P50.9
    intrauterine (in utero) procedure
        P96.5
    malpresentation (malposition) NEC
        P03.1
    maternal (complication of) (use of)
        alcohol P04.3
        analgesia (maternal) P04.0
        anesthesia (maternal) P04.0
        blood loss P02.1
        circulatory disease P00.3
        condition P00.9
            specified NEC P00.89
        delivery P03.9
            Cesarean P03.4
            forceps P03.2
            vacuum extractor P03.3
        diabetes mellitus (pre-existing) P70.1
        disorder P00.9
            specified NEC P00.89
        drugs (addictive) (illegal) NEC
            P04.49
        ectopic pregnancy P01.4
        gestational diabetes P70.0
        hemorrhage P02.1
        hypertensive disorder P00.0
        incompetent cervix P01.0
        infectious disease P00.2
        injury P00.5
        labor and delivery P03.9
        malpresentation before labor P01.7
        maternal death P01.6
        medical procedure P00.7
        medication P04.1
        multiple pregnancy P01.5
        nutritional disorder P00.4
        oligohydramnios P01.2

369

Newborn (Continued)
  affected by (Continued)
    maternal (Continued)
      parasitic disease P00.2
      periodontal disease P00.81
      placenta previa P02.0
      polyhydramnios P01.3
      precipitate delivery P03.5
      pregnancy P01.9
        specified P01.8
      premature rupture of membranes
        P01.1
      renal disease P00.1
      respiratory disease P00.3
      surgical procedure P00.6
      urinary tract disease P00.1
      uterine contraction (abnormal)
        P03.6
    meconium peritonitis P78.0
    medication (legal) (maternal use)
      (prescribed) P04.1
    membrane abnormalities P02.9
      specified NEC P02.8
    membranitis P02.7
    methamphetamine (s) P04.49
    mixed metabolic and respiratory
      acidosis P84
    neonatal abstinence syndrome
      P96.1
    noxious substances transmitted
      via placenta or breast milk
      P04.9
      specified NEC P04.8
    nutritional supplements P04.5
    placenta previa P02.0
    placental
      abnormality (functional)
        (morphological) P02.20
        specified NEC P02.29
      dysfunction P02.29
      infarction P02.29
      insufficiency P02.29
      separation NEC P02.1
      transfusion syndromes P02.3
    placentitis P02.7
    precipitate delivery P03.5
    prolapsed cord P02.4
    respiratory arrest P28.81
    slow intrauterine growth P05.9
    tobacco P04.2
    twin to twin transplacental
      transfusion P02.3
    umbilical cord (tightly) around neck
      P02.5
    umbilical cord condition P02.60
      short cord P02.69
      specified NEC P02.69
    uterine contractions (abnormal)
      P03.6
    vasa previa P02.69
      from intrauterine blood loss
      P50.0
  apnea P28.3
    obstructive P28.4
    primary P28.3
    specified P28.4
  born in hospital Z38.00
    by cesarean Z38.01
  born outside hospital Z38.1
  breast buds P96.89
  breast engorgement P83.4
  check-up —see Newborn, examination
  convulsion P90
  dehydration P74.1

Newborn (Continued)
  examination
    8 to 28 days old Z00.111
    under 8 days old Z00.110
  fever P81.9
    environmentally-induced P81.0
  hyperbilirubinemia P59.9
    of prematurity P59.0
  hypernatremia P74.2
  hyponatremia P74.2
  infection P39.9
    candidal P37.5
    specified NEC P39.8
    urinary tract P39.3
  jaundice P59.8
    due to
      breast milk inhibitor P59.3
      hepatocellular damage P59.20
        specified NEC P59.29
      preterm delivery P59.0
    of prematurity P59.0
    specified NEC P59.8
  late metabolic acidosis P74.0
  mastitis P39.0
    infective P39.0
    noninfective P83.4
  multiple born NEC Z38.8
    born in hospital Z38.68
      by cesarean Z38.69
    born outside hospital Z38.7
  omphalitis P38.9
    with mild hemorrhage P38.1
    without hemorrhage P38.9
  post-term P08.21
  prolonged gestation (over 42 completed
    weeks) P08.22
  quadruplet Z38.8
    born in hospital Z38.63
      by cesarean Z38.64
    born outside hospital Z38.7
  quintuplet Z38.8
    born in hospital Z38.65
      by cesarean Z38.66
    born outside hospital Z38.7
  seizure P90
  sepsis (congenital) P36.9
    due to
      anaerobes NEC P36.5
      Escherichia coli P36.4
      Staphylococcus P36.30
        aureus P36.2
        specified NEC P36.39
      Streptococcus P36.10
        group B P36.0
        specified NEC P36.19
      specified NEC P36.8
  triplet Z38.8
    born in hospital Z38.61
      by cesarean Z38.62
    born outside hospital Z38.7
  twin Z38.5
    born in hospital Z38.30
      by cesarean Z38.31
    born outside hospital Z38.4
  vomiting P92.09
    bilious P92.01
  weight check Z00.111
Newcastle conjunctivitis or disease B30.8
Nezelof's syndrome (pure
  alymphocytosis) D81.4
Niacin (amide) deficiency E52
Nicolas (-Durand)-Favre disease A55
Nicotine —see Tobacco
Nicotinic acid deficiency E52

Niemann-Pick disease or syndrome
  E75.249
  specified NEC E75.248
  type
    A E75.240
    B E75.241
    C E75.242
    D E75.243
Night
  blindness —see Blindness, night
  sweats R61
  terrors (child) F51.4
Nightmares (REM sleep type) F51.5
Nipple —see condition
Nisbet's chancre A57
Nishimoto (-Takeuchi) disease I67.5
Nitritoid crisis or reaction —see Crisis,
  nitritoid
Nitrosohemoglobinemia D74.8
Njovera A65
Nocardiosis, nocardiasis A43.9
  cutaneous A43.1
  lung A43.0
  pneumonia A43.0
  pulmonary A43.0
  specified site NEC A43.8
Nocturia R35.1
  psychogenic F45.8
Nocturnal —see condition
Nodal rhythm I49.8
Node (s) —see also Nodule
  Bouchard's (with arthropathy) M15.2
  Haygarth's M15.8
  Heberden's (with arthropathy) M15.1
  larynx J38.7
  lymph —see condition
  milker's B08.03
  Osler's I33.0
  Schmorl's —see Schmorl's disease
  singer's J38.2
  teacher's J38.2
  tuberculous —see Tuberculosis, lymph
    gland
  vocal cord J38.2
Nodule (s), nodular
  actinomycotic —see Actinomycosis
  breast NEC N63
  colloid (cystic), thyroid E04.1
  cutaneous —see Swelling, localized
  endometrial (stromal) D26.1
  Haygarth's M15.8
  inflammatory —see Inflammation
  juxta-articular
    syphilitic A52.77
    yaws A66.7
  larynx J38.7
  lung, solitary (subsegmental branch of
    the bronchial tree) R91.1
    multiple R91.8
  milker's B08.03
  prostate N40.2
    with lower urinary tract symptoms
      (LUTS) N40.3
    without lower urinary tract
      symptoms (LUTS) N40.2
  pulmonary, solitary (subsegmental
    branch of the bronchial tree) R91.1
  retrocardiac R09.89
  rheumatoid M06.30
    ankle M06.37-
    elbow M06.32-
    foot joint M06.37-
    hand joint M06.34-
    hip M06.35-

Nodule (s), nodular (Continued)
  rheumatoid (Continued)
    knee M06.36-
    multiple site M06.39
    shoulder M06.31-
    vertebra M06.38
    wrist M06.33-
  scrotum (inflammatory) N49.2
  singer's J38.2
  solitary, lung (subsegmental branch of
      the bronchial tree) R91.1
    multiple R91.8
  subcutaneous —see Swelling, localized
  teacher's J38.2
  thyroid (cold) (gland) (nontoxic) E04.1
    with thyrotoxicosis E05.20
      with thyroid storm E05.21
    toxic or with hyperthyroidism E05.20
      with thyroid storm E05.21
  vocal cord J38.2
Noma (gangrenous) (hospital) (infective)
    A69.0
  auricle I96
  mouth A69.0
  pudendi N76.89
  vulvae N76.89
Nomad, nomadism Z59.0
Nonautoimmune hemolytic anemia D59.4
  drug-induced D59.2
Nonclosure —see also Imperfect, closure
  ductus arteriosus (Botallo's) Q25.0
  foramen
    botalli Q21.1
    ovale Q21.1
Noncompliance Z91.19
  with
    dialysis Z91.15
    dietary regimen Z91.11
    medical treatment Z91.19
    medication regimen NEC Z91.14
      underdosing (see also Table of drugs
        and chemicals, categories
        T36-T50, with final character
        6) Z91.14
        intentional NEC Z91.128
          due to financial hardship of
            patient Z91.120
        unintentional NEC Z91.138
          due to patient's age related
            debility Z91.130
    renal dialysis Z91.15
Nondescent (congenital) —see also
    Malposition, congenital
  cecum Q43.3
  colon Q43.3

Nondescent (Continued)
  testicle Q53.9
    bilateral Q53.20
      abdominal Q53.21
      perineal Q53.22
    unilateral Q53.10
      abdominal Q53.11
      perineal Q53.12
Nondevelopment
  brain Q02
    part of Q04.3
  heart Q24.8
  organ or site, congenital NEC —see
    Hypoplasia
Nonengagement
  head NEC O32.4
    in labor, causing obstructed labor
      O64.8
Nonexanthematous tick fever A93.2
Nonexpansion, lung (newborn) P28.0
Nonfunctioning
  cystic duct (see also Disease,
    gallbladder) K82.8
  gallbladder (see also Disease,
    gallbladder) K82.8
  kidney N28.9
  labyrinth —see subcategory H83.2
Non-Hodgkin lymphoma NEC —see
    Lymphoma, non-Hodgkin
Nonimplantation, ovum N97.2
Noninsufflation, fallopian tube
    N97.1
Non-ketotic hyperglycinemia E72.51
Nonne-Milroy syndrome Q82.0
Nonovulation N97.0
Nonpatent fallopian tube N97.1
Nonpneumatization, lung NEC P28.0
Nonrotation —see Malrotation
Nonsecretion, urine —see Anuria
Nonunion
  fracture —see Fracture, by site
  organ or site, congenital NEC —see
    Imperfect, closure
  symphysis pubis, congenital Q74.2
Nonvisualization, gallbladder R93.2
Nonvital, nonvitalized tooth K04.99
Non-working side interference M26.56
Noonan's syndrome Q87.1
Normocytic anemia (infectional) due to
    blood loss (chronic) D50.0
  acute D62
Norrie's disease (congenital) Q15.8
North American blastomycosis B40.9
Norwegian itch B86
Nose, nasal —see condition

Nosebleed R04.0
Nose-picking F98.8
Nosomania F45.21
Nosophobia F45.22
Nostalgia F43.20
Notch of iris Q13.2
Notching nose, congenital (tip) Q30.2
Nothnagel's
  syndrome —see Strabismus, paralytic,
    third nerve
  vasomotor acroparesthesia I73.89
Novy's relapsing fever A68.9
  louse-borne A68.0
  tick-borne A68.1
Noxious
  foodstuffs, poisoning by —see
    Poisoning, food, noxious, plant
  substances transmitted through
    placenta or breast milk P04.9
Nucleus pulposus —see condition
Numbness R20.0
Nuns' knee —see Bursitis, prepatellar
Nursemaid's elbow S53.03-
Nutcracker esophagus K22.4
Nutmeg liver K76.1
Nutrient element deficiency E61.9
  specified NEC E61.8
Nutrition deficient or insufficient (see also
    Malnutrition) E46
  due to
    insufficient food T73.0
    lack of
      care (child) T76.02
        adult T76.01
      food T73.0
Nutritional stunting E45
Nyctalopia (night blindness) —see
    Blindness, night
Nycturia R35.1
  psychogenic F45.8
Nymphomania F52.8
Nystagmus H55.00
  benign paroxysmal —see Vertigo,
    benign paroxysmal
  central positional H81.4-
  congenital H55.01
  dissociated H55.04
  latent H55.02
  miners' H55.09
  positional
    benign paroxysmal H81.4-
    central H81.4-
  specified form NEC H55.09
  visual deprivation H55.03

O

Obermeyer's relapsing fever (European)
A68.0
Obesity E66.9
with alveolar hyperventilation
E66.2
adrenal E27.8
complicating
childbirth O99.214
pregnancy O99.21-
puerperium O99.215
constitutional E66.8
dietary counseling and surveillance
Z71.3
drug-induced E66.1
due to
drug E66.1
excess calories E66.09
morbid E66.01
severe E66.01
endocrine E66.8
endogenous E66.8
familial E66.8
glandular E66.8
hypothyroid —see Hypothyroidism
morbid E66.01
with alveolar hypoventilation
E66.2
due to excess calories E66.01
nutritional E66.09
pituitary E23.6
severe E66.01
specified type NEC E66.8
Oblique —see condition
Obliteration
appendix (lumen) K38.8
artery I77.1
bile duct (noncalculous) K83.1
common duct (noncalculous)
K83.1
cystic duct —see Obstruction,
gallbladder
disease, arteriolar I77.1
endometrium N85.8
eye, anterior chamber —see Disorder,
globe, hypotony
fallopian tube N97.1
lymphatic vessel I89.0
due to mastectomy I97.2
organ or site, congenital NEC —see
Atresia, by site
ureter N13.5
with infection N13.6
urethra —see Stricture, urethra
vein I87.8
vestibule (oral) K08.8
Observation (following) (for) (without
need for further medical care)
Z04.9
accident NEC Z04.3
at work Z04.2
transport Z04.1
adverse effect of drug Z03.6
alleged rape or sexual assault (victim),
ruled out
adult Z04.41
child Z04.42
criminal assault Z04.8
development state
adolescent Z00.3
period of rapid growth in childhood
Z00.2
puberty Z00.3

Observation (Continued)
disease, specified NEC Z03.89
following work accident Z04.2
growth and development state —see
Observation, development state
injuries (accidental) NEC —see also
Observation, accident
newborn (for suspected condition,
ruled out) —see Newborn, affected
by (suspected to be), maternal
(complication of) (use of)
postpartum
immediately after delivery Z39.0
routine follow-up Z39.2
pregnancy (normal) (without
complication) Z34.9-
high risk O09.9-
suicide attempt, alleged NEC Z03.89
self-poisoning Z03.6
suspected, ruled out —see also
Suspected condition, ruled out
abuse, physical
adult Z04.71
child Z04.72
accident at work Z04.2
adult battering victim Z04.71
child battering victim Z04.72
condition NEC Z03.89
newborn —see Newborn, affected
by (suspected to be), maternal
(complication of) (use of)
drug poisoning or adverse effect
Z03.6
exposure (to)
anthrax Z03.810
biological agent NEC Z03.818
inflicted injury NEC Z04.8
suicide attempt, alleged Z03.89
self-poisoning Z03.6
toxic effects from ingested substance
(drug) (poison) Z03.6
toxic effects from ingested substance
(drug) (poison) Z03.6
Obsession, obsessional state F42
Obsessive-compulsive neurosis or
reaction F42
Obstetric embolism, septic —see
Embolism, obstetric, septic
Obstetrical trauma (complicating
delivery) O71.9
with or following ectopic or molar
pregnancy O08.6
specified type NEC O71.89
Obstipation —see Constipation
Obstruction, obstructed, obstructive
airway J98.8
with
allergic alveolitis J67.9
asthma J45.909
with
exacerbation (acute) J45.901
status asthmaticus J45.902
bronchiectasis J47.9
with
exacerbation (acute) J47.1
lower respiratory infection
J47.0
bronchitis (chronic) J44.9
emphysema J43.9
chronic J44.9
with
allergic alveolitis —
see Pneumonitis,
hypersensitivity

Obstruction, obstructed, obstructive
(Continued)
airway (Continued)
chronic (Continued)
with (Continued)
bronchiectasis J47.9
with
exacerbation (acute) J47.1
lower respiratory infection
J47.0
due to
foreign body —see Foreign body,
by site, causing asphyxia
inhalation of fumes or vapors
J68.9
laryngospasm J38.5
ampulla of Vater K83.1
aortic (heart) (valve) —see Stenosis,
aortic
aortoiliac I74.09
aqueduct of Sylvius G91.1
congenital Q03.0
with spina bifida —see Spina
bifida, by site, with
hydrocephalus
Arnold-Chiari —see Arnold-Chiari
disease
artery (see also Embolism, artery)
I74.9
basilar (complete) (partial) —see
Occlusion, artery, basilar
carotid (complete) (partial) —see
Occlusion, artery, carotid
cerebellar —see Occlusion, artery,
cerebellar
cerebral (anterior) (middle)
(posterior) —see Occlusion,
artery, cerebral
precerebral —see Occlusion, artery,
precerebral
renal N28.0
retinal NEC —see Occlusion, artery,
retina
vertebral (complete) (partial) —see
Occlusion, artery, vertebral
band (intestinal) K56.69
bile duct or passage (common) (hepatic)
(noncalculous) K83.1
with calculus K80.51
congenital (causing jaundice)
Q44.3
biliary (duct) (tract) K83.1
gallbladder K82.0
bladder-neck (acquired) N32.0
congenital Q64.31
due to hyperplasia (hypertrophy)
of prostate —see Hyperplasia,
prostate
bowel —see Obstruction, intestine
bronchus J98.09
canal, ear —see Stenosis, external ear
canal
cardia K22.2
caval veins (inferior) (superior)
I87.1
cecum —see Obstruction, intestine
circulatory I99.8
colon —see Obstruction, intestine
common duct (noncalculous) K83.1
coronary (artery) —see Occlusion,
coronary
cystic duct —see also Obstruction,
gallbladder
with calculus K80.21

Obstruction, obstructed, obstructive
  (*Continued*)
  device, implant or graft (*see also*
      Complications, by site and type,
      mechanical) T85.698
    arterial graft NEC —*see*
        Complication, cardiovascular
        device, mechanical, vascular
    catheter NEC T85.628
      cystostomy T83.090
      dialysis (renal) T82.49
        intraperitoneal T85.691
      infusion NEC T82.594
        spinal (epidural) (subdural)
            T85.690
      urinary, indwelling T83.098
    due to infection T85.79
    gastrointestinal —*see* Complications,
        prosthetic device, mechanical,
        gastrointestinal device
    genital NEC T83.498
      intrauterine contraceptive device
          T83.39
      penile prosthesis T83.490
    heart NEC —*see* Complication,
        cardiovascular device,
        mechanical
    joint prosthesis —*see* Complications,
        joint prosthesis, mechanical,
        specified NEC, by site
    orthopedic NEC —*see* Complication,
        orthopedic, device, mechanical
    specified NEC T85.628
    urinary NEC —*see also* Complication,
        genitourinary, device, urinary,
        mechanical
      graft T83.29
    vascular NEC —*see* Complication,
        cardiovascular device,
        mechanical
    ventricular intracranial shunt T85.09
  due to foreign body accidentally left in
      operative wound T81.529
  duodenum K31.5
  ejaculatory duct N50.8
  esophagus K22.2
  eustachian tube (complete) (partial)
      H68.10-
    cartilagenous (extrinsic) H68.13-
      intrinsic H68.12-
    osseous H68.11-
  fallopian tube (bilateral) N97.1
  fecal K56.41
    with hernia —*see* Hernia, by site, with
        obstruction
  foramen of Monro (congenital) Q03.8
    with spina bifida —*see* Spina bifida,
        by site, with hydrocephalus
  foreign body —*see* Foreign body
  gallbladder K82.0
    with calculus, stones K80.21
    congenital Q44.1
  gastric outlet K31.1
  gastrointestinal —*see* Obstruction,
      intestine
  hepatic K76.89
    duct (noncalculous) K83.1
  ileum —*see* Obstruction, intestine
  iliofemoral (artery) I74.5
  intestine K56.60
    with
      adhesions (intestinal) (peritoneal)
          K56.5
      adynamic K56.0

Obstruction, obstructed, obstructive
  (*Continued*)
  intestine (*Continued*)
    by gallstone K56.3
    congenital (small) Q41.9
      large Q42.9
        specified part NEC Q42.8
    neurogenic K56.0
      Hirschsprung's disease or
          megacolon Q43.1
    newborn P76.9
      due to
        fecaliths P76.8
        inspissated milk P76.2
        meconium (plug) P76.0
          in mucoviscidosis E84.11
        specified NEC P76.8
    postoperative K91.3
    reflex K56.0
    specified NEC K56.69
    volvulus K56.2
  intracardiac ball valve prosthesis
      T82.09
  jejunum —*see* Obstruction, intestine
  joint prosthesis —*see* Complications,
      joint prosthesis, mechanical,
      specified NEC, by site
  kidney (calices) N28.89
  labor —*see* Delivery
  lacrimal (passages) (duct)
    by
      dacryolith —*see* Dacryolith
      stenosis —*see* Stenosis, lacrimal
    congenital Q10.5
    neonatal H04.53-
  lacrimonasal duct —*see* Obstruction,
      lacrimal
  lacteal, with steatorrhea K90.2
  laryngitis —*see* Laryngitis
  larynx NEC J38.6
    congenital Q31.8
  lung J98.4
    disease, chronic J44.9
  lymphatic I89.0
  meconium (plug)
    newborn P76.0
      due to fecaliths P76.0
      in mucoviscidosis E84.11
  mitral —*see* Stenosis, mitral
  nasal J34.89
  nasolacrimal duct —*see also*
      Obstruction, lacrimal
    congenital Q10.5
  nasopharynx J39.2
  nose J34.89
  organ or site, congenital NEC —*see*
      Atresia, by site
  pancreatic duct K86.8
  parotid duct or gland K11.8
  pelviureteral junction N13.5
    congenital Q62.39
  pharynx J39.2
  portal (circulation) (vein) I81
  prostate —*see also* Hyperplasia,
      prostate
    valve (urinary) N32.0
  pulmonary valve (heart) I37.0
  pyelonephritis (chronic) N11.1
  pylorus
    adult K31.1
    congenital or infantile Q40.0
  rectosigmoid —*see* Obstruction,
      intestine
  rectum K62.4

Obstruction, obstructed, obstructive
  (*Continued*)
  renal N28.89
    outflow N13.8
    pelvis, congenital Q62.39
  respiratory J98.8
    chronic J44.9
  retinal (vessels) H34.9
  salivary duct (any) K11.8
    with calculus K11.5
  sigmoid —*see* Obstruction,
      intestine
  sinus (accessory) (nasal) J34.89
  Stensen's duct K11.8
  stomach NEC K31.89
    acute K31.0
    congenital Q40.2
    due to pylorospasm K31.3
  submandibular duct K11.8
  submaxillary gland K11.8
    with calculus K11.5
  thoracic duct I89.0
  thrombotic —*see* Thrombosis
  trachea J39.8
  tracheostomy airway J95.03
  tricuspid (valve) —*see* Stenosis,
      tricuspid
  upper respiratory, congenital
      Q34.8
  ureter (functional) (pelvic junction)
      NEC N13.5
    with
      hydronephrosis N13.1
        with infection N13.6
      pyelonephritis (chronic)
          N11.1
    congenital Q62.39
    due to calculus —*see* Calculus,
        ureter
  urethra NEC N36.8
    congenital Q64.39
  urinary (moderate) N13.9
    due to hyperplasia (hypertrophy)
        of prostate —*see* Hyperplasia,
        prostate
    organ or tract (lower) N13.9
    prostatic valve N32.0
    specified NEC N13.8
  uropathy N13.9
  uterus N85.8
  vagina N89.5
  valvular —*see* Endocarditis
  vein, venous I87.1
    caval (inferior) (superior) I87.1
    thrombotic —*see* Thrombosis
    vena cava (inferior) (superior) I87.1
  vesical NEC N32.0
  vesicourethral orifice N32.0
    congenital Q64.31
  vessel NEC I99.8
Obturator —*see* condition
Occlusal wear, teeth K03.0
Occlusio pupillae —*see* Membrane,
    pupillary
Occlusion, occluded
  anus K62.4
    congenital Q42.3
      with fistula Q42.2
  aortoiliac (chronic) I74.09
  aqueduct of Sylvius G91.1
    congenital Q03.0
      with spina bifida —*see* Spina
          bifida, by site, with
          hydrocephalus

Occlusion, occluded (*Continued*)
artery (*see also* Embolism, artery) I74.9
  auditory, internal I65.8
  basilar I65.1
    with
      infarction I63.22
        due to
          embolism I63.12
          thrombosis I63.02
  brain or cerebral I66.9
    with infarction (due to) I63.5
      embolism I63.4
      thrombosis I63.3
  carotid I65.2-
    with
      infarction I63.23-
        due to
          embolism I63.13-
          thrombosis I63.03-
  cerebellar (anterior inferior) (posterior
    inferior) (superior) I66.3
    with infarction I63.54-
      due to
        embolism I63.44-
        thrombosis I63.34-
  cerebral I66.9
    with infarction I63.50
      due to
        embolism I63.40
          specified NEC I63.49
        thrombosis I63.30
          specified NEC I63.39
    anterior I66.1-
      with infarction I63.52-
        due to
          embolism I63.42-
          thrombosis I63.32-
    middle I66.0-
      with infarction I63.51-
        due to
          embolism I63.41-
          thrombosis I63.31-
    posterior I66.2-
      with infarction I63.53-
        due to
          embolism I63.43-
          thrombosis I63.33-
    specified NEC I66.8
      with infarction I63.59
        due to
          embolism I63.4
          thrombosis I63.3
  choroidal (anterior) —*see* Occlusion,
    artery, cerebral, specified NEC
  communicating posterior —*see*
    Occlusion, artery, precerebral,
    specified NEC
  complete
    coronary I25.82
    extremities I70.92
  coronary (acute) (thrombotic)
    (without myocardial infarction)
    I24.0
    with myocardial infarction —*see*
      Infarction, myocardium
    chronic total I25.82
    complete I25.82
    healed or old I25.2
    total (chronic) I25.82
  hypophyseal —*see* Occlusion, artery,
    precerebral, specified NEC
  iliac I74.5
  lower extremities due to stenosis or
    stricture I77.1

Occlusion, occluded (*Continued*)
artery (*Continued*)
  mesenteric (embolic) (thrombotic)
    K55.0
  perforating —*see* Occlusion, artery,
    cerebral, specified NEC
  peripheral I77.9
    thrombotic or embolic I74.4
  pontine —*see* Occlusion, artery,
    cerebral, specified NEC
  precerebral I65.9
    with infarction I63.20
      due to
        embolism I63.10
          specified NEC I63.19
        thrombosis I63.00
          specified NEC I63.09
      specified NEC I63.29
    basilar —*see* Occlusion, artery,
      basilar
    carotid —*see* Occlusion, artery,
      carotid
    puerperal O88.23
    specified NEC I65.8
      with infarction I63.29
        due to
          embolism I63.19
          thrombosis I63.00
    vertebral —*see* Occlusion, artery,
      vertebral
  renal N28.0
  retinal
    branch H34.23-
    central H34.1-
    partial H34.21-
    transient H34.0-
  spinal —*see* Occlusion, artery,
    precerebral, vertebral
  total (chronic)
    coronary I25.82
    extremities I70.92
  vertebral I65.0-
    with
      infarction I63.21-
        due to
          embolism I63.11-
          thrombosis I63.01-
basilar artery —*see* Occlusion, artery,
  basilar
bile duct (common) (hepatic)
  (noncalculous) K83.1
bowel —*see* Obstruction, intestine
carotid (artery) (common)
  (internal) —*see* Occlusion,
  artery, carotid
centric (of teeth) M26.59
  maximum intercuspation discrepancy
    M26.55
cerebellar (artery) —*see* Occlusion,
  artery, cerebellar
cerebral (artery) —*see* Occlusion, artery,
  cerebral
cerebrovascular —*see also* Occlusion,
  artery, cerebral
  with infarction I63.5
cervical canal —*see* Stricture, cervix
cervix (uteri) —*see* Stricture, cervix
choanal Q30.0
choroidal (artery) —*see* Occlusion,
  artery, precerebral, specified NEC
colon —*see* Obstruction, intestine
communicating posterior artery —*see*
  Occlusion, artery, precerebral,
  specified NEC

Occlusion, occluded (*Continued*)
coronary (artery) (vein) (thrombotic) —
  see also Infarct, myocardium
  chronic total I25.82
  healed or old I25.2
  not resulting in infarction I24.0
  total (chronic) I25.82
cystic duct —*see* Obstruction,
  gallbladder
embolic —*see* Embolism
fallopian tube N97.1
  congenital Q50.6
gallbladder —*see also* Obstruction,
  gallbladder
  congenital (causing jaundice) Q44.1
gingiva, traumatic K06.2
hymen N89.6
  congenital Q52.3
hypophyseal (artery) —*see* Occlusion,
  artery, precerebral, specified NEC
iliac artery I74.5
intestine —*see* Obstruction, intestine
lacrimal passages —*see* Obstruction,
  lacrimal
lung J98.4
lymph or lymphatic channel I89.0
mammary duct N64.89
mesenteric artery (embolic)
  (thrombotic) K55.0
nose J34.89
  congenital Q30.0
organ or site, congenital NEC —*see*
  Atresia, by site
oviduct N97.1
  congenital Q50.6
peripheral arteries
  due to stricture or stenosis I77.1
  upper extremity I74.2
pontine (artery) —*see* Occlusion, artery,
  precerebral, specified NEC
posterior lingual, of mandibular teeth
  M26.29
precerebral artery —*see* Occlusion,
  artery, precerebral
punctum lacrimale —*see* Obstruction,
  lacrimal
pupil —*see* Membrane, pupillary
pylorus, adult (*see also* Stricture,
  pylorus) K31.1
renal artery N28.0
retina, retinal
  artery —*see* Occlusion, artery, retinal
  vein (central) H34.81-
    engorgement H34.82-
    tributary H34.83-
  vessels H34.9
spinal artery —*see* Occlusion, artery,
  precerebral, vertebral
teeth (mandibular) (posterior lingual)
  M26.29
thoracic duct I89.0
thrombotic —*see* Thrombosis, artery
traumatic
  edentulous (alveolar) ridge K06.2
  gingiva K06.2
  periodontal K05.5
tubal N97.1
ureter (complete) (partial) N13.5
  congenital Q62.10
ureteropelvic junction N13.5
  congenital Q62.11
ureterovesical orifice N13.5
  congenital Q62.12
urethra —*see* Stricture, urethra

Occlusion, occluded (Continued)
uterus N85.8
vagina N89.5
vascular NEC I99.8
vein —see Thrombosis
retinal —see Occlusion, retinal, vein
vena cava (inferior) (superior) —see
Embolism, vena cava
ventricle (brain) NEC G91.1
vertebral (artery) —see Occlusion,
artery, vertebral
vessel (blood) I99.8
vulva N90.5
Occult
blood in feces (stools) R19.5
Occupational
problems NEC Z56.89
Ochlophobia —see Agoraphobia
Ochronosis (endogenous) E70.29
Ocular muscle —see condition
Oculogyric crisis or disturbance H51.8
psychogenic F45.8
Oculomotor syndrome H51.9
Oculopathy
syphilitic NEC A52.71
congenital
early A50.01
late A50.30
early (secondary) A51.43
late A52.71
Oddi's sphincter spasm K83.4
Odontalgia K08.8
Odontoameloblastoma —see Cyst,
calcifying odontogenic
Odontoclasia K03.89
Odontodysplasia, regional K00.4
Odontogenesis imperfecta K00.5
Odontoma (ameloblastic) (complex)
(compound) (fibroameloblastic) —see
Cyst, calcifying odontogenic
Odontomyelitis (closed) (open) K04.0
Odontorrhagia K08.8
Odontosarcoma, ameloblastic C41.1
upper jaw (bone) C41.0
Oedema, oedematous —see Edema
Oesophag (o) —see Esophag (o)-
Oestriasis —see Myiasis
Oguchi's disease H53.63
Ohara's disease —see Tularemia
Oidiomycosis —see Candidiasis
Oidium albicans infection —see
Candidiasis
Old (previous) myocardial infarction I25.2
Old age (without mention of debility) R54-
dementia F03
Olfactory —see condition
Oligemia —see Anemia
Oligoastrocytoma
specified site —see Neoplasm,
malignant, by site
unspecified site C71.9
Oligocythemia D64.9
Oligodendroblastoma
specified site —see Neoplasm,
malignant
unspecified site C71.9
Oligodendroglioma
anaplastic type
specified site —see Neoplasm,
malignant, by site
unspecified site C71.9
specified site —see Neoplasm,
malignant, by site
unspecified site C71.9
Oligodontia —see Anodontia

Oligoencephalon Q02
Oligohidrosis L74.4
Oligohydramnios O41.0-
Oligohydrosis L74.4
Oligomenorrhea N91.5
primary N91.3
secondary N91.4
Oligophrenia —see also Disability,
intellectual
phenylpyruvic E70.0
Oligospermia N46.11
due to
drug therapy N46.121
efferent duct obstruction N46.123
infection N46.122
radiation N46.124
specified cause NEC N46.129
systemic disease N46.125
Oligotrichia —see Alopecia
Oliguria R34
with, complicating or following ectopic
or molar pregnancy O08.4
postprocedural N99.0
Ollier's disease Q78.4
Omenotocele —see Hernia, abdomen,
specified site NEC
Omentitis —see Peritonitis
Omentum, omental —see condition
Omphalitis (congenital) (newborn) P38.9
with mild hemorrhage P38.1
without hemorrhage P38.9
not of newborn L08.82
tetanus A33
Omphalocele Q79.2
Omphalomesenteric duct, persistent Q43.0
Omphalorrhagia, newborn P51.9
Omsk hemorrhagic fever A98.1
Onanism (excessive) F98.8
Onchocerciasis, onchocercosis B73.1
with
eye disease B73.00
endophthalmitis B73.01
eyelid B73.09
glaucoma B73.02
specified NEC B73.09
eye NEC B73.00
eyelid B73.09
Oncocytoma —see Neoplasm, benign, by
site
Oncovirus, as cause of disease classified
elsewhere B97.32
Ondine's curse —see Apnea, sleep
Oneirophrenia F23
Onychauxis L60.2
congenital Q84.5
Onychia —see also Cellulitis, digit
with lymphangitis —see Lymphangitis,
acute, digit
candidal B37.2
dermatophytic B35.1
Onychitis —see also Cellulitis, digit
with lymphangitis —see Lymphangitis,
acute, digit
Onychocryptosis L60.0
Onychodystrophy L60.3
congenital Q84.6
Onychogryphosis, onychogryposis L60.2
Onycholysis L60.1
Onychomadesis L60.8
Onychomalacia L60.3
Onychomycosis (finger) (toe) B35.1
Onycho-osteodysplasia Q79.8
Onychophagia F98.8
Onychophosis L60.8

Onychoptosis L60.8
Onychorrhexis L60.3
congenital Q84.6
Onychoschizia L60.3
Onyxis (finger) (toe) L60.0
Onyxitis —see also Cellulitis, digit
with lymphangitis —see Lymphangitis,
acute, digit
Oophoritis (cystic) (infectional)
(interstitial) N70.92
with salpingitis N70.93
acute N70.02
with salpingitis N70.03
chronic N70.12
with salpingitis N70.13
complicating abortion —see Abortion,
by type, complicated by, oophoritis
Oophorocele N83.4
Opacity, opacities
cornea H17.-
central H17.1-
congenital Q13.3
degenerative —see Degeneration,
cornea
hereditary —see Dystrophy, cornea
inflammatory —see Keratitis
minor H17.81-
peripheral H17.82-
sequelae of trachoma (healed) B94.0
specified NEC H17.89
enamel (teeth) (fluoride) (nonfluoride)
K00.3
lens —see Cataract
snowball —see Deposit, crystalline
vitreous (humor) NEC H43.39-
congenital Q14.0
membranes and strands H43.31-
Opalescent dentin (hereditary) K00.5
Open, opening
abnormal, organ or site, congenital —
see Imperfect, closure
angle with
borderline
findings
high risk H40.02-
low risk H40.01-
intraocular pressure H40.00-
cupping of discs H40.01-
glaucoma (primary) —see Glaucoma,
open angle
bite
anterior M26.220
posterior M26.221
false —see Imperfect, closure
margin on tooth restoration K08.51
restoration margins of tooth K08.51
wound —see Wound, open
Operational fatigue F48.8
Operative —see condition
Operculitis —see Periodontitis
Operculum —see Break, retina
Ophiasis L63.2
Ophthalmia (see also Conjunctivitis) H10.9
actinic rays —see Photokeratitis
allergic (acute) —see Conjunctivitis,
acute, atopic
blennorrhagic (gonococcal)
(neonatorum) A54.31
diphtheritic A36.86
Egyptian A71.1
electrica —see Photokeratitis
gonococcal (neonatorum) A54.31
metastatic —see Endophthalmitis,
purulent

Ophthalmia (*Continued*)
migraine —*see* Migraine,
   ophthalmoplegic
neonatorum, newborn P39.1
   gonococcal A54.31
nodosa H16.24-
purulent —*see* Conjunctivitis, acute,
   mucopurulent
spring —*see* Conjunctivitis, acute,
   atopic
sympathetic —*see* Uveitis, sympathetic
Ophthalmitis —*see* Ophthalmia
Ophthalmocele (congenital) Q15.8
Ophthalmoneuromyelitis G36.0
Ophthalmoplegia —*see also* Strabismus,
   paralytic
anterior internuclear —*see*
   Ophthalmoplegia, internuclear
ataxia-areflexia G61.0
diabetic —*see* E08-E13 with .39
exophthalmic E05.00
   with thyroid storm E05.01
external H49.88-
   progressive H49.4-
      with pigmentary retinopathy —*see*
         Kearns-Sayre syndrome
   total H49.3-
internal (complete) (total) H52.51-
internuclear H51.2-
migraine —*see* Migraine,
   ophthalmoplegic
Parinaud's H49.88-
progressive external —*see*
   Ophthalmoplegia, external,
   progressive
supranuclear, progressive G23.1
total (external) —*see* Ophthalmoplegia,
   external, total
Opioid (s)
abuse —*see* Abuse, drug, opioids
dependence —*see* Dependence, drug,
   opioids
Opisthognathism M26.09
Opisthorchiasis (felineus) (viverrini)
   B66.0
f**Opitz' disease** D73.2
Opiumism —*see* Dependence, drug,
   opioid
Oppenheim's disease G70.2
Oppenheim-Urbach disease (necrobiosis
   lipoidica diabeticorum) —*see*
   E08-E13 with .620
Optic nerve —*see* condition
Orbit —*see* condition
Orchioblastoma C62.9-
Orchitis (gangrenous) (nonspecific)
   (septic) (suppurative) N45.2
blennorrhagic (gonococcal) (acute)
   (chronic) A54.23
chlamydial A56.19
filarial B74.9
gonococcal (acute) (chronic)
   A54.23
mumps B26.0
syphilitic A52.76
tuberculous A18.15
Orf (virus disease) B08.02
Organic —*see also* condition
brain syndrome F09
heart —*see* Disease, heart
mental disorder F09
psychosis F09
Orgasm
anejaculatory N53.13

Oriental
bilharziasis B65.2
schistosomiasis B65.2
Orifice —*see* condition
Origin of both great vessels from right
   ventricle Q20.1
Ormond's disease (with ureteral
   obstruction) N13.5
with infection N13.6
Ornithine metabolism disorder E72.4
Ornithinemia (Type I) (Type II) E72.4
Ornithosis A70
Orotaciduria, oroticaciduria (congenital)
   (hereditary) (pyrimidine deficiency)
   E79.8
anemia D53.0
Orthodontics
adjustment Z46.4
fitting Z46.4
Orthopnea R06.01
Orthopoxvirus B08.09
specified NEC B08.09
Os, uterus —*see* condition
Osgood-Schlatter disease or
   osteochondrosis —*see*
   Osteochondrosis, juvenile, tibia
Osler (-Weber)-Rendu disease I78.0
Osler's nodes I33.0
Osmidrosis L75.0
Osseous —*see* condition
Ossification
artery —*see* Arteriosclerosis
auricle (ear) —*see* Disorder, pinna,
   specified type NEC
bronchial J98.09
cardiac —*see* Degeneration, myocardial
cartilage (senile) —*see* Disorder,
   cartilage, specified type NEC
coronary (artery) —*see* Disease, heart,
   ischemic, atherosclerotic
diaphragm J98.6
ear, middle —*see* Otosclerosis
falx cerebri G96.19
fontanel, premature Q75.0
heart —*see also* Degeneration, myocardial
valve —*see* Endocarditis
larynx J38.7
ligament —*see* Disorder, tendon,
   specified type NEC
   posterior longitudinal —*see*
      Spondylopathy, specified NEC
meninges (cerebral) (spinal) G96.19
multiple, eccentric centers —*see* Disorder,
   bone, development or growth
muscle —*see also* Calcification, muscle
   due to burns —*see* Myositis,
      ossificans, in, burns
   paralytic —*see* Myositis, ossificans, in,
      quadriplegia
   progressive —*see* Myositis, ossificans,
      progressiva
   specified NEC M61.50
    ankle M61.57-
    foot M61.57-
    forearm M61.53-
    hand M61.54-
    lower leg M61.56-
    multiple sites M61.59
    pelvic region M61.55-
    shoulder region M61.51-
    specified site NEC M61.58
    thigh M61.55-
    upper arm M61.52-
   traumatic —*see* Myositis, ossificans,
      traumatica

Ossification (*Continued*)
myocardium, myocardial —*see*
   Degeneration, myocardial
penis N48.89
periarticular —*see* Disorder, joint,
   specified type NEC
pinna —*see* Disorder, pinna, specified
   type NEC
rider's bone —*see* Ossification, muscle,
   specified NEC
sclera H15.89
subperiosteal, post-traumatic M89.8X-
tendon —*see* Disorder, tendon, specified
   type NEC
trachea J39.8
tympanic membrane —*see* Disorder,
   tympanic membrane, specified
   NEC
vitreous (humor) —*see* Deposit,
   crystalline
Osteitis —*see also* Osteomyelitis
alveolar M27.3
condensans M85.30
   ankle M85.37-
   foot M85.37-
   forearm M85.33-
   hand M85.34-
   lower leg M85.36-
   multiple site M85.39
   neck M85.38
   rib M85.38
   shoulder M85.31-
   skull M85.38
   specified site NEC M85.38
   thigh M85.35-
   toe M85.37-
   upper arm M85.32-
   vertebra M85.38
deformans M88.9
   in (due to)
    malignant neoplasm of bone C41.9
      [M90.60]
    neoplastic disease (*see also*
      Neoplasm) D49.9 [M90.60]
     carpus D49.9 [M90.64-]
     clavicle D49.9 [M90.61-]
     femur D49.9 [M90.65-]
     fibula D49.9 [M90.66-]
     finger D49.9 [M90.64-]
     humerus D49.9 [M90.62-]
     ilium D49.9 [M90.65-]
     ischium D49.9 [M90.65-]
     metacarpus D49.9 [M90.64-]
     metatarsus D49.9 [M90.67-]
     multiple sites D49.9 [M90.69]
     neck D49.9 [M90.68]
     radius D49.9 [M90.63-]
     rib D49.9 [M90.68]
     scapula D49.9 [M90.61-]
     skull D49.9 [M90.68]
     tarsus D49.9 [M90.67-]
     tibia D49.9 [M90.66-]
     toe D49.9 [M90.67-]
     ulna D49.9 [M90.63-]
     vertebra D49.9 [M90.68]
   skull M88.0
   specified NEC —*see* Paget's disease,
    bone, by site
   vertebra M88.1
due to yaws A66.6
fibrosa NEC —*see* Cyst, bone, by site
   circumscripta —*see* Dysplasia,
    fibrous, bone NEC
   cystica (generalisata) E21.0

Osteitis (Continued)
  fibrosa NEC (Continued)
    disseminata Q78.1
    osteoplastica E21.0
  fragilitans Q78.0
  Garr's (sclerosing) —see Osteomyelitis,
      specified type NEC
  jaw (acute) (chronic) (lower)
      (suppurative) (upper) M27.2
  parathyroid E21.0
  petrous bone (acute) (chronic) —see
      Petrositis
  sclerotic, nonsuppurative —see
      Osteomyelitis, specified type
      NEC
  tuberculosa A18.09
    cystica D86.89
    multiplex cystoides D86.89
Osteoarthritis M19.90
  ankle M19.07-
  elbow M19.02-
  foot joint M19.07-
  generalized M15.9
    erosive M15.4
    primary M15.0
    specified NEC M15.8
  hand joint M19.04-
    first carpometacarpal joint M18.9-
  hip M16.1-
    bilateral M16.0
    due to hip dysplasia (unilateral)
        M16.3-
      bilateral M16.2
  interphalangeal
    distal (Heberden) M15.1
    proximal (Bouchard) M15.2
  knee M17.9-
    bilateral M17.0
  post-traumatic NEC M19.92
    ankle M19.17-
    elbow M19.12-
    foot joint M19.17-
    hand joint M19.14-
      first carpometacarpal joint M18.3-
        bilateral M18.2
    hip M16.5-
      bilateral M16.4
    knee M17.3-
      bilateral M17.2
    shoulder M19.11-
    wrist M19.13-
  primary M19.91
    ankle M19.07-
    elbow M19.02-
    foot joint M19.07-
    hand joint M19.04-
      first carpometacarpal joint M18.1-
        bilateral M18.0
    hip M16.1-
      bilateral M16.0
    knee M17.1-
      bilateral M17.0
    shoulder M19.01-
    spine —see Spondylosis
    wrist M19.03-
  secondary M19.93
    ankle M19.27-
    elbow M19.22-
    foot joint M19.27-
    hand joint M19.24-
      first carpometacarpal joint M18.5-
        bilateral M18.4
    hip M16.7
      bilateral M16.6

Osteoarthritis (Continued)
  secondary (Continued)
    knee M17.5
      bilateral M17.4
    multiple M15.3
    shoulder M19.21-
    spine —see Spondylosis
    wrist M19.23-
  shoulder M19.01-
  spine —see Spondylosis
  wrist M19.03-
Osteoarthropathy (hypertrophic)
    M19.90
  ankle —see Osteoarthritis, primary,
      ankle
  elbow —see Osteoarthritis, primary,
      elbow
  foot joint —see Osteoarthritis, primary,
      foot
  hand joint —see Osteoarthritis, primary,
      hand joint
  knee joint —see Osteoarthritis, primary,
      knee
  multiple site —see Osteoarthritis,
      primary, multiple joint
  pulmonary —see also Osteoarthropathy,
      specified type NEC
    hypertrophic —see Osteoarthropathy,
        hypertrophic, specified type
        NEC
  secondary —see Osteoarthropathy,
      specified type NEC
  secondary hypertrophic —see
      Osteoarthropathy, specified type
      NEC
  shoulder —see Osteoarthritis, primary,
      shoulder
  specified joint NEC —see Osteoarthritis,
      primary, specified joint NEC
  specified type NEC M89.40
    carpus M89.44-
    clavicle M89.41-
    femur M89.45-
    fibula M89.46-
    finger M89.44-
    humerus M89.42-
    ilium M89.459
    ischium M89.459
    metacarpus M89.44-
    metatarsus M89.47-
    multiple sites M89.49
    neck M89.48
    radius M89.43-
    rib M89.48
    scapula M89.41-
    skull M89.48
    tarsus M89.47-
    tibia M89.46-
    toe M89.47-
    ulna M89.43-
    vertebra M89.48
  spine —see Spondylosis
  wrist —see Osteoarthritis, primary,
      wrist
Osteoarthrosis (degenerative)
    (hypertrophic) (joint) —see also
    Osteoarthritis
  deformans alkaptonurica E70.29
      [M36.8]
  erosive M15.4
  generalized M15.9
    primary M15.0
  polyarticular M15.9
  spine —see Spondylosis

Osteoblastoma —see Neoplasm, bone,
    benign
  aggressive —see Neoplasm, bone,
      uncertain behavior
Osteochondroarthrosis deformans
    endemica —see Disease, Kaschin-
    Beck
Osteochondritis —see also
    Osteochondropathy, by site
  Brailsford's —see Osteochondrosis,
      juvenile, radius
  dissecans M93.20
    ankle M93.27-
    elbow M93.22-
    foot M93.27-
    hand M93.24-
    hip M93.25-
    knee M93.26-
    multiple sites M93.29
    shoulder joint M93.21-
    specified site NEC M93.28
    wrist M93.23-
  juvenile M92.9
    patellar —see Osteochondrosis,
        juvenile, patella
  syphilitic (congenital) (early) A50.02
      [M90.80]
    ankle A50.02 [M90.87-]
    elbow A50.02 [M90.82-]
    foot A50.02 [M90.87-]
    forearm A50.02 [M90.83-]
    hand A50.02 [M90.84-]
    hip A50.02 [M90.85-]
    knee A50.02 [M90.86-]
    multiple sites A50.02 [M90.89]
    shoulder joint A50.02 [M90.81-]
    specified site NEC A50.02
        [M90.88]
Osteochondrodysplasia Q78.9
  with defects of growth of tubular bones
      and spine Q77.9
    specified NEC Q77.8
  specified NEC Q78.8
Osteochondrodystrophy E78.9
Osteochondrolysis —see Osteochondritis,
    dissecans
Osteochondroma —see Neoplasm, bone,
    benign
Osteochondromatosis D48.0
  syndrome Q78.4
Osteochondromyxosarcoma —see
    Neoplasm, bone, malignant
Osteochondropathy M93.90
  ankle M93.97-
  elbow M93.92-
  foot M93.97-
  hand M93.94-
  hip M93.95-
  Kienböck's disease of adults
      M93.1
  knee M93.96-
  multiple joints M93.99
  osteochondritis dissecans —see
      Osteochondritis, dissecans
  osteochondrosis —see Osteochondrosis
  shoulder region M93.91-
  slipped upper femoral epiphysis —see
      Slipped, epiphysis, upper
      femoral
  specified joint NEC M93.98
  specified type NEC M93.80
    ankle M93.87-
    elbow M93.82-
    foot M93.87-

Osteochondropathy *(Continued)*
  specified type NEC *(Continued)*
    hand M93.84-
    hip M93.85-
    knee M93.86-
    multiple joints M93.89
    shoulder region M93.81-
    specified joint NEC M93.88
    wrist M93.83-
  syphilitic, congenital
    early A50.02 *[M90.80]*
    late A50.56 *[M90.80]*
  wrist M93.93-
Osteochondrosarcoma —*see* Neoplasm,
    bone, malignant
Osteochondrosis —*see also*
    Osteochondropathy, by site
  acetabulum (juvenile) M91.0
  adult —*see* Osteochondropathy,
    specified type NEC, by site
  astragalus (juvenile) —*see*
    Osteochondrosis, juvenile, tarsus
  Blount's —*see* Osteochondrosis,
    juvenile, tibia
  Buchanan's M91.0
  Burns' —*see* Osteochondrosis, juvenile,
    ulna
  calcaneus (juvenile) —*see*
    Osteochondrosis, juvenile, tarsus
  capitular epiphysis (femur) (juvenile) —
    see Legg-Calvé-Perthes disease
  carpal (juvenile) (lunate) (scaphoid) —
    see Osteochondrosis, juvenile,
    hand, carpal lunate
    adult M93.1
  coxae juvenilis —*see* Legg-Calvé-
    Perthes disease
  deformans juvenilis, coxae —*see* Legg-
    Calvé-Perthes disease
  Diaz's —*see* Osteochondrosis, juvenile,
    tarsus
  dissecans (knee) (shoulder) —*see*
    Osteochondritis, dissecans
  femoral capital epiphysis (juvenile) —
    see Legg-Calvé-Perthes disease
  femur (head), juvenile —*see* Legg-
    Calvé-Perthes disease
  fibula (juvenile) —*see* Osteochondrosis,
    juvenile, fibula
  foot NEC (juvenile) M92.8
  Freiberg's —*see* Osteochondrosis,
    juvenile, metatarsus
  Haas' (juvenile) —*see* Osteochondrosis,
    juvenile, humerus
  Haglund's —*see* Osteochondrosis,
    juvenile, tarsus
  hip (juvenile) —*see* Legg-Calvé-Perthes
    disease
  humerus (capitulum) (head)
    (juvenile) —*see* Osteochondrosis,
    juvenile, humerus
  ilium, iliac crest (juvenile) M91.0
  ischiopubic synchondrosis M91.0
  Iselin's —*see* Osteochondrosis, juvenile,
    metatarsus
  juvenile, juvenilis M92.9
    after congenital dislocation of
      hip reduction —*see*
      Osteochondrosis, juvenile, hip,
      specified NEC
    arm —*see* Osteochondrosis, juvenile,
      upper limb NEC
    capitular epiphysis (femur) —*see*
      Legg-Calvé-Perthes disease

Osteochondrosis *(Continued)*
  juvenile, juvenilis *(Continued)*
    clavicle, sternal epiphysis —*see*
      Osteochondrosis, juvenile,
      upper limb NEC
    coxae —*see* Legg-Calvé-Perthes disease
    deformans M92.9
    fibula M92.5-
    foot NEC M92.8
    hand M92.20-
      carpal lunate M92.21-
      metacarpal head M92.22-
      specified site NEC M92.29-
    head of femur —*see* Legg-Calvé-
      Perthes disease
    hip and pelvis M91.9-
      coxa plana —*see* Coxa, plana
      femoral head —*see* Legg-Calvé-
        Perthes disease
      pelvis M91.0
      pseudocoxalgia —*see*
        Pseudocoxalgia
      specified NEC M91.8-
    humerus M92.0-
    limb
      lower NEC M92.8
      upper NEC —*see* Osteochondrosis,
        juvenile, upper limb NEC
    medial cuneiform bone —*see*
      Osteochondrosis, juvenile,
      tarsus
    metatarsus M92.7-
    patella M92.4-
    radius M92.1-
    specified site NEC M92.8
    spine M42.00
      cervical region M42.02
      cervicothoracic region M42.03
      lumbar region M42.06
      lumbosacral region M42.07
      multiple sites M42.09
      occipito-atlanto-axial region M42.01
      sacrococcygeal region M42.08
      thoracic region M42.04
      thoracolumbar region M42.05
    tarsus M92.6-
    tibia M92.5-
    ulna M92.1-
    upper limb NEC M92.3-
    vertebra (body) (epiphyseal plates)
      (Calvé's) (Scheuermann's) —*see*
      Osteochondrosis, juvenile,
      spine
  Kienböck's —*see* Osteochondrosis,
    juvenile, hand, carpal lunate
    adult M93.1
  Köhler's
    patellar —*see* Osteochondrosis,
      juvenile, patella
    tarsal navicular —*see*
      Osteochondrosis, juvenile,
      tarsus
  Legg-Perthes (-Calvé's)
    (-Waldenström) —*see* Legg-Calvé-
    Perthes disease
  limb
    lower NEC (juvenile) M92.8
    upper NEC (juvenile) —*see*
      Osteochondrosis, juvenile,
      upper limb NEC
  lunate bone (carpal) (juvenile) —*see also*
    Osteochondrosis, juvenile, hand,
    carpal lunate
    adult M93.1

Osteochondrosis *(Continued)*
  Mauclaire's —*see* Osteochondrosis,
    juvenile, hand, metacarpal
  metacarpal (head) (juvenile) —*see*
    Osteochondrosis, juvenile, hand,
    metacarpal
  metatarsus (fifth) (head) (juvenile)
    (second) —*see* Osteochondrosis,
    juvenile, metatarsus
  navicular (juvenile) —*see*
    Osteochondrosis, juvenile, tarsus
  os
    calcis (juvenile) —*see*
      Osteochondrosis, juvenile,
      tarsus
    tibiale externum (juvenile) —*see*
      Osteochondrosis, juvenile,
      tarsus
  Osgood-Schlatter —*see*
    Osteochondrosis, juvenile, tibia
  Panner's —*see* Osteochondrosis,
    juvenile, humerus
  patellar center (juvenile) (primary)
    (secondary) —*see* Osteochondrosis,
    juvenile, patella
  pelvis (juvenile) M91.0
  Pierson's M91.0
  radius (head) (juvenile) —*see*
    Osteochondrosis, juvenile, radius
  Scheuermann's —*see* Osteochondrosis,
    juvenile, spine
  Sever's —*see* Osteochondrosis, juvenile,
    tarsus
  Sinding-Larsen —*see* Osteochondrosis,
    juvenile, patella
  spine M42.9
    adult M42.10
      cervical region M42.12
      cervicothoracic region M42.13
      lumbar region M42.16
      lumbosacral region M42.17
      multiple sites M42.19
      occipito-atlanto-axial region
        M42.11
      sacrococcygeal region M42.18
      thoracic region M42.14
      thoracolumbar region M42.15
    juvenile —*see* Osteochondrosis,
      juvenile, spine
  symphysis pubis (juvenile) M91.0
  syphilitic (congenital) A50.02
  talus (juvenile) —*see* Osteochondrosis,
    juvenile, tarsus
  tarsus (navicular) (juvenile) —*see*
    Osteochondrosis, juvenile, tarsus
  tibia (proximal) (tubercle) (juvenile) —
    see Osteochondrosis, juvenile, tibia
  tuberculous —*see* Tuberculosis, bone
  ulna (lower) (juvenile) —*see*
    Osteochondrosis, juvenile, ulna
  van Neck's M91.0
  vertebral —*see* Osteochondrosis, spine
Osteoclastoma D48.0
  malignant —*see* Neoplasm, bone,
    malignant
Osteodynia —*see* Disorder, bone,
    specified type NEC
Osteodystrophy Q78.9
  azotemic N25.0
  congenital Q78.9
  parathyroid, secondary E21.1
  renal N25.0
Osteofibroma —*see* Neoplasm, bone,
    benign

Osteofibrosarcoma —*see* Neoplasm, bone, malignant
Osteogenesis imperfecta Q78.0
Osteogenic —*see* condition
Osteolysis M89.50
  carpus M89.54-
  clavicle M89.51-
  femur M89.55-
  fibula M89.56-
  finger M89.54-
  humerus M89.52-
  ilium M89.559
  ischium M89.559
  joint prosthesis (periprosthetic) —*see* Complications, joint prosthesis, mechanical, periprosthetic, osteolysis, by site
  metacarpus M89.54-
  metatarsus M89.57-
  multiple sites M89.59
  neck M89.58
  periprosthetic —*see* Complications, joint prosthesis, mechanical, periprosthetic, osteolysis, by site
  radius M89.53-
  rib M89.58
  scapula M89.51-
  skull M89.58
  tarsus M89.57-
  tibia M89.56-
  toe M89.57-
  ulna M89.53-
  vertebra M89.58
Osteoma —*see also* Neoplasm, bone, benign
  osteoid —*see also* Neoplasm, bone, benign
  giant —*see* Neoplasm, bone, benign
Osteomalacia M83.9
  adult M83.9
    drug-induced NEC M83.5
    due to
      malabsorption (postsurgical) M83.2
      malnutrition M83.3
    specified NEC M83.8
  aluminium-induced M83.4
  infantile —*see* Rickets
  juvenile —*see* Rickets
  oncogenic E83.89
  pelvis M83.8
  puerperal M83.0
  senile M83.1
  vitamin-D-resistant in adults E83.31 *[M90.8-]*
    carpus E83.31 *[M90.84-]*
    clavicle E83.31 *[M90.81-]*
    femur E83.31 *[M90.85-]*
    fibula E83.31 *[M90.86-]*
    finger E83.31 *[M90.84-]*
    humerus E83.31 *[M90.82-]*
    ilium E83.31 *[M90.859]*
    ischium E83.31 *[M90.859]*
    metacarpus E83.31 *[M90.84-]*
    metatarsus E83.31 *[M90.87-]*
    multiple sites E83.31 *[M90.89]*
    neck E83.31 *[M90.88]*
    radius E83.31 *[M90.83-]*
    rib E83.31 *[M90.88]*
    scapula E83.31 *[M90.819]*
    skull E83.31 *[M90.88]*
    tarsus E83.31 *[M90.879]*
    tibia E83.31 *[M90.869]*
    toe E83.31 *[M90.879]*
    ulna E83.31 *[M90.839]*
    vertebra E83.31 *[M90.88]*

Osteomyelitis (general) (infective) (localized) (neonatal) (purulent) (septic) (staphylococcal) (streptococcal) (suppurative) (with periostitis) M86.9
  acute M86.10
    carpus M86.14-
    clavicle M86.11-
    femur M86.15-
    fibula M86.16-
    finger M86.14-
    hematogenous M86.00
      carpus M86.04-
      clavicle M86.01-
      femur M86.05-
      fibula M86.06-
      finger M86.04-
      humerus M86.02-
      ilium M86.059
      ischium M86.059
      mandible M27.2
      metacarpus M86.04-
      metatarsus M86.07-
      multiple sites M86.09
      neck M86.08
      orbit H05.02-
      petrous bone —*see* Petrositis
      radius M86.03-
      rib M86.08
      scapula M86.01-
      skull M86.08
      tarsus M86.07-
      tibia M86.06-
      toe M86.07-
      ulna M86.03-
      vertebra —*see* Osteomyelitis, vertebra
    humerus M86.12-
    ilium M86.159
    ischium M86.159
    mandible M27.2
    metacarpus M86.14-
    metatarsus M86.17-
    multiple sites M86.19
    neck M86.18
    orbit H05.02-
    petrous bone —*see* Petrositis
    radius M86.13-
    rib M86.18
    scapula M86.11-
    skull M86.18
    tarsus M86.17-
    tibia M86.16-
    toe M86.17-
    ulna M86.13-
    vertebra —*see* Osteomyelitis, vertebra
  chronic (or old) M86.60
    with draining sinus M86.40
      carpus M86.44-
      clavicle M86.41-
      femur M86.45-
      fibula M86.46-
      finger M86.44-
      humerus M86.42-
      ilium M86.459
      ischium M86.459
      mandible M27.2
      metacarpus M86.44-
      metatarsus M86.47-
      multiple sites M86.49
      neck M86.48
      orbit H05.02-
      petrous bone —*see* Petrositis

Osteomyelitis *(Continued)*
  chronic *(Continued)*
    with draining sinus *(Continued)*
      radius M86.43-
      rib M86.48
      scapula M86.41-
      skull M86.48
      tarsus M86.47-
      tibia M86.46-
      toe M86.47-
      ulna M86.43-
      vertebra —*see* Osteomyelitis, vertebra
    carpus M86.64-
    clavicle M86.61-
    femur M86.65-
    fibula M86.66-
    finger M86.64-
    hematogenous NEC M86.50
      carpus M86.54-
      clavicle M86.51-
      femur M86.55-
      fibula M86.56-
      finger M86.54-
      humerus M86.52-
      ilium M86.559
      ischium M86.559
      mandible M27.2
      metacarpus M86.54-
      metatarsus M86.57-
      multifocal M86.30
        carpus M86.34-
        clavicle M86.31-
        femur M86.35-
        fibula M86.36-
        finger M86.34-
        humerus M86.32-
        ilium M86.359
        ischium M86.359
        metacarpus M86.34-
        metatarsus M86.37-
        multiple sites M86.39
        neck M86.38
        radius M86.33-
        rib M86.38
        scapula M86.31-
        skull M86.38
        tarsus M86.37-
        tibia M86.36-
        toe M86.37-
        ulna M86.33-
        vertebra —*see* Osteomyelitis, vertebra
      multiple sites M86.59
      neck M86.58
      orbit H05.02-
      petrous bone —*see* Petrositis
      radius M86.53-
      rib M86.58
      scapula M86.51-
      skull M86.58
      tarsus M86.57-
      tibia M86.56-
      toe M86.57-
      ulna M86.53-
      vertebra —*see* Osteomyelitis, vertebra
    humerus M86.62-
    ilium M86.659
    ischium M86.659
    mandible M27.2
    metacarpus M86.64-
    metatarsus M86.67-
    multifocal —*see* Osteomyelitis, chronic, hematogenous, multifocal

Osteomyelitis *(Continued)*
  chronic *(Continued)*
    multiple sites M86.69
    neck M86.68
    orbit H05.02-
    petrous bone —*see* Petrositis
    radius M86.63-
    rib M86.68
    scapula M86.61-
    skull M86.68
    tarsus M86.67-
    tibia M86.66-
    toe M86.67-
    ulna M86.63-
    vertebra —*see* Osteomyelitis,
      vertebra
  echinococcal B67.2
  Garr's —*see* Osteomyelitis, specified
    type NEC
  jaw (acute) (chronic) (lower) (neonatal)
    (suppurative) (upper) M27.2
  nonsuppurating —*see* Osteomyelitis,
    specified type NEC
  orbit H05.02-
  petrous bone —*see* Petrositis
  Salmonella (arizonae) (cholerae-suis)
    (enteritidis) (typhimurium)
    A02.24
  sclerosing, nonsuppurative —*see*
    Osteomyelitis, specified type
    NEC
  specified type NEC (*see also*
    subcategory) M86.8X-
    mandible M27.2
    orbit H05.02-
    petrous bone —*see* Petrositis
    vertebra —*see* Osteomyelitis,
      vertebra
  subacute M86.20
    carpus M86.24-
    clavicle M86.21-
    femur M86.25-
    fibula M86.26-
    finger M86.24-
    humerus M86.22-
    mandible M27.2
    metacarpus M86.24-
    metatarsus M86.27-
    multiple sites M86.29
    neck M86.28
    orbit H05.02-
    petrous bone —*see* Petrositis
    radius M86.23-
    rib M86.28
    scapula M86.21-
    skull M86.28
    tarsus M86.27-
    tibia M86.26-
    toe M86.27-
    ulna M86.23-
    vertebra —*see* Osteomyelitis, vertebra
  syphilitic A52.77
    congenital (early) A50.02 *[M90.80]*
  tuberculous —*see* Tuberculosis, bone
  typhoid A01.05
  vertebra M46.20
    cervical region M46.22
    cervicothoracic region M46.23
    lumbar region M46.26
    lumbosacral region M46.27
    occipito-atlanto-axial region M46.21
    sacrococcygeal region M46.28
    thoracic region M46.24
    thoracolumbar region M46.25

Osteomyelofibrosis D75.89
Osteomyelosclerosis D75.89
Osteonecrosis M87.9
  due to
    drugs —*see* Osteonecrosis, secondary,
      due to, drugs
    trauma —*see* Osteonecrosis,
      secondary, due to, trauma
  idiopathic aseptic M87.00
    ankle M87.07-
    carpus M87.03-
    clavicle M87.01-
    femur M87.05-
    fibula M87.06-
    finger M87.04-
    humerus M87.02-
    ilium M87.050
    ischium M87.050
    metacarpus M87.04-
    metatarsus M87.07-
    multiple sites M87.09
    neck M87.08
    pelvis M87.050
    radius M87.03-
    rib M87.08
    scapula M87.01-
    skull M87.08
    tarsus M87.07-
    tibia M87.06-
    toe M87.07-
    ulna M87.03-
    vertebra M87.08
  secondary NEC M87.30
    carpus M87.33-
    clavicle M87.31-
    due to
      drugs M87.10
        carpus M87.13-
        clavicle M87.11-
        femur M87.15-
        fibula M87.16-
        finger M87.14-
        humerus M87.12-
        ilium M87.159
        ischium M87.159
        jaw M87.180
        metacarpus M87.14-
        metatarsus M87.17-
        multiple sites M87.19
        neck M87.18
        radius M87.13-
        rib M87.18
        scapula M87.11-
        skull M87.18
        tarsus M87.17-
        tibia M87.16-
        toe M87.17-
        ulna M87.13-
        vertebra M87.18
      hemoglobinopathy NEC D58.2
        [M90.50]
        carpus D58.2 *[M90.54-]*
        clavicle D58.2 *[M90.51-]*
        femur D58.2 *[M90.55-]*
        fibula D58.2 *[M90.56-]*
        finger D58.2 *[M90.54-]*
        humerus D58.2 *[M90.52-]*
        ilium D58.2 *[M90.55-]*
        ischium D58.2 *[M90.55-]*
        metacarpus D58.2 *[M90.54-]*
        metatarsus D58.2 *[M90.57-]*
        multiple sites D58.2 *[M90.58]*
        neck D58.2 *[M90.58]*
        radius D58.2 *[M90.53-]*
        rib D58.2 *[M90.58]*

Osteonecrosis *(Continued)*
  secondary NEC *(Continued)*
    due to *(Continued)*
      hemoglobinopathy NEC
        (Continued)
        scapula D58.2 *[M90.51-]*
        skull D58.2 *[M90.58]*
        tarsus D58.2 *[M90.57-]*
        tibia D58.2 *[M90.56-]*
        toe D58.2 *[M90.57-]*
        ulna D58.2 *[M90.53-]*
        vertebra D58.2 *[M90.58]*
      trauma (previous) M87.20
        carpus M87.23-
        clavicle M87.21-
        femur M87.25-
        fibula M87.26-
        finger M87.24-
        humerus M87.22-
        ilium M87.25-
        ischium M87.25-
        metacarpus M87.24-
        metatarsus M87.27-
        multiple sites M87.29
        neck M87.28
        radius M87.23-
        rib M87.28
        scapula M87.21-
        skull M87.28
        tarsus M87.27-
        tibia M87.26-
        toe M87.27-
        ulna M87.23-
        vertebra M87.28
      femur M87.35-
      fibula M87.36-
      finger M87.34-
      humerus M87.32
      ilium M87.350
      in
        caisson disease T70.3 *[M90.50]*
          carpus T70.3 *[M90.54-]*
          clavicle T70.3 *[M90.51-]*
          femur T70.3 *[M90.55-]*
          fibula T70.3 *[M90.56-]*
          finger T70.3 *[M90.54-]*
          humerus T70.3 *[M90.52-]*
          ilium T70.3 *[M90.55-]*
          ischium T70.3 *[M90.55-]*
          metacarpus T70.3 *[M90.54-]*
          metatarsus T70.3 *[M90.57-]*
          multiple sites T70.3 *[M90.59]*
          neck T70.3 *[M90.58]*
          radius T70.3 *[M90.53-]*
          rib T70.3 *[M90.58]*
          scapula T70.3 *[M90.51-]*
          skull T70.3 *[M90.58]*
          tarsus T70.3 *[M90.57-]*
          tibia T70.3 *[M90.56-]*
          toe T70.3 *[M90.57-]*
          ulna T70.3 *[M90.53-]*
          vertebra T70.3 *[M90.58]*
      ischium M87.350
      metacarpus M87.34-
      metatarsus M87.37-
      multiple site M87.39
      neck M87.38
      radius M87.33-
      rib M87.38
      scapula M87.319
      skull M87.38
      tarsus M87.379
      tibia M87.366
      toe M87.379

Osteonecrosis (Continued)
  secondary NEC (Continued)
    ulna M87.33-
    vertebra M87.38
  specified type NEC M87.80
    carpus M87.83-
    clavicle M87.81-
    femur M87.85-
    fibula M87.86-
    finger M87.84-
    humerus M87.82-
    ilium M87.85-
    ischium M87.85-
    metacarpus M87.84-
    metatarsus M87.87-
    multiple sites M87.89
    neck M87.88
    radius M87.83-
    rib M87.88-
    scapula M87.81-
    skull M87.88
    tarsus M87.87-
    tibia M87.86-
    toe M87.87-
    ulna M87.83-
    vertebra M87.88
Osteo-onycho-arthro-dysplasia Q79.8
Osteo-onychodysplasia, hereditary Q79.8
Osteopathia condensans disseminata
    Q78.8
Osteopathy —see also Osteomyelitis,
    Osteonecrosis, Osteoporosis
  after poliomyelitis M89.60
    carpus M89.64-
    clavicle M89.61-
    femur M89.65-
    fibula M89.66-
    finger M89.64-
    humerus M89.62-
    ilium M89.659
    ischium M89.659
    metacarpus M89.64-
    metatarsus M89.67-
    multiple sites M89.69
    neck M89.68
    radius M89.63-
    rib M89.68
    scapula M89.61-
    skull M89.68
    tarsus M89.67-
    tibia M89.66-
    toe M89.67-
    ulna M89.63-
    vertebra M89.68
  in (due to)
    renal osteodystrophy N25.0
    specified diseases classified
        elsewhere —see subcategory
        M90.8
Osteopenia M85.8-
  borderline M85.8-
Osteoperiostitis —see Osteomyelitis,
    specified type NEC
Osteopetrosis (familial) Q78.2
Osteophyte M25.70
  ankle M25.77-
  elbow M25.72-
  foot joint M25.77-
  hand joint M25.74-
  hip M25.75-
  knee M25.76-
  shoulder M25.71-
  spine M25.78
  vertebrae M25.78
  wrist M25.73-

Osteopoikilosis Q78.8
Osteoporosis (female) (male) M81.0
  with current pathological fracture
      M80.00
  age-related M81.0
    with current pathologic fracture
        M80.00
      carpus M80.04-
      clavicle M80.01-
      fibula M80.06-
      finger M80.04-
      humerus M80.02-
      ilium M80.05-
      ischium M80.05-
      metacarpus M80.04-
      metatarsus M80.07-
      pelvis M80.05-
      radius M80.03-
      scapula M80.01-
      tarsus M80.07-
      tibia M80.06-
      toe M80.07-
      ulna M80.03-
      vertebra M80.08
  disuse M81.8
    with current pathological fracture
        M80.80
      carpus M80.84-
      clavicle M80.81-
      fibula M80.86-
      finger M80.84-
      humerus M80.82-
      ilium M80.85-
      ischium M80.85-
      metacarpus M80.84-
      metatarsus M80.87-
      pelvis M80.85-
      radius M80.83-
      scapula M80.81-
      tarsus M80.87-
      tibia M80.86-
      toe M80.87-
      ulna M80.83-
      vertebra M80.88
  drug-induced —see Osteoporosis,
      specified type NEC
  idiopathic —see Osteoporosis, specified
      type NEC
  involutional —see Osteoporosis,
      age-related
  Lequesne M81.6
  localized M81.6
  postmenopausal M81.0
    with pathological fracture
        M80.00
      carpus M80.04-
      clavicle M80.01-
      fibula M80.06-
      finger M80.04-
      humerus M80.02-
      ilium M80.05-
      ischium M80.05-
      metacarpus M80.04-
      metatarsus M80.07-
      pelvis M80.05-
      radius M80.03-
      scapula M80.01-
      tarsus M80.07-
      tibia M80.06-
      toe M80.07-
      ulna M80.03-
      vertebra M80.08
  postoophorectomy —see Osteoporosis,
      specified type NEC

Osteoporosis (Continued)
  postsurgical malabsorption —see
      Osteoporosis, specified type
      NEC
  post-traumatic —see Osteoporosis,
      specified type NEC
  senile —see Osteoporosis, age-related
  specified type NEC M81.8
    with pathological fracture M80.80
      carpus M80.84-
      clavicle M80.81-
      fibula M80.86-
      finger M80.84-
      humerus M80.82-
      ilium M80.85-
      ischium M80.85-
      metacarpus M80.84-
      metatarsus M80.87-
      pelvis M80.85-
      radius M80.83-
      scapula M80.81-
      tarsus M80.87-
      tibia M80.86-
      toe M80.87-
      ulna M80.83-
      vertebra M80.88
Osteopsathyrosis (idiopathica) Q78.0
Osteoradionecrosis, jaw (acute)
    (chronic) (lower) (suppurative)
    (upper) M27.2
Osteosarcoma (any form) —see
    Neoplasm, bone, malignant
Osteosclerosis Q78.2
  acquired M85.8-
  congenita Q77.4
  fragilitas (generalisata) Q78.2
  myelofibrosis D75.81
Osteosclerotic anemia D64.89
Osteosis
  cutis L94.2
  renal fibrocystic N25.0
Österreicher-Turner syndrome Q87.2
Ostium
  atrioventriculare commune Q21.2
  primum (arteriosum) (defect)
      (persistent) Q21.2
  secundum (arteriosum) (defect) (patent)
      (persistent) Q21.1
Ostrum-Furst syndrome Q75.8
Otalgia —see subcategory H92.0
Otitis (acute) H66.90
  with effusion —see also Otitis, media,
      nonsuppurative
    purulent —see Otitis, media,
        suppurative
  adhesive —see subcategory H74.1
  chronic —see also Otitis, media, chronic
    with effusion —see also Otitis, media,
        nonsuppurative, chronic
  externa H60.9-
    abscess —see Abscess, ear, external
    acute (noninfective) H60.50-
      actinic H60.51-
      chemical H60.52-
      contact H60.53-
      eczematoid H60.54-
      infective —see Otitis, externa,
          infective
      reactive H60.55-
      specified NEC H60.59-
    cellulitis —see Cellulitis, ear
    chronic H60.6-
    diffuse —see Otitis, externa, infective,
        diffuse

381

Otitis *(Continued)*
  externa *(Continued)*
    hemorrhagic —*see* Otitis, externa,
        infective, hemorrhagic
    in (due to)
      aspergillosis B44.89
      candidiasis B37.84
      erysipelas A46 *[H62.40]*
      herpes (simplex) virus infection
          B00.1
        zoster B02.8
      impetigo L01.00 *[H62.40]*
      infectious disease NEC B99
          [H62.4-]
      mycosis NEC B36.9 *[H62.40]*
      parasitic disease NEC B89 *[H62.40]*
      viral disease NEC B34.9 *[H62.40]*
      zoster B02.8
    infective NEC H60.39-
      abscess —*see* Abscess, ear, external
      cellulitis —*see* Cellulitis, ear
      diffuse H60.31-
      hemorrhagic H60.32-
      swimmer's ear —*see* Swimmer's,
          ear
    malignant H60.2-
    mycotic B36.9 *[H62.40]*
      necrotizing —*see* Otitis, externa,
          malignant
      Pseudomonas aeruginosa —*see* Otitis,
          externa, malignant
      reactive —*see* Otitis, externa, acute,
          reactive
      specified NEC —*see* subcategory
          H60.8
    tropical B36.8
    insidiosa —*see* Otosclerosis
    interna —*see* subcategory H83.0
    media (hemorrhagic) (staphylococcal)
        (streptococcal) H66.9-
      with effusion (nonpurulent) —*see*
          Otitis, media, nonsuppurative
      acute, subacute H66.90
        allergic —*see* Otitis, media,
            nonsuppurative, acute,
            allergic
        exudative —*see* Otitis, media,
            nonsuppurative, acute
        mucoid —*see* Otitis, media,
            nonsuppurative, acute
        necrotizing —*see also* Otitis, media,
            suppurative, acute
          in
            measles B05.3
            scarlet fever A38.0
        nonsuppurative NEC —*see* Otitis,
            media, nonsuppurative,
            acute
        purulent —*see* Otitis, media,
            suppurative, acute
        sanguinous —*see* Otitis, media,
            nonsuppurative, acute
        secretory —*see* Otitis, media,
            nonsuppurative, acute, serous
        seromucinous —*see* Otitis, media,
            nonsuppurative, acute
        serous —*see* Otitis, media,
            nonsuppurative, acute, serous
        suppurative —*see* Otitis, media,
            suppurative, acute
      allergic —*see* Otitis, media,
          nonsuppurative
      catarrhal —*see* Otitis, media,
          nonsuppurative

Otitis *(Continued)*
  media *(Continued)*
    chronic H66.90
      with effusion (nonpurulent) —*see*
          Otitis, media, nonsuppurative,
          chronic
      allergic —*see* Otitis, media,
          nonsuppurative, chronic,
          allergic
      benign suppurative —*see* Otitis,
          media, suppurative, chronic,
          tubotympanic
      catarrhal —*see* Otitis, media,
          nonsuppurative, chronic,
          serous
      exudative —*see* Otitis, media,
          nonsuppurative, chronic
      mucinous —*see* Otitis, media,
          nonsuppurative, chronic,
          mucoid
      mucoid —*see* Otitis, media,
          nonsuppurative, chronic,
          mucoid
      nonsuppurative NEC —*see* Otitis,
          media, nonsuppurative,
          chronic
      purulent —*see* Otitis, media,
          suppurative, chronic
      secretory —*see* Otitis, media,
          nonsuppurative, chronic,
          mucoid
      seromucinous —*see* Otitis, media,
          nonsuppurative, chronic
      serous —*see* Otitis, media,
          nonsuppurative, chronic,
          serous
      suppurative —*see* Otitis, media,
          suppurative, chronic
      transudative —*see* Otitis, media,
          nonsuppurative, chronic,
          mucoid
    exudative —*see* Otitis, media,
        nonsuppurative
    in (due to) (with)
      influenza —*see* Influenza, with,
          otitis media
      measles B05.3
      scarlet fever A38.0
      tuberculosis A18.6
      viral disease NEC B34.- *[H67.-]*
    mucoid —*see* Otitis, media,
        nonsuppurative
    nonsuppurative H65.9-
      acute or subacute NEC H65.19-
        allergic H65.11-
          recurrent H65.11-
        recurrent H65.19-
        secretory —*see* Otitis, media,
            nonsuppurative, serous
      serous H65.0-
        recurrent H65.0-
      chronic H65.49-
        allergic H65.41-
        mucoid H65.3-
        serous H65.2-
      postmeasles B05.3
      purulent —*see* Otitis, media,
          suppurative
      secretory —*see* Otitis, media,
          nonsuppurative
      seromucinous —*see* Otitis, media,
          nonsuppurative
      serous —*see* Otitis, media,
          nonsuppurative

Otitis *(Continued)*
  media *(Continued)*
    suppurative H66.4-
      acute H66.00-
        with rupture of ear drum H66.01-
        recurrent H66.00-
          with rupture of ear drum
              H66.01-
      chronic (*see also* subcategory) H66.3
        atticoantral H66.2-
        benign —*see* Otitis, media,
            suppurative, chronic,
            tubotympanic
        tubotympanic H66.1-
      transudative —*see* Otitis, media,
          nonsuppurative
    tuberculous A18.6
  Otocephaly Q18.2
  Otolith syndrome —*see* subcategory
      H81.8
  Otomycosis (diffuse) NEC B36.9
      [H62.40]
    in
      aspergillosis B44.89
      candidiasis B37.84
      moniliasis B37.84
  Otoporosis —*see* Otosclerosis
  Otorrhagia (nontraumatic) H92.2-
    traumatic - code by Type of injury
  Otorrhea H92.1-
    cerebrospinal G96.0
  Otosclerosis (general) H80.9-
    cochlear (endosteal) H80.2-
    involving
      otic capsule —*see* Otosclerosis,
          cochlear
      oval window
        nonobliterative H80.0-
        obliterative H80.1-
      round window —*see* Otosclerosis,
          cochlear
    nonobliterative —*see* Otosclerosis,
        involving, oval window,
        nonobliterative
    obliterative —*see* Otosclerosis,
        involving, oval window,
        obliterative
    specified NEC H80.8-
  Otospongiosis —*see* Otosclerosis
  Otto's disease or pelvis M24.7
  Outcome of delivery Z37.9
    multiple births Z37.9
      all liveborn Z37.50
        quadruplets Z37.52
        quintuplets Z37.53
        sextuplets Z37.54
        specified number NEC Z37.59
        triplets Z37.51
      all stillborn Z37.7
      some liveborn Z37.60
        quadruplets Z37.62
        quintuplets Z37.63
        sextuplets Z37.64
        specified number NEC
            Z37.69
        triplets Z37.61
    single NEC Z37.9
      liveborn Z37.0
      stillborn Z37.1
    twins NEC Z37.9
      both liveborn Z37.2
      both stillborn Z37.4
      one liveborn, one stillborn Z37.3
  Outlet —*see* condition

Ovalocytosis (congenital) (hereditary) —
see Elliptocytosis
Ovarian —see Condition
Ovariocele N83.4
Ovaritis (cystic) —see Oophoritis
Ovary, ovarian —see also condition
resistant syndrome E28.39
vein syndrome N13.8
Overactive —see also Hyperfunction
adrenal cortex NEC E27.0
bladder N32.81
hypothalamus E23.3
thyroid —see Hyperthyroidism
Overactivity R46.3
child —see Disorder, attention-deficit
hyperactivity
Overbite (deep) (excessive) (horizontal)
(vertical) M26.29
Overbreathing —see Hyperventilation
Overconscientious personality F60.5
Overdevelopment —see Hypertrophy
Overdistension —see Distension
Overdose, overdosage (drug) —see Table
of drugs and chemicals, by drug,
poisoning
Overeating R63.2
nonorganic origin F50.8
psychogenic F50.8
Overexertion (effects) (exhaustion) T73.3
Overexposure (effects) T73.9
exhaustion T73.2
Overfeeding —see Overeating
newborn P92.4

Overfill, endodontic M27.52
Overgrowth, bone —see Hypertrophy,
bone
Overhanging of dental restorative
material (unrepairable) K08.52
Overheated (places) (effects) —see Heat
Overjet (excessive horizontal) M26.23
Overlaid, overlying (suffocation) —
see Asphyxia, traumatic, due to
mechanical threat
Overlap, excessive horizontal (teeth)
M26.23
Overlapping toe (acquired) —see also
Deformity, toe, specified NEC
congenital (fifth toe) Q66.89
Overload
circulatory, due to transfusion (blood)
(blood components) (TACO)
E87.71
fluid E87.70
due to transfusion (blood) (blood
components) E87.71
specified NEC E87.79
iron, due to repeated red blood cell
transfusions E83.111
potassium (K) E87.5
sodium (Na) E87.0
Overnutrition —see Hyperalimentation
Overproduction —see also Hypersecretion
ACTH E27.0
catecholamine E27.5
growth hormone E22.0

Overprotection, child by parent
Z62.1
Overriding
aorta Q25.4
finger (acquired) —see Deformity,
finger
congenital Q68.1
toe (acquired) —see also Deformity, toe,
specified NEC
congenital Q66.89
Overstrained R53.83
heart —see Hypertrophy, cardiac
Overuse, muscle NEC M70.8-
Overweight E66.3
Overworked R53.83
Oviduct —see condition
Ovotestis Q56.0
Ovulation (cycle)
failure or lack of N97.0
pain N94.0
Ovum —see condition
Owren's disease or syndrome
(parahemophilia) D68.2
Ox heart —see Hypertrophy, cardiac
Oxalosis E72.53
Oxaluria E72.53
Oxycephaly, oxycephalic Q75.0
syphilitic, congenital A50.02
Oxyuriasis B80
Oxyuris vermicularis (infestation)
B80
Ozena J31.0

P

Pachyderma, pachydermia L85.9
  larynx (verrucosa) J38.7
Pachydermatocele (congenital) Q82.8
Pachydermoperiostosis —see also
      Osteoarthropathy, hypertrophic,
      specified type NEC
  clubbed nail M89.40 [L62]
Pachygyria Q04.3
Pachymeningitis (adhesive) (basal)
      (brain) (cervical) (chronic)
      (circumscribed) (external) (fibrous)
      (hemorrhagic) (hypertrophic)
      (internal) (purulent) (spinal)
      (suppurative) —see Meningitis
Pachyonychia (congenital) Q84.5
Pacinian tumor —see Neoplasm, skin,
      benign
Pad, knuckle or Garrod's M72.1
Paget-Schroetter syndrome I82.890
Paget's disease
  with infiltrating duct carcinoma —see
      Neoplasm, breast, malignant
  bone M88.9
    carpus M88.84-
    clavicle M88.81-
    femur M88.85-
    fibula M88.86-
    finger M88.84-
    humerus M88.82-
    ilium M88.85-
    in neoplastic disease —see Osteitis,
        deformans, in neoplastic
        disease
    ischium M88.85-
    metacarpus M88.84-
    metatarsus M88.87-
    multiple sites M88.89
    neck M88.88
    radius M88.83-
    rib M88.88
    scapula M88.81-
    skull M88.0
    tarsus M88.87-
    tibia M88.86-
    toe M88.87-
    ulna M88.83-
    vertebra M88.88
  breast (female) C50.01-
    male C50.02-
  extramammary —see also Neoplasm,
      skin, malignant
    anus C21.0
      margin C44.590
      skin C44.590
  intraductal carcinoma —see Neoplasm,
      breast, malignant
  malignant —see Neoplasm, skin,
      malignant
    breast (female) C50.01-
      male C50.02-
    unspecified site (female) C50.01-
      male C50.02-
  mammary —see Paget's disease,
      breast
  nipple —see Paget's disease, breast
  osteitis deformans —see Paget's disease,
      bone
Pain (s) (see also Painful) R52
  abdominal R10.9
    colic R10.83
    generalized R10.84
      with acute abdomen R10.0

Pain (s) (Continued)
  abdominal (Continued)
    lower R10.30
      left quadrant R10.32
      pelvic or perineal R10.2
      periumbilical R10.33
      right quadrant R10.31
    rebound —see Tenderness,
        abdominal, rebound
    severe with abdominal rigidity
        R10.0
    tenderness —see Tenderness,
        abdominal
    upper R10.10
      epigastric R10.13
      left quadrant R10.12
      right quadrant R10.11
  acute R52
    due to trauma G89.11
    neoplasm related G89.3
    postprocedural NEC G89.18
    post-thoracotomy G89.12
    specified by site — code to Pain,
        by site
  adnexa (uteri) R10.2
  anginoid —see Pain, precordial
  anus K62.89
  arm —see Pain, limb, upper
  axillary (axilla) M79.62-
  back (postural) M54.9
  bladder R39.89
    associated with micturition —see
        Micturition, painful
  bone —see Disorder, bone, specified
      type NEC
  breast N64.4
  broad ligament R10.2
  cancer associated (acute) (chronic)
      G89.3
  cecum —see Pain, abdominal
  cervicobrachial M53.1
  chest (central) R07.9
    anterior wall R07.89
    atypical R07.89
    ischemic I20.9
    musculoskeletal R07.89
    non-cardiac R07.89
    on breathing R07.1
    pleurodynia R07.81
    precordial R07.2
    wall (anterior) R07.89
  chronic G89.29
    associated with significant
        psychosocial dysfunction G89.4
    due to trauma G89.21
    neoplasm related G89.3
    postoperative NEC G89.28
    postprocedural NEC G89.28
    post-thoracotomy G89.22
    specified NEC G89.29
  coccyx M53.3
  colon —see Pain, abdominal
  coronary —see Angina
  costochondral R07.1
  diaphragm R07.1
  due to cancer G89.3
  due to device, implant or graft (see also
      Complications, by site and type,
      specified NEC) T85.84
    arterial graft NEC T82.848
    breast (implant) T85.84
    catheter NEC T85.84
      dialysis (renal) T82.848
      intraperitoneal T85.84

Pain (s) (Continued)
  due to device, implant or graft
      (Continued)
    catheter NEC (Continued)
      infusion NEC T82.848
        spinal (epidural) (subdural)
            T85.84
      urinary (indwelling) T83.84
    electronic (electrode) (pulse
        generator) (stimulator)
      bone T84.84
      cardiac T82.847
      nervous system (brain) (peripheral
          nerve) (spinal) T85.84
      urinary T83.84
    fixation, internal (orthopedic) NEC
        T84.84
    gastrointestinal (bile duct)
        (esophagus) T85.84
    genital NEC T83.84
    heart NEC T82.847
    infusion NEC T85.84
    joint prosthesis T84.84
    ocular (corneal graft) (orbital
        implant) NEC T85.84
    orthopedic NEC T84.84
    specified NEC T85.84
    urinary NEC T83.84
    vascular NEC T82.848
    ventricular intracranial shunt T85.84
  due to malignancy (primary)
      (secondary) G89.3
  ear —see subcategory H92.0
  epigastric, epigastrium R10.13
  eye —see Pain, ocular
  face, facial R51
    atypical G50.1
  female genital organs NEC N94.89
  finger —see Pain, limb, upper
  flank —see Pain, abdominal
  foot —see Pain, limb, lower
  gallbladder K82.9
  gas (intestinal) R14.1
  gastric —see Pain, abdominal
  generalized NOS R52
  genital organ
    female N94.89
    male N50.8
  groin —see Pain, abdominal, lower
  hand —see Pain, limb, upper
  head —see Headache
  heart —see Pain, precordial
  infra-orbital —see Neuralgia, trigeminal
  intercostal R07.82
  intermenstrual N94.0
  jaw R68.84
  joint M25.50
    ankle M25.57-
    elbow M25.52-
    finger M79.64-
    foot M79.67-
    hand M79.64-
    hip M25.55-
    knee M25.56-
    shoulder M25.51-
    toe M79.67-
    wrist M25.53-
  kidney N23
  laryngeal R07.0
  leg —see Pain, limb, lower
  limb M79.609
    lower M79.60-
      foot M79.67-
      lower leg M79.66-

Pain (s) (*Continued*)
limb (*Continued*)
lower (*Continued*)
thigh M79.65-
toe M79.67-
upper M79.60-
axilla M79.62-
finger M79.64-
forearm M79.63-
hand M79.64-
upper arm M79.62-
loin M54.5
low back M54.5
lumbar region M54.5
mandibular R68.84
mastoid —*see* subcategory H92.0
maxilla R68.84
menstrual (*see also* Dysmenorrhea) N94.6
metacarpophalangeal (joint) —*see* Pain, joint, hand
metatarsophalangeal (joint) —*see* Pain, joint, foot
mouth K13.79
muscle —*see* Myalgia
musculoskeletal (*see also* Pain, by site) M79.1
myofascial M79.1
nasal J34.89
nasopharynx J39.2
neck NEC M54.2
nerve NEC —*see* Neuralgia
neuromuscular —*see* Neuralgia
nose J34.89
ocular H57.1-
ophthalmic —*see* Pain, ocular
orbital region —*see* Pain, ocular
ovary N94.89
over heart —*see* Pain, precordial
ovulation N94.0
pelvic (female) R10.2
penis N48.89
pericardial —*see* Pain, precordial
perineal, perineum R10.2
pharynx J39.2
pleura, pleural, pleuritic R07.89
postoperative NOS G89.18
postprocedural NOS G89.18
post-thoracotomy G89.12
precordial (region) R07.2
premenstrual N94.3
psychogenic (persistent) (any site) F45.41
radicular (spinal) —*see* Radiculopathy
rectum K62.89
respiration R07.1
retrosternal R07.2
rheumatoid, muscular —*see* Myalgia
rib R07.81
root (spinal) —*see* Radiculopathy
round ligament (stretch) R10.2
sacroiliac M53.3
sciatic —*see* Sciatica
scrotum N50.8
seminal vesicle N50.8
shoulder M25.51-
spermatic cord N50.8
spinal root —*see* Radiculopathy
spine M54.9
cervical M54.2
low back M54.5
with sciatica M54.4-
thoracic M54.6
stomach —*see* Pain, abdominal
substernal R07.2

Pain (s) (*Continued*)
temporomandibular (joint) M26.62
testis N50.8
thoracic spine M54.6
with radicular and visceral pain M54.14
throat R07.0
tibia —*see* Pain, limb, lower
toe —*see* Pain, limb, lower
tongue K14.6
tooth K08.8
trigeminal —*see* Neuralgia, trigeminal
tumor associated G89.3
ureter N23
urinary (organ) (system) N23
uterus NEC N94.89
vagina R10.2
vertebrogenic (syndrome) M54.89
vesical R39.89
associated with micturition —*see* Micturition, painful
vulva R10.2
Painful —*see also* Pain
coitus
female N94.1
male N53.12
psychogenic F52.6
ejaculation (semen) N53.12
psychogenic F52.6
erection —*see* Priapism
feet syndrome E53.8
joint replacement (hip) (knee) T84.84
menstruation —*see* Dysmenorrhea
psychogenic F45.8
micturition —*see* Micturition, painful
respiration R07.1
scar NEC L90.5
wire sutures T81.89
Painter's colic —*see* subcategory T56.0
Palate —*see* condition
Palatoplegia K13.79
Palatoschisis —*see* Cleft, palate
Palilalia R48.8
Palliative care Z51.5
Pallor R23.1
optic disc, temporal —*see* Atrophy, optic
Palmar —*see also* condition
fascia —*see* condition
Palpable
cecum K63.89
kidney N28.89
ovary N83.8
prostate N42.9
spleen —*see* Splenomegaly
Palpitations (heart) R00.2
psychogenic F45.8
Palsy (*see also* Paralysis) G83.9
atrophic diffuse (progressive) G12.22
Bell's —*see also* Palsy, facial
newborn P11.3
brachial plexus NEC G54.0
newborn (birth injury) P14.3
brain —*see* Palsy, cerebral
bulbar (progressive) (chronic) G12.22
of childhood (Fazio-Londe) G12.1
pseudo NEC G12.29
supranuclear (progressive) G23.1
cerebral (congenital) G80.9
ataxic G80.4
athetoid G80.3
choreathetoid G80.3

Palsy (*Continued*)
cerebral (*Continued*)
diplegic G80.8
spastic G80.1
dyskinetic G80.3
athetoid G80.3
choreathetoid G80.3
distonic G80.3
dystonic G80.3
hemiplegic G80.8
spastic G80.2
mixed G80.8
monoplegic G80.8
spastic G80.1
paraplegic G80.8
spastic G80.1
quadriplegic G80.8
spastic G80.0
spastic G80.1
diplegic G80.1
hemiplegic G80.2
monoplegic G80.1
quadriplegic G80.0
specified NEC G80.1
tetrapelgic G80.0
specified NEC G80.8
syphilitic A52.12
congenital A50.49
tetraplegic G80.8
spastic G80.0
cranial nerve —*see also* Disorder, nerve, cranial
multiple G52.7
in
infectious disease B99 [G53]
neoplastic disease (*see also* Neoplasm) D49.9 [G53]
parasitic disease B89 [G53]
sarcoidosis D86.82
creeping G12.22
diver's T70.3
Erb's P14.0
facial G51.0
newborn (birth injury) P11.3
glossopharyngeal G52.1
Klumpke (-Déjérine) P14.1
lead —*see* subcategory T56.0
median nerve (tardy) G56.1-
nerve G58.9
specified NEC G58.8
peroneal nerve (acute) (tardy) G57.3-
progressive supranuclear G23.1
pseudobulbar NEC G12.29
radial nerve (acute) G56.3-
seventh nerve —*see also* Palsy, facial
newborn P11.3
shaking —*see* Parkinsonism
spastic (cerebral) (spinal) G80.1
ulnar nerve (tardy) G56.2-
wasting G12.29
Paludism —*see* Malaria
Panangiitis M30.0
Panaris, panaritium —*see also* Cellulitis, digit
with lymphangitis —*see* Lymphangitis, acute, digit
Panarteritis nodosa M30.0
brain or cerebral I67.7
Pancake heart R93.1
with cor pulmonale (chronic) I27.81
Pancarditis (acute) (chronic) I51.89
rheumatic I09.89
active or acute I01.8
Pancoast's syndrome or tumor C34.1-

Pancolitis, ulcerative (chronic) K51.00
  with
    abscess K51.014
    complication K51.019
    fistula K51.013
    obstruction K51.012
    rectal bleeding K51.011
    specified complication NEC
      K51.018
Pancreas, pancreatic —*see* condition
Pancreatitis (annular) (apoplectic)
    (calcareous) (edematous)
    (hemorrhagic) (malignant)
    (recurrent) (subacute) (suppurative)
    K85.9
  acute K85.9
    alcohol induced K85.2
    biliary K85.1
    drug induced K85.3
    gallstone K85.1
    idiopathic K85.0
    specified NEC K85.8
  chronic (infectious) K86.1
    alcohol-induced K86.0
    recurrent K86.1
    relapsing K86.1
  cystic (chronic) K86.1
  cytomegaloviral B25.2
  fibrous (chronic) K86.1
  gallstone K85.1
  gangrenous K85.8
  interstitial (chronic) K86.1
    acute K85.8
  mumps B26.3
  recurrent (chronic) K86.1
  relapsing, chronic K86.1
  syphilitic A52.74
Pancreatoblastoma —*see* Neoplasm,
    pancreas, malignant
Pancreolithiasis K86.8
Pancytolysis D75.89
Pancytopenia (acquired) D61.818
  with
    malformations D61.09
    myelodysplastic syndrome —*see*
      Syndrome, myelodysplastic
    antineoplastic chemotherapy induced
      D61.810
  congenital D61.09
  drug-induced NEC D61.811
Panencephalitis, subacute, sclerosing
    A81.1
Panhematopenia D61.9
  congenital D61.09
  constitutional D61.09
  splenic, primary D73.1
Panhemocytopenia D61.9
  congenital D61.09
  constitutional D61.09
Panhypogonadism E29.1
Panhypopituitarism E23.0
  prepubertal E23.0
Panic (attack) (state) F41.0
  reaction to exceptional stress (transient)
    F43.0
Panmyelopathy, familial, constitutional
    D61.09
Panmyelophthisis D61.82
  congenital D61.09
Panmyelosis (acute) (with myelofibrosis)
    C94.4-
Panner's disease —*see* Osteochondrosis,
    juvenile, humerus
Panneuritis endemica E51.11

Panniculitis (nodular) (nonsuppurative)
    M79.3
  back M54.00
    cervical region M54.02
    cervicothoracic region M54.03
    lumbar region M54.06
    lumbosacral region M54.07
    multiple sites M54.09
    occipito-atlanto-axial region M54.01
    sacrococcygeal region M54.08
    thoracic region M54.04
    thoracolumbar region M54.05
  lupus L93.2
  mesenteric K65.4
  neck M54.02
    cervicothoracic region M54.03
    occipito-atlanto-axial region M54.01
  relapsing M35.6
Panniculus adiposus (abdominal) E65
Pannus (allergic) (cornea) (degenerativus)
    (keratic) H16.42-
  abdominal (symptomatic) E65
  trachomatosus, trachomatous (active)
    A71.1
Panophthalmitis H44.01-
Pansinusitis (chronic) (hyperplastic)
    (nonpurulent) (purulent) J32.4
  acute J01.40
    recurrent J01.41
  tuberculous A15.8
Panuveitis (sympathetic) H44.11-
Panvalvular disease I08.9
  specified NEC I08.8
Papanicolaou smear, cervix Z12.4
  as part of routine gynecological
    examination Z01.419
    with abnormal findings Z01.411
  for suspected neoplasm Z12.4
  nonspecific abnormal finding R87.619
  routine Z01.419
    with abnormal findings Z01.411
Papilledema (choked disc) H47.10
  associated with
    decreased ocular pressure H47.12
    increased intracranial pressure
      H47.11
    retinal disorder H47.13
  Foster-Kennedy syndrome H47.14-
Papillitis H46.00
  anus K62.89
  chronic lingual K14.4
  necrotizing, kidney N17.2
  optic H46.0-
  rectum K62.89
  renal, necrotizing N17.2
  tongue K14.0
Papilloma —*see also* Neoplasm, benign,
    by site
  acuminatum (female) (male)
    (anogenital) A63.0
  benign pinta (primary) A67.0
  bladder (urinary) (transitional cell)
    D41.4
  choroid plexus (lateral ventricle) (third
    ventricle) D33.0
    anaplastic C71.5
    fourth ventricle D33.1
    malignant C71.5
  renal pelvis (transitional cell) D41.1-
    benign D30.1-
  Schneiderian
    specified site —*see* Neoplasm,
      benign, by site
    unspecified site D14.0

Papilloma (*Continued*)
  serous surface
    borderline malignancy
      specified site —*see* Neoplasm,
        uncertain behavior, by site
      unspecified site D39.10
    specified site —*see* Neoplasm, benign,
      by site
    unspecified site D27.9
  transitional (cell)
    bladder (urinary) D41.4
    inverted type —*see* Neoplasm,
      uncertain behavior, by site
    renal pelvis D41.1-
    ureter D41.2-
  ureter (transitional cell) D41.2-
    benign D30.2-
  urothelial —*see* Neoplasm, uncertain
    behavior, by site
  villous —*see* Neoplasm, uncertain
    behavior, by site
    adenocarcinoma in —*see* Neoplasm,
      malignant, by site
    in situ —*see* Neoplasm, in situ
  yaws, plantar or palmar A66.1
Papillomata, multiple, of yaws A66.1
Papillomatosis —*see also* Neoplasm,
    benign, by site
  confluent and reticulated L83
  cystic, breast —*see* Mastopathy,
    cystic
  ductal, breast —*see* Mastopathy,
    cystic
  intraductal (diffuse) —*see* Neoplasm,
    benign, by site
  subareolar duct D24-
Papillomavirus, as cause of
    disease classified elsewhere
    B97.7
Papillon-Léage and Psaume syndrome
    Q87.0
Papule (s) R23.8
  carate (primary) A67.0
  fibrous, of nose D22.39
  Gottron's L94.4
  pinta (primary) A67.0
Papulosis
  lymphomatoid C86.6
  malignant I77.89
Papyraceous fetus O31.0-
Para-albuminemia E88.09
Paracephalus Q89.7
Parachute mitral valve Q23.2
Paracoccidioidomycosis B41.9
  disseminated B41.7
  generalized B41.7
  mucocutaneous-lymphangitic
    B41.8
  pulmonary B41.0
  specified NEC B41.8
  visceral B41.8
Paradentosis K05.4
Paraffinoma T88.8
Paraganglioma D44.7
  adrenal D35.0-
    malignant C74.1-
  aortic body D44.7
    malignant C75.5
  carotid body D44.6
    malignant C75.4
  chromaffin —*see also* Neoplasm,
    benign, by site
    malignant —*see* Neoplasm,
      malignant, by site

Paraganglioma (Continued)
extra-adrenal D44.7
malignant C75.5
specified site —see Neoplasm, malignant, by site
unspecified site C75.5
specified site —see Neoplasm, uncertain behavior, by site
unspecified site D44.7
gangliocytic D13.2
specified site —see Neoplasm, benign, by site
unspecified site D13.2
glomus jugulare D44.7
malignant C75.5
jugular D44.7
malignant C75.5
specified site —see Neoplasm, malignant, by site
unspecified site C75.5
nonchromaffin D44.7
malignant C75.5
specified site —see Neoplasm, malignant, by site
unspecified site C75.5
specified site —see Neoplasm, uncertain behavior, by site
unspecified site D44.7
parasympathetic D44.7
specified site —see Neoplasm, uncertain behavior, by site
unspecified site D44.7
specified site —see Neoplasm, uncertain behavior, by site
sympathetic D44.7
specified site —see Neoplasm, uncertain behavior, by site
unspecified site D44.7
unspecified site D44.7
Parageusia R43.2
psychogenic F45.8
Paragonimiasis B66.4
Paragranuloma, Hodgkin —see Lymphoma, Hodgkin, classical, specified NEC
Parahemophilia (see also Defect, coagulation) D68.2
Parakeratosis R23.4
variegata L41.0
Paralysis, paralytic (complete) (incomplete) G83.9
with
syphilis A52.17
abducens, abducent (nerve) —see Strabismus, paralytic, sixth nerve
abductor, lower extremity G57.9-
accessory nerve G52.8
accommodation —see also Paresis, of accommodation
hysterical F44.89
acoustic nerve (except Deafness) —see subcategory H93.3
agitans (see also Parkinsonism) G20
arteriosclerotic G21.4
alternating (oculomotor) G83.89
amyotrophic G12.21
ankle G57.9-
anus (sphincter) K62.89
arm —see Monoplegia, upper limb
ascending (spinal), acute G61.0
association G12.29
asthenic bulbar G70.00
with exacerbation (acute) G70.01
in crisis G70.01

Paralysis, paralytic (Continued)
ataxic (hereditary) G11.9
general (syphilitic) A52.17
atrophic G58.9
infantile, acute —see Poliomyelitis, paralytic
progressive G12.22
spinal (acute) —see Poliomyelitis, paralytic
axillary G54.0
Babinski-Nageotte's G83.89
Bell's G51.0
newborn P11.3
Benedikt's G46.3
birth injury P14.9
spinal cord P11.5
bladder (neurogenic) (sphincter) N31.2
bowel, colon or intestine K56.0
brachial plexus G54.0
birth injury P14.3
newborn (birth injury) P14.3
brain G83.9
diplegia G83.0
triplegia G83.89
bronchial J98.09
Brown-Séquard G83.81
bulbar (chronic) (progressive) G12.22
infantile —see Poliomyelitis, paralytic
poliomyelitic —see Poliomyelitis, paralytic
pseudo G12.29
bulbospinal G70.00
with exacerbation (acute) G70.01
in crisis G70.01
cardiac (see also Failure, heart) I50.9
cerebrocerebellar, diplegic G80.1
cervical
plexus G54.2
sympathetic G90.09
Céstan-Chenais G46.3
Charcot-Marie-Tooth type G60.0
Clark's G80.9
colon K56.0
compressed air T70.3
compression
arm G56.9-
leg G57.9-
lower extremity G57.9-
upper extremity G56.9-
congenital (cerebral) —see Palsy, cerebral
conjugate movement (gaze) (of eye) H51.0
cortical (nuclear) (supranuclear) H51.0
cordis —see Failure, heart
cranial or cerebral nerve G52.9
creeping G12.22
crossed leg G83.89
crutch —see Injury, brachial plexus
deglutition R13.0
hysterical F44.4
dementia A52.17
descending (spinal) NEC G12.29
diaphragm (flaccid) J98.6
due to accidental dissection of phrenic nerve during procedure —see Puncture, accidental complicating surgery
digestive organs NEC K59.8
diplegic —see Diplegia
divergence (nuclear) H51.8
diver's T70.3

Paralysis, paralytic (Continued)
Duchenne's
birth injury P14.0
due to or associated with
motor neuron disease G12.22
muscular dystrophy G71.0
due to intracranial or spinal birth injury —see Palsy, cerebral
embolic (current episode) I63.4
Erb (-Duchenne) (birth) (newborn) P14.0
Erb's syphilitic spastic spinal A52.17
esophagus K22.8
eye muscle (extrinsic) H49.9
intrinsic —see also Paresis, of accommodation
facial (nerve) G51.0
birth injury P11.3
congenital P11.3
following operation NEC — see Puncture, accidental complicating surgery
newborn (birth injury) P11.3
familial (recurrent) (periodic) G72.3
spastic G11.4
fauces J39.2
finger G56.9-
gait R26.1
gastric nerve (nondiabetic) G52.2
gaze, conjugate H51.0
general (progressive) (syphilitic) A52.17
juvenile A50.45
glottis J38.00
bilateral J38.02
unilateral J38.01
gluteal G54.1
Gubler (-Millard) G46.3
hand —see Monoplegia, upper limb
heart —see Arrest, cardiac
hemiplegic —see Hemiplegia
hyperkalemic periodic (familial) G72.3
hypoglossal (nerve) G52.3
hypokalemic periodic G72.3
hysterical F44.4
ileus K56.0
infantile (see also Poliomyelitis, paralytic) A80.30
bulbar —see Poliomyelitis, paralytic
cerebral —see Palsy, cerebral
spastic —see Palsy, cerebral, spastic
infective —see Poliomyelitis, paralytic
inferior nuclear G83.9
internuclear —see Ophthalmoplegia, internuclear
intestine K56.0
iris H57.09
due to diphtheria (toxin) A36.89
ischemic, Volkmann's (complicating trauma) T79.6
Jackson's G83.89
jake —see Poisoning, food, noxious, plant
Jamaica ginger (jake) G62.2
juvenile general A50.45
Klumpke (-Déjérine) (birth) (newborn) P14.1
labioglossal (laryngeal) (pharyngeal) G12.29
Landry's G61.0
laryngeal nerve (recurrent) (superior) (unilateral) J38.00
bilateral J38.02
unilateral J38.01

Paralysis, paralytic (Continued)
- larynx J38.00
  - bilateral J38.02
  - due to diphtheria (toxin) A36.2
  - unilateral J38.01
- lateral G12.21
- lead —see subcategory T56.0
- left side —see Hemiplegia
- leg G83.1-
  - both —see Paraplegia
  - crossed G83.89
  - hysterical F44.4
  - psychogenic F44.4
  - transient or transitory R29.818
    - traumatic NEC —see Injury, nerve, leg
- levator palpebrae superioris —see Blepharoptosis, paralytic
- limb —see Monoplegia
- lip K13.0
- Lissauer's A52.17
- lower limb —see Monoplegia, lower limb
  - both —see Paraplegia
- lung J98.4
- median nerve G56.1-
- medullary (tegmental) G83.89
- mesencephalic NEC G83.89
  - tegmental G83.89
- middle alternating G83.89
- Millard-Gubler-Foville G46.3
- monoplegic —see Monoplegia
- motor G83.9
- muscle, muscular NEC G72.89
  - due to nerve lesion G58.9
  - eye (extrinsic) H49.9
    - intrinsic —see Paresis, of accommodation
    - oblique —see Strabismus, paralytic, fourth nerve
  - iris sphincter H21.9
  - ischemic (Volkmann's) (complicating trauma) T79.6
  - progressive G12.21
  - pseudohypertrophic G71.0
- musculocutaneous nerve G56.9-
- musculospiral G56.9-
- nerve —see also Disorder, nerve
  - abducent —see Strabismus, paralytic, sixth nerve
  - accessory G52.8
  - auditory (except Deafness) —see subcategory H93.3
  - birth injury P14.9
  - cranial or cerebral G52.9
  - facial G51.0
    - birth injury P11.3
    - congenital P11.3
    - newborn (birth injury) P11.3
  - fourth or trochlear —see Strabismus, paralytic, fourth nerve
  - newborn (birth injury) P14.9
  - oculomotor —see Strabismus, paralytic, third nerve
  - phrenic (birth injury) P14.2
  - radial G56.3-
  - seventh or facial G51.0
    - newborn (birth injury) P11.3
  - sixth or abducent —see Strabismus, paralytic, sixth nerve
  - syphilitic A52.15
  - third or oculomotor —see Strabismus, paralytic, third nerve
  - trigeminal G50.9

Paralysis, paralytic (Continued)
- nerve (Continued)
  - trochlear —see Strabismus, paralytic, fourth nerve
  - ulnar G56.2-
- normokalemic periodic G72.3
- ocular H49.9
  - alternating G83.89
- oculofacial, congenital (Moebius) Q87.0
- oculomotor (external bilateral) (nerve) —see Strabismus, paralytic, third nerve
- palate (soft) K13.79
- paratrigeminal G50.9
- periodic (familial) (hyperkalemic) (hypokalemic) (myotonic) (normokalemic) (potassium sensitive) (secondary) G72.3
- peripheral autonomic nervous system —see Neuropathy, peripheral, autonomic
- peroneal (nerve) G57.3-
- pharynx J39.2
- phrenic nerve G56.8-
- plantar nerve (s) G57.6-
- pneumogastric nerve G52.2
- poliomyelitis (current) —see Poliomyelitis, paralytic
- popliteal nerve G57.3-
- postepileptic transitory G83.84
- progressive (atrophic) (bulbar) (spinal) G12.22
  - general A52.17
  - infantile acute —see Poliomyelitis, paralytic
  - supranuclear G23.1
- pseudobulbar G12.29
- pseudohypertrophic (muscle) G71.0
- psychogenic F44.4
- quadriceps G57.9-
- quadriplegic —see Tetraplegia
- radial nerve G56.3-
- rectus muscle (eye) H49.9
- recurrent isolated sleep G47.53
- respiratory (muscle) (system) (tract) R06.81
  - center NEC G93.89
  - congenital P28.89
  - newborn P28.89
- right side —see Hemiplegia
- saturnine —see subcategory T56.0
- sciatic nerve G57.0-
- senile G83.9
- shaking —see Parkinsonism
- shoulder G56.9-
- sleep, recurrent isolated G47.53
- spastic G83.9
  - cerebral —see Palsy, cerebral, spastic
  - congenital (cerebral) —see Palsy, cerebral, spastic
  - familial G11.4
  - hereditary G11.4
  - quadriplegic G80.0
  - syphilitic (spinal) A52.17
- sphincter, bladder —see Paralysis, bladder
- spinal (cord) G83.9
  - accessory nerve G52.8
  - acute —see Poliomyelitis, paralytic
  - ascending acute G61.0
  - atrophic (acute) —see also Poliomyelitis, paralytic
    - spastic, syphilitic A52.17

Paralysis, paralytic (Continued)
- spinal (cord) (Continued)
  - congenital NEC —see Palsy, cerebral
  - hereditary G95.89
  - infantile —see Poliomyelitis, paralytic
  - progressive G12.21
  - sequelae NEC G83.89
- sternomastoid G52.8
- stomach K31.84
  - diabetic —see Diabetes, by type, with gastroparesis
  - nerve G52.2
    - diabetic —see Diabetes, by type, with gastroparesis
- stroke —see Infarct, brain
- subcapsularis G56.8-
- supranuclear (progressive) G23.1
- sympathetic G90.8
  - cervical G90.09
  - nervous system —see Neuropathy, peripheral, autonomic
- syndrome G83.9
  - specified NEC G83.89
- syphilitic spastic spinal (Erb's) A52.17
- thigh G57.9-
- throat J39.2
  - diphtheritic A36.0
  - muscle J39.2
- thrombotic (current episode) I63.3
- thumb G56.9-
- tick —see Toxicity, venom, arthropod, specified NEC
- Todd's (postepileptic transitory paralysis) G83.84
- toe G57.6-
- tongue K14.8
- transient R29.5
  - arm or leg NEC R29.818
  - traumatic NEC —see Injury, nerve
- trapezius G52.8
- traumatic, transient NEC —see Injury, nerve
- trembling —see Parkinsonism
- triceps brachii G56.9-
- trigeminal nerve G50.9
- trochlear (nerve) —see Strabismus, paralytic, fourth nerve
- ulnar nerve G56.2-
- upper limb —see Monoplegia, upper limb
- uremic N18.9 [G99.8]
- uveoparotitic D86.89
- uvula K13.79
  - postdiphtheritic A36.0
- vagus nerve G52.2
- vasomotor NEC G90.8
- velum palati K13.79
- vesical —see Paralysis, bladder
- vestibular nerve (except Vertigo) —see subcategory H93.3
- vocal cords J38.00
  - bilateral J38.02
  - unilateral J38.01
- Volkmann's (complicating trauma) T79.6
- wasting G12.29
- Weber's G46.3
- wrist G56.9-

Paramedial urethrovesical orifice Q64.79

Paramenia N92.6

Parametritis (*see also* Disease, pelvis, inflammatory) N73.2
 acute N73.0
 complicating abortion —*see* Abortion, by type, complicated by, parametritis
Parametrium, parametric —*see* condition
Paramnesia —*see* Amnesia
Paramolar K00.1
Paramyloidosis E85.8
Paramyoclonus multiplex G25.3
Paramyotonia (congenita) G71.19
Parangi —*see* Yaws
Paranoia (querulans) F22
 senile F03
Paranoid
 dementia (senile) F03
  praecox —*see* Schizophrenia
 personality F60.0
 psychosis (climacteric) (involutional) (menopausal) F22
  psychogenic (acute) F23
  senile F03
 reaction (acute) F23
  chronic F22
 schizophrenia F20.0
 state (climacteric) (involutional) (menopausal) (simple) F22
  senile F03
 tendencies F60.0
 traits F60.0
 trends F60.0
 type, psychopathic personality F60.0
Paraparesis —*see* Paraplegia
Paraphasia R47.02
Paraphilia F65.9
Paraphimosis (congenital) N47.2
 chancroidal A57
Paraphrenia, paraphrenic (late) F22
 schizophrenia F20.0
Paraplegia (lower) G82.20
 ataxic —*see* Degeneration, combined, spinal cord
 complete G82.21
 congenital (cerebral) G80.8
  spastic G80.1
 familial spastic G11.4
 functional (hysterical) F44.4
 hereditary, spastic G11.4
 hysterical F44.4
 incomplete G82.22
 Pott's A18.01
 psychogenic F44.4
 spastic
  Erb's spinal, syphilitic A52.17
  hereditary G11.4
  tropical G04.1
 syphilitic (spastic) A52.17
 tropical spastic G04.1
Parapoxvirus B08.60
 specified NEC B08.69
Paraproteinemia D89.2
 benign (familial) D89.2
 monoclonal D47.2
 secondary to malignant disease D47.2
Parapsoriasis L41.9
 en plaques L41.4
 guttata L41.1
 large plaque L41.4
 retiform, retiformis L41.5
 small plaque L41.3
 specified NEC L41.8
 varioliformis (acuta) L41.0

Parasitic —*see also* condition
 disease NEC B89
 stomatitis B37.0
 sycosis (beard) (scalp) B35.0
 twin Q89.4
Parasitism B89
 intestinal B82.9
 skin B88.9
 specified —*see* Infestation
Parasitophobia F40.218
Parasomnia G47.50
 due to
  alcohol
   abuse F10.182
   dependence F10.282
   use F10.982
  amphetamines
   abuse F15.182
   dependence F15.282
   use F15.982
  caffeine
   abuse F15.182
   dependence F15.282
   use F15.982
  cocaine
   abuse F14.182
   dependence F14.282
   use F14.982
  drug NEC
   abuse F19.182
   dependence F19.282
   use F19.982
  opioid
   abuse F11.182
   dependence F11.282
   use F11.982
  psychoactive substance NEC
   abuse F19.182
   dependence F19.282
   use F19.982
  sedative, hypnotic, or anxiolytic
   abuse F13.182
   dependence F13.282
   use F13.982
  stimulant NEC
   abuse F15.182
   dependence F15.282
   use F15.982
 in conditions classified elsewhere G47.54
 nonorganic origin F51.8
 organic G47.50
 specified NEC G47.59
Paraspadias Q54.9
Paraspasmus facialis G51.8
Parasuicide (attempt)
 history of (personal) Z91.5
 in family Z81.8
Parathyroid gland —*see* condition
Parathyroid tetany E20.9
Paratrachoma A74.0
Paratyphilitis —*see* Appendicitis
Paratyphoid (fever) —*see* Fever, paratyphoid
Paratyphus —*see* Fever, paratyphoid
Paraurethral duct Q64.79
 nonorganic origin F51.5
Paraurethritis —*see also* Urethritis
 gonococcal (acute) (chronic) (with abscess) A54.1
Paravaccinia NEC B08.04
Paravaginitis —*see* Vaginitis
Parencephalitis —*see also* Encephalitis
 sequelae G09
Parent-child conflict —*see* Conflict, parent-child
 estrangement NEC Z62.890

Paresis —*see also* Paralysis
 accommodation —*see* Paresis, of accommodation
 Bernhardt's G57.1-
 bladder (sphincter) —*see also* Paralysis, bladder
  tabetic A52.17
 bowel, colon or intestine K56.0
 extrinsic muscle, eye H49.9
 general (progressive) (syphilitic) A52.17
  juvenile A50.45
 heart —*see* Failure, heart
 insane (syphilitic) A52.17
 juvenile (general) A50.45
 of accommodation H52.52-
 peripheral progressive (idiopathic) G60.3
 pseudohypertrophic G71.0
 senile G83.9
 syphilitic (general) A52.17
  congenital A50.45
 vesical NEC N31.2
Paresthesia —*see also* Disturbance, sensation
 Bernhardt G57.1-
Paretic —*see* condition
Parinaud's
 conjunctivitis H10.89
 oculoglandular syndrome H10.89
 ophthalmoplegia H49.88
Parkinsonism (idiopathic) (primary) G20
 with neurogenic orthostatic hypotension (symptomatic) G90.3
 arteriosclerotic G21.4
 dementia G31.83 [F02.80]
  with behavioral disturbance G31.83 [F02.81]
 due to
  drugs NEC G21.19
   neuroleptic G21.11
 neuroleptic induced G21.11
 postencephalitic G21.3
 secondary G21.9
  due to
   arteriosclerosis G21.4
   drugs NEC G21.19
    neuroleptic G21.11
   encephalitis G21.3
   external agents NEC G21.2
   syphilis A52.19
  specified NEC G21.8
 syphilitic A52.19
 treatment-induced NEC G21.19
 vascular G21.4
Parkinson's disease, syndrome or tremor —*see* Parkinsonism
Parodontitis —*see* Periodontitis
Parodontosis K05.4
Paronychia —*see also* Cellulitis, digit
 with lymphangitis —*see* Lymphangitis, acute, digit
 candidal (chronic) B37.2
 tuberculous (primary) A18.4
Parorexia (psychogenic) F50.8
Parosmia R43.1
 psychogenic F45.8
Parotid gland —*see* condition
Parotitis, parotiditis (allergic) (nonspecific toxic) (purulent) (septic) (suppurative) —*see also* Sialoadenitis
 epidemic —*see* Mumps
 infectious —*see* Mumps
 postoperative K91.89
 surgical K91.89
Parrot fever A70

P

Parrot's disease (early congenital
   syphilitic pseudoparalysis) A50.02
Parry-Romberg syndrome G51.8
Parry's disease or syndrome E05.00
   with thyroid storm E05.01
Pars planitis —see Cyclitis
Parsonage (-Aldren)-Turner syndrome
   G54.5
Parson's disease (exophthalmic goiter)
   E05.00
   with thyroid storm E05.01
Particolored infant Q82.8
Parturition —see Delivery
Parulis K04.7
   with sinus K04.6
Parvovirus, as cause of disease classified
   elsewhere B97.6
Pasini and Pierini's atrophoderma L90.3
Passage
   false, urethra N36.5
   meconium (newborn) during delivery
      P03.82
   of sounds or bougies —see Attention to,
      artificial, opening
Passive —see condition
   smoking Z77.22
Pasteurella septica A28.0
Pasteurellosis —see Infection, Pasteurella
PAT (paroxysmal atrial tachycardia) I47.1
Patau's syndrome —see Trisomy, 13
Patches
   mucous (syphilitic) A51.39
      congenital A50.07
   smokers' (mouth) K13.24
Patellar —see condition
Patent —see also Imperfect, closure
   canal of Nuck Q52.4
   cervix N88.3
   ductus arteriosus or Botallo's Q25.0
   foramen
      botalli Q21.1
      ovale Q21.1
   interauricular septum Q21.1
   interventricular septum Q21.0
   omphalomesenteric duct Q43.0
   os (uteri) —see Patent, cervix
   ostium secundum Q21.1
   urachus Q64.4
   vitelline duct Q43.0
Paterson (-Brown)(-Kelly) syndrome or
   web D50.1
Pathologic, pathological —see also
   condition
   asphyxia R09.01
   fire-setting F63.1
   gambling F63.0
   ovum O02.0
   resorption, tooth K03.3
   stealing F63.2
Pathology (of) —see Disease
   periradicular, associated with previous
      endodontic treatment NEC M27.59
Pattern, sleep-wake, irregular G47.23
Patulous —see also Imperfect, closure
   (congenital)
   alimentary tract Q45.8
      lower Q43.8
      upper Q40.8
   eustachian tube H69.0-
Pause, sinoatrial I49.5
Paxton's disease B36.2
Pearl (s)
   enamel K00.2
   Epstein's K09.8

Pearl-worker's disease —see
   Osteomyelitis, specified type NEC
Pectenosis K62.4
Pectoral —see condition
Pectus
   carinatum (congenital) Q67.7
      acquired M95.4
      rachitic sequelae (late effect) E64.3
   excavatum (congenital) Q67.6
      acquired M95.4
      rachitic sequelae (late effect) E64.3
   recurvatum (congenital) Q67.6
Pedatrophia E41
Pederosis F65.4
Pediculosis (infestation) B85.2
   capitis (head-louse) (any site) B85.0
   corporis (body-louse) (any site) B85.1
   eyelid B85.0
   mixed (classifiable to more than one of
      the titles B85.0-B85.3) B85.4
   pubis (pubic louse) (any site) B85.3
   vestimenti B85.1
   vulvae B85.3
Pediculus (infestation) —see Pediculosis
Pedophilia F65.4
Peg-shaped teeth K00.2
Pelade —see Alopecia, areata
Pelger-Huët anomaly or syndrome D72.0
Peliosis (rheumatica) D69.0
   hepatis K76.4
      with toxic liver disease K71.8
Pelizaeus-Merzbacher disease E75.29
Pellagra (alcoholic) (with
   polyneuropathy) E52
Pellagra-cerebellar-ataxia-renal
   aminoaciduria syndrome E72.02
Pellegrini (-Stieda) disease or syndrome —
   see Bursitis, tibial collateral
Pellizzi's syndrome E34.8
Pel's crisis A52.11
Pelvic —see also condition
   examination (periodic) (routine)
      Z01.419
      with abnormal findings Z01.411
   kidney, congenital Q63.2
Pelviolithiasis —see Calculus, kidney
Pelviperitonitis —see also Peritonitis, pelvic
   gonococcal A54.24
   puerperal O85
Pelvis —see condition or type
Pemphigoid L12.9
   benign, mucous membrane L12.1
   bullous L12.0
   cicatricial L12.1
   juvenile L12.2
   ocular L12.1
   specified NEC L12.8
Pemphigus L10.9
   benign familial (chronic) Q82.8
   Brazilian L10.3
   circinatus L13.0
   conjunctiva L12.1
   drug-induced L10.5
   erythematosus L10.4
   foliaceous L10.2
   gangrenous —see Gangrene
   neonatorum L01.03
   ocular L12.1
   paraneoplastic L10.81
   specified NEC L10.89
   syphilitic (congenital) A50.06
   vegetans L10.1
   vulgaris L10.0
   wildfire L10.3

Pendred's syndrome E07.1
Pendulous
   abdomen, in pregnancy —see
      Pregnancy, complicated by,
      abnormal, pelvic organs or tissues
      NEC
   breast N64.89
Penetrating wound —see also Puncture
   with internal injury —see Injury,
      by site
   eyeball —see Puncture, eyeball
   orbit (with or without foreign body) —
      see Puncture, orbit
   uterus by instrument with or following
      ectopic or molar pregnancy O08.6
Penicillosis B48.4
Penis —see condition
Penitis N48.29
Pentalogy of Fallot Q21.8
Pentasomy X syndrome Q97.1
Pentosuria (essential) E74.8
Percreta placenta - O43.23
Peregrinating patient —see Disorder,
   factitious
Perforation, perforated (nontraumatic) (of)
   accidental during procedure (blood
      vessel) (nerve) (organ) —see
      Complication, accidental puncture
      or laceration
   antrum —see Sinusitis, maxillary
   appendix K35.2
   atrial septum, multiple Q21.1
   attic, ear —see Perforation, tympanum,
      attic
   bile duct (common) (hepatic) K83.2
      cystic K82.2
   bladder (urinary)
      with or following ectopic or molar
         pregnancy O08.6
      obstetrical trauma O71.5
      traumatic S37.29
         at delivery O71.5
   bowel K63.1
      with or following ectopic or molar
         pregnancy O08.6
      newborn P78.0
      obstetrical trauma O71.5
      traumatic —see Laceration, intestine
   broad ligament N83.8
      with or following ectopic or molar
         pregnancy O08.6
      obstetrical trauma O71.6
   by
      device, implant or graft (see also
         Complications, by site and type,
         mechanical) T85.628
         arterial graft NEC —see
            Complication, cardiovascular
            device, mechanical, vascular
         breast (implant) T85.49
         catheter NEC T85.698
            cystostomy T83.090
            dialysis (renal) T82.49
               intraperitoneal T85.691
            infusion NEC T82.594
               spinal (epidural) (subdural)
                  T85.690
         electronic (electrode) (pulse
            generator) (stimulator)
            bone T84.390
            cardiac T82.199
               electrode T82.190
               pulse generator T82.191
               specified type NEC T82.198

Perforation, perforated *(Continued)*
　by *(Continued)*
　　device, implant or graft *(Continued)*
　　　electronic *(Continued)*
　　　　nervous system —*see*
　　　　　Complication, prosthetic
　　　　　device, mechanical,
　　　　　electronic nervous system
　　　　　stimulator
　　　　urinary —*see* Complication,
　　　　　genitourinary, device,
　　　　　urinary, mechanical
　　　fixation, internal (orthopedic)
　　　　NEC —*see* Complication,
　　　　fixation device, mechanical
　　　gastrointestinal —*see*
　　　　Complications, prosthetic
　　　　device, mechanical,
　　　　gastrointestinal device
　　　genital NEC T83.498
　　　　intrauterine contraceptive device
　　　　　T83.39
　　　　penile prosthesis T83.490
　　　heart NEC —*see* Complication,
　　　　cardiovascular device,
　　　　mechanical
　　　joint prosthesis —*see*
　　　　Complications, joint
　　　　prosthesis, mechanical,
　　　　specified NEC, by site
　　　ocular NEC —*see* Complications,
　　　　prosthetic device, mechanical,
　　　　ocular device
　　　orthopedic NEC —*see*
　　　　Complication, orthopedic,
　　　　device, mechanical
　　　specified NEC T85.628
　　　urinary NEC —*see also*
　　　　Complication, genitourinary,
　　　　device, urinary, mechanical
　　　　graft T83.29
　　　　urinary, indwelling T83.098
　　　vascular NEC —*see* Complication,
　　　　cardiovascular device,
　　　　mechanical
　　　ventricular intracranial shunt
　　　　T85.09
　　foreign body left accidentally in
　　　operative wound T81.539
　　instrument (any) during a procedure,
　　　accidental —*see* Puncture,
　　　accidental complicating
　　　surgery
　cecum K35.2
　cervix (uteri) N88.8
　　with or following ectopic or molar
　　　pregnancy O08.6
　　obstetrical trauma O71.3
　colon K63.1
　　newborn P78.0
　　obstetrical trauma O71.5
　　traumatic —*see* Laceration, intestine,
　　　large
　common duct (bile) K83.2
　cornea (due to ulceration) —*see* Ulcer,
　　cornea, perforated
　cystic duct K82.2
　diverticulum (intestine) K57.80
　　with bleeding K57.81
　　large intestine K57.20
　　　with
　　　　bleeding K57.21
　　　　small intestine K57.40
　　　　　with bleeding K57.41

Perforation, perforated *(Continued)*
　diverticulum *(Continued)*
　　small intestine K57.00
　　　with
　　　　bleeding K57.01
　　　　large intestine K57.40
　　　　　with bleeding K57.41
　ear drum —*see* Perforation, tympanum
　esophagus K22.3
　ethmoidal sinus —*see* Sinusitis,
　　ethmoidal
　frontal sinus —*see* Sinusitis, frontal
　gallbladder K82.2
　heart valve —*see* Endocarditis
　ileum K63.1
　　newborn P78.0
　　obstetrical trauma O71.5
　　traumatic —*see* Laceration, intestine,
　　　small
　instrumental, surgical (accidental)
　　(blood vessel) (nerve) (organ) —*see*
　　Puncture, accidental complicating
　　surgery
　intestine NEC K63.1
　　with ectopic or molar pregnancy
　　　O08.6
　　newborn P78.0
　　obstetrical trauma O71.5
　　traumatic —*see* Laceration, intestine
　　ulcerative NEC K63.1
　　　newborn P78.0
　jejunum, jejunal K63.1
　　obstetrical trauma O71.5
　　traumatic —*see* Laceration, intestine,
　　　small
　　ulcer —*see* Ulcer, gastrojejunal, with
　　　perforation
　joint prosthesis —*see* Complications,
　　joint prosthesis, mechanical,
　　specified NEC, by site
　mastoid (antrum) (cell) —*see* Disorder,
　　mastoid, specified NEC
　maxillary sinus —*see* Sinusitis,
　　maxillary
　membrana tympani —*see* Perforation,
　　tympanum
　nasal
　　septum J34.89
　　　congenital Q30.3
　　　syphilitic A52.73
　　sinus J34.89
　　　congenital Q30.8
　　　due to sinusitis —*see* Sinusitis
　palate (*see also* Cleft, palate) Q35.9
　　syphilitic A52.79
　palatine vault (*see also* Cleft, palate,
　　hard) Q35.1
　　syphilitic A52.79
　　congenital A50.59
　pars flaccida (ear drum) —*see*
　　Perforation, tympanum, attic
　pelvic
　　floor S31.030
　　　with
　　　　ectopic or molar pregnancy O08.6
　　　　penetration into retroperitoneal
　　　　　space S31.031
　　　　retained foreign body S31.040
　　　　　with penetration into
　　　　　retroperitoneal space
　　　　　S31.041
　　　following ectopic or molar
　　　　pregnancy O08.6
　　　obstetrical trauma O70.1

Perforation, perforated *(Continued)*
　pelvic *(Continued)*
　　organ S37.99
　　　adrenal gland S37.818
　　　bladder —*see* Perforation, bladder
　　　fallopian tube S37.599
　　　　bilateral S37.592
　　　　unilateral S37.591
　　　kidney S37.09-
　　　obstetrical trauma O71.5
　　　ovary S37.499
　　　　bilateral S37.492
　　　　unilateral S37.491
　　　prostate S37.828
　　　specified organ NEC S37.898
　　　ureter —*see* Perforation, ureter
　　　urethra —*see* Perforation, urethra
　　　uterus —*see* Perforation, uterus
　　perineum —*see* Laceration, perineum
　pharynx J39.2
　rectum K63.1
　　newborn P78.0
　　obstetrical trauma O71.5
　　traumatic S36.63
　root canal space due to endodontic
　　treatment M27.51
　sigmoid K63.1
　　newborn P78.0
　　obstetrical trauma O71.5
　　traumatic S36.533
　sinus (accessory) (chronic) (nasal) J34.89
　sphenoidal sinus —*see* Sinusitis,
　　sphenoidal
　surgical (accidental) (by instrument)
　　(blood vessel) (nerve) (organ) —*see*
　　Puncture, accidental complicating
　　surgery
　traumatic
　　external —*see* Puncture
　　eye —*see* Puncture, eyeball
　　internal organ —*see* Injury, by site
　tympanum, tympanic (membrane)
　　(persistent post-traumatic)
　　(postinflammatory) H72.9-
　　attic H72.1-
　　　multiple —*see* Perforation,
　　　　tympanum, multiple
　　　total —*see* Perforation, tympanum,
　　　　total
　　central H72.0-
　　　multiple —*see* Perforation,
　　　　tympanum, multiple
　　　total —*see* Perforation, tympanum,
　　　　total
　　marginal NEC —*see* subcategory
　　　H72.2
　　multiple H72.81-
　　pars flaccida —*see* Perforation,
　　　tympanum, attic
　　total H72.82-
　　traumatic, current episode S09.2-
　typhoid, gastrointestinal —*see* Typhoid
　ulcer —*see* Ulcer, by site, with
　　perforation
　ureter N28.89
　　traumatic S37.19
　urethra N36.8
　　with ectopic or molar pregnancy
　　　O08.6
　　following ectopic or molar pregnancy
　　　O08.6
　　obstetrical trauma O71.5
　　traumatic S37.39
　　　at delivery O71.5

Perforation, perforated (*Continued*)
  uterus
    with ectopic or molar pregnancy
      O08.6
    by intrauterine contraceptive device
      T83.39
    following ectopic or molar pregnancy
      O08.6
    obstetrical trauma O71.1
    traumatic S37.69
      obstetric O71.1
  uvula K13.79
    syphilitic A52.79
  vagina (*see also* Puncture, vagina)
    O71.4
Periadenitis mucosa necrotica recurrens
  K12.0
Periappendicitis (acute) —*see*
  Appendicitis
Periarteritis nodosa (disseminated)
  (infectious) (necrotizing) M30.0
Periarthritis (joint) —*see also*
  Enthesopathy
  Duplay's M75.0-
  gonococcal A54.42
  humeroscapularis —*see* Capsulitis,
    adhesive
  scapulohumeral —*see* Capsulitis,
    adhesive
  shoulder —*see* Capsulitis, adhesive
  wrist M77.2-
Periarthrosis (angioneural) —*see*
  Enthesopathy
Pericapsulitis, adhesive (shoulder) —*see*
  Capsulitis, adhesive
Pericarditis (with decompensation) (with
    effusion) I31.9
  with rheumatic fever (conditions in I00)
    active —*see* Pericarditis, rheumatic
    inactive or quiescent I09.2
  acute (hemorrhagic) (nonrheumatic)
    (Sicca) I30.9
    with chorea (acute) (rheumatic)
      (Sydenham's) I02.0
    benign I30.8
    nonspecific I30.0
    rheumatic I01.0
      with chorea (acute) (Sydenham's)
        I02.0
  adhesive or adherent (chronic)
    (external) (internal) I31.0
  acute —*see* Pericarditis, acute
    rheumatic I09.2
  bacterial (acute) (subacute) (with serous
    or seropurulent effusion) I30.1
  calcareous I31.1
  cholesterol (chronic) I31.8
    acute I30.9
  chronic (nonrheumatic) I31.9
    rheumatic I09.2
  constrictive (chronic) I31.1
  coxsackie B33.23
  fibrinocaseous (tuberculous) A18.84
  fibrinopurulent I30.1
  fibrinous I30.8
  fibrous I31.0
  gonococcal A54.83
  idiopathic I30.0
  in systemic lupus erythematosus M32.12
  infective I30.1
  meningococcal A39.53
  neoplastic (chronic) I31.8
    acute I30.9
  obliterans, obliterating I31.0

Pericarditis (*Continued*)
  plastic I31.0
  pneumococcal I30.1
  postinfarction I24.1
  purulent I30.1
  rheumatic (active) (acute) (with
    effusion) (with pneumonia) I01.0
    with chorea (acute) (rheumatic)
      (Sydenham's) I02.0
    chronic or inactive (with chorea)
      I09.2
  rheumatoid —*see* Rheumatoid, carditis
  septic I30.1
  serofibrinous I30.8
  staphylococcal I30.1
  streptococcal I30.1
  suppurative I30.1
  syphilitic A52.06
  tuberculous A18.84
  uremic N18.9 [I32]
  viral I30.1
Pericardium, pericardial —*see* condition
Pericellulitis —*see* Cellulitis
Pericementitis (chronic) (suppurative) —
    see also Periodontitis
  acute K05.20
    generalized K05.22
    localized K05.21
Perichondritis
  auricle —*see* Perichondritis, ear
  bronchus J98.09
  ear (external) H61.00-
    acute H61.01-
    chronic H61.02-
  external auditory canal —*see*
    Perichondritis, ear
  larynx J38.7
    syphilitic A52.73
    typhoid A01.09
  nose J34.89
  pinna —*see* Perichondritis, ear
  trachea J39.8
Periclasia K05.4
Pericoronitis —*see* Periodontitis
Pericystitis N30.90
  with hematuria N30.91
Peridiverticulitis (intestine) K57.92
  cecum —*see* Diverticulitis, intestine,
    large
  colon —*see* Diverticulitis, intestine,
    large
  duodenum —*see* Diverticulitis,
    intestine, small
  intestine —*see* Diverticulitis, intestine
  jejunum —*see* Diverticulitis, intestine,
    small
  rectosigmoid —*see* Diverticulitis,
    intestine, large
  rectum —*see* Diverticulitis, intestine,
    large
  sigmoid —*see* Diverticulitis, intestine,
    large
Periendocarditis —*see* Endocarditis
Periepididymitis N45.1
Perifolliculitis L01.02
  abscedens, caput, scalp L66.3
  capitis, abscedens (et suffodiens)
    L66.3
  superficial pustular L01.02
Perihepatitis K65.8
Perilabyrinthitis (acute) —*see*
  subcategory H83.0
Perimeningitis —*see* Meningitis
Perimetritis —*see* Endometritis

Perimetrosalpingitis —*see*
  Salpingo-oophoritis
Perineocele N81.81
Perinephric, perinephritic —*see* condition
Perinephritis —*see also* Infection, kidney
  purulent —*see* Abscess, kidney
Perineum, perineal —*see* condition
Perineuritis NEC —*see* Neuralgia
Periodic —*see* condition
Periodontitis (chronic) (complex)
    (compound) (local) (simplex)
    K05.30
  acute K05.20
    generalized K05.22
    localized K05.21
  apical K04.5
    acute (pulpal origin) K04.4
  generalized K05.32
  localized K05.31
Periodontoclasia K05.4
Periodontosis (juvenile) K05.4
Periods —*see also* Menstruation
  heavy N92.0
  irregular N92.6
  shortened intervals (irregular) N92.1
Perionychia —*see also* Cellulitis, digit
  with lymphangitis —*see* Lymphangitis,
    acute, digit
Perioophoritis —*see* Salpingo-oophoritis
Periorchitis N45.2
Periosteum, periosteal —*see* condition
Periostitis (albuminosa) (circumscribed)
    (diffuse) (infective) (monomelic) —
    see also Osteomyelitis
  alveolar M27.3
  alveolodental M27.3
  dental M27.3
  gonorrheal A54.43
  jaw (lower) (upper) M27.2
  orbit H05.03-
  syphilitic A52.77
    congenital (early) A50.02 [M90.80]
    secondary A51.46
  tuberculous —*see* Tuberculosis, bone
  yaws (hypertrophic) (early) (late)
    A66.6 [M90.80]
Periostosis (hyperplastic) —*see also*
  Disorder, bone, specified type
  NEC
  with osteomyelitis —*see* Osteomyelitis,
    specified type NEC
Peripartum
  cardiomyopathy O90.3
Periphlebitis —*see* Phlebitis
Periproctitis K62.89
Periprostatitis —*see* Prostatitis
Perirectal —*see* condition
Perirenal —*see* condition
Perisalpingitis —*see* Salpingo-oophoritis
Perisplenitis (infectional) D73.89
Peristalsis, visible or reversed R19.2
Peritendinitis —*see* Enthesopathy
Peritoneum, peritoneal —*see* condition
Peritonitis (adhesive) (bacterial)
    (fibrinous) (hemorrhagic)
    (idiopathic) (localized) (perforative)
    (primary) (with adhesions) (with
    effusion) K65.9
  with or following
    abscess K65.1
    appendicitis K35.2
      with perforation or rupture K35.2
      generalized K35.2
      localized K35.3

P

Peritonitis *(Continued)*
  with or following *(Continued)*
    diverticular disease (intestine) K57.80
      with bleeding K57.81
      ectopic or molar pregnancy O08.0
      large intestine K57.20
        with
          bleeding K57.21
          small intestine K57.40
            with bleeding K57.41
      small intestine K57.00
        with
          bleeding K57.01
          large intestine K57.40
            with bleeding K57.41
  acute (generalized) K65.0
  aseptic T81.61
  bile, biliary K65.3
  chemical T81.61
  chlamydial A74.81
  chronic proliferative K65.8
  complicating abortion —*see* Abortion,
      by type, complicated by, pelvic
      peritonitis
  congenital P78.1
  diaphragmatic K65.0
  diffuse K65.0
  diphtheritic A36.89
  disseminated K65.0
  due to
    bile K65.3
    foreign
      body or object accidentally
          left during a procedure
          (instrument) (sponge) (swab)
          T81.599
      substance accidentally left during
          a procedure (chemical)
          (powder) (talc) T81.61
    talc T81.61
    urine K65.8
  eosinophilic K65.8
    acute K65.0
  fibrocaseous (tuberculous) A18.31
  fibropurulent K65.0
  following ectopic or molar pregnancy
      O08.0
  general (ized) K65.0
  gonococcal A54.85
  meconium (newborn) P78.0
  neonatal P78.1
    meconium P78.0
  pancreatic K65.0
  paroxysmal, familial E85.0
    benign E85.0
  pelvic
    female N73.5
      acute N73.3
      chronic N73.4
        with adhesions N73.6
    male K65.0
  periodic, familial E85.0
  proliferative, chronic K65.8
  puerperal, postpartum, childbirth O85
  purulent K65.0
  septic K65.0
  specified NEC K65.8
  spontaneous bacterial K65.2
  subdiaphragmatic K65.0
  subphrenic K65.0
  suppurative K65.0
  syphilitic A52.74
    congenital (early) A50.08 *[K67]*
  talc T81.61

Peritonitis *(Continued)*
  tuberculous A18.31
  urine K65.8
Peritonsillar —*see* condition
Peritonsillitis J36
Perityphlitis K37
Periureteritis N28.89
Periurethral —*see* condition
Periurethritis (gangrenous) —*see* Urethritis
Periuterine —*see* condition
Perivaginitis —*see* Vaginitis
Perivasculitis, retinal H35.06-
Perivasitis (chronic) N49.1
Perivesiculitis (seminal) —*see* Vesiculitis
Perlèche NEC K13.0
  due to
    candidiasis B37.83
    moniliasis B37.83
    riboflavin deficiency E53.0
    vitamin B2 (riboflavin) deficiency
        E53.0
Pernicious —*see* condition
Pernio, perniosis T69.1
Perpetrator (of abuse) —*see* Index to
        External Cause of Injury, Perpetrator
Persecution
  delusion F22
  social Z60.5
Perseveration (tonic) R48.8
Persistence, persistent (congenital)
  anal membrane Q42.3
    with fistula Q42.2
  arteria stapedia Q16.3
  atrioventricular canal Q21.2
  branchial cleft Q18.0
  bulbus cordis in left ventricle Q21.8
  canal of Cloquet Q14.0
  capsule (opaque) Q12.8
  cilioretinal artery or vein Q14.8
  cloaca Q43.7
  communication —*see* Fistula, congenital
  convolutions
    aortic arch Q25.4
    fallopian tube Q50.6
    oviduct Q50.6
    uterine tube Q50.6
  double aortic arch Q25.4
  ductus arteriosus (Botalli) Q25.0
  fetal
    circulation P29.3
    form of cervix (uteri) Q51.828
    hemoglobin, hereditary (HPFH) D56.4
  foramen
    Botalli Q21.1
    ovale Q21.1
  Gartner's duct Q52.4
  hemoglobin, fetal (hereditary) (HPFH)
      D56.4
  hyaloid
    artery (generally incomplete) Q14.0
    system Q14.8
  hymen, in pregnancy or childbirth —
      see Pregnancy, complicated by,
      abnormal, vulva
  lanugo Q84.2
  left
    posterior cardinal vein Q26.8
    root with right arch of aorta Q25.4
    superior vena cava Q26.1
  Meckel's diverticulum Q43.0
    malignant —*see* Table of Neoplasms,
        small intestine, malignant
  mucosal disease (middle ear) —*see*
      Otitis, media, suppurative,
      chronic, tubotympanic

Persistence, persistent *(Continued)*
  nail (s), anomalous Q84.6
  omphalomesenteric duct Q43.0
  organ or site not listed —*see* Anomaly,
      by site
  ostium
    atrioventriculare commune Q21.2
    primum Q21.2
    secundum Q21.1
  ovarian rests in fallopian tube Q50.6
  pancreatic tissue in intestinal tract Q43.8
  primary (deciduous)
    teeth K00.6
    vitreous hyperplasia Q14.0
  pupillary membrane Q13.89
  rhesus (Rh)titer —*see* Complication (s),
      transfusion, incompatibility
      reaction, Rh (factor)
  right aortic arch Q25.4
  sinus
    urogenitalis
      female Q52.8
      male Q55.8
    venosus with imperfect incorporation
        in right auricle Q26.8
  thymus (gland) (hyperplasia) E32.0
  thyroglossal duct Q89.2
  thyrolingual duct Q89.2
  truncus arteriosus or communis Q20.0
  tunica vasculosa lentis Q12.2
  umbilical sinus Q64.4
  urachus Q64.4
  vitelline duct Q43.0
Person (with)
  admitted for clinical research, as
      a control subject (normal
      comparison) (participant) Z00.6
  awaiting admission to adequate facility
      elsewhere Z75.1
  concern (normal) about sick person in
      family Z63.6
  consulting on behalf of another Z71.0
  feigning illness Z76.5
  living (in)
    without
      adequate housing (heating) (space)
          Z59.1
      housing (permanent) (temporary)
          Z59.0
      person able to render necessary
          care Z74.2
      shelter Z59.0
    alone Z60.2
    boarding school Z59.3
    residential institution Z59.3
  on waiting list Z75.1
  sick or handicapped in family Z63.6
Personality (disorder) F60.9
  accentuation of traits (type A pattern)
      Z73.1
  affective F34.0
  aggressive F60.3
  amoral F60.2
  anacastic, anankastic F60.5
  antisocial F60.2
  anxious F60.6
  asocial F60.2
  asthenic F60.7
  avoidant F60.6
  borderline F60.3
  change due to organic condition
      (enduring) F07.0
  compulsive F60.5
  cycloid F34.0
  cyclothymic F34.0

Personality *(Continued)*
dependent F60.7
depressive F34.1
dissocial F60.2
dual F44.81
eccentric F60.89
emotionally unstable F60.3
expansive paranoid F60.0
explosive F60.3
fanatic F60.0
haltlose type F60.89
histrionic F60.4
hyperthymic F34.0
hypothymic F34.1
hysterical F60.4
immature F60.89
inadequate F60.7
labile (emotional) F60.3
mixed (nonspecific) F60.81
morally defective F60.2
multiple F44.81
narcissistic F60.81
obsessional F60.5
obsessive (-compulsive) F60.5
organic F07.0
overconscientious F60.5
paranoid F60.0
passive (-dependent) F60.7
passive-aggressive F60.89
pathologic F60.9
pattern defect or disturbance F60.9
pseudopsychopathic (organic) F07.0
pseudoretarded (organic) F07.0
psychoinfantile F60.4
psychoneurotic NEC F60.89
psychopathic F60.2
querulant F60.0
sadistic F60.89
schizoid F60.1
self-defeating F60.7
sensitive paranoid F60.0
sociopathic (amoral) (antisocial)
(asocial) (dissocial) F60.2
specified NEC F60.89
type A Z73.1
unstable (emotional) F60.3
Perthes' disease —*see* Legg-Calvé-Perthes
disease
Pertussis *(see also* Whooping cough) A37.90
Perversion, perverted
appetite F50.8
psychogenic F50.8
function
pituitary gland E23.2
posterior lobe E22.2
sense of smell and taste R43.8
psychogenic F45.8
sexual —*see* Deviation, sexual
Pervious, congenital —*see also* Imperfect,
closure
ductus arteriosus Q25.0
Pes (congenital) —*see also* Talipes
acquired —*see also* Deformity, limb,
foot, specified NEC
planus —*see* Deformity, limb, flat foot
adductus Q66.89
cavus Q66.7
deformity NEC, acquired —*see*
Deformity, limb, foot, specified
NEC
planus (acquired) (any degree) —*see
also* Deformity, limb, flat foot
rachitic sequelae (late effect) E64.3
valgus Q66.6

Pest, pestis —*see* Plague
Petechia, petechiae R23.3
newborn P54.5
Petechial typhus A75.9
Peter's anomaly Q13.4
Petit mal seizure —*see* Epilepsy,
generalized, specified NEC
Petit's hernia —*see* Hernia, abdomen,
specified site NEC
Petrellidosis B48.2
Petrositis H70.20-
acute H70.21-
chronic H70.22-
Peutz-Jeghers disease or syndrome Q85.8
Peyronie's disease N48.6
Pfeiffer's disease —*see* Mononucleosis,
infectious
Phagedena (dry) (moist) (sloughing) —*see
also* Gangrene
geometric L88
penis N48.29
tropical —*see* Ulcer, skin
vulva N76.6
Phagedenic —*see* condition
Phakoma H35.89
Phakomatosis *(see also* specific eponymous
syndromes) Q85.9
Bourneville's Q85.1
specified NEC Q85.8
Phantom limb syndrome (without pain)
G54.7
with pain G54.6
Pharyngeal pouch syndrome D82.1
Pharyngitis (acute) (catarrhal)
(gangrenous) (infective) (malignant)
(membranous) (phlegmonous)
(pseudomembranous) (simple)
(subacute) (suppurative) (ulcerative)
(viral) J02.9
with influenza, flu, or grippe —*see*
Influenza, with, pharyngitis
aphthous B08.5
atrophic J31.2
chlamydial A56.4
chronic (atrophic) (granular)
(hypertrophic) J31.2
coxsackievirus B08.5
diphtheritic A36.0
enteroviral vesicular B08.5
follicular (chronic) J31.2
fusospirochetal A69.1
gonococcal A54.5
granular (chronic) J31.2
herpesviral B00.2
hypertrophic J31.2
infectional, chronic J31.2
influenzal —*see* Influenza, with,
respiratory manifestations NEC
lymphonodular, acute (enteroviral) B08.8
pneumococcal J02.8
purulent J02.9
putrid J02.9
septic J02.0
sicca J31.2
specified organism NEC J02.8
staphylococcal J02.8
streptococcal J02.0
syphilitic, congenital (early) A50.03
tuberculous A15.8
vesicular, enteroviral B08.5
viral NEC J02.8
Pharyngoconjunctivitis, viral B30.2
Pharyngolaryngitis (acute) J06.0
chronic J37.0

Pharyngoplegia J39.2
Pharyngotonsillitis, herpesviral B00.2
Pharyngotracheitis, chronic J42
Pharynx, pharyngeal —*see* condition
Phenomenon
Arthus' —*see* Arthus' phenomenon
jaw-winking Q07.8
lupus erythematosus (LE) cell M32.9
Raynaud's (secondary) I73.00
with gangrene I73.01
vasomotor R55
vasospastic I73.9
vasovagal R55
Wenckebach's I44.1
Phenylketonuria E70.1
classical E70.0
maternal E70.1
Pheochromoblastoma
specified site —*see* Neoplasm,
malignant, by site
unspecified site C74.10
Pheochromocytoma
malignant
specified site —*see* Neoplasm,
malignant, by site
unspecified site C74.10
specified site —*see* Neoplasm, benign,
by site
unspecified site D35.00
Pheohyphomycosis —*see* Chromomycosis
Pheomycosis —*see* Chromomycosis
Phimosis (congenital) (due to infection)
N47.1
chancroidal A57
Phlebectasia —*see also* Varix
congenital Q27.4
Phlebitis (infective) (pyemic) (septic)
(suppurative) I80.9
antepartum —*see* Thrombophlebitis,
antepartum
blue —*see* Phlebitis, leg, deep
breast, superficial I80.8
cavernous (venous) sinus —*see*
Phlebitis, intracranial (venous)
sinus
cerebral (venous) sinus —*see* Phlebitis,
intracranial (venous) sinus
chest wall, superficial I80.8
cranial (venous) sinus —*see* Phlebitis,
intracranial (venous) sinus
deep (vessels) —*see* Phlebitis, leg, deep
due to implanted device —*see*
Complications, by site and type,
specified NEC
during or resulting from a procedure
T81.72
femoral vein (superficial) I80.1-
femoropopliteal vein I80.0-
gestational —*see* Phlebopathy,
gestational
hepatic veins I80.8
iliofemoral —*see* Phlebitis, femoral
vein
intracranial (venous) sinus (any)
G08
nonpyogenic I67.6
intraspinal venous sinuses and veins
G08
nonpyogenic G95.19
lateral (venous) sinus —*see* Phlebitis,
intracranial (venous) sinus
leg I80.3
antepartum —*see* Thrombophlebitis,
antepartum

Phlebitis *(Continued)*
  leg *(Continued)*
    deep (vessels) NEC I80.20-
      iliac I80.21-
      popliteal vein I80.22-
      specified vessel NEC I80.29-
      tibial vein I80.23-
    femoral vein (superficial) I80.1-
    superficial (vessels) I80.0-
    longitudinal sinus —*see* Phlebitis, intracranial (venous) sinus
    lower limb —*see* Phlebitis, leg
    migrans, migrating (superficial) I82.1
    pelvic
      with ectopic or molar pregnancy O08.0
      following ectopic or molar pregnancy O08.0
      puerperal, postpartum O87.1
    popliteal vein —*see* Phlebitis, leg, deep, popliteal
    portal (vein) K75.1
    postoperative T81.72
    pregnancy —*see* Thrombophlebitis, antepartum
    puerperal, postpartum, childbirth O87.0
      deep O87.1
      pelvic O87.1
      superficial O87.0
    retina —*see* Vasculitis, retina
    saphenous (accessory) (great) (long) (small) —*see* Phlebitis, leg, superficial
    sinus (meninges) —*see* Phlebitis, intracranial (venous) sinus
    specified site NEC I80.8
    syphilitic A52.09
    tibial vein —*see* Phlebitis, leg, deep, tibial
    ulcerative I80.9
      leg —*see* Phlebitis, leg
    umbilicus I80.8
    uterus (septic) —*see* Endometritis
    varicose (leg) (lower limb) —*see* Varix, leg, with, inflammation
Phlebofibrosis I87.8
Phleboliths I87.8
Phlebopathy,
  gestational O22.9-
  puerperal O87.9
Phlebosclerosis I87.8
Phlebothrombosis —*see also* Thrombosis
  antepartum —*see* Thrombophlebitis, antepartum
  pregnancy —*see* Thrombophlebitis, antepartum
  puerperal —*see* Thrombophlebitis, puerperal
Phlebotomus fever A93.1
Phlegmasia
  alba dolens O87.1
    nonpuerperal —*see* Phlebitis, femoral vein
  cerulea dolens —*see* Phlebitis, leg, deep
Phlegmon —*see* Abscess
Phlegmonous —*see* condition
Phlyctenulosis (allergic) (keratoconjunctivitis) (nontuberculous) —*see also* Keratoconjunctivitis
  cornea —*see* Keratoconjunctivitis
  tuberculous A18.52

Phobia, phobic F40.9
  animal F40.218
    spiders F40.210
  examination F40.298
  reaction F40.9
  simple F40.298
  social F40.10
    generalized F40.11
  specific (isolated) F40.298
    animal F40.218
      spiders F40.210
    blood F40.230
    injection F40.231
    injury F40.233
    men F40.290
    natural environment F40.228
      thunderstorms F40.220
    situational F40.248
      bridges F40.242
      closed in spaces F40.240
      flying F40.243
      heights F40.241
    specified focus NEC F40.298
    transfusion F40.231
    women F40.291
  specified NEC F40.8
    medical care NEC F40.232
  state F40.9
Phocas' disease —*see* Mastopathy, cystic
Phocomelia Q73.1
  lower limb —*see* Agenesis, leg, with foot present
  upper limb —*see* Agenesis, arm, with hand present
Phoria H50.50
Phosphate-losing tubular disorder N25.0
Phosphatemia E83.39
Phosphaturia E83.39
Photodermatitis (sun) L56.8
  chronic L57.8
  due to drug L56.8
  light other than sun L59.8
Photokeratitis H16.13-
Photophobia H53.14-
Photophthalmia —*see* Photokeratitis
Photopsia H53.19
Photoretinitis —*see* Retinopathy, solar
Photosensitivity, photosensitization (sun) skin L56.8
  light other than sun L59.8
Phrenitis —*see* Encephalitis
Phrynoderma (vitamin A deficiency) E50.8
Phthiriasis (pubis) B85.3
  with any infestation classifiable to B85.0-B85.2 B85.4
Phthirus infestation —*see* Phthiriasis
Phthisis —*see also* Tuberculosis
  bulbi (infectional) —*see* Disorder, globe, degenerated condition, atrophy
  eyeball (due to infection) —*see* Disorder, globe, degenerated condition, atrophy
Phycomycosis —*see* Zygomycosis
Physalopteriasis B81.8
Physical restraint status Z78.1
Phytobezoar T18.9
  intestine T18.3
  stomach T18.2
Pian —*see* Yaws
Pianoma A66.1
Pica F50.8
  in adults F50.8
  infant or child F98.3
Picking, nose F98.8

Pick-Niemann disease —*see* Niemann-Pick disease or syndrome
Pick's
  cerebral atrophy G31.01 *[F02.80]*
    with behavioral disturbance G31.01 *[F02.81]*
  disease or syndrome (brain) G31.01 *[F02.80]*
    with behavioral disturbance G31.01 *[F02.81]*
Pickwickian syndrome E66.2
Piebaldism E70.39
Piedra (beard) (scalp) B36.8
  black B36.3
  white B36.2
Pierre Robin deformity or syndrome Q87.0
Pierson's disease or osteochondrosis M91.0
Pig-bel A05.2
Pigeon
  breast or chest (acquired) M95.4
    congenital Q67.7
    rachitic sequelae (late effect) E64.3
  breeder's disease or lung J67.2
  fancier's disease or lung J67.2
  toe —*see* Deformity, toe, specified NEC
Pigmentation (abnormal) (anomaly) L81.9
  conjunctiva H11.13-
  cornea (anterior) H18.01-
    posterior H18.05-
    stromal H18.06-
  diminished melanin formation NEC L81.6
  iron L81.8
  lids, congenital Q82.8
  limbus corneae —*see* Pigmentation, cornea
  metals L81.8
  optic papilla, congenital Q14.2
  retina, congenital (grouped) (nevoid) Q14.1
  scrotum, congenital Q82.8
  tattoo L81.8
Piles (see also Hemorrhoids) K64.9
Pili
  annulati or torti (congenital) Q84.1
  incarnati L73.1
Pill roller hand (intrinsic) —*see* Parkinsonism
Pilomatrixoma —*see* Neoplasm, skin, benign
  malignant —*see* Neoplasm, skin, malignant
Pilonidal —*see* condition
Pimple R23.8
Pinched nerve —*see* Neuropathy, entrapment
Pindborg tumor —*see* Cyst, calcifying odontogenic
Pineal body or gland —*see* condition
Pinealoblastoma C75.3
Pinealoma D44.5
  malignant C75.3
Pineoblastoma C75.3
Pineocytoma D44.5
Pinguecula H11.15-
Pingueculitis H10.81-
Pinhole meatus (see also Stricture, urethra) N35.9
Pink
  disease —*see* subcategory T56.1
  eye —*see* Conjunctivitis, acute, mucopurulent

Pinkus' disease (lichen nitidus) L44.1
Pinpoint
  meatus —*see* Stricture, urethra
  os (uteri) —*see* Stricture, cervix
Pins and needles R20.2
Pinta A67.9
  cardiovascular lesions A67.2
  chancre (primary) A67.0
  erythematous plaques A67.1
  hyperchromic lesions A67.1
  hyperkeratosis A67.1
  lesions A67.9
    cardiovascular A67.2
    hyperchromic A67.1
    intermediate A67.1
    late A67.2
    mixed A67.3
    primary A67.0
    skin (achromic) (cicatricial)
      (dyschromic) A67.2
      hyperchromic A67.1
      mixed (achromic and
        hyperchromic) A67.3
  papule (primary) A67.0
  skin lesions (achromic) (cicatricial)
    (dyschromic) A67.2
    hyperchromic A67.1
    mixed (achromic and hyperchromic)
      A67.3
  vitiligo A67.2
Pintids A67.1
Pinworm (disease) (infection) (infestation)
  B80
Piroplasmosis B60.0
Pistol wound —*see* Gunshot wound
Pitchers' elbow —*see* Derangement,
  joint, specified type NEC,
  elbow
Pithecoid pelvis Q74.2
  with disproportion (fetopelvic)
    O33.0
    causing obstructed labor O65.0
Pithiatism F48.8
Pitted —*see* Pitting
Pitting —*see also* Edema R60.9
  lip R60.0
  nail L60.8
  teeth K00.4
Pituitary gland —*see* condition
Pituitary-snuff-taker's disease J67.8
Pityriasis (capitis) L21.0
  alba L30.5
  circinata (et maculata) L42
  furfuracea L21.0
  Hebra's L26
  lichenoides L41.0
    chronica L41.1
    et varioliformis (acuta) L41.0
  maculata (et circinata) L30.5
  nigra B36.1
  pilaris, Hebra's L44.0
  rosea L42
  rotunda L44.8
  rubra (Hebra) pilaris L44.0
  simplex L30.5
  specified type NEC L30.5
  streptogenes L30.5
  versicolor (scrotal) B36.0
Placenta, placental —*see* Pregnancy,
  complicated by (care of)
  (management affected by),
  specified condition
Placentitis O41.14-
Plagiocephaly Q67.3

Plague A20.9
  abortive A20.8
  ambulatory A20.8
  asymptomatic A20.8
  bubonic A20.0
  cellulocutaneous A20.1
  cutaneobubonic A20.1
  lymphatic gland A20.0
  meningitis A20.3
  pharyngeal A20.8
  pneumonic (primary) (secondary) A20.2
  pulmonary, pulmonic A20.2
  septicemic A20.7
  tonsillar A20.8
    septicemic A20.7
Planning, family
  contraception Z30.9
  procreation Z31.69
Plaque (s)
  artery, arterial —*see* Arteriosclerosis
  calcareous —*see* Calcification
  coronary, lipid rich I25.83
  epicardial I31.8
  erythematous, of pinta A67.1
  Hollenhorst's —*see* Occlusion, artery,
    retina
  lipid rich, coronary I25.83
  pleural (without asbestos) J92.9
    with asbestos J92.0
  tongue K13.29
Plasmacytoma C90.3-
  extramedullary C90.2-
  medullary C90.0-
  solitary C90.3-
Plasmacytopenia D72.818
Plasmacytosis D72.822
Plaster ulcer —*see* Ulcer, pressure, by site
Plateau iris syndrome (post-iridectomy)
    (postprocedural) (without glaucoma)
    H21.82
  with glaucoma H40.22-
Platybasia Q75.8
Platyonychia (congenital) Q84.6
  acquired L60.8
Platypelloid pelvis M95.5
  with disproportion (fetopelvic) O33.0
    causing obstructed labor O65.0
  congenital Q74.2
Platyspondylisis Q76.49
Plaut (-Vincent) disease (*see also*
  Vincent's) A69.1
Plethora R23.2
  newborn P61.1
Pleura, pleural —*see* condition
Pleuralgia R07.89
Pleurisy (acute) (adhesive) (chronic)
    (costal) (diaphragmatic) (double)
    (dry) (fibrinous) (fibrous) (interlobar)
    (latent) (plastic) (primary)
    (residual) (sicca) (sterile) (subacute)
    (unresolved) R09.1
  with
    adherent pleura J86.0
    effusion J90
      chylous, chyliform J94.0
      tuberculous (non primary)
        A15.6
        primary (progressive) A15.7
    tuberculosis —*see* Pleurisy,
      tuberculous (non primary)
  encysted —*see* Pleurisy, with effusion
  exudative —*see* Pleurisy, with effusion
  fibrinopurulent, fibropurulent —*see*
    Pyothorax

Pleurisy (*Continued*)
  hemorrhagic —*see* Hemothorax
  pneumococcal J90
  purulent —*see* Pyothorax
  septic —*see* Pyothorax
  serofibrinous —*see* Pleurisy, with
    effusion
  seropurulent —*see* Pyothorax
  serous —*see* Pleurisy, with effusion
  staphylococcal J86.9
  streptococcal J90
  suppurative —*see* Pyothorax
  traumatic (post) (current) —*see* Injury,
    intrathoracic, pleura
  tuberculous (with effusion) (non
    primary) A15.6
    primary (progressive) A15.7
Pleuritis sicca —*see* Pleurisy
Pleurobronchopneumonia —*see*
  Pneumonia, broncho
Pleurodynia R07.81
  epidemic B33.0
  viral B33.0
Pleuropericarditis —*see also* Pericarditis
  acute I30.9
Pleuropneumonia (acute) (bilateral)
    (double) (septic) (*see also* Pneumonia)
    J18.8
  chronic —*see* Fibrosis, lung
Pleuro-pneumonia-like-organism
    (PPLO), as cause of disease
    classified elsewhere B96.0
Pleurorrhea —*see* Pleurisy, with effusion
Plexitis, brachial G54.0
Plica
  polonica B85.0
  syndrome, knee M67.5
  tonsil J35.8
Plicated tongue K14.5
Plug
  bronchus NEC J98.09
  meconium (newborn) NEC syndrome
    P76.0
  mucus —*see* Asphyxia, mucus
Plumbism —*see* subcategory T56.0
Plummer's disease E05.20
  with thyroid storm E05.21
Plummer-Vinson syndrome D50.1
Pluricarential syndrome of infancy E40
Plus (and minus) hand (intrinsic) —*see*
  Deformity, limb, specified type NEC,
  forearm
Pneumathemia —*see* Air, embolism
Pneumatic hammer (drill) syndrome
  T75.21
Pneumatocele (lung) J98.4
  intracranial G93.89
  tension J44.9
Pneumatosis
  cystoides intestinalis K63.89
  intestinalis K63.89
  peritonei K66.8
Pneumaturia R39.89
Pneumoblastoma —*see* Neoplasm, lung,
  malignant
Pneumocephalus G93.89
Pneumococcemia A40.3
Pneumococcus, pneumococcal —*see*
  condition
Pneumoconiosis (due to) (inhalation of)
  J64
  with tuberculosis (any type in A15) J65
  aluminum J63.0
  asbestos J61

Pneumoconiosis (Continued)
bagasse, bagassosis J67.1
bauxite J63.1
beryllium J63.2
coal miners' (simple) J60
coalworkers' (simple) J60
collier's J60
cotton dust J66.0
diatomite (diatomaceous earth) J62.8
dust
  inorganic NEC J63.6
  lime J62.8
  marble J62.8
  organic NEC J66.8
fumes or vapors (from silo) J68.9
graphite J63.3
grinder's J62.8
kaolin J62.8
mica J62.8
millstone maker's J62.8
mineral fibers NEC J61
miner's J60
moldy hay J67.0
potter's J62.8
rheumatoid —see Rheumatoid, lung
sandblaster's J62.8
silica, silicate NEC J62.8
  with carbon J60
stonemason's J62.8
talc (dust) J62.0
Pneumocystis carinii pneumonia
  B59
Pneumocystis jiroveci (pneumonia)
  B59
Pneumocystosis (with pneumonia)
  B59
Pneumohemopericardium I31.2
Pneumohemothorax J94.2
traumatic S27.2
Pneumohydropericardium —see
  Pericarditis
Pneumohydrothorax —see Hydrothorax
Pneumomediastinum J98.2
congenital or perinatal P25.2
Pneumomycosis B49 [J99]
Pneumonia (acute) (double) (migratory)
  (purulent) (septic) (unresolved)
  J18.9
with
  influenza —see Influenza, with,
    pneumonia
  lung abscess J85.1
    due to specified organism —see
      Pneumonia, in (due to)
adenoviral J12.0
adynamic J18.2
alba A50.04
allergic (eosinophilic) J82
alveolar —see Pneumonia, lobar
anaerobes J15.8
anthrax A22.1
apex, apical —see Pneumonia, lobar
Ascaris B77.81
aspiration J69.0
  due to
    aspiration of microorganisms
      bacterial J15.9
      viral J12.9
    food (regurgitated) J69.0
    gastric secretions J69.0
    milk (regurgitated) J69.0
    oils, essences J69.1
    solids, liquids NEC J69.8
    vomitus J69.0

Pneumonia (Continued)
aspiration (Continued)
  newborn P24.81
    amniotic fluid (clear) P24.11
    blood P24.21
    food (regurgitated) P24.31
    liquor (amnii) P24.11
    meconium P24.01
    milk P24.31
    mucus P24.11
    specified NEC P24.81
    stomach contents P24.31
  postprocedural J95.4
atypical NEC J18.9
bacillus J15.9
  specified NEC J15.8
bacterial J15.9
  specified NEC J15.8
Bacteroides (fragilis) (oralis)
  (melaninogenicus) J15.8
basal, basic, basilar —see Pneumonia,
  by type
bronchiolitis obliterans organized
  (BOOP) J84.89
broncho-, bronchial (confluent)
  (croupous) (diffuse) (disseminated)
  (hemorrhagic) (involving lobes)
  (lobar) (terminal) J18.0
  allergic (eosinophilic) J82
  aspiration —see Pneumonia,
    aspiration
  bacterial J15.9
    specified NEC J15.8
  chronic —see Fibrosis, lung
  diplococcal J13
  Eaton's agent J15.7
  Escherichia coli (E. coli) J15.5
  Friedländer's bacillus J15.0
  Hemophilus influenzae J14
  hypostatic J18.2
  inhalation (see also Pneumonia,
    aspiration
    due to fumes or vapors (chemical)
      J68.0
    of oils or essences J69.1
  Klebsiella (pneumoniae) J15.0
  lipid, lipoid J69.1
    endogenous J84.89
  Mycoplasma (pneumoniae) J15.7
  pleuro-pneumonia-like-organisms
    (PPLO) J15.7
  pneumococcal J13
  Proteus J15.6
  Pseudomonas J15.1
  Serratia marcescens J15.6
  specified organism NEC J16.8
  staphylococcal —see Pneumonia,
    staphylococcal
  streptococcal NEC J15.4
    group B J15.3
    pneumoniae J13
  viral, virus —see Pneumonia, viral
Butyrivibrio (fibriosolvens) J15.8
Candida B37.1
caseous —see Tuberculosis, pulmonary
catarrhal —see Pneumonia, broncho
chlamydial J16.0
  congenital P23.1
cholesterol J84.89
cirrhotic (chronic) —see Fibrosis,
  lung
Clostridium (haemolyticum) (novyi)
  J15.8
confluent —see Pneumonia, broncho

Pneumonia (Continued)
congenital (infective) P23.9
due to
  bacterium NEC P23.6
  Chlamydia P23.1
  Escherichia coli P23.4
  Haemophilus influenzae P23.6
  infective organism NEC P23.8
  Klebsiella pneumoniae P23.6
  Mycoplasma P23.6
  Pseudomonas P23.5
  Staphylococcus P23.2
  Streptococcus (except group B)
    P23.6
    group B P23.3
  viral agent P23.0
  specified NEC P23.8
croupous —see Pneumonia, lobar
cryptogenic organizing J84.116
cytomegalic inclusion B25.0
cytomegaloviral B25.0
deglutition —see Pneumonia, aspiration
desquamative interstitial J84.117
diffuse —see Pneumonia, broncho
diplococcal, diplococcus (broncho-)
  (lobar) J13
disseminated (focal) —see Pneumonia,
  broncho
Eaton's agent J15.7
embolic, embolism —see Embolism,
  pulmonary
Enterobacter J15.6
eosinophilic J82
Escherichia coli (E. coli) J15.5
Eubacterium J15.8
fibrinous —see Pneumonia, lobar
fibroid, fibrous (chronic) —see Fibrosis,
  lung
Friedländer's bacillus J15.0
Fusobacterium (nucleatum) J15.8
gangrenous J85.0
giant cell (measles) B05.2
gonococcal A54.84
gram-negative bacteria NEC J15.6
  anaerobic J15.8
Hemophilus influenzae (broncho)
  (lobar) J14
human metapneumovirus J12.3
hypostatic (broncho) (lobar) J18.2
in (due to)
  actinomycosis A42.0
  adenovirus J12.0
  anthrax A22.1
  ascariasis B77.81
  aspergillosis B44.9
  Bacillus anthracis A22.1
  Bacterium anitratum J15.6
  candidiasis B37.1
  chickenpox B01.2
  Chlamydia J16.0
    neonatal P23.1
  coccidioidomycosis B38.2
    acute B38.0
    chronic B38.1
  cytomegalovirus disease B25.0
  Diplococcus (pneumoniae) J13
  Eaton's agent J15.7
  Enterobacter J15.6
  Escherichia coli (E. coli) J15.5
  Friedländer's bacillus J15.0
  fumes and vapors (chemical)
    (inhalation) J68.0
  gonorrhea A54.84
  Hemophilus influenzae
    (H. influenzae) J14

Pneumonia *(Continued)*
  in (due to) *(Continued)*
    Herellea J15.6
    histoplasmosis B39.2
      acute B39.0
      chronic B39.1
    human metapneumovirus J12.3
    Klebsiella (pneumoniae) J15.0
    measles B05.2
    Mycoplasma (pneumoniae) J15.7
    nocardiosis, nocardiasis A43.0
    ornithosis A70
    parainfluenza virus J12.2
    pleuro-pneumonia-like-organism
        (PPLO) J15.7
    pneumococcus J13
    pneumocystosis (Pneumocystis carinii)
      (Pneumocystis jiroveci) B59
    Proteus J15.6
    Pseudomonas NEC J15.1
      pseudomallei A24.1
    psittacosis A70
    Q fever A78
    respiratory syncytial virus J12.1
    rheumatic fever I00 *[J17]*
    rubella B06.81
    Salmonella (infection) A02.22
      typhi A01.03
    schistosomiasis B65.9 *[J17]*
    Serratia marcescens J15.6
    specified
      bacterium NEC J15.8
      organism NEC J16.8
    spirochetal NEC A69.8
    Staphylococcus J15.20
      aureus (methicillin susceptible)
        (MSSA) J15.211
        methicillin resistant (MRSA)
          J15.212
      specified NEC J15.29
    Streptococcus J15.4
      group B J15.3
      pneumoniae J13
      specified NEC J15.4
    toxoplasmosis B58.3
    tularemia A21.2
    typhoid (fever) A01.03
    varicella B01.2
    virus —*see* Pneumonia, viral
    whooping cough A37.91
      due to
        Bordetella parapertussis A37.11
        Bordetella pertussis A37.01
        specified NEC A37.81
    Yersinia pestis A20.2
  inhalation of food or vomit —*see*
    Pneumonia, aspiration
  interstitial J84.9
    chronic J84.111
    desquamative J84.117
    due to
      collagen vascular disease J84.17
      known underlying cause J84.17
    idiopathic NOS J84.111
    in disease classified elsewhere
      J84.17
    lymphocytic (due to collagen
      vascular disease) (in diseases
      classified elsewhere) J84.17
    lymphoid J84.2
    non-specific J84.89
      due to
        collagen vascular disease J84.17
        known underlying cause J84.17

Pneumonia *(Continued)*
  interstitial *(Continued)*
    non-specific *(Continued)*
      idiopathic J84.113
      in diseases classified elsewhere
        J84.17
      plasma cell B59
      pseudomonas J15.1
      usual J84.112
        due to collagen vascular disease
          J84.17
        idiopathic J84.112
        in diseases classified elsewhere
          J84.17
  Klebsiella (pneumoniae) J15.0
  lipid, lipoid (exogenous) J69.1
    endogenous J84.89
  lobar (disseminated) (double)
    (interstitial) J18.1
    bacterial J15.9
      specified NEC J15.8
    chronic —*see* Fibrosis, lung
    Escherichia coli (E. coli) J15.5
    Friedländer's bacillus J15.0
    Hemophilus influenzae J14
    hypostatic J18.2
    Klebsiella (pneumoniae) J15.0
    pneumococcal J13
    Proteus J15.6
    Pseudomonas J15.1
    specified organism NEC J16.8
    staphylococcal —*see* Pneumonia,
      staphylococcal
    streptococcal NEC J15.4
    Streptococcus pneumoniae J13
    viral, virus —*see* Pneumonia, viral
  lobular —*see* Pneumonia, broncho
  Löffler's J82
  lymphoid interstitial J84.2
  massive —*see* Pneumonia, lobar
  meconium P24.01
  MSSA (methicillin susceptible
    Staphylococcus aureus) J15.211
  multilobar —*see* Pneumonia, by type
  Mycoplasma (pneumoniae) J15.7
  necrotic J85.0
  neonatal P23.9
    aspiration —*see* Aspiration, by
      substance, with pneumonia
  nitrogen dioxide J68.9
  organizing J84.89
    due to
      collagen vascular disease J84.17
      known underlying cause J84.17
    in diseases classified elsewhere J84.17
  orthostatic J18.2
  parainfluenza virus J12.2
  parenchymatous —*see* Fibrosis, lung
  passive J18.2
  patchy —*see* Pneumonia, broncho
  Peptococcus J15.8
  Peptostreptococcus J15.8
  plasma cell (of infants) B59
  pleurolobar —*see* Pneumonia, lobar
  pleuro-pneumonia-like organism
    (PPLO) J15.7
  pneumococcal (broncho) (lobar) J13
  Pneumocystis (carinii) (jiroveci) B59
  postinfectional NEC B99 *[J17]*
  postmeasles B05.2
  Proteus J15.6
  Pseudomonas J15.1
  psittacosis A70
  radiation J70.0

Pneumonia *(Continued)*
  respiratory syncytial virus J12.1
  resulting from a procedure J95.89
  rheumatic I00 *[J17]*
  Salmonella (arizonae) (cholerae-suis)
    (enteritidis) (typhimurium)
    A02.22
    typhi A01.03
    typhoid fever A01.03
  SARS-associated coronavirus J12.81
  segmented, segmental —*see*
    Pneumonia, broncho-
  Serratia marcescens J15.6
  specified NEC J18.8
    bacterium NEC J15.8
    organism NEC J16.8
    virus NEC J12.89
  spirochetal NEC A69.8
  staphylococcal (broncho) (lobar) J15.20
    aureus (methicillin susceptible)
      (MSSA) J15.211
      methicillin resistant (MRSA)
        J15.212
    specified NEC J15.29
  static, stasis J18.2
  streptococcal NEC (broncho) (lobar) J15.4
    group
      A J15.4
      B J15.3
      specified NEC J15.4
  Streptococcus pneumoniae J13
  syphilitic, congenital (early) A50.04
  traumatic (complication) (early)
    (secondary) T79.8
  tuberculous (any) —*see* Tuberculosis,
    pulmonary
  tularemic A21.2
  varicella B01.2
  Veillonella J15.8
  ventilator associated J95.851
  viral, virus (broncho) (interstitial)
    (lobar) J12.9
    adenoviral J12.0
    congenital P23.0
    human metapneumovirus J12.3
    parainfluenza J12.2
    respiratory syncytial J12.1
    SARS-associated coronavirus J12.81
    specified NEC J12.89
  white (congenital) A50.04
Pneumonic —*see* condition
Pneumonitis (acute) (primary) —*see also*
  Pneumonia
  air-conditioner J67.7
  allergic (due to) J67.9
    organic dust NEC J67.8
    red cedar dust J67.8
    sequoiosis J67.8
    wood dust J67.8
  aspiration J69.0
    due to
      anesthesia J95.4
        during
          labor and delivery O74.0
          pregnancy O29.01-
          puerperium O89.01
      fumes or gases J68.0
      obstetric O74.0
  chemical (due to gases, fumes or
    vapors) (inhalation) J68.0
    due to anesthesia J95.4
  cholesterol J84.89
  chronic —*see* Fibrosis, lung
  congenital rubella P35.0

Pneumonitis *(Continued)*
crack (cocaine) J68.0
due to
beryllium J68.0
cadmium J68.0
crack (cocaine) J68.0
detergent J69.8
fluorocarbon-polymer J68.0
food, vomit (aspiration) J69.0
fumes or vapors J68.0
gases, fumes or vapors (inhalation)
J68.0
inhalation
blood J69.8
essences J69.1
food (regurgitated), milk, vomit
J69.0
oils, essences J69.1
saliva J69.0
solids, liquids NEC J69.8
manganese J68.0
nitrogen dioxide J68.0
oils, essences J69.1
solids, liquids NEC J69.8
toxoplasmosis (acquired) B58.3
congenital P37.1
vanadium J68.0
ventilator J95.851
eosinophilic J82
hypersensitivity J67.9
air conditioner lung J67.7
bagassosis J67.1
bird fancier's lung J67.2
farmer's lung J67.0
maltworker's lung J67.4
maple bark-stripper's lung J67.6
mushroom worker's lung J67.5
specified organic dust NEC J67.8
suberosis J67.3
interstitial (chronic) J84.89
acute J84.114
lymphoid J84.2
non-specific J84.89
idiopathic J84.113
lymphoid, interstitial J84.2
meconium P24.01
postanesthetic J95.4
correct substance properly
administered —*see* Table of
drugs and chemcials, by drug,
adverse effect
in labor and delivery O74.0
in pregnancy O29.01-
obstetric O74.0
overdose or wrong substance given
or taken (by accident) —*see*
Table of drugs and chemicals, by
drug, poisoning
postpartum, puerperal O89.01
postoperative J95.4
obstetric O74.0
radiation J70.0
rubella, congenital P35.0
ventilation (air-conditioning) J67.7
ventilator associated J95.851
wood-dust J67.8
Pneumonoconiosis —*see* Pneumoconiosis
Pneumoparotid K11.8
Pneumopathy NEC J98.4
alveolar J84.09
due to organic dust NEC J66.8
parietoalveolar J84.09
Pneumopericarditis —*see also* Pericarditis
acute I30.9

Pneumopericardium —*see also*
Pericarditis
congenital P25.3
newborn P25.3
traumatic (post) —*see* Injury, heart
Pneumophagia (psychogenic) F45.8
Pneumopleurisy, pneumopleuritis *(see
also* Pneumonia) J18.8
Pneumopyopericardium I30.1
Pneumopyothorax —*see*
Pyopneumothorax
with fistula J86.0
Pneumorrhagia —*see also* Hemorrhage,
lung
tuberculous —*see* Tuberculosis,
pulmonary
Pneumothorax NOS J93.9
acute J93.83
chronic J93.81
congenital P25.1
perinatal period P25.1
postprocedural J95.811
specified NEC J93.83
spontaneous NOS J93.83
newborn P25.1
primary J93.11
secondary J93.12
tension J93.0
tense valvular, infectional J93.0
tension (spontaneous) J93.0
traumatic S27.0
with hemothorax S27.2
tuberculous —*see* Tuberculosis,
pulmonary
Podagra *(see also* Gout) M10.9
Podencephalus Q01.9
Poikilocytosis R71.8
Poikiloderma L81.6
Civatte's L57.3
congenital Q82.8
vasculare atrophicans L94.5
Poikilodermatomyositis M33.10
with
myopathy M33.12
respiratory involvement M33.11
specified organ involvement NEC
M33.19
Pointed ear (congenital) Q17.3
Poison ivy, oak, sumac or other plant
dermatitis (allergic) (contact)
L23.7
Poisoning (acute) —*see also* Table of drugs
and chemicals
algae and toxins T65.82-
Bacillus B (aertrycke) (cholerae (suis))
(paratyphosus) (suipestifer)
A02.9
botulinus A05.1
bacterial toxins A05.9
berries, noxious —*see* Poisoning, food,
noxious, berries
botulism A05.1
ciguatera fish T61.0-
Clostridium botulinum A05.1
death-cap (Amanita phalloides)
(Amanita verna) —*see*
Poisoning, food, noxious,
mushrooms
drug —*see* Table of drugs and
chemicals, by drug, poisoning
epidemic, fish (noxious) —*see*
Poisoning, seafood
bacterial A05.9
fava bean D55.0

Poisoning *(Continued)*
fish (noxious) T61.9-
bacterial —*see* Intoxication,
foodborne, by agent
ciguatera fish —*see* Poisoning,
ciguatera fish
scombroid fish —*see* Poisoning,
scombroid fish
specified type NEC T61.77-
food (acute) (diseased) (infected)
(noxious) NEC T62.9-
bacterial —*see* Intoxication,
foodborne, by agent
due to
Bacillus (aertrycke) (choleraesuis)
(paratyphosus) (suipestifer)
A02.9
botulinus A05.1
Clostridium (perfringens) (Welchii)
A05.2
salmonella (aertrycke) (callinarum)
(choleraesuis) (enteritidis)
(paratyphi) (suipestifer)
A02.9
with
gastroenteritis A02.0
sepsis A02.1
staphylococcus A05.0
Vibrio
parahaemolyticus A05.3
vulnificus A05.5
noxious or naturally toxic T62.9-
berries —*see* subcategory T62.1-
fish —*see* Poisoning, seafood
mushrooms —*see* subcategory
T62.0X-
plants NEC —*see* subcategory
T62.2X-
seafood —*see* Poisoning, seafood
specified NEC —*see* subcategory
T62.8X-
ichthyotoxism —*see* Poisoning, seafood
kreotoxism, food A05.9
latex T65.81-
lead T56.0-
mushroom —*see* Poisoning, food,
noxious, mushroom
mussels —*see also* Poisoning, shellfish
bacterial —*see* Intoxication,
foodborne, by agent
nicotine (tobacco) T65.2-
noxious foodstuffs —*see* Poisoning,
food, noxious
plants, noxious —*see* Poisoning, food,
noxious, plants NEC
ptomaine —*see* Poisoning, food
radiation J70.0
Salmonella (arizonae) (cholerae-suis)
(enteritidis) (typhimurium) A02.9
scombroid fish T61.1-
seafood (noxious) T61.9-
bacterial —*see* Intoxication,
foodborne, by agent
fish —*see* Poisoning, fish
shellfish —*see* Poisoning, shellfish
specified NEC —*see* subcategory
T61.8X-
shellfish (amnesic) (azaspiracid)
(diarrheic) (neurotoxic) (noxious)
(paralytic) T61.78-
bacterial —*see* Intoxication,
foodborne, by agent
ciguatera mollusk —*see* Poisoning,
ciguatera fish

Poisoning *(Continued)*
  specified substance NEC T65.891
  Staphylococcus, food A05.0
  tobacco (nicotine) T65.2-
  water E87.79
Poker spine —*see* Spondylitis, ankylosing
Poland syndrome Q79.8
Polioencephalitis (acute) (bulbar)
      A80.9
  inferior G12.22
  influenzal —*see* Influenza, with,
      encephalopathy
  superior hemorrhagic (acute)
      (Wernicke's) E51.2
  Wernicke's E51.2
Polioencephalomyelitis (acute) (anterior)
      A80.9
  with beriberi E51.2
Polioencephalopathy, superior
      hemorrhagic E51.2
  with
      beriberi E51.11
      pellagra E52
Poliomeningoencephalitis —*see*
      Meningoencephalitis
Poliomyelitis (acute) (anterior) (epidemic)
      A80.9
  with paralysis (bulbar) —*see*
      Poliomyelitis, paralytic
  abortive A80.4
  ascending (progressive) —*see*
      Poliomyelitis, paralytic
  bulbar (paralytic) —*see* Poliomyelitis,
      paralytic
  congenital P35.8
  nonepidemic A80.9
  nonparalytic A80.4
  paralytic A80.30
      specified NEC A80.39
      vaccine-associated A80.0
      wild virus
          imported A80.1
          indigenous A80.2
  spinal, acute A80.9
Poliosis (eyebrow) (eyelashes) L67.1
  circumscripta, acquired L67.1
Pollakiuria R35.0
  psychogenic F45.8
Pollinosis J30.1
Pollitzer's disease L73.2
Polyadenitis —*see also* Lymphadenitis
  malignant A20.0
Polyalgia M79.89
Polyangiitis M30.0
  microscopic M31.7
  overlap syndrome M30.8
Polyarteritis
  microscopic M31.7
  nodosa M30.0
      with lung involvement M30.1
      juvenile M30.2
      related condition NEC M30.8
Polyarthralgia —*see* Pain, joint
Polyarthritis, polyarthropathy (*see also*
      Arthritis) M13.0
  due to or associated with other
      specified conditions —*see* Arthritis
  epidemic (Australian) (with exanthema)
      B33.1
  infective —*see* Arthritis, pyogenic or
      pyemic
  inflammatory M06.4
  juvenile (chronic) (seronegative) M08.3
  migratory —*see* Fever, rheumatic
  rheumatic, acute —*see* Fever, rheumatic

Polyarthrosis M15.9
  post-traumatic M15.3
  primary M15.0
  specified NEC M15.8
Polycarential syndrome of infancy
      E40
Polychondritis (atrophic) (chronic) —*see
      also* Disorder, cartilage, specified
      type NEC
  relapsing M94.1
Polycoria Q13.2
Polycystic (disease)
  degeneration, kidney Q61.3
      autosomal dominant (adult type)
          Q61.2
      autosomal recessive (infantile type)
          NEC Q61.19
  kidney Q61.3
      autosomal
          dominant Q61.2
          recessive NEC Q61.19
      autosomal dominant (adult type)
          Q61.2
      autosomal recessive (childhood type)
          NEC Q61.19
      infantile type NEC Q61.19
  liver Q44.6
  lung J98.4
      congenital Q33.0
  ovary, ovaries E28.2
  spleen Q89.09
Polycythemia (secondary) D75.1
  acquired D75.1
  benign (familial) D75.0
  due to
      donor twin P61.1
      erythropoietin D75.1
      fall in plasma volume D75.1
      high altitude D75.1
      maternal-fetal transfusion P61.1
      stress D75.1
  emotional D75.1
  erythropoietin D75.1
  familial (benign) D75.0
  Gaisböck's (hypertonica) D75.1
  high altitude D75.1
  hypertonica D75.1
  hypoxemic D75.1
  neonatorum P61.1
  nephrogenous D75.1
  relative D75.1
  secondary D75.1
  spurious D75.1
  stress D75.1
  vera D45
Polycytosis cryptogenica D75.1
Polydactylism, polydactyly Q69.9
  toes Q69.2
Polydipsia R63.1
Polydystrophy, pseudo-Hurler E77.0
Polyembryoma —*see* Neoplasm,
      malignant, by site
Polyglandular
  deficiency E31.0
  dyscrasia E31.9
  dysfunction E31.9
  syndrome E31.8
Polyhydramnios O40.-
Polymastia Q83.1
Polymenorrhea N92.0
Polymyalgia M35.3
  arteritica, giant cell M31.5
  rheumatica M35.3
      with giant cell arteritis M31.5

Polymyositis (acute) (chronic)
      (hemorrhagic) M33.20
  with
      myopathy M33.22
      respiratory involvement M33.21
      skin involvement —*see*
          Dermatopolymyositis
      specified organ involvement NEC
          M33.29
  ossificans (generalisata) (progressiva) —
      see Myositis, ossificans,
      progressiva
Polyneuritis, polyneuritic —*see also*
      Polyneuropathy
  acute (post-)infective G61.0
  alcoholic G62.1
  cranialis G52.7
  demyelinating, chronic inflammatory
      (CIDP) G61.81
  diabetic —*see* Diabetes, polyneuropathy
  diphtheritic A36.83
  due to lack of vitamin NEC E56.9
      [G63]
  endemic E51.11
  erythredema —*see* subcategory
      T56.1
  febrile, acute G61.0
  hereditary ataxic G60.1
  idiopathic, acute G61.0
  infective (acute) G61.0
  inflammatory, chronic demyelinating
      (CIDP) G61.81
  nutritional E63.9 *[G63]*
  postinfective (acute) G61.0
  specified NEC G62.89
Polyneuropathy (peripheral) G62.9
  alcoholic G62.1
  amyloid (Portuguese) E85.1 *[G63]*
  arsenical G62.2
  critical illness G62.81
  demyelinating, chronic inflammatory
      (CIDP) G61.81
  diabetic —*see* Diabetes, polyneuropathy
  drug-induced G62.0
  hereditary G60.9
      specified NEC G60.8
  idiopathic G60.9
      progressive G60.3
  in (due to)
      alcohol G62.1
          sequelae G65.2
      amyloidosis, familial (Portuguese)
          E85.1 *[G63]*
      antitetanus serum G61.1
      arsenic G62.2
          sequelae G65.2
      avitaminosis NEC E56.9 *[G63]*
      beriberi E51.11
      collagen vascular disease NEC M35.9
          [G63]
      deficiency (of)
          B (-complex) vitamins E53.9 *[G63]*
          vitamin B6 E53.1 *[G63]*
      diabetes —*see* Diabetes,
          polyneuropathy
      diphtheria A36.83
      drug or medicament G62.0
          correct substance properly
              administered —*see* Table of
              drugs and chemicals, by drug,
              adverse effect
          overdose or wrong substance
              given or taken —*see* Table of
              drugs and chemicals, by drug,
              poisoning

Polyneuropathy (Continued)
  in (due to) (Continued)
    endocrine disease NEC E34.9 [G63]
    herpes zoster B02.23
    hypoglycemia E16.2 [G63]
    infectious
      disease NEC B99 [G63]
      mononucleosis B27.91
    lack of vitamin NEC E56.9 [G63]
    lead G62.2
      sequelae G65.2
    leprosy A30.9 [G63]
    Lyme disease A69.22
    metabolic disease NEC E88.9 [G63]
    microscopic polyangiitis M31.7 [G63]
    mumps B26.84
    neoplastic disease (see also Neoplasm)
      D49.9 [G63]
    nutritional deficiency NEC E63.9
      [G63]
    organophosphate compounds
      G62.2
      sequelae G65.2
    parasitic disease NEC B89 [G63]
    pellagra E52 [G63]
    polyarteritis nodosa M30.0
    porphyria E80.20 [G63]
    radiation G62.82
    rheumatoid arthritis —see
      Rheumatoid, polyneuropathy
    sarcoidosis D86.89
    serum G61.1
    syphilis (late) A52.15
      congenital A50.43
    systemic
      connective tissue disorder M35.9
        [G63]
      lupus erythematosus M32.19
    toxic agent NEC G62.2
      sequelae G65.2
    triorthocresyl phosphate G62.2
      sequelae G65.2
    tuberculosis A17.89
    uremia N18.9 [G63]
    vitamin B12 deficiency E53.8 [G63]
      with anemia (pernicious) D51.0
        [G63]
        due to dietary deficiency D51.3
          [G63]
    zoster B02.23
  inflammatory G61.9
    chronic demyelinating (CIDP)
      G61.81
    sequelae G65.1
    specified NEC G61.89
  lead G62.2
    sequelae G65.2
  nutritional NEC E63.9 [G63]
  postherpetic (zoster) B02.23
  progressive G60.3
  radiation-induced G62.82
  sensory (hereditary) (idiopathic)
    G60.8
  specified NEC G62.89
  syphilitic (late) A52.15
    congenital A50.43
Polyopia H53.8
Polyorchism, polyorchidism Q55.21
Polyosteoarthritis (see also Osteoarthritis,
  generalized) M15.9
  post-traumatic M15.3
  specified NEC M15.8
Polyostotic fibrous dysplasia Q78.1
Polyotia Q17.0

Polyp, polypus
  accessory sinus J33.8
  adenocarcinoma in —see Neoplasm,
    malignant, by site
  adenocarcinoma in situ in —see
    Neoplasm, in situ, by site
  adenoid tissue J33.0
  adenomatous —see also Neoplasm,
    benign, by site
    adenocarcinoma in —see Neoplasm,
      malignant, by site
    adenocarcinoma in situ in —see
      Neoplasm, in situ, by site
    carcinoma in —see Neoplasm,
      malignant, by site
    carcinoma in situ in —see Neoplasm,
      in situ, by site
    multiple —see Neoplasm, benign
      adenocarcinoma in —see
        Neoplasm, malignant, by site
      adenocarcinoma in situ in —see
        Neoplasm, in situ, by site
  antrum J33.8
  anus, anal (canal) K62.0
  Bartholin's gland N84.3
  bladder D41.4
  carcinoma in —see Neoplasm,
    malignant, by site
  carcinoma in situ in —see Neoplasm, in
    situ, by site
  cecum D12.0
  cervix (uteri) N84.1
    in pregnancy or childbirth —see
      Pregnancy, complicated by,
      abnormal, cervix
    mucous N84.1
    nonneoplastic N84.1
  choanal J33.0
  cholesterol K82.4
  clitoris N84.3
  colon K63.5
    adenomatous D12.6
    ascending D12.2
    cecum D12.0
    descending D12.4
    inflammatory K51.40
      with
        abscess K51.414
        complication K51.419
          specified NEC K51.418
        fistula K51.413
        intestinal obstruction K51.412
        rectal bleeding K51.411
    sigmoid D12.5
    transverse D12.3
  corpus uteri N84.0
  dental K04.0
  duodenum K31.7
  ear (middle) H74.4-
  endometrium N84.0
  ethmoidal (sinus) J33.8
  fallopian tube N84.8
  female genital tract N84.9
    specified NEC N84.8
  frontal (sinus) J33.8
  gallbladder K82.4
  gingiva, gum K06.8
  labia, labium (majus) (minus) N84.3
  larynx (mucous) J38.1
    adenomatous D14.1
  malignant —see Neoplasm, malignant,
    by site
  maxillary (sinus) J33.8
  middle ear —see Polyp, ear (middle)

Polyp, polypus (Continued)
  myometrium N84.0
  nares
    anterior J33.9
    posterior J33.0
  nasal (mucous) J33.9
    cavity J33.0
    septum J33.0
  nasopharyngeal J33.0
  nose (mucous) J33.9
  oviduct N84.8
  pharynx J39.2
  placenta O90.89
  prostate —see Enlargement, enlarged,
    prostate
  pudenda, pudendum N84.3
  pulpal (dental) K04.0
  rectum (nonadenomatous) K62.1
    adenomatous —see Polyp,
      adenomatous
  septum (nasal) J33.0
  sinus (accessory) (ethmoidal) (frontal)
    (maxillary) (sphenoidal) J33.8
  sphenoidal (sinus) J33.8
  stomach K31.7
    adenomatous D13.1
  tube, fallopian N84.8
  turbinate, mucous membrane J33.8
  umbilical, newborn P83.6
  ureter N28.89
  urethra N36.2
  uterus (body) (corpus) (mucous) N84.0
    cervix N84.1
    in pregnancy or childbirth —see
      Pregnancy, complicated by,
      tumor, uterus
  vagina N84.2
  vocal cord (mucous) J38.1
  vulva N84.3
Polyphagia R63.2
Polyploidy Q92.7
Polypoid —see condition
Polyposis —see also Polyp
  coli (adenomatous) D12.6
    adenocarcinoma in C18.9
    adenocarcinoma in situ in —see
      Neoplasm, in situ, by site
    carcinoma in C18.9
  colon (adenomatous) D12.6
  familial D12.6
    adenocarcinoma in situ in —see
      Neoplasm, in situ, by site
  intestinal (adenomatous) D12.6
    malignant lymphomatous C83.1
  multiple, adenomatous (see also
    Neoplasm, benign) D36.9
Polyradiculitis —see Polyneuropathy
Polyradiculoneuropathy (acute)
  (postinfective) (segmentally
  demyelinating) G61.0
Polyserositis
  due to pericarditis I31.1
  pericardial I31.1
  periodic, familial E85.0
  tuberculous A19.9
    acute A19.1
    chronic A19.8
Polysplenia syndrome Q89.09
Polysyndactyly (see also Syndactylism,
  syndactyly) Q70.4
Polytrichia L68.3
Polyunguia Q84.6
Polyuria R35.8
  nocturnal R35.1
  psychogenic F45.8

Pompe's disease (glycogen storage) E74.02
Pompholyx L30.1
Poncet's disease (tuberculous rheumatism) A18.09
Pond fracture —*see* Fracture, skull
Ponos B55.0
Pons, pontine —*see* condition
Poor
  aesthetic of existing restoration of tooth K08.56
  contractions, labor O62.2
  gingival margin to tooth restoration K08.51
  personal hygiene R46.0
  prenatal care, affecting management of pregnancy —*see* Pregnancy, complicated by, insufficient, prenatal care
  sucking reflex (newborn) R29.2
  urinary stream R39.12
  vision NEC H54.7
Poradenitis, nostras inguinalis or venerea A55
Porencephaly (congenital) (developmental) (true) Q04.6
  acquired G93.0
  nondevelopmental G93.0
  traumatic (post) F07.89
Porocephaliasis B88.8
Porokeratosis Q82.8
Poroma, eccrine —*see* Neoplasm, skin, benign
Porphyria (South African) E80.20
  acquired E80.20
  acute intermittent (hepatic) (Swedish) E80.21
  cutanea tarda (hereditary) (symptomatic) E80.1
  due to drugs E80.20
    correct substance properly administered —*see* Table of drugs and chemicals, by drug, adverse effect
    overdose or wrong substance given or taken —*see* Table of drugs and chemicals, by drug, poisoning
  erythropoietic (congenital) (hereditary) E80.0
  hepatocutaneous type E80.1
  secondary E80.20
  toxic NEC E80.20
  variegata E80.20
Porphyrinuria —*see* Porphyria
Porphyruria —*see* Porphyria
Port wine nevus, mark, or stain Q82.5
Portal —*see* condition
Posadas-Wernicke disease B38.9
Positive
  culture (nonspecific)
    blood R78.81
    bronchial washings R84.5
    cerebrospinal fluid R83.5
    cervix uteri R87.5
    nasal secretions R84.5
    nipple discharge R89.5
    nose R84.5
      staphylococcus (Methicillin susceptible) Z22.321
        Methicillin resistant Z22.322
    peritoneal fluid R85.5
    pleural fluid R84.5
    prostatic secretions R86.5
    saliva R85.5

Positive *(Continued)*
  culture *(Continued)*
    seminal fluid R86.5
    sputum R84.5
    synovial fluid R89.5
    throat scrapings R84.5
    urine R82.7
    vagina R87.5
    vulva R87.5
    wound secretions R89.5
  PPD (skin test) R76.11
  serology for syphilis A53.0
    with signs or symptoms - code as Syphilis, by site and stage
    false R76.8
  skin test, tuberculin (without active tuberculosis) R76.11
  test, human immunodeficiency virus (HIV) R75
  VDRL A53.0
    with signs or symptoms - code by site and stage under Syphilis A53.9
  Wassermann reaction A53.0
Postcardiotomy syndrome I97.0
Postcaval ureter Q62.62
Postcholecystectomy syndrome K91.5
Postclimacteric bleeding N95.0
Postcommissurotomy syndrome I97.0
Postconcussional syndrome F07.81
Postcontusional syndrome F07.81
Postcricoid region —*see* condition
Post-dates (40-42 weeks) (pregnancy) (mother) O48.0
  more than 42 weeks gestation O48.1
Postencephalitic syndrome F07.89
Posterior —*see* condition
Posterolateral sclerosis (spinal cord) —*see* Degeneration, combined
Postexanthematous —*see* condition
Postfebrile —*see* condition
Postgastrectomy dumping syndrome K91.1
Posthemiplegic chorea —*see* Monoplegia
Posthemorrhagic anemia (chronic) D50.0
  acute D62
  newborn P61.3
Postherpetic neuralgia (zoster) B02.29
  trigeminal B02.22
Posthitis N47.7
Postimmunization complication or reaction —*see* Complications, vaccination
Postinfectious —*see* condition
Postlaminectomy syndrome NEC M96.1
Postleukotomy syndrome F07.0
Postmastectomy lymphedema (syndrome) I97.2
Postmaturity, postmature (over 42 weeks)
  maternal (over 42 weeks gestation) O48.1
  newborn P08.22
Postmeasles complication NEC (*see also* condition) B05.89
Postmenopausal
  endometrium (atrophic) N95.8
    suppurative (*see also* Endometritis) N71.9
  osteoporosis —*see* Osteoporosis, postmenopausal

Postnasal drip R09.82
  due to
    allergic rhinitis —*see* Rhinitis, allergic
    common cold J00
    gastroesophageal reflux —*see* Reflux, gastroesophageal
    nasopharyngitis —*see* Nasopharyngitis
    other know condition — code to condition
    sinusitis —*see* Sinusitis
Postnatal —*see* condition
Postoperative (postprocedural) —*see* Complication, postoperative
  pneumothorax, therapeutic Z98.3
  state NEC Z98.89
Postpancreatectomy hyperglycemia E89.1
Postpartum —*see* Puerperal
Postphlebitic syndrome —*see* Syndrome, postthrombotic
Postpolio (myelitic) syndrome G14
Postpoliomyelitic —*see also* condition
  osteopathy —*see* Osteopathy, after poliomyelitis
Postprocedural —*see also* Postoperative
  hypoinsulinemia E89.1
Postschizophrenic depression F32.8
Postsurgery status —*see also* Status (post)
  pneumothorax, therapeutic Z98.3
Post-term (40-42 weeks) (pregnancy) (mother) O48.0
  infant P08.21
  more than 42 weeks gestation (mother) O48.1
Post-traumatic brain syndrome, nonpsychotic F07.81
Post-typhoid abscess A01.09
Postures, hysterical F44.2
Postvaccinal reaction or complication —*see* Complications, vaccination
Postvalvulotomy syndrome I97.0
Potain's
  disease (pulmonary edema) —*see* Edema, lung
  syndrome (gastrectasis with dyspepsia) K31.0
Potter's
  asthma J62.8
  facies Q60.6
  lung J62.8
  syndrome (with renal agenesis) Q60.6
Pott's
  curvature (spinal) A18.01
  disease or paraplegia A18.01
  spinal curvature A18.01
  tumor, puffy —*see* Osteomyelitis, specified type NEC
Pouch
  bronchus Q32.4
  Douglas' —*see* condition
  esophagus, esophageal, congenital Q39.6
    acquired K22.5
  gastric K31.4
  Hartmann's K82.8
  pharynx, pharyngeal (congenital) Q38.7
Pouchitis K91.850
Poultrymen's itch B88.0
Poverty NEC Z59.6
  extreme Z59.5
Poxvirus NEC B08.8
Prader-Willi syndrome Q87.1

Preauricular appendage or tag Q17.0
Prebetalipoproteinemia (acquired)
(essential) (familial) (hereditary)
(primary) (secondary) E78.1
with chylomicronemia E78.3
Precipitate labor or delivery O62.3
Preclimacteric bleeding (menorrhagia)
N92.4
Precocious
adrenarche E30.1
menarche E30.1
menstruation E30.1
pubarche E30.1
puberty E30.1
central E22.8
sexual development NEC E30.1
thelarche E30.8
Precocity, sexual (constitutional)
(cryptogenic) (female) (idiopathic)
(male) E30.1
with adrenal hyperplasia E25.9
congenital E25.0
Precordial pain R07.2
Predeciduous teeth K00.2
Prediabetes, prediabetic R73.09
complicating
pregnancy —see Pregnancy,
complicated by, diseases of,
specified type or system NEC
puerperium O99.89
Predislocation status of hip at birth
Q65.6
Pre-eclampsia O14.9-
with pre-existing hypertension —see
Hypertension, complicating
pregnancy, pre-existing, with,
pre-eclampsia
mild O14.0-
moderate O14.0-
severe O14.1-
with hemolysis, elevated liver
enzymes and low platelet count
(HELLP) O14.2-
Pre-eruptive color change, teeth, tooth
K00.8
Pre-excitation atrioventricular
conduction I45.6
Preglaucoma H40.00-
Pregnancy (single) (uterine) —see also
Delivery and Puerperal

Note: The Tabular must be reviewed
for assignment of the appropriate
character indicating the trimester of the
pregnancy

Note: The Tabular must be reviewed
for assignment of appropriate seventh
character for multiple gestation codes
in Chapter 15

abdominal (ectopic) O00.0
with viable fetus O36.7-
ampullar O00.1
biochemical O02.81
broad ligament O00.8
cervical O00.8
chemical O02.81
complicated NOS O26.9-
complicated by (care of) (management
affected by)
abnormal, abnormality
cervix O34.4-
causing obstructed labor O65.5
cord (umbilical) O69.9

Pregnancy (Continued)
complicated by (Continued)
abnormal, abnormality (Continued)
findings on antenatal screening of
mother O28.9
biochemical O28.1
chromosomal O28.5
cytological O28.2
genetic O28.5
hematological O28.0
radiological O28.4
specified NEC O28.8
ultrasonic O28.3
glucose (tolerance) NEC O99.810
pelvic organs O34.9-
specified NEC O34.8-
causing obstructed labor O65.5
pelvis (bony) (major) NEC O33.0
perineum O34.7-
position
placenta O44.1-
without hemorrhage O44.0-
uterus O34.59-
uterus O34.59-
causing obstructed labor O65.5
congenital O34.0-
vagina O34.6-
causing obstructed labor O65.5
vulva O34.7-
causing obstructed labor O65.5
abruptio placentae —see Abruptio
placentae
abscess or cellulitis
bladder O23.1-
breast O91.11-
genital organ or tract O23.9-
abuse
physical O9A.31
psychological O9A.51
sexual O9A.41
adverse effect anesthesia O29.9-
aspiration pneumonitis O29.01-
cardiac arrest O29.11-
cardiac complication NEC O29.19-
cardiac failure O29.12-
central nervous system
complication NEC O29.29-
cerebral anoxia O29.21-
failed or difficult intubation O29.6-
inhalation of stomach contents or
secretions NOS O29.01-
local, toxic reaction O29.3X
Mendelson's syndrome O29.01-
pressure collapse of lung O29.02-
pulmonary complications NEC
O29.09-
specified NEC O29.8X
spinal and epidural type NEC
O29.5X
induced headache O29.4-
albuminuria O12.1-
alcohol use O99.31-
amnionitis O41.12-
anaphylactoid syndrome of pregnancy
O88.01-
anemia (conditions in D50-D64) (pre-
existing) O99.01-
complicating the puerperium
O99.03
antepartum hemorrhage O46.9-
with coagulation defect —see
Hemorrhage, antepartum,
with coagulation defect
specified NEC O46.8X-

Pregnancy (Continued)
complicated by (Continued)
appendicitis O99.61-
atrophy (yellow) (acute) liver
(subacute) O26.61-
bariatric surgery status O99.84⬟
bicornis or bicornuate uterus O34.59-
biliary tract problems O26.61-
breech presentation O32.1
cardiovascular diseases (conditions in
I00-I09, I20-I52, I70-I99) O99.41-
cerebrovascular disorders (conditions
in I60-I69) O99.41-
cervical shortening O26.87-
cervicitis O23.51-
chloasma (gravidarum) O26.89-
cholecystitis O99.61-
cholestasis (intrahepatic) O26.61-
chorioamnionitis O41.12-
circulatory system disorder
(conditions in I00-I09,
I20-I99, O99.41-)
compound presentation O32.6
conjoined twins O30.02-
connective system disorders
(conditions in M00-M99) O99.89
contracted pelvis (general) O33.1
inlet O33.2
outlet O33.3
convulsions (eclamptic) (uremic) (see
also Eclampsia) O15.9
cracked nipple O92.11-
cystitis O23.1-
cystocele O34.8-
death of fetus (near term) O36.4
early pregnancy O02.1
of one fetus or more in multiple
gestation O31.2-
deciduitis O41.14-
decreased fetal movement O36.81-
dental problems O99.61-
diabetes (mellitus) O24.91-
gestational (pregnancy induced) —
see Diabetes, gestational
pre-existing O24.31-
specified NEC O24.81-
type 1 O24.01-
type 2 O24.11-
digestive system disorders
(conditions in K00-K93) O99.61-
diseases of —see Pregnancy,
complicated by, specified body
system disease
biliary tract O26.61-
blood NEC (conditions in D65-D77)
O99.11-
liver O26.61-
specified NEC O99.89
disorders of —see Pregnancy,
complicated by, specified body
system disorder
amniotic fluid and membranes
O41.9-
specified NEC O41.8X-
biliary tract O26.61-
ear and mastoid process
(conditions in H60-H95)
O99.89
eye and adnexa (conditions in
H00-H59) O99.89
liver O26.61-
skin (conditions in L00-L99)
O99.71-
specified NEC O99.89

Pregnancy *(Continued)*
  complicated by *(Continued)*
    displacement, uterus NEC O34.59-
      causing obstructed labor O65.5
    disproportion (due to) O33.9
      fetal deformities NEC O33.7
      generally contracted pelvis O33.1
      hydrocephalic fetus O33.6
      inlet contraction of pelvis O33.2
      mixed maternal and fetal origin
        O33.4
      specified NEC O33.8
    double uterus O34.59-
      causing obstructed labor O65.5
    drug use (conditions in F11-F19)
      O99.32-
    eclampsia, eclamptic (coma)
      (convulsions) (delirium)
      (nephritis) (uremia) *(see also*
      Eclampsia) O15-
    ectopic pregnancy —*see* Pregnancy,
      ectopic
    edema O12.0-
      with
        gestational hypertension, mild
          (see also Preeclampsia)
          O14.0-
        proteinuria O12.2-
    effusion, amniotic fluid —*see*
      Pregnancy, complicated
      by, premature rupture of
      membranes
    elderly
      multigravida O09.52-
      primigravida O09.51-
    embolism *(see also* Embolism,
      obstetric, pregnancy) O88.-
    endocrine diseases NEC O99.28-
    endometritis O86.12
    excessive weight gain O26.0-
    exhaustion O26.81-
      during labor and delivery
        O75.81
    face presentation O32.3
    failed induction of labor O61.9
      failed or difficult intubation for
        anesthesia O29.6-
      instrumental O61.1
      mechanical O61.1
      medical O61.0
      specified NEC O61.8
      surgical O61.1
    false labor (pains) O47.9
      at or after 37 completed weeks of
        pregnancy O47.1
      before 37 completed weeks of
        pregnancy O47.0-
    fatigue O26.81-
      during labor and delivery O75.81
    fatty metamorphosis of liver O26.61-
    female genital mutilation
      O34.8- *[N90.81-]*
    fetal (maternal care for)
      abnormality or damage O35.9
        acid-base balance O68
        specified type NEC O35.8
      acidemia O68
      acidosis O68
      alkalosis O68
      anemia and thrombocytopenia
        O36.82-
      anencephaly O35.0
      chromosomal abnormality
        (conditions in Q90-Q99) O35.1
      conjoined twins O30.02-

Pregnancy *(Continued)*
  complicated by *(Continued)*
    fetal *(Continued)*
      damage from
        amniocentesis O35.7
        biopsy procedures O35.7
        drug addiction O35.5
        hematological investigation O35.7
        intrauterine contraceptive device
          O35.7
        maternal
          alcohol addiction O35.4
          cytomegalovirus infection O35.3
          disease NEC O35.8
          drug addiction O35.5
          listeriosis O35.8
          rubella O35.3
          toxoplasmosis O35.8
          viral infection O35.3
        medical procedure NEC O35.7
        radiation O35.6
      death (near term) O36.4
        early pregnancy O02.1
      decreased movement O36.81-
      disproportion due to deformity
        (fetal) O33.7
      excessive growth (large for dates)
        O36.6-
      growth retardation O36.59-
        light for dates O36.59-
        small for dates O36.59-
      heart rate irregularity (bradycardia)
        (decelerations) (tachycardia)
        O76
      hereditary disease O35.2
      hydrocephalus O35.0
      intrauterine death O36.4
      poor growth O36.59-
        light for dates O36.59-
        small for dates O36.59-
      problem O36.9-
        specified NEC O36.89-
      reduction (elective) O31.3-
      selective termination O31.3-
      spina bifida O35.0
      thrombocytopenia O36.82-
    fibroid (tumor) (uterus) O34.1-
    fissure of nipple O92.11-
    gallstones O99.61-
    gastric banding status O99.84-
    gastric bypass status O99.84-
    genital herpes (asymptomatic)
      (history of) (inactive) O98.51-
    genital tract infection O23.9-
    glomerular diseases (conditions in
      N00-N07) O26.83-
      with hypertension, pre-
        existing —*see* Hypertension,
        complicating, pregnancy, pre-
        existing, with, renal disease
    gonorrhea O98.21-
    grand multiparity O09.4
    habitual aborter —*see* Pregnancy,
      complicated by, recurrent
      pregnancy loss
    HELLP syndrome (hemolysis,
      elevated liver enzymes and low
      platelet count) O14.2-
    hemorrhage
      antepartum —*see* Hemorrhage,
        antepartum
      before 20 completed weeks
        gestation O20.9
        specified NEC O20.8

Pregnancy *(Continued)*
  complicated by *(Continued)*
    hemorrhage *(Continued)*
      due to premature separation,
        placenta *(see also* Abruptio
        placentae) O45.9-
      early O20.9
        specified NEC O20.8
      threatened abortion O20.0
    hemorrhoids O22.4-
    hepatitis (viral) O98.41-
    herniation of uterus O34.59-
    high
      head at term O32.4
      risk —*see* Supervision (of) (for),
        high-risk
    history of in utero procedure during
      previous pregnancy O09.82-
    HIV O98.71-
    human immunodeficiency virus
      (HIV) disease O98.71-
    hydatidiform mole *(see also* Mole,
      hydatidiform) O01.9
    hydramnios O40.-
    hydrocephalic fetus (disproportion)
      O33.6
    hydrops
      amnii O40.-
      fetalis O36.2-
        associated with isoimmunization
          (see also Pregnancy,
          complicated by,
          isoimmunization) O36.11-
    hydrorrhea O42.90
    hyperemesis (gravidarum) (mild) *(see*
      also Hyperemesis, gravidarum)
      O21.0
    hypertension —*see* Hypertension,
      complicating pregnancy
    hypertensive
      heart and renal disease, pre-
        existing —*see* Hypertension,
        complicating, pregnancy, pre-
        existing, with, heart disease,
        with renal disease
      heart disease, pre-existing —*see*
        Hypertension, complicating,
        pregnancy, pre-existing, with,
        heart disease
      renal disease, pre-existing —*see*
        Hypertension, complicating,
        pregnancy, pre-existing, with,
        renal disease
    hypotension O26.5-
    immune disorders NEC (conditions
      in D80-D89) O99.11-
    incarceration, uterus O34.51-
    incompetent cervix O34.3-
    inconclusive fetal viability O36.80
    infection (s) O98.91-
      amniotic fluid or sac O41.10-
      bladder O23.1-
      carrier state NEC O99.830
        streptococcus B O99.820
      genital organ or tract O23.9-
        specified NEC O23.59-
      genitourinary tract O23.9-
      gonorrhea O98.21-
      hepatitis (viral) O98.41-
      HIV O98.71-
      human immunodeficiency virus
        (HIV) O98.71-
      kidney O23.0-
      nipple O91.01-
      parasitic disease O98.91-
        specified NEC O98.81-

Pregnancy *(Continued)*
  complicated by *(Continued)*
    infection (s) *(Continued)*
      protozoal disease O98.61-
      sexually transmitted NEC
        O98.31-
      specified type NEC O98.81-
      syphilis O98.11-
      tuberculosis O98.01-
      urethra O23.2-
      urinary (tract) O23.4-
        specified NEC O23.3-
      viral disease O98.51-
    injury or poisoning (conditions in
      S00-T88) O9A.21-
      due to abuse
        physical O9A.31-
        psychological O9A.51-
        sexual O9A.41-
    insufficient
      prenatal care O09.3-
      weight gain O26.1-
    insulin resistance O26.89
    intrauterine fetal death (near term)
      O36.4
      early pregnancy O02.1
      multiple gestation (one fetus or
        more) O31.2-
    isoimmunization O36.11-
      anti-A sensitization O36.11-
      anti-B sensitization O36.19-
      Rh O36.09-
        anti-D antibody O36.01-
      specified NEC O36.19-
    laceration of uterus NEC O71.81
    malformation
      placenta, placental (vessel) O43.10-
        specified NEC O43.19-
      uterus (congenital) O34.0-
    malnutrition (conditions in E40-E46)
      O25.1-
    maternal hypotension syndrome O26.5-
    mental disorders (conditions in
      F01-F09, F20-F99) O99.34-
      alcohol use O99.31-
      drug use O99.32-
      smoking O99.33-
    mentum presentation O32.3
    metabolic disorders O99.28-
    missed
      abortion O02.1
      delivery O36.4
    multiple gestations O30.9-
      conjoined twins O30.02-
      quadruplet —*see* Pregnancy,
        quadruplet
      specified complication NEC
        O31.8X-
      specified number of multiples
        NEC —*see* Pregnancy,
        multiple (gestation), specified
        NEC
      triplet —*see* Pregnancy, triplet
      twin —*see* Pregnancy, twin
    musculoskeletal condition
      (conditions is M00-M99) O99.89
    necrosis, liver (conditions in K72)
      O26.61-
    neoplasm
      benign
        cervix O34.4-
        corpus uteri O34.1-
        uterus O34.1-
      malignant O9A.11-

Pregnancy *(Continued)*
  complicated by *(Continued)*
    nephropathy NEC O26.83-
    nervous system condition (conditions
      in G00-G99) O99.35-
    nutritional diseases NEC O99.28-
    obesity (pre-existing) O99.21-
    obesity surgery status O99.84-
    oblique lie or presentation O32.2
    older mother —*see* Pregnancy,
      complicated by, elderly
    oligohydramnios O41.0-
      with premature rupture of
        membranes (*see also*
        Pregnancy, complicated
        by, premature rupture of
        membranes) O42-
    onset (spontaneous) of labor after 37
      completed weeks of gestation
      but before 39 completed weeks
      gestation, with delivery by
      (planned) cesarean section
      O75.82
    oophoritis O23.52-
    overdose, drug (*see also* Table of
      drugs and chemicals, by drug,
      poisoning) O9A.21–
    oversize fetus O33.5
    papyraceous fetus O31.0-
    pelvic inflammatory disease O99.89
    periodontal disease O99.61-
    peripheral neuritis O26.82-
    peritoneal (pelvic) adhesions
      O99.89
    phlebitis O22.9-
    phlebopathy O22.9-
    phlebothrombosis (superficial)
      O22.2-
      deep O22.3-
    placenta accreta O43.21-
    placenta increta O43.22-
    placenta percreta O43.23-
    placenta previa O44.1-
      without hemorrhage O44.0-
    placental disorder O43.9-
      specified NEC O43.89-
    placental dysfunction O43.89-
    placental infarction O43.81-
    placental insufficiency O36.51-
    placental transfusion syndromes
      fetomaternal O43.01-
      fetus to fetus O43.02-
      maternofetal O43.01-
    placentitis O41.14-
    pneumonia O99.51-
    poisoning (*see also* Table of drugs and
      chemicals) O9A.21-
    polyhydramnios O40-
    polymorphic eruption of pregnancy
      O26.86
    poor obstetric history NEC O09.29-
    postmaturity (post-term) (40 to 42
      weeks) O48.0
      more than 42 completed weeks
        gestation (prolonged) O48.1
    pre-eclampsia O14.9-
      mild O14.0-
      moderate O14.0-
      severe O14.1-
        with hemolysis, elevated liver
          enzymes and low platelet
          count (HELLP) O14.2-
    premature labor —*see* Pregnancy,
      complicated by, preterm labor

Pregnancy *(Continued)*
  complicated by *(Continued)*
    premature rupture of membranes
      O42.90
      with onset of labor
        within 24 hours O42.00
          after 37 weeks gestation O42.02
          pre-term (before 37 completed
            weeks of gestation) O42.01-
        after 24 hours O42.10
          after 37 weeks gestation O42.12
          pre-term (before 37 completed
            weeks of gestation) O42.11-
      after 37 weeks gestation O42.92
      full-term O42.92
      pre-term (before 37 completed
        weeks of gestation) O42.91-
    premature separation of placenta - (*see
      also* Abruptio placentae) O45.9-
    presentation, fetal —*see* Delivery
      (childbirth) (labor) (complicated
      by)
    preterm delivery O60.10
    preterm labor
      with delivery O60.10
        preterm O60.10
        term O60.20
      second trimester
        with preterm delivery
          second trimester O60.12
          third trimester O60.13
        with term delivery O60.22
        without delivery O60.02
      third trimester
        with term delivery O60.23
        with third trimester preterm
          delivery O60.14
        without delivery O60.03
      without delivery O60.00
        second trimester O60.02
        third trimester O60.03
    previous history of —*see* Pregnancy,
      supervision of, high-risk
    prolapse, uterus O34.52-
    proteinuria (gestational) O12.1-
      with edema O12.2-
    pruritic urticarial papules and
      plaques of pregnancy (PUPPP)
      O26.86
    pruritus (neurogenic) O26.89-
    psychosis or psychoneurosis
      (puerperal) F53
    ptyalism O26.89-
    PUPPP (pruritic urticarial papules and
      plaques of pregnancy) O26.86
    pyelitis O23.0-
    recurrent pregnancy loss O26.2-
    renal disease or failure NEC O26.83-
      with secondary hypertension,
        pre-existing —*see*
        Hypertension, complicating,
        pregnancy, pre-existing,
        secondary
      hypertensive, pre-existing —*see*
        Hypertension, complicating,
        pregnancy, pre-existing, with,
        renal disease
    respiratory condition (conditions in
      J00-J99) O99.51-
    retained, retention
      dead ovum O02.0
      intrauterine contraceptive device
        O26.3-
    retroversion, uterus O34.53-

Pregnancy *(Continued)*
  complicated by *(Continued)*
    Rh immunization, incompatibility or
      sensitization NEC O36.09-
      anti-D antibody O36.01-
    rupture
      amnion (premature) *(see also*
        Pregnancy, complicated
        by, premature rupture of
        membranes) O42-
      membranes (premature) *(see also*
        Pregnancy, complicated
        by, premature rupture of
        membranes) O42-
      uterus (during labor) O71.1
        before onset of labor O71.0-
    salivation (excessive) O26.89-
    salpingitis O23.52-
    salpingo-oophoritis O23.52-
    sepsis (conditions in A40, A41) O98.81-
    size date discrepancy (uterine) O26.84-
    skin condition (conditions in
      L00-L99) O99.71-
    smoking (tobacco) O99.33-
    social problem O09.7-
    specified condition NEC O26.89-
    spotting O26.85-
    streptococcus B carrier state O99.820
    subluxation of symphysis (pubis)
      O26.71-
    syphilis (conditions in A50-A53)
      O98.11-
    threatened
      abortion O20.0
      labor O47.9
        at or after 37 completed weeks of
          gestation O47.1
        before 37 completed weeks of
          gestation O47.0-
    thrombophlebitis (superficial)
      O22.2-
    thrombosis O22.9-
      cerebral venous O22.5-
      cerebrovenous sinus O22.5-
      deep O22.3-
    torsion of uterus O34.59-
    toxemia O14.9-
    transverse lie or presentation O32.2
    tuberculosis (conditions in A15-A19)
      O98.01-
    tumor (benign)
      cervix O34.4-
      malignant - O9A.11-
      uterus O34.1-
    unstable lie O32.0
    upper respiratory infection O99.51-
    urethritis O23.2-
    uterine size date discrepancy
      O26.84-
    vaginitis or vulvitis O23.59-
    varicose veins (lower extremities)
      O22.0-
      genitals O22.1-
      legs O22.0-
      perineal O22.1-
      vaginal or vulval O22.1-
    venereal disease NEC (conditions in
      A63.8) O98.31-
    venous disorders O22.9-
      specified NEC O22.8X-
    very young mother —*see* Pregnancy,
      complicated by, young mother
    viral diseases (conditions in A80-B09,
      B25-B34) O98.51-

Pregnancy *(Continued)*
  complicated by *(Continued)*
    vomiting O21.9
      due to diseases classified elsewhere
        O21.8
      hyperemesis gravidarum (mild)
        (see also Hyperemesis,
        gravidarum) O21.0-
      late (occurring after 20 weeks of
        gestation) O21.2
    young mother
      multigravida O09.62-
      primigravida O09.61-
  concealed O09.3-
  continuing following
    elective fetal reduction of one or more
      fetus O31.3-
    intrauterine death of one or more
      fetus O31.2-
    spontaneous abortion of one or more
      fetus O31.1-
  cornual O00.8
  ectopic (ruptured) O00.9
    abdominal O00.0
      with viable fetus O36.7-
    cervical O00.8
    complicated (by) O07.30
      afibrinogenemia O07.1
      cardiac arrest O07.39
      chemical damage of pelvic
        organ (s) O07.39
      circulatory collapse O07.39
      defibrination syndrome O07.1
      electrolyte imbalance O07.33
      embolism (amniotic fluid) (blood
        clot) (pulmonary) (septic)
        O07.2
      endometritis O07.0
      genital tract and pelvic infection
        O07.0
      hemorrhage (delayed) (excessive)
        O07.1
      infection
        genital tract or pelvic O07.0
        urinary tract O07.39
      intravascular coagulation O07.1
      laceration of pelvic organ (s)
        O07.39
      metabolic disorder O07.33
      oliguria O07.39
      oophoritis O07.0
      parametritis O07.0
      pelvic peritonitis O07.0
      perforation of pelvic organ (s)
        O07.39
      renal failure or shutdown O07.39
      salpingitis or salpingo-oophoritis
        O07.0
      sepsis O07.0
      shock O07.39
        septic O07.0
      specified condition NEC O07.39
      tubular necrosis (renal) O07.39
      uremia O07.39
      urinary infection O07.39
      venous complication NEC
        O07.39
        embolism O07.2
    cornual O00.8
    intraligamentous O00.8
    mural O00.8
    ovarian O00.2
    specified site NEC O00.8
    tubal (ruptured) O00.1

Pregnancy *(Continued)*
  examination (normal) Z34.9-
    first Z34.0-
    high-risk —*see* Pregnancy,
      supervision of, high-risk
    specified Z34.8-
  extrauterine —*see* Pregnancy, ectopic
  fallopian O00.1
  false F45.8
  hidden O09.3-
  high-risk —*see* Pregnancy, supervision
    of, high-risk
  incidental finding Z33.1
  interstitial O00.8
  intraligamentous O00.8
  intramural O00.8
  intraperitoneal O00.0
  isthmian O00.1
  mesometric (mural) O00.8
  molar NEC O02.0
    complicated (by) O07.30
      afibrinogenemia O07.1
      cardiac arrest O07.39
      chemical damage of pelvic
        organ (s) O07.39
      circulatory collapse O07.39
      defibrination syndrome O07.1
      electrolyte imbalance O07.33
      embolism (amniotic fluid) (blood
        clot) (pulmonary) (septic)
        O07.2
      endometritis O07.0
      genital tract and pelvic infection
        O07.0
      hemorrhage (delayed) (excessive)
        O07.1
      infection
        genital tract or pelvic O07.0
        urinary tract O07.39
      intravascular coagulation O07.1
      laceration of pelvic organ (s)
        O07.39
      metabolic disorder O07.33
      oliguria O07.39
      oophoritis O07.0
      parametritis O07.0
      pelvic peritonitis O07.0
      perforation of pelvic organ (s)
        O07.39
      renal failure or shutdown O07.39
      salpingitis or salpingo-oophoritis
        O07.0
      sepsis O07.0
      shock O07.39
        septic O07.0
      specified condition NEC
        O07.39
      tubular necrosis (renal) O07.39
      uremia O07.39
      urinary infection O07.39
      venous complication NEC O07.39
        embolism O07.2
  hydatidiform *(see also* Mole,
    hydatidiform) O01.9
  multiple (gestation) O30.9-
    greater than quadruplets —*see*
      Pregnancy, multiple (gestation),
      specified NEC
    specified NEC O30.80-
      with
        two or more monoamniotic
          fetuses O30.82-
        two or more monochorionic
          fetuses O30.81-

Pregnancy *(Continued)*
  multiple *(Continued)*
    specified NEC *(Continued)*
      two or more monoamniotic fetuses O30.82-
      two or more monochorionic fetuses O30.81-
      unable to determine number of placenta and number of amniotic sacs O30.89-
      unspecified number of placenta and unspecified number of amniotic sacs O30.80-
  mural O00.8
  normal (supervision of) Z34.9-
    first Z34.0-
    high-risk —*see* Pregnancy, supervision of, high-risk
    specified Z34.8-
  ovarian O00.2
  postmature (40 to 42 weeks) O48.0
    more than 42 weeks gestation O48.1
  post-term (40 to 42 weeks) O48.0
  prenatal care only Z34.9-
    first Z34.0-
    high-risk —*see* Pregnancy, supervision of, high-risk
    specified Z34.8-
  prolonged (more than 42 weeks gestation) O48.1
  quadruplet O30.20-
    with
      two or more monoamniotic fetuses O30.22-
      two or more monochorionic fetuses O30.21-
    two or more monoamniotic fetuses O30.22-
    two or more monochorionic fetuses O30.21-
    unable to determine number of placenta and number of amniotic sacs O30.29-
    unspecified number of placenta and unspecified number of amniotic sacs O30.20-
  quintuplet —*see* Pregnancy, multiple (gestation), specified NEC
  sextuplet —*see* Pregnancy, multiple (gestation), specified NEC
  supervision of
    concealed pregnancy O09.3-
    elderly mother
      multigravida O09.52-
      primigravida O09.51-
    hidden pregnancy O09.3-
    high-risk O09.9-
      due to (history of)
        ectopic pregnancy O09.1-
        elderly —*see* Pregnancy, supervision, elderly mother
        grand multiparity O09.4
        infertility O09.0-
        insufficient prenatal care O09.3-
        in utero procedure during previous pregnancy O09.82-
        in vitro fertilization O09.81-
        molar pregnancy O09.1-
        multiple previous pregnancies O09.4-
        older mother —*see* Pregnancy, supervision of, elderly mother

Pregnancy *(Continued)*
  supervision of *(Continued)*
    high-risk *(Continued)*
      due to *(Continued)*
        poor reproductive or obstetric history NEC O09.29-
        pre-term labor O09.21-
        previous
          neonatal death O09.29-
        social problems O09.7-
        specified NEC O09.89-
        very young mother —*see* Pregnancy, supervision, young mother
      resulting from in vitro fertilization O09.81-
    normal Z34.9-
      first Z34.0-
      specified NEC Z34.8-
    young mother
      multigravida O09.62-
      primigravida O09.61-
  triplet O30.10-
    with
      two or more monoamniotic fetuses O30.12-
      two or more monochorionic fetuses O30.11-
    two or more monoamniotic fetuses O30.12-
    two or more monochorionic fetuses O30.11-
    unable to determine number of placenta and number of amniotic sacs O30.19-
    unspecified number of placenta and unspecified number of amniotic sacs O30.10-
  tubal (with abortion) (with rupture) O00.1
  twin O30.00-
    conjoined O30.02-
    dichorionic/diamniotic (two placenta, two amniotic sacs) O30.04-
    monochorionic/diamniotic (one placenta, two amniotic sacs) O30.03-
    monochorionic/monoamniotic (one placenta, one amniotic sac) O30.01-
    unable to determine number of placenta and number of amniotic sacs O30.09-
    unspecified number of placenta and unspecified number of amniotic sacs O30.00-
  unwanted Z64.0
  weeks of gestation
    8 weeks Z3A.08
    9 weeks Z3A.09
    10 weeks Z3A.10
    11 weeks Z3A.11
    12 weeks Z3A.12
    13 weeks Z3A.13
    14 weeks Z3A.14
    15 weeks Z3A.15
    16 weeks Z3A.16
    17 weeks Z3A.17
    18 weeks Z3A.18
    19 weeks Z3A.19
    20 weeks Z3A.20
    21 weeks Z3A.21
    22 weeks Z3A.22
    23 weeks Z3A.23

Pregnancy *(Continued)*
  weeks of gestation *(Continued)*
    24 weeks Z3A.24
    25 weeks Z3A.25
    26 weeks Z3A.26
    27 weeks Z3A.27
    28 weeks Z3A.28
    29 weeks Z3A.29
    30 weeks Z3A.30
    31 weeks Z3A.31
    32 weeks Z3A.32
    33 weeks Z3A.33
    34 weeks Z3A.34
    35 weeks Z3A.35
    36 weeks Z3A.36
    37 weeks Z3A.37
    38 weeks Z3A.38
    39 weeks Z3A.39
    40 weeks Z3A.40
    41 weeks Z3A.41
    42 weeks Z3A.42
    greater than 42 weeks Z3A.49
    less than 8 weeks Z3A.01
    not specified Z3A.00
Preiser's disease —*see* Osteonecrosis, secondary, due to, trauma, metacarpus
Pre-kwashiorkor —*see* Malnutrition, severe
Preleukemia (syndrome) D46.9
Preluxation, hip, congenital Q65.6
Premature —*see also* condition
  adrenarche E27.0
  aging E34.8
  beats I49.40
    atrial I49.1
    auricular I49.1
    supraventricular I49.1
  birth NEC —*see* Preterm, newborn
  closure, foramen ovale Q21.8
  contraction
    atrial I49.1
    atrioventricular I49.49
    auricular I49.1
    auriculoventricular I49.2
    heart (extrasystole) I49.49
    junctional I49.2
    ventricular I49.3
  delivery (*see also* Pregnancy, complicated by, preterm labor) O60.10
  ejaculation F52.4
  infant NEC —*see* Preterm, newborn
    light-for-dates —*see* Light for dates
  labor —*see* Pregnancy, complicated by, preterm labor
  lungs P28.0
  menopause E28.319
    asymptomatic E28.319
    symptomatic E28.310
  newborn
    extreme (less than 28 completed weeks) —*see* Immaturity, extreme
    less than 37 completed weeks —*see* Preterm, newborn
  puberty E30.1
  rupture membranes or amnion —*see* Pregnancy, complicated by, premature rupture of membranes
  senility E34.8
  thelarche E30.8
  ventricular systole I49.3

Prematurity NEC (less than 37 completed weeks) —see Preterm, newborn
   extreme (less than 28 completed weeks) —see Immaturity, extreme
Premenstrual
   dysphoric disorder (PMDD) N94.3
   tension (syndrome) N94.3
Premolarization, cuspids K00.2
Prenatal
   care, normal pregnancy —see Pregnancy, normal
   screening of mother Z36
   teeth K00.6
Preparatory care for subsequent treatment NEC
   for dialysis Z49.01
      peritoneal Z49.02
Prepartum —see condition
Preponderance, left or right ventricular I51.7
Prepuce —see condition
PRES (posterior reversible encephalopathy syndrome) I67.83
Presbycardia R54
Presbycusis, presbyacusia H91.1-
Presbyesophagus K22.8
Presbyophrenia F03
Presbyopia H52.4
Prescription of contraceptives (initial) Z30.019
   emergency (postcoital) Z30.012
   implantable subdermal Z30.019
   injectable Z30.013
   intrauterine contraceptive device Z30.014
   pills Z30.011
   postcoital (emergency) Z30.012
   repeat Z30.40
      implantable subdermal Z30.49
      injectable Z30.42
      pills Z30.41
      specified type NEC Z30.49
   specified type NEC Z30.018
Presence (of)
   ankle-joint implant (functional) (prosthesis) Z96.66-
   aortocoronary (bypass) graft Z95.1
   arterial-venous shunt (dialysis) Z99.2
   artificial
      eye (globe) Z97.0
      heart (fully implantable) (mechanical) Z95.812
         valve Z95.2
      larynx Z96.3
      lens (intraocular) Z96.1
      limb (complete) (partial) Z97.1-
         arm Z97.1-
            bilateral Z97.15
         leg Z97.1-
            bilateral Z97.16
   audiological implant (functional) Z96.29
   bladder implant (functional) Z96.0
   bone
      conduction hearing device Z96.29
      implant (functional) NEC Z96.7
      joint (prosthesis) —see Presence, joint implant
   cardiac
      defibrillator (functional) (with synchronous cardiac pacemaker) Z95.810
      implant or graft Z95.9
         specified type NEC Z95.818
      pacemaker Z95.0

Presence (of) (Continued)
   cerebrospinal fluid drainage device Z98.2
   cochlear implant (functional) Z96.21
   contact lens (es) Z97.3
   coronary artery graft or prosthesis Z95.5
   CSF shunt Z98.2
   dental prosthesis device Z97.2
   dentures Z97.2
   device (external) NEC Z97.8
      cardiac NEC Z95.818
      heart assist Z95.811
      implanted (functional) Z96.9
         specified NEC Z96.89
      prosthetic Z97.8
   ear implant Z96.20
      cochlear implant Z96.21
      myringotomy tube Z96.22
      specified type NEC Z96.29
   elbow-joint implant (functional) (prosthesis) Z96.62-
   endocrine implant (functional) NEC Z96.49
   eustachian tube stent or device (functional) Z96.29
   external hearing-aid or device Z97.4
   finger-joint implant (functional) (prosthetic) Z96.69-
   functional implant Z96.9
      specified NEC Z96.89
   graft
      cardiac NEC Z95.818
      vascular NEC Z95.828
   hearing-aid or device (external) Z97.4
      implant (bone) (cochlear) (functional) Z96.21
   heart assist device Z95.811
   heart valve implant (functional) Z95.2
      prosthetic Z95.2
      specified type NEC Z95.4
      xenogenic Z95.3
   hip-joint implant (functional) (prosthesis) Z96.64-
   implanted device (artificial) (functional) (prosthetic) Z96.9
      automatic cardiac defibrillator (with synchronous cardiac pacemaker) Z95.810
      cardiac pacemaker Z95.0
      cochlear Z96.21
      dental Z96.5
      heart Z95.812
      heart valve Z95.2
         prosthetic Z95.2
         specified NEC Z95.4
         xenogenic Z95.3
      insulin pump Z96.41
      intraocular lens Z96.1
      joint Z96.60
         ankle Z96.66-
         elbow Z96.62-
         finger Z96.69-
         hip Z96.64-
         knee Z96.65-
         shoulder Z96.61-
         specified NEC Z96.698
         wrist Z96.63-
      larynx Z96.3
      myringotomy tube Z96.22
      otological Z96.20
         cochlear Z96.21
         eustachian stent Z96.29
         myringotomy Z96.22
         specified NEC Z96.29
         stapes Z96.29

Presence (of) (Continued)
   implanted device (Continued)
      skin Z96.81
      skull plate Z96.7
      specified NEC Z96.89
      urogenital Z96.0
   insulin pump (functional) Z96.41
   intestinal bypass or anastomosis Z98.0
   intraocular lens (functional) Z96.1
   intrauterine contraceptive device (IUD) Z97.5
   intravascular implant (functional) (prosthetic) NEC Z95.9
      coronary artery Z95.5
      defibrillator (with synchronous cardiac pacemaker) Z95.810
      peripheral vessel (with angioplasty) Z95.820
   joint implant (prosthetic) (any) Z96.60
      ankle —see Presence, ankle joint implant
      elbow —see Presence, elbow joint implant
      finger —see Presence, finger joint implant
      hip —see Presence, hip joint implant
      knee —see Presence, knee joint implant
      shoulder —see Presence, shoulder joint implant
      specified joint NEC Z96.698
      wrist —see Presence, wrist joint implant
   knee-joint implant (functional) (prosthesis) Z96.65-
   laryngeal implant (functional) Z96.3
   mandibular implant (dental) Z96.5
   myringotomy tube (s) Z96.22
   orthopedic-joint implant (prosthetic) (any) —see Presence, joint implant
   otological implant (functional) Z96.29
   shoulder-joint implant (functional) (prosthesis) Z96.61-
   skull-plate implant Z96.7
   spectacles Z97.3
   stapes implant (functional) Z96.29
   systemic lupus erythematosus [SLE] inhibitor D68.62
   tendon implant (functional) (graft) Z96.7
   tooth root (s) implant Z96.5
   ureteral stent Z96.0
   urethral stent Z96.0
   urogenital implant (functional) Z96.0
   vascular implant or device Z95.9
      access port device Z95.828
      specified type NEC Z95.828
   wrist-joint implant (functional) (prosthesis) Z96.63-
Presenile —see also condition
   dementia F03
   premature aging E34.8
Presentation, fetal —see Delivery (childbirth) (labor) (complicated by), malposition, malpresentation
Prespondylolisthesis (congenital) Q76.2
Pressure
   area, skin —see Ulcer, pressure, by site
   brachial plexus G54.0
   brain G93.5
      injury at birth NEC P11.1
   cerebral —see Pressure, brain
   chest R07.89
   cone, tentorial G93.5

Pressure (Continued)
 hyposystolic —see also Hypotension
  incidental reading, without diagnosis
   of hypotension R03.1
 increased
  intracranial (benign) G93.2
   injury at birth P11.0
  intraocular H40.05-
 lumbosacral plexus G54.1
 mediastinum J98.5
 necrosis (chronic) —see Ulcer, pressure,
  by site
 parental, inappropriate (excessive) Z62.6
 sore (chronic) —see Ulcer, pressure, by
  site
 spinal cord G95.20
 ulcer (chronic) —see Ulcer, pressure,
  by site
 venous, increased I87.8
Pre-syncope R55
Preterm
 delivery (see also Pregnancy, complicated
  by, preterm labor) O60.10
 labor —see Pregnancy, complicated by,
  preterm labor
 newborn (infant) P07.30
  gestational age
   28 completed weeks (28 weeks,
    0 days through 28 weeks,
    6 days) P07.31
   29 completed weeks (29 weeks,
    0 days through 29 weeks,
    6 days) P07.32
   30 completed weeks (30 weeks,
    0 days through 30 weeks,
    6 days) P07.33
   31 completed weeks (31 weeks,
    0 days through 31 weeks,
    6 days) P07.34
   32 completed weeks (32 weeks,
    0 days through 32 weeks,
    6 days) P07.35
   33 completed weeks (33 weeks,
    0 days through 33 weeks,
    6 days) P07.36
   34 completed weeks (34 weeks,
    0 days through 34 weeks,
    6 days) P07.37
   35 completed weeks (35 weeks,
    0 days through 35 weeks,
    6 days) P07.38
   36 completed weeks (36 weeks,
    0 days through 36 weeks,
    6 days) P07.39
Previa
 placenta (low) (marginal) (partial)
  (total) (with hemorrhage) O44.1-
  without hemorrhage O44.0-
 vasa O69.4
Priapism N48.30
 due to
  disease classified elsewhere N48.32
  drug N48.33
  specified cause NEC N48.39
  trauma N48.31
Prickling sensation (skin) R20.2
Prickly heat L74.0
Primary —see condition
Primigravida
 elderly, affecting management of
  pregnancy, labor and delivery
  (supervision only) —see
  Pregnancy, complicated by, elderly,
  primigravida

Primigravida (Continued)
 older, affecting management of
  pregnancy, labor and delivery
  (supervision only) —see
  Pregnancy, complicated by,
  elderly, primigravida
 very young, affecting management of
  pregnancy, labor and delivery
  (supervision only) —see
  Pregnancy, complicated by, young
  mother, primigravida
Primipara
 elderly, affecting management of
  pregnancy, labor and delivery
  (supervision only) —see
  Pregnancy, complicated by, elderly,
  primigravida
 older, affecting management of
  pregnancy, labor and delivery
  (supervision only) —see
  Pregnancy, complicated by,
  elderly, primigravida
 very young, affecting management of
  pregnancy, labor and delivery
  (supervision only) —see
  Pregnancy, complicated by, young
  mother, primigravida
Primus varus (bilateral) Q66.2
PRIND (Prolonged reversible ischemic
  neurologic deficit) I63.9
Pringle's disease (tuberous sclerosis)Q85.1
Prinzmetal angina I20.1
Prizefighter ear —see Cauliflower ear
Problem (with) (related to)
 academic Z55.8
 acculturation Z60.3
 adjustment (to)
  change of job Z56.1
  life-cycle transition Z60.0
  pension Z60.0
  retirement Z60.0
 adopted child Z62.821
 alcoholism in family Z63.72
 atypical parenting situation Z62.9
 bankruptcy Z59.8
 behavioral (adult) F69
  drug seeking Z72.89
 birth of sibling affecting child Z62.898
 care (of)
  provider dependency Z74.9
   specified NEC Z74.8
  sick or handicapped person in family
   or household Z63.6
 child
  abuse (affecting the child) —see
   Maltreatment, child
  custody or support proceedings Z65.3
  in care of non-parental family
   member Z62.21
  in foster care Z62.21
  in welfare custody Z62.21
  living in orphanage or group home
   Z62.22
 child-rearing Z62.9
  specified NEC Z62.898
 communication (developmental) F80.9
 conflict or discord (with)
  boss Z56.4
  classmates Z55.4
  counselor Z64.4
  employer Z56.4
  family Z63.9
   specified NEC Z63.8
  probation officer Z64.4

Problem (Continued)
 conflict or discord (Continued)
  social worker Z64.4
  teachers Z55.4
  workmates Z56.4
 conviction in legal proceedings Z65.0
  with imprisonment Z65.1
 counselor Z64.4
 creditors Z59.8
 digestive K92.9
 drug addict in family Z63.72
 ear —see Disorder, ear
 economic Z59.9
  affecting care Z59.9
  specified NEC Z59.8
 education Z55.9
  specified NEC Z55.8
 employment Z56.9
  change of job Z56.1
  discord Z56.4
  environment Z56.5
  sexual harassment Z56.81
  specified NEC Z56.89
  stress NEC Z56.6
  stressful schedule Z56.3
  threat of job loss Z56.2
  unemployment Z56.0
 enuresis, child F98.0
 eye H57.9
 failed examinations (school) Z55.2
 falling Z91.81
 family (see also Disruption, family
  specified NEC) Z63.9
 feeding (elderly) (infant) R63.3
  newborn P92.9
   breast P92.5
   overfeeding P92.4
   slow P92.2
   specified NEC P92.8
   underfeeding P92.3
  nonorganic F50.8
 finance Z59.9
  specified NEC Z59.8
 foreclosure on loan Z59.8
 foster child Z62.822
 frightening experience (s) in childhood
  Z62.898
 genital NEC
  female N94.9
  male N50.9
 health care Z75.9
  specified NEC Z75.8
 hearing —see Deafness
 homelessness Z59.0
 housing Z59.9
  inadequate Z59.1
  isolated Z59.8
  specified NEC Z59.8
 identity (of childhood) F93.8
 illegitimate pregnancy (unwanted) Z64.0
 illiteracy Z55.0
 impaired mobility Z74.09
 imprisonment or incarceration Z65.1
 inadequate teaching affecting education
  Z55.8
 inappropriate (excessive) parental
  pressure Z62.6
 influencing health status NEC Z78.9
 in-law Z63.1
 institutionalization, affecting child
  Z62.22
 intrafamilial communication Z63.8
 jealousy, child F93.8
 landlord Z59.2

Problem *(Continued)*
language (developmental) F80.9
learning (developmental) F81.9
legal Z65.3
conviction without imprisonment Z65.0
imprisonment Z65.1
release from prison Z65.2
life-management Z73.9
specified NEC Z73.89
life-style Z72.9
gambling Z72.6
high-risk sexual behavior (heterosexual) Z72.51
bisexual Z72.53
homosexual Z72.52
inappropriate eating habits Z72.4
self-damaging behavior NEC Z72.89
specified NEC Z72.89
tobacco use Z72.0
literacy Z55.9
low level Z55.0
specified NEC Z55.8
living alone Z60.2
lodgers Z59.2
loss of love relationship in childhood Z62.898
marital Z63.0
involving
divorce Z63.5
estrangement Z63.5
gender identity F66
mastication K08.8
medical
care, within family Z63.6
facilities Z75.9
specified NEC Z75.8
mental F48.9
multiparity Z64.1
negative life events in childhood Z62.9
altered pattern of family relationships Z62.898
frightening experience Z62.898
loss of
love relationship Z62.898
self-esteem Z62.898
physical abuse (alleged) —*see* Maltreatment, child
removal from home Z62.29
specified event NEC Z62.898
neighbor Z59.2
neurological NEC R29.818
new step-parent affecting child Z62.898
none (feared complaint unfounded) Z71.1
occupational NEC Z56.89
parent-child —*see* Conflict, parent-child
personal hygiene Z91.89
personality F69
phase-of-life transition, adjustment Z60.0
presence of sick or disabled person in family or household Z63.79
needing care Z63.6
primary support group (family) Z63.9
specified NEC Z63.8
probation officer Z64.4
psychiatric F99
psychosexual (development) F66
psychosocial Z65.9
specified NEC Z65.8
relationship Z63.9
childhood F93.8
release from prison Z65.2

Problem *(Continued)*
removal from home affecting child Z62.29
seeking and accepting known hazardous and harmful
behavioral or psychological interventions Z65.8
chemical, nutritional or physical interventions Z65.8
sexual function (nonorganic) F52.9
sight H54.7
sleep disorder, child F51.9
smell —*see* Disturbance, sensation, smell
social
environment Z60.9
specified NEC Z60.8
exclusion and rejection Z60.4
worker Z64.4
speech R47.9
developmental F80.9
specified NEC R47.89
swallowing —*see* Dysphagia
taste —*see* Disturbance, sensation, taste
tic, child F95.0
underachievement in school Z55.3
unemployment Z56.0
threatened Z56.2
unwanted pregnancy Z64.0
upbringing Z62.9
specified NEC Z62.898
urinary N39.9
voice production R47.89
work schedule (stressful) Z56.3
Procedure (surgical)
for purpose other than remedying health state Z41.9
specified NEC Z41.8
not done Z53.9
because of
administrative reasons Z53.8
contraindication Z53.09
smoking Z53.01
patient's decision Z53.20
for reasons of belief or group pressure Z53.1
left against medical advice (AMA) Z53.21
specified reason NEC Z53.29
specified reason NEC Z53.8
Procidentia (uteri) N81.3
Proctalgia K62.89
fugax K59.4
spasmodic K59.4
Proctitis K62.89
amebic (acute) A06.0
chlamydial A56.3
gonococcal A54.6
granulomatous —*see* Enteritis, regional, large intestine
herpetic A60.1
radiation K62.7
tuberculous A18.32
ulcerative (chronic) K51.20
with
complication K51.219
abscess K51.214
fistula K51.213
obstruction K51.212
rectal bleeding K51.211
specified NEC K51.218
Proctocele
female (without uterine prolapse) N81.6
with uterine prolapse N81.2
complete N81.3
male K62.3

Proctocolitis, mucosal —*see* Rectosigmoiditis, ulcerative
Proctoptosis K62.3
Proctorrhagia K62.5
Proctosigmoiditis K63.89
ulcerative (chronic) —*see* Rectosigmoiditis, ulcerative
Proctospasm K59.4
psychogenic F45.8
Profichet's disease —*see* Disorder, soft tissue, specified type NEC
Progeria E34.8
Prognathism (mandibular) (maxillary) M26.19
Progonoma (melanotic) —*see* Neoplasm, benign, by site
Progressive —*see* condition
Prolactinoma
specified site —*see* Neoplasm, benign, by site
unspecified site D35.2
Prolapse, prolapsed
anus, anal (canal) (sphincter) K62.2
arm or hand O32.2
causing obstructed labor O64.4
bladder (mucosa) (sphincter) (acquired)
congenital Q79.4
female —*see* Cystocele
male N32.89
breast implant (prosthetic) T85.49
cecostomy K94.09
cecum K63.4
cervix, cervical (hypertrophied) N81.2
anterior lip, obstructing labor O65.5
congenital Q51.828
postpartal, old N81.2
stump N81.85
ciliary body (traumatic) —*see* Laceration, eye(ball), with prolapse or loss of interocular tissue
colon (pedunculated) K63.4
colostomy K94.09
disc (intervertebral) —*see* Displacement, intervertebral disc
eye implant (orbital) T85.398
lens (ocular) —*see* Complications, intraocular lens
fallopian tube N83.4
gastric (mucosa) K31.89
genital, female N81.9
specified NEC N81.89
globe, nontraumatic —*see* Luxation, globe
ileostomy bud K94.19
intervertebral disc —*see* Displacement, intervertebral disc
intestine (small) K63.4
iris (traumatic) —*see* Laceration, eye(ball), with prolapse or loss of interocular tissue
nontraumatic H21.89
kidney N28.83
congenital Q63.2
laryngeal muscles or ventricle J38.7
liver K76.89
meatus urinarius N36.8
mitral (valve) I34.1
ocular lens implant —*see* Complications, intraocular lens
organ or site, congenital NEC —*see* Malposition, congenital
ovary N83.4
pelvic floor, female N81.89

Prolapse, prolapsed (Continued)
perineum, female N81.89
rectum (mucosa) (sphincter) K62.3
due to trichuris trichuria B79
spleen D73.89
stomach K31.89
umbilical cord
complicating delivery O69.0
urachus, congenital Q64.4
ureter N28.89
with obstruction N13.5
with infection N13.6
ureterovesical orifice N28.89
urethra (acquired) (infected) (mucosa)
N36.8
congenital Q64.71
urinary meatus N36.8
congenital Q64.72
uterovaginal N81.4
complete N81.3
incomplete N81.2
uterus (with prolapse of vagina) N81.4
complete N81.3
congenital Q51.818
first degree N81.2
in pregnancy or childbirth —see
Pregnancy, complicated by,
abnormal, uterus
incomplete N81.2
postpartal (old) N81.4
second degree N81.2
third degree N81.3
uveal (traumatic) —see Laceration,
eye(ball), with prolapse or loss of
interocular tissue
vagina (anterior) (wall) —see Cystocele
with prolapse of uterus N81.4
complete N81.3
incomplete N81.2
posterior wall N81.6
posthysterectomy N99.3
vitreous (humor) H43.0-
in wound —see Laceration, eye(ball),
with prolapse or loss of
interocular tissue
womb —see Prolapse, uterus
Prolapsus, female N81.9
specified NEC N81.89
Proliferation (s)
primary cutaneous CD30-positive large
T-cell C86.6
Proliferative —see condition
Prolonged, prolongation (of)
bleeding (time) (idiopathic) R79.1
coagulation (time) R79.1
gestation (over 42 completed weeks)
mother O48.1
newborn P08.22
interval I44.0
labor O63.9
first stage O63.0
second stage O63.1
partial thromboplastin time (PTT) R79.1
pregnancy (more than 42 weeks
gestation) O48.1
prothrombin time R79.1
QT interval I45.81
uterine contractions in labor O62.4
Prominence, prominent
with disproportion (fetopelvic) O33.0
causing obstructed labor O65.0
auricle (congenital) (ear) Q17.5
ischial spine or sacral promontory
nose (congenital) acquired M95.0

Promiscuity —see High, risk, sexual
behavior
Pronation
ankle —see Deformity, limb, foot,
specified NEC
foot —see also Deformity, limb, foot,
specified NEC
congenital Q74.2
Prophylactic
administration of
antibiotics, long-term Z79.2
short-term use - omit code
drug (see also Long-term (current)
drug therapy
(use of)) Z79.899
medication Z79.899
organ removal (for neoplasia
management) Z40.00
breast Z40.01
ovary Z40.02
specified site NEC Z40.09
surgery Z40.9
for risk factors related to malignant
neoplasm —see Prophylactic,
organ removal
specified NEC Z40.8
vaccination Z23
Propionic acidemia E71.121
Proptosis (ocular) —see also
Exophthalmos
thyroid —see Hyperthyroidism, with
goiter
Prosecution, anxiety concerning Z65.3
Prosopagnosia R48.3
Prostadynia N42.81
Prostate, prostatic —see condition
Prostatism —see Hyperplasia, prostate
Prostatitis (congestive) (suppurative)
(with cystitis) N41.9
acute N41.0
cavitary N41.8
chronic N41.1
diverticular N41.8
due to Trichomonas (vaginalis) A59.02
fibrous N41.10
with hematuria N41.11
gonococcal (acute) (chronic) A54.22
granulomatous N41.4
hypertrophic N41.10
with hematuria N41.11
subacute N41.10
with hematuria N41.11
trichomonal A59.02
tuberculous A18.14
Prostatocystitis N41.3
Prostatorrhea N42.89
Prostatosis N42.82
Prostration R53.83
heat —see also Heat, exhaustion
anhydrotic T67.3
due to
salt (and water) depletion T67.4
water depletion T67.3
nervous F48.8
senile R54
Protanomaly (anomalous trichromat)
H53.54
Protanopia (complete) (incomplete)
H53.54
Protection (against) (from) —see
Prophylactic
Protein
deficiency NEC —see Malnutrition
malnutrition —see Malnutrition

Protein (Continued)
sickness (see also Reaction, serum)
T80.69
Proteinemia R77.9
Proteinosis
alveolar (pulmonary) J84.01
lipid or lipoid (of Urbach) E78.89
Proteinuria R80.9
Bence Jones R80.3
complicating pregnancy —see
Proteinuria, gestational
gestational O12.1-
with edema O12.2-
idiopathic R80.0
isolated R80.0
with glomerular lesion N06.9
dense deposit disease N06.6
diffuse
crescentic glomerulonephritis
N06.7
endocapillary proliferative
glomerulonephritis N06.4
mesangiocapillary
glomerulonephritis N06.5
focal and segmental hyalinosis or
sclerosis N06.1
membranous (diffuse) N06.2
mesangial proliferative (diffuse)
N06.3
minimal change N06.0
specified pathology NEC N06.8
orthostatic R80.2
with glomerular lesion —see
Proteinuria, isolated, with
glomerular lesion
persistent R80.1
with glomerular lesion —see
Proteinuria, isolated, with
glomerular lesion
postural R80.2
with glomerular lesion —see
Proteinuria, isolated, with
glomerular lesion
pre-eclamptic —see Pre-eclampsia
specified type NEC R80.8
Proteolysis, pathologic D65
Proteus (mirabilis) (morganii), as cause
of disease classified elsewhere
B96.4
Prothrombin gene mutation
D68.52
Protoporphyria, erythropoietic
E80.0
Protozoal —see also condition
disease B64
specified NEC B60.8
Protrusion, protrusio
acetabuli M24.7
acetabulum (into pelvis) M24.7
device, implant or graft (see also
Complications, by site and type,
mechanical) T85.698
arterial graft NEC —see
Complication, cardiovascular
device, mechanical, vascular
breast (implant) T85.49
catheter NEC T85.698
cystostomy T83.090
dialysis (renal) T82.49
intraperitoneal T85.691
infusion NEC T82.594
spinal (epidural) (subdural)
T85.690
urinary, indwelling T83.098

Protrusion, protrusio (Continued)
  device, implant or graft (Continued)
    electronic (electrode) (pulse
      generator) (stimulator)
      bone T84.390
        nervous system —see Complication,
          prosthetic device, mechanical,
          electronic nervous system
          stimulator
    fixation, internal (orthopedic) NEC —
      see Complication, fixation
      device, mechanical
    gastrointestinal —see Complications,
      prosthetic device, mechanical,
      gastrointestinal device
    genital NEC T83.498
      intrauterine contraceptive device
        T83.39
      penile prosthesis T83.490
    heart NEC —see Complication,
      cardiovascular device,
      mechanical
    joint prosthesis —see Complications,
      joint prosthesis, mechanical,
      specified NEC, by site
    ocular NEC —see Complications,
      prosthetic device, mechanical,
      ocular device
    orthopedic NEC —see Complication,
      orthopedic, device, mechanical
    specified NEC T85.628
    urinary NEC —see also Complication,
      genitourinary, device, urinary,
      mechanical
      graft T83.29
    vascular NEC —see Complication,
      cardiovascular device,
      mechanical
    ventricular intracranial shunt T85.09
  intervertebral disc —see Displacement,
    intervertebral disc
  joint prosthesis —see Complications,
    joint prosthesis, mechanical,
    specified NEC, by site
  nucleus pulposus —see Displacement,
    intervertebral disc
Prune belly (syndrome) Q79.4
Prurigo (ferox) (gravis) (Hebrae) (Hebra's)
  (mitis) (simplex) L28.2
  Besnier's L20.0
  estivalis L56.4
  nodularis L28.1
  psychogenic F45.8
Pruritus, pruritic (essential) L29.9
  ani, anus L29.0
    psychogenic F45.8
  anogenital L29.3
    psychogenic F45.8
  due to onchocerca volvulus B73.1
  gravidarum —see Pregnancy,
    complicated by, specified
    pregnancy-related condition
    NEC
  hiemalis L29.8
  neurogenic (any site) F45.8
  perianal L29.0
  psychogenic (any site) F45.8
  scroti, scrotum L29.1
    psychogenic F45.8
  senile, senilis L29.8
  specified NEC L29.8
    psychogenic F45.8
  Trichomonas A59.9
  vulva, vulvae L29.2
    psychogenic F45.8

Pseudarthrosis, pseudoarthrosis
  (bone) —see Nonunion, fracture
  clavicle, congenital Q74.0
  joint, following fusion or arthrodesis
    M96.0
Pseudoaneurysm —see Aneurysm
Pseudoangina (pectoris) —see Angina
Pseudoangioma I81
Pseudoarteriosus Q28.8
Pseudoarthrosis —see Pseudarthrosis
Pseudobulbar affect (PBA) F48.8
Pseudochromhidrosis L67.8
Pseudocirrhosis, liver, pericardial
  I31.1
Pseudocowpox B08.03
Pseudocoxalgia M91.3-
Pseudocroup J38.5
Pseudo-Cushing's syndrome, alcohol-
  induced E24.4
Pseudocyesis F45.8
Pseudocyst
  lung J98.4
  pancreas K86.3
  retina —see Cyst, retina
Pseudoelephantiasis neuroarthritica
  Q82.0
Pseudoexfoliation, capsule (lens) —see
  Cataract, specified NEC
Pseudofolliculitis barbae L73.1
Pseudoglioma H44.89
Pseudohemophilia (Bernuth's)
  (hereditary) (type B) D68.0
  Type A D69.8
  vascular D69.8
Pseudohermaphroditism Q56.3
  adrenal E25.8
  female Q56.2
    with adrenocortical disorder E25.8
    without adrenocortical disorder
      Q56.2
    adrenal, congenital E25.0
  male Q56.1
    with
      adrenocortical disorder E25.8
      androgen resistance E34.51
      cleft scrotum Q56.1
      feminizing testis E34.51
      5-alpha-reductase deficiency
        E29.1
    without gonadal disorder Q56.1
    adrenal E25.8
Pseudo-Hurler's polydystrophy E77.0
Pseudohydrocephalus G93.2
Pseudohypertrophic muscular dystrophy
  (Erb's) G71.0
Pseudohypertrophy, muscle G71.0
Pseudohypoparathyroidism E20.1
Pseudoinsomnia F51.03
Pseudoleukemia, infantile D64.89
Pseudomembranous —see condition
Pseudomeningocele (cerebral) (infective)
  (post-traumatic) G96.19
  postprocedural (spinal) G97.82
Pseudomenses (newborn) P54.6
Pseudomenstruation (newborn) P54.6
Pseudomonas
  aeruginosa, as cause of disease
    classified elsewhere B96.5
  mallei infection A24.0
    as cause of disease classified
      elsewhere B96.5
  pseudomallei, as cause of disease
    classified elsewhere B96.5
Pseudomyotonia G71.19

Pseudomyxoma peritonei C78.6
Pseudoneuritis, optic (nerve) (disc)
  (papilla), congenital Q14.2
Pseudo-obstruction intestine (acute)
  (chronic) (idiopathic) (intermittent
  secondary) (primary) K59.8
Pseudopapilledema H47.33-
  congenital Q14.2
Pseudoparalysis
  arm or leg R29.818
  atonic, congenital P94.2
Pseudopelade L66.0
Pseudophakia Z96.1
Pseudopolyarthritis, rhizomelic
  M35.3
Pseudopolycythemia D75.1
Pseudopseudohypoparathyroidism
  E20.1
Pseudopterygium H11.81-
Pseudoptosis (eyelid) —see
  Blepharochalasis
Pseudopuberty, precocious
  female heterosexual E25.8
  male isosexual E25.8
Pseudorickets (renal) N25.0
Pseudorubella B08.20
Pseudosclerema, newborn P83.8
Pseudosclerosis (brain)
  Jakob's —see Creutzfeldt-Jakob disease
    or syndrome
  of Westphal (Strüümpell) E83.01
  spastic —see Creutzfeldt-Jakob disease
    or syndrome
Pseudotetanus —see Convulsions
Pseudotetany R29.0
  hysterical F44.5
Pseudotruncus arteriosus Q25.4
Pseudotuberculosis A28.2
  enterocolitis A04.8
  pasteurella (infection) A28.0
Pseudotumor
  cerebri G93.2
  orbital —see Inflammation, orbit
Pseudoxanthoma elasticum Q82.8
Psilosis (sprue) (tropical) K90.1
  nontropical K90.0
Psittacosis A70
Psoitis M60.88
Psoriasis L40.9
  arthropathic L40.50
    arthritis mutilans L40.52
    distal interphalangeal L40.51
    juvenile L40.54
    other specified L40.59
    spondylitis L40.53
  buccal K13.29
  flexural L40.8
  guttate L40.4
  mouth K13.29
  nummular L40.0
  plaque L40.0
  psychogenic F54
  pustular (generalized) L40.1
    palmaris et plantaris L40.3
  specified NEC L40.8
  vulgaris L40.0
Psychasthenia F48.8
Psychiatric disorder or problem
  F99
Psychogenic —see also condition
  factors associated with physical
  conditions F54
Psychological and behavioral factors
  affecting medical condition F59

Psychosyndrome, organic F07.9
Psychotic episode due to or associated
with physical condition F06.8
Pterygium (eye) H11.00-
   amyloid H11.01-
   central H11.02-
   colli Q18.3
   double H11.03-
   peripheral
      progressive H11.05-
      stationary H11.04-
   recurrent H11.06-
Ptilosis (eyelid) —see Madarosis
Ptomaine (poisoning) —see Poisoning,
   food
Ptosis —see also Blepharoptosis
   adiposa (false) —see Blepharoptosis
   breast N64.81
   cecum K63.4
   colon K63.4
   congenital (eyelid) Q10.0
      specified site NEC —see Anomaly,
         by site
   eyelid —see Blepharoptosis
      congenital Q10.0
   gastric K31.89
   intestine K63.4
   kidney N28.83
   liver K76.89
   renal N28.83
   splanchnic K63.4
   spleen D73.89
   stomach K31.89
   viscera K63.4
PTP D69.51
Ptyalism (periodic) K11.7
   hysterical F45.8
   pregnancy —see Pregnancy,
      complicated by, specified
         pregnancy-related condition NEC
   psychogenic F45.8
Ptyalolithiasis K11.5
Pubarche, precocious E30.1
Pubertas praecox E30.1
Puberty (development state) Z00.3
   bleeding (excessive) N92.2
   delayed E30.0
   precocious (constitutional)
      (cryptogenic) (idiopathic) E30.1
      central E22.8
      due to
         ovarian hyperfunction E28.1
            estrogen E28.0
         testicular hyperfunction E29.0
   premature E30.1
      due to
         adrenal cortical hyperfunction
            E25.8
         pineal tumor E34.8
         pituitary (anterior) hyperfunction
            E22.8
Puckering, macula —see Degeneration,
   macula, puckering
Pudenda, pudendum —see condition
Puente's disease (simple glandular
   cheilitis) K13.0
Puerperal, puerperium (complicated by,
   complications)
   abnormal glucose (tolerance test)
      O99.815
   abscess
      areola O91.02
         associated with lactation O91.03
      Bartholin's gland O86.19

Puerperal, puerperium (Continued)
   abscess (Continued)
      breast O91.12
         associated with lactation O91.13
      cervix (uteri) O86.11
      genital organ NEC O86.19
      kidney O86.21
      mammary O91.12
         associated with lactation O91.13
      nipple O91.02
         associated with lactation
            O91.03
      peritoneum O85
      subareolar O91.12
         associated with lactation O91.13
      urinary tract —see Puerperal,
         infection, urinary
      uterus O86.12
      vagina (wall) O86.13
      vaginorectal O86.13
      vulvovaginal gland O86.13
   adnexitis O86.19
   afibrinogenemia, or other coagulation
      defect O72.3
   albuminuria (acute) (subacute) —see
      Proteinuria, gestational
   alcohol use O99.315
   anemia O90.81
      pre-existing (pre-pregnancy) O99.03
   anesthetic death O89.8
   apoplexy O99.43
   bariatric surgery status O99.845
   blood disorder NEC O99.13
   blood dyscrasia O72.3
   cardiomyopathy O90.3
   cerebrovascular disorder (conditions in
      I60-I69) O99.43
   cervicitis O86.11
   circulatory system disorder O99.43
   coagulopathy (any) O72.3
   complications O90.9
      specified NEC O90.89
   convulsions —see Eclampsia
   cystitis O86.22
   cystopyelitis O86.29
   delirium NEC F05
   diabetes O24.93
      gestational —see Puerperal,
         gestational diabetes
      pre-existing O24.33
         specified NEC O24.83
         type 1 O24.03
         type 2 O24.13
   digestive system disorder O99.63
   disease O90.9
      breast NEC O92.29
      cerebrovascular (acute) O99.43
      nonobstetric NEC O99.89
      tubo-ovarian O86.19
      Valsuani's O99.03
   disorder O90.9
      biliary tract O26.63
      lactation O92.79
      liver O26.63
      nonobstetric NEC O99.89
   disruption
      cesarean wound O90.0
      episiotomy wound O90.1
      perineal laceration wound O90.1
   drug use O99.325
   eclampsia (with pre-existing
      hypertension) O15.2
   embolism (pulmonary) (blood clot) —
      see Embolism, obstetric, puerperal

Puerperal, puerperium (Continued)
   endocrine, nutritional or metabolic
      disease NEC O99.285
   endophlebitis —see Puerperal, phlebitis
   endotrachelitis O86.19
   failure
      lactation (complete) O92.3
         partial O92.4
      renal, acute O90.4
   fever (of unknown origin) O86.4
      septic O85
   fissure, nipple O92.12
      associated with lactation O92.13
   fistula
      breast (due to mastitis) O91.12
         associated with lactation O91.13
      nipple O91.02
         associated with lactation O91.03
   galactophoritis O91.22
      associated with lactation O91.23
   galactorrhea O92.6
   gastric banding status O99.845
   gastric bypass status O99.845
   gastrointestinal disease NEC O99.63
   gestational diabetes O24.439
      diet controlled O24.430
      insulin (and diet) controlled O24.434
   gonorrhea O98.23
   hematoma, subdural O99.43
   hemiplegia, cerebral O99.355-
      due to cerebrovascular disorder
         O99.43
   hemorrhage O72.1
      brain O99.43
      bulbar O99.43
      cerebellar O99.43
      cerebral O99.43
      cortical O99.43
      delayed or secondary O72.2
      extradural O99.43
      internal capsule O99.43
      intracranial O99.43
      intrapontine O99.43
      meningeal O99.43
      pontine O99.43
      retained placenta O72.0
      subarachnoid O99.43
      subcortical O99.43
      subdural O99.43
      third stage O72.0
      uterine, delayed O72.2
      ventricular O99.43
   hemorrhoids O87.2
   hepatorenal syndrome O90.4
   hypertension —see Hypertension,
      complicating, puerperium
   hypertrophy, breast O92.29
   induration breast (fibrous) O92.29
   infection O86.4
      cervix O86.11
      generalized O85
      genital tract NEC O86.19
         obstetric surgical wound O86.0
      kidney (bacillus coli) O86.21
      maternal O98.93
         carrier state NEC O99.835
         gonorrhea O98.23
         human immunodeficiency virus
            (HIV) O98.73
         protozoal O98.63
         sexually transmitted NEC O98.33
         specified NEC O98.83
         streptococcus B carrier state
            O99.825

Puerperal, puerperium (Continued)
  infection (Continued)
    maternal (Continued)
      syphilis O98.13
      tuberculosis O98.03
      viral hepatitis O98.43
      viral NEC O98.53
    nipple O91.02
      associated with lactation O91.03
    peritoneum O85
    renal O86.21
    specified NEC O86.89
    urinary (asymptomatic) (tract) NEC
      O86.20
      bladder O86.22
      kidney O86.21
      specified site NEC O86.29
      urethra O86.22
    vagina O86.13
    vein —see Puerperal, phlebitis
  ischemia, cerebral O99.43
  lymphangitis O86.89
    breast O91.22
      associated with lactation O91.23
  malignancy O9A.13
  malnutrition O25.3
  mammillitis O91.02
    associated with lactation O91.03
  mammitis O91.22
    associated with lactation O91.23
  mania F30.8
  mastitis O91.22
    associated with lactation O91.23
    purulent O91.12
      associated with lactation O91.13
  melancholia —see Disorder, depressive
  mental disorder NEC O99.345
  metroperitonitis O85
  metrorrhagia —see Hemorrhage,
    postpartum
  metrosalpingitis O86.19
  metrovaginitis O86.13
  milk leg O87.1
  monoplegia, cerebral O99.43
  mood disturbance O90.6
  necrosis, liver (acute) (subacute)
    (conditions in subcategory K72.0)
    O26.63
    with renal failure O90.4
  nervous system disorder O99.355
  obesity (pre-existing prior to
    pregnancy) O99.215
  obesity surgery status O99.845
  occlusion, precerebral artery O99.43
  paralysis
    bladder (sphincter) O90.89
    cerebral O99.43
  paralytic stroke O99.43
  parametritis O85
  paravaginitis O86.13
  pelviperitonitis O85
  perimetritis O86.19
  perimetrosalpingitis O86.19
  perinephritis O86.21
  periphlebitis —see Puerperal phlebitis
  peritoneal infection O85
  peritonitis (pelvic) O85
  perivaginitis O86.13
  phlebitis O87.0
    deep O87.1
    pelvic O87.1
    superficial O87.0
  phlebothrombosis, deep O87.1
  phlegmasia alba dolens O87.1

Puerperal, puerperium (Continued)
  placental polyp O90.89
  pneumonia, embolic —see Embolism,
    obstetric, puerperal
  pre-eclampsia —see Pre-eclampsia
  psychosis F53
  pyelitis O86.21
  pyelocystitis O86.29
  pyelonephritis O86.21
  pyelonephrosis O86.21
  pyemia O85
  pyocystitis O86.29
  pyohemia O85
  pyometra O86.19
  pyonephritis O86.21
  pyosalpingitis O86.19
  pyrexia (of unknown origin) O86.4
  renal
    disease NEC O90.89
    failure O90.4
  respiratory disease NEC O99.53
  retention
    decidua —see Retention, decidua
    placenta O72.0
    secundines —see Retention,
      secundines
  retrated nipple O92.02
  salpingo-ovaritis O86.19
  salpingoperitonitis O85
  secondary perineal tear O90.1
  sepsis O85
  sepsis (pelvic) O85
  septic thrombophlebitis O86.81
  skin disorder NEC O99.73
  specified condition NEC O99.89
  stroke O99.43
  subinvolution (uterus) O90.89
  subluxation of symphysis (pubis)
    O26.73
  suppuration —see Puerperal, abscess
  tetanus A34
  thelitis O91.02
    associated with lactation O91.03
  thrombocytopenia O72.3
  thrombophlebitis (superficial) O87.0
    deep O87.1
    pelvic O87.1
    septic O86.81
  thrombosis (venous) —see Thrombosis,
    puerperal
  thyroiditis O90.5
  toxemia (eclamptic) (pre-eclamptic)
    (with convulsions) O15.2
  trauma, non-obstetric O9A.23
    caused by abuse (physical)
      (suspected) O9A.33
      confirmed O9A.33
    psychological (suspected)
      O9A.53
      confirmed O9A.53
    sexual (suspected) O9A.43
      confirmed O9A.43
  uremia (due to renal failure) O90.4
  urethritis O86.22
  vaginitis O86.13
  varicose veins (legs) O87.4
    vulva or perineum O87.8
  venous O87.9
  vulvitis O86.19
  vulvovaginitis O86.13
  white leg O87.1
Puerperium —see Puerperal
Pulmolithiasis J98.4
Pulmonary —see condition

Pulpitis (acute) (anachoretic) (chronic)
  (hyperplastic) (irreversible)
  (putrescent) (reversible)
  (suppurative) (ulcerative) K04.0
Pulpless tooth K04.99
Pulse
  alternating R00.8
  bigeminal R00.8
  fast R00.0
  feeble, rapid due to shock following
    injury T79.4
  rapid R00.0
  weak R09.89
Pulsus alternans or trigeminus R00.8
Punch drunk F07.81
Punctum lacrimale occlusion —see
  Obstruction, lacrimal
Puncture
  abdomen, abdominal
    wall S31.139
      with
        foreign body S31.149
        penetration into peritoneal cavity
          S31.639
          with foreign body S31.649
    epigastric region S31.132
      with
        foreign body S31.142
        penetration into peritoneal
          cavity S31.632
          with foreign body S31.642
    left
      lower quadrant S31.134
        with
          foreign body S31.144
          penetration into peritoneal
            cavity S31.634
            with foreign body S31.644
      upper quadrant S31.131
        with
          foreign body S31.141
          penetration into peritoneal
            cavity S31.631
            with foreign body S31.641
    periumbilic region S31.135
      with
        foreign body S31.145
        penetration into peritoneal
          cavity S31.635
          with foreign body S31.645
    right
      lower quadrant S31.133
        with
          foreign body S31.143
          penetration into peritoneal
            cavity S31.633
            with foreign body S31.643
      upper quadrant S31.130
        with
          foreign body S31.140
          penetration into peritoneal
            cavity S31.630
            with foreign body S31.640
  accidental, complicating surgery —see
    Complication, accidental puncture
    or laceration
  alveolar (process) —see Puncture, oral
    cavity
  ankle S91.039
    with
      foreign body S91.049
    left S91.032
      with
        foreign body S91.042

Puncture *(Continued)*
  genital organs, external *(Continued)*
    male S31.531
      with foreign body S31.541
      penis —*see* Puncture, penis
      scrotum —*see* Puncture, scrotum
      testis —*see* Puncture, testis
  groin —*see* Puncture, abdomen, wall
  gum —*see* Puncture, oral cavity
  hand S61.439
    with
      foreign body S61.449
    finger —*see* Puncture, finger
    left S61.432
      with
        foreign body S61.442
    right S61.431
      with
        foreign body S61.441
    thumb —*see* Puncture, thumb
  head S01.93
    with foreign body S01.94
    cheek —*see* Puncture, cheek
    ear —*see* Puncture, ear
    eyelid —*see* Puncture, eyelid
    lip —*see* Puncture, oral cavity
    nose —*see* Puncture, nose
    oral cavity —*see* Puncture, oral cavity
    scalp S01.03
      with foreign body S01.04
    specified site NEC S01.83
      with foreign body S01.84
    temporomandibular area —*see*
      Puncture, cheek
  heart S26.99
    with hemopericardium S26.09
    without hemopericardium S26.19
  heel —*see* Puncture, foot
  hip S71.039
    with foreign body S71.049
    left S71.032
      with foreign body S71.042
    right S71.031
      with foreign body S71.041
  hymen —*see* Puncture, vagina
  hypochondrium —*see* Puncture,
    abdomen, wall
  hypogastric region —*see* Puncture,
    abdomen, wall
  inguinal region —*see* Puncture,
    abdomen, wall
  instep —*see* Puncture, foot
  internal organs —*see* Injury, by site
  interscapular region —*see* Puncture,
    thorax, back
  intestine
    large
      colon S36.599
        ascending S36.590
        descending S36.592
        sigmoid S36.593
        specified site NEC S36.598
        transverse S36.591
      rectum S36.69
    small S36.499
      duodenum S36.490
      specified site NEC S36.498
  intra-abdominal organ S36.99
    gallbladder S36.128
    intestine —*see* Puncture, intestine
    liver S36.118
    pancreas —*see* Puncture, pancreas
    peritoneum S36.81
    specified site NEC S36.898

Puncture *(Continued)*
  intra-abdominal organ *(Continued)*
    spleen S36.09
    stomach S36.39
  jaw —*see* Puncture, head, specified site
    NEC
  knee S81.039
    with foreign body S81.049
    left S81.032
      with foreign body S81.042
    right S81.031
      with foreign body S81.041
  labium (majus) (minus) —*see* Puncture,
    vulva
  lacrimal duct —*see* Puncture, eyelid
  larynx S11.013
    with foreign body S11.014
  leg (lower) S81.839
    with foreign body S81.849
    foot —*see* Puncture, foot
    knee —*see* Puncture, knee
    left S81.832
      with foreign body S81.842
    right S81.831
      with foreign body S81.841
    upper —*see* Puncture, thigh
  lip S01.531
    with foreign body S01.541
  loin —*see* Puncture, abdomen, wall
  lower back —*see* Puncture, back, lower
  lumbar region —*see* Puncture, back,
    lower
  malar region —*see* Puncture, head,
    specified site NEC
  mammary —*see* Puncture, breast
  mastoid region —*see* Puncture, head,
    specified site NEC
  mouth —*see* Puncture, oral cavity
  nail
    finger —*see* Puncture, finger, with
      damage to nail
    toe —*see* Puncture, toe, with damage
      to nail
  nasal (septum) (sinus) —*see* Puncture,
    nose
  nasopharynx —*see* Puncture, head,
    specified site NEC
  neck S11.93
    with foreign body S11.94
    involving
      cervical esophagus —*see* Puncture,
        cervical esophagus
      larynx —*see* Puncture, larynx
      pharynx —*see* Puncture, pharynx
      thyroid gland —*see* Puncture,
        thyroid gland
      trachea —*see* Puncture, trachea
    specified site NEC S11.83
      with foreign body S11.84
  nose (septum) (sinus) S01.23
    with foreign body S01.24
  ocular —*see* Puncture, eyeball - oral
    cavity S01.532
    with foreign body S01.542
  orbit S05.4-
  palate —*see* Puncture, oral cavity
  palm —*see* Puncture, hand
  pancreas S36.299
    body S36.291
    head S36.290
    tail S36.292
  pelvis —*see* Puncture, back, lower
  penis S31.23
    with foreign body S31.24

Puncture *(Continued)*
  perineum
    female S31.43
      with foreign body S31.44
    male S31.139
      with foreign body S31.149
  periocular area (with or without lacrimal
    passages) —*see* Puncture, eyelid
  phalanges
    finger —*see* Puncture, finger
    toe —*see* Puncture, toe
  pharynx S11.23
    with foreign body S11.24
  pinna —*see* Puncture, ear
  popliteal space —*see* Puncture, knee
  prepuce —*see* Puncture, penis
  pubic region S31.139
    with foreign body S31.149
  pudendum —*see* Puncture, genital
    organs, external
  rectovaginal septum —*see* Puncture,
    vagina
  sacral region —*see* Puncture, back,
    lower
  sacroiliac region —*see* Puncture, back,
    lower
  salivary gland —*see* Puncture, oral
    cavity
  scalp S01.03
    with foreign body S01.04
  scapular region —*see* Puncture,
    shoulder
  scrotum S31.33
    with foreign body S31.34
  shin —*see* Puncture, leg
  shoulder S41.039
    with foreign body S41.049
    left S41.032
      with foreign body S41.042
    right S41.031
      with foreign body S41.041
  spermatic cord —*see* Puncture, testis
  sternal region —*see* Puncture, thorax,
    front
  submaxillary region —*see* Puncture,
    head, specified site NEC
  submental region —*see* Puncture, head,
    specified site NEC
  subungual
    finger (s) —*see* Puncture, finger, with
      damage to nail
    toe —*see* Puncture, toe, with damage
      to nail
  supraclavicular fossa —*see* Puncture,
    neck, specified site NEC
  temple, temporal region —*see* Puncture,
    head, specified site NEC
  temporomandibular area —*see*
    Puncture, cheek
  testis S31.33
    with foreign body S31.34
  thigh S71.139
    with foreign body S71.149
    left S71.132
      with foreign body S71.142
    right S71.131
      with foreign body S71.141
  thorax, thoracic (wall) S21.93
    with foreign body S21.94
    back S21.23-
      with
        foreign body S21.24-
          with penetration S21.44
        penetration S21.43

Puncture *(Continued)*
  thorax, thoracic *(Continued)*
    breast —*see* Puncture, breast
    front S21.13-
      with
        foreign body S21.14-
          with penetration
            S21.34
        penetration S21.33
  throat —*see* Puncture, neck
  thumb S61.039
    with
      damage to nail S61.139
        with
          foreign body S61.149
      foreign body S61.049
    left S61.032
      with
        damage to nail S61.132
          with
            foreign body S61.142
        foreign body S61.042
    right S61.031
      with
        damage to nail S61.131
          with
            foreign body S61.141
        foreign body S61.041
  thyroid gland S11.13
    with foreign body S11.14
  toe (s) S91.139
    with
      damage to nail S91.239
        with
          foreign body S91.249
      foreign body S91.149
    great S91.133
      with
        damage to nail S91.233
          with
            foreign body S91.243
        foreign body S91.143
    left S91.132
      with
        damage to nail S91.232
          with
            foreign body
              S91.242
        foreign body S91.142
    right S91.131
      with
        damage to nail S91.231
          with
            foreign body S91.241
        foreign body S91.141
    lesser S91.136
      with
        damage to nail S91.236
          with
            foreign body S91.246
        foreign body S91.146
    left S91.135
      with
        damage to nail S91.235
          with
            foreign body S91.245
        foreign body S91.145
    right S91.134
      with
        damage to nail S91.234
          with
            foreign body S91.244
        foreign body S91.144
  tongue —*see* Puncture, oral cavity

Puncture *(Continued)*
  trachea S11.023
    with foreign body S11.024
  tunica vaginalis —*see* Puncture, testis
  tympanum, tympanic membrane S09.2-
  umbilical region S31.135
    with foreign body S31.145
  uvula —*see* Puncture, oral cavity
  vagina S31.43
    with foreign body S31.44
  vocal cords S11.033
    with foreign body S11.034
  vulva S31.43
    with foreign body S31.44
  wrist S61.539
    with
      foreign body S61.549
    left S61.532
      with
        foreign body S61.542
    right S61.531
      with
        foreign body S61.541
PUO (pyrexia of unknown origin) R50.9
Pupillary membrane (persistent) Q13.89
Pupillotonia —*see* Anomaly, pupil,
    function, tonic pupil
Purpura D69.2
  abdominal D69.0
  allergic D69.0
  anaphylactoid D69.0
  annularis telangiectodes L81.7
  arthritic D69.0
  autoerythrocyte sensitization D69.2
  autoimmune D69.0
  bacterial D69.0
  Bateman's (senile) D69.2
  capillary fragility (hereditary)
    (idiopathic)D69.8
  cryoglobulinemic D89.1
  Devil's pinches D69.2
  fibrinolytic —*see* Fibrinolysis
  fulminans, fulminous D65
  gangrenous D65
  hemorrhagic, hemorrhagica D69.3
    not due to thrombocytopenia D69.0
  Henoch (-Schönlein) (allergic) D69.0
  hypergammaglobulinemic (benign)
    (Waldenström's) D89.0
  idiopathic (thrombocytopenic) D69.3
    nonthrombocytopenic D69.0
  immune thrombocytopenic D69.3
  infectious D69.0
  malignant D69.0
  neonatorum P54.5
  nervosa D69.0
  newborn P54.5
  nonthrombocytopenic D69.2
    hemorrhagic D69.0
    idiopathic D69.0
  nonthrombopenic D69.2
  peliosis rheumatica D69.0
  posttransfusion (post-transfusion)
    (from (fresh) whole blood or blood
      products) D69.51
  primary D69.49
  red cell membrane sensitivity D69.2
  rheumatica D69.0
  Schönlein (-Henoch) (allergic) D69.0
  scorbutic E54 [D77]
  senile D69.2
  simplex D69.2
  symptomatica D69.0
  telangiectasia annularis L81.7

Purpura *(Continued)*
  thrombocytopenic D69.49
    congenital D69.42
    hemorrhagic D69.3
    hereditary D69.42
    idiopathic D69.3
    immune D69.3
    neonatal, transitory P61.0
    thrombotic M31.1
  thrombohemolytic —*see* Fibrinolysis
  thrombolytic —*see* Fibrinolysis
  thrombopenic D69.49
  thrombotic, thrombocytopenic M31.1
  toxic D69.0
  vascular D69.0
  visceral symptoms D69.0
Purpuric spots R23.3
Purulent —*see* condition
Pus
  in
    stool R19.5
    urine N39.0
  tube (rupture) —*see* Salpingo-oophoritis
Pustular rash L08.0
Pustule (nonmalignant) L08.9
  malignant A22.0
Pustulosis palmaris et plantaris L40.3
Putnam (-Dana) disease or syndrome —
    see Degeneration, combined
Putrescent pulp (dental) K04.1
Pyarthritis, pyarthrosis —*see* Arthritis,
    pyogenic or pyemic
  tuberculous —*see* Tuberculosis, joint
Pyelectasis —*see* Hydronephrosis
Pyelitis (congenital) (uremic) —*see also*
    Pyelonephritis
  with
    calculus —*see* category N20
      with hydronephrosis N13.2
    contracted kidney N11.9
  acute N10
  chronic N11.9
    with calculus —*see* category N20
      with hydronephrosis N13.2
  cystica N28.84
  puerperal (postpartum) O86.21
  tuberculous A18.11
Pyelocystitis —*see* Pyelonephritis
Pyelonephritis —*see also* Nephritis,
    tubulo-interstitial
  with
    calculus —*see* category N20
      with hydronephrosis N13.2
    contracted kidney N11.9
  acute N10
  calculus —*see* category N20
    with hydronephrosis N13.2
  chronic N11.9
    with calculus —*see* category N20
      with hydronephrosis N13.2
    associated with ureteral obstruction
      or stricture N11.1
    nonobstructive N11.8
      with reflux (vesicoureteral) N11.0
    obstructive N11.1
    specified NEC N11.8
  in (due to)
    brucellosis A23.9 [N16]
    cryoglobulinemia (mixed) D89.1
      [N16]
    cystinosis E72.04
    diphtheria A36.84
    glycogen storage disease E74.09
      [N16]

P

Pyelonephritis *(Continued)*
  in (due to) *(Continued)*
    leukemia NEC C95.9- *[N16]*
    lymphoma NEC C85.90 *[N16]*
    multiple myeloma C90.0- *[N16]*
    obstruction N11.1
    Salmonella infection A02.25
    sarcoidosis D86.84
    sepsis A41.9 *[N16]*
    Sjögren's disease M35.04
    toxoplasmosis B58.83
    transplant rejection T86.91 *[N16]*
    Wilson's disease E83.01 *[N16]*
   nonobstructive N12
    with reflux (vesicoureteral) N11.0
    chronic N11.8
   syphilitic A52.75
Pyelonephrosis (obstructive) N11.1
  chronic N11.9
Pyelophlebitis I80.8
Pyeloureteritis cystica N28.85
Pyemia, pyemic (fever) (infection) (purulent) —*see also* Sepsis
  joint —*see* Arthritis, pyogenic or pyemic
  liver K75.1
  pneumococcal A40.3
  portal K75.1
  postvaccinal T88.0
  puerperal, postpartum, childbirth O85
  specified organism NEC A41.89
  tuberculous —*see* Tuberculosis, miliary
Pygopagus Q89.4
Pyknoepilepsy (idiopathic) —*see* Pyknolepsy

Pyknolepsy G40.A09
  intractable G40.A19
    with status epilepticus G40.A11
    without status epilepticus G40.A19
  not intractable G40.A09
    with status epilepticus G40.A01
    without status epilepticus G40.A09
Pylephlebitis K75.1
Pyle's syndrome Q78.5
Pylethrombophlebitis K75.1
Pylethrombosis K75.1
Pyloritis K29.90
  with bleeding K29.91
Pylorospasm (reflex) NEC K31.3
  congenital or infantile Q40.0
  neurotic F45.8
  newborn Q40.0
  psychogenic F45.8
Pylorus, pyloric —*see* condition
Pyoarthrosis —*see* Arthritis, pyogenic or pyemic
Pyocele
  mastoid —*see* Mastoiditis, acute
  sinus (accessory) —*see* Sinusitis
  turbinate (bone) J32.9
  urethra (*see also* Urethritis) N34.0
Pyocolpos —*see* Vaginitis
Pyocystitis N30.80
  with hematuria N30.81
Pyoderma, pyodermia L08.0
  gangrenosum L88
  newborn P39.4
  phagedenic L88
  vegetans L08.81
Pyodermatitis L08.0
  vegetans L08.81
Pyogenic —*see* condition

Pyohydronephrosis N13.6
Pyometra, pyometrium, pyometritis —*see* Endometritis
Pyomyositis (tropical) —*see* Myositis, infective
Pyonephritis N12
Pyonephrosis N13.6
  tuberculous A18.11
Pyo-oophoritis —*see* Salpingo-oophoritis
Pyo-ovarium —*see* Salpingo-oophoritis
Pyopericarditis, pyopericardium I30.1
Pyophlebitis —*see* Phlebitis
Pyopneumopericardium I30.1
Pyopneumothorax (infective) J86.9
  with fistula J86.0
  tuberculous NEC A15.6
Pyosalpinx, pyosalpingitis —*see also* Salpingo-oophoritis
Pyothorax J86.9
  with fistula J86.0
  tuberculous NEC A15.6
Pyoureter N28.89
  tuberculous A18.11
Pyramidopallidonigral syndrome G20
Pyrexia (of unknown origin) R50.9
  atmospheric T67.0
  during labor NEC O75.2
  heat T67.0
  newborn P81.9
    environmentally-induced P81.0
  persistent R50.9
  puerperal O86.4
Pyroglobulinemia NEC E88.09
Pyromania F63.1
Pyrosis R12
Pyuria (bacterial) N39.0

Q

Q fever A78
  with pneumonia A78
Quadricuspid aortic valve Q23.8
Quadrilateral fever A78
Quadriparesis —*see* Quadriplegia
  meaning muscle weakness M62.81
Quadriplegia G82.50-
  complete
    C1-C4 level G82.51
    C5-C7 level G82.53
  congenital (cerebral) (spinal) G80.8
    spastic G80.0

Quadriplegia (*Continued*)
  embolic (current episode) I63.4
  functional R53.2
  incomplete
    C1-C4 level G82.52
    C5-C7 level G82.54
  thrombotic (current episode) I63.3
  traumatic — code to injury with
    seventh character S
    current episode —*see* Injury, spinal
      (cord), cervical
Quadruplet, pregnancy —*see* Pregnancy,
  quadruplet
Quarrelsomeness F60.3

Queensland fever A77.3
Quervain's disease M65.4
  thyroid E06.1
Queyrat's erythroplasia D07.4
  penis D07.4
  specified site —*see* Neoplasm, skin, in
    situ
  unspecified site D07.4
Quincke's disease or edema T78.3
  hereditary D84.1
Quinsy (gangrenous) J36
Quintan fever A79.0
Quintuplet, pregnancy —*see* Pregnancy,
  quintuplet

R

Rabbit fever —*see* Tularemia
Rabies A82.9
  contact Z20.3
  exposure to Z20.3
  inoculation reaction —*see*
      Complications, vaccination
  sylvatic A82.0
  urban A82.1
Rachischisis —*see* Spina bifida
Rachitic —*see also* condition
  deformities of spine (late effect)
      (sequelae) E64.3
  pelvis (late effect) (sequelae) E64.3
    with disproportion (fetopelvic)
      O33.0
      causing obstructed labor O65.0
Rachitis, rachitism (acute) (tarda) —*see
  also* Rickets
  renalis N25.0
  sequelae E64.3
Radial nerve —*see* condition
Radiation
  burn —*see* Burn
  effects NOS T66
  sickness NOS T66
  therapy, encounter for Z51.0
Radiculitis (pressure) (vertebrogenic) —
  see Radiculopathy
Radiculomyelitis —*see also* Encephalitis
  toxic, due to
    Clostridium tetani A35
    Corynebacterium diphtheriae
      A36.82
Radiculopathy M54.10
  cervical region M54.12
  cervicothoracic region M54.13
  due to displacement of intervertebral
    disc —*see* Disorder, disc, with,
    radiculopathy
  leg M54.1-
  lumbar region M54.16
  lumbosacral region M54.17
  occipito-atlanto-axial region M54.11
  postherpetic B02.29
  sacrococcygeal region M54.18
  syphilitic A52.11
  thoracic region (with visceral pain)
    M54.14
  thoracolumbar region M54.15
Radiodermal burns (acute, chronic, or
  occupational) —*see* Burn
Radiodermatitis L58.9
  acute L58.0
  chronic L58.1
Radiotherapy session Z51.0
Rage, meaning rabies —*see* Rabies
Ragpicker's disease A22.1
Ragsorter's disease A22.1
Raillietiniasis B71.8
Railroad neurosis F48.8
Railway spine F48.8
Raised —*see also* Elevated
  antibody titer R76.0
Rake teeth, tooth M26.39
Rales R09.89
Ramifying renal pelvis Q63.8
Ramsay-Hunt disease or syndrome (*see
  also* Hunt's disease) B02.21
  meaning dyssynergia cerebellaris
    myoclonica G11.1
Ranula K11.6
  congenital Q38.4

Rape
  adult
    confirmed T74.21
    suspected T76.21
  alleged, observation or examination,
    ruled out
    adult Z04.41
    child Z04.42
  child
    confirmed T74.22
    suspected T76.22
Rapid
  feeble pulse, due to shock, following
    injury T79.4
  heart (beat) R00.0
    psychogenic F45.8
  second stage (delivery) O62.3
  time-zone change syndrome —*see*
    Disorder, sleep, circadian rhythm,
    psychogenic
Rarefaction, bone —*see* Disorder, bone,
  density and structure, specified NEC
Rash (toxic) R21
  canker A38.9
  diaper L22
  drug (internal use) L27.0
    contact (*see also* Dermatitis, due to,
      drugs, external) L25.1
  following immunization T88.1
  food —*see* Dermatitis, due to, food
  heat L74.0
  napkin (psoriasiform) L22
  nettle —*see* Urticaria
  pustular L08.0
  rose R21
    epidemic B06.9
  scarlet A38.9
  serum (*see also* Reaction, serum) T80.69
  wandering tongue K14.1
Rasmussen aneurysm —*see* Tuberculosis,
  pulmonary
Rasmussen encephalitis G04.81
Rat-bite fever A25.9
  due to Streptobacillus moniliformis
    A25.1
  spirochetal (morsus muris) A25.0
Rathke's pouch tumor D44.3
Raymond (-Céstan) **syndrome** I65.8
**Raynaud's disease, phenomenon or
  syndrome** (secondary) I73.00
  with gangrene (symmetric) I73.01
RDS (newborn) (type I) P22.0
  type II P22.1
Reaction —*see also* Disorder
  adaptation —*see* Disorder, adjustment
  adjustment (anxiety) (conduct disorder)
    (depressiveness) (distress) —*see*
    Disorder, adjustment
    with
      mutism, elective (child)
        (adolescent) F94.0
  adverse
    food (any) (ingested) NEC T78.1
    anaphylactic —*see* Shock,
      anaphylactic, due to food
  anaphylactoid —*see* Shock, anaphylactic
  affective —*see* Disorder, mood
  allergic —*see* Allergy
  anaphylactic —*see* Shock, anaphylactic
  anesthesia —*see* Anesthesia,
    complication
  antitoxin (prophylactic) (therapeutic) —
    see Complications, vaccination
  anxiety F41.1
  Arthus —*see* Arthus' phenomenon

Reaction (*Continued*)
  asthenic F48.8
  combat and operational stress F43.0
  compulsive F42
  conversion F44.9
  crisis, acute F43.0
  deoxyribonuclease (DNA) (DNase)
    hypersensitivity D69.2
  depressive (single episode) F32.9
    affective (single episode) F31.4
      recurrent episode F33.9
    neurotic F34.1
    psychoneurotic F34.1
    psychotic F32.3
    recurrent —*see* Disorder, depressive,
      recurrent
  dissociative F44.9
  drug NEC T88.7
    addictive —*see* Dependence, drug
      transmitted via placenta or breast
      milk —*see* Absorption, drug,
      addictive, through placenta
    allergic —*see* Allergy, drug
    lichenoid L43.2
    newborn P93.8
      gray baby syndrome P93.0
    overdose or poisoning (by
      accident) —*see* Table of drugs
      and chemicals, by drug,
      poisoning
    photoallergic L56.1
    phototoxic L56.0
    withdrawal —*see* Dependence, by
      drug, with, withdrawal
      infant of dependent mother P96.1
      newborn P96.1
    wrong substance given or taken
      (by accident) —*see* Table of
      drugs and chemicals, by drug,
      poisoning
  fear F40.9
    child (abnormal) F93.8
  febrile nonhemolytic transfusion
    (FNHTR) R50.84
  fluid loss, cerebrospinal G97.1
  foreign
    body NEC —*see* Granuloma, foreign
      body
      in operative wound (inadvertently
        left) —*see* Foreign body,
        accidentally left during a
        procedure
      substance accidentally left during a
        procedure (chemical) (powder)
        (talc) T81.60
        aseptic peritonitis T81.61
        body or object (instrument)
          (sponge) (swab) —*see* Foreign
          body, accidentally left during
          a procedure
        specified reaction NEC T81.69
  grief —*see* Disorder, adjustment
  Herxheimer's R68.89
  hyperkinetic —*see* Hyperkinesia
  hypochondriacal F45.20
  hypoglycemic, due to insulin E16.0
    with coma (diabetic) —*see* Diabetes,
      coma
      nondiabetic E15
    therapeutic misadventure —*see*
      subcategory T38.3
  hypomanic F30.8
  hysterical F44.9
  immunization —*see* Complications,
    vaccination

Reaction *(Continued)*
 incompatibility
  ABO blood group (infusion) (transfusion) —*see* Complication (s), transfusion, incompatibility reaction, ABO
   delayed serologic T80.39
   minor blood group (Duffy) (E) (K(ell)) (Kidd) (Lewis) (M) (N) (P) (S) T80.89
   Rh (factor) (infusion) (transfusion) —*see* Complication (s), transfusion, incompatibility reaction, Rh (factor)
 inflammatory —*see* Infection
 infusion —*see* Complications, infusion
 inoculation (immune serum) —*see* Complications, vaccination
 insulin T38.3-
 involutional psychotic —*see* Disorder, depressive
 leukemoid D72.823
  basophilic D72.823
  lymphocytic D72.823
  monocytic D72.823
  myelocytic D72.823
  neutrophilic D72.823
 LSD (acute)
  due to drug abuse —*see* Abuse, drug, hallucinogen
  due to drug dependence —*see* Dependence, drug, hallucinogen
 lumbar puncture G97.1
 manic-depressive —*see* Disorder, bipolar
 neurasthenic F48.8
 neurogenic —*see* Neurosis
 neurotic F48.9
 neurotic-depressive F34.1
 nitritoid —*see* Crisis, nitritoid - obsessive-compulsive F42
 nonspecific
  to
   cell mediated immunity measurement of gamma interferon antigen response without active tuberculosis R76.12
   QuantiFERON-TB test (QFT) without active tuberculosis R76.12
   tuberculin test (*see also* Reaction, tuberculin skin test) R76.11
 obsessive-compulsive F42
 organic, acute or subacute —*see* Delirium
 paranoid (acute) F23
  chronic F22
  senile F03
 passive dependency F60.7
 phobic F40.9
 post-traumatic stress, uncomplicated Z73.3
 psychogenic F99
 psychoneurotic —*see also* Neurosis
  compulsive F42
  depersonalization F48.1
  depressive F34.1
  hypochondriacal F45.20
  neurasthenic F48.8
  obsessive F42
 psychophysiologic —*see* Disorder, somatoform

Reaction *(Continued)*
 psychosomatic —*see* Disorder, somatoform
 psychotic —*see* Psychosis
 scarlet fever toxin —*see* Complications, vaccination
 schizophrenic F23
  acute (brief) (undifferentiated) F23
  latent F21
  undifferentiated (acute) (brief) F23
 serological for syphilis —*see* Serology for syphilis
 serum T80.69
  anaphylactic (immediate) (*see also* Shock, anaphylactic) T80.59
  specified reaction NEC
   due to
    administration of blood and blood products T80.61
    immunization T80.62
    serum specified NEC T80.69
    vaccination T80.62
 situational —*see* Disorder, adjustment
 somatization —*see* Disorder, somatoform
 spinal puncture G97.1
 stress (severe) F43.9
  acute (agitation) ("daze") (disorientation) (disturbance of consciousness) (flight reaction) (fugue) F43.0
  specified NEC F43.8
 surgical procedure —*see* Complications, surgical procedure
 tetanus antitoxin —*see* Complications, vaccination
 toxic, to local anesthesia T81.89
  in labor and delivery O74.4
  in pregnancy O29.3X-
  postpartum, puerperal O89.3
 toxin-antitoxin —*see* Complications, vaccination
 transfusion (blood) (bone marrow) (lymphocytes) (allergic) —*see* Complications, transfusion
 tuberculin skin test, abnormal R76.11
 vaccination (any) —*see* Complications, vaccination
 withdrawing, child or adolescent F93.8
Reactive airway disease —*see* Asthma
Reactive depression —*see* Reaction, depressive
Rearrangement
 chromosomal
  balanced (in) Q95.9
   abnormal individual (autosomal) Q95.2
   non-sex (autosomal) chromosomes Q95.2
   sex/non-sex chromosomes Q95.3
  specified NEC Q95.8
Recalcitrant patient —*see* Noncompliance
Recanalization, thrombus —*see* Thrombosis
Recession, receding
 chamber angle (eye) H21.55-
 chin M26.09
 gingival (generalized) (localized) (postinfective) (postoperative) K06.0
Recklinghausen's disease Q85.01
 bones E21.0

Reclus' disease (cystic) —*see* Mastopathy, cystic
Recrudescent typhus (fever) A75.1
Recruitment, auditory H93.21-
Rectalgia K62.89
Rectitis K62.89
Rectocele
 female (without uterine prolapse) N81.6
  with uterine prolapse N81.4
   incomplete N81.2
 in pregnancy —*see* Pregnancy, complicated by, abnormal, pelvic organs or tissues NEC
 male K62.3
Rectosigmoid junction —*see* condition
Rectosigmoiditis K63.89
 ulcerative (chronic) K51.30
  with
   complication K51.319
    abscess K51.314
    fistula K51.313
    obstruction K51.312
    rectal bleeding K51.311
    specified NEC K51.318
Rectourethral —*see* condition
Rectovaginal —*see* condition
Rectovesical —*see* condition
Rectum, rectal —*see* condition
Recurrent —*see* condition
 pregnancy loss —*see* Loss (of), pregnancy, recurrent
Red bugs B88.0
Red-cedar lung or pneumonitis J67.8
Red tide (*see also* Table of Drugs and Chemicals) T65.82-
Reduced
 mobility Z74.09
 ventilatory or vital capacity R94.2
Redundant, redundancy
 anus (congenital) Q43.8
 clitoris N90.89
 colon (congenital) Q43.8
 foreskin (congenital) N47.8
 intestine (congenital) Q43.8
 labia N90.6
 organ or site, congenital NEC —*see* Accessory
 panniculus (abdominal) E65
 prepuce (congenital) N47.8
 pylorus K31.89
 rectum (congenital) Q43.8
 scrotum N50.8
 sigmoid (congenital) Q43.8
 skin (of face) L57.4
  eyelids —*see* Blepharochalasis
 stomach K31.89
Reduplication —*see* Duplication
Reflex R29.2
 hyperactive gag J39.2
 pupillary, abnormal —*see* Anomaly, pupil, function
 vasoconstriction I73.9
 vasovagal R55
Reflux K21.9
 acid K21.9
 esophageal K21.9
  with esophagitis K21.0
  newborn P78.83
 gastroesophageal K21.9
  with esophagitis K21.0
 mitral —*see* Insufficiency, mitral
 ureteral —*see* Reflux, vesicoureteral

Replacement by artificial or mechanical
    device or prosthesis of (Continued)
  intestine Z96.89
  joint Z96.60
    hip —see Presence, hip joint implant
    knee —see Presence, knee joint
      implant
    specified site NEC Z96.698
  larynx Z96.3
  lens Z96.1
  limb (s) —see Presence, artificial,
    limb
  mandible NEC (for tooth root
    implant (s)) Z96.5
  organ NEC Z96.89
  peripheral vessel NEC Z95.828
  stapes Z96.29
  teeth Z97.2
  tendon Z96.7
  tissue NEC Z96.89
  tooth root (s) Z96.5
  vessel NEC Z95.828
    coronary (artery) Z95.5
Request for expert evidence Z04.8
Reserve, decreased or low
  cardiac —see Disease, heart
  kidney N28.89
Residual —see also condition - ovary
    syndrome N99.83
  state, schizophrenic F20.5
  urine R39.19
Resistance, resistant (to)
  activated protein C D68.51
  complicating pregnancy O26.89
  insulin E88.81
  organism (s)
    to
      drug
        aminoglycosides Z16.29
        amoxicillin Z16.11
        ampicillin Z16.11
        antibiotic (s) Z16.20
          multiple Z16.24
          specified NEC Z16.29
        antifungal Z16.32
        antimicrobial (single) Z16.30
          multiple Z16.35
          specified NEC Z16.39
        antimycbacterial (single)
          Z16.341
          multiple Z16.342
        antiparasitic Z16.31
        antiviral Z16.33
        beta lactam antibiotics Z16.10
          specified NEC Z16.19
        cephalosporins Z16.19
        extended beta lactamase (ESBL)
          Z16.12
        fluoroquinolones Z16.23
        macrolides Z16.29
        methicillin —see MRSA
        multiple drugs (MDRO)
          antibiotics Z16.24
        penicillins Z16.11
        quinine (and related compounds)
          Z16.31
        quinolones Z16.23
        sulfonamides Z16.29
        tetracyclines Z16.29
        tuberculostatics (single) Z16.341
          multiple Z16.342
        vancomycin Z16.21
          related antibiotics Z16.22
  thyroid hormone E07.89

Resorption
  dental (roots) K03.3
    alveoli M26.79
  teeth (external) (internal) (pathological)
    (roots) K03.3
Respiration
  Cheyne-Stokes R06.3
  decreased due to shock, following
    injury T79.4
  disorder of, psychogenic F45.8
  insufficient, or poor R06.89
    newborn P28.5
  painful R07.1
  sighing, psychogenic F45.8
Respiratory —see also condition
  distress syndrome (newborn) (type I)
    P22.0
    type II P22.1
  syncytial virus, as cause of disease
    classified elsewhere B97.4
Respite care Z75.5
Response (drug)
  photoallergic L56.1
  phototoxic L56.0
Restless legs (syndrome) G25.81
Restlessness R45.1
Restoration (of)
  dental
    aesthetically inadequate or
      displeasing K08.56
    defective K08.50
      specified NEC K08.59
    failure of marginal integrity K08.51
    failure of periodontal anatomical
      intergrity K08.54
  organ continuity from previous
    sterilization (tuboplasty)
    (vasoplasty) Z31.0
    aftercare Z31.42
  tooth (existing)
    contours biologically incompatible
      with oral health K08.54
    open margins K08.51
    overhanging K08.52
    poor aesthetic K08.56
    poor gingival margins K08.51
  unsatisfactory, of tooth K08.50
    specified NEC K08.59
Restorative material (dental)
  allergy to K08.55
  fractured K08.539
    with loss of material K08.531
    without loss of material K08.530
  unrepairable overhanging of K08.52
Restriction of housing space Z59.1
Rests, ovarian, in fallopian tube Q50.6
Restzustand (schizophrenic) F20.5
Retained —see also Retention
  cholelithiasis following
    cholecystectomy K91.86
  foreign body fragments (type of) Z18.9
    acrylics Z18.2
    animal quill (s) or spines Z18.31
    cement Z18.83
    concrete Z18.83
    crystalline Z18.83
    depleted isotope Z18.09
    depleted uranium Z18.01
    diethylhexylphthalates Z18.2
    glass Z18.81
    isocyanate Z18.2
    magnetic metal Z18.11
    metal Z18.10
    nonmagnetic metal Z18.12
    nontherapeutic radioactive Z18.09

Retained (Continued)
  foreign body fragments (Continued)
    organic NEC Z18.39
    plastic Z18.2
    quill (s) (animal) Z18.31
    radioactive (nontherapeutic) NEC
      Z18.09
    specified NEC Z18.89
    spine (s) (animal) Z18.31
    stone Z18.83
    tooth (teeth) Z18.32
    wood Z18.33
  fragments (type of) Z18.9
    acrylics Z18.2
    animal quill (s) or spines Z18.31
    cement Z18.83
    concrete Z18.83
    crystalline Z18.83
    depleted isotope Z18.09
    depleted uranium Z18.01
    diethylhexylphthalates Z18.2
    glass Z18.81
    isocyanate Z18.2
    magnetic metal Z18.11
    metal Z18.10
    nonmagnectic metal Z18.12
    nontherapeutic radioactive Z18.09
    organic NEC Z18.39
    plastic Z18.2
    quill (s) (animal) Z18.31
    radioactive (nontherapeutic) NEC
      Z18.09
    specified NEC Z18.89
    spine (s) (animal) Z18.31
    stone Z18.83
    tooth (teeth) Z18.32
    wood Z18.33
  gallstones, following cholecystectomy
    K91.86
Retardation
  development, developmental,
    specific —see Disorder,
    developmental
  endochondral bone growth —see
    Disorder, bone, development or
    growth
  growth R62.50
    due to malnutrition E45
  mental —see Disability, intellectual
  motor function, specific F82
  physical (child) R62.52
    due to malnutrition E45
  reading (specific) F81.0
  spelling (specific) (without reading
    disorder) F81.81
Retching —see Vomiting
Retention —see also Retained
  bladder —see Retention, urine
  carbon dioxide E87.2
  cholelithiasis following
    cholecystectomy K91.86
  cyst —see Cyst
  dead
    fetus (at or near term) (mother) O36.4
      early fetal death O02.1
    ovum O02.0
  decidua (fragments) (following
    delivery) (with hemorrhage) O72.2
    without hemorrhage O73.1
  deciduous tooth K00.6
  dental root K08.3
  fecal —see Constipation
  fetus
    dead O36.4
      early O02.1

R

Retention (*Continued*)
fluid R60.9
foreign body —*see also* Foreign body, retained
current trauma - code as Foreign body, by site or type
gallstones, following cholecystectomy K91.86
gastric K31.89
intrauterine contraceptive device, in pregnancy —*see* Pregnancy, complicated by, retention, intrauterine device
membranes (complicating delivery) (with hemorrhage) O72.2
with abortion —*see* Abortion, by type
without hemorrhage O73.1
meniscus —*see* Derangement, meniscus
menses N94.89
milk (puerperal, postpartum) O92.79
nitrogen, extrarenal R39.2
ovary syndrome N99.83
placenta (total) (with hemorrhage) O72.0
without hemorrhage O73.0
portions or fragments (with hemorrhage) O72.2
without hemorrhage O73.1
products of conception
early pregnancy (dead fetus) O02.1
following
delivery (with hemorrhage) O72.2
without hemorrhage O73.1
secundines (following delivery) (with hemorrhage) O72.0
without hemorrhage O73.0
complicating puerperium (delayed hemorrhage) O72.2
partial O72.2
without hemorrhage O73.1
smegma, clitoris N90.89
urine R33.9
drug-induced R33.0
due to hyperplasia (hypertrophy) of prostate —*see* Hyperplasia, prostate
organic R33.8
drug-induced R33.0
psychogenic F45.8
specified NEC R33.8
water (in tissues) —*see* Edema
Reticulation, dust —*see* Pneumoconiosis
Reticulocytosis R70.1
Reticuloendotheliosis
acute infantile C96.0
leukemic C91.4-
malignant C96.9
nonlipid C96.0
Reticulohistiocytoma (giant-cell) D76.3
Reticuloid, actinic L57.1
Reticulosis (skin)
acute of infancy C96.0
hemophagocytic, familial D76.1
histiocytic medullary C96.9
lipomelanotic I89.8
malignant (midline) C86.0
nonlipid C96.0
polymorphic C83.8-
Sézary —*see* Sézary disease
Retina, retinal —*see also* condition
dark area D49.81
Retinitis —*see also* Inflammation, chorioretinal
albuminurica N18.9 *[H32]*
diabetic —*see* Diabetes, retinitis

Retinitis (*Continued*)
disciformis —*see* Degeneration, macula
focal —*see* Inflammation, chorioretinal, focal
gravidarum —*see* Pregnancy, complicated by, specified pregnancy-related condition NEC
juxtapapillaris —*see* Inflammation, chorioretinal, focal, juxtapapillary
luetic —*see* Retinitis, syphilitic
pigmentosa H35.52
proliferans —*see* Disorder, globe, degenerative, specified type NEC
proliferating —*see* Disorder, globe, degenerative, specified type NEC
renal N18.9 *[H32]*
syphilitic (early) (secondary) A51.43
central, recurrent A52.71
congenital (early) A50.01 *[H32]*
late A52.71
tuberculous A18.53
Retinoblastoma C69.2-
differentiated C69.2-
undifferentiated C69.2-
Retinochoroiditis —*see also* Inflammation, chorioretinal
disseminated —*see* Inflammation, chorioretinal, disseminated
syphilitic A52.71
focal —*see* Inflammation, chorioretinal
juxtapapillaris —*see* Inflammation, chorioretinal, focal, juxtapapillary
Retinopathy (background) H35.00
arteriosclerotic I70.8 *[H35.0-]*
atherosclerotic I70.8 *[H35.0-]*
central serous —*see* Chorioretinopathy, central serous
Coats H35.02-
diabetic —*see* Diabetes, retinopathy
exudative H35.02-
hypertensive H35.03-
in (due to)
diabetes —*see* Diabetes, retinopathy
sickle-cell disorders D57.- *[H36]*
of prematurity H35.10-
stage 0 H35.11-
stage 1 H35.12-
stage 2 H35.13-
stage 3 H35.14-
stage 4 H35.15-
stage 5 H35.16-
pigmentary, congenital —*see* Dystrophy, retina
proliferative NEC H35.2-
diabetic —*see* Diabetes, retinopathy, proliferative
sickle-cell D57.- *[H36]*
solar H31.02-
Retinoschisis H33.10-
congenital Q14.1
specified type NEC H33.19-
Retortamoniasis A07.8
Retractile testis Q55.22
Retraction
cervix —*see* Retroversion, uterus
drum (membrane) —*see* Disorder, tympanic membrane, specified NEC
finger —*see* Deformity, finger
lid H02.539
left H02.536
lower H02.535
upper H02.534

Retraction (*Continued*)
lid (*Continued*)
right H02.533
lower H02.532
upper H02.531
lung J98.4
mediastinum J98.5
nipple N64.53
associated with
lactation O92.03
pregnancy O92.01-
puerperium O92.02
congenital Q83.8
palmar fascia M72.0
pleura —*see* Pleurisy
ring, uterus (Bandl's) (pathological) O62.4
sternum (congenital) Q76.7
acquired M95.4
uterus —*see* Retroversion, uterus
valve (heart) —*see* Endocarditis
Retrobulbar —*see* condition
Retrocecal —*see* condition
Retrocession —*see* Retroversion
Retrodisplacement —*see* Retroversion
Retroflection, retroflexion —*see* Retroversion
Retrognathia, retrognathism (mandibular) (maxillary) M26.19
Retrograde menstruation N92.5
Retroperineal —*see* condition
Retroperitoneal —*see* condition
Retroperitonitis K68.9
Retropharyngeal —*see* condition
Retroplacental —*see* condition
Retroposition —*see* Retroversion
Retroprosthetic membrane T85.398
Retrosternal thyroid (congenital) Q89.2
Retroversion, retroverted
cervix —*see* Retroversion, uterus
female NEC —*see* Retroversion, uterus
iris H21.89
testis (congenital) Q55.29
uterus (acquired) (acute) (any degree) (asymptomatic) (cervix) (postinfectional) (postpartal, old) N85.4
congenital Q51.818
in pregnancy O34.53-
Retrovirus, as cause of disease classified elsewhere B97.30
human
immunodeficiency, type 2 (HIV 2) B97.35
T-cell lymphotropic
type I (HTLV-I) B97.33
type II (HTLV-II) B97.34
lentivirus B97.31
oncovirus B97.32
specified NEC B97.39
Retrusion, premaxilla (developmental) M26.09
Rett's disease or syndrome F84.2
Reverse peristalsis R19.2
Reye's syndrome G93.7
Rh (factor)
hemolytic disease (newborn) P55.0
incompatibility, immunization or sensitization
affecting management of pregnancy NEC O36.09-
anti-D antibody O36.01-
newborn P55.0

Rh (Continued)
  incompatibility, immunization or
    sensitization (Continued)
      transfusion reaction —see
        Complication (s), transfusion,
        incompatibility reaction, Rh
        (factor)
      negative mother affecting newborn P55.0
      titer elevated —see Complication (s),
        transfusion, incompatibility
        reaction, Rh (factor)
      transfusion reaction —see
        Complication (s), transfusion,
        incompatibility reaction, Rh
        (factor)
Rhabdomyolysis (idiopathic) NEC
  M62.82
  traumatic T79.6
Rhabdomyoma —see also Neoplasm,
  connective tissue, benign
  adult —see Neoplasm, connective
    tissue, benign
  fetal —see Neoplasm, connective tissue,
    benign
  glycogenic —see Neoplasm, connective
    tissue, benign
Rhabdomyosarcoma (any type) —see
  Neoplasm, connective tissue,
  malignant
Rhabdosarcoma —see
  Rhabdomyosarcoma
Rhesus (factor) **incompatibility** —see Rh,
  incompatibility
Rheumatic (acute) (subacute) (chronic)
  adherent pericardium I09.2
  coronary arteritis I01.9
  degeneration, myocardium I09.0
  fever (acute) —see Fever, rheumatic
  heart —see Disease, heart, rheumatic
  myocardial degeneration —see
    Degeneration, myocardium
  myocarditis (chronic) (inactive)
    (with chorea) I09.0
    with chorea (acute) (rheumatic)
      (Sydenham's) I02.0
    active or acute I01.2
  pancarditis, acute I01.8
    with chorea (acute (rheumatic)
      Sydenham's) I02.0
  pericarditis (active) (acute) (with
    effusion) (with pneumonia) I01.0
    with chorea (acute) (rheumatic)
      (Sydenham's) I02.0
    chronic or inactive I09.2
  pneumonia I00 [J17]
  torticollis M43.6
  typhoid fever A01.09
Rheumatism (articular) (neuralgic)
  (nonarticular) M79.0
  gout —see Arthritis, rheumatoid
  intercostal, meaning Tietze's disease
    M94.0
  palindromic (any site) M12.30
    ankle M12.37-
    elbow M12.32-
    foot joint M12.37-
    hand joint M12.34-
    hip M12.35-
    knee M12.36-
    multiple site M12.39
    shoulder M12.31-
    specified joint NEC M12.38
    wrist M12.33-
  sciatic M54.4-

Rheumatoid —see also condition
  arthritis —see also Arthritis,
    rheumatoid
    with involvement of organs NEC
      M05.60
      ankle M05.67-
      elbow M05.62-
      foot joint M05.67-
      hand joint M05.64-
      hip M05.65-
      knee M05.66-
      multiple site M05.69
      shoulder M05.61-
      vertebra —see Spondylitis,
        ankylosing
      wrist M05.63-
    seronegative —see Arthritis,
      rheumatoid, seronegative
    seropositive —see Arthritis,
      rheumatoid, seropositive
  carditis M05.30
    ankle M05.37-
    elbow M05.32-
    foot joint M05.37-
    hand joint M05.34-
    hip M05.35-
    knee M05.36-
    multiple site M05.39
    shoulder M05.31-
    vertebra —see Spondylitis, ankylosing
    wrist M05.33-
  endocarditis —see Rheumatoid, carditis
  lung (disease) M05.10
    ankle M05.17-
    elbow M05.12-
    foot joint M05.17-
    hand joint M05.14-
    hip M05.15-
    knee M05.16-
    multiple site M05.19
    shoulder M05.11-
    vertebra —see Spondylitis, ankylosing
    wrist M05.13-
  myocarditis —see Rheumatoid, carditis
  myopathy M05.40
    ankle M05.47-
    elbow M05.42-
    foot joint M05.47-
    hand joint M05.44-
    hip M05.45-
    knee M05.46-
    multiple site M05.49
    shoulder M05.41-
    vertebra —see Spondylitis, ankylosing
    wrist M05.43-
  pericarditis —see Rheumatoid, carditis
  polyarthritis —see Arthritis, rheumatoid
  polyneuropathy M05.50
    ankle M05.57-
    elbow M05.52-
    foot joint M05.57-
    hand joint M05.54-
    hip M05.55-
    knee M05.56-
    multiple site M05.59
    shoulder M05.51-
    vertebra —see Spondylitis, ankylosing
    wrist M05.53-
  vasculitis M05.20
    ankle M05.27-
    elbow M05.22-
    foot joint M05.27-
    hand joint M05.24-
    hip M05.25-

Rheumatoid (Continued)
  vasculitis (Continued)
    knee M05.26-
    multiple site M05.29
    shoulder M05.21-
    vertebra —see Spondylitis,
      ankylosing
    wrist M05.23-
Rhinitis (atrophic) (catarrhal)
  (chronic) (croupous) (fibrinous)
  (granulomatous) (hyperplastic)
  (hypertrophic) (membranous)
  (obstructive) (purulent)
  (suppurative) (ulcerative) J31.0
  with
    sore throat —see Nasopharyngitis
  acute J00
  allergic J30.9
    with asthma J45.909
      with
        exacerbation (acute) J45.901
        status asthmaticus J45.902
    due to
      food J30.5
      pollen J30.1
    nonseasonal J30.89
    perennial J30.89
    seasonal NEC J30.2
    specified NEC J30.89
  infective J00
  pneumococcal J00
  syphilitic A52.73
    congenital A50.05 [J99]
  tuberculous A15.8
  vasomotor J30.0
Rhinoantritis (chronic) —see Sinusitis,
  maxillary
Rhinodacryolith —see Dacryolith
Rhinolith (nasal sinus) J34.89
Rhinomegaly J34.89
Rhinopharyngitis (acute) (subacute) —see
  also Nasopharyngitis
  chronic J31.1
  destructive ulcerating A66.5
  mutilans A66.5
Rhinophyma L71.1
Rhinorrhea J34.89
  cerebrospinal (fluid) G96.0
  paroxysmal —see Rhinitis, allergic
  spasmodic —see Rhinitis, allergic
Rhinosalpingitis —see Salpingitis,
  eustachian
Rhinoscleroma A48.8
Rhinosporidiosis B48.1
Rhinovirus infection NEC B34.8
Rhizomelic chondrodysplasia punctata
  E71.540
Rhythm
  atrioventricular nodal I49.8
  disorder I49.9
    coronary sinus I49.8
    ectopic I49.8
    nodal I49.8
  escape I49.9
  heart, abnormal I49.9
  idioventricular I44.2
  nodal I49.8
  sleep, inversion G47.2-
    nonorganic origin —see Disorder,
      sleep, circadian rhythm,
      psychogenic
Rhytidosis facialis L98.8
Rib —see also condition
  cervical Q76.5
Riboflavin deficiency E53.0

Rice bodies —*see also* Loose, body, joint
  knee M23.4-
Richter syndrome —*see* Leukemia,
  chronic lymphocytic, B-cell type
Richter's hernia —*see* Hernia, abdomen,
  with obstruction
Ricinism —*see* Poisoning, food, noxious,
  plant
Rickets (active) (acute) (adolescent) (chest
  wall) (congenital) (current) (infantile)
  (intestinal) E55.0
  adult —*see* Osteomalacia
  celiac K90.0
  hypophosphatemic with nephrotic-
    glycosuric dwarfism E72.09
  inactive E64.3
  kidney N25.0
  renal N25.0
  sequelae, any E64.3
  vitamin-D-resistant E83.31 [M90.80]
Rickettsial disease A79.9
  specified type NEC A79.89
Rickettsialpox (Rickettsia akari) A79.1
Rickettsiosis A79.9
  due to
    Ehrlichia sennetsu A79.81
    Rickettsia akari (rickettsialpox) A79.1
  specified type NEC A79.89
  tick-borne A77.9
  vesicular A79.1
Rider's bone —*see* Ossification, muscle,
  specified NEC
Ridge, alveolus —*see also* condition
  flabby K06.8
Ridged ear, congenital Q17.3
Riedel's
  lobe, liver Q44.7
  struma, thyroiditis or disease E06.5
Rieger's anomaly or syndrome Q13.81
Riehl's melanosis L81.4
Rietti-Greppi-Micheli anemia D56.9
Rieux's hernia —*see* Hernia, abdomen,
  specified site NEC
Riga (-Fede) disease K14.0
Riggs' disease —*see* Periodontitis
Right middle lobe syndrome J98.11
Rigid, rigidity —*see also* condition
  abdominal R19.30
    with severe abdominal pain R10.0
    epigastric R19.36
    generalized R19.37
    left lower quadrant R19.34
    left upper quadrant R19.32
    periumbilic R19.35
    right lower quadrant R19.33
    right upper quadrant R19.31
  articular, multiple, congenital Q68.8
  cervix (uteri) in pregnancy —*see*
    Pregnancy, complicated by,
    abnormal, cervix
  hymen (acquired) (congenital) N89.6
  nuchal R29.1
  pelvic floor in pregnancy —*see*
    Pregnancy, complicated by,
    abnormal, pelvic organs or
    tissues NEC
  perineum or vulva in pregnancy —
    see Pregnancy, complicated by,
    abnormal, vulva
  spine —*see* Dorsopathy, specified NEC
  vagina in pregnancy —*see* Pregnancy,
    complicated by, abnormal, vagina
Rigors R68.89
  with fever R50.9

Riley-Day syndrome G90.1
RIND (reversible ischemic neurologic
  deficit) I63.9
Ring (s)
  aorta (vascular) Q25.4
  Bandl's O62.4
  contraction, complicating delivery O62.4
  esophageal, lower (muscular) K22.2
  Fleischer's (cornea) H18.04-
  hymenal, tight (acquired) (congenital)
    N89.6
  Kayser-Fleischer (cornea) H18.04-
  retraction, uterus, pathological O62.4
  Schatzki's (esophagus) (lower) K22.2
    congenital Q39.3
  Soemmerring's —*see* Cataract, secondary
  vascular (congenital) Q25.8
    aorta Q25.4
Ringed hair (congenital) Q84.1
Ringworm B35.9
  beard B35.0
  black dot B35.0
  body B35.4
  Burmese B35.5
  corporeal B35.4
  foot B35.3
  groin B35.6
  hand B35.2
  honeycomb B35.0
  nails B35.1
  perianal (area) B35.6
  scalp B35.0
  specified NEC B35.8
  Tokelau B35.5
Rise, venous pressure I87.8
Risk, suicidal
  meaning personal history of attempted
    suicide Z91.5
  meaning suicidal ideation —*see*
    Ideation, suicidal
Ritter's disease L00
Rivalry, sibling Z62.891
Rivalta's disease A42.2
River blindness B73.01
Robert's pelvis Q74.2
  with disproportion (fetopelvic) O33.0
    causing obstructed labor O65.0
Robin (-Pierre) syndrome Q87.0
Robinow-Silvermann-Smith syndrome
  Q87.1
Robinson's (hidrotic) ectodermal
  dysplasia or syndrome Q82.4
Robles' disease B73.01
Rocky Mountain (spotted) fever A77.0
Roetheln —*see* Rubella
Roger's disease Q21.0
Rokitansky-Aschoff sinuses
  (gallbladder) K82.8
Rolando's fracture (displaced) S62.22-
  nondisplaced S62.22-
Romano-Ward (prolonged QT interval)
  syndrome I45.81
Romberg's disease or syndrome G51.8
Roof, mouth —*see* condition
Rosacea L71.9
  acne L71.9
  keratitis L71.8
  specified NEC L71.8
Rosary, rachitic E55.0
Rose
  cold J30.1
  fever J30.1
  rash R21
    epidemic B06.9

Rosenbach's erysipeloid A26.0
Rosenthal's disease or syndrome D68.1
Roseola B09
  infantum B08.20
    due to human herpesvirus 6 B08.21
    due to human herpesvirus 7 B08.22
Ross River disease or fever B33.1
Rossbach's disease K31.89
  psychogenic F45.8
Rostan's asthma (cardiac) —*see* Failure,
  ventricular, left
Rotation
  anomalous, incomplete or insufficient,
    intestine Q43.3
  cecum (congenital) Q43.3
  colon (congenital) Q43.3
  spine, incomplete or insufficient —*see*
    Dorsopathy, deforming, specified
    NEC
  tooth, teeth, fully erupted M26.35
  vertebra, incomplete or insufficient —
    see Dorsopathy, deforming,
    specified NEC
Rotes Quérol disease or syndrome —*see*
  Hyperostosis, ankylosing
Roth (-Bernhardt) disease or syndrome —
  see Meralgia paraesthetica
Rothmund (-Thomson) syndrome Q82.8
Rotor's disease or syndrome E80.6
Round
  back (with wedging of vertebrae) —*see*
    Kyphosis
  sequelae (late effect) of rickets E64.3
  worms (large) (infestation) NEC B82.0
    Ascariasis (*see also* Ascariasis) B77.9
Roussy-Lévy syndrome G60.0
Rubella (German measles) B06.9
  complication NEC B06.09
    neurological B06.00
  congenital P35.0
  contact Z20.4
  exposure to Z20.4
  maternal
    care for (suspected) damage to fetus
      O35.3
    manifest rubella in infant P35.0
    suspected damage to fetus affecting
      management of pregnancy O35.3
  specified complications NEC B06.89
Rubeola (meaning measles) —*see*
  Measles
  meaning rubella —*see* Rubella
Rubeosis, iris —*see* Disorder, iris,
  vascular
Rubinstein-Taybi syndrome Q87.2
Rudimentary (congenital) —*see also*
  Agenesis
  arm —*see* Defect, reduction, upper limb
  bone Q79.9
  cervix uteri Q51.828
  eye Q11.2
  lobule of ear Q17.3
  patella Q74.1
  respiratory organs in thoracopagus
    Q89.4
  tracheal bronchus Q32.4
  uterus Q51.818
    in male Q56.1
  vagina Q52.0
Ruled out condition —*see* Observation,
  suspected
Rumination R11.10
  with nausea R11.2
  disorder of infancy F98.21
  neurotic F42

427

Rumination (*Continued*)
  newborn P92.1
  obsessional F42
  psychogenic F42
Runeberg's disease D51.0
Runny nose R09.89
Rupia (syphilitic) A51.39
  congenital A50.06
  tertiary A52.79
Rupture, ruptured
  abscess (spontaneous) - code by site
      under Abscess
  aneurysm —*see* Aneurysm
  anus (sphincter) —*see* Laceration,
      anus
  aorta, aortic I71.8
    abdominal I71.3
    arch I71.1
    ascending I71.1
    descending I71.8
      abdominal I71.3
      thoracic I71.1
    syphilitic A52.01
    thoracoabdominal I71.5
    thorax, thoracic I71.1
    transverse I71.1
    traumatic —*see* Injury, aorta,
        laceration, major
    valve or cusp (*see also* Endocarditis,
        aortic) I35.8
  appendix (with peritonitis) K35.2
  arteriovenous fistula, brain I60.8
  artery I77.2
    brain —*see* Hemorrhage, intracranial,
        intracerebral
    coronary —*see* Infarct, myocardium
    heart —*see* Infarct, myocardium
    pulmonary I28.8
    traumatic (complication) —*see* Injury,
        blood vessel
  bile duct (common) (hepatic) K83.2
    cystic K82.2
  bladder (sphincter) (nontraumatic)
      (spontaneous) N32.89
    following ectopic or molar pregnancy
        O08.6
    obstetrical trauma O71.5
    traumatic S37.29
  blood vessel —*see also* Hemorrhage
    brain —*see* Hemorrhage, intracranial,
        intracerebral
    heart —*see* Infarct, myocardium
    traumatic (complication) —*see* Injury,
        blood vessel, laceration, major,
        by site
  bone —*see* Fracture
  bowel (nontraumatic) K63.1
  brain
    aneurysm (congenital) —*see also*
        Hemorrhage, intracranial,
        subarachnoid
      syphilitic A52.05
    hemorrhagic —*see* Hemorrhage,
        intracranial, intracerebral
  capillaries I78.8
  cardiac (auricle) (ventricle) (wall)
      I23.3
    with hemopericardium I23.0
    infectional I40.9
    traumatic —*see* Injury, heart
  cartilage (articular) (current) —*see also*
        Sprain
    knee S83.3-
    semilunar —*see* Tear, meniscus

Rupture, ruptured (*Continued*)
  cecum (with peritonitis) K65.0
    with peritoneal abscess K35.3
    traumatic S36.598
  celiac artery, traumatic —*see* Injury,
      blood vessel, celiac artery,
      laceration, major
  cerebral aneurysm (congenital) (*see*
      Hemorrhage, intracranial,
      subarachnoid)
  cervix (uteri)
    with ectopic or molar pregnancy O08.6
    following ectopic or molar pregnancy
        O08.6
    obstetrical trauma O71.3
    traumatic S37.69
  chordae tendineae NEC I51.1
    concurrent with acute myocardial
        infarction —*see* Infarct,
        myocardium
    following acute myocardial infarction
        (current complication) I23.4
  choroid (direct) (indirect) (traumatic)
      H31.32-
  circle of Willis I60.6
  colon (nontraumatic) K63.1
    traumatic —*see* Injury, intestine, large
  cornea (traumatic) —*see* Injury, eye,
      laceration
  coronary (artery) (thrombotic) —*see*
      Infarct, myocardium
  corpus luteum (infected) (ovary) N83.1
  cyst —*see* Cyst
  cystic duct K82.2
  Descemet's membrane —*see* Change,
      corneal membrane, Descemet's,
      rupture
    traumatic —*see* Injury, eye, laceration
  diaphragm, traumatic —*see* Injury,
      intrathoracic, diaphragm
  disc —*see* Rupture, intervertebral disc
  diverticulum (intestine) K57.80
    with bleeding K57.81
    bladder N32.3
    large intestine K57.20
      with
        bleeding K57.21
        small intestine K57.40
          with bleeding K57.41
    small intestine K57.00
      with
        bleeding K57.01
        large intestine K57.40
          with bleeding K57.41
  duodenal stump K31.89
  ear drum (nontraumatic) —*see also*
      Perforation, tympanum
    traumatic S09.2-
      due to blast injury —*see* Injury,
          blast, ear
  esophagus K22.3
  eye (without prolapse or loss of
      intraocular tissue) —*see* Injury,
      eye, laceration
  fallopian tube NEC (nonobstetric)
      (nontraumatic) N83.8
    due to pregnancy O00.1
  fontanel P13.1
  gallbladder K82.2
    traumatic S36.128
  gastric —*see also* Rupture, stomach
    vessel K92.2
  globe (eye) (traumatic) —*see* Injury, eye,
      laceration
  graafian follicle (hematoma) N83.0

Rupture, ruptured (*Continued*)
  heart —*see* Rupture, cardiac
  hymen (nontraumatic) (nonintentional)
      N89.8
  internal organ, traumatic —*see* Injury,
      by site
  intervertebral disc —*see* Displacement,
      intervertebral disc
    traumatic —*see* Rupture, traumatic,
        intervertebral disc
  intestine NEC (nontraumatic) K63.1
    traumatic —*see* Injury, intestine
  iris —*see also* Abnormality, pupillary
    traumatic —*see* Injury, eye, laceration
  joint capsule, traumatic —*see* Sprain
  kidney (traumatic) S37.06-
    birth injury P15.8
    nontraumatic N28.89
  lacrimal duct (traumatic) —*see* Injury,
      eye, specified site NEC
  lens (cataract) (traumatic) —*see*
      Cataract, traumatic
  ligament, traumatic —*see* Rupture,
      traumatic, ligament, by site
  liver S36.116
    birth injury P15.0
  lymphatic vessel I89.8
  marginal sinus (placental) (with
      hemorrhage) —*see* Hemorrhage,
      antepartum, specified cause NEC
  membrana tympani (nontraumatic) —
      see Perforation, tympanum
  membranes (spontaneous)
    artificial
      delayed delivery following O75.5
    delayed delivery following —*see*
        Pregnancy, complicated
        by, premature rupture of
        membranes
  meningeal artery I60.8
  meniscus (knee) —*see also* Tear,
      meniscus
    old —*see* Derangement, meniscus
    site other than knee - code as Sprain
  mesenteric artery, traumatic —*see* Injury,
      mesenteric, artery, laceration, major
  mesentery (nontraumatic) K66.8
    traumatic —*see* Injury, intra-
        abdominal, specified, site NEC
  mitral (valve) I34.8
  muscle (traumatic) —*see also* Strain
    diastasis —*see* Diastasis, muscle
    nontraumatic M62.10
      ankle M62.17-
      foot M62.17-
      forearm M62.13-
      hand M62.14-
      lower leg M62.16-
      pelvic region M62.15-
      shoulder region M62.11-
      specified site NEC M62.18
      thigh M62.15-
      upper arm M62.12-
    traumatic —*see* Strain, by site
  musculotendinous junction NEC,
      nontraumatic —*see* Rupture,
      tendon, spontaneous
  mycotic aneurysm causing cerebral
      hemorrhage —*see* Hemorrhage,
      intracranial, subarachnoid
  myocardium, myocardial —*see* Rupture,
      cardiac
    traumatic —*see* Injury, heart
  nontraumatic, meaning hernia —*see*
      Hernia

Rupture, ruptured (Continued)
  obstructed —see Hernia, by site,
    obstructed
  operation wound —see Disruption,
    wound, operation
  ovary, ovarian N83.8
    corpus luteum cyst N83.1
    follicle (graafian) N83.0
  oviduct (nonobstetric) (nontraumatic)
    N83.8
    due to pregnancy O00.1
  pancreas (nontraumatic) K86.8
    traumatic S36.299
  papillary muscle NEC I51.2
    following acute myocardial infarction
      (current complication) I23.5
  pelvic
    floor, complicating delivery O70.1
    organ NEC, obstetrical trauma
      O71.5
  perineum (nonobstetric) (nontraumatic)
    N90.89
    complicating delivery —see Delivery,
      complicated, by, laceration, anus
      (sphincter)
  postoperative wound —see Disruption,
    wound, operation
  prostate (traumatic) S37.828
  pulmonary
    artery I28.8
    valve (heart) I37.8
    vein I28.8
    vessel I28.8
  pus tube —see Salpingitis
  pyosalpinx —see Salpingitis
  rectum (nontraumatic) K63.1
    traumatic S36.69
  retina, retinal (traumatic) (without
    detachment) —see also Break,
    retina
    with detachment —see Detachment,
      retina, with retinal, break
  rotator cuff (nontraumatic) M75.10-
    complete M75.12-
    incomplete M75.11-
  sclera —see Injury, eye, laceration
  sigmoid (nontraumatic) K63.1
    traumatic S36.593
  spinal cord —see also Injury, spinal cord,
    by region
    due to injury at birth P11.5
    newborn (birth injury) P11.5
  spleen (traumatic) S36.09
    birth injury P15.1
    congenital (birth injury) P15.1
    due to P. vivax malaria B51.0
    nontraumatic D73.5
    spontaneous D73.5
  splenic vein R58
    traumatic —see Injury, blood vessel,
      portal vein
  stomach (nontraumatic) (spontaneous)
    K31.89
    traumatic S36.39
  supraspinatus (complete) (incomplete)
    (nontraumatic) —see Tear, rotator
    cuff
  symphysis pubis
    obstetric O71.6
    traumatic S33.4
  synovium (cyst) M66.10
    ankle M66.17-
    elbow M66.12-
    finger M66.14-

Rupture, ruptured (Continued)
  synovium (Continued)
    foot M66.17-
    forearm M66.13-
    hand M66.14-
    pelvic region M66.15-
    shoulder region M66.11-
      specified site NEC M66.18
    thigh M66.15-
    toe M66.17-
    upper arm M66.12-
    wrist M66.13-
  tendon (traumatic) —see Strain
    nontraumatic (spontaneous) M66.9
      ankle M66.87-
      extensor M66.20
        ankle M66.27-
        foot M66.27-
        forearm M66.23-
        hand M66.24-
        lower leg M66.26-
        multiple sites M66.29
        pelvic region M66.25-
        shoulder region M66.21-
        specified site NEC M66.28
        thigh M66.25-
        upper arm M66.22-
      flexor M66.30
        ankle M66.37-
        foot M66.37-
        forearm M66.33-
        hand M66.34-
        lower leg M66.36-
        multiple sites M66.39
        pelvic region M66.35-
        shoulder region M66.31-
        specified site NEC M66.38
        thigh M66.35-
        upper arm M66.32-
      foot M66.87-
      forearm M66.83-
      hand M66.84-
      lower leg M66.86-
      multiple sites M66.89
      pelvic region M66.85-
      shoulder region M66.81-
      specified
        site NEC M66.88
        tendon M66.80
      thigh M66.85-
      upper arm M66.82-
  thoracic duct I89.8
  tonsil J35.8
  traumatic
    aorta —see Injury, aorta, laceration,
      major
    diaphragm —see Injury, intrathoracic,
      diaphragm
    external site —see Wound, open,
      by site
    eye —see Injury, eye, laceration
    internal organ —see Injury, by site
    intervertebral disc
      cervical S13.0
      lumbar S33.0
      thoracic S23.0
    kidney S37.06-
    ligament —see also Sprain
      ankle —see Sprain, ankle
      carpus —see Rupture, traumatic,
        ligament, wrist
      collateral (hand) —see Rupture,
        traumatic, ligament, finger,
        collateral

Rupture, ruptured (Continued)
  traumatic (Continued)
    ligament (Continued)
      finger (metacarpophalangeal)
        (interphalangeal) S63.40-
        collateral S63.41-
          index S63.41-
          little S63.41-
          middle S63.41-
          ring S63.41-
        index S63.40-
        little S63.40-
        middle S63.40-
        palmar S63.42-
          index S63.42-
          little S63.42-
          middle S63.42-
          ring S63.42-
        ring S63.40-
        specified site NEC S63.499
          index S63.49-
          little S63.49-
          middle S63.49-
          ring S63.49-
        volar plate S63.43-
          index S63.43-
          little S63.43-
          middle S63.43-
          ring S63.43-
      foot —see Sprain, foot
      radial collateral S53.2-
      radiocarpal —see Rupture, traumatic,
        ligament, wrist, radiocarpal
      ulnar collateral S53.3-
      ulnocarpal —see Rupture, traumatic,
        ligament, wrist, ulnocarpal
      wrist S63.30-
        collateral S63.31-
        radiocarpal S63.32-
        specified site NEC S63.39-
        ulnocarpal (palmar) S63.33-
    liver S36.116
    membrana tympani —see Rupture,
      ear drum, traumatic
    muscle or tendon —see Strain
    myocardium —see Injury, heart
    pancreas S36.299
    rectum S36.69
    sigmoid S36.593
    spleen S36.09
    stomach S36.39
    symphysis pubis S33.4
    tympanum, tympanic (membrane) —
      see Rupture, ear drum, traumatic
    ureter S37.19
    uterus S37.69
    vagina —see Injury, vagina
    vena cava —see Injury, vena cava,
      laceration, major
  tricuspid (heart) (valve) I07.8
  tube, tubal (nonobstetric)
    (nontraumatic) N83.8
    abscess —see Salpingitis
    due to pregnancy O00.1
  tympanum, tympanic (membrane)
    (nontraumatic) (see also
    Perforation, tympanic
    membrane) H72.9-
    traumatic —see Rupture, ear drum,
      traumatic
  umbilical cord, complicating delivery
    O69.89
  ureter (traumatic) S37.19
    nontraumatic N28.89

Rupture, ruptured *(Continued)*
  urethra (nontraumatic) N36.8
    with ectopic or molar pregnancy O08.6
    following ectopic or molar pregnancy O08.6
    obstetrical trauma O71.5
    traumatic S37.39
  uterosacral ligament (nonobstetric) (nontraumatic) N83.8
  uterus (traumatic) S37.69
    before labor O71.0-
    during or after labor O71.1
    nonpuerperal, nontraumatic N85.8

Rupture, ruptured *(Continued)*
  uterus *(Continued)*
    pregnant (during labor) O71.1
      before labor O71.0-
  vagina —*see* Injury, vagina
  valve, valvular (heart) —*see* Endocarditis
  varicose vein —*see* Varix
  varix —*see* Varix
  vena cava R58
    traumatic —*see* Injury, vena cava, laceration, major
  vesical (urinary) N32.89

Rupture, ruptured *(Continued)*
  vessel (blood) R58
    pulmonary I28.8
    traumatic —*see* Injury, blood vessel
  viscus R19.8
  vulva complicating delivery O70.0
Russell-Silver syndrome Q87.1
Russian spring-summer type encephalitis A84.0
Rust's disease (tuberculous cervical spondylitis) A18.01
Ruvalcaba-Myhre-Smith syndrome E71.440
Rytand-Lipsitch syndrome I44.2

S

Saber, sabre shin or tibia (syphilitic) A50.56 [M90.8-]
Sac lacrimal—see condition
Saccharomyces infection B37.9
Saccharopinuria E72.3
Saccular—see condition
Sacculation
  aorta (nonsyphilitic) —see Aneurysm, aorta
  bladder N32.3
  intralaryngeal (congenital) (ventricular) Q31.3
  larynx (congenital) (ventricular) Q31.3
  organ or site, congenital —see Distortion
  pregnant uterus —see Pregnancy, complicated by, abnormal, uterus
  ureter N28.89
  urethra N36.1
  vesical N32.3
Sachs' amaurotic familial idiocy or disease E75.02
Sachs-Tay disease E75.02
Sacks-Libman disease M32.11
Sacralgia M53.3
Sacralization Q76.49
Sacrodynia M53.3
Sacroiliac joint—see condition
Sacroiliitis NEC M46.1
Sacrum—see condition
Saddle
  back—see Lordosis
  embolus
    abdominal aorta I74.01
    pulmonary artery I26.92
      with acute cor pulmonale I26.02
  injury — code to condition
  nose M95.0
    due to syphilis A50.57
Sadism (sexual) F65.52
Sadness, postpartal O90.6
Sadomasochism F65.50
Saemisch's ulcer (cornea) —see Ulcer, cornea, central
Sahib disease B55.0
Sailors' skin L57.8
Saint
  Anthony's fire —see Erysipelas
  triad —see Hernia, diaphragm
  Vitus' dance —see Chorea, Sydenham's
Salaam
  attack (s) —see Epilepsy, spasms
  tic R25.8
Salicylism
  abuse F55.8
  overdose or wrong substance given — see Table of drugs and chemicals, by drug, poisoning
Salivary duct or gland —see condition
Salivation, excessive K11.7
Salmonella —see Infection, Salmonella
Salmonellosis A02.0
Salpingitis (catarrhal) (fallopian tube) (nodular) (pseudofollicular) (purulent) (septic) N70.91
  with oophoritis N70.93
  acute N70.01
    with oophoritis N70.03
  chlamydial A56.11
  chronic N70.11
    with oophoritis N70.13
  complicating abortion —see Abortion, by type, complicated by, salpingitis

Salpingitis (Continued)
  ear —see Salpingitis, eustachian
  eustachian (tube) H68.00-
    acute H68.01-
    chronic H68.02-
  follicularis N70.11
    with oophoritis N70.13
  gonococcal (acute) (chronic) A54.24
  interstitial, chronic N70.11
    with oophoritis N70.13
  isthmica nodosa N70.11
    with oophoritis N70.13
  specific (gonococcal) (acute) (chronic) A54.24
  tuberculous (acute) (chronic) A18.17
  venereal (gonococcal) (acute) (chronic) A54.24
Salpingocele N83.4
Salpingo-oophoritis (catarrhal) (purulent) (ruptured) (septic) (suppurative) N70.93
  acute N70.03
    with ectopic or molar pregnancy O08.0
    following ectopic or molar pregnancy O08.0
    gonococcal A54.24
  chronic N70.13
  following ectopic or molar pregnancy O08.0
  gonococcal (acute) (chronic) A54.24
  puerperal O86.19
  specific (gonococcal) (acute) (chronic) A54.24
  subacute N70.03
  tuberculous (acute) (chronic) A18.17
  venereal (gonococcal) (acute) (chronic) A54.24
Salpingo-ovaritis —see Salpingo-oophoritis
Salpingoperitonitis —see Salpingo-oophoritis
Salzmann's nodular dystrophy —see Degeneration, cornea, nodular
Sampson's cyst or tumor N80.1
San Joaquin (Valley) fever B38.0
Sandblaster's asthma, lung or pneumoconiosis J62.8
Sander's disease (paranoia) F22
Sandfly fever A93.1
Sandhoff's disease E75.01
Sanfilippo (Type B) (Type C) (Type D) syndrome E76.22
Sanger-Brown ataxia G11.2
Sao Paulo fever or typhus A77.0
Saponification, mesenteric K65.8
Sarcocele (benign)
  syphilitic A52.76
    congenital A50.59
Sarcocystosis A07.8
Sarcoepiplocele —see Hernia
Sarcoepiplomphalocele Q79.2
Sarcoid —see also Sarcoidosis
  arthropathy D86.86
  Boeck's D86.9
  Darier-Roussy D86.3
  iridocyclitis D86.83
  meningitis D86.81
  myocarditis D86.85
  myositis D86.87
  pyelonephritis D86.84
  Spiegler-Fendt L08.89

Sarcoidosis D86.9
  with
    cranial nerve palsies D86.82
    hepatic granuloma D86.89
    polyarthritis D86.86
    tubulo-interstitial nephropathy D86.84
  combined sites NEC D86.89
  lung D86.0
    and lymph nodes D86.2
  lymph nodes D86.1
    and lung D86.2
  meninges D86.81
  skin D86.3
  specified type NEC D86.89
Sarcoma (of) —see also Neoplasm, connective tissue, malignant
  alveolar soft part —see Neoplasm, connective tissue, malignant
  ameloblastic C41.1
    upper jaw (bone) C41.0
  botryoid —see Neoplasm, connective tissue, malignant
  botryoides —see Neoplasm, connective tissue, malignant
  cerebellar C71.6
    circumscribed (arachnoidal) C71.6
  circumscribed (arachnoidal) cerebellar C71.6
  clear cell —see also Neoplasm, connective tissue, malignant
    kidney C64.-
  dendritic cells (accessory cells) C96.4
  embryonal —see Neoplasm, connective tissue, malignant
  endometrial (stromal) C54.1
    isthmus C54.0
  epithelioid (cell) —see Neoplasm, connective tissue, malignant
  Ewing's —see Neoplasm, bone, malignant
  follicular dendritic cell C96.4
  germinoblastic (diffuse) —see Lymphoma, diffuse, large cell
    follicular —see Lymphoma, follicular, specified NEC
  giant cell (except of bone) —see also Neoplasm, connective tissue, malignant
    bone —see Neoplasm, bone, malignant
  glomoid —see Neoplasm, connective tissue, malignant
  granulocytic C92.3-
  hemangioendothelial —see Neoplasm, connective tissue, malignant
  hemorrhagic, multiple —see Sarcoma, Kaposi's
  histiocytic C96.A
  Hodgkin —see Lymphoma, Hodgkin
  immunoblastic (diffuse) —see Lymphoma, diffuse large cell
  interdigitating dendritic cell C96.4
  Kaposi's
    colon C46.4
    connective tissue C46.1
    gastrointestinal organ C46.4
    lung C46.5-
    lymph node (s) C46.3
    palate (hard) (soft) C46.2
    rectum C46.4
    skin C46.0
    specified site NEC C46.7
    stomach C46.4
    unspecified site C46.9

Sarcoma (*Continued*)
  Kupffer cell C22.3
  Langerhans cell C96.4
  leptomeningeal —*see* Neoplasm,
    meninges, malignant
  liver NEC C22.4
  lymphangioendothelial —*see*
    Neoplasm, connective tissue,
    malignant
  lymphoblastic —*see* Lymphoma,
    lymphoblastic (diffuse)
  lymphocytic —*see* Lymphoma, small
    cell B-cell
  mast cell C96.2
  melanotic —*see* Melanoma
  meningeal —*see* Neoplasm, meninges,
    malignant
  meningothelial —*see* Neoplasm,
    meninges, malignant
  mesenchymal —*see also* Neoplasm,
    connective tissue, malignant
    mixed —*see* Neoplasm, connective
      tissue, malignant
  mesothelial —*see* Mesothelioma
  monstrocellular
    specified site —*see* Neoplasm,
      malignant, by site
    unspecified site C71.9
  myeloid C92.3-
  neurogenic —*see* Neoplasm, nerve,
    malignant
  odontogenic C41.1
    upper jaw (bone) C41.0
  osteoblastic —*see* Neoplasm, bone,
    malignant
  osteogenic —*see also* Neoplasm, bone,
    malignant
    juxtacortical —*see* Neoplasm, bone,
      malignant
    periosteal —*see* Neoplasm, bone,
      malignant
  periosteal —*see also* Neoplasm, bone,
    malignant
    osteogenic —*see* Neoplasm, bone,
      malignant
  pleomorphic cell —*see* Neoplasm,
    connective tissue, malignant
  reticulum cell (diffuse) —*see*
    Lymphoma, diffuse large cell
    nodular —*see* Lymphoma,
      follicular
    pleomorphic cell type —*see*
      Lymphoma, diffuse large
      cell
  rhabdoid —*see* Neoplasm, malignant,
    by site
  round cell —*see* Neoplasm, connective
    tissue, malignant
  small cell —*see* Neoplasm, connective
    tissue, malignant
  soft tissue —*see* Neoplasm, connective
    tissue, malignant
  spindle cell —*see* Neoplasm, connective
    tissue, malignant
  stromal (endometrial) C54.1
    isthmus C54.0
  synovial —*see also* Neoplasm,
    connective tissue, malignant
    biphasic —*see* Neoplasm, connective
      tissue, malignant
    epithelioid cell —*see* Neoplasm,
      connective tissue, malignant
    spindle cell —*see* Neoplasm,
      connective tissue, malignant

Sarcomatosis
  meningeal —*see* Neoplasm, meninges,
    malignant
  specified site NEC —*see* Neoplasm,
    connective tissue, malignant
  unspecified site C80.1
Sarcosinemia E72.59
Sarcosporidiosis (intestinal) A07.8
Satiety, early R68.81
Saturnine —*see* condition
Saturnism
  overdose or wrong substance given
    or taken —*see* Table of drugs and
    chemicals, by drug, poisoning
Satyriasis F52.8
Sauriasis —*see* Ichthyosis
SBE (subacute bacterial endocarditis)
  I33.0
Scabies (any site) B86
Scabs R23.4
Scaglietti-Dagnini syndrome E22.0
Scald —*see* Burn
Scalenus anticus (anterior) syndrome G54.0
Scales R23.4
Scaling, skin R23.4
Scalp —*see* condition
Scapegoating affecting child Z62.3
Scaphocephaly Q75.0
Scapulalgia M89.8X1
Scapulohumeral myopathy G71.0
Scar, scarring (*see also* Cicatrix) L90.5
  adherent L90.5
  atrophic L90.5
  cervix
    in pregnancy or childbirth —*see*
      Pregnancy, complicated by,
      abnormal cervix
  cheloid L91.0
  chorioretinal H31.00-
    posterior pole macula H31.01-
    postsurgical H59.81-
    solar retinopathy H31.02-
    specified type NEC H31.09-
  choroid —*see* Scar, chorioretinal
  conjunctiva H11.24-
  cornea H17.9
    xerophthalmic —*see also* Opacity,
      cornea
    vitamin A deficiency E50.6
  duodenum, obstructive K31.5
  hypertrophic L91.0
  keloid L91.0
  labia N90.89
  lung (base) J98.4
  macula —*see* Scar, chorioretinal,
    posterior pole
  muscle M62.89
  myocardium, myocardial I25.2
  painful L90.5
  posterior pole (eye) —*see* Scar,
    chorioretinal, posterior pole
  retina —*see* Scar, chorioretinal
  trachea J39.8
  uterus N85.8
    in pregnancy O34.29
  vagina N89.8
    postoperative N99.2
  vulva N90.89
Scarabiasis B88.2
Scarlatina (anginosa) (maligna) (ulcerosa)
  A38.9
  myocarditis (acute) A38.1
    old —*see* Myocarditis
  otitis media A38.0

Scarlet fever (albuminuria) (angina) A38.9
Schamberg's disease (progressive
  pigmentary dermatosis) L81.7
Schatzki's ring (acquired) (esophagus)
  (lower) K22.2
  congenital Q39.3
Schaufenster krankheit I20.8
Schaumann's
  benign lymphogranulomatosis
    D86.1
  disease or syndrome —*see* Sarcoidosis
Scheie's syndrome E76.03
Schenck's disease B42.1
Scheuermann's disease or
  osteochondrosis —*see*
  Osteochondrosis, juvenile, spine
Schilder (-Flatau) disease G37.0
Schilling-type monocytic leukemia
  C93.0-
Schimmelbusch's disease, cystic mastitis,
  or hyperplasia —*see* Mastopathy,
  cystic
Schistosoma infestation —*see* Infestation,
  Schistosoma
Schistosomiasis B65.9
  with muscle disorder B65.9 [*M63.80*]
    ankle B65.9 [*M63.87-*]
    foot B65.9 [*M63.87-*]
    forearm B65.9 [*M63.83-*]
    hand B65.9 [*M63.84-*]
    lower leg B65.9 [*M63.86-*]
    multiple sites B65.9 [*M63.89*]
    pelvic region B65.9 [*M63.85-*]
    shoulder region B65.9 [*M63.81-*]
    specified site NEC B65.9 [*M63.88*]
    thigh B65.9 [*M63.85-*]
    upper arm B65.9 [*M63.82-*]
  Asiatic B65.2
  bladder B65.0
  chestermani B65.8
  colon B65.1
  cutaneous B65.3
  due to
    S. haematobium B65.0
    S. japonicum B65.2
    S. mansoni B65.1
    S. mattheii B65.8
  Eastern B65.2
  genitourinary tract B65.0
  intestinal B65.1
  lung NEC B65.9 [*J99*]
    pneumonia B65.9 [*J17*]
  Manson's (intestinal) B65.1
  oriental B65.2
  pulmonary NEC B65.9 [*J99*]
    pneumonia B65.9
  Schistosoma
    haematobium B65.0
    japonicum B65.2
    mansoni B65.1
  specified type NEC B65.8
  urinary B65.0
  vesical B65.0
Schizencephaly Q04.6
Schizoaffective psychosis F25.9
Schizodontia K00.2
Schizoid personality F60.1
Schizophrenia, schizophrenic F20.9
  acute (brief) (undifferentiated) F23
  atypical (form) F20.3
  borderline F21
  catalepsy F20.2
  catatonic (type) (excited) (withdrawn)
    F20.2

S

Schizophrenia, schizophrenic *(Continued)*
cenesthopathic, cenesthesiopathic F20.89
childhood type F84.5
chronic undifferentiated F20.5
cyclic F25.0
disorganized (type) F20.1
flexibilitas cerea F20.2
hebephrenic (type) F20.1
incipient F21
latent F21
negative type F20.5
paranoid (type) F20.0
paraphrenic F20.0
post-psychotic depression F32.8
prepsychotic F21
prodromal F21
pseudoneurotic F21
pseudopsychopathic F21
reaction F23
residual (state) (type) F20.5
restzustand F20.5
schizoaffective (type) —*see* Psychosis,
schizoaffective
simple (type) F20.89
simplex F20.89
specified type NEC F20.89
stupor F20.2
syndrome of childhood F84.5
undifferentiated (type) F20.3
chronic F20.5
Schizothymia (persistent) F60.1
Schlatter-Osgood disease or
osteochondrosis —*see*
Osteochondrosis, juvenile, tibia
Schlatter's tibia —*see* Osteochondrosis,
juvenile, tibia
Schmidt's syndrome (polyglandular,
autoimmune) E31.0
Schmincke's carcinoma or tumor —
see Neoplasm, nasopharynx,
malignant
Schmitz (-Stutzer) dysentery A03.0
Schmorl's disease or nodes
lumbar region M51.46
lumbosacral region M51.47
sacrococcygeal region M53.3
thoracic region M51.44
thoracolumbar region M51.45
Schneiderian
papilloma —*see* Neoplasm,
nasopharynx benign
specified site —*see* Neoplasm, benign,
by site
unspecified site D14.0
specified site —*see* Neoplasm,
malignant, by site
unspecified site C30.0
Scholte's syndrome (malignant carcinoid)
E34.0
Scholz (-Bielchowsky-Henneberg)
disease or syndrome E75.25
Schönlein (-Henoch) disease or purpura
(primary) (rheumatic) D69.0
Schottmuller's disease A01.4
Schroeder's syndrome (endocrine
hypertensive) E27.0
Schüller-Christian disease or syndrome
C96.5
Schultze's type acroparesthesia, simple
I73.89
Schultz's disease or syndrome —*see*
Agranulocytosis
Schwalbe-Ziehen-Oppenheim disease
G24.1

Schwannoma —*see also* Neoplasm, nerve,
benign
malignant —*see also* Neoplasm, nerve,
malignant
with rhabdomyoblastic
differentiation —*see* Neoplasm,
nerve, malignant
melanocytic —*see* Neoplasm, nerve,
benign
pigmented —*see* Neoplasm, nerve,
benign
Schwannomatosis Q85.03
Schwartz (-Jampel) syndrome G71.13
Schwartz-Bartter syndrome E22.2
Schweniger-Buzzi anetoderma L90.1
Sciatic —*see* condition
Sciatica (infective)
with lumbago M54.4-
due to intervertebral disc disorder —
see Disorder, disc, with,
radiculopathy
due to displacement of intervertebral
disc (with lumbago) —*see*
Disorder, disc, with, radiculopathy
wallet M54.3-
Scimitar syndrome Q26.8
Sclera —*see* condition
Sclerectasia H15.84-
Scleredema
adultorum —*see* Sclerosis, systemic
Buschke's —*see* Sclerosis, systemic
newborn P83.0
Sclerema (adiposum) (edematosum)
(neonatorum) (newborn) P83.0
adultorum —*see* Sclerosis, systemic
Scleriasis —*see* Scleroderma
Scleritis H15.00-
with corneal involvement H15.04-
anterior H15.01-
brawny H15.02-
in (due to) zoster B02.34
posterior H15.03-
specified type NEC H15.09-
syphilitic A52.71
tuberculous (nodular) A18.51
Sclerochoroiditis H31.8
Scleroconjunctivitis —*see* Scleritis
Sclerocystic ovary syndrome E28.2
Sclerodactyly, sclerodactylia L94.3
Scleroderma, sclerodermia (acrosclerotic)
(diffuse) (generalized) (progressive)
(pulmonary) (*see also* Sclerosis,
systemic) M34.9
circumscribed L94.0
linear L94.1
localized L94.0
newborn P83.8
systemic M34.9
Sclerokeratitis H16.8
tuberculous A18.52
Scleroma nasi A48.8
Scleromalacia (perforans) H15.05-
Scleromyxedema L98.5
Sclérose en plaques G35
Sclerosis, sclerotic
adrenal (gland) E27.8
Alzheimer's —*see* Disease,
Alzheimer's
amyotrophic (lateral) G12.21
aorta, aortic I70.0
valve —*see* Endocarditis, aortic
artery, arterial, arteriolar,
arteriovascular —*see*
Arteriosclerosis
ascending multiple G35

Sclerosis, sclerotic *(Continued)*
brain (generalized) (lobular) G37.9
artery, arterial I67.2
diffuse G37.0
disseminated G35
insular G35
Krabbe's E75.23
miliary G35
multiple G35
presenile (Alzheimer's) —*see* Disease,
Alzheimer's, early onset
senile (arteriosclerotic) I67.2
stem, multiple G35
tuberous Q85.1
bulbar, multiple G35
bundle of His I44.39
cardiac —*see* Disease, heart, ischemic,
atherosclerotic
cardiorenal —*see* Hypertension,
cardiorenal
cardiovascular —*see also* Disease,
cardiovascular
renal —*see* Hypertension,
cardiorenal
cerebellar —*see* Sclerosis, brain
cerebral —*see* Sclerosis, brain
cerebrospinal (disseminated) (multiple)
G35
cerebrovascular I67.2
choroid —*see* Degeneration, choroid
combined (spinal cord) —*see also*
Degeneration, combined
multiple G35
concentric (Balo) G37.5
cornea —*see* Opacity, cornea
coronary (artery) I25.10
with angina pectoris —*see*
Arteriosclerosis, coronary
(artery),
corpus cavernosum
female N90.89
male N48.6
diffuse (brain) (spinal cord) G37.0
disseminated G35
dorsal G35
dorsolateral (spinal cord) —*see*
Degeneration, combined
endometrium N85.5
extrapyramidal G25.9
eye, nuclear (senile) —*see* Cataract,
senile, nuclear
focal and segmental (glomerular)
(*see also* N00-N07 with fourth
character .1) N05.1
Friedreich's (spinal cord) G11.1
funicular (spermatic cord) N50.8
general (vascular) —*see* Arteriosclerosis
gland (lymphatic) I89.8
hepatic K74.1
alcoholic K70.2
hereditary
cerebellar G11.9
spinal (Friedreich's ataxia) G11.1
hippocampal G93.81
insular G35
kidney —*see* Sclerosis, renal
larynx J38.7
lateral (amyotrophic) (descending)
(primary) (spinal) G12.21
lens, senile nuclear —*see* Cataract,
senile, nuclear
liver K74.1
with fibrosis K74.2
alcoholic K70.2
alcoholic K70.2
cardiac K76.1

Sclerosis, sclerotic *(Continued)*
lung —*see* Fibrosis, lung
mastoid —*see* Mastoiditis, chronic
mesial temporal G93.81
mitral I05.8
Mönckeberg's (medial) —*see*
    Arteriosclerosis, extremities
multiple (brain stem) (cerebral)
    (generalized) (spinal cord) G35
myocardium, myocardial —*see* Disease,
    heart, ischemic, atherosclerotic
nuclear (senile), eye —*see* Cataract,
    senile, nuclear
ovary N83.8
pancreas K86.8
penis N48.6
peripheral arteries —*see*
    Arteriosclerosis, extremities
plaques G35
pluriglandular E31.8
polyglandular E31.8
posterolateral (spinal cord) —*see*
    Degeneration, combined
presenile (Alzheimer's) —*see* Disease,
    Alzheimer's, early onset
primary, lateral G12.29
progressive, systemic M34.0
pulmonary —*see* Fibrosis, lung
    artery I27.0
    valve (heart) —*see* Endocarditis,
        pulmonary
renal N26.9
    with
        cystine storage disease E72.09
        hypertensive heart disease
            (conditions in I11) —*see*
            Hypertension, cardiorenal
    arteriolar (hyaline) (hyperplastic) —
        see Hypertension, kidney
retina (senile) (vascular) H35.00
senile (vascular) —*see* Arteriosclerosis
spinal (cord) (progressive) G95.89
    ascending G61.0
    combined —*see also* Degeneration,
        combined
        multiple G35
        syphilitic A52.11
    disseminated G35
    dorsolateral —*see* Degeneration,
        combined
    hereditary (Friedreich's) (mixed
        form) G11.1
    lateral (amyotrophic) G12.21
    multiple G35
    posterior (syphilitic) A52.11
stomach K31.89
subendocardial, congenital I42.4
systemic M34.9
    with
        lung involvement M34.81
        myopathy M34.82
        polyneuropathy M34.83
    drug-induced M34.2
    due to chemicals NEC M34.2
    progressive M34.0
    specified NEC M34.89
temporal (mesial) G93.81
tricuspid (heart) (valve) I07.8
tuberous (brain) Q85.1
tympanic membrane —*see* Disorder,
    tympanic membrane, specified
    NEC
valve, valvular (heart) —*see*
    Endocarditis
vascular —*see* Arteriosclerosis
vein I87.8

Scoliosis (acquired) (postural) M41.9
adolescent (idiopathic) —*see* Scoliosis,
    idiopathic, juvenile
congenital Q67.5
    due to bony malformation Q76.3
    failure of segmentation
        (hemivertebra) Q76.3
    hemivertebra fusion Q76.3
    postural Q67.5
idiopathic M41.20
    adolescent M41.129
        cervical region M41.122
        cervicothoracic region M41.123
        lumbar region M41.126
        lumbosacral region M41.127
        thoracic region M41.124
        thoracolumbar region M41.125
    cervical region M41.22
    cervicothoracic region M41.23
    infantile M41.00
        cervical region M41.02
        cervicothoracic region M41.03
        lumbar region M41.06
        lumbosacral region M41.07
        sacrococcygeal region M41.08
        thoracic region M41.04
        thoracolumbar region M41.05
    juvenile M41.119
        cervical region M41.112
        cervicothoracic region M41.113
        lumbar region M41.116
        lumbosacral region M41.117
        thoracic region M41.114
        thoracolumbar region M41.115
    lumbar region M41.26
    lumbosacral region M41.27
    thoracic region M41.24
    thoracolumbar region M41.25
neuromuscular M41.40
    cervical region M41.42
    cervicothoracic region M41.43
    lumbar region M41.46
    lumbosacral region M41.47
    occipito-atlanto-axial region
        M41.41
    thoracic region M41.44
    thoracolumbar region M41.45
paralytic —*see* Scoliosis, neuromuscular
postradiation therapy M96.5
rachitic (late effect or sequelae) E64.3
    [M49.80]
    cervical region E64.3 [M49.82]
    cervicothoracic region E64.3 [M49.83]
    lumbar region E64.3 [M49.86]
    lumbosacral region E64.3 [M49.87]
    multiple sites E64.3 [M49.89]
    occipito-atlanto-axial region E64.3
        [M49.81]
    sacrococcygeal region E64.3
        [M49.88]
    thoracic region E64.3 [M49.84]
    thoracolumbar region E64.3
        [M49.85]
sciatic M54.4-
secondary (to) NEC M41.50
    cerebral palsy, Friedreich's ataxia,
        poliomyelitis, neuromuscular
        disorders —*see* Scoliosis,
        neuromuscular
    cervical region M41.52
    cervicothoracic region M41.53
    lumbar region M41.56
    lumbosacral region M41.57
    thoracic region M41.54
    thoracolumbar region M41.55

Scoliosis *(Continued)*
specified form NEC M41.80
    cervical region M41.82
    cervicothoracic region M41.83
    lumbar region M41.86
    lumbosacral region M41.87
    thoracic region M41.84
    thoracolumbar region M41.85
thoracogenic M41.30
    thoracic region M41.34
    thoracolumbar region M41.35
tuberculous A18.01
Scoliotic pelvis
with disproportion (fetopelvic) O33.0
    causing obstructed labor O65.0
Scorbutus, scorbutic—*see also* Scurvy
anemia D53.2
Scotoma (arcuate) (Bjerrum) (central)
    (ring) —*see also* Defect, visual field,
    localized, scotoma
scintillating H53.19
Scratch—*see* Abrasion
Scratchy throat R09.89
Screening (for) Z13.9
alcoholism Z13.89
anemia Z13.0
anomaly, congenital Z13.89
antenatal, of mother Z36
arterial hypertension Z13.6
arthropod-borne viral disease NEC
    Z11.59
bacteriuria, asymptomatic Z13.89
behavioral disorder Z13.89
brain injury, traumatic Z13.850
bronchitis, chronic Z13.83
brucellosis Z11.2
cardiovascular disorder Z13.6
cataract Z13.5
chlamydial diseases Z11.8
cholera Z11.0
chromosomal abnormalities
    (nonprocreative) NEC Z13.79
colonoscopy Z12.11
congenital
    dislocation of hip Z13.89
    eye disorder Z13.5
    malformation or deformation Z13.89
contamination NEC Z13.88
cystic fibrosis Z13.228
dengue fever Z11.59
dental disorder Z13.84
depression Z13.89
developmental handicap Z13.4
    in early childhood Z13.4
diabetes mellitus Z13.1
diphtheria Z11.2
disability, intellectual Z13.4
disease or disorder Z13.9
    bacterial NEC Z11.2
        intestinal infectious Z11.0
        respiratory tuberculosis Z11.1
    blood or blood-forming organ Z13.0
    cardiovascular Z13.6
    Chagas' Z11.6
    chlamydial Z11.8
    dental Z13.89
    developmental Z13.4
    digestive tract NEC Z13.818
        lower GI Z13.811
        upper GI Z13.810
    ear Z13.5
    endocrine Z13.29
    eye Z13.5
    genitourinary Z13.89
    heart Z13.6

Screening *(Continued)*
  disease or disorder *(Continued)*
    human immunodeficiency virus
      (HIV) infection Z11.4
    immunity Z13.0
    infection
      intestinal Z11.0
        specified NEC Z11.6
    infectious Z11.9
    mental Z13.89
    metabolic Z13.228
    neurological Z13.89
    nutritional Z13.21
      metabolic Z13.228
        lipoid disorders Z13.220
    protozoal Z11.6
      intestinal Z11.0
    respiratory Z13.83
    rheumatic Z13.828
    rickettsial Z11.8
    sexually-transmitted NEC Z11.3
      human immunodeficiency virus
        (HIV) Z11.4
    sickle-cell (trait) Z13.0
    skin Z13.89
    specified NEC Z13.89
    spirochetal Z11.8
    thyroid Z13.29
    vascular Z13.6
    venereal Z11.3
    viral NEC Z11.59
      human immunodeficiency virus
        (HIV) Z11.4
      intestinal Z11.0
  elevated titer Z13.89
  emphysema Z13.83
  encephalitis, viral (mosquito- or tick-
    borne) Z11.59
  exposure to contaminants (toxic) Z13.88
  fever
    dengue Z11.59
    hemorrhagic Z11.59
    yellow Z11.59
  filariasis Z11.6
  galactosemia Z13.228
  gastrointestinal condition Z13.818
  genetic (nonprocreative)- for
    procreative management —*see*
    Testing, genetic, for procreative
    management
    disease carrier status (nonprocreative)
      Z13.71
    specified NEC (nonprocreative) Z13.79
  genitourinary condition Z13.89
  glaucoma Z13.5
  gonorrhea Z11.3
  gout Z13.89
  helminthiasis (intestinal) Z11.6
  hematopoietic malignancy Z12.89
  hemoglobinopathies NEC Z13.0
  hemorrhagic fever Z11.59
  Hodgkin disease Z12.89
  human immunodeficiency virus (HIV)
    Z11.4
  human papillomavirus Z11.51
  hypertension Z13.6
  immunity disorders Z13.0
  infection
    mycotic Z11.8
    parasitic Z11.8
  ingestion of radioactive substance Z13.88
  intellectual disability Z13.4
  intestinal
    helminthiasis Z11.6
    infectious disease Z11.0

Screening *(Continued)*
  leishmaniasis Z11.6
  leprosy Z11.2
  leptospirosis Z11.8
  leukemia Z12.89
  lymphoma Z12.89
  malaria Z11.6
  malnutrition Z13.29
    metabolic Z13.228
    nutritional Z13.21
  measles Z11.59
  mental disorder Z13.89
  metabolic errors, inborn Z13.228
  multiphasic Z13.89
  musculoskeletal disorder Z13.828
    osteoporosis Z13.820
  mycoses Z11.8
  myocardial infarction (acute)
    Z13.6
  neoplasm (malignant) (of) Z12.9
    bladder Z12.6
    blood Z12.89
    breast Z12.39
      routine mammogram Z12.31
    cervix Z12.4
    colon Z12.11
    genitourinary organs NEC
      Z12.79
      bladder Z12.6
      cervix Z12.4
      ovary Z12.73
      prostate Z12.5
      testis Z12.71
      vagina Z12.72
    hematopoietic system Z12.89
    intestinal tract Z12.10
      colon Z12.11
      rectum Z12.12
      small intestine Z12.13
    lung Z12.2
    lymph (glands) Z12.89
    nervous system Z12.82
    oral cavity Z12.81
    prostate Z12.5
    rectum Z12.12
    respiratory organs Z12.2
    skin Z12.83
    small intestine Z12.13
    specified site NEC Z12.89
    stomach Z12.0
  nephropathy Z13.89
  nervous system disorders NEC
    Z13.858
  neurological condition Z13.89
  osteoporosis Z13.820
  parasitic infestation Z11.9
    specified NEC Z11.8
  phenylketonuria Z13.228
  plague Z11.2
  poisoning (chemical) (heavy metal)
    Z13.88
  poliomyelitis Z11.59
  postnatal, chromosomal abnormalities
    Z13.89
  prenatal, of mother Z36
  protozoal disease Z11.6
    intestinal Z11.0
  pulmonary tuberculosis Z11.1
  radiation exposure Z13.88
  respiratory condition Z13.83
  respiratory tuberculosis Z11.1
  rheumatoid arthritis Z13.828
  rubella Z11.59
  schistosomiasis Z11.6

Screening *(Continued)*
  sexually-transmitted disease NEC Z11.3
    human immunodeficiency virus
      (HIV) Z11.4
  sickle-cell disease or trait Z13.0
  skin condition Z13.89
  sleeping sickness Z11.6
  special Z13.9
    specified NEC Z13.89
  syphilis Z11.3
  tetanus Z11.2
  trachoma Z11.8
  traumatic brain injury Z13.850
  trypanosomiasis Z11.6
  tuberculosis, respiratory Z11.1
  venereal disease Z11.3
  viral encephalitis (mosquito- or tick-
    borne) Z11.59
  whooping cough Z11.2
  worms, intestinal Z11.6
  yaws Z11.8
  yellow fever Z11.59
Scrofula, scrofulosis (tuberculosis of
  cervical lymph glands) A18.2
Scrofulide (primary) (tuberculous) A18.4
Scrofuloderma, scrofulodermia (any site)
  (primary) A18.4
Scrofulosus lichen (primary)
  (tuberculous) A18.4
Scrofulous —*see* condition
Scrotal tongue K14.5
Scrotum —*see* condition
Scurvy, scorbutic E54
  anemia D53.2
  gum E54
  infantile E54
  rickets E55.0 *[M90.80]*
Sealpox B08.62
Seasickness T75.3
Seatworm (infection) (infestation) B80
Sebaceous —*see also* condition
  cyst —*see* Cyst, sebaceous
Seborrhea, seborrheic L21.9
  capillitii R23.8
  capitis L21.0
  dermatitis L21.9
    infantile L21.1
  eczema L21.9
    infantile L21.1
  sicca L21.0
Seckel's syndrome Q87.1
Seclusion, pupil —*see* Membrane,
  pupillary
Second hand tobacco smoke exposure
  (acute) (chronic) Z77.22
  in the perinatal period P96.81
Secondary
  dentin (in pulp) K04.3
  neoplasm, secondaries —*see* Table of
    Neoplasms, secondary
Secretion
  antidiuretic hormone, inappropriate
    E22.2
  catecholamine, by pheochromocytoma
    E27.5
  hormone
    antidiuretic, inappropriate
      (syndrome) E22.2
    by
      carcinoid tumor E34.0
      pheochromocytoma E27.5
    ectopic NEC E34.2
  urinary
    excessive R35.8
    suppression R34

Section
nerve, traumatic —*see* Injury, nerve
Segmentation, incomplete (congenital) —
see also Fusion
bone NEC Q78.8
lumbosacral (joint) (vertebra) Q76.49
Seitelberger's syndrome (infantile
neuraxonal dystrophy) G31.89
Seizure (s) (*see also* Convulsions) R56.9
akinetic —*see* Epilepsy, generalized,
specified NEC
atonic —*see* Epilepsy, generalized,
specified NEC
autonomic (hysterical) F44.5
convulsive —*see* Convulsions
cortical (focal) (motor) —*see* Epilepsy,
localization-related, symptomatic,
with simple partial seizures
disorder (*see also* Epilepsy) G40.909
due to stroke —*see* Sequelae (of),
disease, cerebrovascular, by type,
specified NEC
epileptic —*see* Epilepsy
febrile (simple) R56.00
with status epilepticus G40.901
complex (atypical) (complicated) R56.01
with status epilepticus G40.901
grand mal G40.409
intractable G40.419
with status epilepticus G40.411
without status epilepticus G40.419
not intractable G40.409
with status epilepticus G40.401
without status epilepticus G40.409
heart —*see* Disease, heart
hysterical F44.5
intractable G40.919
with status epilepticus G40.911
Jacksonian (focal) (motor type) (sensory
type) —*see* Epilepsy, localization-
related, symptomatic, with simple
partial seizures
newborn P90
nonspecific epileptic
atonic —*see* Epilepsy, generalized,
specified NEC
clonic —*see* Epilepsy, generalized,
specified NEC
myoclonic —*see* Epilepsy,
generalized, specified NEC
tonic —*see* Epilepsy, generalized,
specified NEC
tonic-clonic —*see* Epilepsy,
generalized, specified NEC
partial, developing into secondarily
generalized seizures
complex —*see* Epilepsy, localization-
related, symptomatic, with
complex partial seizures
simple —*see* Epilepsy, localization-
related, symptomatic, with
simple partial seizures
petit mal G40.409
intractable G40.419
with status epilepticus G40.411
without status epilepticus G40.419
not intractable G40.409
with status epilepticus G40.401
without status epilepticus G40.409
post traumatic R56.1
recurrent G40.909
specified NEC G40.89
uncinate —*see* Epilepsy, localization-
related, symptomatic, with
complex partial seizures

Selenium deficiency, dietary E59
Self-damaging behavior (life-style) Z72.89
Self-harm (attempted)
history (personal) Z91.5
in family Z81.8
Self-mutilation (attempted)
history (personal) Z91.5
in family Z81.8
Self-poisoning
history (personal) Z91.5
in family Z81.8
observation following (alleged) attempt
Z03.6
Semicoma R40.1
Seminal vesiculitis N49.0
Seminoma C62.9-
specified site —*see* Neoplasm,
malignant, by site
Senear-Usher disease or syndrome
L10.4
Senectus R54
Senescence (without mention of
psychosis) R54
Senile, senility (*see also* condition) R41.81
with
acute confusional state F05
mental changes NOS F03
psychosis NEC —*see* Psychosis, senile
asthenia R54
cervix (atrophic) N88.8
debility R54
endometrium (atrophic) N85.8
fallopian tube (atrophic) —*see* Atrophy,
fallopian tube
heart (failure) R54
ovary (atrophic) —*see* Atrophy, ovary
premature E34.8
vagina, vaginitis (atrophic) N95.2
wart L82.1
Sensation
burning (skin) R20.8
tongue K14.6
loss of R20.8
prickling (skin) R20.2
tingling (skin) R20.2
Sense loss
smell —*see* Disturbance, sensation,
smell
taste —*see* Disturbance, sensation,
taste
touch R20.8
Sensibility disturbance (cortical) (deep)
(vibratory) R20.9
Sensitive, sensitivity —*see also* Allergy
carotid sinus G90.01
child (excessive) F93.8
cold, autoimmune D59.1
dentin K03.89
latex Z91.040
methemoglobin D74.8
tuberculin, without clinical or
radiological symptoms R76.11
visual
glare H53.71
impaired contrast H53.72
Sensitiver Beziehungswahn F22
Sensitization, auto-erythrocytic
D69.2
Separation
anxiety, abnormal (of childhood)
F93.0
apophysis, traumatic - code as Fracture,
by site
choroid —*see* Detachment, choroid

Separation (*Continued*)
epiphysis, epiphyseal
nontraumatic —*see also*
Osteochondropathy, specified
type NEC
upper femoral —*see* Slipped,
epiphysis, upper femoral
traumatic - code as Fracture, by site
fracture —*see* Fracture
infundibulum cardiac from right
ventricle by a partition Q24.3
joint (traumatic) (current) - code by site
under Dislocation
pubic bone, obstetrical trauma O71.6
retina, retinal —*see* Detachment, retina
symphysis pubis, obstetrical trauma
O71.6
tracheal ring, incomplete, congenital
Q32.1
Sepsis (generalized) (unspecified
organism) A41.9
with
organ dysfunction (acute) (multiple)
R65.20
with septic shock R65.21
actinomycotic A42.7
adrenal hemorrhage syndrome
(meningococcal) A39.1
anaerobic A41.4
Bacillus anthracis A22.7
Brucella (*see also* Brucellosis) A23.9
candidal B37.7
cryptogenic A41.9
due to device, implant or graft T85.79
arterial graft NEC T82.7
breast (implant) T85.79
catheter NEC T85.79
dialysis (renal) T82.7
intraperitoneal T85.71
infusion NEC T82.7
spinal (epidural) (subdural)
T85.79
urinary (indwelling) T83.51
ectopic or molar pregnancy O08.82
electronic (electrode) (pulse
generator) (stimulator)
bone T84.7
cardiac T82.7
nervous system (brain) (peripheral
nerve) (spinal) T85.79
urinary T83.59
fixation, internal (orthopedic) —*see*
Complication, fixation device,
infection
gastrointestinal (bile duct)
(esophagus) T85.79
genital T83.6
heart NEC T82.7
valve (prosthesis) T82.6
graft T82.7
joint prosthesis —*see* Complication,
joint prosthesis, infection
ocular (corneal graft) (orbital
implant) T85.79
orthopedic NEC T84.7
fixation device, internal —*see*
Complication, fixation device,
infection
specified NEC T85.79
vascular T82.7
ventricular intracranial shunt
T85.79
during labor O75.3
Enterococcus A41.81

Sepsis *(Continued)*
Erysipelothrix (rhusiopathiae)
(erysipeloid) A26.7
Escherichia coli (E. coli) A41.5
extraintestinal yersiniosis A28.2
following
abortion (subsequent episode) O08.0
current episode —*see* Abortion
ectopic or molar pregnancy O08.82
immunization T88.0
infusion, therapeutic injection or
transfusion NEC T80.29
gangrenous A41.9
gonococcal A54.86
Gram-negative (organism) A41.5
anaerobic A41.4
Haemophilus influenzae A41.3
herpesviral B00.7
intra-abdominal K65.1
intraocular —*see* Endophthalmitis,
purulent
Listeria monocytogenes A32.7
localized — code to specific localized
infection
in operation wound T81.4
skin —*see* Abscess
malleus A24.0
melioidosis A24.1
meningeal —*see* Meningitis
meningococcal A39.4
acute A39.2
chronic A39.3
MSSA (Methicillin susceptible
Staphylococcus aureus) A41.01
newborn P36.9
due to
anaerobes NEC P36.5
Escherichia coli P36.4
Staphylococcus P36.30
aureus P36.2
specified NEC P36.39
Streptococcus P36.10
group B P36.0
specified NEC P36.19
specified NEC P36.8
Pasteurella multocida A28.0
pelvic, puerperal, postpartum,
childbirth O85
pneumococcal A40.3
postprocedural T81.4
puerperal, postpartum, childbirth
(pelvic) O85
Salmonella (arizonae) (cholerae-suis)
(enteritidis) (typhimurium) A02.1
severe R65.20
with septic shock R65.21
Shigella (*see also* Dysentery, bacillary)
A03.9
skin, localized —*see* Abscess
specified organism NEC A41.89
Staphylococcus, staphylococcal A41.2
aureus (methicillin susceptible)
(MSSA) A41.01
methicillin resistant (MRSA)
A41.02
coagulase-negative A41.1
specified NEC A41.1
Streptococcus, streptococcal A40.9
agalactiae A40.1
group
A A40.0
B A40.1
D A41.81
neonatal P36.10
group B P36.0
specified NEC P36.19
pneumoniae A40.3

Sepsis *(Continued)*
MSSA *(Continued)*
Streptococcus, streptococcal
(Continued)
pyogenes A40.0
specified NEC A40.8
tracheostomy stoma J95.02
tularemic A21.7
umbilical, umbilical cord
(newborn) —*see* Sepsis, newborn
Yersinia pestis A20.7
Septate —*see* Septum
Septic —*see* condition
arm —*see* Cellulitis, upper limb
with lymphangitis —*see*
Lymphangitis, acute, upper limb
embolus —*see* Embolism
finger —*see* Cellulitis, digit
with lymphangitis —*see*
Lymphangitis, acute, digit
foot —*see* Cellulitis, lower limb
with lymphangitis —*see*
Lymphangitis, acute, lower limb
gallbladder (acute) K81.0
hand —*see* Cellulitis, upper limb
with lymphangitis —*see*
Lymphangitis, acute, upper limb
joint —*see* Arthritis, pyogenic or pyemic
leg —*see* Cellulitis, lower limb
with lymphangitis —*see*
Lymphangitis, acute, lower limb
nail —*see also* Cellulitis, digit
with lymphangitis —*see*
Lymphangitis, acute, digit
sore —*see also* Abscess
throat J02.0
streptococcal J02.0
spleen (acute) D73.89
teeth, tooth (pulpal origin) K04.4
throat —*see* Pharyngitis
thrombus —*see* Thrombosis
toe —*see* Cellulitis, digit
with lymphangitis —*see*
Lymphangitis, acute, digit
tonsils, chronic J35.01
with adenoiditis J35.03
uterus —*see* Endometritis
Septicemia A41.9
meaning sepsis —*see* Sepsis
Septum, septate (congenital) —*see also*
Anomaly, by site
anal Q42.3
with fistula Q42.2
aqueduct of Sylvius Q03.0
with spina bifida —*see* Spina bifida,
by site, with hydrocephalus
uterus (complete) (partial) Q51.2
vagina Q52.10
in pregnancy —*see* Pregnancy,
complicated by, abnormal vagina
causing obstructed labor O65.5
longitudinal (with or without
obstruction) Q52.12
transverse Q52.11
Sequelae (of) —*see also* condition
abscess, intracranial or intraspinal
(conditions in G06) G09
amputation — code to injury with
seventh character S
burn and corrosion — code to injury
with seventh character S
calcium deficiency E64.8
cerebrovascular disease —*see* Sequelae,
disease, cerebrovascular
childbirth O94

Sequelae (of) *(Continued)*
contusion — code to injury with
seventh character S
corrosion —*see* Sequelae, burn and
corrosion
crushing injury — code to injury with
seventh character S
disease
cerebrovascular I69.90
alteration of sensation
I69.998
aphasia I69.920
apraxia I69.990
ataxia I69.993
cognitive deficits I69.91
disturbance of vision I69.998
dysarthria I69.922
dysphagia I69.991
dysphasia I69.921
facial droop I69.992
facial weakness I69.992
fluency disorder I69.923
hemiplegia I69.95-
hemorrhage
intracerebral —*see* Sequelae,
hemorrhage, intracerebral
intracranial, nontraumatic
NEC —*see* Sequelae,
hemorrhage, intracranial,
nontraumatic
subarachnoid —*see* Sequelae,
hemorrhage, subarachnoid
language deficit I69.928
monoplegia
lower limb I69.84-
upper limb I69.93-
paralytic syndrome I69.96-
specified effect NEC I69.998
specified type NEC I69.80
alteration of sensation I69.898
aphasia I69.820
apraxia I69.890
ataxia I69.893
cognitive deficits I69.81
disturbance of vision I69.898
dysarthria I69.822
dysphagia I69.891
dysphasia I69.821
facial droop I69.892
facial weakness I69.892
fluency disorder I69.823
hemiplegia I69.85-
language deficit I69.828
monoplegia
lower limb I69.84-
upper limb I69.83-
paralytic syndrome I69.86-
specified effect NEC I69.898
speech deficit I69.928
speech deficit I69.828
stroke NOS —*see* Sequelae, stroke
NOS
dislocation — code to injury with
seventh character S
encephalitis or encephalomyelitis
(conditions in G04) G09
in infectious disease NEC B94.8
viral B94.1
external cause — code to injury with
seventh character S
foreign body entering natural orifice —
code to injury with seventh
character S
fracture — code to injury with seventh
character S

S

Sequelae(of) (Continued)
  frostbite — code to injury with seventh
    character S
  Hansen's disease B92
  hemorrhage
    intracerebral I69.10
      alteration of sensation I69.198
      aphasia I69.120
      apraxia I69.190
      ataxia I69.193
      cognitive deficits I69.11
      disturbance of vision I69.198
      dysarthria I69.122
      dysphagia I69.191
      dysphasia I69.121
      facial droop I69.192
      facial weakness I69.192
      fluency disorder I69.123
      hemiplegia I69.15-
      language deficit NEC I69.128
      monoplegia
        lower limb I69.14-
        upper limb I69.13-
      paralytic syndrome I69.16-
      specified effect NEC I69.198
      speech deficit NEC I69.128
    intracranial, nontraumatic NEC I69.20
      alteration of sensation I69.298
      aphasia I69.220
      apraxia I69.290
      ataxia I69.293
      cognitive deficits I69.21
      disturbance of vision I69.298
      dysarthria I69.222
      dysphagia I69.291
      dysphasia I69.221
      facial droop I69.292
      facial weakness I69.292
      fluency disorder I69.223
      hemiplegia I69.25-
      language deficit NEC I69.228
      monoplegia
        lower limb I69.24-
        upper limb I69.23-
      paralytic syndrome I69.26-
      specified effect NEC I69.298
      speech deficit NEC I69.228
    subarachnoid I69.00
      alteration of sensation I69.098
      aphasia I69.020
      apraxia I69.090
      ataxia I69.093
      cognitive deficits I69.01
      disturbance of vision I69.098
      dysarthria I69.022
      dysphagia I69.091
      dysphasia I69.021
      facial droop I69.092
      facial weakness I69.092
      fluency disorder I69.023
      hemiplegia I69.05-
      language deficit NEC I69.028
      monoplegia
        lower limb I69.04-
        upper limb I69.03-
      paralytic syndrome I69.06-
      specified effect NEC I69.098
      speech deficit NEC I69.028
  hepatitis, viral B94.2
  hyperalimentation E68
  infarction
    cerebral I69.30
      alteration of sensation I69.398
      aphasia I69.320
      apraxia I69.390

Sequelae(of) (Continued)
  infarction (Continued)
    cerebral (Continued)
      ataxia I69.393
      cognitive deficits I69.31
      disturbance of vision I69.398
      dysarthria I69.322
      dysphagia I69.391
      dysphasia I69.321
      facial droop I69.392
      facial weakness I69.392
      fluency disorder I69.323
      hemiplegia I69.35-
      language deficit NEC I69.328
      monoplegia
        lower limb I69.34-
        upper limb I69.33-
      paralytic syndrome I69.36-
      specified effect NEC I69.398
      speech deficit NEC I69.328
  infection, pyogenic, intracranial or
    intraspinal G09
  infectious disease B94.9
    specified NEC B94.8
  injury — code to injury with seventh
    character S
  leprosy B92
  meningitis
    bacterial (conditions in G00) G09
    other or unspecified cause
      (conditions in G03) G09
  muscle (and tendon) injury — code to
    injury with seventh character S
  myelitis —see Sequelae, encephalitis
  niacin deficiency E64.8
  nutritional deficiency E64.9
    specified NEC E64.8
  obstetrical condition O94
  parasitic disease B94.9
  phlebitis or thrombophlebitis of
    intracranial or intraspinal venous
    sinuses and veins (conditions in
    G08) G09
  poisoning — code to poisoning with
    seventh character S
    nonmedicinal substance —see
      Sequelae, toxic effect,
      nonmedicinal substance
  poliomyelitis (acute) B91
  pregnancy O94
  protein-energy malnutrition E64.0
  puerperium O94
  rickets E64.3
  selenium deficiency E64.8
  sprain and strain — code to injury with
    seventh character S
  stroke NOS I69.30
    alteration in sensation I69.398
    aphasia I69.320
    apraxia I69.390
    ataxia I69.393
    cognitive deficits I69.31
    disturbance of vision I69.398
    dysarthria I69.322
    dysphagia I69.391
    dysphasia I69.321
    facial droop I69.392
    facial weakness I69.392
    hemiplegia I69.35-
    language deficit NEC
      I69.328
    monoplegia
      lower limb I69.34-
      upper limb I69.33-
    paralytic syndrome I69.36-

Sequelae(of) (Continued)
  stroke NOS (Continued)
    specified effect NEC I69.398
    speech deficit NEC I69.328
  tendon and muscle injury — code to
    injury with seventh character S
  thiamine deficiency E64.8
  trachoma B94.0
  tuberculosis B90.9
    bones and joints B90.2
    central nervous system B90.0
    genitourinary B90.1
    pulmonary (respiratory) B90.9
    specified organs NEC B90.8
  viral
    encephalitis B94.1
    hepatitis B94.2
  vitamin deficiency NEC E64.8
    A E64.1
    B E64.8
    C E64.2
  wound, open — code to injury with
    seventh character S
Sequestration—see also Sequestrum
  lung, congenital Q33.2
Sequestrum
  bone —see Osteomyelitis, chronic
  dental M27.2
  jaw bone M27.2
  orbit —see Osteomyelitis, orbit
  sinus (accessory) (nasal) —see Sinusitis
Sequoiosis lung or pneumonitis
  J67.8
Serology for syphilis
  doubtful
    with signs or symptoms - code
      by site and stage under
      Syphilis
    follow-up of latent syphilis —see
      Syphilis, latent
  negative, with signs or symptoms —
    code by site and stage under
    Syphilis
  positive A53.0
    with signs or symptoms - code by site
      and stage under Syphilis
  reactivated A53.0
Seroma—see also Hematoma
  traumatic, secondary and recurrent
    T79.2
Seropurulent—see condition
Serositis, multiple K65.8
  pericardial I31.1
  peritoneal K65.8
Serous—see condition
Sertoli cell
  adenoma
    specified site —see Neoplasm, benign,
      by site
    unspecified site
      female D27.9
      male D29.20
  carcinoma
    specified site —see Neoplasm,
      malignant, by site
    unspecified site (male) C62.9-
    female C56.9
  tumor
    with lipid storage
      specified site —see Neoplasm,
        benign, by site
      unspecified site
        female D27.9
        male D29.20

Sertoli cell (Continued)
  tumor (Continued)
    specified site —see Neoplasm, benign,
      by site
    unspecified site
      female D27.9
      male D29.20
Sertoli-Leydig cell tumor—see
  Neoplasm, benign, by site
  specified site —see Neoplasm, benign,
    by site
  unspecified site
    female D27.9
    male D29.20
Serum
  allergy, allergic reaction (see also
    Reaction, serum) T80.69
    shock (see also Shock, anaphylactic)
      T80.59
  arthritis (see also Reaction, serum)
    T80.69
  complication or reaction NEC (see also
    Reaction, serum) T80.69
  disease NEC (see also Reaction, serum)
    T80.69
  hepatitis —see also Hepatitis, viral,
    type B
    carrier (suspected) of Z22.51
  intoxication (see also Reaction, serum)
    T80.69
  neuritis (see also Reaction, serum)
    T80.69
  neuropathy G61.1
  poisoning NEC (see also Reaction,
    serum) T80.69
  rash NEC (see also Reaction, serum)
    T80.69
  reaction NEC (see also Reaction, serum)
    T80.69
  sickness NEC (see also Reaction, serum)
    T80.69
  urticaria (see also Reaction, serum)
    T80.69
Sesamoiditis—see Osteomyelitis,
  specified type NEC
Sever's disease or osteochondrosis—
  see Osteochondrosis, juvenile,
  tarsus
Severe sepsis R65.20
  with septic shock R65.21
Sex
  chromosome mosaics Q97.8
    lines with various numbers of X
      chromosomes Q97.2
  education Z70.8
  reassignment surgery status Z87.890
Sextuplet pregnancy—see Pregnancy,
  sextuplet
Sexual
  function, disorder of (psychogenic)
    F52.9
  immaturity (female) (male) E30.0
  impotence (psychogenic) organic origin
    NEC —see Dysfunction, sexual,
    male
  precocity (constitutional) (cryptogenic)
    (female) (idiopathic) (male)
    E30.1
Sexuality, pathologic—see Deviation,
  sexual
Sézary disease C84.1-
Shadow, lung R91.8
Shaking palsy or paralysis—see
  Parkinsonism

Shallowness, acetabulum—see
  Derangement, joint, specified type
  NEC, hip
Shaver's disease J63.1
Sheath (tendon) —see condition
Sheathing, retinal vessels H35.01-
Shedding
  nail L60.8
  premature, primary (deciduous) teeth
    K00.6
Sheehan's disease or syndrome
  E23.0
Shelf, rectal K62.89
Shell teeth K00.5
Shellshock (current) F43.0
  lasting state —see Disorder, post-
    traumatic stress
Shield kidney Q63.1
Shift
  auditory threshold (temporary)
    H93.24-
  mediastinal R93.8
Shifting sleep-work schedule (affecting
  sleep) G47.26
Shiga (-Kruse) dysentery A03.0
Shiga's bacillus A03.0
Shigella (dysentery) —see Dysentery,
  bacillary
Shigellosis A03.9
  Group A A03.0
  Group B A03.1
  Group C A03.2
  Group D A03.3
Shin splints T79.6
Shingles—see Herpes, zoster
Shipyard disease or eye B30.0
Shirodkar suture, in pregnancy—
  see Pregnancy, complicated by,
  incompetent cervix
Shock R57.9
  with ectopic or molar pregnancy
    O08.3
  adrenal (cortical) (Addisonian)
    E27.2
  adverse food reaction (anaphylactic) —
    see Shock, anaphylactic, due to
    food
  allergic —see Shock, anaphylactic
  anaphylactic T78.2
    chemical —see Table of drugs and
      chemicals
    due to drug or medicinal substance
      correct substance properly
        administered T88.6
      overdose or wrong substance given
        or taken (by accident) —see
        Table of drugs and chemicals,
        by drug, poisoning
    due to food (nonpoisonous) T78.00
      additives T78.06
      dairy products T78.07
      eggs T78.08
      fish T78.03
        shellfish T78.02
      fruit T78.04
      milk T78.07
      nuts T78.05
        peanuts T78.01
      peanuts T78.01
      seeds T78.05
      specified type NEC T78.09
      vegetable T78.04
    following sting (s) —see Venom
    immunization T80.52

Shock (Continued)
  anaphylactic (Continued)
    serum T80.59
      blood and blood products T80.51
      immunization T80.52
      specified NEC T80.59
      vaccination T80.52
  anaphylactoid —see Shock, anaphylactic
  anesthetic
    correct substance properly
      administered T88.2
    overdose or wrong substance
      given or taken —see Table of
      drugs and chemicals, by drug,
      poisoning
    specified anesthetic —see Table of
      drugs and chemicals, by drug,
      poisoning
  cardiogenic R57.0
  chemical substance —see Table of drugs
    and chemicals
  complicating ectopic or molar
    pregnancy O08.3
  culture —see Disorder, adjustment
  drug
    due to correct substance properly
      administered T88.6
    overdose or wrong substance given
      or taken (by accident) —see
      Table of drugs and chemicals, by
      drug, poisoning
  during or after labor and delivery O75.1
  electric T75.4
    (taser) T75.4
  endotoxic R65.21
    postprocedural (during or resulting
      from a procedure, not elsewhere
      classified) T81.12
  following
    ectopic or molar pregnancy O08.3
    injury (immediate) (delayed) T79.4
    labor and delivery O75.1
  food (anaphylactic) —see Shock,
    anaphylactic, due to food
  from electroshock gun (taser) T75.4
  gram-negative R65.21
    postprocedural (during or resulting
      from a procedure, not elsewhere
      classified) T81.12
  hematologic R57.8
  hemorrhagic
    surgery (intraoperative)
      (postoperative) T81.19
    trauma T79.4
  hypovolemic R57.1
    surgical T81.19
    traumatic T79.4
  insulin E15
    therapeutic misadventure —see
      subcategory T38.3
  kidney N17.0
    traumatic (following crushing) T79.5
  lightning T75.01
  lung J80
  obstetric O75.1
    with ectopic or molar pregnancy
      O08.3
    following ectopic or molar pregnancy
      O08.3
  pleural (surgical) T81.19
    due to trauma T79.4
  postprocedural (postoperative) T81.10
    with ectopic or molar pregnancy O08.3
    cardiogenic T81.11

Simple, simplex —*see* condition
Simulation, conscious (of illness) Z76.5
Simultanagnosia (asimultagnosia) R48.3
Sin Nombre virus disease (Hantavirus)
    (cardio)-pulmonary syndrome) B33.4
Sinding-Larsen disease or
    osteochondrosis —*see*
    Osteochondrosis, juvenile, patella
Singapore hemorrhagic fever A91
Singer's node or nodule J38.2
Single
  atrium Q21.2
  coronary artery Q24.5
  umbilical artery Q27.0
  ventricle Q20.4
Singultus R06.6
  epidemicus B33.0
Sinus —*see also* Fistula
  abdominal K63.89
  arrest I45.5
  arrhythmia I49.8
  bradycardia R00.1
  branchial cleft (internal) (external)
    Q18.0
  coccygeal —*see* Sinus, pilonidal
  dental K04.6
  dermal (congenital) Q06.8
    with abscess Q06.8
    coccygeal, pilonidal —*see* Sinus,
     coccygeal
  infected, skin NEC L08.89
  marginal, ruptured or bleeding —
    see Hemorrhage, antepartum,
    specified cause NEC
  medial, face and neck Q18.8
  pause I45.5
  pericranii Q01.9
  pilonidal (infected) (rectum) L05.92
    with abscess L05.02
  preauricular Q18.1
  rectovaginal N82.3
  Rokitansky-Aschoff (gallbladder)
    K82.8
  sacrococcygeal (dermoid) (infected) —
    see Sinus, pilonidal
  tachycardia R00.0
    paroxysmal I47.1
  tarsi syndrome —*see* Syndrome, tarsal
    tunnel
  testis N50.8
  tract (postinfective) —*see* Fistula
  urachus Q64.4
Sinusitis (accessory) (chronic)
    (hyperplastic) (nasal) (nonpurulent)
    (purulent) J32.9
  acute J01.90
    ethmoidal J01.20
     recurrent J01.21
    frontal J01.10
     recurrent J01.11
    involving more than one sinus, other
     than pansinusitis J01.80
     recurrent J01.81
    maxillary J01.00
     recurrent J01.01
    pansinusitis J01.40
     recurrent J01.41
    recurrent J01.91
    specified NEC J01.80
     recurrent J01.81
    sphenoidal J01.30
     recurrent J01.31
  allergic —*see* Rhinitis, allergic
  due to high altitude T70.1

Sinusitis *(Continued)*
  ethmoidal J32.2
    acute J01.20
     recurrent J01.21
  frontal J32.1
    acute J01.10
     recurrent J01.11
  influenzal —*see* Influenza, with,
    respiratory manifestations NEC
  involving more than one sinus but not
    pansinusitis J32.8
    acute J01.80
     recurrent J01.81
  maxillary J32.0
    acute J01.00
     recurrent J01.01
  sphenoidal J32.3
    acute J01.30
     recurrent J01.31
  tuberculous, any sinus A15.8
Sinusitis-bronchiectasis-situs inversus
    (syndrome) (triad) Q89.3
Sipple's syndrome E31.22
Sirenomelia (syndrome) Q87.2
Siriasis T67.0
Sirkari's disease B55.0
Siti A65
Situation, psychiatric F99
Situational
  disturbance (transient) —*see* Disorder,
    adjustment
    acute F43.0
  maladjustment —*see* Disorder,
    adjustment
  reaction —*see* Disorder, adjustment
    acute F43.0
Situs inversus or transversus
    (abdominalis) (thoracis) Q89.3
Sixth disease B08.20
  due to human herpesvirus 6 B08.21
  due to human herpesvirus 7 B08.22
Sjögren-Larsson syndrome Q87.1
Sjögren's syndrome or disease —*see* Sicca
    syndrome
Skeletal —*see* condition
Skene's gland —*see* condition
Skenitis —*see* Urethritis
Skerljevo A65
Skevas-Zerfus disease —*see* Toxicity,
    venom, marine animal, sea anemone
Skin —*see also* condition
  clammy R23.1
  donor —*see* Donor, skin
  hidebound M35.9
Slate-dressers' or slate-miners' lung J62.8
Sleep
  apnea —*see* Apnea, sleep
  deprivation Z72.820
  disorder or disturbance G47.9
    child F51.9
     nonorganic origin F51.9
     specified NEC G47.8
    disturbance G47.9
     nonorganic origin F51.9
    drunkenness F51.9
    rhythm inversion G47.2-
    terrors F51.4
    walking F51.3
     hysterical F44.89
Sleep hygiene
  abuse Z72.821
  inadequate Z72.821
  poor Z72.821
Sleeping sickness —*see* Sickness, sleeping

Sleeplessness —*see* Insomnia
  menopausal N95.11
Sleep-wake schedule disorder G47.20
Slim disease (in HIV infection) B20
Slipped, slipping
  epiphysis (traumatic) —*see also*
    Osteochondropathy, specified type
    NEC
    capital femoral (traumatic)
     acute (on chronic) S79.01-
    current traumatic - code as Fracture,
     by site
    upper femoral (nontraumatic) M93.00-
     acute M93.01-
      on chronic M93.03-
     chronic M93.02-
  intervertebral disc —*see* Displacement,
    intervertebral disc
  ligature, umbilical P51.8
  patella —*see* Disorder, patella,
    derangement NEC
  rib M89.8X8
  sacroiliac joint —*see* subcategory M53.2
  tendon —*see* Disorder, tendon
  ulnar nerve, nontraumatic —*see* Lesion,
    nerve, ulnar
  vertebra NEC —*see* Spondylolisthesis
Slocumb's syndrome E27.0
Sloughing (multiple) (phagedena)
    (skin) —*see also* Gangrene
  abscess —*see* Abscess
  appendix K38.8
  fascia —*see* Disorder, soft tissue,
    specified type NEC
  scrotum N50.8
  tendon —*see* Disorder, tendon
  transplanted organ —*see* Rejection,
    transplant
  ulcer —*see* Ulcer, skin
Slow
  feeding, newborn P92.2
  flow syndrome, coronary I20.8
  heart(beat) R00.1
Slowing, urinary stream R39.19
Sluder's neuralgia (syndrome) G44.89
Slurred, slurring speech R47.81
Small (ness)
  for gestational age —*see* Small for dates
  introitus, vagina N89.6
  kidney (unknown cause) N27.9
    bilateral N27.1
    unilateral N27.0
  ovary (congenital) Q50.39
  pelvis
    with disproportion (fetopelvic) O33.1
     causing obstructed labor O65.1
  uterus N85.8
  white kidney N03.9
Small-and-light-for-dates —*see* Small for
    dates
Small-for-dates (infant) P05.10
  with weight of
    499 grams or less P05.11
    500-749 grams P05.12
    750-999 grams P05.13
    1000-1249 grams P05.14
    1250-1499 grams P05.15
    1500-1749 grams P05.16
    1750-1999 grams P05.17
    2000-2499 grams P05.18
Smallpox B03
Smearing, fecal R15.1
Smith-Lemli-Opitz syndrome E78.72
Smith's fracture S52.54-
Smoker —*see* Dependence, drug, nicotine

Smoker's
  bronchitis J41.0
  cough J41.0
  palate K13.24
  throat J31.2
  tongue K13.24
Smoking
  passive Z77.22
Smothering spells R06.81
Snaggle teeth, tooth M26.39
Snapping
  finger —see Trigger finger
  hip —see Derangement, joint, specified
      type NEC, hip
  involving the iliotiblial band M76.3-
  knee —see Derangement, knee
      involving the iliotiblial band
      M76.3-
Sneddon-Wilkinson disease or
      syndrome (sub-corneal pustular
      dermatosis) L13.1
Sneezing (intractable) R06.7
Sniffing
  cocaine
      abuse —see Abuse, drug, cocaine
      dependence —see Dependence, drug,
          cocaine
  gasoline
      abuse —see Abuse, drug, inhalant
      dependence —see Dependence, drug,
          inhalant
  glue (airplane)
      abuse —see Abuse, drug, inhalant
      drug dependence —see Dependence,
          drug, inhalant
Sniffles
  newborn P28.89
Snoring R06.83
Snow blindness —see Photokeratitis
Snuffles (non-syphilitic) R06.5
  newborn P28.89
  syphilitic (infant) A50.05 [J99]
Social
  exclusion Z60.4
      due to discrimination or persecution
          (perceived) Z60.5
  migrant Z59.0
      acculturation difficulty Z60.3
  rejection Z60.4
      due to discrimination or persecution
          Z60.5
  role conflict NEC Z73.5
  skills inadequacy NEC Z73.4
  transplantation Z60.3
Sodoku A25.0
Soemmerring's ring —see Cataract,
      secondary
Soft —see also condition
  nails L60.3
Softening
  bone —see Osteomalacia
  brain (necrotic) (progressive) G93.89
      congenital Q04.8
      embolic I63.4
      hemorrhagic —see Hemorrhage,
          intracranial, intracerebral
      occlusive I63.5
      thrombotic I63.3
  cartilage M94.2-
      patella M22.4-
  cerebellar —see Softening, brain
  cerebral —see Softening, brain
  cerebrospinal —see Softening, brain
  myocardial, heart —see Degeneration,
      myocardial

Softening (Continued)
  spinal cord G95.89
  stomach K31.89
Soldier's
  heart F45.8
  patches I31.0
Solitary
  cyst, kidney N28.1
  kidney, congenital Q60.0
Solvent abuse —see Abuse, drug,
      inhalant
  dependence —see Dependence, drug,
      inhalant
Somatization reaction, somatic
      reaction —see Disorder, somatoform
Somnambulism F51.3
  hysterical F44.89
Somnolence R40.0
  nonorganic origin F51.11
Sonne dysentery A03.3
Soor B37.0
Sore
  bed —see Ulcer, pressure, by site
  chiclero B55.1
  Delhi B55.1
  desert —see Ulcer, skin
  eye H57.1-
  Lahore B55.1
  mouth K13.79
      canker K12.0
  muscle M79.1
  Naga —see Ulcer, skin
  of skin —see Ulcer, skin - oriental B55.1
  pressure —see Ulcer, pressure, by site
  skin L98.9
  soft A57
  throat (acute) —see also Pharyngitis
      with influenza, flu, or grippe —see
          Influenza, with, respiratory
          manifestations NEC
      chronic J31.2
      coxsackie (virus) B08.5
      diphtheritic A36.0
      herpesviral B00.2
      influenzal —see Influenza, with,
          respiratory manifestations NEC
      septic J02.0
      streptococcal (ulcerative) J02.0
      viral NEC J02.8
          coxsackie B08.5
  tropical —see Ulcer, skin
  veldt —see Ulcer, skin
Soto's syndrome (cerebral gigantism)
      Q87.3
South African cardiomyopathy
      syndrome I42.8
Southeast Asian hemorrhagic fever
      A91
Spacing
  abnormal, tooth, teeth, fully erupted
      M26.30
  excessive, tooth, fully erupted M26.32
Spade-like hand (congenital) Q68.1
Spading nail L60.8
  congenital Q84.6
Spanish collar N47.1
Sparganosis B70.1
Spasm(s), spastic, spasticity (see also
      condition) R25.2
  accommodation —see Spasm, of
      accommodation
  ampulla of Vater K83.4
  anus, ani (sphincter) (reflex) K59.4
      psychogenic F45.8

Spasm(s), spastic, spasticity (Continued)
  artery I73.9
      cerebral G45.9
  Bell's G51.3
  bladder (sphincter, external or internal)
      N32.89
      psychogenic F45.8
  bronchus, bronchiole J98.01
  cardia K22.0
  cardiac I20.1
  carpopedal —see Tetany
  cerebral (arteries) (vascular) G45.9
  cervix, complicating delivery O62.4
  ciliary body (of accommodation) —see
      Spasm, of accommodation
  colon K58.9
      with diarrhea K58.0
      psychogenic F45.8
  common duct K83.8
  compulsive —see Tic
  conjugate H51.8
  coronary (artery) I20.1
  diaphragm (reflex) R06.6
      epidemic B33.0
      psychogenic F45.8
  duodenum K59.8
  epidemic diaphragmatic (transient)
      B33.0
  esophagus (diffuse) K22.4
      psychogenic F45.8
  facial G51.3
  fallopian tube N83.8
  gastrointestinal (tract) K31.89
      psychogenic F45.8
  glottis J38.5
      hysterical F44.4
      psychogenic F45.8
          conversion reaction F44.4
      reflex through recurrent laryngeal
          nerve J38.5
  habit —see Tic
  heart I20.1
  hemifacial (clonic) G51.3
  hourglass —see Contraction, hourglass
  hysterical F44.4
  infantile —see Epilepsy, spasms
  inferior oblique, eye H51.8
  intestinal (see also Syndrome, irritable
      bowel) K58.9
      psychogenic F45.8
  larynx, laryngeal J38.5
      hysterical F44.4
      psychogenic F45.8
          conversion reaction F44.4
  levator palpebrae superioris —see
      Disorder, eyelid function
  muscle NEC M62.838
      back M62.830
  nerve, trigeminal G51.0
  nervous F45.8
  nodding F98.4
  occupational F48.8
  oculogyric H51.8
      psychogenic F45.8
  of accommodation H52.53-
  ophthalmic artery —see Occlusion,
      artery, retina
  perineal, female N94.89
  peroneo-extensor —see also Deformity,
      limb, flat foot
  pharynx (reflex) J39.2
      hysterical F45.8
      psychogenic F45.8
  psychogenic F45.8

Spasm(s), spastic, spasticity (Continued)
  pylorus NEC K31.3
    adult hypertrophic K31.89
    congenital or infantile Q40.0
    psychogenic F45.8
  rectum (sphincter) K59.4
    psychogenic F45.8
  retinal (artery) —see Occlusion, artery,
    retina
  sigmoid (see also Syndrome, irritable
    bowel) K58.9
    psychogenic F45.8
  sphincter of Oddi K83.4
  stomach K31.89
    neurotic F45.8
  throat J39.2
    hysterical F45.8
    psychogenic F45.8
  tic F95.9
    chronic F95.1
    transient of childhood F95.0
  tongue K14.8
  torsion (progressive) G24.1
  trigeminal nerve —see Neuralgia,
    trigeminal
  ureter N13.5
  urethra (sphincter) N35.9
  uterus N85.8
    complicating labor O62.4
  vagina N94.2
    psychogenic F52.5
  vascular I73.9
  vasomotor I73.9
  vein NEC I87.8
  viscera —see Pain, abdominal
Spasmodic —see condition
Spasmophilia —see Tetany
Spasmus nutans F98.4
Spastic, spasticity —see also Spasm
  child (cerebral) (congenital) (paralysis)
    G80.1
Speaker's throat R49.8
Specific, specified —see condition
Speech
  defect, disorder, disturbance,
    impediment R47.9
    psychogenic, in childhood and
     adolescence F98.8
    slurring R47.81
    specified NEC R47.89
Spencer's disease A08.19
Spens' syndrome (syncope with heart
  block) I45.9
Sperm counts (fertility testing) Z31.41
  postvasectomy Z30.8
  reversal Z31.42
Spermatic cord —see condition
Spermatocele N43.40
  congenital Q55.4
  multiple N43.42
  single N43.41
Spermatocystitis N49.0
Spermatocytoma C62.9-
  specified site —see Neoplasm,
    malignant, by site
Spermatorrhea N50.8
Sphacelus —see Gangrene
Sphenoidal —see condition
Sphenoiditis (chronic) —see Sinusitis,
  sphenoidal
Sphenopalatine ganglion neuralgia
  G90.09
Sphericity, increased, lens (congenital)
  Q12.4

Spherocytosis (congenital) (familial)
  (hereditary) D58.0
  hemoglobin disease D58.0
  sickle-cell (disease) D57.8-
Spherophakia Q12.4
Sphincter —see condition
Sphincteritis, sphincter of Oddi —see
  Cholangitis
Sphingolipidosis E75.3
  specified NEC E75.29
Sphingomyelinosis E75.3
Spicule tooth K00.2
Spider
  bite —see Toxicity, venom, spider
  fingers —see Syndrome, Marfan's
  nevus I78.1
  toes —see Syndrome, Marfan's
  vascular I78.1
Spiegler-Fendt
  benign lymphocytoma L98.8
  sarcoid L08.89
Spielmeyer-Vogt disease E75.4
Spina bifida (aperta) Q05.9
  with hydrocephalus NEC Q05.4
  cervical Q05.5
    with hydrocephalus Q05.0
  dorsal Q05.6
    with hydrocephalus Q05.1
  lumbar Q05.7
    with hydrocephalus Q05.2
  lumbosacral Q05.7
    with hydrocephalus Q05.2
  occulta Q76.0
  sacral Q05.8
    with hydrocephalus Q05.3
  thoracic Q05.6
    with hydrocephalus Q05.1
  thoracolumbar Q05.6
    with hydrocephalus Q05.1
Spindle, Krukenberg's —see
  Pigmentation, cornea, posterior
Spine, spinal —see condition
Spiradenoma (eccrine) —see Neoplasm,
  skin, benign
Spirillosis A25.0
Spirillum
  minus A25.0
  obermeieri infection A68.0
Spirochetal —see condition
Spirochetosis A69.9
  arthritic, arthritica A69.9
  bronchopulmonary A69.8
  icterohemorrhagic A27.0
  lung A69.8
Spirometrosis B70.1
Spitting blood —see Hemoptysis
Splanchnoptosis K63.4
Spleen, splenic —see condition
Splenectasis —see Splenomegaly
Splenitis (interstitial) (malignant)
  (nonspecific) D73.89
  malarial B54
  tuberculous A18.85
Splenocele D73.89
Splenomegaly, splenomegalia (Bengal)
  (cryptogenic) (idiopathic) (tropical)
  R16.1
  with hepatomegaly R16.2
  cirrhotic D73.2
  congenital Q89.09
  congestive, chronic D73.2
  Egyptian B65.1
  Gaucher's E75.22
  malarial (see also Malaria) B54 [D77]
  neutropenic D73.81

Splenomegaly, splenomegalia
  (Continued)
  Niemann-Pick —see Niemann-Pick
    disease or syndrome
  siderotic D73.2
  syphilitic A52.79
    congenital (early) A50.08 [D77]
Splenopathy D73.9
Splenoptosis D73.89
Splenosis D73.89
Splinter —see Foreign body, superficial,
  by site
Split, splitting
  foot Q72.7-
  heart sounds R01.2
  lip, congenital —see Cleft, lip
  nails L60.3
  urinary stream R39.13
Spondylarthrosis —see Spondylosis
Spondylitis (chronic) —see also
  Spondylopathy, inflammatory
  ankylopoietica —see Spondylitis,
    ankylosing
  ankylosing (chronic) M45.9
    with lung involvement M45.9 [J99]
    cervical region M45.2
    cervicothoracic region M45.3
    juvenile M08.1
    lumbar region M45.6
    lumbosacral region M45.7
    multiple sites M45.0
    occipito-atlanto-axial region M45.1
    sacrococcygeal region M45.8
    thoracic region M45.4
    thoracolumbar region M45.5
  atrophic (ligamentous) —see
    Spondylitis, ankylosing
  deformans (chronic) —see Spondylosis
  gonococcal A54.41
  gouty M10.08
  in (due to)
    brucellosis A23.9 [M49.80]
     cervical region A23.9 [M49.82]
     cervicothoracic region A23.9
      [M49.83]
     lumbar region A23.9 [M49.86]
     lumbosacral region A23.9
      [M49.87]
     multiple sites A23.9 [M49.89]
     occipito-atlanto-axial region A23.9
      [M49.81]
     sacrococcygeal region A23.9
      [M49.88]
     thoracic region A23.9 [M49.84]
     thoracolumbar region A23.9
      [M49.85]
    enterobacteria (see also subcategory
     M49.8) A04.9
    tuberculosis A18.01
  infectious NEC —see Spondylopathy,
    infective
  juvenile ankylosing (chronic) M08.1
  Kümmell's —see Spondylopathy,
    traumatic
  Marie-Strümpell —see Spondylitis,
    ankylosing
  muscularis —see Spondylopathy,
    specified NEC
  psoriatic L40.53
  rheumatoid —see Spondylitis,
    ankylosing
  rhizomelica —see Spondylitis,
    ankylosing
  sacroiliac NEC M46.1

Spondylitis (*Continued*)
  senescent, senile —*see* Spondylosis
  traumatic (chronic) or post-traumatic —
      see Spondylopathy, traumatic
  tuberculous A18.01
  typhosa A01.05
Spondylolisthesis (acquired)
      (degenerative) M43.10
  with disproportion (fetopelvic)
      O33.0
    causing obstructed labor O65.0
  cervical region M43.12
  cervicothoracic region M43.13
  congenital Q76.2
  lumbar region M43.16
  lumbosacral region M43.17
  multiple sites M43.19
  occipito-atlanto-axial region M43.11
  sacrococcygeal region M43.18
  thoracic region M43.14
  thoracolumbar region M43.15
  traumatic (old) M43.10
    acute
      fifth cervical (displaced) S12.430
        nondisplaced S12.431
        specified type NEC (displaced)
          S12.450
          nondisplaced S12.451
        type III S12.44
      fourth cervical (displaced)
          S12.330
        nondisplaced S12.331
        specified type NEC (displaced)
          S12.350
          nondisplaced S12.351
        type III S12.34
      second cervical (displaced)
          S12.130
        nondisplaced S12.131
        specified type NEC (displaced)
          S12.150
          nondisplaced S12.151
        type III S12.14
      seventh cervical (displaced) S12.630
        nondisplaced S12.631
        specified type NEC (displaced)
          S12.650
          nondisplaced S12.651
        type III S12.64
      sixth cervical (displaced) S12.530
        nondisplaced S12.531
        specified type NEC (displaced)
          S12.550
          nondisplaced S12.551
        type III S12.54
      third cervical (displaced)
          S12.230
        nondisplaced S12.231
        specified type NEC (displaced)
          S12.250
          nondisplaced S12.251
        type III S12.24
Spondylolysis (acquired) M43.00
  cervical region M43.02
  cervicothoracic region M43.03
  congenital Q76.2
  lumbar region M43.06
  lumbosacral region M43.07
    with disproportion (fetopelvic)
        O33.0
      causing obstructed labor O65.8
  multiple sites M43.09
  occipito-atlanto-axial region M43.01
  sacrococcygeal region M43.08

Spondylolysis (*Continued*)
  thoracic region M43.04
  thoracolumbar region M43.05
Spondylopathy M48.9
  infective NEC M46.50
    cervical region M46.52
    cervicothoracic region M46.53
    lumbar region M46.56
    lumbosacral region M46.57
    multiple sites M46.59
    occipito-atlanto-axial region M46.51
    sacrococcygeal region M46.58
    thoracic region M46.54
    thoracolumbar region M46.55
  inflammatory M46.90
    cervical region M46.92
    cervicothoracic region M46.93
    lumbar region M46.96
    lumbosacral region M46.97
    multiple sites M46.99
    occipito-atlanto-axial region M46.91
    sacrococcygeal region M46.98
    specified type NEC M46.80
      cervical region M46.82
      cervicothoracic region
          M46.83
      lumbar region M46.86
      lumbosacral region M46.87
      multiple sites M46.89
      occipito-atlanto-axial region
          M46.81
      sacrococcygeal region M46.88
      thoracic region M46.84
      thoracolumbar region M46.85
    thoracic region M46.94
    thoracolumbar region M46.95
  neuropathic, in
    syringomyelia and syringobulbia
        G95.0
    tabes dorsalis A52.11
  specified NEC —*see* subcategory M48.8
  traumatic M48.30
    cervical region M48.32
    cervicothoracic region M48.33
    lumbar region M48.36
    lumbosacral region M48.37
    occipito-atlanto-axial region
        M48.31
    sacrococcygeal region M48.38
    thoracic region M48.34
    thoracolumbar region M48.35
Spondylosis M47.9
  with
    disproportion (fetopelvic) O33.0
      causing obstructed labor O65.0
    myelopathy NEC M47.10
      cervical region M47.12
      cervicothoracic region M47.13
      lumbar region M47.16
      lumbosacral region M47.17
      occipito-atlanto-axial region
          M47.11
      sacrococcygeal region M47.18
      thoracic region M47.14
      thoracolumbar region M47.15
    radiculopathy M47.20
      cervical region M47.22
      cervicothoracic region M47.23
      lumbar region M47.26
      lumbosacral region M47.27
      occipito-atlanto-axial region M47.21
      sacrococcygeal region M47.28
      thoracic region M47.24
      thoracolumbar region M47.25

Spondylosis (*Continued*)
  without myelopathy or radiculopathy
      M47.819
    cervical region M47.812
    cervicothoracic region M47.813
    lumbar region M47.816
    lumbosacral region M47.817
    occipito-atlanto-axial region
        M47.811
    sacrococcygeal region M47.818
    thoracic region M47.814
    thoracolumbar region M47.815
  specified NEC M47.899
    cervical region M47.892
    cervicothoracic region M47.893
    lumbar region M47.896
    lumbosacral region M47.897
    occipito-atlanto-axial region
        M47.891
    sacrococcygeal region M47.898
    thoracic region M47.894
    thoracolumbar region M47.895
  traumatic —*see* Spondylopathy,
      traumatic
Sponge
  inadvertently left in operation
      wound —*see* Foreign body,
      accidentally left during a
      procedure
  kidney (medullary) Q61.5
Sponge-diver's disease —*see* Toxicity,
    venom, marine animal, sea anemone
Spongioblastoma (any type) —*see*
    Neoplasm, malignant, by site
  specified site —*see* Neoplasm,
    malignant, by site
  unspecified site C71.9
Spongioneuroblastoma —*see* Neoplasm,
    malignant, by site
Spontaneous —*see also* condition
  fracture (cause unknown) —*see*
      Fracture, pathological
Spoon nail L60.3
  congenital Q84.6
Sporadic —*see* condition
Sporothrix schenckii infection —*see*
    Sporotrichosis
Sporotrichosis B42.9
  arthritis B42.82
  disseminated B42.7
  generalized B42.7
  lymphocutaneous (fixed) (progressive)
      B42.1
  pulmonary B42.0
  specified NEC B42.89
Spots, spotting (in) (of)
  Bitot's —*see also* Pigmentation,
    conjunctiva
    in the young child E50.1
    vitamin A deficiency E50.1
  café, au lait L81.3
  Cayenne pepper I78.1
  cotton wool, retina —*see* Occlusion,
    artery, retina
  de Morgan's (senile angiomas) I78.1
  Fuchs' black (myopic) H44.2-
  intermenstrual (regular) N92.0
    irregular N92.1
  Koplik's B05.9
  liver L81.4
  pregnancy O26.85-
  purpuric R23.3
  ruby I78.1
Spotted fever (*see* Fever, spotted) N92.3

Sprain (joint) (ligament)
  acromioclavicular joint or ligament S43.5-
  ankle S93.40-
    calcaneofibular ligament S93.41-
    deltoid ligament S93.42-
    internal collateral ligament —*see* Sprain, ankle, specified ligament NEC
    specified ligament NEC S93.49-
    talofibular ligament —*see* Sprain, ankle, specified ligament NEC
    tibiofibular ligament S93.43-
  anterior longitudinal, cervical S13.4
  atlas, atlanto-axial, atlanto-occipital S13.4
  breast bone —*see* Sprain, sternum
  calcaneofibular —*see* Sprain, ankle
  carpal —*see* Sprain, wrist
  carpometacarpal —*see* Sprain, hand, specified site NEC
  cartilage
    costal S23.41
    semilunar (knee) —*see* Sprain, knee, specified site NEC
      with current tear —*see* Tear, meniscus
    thyroid region S13.5
    xiphoid —*see* Sprain, sternum
  cervical, cervicodorsal, cervicothoracic S13.4
  chondrosternal S23.421
  coracoclavicular S43.8-
  coracohumeral S43.41-
  coronary, knee —*see* Sprain, knee, specified site NEC
  costal cartilage S23.41
  cricoarytenoid articulation or ligament S13.5
  cricothyroid articulation S13.5
  cruciate, knee —*see* Sprain, knee, cruciate
  deltoid, ankle —*see* Sprain, ankle
  dorsal (spine) S23.3
  elbow S53.40-
    radial collateral ligament S53.43-
    radiohumeral S53.41-
    rupture
      radial collateral ligament —*see* Rupture, traumatic, ligament, radial collateral
      ulnar collateral ligament —*see* Rupture, traumatic, ligament, ulnar collateral
    specified type NEC S53.49-
    ulnar collateral ligament S53.44-
    ulnohumeral S53.42-
  femur, head —*see* Sprain, hip
  fibular collateral, knee —*see* Sprain, knee, collateral
  fibulocalcaneal —*see* Sprain, ankle
  finger (s) S63.61-
    index S63.61-
    interphalangeal (joint) S63.63-
      index S63.63-
      little S63.63-
      middle S63.63-
      ring S63.63-
    little S63.61-
    metacarpophalangeal (joint) S63.65-
    middle S63.61-
    ring S63.61-

Sprain (Continued)
  finger (s) (Continued)
    specified site NEC S63.69-
      index S63.69-
      little S63.69-
      middle S63.69-
      ring S63.69-
  foot S93.60-
    specified ligament NEC S93.69-
    tarsal ligament S93.61-
    tarsometatarsal ligament S93.62-
    toe —*see* Sprain, toe
  hand S63.9-
    finger —*see* Sprain, finger
    specified site NEC —*see* subcategory S63.8
    thumb —*see* Sprain, thumb
  head S03.9
  hip S73.10-
    iliofemoral ligament S73.11-
    ischiocapsular (ligament) S73.12-
    specified NEC S73.19-
  iliofemoral —*see* Sprain, hip
  innominate
    acetabulum —*see* Sprain, hip
    sacral junction S33.6
  internal
    collateral, ankle —*see* Sprain, ankle
    semilunar cartilage —*see* Sprain, knee, specified site NEC
  interphalangeal
    finger —*see* Sprain, finger, interphalangeal (joint)
    toe —*see* Sprain, toe, interphalangeal joint
  ischiocapsular —*see* Sprain, hip
  ischiofemoral —*see* Sprain, hip
  jaw (articular disc) (cartilage) (meniscus) S03.4
    old M26.69
  knee S83.9-
    collateral ligament S83.40-
      lateral (fibular) S83.42-
      medial (tibial) S83.41-
    cruciate ligament S83.50-
      anterior S83.51-
      posterior S83.52-
    lateral (fibular) collateral ligament S83.42-
    medial (tibial) collateral ligament S83.41-
    patellar ligament S76.11-
    specified site NEC S83.8X-
    superior tibiofibular joint (ligament) S83.6-
  lateral collateral, knee —*see* Sprain, knee, collateral
  lumbar (spine) S33.5
  lumbosacral S33.9
  mandible (articular disc) S03.4
    old M26.69
  medial collateral, knee —*see* Sprain, knee, collateral
  meniscus
    jaw S03.4
      old M26.69
    knee —*see* Sprain, knee, specified site NEC
      with current tear —*see* Tear, meniscus
      old —*see* Derangement, knee, meniscus, due to old tear
    mandible S03.4
      old M26.69

Sprain (Continued)
  metacarpal (distal) (proximal) —*see* Sprain, hand, specified site NEC
  metacarpophalangeal —*see* Sprain, finger, metacarpophalangeal (joint)
  metatarsophalangeal —*see* Sprain, toe, metatarsophalangeal joint
  midcarpal —*see* Sprain, hand, specified site NEC
  midtarsal —*see* Sprain, foot, specified site NEC
  neck S13.9
    anterior longitudinal cervical ligament S13.4
    atlanto-axial joint S13.4
    atlanto-occipital joint S13.4
    cervical spine S13.4
    cricoarytenoid ligament S13.5
    cricothyroid ligament S13.5
    specified site NEC S13.8
    thyroid region (cartilage) S13.5
  nose S03.8
  orbicular, hip —*see* Sprain, hip
  patella —*see* Sprain, knee, specified site NEC
  patellar ligament S76.11-
  pelvis NEC S33.8
  phalanx
    finger —*see* Sprain, finger
    toe —*see* Sprain, toe
  pubofemoral —*see* Sprain, hip
  radiocarpal —*see* Sprain, wrist
  radiohumeral —*see* Sprain, elbow
  radius, collateral —*see* Rupture, traumatic, ligament, radial collateral
  rib (cage) S23.41
  rotator cuff (capsule) S43.42-
  sacroiliac (region)
    chronic or old —*see* subcategory M53.2
    joint S33.6
  scaphoid (hand) —*see* Sprain, hand, specified site NEC
  scapula (r) —*see* Sprain, shoulder girdle, specified site NEC
  semilunar cartilage (knee) —*see* Sprain, knee, specified site NEC
    with current tear —*see* Tear, meniscus
    old —*see* Derangement, knee, meniscus, due to old tear
  shoulder joint S43.40-
    acromioclavicular joint (ligament) —*see* Sprain, acromioclavicular joint
    blade —*see* Sprain, shoulder, girdle, specified site NEC
    coracoclavicular joint (ligament) —*see* Sprain, coracoclavicular joint
    coracohumeral ligament —*see* Sprain, coracohumeral joint
    girdle S43.9-
      specified site NEC S43.8-
    rotator cuff —*see* Sprain, rotator cuff
    specified site NEC S43.49-
    sternoclavicular joint (ligament) —*see* Sprain, sternoclavicular joint
  spine
    cervical S13.4
    lumbar S33.5
    thoracic S23.3
  sternoclavicular joint S43.6-

Sprain *(Continued)*
  sternum S23.429
    chondrosternal joint S23.421
    specified site NEC S23.428
    sternoclavicular (joint) (ligament)
      S23.420
  symphysis
    jaw S03.4
      old M26.69
    mandibular S03.4
      old M26.69
  talofibular —*see* Sprain, ankle
  tarsal —*see* Sprain, foot, specified site
    NEC
  tarsometatarsal —*see* Sprain, foot,
    specified site NEC
  temporomandibular S03.4
    old M26.69
  thorax S23.9
    ribs S23.41
    specified site NEC S23.8
    spine S23.3
    sternum —*see* Sprain, sternum
  thumb S63.60-
    interphalangeal (joint) S63.62-
    metacarpophalangeal (joint)
      S63.64-
    specified site NEC S63.68-
  thyroid cartilage or region S13.5
  tibia (proximal end) —*see* Sprain, knee,
    specified site NEC
  tibial collateral, knee —*see* Sprain, knee,
    collateral
  tibiofibular
    distal —*see* Sprain, ankle
    superior —*see* Sprain, knee, specified
      site NEC
  toe (s) S93.50-
    great S93.50-
    interphalangeal joint S93.51-
      great S93.51-
      lesser S93.51-
    lesser S93.50-
    metatarsophalangeal joint
      S93.52-
      great S93.52-
      lesser S93.52-
  ulna, collateral —*see* Rupture,
    traumatic, ligament, ulnar
    collateral
  ulnohumeral —*see* Sprain, elbow
  wrist S63.50-
    carpal S63.51-
    radiocarpal S63.52-
    specified site NEC S63.59-
  xiphoid cartilage —*see* Sprain,
    sternum
Sprengel's deformity (congenital)
  Q74.0
Sprue (tropical) K90.1
  celiac K90.0
  idiopathic K90.0
  meaning thrush B37.0
  nontropical K90.0
Spur, bone —*see also* Enthesopathy
  calcaneal M77.3-
  iliac crest M76.2-
  nose (septum) J34.89
Spurway's syndrome Q78.0
Sputum
  abnormal (amount) (color) (odor)
    (purulent) R09.3
  blood-stained R04.2
  excessive (cause unknown) R09.3

Squamous —*see also* condition
  epithelium in
    cervical canal (congenital)
      Q51.828
    uterine mucosa (congenital)
      Q51.818
Squashed nose M95.0
  congenital Q67.4
Squeeze, diver's T70.3
Squint —*see also* Strabismus
  accommodative —*see* Strabismus,
    convergent concomitant
St. Hubert's disease A82.9
Stab —*see also* Laceration
  internal organs —*see* Injury, by site
Stafne's cyst or cavity M27.0
Staggering gait R26.0
  hysterical F44.4
Staghorn calculus —*see* Calculus,
  kidney
Stähli's line (cornea) (pigment) —*see*
  Pigmentation, cornea, anterior
Stain, staining
  meconium (newborn) P96.83
  port wine Q82.5
  tooth, teeth (hard tissues) (extrinsic)
    K03.6
    due to
      accretions K03.6
      deposits (betel) (black) (green)
        (materia alba) (orange) (soft)
        (tobacco) K03.6
      metals (copper) (silver) K03.7
      nicotine K03.6
      pulpal bleeding K03.7
      tobacco K03.6
    intrinsic K00.8
Stammering (*see also* Disorder, fluency)
  F80.81
Standstill
  auricular I45.5
  cardiac —*see* Arrest, cardiac
  sinoatrial I45.5
  ventricular —*see* Arrest, cardiac
Stannosis J63.5
Stanton's disease —*see* Melioidosis
Staphylitis (acute) (catarrhal)
  (chronic) (gangrenous)
  (membranous) (suppurative)
  (ulcerative) K12.2
Staphylococcal scalded skin syndrome
  L00
Staphylococcemia A41.2
Staphylococcus, staphylococcal —*see also*
  condition
  as cause of disease classified elsewhere
    B95.8
  aureus (methicillin susceptible)
    (MSSA) B95.61
    methicillin resistant (MRSA)
      B95.62
  specified NEC, as cause of disease
    classified elsewhere B95.7
Staphyloma (sclera)
  cornea H18.72-
  equatorial H15.81-
  localized (anterior) H15.82-
  posticum H15.83-
  ring H15.85-
Stargardt's disease —*see* Dystrophy,
  retina
Starvation (inanition) (due to lack of
  food) T73.0
  edema —*see* Malnutrition, severe

Stasis
  bile (noncalculous) K83.1
  bronchus J98.09
    with infection —*see* Bronchitis
  cardiac —*see* Failure, heart, congestive
  cecum K59.8
  colon K59.8
  dermatitis —*see* Varix, leg, with,
    inflammation
  duodenal K31.5
  eczema —*see* Varix, leg, with,
    inflammation
  edema —*see* Hypertension, venous
    (chronic), idiopathic
  foot T69.0-
  ileocecal coil K59.8
  ileum K59.8
  intestinal K59.8
  jejunum K59.8
  kidney N19
  liver (cirrhotic) K76.1
  lymphatic I89.8
  pneumonia J18.2
  pulmonary —*see* Edema, lung
  rectal K59.8
  renal N19
    tubular N17.0
  ulcer —*see* Varix, leg, with, ulcer
    without varicose veins I87.2
  urine —*see* Retention, urine
  venous I87.8
State (of)
  affective and paranoid, mixed, organic
    psychotic F06.8
  agitated R45.1
    acute reaction to stress F43.0
  anxiety (neurotic) F41.1
  apprehension F41.1
  burn-out Z73.0
  climacteric, female Z78.0
    symptomatic N95.1
  compulsive F42
    mixed with obsessional thoughts F42
  confusional (psychogenic) F44.89
    acute —*see also* Delirium
      with
        arteriosclerotic dementia F01.50
          with behavioral disturbance
            F01.51
        senility or dementia F05
      alcoholic F10.231
      epileptic F05
    reactive (from emotional stress,
      psychological trauma) F44.89
    subacute —*see* Delirium
  convulsive —*see* Convulsions
  crisis F43.0
  depressive F32.9
    neurotic F34.1
  dissociative F44.9
  emotional shock (stress) R45.7
  hypercoagulation —*see*
    Hypercoagulable
  locked-in G83.5
  menopausal Z78.0
    symptomatic N95.1
  neurotic F48.9
    with depersonalization F48.1
  obsessional F42
  oneiroid (schizophrenia-like) F23
  organic
    hallucinatory (nonalcoholic) F06.0
    paranoid (-hallucinatory) F06.2
  panic F41.0

State(of) (Continued)
  paranoid F22
    climacteric F22
    involutional F22
    menopausal F22
    organic F06.2
    senile F03
    simple F22
  persistent vegetative R40.3
  phobic F40.9
  postleukotomy F07.0
  pregnant, incidental Z33.1
  psychogenic, twilight F44.89
  psychopathic (constitutional) F60.2
  psychotic, organic —see also Psychosis,
      organic
    mixed paranoid and affective F06.8
    senile or presenile F03
    transient NEC F06.8
      with
        depression F06.31
        hallucinations F06.0
  residual schizophrenic F20.5
  restlessness R45.1
  stress (emotional) R45.7
  tension (mental) F48.9
    specified NEC F48.8
  transient organic psychotic NEC
      F06.8
    depressive type F06.31
    hallucinatory type F06.30
  twilight
    epileptic F05
    psychogenic F44.89
  vegetative, persistent R40.3
  vital exhaustion Z73.0
  withdrawal —see Withdrawal, state
Status(post) —see also Presence (of)
  absence, epileptic —see Epilepsy, by
      type, with status epilepticus
  administration of tPA (rtPA) in a
      different facility within the last
      24 hours prior to admission to the
      current facility Z92.82
  adrenalectomy (unilateral) (bilateral)
      E89.6
  anastomosis Z98.0
  anginosus I20.9
  angioplasty (peripheral) Z98.62
    with implant Z95.820
    coronary artery Z98.61
      with implant Z95.5
  aortocoronary bypass Z95.1
  arthrodesis Z98.1
  artificial opening (of) Z93.9
    gastrointestinal tract Z93.4
    specified NEC Z93.8
    urinary tract Z93.6
    vagina Z93.8
  asthmaticus —see Asthma, by type,
      with status asthmaticus
  awaiting organ transplant Z76.82
  bariatric surgery Z98.84
  bed confinement Z74.01
  bleb, filtering (vitreous), after glaucoma
      surgery Z98.83
  breast implant Z98.82
    removal Z98.86
  cataract extraction Z98.4-
  cholecystectomy Z90.49
  clitorectomy N90.811
    with excision of labia minora N90.812
  colectomy (complete) (partial) Z90.49
  colonization —see Carrier (suspected) of

Status(Continued)
  colostomy Z93.3
  convulsivus idiopathicus —see Epilepsy,
      by type, with status epilepticus
  coronary artery angioplasty —see
      Status, angioplasty, coronary
      artery
  cystectomy (urinary bladder) Z90.6
  cystostomy Z93.50
    appendico-vesicostomy Z93.52
    cutaneous Z93.51
    specified NEC Z93.59
  delinquent immunization Z28.3
  dental Z98.818
    crown Z98.811
    fillings Z98.811
    restoration Z98.811
    sealant Z98.810
    specified NEC Z98.818
  deployment (current) (military) Z56.82
  dialysis (hemodialysis) (peritoneal) Z99.2
  do not resuscitate (DNR) Z66
  donor —see Donor
  embedded fragments —see Retained,
      foreign body fragments (type of)
  embedded splinter —see Retained,
      foreign body fragments (type of)
  enterostomy Z93.4
  epileptic, epilepticus (see also Epilepsy,
      by type, with status epilepticus)
      G40.901
  estrogen receptor
    negative Z17.0
    positive Z17.1
  female genital cutting —see Female
      genital mutilation status
  female genital mutilation —see Female
      genital mutilation status
  filtering (vitreous) bleb after glaucoma
      surgery Z98.83
  gastrectomy (complete) (partial) Z90.3
  gastric banding Z98.84
  gastric bypass for obesity Z98.84
  gastrostomy Z93.1
  human immunodeficiency virus (HIV)
      infection, asymptomatic Z21
  hysterectomy (complete) (total) Z90.710
    partial (with remaining cervial
        stump) Z90.711
  ileostomy Z93.2
  implant
    breast Z98.82
  infibulation N90.813
  intestinal bypass Z98.0
  jejunostomy Z93.4
  lapsed immunization schedule Z28.3
  laryngectomy Z90.02
  lymphaticus E32.8
  marmoratus G80.3
  mastectomy (unilateral) (bilateral)
      Z90.1-
  military deployment status (current)
      Z56.82
    in theater or in support of military
        war, peacekeeping and
        humanitarian operations
        Z56.82
  nephrectomy (unilateral) (bilateral)
      Z90.5
  nephrostomy Z93.6
  obesity surgery Z98.84
  oophorectomy
    bilateral Z90.722
    unilateral Z90.721

Status(Continued)
  organ replacement
    by artificial or mechanical device or
        prosthesis of
      artery Z95.828
      bladder Z96.0
      blood vessel Z95.828
      breast Z97.8
      eye globe Z97.0
      heart Z95.812
        valve Z95.2
      intestine Z97.8
      joint Z96.60
        hip —see Presence, hip joint
            implant
        knee —see Presence, knee joint
            implant
        specified site NEC Z96.698
      kidney Z97.8
      larynx Z96.3
      lens Z96.1
      limbs —see Presence, artificial, limb
      liver Z97.8
      lung Z97.8
      pancreas Z97.8
    by organ transplant (heterologous)
        (homologous) —see Transplant
  pacemaker
    brain Z96.89
    cardiac Z95.0
    specified NEC Z96.89
  pancreatectomy Z90.410
    complete Z90.410
    partial Z90.411
    total Z90.410
  pneumonectomy (complete) (partial)
      Z90.2
  pneumothorax, therapeutic Z98.3
  postcommotio cerebri F07.81
  postoperative (postprocedural) NEC
      Z98.89
    breast implant Z98.82
    dental Z98.818
      crown Z98.811
      fillings Z98.811
      restoration Z98.811
      sealant Z98.810
      specified NEC Z98.818
    pneumothorax, therapeutic Z98.3
  postpartum (routine follow-up) Z39.2
    care immediately after delivery Z39.0
  postsurgical (postprocedural) NEC
      Z98.89
    pneumothorax, therapeutic Z98.3
  pregnancy, incidental Z33.1
  prosthesis coronary angioplasty Z95.5
  pseudophakia Z96.1
  renal dialysis (hemodialysis)
      (peritoneal) Z99.2
  retained foreign body —see Retained,
      foreign body fragments (type of)
  reversed jejunal transposition (for
      bypass Z98.0
  salpingo-oophorectomy
    bilateral Z90.722
    unilateral Z90.721
  sex reassignment surgery status Z87.890
  shunt
    arteriovenous (for dialysis) Z99.2
    cerebrospinal fluid Z98.2
    ventricular (communicating) (for
        drainage) Z98.2
  splenectomy Z90.81
  thymicolymphaticus E32.8
  thymicus E32.8

S

Status (Continued)
  thymolymphaticus E32.8
  thyroidectomy (hypothyroidism) E89.0
  tooth (teeth) extraction (see also
    Absence, teeth, acquired) K08.409
  tPA (rtPA) administration in a different
    facility within the last 24 hours
    prior to admission to current
    facility Z92.82
  tracheostomy Z93.0
  transplant —see Transplant
    organ removed Z98.85
  tubal ligation Z98.51
  underimmunization Z28.3
  ureterostomy Z93.6
  urethrostomy Z93.6
  vagina, artificial Z93.8
  vasectomy Z98.52
  wheelchair confinement Z99.3
Stealing
  child problem F91.8
    in company with others Z72.810
  pathological (compulsive) F63.2
Steam burn —see Burn
Steatocystoma multiplex L72.2
Steatohepatitis (nonalcoholic) (NASH)
  K75.81
Steatoma L72.3
  eyelid (cystic) —see Dermatosis, eyelid
    infected —see Hordeolum
Steatorrhea (chronic) K90.4
  with lacteal obstruction K90.2
  idiopathic (adult) (infantile) K90.0
  pancreatic K90.3
  primary K90.0
  tropical K90.1
Steatosis E88.89
  heart —see Degeneration, myocardial
  kidney N28.89
  liver NEC K76.0
Steele-Richardson-Olszewski disease or
  syndrome G23.1
Steinbrocker's syndrome G90.8
Steinert's disease G71.11
Stein-Leventhal syndrome E28.2
Stein's syndrome E28.2
STEMI (see also - Infarct, myocardium, ST
  elevation) I21.3
Stenocardia I20.8
Stenocephaly Q75.8
Stenosis, stenotic (cicatricial) —see also
  Stricture
  ampulla of Vater K83.1
  anus, anal (canal) (sphincter) K62.4
    and rectum K62.4
    congenital Q42.3
      with fistula Q42.2
  aorta (ascending) (supraventricular)
    (congenital) Q25.3
    arteriosclerotic I70.0
    calcified I70.0
  aortic (valve) I35.0
    with insufficiency I35.2
    congenital Q23.0
    rheumatic I06.0
      with
        incompetency, insufficiency or
          regurgitation I06.2
          with mitral (valve) disease I08.0
            with tricuspid (valve)
              disease I08.3
        mitral (valve) disease I08.0
          with tricuspid (valve) disease
            I08.3

Stenosis, stenotic (Continued)
  aortic (Continued)
    rheumatic (Continued)
      with (Continued)
        tricuspid (valve) disease I08.2
          with mitral (valve) disease
            I08.3
    specified cause NEC I35.0
    syphilitic A52.03
  aqueduct of Sylvius (congenital) Q03.0
    with spina bifida —see Spina bifida,
      by site, with hydrocephalus
    acquired G91.1
  artery NEC (see also Arteriosclerosis) I77.1
    celiac I77.4
    cerebral —see Occlusion, artery,
      cerebral
    extremities —see Arteriosclerosis,
      extremities
    precerebral —see Occlusion, artery,
      precerebral
    pulmonary (congenital) Q25.6
      acquired I28.8
    renal I70.1
  bile duct (common) (hepatic) K83.1
    congenital Q44.3
  bladder-neck (acquired) N32.0
    congenital Q64.31
  brain G93.89
  bronchus J98.09
    congenital Q32.3
    syphilitic A52.72
  cardia (stomach) K22.2
    congenital Q39.3
  cardiovascular —see Disease,
    cardiovascular
  caudal M48.08
  cervix, cervical (canal) N88.2
    congenital Q51.828
    in pregnancy or childbirth —see
      Pregnancy, complicated by,
      abnormal cervix
  colon —see also Obstruction, intestine
    congenital Q42.9
      specified NEC Q42.8
  colostomy K94.03
  common (bile) duct K83.1
    congenital Q44.3
  coronary (artery) —see Disease, heart,
    ischemic, atherosclerotic
  cystic duct —see Obstruction,
    gallbladder
  due to presence of device, implant
    or graft (see also Complications,
    by site and type, specified NEC)
    T85.85
    arterial graft NEC T82.858
    breast (implant) T85.85
    catheter T85.85
      dialysis (renal) T82.858
        intraperitoneal T85.85
      infusion NEC T82.858
        spinal (epidural) (subdural)
          T85.85
      urinary (indwelling) T83.85
    fixation, internal (orthopedic) NEC
      T84.85
    gastrointestinal (bile duct)
      (esophagus) T85.85
    genital NEC T83.85
    heart NEC T82.857
    joint prosthesis T84.85
    ocular (corneal graft) (orbital
      implant) NEC T85.85

Stenosis, stenotic (Continued)
  due to presence of device, implant or
    graft (Continued)
    orthopedic NEC T84.85
    specified NEC T85.85
    urinary NEC T83.85
    vascular NEC T82.858
    ventricular intracranial shunt
      T85.85
  duodenum K31.5
    congenital Q41.0
  ejaculatory duct NEC N50.8
  endocervical os —see Stenosis, cervix
  enterostomy K94.13
  esophagus K22.2
    congenital Q39.3
    syphilitic A52.79
      congenital A50.59 [K23]
  eustachian tube —see Obstruction,
    eustachian tube
  external ear canal (acquired) H61.30-
    congenital Q16.1
    due to
      inflammation H61.32-
      trauma H61.31-
    postprocedural H95.81-
    specified cause NEC H61.39-
  gallbladder —see Obstruction,
    gallbladder
  glottis J38.6
  heart valve (congenital) Q24.8
    aortic Q23.0
    mitral Q23.2
    pulmonary Q22.1
    tricuspid Q22.4
  hepatic duct K83.1
  hymen N89.6
  hypertrophic subaortic (idiopathic)
    I42.1
  ileum K56.69
    congenital Q41.2
  infundibulum cardia Q24.3
  intervertebral foramina —see also
    Lesion, biomechanical, specified
    NEC
    connective tissue M99.79
      abdomen M99.79
      cervical region M99.71
      cervicothoracic M99.71
      head region M99.70
      lumbar region M99.73
      lumbosacral M99.73
      occipitocervical M99.70
      sacral region M99.74
      sacrococcygeal M99.74
      sacroiliac M99.74
      specified NEC M99.79
      thoracic region M99.72
      thoracolumbar M99.72
    disc M99.79
      abdomen M99.79
      cervical region M99.71
      cervicothoracic M99.71
      head region M99.70
      lower extremity M99.76
      lumbar region M99.73
      lumbosacral M99.73
      occipitocervical M99.70
      pelvic M99.75
      rib cage M99.78
      sacral region M99.74
      sacrococcygeal M99.74
      sacroiliac M99.74
      specified NEC M99.79

Stenosis, stenotic (Continued)
  intervertebral foramina (Continued)
    disc (Continued)
      thoracic region M99.72
      thoracolumbar M99.72
      upper extremity M99.77
    osseous M99.69
      abdomen M99.69
      cervical region M99.61
      cervicothoracic M99.61
      head region M99.60
      lower extremity M99.66
      lumbar region M99.63
      lumbosacral M99.63
      occipitocervical M99.60
      pelvic M99.65
      rib cage M99.68
      sacral region M99.64
      sacrococcygeal M99.64
      sacroiliac M99.64
      specified NEC M99.69
      thoracic region M99.62
      thoracolumbar M99.62
      upper extremity M99.67
    subluxation —see Stenosis,
      intervertebral foramina, osseous
  intestine —see also Obstruction,
    intestine
    congenital (small) Q41.9
      large Q42.9
        specified NEC Q42.8
      specified NEC Q41.8
  jejunum K56.69
    congenital Q41.1
  lacrimal (passage)
    canaliculi H04.54-
    congenital Q10.5
    duct H04.55-
    punctum H04.56-
    sac H04.57-
  lacrimonasal duct —see Stenosis,
    lacrimal, duct
    congenital Q10.5
  larynx J38.6
    congenital NEC Q31.8
      subglottic Q31.1
    syphilitic A52.73
      congenital A50.59 [J99]
  mitral (chronic) (inactive) (valve) I05.0
    with
      aortic valve disease I08.0
      incompetency, insufficiency or
        regurgitation I05.2
    active or acute I01.1
      with rheumatic or Sydenham's
        chorea I02.0
    congenital Q23.2
    specified cause, except rheumatic
      I34.2
    syphilitic A52.03
  myocardium, myocardial —see also
    Degeneration, myocardial
    hypertrophic subaortic (idiopathic)
      I42.1
  nares (anterior) (posterior) J34.89
    congenital Q30.0
  nasal duct —see also Stenosis, lacrimal,
    duct
    congenital Q10.5
  nasolacrimal duct —see also Stenosis,
    lacrimal, duct
    congenital Q10.5
  neural canal —see also Lesion,
    biomechanical, specified NEC

Stenosis, stenotic (Continued)
  neural canal (Continued)
    connective tissue M99.49
      abdomen M99.49
      cervical region M99.41
      cervicothoracic M99.41
      head region M99.40
      lower extremity M99.46
      lumbar region M99.43
      lumbosacral M99.43
      occipitocervical M99.40
      pelvic M99.45
      rib cage M99.48
      sacral region M99.44
      sacrococcygeal M99.44
      sacroiliac M99.44
      specified NEC M99.49
      thoracic region M99.42
      thoracolumbar M99.42
      upper extremity M99.47
    intervertebral disc M99.59
      abdomen M99.59
      cervical region M99.51
      cervicothoracic M99.51
      head region M99.50
      lower extremity M99.56
      lumbar region M99.53
      lumbosacral M99.53
      occipitocervical M99.50
      pelvic M99.55
      rib cage M99.58
      sacral region M99.54
      sacrococcygeal M99.54
      sacroiliac M99.54
      specified NEC M99.59
      thoracic region M99.52
      thoracolumbar M99.52
      upper extremity M99.57
    osseous M99.39
      abdomen M99.39
      cervical region M99.31
      cervicothoracic M99.31
      head region M99.30
      lower extremity M99.36
      lumbar region M99.33
      lumbosacral M99.33
      occipitocervical M99.30
      pelvic M99.35
      rib cage M99.38
      sacral region M99.34
      sacrococcygeal M99.34
      sacroiliac M99.34
      specified NEC M99.39
      thoracic region M99.32
      thoracolumbar M99.32
      upper extremity M99.37
    subluxation M99.29
      cervical region M99.21
      cervicothoracic M99.21
      head region M99.20
      lower extremity M99.26
      lumbar region M99.23
      lumbosacral M99.23
      occipitocervical M99.20
      pelvic M99.25
      rib cage M99.28
      sacral region M99.24
      sacrococcygeal M99.24
      sacroiliac M99.24
      specified NEC M99.29
      thoracic region M99.22
      thoracolumbar M99.22
      upper extremity M99.27
  oesophagus —see Stenosis, esophagus

Stenosis, stenotic (Continued)
  organ or site, congenital NEC —see
    Atresia, by site
  papilla of Vater K83.1
  pulmonary (artery) (congenital) Q25.6
    with ventricular septal defect,
      transposition of aorta, and
      hypertrophy of right ventricle
      Q21.3
    acquired I28.8
    in tetralogy of Fallot Q21.3
    infundibular Q24.3
    subvalvular Q24.3
    supravalvular Q25.6
    valve I37.0
      with insufficiency I37.2
      congenital Q22.1
      rheumatic I09.89
        with aortic, mitral or tricuspid
        (valve) disease I08.8
    vein, acquired I28.8
    vessel NEC I28.8
  pulmonic (congenital) Q22.1
    infundibular Q24.3
    subvalvular Q24.3
  pylorus (hypertrophic) (acquired) K31.1
    adult K31.1
    congenital Q40.0
    infantile Q40.0
  rectum (sphincter) —see Stricture,
    rectum
  renal artery I70.1
    congenital Q27.1
  salivary duct (any) K11.8
  sphincter of Oddi K83.1
  spinal M48.00
    cervical region M48.02
    cervicothoracic region M48.03
    lumbar region M48.06
    lumbosacral region M48.07
    occipito-atlanto-axial region
      M48.01
    sacrococcygeal region M48.08
    thoracic region M48.04
    thoracolumbar region M48.05
  stomach, hourglass K31.2
  subaortic (congenital) Q24.4
    hypertrophic (idiopathic) I42.1
  subglottic J38.6
    congenital Q31.1
    postprocedural J95.5
  trachea J39.8
    congenital Q32.1
    syphilitic A52.73
    tuberculous NEC A15.5
  tracheostomy J95.03
  tricuspid (valve) I07.0
    with
      aortic (valve) disease I08.2
      incompetency, insufficiency or
        regurgitation I07.2
        with aortic (valve) disease I08.2
          with mitral (valve) disease
          I08.3
        mitral (valve) disease I08.1
          with aortic (valve) disease
          I08.3
    congenital Q22.4
    nonrheumatic I36.0
      with insufficiency I36.2
  tubal N97.1
  ureter —see Atresia, ureter
  ureteropelvic junction, congenital
    Q62.11

Stenosis, stenotic *(Continued)*
  ureterovesical orifice, congenital
    Q62.12
  urethra (valve) —*see also* Stricture,
    urethra
    congenital Q64.32
  urinary meatus, congenital Q64.33
  vagina N89.5
    congenital Q52.4
    in pregnancy —*see* Pregnancy,
      complicated by, abnormal
      vagina
      causing obstructed labor O65.5
  valve (cardiac) (heart) (*see also*
    Endocarditis) I38
    congenital Q24.8
      aortic Q23.0
      mitral Q23.2
      pulmonary Q22.1
      tricuspid Q22.4
  vena cava (inferior) (superior) I87.1
    congenital Q26.0
  vesicourethral orifice Q64.31
  vulva N90.5
Stent jail T82.897
Stercolith (impaction) K56.41
  appendix K38.1
Stercoraceous, stercoral ulcer K63.3
  anus or rectum K62.6
Stereotypies NEC F98.4
Sterility —*see* Infertility
Sterilization —*see* Encounter (for),
  sterilization
Sternalgia —*see* Angina
Sternopagus Q89.4
Sternum bifidum Q76.7
Steroid
  effects (adverse) (adrenocortical)
    (iatrogenic)
    cushingoid E24.2
      correct substance properly
        administered —*see* Table of
        drugs and chemicals, by drug,
        adverse effect
      overdose or wrong substance
        given or taken —*see* Table of
        drugs and chemicals, by drug,
        poisoning
    diabetes —*see* category E09
      correct substance properly
        administered – Table of drugs
        and chemicals, by drug,
        adverse effect
      overdose or wrong substance
        given or taken —*see* Table of
        drugs and chemicals, by drug,
        poisoning
    fever R50.2
    insufficiency E27.3
      correct substance properly
        administered —*see* Table of
        drugs and chemicals, by drug,
        adverse effect
      overdose or wrong substance
        given or taken —*see* Table of
        drugs and chemicals, by drug,
        poisoning
  responder H40.04-
Stevens-Johnson disease or syndrome
  L51.1
  toxic epidermal necrolysis overlap
    L51.3
Stewart-Morel syndrome M85.2
Sticker's disease B08.3

Sticky eye —*see* Conjunctivitis, acute,
  mucopurulent
Stieda's disease —*see* Bursitis, tibial
  collateral
Stiff neck —*see* Torticollis
Stiff-man syndrome G25.82
Stiffness, joint NEC M25.60
  ankle M25.67-
  ankylosis —*see* Ankylosis, joint
  contracture —*see* Contraction, joint
  elbow M25.6-
  foot M25.6-
  hand M25.6-
  hip M25.6-
  knee M25.6-
  shoulder M25.1-
  wrist M25.3-
Stigmata congenital syphilis A50.59
Stillbirth P95
Still-Felty syndrome —*see* Felty's
  syndrome
Still's disease or syndrome (juvenile)
  M08.20
  adult-onset M06.1
  ankle M08.27-
  elbow M08.22-
  foot joint M08.27-
  hand joint M08.24-
  hip M08.25-
  knee M08.26-
  multiple site M08.29
  shoulder M08.21-
  vertebra M08.28
  wrist M08.23-
Stimulation, ovary E28.1
Sting (venomous) (with allergic or
  anaphylactic shock) —*see* Table of
  drugs and chemicals, by animal or
  substance, poisoning
Stippled epiphyses Q78.8
Stitch
  abscess T81.4
  burst (in operation wound) —*see*
    Disruption, wound, operation
Stokes-Adams disease or syndrome I45.9
Stokes' disease E05.00
  with thyroid storm E05.01
Stokvis (-Talma) disease D74.8BD>
Stoma malfunction
  colostomy K94.03
  enterostomy K94.13
  gastrostomy K94.23
  ileostomy K94.13
  tracheostomy J95.03
Stomach —*see* condition
Stomatitis (denture) (ulcerative) K12.1
  angular K13.0
    due to dietary or vitamin deficiency
      E53.0
  aphthous K12.0
  bovine B08.61
  candidal B37.0
  catarrhal K12.1
  diphtheritic A36.89
  due to
    dietary deficiency E53.0
    thrush B37.0
    vitamin deficiency
      B group NEC E53.9
      B2 (riboflavin) E53.0
  epidemic B08.8
  epizootic B08.8
  follicular K12.1
  gangrenous A69.0

Stomatitis *(Continued)*
  Geotrichum B48.3
  herpesviral, herpetic B00.2
  herpetiformis K12.0
  malignant K12.1
  membranous acute K12.1
  monilial B37.0
  mycotic B37.0
  necrotizing ulcerative A69.0
  parasitic B37.0
  septic K12.1
  spirochetal A69.1
  suppurative (acute) K12.2
  ulceromembranous A69.1
  vesicular K12.1
    with exanthem (enteroviral) B08.4
    virus disease A93.8
  Vincent's A69.1
Stomatocytosis D58.8
Stomatomycosis B37.0
Stomatorrhagia K13.79
Stone (s) —*see also* Calculus
  bladder (diverticulum) N21.0
  cystine E72.09
  heart syndrome I50.1
  kidney N20.0
  prostate N42.0
  pulpal (dental) K04.2
  renal N20.0
  salivary gland or duct (any) K11.5
  urethra (impacted) N21.1
  urinary (duct) (impacted) (passage)
    N20.9
    bladder (diverticulum) N21.0
    lower tract N21.9
    specified NEC N21.8
  xanthine E79.8 [N22]
Stonecutter's lung J62.8
Stonemason's asthma, disease, lung or
  pneumoconiosis J62.8
Stoppage
  heart —*see* Arrest, cardiac
  urine —*see* Retention, urine
Storm, thyroid —*see* Thyrotoxicosis
Strabismus (congenital) (nonparalytic)
  H50.9
  concomitant H50.40
    convergent —*see* Strabismus,
      convergent concomitant
    divergent —*see* Strabismus, divergent
      concomitant
  convergent concomitant H50.00
    accommodative component H50.43
    alternating H50.05
      with
        A pattern H50.06
        specified nonconcomitances
          NEC H50.08
        V pattern H50.07
    monocular H50.01-
      with
        A pattern H50.02-
        specified nonconcomitances
          NEC H50.04-
        V pattern H50.03-
      intermittent H50.31-
        alternating H50.32
  cyclotropia H50.1-
  divergent concomitant H50.10
    alternating H50.15
      with
        A pattern H50.16
        specified noncomitances NEC
          H50.18
        V pattern H50.17

S

Strabismus *(Continued)*
  divergent concomitant *(Continued)*
    monocular H50.11-
      with
        A pattern H50.12-
        specified noncomitances NEC
          H50.14-
        V pattern H50.13-
      intermittent H50.33-
      alternating H50.34
  Duane's syndrome H50.81-
  due to adhesions, scars H50.69
  heterophoria H50.50
    alternating H50.55
    cyclophoria H50.54
    esophoria H50.51
    exophoria H50.52
    vertical H50.53
  heterotropia H50.40
    intermittent H50.30
  hypertropia H50.2-
  hypotropia —*see* Hypertropia
  latent H50.50
  mechanical H50.60
    Brown's sheath syndrome H50.61-
    specified type NEC H50.69
  monofixation syndrome H50.42
  paralytic H49.9
    abducens nerve H49.2-
    fourth nerve H49.1-
    Kearns-Sayre syndrome H49.81-
    ophthalmoplegia (external)
      progressive H49.4-
        with pigmentary retinopathy
          H49.81-
      total H49.3-
    sixth nerve H49.2-
    specified type NEC H49.88-
    third nerve H49.0-
    trochlear nerve H49.1-
  specified type NEC H50.89
  vertical H50.2-
Strain
  back S39.012
  cervical S16.1
  eye NEC —*see* Disturbance, vision,
    subjective
  heart —*see* Disease, heart
  low back S39.012
  mental NOS Z73.3
    work-related Z56.6
  muscle (tendon) —*see* Injury, muscle,
    by site, strain
  neck S16.1
  physical NOS Z73.3
    work-related Z56.6
  postural —*see also* Disorder, soft tissue,
    due to use
  psychological NEC Z73.3
  tendon —*see* Injury, muscle, by site, strain
Straining, on urination R39.16
Strand, vitreous —*see* Opacity, vitreous,
  membranes and strands
Strangulation, strangulated —*see also*
  Asphyxia, traumatic
  appendix K38.8
  bladder-neck N32.0
  bowel or colon K56.2
  food or foreign body —*see* Foreign body,
    by site
  hemorrhoids —*see* Hemorrhoids, with
    complication
  hernia —*see also* Hernia, by site, with
    obstruction

Strangulation, strangulated *(Continued)*
  hernia *(Continued)*
    with gangrene —*see* Hernia, by site,
      with gangrene
    intestine (large) (small) K56.2
      with hernia —*see also* Hernia, by site,
        with obstruction
        with gangrene —*see* Hernia, by site,
          with gangrene
    mesentery K56.2
    mucus —*see* Asphyxia, mucus
    omentum K56.2
    organ or site, congenital NEC —*see*
      Atresia, by site
    ovary —*see* Torsion, ovary
    penis N48.89
      foreign body T19.4
    rupture —*see* Hernia, by site, with
      obstruction
    stomach due to hernia —*see also* Hernia,
      by site, with obstruction
      with gangrene —*see* Hernia, by site,
        with gangrene
    vesicourethral orifice N32.0
Strangury R30.0
Straw itch B88.0
Strawberry
  gallbladder K82.4
  mark Q82.5
  tongue (red) (white) K14.3
Streak(s)
  macula, angioid H35.33
  ovarian Q50.32
Strephosymbolia F81.0
  secondary to organic lesion R48.8
Streptobacillary fever A25.1
Streptobacillosis A25.1
Streptobacillus moniliformis A25.1
Streptococcus, streptococcal —*see also*
  condition
  as cause of disease classified elsewhere
    B95.5
  group
    A, as cause of disease classified
      elsewhere B95.0
    B, as cause of disease classified
      elsewhere B95.1
    D, as cause of disease classified
      elsewhere B95.2
  pneumoniae, as cause of disease
    classified elsewhere B95.3
  specified NEC, as cause of disease
    classified elsewhere B95.4
Streptomycosis B47.1
Streptotrichosis A48.8
Stress F43.9
  family —*see* Disruption, family
  fetal P84
    complicating pregnancy O77.9
    due to drug administration O77.1
  mental NEC Z73.3
    work-related Z56.6
  physical NEC Z73.3
    work-related Z56.6
  polycythemia D75.1
  reaction (see also Reaction, stress)
    F43.9
  work schedule Z56.3
Stretching, nerve —*see* Injury, nerve
Striae albicantes, atrophicae or distensae
  (cutis) L90.6
Stricture —*see also* Stenosis
  ampulla of Vater K83.1
  anus (sphincter) K62.4

Stricture *(Continued)*
  anus *(Continued)*
    congenital Q42.3
      with fistula Q42.2
    infantile Q42.3
      with fistula Q42.2
  aorta (ascending) (congenital) Q25.3
    arteriosclerotic I70.0
    calcified I70.0
    supravalvular, congenital Q25.3
  aortic (valve) —*see* Stenosis, aortic
  aqueduct of Sylvius (congenital)
    Q03.0
    with spina bifida —*see* Spina bifida,
      by site, with hydrocephalus
    acquired G91.1
  artery I77.1
    basilar —*see* Occlusion, artery, basilar
    carotid —*see* Occlusion, artery, carotid
    celiac I77.4
    congenital (peripheral) Q27.8
      cerebral Q28.3
      coronary Q24.5
      digestive system Q27.8
      lower limb Q27.8
      retinal Q14.1
      specified site NEC Q27.8
      umbilical Q27.0
      upper limb Q27.8
    coronary —*see* Disease, heart,
      ischemic, atherosclerotic
      congenital Q24.5
    precerebral —*see* Occlusion, artery,
      precerebral
    pulmonary (congenital) Q25.6
      acquired I28.8
    renal I70.1
    vertebral —*see* Occlusion, artery,
      vertebral
  auditory canal (external) (congenital)
    acquired —*see* Stenosis, external ear
      canal
  bile duct (common) (hepatic) K83.1
    congenital Q44.3
    postoperative K91.89
  bladder N32.89
    neck N32.0
  bowel —*see* Obstruction, intestine
  brain G93.89
  bronchus J98.09
    congenital Q32.3
    syphilitic A52.72
  cardia (stomach) K22.2
    congenital Q39.3
  cardiac —*see also* Disease, heart
    orifice (stomach) K22.2
  cecum —*see* Obstruction, intestine
  cervix, cervical (canal) N88.2
    congenital Q51.828
    in pregnancy —*see* Pregnancy,
      complicated by, abnormal cervix
      causing obstructed labor O65.5
  colon —*see also* Obstruction, intestine
    congenital Q42.9
      specified NEC Q42.8
  colostomy K94.03
  common (bile) duct K83.1
  coronary (artery) —*see* Disease, heart,
    ischemic, atherosclerotic
  cystic duct —*see* Obstruction,
    gallbladder
  digestive organs NEC, congenital Q45.8
  duodenum K31.5
    congenital Q41.0

S

Stricture *(Continued)*
    ear canal (external) (congenital)
        Q16.1
        acquired —*see* Stricture, auditory
            canal, acquired
    ejaculatory duct N50.8
    enterostomy K94.13
    esophagus K22.2
        congenital Q39.3
        syphilitic A52.79
            congenital A50.59 *[K23]*
    eustachian tube —*see also* Obstruction,
        eustachian tube
        congenital Q17.8
    fallopian tube N97.1
        gonococcal A54.24
        tuberculous A18.17
    gallbladder —*see* Obstruction,
        gallbladder
    glottis J38.6
    heart —*see also* Disease, heart
        valve *(see also* Endocarditis) I38
            aortic Q23.0
            mitral Q23.4
            pulmonary Q22.1
            tricuspid Q22.4
    hepatic duct K83.1
    hourglass, of stomach K31.2
    hymen N89.6
    hypopharynx J39.2
    ileum K56.69
        congenital Q41.2
    intestine —*see also* Obstruction,
        intestine
        congenital (small) Q41.9
            large Q42.9
                specified NEC Q42.8
            specified NEC Q41.8
        ischemic K55.1
    jejunum K56.69
        congenital Q41.1
    lacrimal passages —*see also* Stenosis,
        lacrimal
        congenital Q10.5
    larynx J38.6
        congenital NEC Q31.8
            subglottic Q31.1
        syphilitic A52.73
            congenital A50.59 *[J99]*
    meatus
        ear (congenital) Q16.1
            acquired —*see* Stricture, auditory
                canal, acquired
        osseous (ear) (congenital) Q16.1
            acquired —*see* Stricture, auditory
                canal, acquired
        urinarius —*see also* Stricture, urethra
            congenital Q64.33
    mitral (valve) —*see* Stenosis, mitral
    myocardium, myocardial I51.5
        hypertrophic subaortic (idiopathic)
            I42.1
    nares (anterior) (posterior) J34.89
        congenital Q30.0
    nasal duct —*see also* Stenosis, lacrimal,
        duct
        congenital Q10.5
    nasolacrimal duct —*see also* Stenosis,
        lacrimal, duct
        congenital Q10.5
    nasopharynx J39.2
        syphilitic A52.73
    nose J34.89
        congenital Q30.0

Stricture *(Continued)*
    nostril (anterior) (posterior) J34.89
        congenital Q30.0
        syphilitic A52.73
            congenital A50.59 *[J99]*
    oesophagus —*see* Stricture, esophagus
    organ or site, congenital NEC —*see*
        Atresia, by site
    os uteri —*see* Stricture, cervix
    osseous meatus (ear) (congenital)
        Q16.1
        acquired —*see* Stricture, auditory
            canal, acquired
    oviduct —*see* Stricture, fallopian tube
    pelviureteric junction (congenital)
        Q62.11
    penis, by foreign body T19.4
    pharynx J39.2
    prostate N42.89
    pulmonary, pulmonic
        artery (congenital) Q25.6
            acquired I28.8
            noncongenital I28.8
        infundibulum (congenital) Q24.3
        valve I37.0
            congenital Q22.1
        vein, acquired I28.8
        vessel NEC I28.8
    punctum lacrimale —*see also* Stenosis,
        lacrimal, punctum
        congenital Q10.5
    pylorus (hypertrophic) K31.1
        adult K31.1
        congenital Q40.0
        infantile Q40.0
    rectosigmoid K56.69
    rectum (sphincter) K62.4
        congenital Q42.1
            with fistula Q42.0
        due to
            chlamydial lymphogranuloma A55
            irradiation K91.89
            lymphogranuloma venereum A55
        gonococcal A54.6
        inflammatory (chlamydial) A55
        syphilitic A52.74
        tuberculous A18.32
    renal artery I70.1
        congenital Q27.1
    salivary duct or gland (any) K11.8
    sigmoid (flexure) —*see* Obstruction,
        intestine
    spermatic cord N50.8
    stoma (following) (of)
        colostomy K94.03
        enterostomy K94.13
        gastrostomy K94.23
        ileostomy K94.13
        tracheostomy J95.03
    stomach K31.89
        congenital Q40.2
        hourglass K31.2
    subaortic Q24.4
        hypertrophic (acquired) (idiopathic)
            I42.1
    subglottic J38.6
    syphilitic NEC A52.79
    trachea J39.8
        congenital Q32.1
        syphilitic A52.73
        tuberculous NEC A15.5
    tracheostomy J95.03
    tricuspid (valve) —*see* Stenosis, tricuspid
    tunica vaginalis N50.8

Stricture *(Continued)*
    ureter (postoperative) N13.5
        with
            hydronephrosis N13.1
                with infection N13.6
            pyelonephritis (chronic) N11.1
        congenital —*see* Atresia, ureter
        tuberculous A18.11
    ureteropelvic junction (congenital)
        Q62.11
    ureterovesical orifice N13.5
        with infection N13.6
    urethra (organic) (spasmodic) N35.9
        associated with schistosomiasis
            B65.0 *[N37]*
        congenital Q64.39
            valvular (posterior) Q64.2
        due to
            infection —*see* Stricture, urethra,
                postinfective
            trauma —*see* Stricture, urethra,
                post-traumatic
        gonococcal, gonorrheal A54.01
        infective NEC —*see* Stricture, urethra,
            postinfective
        late effect (sequelae) of injury —*see*
            Stricture, urethra, post-traumatic
        postcatheterization —*see* Stricture,
            urethra, postprocedural
        postinfective NEC
            female N35.12
            male N35.119
                anterior urethra N35.114
                bulbous urethra N35.112
                meatal N35.111
                membranous urethra N35.113
        postobstetric N35.021
        postoperative —*see* Stricture, urethra,
            postprocedural
        postprocedural
            female N99.12
            male N99.114
                anterior urethra N99.113
                bulbous urethra N99.111
                meatal N99.110
                membranous urethra N99.112
        post-traumatic
            female N35.028
                due to childbirth N35.021
            male N35.014
                anterior urethra N35.013
                bulbous urethra N35.011
                meatal N35.010
                membranous urethra N35.012
        sequela (late effect) of
            childbirth N35.021
            injury —*see* Stricture, urethra,
                post-traumatic
        specified cause NEC N35.8
        syphilitic A52.76
        traumatic —*see* Stricture, urethra,
            post-traumatic
        valvular (posterior), congenital Q64.2
    urinary meatus —*see* Stricture, urethra
    uterus, uterine (synechiae) N85.6
        os (external) (internal) —*see* Stricture,
            cervix
    vagina (outlet) —*see* Stenosis, vagina
    valve (cardiac) (heart) —*see also*
        Endocarditis
        congenital
            aortic Q23.0
            mitral Q23.2
            pulmonary Q22.1
            tricuspid Q22.4

Stricture *(Continued)*
vas deferens N50.8
congenital Q55.4
vein I87.1
vena cava (inferior) (superior) NEC
I87.1
congenital Q26.0
vesicourethral orifice N32.0
congenital Q64.31
vulva (acquired) N90.5
Stridor R06.1
congenital (larynx) P28.89
Stridulous —*see* condition
Stroke (apoplectic) (brain) (embolic)
(ischemic) (paralytic) (thrombotic)
I63.9
epileptic —*see* Epilepsy
heat T67.0
in evolution I63.9
intraoperative
during cardiac surgery I97.810
during other surgery I97.811
lightning —*see* Lightning
meaning
cerebral hemorrhage — code to
Hemorrhage, intracranial
cerebral infarction — code to
Infarction, cerebral
postprocedural
following cardiac surgery I97.820
following other surgery I97.821
unspecified (NOS) I63.9
Stromatosis, endometrial D39.0
Strongyloidiasis, strongyloidosis B78.9
cutaneous B78.1
disseminated B78.7
intestinal B78.0
Strophulus pruriginosus L28.2
Struck by lightning —*see* Lightning
Struma —*see also* Goiter
Hashimoto E06.3
lymphomatosa E06.3
nodosa (simplex) E04.9
endemic E01.2
multinodular E01.1
multinodular E04.2
iodine-deficiency related E01.1
toxic or with hyperthyroidism E05.20
with thyroid storm E05.21
multinodular E05.20
with thyroid storm E05.21
uninodular E05.10
with thyroid storm E05.11
toxicosa E05.20
with thyroid storm E05.21
multinodular E05.20
with thyroid storm E05.21
uninodular E05.10
with thyroid storm E05.11
uninodular E04.1
ovarii D27.-
Riedel's E06.5
Strumipriva cachexia E03.4
Strümpell-Marie spine —*see* Spondylitis,
ankylosing
Strümpell-Westphal pseudosclerosis
E83.01
Stuart deficiency disease (factor X) D68.2
Stuart-Prower factor deficiency (factor
X) D68.2
Student's elbow —*see* Bursitis, elbow,
olecranon
Stump —*see* Amputation
Stunting, nutritional E45

Stupor (catatonic) R40.1
depressive F32.8
dissociative F44.2
manic F30.2
manic-depressive F31.89
psychogenic (anergic) F44.2
reaction to exceptional stress (transient)
F43.0
Sturge (-Weber) (-Dimitri) (-Kalischer)
disease or syndrome Q85.8
Stuttering F80.81
adult onset F98.5
childhood onset F80.81
following cerebrovascular disease —
see Disorder, fluency, following
cerebrovascular disease
in conditions classified elsewhere
R47.82
Sty, stye (external) (internal) (meibomian)
(zeisian) —*see* Hordeolum
Subacidity, gastric K31.89
psychogenic F45.8
Subacute —*see* condition
Subarachnoid —*see* condition
Subcortical —*see* condition
Subcostal syndrome, nerve
compression —*see* Mononeuropathy,
upper limb, specified site NEC
Subcutaneous, subcuticular —*see*
condition
Subdural —*see* condition
Subendocardium —*see* condition
Subependymoma
specified site —*see* Neoplasm, uncertain
behavior, by site
unspecified site D43.2
Suberosis J67.3
Subglossitis —*see* Glossitis
Subhemophilia D66
Subinvolution
breast (postlactational) (postpuerperal)
N64.89
puerperal O90.89
uterus (chronic) (nonpuerperal)
N85.3
puerperal O90.89
Sublingual —*see* condition
Sublinguitis —*see* Sialoadenitis
Subluxatable hip Q65.6
Subluxation —*see also* Dislocation
acromioclavicular S43.11-
ankle S93.0-
atlantoaxial, recurrent M43.4
with myelopathy M43.3
carpometacarpal (joint) NEC S63.05-
thumb S63.04-
complex, vertebral —*see* Complex,
subluxation
congenital —*see also* Malposition,
congenital
hip —*see* Dislocation, hip, congenital,
partial
joint (excluding hip)
lower limb Q68.8
shoulder Q68.8
upper limb Q68.8
elbow (traumatic) S53.10-
anterior S53.11-
lateral S53.14-
medial S53.13-
posterior S53.12-
specified type NEC S53.19-
finger S63.20-
index S63.20-

Subluxation *(Continued)*
finger *(Continued)*
interphalangeal S63.22-
distal S63.24-
index S63.24-
little S63.24-
middle S63.24-
ring S63.24-
index S63.22-
little S63.22-
middle S63.22-
proximal S63.23-
index S63.23-
little S63.23-
middle S63.23-
ring S63.23-
ring S63.22-
little S63.20-
metacarpophalangeal S63.21-
index S63.21-
little S63.21-
middle S63.21-
ring S63.21-
middle S63.20-
ring S63.20-
foot S93.30-
specified site NEC S93.33-
tarsal joint S93.31-
tarsometatarsal joint S93.32-
toe —*see* Subluxation, toe
hip S73.00-
anterior S73.03-
obturator S73.02-
central S73.04-
posterior S73.01-
interphalangeal (joint)
finger S63.22-
distal joint S63.24-
index S63.24-
little S63.24-
middle S63.24-
ring S63.24-
index S63.22-
little S63.22-
middle S63.22-
proximal joint S63.23-
index S63.23-
little S63.23-
middle S63.23-
ring S63.23-
ring S63.22-
thumb S63.12-
distal joint S63.14-
proximal joint S63.13-
toe S93.13-
great S93.13-
lesser S93.13-
joint prosthesis —*see* Complications,
joint prosthesis, mechanical,
displacement, by site
knee S83.10-
cap —*see* Subluxation, patella
patella —*see* Subluxation, patella
proximal tibia
anteriorly S83.11-
laterally S83.14-
medially S83.13-
posteriorly S83.12-
specified type NEC S83.19-
lens —*see* Dislocation, lens, partial
ligament, traumatic —*see* Sprain,
by site
metacarpal (bone)
proximal end S63.06-

453

Subluxation *(Continued)*
  metacarpophalangeal (joint)
    finger S63.21-
      index S63.21-
      little S63.21-
      middle S63.21-
      ring S63.21-
      thumb S63.11-
  metatarsophalangeal joint S93.14-
    great toe S93.14-
    lesser toe S93.14-
  midcarpal (joint) S63.03-
  patella S83.00-
    lateral S83.01-
    recurrent (nontraumatic) —*see*
        Dislocation, patella, recurrent,
        incomplete
    specified type NEC S83.09-
  pathological —*see* Dislocation,
      pathological
  radial head S53.00-
    anterior S53.01-
    nursemaid's elbow S53.03-
    posterior S53.02-
    specified type NEC S53.09-
  radiocarpal (joint) S63.02-
  radioulnar (joint)
    distal S63.01-
    proximal —*see* Subluxation,
        elbow
  shoulder
    congenital Q68.8
    girdle S43.30-
      scapula S43.31-
      specified site NEC S43.39-
    traumatic S43.00-
      anterior S43.01-
      inferior S43.03-
      posterior S43.02-
      specified type NEC S43.08-
  sternoclavicular (joint) S43.20-
    anterior S43.21-
    posterior S43.22-
  symphysis (pubis)
  thumb S63.103
    interphalangeal joint —*see*
        Subluxation, interphalangeal
        (joint), thumb
    metacarpophalangeal
        joint —*see* Subluxation,
        metacarpophalangeal
        (joint), thumb
  toe (s) S93.10-
    great S93.10-
      interphalangeal joint S93.13-
      metatarsophalangeal joint
          S93.14-
    interphalangeal joint S93.13-
    lesser S93.10-
      interphalangeal joint S93.13-
      metatarsophalangeal joint
          S93.14-
    metatarsophalangeal joint
        S93.149
  ulnohumeral joint —*see* Subluxation,
      elbow
  vertebral
    recurrent NEC —*see* subcategory
        M43.5
    traumatic
      cervical S13.100
        atlantoaxial joint S13.120
        atlantooccipital joint S13.110
        atloidooccipital joint S13.110

Subluxation *(Continued)*
  vertebral *(Continued)*
    traumatic *(Continued)*
      cervical *(Continued)*
        joint between
          C0 and C1 S13.110
          C1 and C2 S13.120
          C2 and C3 S13.130
          C3 and C4 S13.140
          C4 and C5 S13.150
          C5 and C6 S13.160
          C6 and C7 S13.170
          C7 and T1 S13.180
        occipitoatloid joint S13.110
      lumbar S33.100
        joint between
          L1 and L2 S33.110
          L2 and L3 S33.120
          L3 and L4 S33.130
          L4 and L5 S33.140
      thoracic S23.100
        joint between
          T1 and T2 S23.110
          T2 and T3 S23.120
          T3 and T4 S23.122
          T4 and T5 S23.130
          T5 and T6 S23.132
          T6 and T7 S23.140
          T7 and T8 S23.142
          T8 and T9 S23.150
          T9 and T10 S23.152
          T10 and T11 S23.160
          T11 and T12 S23.162
          T12 and L1 S23.170
  ulna
    distal end S63.07-
    proximal end —*see* Subluxation,
        elbow
  wrist (carpal bone) S63.00-
    carpometacarpal joint —*see*
        Subluxation, carpometacarpal
        (joint)
    distal radioulnar joint —*see*
        Subluxation, radioulnar
        (joint), distal
    metacarpal bone, proximal —*see*
        Subluxation, metacarpal (bone),
        proximal end
    midcarpal —*see* Subluxation,
        midcarpal (joint)
    radiocarpal joint —*see* Subluxation,
        radiocarpal (joint)
    recurrent —*see* Dislocation, recurrent,
        wrist
    specified site NEC S63.09-
    ulna —*see* Subluxation, ulna, distal
        end
Submaxillary —*see* condition
Submersion (fatal) (nonfatal) T75.1
Submucous —*see* condition
Subnormal, subnormality
  accommodation (old age) H52.4
  mental —*see* Disability, intellectual
  temperature (accidental) T68
Subphrenic —*see* condition
Subscapular nerve —*see* condition
Subseptus uterus Q51.2
Subsiding appendicitis K36
Substernal thyroid E04.9
  congenital Q89.2
Substitution disorder F44.9
Subtentorial —*see* condition
Subthyroidism (acquired) —*see also*
    Hypothyroidism
  congenital E03.1

Succenturiate placenta O43.19-
Sucking thumb, child (excessive) F98.8
Sudamen, sudamina L74.1
Sudanese kala-azar B55.0
Sudden
  hearing loss —*see* Deafness, sudden
  heart failure —*see* Failure, heart
Sudeck's atrophy, disease, or
    syndrome—*see* Algoneurodystrophy
Suffocation—*see* Asphyxia, traumatic
Sugar
  blood
    high (transient) R73.9
    low (transient) E16.2
  in urine R81
Suicide, suicidal (attempted) T14.91
  by poisoning —*see* Table of drugs and
      chemicals
  history of (personal) Z91.5
    in family Z81.8
  ideation —*see* Ideation, suicidal
  risk
    meaning personal history of
        attempted suicide Z91.5
    meaning suicidal ideation —*see*
        Ideation, suicidal
  tendencies
    meaning personal history of
        attempted suicide Z91.5
    meaning suicidal ideation —*see*
        Ideation, suicidal
  trauma —*see* nature of injury by site
Suipestifer infection—*see* Infection,
    salmonella
Sulfhemoglobinemia,
    sulphemoglobinemia (acquired)
    (with methemoglobinemia) D74.8
Sumatran mite fever A75.3
Summer—*see* condition
Sunburn L55.9
  first degree L55.0
  second degree L55.1
  third degree L55.2
SUNCT (short lasting unilateral
    neuralgiform headache with
    conjunctival injection and tearing)
    G44.059
  intractable G44.051
  not intractable G44.059
Sunken acetabulum—*see* Derangement,
    joint, specified type NEC, hip
Sunstroke T67.0
Superfecundation—*see* Pregnancy,
    multiple
Superfetation—*see* Pregnancy, multiple
Superinvolution (uterus) N85.8
Supernumerary (congenital)
  aortic cusps Q23.8
  auditory ossicles Q16.3
  bone Q79.8
  breast Q83.1
  carpal bones Q74.0
  cusps, heart valve NEC Q24.8
    aortic Q23.8
    mitral Q23.2
    pulmonary Q22.3
  digit (s) Q69.9
  ear (lobule) Q17.0
  fallopian tube Q50.6
  finger Q69.0
  hymen Q52.4
  kidney Q63.0
  lacrimonasal duct Q10.6
  lobule (ear) Q17.0
  mitral cusps Q23.2

Supernumerary (Continued)
muscle Q79.8
nipple (s) Q83.3
organ or site not listed —see Accessory
ossicles, auditory Q16.3
ovary Q50.31
oviduct Q50.6
pulmonary, pulmonic cusps Q22.3
rib Q76.6
cervical or first (syndrome) Q76.5
roots (of teeth) K00.2
spleen Q89.09
tarsal bones Q74.2
teeth K00.1
testis Q55.29
thumb Q69.1
toe Q69.2
uterus Q51.2
vagina Q52.1
vertebra Q76.49
Supervision (of)
contraceptive —see Prescription,
contraceptives
dietary (for) Z71.3
allergy (food) Z71.3
colitis Z71.3
diabetes mellitus Z71.3
food allergy or intolerance Z71.3
gastritis Z71.3
hypercholesterolemia Z71.3
hypoglycemia Z71.3
intolerance (food) Z71.3
obesity Z71.3
specified NEC Z71.3
healthy infant or child Z76.2
foundling Z76.1
high-risk pregnancy —see Pregnancy,
complicated by, high, risk
lactation Z39.1
pregnancy —see Pregnancy, supervision
of
Supplemental teeth K00.1
Suppression
binocular vision H53.34
lactation O92.5
menstruation N94.89
ovarian secretion E28.39
renal N28.9
urine, urinary secretion R34
Suppuration, suppurative —see also
condition
accessory sinus (chronic) —see Sinusitis
adrenal gland
antrum (chronic) —see Sinusitis,
maxillary
bladder —see Cystitis
brain G06.0
sequelae G09
breast N61
puerperal, postpartum or
gestational —see Mastitis,
obstetric,
purulent
dental periosteum M27.3
ear (middle) —see also Otitis, media
external NEC —see Otitis, externa,
infective
internal —see subcategory H83.0
ethmoidal (chronic) (sinus) —see
Sinusitis, ethmoidal
fallopian tube —see Salpingo-
oophoritis
frontal (chronic) (sinus) —see Sinusitis,
frontal

Suppuration, suppurative (Continued)
gallbladder (acute) K81.0
gum K05.20
generalized K05.22
localized K05.21
intracranial G06.0
joint —see Arthritis, pyogenic or pyemic
labyrinthine —see subcategory H83.0
lung —see Abscess, lung
mammary gland N61
puerperal, postpartum O91.12
associated with lactation O91.13
maxilla, maxillary M27.2
sinus (chronic) —see Sinusitis,
maxillary
muscle —see Myositis, infective
nasal sinus (chronic) —see Sinusitis
pancreas, acute K85.8
parotid gland —see Sialoadenitis
pelvis, pelvic
female —see Disease, pelvis,
inflammatory
male K65.0
pericranial —see Osteomyelitis
salivary duct or gland (any) —see
Sialoadenitis
sinus (accessory) (chronic) (nasal) —see
Sinusitis
sphenoidal sinus (chronic) —see
Sinusitis, sphenoidal
thymus (gland) E32.1
thyroid (gland) E06.0
tonsil —see Tonsillitis
uterus —see Endometritis
Supraeruption of tooth (teeth) M26.34
Supraglottitis J04.30
with obstruction J04.31
Suprarenal (gland) —see condition
Suprascapular nerve —see condition
Suprasellar —see condition
Surfer's knots or nodules S89.8-
Surgical
emphysema T81.82
procedures, complication or
misadventure —see Complications,
surgical procedures
shock T81.10
Surveillance (of) (for) —see also
Observation
alcohol abuse Z71.41
contraceptive —see Prescription,
contraceptives
dietary Z71.3
drug abuse Z71.51
Susceptibility to disease, genetic
Z15.89
malignant neoplasm Z15.09
breast Z15.01
endometrium Z15.04
ovary Z15.02
prostate Z15.03
specified NEC Z15.09
multiple endocrine neoplasia
Z15.81
Suspected condition, ruled out —see also
Observation, suspected
amniotic cavity and membrane Z03.71
cervical shortening Z03.75
fetal anomaly Z03.73
fetal growth Z03.74
maternal and fetal conditions NEC Z03.79
oligohydramnios Z03.71
placental problem Z03.72
polyhydramnios Z03.71

Suspended uterus
in pregnancy or childbirth —see
Pregnancy, complicated by,
abnormal uterus
Sutton's nevus D22.9
Suture
burst (in operation wound) T81.31
external operation wound T81.31
internal operation wound T81.32
inadvertently left in operation
wound —see Foreign body,
accidentally left during a
procedure
removal Z48.02
**Swab inadvertently left in operation
wound** —see Foreign body,
accidentally left during a procedure
Swallowed, swallowing
difficulty —see Dysphagia
foreign body —see Foreign body,
alimentary tract
Swan-neck deformity (finger) —see
Deformity, finger, swan-neck
Swearing, compulsive F42
in Gilles de la Tourette's syndrome F95.2
Sweat, sweats
fetid L75.0
night R61
Sweating, excessive R61
Sweeley-Klionsky disease E75.21
Sweet's disease or dermatosis L98.2
Swelling (of) R60.9
abdomen, abdominal (not referable to
any particular organ) —see Mass,
abdominal
ankle —see Effusion, joint, ankle
arm M79.89
forearm M79.89
breast N63
Calabar B74.3
cervical gland R59.0
chest, localized R22.2
ear H93.8-
extremity (lower) (upper) —see
Disorder, soft tissue, specified type
NEC
finger M79.89
foot M79.89
glands R59.9
generalized R59.1
localized R59.0
hand M79.89
head (localized) R22.0
inflammatory —see Inflammation
intra-abdominal —see Mass,
abdominal
joint —see Effusion, joint
leg M79.89
lower M79.89
limb —see Disorder, soft tissue,
specified type NEC
localized (skin) R22.9
chest R22.2
head R22.0
limb
lower —see Mass, localized, limb,
lower
upper —see Mass, localized, limb,
upper
neck R22.1
trunk R22.2
neck (localized) R22.1
pelvic —see Mass, abdominal
scrotum N50.8

Swelling (Continued)
splenic —see Splenomegaly
testis N50.8
toe M79.89
umbilical R19.09
wandering, due to Gnathostoma (spinigerum) B83.1
white —see Tuberculosis, arthritis
Swift (-Feer) disease
overdose or wrong substance given or taken —see Table of drugs and chemicals, by drug, poisoning
Swimmer's
cramp T75.1
ear H60.33-
itch B65.3
Swimming in the head R42
Swollen —see Swelling
Swyer syndrome Q99.1
Sycosis L73.8
barbae (not parasitic) L73.8
contagiosa (mycotic) B35.0
lupoides L73.8
mycotic B35.0
parasitic B35.0
vulgaris L73.8
Sydenham's chorea —see Chorea, Sydenham's
Sylvatic yellow fever A95.0
Sylvest's disease B33.0
Symblepharon H11.23-
congenital Q10.3
Symond's syndrome G93.2
Sympathetic —see condition
Sympatheticotonia G90.8
Sympathicoblastoma
specified site —see Neoplasm, malignant, by site
unspecified site C74.90
Sympathogonioma —see Sympathicoblastoma
Symphalangy (fingers) (toes) Q70.9
Symptoms NEC R68.89
breast NEC N64.59
development NEC R63.8
factitious, self-induced —see Disorder, factitious
genital organs, female R10.2
involving
abdomen NEC R19.8
appearance NEC R46.89
awareness R41.9
altered mental status R41.82
amnesia —see Amnesia
borderline intellectual functioning R41.83
coma —see Coma
disorientation R41.0
neurologic neglect syndrome R41.4
senile cognitive decline R41.81
specified symptom NEC R41.89
behavior NEC R46.89
cardiovascular system NEC R09.89
chest NEC R09.89
circulatory system NEC R09.89
cognitive functions R41.9
altered mental status R41.82
amnesia —see Amnesia
borderline intellectual functioning R41.83
coma —see Coma
disorientation R41.0
neurologic neglect syndrome R41.4
senile cognitive decline R41.81
specified symptom NEC R41.89

Symptoms NEC (Continued)
involving (Continued)
development NEC R62.50
digestive system NEC R19.8
emotional state NEC R45.89
emotional lability R45.86
food and fluid intake R63.8
general perceptions and sensations R44.9
specified NEC R44.8
musculoskeletal system R29.91
specified NEC R29.898
nervous system R29.90
specified NEC R29.818
pelvis NEC R19.8
respiratory system NEC R09.89
skin and integument R23.9
urinary system R39.9
menopausal N95.1
metabolism NEC R63.8
neurotic F48.8
of infancy R68.19
pelvis NEC, female R10.2
skin and integument NEC R23.8
subcutaneous tissue NEC R23.8
Sympus Q74.2
Syncephalus Q89.4
Synchondrosis
abnormal (congenital) Q78.8
ischiopubic M91.0
Synchysis (scintillans) (senile) (vitreous body) H43.89
Syncope (near) (pre-) R55
anginosa I20.8
bradycardia R00.1
cardiac R55
carotid sinus G90.01
due to spinal (lumbar) puncture G97.1
heart R55
heat T67.1
laryngeal R05
psychogenic F48.8
tussive R05
vasoconstriction R55
vasodepressor R55
vasomotor R55
vasovagal R55
Syndactylism, syndactyly Q70.9
complex (with synostosis)
fingers Q70.0-
toes Q70.2-
simple (without synostosis)
fingers Q70.1-
toes Q70.3-
Syndrome —see also Disease
5q minus NOS D46.C
48,XXXX Q97.1
49,XXXXX Q97.1
abdominal
acute R10.0
muscle deficiency Q79.4
abnormal innervation H02.519
left H02.516
lower H02.515
upper H02.514
right H02.513
lower H02.512
upper H02.511
abstinence, neonatal P96.1
acid pulmonary aspiration, obstetric O74.0
acquired immunodeficiency —see Human, immunodeficiency virus (HIV) disease

Syndrome (Continued)
acute abdominal R10.0
acute respiratory distress (adult) (child) J80
Adair-Dighton Q78.0
Adams-Stokes (-Morgagni) I45.9
adiposogenital E23.6
adrenal
hemorrhage (meningococcal) A39.1
meningococcic A39.1
adrenocortical —see Cushing's, syndrome
adrenogenital E25.9
congenital, associated with enzyme deficiency E25.0
afferent loop NEC K91.89
Alagille's Q44.7
alcohol withdrawal (without convulsions) —see Dependence, alcohol, with, withdrawal
Alder's D72.0
Aldrich (-Wiskott) D82.0
alien hand R41.4
Alport Q87.81
alveolar hypoventilation E66.2
alveolocapillary block J84.10
amnesic, amnestic (confabulatory) (due to) —see Disorder, amnesic
amyostatic (Wilson's disease) E83.01
androgen insensitivity E34.50
complete E34.51
partial E34.52
androgen resistance (see also Syndrome, androgen insensitivity) E34.50
Angelman Q93.5
anginal —see Angina
ankyloglossia superior Q38.1
anterior
chest wall R07.89
cord G83.82
spinal artery G95.19
compression M47.019
cervical region M47.012
cervicothoracic region M47.013
lumbar region M47.016
occipito-atlanto-axial region M47.011
thoracic region M47.014
thoracolumbar region M47.015
tibial M76.81-
antibody deficiency D80.9
agammaglobulinemic D80.1
hereditary D80.0
congenital D80.0
hypogammaglobulinemic D80.1
hereditary D80.0
anticardiolipin (-antibody) D68.61
antiphospholipid (-antibody) D68.61
aortic
arch M31.4
bifurcation I74.09
aortomesenteric duodenum occlusion K31.5
apical ballooning (transient left ventricular) I51.81
arcuate ligament I77.4
argentaffin, argintaffinoma E34.0
Arnold-Chiari —see Arnold-Chiari disease
Arrillaga-Ayerza I27.0
Asherman's N85.6
aspiration, of newborn —see Aspiration, by substance, with pneumonia
meconium P24.01

Syndrome *(Continued)*
  ataxia-telangiectasia G11.3
  auriculotemporal G50.8
  autoerythrocyte sensitization (Gardner-
    Diamond) D69.2
  autoimmune lymphoproliferative
    [ALPS] D89.82
  autoimmune polyglandular E31.0
  autosomal —*see* Abnormal, autosomes
  Avellis' G46.8
  Ayerza (-Arrillaga) I27.0
  Babinski-Nageotte G83.89
  Bakwin-Krida Q79.8
  bare lymphocyte D81.6
  Barré-Guillain G61.0
  Barré-Liéou M53.0
  Barrett's —*see* Barrett's, esophagus
  Barsony-Polgar K22.4
  Barsony-Teschendorf K22.4
  Barth E78.71
  Bartter's E26.81
  basal cell nevus Q87.89
  Basedow's E05.00
    with thyroid storm E05.01
  basilar artery G45.0
  Batten-Steinert G71.11
  battered
    baby or child —*see* Maltreatment,
      child, physical abuse
    spouse —*see* Maltreatment, adult,
      physical abuse
  Beals Q87.40
  Beau's I51.5
  Beck's I65.8
  Benedikt's G46.3
  Béquez César (-Steinbrinck-Chédiak-
    Higashi) D70.330
  Bernhardt-Roth —*see* Meralgia
    paresthetica
  Bernheim's I50.9
  big spleen D73.1
  bilateral polycystic ovarian E28.2
  Bing-Horton's —*see* Horton's headache
  Birt-Hogg-Dube syndrome Q87.89
  Björck (-Thorsen) E34.0
  black
    lung J60
    widow spider bite —*see* Toxicity,
      venom, spider, black widow
  Blackfan-Diamond D61.01
  blind loop K90.2
    congenital Q43.8
    postsurgical K91.2
  blue sclera Q78.0
  blue toe I75.02-
  Boder-Sedgewick G11.3
  Boerhaave's K22.3
  Borjeson Forssman Lehmann Q89.8
  Bouillaud's I01.9
  Bourneville (-Pringle) Q85.1
  Bouveret (-Hoffman) I47.9
  brachial plexus G54.0
  bradycardia-tachycardia I49.5
  brain (nonpsychotic) F09
    with psychosis, psychotic reaction
      F09
    acute or subacute —*see* Delirium
    congenital —*see* Disability,
      intellectual
    organic F09
      post-traumatic (nonpsychotic)
        F07.81
        psychotic F09
      personality change F07.0

Syndrome *(Continued)*
  brain *(Continued)*
    postcontusional F07.81
    post-traumatic, nonpsychotic
      F07.81
    psycho-organic F09
    psychotic F06.8
  brain stem stroke G46.3
  Brandt's (acrodermatitis enteropathica)
    E83.2
  broad ligament laceration N83.8
  Brock's J98.11
  bronze baby P83.8
  Brown-Sequard G83.81
  bubbly lung P27.0
  Buchem's M85.2
  Budd-Chiari I82.0
  bulbar (progressive) G12.22
  Bürger-Grütz E78.3
  Burke's K86.8
  Burnett's (milk-alkali) E83.52
  burning feet E53.9
  Bywaters' T79.5
  Call-Fleming I67.841
  carbohydrate-deficient glycoprotein
    (CDGS) E77.8
  carcinogenic thrombophlebitis I82.1
  carcinoid E34.0
  cardiac asthma I50.1
  cardiacos negros I27.0
  cardiofaciocutaneous Q87.89
  cardiopulmonary-obesity E66.2
  cardiorenal —*see* Hypertension,
    cardiorenal
  cardiorespiratory distress (idiopathic),
    newborn P22.0
  cardiovascular renal —*see*
    Hypertension, cardiorenal
  carotid
    artery (hemispheric) (internal)
      G45.1
    body G90.01
    sinus G90.01
  carpal tunnel G56.0-
  Cassidy (-Scholte) E34.0
  cat-cry Q93.4
  cat eye Q92.8
  cauda equina G83.4
  causalgia —*see* Causalgia
  celiac K90.0
    artery compression I77.4
    axis I77.4
  central pain G89.0
  cerebellar
    hereditary G11.9
    stroke G46.4
  cerebellomedullary malformation —*see*
    Spina bifida
  cerebral
    artery
      anterior G46.1
      middle G46.0
      posterior G46.2
    gigantism E22.0
  cervical (root) M53.1
    disc —*see* Disorder, disc, cervical,
      with neuritis
    fusion Q76.1
    posterior, sympathicus M53.0
    rib Q76.5
    sympathetic paralysis G90.2
  cervicobrachial (diffuse) M53.1
  cervicocranial M53.0
  cervicodorsal outlet G54.2

Syndrome *(Continued)*
  cervicothoracic outlet G54.0
  Céstan (-Raymond) I65.8
  Charcot's (angina cruris) (intermittent
    claudication) I73.9
  Charcot-Weiss-Baker G90.09
  CHARGE Q89.8
  Chédiak-Higashi (-Steinbrinck) E70.330
  chest wall R07.1
  Chiari's (hepatic vein thrombosis) I82.0
  Chilaiditi's Q43.3
  child maltreatment —*see* Maltreatment,
    child
  chondrocostal junction M94.0
  chondroectodermal dysplasia Q77.6
  chromosome 4 short arm deletion Q93.3
  chromosome 5 short arm deletion Q93.4
  chronic
    pain G89.4
      personality F68.8
  Clarke-Hadfield K86.8
  Clerambault's automatism G93.89
  Clouston's (hidrotic ectodermal
    dysplasia) Q82.4
  clumsiness, clumsy child F82
  cluster headache G44.009
    intractable G44.001
    not intractable G44.009
  Coffin-Lowry Q89.8
  cold injury (newborn) P80.0
  combined immunity deficiency D81.9
  compartment (deep) (posterior)
    (traumatic) T79.A0
    abdomen T79.A3
    lower extremity (hip, buttock, thigh,
      leg, foot, toes) T79.A2
    nontraumatic
      abdomen M79.A3
      lower extremity (hip, buttock,
        thigh, leg, foot, toes) M79.A2-
      specified site NEC M79.A9
      upper extremity (shoulder, arm,
        forearm, wrist, hand, fingers)
        M79.A1-
    postprocedural —*see* Syndrome
      compartment, nontraumatic
    specified site NEC T79.A9
    upper extremity (shoulder, arm,
      forearm, wrist, hand, fingers)
      T79.A1
  complex regional pain —*see* Syndrome,
    pain, complex regional
  compression T79.5
    anterior spinal —*see* Syndrome,
      anterior, spinal artery,
      compression
    cauda equina G83.4
    celiac artery I77.4
    vertebral artery M47.029
      cervical region M47.022
      occipito-atlanto-axial region
        M47.021
  concussion F07.81
  congenital
    affecting multiple systems NEC
      Q87.89
    central alveolar hypoventilation
      G47.35
    facial diplegia Q87.0
    muscular hypertrophy-cerebral Q87.89
    oculo-auriculovertebral Q87.0
    oculofacial diplegia (Moebius) Q87.0
    rubella (manifest) P35.0
  congestion-fibrosis (pelvic), female
    N94.89

Syndrome *(Continued)*
  congestive dysmenorrhea N94.6
  Conn's E26.01
  connective tissue M35.9
    overlap NEC M35.1
  conus medullaris G95.81
  cord
    anterior G83.82
    posterior G83.83
  coronary
    acute NEC I24.9
    insufficiency or intermediate I20.0
    slow flow I20.8
  Costen's (complex) M26.69
  costochondral junction M94.0
  costoclavicular G54.0
  costovertebral E22.0
  Cowden Q85.8
  craniovertebral M53.0
  Creutzfeldt-Jakob —*see* Creutzfeldt-
    Jakob disease or syndrome
  cri-du-chat Q93.4
  crib death R99
  cricopharyngeal —*see* Dysphagia
  croup J05.0
  CRPS I —*see* Syndrome, pain, complex
    regional I
  crush T79.5
  cryptophthalmos Q87.0
  cubital tunnel —*see* Lesion, nerve, ulnar
  Curschmann (-Batten) (-Steinert) G71.11
  Cushing's E24.9
    alcohol-induced E24.4
    drug-induced E24.2
    due to
      alcohol
        drugs E24.2
      ectopic ACTH E24.3
      overproduction of pituitary ACTH
        E24.0
    overdose or wrong substance
      given or taken —*see* Table of
        drugs and chemicals, by drug,
        poisoning
    pituitary-dependent E24.0
    specified type NEC E24.8
  cystic duct stump K91.5
  Dana-Putnam D51.0
  Danbolt (-Cross) (acrodermatitis
    enteropathica) E83.2
  Dandy-Walker Q03.1
    with spina bifida Q07.01
  Danlos' Q79.8
  defibrination —*see also* Fibrinolysis
    with
      antepartum hemorrhage —*see*
        Hemorrhage, antepartum,
        with coagulation defect
      intrapartum hemorrhage —*see*
        Hemorrhage, complicating,
        delivery
      newborn P60
      postpartum O72.3
  Degos' I77.8
  Déjérine-Roussy G89.0
  delayed sleep phase G47.21
  demyelinating G37.9
  dependence —*see* F10-F19 with fourth
    character .2
  depersonalization (-derealization)
    F48.1
  De Quervain E34.51
  de Toni-Fanconi (-Debré) E72.09
    with cystinosis E72.04

Syndrome *(Continued)*
  diabetes mellitus-hypertension-
    nephrosis —*see* Diabetes,
    nephrosis
  diabetes mellitus in newborn infant
    P70.2
  diabetes-nephrosis —*see* Diabetes,
    nephrosis
  diabetic amyotrophy —*see* Diabetes,
    amyotrophy
  Diamond-Blackfan D61.01
  Diamond-Gardener D69.2
  DIC (diffuse or disseminated
    intravascular coagulopathy) D65
  di George's D82.1
  Dighton's Q78.0
  disequilibrium E87.8
  Döhle body-panmyelopathic D72.0
  dorsolateral medullary G46.4
  double athetosis G80.3
  Down (*see also* Down syndrome) Q90.9
  Dresbach's (elliptocytosis) D58.1
  Dressler's (postmyocardial infarction)
    I24.1
    postcardiotomy I97.0
  drug withdrawal, infant of dependent
    mother P96.1
  dry eye H04.12-
  due to abnormality
    chromosomal Q99.9
      sex
        female phenotype Q97.9
        male phenotype Q98.9
      specified NEC Q99.8
  dumping (postgastrectomy) K91.1
    nonsurgical K31.89
  Dupré's (meningism) R29.1
  dysmetabolic X E88.81
  dyspraxia, developmental F82
  Eagle-Barrett Q79.4
  Eaton-Lambert —*see* Syndrome,
    Lambert-Eaton
  Ebstein's Q22.5
  ectopic ACTH E24.3
  eczema-thrombocytopenia D82.0
  Eddowes' Q78.0
  effort (psychogenic) F45.8
  Ehlers-Danlos Q79.6
  Eisenmenger's I27.89
  Ekman's Q78.0
  electric feet E53.8
  Ellis-van Creveld Q77.6
  empty nest Z60.0
  endocrine-hypertensive E27.0
  entrapment —*see* Neuropathy,
    entrapment
  eosinophilia-myalgia M35.8
  epileptic —*see also* Epilepsy, by type
    absence G40.A09
      intractable G40.A19
        with status epilepticus G40.A11
        without status epilepticus
          G40.A19
      not intractable G40.A09
        with status epilepticus G40.A01
        without status epilepticus
          G40.A09
  Erdheim-Chester (ECD) E88.89
  Erdheim's E22.0
  erythrocyte fragmentation D59.4
  Evans D69.41
  exhaustion F48.8
  extrapyramidal G25.9
    specified NEC G25.89

Syndrome *(Continued)*
  eye retraction —*see* Strabismus
  eyelid-malar-mandible Q87.0
  Faber's D50.9
  facial pain, paroxysmal G50.0
  Fallot's Q21.3
  familial eczema-thrombocytopenia
    (Wiskott-Aldrich) D82.0
  Fanconi (-de Toni) (-Debré) E72.09
    with cystinosis E72.04
  Fanconi's (anemia) (congenital
    pancytopenia) D61.09
  fatigue
    chronic R53.82
    psychogenic F48.8
  faulty bowel habit K59.3
  Feil-Klippel (brevicollis) Q76.1
  Felty's —*see* Felty's syndrome
  fertile eunuch E23.0
  fetal
    alcohol (dysmorphic) Q86.0
    hydantoin Q86.1
  Fiedler's I40.1
  first arch Q87.0
  fish odor E72.8
  Fisher's G61.0
  Fitzhugh-Curtis
    due to
      Chlamydia trachomatis A74.81
      Neisseria gonorrhorea (gonococcal
        peritonitis) A54.85
  Fitz's K85.8
  Flajani (-Basedow) E05.00
    with thyroid storm E05.01
  flatback —*see* Flatback syndrome
  floppy
    baby P94.2
    iris (intraoeprative) (IFIS) H21.81
    mitral valve I34.1
  flush E34.0
  Foix-Alajouanine G95.19
  Fong's Q79.8
  foramen magnum G93.5
  Foster-Kennedy H47.14-
  Foville's (peduncular) G46.3
  fragile X Q99.2
  Franceschetti Q75.4
  Frey's
    auriculotemporal G50.8
    hyperhidrosis L74.52
  Friderichsen-Waterhouse A39.1
  Froin's G95.89
  frontal lobe F07.0
  Fukuhara E88.49
  functional
    bowel K59.9
    prepubertal castrate E29.1
  Gaisböck's D75.1
  ganglion (basal ganglia brain) G25.9
    geniculi G51.1
  Gardner-Diamond D69.2
  gastroesophageal
    junction K22.0
    laceration-hemorrhage K22.6
  gastrojejunal loop obstruction K91.89
  Gee-Herter-Heubner K90.0
  Gelineau's G47.419
    with cataplexy G47.411
  genito-anorectal A55
  Gerstmann-Sträussler-Scheinker (GSS)
    A81.82
  Gianotti-Crosti L44.4
  giant platelet (Bernard-Soulier) D69.1
  Gilles de la Tourette's F95.2

Syndrome(Continued)

goiter-deafness E07.1
Goldberg Q89.8
Goldberg-Maxwell E34.51
Good's D83.8
Gopalan' (burning feet) E53.8
Gorlin's Q87.89
Gougerot-Blum L81.7
Gouley's I31.1
Gower's R55
gray or grey (newborn) P93.0
    platelet D69.1
Gubler-Millard G46.3
Guillain-Barré (-Strohl) G61.0
gustatory sweating G50.8
Hadfield-Clarke K86.8
hair tourniquet —see Constriction,
    external, by site
Hamman's J98.19
hand-foot L27.1
hand-shoulder G90.8
hantavirus (cardio)-pulmonary (HPS)
    (HCPS) B33.4
happy puppet Q93.5
Harada's H30.81-
Hayem-Faber D50.9
headache NEC G44.89
    complicated NEC G44.59
Heberden's I20.8
Hedinger's E34.0
Hegglin's D72.0
HELLP (hemolysis, elevated liver
    enzymes and low platelet count)
    O14.2-
hemolytic-uremic D59.3
hemophagocytic, infection-associated
    D76.2
Henoch-Schönlein D69.0
hepatic flexure K59.8
hepatopulmonary K76.81
hepatorenal K76.7
    following delivery O90.4
    postoperative or postprocedural
        K91.83
    postpartum, puerperal O90.4
hepatourologic K76.7
Herter (-Gee) (nontropical sprue) K90.0
Heubner-Herter K90.0
Heyd's K76.7
Hilger's G90.09
histamine-like (fish poisoning) —see
    Poisoning, fish
histiocytic D76.3
histiocytosis NEC D76.3
HIV infection, acute B20
Hoffmann-Werdnig G12.0
Hollander-Simons E88.1
Hoppe-Goldflam G70.00
    with exacerbation (acute) G70.01
    in crisis G70.01
Horner's G90.2
hungry bone E83.81
hunterian glossitis D51.0
Hutchinson's triad A50.53
hyperabduction G54.0
hyperammonemia-hyperornithinemia-
    homocitrullinemia E72.4
hypereosinophilic (idiopathic) D72.1
hyperimmunoglobulin E (IgE) D82.4
hyperkalemic E87.5
hyperkinetic —see Hyperkinesia
hypermobility M35.7
hypernatremia E87.0
hyperosmolarity E87.0

Syndrome(Continued)

hyperperfusion G97.82
hypersplenic D73.1
hypertransfusion, newborn P61.1
hyperventilation F45.8
hyperviscosity (of serum)
    polycythemic D75.1
    sclerothymic D58.8
hypoglycemic (familial) (neonatal) E16.2
hypokalemic E87.6
hyponatremic E87.1
hypopituitarism E23.0
hypoplastic left-heart Q23.4
hypopotassemia E87.6
hyposmolality E87.1
hypotension, maternal O26.5-
hypothenar hammer I73.89
ICF (intravascular coagulation-
    fibrinolysis) D65
idiopathic
    cardiorespiratory distress, newborn
        P22.0
    nephrotic (infantile) N04.9
iliotibial band M76.3-
immobility, immobilization (paraplegic)
    M62.3
immune reconstitution D89.3
immune reconstitution inflammatory
    [IRIS] D89.3
immunity deficiency, combined
    D81.9
immunodeficiency
    acquired —see Human,
        immunodeficiency
        virus (HIV) disease
    combined D81.9
impending coronary I20.0
impingement, shoulder M75.4-
inappropriate secretion of antidiuretic
    hormone E22.2
infant
    gestational diabetes P70.0
    of diabetic mother P70.1
infantilism (pituitary) E23.0
inferior vena cava I87.1
inspissated bile (newborn) P59.1
institutional (childhood) F94.2
insufficient sleep F51.12
intermediate coronary (artery) I20.0
interspinous ligament —see
        Spondylopathy, specified NEC
intestinal
    carcinoid E34.0
    knot K56.2
intravascular coagulation-fibrinolysis
    (ICF) D65
iodine-deficiency, congenital E00.9
    type
        mixed E00.2
        myxedematous E00.1
        neurological E00.0
IRDS (idiopathic respiratory distress,
    newborn) P22.0
irritable
    bowel K58.9
        with diarrhea K58.0
        psychogenic F45.8
    heart (psychogenic) F45.8
    weakness F48.8
ischemic bowel (transient) K55.9
    chronic K55.1
    due to mesenteric artery insufficiency
        K55.1
IVC (intravascular coagulopathy) D65

Syndrome(Continued)

Ivemark's Q89.01
Jaccoud's —see Arthropathy,
        postrheumatic, chronic
Jackson's G83.89
Jakob-Creutzfeldt —see Creutzfeldt-
        Jakob disease or syndrome
jaw-winking Q07.8
Jervell-Lange-Nielsen I45.81
jet lag G47.25
Job's D71
Joseph-Diamond-Blackfan D61.01
jugular foramen G52.7
Kabuki Q89.8
Kanner's (autism) F84.0
Kartagener's Q89.3
Kelly's D50.1
Kimmelstiel-Wilson —see Diabetes,
        specified type, with Kimmelstiel-
        Wilson disease
Klein (e)-Levine G47.13
Klippel-Feil (brevicollis) Q76.1
Köhler-Pellegrini-Steida —see Bursitis,
        tibial collateral
König's K59.8
Korsakoff (-Wernicke) (nonalcoholic)
        F04
    alcoholic F10.26
Kostmann's D70.0
Krabbe's congenital muscle hypoplasia
        Q79.8
labyrinthine —see subcategory H83.2
lacunar NEC G46.7
Lambert-Eaton G70.80
    in
        neoplastic disease G73.1
        specified disease NEC G70.81
Landau-Kleffner —see Epilepsy,
        specified NEC
Larsen's Q74.8
lateral
    cutaneous nerve of thigh G57.1-
    medullary G46.4
Launois' E22.0
lazy
    leukocyte D70.8
    posture M62.3
Lemiere I80.8
Lennox-Gastaut G40.812
    intractable G40.814
        with status epilepticus G40.813
        without status epilepticus
            G40.814
    not intractable G40.812
        with status epilepticus G40.811
        without status epilepticus
            G40.812
lenticular, progressive E83.01
Leopold-Levi's E05.90
Lev's I44.2
Li-Fraumeni Z15.01
Lichtheim's D51.0
Lightwood's N25.89
Lignac (de Toni) (-Fanconi) (-Debré)
        E72.09
    with cystinosis E72.04
Likoff's I20.8
limbic epilepsy personality F07.0
liver-kidney K76.7
lobotomy F07.0
Loffler's J82
long arm 18 or 21 deletion Q93.89
long QT I45.81
Louis-Barré G11.3

459

Syndrome *(Continued)*

low
  atmospheric pressure T70.29
  back M54.5
  output (cardiac) I50.9
lower radicular, newborn (birth injury)
  P14.8
Luetscher's (dehydration) E86.0
Lupus anticoagulant D68.62
Lutembacher's Q21.1
macrophage activation D76.1
  due to infection D76.2
magnesium-deficiency R29.0
Mal de Debarquement R42
malabsorption K90.9
  postsurgical K91.2
malformation, congenital, due to
  alcohol Q86.0
  exogenous cause NEC Q86.8
  hydantoin Q86.1
  warfarin Q86.2
malignant
  carcinoid E34.0
  neuroleptic G21.0
Mallory-Weiss K22.6
mandibulofacial dysostosis Q75.4
manic-depressive —*see* Disorder,
  bipolar, affective
maple-syrup-urine E71.0
Marable's I77.4
Marfan's Q87.40
  with
    cardiovascular manifestations
      Q87.418
      aortic dilation Q87.410
    ocular manifestations Q87.42
    skeletal manifestations Q87.43
Marie's (acromegaly) E22.0
maternal hypotension —*see* Syndrome,
  hypotension, maternal
May (-Hegglin) D72.0
McArdle (-Schmidt) (-Pearson) E74.04
McQuarrie's E16.2
meconium plug (newborn) P76.0
median arcuate ligament I77.4
Meekeren-Ehlers-Danlos Q79.6
megavitamin-B6 E67.2
Meige G24.4
MELAS E88.41
Mendelson's O74.0
MERRF (myoclonic epilepsy associated
  with ragged-red fibers) E88.42
mesenteric
  artery (superior) K55.1
  vascular insufficiency K55.1
metabolic E88.81
metastatic carcinoid E34.0
micrognathia-glossoptosis Q87.0
midbrain NEC G93.89
middle lobe (lung) J98.19
middle radicular G54.0
migraine (*see also* Migraine) G43.909
Mikulicz' K11.8
milk-alkali E83.52
Millard-Gubler G46.3
Miller-Dieker Q93.88
Miller-Fisher G61.0
Minkowski-Chauffard D58.0
Mirizzi's K83.1
MNGIE (Mitochondrial
  Neurogastrointestinal
  Encephalopathy) E88.49
Möbius, ophthalmoplegic migraine —
  see Migraine, ophthalmoplegic

Syndrome *(Continued)*

monofixation H50.42
Morel-Moore M85.2
Morel-Morgagni M85.2
Morgagni (-Morel) (-Stewart) M85.2
Morgagni-Adams-Stokes I45.9
Mounier-Kuhn Q32.4
  with bronchiectasis J47.9
    with
      exacerbation (acute) J47.1
      lower respiratory infection J47.0
  acquired J98.09
    with bronchiectasis J47.9
      with
        exacerbation (acute) J47.1
        lower respiratory infection
          J47.0
mucocutaneous lymph node (acute
  febrile) (MCLS) M30.3
multiple endocrine neoplasia (MEN) —
  see Neoplasia, endocrine, multiple
  (MEN}
multiple operations —*see* Disorder,
  factitious
myasthenic G70.9
  in
    diabetes mellitus —*see* Diabetes,
      amyotrophy
    endocrine disease NEC E34.9 *[G73.3]*
    neoplastic disease (*see also*
      Neoplasm) D49.9 *[G73.3]*
    thyrotoxicosis (hyperthyroidism)
      E05.90 *[G73.3]*
      with thyroid storm E05.91 *[G73.3]*
myelodysplastic D46.9
  with
    5q deletion D46.C
    isolated del (5q) chromosomal
      abnormality D46.C
  lesions, low grade D46.20
  specified NEC D46.Z
myelopathic pain G89.0
myeloproliferative (chronic) D47.1
myofascial pain M79.1
Naffziger's G54.0
nail patella Q87.2
NARP (Neuropathy, Ataxia and
  Retinitis pigmentosa) E88.49
neonatal abstinence P96.1
nephritic —*see also* Nephritis
  with edema —*see* Nephrosis
  acute N00.9
  chronic N03.9
  rapidly progressive N01.9
nephrotic (congenital) (*see also*
  Nephrosis) N04.9
  with
    dense deposit disease N04.6
    diffuse
      crescentic glomerulonephritis
        N04.7
      endocapillary proliferative
        glomerulonephritis N04.4
      membranous glomerulonephritis
        N04.2
      mesangial proliferative
        glomerulonephritis N04.3
      mesangiocapillary
        glomerulonephritis N04.5
    focal and segmental glomerular
      lesions N04.1
    minor glomerular abnormality
      N04.0
    specified morphological changes
      NEC N04.8
  diabetic —*see* Diabetes, nephrosis

Syndrome *(Continued)*

neurologic neglect R41.4
Nezelof's D81.4
Nonne-Milroy-Meige Q82.0
Nothnagel's vasomotor acroparesthesia
  I73.89
oculomotor H51.9
ophthalmoplegia-cerebellar ataxia —*see*
  Strabismus, paralytic, third nerve
oral-facial-digital Q87.0
organic
  affective F06.30
  amnesic (not alcohol- or drug-
    induced) F04
  brain F09
  depressive F06.31
  hallucinosis F06.0
  personality F07.0
Ormond's N13.5
oro-facial-digital Q87.0
os trigonum Q68.8
Osler-Weber-Rendu I78.0
osteoporosis-osteomalacia M83.8
Osterreicher-Turner Q79.8
otolith —*see* subcategory H81.8
oto-palatal-digital Q87.0
outlet (thoracic) G54.0
ovary
  polycystic E28.2
  resistant E28.39
  sclerocystic E28.2
Owren's D68.2
Paget-Schroetter I82.890
pain —*see also* Pain
  complex regional I G90.50
    lower limb G90.52-
    specified site NEC G90.59
    upper limb G90.51-
  complex regional II —*see* Causalgia
painful
  bruising D69.2
  feet E53.8
  prostate N42.81
paralysis agitans —*see* Parkinsonism
paralytic G83.9
  specified NEC G83.89
Parinaud's H51.0
parkinsonian —*see* Parkinsonism
Parkinson's —*see* Parkinsonism
paroxysmal facial pain G50.0
Parry's E05.00
  with thyroid storm E05.01
Parsonage (-Aldren)-Turner G54.5
patella clunk M25.86-
Paterson (-Brown) (-Kelly) D50.1
pectoral girdle I77.89
pectoralis minor I77.89
Pelger-Huet D72.0
pellagra-cerebellar ataxia-renal
  aminoaciduria E72.02
pellagroid E52
Pellegrini-Stieda —*see* Bursitis, tibial
  collateral
pelvic congestion-fibrosis, female
  N94.89
penta X Q97.1
peptic ulcer —*see* Ulcer, peptic
perabduction I77.89
periodic headache, in adults and
  children —*see* Headache, periodic
  syndromes in adults and children
periurethral fibrosis N13.5
phantom limb (without pain) G54.7
  with pain G54.6
pharyngeal pouch D82.1

Syndrome *(Continued)*
Pick's (heart) (liver) I31.1
Pickwickian E66.2
PIE (pulmonary infiltration with
    eosinophilia) J82
pigmentary pallidal degeneration
    (progressive) G23.0
pineal E34.8
pituitary E22.0
placental transfusion —*see* Pregnancy,
    complicated by, placental
    transfusion syndromes
plantar fascia M72.2
plateau iris (post-iridectomy)
    (postprocedural) H21.82
Plummer-Vinson D50.1
pluricarential of infancy E40
plurideficiency E40
pluriglandular (compensatory) E31.8
    autoimmune E31.0
pneumatic hammer T75.21
polyangiitis overlap M30.8
polycarential of infancy E40
polyglandular E31.8
    autoimmune E31.0
polysplenia Q89.09
pontine NEC G93.89
popliteal
    artery entrapment I77.89
    web Q87.89
post chemoembolization — code to
    associated conditions
postcardiac injury
    postcardiotomy I97.0
    postmyocardial infarction I24.1
postcardiotomy I97.0
postcholecystectomy K91.5
postcommissurotomy I97.0
postconcussional F07.81
postcontusional F07.81
postencephalitic F07.89
posterior
    cervical sympathetic M53.0
    cord G83.83
    fossa compression G93.5
    reversible encephalopathy (PRES)
        I67.83
postgastrectomy (dumping) K91.1
postgastric surgery K91.1
postinfarction I24.1
postlaminectomy NEC M96.1
postleukotomy F07.0
postmastectomy lymphedema I97.2
postmyocardial infarction I24.1
postoperative NEC T81.9
    blind loop K90.2
postpartum panhypopituitary
    (Sheehan) E23.0
postpolio (myelitic) G14
postthrombotic I87.009
    with
        inflammation I87.02-
            with ulcer I87.03-
        specified complication NEC
            I87.09-
        ulcer I87.01-
            with inflammation I87.03-
    asymptomatic I87.00-
postvagotomy K91.1
postvalvulotomy I97.0
postviral NEC G93.3
    fatigue G93.3
Potain's K31.0
potassium intoxication E87.5

Syndrome *(Continued)*
precerebral artery (multiple) (bilateral)
    G45.2
preinfarction I20.0
preleukemic D46.9
premature senility E34.8
premenstrual dysphoric N94.3
premenstrual tension N94.3
Prinzmetal-Massumi R07.1
prune belly Q79.4
pseudocarpal tunnel (sublimis) —*see*
    Syndrome, carpal tunnel
pseudoparalytica G70.00
    with exacerbation (acute) G70.01
    in crisis G70.01
pseudo -Turner's Q87.1
psycho-organic (nonpsychotic severity)
    F07.9
    acute or subacute F05
    depressive type F06.31
    hallucinatory type F06.0
    nonpsychotic severity F07.0
    specified NEC F07.89
pulmonary
    arteriosclerosis I27.0
    dysmaturity (Wilson-Mikity)
        P27.0
    hypoperfusion (idiopathic) P22.0
    renal (hemorrhagic) (Goodpasture's)
        M31.0
pure
    motor lacunar G46.5
    sensory lacunar G46.6
Putnam-Dana D51.0
pyramidopallidonigral G20
pyriformis —*see* Lesion, nerve, sciatic
QT interval prolongation I45.81
radicular NEC —*see* Radiculopathy
    upper limbs, newborn (birth injury)
        P14.3
rapid time-zone change G47.25
Rasmussen G04.81
Raymond (-Céstan) I65.8
Raynaud's I73.00
    with gangrene I73.01
RDS (respiratory distress syndrome,
    newborn) P22.0
reactive airways dysfunction J68.3
Refsum's G60.1
Reifenstein E34.52
renal glomerulohyalinosis-diabetic —
    see Diabetes, nephrosis
Rendu-Osler-Weber I78.0
residual ovary N99.83
resistant ovary E28.39
respiratory
    distress
        acute J80
        adult J80
        child J80
        newborn (idiopathic) (type I) P22.0
        type II P22.1
restless legs G25.81
retinoblastoma (familial) C69.2
retroperitoneal fibrosis N13.5
retroviral seroconversion (acute) Z21
Reye's G93.7
Richter —*see* Leukemia, chronic
    lymphocytic, B-cell type
Ridley's I50.1
right
    heart, hypoplastic Q22.6
    ventricular obstruction —*see* Failure,
        heart, congestive

Syndrome *(Continued)*
Romano-Ward (prolonged QT interval)
    I45.81
rotator cuff, shoulder (*see also* Tear,
    rotator cuff) M75.10-
Rotes Quérol —*see* Hyperostosis,
    ankylosing
Roth —*see* Meralgia paresthetica
rubella (congenital) P35.0
Ruvalcaba-Myhre-Smith E71.440
Rytand-Lipsitch I44.2
salt
    depletion E87.1
        due to heat NEC T67.8
            causing heat exhaustion or
                prostration T67.4
    low E87.1
salt-losing N28.89
Scaglietti-Dagnini E22.0
scalenus anticus (anterior) G54.0
scapulocostal —*see* Mononeuropathy,
    upper limb, specified site NEC
scapuloperoneal G71.0
schizophrenic, of childhood NEC
    F84.5
Schnitzler D47.2
Scholte's E34.0
Schroeder's E27.0
Schüller-Christian C96.5
Schwachman's —*see* Syndrome,
    Shwachman's
Schwartz (-Jampel) G71.13
Schwartz-Bartter E22.2
scimitar Q26.8
sclerocystic ovary E28.2
Seitelberger's G31.89
septicemic adrenal hemorrhage A39.1
seroconversion, retroviral (acute) Z21
serous meningitis G93.2
severe acute respiratory (SARS) J12.81
shaken infant T74.4
shock (traumatic) T79.4
    kidney N17.0
        following crush injury T79.5
    toxic A48.3
shock-lung J80
Shone's — code to specific anomalies
short
    bowel K91.2
    rib Q77.2
shoulder-hand —*see*
    Algoneurodystrophy
Shwachman's D70.4
sicca —*see* Sicca syndrome
sick
    cell E87.1
    sinus I49.5
sick-euthyroid E07.81
sideropenic D50.1
Siemens' ectodermal dysplasia Q82.4
Silfverskiöld's Q78.9
Simons' E88.1
sinus tarsi —*see* Syndrome, tarsal
    tunnel
sinusitis-bronchiectasis-situs inversus
    Q89.3
Sipple's E31.22
sirenomelia Q87.2
Slocumb's E27.0
slow flow, coronary I20.8
Sluder's G44.89
Smith-Magenis Q93.88
Sneddon-Wilkinson L13.1
Sotos' E22.0
South African cardiomyopathy I42.8

Syndrome (Continued)
  spasmodic
    upward movement, eyes H51.8
    winking F95.8
  Spen's I45.9
  splenic
    agenesis Q89.01
    flexure K59.8
    neutropenia D73.81
  Spurway's Q78.0
  staphylococcal scalded skin L00
  Stein-Leventhal E28.2
  Stein's E28.2
  Stevens-Johnson syndrome L51.1
    toxic epidermal necrolysis overlap
      L51.3
  Stewart-Morel M85.2
  Stickler Q89.8
  stiff baby Q89.8
  stiff man G25.82
  Still-Felty —see Felty's syndrome
  Stokes (-Adams) I45.9
  stone heart I50.1
  straight back, congenital Q76.49
  subclavian steal G45.8
  subcoracoid-pectoralis minor G54.0
  subcostal nerve compression I77.89
  subphrenic interposition Q43.3
  superior
    cerebellar artery I63.8
    mesenteric artery K55.1
    semi-circular canal dehiscence
      H83.8X-
    vena cava I87.1
  supine hypotensive (maternal) —see
    Syndrome, hypotension, maternal
  suprarenal cortical E27.0
  supraspinatus (see also Tear, rotator cuff)
    M75.10-
  Susac G93.49
  swallowed blood P78.2
  sweat retention L74.0
  Swyer Q99.1
  Symond's G93.2
  sympathetic
    cervical paralysis G90.2
    pelvic, female N94.89
  systemic inflammatory response (SIRS),
    of non-infectious origin (without
    organ dysfunction) R65.10
    with acute organ dysfunction
      R65.11
  tachycardia-bradycardia I49.5
  takotsubo I51.81
  TAR (thrombocytopenia with absent
    radius) Q87.2
  tarsal tunnel G57.5-
  teething K00.7
  tegmental G93.89
  telangiectasic-pigmentation-cataract
    Q82.8
  temporal pyramidal apex —see Otitis,
    media, suppurative, acute
  temporomandibular joint-pain-
    dysfunction M26.62
  Terry's H44.2-
  testicular feminization (see
    also Syndrome, androgen
    insensitivity) E34.51
  thalamic pain (hyperesthetic) G89.0
  thoracic outlet (compression) G54.0
  Thorson-Björck E34.0
  thrombocytopenia with absent radius
    (TAR) Q87.2

Syndrome (Continued)
  thyroid-adrenocortical insufficiency E31.0
  tibial
    anterior M76.81-
    posterior M76.82-
  Tietze's M94.0
  time-zone (rapid) G47.25
  Toni-Fanconi E72.09
    with cystinosis E72.04
  Touraine's Q79.8
  tourniquet —see Constriction, external,
    by site
  toxic shock A48.3
  transient left ventricular apical
    ballooning I51.81
  traumatic vasospastic T75.22
  Treacher Collins Q75.4
  triple X, female Q97.0
  trisomy Q92.9
    13 Q91.7
      meiotic nondisjunction Q91.4
      mitotic nondisjunction Q91.5
      mosaicism Q91.5
      translocation Q91.6
    18 Q91.3
      meiotic nondisjunction Q91.0
      mitotic nondisjunction Q91.1
      mosaicism Q91.1
      translocation Q91.2
    20 (q)(p) Q92.8
    21 Q90.9
      meiotic nondisjunction Q90.0
      mitotic nondisjunction Q90.1
      mosaicism Q90.1
      translocation Q90.2
    22 Q92.8
  tropical wet feet T69.0-
  Trousseau's I82.1
  tumor lysis (following antineoplastic
    chemotherapy) (spontaneous)
    NEC E88.3
  Twiddler's (due to)
    automatic implantable defibrillator
      T82.198
    cardiac pacemaker T82.198
  Unverricht (-Lundborg) —see Epilepsy,
    generalized, idiopathic
  upward gaze H51.8
  uremia, chronic (see also Disease,
    kidney, chronic) N18.9
  urethral N34.3
  urethro-oculo-articular —see Reiter's
    disease
  urohepatic K76.7
  vago-hypoglossal G52.7
  van Buchem's M85.2
  van der Hoeve's Q78.0
  vascular NEC in cerebrovascular
    disease G46.8
  vasoconstriction, reversible
    cerebrovascular I67.841
  vasomotor I73.9
  vasospastic (traumatic) T75.22
  vasovagal R55
  VATER Q87.2
  velo-cardio-facial Q93.81
  vena cava (inferior) (superior)
    (obstruction) I87.1
  vertebral
    artery G45.0
      compression —see Syndrome,
        anterior, spinal artery,
        compression
    steal G45.0

Syndrome (Continued)
  vertebro-basilar artery G45.0
  vertebrogenic (pain) M54.89
  vertiginous —see Disorder, vestibular
    function
  Vinson-Plummer D50.1
  virus B34.9
  visceral larva migrans B83.0
  visual disorientation H53.8
  vitamin B6 deficiency E53.1
  vitreal corneal H59.01-
  vitreous (touch) H59.01-
  Vogt-Koyanagi H20.82-
  Volkmann's T79.6
  von Schroetter's I82.890
  von Willebrand (-Jürgen) D68.0
  Waldenström-Kjellberg D50.1
  Wallenberg's G46.3
  water retention E87.79
  Waterhouse (-Friderichsen) A39.1
  Weber-Gubler G46.3
  Weber-Leyden G46.3
  Weber's G46.3
  Wegener's M31.30
    with
      kidney involvement M31.31
      lung involvement M31.30
        with kidney involvement M31.31
  Weingarten's (tropical eosinophilia)
    J82
  Weiss-Baker G90.09
  Werdnig-Hoffman G12.0
  Wermer's E31.21
  Werner's E34.8
  Wernicke-Korsakoff (nonalcoholic) F04
    alcoholic F10.26
  West's —see Epilepsy, spasms
  Westphal-Strümpell E83.01
  wet
    feet (maceration) (tropical) T69.0-
    lung, newborn P22.1
  whiplash S13.4
  whistling face Q87.0
  Wilkie's K55.1
  Wilkinson-Sneddon L13.1
  Willebrand (-Jürgens) D68.0
  Wilson's (hepatolenticular
    degeneration) E83.01
  Wiskott-Aldrich D82.0
  withdrawal —see Withdrawal, state
    drug
      infant of dependent mother P96.1
      therapeutic use, newborn P96.2
  Woakes' (ethmoiditis) J33.1
  Wright's (hyperabduction) I77.89
  X I20.9
  XXXX Q97.1
  XXXXX Q97.1
  XXXXY Q98.1
  XXY Q98.0
  yellow nail L60.5
  Zahorsky's B08.5
  Zellweger syndrome E71.510
  Zellweger-like syndrome E71.541
Synechia (anterior) (iris) (posterior)
  (pupil) —see also Adhesions, iris
  intra-uterine (traumatic) N85.6
Synesthesia R20.8
Syngamiasis, syngamosis B83.3
Synodontia K00.2
Synorchidism, synorchism Q55.1
Synostosis (congenital) Q78.8
  astragalo-scaphoid Q74.2
  radioulnar Q74.0

Synovial sarcoma —*see* Neoplasm, connective tissue, malignant

Synovioma (malignant) —*see also* Neoplasm, connective tissue, malignant
- benign —*see* Neoplasm, connective tissue, benign

Synoviosarcoma —*see* Neoplasm, connective tissue, malignant

Synovitis —*see also* Tenosynovitis
- crepitant
  - hand M70.0-
  - wrist M70.03-
- gonococcal A54.49
- gouty —*see* Gout, idiopathic
- in (due to)
  - crystals M65.8-
  - gonorrhea A54.49
  - syphilis (late) A52.78
  - use, overuse, pressure —*see* Disorder, soft tissue, due to use
- infective NEC —*see* Tenosynovitis, infective NEC
- specified NEC —*see* Tenosynovitis, specified type NEC
- syphilitic A52.78
  - congenital (early) A50.02
- toxic —*see* Synovitis, transient
- transient M67.3-
  - ankle M67.37-
  - elbow M67.32-
  - foot joint M67.37-
  - hand joint M67.34-
  - hip M67.35-
  - knee M67.36-
  - multiple site M67.39
  - pelvic region M67.35-
  - shoulder M67.31-
  - specified joint NEC M67.38
  - wrist M67.33-
- traumatic, current —*see* Sprain
- tuberculous —*see* Tuberculosis, synovitis
- villonodular (pigmented) M12.2-
  - ankle M12.27-
  - elbow M12.22-
  - foot joint M12.27-
  - hand joint M12.24-
  - hip M12.25-
  - knee M12.26-
  - multiple site M12.29
  - pelvic region M12.25-
  - shoulder M12.21-
  - specified joint NEC M12.28
  - wrist M12.23-

Syphilid A51.39
- congenital A50.06
- newborn A50.06
- tubercular (late) A52.79

Syphilis, syphilitic (acquired) A53.9
- abdomen (late) A52.79
- acoustic nerve A52.15
- adenopathy (secondary) A51.49
- adrenal (gland) (with cortical hypofunction) A52.79
- age under 2 years NOS —*see also* Syphilis, congenital, early
  - acquired A51.9
- alopecia (secondary) A51.32
- anemia (late) A52.79 [D63.8]
- aneurysm (aorta) (ruptured) A52.01
  - central nervous system A52.05
  - congenital A50.54 [I79.0]

Syphilis, syphilitic (Continued)
- anus (late) A52.74
  - primary A51.1
  - secondary A51.39
- aorta (arch) (abdominal) (thoracic) A52.02
  - aneurysm A52.01
- aortic (insufficiency) (regurgitation) (stenosis) A52.03
  - aneurysm A52.01
- arachnoid (adhesive) (cerebral) (spinal) A52.13
- asymptomatic —*see* Syphilis, latent
- ataxia (locomotor) A52.11
- atrophoderma maculatum A51.39
- auricular fibrillation A52.06
- bladder (late) A52.76
- bone A52.77
  - secondary A51.46
- brain A52.17
- breast (late) A52.79
- bronchus (late) A52.72
- bubo (primary) A51.0
- bulbar palsy A52.19
- bursa (late) A52.78
- cardiac decompensation A52.06
- cardiovascular A52.00
- central nervous system (late) (recurrent) (relapse) (tertiary) A52.3
  - with
    - ataxia A52.11
    - general paralysis A52.17
      - juvenile A50.45
    - paresis (general) A52.17
      - juvenile A50.45
    - tabes (dorsalis) A52.11
      - juvenile A50.45
    - taboparesis A52.17
      - juvenile A50.45
  - aneurysm A52.05
  - congenital A50.40
  - juvenile A50.40
  - remission in (sustained) A52.3
  - serology doubtful, negative, or positive A52.3
  - specified nature or site NEC A52.19
  - vascular A52.05
- cerebral A52.17
  - meningovascular A52.13
  - nerves (multiple palsies) A52.15
  - sclerosis A52.17
  - thrombosis A52.05
- cerebrospinal (tabetic type) A52.12
- cerebrovascular A52.05
- cervix (late) A52.76
- chancre (multiple) A51.0
  - extragenital A51.2
  - Rollet's A51.0
- Charcot's joint A52.16
- chorioretinitis A51.43
  - congenital A50.01
  - late A52.71
  - prenatal A50.01
- choroiditis —*see* Syphilitic chorioretinitis
- choroidoretinitis —*see* Syphilitic chorioretinitis
- ciliary body (secondary) A51.43
  - late A52.71
- colon (late) A52.74
- combined spinal sclerosis A52.11
- condyloma (latum) A51.31

Syphilis, syphilitic (Continued)
- congenital A50.9
  - with
    - paresis (general) A50.45
    - tabes (dorsalis) A50.45
    - taboparesis A50.45
  - chorioretinitis, choroiditis A50.01 [H32]
  - early, or less than 2 years after birth NEC A50.2
    - with manifestations —*see* Syphilis, congenital, early, symptomatic
    - latent (without manifestations) A50.1
      - negative spinal fluid test A50.1
      - serology positive A50.1
    - symptomatic A50.09
      - cutaneous A50.06
      - mucocutaneous A50.07
      - oculopathy A50.01
      - osteochondropathy A50.02
      - pharyngitis A50.03
      - pneumonia A50.04
      - rhinitis A50.05
      - visceral A50.08
  - interstitial keratitis A50.31
  - juvenile neurosyphilis A50.45
  - late, or 2 years or more after birth NEC A50.7
    - chorioretinitis, choroiditis A50.32
    - interstitial keratitis A50.31
    - juvenile neurosyphilis A50.45
    - latent (without manifestations) A50.6
      - negative spinal fluid test A50.6
      - serology positive A50.6
    - symptomatic or with manifestations NEC A50.59
      - arthropathy A50.55
      - cardiovascular A50.54
      - Clutton's joints A50.51
      - Hutchinson's teeth A50.52
      - Hutchinson's triad A50.53
      - osteochondropathy A50.56
      - saddle nose A50.57
- conjugal A53.9
  - tabes A52.11
- conjunctiva (late) A52.71
- contact Z20.2
- cord bladder A52.19
- cornea, late A52.71
- coronary (artery) (sclerosis) A52.06
- coryza, congenital A50.05
- cranial nerve A52.15
  - multiple palsies A52.15
- cutaneous —*see* Syphilis, skin
- dacryocystitis (late) A52.71
- degeneration, spinal cord A52.12
- dementia paralytica A52.17
  - juvenilis A50.45
- destruction of bone A52.77
- dilatation, aorta A52.01
- due to blood transfusion A53.9
- dura mater A52.13
- ear A52.79
  - inner A52.79
    - nerve (eighth) A52.15
    - neurorecurrence A52.15
- early A51.9
  - cardiovascular A52.00
  - central nervous system A52.3
  - latent (without manifestations) (less than 2 years after infection) A51.5
    - negative spinal fluid test A51.5
    - serological relapse after treatment A51.5
    - serology positive A51.5

Syphilis, syphilitic (Continued)
   early (Continued)
      relapse (treated, untreated)
         A51.9
      skin A51.39
      symptomatic A51.9
         extragenital chancre A51.2
         primary, except extragenital
           chancre A51.0
         secondary (see also Syphilis,
           secondary) A51.39
           relapse (treated, untreated)
              A51.49
      ulcer A51.39
   eighth nerve (neuritis) A52.15
   endemic A65
   endocarditis A52.03
      aortic A52.03
      pulmonary A52.03
   epididymis (late) A52.76
   epiglottis (late) A52.73
   epiphysitis (congenital) (early)
      A50.02
   episcleritis (late) A52.71
   esophagus A52.79
   eustachian tube A52.73
   exposure to Z20.2
   eye A52.71
   eyelid (late) (with gumma) A52.71
   fallopian tube (late) A52.76
   fracture A52.77
   gallbladder (late) A52.74
   gastric (polyposis) (late) A52.74
   general A53.9
      paralysis A52.17
         juvenile A50.45
   genital (primary) A51.0
   glaucoma A52.71
   gumma NEC A52.79
      cardiovascular system A52.00
      central nervous system A52.3
      congenital A50.59
   heart (block) (decompensation)
      (disease) (failure) A52.06 [I52]
      valve NEC A52.03
   hemianesthesia A52.19
   hemianopsia A52.71
   hemiparesis A52.17
   hemiplegia A52.17
   hepatic artery A52.09
   hepatis A52.74
   hepatomegaly, congenital A50.08
   hereditaria tarda —see Syphilis,
      congenital, late
   hereditary —see Syphilis, congenital
   Hutchinson's teeth A50.52
   hyalitis A52.71
   inactive —see Syphilis, latent
   infantum —see Syphilis, congenital
   inherited —see Syphilis, congenital
   internal ear A52.79
   intestine (late) A52.74
   iris, iritis (secondary) A51.43
      late A52.71
   joint (late) A52.77
   keratitis (congenital) (interstitial) (late)
      A50.31
   kidney (late) A52.75
   lacrimal passages (late) A52.71
   larynx (late) A52.73
   late A52.9
      cardiovascular A52.00
      central nervous system A52.3
      kidney A52.75

Syphilis, syphilitic (Continued)
   late (Continued)
      latent or 2 years or more
         after infection (without
         manifestations) A52.8
         negative spinal fluid test A52.8
         serology positive A52.8
      paresis A52.17
      specified site NEC A52.79
      symptomatic or with manifestations
         A52.79
      tabes A52.11
   latent A53.0
      with signs or symptoms - code by site
         and stage under Syphilis
      central nervous system A52.2
      date of infection unspecified A53.0
      early, or less than 2 years after
         infection A51.5
      follow-up of latent syphilis A53.0
         date of infection unspecified
           A53.0
         late, or 2 years or more after
           infection A52.8
      late, or 2 years or more after infection
         A52.8
      positive serology (only finding) A53.0
         date of infection unspecified A53.0
         early, or less than 2 years after
           infection A51.5
         late, or 2 years or more after
           infection A52.8
   lens (late) A52.71
   leukoderma A51.39
      late A52.79
   lienitis A52.79
   lip A51.39
      chancre (primary) A51.2
      late A52.79
   Lissauer's paralysis A52.17
   liver A52.74
   locomotor ataxia A52.11
   lung A52.72
   lymph gland (early) (secondary) A51.49
      late A52.79
   lymphadenitis (secondary) A51.49
   macular atrophy of skin A51.39
      striated A52.79
   mediastinum (late) A52.73
   meninges (adhesive) (brain) (spinal
      cord) A52.13
   meningitis A52.13
      acute (secondary) A51.41
      congenital A50.41
   meningoencephalitis A52.14
   meningovascular A52.13
      congenital A50.41
   mesarteritis A52.09
      brain A52.04
   middle ear A52.77
   mitral stenosis A52.03
   monoplegia A52.17
   mouth (secondary) A51.39
      late A52.79
   mucocutaneous (secondary) A51.39
      late A52.79
   mucous
      membrane (secondary) A51.39
         late A52.79
      patches A51.39
         congenital A50.07
   mulberry molars A50.52
   muscle A52.78
   myocardium A52.06

Syphilis, syphilitic (Continued)
   nasal sinus (late) A52.73
   neonatorum —see Syphilis, congenital
   nephrotic syndrome (secondary)
      A51.44
   nerve palsy (any cranial nerve) A52.15
      multiple A52.15
   nervous system, central A52.3
   neuritis A52.15
      acoustic A52.15
   neurorecidive of retina A52.19
   neuroretinitis A52.19
   newborn —see Syphilis, congenital
   nodular superficial (late) A52.79
   nonvenereal A65
   nose (late) A52.73
      saddle back deformity A50.57
   occlusive arterial disease A52.09
   oculopathy A52.71
   oesophagus (late) A52.79
   ophthalmic (late) A52.71
   optic nerve (atrophy) (neuritis) (papilla)
      A52.15
   orbit (late) A52.71
   organic A53.9
   osseous (late) A52.77
   osteochondritis (congenital) (early)
      A50.02 [M90.80]
   osteoporosis A52.77
   ovary (late) A52.76
   oviduct (late) A52.76
   palate (late) A52.79
   pancreas (late) A52.74
   paralysis A52.17
      general A52.17
         juvenile A50.45
   paresis (general) A52.17
      juvenile A50.45
   paresthesia A52.19
   Parkinson's disease or syndrome A52.19
   paroxysmal tachycardia A52.06
   pemphigus (congenital) A50.06
   penis (chancre) A51.0
      late A52.76
   pericardium A52.06
   perichondritis, larynx (late) A52.73
   periosteum (late) A52.77
      congenital (early) A50.02 [M90.80]
      early (secondary) A51.46
   peripheral nerve A52.79
   petrous bone (late) A52.77
   pharynx (late) A52.73
      secondary A51.39
   pituitary (gland) A52.79
   pleura (late) A52.73
   pneumonia, white A50.04
   pontine lesion A52.17
   portal vein A52.09
   primary A51.0
      anal A51.1
      and secondary —see Syphilis,
         secondary
      central nervous system A52.3
      extragenital chancre NEC A51.2
      fingers A51.2
      genital A51.0
      lip A51.2
      specified site NEC A51.2
      tonsils A51.2
   prostate (late) A52.76
   ptosis (eyelid) A52.71
   pulmonary (late) A52.72
      artery A52.09
   pyelonephritis (late) A52.75

Syphilis, syphilitic *(Continued)*
  recently acquired, symptomatic A51.9
  rectum (late) A52.74
  respiratory tract (late) A52.73
  retina, late A52.71
  retrobulbar neuritis A52.15
  salpingitis A52.76
  sclera (late) A52.71
  sclerosis
    cerebral A52.17
    coronary A52.06
    multiple A52.11
  scotoma (central) A52.71
  scrotum (late) A52.76
  secondary (and primary) A51.49
    adenopathy A51.49
    anus A51.39
    bone A51.46
    chorioretinitis, choroiditis A51.43
    hepatitis A51.45
    liver A51.45
    lymphadenitis A51.49
    meningitis (acute) A51.41
    mouth A51.39
    mucous membranes A51.39
    periosteum, periostitis A51.46
    pharynx A51.39
    relapse (treated, untreated) A51.49
    skin A51.39
    specified form NEC A51.49
    tonsil A51.39
    ulcer A51.39
    viscera NEC A51.49
    vulva A51.39
  seminal vesicle (late) A52.76
  seronegative with signs or symptoms - code by site and stage under Syphilis
  seropositive
    with signs or symptoms - code by site and stage under Syphilis
    follow-up of latent syphilis —*see* Syphilis, latent
    only finding —*see* Syphilis, latent
  seventh nerve (paralysis) A52.15
  sinus, sinusitis (late) A52.73
  skeletal system A52.77

Syphilis, syphilitic *(Continued)*
  skin (with ulceration) (early) (secondary) A51.39
    late or tertiary A52.79
  small intestine A52.74
  spastic spinal paralysis A52.17
  spermatic cord (late) A52.76
  spinal (cord) A52.12
  spleen A52.79
  splenomegaly A52.79
  spondylitis A52.77
  staphyloma A52.71
  stigmata (congenital) A50.59
  stomach A52.74
  synovium A52.78
  tabes dorsalis (late) A52.11
    juvenile A50.45
  tabetic type A52.11
    juvenile A50.45
  taboparesis A52.17
    juvenile A50.45
  tachycardia A52.06
  tendon (late) A52.78
  tertiary A52.9
    with symptoms NEC A52.79
    cardiovascular A52.00
    central nervous system A52.3
    multiple NEC A52.79
    specified site NEC A52.79
  testis A52.76
  thorax A52.73
  throat A52.73
  thymus (gland) (late) A52.79
  thyroid (late) A52.79
  tongue (late) A52.79
  tonsil (lingual) (late) A52.73
    primary A51.2
    secondary A51.39
  trachea (late) A52.73
  tunica vaginalis (late) A52.76
  ulcer (any site) (early) (secondary) A51.39
    late A52.79
    perforating A52.79
      foot A52.11
  urethra (late) A52.76
  urogenital (late) A52.76
  uterus (late) A52.76
  uveal tract (secondary) A51.43
    late A52.71

Syphilis, syphilitic *(Continued)*
  uveitis (secondary) A51.43
    late A52.71
  uvula (late) (perforated) A52.79
  vagina A51.0
    late A52.76
  valvulitis NEC A52.03
  vascular A52.00
    brain (cerebral) A52.05
  ventriculi A52.74
  vesicae urinariae (late) A52.76
  viscera (abdominal) (late) A52.74
    secondary A51.49
  vitreous (opacities) (late) A52.71
    hemorrhage A52.71
  vulva A51.0
    late A52.76
    secondary A51.39
Syphiloma A52.79
  cardiovascular system A52.00
  central nervous system A52.3
  circulatory system A52.00
  congenital A50.59
Syphilophobia F45.29
Syringadenoma —*see also* Neoplasm, skin, benign
  papillary —*see* Neoplasm, skin, benign
Syringobulbia G95.0
Syringocystadenoma —*see* Neoplasm, skin, benign
  papillary —*see* Neoplasm, skin, benign
Syringoma —*see also* Neoplasm, skin, benign
  chondroid —*see* Neoplasm, skin, benign
Syringomyelia G95.0
Syringomyelitis —*see* Encephalitis
Syringomyelocele —*see* Spina bifida
Syringopontia G95.0
System, systemic —*see also* condition
  disease, combined —*see* Degeneration, combined
  inflammatory response syndrome (SIRS) of non-infectious origin (without organ dysfunction) R65.10
    with acute organ dysfunction R65.11
  lupus erythematosus M32.9
    inhibitor present D68.62

T

Tabacism, tabacosis, tabagism —see also
    Poisioning, tobacco
  meaning dependence (without
    remission) F17.200
    with
      disorder F17.299
        remission F17.211
        specified disorder NEC F17.298
        withdrawal F17.203
Tabardillo A75.9
  flea-borne A75.2
  louse-borne A75.0
Tabes, tabetic A52.10
  with
    central nervous system syphilis
      A52.10
    Charcot's joint A52.16
    cord bladder A52.19
    crisis, viscera (any) A52.19
    paralysis, general A52.17
    paresis (general) A52.17
    perforating ulcer (foot) A52.19
  arthropathy (Charcot) A52.16
  bladder A52.19
  bone A52.11
  cerebrospinal A52.12
  congenital A50.45
  conjugal A52.10
  dorsalis A52.11
    juvenile A50.49
  juvenile A50.49
  latent A52.19
  mesenterica A18.39
  paralysis, insane, general A52.17
  spasmodic A52.17
  syphilis (cerebrospinal) A52.12
Taboparalysis A52.17
Taboparesis (remission) A52.17
  juvenile A50.45
TAC (trigeminal autonomic cephalgia)
  NEC G44.099
  intractable G44.091
  not intractable G44.099
Tache noir S60.22-
Tachyalimentation K91.2
Tachyarrhythmia, tachyrhythmia —see
  Tachycardia
Tachycardia R00.0
  atrial (paroxysmal) I47.1
  auricular I47.1
  AV nodal re-entry (re-entrant) I47.1
  junctional (paroxysmal) I47.1
  newborn P29.11
  nodal (paroxysmal) I47.1
  non-paroxysmal AV nodal I45.89
  paroxysmal (sustained) (nonsustained)
    I47.9
    with sinus bradycardia I49.5
    atrial (PAT) I47.1
    atrioventricular (AV) (re-entrant)
      I47.1
      psychogenic F54
    junctional I47.1
      ectopic I47.1
    nodal I47.1
    psychogenic (atrial) (supraventricular)
      (ventricular) F54
    supraventricular (sustained) I47.1
      psychogenic F54
    ventricular I47.2
      psychogenic F54
  psychogenic F45.8
  sick sinus I49.5

Tachycardia (Continued)
  sinoauricular NOS R00.0
    paroxysmal I47.1
  sinus [sinusal] NOS R00.0
    paroxysmal I47.1
  supraventricular I47.1
  ventricular (paroxysmal) (sustained) I47.2
    psychogenic F54
Tachygastria K31.89
Tachypnea R06.82
  hysterical F45.8
  newborn (idiopathic) (transitory) P22.1
  psychogenic F45.8
  transitory, of newborn P22.1
TACO (transfusion associated circulatory
  overload) E87.71
Taenia (infection) (infestation) B68.9
  diminuta B71.0
  echinococcal infestation B67.90
  mediocanellata B68.1
  nana B71.0
  saginata B68.1
  solium (intestinal form) B68.0
    larval form —see Cysticercosis
Taeniasis (intestine) —see Taenia
Tag (hypertrophied skin) (infected) L91.8
  adenoid J35.8
  anus K64.4
  hemorrhoidal K64.4
  hymen N89.8
  perineal N90.89
  preauricular Q17.0
  sentinel K64.4
  skin L91.8
    accessory (congenital) Q82.8
    anus K64.4
    congenital Q82.8
    preauricular Q17.0
  tonsil J35.8
  urethra, urethral N36.8
  vulva N90.89
Tahyna fever B33.8
Takahara's disease E80.3
Takayasu's disease or syndrome M31.4
Talcosis (pulmonary) J62.0
Talipes (congenital) Q66.89
  acquired, planus —see Deformity, limb,
    flat foot
  asymmetric Q66.89
  calcaneovalgus Q66.4
  calcaneovarus Q66.1
  calcaneus Q66.89
  cavus Q66.7
  equinovalgus Q66.6
  equinovarus Q66.0
  equinus Q66.89
  percavus Q66.7
  planovalgus Q66.6
  planus (acquired) (any degree) —see
    also Deformity, limb, flat foot
    congenital Q66.5-
    due to rickets (sequelae) E64.3
  valgus Q66.6
  varus Q66.3
Tall stature, constitutional E34.4
Talma's disease M62.89
Talon noir S90.3-
  hand S60.22-
  heel S90.3-
  toe S90.1-
Tamponade, heart I31.4
Tanapox (virus disease) B08.71
Tangier disease E78.6
Tantrum, child problem F91.8

Tapeworm (infection) (infestation) —see
  Infestation, tapeworm
Tapia's syndrome G52.7
TAR (thrombocytopenia with absent
  radius) syndrome Q87.2
Tarral-Besnier disease L44.0
Tarsal tunnel syndrome —see Syndrome,
  tarsal tunnel
Tarsalgia —see Pain, limb, lower
Tarsitis (eyelid) H01.8
  syphilitic A52.71
  tuberculous A18.4
Tartar (teeth) (dental calculus) K03.6
Tattoo (mark) L81.8
Tauri's disease E74.09
Taurodontism K00.2
Taussig-Bing syndrome Q20.1
Taybi's syndrome Q87.2
Tay-Sachs amaurotic familial idiocy or
  disease E75.02
TBI (traumatic brain injury) —see
  category S06
Teacher's node or nodule J38.2
Tear, torn (traumatic) —see also Laceration
  with abortion —see Abortion
  annular fibrosis M51.35
  anus, anal (sphincter) S31.831
    complicating delivery
      with third degree perineal
        laceration O70.2
        with mucosa O70.3
      without third degree perineal
        laceration O70.4
    nontraumatic (healed) (old) K62.81
  articular cartilage, old —see
    Derangement, joint, articular
    cartilage, by site
  bladder
    with ectopic or molar pregnancy
      O08.6
    following ectopic or molar pregnancy
      O08.6
    obstetrical O71.5
    traumatic —see Injury, bladder
  bowel
    with ectopic or molar pregnancy O08.6
    following ectopic or molar pregnancy
      O08.6
    obstetrical trauma O71.5
  broad ligament
    with ectopic or molar pregnancy O08.6
    following ectopic or molar pregnancy
      O08.6
    obstetrical trauma O71.6
  bucket handle (knee) (meniscus) —see
    Tear, meniscus
  capsule, joint —see Sprain
  cartilage —see also Sprain
    articular, old —see Derangement,
      joint, articular cartilage, by site
  cervix
    with ectopic or molar pregnancy O08.6
    following ectopic or molar pregnancy
      O08.6
    obstetrical trauma (current) O71.3
    old N88.1
    traumatic —see Injury, uterus
  dural G97.41
    nontraumatic G96.11
  internal organ —see Injury, by site
  knee cartilage
    articular (current) S83.3-
    old —see Derangement, knee,
      meniscus, due to old tear

Tension (*Continued*)
  pneumothorax J93.0
  premenstrual N94.3
  state (mental) F48.9
Tentorium —*see* condition
Teratencephalus Q89.8
Teratism Q89.7
Teratoblastoma (malignant) —*see*
  Neoplasm, malignant, by site
Teratocarcinoma —*see also* Neoplasm,
  malignant, by site
  liver C22.7
Teratoma (solid) —*see also* Neoplasm,
  uncertain behavior, by site
  with embryonal carcinoma, mixed —
    see Neoplasm, malignant,
    by site
  with malignant transformation —*see*
    Neoplasm, malignant, by site
  adult (cystic) —*see* Neoplasm, benign,
    by site
  benign —*see* Neoplasm, benign,
    by site
  combined with choriocarcinoma —*see*
    Neoplasm, malignant, by site
  cystic (adult) —*see* Neoplasm, benign,
    by site
  differentiated —*see* Neoplasm, benign,
    by site
  embryonal —*see also* Neoplasm,
    malignant, by site
    liver C22.7
  immature —*see* Neoplasm, malignant,
    by site
    liver C22.7
  adult, benign, cystic, differentiated
    type or mature D13.4
  malignant —*see also* Neoplasm,
    malignant, by site
    anaplastic —*see* Neoplasm,
      malignant, by site
    intermediate —*see* Neoplasm,
      malignant, by site
      specified site —*see* Neoplasm,
        malignant, by site
      unspecified site C62.90
    undifferentiated —*see* Neoplasm,
      malignant, by site
  mature —*see* Neoplasm, uncertain
    behavior, by site
    malignant —*see* Neoplasm, by site,
      malignant, by site
  ovary D27.-
    embryonal, immature or malignant
      C56-
  solid —*see* Neoplasm, uncertain
    behavior, by site
  testis C62.9-
    adult, benign, cystic, differentiated
      type or mature D29.2-
    scrotal C62.1-
    undescended C62.0-
Termination
  anomalous —*see also* Malposition,
    congenital
    right pulmonary vein Q26.3
  pregnancy, elective Z33.2
Ternidens diminutus infestation
  B81.8
Ternidensiasis B81.8
Terror (s) night (child) F51.4
Terrorism, victim of Z65.4
Terry's syndrome H44.2-
Tertiary —*see* condition

Test, tests, testing (for)
  adequacy (for dialysis)
    hemodialysis Z49.31
    peritoneal Z49.32
  blood pressure Z01.30
    abnormal reading —*see* Blood,
      pressure
  blood typing Z01.83
    Rh typing Z01.83
  blood-alcohol Z04.8
    positive —*see* Findings, abnormal, in
      blood
  blood-drug Z04.8
    positive —*see* Findings, abnormal, in
      blood
  cardiac pulse generator (battery) Z45.010
  fertility Z31.41
  genetic
    disease carrier status for procreative
      management
      female Z31.430
      male Z31.440
    male partner of patient with recurrent
      pregnancy loss Z31.441
    procreative management NEC
      female Z31.438
      male Z31.448
  hearing Z01.10
    with abnormal findings NEC Z01.118
  HIV (human immunodeficiency virus)
    nonconclusive (in infants) R75
    positive Z21
    seropositive Z21
  immunity status Z01.84
  intelligence NEC Z01.89
  laboratory (as part of a general medical
    examination) Z00.00
    with abnormal finding Z00.01
    for medicolegal reason NEC Z04.8
  male partner of patient with recurrent
    pregnancy loss Z31.441
  Mantoux (for tuberculosis) Z11.1
    abnormal result R76.11
  pregnancy, positive first pregnancy —
    see Pregnancy, normal, first
  procreative Z31.49
    fertility Z31.41
  skin, diagnostic
    allergy Z01.82
      special screening examination —*see*
        Screening, by name of disease
    Mantoux Z11.1
    tuberculin Z11.1
  specified NEC Z01.89
  tuberculin Z11.1
    abnormal result R76.11
  vision Z01.00
    with abnormal findings Z01.01
  Wassermann Z11.3
    positive —*see* Serology for syphilis,
      positive
Testicle, testicular, testis —*see also*
  condition
  feminization syndrome (*see also*
    Syndrome, androgen insensitivity)
    E34.51
  migrans Q55.29
Tetanus, tetanic (cephalic) (convulsions)
  A35
  with
    abortion A34
    ectopic or molar pregnancy O08.0
  following ectopic or molar pregnancy
    O08.0

Tetanus, tetanic (*Continued*)
  inoculation reaction (due to serum) —
    see Complications, vaccination
  neonatorum A33
  obstetrical A34
  puerperal, postpartum, childbirth A34
Tetany (due to) R29.0
  alkalosis E87.3
  associated with rickets E55.0
  convulsions R29.0
    hysterical F44.5
  functional (hysterical) F44.5
  hyperkinetic R29.0
    hysterical F44.5
  hyperpnea R06.4
    hysterical F44.5
    psychogenic F45.8
  hyperventilation (*see also*
    Hyperventilation) R06.4
    hysterical F44.5
  neonatal (without calcium or
    magnesium deficiency) P71.3
  parathyroid (gland) E20.9
  parathyroprival E89.2
  post- (para)thyroidectomy E89.2
  postoperative E89.2
  pseudotetany R29.0
  psychogenic (conversion reaction) F44.5
Tetralogy of Fallot Q21.3
Tetraplegia (chronic) (*see also*
  Quadriplegia) G82.50-
Thailand hemorrhagic fever A91
Thalassanemia —*see* Thalassemia
Thalassemia (anemia) (disease) D56.9
  with other hemoglobinopathy D56.8
  alpha (major) (severe) (triple gene
    defect) D56.0
    minor D56.3
    silent carrier D56.3
    trait D56.3
  beta (severe) D56.1
    homozygous D56.1
    major D56.1
    minor D56.3
    trait D56.3
  delta-beta (homozygous) D56.2
    minor D56.3
    trait D56.3
  dominant D56.8
  hemoglobin
    C D56.8
    E-beta D56.5
  intermedia D56.1
  major D56.1
  minor D56.3
  mixed D56.8
  sickle-cell —*see* Disease, sickle-cell,
    thalassemia
  specified type NEC D56.8
  trait D56.3
  variants D56.8
Thanatophoric dwarfism or short stature
  Q77.1
Thaysen-Gee disease (nontropical sprue)
  K90.0
Thaysen's disease K90.0
Thecoma D27-
  luteinized D27-
  malignant C56-
Thelarche, premature E30.8
Thelaziasis B83.8
Thelitis N61
  puerperal, postpartum or gestational —
    see Infection, nipple

Therapeutic —*see* condition
Therapy
  drug, long-term (current) (prophylactic)
    agents affecting estrogen receptors
        and estrogen levels NEC Z79.818
    anastrozole (Arimidex) Z79.811
    antibiotics Z79.2
      short-term use - omit code
    anticoagulants Z79.01
    anti-inflammatory Z79.1
    antiplatelet Z79.02
    antithrombotics Z79.02
    aromatase inhibitors Z79.811
    aspirin Z79.82
    birth control pill or patch Z79.3
    bisphosphonates Z79.83
    contraceptive, oral Z79.3
  drug, long-term (*Continued*)
    drug, specified NEC Z79.899
    estrogen receptor downregulators
        Z79.818
    Evista Z79.810
    exemestane (Aromasin) Z79.811
    Fareston Z79.810
    fulvestrant (Faslodex) Z79.818
    gonadotropin-releasing hormone
        (GnRH) agonist Z79.818
    goserelin acetate (Zoladex) Z79.818
    hormone replacement
        (postmenopausal) Z79.890
    insulin Z79.4
    letrozole (Femara) Z79.811
    leuprolide acetate (leuprorelin)
        (Lupron) Z79.818
    megestrol acetate (Megace) Z79.818
    methadone
      for pain management Z79.891
      maintenance therapy F11.20
    Nolvadex Z79.810
    opiate analgesic Z79.891
    oral contraceptive Z79.3
    raloxifene (Evista) Z79.810
    selective estrogen receptor
        modulators (SERMs) Z79.810
    short term - omit code
    steroids
      inhaled Z79.51
      systemic Z79.52
    tamoxifen (Nolvadex) Z79.810
    toremifene (Fareston) Z79.810
Thermic —*see* condition
Thermography (abnormal) (*see also*
    Abnormal, diagnostic imaging) R93.8
  breast R92.8
Thermoplegia T67.0
Thesaurismosis, glycogen —*see* Disease,
    glycogen storage
Thiamin deficiency E51.9
  specified NEC E51.8
Thiaminic deficiency with beriberi
    E51.11
Thibierge-Weissenbach syndrome —*see*
    Sclerosis, systemic
Thickening
  bone —*see* Hypertrophy, bone
  breast N64.59
  endometrium R93.8
  epidermal L85.9
    specified NEC L85.8
  hymen N89.6
  larynx J38.7
  nail L60.2
    congenital Q84.5
  periosteal —*see* Hypertrophy, bone

Thickening (*Continued*)
  pleura J92.9
    with asbestos J92.0
  skin R23.4
  subepiglottic J38.7
  tongue K14.8
  valve, heart —*see* Endocarditis
Thigh —*see* condition
Thinning vertebra —*see* Spondylopathy,
    specified NEC
Thirst, excessive R63.1
  due to deprivation of water T73.1
Thomsen disease G71.12
Thoracic —*see also* condition
  kidney Q63.2
  outlet syndrome G54.0
Thoracogastroschisis (congenital) Q79.8
Thoracopagus Q89.4
Thorax —*see* condition
Thorn's syndrome N28.89
Thorson-Björck syndrome E34.0
Threadworm (infection) (infestation)
    B80
Threatened
  abortion O20.0
    with subsequent abortion O03.9
  job loss, anxiety concerning Z56.2
  labor (without delivery) O47.9
    after 37 completed weeks of gestation
        O47.1
    before 37 completed weeks of
        gestation O47.0-
  loss of job, anxiety concerning Z56.2
  miscarriage O20.0
  unemployment, anxiety concerning
      Z56.2
Three-day fever A93.1
ThresHers' lung J67.0
Thrix annulata (congenital) Q84.1
Throat —*see* condition
Thrombasthenia (Glanzmann)
    (hemorrhagic) (hereditary) D69.1
Thromboangiitis I73.1
  obliterans (general) I73.1
    cerebral I67.89
    vessels
      brain I67.89
      spinal cord I67.89
Thromboarteritis —*see* Arteritis
Thromboasthenia (Glanzmann)
    (hemorrhagic) (hereditary)
    D69.1
Thrombocytasthenia (Glanzmann)
    D69.1
Thrombocythemia (essential)
    (hemorrhagic) (idiopathic)
    (primary) D47.3
Thrombocytopathy (dystrophic)
    (granulopenic) D69.1
Thrombocytopenia, thrombocytopenic
    D69.6
  with absent radius (TAR) Q87.2
  congenital D69.42
  dilutional D69.59
  due to
    drugs D69.59
    extracorporeal circulation of blood
        D69.59
    (massive)blood transfusion D69.59
    platelet alloimmunization D69.59
  essential D69.3
  heparin induced (HIT) D75.82
  hereditary D69.42
  idiopathic D69.3

Thrombocytopenia, thrombocytopenic
    (*Continued*)
  neonatal, transitory P61.0
    due to
      exchange transfusion P61.0
      idiopathic maternal
          thrombocytopenia P61.0
      isoimmunization P61.0
  primary NEC D69.49
    idiopathic D69.3
  puerperal, postpartum O72.3
  secondary D69.59
  transient neonatal P61.0
Thrombocytosis, essential
    D47.3
  primary D47.3
Thromboembolism —*see* Embolism
Thrombopathy (Bernard-Soulier)
    D69.1
  constitutional D68.0
  Willebrand-Jurgens D68.0
Thrombopenia —*see* Thrombocytopenia
Thrombophilia D68.59
  primary NEC D68.59
  secondary NEC D68.69
  specified NEC D68.69
Thrombophlebitis I80.9
  antepartum O22.2-
    deep O22.3-
    superficial O22.2-
  cavernous (venous) sinus G08
    complicating pregnancy
        O22.5-
    nonpyogenic I67.6
  cerebral (sinus) (vein) G08
    nonpyogenic I67.6
    sequelae G09
  due to implanted device —*see*
      Complications, by site and type,
      specified NEC
  during or resulting from a procedure
      NEC T81.72
  femoral vein (superficial) I80.1-
  femoropopliteal vein I80.0-
  hepatic (vein) I80.8
  idiopathic, recurrent I82.1
  iliofemoral I80.1-
  intracranial venous sinus (any)
      G08
    nonpyogenic I67.6
    sequelae G09
  intraspinal venous sinuses and veins
      G08
    nonpyogenic G95.19
  lateral (venous) sinus G08
    nonpyogenic I67.6
  leg I80.299
    superficial I80.0-
  longitudinal (venous) sinus G08
    nonpyogenic I67.6
  lower extremity I80.299
  migrans, migrating I82.1
  pelvic
    with ectopic or molar pregnancy
        O08.0
    following ectopic or molar pregnancy
        O08.0
    puerperal O87.1
  popliteal vein —*see* Phlebitis, leg, deep,
      popliteal
  portal (vein) K75.1
  postoperative T81.72
  pregnancy —*see* Thrombophlebitis,
      antepartum

Thrombophlebitis (*Continued*)
  puerperal, postpartum, childbirth O87.0
    deep O87.1
    pelvic O87.1
    septic O86.81
    superficial O87.0
  saphenous (greater) (lesser) I80.0-
  sinus (intracranial) G08
    nonpyogenic I67.6
  specified site NEC I80.8
  tibial vein I80.23-
Thrombosis, thrombotic (bland) (multiple) (progressive) (silent) (vessel) I82.90
  anal K64.5
  antepartum —*see* Thrombophlebitis, antepartum
  aorta, aortic I74.10
    abdominal I74.09
      saddle I74.01
    bifurcation I74.09
    saddle I74.01
    specified site NEC I74.19
    terminal I74.09
    thoracic I74.11
    valve —*see* Endocarditis, aortic
  apoplexy I63.3
  artery, arteries (postinfectional) I74.9
    auditory, internal —*see* Occlusion, artery, precerebral, specified NEC
    basilar —*see* Occlusion, artery, basilar
    carotid (common) (internal) —*see* Occlusion, artery, carotid
  artery, arteries (*Continued*)
    cerebellar (anterior inferior) (posterior inferior) (superior) —*see* Occlusion, artery, cerebellar
    cerebral —*see* Occlusion, artery, cerebral
    choroidal (anterior) —*see* Occlusion, artery, cerebral, specified NEC
    communicating, posterior —*see* Occlusion, artery, cerebral, specified NEC
    coronary —*see also* Infarct, myocardium
      not resulting in infarction I24.0
    hepatic I74.8
    hypophyseal —*see* Occlusion, artery, cerebral, specified NEC
    iliac I74.5
    limb I74.4
      lower I74.3
      upper I74.2
    meningeal, anterior or posterior —*see* Occlusion, artery, cerebral, specified NEC
    mesenteric (with gangrene) K55.0
    ophthalmic —*see* Occlusion, artery, retina
    pontine —*see* Occlusion, artery, cerebral, specified NEC
    precerebral —*see* Occlusion, artery, precerebral
    pulmonary (iatrogenic) —*see* Embolism, pulmonary
    renal N28.0
    retinal —*see* Occlusion, artery, retina
    spinal, anterior or posterior G95.11
    traumatic NEC T14.8
    vertebral —*see* Occlusion, artery, vertebral

Thrombosis, thrombotic (*Continued*)
  atrium, auricular —*see also* Infarct, myocardium
    following acute myocardial infarction (current complication) I23.6
    not resulting in infarction I24.0
  basilar (artery) —*see* Occlusion, artery, basilar
  brain (artery) (stem) —*see also* Occlusion, artery, cerebral
    due to syphilis A52.05
    puerperal O99.43
    sinus —*see* Thrombosis, intracranial venous sinus
  capillary I78.8
  cardiac —*see also* Infarct, myocardium
    not resulting in infarction I24.0
    valve —*see* Endocarditis
  carotid (artery) (common) (internal) —*see* Occlusion, artery, carotid
  cavernous (venous) sinus —*see* Thrombosis, intracranial venous sinus
  cerebellar artery (anterior inferior) (posterior inferior) (superior) I66.3
  cerebral (artery) —*see* Occlusion, artery, cerebral
  cerebrovenous sinus —*see also* Thrombosis, intracranial venous sinus
    puerperium O87.3
  chronic I82.91
  coronary (artery) (vein) —*see also* Infarct, myocardium
    not resulting in infarction I24.0
  corpus cavernosum N48.89
  cortical I66.9
  deep —*see* Embolism, vein, lower extremity
  due to device, implant or graft (*see also* Complications, by site and type, specified NEC) T85.86
    arterial graft NEC T82.868
    breast (implant) T85.86
    catheter NEC T85.86
      dialysis (renal) T82.868
        intraperitoneal T85.86
      infusion NEC T82.868
        spinal (epidural) (subdural) T85.86
      urinary (indwelling) T83.86
    electronic (electrode) (pulse generator) (stimulator)
      bone T84.86
      cardiac T82.867
      nervous system (brain) (peripheral nerve) (spinal) T85.86
      urinary T83.86
    fixation, internal (orthopedic) NEC T84.86
    gastrointestinal (bile duct) (esophagus) T85.86
    genital NEC T83.86
    heart T82.867
    joint prosthesis T84.86
    ocular (corneal graft) (orbital implant) NEC T85.86
    orthopedic NEC T84.86
    specified NEC T85.86
    urinary NEC T83.86
    vascular NEC T82.868
    ventricular intracranial shunt T85.86
  during the puerperium —*see* Thrombosis, puerperal

Thrombosis, thrombotic (*Continued*)
  endocardial —*see also* Infarct, myocardium
    not resulting in infarction I24.0
  eye —*see* Occlusion, retina
  genital organ
    female NEC N94.89
      pregnancy —*see* Thrombophlebitis, antepartum
    male N50.1
  gestational —*see* Phlebopathy, gestational
  heart (chamber) —*see also* Infarct, myocardium
    not resulting in infarction I24.0
  hepatic (vein) I82.0
    artery I74.8
  history (of) Z86.718
  intestine (with gangrene) K55.0
  intracardiac NEC (apical) (atrial) (auricular) (ventricular) (old) I51.3
  intracranial (arterial) I66.9
    venous sinus (any) G08
      nonpyogenic origin I67.6
      puerperium O87.3
  intramural —*see also* Infarct, myocardium
    not resulting in infarction I24.0
  intraspinal venous sinuses and veins G08
    nonpyogenic G95.19
  kidney (artery) N28.0
  lateral (venous) sinus —*see* Thrombosis, intracranial venous sinus
  leg —*see* Thrombosis, vein, lower extremity
    arterial I74.3
  liver (venous) I82.0
    artery I74.8
    portal vein I81
  longitudinal (venous) sinus —*see* Thrombosis, intracranial venous sinus
  lower limb —*see* Thrombosis, vein, lower extremity
  lung (iatrogenic) (postoperative) —*see* Embolism, pulmonary
  meninges (brain) (arterial) I66.8
  mesenteric (artery) (with gangrene) K55.0
    vein (inferior) (superior) I81
  mitral I34.8
  mural —*see also* Infarct, myocardium
    due to syphilis A52.06
    not resulting in infarction I24.0
  omentum (with gangrene) K55.0
  ophthalmic —*see* Occlusion, retina
  pampiniform plexus (male) N50.1
  parietal —*see also* Infarct, myocardium
    not resulting in infarction I24.0
  penis, superficial vein N48.81
  perianal venous K64.5
  peripheral arteries I74.4
    upper I74.2
  personal history (of) Z86.718
  portal I81
    due to syphilis A52.09
  precerebral artery —*see* Occlusion, artery, precerebral
  puerperal, postpartum O87.0
    brain (artery) O99.43
      venous (sinus) O87.3
    cardiac O99.43
    cerebral (artery) O99.43
      venous (sinus) O87.3
    superficial O87.0

Thrombosis, thrombotic (Continued)
pulmonary (artery) (iatrogenic)
(postoperative) (vein) —see
Embolism, pulmonary
renal (artery) N28.0
vein I82.3
resulting from presence of device,
implant or graft —see
Complications, by site and type,
specified NEC
retina, retinal —see Occlusion, retina
scrotum N50.1
seminal vesicle N50.1
sigmoid (venous) sinus —see
Thrombosis, intracranial venous
sinus
sinus, intracranial (any) —see
Thrombosis, intracranial venous
sinus
specified site NEC I82.890
chronic I82.891
spermatic cord N50.1
spinal cord (arterial) G95.11
due to syphilis A52.09
pyogenic origin G06.1
spleen, splenic D73.5
artery I74.8
testis N50.1
traumatic NEC T14.8
tricuspid I07.8
tumor —see Neoplasm, by site
tunica vaginalis N50.1
umbilical cord (vessels), complicating
delivery O69.5
vas deferens N50.1
vein (acute) I82.90
antecubital I82.61-
chronic I82.71-
axillary I82.A1-
chronic I82.A2-
basilic I82.61-
chronic I82.71-
brachial I82.62-
chronic I82.72-
brachiocephalic (innominate) I82.290
chronic I82.291
cerebral, nonpyogenic I67.6
cephalic I82.61-
chronic I82.71-
chronic I82.91
deep (DVT) I82.40-
calf I82.4Z-
chronic I82.5Z-
lower leg I82.4Z-
chronic I82.5Z-
thigh I82.4Y-
chronic I82.5Y-
upper leg I82.4Y
chronic I82.5y-
femoral I82.41-
chronic I82.51-
iliac (iliofemoral) I82.42-
chronic I82.52-
innominate I82.290
chronic I82.291
internal jugular I82.C1-
chronic I82.C2-
lower extremity
deep I82.40-
chronic I82.50-
specified NEC I82.49-
chronic NEC I82.59-
distal
deep I82.4Z-

Thrombosis, thrombotic (Continued)
vein (Continued)
lower extremity (Continued)
proximal
deep I82.4Y-
chronic I82.5Y-
superficial I82.81-
perianal K64.5
popliteal I82.43-
chronic I82.53-
radial I82.62-
chronic I82.72-
renal I82.3
saphenous (greater) (lesser) I82.81-
specified NEC I82.890
chronic NEC I82.891
subclavian I82.B1-
chronic I82.B2-
thoracic NEC I82.290
chronic I82.291
tibial I82.44-
chronic I82.54-
ulnar I82.62-
chronic I82.72-
upper extremity I82.60-
chronic I82.70-
deep I82.62-
chronic I82.72-
superficial I82.61-
chronic I82.71-
vena cava
inferior I82.220
chronic I82.221
superior I82.210
chronic I82.211
venous, perianal K64.5
ventricle —see also Infarct, myocardium
following acute myocardial infarction
(current complication) I23.6
not resulting in infarction I24.0
Thrombus —see Thrombosis
Thrush —see also Candidiasis
newborn P37.5
oral B37.0
vaginal B37.3
Thumb —see also condition
sucking (child problem) F98.8
Thymitis E32.8
Thymoma (benign) D15.0
malignant C37
Thymus, thymic (gland) —see condition
Thyrocele —see Goiter
Thyroglossal —see also condition
cyst Q89.2
duct, persistent Q89.2
Thyroid (gland) (body) —see also
condition
hormone resistance E07.89
lingual Q89.2
nodule (cystic) (nontoxic) (single) E04.1
Thyroiditis E06.9
acute (nonsuppurative) (pyogenic)
(suppurative) E06.0
autoimmune E06.3
chronic (nonspecific) (sclerosing)
E06.5
with thyrotoxicosis, transient E06.2
fibrous E06.5
lymphadenoid E06.3
lymphocytic E06.3
lymphoid E06.3
de Quervain's E06.1
drug-induced E06.4
fibrous (chronic) E06.5

Thyroiditis (Continued)
giant-cell (follicular) E06.1
granulomatous (de Quervain)
(subacute) E06.1
Hashimoto's (struma lymphomatosa)
E06.3
iatrogenic E06.4
ligneous E06.5
lymphocytic (chronic) E06.3
lymphoid E06.3
lymphomatous E06.3
nonsuppurative E06.1
postpartum, puerperal O90.5
pseudotuberculous E06.1
pyogenic E06.0
radiation E06.4
Riedel's E06.5
subacute (granulomatous) E06.1
suppurative E06.0
tuberculous A18.81
viral E06.1
woody E06.5
Thyrolingual duct, persistent Q89.2
Thyromegaly E01.0
Thyrotoxic
crisis —see Thyrotoxicosis
heart disease or failure (see also
Thyrotoxicosis) E05.90 [I43]
with thyroid storm E05.91 [I43]
storm —see Thyrotoxicosis
Thyrotoxicosis (recurrent) E05.90
with
goiter (diffuse) E05.00
with thyroid storm E05.01
adenomatous uninodular E05.10
with thyroid storm E05.11
multinodular E05.20
with thyroid storm E05.21
nodular E05.20
with thyroid storm E05.21
uninodular E05.10
with thyroid storm E05.11
infiltrative
dermopathy E05.00
with thyroid storm E05.01
ophthalmopathy E05.00
with thyroid storm E05.01
single thyroid nodule E05.10
with thyroid storm E05.11
thyroid storm E05.91
due to
ectopic thyroid nodule or tissue E05.30
with thyroid storm E05.31
ingestion of (excessive) thyroid
material E05.40
with thyroid storm E05.41
overproduction of thyroid-
stimulating hormone E05.80
with thyroid storm E05.81
specified cause NEC E05.80
with thyroid storm E05.81
factitia E05.40
with thyroid storm E05.41
heart E05.90 [I43]
with thyroid storm E05.91 [I43]
failure E05.90 [I43]
neonatal (transient) P72.1
transient with chronic thyroiditis E06.2
Tibia vara —see Osteochondrosis,
juvenile, tibia
Tic (disorder) F95.9
breathing F95.8
child problem F95.0
compulsive F95.1

Tic *(Continued)*
de la Tourette F95.2
degenerative (generalized) (localized)
G25.69
facial G25.69
disorder
chronic
motor F95.1
vocal F95.1
combined vocal and multiple motor
F95.2
transient F95.0
douloureux G50.0
atypical G50.1
postherpetic, postzoster B02.22
drug-induced G25.61
eyelid F95.8
habit F95.9
chronic F95.1
transient of childhood F95.0
lid, transient of childhood F95.0
motor-verbal F95.2
occupational F48.8
orbicularis F95.8
transient of childhood F95.0
organic origin G25.69
postchoreic G25.69
psychogenic, compulsive F95.1
salaam R25.8
spasm (motor or vocal) F95.9
chronic F95.1
transient of childhood F95.0
specified NEC F95.8
Tick-borne —*see* condition
Tietze's disease or syndrome M94.0
Tight, tightness
anus K62.89
chest R07.89
fascia (lata) M62.89
foreskin (congenital) N47.1
hymen, hymenal ring N89.6
introitus (acquired) (congenital) N89.6
rectal sphincter K62.89
tendon —*see* Short, tendon
urethral sphincter N35.9
Tilting vertebra —*see* Dorsopathy,
deforming, specified NEC
Timidity, child F93.8
Tin-miner's lung J63.5
Tinea (intersecta) (tarsi) B35.9
amiantacea L44.8
asbestina B35.0
barbae B35.0
beard B35.0
black dot B35.0
blanca B36.2
capitis B35.0
corporis B35.4
cruris B35.6
flava B36.0
foot B35.3
furfuracea B36.0
imbricata (Tokelau) B35.5
kerion B35.0
manuum B35.2
microsporic —*see* Dermatophytosis
nigra B36.1
nodosa —*see* Piedra
pedis B35.3
scalp B35.0
specified site NEC B35.8
sycosis B35.0
tonsurans B35.0
trichophytic —*see* Dermatophytosis

Tinea *(Continued)*
unguium B35.1
versicolor B36.0
Tingling sensation (skin) R20.2
Tinnitus (audible) (aurium)
(subjective) —*see* subcategory H93.1
Tipped tooth (teeth) M26.33
Tipping
pelvis M95.5
with disproportion (fetopelvic) O33.0
causing obstructed labor O65.0
tooth (teeth), fully erupted M26.33
Tiredness R53.83
Tissue —*see* condition
Tobacco (nicotine)
dependence —*see* Dependence, drug,
nicotine
harmful use Z72.0
heart —*see* Tobacco, toxic effect
maternal use, affecting newborn
P04.2
toxic effect —*see* Table of drugs
and chemicals, by substance,
poisoning
chewing tobacco —*see* Table of drugs
and chemicals, by substance,
poisoning
cigarettes —*see* Table of drugs
and chemicals, by substance,
poisoning
use Z72.0
complicating
childbirth O99.334
pregnancy O99.33-
puerperium O99.335
counseling and surveillance Z71.6
withdrawal state —*see* Dependence,
drug, nicotine
Tocopherol deficiency E56.0
Todd's
cirrhosis K74.3
paralysis (postepileptic) (transitory)
G83.84
Toe —*see* condition
Toilet, artificial opening —*see* Attention
to, artificial, opening
Tokelau (ringworm) B35.5
Tollwut —*see* Rabies
Tommaselli's disease R31.9
correct substance properly
administered —*see* Table of drugs
and chemicals, by drug, adverse
effect
overdose or wrong substance given
or taken —*see* Table of drugs and
chemicals, by drug, poisoning
Tongue —*see also* condition
tie Q38.1
Tonic pupil —*see* Anomaly, pupil,
function, tonic pupil
Toni-Fanconi syndrome (cystinosis) E72.09
with cystinosis E72.04
Tonsil —*see* condition
Tonsillitis (acute) (catarrhal) (croupous)
(follicular) (gangrenous) (infective)
(lacunar) (lingual) (malignant)
(membranous) (parenchymatous)
(phlegmonous) (pseudomembranous)
(purulent) (septic) (subacute)
(suppurative) (toxic) (ulcerative)
(vesicular) (viral) J03.90
chronic J35.01
with adenoiditis J35.03
diphtheritic A36.0

Tonsillitis *(Continued)*
hypertrophic J35.01
with adenoiditis J35.03
recurrent J03.91
specified organism NEC J03.80
recurrent J03.81
staphylococcal J03.80
recurrent J03.81
streptococcal J03.00
recurrent J03.01
tuberculous A15.8
Vincent's A69.1
Tooth, teeth —*see* condition
Toothache K08.8
Topagnosis R20.8
Tophi —*see* Gout
TORCH infection —*see* Infection,
congenital
without active infection P00.2
Torn —*see* Tear
Tornwaldt's cyst or disease J39.2
Torsion
accessory tube —*see* Torsion, fallopian
tube
adnexa (female) —*see* Torsion, fallopian
tube
aorta, acquired I77.1
appendix epididymis N44.04
appendix testis N44.03
bile duct (common) (hepatic) K83.8
congenital Q44.5
bowel, colon or intestine K56.2
cervix —*see* Malposition, uterus
cystic duct K82.8
dystonia —*see* Dystonia, torsion
epididymis (appendix) N44.04
fallopian tube N83.52
with ovary N83.53
gallbladder K82.8
congenital Q44.1
hydatid of Morgagni
female N83.52
male N44.03
kidney (pedicle) (leading to infarction)
N28.0
Meckel's diverticulum (congenital)
Q43.0
malignant —*see* Table of Neoplasms,
small intestine, malignant
mesentery K56.2
omentum K56.2
organ or site, congenital NEC —*see*
Anomaly, by site
ovary (pedicle) N83.51
with fallopian tube N83.53
congenital Q50.2
oviduct —*see* Torsion, fallopian tube
penis (acquired) N48.82
congenital Q55.63
spasm —*see* Dystonia, torsion
spermatic cord N44.02
extravaginal N44.01
intravaginal N44.02
spleen D73.5
testis, testicle N44.00
appendix N44.03
tibia —*see* Deformity, limb, specified
type NEC, lower leg
uterus —*see* Malposition, uterus
Torticollis (intermittent) (spastic) M43.6
congenital (sternomastoid) Q68.0
due to birth injury P15.8
hysterical F44.4
ocular R29.891

Torticollis *(Continued)*
   psychogenic F45.8
      conversion reaction F44.4
   rheumatic M43.6
   rheumatoid M06.88
   spasmodic G24.3
   traumatic, current S13.4
Tortipelvis G24.1
Tortuous
   artery I77.1
   organ or site, congenital NEC —*see*
      Distortion
   retinal vessel, congenital Q14.1
   ureter N13.8
   urethra N36.8
   vein —*see* Varix
Torture, victim of Z65.4
Torula, torular (histolytica) (infection) —
   see Cryptococcosis
Torulosis —*see* Cryptococcosis
Torus (mandibularis) (palatinus)
   M27.0
   fracture —*see* Fracture, by site,
      torus
Touraine's syndrome Q79.8
Tourette's syndrome F95.2
Tourniquet syndrome —*see* Constriction,
   external, by site
Tower skull Q75.0
   with exophthalmos Q87.0
Toxemia R68.89
   bacterial —*see* Sepsis
   burn —*see* Burn
   eclamptic (with pre-existing
      hypertension) —*see* Eclampsia
   erysipelatous —*see* Erysipelas
   fatigue R68.89
   food —*see* Poisoning, food
   gastrointestinal K52.1
   intestinal K52.1
   kidney —*see* Uremia
   malarial —*see* Malaria
   myocardial —*see* Myocarditis, toxic
   of pregnancy —*see* Pre-eclampsia
   pre-eclamptic —*see* Pre-eclampsia
   small intestine K52.1
   staphylococcal, due to food A05.0
   stasis R68.89
   uremic —*see* Uremia
   urinary —*see* Uremia
Toxemica cerebropathia psychica
   (nonalcoholic) F04
   alcoholic —*see* Alcohol, amnestic
      disorder
Toxic (poisoning) —*see also* condition
   T65.91
   effect —*see* Table of drugs and
      chemicals, by substance,
      poisoning
   shock syndrome A48.3
   thyroid (gland) —*see* Thyrotoxicosis
Toxicemia —*see* Toxemia
Toxicity —*see* Table of drugs and
   chemicals, by substance,
   poisoning
   fava bean D55.0
   food, noxious —*see* Poisoning, food
   from drug or nonmedicinal
      substance —*see* Table of drugs and
      chemicals, by drug
Toxicosis —*see also* Toxemia
   capillary, hemorrhagic D69.0
Toxinfection, gastrointestinal K52.1
Toxocariasis B83.0

Toxoplasma, toxoplasmosis (acquired)
   B58.9
   with
      hepatitis B58.1
      meningoencephalitis B58.2
      ocular involvement B58.00
      other organ involvement B58.89
      pneumonia, pneumonitis B58.3
   congenital (acute) (subacute) (chronic)
      P37.1
   maternal, manifest toxoplasmosis in
      infant (acute) (subacute) (chronic)
      P37.1
tPA (rtPA) administation in a different
   facility within the last 24 hours
   prior to admission to current facility
   Z92.82
Trabeculation, bladder N32.89
Trachea —*see* condition
Tracheitis (catarrhal) (infantile)
   (membranous) (plastic) (septal)
   (suppurative) (viral) J04.10
   with
      bronchitis (15 years of age and above)
         J40
         acute or subacute —*see* Bronchitis,
            acute
         chronic J42
         tuberculous NEC A15.5
         under 15 years of age J20.9
      laryngitis (acute) J04.2
         chronic J37.1
         tuberculous NEC A15.5
   acute J04.10
      with obstruction J04.11
   chronic J42
      with
         bronchitis (chronic) J42
         laryngitis (chronic) J37.1
   diphtheritic (membranous) A36.89
   due to external agent —*see*
      Inflammation, respiratory, upper,
      due to
   syphilitic A52.73
   tuberculous A15.5
Trachelitis (nonvenereal) —*see* Cervicitis
Tracheobronchial —*see* condition
Tracheobronchitis (15 years of age and
   above) —*see also* Bronchitis
   due to
      Bordetella bronchiseptica A37.80
         with pneumonia A37.81
      Francisella tularensis A21.8
Tracheobronchomegaly Q32.4
   with bronchiectasis J47.9
      with
         exacerbation (acute) J47.1
         lower respiratory infection J47.0
   acquired J98.09
      with bronchiectasis J47.9
         with
            exacerbation (acute) J47.1
            lower respiratory infection J47.0
Tracheobronchopneumonitis —*see*
   Pneumonia, broncho-
Tracheocele (external) (internal) J39.8
   congenital Q32.1
Tracheomalacia J39.8
   congenital Q32.0
Tracheopharyngitis (acute) J06.9
   chronic J42
   due to external agent —*see*
      Inflammation, respiratory, upper,
      due to
Tracheostenosis J39.8

Tracheostomy
   complication —*see* Complication,
      tracheostomy
   status Z93.0
      attention to Z43.0
      malfunctioning J95.03
Trachoma, trachomatous A71.9
   active (stage) A71.1
   contraction of conjunctiva A71.1
   dubium A71.0
   healed or sequelae B94.0
   initial (stage) A71.0
   pannus A71.1
   Türck's J37.0
Traction, vitreomacular H43.82-
Train sickness T75.3
Trait (s)
   Hb-S D57.3
   hemoglobin
      abnormal NEC D58.2
         with thalassemia D56.3
      C —*see* Disease, hemoglobin C
      S (Hb-S) D57.3
   Lepore D56.3
   personality, accentuated Z73.1
   sickle-cell D57.3
      with elliptocytosis or spherocytosis
         D57.3
   type A personality Z73.1
Tramp Z59.0
Trance R41.89
   hysterical F44.89
Transaminasemia R74.0
Transection
   abdomen (partial) S38.3
   aorta (incomplete) —*see also* Injury,
      aorta
      complete —*see* Injury, aorta,
         laceration, major
   carotid artery (incomplete) —*see also*
      Injury, blood vessel, carotid,
      laceration
      complete —*see* Injury, blood
         vessel, carotid, laceration,
         major
   celiac artery (incomplete) S35.211
      branch (incomplete) S35.291
         complete S35.292
      complete S35.212
   innominate
      artery (incomplete) —*see also*
         Injury, blood vessel, thoracic,
         innominate, artery, laceration
         complete —*see* Injury, blood vessel,
            thoracic, innominate, artery,
            laceration, major
      vein (incomplete) —*see also* Injury,
         blood vessel, thoracic,
         innominate, vein, laceration
         complete —*see* Injury, blood vessel,
            thoracic, innominate, vein,
            laceration, major
   jugular vein (external) (incomplete) —
      see also Injury, blood vessel, jugular
      vein, laceration
      complete —*see* Injury, blood vessel,
         jugular vein, laceration,
         major
      internal (incomplete) —*see also* Injury,
         blood vessel, jugular vein,
         internal, laceration
         complete —*see* Injury, blood
            vessel, jugular vein, internal,
            laceration, major

Transection (Continued)
  mesenteric artery (incomplete) —see also
      Injury, mesenteric, artery, laceration
    complete —see Injury, mesenteric
      artery, laceration, major
  pulmonary vessel (incomplete) —see
      also Injury, blood vessel, thoracic,
      pulmonary, laceration
    complete —see Injury, blood vessel,
      thoracic, pulmonary, laceration,
      major
  subclavian —see Transection,
      innominate
  vena cava (incomplete) —see also Injury,
      vena cava
    complete —see Injury, vena cava,
      laceration, major
  vertebral artery (incomplete) —see also
      Injury, blood vessel, vertebral,
      laceration
    complete —see Injury, blood vessel,
      vertebral, laceration, major
Transfusion
  associated (red blood cell)
      hemochromatosis E83.111
  blood
    ABO incompatible —see
        Complication (s), transfusion,
        incompatibility reaction, ABO
    minor blood group (Duffy) (E)
        (K(ell)) (Kidd) (Lewis) (M) (N)
        (P) (S) T80.89
    reaction or complication —see
        Complications, transfusion
  fetomaternal (mother) —see Pregnancy,
      complicated by, placenta,
      transfusion syndrome
  maternofetal (mother) —see Pregnancy,
      complicated by, placenta,
      transfusion syndrome
  placental (syndrome) (mother) —see
      Pregnancy, complicated by,
      placenta, transfusion syndrome
  reaction (adverse) —see Complications,
      transfusion
  related acute lung injury (TRALI) J95.84
  twin-to-twin —see Pregnancy,
      complicated by, placenta,
      transfusion syndrome, fetus to
      fetus
Transient (meaning homeless) (see also
      condition) Z59.0
Translocation
  balanced autosomal Q95.9
    in normal individual Q95.0
  chromosomes NEC Q99.8
    balanced and insertion in normal
        individual Q95.0
  Down's syndrome Q90.2
  trisomy
    13 Q91.6
    18 Q91.2
    21 Q90.2
Translucency, iris —see Degeneration, iris
Transmission of chemical substances
      through the placenta —see
      Absorption, chemical, through
      placenta
Transparency, lung, unilateral J43.0
Transplant (ed) (status) Z94.9
  awaiting organ Z76.82
  bone Z94.6
    marrow Z94.81
  candidate Z76.82

Transplant (Continued)
  complication —see Complication,
      transplant
  cornea Z94.7
  heart Z94.1
    and lung (s) Z94.3
    valve Z95.2
      prosthetic Z95.2
      specified NEC Z95.4
      xenogenic Z95.3
  intestine Z94.82
  kidney Z94.0
  liver Z94.4
  lung (s) Z94.2
    and heart Z94.3
  organ (failure) (infection) (rejection)
      Z94.9
    removal status Z98.85
  pancreas Z94.83
  skin Z94.5
  social Z60.3
  specified organ or tissue NEC Z94.89
  stem cells Z94.84
  tissue Z94.9
Transplants, ovarian, endometrial N80.1
Transposed —see Transposition
Transposition (congenital) —see also
      Malposition, congenital
  abdominal viscera Q89.3
  aorta (dextra) Q20.3
  appendix Q43.8
  colon Q43.8
  corrected Q20.5
  great vessels (complete) (partial) Q20.3
  heart Q24.0
    with complete transposition of
        viscera Q89.3
  intestine (large) (small) Q43.8
  reversed jejunal (for bypass) (status)
      Z98.0
  scrotum Q55.23
  stomach Q40.2
    with general transposition of viscera
        Q89.3
  tooth, teeth, fully erupted M26.30
  vessels, great (complete) (partial)
      Q20.3
  viscera (abdominal) (thoracic) Q89.3
Transsexualism F64.1
Transverse —see also condition
  arrest (deep), in labor O64.0
  lie (mother) O32.2
    causing obstructed labor O64.8
Transvestism, transvestitism (dual-role)
      F64.1
  fetishistic F65.1
Trapped placenta (with hemorrhage)
      O72.0
  without hemorrhage O73.0
Trauma, traumatism —see also Injury
  acoustic —see subcategory H83.3
  birth —see Birth, injury
  complicating ectopic or molar
      pregnancy O08.6
  during delivery O71.9
  following ectopic or molar pregnancy
      O08.6
  obstetric O71.9
    specified NEC O71.89
Traumatic —see also condition
  brain injury —see category S06
Treacher Collins syndrome Q75.4
Treitz's hernia —see Hernia, abdomen,
      specified site NEC

Trematode infestation —see Infestation,
      fluke
Trematodiasis —see Infestation, fluke
Trembling paralysis —see Parkinsonism
Tremor (s) R25.1
  drug induced G25.1
  essential (benign) G25.0
  familial G25.0
  hereditary G25.0
  hysterical F44.4
  intention G25.2
  medication induced postural
      G25.1
  mercurial —see subcategory T56.1
  Parkinson's —see Parkinsonism
  psychogenic (conversion reaction)
      F44.4
  senilis R54
  specified type NEC G25.2
Trench
  fever A79.0
  foot —see Immersion, foot
  mouth A69.1
Treponema pallidum infection —see
      Syphilis
Treponematosis
  due to
    T. pallidum —see Syphilis
    T. pertenue —see Yaws
Triad
  Hutchinson's (congenital syphilis)
      A50.53
  Kartagener's Q89.3
  Saint's —see Hernia, diaphragm
Trichiasis (eyelid) H02.059
  with entropion —see Entropion
  left H02.056
    lower H02.055
    upper H02.054
  right H02.053
    lower H02.052
    upper H02.051
Trichinella spiralis (infection)
      (infestation) B75
Trichinellosis, trichiniasis,
      trichinelliasis, trichinosis
      B75
  with muscle disorder B75 [M63.80]
    ankle B75 [M63.87-]
    foot B75 [M63.87-]
    forearm B75 [M63.83-]
    hand B75 [M63.84-]
    lower leg B75 [M63.86-]
    multiple sites B75 [M63.89]
    pelvic region B75 [M63.85-]
    shoulder region B75 [M63.81-]
    specified site NEC B75 [M63.88]
    thigh B75 [M63.85-]
    upper arm B75 [M63.82-]
Trichobezoar T18.9
  intestine T18.3
  stomach T18.2
Trichocephaliasis, trichocephalosis
      B79
Trichocephalus infestation B79
Trichoclasis L67.8
Trichoepithelioma —see also Neoplasm,
      skin, benign
  malignant —see Neoplasm, skin,
      malignant
Trichofolliculoma —see Neoplasm, skin,
      benign
Tricholemmoma —see Neoplasm, skin,
      benign

Trichomoniasis A59.9
  bladder A59.03
  cervix A59.09
  intestinal A07.8
  prostate A59.02
  seminal vesicles A59.09
  specified site NEC A59.8
  urethra A59.03
  urogenitalis A59.00
  vagina A59.01
  vulva A59.01
Trichomycosis
  axillaris A48.8
  nodosa, nodularis B36.8
Trichonodosis L67.8
Trichophytid, trichophyton infection —
    see Dermatophytosis
Trichophytobezoar T18.9
  intestine T18.3
  stomach T18.2
Trichophytosis —see Dermatophytosis
Trichoptilosis L67.8
Trichorrhexis (nodosa) (invaginata)
    L67.0
Trichosis axillaris A48.8
Trichosporosis nodosa B36.2
Trichostasis spinulosa (congenital)
    Q84.1
Trichostrongyliasis, trichostrongylosis
    (small intestine) B81.2
Trichostrongylus infection B81.2
Trichotillomania F63.3
Trichromat, trichromatopsia, anomalous
    (congenital) H53.55
Trichuriasis B79
Trichuris trichiura (infection) (infestation)
    (any site) B79
Tricuspid (valve) —see condition
Trifid —see also Accessory
  kidney (pelvis) Q63.8
  tongue Q38.3
Trigeminal neuralgia —see Neuralgia,
    trigeminal
Trigeminy R00.8
Trigger finger (acquired) M65.30
  congenital Q74.0
  index finger M65.32-
  little finger M65.35-
  middle finger M65.33-
  ring finger M65.34-
  thumb M65.31-
Trigonitis (bladder) (chronic)
    (pseudomembranous) N30.30
  with hematuria N30.31
Trigonocephaly Q75.0
Trilocular heart —see Cor triloculare
Trimethylaminuria E72.52
Tripartite placenta O43.19-
Triphalangeal thumb Q74.0
Triple —see also Accessory
  kidneys Q63.0
  uteri Q51.818
  X, female Q97.0
Triplegia G83.89
  congenital G80.8
Triplet (newborn) —see also Newborn,
    triplet
  complicating pregnancy —see
    Pregnancy, triplet
Triplication —see Accessory
Triploidy Q92.7
Trismus R25.2
  neonatorum A33
  newborn A33

Trisomy (syndrome) Q92.9
  13 (partial) Q91.7
    meiotic nondisjunction Q91.4
    mitotic nondisjunction Q91.5
    mosaicism Q91.5
    translocation Q91.6
  18 (partial) Q91.3
    meiotic nondisjunction Q91.0
    mitotic nondisjunction Q91.1
    mosaicism Q91.1
    translocation Q91.2
  20 Q92.8
  21 (partial) Q90.9
    meiotic nondisjunction Q90.0
    mitotic nondisjunction Q90.1
    mosaicism Q90.1
    translocation Q90.2
  22 Q92.8
  autosomes Q92.9
  chromosome specified NEC
      Q92.8
    partial Q92.2
      due to unbalanced translocation
        Q92.5
    specified NEC Q92.8
    whole (nonsex chromosome)
      meiotic nondisjunction Q92.0
      mitotic nondisjunction Q92.1
      mosaicism Q92.1
  due to
    dicentrics —see Extra, marker
        chromosomes
    extra rings —see Extra, marker
        chromosomes
    isochromosomes —see Extra, marker
        chromosomes
  specified NEC Q92.8
  whole chromosome Q92.9
    meiotic nondisjunction Q92.0
    mitotic nondisjunction Q92.1
    mosaicism Q92.1
    partial Q92.9
    specified NEC Q92.8
Tritanomaly, tritanopia H53.55
Trombiculosis, trombiculiasis,
    trombidiosis B88.0
Trophedema (congenital) (hereditary)
    Q82.0
Trophoblastic disease (see also Mole,
    hydatidiform) O01.9
Tropholymphedema Q82.0
Trophoneurosis NEC G96.8
  disseminated M34.9
Tropical —see condition
Trouble —see also Disease
  heart —see Disease, heart
  kidney —see Disease, renal
  nervous R45.0
  sinus —see Sinusitis
Trousseau's syndrome (thrombophlebitis
    migrans) I82.1
Truancy, childhood
  from school Z72.810
Truncus
  arteriosus (persistent) Q20.0
  communis Q20.0
Trunk —see condition
Trypanosomiasis
  African B56.9
    by Trypanosoma brucei
      gambiense B56.0
      rhodesiense B56.1
  American —see Chagas' disease
  Brazilian —see Chagas' disease

Trypanosomiasis (Continued)
  by Trypanosoma
    brucei gambiense B56.0
    brucei rhodesiense B56.1
    cruzi —see Chagas' disease
  gambiensis, Gambian B56.0
  rhodesiensis, Rhodesian B56.1
  South American —see Chagas' disease
  where
    African trypanosomiasis is prevalent
      B56.9
    Chagas' disease is prevalent B57.2
T-shaped incisors K00.2
Tsutsugamushi (disease) (fever) A75.3
Tube, tubal, tubular —see condition
Tubercle —see also Tuberculosis
  brain, solitary A17.81
  Darwin's Q17.8
  Ghon, primary infection A15.7
Tuberculid, tuberculide (indurating,
    subcutaneous) (lichenoid) (miliary)
    (papulonecrotic) (primary) (skin)
    A18.4
Tuberculoma —see also Tuberculosis
  brain A17.81
  meninges (cerebral) (spinal) A17.1
  spinal cord A17.81
Tuberculosis, tubercular, tuberculous
    (calcification) (calcified) (caseous)
    (chromogenic acid-fast bacilli)
    (degeneration) (fibrocaseous)
    (fistula) (interstitial) (isolated
    circumscribed lesions) (necrosis)
    (parenchymatous) (ulcerative) A15.9
  with pneumoconiosis (any condition in
    J60-J64) J65
  abdomen (lymph gland) A18.39
  abscess (respiratory) A15.9
    bone A18.03
      hip A18.02
      knee A18.02
      sacrum A18.01
      specified site NEC A18.03
      spinal A18.01
      vertebra A18.01
    brain A17.81
    breast A18.89
    Cowper's gland A18.15
    dura (mater) (cerebral) (spinal)
      A17.81
    epidural (cerebral) (spinal) A17.81
    female pelvis A18.17
    frontal sinus A15.8
    genital organs NEC A18.10
    genitourinary A18.10
    gland (lymphatic) —see Tuberculosis,
      lymph gland
    hip A18.02
    intestine A18.32
    ischiorectal A18.32
    joint NEC A18.02
      hip A18.02
      knee A18.02
      specified NEC A18.02
      vertebral A18.01
    kidney A18.11
    knee A18.02
    latent R76.11
    lumbar (spine) A18.01
    lung —see Tuberculosis, pulmonary
    meninges (cerebral) (spinal) A17.0
    muscle A18.09
    perianal (fistula) A18.32
    perinephritic A18.11

Tuberculosis, tubercular, tuberculous
(Continued)
abscess (Continued)
  perirectal A18.32
  rectum A18.32
  retropharyngeal A15.8
  sacrum A18.01
  scrofulous A18.2
  scrotum A18.15
  skin (primary) A18.4
  spinal cord A17.81
  spine or vertebra (column) A18.01
  subdiaphragmatic A18.31
  testis A18.15
  urinary A18.13
  uterus A18.17
accessory sinus —see Tuberculosis,
  sinus
Addison's disease A18.7
adenitis —see Tuberculosis, lymph
  gland
adenoids A15.8
adenopathy —see Tuberculosis, lymph
  gland
adherent pericardium A18.84
adnexa (uteri) A18.17
adrenal (capsule) (gland) A18.7
alimentary canal A18.32
anemia A18.89
ankle (joint) (bone) A18.02
anus A18.32
apex, apical —see Tuberculosis,
  pulmonary
appendicitis, appendix A18.32
arachnoid A17.0
artery, arteritis A18.89
  cerebral A18.89
arthritis (chronic) (synovial) A18.02
  spine or vertebra (column) A18.01
articular —see Tuberculosis, joint
ascites A18.31
asthma —see Tuberculosis, pulmonary
axilla, axillary (gland) A18.2
bladder A18.12
bone A18.03
  hip A18.02
  knee A18.02
  limb NEC A18.03
  sacrum A18.01
  spine or vertebral column A18.01
bowel (miliary) A18.32
brain A17.81
breast A18.89
broad ligament A18.17
bronchi, bronchial, bronchus A15.5
  ectasia, ectasis (bronchiectasis) —see
    Tuberculosis, pulmonary
  fistula A15.5
    primary (progressive) A15.7
  gland or node A15.4
    primary (progressive) A15.7
  lymph gland or node A15.4
    primary (progressive) A15.7
bronchiectasis —see Tuberculosis,
  pulmonary
bronchitis A15.5
bronchopleural A15.6
bronchopneumonia,
    bronchopneumonic —see
    Tuberculosis, pulmonary
bronchorrhagia A15.5
bronchotracheal A15.5
bronze disease A18.7
buccal cavity A18.83

Tuberculosis, tubercular, tuberculous
(Continued)
bulbourethral gland A18.15
bursa A18.09
cachexia A15.9
cardiomyopathy A18.84
caries —see Tuberculosis, bone
cartilage A18.02
  intervertebral A18.01
catarrhal —see Tuberculosis, respiratory
cecum A18.32
cellulitis (primary) A18.4
cerebellum A17.81
cerebral, cerebrum A17.81
cerebrospinal A17.81
  meninges A17.0
cervical (lymph gland or node) A18.2
cervicitis, cervix (uteri) A18.16
chest —see Tuberculosis, respiratory
chorioretinitis A18.53
choroid, choroiditis A18.53
ciliary body A18.54
colitis A18.32
collier's J65
colliquativa (primary) A18.4
colon A18.32
complex, primary A15.7
congenital P37.0
conjunctiva A18.59
connective tissue (systemic) A18.89
contact Z20.1
cornea (ulcer) A18.52
Cowper's gland A18.15
coxae A18.02
coxalgia A18.02
cul-de-sac of Douglas A18.17
curvature, spine A18.01
cutis (colliquativa) (primary) A18.4
cyst, ovary A18.18
cystitis A18.12
dactylitis A18.03
diarrhea A18.32
diffuse —see Tuberculosis, miliary
digestive tract A18.32
disseminated —see Tuberculosis,
  miliary
duodenum A18.32
dura (mater) (cerebral) (spinal) A17.0
  abscess (cerebral) (spinal) A17.81
dysentery A18.32
ear (inner) (middle) A18.6
  bone A18.03
  external (primary) A18.4
  skin (primary) A18.4
elbow A18.02
emphysema —see Tuberculosis,
  pulmonary
empyema A15.6
encephalitis A17.82
endarteritis A18.89
endocarditis A18.84
  aortic A18.84
  mitral A18.84
  pulmonary A18.84
  tricuspid A18.84
endocrine glands NEC A18.82
endometrium A18.17
enteric, enterica, enteritis A18.32
enterocolitis A18.32
epididymis, epididymitis A18.15
epidural abscess (cerebral) (spinal)
  A17.81
epiglottis A15.5
episcleritis A18.51

Tuberculosis, tubercular, tuberculous
(Continued)
erythema (induratum) (nodosum)
    (primary) A18.4
esophagus A18.83
eustachian tube A18.6
exposure (to) Z20.1
exudative —see Tuberculosis,
  pulmonary
eye A18.50
eyelid (primary) (lupus) A18.4
fallopian tube (acute) (chronic) A18.17
fascia A18.09
fauces A15.8
female pelvic inflammatory disease
    A18.17
finger A18.03
first infection A15.7
gallbladder A18.83
ganglion A18.09
gastritis A18.83
gastrocolic fistula A18.32
gastroenteritis A18.32
gastrointestinal tract A18.32
general, generalized —see Tuberculosis,
  miliary
genital organs A18.10
genitourinary A18.10
genu A18.02
glandula suprarenalis A18.7
glandular, general A18.2
glottis A15.5
grinder's J65
gum A18.83
hand A18.03
heart A18.84
hematogenous —see Tuberculosis,
  miliary
hemoptysis —see Tuberculosis,
  pulmonary
hemorrhage NEC —see Tuberculosis,
  pulmonary
hemothorax A15.6
hepatitis A18.83
hilar lymph nodes A15.4
  primary (progressive) A15.7
hip (joint) (disease) (bone) A18.02
hydropneumothorax A15.6
hydrothorax A15.6
hypoadrenalism A18.7
hypopharynx A15.8
ileocecal (hyperplastic) A18.32
ileocolitis A18.32
ileum A18.32
iliac spine (superior) A18.03
immunological findings only A15.7
indurativa (primary) A18.4
infantile A15.7
infection A15.9
  without clinical manifestations A15.7
infraclavicular gland A18.2
inguinal gland A18.2
inguinalis A18.2
intestine (any part) A18.32
iridocyclitis A18.54
iris, iritis A18.54
ischiorectal A18.32
jaw A18.03
jejunum A18.32
joint A18.02
  vertebral A18.01
keratitis (interstitial) A18.52
keratoconjunctivitis A18.52
kidney A18.11

Tuberculosis, tubercular, tuberculous
  (Continued)
 knee (joint) A18.02
 kyphosis, kyphoscoliosis A18.01
 laryngitis A15.5
 larynx A15.5
 leptomeninges, leptomeningitis
     (cerebral) (spinal) A17.0
 lichenoides (primary) A18.4
 linguae A18.83
 lip A18.83
 liver A18.83
 lordosis A18.01
 lung —see Tuberculosis, pulmonary
 lupus vulgaris A18.4
 lymph gland or node (peripheral) A18.2
     abdomen A18.39
     bronchial A15.4
         primary (progressive) A15.7
     cervical A18.2
     hilar A15.4
         primary (progressive) A15.7
     intrathoracic A15.4
         primary (progressive) A15.7
     mediastinal A15.4
         primary (progressive) A15.7
     mesenteric A18.39
     retroperitoneal A18.39
     tracheobronchial A15.4
         primary (progressive) A15.7
 lymphadenitis —see Tuberculosis,
     lymph gland
 lymphangitis —see Tuberculosis, lymph
     gland
 lymphatic (gland) (vessel) —see
     Tuberculosis, lymph gland
 mammary gland A18.89
 marasmus A15.9
 mastoiditis A18.03
 mediastinal lymph gland or node A15.4
     primary (progressive) A15.7
 mediastinitis A15.8
     primary (progressive) A15.7
 mediastinum A15.8
     primary (progressive) A15.7
 medulla A17.81
 melanosis, Addisonian A18.7
 meninges, meningitis (basilar) (cerebral)
     (cerebrospinal) (spinal) A17.0
 meningoencephalitis A17.82
 mesentery, mesenteric (gland or node)
     A18.39
 miliary A19.9
     acute A19.2
         multiple sites A19.1
         single specified site A19.0
     chronic A19.8
     specified NEC A19.8
 millstone makers' J65
 miner's J65
 molder's J65
 mouth A18.83
 multiple A19.9
     acute A19.1
     chronic A19.8
 muscle A18.09
 myelitis A17.82
 myocardium, myocarditis A18.84
 nasal (passage) (sinus) A15.8
 nasopharynx A15.8
 neck gland A18.2
 nephritis A18.11
 nerve (mononeuropathy) A17.83
 nervous system A17.9

Tuberculosis, tubercular, tuberculous
  (Continued)
 nose (septum) A15.8
 ocular A18.50
 omentum A18.31
 oophoritis (acute) (chronic) A18.17
 optic (nerve trunk) (papilla) A18.59
 orbit A18.59
 orchitis A18.15
 organ, specified NEC A18.89
 osseous —see Tuberculosis, bone
 osteitis —see Tuberculosis, bone
 osteomyelitis —see Tuberculosis, bone
 otitis media A18.6
 ovary, ovaritis (acute) (chronic) A18.17
 oviduct (acute) (chronic) A18.17
 pachymeningitis A17.0
 palate (soft) A18.83
 pancreas A18.83
 papulonecrotic (a) (primary) A18.4
 parathyroid glands A18.82
 paronychia (primary) A18.4
 parotid gland or region A18.83
 pelvis (bony) A18.03
 penis A18.15
 peribronchitis A15.5
 pericardium, pericarditis A18.84
 perichondritis, larynx A15.5
 periostitis —see Tuberculosis, bone
 perirectal fistula A18.32
 peritoneum NEC A18.31
 peritonitis A18.31
 pharynx, pharyngitis A15.8
 phlyctenulosis (keratoconjunctivitis)
     A18.52
 phthisis NEC —see Tuberculosis,
     pulmonary
 pituitary gland A18.82
 pleura, pleural, pleurisy, pleuritis
     (fibrinous) (obliterative) (purulent)
     (simple plastic) (with effusion)
     A15.6
     primary (progressive) A15.7
 pneumonia, pneumonic —see
     Tuberculosis, pulmonary
 pneumothorax (spontaneous) (tense
     valvular) —see Tuberculosis,
     pulmonary
 polyneuropathy A17.89
 polyserositis A19.9
     acute A19.1
     chronic A19.8
 potter's J65
 prepuce A18.15
 primary (complex) A15.7
 proctitis A18.32
 prostate, prostatitis A18.14
 pulmonalis —see Tuberculosis,
     pulmonary
 pulmonary (cavitated) (fibrotic)
     (infiltrative) (nodular) A15.0
     childhood type or first infection
         A15.7
     primary (complex) A15.7
 pyelitis A18.11
 pyelonephritis A18.11
 pyemia —see Tuberculosis, miliary
 pyonephrosis A18.11
 pyopneumothorax A15.6
 pyothorax A15.6
 rectum (fistula) (with abscess) A18.32
 reinfection stage —see Tuberculosis,
     pulmonary
 renal A18.11

Tuberculosis, tubercular, tuberculous
  (Continued)
 renis A18.11
 respiratory A15.9
     primary A15.7
     specified site NEC A15.8
 retina, retinitis A18.53
 retroperitoneal (lymph gland or node)
     A18.39
 rheumatism NEC A18.09
 rhinitis A15.8
 sacroiliac (joint) A18.01
 sacrum A18.01
 salivary gland A18.83
 salpingitis (acute) (chronic) A18.17
 sandblaster's J65
 sclera A18.51
 scoliosis A18.01
 scrofulous A18.2
 scrotum A18.15
 seminal tract or vesicle A18.15
 senile A15.9
 septic —see Tuberculosis, miliary
 shoulder (joint) A18.02
     blade A18.03
 sigmoid A18.32
 sinus (any nasal) A15.8
     bone A18.03
     epididymis A18.15
 skeletal NEC A18.03
 skin (any site) (primary) A18.4
 small intestine A18.32
 soft palate A18.83
 spermatic cord A18.15
 spine, spinal (column) A18.01
     cord A17.81
     medulla A17.81
     membrane A17.0
     meninges A17.0
 spleen, splenitis A18.85
 spondylitis A18.01
 sternoclavicular joint A18.02
 stomach A18.83
 stonemason's J65
 subcutaneous tissue (cellular) (primary)
     A18.4
 subcutis (primary) A18.4
 subdeltoid bursa A18.83
 submaxillary (region) A18.83
 supraclavicular gland A18.2
 suprarenal (capsule) (gland)
     A18.7
 swelling, joint (see also category M01)
     (see also Tuberculosis, joint)
     A18.02
 symphysis pubis A18.02
 synovitis A18.09
     articular A18.02
     spine or vertebra A18.01
 systemic —see Tuberculosis, miliary
 tarsitis A18.4
 tendon (sheath) —see Tuberculosis,
     tenosynovitis
 tenosynovitis A18.09
     spine or vertebra A18.01
 testis A18.15
 throat A15.8
 thymus gland A18.82
 thyroid gland A18.81
 tongue A18.83
 tonsil, tonsillitis A15.8
 trachea, tracheal A15.5
     lymph gland or node A15.4
         primary (progressive) A15.7

Tuberculosis, tubercular, tuberculous
(Continued)
  tracheobronchial A15.5
    lymph gland or node A15.4
      primary (progressive) A15.7
  tubal (acute) (chronic) A18.17
  tunica vaginalis A18.15
  ulcer (skin) (primary) A18.4
    bowel or intestine A18.32
    specified NEC - code under
      Tuberculosis, by site
  unspecified site A15.9
  ureter A18.11
  urethra, urethral (gland)
    A18.13
  urinary organ or tract A18.13
  uterus A18.17
  uveal tract A18.54
  uvula A18.83
  vagina A18.18
  vas deferens A18.15
  verruca, verrucosa (cutis) (primary)
    A18.4
  vertebra (column) A18.01
  vesiculitis A18.15
  vulva A18.18
  wrist (joint) A18.02
Tuberculum
  Carabelli (*see* Note at) K00.2
  occlusal (*see* Note at) K00.2
  paramolare K00.2
Tuberosity, enitre maxillary
  M26.07
Tuberous sclerosis (brain) Q85.1
Tubo-ovarian —*see* condition
Tuboplasty, after previous sterilization
  Z31.0
  aftercare Z31.42
Tubotympanitis, catarrhal (chronic) —
  see Otitis, media, nonsuppurative,
  chronic, serous
Tularemia A21.9
  with
    conjunctivitis A21.1
    pneumonia A21.2
  abdominal A21.3
  bronchopneumonic A21.2
  conjunctivitis A21.1
  cryptogenic A21.3
  enteric A21.3
  gastrointestinal A21.3
  generalized A21.7
  ingestion A21.3
  intestinal A21.3
  oculoglandular A21.1
  ophthalmic A21.1
  pneumonia (any), pneumonic
    A21.2
  pulmonary A21.2
  sepsis A21.7
  specified NEC A21.8
  typhoidal A21.7
  ulceroglandular A21.0
Tularensis conjunctivitis A21.1
Tumefaction —*see also* Swelling
  liver —*see* Hypertrophy, liver
Tumor —*see also* Neoplasm, unspecified
  behavior, by site
  acinar cell —*see* Neoplasm, uncertain
    behavior, by site
  acinic cell —*see* Neoplasm, uncertain
    behavior, by site
  adenocarcinoid —*see* Neoplasm,
    malignant, by site

Tumor *(Continued)*
  adenomatoid —*see also* Neoplasm,
    benign, by site
  odontogenic —*see* Cyst, calcifying
    odontogenic
  adnexal (skin) —*see* Neoplasm, skin,
    benign, by site
  adrenal
    cortical (benign) D35.0-
      malignant C74.0-
    rest —*see* Neoplasm, benign, by site
  alpha-cell
    malignant
      pancreas C25.4
      specified site NEC —*see* Neoplasm,
        malignant, by site
      unspecified site C25.4
    pancreas D13.7
    specified site NEC —*see* Neoplasm,
      benign, by site
    unspecified site D13.7
  aneurysmal —*see* Aneurysm
  aortic body D44.7
    malignant C75.5
  Askin's —*see* Neoplasm, connective
    tissue, malignant
  basal cell (*see also* Neoplasm, skin,
    uncertain behavior) D48.5
  Bednar —*see* Neoplasm, skin, malignant
  benign (unclassified) —*see* Neoplasm,
    benign, by site
  beta-cell
    malignant
      pancreas C25.4
      specified site NEC —*see* Neoplasm,
        malignant, by site
      unspecified site C25.4
    pancreas D13.7
    specified site NEC —*see* Neoplasm,
      benign, by site
    unspecified site D13.7
  Brenner D27.9
    borderline malignancy D39.1-
    malignant C56-
    proliferating D39.1
  bronchial alveolar, intravascular D38.1
  Brooke's —*see* Neoplasm, skin, benign
  brown fat —*see* Lipoma
  Burkitt —*see* Lymphoma, Burkitt
  calcifying epithelial odontogenic —*see*
    Cyst, calcifying odontogenic
  carcinoid
    benign D3A.00
      appendix D3A.020
      ascending colon D3A.022
      bronchus (lung) D3A.090
      cecum D3A.021
      colon D3A.029
      descending colon D3A.024
      duodenum D3A.010
      foregut NOS D3A.094
      hindgut NOS D3A.096
      ileum D3A.012
      jejunum D3A.011
      kidney D3A.093
      large intestine D3A.029
      lung (bronchus) D3A.090
      midgut NOS D3A.095
      rectum D3A.026
      sigmoid colon D3A.025
      small intestine D3A.019
      specified NEC D3A.098
      stomach D3A.092
      thymus D3A.091
      transverse colon D3A.023

Tumor *(Continued)*
  carcinoid *(Continued)*
    malignant C7A.00
      appendix C7A.020
      ascending colon C7A.022
      bronchus (lung) C7A.090
      cecum C7A.021
      colon C7A.029
      descending colon C7A.024
      duodenum C7A.010
      foregut NOS C7A.094
      hindgut NOS C7A.096
      ileum C7A.012
      jejunum C7A.011
      kidney C7A.093
      large intestine C7A.029
      lung (bronchus) C7A.090
      midgut NOS C7A.095
      rectum C7A.026
      sigmoid colon C7A.025
      small intestine C7A.019
      specified NEC C7A.098
      stomach C7A.092
      thymus C7A.091
      transverse colon C7A.023
    mesentary metastasis C7B.04
    secondary C7B.00
      bone C7B.03
      distant lymph nodes
        C7B.01
      liver C7B.02
      peritoneum C7B.04
      specified NEC C7B.09
  carotid body D44.6
    malignant C75.4
  cells —*see also* Neoplasm, unspecified
    behavior, by site
    benign —*see* Neoplasm, benign, by
      site
    malignant —*see* Neoplasm,
      malignant, by site
    uncertain whether benign or
      malignant —*see* Neoplasm,
      uncertain behavior, by site
  cervix, in pregnancy or childbirth —*see*
    Pregnancy, complicated by, tumor,
    cervix
  chondromatous giant cell —*see*
    Neoplasm, bone, benign
  chromaffin —*see also* Neoplasm, benign,
    by site
    malignant —*see* Neoplasm,
      malignant, by site
  Cock's peculiar L72.3
  Codman's —*see* Neoplasm, bone,
    benign
  dentigerous, mixed —*see* Cyst,
    calcifying odontogenic
  dermoid —*see* Neoplasm, benign, by
    site
    with malignant transformation
      C56-
  desmoid (extra-abdominal) —*see also*
    Neoplasm, connective tissue,
    uncertain behavior
    abdominal —*see* Neoplasm,
      connective tissue, uncertain
      behavior
  embolus —*see* Neoplasm, secondary,
    by site
  embryonal (mixed) —*see also*
    Neoplasm, uncertain behavior,
    by site
    liver C22.7

Tumor *(Continued)*
  endodermal sinus
    specified site —*see* Neoplasm,
      malignant, by site
    unspecified site
      female C56.-
      male C62.90
  epithelial
    benign —*see* Neoplasm, benign,
      by site
    malignant —*see* Neoplasm,
      malignant, by site
  Ewing's —*see* Neoplasm, bone,
    malignant, by site
  fatty —*see* Lipoma
  fibroid —*see* Leiomyoma
  G cell
    malignant
      pancreas C25.4
      specified site NEC —*see* Neoplasm,
        malignant, by site
      unspecified site C25.4
    specified site —*see* Neoplasm,
      uncertain behavior, by site
    unspecified site D37.8
  germ cell —*see also* Neoplasm,
    malignant, by site
    mixed —*see* Neoplasm, malignant,
      by site
  ghost cell, odontogenic —*see* Cyst,
    calcifying odontogenic
  giant cell —*see also* Neoplasm, uncertain
    behavior, by site
    bone D48.0
      malignant —*see* Neoplasm, bone,
        malignant
      chondromatous —*see* Neoplasm,
        bone, benign
      malignant —*see* Neoplasm,
        malignant, by site
    soft parts —*see* Neoplasm,
      connective tissue, uncertain
      behavior
      malignant —*see* Neoplasm,
        connective tissue,
        malignant
  glomus D18.00
    intra-abdominal D18.03
    intracranial D18.02
    jugulare D44.7
      malignant C75.5
    skin D18.01
    specified site NEC D18.09
  gonadal stromal —*see* Neoplasm,
    uncertain behavior, by site
  granular cell —*see also* Neoplasm,
    connective tissue, benign
    malignant —*see* Neoplasm,
      connective tissue,
      malignant
  granulosa cell D39.1-
    juvenile D39.1-
    malignant C56-
  granulosa cell-theca cell D39.1-
    malignant C56-
  Grawitz's C64-
  hemorrhoidal —*see* Hemorrhoids
  hilar cell D27-
  hilus cell D27-
  Hurthle cell (benign) D34
    malignant C73
  hydatid —*see* Echinococcus
  hypernephroid —*see also* Neoplasm,
    uncertain behavior, by site

Tumor *(Continued)*
  interstitial cell —*see also* Neoplasm,
    uncertain behavior, by site
    benign —*see* Neoplasm, benign,
      by site
    malignant —*see* Neoplasm,
      malignant, by site
  intravascular bronchial alveolar
    D38.1
  islet cell —*see* Neoplasm, benign, by site
    malignant —*see* Neoplasm,
      malignant, by site
      pancreas C25.4
      specified site NEC —*see* Neoplasm,
        malignant, by site
      unspecified site C25.4
    pancreas D13.7
    specified site NEC —*see* Neoplasm,
      benign, by site
    unspecified site D13.7
  juxtaglomerular D41.0-
  Klatskin's C22.1
  Krukenberg's C79.6-
  Leydig cell —*see* Neoplasm, uncertain
    behavior, by site
    benign —*see* Neoplasm, benign, by
      site
      specified site —*see* Neoplasm,
        benign, by site
      unspecified site
        female D27.9
        male D29.20
    malignant —*see* Neoplasm,
      malignant, by site
      specified site —*see* Neoplasm,
        malignant, by site
      unspecified site
        female C56.9
        male C62.90
    specified site —*see* Neoplasm,
      uncertain behavior, by site
    unspecified site
      female D39.10
      male D40.10
  lipid cell, ovary D27-
  lipoid cell, ovary D27-
  malignant (*see also* Neoplasm,
    malignant, by site) C80.1
    fusiform cell (type) C80.1
    giant cell (type) C80.1
    localized, plasma cell —*see*
      Plasmacytoma, solitary
    mixed NEC C80.1
    small cell (type) C80.1
    spindle cell (type) C80.1
    unclassified C80.1
  mast cell D47.0
    malignant C96.2
  melanotic, neuroectodermal —*see*
    Neoplasm, benign, by site
  Merkel cell —*see* Carcinoma, Merkel
    cell
  mesenchymal
    malignant —*see* Neoplasm, connec-
      tive tissue, malignant
    mixed —*see* Neoplasm, connective
      tissue, uncertain behavior
  mesodermal, mixed —*see also*
    Neoplasm, malignant, by site
    liver C22.4
  mesonephric —*see also* Neoplasm,
    uncertain behavior, by site
    malignant —*see* Neoplasm,
      malignant, by site

Tumor *(Continued)*
  metastatic
    from specified site —*see* Neoplasm,
      malignant, by site
    of specified site —*see* Neoplasm,
      malignant, by site
    to specified site —*see* Neoplasm,
      secondary, by site
  mixed NEC —*see also* Neoplasm,
    benign, by site
    malignant —*see* Neoplasm,
      malignant, by site
  mucinous of low malignant potential
    specified site —*see* Neoplasm,
      malignant, by site
    unspecified site C56.9
  mucocarcinoid
    specified site —*see* Neoplasm,
      malignant, by site
    unspecified site C18.1
  mucoepidermoid —*see* Neoplasm,
    uncertain behavior, by site
  Müllerian, mixed
    specified site —*see* Neoplasm,
      malignant, by site
    unspecified site C54.9
  myoepithelial —*see* Neoplasm, benign,
    by site
  neuroectodermal (peripheral) —*see*
    Neoplasm, malignant, by site
    primitive
      specified site —*see* Neoplasm,
        malignant, by site
      unspecified site C71.9
  neuroendocrine D3A.8
    malignant poorly differentiated C7A.1
    secondary NEC C7B.8
    specified NEC C7A.8
  neurogenic olfactory C30.0
  nonencapsulated sclerosing C73
  odontogenic (adenomatoid) (benign)
    (calcifying epithelial) (keratocystic)
    (squamous) —*see* Cyst, calcifying
    odontogenic
    malignant C41.1
      upper jaw (bone) C41.0
  ovarian stromal D39.1-
  ovary, in pregnancy —*see* Pregnancy,
    complicated by
  pacinian —*see* Neoplasm, skin, benign
  Pancoast's —*see* Pancoast's
    syndrome
  papillary —*see also* Papilloma
    cystic D37.9
    mucinous of low malignant potential
      C56-
      specified site —*see* Neoplasm,
        malignant, by site
      unspecified site C56.9
    serous of low malignant potential
      specified site —*see* Neoplasm,
        malignant, by site
      unspecified site C56.9
  pelvic, in pregnancy or childbirth —*see*
    Pregnancy, complicated by
  phantom F45.8
  phyllodes D48.6-
    benign D24-
    malignant —*see* Neoplasm, breast,
      malignant
  Pindborg —*see* Cyst, calcifying
    odontogenic
  placental site trophoblastic D39.2
  plasma cell (malignant) (localized) —*see*
    Plasmacytoma, solitary

479

Tumor *(Continued)*
  polyvesicular vitelline
    specified site —*see* Neoplasm,
      malignant, by site
    unspecified site
      female C56.9
      male C62.90
  Pott's puffy —*see* Osteomyelitis,
    specified NEC
  Rathke's pouch D44.3
  retinal anlage —*see* Neoplasm, benign,
    by site
  salivary gland type, mixed —*see*
    Neoplasm, salivary gland,
    benign
    malignant —*see* Neoplasm, salivary
      gland, malignant
  Sampson's N80.1
  Schmincke's —*see* Neoplasm,
    nasopharynx, malignant
  sclerosing stromal D27-
  sebaceous —*see* Cyst, sebaceous
  secondary —*see* Neoplasm, secondary,
    by site
    carcinoid C7B.00
      bone C7B.03
      distant lymph nodes C7B.01
      liver C7B.02
      peritoneum C7B.04
      specified NEC C7B.09
    neuroendocrine NEC C7B.8
  serous of low malignant potential
    specified site —*see* Neoplasm,
      malignant, by site
    unspecified site C56.9
  Sertoli cell —*see* Neoplasm, benign, by
    site
    with lipid storage
      specified site —*see* Neoplasm,
        benign, by site
      unspecified site
        female D27.9
        male D29.20
    specified site —*see* Neoplasm, benign,
      by site
    unspecified site
      female D27.9
      male D29.20
  Sertoli-Leydig cell —*see* Neoplasm,
    benign, by site
    specified site —*see* Neoplasm, benign,
      by site
    unspecified site
      female D27.9
      male D29.20
  sex cord(-stromal) —*see* Neoplasm,
    uncertain behavior, by site
    with annular tubules D39.1-
  skin appendage —*see* Neoplasm, skin,
    benign
  smooth muscle —*see* Neoplasm,
    connective tissue, uncertain
    behavior
  soft tissue
    benign —*see* Neoplasm, connective
      tissue, benign
    malignant —*see* Neoplasm,
      connective tissue, malignant
  sternomastoid (congenital) Q68.0
  stromal
    endometrial D39.0
    gastric D48.1
      benign D21.4
      malignant C16.9
      uncertain behavior D48.1

Tumor *(Continued)*
  stromal *(Continued)*
    gastrointestinal
      benign D21.4
      malignant C49.4
      uncertain behavior D48.1
    intestine
      benign D21.4
      malignant C49.4
      uncertain behavior D48.1
    ovarian D39.1-
    stomach
      benign D21.4
      malignant C16.9
      uncertain behavior D48.1
  sweat gland —*see also* Neoplasm, skin,
    uncertain behavior
    benign —*see* Neoplasm, skin, benign
    malignant —*see* Neoplasm, skin,
      malignant
  syphilitic, brain A52.17
  testicular D40.10
  testicular stromal D40.1-
  theca cell D27.-
  theca cell-granulosa cell D39.1-
  Triton, malignant —*see* Neoplasm,
    nerve, malignant
  trophoblastic, placental site D39.2
  turban D23.4
  uterus (body), in pregnancy or
    childbirth —*see* Pregnancy,
    complicated by, tumor, uterus
  vagina, in pregnancy or childbirth —*see*
    Pregnancy, complicated by
  varicose —*see* Varix
  von Recklinghausen's —*see*
    Neurofibromatosis
  vulva or perineum, in pregnancy
    or childbirth —*see* Pregnancy,
    complicated by
    causing obstructed labor O65.5
  Warthin's —*see* Neoplasm, salivary
    gland, benign
  Wilms' C64-
  yolk sac —*see* Neoplasm, malignant,
    by site
    specified site —*see* Neoplasm,
      malignant, by site
    unspecified site
      female C56.9
      male C62.90
Tumor lysis syndrome (following
  antineoplastic chemotherapy)
  (spontaneous) NEC E88.3
Tumorlet —*see* Neoplasm, uncertain
  behavior, by site
Tungiasis B88.1
Tunica vasculosa lentis Q12.2
Turban tumor D23.4
Türck's trachoma J37.0
Turner-Kieser syndrome Q79.8
Turner-like syndrome Q87.1
Turner's
  hypoplasia (tooth) K00.4
  syndrome Q96.9
    specified NEC Q96.8
  tooth K00.4
Turner-Ullrich syndrome Q96.9
Tussis convulsiva —*see* Whooping
  cough
Twiddler's syndrome (due to)
  automatic implantable defibrillator
    T82.198
  cardiac pacemaker T82.198

Twilight state
  epileptic F05
  psychogenic F44.89
Twin (newborn) —*see also* Newborn, twin
  conjoined Q89.4
  pregnancy —*see* Pregnancy, twin,
    conjoined
Twinning, teeth K00.2
Twist, twisted
  bowel, colon or intestine K56.2
  hair (congenital) Q84.1
  mesentery K56.2
  omentum K56.2
  organ or site, congenital NEC —*see*
    Anomaly, by site
  ovarian pedicle —*see* Torsion, ovary
Twitching R25.3
Tylosis (acquired) L84
  buccalis K13.29
  linguae K13.29
  palmaris et plantaris (congenital)
    (inherited) Q82.8
  acquired L85.1
Tympanism R14.0
Tympanites (abdominal) (intestinal)
  R14.0
Tympanitis —*see* Myringitis
Tympanosclerosis —*see* subcategory
  H74.0
Tympanum —*see* condition
Tympany
  abdomen R14.0
  chest R09.89
Type A behavior pattern Z73.1
Typhlitis —*see* Appendicitis
Typhoenteritis —*see* Typhoid
Typhoid (abortive) (ambulant) (any
  site) (clinical) (fever) (hemorrhagic)
  (infection) (intermittent) (malignant)
  (rheumatic) (Widal negative) A01.00
  with pneumonia A01.03
  abdominal A01.09
  arthritis A01.04
  carrier (suspected) of Z22.0
  cholecystitis (current) A01.09
  endocarditis A01.02
  heart involvement A01.02
  inoculation reaction —*see*
    Complications, vaccination
  meningitis A01.01
  mesenteric lymph nodes A01.09
  myocarditis A01.02
  osteomyelitis A01.05
  perichondritis, larynx A01.09
  pneumonia A01.03
  specified NEC A01.09
  spine A01.05
  ulcer (perforating) A01.09
Typhomalaria (fever) —*see* Malaria
Typhomania A01.00
Typhoperitonitis A01.09
Typhus (fever) A75.9
  abdominal, abdominalis —*see* Typhoid
  African tick A77.1
  amarillic A95.9
  brain A75.9 *[G94]*
  cerebral A75.9 *[G94]*
  classical A75.0
  due to Rickettsia
    prowazekii A75.0
      recrudescent A75.1
    tsutsugamushi A75.3
    typhi A75.2
  endemic (flea-borne) A75.2

Typhus *(Continued)*
  epidemic (louse-borne) A75.0
  exanthematic NEC A75.0
  exanthematicus SAI A75.0
    brillii SAI A75.1
    mexicanus SAI A75.2
    typhus murinus A75.2
  flea-borne A75.2
  India tick A77.1
  Kenya (tick) A77.1
  louse-borne A75.0

Typhus *(Continued)*
  Mexican A75.2
  mite-borne A75.3
  murine A75.2
  North Asian tick-borne A77.2
  petechial A75.9
  Queensland tick A77.3
  rat A75.2
  recrudescent A75.1
  recurrens —*see* Fever, relapsing
  Sao Paulo A77.0

Typhus *(Continued)*
  scrub (China) (India) (Malaysia) (New
    Guinea) A75.3
  shop (of Malaysia) A75.2
  Siberian tick A77.2
  tick-borne A77.9
  tropical (mite-borne) A75.3
Tyrosinemia E70.21
  newborn, transitory P74.5
Tyrosinosis E70.21
Tyrosinuria E70.29

U

Uhl's anomaly or disease Q24.8
Ulcer, ulcerated, ulcerating, ulceration, ulcerative
  alveolar process M27.3
  amebic (intestine) A06.1
    skin A06.7
  anastomotic —see Ulcer, gastrojejunal
  anorectal K62.6
  antral —see Ulcer, stomach
  anus (sphincter) (solitary) K62.6
  aorta —see Aneurysm
  aphthous (oral) (recurrent) K12.0
    genital organ (s)
      female N76.6
      male N50.8
  artery I77.2
  atrophic —see Ulcer, skin
    decubitus —see Ulcer, pressure, by site
  back L98.429
    with
      bone necrosis L98.424
      exposed fat layer L98.422
      muscle necrosis L98.423
      skin breakdown only L98.421
  Barrett's (esophagus) K22.10
    with bleeding K22.11
  bile duct (common) (hepatic) K83.8
  bladder (solitary) (sphincter) NEC N32.89
    bilharzial B65.9 [N33]
    in schistosomiasis (bilharzial) B65.9 [N33]
    submucosal —see Cystitis, interstitial
    tuberculous A18.12
  bleeding K27.4
  bone —see Osteomyelitis, specified type NEC
  bowel —see Ulcer, intestine
  breast N61
  bronchus J98.09
  buccal (cavity) (traumatic) K12.1
  Buruli A31.1
  buttock L98.419
    with
      bone necrosis L98.414
      exposed fat layer L98.412
      muscle necrosis L98.413
      skin breakdown only L98.411
  cancerous —see Neoplasm, malignant, by site
  cardia K22.10
    with bleeding K22.11
  cardioesophageal (peptic) K22.10
    with bleeding K22.11
  cecum —see Ulcer, intestine
  cervix (uteri) (decubitus) (trophic) N86
    with cervicitis N72
  chancroidal A57
  chiclero B55.1
  chronic (cause unknown) —see Ulcer, skin
  Cochin-China B55.1
  colon —see Ulcer, intestine
  conjunctiva H10.89
  cornea H16.00-
    with hypopyon H16.03-
    central H16.01-
    dendritic (herpes simplex) B00.52
    marginal H16.04-
    Mooren's H16.05-
    mycotic H16.06-

Ulcer, ulcerated, ulcerating, ulceration, ulcerative (Continued)
  cornea (Continued)
    perforated H16.07-
    ring H16.02-
    tuberculous (phlyctenular) A18.52
  corpus cavernosum (chronic) N48.5
  crural —see Ulcer, lower limb
  Curling's —see Ulcer, peptic, acute
  Cushing's —see Ulcer, peptic, acute
  cystic duct K82.8
  cystitis (interstitial) —see Cystitis, interstitial
  decubitus —see Ulcer, pressure, by site
  dendritic, cornea (herpes simplex) B00.52
  diabetes, diabetic —see Diabetes, ulcer
  Dieulafoy's K25.0
  due to
    infection NEC —see Ulcer, skin
    radiation NEC L59.8
    trophic disturbance (any region) —see Ulcer, skin
    X-ray L58.1
  duodenum, duodenal (eroded) (peptic) K26.9
    with
      hemorrhage K26.4
        and perforation K26.6
      perforation K26.5
    acute K26.3
      with
        hemorrhage K26.0
          and perforation K26.2
        perforation K26.1
    chronic K26.7
      with
        hemorrhage K26.4
          and perforation K26.6
        perforation K26.5
  dysenteric A09
  elusive —see Cystitis, interstitial
  endocarditis (acute) (chronic) (subacute) I28.8
  epiglottis J38.7
  esophagus (peptic) K22.10
    with bleeding K22.11
    due to
      aspirin K22.10
        with bleeding K22.11
      gastrointestinal reflux disease K21.0
      ingestion of chemical or medicament K22.10
        with bleeding K22.11
    fungal K22.10
      with bleeding K22.11
    infective K22.10
      with bleeding K22.11
    varicose —see Varix, esophagus
  eyelid (region) H01.8
  fauces J39.2
  Fenwick (-Hunner) (solitary) —see Cystitis, interstitial
  fistulous —see Ulcer, skin
  foot (indolent) (trophic) —see Ulcer, lower limb
  frambesial, initial A66.0
  frenum (tongue) K14.0
  gallbladder or duct K82.8
  gangrenous —see Gangrene
  gastric —see Ulcer, stomach

Ulcer, ulcerated, ulcerating, ulceration, ulcerative (Continued)
  gastrocolic —see Ulcer, gastrojejunal
  gastroduodenal —see Ulcer, peptic
  gastroesophageal —see Ulcer, stomach
  gastrointestinal —see Ulcer, gastrojejunal
  gastrojejunal (peptic) K28.9
    with
      hemorrhage K28.4
        and perforation K28.6
      perforation K28.5
    acute K28.3
      with
        hemorrhage K28.0
          and perforation K28.2
        perforation K28.1
    chronic K28.7
      with
        hemorrhage K28.4
          and perforation K28.6
        perforation K28.5
  gastrojejunocolic —see Ulcer, gastrojejunal
  gingiva K06.8
  gingivitis K05.10
    nonplaque induced K05.11
    plaque induced K05.10
  glottis J38.7
  granuloma of pudenda A58
  gum K06.8
  gumma, due to yaws A66.4
  heel —see Ulcer, lower limb
  hemorrhoid (see also Hemorrhoids, by degree) K64.8
  Hunner's —see Cystitis, interstitial
  hypopharynx J39.2
  hypopyon (chronic) (subacute) —see Ulcer, cornea, with hypopyon
  hypostaticum —see Ulcer, varicose
  ileum —see Ulcer, intestine
  intestine, intestinal K63.3
    with perforation K63.1
    amebic A06.1
    duodenal —see Ulcer, duodenum
    granulocytopenic (with hemorrhage) —see Neutropenia
    marginal —see Ulcer, gastrojejunal
    perforating K63.1
      newborn P78.0
    primary, small intestine K63.3
    rectum K62.6
    stercoraceous, stercoral K63.3
    tuberculous A18.32
    typhoid (fever) —see Typhoid
    varicose I86.8
  jejunum, jejunal —see Ulcer, gastrojejunal
  keratitis —see Ulcer, cornea
  knee —see Ulcer, lower limb
  labium (majus) (minus) N76.6
  laryngitis —see Laryngitis
  larynx (aphthous) (contact) J38.7
    diphtheritic A36.2
  leg —see Ulcer, lower limb
  lip K13.0
  Lipschütz's N76.6
  lower limb (atrophic) (chronic) (neurogenic) (perforating) (pyogenic) (trophic) (tropical) L97.909
    with
      bone necrosis L97.904
      exposed fat layer L97.902
      muscle necrosis L97.903
      skin breakdown only L97.901

Ulcer, ulcerated, ulcerating, ulceration, ulcerative *(Continued)*
lower limb *(Continued)*
ankle L97.309
with
bone necrosis L97.304
exposed fat layer L97.302
muscle necrosis L97.303
skin breakdown only L97.301
left L97.329
with
bone necrosis L97.324
exposed fat layer L97.322
muscle necrosis L97.323
skin breakdown only L97.321
right L97.319
with
bone necrosis L97.314
exposed fat layer L97.312
muscle necrosis L97.313
skin breakdown only L97.311
calf L97.209
with
bone necrosis L97.204
exposed fat layer L97.202
muscle necrosis L97.203
skin breakdown only L97.201
left L97.229
with
bone necrosis L97.224
exposed fat layer L97.222
muscle necrosis L97.223
skin breakdown only L97.221
right L97.219
with
bone necrosis L97.214
exposed fat layer L97.212
muscle necrosis L97.213
skin breakdown only L97.211
decubitus —*see* Ulcer, pressure, by site
foot specified NEC L97.509
with
bone necrosis L97.504
exposed fat layer L97.502
muscle necrosis L97.503
skin breakdown only L97.501
left L97.529
with
bone necrosis L97.524
exposed fat layer L97.522
muscle necrosis L97.523
skin breakdown only L97.521
right L97.519
with
bone necrosis L97.514
exposed fat layer L97.512
muscle necrosis L97.513
skin breakdown only L97.511
heel L97.409
with
bone necrosis L97.404
exposed fat layer L97.402
muscle necrosis L97.403
skin breakdown only L97.401
left L97.429
with
bone necrosis L97.424
exposed fat layer L97.422
muscle necrosis L97.423
skin breakdown only L97.421
right L97.419
with
bone necrosis L97.414
exposed fat layer L97.412
muscle necrosis L97.413
skin breakdown only L97.411

Ulcer, ulcerated, ulcerating, ulceration, ulcerative *(Continued)*
lower limb *(Continued)*
left L97.929
with
bone necrosis L97.924
exposed fat layer L97.922
muscle necrosis L97.923
skin breakdown only L97.921
lower leg NOS L97.909
with
bone necrosis L97.904
exposed fat layer L97.902
muscle necrosis L97.903
skin breakdown only L97.901
left L97.929
with
bone necrosis L97.924
exposed fat layer L97.922
muscle necrosis L97.923
skin breakdown only
L97.921
right L97.919
with
bone necrosis L97.914
exposed fat layer L97.912
muscle necrosis L97.913
skin breakdown only L97.911
specified site NEC L97.809
with
bone necrosis L97.804
exposed fat layer L97.802
muscle necrosis L97.803
skin breakdown only L97.801
left L97.829
with
bone necrosis L97.824
exposed fat layer L97.822
muscle necrosis L97.823
skin breakdown only
L97.821
right L97.819
with
bone necrosis L97.814
exposed fat layer L97.812
muscle necrosis L97.813
skin breakdown only
L97.811
midfoot L97.409
with
bone necrosis L97.404
exposed fat layer L97.402
muscle necrosis L97.403
skin breakdown only L97.401
left L97.429
with
bone necrosis L97.424
exposed fat layer L97.422
muscle necrosis L97.423
skin breakdown only
L97.421
right L97.419
with
bone necrosis L97.414
exposed fat layer L97.412
muscle necrosis L97.413
skin breakdown only
L97.411
right L97.919
with
bone necrosis L97.914
exposed fat layer L97.912
muscle necrosis L97.913
skin breakdown only L97.911

Ulcer, ulcerated, ulcerating, ulceration, ulcerative *(Continued)*
lower limb *(Continued)*
thigh L97.109
with
bone necrosis L97.104
exposed fat layer L97.102
muscle necrosis L97.103
skin breakdown only L97.101
left L97.129
with
bone necrosis L97.124
exposed fat layer L97.122
muscle necrosis L97.123
skin breakdown only L97.121
right L97.119
with
bone necrosis L97.114
exposed fat layer L97.112
muscle necrosis L97.113
skin breakdown only L97.111
toe L97.509
with
bone necrosis L97.504
exposed fat layer L97.502
muscle necrosis L97.503
skin breakdown only L97.501
left L97.529
with
bone necrosis L97.524
exposed fat layer L97.522
muscle necrosis L97.523
skin breakdown only L97.521
right L97.519
with
bone necrosis L97.514
exposed fat layer L97.512
muscle necrosis L97.513
skin breakdown only L97.511
leprous A30.1
syphilitic A52.19
varicose —*see* Varix, leg, with, ulcer
luetic —*see* Ulcer, syphilitic
lung J98.4
tuberculous —*see* Tuberculosis,
pulmonary
malignant —*see* Neoplasm, malignant,
by site
marginal NEC —*see* Ulcer,
gastrojejunal
meatus (urinarius) N34.2
Meckel's diverticulum Q43.0
malignant —*see* Table of Neoplasms,
small intestine, malignant
Meleney's (chronic undermining) —*see*
Ulcer, skin
Mooren's (cornea) —*see* Ulcer, cornea,
Mooren's
mycobacterial (skin) A31.1
nasopharynx J39.2
neck, uterus N86
neurogenic NEC —*see* Ulcer, skin
nose, nasal (passage) (infective)
(septum) J34.0
skin —*see* Ulcer, skin
spirochetal A69.8
varicose (bleeding) I86.8
oral mucosa (traumatic) K12.1
palate (soft) K12.1
penis (chronic) N48.5
peptic (site unspecified) K27.9
with
hemorrhage K27.4
and perforation K27.6
perforation K27.5

Ulcer, ulcerated, ulcerating, ulceration,
ulcerative (Continued)
peptic (Continued)
acute K27.3
with
hemorrhage K27.0
and perforation K27.2
perforation K27.1
chronic K27.7
with
hemorrhage K27.4
and perforation K27.6
perforation K27.5
esophagus K22.10
with bleeding K22.11
newborn P78.82
perforating K27.5
skin —see Ulcer, skin
peritonsillar J35.8
phagedenic (tropical) —see Ulcer, skin
pharynx J39.2
phlebitis —see Phlebitis
plaster —see Ulcer, pressure, by site
popliteal space —see Ulcer, lower limb
postpyloric —see Ulcer, duodenum
prepuce N47.7
prepyloric —see Ulcer, stomach
pressure (pressure area) L89.9-
ankle L89.5-
back L89.1-
buttock L89.3-
coccyx L89.15-
contiguous site of back, buttock, hip
L89.4-
elbow L89.0-
face L89.81-
head L89.81-
heel L89.6-
hip L89.2-
sacral region (tailbone) L89.15-
specified site NEC L89.89-
stage 1 (healing) (pre-ulcer skin
changes limited to persistent focal
edema)
ankle L89.5-
back L89.1-
buttock L89.3-
coccyx L89.15-
contiguous site of back, buttock,
hip L89.4-
elbow L89.0-
face L89.81-
head L89.81-
heel L89.6-
hip L89.2-
sacral region (tailbone) L89.15-
specified site NEC L89.89-
stage 2 (healing) (abrasion, blister,
partial thickness skin loss
involving epidermis and/or
dermis)
ankle L89.5-
back L89.1-
buttock L89.3-
coccyx L89.15-
contiguous site of back, buttock,
hip L89.4-
elbow L89.0-
face L89.81-
head L89.81-
heel L89.6-
hip L89.2-
sacral region (tailbone) L89.15-
specified site NEC L89.89-

Ulcer, ulcerated, ulcerating, ulceration,
ulcerative (Continued)
pressure (Continued)
stage 3 (healing) (full thickness
skin loss involving damage or
necrosis of subcutaneous tissue)
ankle L89.5-
back L89.1-
buttock L89.3-
coccyx L89.15-
contiguous site of back, buttock,
hip L89.4-
elbow L89.0-
face L89.81-
head L89.81-
heel L89.6-
hip L89.2-
sacral region (tailbone) L89.15-
specified site NEC L89.89-
stage 4 (healing) (necrosis of soft
tissues through to underlying
muscle, tendon, or bone)
ankle L89.5-
back L89.1-
buttock L89.3-
coccyx L89.15-
contiguous site of back, buttock,
hip L89.4-
elbow L89.0-
face L89.81-
head L89.81-
heel L89.6-
hip L89.2-
sacral region (tailbone) L89.15-
specified site NEC L89.89-
unspecified stage
ankle L89.5-
back L89.1-
buttock L89.3-
coccyx L89.15-
contiguous site of back, buttock,
hip L89.4-
elbow L89.0-
face L89.81-
head L89.81-
heel L89.6-
hip L89.2-
sacral region (tailbone) L89.15-
specified site NEC L89.89-
unstageable
ankle L89.5-
back L89.1-
buttock L89.3-
coccyx L89.15-
contiguous site of back, buttock,
hip L89.4-
elbow L89.0-
face L89.81-
head L89.81-
heel L89.6-
hip L89.2-
sacral region (tailbone) L89.15-
specified site NEC L89.89-
primary of intestine K63.3
with perforation K63.1
prostate N41.9
pyloric —see Ulcer, stomach
rectosigmoid K63.3
with perforation K63.1
rectum (sphincter) (solitary) K62.6
stercoraceous, stercoral K62.6
retina —see Inflammation, chorioretinal
rodent —see also Neoplasm, skin,
malignant

Ulcer, ulcerated, ulcerating, ulceration,
ulcerative (Continued)
sclera —see Scleritis
scrofulous (tuberculous) A18.2
scrotum N50.8
tuberculous A18.15
varicose I86.1
seminal vesicle N50.8
sigmoid —see Ulcer, intestine
skin (atrophic) (chronic) (neurogenic)
(non-healing) (perforating)
(pyogenic) (trophic) (tropical)
L98.499
with gangrene —see Gangrene
amebic A06.7
back —see Ulcer, back
buttock —see Ulcer, buttock
decubitus —see Ulcer, pressure
lower limb —see Ulcer, lower limb
mycobacterial A31.1
specified site NEC L98.499
with
bone necrosis L98.494
exposed fat layer L98.492
muscle necrosis L98.493
skin breakdown only L98.491
tuberculous (primary) A18.4
varicose —see Ulcer, varicose
sloughing —see Ulcer, skin
solitary, anus or rectum (sphincter)
K62.6
sore throat J02.9
streptococcal J02.0
spermatic cord N50.8
spine (tuberculous) A18.01
stasis (venous) —see Varix, leg, with,
ulcer
without varicose veins I87.2
stercoraceous, stercoral K63.3
with perforation K63.1
anus or rectum K62.6
stoma, stomal —see Ulcer, gastrojejunal
stomach (eroded) (peptic) (round) K25.9
with
hemorrhage K25.4
and perforation K25.6
perforation K25.5
acute K25.3
with
hemorrhage K25.0
and perforation K25.2
perforation K25.1
chronic K25.7
with
hemorrhage K25.4
and perforation K25.6
perforation K25.5
stomal —see Ulcer, gastrojejunal
stomatitis K12.1
stress —see Ulcer, peptic
strumous (tuberculous) A18.2
submucosal, bladder —see Cystitis,
interstitial
syphilitic (any site) (early) (secondary)
A51.39
late A52.79
perforating A52.79
foot A52.11
testis N50.8
thigh —see Ulcer, lower limb
throat J39.2
diphtheritic A36.0
toe —see Ulcer, lower limb
tongue (traumatic) K14.0

Ulcer, ulcerated, ulcerating, ulceration,
    ulcerative *(Continued)*
  tonsil J35.8
    diphtheritic A36.0
  trachea J39.8
  trophic —*see* Ulcer, skin
  tropical —*see* Ulcer, skin
  tuberculous —*see* Tuberculosis, ulcer
  tunica vaginalis N50.8
  turbinate J34.89
  typhoid (perforating) —*see* Typhoid
  unspecified site —*see* Ulcer, skin
  urethra (meatus) —*see* Urethritis
  uterus N85.8
    cervix N86
      with cervicitis N72
    neck N86
      with cervicitis N72
  vagina N76.5
    in Behçet's disease M35.2 *[N77.0]*
    pessary N89.8
  valve, heart I33.0
  varicose (lower limb, any part) —*see
      also* Varix, leg, with, ulcer
    broad ligament I86.2
    esophagus —*see* Varix, esophagus
    inflamed or infected —*see* Varix, leg,
        with ulcer, with inflammation
    nasal septum I86.8
    perineum I86.3
    scrotum I86.1
    specified site NEC I86.8
    sublingual I86.0
    vulva I86.3
  vas deferens N50.8
  vulva (acute) (infectional) N76.6
    in (due to)
      Behçet's disease M35.2 *[N77.0]*
      herpesviral (herpes simplex)
          infection A60.04
      tuberculosis A18.18
  vulvobuccal, recurring N76.6
  X-ray L58.1
  yaws A66.4
Ulcerosa scarlatina A38.8
Ulcus —*see also* Ulcer
  cutis tuberculosum A18.4
  duodeni —*see* Ulcer, duodenum
  durum (syphilitic) A51.0
    extragenital A51.2
  gastrojejunale —*see* Ulcer,
      gastrojejunal
  hypostaticum —*see* Ulcer, varicose
  molle (cutis) (skin) A57
  serpens corneae —*see* Ulcer, cornea,
      central
  ventriculi —*see* Ulcer, stomach
Ulegyria Q04.8
Ulerythema
  ophryogenes, congenital Q84.2
  sycosiforme L73.8
Ullrich(-Bonnevie)(-Turner) syndrome
    Q87.1
Ullrich-Feichtiger syndrome Q87.0
Ulnar —*see* condition
Ulorrhagia, ulorrhea K06.8
Umbilicus, umbilical —*see* condition
Unacceptable
  contours of tooth K08.54
  morphology of tooth K08.54
Unavailability (of)
  bed at medical facility Z75.1
  health service-related agencies
      Z75.4

Unavailability *(Continued)*
  medical facilities (at) Z75.3
    due to
      investigation by social service
          agency Z75.2
      lack of services at home Z75.0
      remoteness from facility Z75.3
      waiting list Z75.1
    home Z75.0
    outpatient clinic Z75.3
  schooling Z55.1
  social service agencies Z75.4
Uncinaria americana infestation
    B76.1
Uncinariasis B76.9
Uncongenial work Z56.5
Unconscious (ness) —*see* Coma
Under observation —*see* Observation
Underachievement in school Z55.3
Underdevelopment —*see also*
    Undeveloped
  nose Q30.1
  sexual E30.0
Underdosing (*see also* Table of drugs and
    chemicals, categories T36-T50, with
    final character 6) Z91.14
  intentional NEC Z91.128
    due to financial hardship of patient
        Z91.120
  unintentional NEC Z91.138
    due to patient's age related debility
        Z91.130
Underfeeding, newborn P92.3
Underfill, endodontic M27.53
Underimmunization status Z28.3
Undernourishment —*see* Malnutrition
Undernutrition —*see* Malnutrition
Underweight R63.6
  for gestational age —*see* Light for dates
Underwood's disease P83.0
Undescended —*see also* Malposition,
    congenital
  cecum Q43.3
  colon Q43.3
  testicle —*see* Cryptorchid
Undeveloped, undevelopment —*see also*
    Hypoplasia
  brain (congenital) Q02
  cerebral (congenital) Q02
  heart Q24.8
  lung Q33.6
  testis E29.1
  uterus E30.0
Undiagnosed (disease) R69
Undulant fever —*see* Brucellosis
Unemployment, anxiety concerning Z56.0
  threatened Z56.2
Unequal length (acquired) (limb) —*see
    also* Deformity, limb, unequal length
  leg —*see also* Deformity, limb, unequal
      length
    congenital Q72.9-
Unextracted dental root K08.3
Unguis incarnatus L60.0
Unhappiness R45.2
Unicornate uterus Q51.4
Unilateral —*see also* condition
  development, breast N64.89
  organ or site, congenital NEC —*see*
      Agenesis, by site
Unilocular heart Q20.8
Union, abnormal —*see also* Fusion
  larynx and trachea Q34.8
Universal mesentery Q43.3

Unrepairable overhanging of dental
    restorative materials K08.52
Unsatisfactory
  restoration of tooth K08.50
    specified NEC K08.59
  sample of cytologic smear
    anus R85.615
    cervix R87.615
    vagina R87.625
  surroundings Z59.1
  work Z56.5
Unsoundness of mind —*see* Psychosis
Unstable
  back NEC —*see* Instability, joint,
      spine
  hip (congenital) Q65.6
    acquired —*see* Derangement, joint,
        specified type NEC, hip
  joint —*see* Instability, joint
    secondary to removal of joint
        prosthesis M96.89
  lie (mother) O32.0
  lumbosacral joint (congenital)
    acquired —*see* subcategory M53.2
  sacroiliac —*see* subcategory M53.2
  spine NEC —*see* Instability, joint, spine
Unsteadiness on feet R26.81
Untruthfulness, child problem F91.8
Unverricht(-Lundborg) disease or
    epilepsy —*see* Epilepsy, generalized,
    idiopathic
Unwanted pregnancy Z64.0
Upbringing, institutional Z62.22
  away from parents NEC Z62.29
  in care of non-parental family member
      Z62.21
  in foster care Z62.21
  in orphanage or group home Z62.22
  in welfare custody Z62.21
Upper respiratory —*see* condition
Upset
  gastric K30
  gastrointestinal K30
    psychogenic F45.8
  intestinal (large) (small) K59.9
    psychogenic F45.8
  menstruation N93.9
  mental F48.9
  stomach K30
    psychogenic F45.8
Urachus —*see also* condition
  patent or persistent Q64.4
Urbach-Oppenheim disease (necrobiosis
    lipoidica diabeticorum) —*see*
    E08-E13 with .620
Urbach-Wiethe disease E78.89
Urbach's lipoid proteinosis E78.89
Urban yellow fever A95.1
Urea
  blood, high —*see* Uremia
  cycle metabolism disorder —*see*
      Disorder, urea cycle metabolism
Uremia, uremic N19
  with
    ectopic or molar pregnancy O08.4
    polyneuropathy N18.9 *[G63]*
  chronic (*see also* Disease, kidney,
      chronic) N18.9
    due to hypertension —*see*
        Hypertensive, kidney
  complicating
    ectopic or molar pregnancy O08.4
  congenital P96.0
  extrarenal R39.2

Uremia, uremic (*Continued*)
- following ectopic or molar pregnancy O08.4
- newborn P96.0
- prerenal R39.2

Ureter, ureteral —*see* condition
Ureteralgia N23
Ureterectasis —*see* Hydroureter
Ureteritis N28.89
- cystica N28.86
- due to calculus N20.1
  - with calculus, kidney N20.2
    - with hydronephrosis N13.2
- gonococcal (acute) (chronic) A54.21
- nonspecific N28.89

Ureterocele N28.89
- congenital (orthotopic) Q62.31
  - ectopic Q62.32

Ureterolith, ureterolithiasis —*see* Calculus, ureter
Ureterostomy
- attention to Z43.6
- status Z93.6

Urethra, urethral —*see* condition
Urethralgia R39.89
Urethritis (anterior) (posterior) N34.2
- calculous N21.1
- candidal B37.41
- chlamydial A56.01
- diplococcal (gonococcal) A54.01
  - with abscess (accessory gland) (periurethral) A54.1
- gonococcal A54.01
  - with abscess (accessory gland) (periurethral) A54.1
- nongonococcal N34.1
  - Reiter's —*see* Reiter's disease
- nonspecific N34.1
- nonvenereal N34.1
- postmenopausal N34.2
- puerperal O86.29
- Reiter's —*see* Reiter's disease
- specified NEC N34.2
- trichomonal or due to Trichomonas (vaginalis) A59.03

Urethrocele N81.0
- with
  - cystocele —*see* Cystocele
  - prolapse of uterus —*see* Prolapse, uterus

Urethrolithiasis (with colic or infection) N21.1
Urethrorectal —*see* condition
Urethrorrhagia N36.8
Urethrorrhea R36.9
Urethrostomy
- attention to Z43.6
- status Z93.6

Urethrotrigonitis —*see* Trigonitis
Urethrovaginal —*see* condition
Urgency
- fecal R15.2
- hypertensive —*see* Hypertension
- urinary N39.41

Urhidrosis, uridrosis L74.8
Uric acid in blood (increased) E79.0
Uricacidemia (asymptomatic) E79.0
Uricemia (asymptomatic) E79.0
Uricosuria R82.99
Urinary —*see* condition
Urination
- frequent R35.0
- painful R30.9

Urine
- blood in —*see* Hematuria
- discharge, excessive R35.8
- enuresis, nonorganic origin F98.0
- extravasation R39.0
- frequency R35.0
- incontinence R32
  - nonorganic origin F98.0
- intermittent stream R39.19
- pus in N39.0
- retention or stasis R33.9
  - organic R33.8
    - drug-induced R33.0
  - psychogenic F45.8
- secretion
  - deficient R34
  - excessive R35.8
  - frequency R35.0
- stream
  - intermittent R39.19
  - slowing R39.19
  - splitting R39.13
  - weak R39.12

Urinemia —*see* Uremia
Urinoma, urethra N36.8
Uroarthritis, infectious (Reiter's) —*see* Reiter's disease
Urodialysis R34
Urolithiasis —*see* Calculus, urinary
Uronephrosis —*see* Hydronephrosis
Uropathy N39.9
- obstructive N13.9
  - specified NEC N13.8
- reflux N13.9
  - specified NEC N13.8
- vesicoureteral reflux-associated —*see* Reflux, vesicoureteral

Urosepsis — code to condition
Urticaria L50.9
- with angioneurotic edema T78.3
  - hereditary D84.1
- allergic L50.0
- cholinergic L50.5
- chronic L50.8
- cold, familial L50.2
- contact L50.6
- dermatographic L50.3
- due to
  - cold or heat L50.2
  - drugs L50.0
  - food L50.0
  - inhalants L50.0
  - plants L50.6
  - serum (*see also* Reaction, serum) T80.69
- factitial L50.3
- giant T78.3
  - hereditary D84.1
- gigantea T78.3
- idiopathic L50.1
- larynx T78.3
  - hereditary D84.1
- neonatorum P83.8
- nonallergic L50.1
- papulosa (Hebra) L28.2
- pigmentosa Q82.2
- recurrent periodic L50.8
- serum (*see also* Reaction, serum) T80.69
- solar L56.3
- specified type NEC L50.8
- thermal (cold) (heat) L50.2
- vibratory L50.4
- xanthelasmoidea Q82.2

Use (of)
- alcohol F10.99
  - with sleep disorder F10.982
  - harmful —*see* Abuse, alcohol
- amphetamines —*see* Use, stimulant NEC
- caffeine —*see* Use, stimulant NEC
- cannabis F12.90
  - with
    - anxiety disorder F12.980
    - intoxication F12.929
      - with
        - delirium F12.921
        - perceptual disturbance F12.922
      - uncomplicated F12.920
    - other specified disorder F12.988
    - psychosis F12.959
      - delusions F12.950
      - hallucinations F12.951
    - unspecified disorder F12.99
- cocaine F14.90
  - with
    - anxiety disorder F14.980
    - intoxication F14.929
      - with
        - delirium F14.921
        - perceptual disturbance F14.922
      - uncomplicated F14.920
    - other specified disorder F14.988
    - psychosis F14.959
      - delusions F14.950
      - hallucinations F14.951
    - sexual dysfunction F14.981
    - sleep disorder F14.982
    - unspecified disorder F14.99
  - harmful —*see* Abuse, drug, cocaine
- drug (s) NEC F19.90
  - with sleep disorder F19.982
  - harmful —*see* Abuse, drug, by type
- hallucinogen NEC F16.90
  - with
    - anxiety disorder F16.980
    - intoxication F16.929
      - with
        - delirium F16.921
      - uncomplicated F16.920
    - mood disorder F16.94
    - other specified disorder F16.988
    - perception disorder (flashbacks) F16.983
    - psychosis F16.959
      - delusions F16.950
      - hallucinations F16.951
    - unspecified disorder F16.99
  - harmful —*see* Abuse, drug, hallucinogen NEC
- inhalants F18.90
  - with
    - anxiety disorder F18.980
    - intoxication F18.929
      - with delirium F18.921
      - uncomplicated F18.920
    - mood disorder F18.94
    - other specified disorder F18.988
    - persisting dementia F18.97
    - psychosis F18.959
      - delusions F18.950
      - hallucinations F18.951
    - unspecified disorder F18.99
  - harmful —*see* Abuse, drug, inhalant
- methadone F11.20
- nonprescribed drugs F19.90
  - harmful —*see* Abuse, nonpsychoactive substance

Use *(Continued)*
 opioid F11.90
  with
   disorder F11.99
    mood F11.94
    sleep F11.982
    specified type NEC F11.988
   intoxication F11.929
    with
     delirium F11.921
     perceptual disturbance F11.922
    uncomplicated F11.920
   withdrawal F11.93
  harmful —*see* Abuse, drug, opioid
 patent medicines F19.90
  harmful —*see* Abuse, non-
   psychoactive substance
 psychoactive drug NEC F19.90
  with
   anxiety disorder F19.980
   intoxication F19.929
    with
     delirium F19.921
     perceptual disturbance F19.922
    uncomplicated F19.920
   mood disorder F19.94
   other specified disorder F19.988
   persisting
    amnestic disorder F19.96
    dementia F19.97
   psychosis F19.959
    delusions F19.950
    hallucinations F19.951
   sexual dysfunction F19.981
   sleep disorder F19.982
   unspecified disorder F19.99
   withdrawal F19.939
    with
     delirium F19.931
     perceptual disturbance F19.932
    uncomplicated F19.930
  harmful —*see* Abuse, drug NEC,
   psychoactive NEC

Use *(Continued)*
 sedative, hypnotic, or anxiolytic
  F13.90
  with
   anxiety disorder F13.980
   intoxication F13.929
    with
     delirium F13.921
    uncomplicated F13.920
   other specified disorder F13.988
   persisting
    amnestic disorder F13.96
    dementia F13.97
   psychosis F13.959
    delusions F13.950
    hallucinations F13.951
   sexual dysfunction F13.981
   sleep disorder F13.982
   unspecified disorder F13.99
  harmful —*see* Abuse, drug,
   sedative, hypnotic, or
   anxiolytic
 stimulant NEC F15.90
  with
   anxiety disorder F15.980
   intoxication F15.929
    with
     delirium F15.921
     perceptual disturbance
      F15.922
    uncomplicated F15.920
   mood disorder F15.94
   other specified disorder F15.988
   psychosis F15.959
    delusions F15.950
    hallucinations F15.951
   sexual dysfunction F15.981
   sleep disorder F15.982
   unspecified disorder F15.99
   withdrawal F15.93
  harmful —*see* Abuse, drug, stimulant
   NEC

Use *(Continued)*
 tobacco Z72.0
  with dependence —*see* Dependence,
   drug, nicotine
 volatile solvents (*see also* Use, inhalant)
  F18.90
  harmful —*see* Abuse, drug, inhalant
Usher-Senear disease or syndrome
 L10.4
Uta B55.1
Uteromegaly N85.2
Uterovaginal —*see* condition
Uterovesical —*see* condition
Uveal —*see* condition
Uveitis (anterior) —*see also*
 Iridocyclitis
 acute —*see* Iridocyclitis, acute
 chronic —*see* Iridocyclitis, chronic
 due to toxoplasmosis (acquired)
  B58.09
  congenital P37.1
 granulomatous —*see* Iridocyclitis,
  chronic
 heterochromic —*see* Cyclitis, Fuchs'
  heterochromic
 lens-induced —*see* Iridocyclitis,
  lens-induced
 posterior —*see* Chorioretinitis
 sympathetic H44.13-
 syphilitic (secondary) A51.43
  congenital (early) A50.01
  late A52.71
 tuberculous A18.54
Uveoencephalitis —*see* Inflammation,
 chorioretinal
Uveokeratitis —*see* Iridocyclitis
Uveoparotitis D86.89
Uvula —*see* condition
Uvulitis (acute) (catarrhal) (chronic)
 (membranous) (suppurative)
 (ulcerative) K12.2

V

Vaccination (prophylactic)
  complication or reaction —*see*
    Complications, vaccination
  delayed Z28.9
  encounter for Z23
  not done —*see* Immunization, not done,
    because (of)
Vaccinia (generalized) (localized) T88.1
  without vaccination B08.011
  congenital P35.8
Vacuum, in sinus (accessory) (nasal)
  J34.89
Vagabond, vagabondage Z59.0
Vagabond's disease B85.1
Vagina, vaginal —*see* condition
Vaginalitis (tunica) (testis) N49.1
Vaginismus (reflex) N94.2
  functional F52.5
  nonorganic F52.5
  psychogenic F52.5
  secondary N94.2
Vaginitis (acute) (circumscribed) (diffuse)
    (emphysematous) (nonvenereal)
    (ulcerative) N76.0
  with ectopic or molar pregnancy O08.0
  amebic A06.82
  atrophic, postmenopausal N95.2
  bacterial N76.0
  blennorrhagic (gonococcal) A54.02
  candidal B37.3
  chlamydial A56.02
  chronic N76.1
  due to Trichomonas (vaginalis) A59.01
  following ectopic or molar pregnancy
    O08.0
  gonococcal A54.02
    with abscess (accessory gland)
      (periurethral) A54.1
  granuloma A58
  in (due to)
    candidiasis B37.3
    herpesviral (herpes simplex) infection
      A60.04
    pinworm infection B80 [N77.1]
  monilial B37.3
  mycotic (candidal) B37.3
  postmenopausal atrophic N95.2
  puerperal (postpartum) O86.13
  senile (atrophic) N95.2
  subacute or chronic N76.1
  syphilitic (early) A51.0
    late A52.76
  trichomonal A59.01
  tuberculous A18.18
Vaginosis —*see* Vaginitis
Vagotonia G52.2
Vagrancy Z59.0
VAIN —*see* Neoplasia, intraepithelial,
  vagina
Vallecula —*see* condition
Valley fever B38.0
Valsuani's disease —*see* Anemia, obstetric
Valve, valvular (formation) —*see also*
    condition
  cerebral ventricle (communicating) in
    situ Z98.2
  cervix, internal os Q51.828
  congenital NEC —*see* Atresia, by site
  ureter (pelvic junction) (vesical orifice)
    Q62.39
  urethra (congenital) (posterior) Q64.2
Valvulitis (chronic) —*see* Endocarditis

Valvulopathy —*see* Endocarditis
Van Bogaert's leukoencephalopathy
  (sclerosing) (subacute) A81.1
Van Bogaert-Scherer-Epstein disease or
  syndrome E75.5
Van Buchem's syndrome M85.2
Van Creveld-von Gierke disease E74.01
Van der Hoeve (-de Kleyn) syndrome
  Q78.0
Van der Woude's syndrome Q38.0
Van Neck's disease or osteochondrosis
  M91.0
Vanishing lung J44.9
Vapor asphyxia or suffocation T59.9
  specified agent —*see* Table of drugs and
    chemicals
Variance, lethal ball, prosthetic heart
    valve T82.09
Variants, thalassemic D56.8
Variations in hair color L67.1
Varicella B01.9
  with
    complications NEC B01.89
    encephalitis B01.11
    encephalomyelitis B01.11
    meningitis B01.0
    myelitis B01.12
    pneumonia B01.2
  congenital P35.8
Varices —*see* Varix
Varicocele (scrotum) (thrombosed)
  I86.1
  ovary I86.2
  perineum I86.3
  spermatic cord (ulcerated) I86.1
Varicose
  aneurysm (ruptured) I77.0
  dermatitis —*see* Varix, leg, with,
    inflammation
  eczema —*see* Varix, leg, with,
    inflammation
  phlebitis —*see* Varix, with,
    inflammation
  tumor —*see* Varix
  ulcer (lower limb, any part) —*see also*
    Varix, leg, with, ulcer
    anus (see also Hemorrhoids) K64.8
    esophagus —*see* Varix, esophagus
    inflamed or infected —*see* Varix, leg,
      with ulcer, with inflammation
    nasal septum I86.8
    perineum I86.3
    scrotum I86.1
    specified site NEC I86.8
  vein —*see* Varix
  vessel —*see* Varix, leg
Varicosis, varicosities, varicosity —*see*
  Varix
Variola (major) (minor) B03
Varioloid B03
Varix (lower limb) (ruptured) I83.90
  with
    edema I83.899
    inflammation I83.10
      with ulcer (venous) I83.209
    pain I83.819
    specified complication NEC I83.899
    stasis dermatitis I83.10
      with ulcer (venous) I83.209
    swelling I83.899
    ulcer I83.009
      with inflammation I83.209
  aneurysmal I77.0
  asymptomatic I83.9-

Varix (*Continued*)
  bladder I86.2
  broad ligament I86.2
  complicating
    childbirth (lower extremity) O87.4
      anus or rectum O87.2
      genital (vagina, vulva or perineum)
        O87.8
    pregnancy (lower extremity) O22.0-
      anus or rectum O22.4-
      genital (vagina, vulva or perineum)
        O22.1-
    puerperium (lower extremity) O87.4
      anus or rectum O87.2
      genital (vagina, vulva, perineum)
        O87.8
  congenital (any site) Q27.8
  esophagus (idiopathic) (primary)
    (ulcerated) I85.00
    bleeding I85.01
    congenital Q27.8
    in (due to)
      alcoholic liver disease I85.10
        bleeding I85.11
      cirrhosis of liver I85.10
        bleeding I85.11
      portal hypertension I85.10
        bleeding I85.11
      schistosomiasis I85.10
        bleeding I85.11
      toxic liver disease I85.10
        bleeding I85.11
    secondary I85.10
      bleeding I85.11
  gastric I86.4
  inflamed or infected I83.10
    ulcerated I83.209
  labia (majora) I86.3
  leg (asymptomatic) I83.90
    with
      edema I83.899
      inflammation I83.10
        with ulcer —*see* Varix, leg, with,
          ulcer, with inflammation
          by site
      pain I83.819
      specified complication NEC
        I83.899
      swelling I83.899
      ulcer I83.009
        with inflammation I83.209
        ankle I83.003
          with inflammation I83.203
        calf I83.002
          with inflammation I83.202
        foot NEC I83.005
          with inflammation I83.205
        heel I83.004
          with inflammation I83.204
        lower leg NEC I83.008
          with inflammation I83.208
        midfoot I83.004
          with inflammation I83.204
        thigh I83.001
          with inflammation I83.201
    bilateral (asymptomatic) I83.93
      with
        edema I83.893
        pain I83.813
        specified complication NEC
          I83.893
        swelling I83.893
        ulcer I83.009
          with inflammation I83.209

Vertigo (Continued)
  hysterical F44.89
  infrasound T75.23
  labyrinthine —see subcategory H81.0
  laryngeal R05
  malignant positional H81.4-
  Ménière's —see subcategory H81.40
  menopausal N95.11
  otogenic —see Vertigo, aural
  paroxysmal positional, benign —see
      Vertigo, benign paroxysmal
  Pedersen's (epidemic) —see Neuronitis,
      vestibular
  peripheral NEC H81.39-
  positional
      benign paroxysmal —see Vertigo,
          benign paroxysmal
      malignant H81.4-
Very-low-density-lipoprotein-type
    (VLDL) hyperlipoproteinemia
    E78.1
Vesania —see Psychosis
Vesical —see condition
Vesicle
  cutaneous R23.8
  seminal —see condition
  skin R23.8
Vesicocolic —see condition
Vesicoperineal —see condition
Vesicorectal —see condition
Vesicourethrorectal —see condition
Vesicovaginal —see condition
Vesicular —see condition
Vesiculitis (seminal) N49.0
  amebic A06.82
  gonorrheal (acute) (chronic)
      A54.23
  trichomonal A59.09
  tuberculous A18.15
Vestibulitis (ear) (see also subcategory)
    H83.0
  nose (external) J34.89
  vulvar N94.810
Vestibulopathy, acute peripheral
    (recurrent) —see Neuronitis,
    vestibular
Vestige, vestigial —see also Persistence
  branchial Q18.0
  structures in vitreous Q14.0
Vibration
  adverse effects T75.20
      pneumatic hammer syndrome
          T75.21
      specified effect NEC T75.29
      vasospastic syndrome T75.22
      vertigo from infrasound T75.23
  exposure (occupational) Z57.7
  vertigo T75.23
Vibriosis A28.9
Victim (of)
  crime Z65.4
  disaster Z65.5
  terrorism Z65.4
  torture Z65.4
  war Z65.5
Vidal's disease L28.0
Villaret's syndrome G52.7
Villous —see condition
VIN —see Neoplasia, intraepithelial,
    vulva
Vincent's infection (angina) (gingivitis)
    A69.1
  stomatitis NEC A69.1
Vinson-Plummer syndrome D50.1

Violence, physical R45.6
Viosterol deficiency —see Deficiency,
    calciferol
Vipoma —see Neoplasm, malignant, by site
Viremia B34.9
Virilism (adrenal) E25.9
  congenital E25.0
Virilization (female) (suprarenal)
    E25.9
  congenital E25.0
  isosexual E28.2
Virulent bubo A57
Virus, viral —see also condition
  as cause of disease classified elsewhere
      B97.89
  cytomegalovirus B25.9
  human immunodeficiency (HIV) —see
      Human, immunodeficiency virus
      (HIV) disease
  infection —see Infection, virus
  specified NEC B34.8
  swine influenza (viruses that normally
      cause infections in pigs) (see also
      Influenza, due to, identified novel
      influenza A virus) J09.X2
  West Nile (fever) A92.30
      with
          complications NEC A92.39
          cranial nerve disorders A92.32
          encephalitis A92.31
          encephalomyelitis A92.31
          neurologic manifestation NEC
              A92.32
          optic neuritis A92.32
          polyradiculitis A92.32
Viscera, visceral —see condition
Visceroptosis K63.4
Visible peristalsis R19.2
Vision, visual
  binocular, suppression H53.34
  blurred, blurring H53.8
      hysterical F44.6
  defect, defective NEC H54.7
  disorientation (syndrome) H53.8
  disturbance H53.9
      hysterical F44.6
  double H53.2
  examination Z01.00
      with abnormal findings Z01.01
  field, limitation (defect) —see Defect,
      visual field
  hallucinations R44.1
  halos H53.19
  loss —see Loss, vision
      sudden —see Disturbance, vision,
          subjective, loss, sudden
  low (both eyes) —see Low, vision
  perception, simultaneous without
      fusion H53.33
Vitality, lack or want of R53.83
  newborn P96.89
Vitamin deficiency —see Deficiency,
    vitamin
Vitelline duct, persistent Q43.0
Vitiligo L80
  eyelid H02.739
      left H02.736
          lower H02.735
          upper H02.734
      right H02.733
          lower H02.732
          upper H02.731
  pinta A67.2
  vulva N90.89

Vitreal corneal syndrome H59.01-
Vitreoretinopathy, proliferative —see also
    Retinopathy, proliferative
  with retinal detachment —see
      Detachment, retina, traction
Vitreous —see also condition
  touch syndrome —see Complication,
      postprocedural, following cataract
      surgery
Vocal cord —see condition
Vogt-Koyanagi syndrome H20.82-
Vogt's disease or syndrome G80.3
Vogt-Spielmeyer amaurotic idiocy or
    disease E75.4
Voice
  change R49.9
      specified NEC R49.8
  loss —see Aphonia
Volhynian fever A79.0
Volkmann's ischemic contracture or
    paralysis (complicating trauma)
    T79.6
Volvulus (bowel) (colon) (duodenum)
    (intestine) K56.2
  with perforation K56.2
  congenital Q43.8
  fallopian tube —see Torsion, fallopian
      tube
  oviduct —see Torsion, fallopian tube
  stomach (due to absence of gastrocolic
      ligament) K31.89
Vomiting R11.10
  with nausea R11.2
  without nausea R11.11
  asphyxia —see Foreign body, by site,
      causing asphyxia, gastric
      contents
  bilious (cause unknown) R11.14
      following gastro-intestinal surgery
          K91.0
      in newborn P92.01
  blood —see Hematemesis
  causing asphyxia, choking, or
      suffocation —see Foreign body, by
      site
  cyclical G43.A0
      with refractory migraine G43.A1
      intractable G43.A1
      not intractable G43.A0
      psychogenic F50.8
      without refractory migraine
          G43.A0
  fecal mater R11.13
  following gastrointestinal surgery
      K91.0
      psychogenic F50.8
  functional K31.89
  hysterical F50.8
  nervous F50.8
  neurotic F50.8
  newborn NEC P92.09
      bilious P92.01
  periodic R11.10
      psychogenic F50.8
  projectile R11.12
  psychogenic F50.8
  uremic —see Uremia
Vomito negro —see Fever, yellow
Von Bezold's abscess —see Mastoiditis,
    acute
Von Economo-Cruchet disease
    A85.8
Von Eulenburg's disease G71.19
Von Gierke's disease E74.01

Von Hippel (-Lindau) disease or
   syndrome Q85.8
Von Jaksch's anemia or disease
   D64.89
Von Recklinghausen
   disease (neurofibromatosis) Q85.01
     bones E21.0
Von Schroetter's syndrome I82.890
Von Willebrand (-Jurgens)(-Minot)
   disease or syndrome D68.0
Von Zumbusch's disease L40.1
Voyeurism F65.3
Vrolik's disease Q78.0
Vulva —*see* condition
Vulvismus N94.2

Vulvitis (acute) (allergic) (atrophic)
   (hypertrophic) (intertriginous)
   (senile) N76.2
with ectopic or molar pregnancy O08.0
adhesive, congenital Q52.79
blennorrhagic (gonococcal) A54.02
candidal B37.3
chlamydial A56.02
due to Haemophilus ducreyi A57
following ectopic or molar pregnancy
   O08.0
gonococcal A54.02
   with abscess (accessory gland)
     (periurethral) A54.1

Vulvitis *(Continued)*
   herpesviral A60.04
   leukoplakic N90.4
   monilial B37.3
   puerperal (postpartum) O86.19
   subacute or chronic N76.3
   syphilitic (early) A51.0
     late A52.76
   trichomonal A59.01
   tuberculous A18.18
Vulvodynia N94.819
   specified NEC N94.818
Vulvorectal —*see* condition
Vulvovaginitis (acute) —*see* Vaginitis

W

Waiting list, person on Z75.1
  for organ transplant Z76.82
  undergoing social agency investigation Z75.2
Waldenström
  hypergammaglobulinemia D89.0
  syndrome or macroglobulinemia C88.0
Waldenström-Kjellberg syndrome D50.1
Walking
  difficulty R26.2
    psychogenic F44.4
  sleep F51.3
    hysterical F44.89
Wall, abdominal —see condition
Wallenberg's disease or syndrome G46.3
Wallgren's disease I87.8
Wandering
  gallbladder, congenital Q44.1
  in diseases classified elsewhere Z91.83
  kidney, congenital Q63.8
  organ or site, congenital NEC —see Malposition, congenital, by site
  pacemaker (heart) I49.8
  spleen D73.89
War neurosis F48.8
Wart (due to HPV) (filiform) (infectious) (viral) B07.9
  anogenital region (venereal) A63.0
  common B07.8
  external genital organs (venereal) A63.0
  flat B07.8
  Hassal-Henle's (of cornea) H18.49
  Peruvian A44.1
  plantar B07.0
  prosector (tuberculous) A18.4
  seborrheic L82.1
    inflamed L82.0
  senile (seborrheic) L82.1
    inflamed L82.0
  tuberculous A18.4
  venereal A63.0
Warthin's tumor —see Neoplasm, salivary gland, benign
Wassilieff's disease A27.0
Wasting
  disease R64
    due to malnutrition E41
  extreme (due to malnutrition) E41
  muscle NEC —see Atrophy, muscle
Water
  clefts (senile cataract) —see Cataract, senile, incipient
  deprivation of T73.1
  intoxication E87.79
  itch B76.9
  lack of T73.1
  loading E87.70
  on
    brain —see Hydrocephalus
    chest J94.8
  poisoning E87.79
Waterbrash R12
Waterhouse(-Friderichsen) syndrome or disease (meningococcal) A39.1
Water-losing nephritis N25.89
Watermelon stomach K31.819
  with hemorrhage K31.811
  without hemorrhage K31.819
Watsoniasis B66.8

Wax in ear —see Impaction, cerumen
Weak, weakening, weakness (generalized) R53.1
  arches (acquired) —see also Deformity, limb, flat foot
  bladder (sphincter) R32
  facial R29.810
    following
      cerebrovascular disease I69.992
        cerebral infarction I69.392
        intracerebral hemorrhage I69.192
        nontraumatic intracranial hemorrhage NEC I69.292
        specified disease NEC I69.892
        stroke I69.392
        subarachnoid hemorrhage I69.092
  foot (double) —see Weak, arches
  heart, cardiac —see Failure, heart
  mind F70
  muscle M62.81
  myocardium —see Failure, heart
  newborn P96.89
  pelvic fundus N81.89
  pubocervical tissue N81.82
  rectovaginal tissue N81.83
  senile R54
  urinary stream R39.12
  valvular —see Endocarditis
Wear, worn (with normal or routine use)
  articular bearing surface of
    internal joint prosthesis —see Complications, joint prosthesis, mechanical, wear of articular bearing surfaces, by site
  device, implant or graft —see Complications, by site, mechanical complication
  tooth, teeth (approximal) (hard tissues) (interproximal) (occlusal) K03.0
Weather, weathered
  effects of
    cold T69.9
      specified effect NEC T69.8
    hot —see Heat
  skin L57.8
Weaver's syndrome Q87.3
Web, webbed (congenital)
  duodenal Q43.8
  esophagus Q39.4
  fingers Q70.1
  larynx (glottic) (subglottic) Q31.0
  neck (pterygium colli) Q18.3
  Paterson-Kelly D50.1
  popliteal syndrome Q87.89
  toes Q70.3
Weber-Christian disease M35.6
Weber-Cockayne syndrome (epidermolysis bullosa) Q81.8
Weber-Gubler syndrome G46.3
Weber-Leyden syndrome G46.3
Weber-Osler syndrome I78.0
Weber's paralysis or syndrome G46.3
Wedge-shaped or wedging vertebra —see Collapse, vertebra NEC
Wegener's granulomatosis or syndrome M31.30
  with
    kidney involvement M31.31
    lung involvement M31.30
      with kidney involvement M31.31
Wegner's disease A50.02
Weight
  1000-2499 grams at birth (low) —see Low, birthweight

Weight (Continued)
  999 grams or less at birth (extremely low) —see Low, birthweight, extreme
  gain (abnormal) (excessive) R63.5
    in pregnancy —see Pregnancy, complicated by, excessive weight gain
    low —see Pregnancy, complicated by, insufficient, weight gain
  loss (abnormal) (cause unknown) R63.4
Weightlessness (effect of) T75.82
Weil (l)-Marchesani syndrome Q87.1
Weil's disease A27.0
Weingarten's syndrome J82
Weir Mitchell's disease I73.81
Weiss-Baker syndrome G90.09
Wells' disease L98.3
Wen —see Cyst, sebaceous
Wenckebach's block or phenomenon I44.1
Werdnig-Hoffmann syndrome (muscular atrophy) G12.0
Werlhof's disease D69.3
Werner-His disease A79.0
Wermer's disease or syndrome E31.21
Werner's disease or syndrome E34.8
Wernicke-Korsakoff's syndrome or psychosis (alcoholic) F10.96
  with dependence F10.26
  drug-induced
    due to drug abuse —see Abuse, drug, by type, with amnestic disorder
    due to drug dependence —see Dependence, drug, by type, with amnestic disorder
  nonalcoholic F04
Wernicke-Posadas disease B38.9
Wernicke's
  developmental aphasia F80.2
  disease or syndrome E51.2
  encephalopathy E51.2
  polioencephalitis, superior E51.2
West African fever B50.8
Westphal-Strümpell syndrome E83.01
West's syndrome —see Epilepsy, spasms
Wet
  feet, tropical (maceration) (syndrome) —see Immersion, foot
  lung (syndrome), newborn P22.1
Wharton's duct —see condition
Wheal —see Urticaria
Wheezing R06.2
Whiplash injury S13.4
Whipple's disease (see also subcategory M14.8-) K90.81
Whipworm (disease) (infection) (infestation) B79
Whistling face Q87.0
White —see also condition
  kidney, small N03.9
  leg, puerperal, postpartum, childbirth O87.1
  mouth B37.0
  patches of mouth K13.29
  spot lesions, teeth
    chewing surface K02.51
    pit and fissure surface K02.51
    smooth surface K02.61
Whitehead L70.0
Whitlow —see also Cellulitis, digit
  with lymphangitis —see Lymphangitis, acute, digit
  herpesviral B00.89
Whitmore's disease or fever —see Melioidosis

Whooping cough A37.90
  with pneumonia A37.91
    due to Bordetella
      bronchiseptica A37.81
      parapertussis A37.11
      pertussis A37.01
    specified organism NEC A37.81
  due to
    Bordetella
      bronchiseptica A37.80
        with pneumonia A37.81
      parapertussis A37.10
        with pneumonia A37.11
      pertussis A37.00
        with pneumonia A37.01
    specified NEC A37.80
      with pneumonia A37.81
Wichman's asthma J38.5
Wide cranial sutures, newborn P96.3
Widening aorta —*see* Ectasia, aorta
  with aneurysm —*see* Aneurysm, aorta
Wilkie's disease or syndrome K55.1
Wilkinson-Sneddon disease or
  syndrome L13.1
Willebrand (-Jürgens) thrombopathy D68.0
Willige-Hunt disease or syndrome G23.1
Wilms' tumor C64-
Wilson's
  disease or syndrome E83.01
  hepatolenticular degeneration E83.01
  lichen ruber L43.9
Wilson-Mikity syndrome P27.0
Window —*see also* Imperfect, closure
  aorticopulmonary Q21.4
Winter —*see* condition
Wiskott-Aldrich syndrome D82.0
Withdrawal state —*see also* Dependence,
  drug by type, with withdrawal
  newborn
    correct therapeutic substance
      properly administered P96.2
    infant of dependent mother P96.1
    therapeutic substance, neonatal P96.2
Witts' anemia D50.8
Witzelsucht F07.0
Woakes' ethmoiditis or syndrome J33.1
Wolff-Hirschorn syndrome Q93.3
Wolff-Parkinson-White syndrome I45.6
Wolhynian fever A79.0
Wolman's disease E75.5
Wood lung or pneumonitis J67.8
Woolly, wooly hair (congenital) (nevus)
  Q84.1
Woolsorter's disease A22.1
Word
  blindness (congenital) (developmental)
    F81.0
  deafness (congenital) (developmental)
    H93.25
Worm (s) (infection) (infestation) —*see also*
  Infestation, helminth
  guinea B72
  in intestine NEC B82.0
Worm-eaten soles A66.3
Worn out —*see* Exhaustion
  cardiac
    defibrillator (with synchronous
      cardiac pacemaker) Z45.02
    pacemaker
      battery Z45.010
      lead Z45.018
  device, implant or graft —*see*
    Complications, by site, mechanical
Worried well Z71.1

Worries R45.82
Wound, open
  abdomen, abdominal
    wall S31.109
      with penetration into peritoneal
        cavity S31.609
      bite —*see* Bite, abdomen, wall
      epigastric region S31.102
        with penetration into peritoneal
          cavity S31.602
        bite —*see* Bite, abdomen, wall,
          epigastric region
        laceration —*see* Laceration,
          abdomen, wall, epigastric
          region
        puncture —*see* Puncture,
          abdomen, wall, epigastric
          region
      laceration —*see* Laceration,
        abdomen, wall
      left
        lower quadrant S31.104
          with penetration into peritoneal
            cavity S31.604
          bite —*see* Bite, abdomen, wall,
            left, lower quadrant
          laceration —*see* Laceration,
            abdomen, wall, left,
            lower quadrant
          puncture —*see* Puncture,
            abdomen, wall, left,
            lower quadrant
        upper quadrant S31.101
          with penetration into
            peritoneal cavity
            S31.601
          bite —*see* Bite, abdomen, wall,
            left, upper quadrant
          laceration —*see* Laceration,
            abdomen, wall, left,
            upper quadrant
          puncture —*see* Puncture,
            abdomen, wall, left,
            upper quadrant
      periumbilic region S31.105
        with penetration into peritoneal
          cavity S31.605
        bite —*see* Bite, abdomen, wall,
          periumbilic region
        laceration —*see* Laceration,
          abdomen, wall, periumbilic
          region
        puncture —*see* Puncture,
          abdomen, wall, periumbilic
          region
      puncture —*see* Puncture, abdomen,
        wall
      right
        lower quadrant S31.103
          with penetration into
            peritoneal cavity S31.603
          bite —*see* Bite, abdomen, wall,
            right, lower quadrant
          laceration —*see* Laceration,
            abdomen, wall, right,
            lower quadrant
          puncture —*see* Puncture,
            abdomen, wall, right,
            lower quadrant
        upper quadrant S31.100
          with penetration into
            peritoneal cavity S31.600
          bite —*see* Bite, abdomen, wall,
            right, upper quadrant
          laceration —*see* Laceration,
            abdomen, wall, right,
            upper quadrant

Wound, open *(Continued)*
  abdomen, abdominal *(Continued)*
    wall *(Continued)*
      right *(Continued)*
        upper quadrant *(Continued)*
          puncture —*see* Puncture,
            abdomen, wall, right,
            upper quadrant
  alveolar (process) —*see* Wound, open,
    oral cavity
  ankle S91.00-
    bite —*see* Bite, ankle
    laceration —*see* Laceration, ankle
    puncture —*see* Puncture, ankle
  antecubital space —*see* Wound, open,
    elbow
  anterior chamber, eye —*see* Wound,
    open, ocular
  anus S31.839
    bite S31.835
    laceration —*see* Laceration, anus
    puncture —*see* Puncture, anus
  arm (upper) S41.10-
    with amputation —*see* Amputation,
      traumatic, arm
    bite —*see* Bite, arm
    forearm —*see* Wound, open, forearm
    laceration —*see* Laceration, arm
    puncture —*see* Puncture, arm
  auditory canal (external) (meatus) —*see*
    Wound, open, ear
  auricle, ear —*see* Wound, open, ear
  axilla —*see* Wound, open, arm
  back —*see also* Wound, open, thorax,
    back
    lower S31.000
      with penetration into
        retroperitoneal space S31.001
      bite —*see* Bite, back, lower
      laceration —*see* Laceration, back,
        lower
      puncture —*see* Puncture, back,
        lower
  bite —*see* Bite
  blood vessel —*see* Injury, blood vessel
  breast S21.00-
    with amputation —*see* Amputation,
      traumatic, breast
    bite —*see* Bite, breast
    laceration —*see* Laceration, breast
    puncture —*see* Puncture, breast
  buttock S31.809
    bite —*see* Bite, buttock
    laceration —*see* Laceration, buttock
    left S31.829
    puncture —*see* Puncture, buttock
    right S31.819
  calf —*see* Wound, open, leg
  canaliculus lacrimalis —*see* Wound,
    open, eyelid
  canthus, eye —*see* Wound, open, eyelid
  cervical esophagus S11.20
    bite S11.25
    laceration —*see* Laceration,
      esophagus, traumatic, cervical
    puncture —*see* Puncture, cervical
      esophagus
  cheek (external) S01.40-
    bite —*see* Bite, cheek
    internal —*see* Wound, open, oral
      cavity
    laceration —*see* Laceration, cheek
    puncture —*see* Puncture, cheek
  chest wall —*see* Wound, open, thorax

Wound, open *(Continued)*
  chin —*see* Wound, open, head, specified
      site NEC
  choroid —*see* Wound, open, ocular
  ciliary body (eye) —*see* Wound, open,
      ocular
  clitoris S31.40
      with amputation —*see* Amputation,
          traumatic, clitoris
      bite S31.45
      laceration —*see* Laceration, vulva
      puncture —*see* Puncture, vulva
  conjunctiva —*see* Wound, open,
      ocular
  cornea —*see* Wound, open, ocular
  costal region —*see* Wound, open,
      thorax
  Descemet's membrane —*see* Wound,
      open, ocular
  digit (s)
      foot —*see* Wound, open, toe
      hand —*see* Wound, open, finger
  ear (canal) (external) S01.30-
      with amputation —*see* Amputation,
          traumatic, ear
      bite —*see* Bite, ear
      drum S09.2-
      laceration —*see* Laceration, ear
      puncture —*see* Puncture, ear
  elbow S51.00-
      bite —*see* Bite, elbow
      laceration —*see* Laceration, elbow
      puncture —*see* Puncture, elbow
  epididymis —*see* Wound, open, testis
  epigastric region S31.102
      with penetration into peritoneal
          cavity S31.602
      bite —*see* Bite, abdomen, wall,
          epigastric region
      laceration —*see* Laceration, abdomen,
          wall, epigastric region
      puncture —*see* Puncture, abdomen,
          wall, epigastric region
  epiglottis —*see* Wound, open, neck,
      specified site NEC
  esophagus (thoracic) S27.819
      cervical —*see* Wound, open, cervical
          esophagus
      laceration S27.813
      specified type NEC S27.818
  eye —*see* Wound, open, ocular
  eyeball —*see* Wound, open, ocular
  eyebrow —*see* Wound, open, eyelid
  eyelid S01.10-
      bite —*see* Bite, eyelid
      laceration —*see* Laceration, eyelid
      puncture —*see* Puncture, eyelid
  face NEC —*see* Wound, open, head,
      specified site NEC
  finger (s) S61.209
      with
          amputation —*see* Amputation,
              traumatic, finger
          damage to nail S61.309
      bite —*see* Bite, finger
      index S61.208
          with
              damage to nail S61.308
          left S61.201
              with
                  damage to nail S61.301
          right S61.200
              with
                  damage to nail S61.300

Wound, open *(Continued)*
  finger (s) *(Continued)*
      laceration —*see* Laceration, finger
      little S61.208
          with
              damage to nail S61.308
          left S61.207
              with damage to nail S61.307
          right S61.206
              with damage to nail S61.306
      middle S61.208
          with
              damage to nail S61.308
          left S61.203
              with damage to nail S61.303
          right S61.202
              with damage to nail S61.302
      puncture —*see* Puncture, finger
      ring S61.208
          with
              damage to nail S61.308
          left S61.205
              with damage to nail S61.305
          right S61.204
              with damage to nail S61.304
  flank —*see* Wound, open, abdomen,
      wall
  foot (except toe (s) alone) S91.30-
      with amputation —*see* Amputation,
          traumatic, foot
      bite —*see* Bite, foot
      laceration —*see* Laceration, foot
      puncture —*see* Puncture, foot
      toe —*see* Wound, open, toe
  forearm S51.80-
      with
          amputation —*see* Amputation,
              traumatic, forearm
      bite —*see* Bite, forearm
      elbow only —*see* Wound, open,
          elbow
      laceration —*see* Laceration, forearm
      puncture —*see* Puncture, forearm
  forehead —*see* Wound, open, head,
      specified site NEC
  genital organs, external
      with amputation —*see* Amputation,
          traumatic, genital organs
      bite —*see* Bite, genital organ
      female S31.502
          vagina S31.40
          vulva S31.40
      laceration —*see* Laceration, genital
          organ
      male S31.501
          penis S31.20
          scrotum S31.30
          testes S31.30
      puncture —*see* Puncture, genital
          organ
  globe (eye) —*see* Wound, open,
      ocular
  groin —*see* Wound, open, abdomen,
      wall
  gum —*see* Wound, open, oral cavity
  hand S61.40-
      with
          amputation —*see* Amputation,
              traumatic, hand
      bite —*see* Bite, hand
      finger (s) —*see* Wound, open, finger
      laceration —*see* Laceration, hand
      puncture —*see* Puncture, hand
      thumb —*see* Wound, open, thumb

Wound, open *(Continued)*
  head S01.90
      bite —*see* Bite, head
      cheek —*see* Wound, open, cheek
      ear —*see* Wound, open, ear
      eyelid —*see* Wound, open, eyelid
      laceration —*see* Laceration, head
      lip —*see* Wound, open, lip
      nose S01.20
      oral cavity —*see* Wound, open, oral
          cavity
      puncture —*see* Puncture, head
      scalp —*see* Wound, open, scalp
      specified site NEC S01.80
      temporomandibular area —*see*
          Wound, open, cheek
  heel —*see* Wound, open, foot
  hip S71.00-
      with amputation —*see* Amputation,
          traumatic, hip
      bite —*see* Bite, hip
      laceration —*see* Laceration, hip
      puncture —*see* Puncture, hip
  hymen S31.40
      bite —*see* Bite, vulva
      laceration —*see* Laceration, vagina
      puncture —*see* Puncture, vagina
  hypochondrium S31.109
      bite —*see* Bite, hypochondrium
      laceration —*see* Laceration,
          hypochondrium
      puncture —*see* Puncture,
          hypochondrium
  hypogastric region S31.109
      bite —*see* Bite, hypogastric region
      laceration —*see* Laceration,
          hypogastric region
      puncture —*see* Puncture, hypogastric
          region
  iliac (region) —*see* Wound, open,
      inguinal region
  inguinal region S31.109
      bite —*see* Bite, abdomen, wall, lower
          quadrant
      laceration —*see* Laceration, inguinal
          region
      puncture —*see* Puncture, inguinal
          region
  instep —*see* Wound, open, foot
  interscapular region —*see* Wound,
      open, thorax, back
  intraocular —*see* Wound, open, ocular
  iris —*see* Wound, open, ocular
  jaw —*see* Wound, open, head, specified
      site NEC
  knee S81.00-
      bite —*see* Bite, knee
      laceration —*see* Laceration, knee
      puncture —*see* Puncture, knee
  labium (majus) (minus) —*see* Wound,
      open, vulva
  laceration —*see* Laceration, by site
  lacrimal duct —*see* Wound, open,
      eyelid
  larynx S11.019
      bite —*see* Bite, larynx
      laceration —*see* Laceration, larynx
      puncture —*see* Puncture, larynx
  left
      lower quadrant S31.104
          with penetration into peritoneal
              cavity S31.604
          bite —*see* Bite, abdomen, wall, left,
              lower quadrant

Wound, open (*Continued*)
  left (*Continued*)
    lower quadrant (*Continued*)
      laceration —*see* Laceration, abdomen, wall, left, lower quadrant
      puncture —*see* Puncture, abdomen, wall, left, lower quadrant
    upper quadrant S31.101
      with penetration into peritoneal cavity S31.601
      bite —*see* Bite, abdomen, wall, left, upper quadrant
      laceration —*see* Laceration, abdomen, wall, left, upper quadrant
      puncture —*see* Puncture, abdomen, wall, left, upper quadrant
  leg (lower) S81.80-
    with amputation —*see* Amputation, traumatic, leg
    ankle —*see* Wound, open, ankle
    bite —*see* Bite, leg
    foot —*see* Wound, open, foot
    knee —*see* Wound, open, knee
    laceration —*see* Laceration, leg
    puncture —*see* Puncture, leg
    toe —*see* Wound, open, toe
    upper —*see* Wound, open, thigh
  lip S01.501
    bite —*see* Bite, lip
    laceration —*see* Laceration, lip
    puncture —*see* Puncture, lip
  loin S31.109
    bite —*see* Bite, abdomen, wall
    laceration —*see* Laceration, loin
    puncture —*see* Puncture, loin
  lower back —*see* Wound, open, back, lower
  lumbar region —*see* Wound, open, back, lower
  malar region —*see* Wound, open, head, specified site NEC
  mammary —*see* Wound, open, breast
  mastoid region —*see* Wound, open, head, specified site NEC
  mouth —*see* Wound, open, oral cavity
  nail
    finger —*see* Wound, open, finger, with damage to nail
    toe —*see* Wound, open, toe, with damage to nail
  nape (neck) —*see* Wound, open, neck
  nasal (septum) (sinus) —*see* Wound, open, nose
  nasopharynx —*see* Wound, open, head, specified site NEC
  neck S11.90
    bite —*see* Bite, neck
    involving
      cervical esophagus S11.20
      larynx —*see* Wound, open, larynx
      pharynx S11.20
      thyroid S11.10
      trachea (cervical) S11.029
        bite —*see* Bite, trachea
        laceration S11.021
          with foreign body S11.022
        puncture S11.023
          with foreign body S11.024
    laceration —*see* Laceration, neck
    puncture —*see* Puncture, neck
    specified site NEC S11.80
      specified type NEC S11.89

Wound, open (*Continued*)
  nose (septum) (sinus) S01.20
    with amputation —*see* Amputation, traumatic, nose
    bite —*see* Bite, nose
    laceration —*see* Laceration, nose
    puncture —*see* Puncture, nose
  ocular S05.90
    avulsion (traumatic enucleation) S05.7-
    eyeball S05.6-
      with foreign body S05.5-
    eyelid —*see* Wound, open, eyelid
    laceration and rupture S05.3-
      with prolapse or loss of intraocular tissue S05.2-
    orbit (penetrating) (with or without foreign body) S05.4-
    periocular area —*see* Wound, open, eyelid
    specified NEC S05.8X-
  oral cavity S01.502
    bite S01.552
    laceration —*see* Laceration, oral cavity
    puncture —*see* Puncture, oral cavity
  orbit —*see* Wound, open, ocular, orbit
  palate —*see* Wound, open, oral cavity
  palm —*see* Wound, open, hand
  pelvis, pelvic —*see also* Wound, open, back, lower
    girdle —*see* Wound, open, hip
  penetrating —*see* Puncture, by site
  penis S31.20
    with amputation —*see* Amputation, traumatic, penis
    bite S31.25
    laceration —*see* Laceration, penis
    puncture —*see* Puncture, penis
  perineum
    bite —*see* Bite, perineum
    female S31.502
    laceration —*see* Laceration, perineum
    male S31.501
    puncture —*see* Puncture, perineum
  periocular area (with or without lacrimal passages) —*see* Wound, open, eyelid
  periumbilic region S31.105
    with penetration into peritoneal cavity S31.605
    bite —*see* Bite, abdomen, wall, periumbilic region
    laceration —*see* Laceration, abdomen, wall, periumbilic region
    puncture —*see* Puncture, abdomen, wall, periumbilic region
  phalanges
    finger —*see* Wound, open, finger
    toe —*see* Wound, open, toe
  pharynx S11.20
  pinna —*see* Wound, open, ear
  popliteal space —*see* Wound, open, knee
  prepuce —*see* Wound, open, penis
  pubic region —*see* Wound, open, back, lower
  pudendum —*see* Wound, open, genital organs, external
  puncture wound —*see* Puncture
  rectovaginal septum —*see* Wound, open, vagina

Wound, open (*Continued*)
  right
    lower quadrant S31.103
      with penetration into peritoneal cavity S31.603
      bite —*see* Bite, abdomen, wall, right, lower quadrant
      laceration —*see* Laceration, abdomen, wall, right, lower quadrant
      puncture —*see* Puncture, abdomen, wall, right, lower quadrant
    upper quadrant S31.100
      with penetration into peritoneal cavity S31.600
      bite —*see* Bite, abdomen, wall, right, upper quadrant
      laceration —*see* Laceration, abdomen, wall, right, upper quadrant
      puncture —*see* Puncture, abdomen, wall, right, upper quadrant
  sacral region —*see* Wound, open, back, lower
  sacroiliac region —*see* Wound, open, back, lower
  salivary gland —*see* Wound, open, oral cavity
  scalp S01.00
    bite S01.05
    laceration —*see* Laceration, scalp
    puncture —*see* Puncture, scalp
  scalpel, newborn (birth injury) P15.8
  scapular region —*see* Wound, open, shoulder
  sclera —*see* Wound, open, ocular
  scrotum S31.30
    with amputation —*see* Amputation, traumatic, scrotum
    bite S31.35
    laceration —*see* Laceration, scrotum
    puncture —*see* Puncture, scrotum
  shin —*see* Wound, open, leg
  shoulder S41.00-
    with amputation —*see* Amputation, traumatic, arm
    bite —*see* Bite, shoulder
    laceration —*see* Laceration, shoulder
    puncture —*see* Puncture, shoulder
  skin NOS T14.8
  spermatic cord —*see* Wound, open, testis
  sternal region —*see* Wound, open, thorax, front wall
  submaxillary region —*see* Wound, open, head, specified site NEC
  submental region —*see* Wound, open, head, specified site NEC
  subungual
    finger (s) —*see* Wound, open, finger
    toe (s) —*see* Wound, open, toe
  supraclavicular region —*see* Wound, open, neck, specified site NEC
  temple, temporal region —*see* Wound, open, head, specified site NEC
  temporomandibular area —*see* Wound, open, cheek
  testis S31.30
    with amputation —*see* Amputation, traumatic, testes
    bite S31.35
    laceration —*see* Laceration, testis
    puncture —*see* Puncture, testis

Wound, open *(Continued)*
 thigh S71.10-
  with amputation —*see* Amputation,
   traumatic, hip
  bite —*see* Bite, thigh
  laceration —*see* Laceration, thigh
  puncture —*see* Puncture, thigh
 thorax, thoracic (wall) S21.90
  back S21.20-
   with penetration S21.40
  bite —*see* Bite, thorax
  breast —*see* Wound, open, breast
  front S21.10-
   with penetration S21.30
  laceration —*see* Laceration,
   thorax
  puncture —*see* Puncture, thorax
 throat —*see* Wound, open, neck
 thumb S61.009
  with
   amputation —*see* Amputation,
    traumatic, thumb
   damage to nail S61.109
  bite —*see* Bite, thumb
  laceration —*see* Laceration,
   thumb
  left S61.002
   with
    damage to nail S61.102
  puncture —*see* Puncture, thumb
  right S61.001
   with
    damage to nail S61.101
 thyroid (gland) —*see* Wound, open,
  neck, thyroid
 toe (s) S91.109
  with
   amputation —*see* Amputation,
    traumatic, toe
   damage to nail S91.209

Wound, open *(Continued)*
 toe (s) *(Continued)*
  bite —*see* Bite, toe
  great S91.103
   with
    damage to nail S91.203
   left S91.102
    with
     damage to nail S91.202
   right S91.101
    with
     damage to nail S91.201
  laceration —*see* Laceration, toe
  lesser S91.106
   with
    damage to nail S91.206
   left S91.105
    with
     damage to nail S91.205
   right S91.104
    with
     damage to nail S91.204
  puncture —*see* Puncture, toe
 tongue —*see* Wound, open, oral
  cavity
 trachea (cervical region) —*see* Wound,
  open, neck, trachea
 tunica vaginalis —*see* Wound, open,
  testis
 tympanum, tympanic membrane
  S09.2-
  laceration —*see* Laceration, ear,
   drum
  puncture —*see* Puncture,
   tympanum
 umbilical region —*see* Wound, open,
  abdomen, wall, periumbilic
  region

Wound, open *(Continued)*
 uvula —*see* Wound, open, oral
  cavity
 vagina S31.40
  bite S31.45
  laceration —*see* Laceration,
   vagina
  puncture —*see* Puncture, vagina
 vitreous (humor) —*see* Wound, open,
  ocular
 vocal cord S11.039
  bite —*see* Bite, vocal cord
  laceration S11.031
   with foreign body S11.032
  puncture S11.033
   with foreign body S11.034
 vulva S31.40
  with amputation —*see* Amputation,
   traumatic, vulva
  bite S31.45
  laceration —*see* Laceration, vulva
  puncture —*see* Puncture, vulva
 wrist S61.50-
  bite —*see* Bite, wrist
  laceration —*see* Laceration, wrist
  puncture —*see* Puncture, wrist
Wound, superficial —*see* Injury (*see also*
 specified injury type)
Wright's syndrome G54.0
Wrist —*see* condition
Wrong drug (by accident) (given in
 error) —*see* Table of drugs and
 chemicals, by drug, poisoning
Wry neck —*see* Torticollis
Wuchereria (bancrofti) infestation
 B74.0
Wuchereriasis B74.0
Wuchernde Struma Langhans C73

X

Xanthelasma (eyelid) (palpebrarum)
    H02.60
    left H02.66
       lower H02.65
       upper H02.64
    right H02.63
       lower H02.62
       upper H02.61
Xanthelasmatosis (essential) E78.2
Xanthinuria, hereditary E79.8
Xanthoastrocytoma
    specified site —*see* Neoplasm,
       malignant, by site
    unspecified site C71.9
Xanthofibroma —*see* Neoplasm,
    connective tissue, benign
Xanthogranuloma D76.3
Xanthoma (s), xanthomatosis (primary)
    (familial) (hereditary) E75.5
    with
       hyperlipoproteinemia
          Type I E78.3
          Type III E78.2
          Type IV E78.1
          Type V E78.3
    cerebrotendinous E75.5
    cutaneotendinous E75.5
    disseminatum (skin) E78.2

Xanthoma (s), xanthomatosis (*Continued*)
    eruptive E78.2
    hypercholesterinemic E78.0
    hypercholesterolemic E78.0
    hyperlipidemic E78.5
    joint E75.5
    multiple (skin) E78.2
    tendon (sheath) E75.5
    tuberosum E78.2
    tuberous E78.2
    tubo-eruptive E78.2
    verrucous, oral mucosa K13.4
Xanthosis R23.8
Xenophobia F40.10
Xeroderma —*see also* Ichthyosis
    acquired L85.0
       eyelid H01.149
          left H01.146
             lower H01.145
             upper H01.144
          right H01.143
             lower H01.142
             upper H01.141
    pigmentosum Q82.1
    vitamin A deficiency E50.8
Xerophthalmia (vitamin A deficiency)
    E50.7
    unrelated to vitamin A deficiency —*see*
       Keratoconjunctivitis

Xerosis
    conjunctiva H11.14-
       with Bitot's spots —*see also*
          Pigmentation, conjunctiva
          vitamin A deficiency E50.1
       vitamin A deficiency E50.0
    cornea H18.89-
       with ulceration —*see* Ulcer, cornea
          vitamin A deficiency E50.3
       vitamin A deficiency E50.2
    cutis L85.3
    skin L85.3
Xerostomia K11.7
Xiphopagus Q89.4
XO syndrome Q96.9
X-ray (of)
    abnormal findings —*see* Abnormal,
       diagnostic imaging
    breast (mammogram) (routine)
       Z12.31
    chest
       routine (as part of a general medical
          examination) Z00.00
       with abnormal findings Z00.01
    routine (as part of a general medical
       examination) Z00.00
       with abnormal findings Z00.01
XXXXY syndrome Q98.1
XXY syndrome Q98.0

X

Y

Yaba pox virus disease B08.72
Yatapoxvirus B08.70
  specified NEC B08.79
Yawning R06.89
  psychogenic F45.8
Yaws A66.9
  bone lesions A66.6
  butter A66.1
  chancre A66.0
  cutaneous, less than five years after
      infection A66.2
  early (cutaneous) (macular)
      (maculopapular) (micropapular)
      (papular) A66.2
    frambeside A66.2
    skin lesions NEC A66.2
  eyelid A66.2
  ganglion A66.6
  gangosis, gangosa A66.5
  gumma, gummata A66.4
    bone A66.6
  gummatous
    frambeside A66.4
    osteitis A66.6
    periostitis A66.6
  hydrarthrosis (see also subcategory
      M14.8-) A66.6

Yaws (Continued)
  hyperkeratosis (early) (late) A66.3
  initial lesions A66.0
  joint lesions (see also subcategory
      M14.8-) A66.6
  juxta-articular nodules A66.7
  late nodular (ulcerated) A66.4
  latent (without clinical manifestations)
      (with positive serology) A66.8
  mother A66.0
  mucosal A66.7
  multiple papillomata A66.1
  nodular, late (ulcerated) A66.4
  osteitis A66.6
  papilloma, plantar or palmar A66.1
  periostitis (hypertrophic) A66.6
  specified NEC A66.7
  ulcers A66.4
  wet crab A66.1
Yeast infection (see also Candidiasis) B37.9
Yellow
  atrophy (liver) —see Failure, hepatic
  fever —see Fever, yellow
  jack —see Fever, yellow
  jaundice —see Jaundice
  nail syndrome L60.5
Yersiniosis —see also Infection, Yersinia
  extraintestinal A28.2
  intestinal A04.6

Z

Zahorsky's syndrome (herpangina)
    B08.5
Zellweger's syndrome Q87.89
Zenker's diverticulum (esophagus)
    K22.5
Ziehen-Oppenheim disease G24.1
Zieve's syndrome K70.0
Zinc
  deficiency, dietary E60
  metabolism disorder E83.2
Zollinger-Ellison syndrome E16.4
Zona —see Herpes, zoster
Zoophobia F40.218
Zoster (herpes) —see Herpes, zoster
Zygomycosis B46.9
  specified NEC B46.8
Zymotic —see condition

ICD-10-CM
Table of Neoplasms

	Malignant Primary	Malignant Secondary	Ca in situ	Benign	Uncertain Behavior	Unspecified Behavior

The list below gives the code numbers for neoplasms by anatomical site. For each site there are six possible code numbers according to whether the neoplasm in question is malignant, benign, in situ, of uncertain behavior, or of unspecified nature. The description of the neoplasm will often indicate which of the six columns is appropriate; e.g., malignant melanoma of skin, benign fibroadenoma of breast, carcinoma in situ of cervix uteri.

Where such descriptors are not present, the remainder of the Index should be consulted where guidance is given to the appropriate column for each morphological (histological) variety listed; e.g., Mesonephroma — *see Neoplasm, malignant;* Embryoma — *see also Neoplasm, uncertain behavior;* Disease, Bowen's — *see Neoplasm, skin, in situ.* However, the guidance in the Index can be overridden if one of the descriptors mentioned above is present; e.g., malignant adenoma of colon is coded to C18.9 and not to D12.6 as the adjective "malignant" overrides the Index entry "Adenoma — *see also Neoplasm, benign.*"

Codes listed with a dash -, following the code have a required additional character for laterality. The tablular must be reviewed for the complete code.

	Malignant Primary	Malignant Secondary	Ca in situ	Benign	Uncertain Behavior	Unspecified Behavior
Neoplasm, neoplastic	C80.1	C79.9	D09.9	D36.9	D48.9	D49.9
abdomen, abdominal	C76.2	C79.8-	D09.8	D36.7	D48.7	D49.89
cavity	C76.2	C79.8-	D09.8	D36.7	D48.7	D49.89
organ	C76.2	C79.8-	D09.8	D36.7	D48.7	D49.89
viscera	C76.2	C79.8-	D09.8	D36.7	D48.7	D49.89
wall — *see also Neoplasm, abdomen, wall, skin*	C44.509	C79.2-	D04.5	D23.5	D48.5	D49.2
connective tissue	C49.4	C79.8-	—	D21.4	D48.1	D49.2
skin	C44.509					
basal cell carcinoma	C44.519	—	—	—	—	—
specified type NEC	C44.599	—	—	—	—	—
squamous cell carcinoma	C44.529	—	—	—	—	—
abdominopelvic	C76.8	C79.8-	—	D36.7	D48.7	D49.89
accessory sinus — *see Neoplasm, sinus*						
acoustic nerve	C72.4-	C79.49	—	D33.3	D43.3	D49.7
adenoid (pharynx) (tissue)	C11.1	C79.89	D00.08	D10.6	D37.05	D49.0
adipose tissue — *see also Neoplasm, connective tissue*	C49.4	C79.89	—	D21.9	D48.1	D49.2
adnexa (uterine)	C57.4	C79.89	D07.39	D28.7	D39.8	D49.5
adrenal	C74.9-	C79.7-	D09.3	D35.0-	D44.1-	D49.7
capsule	C74.9-	C79.7-	D09.3	D35.0-	D44.1-	D49.7
cortex	C74.0-	C79.7-	D09.3	D35.0-	D44.1-	D49.7
gland	C74.9-	C79.7-	D09.3	D35.0-	D44.1-	D49.7
medulla	C74.1-	C79.7-	D09.3	D35.0-	D44.1-	D49.7
ala nasi (external) — *see also Neoplasm, skin, nose*	C44.301	C79.2	D04.39	D23.39	D48.5	D49.2
alimentary canal or tract NEC	C26.9	C78.80	D01.9	D13.9	D37.9	D49.0
alveolar	C03.9	C79.89	D00.03	D10.39	D37.09	D49.0
mucosa	C03.9	C79.89	D00.03	D10.39	D37.09	D49.0
lower	C03.1	C79.89	D00.03	D10.39	D37.09	D49.0
upper	C03.0	C79.89	D00.03	D10.39	D37.09	D49.0
ridge or process	C41.1	C79.51	—	D16.5-	D48.0	D49.2
carcinoma	C03.9	C79.8-	—	—	—	—
lower	C03.1	C79.8-	—	—	—	—
upper	C03.0	C79.8-	—	—	—	—

TABLE OF NEOPLASMS

	Malignant Primary	Malignant Secondary	Ca in situ	Benign	Uncertain Behavior	Unspecified Behavior
alveolar (Continued)						
ridge or process (Continued)						
lower	C41.1	C79.51	—	D16.5-	D48.0	D49.2
mucosa	C03.9	C79.89	D00.03	D10.39	D37.09	D49.0
lower	C03.1	C79.89	D00.03	D10.39	D37.09	D49.0
upper	C03.0	C79.89	D00.03	D10.39	D37.09	D49.0
upper	C41.0	C79.51	—	D16.4-	D48.0	D49.2
sulcus	C06.1	C79.89	D00.02	D10.39	D37.09	D49.0
alveolus	C03.9	C79.89	D00.03	D10.39	D37.09	D49.0
lower	C03.1	C79.89	D00.03	D10.39	D37.09	D49.0
upper	C03.0	C79.89	D00.03	D10.39	D37.09	D49.0
ampulla of Vater	C24.1	C78.89	D01.5	D13.5	D37.6	D49.0
ankle NEC	C76.5-	C79.89	D04.7-	D36.7	D48.7	D49.89
anorectum, anorectal (junction)	C21.8	C78.5	D01.3	D12.9	D37.8	D49.0
antecubital fossa or space	C76.4-	C79.89	D04.6-	D36.7	D48.7	D49.89
antrum (Highmore) (maxillary)	C31.0	C78.39	D02.3	D14.0	D38.5	D49.1
pyloric	C16.3	C78.89	D00.2	D13.1	D37.1	D49.0
tympanicum	C30.1	C78.39	D02.3	D14.0	D38.5	D49.1
anus, anal	C21.0	C78.5	D01.3	D12.9	D37.8	D49.0
canal	C21.1	C78.5	D01.3	D12.9	D37.8	D49.0
cloacogenic zone	C21.2	C78.5	D01.3	D12.9	D37.8	D49.0
margin — see also Neoplasm, anus, skin	C44.500	C79.2	D04.5	D23.5	D48.5	D49.2
overlapping lesion with rectosigmoid junction or rectum	C21.8	—	—	—	—	—
skin	C44.500	C79.2	D04.5	D23.5	D48.5	D49.2
basal cell carcinoma	C44.510	—	—	—	—	—
specified type NEC	C44.590	—	—	—	—	—
squamous cell carcinoma	C44.520	—	—	—	—	—
sphincter	C21.1	C78.5	D01.3	D12.9	D37.8	D49.0
aorta (thoracic)	C49.3	C79.89	—	D21.3	D48.1	D49.2
abdominal	C49.4	C79.89	—	D21.4	D48.1	D49.2
aortic body	C75.5	C79.89	—	D35.6	D44.7	D49.7
aponeurosis	C49.9	C79.89	—	D21.9	D48.1	D49.2
palmar	C49.1-	C79.89	—	D21.1-	D48.1	D49.2
plantar	C49.2-	C79.89	—	D21.2-	D48.1	D49.2
appendix	C18.1	C78.5	D01.0	D12.1	D37.3	D49.0
arachnoid	C70.9	C79.49	—	D32.9	D42.9	D49.7
cerebral	C70.0	C79.32	—	D32.0	D42.0	D49.7
spinal	C70.1	C79.49	—	D32.1	D42.1	D49.7
areola	C50.0-	C79.81	D05.-	D24.-	D48.6-	D49.3
arm NEC	C76.4-	C79.89	D04.6-	D36.7	D48.7	D49.89
artery — see Neoplasm, connective tissue						

	Malignant Primary	Malignant Secondary	Ca in situ	Benign	Uncertain Behavior	Unspecified Behavior
aryepiglottic fold	C13.1	C79.89	D00.08	D10.7	D37.05	D49.0
hypopharyngeal aspect	C13.1	C79.89	D00.08	D10.7	D37.05	D49.0
laryngeal aspect	C32.1	C78.39	D02.0	D14.1	D38.0	D49.1
marginal zone	C13.1	C79.89	D00.08	D10.7	D37.05	D49.0
arytenoid (cartilage)	C32.3	C78.39	D02.0	D14.1	D38.0	D49.1
fold — *see Neoplasm, aryepiglottic*						
associated with transplanted organ	C80.2	—	—	—	—	—
atlas	C41.2	C79.51	—	D16.6	D48.0	D49.2
atrium, cardiac	C38.0	C79.89	—	D15.1	D48.7	D49.89
auditory						
canal (external) (skin) A81	C44.20-	C79.2	D04.2-	D23.2-	D48.5	D49.2
internal	C30.1	C78.39	D02.3	D14.0	D38.5	D49.1
nerve	C72.4-	C79.49	—	D33.3	D43.3	D49.7
tube	C30.1	C78.39	D02.3	D14.0	D38.5	D49.1
opening	C11.2	C79.89	D00.08	D10.6	D37.05	D49.0
auricle, ear — *see also Neoplasm, skin, ear*	C44.20-	C79.2	D04.2-	D23.2-	D48.5	D49.2
auricular canal (external) — *see also Neoplasm, skin, ear*	C44.20-	C79.2	D04.2-	D23.2-	D48.5	D49.2
internal	C30.1	C78.39	D02.3	D14.0	D38.5	D49.2
autonomic nerve or nervous system NEC (*see Neoplasm, nerve, peripheral*)						
axilla, axillary	C76.1	C79.89	D09.8	D36.7	D48.7	D49.89
fold — *see also Neoplasm, skin, trunk*	C44.509	C79.2	D04.5	D23.5	D48.5	D49.2
back NEC	C76.8	C79.89	D04.5	D36.7	D48.7	D49.89
Bartholin's gland	C51.0	C79.82	D07.1	D28.0	D39.8	D49.5
basal ganglia	C71.0	C79.31	—	D33.0	D43.0	D49.6
basis pedunculi	C71.7	C79.31	—	D33.1	D43.1	D49.6
bile or biliary (tract)	C24.9	C78.89	D01.5	D13.5	D37.6	D49.0
canaliculi (biliferi) (intrahepatic)	C22.1	C78.7	D01.5	D13.4	D37.6	D49.0
canals, interlobular	C22.1	C78.89	D01.5	D13.4	D37.6	D49.0
duct or passage (common) (cystic) (extrahepatic)	C24.0	C78.89	D01.5	D13.5	D37.6	D49.0
interlobular	C22.1	C78.89	D01.5	D13.4	D37.6	D49.0
intrahepatic	C22.1	C78.7	D01.5	D13.4	D37.6	D49.0
and extrahepatic	C24.8	C78.89	D01.5	D13.5	D37.6	D49.0
bladder (urinary)	C67.9	C79.11	D09.0	D30.3	D41.4	D49.4
dome	C67.1	C79.11	D09.0	D30.3	D41.4	D49.4
neck	C67.5	C79.11	D09.0	D30.3	D41.4	D49.4
orifice	C67.9	C79.11	D09.0	D30.3	D41.4	D49.4
ureteric	C67.6	C79.11	D09.0	D30.3	D41.4	D49.4
urethral	C67.5	C79.11	D09.0	D30.3	D41.4	D49.4
overlapping lesion	C67.8	—	—	—	—	—
sphincter	C67.8	C79.11	D09.0	D30.3	D41.4	D49.4
trigone	C67.0	C79.11	D09.0	D30.3	D41.4	D49.4
urachus	C67.7	C79.11	D09.0	D30.3	D41.4	D49.4

	Malignant Primary	Malignant Secondary	Ca in situ	Benign	Uncertain Behavior	Unspecified Behavior
bladder (urinary) *(Continued)*						
wall	C67.9	C79.11	D09.0	D30.3	D41.4	D49.4
anterior	C67.3	C79.11	D09.0	D30.3	D41.4	D49.4
lateral	C67.2	C79.11	D09.0	D30.3	D41.4	D49.4
posterior	C67.4	C79.11	D09.0	D30.3	D41.4	D49.4
blood vessel—*see Neoplasm, connective tissue*						
bone (periosteum)	C41.9	C79.51	—	D16.9-	D48.0	D49.2
acetabulum	C41.4	C79.51	—	D16.8-	D48.0	D49.2
ankle	C40.3-	C79.51	—	D16.3-	—	—
arm NEC	C40.0-	C79.51	—	D16.0-	—	—
astragalus	C40.3-	C79.51	—	D16.3-	—	—
atlas	C41.2	C79.51	—	D16.6-	D48.0	D49.2
axis	C41.2	C79.51	—	D16.6-	D48.0	D49.2
back NEC	C41.2	C79.51	—	D16.6-	D48.0	D49.2
calcaneus	C40.3-	C79.51	—	D16.3-	—	—
calvarium	C41.0	C79.51	—	D16.4-	D48.0	D49.2
carpus (any)	C40.1-	C79.51	—	D16.1-	—	—
cartilage NEC	C41.9	C79.51	—	D16.9-	D48.0	D49.2
clavicle	C41.3	C79.51	—	D16.7-	D48.0	D49.2
clivus	C41.0	C79.51	—	D16.4-	D48.0	D49.2
coccygeal vertebra	C41.4	C79.51	—	D16.8-	D48.0	D49.2
coccyx	C41.4	C79.51	—	D16.8-	D48.0	D49.2
costal cartilage	C41.3	C79.51	—	D16.7-	D48.0	D49.2
costovertebral joint	C41.3	C79.51	—	D16.7-	D48.0	D49.2
cranial	C41.0	C79.51	—	D16.4-	D48.0	D49.2
cuboid	C40.3-	C79.51	—	D16.3-	—	—
cuneiform	C41.9	C79.51	—	D16.9-	D48.0	D49.2
elbow	C40.0-	C79.51	—	D16.0-	—	—
ethmoid (labyrinth)	C41.0	C79.51	—	D16.4-	D48.0	D49.2
face	C41.0	C79.51	—	D16.4-	D48.0	D49.2
femur (any part)	C40.2-	C79.51	—	D16.2-	—	—
fibula (any part)	C40.2-	C79.51	—	D16.2-	—	—
finger (any)	C40.1-	C79.51	—	D16.1-	—	—
foot	C40.3-	C79.51	—	D16.3-	—	—
forearm	C40.0-	C79.51	—	D16.0-	—	—
frontal	C41.0	C79.51	—	D16.4-	D48.0	D49.2
hand	C40.1-	C79.51	—	D16.1-	—	—
heel	C40.3-	C79.51	—	D16.3-	—	—
hip	C41.4	C79.51	—	D16.8-	D48.0	D49.2
humerus (any part)	C40.0-	C79.51	—	D16.0-	—	—
hyoid	C41.0	C79.51	—	D16.4-	D48.0	D49.2
ilium	C41.4	C79.51	—	D16.8-	D48.0	D49.2
innominate	C41.4	C79.51	—	D16.8-	D48.0	D49.2

	Malignant Primary	Malignant Secondary	Ca in situ	Benign	Uncertain Behavior	Unspecified Behavior
bone *(Continued)*						
intervertebral cartilage or disc	C41.2	C79.51	—	D16.6-	D48.0	D49.2
ischium	C41.4	C79.51	—	D16.8-	D48.0	D49.2
jaw (lower)	C41.1	C79.51	—	D16.5-	D48.0	D49.2
knee	C40.2-	C79.51	—	D16.2-	—	—
leg NEC	C40.2-	C79.51	—	D16.2-	—	—
limb NEC	C40.9-	C79.51	—	D16.9-	—	—
lower (long bones)	C40.2-	C79.51	—	D16.2-	—	—
short bones	C40.3-	C79.51	—	D16.3-	—	—
upper (long bones)	C40.0-	C79.51	—	D16.0-	—	—
short bones	C40.1-	C79.51	—	D16.1-	—	—
malar	C41.0	C79.51	—	D16.4-	D48.0	D49.2
mandible	C41.1	C79.51	—	D16.5-	D48.0	D49.2
marrow NEC (any bone)	C96.9	C79.52	—	—	D47.9	D49.89
mastoid	C41.0	C79.51	—	D16.4-	D48.0	D49.2
maxilla, maxillary (superior)	C41.0	C79.51	—	D16.4-	D48.0	D49.2
inferior	C41.1	C79.51	—	D16.5-	D48.0	D49.2
metacarpus (any)	C40.1-	C79.51	—	D16.1-	—	—
metatarsus (any)	C40.3-	C79.51	—	D16.3-	—	—
overlapping sites	C40.8-	—	—	—	—	—
navicular						
ankle	C40.3-	C79.51	—	—	—	—
hand	C40.1-	C79.51	—	—	—	—
nose, nasal	C41.0	C79.51	—	D16.4-	D48.0	D49.2
occipital	C41.0	C79.51	—	D16.4-	D48.0	D49.2
orbit	C41.0	C79.51	—	D16.4-	D48.0	D49.2
parietal	C41.0	C79.51	—	D16.4-	D48.0	D49.2
patella	C40.2-	C79.51	—	—	—	—
pelvic	C41.4	C79.51	—	D16.8	D48.0	D49.2
phalanges						
foot	C40.3-	C79.51	—	—	—	—
hand	C40.1-	C79.51	—	—	—	—
pubic	C41.4	C79.51	—	D16.8	D48.0	D49.2
radius (any part)	C40.0-	C79.51	—	D16.0-	—	—
rib	C41.3	C79.51	—	D16.7	D48.0	D49.2
sacral vertebra	C41.4	C79.51	—	D16.8	D48.0	D49.2
sacrum	C41.4	C79.51	—	D16.8	D48.0	D49.2
scaphoid					—	—
of ankle	C40.3-	C79.51	—	—	—	—
of hand	C40.1-	C79.51	—	—	—	—
scapula (any part)	C40.0-	C79.51	—	D16.0-	—	—
sella turcica	C41.0	C79.51	—	D16.4-	D48.0	D49.2
shoulder	C40.0-	C79.51	—	D16.0-	—	—

	Malignant Primary	Malignant Secondary	Ca in situ	Benign	Uncertain Behavior	Unspecified Behavior
bone *(Continued)*						
skull	C41.0	C79.51	—	D16.4-	D48.0	D49.2
sphenoid	C41.0	C79.51	—	D16.4-	D48.0	D49.2
spine, spinal (column)	C41.2	C79.51	—	D16.6	D48.0	D49.2
coccyx	C41.4	C79.51	—	D16.8	D48.0	D49.2
sacrum	C41.4	C79.51	—	D16.8	D48.0	D49.2
sternum	C41.3	C79.51	—	D16.7	D48.0	D49.2
tarsus (any)	C40.3-	C79.51	—	—	—	—
temporal	C41.0	C79.51	—	D16.4-	D48.0	D49.2
thumb	C40.1-	C79.51	—	—	—	—
tibia (any part)	C40.2-	C79.51	—	—	—	—
toe (any)	C40.3-	C79.51	—	—	—	—
trapezium	C40.1-	C79.51	—	—	—	—
trapezoid	C40.1-	C79.51	—	—	—	—
turbinate	C41.0	C79.51	—	D16.4-	D48.0	D49.2
ulna (any part)	C40.0-	C79.51	—	D16.0-	—	—
unciform	C40.1-	C79.51	—	—	—	—
vertebra (column)	C41.2	C79.51	—	D16.6	D48.0	D49.2
coccyx	C41.4	C79.51	—	D16.8	D48.0	D49.2
sacrum	C41.4	C79.51	—	D16.8	D48.0	D49.2
vomer	C41.0	C79.51	—	D16.4-	D48.0	D49.2
wrist	C40.1-	C79.51	—	—	—	—
xiphoid process	C41.3	C79.51	—	D16.7	D48.0	D49.2
zygomatic	C41.0	C79.51	—	D16.4-	D48.0	D49.2
book-leaf (mouth)	C06.89	C79.89	D00.00	D10.39	D37.09	D49.0
bowel — *see Neoplasm, intestine*						
brachial plexus	C47.1-	C79.89	—	D36.12	D48.2	D49.2
brain NEC	C71.9	C79.31	—	D33.2	D43.2	D49.6
basal ganglia	C71.0	C79.31	—	D33.0	D43.0	D49.6
cerebellopontine angle	C71.6	C79.31	—	D33.1	D43.1	D49.6
cerebellum NOS	C71.6	C79.31	—	D33.1	D43.1	D49.6
cerebrum	C71.0	C79.31	—	D33.0	D43.0	D49.6
choroid plexus	C71.7	C79.31	—	D33.1	D43.1	D49.6
corpus callosum	C71.8	C79.31	—	D33.2	D43.2	D49.6
corpus striatum	C71.0	C79.31	—	D33.0	D43.0	D49.6
cortex (cerebral)	C71.0	C79.31	—	D33.0	D43.0	D49.6
frontal lobe	C71.1	C79.31	—	D33.0	D43.0	D49.6
globus pallidus	C71.0	C79.31	—	D33.0	D43.0	D49.6
hippocampus	C71.2	C79.31	—	D33.0	D43.0	D49.6
hypothalamus	C71.0	C79.31	—	D33.0	D43.0	D49.6
internal capsule	C71.0	C79.31	—	D33.0	D43.0	D49.6
medulla oblongata	C71.7	C79.31	—	D33.1	D43.1	D49.6
meninges	C70.0	C79.32	—	D32.0	D42.0	D49.7

	Malignant Primary	Malignant Secondary	Ca in situ	Benign	Uncertain Behavior	Unspecified Behavior
brain NEC *(Continued)*						
midbrain	C71.7	C79.31	—	D33.1	D43.1	D49.6
occipital lobe	C71.4	C79.31	—	D33.0	D43.0	D49.6
overlapping lesion	C71.8	C79.31	—	—	—	—
parietal lobe	C71.3	C79.31	—	D33.0	D43.0	D49.6
peduncle	C71.7	C79.31	—	D33.1	D43.1	D49.6
pons	C71.7	C79.31	—	D33.1	D43.1	D49.6
stem	C71.7	C79.31	—	D33.1	D43.1	D49.6
tapetum	C71.8	C79.31	—	D33.2	D43.2	D49.6
temporal lobe	C71.2	C79.31	—	D33.0	D43.0	D49.6
thalamus	C71.0	C79.31	—	D33.0	D43.0	D49.6
uncus	C71.2	C79.31	—	D33.0	D43.0	D49.6
ventricle (floor)	C71.5	C79.31	—	D33.0	D43.0	D49.6
fourth	C71.7	C79.31	—	D33.1	D43.1	D49.6
branchial (cleft) (cyst) (vestiges)	C10.4	C79.89	D00.08	D10.5	D37.05	D49.0
breast (connective tissue) (glandular tissue) (soft parts)	C50.9-	C79.81	D05.-	D24.-	D48.6-	D49.3
areola	C50.0-	C79.81	D05.-	D24.-	D48.6-	D49.3
axillary tail	C50.6-	C79.81	D05.-	D24.-	D48.6-	D49.3
central portion	C50.1-	C79.81	D05.-	D24.-	D48.6-	D49.3
inner	C50.8-	C79.81	D05.-	D24.-	D48.6-	D49.3
lower	C50.8-	C79.81	D05.-	D24.-	D48.6-	D49.3
lower-inner quadrant	C50.3-	C79.81	D05.-	D24.-	D48.6-	D49.3
lower-outer quadrant	C50.5-	C79.81	D05.-	D24.-	D48.6-	D49.3
mastectomy site (skin) — *see also Neoplasm, breast, skin*	C44.501	C79.2	—	—	—	—
specified as breast tissue	C50.8-	C79.81	—	—	—	—
midline	C50.8-	C79.81	D05.-	D24.-	D48.6-	D49.3
nipple	C50.0-	C79.81	D05.-	D24.-	D48.6-	D49.3
outer	C50.8-	C79.81	D05.-	D24.-	D48.6-	D49.3
overlapping lesion	C50.8-	—	—	—	—	—
skin	C44.501	C79.2	D04.5	D23.5	D48.5	D49.2
basal cell carcinoma	C44.511	—	—	—	—	—
specified type NEC	C44.591	—	—	—	—	—
squamous cell carcinoma	C44.521	—	—	—	—	—
tail (axillary)	C50.6-	C79.81	D05.-	D24.-	D48.6-	D49.3
upper	C50.8-	C79.81	D05.-	D24.-	D48.6-	D49.3
upper-inner quadrant	C50.2-	C79.81	D05.-	D24.-	D48.6-	D49.3
upper-outer quadrant	C50.4-	C79.81	D05.-	D24.-	D48.6-	D49.3
broad ligament	C57.1	C79.82	D07.39	D28.2	D39.8	D49.5
bronchiogenic, bronchogenic (lung)	C34.9-	C78.0-	D02.2-	D14.3-	D38.1	D49.1
bronchiole	C34.9-	C78.0-	D02.2-	D14.3-	D38.1	D49.1
bronchus	C34.9-	C78.0-	D02.2-	D14.3-	D38.1	D49.1
carina	C34.0-	C78.0-	D02.2-	D14.3-	D38.1	D49.1
lower lobe of lung	C34.3-	C78.0-	D02.2-	D14.3-	D38.1	D49.1

	Malignant Primary	Malignant Secondary	Ca in situ	Benign	Uncertain Behavior	Unspecified Behavior
bronchus *(Continued)*						
main	C34.0-	C78.0-	D02.2-	D14.3-	D38.1	D49.1
middle lobe of lung	C34.2	C78.0-	D02.21	D14.31	D38.1	D49.1
overlapping lesion	C34.8-	—	—	—	—	—
upper lobe of lung	C34.1-	C78.0-	D02.2-	D14.3-	D38.1	D49.1
brow	C44.309	C79.2	D04.39	D23.39	D48.5	D49.2
basal cell carcinoma	C44.319	—	—	—	—	—
specified type NEC	C44.399	—	—	—	—	—
squamous cell carcinoma	C44.329	—	—	—	—	—
buccal (cavity)	C06.9	C79.89	D00.00	D10.39	D37.09	D49.0
commissure	C06.0	C79.89	D00.02	D10.39	D37.09	D49.0
groove (lower) (upper)	C06.1	C79.89	D00.02	D10.39	D37.09	D49.0
mucosa	C06.0	C79.89	D00.02	D10.39	D37.09	D49.0
sulcus (lower) (upper)	C06.1	C79.89	D00.02	D10.39	D37.09	D49.0
bulbourethral gland	C68.0	C79.19	D09.19	D30.4	D41.3	D49.5
bursa — *see Neoplasm, connective tissue*						
buttock NEC	C76.3	C79.89	D04.5	D36.7	D48.7	D49.89
calf	C76.5-	C79.89	D04.7-	D36.7	D48.7	D49.89
calvarium	C41.0	C79.51	—	D16.4-	D48.0	D49.2
calyx, renal	C65.-	C79.0-	D09.19	D30.1-	D41.1-	D49.5
canal						
anal	C21.1	C78.5	D01.3	D12.9	D37.8	D49.0
auditory (external) — *see also Neoplasm, skin, ear*	C44.20-	C79.2	D04.2-	D23.2-	D48.5	D49.2
auricular (external) — *see also Neoplasm, skin, ear*	C44.20-	C79.2	D04.2-	D23.2-	D48.5	D49.2
canaliculi, biliary (biliferi) (intrahepatic)	C22.1	C78.7	D01.5	D13.4	D37.6	D49.0
canthus (eye) (inner) (outer)	C44.10-	C79.2	D04.1-	D23.1-	D48.5	D49.2
basal cell carcinoma	C44.11-	—	—	—	—	—
specified type NEC	C44.19-	—	—	—	—	—
squamous cell carcinoma	C44.12-	—	—	—	—	—
capillary — *see Neoplasm, connective tissue*						
caput coli	C18.0	C78.5	D01.0	D12.0	D37.4	D49.0
carcinoid — *see Tumor, carcinoid*						
cardia (gastric)	C16.0	C78.89	D00.2	D13.1	D37.1	D49.0
cardiac orifice (stomach)	C16.0	C78.89	D00.2	D13.1	D37.1	D49.0
cardio-esophageal junction	C16.0	C78.89	D00.2	D13.1	D37.1	D49.0
cardio-esophagus	C16.0	C78.89	D00.2	D13.1	D37.1	D49.0
carina (bronchus)	C34.0-	C78.0-	D02.2-	D14.3-	D38.1	D49.1
carotid (artery)	C49.0	C79.89	—	D21.0	D48.1	D49.2
body	C75.4	C79.89	—	D35.5	D44.6	D49.7
carpus (any bone)	C40.1-	C79.51	—	D16.1-	—	—
cartilage (articular) (joint) NEC — *see also Neoplasm, bone*	C41.9	C79.51	—	D16.9-	D48.0	D49.2
arytenoid	C32.3	C78.39	D02.0	D14.1	D38.0	D49.1
auricular	C49.0	C79.89	—	D21.0	D48.1	D49.2

	Malignant Primary	Malignant Secondary	Ca in situ	Benign	Uncertain Behavior	Unspecified Behavior
cartilage NEC *(Continued)*						
bronchi	C34.0-	C78.39	—	D14.3-	D38.1	D49.1
costal	C41.3	C79.51	—	D16.7	D48.0	D49.2
cricoid	C32.3	C78.39	D02.0	D14.1	D38.0	D49.1
cuneiform	C32.3	C78.39	D02.0	D14.1	D38.0	D49.1
ear (external)	C49.0	C79.89	—	D21.0	D48.1	D49.2
ensiform	C41.3	C79.51	—	D16.7	D48.0	D49.2
epiglottis	C32.1	C78.39	D02.0	D14.1	D38.0	D49.1
anterior surface	C10.1	C79.89	D00.08	D10.5	D37.05	D49.0
eyelid	C49.0	C79.89	—	D21.0	D48.1	D49.2
intervertebral	C41.2	C79.51	—	D16.6	D48.0	D49.2
larynx, laryngeal	C32.3	C78.39	D02.0	D14.1	D38.0	D49.1
nose, nasal	C30.0	C78.39	D02.3	D14.0	D38.5	D49.1
pinna	C49.0	C79.89	—	D21.0	D48.1	D49.2
rib	C41.3	C79.51	—	D16.7	D48.0	D49.2
semilunar (knee)	C40.2-	C79.51	—	D16.2-	D48.0	D49.2
thyroid	C32.3	C78.39	D02.0	D14.1	D38.0	D49.1
trachea	C33	C78.39	D02.1	D14.2	D38.1	D49.1
cauda equina	C72.1	C79.49	—	D33.4	D43.4	D49.7
cavity						
buccal	C06.9	C79.89	D00.00	D10.30	D37.09	D49.0
nasal	C30.0	C78.39	D02.3	D14.0	D38.5	D49.1
oral	C06.9	C79.89	D00.00	D10.30	D37.09	D49.0
peritoneal	C48.2	C78.6	—	D20.1	D48.4	D49.0
tympanic	C30.1	C78.39	D02.3	D14.0	D38.5	D49.1
cecum	C18.0	C78.5	D01.0	D12.0	D37.4	D49.0
central nervous system	C72.9	C79.40	—	—	—	—
cerebellopontine (angle)	C71.6	C79.31	—	D33.1	D43.1	D49.6
cerebellum, cerebellar	C71.6	C79.31	—	D33.1	D43.1	D49.6
cerebrum, cerebral (cortex) (hemisphere) (white matter)	C71.0	C79.31	—	D33.0	D43.0	D49.6
meninges	C70.0	C79.32	—	D32.0	D42.0	D49.7
peduncle	C71.7	C79.31	—	D33.1	D43.1	D49.6
ventricle	C71.5	C79.31	—	D33.0	D43.0	D49.6
fourth	C71.7	C79.31	—	D33.1	D43.1	D49.6
cervical region	C76.0	C79.89	D09.8	D36.7	D48.7	D49.89
cervix (cervical) (uteri) (uterus)	C53.9	C79.82	D06.9	D26.0	D39.0	D49.5
canal	C53.0	C79.82	D06.0	D26.0	D39.0	D49.5
endocervix (canal) (gland)	C53.0	C79.82	D06.0	D26.0	D39.0	D49.5
exocervix	C53.1	C79.82	D06.1	D26.0	D39.0	D49.5
external os	C53.1	C79.82	D06.1	D26.0	D39.0	D49.5
internal os	C53.0	C79.82	D06.0	D26.0	D39.0	D49.5
nabothian gland	C53.0	C79.82	D06.0	D26.0	D39.0	D49.5
overlapping lesion	C53.8	—	—	—	—	—

	Malignant Primary	Malignant Secondary	Ca in situ	Benign	Uncertain Behavior	Unspecified Behavior
cervix *(Continued)*						
squamocolumnar junction	C53.8	C79.82	D06.7	D26.0	D39.0	D49.5
stump	C53.8	C79.82	D06.7	D26.0	D39.0	D49.5
cheek	C76.0	C79.89	D09.8	D36.7	D48.7	D49.89
external	C44.309	C79.2	D04.39	D23.39	D48.5	D49.2
basal cell carcinoma	C44.319	—	—	—	—	—
specified type NEC	C44.399	—	—	—	—	—
squamous cell carcinoma	C44.329	—	—	—	—	—
inner aspect	C06.0	C79.89	D00.02	D10.39	D37.09	D49.0
internal	C06.0	C79.89	D00.02	D10.39	D37.09	D49.0
mucosa	C06.0	C79.89	D00.02	D10.39	D37.09	D49.0
chest (wall) NEC	C76.1	C79.89	D09.8	D36.7	D48.7	D49.89
chiasma opticum	C72.3-	C79.49	—	D33.3	D43.3	D49.7
chin	C44.309	C79.2	D04.39	D23.39	D48.5	D49.2
basal cell carcinoma	C44.319	—	—	—	—	—
specified type NEC	C44.399	—	—	—	—	—
squamous cell carcinoma	C44.329	—	—	—	—	—
choana	C11.3	C79.89	D00.08	D10.6	D37.05	D49.0
cholangiole	C22.1	C78.89	D01.5	D13.4	D37.6	D49.0
choledochal duct	C24.0	C78.89	D01.5	D13.5	D37.6	D49.0
choroid	C69.3-	C79.49	D09.2-	D31.3-	D48.7	D49.81
plexus	C71.5	C79.31	—	D33.0	D43.0	D49.6
ciliary body	C69.4-	C79.49	D09.2-	D31.4-	D48.7	D49.89
clavicle	C41.3	C79.51	—	D16.7	D48.0	D49.2
clitoris	C51.2	C79.82	D07.1	D28.0	D39.8	D49.5
clivus	C41.0	C79.51	—	D16.4-	D48.0	D49.2
cloacogenic zone	C21.2	C78.5	D01.3	D12.9	D37.8	D49.0
coccygeal						
body or glomus	C75.5	C79.89	—	D35.6	D44.7	D49.7
vertebra	C41.4	C79.51	—	D16.8	D48.0	D49.2
coccyx	C41.4	C79.51	—	D16.8	D48.0	D49.2
colon	C18.9	C78.5	—	—	—	—
with rectum	C19	C78.5	D01.1	D12.7	D37.5	D49.0
column, spinal — *see Neoplasm, spine*						
columnella — *see also Neoplasm, skin, face*	C44.390	C79.2	D04.39	D23.39	D48.5	D49.2
commissure						
labial, lip	C00.6	C79.89	D00.01	D10.39	D37.01	D49.0
laryngeal	C32.0	C78.39	D02.0	D14.1	D38.0	D49.1
common (bile) duct	C24.0	C78.89	D01.5	D13.5	D37.6	D49.0
concha — *see also Neoplasm, skin, ear*	C44.20-	C79.2	D04.2-	D23.2-	D48.5	D49.2
nose	C30.0	C78.39	D02.3	D14.0	D38.5	D49.1
conjunctiva	C69.0-	C79.49	D09.2-	D31.0-	D48.7	D49.89

	Malignant Primary	Malignant Secondary	Ca in situ	Benign	Uncertain Behavior	Unspecified Behavior
Note: For neoplasms of connective tissue (blood vessel, bursa, fascia, ligament, muscle, peripheral nerves, sympathetic and parasympathetic nerves and ganglia, synovia, tendon, etc.) or of morphological types that indicate connective tissue, code according to the list under "Neoplasm, connective tissue". For sites that do not appear in this list, code to neoplasm of that site; e.g., fibrosarcoma, pancreas (C25.9)						
Note: Morphological types that indicate connective tissue appear in their proper place in the alphabetic index with the instruction *"see Neoplasm, connective tissue ...."*						
connective tissue NEC	C49.9	C79.89	—	D21.9	D48.1	D49.2
abdomen	C49.4	C79.89	—	D21.4	D48.1	D49.2
abdominal wall	C49.4	C79.89	—	D21.4	D48.1	D49.2
ankle	C49.2-	C79.89	—	D21.2-	D48.1	D49.2
antecubital fossa or space	C49.1-	C79.89	—	D21.1-	D48.1	D49.2
arm	C49.1-	C79.89	—	D21.1-	D48.1	D49.2
auricle (ear)	C49.0	C79.89	—	D21.0	D48.1	D49.2
axilla	C49.3	C79.89	—	D21.3	D48.1	D49.2
back	C49.6	C79.89	—	D21.6	D48.1	D49.2
breast — *see Neoplasm, breast*						
buttock	C49.5	C79.89	—	D21.5	D48.1	D49.2
calf	C49.2-	C79.89	—	D21.2-	D48.1	D49.2
cervical region	C49.0	C79.89	—	D21.0	D48.1	D49.2
cheek	C49.0	C79.89	—	D21.0	D48.1	D49.2
chest (wall)	C49.3	C79.89	—	D21.3	D48.1	D49.2
chin	C49.0	C79.89	—	D21.0	D48.1	D49.2
diaphragm	C49.3	C79.89	—	D21.3	D48.1	D49.2
ear (external)	C49.0	C79.89	—	D21.0	D48.1	D49.2
elbow	C49.1-	C79.89	—	D21.1-	D48.1	D49.2
extrarectal	C49.5	C79.89	—	D21.5	D48.1	D49.2
extremity	C49.9	C79.89	—	D21.9	D48.1	D49.2
lower	C49.2-	C79.89	—	D21.2-	D48.1	D49.2
upper	C49.1-	C79.89	—	D21.1-	D48.1	D49.2
eyelid	C49.0	C79.89	—	D21.0	D48.1	D49.2
face	C49.0	C79.89	—	D21.0	D48.1	D49.2
finger	C49.1-	C79.89	—	D21.1-	D48.1	D49.2
flank	C49.6	C79.89	—	D21.6	D48.1	D49.2
foot	C49.2-	C79.89	—	D21.2-	D48.1	D49.2
forearm	C49.1-	C79.89	—	D21.1-	D48.1	D49.2
forehead	C49.0	C79.89	—	D21.0	D48.1	D49.2
gastric	C49.4	C79.89	—	D21.4	D48.1	D49.2
gastrointestinal	C49.4	C79.89	—	D21.4	D48.1	D49.2
gluteal region	C49.5	C79.89	—	D21.5	D48.1	D49.2
great vessels NEC	C49.3	C79.89	—	D21.3	D48.1	D49.2
groin	C49.5	C79.89	—	D21.5	D48.1	D49.2
hand	C49.1-	C79.89	—	D21.1-	D48.1	D49.2

	Malignant Primary	Malignant Secondary	Ca in situ	Benign	Uncertain Behavior	Unspecified Behavior
connective tissue NEC *(Continued)*						
head	C49.0	C79.89	—	D21.0	D48.1	D49.2
heel	C49.2-	C79.89	—	D21.2-	D48.1	D49.2
hip	C49.2-	C79.89	—	D21.2-	D48.1	D49.2
hypochondrium	C49.4	C79.89	—	D21.4	D48.1	D49.2
iliopsoas muscle	C49.5	C79.89	—	D21.5	D48.1	D49.2
infraclavicular region	C49.3	C79.89	—	D21.3	D48.1	D49.2
inguinal (canal) (region)	C49.5	C79.89	—	D21.5	D48.1	D49.2
intestinal	C49.4	C79.89	—	D21.4	D48.1	D49.2
intrathoracic	C49.3	C79.89	—	D21.3	D48.1	D49.2
ischiorectal fossa	C49.5	C79.89	—	D21.5	D48.1	D49.2
jaw	C03.9	C79.89	D00.03	D10.39	D48.1	D49.0
knee	C49.2-	C79.89	—	D21.2-	D48.1	D49.2
leg	C49.2-	C79.89	—	D21.2-	D48.1	D49.2
limb NEC	C49.9	C79.89	—	D21.9	D48.1	D49.2
lower	C49.2-	C79.89	—	D21.2-	D48.1	D49.2
upper	C49.1-	C79.89	—	D21.1-	D48.1	D49.2
nates	C49.5	C79.89	—	D21.5	D48.1	D49.2
neck	C49.0	C79.89	—	D21.0	D48.1	D49.2
orbit	C69.6-	C79.49	D09.2-	D31.6-	D48.1	D49.89
overlapping lesion	C49.8	—	—	—	—	—
pararectal	C49.5	C79.89	—	D21.5	D48.1	D49.2
para-urethral	C49.5	C79.89	—	D21.5	D48.1	D49.2
paravaginal	C49.5	C79.89	—	D21.5	D48.1	D49.2
pelvis (floor)	C49.5	C79.89	—	D21.5	D48.1	D49.2
pelvo-abdominal	C49.8	C79.89	—	D21.6	D48.1	D49.2
perineum	C49.5	C79.89	—	D21.5	D48.1	D49.2
perirectal (tissue)	C49.5	C79.89	—	D21.5	D48.1	D49.2
periurethral (tissue)	C49.5	C79.89	—	D21.5	D48.1	D49.2
popliteal fossa or space	C49.2-	C79.89	—	D21.2-	D48.1	D49.2
presacral	C49.5	C79.89	—	D21.5	D48.1	D49.2
psoas muscle	C49.4	C79.89	—	D21.4	D48.1	D49.2
pterygoid fossa	C49.0	C79.89	—	D21.0	D48.1	D49.2
rectovaginal septum or wall	C49.5	C79.89	—	D21.5	D48.1	D49.2
rectovesical	C49.5	C79.89	—	D21.5	D48.1	D49.2
retroperitoneum	C48.0	C78.6	—	D20.0	D48.3	D49.0
sacrococcygeal region	C49.5	C79.89	—	D21.5	D48.1	D49.2
scalp	C49.0	C79.89	—	D21.0	D48.1	D49.2
scapular region	C49.3	C79.89	—	D21.3	D48.1	D49.2
shoulder	C49.1-	C79.89	—	D21.1-	D48.1	D49.2
skin (dermis) NEC — *see also Neoplasm, skin, by site*	C44.90	C79.2	D04.9	D23.9	D48.5	D49.2
stomach	C49.4	C79.89	—	D21.4	D48.1	D49.2
submental	C49.0	C79.89	—	D21.0	D48.1	D49.2

	Malignant Primary	Malignant Secondary	Ca in situ	Benign	Uncertain Behavior	Unspecified Behavior
connective tissue NEC *(Continued)*						
supraclavicular region	C49.0	C79.89	—	D21.0	D48.1	D49.2
temple	C49.0	C79.89	—	D21.0	D48.1	D49.2
temporal region	C49.0	C79.89	—	D21.0	D48.1	D49.2
thigh	C49.2-	C79.89	—	D21.2-	D48.1	D49.2
thoracic (duct) (wall)	C49.3	C79.89	—	D21.3	D48.1	D49.2
thorax	C49.3	C79.89	—	D21.3	D48.1	D49.2
thumb	C49.1-	C79.89	—	D21.1-	D48.1	D49.2
toe	C49.2-	C79.89	—	D21.2-	D48.1	D49.2
trunk	C49.6	C79.89	—	D21.6	D48.1	D49.2
umbilicus	C49.4	C79.89	—	D21.4	D48.1	D49.2
vesicorectal	C49.5	C79.89	—	D21.5	D48.1	D49.2
wrist	C49.1-	C79.89	—	D21.1-	D48.1	D49.2
conus medullaris	C72.0	C79.49	—	D33.4	D43.4	D49.7
cord (true) (vocal)	C32.0	C78.39	D02.0	D14.1	D38.0	D49.1
false	C32.1	C78.39	D02.0	D14.1	D38.0	D49.1
spermatic	C63.1-	C79.82	D07.69	D29.8	D40.8	D49.5
spinal (cervical) (lumbar) (thoracic)	C72.0	C79.49	—	D33.4	D43.4	D49.7
cornea (limbus)	C69.1-	C79.49	D09.2-	D31.1-	D48.7	D49.89
corpus						
albicans	C56.-	C79.6-	D07.39	D27.-	D39.1-	D49.5
callosum, brain	C71.0	C79.31	—	D33.2	D43.2	D49.6
cavernosum	C60.2	C79.82	D07.4	D29.0	D40.8	D49.5
gastric	C16.2-	C78.89	D00.2	D13.1	D37.1	D49.0
overlapping sites	C54.8	—	—	—	—	—
penis	C60.2	C79.82	D07.4	D29.0	D40.8	D49.5
striatum, cerebrum	C71.0	C79.31	—	D33.0	D43.0	D49.6
uteri	C54.9	C79.82	D07.0	D26.1	D39.0	D49.5
isthmus	C54.0	C79.82	D07.0	D26.1	D39.0	D49.5
cortex						
adrenal	C74.0-	C79.7-	D09.3	D35.0-	D44.1-	D49.7
cerebral	C71.0	C79.31	—	D33.0	D43.0	D49.6
costal cartilage	C41.3	C79.51	—	D16.7	D48.0	D49.2
costovertebral joint	C41.3	C79.51	—	D16.7	D48.0	D49.2
Cowper's gland	C68.0	C79.19	D09.19	D30.4	D41.3	D49.5
cranial (fossa, any)	C71.9	C79.31	—	D33.2	D43.2	D49.6
meninges	C70.0	C79.32	—	D32.0	D42.0	D49.7
nerve	C72.50	C79.49	—	D33.3	D43.3	D49.7
specified NEC	C72.59	C79.49	—	D33.3	D43.3	D49.7
craniobuccal pouch	C75.2	C79.89	D09.3	D35.2	D44.3	D49.7
craniopharyngeal (duct) (pouch)	C75.2	C79.89	D09.3	D35.3	D44.4	D49.7
cricoid	C13.0	C79.89	D00.08	D10.7	D37.05	D49.0
cartilage	C32.3	C79.89	D02.0	D14.1	D38.0	D49.1

	Malignant Primary	Malignant Secondary	Ca in situ	Benign	Uncertain Behavior	Unspecified Behavior
cricopharynx	C13.0	C79.89	D00.08	D10.7	D37.05	D49.0
crypt of Morgagni	C21.8	C78.5	D01.3	D12.9	D37.8	D49.0
crystalline lens	C69.4-	C79.49	D09.2-	D31.4-	D48.7	D49.89
cul-de-sac (Douglas')	C48.1	C78.6	—	D20.1	D48.4	D49.0
cuneiform cartilage	C32.3	C78.39	D02.0	D14.1	D38.0	D49.1
cutaneous — see Neoplasm, skin						
cutis — see Neoplasm, skin						
cystic (bile) duct (common)	C24.0	C78.89	D01.5	D13.5	D37.6	D49.0
dermis — see Neoplasm, skin						
diaphragm	C49.3	C79.89	—	D21.3	D48.1	D49.2
digestive organs, system, tube, or tract NEC	C26.9	C78.89	D01.9	D13.9	D37.9	D49.0
disc, intervertebral	C41.2	C79.51		D16.6	D48.0	D49.2
disease, generalized	C80.0	—	—	—	—	—
disseminated	C80.0	—	—	—	—	—
Douglas' cul-de-sac or pouch	C48.1	C78.6	—	D20.1	D48.4	D49.0
duodenojejunal junction	C17.8	C78.4	D01.49	D13.39	D37.2	D49.0
duodenum	C17.0	C78.4	D01.49	D13.2	D37.2	D49.0
dura (cranial) (mater)	C70.9	C79.49	—	D32.9	D42.9	D49.7
cerebral	C70.0	C79.32	—	D32.0	D42.0	D49.7
spinal	C70.1	C79.49	—	D32.1	D42.1	D49.7
ear (external) — see also Neoplasm, skin, ear	C44.20-	C79.2	D04.2-	D23.2-	D48.5	D49.2
auricle or auris — see also Neoplasm, skin, ear	C44.20-	C79.2	D04.2-	D23.2-	D48.5	D49.2
canal, external — see also Neoplasm, skin, ear	C44.20-	C79.2	D04.2-	D23.2-	D48.5	D49.2
cartilage	C49.0	C79.89	—	D21.0	D48.1	D49.2
external meatus — see also Neoplasm, skin, ear	C44.20-	C79.2	D04.2-	D23.2-	D48.5	D49.2
inner	C30.1	C78.39	D02.3	D14.0	D38.5	D49.1
lobule — see also Neoplasm, skin, ear	C44.20-	C79.2	D04.2-	D23.2-	D48.5	D49.2
middle	C30.1	C78.39	D02.3	D14.0	D38.5	D49.1
overlapping lesion with accessory sinuses	C31.8	—	—	—	—	—
skin	C44.20-	C79.2	D04.2-	D23.2-	D48.5	D49.2
basal cell carcinoma	C44.21-	—	—	—	—	—
specified type NEC	C44.29-	—	—	—	—	—
squamous cell carcinoma	C44.22-	—	—	—	—	—
earlobe	C44.20-	C79.2	D04.2-	D23.2-	D48.5	D49.2
basal cell carcinoma	C44.21-	—	—	—	—	—
specified type NEC	C44.29-	—	—	—	—	—
squamous cell carcinoma	C44.22-	—	—	—	—	—
ejaculatory duct	C63.7	C79.82	D07.69	D29.8	D40.8	D49.5
elbow NEC	C76.4-	C79.89	D04.6-	D36.7	D48.7	D49.89
endocardium	C38.0	C79.89	—	D15.1	D48.7	D49.89
endocervix (canal) (gland)	C53.0	C79.82	D06.0	D26.0	D39.0	D49.5
endocrine gland NEC	C75.9	C79.89	D09.3	D35.9	D44.9	D49.7
pluriglandular	C75.8	C79.89	D09.3	D35.7	D44.9	D49.7

	Malignant Primary	Malignant Secondary	Ca in situ	Benign	Uncertain Behavior	Unspecified Behavior
endometrium (gland) (stroma)	C54.1	C79.82	D07.0	D26.1	D39.0	D49.5
ensiform cartilage	C41.3	C79.51	—	D16.7	D48.0	D49.2
enteric — see Neoplasm, intestine						
ependyma (brain)	C71.5	C79.31	—	D33.0	D43.0	D49.6
fourth ventricle	C71.7	C79.31	—	D33.1	D43.1	D49.6
epicardium	C38.0	C79.89	—	D15.1	D48.7	D49.89
epididymis	C63.0-	C79.82	D07.69	D29.3-	D40.8	D49.5
epidural	C72.9	C79.49	—	D33.9	D43.9	D49.7
epiglottis	C32.1	C78.39	D02.0	D14.1	D38.0	D49.1
anterior aspect or surface	C10.1	C79.89	D00.08	D10.5	D37.05	D49.0
cartilage	C32.3	C78.39	D02.0	D14.1	D38.0	D49.1
free border (margin)	C10.1	C79.89	D00.08	D10.5	D37.05	D49.0
junctional region	C10.8	C79.89	D00.08	D10.5	D37.05	D49.0
posterior (laryngeal) surface	C32.1	C78.39	D02.0	D14.1	D38.0	D49.1
suprahyoid portion	C32.1	C78.39	D02.0	D14.1	D38.0	D49.1
esophagogastric junction	C16.0	C78.89	D00.2	D13.1	D37.1	D49.0
esophagus	C15.9	C78.89	D00.1	D13.0	D37.8	D49.0
abdominal	C15.5	C78.89	D00.1	D13.0	D37.8	D49.0
cervical	C15.3	C78.89	D00.1	D13.0	D37.8	D49.0
distal (third)	C15.5	C78.89	D00.1	D13.0	D37.8	D49.0
lower (third)	C15.5	C78.89	D00.1	D13.0	D37.8	D49.0
middle (third)	C15.4	C78.89	D00.1	D13.0	D37.8	D49.0
overlapping lesion	C15.8	—	—	—	—	—
proximal (third)	C15.3	C78.89	D00.1	D13.0	D37.8	D49.0
thoracic	C15.4	C78.89	D00.1	D13.0	D37.8	D49.0
upper (third)	C15.3	C78.89	D00.1	D13.0	D37.8	D49.0
ethmoid (sinus)	C31.1	C78.39	D02.3	D14.0	D38.5	D49.1
bone or labyrinth	C41.0	C79.51	—	D16.4-	D48.0	D49.2
eustachian tube	C30.1	C78.39	D02.3	D14.0	D38.5	D49.1
exocervix	C53.1	C79.82	D06.1	D26.0	D39.0	D49.5
external						
meatus (ear) — see also Neoplasm, skin, ear	C44.20-	C79.2	D04.2-	D23.2-	D48.5	D49.2
os, cervix uteri	C53.1	C79.82	D06.1	D26.0	D39.0	D49.5
extradural	C72.9	C79.49	—	D33.9	D43.9	D49.7
extrahepatic (bile) duct	C24.0	C78.89	D01.5	D13.5	D37.6	D49.0
overlapping lesion with gallbladder	C24.8	—	—	—	—	—
extraocular muscle	C69.6-	C79.49	D09.2-	D31.6-	D48.7	D49.89
extrarectal	C76.3	C79.89	D09.8	D36.7	D48.7	D49.89
extremity	C76.8	C79.89	D04.8	D36.7	D48.7	D49.89
lower	C76.5-	C79.89	D04.7-	D36.7	D48.7	D49.89
upper	C76.4-	C79.89	D04.6-	D36.7	D48.7	D49.89
eye NEC	C69.9-	C79.49	D09.2	D31.9	D48.7	D49.89
overlapping sites	C69.8	—	—	—	—	—
eyeball	C69.4-	C79.49	D09.2-	D31.4-	D48.7	D49.89

	Malignant Primary	Malignant Secondary	Ca in situ	Benign	Uncertain Behavior	Unspecified Behavior
eyebrow	C44.309	C79.2	D04.39	D23.39	D48.5	D49.2
basal cell carcinoma	C44.319	—	—	—	—	—
specified type NEC	C44.399	—	—	—	—	—
squamous cell carcinoma	C44.329	—	—	—	—	—
eyelid (lower) (skin) (upper)	C44.10-	—	—	—	—	—
basal cell carcinoma	C44.11-	—	—	—	—	—
cartilage	C49.0	C79.89	—	D21.0	D48.1	D49.2
specified type NEC	C44.19-	—	—	—	—	—
squamous cell carcinoma	C44.12-	—	—	—	—	—
face NEC	C76.0	C79.89	D04.39	D36.7	D48.7	D49.89
fallopian tube (accessory)	C57.0-	C79.82	D07.39	D28.2	D39.8	D49.5
falx (cerebella) (cerebri)	C70.0	C79.32	—	D32.0	D42.0	D49.7
fascia — *see also Neoplasm, connective tissue*						
palmar	C49.1-	C79.89	—	D21.1-	D48.1	D49.2
plantar	C49.2-	C79.89	—	D21.2-	D48.1	D49.2
fatty tissue — *see Neoplasm, connective tissue*						
fauces, faucial NEC	C10.9	C79.89	D00.08	D10.5	D37.05	D49.0
pillars	C09.1	C79.89	D00.08	D10.5	D37.05	D49.0
tonsil	C09.9	C79.89	D00.08	D10.4	D37.05	D49.0
femur (any part)	C40.2-	—	—	D16.2-	—	—
fetal membrane	C58	C79.82	D07.0	D26.7	D39.2	D49.5
fibrous tissue — *see Neoplasm, connective tissue*						
fibula (any part)	C40.2-	C79.51	—	D16.2-	—	—
filum terminale	C72.0	C79.49	—	D33.4	D43.4	D49.7
finger NEC	C76.4-	C79.89	D04.6-	D36.7	D48.7	D49.89
flank NEC	C76.8	C79.89	D04.5	D36.7	D48.7	D49.89
follicle, nabothian	C53.0	C79.82	D06.0	D26.0	D39.0	D49.5
foot NEC	C76.5-	C79.89	D04.7-	D36.7	D48.7	D49.89
forearm NEC	C76.4-	C79.89	D04.6-	D36.7	D48.7	D49.89
forehead (skin)	C44.309	C79.2	D04.39	D23.39	D48.5	D49.2
basal cell carcinoma	C44.319	—	—	—	—	—
specified type NEC	C44.399	—	—	—	—	—
squamous cell carcinoma	C44.329	—	—	—	—	—
foreskin	C60.0	C79.82	D07.4	D29.0	D40.8	D49.5
fornix						
pharyngeal	C11.3	C79.89	D00.08	D10.6	D37.05	D49.0
vagina	C52	C79.82	D07.2	D28.1	D39.8	D49.5
fossa (of)						
anterior (cranial)	C71.9	C79.31	—	D33.2	D43.2	D49.6
cranial	C71.9	C79.31	—	D33.2	D43.2	D49.6
ischiorectal	C76.3	C79.89	D09.8	D36.7	D48.7	D49.89
middle (cranial)	C71.9	C79.31	—	D33.2	D43.2	D49.6
piriform	C12	C79.89	D00.08	D10.7	D37.05	D49.0

	Malignant Primary	Malignant Secondary	Ca in situ	Benign	Uncertain Behavior	Unspecified Behavior
fossa *(Continued)*						
pituitary	C75.1	C79.89	D09.3	D35.2	D44.3	D49.7
posterior (cranial)	C71.9	C79.31	—	D33.2	D43.2	D49.6
pterygoid	C49.0	C79.89	—	D21.0	D48.1	D49.2
pyriform	C12	C79.89	D00.08	D10.7	D37.05	D49.0
Rosenmuller	C11.2	C79.89	D00.08	D10.6	D37.05	D49.0
tonsillar	C09.0	C79.89	D00.08	D10.5	D37.05	D49.0
fourchette	C51.9	C79.82	D07.1	D28.0	D39.8	D49.5
frenulum						
labii — *see* Neoplasm, lip, internal						
linguae	C02.2	C79.89	D00.07	D10.1	D37.02	D49.0
frontal						
bone	C41.0	C79.51	—	D16.4-	D48.0	D49.2
lobe, brain	C71.1	C79.31	—	D33.0	D43.0	D49.6
pole	C71.1	C79.31	—	D33.0	D43.0	D49.6
sinus	C31.2	C78.39	D02.3	D14.0	D38.5	D49.1
fundus						
stomach	C16.1	C78.89	D00.2	D13.1	D37.1	D49.0
uterus	C54.3	C79.82	D07.0	D26.1	D39.0	D49.5
gall duct (extrahepatic)	C24.0	C78.89	D01.5	D13.5	D37.6	D49.0
intrahepatic	C22.1	C78.7	D01.5	D13.4	D37.6	D49.0
gallbladder	C23	C78.89	D01.5	D13.5	D37.6	D49.0
overlapping lesion with extrahepatic bile ducts	C24.8	—	—	—	—	—
ganglia — *see also* Neoplasm, nerve, peripheral	C47.9	C79.89	—	D36.10	D48.2	D49.2
basal	C71.0	C79.31	—	D33.0	D43.0	D49.6
cranial nerve	C72.50	C79.49	—	D33.3	D43.3	D49.7
Gartner's duct	C52	C79.82	D07.2	D28.1	D39.8	D49.5
gastric — *see* Neoplasm, stomach						
gastrocolic	C26.9	C78.89	D01.9	D13.9	D37.9	D49.0
gastroesophageal junction	C16.0	C78.89	D00.2	D13.1	D37.1	D49.0
gastrointestinal (tract) NEC	C26.9	C78.89	D01.9	D13.9	D37.9	D49.0
generalized	C80.0	—	—	—	—	—
genital organ or tract						
female NEC	C57.9	C79.82	D07.30	D28.9	D39.9	D49.5
overlapping lesion	C57.8	—	—	—	—	—
specified site NEC	C57.7	C79.82	D07.39	D28.7	D39.8	D49.5
male NEC	C63.9	C79.82	D07.60	D29.9	D40.9	D49.5
overlapping lesion	C63.8	—	—	—	—	—
specified site NEC	C63.7	C79.82	D07.69	D29.8	D40.8	D49.5
genitourinary tract						
female	C57.9	C79.82	D07.30	D28.9	D39.9	D49.5
male	C63.9	C79.82	D07.60	D29.9	D40.9	D49.5

	Malignant Primary	Malignant Secondary	Ca in situ	Benign	Uncertain Behavior	Unspecified Behavior
gingiva (alveolar) (marginal)	C03.9	C79.89	D00.03	D10.39	D37.09	D49.0
lower	C03.1	C79.89	D00.03	D10.39	D37.09	D49.0
mandibular	C03.1	C79.89	D00.03	D10.39	D37.09	D49.0
maxillary	C03.0	C79.89	D00.03	D10.39	D37.09	D49.0
upper	C03.0	C79.89	D00.03	D10.39	D37.09	D49.0
gland, glandular (lymphatic) (system) — see also Neoplasm, lymph gland						
endocrine NEC	C75.9	C79.89	D09.3	D35.9	D44.9	D49.7
salivary — see Neoplasm, salivary gland						
glans penis	C60.1	C79.82	D07.4	D29.0	D40.8	D49.5
globus pallidus	C71.0	C79.31	—	D33.0	D43.0	D49.6
glomus						
coccygeal	C75.5	C79.89	—	D35.6	D44.7	D49.7
jugularis	C75.5	C79.89	—	D35.6	D44.7	D49.7
glosso-epiglottic fold(s)	C10.1	C79.89	D00.08	D10.5	D37.05	D49.0
glossopalatine fold	C09.1	C79.89	D00.08	D10.5	D37.05	D49.0
glossopharyngeal sulcus	C09.0	C79.89	D00.08	D10.5	D37.05	D49.0
glottis	C32.0	C78.39	D02.0	D14.1	D38.0	D49.1
gluteal region	C76.3	C79.89	D04.5	D36.7	D48.7	D49.89
great vessels NEC	C49.3	C79.89	—	D21.3	D48.1	D49.2
groin NEC	C76.3	C79.89	D04.5	D36.7	D48.7	D49.89
gum	C03.9	C79.89	D00.03	D10.39	D37.09	D49.0
lower	C03.1	C79.89	D00.03	D10.39	D37.09	D49.0
upper	C03.0	C79.89	D00.03	D10.39	D37.09	D49.0
hand NEC	C76.4-	C79.89	D04.6-	D36.7	D48.7	D49.89
head NEC	C76.0	C79.89	D04.4	D36.7	D48.7	D49.89
heart	C38.0	C79.89	—	D15.1	D48.7	D49.89
heel NEC	C76.5-	C79.89	D04.7-	D36.7	D48.7	D49.89
helix — see also Neoplasm, skin, ear	C44.20-	C79.2	D04.2-	D23.2-	D48.5	D49.2
hematopoietic, hemopoietic tissue NEC	C96.9	—	—	—	—	—
specified NEC	C96.Z	—	—	—	—	—
hemisphere, cerebral	C71.0	C79.31	—	D33.0	D43.0	D49.6
hemorrhoidal zone	C21.1	C78.5	D01.3	D12.9	D37.8	D49.0
hepatic — see also Index to disease, by histology	C22.9	C78.7	D01.5	D13.4	D37.6	D49.0
duct (bile)	C24.0	C78.89	D01.5	D13.5	D37.6	D49.0
flexure (colon)	C18.3	C78.5	D01.0	D12.3	D37.4	D49.0
primary	C22.8	C78.7	D01.5	D13.4	D37.6	D49.0
hepatoblastoma	C22.2	C78.7	D01.5	D13.4	D37.6	D49.0
hepatoma	C22.0	C78.7	D01.5	D13.4	D37.6	D49.0
hilus of lung	C34.0-	C78.0-	D02.2-	D14.3-	D38.1	D49.1
hip NEC	C76.5-	C79.89	D04.7-	D36.7	D48.7	D49.89
hippocampus, brain	C71.2	C79.31	—	D33.0	D43.0	D49.6
humerus (any part)	C40.0-	C79.51	—	D16.0-	—	—
hymen	C52	C79.82	D07.2	D28.1	D39.8	D49.5

TABLE OF NEOPLASMS

	Malignant Primary	Malignant Secondary	Ca in situ	Benign	Uncertain Behavior	Unspecified Behavior
hypopharynx, hypopharyngeal NEC	C13.9	C79.89	D00.08	D10.7	D37.05	D49.0
overlapping lesion	C13.8	—	—	—	—	—
postcricoid region	C13.0	C79.89	D00.08	D10.7	D37.05	D49.0
posterior wall	C13.2	C79.89	D00.08	D10.7	D37.05	D49.0
pyriform fossa (sinus)	C12	C79.89	D00.08	D10.7	D37.05	D49.0
hypophysis	C75.1	C79.89	D09.3	D35.2	D44.3	D49.7
hypothalamus	C71.0	C79.31	—	D33.0	D43.0	D49.6
ileocecum, ileocecal (coil) (junction) (valve)	C18.0	C78.5	D01.0	D12.0	D37.4	D49.0
ileum	C17.2	C78.4	D01.49	D13.39	D37.2	D49.0
ilium	C41.4	C79.51	—	D16.8	D48.0	D49.2
immunoproliferative NEC	C88.9	—	—	—	—	—
infraclavicular (region)	C76.1	C79.89	D04.5	D36.7	D48.7	D49.89
inguinal (region)	C76.3	C79.89	D04.5	D36.7	D48.7	D49.89
insula	C71.0	C79.31	—	D33.0	D43.0	D49.6
insular tissue (pancreas)	C25.4	C78.89	D01.7	D13.7	D37.8	D49.0
brain	C71.0	C79.31	—	D33.0	D43.0	D49.6
interarytenoid fold	C13.1	C79.89	D00.08	D10.7	D37.05	D49.0
hypopharyngeal aspect	C13.1	C79.89	D00.08	D10.7	D37.05	D49.0
laryngeal aspect	C32.1	C79.89	D02.0	D14.1	D38.0	D49.1
marginal zone	C13.1	C79.89	D00.08	D10.7	D37.05	D49.0
interdental papillae	C03.9	C79.89	D00.03	D10.39	D37.09	D49.0
lower	C03.1	C79.89	D00.03	D10.39	D37.09	D49.0
upper	C03.0	C79.89	D00.03	D10.39	D37.09	D49.0
internal						
capsule	C71.0	C79.31	—	D33.0	D43.0	D49.6
os (cervix)	C53.0	C79.82	D06.0	D26.0	D39.0	D49.5
intervertebral cartilage or disc	C41.2	C79.51	—	D16.6	D48.0	D49.2
intestine, intestinal	C26.0	C78.80	D01.40	D13.9	D37.8	D49.0
large	C18.9	C78.5	D01.0	D12.6	D37.4	D49.0
appendix	C18.1	C78.5	D01.0	D12.1	D37.3	D49.0
caput coli	C18.0	C78.5	D01.0	D12.0	D37.4	D49.0
cecum	C18.0	C78.5	D01.0	D12.0	D37.4	D49.0
colon	C18.9	C78.5	D01.0	D12.6	D37.4	D49.0
and rectum	C19	C78.5	D01.1	D12.7	D37.5	D49.0
ascending	C18.2	C78.5	D01.0	D12.2	D37.4	D49.0
caput	C18.0	C78.5	D01.0	D12.0	D37.4	D49.0
descending	C18.6	C78.5	D01.0	D12.4	D37.4	D49.0
distal	C18.6	C78.5	D01.0	D12.4	D37.4	D49.0
left	C18.6	C78.5	D01.0	D12.4	D37.4	D49.0
overlapping lesion	C18.8	—	—	—	—	—
pelvic	C18.7	C78.5	D01.0	D12.5	D37.4	D49.0
right	C18.2	C78.5	D01.0	D12.2	D37.4	D49.0
sigmoid (flexure)	C18.7	C78.5	D01.0	D12.5	D37.4	D49.0
transverse	C18.4	C78.5	D01.0	D12.3	D37.4	D49.0

	Malignant Primary	Malignant Secondary	Ca in situ	Benign	Uncertain Behavior	Unspecified Behavior
intestine, intestinal *(Continued)*						
large *(Continued)*						
hepatic flexure	C18.3	C78.5	D01.0	D12.3	D37.4	D49.0
ileocecum, ileocecal (coil) (valve)	C18.0	C78.5	D01.0	D12.0	D37.4	D49.0
overlapping lesion	C18.8	—	—	—	—	—
sigmoid flexure (lower) (upper)	C18.7	C78.5	D01.0	D12.5	D37.4	D49.0
splenic flexure	C18.5	C78.5	D01.0	D12.3	D37.4	D49.0
small	C17.9	C78.4	D01.40	D13.30	D37.2	D49.0
duodenum	C17.0	C78.4	D01.49	D13.2	D37.2	D49.0
ileum	C17.2	C78.4	D01.49	D13.39	D37.2	D49.0
jejunum	C17.1	C78.4	D01.49	D13.39	D37.2	D49.0
overlapping lesion	C17.8	—	—	—	—	—
tract NEC	C26.0	C78.89	D01.40	D13.9	D37.8	D49.0
intra-abdominal	C76.2	C79.89	D09.8	D36.7	D48.7	D49.89
intracranial NEC	C71.9	C79.31	—	D33.2	D43.2	D49.6
intrahepatic (bile) duct	C22.1	C78.7	D01.5	D13.4	D37.6	D49.0
intraocular	C69.4-	C79.49	D09.2-	D31.4-	D48.7	D49.89
intraorbital	C69.6-	C79.49	D09.2-	D31.6-	D48.7	D49.89
intrasellar	C75.1	C79.89	D09.3	D35.2	D44.3	D49.7
intrathoracic (cavity) (organs)	C76.1	C79.89	D09.8	D15.9	D48.7	D49.89
specified NEC	C76.1	C79.89	D09.8	D15.7	—	—
iris	C69.4-	C79.49	D09.2-	D31.4-	D48.7	D49.89
ischiorectal (fossa)	C76.3	C79.89	D09.8	D36.7	D48.7	D49.89
ischium	C41.4	C79.51	—	D16.8	D48.0	D49.2
island of Reil	C71.0	C79.31	—	D33.0	D43.0	D49.6
islands or islets of Langerhans	C25.4	C78.89	D01.7	D13.7	D37.8	D49.0
isthmus uteri	C54.0	C79.82	D07.0	D26.1	D39.0	D49.5
jaw	C76.0	C79.89	D09.8	D36.7	D48.7	D49.89
bone	C41.1	C79.51	—	D16.5-	D48.0	D49.2
lower	C41.1	C79.51	—	D16.5-	—	—
upper	C41.0	C79.51	—	D16.4-	—	—
carcinoma (any type) (lower) (upper)	C76.0	C79.89	—	—	—	—
skin—*see also Neoplasm, skin, face*	C44.309	C79.2	D04.39	D23.39	D48.5	D49.2
soft tissues	C03.9	C79.89	D00.03	D10.39	D37.09	D49.0
lower	C03.1	C79.89	D00.03	D10.39	D37.09	D49.0
upper	C03.0	C79.89	D00.03	D10.39	D37.09	D49.0
jejunum	C17.1	C78.4	D01.49	D13.39	D37.2	D49.0
joint NEC—*see also Neoplasm, bone*	C41.9	C79.51	—	D16.9-	D48.0	D49.2
acromioclavicular	C40.0-	C79.51	—	D16.0-	—	—
bursa or synovial membrane—*see Neoplasm, connective tissue*						
costovertebral	C41.3	C79.51	—	D16.7	D48.0	D49.2
sternocostal	C41.3	C79.51	—	D16.7	D48.0	D49.2
temporomandibular	C41.1	C79.51	—	D16.5-	D48.0	D49.2

TABLE OF NEOPLASMS

	Malignant Primary	Malignant Secondary	Ca in situ	Benign	Uncertain Behavior	Unspecified Behavior
junction						
anorectal	C21.8	C78.5	D01.3	D12.9	D37.8	D49.0
cardioesophageal	C16.0	C78.89	D00.2	D13.1	D37.1	D49.0
esophagogastric	C16.0	C78.89	D00.2	D13.1	D37.1	D49.0
gastroesophageal	C16.0	C78.89	D00.2	D13.1	D37.1	D49.0
hard and soft palate	C05.9	C79.89	D00.00	D10.39	D37.09	D49.0
ileocecal	C18.0	C78.5	D01.0	D12.0	D37.4	D49.0
pelvirectal	C19	C78.5	D01.1	D12.7	D37.5	D49.0
pelviureteric	C65.-	C79.0-	D09.19	D30.1-	D41.1-	D49.5
rectosigmoid	C19	C78.5	D01.1	D12.7	D37.5	D49.0
squamocolumnar, of cervix	C53.8	C79.82	D06.7	D26.0	D39.0	D49.5
Kaposi's sarcoma — see Kaposi's, sarcoma						
kidney (parenchymal)	C64.-	C79.0-	D09.19	D30.0-	D41.0-	D49.5
calyx	C65.-	C79.0-	D09.19	D30.1-	D41.1-	D49.5
hilus	C65.-	C79.0-	D09.19	D30.1-	D41.1-	D49.5
pelvis	C65.-	C79.0-	D09.19	D30.1-	D41.1-	D49.5
knee NEC	C76.5-	C79.89	D04.7-	D36.7	D48.7	D49.89
labia (skin)	C51.9	C79.82	D07.1	D28.0	D39.8	D49.5
majora	C51.0	C79.82	D07.1	D28.0	D39.8	D49.5
minora	C51.1	C79.82	D07.1	D28.0	D39.8	D49.5
labial — see also Neoplasm, lip	C00.9	C79.89	D00.01	D10.0	D37.01	D49.0
sulcus (lower) (upper)	C06.1	C79.89	D00.02	D10.39	D37.09	D49.0
labium (skin)	C51.9	C79.82	D07.1	D28.0	D39.8	D49.5
majus	C51.0	C79.82	D07.1	D28.0	D39.8	D49.5
minus	C51.1	C79.82	D07.1	D28.0	D39.8	D49.5
lacrimal						
canaliculi	C69.5-	C79.49	D09.2-	D31.5-	D48.7	D49.89
duct (nasal)	C69.5-	C79.49	D09.2-	D31.5-	D48.7	D49.89
gland	C69.5-	C79.49	D09.2-	D31.5-	D48.7	D49.89
punctum	C69.5-	C79.49	D09.2-	D31.5-	D48.7	D49.89
sac	C69.5-	C79.49	D09.2-	D31.5-	D48.7	D49.89
Langerhans, islands or islets	C25.4	C78.89	D01.7	D13.7	D37.8	D49.0
laryngopharynx	C13.9	C79.89	D00.08	D10.7	D37.05	D49.0
larynx, laryngeal NEC	C32.9	C78.39	D02.0	D14.1	D38.0	D49.1
aryepiglottic fold	C32.1	C78.39	D02.0	D14.1	D38.0	D49.1
cartilage (arytenoid) (cricoid) (cuneiform) (thyroid)	C32.3	C78.39	D02.0	D14.1	D38.0	D49.1
commissure (anterior) (posterior)	C32.0	C78.39	D02.0	D14.1	D38.0	D49.1
extrinsic NEC	C32.1	C78.39	D02.0	D14.1	D38.0	D49.1
meaning hypopharynx	C13.9	C79.89	D00.08	D10.7	D37.05	D49.0
interarytenoid fold	C32.1	C78.39	D02.0	D14.1	D38.0	D49.1
intrinsic	C32.0	C78.39	D02.0	D14.1	D38.0	D49.1
overlapping lesion	C32.8	—	—	—	—	—
ventricular band	C32.1	C78.39	D02.0	D14.1	D38.0	D49.1
leg NEC	C76.5-	C79.89	D04.7-	D36.7	D48.7	D49.89

	Malignant Primary	Malignant Secondary	Ca in situ	Benign	Uncertain Behavior	Unspecified Behavior
lens, crystalline	C69.4-	C79.49	D09.2-	D31.4-	D48.7	D49.89
lid (lower) (upper)	C44.10-	C79.2	D04.1-	D23.1-	D48.5	D49.2
basal cell carcinoma	C44.11-	—	—	—	—	—
specified type NEC	C44.19-	—	—	—	—	—
squamous cell carcinoma	C44.12-	—	—	—	—	—
ligament — see also Neoplasm, connective tissue						
broad	C57.1	C79.82	D07.39	D28.2	D39.8	D49.5
Mackenrodt's	C57.7	C79.82	D07.39	D28.7	D39.8	D49.5
non-uterine — see Neoplasm, connective tissue						
round	C57.2	C79.82	—	D28.2	D39.8	D49.5
sacro-uterine	C57.3	C79.82	—	D28.2	D39.8	D49.5
uterine	C57.3	C79.82	—	D28.2	D39.8	D49.5
utero-ovarian	C57.7	C79.82	D07.39	D28.2	D39.8	D49.5
uterosacral	C57.3	C79.82	—	D28.2	D39.8	D49.5
limb	C76.8	C79.89	D04.8	D36.7	D48.7	D49.89
lower	C76.5-	C79.89	D04.7-	D36.7	D48.7	D49.89
upper	C76.4-	C79.89	D04.6-	D36.7	D48.7	D49.89
limbus of cornea	C69.1-	C79.49	D09.2-	D31.1-	D48.7	D49.89
lingual NEC — see also Neoplasm, tongue	C02.9	C79.89	D00.07	D10.1	D37.02	D49.0
lingula, lung	C34.1-	C78.0-	D02.2-	D14.3-	D38.1	D49.1
lip	C00.9	C79.89	D00.01	D10.0	D37.01	D49.0
buccal aspect — see Neoplasm, lip, internal						
commissure	C00.6	C79.89	D00.01	D10.0	D37.01	D49.0
external	C00.2	C79.89	D00.01	D10.0	D37.01	D49.0
lower	C00.1	C79.89	D00.01	D10.0	D37.01	D49.0
upper	C00.0	C79.89	D00.01	D10.0	D37.01	D49.0
frenulum — see Neoplasm, lip, internal						
inner aspect — see Neoplasm, lip, internal						
internal	C00.5	C79.89	D00.01	D10.0	D37.01	D49.0
lower	C00.4	C79.89	D00.01	D10.0	D37.01	D49.0
upper	C00.3	C79.89	D00.01	D10.0	D37.01	D49.0
lipstick area	C00.2	C79.89	D00.01	D10.0	D37.01	D49.0
lower	C00.1	C79.89	D00.01	D10.0	D37.01	D49.0
upper	C00.0	C79.89	D00.01	D10.0	D37.01	D49.0
lower	C00.1	C79.89	D00.01	D10.0	D37.01	D49.0
internal	C00.4	C79.89	D00.01	D10.0	D37.01	D49.0
mucosa — see Neoplasm, lip, internal						
oral aspect — see Neoplasm, lip, internal						
overlapping lesion	C00.8	—	—	—	—	—
with oral cavity or pharynx	C14.8	—	—	—	—	—
skin (commissure) (lower) (upper)	C44.00	C79.2	D04.0	D23.0	D48.5	D49.2
basal cell carcinoma	C44.01	—	—	—	—	—
specified type NEC	C44.09	—	—	—	—	—
squamous cell carcinoma	C44.02	—	—	—	—	—

	Malignant Primary	Malignant Secondary	Ca in situ	Benign	Uncertain Behavior	Unspecified Behavior
lip *(Continued)*						
upper	C00.0	C79.89	D00.01	D10.0	D37.01	D49.0
internal	C00.3	C79.89	D00.01	D10.0	D37.01	D49.0
vermilion border	C00.2	C79.89	D00.01	D10.0	D37.01	D49.0
lower	C00.1	C79.89	D00.01	D10.0	D37.01	D49.0
upper	C00.0	C79.89	D00.01	D10.0	D37.01	D49.0
lipomatous — *see Lipoma, by site*						
liver — *see also Index to disease, by histology*	C22.9	C78.7	D01.5	D13.4	D37.6	D49.0
primary	C22.8	C78.7	D01.5	D13.4	D37.6	D49.0
lumbosacral plexus	C47.5	C79.89	—	D36.16	D48.2	D49.2
lung	C34.9-	C78.0-	D02.2-	D14.3-	D38.1	D49.1
azygos lobe	C34.1-	C78.0-	D02.2-	D14.3-	D38.1	D49.1
carina	C34.0-	C78.0-	D02.2-	D14.3-	D38.1	D49.1
hilus	C34.0-	C78.0-	D02.2-	D14.3-	D38.1	D49.1
lingula	C34.1-	C78.0-	D02.2-	D14.3-	D38.1	D49.1
lobe NEC	C34.9-	C78.0-	D02.2-	D14.3-	D38.1	D49.1
lower lobe	C34.3-	C78.0-	D02.2-	D14.3-	D38.1	D49.1
main bronchus	C34.0-	C78.0-	D02.2-	D14.3-	D38.1	D49.1
mesothelioma — *see Mesothelioma*						
middle lobe	C34.2	C78.0-	D02.21	D14.31	D38.1	D49.1
overlapping lesion	C34.8-	—	—	—	—	—
upper lobe	C34.1-	C78.0-	D02.2-	D14.3-	D38.1	D49.1
lymph, lymphatic channel NEC	C49.9	C79.89	—	D21.9	D48.1	D49.2
gland (secondary)	—	C77.9	—	D36.0	D48.7	D49.89
abdominal	—	C77.2	—	D36.0	D48.7	D49.89
aortic	—	C77.2	—	D36.0	D48.7	D49.89
arm	—	C77.3	—	D36.0	D48.7	D49.89
auricular (anterior) (posterior)	—	C77.0	—	D36.0	D48.7	D49.89
axilla, axillary	—	C77.3	—	D36.0	D48.7	D49.89
brachial	—	C77.3	—	D36.0	D48.7	D49.89
bronchial	—	C77.1	—	D36.0	D48.7	D49.89
bronchopulmonary	—	C77.1	—	D36.0	D48.7	D49.89
celiac	—	C77.2	—	D36.0	D48.7	D49.89
cervical	—	C77.0	—	D36.0	D48.7	D49.89
cervicofacial	—	C77.0	—	D36.0	D48.7	D49.89
Cloquet	—	C77.4	—	D36.0	D48.7	D49.89
colic	—	C77.2	—	D36.0	D48.7	D49.89
common duct	—	C77.2	—	D36.0	D48.7	D49.89
cubital	—	C77.3	—	D36.0	D48.7	D49.89
diaphragmatic	—	C77.1	—	D36.0	D48.7	D49.89
epigastric, inferior	—	C77.1	—	D36.0	D48.7	D49.89
epitrochlear	—	C77.3	—	D36.0	D48.7	D49.89
esophageal	—	C77.1	—	D36.0	D48.7	D49.89
face	—	C77.0	—	D36.0	D48.7	D49.89

	Malignant Primary	Malignant Secondary	Ca in situ	Benign	Uncertain Behavior	Unspecified Behavior
lymph, lymphatic channel NEC *(Continued)*						
gland *(Continued)*						
femoral	—	C77.4	—	D36.0	D48.7	D49.89
gastric	—	C77.2	—	D36.0	D48.7	D49.89
groin	—	C77.4	—	D36.0	D48.7	D49.89
head	—	C77.0	—	D36.0	D48.7	D49.89
hepatic	—	C77.2	—	D36.0	D48.7	D49.89
hilar (pulmonary)	—	C77.1	—	D36.0	D48.7	D49.89
splenic	—	C77.2	—	D36.0	D48.7	D49.89
hypogastric	—	C77.5	—	D36.0	D48.7	D49.89
ileocolic	—	C77.2	—	D36.0	D48.7	D49.89
iliac	—	C77.5	—	D36.0	D48.7	D49.89
infraclavicular	—	C77.3	—	D36.0	D48.7	D49.89
inguina, inguinal	—	C77.4	—	D36.0	D48.7	D49.89
innominate	—	C77.1	—	D36.0	D48.7	D49.89
intercostal	—	C77.1	—	D36.0	D48.7	D49.89
intestinal	—	C77.2	—	D36.0	D48.7	D49.89
intrabdominal	—	C77.2	—	D36.0	D48.7	D49.89
intrapelvic	—	C77.5	—	D36.0	D48.7	D49.89
intrathoracic	—	C77.1	—	D36.0	D48.7	D49.89
jugular	—	C77.0	—	D36.0	D48.7	D49.89
leg	—	C77.4	—	D36.0	D48.7	D49.89
limb						
lower	—	C77.4	—	D36.0	D48.7	D49.89
upper	—	C77.3	—	D36.0	D48.7	D49.89
lower limb	—	C77.4	—	D36.0	D48.7	D49.89
lumbar	—	C77.2	—	D36.0	D48.7	D49.89
mandibular	—	C77.0	—	D36.0	D48.7	D49.89
mediastinal	—	C77.1	—	D36.0	D48.7	D49.89
mesenteric (inferior) (superior)	—	C77.2	—	D36.0	D48.7	D49.89
midcolic	—	C77.2	—	D36.0	D48.7	D49.89
multiple sites in categories C77.0 - C77.5	—	C77.8	—	D36.0	D48.7	D49.89
neck	—	C77.0	—	D36.0	D48.7	D49.89
obturator	—	C77.5	—	D36.0	D48.7	D49.89
occipital	—	C77.0	—	D36.0	D48.7	D49.89
pancreatic	—	C77.2	—	D36.0	D48.7	D49.89
para-aortic	—	C77.2	—	D36.0	D48.7	D49.89
paracervical	—	C77.5	—	D36.0	D48.7	D49.89
parametrial	—	C77.5	—	D36.0	D48.7	D49.89
parasternal	—	C77.1	—	D36.0	D48.7	D49.89
parotid	—	C77.0	—	D36.0	D48.7	D49.89
pectoral	—	C77.3	—	D36.0	D48.7	D49.89
pelvic	—	C77.5	—	D36.0	D48.7	D49.89

	Malignant Primary	Malignant Secondary	Ca in situ	Benign	Uncertain Behavior	Unspecified Behavior
lymph, lymphatic channel NEC *(Continued)*						
gland *(Continued)*						
peri-aortic	—	C77.2	—	D36.0	D48.7	D49.89
peripancreatic	—	C77.2	—	D36.0	D48.7	D49.89
popliteal	—	C77.4	—	D36.0	D48.7	D49.89
porta hepatis	—	C77.2	—	D36.0	D48.7	D49.89
portal	—	C77.2	—	D36.0	D48.7	D49.89
preauricular	—	C77.0	—	D36.0	D48.7	D49.89
prelaryngeal	—	C77.0	—	D36.0	D48.7	D49.89
presymphysial	—	C77.5	—	D36.0	D48.7	D49.89
pretracheal	—	C77.0	—	D36.0	D48.7	D49.89
primary (any site) NEC	C96.9	—	—	—	—	—
pulmonary (hiler)	—	C77.1	—	D36.0	D48.7	D49.89
pyloric	—	C77.2	—	D36.0	D48.7	D49.89
retroperitoneal	—	C77.2	—	D36.0	D48.7	D49.89
retropharyngeal	—	C77.0	—	D36.0	D48.7	D49.89
Rosenmuller's	—	C77.4	—	D36.0	D48.7	D49.89
sacral	—	C77.5	—	D36.0	D48.7	D49.89
scalene	—	C77.0	—	D36.0	D48.7	D49.89
site NEC	—	C77.9	—	D36.0	D48.7	D49.89
splenic (hilar)	—	C77.2	—	D36.0	D48.7	D49.89
subclavicular	—	C77.3	—	D36.0	D48.7	D49.89
subinguinal	—	C77.4	—	D36.0	D48.7	D49.89
sublingual	—	C77.0	—	D36.0	D48.7	D49.89
submandibular	—	C77.0	—	D36.0	D48.7	D49.89
submaxillary	—	C77.0	—	D36.0	D48.7	D49.89
submental	—	C77.0	—	D36.0	D48.7	D49.89
subscapular	—	C77.3	—	D36.0	D48.7	D49.89
supraclavicular	—	C77.0	—	D36.0	D48.7	D49.89
thoracic	—	C77.1	—	D36.0	D48.7	D49.89
tibial	—	C77.4	—	D36.0	D48.7	D49.89
tracheal	—	C77.1	—	D36.0	D48.7	D49.89
tracheobronchial	—	C77.1	—	D36.0	D48.7	D49.89
upper limb	—	C77.3	—	D36.0	D48.7	D49.89
Virchow's	—	C77.0	—	D36.0	D48.7	D49.89
node — *see also Neoplasm, lymph gland*						
primary NEC	C96.9	—	—	—	—	—
vessel — *see also Neoplasm, connective tissue*	C49.9	C79.89	—	D21.9	D48.1	D49.2
Mackenrodt's ligament	C57.7	C79.82	D07.39	D28.7	D39.8	D49.5
malar	C41.0	C79.51	—	D16.4-	D48.0	D49.2
region — *see Neoplasm, cheek*						
mammary gland — *see Neoplasm, breast*						

TABLE OF NEOPLASMS

	Malignant Primary	Malignant Secondary	Ca in situ	Benign	Uncertain Behavior	Unspecified Behavior
mandible	C41.1	C79.51	—	D16.5-	D48.0	D49.2
alveolar						
mucosa (carcinoma)	C03.1	C79.89	D00.03	D10.39	D37.09	D49.0
ridge or process	C41.1	C79.51	—	D16.5-	D48.0	D49.2
marrow (bone) NEC	C96.9	C79.52	—	—	D47.9	D49.89
mastectomy site (skin) — see also Neoplasm, breast, skin	C44.501	C79.2	—	—	—	—
specified as breast tissue	C50.8-	C79.81	—	—	—	—
mastoid (air cells) (antrum) (cavity)	C30.1	C78.39	D02.3	D14.0	D38.5	D49.1
bone or process	C41.0	C79.51	—	D16.4-	D48.0	D49.2
maxilla, maxillary (superior)	C41.0	C79.51	—	D16.4-	D48.0	D49.2
alveolar						
mucosa	C03.0	C79.89	D00.03	D10.39	D37.09	D49.0
ridge or process (carcinoma)	C41.0	C79.51	—	D16.4-	D48.0	D49.2
antrum	C31.0	C78.39	D02.3	D14.0	D38.5	D49.1
carcinoma	C03.0	C79.51	—	—	—	—
inferior — see Neoplasm, mandible						
sinus	C31.0	C78.39	D02.3	D14.0	D38.5	D49.1
meatus external (ear) — see also Neoplasm, skin, ear	C44.20-	C79.2	D04.2-	D23.2-	D48.5	D49.2
Meckel diverticulum, malignant	C17.3	C78.4	D01.49	D13.39	D37.2	D49.0
mediastinum, mediastinal	C38.3	C78.1	—	D15.2	D38.3	D49.89
anterior	C38.1	C78.1	—	D15.2	D38.3	D49.89
posterior	C38.2	C78.1	—	D15.2	D38.3	D49.89
medulla						
adrenal	C74.1-	C79.7-	D09.3	D35.0-	D44.1-	D49.7
oblongata	C71.7	C79.31	—	D33.1	D43.1	D49.6
meibomian gland	C44.10-	C79.2	D04.1-	D23.1-	D48.5	D49.2
basal cell carcinoma	C44.11-	—	—	—	—	—
specified type NEC	C44.19-	—	—	—	—	—
squamous cell carcinoma	C44.12-	—	—	—	—	—
melanoma — see Melanoma						
meninges	C70.9	C79.49	—	D32.9	D42.9	D49.7
brain	C70.0	C79.32	—	D32.0	D42.0	D49.7
cerebral	C70.0	C79.32	—	D32.0	D42.0	D49.7
crainial	C70.0	C79.32	—	D32.0	D42.0	D49.7
intracranial	C70.0	C79.32	—	D32.0	D42.0	D49.7
spinal (cord)	C70.1	C79.49	—	D32.1	D42.1	D49.7
meniscus, knee joint (lateral) (medial)	C40.2-	C79.51	—	D16.2-	D48.0	D49.2
Merkel cell — see Carcinoma, Merkel cell						
mesentery, mesenteric	C48.1	C78.6	—	D20.1	D48.4	D49.0
mesoappendix	C48.1	C78.6	—	D20.1	D48.4	D49.0
mesocolon	C48.1	C78.6	—	D20.1	D48.4	D49.0
mesopharynx — see Neoplasm, oropharynx						
mesosalpinx	C57.1	C79.82	D07.39	D28.2	D39.8	D49.5

	Malignant Primary	Malignant Secondary	Ca in situ	Benign	Uncertain Behavior	Unspecified Behavior
mesothelial tissue — *see Mesothelioma*						
mesothelioma — *see Mesothelioma*						
mesovarium	C57.1	C79.82	D07.39	D28.2	D39.8	D49.5
metacarpus (any bone)	C40.1-	C79.51	—	D16.1-	—	—
metastatic NEC — *see also Neoplasm, by site, secondary*	—	C79.9	—	—	—	—
metatarsus (any bone)	C40.3-	C79.51	—	D16.3-	—	—
midbrain	C71.7	C79.31	—	D33.1	D43.1	D49.6
milk duct — *see Neoplasm, breast*						
mons						
pubis	C51.9	C79.82	D07.1	D28.0	D39.8	D49.5
veneris	C51.9	C79.82	D07.1	D28.0	D39.8	D49.5
motor tract	C72.9	C79.49	—	D33.9	D43.9	D49.7
brain	C71.9	C79.31	—	D33.2	D43.2	D49.6
cauda equina	C72.1	C79.49	—	D33.4	D43.4	D49.7
spinal	C72.0	C79.49	—	D33.4	D43.4	D49.7
mouth	C06.9	C79.89	D00.00	D10.30	D37.09	D49.0
book-leaf	C06.89	C79.89	—	—	—	—
floor	C04.9	C79.89	D00.06	D10.2	D37.09	D49.0
anterior portion	C04.0	C79.89	D00.06	D10.2	D37.09	D49.0
lateral portion	C04.1	C79.89	D00.06	D10.2	D37.09	D49.0
overlapping lesion	C04.8	—	—	—	—	—
overlapping NEC	C06.80	—	—	—	—	—
roof	C05.9	C79.89	D00.00	D10.39	D37.09	D49.0
specified part NEC	C06.89	C79.89	D00.00	D10.39	D37.09	D49.0
vestibule	C06.1	C79.89	D00.00	D10.39	D37.09	D49.0
mucosa						
alveolar (ridge or process)	C03.9	C79.89	D00.03	D10.39	D37.09	D49.0
lower	C03.1	C79.89	D00.03	D10.39	D37.09	D49.0
upper	C03.0	C79.89	D00.03	D10.39	D37.09	D49.0
buccal	C06.0	C79.89	D00.02	D10.39	D37.09	D49.0
cheek	C06.0	C79.89	D00.02	D10.39	D37.09	D49.0
lip — *see Neoplasm, lip, internal*						
nasal	C30.0	C78.39	D02.3	D14.0	D38.5	D49.1
oral	C06.0	C79.89	D00.02	D10.39	D37.09	D49.0
Mullerian duct						
female	C57.7	C79.82	D07.39	D28.7	D39.8	D49.5
male	C63.7	C79.82	D07.69	D29.8	D40.8	D49.5
muscle — *see also Neoplasm, connective tissue*						
extraocular	C69.6-	C79.49	D09.2-	D31.6-	D48.7	D49.89
myocardium	C38.0	C79.89	—	D15.1	D48.7	D49.89
myometrium	C54.2	C79.82	D07.0	D26.1	D39.0	D49.5
myopericardium	C38.0	C79.89	—	D15.1	D48.7	D49.89
nabothian gland (follicle)	C53.0	C79.82	D06.0	D26.0	D39.0	D49.5

TABLE OF NEOPLASMS

	Malignant Primary	Malignant Secondary	Ca in situ	Benign	Uncertain Behavior	Unspecified Behavior
nail — *see also Neoplasm, skin, limb*	C44.90	C79.2	D04.9	D23.9	D48.5	D49.2
finger — *see also Neoplasm, skin, limb, upper*	C44.60-	C79.2	D04.6-	D23.6-	D48.5	D49.2
toe — *see also Neoplasm, skin, limb, lower*	C44.70-	C79.2	D04.7-	D23.7-	D48.5	D49.2
nares, naris (anterior) (posterior)	C30.0	C78.39	D02.3	D14.0	D38.5	D49.1
nasal — *see Neoplasm, nose*						
nasolabial groove — *see also Neoplasm, skin, face*	C44.309	C79.2	D04.39	D23.39	D48.5	D49.2
nasolacrimal duct	C69.5-	C79.49	D09.2-	D31.5-	D48.7	D49.89
nasopharynx, nasopharyngeal	C11.9	C79.89	D00.08	D10.6	D37.05	D49.0
floor	C11.3	C79.89	D00.08	D10.6	D37.05	D49.0
overlapping lesion	C11.8	—	—	—	—	—
roof	C11.0	C79.89	D00.08	D10.6	D37.05	D49.0
wall	C11.9	C79.89	D00.08	D10.6	D37.05	D49.0
anterior	C11.3	C79.89	D00.08	D10.6	D37.05	D49.0
lateral	C11.2	C79.89	D00.08	D10.6	D37.05	D49.0
posterior	C11.1	C79.89	D00.08	D10.6	D37.05	D49.0
superior	C11.0	C79.89	D00.08	D10.6	D37.05	D49.0
nates — *see also Neoplasm, skin, trunk*	C44.509	C79.2	D04.5	D23.5	D48.5	D49.2
neck NEC	C76.0	C79.89	D09.8	D36.7	D48.7	D49.89
skin	C44.40	—	—	—	—	—
basal cell carcinoma	C44.41	—	—	—	—	—
specified type NEC	C44.49	—	—	—	—	—
squamous cell carcinoma	C44.42	—	—	—	—	—
nerve (ganglion)	C47.9	C79.89	—	D36.10	D48.2	D49.2
abducens	C72.59	C79.49	—	D33.3	D43.3	D49.7
accessory (spinal)	C72.59	C79.49	—	D33.3	D43.3	D49.7
acoustic	C72.4-	C79.49	—	D33.3	D43.3	D49.7
auditory	C72.4-	C79.49	—	D33.3	D43.3	D49.7
autonomic NEC — *see also Neoplasm, nerve, peripheral*	C47.9	C79.89	—	D36.10	D48.2	D49.2
brachial	C47.1-	C79.89	—	D36.12	D48.2	D49.2
cranial	C72.50	C79.49	—	D33.3	D43.3	D49.7
specified NEC	C72.59	C79.49	—	D33.3	D43.3	D49.7
facial	C72.59	C79.49	—	D33.3	D43.3	D49.7
femoral	C47.2-	C79.89	—	D36.13	D48.2	D49.2
ganglion NEC — *see also Neoplasm, nerve, peripheral*	C47.9	C79.89	—	D36.10	D48.2	D49.2
glossopharyngeal	C72.59	C79.49	—	D33.3	D43.3	D49.7
hypoglossal	C72.59	C79.49	—	D33.3	D43.3	D49.7
intercostal	C47.3	C79.89	—	D36.14	D48.2	D49.2
lumbar	C47.6	C79.89	—	D36.17	D48.2	D49.2
median	C47.1-	C79.89	—	D36.12	D48.2	D49.2
obturator	C47.2-	C79.89	—	D36.13	D48.2	D49.2
oculomotor	C72.59	C79.49	—	D33.3	D43.3	D49.7
olfactory	C47.2-	C79.49	—	D33.3	D43.3	D49.7
optic	C72.3-	C79.49	—	D33.3	D43.3	D49.7
parasympathetic NEC	C47.9	C79.89	—	D36.10	D48.2	D49.2

	Malignant Primary	Malignant Secondary	Ca in situ	Benign	Uncertain Behavior	Unspecified Behavior
nerve *(Continued)*						
peripheral NEC	C47.9	C79.89	—	D36.10	D48.2	D49.2
abdomen	C47.4	C79.89	—	D36.15	D48.2	D49.2
abdominal wall	C47.4	C79.89	—	D36.15	D48.2	D49.2
ankle	C47.2-	C79.89	—	D36.13	D48.2	D49.2
antecubital fossa or space	C47.1-	C79.89	—	D36.12	D48.2	D49.2
arm	C47.1-	C79.89	—	D36.12	D48.2	D49.2
auricle (ear)	C47.0	C79.89	—	D36.11	D48.2	D49.2
axilla	C47.3	C79.89	—	D36.12	D48.2	D49.2
back	C47.6	C79.89	—	D36.17	D48.2	D49.2
buttock	C47.5	C79.89	—	D36.16	D48.2	D49.2
calf	C47.2-	C79.89	—	D36.13	D48.2	D49.2
cervical region	C47.0	C79.89	—	D36.11	D48.2	D49.2
cheek	C47.0	C79.89	—	D36.11	D48.2	D49.2
chest (wall)	C47.3	C79.89	—	D36.14	D48.2	D49.2
chin	C47.0	C79.89	—	D36.11	D48.2	D49.2
ear (external)	C47.0	C79.89	—	D36.11	D48.2	D49.2
elbow	C47.1-	C79.89	—	D36.12	D48.2	D49.2
extrarectal	C47.5	C79.89	—	D36.16	D48.2	D49.2
extremity	C47.9	C79.89	—	D36.10	D48.2	D49.2
lower	C47.2-	C79.89	—	D36.13	D48.2	D49.2
upper	C47.1-	C79.89	—	D36.12	D48.2	D49.2
eyelid	C47.0	C79.89	—	D36.11	D48.2	D49.2
face	C47.0	C79.89	—	D36.11	D48.2	D49.2
finger	C47.1-	C79.89	—	D36.12	D48.2	D49.2
flank	C47.6	C79.89	—	D36.17	D48.2	D49.2
foot	C47.2-	C79.89	—	D36.13	D48.2	D49.2
forearm	C47.1-	C79.89	—	D36.12	D48.2	D49.2
forehead	C47.0	C79.89	—	D36.11	D48.2	D49.2
gluteal region	C47.5	C79.89	—	D36.16	D48.2	D49.2
groin	C47.5	C79.89	—	D36.16	D48.2	D49.2
hand	C47.1-	C79.89	—	D36.12	D48.2	D49.2
head	C47.0	C79.89	—	D36.11	D48.2	D49.2
heel	C47.2-	C79.89	—	D36.13	D48.2	D49.2
hip	C47.2-	C79.89	—	D36.13	D48.2	D49.2
infraclavicular region	C47.3	C79.89	—	D36.14	D48.2	D49.2
inguinal (canal) (region)	C47.5	C79.89	—	D36.16	D48.2	D49.2
intrathoracic	C47.3	C79.89	—	D36.14	D48.2	D49.2
ischiorectal fossa	C47.5	C79.89	—	D36.16	D48.2	D49.2
knee	C47.2-	C79.89	—	D36.13	D48.2	D49.2
leg	C47.2-	C79.89	—	D36.13	D48.2	D49.2
limb NEC	C47.9	C79.89	—	D36.10	D48.2	D49.2
lower	C47.2-	C79.89	—	D36.13	D48.2	D49.2
upper	C47.1-	C79.89	—	D36.12	D48.2	D49.2

	Malignant Primary	Malignant Secondary	Ca in situ	Benign	Uncertain Behavior	Unspecified Behavior
nerve *(Continued)*						
peripheral NEC *(Continued)*						
nates	C47.5	C79.89	—	D36.16	D48.2	D49.2
neck	C47.0	C79.89	—	D36.11	D48.2	D49.2
orbit	C69.6-	C79.49	—	D31.6-	D48.7	D49.2
pararectal	C47.5	C79.89	—	D36.16	D48.2	D49.2
paraurethral	C47.5	C79.89	—	D36.16	D48.2	D49.2
paravaginal	C47.5	C79.89	—	D36.16	D48.2	D49.2
pelvis (floor)	C47.5	C79.89	—	D36.16	D48.2	D49.2
pelvoabdominal	C47.8	C79.89	—	D36.17	D48.2	D49.2
perineum	C47.5	C79.89	—	D36.16	D48.2	D49.2
perirectal (tissue)	C47.5	C79.89	—	D36.16	D48.2	D49.2
periurethral (tissue)	C47.5	C79.89	—	D36.16	D48.2	D49.2
popliteal fossa or space	C47.2-	C79.89	—	D36.13	D48.2	D49.2
presacral	C47.5	C79.89	—	D36.16	D48.2	D49.2
pterygoid fossa	C47.0	C79.89	—	D36.11	D48.2	D49.2
rectovaginal septum or wall	C47.5	C79.89	—	D36.16	D48.2	D49.2
rectovesical	C47.5	C79.89	—	D36.16	D48.2	D49.2
sacrococcygeal region	C47.5	C79.89	—	D36.16	D48.2	D49.2
scalp	C47.0	C79.89	—	D36.11	D48.2	D49.2
scapular region	C47.3	C79.89	—	D36.14	D48.2	D49.2
shoulder	C47.1-	C79.89	—	D36.12	D48.2	D49.2
submental	C47.0	C79.89	—	D36.11	D48.2	D49.2
supraclavicular region	C47.0	C79.89	—	D36.11	D48.2	D49.2
temple	C47.0	C79.89	—	D36.11	D48.2	D49.2
temporal region	C47.0	C79.89	—	D36.11	D48.2	D49.2
thigh	C47.2-	C79.89	—	D36.13	D48.2	D49.2
thoracic (duct) (wall)	C47.3	C79.89	—	D36.14	D48.2	D49.2
thorax	C47.3	C79.89	—	D36.14	D48.2	D49.2
thumb	C47.1-	C79.89	—	D36.12	D48.2	D49.2
toe	C47.2-	C79.89	—	D36.13	D48.2	D49.2
trunk	C47.6	C79.89	—	D36.17	D48.2	D49.2
umbilicus	C47.4	C79.89	—	D36.15	D48.2	D49.2
vesicorectal	C47.5	C79.89	—	D36.16	D48.2	D49.2
wrist	C47.1-	C79.89	—	D36.12	D48.2	D49.2
radial	C47.1-	C79.89	—	D36.12	D48.2	D49.2
sacral	C47.5	C79.89	—	D36.16	D48.2	D49.2
sciatic	C47.2-	C79.89	—	D36.13	D48.2	D49.2
spinal NEC	C47.9	C79.89	—	D36.10	D48.2	D49.2
accessory	C72.59	C79.49	—	D33.3	D43.3	D49.7
sympathetic NEC — *see also Neoplasm, nerve, peripheral*	C47.9	C79.89	—	D36.10	D48.2	D49.2
trigeminal	C72.59	C79.49	—	D33.3	D43.3	D49.7
trochlear	C72.59	C79.49	—	D33.3	D43.3	D49.7

	Malignant Primary	Malignant Secondary	Ca in situ	Benign	Uncertain Behavior	Unspecified Behavior
nerve *(Continued)*						
ulnar	C47.1-	C79.89	—	D36.12	D48.2	D49.2
vagus	C72.59	C79.49	—	D33.3	D43.3	D49.7
nervous system (central)	C72.9	C79.40	—	D33.9	D43.9	D49.7
autonomic — *see Neoplasm, nerve, peripheral*						
parasympathetic — *see Neoplasm, nerve, peripheral*						
specified site NEC	—	C79.49	—	D33.7	D43.8	—
sympathetic — *see Neoplasm, nerve, peripheral*						
nevus — *see Nevus*						
nipple	C50.0-	C79.81	D05.-	D24.-	—	—
nose, nasal	C76.0	C79.89	D09.8	D36.7	D48.7	D49.89
ala (external) (nasi) — *see also Neoplasm, nose, skin*	C44.301	C79.2	D04.39	D23.39	D48.5	D49.2
bone	C41.0	C79.51	—	D16.4-	D48.0	D49.2
cartilage	C30.0	C78.39	D02.3	D14.0	D38.5	D49.1
cavity	C30.0	C78.39	D02.3	D14.0	D38.5	D49.1
choana	C11.3	C79.89	D00.08	D10.6	D37.05	D49.0
external (skin) — *see also Neoplasm, nose, skin*	C44.301	C79.2	D04.39	D23.39	D48.5	D49.2
fossa	C30.0	C78.39	D02.3	D14.0	D38.5	D49.1
internal	C30.0	C78.39	D02.3	D14.0	D38.5	D49.1
mucosa	C30.0	C78.39	D02.3	D14.0	D38.5	D49.1
septum	C30.0	C78.39	D02.3	D14.0	D38.5	D49.1
posterior margin	C11.3	C79.89	D00.08	D10.6	D37.05	D49.0
sinus — *see Neoplasm, sinus*						
skin	C44.301	C79.2	D04.39	D23.39	D48.5	D49.2
basal cell carcinoma	C44.311	—	—	—	—	—
specified type NEC	C44.391	—	—	—	—	—
squamous cell carcinoma	C44.321	—	—	—	—	—
turbinate (mucosa)	C30.0	C78.39	D02.3	D14.0	D38.5	D49.1
bone	C41.0	C79.51	—	D16.4-	D48.0	D49.2
vestibule	C30.0	C78.39	D02.3	D14.0	D38.5	D49.1
nostril	C30.0	C78.39	D02.3	D14.0	D38.5	D49.1
nucleus pulposus	C41.2	C79.51	—	D16.6	D48.0	D49.2
occipital						
bone	C41.0	C79.51	—	D16.4-	D48.0	D49.2
lobe or pole, brain	C71.4	C79.31	—	D33.0	D43.0	D49.6
odontogenic — *see Neoplasm, jaw bone*						
olfactory nerve or bulb	C72.2-	C79.49	—	D33.3	D43.3	D49.7
olive (brain)	C71.7	C79.31	—	D33.1	D43.1	D49.6
omentum	C48.1	C78.6	—	D20.1	D48.4	D49.0
operculum (brain)	C71.0	C79.31	—	D33.0	D43.0	D49.6
optic nerve, chiasm, or tract	C72.3-	C79.49	—	D33.3	D43.3	D49.7
oral (cavity)	C06.9	C79.89	D00.00	D10.30	D37.09	D49.0
ill-defined	C14.8	C79.89	D00.00	D10.30	D37.09	D49.0
mucosa	C06.0	C79.89	D00.02	D10.39	D37.09	D49.0

	Malignant Primary	Malignant Secondary	Ca in situ	Benign	Uncertain Behavior	Unspecified Behavior
orbit	C69.6-	C79.49	D09.2-	D31.6-	D48.7	D49.89
autonomic nerve	C69.6-	C79.49	—	D31.6-	D48.7	D49.2
bone	C41.0	C79.51	—	D16.4-	D48.0	D49.2
eye	C69.6-	C79.49	D09.2-	D31.6-	D48.7	D49.89
peripheral nerves	C69.6-	C79.49	—	D31.6-	D48.7	D49.2
soft parts	C69.6-	C79.49	D09.2-	D31.6-	D48.7	D49.89
organ of Zuckerkandl	C75.5	C79.89	—	D35.6	D44.7	D49.7
oropharynx	C10.9	C79.89	D00.08	D10.5	D37.05	D49.0
branchial cleft (vestige)	C10.4	C79.89	D00.08	D10.5	D37.05	D49.0
junctional region	C10.8	C79.89	D00.08	D10.5	D37.05	D49.0
lateral wall	C10.2	C79.89	D00.08	D10.5	D37.05	D49.0
overlapping lesion	C10.8	—	—	—	—	—
pillars or fauces	C09.1	C79.89	D00.08	D10.5	D37.05	D49.0
posterior wall	C10.3	C79.89	D00.08	D10.5	D37.05	D49.0
vallecula	C10.0	C79.89	D00.08	D10.5	D37.05	D49.0
os						
external	C53.1	C79.82	D06.1	D26.0	D39.0	D49.5
internal	C53.0	C79.82	D06.0	D26.0	D39.0	D49.5
ovary	C56.-	C79.6-	D07.39	D27.-	D39.1-	D49.5
oviduct	C57.0-	C79.82	D07.39	D28.2	D39.8	D49.5
palate	C05.9	C79.89	D00.00	D10.39	D37.09	D49.0
hard	C05.0	C79.89	D00.05	D10.39	D37.09	D49.0
junction of hard and soft palate	C05.9	C79.89	D00.00	D10.39	D37.09	D49.0
overlapping lesions	C05.8	—	—	—	—	—
soft	C05.1	C79.89	D00.04	D10.39	D37.09	D49.0
nasopharyngeal surface	C11.3	C79.89	D00.08	D10.6	D37.05	D49.0
posterior surface	C11.3	C79.89	D00.08	D10.6	D37.05	D49.0
superior surface	C11.3	C79.89	D00.08	D10.6	D37.05	D49.0
palatoglossal arch	C09.1	C79.89	D00.00	D10.5	D37.09	D49.0
palatopharyngeal arch	C09.1	C79.89	D00.00	D10.5	D37.09	D49.0
pallium	C71.0	C79.31	—	D33.0	D43.0	D49.6
palpebra	C44.10-	C79.2	D04.1-	D23.1-	D48.5	D49.2
basal cell carcinoma	C44.11-	—	—	—	—	—
specified type NEC	C44.19-	—	—	—	—	—
squamous cell carcinoma	C44.12-	—	—	—	—	—
pancreas	C25.9	C78.89	D01.7	D13.6	D37.8	D49.0
body	C25.1	C78.89	D01.7	D13.6	D37.8	D49.0
duct (of Santorini) (of Wirsung)	C25.3	C78.89	D01.7	D13.6	D37.8	D49.0
ectopic tissue	C25.7	C78.89	—	D13.6	D37.8	D49.0
head	C25.0	C78.89	D01.7	D13.6	D37.8	D49.0
islet cells	C25.4	C78.89	D01.7	D13.7	D37.8	D49.0
neck	C25.7	C78.89	D01.7	D13.6	D37.8	D49.0
overlapping lesion	C25.8	—	—	—	—	—
tail	C25.2	C78.89	D01.7	D13.6	D37.8	D49.0

	Malignant Primary	Malignant Secondary	Ca in situ	Benign	Uncertain Behavior	Unspecified Behavior
para-aortic body	C75.5	C79.89	—	D35.6	D44.7	D49.7
paraganglion NEC	C75.5	C79.89	—	D35.6	D44.7	D49.7
parametrium	C57.3	C79.82	—	D28.2	D39.8	D49.5
paranephric	C48.0	C78.6	—	D20.0	D48.3	D49.0
pararectal	C76.3	C79.89	—	D36.7	D48.7	D49.89
parasagittal (region)	C76.0	C79.89	D09.8	D36.7	D48.7	D49.89
parasellar	C72.9	C79.49	—	D33.9	D43.8	D49.7
parathyroid (gland)	C75.0	C79.89	D09.3	D35.1	D44.2	D49.7
paraurethral	C76.3	C79.89	—	D36.7	D48.7	D49.89
gland	C68.1	C79.19	D09.19	D30.8	D41.8	D49.5
paravaginal	C76.3	C79.89	—	D36.7	D48.7	D49.89
parenchyma, kidney	C64.-	C79.0-	D09.19	D30.0-	D41.0-	D49.5
parietal						
bone	C41.0	C79.51	—	D16.4-	D48.0	D49.2
lobe, brain	C71.3	C79.31	—	D33.0	D43.0	D49.6
paroophoron	C57.1	C79.82	D07.39	D28.2	D39.8	D49.5
parotid (duct) (gland)	C07	C79.89	D00.00	D11.0	D37.030	D49.0
parovarium	C57.1	C79.82	D07.39	D28.2	D39.8	D49.5
patella	C40.20	C79.51	—	—	—	—
peduncle, cerebral	C71.7	C79.31	—	D33.1	D43.1	D49.6
pelvirectal junction	C19	C78.5	D01.1	D12.7	D37.5	D49.0
pelvis, pelvic	C76.3	C79.89	D09.8	D36.7	D48.7	D49.89
bone	C41.4	C79.51	—	D16.8	D48.0	D49.2
floor	C76.3	C79.89	D09.8	D36.7	D48.7	D49.89
renal	C65.-	C79.0-	D09.19	D30.1-	D41.1-	D49.5
viscera	C76.3	C79.89	D09.8	D36.7	D48.7	D49.89
wall	C76.3	C79.89	D09.8	D36.7	D48.7	D49.89
pelvo-abdominal	C76.8	C79.89	D09.8	D36.7	D48.7	D49.89
penis	C60.9	C79.82	D07.4	D29.0	D40.8	D49.5
body	C60.2	C79.82	D07.4	D29.0	D40.8	D49.5
corpus (cavernosum)	C60.2	C79.82	D07.4	D29.0	D40.8	D49.5
glans	C60.1	C79.82	D07.4	D29.0	D40.8	D49.5
overlapping sites	C60.8	—	—	—	—	—
skin NEC	C60.9	C79.82	D07.4	D29.0	D40.8	D49.5
periadrenal (tissue)	C48.0	C78.6	—	D20.0	D48.3	D49.0
perianal (skin) — see also Neoplasm, anus, skin	C44.500	C79.2	D04.5	D23.5	D48.5	D49.2
pericardium	C38.0	C79.89	—	D15.1	D48.7	D49.89
perinephric	C48.0	C78.6	—	D20.0	D48.3	D49.0
perineum	C76.3	C79.89	D09.8	D36.7	D48.7	D49.89
periodontal tissue NEC	C03.9	C79.89	D00.03	D10.39	D37.09	D49.0
periosteum — see Neoplasm, bone						
peripancreatic	C48.0	C78.6	—	D20.0	D48.3	D49.0
peripheral nerve NEC	C47.9	C79.89	—	D36.10	D48.2	D49.2
perirectal (tissue)	C76.3	C79.89	—	D36.7	D48.7	D49.89

533

	Malignant Primary	Malignant Secondary	Ca in situ	Benign	Uncertain Behavior	Unspecified Behavior
perirenal (tissue)	C48.0	C78.6	—	D20.0	D48.3	D49.0
peritoneum, peritoneal (cavity)	C48.2	C78.6	—	D20.1	D48.4	D49.0
benign mesothelial tissue — see Mesothelioma, benign						
overlapping lesion	C48.8	—	—	—	—	—
with digestive organs	C26.9	—	—	—	—	—
parietal	C48.1	C78.6	—	D20.1	D48.4	D49.0
pelvic	C48.1	C78.6	—	D20.1	D48.4	D49.0
specified part NEC	C48.1	C78.6	—	D20.1	D48.4	D49.0
peritonsillar (tissue)	C76.0	C79.89	D09.8	D36.7	D48.7	D49.89
periurethral tissue	C76.3	C79.89	—	D36.7	D48.7	D49.89
phalanges						
foot	C40.3-	C79.51	—	D16.3-	—	—
hand	C40.1-	C79.51	—	D16.1-	—	—
pharynx, pharyngeal	C14.0	C79.89	D00.08	D10.9	D37.05	D49.0
bursa	C11.1	C79.89	D00.08	D10.6	D37.05	D49.0
fornix	C11.3	C79.89	D00.08	D10.6	D37.05	D49.0
recess	C11.2	C79.89	D00.08	D10.6	D37.05	D49.0
region	C14.0	C79.89	D00.08	D10.9	D37.05	D49.0
tonsil	C11.1	C79.89	D00.08	D10.6	D37.05	D49.0
wall (lateral) (posterior)	C14.0	C79.89	D00.08	D10.9	D37.05	D49.0
pia mater	C70.9	C79.40	—	D32.9	D42.9	D49.7
cerebral	C70.0	C79.32	—	D32.0	D42.0	D49.7
cranial	C70.0	C79.32	—	D32.0	D42.0	D49.7
spinal	C70.1	C79.49	—	D32.1	D42.1	D49.7
pillars of fauces	C09.1	C79.89	D00.08	D10.5	D37.05	D49.0
pineal (body) (gland)	C75.3	C79.89	D09.3	D35.4	D44.5	D49.7
pinna (ear) NEC — see also Neoplasm, skin, ear	C44.20-	C79.2	D04.2-	D23.2-	D48.5	D49.2
piriform fossa or sinus	C12	C79.89	D00.08	D10.7	D37.05	D49.0
pituitary (body) (fossa) (gland) (lobe)	C75.1	C79.89	D09.3	D35.2	D44.3	D49.7
placenta	C58	C79.82	D07.0	D26.7	D39.2	D49.5
pleura, pleural (cavity)	C38.4	C78.2	—	D19.0	D38.2	D49.1
overlapping lesion with heart or mediastinum	C38.8	—	—	—	—	—
parietal	C38.4	C78.2	—	D19.0	D38.2	D49.1
visceral	C38.4	C78.2	—	D19.0	D38.2	D49.1
plexus						
brachial	C47.1-	C79.89	—	D36.12	D48.2	D49.2
cervical	C47.0	C79.89	—	D36.11	D48.2	D49.2
choroid	C71.5	C79.31	—	D33.0	D43.0	D49.6
lumbosacral	C47.5	C79.89	—	D36.16	D48.2	D49.2
sacral	C47.5	C79.89	—	D36.16	D48.2	D49.2
pluriendocrine	C75.8	C79.89	D09.3	D35.7	D44.9	D49.7
pole						
frontal	C71.1	C79.31	—	D33.0	D43.0	D49.6
occipital	C71.4	C79.31	—	D33.0	D43.0	D49.6

	Malignant Primary	Malignant Secondary	Ca in situ	Benign	Uncertain Behavior	Unspecified Behavior
pons (varolii)	C71.7	C79.31	—	D33.1	D43.1	D49.6
popliteal fossa or space	C76.5-	C79.89	D04.7-	D36.7	D48.7	D49.89
postcricoid (region)	C13.0	C79.89	D00.08	D10.7	D37.05	D49.0
posterior fossa (cranial)	C71.9	C79.31	—	D33.2	D43.2	D49.6
postnasal space	C11.9	C79.89	D00.08	D10.6	D37.05	D49.0
prepuce	C60.0	C79.82	D07.4	D29.0	D40.8	D49.5
prepylorus	C16.4	C78.89	D00.2	D13.1	D37.1	D49.0
presacral (region)	C76.3	C79.89	—	D36.7	D48.7	D49.89
prostate (gland)	C61	C79.82	D07.5	D29.1	D40.0	D49.5
utricle	C68.0	C79.19	D09.19	D30.4	D41.3	D49.5
pterygoid fossa	C49.0	C79.89	—	D21.0	D48.1	D49.2
pubic bone	C41.4	C79.51	—	D16.8	D48.0	D49.2
pudenda, pudendum (female)	C51.9	C79.82	D07.1	D28.0	D39.8	D49.5
pulmonary — see also Neoplasm, lung	C34.9-	C78.0-	D02.2-	D14.3-	D38.1	D49.1
putamen	C71.0	C79.31	—	D33.0	D43.0	D49.6
pyloric						
antrum	C16.3	C78.89	D00.2	D13.1	D37.1	D49.0
canal	C16.4	C78.89	D00.2	D13.1	D37.1	D49.0
pylorus	C16.4	C78.89	D00.2	D13.1	D37.1	D49.0
pyramid (brain)	C71.7	C79.31	—	D33.1	D43.1	D49.6
pyriform fossa or sinus	C12	C79.89	D00.08	D10.7	D37.05	D49.0
radius (any part)	C40.0-	C79.51	—	D16.0-	—	—
Rathke's pouch	C75.1	C79.89	D09.3	D35.2	D44.3	D49.7
rectosigmoid (junction)	C19	C78.5	D01.1	D12.7	D37.5	D49.0
overlapping lesion with anus or rectum	C21.8	—	—	—	—	—
rectouterine pouch	C48.1	C78.6	—	D20.1	D48.4	D49.0
rectovaginal septum or wall	C76.3	C79.89	D09.8	D36.7	D48.7	D49.89
rectovesical septum	C76.3	C79.89	D09.8	D36.7	D48.7	D49.89
rectum (ampulla)	C20	C78.5	D01.2	D12.8	D37.5	D49.0
and colon	C19	C78.5	D01.1	D12.7	D37.5	D49.0
overlapping lesion with anus or rectosigmoid junction	C21.8	—	—	—	—	—
renal	C64.-	C79.0-	D09.19	D30.0-	D41.0-	D49.5
calyx	C65.-	C79.0-	D09.19	D30.1-	D41.1-	D49.5
hilus	C65.-	C79.0-	D09.19	D30.1-	D41.1-	D49.5
parenchyma	C64.-	C79.0-	D09.19	D30.0-	D41.0-	D49.5
pelvis	C65.-	C79.0-	D09.19	D30.1-	D41.1-	D49.5
respiratory						
organs or system NEC	C39.9	C78.30	D02.4	D14.4	D38.6	D49.1
tract NEC	C39.9	C78.30	D02.4	D14.4	D38.5	D49.1
upper	C39.0	C78.30	D02.4	D14.4	D38.5	D49.1
retina	C69.2-	C79.49	D09.2-	D31.2-	D48.7	D49.81
retrobulbar	C69.6-	C79.49	—	D31.6-	D48.7	D49.89
retrocecal	C48.0	C78.6	—	D20.0	D48.3	D49.0
retromolar (area) (triangle) (trigone)	C06.2	C79.89	D00.00	D10.39	D37.09	D49.0

	Malignant Primary	Malignant Secondary	Ca in situ	Benign	Uncertain Behavior	Unspecified Behavior
retro-orbital	C76.0	C79.89	D09.8	D36.7	D48.7	D49.89
retroperitoneal (space) (tissue)	C48.0	C78.6	—	D20.0	D48.3	D49.0
retroperitoneum	C48.0	C78.6	—	D20.0	D48.3	D49.0
retropharyngeal	C14.0	C79.89	D00.08	D10.9	D37.05	D49.0
retrovesical (septum)	C76.3	C79.89	D09.8	D36.7	D48.7	D49.89
rhinencephalon	C71.0	C79.31	—	D33.0	D43.0	D49.6
rib	C41.3	C79.51	—	D16.7	D48.0	D49.2
Rosenmuller's fossa	C11.2	C79.89	D00.08	D10.6	D37.05	D49.0
round ligament	C57.2	C79.82	—	D28.2	D39.8	D49.5
sacrococcyx, sacrococcygeal	C41.4	C79.51	—	D16.8	D48.0	D49.2
region	C76.3	C79.89	D09.8	D36.7	D48.7	D49.89
sacrouterine ligament	C57.3	C79.82	—	D28.2	D39.8	D49.5
sacrum, sacral (vertebra)	C41.4	C79.51	—	D16.8	D48.0	D49.2
salivary gland or duct (major)	C08.9	C79.89	D00.00	D11.9	D37.039	D49.0
minor NEC	C06.9	C79.89	D00.00	D10.39	D37.04	D49.0
overlapping lesion	C08.9	—	—	—	—	—
parotid	C07	C79.89	D00.00	D11.0	D37.030	D49.0
pluriglandular	C08.9	C79.89	D00.00	D11.9	D37.039	D49.0
sublingual	C08.1	C79.89	D00.00	D11.7	D37.031	D49.0
submandibular	C08.0	C79.89	D00.00	D11.7	D37.032	D49.0
submaxillary	C08.0	C79.89	D00.00	D11.7	D37.032	D49.0
salpinx (uterine)	C57.0-	C79.82	D07.39	D28.2	D39.8	D49.5
Santorini's duct	C25.3	C78.89	D01.7	D13.6	D37.8	D49.0
scalp	C44.40	C79.2	D04.4	D23.4	D48.5	D49.2
basal cell carcinoma	C44.41	—	—	—	—	—
specified type NEC	C44.49	—	—	—	—	—
squamous cell carcinoma	C44.42	—	—	—	—	—
scapula (any part)	C40.0-	C79.51	—	D16.0-	—	—
scapular region	C76.1	C79.89	D09.8	D36.7	D48.7	D49.89
scar NEC — see also Neoplasm, skin, by site	C44.90	C79.2	D04.9	D23.9	D48.5	D49.2
sciatic nerve	C47.2-	C79.89	—	D36.13	D48.2	D49.2
sclera	C69.4-	C79.49	D09.2-	D31.4-	D48.7	D49.89
scrotum (skin)	C63.2	C79.82	D07.61	D29.4	D40.8	D49.5
sebaceous gland — see Neoplasm, skin						
sella turcica	C75.1	C79.89	D09.3	D35.2	D44.3	D49.7
bone	C41.0	C79.51	—	D16.4-	D48.0	D49.2
semilunar cartilage (knee)	C40.2-	C79.51	—	D16.2-	D48.0	D49.2
seminal vesicle	C63.7	C79.82	D07.69	D29.8	D40.8	D49.5
septum						
nasal	C30.0	C78.39	D02.3	D14.0	D38.5	D49.1
posterior margin	C11.3	C79.89	D00.08	D10.6	D37.05	D49.0
rectovaginal	C76.3	C79.89	D09.8	D36.7	D48.7	D49.89
rectovesical	C76.3	C79.89	D09.8	D36.7	D48.7	D49.89

TABLE OF NEOPLASMS

	Malignant Primary	Malignant Secondary	Ca in situ	Benign	Uncertain Behavior	Unspecified Behavior
septum *(Continued)*						
urethrovaginal	C57.9	C79.82	D07.30	D28.9	D39.9	D49.5
vesicovaginal	C57.9	C79.82	D07.30	D28.9	D39.9	D49.5
shoulder NEC	C76.4-	C79.89	D04.6-	D36.7	D48.7	D49.89
sigmoid flexure (lower) (upper)	C18.7	C78.5	D01.0	D12.5	D37.4	D49.0
sinus (accessory)	C31.9	C78.39	D02.3	D14.0	D38.5	D49.1
bone (any)	C41.0	C79.51	—	D16.4-	D48.0	D49.2
ethmoidal	C31.1	C78.39	D02.3	D14.0	D38.5	D49.1
frontal	C31.2	C78.39	D02.3	D14.0	D38.5	D49.1
maxillary	C31.0	C78.39	D02.3	D14.0	D38.5	D49.1
nasal, paranasal NEC	C31.9	C78.39	D02.3	D14.0	D38.5	D49.1
overlapping lesion	C31.8	—	—	—	—	—
pyriform	C12	C79.89	D00.08	D10.7	D37.05	D49.0
sphenoid	C31.3	C78.39	D02.3	D14.0	D38.5	D49.1
skeleton, skeletal NEC	C41.9	C79.51	—	D16.9-	D48.0	D49.2
Skene's gland	C68.1	C79.19	D09.19	D30.8	D41.8	D49.5
skin NOS	C44.90	C79.2	D04.9	D23.9	D48.5	D49.2
abdominal wall	C44.509	C79.2	D04.5	D23.5	D48.5	D49.2
basal cell carcinoma	C44.519	—	—	—	—	—
specified type NEC	C44.599	—	—	—	—	—
squamous cell carcinoma	C44.529	—	—	—	—	—
ala nasi — *see also Neoplasm, nose, skin*	C44.301	C79.2	D04.39	D23.39	D48.5	D49.2
ankle — *see also Neoplasm, skin, limb, lower*	C44.70-	C79.2	D04.7-	D23.7-	D48.5	D49.2
antecubital space — *see also Neoplasm, skin, limb, upper*	C44.60-	C79.2	D04.6-	D23.6-	D48.5	D49.2
anus	C44.500	C79.2	D04.5	D23.5	D48.5	D49.2
basal cell carcinoma	C44.510	—	—	—	—	—
specified type NEC	C44.590	—	—	—	—	—
squamous cell carcinoma	C44.520	—	—	—	—	—
arm — *see also Neoplasm, skin, limb, upper*	C44.60-	C79.2	D04.6-	D23.6-	D48.5	D49.2
auditory canal (external) — *see also Neoplasm, skin, ear*	C44.20-	C79.2	D04.2-	D23.2-	D48.5	D49.2
auricle (ear) — *see also Neoplasm, skin, ear*	C44.20-	C79.2	D04.2-	D23.2-	D48.5	D49.2
auricular canal (external) — *see also Neoplasm, skin, ear*	C44.20-	C79.2	D04.2-	D23.2-	D48.5	D49.2
axilla, axillary fold — *see also Neoplasm, skin, trunk*	C44.509	C79.2	D04.5	D23.5	D48.5	D49.2
back — *see also Neoplasm, skin, trunk*	C44.509	C79.2	D04.5	D23.5	D48.5	D49.2
basal cell carcinoma	C44.91					
breast	C44.501	C79.2	D04.5	D23.5	D48.5	D49.2
basal cell carcinoma	C44.511	—	—	—	—	—
specified type NEC	C44.591	—	—	—	—	—
squamous cell carcinoma	C44.521	—	—	—	—	—
brow — *see also Neoplasm, skin, face*	C44.309	C79.2	D04.39	D23.39	D48.5	D49.2
buttock — *see also Neoplasm, skin, trunk*	C44.509	C79.2	D04.5	D23.5	D48.5	D49.2
calf — *see also Neoplasm, skin, limb, lower*	C44.70-	C79.2	D04.7-	D23.7-	D48.5	D49.2

	Malignant Primary	Malignant Secondary	Ca in situ	Benign	Uncertain Behavior	Unspecified Behavior
skin NOS *(Continued)*						
canthus (eye) (inner) (outer)	C44.10-	C79.2	D04.1-	D23.1-	D48.5	D49.2
basal cell carcinoma	C44.11-	—	—	—	—	—
specified type NEC	C44.19-	—	—	—	—	—
squamous cell carcinoma	C44.12-	—	—	—	—	—
cervical region — *see also Neoplasm, skin, neck*	C44.40	C79.2	D04.4	D23.4	D48.5	D49.2
cheek (external) — *see also Neoplasm, skin, face*	C44.309	C79.2	D04.39	D23.39	D48.5	D49.2
chest (wall) — *see also Neoplasm, skin, trunk*	C44.509	C79.2	D04.5	D23.5	D48.5	D49.2
chin — *see also Neoplasm, skin, face*	C44.309	C79.2	D04.39	D23.39	D48.5	D49.2
clavicular area — *see also Neoplasm, skin, trunk*	C44.509	C79.2	D04.5	D23.5	D48.5	D49.2
clitoris	C51.2	C79.82	D07.1	D28.0	D39.8	D49.5
columnella — *see also Neoplasm, skin, face*	C44.309	C79.2	D04.39	D23.39	D48.5	D49.2
concha — *see also Neoplasm, skin, ear*	C44.20-	C79.2	D04.2-	D23.2-	D48.5	D49.2
ear (external)	C44.20-	C79.2	D04.2-	D23.2-	D48.5	D49.2
basal cell carcinoma	C44.21-	—	—	—	—	—
specified type NEC	C44.29-	—	—	—	—	—
squamous cell carcinoma	C44.22-	—	—	—	—	—
elbow — *see also Neoplasm, skin, limb, upper*	C44.60-	C79.2	D04.6-	D23.6-	D48.5	D49.2
eyebrow — *see also Neoplasm, skin, face*	C44.309	C79.2	D04.39	D23.39	D48.5	D49.2
eyelid	C44.10-	C79.2	D04.1-	D23.1-	D48.5	D49.2
basal cell carcinoma	C44.11-	—	—	—	—	—
specified type NEC	C44.19-	—	—	—	—	—
squamous cell carcinoma	C44.12-	—	—	—	—	—
face NOS	C44.300	C79.2	D04.30	D23.30	D48.5	D49.2
basal cell carcinoma	C44.310	—	—	—	—	—
specified type NEC	C44.390	—	—	—	—	—
squamous cell carcinoma	C44.320	—	—	—	—	—
female genital organs (external)	C51.9	C79.82	D07.1	D28.0	D39.8	D49.5
clitoris	C51.2	C79.82	D07.1	D28.0	D39.8	D49.5
labium NEC	C51.9	C79.82	D07.1	D28.0	D39.8	D49.5
majus	C51.0	C79.82	D07.1	D28.0	D39.8	D49.5
minus	C51.1	C79.82	D07.1	D28.0	D39.8	D49.5
pudendum	C51.9	C79.82	D07.1	D28.0	D39.8	D49.5
vulva	C51.9	C79.82	D07.1	D28.0	D39.8	D49.5
finger — *see also Neoplasm, skin, limb, upper*	C44.60-	C79.2	D04.6-	D23.6-	D48.5	D49.2
flank — *see also Neoplasm, skin, trunk*	C44.509	C79.2	D04.5	D23.5	D48.5	D49.2
foot — *see also Neoplasm, skin, limb, lower*	C44.70-	C79.2	D04.7-	D23.7-	D48.5	D49.2
forearm — *see also Neoplasm, skin, limb, upper*	C44.60-	C79.2	D04.6-	D23.6-	D48.5	D49.2
forehead — *see also Neoplasm, skin, face*	C44.309	C79.2	D04.39	D23.39	D48.5	D49.2
glabella — *see also Neoplasm, skin, face*	C44.309	C79.2	D04.39	D23.39	D48.5	D49.2
gluteal region — *see also Neoplasm, skin, trunk*	C44.509	C79.2	D04.5	D23.5	D48.5	D49.2
groin — *see also Neoplasm, skin, trunk*	C44.509	C79.2	D04.5	D23.5	D48.5	D49.2
hand — *see also Neoplasm, skin, limb, upper*	C44.60-	C79.2	D04.6-	D23.6-	D48.5	D49.2

	Malignant Primary	Malignant Secondary	Ca in situ	Benign	Uncertain Behavior	Unspecified Behavior
skin NOS *(Continued)*						
head NEC — *see also Neoplasm, skin, scalp*	C44.40	C79.2	D04.4	D23.4	D48.5	D49.2
heel — *see also Neoplasm, skin, limb, lower*	C44.70-	C79.2	D04.7-	D23.7-	D48.5	D49.2
helix — *see also Neoplasm, skin, ear*	C44.20-	C79.2	D04.2-	D23.2-	D48.5	D49.2
hip — *see also Neoplasm, skin, limb, lower*	C44.70-	C79.2	D04.7-	D23.7-	D48.5	D49.2
infraclavicular region — *see also Neoplasm, skin, trunk*	C44.509	C79.2	D04.5	D23.5	D48.5	D49.2
inguinal region — *see also Neoplasm, skin, trunk*	C44.509	C79.2	D04.5	D23.5	D48.5	D49.2
jaw — *see also Neoplasm, skin, face*	C44.309	C79.2	D04.39	D23.39	D48.5	D49.2
Kaposi's sarcoma — *see Kaposi's, sarcoma, skin*						
knee — *see also Neoplasm, skin, limb, lower*	C44.70-	C79.2	D04.7-	D23.7-	D48.5	D49.2
labia						
majora	C51.0	C79.82	D07.1	D28.0	D39.8	D49.5
minora	C51.1	C79.82	D07.1	D28.0	D39.8	D49.5
leg — *see also Neoplasm, skin, limb, lower*	C44.70-	C79.2	D04.7-	D23.7-	D48.5	D49.2
lid (lower) (upper)	C44.10-	C79.2	D04.1-	D23.1-	D48.5	D49.2
basal cell carcinoma	C44.11-	—	—	—	—	—
specified type NEC	C44.19-	—	—	—	—	—
squamous cell carcinoma	C44.12-	—	—	—	—	—
limb NEC	C44.90	C79.2	D04.9	D23.9	D48.5	D49.2
basal cell carcinoma	C44.91					
lower	C44.70-	C79.2	D04.7-	D23.7-	D48.5	D49.2
basal cell carcinoma	C44.71-	—	—	—	—	—
specified type NEC	C44.79-	—	—	—	—	—
squamous cell carcinoma	C44.72-	—	—	—	—	—
upper	C44.60-	C79.2	D04.6-	D23.6-	D48.5	D49.2
basal cell carcinoma	C44.61-	—	—	—	—	—
specified type NEC	C44.69-	—	—	—	—	—
squamous cell carcinoma	C44.62-	—	—	—	—	—
lip (lower) (upper)	C44.00	C79.2	D04.0	D23.0	D48.5	D49.2
basal cell carcinoma	C44.01	—	—	—	—	—
specified type NEC	C44.09	—	—	—	—	—
squamous cell carcinoma	C44.02	—	—	—	—	—
male genital organs	C63.9	C79.82	D07.60	D29.9	D40.8	D49.5
penis	C60.9	C79.82	D07.4	D29.0	D40.8	D49.5
prepuce	C60.0	C79.82	D07.4	D29.0	D40.8	D49.5
scrotum	C63.2	C79.82	D07.61	D29.4	D40.8	D49.5
mastectomy site (skin) — *see also Neoplasm, skin, breast*	C44.501	C79.2	—	—	—	—
specified as breast tissue	C50.8-	C79.81	—	—	—	—
meatus, acoustic (external) — *see also Neoplasm, skin, ear*	C44.20-	C79.2	D04.2-	D23.2-	D48.5	D49.2
melanotic — *see Melanoma*						
Merkel cell — *see Carcinoma, Merkel cell*						
nates — *see also Neoplasm, skin, trunk*	C44.509	C79.2	D04.5	D23.5	D48.5	D49.2

	Malignant Primary	Malignant Secondary	Ca in situ	Benign	Uncertain Behavior	Unspecified Behavior
skin NOS *(Continued)*						
neck	C44.40	C79.2	D04.4	D23.4	D48.5	D49.2
basal cell carcinoma	C44.41	—	—	—	—	—
specified type NEC	C44.49	—	—	—	—	—
squamous cell carcinoma	C44.42	—	—	—	—	—
nevus — *see Nevus, skin*						
nose (external) — *see also Neoplasm, nose, skin*	C44.301	C79.2	D04.39	D23.39	D48.5	D49.2
overlapping lesion	C44.80					
basal cell carcinoma	C44.81	—	—	—	—	—
specified type NEC	C44.89	—	—	—	—	—
squamous cell carcinoma	C44.82	—	—	—	—	—
palm — *see also Neoplasm, skin, limb, upper*	C44.60-	C79.2	D04.6-	D23.6-	D48.5	D49.2
palpebra	C44.10-	C79.2	D04.1-	D23.1-	D48.5	D49.2
basal cell carcinoma	C44.11-	—	—	—	—	—
specified type NEC	C44.19-	—	—	—	—	—
squamous cell carcinoma	C44.12-	—	—	—	—	—
penis NEC	C60.9	C79.82	D07.4	D29.0	D40.8	D49.5
perianal — *see also Neoplasm, skin, anus*	C44.500	C79.2	D04.5	D23.5	D48.5	D49.2
perineum — *see also Neoplasm, skin, anus*	C44.500	C79.2	D04.5	D23.5	D48.5	D49.2
pinna — *see also Neoplasm, skin, ear*	C44.20-	C79.2	D04.2-	D23.2-	D48.5	D49.2
plantar — *see also Neoplasm, skin, limb, lower*	C44.70-	C79.2	D04.7-	D23.7-	D48.5	D49.2
popliteal fossa or space — *see also Neoplasm, skin, limb, lower*	C44.70-	C79.2	D04.7-	D23.7-	D48.5	D49.2
prepuce	C60.0	C79.82	D07.4	D29.0	D40.8	D49.5
pubes — *see also Neoplasm, skin, trunk*	C44.509	C79.2	D04.5	D23.5	D48.5	D49.2
sacrococcygeal region — *see also Neoplasm, skin, trunk*	C44.509	C79.2	D04.5	D23.5	D48.5	D49.2
scalp	C44.40	C79.2	D04.4	D23.4	D48.5	D49.2
basal cell carcinoma	C44.41	—	—	—	—	—
specified type NEC	C44.49	—	—	—	—	—
squamous cell carcinoma	C44.42	—	—	—	—	—
scapular region — *see also Neoplasm, skin, trunk*	C44.509	C79.2	D04.5	D23.5	D48.5	D49.2
scrotum	C63.2	C79.82	D07.61	D29.4	D40.8	D49.5
shoulder — *see also Neoplasm, skin, limb, upper*	C44.60-	C79.2	D04.6-	D23.6-	D48.5	D49.2
sole (foot) — *see also Neoplasm, skin, limb, lower*	C44.70-	C79.2	D04.7-	D23.7-	D48.5	D49.2
specified sites NEC	C44.80	C79.2	D04.8	D23.9	D48.5	D49.2
basal cell carcinoma	C44.81	—	—	—	—	—
specified type NEC	C44.89	—	—	—	—	—
squamous cell carcinoma	C44.82	—	—	—	—	—
specified type NEC	C44.99	—	—	—	—	—
squamous cell carcinoma	C44.92	—	—	—	—	—
submammary fold — *see also Neoplasm, skin, trunk*	C44.509	C79.2	D04.5	D23.5	D48.5	D49.2
supraclavicular region — *see also Neoplasm, skin, neck*	C44.40	C79.2	D04.4	D23.4	D48.5	D49.2
temple — *see also Neoplasm, skin, face*	C44.309	C79.2	D04.39	D23.39	D48.5	D49.2
thigh — *see also Neoplasm, skin, limb, lower*	C44.70-	C79.2	D04.7-	D23.7-	D48.5	D49.2
thoracic wall — *see also Neoplasm, skin, trunk*	C44.509	C79.2	D04.5	D23.5	D48.5	D49.2

540

	Malignant Primary	Malignant Secondary	Ca in situ	Benign	Uncertain Behavior	Unspecified Behavior
skin NOS *(Continued)*						
thumb—*see also Neoplasm, skin, limb, upper*	C44.60-	C79.2	D04.6-	D23.6-	D48.5	D49.2
toe—*see also Neoplasm, skin, limb, lower*	C44.70-	C79.2	D04.7-	D23.7-	D48.5	D49.2
tragus—*see also Neoplasm, skin, ear*	C44.20-	C79.2	D04.2-	D23.2-	D48.5	D49.2
trunk	C44.509	C79.2	D04.5	D23.5	D48.5	D49.2
basal cell carcinoma	C44.519	—	—	—	—	—
specified type NEC	C44.599	—	—	—	—	—
squamous cell carcinoma	C44.529	—	—	—	—	—
umbilicus—*see also Neoplasm, skin, trunk*	C44.509	C79.2	D04.5	D23.5	D48.5	D49.2
vulva	C51.9	C79.82	D07.1	D28.0	D39.8	D49.5
overlapping lesion	C51.8	—	—	—	—	—
wrist—*see also Neoplasm, skin, limb, upper*	C44.60-	C79.2	D04.6-	D23.6-	D48.5	D49.2
skull	C41.0	C79.51	—	D16.4-	D48.0	D49.2
soft parts or tissues—*see Neoplasm, connective tissue*						
specified site NEC	C76.8	C79.89	D09.8	D36.7	D48.7	D49.89
spermatic cord	C63.1-	C79.82	D07.69	D29.8	D40.8	D49.5
sphenoid	C31.3	C78.39	D02.3	D14.0	D38.5	D49.1
bone	C41.0	C79.51	—	D16.4-	D48.0	D49.2
sinus	C31.3	C78.39	D02.3	D14.0	D38.5	D49.1
sphincter						
anal	C21.1	C78.5	D01.3	D12.9	D37.8	D49.0
of Oddi	C24.0	C78.89	D01.5	D13.5	D37.6	D49.0
spine, spinal (column)	C41.2	C79.51	—	D16.6	D48.0	D49.2
bulb	C71.7	C79.31	—	D33.1	D43.1	D49.6
coccyx	C41.4	C79.51	—	D16.8	D48.0	D49.2
cord (cervical) (lumbar) (sacral) (thoracic)	C72.0	C79.49	—	D33.4	D43.4	D49.7
dura mater	C70.1	C79.49	—	D32.1	D42.1	D49.7
lumbosacral	C41.2	C79.51	—	D16.6	D48.0	D49.2
marrow NEC	C96.9	C79.52	—	—	D47.9	D49.89
membrane	C70.1	C79.49	—	D32.1	D42.1	D49.7
meninges	C70.1	C79.49	—	D32.1	D42.1	D49.7
nerve (root)	C47.9	C79.89	—	D36.10	D48.2	D49.2
pia mater	C70.1	C79.49	—	D32.1	D42.1	D49.7
root	C47.9	C79.89	—	D36.10	D48.2	D49.2
sacrum	C41.4	C79.51	—	D16.8	D48.0	D49.2
spleen, splenic NEC	C26.1	C78.89	D01.7	D13.9	D37.8	D49.0
flexure (colon)	C18.5	C78.5	D01.0	D12.3	D37.4	D49.0
stem, brain	C71.7	C79.31	—	D33.1	D43.1	D49.6
Stensen's duct	C07	C79.89	D00.00	D11.0	D37.030	D49.0
sternum	C41.3	C79.51	—	D16.7	D48.0	D49.2
stomach	C16.9	C78.89	D00.2	D13.1	D37.1	D49.0
antrum (pyloric)	C16.3	C78.89	D00.2	D13.1	D37.1	D49.0
body	C16.2	C78.89	D00.2	D13.1	D37.1	D49.0
cardia	C16.0	C78.89	D00.2	D13.1	D37.1	D49.0

	Malignant Primary	Malignant Secondary	Ca in situ	Benign	Uncertain Behavior	Unspecified Behavior
stomach *(Continued)*						
cardiac orifice	C16.0	C78.89	D00.2	D13.1	D37.1	D49.0
corpus	C16.2	C78.89	D00.2	D13.1	D37.1	D49.0
fundus	C16.1	C78.89	D00.2	D13.1	D37.1	D49.0
greater curvature NEC	C16.6	C78.89	D00.2	D13.1	D37.1	D49.0
lesser curvature NEC	C16.5	C78.89	D00.2	D13.1	D37.1	D49.0
overlapping lesion	C16.8	—	—	—	—	—
prepylorus	C16.4	C78.89	D00.2	D13.1	D37.1	D49.0
pylorus	C16.4	C78.89	D00.2	D13.1	D37.1	D49.0
wall NEC	C16.9	C78.89	D00.2	D13.1	D37.1	D49.0
anterior NEC	C16.8	C78.89	D00.2	D13.1	D37.1	D49.0
posterior NEC	C16.8	C78.89	D00.2	D13.1	D37.1	D49.0
stroma, endometrial	C54.1	C79.82	D07.0	D26.1	D39.0	D49.5
stump, cervical	C53.8	C79.82	D06.7	D26.0	D39.0	D49.5
subcutaneous (nodule) (tissue) NEC — *see Neoplasm, connective tissue*						
subdural	C70.9	C79.32	—	D32.9	D42.9	D49.7
subglottis, subglottic	C32.2	C78.39	D02.0	D14.1	D38.0	D49.1
sublingual	C04.9	C79.89	D00.06	D10.2	D37.09	D49.0
gland or duct	C08.1	C79.89	D00.00	D11.7	D37.031	D49.0
submandibular gland	C08.0	C79.89	D00.00	D11.7	D37.032	D49.0
submaxillary gland or duct	C08.0	C79.89	D00.00	D11.7	D37.032	D49.0
submental	C76.0	C79.89	D09.8	D36.7	D48.7	D49.89
subpleural	C34.9-	C78.0-	D02.2-	D14.3-	D38.1	D49.1
substernal	C38.1	C78.1	—	D15.2	D38.3	D49.89
sudoriferous, sudoriparous gland, site unspecified	C44.90	C79.2	D04.9	D23.9	D48.5	D49.2
specified site — *see Neoplasm, skin*						
supraclavicular region	C76.0	C79.89	D09.8	D36.7	D48.7	D49.89
supraglottis	C32.1	C78.39	D02.0	D14.1	D38.0	D49.1
suprarenal	C74.9-	C79.7-	D09.3	D35.0-	D44.1-	D49.7
capsule	C74.9-	C79.7-	D09.3	D35.0-	D44.1-	D49.7
cortex	C74.0-	C79.7-	D09.3	D35.0-	D44.1-	D49.7
gland	C74.9-	C79.7-	D09.3	D35.0-	D44.1-	D49.7
medulla	C74.1-	C79.7-	D09.3	D35.0-	D44.1-	D49.7
suprasellar (region)	C71.9	C79.31	—	D33.2	D43.2	D49.6
supratentorial (brain) NEC	C71.0	C79.31	—	D33.0	D43.0	D49.6
sweat gland (apocrine) (eccrine), site unspecified	C44.90	C79.2	D04.9	D23.9	D48.5	D49.2
specified site — *see Neoplasm, skin*						
sympathetic nerve or nervous system NEC	C47.9	C79.89	—	D36.10	D48.2	D49.2
symphysis pubis	C41.4	C79.51	—	D16.8	D48.0	D49.2
synovial membrane — *see Neoplasm, connective tissue*						
tapetum, brain	C71.8	C79.31	—	D33.2	D43.2	D49.6
tarsus (any bone)	C40.3-	C79.51	—	D16.3-	—	—
temple (skin) — *see also Neoplasm, skin, face*	C44.309	C79.2	D04.39	D23.39	D48.5	D49.2

	Malignant Primary	Malignant Secondary	Ca in situ	Benign	Uncertain Behavior	Unspecified Behavior
temporal						
bone	C41.0	C79.51	—	D16.4-	D48.0	D49.2
lobe or pole	C71.2	C79.31	—	D33.0	D43.0	D49.6
region	C76.0	C79.89	D09.8	D36.7	D48.7	D49.89
skin — see also Neoplasm, skin, face	C44.309	C79.2	D04.39	D23.39	D48.5	D49.2
tendon (sheath) — see Neoplasm, connective tissue						
tentorium (cerebelli)	C70.0	C79.32	—	D32.0	D42.0	D49.7
testis, testes	C62.9-	C79.82	D07.69	D29.2-	D40.1-	D49.5
descended	C62.1-	C79.82	D07.69	D29.2-	D40.1-	D49.5
ectopic	C62.0-	C79.82	D07.69	D29.2-	D40.1-	D49.5
retained	C62.0-	C79.82	D07.69	D29.2-	D40.1-	D49.5
scrotal	C62.1-	C79.82	D07.69	D29.2-	D40.1-	D49.5
undescended	C62.0-	C79.82	D07.69	D29.2-	D40.1-	D49.5
unspecified whether descended or undescended	C62.9-	C79.82	D07.69	D29.2-	D40.1-	D49.5
thalamus	C71.0	C79.31	—	D33.0	D43.0	D49.6
thigh NEC	C76.5-	C79.89	D04.7-	D36.7	D48.7	D49.89
thorax, thoracic (cavity) (organs NEC)	C76.1	C79.89	D09.8	D36.7	D48.7	D49.89
duct	C49.3	C79.89	—	D21.3	D48.1	D49.2
wall NEC	C76.1	C79.89	D09.8	D36.7	D48.7	D49.89
throat	C14.0	C79.89	D00.08	D10.9	D37.05	D49.0
thumb NEC	C76.4-	C79.89	D04.6-	D36.7	D48.7	D49.89
thymus (gland)	C37	C79.89	D09.3	D15.0	D38.4	D49.89
thyroglossal duct	C73	C79.89	D09.3	D34	D44.0	D49.7
thyroid (gland)	C73	C79.89	D09.3	D34	D44.0	D49.7
cartilage	C32.3	C78.39	D02.0	D14.1	D38.0	D49.1
tibia (any part)	C40.2-	C79.51	—	D16.2-	—	—
toe NEC	C76.5-	C79.89	D04.7-	D36.7	D48.7	D49.89
tongue	C02.9	C79.89	D00.07	D10.1	D37.02	D49.0
anterior (two-thirds) NEC	C02.3	C79.89	D00.07	D10.1	D37.02	D49.0
dorsal surface	C02.0	C79.89	D00.07	D10.1	D37.02	D49.0
ventral surface	C02.2	C79.89	D00.07	D10.1	D37.02	D49.0
base (dorsal surface)	C01	C79.89	D00.07	D10.1	D37.02	D49.0
border (lateral)	C02.1	C79.89	D00.07	D10.1	D37.02	D49.0
dorsal surface NEC	C02.0	C79.89	D00.07	D10.1	D37.02	D49.0
fixed part NEC	C01	C79.89	D00.07	D10.1	D37.02	D49.0
foreamen cecum	C02.0	C79.89	D00.07	D10.1	D37.02	D49.0
frenulum linguae	C02.2	C79.89	D00.07	D10.1	D37.02	D49.0
junctional zone	C02.8	C79.89	D00.07	D10.1	D37.02	D49.0
margin (lateral)	C02.1	C79.89	D00.07	D10.1	D37.02	D49.0
midline NEC	C02.0	C79.89	D00.07	D10.1	D37.02	D49.0
mobile part NEC	C02.3	C79.89	D00.07	D10.1	D37.02	D49.0
overlapping lesion	C02.8	—	—	—	—	—
posterior (third)	C01	C79.89	D00.07	D10.1	D37.02	D49.0

	Malignant Primary	Malignant Secondary	Ca in situ	Benign	Uncertain Behavior	Unspecified Behavior
tongue *(Continued)*						
root	C01	C79.89	D00.07	D10.1	D37.02	D49.0
surface (dorsal)	C02.0	C79.89	D00.07	D10.1	D37.02	D49.0
base	C01	C79.89	D00.07	D10.1	D37.02	D49.0
ventral	C02.2	C79.89	D00.07	D10.1	D37.02	D49.0
tip	C02.1	C79.89	D00.07	D10.1	D37.02	D49.0
tonsil	C02.4	C79.89	D00.07	D10.1	D37.02	D49.0
tonsil	C09.9	C79.89	D00.08	D10.4	D37.05	D49.0
fauces, faucial	C09.9	C79.89	D00.08	D10.4	D37.05	D49.0
lingual	C02.4	C79.89	D00.07	D10.1	D37.02	D49.0
overlapping sites	C09.8	—	—	—	—	—
palatine	C09.9	C79.89	D00.08	D10.4	D37.05	D49.0
pharyngeal	C11.1	C79.89	D00.08	D10.6	D37.05	D49.0
pillar (anterior) (posterior)	C09.1	C79.89	D00.08	D10.5	D37.05	D49.0
tonsillar fossa	C09.0	C79.89	D00.08	D10.5	D37.05	D49.0
tooth socket NEC	C03.9	C79.89	D00.03	D10.39	D37.09	D49.0
trachea (cartilage) (mucosa)	C33	C78.39	D02.1	D14.2	D38.1	D49.1
overlapping lesion with bronchus or lung	C34.8-	—	—	—	—	—
tracheobronchial	C34.8-	C78.39	D02.1	D14.2	D38.1	D49.1
overlapping lesion with lung	C34.8-	—	—	—	—	—
tragus — *see also Neoplasm, skin, ear*	C44.20-	C79.2	D04.2-	D23.2-	D48.5	D49.2
trunk NEC	C76.8	C79.89	D04.5	D36.7	D48.7	D49.89
tubo-ovarian	C57.8	C79.82	D07.39	D28.7	D39.8	D49.5
tunica vaginalis	C63.7	C79.82	D07.69	D29.8	D40.8	D49.5
turbinate (bone)	C41.0	C79.51	—	D16.4-	D48.0	D49.2
nasal	C30.0	C78.39	D02.3	D14.0	D38.5	D49.1
tympanic cavity	C30.1	C78.39	D02.3	D14.0	D38.5	D49.1
ulna (any part)	C40.0-	C79.51	—	D16.0-	—	—
umbilicus, umbilical — *see also Neoplasm, skin, trunk*	C44.509	C79.2	D04.5	D23.5	D48.5	D49.2
uncus, brain	C71.2	C79.31	—	D33.0	D43.0	D49.6
unknown site or unspecified	C80.1	C79.9	D09.9	D36.9	D48.9	D49.9
urachus	C67.7	C79.11	D09.0	D30.3	D41.4	D49.4
ureter, ureteral	C66.-	C79.19	D09.19	D30.2-	D41.2-	D49.5
orifice (bladder)	C67.6	C79.11	D09.0	D30.3	D41.4	D49.4
ureter-bladder (junction)	C67.6	C79.11	D09.0	D30.3	D41.4	D49.4
urethra, urethral (gland)	C68.0	C79.19	D09.19	D30.4	D41.3	D49.5
orifice, internal	C67.5	C79.11	D09.0	D30.3	D41.4	D49.4
urethrovaginal (septum)	C57.9	C79.82	D07.30	D28.9	D39.8	D49.5
urinary organ or system	C68.9	C79.10	D09.10	D30.9	D41.9	D49.5
bladder — *see Neoplasm, bladder*						
overlapping lesion	C68.8	—	—	—	—	—
specified sites NEC	C68.8	C79.19	D09.19	D30.8	D41.8	D49.5

TABLE OF NEOPLASMS

	Malignant Primary	Malignant Secondary	Ca in situ	Benign	Uncertain Behavior	Unspecified Behavior
utero-ovarian	C57.8	C79.82	D07.39	D28.7	D39.8	D49.5
ligament	C57.1	C79.82	D07.39	D28.2	D39.8	D49.5
uterosacral ligament	C57.3	C79.82	—	D28.2	D39.8	D49.5
uterus, uteri, uterine	C55	C79.82	D07.0	D26.9	D39.0	D49.5
adnexa NEC	C57.4	C79.82	D07.39	D28.7	D39.8	D49.5
body	C54.9	C79.82	D07.0	D26.1	D39.0	D49.5
cervix	C53.9	C79.82	D06.9	D26.0	D39.0	D49.5
cornu	C54.9	C79.82	D07.0	D26.1	D39.0	D49.5
corpus	C54.9	C79.82	D07.0	D26.1	D39.0	D49.5
endocervix (canal) (gland)	C53.0	C79.82	D06.0	D26.0	D39.0	D49.5
endometrium	C54.1	C79.82	D07.0	D26.1	D39.0	D49.5
exocervix	C53.1	C79.82	D06.1	D26.0	D39.0	D49.5
external os	C53.1	C79.82	D06.1	D26.0	D39.0	D49.5
fundus	C54.3	C79.82	D07.0	D26.1	D39.0	D49.5
internal os	C53.0	C79.82	D06.0	D26.0	D39.0	D49.5
isthmus	C54.0	C79.82	D07.0	D26.1	D39.0	D49.5
ligament	C57.3	C79.82	—	D28.2	D39.8	D49.5
broad	C57.1	C79.82	D07.39	D28.2	D39.8	D49.5
round	C57.2	C79.82	—	D28.2	D39.8	D49.5
lower segment	C54.0	C79.82	D07.0	D26.1	D39.0	D49.5
myometrium	C54.2	C79.82	D07.0	D26.1	D39.0	D49.5
overlapping sites	C54.8	—	—	—	—	—
squamocolumnar junction	C53.8	C79.82	D06.7	D26.0	D39.0	D49.5
tube	C57.0-	C79.82	D07.39	D28.2	D39.8	D49.5
utricle, prostatic	C68.0	C79.19	D09.19	D30.4	D41.3	D49.5
uveal tract	C69.4-	C79.49	D09.2-	D31.4-	D48.7	D49.89
uvula	C05.2	C79.89	D00.04	D10.39	D37.09	D49.0
vagina, vaginal (fornix) (vault) (wall)	C52	C79.82	D07.2	D28.1	D39.8	D49.5
vaginovesical	C57.9	C79.82	D07.30	D28.9	D39.9	D49.5
septum	C57.9	C79.82	D07.30	D28.9	D39.9	D49.5
vallecula (epigiottis)	C10.0	C79.89	D00.08	D10.5	D37.05	D49.0
vas deferens	C63.1-	C79.82	D07.69	D29.8	D40.8	D49.5
vascular — *see Neoplasm, connective tissue*						
Vater's ampulla	C24.1	C78.89	D01.5	D13.5	D37.6	D49.0
vein, venous — *see Neoplasm, connective tissue*						
vena cava (abdominal) (inferior)	C49.4	C79.89	—	D21.4	D48.1	D49.2
superior	C49.3	C79.89	—	D21.3	D48.1	D49.2
ventricle (cerebral) (floor) (lateral) (third)	C71.5	C79.31	—	D33.0	D43.0	D49.6
cardiac (left) (right)	C38.0	C79.89	—	D15.1	D48.7	D49.89
fourth	C71.7	C79.31	—	D33.1	D43.1	D49.6
ventricular band of larynx	C32.1	C78.39	D02.0	D14.1	D38.0	D49.1
ventriculus — *see Neoplasm, stomach*						

	Malignant Primary	Malignant Secondary	Ca in situ	Benign	Uncertain Behavior	Unspecified Behavior
vermillion border — see Neoplasm, lip						
vermis, cerebellum	C71.6	C79.31	—	D33.1	D43.1	D49.6
vertebra (column)	C41.2	C79.51	—	D16.6	D48.0	D49.2
coccyx	C41.4	C79.51	—	D16.8-	D48.0	D49.2
marrow NEC	C96.9	C79.52	—	—	D47.9	D49.89
sacrum	C41.4	C79.51	—	D16.8-	D48.0	D49.2
vesical — see Neoplasm, bladder						
vesicle, seminal	C63.7	C79.82	D07.69	D29.8	D40.8	D49.5
vesicocervical tissue	C57.9	C79.82	D07.30	D28.9	D39.9	D49.5
vesicorectal	C76.3	C79.82	D09.8	D36.7	D48.7	D49.89
vesicovaginal	C57.9	C79.82	D07.30	D28.9	D39.9	D49.5
septum	C57.9	C79.82	D07.30	D28.9	D39.8	D49.5
vessel (blood) — see Neoplasm, connective tissue						
vestibular gland, greater	C51.0	C79.82	D07.1	D28.0	D39.8	D49.5
vestibule						
mouth	C06.1	C79.89	D00.00	D10.39	D37.09	D49.0
nose	C30.0	C78.39	D02.3	D14.0	D38.5	D49.1
Virchow's gland	C77.0	C77.0	—	D36.0	D48.7	D49.89
viscera NEC	C76.8	C79.89	D09.8	D36.7	D48.7	D49.89
vocal cords (true)	C32.0	C78.39	D02.0	D14.1	D38.0	D49.1
false	C32.1	C78.39	D02.0	D14.1	D38.0	D49.1
vomer	C41.0	C79.51	—	D16.4-	D48.0	D49.2
vulva	C51.9	C79.82	D07.1	D28.0	D39.8	D49.5
vulvovaginal gland	C51.0	C79.82	D07.1	D28.0	D39.8	D49.5
Waldeyer's ring	C14.2	C79.89	D00.08	D10.9	D37.05	D49.0
Wharton's duct	C08.0	C79.89	D00.00	D11.7	D37.032	D49.0
white matter (central) (cerebral)	C71.0	C79.31	—	D33.0	D43.0	D49.6
windpipe	C33	C78.39	D02.1	D14.2	D38.1	D49.1
Wirsung's duct	C25.3	C78.89	D01.7	D13.6	D37.8	D49.0
wolffian (body) (duct)						
female	C57.7	C79.82	D07.39	D28.7	D39.8	D49.5
male	C63.7	C79.82	D07.69	D29.8	D40.8	D49.5
womb — see Neoplasm, uterus						
wrist NEC	C76.4-	C79.89	D04.6-	D36.7	D48.7	D49.89
xiphoid process	C41.3	C79.51	—	D16.7	D48.0	D49.2
Zuckerkandl organ	C75.5	C79.89	—	D35.6	D44.7	D49.7

ICD-10-CM
Table of Drugs
and Chemicals

Substance	External Cause (T-Code)					
	Poisoning, Accidental (Unintentional)	Poisoning, Intentional Self-Harm	Poisoning, Assault	Poisoning, Undetermined	Adverse Effect	Underdosing
#						
1-propanol	T51.3X1	T51.3X2	T51.3X3	T51.3X4	—	—
2-propanol	T51.2X1	T51.2X2	T51.2X3	T51.2X4	—	—
2,4-D (dichlorophen-oxyacetic acid)	T60.3X1	T60.3X2	T60.3X3	T60.3X4	—	—
2,4-toluene diisocyanate	T65.0X1	T65.0X2	T65.0X3	T65.0X4	—	—
2,4,5-T (trichloro-phenoxyacetic acid)	T60.1X1	T60.1X2	T60.1X3	T60.1X4	—	—
14-hydroxydihydro-morphinone	T40.2X1	T40.2X2	T40.2X3	T40.2X4	T40.2X5	T40.2X6
A						
ABOB	T37.5X1	T37.5X2	T37.5X3	T37.5X4	T37.5X5	T37.5X6
Abrine	T62.2X1	T62.2X2	T62.2X3	T62.2X4	—	—
Abrus (seed)	T62.2X1	T62.2X2	T62.2X3	T62.2X4	—	—
Absinthe	T51.0X1	T51.0X2	T51.0X3	T51.0X4	—	—
beverage	T51.0X1	T51.0X2	T51.0X3	T51.0X4	—	—
Acaricide	T60.8X1	T60.8X2	T60.8X3	T60.8X4	—	—
Acebutolol	T44.7X1	T44.7X2	T44.7X3	T44.7X4	T44.7X5	T44.7X6
Acecarbromal	T42.6X1	T42.6X2	T42.6X3	T42.6X4	T42.6X5	T42.6X6
Aceclidine	T44.1X1	T44.1X2	T44.1X3	T44.1X4	T44.1X5	T44.1X6
Acedapsone	T37.0X1	T37.0X2	T37.0X3	T37.0X4	T37.0X5	T37.0X6
Acefylline piperazine	T48.6X1	T48.6X2	T48.6X3	T48.6X4	T48.6X5	T48.6X6
Acemorphan	T40.2X1	T40.2X2	T40.2X3	T40.2X4	T40.2X5	T40.2X6
Acenocoumarin	T45.511	T45.512	T45.513	T45.514	T45.515	T45.516
Acenocoumarol	T45.511	T45.512	T45.513	T45.514	T45.515	T45.516
Acepifylline	T48.6X1	T48.6X2	T48.6X3	T48.6X4	T48.6X5	T48.6X6
Acepromazine	T43.3X1	T43.3X2	T43.3X3	T43.3X4	T43.3X5	T43.3X6
Acesulfamethoxypyridazine	T37.0X1	T37.0X2	T37.0X3	T37.0X4	T37.0X5	T37.0X6
Acetal	T52.8X1	T52.8X2	T52.8X3	T52.8X4	—	—
Acetaldehyde (vapor)	T52.8X1	T52.8X2	T52.8X3	T52.8X4	—	—
liquid	T65.891	T65.892	T65.893	T65.894	—	—
P-Acetamidophenol	T39.1X1	T39.1X2	T39.1X3	T39.1X4	T39.1X5	T39.1X6
Acetaminophen	T39.1X1	T39.1X2	T39.1X3	T39.1X4	T39.1X5	T39.1X6
Acetaminosalol	T39.1X1	T39.1X2	T39.1X3	T39.1X4	T39.1X5	T39.1X6
Acetanilide	T39.1X1	T39.1X2	T39.1X3	T39.1X4	T39.1X5	T39.1X6
Acetarsol	T37.3X1	T37.3X2	T37.3X3	T37.3X4	T37.3X5	T37.3X6
Acetazolamide	T50.2X1	T50.2X2	T50.2X3	T50.2X4	T50.2X5	T50.2X6
Acetiamine	T45.2X1	T45.2X2	T45.2X3	T45.2X4	T45.2X5	T45.2X6
Acetic						
acid	T54.2X1	T54.2X2	T54.2X3	T54.2X4	—	—
with sodium acetate (ointment)	T49.3X1	T49.3X2	T49.3X3	T49.3X4	T49.3X5	T49.3X6
ester (solvent) (vapor)	T52.8X1	T52.8X2	T52.8X3	T52.8X4	—	—

TABLE OF DRUGS AND CHEMICALS

Substance	Poisoning, Accidental (Unintentional)	Poisoning, Intentional Self-Harm	Poisoning, Assault	Poisoning, Undetermined	Adverse Effect	Underdosing
Acetic (Continued)						
acid (Continued)						
irrigating solution	T50.3X1	T50.3X2	T50.3X3	T50.3X4	T50.3X5	T50.3X6
medicinal (lotion)	T49.2X1	T49.2X2	T49.2X3	T49.2X4	T49.2X5	T49.2X6
anhydride	T65.891	T65.892	T65.893	T65.894	—	—
ether (vapor)	T52.8X1	T52.8X2	T52.8X3	T52.8X4	—	—
Acetohexamide	T38.3X1	T38.3X2	T38.3X3	T38.3X4	T38.3X5	T38.3X6
Acetohydroxamic acid	T50.991	T50.992	T50.993	T50.994	T50.995	T50.996
Acetomenaphthone	T45.7X1	T45.7X2	T45.7X3	T45.7X4	T45.7X5	T45.7X6
Acetomorphine	T40.1X1	T40.1X2	T40.1X3	T40.1X4	T40.1X5	—
Acetone (oils)	T52.4X1	T52.4X2	T52.4X3	T52.4X4	—	—
chlorinated	T52.4X1	T52.4X2	T52.4X3	T52.4X4	—	—
vapor	T52.4X1	T52.4X2	T52.4X3	T52.4X4	—	—
Acetonitrile	T52.8X1	T52.8X2	T52.8X3	T52.8X4	—	—
Acetophenazine	T43.3X1	T43.3X2	T43.3X3	T43.3X4	T43.3X5	T43.3X6
Acetophenetedin	T39.1X1	T39.1X2	T39.1X3	T39.1X4	T39.1X5	T39.1X6
Acetophenone	T52.4X1	T52.4X2	T52.4X3	T52.4X4		
Acetorphine	T40.2X1	T40.2X2	T40.2X3	T40.2X4		
Acetosulfone (sodium)	T37.1X1	T37.1X2	T37.1X3	T37.1X4	T37.1X5	T37.1X6
Acetrizoate (sodium)	T50.8X1	T50.8X2	T50.8X3	T50.8X4	T50.8X5	T50.8X6
Acetylcarbromal	T42.6X1	T42.6X2	T42.6X3	T42.6X4	T42.6X5	T42.6X6
Acetrizoic acid	T50.8X1	T50.8X2	T50.8X3	T50.8X4	T50.8X5	T50.8X6
Acetyl						
bromide	T53.6X1	T53.6X2	T53.6X3	T53.6X4	—	—
chloride	T53.6X1	T53.6X2	T53.6X3	T53.6X4	—	—
Acetylcholine						
chloride	T44.1X1	T44.1X2	T44.1X3	T44.1X4	T44.1X5	T44.1X6
derivative	T44.1X1	T44.1X2	T44.1X3	T44.1X4	T44.1X5	T44.1X6
Acetylcysteine	T48.4X1	T48.4X2	T48.4X3	T48.4X4	T48.4X5	T48.4X6
Acetyldigitoxin	T46.0X1	T46.0X2	T46.0X3	T46.0X4	T46.0X5	T46.0X6
Acetyldigoxin	T46.0X1	T46.0X2	T46.0X3	T46.0X4	T46.0X5	T46.0X6
Acetyldihydrocodeine	T40.2X1	T40.2X2	T40.2X3	T40.2X4	—	—
Acetyldihydrocodeinone	T40.2X1	T40.2X2	T40.2X3	T40.2X4	—	—
Acetylene (gas)	T59.891	T59.892	T59.893	T59.894	—	—
dichloride	T53.6X1	T53.6X2	T53.6X3	T53.6X4	—	—
incomplete combustion of	T58.11	T58.12	T58.13	T58.14	—	—
industrial	T59.891	T59.892	T59.893	T59.894	—	—
tetrachloride	T53.6X1	T53.6X2	T53.6X3	T53.6X4	—	—
vapor	T53.6X1	T53.6X2	T53.6X3	T53.6X4	—	—
Acetylphenylhydrazine	T39.8X1	T39.8X2	T39.8X3	T39.8X4	T39.8X5	T39.8X6

Substance	Poisoning, Accidental (Unintentional)	Poisoning, Intentional Self-Harm	Poisoning, Assault	Poisoning, Undetermined	Adverse Effect	Underdosing
	External Cause (T-Code)					
Acetylpheneturide	T42.6X1	T42.6X2	T42.6X3	T42.6X4	T42.6X5	T42.6X6
Acetylsalicylic acid (salts)	T39.011	T39.012	T39.013	T39.014	T39.015	T39.016
enteric coated	T39.011	T39.012	T39.013	T39.014	T39.015	T39.016
Acetylsulfamethoxypyridazine	T37.0X1	T37.0X2	T37.0X3	T37.0X4	T37.0X5	T37.0X6
Achromycin	T36.4X1	T36.4X2	T36.4X3	T36.4X4	T36.4X5	T36.4X6
ophthalmic preparation	T49.5X1	T49.5X2	T49.5X3	T49.5X4	T49.5X5	T49.5X6
topical NEC	T49.0X1	T49.0X2	T49.0X3	T49.0X4	T49.0X5	T49.0X6
Aciclovir	T37.5X1	T37.5X2	T37.5X3	T37.5X4	T37.5X5	T37.5X6
Acid (corrosive) NEC	T54.2X1	T54.2X2	T54.2X3	T54.2X4	—	—
Acidifying agent NEC	T50.901	T50.902	T50.903	T50.904	T50.905	T50.906
Acipimox	T46.6X1	T46.6X2	T46.6X3	T46.6X4	T46.6X5	T46.6X6
Acitretin	T50.991	T50.992	T50.993	T50.994	T50.995	T50.996
Aclarubicin	T45.1X1	T45.1X2	T45.1X3	T45.1X4	T45.1X5	T45.1X6
Aclatonium napadisilate	T48.1X1	T48.1X2	T48.1X3	T48.1X4	T48.1X5	T48.1X6
Aconite (wild)	T46.991	T46.992	T46.993	T46.994	T46.995	T46.996
Aconitine	T46.991	T46.992	T46.993	T46.994	T46.995	T46.996
Aconitum ferox	T46.991	T46.992	T46.993	T46.994	T46.995	T46.996
Acridine	T65.6X1	T65.6X2	T65.6X3	T65.6X4	—	—
vapor	T59.891	T59.892	T59.893	T59.894	—	—
Acriflavine	T37.91	T37.92	T37.93	T37.94	T37.95	T37.96
Acriflavinium chloride	T49.0X1	T49.0X2	T49.0X3	T49.0X4	T49.0X5	T49.0X6
Acrinol	T49.0X1	T49.0X2	T49.0X3	T49.0X4	T49.0X5	T49.0X6
Acrisorcin	T49.0X1	T49.0X2	T49.0X3	T49.0X4	T49.0X5	T49.0X6
Acrivastine	T45.0X1	T45.0X2	T45.0X3	T45.0X4	T45.0X5	T45.0X6
Acrolein (gas)	T59.891	T59.892	T59.893	T59.894	—	—
liquid	T54.1X1	T54.1X2	T54.1X3	T54.1X4	—	—
Acrylamide	T65.891	T65.892	T65.893	T65.894	—	—
Acrylic resin	T49.3X1	T49.3X2	T49.3X3	T49.3X4	T49.3X5	T49.3X6
Acrylonitrile	T65.891	T65.892	T65.893	T65.894	—	—
Actaea spicata	T62.2X1	T62.2X2	T62.2X3	T62.2X4	—	—
berry	T62.1X1	T62.1X2	T62.1X3	T62.1X4	—	—
Acterol	T37.3X1	T37.3X2	T37.3X3	T37.3X4	T37.3X5	T37.3X6
ACTH	T38.811	T38.812	T38.813	T38.814	T38.815	T38.816
Actinomycin C	T45.1X1	T45.1X2	T45.1X3	T45.1X4	T45.1X5	T45.1X6
Actinomycin D	T45.1X1	T45.1X2	T45.1X3	T45.1X4	T45.1X5	T45.1X6
Activated charcoal — see also Charcoal, medicinal	T47.6X1	T47.6X2	T47.6X3	T47.6X4	T47.6X5	T47.6X6
Acyclovir	T37.5X1	T37.5X2	T37.5X3	T37.5X4	T37.5X5	T37.5X6
Adenine	T45.2X1	T45.2X2	T45.2X3	T45.2X4	T45.2X5	T45.2X6
arabinoside	T37.5X1	T37.5X2	T37.5X3	T37.5X4	T37.5X5	T37.5X6
Adenosine (phosphate)	T46.2X1	T46.2X2	T46.2X3	T46.2X4	T46.2X5	T46.2X6

TABLE OF DRUGS AND CHEMICALS

Substance	External Cause (T-Code)					
	Poisoning, Accidental (Unintentional)	Poisoning, Intentional Self-Harm	Poisoning, Assault	Poisoning, Undetermined	Adverse Effect	Underdosing
ADH	T38.891	T38.892	T38.893	T38.894	T38.895	T38.896
Adhesive NEC	T65.891	T65.892	T65.893	T65.894	—	—
Adicillin	T36.0X1	T36.0X2	T36.0X3	T36.0X4	T36.0X5	T36.0X6
Adiphenine	T44.3X1	T44.3X2	T44.3X3	T44.3X4	T44.3X5	T44.3X6
Adipiodone	T50.8X1	T50.8X2	T50.8X3	T50.8X4	T50.8X5	T50.8X6
Adjunct, pharmaceutical	T50.901	T50.902	T50.903	T50.904	T50.905	T50.906
Adrenal (extract, cortex or medulla) (glucocorticoids) (hormones) (mineralocorticoids)	T38.0X1	T38.0X2	T38.0X3	T38.0X4	T38.0X5	T38.0X6
ENT agent	T49.6X1	T49.6X2	T49.6X3	T49.6X4	T49.6X5	T49.6X6
ophthalmic preparation	T49.5X1	T49.5X2	T49.5X3	T49.5X4	T49.5X5	T49.5X6
topical NEC	T49.0X1	T49.0X2	T49.0X3	T49.0X4	T49.0X5	T49.0X6
Adrenaline	T44.5X1	T44.5X2	T44.5X3	T44.5X4	T44.5X5	T44.5X6
Adrenalin — see Adrenaline						
Adrenergic NEC	T44.901	T44.902	T44.903	T44.904	T44.905	T44.906
blocking agent NEC	T44.8X1	T44.8X2	T44.8X3	T44.8X4	T44.8X5	T44.8X6
beta, heart	T44.7X1	T44.7X2	T44.7X3	T44.7X4	T44.7X5	T44.7X6
specified NEC	T44.991	T44.992	T44.993	T44.994	T44.995	T44.996
Adrenochrome						
(mono) semicarbazone	T46.991	T46.992	T46.993	T46.994	T46.995	T46.996
derivative	T46.991	T46.992	T46.993	T46.994	T46.995	T46.996
Adrenocorticotrophic hormone	T38.811	T38.812	T38.813	T38.814	T38.815	T38.816
Adrenocorticotrophin	T38.811	T38.812	T38.813	T38.814	T38.815	T38.816
Adriamycin	T45.1X1	T45.1X2	T45.1X3	T45.1X4	T45.1X5	T45.1X6
Aerosol spray NEC	T65.91	T65.92	T65.93	T65.94	—	—
Aerosporin	T36.8X1	T36.8X2	T36.8X3	T36.8X4	T36.8X5	T36.8X6
ENT agent	T49.6X1	T49.6X2	T49.6X3	T49.6X4	T49.6X5	T49.6X6
ophthalmic preparation	T49.5X1	T49.5X2	T49.5X3	T49.5X4	T49.5X5	T49.5X6
topical NEC	T49.0X1	T49.0X2	T49.0X3	T49.0X4	T49.0X5	T49.0X6
Aethusa cynapium	T62.2X1	T62.2X2	T62.2X3	T62.2X4	—	—
Afghanistan black	T40.7X1	T40.7X2	T40.7X3	T40.7X4	T40.7X5	T40.7X6
Aflatoxin	T64.01	T64.02	T64.03	T64.04	—	—
Afloqualone	T42.8X1	T42.8X2	T42.8X3	T42.8X4	T42.8X5	T42.8X6
African boxwood	T62.2X1	T62.2X2	T62.2X3	T62.2X4	—	—
Agar	T47.4X1	T47.4X2	T47.4X3	T47.4X4	T47.4X5	T47.4X6
Agonist						
predominantly						
alpha-adrenoreceptor	T44.4X1	T44.4X2	T44.4X3	T44.4X4	T44.4X5	T44.4X6
beta-adrenoreceptor	T44.5X1	T44.5X2	T44.5X3	T44.5X4	T44.5X5	T44.5X6
Agricultural agent NEC	T65.91	T65.92	T65.93	T65.94	—	—
Agrypnal	T42.3X1	T42.3X2	T42.3X3	T42.3X4	T42.3X5	T42.3X6

Substance	External Cause (T-Code)					
	Poisoning, Accidental (Unintentional)	Poisoning, Intentional Self-Harm	Poisoning, Assault	Poisoning, Undetermined	Adverse Effect	Underdosing
AHLG	T50.Z11	T50.Z12	T50.Z13	T50.Z14	T50.Z15	T50.Z16
Air contaminant(s), source/type NOS	T65.91	T65.92	T65.93	T65.94	—	—
Ajmaline	T46.2X1	T46.2X2	T46.2X3	T46.2X4	T46.2X5	T46.2X6
Akritoin	T37.8X1	T37.8X2	T37.8X3	T37.8X4	T37.8X5	T37.8X6
Akee	T62.1X1	T62.1X2	T62.1X3	T62.1X4	—	—
Akrinol	T49.0X1	T49.0X2	T49.0X3	T49.0X4	T49.0X5	T49.0X6
Alacepril	T46.4X1	T46.4X2	T46.4X3	T46.4X4	T46.4X5	T46.4X6
Alantolactone	T37.4X1	T37.4X2	T37.4X3	T37.4X4	T37.4X5	T37.4X6
Albamycin	T36.8X1	T36.8X2	T36.8X3	T36.8X4	T36.8X5	T36.8X6
Albendazole	T37.4X1	T37.4X2	T37.4X3	T37.4X4	T37.4X5	T37.4X6
Albumin						
bovine	T45.8X1	T45.8X2	T45.8X3	T45.8X4	T45.8X5	T45.8X6
human serum	T45.8X1	T45.8X2	T45.8X3	T45.8X4	T45.8X5	T45.8X6
salt-poor	T45.8X1	T45.8X2	T45.8X3	T45.8X4	T45.8X5	T45.8X6
normal human serum	T45.8X1	T45.8X2	T45.8X3	T45.8X4	T45.8X5	T45.8X6
Albuterol	T48.6X1	T48.6X2	T48.6X3	T48.6X4	T48.6X5	T48.6X6
Albutoin	T42.0X1	T42.0X2	T42.0X3	T42.0X4	T42.0X5	T42.0X6
Alclometasone	T49.0X1	T49.0X2	T49.0X3	T49.0X4	T49.0X5	T49.0X6
Alcohol	T51.91	T51.92	T51.93	T51.94	—	—
absolute	T51.0X1	T51.0X2	T51.0X3	T51.0X4	—	—
beverage	T51.0X1	T51.0X2	T51.0X3	T51.0X4	—	—
allyl	T51.8X1	T51.8X2	T51.8X3	T51.8X4	—	—
amyl	T51.3X1	T51.3X2	T51.3X3	T51.3X4	—	—
antifreeze	T51.1X1	T51.1X2	T51.1X3	T51.1X4	—	—
beverage	T51.0X1	T51.0X2	T51.0X3	T51.0X4	—	—
butyl	T51.3X1	T51.3X2	T51.3X3	T51.3X4	—	—
dehydrated	T51.0X1	T51.0X2	T51.0X3	T51.0X4	—	—
beverage	T51.0X1	T51.0X2	T51.0X3	T51.0X4	—	—
denatured	T51.0X1	T51.0X2	T51.0X3	T51.0X4	—	—
deterrent NEC	T50.6X1	T50.6X2	T50.6X3	T50.6X4	T50.6X5	T50.6X6
diagnostic (gastric function)	T50.8X1	T50.8X2	T50.8X3	T50.8X4	T50.8X5	T50.8X6
ethyl	T51.0X1	T51.0X2	T51.0X3	T51.0X4	—	—
beverage	T51.0X1	T51.0X2	T51.0X3	T51.0X4	—	—
grain	T51.0X1	T51.0X2	T51.0X3	T51.0X4	—	—
beverage	T51.0X1	T51.0X2	T51.0X3	T51.0X4	—	—
industrial	T51.0X1	T51.0X2	T51.0X3	T51.0X4	—	—
isopropyl	T51.2X1	T51.2X2	T51.2X3	T51.2X4	—	—
methyl	T51.1X1	T51.1X2	T51.1X3	T51.1X4	—	—
preparation for consumption	T51.0X1	T51.0X2	T51.0X3	T51.0X4	—	—

TABLE OF DRUGS AND CHEMICALS

Substance	Poisoning, Accidental (Unintentional)	Poisoning, Intentional Self-Harm	Poisoning, Assault	Poisoning, Undetermined	Adverse Effect	Underdosing
			External Cause (T-Code)			
Alcohol *(Continued)*						
propyl	T51.3X1	T51.3X2	T51.3X3	T51.3X4	—	—
secondary	T51.2X1	T51.2X2	T51.2X3	T51.2X4	—	—
radiator	T51.1X1	T51.1X2	T51.1X3	T51.1X4	—	—
rubbing	T51.2X1	T51.2X2	T51.2X3	T51.2X4	—	—
specified type NEC	T51.8X1	T51.8X2	T51.8X3	T51.8X4	—	—
surgical	T51.0X1	T51.0X2	T51.0X3	T51.0X4	—	—
vapor (from any type of Alcohol)	T59.891	T59.892	T59.893	T59.894		
wood	T51.1X1	T51.1X2	T51.1X3	T51.1X4		
Alcuronium (chloride)	T48.1X1	T48.1X2	T48.1X3	T48.1X4	T48.1X5	T48.1X6
Aldactone	T50.0X1	T50.0X2	T50.0X3	T50.0X4	T50.0X5	T50.0X6
Aldesulfone sodium	T37.1X1	T37.1X2	T37.1X3	T37.1X4	T37.1X5	T37.1X6
Aldicarb	T60.0X1	T60.0X2	T60.0X3	T60.0X4	—	—
Aldomet	T46.5X1	T46.5X2	T46.5X3	T46.5X4	T46.5X5	T46.5X6
Aldosterone	T50.0X1	T50.0X2	T50.0X3	T50.0X4	T50.0X5	T50.0X6
Aldrin (dust)	T60.1X1	T60.1X2	T60.1X3	T60.1X4	—	—
Aleve — *see Naproxen*						
Alexitol sodium	T47.1X1	T47.1X2	T47.1X3	T47.1X4	T47.1X5	T47.1X6
Alfacalcidol	T45.2X1	T45.2X2	T45.2X3	T45.2X4	T45.2X5	T45.2X6
Alfadolone	T41.1X1	T41.1X2	T41.1X3	T41.1X4	T41.1X5	T41.1X6
Alfaxalone	T41.1X1	T41.1X2	T41.1X3	T41.1X4	T41.1X5	T41.1X6
Alfentanil	T40.4X1	T40.4X2	T40.4X3	T40.4X4	T40.4X5	T40.4X6
Alfuzosin (hydrochloride)	T44.8X1	T44.8X2	T44.8X3	T44.8X4	T44.8X5	T44.8X6
Algae (harmful) (toxin)	T65.821	T65.822	T65.823	T65.824	—	—
Algeldrate	T47.1X1	T47.1X2	T47.1X3	T47.1X4	T47.1X5	T47.1X6
Algin	T47.8X1	T47.8X2	T47.8X3	T47.8X4	T47.8X5	T47.8X6
Alglucerase	T45.3X1	T45.3X2	T45.3X3	T45.3X4	T45.3X5	T45.3X6
Alidase	T45.3X1	T45.3X2	T45.3X3	T45.3X4	T45.3X5	T45.3X6
Alimemazine	T43.3X1	T43.3X2	T43.3X3	T43.3X4	T43.3X5	T43.3X6
Aliphatic thiocyanates	T65.0X1	T65.0X2	T65.0X3	T65.0X4	—	—
Alizapride	T45.0X1	T45.0X2	T45.0X3	T45.0X4	T45.0X5	T45.0X6
Alkali (caustic)	T54.3X1	T54.3X2	T54.3X3	T54.3X4	—	—
Alkalizing agent NEC	T50.901	T50.902	T50.903	T50.904	T50.905	T50.906
Alkaline antiseptic solution (aromatic)	T49.6X1	T49.6X2	T49.6X3	T49.6X4	T49.6X5	T49.6X6
Alkalinizing agents (medicinal)	T50.901	T50.902	T50.903	T50.904	T50.905	T50.906
Alka-seltzer	T39.011	T39.012	T39.013	T39.014	T39.015	T39.016
Alkavervir	T46.5X1	T46.5X2	T46.5X3	T46.5X4	T46.5X5	T46.5X6
Alkonium (bromide)	T49.0X1	T49.0X2	T49.0X3	T49.0X4	T49.0X5	T49.0X6
Alkylating drug NEC	T45.1X1	T45.1X2	T45.1X3	T45.1X4	T45.1X5	T45.1X6
antimyeloproliferative	T45.1X1	T45.1X2	T45.1X3	T45.1X4	T45.1X5	T45.1X6
lymphatic	T45.1X1	T45.1X2	T45.1X3	T45.1X4	T45.1X5	T45.1X6

Substance	External Cause (T-Code)					
	Poisoning, Accidental (Unintentional)	Poisoning, Intentional Self-Harm	Poisoning, Assault	Poisoning, Undetermined	Adverse Effect	Underdosing
Alkylisocyanate	T65.0X1	T65.0X2	T65.0X3	T65.0X4	—	—
Allantoin	T49.411	T49.412	T49.413	T49.414	T49.415	T49.416
Allegron	T43.0X1	T43.0X2	T43.0X3	T43.0X4	T43.0X5	T43.0X6
Allethrin	T49.0X1	T49.0X2	T49.0X3	T49.0X4	T49.0X5	T49.0X6
Allobarbital	T42.3X1	T42.3X2	T42.3X3	T42.3X4	T42.3X5	T42.3X6
Allopurinol	T50.4X1	T50.4X2	T50.4X3	T50.4X4	T50.4X5	T50.4X6
Allyl						
alcohol	T51.8X1	T51.8X2	T51.8X3	T51.8X4	—	—
disulfide	T46.6X1	T46.6X2	T46.6X3	T46.6X4	T46.6X5	T46.6X6
Allylestrenol	T38.5X1	T38.5X2	T38.5X3	T38.5X4	T38.5X5	T38.5X6
Allylisopropylacetylurea	T42.6X1	T42.6X2	T42.6X3	T42.6X4	T42.6X5	T42.6X6
Allylisopropylmalonylurea	T42.3X1	T42.3X2	T42.3X3	T42.3X4	T42.3X5	T42.3X6
Allylthiourea	T49.3X1	T49.3X2	T49.3X3	T49.3X4	T49.3X5	T49.3X6
Allyltribromide	T42.6X1	T42.6X2	T42.6X3	T42.6X4	T42.6X5	T42.6X6
Allypropymal	T42.3X1	T42.3X2	T42.3X3	T42.3X4	T42.3X5	T42.3X6
Almagate	T47.1X1	T47.1X2	T47.1X3	T47.1X4	T47.1X5	T47.1X6
Almasilate	T47.1X1	T47.1X2	T47.1X3	T47.1X4	T47.1X5	T47.1X6
Almitrine	T50.7X1	T50.7X2	T50.7X3	T50.7X4	T50.7X5	T50.7X6
Aloes	T47.2X1	T47.2X2	T47.2X3	T47.2X4	T47.2X5	T47.2X6
Aloglutamol	T47.1X1	T47.1X2	T47.1X3	T47.1X4	T47.1X5	T47.1X6
Aloin	T47.2X1	T47.2X2	T47.2X3	T47.2X4	T47.2X5	T47.2X6
Aloxidone	T42.2X1	T42.2X2	T42.2X3	T42.2X4	T42.2X5	T42.2X6
Alpha						
acetyldigoxin	T46.0X1	T46.0X2	T46.0X3	T46.0X4	T46.0X5	T46.0X6
adrenergic blocking drug	T44.6X1	T44.6X2	T44.6X3	T44.6X4	T44.6X5	T44.6X6
amylase	T45.3X1	T45.3X2	T45.3X3	T45.3X4	T45.3X5	T45.3X6
tocoferol (acetate)	T45.2X1	T45.2X2	T45.2X3	T45.2X4	T45.2X5	T45.2X6
tocopherol	T45.2X1	T45.2X2	T45.2X3	T45.2X4	T45.2X5	T45.2X6
Alphadolone	T41.1X1	T41.1X2	T41.1X3	T41.1X4	T41.1X5	T41.1X6
Alphaprodine	T40.4X1	T40.4X2	T40.4X3	T40.4X4	T40.4X5	T40.4X6
Alphaxalone	T41.1X1	T41.1X2	T41.1X3	T41.1X4	T41.1X5	T41.1X6
Alprazolam	T42.4X1	T42.4X2	T42.4X3	T42.4X4	T42.4X5	T42.4X6
Alprenolol	T44.7X1	T44.7X2	T44.7X3	T44.7X4	T44.7X5	T44.7X6
Alprostadil	T46.7X1	T46.7X2	T46.7X3	T46.7X4	T46.7X5	T46.7X6
Alsactide	T38.811	T38.812	T38.813	T38.814	T38.815	T38.816
Alseroxylon	T46.5X1	T46.5X2	T46.5X3	T46.5X4	T46.5X5	T46.5X6
Alteplase	T45.611	T45.612	T45.613	T45.614	T45.615	T45.616
Altizide	T50.2X1	T50.2X2	T50.2X3	T50.2X4	T50.2X5	T50.2X6
Altretamine	T45.1X1	T45.1X2	T45.1X3	T45.1X4	T45.1X5	T45.1X6

Substance	External Cause (T-Code)					
	Poisoning, Accidental (Unintentional)	Poisoning, Intentional Self-Harm	Poisoning, Assault	Poisoning, Undetermined	Adverse Effect	Underdosing
Alum (medicinal)	T49.4X1	T49.4X2	T49.4X3	T49.4X4	T49.4X5	T49.4X6
nonmedicinal (ammonium) (potassium)	T56.891	T56.892	T56.893	T56.894	—	—
Aluminium, aluminum						
acetate	T49.2X1	T49.2X2	T49.2X3	T49.2X4	T49.2X5	T49.2X6
solution	T49.0X1	T49.0X2	T49.0X3	T49.0X4	T49.0X5	T49.0X6
aspirin	T39.011	T39.012	T39.013	T39.014	T39.015	T39.016
bis (acetylsalicylate)	T39.011	T39.012	T39.013	T39.014	T39.015	T39.016
carbonate (gel, basic)	T47.1X1	T47.1X2	T47.1X3	T47.1X4	T47.1X5	T47.1X6
chlorhydroxide-complex	T47.1X1	T47.1X2	T47.1X3	T47.1X4	T47.1X5	T47.1X6
chloride	T49.2X1	T49.2X2	T49.2X3	T49.2X4	T49.2X5	T49.2X6
clofibrate	T46.6X1	T46.6X2	T46.6X3	T46.6X4	T46.6X5	T46.6X6
diacetate	T49.2X1	T49.2X2	T49.2X3	T49.2X4	T49.2X5	T49.2X6
glycinate	T47.1X1	T47.1X2	T47.1X3	T47.1X4	T47.1X5	T47.1X6
hydroxide (gel)	T47.1X1	T47.1X2	T47.1X3	T47.1X4	T47.1X5	T47.1X6
hydroxide-magnesium carb. gel	T47.1X1	T47.1X2	T47.1X3	T47.1X4	T47.1X5	T47.1X6
magnesium silicate	T47.1X1	T47.1X2	T47.1X3	T47.1X4	T47.1X5	T47.1X6
nicotinate	T46.7X1	T46.7X2	T46.7X3	T46.7X4	T46.7X5	T46.7X6
ointment (surgical) (topical)	T49.3X1	T49.3X2	T49.3X3	T49.3X4	T49.3X5	T49.3X6
phosphate	T47.1X1	T47.1X2	T47.1X3	T47.1X4	T47.1X5	T47.1X6
salicylate	T39.091	T39.092	T39.093	T39.094	T39.095	T39.096
silicate	T47.1X1	T47.1X2	T47.1X3	T47.1X4	T47.1X5	T47.1X6
sodium silicate	T47.1X1	T47.1X2	T47.1X3	T47.1X4	T47.1X5	T47.1X6
subacetate	T49.2X1	T49.2X2	T49.2X3	T49.2X4	T49.2X5	T49.2X6
sulfate	T49.0X1	T49.0X2	T49.0X3	T49.0X4	T49.0X5	T49.0X6
tannate	T47.6X1	T47.6X2	T47.6X3	T47.6X4	T47.6X5	T47.6X6
topical NEC	T49.3X1	T49.3X2	T49.3X3	T49.3X4	T49.3X5	T49.3X6
Alurate	T42.3X1	T42.3X2	T42.3X3	T42.3X4	T42.3X5	T42.3X6
Alverine	T44.3X1	T44.3X2	T44.3X3	T44.3X4	T44.3X5	T44.3X6
Alvodine	T40.2X1	T40.2X2	T40.2X3	T40.2X4	T40.2X5	T40.2X6
Amanita phalloides	T62.0X1	T62.0X2	T62.0X3	T62.0X4	—	—
Amanitine	T62.0X1	T62.0X2	T62.0X3	T62.0X4	—	—
Amantadine	T42.8X1	T42.8X2	T42.8X3	T42.8X4	T42.8X5	T42.8X6
Ambazone	T49.6X1	T49.6X2	T49.6X3	T49.6X4	T49.6X5	T49.6X6
Ambenonium (chloride)	T44.0X1	T44.0X2	T44.0X3	T44.0X4	T44.0X5	T44.0X6
Ambroxol	T48.4X1	T48.4X2	T48.4X3	T48.4X4	T48.4X5	T48.4X6
Ambuphylline	T48.6X1	T48.6X2	T48.6X3	T48.6X4	T48.6X5	T48.6X6
Ambutonium bromide	T44.3X1	T44.3X2	T44.3X3	T44.3X4	T44.3X5	T44.3X6
Amcinonide	T49.0X1	T49.0X2	T49.0X3	T49.0X4	T49.0X5	T49.0X6
Amdinocilline	T36.0X1	T36.0X2	T36.0X3	T36.0X4	T36.0X5	T36.0X6

Substance	Poisoning, Accidental (Unintentional)	Poisoning, Intentional Self-Harm	Poisoning, Assault	Poisoning, Undetermined	Adverse Effect	Underdosing
Ametazole	T50.8X1	T50.8X2	T50.8X3	T50.8X4	T50.8X5	T50.8X6
Amethocaine	T41.3X1	T41.3X2	T41.3X3	T41.3X4	T41.3X5	T41.3X6
regional	T41.3X1	T41.3X2	T41.3X3	T41.3X4	T41.3X5	T41.3X6
spinal	T41.3X1	T41.3X2	T41.3X3	T41.3X4	T41.3X5	T41.3X6
Amethopterin	T45.1X1	T45.1X2	T45.1X3	T45.1X4	T45.1X5	T45.1X6
Amezinium metilsulfate	T44.991	T44.992	T44.993	T44.994	T44.995	T44.996
Amfebutamone	T43.291	T43.292	T43.293	T43.294	T43.295	T43.296
Amfepramone	T50.5X1	T50.5X2	T50.5X3	T50.5X4	T50.5X5	T50.5X6
Amfetamine	T43.621	T43.622	T43.623	T43.624	T43.625	T43.626
Amfetaminil	T43.621	T43.622	T43.623	T43.624	T43.625	T43.626
Amfomycin	T36.8X1	T36.8X2	T36.8X3	T36.8X4	T36.8X5	T36.8X6
Amidefrine mesilate	T48.5X1	T48.5X2	T48.5X3	T48.5X4	T48.5X5	T48.5X6
Amidone	T40.3X1	T40.3X2	T40.3X3	T40.3X4	T40.3X5	T40.3X6
Amidopyrine	T39.2X1	T39.2X2	T39.2X3	T39.2X4	T39.2X5	T39.2X6
Amidotrizoate	T50.8X1	T50.8X2	T50.8X3	T50.8X4	T50.8X5	T50.8X6
Amiflamine	T43.1X1	T43.1X2	T43.1X3	T43.1X4	T43.1X5	T43.1X6
Amikacin	T36.5X1	T36.5X2	T36.5X3	T36.5X4	T36.5X5	T36.5X6
Amikhelline	T46.3X1	T46.3X2	T46.3X3	T46.3X4	T46.3X5	T46.3X6
Amiloride	T50.2X1	T50.2X2	T50.2X3	T50.2X4	T50.2X5	T50.2X6
Aminacrine	T49.0X1	T49.0X2	T49.0X3	T49.0X4	T49.0X5	T49.0X6
Amineptine	T43.011	T43.012	T43.013	T43.014	T43.015	T43.016
Aminitrozole	T37.3X1	T37.3X2	T37.3X3	T37.3X4	T37.3X5	T37.3X6
Aminoacetic acid (derivatives)	T50.3X1	T50.3X2	T50.3X3	T50.3X4	T50.3X5	T50.3X6
Amino acids	T50.3X1	T50.3X2	T50.3X3	T50.3X4	T50.3X5	T50.3X6
Aminoacridine	T49.0X1	T49.0X2	T49.0X3	T49.0X4	T49.0X5	T49.0X6
Aminobenzoic acid (-p)	T49.3X1	T49.3X2	T49.3X3	T49.3X4	T49.3X5	T49.3X6
4-Aminobutyric acid	T43.8X1	T43.8X2	T43.8X3	T43.8X4	T43.8X5	T43.8X6
Aminocaproic acid	T45.621	T45.622	T45.623	T45.624	T45.625	T45.626
Aminofenazone	T39.2X1	T39.2X2	T39.2X3	T39.2X4	T39.2X5	T39.2X6
Aminoethylisothiourium	T45.8X1	T45.8X2	T45.8X3	T45.8X4	T45.8X5	T45.8X6
Aminoglutethimide	T45.1X1	T45.1X2	T45.1X3	T45.1X4	T45.1X5	T45.1X6
Aminohippuric acid	T50.8X1	T50.8X2	T50.8X3	T50.8X4	T50.8X5	T50.8X6
Aminomethylbenzoic acid	T45.691	T45.692	T45.693	T45.694	T45.695	T45.696
Aminometradine	T50.2X1	T50.2X2	T50.2X3	T50.2X4	T50.2X5	T50.2X6
Aminopentamide	T44.3X1	T44.3X2	T44.3X3	T44.3X4	T44.3X5	T44.3X6
Aminophenazone	T39.2X1	T39.2X2	T39.2X3	T39.2X4	T39.2X5	T39.2X6
Aminophenol	T54.0X1	T54.0X2	T54.0X3	T54.0X4	—	—
4-Aminophenol derivatives	T39.1X1	T39.1X2	T39.1X3	T39.1X4	T39.1X5	T39.1X6
Aminophenylpyridone	T43.591	T43.592	T43.593	T43.594	T43.595	T43.596

TABLE OF DRUGS AND CHEMICALS

Substance	Poisoning, Accidental (Unintentional)	Poisoning, Intentional Self-Harm	Poisoning, Assault	Poisoning, Undetermined	Adverse Effect	Underdosing
Aminophylline	T48.6X1	T48.6X2	T48.6X3	T48.6X4	T48.6X5	T48.6X6
Aminopterin sodium	T45.1X1	T45.1X2	T45.1X3	T45.1X4	T45.1X5	T45.1X6
Aminopyrine	T39.2X1	T39.2X2	T39.2X3	T39.2X4	T39.2X5	T39.2X6
8-Aminoquinoline drugs	T37.2X1	T37.2X2	T37.2X3	T37.2X4	T37.2X5	T37.2X6
Aminorex	T50.5X1	T50.5X2	T50.5X3	T50.5X4	T50.5X5	T50.5X6
Aminosalicylic acid	T37.1X1	T37.1X2	T37.1X3	T37.1X4	T37.1X5	T37.1X6
Aminosalylum	T37.1X1	T37.1X2	T37.1X3	T37.1X4	T37.1X5	T37.1X6
Amiodarone	T46.2X1	T46.2X2	T46.2X3	T46.2X4	T46.2X5	T46.2X6
Amiphenazole	T50.7X1	T50.7X2	T50.7X3	T50.7X4	T50.7X5	T50.7X6
Amiquinsin	T46.5X1	T46.5X2	T46.5X3	T46.5X4	T46.5X5	T46.5X6
Amisometradine	T50.2X1	T50.2X2	T50.2X3	T50.2X4	T50.2X5	T50.2X6
Amisulpride	T43.591	T43.592	T43.593	T43.594	T43.595	T43.596
Amitriptyline	T43.021	T43.022	T43.023	T43.024	T43.025	T43.026
Amitriptylinoxide	T43.021	T43.022	T43.023	T43.024	T43.025	T43.026
Amlexanox	T48.6X1	T48.6X2	T48.6X3	T48.6X4	T48.6X5	T48.6X6
Ammonia (fumes) (gas) (vapor)	T59.891	T59.892	T59.893	T59.894	—	—
aromatic spirit	T48.991	T48.992	T48.993	T48.994	T48.995	T48.996
liquid (household)	T54.3X1	T54.3X2	T54.3X3	T54.3X4	—	—
Ammoniated mercury	T49.0X1	T49.0X2	T49.0X3	T49.0X4	T49.0X5	T49.0X6
Ammonium						
acid tartrate	T49.5X1	T49.5X2	T49.5X3	T49.5X4	T49.5X5	T49.5X6
bromide	T42.6X1	T42.6X2	T42.6X3	T42.6X4	T42.6X5	T42.6X6
carbonate	T54.3X1	T54.3X2	T54.3X3	T54.3X4	—	—
chloride	T50.991	T50.992	T50.993	T50.994	T50.995	T50.996
expectorant	T48.4X1	T48.4X2	T48.4X3	T48.4X4	T48.4X5	T48.4X6
compounds (household) NEC	T54.3X1	T54.3X2	T54.3X3	T54.3X4	—	—
fumes (any usage)	T59.891	T59.892	T59.893	T59.894	—	—
industrial	T54.3X1	T54.3X2	T54.3X3	T54.3X4	—	—
ichthyosulronate	T49.4X1	T49.4X2	T49.4X3	T49.4X4	T49.4X5	T49.4X6
mandelate	T37.91	T37.92	T37.93	T37.94	T37.95	T37.96
sulfamate	T60.3X1	T60.3X2	T60.3X3	T60.3X4	—	—
sulfonate resin	T47.8X1	T47.8X2	T47.8X3	T47.8X4	T47.8X5	T47.8X6
Amobarbital (sodium)	T42.3X1	T42.3X2	T42.3X3	T42.3X4	T42.3X5	T42.3X6
Amodiaquine	T37.2X1	T37.2X2	T37.2X3	T37.2X4	T37.2X5	T37.2X6
Amopyroquin(e)	T37.2X1	T37.2X2	T37.2X3	T37.2X4	T37.2X5	T37.2X6
Amoxapine	T43.011	T43.012	T43.013	T43.014	T43.015	T43.016
Amoxicillin	T36.0X1	T36.0X2	T36.0X3	T36.0X4	T36.0X5	T36.0X6
Amperozide	T43.591	T43.592	T43.593	T43.594	T43.595	T43.596
Amphenidone	T43.591	T43.592	T43.593	T43.594	T43.595	T43.596
Amphetamine NEC	T43.621	T43.622	T43.623	T43.624	T43.625	T43.626

Substance	External Cause (T-Code)					
	Poisoning, Accidental (Unintentional)	Poisoning, Intentional Self-Harm	Poisoning, Assault	Poisoning, Undetermined	Adverse Effect	Underdosing
Amphomycin	T36.8X1	T36.8X2	T36.8X3	T36.8X4	T36.8X5	T36.8X6
Amphotalide	T37.4X1	T37.4X2	T37.4X3	T37.4X4	T37.4X5	T37.4X6
Amphotericin B	T36.7X1	T36.7X2	T36.7X3	T36.7X4	T36.7X5	T36.7X6
topical	T49.0X1	T49.0X2	T49.0X3	T49.0X4	T49.0X5	T49.0X6
Ampicillin	T36.0X1	T36.0X2	T36.0X3	T36.0X4	T36.0X5	T36.0X6
Amprotropine	T44.3X1	T44.3X2	T44.3X3	T44.3X4	T44.3X5	T44.3X6
Amsacrine	T45.1X1	T45.1X2	T45.1X3	T45.1X4	T45.1X5	T45.1X6
Amygdaline	T62.2X1	T62.2X2	T62.2X3	T62.2X4	—	—
Amyl						
acetate	T52.8X1	T52.8X2	T52.8X3	T52.8X4	—	—
vapor	T59.891	T59.892	T59.893	T59.894	—	—
alcohol	T51.3X1	T51.3X2	T51.3X3	T51.3X4	—	—
chloride	T53.6X1	T53.6X2	T53.6X3	T53.6X4	—	—
formate	T52.8X1	T52.8X2	T52.8X3	T52.8X4	—	—
nitrite	T46.3X1	T46.3X2	T46.3X3	T46.3X4	T46.3X5	T46.3X6
propionate	T65.891	T65.892	T65.893	T65.894	—	—
Amylase	T47.5X1	T47.5X2	T47.5X3	T47.5X4	T47.5X5	T47.5X6
Amyleine, regional	T41.3X1	T41.3X2	T41.3X3	T41.3X4	T41.3X5	T41.3X6
Amylene						
dichloride	T53.6X1	T53.6X2	T53.6X3	T53.6X4	—	—
hydrate	T51.3X1	T51.3X2	T51.3X3	T51.3X4	—	—
Amylmetacresol	T49.6X1	T49.6X2	T49.6X3	T49.6X4	T49.6X5	T49.6X6
Amylobarbitone	T42.3X1	T42.3X2	T42.3X3	T42.3X4	T42.3X5	T42.3X6
Amylocaine, regional	T41.3X1	T41.3X2	T41.3X3	T41.3X4	T41.3X5	T41.3X6
infiltration (subcutaneous)	T41.3X1	T41.3X2	T41.3X3	T41.3X4	T41.3X5	T41.3X6
nerve block (peripheral) (plexus)	T41.3X1	T41.3X2	T41.3X3	T41.3X4	T41.3X5	T41.3X6
spinal	T41.3X1	T41.3X2	T41.3X3	T41.3X4	T41.3X5	T41.3X6
topical (surface)	T41.3X1	T41.3X2	T41.3X3	T41.3X4	T41.3X5	T41.3X6
Amylopectin	T47.6X1	T47.6X2	T47.6X3	T47.6X4	T47.6X5	T47.6X6
Amytal (sodium)	T42.3X1	T42.3X2	T42.3X3	T42.3X4	T42.3X5	T42.3X6
Anabolic steroid	T38.7X1	T38.7X2	T38.7X3	T38.7X4	T38.7X5	T38.7X6
Analeptic NEC	T50.7X1	T50.7X2	T50.7X3	T50.7X4	T50.7X5	T50.7X6
Analgesic	T39.91	T39.92	T39.93	T39.94	T39.95	T39.96
anti-inflammatory NEC	T39.91	T39.92	T39.93	T39.94	T39.95	T39.96
propionic acid derivative	T39.311	T39.312	T39.313	T39.314	T39.315	T39.316
antirheumatic NEC	T39.4X1	T39.4X2	T39.4X3	T39.4X4	T39.4X5	T39.4X6
aromatic NEC	T39.1X1	T39.1X2	T39.1X3	T39.1X4	T39.1X5	T39.1X6
narcotic NEC	T40.601	T40.602	T40.603	T40.604	T40.605	T40.606
combination	T40.601	T40.602	T40.603	T40.604	T40.605	T40.606
obstetric	T40.601	T40.602	T40.603	T40.604	T40.605	T40.606

Substance	Poisoning, Accidental (Unintentional)	Poisoning, Intentional Self-Harm	Poisoning, Assault	Poisoning, Undetermined	Adverse Effect	Underdosing
External Cause (T-Code)						
Analgesic *(Continued)*						
non-narcotic NEC	T39.91	T39.92	T39.93	T39.94	T39.95	T39.96
combination	T39.91	T39.92	T39.93	T39.94	T39.95	T39.96
pyrazole	T39.2X1	T39.2X2	T39.2X3	T39.2X4	T39.2X5	T39.2X6
specified NEC	T39.8X1	T39.8X2	T39.8X3	T39.8X4	T39.8X5	T39.8X6
Analgin	T39.2X1	T39.2X2	T39.2X3	T39.2X4	T39.2X5	T39.2X6
Anamirta cocculus	T62.1X1	T62.1X2	T62.1X3	T62.1X4	—	—
Ancillin	T36.0X1	T36.0X2	T36.0X3	T36.0X4	T36.0X5	T36.0X6
Ancrod	T45.691	T45.692	T45.693	T45.694	T45.695	T45.696
Androgen	T38.7X1	T38.7X2	T38.7X3	T38.7X4	T38.7X5	T38.7X6
Androgen-estrogen mixture	T38.7X1	T38.7X2	T38.7X3	T38.7X4	T38.7X5	T38.7X6
Androstalone	T38.7X1	T38.7X2	T38.7X3	T38.7X4	T38.7X5	T38.7X6
Androstanolone	T38.7X1	T38.7X2	T38.7X3	T38.7X4	T38.7X5	T38.7X6
Androsterone	T38.7X1	T38.7X2	T38.7X3	T38.7X4	T38.7X5	T38.7X6
Anemone pulsatilla	T62.2X1	T62.2X2	T62.2X3	T62.2X4	—	—
Anesthesia						
caudal	T41.3X1	T41.3X2	T41.3X3	T41.3X4	T41.3X5	T41.3X6
endotracheal	T41.0X1	T41.0X2	T41.0X3	T41.0X4	T41.0X5	T41.0X6
epidural	T41.3X1	T41.3X2	T41.3X3	T41.3X4	T41.3X5	T41.3X6
inhalation	T41.0X1	T41.0X2	T41.0X3	T41.0X4	T41.0X5	T41.0X6
local	T41.3X1	T41.3X2	T41.3X3	T41.3X4	T41.3X5	T41.3X6
mucosal	T41.3X1	T41.3X2	T41.3X3	T41.3X4	T41.3X5	T41.3X6
muscle relaxation	T48.1X1	T48.1X2	T48.1X3	T48.1X4	T48.1X5	T48.1X6
nerve blocking	T41.3X1	T41.3X2	T41.3X3	T41.3X4	T41.3X5	T41.3X6
plexus blocking	T41.3X1	T41.3X2	T41.3X3	T41.3X4	T41.3X5	T41.3X6
potentiated	T41.201	T41.202	T41.203	T41.204	T41.205	T41.206
rectal	T41.201	T41.202	T41.203	T41.204	T41.205	T41.206
general	T41.201	T41.202	T41.203	T41.204	T41.205	T41.206
local	T41.3X1	T41.3X2	T41.3X3	T41.3X4	T41.3X5	T41.3X6
regional	T41.3X1	T41.3X2	T41.3X3	T41.3X4	T41.3X5	T41.3X6
surface	T41.3X1	T41.3X2	T41.3X3	T41.3X4	T41.3X5	T41.3X6
Anesthetic NEC—*see also* Anesthesia	T41.41	T41.42	T41.43	T41.44	T41.45	T41.46
with muscle relaxant	T41.201	T41.202	T41.203	T41.204	T41.205	T41.206
general	T41.201	T41.202	T41.203	T41.204	T41.205	T41.206
local	T41.3X1	T41.3X2	T41.3X3	T41.3X4	T41.3X5	T41.3X6
gaseous NEC	T41.0X1	T41.0X2	T41.0X3	T41.0X4	T41.0X5	T41.0X6
general NEC	T41.201	T41.202	T41.203	T41.204	T41.205	T41.206
halogenated hydrocarbon derivatives NEC	T41.0X1	T41.0X2	T41.0X3	T41.0X4	T41.0X5	T41.0X6
infiltration NEC	T41.3X1	T41.3X2	T41.3X3	T41.3X4	T41.3X5	T41.3X6
intravenous NEC	T41.1X1	T41.1X2	T41.1X3	T41.1X4	T41.1X5	T41.1X6

Substance	Poisoning, Accidental (Unintentional)	Poisoning, Intentional Self-Harm	Poisoning, Assault	Poisoning, Undetermined	Adverse Effect	Underdosing
Anesthetic NEC *(Continued)*						
local NEC	T41.3X1	T41.3X2	T41.3X3	T41.3X4	T41.3X5	T41.3X6
rectal	T41.201	T41.202	T41.203	T41.204	T41.205	T41.206
general	T41.201	T41.202	T41.203	T41.204	T41.205	T41.206
local	T41.3X1	T41.3X2	T41.3X3	T41.3X4	T41.3X5	T41.3X6
regional NEC	T41.3X1	T41.3X2	T41.3X3	T41.3X4	T41.3X5	T41.3X6
spinal NEC	T41.3X1	T41.3X2	T41.3X3	T41.3X4	T41.3X5	T41.3X6
thiobarbiturate	T41.1X1	T41.1X2	T41.1X3	T41.1X4	T41.1X5	T41.1X6
topical	T41.3X1	T41.3X2	T41.3X3	T41.3X4	T41.3X5	T41.3X6
Aneurine	T45.2X1	T45.2X2	T45.2X3	T45.2X4	T45.2X5	T45.2X6
Angio-Conray	T50.8X1	T50.8X2	T50.8X3	T50.8X4	T50.8X5	T50.8X6
Angiotensin	T44.5X1	T44.5X2	T44.5X3	T44.5X4	T44.5X5	T44.5X6
Angiotensinamide	T44.991	T44.992	T44.993	T44.994	T44.995	T44.996
Anhydrohydroxy-progesterone	T38.5X1	T38.5X2	T38.5X3	T38.5X4	T38.5X5	T38.5X6
Anhydron	T50.2X1	T50.2X2	T50.2X3	T50.2X4	T50.2X5	T50.2X6
Anileridine	T40.4X1	T40.4X2	T40.4X3	T40.4X4	T40.4X5	T40.4X6
Aniline (dye) (liquid)	T65.3X1	T65.3X2	T65.3X3	T65.3X4	—	—
analgesic	T39.1X1	T39.1X2	T39.1X3	T39.1X4	T39.1X5	T39.1X6
derivatives, therapeutic NEC	T39.1X1	T39.1X2	T39.1X3	T39.1X4	T39.1X5	T39.1X6
vapor	T65.3X1	T65.3X2	T65.3X3	T65.3X4	—	—
Anise oil	T47.5X1	T47.5X2	T47.5X3	T47.5X4	T47.5X5	T47.5X6
Aniscoropine	T44.3X1	T44.3X2	T44.3X3	T44.3X4	T44.3X5	T44.3X6
Anisidine	T65.3X1	T65.3X2	T65.3X3	T65.3X4	—	—
Anisindione	T45.511	T45.512	T45.513	T45.514	T45.515	T45.516
Anisotropine methyl-bromide	T44.3X1	T44.3X2	T44.3X3	T44.3X4	T44.3X5	T44.3X6
Anistreplase	T45.611	T45.612	T45.613	T45.614	T45.615	T45.616
Anorexiant (central)	T50.5X1	T50.5X2	T50.5X3	T50.5X4	T50.5X5	T50.5X6
Anorexic agents	T50.5X1	T50.5X2	T50.5X3	T50.5X4	T50.5X5	T50.5X6
Ansamycin	T36.6X1	T36.6X2	T36.6X3	T36.6X4	T36.6X5	T36.6X6
Ant (bite) (sting)	T63.421	T63.422	T63.423	T63.424	—	—
Antabuse	T50.6X1	T50.6X2	T50.6X3	T50.6X4	T50.6X5	T50.6X6
Ant poison — *see Insecticide*						
Antacid NEC	T47.1X1	T47.1X2	T47.1X3	T47.1X4	T47.1X5	T47.1X6
Antagonist						
Aldosterone	T50.0X1	T50.0X2	T50.0X3	T50.0X4	T50.0X5	T50.0X6
alpha-adrenoreceptor	T44.6X1	T44.6X2	T44.6X3	T44.6X4	T44.6X5	T44.6X6
anticoagulant	T45.7X1	T45.7X2	T45.7X3	T45.7X4	T45.7X5	T45.7X6
beta-adrenoreceptor	T44.7X1	T44.7X2	T44.7X3	T44.7X4	T44.7X5	T44.7X6
extrapyramidal NEC	T44.3X1	T44.3X2	T44.3X3	T44.3X4	T44.3X5	T44.3X6
folic acid	T45.1X1	T45.1X2	T45.1X3	T45.1X4	T45.1X5	T45.1X6

Substance	Poisoning, Accidental (Unintentional)	Poisoning, Intentional Self-Harm	Poisoning, Assault	Poisoning, Undetermined	Adverse Effect	Underdosing
Antagonist *(Continued)*						
H2 receptor	T47.0X1	T47.0X2	T47.0X3	T47.0X4	T47.0X5	T47.0X6
heavy metal	T45.8X1	T45.8X2	T45.8X3	T45.8X4	T45.8X5	T45.8X6
narcotic analgesic	T50.7X1	T50.7X2	T50.7X3	T50.7X4	T50.7X5	T50.7X6
opiate	T50.7X1	T50.7X2	T50.7X3	T50.7X4	T50.7X5	T50.7X6
pyrimidine	T45.1X1	T45.1X2	T45.1X3	T45.1X4	T45.1X5	T45.1X6
serotonin	T46.5X1	T46.5X2	T46.5X3	T46.5X4	T46.5X5	T46.5X6
Antazolin(e)	T45.0X1	T45.0X2	T45.0X3	T45.0X4	T45.0X5	T45.0X6
Anterior pituitary hormone NEC	T38.811	T38.812	T38.813	T38.814	T38.815	T38.816
Anthelmintic NEC	T37.4X1	T37.4X2	T37.4X3	T37.4X4	T37.4X5	T37.4X6
Anthiolimine	T37.4X1	T37.4X2	T37.4X3	T37.4X4	T37.4X5	T37.4X6
Anthralin	T49.4X1	T49.4X2	T49.4X3	T49.4X4	T49.4X5	T49.4X6
Anthramycin	T45.1X1	T45.1X2	T45.1X3	T45.1X4	T45.1X5	T45.1X6
Antiadrenergic NEC	T44.8X1	T44.8X2	T44.8X3	T44.8X4	T44.8X5	T44.8X6
Antiallergic NEC	T45.0X1	T45.0X2	T45.0X3	T45.0X4	T45.0X5	T45.0X6
Anti-anemic (drug) (preparation)	T45.8X1	T45.8X2	T45.8X3	T45.8X4	T45.8X5	T45.8X6
Antiandrogen NEC	T38.6X1	T38.6X2	T38.6X3	T38.6X4	T38.6X5	T38.6X6
Antianxiety drug NEC	T43.501	T43.502	T43.503	T43.504	T43.505	T43.506
Antiaris toxicaria	T65.891	T65.892	T65.893	T65.894	—	—
Antiarteriosclerotic drug	T46.6X1	T46.6X2	T46.6X3	T46.6X4	T46.6X5	T46.6X6
Antiasthmatic drug NEC	T48.6X1	T48.6X2	T48.6X3	T48.6X4	T48.6X5	T48.6X6
Antibiotic NEC	T36.91	T36.92	T36.93	T36.94	T36.95	T36.96
aminoglycoside	T36.5X1	T36.5X2	T36.5X3	T36.5X4	T36.5X5	T36.5X6
anticancer	T45.1X1	T45.1X2	T45.1X3	T45.1X4	T45.1X5	T45.1X6
antifungal	T36.7X1	T36.7X2	T36.7X3	T36.7X4	T36.7X5	T36.7X6
antimycobacterial	T36.5X1	T36.5X2	T36.5X3	T36.5X4	T36.5X5	T36.5X6
antineoplastic	T45.1X1	T45.1X2	T45.1X3	T45.1X4	T45.1X5	T45.1X6
cephalosporin (group)	T36.1X1	T36.1X2	T36.1X3	T36.1X4	T36.1X5	T36.1X6
chloramphenicol (group)	T36.2X1	T36.2X2	T36.2X3	T36.2X4	T36.2X5	T36.2X6
ENT	T49.6X1	T49.6X2	T49.6X3	T49.6X4	T49.6X5	T49.6X6
eye	T49.5X1	T49.5X2	T49.5X3	T49.5X4	T49.5X5	T49.5X6
fungicidal (local)	T49.0X1	T49.0X2	T49.0X3	T49.0X4	T49.0X5	T49.0X6
intestinal	T36.8X1	T36.8X2	T36.8X3	T36.8X4	T36.8X5	T36.8X6
b-lactam NEC	T36.1X1	T36.1X2	T36.1X3	T36.1X4	T36.1X5	T36.1X6
local	T49.0X1	T49.0X2	T49.0X3	T49.0X4	T49.0X5	T49.0X6
macrolides	T36.3X1	T36.3X2	T36.3X3	T36.3X4	T36.3X5	T36.3X6
polypeptide	T36.8X1	T36.8X2	T36.8X3	T36.8X4	T36.8X5	T36.8X6
specified NEC	T36.8X1	T36.8X2	T36.8X3	T36.8X4	T36.8X5	T36.8X6
tetracycline (group)	T36.4X1	T36.4X2	T36.4X3	T36.4X4	T36.4X5	T36.4X6
throat	T49.6X1	T49.6X2	T49.6X3	T49.6X4	T49.6X5	T49.6X6

Substance	Poisoning, Accidental (Unintentional)	Poisoning, Intentional Self-Harm	Poisoning, Assault	Poisoning, Undetermined	Adverse Effect	Underdosing
			External Cause (T-Code)			
Anticancer agents NEC	T45.1X1	T45.1X2	T45.1X3	T45.1X4	T45.1X5	T45.1X6
Anticholesterolemic drug NEC	T46.6X1	T46.6X2	T46.6X3	T46.6X4	T46.6X5	T46.6X6
Anticholinergic NEC	T44.3X1	T44.3X2	T44.3X3	T44.3X4	T44.3X5	T44.3X6
Anticholinesterase	T44.0X1	T44.0X2	T44.0X3	T44.0X4	T44.0X5	T44.0X6
organophosphorus	T44.0X1	T44.0X2	T44.0X3	T44.0X4	T44.0X5	T44.0X6
insecticide	T60.0X1	T60.0X2	T60.0X3	T60.0X4	—	—
nerve gas	T59.891	T59.892	T59.893	T59.894	—	—
reversible	T44.0X1	T44.0X2	T44.0X3	T44.0X4	T44.0X5	T44.0X6
ophthalmological	T49.5X1	T49.5X2	T49.5X3	T49.5X4	T49.5X5	T49.5X6
Anticoagulant NEC	T45.511	T45.512	T45.513	T45.514	T45.515	T45.516
Antagonist	T45.7X1	T45.7X2	T45.7X3	T45.7X4	T45.7X5	T45.7X6
Anti-common-cold drug NEC	T48.5X1	T48.5X2	T48.5X3	T48.5X4	T48.5X5	T48.5X6
Anticonvulsant	T42.71	T42.72	T42.73	T42.74	T42.75	T42.76
barbiturate	T42.3X1	T42.3X2	T42.3X3	T42.3X4	T42.3X5	T42.3X6
combination (with barbiturate)	T42.3X1	T42.3X2	T42.3X3	T42.3X4	T42.3X5	T42.3X6
hydantoin	T42.0X1	T42.0X2	T42.0X3	T42.0X4	T42.0X5	T42.0X6
hypnotic NEC	T42.6X1	T42.6X2	T42.6X3	T42.6X4	T42.6X5	T42.6X6
oxazolidinedione	T42.2X1	T42.2X2	T42.2X3	T42.2X4	T42.2X5	T42.2X6
pyrimidinedione	T42.6X1	T42.6X2	T42.6X3	T42.6X4	T42.6X5	T42.6X6
specified NEC	T42.6X1	T42.6X2	T42.6X3	T42.6X4	T42.6X5	T42.6X6
succinimide	T42.2X1	T42.2X2	T42.2X3	T42.2X4	T42.2X5	T42.2X6
Anti-D immunoglobulin (human)	T50.Z11	T50.Z12	T50.Z13	T50.Z14	T50.Z15	T50.Z16
Antidepressant NEC	T43.201	T43.202	T43.203	T43.204	T43.205	T43.206
monoamine oxidase inhibitor	T43.1X1	T43.1X2	T43.1X3	T43.1X4	T43.1X5	T43.1X6
selective serotonin norepinephrine reuptake inhibitor	T43.211	T43.212	T43.213	T43.214	T43.215	T43.216
selective serotonin reuptake inhibitor	T43.221	T43.222	T43.223	T43.224	T43.225	T43.226
specified NEC	T43.291	T43.292	T43.293	T43.294	T43.295	T43.296
tetracyclic	T43.021	T43.022	T43.023	T43.024	T43.025	T43.026
triazolopyridine	T43.221	T43.222	T43.223	T43.224	T43.225	T43.226
tricyclic	T43.011	T43.012	T43.013	T43.014	T43.015	T43.016
Antidiabetic NEC	T38.3X1	T38.3X2	T38.3X3	T38.3X4	T38.3X5	T38.3X6
biguanide	T38.3X1	T38.3X2	T38.3X3	T38.3X4	T38.3X5	T38.3X6
and sulfonyl combined	T38.3X1	T38.3X2	T38.3X3	T38.3X4	T38.3X5	T38.3X6
combined	T38.3X1	T38.3X2	T38.3X3	T38.3X4	T38.3X5	T38.3X6
sulfonylurea	T38.3X1	T38.3X2	T38.3X3	T38.3X4	T38.3X5	T38.3X6
Antidiarrheal drug NEC	T47.6X1	T47.6X2	T47.6X3	T47.6X4	T47.6X5	T47.6X6
absorbent	T47.6X1	T47.6X2	T47.6X3	T47.6X4	T47.6X5	T47.6X6
Antidiphtheria serum	T50.Z11	T50.Z12	T50.Z13	T50.Z14	T50.Z15	T50.Z16
Antidiuretic hormone	T38.891	T38.892	T38.893	T38.894	T38.895	T38.896

Substance	Poisoning, Accidental (Unintentional)	Poisoning, Intentional Self-Harm	Poisoning, Assault	Poisoning, Undetermined	Adverse Effect	Underdosing
Antidote NEC	T50.6X1	T50.6X2	T50.6X3	T50.6X4	T50.6X5	T50.6X6
heavy metal	T45.8X1	T45.8X2	T45.8X3	T45.8X4	T45.8X5	T45.8X6
Antidysrhythmic NEC	T46.2X1	T46.2X2	T46.2X3	T46.2X4	T46.2X5	T46.2X6
Antiemetic drug	T45.0X1	T45.0X2	T45.0X3	T45.0X4	T45.0X5	T45.0X6
Antiepilepsy agent	T42.71	T42.72	T42.73	T42.74	T42.75	T42.76
combination	T42.5X1	T42.5X2	T42.5X3	T42.5X4	T42.5X5	T42.5X6
mixed	T42.5X1	T42.5X2	T42.5X3	T42.5X4	T42.5X5	T42.5X6
specified, NEC	T42.6X1	T42.6X2	T42.6X3	T42.6X4	T42.6X5	T42.6X6
Antiestrogen NEC	T38.6X1	T38.6X2	T38.6X3	T38.6X4	T38.6X5	T38.6X6
Antifertility pill	T38.4X1	T38.4X2	T38.4X3	T38.4X4	T38.4X5	T38.4X6
Antifibrinolytic drug	T45.621	T45.622	T45.623	T45.624	T45.625	T45.626
Antifilarial drug	T37.4X1	T37.4X2	T37.4X3	T37.4X4	T37.4X5	T37.4X6
Antiflatulent	T47.5X1	T47.5X2	T47.5X3	T47.5X4	T47.5X5	T47.5X6
Antifreeze	T65.91	T65.92	T65.93	T65.94	—	—
alcohol	T51.1X1	T51.1X2	T51.1X3	T51.1X4	—	—
ethylene glycol	T51.8X1	T51.8X2	T51.8X3	T51.8X4	—	—
Antifungal						
antibiotic (systemic)	T36.7X1	T36.7X2	T36.7X3	T36.7X4	T36.7X5	T36.7X6
anti-infective NEC	T37.91	T37.92	T37.93	T37.94	T37.95	T37.96
disinfectant, local	T49.0X1	T49.0X2	T49.0X3	T49.0X4	T49.0X5	T49.0X6
nonmedicinal (spray)	T60.3X1	T60.3X2	T60.3X3	T60.3X4	—	—
topical	T49.0X1	T49.0X2	T49.0X3	T49.0X4	T49.0X5	T49.0X6
Anti-gastric-secretion drug NEC	T47.1X1	T47.1X2	T47.1X3	T47.1X4	T47.1X5	T47.1X6
Antigonadotrophin NEC	T38.6X1	T38.6X2	T38.6X3	T38.6X4	T38.6X5	T38.6X6
Antihallucinogen	T43.501	T43.502	T43.503	T43.504	T43.505	T43.506
Antihelmintics	T37.4X1	T37.4X2	T37.4X3	T37.4X4	T37.4X5	T37.4X6
Antihemophilic						
factor	T45.8X1	T45.8X2	T45.8X3	T45.8X4	T45.8X5	T45.8X6
fraction	T45.8X1	T45.8X2	T45.8X3	T45.8X4	T45.8X5	T45.8X6
globulin concentrate	T45.7X1	T45.7X2	T45.7X3	T45.7X4	T45.7X5	T45.7X6
human plasma	T45.8X1	T45.8X2	T45.8X3	T45.8X4	T45.8X5	T45.8X6
plasma, dried	T45.7X1	T45.7X2	T45.7X3	T45.7X4	T45.7X5	T45.7X6
Antihemorrhoidal preparation	T49.2X1	T49.2X2	T49.2X3	T49.2X4	T49.2X5	T49.2X6
Antiheparin drug	T45.7X1	T45.7X2	T45.7X3	T45.7X4	T45.7X5	T45.7X6
Antihistamine	T45.0X1	T45.0X2	T45.0X3	T45.0X4	T45.0X5	T45.0X6
Antihookworm drug	T37.4X1	T37.4X2	T37.4X3	T37.4X4	T37.4X5	T37.4X6
Anti-human lymphocytic globulin	T50.Z11	T50.Z12	T50.Z13	T50.Z14	T50.Z15	T50.Z16
Antihyperlipidemic drug	T46.6X1	T46.6X2	T46.6X3	T46.6X4	T46.6X5	T46.6X6
Antihypertensive drug NEC	T46.5X1	T46.5X2	T46.5X3	T46.5X4	T46.5X5	T46.5X6

Substance	External Cause (T-Code)					
	Poisoning, Accidental (Unintentional)	Poisoning, Intentional Self-Harm	Poisoning, Assault	Poisoning, Undetermined	Adverse Effect	Underdosing
Anti-infective NEC	T37.91	T37.92	T37.93	T37.94	T37.95	T37.96
anthelmintic	T37.4X1	T37.4X2	T37.4X3	T37.4X4	T37.4X5	T37.4X6
antibiotics	T36.91	T36.92	T36.93	T36.94	T36.95	T36.96
specified NEC	T36.8X1	T36.8X2	T36.8X3	T36.8X4	T36.8X5	T36.8X6
antimalarial	T37.2X1	T37.2X2	T37.2X3	T37.2X4	T37.2X5	T37.2X6
antimycobacterial NEC	T37.1X1	T37.1X2	T37.1X3	T37.1X4	T37.1X5	T37.1X6
antibiotics	T36.5X1	T36.5X2	T36.5X3	T36.5X4	T36.5X5	T36.5X6
antiprotozoal NEC	T37.3X1	T37.3X2	T37.3X3	T37.3X4	T37.3X5	T37.3X6
blood	T37.2X1	T37.2X2	T37.2X3	T37.2X4	T37.2X5	T37.2X6
antiviral	T37.5X1	T37.5X2	T37.5X3	T37.5X4	T37.5X5	T37.5X6
arsenical	T37.8X1	T37.8X2	T37.8X3	T37.8X4	T37.8X5	T37.8X6
bismuth, local	T49.0X1	T49.0X2	T49.0X3	T49.0X4	T49.0X5	T49.0X6
ENT	T49.6X1	T49.6X2	T49.6X3	T49.6X4	T49.6X5	T49.6X6
eye NEC	T49.5X1	T49.5X2	T49.5X3	T49.5X4	T49.5X5	T49.5X6
heavy metals NEC	T37.8X1	T37.8X2	T37.8X3	T37.8X4	T37.8X5	T37.8X6
local NEC	T49.0X1	T49.0X2	T49.0X3	T49.0X4	T49.0X5	T49.0X6
specified NEC	T49.0X1	T49.0X2	T49.0X3	T49.0X4	T49.0X5	T49.0X6
mixed	T37.91	T37.92	T37.93	T37.94	T37.95	T37.96
ophthalmic preparation	T49.5X1	T49.5X2	T49.5X3	T49.5X4	T49.5X5	T49.5X6
topical NEC	T49.0X1	T49.0X2	T49.0X3	T49.0X4	T49.0X5	T49.0X6
Anti-inflammatory drug NEC	T49.0X1	T49.0X2	T49.0X3	T49.0X4	T49.0X5	T49.0X6
local	T49.0X1	T49.0X2	T49.0X3	T49.0X4	T49.0X5	T49.0X6
nonsteroidal NEC	T39.391	T39.392	T39.393	T39.394	T39.395	T39.396
propionic acid derivative	T39.311	T39.312	T39.313	T39.314	T39.315	T39.316
specified NEC	T39.391	T39.392	T39.393	T39.394	T39.395	T39.396
Antikaluretic	T50.3X1	T50.3X2	T50.3X3	T50.3X4	T50.3X5	T50.3X6
Antiknock (tetraethyl lead)	T56.0X1	T56.0X2	T56.0X3	T56.0X4	—	—
Antilipemic drug NEC	T46.6X1	T46.6X2	T46.6X3	T46.6X4	T46.6X5	T46.6X6
Antimalarial	T37.2X1	T37.2X2	T37.2X3	T37.2X4	T37.2X5	T37.2X6
prophylactic NEC	T37.2X1	T37.2X2	T37.2X3	T37.2X4	T37.2X5	T37.2X6
pyrimidine derivative	T37.2X1	T37.2X2	T37.2X3	T37.2X4	T37.2X5	T37.2X6
Antimetabolite	T45.1X1	T45.1X2	T45.1X3	T45.1X4	T45.1X5	T45.1X6
Antimitotic agent	T45.1X1	T45.1X2	T45.1X3	T45.1X4	T45.1X5	T45.1X6
Antimony (compounds) (vapor) NEC	T56.891	T56.892	T56.893	T56.894	—	—
anti-infectives	T37.8X1	T37.8X2	T37.8X3	T37.8X4	T37.8X5	T37.8X6
dimercaptosuccinate	T37.3X1	T37.3X2	T37.3X3	T37.3X4	T37.3X5	T37.3X6
hydride	T56.891	T56.892	T56.893	T56.894	—	—
pesticide (vapor)	T60.8X1	T60.8X2	T60.8X3	T60.8X4	—	—
potassium (sodium) tartrate	T37.8X1	T37.8X2	T37.8X3	T37.8X4	T37.8X5	T37.8X6

Substance	External Cause (T-Code)					
	Poisoning, Accidental (Unintentional)	Poisoning, Intentional Self-Harm	Poisoning, Assault	Poisoning, Undetermined	Adverse Effect	Underdosing
Antimony NEC *(Continued)*						
sodium dimercaptosuccinate	T37.3X1	T37.3X2	T37.3X3	T37.3X4	T37.3X5	T37.3X6
tartrated	T37.8X1	T37.8X2	T37.8X3	T37.8X4	T37.8X5	T37.8X6
Antimuscarinic NEC	T44.3X1	T44.3X2	T44.3X3	T44.3X4	T44.3X5	T44.3X6
Antimycobacterial drug NEC	T37.1X1	T37.1X2	T37.1X3	T37.1X4	T37.1X5	T37.1X6
antibiotics	T36.5X1	T36.5X2	T36.5X3	T36.5X4	T36.5X5	T36.5X6
combination	T37.1X1	T37.1X2	T37.1X3	T37.1X4	T37.1X5	T37.1X6
Antinausea drug	T45.0X1	T45.0X2	T45.0X3	T45.0X4	T45.0X5	T45.0X6
Antinematode drug	T37.4X1	T37.4X2	T37.4X3	T37.4X4	T37.4X5	T37.4X6
Antineoplastic NEC	T45.1X1	T45.1X2	T45.1X3	T45.1X4	T45.1X5	T45.1X6
alkaloidal	T45.1X1	T45.1X2	T45.1X3	T45.1X4	T45.1X5	T45.1X6
antibiotics	T45.1X1	T45.1X2	T45.1X3	T45.1X4	T45.1X5	T45.1X6
combination	T45.1X1	T45.1X2	T45.1X3	T45.1X4	T45.1X5	T45.1X6
estrogen	T38.5X1	T38.5X2	T38.5X3	T38.5X4	T38.5X5	T38.5X6
steroid	T38.7X1	T38.7X2	T38.7X3	T38.7X4	T38.7X5	T38.7X6
Antiparasitic drug (systemic)	T37.91	T37.92	T37.93	T37.94	T37.95	T37.96
local	T49.0X1	T49.0X2	T49.0X3	T49.0X4	T49.0X5	T49.0X6
specified NEC	T37.8X1	T37.8X2	T37.8X3	T37.8X4	T37.8X5	T37.8X6
Antiparkinsonism drug NEC	T42.8X1	T42.8X2	T42.8X3	T42.8X4	T42.8X5	T42.8X6
Antiperspirant NEC	T49.2X1	T49.2X2	T49.2X3	T49.2X4	T49.2X5	T49.2X6
Antiphlogistic NEC	T39.4X1	T39.4X2	T39.4X3	T39.4X4	T39.4X5	T39.4X6
Antiplatyhelmintic drug	T37.4X1	T37.4X2	T37.4X3	T37.4X4	T37.4X5	T37.4X6
Antiprotozoal drug NEC	T37.3X1	T37.3X2	T37.3X3	T37.3X4	T37.3X5	T37.3X6
blood	T37.2X1	T37.2X2	T37.2X3	T37.2X4	T37.2X5	T37.2X6
local	T49.0X1	T49.0X2	T49.0X3	T49.0X4	T49.0X5	T49.0X6
Antipruritic drug NEC	T49.1X1	T49.1X2	T49.1X3	T49.1X4	T49.1X5	T49.1X6
Antipsychotic drug	T43.501	T43.502	T43.503	T43.504	T43.505	T43.506
specified NEC	T43.591	T43.592	T43.593	T43.594	T43.595	T43.596
Antipyretic	T39.91	T39.92	T39.93	T39.94	T39.95	T39.96
specified NEC	T39.8X1	T39.8X2	T39.8X3	T39.8X4	T39.8X5	T39.8X6
Antipyrine	T39.2X1	T39.2X2	T39.2X3	T39.2X4	T39.2X5	T39.2X6
Antirabies hyperimmune serum	T50.Z11	T50.Z12	T50.Z13	T50.Z14	T50.Z15	T50.Z16
Antirheumatic NEC	T39.4X1	T39.4X2	T39.4X3	T39.4X4	T39.4X5	T39.4X6
Antirigidity drug NEC	T42.8X1	T42.8X2	T42.8X3	T42.8X4	T42.8X5	T42.8X6
Antischistosomal drug	T37.4X1	T37.4X2	T37.4X3	T37.4X4	T37.4X5	T37.4X6
Antiscorpion sera	T50.Z11	T50.Z12	T50.Z13	T50.Z14	T50.Z15	T50.Z16
Antiseborrheics	T49.4X1	T49.4X2	T49.4X3	T49.4X4	T49.4X5	T49.4X6
Antiseptics (external) (medicinal)	T49.0X1	T49.0X2	T49.0X3	T49.0X4	T49.0X5	T49.0X6
Antistine	T45.0X1	T45.0X2	T45.0X3	T45.0X4	T45.0X5	T45.0X6
Antitapeworm drug	T37.4X1	T37.4X2	T37.4X3	T37.4X4	T37.4X5	T37.4X6

Substance	External Cause (T-Code)					
	Poisoning, Accidental (Unintentional)	Poisoning, Intentional Self-Harm	Poisoning, Assault	Poisoning, Undetermined	Adverse Effect	Underdosing
Antitetanus immunoglobulin	T50.Z11	T50.Z12	T50.Z13	T50.Z14	T50.Z15	T50.Z16
Antithyroid drug NEC	T38.2X1	T38.2X2	T38.2X3	T38.2X4	T38.2X5	T38.2X6
Antitoxin	T50.Z11	T50.Z12	T50.Z13	T50.Z14	T50.Z15	T50.Z16
diphtheria	T50.Z11	T50.Z12	T50.Z13	T50.Z14	T50.Z15	T50.Z16
gas gangrene	T50.Z11	T50.Z12	T50.Z13	T50.Z14	T50.Z15	T50.Z16
tetanus	T50.Z11	T50.Z12	T50.Z13	T50.Z14	T50.Z15	T50.Z16
Antitoxin, any	T50.901	T50.902	T50.903	T50.904	T50.905	T50.906
Antitrichomonal drug	T37.3X1	T37.3X2	T37.3X3	T37.3X4	T37.3X5	T37.3X6
Antituberculars	T37.1X1	T37.1X2	T37.1X3	T37.1X4	T37.1X5	T37.1X6
antibiotics	T36.5X1	T36.5X2	T36.5X3	T36.5X4	T36.5X5	T36.5X6
Antitussive NEC	T48.3X1	T48.3X2	T48.3X3	T48.3X4	T48.3X5	T48.3X6
codeine mixture	T40.2X1	T40.2X2	T40.2X3	T40.2X4	T40.2X5	T40.2X6
opiate	T40.2X1	T40.2X2	T40.2X3	T40.2X4	T40.2X5	T40.2X6
Antivaricose drug	T46.8X1	T46.8X2	T46.8X3	T46.8X4	T46.8X5	T46.8X6
Antivenin, antivenom (sera)	T50.Z11	T50.Z12	T50.Z13	T50.Z14	T50.Z15	T50.Z16
crotaline	T50.Z11	T50.Z12	T50.Z13	T50.Z14	T50.Z15	T50.Z16
spider bite	T50.Z11	T50.Z12	T50.Z13	T50.Z14	T50.Z15	T50.Z16
Antivertigo drug	T45.0X1	T45.0X2	T45.0X3	T45.0X4	T45.0X5	T45.0X6
Antiviral drug NEC	T37.5X1	T37.5X2	T37.5X3	T37.5X4	T37.5X5	T37.5X6
eye	T49.5X1	T49.5X2	T49.5X3	T49.5X4	T49.5X5	T49.5X6
Antiwhipworm drug	T37.4X1	T37.4X2	T37.4X3	T37.4X4	T37.4X5	T37.4X6
Ant poisons — see Pesticides						
Antrol — see also by specific chemical substance	T60.91	T60.92	T60.93	T60.94	—	—
fungicide	T60.91	T60.92	T60.93	T60.94	—	—
ANTU (alpha naphthylthiourea)	T60.4X1	T60.4X2	T60.4X3	T60.4X4	—	—
Apalcillin	T36.0X1	T36.0X2	T36.0X3	T36.0X4	T36.0X5	T36.0X6
APC	T48.5X1	T48.5X2	T48.5X3	T48.5X4	T48.5X5	T48.5X6
Aplonidine	T44.4X1	T44.4X2	T44.4X3	T44.4X4	T44.4X5	T44.4X6
Apomorphine	T47.7X1	T47.7X2	T47.7X3	T47.7X4	T47.7X5	T47.7X6
Appetite depressants, central	T50.5X1	T50.5X2	T50.5X3	T50.5X4	T50.5X5	T50.5X6
Apraclonidine (hydrochloride)	T44.4X1	T44.4X2	T44.4X3	T44.4X4	T44.4X5	T44.4X6
Apresoline	T46.5X1	T46.5X2	T46.5X3	T46.5X4	T46.5X5	T46.5X6
Aprindine	T46.2X1	T46.2X2	T46.2X3	T46.2X4	T46.2X5	T46.2X6
Aprobarbital	T42.3X1	T42.3X2	T42.3X3	T42.3X4	T42.3X5	T42.3X6
Apronalide	T42.6X1	T42.6X2	T42.6X3	T42.6X4	T42.6X5	T42.6X6
Aprotinin	T45.621	T45.622	T45.623	T45.624	T45.625	T45.626
Aptocaine	T41.3X1	T41.3X2	T41.3X3	T41.3X4	T41.3X5	T41.3X6
Aqua fortis	T54.2X1	T54.2X2	T54.2X3	T54.2X4	—	—
Ara-A	T37.5X1	T37.5X2	T37.5X3	T37.5X4	T37.5X5	T37.5X6
Ara-C	T45.1X1	T45.1X2	T45.1X3	T45.1X4	T45.1X5	T45.1X6

Substance	Poisoning, Accidental (Unintentional)	Poisoning, Intentional Self-Harm	Poisoning, Assault	Poisoning, Undetermined	Adverse Effect	Underdosing
Arachis oil	T49.3X1	T49.3X2	T49.3X3	T49.3X4	T49.3X5	T49.3X6
cathartic	T47.4X1	T47.4X2	T47.4X3	T47.4X4	T47.4X5	T47.4X6
Aralen	T37.2X1	T37.2X2	T37.2X3	T37.2X4	T37.2X5	T37.2X6
Arecoline	T44.1X1	T44.1X2	T44.1X3	T44.1X4	T44.1X5	T44.1X6
Arginine	T50.991	T50.992	T50.993	T50.994	T50.995	T50.996
glutamate	T50.991	T50.992	T50.993	T50.994	T50.995	T50.996
Argyrol	T49.0X1	T49.0X2	T49.0X3	T49.0X4	T49.0X5	T49.0X6
ENT agent	T49.6X1	T49.6X2	T49.6X3	T49.6X4	T49.6X5	T49.6X6
ophthalmic preparation	T49.5X1	T49.5X2	T49.5X3	T49.5X4	T49.5X5	T49.5X6
Aristocort	T38.0X1	T38.0X2	T38.0X3	T38.0X4	T38.0X5	T38.0X6
ENT agent	T49.6X1	T49.6X2	T49.6X3	T49.6X4	T49.6X5	T49.6X6
ophthalmic preparation	T49.5X1	T49.5X2	T49.5X3	T49.5X4	T49.5X5	T49.5X6
topical NEC	T49.0X1	T49.0X2	T49.0X3	T49.0X4	T49.0X5	T49.0X6
Aromatics, corrosive	T54.1X1	T54.1X2	T54.1X3	T54.1X4	—	—
disinfectants	T54.1X1	T54.1X2	T54.1X3	T54.1X4	—	—
Arsenate of lead	T57.0X1	T57.0X2	T57.0X3	T57.0X4	—	—
herbicide	T57.0X1	T57.0X2	T57.0X3	T57.0X4	—	—
Arsenic, arsenicals (compounds) (dust) (vapor) NEC	T57.0X1	T57.0X2	T57.0X3	T57.0X4	—	—
anti-infectives	T37.8X1	T37.8X2	T37.8X3	T37.8X4	T37.8X5	T37.8X6
pesticide (dust) (fumes)	T57.0X1	T57.0X2	T57.0X3	T57.0X4	—	—
Arsine (gas)	T57.0X1	T57.0X2	T57.0X3	T57.0X4	—	—
Arsphenamine (silver)	T37.8X1	T37.8X2	T37.8X3	T37.8X4	T37.8X5	T37.8X6
Arsthinol	T37.3X1	T37.3X2	T37.3X3	T37.3X4	T37.3X5	T37.3X6
Artane	T44.3X1	T44.3X2	T44.3X3	T44.3X4	T44.3X5	T44.3X6
Arthropod (venomous) NEC	T63.481	T63.482	T63.483	T63.484	—	—
Articaine	T41.3X1	T41.3X2	T41.3X3	T41.3X4	T41.3X5	T41.3X6
Asbestos	T57.8X1	T57.8X2	T57.8X3	T57.8X4	—	—
Ascaridole	T37.4X1	T37.4X2	T37.4X3	T37.4X4	T37.4X5	T37.4X6
Ascorbic acid	T45.2X1	T45.2X2	T45.2X3	T45.2X4	T45.2X5	T45.2X6
Asiaticoside	T49.0X1	T49.0X2	T49.0X3	T49.0X4	T49.0X5	T49.0X6
Asparaginase	T45.1X1	T45.1X2	T45.1X3	T45.1X4	T45.1X5	T45.1X6
Aspidium (oleoresin)	T37.4X1	T37.4X2	T37.4X3	T37.4X4	T37.4X5	T37.4X6
Aspirin (aluminum) (soluble)	T39.011	T39.012	T39.013	T39.014	T39.015	T39.016
Aspoxicillin	T36.0X1	T36.0X2	T36.0X3	T36.0X4	T36.0X5	T36.0X6
Astemizole	T45.0X1	T45.0X2	T45.0X3	T45.0X4	T45.0X5	T45.0X6
Astringent (local)	T49.2X1	T49.2X2	T49.2X3	T49.2X4	T49.2X5	T49.2X6
specified NEC	T49.2X1	T49.2X2	T49.2X3	T49.2X4	T49.2X5	T49.2X6
Astromicin	T36.5X1	T36.5X2	T36.5X3	T36.5X4	T36.5X5	T36.5X6
Ataractic drug NEC	T43.501	T43.502	T43.503	T43.504	T43.505	T43.506

Substance	External Cause (T-Code)					
	Poisoning, Accidental (Unintentional)	Poisoning, Intentional Self-Harm	Poisoning, Assault	Poisoning, Undetermined	Adverse Effect	Underdosing
Atenolol	T44.7X1	T44.7X2	T44.7X3	T44.7X4	T44.7X5	T44.7X6
Atonia drug, intestinal	T47.4X1	T47.4X2	T47.4X3	T47.4X4	T47.4X5	T47.4X6
Atophan	T50.4X1	T50.4X2	T50.4X3	T50.4X4	T50.4X5	T50.4X6
Atracurium besilate	T48.1X1	T48.1X2	T48.1X3	T48.1X4	T48.1X5	T48.1X6
Atropine	T44.3X1	T44.3X2	T44.3X3	T44.3X4	T44.3X5	T44.3X6
derivative	T44.3X1	T44.3X2	T44.3X3	T44.3X4	T44.3X5	T44.3X6
methonitrate	T44.3X1	T44.3X2	T44.3X3	T44.3X4	T44.3X5	T44.3X6
Attapulgite	T47.6X1	T47.6X2	T47.6X3	T47.6X4	T47.6X5	T47.6X6
Attenuvax	T50.991	T50.992	T50.993	T50.994	T50.995	T50.996
Auramine	T65.891	T65.892	T65.893	T65.894	—	—
dye	T65.6X1	T65.6X2	T65.6X3	T65.6X4	—	—
fungicide	T60.3X1	T60.3X2	T60.3X3	T60.3X4	—	—
Auranofin	T39.4X1	T39.4X2	T39.4X3	T39.4X4	T39.4X5	T39.4X6
Aurantiin	T46.991	T46.992	T46.993	T46.994	T46.995	T46.996
Aureomycin	T36.4X1	T36.4X2	T36.4X3	T36.4X4	T36.4X5	T36.4X6
ophthalmic preparation	T49.5X1	T49.5X2	T49.5X3	T49.5X4	T49.5X5	T49.5X6
topical NEC	T49.0X1	T49.0X2	T49.0X3	T49.0X4	T49.0X5	T49.0X6
Aurothioglucose	T39.4X1	T39.4X2	T39.4X3	T39.4X4	T39.4X5	T39.4X6
Aurothioglycanide	T39.4X1	T39.4X2	T39.4X3	T39.4X4	T39.4X5	T39.4X6
Aurothiomalate sodium	T39.4X1	T39.4X2	T39.4X3	T39.4X4	T39.4X5	T39.4X6
Aurotioprol	T39.4X1	T39.4X2	T39.4X3	T39.4X4	T39.4X5	T39.4X6
Automobile fuel	T52.0X1	T52.0X2	T52.0X3	T52.0X4	—	—
Autonomic nervous system agent NEC	T44.901	T44.902	T44.903	T44.904	T44.905	T44.906
Avlosulfon	T37.1X1	T37.1X2	T37.1X3	T37.1X4	T37.1X5	T37.1X6
Avomine	T42.6X1	T42.6X2	T42.6X3	T42.6X4	T42.6X5	T42.6X6
Axerophthol	T45.2X1	T45.2X2	T45.2X3	T45.2X4	T45.2X5	T45.2X6
Azacitidine	T45.1X1	T45.1X2	T45.1X3	T45.1X4	T45.1X5	T45.1X6
Azacyclonol	T43.591	T43.592	T43.593	T43.594	T43.595	T43.596
Azadirachta	T60.2X1	T60.2X2	T60.2X3	T60.2X4	—	—
Azanidazole	T37.3X1	T37.3X2	T37.3X3	T37.3X4	T37.3X5	T37.3X6
Azapetine	T46.7X1	T46.7X2	T46.7X3	T46.7X4	T46.7X5	T46.7X6
Azapropazone	T39.2X1	T39.2X2	T39.2X3	T39.2X4	T39.2X5	T39.2X6
Azaribine	T45.1X1	T45.1X2	T45.1X3	T45.1X4	T45.1X5	T45.1X6
Azaserine	T45.1X1	T45.1X2	T45.1X3	T45.1X4	T45.1X5	T45.1X6
Azatadine	T45.0X1	T45.0X2	T45.0X3	T45.0X4	T45.0X5	T45.0X6
Azatepa	T45.1X1	T45.1X2	T45.1X3	T45.1X4	T45.1X5	T45.1X6
Azathioprine	T45.1X1	T45.1X2	T45.1X3	T45.1X4	T45.1X5	T45.1X6
Azelaic acid	T49.0X1	T49.0X2	T49.0X3	T49.0X4	T49.0X5	T49.0X6
Azelastine	T45.0X1	T45.0X2	T45.0X3	T45.0X4	T45.0X5	T45.0X6

TABLE OF DRUGS AND CHEMICALS

Substance	External Cause (T-Code)					
	Poisoning, Accidental (Unintentional)	Poisoning, Intentional Self-Harm	Poisoning, Assault	Poisoning, Undetermined	Adverse Effect	Underdosing
Azidocillin	T36.0X1	T36.0X2	T36.0X3	T36.0X4	T36.0X5	T36.0X6
Azidothymidine	T37.5X1	T37.5X2	T37.5X3	T37.5X4	T37.5X5	T37.5X6
Azinphos (ethyl) (methyl)	T60.0X1	T60.0X2	T60.0X3	T60.0X4	—	—
Aziridine (chelating)	T54.1X1	T54.1X2	T54.1X3	T54.1X4	—	—
Azithromycin	T36.3X1	T36.3X2	T36.3X3	T36.3X4	T36.3X5	T36.3X6
Azlocillin	T36.01	T36.02	T36.03	T36.04	T36.05	T36.06
Azobenzene smoke	T65.3X1	T65.3X2	T65.3X3	T65.3X4	—	—
acaricide	T60.8X1	T60.8X2	T60.8X3	T60.8X4	—	—
Azosulfamide	T37.0X1	T37.0X2	T37.0X3	T37.0X4	T37.0X5	T37.0X6
AZT	T37.5X1	T37.5X2	T37.5X3	T37.5X4	T37.5X5	T37.5X6
Aztreonam	T36.1X1	T36.1X2	T36.1X3	T36.1X4	T36.1X5	T36.1X6
Azulfidine	T37.0X1	T37.0X2	T37.0X3	T37.0X4	T37.0X5	T37.0X6
Azuresin	T50.8X1	T50.8X2	T50.8X3	T50.8X4	T50.8X5	T50.8X6
B						
Bacampicillin	T36.0X1	T36.0X2	T36.0X3	T36.0X4	T36.0X5	T36.0X6
Bacillus						
lactobacillus	T47.8X1	T47.8X2	T47.8X3	T47.8X4	T47.8X5	T47.8X6
subtilis	T47.6X1	T47.6X2	T47.6X3	T47.6X4	T47.6X5	T47.6X6
Bacimycin	T49.0X1	T49.0X2	T49.0X3	T49.0X4	T49.0X5	T49.0X6
ophthalmic preparation	T49.5X1	T49.5X2	T49.5X3	T49.5X4	T49.5X5	T49.5X6
Bacitracin zinc	T49.0X1	T49.0X2	T49.0X3	T49.0X4	T49.0X5	T49.0X6
with neomycin	T49.0X1	T49.0X2	T49.0X3	T49.0X4	T49.0X5	T49.0X6
ENT agent	T49.6X1	T49.6X2	T49.6X3	T49.6X4	T49.6X5	T49.6X6
ophthalmic preparation	T49.5X1	T49.5X2	T49.5X3	T49.5X4	T49.5X5	T49.5X6
topical NEC	T49.0X1	T49.0X2	T49.0X3	T49.0X4	T49.0X5	T49.0X6
Baclofen	T42.8X1	T42.8X2	T42.8X3	T42.8X4	T42.8X5	T42.8X6
Baking soda	T50.991	T50.992	T50.993	T50.994	T50.995	T50.996
BAL	T45.8X1	T45.8X2	T45.8X3	T45.8X4	T45.8X5	T45.8X6
Bambuterol	T48.6X1	T48.6X2	T48.6X3	T48.6X4	T48.6X5	T48.6X6
Bamethan (sulfate)	T46.7X1	T46.7X2	T46.7X3	T46.7X4	T46.7X5	T46.7X6
Bamifylline	T48.6X1	T48.6X2	T48.6X3	T48.6X4	T48.6X5	T48.6X6
Bamipine	T45.0X1	T45.0X2	T45.0X3	T45.0X4	T45.0X5	T45.0X6
Baneberry — see Actaea spicata						
Banewort — see Belladonna						
Barbenyl	T42.3X1	T42.3X2	T42.3X3	T42.3X4	T42.3X5	T42.3X6
Barbexaclone	T42.6X1	T42.6X2	T42.6X3	T42.6X4	T42.6X5	T42.6X6
Barbital	T42.3X1	T42.3X2	T42.3X3	T42.3X4	T42.3X5	T42.3X6
sodium	T42.3X1	T42.3X2	T42.3X3	T42.3X4	T42.3X5	T42.3X6
Barbitone	T42.3X1	T42.3X2	T42.3X3	T42.3X4	T42.3X5	T42.3X6

Substance	Poisoning, Accidental (Unintentional)	Poisoning, Intentional Self-Harm	Poisoning, Assault	Poisoning, Undetermined	Adverse Effect	Underdosing
			External Cause (T-Code)			
Barbiturate NEC	T42.3X1	T42.3X2	T42.3X3	T42.3X4	T42.3X5	T42.3X6
with tranquilizer	T42.3X1	T42.3X2	T42.3X3	T42.3X4	T42.3X5	T42.3X6
anesthetic (intravenous)	T41.1X1	T41.1X2	T41.1X3	T41.1X4	T41.1X5	T41.1X6
Barium (carbonate) (chloride) (sulfite)	T57.8X1	T57.8X2	T57.8X3	T57.8X4	—	—
diagnostic agent	T50.8X1	T50.8X2	T50.8X3	T50.8X4	T50.8X5	T50.8X6
pesticide	T60.4X1	T60.4X2	T60.4X3	T60.4X4	—	—
rodenticide	T60.4X1	T60.4X2	T60.4X3	T60.4X4	—	—
sulfate (medicinal)	T50.8X1	T50.8X2	T50.8X3	T50.8X4	T50.8X5	T50.8X6
Barrier cream	T49.3X1	T49.3X2	T49.3X3	T49.3X4	T49.3X5	T49.3X6
Basic fuchsin	T49.0X1	T49.0X2	T49.0X3	T49.0X4	T49.0X5	T49.0X6
Battery acid or fluid	T54.2X1	T54.2X2	T54.2X3	T54.2X4	—	—
Bay rum	T51.8X1	T51.8X2	T51.8X3	T51.8X4	—	—
BCG (vaccine)	T50.A91	T50.A92	T50.A93	T50.A94	T50.A95	T50.A96
BCNU	T45.1X1	T45.1X2	T45.1X3	T45.1X4	T45.1X5	T45.1X6
Bearsfoot	T62.2X1	T62.2X2	T62.2X3	T62.2X4	—	—
Beclamide	T42.6X1	T42.6X2	T42.6X3	T42.6X4	T42.6X5	T42.6X6
Beclomethasone	T44.5X1	T44.5X2	T44.5X3	T44.5X4	T44.5X5	T44.5X6
Bee (sting) (venom)	T63.441	T63.442	T63.443	T63.444	—	—
Befunolol	T49.5X1	T49.5X2	T49.5X3	T49.5X4	T49.5X5	T49.5X6
Bekanamycin	T36.5X1	T36.5X2	T36.5X3	T36.5X4	T36.5X5	T36.5X6
Belladonna — see also Nightshade						
alkaloids	T44.3X1	T44.3X2	T44.3X3	T44.3X4	T44.3X5	T44.3X6
extract	T44.3X1	T44.3X2	T44.3X3	T44.3X4	T44.3X5	T44.3X6
herb	T44.3X1	T44.3X2	T44.3X3	T44.3X4	T44.3X5	T44.3X6
Bemegride	T50.7X1	T50.7X2	T50.7X3	T50.7X4	T50.7X5	T50.7X6
Benactyzine	T44.3X1	T44.3X2	T44.3X3	T44.3X4	T44.3X5	T44.3X6
Benadryl	T45.0X1	T45.0X2	T45.0X3	T45.0X4	T45.0X5	T45.0X6
Benaprizine	T44.3X1	T44.3X2	T44.3X3	T44.3X4	T44.3X5	T44.3X6
Benazepril	T46.4X1	T46.4X2	T46.4X3	T46.4X4	T46.4X5	T46.4X6
Bencyclane	T46.7X1	T46.7X2	T46.7X3	T46.7X4	T46.7X5	T46.7X6
Bendazol	T46.3X1	T46.3X2	T46.3X3	T46.3X4	T46.3X5	T46.3X6
Bendrofluazide	T50.2X1	T50.2X2	T50.2X3	T50.2X4	T50.2X5	T50.2X6
Bendroflumethiazide	T50.2X1	T50.2X2	T50.2X3	T50.2X4	T50.2X5	T50.2X6
Benemid	T50.4X1	T50.4X2	T50.4X3	T50.4X4	T50.4X5	T50.4X6
Benethamine penicillin	T36.0X1	T36.0X2	T36.0X3	T36.0X4	T36.0X5	T36.0X6
Benisone	T49.0X1	T49.0X2	T49.0X3	T49.0X4	T49.0X5	T49.0X6
Benexate	T47.1X1	T47.1X2	T47.1X3	T47.1X4	T47.1X5	T47.1X6
Benfluorex	T46.6X1	T46.6X2	T46.6X3	T46.6X4	T46.6X5	T46.6X6
Benfotiamine	T45.2X1	T45.2X2	T45.2X3	T45.2X4	T45.2X5	T45.2X6
Benomyl	T60.0X1	T60.0X2	T60.0X3	T60.0X4	—	—

TABLE OF DRUGS AND CHEMICALS

Substance	External Cause (T-Code)					
	Poisoning, Accidental (Unintentional)	Poisoning, Intentional Self-Harm	Poisoning, Assault	Poisoning, Undetermined	Adverse Effect	Underdosing
Benoquin	T49.8X1	T49.8X2	T49.8X3	T49.8X4	T49.8X5	T49.8X6
Benoxinate	T41.3X1	T41.3X2	T41.3X3	T41.3X4	T41.3X5	T41.3X6
Benperidol	T43.4X1	T43.4X2	T43.4X3	T43.4X4	T43.4X5	T43.4X6
Benproperine	T48.3X1	T48.3X2	T48.3X3	T48.3X4	T48.3X5	T48.3X6
Benserazide	T42.8X1	T42.8X2	T42.8X3	T42.8X4	T42.8X5	T42.8X6
Bentazepam	T42.4X1	T42.4X2	T42.4X3	T42.4X4	T42.4X5	T42.4X6
Bentiromide	T50.8X1	T50.8X2	T50.8X3	T50.8X4	T50.8X5	T50.8X6
Bentonite	T49.3X1	T49.3X2	T49.3X3	T49.3X4	T49.3X5	T49.3X6
Benzalbutyramide	T46.6X1	T46.6X2	T46.6X3	T46.6X4	T46.6X5	T46.6X6
Benzalkonium (chloride)	T49.0X1	T49.0X2	T49.0X3	T49.0X4	T49.0X5	T49.0X6
ophthalmic preparation	T49.5X1	T49.5X2	T49.5X3	T49.5X4	T49.5X5	T49.5X6
Benzamine	T41.3X1	T41.3X2	T41.3X3	T41.3X4	T41.3X5	T41.3X6
lactate	T49.1X1	T49.1X2	T49.1X3	T49.1X4	T49.1X5	T49.1X6
Benzamidosalicylate (calcium)	T37.1X1	T37.1X2	T37.1X3	T37.1X4	T37.1X5	T37.1X6
Benzamphetamine	T50.5X1	T50.5X2	T50.5X3	T50.5X4	T50.5X5	T50.5X6
Benzapril hydrochloride	T46.5X1	T46.5X2	T46.5X3	T46.5X4	T46.5X5	T46.5X6
Benzathine benzylpenicillin	T36.0X1	T36.0X2	T36.0X3	T36.0X4	T36.0X5	T36.0X6
Benzathine penicillin	T36.0X1	T36.0X2	T36.0X3	T36.0X4	T36.0X5	T36.0X6
Benzatropine	T42.8X1	T42.8X2	T42.8X3	T42.8X4	T42.8X5	T42.8X6
Benzbromarone	T50.4X1	T50.4X2	T50.4X3	T50.4X4	T50.4X5	T50.4X6
Benzcarbimine	T45.1X1	T45.1X2	T45.1X3	T45.1X4	T45.1X5	T45.1X6
Benzedrex	T44.991	T44.992	T44.993	T44.994	T44.995	T44.996
Benzedrine (amphetamine)	T43.621	T43.622	T43.623	T43.624	T43.625	T43.626
Benzenamine	T65.3X1	T65.3X2	T65.3X3	T65.3X4	—	—
Benzene	T52.1X1	T52.1X2	T52.1X3	T52.1X4	—	—
homologues (acetyl) (dimethyl) (methyl) (solvent)	T52.2X1	T52.2X2	T52.2X3	T52.2X4	—	—
Benzethonium (chloride)	T49.0X1	T49.0X2	T49.0X3	T49.0X4	T49.0X5	T49.0X6
Benzfetamine	T50.5X1	T50.5X2	T50.5X3	T50.5X4	T50.5X5	T50.5X6
Benzhexol	T44.3X1	T44.3X2	T44.3X3	T44.3X4	T44.3X5	T44.3X6
Benzhydramine (chloride)	T45.0X1	T45.0X2	T45.0X3	T45.0X4	T45.0X5	T45.0X6
Benzidine	T65.891	T65.892	T65.893	T65.894	—	—
Benzilonium bromide	T44.3X1	T44.3X2	T44.3X3	T44.3X4	T44.3X5	T44.3X6
Benzimidazole	T60.3X1	T60.3X2	T60.3X3	T60.3X4	—	—
Benzin(e) — see Ligroin						
Benziodarone	T46.3X1	T46.3X2	T46.3X3	T46.3X4	T46.3X5	T46.3X6
Benznidazole	T37.3X1	T37.3X2	T37.3X3	T37.3X4	T37.3X5	T37.3X6
Benzocaine	T41.3X1	T41.3X2	T41.3X3	T41.3X4	T41.3X5	T41.3X6
Benzoctamine	T43.0X1	T43.0X2	T43.0X3	T43.0X4	T43.0X5	T43.0X6
Benzodiapin	T42.4X1	T42.4X2	T42.4X3	T42.4X4	T42.4X5	T42.4X6
Benzodiazepine NEC	T42.4X1	T42.4X2	T42.4X3	T42.4X4	T42.4X5	T42.4X6

Substance	Poisoning, Accidental (Unintentional)	Poisoning, Intentional Self-Harm	Poisoning, Assault	Poisoning, Undetermined	Adverse Effect	Underdosing
Benzoic acid	T49.0X1	T49.0X2	T49.0X3	T49.0X4	T49.0X5	T49.0X6
with salicylic acid	T49.0X1	T49.0X2	T49.0X3	T49.0X4	T49.0X5	T49.0X6
Benzoin (tincture)	T48.5X1	T48.5X2	T48.5X3	T48.5X4	T48.5X5	T48.5X6
Benzol (benzene)	T52.1X1	T52.1X2	T52.1X3	T52.1X4	—	—
vapor	T52.0X1	T52.0X2	T52.0X3	T52.0X4	—	—
Benzomorphan	T40.2X1	T40.2X2	T40.2X3	T40.2X4	T40.2X5	T40.2X6
Benzonatate	T48.3X1	T48.3X2	T48.3X3	T48.3X4	T48.3X5	T48.3X6
Benzophenones	T49.3X1	T49.3X2	T49.3X3	T49.3X4	T49.3X5	T49.3X6
Benzopyrone	T46.991	T46.992	T46.993	T46.994	T46.995	T46.996
Benzothiadiazides	T50.2X1	T50.2X2	T50.2X3	T50.2X4	T50.2X5	T50.2X6
Benzoxonium chloride	T49.0X1	T49.0X2	T49.0X3	T49.0X4	T49.0X5	T49.0X6
Benzoyl peroxide	T49.0X1	T49.0X2	T49.0X3	T49.0X4	T49.0X5	T49.0X6
Benzoylpas calcium	T37.1X1	T37.1X2	T37.1X3	T37.1X4	T37.1X5	T37.1X6
Benzperidin	T43.591	T43.592	T43.593	T43.594	T43.595	T43.596
Benzperidol	T43.591	T43.592	T43.593	T43.594	T43.595	T43.596
Benzphetamine	T50.5X1	T50.5X2	T50.5X3	T50.5X4	T50.5X5	T50.5X6
Benzpyrinium bromide	T44.1X1	T44.1X2	T44.1X3	T44.1X4	T44.1X5	T44.1X6
Benzquinamide	T45.0X1	T45.0X2	T45.0X3	T45.0X4	T45.0X5	T45.0X6
Benzthiazide	T50.2X1	T50.2X2	T50.2X3	T50.2X4	T50.2X5	T50.2X6
Benztropine						
anticholinergic	T44.3X1	T44.3X2	T44.3X3	T44.3X4	T44.3X5	T44.3X6
antiparkinson	T42.8X1	T42.8X2	T42.8X3	T42.8X4	T42.8X5	T42.8X6
Benzydamine	T49.0X1	T49.0X2	T49.0X3	T49.0X4	T49.0X5	T49.0X6
Benzyl						
acetate	T52.8X1	T52.8X2	T52.8X3	T52.8X4	—	—
alcohol	T49.0X1	T49.0X2	T49.0X3	T49.0X4	T49.0X5	T49.0X6
benzoate	T49.0X1	T49.0X2	T49.0X3	T49.0X4	T49.0X5	T49.0X6
Benzoic acid	T49.0X1	T49.0X2	T49.0X3	T49.0X4	T49.0X5	T49.0X6
morphine	T40.2X1	T40.2X2	T40.2X3	T40.2X4	—	—
nicotinate	T46.6X1	T46.6X2	T46.6X3	T46.6X4	T46.6X5	T46.6X6
penicillin	T36.0X1	T36.0X2	T36.0X3	T36.0X4	T36.0X5	T36.0X6
Benzylhydrochlorthia-zide	T50.2X1	T50.2X2	T50.2X3	T50.2X4	T50.2X5	T50.2X6
Benzylpenicillin	T36.0X1	T36.0X2	T36.0X3	T36.0X4	T36.0X5	T36.0X6
Benzylthiouracil	T38.2X1	T38.2X2	T38.2X3	T38.2X4	T38.2X5	T38.2X6
Bephenium hydroxy-naphthoate	T37.4X1	T37.4X2	T37.4X3	T37.4X4	T37.4X5	T37.4X6
Bepridil	T46.1X1	T46.1X2	T46.1X3	T46.1X4	T46.1X5	T46.1X6
Bergamot oil	T65.891	T65.892	T65.893	T65.894	—	—
Bergapten	T50.991	T50.992	T50.993	T50.994	T50.995	T50.996
Berries, poisonous	T62.1X1	T62.1X2	T62.1X3	T62.1X4	—	—
Beryllium (compounds)	T56.7X1	T56.7X2	T56.7X3	T56.7X4	—	—

TABLE OF DRUGS AND CHEMICALS (sidebar)

Substance	Poisoning, Accidental (Unintentional)	Poisoning, Intentional Self-Harm	Poisoning, Assault	Poisoning, Undetermined	Adverse Effect	Underdosing
b-acetyldigoxin	T46.0X1	T46.0X2	T46.0X3	T46.0X4	T46.0X5	T46.0X6
beta adrenergic blocking agent, heart	T44.7X1	T44.7X2	T44.7X3	T44.7X4	T44.7X5	T44.7X6
b-benzalbutyramide	T46.6X1	T46.6X2	T46.6X3	T46.6X4	T46.6X5	T46.6X6
Betacarotene	T45.2X1	T45.2X2	T45.2X3	T45.2X4	T45.2X5	T45.2X6
b-eucaine	T49.1X1	T49.1X2	T49.1X3	T49.1X4	T49.1X5	T49.1X6
Beta-Chlor	T42.6X1	T42.6X2	T42.6X3	T42.6X4	T42.6X5	T42.6X6
b-galactosidase	T47.5X1	T47.5X2	T47.5X3	T47.5X4	T47.5X5	T47.5X6
Betahistine	T46.7X1	T46.7X2	T46.7X3	T46.7X4	T46.7X5	T46.7X6
Betaine	T47.5X1	T47.5X2	T47.5X3	T47.5X4	T47.5X5	T47.5X6
Betamethasone	T49.0X1	T49.0X2	T49.0X3	T49.0X4	T49.0X5	T49.0X6
topical	T49.0X1	T49.0X2	T49.0X3	T49.0X4	T49.0X5	T49.0X6
Betamicin	T36.8X1	T36.8X2	T36.8X3	T36.8X4	T36.8X5	T36.8X6
Betanidine	T46.5X1	T46.5X2	T46.5X3	T46.5X4	T46.5X5	T46.5X6
b-sitosterol(s)	T46.6X1	T46.6X2	T46.6X3	T46.6X4	T46.6X5	T46.6X6
Betaxolol	T44.7X1	T44.7X2	T44.7X3	T44.7X4	T44.7X5	T44.7X6
Betazole	T50.8X1	T50.8X2	T50.8X3	T50.8X4	T50.8X5	T50.8X6
Bethanechol	T44.1X1	T44.1X2	T44.1X3	T44.1X4	T44.1X5	T44.1X6
chloride	T44.1X1	T44.1X2	T44.1X3	T44.1X4	T44.1X5	T44.1X6
Bethanidine	T46.5X1	T46.5X2	T46.5X3	T46.5X4	T46.5X5	T46.5X6
Betoxycaine	T41.3X1	T41.3X2	T41.3X3	T41.3X4	T41.3X5	T41.3X6
Betula oil	T49.3X1	T49.3X2	T49.3X3	T49.3X4	T49.3X5	T49.3X6
Bevantolol	T44.7X1	T44.7X2	T44.7X3	T44.7X4	T44.7X5	T44.7X6
Bevonium metilsulfate	T44.3X1	T44.3X2	T44.3X3	T44.3X4	T44.3X5	T44.3X6
Bezafibrate	T46.6X1	T46.6X2	T46.6X3	T46.6X4	T46.6X5	T46.6X6
Bezitramide	T40.4X1	T40.4X2	T40.4X3	T40.4X4	T40.4X5	T40.4X6
BHA	T50.991	T50.992	T50.993	T50.994	T50.995	T50.996
Bhang	T40.7X1	T40.7X2	T40.7X3	T40.7X4	T40.7X5	T40.7X6
BHC (medicinal)	T49.0X1	T49.0X2	T49.0X3	T49.0X4	T49.0X5	T49.0X6
nonmedicinal (vapor)	T53.6X1	T53.6X2	T53.6X3	T53.6X4	—	—
Bialamicol	T37.3X1	T37.3X2	T37.3X3	T37.3X4	T37.3X5	T37.3X6
Bibenzonium bromide	T48.3X1	T48.3X2	T48.3X3	T48.3X4	T48.3X5	T48.3X6
Bibrocathol	T49.5X1	T49.5X2	T49.5X3	T49.5X4	T49.5X5	T49.5X6
Bichloride of mercury — see Mercury, chloride						
Bichromates (calcium) (potassium) (sodium) (crystals)	T57.8X1	T57.8X2	T57.8X3	T57.8X4	—	—
fumes	T56.2X1	T56.2X2	T56.2X3	T56.2X4	—	—
Biclotymol	T49.6X1	T49.6X2	T49.6X3	T49.6X4	T49.6X5	T49.6X6
Bicucculine	T50.7X1	T50.7X2	T50.7X3	T50.7X4	T50.7X5	T50.7X6
Bifemelane	T43.291	T43.292	T43.293	T43.294	T43.295	T43.296
Biguanide derivatives, oral	T38.3X1	T38.3X2	T38.3X3	T38.3X4	T38.3X5	T38.3X6

Substance	External Cause (T-Code)					
	Poisoning, Accidental (Unintentional)	Poisoning, Intentional Self-Harm	Poisoning, Assault	Poisoning, Undetermined	Adverse Effect	Underdosing
Biligrafin	T50.8X1	T50.8X2	T50.8X3	T50.8X4	T50.8X5	T50.8X6
Bile salts	T47.5X1	T47.5X2	T47.5X3	T47.5X4	T47.5X5	T47.5X6
Bilopaque	T50.8X1	T50.8X2	T50.8X3	T50.8X4	T50.8X5	T50.8X6
Binifibrate	T46.6X1	T46.6X2	T46.6X3	T46.6X4	T46.6X5	T46.6X6
Binitrobenzol	T65.3X1	T65.3X2	T65.3X3	T65.3X4	—	—
Bioflavonoid(s)	T46.991	T46.992	T46.993	T46.994	T46.995	T46.996
Biological substance NEC	T50.901	T50.902	T50.903	T50.904	T50.905	T50.906
Biotin	T45.2X1	T45.2X2	T45.2X3	T45.2X4	T45.2X5	T45.2X6
Biperiden	T44.3X1	T44.3X2	T44.3X3	T44.3X4	T44.3X5	T44.3X6
Bisacodyl	T47.2X1	T47.2X2	T47.2X3	T47.2X4	T47.2X5	T47.2X6
Bisbentiamine	T45.2X1	T45.2X2	T45.2X3	T45.2X4	T45.2X5	T45.2X6
Bisbutiamine	T45.2X1	T45.2X2	T45.2X3	T45.2X4	T45.2X5	T45.2X6
Bisdequalinium (salts) (diacetate)	T49.6X1	T49.6X2	T49.6X3	T49.6X4	T49.6X5	T49.6X6
Bishydroxycoumarin	T45.511	T45.512	T45.513	T45.514	T45.515	T45.516
Bismarsen	T37.8X1	T37.8X2	T37.8X3	T37.8X4	T37.8X5	T37.8X6
Bismuth salts	T47.6X1	T47.6X2	T47.6X3	T47.6X4	T47.6X5	T47.6X6
aluminate	T47.1X1	T47.1X2	T47.1X3	T47.1X4	T47.1X5	T47.1X6
anti-infectives	T37.8X1	T37.8X2	T37.8X3	T37.8X4	T37.8X5	T37.8X6
formic iodide	T49.0X1	T49.0X2	T49.0X3	T49.0X4	T49.0X5	T49.0X6
glycolylarsenate	T49.0X1	T49.0X2	T49.0X3	T49.0X4	T49.0X5	T49.0X6
nonmedicinal (compounds) NEC	T65.91	T65.92	T65.93	T65.94	—	—
subcarbonate	T47.6X1	T47.6X2	T47.6X3	T47.6X4	T47.6X5	T47.6X6
subsalicylate	T37.8X1	T37.8X2	T37.8X3	T37.8X4	T37.8X5	T37.8X6
sulfarsphenamine	T37.8X1	T37.8X2	T37.8X3	T37.8X4	T37.8X5	T37.8X6
Bisoprolol	T44.7X1	T44.7X2	T44.7X3	T44.7X4	T44.7X5	T44.7X6
Bisoxatin	T47.2X1	T47.2X2	T47.2X3	T47.2X4	T47.2X5	T47.2X6
Bisulepin (hydrochloride)	T45.0X1	T45.0X2	T45.0X3	T45.0X4	T45.0X5	T45.0X6
Bithionol	T37.8X1	T37.8X2	T37.8X3	T37.8X4	T37.8X5	T37.8X6
anthelminthic	T37.4X1	T37.4X2	T37.4X3	T37.4X4	T37.4X5	T37.4X6
Bitolterol	T48.6X1	T48.6X2	T48.6X3	T48.6X4	T48.6X5	T48.6X6
Bitoscanate	T37.4X1	T37.4X2	T37.4X3	T37.4X4	T37.4X5	T37.4X6
Bitter almond oil	T62.8X1	T62.8X2	T62.8X3	T62.8X4	—	—
Bittersweet	T62.2X1	T62.2X2	T62.2X3	T62.2X4	—	—
Black						
flag	T60.91	T60.92	T60.93	T60.94	—	—
henbane	T62.2X1	T62.2X2	T62.2X3	T62.2X4	—	—
leaf (40)	T60.91	T60.92	T60.93	T60.94	—	—
widow spider (bite)	T63.311	T63.312	T63.313	T63.314	—	—
antivenin	T50.Z11	T50.Z12	T50.Z13	T50.Z14	T50.Z15	T50.Z16
Blast furnace gas (carbon monoxide from)	T58.8X1	T58.8X2	T58.8X3	T58.8X4	—	—

Substance	External Cause (T-Code)					
	Poisoning, Accidental (Unintentional)	Poisoning, Intentional Self-Harm	Poisoning, Assault	Poisoning, Undetermined	Adverse Effect	Underdosing
Bleach	T54.91	T54.92	T54.93	T54.94	—	—
Bleaching agent (medicinal)	T49.4X1	T49.4X2	T49.4X3	T49.4X4	T49.4X5	T49.4X6
Bleomycin	T45.1X1	T45.1X2	T45.1X3	T45.1X4	T45.1X5	T45.1X6
Blockain	T41.3X1	T41.3X2	T41.3X3	T41.3X4	T41.3X5	T41.3X6
infiltration (subcutaneous)	T41.3X1	T41.3X2	T41.3X3	T41.3X4	T41.3X5	T41.3X6
nerve block (peripheral) (plexus)	T41.3X1	T41.3X2	T41.3X3	T41.3X4	T41.3X5	T41.3X6
topical (surface)	T41.3X1	T41.3X2	T41.3X3	T41.3X4	T41.3X5	T41.3X6
Blockers, calcium channel	T46.1X1	T46.1X2	T46.1X3	T46.1X4	T46.1X5	T46.1X6
Blood (derivatives) (natural) (plasma) (whole)	T45.8X1	T45.8X2	T45.8X3	T45.8X4	T45.8X5	T45.8X6
dried	T45.8X1	T45.8X2	T45.8X3	T45.8X4	T45.8X5	T45.8X6
drug affecting NEC	T45.91	T45.92	T45.93	T45.94	T45.95	T45.96
expander NEC	T45.8X1	T45.8X2	T45.8X3	T45.8X4	T45.8X5	T45.8X6
fraction NEC	T45.8X1	T45.8X2	T45.8X3	T45.8X4	T45.8X5	T45.8X6
substitute (macromolecular)	T45.8X1	T45.8X2	T45.8X3	T45.8X4	T45.8X5	T45.8X6
Blue velvet	T40.2X1	T40.2X2	T40.2X3	T40.2X4	—	—
Bone meal	T62.8X1	T62.8X2	T62.8X3	T62.8X4	—	—
Bonine	T45.0X1	T45.0X2	T45.0X3	T45.0X4	T45.0X5	T45.0X6
Bopindolol	T44.7X1	T44.7X2	T44.7X3	T44.7X4	T44.7X5	T44.7X6
Boracic acid	T49.0X1	T49.0X2	T49.0X3	T49.0X4	T49.0X5	T49.0X6
ENT agent	T49.6X1	T49.6X2	T49.6X3	T49.6X4	T49.6X5	T49.6X6
ophthalmic preparation	T49.5X1	T49.5X2	T49.5X3	T49.5X4	T49.5X5	T49.5X6
Borane complex	T57.8X1	T57.8X2	T57.8X3	T57.8X4	—	—
Borate(s)	T57.8X1	T57.8X2	T57.8X3	T57.8X4	—	—
buffer	T50.991	T50.992	T50.993	T50.994	T50.995	T50.996
cleanser	T54.91	T54.92	T54.93	T54.94	—	—
sodium	T57.8X1	T57.8X2	T57.8X3	T57.8X4	—	—
Borax (cleanser)	T54.91	T54.92	T54.93	T54.94	—	—
Bordeaux mixture	T60.3X1	T60.3X2	T60.3X3	T60.3X4	—	—
Boric acid	T49.0X1	T49.0X2	T49.0X3	T49.0X4	T49.0X5	T49.0X6
ENT agent	T49.6X1	T49.6X2	T49.6X3	T49.6X4	T49.6X5	T49.6X6
ophthalmic preparation	T49.5X1	T49.5X2	T49.5X3	T49.5X4	T49.5X5	T49.5X6
Bornaprine	T44.3X1	T44.3X2	T44.3X3	T44.3X4	T44.3X5	T44.3X6
Boron	T57.8X1	T57.8X2	T57.8X3	T57.8X4	—	—
hydride NEC	T57.8X1	T57.8X2	T57.8X3	T57.8X4	—	—
fumes or gas	T57.8X1	T57.8X2	T57.8X3	T57.8X4	—	—
trifluoride	T59.891	T59.892	T59.893	T59.894	—	—
Botox	T48.291	T48.292	T48.293	T48.294	T48.295	T48.296
Botulinus anti-toxin (type A, B)	T50.Z11	T50.Z12	T50.Z13	T50.Z14	T50.Z15	T50.Z16
Brake fluid vapor	T59.891	T59.892	T59.893	T59.894	—	—
Brallobarbital	T42.3X1	T42.3X2	T42.3X3	T42.3X4	T42.3X5	T42.3X6

Substance	External Cause (T-Code)					
	Poisoning, Accidental (Unintentional)	Poisoning, Intentional Self-Harm	Poisoning, Assault	Poisoning, Undetermined	Adverse Effect	Underdosing
Bran (wheat)	T47.4X1	T47.4X2	T47.4X3	T47.4X4	T47.4X5	T47.4X6
Brass (fumes)	T56.891	T56.892	T56.893	T56.894	—	—
Brasso	T52.0X1	T52.0X2	T52.0X3	T52.0X4	—	—
Bretylium tosilate	T46.2X1	T46.2X2	T46.2X3	T46.2X4	T46.2X5	T46.2X6
Brevital (sodium)	T41.1X1	T41.1X2	T41.1X3	T41.1X4	T41.1X5	T41.1X6
Brinase	T45.3X1	T45.3X2	T45.3X3	T45.3X4	T45.3X5	T45.3X6
British antilewisite	T45.8X1	T45.8X2	T45.8X3	T45.8X4	T45.8X5	T45.8X6
Brodifacoum	T60.4X1	T60.4X2	T60.4X3	T60.4X4	—	—
Bromal (hydrate)	T42.6X1	T42.6X2	T42.6X3	T42.6X4	T42.6X5	T42.6X6
Bromazepam	T42.4X1	T42.4X2	T42.4X3	T42.4X4	T42.4X5	T42.4X6
Bromazine	T45.0X1	T45.0X2	T45.0X3	T45.0X4	T45.0X5	T45.0X6
Brombenzylcyanide	T59.3X1	T59.3X2	T59.3X3	T59.3X4	—	—
Bromelains	T45.3X1	T45.3X2	T45.3X3	T45.3X4	T45.3X5	T45.3X6
Bromethalin	T60.4X1	T60.4X2	T60.4X3	T60.4X4	—	—
Bromhexine	T48.4X1	T48.4X2	T48.4X3	T48.4X4	T48.4X5	T48.4X6
Bromide salts	T42.6X1	T42.6X2	T42.6X3	T42.6X4	T42.6X5	T42.6X6
Bromindione	T45.511	T45.512	T45.513	T45.514	T45.515	T45.516
Bromine						
compounds (medicinal)	T42.6X1	T42.6X2	T42.6X3	T42.6X4	T42.6X5	T42.6X6
sedative	T42.6X1	T42.6X2	T42.6X3	T42.6X4	T42.6X5	T42.6X6
vapor	T59.891	T59.892	T59.893	T59.894	—	—
Bromisovalum	T42.6X1	T42.6X2	T42.6X3	T42.6X4	T42.6X5	T42.6X6
Bromisoval	T42.6X1	T42.6X2	T42.6X3	T42.6X4	T42.6X5	T42.6X6
Bromobenzylcyanide	T59.3X1	T59.3X2	T59.3X3	T59.3X4	—	—
Bromochlorosalicylani-lide	T49.0X1	T49.0X2	T49.0X3	T49.0X4	T49.0X5	T49.0X6
Bromocriptine	T42.8X1	T42.8X2	T42.8X3	T42.8X4	T42.8X5	T42.8X6
Bromodiphenhydramine	T45.0X1	T45.0X2	T45.0X3	T45.0X4	T45.0X5	T45.0X6
Bromoform	T42.6X1	T42.6X2	T42.6X3	T42.6X4	T42.6X5	T42.6X6
Bromophenol blue reagent	T50.991	T50.992	T50.993	T50.994	T50.995	T50.996
Bromopride	T47.8X1	T47.8X2	T47.8X3	T47.8X4	T47.8X5	T47.8X6
Bromosalicylchloranitide	T49.0X1	T49.0X2	T49.0X3	T49.0X4	T49.0X5	T49.0X6
Bromosalicylhydroxamic acid	T37.1X1	T37.1X2	T37.1X3	T37.1X4	T37.1X5	T37.1X6
Bromo-seltzer	T39.1X1	T39.1X2	T39.1X3	T39.1X4	T39.1X5	T39.1X6
Bromoxynil	T60.3X1	T60.3X2	T60.3X3	T60.3X4	—	—
Bromperidol	T43.4X1	T43.4X2	T43.4X3	T43.4X4	T43.4X5	T43.4X6
Brompheniramine	T45.0X1	T45.0X2	T45.0X3	T45.0X4	T45.0X5	T45.0X6
Bromsulfophthalein	T50.8X1	T50.8X2	T50.8X3	T50.8X4	T50.8X5	T50.8X6
Bromural	T42.6X1	T42.6X2	T42.6X3	T42.6X4	T42.6X5	T42.6X6
Bromvaletone	T42.6X1	T42.6X2	T42.6X3	T42.6X4	T42.6X5	T42.6X6
Bronchodilator NEC	T48.6X1	T48.6X2	T48.6X3	T48.6X4	T48.6X5	T48.6X6

TABLE OF DRUGS AND CHEMICALS

Substance	External Cause (T-Code)					
	Poisoning, Accidental (Unintentional)	Poisoning, Intentional Self-Harm	Poisoning, Assault	Poisoning, Undetermined	Adverse Effect	Underdosing
Brotizolam	T42.4X1	T42.4X2	T42.4X3	T42.4X4	T42.4X5	T42.4X6
Brovincamine	T46.7X1	T46.7X2	T46.7X3	T46.7X4	T46.7X5	T46.7X6
Brown spider (bite) (venom)	T63.391	T63.392	T63.393	T63.394	—	—
Brown recluse spider (bite) (venom)	T63.331	T63.332	T63.333	T63.334	—	—
Broxaterol	T48.6X1	T48.6X2	T48.6X3	T48.6X4	T48.6X5	T48.6X6
Broxuridine	T45.1X1	T45.1X2	T45.1X3	T45.1X4	T45.1X5	T45.1X6
Broxyquinoline	T37.8X1	T37.8X2	T37.8X3	T37.8X4	T37.8X5	T37.8X6
Bruceine	T48.291	T48.292	T48.293	T48.294	T48.295	T48.296
Brucia	T62.2X1	T62.2X2	T62.2X3	T62.2X4	—	—
Brucine	T65.1X1	T65.1X2	T65.1X3	T65.1X4	—	—
Brunswick green — see Copper						
Bruten — see Ibuprofen						
Bryonia	T47.2X1	T47.2X2	T47.2X3	T47.2X4	T47.2X5	T47.2X6
Buclizine	T45.0X1	T45.0X2	T45.0X3	T45.0X4	T45.0X5	T45.0X6
Buclosamide	T49.0X1	T49.0X2	T49.0X3	T49.0X4	T49.0X5	T49.0X6
Budesonide	T44.5X1	T44.5X2	T44.5X3	T44.5X4	T44.5X5	T44.5X6
Budralazine	T46.5X1	T46.5X2	T46.5X3	T46.5X4	T46.5X5	T46.5X6
Bufferin	T39.011	T39.012	T39.013	T39.014	T39.015	T39.016
Buflomedil	T46.7X1	T46.7X2	T46.7X3	T46.7X4	T46.7X5	T46.7X6
Buformin	T38.3X1	T38.3X2	T38.3X3	T38.3X4	T38.3X5	T38.3X6
Bufotenine	T40.991	T40.992	T40.993	T40.994	—	—
Bufrolin	T48.6X1	T48.6X2	T48.6X3	T48.6X4	T48.6X5	T48.6X6
Bufylline	T48.6X1	T48.6X2	T48.6X3	T48.6X4	T48.6X5	T48.6X6
Bulk filler	T50.5X1	T50.5X2	T50.5X3	T50.5X4	T50.5X5	T50.5X6
cathartic	T47.4X1	T47.4X2	T47.4X3	T47.4X4	T47.4X5	T47.4X6
Bumetanide	T50.1X1	T50.1X2	T50.1X3	T50.1X4	T50.1X5	T50.1X6
Bunaftine	T46.2X1	T46.2X2	T46.2X3	T46.2X4	T46.2X5	T46.2X6
Bunamiodyl	T50.8X1	T50.8X2	T50.8X3	T50.8X4	T50.8X5	T50.8X6
Bunazosin	T44.6X1	T44.6X2	T44.6X3	T44.6X4	T44.6X5	T44.6X6
Bunitrolol	T44.7X1	T44.7X2	T44.7X3	T44.7X4	T44.7X5	T44.7X6
Buphenine	T46.7X1	T46.7X2	T46.7X3	T46.7X4	T46.7X5	T46.7X6
Bupivacaine	T41.3X1	T41.3X2	T41.3X3	T41.3X4	T41.3X5	T41.3X6
infiltration (subcutaneous)	T41.3X1	T41.3X2	T41.3X3	T41.3X4	T41.3X5	T41.3X6
nerve block (peripheral) (plexus)	T41.3X1	T41.3X2	T41.3X3	T41.3X4	T41.3X5	T41.3X6
spinal	T41.3X1	T41.3X2	T41.3X3	T41.3X4	T41.3X5	T41.3X6
Bupranolol	T44.7X1	T44.7X2	T44.7X3	T44.7X4	T44.7X5	T44.7X6
Buprenorphine	T40.4X1	T40.4X2	T40.4X3	T40.4X4	T40.4X5	T40.4X6
Bupropion	T43.291	T43.292	T43.293	T43.294	T43.295	T43.296
Burimamide	T47.1X1	T47.1X2	T47.1X3	T47.1X4	T47.1X5	T47.1X6
Buserelin	T38.891	T38.892	T38.893	T38.894	T38.895	T38.896

Substance	External Cause (T-Code)					
	Poisoning, Accidental (Unintentional)	Poisoning, Intentional Self-Harm	Poisoning, Assault	Poisoning, Undetermined	Adverse Effect	Underdosing
Buspirone	T43.591	T43.592	T43.593	T43.594	T43.595	T43.596
Busulfan, busulphan	T45.1X1	T45.1X2	T45.1X3	T45.1X4	T45.1X5	T45.1X6
Butabarbital (sodium)	T42.3X1	T42.3X2	T42.3X3	T42.3X4	T42.3X5	T42.3X6
Butabarbitone	T42.3X1	T42.3X2	T42.3X3	T42.3X4	T42.3X5	T42.3X6
Butabarpal	T42.3X1	T42.3X2	T42.3X3	T42.3X4	T42.3X5	T42.3X6
Butacaine	T41.3X1	T41.3X2	T41.3X3	T41.3X4	T41.3X5	T41.3X6
Butalamine	T46.7X1	T46.7X2	T46.7X3	T46.7X4	T46.7X5	T46.7X6
Butalbital	T42.3X1	T42.3X2	T42.3X3	T42.3X4	T42.3X5	T42.3X6
Butallylonal	T42.3X1	T42.3X2	T42.3X3	T42.3X4	T42.3X5	T42.3X6
Butamben	T41.3X1	T41.3X2	T41.3X3	T41.3X4	T41.3X5	T41.3X6
Butamirate	T48.3X1	T48.3X2	T48.3X3	T48.3X4	T48.3X5	T48.3X6
Butane (distributed in mobile container)	T59.891	T59.892	T59.893	T59.894	—	—
distributed through pipes	T59.891	T59.892	T59.893	T59.894	—	—
incomplete combustion	T58.11	T58.12	T58.13	T58.14	—	—
Butanilicaine	T41.3X1	T41.3X2	T41.3X3	T41.3X4	T41.3X5	T41.3X6
Butanol	T51.3X1	T51.3X2	T51.3X3	T51.3X4	—	—
Butanone, 2-butanone	T52.4X1	T52.4X2	T52.4X3	T52.4X4	—	—
Butantrone	T49.4X1	T49.4X2	T49.4X3	T49.4X4	T49.4X5	T49.4X6
Butaperazine	T43.3X1	T43.3X2	T43.3X3	T43.3X4	T43.3X5	T43.3X6
Butazolidin	T39.2X1	T39.2X2	T39.2X3	T39.2X4	T39.2X5	T39.2X6
Butetamate	T48.6X1	T48.6X2	T48.6X3	T48.6X4	T48.6X5	T48.6X6
Butethal	T42.3X1	T42.3X2	T42.3X3	T42.3X4	T42.3X5	T42.3X6
Butethamate	T44.3X1	T44.3X2	T44.3X3	T44.3X4	T44.3X5	T44.3X6
Buthalitone (sodium)	T41.1X1	T41.1X2	T41.1X3	T41.1X4	T41.1X5	T41.1X6
Butisol (sodium)	T42.3X1	T42.3X2	T42.3X3	T42.3X4	T42.3X5	T42.3X6
Butizide	T50.2X1	T50.2X2	T50.2X3	T50.2X4	T50.2X5	T50.2X6
Butobarbital	T42.3X1	T42.3X2	T42.3X3	T42.3X4	T42.3X5	T42.3X6
sodium	T42.3X1	T42.3X2	T42.3X3	T42.3X4	T42.3X5	T42.3X6
Butobarbitone	T42.3X1	T42.3X2	T42.3X3	T42.3X4	T42.3X5	T42.3X6
Butoconazole (nitrate)	T49.0X1	T49.0X2	T49.0X3	T49.0X4	T49.0X5	T49.0X6
Butorphanol	T40.4X1	T40.4X2	T40.4X3	T40.4X4	T40.4X5	T40.4X6
Butriptyline	T43.011	T43.012	T43.013	T43.014	T43.015	T43.016
Butropium bromide	T44.3X1	T44.3X2	T44.3X3	T44.3X4	T44.3X5	T44.3X6
Buttercups	T62.2X1	T62.2X2	T62.2X3	T62.2X4	—	—
Butter of antimony — see Antimony						
Butyl						
acetate (secondary)	T52.8X1	T52.8X2	T52.8X3	T52.8X4	—	—
alcohol	T51.3X1	T51.3X2	T51.3X3	T51.3X4	—	—
aminobenzoate	T41.3X1	T41.3X2	T41.3X3	T41.3X4	T41.3X5	T41.3X6
butyrate	T52.8X1	T52.8X2	T52.8X3	T52.8X4	—	—

Substance	External Cause (T-Code)					
	Poisoning, Accidental (Unintentional)	Poisoning, Intentional Self-Harm	Poisoning, Assault	Poisoning, Undetermined	Adverse Effect	Underdosing
Butyl *(Continued)*						
carbinol	T51.3X1	T51.3X2	T51.3X3	T51.3X4	—	—
carbitol	T52.3X1	T52.3X2	T52.3X3	T52.3X4	—	—
cellosolve	T52.3X1	T52.3X2	T52.3X3	T52.3X4	—	—
chloral (hydrate)	T42.6X1	T42.6X2	T42.6X3	T42.6X4	T42.6X5	T42.6X6
formate	T52.8X1	T52.8X2	T52.8X3	T52.8X4	—	—
lactate	T52.8X1	T52.8X2	T52.8X3	T52.8X4	—	—
propionate	T52.8X1	T52.8X2	T52.8X3	T52.8X4	—	—
scopolamine bromide	T44.3X1	T44.3X2	T44.3X3	T44.3X4	T44.3X5	T44.3X6
thiobarbital sodium	T41.1X1	T41.1X2	T41.1X3	T41.1X4	T41.1X5	T41.1X6
Butylated hydroxy-anisole	T50.991	T50.992	T50.993	T50.994	T50.995	T50.996
Butylchloral hydrate	T42.6X1	T42.6X2	T42.6X3	T42.6X4	T42.6X5	T42.6X6
Butyltoluene	T52.2X1	T52.2X2	T52.2X3	T52.2X4	—	—
Butyn	T41.3X1	T41.3X2	T41.3X3	T41.3X4	T41.3X5	T41.3X6
Butyrophenone (-based tranquilizers)	T43.4X1	T43.4X2	T43.4X3	T43.4X4	T43.4X5	T43.4X6
C						
Cabergoline	T42.8X1	T42.8X2	T42.8X3	T42.8X4	T42.8X5	T42.8X6
Cacodyl, cacodylic acid	T57.0X1	T57.0X2	T57.0X3	T57.0X4	—	—
Cactinomycin	T45.1X1	T45.1X2	T45.1X3	T45.1X4	T45.1X5	T45.1X6
Cade oil	T49.4X1	T49.4X2	T49.4X3	T49.4X4	T49.4X5	T49.4X6
Cadexomer iodine	T49.0X1	T49.0X2	T49.0X3	T49.0X4	T49.0X5	T49.0X6
Cadmium (chloride) (fumes) (oxide)	T56.3X1	T56.3X2	T56.3X3	T56.3X4	—	—
sulfide (medicinal) NEC	T49.4X1	T49.4X2	T49.4X3	T49.4X4	T49.4X5	T49.4X6
Cadralazine	T46.5X1	T46.5X2	T46.5X3	T46.5X4	T46.5X5	T46.5X6
Caffeine	T43.611	T43.612	T43.613	T43.614	T43.615	T43.616
Calabar bean	T62.2X1	T62.2X2	T62.2X3	T62.2X4	—	—
Caladium seguinum	T62.2X1	T62.2X2	T62.2X3	T62.2X4	—	—
Calamine (lotion)	T49.3X1	T49.3X2	T49.3X3	T49.3X4	T49.3X5	T49.3X6
Calcifediol	T45.2X1	T45.2X2	T45.2X3	T45.2X4	T45.2X5	T45.2X6
Calciferol	T45.2X1	T45.2X2	T45.2X3	T45.2X4	T45.2X5	T45.2X6
Calcitonin	T50.991	T50.992	T50.993	T50.994	T50.995	T50.996
Calcitriol	T45.2X1	T45.2X2	T45.2X3	T45.2X4	T45.2X5	T45.2X6
Calcium	T50.3X1	T50.3X2	T50.3X3	T50.3X4	T50.3X5	T50.3X6
actylsalicylate	T39.011	T39.012	T39.013	T39.014	T39.015	T39.016
benzamidosalicylate	T37.1X1	T37.1X2	T37.1X3	T37.1X4	T37.1X5	T37.1X6
bromide	T42.6X1	T42.6X2	T42.6X3	T42.6X4	T42.6X5	T42.6X6
bromolactobionate	T42.6X1	T42.6X2	T42.6X3	T42.6X4	T42.6X5	T42.6X6
carbaspirin	T39.011	T39.012	T39.013	T39.014	T39.015	T39.016
carbimide	T50.6X1	T50.6X2	T50.6X3	T50.6X4	T50.6X5	T50.6X6

Substance	Poisoning, Accidental (Unintentional)	Poisoning, Intentional Self-Harm	Poisoning, Assault	Poisoning, Undetermined	Adverse Effect	Underdosing
External Cause (T-Code)						
Calcium *(Continued)*						
carbonate	T47.1X1	T47.1X2	T47.1X3	T47.1X4	T47.1X5	T47.1X6
chloride	T50.991	T50.992	T50.993	T50.994	T50.995	T50.996
anhydrous	T50.991	T50.992	T50.993	T50.994	T50.995	T50.996
cyanide	T57.8X1	T57.8X2	T57.8X3	T57.8X4	—	—
dioctyl sulfosuccinate	T47.4X1	T47.4X2	T47.4X3	T47.4X4	T47.4X5	T47.4X6
disodium edathamil	T45.8X1	T45.8X2	T45.8X3	T45.8X4	T45.8X5	T45.8X6
disodium edetate	T45.8X1	T45.8X2	T45.8X3	T45.8X4	T45.8X5	T45.8X6
dobesilate	T46.991	T46.992	T46.993	T46.994	T46.995	T46.996
EDTA	T45.8X1	T45.8X2	T45.8X3	T45.8X4	T45.8X5	T45.8X6
ferrous citrate	T45.4X1	T45.4X2	T45.4X3	T45.4X4	T45.4X5	T45.4X6
folinate	T45.8X1	T45.8X2	T45.8X3	T45.8X4	T45.8X5	T45.8X6
glubionate	T50.3X1	T50.3X2	T50.3X3	T50.3X4	T50.3X5	T50.3X6
gluconate	T50.3X1	T50.3X2	T50.3X3	T50.3X4	T50.3X5	T50.3X6
gluconogalactogluconate	T50.3X1	T50.3X2	T50.3X3	T50.3X4	T50.3X5	T50.3X6
hydrate, hydroxide	T54.3X1	T54.3X2	T54.3X3	T54.3X4	—	—
hypochlorite	T54.3X1	T54.3X2	T54.3X3	T54.3X4	—	—
iodide	T48.4X1	T48.4X2	T48.4X3	T48.4X4	T48.4X5	T48.4X6
ipodate	T50.8X1	T50.8X2	T50.8X3	T50.8X4	T50.8X5	T50.8X6
lactate	T50.3X1	T50.3X2	T50.3X3	T50.3X4	T50.3X5	T50.3X6
leucovorin	T45.8X1	T45.8X2	T45.8X3	T45.8X4	T45.8X5	T45.8X6
mandelate	T37.91	T37.92	T37.93	T37.94	T37.95	T37.96
oxide	T54.3X1	T54.3X2	T54.3X3	T54.3X4	—	—
pantothenate	T45.2X1	T45.2X2	T45.2X3	T45.2X4	T45.2X5	T45.2X6
phosphate	T50.3X1	T50.3X2	T50.3X3	T50.3X4	T50.3X5	T50.3X6
salicylate	T39.091	T39.092	T39.093	T39.094	T39.095	T39.096
salts	T50.3X1	T50.3X2	T50.3X3	T50.3X4	T50.3X5	T50.3X6
Calculus-dissolving drug	T50.991	T50.992	T50.993	T50.994	T50.995	T50.996
Calomel	T49.0X1	T49.0X2	T49.0X3	T49.0X4	T49.0X5	T49.0X6
Caloric agent	T50.3X1	T50.3X2	T50.3X3	T50.3X4	T50.3X5	T50.3X6
Calusterone	T38.7X1	T38.7X2	T38.7X3	T38.7X4	T38.7X5	T38.7X6
Camazepam	T42.4X1	T42.4X2	T42.4X3	T42.4X4	T42.4X5	T42.4X6
Camomile	T49.0X1	T49.0X2	T49.0X3	T49.0X4	T49.0X5	T49.0X6
Camoquin	T37.2X1	T37.2X2	T37.2X3	T37.2X4	T37.2X5	T37.2X6
Camphor						
insecticide	T60.2X1	T60.2X2	T60.2X3	T60.2X4	—	—
medicinal	T49.8X1	T49.8X2	T49.8X3	T49.8X4	T49.8X5	T49.8X6
Camylofin	T44.3X1	T44.3X2	T44.3X3	T44.3X4	T44.3X5	T44.3X6
Cancer chemotherapy drug regimen	T45.1X1	T45.1X2	T45.1X3	T45.1X4	T45.1X5	T45.1X6
Candeptin	T49.0X1	T49.0X2	T49.0X3	T49.0X4	T49.0X5	T49.0X6

Substance	External Cause (T-Code)					
	Poisoning, Accidental (Unintentional)	Poisoning, Intentional Self-Harm	Poisoning, Assault	Poisoning, Undetermined	Adverse Effect	Underdosing
Candicidin	T49.0X1	T49.0X2	T49.0X3	T49.0X4	T49.0X5	T49.0X6
Cannabinol	T40.7X1	T40.7X2	T40.7X3	T40.7X4	T40.7X5	T40.7X6
Cannabis (derivatives)	T40.7X1	T40.7X2	T40.7X3	T40.7X4	T40.7X5	T40.7X6
Canned heat	T51.1X1	T51.1X2	T51.1X3	T51.1X4	—	—
Canrenoic acid	T50.0X1	T50.0X2	T50.0X3	T50.0X4	T50.0X5	T50.0X6
Canrenone	T50.0X1	T50.0X2	T50.0X3	T50.0X4	T50.0X5	T50.0X6
Cantharides, cantharidin, cantharis	T49.8X1	T49.8X2	T49.8X3	T49.8X4	T49.8X5	T49.8X6
Canthaxanthin	T50.991	T50.992	T50.993	T50.994	T50.995	T50.996
Capillary-active drug NEC	T46.901	T46.902	T46.903	T46.904	T46.905	T46.906
Capreomycin	T36.8X1	T36.8X2	T36.8X3	T36.8X4	T36.8X5	T36.8X6
Capsicum	T49.4X1	T49.4X2	T49.4X3	T49.4X4	T49.4X5	T49.4X6
Captafol	T60.3X1	T60.3X2	T60.3X3	T60.3X4	—	—
Captan	T60.3X1	T60.3X2	T60.3X3	T60.3X4	—	—
Captodiame, captodiamine	T43.591	T43.592	T43.593	T43.594	T43.595	T43.596
Captopril	T46.4X1	T46.4X2	T46.4X3	T46.4X4	T46.4X5	T46.4X6
Caramiphen	T44.3X1	T44.3X2	T44.3X3	T44.3X4	T44.3X5	T44.3X6
Carazolol	T44.7X1	T44.7X2	T44.7X3	T44.7X4	T44.7X5	T44.7X6
Carbachol	T44.1X1	T44.1X2	T44.1X3	T44.1X4	T44.1X5	T44.1X6
Carbacrylamine (resin)	T50.3X1	T50.3X2	T50.3X3	T50.3X4	T50.3X5	T50.3X6
Carbamate (insecticide)	T60.0X1	T60.0X2	T60.0X3	T60.0X4	—	—
Carbamate (sedative)	T42.6X1	T42.6X2	T42.6X3	T42.6X4	T42.6X5	T42.6X6
herbicide	T60.0X1	T60.0X2	T60.0X3	T60.0X4	—	—
insecticide	T60.0X1	T60.0X2	T60.0X3	T60.0X4	—	—
Carbamazepine	T42.1X1	T42.1X2	T42.1X3	T42.1X4	T42.1X5	T42.1X6
Carbamide	T47.3X1	T47.3X2	T47.3X3	T47.3X4	T47.3X5	T47.3X6
peroxide	T49.0X1	T49.0X2	T49.0X3	T49.0X4	T49.0X5	T49.0X6
topical	T49.8X1	T49.8X2	T49.8X3	T49.8X4	T49.8X5	T49.8X6
Carbamylcholine chloride	T44.1X1	T44.1X2	T44.1X3	T44.1X4	T44.1X5	T44.1X6
Carbaril	T60.0X1	T60.0X2	T60.0X3	T60.0X4	—	—
Carbarsone	T37.3X1	T37.3X2	T37.3X3	T37.3X4	T37.3X5	T37.3X6
Carbaryl	T60.0X1	T60.0X2	T60.0X3	T60.0X4	—	—
Carbaspirin	T39.011	T39.012	T39.013	T39.014	T39.015	T39.016
Carbazochrome (salicylate) (sodium sulfonate)	T49.4X1	T49.4X2	T49.4X3	T49.4X4	T49.4X5	T49.4X6
Carbenicillin	T36.0X1	T36.0X2	T36.0X3	T36.0X4	T36.0X5	T36.0X6
Carbenoxolone	T47.1X1	T47.1X2	T47.1X3	T47.1X4	T47.1X5	T47.1X6
Carbetapentane	T48.3X1	T48.3X2	T48.3X3	T48.3X4	T48.3X5	T48.3X6
Carbethyl salicylate	T39.091	T39.092	T39.093	T39.094	T39.095	T39.096
Carbidopa (with levodopa)	T42.8X1	T42.8X2	T42.8X3	T42.8X4	T42.8X5	T42.8X6
Carbimazole	T38.2X1	T38.2X2	T38.2X3	T38.2X4	T38.2X5	T38.2X6

Substance	Poisoning, Accidental (Unintentional)	Poisoning, Intentional Self-Harm	Poisoning, Assault	Poisoning, Undetermined	Adverse Effect	Underdosing
			External Cause (T-Code)			
Carbinol	T51.1X1	T51.1X2	T51.1X3	T51.1X4	—	—
Carbinoxamine	T45.0X1	T45.0X2	T45.0X3	T45.0X4	T45.0X5	T45.0X6
Carbiphene	T39.8X1	T39.8X2	T39.8X3	T39.8X4	T39.8X5	T39.8X6
Carbitol	T52.3X1	T52.3X2	T52.3X3	T52.3X4	—	—
Carbocaine	T41.3X1	T41.3X2	T41.3X3	T41.3X4	T41.3X5	T41.3X6
infiltration (subcutaneous)	T41.3X1	T41.3X2	T41.3X3	T41.3X4	T41.3X5	T41.3X6
nerve block (peripheral) (plexus)	T41.3X1	T41.3X2	T41.3X3	T41.3X4	T41.3X5	T41.3X6
topical (surface)	T41.3X1	T41.3X2	T41.3X3	T41.3X4	T41.3X5	T41.3X6
Carbo medicinalis	T47.6X1	T47.6X2	T47.6X3	T47.6X4	T47.6X5	T47.6X6
Carbomycin	T36.8X1	T36.8X2	T36.8X3	T36.8X4	T36.8X5	T36.8X6
Carbocisteine	T48.4X1	T48.4X2	T48.4X3	T48.4X4	T48.4X5	T48.4X6
Carbocromen	T46.3X1	T46.3X2	T46.3X3	T46.3X4	T46.3X5	T46.3X6
Carbol fuchsin	T49.0X1	T49.0X2	T49.0X3	T49.0X4	T49.0X5	T49.0X6
Carbolic acid — see also Phenol	T54.0X1	T54.0X2	T54.0X3	T54.0X4	—	—
Carbolonium (bromide)	T48.1X1	T48.1X2	T48.1X3	T48.1X4	T48.1X5	T48.1X6
Carbon						
bisulfide (liquid)	T65.4X1	T65.4X2	T65.4X3	T65.4X4	—	—
vapor	T65.4X1	T65.4X2	T65.4X3	T65.4X4	—	—
dioxide (gas)	T59.7X1	T59.7X2	T59.7X3	T59.7X4	—	—
medicinal	T41.5X1	T41.5X2	T41.5X3	T41.5X4	T41.5X5	T41.5X6
nonmedicinal	T59.7X1	T59.7X2	T59.7X3	T59.7X4	—	—
snow	T49.4X1	T49.4X2	T49.4X3	T49.4X4	T49.4X5	T49.4X6
disulfide (liquid)	T65.4X1	T65.4X2	T65.4X3	T65.4X4	—	—
vapor	T65.4X1	T65.4X2	T65.4X3	T65.4X4	—	—
monoxide (from incomplete combustion)	T58.91	T58.92	T58.93	T58.94	—	—
blast furnace gas	T58.8X1	T58.8X2	T58.8X3	T58.8X4	—	—
butane (distributed in mobile container)	T58.11	T58.12	T58.13	T58.14	—	—
distributed through pipes	T58.11	T58.12	T58.13	T58.14	—	—
charcoal fumes	T58.2X1	T58.2X2	T58.2X3	T58.2X4	—	—
coal	T58.2X1	T58.2X2	T58.2X3	T58.2X4	—	—
coke (in domestic stoves, fireplaces)	T58.2X1	T58.2X2	T58.2X3	T58.2X4	—	—
gas (piped)	T58.11	T58.12	T58.13	T58.14	—	—
solid (in domestic stoves, fireplaces)	T58.2X1	T58.2X2	T58.2X3	T58.2X4	—	—
exhaust gas (motor) not in transit	T58.01	T58.02	T58.03	T58.04	—	—
combustion engine, any not in watercraft	T58.01	T58.02	T58.03	T58.04	—	—
farm tractor, not in transit	T58.01	T58.02	T58.03	T58.04	—	—
gas engine	T58.01	T58.02	T58.03	T58.04	—	—
motor pump	T58.01	T58.02	T58.03	T58.04	—	—
motor vehicle, not in transit	T58.01	T58.02	T58.03	T58.04	—	—

Substance	Poisoning, Accidental (Unintentional)	Poisoning, Intentional Self-Harm	Poisoning, Assault	Poisoning, Undetermined	Adverse Effect	Underdosing
	External Cause (T-Code)					
Carbon *(Continued)*						
monoxide *(Continued)*						
fuel (in domestic use)	T58.2X1	T58.2X2	T58.2X3	T58.2X4	—	—
gas (piped)	T58.11	T58.12	T58.13	T58.14	—	—
in mobile container	T58.11	T58.12	T58.13	T58.14	—	—
utility	T58.11	T58.12	T58.13	T58.14	—	—
in mobile container	T58.11	T58.12	T58.13	T58.14	—	—
piped (natural)	T58.11	T58.12	T58.13	T58.14	—	—
illuminating gas	T58.11	T58.12	T58.13	T58.14	—	—
industrial fuels or gases, any	T58.8X1	T58.8X2	T58.8X3	T58.8X4	—	—
kerosene (in domestic stoves, fireplaces)	T58.2X1	T58.2X2	T58.2X3	T58.2X4	—	—
kiln gas or vapor	T58.8X1	T58.8X2	T58.8X3	T58.8X4	—	—
motor exhaust gas, not in transit	T58.01	T58.02	T58.03	T58.04	—	—
piped gas (manufactured) (natural)	T58.11	T58.12	T58.13	T58.14	—	—
producer gas	T58.8X1	T58.8X2	T58.8X3	T58.8X4	—	—
propane (distributed in mobile container)	T58.11	T58.12	T58.13	T58.14	—	—
distributed through pipes	T58.11	T58.12	T58.13	T58.14	—	—
specified source NEC	T58.8X1	T58.8X2	T58.8X3	T58.8X4	—	—
stove gas	T58.11	T58.12	T58.13	T58.14	—	—
piped	T58.11	T58.12	T58.13	T58.14	—	—
utility gas	T58.11	T58.12	T58.13	T58.14	—	—
piped	T58.11	T58.12	T58.13	T58.14	—	—
water gas	T58.1X1	T58.1X2	T58.1X3	T58.1X4	—	—
wood (in domestic stoves, fireplaces)	T58.2X1	T58.2X2	T58.2X3	T58.2X4	—	—
tetrachloride (vapor) NEC	T53.0X1	T53.0X2	T53.0X3	T53.0X4	—	—
liquid (cleansing agent) NEC	T53.0X1	T53.0X2	T53.0X3	T53.0X4	—	—
solvent	T53.0X1	T53.0X2	T53.0X3	T53.0X4	—	—
Carbonic acid gas	T59.7X1	T59.7X2	T59.7X3	T59.7X4	—	—
anhydrase inhibitor NEC	T50.2X1	T50.2X2	T50.2X3	T50.2X4	T50.2X5	T50.2X6
Carbophenothion	T60.0X1	T60.0X2	T60.0X3	T60.0X4	—	—
Carboplatin	T45.1X1	T45.1X2	T45.1X3	T45.1X4	T45.1X5	T45.1X6
Carboprost	T48.0X1	T48.0X2	T48.0X3	T48.0X4	T48.0X5	T48.0X6
Carboquone	T45.1X1	T45.1X2	T45.1X3	T45.1X4	T45.1X5	T45.1X6
Carbowax	T49.3X1	T49.3X2	T49.3X3	T49.3X4	T49.3X5	T49.3X6
Carboxymethyl-cellulose	T47.4X1	T47.4X2	T47.4X3	T47.4X4	T47.4X5	T47.4X6
S-Carboxymethyl-cysteine	T48.4X1	T48.4X2	T48.4X3	T48.4X4	T48.4X5	T48.4X6
Carbrital	T42.3X1	T42.3X2	T42.3X3	T42.3X4	T42.3X5	T42.3X6
Carbromal	T42.6X1	T42.6X2	T42.6X3	T42.6X4	T42.6X5	T42.6X6
Carbutamide	T38.3X1	T38.3X2	T38.3X3	T38.3X4	T38.3X5	T38.3X6
Carbuterol	T48.6X1	T48.6X2	T48.6X3	T48.6X4	T48.6X5	T48.6X6

Substance	External Cause (T-Code)					
	Poisoning, Accidental (Unintentional)	Poisoning, Intentional Self-Harm	Poisoning, Assault	Poisoning, Undetermined	Adverse Effect	Underdosing
Cardiac						
depressants	T46.2X1	T46.2X2	T46.2X3	T46.2X4	T46.2X5	T46.2X6
rhythm regulator	T46.2X1	T46.2X2	T46.2X3	T46.2X4	T46.2X5	T46.2X6
specified NEC	T46.2X1	T46.2X2	T46.2X3	T46.2X4	T46.2X5	T46.2X6
Cardiografin	T50.8X1	T50.8X2	T50.8X3	T50.8X4	T50.8X5	T50.8X6
Cardio-green	T50.8X1	T50.8X2	T50.8X3	T50.8X4	T50.8X5	T50.8X6
Cardiotonic (glycoside) NEC	T46.0X1	T46.0X2	T46.0X3	T46.0X4	T46.0X5	T46.0X6
Cardiovascular drug NEC	T46.901	T46.902	T46.903	T46.904	T46.905	T46.906
Cardrase	T50.2X1	T50.2X2	T50.2X3	T50.2X4	T50.2X5	T50.2X6
Carfusin	T49.0X1	T49.0X2	T49.0X3	T49.0X4	T49.0X5	T49.0X6
Carfecillin	T36.0X1	T36.0X2	T36.0X3	T36.0X4	T36.0X5	T36.0X6
Carfenazine	T43.3X1	T43.3X2	T43.3X3	T43.3X4	T43.3X5	T43.3X6
Carindacillin	T36.0X1	T36.0X2	T36.0X3	T36.0X4	T36.0X5	T36.0X6
Carisoprodol	T42.8X1	T42.8X2	T42.8X3	T42.8X4	T42.8X5	T42.8X6
Carmellose	T47.4X1	T47.4X2	T47.4X3	T47.4X4	T47.4X5	T47.4X6
Carminative	T47.5X1	T47.5X2	T47.5X3	T47.5X4	T47.5X5	T47.5X6
Carmofur	T45.1X1	T45.1X2	T45.1X3	T45.1X4	T45.1X5	T45.1X6
Carmustine	T45.1X1	T45.1X2	T45.1X3	T45.1X4	T45.1X5	T45.1X6
Carotene	T45.2X1	T45.2X2	T45.2X3	T45.2X4	T45.2X5	T45.2X6
Carphenazine	T43.3X1	T43.3X2	T43.3X3	T43.3X4	T43.3X5	T43.3X6
Carpipramine	T42.4X1	T42.4X2	T42.4X3	T42.4X4	T42.4X5	T42.4X6
Carprofen	T39.311	T39.312	T39.313	T39.314	T39.315	T39.316
Carpronium chloride	T44.3X1	T44.3X2	T44.3X3	T44.3X4	T44.3X5	T44.3X6
Carrageenan	T47.8X1	T47.8X2	T47.8X3	T47.8X4	T47.8X5	T47.8X6
Carteolol	T44.7X1	T44.7X2	T44.7X3	T44.7X4	T44.7X5	T44.7X6
Carter's Little Pills	T47.2X1	T47.2X2	T47.2X3	T47.2X4	T47.2X5	T47.2X6
Cascara (sagrada)	T47.2X1	T47.2X2	T47.2X3	T47.2X4	T47.2X5	T47.2X6
Cassava	T62.2X1	T62.2X2	T62.2X3	T62.2X4	—	—
Castellani's paint	T49.0X1	T49.0X2	T49.0X3	T49.0X4	T49.0X5	T49.0X6
Castor						
bean	T62.2X1	T62.2X2	T62.2X3	T62.2X4	—	—
oil	T47.2X1	T47.2X2	T47.2X3	T47.2X4	T47.2X5	T47.2X6
Catalase	T45.3X1	T45.3X2	T45.3X3	T45.3X4	T45.3X5	T45.3X6
Caterpillar (sting)	T63.431	T63.432	T63.433	T63.434	—	—
Catha (edulis) (tea)	T43.691	T43.692	T43.693	T43.694	—	—
Cathartic NEC	T47.4X1	T47.4X2	T47.4X3	T47.4X4	T47.4X5	T47.4X6
anthacene derivative	T47.2X1	T47.2X2	T47.2X3	T47.2X4	T47.2X5	T47.2X6
bulk	T47.4X1	T47.4X2	T47.4X3	T47.4X4	T47.4X5	T47.4X6
contact	T47.2X1	T47.2X2	T47.2X3	T47.2X4	T47.2X5	T47.2X6
emollient NEC	T47.4X1	T47.4X2	T47.4X3	T47.4X4	T47.4X5	T47.4X6

Substance	Poisoning, Accidental (Unintentional)	Poisoning, Intentional Self-Harm	Poisoning, Assault	Poisoning, Undetermined	Adverse Effect	Underdosing
External Cause (T-Code)						
Cathartic NEC *(Continued)*						
irritant NEC	T47.2X1	T47.2X2	T47.2X3	T47.2X4	T47.2X5	T47.2X6
mucilage	T47.4X1	T47.4X2	T47.4X3	T47.4X4	T47.4X5	T47.4X6
saline	T47.3X1	T47.3X2	T47.3X3	T47.3X4	T47.3X5	T47.3X6
vegetable	T47.2X1	T47.2X2	T47.2X3	T47.2X4	T47.2X5	T47.2X6
Cathine	T50.5X1	T50.5X2	T50.5X3	T50.5X4	T50.5X5	T50.5X6
Cathomycin	T36.8X1	T36.8X2	T36.8X3	T36.8X4	T36.8X5	T36.8X6
Cation exchange resin	T50.3X1	T50.3X2	T50.3X3	T50.3X4	T50.3X5	T50.3X6
Caustic(s) NEC	T54.91	T54.92	T54.93	T54.94	—	—
alkali	T54.3X1	T54.3X2	T54.3X3	T54.3X4	—	—
hydroxide	T54.3X1	T54.3X2	T54.3X3	T54.3X4	—	—
potash	T54.3X1	T54.3X2	T54.3X3	T54.3X4	—	—
soda	T54.3X1	T54.3X2	T54.3X3	T54.3X4	—	—
specified NEC	T54.91	T54.92	T54.93	T54.94	—	—
Ceepryn	T49.0X1	T49.0X2	T49.0X3	T49.0X4	T49.0X5	T49.0X6
ENT agent	T49.6X1	T49.6X2	T49.6X3	T49.6X4	T49.6X5	T49.6X6
lozenges	T49.6X1	T49.6X2	T49.6X3	T49.6X4	T49.6X5	T49.6X6
Cefacetrile	T36.1X1	T36.1X2	T36.1X3	T36.1X4	T36.1X5	T36.1X6
Cefaclor	T36.1X1	T36.1X2	T36.1X3	T36.1X4	T36.1X5	T36.1X6
Cefadroxil	T36.1X1	T36.1X2	T36.1X3	T36.1X4	T36.1X5	T36.1X6
Cefalexin	T36.1X1	T36.1X2	T36.1X3	T36.1X4	T36.1X5	T36.1X6
Cefaloglycin	T36.1X1	T36.1X2	T36.1X3	T36.1X4	T36.1X5	T36.1X6
Cefaloridine	T36.1X1	T36.1X2	T36.1X3	T36.1X4	T36.1X5	T36.1X6
Cefalosporins	T36.1X1	T36.1X2	T36.1X3	T36.1X4	T36.1X5	T36.1X6
Cefalotin	T36.1X1	T36.1X2	T36.1X3	T36.1X4	T36.1X5	T36.1X6
Cefamandole	T36.1X1	T36.1X2	T36.1X3	T36.1X4	T36.1X5	T36.1X6
Cefamycin antibiotic	T36.1X1	T36.1X2	T36.1X3	T36.1X4	T36.1X5	T36.1X6
Cefapirin	T36.1X1	T36.1X2	T36.1X3	T36.1X4	T36.1X5	T36.1X6
Cefatrizine	T36.1X1	T36.1X2	T36.1X3	T36.1X4	T36.1X5	T36.1X6
Cefazedone	T36.1X1	T36.1X2	T36.1X3	T36.1X4	T36.1X5	T36.1X6
Cefazolin	T36.1X1	T36.1X2	T36.1X3	T36.1X4	T36.1X5	T36.1X6
Cefbuperazone	T36.1X1	T36.1X2	T36.1X3	T36.1X4	T36.1X5	T36.1X6
Cefetamet	T36.1X1	T36.1X2	T36.1X3	T36.1X4	T36.1X5	T36.1X6
Cefixime	T36.1X1	T36.1X2	T36.1X3	T36.1X4	T36.1X5	T36.1X6
Cefmenoxime	T36.1X1	T36.1X2	T36.1X3	T36.1X4	T36.1X5	T36.1X6
Cefmetazole	T36.1X1	T36.1X2	T36.1X3	T36.1X4	T36.1X5	T36.1X6
Cefminox	T36.1X1	T36.1X2	T36.1X3	T36.1X4	T36.1X5	T36.1X6
Cefonicid	T36.1X1	T36.1X2	T36.1X3	T36.1X4	T36.1X5	T36.1X6
Cefoperazone	T36.1X1	T36.1X2	T36.1X3	T36.1X4	T36.1X5	T36.1X6

Substance	Poisoning, Accidental (Unintentional)	Poisoning, Intentional Self-Harm	Poisoning, Assault	Poisoning, Undetermined	Adverse Effect	Underdosing
	External Cause (T-Code)					
Ceforanide	T36.1X1	T36.1X2	T36.1X3	T36.1X4	T36.1X5	T36.1X6
Cefotaxime	T36.1X1	T36.1X2	T36.1X3	T36.1X4	T36.1X5	T36.1X6
Cefotetan	T36.1X1	T36.1X2	T36.1X3	T36.1X4	T36.1X5	T36.1X6
Cefotiam	T36.1X1	T36.1X2	T36.1X3	T36.1X4	T36.1X5	T36.1X6
Cefoxitin	T36.1X1	T36.1X2	T36.1X3	T36.1X4	T36.1X5	T36.1X6
Cefpimizole	T36.1X1	T36.1X2	T36.1X3	T36.1X4	T36.1X5	T36.1X6
Cefpiramide	T36.1X1	T36.1X2	T36.1X3	T36.1X4	T36.1X5	T36.1X6
Cefradine	T36.1X1	T36.1X2	T36.1X3	T36.1X4	T36.1X5	T36.1X6
Cefroxadine	T36.1X1	T36.1X2	T36.1X3	T36.1X4	T36.1X5	T36.1X6
Cefsulodin	T36.1X1	T36.1X2	T36.1X3	T36.1X4	T36.1X5	T36.1X6
Ceftazidime	T36.1X1	T36.1X2	T36.1X3	T36.1X4	T36.1X5	T36.1X6
Cefteram	T36.1X1	T36.1X2	T36.1X3	T36.1X4	T36.1X5	T36.1X6
Ceftezole	T36.1X1	T36.1X2	T36.1X3	T36.1X4	T36.1X5	T36.1X6
Ceftizoxime	T36.1X1	T36.1X2	T36.1X3	T36.1X4	T36.1X5	T36.1X6
Ceftriaxone	T36.1X1	T36.1X2	T36.1X3	T36.1X4	T36.1X5	T36.1X6
Cefuroxime	T36.1X1	T36.1X2	T36.1X3	T36.1X4	T36.1X5	T36.1X6
Cefuzonam	T36.1X1	T36.1X2	T36.1X3	T36.1X4	T36.1X5	T36.1X6
Celestone	T38.0X1	T38.0X2	T38.0X3	T38.0X4	T38.0X5	T38.0X6
topical	T49.0X1	T49.0X2	T49.0X3	T49.0X4	T49.0X5	T49.0X6
Celiprolol	T44.7X1	T44.7X2	T44.7X3	T44.7X4	T44.7X5	T44.7X6
Cellosolve	T52.91	T52.92	T52.93	T52.94	—	—
Cell stimulants and proliferants	T49.8X1	T49.8X2	T49.8X3	T49.8X4	T49.8X5	T49.8X6
Cellulose						
cathartic	T47.4X1	T47.4X2	T47.4X3	T47.4X4	T47.4X5	T47.4X6
hydroxyethyl	T47.4X1	T47.4X2	T47.4X3	T47.4X4	T47.4X5	T47.4X6
nitrates (topical)	T49.3X1	T49.3X2	T49.3X3	T49.3X4	T49.3X5	T49.3X6
oxidized	T49.4X1	T49.4X2	T49.4X3	T49.4X4	T49.4X5	T49.4X6
Centipede (bite)	T63.411	T63.412	T63.413	T63.414	—	—
Central nervous system						
depressants	T42.71	T42.72	T42.73	T42.74	T42.75	T42.76
anesthetic (general) NEC	T41.201	T41.202	T41.203	T41.204	T41.205	T41.206
gases NEC	T41.0X1	T41.0X2	T41.0X3	T41.0X4	T41.0X5	T41.0X6
intravenous	T41.1X1	T41.1X2	T41.1X3	T41.1X4	T41.1X5	T41.1X6
barbiturates	T42.3X1	T42.3X2	T42.3X3	T42.3X4	T42.3X5	T42.3X6
benzodiazepines	T42.4X1	T42.4X2	T42.4X3	T42.4X4	T42.4X5	T42.4X6
bromides	T42.6X1	T42.6X2		T42.6X4	T42.6X5	T42.6X6
cannabis sativa	T40.7X1	T40.7X2	T40.7X3	T40.7X4	T40.7X5	T40.7X6
chloral hydrate	T42.6X1	T42.6X2	T42.6X3	T42.6X4	T42.6X5	T42.6X6
ethanol	T51.0X1	T51.0X2	T51.0X3	T51.0X4	—	—

	External Cause (T-Code)					
Substance	Poisoning, Accidental (Unintentional)	Poisoning, Intentional Self-Harm	Poisoning, Assault	Poisoning, Undetermined	Adverse Effect	Underdosing
Central nervous system *(Continued)*						
depressants *(Continued)*						
hallucinogenics	T40.901	T40.902	T40.903	T40.904	T40.905	T40.906
hypnotics	T42.71	T42.72	T42.73	T42.74	T42.75	T42.76
specified NEC	T42.6X1	T42.6X2	T42.6X3	T42.6X4	T42.6X5	T42.6X6
muscle relaxants	T42.8X1	T42.8X2	T42.8X3	T42.8X4	T42.8X5	T42.8X6
paraldehyde	T42.6X1	T42.6X2	T42.6X3	T42.6X4	T42.6X5	T42.6X6
sedatives; sedative-hypnotics	T42.71	T42.72	T42.73	T42.74	T42.75	T42.76
mixed NEC	T42.6X1	T42.6X2	T42.6X3	T42.6X4	T42.6X5	T42.6X6
specified NEC	T42.6X1	T42.6X2	T42.6X3	T42.6X4	T42.6X5	T42.6X6
muscle-tone depressants	T42.8X1	T42.8X2	T42.8X3	T42.8X4	T42.8X5	T42.8X6
stimulants	T43.601	T43.602	T43.603	T43.604	T43.605	T43.606
amphetamines	T43.621	T43.622	T43.623	T43.624	T43.625	T43.626
analeptics	T50.7X1	T50.7X2	T50.7X3	T50.7X4	T50.7X5	T50.7X6
antidepressants	T43.201	T43.202	T43.203	T43.204	T43.205	T43.206
opiate antagonists	T50.7X1	T50.7X2	T50.7X3	T50.7X4	T50.7X5	T50.7X6
specified NEC	T43.691	T43.692	T43.693	T43.694	T43.695	T43.696
Cephalexin	T36.1X1	T36.1X2	T36.1X3	T36.1X4	T36.1X5	T36.1X6
Cephaloglycin	T36.1X1	T36.1X2	T36.1X3	T36.1X4	T36.1X5	T36.1X6
Cephaloridine	T36.1X1	T36.1X2	T36.1X3	T36.1X4	T36.1X5	T36.1X6
Cephalosporins	T36.1X1	T36.1X2	T36.1X3	T36.1X4	T36.1X5	T36.1X6
N (adicillin)	T36.0X1	T36.0X2	T36.0X3	T36.0X4	T36.0X5	T36.0X6
Cephalothin	T36.1X1	T36.1X2	T36.1X3	T36.1X4	T36.1X5	T36.1X6
Cephalotin	T36.1X1	T36.1X2	T36.1X3	T36.1X4	T36.1X5	T36.1X6
Cephradine	T36.1X1	T36.1X2	T36.1X3	T36.1X4	T36.1X5	T36.1X6
Cerbera (odallam)	T62.2X1	T62.2X2	T62.2X3	T62.2X4	—	—
Cerberin	T46.0X1	T46.0X2	T46.0X3	T46.0X4	T46.0X5	T46.0X6
Cerebral stimulants	T43.601	T43.602	T43.603	T43.604	T43.605	T43.606
psychotherapeutic	T43.601	T43.602	T43.603	T43.604	T43.605	T43.606
specified NEC	T43.691	T43.692	T43.693	T43.694	T43.695	T43.696
Cerium oxalate	T45.0X1	T45.0X2	T45.0X3	T45.0X4	T45.0X5	T45.0X6
Cerous oxalate	T45.0X1	T45.0X2	T45.0X3	T45.0X4	T45.0X5	T45.0X6
Ceruletide	T50.8X1	T50.8X2	T50.8X3	T50.8X4	T50.8X5	T50.8X6
Cetalkonium (chloride)	T49.0X1	T49.0X2	T49.0X3	T49.0X4	T49.0X5	T49.0X6
Cethexonium chloride	T49.0X1	T49.0X2	T49.0X3	T49.0X4	T49.0X5	T49.0X6
Cetiedil	T46.7X1	T46.7X2	T46.7X3	T46.7X4	T46.7X5	T46.7X6
Cetirizine	T45.0X1	T45.0X2	T45.0X3	T45.0X4	T45.0X5	T45.0X6
Cetomacrogol	T50.991	T50.992	T50.993	T50.994	T50.995	T50.996
Cetotiamine	T45.2X1	T45.2X2	T45.2X3	T45.2X4	T45.2X5	T45.2X6

Substance	Poisoning, Accidental (Unintentional)	Poisoning, Intentional Self-Harm	Poisoning, Assault	Poisoning, Undetermined	Adverse Effect	Underdosing
Cetoxime	T45.0X1	T45.0X2	T45.0X3	T45.0X4	T45.0X5	T45.0X6
Cetraxate	T47.1X1	T47.1X2	T47.1X3	T47.1X4	T47.1X5	T47.1X6
Cetrimide	T49.0X1	T49.0X2	T49.0X3	T49.0X4	T49.0X5	T49.0X6
Cetrimonium (bromide)	T49.0X1	T49.0X2	T49.0X3	T49.0X4	T49.0X5	T49.0X6
Cetylpyridinium chloride	T49.0X1	T49.0X2	T49.0X3	T49.0X4	T49.0X5	T49.0X6
ENT agent	T49.6X1	T49.6X2	T49.6X3	T49.6X4	T49.6X5	T49.6X6
lozenges	T49.6X1	T49.6X2	T49.6X3	T49.6X4	T49.6X5	T49.6X6
Cevadillasee Sabadilla						
Cevitamic acid	T45.2X1	T45.2X2	T45.2X3	T45.2X4	T45.2X5	T45.2X6
Chalk, precipitated	T47.1X1	T47.1X2	T47.1X3	T47.1X4	T47.1X5	T47.1X6
Chamomile	T49.0X1	T49.0X2	T49.0X3	T49.0X4	T49.0X5	T49.0X6
Ch'an su	T46.0X1	T46.0X2	T46.0X3	T46.0X4	T46.0X5	T46.0X6
Charcoal	T47.6X1	T47.6X2	T47.6X3	T47.6X4	T47.6X5	T47.6X6
activated — see also Charcoal, medicinal	T47.6X1	T47.6X2	T47.6X3	T47.6X4	T47.6X5	T47.6X6
fumes (Carbon monoxide)	T58.2X1	T58.2X2	T58.2X3	T58.2X4	—	—
industrial	T58.8X1	T58.8X2	T58.8X3	T58.8X4	—	—
medicinal (activated)	T47.6X1	T47.6X2	T47.6X3	T47.6X4	T47.6X5	T47.6X6
antidiarrheal	T47.6X1	T47.6X2	T47.6X3	T47.6X4	T47.6X5	T47.6X6
poison control	T47.8X1	T47.8X2	T47.8X3	T47.8X4	T47.8X5	T47.8X6
specified use other than for diarrhea	T47.8X1	T47.8X2	T47.8X3	T47.8X4	T47.8X5	T47.8X6
topical	T49.8X1	T49.8X2	T49.8X3	T49.8X4	T49.8X5	T49.8X6
Chaulmosulfone	T37.1X1	T37.1X2	T37.1X3	T37.1X4	T37.1X5	T37.1X6
Chelating agent NEC	T50.6X1	T50.6X2	T50.6X3	T50.6X4	T50.6X5	T50.6X6
Chelidonium majus	T62.2X1	T62.2X2	T62.2X3	T62.2X4	—	—
Chemical substance NEC	T65.91	T65.92	T65.93	T65.94	—	—
Chenodeoxycholic acid	T47.5X1	T47.5X2	T47.5X3	T47.5X4	T47.5X5	T47.5X6
Chenodiol	T47.5X1	T47.5X2	T47.5X3	T47.5X4	T47.5X5	T47.5X6
Chenopodium	T37.4X1	T37.4X2	T37.4X3	T37.4X4	T37.4X5	T37.4X6
Cherry laurel	T62.2X1	T62.2X2	T62.2X3	T62.2X4	—	—
Chinidin(e)	T46.2X1	T46.2X2	T46.2X3	T46.2X4	T46.2X5	T46.2X6
Chiniofon	T37.8X1	T37.8X2	T37.8X3	T37.8X4	T37.8X5	T37.8X6
Chlophedianol	T48.3X1	T48.3X2	T48.3X3	T48.3X4	T48.3X5	T48.3X6
Chloral	T42.6X1	T42.6X2	T42.6X3	T42.6X4	T42.6X5	T42.6X6
derivative	T42.6X1	T42.6X2	T42.6X3	T42.6X4	T42.6X5	T42.6X6
hydrate	T42.6X1	T42.6X2	T42.6X3	T42.6X4	T42.6X5	T42.6X6
Chloralamide	T42.6X1	T42.6X2	T42.6X3	T42.6X4	T42.6X5	T42.6X6
Chloralodol	T42.6X1	T42.6X2	T42.6X3	T42.6X4	T42.6X5	T42.6X6
Chloralose	T60.4X1	T60.4X2	T60.4X3	T60.4X4	—	—
Chlorambucil	T45.1X1	T45.1X2	T45.1X3	T45.1X4	T45.1X5	T45.1X6

Substance	External Cause (T-Code)					
	Poisoning, Accidental (Unintentional)	Poisoning, Intentional Self-Harm	Poisoning, Assault	Poisoning, Undetermined	Adverse Effect	Underdosing
Chloramine	T57.8X1	T57.8X2	T57.8X3	T57.8X4	—	—
T	T49.0X1	T49.0X2	T49.0X3	T49.0X4	T49.0X5	T49.0X6
topical	T49.0X1	T49.0X2	T49.0X3	T49.0X4	T49.0X5	T49.0X6
Chloramphenicol	T36.2X1	T36.2X2	T36.2X3	T36.2X4	T36.2X5	T36.2X6
ENT agent	T49.6X1	T49.6X2	T49.6X3	T49.6X4	T49.6X5	T49.6X6
ophthalmic preparation	T49.5X1	T49.5X2	T49.5X3	T49.5X4	T49.5X5	T49.5X6
topical NEC	T49.0X1	T49.0X2	T49.0X3	T49.0X4	T49.0X5	T49.0X6
Chlorate (potassium) (sodium) NEC	T60.3X1	T60.3X2	T60.3X3	T60.3X4	—	—
herbicide	T60.3X1	T60.3X2	T60.3X3	T60.3X4	—	—
Chlorazanil	T50.2X1	T50.2X2	T50.2X3	T50.2X4	T50.2X5	T50.2X6
Chlorbenzene, chlorbenzol	T53.7X1	T53.7X2	T53.7X3	T53.7X4	—	—
Chlorbenzoxamine	T44.3X1	T44.3X2	T44.3X3	T44.3X4	T44.3X5	T44.3X6
Chlorbutol	T42.6X1	T42.6X2	T42.6X3	T42.6X4	T42.6X5	T42.6X6
Chlorcyclizine	T45.0X1	T45.0X2	T45.0X3	T45.0X4	T45.0X5	T45.0X6
Chlordan(e) (dust)	T60.1X1	T60.1X2	T60.1X3	T60.1X4	—	—
Chlordantoin	T49.0X1	T49.0X2	T49.0X3	T49.0X4	T49.0X5	T49.0X6
Chlordiazepoxide	T42.4X1	T42.4X2	T42.4X3	T42.4X4	T42.4X5	T42.4X6
Chlordiethyl benzamide	T49.3X1	T49.3X2	T49.3X3	T49.3X4	T49.3X5	T49.3X6
Chloresium	T49.8X1	T49.8X2	T49.8X3	T49.8X4	T49.8X5	T49.8X6
Chlorethiazol	T42.6X1	T42.6X2	T42.6X3	T42.6X4	T42.6X5	T42.6X6
Chlorethyl — see Ethyl chloride						
Chloretone	T42.6X1	T42.6X2	T42.6X3	T42.6X4	T42.6X5	T42.6X6
Chlorex	T53.6X1	T53.6X2	T53.6X3	T53.6X4	—	—
insecticide	T60.1X1	T60.1X2	T60.1X3	T60.1X4	—	—
Chlorfenvinphos	T60.0X1	T60.0X2	T60.0X3	T60.0X4	—	—
Chlorhexadol	T42.6X1	T42.6X2	T42.6X3	T42.6X4	T42.6X5	T42.6X6
Chlorhexamide	T45.1X1	T45.1X2	T45.1X3	T45.1X4	T45.1X5	T45.1X6
Chlorhexidine	T49.0X1	T49.0X2	T49.0X3	T49.0X4	T49.0X5	T49.0X6
Chlorhydroxyquinolin	T49.0X1	T49.0X2	T49.0X3	T49.0X4	T49.0X5	T49.0X6
Chloride of lime (bleach)	T54.3X1	T54.3X2	T54.3X3	T54.3X4	—	—
Chlorimipramine	T43.011	T43.012	T43.013	T43.014	T43.015	T43.016
Chlorinated						
camphene	T53.6X1	T53.6X2	T53.6X3	T53.6X4	—	—
diphenyl	T53.7X1	T53.7X2	T53.7X3	T53.7X4	—	—
hydrocarbons NEC	T53.91	T53.92	T53.93	T53.94	—	—
solvents	T53.91	T53.92	T53.93	T53.94	—	—
lime (bleach)	T54.3X1	T54.3X2	T54.3X3	T54.3X4	—	—
and boric acid solution	T49.0X1	T49.0X2	T49.0X3	T49.0X4	T49.0X5	T49.0X6
naphthalene (insecticide)	T60.1X1	T60.1X2	T60.1X3	T60.1X4	—	—
industrial (non-pesticide)	T53.7X1	T53.7X2	T53.7X3	T53.7X4	—	—

	External Cause (T-Code)					
Substance	Poisoning, Accidental (Unintentional)	Poisoning, Intentional Self-Harm	Poisoning, Assault	Poisoning, Undetermined	Adverse Effect	Underdosing
Chlorinated *(Continued)*						
pesticide NEC	T60.8X1	T60.8X2	T60.8X3	T60.8X4	—	—
soda — *see also sodium hypochlorite*						
solution	T49.0X1	T49.0X2	T49.0X3	T49.0X4	T49.0X5	T49.0X6
Chlorine (fumes) (gas)	T59.4X1	T59.4X2	T59.4X3	T59.4X4	—	—
bleach	T54.3X1	T54.3X2	T54.3X3	T54.3X4	—	—
compound gas NEC	T59.4X1	T59.4X2	T59.4X3	T59.4X4	—	—
disinfectant	T59.4X1	T59.4X2	T59.4X3	T59.4X4	—	—
releasing agents NEC	T59.4X1	T59.4X2	T59.4X3	T59.4X4	—	—
Chlorisondamine chloride	T46.991	T46.992	T46.993	T46.994	T46.995	T46.996
Chlormadinone	T38.5X1	T38.5X2	T38.5X3	T38.5X4	T38.5X5	T38.5X6
Chlormephos	T60.0X1	T60.0X2	T60.0X3	T60.0X4	—	—
Chlormerodrin	T50.2X1	T50.2X2	T50.2X3	T50.2X4	T50.2X5	T50.2X6
Chlormethiazole	T42.6X1	T42.6X2	T42.6X3	T42.6X4	T42.6X5	T42.6X6
Chlormethine	T45.1X1	T45.1X2	T45.1X3	T45.1X4	T45.1X5	T45.1X6
Chlormethylenecycline	T36.4X1	T36.4X2	T36.4X3	T36.4X4	T36.4X5	T36.4X6
Chlormezanone	T42.6X1	T42.6X2	T42.6X3	T42.6X4	T42.6X5	T42.6X6
Chloroacetic acid	T60.3X1	T60.3X2	T60.3X3	T60.3X4	—	—
Chloroacetone	T59.3X1	T59.3X2	T59.3X3	T59.3X4	—	—
Chloroacetophenone	T59.3X1	T59.3X2	T59.3X3	T59.3X4	—	—
Chloroaniline	T53.7X1	T53.7X2	T53.7X3	T53.7X4	—	—
Chlorobenzene, chlorobenzol	T53.7X1	T53.7X2	T53.7X3	T53.7X4	—	—
Chlorobromomethane (fire extinguisher)	T53.6X1	T53.6X2	T53.6X3	T53.6X4	—	—
Chlorobutanol	T49.0X1	T49.0X2	T49.0X3	T49.0X4	T49.0X5	T49.0X6
Chlorocresol	T49.0X1	T49.0X2	T49.0X3	T49.0X4	T49.0X5	T49.0X6
Chlorodehydro-methyltestosterone	T38.7X1	T38.7X2	T38.7X3	T38.7X4	T38.7X5	T38.7X6
Chlorodinitrobenzene	T53.7X1	T53.7X2	T53.7X3	T53.7X4	—	—
dust or vapor	T53.7X1	T53.7X2	T53.7X3	T53.7X4	—	—
Chlorodiphenyl	T53.7X1	T53.7X2	T53.7X3	T53.7X4	—	—
Chloroethane — *see Ethyl chloride*						
Chloroethylene	T53.6X1	T53.6X2	T53.6X3	T53.6X4	—	—
Chlorofluorocarbons	T53.5X1	T53.5X2	T53.5X3	T53.5X4	—	—
Chloroform (fumes) (vapor)	T53.1X1	T53.1X2	T53.1X3	T53.1X4	—	—
anesthetic	T41.0X1	T41.0X2	T41.0X3	T41.0X4	T41.0X5	T41.0X6
solvent	T53.1X1	T53.1X2	T53.1X3	T53.1X4	—	—
water, concentrated	T41.0X1	T41.0X2	T41.0X3	T41.0X4	T41.0X5	T41.0X6
Chloroguanide	T37.2X1	T37.2X2	T37.2X3	T37.2X4	T37.2X5	T37.2X6
Chloromycetin	T36.2X1	T36.2X2	T36.2X3	T36.2X4	T36.2X5	T36.2X6
ENT agent	T49.6X1	T49.6X2	T49.6X3	T49.6X4	T49.6X5	T49.6X6
ophthalmic preparation	T49.5X1	T49.5X2	T49.5X3	T49.5X4	T49.5X5	T49.5X6

TABLE OF DRUGS AND CHEMICALS

Substance	Poisoning, Accidental (Unintentional)	Poisoning, Intentional Self-Harm	Poisoning, Assault	Poisoning, Undetermined	Adverse Effect	Underdosing
			External Cause (T-Code)			
Chloromycetin *(Continued)*						
otic solution	T49.6X1	T49.6X2	T49.6X3	T49.6X4	T49.6X5	T49.6X6
topical NEC	T49.0X1	T49.0X2	T49.0X3	T49.0X4	T49.0X5	T49.0X6
Chloronitrobenzene	T53.7X1	T53.7X2	T53.7X3	T53.7X4	—	—
dust or vapor	T53.7X1	T53.7X2	T53.7X3	T53.7X4	—	—
Chlorophacinone	T60.4X1	T60.4X2	T60.4X3	T60.4X4	—	—
Chlorophenol	T53.7X1	T53.7X2	T53.7X3	T53.7X4	—	—
Chlorophenothane	T60.1X1	T60.1X2	T60.1X3	T60.1X4	—	—
Chlorophyll	T50.991	T50.992	T50.993	T50.994	T50.995	T50.996
Chloropicrin (fumes)	T53.6X1	T53.6X2	T53.6X3	T53.6X4	—	—
fumigant	T60.8X1	T60.8X2	T60.8X3	T60.8X4	—	—
fungicide	T60.3X1	T60.3X2	T60.3X3	T60.3X4	—	—
pesticide	T60.8X1	T60.8X2	T60.8X3	T60.8X4	—	—
Chloroprocaine	T41.3X1	T41.3X2	T41.3X3	T41.3X4	T41.3X5	T41.3X6
infiltration (subcutaneous)	T41.3X1	T41.3X2	T41.3X3	T41.3X4	T41.3X5	T41.3X6
nerve block (peripheral) (plexus)	T41.3X1	T41.3X2	T41.3X3	T41.3X4	T41.3X5	T41.3X6
spinal	T41.3X1	T41.3X2	T41.3X3	T41.3X4	T41.3X5	T41.3X6
Chloroptic	T49.5X1	T49.5X2	T49.5X3	T49.5X4	T49.5X5	T49.5X6
Chloropurine	T45.1X1	T45.1X2	T45.1X3	T45.1X4	T45.1X5	T45.1X6
Chloropyramine	T45.0X1	T45.0X2	T45.0X3	T45.0X4	T45.0X5	T45.0X6
Chloropyrifos	T60.0X1	T60.0X2	T60.0X3	T60.0X4	—	—
Chloropyrilene	T45.0X1	T45.0X2	T45.0X3	T45.0X4	T45.0X5	T45.0X6
Chloroquine	T37.2X1	T37.2X2	T37.2X3	T37.2X4	T37.2X5	T37.2X6
Chlorothalonil	T60.3X1	T60.3X2	T60.3X3	T60.3X4	—	—
Chlorothen	T45.0X1	T45.0X2	T45.0X3	T45.0X4	T45.0X5	T45.0X6
Chlorothiazide	T50.2X1	T50.2X2	T50.2X3	T50.2X4	T50.2X5	T50.2X6
Chlorothymol	T49.4X1	T49.4X2	T49.4X3	T49.4X4	T49.4X5	T49.4X6
Chlorotrianisene	T38.5X1	T38.5X2	T38.5X3	T38.5X4	T38.5X5	T38.5X6
Chlorovinyldichloro-arsine, not in war	T57.0X1	T57.0X2	T57.0X3	T57.0X4	—	—
Chloroxine	T49.4X1	T49.4X2	T49.4X3	T49.4X4	T49.4X5	T49.4X6
Chloroxylenol	T49.0X1	T49.0X2	T49.0X3	T49.0X4	T49.0X5	T49.0X6
Chlorphenamine	T45.0X1	T45.0X2	T45.0X3	T45.0X4	T45.0X5	T45.0X6
Chlorphenesin	T42.8X1	T42.8X2	T42.8X3	T42.8X4	T42.8X5	T42.8X6
topical (antifungal)	T49.0X1	T49.0X2	T49.0X3	T49.0X4	T49.0X5	T49.0X6
Chlorpheniramine	T45.0X1	T45.0X2	T45.0X3	T45.0X4	T45.0X5	T45.0X6
Chlorphenoxamine	T45.0X1	T45.0X2	T45.0X3	T45.0X4	T45.0X5	T45.0X6
Chlorphentermine	T50.5X1	T50.5X2	T50.5X3	T50.5X4	T50.5X5	T50.5X6
Chlorprocaine — *see Chloroprocaine*						
Chlorproguanil	T37.2X1	T37.2X2	T37.2X3	T37.2X4	T37.2X5	T37.2X6
Chlorpromazine	T43.3X1	T43.3X2	T43.3X3	T43.3X4	T43.3X5	T43.3X6

Substance	External Cause (T-Code)					
	Poisoning, Accidental (Unintentional)	Poisoning, Intentional Self-Harm	Poisoning, Assault	Poisoning, Undetermined	Adverse Effect	Underdosing
Chlorpropamide	T38.3X1	T38.3X2	T38.3X3	T38.3X4	T38.3X5	T38.3X6
Chlorprothixene	T43.4X1	T43.4X2	T43.4X3	T43.4X4	T43.4X5	T43.4X6
Chlorquinaldol	T49.0X1	T49.0X2	T49.0X3	T49.0X4	T49.0X5	T49.0X6
Chlorquinol	T49.0X1	T49.0X2	T49.0X3	T49.0X4	T49.0X5	T49.0X6
Chlortalidone	T50.2X1	T50.2X2	T50.2X3	T50.2X4	T50.2X5	T50.2X6
Chlortetracycline	T36.4X1	T36.4X2	T36.4X3	T36.4X4	T36.4X5	T36.4X6
Chlorthalidone	T50.2X1	T50.2X2	T50.2X3	T50.2X4	T50.2X5	T50.2X6
Chlorthiophos	T60.0X1	T60.0X2	T60.0X3	T60.0X4	—	—
Chlorotrianisene	T38.5X1	T38.5X2	T38.5X3	T38.5X4	T38.5X5	T38.5X6
Chlor-Trimeton	T45.0X1	T45.0X2	T45.0X3	T45.0X4	T45.0X5	T45.0X6
Chlorthion	T60.0X1	T60.0X2	T60.0X3	T60.0X4	—	—
Chlorzoxazone	T42.8X1	T42.8X2	T42.8X3	T42.8X4	T42.8X5	T42.8X6
Choke damp	T59.7X1	T59.7X2	T59.7X3	T59.7X4	—	—
Cholagogues	T47.5X1	T47.5X2	T47.5X3	T47.5X4	T47.5X5	T47.5X6
Cholebrine	T50.8X1	T50.8X2	T50.8X3	T50.8X4	T50.8X5	T50.8X6
Cholecalciferol	T45.2X1	T45.2X2	T45.2X3	T45.2X4	T45.2X5	T45.2X6
Cholecystokinin	T50.8X1	T50.8X2	T50.8X3	T50.8X4	T50.8X5	T50.8X6
Cholera vaccine	T50.A91	T50.A92	T50.A93	T50.A94	T50.A95	T50.A96
Choleretic	T47.5X1	T47.5X2	T47.5X3	T47.5X4	T47.5X5	T47.5X6
Cholesterol-lowering agents	T46.6X1	T46.6X2	T46.6X3	T46.6X4	T46.6X5	T46.6X6
Cholestyramine (resin)	T46.6X1	T46.6X2	T46.6X3	T46.6X4	T46.6X5	T46.6X6
Cholic acid	T47.5X1	T47.5X2	T47.5X3	T47.5X4	T47.5X5	T47.5X6
Choline	T48.6X1	T48.6X2	T48.6X3	T48.6X4	T48.6X5	T48.6X6
chloride	T50.991	T50.992	T50.993	T50.994	T50.995	T50.996
dihydrogen citrate	T50.991	T50.992	T50.993	T50.994	T50.995	T50.996
salicylate	T39.091	T39.092	T39.093	T39.094	T39.095	T39.096
theophyllinate	T48.6X1	T48.6X2	T48.6X3	T48.6X4	T48.6X5	T48.6X6
Cholinergic (drug) NEC	T44.1X1	T44.1X2	T44.1X3	T44.1X4	T44.1X5	T44.1X6
muscle tone enhancer	T44.1X1	T44.1X2	T44.1X3	T44.1X4	T44.1X5	T44.1X6
organophosphorus	T44.0X1	T44.0X2	T44.0X3	T44.0X4	T44.0X5	T44.0X6
insecticide	T60.0X1	T60.0X2	T60.0X3	T60.0X4	—	—
nerve gas	T59.891	T59.892	T59.893	T59.894	—	—
trimethyl ammonium propanediol	T44.1X1	T44.1X2	T44.1X3	T44.1X4	T44.1X5	T44.1X6
Cholinesterase reactivator	T50.6X1	T50.6X2	T50.6X3	T50.6X4	T50.6X5	T50.6X6
Cholografin	T50.8X1	T50.8X2	T50.8X3	T50.8X4	T50.8X5	T50.8X6
Chorionic gonadotropin	T38.891	T38.892	T38.893	T38.894	T38.895	T38.896
Chromate	T56.2X1	T56.2X2	T56.2X3	T56.2X4	—	—
dust or mist	T56.2X1	T56.2X2	T56.2X3	T56.2X4	—	—
lead — see also lead	T56.0X1	T56.0X2	T56.0X3	T56.0X4	—	—
paint	T56.0X1	T56.0X2	T56.0X3	T56.0X4	—	—

TABLE OF DRUGS AND CHEMICALS

Substance	Poisoning, Accidental (Unintentional)	Poisoning, Intentional Self-Harm	Poisoning, Assault	Poisoning, Undetermined	Adverse Effect	Underdosing
Chromic						
acid	T56.2X1	T56.2X2	T56.2X3	T56.2X4	—	—
dust or mist	T56.2X1	T56.2X2	T56.2X3	T56.2X4	—	—
phosphate 32P	T45.1X1	T45.1X2	T45.1X3	T45.1X4	T45.1X5	T45.1X6
Chromium	T56.2X1	T56.2X2	T56.2X3	T56.2X4	—	—
compounds — see Chromate						
sesquioxide	T50.8X1	T50.8X2	T50.8X3	T50.8X4	T50.8X5	T50.8X6
Chromomycin A3	T45.1X1	T45.1X2	T45.1X3	T45.1X4	T45.1X5	T45.1X6
Chromonar	T46.3X1	T46.3X2	T46.3X3	T46.3X4	T46.3X5	T46.3X6
Chromyl chloride	T56.2X1	T56.2X2	T56.2X3	T56.2X4	—	—
Chrysarobin	T49.4X1	T49.4X2	T49.4X3	T49.4X4	T49.4X5	T49.4X6
Chrysazin	T47.2X1	T47.2X2	T47.2X3	T47.2X4	T47.2X5	T47.2X6
Chymar	T45.3X1	T45.3X2	T45.3X3	T45.3X4	T45.3X5	T45.3X6
ophthalmic preparation	T49.5X1	T49.5X2	T49.5X3	T49.5X4	T49.5X5	T49.5X6
Chymopapain	T45.3X1	T45.3X2	T45.3X3	T45.3X4	T45.3X5	T45.3X6
Chymotrypsin	T45.3X1	T45.3X2	T45.3X3	T45.3X4	T45.3X5	T45.3X6
ophthalmic preparation	T49.5X1	T49.5X2	T49.5X3	T49.5X4	T49.5X5	T49.5X6
Cianidanol	T50.991	T50.992	T50.993	T50.994	T50.995	T50.996
Cianopramine	T43.011	T43.012	T43.013	T43.014	T43.015	T43.016
Cibenzoline	T46.2X1	T46.2X2	T46.2X3	T46.2X4	T46.2X5	T46.2X6
Ciclacillin	T36.0X1	T36.0X2	T36.0X3	T36.0X4	T36.0X5	T36.0X6
Ciclobarbital — see Hexobarbital						
Ciclonicate	T46.7X1	T46.7X2	T46.7X3	T46.7X4	T46.7X5	T46.7X6
Ciclopirox (olamine)	T49.0X1	T49.0X2	T49.0X3	T49.0X4	T49.0X5	T49.0X6
Ciclosporin	T45.1X1	T45.1X2	T45.1X3	T45.1X4	T45.1X5	T45.1X6
Cicuta maculata or virosa	T62.2X1	T62.2X2	T62.2X3	T62.2X4	—	—
Cicutoxin	T62.2X1	T62.2X2	T62.2X3	T62.2X4	—	—
Cigarette lighter fluid	T52.0X1	T52.0X2	T52.0X3	T52.0X4	—	—
Cigarettes (tobacco)	T65.221	T65.222	T65.223	T65.224	—	—
Ciguatoxin	T61.01	T61.02	T61.03	T61.04	—	—
Cilazapril	T46.4X1	T46.4X2	T46.4X3	T46.4X4	T46.4X5	T46.4X6
Cimetidine	T47.0X1	T47.0X2	T47.0X3	T47.0X4	T47.0X5	T47.0X6
Cimetropium bromide	T44.3X1	T44.3X2	T44.3X3	T44.3X4	T44.3X5	T44.3X6
Cinchocaine	T41.3X1	T41.3X2	T41.3X3	T41.3X4	T41.3X5	T41.3X6
topical (surface)	T41.3X1	T41.3X2	T41.3X3	T41.3X4	T41.3X5	T41.3X6
Cinchona	T37.2X1	T37.2X2	T37.2X3	T37.2X4	T37.2X5	T37.2X6
Cinchonine alkaloids	T37.2X1	T37.2X2	T37.2X3	T37.2X4	T37.2X5	T37.2X6
Cinchophen	T50.4X1	T50.4X2	T50.4X3	T50.4X4	T50.4X5	T50.4X6
Cinepazide	T46.7X1	T46.7X2	T46.7X3	T46.7X4	T46.7X5	T46.7X6
Cinnamedrine	T48.5X1	T48.5X2	T48.5X3	T48.5X4	T48.5X5	T48.5X6

Substance	External Cause (T-Code)					
	Poisoning, Accidental (Unintentional)	Poisoning, Intentional Self-Harm	Poisoning, Assault	Poisoning, Undetermined	Adverse Effect	Underdosing
Cinnarizine	T45.0X1	T45.0X2	T45.0X3	T45.0X4	T45.0X5	T45.0X6
Cinoxacin	T37.8X1	T37.8X2	T37.8X3	T37.8X4	T37.8X5	T37.8X6
Ciprofibrate	T46.6X1	T46.6X2	T46.6X3	T46.6X4	T46.6X5	T46.6X6
Ciprofloxacin	T36.8X1	T36.8X2	T36.8X3	T36.8X4	T36.8X5	T36.8X6
Cisapride	T47.8X1	T47.8X2	T47.8X3	T47.8X4	T47.8X5	T47.8X6
Cisplatin	T45.1X1	T45.1X2	T45.1X3	T45.1X4	T45.1X5	T45.1X6
Citalopram	T43.221	T43.222	T43.223	T43.224	T43.225	T43.226
Citanest	T41.3X1	T41.3X2	T41.3X3	T41.3X4	T41.3X5	T41.3X6
infiltration (subcutaneous)	T41.3X1	T41.3X2	T41.3X3	T41.3X4	T41.3X5	T41.3X6
nerve block (peripheral) (plexus)	T41.3X1	T41.3X2	T41.3X3	T41.3X4	T41.3X5	T41.3X6
Citric acid	T47.5X1	T47.5X2	T47.5X3	T47.5X4	T47.5X5	T47.5X6
Citrovorum (factor)	T45.8X1	T45.8X2	T45.8X3	T45.8X4	T45.8X5	T45.8X6
Claviceps purpurea	T62.2X1	T62.2X2	T62.2X3	T62.2X4	—	—
Clavulanic acid	T36.1X1	T36.1X2	T36.1X3	T36.1X4	T36.1X5	T36.1X6
Cleaner, cleansing agent, type not specified	T65.891	T65.892	T65.893	T65.894	—	—
of paint or varnish	T52.91	T52.92	T52.93	T52.94	—	—
specified type NEC	T65.891	T65.892	T65.893	T65.894	—	—
Clebopride	T47.8X1	T47.8X2	T47.8X3	T47.8X4	T47.8X5	T47.8X6
Clefamide	T37.3X1	T37.3X2	T37.3X3	T37.3X4	T37.3X5	T37.3X6
Clemastine	T45.0X1	T45.0X2	T45.0X3	T45.0X4	T45.0X5	T45.0X6
Clematis vitalba	T62.2X1	T62.2X2	T62.2X3	T62.2X4	—	—
Clemizole	T45.0X1	T45.0X2	T45.0X3	T45.0X4	T45.0X5	T45.0X6
penicillin	T36.0X1	T36.0X2	T36.0X3	T36.0X4	T36.0X5	T36.0X6
Clenbuterol	T48.6X1	T48.6X2	T48.6X3	T48.6X4	T48.6X5	T48.6X6
Clidinium bromide	T44.3X1	T44.3X2	T44.3X3	T44.3X4	T44.3X5	T44.3X6
Clindamycin	T36.8X1	T36.8X2	T36.8X3	T36.8X4	T36.8X5	T36.8X6
Clinofibrate	T46.6X1	T46.6X2	T46.6X3	T46.6X4	T46.6X5	T46.6X6
Clioquinol	T37.8X1	T37.8X2	T37.8X3	T37.8X4	T37.8X5	T37.8X6
Cliradon	T40.2X1	T40.2X2	T40.2X3	T40.2X4	—	—
Clobazam	T42.4X1	T42.4X2	T42.4X3	T42.4X4	T42.4X5	T42.4X6
Clobenzorex	T50.5X1	T50.5X2	T50.5X3	T50.5X4	T50.5X5	T50.5X6
Clobetasol	T49.0X1	T49.0X2	T49.0X3	T49.0X4	T49.0X5	T49.0X6
Clobetasone	T49.0X1	T49.0X2	T49.0X3	T49.0X4	T49.0X5	T49.0X6
Clobutinol	T48.3X1	T48.3X2	T48.3X3	T48.3X4	T48.3X5	T48.3X6
Clocapramine	T43.0X1	T43.0X2	T43.0X3	T43.0X4	T43.0X5	T43.0X6
Clocortolone	T38.0X1	T38.0X2	T38.0X3	T38.0X4	T38.0X5	T38.0X6
Clodantoin	T49.0X1	T49.0X2	T49.0X3	T49.0X4	T49.0X5	T49.0X6
Clodronic acid	T50.991	T50.992	T50.993	T50.994	T50.995	T50.996
Clofazimine	T37.1X1	T37.1X2	T37.1X3	T37.1X4	T37.1X5	T37.1X6
Clofedanol	T48.3X1	T48.3X2	T48.3X3	T48.3X4	T48.3X5	T48.3X6

Substance	External Cause (T-Code)					
	Poisoning, Accidental (Unintentional)	Poisoning, Intentional Self-Harm	Poisoning, Assault	Poisoning, Undetermined	Adverse Effect	Underdosing
Clofenamide	T50.2X1	T50.2X2	T50.2X3	T50.2X4	T50.2X5	T50.2X6
Clofenotane	T49.0X1	T49.0X2	T49.0X3	T49.0X4	T49.0X5	T49.0X6
Clofezone	T39.2X1	T39.2X2	T39.2X3	T39.2X4	T39.2X5	T39.2X6
Clofibrate	T46.6X1	T46.6X2	T46.6X3	T46.6X4	T46.6X5	T46.6X6
Clofibride	T46.6X1	T46.6X2	T46.6X3	T46.6X4	T46.6X5	T46.6X6
Cloforex	T50.5X1	T50.5X2	T50.5X3	T50.5X4	T50.5X5	T50.5X6
Clomacran	T43.0X1	T43.0X2	T43.0X3	T43.0X4	T43.0X5	T43.0X6
Clomethiazole	T42.6X1	T42.6X2	T42.6X3	T42.6X4	T42.6X5	T42.6X6
Clometocillin	T36.0X1	T36.0X2	T36.0X3	T36.0X4	T36.0X5	T36.0X6
Clomifene	T38.5X1	T38.5X2	T38.5X3	T38.5X4	T38.5X5	T38.5X6
Clomiphene	T38.5X1	T38.5X2	T38.5X3	T38.5X4	T38.5X5	T38.5X6
Clomipramine	T43.011	T43.012	T43.013	T43.014	T43.015	T43.016
Clomocycline	T36.4X1	T36.4X2	T36.4X3	T36.4X4	T36.4X5	T36.4X6
Clonazepam	T42.4X1	T42.4X2	T42.4X3	T42.4X4	T42.4X5	T42.4X6
Clonidine	T46.5X1	T46.5X2	T46.5X3	T46.5X4	T46.5X5	T46.5X6
Clonixin	T39.8X1	T39.8X2	T39.8X3	T39.8X4	T39.8X5	T39.8X6
Clopamide	T50.2X1	T50.2X2	T50.2X3	T50.2X4	T50.2X5	T50.2X6
Clopenthixol	T43.4X1	T43.4X2	T43.4X3	T43.4X4	T43.4X5	T43.4X6
Cloperastine	T48.3X1	T48.3X2	T48.3X3	T48.3X4	T48.3X5	T48.3X6
Clophedianol	T48.3X1	T48.3X2	T48.3X3	T48.3X4	T48.3X5	T48.3X6
Cloponone	T36.2X1	T36.2X2	T36.2X3	T36.2X4	T36.2X5	T36.2X6
Cloprednol	T38.0X1	T38.0X2	T38.0X3	T38.0X4	T38.0X5	T38.0X6
Cloral betaine	T42.6X1	T42.6X2	T42.6X3	T42.6X4	T42.6X5	T42.6X6
Cloramfenicol	T36.2X1	T36.2X2	T36.2X3	T36.2X4	T36.2X5	T36.2X6
Clorazepate (dipotassium)	T42.4X1	T42.4X2	T42.4X3	T42.4X4	T42.4X5	T42.4X6
Clorexolone	T50.2X1	T50.2X2	T50.2X3	T50.2X4	T50.2X5	T50.2X6
Clorox (bleach)	T54.91	T54.92	T54.93	T54.94	—	—
Clorfenamine	T45.0X1	T45.0X2	T45.0X3	T45.0X4	T45.0X5	T45.0X6
Clorgiline	T43.1X1	T43.1X2	T43.1X3	T43.1X4	T43.1X5	T43.1X6
Clorotepine	T44.3X1	T44.3X2	T44.3X3	T44.3X4	T44.3X5	T44.3X6
Clorprenaline	T48.6X1	T48.6X2	T48.6X3	T48.6X4	T48.6X5	T48.6X6
Clortermine	T50.5X1	T50.5X2	T50.5X3	T50.5X4	T50.5X5	T50.5X6
Clotiapine	T43.591	T43.592	T43.593	T43.594	T43.595	T43.596
Clotiazepam	T42.4X1	T42.4X2	T42.4X3	T42.4X4	T42.4X5	T42.4X6
Clotibric acid	T46.6X1	T46.6X2	T46.6X3	T46.6X4	T46.6X5	T46.6X6
Clotrimazole	T49.0X1	T49.0X2	T49.0X3	T49.0X4	T49.0X5	T49.0X6
Cloxacillin	T36.0X1	T36.0X2	T36.0X3	T36.0X4	T36.0X5	T36.0X6
Cloxazolam	T42.4X1	T42.4X2	T42.4X3	T42.4X4	T42.4X5	T42.4X6
Cloxiquine	T49.0X1	T49.0X2	T49.0X3	T49.0X4	T49.0X5	T49.0X6
Clozapine	T42.4X1	T42.4X2	T42.4X3	T42.4X4	T42.4X5	T42.4X6

Substance	External Cause (T-Code)					
	Poisoning, Accidental (Unintentional)	Poisoning, Intentional Self-Harm	Poisoning, Assault	Poisoning, Undetermined	Adverse Effect	Underdosing
Coagulant NEC	T45.7X1	T45.7X2	T45.7X3	T45.7X4	T45.7X5	T45.7X6
Coal (carbon monoxide from) — see also Carbon, monoxide, coal	T58.2X1	T58.2X2	T58.2X3	T58.2X4	—	—
oil — see Kerosene						
tar	T49.1X1	T49.1X2	T49.1X3	T49.1X4	T49.1X5	T49.1X6
fumes	T59.891	T59.892	T59.893	T59.894	—	—
medicinal (ointment)	T49.4X1	T49.4X2	T49.4X3	T49.4X4	T49.4X5	T49.4X6
analgesics NEC	T39.2X1	T39.2X2	T39.2X3	T39.2X4	T39.2X5	T39.2X6
naphtha (solvent)	T52.0X1	T52.0X2	T52.0X3	T52.0X4		
Cobalamine	T45.2X1	T45.2X2	T45.2X3	T45.2X4	T45.2X5	T45.2X6
Cobalt (nonmedicinal) (fumes) (industrial)	T56.891	T56.892	T56.893	T56.894		
medicinal (trace) (chloride)	T45.8X1	T45.8X2	T45.8X3	T45.8X4	T45.8X5	T45.8X6
Cobra (venom)	T63.041	T63.042	T63.043	T63.044		
Coca (leaf)	T40.5X1	T40.5X2	T40.5X3	T40.5X4	T40.5X5	T40.5X6
Cocaine	T40.5X1	T40.5X2	T40.5X3	T40.5X4	T40.5X5	T40.5X6
topical anesthetic	T41.3X1	T41.3X2	T41.3X3	T41.3X4	T41.3X5	T41.3X6
Cocarboxylase	T45.3X1	T45.3X2	T45.3X3	T45.3X4	T45.3X5	T45.3X6
Coccidioidin	T50.8X1	T50.8X2	T50.8X3	T50.8X4	T50.8X5	T50.8X6
Cocculus indicus	T62.1X1	T62.1X2	T62.1X3	T62.1X4		
Cochineal	T65.6X1	T65.6X2	T65.6X3	T65.6X4		
medicinal products	T50.991	T50.992	T50.993	T50.994	T50.995	T50.996
Codeine	T40.2X1	T40.2X2	T40.2X3	T40.2X4	T40.2X5	T40.2X6
Cod-liver oil	T45.2X1	T45.2X2	T45.2X3	T45.2X4	T45.2X5	T45.2X6
Coenzyme A	T50.991	T50.992	T50.993	T50.994	T50.995	T50.996
Coffee	T62.8X1	T62.8X2	T62.8X3	T62.8X4	—	—
Cogalactoisomerase	T50.991	T50.992	T50.993	T50.994	T50.995	T50.996
Cogentin	T44.3X1	T44.3X2	T44.3X3	T44.3X4	T44.3X5	T44.3X6
Coke fumes or gas (carbon monoxide)	T58.2X1	T58.2X2	T58.2X3	T58.2X4	—	—
industrial use	T58.8X1	T58.8X2	T58.8X3	T58.8X4	—	—
Colace	T47.4X1	T47.4X2	T47.4X3	T47.4X4	T47.4X5	T47.4X6
Colaspase	T45.1X1	T45.1X2	T45.1X3	T45.1X4	T45.1X5	T45.1X6
Colchicine	T50.4X1	T50.4X2	T50.4X3	T50.4X4	T50.4X5	T50.4X6
Colchicum	T62.2X1	T62.2X2	T62.2X3	T62.2X4	—	—
Cold cream	T49.3X1	T49.3X2	T49.3X3	T49.3X4	T49.3X5	T49.3X6
Colecalciferol	T45.2X1	T45.2X2	T45.2X3	T45.2X4	T45.2X5	T45.2X6
Colestipol	T46.6X1	T46.6X2	T46.6X3	T46.6X4	T46.6X5	T46.6X6
Colestyramine	T46.6X1	T46.6X2	T46.6X3	T46.6X4	T46.6X5	T46.6X6
Colimycin	T36.8X1	T36.8X2	T36.8X3	T36.8X4	T36.8X5	T36.8X6
Colistimethate	T36.8X1	T36.8X2	T36.8X3	T36.8X4	T36.8X5	T36.8X6
Colistin	T36.8X1	T36.8X2	T36.8X3	T36.8X4	T36.8X5	T36.8X6
sulfate (eye preparation)	T49.5X1	T49.5X2	T49.5X3	T49.5X4	T49.5X5	T49.5X6

TABLE OF DRUGS AND CHEMICALS

Substance	External Cause (T-Code)					
	Poisoning, Accidental (Unintentional)	Poisoning, Intentional Self-Harm	Poisoning, Assault	Poisoning, Undetermined	Adverse Effect	Underdosing
Collagen	T50.991	T50.992	T50.993	T50.994	T50.995	T50.996
Collagenase	T49.4X1	T49.4X2	T49.4X3	T49.4X4	T49.4X5	T49.4X6
Collodion	T49.3X1	T49.3X2	T49.3X3	T49.3X4	T49.3X5	T49.3X6
Colocynth	T47.2X1	T47.2X2	T47.2X3	T47.2X4	T47.2X5	T47.2X6
Colophony adhesive	T49.3X1	T49.3X2	T49.3X3	T49.3X4	T49.3X5	T49.3X6
Colorant — see also Dye	T50.991	T50.992	T50.993	T50.994	T50.995	T50.996
Coloring matter — see Dye(s)						
Combustion gas (after combustion) — see Carbon, monoxide						
prior to combustion	T59.891	T59.892	T59.893	T59.894	—	—
Compazine	T43.3X1	T43.3X2	T43.3X3	T43.3X4	T43.3X5	T43.3X6
Compound						
42 (warfarin)	T60.4X1	T60.4X2	T60.4X3	T60.4X4	—	—
269 (endrin)	T60.1X1	T60.1X2	T60.1X3	T60.1X4	—	—
497 (dieldrin)	T60.1X1	T60.1X2	T60.1X3	T60.1X4	—	—
1080 (sodium fluoroacetate)	T60.4X1	T60.4X2	T60.4X3	T60.4X4	—	—
3422 (parathion)	T60.0X1	T60.0X2	T60.0X3	T60.0X4	—	—
3911 (phorate)	T60.0X1	T60.0X2	T60.0X3	T60.0X4	—	—
3956 (toxaphene)	T60.1X1	T60.1X2	T60.1X3	T60.1X4	—	—
4049 (malathion)	T60.0X1	T60.0X2	T60.0X3	T60.0X4	—	—
4069 (malathion)	T60.0X1	T60.0X2	T60.0X3	T60.0X4	—	—
4124 (dicapthon)	T60.0X1	T60.0X2	T60.0X3	T60.0X4	—	—
E (cortisone)	T38.0X1	T38.0X2	T38.0X3	T38.0X4	T38.0X5	T38.0X6
F (hydrocortisone)	T38.0X1	T38.0X2	T38.0X3	T38.0X4	T38.0X5	T38.0X6
Congener, anabolic	T38.7X1	T38.7X2	T38.7X3	T38.7X4	T38.7X5	T38.7X6
Congo red	T50.8X1	T50.8X2	T50.8X3	T50.8X4	T50.8X5	T50.8X6
Coniine, conine	T62.2X1	T62.2X2	T62.2X3	T62.2X4	—	—
Conium (maculatum)	T62.2X1	T62.2X2	T62.2X3	T62.2X4	—	—
Conjugated estrogenic substances	T38.5X1	T38.5X2	T38.5X3	T38.5X4	T38.5X5	T38.5X6
Contac	T48.5X1	T48.5X2	T48.5X3	T48.5X4	T48.5X5	T48.5X6
Contact lens solution	T49.5X1	T49.5X2	T49.5X3	T49.5X4	T49.5X5	T49.5X6
Contraceptive (oral)	T38.4X1	T38.4X2	T38.4X3	T38.4X4	T38.4X5	T38.4X6
vaginal	T49.8X1	T49.8X2	T49.8X3	T49.8X4	T49.8X5	T49.8X6
Contrast medium, radiography	T50.8X1	T50.8X2	T50.8X3	T50.8X4	T50.8X5	T50.8X6
Convallaria glycosides	T46.0X1	T46.0X2	T46.0X3	T46.0X4	T46.0X5	T46.0X6
Convallaria majalis	T62.2X1	T62.2X2	T62.2X3	T62.2X4	—	—
berry	T62.1X1	T62.1X2	T62.1X3	T62.1X4	—	—
Copper (dust) (fumes) (nonmedicinal) NEC	T56.4X1	T56.4X2	T56.4X3	T56.4X4	—	—
arsenate, arsenite	T57.0X1	T57.0X2	T57.0X3	T57.0X4	—	—
insecticide	T60.2X1	T60.2X2	T60.2X3	T60.2X4	—	—

Substance	External Cause (T-Code)					
	Poisoning, Accidental (Unintentional)	Poisoning, Intentional Self-Harm	Poisoning, Assault	Poisoning, Undetermined	Adverse Effect	Underdosing
Copper NEC *(Continued)*						
emetic	T47.7X1	T47.7X2	T47.7X3	T47.7X4	T47.7X5	T47.7X6
fungicide	T60.3X1	T60.3X2	T60.3X3	T60.3X4	—	—
gluconate	T49.0X1	T49.0X2	T49.0X3	T49.0X4	T49.0X5	T49.0X6
insecticide	T60.2X1	T60.2X2	T60.2X3	T60.2X4		
medicinal (trace)	T45.8X1	T45.8X2	T45.8X3	T45.8X4	T45.8X5	T45.8X6
oleate	T49.0X1	T49.0X2	T49.0X3	T49.0X4	T49.0X5	T49.0X6
sulfate	T56.4X1	T56.4X2	T56.4X3	T56.4X4	—	—
cupric	T56.4X1	T56.4X2	T56.4X3	T56.4X4	—	—
fungicide	T60.3X1	T60.3X2	T60.3X3	T60.3X4	—	—
medicinal						
ear	T49.6X1	T49.6X2	T49.6X3	T49.6X4	T49.6X5	T49.6X6
emetic	T47.7X1	T47.7X2	T47.7X3	T47.7X4	T47.7X5	T47.7X6
eye	T49.5X1	T49.5X2	T49.5X3	T49.5X4	T49.5X5	T49.5X6
cuprous	T56.4X1	T56.4X2	T56.4X3	T56.4X4	—	—
fungicide	T60.3X1	T60.3X2	T60.3X3	T60.3X4	—	—
medicinal						
ear	T49.6X1	T49.6X2	T49.6X3	T49.6X4	T49.6X5	T49.6X6
emetic	T47.7X1	T47.7X2	T47.7X3	T47.7X4	T47.7X5	T47.7X6
eye	T49.5X1	T49.5X2	T49.5X3	T49.5X4	T49.5X5	T49.5X6
Copperhead snake (bite) (venom)	T63.061	T63.062	T63.063	T63.064	—	—
Coral (sting)	T63.691	T63.692	T63.693	T63.694	—	—
snake (bite) (venom)	T63.021	T63.022	T63.023	T63.024	—	—
Corbadrine	T49.6X1	T49.6X2	T49.6X3	T49.6X4	T49.6X5	T49.6X6
Cordran	T49.0X1	T49.0X2	T49.0X3	T49.0X4	T49.0X5	T49.0X6
Cordite	T65.891	T65.892	T65.893	T65.894	—	—
vapor	T59.891	T59.892	T59.893	T59.894	—	—
Corn cures	T49.4X1	T49.4X2	T49.4X3	T49.4X4	T49.4X5	T49.4X6
Cornhusker's lotion	T49.3X1	T49.3X2	T49.3X3	T49.3X4	T49.3X5	T49.3X6
Corn starch	T49.3X1	T49.3X2	T49.3X3	T49.3X4	T49.3X5	T49.3X6
Coronary vasodilator NEC	T46.3X1	T46.3X2	T46.3X3	T46.3X4	T46.3X5	T46.3X6
Corrosive NEC	T54.91	T54.92	T54.93	T54.94	—	—
acid NEC	T54.2X1	T54.2X2	T54.2X3	T54.2X4	—	—
aromatics	T54.1X1	T54.1X2	T54.1X3	T54.1X4	—	—
disinfectant	T54.1X1	T54.1X2	T54.1X3	T54.1X4	—	—
fumes NEC	T54.91	T54.92	T54.93	T54.94	—	—
specified NEC	T54.91	T54.92	T54.93	T54.94	—	—
sublimate	T56.1X1	T56.1X2	T56.1X3	T56.1X4	—	—
Cortate	T38.0X1	T38.0X2	T38.0X3	T38.0X4	T38.0X5	T38.0X6

Substance	Poisoning, Accidental (Unintentional)	External Cause (T-Code)				
		Poisoning, Intentional Self-Harm	Poisoning, Assault	Poisoning, Undetermined	Adverse Effect	Underdosing
Cort-Dome	T38.0X1	T38.0X2	T38.0X3	T38.0X4	T38.0X5	T38.0X6
ENT agent	T49.6X1	T49.6X2	T49.6X3	T49.6X4	T49.6X5	T49.6X6
ophthalmic preparation	T49.5X1	T49.5X2	T49.5X3	T49.5X4	T49.5X5	T49.5X6
topical NEC	T49.0X1	T49.0X2	T49.0X3	T49.0X4	T49.0X5	T49.0X6
Cortef	T38.0X1	T38.0X2	T38.0X3	T38.0X4	T38.0X5	T38.0X6
ENT agent	T49.6X1	T49.6X2	T49.6X3	T49.6X4	T49.6X5	T49.6X6
ophthalmic preparation	T49.5X1	T49.5X2	T49.5X3	T49.5X4	T49.5X5	T49.5X6
topical NEC	T49.0X1	T49.0X2	T49.0X3	T49.0X4	T49.0X5	T49.0X6
Corticosteroid	T38.0X1	T38.0X2	T38.0X3	T38.0X4	T38.0X5	T38.0X6
ENT agent	T49.6X1	T49.6X2	T49.6X3	T49.6X4	T49.6X5	T49.6X6
mineral	T50.0X1	T50.0X2	T50.0X3	T50.0X4	T50.0X5	T50.0X6
ophthalmic	T49.5X1	T49.5X2	T49.5X3	T49.5X4	T49.5X5	T49.5X6
topical NEC	T49.0X1	T49.0X2	T49.0X3	T49.0X4	T49.0X5	T49.0X6
Corticotropin	T38.811	T38.812	T38.813	T38.814	T38.815	T38.816
Cortisol	T49.0X1	T49.0X2	T49.0X3	T49.0X4	T49.0X5	T49.0X6
ENT agent	T49.6X1	T49.6X2	T49.6X3	T49.6X4	T49.6X5	T49.6X6
ophthalmic preparation	T49.5X1	T49.5X2	T49.5X3	T49.5X4	T49.5X5	T49.5X6
topical NEC	T49.0X1	T49.0X2	T49.0X3	T49.0X4	T49.0X5	T49.0X6
Cortisone (acetate)	T38.0X1	T38.0X2	T38.0X3	T38.0X4	T38.0X5	T38.0X6
ENT agent	T49.6X1	T49.6X2	T49.6X3	T49.6X4	T49.6X5	T49.6X6
ophthalmic preparation	T49.5X1	T49.5X2	T49.5X3	T49.5X4	T49.5X5	T49.5X6
topical NEC	T49.0X1	T49.0X2	T49.0X3	T49.0X4	T49.0X5	T49.0X6
Cortivazol	T38.0X1	T38.0X2	T38.0X3	T38.0X4	T38.0X5	T38.0X6
Cortogen	T38.0X1	T38.0X2	T38.0X3	T38.0X4	T38.0X5	T38.0X6
ENT agent	T49.6X1	T49.6X2	T49.6X3	T49.6X4	T49.6X5	T49.6X6
ophthalmic preparation	T49.5X1	T49.5X2	T49.5X3	T49.5X4	T49.5X5	T49.5X6
Cortone	T38.0X1	T38.0X2	T38.0X3	T38.0X4	T38.0X5	T38.0X6
ENT agent	T49.6X1	T49.6X2	T49.6X3	T49.6X4	T49.6X5	T49.6X6
ophthalmic preparation	T49.5X1	T49.5X2	T49.5X3	T49.5X4	T49.5X5	T49.5X6
Cortril	T38.0X1	T38.0X2	T38.0X3	T38.0X4	T38.0X5	T38.0X6
ENT agent	T49.6X1	T49.6X2	T49.6X3	T49.6X4	T49.6X5	T49.6X6
ophthalmic preparation	T49.5X1	T49.5X2	T49.5X3	T49.5X4	T49.5X5	T49.5X6
topical NEC	T49.0X1	T49.0X2	T49.0X3	T49.0X4	T49.0X5	T49.0X6
Corynebacterium parvum	T45.1X1	T45.1X2	T45.1X3	T45.1X4	T45.1X5	T45.1X6
Cosmetic preparation	T49.8X1	T49.8X2	T49.8X3	T49.8X4	T49.8X5	T49.8X6
Cosmetics	T49.8X1	T49.8X2	T49.8X3	T49.8X4	T49.8X5	T49.8X6
Cosyntropin	T38.811	T38.812	T38.813	T38.814	T38.815	T38.816
Cotarnine	T45.7X1	T45.7X2	T45.7X3	T45.7X4	T45.7X5	T45.7X6
Co-trimoxazole	T36.8X1	T36.8X2	T36.8X3	T36.8X4	T36.8X5	T36.8X6
Cottonseed oil	T49.3X1	T49.3X2	T49.3X3	T49.3X4	T49.3X5	T49.3X6

Substance	External Cause (T-Code)					
	Poisoning, Accidental (Unintentional)	Poisoning, Intentional Self-Harm	Poisoning, Assault	Poisoning, Undetermined	Adverse Effect	Underdosing
Cough mixture (syrup)	T48.4X1	T48.4X2	T48.4X3	T48.4X4	T48.4X5	T48.4X6
containing opiates	T40.2X1	T40.2X2	T40.2X3	T40.2X4	T40.2X5	T40.2X6
expectorants	T48.4X1	T48.4X2	T48.4X3	T48.4X4	T48.4X5	T48.4X6
Coumadin	T45.511	T45.512	T45.513	T45.514	T45.515	T45.516
rodenticide	T60.4X1	T60.4X2	T60.4X3	T60.4X4	—	—
Coumaphos	T60.0X1	T60.0X2	T60.0X3	T60.0X4	—	—
Coumarin	T45.511	T45.512	T45.513	T45.514	T45.515	T45.516
Coumetarol	T45.511	T45.512	T45.513	T45.514	T45.515	T45.516
Cowbane	T62.2X1	T62.2X2	T62.2X3	T62.2X4	—	—
Cozyme	T45.2X1	T45.2X2	T45.2X3	T45.2X4	T45.2X5	T45.2X6
Crack	T40.5X1	T40.5X2	T40.5X3	T40.5X4	—	—
Crataegus extract	T46.0X1	T46.0X2	T46.0X3	T46.0X4	T46.0X5	T46.0X6
Creolin	T54.1X1	T54.1X2	T54.1X3	T54.1X4	—	—
disinfectant	T54.1X1	T54.1X2	T54.1X3	T54.1X4	—	—
Creosol (compound)	T49.0X1	T49.0X2	T49.0X3	T49.0X4	T49.0X5	T49.0X6
Creosote (coal tar) (beechwood)	T49.0X1	T49.0X2	T49.0X3	T49.0X4	T49.0X5	T49.0X6
medicinal (expectorant)	T48.4X1	T48.4X2	T48.4X3	T48.4X4	T48.4X5	T48.4X6
syrup	T48.4X1	T48.4X2	T48.4X3	T48.4X4	T48.4X5	T48.4X6
Cresol(s)	T49.0X1	T49.0X2	T49.0X3	T49.0X4	T49.0X5	T49.0X6
and soap solution	T49.0X1	T49.0X2	T49.0X3	T49.0X4	T49.0X5	T49.0X6
Cresyl acetate	T49.0X1	T49.0X2	T49.0X3	T49.0X4	T49.0X5	T49.0X6
Cresylic acid	T49.0X1	T49.0X2	T49.0X3	T49.0X4	T49.0X5	T49.0X6
Crimidine	T60.4X1	T60.4X2	T60.4X3	T60.4X4	—	—
Croconazole	T37.8X1	T37.8X2	T37.8X3	T37.8X4	T37.8X5	T37.8X6
Cromoglicic acid	T48.6X1	T48.6X2	T48.6X3	T48.6X4	T48.6X5	T48.6X6
Cromolyn	T48.6X1	T48.6X2	T48.6X3	T48.6X4	T48.6X5	T48.6X6
Cromonar	T46.3X1	T46.3X2	T46.3X3	T46.3X4	T46.3X5	T46.3X6
Cropropamide	T39.8X1	T39.8X2	T39.8X3	T39.8X4	T39.8X5	T39.8X6
with crotethamide	T50.7X1	T50.7X2	T50.7X3	T50.7X4	T50.7X5	T50.7X6
Crotamiton	T49.0X1	T49.0X2	T49.0X3	T49.0X4	T49.0X5	T49.0X6
Crotethamide	T39.8X1	T39.8X2	T39.8X3	T39.8X4	T39.8X5	T39.8X6
with cropropamide	T50.7X1	T50.7X2	T50.7X3	T50.7X4	T50.7X5	T50.7X6
Croton (oil)	T47.2X1	T47.2X2	T47.2X3	T47.2X4	T47.2X5	T47.2X6
chloral	T42.6X1	T42.6X2	T42.6X3	T42.6X4	T42.6X5	T42.6X6
Crude oil	T52.0X1	T52.0X2	T52.0X3	T52.0X4	—	—
Cryogenine	T39.8X1	T39.8X2	T39.8X4	T39.8X4	T39.8X5	T39.8X6
Cryolite (vapor)	T60.1X1	T60.1X2	T60.1X3	T60.1X4	—	—
insecticide	T60.1X1	T60.1X2	T60.1X3	T60.1X4	—	—
Cryptenamine (tannates)	T46.5X1	T46.5X2	T46.5X3	T46.5X4	T46.5X5	T46.5X6
Crystal violet	T49.0X1	T49.0X2	T49.0X3	T49.0X4	T49.0X5	T49.0X6

Substance	Poisoning, Accidental (Unintentional)	Poisoning, Intentional Self-Harm	Poisoning, Assault	Poisoning, Undetermined	Adverse Effect	Underdosing
	External Cause (T-Code)					
Cuckoopint	T62.2X1	T62.2X2	T62.2X3	T62.2X4	—	—
Cumetharol	T45.511	T45.512	T45.513	T45.514	T45.515	T45.516
Cupric						
acetate	T60.3X1	T60.3X2	T60.3X3	T60.3X4	—	—
acetoarsenite	T57.0X1	T57.0X2	T57.0X3	T57.0X4	—	—
arsenate	T57.0X1	T57.0X2	T57.0X3	T57.0X4	—	—
gluconate	T49.0X1	T49.0X2	T49.0X3	T49.0X4	T49.0X5	T49.0X6
oleate	T49.0X1	T49.0X2	T49.0X3	T49.0X4	T49.0X5	T49.0X6
sulfate	T56.4X1	T56.4X2	T56.4X3	T56.4X4	—	—
Cuprous sulfate — see also Copper sulfate	T56.4X1	T56.4X2	T56.4X3	T56.4X4	—	—
Curare, curarine	T48.1X1	T48.1X2	T48.1X3	T48.1X4	T48.1X5	T48.1X6
Cyamemazine	T43.3X1	T43.3X2	T43.3X3	T43.3X4	T43.3X5	T43.3X6
Cyamopsis tetragono-loba	T46.6X1	T46.6X2	T46.6X3	T46.6X4	T46.6X5	T46.6X6
Cyanacetyl hydrazide	T37.1X1	T37.1X2	T37.1X3	T37.1X4	T37.1X5	T37.1X6
Cyanic acid (gas)	T59.891	T59.892	T59.893	T59.894	—	—
Cyanide(s) (compounds) (potassium) (sodium) NEC	T65.0X1	T65.0X2	T65.0X3	T65.0X4	—	—
dust or gas (inhalation) NEC	T57.3X1	T57.3X2	T57.3X3	T57.3X4	—	—
fumigant	T65.0X1	T65.0X2	T65.0X3	T65.0X4	—	—
hydrogen	T57.3X1	T57.3X2	T57.3X3	T57.3X4	—	—
mercuric — see Mercury						
pesticide (dust) (fumes)	T65.0X1	T65.0X2	T65.0X3	T65.0X4	—	—
Cyanoacrylate adhesive	T49.3X1	T49.3X2	T49.3X3	T49.3X4	T49.3X5	T49.3X6
Cyanocobalamin	T45.8X1	T45.8X2	T45.8X3	T45.8X4	T45.8X5	T45.8X6
Cyanogen (chloride) (gas) NEC	T59.891	T59.892	T59.893	T59.894	—	—
Cyclacillin	T36.0X1	T36.0X2	T36.0X3	T36.0X4	T36.0X5	T36.0X6
Cyclaine	T41.3X1	T41.3X2	T41.3X3	T41.3X4	T41.3X5	T41.3X6
Cyclamate	T50.991	T50.992	T50.993	T50.994	T50.995	T50.996
Cyclamen europaeum	T62.2X1	T62.2X2	T62.2X3	T62.2X4	—	—
Cyclandelate	T46.7X1	T46.7X2	T46.7X3	T46.7X4	T46.7X5	T46.7X6
Cyclazocine	T50.7X1	T50.7X2	T50.7X3	T50.7X4	T50.7X5	T50.7X6
Cyclizine	T45.0X1	T45.0X2	T45.0X3	T45.0X4	T45.0X5	T45.0X6
Cyclobarbital	T42.3X1	T42.3X2	T42.3X3	T42.3X4	T42.3X5	T42.3X6
Cyclobarbitone	T42.3X1	T42.3X2	T42.3X3	T42.3X4	T42.3X5	T42.3X6
Cyclobenzaprine	T48.1X1	T48.1X2	T48.1X3	T48.1X4	T48.1X5	T48.1X6
Cyclodrine	T44.3X1	T44.3X2	T44.3X3	T44.3X4	T44.3X5	T44.3X6
Cycloguanil embonate	T37.2X1	T37.2X2	T37.2X3	T37.2X4	T37.2X5	T37.2X6
Cycloheptadiene	T43.291	T43.292	T43.293	T43.294	T43.295	T43.296
Cyclohexane	T52.8X1	T52.8X2	T52.8X3	T52.8X4	—	—
Cyclohexanol	T51.8X1	T51.8X2	T51.8X3	T51.8X4	—	—
Cyclohexanone	T52.4X1	T52.4X2	T52.4X3	T52.4X4	—	—

Substance	External Cause (T-Code)					
	Poisoning, Accidental (Unintentional)	Poisoning, Intentional Self-Harm	Poisoning, Assault	Poisoning, Undetermined	Adverse Effect	Underdosing
Cycloheximide	T60.3X1	T60.3X2	T60.3X3	T60.3X4	—	—
Cyclohexyl acetate	T52.8X1	T52.8X2	T52.8X3	T52.8X4	—	—
Cycloleucin	T45.1X1	T45.1X2	T45.1X3	T45.1X4	T45.1X5	T45.1X6
Cyclomethycaine	T41.3X1	T41.3X2	T41.3X3	T41.3X4	T41.3X5	T41.3X6
Cyclopentamine	T44.4X1	T44.4X2	T44.4X3	T44.4X4	T44.4X5	T44.4X6
Cyclopenthiazide	T50.2X1	T50.2X2	T50.2X3	T50.2X4	T50.2X5	T50.2X6
Cyclopentolate	T44.3X1	T44.3X2	T44.3X3	T44.3X4	T44.3X5	T44.3X6
Cyclophosphamide	T45.1X1	T45.1X2	T45.1X3	T45.1X4	T45.1X5	T45.1X6
Cycloplegic drug	T49.5X1	T49.5X2	T49.5X3	T49.5X4	T49.5X5	T49.5X6
Cyclopropane	T41.291	T41.292	T41.293	T41.294	T41.295	T41.296
Cyclopyrabital	T39.8X1	T39.8X2	T39.8X3	T39.8X4	T39.8X5	T39.8X6
Cycloserine	T37.1X1	T37.1X2	T37.1X3	T37.1X4	T37.1X5	T37.1X6
Cyclosporin	T45.1X1	T45.1X2	T45.1X3	T45.1X4	T45.1X5	T45.1X6
Cyclothiazide	T50.2X1	T50.2X2	T50.2X3	T50.2X4	T50.2X5	T50.2X6
Cycrimine	T44.3X1	T44.3X2	T44.3X3	T44.3X4	T44.3X5	T44.3X6
Cyhalothrin	T60.1X1	T60.1X2	T60.1X3	T60.1X4	—	—
Cymarin	T46.0X1	T46.0X2	T46.0X3	T46.0X4	T46.0X5	T46.0X6
Cypermethrin	T60.1X1	T60.1X2	T60.1X3	T60.1X4	—	—
Cyphenothrin	T60.2X1	T60.2X2	T60.2X3	T60.2X4		
Cyproheptadine	T45.0X1	T45.0X2	T45.0X3	T45.0X4	T45.0X5	T45.0X6
Cyprolidol	T43.291	T43.292	T43.293	T43.294	T43.295	T43.296
Cyproterone	T38.6X1	T38.6X2	T38.6X3	T38.6X4	T38.6X5	T38.6X6
Cysteamine	T50.6X1	T50.6X2	T50.6X3	T50.6X4	T50.6X5	T50.6X6
Cytarabine	T45.1X1	T45.1X2	T45.1X3	T45.1X4	T45.1X5	T45.1X6
Cytisus						
laburnum	T62.2X1	T62.2X2	T62.2X3	T62.2X4	—	—
scoparius	T62.2X1	T62.2X2	T62.2X3	T62.2X4	—	—
Cytochrome C	T47.5X1	T47.5X2	T47.5X3	T47.5X4	T47.5X5	T47.5X6
Cytomel	T38.1X1	T38.1X2	T38.1X3	T38.1X4	T38.1X5	T38.1X6
Cytosine arabinoside	T45.1X1	T45.1X2	T45.1X3	T45.1X4	T45.1X5	T45.1X6
Cytoxan	T45.1X1	T45.1X2	T45.1X3	T45.1X4	T45.1X5	T45.1X6
Cytozyme	T45.7X1	T45.7X2	T45.7X3	T45.7X4	T45.7X5	T45.7X6
2,4-D	T60.3X1	T60.3X2	T60.3X3	T60.3X4	—	—
D						
Dacarbazine	T45.1X1	T45.1X2	T45.1X3	T45.1X4	T45.1X5	T45.1X6
Dactinomycin	T45.1X1	T45.1X2	T45.1X3	T45.1X4	T45.1X5	T45.1X6
DADPS	T37.1X1	T37.1X2	T37.1X3	T37.1X4	T37.1X5	T37.1X6
Dakin's solution	T49.0X1	T49.0X2	T49.0X3	T49.0X4	T49.0X5	T49.0X6
Dalapon (sodium)	T60.3X1	T60.3X2	T60.3X3	T60.3X4	—	—

Substance	Poisoning, Accidental (Unintentional)	Poisoning, Intentional Self-Harm	Poisoning, Assault	Poisoning, Undetermined	Adverse Effect	Underdosing
			External Cause (T-Code)			
Dalmane	T42.4X1	T42.4X2	T42.4X3	T42.4X4	T42.4X5	T42.4X6
Danazol	T38.6X1	T38.6X2	T38.6X3	T38.6X4	T38.6X5	T38.6X6
Danilone	T45.511	T45.512	T45.513	T45.514	T45.515	T45.516
Danthron	T47.2X1	T47.2X2	T47.2X3	T47.2X4	T47.2X5	T47.2X6
Dantrolene	T42.8X1	T42.8X2	T42.8X3	T42.8X4	T42.8X5	T42.8X6
Dantron	T47.2X1	T47.2X2	T47.2X3	T47.2X4	T47.2X5	T47.2X6
Daphne (gnidium) (mezereum)	T62.2X1	T62.2X2	T62.2X3	T62.2X4	—	—
berry	T62.1X1	T62.1X2	T62.1X3	T62.1X4	—	—
Dapsone	T37.1X1	T37.1X2	T37.1X3	T37.1X4	T37.1X5	T37.1X6
Daraprim	T37.2X1	T37.2X2	T37.2X3	T37.2X4	T37.2X5	T37.2X6
Darnel	T62.2X1	T62.2X2	T62.2X3	T62.2X4	—	—
Darvon	T39.8X1	T39.8X2	T39.8X3	T39.8X4	T39.8X5	T39.8X6
Daunomycin	T45.1X1	T45.1X2	T45.1X3	T45.1X4	T45.1X5	T45.1X6
Daunorubicin	T45.1X1	T45.1X2	T45.1X3	T45.1X4	T45.1X5	T45.1X6
DBI	T38.3X1	T38.3X2	T38.3X3	T38.3X4	T38.3X5	T38.3X6
D-Con	T60.91	T60.92	T60.93	T60.94	—	—
insecticide	T60.2X1	T60.2X2	T60.2X3	T60.2X4	—	—
rodenticide	T60.4X1	T60.4X2	T60.4X3	T60.4X4	—	—
DDAVP	T38.891	T38.892	T38.893	T38.894	T38.895	T38.896
DDE (bis(chlorophenyl)-dichloroethylene)	T60.2X1	T60.2X2	T60.2X3	T60.2X4	—	—
DDS	T37.1X1	T37.1X2	T37.1X3	T37.1X4	T37.1X5	T37.1X6
DDT (dust)	T60.1X1	T60.1X2	T60.1X3	T60.1X4	—	—
Deadly nightshade—*see also Belladonna*	T62.2X1	T62.2X2	T62.2X3	T62.2X4	—	—
berry	T62.1X1	T62.1X2	T62.1X3	T62.1X4	—	—
Deamino-D-arginine vasopressin	T38.891	T38.892	T38.893	T38.894	T38.895	T38.896
Deanol (aceglumate)	T50.991	T50.992	T50.993	T50.994	T50.995	T50.996
Debrisoquine	T46.5X1	T46.5X2	T46.5X3	T46.5X4	T46.5X5	T46.5X6
Decaborane	T57.8X1	T57.8X2	T57.8X3	T57.8X4	—	—
fumes	T59.891	T59.892	T59.893	T59.894	—	—
Decadron	T38.0X1	T38.0X2	T38.0X3	T38.0X4	T38.0X5	T38.0X6
ENT agent	T49.6X1	T49.6X2	T49.6X3	T49.6X4	T49.6X5	T49.6X6
ophthalmic preparation	T49.5X1	T49.5X2	T49.5X3	T49.5X4	T49.5X5	T49.5X6
topical NEC	T49.0X1	T49.0X2	T49.0X3	T49.0X4	T49.0X5	T49.0X6
Decahydronaphthalene	T52.8X1	T52.8X2	T52.8X3	T52.8X4	—	—
Decalin	T52.8X1	T52.8X2	T52.8X3	T52.8X4	—	—
Decamethonium (bromide)	T48.1X1	T48.1X2	T48.1X3	T48.1X4	T48.1X5	T48.1X6
Decholin	T47.5X1	T47.5X2	T47.5X3	T47.5X4	T47.5X5	T47.5X6
Declomycin	T36.4X1	T36.4X2	T36.4X3	T36.4X4	T36.4X5	T36.4X6
Decongestant, nasal (mucosa)	T48.5X1	T48.5X2	T48.5X3	T48.5X4	T48.5X5	T48.5X6
combination	T48.5X1	T48.5X2	T48.5X3	T48.5X4	T48.5X5	T48.5X6

Substance	External Cause (T-Code)					
	Poisoning, Accidental (Unintentional)	Poisoning, Intentional Self-Harm	Poisoning, Assault	Poisoning, Undetermined	Adverse Effect	Underdosing
Deet	T60.8X1	T60.8X2	T60.8X3	T60.8X4	—	—
Deferoxamine	T45.8X1	T45.8X2	T45.8X3	T45.8X4	T45.8X5	T45.8X6
Deflazacort	T38.0X1	T38.0X2	T38.0X3	T38.0X4	T38.0X5	T38.0X6
Deglycyrrhizinized extract of licorice	T48.4X1	T48.4X2	T48.4X3	T48.4X4	T48.4X5	T48.4X6
Dehydrocholic acid	T47.5X1	T47.5X2	T47.5X3	T47.5X4	T47.5X5	T47.5X6
Dehydroemetine	T37.3X1	T37.3X2	T37.3X3	T37.3X4	T37.3X5	T37.3X6
Dekalin	T52.8X1	T52.8X2	T52.8X3	T52.8X4	—	—
Delalutin	T38.5X1	T38.5X2	T38.5X3	T38.5X4	T38.5X5	T38.5X6
Delphinium	T62.2X1	T62.2X2	T62.2X3	T62.2X4	—	—
Deltasone	T38.0X1	T38.0X2	T38.0X3	T38.0X4	T38.0X5	T38.0X6
Deltra	T38.0X1	T38.0X2	T38.0X3	T38.0X4	T38.0X5	T38.0X6
Delvinal	T42.3X1	T42.3X2	T42.3X3	T42.3X4	T42.3X5	T42.3X6
Delorazepam	T42.4X1	T42.4X2	T42.4X3	T42.4X4	T42.4X5	T42.4X6
Deltamethrin	T60.1X1	T60.1X2	T60.1X3	T60.1X4	—	—
Demecarium (bromide)	T49.5X1	T49.5X2	T49.5X3	T49.5X4	T49.5X5	T49.5X6
Demeclocycline	T36.4X1	T36.4X2	T36.4X3	T36.4X4	T36.4X5	T36.4X6
Demecolcine	T45.1X1	T45.1X2	T45.1X3	T45.1X4	T45.1X5	T45.1X6
Demegestone	T38.5X1	T38.5X2	T38.5X3	T38.5X4	T38.5X5	T38.5X6
Demelanizing agents	T49.8X1	T49.8X2	T49.8X3	T49.8X4	T49.8X5	T49.8X6
Demephion -O and -S	T60.0X1	T60.0X2	T60.0X3	T60.0X4	—	—
Demerol	T40.2X1	T40.2X2	T40.2X3	T40.2X4	T40.2X5	T40.2X6
Demethylchlortetracycline	T36.4X1	T36.4X2	T36.4X3	T36.4X4	T36.4X5	T36.4X6
Demethyltetracycline	T36.4X1	T36.4X2	T36.4X3	T36.4X4	T36.4X5	T36.4X6
Demeton -O and -S	T60.0X1	T60.0X2	T60.0X3	T60.0X4	—	—
Demulcent (external)	T49.3X1	T49.3X2	T49.3X3	T49.3X4	T49.3X5	T49.3X6
specified NEC	T49.3X1	T49.3X2	T49.3X3	T49.3X4	T49.3X5	T49.3X6
Demulen	T38.4X1	T38.4X2	T38.4X3	T38.4X4	T38.4X5	T38.4X6
Denatured alcohol	T51.0X1	T51.0X2	T51.0X3	T51.0X4	—	—
Dendrid	T49.5X1	T49.5X2	T49.5X3	T49.5X4	T49.5X5	T49.5X6
Dental drug, topical application NEC	T49.7X1	T49.7X2	T49.7X3	T49.7X4	T49.7X5	T49.7X6
Dentifrice	T49.7X1	T49.7X2	T49.7X3	T49.7X4	T49.7X5	T49.7X6
Deodorant spray (feminine hygiene)	T49.8X1	T49.8X2	T49.8X3	T49.8X4	T49.8X5	T49.8X6
Deoxycortone	T50.0X1	T50.0X2	T50.0X3	T50.0X4	T50.0X5	T50.0X6
2-Deoxy-5-fluorouridine	T45.1X1	T45.1X2	T45.1X3	T45.1X4	T45.1X5	T45.1X6
5-Deoxy-5-fluorouridine	T45.1X1	T45.1X2	T45.1X3	T45.1X4	T45.1X5	T45.1X6
Deoxyribonuclease (pancreatic)	T45.3X1	T45.3X2	T45.3X3	T45.3X4	T45.3X5	T45.3X6
Depilatory	T49.4X1	T49.4X2	T49.4X3	T49.4X4	T49.4X5	T49.4X6
Deprenalin	T42.8X1	T42.8X2	T42.8X3	T42.8X4	T42.8X5	T42.8X6
Deprenyl	T42.8X1	T42.8X2	T42.8X3	T42.8X4	T42.8X5	T42.8X6

TABLE OF DRUGS AND CHEMICALS

Substance	External Cause (T-Code)					
	Poisoning, Accidental (Unintentional)	Poisoning, Intentional Self-Harm	Poisoning, Assault	Poisoning, Undetermined	Adverse Effect	Underdosing
Depressant, appetite	T50.5X1	T50.5X2	T50.5X3	T50.5X4	T50.5X5	T50.5X6
Depressant						
appetite, central	T50.5X1	T50.5X2	T50.5X3	T50.5X4	T50.5X5	T50.5X6
cardiac	T46.2X1	T46.2X2	T46.2X3	T46.2X4	T46.2X5	T46.2X6
central nervous system (anesthetic) — see also Central nervous system, depressants	T42.71	T42.72	T42.73	T42.74	T42.75	T42.76
general anesthetic	T41.201	T41.202	T41.203	T41.204	T41.205	T41.206
muscle tone	T42.8X1	T42.8X2	T42.8X3	T42.8X4	T42.8X5	T42.8X6
muscle tone, central	T42.8X1	T42.8X2	T42.8X3	T42.8X4	T42.8X5	T42.8X6
psychotherapeutic	T43.501	T43.502	T43.503	T43.504	T43.505	T43.506
Deptropine	T45.0X1	T45.0X2	T45.0X3	T45.0X4	T45.0X5	T45.0X6
Dequalinium (chloride)	T49.0X1	T49.0X2	T49.0X3	T49.0X4	T49.0X5	T49.0X6
Derris root	T60.2X1	T60.2X2	T60.2X3	T60.2X4	—	—
Deserpidine	T43.011	T43.012	T43.013	T43.014	T43.015	T43.016
Desferrioxamine	T45.8X1	T45.8X2	T45.8X3	T45.8X4	T45.8X5	T45.8X6
Desipramine	T43.0X1	T43.0X2	T43.0X3	T43.0X4	T43.0X5	T43.0X6
Deslanoside	T46.0X1	T46.0X2	T46.0X3	T46.0X4	T46.0X5	T46.0X6
Desloughing agent	T49.4X1	T49.4X2	T49.4X3	T49.4X4	T49.4X5	T49.4X6
Desmethylimipramine	T43.011	T43.012	T43.013	T43.014	T43.015	T43.016
Desmopressin	T38.891	T38.892	T38.893	T38.894	T38.895	T38.896
Desocodeine	T40.2X1	T40.2X2	T40.2X3	T40.2X4	T40.2X5	T40.2X6
Desogestrel	T38.5X1	T38.5X2	T38.5X3	T38.5X4	T38.5X5	T38.5X6
Desomorphine	T40.2X1	T40.2X2	T40.2X3	T40.2X4	—	—
Desonide	T49.0X1	T49.0X2	T49.0X3	T49.0X4	T49.0X5	T49.0X6
Desoximetasone	T49.0X1	T49.0X2	T49.0X3	T49.0X4	T49.0X5	T49.0X6
Desoxycorticosteroid	T50.0X1	T50.0X2	T50.0X3	T50.0X4	T50.0X5	T50.0X6
Desoxycortone	T50.0X1	T50.0X2	T50.0X3	T50.0X4	T50.0X5	T50.0X6
Desoxyephedrine	T43.621	T43.622	T43.623	T43.624	T43.625	T43.626
Detaxtran	T46.6X1	T46.6X2	T46.6X3	T46.6X4	T46.6X5	T46.6X6
Detergent	T49.2X1	T49.2X2	T49.2X3	T49.2X4	T49.2X5	T49.2X6
external medication	T49.2X1	T49.2X2	T49.2X3	T49.2X4	T49.2X5	T49.2X6
local	T49.2X1	T49.2X2	T49.2X3	T49.2X4	T49.2X5	T49.2X6
medicinal	T49.2X1	T49.2X2	T49.2X3	T49.2X4	T49.2X5	T49.2X6
nonmedicinal	T55.1X1	T55.1X2	T55.1X3	T55.1X4	—	—
specified NEC	T55.1X1	T55.1X2	T55.1X3	T55.1X4	T55.1X5	T55.1X6
Deterrent, alcohol	T50.6X1	T50.6X2	T50.6X3	T50.6X4	T50.6X5	T50.6X6
Detoxifying agent	T50.6X1	T50.6X2	T50.6X3	T50.6X4	T50.6X5	T50.6X6
Detrothyronine	T38.1X1	T38.1X2	T38.1X3	T38.1X4	T38.1X5	T38.1X6
Dettol (external medication)	T49.0X1	T49.0X2	T49.0X3	T49.0X4	T49.0X5	T49.0X6

Substance	External Cause (T-Code)					
	Poisoning, Accidental (Unintentional)	Poisoning, Intentional Self-Harm	Poisoning, Assault	Poisoning, Undetermined	Adverse Effect	Underdosing
Dexamethasone	T38.0X1	T38.0X2	T38.0X3	T38.0X4	T38.0X5	T38.0X6
ENT agent	T49.6X1	T49.6X2	T49.6X3	T49.6X4	T49.6X5	T49.6X6
ophthalmic preparation	T49.5X1	T49.5X2	T49.5X3	T49.5X4	T49.5X5	T49.5X6
topical NEC	T49.0X1	T49.0X2	T49.0X3	T49.0X4	T49.0X5	T49.0X6
Dexamfetamine	T43.621	T43.622	T43.623	T43.624	T43.625	T43.626
Dexamphetamine	T43.621	T43.622	T43.623	T43.624	T43.625	T43.626
Dexbrompheniramine	T45.0X1	T45.0X2	T45.0X3	T45.0X4	T45.0X5	T45.0X6
Dexchlorpheniramine	T45.0X1	T45.0X2	T45.0X3	T45.0X4	T45.0X5	T45.0X6
Dexedrine	T43.621	T43.622	T43.623	T43.624	T43.625	T43.626
Dexetimide	T44.3X1	T44.3X2	T44.3X3	T44.3X4	T44.3X5	T44.3X6
Dexfenfluramine	T50.5X1	T50.5X2	T50.5X3	T50.5X4	T50.5X5	T50.5X6
Dexpanthenol	T45.2X1	T45.2X2	T45.2X3	T45.2X4	T45.2X5	T45.2X6
Dextran (40) (70) (150)	T45.8X1	T45.8X2	T45.8X3	T45.8X4	T45.8X5	T45.8X6
Dextriferron	T45.4X1	T45.4X2	T45.4X3	T45.4X4	T45.4X5	T45.4X6
Dextroamphetamine	T43.621	T43.622	T43.623	T43.624	T43.625	T43.626
Dextro calcium pantothenate	T45.2X1	T45.2X2	T45.2X3	T45.2X4	T45.2X5	T45.2X6
Dextromethorphan	T48.3X1	T48.3X2	T48.3X3	T48.3X4	T48.3X5	T48.3X6
Dextromoramide	T40.4X1	T40.4X2	T40.4X3	T40.4X4	—	—
topical	T49.8X1	T49.8X2	T49.8X3	T49.8X4	T49.8X5	T49.8X6
Dextro pantothenyl alcohol	T45.2X1	T45.2X2	T45.2X3	T45.2X4	T45.2X5	T45.2X6
Dextropropoxyphene	T40.4X1	T40.4X2	T40.4X3	T40.4X4	T40.4X5	T40.4X6
Dextrorphan	T40.2X1	T40.2X2	T40.2X3	T40.2X4	T40.2X5	T40.2X6
Dextrose	T50.3X1	T50.3X2	T50.3X3	T50.3X4	T50.3X5	T50.3X6
concentrated solution, intravenous	T46.8X1	T46.8X2	T46.8X3	T46.8X4	T46.8X5	T46.8X6
Dextrothyroxin	T38.1X1	T38.1X2	T38.1X3	T38.1X4	T38.1X5	T38.1X6
Dextrothyroxine sodium	T38.1X1	T38.1X2	T38.1X3	T38.1X4	T38.1X5	T38.1X6
DFP	T44.0X1	T44.0X2	T44.0X3	T44.0X4	T44.0X5	T44.0X6
DHE	T37.3X1	T37.3X2	T37.3X3	T37.3X4	T37.3X5	T37.3X6
45	T46.5X1	T46.5X2	T46.5X3	T46.5X4	T46.5X5	T46.5X6
Diabinese	T38.3X1	T38.3X2	T38.3X3	T38.3X4	T38.3X5	T38.3X6
Diacetone alcohol	T52.4X1	T52.4X2	T52.4X3	T52.4X4	—	—
Diacetyl monoxime	T50.991	T50.992	T50.993	T50.994	—	—
Diacetylmorphine	T40.1X1	T40.1X2	T40.1X3	T40.1X4	T40.1X5	—
Diachylon plaster	T49.4X1	T49.4X2	T49.4X3	T49.4X4	T49.4X5	T49.4X6
Diaethylstilboestrolum	T38.5X1	T38.5X2	T38.5X3	T38.5X4	T38.5X5	T38.5X6
Diagnostic agent NEC	T50.8X1	T50.8X2	T50.8X3	T50.8X4	T50.8X5	T50.8X6
Dial (soap)	T49.2X1	T49.2X2	T49.2X3	T49.2X4	T49.2X5	T49.2X6
sedative	T42.3X1	T42.3X2	T42.3X3	T42.3X4	T42.3X5	T42.3X6
Dialkyl carbonate	T52.91	T52.92	T52.93	T52.94	—	—

TABLE OF DRUGS AND CHEMICALS

Substance	Poisoning, Accidental (Unintentional)	Poisoning, Intentional Self-Harm	Poisoning, Assault	Poisoning, Undetermined	Adverse Effect	Underdosing
	External Cause (T-Code)					
Diallylbarbituric acid	T42.3X1	T42.3X2	T42.3X3	T42.3X4	T42.3X5	T42.3X6
Diallymal	T42.3X1	T42.3X2	T42.3X3	T42.3X4	T42.3X5	T42.3X6
Dialysis solution (intraperitoneal)	T50.3X1	T50.3X2	T50.3X3	T50.3X4	T50.3X5	T50.3X6
Diaminodiphenylsulfone	T37.1X1	T37.1X2	T37.1X3	T37.1X4	T37.1X5	T37.1X6
Diamorphine	T40.1X1	T40.1X2	T40.1X3	T40.1X4	T40.1X5	—
Diamox	T50.2X1	T50.2X2	T50.2X3	T50.2X4	T50.2X5	T50.2X6
Diamthazole	T49.0X1	T49.0X2	T49.0X3	T49.0X4	T49.0X5	T49.0X6
Dianthone	T47.2X1	T47.2X2	T47.2X3	T47.2X4	T47.2X5	T47.2X6
Diaphenylsulfone	T37.0X1	T37.0X2	T37.0X3	T37.0X4	T37.0X5	T37.0X6
Diasone (sodium)	T37.1X1	T37.1X2	T37.1X3	T37.1X4	T37.1X5	T37.1X6
Diastase	T47.5X1	T47.5X2	T47.5X3	T47.5X4	T47.5X5	T47.5X6
Diatrizoate	T50.8X1	T50.8X2	T50.8X3	T50.8X4	T50.8X5	T50.8X6
Diazepam	T42.4X1	T42.4X2	T42.4X3	T42.4X4	T42.4X5	T42.4X6
Diazinon	T60.0X1	T60.0X2	T60.0X3	T60.0X4	—	—
Diazomethane (gas)	T59.891	T59.892	T59.893	T59.894	—	—
Diazoxide	T46.5X1	T46.5X2	T46.5X3	T46.5X4	T46.5X5	T46.5X6
Dibekacin	T36.5X1	T36.5X2	T36.5X3	T36.5X4	T36.5X5	T36.5X6
Dibenamine	T44.6X1	T44.6X2	T44.6X3	T44.6X4	T44.6X5	T44.6X6
Dibenzepin	T43.011	T43.012	T43.013	T43.014	T43.015	T43.016
Dibenzheptropine	T45.0X1	T45.0X2	T45.0X3	T45.0X4	T45.0X5	T45.0X6
Dibenzyline	T44.6X1	T44.6X2	T44.6X3	T44.6X4	T44.6X5	T44.6X6
Diborane (gas)	T59.891	T59.892	T59.893	T59.894	—	—
Dibromochloropropane	T60.8X1	T60.8X2	T60.8X3	T60.8X4	—	—
Dibromodulcitol	T45.1X1	T45.1X2	T45.1X3	T45.1X4	T45.1X5	T45.1X6
Dibromoethane	T53.6X1	T53.6X2	T53.6X3	T53.6X4	—	—
Dibromomannitol	T45.1X1	T45.1X2	T45.1X3	T45.1X4	T45.1X5	T45.1X6
Dibromopropamidine isethionate	T49.0X1	T49.0X2	T49.0X3	T49.0X4	T49.0X5	T49.0X6
Dibrompropamidine	T49.0X1	T49.0X2	T49.0X3	T49.0X4	T49.0X5	T49.0X6
Dibucaine	T41.3X1	T41.3X2	T41.3X3	T41.3X4	T41.3X5	T41.3X6
topical (surface)	T41.3X1	T41.3X2	T41.3X3	T41.3X4	T41.3X5	T41.3X6
Dibunate sodium	T48.3X1	T48.3X2	T48.3X3	T48.3X4	T48.3X5	T48.3X6
Dibutoline sulfate	T44.3X1	T44.3X2	T44.3X3	T44.3X4	T44.3X5	T44.3X6
Dicamba	T60.3X1	T60.3X2	T60.3X3	T60.3X4	—	—
Dicapthon	T60.0X1	T60.0X2	T60.0X3	T60.0X4	—	—
Dichlobenil	T60.3X1	T60.3X2	T60.3X3	T60.3X4	—	—
Dichlone	T60.3X1	T60.3X2	T60.3X3	T60.3X4	—	—
Dichloralphenozone	T42.6X1	T42.6X2	T42.6X3	T42.6X4	T42.6X5	T42.6X6
Dichlorbenzidine	T65.3X1	T65.3X2	T65.3X3	T65.3X4	—	—
Dichlorhydrin	T52.8X1	T52.8X2	T52.8X3	T52.8X4	—	—
Dichlorhydroxyquinoline	T37.8X1	T37.8X2	T37.8X3	T37.8X4	T37.8X5	T37.8X6

Substance	External Cause (T-Code)					
	Poisoning, Accidental (Unintentional)	Poisoning, Intentional Self-Harm	Poisoning, Assault	Poisoning, Undetermined	Adverse Effect	Underdosing
Dichlorobenzene	T53.7X1	T53.7X2	T53.7X3	T53.7X4	—	—
Dichlorobenzyl alcohol	T49.6X1	T49.6X2	T49.6X3	T49.6X4	T49.6X5	T49.6X6
Dichlorodifluoromethane	T53.5X1	T53.5X2	T53.5X3	T53.5X4	—	—
Dichloroethane	T52.8X1	T52.8X2	T52.8X3	T52.8X4	—	—
Sym-Dichloroethyl ether	T53.6X1	T53.6X2	T53.6X3	T53.6X4	—	—
Dichloroethyl sulfide, not in war	T59.891	T59.892	T59.893	T59.894	—	—
Dichloroethylene	T53.6X1	T53.6X2	T53.6X3	T53.6X4	—	—
Dichloroformoxine, not in war	T59.891	T59.892	T59.893	T59.894	—	—
Dichlorohydrin, alpha-dichlorohydrin	T52.8X1	T52.8X2	T52.8X3	T52.8X4	—	—
Dichloromethane (solvent)	T53.4X1	T53.4X2	T53.4X3	T53.4X4	—	—
vapor	T53.4X1	T53.4X2	T53.4X3	T53.4X4	—	—
Dichloronaphthoquinone	T60.3X1	T60.3X2	T60.3X3	T60.3X4	—	—
Dichlorophen	T37.4X1	T37.4X2	T37.4X3	T37.4X4	T37.4X5	T37.4X6
2,4-Dichlorophenoxy-acetic acid	T60.3X1	T60.3X2	T60.3X3	T60.3X4	—	—
Dichloropropene	T60.3X1	T60.3X2	T60.3X3	T60.3X4	—	—
Dichloropropionic acid	T60.3X1	T60.3X2	T60.3X3	T60.3X4	—	—
Dichlorphenamide	T50.2X1	T50.2X2	T50.2X3	T50.2X4	T50.2X5	T50.2X6
Dichlorvos	T60.0X1	T60.0X2	T60.0X3	T60.0X4	—	—
Diclofenac	T39.391	T39.392	T39.393	T39.394	T39.395	T39.396
Diclofenamide	T50.2X1	T50.2X2	T50.2X3	T50.2X4	T50.2X5	T50.2X6
Diclofensine	T43.291	T43.292	T43.293	T43.294	T43.295	T43.296
Diclonixine	T39.8X1	T39.8X2	T39.8X3	T39.8X4	T39.8X5	T39.8X6
Dicloxacillin	T36.0X1	T36.0X2	T36.0X3	T36.0X4	T36.0X5	T36.0X6
Dicophane	T49.0X1	T49.0X2	T49.0X3	T49.0X4	T49.0X5	T49.0X6
Dicoumarol, dicoumarin, dicumarol	T45.511	T45.512	T45.513	T45.514	T45.515	T45.516
Dicrotophos	T60.0X1	T60.0X2	T60.0X3	T60.0X4	—	—
Dicyanogen (gas)	T65.0X1	T65.0X2	T65.0X3	T65.0X4	—	—
Dicyclomine	T44.3X1	T44.3X2	T44.3X3	T44.3X4	T44.3X5	T44.3X6
Dicycloverine	T44.3X1	T44.3X2	T44.3X3	T44.3X4	T44.3X5	T44.3X6
Dideoxycytidine	T37.5X1	T37.5X2	T37.5X3	T37.5X4	T37.5X5	T37.5X6
Dideoxyinosine	T37.5X1	T37.5X2	T37.5X3	T37.5X4	T37.5X5	T37.5X6
Dieldrin (vapor)	T60.1X1	T60.1X2	T60.1X3	T60.1X4	—	—
Diemal	T42.3X1	T42.3X2	T42.3X3	T42.3X4	T42.3X5	T42.3X6
Dienestrol	T38.5X1	T38.5X2	T38.5X3	T38.5X4	T38.5X5	T38.5X6
Dienoestrol	T38.5X1	T38.5X2	T38.5X3	T38.5X4	T38.5X5	T38.5X6
Dietetic drug NEC	T50.901	T50.902	T50.903	T50.904	T50.905	T50.906
Diethazine	T42.8X1	T42.8X2	T42.8X3	T42.8X4	T42.8X5	T42.8X6
Diethyl						
barbituric acid	T42.3X1	T42.3X2	T42.3X3	T42.3X4	T42.3X5	T42.3X6
carbamazine	T37.4X1	T37.4X2	T37.4X3	T37.4X4	T37.4X5	T37.4X6

Substance	Poisoning, Accidental (Unintentional)	Poisoning, Intentional Self-Harm	Poisoning, Assault	Poisoning, Undetermined	Adverse Effect	Underdosing
Diethyl *(Continued)*						
carbinol	T51.3X1	T51.3X2	T51.3X3	T51.3X4	—	—
carbonate	T52.8X1	T52.8X2	T52.8X3	T52.8X4	—	—
ether (vapor) — *see also ether*	T41.0X1	T41.0X2	T41.0X3	T41.0X4	T41.0X5	T41.0X6
oxide	T52.8X1	T52.8X2	T52.8X3	T52.8X4	—	—
propion	T50.5X1	T50.5X2	T50.5X3	T50.5X4	T50.5X5	T50.5X6
stilbestrol	T38.5X1	T38.5X2	T38.5X3	T38.5X4	T38.5X5	T38.5X6
toluamide (nonmedicinal)	T60.8X1	T60.8X2	T60.8X3	T60.8X4	—	—
medicinal	T49.3X1	T49.3X2	T49.3X3	T49.3X4	T49.3X5	T49.3X6
Diethylcarbamazine	T37.4X1	T37.4X2	T37.4X3	T37.4X4	T37.4X5	T37.4X6
Diethylene						
dioxide	T52.8X1	T52.8X2	T52.8X3	T52.8X4	—	—
glycol (monoacetate) (monobutyl ether) (monoethyl ether)	T52.3X1	T52.3X2	T52.3X3	T52.3X4	—	—
Diethylhexylphthalate	T65.891	T65.892	T65.893	T65.894	—	—
Diethylpropion	T50.5X1	T50.5X2	T50.5X3	T50.5X4	T50.5X5	T50.5X6
Diethylstilbestrol	T38.5X1	T38.5X2	T38.5X3	T38.5X4	T38.5X5	T38.5X6
Diethylstilboestrol	T38.5X1	T38.5X2	T38.5X3	T38.5X4	T38.5X5	T38.5X6
Diethylsulfone-diethylmethane	T42.6X1	T42.6X2	T42.6X3	T42.6X4	T42.6X5	T42.6X6
Diethyltoluamide	T49.0X1	T49.0X2	T49.0X3	T49.0X4	T49.0X5	T49.0X6
Diethyltryptamine (DET)	T40.991	T40.992	T40.993	T40.994	—	—
Difebarbamate	T42.3X1	T42.3X2	T42.3X3	T42.3X4	T42.3X5	T42.3X6
Difencloxazine	T40.2X1	T40.2X2	T40.2X3	T40.2X4	T40.2X5	T40.2X6
Difenidol	T45.0X1	T45.0X2	T45.0X3	T45.0X4	T45.0X5	T45.0X6
Difenoxin	T47.6X1	T47.6X2	T47.6X3	T47.6X4	T47.6X5	T47.6X6
Difetarsone	T37.3X1	T37.3X2	T37.3X3	T37.3X4	T37.3X5	T37.3X6
Diffusin	T45.3X1	T45.3X2	T45.3X3	T45.3X4	T45.3X5	T45.3X6
Diflorasone	T49.0X1	T49.0X2	T49.0X3	T49.0X4	T49.0X5	T49.0X6
Diflubenzuron	T60.1X1	T60.1X2	T60.1X3	T60.1X4	—	—
Diflos	T44.0X1	T44.0X2	T44.0X3	T44.0X4	T44.0X5	T44.0X6
Diflucortolone	T49.0X1	T49.0X2	T49.0X3	T49.0X4	T49.0X5	T49.0X6
Diflunisal	T39.091	T39.092	T39.093	T39.094	T39.095	T39.096
Difluoromethyldopa	T42.8X1	T42.8X2	T42.8X3	T42.8X4	T42.8X5	T42.8X6
Difluorophate	T44.0X1	T44.0X2	T44.0X3	T44.0X4	T44.0X5	T44.0X6
Digestant NEC	T47.5X1	T47.5X2	T47.5X3	T47.5X4	T47.5X5	T47.5X6
Digitalin(e)	T46.0X1	T46.0X2	T46.0X3	T46.0X4	T46.0X5	T46.0X6
Digitalis (leaf) (glycoside)	T46.0X1	T46.0X2	T46.0X3	T46.0X4	T46.0X5	T46.0X6
lanata	T46.0X1	T46.0X2	T46.0X3	T46.0X4	T46.0X5	T46.0X6
purpurea	T46.0X1	T46.0X2	T46.0X3	T46.0X4	T46.0X5	T46.0X6
Digitoxin	T46.0X1	T46.0X2	T46.0X3	T46.0X4	T46.0X5	T46.0X6

Substance	Poisoning, Accidental (Unintentional)	Poisoning, Intentional Self-Harm	Poisoning, Assault	Poisoning, Undetermined	Adverse Effect	Underdosing
	External Cause (T-Code)					
Digitoxose	T46.0X1	T46.0X2	T46.0X3	T46.0X4	T46.0X5	T46.0X6
Digoxin	T46.0X1	T46.0X2	T46.0X3	T46.0X4	T46.0X5	T46.0X6
Digoxine	T46.0X1	T46.0X2	T46.0X3	T46.0X4	T46.0X5	T46.0X6
Dihydralazine	T46.5X1	T46.5X2	T46.5X3	T46.5X4	T46.5X5	T46.5X6
Dihydrazine	T46.5X1	T46.5X2	T46.5X3	T46.5X4	T46.5X5	T46.5X6
Dihydrocodeinone	T40.2X1	T40.2X2	T40.2X3	T40.2X4	T40.2X5	T40.2X6
Dihydroergocornine	T46.7X1	T46.7X2	T46.7X3	T46.7X4	T46.7X5	T46.7X6
Dihydroergocristine (mesilate)	T46.7X1	T46.7X2	T46.7X3	T46.7X4	T46.7X5	T46.7X6
Dihydroergokryptine	T46.7X1	T46.7X2	T46.7X3	T46.7X4	T46.7X5	T46.7X6
Dihydroergotamine	T46.5X1	T46.5X2	T46.5X3	T46.5X4	T46.5X5	T46.5X6
Dihydroergotoxine	T46.7X1	T46.7X2	T46.7X3	T46.7X4	T46.7X5	T46.7X6
mesilate	T46.7X1	T46.7X2	T46.7X3	T46.7X4	T46.7X5	T46.7X6
Dihydrohydroxycodein-one	T40.2X1	T40.2X2	T40.2X3	T40.2X4	T40.2X5	T40.2X6
Dihydrohydroxymorphinone	T40.2X1	T40.2X2	T40.2X3	T40.2X4	T40.2X5	T40.2X6
Dihydroisocodeine	T40.2X1	T40.2X2	T40.2X3	T40.2X4	T40.2X5	T40.2X6
Dihydromorphine	T40.2X1	T40.2X2	T40.2X3	T40.2X4	—	—
Dihydromorphinone	T40.2X1	T40.2X2	T40.2X3	T40.2X4	T40.2X5	T40.2X6
Dihydrostreptomycin	T36.5X1	T36.5X2	T36.5X3	T36.5X4	T36.5X5	T36.5X6
Dihydrotachysterol	T45.2X1	T45.2X2	T45.2X3	T45.2X4	T45.2X5	T45.2X6
Dihydroxyaluminum aminoacetate	T47.1X1	T47.1X2	T47.1X3	T47.1X4	T47.1X5	T47.1X6
Dihydroxyaluminum sodium carbonate	T47.1X1	T47.1X2	T47.1X3	T47.1X4	T47.1X5	T47.1X6
Dihydroxyanthraquinone	T47.2X1	T47.2X2	T47.2X3	T47.2X4	T47.2X5	T47.2X6
Dihydroxycodeinone	T40.2X1	T40.2X2	T40.2X3	T40.2X4	T40.2X5	T40.2X6
Dihydroxypropyl theophylline	T50.2X1	T50.2X2	T50.2X3	T50.2X4	T50.2X5	T50.2X6
Diiodohydroxyquin	T37.8X1	T37.8X2	T37.8X3	T37.8X4	T37.8X5	T37.8X6
topical	T49.0X1	T49.0X2	T49.0X3	T49.0X4	T49.0X5	T49.0X6
Diiodohydroxyquinoline	T37.8X1	T37.8X2	T37.8X3	T37.8X4	T37.8X5	T37.8X6
Diiodotyrosine	T38.2X1	T38.2X2	T38.2X3	T38.2X4	T38.2X5	T38.2X6
Diisopromine	T44.3X1	T44.3X2	T44.3X3	T44.3X4	T44.3X5	T44.3X6
Diisopropylamine	T46.3X1	T46.3X2	T46.3X3	T46.3X4	T46.3X5	T46.3X6
Diisopropylfluorophosphonate	T44.0X1	T44.0X2	T44.0X3	T44.0X4	T44.0X5	T44.0X6
Dilantin	T42.0X1	T42.0X2	T42.0X3	T42.0X4	T42.0X5	T42.0X6
Dilaudid	T40.2X1	T40.2X2	T40.2X3	T40.2X4	T40.2X5	T40.2X6
Dilazep	T46.3X1	T46.3X2	T46.3X3	T46.3X4	T46.3X5	T46.3X6
Dill	T47.5X1	T47.5X2	T47.5X3	T47.5X4	T47.5X5	T47.5X6
Diloxanide	T37.3X1	T37.3X2	T37.3X3	T37.3X4	T37.3X5	T37.3X6
Diltiazem	T46.1X1	T46.1X2	T46.1X3	T46.1X4	T46.1X5	T46.1X6
Dimazole	T49.0X1	T49.0X2	T49.0X3	T49.0X4	T49.0X5	T49.0X6
Dimefline	T50.7X1	T50.7X2	T50.7X3	T50.7X4	T50.7X5	T50.7X6

TABLE OF DRUGS AND CHEMICALS

Substance	Poisoning, Accidental (Unintentional)	Poisoning, Intentional Self-Harm	Poisoning, Assault	Poisoning, Undetermined	Adverse Effect	Underdosing
			External Cause (T-Code)			
Dimefox	T60.0X1	T60.0X2	T60.0X3	T60.0X4	—	—
Dimemorfan	T48.3X1	T48.3X2	T48.3X3	T48.3X4	T48.3X5	T48.3X6
Dimenhydrinate	T45.0X1	T45.0X2	T45.0X3	T45.0X4	T45.0X5	T45.0X6
Dimercaprol (British anti-lewisite)	T45.8X1	T45.8X2	T45.8X3	T45.8X4	T45.8X5	T45.8X6
Dimercaptopropanol	T45.8X1	T45.8X2	T45.8X3	T45.8X4	T45.8X5	T45.8X6
Dimestrol	T38.5X1	T38.5X2	T38.5X3	T38.5X4	T38.5X5	T38.5X6
Dimetane	T45.0X1	T45.0X2	T45.0X3	T45.0X4	T45.0X5	T45.0X6
Dimethicone	T47.1X1	T47.1X2	T47.1X3	T47.1X4	T47.1X5	T47.1X6
Dimethindene	T45.0X1	T45.0X2	T45.0X3	T45.0X4	T45.0X5	T45.0X6
Dimethisoquin	T49.1X1	T49.1X2	T49.1X3	T49.1X4	T49.1X5	T49.1X6
Dimethisterone	T38.5X1	T38.5X2	T38.5X3	T38.5X4	T38.5X5	T38.5X6
Dimethoate	T60.0X1	T60.0X2	T60.0X3	T60.0X4	—	—
Dimethocaine	T41.3X1	T41.3X2	T41.3X3	T41.3X4	T41.3X5	T41.3X6
Dimethoxanate	T48.3X1	T48.3X2	T48.3X3	T48.3X4	T48.3X5	T48.3X6
Dimethyl						
arsine, arsinic acid	T57.0X1	T57.0X2	T57.0X3	T57.0X4	—	—
carbinol	T51.2X1	T51.2X2	T51.2X3	T51.2X4	—	—
carbonate	T52.8X1	T52.8X2	T52.8X3	T52.8X4	—	—
diguanide	T38.3X1	T38.3X2	T38.3X3	T38.3X4	T38.3X5	T38.3X6
ketone	T52.4X1	T52.4X2	T52.4X3	T52.4X4	—	—
vapor	T52.4X1	T52.4X2	T52.4X3	T52.4X4	—	—
meperidine	T40.2X1	T40.2X2	T40.2X3	T40.2X4	T40.2X5	T40.2X6
parathion	T60.0X1	T60.0X2	T60.0X3	T60.0X4	—	—
phthlate	T49.3X1	T49.3X2	T49.3X3	T49.3X4	T49.3X5	T49.3X6
polysiloxane	T47.8X1	T47.8X2	T47.8X3	T47.8X4	T47.8X5	T47.8X6
sulfate (fumes)	T59.891	T59.892	T59.893	T59.894	—	—
liquid	T65.891	T65.892	T65.893	T65.894	—	—
sulfoxide (nonmedicinal)	T52.8X1	T52.8X2	T52.8X3	T52.8X4	—	—
medicinal	T49.4X1	T49.4X2	T49.4X3	T49.4X4	T49.4X5	T49.4X6
tryptamine	T40.991	T40.992	T40.993	T40.994	—	—
tubocurarine	T48.1X1	T48.1X2	T48.1X3	T48.1X4	T48.1X5	T48.1X6
Dimethylamine sulfate	T49.4X1	T49.4X2	T49.4X3	T49.4X4	T49.4X5	T49.4X6
Dimethylformamide	T52.8X1	T52.8X2	T52.8X3	T52.8X4	—	—
Dimethyltubocurarinium chloride	T48.1X1	T48.1X2	T48.1X3	T48.1X4	T48.1X5	T48.1X6
Dimeticone	T47.1X1	T47.1X2	T47.1X3	T47.1X4	T47.1X5	T47.1X6
Dimetilan	T60.0X1	T60.0X2	T60.0X3	T60.0X4	—	—
Dimetindene	T45.0X1	T45.0X2	T45.0X3	T45.0X4	T45.0X5	T45.0X6
Dimetotiazine	T43.3X1	T43.3X2	T43.3X3	T43.3X4	T43.3X5	T43.3X6

Substance	External Cause (T-Code)					
	Poisoning, Accidental (Unintentional)	Poisoning, Intentional Self-Harm	Poisoning, Assault	Poisoning, Undetermined	Adverse Effect	Underdosing
Dimorpholamine	T50.7X1	T50.7X2	T50.7X3	T50.7X4	T50.7X5	T50.7X6
Dimoxyline	T46.3X1	T46.3X2	T46.3X3	T46.3X4	T46.3X5	T46.3X6
Dinitrobenzene	T65.3X1	T65.3X2	T65.3X3	T65.3X4	—	—
vapor	T59.891	T59.892	T59.893	T59.894	—	—
Dinitrobenzol	T65.3X1	T65.3X2	T65.3X3	T65.3X4	—	—
vapor	T59.891	T59.892	T59.893	T59.894	—	—
Dinitrobutylphenol	T65.3X1	T65.3X2	T65.3X3	T65.3X4	—	—
Dinitro (-ortho-)cresol (pesticide) (spray)	T65.3X1	T65.3X2	T65.3X3	T65.3X4	—	—
Dinitrocyclohexylphenol	T65.3X1	T65.3X2	T65.3X3	T65.3X4	—	—
Dinitrophenol	T65.3X1	T65.3X2	T65.3X3	T65.3X4	—	—
Dinoprost	T48.0X1	T48.0X2	T48.0X3	T48.0X4	T48.0X5	T48.0X6
Dinoprostone	T48.0X1	T48.0X2	T48.0X3	T48.0X4	T48.0X5	T48.0X6
Dinoseb	T60.3X1	T60.3X2	T60.3X3	T60.3X4	—	—
Dioctyl sulfosuccinate (calcium) (sodium)	T47.4X1	T47.4X2	T47.4X3	T47.4X4	T47.4X5	T47.4X6
Diodone	T50.8X1	T50.8X2	T50.8X3	T50.8X4	T50.8X5	T50.8X6
Diodoquin	T37.8X1	T37.8X2	T37.8X3	T37.8X4	T37.8X5	T37.8X6
Dionin	T40.2X1	T40.2X2	T40.2X3	T40.2X4	T40.2X5	T40.2X6
Diosmin	T46.991	T46.992	T46.993	T46.994	T46.995	T46.996
Dioxane	T52.8X1	T52.8X2	T52.8X3	T52.8X4	—	—
Dioxathion	T60.0X1	T60.0X2	T60.0X3	T60.0X4	—	—
Dioxin	T53.7X1	T53.7X2	T53.7X3	T53.7X4	—	—
Dioxopromethazine	T43.3X1	T43.3X2	T43.3X3	T43.3X4	T43.3X5	T43.3X6
Dioxyline	T46.3X1	T46.3X2	T46.3X3	T46.3X4	T46.3X5	T46.3X6
Dipentene	T52.8X1	T52.8X2	T52.8X3	T52.8X4	—	—
Diperodon	T41.3X1	T41.3X2	T41.3X3	T41.3X4	T41.3X5	T41.3X6
Diphacinone	T60.4X1	T60.4X2	T60.4X3	T60.4X4	—	—
Diphemanil	T44.3X1	T44.3X2	T44.3X3	T44.3X4	T44.3X5	T44.3X6
metilsulfate	T44.3X1	T44.3X2	T44.3X3	T44.3X4	T44.3X5	T44.3X6
Diphenadione	T45.511	T45.512	T45.513	T45.514	T45.515	T45.516
rodenticide	T60.4X1	T60.4X2	T60.4X3	T60.4X4	—	—
Diphenhydramine	T45.0X1	T45.0X2	T45.0X3	T45.0X4	T45.0X5	T45.0X6
Diphenidol	T45.0X1	T45.0X2	T45.0X3	T45.0X4	T45.0X5	T45.0X6
Diphenoxylate	T47.6X1	T47.6X2	T47.6X3	T47.6X4	T47.6X5	T47.6X6
Diphenylamine	T65.3X1	T65.3X2	T65.3X3	T65.3X4	—	—
Diphenylbutazone	T39.2X1	T39.2X2	T39.2X3	T39.2X4	T39.2X5	T39.2X6
Diphenylchloroarsine, not in war	T57.0X1	T57.0X2	T57.0X3	T57.0X4	—	—
Diphenylhydantoin	T42.0X1	T42.0X2	T42.0X3	T42.0X4	T42.0X5	T42.0X6
Diphenylmethane dye	T52.1X1	T52.1X2	T52.1X3	T52.1X4		

TABLE OF DRUGS AND CHEMICALS

Substance	External Cause (T-Code)					
	Poisoning, Accidental (Unintentional)	Poisoning, Intentional Self-Harm	Poisoning, Assault	Poisoning, Undetermined	Adverse Effect	Underdosing
Diphenylpyraline	T45.0X1	T45.0X2	T45.0X3	T45.0X4	T45.0X5	T45.0X6
Diphtheria						
antitoxin	T50.Z11	T50.Z12	T50.Z13	T50.Z14	T50.Z15	T50.Z16
toxoid	T50.A91	T50.A92	T50.A93	T50.A94	T50.A95	T50.A96
with tetanus toxoid	T50.A21	T50.A22	T50.A23	T50.A24	T50.A25	T50.A26
with pertussis component	T50.A11	T50.A12	T50.A13	T50.A14	T50.A15	T50.A16
vaccine (combination)	T50.A91	T50.A92	T50.A93	T50.A94	T50.A95	T50.A96
combination						
including pertussis	T50.A11	T50.A12	T50.A13	T50.A14	T50.A15	T50.A16
without pertussis	T50.A21	T50.A22	T50.A23	T50.A24	T50.A25	T50.A26
Diphylline	T50.2X1	T50.2X2	T50.2X3	T50.2X4	T50.2X5	T50.2X6
Dipipanone	T40.4X1	T40.4X2	T40.4X3	T40.4X4	—	—
Dipivefrine	T49.5X1	T49.5X2	T49.5X3	T49.5X4	T49.5X5	T49.5X6
Diplovax	T50.B91	T50.B92	T50.B93	T50.B94	T50.B95	T50.B96
Diprophylline	T50.2X1	T50.2X2	T50.2X3	T50.2X4	T50.2X5	T50.2X6
Dipropyline	T48.291	T48.292	T48.293	T48.294	T48.295	T48.296
Dipyridamole	T46.3X1	T46.3X2	T46.3X3	T46.3X4	T46.3X5	T46.3X6
Dipyrone	T39.2X1	T39.2X2	T39.2X3	T39.2X4	T39.2X5	T39.2X6
Diquat (dibromide)	T60.3X1	T60.3X2	T60.3X3	T60.3X4	—	—
Disinfectant	T65.891	T65.892	T65.893	T65.894	—	—
alkaline	T54.3X1	T54.3X2	T54.3X3	T54.3X4	—	—
aromatic	T54.1X1	T54.1X2	T54.1X3	T54.1X4	—	—
intestinal	T37.8X1	T37.8X2	T37.8X3	T37.8X4	T37.8X5	T37.8X6
Disipal	T42.8X1	T42.8X2	T42.8X3	T42.8X4	T42.8X5	T42.8X6
Disodium edetate	T50.6X1	T50.6X2	T50.6X3	T50.6X4	T50.6X5	T50.6X6
Disoprofol	T41.291	T41.292	T41.293	T41.294	T41.295	T41.296
Disopyramide	T46.2X1	T46.2X2	T46.2X3	T46.2X4	T46.2X5	T46.2X6
Distigmine (bromide)	T44.0X1	T44.0X2	T44.0X3	T44.0X4	T44.0X5	T44.0X6
Disulfamide	T50.2X1	T50.2X2	T50.2X3	T50.2X4	T50.2X5	T50.2X6
Disulfanilamide	T37.0X1	T37.0X2	T37.0X3	T37.0X4	T37.0X5	T37.0X6
Disulfiram	T50.6X1	T50.6X2	T50.6X3	T50.6X4	T50.6X5	T50.6X6
Disulfoton	T60.0X1	T60.0X2	T60.0X3	T60.0X4	—	—
Dithiazanine iodide	T37.4X1	T37.4X2	T37.4X3	T37.4X4	T37.4X5	T37.4X6
Dithiocarbamate	T60.0X1	T60.0X2	T60.0X3	T60.0X4	—	—
Dithranol	T49.4X1	T49.4X2	T49.4X3	T49.4X4	T49.4X5	T49.4X6
Diucardin	T50.2X1	T50.2X2	T50.2X3	T50.2X4	T50.2X5	T50.2X6
Diupres	T50.2X1	T50.2X2	T50.2X3	T50.2X4	T50.2X5	T50.2X6
Diuretic NEC	T50.2X1	T50.2X2	T50.2X3	T50.2X4	T50.2X5	T50.2X6
benzothiadiazine	T50.2X1	T50.2X2	T50.2X3	T50.2X4	T50.2X5	T50.2X6
carbonic acid anhydrase inhibitors	T50.2X1	T50.2X2	T50.2X3	T50.2X4	T50.2X5	T50.2X6

Substance	External Cause (T-Code)					
	Poisoning, Accidental (Unintentional)	Poisoning, Intentional Self-Harm	Poisoning, Assault	Poisoning, Undetermined	Adverse Effect	Underdosing
Diuretic NEC *(Continued)*						
furfuryl NEC	T50.2X1	T50.2X2	T50.2X3	T50.2X4	T50.2X5	T50.2X6
loop (high-ceiling)	T50.1X1	T50.1X2	T50.1X3	T50.1X4	T50.1X5	T50.1X6
mercurial NEC	T50.2X1	T50.2X2	T50.2X3	T50.2X4	T50.2X5	T50.2X6
osmotic	T50.2X1	T50.2X2	T50.2X3	T50.2X4	T50.2X5	T50.2X6
purine NEC	T50.2X1	T50.2X2	T50.2X3	T50.2X4	T50.2X5	T50.2X6
saluretic NEC	T50.2X1	T50.2X2	T50.2X3	T50.2X4	T50.2X5	T50.2X6
sulfonamide	T50.2X1	T50.2X2	T50.2X3	T50.2X4	T50.2X5	T50.2X6
thiazide NEC	T50.2X1	T50.2X2	T50.2X3	T50.2X4	T50.2X5	T50.2X6
xanthine	T50.2X1	T50.2X2	T50.2X3	T50.2X4	T50.2X5	T50.2X6
Diurgin	T50.2X1	T50.2X2	T50.2X3	T50.2X4	T50.2X5	T50.2X6
Diuril	T50.2X1	T50.2X2	T50.2X3	T50.2X4	T50.2X5	T50.2X6
Diuron	T60.3X1	T60.3X2	T60.3X3	T60.3X4	—	—
Divalproex	T42.6X1	T42.6X2	T42.6X3	T42.6X4	T42.6X5	T42.6X6
Divinyl ether	T41.0X1	T41.0X2	T41.0X3	T41.0X4	T41.0X5	T41.0X6
Dixanthogen	T49.0X1	T49.0X2	T49.0X3	T49.0X4	T49.0X5	T49.0X6
Dixyrazine	T43.3X1	T43.3X2	T43.3X3	T43.3X4	T43.3X5	T43.3X6
D-lysergic acid diethylamide	T40.8X1	T40.8X2	T40.8X3	T40.8X4	T40.8X5	—
DMCT	T36.4X1	T36.4X2	T36.4X3	T36.4X4	T36.4X5	T36.4X6
DMSO — *see Dimethyl sulfoxide*						
DNBP	T60.3X1	T60.3X2	T60.3X3	T60.3X4	—	—
DNOC	T65.3X1	T65.3X2	T65.3X3	T65.3X4	—	—
DOCA	T38.0X1	T38.0X2	T38.0X3	T38.0X4	T38.0X5	T38.0X6
Dobutamine	T44.5X1	T44.5X2	T44.5X3	T44.5X4	T44.5X5	T44.5X6
Docusate sodium	T47.4X1	T47.4X2	T47.4X3	T47.4X4	T47.4X5	T47.4X6
Dodicin	T49.0X1	T49.0X2	T49.0X3	T49.0X4	T49.0X5	T49.0X6
Dofamium chloride	T49.0X1	T49.0X2	T49.0X3	T49.0X4	T49.0X5	T49.0X6
Dolophine	T40.3X1	T40.3X2	T40.3X3	T40.3X4	T40.3X5	T40.3X6
Doloxene	T39.8X1	T39.8X2	T39.8X3	T39.8X4	T39.8X5	T39.8X6
Domestic gas (after combustion) — *see Gas, utility*						
prior to combustion	T59.891	T59.892	T59.893	T59.894	—	—
Domiodol	T48.4X1	T48.4X2	T48.4X3	T48.4X4	T48.4X5	T48.4X6
Domiphen (bromide)	T49.0X1	T49.0X2	T49.0X3	T49.0X4	T49.0X5	T49.0X6
Domperidone	T45.0X1	T45.0X2	T45.0X3	T45.0X4	T45.0X5	T45.0X6
Dopa	T42.8X1	T42.8X2	T42.8X3	T42.8X4	T42.8X5	T42.8X6
Dopamine	T44.991	T44.992	T44.993	T44.994	T44.995	T44.996
Doriden	T42.6X1	T42.6X2	T42.6X3	T42.6X4	T42.6X5	T42.6X6
Dormiral	T42.3X1	T42.3X2	T42.3X3	T42.3X4	T42.3X5	T42.3X6
Dormison	T42.6X1	T42.6X2	T42.6X3	T42.6X4	T42.6X5	T42.6X6
Dornase	T48.4X1	T48.4X2	T48.4X3	T48.4X4	T48.4X5	T48.4X6

Substance	Poisoning, Accidental (Unintentional)	Poisoning, Intentional Self-Harm	Poisoning, Assault	Poisoning, Undetermined	Adverse Effect	Underdosing
	External Cause (T-Code)					
Dorsacaine	T41.3X1	T41.3X2	T41.3X3	T41.3X4	T41.3X5	T41.3X6
Dosulepin	T43.011	T43.012	T43.013	T43.014	T43.015	T43.016
Dothiepin	T43.011	T43.012	T43.013	T43.014	T43.015	T43.016
Doxantrazole	T48.6X1	T48.6X2	T48.6X3	T48.6X4	T48.6X5	T48.6X6
Doxapram	T50.7X1	T50.7X2	T50.7X3	T50.7X4	T50.7X5	T50.7X6
Doxazosin	T44.6X1	T44.6X2	T44.6X3	T44.6X4	T44.6X5	T44.6X6
Doxepin	T43.011	T43.012	T43.013	T43.014	T43.015	T43.016
Doxifluridine	T45.1X1	T45.1X2	T45.1X3	T45.1X4	T45.1X5	T45.1X6
Doxorubicin	T45.1X1	T45.1X2	T45.1X3	T45.1X4	T45.1X5	T45.1X6
Doxycycline	T36.4X1	T36.4X2	T36.4X3	T36.4X4	T36.4X5	T36.4X6
Doxylamine	T45.0X1	T45.0X2	T45.0X3	T45.0X4	T45.0X5	T45.0X6
Dramamine	T45.0X1	T45.0X2	T45.0X3	T45.0X4	T45.0X5	T45.0X6
Drano (drain cleaner)	T54.3X1	T54.3X2	T54.3X3	T54.3X4	—	—
Dressing, live pulp	T49.7X1	T49.7X2	T49.7X3	T49.7X4	T49.7X5	T49.7X6
Drocode	T40.2X1	T40.2X2	T40.2X3	T40.2X4	T40.2X5	T40.2X6
Dromoran	T40.2X1	T40.2X2	T40.2X3	T40.2X4	T40.2X5	T40.2X6
Dromostanolone	T38.7X1	T38.7X2	T38.7X3	T38.7X4	T38.7X5	T38.7X6
Dronabinol	T40.7X1	T40.7X2	T40.7X3	T40.7X4	T40.7X5	T40.7X6
Droperidol	T43.591	T43.592	T43.593	T43.594	T43.595	T43.596
Dropropizine	T48.3X1	T48.3X2	T48.3X3	T48.3X4	T48.3X5	T48.3X6
Drostanolone	T38.7X1	T38.7X2	T38.7X3	T38.7X4	T38.7X5	T38.7X6
Drotaverine	T44.3X1	T44.3X2	T44.3X3	T44.3X4	T44.3X5	T44.3X6
Drotrecogin alfa	T45.511	T45.512	T45.513	T45.514	T45.515	T45.516
Drug NEC	T50.901	T50.902	T50.903	T50.904	T50.905	T50.906
specified NEC	T50.991	T50.992	T50.993	T50.994	T50.995	T50.996
DTIC	T45.1X1	T45.1X2	T45.1X3	T45.1X4	T45.1X5	T45.1X6
Duboisine	T44.3X1	T44.3X2	T44.3X3	T44.3X4	T44.3X5	T44.3X6
Dulcolax	T47.2X1	T47.2X2	T47.2X3	T47.2X4	T47.2X5	T47.2X6
Duponol (C) (EP)	T49.2X1	T49.2X2	T49.2X3	T49.2X4	T49.2X5	T49.2X6
Durabolin	T38.7X1	T38.7X2	T38.7X3	T38.7X4	T38.7X5	T38.7X6
Dyclone	T41.3X1	T41.3X2	T41.3X3	T41.3X4	T41.3X5	T41.3X6
Dyclonine	T41.3X1	T41.3X2	T41.3X3	T41.3X4	T41.3X5	T41.3X6
Dydrogesterone	T38.5X1	T38.5X2	T38.5X3	T38.5X4	T38.5X5	T38.5X6
Dye NEC	T65.6X1	T65.6X2	T65.6X3	T65.6X4	—	—
antiseptic	T49.0X1	T49.0X2	T49.0X3	T49.0X4	T49.0X5	T49.0X6
diagnostic agents	T50.8X1	T50.8X2	T50.8X3	T50.8X4	T50.8X5	T50.8X6
pharmaceutical NEC	T50.901	T50.902	T50.903	T50.904	T50.905	T50.906
Dyflos	T44.0X1	T44.0X2	T44.0X3	T44.0X4	T44.0X5	T44.0X6
Dymelor	T38.3X1	T38.3X2	T38.3X3	T38.3X4	T38.3X5	T38.3X6

Substance	External Cause (T-Code)					
	Poisoning, Accidental (Unintentional)	Poisoning, Intentional Self-Harm	Poisoning, Assault	Poisoning, Undetermined	Adverse Effect	Underdosing
Dynamite	T65.3X1	T65.3X2	T65.3X3	T65.3X4	—	—
fumes	T59.891	T59.892	T59.893	T59.894	—	—
Dyphylline	T44.3X1	T44.3X2	T44.3X3	T44.3X4	T44.3X5	T44.3X6
E						
Ear drug NEC	T49.6X1	T49.6X2	T49.6X3	T49.6X4	T49.6X5	T49.6X6
Ear preparations	T49.6X1	T49.6X2	T49.6X3	T49.6X4	T49.6X5	T49.6X6
Econazole	T49.0X1	T49.0X2	T49.0X3	T49.0X4	T49.0X5	T49.0X6
Ecothiopate iodide	T49.5X1	T49.5X2	T49.5X3	T49.5X4	T49.5X5	T49.5X6
Echothiophate, echothiopate, ecothiopate	T49.5X1	T49.5X2	T49.5X3	T49.5X4	T49.5X5	T49.5X6
Ecstasy	T43.621	T43.622	T43.623	T43.624	T43.625	T43.626
Ectylurea	T42.6X1	T42.6X2	T42.6X3	T42.6X4	T42.6X5	T42.6X6
Edathamil disodium	T45.8X1	T45.8X2	T45.8X3	T45.8X4	T45.8X5	T45.8X6
Edecrin	T50.1X1	T50.1X2	T50.1X3	T50.1X4	T50.1X5	T50.1X6
Edetate, disodium (calcium)	T45.8X1	T45.8X2	T45.8X3	T45.8X4	T45.8X5	T45.8X6
Edoxudine	T49.5X1	T49.5X2	T49.5X3	T49.5X4	T49.5X5	T49.5X6
Edrophonium	T44.0X1	T44.0X2	T44.0X3	T44.0X4	T44.0X5	T44.0X6
chloride	T44.0X1	T44.0X2	T44.0X3	T44.0X4	T44.0X5	T44.0X6
EDTA	T50.6X1	T50.6X2	T50.6X3	T50.6X4	T50.6X5	T50.6X6
Eflornithine	T37.2X1	T37.2X2	T37.2X3	T37.2X4	T37.2X5	T37.2X6
Efloxate	T46.3X1	T46.3X2	T46.3X3	T46.3X4	T46.3X5	T46.3X6
Elase	T49.8X1	T49.8X2	T49.8X3	T49.8X4	T49.8X5	T49.8X6
Elastase	T47.5X1	T47.5X2	T47.5X3	T47.5X4	T47.5X5	T47.5X6
Elaterium	T47.2X1	T47.2X2	T47.2X3	T47.2X4	T47.2X5	T47.2X6
Elcatonin	T50.991	T50.992	T50.993	T50.994	T50.995	T50.996
Elder	T62.2X1	T62.2X2	T62.2X3	T62.2X4	—	—
berry (unripe)	T62.1X1	T62.1X2	T62.1X3	T62.1X4	—	—
Electrolyte balance drug	T50.3X1	T50.3X2	T50.3X3	T50.3X4	T50.3X5	T50.3X6
Electrolytes NEC	T50.3X1	T50.3X2	T50.3X3	T50.3X4	T50.3X5	T50.3X6
Electrolytic agent NEC	T50.3X1	T50.3X2	T50.3X3	T50.3X4	T50.3X5	T50.3X6
Elemental diet	T50.901	T50.902	T50.903	T50.904	T50.905	T50.906
Elliptinium acetate	T45.1X1	T45.1X2	T45.1X3	T45.1X4	T45.1X5	T45.1X6
Embramine	T45.0X1	T45.0X2	T45.0X3	T45.0X4	T45.0X5	T45.0X6
Emepronium (salts)	T44.3X1	T44.3X2	T44.3X3	T44.3X4	T44.3X5	T44.3X6
bromide	T44.3X1	T44.3X2	T44.3X3	T44.3X4	T44.3X5	T44.3X6
Emetic NEC	T47.7X1	T47.7X2	T47.7X3	T47.7X4	T47.7X5	T47.7X6
Emetine	T37.3X1	T37.3X2	T37.3X3	T37.3X4	T37.3X5	T37.3X6
Emollient NEC	T49.3X1	T49.3X2	T49.3X3	T49.3X4	T49.3X5	T49.3X6
Emorfazone	T39.8X1	T39.8X2	T39.8X3	T39.8X4	T39.8X5	T39.8X6

Substance	External Cause (T-Code)					
	Poisoning, Accidental (Unintentional)	Poisoning, Intentional Self-Harm	Poisoning, Assault	Poisoning, Undetermined	Adverse Effect	Underdosing
Emylcamate	T43.591	T43.592	T43.593	T43.594	T43.595	T43.596
Enalapril	T46.4X1	T46.4X2	T46.4X3	T46.4X4	T46.4X5	T46.4X6
Enalaprilat	T46.4X1	T46.4X2	T46.4X3	T46.4X4	T46.4X5	T46.4X6
Encainide	T46.2X1	T46.2X2	T46.2X3	T46.2X4	T46.2X5	T46.2X6
Endocaine	T41.3X1	T41.3X2	T41.3X3	T41.3X4	T41.3X5	T41.3X6
Endosulfan	T60.2X1	T60.2X2	T60.2X3	T60.2X4	—	—
Endothall	T60.3X1	T60.3X2	T60.3X3	T60.3X4	—	—
Endralazine	T46.5X1	T46.5X2	T46.5X3	T46.5X4	T46.5X5	T46.5X6
Endrin	T60.1X1	T60.1X2	T60.1X3	T60.1X4	—	—
Enflurane	T41.0X1	T41.0X2	T41.0X3	T41.0X4	T41.0X5	T41.0X6
Enhexymal	T42.3X1	T42.3X2	T42.3X3	T42.3X4	T42.3X5	T42.3X6
Enocitabine	T45.1X1	T45.1X2	T45.1X3	T45.1X4	T45.1X5	T45.1X6
Enovid	T38.4X1	T38.4X2	T38.4X3	T38.4X4	T38.4X5	T38.4X6
Enoxacin	T36.8X1	T36.8X2	T36.8X3	T36.8X4	T36.8X5	T36.8X6
Enoxaparin (sodium)	T45.511	T45.512	T45.513	T45.514	T45.515	T45.516
Enpiprazole	T43.591	T43.592	T43.593	T43.594	T43.595	T43.596
Enprofylline	T48.6X1	T48.6X2	T48.6X3	T48.6X4	T48.6X5	T48.6X6
Enprostil	T47.1X1	T47.1X2	T47.1X3	T47.1X4	T47.1X5	T47.1X6
ENT preparations (anti-infectives)	T49.6X1	T49.6X2	T49.6X3	T49.6X4	T49.6X5	T49.6X6
Enviomycin	T36.8X1	T36.8X2	T36.8X3	T36.8X4	T36.8X5	T36.8X6
Enzodase	T45.3X1	T45.3X2	T45.3X3	T45.3X4	T45.3X5	T45.3X6
Enzyme NEC	T45.3X1	T45.3X2	T45.3X3	T45.3X4	T45.3X5	T45.3X6
depolymerizing	T49.8X1	T49.8X2	T49.8X3	T49.8X4	T49.8X5	T49.8X6
fibrolytic	T45.3X1	T45.3X2	T45.3X3	T45.3X4	T45.3X5	T45.3X6
gastric	T47.5X1	T47.5X2	T47.5X3	T47.5X4	T47.5X5	T47.5X6
intestinal	T47.5X1	T47.5X2	T47.5X3	T47.5X4	T47.5X5	T47.5X6
local action	T49.4X1	T49.4X2	T49.4X3	T49.4X4	T49.4X5	T49.4X6
proteolytic	T49.4X1	T49.4X2	T49.4X3	T49.4X4	T49.4X5	T49.4X6
thrombolytic	T45.3X1	T45.3X2	T45.3X3	T45.3X4	T45.3X5	T45.3X6
EPAB	T41.3X1	T41.3X2	T41.3X3	T41.3X4	T41.3X5	T41.3X6
Epanutin	T42.0X1	T42.0X2	T42.0X3	T42.0X4	T42.0X5	T42.0X6
Ephedra	T44.991	T44.992	T44.993	T44.994	T44.995	T44.996
Ephedrine	T44.991	T44.992	T44.993	T44.994	T44.995	T44.996
Epichlorhydrin, epichlorohydrin	T52.8X1	T52.8X2	T52.8X3	T52.8X4	—	—
Epicillin	T36.0X1	T36.0X2	T36.0X3	T36.0X4	T36.0X5	T36.0X6
Epiestriol	T38.5X1	T38.5X2	T38.5X3	T38.5X4	T38.5X5	T38.5X6
Epilim — see Sodium valproate						
Epimestrol	T38.5X1	T38.5X2	T38.5X3	T38.5X4	T38.5X5	T38.5X6
Epinephrine	T44.5X1	T44.5X2	T44.5X3	T44.5X4	T44.5X5	T44.5X6

Substance	Poisoning, Accidental (Unintentional)	Poisoning, Intentional Self-Harm	Poisoning, Assault	Poisoning, Undetermined	Adverse Effect	Underdosing
	External Cause (T-Code)					
Epirubicin	T45.1X1	T45.1X2	T45.1X3	T45.1X4	T45.1X5	T45.1X6
Epitiostanol	T38.7X1	T38.7X2	T38.7X3	T38.7X4	T38.7X5	T38.7X6
Epitizide	T50.2X1	T50.2X2	T50.2X3	T50.2X4	T50.2X5	T50.2X6
EPN	T60.0X1	T60.0X2	T60.0X3	T60.0X4	—	—
EPO	T45.8X1	T45.8X2	T45.8X3	T45.8X4	T45.8X5	T45.8X6
Epoetin alpha	T45.8X1	T45.8X2	T45.8X3	T45.8X4	T45.8X5	T45.8X6
Epomediol	T50.991	T50.992	T50.993	T50.994	T50.995	T50.996
Epoprostenol	T45.521	T45.522	T45.523	T45.524	T45.525	T45.526
Epoxy resin	T65.891	T65.892	T65.893	T65.894	—	—
Eprazinone	T48.4X1	T48.4X2	T48.4X3	T48.4X4	T48.4X5	T48.4X6
Epsilon amino-caproic acid	T45.621	T45.622	T45.623	T45.624	T45.625	T45.626
Epsom salt	T47.3X1	T47.3X2	T47.3X3	T47.3X4	T47.3X5	T47.3X6
Eptazocine	T40.4X1	T40.4X2	T40.4X3	T40.4X4	T40.4X5	T40.4X6
Equanil	T43.591	T43.592	T43.593	T43.594	T43.595	T43.596
Equisetum	T62.2X1	T62.2X2	T62.2X3	T62.2X4	—	—
diuretic	T50.2X1	T50.2X2	T50.2X3	T50.2X4	T50.2X5	T50.2X6
Ergobasine	T48.0X1	T48.0X2	T48.0X3	T48.0X4	T48.0X5	T48.0X6
Ergocalciferol	T45.2X1	T45.2X2	T45.2X3	T45.2X4	T45.2X5	T45.2X6
Ergoloid mesylates	T46.7X1	T46.7X2	T46.7X3	T46.7X4	T46.7X5	T46.7X6
Ergometrine	T48.0X1	T48.0X2	T48.0X3	T48.0X4	T48.0X5	T48.0X6
Ergonovine	T48.0X1	T48.0X2	T48.0X3	T48.0X4	T48.0X5	T48.0X6
Ergot NEC	T64.81	T64.82	T64.83	T64.84	—	—
derivative	T48.0X1	T48.0X2	T48.0X3	T48.0X4	T48.0X5	T48.0X6
medicinal (alkaloids)	T48.0X1	T48.0X2	T48.0X3	T48.0X4	T48.0X5	T48.0X6
prepared	T48.0X1	T48.0X2	T48.0X3	T48.0X4	T48.0X5	T48.0X6
Ergotamine	T46.5X1	T46.5X2	T46.5X3	T46.5X4	T46.5X5	T46.5X6
Ergotocine	T48.0X1	T48.0X2	T48.0X3	T48.0X4	T48.0X5	T48.0X6
Ergotrate	T48.0X1	T48.0X2	T48.0X3	T48.0X4	T48.0X5	T48.0X6
Eritrityl tetranitrate	T46.3X1	T46.3X2	T46.3X3	T46.3X4	T46.3X5	T46.3X6
Erythrityl tetranitrate	T46.3X1	T46.3X2	T46.3X3	T46.3X4	T46.3X5	T46.3X6
Erythrol tetranitrate	T46.3X1	T46.3X2	T46.3X3	T46.3X4	T46.3X5	T46.3X6
Erythromycin (salts)	T36.3X1	T36.3X2	T36.3X3	T36.3X4	T36.3X5	T36.3X6
ophthalmic preparation	T49.5X1	T49.5X2	T49.5X3	T49.5X4	T49.5X5	T49.5X6
topical NEC	T49.0X1	T49.0X2	T49.0X3	T49.0X4	T49.0X5	T49.0X6
Erythropoietin	T45.8X1	T45.8X2	T45.8X3	T45.8X4	T45.8X5	T45.8X6
human	T45.8X1	T45.8X2	T45.8X3	T45.8X4	T45.8X5	T45.8X6
Escin	T46.991	T46.992	T46.993	T46.994	T46.995	T46.996
Esculin	T45.2X1	T45.2X2	T45.2X3	T45.2X4	T45.2X5	T45.2X6
Esculoside	T45.2X1	T45.2X2	T45.2X3	T45.2X4	T45.2X5	T45.2X6

Substance	External Cause (T-Code)					
	Poisoning, Accidental (Unintentional)	Poisoning, Intentional Self-Harm	Poisoning, Assault	Poisoning, Undetermined	Adverse Effect	Underdosing
ESDT (ether-soluble tar distillate)	T49.1X1	T49.1X2	T49.1X3	T49.1X4	T49.1X5	T49.1X6
Eserine	T49.5X1	T49.5X2	T49.5X3	T49.5X4	T49.5X5	T49.5X6
Esflurbiprofen	T39.311	T39.312	T39.313	T39.314	T39.315	T39.316
Eskabarb	T42.3X1	T42.3X2	T42.3X3	T42.3X4	T42.3X5	T42.3X6
Eskalith	T43.8X1	T43.8X2	T43.8X3	T43.8X4	T43.8X5	T43.8X6
Esmolol	T44.7X1	T44.7X2	T44.7X3	T44.7X4	T44.7X5	T44.7X6
Estanozolol	T38.7X1	T38.7X2	T38.7X3	T38.7X4	T38.7X5	T38.7X6
Estazolam	T42.4X1	T42.4X2	T42.4X3	T42.4X4	T42.4X5	T42.4X6
Estradiol	T38.5X1	T38.5X2	T38.5X3	T38.5X4	T38.5X5	T38.5X6
with testosterone	T38.7X1	T38.7X2	T38.7X3	T38.7X4	T38.7X5	T38.7X6
benzoate	T38.5X1	T38.5X2	T38.5X3	T38.5X4	T38.5X5	T38.5X6
Estramustine	T45.1X1	T45.1X2	T45.1X3	T45.1X4	T45.1X5	T45.1X6
Estriol	T38.5X1	T38.5X2	T38.5X3	T38.5X4	T38.5X5	T38.5X6
Estrogen	T38.5X1	T38.5X2	T38.5X3	T38.5X4	T38.5X5	T38.5X6
with progesterone	T38.5X1	T38.5X2	T38.5X3	T38.5X4	T38.5X5	T38.5X6
conjugated	T38.5X1	T38.5X2	T38.5X3	T38.5X4	T38.5X5	T38.5X6
Estrone	T38.5X1	T38.5X2	T38.5X3	T38.5X4	T38.5X5	T38.5X6
Estropipate	T38.5X1	T38.5X2	T38.5X3	T38.5X4	T38.5X5	T38.5X6
Etacrynate sodium	T50.1X1	T50.1X2	T50.1X3	T50.1X4	T50.1X5	T50.1X6
Etacrynic acid	T50.1X1	T50.1X2	T50.1X3	T50.1X4	T50.1X5	T50.1X6
Etafedrine	T48.6X1	T48.6X2	T48.6X3	T48.6X4	T48.6X5	T48.6X6
Etafenone	T46.3X1	T46.3X2	T46.3X3	T46.3X4	T46.3X5	T46.3X6
Etambutol	T37.1X1	T37.1X2	T37.1X3	T37.1X4	T37.1X5	T37.1X6
Etamiphyllin	T48.6X1	T48.6X2	T48.6X3	T48.6X4	T48.6X5	T48.6X6
Etamivan	T50.7X1	T50.7X2	T50.7X3	T50.7X4	T50.7X5	T50.7X6
Etamsylate	T45.7X1	T45.7X2	T45.7X3	T45.7X4	T45.7X5	T45.7X6
Etebenecid	T50.4X1	T50.4X2	T50.4X3	T50.4X4	T50.4X5	T50.4X6
Ethacridine	T49.0X1	T49.0X2	T49.0X3	T49.0X4	T49.0X5	T49.0X6
Ethacrynic acid	T50.1X1	T50.1X2	T50.1X3	T50.1X4	T50.1X5	T50.1X6
Ethadione	T42.2X1	T42.2X2	T42.2X3	T42.2X4	T42.2X5	T42.2X6
Ethambutol	T37.1X1	T37.1X2	T37.1X3	T37.1X4	T37.1X5	T37.1X6
Ethamide	T50.2X1	T50.2X2	T50.2X3	T50.2X4	T50.2X5	T50.2X6
Ethamivan	T50.7X1	T50.7X2	T50.7X3	T50.7X4	T50.7X5	T50.7X6
Ethamsylate	T45.7X1	T45.7X2	T45.7X3	T45.7X4	T45.7X5	T45.7X6
Ethanol	T51.0X1	T51.0X2	T51.0X3	T51.0X4	—	—
beverage	T51.0X1	T51.0X2	T51.0X3	T51.0X4	—	—
Ethanolamine oleate	T46.8X1	T46.8X2	T46.8X3	T46.8X4	T46.8X5	T46.8X6
Ethaverine	T44.3X1	T44.3X2	T44.3X3	T44.3X4	T44.3X5	T44.3X6
Ethchlorvynol	T42.6X1	T42.6X2	T42.6X3	T42.6X4	T42.6X5	T42.6X6
Ethebenecid	T50.4X1	T50.4X2	T50.4X3	T50.4X4	T50.4X5	T50.4X6

Substance	Poisoning, Accidental (Unintentional)	Poisoning, Intentional Self-Harm	Poisoning, Assault	Poisoning, Undetermined	Adverse Effect	Underdosing
	External Cause (T-Code)					
Ether (vapor)	T41.0X1	T41.0X2	T41.0X3	T41.0X4	T41.0X5	T41.0X6
anesthetic	T41.0X1	T41.0X2	T41.0X3	T41.0X4	T41.0X5	T41.0X6
divinyl	T41.0X1	T41.0X2	T41.0X3	T41.0X4	T41.0X5	T41.0X6
ethyl (medicinal)	T41.0X1	T41.0X2	T41.0X3	T41.0X4	T41.0X5	T41.0X6
nonmedicinal	T52.8X1	T52.8X2	T52.8X3	T52.8X4	—	—
petroleum — *see Ligroin*						
solvent	T52.8X1	T52.8X2	T52.8X3	T52.8X4	—	—
Ethiazide	T50.2X1	T50.2X2	T50.2X3	T50.2X4	T50.2X5	T50.2X6
Ethidium chloride (vapor)	T59.891	T59.892	T59.893	T59.894	—	—
Ethinamate	T42.6X1	T42.6X2	T42.6X3	T42.6X4	T42.6X5	T42.6X6
Ethinylestradiol, ethinyloestradiol	T38.5X1	T38.5X2	T38.5X3	T38.5X4	T38.5X5	T38.5X6
with						
levonorgestrel	T38.4X1	T38.4X2	T38.4X3	T38.4X4	T38.4X5	T38.4X6
norethisterone	T38.4X1	T38.4X2	T38.4X3	T38.4X4	T38.4X5	T38.4X6
Ethiodized oil (131 I)	T50.8X1	T50.8X2	T50.8X3	T50.8X4	T50.8X5	T50.8X6
Ethion	T60.0X1	T60.0X2	T60.0X3	T60.0X4	—	—
Ethionamide	T37.1X1	T37.1X2	T37.1X3	T37.1X4	T37.1X5	T37.1X6
Ethioniamide	T37.1X1	T37.1X2	T37.1X3	T37.1X4	T37.1X5	T37.1X6
Ethisterone	T38.5X1	T38.5X2	T38.5X3	T38.5X4	T38.5X5	T38.5X6
Ethobral	T42.3X1	T42.3X2	T42.3X3	T42.3X4	T42.3X5	T42.3X6
Ethocaine (infiltration) (topical)	T41.3X1	T41.3X2	T41.3X3	T41.3X4	T41.3X5	T41.3X6
nerve block (peripheral) (plexus)	T41.3X1	T41.3X2	T41.3X3	T41.3X4	T41.3X5	T41.3X6
spinal	T41.3X1	T41.3X2	T41.3X3	T41.3X4	T41.3X5	T41.3X6
Ethoheptazine	T40.4X1	T40.4X2	T40.4X3	T40.4X4	T40.4X5	T40.4X6
Ethopropazine	T44.3X1	T44.3X2	T44.3X3	T44.3X4	T44.3X5	T44.3X6
Ethosuximide	T42.2X1	T42.2X2	T42.2X3	T42.2X4	T42.2X5	T42.2X6
Ethotoin	T42.0X1	T42.0X2	T42.0X3	T42.0X4	T42.0X5	T42.0X6
Ethoxazene	T37.91	T37.92	T37.93	T37.94	T37.95	T37.96
Ethoxazorutoside	T46.991	T46.992	T46.993	T46.994	T46.995	T46.996
2-Ethoxyethanol	T52.3X1	T52.3X2	T52.3X3	T52.3X4	—	—
Ethoxzolamide	T50.2X1	T50.2X2	T50.2X3	T50.2X4	T50.2X5	T50.2X6
Ethyl						
acetate	T52.8X1	T52.8X2	T52.8X3	T52.8X4	—	—
alcohol	T51.0X1	T51.0X2	T51.0X3	T51.0X4	—	—
beverage	T51.0X1	T51.0X2	T51.0X3	T51.0X4	—	—
aldehyde (vapor)	T59.891	T59.892	T59.893	T59.894	—	—
liquid	T52.8X1	T52.8X2	T52.8X3	T52.8X4	—	—
aminobenzoate	T41.3X1	T41.3X2	T41.3X3	T41.3X4	T41.3X5	T41.3X6
aminophenothiazine	T43.3X1	T43.3X2	T43.3X3	T43.3X4	T43.3X5	T43.3X6
benzoate	T52.8X1	T52.8X2	T52.8X3	T52.8X4	—	—

| | External Cause (T-Code) | | | | | |
Substance	Poisoning, Accidental (Unintentional)	Poisoning, Intentional Self-Harm	Poisoning, Assault	Poisoning, Undetermined	Adverse Effect	Underdosing
Ethyl *(Continued)*						
biscoumacetate	T45.511	T45.512	T45.513	T45.514	T45.515	T45.516
bromide (anesthetic)	T41.0X1	T41.0X2	T41.0X3	T41.0X4	T41.0X5	T41.0X6
carbamate	T45.1X1	T45.1X2	T45.1X3	T45.1X4	T45.1X5	T45.1X6
carbinol	T51.3X1	T51.3X2	T51.3X3	T51.3X4	—	—
carbonate	T52.8X1	T52.8X2	T52.8X3	T52.8X4	—	—
chaulmoograte	T37.1X1	T37.1X2	T37.1X3	T37.1X4	T37.1X5	T37.1X6
chloride (anesthetic)	T41.0X1	T41.0X2	T41.0X3	T41.0X4	T41.0X5	T41.0X6
anesthetic (local)	T41.3X1	T41.3X2	T41.3X3	T41.3X4	T41.3X5	T41.3X6
inhaled	T41.0X1	T41.0X2	T41.0X3	T41.0X4	T41.0X5	T41.0X6
local	T49.4X1	T49.4X2	T49.4X3	T49.4X4	T49.4X5	T49.4X6
solvent	T53.6X1	T53.6X2	T53.6X3	T53.6X4	—	—
dibunate	T48.3X1	T48.3X2	T48.3X3	T48.3X4	T48.3X5	T48.3X6
dichloroarsine (vapor)	T57.0X1	T57.0X2	T57.0X3	T57.0X4	—	—
estranol	T38.7X1	T38.7X2	T38.7X3	T38.7X4	T38.7X5	T38.7X6
ether — *see also ether*	T52.8X1	T52.8X2	T52.8X3	T52.8X4	—	—
formate NEC (solvent)	T52.0X1	T52.0X2	T52.0X3	T52.0X4	—	—
fumarate	T49.4X1	T49.4X2	T49.4X3	T49.4X4	T49.4X5	T49.4X6
hydroxyisobutyrate NEC (solvent)	T52.8X1	T52.8X2	T52.8X3	T52.8X4	—	—
iodoacetate	T59.3X1	T59.3X2	T59.3X3	T59.3X4	—	—
lactate NEC (solvent)	T52.8X1	T52.8X2	T52.8X3	T52.8X4	—	—
loflazepate	T42.4X1	T42.4X2	T42.4X3	T42.4X4	T42.4X5	T42.4X6
mercuric chloride	T56.1X1	T56.1X2	T56.1X3	T56.1X4	—	—
methylcarbinol	T51.8X1	T51.8X2	T51.8X3	T51.8X4	—	—
morphine	T40.2X1	T40.2X2	T40.2X3	T40.2X4	T40.2X5	T40.2X6
noradrenaline	T48.6X1	T48.6X2	T48.6X3	T48.6X4	T48.6X5	T48.6X6
oxybutyrate NEC (solvent)	T52.8X1	T52.8X2	T52.8X3	T52.8X4	—	—
Ethylene (gas)	T59.891	T59.892	T59.893	T59.894	—	—
anesthetic (general)	T41.0X1	T41.0X2	T41.0X3	T41.0X4	T41.0X5	T41.0X6
chlorohydrin	T52.8X1	T52.8X2	T52.8X3	T52.8X4	—	—
vapor	T53.6X1	T53.6X2	T53.6X3	T53.6X4	—	—
dichloride	T52.8X1	T52.8X2	T52.8X3	T52.8X4	—	—
vapor	T53.6X1	T53.6X2	T53.6X3	T53.6X4	—	—
dinitrate	T52.3X1	T52.3X2	T52.3X3	T52.3X4	—	—
glycol(s)	T52.8X1	T52.8X2	T52.8X3	T52.8X4	—	—
dinitrate	T52.3X1	T52.3X2	T52.3X3	T52.3X4	—	—
monobutyl ether	T52.3X1	T52.3X2	T52.3X3	T52.3X4	—	—
imine	T54.1X1	T54.1X2	T54.1X3	T54.1X4	—	—
oxide (fumigant) (nonmedicinal)	T59.891	T59.892	T59.893	T59.894	—	—
medicinal	T49.0X1	T49.0X2	T49.0X3	T49.0X4	T49.0X5	T49.0X6

Substance	External Cause (T-Code)					
	Poisoning, Accidental (Unintentional)	Poisoning, Intentional Self-Harm	Poisoning, Assault	Poisoning, Undetermined	Adverse Effect	Underdosing
Ethylenediamine theophylline	T48.6X1	T48.6X2	T48.6X3	T48.6X4	T48.6X5	T48.6X6
Ethylenediaminetetra-acetic acid	T50.6X1	T50.6X2	T50.6X3	T50.6X4	T50.6X5	T50.6X6
Ethylenedinitrilotetra-acetate	T50.6X1	T50.6X2	T50.6X3	T50.6X4	T50.6X5	T50.6X6
Ethylestrenol	T38.7X1	T38.7X2	T38.7X3	T38.7X4	T38.7X5	T38.7X6
Ethylhydroxycellulose	T47.4X1	T47.4X2	T47.4X3	T47.4X4	T47.4X5	T47.4X6
Ethylidene						
chloride NEC	T53.6X1	T53.6X2	T53.6X3	T53.6X4	—	—
diacetate	T60.3X1	T60.3X2	T60.3X3	T60.3X4	—	—
dicoumarin	T45.511	T45.512	T45.513	T45.514	T45.515	T45.516
dicoumarol	T45.511	T45.512	T45.513	T45.514	T45.515	T45.516
diethyl ether	T52.0X1	T52.0X2	T52.0X3	T52.0X4	—	—
Ethylmorphine	T40.2X1	T40.2X2	T40.2X3	T40.2X4	T40.2X5	T40.2X6
Ethylnorepinephrine	T48.6X1	T48.6X2	T48.6X3	T48.6X4	T48.6X5	T48.6X6
Ethylparachlorophen-oxyisobutyrate	T46.6X1	T46.6X2	T46.6X3	T46.6X4	T46.6X5	T46.6X6
Ethynodiol	T38.4X1	T38.4X2	T38.4X3	T38.4X4	T38.4X5	T38.4X6
with mestranol diacetate	T38.4X1	T38.4X2	T38.4X3	T38.4X4	T38.4X5	T38.4X6
Etidocaine	T41.3X1	T41.3X2	T41.3X3	T41.3X4	T41.3X5	T41.3X6
infiltration (subcutaneous)	T41.3X1	T41.3X2	T41.3X3	T41.3X4	T41.3X5	T41.3X6
nerve (peripheral) (plexus)	T41.3X1	T41.3X2	T41.3X3	T41.3X4	T41.3X5	T41.3X6
Etidronate	T50.991	T50.992	T50.993	T50.994	T50.995	T50.996
Etidronic acid (disodium salt)	T50.991	T50.992	T50.993	T50.994	T50.995	T50.996
Etifoxine	T42.6X1	T42.6X2	T42.6X3	T42.6X4	T42.6X5	T42.6X6
Etilefrine	T44.4X1	T44.4X2	T44.4X3	T44.4X4	T44.4X5	T44.4X6
Etilfen	T42.3X1	T42.3X2	T42.3X3	T42.3X4	T42.3X5	T42.3X6
Etinodiol	T38.4X1	T38.4X2	T38.4X3	T38.4X4	T38.4X5	T38.4X6
Etiroxate	T46.6X1	T46.6X2	T46.6X3	T46.6X4	T46.6X5	T46.6X6
Etizolam	T42.4X1	T42.4X2	T42.4X3	T42.4X4	T42.4X5	T42.4X6
Etodolac	T39.391	T39.392	T39.393	T39.394	T39.395	T39.396
Etofamide	T37.3X1	T37.3X2	T37.3X3	T37.3X4	T37.3X5	T37.3X6
Etofibrate	T46.6X1	T46.6X2	T46.6X3	T46.6X4	T46.6X5	T46.6X6
Etofylline	T46.7X1	T46.7X2	T46.7X3	T46.7X4	T46.7X5	T46.7X6
clofibrate	T46.6X1	T46.6X2	T46.6X3	T46.6X4	T46.6X5	T46.6X6
Etoglucid	T45.1X1	T45.1X2	T45.1X3	T45.1X4	T45.1X5	T45.1X6
Etomidate	T41.1X1	T41.1X2	T41.1X3	T41.1X4	T41.1X5	T41.1X6
Etomide	T39.8X1	T39.8X2	T39.8X3	T39.8X4	T39.8X5	T39.8X6
Etomidoline	T44.3X1	T44.3X2	T44.3X3	T44.3X4	T44.3X5	T44.3X6
Etoposide	T45.1X1	T45.1X2	T45.1X3	T45.1X4	T45.1X5	T45.1X6
Etorphine	T40.2X1	T40.2X2	T40.2X3	T40.2X4	T40.2X5	T40.2X6
Etoval	T42.3X1	T42.3X2	T42.3X3	T42.3X4	T42.3X5	T42.3X6
Etozolin	T50.1X1	T50.1X2	T50.1X3	T50.1X4	T50.1X5	T50.1X6

	External Cause (T-Code)					
Substance	Poisoning, Accidental (Unintentional)	Poisoning, Intentional Self-Harm	Poisoning, Assault	Poisoning, Undetermined	Adverse Effect	Underdosing
Etretinate	T50.991	T50.992	T50.993	T50.994	T50.995	T50.996
Etryptamine	T43.691	T43.692	T43.693	T43.694	T43.695	T43.696
Etybenzatropine	T44.3X1	T44.3X2	T44.3X3	T44.3X4	T44.3X5	T44.3X6
Etynodiol	T38.4X1	T38.4X2	T38.4X3	T38.4X4	T38.4X5	T38.4X6
Eucaine	T41.3X1	T41.3X2	T41.3X3	T41.3X4	T41.3X5	T41.3X6
Eucalyptus oil	T49.7X1	T49.7X2	T49.7X3	T49.7X4	T49.7X5	T49.7X6
Eucatropine	T49.5X1	T49.5X2	T49.5X3	T49.5X4	T49.5X5	T49.5X6
Eucodal	T40.2X1	T40.2X2	T40.2X3	T40.2X4	T40.2X5	T40.2X6
Euneryl	T42.3X1	T42.3X2	T42.3X3	T42.3X4	T42.3X5	T42.3X6
Euphthalmine	T44.3X1	T44.3X2	T44.3X3	T44.3X4	T44.3X5	T44.3X6
Eurax	T49.0X1	T49.0X2	T49.0X3	T49.0X4	T49.0X5	T49.0X6
Euresol	T49.4X1	T49.4X2	T49.4X3	T49.4X4	T49.4X5	T49.4X6
Euthroid	T38.1X1	T38.1X2	T38.1X3	T38.1X4	T38.1X5	T38.1X6
Evans blue	T50.8X1	T50.8X2	T50.8X3	T50.8X4	T50.8X5	T50.8X6
Evipal	T42.3X1	T42.3X2	T42.3X3	T42.3X4	T42.3X5	T42.3X6
sodium	T41.1X1	T41.1X2	T41.1X3	T41.1X4	T41.1X5	T41.1X6
Evipan	T42.3X1	T42.3X2	T42.3X3	T42.3X4	T42.3X5	T42.3X6
sodium	T41.1X1	T41.1X2	T41.1X3	T41.1X4	T41.1X5	T41.1X6
Exalamide	T49.0X1	T49.0X2	T49.0X3	T49.0X4	T49.0X5	T49.0X6
Exalgin	T39.1X1	T39.1X2	T39.1X3	T39.1X4	T39.1X5	T39.1X6
Excipients, pharmaceutical	T50.901	T50.902	T50.903	T50.904	T50.905	T50.906
Exhaust gas (engine) (motor vehicle)	T58.01	T58.02	T58.03	T58.04	—	—
Ex-Lax (phenolphthalein)	T47.2X1	T47.2X2	T47.2X3	T47.2X4	T47.2X5	T47.2X6
Expectorant NEC	T48.4X1	T48.4X2	T48.4X3	T48.4X4	T48.4X5	T48.4X6
Extended insulin zinc suspension	T38.3X1	T38.3X2	T38.3X3	T38.3X4	T38.3X5	T38.3X6
External medications (skin) (mucous membrane)	T49.91	T49.92	T49.93	T49.94	T49.95	T49.96
dental agent	T49.7X1	T49.7X2	T49.7X3	T49.7X4	T49.7X5	T49.7X6
ENT agent	T49.6X1	T49.6X2	T49.6X3	T49.6X4	T49.6X5	T49.6X6
ophthalmic preparation	T49.5X1	T49.5X2	T49.5X3	T49.5X4	T49.5X5	T49.5X6
specified NEC	T49.8X1	T49.8X2	T49.8X3	T49.8X4	T49.8X5	T49.8X6
Extrapyramidal antagonist NEC	T44.3X1	T44.3X2	T44.3X3	T44.3X4	T44.3X5	T44.3X6
Eye agents (anti-infective)	T49.5X1	T49.5X2	T49.5X3	T49.5X4	T49.5X5	T49.5X6
Eye drug NEC	T49.5X1	T49.5X2	T49.5X3	T49.5X4	T49.5X5	T49.5X6
F						
FAC (fluorouracil + doxorubicin + cyclophosphamide)	T45.1X1	T45.1X2	T45.1X3	T45.1X4	T45.1X5	T45.1X6
Factor						
I (fibrinogen)	T45.8X1	T45.8X2	T45.8X3	T45.8X4	T45.8X5	T45.8X6
III (thromboplastin)	T45.8X1	T45.8X2	T45.8X3	T45.8X4	T45.8X5	T45.8X6
VIII (antihemophilic Factor) (Concentrate)	T45.8X1	T45.8X2	T45.8X3	T45.8X4	T45.8X5	T45.8X6

Substance	Poisoning, Accidental (Unintentional)	Poisoning, Intentional Self-Harm	Poisoning, Assault	Poisoning, Undetermined	Adverse Effect	Underdosing
External Cause (T-Code)						
Factor *(Continued)*						
IX complex	T45.7X1	T45.7X2	T45.7X3	T45.7X4	T45.7X5	T45.7X6
human	T45.8X1	T45.8X2	T45.8X3	T45.8X4	T45.8X5	T45.8X6
Famotidine	T47.0X1	T47.0X2	T47.0X3	T47.0X4	T47.0X5	T47.0X6
Fat suspension, intravenous	T50.991	T50.992	T50.993	T50.994	T50.995	T50.996
Fazadinium bromide	T48.1X1	T48.1X2	T48.1X3	T48.1X4	T48.1X5	T48.1X6
Febarbamate	T42.3X1	T42.3X2	T42.3X3	T42.3X4	T42.3X5	T42.3X6
Fecal softener	T47.4X1	T47.4X2	T47.4X3	T47.4X4	T47.4X5	T47.4X6
Fedrilate	T48.3X1	T48.3X2	T48.3X3	T48.3X4	T48.3X5	T48.3X6
Felodipine	T46.1X1	T46.1X2	T46.1X3	T46.1X4	T46.1X5	T46.1X6
Felypressin	T38.891	T38.892	T38.893	T38.894	T38.895	T38.896
Femoxetine	T43.221	T43.222	T43.223	T43.224	T43.225	T43.226
Fenalcomine	T46.3X1	T46.3X2	T46.3X3	T46.3X4	T46.3X5	T46.3X6
Fenamisal	T37.1X1	T37.1X2	T37.1X3	T37.1X4	T37.1X5	T37.1X6
Fenazone	T39.2X1	T39.2X2	T39.2X3	T39.2X4	T39.2X5	T39.2X6
Fenbendazole	T37.4X1	T37.4X2	T37.4X3	T37.4X4	T37.4X5	T37.4X6
Fenbutrazate	T50.5X1	T50.5X2	T50.5X3	T50.5X4	T50.5X5	T50.5X6
Fencamfamine	T43.691	T43.692	T43.693	T43.694	T43.695	T43.696
Fendiline	T46.1X1	T46.1X2	T46.1X3	T46.1X4	T46.1X5	T46.1X6
Fenetylline	T43.691	T43.692	T43.693	T43.694	T43.695	T43.696
Fenflumizole	T39.391	T39.392	T39.393	T39.394	T39.395	T39.396
Fenfluramine	T50.5X1	T50.5X2	T50.5X3	T50.5X4	T50.5X5	T50.5X6
Fenobarbital	T42.3X1	T42.3X2	T42.3X3	T42.3X4	T42.3X5	T42.3X6
Fenofibrate	T46.6X1	T46.6X2	T46.6X3	T46.6X4	T46.6X5	T46.6X6
Fenoprofen	T39.311	T39.312	T39.313	T39.314	T39.315	T39.316
Fenoterol	T48.6X1	T48.6X2	T48.6X3	T48.6X4	T48.6X5	T48.6X6
Fenoverine	T44.3X1	T44.3X2	T44.3X3	T44.3X4	T44.3X5	T44.3X6
Fenoxazoline	T48.5X1	T48.5X2	T48.5X3	T48.5X4	T48.5X5	T48.5X6
Fenproporex	T50.5X1	T50.5X2	T50.5X3	T50.5X4	T50.5X5	T50.5X6
Fenquizone	T50.2X1	T50.2X2	T50.2X3	T50.2X4	T50.2X5	T50.2X6
Fentanyl	T40.4X1	T40.4X2	T40.4X3	T40.4X4	T40.4X5	T40.4X6
Fentazin	T43.3X1	T43.3X2	T43.3X3	T43.3X4	T43.3X5	T43.3X6
Fenthion	T60.0X1	T60.0X2	T60.0X3	T60.0X4	—	—
Fenticlor	T49.0X1	T49.0X2	T49.0X3	T49.0X4	T49.0X5	T49.0X6
Fenylbutazone	T39.2X1	T39.2X2	T39.2X3	T39.2X4	T39.2X5	T39.2X6
Feprazone	T39.2X1	T39.2X2	T39.2X3	T39.2X4	T39.2X5	T39.2X6
Fer de lance (bite) (venom)	T63.061	T63.062	T63.063	T63.064	—	—
Ferric — *see also Iron*						
chloride	T45.4X1	T45.4X2	T45.4X3	T45.4X4	T45.4X5	T45.4X6
citrate	T45.4X1	T45.4X2	T45.4X3	T45.4X4	T45.4X5	T45.4X6

Substance	External Cause (T-Code)					
	Poisoning, Accidental (Unintentional)	Poisoning, Intentional Self-Harm	Poisoning, Assault	Poisoning, Undetermined	Adverse Effect	Underdosing
Ferric (Continued)						
hydroxide						
colloidal	T45.4X1	T45.4X2	T45.4X3	T45.4X4	T45.4X5	T45.4X6
polymaltose	T45.4X1	T45.4X2	T45.4X3	T45.4X4	T45.4X5	T45.4X6
pyrophosphate	T45.4X1	T45.4X2	T45.4X3	T45.4X4	T45.4X5	T45.4X6
Ferritin	T45.4X1	T45.4X2	T45.4X3	T45.4X4	T45.4X5	T45.4X6
Ferrocholinate	T45.4X1	T45.4X2	T45.4X3	T45.4X4	T45.4X5	T45.4X6
Ferrodextrane	T45.4X1	T45.4X2	T45.4X3	T45.4X4	T45.4X5	T45.4X6
Ferropolimaler	T45.4X1	T45.4X2	T45.4X3	T45.4X4	T45.4X5	T45.4X6
Ferrous — see also Iron						
phosphate	T45.4X1	T45.4X2	T45.4X3	T45.4X4	T45.4X5	T45.4X6
salt	T45.4X1	T45.4X2	T45.4X3	T45.4X4	T45.4X5	T45.4X6
with folic acid	T45.4X1	T45.4X2	T45.4X3	T45.4X4	T45.4X5	T45.4X6
Ferrous fumerate, gluconate, lactate, salt NEC, sulfate (medicinal)	T45.4X1	T45.4X2	T45.4X3	T45.4X4	T45.4X5	T45.4X6
Ferrovanadium (fumes)	T59.891	T59.892	T59.893	T59.894	—	—
Ferrum — see Iron						
Fertilizers NEC	T65.891	T65.892	T65.893	T65.894	—	—
with herbicide mixture	T60.3X1	T60.3X2	T60.3X3	T60.3X4	—	—
Fetoxilate	T47.6X1	T47.6X2	T47.6X3	T47.6X4	T47.6X5	T47.6X6
Fiber, dietary	T47.4X1	T47.4X2	T47.4X3	T47.4X4	T47.4X5	T47.4X6
Fibrinogen (human)	T45.8X1	T45.8X2	T45.8X3	T45.8X4	T45.8X5	T45.8X6
Fibrinolysin (human)	T45.691	T45.692	T45.693	T45.694	T45.695	T45.696
Fibrinolysis						
affecting drug	T45.601	T45.602	T45.603	T45.604	T45.605	T45.606
inhibitor NEC	T45.621	T45.622	T45.623	T45.624	T45.625	T45.626
Fibrinolytic drug	T45.611	T45.612	T45.613	T45.614	T45.615	T45.616
Filix mas	T37.4X1	T37.4X2	T37.4X3	T37.4X4	T37.4X5	T37.4X6
Filtering cream	T49.3X1	T49.3X2	T49.3X3	T49.3X4	T49.3X5	T49.3X6
Fiorinal	T39.011	T39.012	T39.013	T39.014	T39.015	T39.016
Firedamp	T59.891	T59.892	T59.893	T59.894	—	—
Fish, noxious, nonbacterial	T61.91	T61.92	T61.93	T61.94	—	—
ciguatera	T61.01	T61.02	T61.03	T61.04	—	—
scombroid	T61.11	T61.12	T61.13	T61.14	—	—
shell	T61.781	T61.782	T61.783	T61.784	—	—
specified NEC	T61.771	T61.772	T61.773	T61.774	—	—
Flagyl	T37.3X1	T37.3X2	T37.3X3	T37.3X4	T37.3X5	T37.3X6
Flavine adenine dinucleotide	T45.2X1	T45.2X2	T45.2X3	T45.2X4	T45.2X5	T45.2X6
Flavodic acid	T46.991	T46.992	T46.993	T46.994	T46.995	T46.996
Flavoxate	T44.3X1	T44.3X2	T44.3X3	T44.3X4	T44.3X5	T44.3X6

Substance	External Cause (T-Code)					
	Poisoning, Accidental (Unintentional)	Poisoning, Intentional Self-Harm	Poisoning, Assault	Poisoning, Undetermined	Adverse Effect	Underdosing
Flaxedil	T48.1X1	T48.1X2	T48.1X3	T48.1X4	T48.1X5	T48.1X6
Flaxseed (medicinal)	T49.3X1	T49.3X2	T49.3X3	T49.3X4	T49.3X5	T49.3X6
Flecainide	T46.2X1	T46.2X2	T46.2X3	T46.2X4	T46.2X5	T46.2X6
Fleroxacin	T36.8X1	T36.8X2	T36.8X3	T36.8X4	T36.8X5	T36.8X6
Floctafenine	T39.8X1	T39.8X2	T39.8X3	T39.8X4	T39.8X5	T39.8X6
Flomax	T44.6X1	T44.6X2	T44.6X3	T44.6X4	T44.6X5	T44.6X6
Flomoxef	T36.1X1	T36.1X2	T36.1X3	T36.1X4	T36.1X5	T36.1X6
Flopropione	T44.3X1	T44.3X2	T44.3X3	T44.3X4	T44.3X5	T44.3X6
Florantyrone	T47.5X1	T47.5X2	T47.5X3	T47.5X4	T47.5X5	T47.5X6
Floraquin	T37.8X1	T37.8X2	T37.8X3	T37.8X4	T37.8X5	T37.8X6
Florinef	T38.0X1	T38.0X2	T38.0X3	T38.0X4	T38.0X5	T38.0X6
ENT agent	T49.6X1	T49.6X2	T49.6X3	T49.6X4	T49.6X5	T49.6X6
ophthalmic preparation	T49.5X1	T49.5X2	T49.5X3	T49.5X4	T49.5X5	T49.5X6
topical NEC	T49.0X1	T49.0X2	T49.0X3	T49.0X4	T49.0X5	T49.0X6
Flowers of sulfur	T49.4X1	T49.4X2	T49.4X3	T49.4X4	T49.4X5	T49.4X6
Floxuridine	T45.1X1	T45.1X2	T45.1X3	T45.1X4	T45.1X5	T45.1X6
Fluanisone	T43.4X1	T43.4X2	T43.4X3	T43.4X4	T43.4X5	T43.4X6
Flubendazole	T37.4X1	T37.4X2	T37.4X3	T37.4X4	T37.4X5	T37.4X6
Fluclorolone acetonide	T49.0X1	T49.0X2	T49.0X3	T49.0X4	T49.0X5	T49.0X6
Flucloxacillin	T36.0X1	T36.0X2	T36.0X3	T36.0X4	T36.0X5	T36.0X6
Fluconazole	T37.8X1	T37.8X2	T37.8X3	T37.8X4	T37.8X5	T37.8X6
Flucytosine	T37.8X1	T37.8X2	T37.8X3	T37.8X4	T37.8X5	T37.8X6
Fludeoxyglucose (18F)	T50.8X1	T50.8X2	T50.8X3	T50.8X4	T50.8X5	T50.8X6
Fludiazepam	T42.4X1	T42.4X2	T42.4X3	T42.4X4	T42.4X5	T42.4X6
Fludrocortisone	T50.0X1	T50.0X2	T50.0X3	T50.0X4	T50.0X5	T50.0X6
ENT agent	T49.6X1	T49.6X2	T49.6X3	T49.6X4	T49.6X5	T49.6X6
ophthalmic preparation	T49.5X1	T49.5X2	T49.5X3	T49.5X4	T49.5X5	T49.5X6
topical NEC	T49.0X1	T49.0X2	T49.0X3	T49.0X4	T49.0X5	T49.0X6
Fludroxycortide	T49.0X1	T49.0X2	T49.0X3	T49.0X4	T49.0X5	T49.0X6
Flufenamic acid	T39.391	T39.392	T39.393	T39.394	T39.395	T39.396
Fluindione	T45.511	T45.512	T45.513	T45.514	T45.515	T45.516
Flumequine	T37.8X1	T37.8X2	T37.8X3	T37.8X4	T37.8X5	T37.8X6
Flumethasone	T49.0X1	T49.0X2	T49.0X3	T49.0X4	T49.0X5	T49.0X6
Flumethiazide	T50.2X1	T50.2X2	T50.2X3	T50.2X4	T50.2X5	T50.2X6
Flumidin	T37.5X1	T37.5X2	T37.5X3	T37.5X4	T37.5X5	T37.5X6
Flunarizine	T46.7X1	T46.7X2	T46.7X3	T46.7X4	T46.7X5	T46.7X6
Flunidazole	T37.8X1	T37.8X2	T37.8X3	T37.8X4	T37.8X5	T37.8X6
Flunisolide	T48.6X1	T48.6X2	T48.6X3	T48.6X4	T48.6X5	T48.6X6
Flunitrazepam	T42.4X1	T42.4X2	T42.4X3	T42.4X4	T42.4X5	T42.4X6

TABLE OF DRUGS AND CHEMICALS

627

Substance	Poisoning, Accidental (Unintentional)	Poisoning, Intentional Self-Harm	Poisoning, Assault	Poisoning, Undetermined	Adverse Effect	Underdosing
	External Cause (T-Code)					
Fluocinolone (acetonide)	T49.0X1	T49.0X2	T49.0X3	T49.0X4	T49.0X5	T49.0X6
Fluocinonide	T49.0X1	T49.0X2	T49.0X3	T49.0X4	T49.0X5	T49.0X6
Fluocortin (butyl)	T49.0X1	T49.0X2	T49.0X3	T49.0X4	T49.0X5	T49.0X6
Fluocortolone	T49.0X1	T49.0X2	T49.0X3	T49.0X4	T49.0X5	T49.0X6
Fluohydrocortisone	T38.0X1	T38.0X2	T38.0X3	T38.0X4	T38.0X5	T38.0X6
ENT agent	T49.6X1	T49.6X2	T49.6X3	T49.6X4	T49.6X5	T49.6X6
ophthalmic preparation	T49.5X1	T49.5X2	T49.5X3	T49.5X4	T49.5X5	T49.5X6
topical NEC	T49.0X1	T49.0X2	T49.0X3	T49.0X4	T49.0X5	T49.0X6
Fluonid	T49.0X1	T49.0X2	T49.0X3	T49.0X4	T49.0X5	T49.0X6
Fluopromazine	T43.3X1	T43.3X2	T43.3X3	T43.3X4	T43.3X5	T43.3X6
Fluoroacetate	T60.8X1	T60.8X2	T60.8X3	T60.8X4	—	—
Fluorescein	T50.8X1	T50.8X2	T50.8X3	T50.8X4	T50.8X5	T50.8X6
Fluorhydrocortisone	T50.0X1	T50.0X2	T50.0X3	T50.0X4	T50.0X5	T50.0X6
Fluoride (nonmedicinal) (pesticide) (sodium) NEC	T60.8X1	T60.8X2	T60.8X3	T60.8X4	—	—
hydrogen — see Hydrofluoric acid						
medicinal NEC	T50.991	T50.992	T50.993	T50.994	T50.995	T50.996
dental use	T49.7X1	T49.7X2	T49.7X3	T49.7X4	T49.7X5	T49.7X6
not pesticide NEC	T54.91	T54.92	T54.93	T54.94	—	—
stannous	T49.7X1	T49.7X2	T49.7X3	T49.7X4	T49.7X5	T49.7X6
Fluorinated corticosteroids	T38.0X1	T38.0X2	T38.0X3	T38.0X4	T38.0X5	T38.0X6
Fluorine (gas)	T59.5X1	T59.5X2	T59.5X3	T59.5X4	—	—
salt — see Fluoride(s)						
Fluoristan	T49.7X1	T49.7X2	T49.7X3	T49.7X4	T49.7X5	T49.7X6
Fluormetholone	T49.0X1	T49.0X2	T49.0X3	T49.0X4	T49.0X5	T49.0X6
Fluoroacetate	T60.8X1	T60.8X2	T60.8X3	T60.8X4	—	—
Fluorocarbon monomer	T53.6X1	T53.6X2	T53.6X3	T53.6X4	—	—
Fluorocytosine	T37.8X1	T37.8X2	T37.8X3	T37.8X4	T37.8X5	T37.8X6
Fluorodeoxyuridine	T45.1X1	T45.1X2	T45.1X3	T45.1X4	T45.1X5	T45.1X6
Fluorometholone	T49.0X1	T49.0X2	T49.0X3	T49.0X4	T49.0X5	T49.0X6
ophthalmic preparation	T49.5X1	T49.5X2	T49.5X3	T49.5X4	T49.5X5	T49.5X6
Fluorophosphate insecticide	T60.0X1	T60.0X2	T60.0X3	T60.0X4	—	—
Fluorosol	T46.3X1	T46.3X2	T46.3X3	T46.3X4	T46.3X5	T46.3X6
Fluorouracil	T45.1X1	T45.1X2	T45.1X3	T45.1X4	T45.1X5	T45.1X6
Fluorphenylalanine	T49.5X1	T49.5X2	T49.5X3	T49.5X4	T49.5X5	T49.5X6
Fluothane	T41.0X1	T41.0X2	T41.0X3	T41.0X4	T41.0X5	T41.0X6
Fluoxetine	T43.221	T43.222	T43.223	T43.224	T43.225	T43.226
Fluoxymesterone	T38.7X1	T38.7X2	T38.7X3	T38.7X4	T38.7X5	T38.7X6
Flupenthixol	T43.4X1	T43.4X2	T43.4X3	T43.4X4	T43.4X5	T43.4X6
Flupentixol	T43.4X1	T43.4X2	T43.4X3	T43.4X4	T43.4X5	T43.4X6
Fluphenazine	T43.3X1	T43.3X2	T43.3X3	T43.3X4	T43.3X5	T43.3X6

Substance	External Cause (T-Code)					
	Poisoning, Accidental (Unintentional)	Poisoning, Intentional Self-Harm	Poisoning, Assault	Poisoning, Undetermined	Adverse Effect	Underdosing
Fluprednidene	T49.0X1	T49.0X2	T49.0X3	T49.0X4	T49.0X5	T49.0X6
Fluprednisolone	T38.0X1	T38.0X2	T38.0X3	T38.0X4	T38.0X5	T38.0X6
Fluradoline	T39.8X1	T39.8X2	T39.8X3	T39.8X4	T39.8X5	T39.8X6
Flurandrenolide	T49.0X1	T49.0X2	T49.0X3	T49.0X4	T49.0X5	T49.0X6
Flurandrenolone	T49.0X1	T49.0X2	T49.0X3	T49.0X4	T49.0X5	T49.0X6
Flurazepam	T42.4X1	T42.4X2	T42.4X3	T42.4X4	T42.4X5	T42.4X6
Flurbiprofen	T39.311	T39.312	T39.313	T39.314	T39.315	T39.316
Flurobate	T49.0X1	T49.0X2	T49.0X3	T49.0X4	T49.0X5	T49.0X6
Flurotyl	T43.291	T43.292	T43.293	T43.294	T43.295	T43.296
Fluroxene	T41.0X1	T41.0X2	T41.0X3	T41.0X4	T41.0X5	T41.0X6
Fluspirilene	T43.591	T43.592	T43.593	T43.594	T43.595	T43.596
Flutamide	T38.6X1	T38.6X2	T38.6X3	T38.6X4	T38.6X5	T38.6X6
Flutazolam	T42.4X1	T42.4X2	T42.4X3	T42.4X4	T42.4X5	T42.4X6
Fluticasone propionate	T49.1X1	T49.1X2	T49.1X3	T49.1X4	T49.1X5	T49.1X6
Flutoprazepam	T42.4X1	T42.4X2	T42.4X3	T42.4X4	T42.4X5	T42.4X6
Flutropium bromide	T48.6X1	T48.6X2	T48.6X3	T48.6X4	T48.6X5	T48.6X6
Fluvoxamine	T43.221	T43.222	T43.223	T43.224	T43.225	T43.226
Folacin	T45.8X1	T45.8X2	T45.8X3	T45.8X4	T45.8X5	T45.8X6
Folic acid	T45.8X1	T45.8X2	T45.8X3	T45.8X4	T45.8X5	T45.8X6
with ferrous salt	T45.2X1	T45.2X2	T45.2X3	T45.2X4	T45.2X5	T45.2X6
antagonist	T45.1X1	T45.1X2	T45.1X3	T45.1X4	T45.1X5	T45.1X6
Folinic acid	T45.8X1	T45.8X2	T45.8X3	T45.8X4	T45.8X5	T45.8X6
Folium stramoniae	T48.6X1	T48.6X2	T48.6X3	T48.6X4	T48.6X5	T48.6X6
Follicle-stimulating hormone, human	T38.811	T38.812	T38.813	T38.814	T38.815	T38.816
Folpet	T60.3X1	T60.3X2	T60.3X3	T60.3X4	—	—
Fominoben	T48.3X1	T48.3X2	T48.3X3	T48.3X4	T48.3X5	T48.3X6
Food, foodstuffs, noxious, nonbacterial, NEC	T62.91	T62.92	T62.93	T62.94	—	—
berries	T62.1X1	T62.1X2	T62.1X3	T62.1X4	—	—
fish—see also Fish	T61.91	T61.92	T61.93	T61.94	—	—
mushrooms	T62.0X1	T62.0X2	T62.0X3	T62.0X4	—	—
plants	T62.2X1	T62.2X2	T62.2X3	T62.2X4	—	—
seafood	T61.91	T61.92	T61.93	T61.94	—	—
specified NEC	T61.8X1	T61.8X2	T61.8X3	T61.8X4	—	—
seeds	T62.2X1	T62.2X2	T62.2X3	T62.2X4	—	—
shellfish	T61.781	T61.782	T61.783	T61.784	—	—
specified NEC	T62.8X1	T62.8X2	T62.8X3	T62.8X4	—	—
Fool's parsley	T62.2X1	T62.2X2	T62.2X3	T62.2X4	—	—
Formaldehyde (solution), gas or vapor	T59.2X1	T59.2X2	T59.2X3	T59.2X4	—	—
fungicide	T60.3X1	T60.3X2	T60.3X3	T60.3X4	—	—

Substance	Poisoning, Accidental (Unintentional)	Poisoning, Intentional Self-Harm	Poisoning, Assault	Poisoning, Undetermined	Adverse Effect	Underdosing
Formalin	T59.2X1	T59.2X2	T59.2X3	T59.2X4	—	—
fungicide	T60.3X1	T60.3X2	T60.3X3	T60.3X4	—	—
vapor	T59.2X1	T59.2X2	T59.2X3	T59.2X4	—	—
Formic acid	T54.2X1	T54.2X2	T54.2X3	T54.2X4	—	—
vapor	T59.891	T59.892	T59.893	T59.894	—	—
Foscarnet sodium	T37.5X1	T37.5X2	T37.5X3	T37.5X4	T37.5X5	T37.5X6
Fosfestrol	T38.5X1	T38.5X2	T38.5X3	T38.5X4	T38.5X5	T38.5X6
Fosfomycin	T36.8X1	T36.8X2	T36.8X3	T36.8X4	T36.8X5	T36.8X6
Fosfonet sodium	T37.5X1	T37.5X2	T37.5X3	T37.5X4	T37.5X5	T37.5X6
Fosinopril	T46.4X1	T46.4X2	T46.4X3	T46.4X4	T46.4X5	T46.4X6
sodium	T46.4X1	T46.4X2	T46.4X3	T46.4X4	T46.4X5	T46.4X6
Fowler's solution	T57.0X1	T57.0X2	T57.0X3	T57.0X4	—	—
Foxglove	T62.2X1	T62.2X2	T62.2X3	T62.2X4	—	—
Framycetin	T36.5X1	T36.5X2	T36.5X3	T36.5X4	T36.5X5	T36.5X6
Frangula	T47.2X1	T47.2X2	T47.2X3	T47.2X4	T47.2X5	T47.2X6
extract	T47.2X1	T47.2X2	T47.2X3	T47.2X4	T47.2X5	T47.2X6
Frei antigen	T50.8X1	T50.8X2	T50.8X3	T50.8X4	T50.8X5	T50.8X6
Freon	T53.5X1	T53.5X2	T53.5X3	T53.5X4	—	—
Fructose	T50.3X1	T50.3X2	T50.3X3	T50.3X4	T50.3X5	T50.3X6
Frusemide	T50.1X1	T50.1X2	T50.1X3	T50.1X4	T50.1X5	T50.1X6
FSH	T38.811	T38.812	T38.813	T38.814	T38.815	T38.816
Ftorafur	T45.1X1	T45.1X2	T45.1X3	T45.1X4	T45.1X5	T45.1X6
Fuel						
automobile	T52.0X1	T52.0X2	T52.0X3	T52.0X4	—	—
exhaust gas, not in transit	T58.01	T58.02	T58.03	T58.04	—	—
vapor NEC	T52.0X1	T52.0X2	T52.0X3	T52.0X4	—	—
gas (domestic use) — see also Carbon, monoxide, fuel, utility	T59.891	T59.892	T59.893	T59.894		
utility	T59.891	T59.892	T59.893	T59.894	—	—
in mobile container	T59.891	T59.892	T59.893	T59.894		
incomplete combustion of — see Carbon, monoxide, fuel, utility						
piped (natural)	T59.891	T59.892	T59.893	T59.894	—	
industrial, incomplete combustion	T58.8X1	T58.8X2	T58.8X3	T58.8X4	—	—
Fugillin	T36.8X1	T36.8X2	T36.8X3	T36.8X4	T36.8X5	T36.8X6
Fulminate of mercury	T56.1X1	T56.1X2	T56.1X3	T56.1X4	—	—
Fulvicin	T36.7X1	T36.7X2	T36.7X3	T36.7X4	T36.7X5	T36.7X6
Fumadil	T36.8X1	T36.8X2	T36.8X3	T36.8X4	T36.8X5	T36.8X6
Fumagillin	T36.8X1	T36.8X2	T36.8X3	T36.8X4	T36.8X5	T36.8X6
Fumaric acid	T49.4X1	T49.4X2	T49.4X3	T49.4X4	T49.4X5	T49.4X6
Fumes (from)	T59.91	T59.92	T59.93	T59.94	—	—
carbon monoxide — see Carbon, monoxide						
charcoal (domestic use) — see Charcoal, fumes						

Substance	External Cause (T-Code)					
	Poisoning, Accidental (Unintentional)	Poisoning, Intentional Self-Harm	Poisoning, Assault	Poisoning, Undetermined	Adverse Effect	Underdosing
Fumes *(Continued)*						
chloroform — *see Chloroform*						
coke (in domestic stoves, fireplaces) — *see Coke, fumes*						
corrosive NEC	T54.91	T54.92	T54.93	T54.94	—	—
ether — *see ether*						
freons	T53.5X1	T53.5X2	T53.5X3	T53.5X4	—	—
hydrocarbons	T59.891	T59.892	T59.893	T59.894	—	—
petroleum (liquefied)	T59.891	T59.892	T59.893	T59.894	—	—
distributed through pipes (pure or mixed with air)	T59.891	T59.892	T59.893	T59.894	—	—
lead — *see lead*						
metal — *see Metals, or the specified metal*						
nitrogen dioxide	T59.0X1	T59.0X2	T59.0X3	T59.0X4	—	—
pesticides — *see Pesticides*						
petroleum (liquefied)	T59.891	T59.892	T59.893	T59.894	—	—
distributed through pipes (pure or mixed with air)	T59.891	T59.892	T59.893	T59.894	—	—
polyester	T59.891	T59.892	T59.893	T59.894	—	—
specified source NEC — *see also substance specified*	T59.891	T59.892	T59.893	T59.894	—	—
sulfur dioxide	T59.1X1	T59.1X2	T59.1X3	T59.1X4	—	—
Fumigant NEC	T60.91	T60.92	T60.93	T60.94	—	—
Fungi, noxious, used as food	T62.0X1	T62.0X2	T62.0X3	T62.0X4	—	—
Fungicide NEC (nonmedicinal)	T60.3X1	T60.3X2	T60.3X3	T60.3X4	—	—
Fungizone	T36.7X1	T36.7X2	T36.7X3	T36.7X4	T36.7X5	T36.7X6
topical	T49.0X1	T49.0X2	T49.0X3	T49.0X4	T49.0X5	T49.0X6
Furacin	T49.0X1	T49.0X2	T49.0X3	T49.0X4	T49.0X5	T49.0X6
Furadantin	T37.91	T37.92	T37.93	T37.94	T37.95	T37.96
Furazolidone	T37.8X1	T37.8X2	T37.8X3	T37.8X4	T37.8X5	T37.8X6
Furazolium chloride	T49.0X1	T49.0X2	T49.0X3	T49.0X4	T49.0X5	T49.0X6
Furfural	T52.8X1	T52.8X2	T52.8X3	T52.8X4	—	—
Furnace (coal burning) (domestic), gas from industrial	T58.2X1	T58.2X2	T58.2X3	T58.2X4	—	—
industrial	T58.8X1	T58.8X2	T58.8X3	T58.8X4	—	—
Furniture polish	T65.891	T65.892	T65.893	T65.894	—	—
Furosemide	T50.1X1	T50.1X2	T50.1X3	T50.1X4	T50.1X5	T50.1X6
Furoxone	T37.91	T37.92	T37.93	T37.94	T37.95	T37.96
Fursultiamine	T45.2X1	T45.2X2	T45.2X3	T45.2X4	T45.2X5	T45.2X6
Fusafungine	T36.8X1	T36.8X2	T36.8X3	T36.8X4	T36.8X5	T36.8X6
Fusel oil (any) (amyl) (butyl) (propyl), vapor	T51.3X1	T51.3X2	T51.3X3	T51.3X4	—	—
Fusidate (ethanolamine) (sodium)	T36.8X1	T36.8X2	T36.8X3	T36.8X4	T36.8X5	T36.8X6
Fusidic acid	T36.8X1	T36.8X2	T36.8X3	T36.8X4	T36.8X5	T36.8X6
Fytic acid, nonasodium	T50.6X1	T50.6X2	T50.6X3	T50.6X4	T50.6X5	T50.6X6

Substance	External Cause (T-Code)					
	Poisoning, Accidental (Unintentional)	Poisoning, Intentional Self-Harm	Poisoning, Assault	Poisoning, Undetermined	Adverse Effect	Underdosing
G						
GABA	T43.8X1	T43.8X2	T43.8X3	T43.8X4	T43.8X5	T43.8X6
Gadopentetic acid	T50.8X1	T50.8X2	T50.8X3	T50.8X4	T50.8X5	T50.8X6
Galactose	T50.3X1	T50.3X2	T50.3X3	T50.3X4	T50.3X5	T50.3X6
b-Galactosidase	T47.5X1	T47.5X2	T47.5X3	T47.5X4	T47.5X5	T47.5X6
Galantamine	T44.0X1	T44.0X2	T44.0X3	T44.0X4	T44.0X5	T44.0X6
Gallamine (triethiodide)	T48.1X1	T48.1X2	T48.1X3	T48.1X4	T48.1X5	T48.1X6
Gallium citrate	T50.991	T50.992	T50.993	T50.994	T50.995	T50.996
Gallopamil	T46.1X1	T46.1X2	T46.1X3	T46.1X4	T46.1X5	T46.1X6
Gamboge	T47.2X1	T47.2X2	T47.2X3	T47.2X4	T47.2X5	T47.2X6
Gamimune	T50.Z11	T50.Z12	T50.Z13	T50.Z14	T50.Z15	T50.Z16
Gamma-aminobutyric acid	T43.8X1	T43.8X2	T43.8X3	T43.8X4	T43.8X5	T43.8X6
Gamma-benzene hexachloride (medicinal)	T49.0X1	T49.0X2	T49.0X3	T49.0X4	T49.0X5	T49.0X6
nonmedicinal, vapor	T53.6X1	T53.6X2	T53.6X3	T53.6X4	—	—
Gamma-BHC (medicinal) — *see also Gamma-benzene hexachloride*	T49.0X1	T49.0X2	T49.0X3	T49.0X4	T49.0X5	T49.0X6
Gamma globulin	T50.Z11	T50.Z12	T50.Z13	T50.Z14	T50.Z15	T50.Z16
Gamulin	T50.Z11	T50.Z12	T50.Z13	T50.Z14	T50.Z15	T50.Z16
Ganciclovir (sodium)	T37.5X1	T37.5X2	T37.5X3	T37.5X4	T37.5X5	T37.5X6
Ganglionic blocking drug NEC	T44.2X1	T44.2X2	T44.2X3	T44.2X4	T44.2X5	T44.2X6
specified NEC	T44.2X1	T44.2X2	T44.2X3	T44.2X4	T44.2X5	T44.2X6
Ganja	T40.7X1	T40.7X2	T40.7X3	T40.7X4	T40.7X5	T40.7X6
Garamycin	T36.5X1	T36.5X2	T36.5X3	T36.5X4	T36.5X5	T36.5X6
ophthalmic preparation	T49.5X1	T49.5X2	T49.5X3	T49.5X4	T49.5X5	T49.5X6
topical NEC	T49.0X1	T49.0X2	T49.0X3	T49.0X4	T49.0X5	T49.0X6
Gardenal	T42.3X1	T42.3X2	T42.3X3	T42.3X4	T42.3X5	T42.3X6
Gardepanyl	T42.3X1	T42.3X2	T42.3X3	T42.3X4	T42.3X5	T42.3X6
Gas	T59.91	T59.92	T59.93	T59.94	—	—
acetylene	T59.891	T59.892	T59.893	T59.894	—	—
incomplete combustion of	T58.11	T58.12	T58.13	T58.14	—	—
air contaminants, source or type not specified	T59.91	T59.92	T59.93	T59.94	—	—
anesthetic	T41.0X1	T41.0X2	T41.0X3	T41.0X4	T41.0X5	T41.0X6
blast furnace	T58.8X1	T58.8X2	T58.8X3	T58.8X4	—	—
butane — *see butane*						
carbon monoxide — *see Carbon, monoxide*						
chlorine	T59.4X1	T59.4X2	T59.4X3	T59.4X4	—	—
coal	T58.2X1	T58.2X2	T58.2X3	T58.2X4	—	—
cyanide	T57.3X1	T57.3X2	T57.3X3	T57.3X4	—	—
dicyanogen	T65.0X1	T65.0X2	T65.0X3	T65.0X4	—	—
domestic — *see Domestic gas*	T57.91	T57.92	T57.93	T57.94	—	—

TABLE OF DRUGS AND CHEMICALS

Substance	External Cause (T-Code)					
	Poisoning, Accidental (Unintentional)	Poisoning, Intentional Self-Harm	Poisoning, Assault	Poisoning, Undetermined	Adverse Effect	Underdosing
Gas *(Continued)*						
exhaust	T57.91	T57.92	T57.93	T57.94	—	—
from utility (for cooking, heating, or lighting) (after combustion) — *see Carbon, monoxide, fuel, utility*						
prior to combustion	T59.891	T59.892	T59.893	T59.894	—	—
from wood or coal-burning stove or fireplace	T57.91	T57.92	T57.93	T57.94	—	—
fuel (domestic use) (after combustion) — *see also Carbon, monoxide, fuel*	T57.91	T57.92	T57.93	T57.94	—	—
industrial use	T58.8X1	T58.8X2	T58.8X3	T58.8X4	—	—
prior to combustion	T59.891	T59.892	T59.893	T59.894	—	—
utility	T59.891	T59.892	T59.893	T59.894	—	—
in mobile container	T59.891	T59.892	T59.893	T59.894	—	—
incomplete combustion of — *see Carbon, monoxide, fuel, utility*						
piped (natural)	T59.891	T59.892	T59.893	T59.894	—	—
garage	T58.01	T58.02	T58.03	T58.04	—	—
hydrocarbon NEC	T59.891	T59.892	T59.893	T59.894	—	—
incomplete combustion of — *see Carbon, monoxide, fuel, utility*						
liquefied — *see butane*						
piped	T59.891	T59.892	T59.893	T59.894	—	—
hydrocyanic acid	T65.0X1	T65.0X2	T65.0X3	T65.0X4	—	—
illuminating (after combustion)	T58.11	T58.12	T58.13	T58.14	—	—
prior to combustion	T59.891	T59.892	T59.893	T59.894	—	—
incomplete combustion, any — *see Carbon, monoxide*						
kiln	T58.8X1	T58.8X2	T58.8X3	T58.8X4	—	—
lacrimogenic	T59.3X1	T59.3X2	T59.3X3	T59.3X4	—	—
liquefied petroleum — *see butane*						
marsh	T59.891	T59.892	T59.893	T59.894	—	—
motor exhaust, not in transit	T58.01	T58.02	T58.03	T58.04	—	—
mustard, not in war	T59.891	T59.892	T59.893	T59.894	—	—
natural	T59.891	T59.892	T59.893	T59.894	—	—
nerve, not in war	T59.91	T59.92	T59.93	T59.94	—	—
oil	T52.0X1	T52.0X2	T52.0X3	T52.0X4	—	—
petroleum (liquefied) (distributed in mobile containers)	T59.891	T59.892	T59.893	T59.894	—	—
piped (pure or mixed with air)	T59.891	T59.892	T59.893	T59.894	—	—
piped (manufactured) (natural) NEC	T59.891	T59.892	T59.893	T59.894	—	—
producer	T58.8X1	T58.8X2	T58.8X3	T58.8X4	—	—
propane — *see propane*						
refrigerant (chlorofluoro-carbon)	T53.5X1	T53.5X2	T53.5X3	T53.5X4	—	—
not chlorofluoro-carbon	T59.891	T59.892	T59.893	T59.894	—	—
sewer	T59.91	T59.92	T59.93	T59.94	—	—
specified source NEC	T59.91	T59.92	T59.93	T59.94	—	—

Substance	External Cause (T-Code)					
	Poisoning, Accidental (Unintentional)	Poisoning, Intentional Self-Harm	Poisoning, Assault	Poisoning, Undetermined	Adverse Effect	Underdosing
Gas *(Continued)*						
stove (after combustion)	T58.11	T58.12	T58.13	T58.14	—	—
tear	T59.3X1	T59.3X2	T59.3X3	T59.3X4	—	—
therapeutic	T41.5X1	T41.5X2	T41.5X3	T41.5X4	T41.5X5	T41.5X6
utility (for cooking, heating, or lighting) (piped) NEC	T59.891	T59.892	T59.893	T59.894		
in mobile container	T59.891	T59.892	T59.893	T59.894	—	—
incomplete combustion of — *see Carbon, monoxide, fuel, utilty*						
piped (natural)	T59.891	T59.892	T59.893	T59.894		
water	T58.1X1	T58.1X2	T58.1X3	T58.1X4	—	—
incomplete combustion of — *see Carbon, monoxide, fuel, utility*						
Gaseous substance — *see Gas*						
Gasoline	T52.0X1	T52.0X2	T52.0X3	T52.0X4	—	—
vapor	T52.0X1	T52.0X2	T52.0X3	T52.0X4	—	—
Gastric enzymes	T47.5X1	T47.5X2	T47.5X3	T47.5X4	T47.5X5	T47.5X6
Gastrografin	T50.8X1	T50.8X2	T50.8X3	T50.8X4	T50.8X5	T50.8X6
Gastrointestinal drug	T47.91	T47.92	T47.93	T47.94	T47.95	T47.96
biological	T47.8X1	T47.8X2	T47.8X3	T47.8X4	T47.8X5	T47.8X6
specified NEC	T47.8X1	T47.8X2	T47.8X3	T47.8X4	T47.8X5	T47.8X6
Gaultheria procumbens	T62.2X1	T62.2X2	T62.2X3	T62.2X4	—	—
Gelatin (intravenous)	T45.8X1	T45.8X2	T45.8X3	T45.8X4	T45.8X5	T45.8X6
absorbable (sponge)	T45.7X1	T45.7X2	T45.7X3	T45.7X4	T45.7X5	T45.7X6
Gefarnate	T44.3X1	T44.3X2	T44.3X3	T44.3X4	T44.3X5	T44.3X6
Gelfilm	T49.8X1	T49.8X2	T49.8X3	T49.8X4	T49.8X5	T49.8X6
Gelfoam	T45.7X1	T45.7X2	T45.7X3	T45.7X4	T45.7X5	T45.7X6
Gelsemine	T50.991	T50.992	T50.993	T50.994	T50.995	T50.996
Gelsemium (sempervirens)	T62.2X1	T62.2X2	T62.2X3	T62.2X4	—	—
Gemeprost	T48.0X1	T48.0X2	T48.0X3	T48.0X4	T48.0X5	T48.0X6
Gemfibrozil	T46.6X1	T46.6X2	T46.6X3	T46.6X4	T46.6X5	T46.6X6
Gemonil	T42.3X1	T42.3X2	T42.3X3	T42.3X4	T42.3X5	T42.3X6
Gentamicin	T36.5X1	T36.5X2	T36.5X3	T36.5X4	T36.5X5	T36.5X6
ophthalmic preparation	T49.5X1	T49.5X2	T49.5X3	T49.5X4	T49.5X5	T49.5X6
topical NEC	T49.0X1	T49.0X2	T49.0X3	T49.0X4	T49.0X5	T49.0X6
Gentian	T47.5X1	T47.5X2	T47.5X3	T47.5X4	T47.5X5	T47.5X6
violet	T49.0X1	T49.0X2	T49.0X3	T49.0X4	T49.0X5	T49.0X6
Gepefrine	T44.4X1	T44.4X2	T44.4X3	T44.4X4	T44.4X5	T44.4X6
Gestonorone caproate	T38.5X1	T38.5X2	T38.5X3	T38.5X4	T38.5X5	T38.5X6
Gexane	T49.0X1	T49.0X2	T49.0X3	T49.0X4	T49.0X5	T49.0X6
Gila monster (venom)	T63.111	T63.112	T63.113	T63.114	—	—
Ginger	T47.5X1	T47.5X2	T47.5X3	T47.5X4	T47.5X5	T47.5X6
Jamaica — *see Jamaica, ginger*						

Substance	Poisoning, Accidental (Unintentional)	Poisoning, Intentional Self-Harm	Poisoning, Assault	Poisoning, Undetermined	Adverse Effect	Underdosing
Gitalin	T46.0X1	T46.0X2	T46.0X3	T46.0X4	T46.0X5	T46.0X6
amorphous	T46.0X1	T46.0X2	T46.0X3	T46.0X4	T46.0X5	T46.0X6
Gitaloxin	T46.0X1	T46.0X2	T46.0X3	T46.0X4	T46.0X5	T46.0X6
Gitoxin	T46.0X1	T46.0X2	T46.0X3	T46.0X4	T46.0X5	T46.0X6
Glafenine	T39.8X1	T39.8X2	T39.8X3	T39.8X4	T39.8X5	T39.8X6
Glandular extract (medicinal) NEC	T50.Z91	T50.Z92	T50.Z93	T50.Z94	T50.Z95	T50.Z96
Glaucarubin	T37.3X1	T37.3X2	T37.3X3	T37.3X4	T37.3X5	T37.3X6
Glibenclamide	T38.3X1	T38.3X2	T38.3X3	T38.3X4	T38.3X5	T38.3X6
Glibornuride	T38.3X1	T38.3X2	T38.3X3	T38.3X4	T38.3X5	T38.3X6
Gliclazide	T38.3X1	T38.3X2	T38.3X3	T38.3X4	T38.3X5	T38.3X6
Glimidine	T38.3X1	T38.3X2	T38.3X3	T38.3X4	T38.3X5	T38.3X6
Glipizide	T38.3X1	T38.3X2	T38.3X3	T38.3X4	T38.3X5	T38.3X6
Gliquidone	T38.3X1	T38.3X2	T38.3X3	T38.3X4	T38.3X5	T38.3X6
Glisolamide	T38.3X1	T38.3X2	T38.3X3	T38.3X4	T38.3X5	T38.3X6
Glisoxepide	T38.3X1	T38.3X2	T38.3X3	T38.3X4	T38.3X5	T38.3X6
Globin zinc insulin	T38.3X1	T38.3X2	T38.3X3	T38.3X4	T38.3X5	T38.3X6
Globulin						
antilymphocytic	T50.Z11	T50.Z12	T50.Z13	T50.Z14	T50.Z15	T50.Z16
antirhesus	T50.Z11	T50.Z12	T50.Z13	T50.Z14	T50.Z15	T50.Z16
antivenin	T50.Z11	T50.Z12	T50.Z13	T50.Z14	T50.Z15	T50.Z16
antiviral	T50.Z11	T50.Z12	T50.Z13	T50.Z14	T50.Z15	T50.Z16
Glucagon	T38.3X1	T38.3X2	T38.3X3	T38.3X4	T38.3X5	T38.3X6
Glucocorticoids	T38.0X1	T38.0X2	T38.0X3	T38.0X4	T38.0X5	T38.0X6
Glucocorticosteroid	T38.0X1	T38.0X2	T38.0X3	T38.0X4	T38.0X5	T38.0X6
Gluconic acid	T50.991	T50.992	T50.993	T50.994	T50.995	T50.996
Glucosamine sulfate	T39.4X1	T39.4X2	T39.4X3	T39.4X4	T39.4X5	T39.4X6
Glucose	T50.3X1	T50.3X2	T50.3X3	T50.3X4	T50.3X5	T50.3X6
with sodium chloride	T50.3X1	T50.3X2	T50.3X3	T50.3X4	T50.3X5	T50.3X6
Glucosulfone sodium	T37.1X1	T37.1X2	T37.1X3	T37.1X4	T37.1X5	T37.1X6
Glucurolactone	T47.8X1	T47.8X2	T47.8X3	T47.8X4	T47.8X5	T47.8X6
Glue NEC	T52.8X1	T52.8X2	T52.8X3	T52.8X4	—	—
Glutamic acid	T47.5X1	T47.5X2	T47.5X3	T47.5X4	T47.5X5	T47.5X6
Glutaral (medicinal)	T49.0X1	T49.0X2	T49.0X3	T49.0X4	T49.0X5	T49.0X6
nonmedicinal	T65.891	T65.892	T65.893	T65.894	—	—
Glutaraldehyde (nonmedicinal)	T65.891	T65.892	T65.893	T65.894	—	—
medicinal	T49.0X1	T49.0X2	T49.0X3	T49.0X4	T49.0X5	T49.0X6
Glutathione	T50.6X1	T50.6X2	T50.6X3	T50.6X4	T50.6X5	T50.6X6
Glutethimide	T42.6X1	T42.6X2	T42.6X3	T42.6X4	T42.6X5	T42.6X6
Glyburide	T38.3X1	T38.3X2	T38.3X3	T38.3X4	T38.3X5	T38.3X6

Substance	Poisoning, Accidental (Unintentional)	Poisoning, Intentional Self-Harm	Poisoning, Assault	Poisoning, Undetermined	Adverse Effect	Underdosing
			External Cause (T-Code)			
Glycerin	T47.4X1	T47.4X2	T47.4X3	T47.4X4	T47.4X5	T47.4X6
Glycerol	T47.4X1	T47.4X2	T47.4X3	T47.4X4	T47.4X5	T47.4X6
borax	T49.6X1	T49.6X2	T49.6X3	T49.6X4	T49.6X5	T49.6X6
intravenous	T50.3X1	T50.3X2	T50.3X3	T50.3X4	T50.3X5	T50.3X6
iodinated	T48.4X1	T48.4X2	T48.4X3	T48.4X4	T48.4X5	T48.4X6
Glycerophosphate	T50.991	T50.992	T50.993	T50.994	T50.995	T50.996
Glyceryl						
gualacolate	T48.4X1	T48.4X2	T48.4X3	T48.4X4	T48.4X5	T48.4X6
nitrate	T46.3X1	T46.3X2	T46.3X3	T46.3X4	T46.3X5	T46.3X6
triacetate (topical)	T49.0X1	T49.0X2	T49.0X3	T49.0X4	T49.0X5	T49.0X6
trinitrate	T46.3X1	T46.3X2	T46.3X3	T46.3X4	T46.3X5	T46.3X6
Glycine	T50.3X1	T50.3X2	T50.3X3	T50.3X4	T50.3X5	T50.3X6
Glyclopyramide	T38.3X1	T38.3X2	T38.3X3	T38.3X4	T38.3X5	T38.3X6
Glycobiarsol	T37.3X1	T37.3X2	T37.3X3	T37.3X4	T37.3X5	T37.3X6
Glycols (ether)	T52.3X1	T52.3X2	T52.3X3	T52.3X4	—	—
Glyconiazide	T37.1X1	T37.1X2	T37.1X3	T37.1X4	T37.1X5	T37.1X6
Glycopyrrolate	T44.3X1	T44.3X2	T44.3X3	T44.3X4	T44.3X5	T44.3X6
Glycopyrronium	T44.3X1	T44.3X2	T44.3X3	T44.3X4	T44.3X5	T44.3X6
bromide	T44.3X1	T44.3X2	T44.3X3	T44.3X4	T44.3X5	T44.3X6
Glycoside, cardiac (stimulant)	T46.0X1	T46.0X2	T46.0X3	T46.0X4	T46.0X5	T46.0X6
Glycyclamide	T38.3X1	T38.3X2	T38.3X3	T38.3X4	T38.3X5	T38.3X6
Glycyrrhiza extract	T48.4X1	T48.4X2	T48.4X3	T48.4X4	T48.4X5	T48.4X6
Glycyrrhizic acid	T48.4X1	T48.4X2	T48.4X3	T48.4X4	T48.4X5	T48.4X6
Glycyrrhizinate potassium	T48.4X1	T48.4X2	T48.4X3	T48.4X4	T48.4X5	T48.4X6
Glymidine sodium	T38.3X1	T38.3X2	T38.3X3	T38.3X4	T38.3X5	T38.3X6
Glyphosate	T60.3X1	T60.3X2	T60.3X3	T60.3X4	—	—
Glyphylline	T48.6X1	T48.6X2	T48.6X3	T48.6X4	T48.6X5	T48.6X6
Gold						
colloidal (l98Au)	T45.1X1	T45.1X2	T45.1X3	T45.1X4	T45.1X5	T45.1X6
salts	T39.4X1	T39.4X2	T39.4X3	T39.4X4	T39.4X5	T39.4X6
Golden sulfide of antimony	T56.891	T56.892	T56.893	T56.894	—	—
Goldylocks	T62.2X1	T62.2X2	T62.2X3	T62.2X4	—	—
Gonadal tissue extract	T38.901	T38.902	T38.903	T38.904	T38.905	T38.906
female	T38.5X1	T38.5X2	T38.5X3	T38.5X4	T38.5X5	T38.5X6
male	T38.7X1	T38.7X2	T38.7X3	T38.7X4	T38.7X5	T38.7X6
Gonadorelin	T38.891	T38.892	T38.893	T38.894	T38.895	T38.896
Gonadotropin	T38.891	T38.892	T38.893	T38.894	T38.895	T38.896
chorionic	T38.891	T38.892	T38.893	T38.894	T38.895	T38.896
pituitary	T38.811	T38.812	T38.813	T38.814	T38.815	T38.816
Goserelin	T45.1X1	T45.1X2	T45.1X3	T45.1X4	T45.1X5	T45.1X6

Substance	External Cause (T-Code)					
	Poisoning, Accidental (Unintentional)	Poisoning, Intentional Self-Harm	Poisoning, Assault	Poisoning, Undetermined	Adverse Effect	Underdosing
Grain alcohol	T51.0X1	T51.0X2	T51.0X3	T51.0X4	—	—
Gramicidin	T49.0X1	T49.0X2	T49.0X3	T49.0X4	T49.0X5	T49.0X6
Granisetron	T45.0X1	T45.0X2	T45.0X3	T45.0X4	T45.0X5	T45.0X6
Gratiola officinalis	T62.2X1	T62.2X2	T62.2X3	T62.2X4	—	—
Grease	T65.891	T65.892	T65.893	T65.894	—	—
Green hellebore	T62.2X1	T62.2X2	T62.2X3	T62.2X4	—	—
Green soap	T49.2X1	T49.2X2	T49.2X3	T49.2X4	T49.2X5	T49.2X6
Grifulvin	T36.7X1	T36.7X2	T36.7X3	T36.7X4	T36.7X5	T36.7X6
Griseofulvin	T36.7X1	T36.7X2	T36.7X3	T36.7X4	T36.7X5	T36.7X6
Growth hormone	T38.811	T38.812	T38.813	T38.814	T38.815	T38.816
Guaiacol derivatives	T48.4X1	T48.4X2	T48.4X3	T48.4X4	T48.4X5	T48.4X6
Guaiac reagent	T50.991	T50.992	T50.993	T50.994	T50.995	T50.996
Guaifenesin	T48.4X1	T48.4X2	T48.4X3	T48.4X4	T48.4X5	T48.4X6
Guaimesal	T48.4X1	T48.4X2	T48.4X3	T48.4X4	T48.4X5	T48.4X6
Guaiphenesin	T48.4X1	T48.4X2	T48.4X3	T48.4X4	T48.4X5	T48.4X6
Guamecycline	T36.4X1	T36.4X2	T36.4X3	T36.4X4	T36.4X5	T36.4X6
Guanabenz	T46.5X1	T46.5X2	T46.5X3	T46.5X4	T46.5X5	T46.5X6
Guanacline	T46.5X1	T46.5X2	T46.5X3	T46.5X4	T46.5X5	T46.5X6
Guanadrel	T46.5X1	T46.5X2	T46.5X3	T46.5X4	T46.5X5	T46.5X6
Guanatol	T37.2X1	T37.2X2	T37.2X3	T37.2X4	T37.2X5	T37.2X6
Guanethidine	T46.5X1	T46.5X2	T46.5X3	T46.5X4	T46.5X5	T46.5X6
Guanfacine	T46.5X1	T46.5X2	T46.5X3	T46.5X4	T46.5X5	T46.5X6
Guano	T65.891	T65.892	T65.893	T65.894	—	—
Guanochlor	T46.5X1	T46.5X2	T46.5X3	T46.5X4	T46.5X5	T46.5X6
Guanoclor	T46.5X1	T46.5X2	T46.5X3	T46.5X4	T46.5X5	T46.5X6
Guanoctine	T46.5X1	T46.5X2	T46.5X3	T46.5X4	T46.5X5	T46.5X6
Guanoxabenz	T46.5X1	T46.5X2	T46.5X3	T46.5X4	T46.5X5	T46.5X6
Guanoxan	T46.5X1	T46.5X2	T46.5X3	T46.5X4	T46.5X5	T46.5X6
Guar gum (medicinal)	T46.6X1	T46.6X2	T46.6X3	T46.6X4	T46.6X5	T46.6X6
H						
Hachimycin	T36.7X1	T36.7X2	T36.7X3	T36.7X4	T36.7X5	T36.7X6
Hair						
dye	T49.4X1	T49.4X2	T49.4X3	T49.4X4	T49.4X5	T49.4X6
preparation NEC	T49.4X1	T49.4X2	T49.4X3	T49.4X4	T49.4X5	T49.4X6
Halazepam	T42.4X1	T42.4X2	T42.4X3	T42.4X4	T42.4X5	T42.4X6
Halcinolone	T49.0X1	T49.0X2	T49.0X3	T49.0X4	T49.0X5	T49.0X6
Halcinonide	T49.0X1	T49.0X2	T49.0X3	T49.0X4	T49.0X5	T49.0X6
Halethazole	T49.0X1	T49.0X2	T49.0X3	T49.0X4	T49.0X5	T49.0X6
Hallucinogen NEC	T40.901	T40.902	T40.903	T40.904	T40.905	T40.906

Substance	External Cause (T-Code)					
	Poisoning, Accidental (Unintentional)	Poisoning, Intentional Self-Harm	Poisoning, Assault	Poisoning, Undetermined	Adverse Effect	Underdosing
Halofantrine	T37.2X1	T37.2X2	T37.2X3	T37.2X4	T37.2X5	T37.2X6
Halofenate	T46.6X1	T46.6X2	T46.6X3	T46.6X4	T46.6X5	T46.6X6
Halometasone	T49.0X1	T49.0X2	T49.0X3	T49.0X4	T49.0X5	T49.0X6
Haloperidol	T43.4X1	T43.4X2	T43.4X3	T43.4X4	T43.4X5	T43.4X6
Haloprogin	T49.0X1	T49.0X2	T49.0X3	T49.0X4	T49.0X5	T49.0X6
Halotex	T49.0X1	T49.0X2	T49.0X3	T49.0X4	T49.0X5	T49.0X6
Halothane	T41.0X1	T41.0X2	T41.0X3	T41.0X4	T41.0X5	T41.0X6
Haloxazolam	T42.4X1	T42.4X2	T42.4X3	T42.4X4	T42.4X5	T42.4X6
Halquinols	T49.0X1	T49.0X2	T49.0X3	T49.0X4	T49.0X5	T49.0X6
Hamamelis	T49.2X1	T49.2X2	T49.2X3	T49.2X4	T49.2X5	T49.2X6
Haptendextran	T45.8X1	T45.8X2	T45.8X3	T45.8X4	T45.8X5	T45.8X6
Harmonyl	T46.5X1	T46.5X2	T46.5X3	T46.5X4	T46.5X5	T46.5X6
Hartmann's solution	T50.3X1	T50.3X2	T50.3X3	T50.3X4	T50.3X5	T50.3X6
Hashish	T40.7X1	T40.7X2	T40.7X3	T40.7X4	T40.7X5	T40.7X6
Hawaiian Woodrose seeds	T40.991	T40.992	T40.993	T40.994	—	—
HCB	T60.3X1	T60.3X2	T60.3X3	T60.3X4		
HCH	T53.6X1	T53.6X2	T53.6X3	T53.6X4	—	
medicinal	T49.0X1	T49.0X2	T49.0X3	T49.0X4	T49.0X5	T49.0X6
HCN	T57.3X1	T57.3X2	T57.3X3	T57.3X4	—	
Headache cures, drugs, powders NEC	T50.901	T50.902	T50.903	T50.904	T50.905	T50.906
Heavenly Blue (morning glory)	T40.991	T40.992	T40.993	T40.994	—	—
Heavy metal antidote	T45.8X1	T45.8X2	T45.8X3	T45.8X4	T45.8X5	T45.8X6
Hedaquinium	T49.0X1	T49.0X2	T49.0X3	T49.0X4	T49.0X5	T49.0X6
Hedge hyssop	T62.2X1	T62.2X2	T62.2X3	T62.2X4	—	—
Heet	T49.8X1	T49.8X2	T49.8X3	T49.8X4	T49.8X5	T49.8X6
Helium	T48.991	T48.992	T48.993	T48.994	T48.995	T48.996
Helenin	T37.4X1	T37.4X2	T37.4X3	T37.4X4	T37.4X5	T37.4X6
Hellebore (black) (green) (white)	T62.2X1	T62.2X2	T62.2X3	T62.2X4	—	—
Helium (nonmedicinal) NEC	T59.891	T59.892	T59.893	T59.894	—	—
medicinal	T48.991	T48.992	T48.993	T48.994	T48.995	T48.996
Hematin	T45.8X1	T45.8X2	T45.8X3	T45.8X4	T45.8X5	T45.8X6
Hematinic preparation	T45.8X1	T45.8X2	T45.8X3	T45.8X4	T45.8X5	T45.8X6
Hemlock	T62.2X1	T62.2X2	T62.2X3	T62.2X4	—	—
Hemostatic	T45.621	T45.622	T45.623	T45.624	T45.625	T45.626
drug, systemic	T45.621	T45.622	T45.623	T45.624	T45.625	T45.626
Hemostyptic	T49.4X1	T49.4X2	T49.4X3	T49.4X4	T49.4X5	T49.4X6
Henbane	T62.2X1	T62.2X2	T62.2X3	T62.2X4	—	—
Heparin (sodium)	T45.511	T45.512	T45.513	T45.514	T45.515	T45.516
action reverser	T45.7X1	T45.7X2	T45.7X3	T45.7X4	T45.7X5	T45.7X6
Heparin-fraction	T45.511	T45.512	T45.513	T45.514	T45.515	T45.516

Substance	External Cause (T-Code)					
	Poisoning, Accidental (Unintentional)	Poisoning, Intentional Self-Harm	Poisoning, Assault	Poisoning, Undetermined	Adverse Effect	Underdosing
Heparinoid (systemic)	T45.511	T45.512	T45.513	T45.514	T45.515	T45.516
Hepatic secretion stimulant	T47.8X1	T47.8X2	T47.8X3	T47.8X4	T47.8X5	T47.8X6
Hepatitis B						
immune globulin	T50.Z11	T50.Z12	T50.Z13	T50.Z14	T50.Z15	T50.Z16
vaccine	T50.B91	T50.B92	T50.B93	T50.B94	T50.B95	T50.B96
Hepronicate	T46.7X1	T46.7X2	T46.7X3	T46.7X4	T46.7X5	T46.7X6
Heptabarb	T42.3X1	T42.3X2	T42.3X3	T42.3X4	T42.3X5	T42.3X6
Heptabarbitone	T42.3X1	T42.3X2	T42.3X3	T42.3X4	T42.3X5	T42.3X6
Heptabarbital	T42.3X1	T42.3X2	T42.3X3	T42.3X4	T42.3X5	T42.3X6
Heptachlor	T60.1X1	T60.1X2	T60.1X3	T60.1X4	—	—
Heptalgin	T40.2X1	T40.2X2	T40.2X3	T40.2X4	T40.2X5	T40.2X6
Heptaminol	T46.3X1	T46.3X2	T46.3X3	T46.3X4	T46.3X5	T46.3X6
Herbicide NEC	T60.3X1	T60.3X2	T60.3X3	T60.3X4	—	—
Heroin	T40.1X1	T40.1X2	T40.1X3	T40.1X4	T40.1X5	—
Herplex	T49.5X1	T49.5X2	T49.5X3	T49.5X4	T49.5X5	T49.5X6
HES	T45.8X1	T45.8X2	T45.8X3	T45.8X4	T45.8X5	T45.8X6
Hesperidin	T46.991	T46.992	T46.993	T46.994	T46.995	T46.996
Hetacillin	T36.0X1	T36.0X2	T36.0X3	T36.0X4	T36.0X5	T36.0X6
Hetastarch	T45.8X1	T45.8X2	T45.8X3	T45.8X4	T45.8X5	T45.8X6
HETP	T60.0X1	T60.0X2	T60.0X3	T60.0X4	—	—
Hexachlorobenzene (vapor)	T60.3X1	T60.3X2	T60.3X3	T60.3X4	—	—
Hexachlorocyclohexane	T53.6X1	T53.6X2	T53.6X3	T53.6X4	—	—
Hexachlorophene	T49.0X1	T49.0X2	T49.0X3	T49.0X4	T49.0X5	T49.0X6
Hexadiline	T46.3X1	T46.3X2	T46.3X3	T46.3X4	T46.3X5	T46.3X6
Hexadimethrine (bromide)	T45.7X1	T45.7X2	T45.7X3	T45.7X4	T45.7X5	T45.7X6
Hexadylamine	T46.3X1	T46.3X2	T46.3X3	T46.3X4	T46.3X5	T46.3X6
Hexaethyl tetraphosphate	T60.0X1	T60.0X2	T60.0X3	T60.0X4	—	—
Hexafluorenium bromide	T48.1X1	T48.1X2	T48.1X3	T48.1X4	T48.1X5	T48.1X6
Hexafluorodiethyl ether	T43.291	T43.292	T43.293	T43.294	T43.295	T43.296
Hexafluronium (bromide)	T48.1X1	T48.1X2	T48.1X3	T48.1X4	T48.1X5	T48.1X6
Hexahydrobenzol	T52.8X1	T52.8X2	T52.8X3	T52.8X4	—	—
Hexahydrocresol(s)	T51.8X1	T51.8X2	T51.8X3	T51.8X4	—	—
arsenide	T57.0X1	T57.0X2	T57.0X3	T57.0X4	—	—
arseniurated	T57.0X1	T57.0X2	T57.0X3	T57.0X4	—	—
cyanide	T57.3X1	T57.3X2	T57.3X3	T57.3X4	—	—
gas	T59.891	T59.892	T59.893	T59.894		
Fluoride (liquid)	T57.8X1	T57.8X2	T57.8X3	T57.8X4	—	—
vapor	T59.891	T59.892	T59.893	T59.894		
phophorated	T60.0X1	T60.0X2	T60.0X3	T60.0X4	—	—
sulfate	T57.8X1	T57.8X2	T57.8X3	T57.8X4	—	—

Substance	External Cause (T-Code)					
	Poisoning, Accidental (Unintentional)	Poisoning, Intentional Self-Harm	Poisoning, Assault	Poisoning, Undetermined	Adverse Effect	Underdosing
Hexahydrocresol(s) *(Continued)*						
sulfide (gas)	T59.6X1	T59.6X2	T59.6X3	T59.6X4	—	—
arseniurated	T57.0X1	T57.0X2	T57.0X3	T57.0X4	—	—
sulfurated	T57.8X1	T57.8X2	T57.8X3	T57.8X4	—	—
Hexahydrophenol	T51.8X1	T51.8X2	T51.8X3	T51.8X4	—	—
Hexa-germ	T49.2X1	T49.2X2	T49.2X3	T49.2X4	T49.2X5	T49.2X6
Hexalen	T51.8X1	T51.8X2	T51.8X3	T51.8X4	—	—
Hexamethonium bromide	T44.2X1	T44.2X2	T44.2X3	T44.2X4	T44.2X5	T44.2X6
Hexamethylene	T52.8X1	T52.8X2	T52.8X3	T52.8X4	—	—
Hexamethylmelamine	T45.1X1	T45.1X2	T45.1X3	T45.1X4	T45.1X5	T45.1X6
Hexamidine	T49.0X1	T49.0X2	T49.0X3	T49.0X4	T49.0X5	T49.0X6
Hexamine (mandelate)	T37.8X1	T37.8X2	T37.8X3	T37.8X4	T37.8X5	T37.8X6
Hexanone, 2-hexanone	T52.4X1	T52.4X2	T52.4X3	T52.4X4	—	—
Hexanuorenium	T48.1X1	T48.1X2	T48.1X3	T48.1X4	T48.1X5	T48.1X6
Hexapropymate	T42.6X1	T42.6X2	T42.6X3	T42.6X4	T42.6X5	T42.6X6
Hexasonium iodide	T44.3X1	T44.3X2	T44.3X3	T44.3X4	T44.3X5	T44.3X6
Hexcarbacholine bromide	T48.1X1	T48.1X2	T48.1X3	T48.1X4	T48.1X5	T48.1X6
Hexemal	T42.3X1	T42.3X2	T42.3X3	T42.3X4	T42.3X5	T42.3X6
Hexestrol	T38.5X1	T38.5X2	T38.5X3	T38.5X4	T38.5X5	T38.5X6
Hexethal (sodium)	T42.3X1	T42.3X2	T42.3X3	T42.3X4	T42.3X5	T42.3X6
Hexetidine	T37.8X1	T37.8X2	T37.8X3	T37.8X4	T37.8X5	T37.8X6
Hexobarbital	T42.3X1	T42.3X2	T42.3X3	T42.3X4	T42.3X5	T42.3X6
rectal	T41.291	T41.292	T41.293	T41.294	T41.295	T41.296
sodium	T41.1X1	T41.1X2	T41.1X3	T41.1X4	T41.1X5	T41.1X6
Hexobendine	T46.3X1	T46.3X2	T46.3X3	T46.3X4	T46.3X5	T46.3X6
Hexocyclium	T44.3X1	T44.3X2	T44.3X3	T44.3X4	T44.3X5	T44.3X6
metilsulfate	T44.3X1	T44.3X2	T44.3X3	T44.3X4	T44.3X5	T44.3X6
Hexoestrol	T38.5X1	T38.5X2	T38.5X3	T38.5X4	T38.5X5	T38.5X6
Hexone	T52.4X1	T52.4X2	T52.4X3	T52.4X4	—	—
Hexoprenaline	T48.6X1	T48.6X2	T48.6X3	T48.6X4	T48.6X5	T48.6X6
Hexylcaine	T41.3X1	T41.3X2	T41.3X3	T41.3X4	T41.3X5	T41.3X6
Hexylresorcinol	T52.2X1	T52.2X2	T52.2X3	T52.2X4	—	—
HGH (human growth hormone)	T38.811	T38.812	T38.813	T38.814	T38.815	T38.816
Hinkle's pills	T47.2X1	T47.2X2	T47.2X3	T47.2X4	T47.2X5	T47.2X6
Histalog	T50.8X1	T50.8X2	T50.8X3	T50.8X4	T50.8X5	T50.8X6
Histamine (phosphate)	T50.8X1	T50.8X2	T50.8X3	T50.8X4	T50.8X5	T50.8X6
Histoplasmin	T50.8X1	T50.8X2	T50.8X3	T50.8X4	T50.8X5	T50.8X6
Holly berries	T62.2X1	T62.2X2	T62.2X3	T62.2X4	—	—
Homatropine	T44.3X1	T44.3X2	T44.3X3	T44.3X4	T44.3X5	T44.3X6
methylbromide	T44.3X1	T44.3X2	T44.3X3	T44.3X4	T44.3X5	T44.3X6

Substance	Poisoning, Accidental (Unintentional)	Poisoning, Intentional Self-Harm	Poisoning, Assault	Poisoning, Undetermined	Adverse Effect	Underdosing
	External Cause (T-Code)					
Homochlorcyclizine	T45.0X1	T45.0X2	T45.0X3	T45.0X4	T45.0X5	T45.0X6
Homosalate	T49.3X1	T49.3X2	T49.3X3	T49.3X4	T49.3X5	T49.3X6
Homo-tet	T50.Z11	T50.Z12	T50.Z13	T50.Z14	T50.Z15	T50.Z16
Hormone	T38.801	T38.802	T38.803	T38.804	T38.805	T38.806
adrenal cortical steroids	T38.0X1	T38.0X2	T38.0X3	T38.0X4	T38.0X5	T38.0X6
androgenic	T38.7X1	T38.7X2	T38.7X3	T38.7X4	T38.7X5	T38.7X6
anterior pituitary NEC	T38.811	T38.812	T38.813	T38.814	T38.815	T38.816
antidiabetic agents	T38.3X1	T38.3X2	T38.3X3	T38.3X4	T38.3X5	T38.3X6
antidiuretic	T38.891	T38.892	T38.893	T38.894	T38.895	T38.896
cancer therapy	T45.1X1	T45.1X2	T45.1X3	T45.1X4	T45.1X5	T45.1X6
follicle stimulating	T38.811	T38.812	T38.813	T38.814	T38.815	T38.816
gonadotropic	T38.891	T38.892	T38.893	T38.894	T38.895	T38.896
pituitary	T38.811	T38.812	T38.813	T38.814	T38.815	T38.816
growth	T38.811	T38.812	T38.813	T38.814	T38.815	T38.816
luteinizing	T38.811	T38.812	T38.813	T38.814	T38.815	T38.816
ovarian	T38.5X1	T38.5X2	T38.5X3	T38.5X4	T38.5X5	T38.5X6
oxytocic	T48.0X1	T48.0X2	T48.0X3	T48.0X4	T48.0X5	T48.0X6
parathyroid (derivatives)	T50.991	T50.992	T50.993	T50.994	T50.995	T50.996
pituitary (posterior) NEC	T38.891	T38.892	T38.893	T38.894	T38.895	T38.896
anterior	T38.811	T38.812	T38.813	T38.814	T38.815	T38.816
specified, NEC	T38.891	T38.892	T38.893	T38.894	T38.895	T38.896
thyroid	T38.1X1	T38.1X2	T38.1X3	T38.1X4	T38.1X5	T38.1X6
Hornet (sting)	T63.451	T63.452	T63.453	T63.454	—	—
Horse anti-human lymphocytic serum	T50.Z11	T50.Z12	T50.Z13	T50.Z14	T50.Z15	T50.Z16
Horticulture agent NEC	T65.91	T65.92	T65.93	T65.94	—	—
with pesticide	T60.91	T60.92	T60.93	T60.94	—	—
Human						
albumin	T45.8X1	T45.8X2	T45.8X3	T45.8X4	T45.8X5	T45.8X6
growth hormone (HGH)	T38.811	T38.812	T38.813	T38.814	T38.815	T38.816
immune serum	T50.Z11	T50.Z12	T50.Z13	T50.Z14	T50.Z15	T50.Z16
Hyaluronidase	T45.3X1	T45.3X2	T45.3X3	T45.3X4	T45.3X5	T45.3X6
Hyazyme	T45.3X1	T45.3X2	T45.3X3	T45.3X4	T45.3X5	T45.3X6
Hycodan	T40.2X1	T40.2X2	T40.2X3	T40.2X4	T40.2X5	T40.2X6
Hydantoin derivative NEC	T42.0X1	T42.0X2	T42.0X3	T42.0X4	T42.0X5	T42.0X6
Hydeltra	T38.0X1	T38.0X2	T38.0X3	T38.0X4	T38.0X5	T38.0X6
Hydergine	T44.6X1	T44.6X2	T44.6X3	T44.6X4	T44.6X5	T44.6X6
Hydrabamine penicillin	T36.0X1	T36.0X2	T36.0X3	T36.0X4	T36.0X5	T36.0X6
Hydralazine	T46.5X1	T46.5X2	T46.5X3	T46.5X4	T46.5X5	T46.5X6
Hydrargaphen	T49.0X1	T49.0X2	T49.0X3	T49.0X4	T49.0X5	T49.0X6

TABLE OF DRUGS AND CHEMICALS

Substance	Poisoning, Accidental (Unintentional)	Poisoning, Intentional Self-Harm	Poisoning, Assault	Poisoning, Undetermined	Adverse Effect	Underdosing
	External Cause (T-Code)					
Hydrargyri amino-chloridum	T49.0X1	T49.0X2	T49.0X3	T49.0X4	T49.0X5	T49.0X6
Hydrastine	T48.291	T48.292	T48.293	T48.294	T48.295	T48.296
Hydrazine	T54.1X1	T54.1X2	T54.1X3	T54.1X4	—	—
monoamine oxidase inhibitors	T43.1X1	T43.1X2	T43.1X3	T43.1X4	T43.1X5	T43.1X6
Hydrazoic acid, azides	T54.2X1	T54.2X2	T54.2X3	T54.2X4	—	—
Hydriodic acid	T48.4X1	T48.4X2	T48.4X3	T48.4X4	T48.4X5	T48.4X6
Hydrocarbon gas	T59.891	T59.892	T59.893	T59.894	—	—
incomplete combustion of—*see Carbon, monoxide, fuel, utility*						
liquefied (mobile container)	T59.891	T59.892	T59.893	T59.894	—	—
piped (natural)	T59.891	T59.892	T59.893	T59.894	—	—
Hydrochloric acid (liquid)	T54.2X1	T54.2X2	T54.2X3	T54.2X4		
medicinal (digestant)	T47.5X1	T47.5X2	T47.5X3	T47.5X4	T47.5X5	T47.5X6
vapor	T59.891	T59.892	T59.893	T59.894	—	—
Hydrochlorothiazide	T50.2X1	T50.2X2	T50.2X3	T50.2X4	T50.2X5	T50.2X6
Hydrocodone	T40.2X1	T40.2X2	T40.2X3	T40.2X4	T40.2X5	T40.2X6
Hydrocortisone (derivatives)	T49.0X1	T49.0X2	T49.0X3	T49.0X4	T49.0X5	T49.0X6
aceponate	T49.0X1	T49.0X2	T49.0X3	T49.0X4	T49.0X5	T49.0X6
ENT agent	T49.6X1	T49.6X2	T49.6X3	T49.6X4	T49.6X5	T49.6X6
ophthalmic preparation	T49.5X1	T49.5X2	T49.5X3	T49.5X4	T49.5X5	T49.5X6
topical NEC	T49.0X1	T49.0X2	T49.0X3	T49.0X4	T49.0X5	T49.0X6
Hydrocortone	T38.0X1	T38.0X2	T38.0X3	T38.0X4	T38.0X5	T38.0X6
ENT agent	T49.6X1	T49.6X2	T49.6X3	T49.6X4	T49.6X5	T49.6X6
ophthalmic preparation	T49.5X1	T49.5X2	T49.5X3	T49.5X4	T49.5X5	T49.5X6
topical NEC	T49.0X1	T49.0X2	T49.0X3	T49.0X4	T49.0X5	T49.0X6
Hydrocyanic acid (liquid)	T57.3X1	T57.3X2	T57.3X3	T57.3X4	—	—
gas	T65.0X1	T65.0X2	T65.0X3	T65.0X4	—	—
Hydroflumethiazide	T50.2X1	T50.2X2	T50.2X3	T50.2X4	T50.2X5	T50.2X6
Hydrofluoric acid (liquid)	T54.2X1	T54.2X2	T54.2X3	T54.2X4	—	—
vapor	T59.891	T59.892	T59.893	T59.894	—	—
Hydrogen	T59.891	T59.892	T59.893	T59.894	—	—
arsenide	T57.0X1	T57.0X2	T57.0X3	T57.0X4	—	—
arseniureted	T57.0X1	T57.0X2	T57.0X3	T57.0X4	—	—
chloride	T57.8X1	T57.8X2	T57.8X3	T57.8X4	—	—
cyanide (salts)	T57.3X1	T57.3X2	T57.3X3	T57.3X4	—	—
gas	T57.3X1	T57.3X2	T57.3X3	T57.3X4	—	—
Fluoride	T59.5X1	T59.5X2	T59.5X3	T59.5X4	—	—
vapor	T59.5X1	T59.5X2	T59.5X3	T59.5X4	—	—
peroxide	T49.0X1	T49.0X2	T49.0X3	T49.0X4	T49.0X5	T49.0X6
phosphureted	T57.1X1	T57.1X2	T57.1X3	T57.1X4	—	—

Substance	External Cause (T-Code)					
	Poisoning, Accidental (Unintentional)	Poisoning, Intentional Self-Harm	Poisoning, Assault	Poisoning, Undetermined	Adverse Effect	Underdosing
Hydrogen *(Continued)*						
sulfide	T59.6X1	T59.6X2	T59.6X3	T59.6X4	—	—
arseniureted	T57.0X1	T57.0X2	T57.0X3	T57.0X4	—	—
sulfureted	T59.6X1	T59.6X2	T59.6X3	T59.6X4	—	—
Hydromethylpyridine	T46.7X1	T46.7X2	T46.7X3	T46.7X4	T46.7X5	T46.7X6
Hydromorphinol	T40.2X1	T40.2X2	T40.2X3	T40.2X4	—	—
Hydromorphinone	T40.2X1	T40.2X2	T40.2X3	T40.2X4	T40.2X5	T40.2X6
Hydromorphone	T40.2X1	T40.2X2	T40.2X3	T40.2X4	T40.2X5	T40.2X6
Hydromox	T50.2X1	T50.2X2	T50.2X3	T50.2X4	T50.2X5	T50.2X6
Hydrophilic lotion	T49.3X1	T49.3X2	T49.3X3	T49.3X4	T49.3X5	T49.3X6
Hydroquinidine	T46.2X1	T46.2X2	T46.2X3	T46.2X4	T46.2X5	T46.2X6
Hydroquinone	T52.2X1	T52.2X2	T52.2X3	T52.2X4	—	—
vapor	T59.891	T59.892	T59.893	T59.894	—	—
Hydrosulfuric acid (gas)	T59.6X1	T59.6X2	T59.6X3	T59.6X4	—	—
Hydrotalcite	T47.1X1	T47.1X2	T47.1X3	T47.1X4	T47.1X5	T47.1X6
Hydrous wool fat	T49.3X1	T49.3X2	T49.3X3	T49.3X4	T49.3X5	T49.3X6
Hydroxide, caustic	T54.3X1	T54.3X2	T54.3X3	T54.3X4	—	—
Hydroxocobalamin	T45.8X1	T45.8X2	T45.8X3	T45.8X4	T45.8X5	T45.8X6
Hydroxyamphetamine	T49.5X1	T49.5X2	T49.5X3	T49.5X4	T49.5X5	T49.5X6
Hydroxycarbamide	T45.1X1	T45.1X2	T45.1X3	T45.1X4	T45.1X5	T45.1X6
Hydroxychloroquine	T37.8X1	T37.8X2	T37.8X3	T37.8X4	T37.8X5	T37.8X6
Hydroxydihydrocodeinone	T40.2X1	T40.2X2	T40.2X3	T40.2X4	T40.2X5	T40.2X6
Hydroxyestrone	T38.5X1	T38.5X2	T38.5X3	T38.5X4	T38.5X5	T38.5X6
Hydroxyethyl starch	T45.8X1	T45.8X2	T45.8X3	T45.8X4	T45.8X5	T45.8X6
Hydroxymethylpentanone	T52.4X1	T52.4X2	T52.4X3	T52.4X4	—	—
Hydroxyphenamate	T43.591	T43.592	T43.593	T43.594	T43.595	T43.596
Hydroxyphenylbutazone	T39.2X1	T39.2X2	T39.2X3	T39.2X4	T39.2X5	T39.2X6
Hydroxyprogesterone	T38.5X1	T38.5X2	T38.5X3	T38.5X4	T38.5X5	T38.5X6
caproate	T38.5X1	T38.5X2	T38.5X3	T38.5X4	T38.5X5	T38.5X6
Hydroxyquinoline (derivatives) NEC	T37.8X1	T37.8X2	T37.8X3	T37.8X4	T37.8X5	T37.8X6
Hydroxystilbamidine	T37.3X1	T37.3X2	T37.3X3	T37.3X4	T37.3X5	T37.3X6
Hydroxytoluene (nonmedicinal)	T54.0X1	T54.0X2	T54.0X3	T54.0X4	—	—
medicinal	T49.0X1	T49.0X2	T49.0X3	T49.0X4	T49.0X5	T49.0X6
Hydroxyurea	T45.1X1	T45.1X2	T45.1X3	T45.1X4	T45.1X5	T45.1X6
Hydroxyzine	T43.591	T43.592	T43.593	T43.594	T43.595	T43.596
Hyoscine	T44.3X1	T44.3X2	T44.3X3	T44.3X4	T44.3X5	T44.3X6
Hyoscyamine	T44.3X1	T44.3X2	T44.3X3	T44.3X4	T44.3X5	T44.3X6
Hyoscyamus	T44.3X1	T44.3X2	T44.3X3	T44.3X4	T44.3X5	T44.3X6
dry extract	T44.3X1	T44.3X2	T44.3X3	T44.3X4	T44.3X5	T44.3X6

TABLE OF DRUGS AND CHEMICALS

Substance	External Cause (T-Code)					
	Poisoning, Accidental (Unintentional)	Poisoning, Intentional Self-Harm	Poisoning, Assault	Poisoning, Undetermined	Adverse Effect	Underdosing
Hypaque	T50.8X1	T50.8X2	T50.8X3	T50.8X4	T50.8X5	T50.8X6
Hypertussis	T50.Z11	T50.Z12	T50.Z13	T50.Z14	T50.Z15	T50.Z16
Hypnotic	T42.71	T42.72	T42.73	T42.74	T42.75	T42.76
anticonvulsant	T42.71	T42.72	T42.73	T42.74	T42.75	T42.76
specified NEC	T42.6X1	T42.6X2	T42.6X3	T42.6X4	T42.6X5	T42.6X6
Hypochlorite	T49.0X1	T49.0X2	T49.0X3	T49.0X4	T49.0X5	T49.0X6
Hypophysis, posterior	T38.891	T38.892	T38.893	T38.894	T38.895	T38.896
Hypotensive NEC	T46.5X1	T46.5X2	T46.5X3	T46.5X4	T46.5X5	T46.5X6
Hypromellose	T49.5X1	T49.5X2	T49.5X3	T49.5X4	T49.5X5	T49.5X6
I						
Ibacitabine	T37.5X1	T37.5X2	T37.5X3	T37.5X4	T37.5X5	T37.5X6
Ibopamine	T44.991	T44.992	T44.993	T44.994	T44.995	T44.996
Ibufenac	T39.311	T39.312	T39.313	T39.314	T39.315	T39.316
Ibuprofen	T39.311	T39.312	T39.313	T39.314	T39.315	T39.316
Ibuproxam	T39.311	T39.312	T39.313	T39.314	T39.315	T39.316
Ibuterol	T48.6X1	T48.6X2	T48.6X3	T48.6X4	T48.6X5	T48.6X6
Ichthammol	T49.0X1	T49.0X2	T49.0X3	T49.0X4	T49.0X5	T49.0X6
Ichthyol	T49.4X1	T49.4X2	T49.4X3	T49.4X4	T49.4X5	T49.4X6
Idarubicin	T45.1X1	T45.1X2	T45.1X3	T45.1X4	T45.1X5	T45.1X6
Idrocilamide	T42.8X1	T42.8X2	T42.8X3	T42.8X4	T42.8X5	T42.8X6
Ifenprodil	T46.7X1	T46.7X2	T46.7X3	T46.7X4	T46.7X5	T46.7X6
Ifosfamide	T45.1X1	T45.1X2	T45.1X3	T45.1X4	T45.1X5	T45.1X6
Iletin	T38.3X1	T38.3X2	T38.3X3	T38.3X4	T38.3X5	T38.3X6
Ilex	T62.2X1	T62.2X2	T62.2X3	T62.2X4	—	—
Illuminating gas (after combustion)	T58.11	T58.12	T58.13	T58.14	—	—
prior to combustion	T59.891	T59.892	T59.893	T59.894	—	—
Ilopan	T45.2X1	T45.2X2	T45.2X3	T45.2X4	T45.2X5	T45.2X6
Iloprost	T46.7X1	T46.7X2	T46.7X3	T46.7X4	T46.7X5	T46.7X6
Ilotycin	T36.3X1	T36.3X2	T36.3X3	T36.3X4	T36.3X5	T36.3X6
ophthalmic preparation	T49.5X1	T49.5X2	T49.5X3	T49.5X4	T49.5X5	T49.5X6
topical NEC	T49.0X1	T49.0X2	T49.0X3	T49.0X4	T49.0X5	T49.0X6
Imidazole-4-carboxamide	T45.1X1	T45.1X2	T45.1X3	T45.1X4	T45.1X5	T45.1X6
Imipenem	T36.0X1	T36.0X2	T36.0X3	T36.0X4	T36.0X5	T36.0X6
Imipramine	T43.011	T43.012	T43.013	T43.014	T43.015	T43.016
Iminostilbene	T42.1X1	T42.1X2	T42.1X3	T42.1X4	T42.1X5	T42.1X6
Immu-G	T50.Z11	T50.Z12	T50.Z13	T50.Z14	T50.Z15	T50.Z16
Immuglobin	T50.Z11	T50.Z12	T50.Z13	T50.Z14	T50.Z15	T50.Z16
Immune						
globulin	T50.Z11	T50.Z12	T50.Z13	T50.Z14	T50.Z15	T50.Z16
serum globulin	T50.Z11	T50.Z12	T50.Z13	T50.Z14	T50.Z15	T50.Z16

Substance	External Cause (T-Code)					
	Poisoning, Accidental (Unintentional)	Poisoning, Intentional Self-Harm	Poisoning, Assault	Poisoning, Undetermined	Adverse Effect	Underdosing
Immunoglobin human (intravenous) (normal)	T50.Z11	T50.Z12	T50.Z13	T50.Z14	T50.Z15	T50.Z16
unmodified	T50.Z11	T50.Z12	T50.Z13	T50.Z14	T50.Z15	T50.Z16
Immunosuppressive drug	T45.1X1	T45.1X2	T45.1X3	T45.1X4	T45.1X5	T45.1X6
Immu-tetanus	T50.Z11	T50.Z12	T50.Z13	T50.Z14	T50.Z15	T50.Z16
Indalpine	T43.221	T43.222	T43.223	T43.224	T43.225	T43.226
Indanazoline	T48.5X1	T48.5X2	T48.5X3	T48.5X4	T48.5X5	T48.5X6
Indandione (derivatives)	T45.511	T45.512	T45.513	T45.514	T45.515	T45.516
Indapamide	T46.5X1	T46.5X2	T46.5X3	T46.5X4	T46.5X5	T46.5X6
Indendione (derivatives)	T45.511	T45.512	T45.513	T45.514	T45.515	T45.516
Indenolol	T44.7X1	T44.7X2	T44.7X3	T44.7X4	T44.7X5	T44.7X6
Inderal	T44.7X1	T44.7X2	T44.7X3	T44.7X4	T44.7X5	T44.7X6
Indian						
hemp	T40.7X1	T40.7X2	T40.7X3	T40.7X4	T40.7X5	T40.7X6
tobacco	T62.291	T62.292	T62.293	T62.294	—	—
Indigo carmine	T50.8X1	T50.8X2	T50.8X3	T50.8X4	T50.8X5	T50.8X6
Indobufen	T45.521	T45.522	T45.523	T45.524	T45.525	T45.526
Indocin	T39.2X1	T39.2X2	T39.2X3	T39.2X4	T39.2X5	T39.2X6
Indocyanine green	T50.8X1	T50.8X2	T50.8X3	T50.8X4	T50.8X5	T50.8X6
Indometacin	T39.391	T39.392	T39.393	T39.394	T39.395	T39.396
Indomethacin	T39.391	T39.392	T39.393	T39.394	T39.395	T39.396
farnesil	T39.4X1	T39.4X2	T39.4X3	T39.4X4	T39.4X5	T39.4X6
Indoramin	T44.6X1	T44.6X2	T44.6X3	T44.6X4	T44.6X5	T44.6X6
Industrial						
alcohol	T51.0X1	T51.0X2	T51.0X3	T51.0X4	—	—
fumes	T59.891	T59.892	T59.893	T59.894	—	—
solvents (fumes) (vapors)	T52.91	T52.92	T52.93	T52.94	—	—
Influenza vaccine	T50.B91	T50.B92	T50.B93	T50.B94	T50.B95	T50.B96
Ingested substance NEC	T65.91	T65.92	T65.93	T65.94	—	—
INH	T37.1X1	T37.1X2	T37.1X3	T37.1X4	T37.1X5	T37.1X6
Inhalation, gas (noxious) — see Gas						
Inhibitor						
angiotensin-converting enzyme	T46.4X1	T46.4X2	T46.4X3	T46.4X4	T46.4X5	T46.4X6
carbonic anhydrase	T50.2X1	T50.2X2	T50.2X3	T50.2X4	T50.2X5	T50.2X6
fibrinolysis	T45.621	T45.622	T45.623	T45.624	T45.625	T45.626
monoamine oxidase NEC	T43.1X1	T43.1X2	T43.1X3	T43.1X4	T43.1X5	T43.1X6
hydrazine	T43.1X1	T43.1X2	T43.1X3	T43.1X4	T43.1X5	T43.1X6
postsynaptic	T43.8X1	T43.8X2	T43.8X3	T43.8X4	T43.8X5	T43.8X6
prothrombin synthesis	T45.511	T45.512	T45.513	T45.514	T45.515	T45.516
Ink	T65.891	T65.892	T65.893	T65.894		—
Innovar	T42.71	T42.72	T42.73	T42.74	T42.75	T42.76

TABLE OF DRUGS AND CHEMICALS

Substance	Poisoning, Accidental (Unintentional)	Poisoning, Intentional Self-Harm	Poisoning, Assault	Poisoning, Undetermined	Adverse Effect	Underdosing
Inosine pranobex	T37.5X1	T37.5X2	T37.5X3	T37.5X4	T37.5X5	T37.5X6
Inositol	T50.991	T50.992	T50.993	T50.994	T50.995	T50.996
nicotinate	T46.7X1	T46.7X2	T46.7X3	T46.7X4	T46.7X5	T46.7X6
Inproquone	T45.1X1	T45.1X2	T45.1X3	T45.1X4	T45.1X5	T45.1X6
Insect (sting), venomous	T63.481	T63.482	T63.483	T63.484	—	—
ant	T63.421	T63.422	T63.423	T63.424	—	—
bee	T63.441	T63.442	T63.443	T63.444	—	—
caterpillar	T63.431	T63.432	T63.433	T63.434	—	—
hornet	T63.451	T63.452	T63.453	T63.454	—	—
wasp	T63.461	T63.462	T63.463	T63.464	—	—
Insecticide NEC	T60.91	T60.92	T60.93	T60.94	—	—
carbamate	T60.0X1	T60.0X2	T60.0X3	T60.0X4	—	—
chlorinated	T60.1X1	T60.1X2	T60.1X3	T60.1X4	—	—
mixed	T60.91	T60.92	T60.93	T60.94	—	—
organochlorine	T60.1X1	T60.1X2	T60.1X3	T60.1X4	—	—
organophosphorus	T60.0X1	T60.0X2	T60.0X3	T60.0X4	—	—
Insular tissue extract	T38.3X1	T38.3X2	T38.3X3	T38.3X4	T38.3X5	T38.3X6
Insulin (amorphous) (globin) (isophane) (Lente) (NPH) (Semilente) (Ultralente)	T38.3X1	T38.3X2	T38.3X3	T38.3X4	T38.3X5	T38.3X6
defalan	T38.3X1	T38.3X2	T38.3X3	T38.3X4	T38.3X5	T38.3X6
human	T38.3X1	T38.3X2	T38.3X3	T38.3X4	T38.3X5	T38.3X6
injection, soluble	T38.3X1	T38.3X2	T38.3X3	T38.3X4	T38.3X5	T38.3X6
biphasic	T38.3X1	T38.3X2	T38.3X3	T38.3X4	T38.3X5	T38.3X6
intermediate acting	T38.3X1	T38.3X2	T38.3X3	T38.3X4	T38.3X5	T38.3X6
protamine zinc	T38.3X1	T38.3X2	T38.3X3	T38.3X4	T38.3X5	T38.3X6
slow acting	T38.3X1	T38.3X2	T38.3X3	T38.3X4	T38.3X5	T38.3X6
zinc						
protamine injection	T38.3X1	T38.3X2	T38.3X3	T38.3X4	T38.3X5	T38.3X6
suspension (amorphous) (crystalline)	T38.3X1	T38.3X2	T38.3X3	T38.3X4	T38.3X5	T38.3X6
Interferon (alpha) (beta) (gamma)	T37.5X1	T37.5X2	T37.5X3	T37.5X4	T37.5X5	T37.5X6
Intestinal motility control drug	T47.6X1	T47.6X2	T47.6X3	T47.6X4	T47.6X5	T47.6X6
biological	T47.8X1	T47.8X2	T47.8X3	T47.8X4	T47.8X5	T47.8X6
Intranarcon	T41.1X1	T41.1X2	T41.1X3	T41.1X4	T41.1X5	T41.1X6
Intravenous						
amino acids	T50.991	T50.992	T50.993	T50.994	T50.995	T50.996
fat suspension	T50.991	T50.992	T50.993	T50.994	T50.995	T50.996
Inulin	T50.8X1	T50.8X2	T50.8X3	T50.8X4	T50.8X5	T50.8X6
Invert sugar	T50.3X1	T50.3X2	T50.3X3	T50.3X4	T50.3X5	T50.3X6
Inza — *see* Naproxen						
Iobenzamic acid	T50.8X1	T50.8X2	T50.8X3	T50.8X4	T50.8X5	T50.8X6
Iocarmic acid	T50.8X1	T50.8X2	T50.8X3	T50.8X4	T50.8X5	T50.8X6

Substance	External Cause (T-Code)					
	Poisoning, Accidental (Unintentional)	Poisoning, Intentional Self-Harm	Poisoning, Assault	Poisoning, Undetermined	Adverse Effect	Underdosing
Iocetamic acid	T50.8X1	T50.8X2	T50.8X3	T50.8X4	T50.8X5	T50.8X6
Iodamide	T50.8X1	T50.8X2	T50.8X3	T50.8X4	T50.8X5	T50.8X6
Iodide NEC — *see also Iodine*	T49.0X1	T49.0X2	T49.0X3	T49.0X4	T49.0X5	T49.0X6
mercury (ointment)	T49.0X1	T49.0X2	T49.0X3	T49.0X4	T49.0X5	T49.0X6
methylate	T49.0X1	T49.0X2	T49.0X3	T49.0X4	T49.0X5	T49.0X6
potassium (expectorant) NEC	T48.4X1	T48.4X2	T48.4X3	T48.4X4	T48.4X5	T48.4X6
Iodinated						
contrast medium	T50.8X1	T50.8X2	T50.8X3	T50.8X4	T50.8X5	T50.8X6
glycerol	T48.4X1	T48.4X2	T48.4X3	T48.4X4	T48.4X5	T48.4X6
human serum albumin (131I)	T50.8X1	T50.8X2	T50.8X3	T50.8X4	T50.8X5	T50.8X6
Iodine (antiseptic, external) (tincture) NEC	T49.0X1	T49.0X2	T49.0X3	T49.0X4	T49.0X5	T49.0X6
125 — *see also Radiation sickness, and Exposure to radioactivce isotopes*	T50.8X1	T50.8X2	T50.8X3	T50.8X4	T50.8X5	T50.8X6
therapeutic	T50.991	T50.992	T50.993	T50.994	T50.995	T50.996
131 — *see also Radiation sickness, and Exposure to radioactivce isotopes*	T50.8X1	T50.8X2	T50.8X3	T50.8X4	T50.8X5	T50.8X6
therapeutic	T38.2X1	T38.2X2	T38.2X3	T38.2X4	T38.2X5	T38.2X6
diagnostic	T50.8X1	T50.8X2	T50.8X3	T50.8X4	T50.8X5	T50.8X6
for thyroid conditions (antithyroid)	T38.2X1	T38.2X2	T38.2X3	T38.2X4	T38.2X5	T38.2X6
solution	T49.0X1	T49.0X2	T49.0X3	T49.0X4	T49.0X5	T49.0X6
vapor	T59.891	T59.892	T59.893	T59.894	—	—
Iodipamide	T50.8X1	T50.8X2	T50.8X3	T50.8X4	T50.8X5	T50.8X6
Iodized (poppy seed) oil	T50.8X1	T50.8X2	T50.8X3	T50.8X4	T50.8X5	T50.8X6
Iodobismitol	T37.8X1	T37.8X2	T37.8X3	T37.8X4	T37.8X5	T37.8X6
Iodochlorhydroxyquin	T37.8X1	T37.8X2	T37.8X3	T37.8X4	T37.8X5	T37.8X6
topical	T49.0X1	T49.0X2	T49.0X3	T49.0X4	T49.0X5	T49.0X6
Iodochlorhydroxyquino-line	T37.8X1	T37.8X2	T37.8X3	T37.8X4	T37.8X5	T37.8X6
Iodocholesterol (131I)	T50.8X1	T50.8X2	T50.8X3	T50.8X4	T50.8X5	T50.8X6
Iodoform	T49.0X1	T49.0X2	T49.0X3	T49.0X4	T49.0X5	T49.0X6
Iodohippuric acid	T50.8X1	T50.8X2	T50.8X3	T50.8X4	T50.8X5	T50.8X6
Iodopanoic acid	T50.8X1	T50.8X2	T50.8X3	T50.8X4	T50.8X5	T50.8X6
Iodophthalein (sodium)	T50.8X1	T50.8X2	T50.8X3	T50.8X4	T50.8X5	T50.8X6
Iodopyracet	T50.8X1	T50.8X2	T50.8X3	T50.8X4	T50.8X5	T50.8X6
Iodoquinol	T37.8X1	T37.8X2	T37.8X3	T37.8X4	T37.8X5	T37.8X6
Iodoxamic acid	T50.8X1	T50.8X2	T50.8X3	T50.8X4	T50.8X5	T50.8X6
Iofendylate	T50.8X1	T50.8X2	T50.8X3	T50.8X4	T50.8X5	T50.8X6
Ioglycamic acid	T50.8X1	T50.8X2	T50.8X3	T50.8X4	T50.8X5	T50.8X6
Iohexol	T50.8X1	T50.8X2	T50.8X3	T50.8X4	T50.8X5	T50.8X6
Ion exchange resin						
anion	T47.8X1	T47.8X2	T47.8X3	T47.8X4	T47.8X5	T47.8X6
cation	T50.3X1	T50.3X2	T50.3X3	T50.3X4	T50.3X5	T50.3X6

Substance	Poisoning, Accidental (Unintentional)	Poisoning, Intentional Self-Harm	Poisoning, Assault	Poisoning, Undetermined	Adverse Effect	Underdosing
Ion exchange resin *(Continued)*						
cholestyramine	T46.6X1	T46.6X2	T46.6X3	T46.6X4	T46.6X5	T46.6X6
intestinal	T47.8X1	T47.8X2	T47.8X3	T47.8X4	T47.8X5	T47.8X6
Iopamidol	T50.8X1	T50.8X2	T50.8X3	T50.8X4	T50.8X5	T50.8X6
Iopanoic acid	T50.8X1	T50.8X2	T50.8X3	T50.8X4	T50.8X5	T50.8X6
Iophenoic acid	T50.8X1	T50.8X2	T50.8X3	T50.8X4	T50.8X5	T50.8X6
Iopodate, sodium	T50.8X1	T50.8X2	T50.8X3	T50.8X4	T50.8X5	T50.8X6
Iopodic acid	T50.8X1	T50.8X2	T50.8X3	T50.8X4	T50.8X5	T50.8X6
Iopromide	T50.8X1	T50.8X2	T50.8X3	T50.8X4	T50.8X5	T50.8X6
Iopydol	T50.8X1	T50.8X2	T50.8X3	T50.8X4	T50.8X5	T50.8X6
Iotalamic acid	T50.8X1	T50.8X2	T50.8X3	T50.8X4	T50.8X5	T50.8X6
Iothalamate	T50.8X1	T50.8X2	T50.8X3	T50.8X4	T50.8X5	T50.8X6
Iothiouracil	T38.2X1	T38.2X2	T38.2X3	T38.2X4	T38.2X5	T38.2X6
Iotrol	T50.8X1	T50.8X2	T50.8X3	T50.8X4	T50.8X5	T50.8X6
Iotrolan	T50.8X1	T50.8X2	T50.8X3	T50.8X4	T50.8X5	T50.8X6
Iotroxate	T50.8X1	T50.8X2	T50.8X3	T50.8X4	T50.8X5	T50.8X6
Iotroxic acid	T50.8X1	T50.8X2	T50.8X3	T50.8X4	T50.8X5	T50.8X6
Ioversol	T50.8X1	T50.8X2	T50.8X3	T50.8X4	T50.8X5	T50.8X6
Ioxaglate	T50.8X1	T50.8X2	T50.8X3	T50.8X4	T50.8X5	T50.8X6
Ioxaglic acid	T50.8X1	T50.8X2	T50.8X3	T50.8X4	T50.8X5	T50.8X6
Ioxitalamic acid	T50.8X1	T50.8X2	T50.8X3	T50.8X4	T50.8X5	T50.8X6
Ipecac	T47.7X1	T47.7X2	T47.7X3	T47.7X4	T47.7X5	T47.7X6
Ipecacuanha	T48.4X1	T48.4X2	T48.4X3	T48.4X4	T48.4X5	T48.4X6
Ipodate, calcium	T50.8X1	T50.8X2	T50.8X3	T50.8X4	T50.8X5	T50.8X6
Ipral	T42.3X1	T42.3X2	T42.3X3	T42.3X4	T42.3X5	T42.3X6
Ipratropium (bromide)	T48.6X1	T48.6X2	T48.6X3	T48.6X4	T48.6X5	T48.6X6
Ipriflavone	T46.3X1	T46.3X2	T46.3X3	T46.3X4	T46.3X5	T46.3X6
Iprindole	T43.011	T43.012	T43.013	T43.014	T43.015	T43.016
Iproclozide	T43.1X1	T43.1X2	T43.1X3	T43.1X4	T43.1X5	T43.1X6
Iprofenin	T50.8X1	T50.8X2	T50.8X3	T50.8X4	T50.8X5	T50.8X6
Iproheptine	T49.2X1	T49.2X2	T49.2X3	T49.2X4	T49.2X5	T49.2X6
Iproniazid	T43.1X1	T43.1X2	T43.1X3	T43.1X4	T43.1X5	T43.1X6
Iproplatin	T45.1X1	T45.1X2	T45.1X3	T45.1X4	T45.1X5	T45.1X6
Iproveratril	T46.1X1	T46.1X2	T46.1X3	T46.1X4	T46.1X5	T46.1X6
Iron (compounds) (medicinal) NEC	T45.4X1	T45.4X2	T45.4X3	T45.4X4	T45.4X5	T45.4X6
ammonium	T45.4X1	T45.4X2	T45.4X3	T45.4X4	T45.4X5	T45.4X6
dextran injection	T45.4X1	T45.4X2	T45.4X3	T45.4X4	T45.4X5	T45.4X6
nonmedicinal	T56.891	T56.892	T56.893	T56.894	—	—

Substance	External Cause (T-Code)					
	Poisoning, Accidental (Unintentional)	Poisoning, Intentional Self-Harm	Poisoning, Assault	Poisoning, Undetermined	Adverse Effect	Underdosing
Iron NEC *(Continued)*						
salts	T45.4X1	T45.4X2	T45.4X3	T45.4X4	T45.4X5	T45.4X6
sorbitex	T45.4X1	T45.4X2	T45.4X3	T45.4X4	T45.4X5	T45.4X6
sorbitol citric acid complex	T45.4X1	T45.4X2	T45.4X3	T45.4X4	T45.4X5	T45.4X6
Irrigating fluid (vaginal)	T49.8X1	T49.8X2	T49.8X3	T49.8X4	T49.8X5	T49.8X6
eye	T49.5X1	T49.5X2	T49.5X3	T49.5X4	T49.5X5	T49.5X6
Isepamicin	T36.5X1	T36.5X2	T36.5X3	T36.5X4	T36.5X5	T36.5X6
Isoaminile (citrate)	T48.3X1	T48.3X2	T48.3X3	T48.3X4	T48.3X5	T48.3X6
Isoamyl nitrite	T46.3X1	T46.3X2	T46.3X3	T46.3X4	T46.3X5	T46.3X6
Isobenzan	T60.1X1	T60.1X2	T60.1X3	T60.1X4	—	—
Isobutyl acetate	T52.8X1	T52.8X2	T52.8X3	T52.8X4	—	—
Isocarboxazid	T43.1X1	T43.1X2	T43.1X3	T43.1X4	T43.1X5	T43.1X6
Isoconazole	T49.0X1	T49.0X2	T49.0X3	T49.0X4	T49.0X5	T49.0X6
Isocyanate	T65.0X1	T65.0X2	T65.0X3	T65.0X4	—	—
Isoephedrine	T44.991	T44.992	T44.993	T44.994	T44.995	T44.996
Isoetarine	T48.6X1	T48.6X2	T48.6X3	T48.6X4	T48.6X5	T48.6X6
Isoethadione	T42.2X1	T42.2X2	T42.2X3	T42.2X4	T42.2X5	T42.2X6
Isoetharine	T44.5X1	T44.5X2	T44.5X3	T44.5X4	T44.5X5	T44.5X6
Isoflurane	T41.0X1	T41.0X2	T41.0X3	T41.0X4	T41.0X5	T41.0X6
Isoflurophate	T44.0X1	T44.0X2	T44.0X3	T44.0X4	T44.0X5	T44.0X6
Isomaltose, ferric complex	T45.4X1	T45.4X2	T45.4X3	T45.4X4	T45.4X5	T45.4X6
Isometheptene	T44.3X1	T44.3X2	T44.3X3	T44.3X4	T44.3X5	T44.3X6
Isoniazid	T37.1X1	T37.1X2	T37.1X3	T37.1X4	T37.1X5	T37.1X6
with						
rifampicin	T36.6X1	T36.6X2	T36.6X3	T36.6X4	T36.6X5	T36.6X6
thioacetazone	T37.1X1	T37.1X2	T37.1X3	T37.1X4	T37.1X5	T37.1X6
Isonicotinic acid hydrazide	T37.1X1	T37.1X2	T37.1X3	T37.1X4	T37.1X5	T37.1X6
Isonipecaine	T40.4X1	T40.4X2	T40.4X3	T40.4X4	T40.4X5	T40.4X6
Isopentaquine	T37.2X1	T37.2X2	T37.2X3	T37.2X4	T37.2X5	T37.2X6
Isophane insulin	T38.3X1	T38.3X2	T38.3X3	T38.3X4	T38.3X5	T38.3X6
Isophorone	T65.891	T65.892	T65.893	T65.894	—	—
Isophosphamide	T45.1X1	T45.1X2	T45.1X3	T45.1X4	T45.1X5	T45.1X6
Isopregnenone	T38.5X1	T38.5X2	T38.5X3	T38.5X4	T38.5X5	T38.5X6
Isoprenaline	T48.6X1	T48.6X2	T48.6X3	T48.6X4	T48.6X5	T48.6X6
Isopromethazine	T43.3X1	T43.3X2	T43.3X3	T43.3X4	T43.3X5	T43.3X6
Isopropamide	T44.3X1	T44.3X2	T44.3X3	T44.3X4	T44.3X5	T44.3X6
iodide	T44.3X1	T44.3X2	T44.3X3	T44.3X4	T44.3X5	T44.3X6
Isopropanol	T51.2X1	T51.2X2	T51.2X3	T51.2X4	—	—

Substance	Poisoning, Accidental (Unintentional)	Poisoning, Intentional Self-Harm	Poisoning, Assault	Poisoning, Undetermined	Adverse Effect	Underdosing
Isopropyl						
acetate	T52.8X1	T52.8X2	T52.8X3	T52.8X4	—	—
alcohol	T51.2X1	T51.2X2	T51.2X3	T51.2X4	—	—
medicinal	T49.4X1	T49.4X2	T49.4X3	T49.4X4	T49.4X5	T49.4X6
ether	T52.8X1	T52.8X2	T52.8X3	T52.8X4	—	—
Isopropylaminophena-zone	T39.2X1	T39.2X2	T39.2X3	T39.2X4	T39.2X5	T39.2X6
Isoproterenol	T48.6X1	T48.6X2	T48.6X3	T48.6X4	T48.6X5	T48.6X6
Isosorbide dinitrate	T46.3X1	T46.3X2	T46.3X3	T46.3X4	T46.3X5	T46.3X6
Isothipendyl	T45.0X1	T45.0X2	T45.0X3	T45.0X4	T45.0X5	T45.0X6
Isotretinoin	T50.991	T50.992	T50.993	T50.994	T50.995	T50.996
Isoxazolyl penicillin	T36.0X1	T36.0X2	T36.0X3	T36.0X4	T36.0X5	T36.0X6
Isoxicam	T39.391	T39.392	T39.393	T39.394	T39.395	T39.396
Isoxsuprine	T46.7X1	T46.7X2	T46.7X3	T46.7X4	T46.7X5	T46.7X6
Ispagula	T47.4X1	T47.4X2	T47.4X3	T47.4X4	T47.4X5	T47.4X6
husk	T47.4X1	T47.4X2	T47.4X3	T47.4X4	T47.4X5	T47.4X6
Isradipine	T46.1X1	T46.1X2	T46.1X3	T46.1X4	T46.1X5	T46.1X6
l-thyroxine sodium	T38.1X1	T38.1X2	T38.1X3	T38.1X4	T38.1X5	T38.1X6
Itraconazole	T37.8X1	T37.8X2	T37.8X3	T37.8X4	T37.8X5	T37.8X6
Itramin tosilate	T46.3X1	T46.3X2	T46.3X3	T46.3X4	T46.3X5	T46.3X6
Ivermectin	T37.4X1	T37.4X2	T37.4X3	T37.4X4	T37.4X5	T37.4X6
Izoniazid	T37.1X1	T37.1X2	T37.1X3	T37.1X4	T37.1X5	T37.1X6
with thioacetazone	T37.1X1	T37.1X2	T37.1X3	T37.1X4	T37.1X5	T37.1X6
J						
Jalap	T47.2X1	T47.2X2	T47.2X3	T47.2X4	T47.2X5	T47.2X6
Jamaica						
dogwood (bark)	T39.8X1	T39.8X2	T39.8X3	T39.8X4	T39.8X5	T39.8X6
ginger	T65.891	T65.892	T65.893	T65.894	—	—
root	T62.2X1	T62.2X2	T62.2X3	T62.2X4	—	—
Jatropha	T62.2X1	T62.2X2	T62.2X3	T62.2X4	—	—
curcas	T62.2X1	T62.2X2	T62.2X3	T62.2X4	—	—
Jectofer	T45.4X1	T45.4X2	T45.4X3	T45.4X4	T45.4X5	T45.4X6
Jellyfish (sting)	T63.621	T63.622	T63.623	T63.624		
Jequirity (bean)	T62.2X1	T62.2X2	T62.2X3	T62.2X4	—	—
Jimson weed (stramonium)	T62.2X1	T62.2X2	T62.2X3	T62.2X4	—	—
seeds	T62.2X1	T62.2X2	T62.2X3	T62.2X4	—	—
Josamycin	T36.3X1	T36.3X2	T36.3X3	T36.3X4	T36.3X5	T36.3X6
Juniper tar	T49.1X1	T49.1X2	T49.1X3	T49.1X4	T49.1X5	T49.1X6

Substance	External Cause (T-Code)					
	Poisoning, Accidental (Unintentional)	Poisoning, Intentional Self-Harm	Poisoning, Assault	Poisoning, Undetermined	Adverse Effect	Underdosing
K						
Kallidinogenase	T46.7X1	T46.7X2	T46.7X3	T46.7X4	T46.7X5	T46.7X6
Kallikrein	T46.7X1	T46.7X2	T46.7X3	T46.7X4	T46.7X5	T46.7X6
Kanamycin	T36.5X1	T36.5X2	T36.5X3	T36.5X4	T36.5X5	T36.5X6
Kantrex	T36.5X1	T36.5X2	T36.5X3	T36.5X4	T36.5X5	T36.5X6
Kaolin	T47.6X1	T47.6X2	T47.6X3	T47.6X4	T47.6X5	T47.6X6
light	T47.6X1	T47.6X2	T47.6X3	T47.6X4	T47.6X5	T47.6X6
Karaya (gum)	T47.4X1	T47.4X2	T47.4X3	T47.4X4	T47.4X5	T47.4X6
Kebuzone	T39.2X1	T39.2X2	T39.2X3	T39.2X4	T39.2X5	T39.2X6
Kelevan	T60.1X1	T60.1X2	T60.1X3	T60.1X4	—	—
Kemithal	T41.1X1	T41.1X2	T41.1X3	T41.1X4	T41.1X5	T41.1X6
Kenacort	T38.0X1	T38.0X2	T38.0X3	T38.0X4	T38.0X5	T38.0X6
Keratolytic drug NEC	T49.4X1	T49.4X2	T49.4X3	T49.4X4	T49.4X5	T49.4X6
anthracene	T49.4X1	T49.4X2	T49.4X3	T49.4X4	T49.4X5	T49.4X6
Keratoplastic NEC	T49.4X1	T49.4X2	T49.4X3	T49.4X4	T49.4X5	T49.4X6
Kerosene, kerosine (fuel) (solvent) NEC	T52.0X1	T52.0X2	T52.0X3	T52.0X4	—	—
insecticide	T52.0X1	T52.0X2	T52.0X3	T52.0X4	—	—
vapor	T52.0X1	T52.0X2	T52.0X3	T52.0X4	—	—
Ketamine	T41.291	T41.292	T41.293	T41.294	T41.295	T41.296
Ketazolam	T42.4X1	T42.4X2	T42.4X3	T42.4X4	T42.4X5	T42.4X6
Ketazon	T39.2X1	T39.2X2	T39.2X3	T39.2X4	T39.2X5	T39.2X6
Ketobemidone	T40.4X1	T40.4X2	T40.4X3	T40.4X4	—	—
Ketoconazole	T49.0X1	T49.0X2	T49.0X3	T49.0X4	T49.0X5	T49.0X6
Ketols	T52.4X1	T52.4X2	T52.4X3	T52.4X4	—	—
Ketone oils	T52.4X1	T52.4X2	T52.4X3	T52.4X4	—	—
Ketoprofen	T39.311	T39.312	T39.313	T39.314	T39.315	T39.316
Ketorolac	T39.8X1	T39.8X2	T39.8X3	T39.8X4	T39.8X5	T39.8X6
Ketotifen	T45.0X1	T45.0X2	T45.0X3	T45.0X4	T45.0X5	T45.0X6
Khat	T43.691	T43.692	T43.693	T43.694	—	—
Khellin	T46.3X1	T46.3X2	T46.3X3	T46.3X4	T46.3X5	T46.3X6
Khelloside	T46.3X1	T46.3X2	T46.3X3	T46.3X4	T46.3X5	T46.3X6
Kiln gas or vapor (carbon monoxide)	T58.8X1	T58.8X2	T58.8X3	T58.8X4	—	—
Kitasamycin	T36.3X1	T36.3X2	T36.3X3	T36.3X4	T36.3X5	T36.3X6
Konsyl	T47.4X1	T47.4X2	T47.4X3	T47.4X4	T47.4X5	T47.4X6
Kosam seed	T62.2X1	T62.2X2	T62.2X3	T62.2X4	—	—
Krait (venom)	T63.091	T63.092	T63.093	T63.094	—	—
Kwell (insecticide)	T60.1X1	T60.1X2	T60.1X3	T60.1X4	—	—
anti-infective (topical)	T49.0X1	T49.0X2	T49.0X3	T49.0X4	T49.0X5	T49.0X6

TABLE OF DRUGS AND CHEMICALS

Substance	External Cause (T-Code)					
	Poisoning, Accidental (Unintentional)	Poisoning, Intentional Self-Harm	Poisoning, Assault	Poisoning, Undetermined	Adverse Effect	Underdosing
L						
Labetalol	T44.8X1	T44.8X2	T44.8X3	T44.8X4	T44.8X5	T44.8X6
Laburnum (seeds)	T62.2X1	T62.2X2	T62.2X3	T62.2X4	—	—
leaves	T62.2X1	T62.2X2	T62.2X3	T62.2X4	—	—
Lachesine	T49.5X1	T49.5X2	T49.5X3	T49.5X4	T49.5X5	T49.5X6
Lacidipine	T46.5X1	T46.5X2	T46.5X3	T46.5X4	T46.5X5	T46.5X6
Lacquer	T65.6X1	T65.6X2	T65.6X3	T65.6X4	—	—
Lacrimogenic gas	T59.3X1	T59.3X2	T59.3X3	T59.3X4	—	—
Lactated potassic saline	T50.3X1	T50.3X2	T50.3X3	T50.3X4	T50.3X5	T50.3X6
Lactic acid	T49.8X1	T49.8X2	T49.8X3	T49.8X4	T49.8X5	T49.8X6
Lactobacillus						
acidophilus	T47.6X1	T47.6X2	T47.6X3	T47.6X4	T47.6X5	T47.6X6
compound	T47.6X1	T47.6X2	T47.6X3	T47.6X4	T47.6X5	T47.6X6
bifidus, lyophilized	T47.6X1	T47.6X2	T47.6X3	T47.6X4	T47.6X5	T47.6X6
bulgaricus	T47.6X1	T47.6X2	T47.6X3	T47.6X4	T47.6X5	T47.6X6
sporogenes	T47.6X1	T47.6X2	T47.6X3	T47.6X4	T47.6X5	T47.6X6
Lactoflavin	T45.2X1	T45.2X2	T45.2X3	T45.2X4	T45.2X5	T45.2X6
Lactose (as excipient)	T50.901	T50.902	T50.903	T50.904	T50.905	T50.906
Lactuca (virosa) (extract)	T42.6X1	T42.6X2	T42.6X3	T42.6X4	T42.6X5	T42.6X6
Lactucarium	T42.6X1	T42.6X2	T42.6X3	T42.6X4	T42.6X5	T42.6X6
Lactulose	T47.3X1	T47.3X2	T47.3X3	T47.3X4	T47.3X5	T47.3X6
Laevo — see Levo-						
Lanatosides	T46.0X1	T46.0X2	T46.0X3	T46.0X4	T46.0X5	T46.0X6
Lanolin	T49.3X1	T49.3X2	T49.3X3	T49.3X4	T49.3X5	T49.3X6
Largactil	T43.3X1	T43.3X2	T43.3X3	T43.3X4	T43.3X5	T43.3X6
Larkspur	T62.2X1	T62.2X2	T62.2X3	T62.2X4	—	—
Laroxyl	T43.011	T43.012	T43.013	T43.014	T43.015	T43.016
Lassar's paste	T49.4X1	T49.4X2	T49.4X3	T49.4X4	T49.4X5	T49.4X6
Lasix	T50.1X1	T50.1X2	T50.1X3	T50.1X4	T50.1X5	T50.1X6
Latamoxef	T36.1X1	T36.1X2	T36.1X3	T36.1X4	T36.1X5	T36.1X6
Latex	T65.811	T65.812	T65.813	T65.814	—	—
Lathyrus (seed)	T62.2X1	T62.2X2	T62.2X3	T62.2X4	—	—
Laudanum	T40.0X1	T40.0X2	T40.0X3	T40.0X4	T40.0X5	T40.0X6
Laudexium	T48.1X1	T48.1X2	T48.1X3	T48.1X4	T48.1X5	T48.1X6
Laughing gas	T41.0X1	T41.0X2	T41.0X3	T41.0X4	T41.0X5	T41.0X6
Laurel, black or cherry	T62.2X1	T62.2X2	T62.2X3	T62.2X4	—	—
Laurolinium	T49.0X1	T49.0X2	T49.0X3	T49.0X4	T49.0X5	T49.0X6
Lauryl sulfoacetate	T49.2X1	T49.2X2	T49.2X3	T49.2X4	T49.2X5	T49.2X6

Substance	External Cause (T-Code)					
	Poisoning, Accidental (Unintentional)	Poisoning, Intentional Self-Harm	Poisoning, Assault	Poisoning, Undetermined	Adverse Effect	Underdosing
Laxative NEC	T47.4X1	T47.4X2	T47.4X3	T47.4X4	T47.4X5	T47.4X6
osmotic	T47.3X1	T47.3X2	T47.3X3	T47.3X4	T47.3X5	T47.3X6
saline	T47.3X1	T47.3X2	T47.3X3	T47.3X4	T47.3X5	T47.3X6
stimulant	T47.2X1	T47.2X2	T47.2X3	T47.2X4	T47.2X5	T47.2X6
L-dopa	T42.8X1	T42.8X2	T42.8X3	T42.8X4	T42.8X5	T42.8X6
Lead (dust) (fumes) (vapor) NEC	T56.0X1	T56.0X2	T56.0X3	T56.0X4	—	—
acetate	T49.2X1	T49.2X2	T49.2X3	T49.2X4	T49.2X5	T49.2X6
alkyl (fuel additive)	T56.0X1	T56.0X2	T56.0X3	T56.0X4	—	—
anti-infectives	T37.8X1	T37.8X2	T37.8X3	T37.8X4	T37.8X5	T37.8X6
antiknock compound (tetraethyl)	T56.0X1	T56.0X2	T56.0X3	T56.0X4	—	—
arsenate, arsenite (dust) (herbicide) (insecticide) (vapor)	T57.0X1	T57.0X2	T57.0X3	T57.0X4	—	—
carbonate	T56.0X1	T56.0X2	T56.0X3	T56.0X4	—	—
paint	T56.0X1	T56.0X2	T56.0X3	T56.0X4	—	—
chromate	T56.0X1	T56.0X2	T56.0X3	T56.0X4	—	—
paint	T56.0X1	T56.0X2	T56.0X3	T56.0X4	—	—
dioxide	T56.0X1	T56.0X2	T56.0X3	T56.0X4	—	—
inorganic	T56.0X1	T56.0X2	T56.0X3	T56.0X4	—	—
iodide	T56.0X1	T56.0X2	T56.0X3	T56.0X4	—	—
pigment (paint)	T56.0X1	T56.0X2	T56.0X3	T56.0X4	—	—
monoxide (dust)	T56.0X1	T56.0X2	T56.0X3	T56.0X4	—	—
paint	T56.0X1	T56.0X2	T56.0X3	T56.0X4	—	—
organic	T56.0X1	T56.0X2	T56.0X3	T56.0X4	—	—
oxide	T56.0X1	T56.0X2	T56.0X3	T56.0X4	—	—
paint	T56.0X1	T56.0X2	T56.0X3	T56.0X4	—	—
paint	T56.0X1	T56.0X2	T56.0X3	T56.0X4	—	—
salts	T56.0X1	T56.0X2	T56.0X3	T56.0X4	—	—
specified compound NEC	T56.0X1	T56.0X2	T56.0X3	T56.0X4	—	—
tetra-ethyl	T56.0X1	T56.0X2	T56.0X3	T56.0X4	—	—
Lebanese red	T40.7X1	T40.7X2	T40.7X3	T40.7X4	T40.7X5	T40.7X6
Lefetamine	T39.8X1	T39.8X2	T39.8X3	T39.8X4	T39.8X5	T39.8X6
Lenperone	T43.4X1	T43.4X2	T43.4X3	T43.4X4	T43.4X5	T43.4X6
Lente lietin (insulin)	T38.3X1	T38.3X2	T38.3X3	T38.3X4	T38.3X5	T38.3X6
Leptazol	T50.7X1	T50.7X2	T50.7X3	T50.7X4	T50.7X5	T50.7X6
Leptophos	T60.0X1	T60.0X2	T60.0X3	T60.0X4	—	—
Leritine	T40.2X1	T40.2X2	T40.2X3	T40.2X4	T40.2X5	T40.2X6
Letosteine	T48.4X1	T48.4X2	T48.4X3	T48.4X4	T48.4X5	T48.4X6
Letter	T38.1X1	T38.1X2	T38.1X3	T38.1X4	T38.1X5	T38.1X6
Lettuce opium	T42.6X1	T42.6X2	T42.6X3	T42.6X4	T42.6X5	T42.6X6
Leucinocaine	T41.3X1	T41.3X2	T41.3X3	T41.3X4	T41.3X5	T41.3X6

External Cause (T-Code)

Substance	Poisoning, Accidental (Unintentional)	Poisoning, Intentional Self-Harm	Poisoning, Assault	Poisoning, Undetermined	Adverse Effect	Underdosing
Leucocianidol	T46.991	T46.992	T46.993	T46.994	T46.995	T46.996
Leucovorin (factor)	T45.8X1	T45.8X2	T45.8X3	T45.8X4	T45.8X5	T45.8X6
Leukeran	T45.1X1	T45.1X2	T45.1X3	T45.1X4	T45.1X5	T45.1X6
Leuprolide	T38.891	T38.892	T38.893	T38.894	T38.895	T38.896
Levalbuterol	T48.6X1	T48.6X2	T48.6X3	T48.6X4	T48.6X5	T48.6X6
Levallorphan	T50.7X1	T50.7X2	T50.7X3	T50.7X4	T50.7X5	T50.7X6
Levamisole	T37.4X1	T37.4X2	T37.4X3	T37.4X4	T37.4X5	T37.4X6
Levanil	T42.6X1	T42.6X2	T42.6X3	T42.6X4	T42.6X5	T42.6X6
Levarterenol	T44.4X1	T44.4X2	T44.4X3	T44.4X4	T44.4X5	T44.4X6
Levdropropizine	T48.3X1	T48.3X2	T48.3X3	T48.3X4	T48.3X5	T48.3X6
Levobunolol	T49.5X1	T49.5X2	T49.5X3	T49.5X4	T49.5X5	T49.5X6
Levocabastine (hydrochloride)	T45.0X1	T45.0X2	T45.0X3	T45.0X4	T45.0X5	T45.0X6
Levocarnitine	T50.991	T50.992	T50.993	T50.994	T50.995	T50.996
Levodopa	T42.8X1	T42.8X2	T42.8X3	T42.8X4	T42.8X5	T42.8X6
with carbidopa	T42.8X1	T42.8X2	T42.8X3	T42.8X4	T42.8X5	T42.8X6
Levo-dromoran	T40.2X1	T40.2X2	T40.2X3	T40.2X4	T40.2X5	T40.2X6
Levoglutamide	T50.991	T50.992	T50.993	T50.994	T50.995	T50.996
Levoid	T38.1X1	T38.1X2	T38.1X3	T38.1X4	T38.1X5	T38.1X6
Levo-iso-methadone	T40.3X1	T40.3X2	T40.3X3	T40.3X4	T40.3X5	T40.3X6
Levomepromazine	T43.3X1	T43.3X2	T43.3X3	T43.3X4	T43.3X5	T43.3X6
Levonordefrin	T49.6X1	T49.6X2	T49.6X3	T49.6X4	T49.6X5	T49.6X6
Levonorgestrel	T38.4X1	T38.4X2	T38.4X3	T38.4X4	T38.4X5	T38.4X6
with ethinylestradiol	T38.5X1	T38.5X2	T38.5X3	T38.5X4	T38.5X5	T38.5X6
Levopromazine	T43.3X1	T43.3X2	T43.3X3	T43.3X4	T43.3X5	T43.3X6
Levoprome	T42.6X1	T42.6X2	T42.6X3	T42.6X4	T42.6X5	T42.6X6
Levopropoxyphene	T40.4X1	T40.4X2	T40.4X3	T40.4X4	T40.4X5	T40.4X6
Levopropylhexedrine	T50.5X1	T50.5X2	T50.5X3	T50.5X4	T50.5X5	T50.5X6
Levoproxyphylline	T48.6X1	T48.6X2	T48.6X3	T48.6X4	T48.6X5	T48.6X6
Levorphanol	T40.4X1	T40.4X2	T40.4X3	T40.4X4	T40.4X5	T40.4X6
Levothyroxine	T38.1X1	T38.1X2	T38.1X3	T38.1X4	T38.1X5	T38.1X6
sodium	T38.1X1	T38.1X2	T38.1X3	T38.1X4	T38.1X5	T38.1X6
Levsin	T44.3X1	T44.3X2	T44.3X3	T44.3X4	T44.3X5	T44.3X6
Levulose	T50.3X1	T50.3X2	T50.3X3	T50.3X4	T50.3X5	T50.3X6
Lewisite (gas), not in war	T57.0X1	T57.0X2	T57.0X3	T57.0X4	—	—
Librium	T42.4X1	T42.4X2	T42.4X3	T42.4X4	T42.4X5	T42.4X6
Lidex	T49.0X1	T49.0X2	T49.0X3	T49.0X4	T49.0X5	T49.0X6
Lidocaine	T41.3X1	T41.3X2	T41.3X3	T41.3X4	T41.3X5	T41.3X6
regional	T41.3X1	T41.3X2	T41.3X3	T41.3X4	T41.3X5	T41.3X6
spinal	T41.3X1	T41.3X2	T41.3X3	T41.3X4	T41.3X5	T41.3X6
Lidofenin	T50.8X1	T50.8X2	T50.8X3	T50.8X4	T50.8X5	T50.8X6

Substance	External Cause (T-Code)					
	Poisoning, Accidental (Unintentional)	Poisoning, Intentional Self-Harm	Poisoning, Assault	Poisoning, Undetermined	Adverse Effect	Underdosing
Lidoflazine	T46.1X1	T46.1X2	T46.1X3	T46.1X4	T46.1X5	T46.1X6
Lighter fluid	T52.0X1	T52.0X2	T52.0X3	T52.0X4	—	—
Lignin hemicellulose	T47.6X1	T47.6X2	T47.6X3	T47.6X4	T47.6X5	T47.6X6
Lignocaine	T41.3X1	T41.3X2	T41.3X3	T41.3X4	T41.3X5	T41.3X6
regional	T41.3X1	T41.3X2	T41.3X3	T41.3X4	T41.3X5	T41.3X6
spinal	T41.3X1	T41.3X2	T41.3X3	T41.3X4	T41.3X5	T41.3X6
Ligroin(e) (solvent)	T52.0X1	T52.0X2	T52.0X3	T52.0X4	—	—
vapor	T59.891	T59.892	T59.893	T59.894	—	—
Ligustrum vulgare	T62.2X1	T62.2X2	T62.2X3	T62.2X4	—	—
Lily of the valley	T62.2X1	T62.2X2	T62.2X3	T62.2X4	—	—
Lime (chloride)	T54.3X1	T54.3X2	T54.3X3	T54.3X4	—	—
Limonene	T52.8X1	T52.8X2	T52.8X3	T52.8X4	—	—
Lincomycin	T36.8X1	T36.8X2	T36.8X3	T36.8X4	T36.8X5	T36.8X6
Lindane (insecticide) (nonmedicinal) (vapor)	T53.6X1	T53.6X2	T53.6X3	T53.6X4	—	—
medicinal	T49.0X1	T49.0X2	T49.0X3	T49.0X4	T49.0X5	T49.0X6
Liniments NEC	T49.91	T49.92	T49.93	T49.94	T49.95	T49.96
Linoleic acid	T46.6X1	T46.6X2	T46.6X3	T46.6X4	T46.6X5	T46.6X6
Linolenic acid	T46.6X1	T46.6X2	T46.6X3	T46.6X4	T46.6X5	T46.6X6
Linseed	T47.4X1	T47.4X2	T47.4X3	T47.4X4	T47.4X5	T47.4X6
Liothyronine	T38.1X1	T38.1X2	T38.1X3	T38.1X4	T38.1X5	T38.1X6
Liotrix	T38.1X1	T38.1X2	T38.1X3	T38.1X4	T38.1X5	T38.1X6
Lipancreatin	T47.5X1	T47.5X2	T47.5X3	T47.5X4	T47.5X5	T47.5X6
Lipo-alprostadil	T46.7X1	T46.7X2	T46.7X3	T46.7X4	T46.7X5	T46.7X6
Lipo-Lutin	T38.5X1	T38.5X2	T38.5X3	T38.5X4	T38.5X5	T38.5X6
Lipotropic drug NEC	T50.901	T50.902	T50.903	T50.904	T50.905	T50.906
Liquefied petroleum gases	T59.891	T59.892	T59.893	T59.894	—	—
piped (pure or mixed with air)	T59.891	T59.892	T59.893	T59.894	—	—
Liquid						
paraffin	T47.4X1	T47.4X2	T47.4X3	T47.4X4	T47.4X5	T47.4X6
petrolatum	T47.4X1	T47.4X2	T47.4X3	T47.4X4	T47.4X5	T47.4X6
topical	T49.3X1	T49.3X2	T49.3X3	T49.3X4	T49.3X5	T49.3X6
specified NEC	T65.891	T65.892	T65.893	T65.894	—	—
substance	T65.91	T65.92	T65.93	T65.94	—	—
Liquor creosolis compositus	T65.891	T65.892	T65.893	T65.894	—	—
Liquorice	T48.4X1	T48.4X2	T48.4X3	T48.4X4	T48.4X5	T48.4X6
extract	T47.8X1	T47.8X2	T47.8X3	T47.8X4	T47.8X5	T47.8X6
Lirugen	T50.991	T50.992	T50.993	T50.994	T50.995	T50.996
Lisinopril	T46.4X1	T46.4X2	T46.4X3	T46.4X4	T46.4X5	T46.4X6
Lisuride	T42.8X1	T42.8X2	T42.8X3	T42.8X4	T42.8X5	T42.8X6
Lithane	T43.8X1	T43.8X2	T43.8X3	T43.8X4	T43.8X5	T43.8X6

Substance	Poisoning, Accidental (Unintentional)	Poisoning, Intentional Self-Harm	Poisoning, Assault	Poisoning, Undetermined	Adverse Effect	Underdosing
Lithium	T56.891	T56.892	T56.893	T56.894	—	—
gluconate	T43.591	T43.592	T43.593	T43.594	T43.595	T43.596
salts (carbonate)	T43.591	T43.592	T43.593	T43.594	T43.595	T43.596
Lithonate	T43.8X1	T43.8X2	T43.8X3	T43.8X4	T43.8X5	T43.8X6
Liver						
extract	T45.8X1	T45.8X2	T45.8X3	T45.8X4	T45.8X5	T45.8X6
for parenteral use	T45.8X1	T45.8X2	T45.8X3	T45.8X4	T45.8X5	T45.8X6
fraction 1	T45.8X1	T45.8X2	T45.8X3	T45.8X4	T45.8X5	T45.8X6
hydrolysate	T45.8X1	T45.8X2	T45.8X3	T45.8X4	T45.8X5	T45.8X6
Lizard (bite) (venom)	T63.121	T63.122	T63.123	T63.124	—	—
LMD	T45.8X1	T45.8X2	T45.8X3	T45.8X4	T45.8X5	T45.8X6
Lobelia	T62.2X1	T62.2X2	T62.2X3	T62.2X4	—	—
Lobeline	T50.7X1	T50.7X2	T50.7X3	T50.7X4	T50.7X5	T50.7X6
Local action drug NEC	T49.8X1	T49.8X2	T49.8X3	T49.8X4	T49.8X5	T49.8X6
Locorten	T49.0X1	T49.0X2	T49.0X3	T49.0X4	T49.0X5	T49.0X6
Lofepramine	T43.011	T43.012	T43.013	T43.014	T43.015	T43.016
Lolium temulentum	T62.2X1	T62.2X2	T62.2X3	T62.2X4	—	—
Lomotil	T47.6X1	T47.6X2	T47.6X3	T47.6X4	T47.6X5	T47.6X6
Lomustine	T45.1X1	T45.1X2	T45.1X3	T45.1X4	T45.1X5	T45.1X6
Lonidamine	T45.1X1	T45.1X2	T45.1X3	T45.1X4	T45.1X5	T45.1X6
Loperamide	T47.6X1	T47.6X2	T47.6X3	T47.6X4	T47.6X5	T47.6X6
Loprazolam	T42.4X1	T42.4X2	T42.4X3	T42.4X4	T42.4X5	T42.4X6
Lorajmine	T46.2X1	T46.2X2	T46.2X3	T46.2X4	T46.2X5	T46.2X6
Loratidine	T45.0X1	T45.0X2	T45.0X3	T45.0X4	T45.0X5	T45.0X6
Lorazepam	T42.4X1	T42.4X2	T42.4X3	T42.4X4	T42.4X5	T42.4X6
Lorcainide	T46.2X1	T46.2X2	T46.2X3	T46.2X4	T46.2X5	T46.2X6
Lormetazepam	T42.4X1	T42.4X2	T42.4X3	T42.4X4	T42.4X5	T42.4X6
Lotions NEC	T49.91	T49.92	T49.93	T49.94	T49.95	T49.96
Lotusate	T42.3X1	T42.3X2	T42.3X3	T42.3X4	T42.3X5	T42.3X6
Lovastatin	T46.6X1	T46.6X2	T46.6X3	T46.6X4	T46.6X5	T46.6X6
Loxapine	T43.591	T43.592	T43.593	T43.594	T43.595	T43.596
Lowila	T49.2X1	T49.2X2	T49.2X3	T49.2X4	T49.2X5	T49.2X6
Lozenges (throat)	T49.6X1	T49.6X2	T49.6X3	T49.6X4	T49.6X5	T49.6X6
LSD	T40.8X1	T40.8X2	T40.8X3	T40.8X4	T40.8X5	—
L-Tryptophan — see amino acid						
Lubricant, eye	T49.5X1	T49.5X2	T49.5X3	T49.5X4	T49.5X5	T49.5X6
Lubricating oil NEC	T52.0X1	T52.0X2	T52.0X3	T52.0X4	—	—
Lucanthone	T37.4X1	T37.4X2	T37.4X3	T37.4X4	T37.4X5	T37.4X6
Luminal	T42.3X1	T42.3X2	T42.3X3	T42.3X4	T42.3X5	T42.3X6
Lung irritant (gas) NEC	T59.91	T59.92	T59.93	T59.94	—	—

Substance	Poisoning, Accidental (Unintentional)	Poisoning, Intentional Self-Harm	Poisoning, Assault	Poisoning, Undetermined	Adverse Effect	Underdosing
			External Cause (T-Code)			
Luteinizing hormone	T38.811	T38.812	T38.813	T38.814	T38.815	T38.816
Lutocylol	T38.5X1	T38.5X2	T38.5X3	T38.5X4	T38.5X5	T38.5X6
Lutromone	T38.5X1	T38.5X2	T38.5X3	T38.5X4	T38.5X5	T38.5X6
Lututrin	T48.291	T48.292	T48.293	T48.294	T48.295	T48.296
Lye (Concentrated)	T54.3X1	T54.3X2	T54.3X3	T54.3X4	—	—
Lygranum (skin test)	T50.8X1	T50.8X2	T50.8X3	T50.8X4	T50.8X5	T50.8X6
Lymecycline	T36.4X1	T36.4X2	T36.4X3	T36.4X4	T36.4X5	T36.4X6
Lymphogranuloma venereum antigen	T50.8X1	T50.8X2	T50.8X3	T50.8X4	T50.8X5	T50.8X6
Lynestrenol	T38.4X1	T38.4X2	T38.4X3	T38.4X4	T38.4X5	T38.4X6
Lypressin	T38.891	T38.892	T38.893	T38.894	T38.895	T38.896
Lyovac Sodium Edecrin	T50.1X1	T50.1X2	T50.1X3	T50.1X4	T50.1X5	T50.1X6
Lysergic acid diethylamide	T40.8X1	T40.8X2	T40.8X3	T40.8X4	T40.8X5	—
Lysergide	T40.8X1	T40.8X2	T40.8X3	T40.8X4	T40.8X5	—
Lysine vasopressin	T38.891	T38.892	T38.893	T38.894	T38.895	T38.896
Lysol	T54.1X1	T54.1X2	T54.1X3	T54.1X4	—	—
Lysozyme	T49.0X1	T49.0X2	T49.0X3	T49.0X4	T49.0X5	T49.0X6
Lytta (vitatta)	T49.8X1	T49.8X2	T49.8X3	T49.8X4	T49.8X5	T49.8X6
M						
Mace	T59.3X1	T59.3X2	T59.3X3	T59.3X4	—	—
Macrogol	T50.991	T50.992	T50.993	T50.994	T50.995	T50.996
Macrolide						
anabolic drug	T38.7X1	T38.7X2	T38.7X3	T38.7X4	T38.7X5	T38.7X6
antibiotic	T36.3X1	T36.3X2	T36.3X3	T36.3X4	T36.3X5	T36.3X6
Mafenide	T49.0X1	T49.0X2	T49.0X3	T49.0X4	T49.0X5	T49.0X6
Magaldrate	T47.1X1	T47.1X2	T47.1X3	T47.1X4	T47.1X5	T47.1X6
Magic mushroom	T40.991	T40.992	T40.993	T40.994	—	—
Magnamycin	T36.8X1	T36.8X2	T36.8X3	T36.8X4	T36.8X5	T36.8X6
Magnesia magma	T47.1X1	T47.1X2	T47.1X3	T47.1X4	T47.1X5	T47.1X6
Magnesium NEC	T56.891	T56.892	T56.893	T56.894	—	—
carbonate	T47.1X1	T47.1X2	T47.1X3	T47.1X4	T47.1X5	T47.1X6
citrate	T47.4X1	T47.4X2	T47.4X3	T47.4X4	T47.4X5	T47.4X6
hydroxide	T47.1X1	T47.1X2	T47.1X3	T47.1X4	T47.1X5	T47.1X6
oxide	T47.1X1	T47.1X2	T47.1X3	T47.1X4	T47.1X5	T47.1X6
peroxide	T49.0X1	T49.0X2	T49.0X3	T49.0X4	T49.0X5	T49.0X6
salicylate	T39.091	T39.092	T39.093	T39.094	T39.095	T39.096
silicofluoride	T50.3X1	T50.3X2	T50.3X3	T50.3X4	T50.3X5	T50.3X6
sulfate	T47.4X1	T47.4X2	T47.4X3	T47.4X4	T47.4X5	T47.4X6
thiosulfate	T45.0X1	T45.0X2	T45.0X3	T45.0X4	T45.0X5	T45.0X6
trisilicate	T47.1X1	T47.1X2	T47.1X3	T47.1X4	T47.1X5	T47.1X6

Substance	Poisoning, Accidental (Unintentional)	External Cause (T-Code)				
		Poisoning, Intentional Self-Harm	Poisoning, Assault	Poisoning, Undetermined	Adverse Effect	Underdosing
Malathion (medicinal)	T49.0X1	T49.0X2	T49.0X3	T49.0X4	T49.0X5	T49.0X6
insecticide	T60.0X1	T60.0X2	T60.0X3	T60.0X4	—	—
Male fern extract	T37.4X1	T37.4X2	T37.4X3	T37.4X4	T37.4X5	T37.4X6
M-AMSA	T45.1X1	T45.1X2	T45.1X3	T45.1X4	T45.1X5	T45.1X6
Mandelic acid	T37.8X1	T37.8X2	T37.8X3	T37.8X4	T37.8X5	T37.8X6
Manganese (dioxide) (salts)	T57.2X1	T57.2X2	T57.2X3	T57.2X4	—	—
medicinal	T50.991	T50.992	T50.993	T50.994	T50.995	T50.996
Mannitol	T47.3X1	T47.3X2	T47.3X3	T47.3X4	T47.3X5	T47.3X6
hexanitrate	T46.3X1	T46.3X2	T46.3X3	T46.3X4	T46.3X5	T46.3X6
Mannomustine	T45.1X1	T45.1X2	T45.1X3	T45.1X4	T45.1X5	T45.1X6
MAO inhibitors	T43.1X1	T43.1X2	T43.1X3	T43.1X4	T43.1X5	T43.1X6
Mapharsen	T37.8X1	T37.8X2	T37.8X3	T37.8X4	T37.8X5	T37.8X6
Maphenide	T49.0X1	T49.0X2	T49.0X3	T49.0X4	T49.0X5	T49.0X6
Maprotiline	T43.021	T43.022	T43.023	T43.024	T43.025	T43.026
Marcaine	T41.3X1	T41.3X2	T41.3X3	T41.3X4	T41.3X5	T41.3X6
infiltration (subcutaneous)	T41.3X1	T41.3X2	T41.3X3	T41.3X4	T41.3X5	T41.3X6
nerve block (peripheral) (plexus)	T41.3X1	T41.3X2	T41.3X3	T41.3X4	T41.3X5	T41.3X6
Marezine	T45.0X1	T45.0X2	T45.0X3	T45.0X4	T45.0X5	T45.0X6
Marihuana	T40.7X1	T40.7X2	T40.7X3	T40.7X4	T40.7X5	T40.7X6
Marijuana	T40.7X1	T40.7X2	T40.7X3	T40.7X4	T40.7X5	T40.7X6
Marine (sting)	T63.691	T63.692	T63.693	T63.694	—	—
animals (sting)	T63.691	T63.692	T63.693	T63.694	—	—
plants (sting)	T63.711	T63.712	T63.713	T63.714	—	—
Marplan	T43.1X1	T43.1X2	T43.1X3	T43.1X4	T43.1X5	T43.1X6
Marsh gas	T59.891	T59.892	T59.893	T59.894	—	—
Marsilid	T43.1X1	T43.1X2	T43.1X3	T43.1X4	T43.1X5	T43.1X6
Matulane	T45.1X1	T45.1X2	T45.1X3	T45.1X4	T45.1X5	T45.1X6
Mazindol	T50.5X1	T50.5X2	T50.5X3	T50.5X4	T50.5X5	T50.5X6
MCPA	T60.3X1	T60.3X2	T60.3X3	T60.3X4	—	—
MDMA	T43.621	T43.622	T43.623	T43.624	T43.625	T43.626
Meadow saffron	T62.2X1	T62.2X2	T62.2X3	T62.2X4	—	—
Measles virus vaccine (attenuated)	T50.B91	T50.B92	T50.B93	T50.B94	T50.B95	T50.B96
Meat, noxious	T62.8X1	T62.8X2	T62.8X3	T62.8X4	—	—
Meballymal	T42.3X1	T42.3X2	T42.3X3	T42.3X4	T42.3X5	T42.3X6
Mebanazine	T43.1X1	T43.1X2	T43.1X3	T43.1X4	T43.1X5	T43.1X6
Mebaral	T42.3X1	T42.3X2	T42.3X3	T42.3X4	T42.3X5	T42.3X6
Mebendazole	T37.4X1	T37.4X2	T37.4X3	T37.4X4	T37.4X5	T37.4X6
Mebeverine	T44.3X1	T44.3X2	T44.3X3	T44.3X4	T44.3X5	T44.3X6
Mebhydrolin	T45.0X1	T45.0X2	T45.0X3	T45.0X4	T45.0X5	T45.0X6
Mebumal	T42.3X1	T42.3X2	T42.3X3	T42.3X4	T42.3X5	T42.3X6

Substance	Poisoning, Accidental (Unintentional)	Poisoning, Intentional Self-Harm	Poisoning, Assault	Poisoning, Undetermined	Adverse Effect	Underdosing
Mebutamate	T43.591	T43.592	T43.593	T43.594	T43.595	T43.596
Mecamylamine	T44.2X1	T44.2X2	T44.2X3	T44.2X4	T44.2X5	T44.2X6
Mechlorethamine	T45.1X1	T45.1X2	T45.1X3	T45.1X4	T45.1X5	T45.1X6
Mecillinam	T36.0X1	T36.0X2	T36.0X3	T36.0X4	T36.0X5	T36.0X6
Meclizine (hydrochloride)	T45.0X1	T45.0X2	T45.0X3	T45.0X4	T45.0X5	T45.0X6
Meclocycline	T36.4X1	T36.4X2	T36.4X3	T36.4X4	T36.4X5	T36.4X6
Meclofenamate	T39.391	T39.392	T39.393	T39.394	T39.395	T39.396
Meclofenamic acid	T39.391	T39.392	T39.393	T39.394	T39.395	T39.396
Meclofenoxate	T43.691	T43.692	T43.693	T43.694	T43.695	T43.696
Meclozine	T45.0X1	T45.0X2	T45.0X3	T45.0X4	T45.0X5	T45.0X6
Mecobalamin	T45.8X1	T45.8X2	T45.8X3	T45.8X4	T45.8X5	T45.8X6
Mecoprop	T60.3X1	T60.3X2	T60.3X3	T60.3X4	—	—
Mecrilate	T49.3X1	T49.3X2	T49.3X3	T49.3X4	T49.3X5	T49.3X6
Mecysteine	T48.4X1	T48.4X2	T48.4X3	T48.4X4	T48.4X5	T48.4X6
Medazepam	T42.4X1	T42.4X2	T42.4X3	T42.4X4	T42.4X5	T42.4X6
Medicament NEC	T50.901	T50.902	T50.903	T50.904	T50.905	T50.906
Medinal	T42.3X1	T42.3X2	T42.3X3	T42.3X4	T42.3X5	T42.3X6
Medomin	T42.3X1	T42.3X2	T42.3X3	T42.3X4	T42.3X5	T42.3X6
Medrogestone	T38.5X1	T38.5X2	T38.5X3	T38.5X4	T38.5X5	T38.5X6
Medroxalol	T44.8X1	T44.8X2	T44.8X3	T44.8X4	T44.8X5	T44.8X6
Medroxyprogesterone acetate (depot)	T38.5X1	T38.5X2	T38.5X3	T38.5X4	T38.5X5	T38.5X6
Medrysone	T49.0X1	T49.0X2	T49.0X3	T49.0X4	T49.0X5	T49.0X6
Mefenamic acid	T39.391	T39.392	T39.393	T39.394	T39.395	T39.396
Mefenorex	T50.5X1	T50.5X2	T50.5X3	T50.5X4	T50.5X5	T50.5X6
Mefloquine	T37.2X1	T37.2X2	T37.2X3	T37.2X4	T37.2X5	T37.2X6
Mefruside	T50.2X1	T50.2X2	T50.2X3	T50.2X4	T50.2X5	T50.2X6
Megahallucinogen	T40.901	T40.902	T40.903	T40.904	T40.905	T40.906
Megestrol	T38.5X1	T38.5X2	T38.5X3	T38.5X4	T38.5X5	T38.5X6
Meglumine						
antimoniate	T37.8X1	T37.8X2	T37.8X3	T37.8X4	T37.8X5	T37.8X6
diatrizoate	T50.8X1	T50.8X2	T50.8X3	T50.8X4	T50.8X5	T50.8X6
iodipamide	T50.8X1	T50.8X2	T50.8X3	T50.8X4	T50.8X5	T50.8X6
iotroxate	T50.8X1	T50.8X2	T50.8X3	T50.8X4	T50.8X5	T50.8X6
MEK (methyl ethyl ketone)	T52.4X1	T52.4X2	T52.4X3	T52.4X4	—	—
Meladrazine	T44.3X1	T44.3X2	T44.3X3	T44.3X4	T44.3X5	T44.3X6
Meladinin	T49.3X1	T49.3X2	T49.3X3	T49.3X4	T49.3X5	T49.3X6
Melaleuca alternifolia oil	T49.0X1	T49.0X2	T49.0X3	T49.0X4	T49.0X5	T49.0X6
Melanizing agents	T49.3X1	T49.3X2	T49.3X3	T49.3X4	T49.3X5	T49.3X6
Melanocyte-stimulating hormone	T38.891	T38.892	T38.893	T38.894	T38.895	T38.896
Melarsonyl potassium	T37.3X1	T37.3X2	T37.3X3	T37.3X4	T37.3X5	T37.3X6

TABLE OF DRUGS AND CHEMICALS

Substance	External Cause (T-Code)					
	Poisoning, Accidental (Unintentional)	Poisoning, Intentional Self-Harm	Poisoning, Assault	Poisoning, Undetermined	Adverse Effect	Underdosing
Melarsoprol	T37.3X1	T37.3X2	T37.3X3	T37.3X4	T37.3X5	T37.3X6
Melia azedarach	T62.2X1	T62.2X2	T62.2X3	T62.2X4	—	—
Melitracen	T43.011	T43.012	T43.013	T43.014	T43.015	T43.016
Mellaril	T43.3X1	T43.3X2	T43.3X3	T43.3X4	T43.3X5	T43.3X6
Meloxine	T49.3X1	T49.3X2	T49.3X3	T49.3X4	T49.3X5	T49.3X6
Melperone	T43.4X1	T43.4X2	T43.4X3	T43.4X4	T43.4X5	T43.4X6
Melphalan	T45.1X1	T45.1X2	T45.1X3	T45.1X4	T45.1X5	T45.1X6
Memantine	T43.8X1	T43.8X2	T43.8X3	T43.8X4	T43.8X5	T43.8X6
Menadiol	T45.7X1	T45.7X2	T45.7X3	T45.7X4	T45.7X5	T45.7X6
sodium sulfate	T45.7X1	T45.7X2	T45.7X3	T45.7X4	T45.7X5	T45.7X6
Menadione	T45.7X1	T45.7X2	T45.7X3	T45.7X4	T45.7X5	T45.7X6
sodium bisulfite	T45.7X1	T45.7X2	T45.7X3	T45.7X4	T45.7X5	T45.7X6
Menaphthone	T45.7X1	T45.7X2	T45.7X3	T45.7X4	T45.7X5	T45.7X6
Menaquinone	T45.7X1	T45.7X2	T45.7X3	T45.7X4	T45.7X5	T45.7X6
Menatetrenone	T45.7X1	T45.7X2	T45.7X3	T45.7X4	T45.7X5	T45.7X6
Meningococcal vaccine	T50.A91	T50.A92	T50.A93	T50.A94	T50.A95	T50.A96
Menningovax (-AC) (-C)	T50.A91	T50.A92	T50.A93	T50.A94	T50.A95	T50.A96
Menotropins	T38.811	T38.812	T38.813	T38.814	T38.815	T38.816
Menthol	T48.5X1	T48.5X2	T48.5X3	T48.5X4	T48.5X5	T48.5X6
Mepacrine	T37.2X1	T37.2X2	T37.2X3	T37.2X4	T37.2X5	T37.2X6
Meparfynol	T42.6X1	T42.6X2	T42.6X3	T42.6X4	T42.6X5	T42.6X6
Mepartricin	T36.7X1	T36.7X2	T36.7X3	T36.7X4	T36.7X5	T36.7X6
Mepazine	T43.3X1	T43.3X2	T43.3X3	T43.3X4	T43.3X5	T43.3X6
Mepenzolate	T44.3X1	T44.3X2	T44.3X3	T44.3X4	T44.3X5	T44.3X6
bromide	T44.3X1	T44.3X2	T44.3X3	T44.3X4	T44.3X5	T44.3X6
Meperidine	T40.4X1	T40.4X2	T40.4X3	T40.4X4	T40.4X5	T40.4X6
Mephebarbital	T42.3X1	T42.3X2	T42.3X3	T42.3X4	T42.3X5	T42.3X6
Mephenamin(e)	T42.8X1	T42.8X2	T42.8X3	T42.8X4	T42.8X5	T42.8X6
Mephenesin	T42.8X1	T42.8X2	T42.8X3	T42.8X4	T42.8X5	T42.8X6
Mephenhydramine	T45.0X1	T45.0X2	T45.0X3	T45.0X4	T45.0X5	T45.0X6
Mephenoxalone	T42.8X1	T42.8X2	T42.8X3	T42.8X4	T42.8X5	T42.8X6
Mephentermine	T44.991	T44.992	T44.993	T44.994	T44.995	T44.996
Mephenytoin	T42.0X1	T42.0X2	T42.0X3	T42.0X4	T42.0X5	T42.0X6
with phenobarbital	T42.3X1	T42.3X2	T42.3X3	T42.3X4	T42.3X5	T42.3X6
Mephobarbital	T42.3X1	T42.3X2	T42.3X3	T42.3X4	T42.3X5	T42.3X6
Mephosfolan	T60.0X1	T60.0X2	T60.0X3	T60.0X4	—	—
Mepindolol	T44.7X1	T44.7X2	T44.7X3	T44.7X4	T44.7X5	T44.7X6
Mepiperphenidol	T44.3X1	T44.3X2	T44.3X3	T44.3X4	T44.3X5	T44.3X6
Mepitiostane	T38.7X1	T38.7X2	T38.7X3	T38.7X4	T38.7X5	T38.7X6

Substance	Poisoning, Accidental (Unintentional)	Poisoning, Intentional Self-Harm	Poisoning, Assault	Poisoning, Undetermined	Adverse Effect	Underdosing
	External Cause (T-Code)					
Mepivacaine	T41.3X1	T41.3X2	T41.3X3	T41.3X4	T41.3X5	T41.3X6
epidural	T41.3X1	T41.3X2	T41.3X3	T41.3X4	T41.3X5	T41.3X6
Meprednisone	T38.0X1	T38.0X2	T38.0X3	T38.0X4	T38.0X5	T38.0X6
Meprobam	T43.591	T43.592	T43.593	T43.594	T43.595	T43.596
Meprobamate	T43.591	T43.592	T43.593	T43.594	T43.595	T43.596
Meproscillarin	T46.0X1	T46.0X2	T46.0X3	T46.0X4	T46.0X5	T46.0X6
Meprylcaine	T41.3X1	T41.3X2	T41.3X3	T41.3X4	T41.3X5	T41.3X6
Meptazinol	T39.8X1	T39.8X2	T39.8X3	T39.8X4	T39.8X5	T39.8X6
Mepyramine	T45.0X1	T45.0X2	T45.0X3	T45.0X4	T45.0X5	T45.0X6
Mequitazine	T43.3X1	T43.3X2	T43.3X3	T43.3X4	T43.3X5	T43.3X6
Meralluride	T50.2X1	T50.2X2	T50.2X3	T50.2X4	T50.2X5	T50.2X6
Merbaphen	T50.2X1	T50.2X2	T50.2X3	T50.2X4	T50.2X5	T50.2X6
Merbromin	T49.0X1	T49.0X2	T49.0X3	T49.0X4	T49.0X5	T49.0X6
Mercaptobenzothiazole salts	T49.0X1	T49.0X2	T49.0X3	T49.0X4	T49.0X5	T49.0X6
Mercaptomerin	T50.2X1	T50.2X2	T50.2X3	T50.2X4	T50.2X5	T50.2X6
Mercaptopurine	T45.1X1	T45.1X2	T45.1X3	T45.1X4	T45.1X5	T45.1X6
Mercumatilin	T50.2X1	T50.2X2	T50.2X3	T50.2X4	T50.2X5	T50.2X6
Mercuramide	T50.2X1	T50.2X2	T50.2X3	T50.2X4	T50.2X5	T50.2X6
Mercurochrome	T49.0X1	T49.0X2	T49.0X3	T49.0X4	T49.0X5	T49.0X6
Mercurophylline	T50.2X1	T50.2X2	T50.2X3	T50.2X4	T50.2X5	T50.2X6
Mercury, mercurial, mercuric, mercurous (compounds) (cyanide) (fumes) (nonmedicinal) (vapor) NEC	T56.1X1	T56.1X2	T56.1X3	T56.1X4	—	—
ammoniated	T49.0X1	T49.0X2	T49.0X3	T49.0X4	T49.0X5	T49.0X6
anti-infective						
local	T49.0X1	T49.0X2	T49.0X3	T49.0X4	T49.0X5	T49.0X6
systemic	T37.8X1	T37.8X2	T37.8X3	T37.8X4	T37.8X5	T37.8X6
topical	T49.0X1	T49.0X2	T49.0X3	T49.0X4	T49.0X5	T49.0X6
chloride (ammoniated)	T49.0X1	T49.0X2	T49.0X3	T49.0X4	T49.0X5	T49.0X6
fungicide	T56.1X1	T56.1X2	T56.1X3	T56.1X4	—	—
diuretic NEC	T50.2X1	T50.2X2	T50.2X3	T50.2X4	T50.2X5	T50.2X6
fungicide	T56.1X1	T56.1X2	T56.1X3	T56.1X4	—	—
organic (fungicide)	T56.1X1	T56.1X2	T56.1X3	T56.1X4	—	—
oxide, yellow	T49.0X1	T49.0X2	T49.0X3	T49.0X4	T49.0X5	T49.0X6
Mersalyl	T50.2X1	T50.2X2	T50.2X3	T50.2X4	T50.2X5	T50.2X6
Merthiolate	T49.0X1	T49.0X2	T49.0X3	T49.0X4	T49.0X5	T49.0X6
ophthalmic preparation	T49.5X1	T49.5X2	T49.5X3	T49.5X4	T49.5X5	T49.5X6
Meruvax	T50.B91	T50.B92	T50.B93	T50.B94	T50.B95	T50.B96
Mesalazine	T47.8X1	T47.8X2	T47.8X3	T47.8X4	T47.8X5	T47.8X6
Mescal buttons	T40.991	T40.992	T40.993	T40.994	—	—

TABLE OF DRUGS AND CHEMICALS

TABLE OF DRUGS AND CHEMICALS

Substance	Poisoning, Accidental (Unintentional)	Poisoning, Intentional Self-Harm	Poisoning, Assault	Poisoning, Undetermined	Adverse Effect	Underdosing
Mescaline	T40.991	T40.992	T40.993	T40.994	—	—
Mesna	T48.4X1	T48.4X2	T48.4X3	T48.4X4	T48.4X5	T48.4X6
Mesoglycan	T46.6X1	T46.6X2	T46.6X3	T46.6X4	T46.6X5	T46.6X6
Mesoridazine	T43.3X1	T43.3X2	T43.3X3	T43.3X4	T43.3X5	T43.3X6
Mestanolone	T38.7X1	T38.7X2	T38.7X3	T38.7X4	T38.7X5	T38.7X6
Mesterolone	T38.7X1	T38.7X2	T38.7X3	T38.7X4	T38.7X5	T38.7X6
Mestranol	T38.5X1	T38.5X2	T38.5X3	T38.5X4	T38.5X5	T38.5X6
Mesulergine	T42.8X1	T42.8X2	T42.8X3	T42.8X4	T42.8X5	T42.8X6
Mesulfen	T49.0X1	T49.0X2	T49.0X3	T49.0X4	T49.0X5	T49.0X6
Mesuximide	T42.2X1	T42.2X2	T42.2X3	T42.2X4	T42.2X5	T42.2X6
Metabutethamine	T41.3X1	T41.3X2	T41.3X3	T41.3X4	T41.3X5	T41.3X6
Metactesylacetate	T49.0X1	T49.0X2	T49.0X3	T49.0X4	T49.0X5	T49.0X6
Metacycline	T36.4X1	T36.4X2	T36.4X3	T36.4X4	T36.4X5	T36.4X6
Metaldehyde (snail killer) NEC	T60.8X1	T60.8X2	T60.8X3	T60.8X4	—	—
Metals (heavy) (nonmedicinal)	T56.91	T56.92	T56.93	T56.94	—	—
dust, fumes, or vapor NEC	T56.91	T56.92	T56.93	T56.94	—	—
light NEC	T56.91	T56.92	T56.93	T56.94	—	—
dust, fumes, or vapor NEC	T56.91	T56.92	T56.93	T56.94	—	—
specified NEC	T56.891	T56.892	T56.893	T56.894	—	—
thallium	T56.811	T56.812	T56.813	T56.814	—	—
Metamfetamine	T43.621	T43.622	T43.623	T43.624	T43.625	T43.626
Metamizole sodium	T39.2X1	T39.2X2	T39.2X3	T39.2X4	T39.2X5	T39.2X6
Metampicillin	T36.0X1	T36.0X2	T36.0X3	T36.0X4	T36.0X5	T36.0X6
Metamucil	T47.4X1	T47.4X2	T47.4X3	T47.4X4	T47.4X5	T47.4X6
Metaphen	T49.0X1	T49.0X2	T49.0X3	T49.0X4	T49.0X5	T49.0X6
Metandienone	T38.7X1	T38.7X2	T38.7X3	T38.7X4	T38.7X5	T38.7X6
Metandrostenolone	T38.7X1	T38.7X2	T38.7X3	T38.7X4	T38.7X5	T38.7X6
Metaphos	T60.0X1	T60.0X2	T60.0X3	T60.0X4	—	—
Metapramine	T43.011	T43.012	T43.013	T43.014	T43.015	T43.016
Metaproterenol	T48.291	T48.292	T48.293	T48.294	T48.295	T48.296
Metaraminol	T44.4X1	T44.4X2	T44.4X3	T44.4X4	T44.4X5	T44.4X6
Metaxalone	T42.8X1	T42.8X2	T42.8X3	T42.8X4	T42.8X5	T42.8X6
Metenolone	T38.7X1	T38.7X2	T38.7X3	T38.7X4	T38.7X5	T38.7X6
Metergoline	T42.8X1	T42.8X2	T42.8X3	T42.8X4	T42.8X5	T42.8X6
Metescufylline	T46.991	T46.992	T46.993	T46.994	T46.995	T46.996
Metetoin	T42.0X1	T42.0X2	T42.0X3	T42.0X4	T42.0X5	T42.0X6
Metformin	T38.3X1	T38.3X2	T38.3X3	T38.3X4	T38.3X5	T38.3X6
Methacholine	T44.1X1	T44.1X2	T44.1X3	T44.1X4	T44.1X5	T44.1X6
Methacycline	T36.4X1	T36.4X2	T36.4X3	T36.4X4	T36.4X5	T36.4X6
Methadone	T40.3X1	T40.3X2	T40.3X3	T40.3X4	T40.3X5	T40.3X6

Substance	External Cause (T-Code)					
	Poisoning, Accidental (Unintentional)	Poisoning, Intentional Self-Harm	Poisoning, Assault	Poisoning, Undetermined	Adverse Effect	Underdosing
Methallenestril	T38.5X1	T38.5X2	T38.5X3	T38.5X4	T38.5X5	T38.5X6
Methallenoestril	T38.5X1	T38.5X2	T38.5X3	T38.5X4	T38.5X5	T38.5X6
Methamphetamine	T43.621	T43.622	T43.623	T43.624	T43.625	T43.626
Methampyrone	T39.2X1	T39.2X2	T39.2X3	T39.2X4	T39.2X5	T39.2X6
Methandienone	T38.7X1	T38.7X2	T38.7X3	T38.7X4	T38.7X5	T38.7X6
Methandriol	T38.7X1	T38.7X2	T38.7X3	T38.7X4	T38.7X5	T38.7X6
Methandrostenolone	T38.7X1	T38.7X2	T38.7X3	T38.7X4	T38.7X5	T38.7X6
Methane	T59.891	T59.892	T59.893	T59.894	—	—
Methanethiol	T59.891	T59.892	T59.893	T59.894	—	—
Methaniazide	T37.1X1	T37.1X2	T37.1X3	T37.1X4	T37.1X5	T37.1X6
Methanol (vapor)	T51.1X1	T51.1X2	T51.1X3	T51.1X4	—	—
Methantheline	T44.3X1	T44.3X2	T44.3X3	T44.3X4	T44.3X5	T44.3X6
Methanthelinium bromide	T44.3X1	T44.3X2	T44.3X3	T44.3X4	T44.3X5	T44.3X6
Methaphenilene	T45.0X1	T45.0X2	T45.0X3	T45.0X4	T45.0X5	T45.0X6
Methapyrilene	T45.0X1	T45.0X2	T45.0X3	T45.0X4	T45.0X5	T45.0X6
Methaqualone (compound)	T42.6X1	T42.6X2	T42.6X3	T42.6X4	T42.6X5	T42.6X6
Metharbital	T42.3X1	T42.3X2	T42.3X3	T42.3X4	T42.3X5	T42.3X6
Methazolamide	T50.2X1	T50.2X2	T50.2X3	T50.2X4	T50.2X5	T50.2X6
Methdilazine	T43.3X1	T43.3X2	T43.3X3	T43.3X4	T43.3X5	T43.3X6
Methedrine	T43.621	T43.622	T43.623	T43.624	T43.625	T43.626
Methenamine (mandelate)	T37.8X1	T37.8X2	T37.8X3	T37.8X4	T37.8X5	T37.8X6
Methenolone	T38.7X1	T38.7X2	T38.7X3	T38.7X4	T38.7X5	T38.7X6
Methergine	T48.0X1	T48.0X2	T48.0X3	T48.0X4	T48.0X5	T48.0X6
Methetoin	T42.0X1	T42.0X2	T42.0X3	T42.0X4	T42.0X5	T42.0X6
Methiacil	T38.2X1	T38.2X2	T38.2X3	T38.2X4	T38.2X5	T38.2X6
Methicillin	T36.0X1	T36.0X2	T36.0X3	T36.0X4	T36.0X5	T36.0X6
Methimazole	T38.2X1	T38.2X2	T38.2X3	T38.2X4	T38.2X5	T38.2X6
Methiodal sodium	T50.8X1	T50.8X2	T50.8X3	T50.8X4	T50.8X5	T50.8X6
Methionine	T50.991	T50.992	T50.993	T50.994	T50.995	T50.996
Methisazone	T37.5X1	T37.5X2	T37.5X3	T37.5X4	T37.5X5	T37.5X6
Methisoprinol	T37.5X1	T37.5X2	T37.5X3	T37.5X4	T37.5X5	T37.5X6
Methitural	T42.3X1	T42.3X2	T42.3X3	T42.3X4	T42.3X5	T42.3X6
Methixene	T44.3X1	T44.3X2	T44.3X3	T44.3X4	T44.3X5	T44.3X6
Methobarbital, methobarbitone	T42.3X1	T42.3X2	T42.3X3	T42.3X4	T42.3X5	T42.3X6
Methocarbamol	T42.8X1	T42.8X2	T42.8X3	T42.8X4	T42.8X5	T42.8X6
skeletal muscle relaxant	T48.1X1	T48.1X2	T48.1X3	T48.1X4	T48.1X5	T48.1X6
Methohexital	T41.1X1	T41.1X2	T41.1X3	T41.1X4	T41.1X5	T41.1X6
Methohexitone	T41.1X1	T41.1X2	T41.1X3	T41.1X4	T41.1X5	T41.1X6
Methoin	T42.0X1	T42.0X2	T42.0X3	T42.0X4	T42.0X5	T42.0X6
Methopholine	T39.8X1	T39.8X2	T39.8X3	T39.8X4	T39.8X5	T39.8X6

TABLE OF DRUGS AND CHEMICALS

Substance	External Cause (T-Code)					
	Poisoning, Accidental (Unintentional)	Poisoning, Intentional Self-Harm	Poisoning, Assault	Poisoning, Undetermined	Adverse Effect	Underdosing
Methopromazine	T43.3X1	T43.3X2	T43.3X3	T43.3X4	T43.3X5	T43.3X6
Methorate	T48.3X1	T48.3X2	T48.3X3	T48.3X4	T48.3X5	T48.3X6
Methoserpidine	T46.5X1	T46.5X2	T46.5X3	T46.5X4	T46.5X5	T46.5X6
Methotrexate	T45.1X1	T45.1X2	T45.1X3	T45.1X4	T45.1X5	T45.1X6
Methotrimeprazine	T43.3X1	T43.3X2	T43.3X3	T43.3X4	T43.3X5	T43.3X6
Methoxa-Dome	T49.3X1	T49.3X2	T49.3X3	T49.3X4	T49.3X5	T49.3X6
Methoxamine	T44.4X1	T44.4X2	T44.4X3	T44.4X4	T44.4X5	T44.4X6
Methoxsalen	T50.991	T50.992	T50.993	T50.994	T50.995	T50.996
Methoxyaniline	T65.3X1	T65.3X2	T65.3X3	T65.3X4	—	—
Methoxybenzyl penicillin	T36.0X1	T36.0X2	T36.0X3	T36.0X4	T36.0X5	T36.0X6
Methoxychlor	T53.7X1	T53.7X2	T53.7X3	T53.7X4		
Methoxy-DDT	T53.7X1	T53.7X2	T53.7X3	T53.7X4	—	—
2-Methoxyethanol	T52.3X1	T52.3X2	T52.3X3	T52.3X4	—	—
Methoxyflurane	T41.0X1	T41.0X2	T41.0X3	T41.0X4	T41.0X5	T41.0X6
Methoxyphenamine	T48.6X1	T48.6X2	T48.6X3	T48.6X4	T48.6X5	T48.6X6
Methoxypromazine	T43.3X1	T43.3X2	T43.3X3	T43.3X4	T43.3X5	T43.3X6
5-Methoxypsoralen (5-MOP)	T50.991	T50.992	T50.993	T50.994	T50.995	T50.996
8-Methoxypsoralen (8-MOP)	T50.991	T50.992	T50.993	T50.994	T50.995	T50.996
Methscopolamine bromide	T44.3X1	T44.3X2	T44.3X3	T44.3X4	T44.3X5	T44.3X6
Methsuximide	T42.2X1	T42.2X2	T42.2X3	T42.2X4	T42.2X5	T42.2X6
Methyclothiazide	T50.2X1	T50.2X2	T50.2X3	T50.2X4	T50.2X5	T50.2X6
Methyl						
acetate	T52.4X1	T52.4X2	T52.4X3	T52.4X4	—	—
acetone	T52.4X1	T52.4X2	T52.4X3	T52.4X4	—	—
acrylate	T65.891	T65.892	T65.893	T65.894	—	—
alcohol	T51.1X1	T51.1X2	T51.1X3	T51.1X4	—	—
aminophenol	T65.3X1	T65.3X2	T65.3X3	T65.3X4	—	—
amphetamine	T43.621	T43.622	T43.623	T43.624	T43.625	T43.626
androstanolone	T38.7X1	T38.7X2	T38.7X3	T38.7X4	T38.7X5	T38.7X6
atropine	T44.3X1	T44.3X2	T44.3X3	T44.3X4	T44.3X5	T44.3X6
benzene	T52.2X1	T52.2X2	T52.2X3	T52.2X4	—	—
benzoate	T52.8X1	T52.8X2	T52.8X3	T52.8X4	—	—
benzol	T52.2X1	T52.2X2	T52.2X3	T52.2X4	—	—
bromide (gas)	T59.891	T59.892	T59.893	T59.894	—	—
fumigant	T60.8X1	T60.8X2	T60.8X3	T60.8X4	—	—
butanol	T51.3X1	T51.3X2	T51.3X3	T51.3X4	—	—
carbinol	T51.1X1	T51.1X2	T51.1X3	T51.1X4	—	—
carbonate	T52.8X1	T52.8X2	T52.8X3	T52.8X4	—	—
CCNU	T45.1X1	T45.1X2	T45.1X3	T45.1X4	T45.1X5	T45.1X6
cellosolve	T52.91	T52.92	T52.93	T52.94	—	—

Substance	Poisoning, Accidental (Unintentional)	Poisoning, Intentional Self-Harm	Poisoning, Assault	Poisoning, Undetermined	Adverse Effect	Underdosing
			External Cause (T-Code)			
Methyl *(Continued)*						
cellulose	T47.4X1	T47.4X2	T47.4X3	T47.4X4	T47.4X5	T47.4X6
chloride (gas)	T59.891	T59.892	T59.893	T59.894	—	—
chloroformate	T59.3X1	T59.3X2	T59.3X3	T59.3X4	—	—
cyclohexane	T52.8X1	T52.8X2	T52.8X3	T52.8X4	—	—
cyclohexanol	T51.8X1	T51.8X2	T51.8X3	T51.8X4	—	—
cyclohexanone	T52.8X1	T52.8X2	T52.8X3	T52.8X4	—	—
cyclohexyl acetate	T52.8X1	T52.8X2	T52.8X3	T52.8X4	—	—
demeton	T60.0X1	T60.0X2	T60.0X3	T60.0X4	—	—
dihydromorphinone	T40.2X1	T40.2X2	T40.2X3	T40.2X4	T40.2X5	T40.2X6
ergometrine	T48.0X1	T48.0X2	T48.0X3	T48.0X4	T48.0X5	T48.0X6
ergonovine	T48.0X1	T48.0X2	T48.0X3	T48.0X4	T48.0X5	T48.0X6
ethyl ketone	T52.4X1	T52.4X2	T52.4X3	T52.4X4	—	—
glucamine antimonate	T37.8X1	T37.8X2	T37.8X3	T37.8X4	T37.8X5	T37.8X6
hydrazine	T65.891	T65.892	T65.893	T65.894	—	—
iodide	T65.891	T65.892	T65.893	T65.894	—	—
isobutyl ketone	T52.4X1	T52.4X2	T52.4X3	T52.4X4	—	—
isothiocyanate	T60.3X1	T60.3X2	T60.3X3	T60.3X4	—	—
mercaptan	T59.891	T59.892	T59.893	T59.894	—	—
morphine NEC	T40.2X1	T40.2X2	T40.2X3	T40.2X4	T40.2X5	T40.2X6
nicotinate	T49.4X1	T49.4X2	T49.4X3	T49.4X4	T49.4X5	T49.4X6
paraben	T49.0X1	T49.0X2	T49.0X3	T49.0X4	T49.0X5	T49.0X6
parafynol	T42.6X1	T42.6X2	T42.6X3	T42.6X4	T42.6X5	T42.6X6
parathion	T60.0X1	T60.0X2	T60.0X3	T60.0X4	—	—
peridol	T43.4X1	T43.4X2	T43.4X3	T43.4X4	T43.4X5	T43.4X6
phenidate	T43.631	T43.632	T43.633	T43.634	T43.635	T43.636
prednisolone	T38.0X1	T38.0X2	T38.0X3	T38.0X4	T38.0X5	T38.0X6
ENT agent	T49.6X1	T49.6X2	T49.6X3	T49.6X4	T49.6X5	T49.6X6
ophthalmic preparation	T49.5X1	T49.5X2	T49.5X3	T49.5X4	T49.5X5	T49.5X6
topical NEC	T49.0X1	T49.0X2	T49.0X3	T49.0X4	T49.0X5	T49.0X6
propylcarbinol	T51.3X1	T51.3X2	T51.3X3	T51.3X4	—	—
rosaniline NEC	T49.0X1	T49.0X2	T49.0X3	T49.0X4	T49.0X5	T49.0X6
salicylate	T49.2X1	T49.2X2	T49.2X3	T49.2X4	T49.2X5	T49.2X6
sulfate (fumes)	T59.891	T59.892	T59.893	T59.894	—	—
liquid	T52.8X1	T52.8X2	T52.8X3	T52.8X4	—	—
sulfonal	T42.6X1	T42.6X2	T42.6X3	T42.6X4	T42.6X5	T42.6X6
testosterone	T38.7X1	T38.7X2	T38.7X3	T38.7X4	T38.7X5	T38.7X6
thiouracil	T38.2X1	T38.2X2	T38.2X3	T38.2X4	T38.2X5	T38.2X6
Methylamphetamine	T43.621	T43.622	T43.623	T43.624	T43.625	T43.626
Methylated spirit	T51.1X1	T51.1X2	T51.1X3	T51.1X4	—	—

Substance	External Cause (T-Code)					
	Poisoning, Accidental (Unintentional)	Poisoning, Intentional Self-Harm	Poisoning, Assault	Poisoning, Undetermined	Adverse Effect	Underdosing
Methylatropine nitrate	T44.3X1	T44.3X2	T44.3X3	T44.3X4	T44.3X5	T44.3X6
Methylbenactyzium bromide	T44.3X1	T44.3X2	T44.3X3	T44.3X4	T44.3X5	T44.3X6
Methylbenzethonium chloride	T49.0X1	T49.0X2	T49.0X3	T49.0X4	T49.0X5	T49.0X6
Methylcellulose	T47.4X1	T47.4X2	T47.4X3	T47.4X4	T47.4X5	T47.4X6
laxative	T47.4X1	T47.4X2	T47.4X3	T47.4X4	T47.4X5	T47.4X6
Methylchlorophenoxy-acetic acid	T60.3X1	T60.3X2	T60.3X3	T60.3X4	—	—
Methyldopa	T46.5X1	T46.5X2	T46.5X3	T46.5X4	T46.5X5	T46.5X6
Methyldopate	T46.5X1	T46.5X2	T46.5X3	T46.5X4	T46.5X5	T46.5X6
Methylene						
blue	T50.6X1	T50.6X2	T50.6X3	T50.6X4	T50.6X5	T50.6X6
chloride or dichloride (solvent) NEC	T53.4X1	T53.4X2	T53.4X3	T53.4X4	—	—
Methylenedioxyamphet-amine	T43.621	T43.622	T43.623	T43.624	T43.625	T43.626
Methylenedioxymethamphetamine	T43.621	T43.622	T43.623	T43.624	T43.625	T43.626
Methylergometrine	T48.0X1	T48.0X2	T48.0X3	T48.0X4	T48.0X5	T48.0X6
Methylergonovine	T48.0X1	T48.0X2	T48.0X3	T48.0X4	T48.0X5	T48.0X6
Methylestrenolone	T38.5X1	T38.5X2	T38.5X3	T38.5X4	T38.5X5	T38.5X6
Methylethyl cellulose	T50.991	T50.992	T50.993	T50.994	T50.995	T50.996
Methylhexabital	T42.3X1	T42.3X2	T42.3X3	T42.3X4	T42.3X5	T42.3X6
Methylmorphine	T40.2X1	T40.2X2	T40.2X3	T40.2X4	T40.2X5	T40.2X6
Methylparaben (ophthalmic)	T49.5X1	T49.5X2	T49.5X3	T49.5X4	T49.5X5	T49.5X6
Methylparafynol	T42.6X1	T42.6X2	T42.6X3	T42.6X4	T42.6X5	T42.6X6
Methylpentynol, methylpenthynol	T42.6X1	T42.6X2	T42.6X3	T42.6X4	T42.6X5	T42.6X6
Methylphenidate	T43.631	T43.632	T43.633	T43.634	T43.635	T43.636
Methylphenobarbital	T42.3X1	T42.3X2	T42.3X3	T42.3X4	T42.3X5	T42.3X6
Methylpolysiloxane	T47.1X1	T47.1X2	T47.1X3	T47.1X4	T47.1X5	T47.1X6
Methylprednisolone — see Methyl, prednisolone						
Methylrosaniline	T49.0X1	T49.0X2	T49.0X3	T49.0X4	T49.0X5	T49.0X6
Methylrosanilinium chloride	T49.0X1	T49.0X2	T49.0X3	T49.0X4	T49.0X5	T49.0X6
Methyltestosterone	T38.7X1	T38.7X2	T38.7X3	T38.7X4	T38.7X5	T38.7X6
Methylthionine chloride	T50.6X1	T50.6X2	T50.6X3	T50.6X4	T50.6X5	T50.6X6
Methylthioninium chloride	T50.6X1	T50.6X2	T50.6X3	T50.6X4	T50.6X5	T50.6X6
Methylthiouracil	T38.2X1	T38.2X2	T38.2X3	T38.2X4	T38.2X5	T38.2X6
Methyprylon	T42.6X1	T42.6X2	T42.6X3	T42.6X4	T42.6X5	T42.6X6
Methysergide	T46.5X1	T46.5X2	T46.5X3	T46.5X4	T46.5X5	T46.5X6
Metiamide	T47.1X1	T47.1X2	T47.1X3	T47.1X4	T47.1X5	T47.1X6
Meticillin	T36.0X1	T36.0X2	T36.0X3	T36.0X4	T36.0X5	T36.0X6
Meticrane	T50.2X1	T50.2X2	T50.2X3	T50.2X4	T50.2X5	T50.2X6
Metildigoxin	T46.0X1	T46.0X2	T46.0X3	T46.0X4	T46.0X5	T46.0X6
Metipranolol	T49.5X1	T49.5X2	T49.5X3	T49.5X4	T49.5X5	T49.5X6

Substance	External Cause (T-Code)					
	Poisoning, Accidental (Unintentional)	Poisoning, Intentional Self-Harm	Poisoning, Assault	Poisoning, Undetermined	Adverse Effect	Underdosing
Metirosine	T46.5X1	T46.5X2	T46.5X3	T46.5X4	T46.5X5	T46.5X6
Metisazone	T37.5X1	T37.5X2	T37.5X3	T37.5X4	T37.5X5	T37.5X6
Metixene	T44.3X1	T44.3X2	T44.3X3	T44.3X4	T44.3X5	T44.3X6
Metizoline	T48.5X1	T48.5X2	T48.5X3	T48.5X4	T48.5X5	T48.5X6
Metoclopramide	T45.0X1	T45.0X2	T45.0X3	T45.0X4	T45.0X5	T45.0X6
Metofenazate	T43.3X1	T43.3X2	T43.3X3	T43.3X4	T43.3X5	T43.3X6
Metofoline	T39.8X1	T39.8X2	T39.8X3	T39.8X4	T39.8X5	T39.8X6
Metolazone	T50.2X1	T50.2X2	T50.2X3	T50.2X4	T50.2X5	T50.2X6
Metopon	T40.2X1	T40.2X2	T40.2X3	T40.2X4	T40.2X5	T40.2X6
Metoprine	T45.1X1	T45.1X2	T45.1X3	T45.1X4	T45.1X5	T45.1X6
Metoprolol	T44.7X1	T44.7X2	T44.7X3	T44.7X4	T44.7X5	T44.7X6
Metrifonate	T60.0X1	T60.0X2	T60.0X3	T60.0X4	—	—
Metrizamide	T50.8X1	T50.8X2	T50.8X3	T50.8X4	T50.8X5	T50.8X6
Metrizoic acid	T50.8X1	T50.8X2	T50.8X3	T50.8X4	T50.8X5	T50.8X6
Metronidazole	T37.8X1	T37.8X2	T37.8X3	T37.8X4	T37.8X5	T37.8X6
Metycaine	T41.3X1	T41.3X2	T41.3X3	T41.3X4	T41.3X5	T41.3X6
infiltration (subcutaneous)	T41.3X1	T41.3X2	T41.3X3	T41.3X4	T41.3X5	T41.3X6
nerve block (peripheral) (plexus)	T41.3X1	T41.3X2	T41.3X3	T41.3X4	T41.3X5	T41.3X6
topical (surface)	T41.3X1	T41.3X2	T41.3X3	T41.3X4	T41.3X5	T41.3X6
Metyrapone	T50.8X1	T50.8X2	T50.8X3	T50.8X4	T50.8X5	T50.8X6
Mevinphos	T60.0X1	T60.0X2	T60.0X3	T60.0X4	—	—
Mexazolam	T42.4X1	T42.4X2	T42.4X3	T42.4X4	T42.4X5	T42.4X6
Mexenone	T49.3X1	T49.3X2	T49.3X3	T49.3X4	T49.3X5	T49.3X6
Mexiletine	T46.2X1	T46.2X2	T46.2X3	T46.2X4	T46.2X5	T46.2X6
Mezereon	T62.2X1	T62.2X2	T62.2X3	T62.2X4	—	—
berries	T62.1X1	T62.1X2	T62.1X3	T62.1X4	—	—
Mezlocillin	T36.0X1	T36.0X2	T36.0X3	T36.0X4	T36.0X5	T36.0X6
Mianserin	T43.021	T43.022	T43.023	T43.024	T43.025	T43.026
Micatin	T49.0X1	T49.0X2	T49.0X3	T49.0X4	T49.0X5	T49.0X6
Miconazole	T49.0X1	T49.0X2	T49.0X3	T49.0X4	T49.0X5	T49.0X6
Micronomicin	T36.5X1	T36.5X2	T36.5X3	T36.5X4	T36.5X5	T36.5X6
Midazolam	T42.4X1	T42.4X2	T42.4X3	T42.4X4	T42.4X5	T42.4X6
Midecamycin	T36.3X1	T36.3X2	T36.3X3	T36.3X4	T36.3X5	T36.3X6
Mifepristone	T38.6X1	T38.6X2	T38.6X3	T38.6X4	T38.6X5	T38.6X6
Milk of magnesia	T47.1X1	T47.1X2	T47.1X3	T47.1X4	T47.1X5	T47.1X6
Millipede (tropical) (venomous)	T63.411	T63.412	T63.413	T63.414	—	—
Miltown	T43.591	T43.592	T43.593	T43.594	T43.595	T43.596
Milverine	T44.3X1	T44.3X2	T44.3X3	T44.3X4	T44.3X5	T44.3X6
Minaprine	T43.291	T43.292	T43.293	T43.294	T43.295	T43.296

Substance	External Cause (T-Code)					
	Poisoning, Accidental (Unintentional)	Poisoning, Intentional Self-Harm	Poisoning, Assault	Poisoning, Undetermined	Adverse Effect	Underdosing
Minaxolone	T41.291	T41.292	T41.293	T41.294	T41.295	T41.296
Mineral						
acids	T54.2X1	T54.2X2	T54.2X3	T54.2X4	—	—
oil (laxative) (medicinal)	T47.4X1	T47.4X2	T47.4X3	T47.4X4	T47.4X5	T47.4X6
emulsion	T47.2X1	T47.2X2	T47.2X3	T47.2X4	T47.2X5	T47.2X6
nonmedicinal	T52.0X1	T52.0X2	T52.0X3	T52.0X4	—	—
topical	T49.3X1	T49.3X2	T49.3X3	T49.3X4	T49.3X5	T49.3X6
salt NEC	T50.3X1	T50.3X2	T50.3X3	T50.3X4	T50.3X5	T50.3X6
spirits	T52.0X1	T52.0X2	T52.0X3	T52.0X4	—	—
Mineralocorticosteroid	T50.0X1	T50.0X2	T50.0X3	T50.0X4	T50.0X5	T50.0X6
Minocycline	T36.4X1	T36.4X2	T36.4X3	T36.4X4	T36.4X5	T36.4X6
Minoxidil	T46.7X1	T46.7X2	T46.7X3	T46.7X4	T46.7X5	T46.7X6
Miokamycin	T36.3X1	T36.3X2	T36.3X3	T36.3X4	T36.3X5	T36.3X6
Miotic drug	T49.5X1	T49.5X2	T49.5X3	T49.5X4	T49.5X5	T49.5X6
Mipafox	T60.0X1	T60.0X2	T60.0X3	T60.0X4	—	—
Mirex	T60.1X1	T60.1X2	T60.1X3	T60.1X4	—	—
Mirtazapine	T43.021	T43.022	T43.023	T43.024	T43.025	T43.026
Misonidazole	T37.3X1	T37.3X2	T37.3X3	T37.3X4	T37.3X5	T37.3X6
Misoprostol	T47.1X1	T47.1X2	T47.1X3	T47.1X4	T47.1X5	T47.1X6
Mithramycin	T45.1X1	T45.1X2	T45.1X3	T45.1X4	T45.1X5	T45.1X6
Mitobronitol	T45.1X1	T45.1X2	T45.1X3	T45.1X4	T45.1X5	T45.1X6
Mitoguazone	T45.1X1	T45.1X2	T45.1X3	T45.1X4	T45.1X5	T45.1X6
Mitolactol	T45.1X1	T45.1X2	T45.1X3	T45.1X4	T45.1X5	T45.1X6
Mitomycin	T45.1X1	T45.1X2	T45.1X3	T45.1X4	T45.1X5	T45.1X6
Mitopodozide	T45.1X1	T45.1X2	T45.1X3	T45.1X4	T45.1X5	T45.1X6
Mitotane	T45.1X1	T45.1X2	T45.1X3	T45.1X4	T45.1X5	T45.1X6
Mitoxantrone	T45.1X1	T45.1X2	T45.1X3	T45.1X4	T45.1X5	T45.1X6
Mivacurium chloride	T48.1X1	T48.1X2	T48.1X3	T48.1X4	T48.1X5	T48.1X6
Miyari bacteria	T47.6X1	T47.6X2	T47.6X3	T47.6X4	T47.6X5	T47.6X6
Moclobemide	T43.1X1	T43.1X2	T43.1X3	T43.1X4	T43.1X5	T43.1X6
Moderil	T46.5X1	T46.5X2	T46.5X3	T46.5X4	T46.5X5	T46.5X6
Mofebutazone	T39.2X1	T39.2X2	T39.2X3	T39.2X4	T39.2X5	T39.2X6
Mogadon — see Nitrazepam						
Molindone	T43.591	T43.592	T43.593	T43.594	T43.595	T43.596
Molsidomine	T46.3X1	T46.3X2	T46.3X3	T46.3X4	T46.3X5	T46.3X6
Mometasone	T49.0X1	T49.0X2	T49.0X3	T49.0X4	T49.0X5	T49.0X6
Monistat	T49.0X1	T49.0X2	T49.0X3	T49.0X4	T49.0X5	T49.0X6
Monkshood	T62.2X1	T62.2X2	T62.2X3	T62.2X4	—	—
Monoamine oxidase inhibitor NEC	T43.1X1	T43.1X2	T43.1X3	T43.1X4	T43.1X5	T43.1X6
hydrazine	T43.1X1	T43.1X2	T43.1X3	T43.1X4	T43.1X5	T43.1X6

Substance	External Cause (T-Code)					
	Poisoning, Accidental (Unintentional)	Poisoning, Intentional Self-Harm	Poisoning, Assault	Poisoning, Undetermined	Adverse Effect	Underdosing
Monobenzone	T49.4X1	T49.4X2	T49.4X3	T49.4X4	T49.4X5	T49.4X6
Monochloroacetic acid	T60.3X1	T60.3X2	T60.3X3	T60.3X4	—	—
Monochlorobenzene	T53.7X1	T53.7X2	T53.7X3	T53.7X4	—	—
Monoethanolamine	T46.8X1	T46.8X2	T46.8X3	T46.8X4	T46.8X5	T46.8X6
oleate	T46.8X1	T46.8X2	T46.8X3	T46.8X4	T46.8X5	T46.8X6
Monooctanoin	T50.991	T50.992	T50.993	T50.994	T50.995	T50.996
Monophenylbutazone	T39.2X1	T39.2X2	T39.2X3	T39.2X4	T39.2X5	T39.2X6
Monosodium glutamate	T65.891	T65.892	T65.893	T65.894	—	—
Monosulfiram	T49.0X1	T49.0X2	T49.0X3	T49.0X4	T49.0X5	T49.0X6
Monoxide, carbon — *see Carbon, monoxide*	T57.91	T57.92	T57.93	T57.94	—	
Monoxidine hydrochloride	T46.1X1	T46.1X2	T46.1X3	T46.1X4	T46.1X5	T46.1X6
Monuron	T60.3X1	T60.3X2	T60.3X3	T60.3X4	—	—
Moperone	T43.4X1	T43.4X2	T43.4X3	T43.4X4	T43.4X5	T43.4X6
Mopidamol	T45.1X1	T45.1X2	T45.1X3	T45.1X4	T45.1X5	T45.1X6
MOPP (mechlorethamine + vincristine + prednisone + procarbazine)	T45.1X1	T45.1X2	T45.1X3	T45.1X4	T45.1X5	T45.1X6
Morfin	T40.2X1	T40.2X2	T40.2X3	T40.2X4	T40.2X5	T40.2X6
Morinamide	T37.1X1	T37.1X2	T37.1X3	T37.1X4	T37.1X5	T37.1X6
Morning glory seeds	T40.991	T40.992	T40.993	T40.994	—	—
Moroxydine	T37.5X1	T37.5X2	T37.5X3	T37.5X4	T37.5X5	T37.5X6
Morphazinamide	T37.1X1	T37.1X2	T37.1X3	T37.1X4	T37.1X5	T37.1X6
Morphine	T40.2X1	T40.2X2	T40.2X3	T40.2X4	T40.2X5	T40.2X6
antagonist	T50.7X1	T50.7X2	T50.7X3	T50.7X4	T50.7X5	T50.7X6
Morpholinylethylmorphine	T40.2X1	T40.2X2	T40.2X3	T40.2X4	—	—
Morsuximide	T42.2X1	T42.2X2	T42.2X3	T42.2X4	T42.2X5	T42.2X6
Mosapramine	T43.591	T43.592	T43.593	T43.594	T43.595	T43.596
Moth balls — *see also Pesticides*	T60.2X1	T60.2X2	T60.2X3	T60.2X4		
naphthalene	T60.2X1	T60.2X2	T60.2X3	T60.2X4	—	—
paradichlorobenzene	T60.1X1	T60.1X2	T60.1X3	T60.1X4	—	—
Motor exhaust gas	T58.01	T58.02	T58.03	T58.04	—	—
Mouthwash (antiseptic) (zinc chloride)	T49.6X1	T49.6X2	T49.6X3	T49.6X4	T49.6X5	T49.6X6
Moxastine	T45.0X1	T45.0X2	T45.0X3	T45.0X4	T45.0X5	T45.0X6
Moxaverine	T44.3X1	T44.3X2	T44.3X3	T44.3X4	T44.3X5	T44.3X6
Moxifensine	T43.291	T43.292	T43.293	T43.294	T43.295	T43.296
Moxisylyte	T46.7X1	T46.7X2	T46.7X3	T46.7X4	T46.7X5	T46.7X6
Mucilage, plant	T47.4X1	T47.4X2	T47.4X3	T47.4X4	T47.4X5	T47.4X6
Mucolytic drug	T48.4X1	T48.4X2	T48.4X3	T48.4X4	T48.4X5	T48.4X6
Mucomyst	T48.4X1	T48.4X2	T48.4X3	T48.4X4	T48.4X5	T48.4X6
Mucous membrane agents (external)	T49.91	T49.92	T49.93	T49.94	T49.95	T49.96
specified NEC	T49.8X1	T49.8X2	T49.8X3	T49.8X4	T49.8X5	T49.8X6

Substance	Poisoning, Accidental (Unintentional)	Poisoning, Intentional Self-Harm	Poisoning, Assault	Poisoning, Undetermined	Adverse Effect	Underdosing
Mumps						
immune globulin (human)	T50.Z11	T50.Z12	T50.Z13	T50.Z14	T50.Z15	T50.Z16
skin test antigen	T50.8X1	T50.8X2	T50.8X3	T50.8X4	T50.8X5	T50.8X6
vaccine	T50.B91	T50.B92	T50.B93	T50.B94	T50.B95	T50.B96
Mumpsvax	T50.B91	T50.B92	T50.B93	T50.B94	T50.B95	T50.B96
Mupirocin	T49.0X1	T49.0X2	T49.0X3	T49.0X4	T49.0X5	T49.0X6
Muriatic acid — see Hydrochloric acid						
Muromonab-CD3	T45.1X1	T45.1X2	T45.1X3	T45.1X4	T45.1X5	T45.1X6
Muscle relaxant — see Relaxant, muscle						
Muscle-action drug NEC	T48.201	T48.202	T48.203	T48.204	T48.205	T48.206
Muscle affecting agents NEC	T48.201	T48.202	T48.203	T48.204	T48.205	T48.206
oxytocic	T48.0X1	T48.0X2	T48.0X3	T48.0X4	T48.0X5	T48.0X6
relaxants	T48.201	T48.202	T48.203	T48.204	T48.205	T48.206
central nervous system	T42.8X1	T42.8X2	T42.8X3	T42.8X4	T42.8X5	T42.8X6
skeletal	T48.1X1	T48.1X2	T48.1X3	T48.1X4	T48.1X5	T48.1X6
smooth	T44.3X1	T44.3X2	T44.3X3	T44.3X4	T44.3X5	T44.3X6
Muscle-tone depressant, central NEC	T42.8X1	T42.8X2	T42.8X3	T42.8X4	T42.8X5	T42.8X6
specified NEC	T42.8X1	T42.8X2	T42.8X3	T42.8X4	T42.8X5	T42.8X6
Mushroom, noxious	T62.0X1	T62.0X2	T62.0X3	T62.0X4	—	—
Mussel, noxious	T61.781	T61.782	T61.783	T61.784	—	—
Mustard (emetic)	T47.7X1	T47.7X2	T47.7X3	T47.7X4	T47.7X5	T47.7X6
black	T47.7X1	T47.7X2	T47.7X3	T47.7X4	T47.7X5	T47.7X6
gas, not in war	T59.91	T59.92	T59.93	T59.94	—	—
nitrogen	T45.1X1	T45.1X2	T45.1X3	T45.1X4	T45.1X5	T45.1X6
Mustine	T45.1X1	T45.1X2	T45.1X3	T45.1X4	T45.1X5	T45.1X6
M-vac	T45.1X1	T45.1X2	T45.1X3	T45.1X4	T45.1X5	T45.1X6
Mycifradin	T36.5X1	T36.5X2	T36.5X3	T36.5X4	T36.5X5	T36.5X6
topical	T49.0X1	T49.0X2	T49.0X3	T49.0X4	T49.0X5	T49.0X6
Mycitracin	T36.8X1	T36.8X2	T36.8X3	T36.8X4	T36.8X5	T36.8X6
ophthalmic preparation	T49.5X1	T49.5X2	T49.5X3	T49.5X4	T49.5X5	T49.5X6
Mycostatin	T36.7X1	T36.7X2	T36.7X3	T36.7X4	T36.7X5	T36.7X6
topical	T49.0X1	T49.0X2	T49.0X3	T49.0X4	T49.0X5	T49.0X6
Mycotoxins	T64.81	T64.82	T64.83	T64.84	—	—
aflatoxin	T64.01	T64.02	T64.03	T64.04	—	—
specified NEC	T64.81	T64.82	T64.83	T64.84	—	—
Mydriacyl	T44.3X1	T44.3X2	T44.3X3	T44.3X4	T44.3X5	T44.3X6
Mydriatic drug	T49.5X1	T49.5X2	T49.5X3	T49.5X4	T49.5X5	T49.5X6
Myelobromal	T45.1X1	T45.1X2	T45.1X3	T45.1X4	T45.1X5	T45.1X6
Myleran	T45.1X1	T45.1X2	T45.1X3	T45.1X4	T45.1X5	T45.1X6
Myochrysin(e)	T39.2X1	T39.2X2	T39.2X3	T39.2X4	T39.2X5	T39.2X6

Substance	External Cause (T-Code)					
	Poisoning, Accidental (Unintentional)	Poisoning, Intentional Self-Harm	Poisoning, Assault	Poisoning, Undetermined	Adverse Effect	Underdosing
Myoneural blocking agents	T48.1X1	T48.1X2	T48.1X3	T48.1X4	T48.1X5	T48.1X6
Myralact	T49.0X1	T49.0X2	T49.0X3	T49.0X4	T49.0X5	T49.0X6
Myristica fragrans	T62.2X1	T62.2X2	T62.2X3	T62.2X4	—	—
Myristicin	T65.891	T65.892	T65.893	T65.894	—	—
Mysoline	T42.3X1	T42.3X2	T42.3X3	T42.3X4	T42.3X5	T42.3X6
N						
Nabilone	T40.7X1	T40.7X2	T40.7X3	T40.7X4	T40.7X5	T40.7X6
Nabumetone	T39.391	T39.392	T39.393	T39.394	T39.395	T39.396
Nadolol	T44.7X1	T44.7X2	T44.7X3	T44.7X4	T44.7X5	T44.7X6
Nafcillin	T36.0X1	T36.0X2	T36.0X3	T36.0X4	T36.0X5	T36.0X6
Nafoxidine	T38.6X1	T38.6X2	T38.6X3	T38.6X4	T38.6X5	T38.6X6
Naftazone	T46.991	T46.992	T46.993	T46.994	T46.995	T46.996
Naftidrofuryl (oxalate)	T46.7X1	T46.7X2	T46.7X3	T46.7X4	T46.7X5	T46.7X6
Naftifine	T49.0X1	T49.0X2	T49.0X3	T49.0X4	T49.0X5	T49.0X6
Nail polish remover	T52.91	T52.92	T52.93	T52.94	—	—
Nalbuphine	T40.4X1	T40.4X2	T40.4X3	T40.4X4	T40.4X5	T40.4X6
Naled	T60.0X1	T60.0X2	T60.0X3	T60.0X4	—	—
Nalidixic acid	T37.8X1	T37.8X2	T37.8X3	T37.8X4	T37.8X5	T37.8X6
Nalorphine	T50.7X1	T50.7X2	T50.7X3	T50.7X4	T50.7X5	T50.7X6
Naloxone	T50.7X1	T50.7X2	T50.7X3	T50.7X4	T50.7X5	T50.7X6
Naltrexone	T50.7X1	T50.7X2	T50.7X3	T50.7X4	T50.7X5	T50.7X6
Namenda	T43.8X1	T43.8X2	T43.8X3	T43.8X4	T43.8X5	T43.8X6
Nandrolone	T38.7X1	T38.7X2	T38.7X3	T38.7X4	T38.7X5	T38.7X6
Naphazoline	T48.5X1	T48.5X2	T48.5X3	T48.5X4	T48.5X5	T48.5X6
Naphtha (painters') (petroleum)	T52.0X1	T52.0X2	T52.0X3	T52.0X4	—	—
solvent	T52.0X1	T52.0X2	T52.0X3	T52.0X4	—	—
vapor	T52.0X1	T52.0X2	T52.0X3	T52.0X4	—	—
Naphthalene (non-chlorinated)	T60.2X1	T60.2X2	T60.2X3	T60.2X4	—	—
chlorinated	T60.1X1	T60.1X2	T60.1X3	T60.1X4	—	—
vapor	T60.1X1	T60.1X2	T60.1X3	T60.1X4	—	—
insecticide or moth repellent	T60.2X1	T60.2X2	T60.2X3	T60.2X4	—	—
chlorinated	T60.1X1	T60.1X2	T60.1X3	T60.1X4	—	—
vapor	T60.2X1	T60.2X2	T60.2X3	T60.2X4	—	—
chlorinated	T60.1X1	T60.1X2	T60.1X3	T60.1X4	—	—
Naphthol	T65.891	T65.892	T65.893	T65.894		
Naphthylamine	T65.891	T65.892	T65.893	T65.894	—	—
Naphthylthiourea (ANTU)	T60.4X1	T60.4X2	T60.4X3	T60.4X4	—	—
Naprosyn — see Naproxen						
Naproxen	T39.311	T39.312	T39.313	T39.314	T39.315	T39.316

Substance	External Cause (T-Code)					
	Poisoning, Accidental (Unintentional)	Poisoning, Intentional Self-Harm	Poisoning, Assault	Poisoning, Undetermined	Adverse Effect	Underdosing
Narcotic (drug)	T40.601	T40.602	T40.603	T40.604	T40.605	T40.606
analgesic NEC	T40.601	T40.602	T40.603	T40.604	T40.605	T40.606
antagonist	T50.7X1	T50.7X2	T50.7X3	T50.7X4	T50.7X5	T50.7X6
specified NEC	T40.691	T40.692	T40.693	T40.694	T40.695	T40.696
synthetic	T40.4X1	T40.4X2	T40.4X3	T40.4X4	T40.4X5	T40.4X6
Narcotine	T48.3X1	T48.3X2	T48.3X3	T48.3X4	T48.3X5	T48.3X6
Nardil	T43.1X1	T43.1X2	T43.1X3	T43.1X4	T43.1X5	T43.1X6
Nasal drug NEC	T49.6X1	T49.6X2	T49.6X3	T49.6X4	T49.6X5	T49.6X6
Natamycin	T49.0X1	T49.0X2	T49.0X3	T49.0X4	T49.0X5	T49.0X6
Natrium cyanide — see Cyanide(s)						
Natural gas	T59.891	T59.892	T59.893	T59.894	—	—
incomplete combustion	T57.91	T57.92	T57.93	T57.94	—	—
Natural						
blood (product)	T45.8X1	T45.8X2	T45.8X3	T45.8X4	T45.8X5	T45.8X6
gas (piped)	T59.891	T59.892	T59.893	T59.894	—	—
incomplete combustion	T58.11	T58.12	T58.13	T58.14	—	—
Nealbarbital	T42.3X1	T42.3X2	T42.3X3	T42.3X4	T42.3X5	T42.3X6
Nectadon	T48.3X1	T48.3X2	T48.3X3	T48.3X4	T48.3X5	T48.3X6
Nedocromil	T48.6X1	T48.6X2	T48.6X3	T48.6X4	T48.6X5	T48.6X6
Nefopam	T39.8X1	T39.8X2	T39.8X3	T39.8X4	T39.8X5	T39.8X6
Nematocyst (sting)	T63.691	T63.692	T63.693	T63.694	—	—
Nembutal	T42.3X1	T42.3X2	T42.3X3	T42.3X4	T42.3X5	T42.3X6
Nemonapride	T43.591	T43.592	T43.593	T43.594	T43.595	T43.596
Neoarsphenamine	T37.8X1	T37.8X2	T37.8X3	T37.8X4	T37.8X5	T37.8X6
Neocinchophen	T50.4X1	T50.4X2	T50.4X3	T50.4X4	T50.4X5	T50.4X6
Neomycin (derivatives)	T36.5X1	T36.5X2	T36.5X3	T36.5X4	T36.5X5	T36.5X6
with						
bacitracin	T49.0X1	T49.0X2	T49.0X3	T49.0X4	T49.0X5	T49.0X6
neostigmine	T44.0X1	T44.0X2	T44.0X3	T44.0X4	T44.0X5	T44.0X6
ENT agent	T49.6X1	T49.6X2	T49.6X3	T49.6X4	T49.6X5	T49.6X6
ophthalmic preparation	T49.5X1	T49.5X2	T49.5X3	T49.5X4	T49.5X5	T49.5X6
topical NEC	T49.0X1	T49.0X2	T49.0X3	T49.0X4	T49.0X5	T49.0X6
Neonal	T42.3X1	T42.3X2	T42.3X3	T42.3X4	T42.3X5	T42.3X6
Neoprontosil	T37.0X1	T37.0X2	T37.0X3	T37.0X4	T37.0X5	T37.0X6
Neosalvarsan	T37.8X1	T37.8X2	T37.8X3	T37.8X4	T37.8X5	T37.8X6
Neosilversalvarsan	T37.8X1	T37.8X2	T37.8X3	T37.8X4	T37.8X5	T37.8X6
Neosporin	T36.8X1	T36.8X2	T36.8X3	T36.8X4	T36.8X5	T36.8X6
ENT agent	T49.6X1	T49.6X2	T49.6X3	T49.6X4	T49.6X5	T49.6X6
opthalmic preparation	T49.5X1	T49.5X2	T49.5X3	T49.5X4	T49.5X5	T49.5X6
topical NEC	T49.0X1	T49.0X2	T49.0X3	T49.0X4	T49.0X5	T49.0X6

Substance	External Cause (T-Code)					
	Poisoning, Accidental (Unintentional)	Poisoning, Intentional Self-Harm	Poisoning, Assault	Poisoning, Undetermined	Adverse Effect	Underdosing
Neostigmine bromide	T44.0X1	T44.0X2	T44.0X3	T44.0X4	T44.0X5	T44.0X6
Neraval	T42.3X1	T42.3X2	T42.3X3	T42.3X4	T42.3X5	T42.3X6
Neravan	T42.3X1	T42.3X2	T42.3X3	T42.3X4	T42.3X5	T42.3X6
Nerium oleander	T62.2X1	T62.2X2	T62.2X3	T62.2X4	—	—
Nerve gas, not in war	T59.91	T59.92	T59.93	T59.94	—	—
Nesacaine	T41.3X1	T41.3X2	T41.3X3	T41.3X4	T41.3X5	T41.3X6
infiltration (subcutaneous)	T41.3X1	T41.3X2	T41.3X3	T41.3X4	T41.3X5	T41.3X6
nerve block (peripheral) (plexus)	T41.3X1	T41.3X2	T41.3X3	T41.3X4	T41.3X5	T41.3X6
Netilmicin	T36.5X1	T36.5X2	T36.5X3	T36.5X4	T36.5X5	T36.5X6
Neurobarb	T42.3X1	T42.3X2	T42.3X3	T42.3X4	T42.3X5	T42.3X6
Neuroleptic drug NEC	T43.501	T43.502	T43.503	T43.504	T43.505	T43.506
Neuromuscular blocking drug	T48.1X1	T48.1X2	T48.1X3	T48.1X4	T48.1X5	T48.1X6
Neutral insulin injection	T38.3X1	T38.3X2	T38.3X3	T38.3X4	T38.3X5	T38.3X6
Neutral spirits	T51.0X1	T51.0X2	T51.0X3	T51.0X4	—	—
beverage	T51.0X1	T51.0X2	T51.0X3	T51.0X4	—	—
Niacin	T46.7X1	T46.7X2	T46.7X3	T46.7X4	T46.7X5	T46.7X6
Niacinamide	T45.2X1	T45.2X2	T45.2X3	T45.2X4	T45.2X5	T45.2X6
Nialamide	T43.1X1	T43.1X2	T43.1X3	T43.1X4	T43.1X5	T43.1X6
Niaprazine	T42.6X1	T42.6X2	T42.6X3	T42.6X4	T42.6X5	T42.6X6
Nicametate	T46.7X1	T46.7X2	T46.7X3	T46.7X4	T46.7X5	T46.7X6
Nicardipine	T46.1X1	T46.1X2	T46.1X3	T46.1X4	T46.1X5	T46.1X6
Nicergoline	T46.7X1	T46.7X2	T46.7X3	T46.7X4	T46.7X5	T46.7X6
Nickel (carbonyl) (tetra-carbonyl) (fumes) (vapor)	T56.891	T56.892	T56.893	T56.894	—	—
Nickelocene	T56.891	T56.892	T56.893	T56.894	—	—
Niclosamide	T37.4X1	T37.4X2	T37.4X3	T37.4X4	T37.4X5	T37.4X6
Nicofuranose	T46.7X1	T46.7X2	T46.7X3	T46.7X4	T46.7X5	T46.7X6
Nicomorphine	T40.2X1	T40.2X2	T40.2X3	T40.2X4	—	—
Nicorandil	T46.3X1	T46.3X2	T46.3X3	T46.3X4	T46.3X5	T46.3X6
Nicotiana (plant)	T62.2X1	T62.2X2	T62.2X3	T62.2X4	—	—
Nicotinamide	T45.2X1	T45.2X2	T45.2X3	T45.2X4	T45.2X5	T45.2X6
Nicotine (insecticide) (spray) (sulfate) NEC	T60.2X1	T60.2X2	T60.2X3	T60.2X4	—	—
from tobacco	T65.291	T65.292	T65.293	T65.294	—	—
cigarettes	T65.221	T65.222	T65.223	T65.224	—	—
not insecticide	T65.291	T65.292	T65.293	T65.294	—	—
Nicotinic acid	T46.7X1	T46.7X2	T46.7X3	T46.7X4	T46.7X5	T46.7X6
Nicotinyl alcohol	T46.7X1	T46.7X2	T46.7X3	T46.7X4	T46.7X5	T46.7X6
Nicoumalone	T45.511	T45.512	T45.513	T45.514	T45.515	T45.516
Nifedipine	T46.1X1	T46.1X2	T46.1X3	T46.1X4	T46.1X5	T46.1X6
Nifenazone	T39.2X1	T39.2X2	T39.2X3	T39.2X4	T39.2X5	T39.2X6
Nifuraldezone	T37.91	T37.92	T37.93	T37.94	T37.95	T37.96

Substance	Poisoning, Accidental (Unintentional)	Poisoning, Intentional Self-Harm	Poisoning, Assault	Poisoning, Undetermined	Adverse Effect	Underdosing
			External Cause (T-Code)			
Nifuratel	T37.8X1	T37.8X2	T37.8X3	T37.8X4	T37.8X5	T37.8X6
Nifurtimox	T37.3X1	T37.3X2	T37.3X3	T37.3X4	T37.3X5	T37.3X6
Nifurtoinol	T37.8X1	T37.8X2	T37.8X3	T37.8X4	T37.8X5	T37.8X6
Nightshade, deadly (solanum) — see also Belladonna	T62.2X1	T62.2X2	T62.2X3	T62.2X4	—	—
berry	T62.1X1	T62.1X2	T62.1X3	T62.1X4	—	—
Nikethamide	T50.7X1	T50.7X2	T50.7X3	T50.7X4	T50.7X5	T50.7X6
Nilstat	T36.7X1	T36.7X2	T36.7X3	T36.7X4	T36.7X5	T36.7X6
topical	T49.0X1	T49.0X2	T49.0X3	T49.0X4	T49.0X5	T49.0X6
Nilutamide	T38.6X1	T38.6X2	T38.6X3	T38.6X4	T38.6X5	T38.6X6
Nimesulide	T39.391	T39.392	T39.393	T39.394	T39.395	T39.396
Nimetazepam	T42.4X1	T42.4X2	T42.4X3	T42.4X4	T42.4X5	T42.4X6
Nimodipine	T46.1X1	T46.1X2	T46.1X3	T46.1X4	T46.1X5	T46.1X6
Nimorazole	T37.3X1	T37.3X2	T37.3X3	T37.3X4	T37.3X5	T37.3X6
Nimustine	T45.1X1	T45.1X2	T45.1X3	T45.1X4	T45.1X5	T45.1X6
Niridazole	T37.4X1	T37.4X2	T37.4X3	T37.4X4	T37.4X5	T37.4X6
Nisentil	T40.2X1	T40.2X2	T40.2X3	T40.2X4	T40.2X5	T40.2X6
Nisoldipine	T46.1X1	T46.1X2	T46.1X3	T46.1X4	T46.1X5	T46.1X6
Nitramine	T65.3X1	T65.3X2	T65.3X3	T65.3X4	—	—
Nitrate, organic	T46.3X1	T46.3X2	T46.3X3	T46.3X4	T46.3X5	T46.3X6
Nitrazepam	T42.4X1	T42.4X2	T42.4X3	T42.4X4	T42.4X5	T42.4X6
Nitrefazole	T50.6X1	T50.6X2	T50.6X3	T50.6X4	T50.6X5	T50.6X6
Nitrendipine	T46.1X1	T46.1X2	T46.1X3	T46.1X4	T46.1X5	T46.1X6
Nitric						
acid (liquid)	T54.2X1	T54.2X2	T54.2X3	T54.2X4	—	—
vapor	T59.891	T59.892	T59.893	T59.894	—	—
oxide (gas)	T59.0X1	T59.0X2	T59.0X3	T59.0X4	—	—
Nitrimidazine	T37.3X1	T37.3X2	T37.3X3	T37.3X4	T37.3X5	T37.3X6
Nitrite, amyl (medicinal) (vapor)	T46.3X1	T46.3X2	T46.3X3	T46.3X4	T46.3X5	T46.3X6
Nitroaniline	T65.3X1	T65.3X2	T65.3X3	T65.3X4	—	—
vapor	T59.891	T59.892	T59.893	T59.894	—	—
Nitrobenzene, nitrobenzol	T65.3X1	T65.3X2	T65.3X3	T65.3X4	—	—
vapor	T65.3X1	T65.3X2	T65.3X3	T65.3X4	—	—
Nitrocellulose	T65.891	T65.892	T65.893	T65.894	—	—
lacquer	T65.891	T65.892	T65.893	T65.894	—	—
Nitrodiphenyl	T65.3X1	T65.3X2	T65.3X3	T65.3X4	—	—
Nitrofural	T49.0X1	T49.0X2	T49.0X3	T49.0X4	T49.0X5	T49.0X6
Nitrofurantoin	T37.8X1	T37.8X2	T37.8X3	T37.8X4	T37.8X5	T37.8X6
Nitrofurazone	T49.0X1	T49.0X2	T49.0X3	T49.0X4	T49.0X5	T49.0X6
Nitrogen	T59.0X1	T59.0X2	T59.0X3	T59.0X4	—	—
mustard	T45.1X1	T45.1X2	T45.1X3	T45.1X4	T45.1X5	T45.1X6

TABLE OF DRUGS AND CHEMICALS

Substance	External Cause (T-Code)					
	Poisoning, Accidental (Unintentional)	Poisoning, Intentional Self-Harm	Poisoning, Assault	Poisoning, Undetermined	Adverse Effect	Underdosing
Nitroglycerin, nitro-glycerol (medicinal)	T46.3X1	T46.3X2	T46.3X3	T46.3X4	T46.3X5	T46.3X6
nonmedicinal	T65.5X1	T65.5X2	T65.5X3	T65.5X4	—	—
fumes	T65.5X1	T65.5X2	T65.5X3	T65.5X4	—	—
Nitroglycol	T52.3X1	T52.3X2	T52.3X3	T52.3X4		
Nitrohydrochloric acid	T54.2X1	T54.2X2	T54.2X3	T54.2X4	—	—
Nitromersol	T49.0X1	T49.0X2	T49.0X3	T49.0X4	T49.0X5	T49.0X6
Nitronaphthalene	T65.891	T65.892	T65.893	T65.894		
Nitrophenol	T54.0X1	T54.0X2	T54.0X3	T54.0X4		
Nitropropane	T52.8X1	T52.8X2	T52.8X3	T52.8X4	—	—
Nitroprusside	T46.5X1	T46.5X2	T46.5X3	T46.5X4	T46.5X5	T46.5X6
Nitrosodimethylamine	T65.3X1	T65.3X2	T65.3X3	T65.3X4	—	—
Nitrothiazol	T37.4X1	T37.4X2	T37.4X3	T37.4X4	T37.4X5	T37.4X6
Nitrotoluene, nitrotoluol	T65.3X1	T65.3X2	T65.3X3	T65.3X4	—	—
vapor	T65.3X1	T65.3X2	T65.3X3	T65.3X4	—	—
Nitrous						
acid (liquid)	T54.2X1	T54.2X2	T54.2X3	T54.2X4		
fumes	T59.891	T59.892	T59.893	T59.894	—	—
ether spirit	T46.3X1	T46.3X2	T46.3X3	T46.3X4	T46.3X5	T46.3X6
oxide	T41.0X1	T41.0X2	T41.0X3	T41.0X4	T41.0X5	T41.0X6
Nitroxoline	T37.8X1	T37.8X2	T37.8X3	T37.8X4	T37.8X5	T37.8X6
Nitrozone	T49.0X1	T49.0X2	T49.0X3	T49.0X4	T49.0X5	T49.0X6
Nizatidine	T47.0X1	T47.0X2	T47.0X3	T47.0X4	T47.0X5	T47.0X6
Nizofenone	T43.8X1	T43.8X2	T43.8X3	T43.8X4	T43.8X5	T43.8X6
Noctec	T42.6X1	T42.6X2	T42.6X3	T42.6X4	T42.6X5	T42.6X6
Noludar	T42.6X1	T42.6X2	T42.6X3	T42.6X4	T42.6X5	T42.6X6
Noptil	T42.3X1	T42.3X2	T42.3X3	T42.3X4	T42.3X5	T42.3X6
Nomegestrol	T38.5X1	T38.5X2	T38.5X3	T38.5X4	T38.5X5	T38.5X6
Nomifensine	T43.291	T43.292	T43.293	T43.294	T43.295	T43.296
Nonoxinol	T49.8X1	T49.8X2	T49.8X3	T49.8X4	T49.8X5	T49.8X6
Nonylphenoxy (polyethoxy-ethanol)	T49.8X1	T49.8X2	T49.8X3	T49.8X4	T49.8X5	T49.8X6
Noptil	T42.3X1	T42.3X2	T42.3X3	T42.3X4	T42.3X5	T42.3X6
Noradrenaline	T44.4X1	T44.4X2	T44.4X3	T44.4X4	T44.4X5	T44.4X6
Noramidopyrine	T39.2X1	T39.2X2	T39.2X3	T39.2X4	T39.2X5	T39.2X6
methanesulfonate sodium	T39.2X1	T39.2X2	T39.2X3	T39.2X4	T39.2X5	T39.2X6
Norbormide	T60.4X1	T60.4X2	T60.4X3	T60.4X4	—	—
Nordazepam	T42.4X1	T42.4X2	T42.4X3	T42.4X4	T42.4X5	T42.4X6
Norepinephrine	T44.4X1	T44.4X2	T44.4X3	T44.4X4	T44.4X5	T44.4X6
Norethandrolone	T38.7X1	T38.7X2	T38.7X3	T38.7X4	T38.7X5	T38.7X6
Norethindrone	T38.4X1	T38.4X2	T38.4X3	T38.4X4	T38.4X5	T38.4X6

TABLE OF DRUGS AND CHEMICALS

Substance	External Cause (T-Code)					
	Poisoning, Accidental (Unintentional)	Poisoning, Intentional Self-Harm	Poisoning, Assault	Poisoning, Undetermined	Adverse Effect	Underdosing
Norethisterone (acetate) (enantate)	T38.4X1	T38.4X2	T38.4X3	T38.4X4	T38.4X5	T38.4X6
with ethinylestradiol	T38.5X1	T38.5X2	T38.5X3	T38.5X4	T38.5X5	T38.5X6
Noretynodrel	T38.5X1	T38.5X2	T38.5X3	T38.5X4	T38.5X5	T38.5X6
Norfenefrine	T44.4X1	T44.4X2	T44.4X3	T44.4X4	T44.4X5	T44.4X6
Norfloxacin	T36.8X1	T36.8X2	T36.8X3	T36.8X4	T36.8X5	T36.8X6
Norgestrel	T38.4X1	T38.4X2	T38.4X3	T38.4X4	T38.4X5	T38.4X6
Norgestrienone	T38.4X1	T38.4X2	T38.4X3	T38.4X4	T38.4X5	T38.4X6
Norlestrin	T38.4X1	T38.4X2	T38.4X3	T38.4X4	T38.4X5	T38.4X6
Norlutin	T38.4X1	T38.4X2	T38.4X3	T38.4X4	T38.4X5	T38.4X6
Normal serum albumin (human), salt-poor	T45.8X1	T45.8X2	T45.8X3	T45.8X4	T45.8X5	T45.8X6
Normethandrone	T38.5X1	T38.5X2	T38.5X3	T38.5X4	T38.5X5	T38.5X6
Normison — see Benzodiazepines						
Normorphine	T40.2X1	T40.2X2	T40.2X3	T40.2X4	—	—
Norpseudoephedrine	T50.5X1	T50.5X2	T50.5X3	T50.5X4	T50.5X5	T50.5X6
Nortestosterone (furanpropionate)	T38.7X1	T38.7X2	T38.7X3	T38.7X4	T38.7X5	T38.7X6
Nortriptyline	T43.011	T43.012	T43.013	T43.014	T43.015	T43.016
Noscapine	T48.3X1	T48.3X2	T48.3X3	T48.3X4	T48.3X5	T48.3X6
Nose preparations	T49.6X1	T49.6X2	T49.6X3	T49.6X4	T49.6X5	T49.6X6
Novobiocin	T36.5X1	T36.5X2	T36.5X3	T36.5X4	T36.5X5	T36.5X6
Novocain (infiltration) (topical)	T41.3X1	T41.3X2	T41.3X3	T41.3X4	T41.3X5	T41.3X6
nerve block (peripheral) (plexus)	T41.3X1	T41.3X2	T41.3X3	T41.3X4	T41.3X5	T41.3X6
spinal	T41.3X1	T41.3X2	T41.3X3	T41.3X4	T41.3X5	T41.3X6
Noxious foodstuff	T62.91	T62.92	T62.93	T62.94	—	—
specified NEC	T62.8X1	T62.8X2	T62.8X3	T62.8X4	—	—
Noxiptiline	T43.011	T43.012	T43.013	T43.014	T43.015	T43.016
Noxytiolin	T49.0X1	T49.0X2	T49.0X3	T49.0X4	T49.0X5	T49.0X6
NPH Iletin (insulin)	T38.3X1	T38.3X2	T38.3X3	T38.3X4	T38.3X5	T38.3X6
Numorphan	T40.2X1	T40.2X2	T40.2X3	T40.2X4	T40.2X5	T40.2X6
Nunol	T42.3X1	T42.3X2	T42.3X3	T42.3X4	T42.3X5	T42.3X6
Nupercaine (spinal anesthetic)	T41.3X1	T41.3X2	T41.3X3	T41.3X4	T41.3X5	T41.3X6
topical (surface)	T41.3X1	T41.3X2	T41.3X3	T41.3X4	T41.3X5	T41.3X6
Nutmeg oil (liniment)	T49.3X1	T49.3X2	T49.3X3	T49.3X4	T49.3X5	T49.3X6
Nutritional supplement	T50.901	T50.902	T50.903	T50.904	T50.905	T50.906
Nux vomica	T65.1X1	T65.1X2	T65.1X3	T65.1X4	—	—
Nydrazid	T37.1X1	T37.1X2	T37.1X3	T37.1X4	T37.1X5	T37.1X6
Nylidrin	T46.7X1	T46.7X2	T46.7X3	T46.7X4	T46.7X5	T46.7X6
Nystatin	T36.7X1	T36.7X2	T36.7X3	T36.7X4	T36.7X5	T36.7X6
topical	T49.0X1	T49.0X2	T49.0X3	T49.0X4	T49.0X5	T49.0X6
Nytol	T45.0X1	T45.0X2	T45.0X3	T45.0X4	T45.0X5	T45.0X6

Substance	Poisoning, Accidental (Unintentional)	Poisoning, Intentional Self-Harm	Poisoning, Assault	Poisoning, Undetermined	Adverse Effect	Underdosing
	External Cause (T-Code)					
O						
Obidoxime chloride	T50.6X1	T50.6X2	T50.6X3	T50.6X4	T50.6X5	T50.6X6
Octafonium (chloride)	T49.3X1	T49.3X2	T49.3X3	T49.3X4	T49.3X5	T49.3X6
Octamethyl pyrophos-phoramide	T60.0X1	T60.0X2	T60.0X3	T60.0X4	—	—
Octanoin	T50.991	T50.992	T50.993	T50.994	T50.995	T50.996
Octatropine methyl-bromide	T44.3X1	T44.3X2	T44.3X3	T44.3X4	T44.3X5	T44.3X6
Octotiamine	T45.2X1	T45.2X2	T45.2X3	T45.2X4	T45.2X5	T45.2X6
Octoxinol (9)	T49.8X1	T49.8X2	T49.8X3	T49.8X4	T49.8X5	T49.8X6
Octreotide	T38.991	T38.992	T38.993	T38.994	T38.995	T38.996
Octyl nitrite	T46.3X1	T46.3X2	T46.3X3	T46.3X4	T46.3X5	T46.3X6
Oestradiol	T38.5X1	T38.5X2	T38.5X3	T38.5X4	T38.5X5	T38.5X6
Oestriol	T38.5X1	T38.5X2	T38.5X3	T38.5X4	T38.5X5	T38.5X6
Oestrogen	T38.5X1	T38.5X2	T38.5X3	T38.5X4	T38.5X5	T38.5X6
Oestrone	T38.5X1	T38.5X2	T38.5X3	T38.5X4	T38.5X5	T38.5X6
Ofloxacin	T36.8X1	T36.8X2	T36.8X3	T36.8X4	T36.8X5	T36.8X6
Oil (of)	T65.891	T65.892	T65.893	T65.894	—	—
bitter almond	T62.8X1	T62.8X2	T62.8X3	T62.8X4	—	—
cloves	T49.7X1	T49.7X2	T49.7X3	T49.7X4	T49.7X5	T49.7X6
colors	T65.6X1	T65.6X2	T65.6X3	T65.6X4	—	—
fumes	T59.891	T59.892	T59.893	T59.894	—	—
lubricating	T52.0X1	T52.0X2	T52.0X3	T52.0X4	—	—
Niobe	T52.8X1	T52.8X2	T52.8X3	T52.8X4	—	—
vitriol (liquid)	T54.2X1	T54.2X2	T54.2X3	T54.2X4	—	—
fumes	T54.2X1	T54.2X2	T54.2X3	T54.2X4	—	—
wintergreen (bitter) NEC	T49.3X1	T49.3X2	T49.3X3	T49.3X4	T49.3X5	T49.3X6
Oily preparation (for skin)	T49.3X1	T49.3X2	T49.3X3	T49.3X4	T49.3X5	T49.3X6
Ointment NEC	T49.3X1	T49.3X2	T49.3X3	T49.3X4	T49.3X5	T49.3X6
Olanzapine	T43.591	T43.592	T43.593	T43.594	T43.595	T43.596
Oleander	T62.2X1	T62.2X2	T62.2X3	T62.2X4	—	—
Oleandomycin	T36.3X1	T36.3X2	T36.3X3	T36.3X4	T36.3X5	T36.3X6
Oleandrin	T46.0X1	T46.0X2	T46.0X3	T46.0X4	T46.0X5	T46.0X6
Oleic acid	T46.6X1	T46.6X2	T46.6X3	T46.6X4	T46.6X5	T46.6X6
Oleovitamin A	T45.2X1	T45.2X2	T45.2X3	T45.2X4	T45.2X5	T45.2X6
Oleum ricini	T47.2X1	T47.2X2	T47.2X3	T47.2X4	T47.2X5	T47.2X6
Olive oil (medicinal) NEC	T47.4X1	T47.4X2	T47.4X3	T47.4X4	T47.4X5	T47.4X6
Olivomycin	T45.1X1	T45.1X2	T45.1X3	T45.1X4	T45.1X5	T45.1X6
Olsalazine	T47.8X1	T47.8X2	T47.8X3	T47.8X4	T47.8X5	T47.8X6
Omeprazole	T47.1X1	T47.1X2	T47.1X3	T47.1X4	T47.1X5	T47.1X6

Substance	External Cause (T-Code)					
	Poisoning, Accidental (Unintentional)	Poisoning, Intentional Self-Harm	Poisoning, Assault	Poisoning, Undetermined	Adverse Effect	Underdosing
OMPA	T60.0X1	T60.0X2	T60.0X3	T60.0X4	—	—
Ondansetron	T45.0X1	T45.0X2	T45.0X3	T45.0X4	T45.0X5	T45.0X6
Oncovin	T45.1X1	T45.1X2	T45.1X3	T45.1X4	T45.1X5	T45.1X6
Ophthaine	T41.3X1	T41.3X2	T41.3X3	T41.3X4	T41.3X5	T41.3X6
Ophthetic	T41.3X1	T41.3X2	T41.3X3	T41.3X4	T41.3X5	T41.3X6
Opiate NEC	T40.601	T40.602	T40.603	T40.604	T40.605	T40.606
antagonists	T50.7X1	T50.7X2	T50.7X3	T50.7X4	T50.7X5	T50.7X6
Opioid NEC	T40.2X1	T40.2X2	T40.2X3	T40.2X4	T40.2X5	T40.2X6
Opipramol	T43.011	T43.012	T43.013	T43.014	T43.015	T43.016
Opium alkaloids (total)	T40.0X1	T40.0X2	T40.0X3	T40.0X4	T40.0X5	T40.0X6
standardized powdered	T40.0X1	T40.0X2	T40.0X3	T40.0X4	T40.0X5	T40.0X6
tincture (camphorated)	T40.0X1	T40.0X2	T40.0X3	T40.0X4	T40.0X5	T40.0X6
Oracon	T38.4X1	T38.4X2	T38.4X3	T38.4X4	T38.4X5	T38.4X6
Oragrafin	T50.8X1	T50.8X2	T50.8X3	T50.8X4	T50.8X5	T50.8X6
Oral contraceptives	T38.4X1	T38.4X2	T38.4X3	T38.4X4	T38.4X5	T38.4X6
Oral rehydration salts	T50.3X1	T50.3X2	T50.3X3	T50.3X4	T50.3X5	T50.3X6
Orazamide	T50.991	T50.992	T50.993	T50.994	T50.995	T50.996
Orciprenaline	T48.291	T48.292	T48.293	T48.294	T48.295	T48.296
Organidin	T48.4X1	T48.4X2	T48.4X3	T48.4X4	T48.4X5	T48.4X6
Organonitrate NEC	T46.3X1	T46.3X2	T46.3X3	T46.3X4	T46.3X5	T46.3X6
Organophosphates	T60.0X1	T60.0X2	T60.0X3	T60.0X4	—	—
Orimune	T50.B91	T50.B92	T50.B93	T50.B94	T50.B95	T50.B96
Orinase	T38.3X1	T38.3X2	T38.3X3	T38.3X4	T38.3X5	T38.3X6
Ormeloxifene	T38.6X1	T38.6X2	T38.6X3	T38.6X4	T38.6X5	T38.6X6
Ornidazole	T37.3X1	T37.3X2	T37.3X3	T37.3X4	T37.3X5	T37.3X6
Ornithine aspartate	T50.991	T50.992	T50.993	T50.994	T50.995	T50.996
Ornoprostil	T47.1X1	T47.1X2	T47.1X3	T47.1X4	T47.1X5	T47.1X6
Orphenadrine (hydrochloride)	T42.8X1	T42.8X2	T42.8X3	T42.8X4	T42.8X5	T42.8X6
Ortal (sodium)	T42.3X1	T42.3X2	T42.3X3	T42.3X4	T42.3X5	T42.3X6
Orthoboric acid	T49.0X1	T49.0X2	T49.0X3	T49.0X4	T49.0X5	T49.0X6
ENT agent	T49.6X1	T49.6X2	T49.6X3	T49.6X4	T49.6X5	T49.6X6
ophthalmic preparation	T49.5X1	T49.5X2	T49.5X3	T49.5X4	T49.5X5	T49.5X6
Orthocaine	T41.3X1	T41.3X2	T41.3X3	T41.3X4	T41.3X5	T41.3X6
Orthodichlorobenzene	T53.7X1	T53.7X2	T53.7X3	T53.7X4	—	—
Ortho-Novum	T38.4X1	T38.4X2	T38.4X3	T38.4X4	T38.4X5	T38.4X6
Orthotolidine (reagent)	T54.2X1	T54.2X2	T54.2X3	T54.2X4	—	—
Osmic acid (liquid)	T54.2X1	T54.2X2	T54.2X3	T54.2X4	—	—
fumes	T54.2X1	T54.2X2	T54.2X3	T54.2X4	—	—
Osmotic diuretics	T50.2X1	T50.2X2	T50.2X3	T50.2X4	T50.2X5	T50.2X6
Otilonium bromide	T44.3X1	T44.3X2	T44.3X3	T44.3X4	T44.3X5	T44.3X6

Substance	External Cause (T-Code)					
	Poisoning, Accidental (Unintentional)	Poisoning, Intentional Self-Harm	Poisoning, Assault	Poisoning, Undetermined	Adverse Effect	Underdosing
Otorhinolaryngological drug NEC	T49.6X1	T49.6X2	T49.6X3	T49.6X4	T49.6X5	T49.6X6
Ouabain(e)	T46.0X1	T46.0X2	T46.0X3	T46.0X4	T46.0X5	T46.0X6
Ovarian						
hormone	T38.5X1	T38.5X2	T38.5X3	T38.5X4	T38.5X5	T38.5X6
stimulant	T38.5X1	T38.5X2	T38.5X3	T38.5X4	T38.5X5	T38.5X6
Ovral	T38.4X1	T38.4X2	T38.4X3	T38.4X4	T38.4X5	T38.4X6
Ovulen	T38.4X1	T38.4X2	T38.4X3	T38.4X4	T38.4X5	T38.4X6
Oxacillin	T36.0X1	T36.0X2	T36.0X3	T36.0X4	T36.0X5	T36.0X6
Oxalic acid	T54.2X1	T54.2X2	T54.2X3	T54.2X4	—	—
ammonium salt	T50.991	T50.992	T50.993	T50.994	T50.995	T50.996
Oxamniquine	T37.4X1	T37.4X2	T37.4X3	T37.4X4	T37.4X5	T37.4X6
Oxanamide	T43.591	T43.592	T43.593	T43.594	T43.595	T43.596
Oxandrolone	T38.7X1	T38.7X2	T38.7X3	T38.7X4	T38.7X5	T38.7X6
Oxantel	T37.4X1	T37.4X2	T37.4X3	T37.4X4	T37.4X5	T37.4X6
Oxapium iodide	T44.3X1	T44.3X2	T44.3X3	T44.3X4	T44.3X5	T44.3X6
Oxaprotiline	T43.021	T43.022	T43.023	T43.024	T43.025	T43.026
Oxaprozin	T39.311	T39.312	T39.313	T39.314	T39.315	T39.316
Oxatomide	T45.0X1	T45.0X2	T45.0X3	T45.0X4	T45.0X5	T45.0X6
Oxazepam	T42.4X1	T42.4X2	T42.4X3	T42.4X4	T42.4X5	T42.4X6
Oxazimedrine	T50.5X1	T50.5X2	T50.5X3	T50.5X4	T50.5X5	T50.5X6
Oxazolam	T42.4X1	T42.4X2	T42.4X3	T42.4X4	T42.4X5	T42.4X6
Oxazolidine derivatives	T42.2X1	T42.2X2	T42.2X3	T42.2X4	T42.2X5	T42.2X6
Oxazolidinedione (derivative)	T42.2X1	T42.2X2	T42.2X3	T42.2X4	T42.2X5	T42.2X6
Ox bile extract	T47.5X1	T47.5X2	T47.5X3	T47.5X4	T47.5X5	T47.5X6
Oxcarbazepine	T42.1X1	T42.1X2	T42.1X3	T42.1X4	T42.1X5	T42.1X6
Oxedrine	T44.4X1	T44.4X2	T44.4X3	T44.4X4	T44.4X5	T44.4X6
Oxeladin (citrate)	T48.3X1	T48.3X2	T48.3X3	T48.3X4	T48.3X5	T48.3X6
Oxendolone	T38.5X1	T38.5X2	T38.5X3	T38.5X4	T38.5X5	T38.5X6
Oxetacaine	T41.3X1	T41.3X2	T41.3X3	T41.3X4	T41.3X5	T41.3X6
Oxethazine	T41.3X1	T41.3X2	T41.3X3	T41.3X4	T41.3X5	T41.3X6
Oxetorone	T39.8X1	T39.8X2	T39.8X3	T39.8X4	T39.8X5	T39.8X6
Oxiconazole	T49.0X1	T49.0X2	T49.0X3	T49.0X4	T49.0X5	T49.0X6
Oxidizing agent NEC	T54.91	T54.92	T54.93	T54.94	—	—
Oxipurinol	T50.4X1	T50.4X2	T50.4X3	T50.4X4	T50.4X5	T50.4X6
Oxitriptan	T43.291	T43.292	T43.293	T43.294	T43.295	T43.296
Oxitropium bromide	T48.6X1	T48.6X2	T48.6X3	T48.6X4	T48.6X5	T48.6X6
Oxodipine	T46.1X1	T46.1X2	T46.1X3	T46.1X4	T46.1X5	T46.1X6
Oxolamine	T48.3X1	T48.3X2	T48.3X3	T48.3X4	T48.3X5	T48.3X6
Oxolinic acid	T37.8X1	T37.8X2	T37.8X3	T37.8X4	T37.8X5	T37.8X6
Oxomemazine	T43.3X1	T43.3X2	T43.3X3	T43.3X4	T43.3X5	T43.3X6

TABLE OF DRUGS AND CHEMICALS

Substance	External Cause (T-Code)					
	Poisoning, Accidental (Unintentional)	Poisoning, Intentional Self-Harm	Poisoning, Assault	Poisoning, Undetermined	Adverse Effect	Underdosing
Oxophenarsine	T37.3X1	T37.3X2	T37.3X3	T37.3X4	T37.3X5	T37.3X6
Oxprenolol	T44.7X1	T44.7X2	T44.7X3	T44.7X4	T44.7X5	T44.7X6
Oxsoralen	T49.3X1	T49.3X2	T49.3X3	T49.3X4	T49.3X5	T49.3X6
Oxtriphylline	T48.6X1	T48.6X2	T48.6X3	T48.6X4	T48.6X5	T48.6X6
Oxybate sodium	T41.291	T41.292	T41.293	T41.294	T41.295	T41.296
Oxybuprocaine	T41.3X1	T41.3X2	T41.3X3	T41.3X4	T41.3X5	T41.3X6
Oxybutynin	T44.3X1	T44.3X2	T44.3X3	T44.3X4	T44.3X5	T44.3X6
Oxychlorosene	T49.0X1	T49.0X2	T49.0X3	T49.0X4	T49.0X5	T49.0X6
Oxycodone	T40.2X1	T40.2X2	T40.2X3	T40.2X4	T40.2X5	T40.2X6
Oxyfedrine	T46.3X1	T46.3X2	T46.3X3	T46.3X4	T46.3X5	T46.3X6
Oxygen	T41.5X1	T41.5X2	T41.5X3	T41.5X4	T41.5X5	T41.5X6
Oxylone	T49.0X1	T49.0X2	T49.0X3	T49.0X4	T49.0X5	T49.0X6
ophthalmic preparation	T49.5X1	T49.5X2	T49.5X3	T49.5X4	T49.5X5	T49.5X6
Oxymesterone	T38.7X1	T38.7X2	T38.7X3	T38.7X4	T38.7X5	T38.7X6
Oxymetazoline	T48.5X1	T48.5X2	T48.5X3	T48.5X4	T48.5X5	T48.5X6
Oxymetholone	T38.7X1	T38.7X2	T38.7X3	T38.7X4	T38.7X5	T38.7X6
Oxymorphone	T40.2X1	T40.2X2	T40.2X3	T40.2X4	T40.2X5	T40.2X6
Oxypertine	T43.591	T43.592	T43.593	T43.594	T43.595	T43.596
Oxyphenbutazone	T39.2X1	T39.2X2	T39.2X3	T39.2X4	T39.2X5	T39.2X6
Oxyphencyclimine	T44.3X1	T44.3X2	T44.3X3	T44.3X4	T44.3X5	T44.3X6
Oxyphenisatine	T47.2X1	T47.2X2	T47.2X3	T47.2X4	T47.2X5	T47.2X6
Oxyphenonium bromide	T44.3X1	T44.3X2	T44.3X3	T44.3X4	T44.3X5	T44.3X6
Oxypolygelatin	T45.8X1	T45.8X2	T45.8X3	T45.8X4	T45.8X5	T45.8X6
Oxyquinoline (derivatives)	T37.8X1	T37.8X2	T37.8X3	T37.8X4	T37.8X5	T37.8X6
Oxytetracycline	T36.4X1	T36.4X2	T36.4X3	T36.4X4	T36.4X5	T36.4X6
Oxytocic drug NEC	T48.0X1	T48.0X2	T48.0X3	T48.0X4	T48.0X5	T48.0X6
Oxytocin (synthetic)	T48.0X1	T48.0X2	T48.0X3	T48.0X4	T48.0X5	T48.0X6
Ozone	T59.891	T59.892	T59.893	T59.894	—	—
P						
PABA	T49.3X1	T49.3X2	T49.3X3	T49.3X4	T49.3X5	T49.3X6
Packed red cells	T45.8X1	T45.8X2	T45.8X3	T45.8X4	T45.8X5	T45.8X6
Padimate	T49.3X1	T49.3X2	T49.3X3	T49.3X4	T49.3X5	T49.3X6
Paint NEC	T65.6X1	T65.6X2	T65.6X3	T65.6X4	—	—
cleaner	T52.91	T52.92	T52.93	T52.94	—	—
fumes NEC	T59.891	T59.892	T59.893	T59.894	—	—
lead (fumes)	T56.0X1	T56.0X2	T56.0X3	T56.0X4	—	—
solvent NEC	T52.8X1	T52.8X2	T52.8X3	T52.8X4	—	—
stripper	T52.8X1	T52.8X2	T52.8X3	T52.8X4	—	—
Palfium	T40.2X1	T40.2X2	T40.2X3	T40.2X4	—	—

Substance	Poisoning, Accidental (Unintentional)	Poisoning, Intentional Self-Harm	Poisoning, Assault	Poisoning, Undetermined	Adverse Effect	Underdosing
Palm kernel oil	T50.991	T50.992	T50.993	T50.994	T50.995	T50.996
Paludrine	T37.2X1	T37.2X2	T37.2X3	T37.2X4	T37.2X5	T37.2X6
PAM (pralidoxime)	T50.6X1	T50.6X2	T50.6X3	T50.6X4	T50.6X5	T50.6X6
Pamaquine (naphthoute)	T37.2X1	T37.2X2	T37.2X3	T37.2X4	T37.2X5	T37.2X6
Panadol	T39.1X1	T39.1X2	T39.1X3	T39.1X4	T39.1X5	T39.1X6
Pancreatic						
digestive secretion stimulant	T47.8X1	T47.8X2	T47.8X3	T47.8X4	T47.8X5	T47.8X6
dornase	T45.3X1	T45.3X2	T45.3X3	T45.3X4	T45.3X5	T45.3X6
Pancreatin	T47.5X1	T47.5X2	T47.5X3	T47.5X4	T47.5X5	T47.5X6
Pancrelipase	T47.5X1	T47.5X2	T47.5X3	T47.5X4	T47.5X5	T47.5X6
Pancuronium (bromide)	T48.1X1	T48.1X2	T48.1X3	T48.1X4	T48.1X5	T48.1X6
Pangamic acid	T45.2X1	T45.2X2	T45.2X3	T45.2X4	T45.2X5	T45.2X6
Panthenol	T45.2X1	T45.2X2	T45.2X3	T45.2X4	T45.2X5	T45.2X6
topical	T49.8X1	T49.8X2	T49.8X3	T49.8X4	T49.8X5	T49.8X6
Pantopon	T40.0X1	T40.0X2	T40.0X3	T40.0X4	T40.0X5	T40.0X6
Pantothenic acid	T45.2X1	T45.2X2	T45.2X3	T45.2X4	T45.2X5	T45.2X6
Panwarfin	T45.511	T45.512	T45.513	T45.514	T45.515	T45.516
Papain	T47.5X1	T47.5X2	T47.5X3	T47.5X4	T47.5X5	T47.5X6
digestant	T47.5X1	T47.5X2	T47.5X3	T47.5X4	T47.5X5	T47.5X6
Papaveretum	T40.0X1	T40.0X2	T40.0X3	T40.0X4	T40.0X5	T40.0X6
Papaverine	T44.3X1	T44.3X2	T44.3X3	T44.3X4	T44.3X5	T44.3X6
Para-acetamidophenol	T39.1X1	T39.1X2	T39.1X3	T39.1X4	T39.1X5	T39.1X6
Para-aminobenzoic acid	T49.3X1	T49.3X2	T49.3X3	T49.3X4	T49.3X5	T49.3X6
Para-aminophenol derivatives	T39.1X1	T39.1X2	T39.1X3	T39.1X4	T39.1X5	T39.1X6
Para-aminosalicylic acid	T37.1X1	T37.1X2	T37.1X3	T37.1X4	T37.1X5	T37.1X6
Paracetaldehyde	T42.6X1	T42.6X2	T42.6X3	T42.6X4	T42.6X5	T42.6X6
Paracetamol	T39.1X1	T39.1X2	T39.1X3	T39.1X4	T39.1X5	T39.1X6
Parachlorophenol (camphorated)	T49.0X1	T49.0X2	T49.0X3	T49.0X4	T49.0X5	T49.0X6
Paracodin	T40.2X1	T40.2X2	T40.2X3	T40.2X4	T40.2X5	T40.2X6
Paradione	T42.2X1	T42.2X2	T42.2X3	T42.2X4	T42.2X5	T42.2X6
Paraffin(s) (wax)	T52.0X1	T52.0X2	T52.0X3	T52.0X4	—	—
liquid (medicinal)	T47.4X1	T47.4X2	T47.4X3	T47.4X4	T47.4X5	T47.4X6
nonmedicinal	T52.0X1	T52.0X2	T52.0X3	T52.0X4	—	—
Paraformaldehyde	T60.3X1	T60.3X2	T60.3X3	T60.3X4	—	—
Paraldehyde	T42.6X1	T42.6X2	T42.6X3	T42.6X4	T42.6X5	T42.6X6
Paramethadione	T42.2X1	T42.2X2	T42.2X3	T42.2X4	T42.2X5	T42.2X6
Paramethasone	T38.0X1	T38.0X2	T38.0X3	T38.0X4	T38.0X5	T38.0X6
acetate	T49.0X1	T49.0X2	T49.0X3	T49.0X4	T49.0X5	T49.0X6
Paraoxon	T60.0X1	T60.0X2	T60.0X3	T60.0X4	—	—
Paraquat	T60.3X1	T60.3X2	T60.3X3	T60.3X4	—	—

Substance	External Cause (T-Code)					
	Poisoning, Accidental (Unintentional)	Poisoning, Intentional Self-Harm	Poisoning, Assault	Poisoning, Undetermined	Adverse Effect	Underdosing
Parasympatholytic NEC	T44.3X1	T44.3X2	T44.3X3	T44.3X4	T44.3X5	T44.3X6
Parasympathomimetic drug NEC	T44.1X1	T44.1X2	T44.1X3	T44.1X4	T44.1X5	T44.1X6
Parathion	T60.0X1	T60.0X2	T60.0X3	T60.0X4	—	—
Parathormone	T50.991	T50.992	T50.993	T50.994	T50.995	T50.996
Parathyroid extract	T50.991	T50.992	T50.993	T50.994	T50.995	T50.996
Paratyphoid vaccine	T50.A91	T50.A92	T50.A93	T50.A94	T50.A95	T50.A96
Paredrine	T44.4X1	T44.4X2	T44.4X3	T44.4X4	T44.4X5	T44.4X6
Paregoric	T40.0X1	T40.0X2	T40.0X3	T40.0X4	T40.0X5	T40.0X6
Pargyline	T46.5X1	T46.5X2	T46.5X3	T46.5X4	T46.5X5	T46.5X6
Paris green	T57.0X1	T57.0X2	T57.0X3	T57.0X4	—	—
insecticide	T57.0X1	T57.0X2	T57.0X3	T57.0X4	—	—
Parnate	T43.1X1	T43.1X2	T43.1X3	T43.1X4	T43.1X5	T43.1X6
Paromomycin	T36.5X1	T36.5X2	T36.5X3	T36.5X4	T36.5X5	T36.5X6
Paroxypropione	T45.1X1	T45.1X2	T45.1X3	T45.1X4	T45.1X5	T45.1X6
Parzone	T40.2X1	T40.2X2	T40.2X3	T40.2X4	T40.2X5	T40.2X6
PAS	T37.1X1	T37.1X2	T37.1X3	T37.1X4	T37.1X5	T37.1X6
Pasiniazid	T37.1X1	T37.1X2	T37.1X3	T37.1X4	T37.1X5	T37.1X6
PBB (polybrominated biphenyls)	T65.891	T65.892	T65.893	T65.894	—	—
PCB	T65.891	T65.892	T65.893	T65.894	—	—
PCP						
meaning pentachlorophenol	T60.1X1	T60.1X2	T60.1X3	T60.1X4	—	—
fungicide	T60.3X1	T60.3X2	T60.3X3	T60.3X4	—	—
herbicide	T60.3X1	T60.3X2	T60.3X3	T60.3X4	—	—
insecticide	T60.1X1	T60.1X2	T60.1X3	T60.1X4	—	—
meaning phencyclidine	T40.991	T40.992	T40.993	T40.994	—	—
Peach kernel oil (emulsion)	T47.4X1	T47.4X2	T47.4X3	T47.4X4	T47.4X5	T47.4X6
Peanut oil (emulsion) NEC	T47.4X1	T47.4X2	T47.4X3	T47.4X4	T47.4X5	T47.4X6
topical	T49.3X1	T49.3X2	T49.3X3	T49.3X4	T49.3X5	T49.3X6
Pearly Gates (morning glory seeds)	T40.991	T40.992	T40.993	T40.994	—	—
Pecazine	T43.3X1	T43.3X2	T43.3X3	T43.3X4	T43.3X5	T43.3X6
Pectin	T47.6X1	T47.6X2	T47.6X3	T47.6X4	T47.6X5	T47.6X6
Pefloxacin	T37.8X1	T37.8X2	T37.8X3	T37.8X4	T37.8X5	T37.8X6
Pegademase, bovine	T50.Z91	T50.Z92	T50.Z93	T50.Z94	T50.Z95	T50.Z96
Pelletierine tannate	T37.4X1	T37.4X2	T37.4X3	T37.4X4	T37.4X5	T37.4X6
Pemirolast (potassium)	T48.6X1	T48.6X2	T48.6X3	T48.6X4	T48.6X5	T48.6X6
Pemoline	T50.7X1	T50.7X2	T50.7X3	T50.7X4	T50.7X5	T50.7X6
Pempidine	T44.2X1	T44.2X2	T44.2X3	T44.2X4	T44.2X5	T44.2X6
Penamecillin	T36.0X1	T36.0X2	T36.0X3	T36.0X4	T36.0X5	T36.0X6
Penbutolol	T44.7X1	T44.7X2	T44.7X3	T44.7X4	T44.7X5	T44.7X6
Penethamate	T36.0X1	T36.0X2	T36.0X3	T36.0X4	T36.0X5	T36.0X6

682

Substance	External Cause (T-Code)					
	Poisoning, Accidental (Unintentional)	Poisoning, Intentional Self-Harm	Poisoning, Assault	Poisoning, Undetermined	Adverse Effect	Underdosing
Penfluridol	T43.591	T43.592	T43.593	T43.594	T43.595	T43.596
Penflutizide	T50.2X1	T50.2X2	T50.2X3	T50.2X4	T50.2X5	T50.2X6
Pengitoxin	T46.0X1	T46.0X2	T46.0X3	T46.0X4	T46.0X5	T46.0X6
Penicillamine	T50.6X1	T50.6X2	T50.6X3	T50.6X4	T50.6X5	T50.6X6
Penicillin (any)	T36.0X1	T36.0X2	T36.0X3	T36.0X4	T36.0X5	T36.0X6
Penicillinase	T45.3X1	T45.3X2	T45.3X3	T45.3X4	T45.3X5	T45.3X6
Penicilloyl polylysine	T50.8X1	T50.8X2	T50.8X3	T50.8X4	T50.8X5	T50.8X6
Penimepicycline	T36.4X1	T36.4X2	T36.4X3	T36.4X4	T36.4X5	T36.4X6
Pentachloroethane	T53.6X1	T53.6X2	T53.6X3	T53.6X4	—	—
Pentachloronaphthalene	T53.7X1	T53.7X2	T53.7X3	T53.7X4	—	—
Pentachlorophenol (pesticide)	T60.1X1	T60.1X2	T60.1X3	T60.1X4	—	—
fungicide	T60.3X1	T60.3X2	T60.3X3	T60.3X4	—	—
herbicide	T60.3X1	T60.3X2	T60.3X3	T60.3X4	—	—
insecticide	T60.1X1	T60.1X2	T60.1X3	T60.1X4	—	—
Pentaerythritol tetranitrate	T46.3X1	T46.3X2	T46.3X3	T46.3X4	T46.3X5	T46.3X6
Pentaerythritol	T46.3X1	T46.3X2	T46.3X3	T46.3X4	T46.3X5	T46.3X6
chloral	T42.6X1	T42.6X2	T42.6X3	T42.6X4	T42.6X5	T42.6X6
tetranitrate NEC	T46.3X1	T46.3X2	T46.3X3	T46.3X4	T46.3X5	T46.3X6
Pentagastrin	T50.8X1	T50.8X2	T50.8X3	T50.8X4	T50.8X5	T50.8X6
Pentalin	T53.6X1	T53.6X2	T53.6X3	T53.6X4	—	—
Pentamethonium bromide	T44.2X1	T44.2X2	T44.2X3	T44.2X4	T44.2X5	T44.2X6
Pentamidine	T37.3X1	T37.3X2	T37.3X3	T37.3X4	T37.3X5	T37.3X6
Pentanol	T51.3X1	T51.3X2	T51.3X3	T51.3X4	—	—
Pentapyrrolinium (bitartrate)	T44.2X1	T44.2X2	T44.2X3	T44.2X4	T44.2X5	T44.2X6
Pentaquine	T37.2X1	T37.2X2	T37.2X3	T37.2X4	T37.2X5	T37.2X6
Pentazocine	T40.4X1	T40.4X2	T40.4X3	T40.4X4	T40.4X5	T40.4X6
Pentetrazole	T50.7X1	T50.7X2	T50.7X3	T50.7X4	T50.7X5	T50.7X6
Penthienate bromide	T44.3X1	T44.3X2	T44.3X3	T44.3X4	T44.3X5	T44.3X6
Pentifylline	T46.7X1	T46.7X2	T46.7X3	T46.7X4	T46.7X5	T46.7X6
Pentobarbital	T42.3X1	T42.3X2	T42.3X3	T42.3X4	T42.3X5	T42.3X6
sodium	T42.3X1	T42.3X2	T42.3X3	T42.3X4	T42.3X5	T42.3X6
Pentobarbitone	T42.3X1	T42.3X2	T42.3X3	T42.3X4	T42.3X5	T42.3X6
Pentolonium tartrate	T44.2X1	T44.2X2	T44.2X3	T44.2X4	T44.2X5	T44.2X6
Pentosan polysulfate (sodium)	T39.8X1	T39.8X2	T39.8X3	T39.8X4	T39.8X5	T39.8X6
Pentostatin	T45.1X1	T45.1X2	T45.1X3	T45.1X4	T45.1X5	T45.1X6
Pentothal	T41.1X1	T41.1X2	T41.1X3	T41.1X4	T41.1X5	T41.1X6
Pentoxifylline	T46.7X1	T46.7X2	T46.7X3	T46.7X4	T46.7X5	T46.7X6
Pentoxyverine	T48.3X1	T48.3X2	T48.3X3	T48.3X4	T48.3X5	T48.3X6
Pentrinat	T46.3X1	T46.3X2	T46.3X3	T46.3X4	T46.3X5	T46.3X6
Pentylenetetrazole	T50.7X1	T50.7X2	T50.7X3	T50.7X4	T50.7X5	T50.7X6

Substance	External Cause (T-Code)					
	Poisoning, Accidental (Unintentional)	Poisoning, Intentional Self-Harm	Poisoning, Assault	Poisoning, Undetermined	Adverse Effect	Underdosing
Pentylsalicylamide	T37.1X1	T37.1X2	T37.1X3	T37.1X4	T37.1X5	T37.1X6
Pentymal	T42.3X1	T42.3X2	T42.3X3	T42.3X4	T42.3X5	T42.3X6
Peplomycin	T45.1X1	T45.1X2	T45.1X3	T45.1X4	T45.1X5	T45.1X6
Peppermint (oil)	T47.5X1	T47.5X2	T47.5X3	T47.5X4	T47.5X5	T47.5X6
Pepsin	T47.5X1	T47.5X2	T47.5X3	T47.5X4	T47.5X5	T47.5X6
digestant	T47.5X1	T47.5X2	T47.5X3	T47.5X4	T47.5X5	T47.5X6
Pepstatin	T47.1X1	T47.1X2	T47.1X3	T47.1X4	T47.1X5	T47.1X6
Peptavlon	T50.8X1	T50.8X2	T50.8X3	T50.8X4	T50.8X5	T50.8X6
Perazine	T43.3X1	T43.3X2	T43.3X3	T43.3X4	T43.3X5	T43.3X6
Percaine (spinal)	T41.3X1	T41.3X2	T41.3X3	T41.3X4	T41.3X5	T41.3X6
topical (surface)	T41.3X1	T41.3X2	T41.3X3	T41.3X4	T41.3X5	T41.3X6
Perchloroethylene	T53.3X1	T53.3X2	T53.3X3	T53.3X4	—	—
medicinal	T37.4X1	T37.4X2	T37.4X3	T37.4X4	T37.4X5	T37.4X6
vapor	T53.3X1	T53.3X2	T53.3X3	T53.3X4	—	—
Percodan	T40.2X1	T40.2X2	T40.2X3	T40.2X4	T40.2X5	T40.2X6
Percogesic — see also acetaminophen	T45.0X1	T45.0X2	T45.0X3	T45.0X4	T45.0X5	T45.0X6
Percorten	T38.0X1	T38.0X2	T38.0X3	T38.0X4	T38.0X5	T38.0X6
Pergolide	T42.8X1	T42.8X2	T42.8X3	T42.8X4	T42.8X5	T42.8X6
Pergonal	T38.811	T38.812	T38.813	T38.814	T38.815	T38.816
Perhexilene	T46.3X1	T46.3X2	T46.3X3	T46.3X4	T46.3X5	T46.3X6
Perhexiline (maleate)	T46.3X1	T46.3X2	T46.3X3	T46.3X4	T46.3X5	T46.3X6
Periactin	T45.0X1	T45.0X2	T45.0X3	T45.0X4	T45.0X5	T45.0X6
Periciazine	T43.3X1	T43.3X2	T43.3X3	T43.3X4	T43.3X5	T43.3X6
Periclor	T42.6X1	T42.6X2	T42.6X3	T42.6X4	T42.6X5	T42.6X6
Perindopril	T46.4X1	T46.4X2	T46.4X3	T46.4X4	T46.4X5	T46.4X6
Perisoxal	T39.8X1	T39.8X2	T39.8X3	T39.8X4	T39.8X5	T39.8X6
Peritrate	T46.3X1	T46.3X2	T46.3X3	T46.3X4	T46.3X5	T46.3X6
Peritoneal dialysis solution	T50.3X1	T50.3X2	T50.3X3	T50.3X4	T50.3X5	T50.3X6
Perlapine	T42.4X1	T42.4X2	T42.4X3	T42.4X4	T42.4X5	T42.4X6
Permanganate	T65.891	T65.892	T65.893	T65.894	—	—
Permethrin	T60.1X1	T60.1X2	T60.1X3	T60.1X4	—	—
Pernocton	T42.3X1	T42.3X2	T42.3X3	T42.3X4	T42.3X5	T42.3X6
Pernoston	T42.3X1	T42.3X2	T42.3X3	T42.3X4	T42.3X5	T42.3X6
Peronine	T40.2X1	T40.2X2	T40.2X3	T40.2X4	—	—
Perphenazine	T43.3X1	T43.3X2	T43.3X3	T43.3X4	T43.3X5	T43.3X6
Pertofrane	T43.011	T43.012	T43.013	T43.014	T43.015	T43.016
Pertussis						
immune serum (human)	T50.Z11	T50.Z12	T50.Z13	T50.Z14	T50.Z15	T50.Z16
vaccine (with diphtheria toxoid) (with tetanus toxoid)	T50.A11	T50.A12	T50.A13	T50.A14	T50.A15	T50.A16
Peruvian balsam	T49.0X1	T49.0X2	T49.0X3	T49.0X4	T49.0X5	T49.0X6

Substance	Poisoning, Accidental (Unintentional)	Poisoning, Intentional Self-Harm	Poisoning, Assault	Poisoning, Undetermined	Adverse Effect	Underdosing
Peruvoside	T46.0X1	T46.0X2	T46.0X3	T46.0X4	T46.0X5	T46.0X6
Pesticide (dust) (fumes) (vapor) NEC	T60.91	T60.92	T60.93	T60.94	—	—
arsenic	T57.0X1	T57.0X2	T57.0X3	T57.0X4	—	—
chlorinated	T60.1X1	T60.1X2	T60.1X3	T60.1X4	—	—
cyanide	T65.0X1	T65.0X2	T65.0X3	T65.0X4	—	—
kerosene	T52.0X1	T52.0X2	T52.0X3	T52.0X4	—	—
mixture (of compounds)	T60.91	T60.92	T60.93	T60.94	—	—
naphthalene	T60.2X1	T60.2X2	T60.2X3	T60.2X4	—	—
organochlorine (compounds)	T60.1X1	T60.1X2	T60.1X3	T60.1X4	—	—
petroleum (distillate) (products) NEC	T60.8X1	T60.8X2	T60.8X3	T60.8X4	—	—
specified ingredient NEC	T60.8X1	T60.8X2	T60.8X3	T60.8X4	—	—
strychnine	T65.1X1	T65.1X2	T65.1X3	T65.1X4	—	—
thallium	T60.4X1	T60.4X2	T60.4X3	T60.4X4	—	—
Pethidine	T40.4X1	T40.4X2	T40.4X3	T40.4X4	T40.4X5	T40.4X6
Petrichloral	T42.6X1	T42.6X2	T42.6X3	T42.6X4	T42.6X5	T42.6X6
Petrol	T52.0X1	T52.0X2	T52.0X3	T52.0X4	—	—
vapor	T52.0X1	T52.0X2	T52.0X3	T52.0X4	—	—
Petrolatum	T49.3X1	T49.3X2	T49.3X3	T49.3X4	T49.3X5	T49.3X6
hydrophilic	T49.3X1	T49.3X2	T49.3X3	T49.3X4	T49.3X5	T49.3X6
liquid	T47.4X1	T47.4X2	T47.4X3	T47.4X4	T47.4X5	T47.4X6
topical	T49.3X1	T49.3X2	T49.3X3	T49.3X4	T49.3X5	T49.3X6
nonmedicinal	T52.0X1	T52.0X2	T52.0X3	T52.0X4	—	—
red veterinary	T49.3X1	T49.3X2	T49.3X3	T49.3X4	T49.3X5	T49.3X6
white	T49.3X1	T49.3X2	T49.3X3	T49.3X4	T49.3X5	T49.3X6
Petroleum (products) NEC	T52.0X1	T52.0X2	T52.0X3	T52.0X4	—	—
benzine(s) — see Ligroin						
ether — see Ligroin						
jelly — see Petrolatum						
naphtha — see Ligroin						
pesticide	T60.8X1	T60.8X2	T60.8X3	T60.8X4	—	—
solids	T52.0X1	T52.0X2	T52.0X3	T52.0X4	—	—
solvents	T52.0X1	T52.0X2	T52.0X3	T52.0X4	—	—
vapor	T52.0X1	T52.0X2	T52.0X3	T52.0X4	—	—
Peyote	T40.991	T40.992	T40.993	T40.994	—	—
Phanodorm, phanodorn	T42.3X1	T42.3X2	T42.3X3	T42.3X4	T42.3X5	T42.3X6
Phanquinone	T37.3X1	T37.3X2	T37.3X3	T37.3X4	T37.3X5	T37.3X6
Phanquone	T37.3X1	T37.3X2	T37.3X3	T37.3X4	T37.3X5	T37.3X6
Pharmaceutical						
adjunct NEC	T50.901	T50.902	T50.903	T50.904	T50.905	T50.906
excipient NEC	T50.901	T50.902	T50.903	T50.904	T50.905	T50.906

	External Cause (T-Code)					
Substance	Poisoning, Accidental (Unintentional)	Poisoning, Intentional Self-Harm	Poisoning, Assault	Poisoning, Undetermined	Adverse Effect	Underdosing
Pharmaceutical *(Continued)*						
sweetener	T50.901	T50.902	T50.903	T50.904	T50.905	T50.906
viscous agent	T50.901	T50.902	T50.903	T50.904	T50.905	T50.906
Phemitone	T42.3X1	T42.3X2	T42.3X3	T42.3X4	T42.3X5	T42.3X6
Phenacaine	T41.3X1	T41.3X2	T41.3X3	T41.3X4	T41.3X5	T41.3X6
Phenacemide	T42.6X1	T42.6X2	T42.6X3	T42.6X4	T42.6X5	T42.6X6
Phenacetin	T39.1X1	T39.1X2	T39.1X3	T39.1X4	T39.1X5	T39.1X6
Phenadoxone	T40.2X1	T40.2X2	T40.2X3	T40.2X4	—	—
Phenaglycodol	T43.591	T43.592	T43.593	T43.594	T43.595	T43.596
Phenantoin	T42.0X1	T42.0X2	T42.0X3	T42.0X4	T42.0X5	T42.0X6
Phenaphthazine reagent	T50.991	T50.992	T50.993	T50.994	T50.995	T50.996
Phenazocine	T40.4X1	T40.4X2	T40.4X3	T40.4X4	T40.4X5	T40.4X6
Phenazone	T39.2X1	T39.2X2	T39.2X3	T39.2X4	T39.2X5	T39.2X6
Phenazopyridine	T39.8X1	T39.8X2	T39.8X3	T39.8X4	T39.8X5	T39.8X6
Phenbenicillin	T36.0X1	T36.0X2	T36.0X3	T36.0X4	T36.0X5	T36.0X6
Phenbutrazate	T50.5X1	T50.5X2	T50.5X3	T50.5X4	T50.5X5	T50.5X6
Phencyclidine	T40.991	T40.992	T40.993	T40.994	T40.995	T40.996
Phendimetrazine	T50.5X1	T50.5X2	T50.5X3	T50.5X4	T50.5X5	T50.5X6
Phenelzine	T43.1X1	T43.1X2	T43.1X3	T43.1X4	T43.1X5	T43.1X6
Phenemal	T42.3X1	T42.3X2	T42.3X3	T42.3X4	T42.3X5	T42.3X6
Phenergan	T42.6X1	T42.6X2	T42.6X3	T42.6X4	T42.6X5	T42.6X6
Pheneticillin	T36.0X1	T36.0X2	T36.0X3	T36.0X4	T36.0X5	T36.0X6
Pheneturide	T42.6X1	T42.6X2	T42.6X3	T42.6X4	T42.6X5	T42.6X6
Phenformin	T38.3X1	T38.3X2	T38.3X3	T38.3X4	T38.3X5	T38.3X6
Phenglutarimide	T44.3X1	T44.3X2	T44.3X3	T44.3X4	T44.3X5	T44.3X6
Phenicarbazide	T39.8X1	T39.8X2	T39.8X3	T39.8X4	T39.8X5	T39.8X6
Phenindamine	T45.0X1	T45.0X2	T45.0X3	T45.0X4	T45.0X5	T45.0X6
Phenindione	T45.511	T45.512	T45.513	T45.514	T45.515	T45.516
Pheniprazine	T43.1X1	T43.1X2	T43.1X3	T43.1X4	T43.1X5	T43.1X6
Pheniramine	T45.0X1	T45.0X2	T45.0X3	T45.0X4	T45.0X5	T45.0X6
Phenisatin	T47.2X1	T47.2X2	T47.2X3	T47.2X4	T47.2X5	T47.2X6
Phenmetrazine	T50.5X1	T50.5X2	T50.5X3	T50.5X4	T50.5X5	T50.5X6
Phenobal	T42.3X1	T42.3X2	T42.3X3	T42.3X4	T42.3X5	T42.3X6
Phenobarbital	T42.3X1	T42.3X2	T42.3X3	T42.3X4	T42.3X5	T42.3X6
with						
mephenytoin	T42.3X1	T42.3X2	T42.3X3	T42.3X4	T42.3X5	T42.3X6
phenytoin	T42.3X1	T42.3X2	T42.3X3	T42.3X4	T42.3X5	T42.3X6
sodium	T42.3X1	T42.3X2	T42.3X3	T42.3X4	T42.3X5	T42.3X6
Phenobarbitone	T42.3X1	T42.3X2	T42.3X3	T42.3X4	T42.3X5	T42.3X6

Substance	External Cause (T-Code)					
	Poisoning, Accidental (Unintentional)	Poisoning, Intentional Self-Harm	Poisoning, Assault	Poisoning, Undetermined	Adverse Effect	Underdosing
Phenobutiodil	T50.8X1	T50.8X2	T50.8X3	T50.8X4	T50.8X5	T50.8X6
Phenoctide	T49.0X1	T49.0X2	T49.0X3	T49.0X4	T49.0X5	T49.0X6
Phenol	T49.0X1	T49.0X2	T49.0X3	T49.0X4	T49.0X5	T49.0X6
disinfectant	T54.0X1	T54.0X2	T54.0X3	T54.0X4	—	—
in oil injection	T46.8X1	T46.8X2	T46.8X3	T46.8X4	T46.8X5	T46.8X6
medicinal	T49.1X1	T49.1X2	T49.1X3	T49.1X4	T49.1X5	T49.1X6
nonmedicinal NEC	T54.0X1	T54.0X2	T54.0X3	T54.0X4	—	—
pesticide	T60.8X1	T60.8X2	T60.8X3	T60.8X4	—	—
red	T50.8X1	T50.8X2	T50.8X3	T50.8X4	T50.8X5	T50.8X6
Phenolic preparation	T49.1X1	T49.1X2	T49.1X3	T49.1X4	T49.1X5	T49.1X6
Phenolphthalein	T47.2X1	T47.2X2	T47.2X3	T47.2X4	T47.2X5	T47.2X6
Phenolsulfonphthalein	T50.8X1	T50.8X2	T50.8X3	T50.8X4	T50.8X5	T50.8X6
Phenomorphan	T40.2X1	T40.2X2	T40.2X3	T40.2X4	—	—
Phenonyl	T42.3X1	T42.3X2	T42.3X3	T42.3X4	T42.3X5	T42.3X6
Phenoperidine	T40.4X1	T40.4X2	T40.4X3	T40.4X4	—	—
Phenopyrazone	T46.991	T46.992	T46.993	T46.994	T46.995	T46.996
Phenoquin	T50.4X1	T50.4X2	T50.4X3	T50.4X4	T50.4X5	T50.4X6
Phenothiazine (psychotropic) NEC	T43.3X1	T43.3X2	T43.3X3	T43.3X4	T43.3X5	T43.3X6
insecticide	T60.2X1	T60.2X2	T60.2X3	T60.2X4	—	—
Phenothrin	T49.0X1	T49.0X2	T49.0X3	T49.0X4	T49.0X5	T49.0X6
Phenoxybenzamine	T46.7X1	T46.7X2	T46.7X3	T46.7X4	T46.7X5	T46.7X6
Phenoxyethanol	T49.0X1	T49.0X2	T49.0X3	T49.0X4	T49.0X5	T49.0X6
Phenoxymethyl penicillin	T36.0X1	T36.0X2	T36.0X3	T36.0X4	T36.0X5	T36.0X6
Phenprobamate	T42.8X1	T42.8X2	T42.8X3	T42.8X4	T42.8X5	T42.8X6
Phenprocoumon	T45.511	T45.512	T45.513	T45.514	T45.515	T45.516
Phensuximide	T42.2X1	T42.2X2	T42.2X3	T42.2X4	T42.2X5	T42.2X6
Phentermine	T50.5X1	T50.5X2	T50.5X3	T50.5X4	T50.5X5	T50.5X6
Phenthicillin	T36.0X1	T36.0X2	T36.0X3	T36.0X4	T36.0X5	T36.0X6
Phentolamine	T46.7X1	T46.7X2	T46.7X3	T46.7X4	T46.7X5	T46.7X6
Phenyl						
butazone	T39.2X1	T39.2X2	T39.2X3	T39.2X4	T39.2X5	T39.2X6
enediamine	T65.3X1	T65.3X2	T65.3X3	T65.3X4		
hydrazine	T65.3X1	T65.3X2	T65.3X3	T65.3X4	—	—
antineoplastic	T45.1X1	T45.1X2	T45.1X3	T45.1X4	T45.1X5	T45.1X6
mercuric compounds — *see* Mercury						
salicylate	T49.3X1	T49.3X2	T49.3X3	T49.3X4	T49.3X5	T49.3X6
Phenylalanine mustard	T45.1X1	T45.1X2	T45.1X3	T45.1X4	T45.1X5	T45.1X6
Phenylbutazone	T39.2X1	T39.2X2	T39.2X3	T39.2X4	T39.2X5	T39.2X6
Phenylenediamine	T65.3X1	T65.3X2	T65.3X3	T65.3X4	—	—

Substance	External Cause (T-Code)					
	Poisoning, Accidental (Unintentional)	Poisoning, Intentional Self-Harm	Poisoning, Assault	Poisoning, Undetermined	Adverse Effect	Underdosing
Phenylephrine	T44.4X1	T44.4X2	T44.4X3	T44.4X4	T44.4X5	T44.4X6
Phenylethylbiguanide	T38.3X1	T38.3X2	T38.3X3	T38.3X4	T38.3X5	T38.3X6
Phenylmercuric						
acetate	T49.0X1	T49.0X2	T49.0X3	T49.0X4	T49.0X5	T49.0X6
borate	T49.0X1	T49.0X2	T49.0X3	T49.0X4	T49.0X5	T49.0X6
nitrate	T49.0X1	T49.0X2	T49.0X3	T49.0X4	T49.0X5	T49.0X6
Phenylmethylbarbitone	T42.3X1	T42.3X2	T42.3X3	T42.3X4	T42.3X5	T42.3X6
Phenylpropanol	T47.5X1	T47.5X2	T47.5X3	T47.5X4	T47.5X5	T47.5X6
Phenylpropanolamine	T44.991	T44.992	T44.993	T44.994	T44.995	T44.996
Phenylsulfthion	T60.0X1	T60.0X2	T60.0X3	T60.0X4	—	—
Phenyltoloxamine	T45.0X1	T45.0X2	T45.0X3	T45.0X4	T45.0X5	T45.0X6
Phenyramidol, phenyramidon	T39.8X1	T39.8X2	T39.8X3	T39.8X4	T39.8X5	T39.8X6
Phenytoin	T42.0X1	T42.0X2	T42.0X3	T42.0X4	T42.0X5	T42.0X6
with Phenobarbital	T42.3X1	T42.3X2	T42.3X3	T42.3X4	T42.3X5	T42.3X6
pHisoHex	T49.2X1	T49.2X2	T49.2X3	T49.2X4	T49.2X5	T49.2X6
Pholcodine	T48.3X1	T48.3X2	T48.3X3	T48.3X4	T48.3X5	T48.3X6
Pholedrine	T46.991	T46.992	T46.993	T46.994	T46.995	T46.996
Phorate	T60.0X1	T60.0X2	T60.0X3	T60.0X4	—	—
Phosdrin	T60.0X1	T60.0X2	T60.0X3	T60.0X4	—	—
Phosfolan	T60.0X1	T60.0X2	T60.0X3	T60.0X4	—	—
Phosgene (gas)	T59.891	T59.892	T59.893	T59.894	—	—
Phosphamidon	T60.0X1	T60.0X2	T60.0X3	T60.0X4	—	—
Phosphate	T65.891	T65.892	T65.893	T65.894	—	—
laxative	T47.4X1	T47.4X2	T47.4X3	T47.4X4	T47.4X5	T47.4X6
organic	T60.0X1	T60.0X2	T60.0X3	T60.0X4	—	—
solvent	T52.91	T52.92	T52.93	T52.94	—	—
tricresyl	T65.891	T65.892	T65.893	T65.894	—	—
Phosphine	T57.1X1	T57.1X2	T57.1X3	T57.1X4	—	—
fumigant	T57.1X1	T57.1X2	T57.1X3	T57.1X4	—	—
Phospholine	T49.5X1	T49.5X2	T49.5X3	T49.5X4	T49.5X5	T49.5X6
Phosphoric acid	T54.2X1	T54.2X2	T54.2X3	T54.2X4	—	—
Phosphorus (compound) NEC	T57.1X1	T57.1X2	T57.1X3	T57.1X4	—	—
pesticide	T60.0X1	T60.0X2	T60.0X3	T60.0X4	—	—
Phthalates	T65.891	T65.892	T65.893	T65.894	—	—
Phthalic anhydride	T65.891	T65.892	T65.893	T65.894	—	—
Phthalimidoglutarimide	T42.6X1	T42.6X2	T42.6X3	T42.6X4	T42.6X5	T42.6X6
Phthalylsulfathiazole	T37.0X1	T37.0X2	T37.0X3	T37.0X4	T37.0X5	T37.0X6
Phylloquinone	T45.7X1	T45.7X2	T45.7X3	T45.7X4	T45.7X5	T45.7X6
Physeptone	T40.3X1	T40.3X2	T40.3X3	T40.3X4	T40.3X5	T40.3X6

	External Cause (T-Code)					
Substance	Poisoning, Accidental (Unintentional)	Poisoning, Intentional Self-Harm	Poisoning, Assault	Poisoning, Undetermined	Adverse Effect	Underdosing
Physostigma venenosum	T62.2X1	T62.2X2	T62.2X3	T62.2X4	—	—
Physostigmine	T49.5X1	T49.5X2	T49.5X3	T49.5X4	T49.5X5	T49.5X6
Phytolacca decandra	T62.2X1	T62.2X2	T62.2X3	T62.2X4	—	—
berries	T62.1X1	T62.1X2	T62.1X3	T62.1X4	—	—
Phytomenadione	T45.7X1	T45.7X2	T45.7X3	T45.7X4	T45.7X5	T45.7X6
Phytonadione	T45.7X1	T45.7X2	T45.7X3	T45.7X4	T45.7X5	T45.7X6
Picoperine	T48.3X1	T48.3X2	T48.3X3	T48.3X4	T48.3X5	T48.3X6
Picosulfate (sodium)	T47.2X1	T47.2X2	T47.2X3	T47.2X4	T47.2X5	T47.2X6
Picric (acid)	T54.2X1	T54.2X2	T54.2X3	T54.2X4	—	—
Picrotoxin	T50.7X1	T50.7X2	T50.7X3	T50.7X4	T50.7X5	T50.7X6
Piketoprofen	T49.0X1	T49.0X2	T49.0X3	T49.0X4	T49.0X5	T49.0X6
Pilocarpine	T44.1X1	T44.1X2	T44.1X3	T44.1X4	T44.1X5	T44.1X6
Pilocarpus (jaborandi) extract	T44.1X1	T44.1X2	T44.1X3	T44.1X4	T44.1X5	T44.1X6
Pilsicainide (hydrochloride)	T46.2X1	T46.2X2	T46.2X3	T46.2X4	T46.2X5	T46.2X6
Pimaricin	T36.7X1	T36.7X2	T36.7X3	T36.7X4	T36.7X5	T36.7X6
Pimeclone	T50.7X1	T50.7X2	T50.7X3	T50.7X4	T50.7X5	T50.7X6
Pimelic ketone	T52.8X1	T52.8X2	T52.8X3	T52.8X4	—	—
Pimethixene	T45.0X1	T45.0X2	T45.0X3	T45.0X4	T45.0X5	T45.0X6
Piminodine	T40.2X1	T40.2X2	T40.2X3	T40.2X4	T40.2X5	T40.2X6
Pimozide	T43.591	T43.592	T43.593	T43.594	T43.595	T43.596
Pinacidil	T46.5X1	T46.5X2	T46.5X3	T46.5X4	T46.5X5	T46.5X6
Pinaverium bromide	T44.3X1	T44.3X2	T44.3X3	T44.3X4	T44.3X5	T44.3X6
Pinazepam	T42.4X1	T42.4X2	T42.4X3	T42.4X4	T42.4X5	T42.4X6
Pindolol	T44.7X1	T44.7X2	T44.7X3	T44.7X4	T44.7X5	T44.7X6
Pindone	T60.4X1	T60.4X2	T60.4X3	T60.4X4	—	—
Pine oil (disinfectant)	T65.891	T65.892	T65.893	T65.894	—	—
Pinkroot	T37.4X1	T37.4X2	T37.4X3	T37.4X4	T37.4X5	T37.4X6
Pipadone	T40.2X1	T40.2X2	T40.2X3	T40.2X4	—	—
Pipamazine	T45.0X1	T45.0X2	T45.0X3	T45.0X4	T45.0X5	T45.0X6
Pipamperone	T43.4X1	T43.4X2	T43.4X3	T43.4X4	T43.4X5	T43.4X6
Pipazetate	T48.3X1	T48.3X2	T48.3X3	T48.3X4	T48.3X5	T48.3X6
Pipemidic acid	T37.8X1	T37.8X2	T37.8X3	T37.8X4	T37.8X5	T37.8X6
Pipenzolate bromide	T44.3X1	T44.3X2	T44.3X3	T44.3X4	T44.3X5	T44.3X6
Piperacetazine	T43.3X1	T43.3X2	T43.3X3	T43.3X4	T43.3X5	T43.3X6
Piperacillin	T36.0X1	T36.0X2	T36.0X3	T36.0X4	T36.0X5	T36.0X6
Piperazine	T37.4X1	T37.4X2	T37.4X3	T37.4X4	T37.4X5	T37.4X6
estrone sulfate	T38.5X1	T38.5X2	T38.5X3	T38.5X4	T38.5X5	T38.5X6
Piper cubeba	T62.2X1	T62.2X2	T62.2X3	T62.2X4	—	—
Piperidione	T48.3X1	T48.3X2	T48.3X3	T48.3X4	—	—

Substance	External Cause (T-Code)					
	Poisoning, Accidental (Unintentional)	Poisoning, Intentional Self-Harm	Poisoning, Assault	Poisoning, Undetermined	Adverse Effect	Underdosing
Piperidolate	T44.3X1	T44.3X2	T44.3X3	T44.3X4	T44.3X5	T44.3X6
Piperocaine	T41.3X1	T41.3X2	T41.3X3	T41.3X4	T41.3X5	T41.3X6
infiltration (subcutaneous)	T41.3X1	T41.3X2	T41.3X3	T41.3X4	T41.3X5	T41.3X6
nerve block (peripheral) (plexus)	T41.3X1	T41.3X2	T41.3X3	T41.3X4	T41.3X5	T41.3X6
topical (surface)	T41.3X1	T41.3X2	T41.3X3	T41.3X4	T41.3X5	T41.3X6
Piperonyl butoxide	T60.8X1	T60.8X2	T60.8X3	T60.8X4	—	—
Pipethanate	T44.3X1	T44.3X2	T44.3X3	T44.3X4	T44.3X5	T44.3X6
Pipobroman	T45.1X1	T45.1X2	T45.1X3	T45.1X4	T45.1X5	T45.1X6
Pipofezine	T43.0X1	T43.0X2	T43.0X3	T43.0X4	T43.0X5	T43.0X6
Pipotiazine	T43.3X1	T43.3X2	T43.3X3	T43.3X4	T43.3X5	T43.3X6
Pipoxizine	T45.0X1	T45.0X2	T45.0X3	T45.0X4	T45.0X5	T45.0X6
Pipradrol	T43.691	T43.692	T43.693	T43.694	T43.695	T43.696
Piprinhydrinate	T45.0X1	T45.0X2	T45.0X3	T45.0X4	T45.0X5	T45.0X6
Pirarubicin	T45.1X1	T45.1X2	T45.1X3	T45.1X4	T45.1X5	T45.1X6
Pirazinamide	T37.1X1	T37.1X2	T37.1X3	T37.1X4	T37.1X5	T37.1X6
Pirbuterol	T48.6X1	T48.6X2	T48.6X3	T48.6X4	T48.6X5	T48.6X6
Pirenzepine	T47.1X1	T47.1X2	T47.1X3	T47.1X4	T47.1X5	T47.1X6
Piretanide	T50.1X1	T50.1X2	T50.1X3	T50.1X4	T50.1X5	T50.1X6
Piribedil	T42.8X1	T42.8X2	T42.8X3	T42.8X4	T42.8X5	T42.8X6
Piridoxilate	T46.3X1	T46.3X2	T46.3X3	T46.3X4	T46.3X5	T46.3X6
Piritramide	T40.4X1	T40.4X2	T40.4X3	T40.4X4	—	—
Pirlindole	T43.0X1	T43.0X2	T43.0X3	T43.0X4	T43.0X5	T43.0X6
Piromidic acid	T37.8X1	T37.8X2	T37.8X3	T37.8X4	T37.8X5	T37.8X6
Piroxicam	T39.391	T39.392	T39.393	T39.394	T39.395	T39.396
beta-cyclodextrin complex	T39.8X1	T39.8X2	T39.8X3	T39.8X4	T39.8X5	T39.8X6
Pirozadil	T46.6X1	T46.6X2	T46.6X3	T46.6X4	T46.6X5	T46.6X6
Piscidia (bark) (erythrina)	T39.8X1	T39.8X2	T39.8X3	T39.8X4	T39.8X5	T39.8X6
Pitch	T65.891	T65.892	T65.893	T65.894	—	—
Pitkin's solution	T41.3X1	T41.3X2	T41.3X3	T41.3X4	T41.3X5	T41.3X6
Pitocin	T48.0X1	T48.0X2	T48.0X3	T48.0X4	T48.0X5	T48.0X6
Pitressin (tannate)	T38.891	T38.892	T38.893	T38.894	T38.895	T38.896
Pituitary extracts (posterior)	T38.891	T38.892	T38.893	T38.894	T38.895	T38.896
anterior	T38.811	T38.812	T38.813	T38.814	T38.815	T38.816
Pituitrin	T38.891	T38.892	T38.893	T38.894	T38.895	T38.896
Pivampicillin	T36.0X1	T36.0X2	T36.0X3	T36.0X4	T36.0X5	T36.0X6
Pivmecillinam	T36.0X1	T36.0X2	T36.0X3	T36.0X4	T36.0X5	T36.0X6
Placental hormone	T38.891	T38.892	T38.893	T38.894	T38.895	T38.896
Placidyl	T42.6X1	T42.6X2	T42.6X3	T42.6X4	T42.6X5	T42.6X6
Plague vaccine	T50.A91	T50.A92	T50.A93	T50.A94	T50.A95	T50.A96

Substance	External Cause (T-Code)					
	Poisoning, Accidental (Unintentional)	Poisoning, Intentional Self-Harm	Poisoning, Assault	Poisoning, Undetermined	Adverse Effect	Underdosing
Plant						
food or fertilizer NEC	T65.891	T65.892	T65.893	T65.894	—	—
containing herbicide	T60.3X1	T60.3X2	T60.3X3	T60.3X4	—	—
noxious, used as food	T62.2X1	T62.2X2	T62.2X3	T62.2X4	—	—
berries	T62.1X1	T62.1X2	T62.1X3	T62.1X4	—	—
seeds	T62.2X1	T62.2X2	T62.2X3	T62.2X4	—	—
specified type NEC	T62.2X1	T62.2X2	T62.2X3	T62.2X4	—	—
Plasma	T45.8X1	T45.8X2	T45.8X3	T45.8X4	T45.8X5	T45.8X6
expander NEC	T45.8X1	T45.8X2	T45.8X3	T45.8X4	T45.8X5	T45.8X6
protein fraction (human)	T45.8X1	T45.8X2	T45.8X3	T45.8X4	T45.8X5	T45.8X6
Plasmanate	T45.8X1	T45.8X2	T45.8X3	T45.8X4	T45.8X5	T45.8X6
Plasminogen (tissue) activator	T45.611	T45.612	T45.613	T45.614	T45.615	T45.616
Plaster dressing	T49.3X1	T49.3X2	T49.3X3	T49.3X4	T49.3X5	T49.3X6
Plastic dressing	T49.3X1	T49.3X2	T49.3X3	T49.3X4	T49.3X5	T49.3X6
Plegicil	T43.3X1	T43.3X2	T43.3X3	T43.3X4	T43.3X5	T43.3X6
Plicamycin	T45.1X1	T45.1X2	T45.1X3	T45.1X4	T45.1X5	T45.1X6
Podophyllotoxin	T49.8X1	T49.8X2	T49.8X3	T49.8X4	T49.8X5	T49.8X6
Podophyllum (resin)	T49.4X1	T49.4X2	T49.4X3	T49.4X4	T49.4X5	T49.4X6
Poison NEC	T65.91	T65.92	T65.93	T65.94	—	—
Poisonous berries	T62.1X1	T62.1X2	T62.1X3	T62.1X4	—	—
Pokeweed (any part)	T62.2X1	T62.2X2	T62.2X3	T62.2X4	—	—
Poldine metilsulfate	T44.3X1	T44.3X2	T44.3X3	T44.3X4	T44.3X5	T44.3X6
Polidexide (sulfate)	T46.6X1	T46.6X2	T46.6X3	T46.6X4	T46.6X5	T46.6X6
Polidocanol	T46.8X1	T46.8X2	T46.8X3	T46.8X4	T46.8X5	T46.8X6
Poliomyelitis vaccine	T50.B91	T50.B92	T50.B93	T50.B94	T50.B95	T50.B96
Polish (car) (floor) (furniture) (metal) (porcelain) (silver)	T65.891	T65.892	T65.893	T65.894	—	—
abrasive	T65.891	T65.892	T65.893	T65.894	—	—
porcelain	T65.891	T65.892	T65.893	T65.894	—	—
Poloxalkol	T47.4X1	T47.4X2	T47.4X3	T47.4X4	T47.4X5	T47.4X6
Poloxamer	T47.4X1	T47.4X2	T47.4X3	T47.4X4	T47.4X5	T47.4X6
Polyaminostyrene resins	T50.3X1	T50.3X2	T50.3X3	T50.3X4	T50.3X5	T50.3X6
Polycarbophil	T47.4X1	T47.4X2	T47.4X3	T47.4X4	T47.4X5	T47.4X6
Polychlorinated biphenyl	T65.891	T65.892	T65.893	T65.894	—	—
Polycycline	T36.4X1	T36.4X2	T36.4X3	T36.4X4	T36.4X5	T36.4X6
Polyester fumes	T59.891	T59.892	T59.893	T59.894	—	—
Polyester resin hardener	T52.91	T52.92	T52.93	T52.94	—	—
fumes	T59.891	T59.892	T59.893	T59.894	—	—
Polyestradiol phosphate	T38.5X1	T38.5X2	T38.5X3	T38.5X4	T38.5X5	T38.5X6
Polyethanolamine alkyl sulfate	T49.2X1	T49.2X2	T49.2X3	T49.2X4	T49.2X5	T49.2X6

TABLE OF DRUGS AND CHEMICALS

Substance	External Cause (T-Code)					
	Poisoning, Accidental (Unintentional)	Poisoning, Intentional Self-Harm	Poisoning, Assault	Poisoning, Undetermined	Adverse Effect	Underdosing
Polyethylene adhesive	T49.3X1	T49.3X2	T49.3X3	T49.3X4	T49.3X5	T49.3X6
Polyferose	T45.4X1	T45.4X2	T45.4X3	T45.4X4	T45.4X5	T45.4X6
Polygeline	T45.8X1	T45.8X2	T45.8X3	T45.8X4	T45.8X5	T45.8X6
Polymyxin	T36.8X1	T36.8X2	T36.8X3	T36.8X4	T36.8X5	T36.8X6
B	T36.8X1	T36.8X2	T36.8X3	T36.8X4	T36.8X5	T36.8X6
ENT agent	T49.6X1	T49.6X2	T49.6X3	T49.6X4	T49.6X5	T49.6X6
ophthalmic preparation	T49.5X1	T49.5X2	T49.5X3	T49.5X4	T49.5X5	T49.5X6
topical NEC	T49.0X1	T49.0X2	T49.0X3	T49.0X4	T49.0X5	T49.0X6
E sulfate (eye preparation)	T49.5X1	T49.5X2	T49.5X3	T49.5X4	T49.5X5	T49.5X6
Polynoxylin	T49.0X1	T49.0X2	T49.0X3	T49.0X4	T49.0X5	T49.0X6
Polyoestradiol phosphate	T38.5X1	T38.5X2	T38.5X3	T38.5X4	T38.5X5	T38.5X6
Polyoxymethyleneurea	T49.0X1	T49.0X2	T49.0X3	T49.0X4	T49.0X5	T49.0X6
Polysilane	T47.8X1	T47.8X2	T47.8X3	T47.8X4	T47.8X5	T47.8X6
Polytetrafluoroethylene (inhaled)	T59.891	T59.892	T59.893	T59.894	—	—
Polythiazide	T50.2X1	T50.2X2	T50.2X3	T50.2X4	T50.2X5	T50.2X6
Polyvidone	T45.8X1	T45.8X2	T45.8X3	T45.8X4	T45.8X5	T45.8X6
Polyvinylpyrrolidone	T45.8X1	T45.8X2	T45.8X3	T45.8X4	T45.8X5	T45.8X6
Pontocaine (hydrochloride) (infiltration) (topical)	T41.3X1	T41.3X2	T41.3X3	T41.3X4	T41.3X5	T41.3X6
nerve block (peripheral) (plexus)	T41.3X1	T41.3X2	T41.3X3	T41.3X4	T41.3X5	T41.3X6
spinal	T41.3X1	T41.3X2	T41.3X3	T41.3X4	T41.3X5	T41.3X6
Porfiromycin	T45.1X1	T45.1X2	T45.1X3	T45.1X4	T45.1X5	T45.1X6
Posterior pituitary hormone NEC	T38.891	T38.892	T38.893	T38.894	T38.895	T38.896
Pot	T40.7X1	T40.7X2	T40.7X3	T40.7X4	T40.7X5	T40.7X6
Potash (caustic)	T54.3X1	T54.3X2	T54.3X3	T54.3X4	—	—
Potassic saline injection (lactated)	T50.3X1	T50.3X2	T50.3X3	T50.3X4	T50.3X5	T50.3X6
Potassium (salts) NEC	T50.3X1	T50.3X2	T50.3X3	T50.3X4	T50.3X5	T50.3X6
aminobenzoate	T45.8X1	T45.8X2	T45.8X3	T45.8X4	T45.8X5	T45.8X6
aminosalicylate	T37.1X1	T37.1X2	T37.1X3	T37.1X4	T37.1X5	T37.1X6
antimony 'tartrate'	T37.8X1	T37.8X2	T37.8X3	T37.8X4	T37.8X5	T37.8X6
arsenite (solution)	T57.0X1	T57.0X2	T57.0X3	T57.0X4	—	—
bichromate	T56.2X1	T56.2X2	T56.2X3	T56.2X4	—	—
bisulfate	T47.3X1	T47.3X2	T47.3X3	T47.3X4	T47.3X5	T47.3X6
bromide	T42.6X1	T42.6X2	T42.6X3	T42.6X4	T42.6X5	T42.6X6
canrenoate	T50.0X1	T50.0X2	T50.0X3	T50.0X4	T50.0X5	T50.0X6
carbonate	T54.3X1	T54.3X2	T54.3X3	T54.3X4	—	—
chlorate NEC	T65.891	T65.892	T65.893	T65.894	—	—
chloride	T50.3X1	T50.3X2	T50.3X3	T50.3X4	T50.3X5	T50.3X6
citrate	T50.991	T50.992	T50.993	T50.994	T50.995	T50.996
cyanide	T65.0X1	T65.0X2	T65.0X3	T65.0X4	—	—

Substance	Poisoning, Accidental (Unintentional)	Poisoning, Intentional Self-Harm	Poisoning, Assault	Poisoning, Undetermined	Adverse Effect	Underdosing
Potassium NEC *(Continued)*						
ferric hexacyanoferrate (medicinal)	T50.6X1	T50.6X2	T50.6X3	T50.6X4	T50.6X5	T50.6X6
nonmedicinal	T65.891	T65.892	T65.893	T65.894	—	—
Fluoride	T57.8X1	T57.8X2	T57.8X3	T57.8X4	—	—
glucaldrate	T47.1X1	T47.1X2	T47.1X3	T47.1X4	T47.1X5	T47.1X6
hydroxide	T54.3X1	T54.3X2	T54.3X3	T54.3X4	—	—
iodate	T49.0X1	T49.0X2	T49.0X3	T49.0X4	T49.0X5	T49.0X6
iodide	T48.4X1	T48.4X2	T48.4X3	T48.4X4	T48.4X5	T48.4X6
nitrate	T57.8X1	T57.8X2	T57.8X3	T57.8X4	—	—
oxalate	T65.891	T65.892	T65.893	T65.894	—	—
perchlorate (nonmedicinal) NEC	T65.891	T65.892	T65.893	T65.894	—	—
antithyroid	T38.2X1	T38.2X2	T38.2X3	T38.2X4	T38.2X5	T38.2X6
medicinal	T38.2X1	T38.2X2	T38.2X3	T38.2X4	T38.2X5	T38.2X6
Permanganate (nonmedicinal)	T65.891	T65.892	T65.893	T65.894	—	—
medicinal	T49.0X1	T49.0X2	T49.0X3	T49.0X4	T49.0X5	T49.0X6
sulfate	T47.2X1	T47.2X2	T47.2X3	T47.2X4	T47.2X5	T47.2X6
Potassium-removing resin	T50.3X1	T50.3X2	T50.3X3	T50.3X4	T50.3X5	T50.3X6
Potassium-retaining drug	T50.3X1	T50.3X2	T50.3X3	T50.3X4	T50.3X5	T50.3X6
Povidone	T45.8X1	T45.8X2	T45.8X3	T45.8X4	T45.8X5	T45.8X6
iodine	T49.0X1	T49.0X2	T49.0X3	T49.0X4	T49.0X5	T49.0X6
Practolol	T44.7X1	T44.7X2	T44.7X3	T44.7X4	T44.7X5	T44.7X6
Prajmalium bitartrate	T46.2X1	T46.2X2	T46.2X3	T46.2X4	T46.2X5	T46.2X6
Pralidoxime (iodide)	T50.6X1	T50.6X2	T50.6X3	T50.6X4	T50.6X5	T50.6X6
chloride	T50.6X1	T50.6X2	T50.6X3	T50.6X4	T50.6X5	T50.6X6
Pramiverine	T44.3X1	T44.3X2	T44.3X3	T44.3X4	T44.3X5	T44.3X6
Pramocaine	T49.1X1	T49.1X2	T49.1X3	T49.1X4	T49.1X5	T49.1X6
Pramoxine	T49.1X1	T49.1X2	T49.1X3	T49.1X4	T49.1X5	T49.1X6
Prasterone	T38.7X1	T38.7X2	T38.7X3	T38.7X4	T38.7X5	T38.7X6
Pravastatin	T46.6X1	T46.6X2	T46.6X3	T46.6X4	T46.6X5	T46.6X6
Prazepam	T42.4X1	T42.4X2	T42.4X3	T42.4X4	T42.4X5	T42.4X6
Praziquantel	T37.4X1	T37.4X2	T37.4X3	T37.4X4	T37.4X5	T37.4X6
Prazitone	T43.291	T43.292	T43.293	T43.294	T43.295	T43.296
Prazosin	T44.6X1	T44.6X2	T44.6X3	T44.6X4	T44.6X5	T44.6X6
Prednicarbate	T49.0X1	T49.0X2	T49.0X3	T49.0X4	T49.0X5	T49.0X6
Prednimustine	T45.1X1	T45.1X2	T45.1X3	T45.1X4	T45.1X5	T45.1X6
Prednisolone	T38.0X1	T38.0X2	T38.0X3	T38.0X4	T38.0X5	T38.0X6
ENT agent	T49.6X1	T49.6X2	T49.6X3	T49.6X4	T49.6X5	T49.6X6
ophthalmic preparation	T49.5X1	T49.5X2	T49.5X3	T49.5X4	T49.5X5	T49.5X6
steaglate	T49.0X1	T49.0X2	T49.0X3	T49.0X4	T49.0X5	T49.0X6
topical NEC	T49.0X1	T49.0X2	T49.0X3	T49.0X4	T49.0X5	T49.0X6

External Cause (T-Code)

TABLE OF DRUGS AND CHEMICALS

693

Substance	External Cause (T-Code)					
	Poisoning, Accidental (Unintentional)	Poisoning, Intentional Self-Harm	Poisoning, Assault	Poisoning, Undetermined	Adverse Effect	Underdosing
Prednisone	T38.0X1	T38.0X2	T38.0X3	T38.0X4	T38.0X5	T38.0X6
Prednylidene	T38.0X1	T38.0X2	T38.0X3	T38.0X4	T38.0X5	T38.0X6
Pregnandiol	T38.5X1	T38.5X2	T38.5X3	T38.5X4	T38.5X5	T38.5X6
Pregneninolone	T38.5X1	T38.5X2	T38.5X3	T38.5X4	T38.5X5	T38.5X6
Preludin	T43.691	T43.692	T43.693	T43.694	T43.695	T43.696
Premarin	T38.5X1	T38.5X2	T38.5X3	T38.5X4	T38.5X5	T38.5X6
Premedication anesthetic	T41.201	T41.202	T41.203	T41.204	T41.205	T41.206
Prenalterol	T44.5X1	T44.5X2	T44.5X3	T44.5X4	T44.5X5	T44.5X6
Prenoxdiazine	T48.3X1	T48.3X2	T48.3X3	T48.3X4	T48.3X5	T48.3X6
Prenylamine	T46.3X1	T46.3X2	T46.3X3	T46.3X4	T46.3X5	T46.3X6
Preparation, local	T49.4X1	T49.4X2	T49.4X3	T49.4X4	T49.4X5	T49.4X6
Preparation H	T49.8X1	T49.8X2	T49.8X3	T49.8X4	T49.8X5	T49.8X6
Preservative (nonmedicinal)	T65.891	T65.892	T65.893	T65.894	—	—
medicinal	T50.901	T50.902	T50.903	T50.904	T50.905	T50.906
wood	T60.91	T60.92	T60.93	T60.94	—	—
Prethcamide	T50.7X1	T50.7X2	T50.7X3	T50.7X4	T50.7X5	T50.7X6
Pride of China	T62.2X1	T62.2X2	T62.2X3	T62.2X4	—	—
Pridinol	T44.3X1	T44.3X2	T44.3X3	T44.3X4	T44.3X5	T44.3X6
Prifinium bromide	T44.3X1	T44.3X2	T44.3X3	T44.3X4	T44.3X5	T44.3X6
Prilocaine	T41.3X1	T41.3X2	T41.3X3	T41.3X4	T41.3X5	T41.3X6
infiltration (subcutaneous)	T41.3X1	T41.3X2	T41.3X3	T41.3X4	T41.3X5	T41.3X6
nerve block (peripheral) (plexus)	T41.3X1	T41.3X2	T41.3X3	T41.3X4	T41.3X5	T41.3X6
regional	T41.3X1	T41.3X2	T41.3X3	T41.3X4	T41.3X5	T41.3X6
Primaquine	T37.2X1	T37.2X2	T37.2X3	T37.2X4	T37.2X5	T37.2X6
Primidone	T42.6X1	T42.6X2	T42.6X3	T42.6X4	T42.6X5	T42.6X6
Primula (veris)	T62.2X1	T62.2X2	T62.2X3	T62.2X4	—	—
Prinadol	T40.2X1	T40.2X2	T40.2X3	T40.2X4	T40.2X5	T40.2X6
Priscol, Priscoline	T44.6X1	T44.6X2	T44.6X3	T44.6X4	T44.6X5	T44.6X6
Pristinamycin	T36.3X1	T36.3X2	T36.3X3	T36.3X4	T36.3X5	T36.3X6
Privet	T62.2X1	T62.2X2	T62.2X3	T62.2X4	—	—
berries	T62.1X1	T62.1X2	T62.1X3	T62.1X4	—	—
Privine	T44.4X1	T44.4X2	T44.4X3	T44.4X4	T44.4X5	T44.4X6
Pro-Banthine	T44.3X1	T44.3X2	T44.3X3	T44.3X4	T44.3X5	T44.3X6
Probarbital	T42.3X1	T42.3X2	T42.3X3	T42.3X4	T42.3X5	T42.3X6
Probenecid	T50.4X1	T50.4X2	T50.4X3	T50.4X4	T50.4X5	T50.4X6
Probucol	T46.6X1	T46.6X2	T46.6X3	T46.6X4	T46.6X5	T46.6X6
Procainamide	T46.2X1	T46.2X2	T46.2X3	T46.2X4	T46.2X5	T46.2X6
Procaine	T41.3X1	T41.3X2	T41.3X3	T41.3X4	T41.3X5	T41.3X6
benzylpenicillin	T36.0X1	T36.0X2	T36.0X3	T36.0X4	T36.0X5	T36.0X6
nerve block (periphreal) (plexus)	T41.3X1	T41.3X2	T41.3X3	T41.3X4	T41.3X5	T41.3X6

TABLE OF DRUGS AND CHEMICALS

Substance	Poisoning, Accidental (Unintentional)	Poisoning, Intentional Self-Harm	Poisoning, Assault	Poisoning, Undetermined	Adverse Effect	Underdosing
			External Cause (T-Code)			
Procaine *(Continued)*						
penicillin G	T36.0X1	T36.0X2	T36.0X3	T36.0X4	T36.0X5	T36.0X6
regional	T41.3X1	T41.3X2	T41.3X3	T41.3X4	T41.3X5	T41.3X6
spinal	T41.3X1	T41.3X2	T41.3X3	T41.3X4	T41.3X5	T41.3X6
Procalmidol	T43.591	T43.592	T43.593	T43.594	T43.595	T43.596
Procarbazine	T45.1X1	T45.1X2	T45.1X3	T45.1X4	T45.1X5	T45.1X6
Procaterol	T44.5X1	T44.5X2	T44.5X3	T44.5X4	T44.5X5	T44.5X6
Prochlorperazine	T43.3X1	T43.3X2	T43.3X3	T43.3X4	T43.3X5	T43.3X6
Procyclidine	T44.3X1	T44.3X2	T44.3X3	T44.3X4	T44.3X5	T44.3X6
Producer gas	T58.8X1	T58.8X2	T58.8X3	T58.8X4	—	—
Profadol	T40.4X1	T40.4X2	T40.4X3	T40.4X4	T40.4X5	T40.4X6
Profenamine	T44.3X1	T44.3X2	T44.3X3	T44.3X4	T44.3X5	T44.3X6
Profenil	T44.3X1	T44.3X2	T44.3X3	T44.3X4	T44.3X5	T44.3X6
Proflavine	T49.0X1	T49.0X2	T49.0X3	T49.0X4	T49.0X5	T49.0X6
Progabide	T42.6X1	T42.6X2	T42.6X3	T42.6X4	T42.6X5	T42.6X6
Progestin	T38.5X1	T38.5X2	T38.5X3	T38.5X4	T38.5X5	T38.5X6
oral contraceptive	T38.4X1	T38.4X2	T38.4X3	T38.4X4	T38.4X5	T38.4X6
Progesterone	T38.5X1	T38.5X2	T38.5X3	T38.5X4	T38.5X5	T38.5X6
Progestogen NEC	T38.5X1	T38.5X2	T38.5X3	T38.5X4	T38.5X5	T38.5X6
Progestone	T38.5X1	T38.5X2	T38.5X3	T38.5X4	T38.5X5	T38.5X6
Proglumide	T47.1X1	T47.1X2	T47.1X3	T47.1X4	T47.1X5	T47.1X6
Proguanil	T37.2X1	T37.2X2	T37.2X3	T37.2X4	T37.2X5	T37.2X6
Prolactin	T38.811	T38.812	T38.813	T38.814	T38.815	T38.816
Prolintane	T43.691	T43.692	T43.693	T43.694	T43.695	T43.696
Proloid	T38.1X1	T38.1X2	T38.1X3	T38.1X4	T38.1X5	T38.1X6
Proluton	T38.5X1	T38.5X2	T38.5X3	T38.5X4	T38.5X5	T38.5X6
Promacetin	T37.1X1	T37.1X2	T37.1X3	T37.1X4	T37.1X5	T37.1X6
Promazine	T43.3X1	T43.3X2	T43.3X3	T43.3X4	T43.3X5	T43.3X6
Promedol	T40.2X1	T40.2X2	T40.2X3	T40.2X4	—	—
Promegestone	T38.5X1	T38.5X2	T38.5X3	T38.5X4	T38.5X5	T38.5X6
Promethazine (teoclate)	T43.3X1	T43.3X2	T43.3X3	T43.3X4	T43.3X5	T43.3X6
Promin	T37.1X1	T37.1X2	T37.1X3	T37.1X4	T37.1X5	T37.1X6
Pronase	T45.3X1	T45.3X2	T45.3X3	T45.3X4	T45.3X5	T45.3X6
Pronestyl (hydrochloride)	T46.2X1	T46.2X2	T46.2X3	T46.2X4	T46.2X5	T46.2X6
Pronetalol	T44.7X1	T44.7X2	T44.7X3	T44.7X4	T44.7X5	T44.7X6
Prontosil	T37.0X1	T37.0X2	T37.0X3	T37.0X4	T37.0X5	T37.0X6
Propachlor	T60.3X1	T60.3X2	T60.3X3	T60.3X4	—	—
Propafenone	T46.2X1	T46.2X2	T46.2X3	T46.2X4	T46.2X5	T46.2X6
Propallylonal	T42.3X1	T42.3X2	T42.3X3	T42.3X4	T42.3X5	T42.3X6
Propamidine	T49.0X1	T49.0X2	T49.0X3	T49.0X4	T49.0X5	T49.0X6

Substance	External Cause (T-Code)					
	Poisoning, Accidental (Unintentional)	Poisoning, Intentional Self-Harm	Poisoning, Assault	Poisoning, Undetermined	Adverse Effect	Underdosing
Propane (distributed in mobile container)	T59.891	T59.892	T59.893	T59.894	—	—
distributed through pipes	T59.891	T59.892	T59.893	T59.894	—	—
incomplete combustion	T57.11	T57.12	T57.13	T57.14	—	—
Propanidid	T41.291	T41.292	T41.293	T41.294	T41.295	T41.296
Propanil	T60.3X1	T60.3X2	T60.3X3	T60.3X4	—	—
1-Propanol	T51.3X1	T51.3X2	T51.3X3	T51.3X4	—	—
2-Propanol	T51.2X1	T51.2X2	T51.2X3	T51.2X4	—	—
Propantheline	T44.3X1	T44.3X2	T44.3X3	T44.3X4	T44.3X5	T44.3X6
bromide	T44.3X1	T44.3X2	T44.3X3	T44.3X4	T44.3X5	T44.3X6
Proparacaine	T41.3X1	T41.3X2	T41.3X3	T41.3X4	T41.3X5	T41.3X6
Propatylnitrate	T46.3X1	T46.3X2	T46.3X3	T46.3X4	T46.3X5	T46.3X6
Propicillin	T36.0X1	T36.0X2	T36.0X3	T36.0X4	T36.0X5	T36.0X6
Propiolactone	T49.0X1	T49.0X2	T49.0X3	T49.0X4	T49.0X5	T49.0X6
Propiomazine	T45.0X1	T45.0X2	T45.0X3	T45.0X4	T45.0X5	T45.0X6
Propionaidehyde (medicinal)	T42.6X1	T42.6X2	T42.6X3	T42.6X4	T42.6X5	T42.6X6
Propionate (calcium) (sodium)	T49.0X1	T49.0X2	T49.0X3	T49.0X4	T49.0X5	T49.0X6
Propion gel	T49.0X1	T49.0X2	T49.0X3	T49.0X4	T49.0X5	T49.0X6
Propitocaine	T41.3X1	T41.3X2	T41.3X3	T41.3X4	T41.3X5	T41.3X6
infiltration (subcutaneous)	T41.3X1	T41.3X2	T41.3X3	T41.3X4	T41.3X5	T41.3X6
nerve block (peripheral) (plexus)	T41.3X1	T41.3X2	T41.3X3	T41.3X4	T41.3X5	T41.3X6
Propofol	T41.291	T41.292	T41.293	T41.294	T41.295	T41.296
Propoxur	T60.0X1	T60.0X2	T60.0X3	T60.0X4	—	—
Propoxycaine	T41.3X1	T41.3X2	T41.3X3	T41.3X4	T41.3X5	T41.3X6
infiltration (subcutaneous)	T41.3X1	T41.3X2	T41.3X3	T41.3X4	T41.3X5	T41.3X6
nerve block (peripheral) (plexus)	T41.3X1	T41.3X2	T41.3X3	T41.3X4	T41.3X5	T41.3X6
topical (surface)	T41.3X1	T41.3X2	T41.3X3	T41.3X4	T41.3X5	T41.3X6
Propoxyphene	T40.4X1	T40.4X2	T40.4X3	T40.4X4	T40.4X5	T40.4X6
Propranolol	T44.7X1	T44.7X2	T44.7X3	T44.7X4	T44.7X5	T44.7X6
Propyl						
alcohol	T51.3X1	T51.3X2	T51.3X3	T51.3X4	—	—
carbinol	T51.3X1	T51.3X2	T51.3X3	T51.3X4	—	—
hexadrine	T44.4X1	T44.4X2	T44.4X3	T44.4X4	T44.4X5	T44.4X6
iodone	T50.8X1	T50.8X2	T50.8X3	T50.8X4	T50.8X5	T50.8X6
thiouracil	T38.2X1	T38.2X2	T38.2X3	T38.2X4	T38.2X5	T38.2X6
Propylaminophenothiazine	T43.3X1	T43.3X2	T43.3X3	T43.3X4	T43.3X5	T43.3X6
Propylene	T59.891	T59.892	T59.893	T59.894	—	—
Propylhexedrine	T48.5X1	T48.5X2	T48.5X3	T48.5X4	T48.5X5	T48.5X6
Propyliodone	T50.8X1	T50.8X2	T50.8X3	T50.8X4	T50.8X5	T50.8X6
Propylthiouracil	T38.2X1	T38.2X2	T38.2X3	T38.2X4	T38.2X5	T38.2X6
Propylparaben (ophthalmic)	T49.5X1	T49.5X2	T49.5X3	T49.5X4	T49.5X5	T49.5X6

Substance	External Cause (T-Code)					
	Poisoning, Accidental (Unintentional)	Poisoning, Intentional Self-Harm	Poisoning, Assault	Poisoning, Undetermined	Adverse Effect	Underdosing
Propyphenazone	T39.2X1	T39.2X2	T39.2X3	T39.2X4	T39.2X5	T39.2X6
Proquazone	T39.391	T39.392	T39.393	T39.394	T39.395	T39.396
Proscillaridin	T46.0X1	T46.0X2	T46.0X3	T46.0X4	T46.0X5	T46.0X6
Prostacyclin	T45.521	T45.522	T45.523	T45.524	T45.525	T45.526
Prostaglandin (I2)	T45.521	T45.522	T45.523	T45.524	T45.525	T45.526
E1	T46.7X1	T46.7X2	T46.7X3	T46.7X4	T46.7X5	T46.7X6
E2	T48.0X1	T48.0X2	T48.0X3	T48.0X4	T48.0X5	T48.0X6
F2 alpha	T48.0X1	T48.0X2	T48.0X3	T48.0X4	T48.0X5	T48.0X6
Prostigmin	T44.0X1	T44.0X2	T44.0X3	T44.0X4	T44.0X5	T44.0X6
Prosultiamine	T45.2X1	T45.2X2	T45.2X3	T45.2X4	T45.2X5	T45.2X6
Protamine sulfate	T45.7X1	T45.7X2	T45.7X3	T45.7X4	T45.7X5	T45.7X6
zinc insulin	T38.3X1	T38.3X2	T38.3X3	T38.3X4	T38.3X5	T38.3X6
Protease	T47.5X1	T47.5X2	T47.5X3	T47.5X4	T47.5X5	T47.5X6
Protectant, skin NEC	T49.3X1	T49.3X2	T49.3X3	T49.3X4	T49.3X5	T49.3X6
Protein hydrolysate	T50.991	T50.992	T50.993	T50.994	T50.995	T50.996
Prothiaden — see Dothiepin hydrochloride						
Prothionamide	T37.1X1	T37.1X2	T37.1X3	T37.1X4	T37.1X5	T37.1X6
Prothipendyl	T43.591	T43.592	T43.593	T43.594	T43.595	T43.596
Prothoate	T60.0X1	T60.0X2	T60.0X3	T60.0X4	—	—
Prothrombin						
activator	T45.7X1	T45.7X2	T45.7X3	T45.7X4	T45.7X5	T45.7X6
synthesis inhibitor	T45.511	T45.512	T45.513	T45.514	T45.515	T45.516
Protionamide	T37.1X1	T37.1X2	T37.1X3	T37.1X4	T37.1X5	T37.1X6
Protirelin	T38.891	T38.892	T38.893	T38.894	T38.895	T38.896
Protokylol	T48.6X1	T48.6X2	T48.6X3	T48.6X4	T48.6X5	T48.6X6
Protopam	T50.6X1	T50.6X2	T50.6X3	T50.6X4	T50.6X5	T50.6X6
Protoveratrine(s) (A) (B)	T46.5X1	T46.5X2	T46.5X3	T46.5X4	T46.5X5	T46.5X6
Protriptyline	T43.011	T43.012	T43.013	T43.014	T43.015	T43.016
Provera	T38.5X1	T38.5X2	T38.5X3	T38.5X4	T38.5X5	T38.5X6
Provitamin A	T45.2X1	T45.2X2	T45.2X3	T45.2X4	T45.2X5	T45.2X6
Proxibarbal	T42.3X1	T42.3X2	T42.3X3	T42.3X4	T42.3X5	T42.3X6
Proxymetacaine	T41.3X1	T41.3X2	T41.3X3	T41.3X4	T41.3X5	T41.3X6
Proxyphylline	T48.6X1	T48.6X2	T48.6X3	T48.6X4	T48.6X5	T48.6X6
Prozac — see Fluoxetine hydrochloride						
Prunus						
laurocerasus	T62.2X1	T62.2X2	T62.2X3	T62.2X4	—	—
virginiana	T62.2X1	T62.2X2	T62.2X3	T62.2X4	—	—
Prussian blue						
commercial	T65.891	T65.892	T65.893	T65.894	—	—
therapeutic	T50.6X1	T50.6X2	T50.6X3	T50.6X4	T50.6X5	T50.6X6

Substance	Poisoning, Accidental (Unintentional)	Poisoning, Intentional Self-Harm	Poisoning, Assault	Poisoning, Undetermined	Adverse Effect	Underdosing
Prussic acid	T65.0X1	T65.0X2	T65.0X3	T65.0X4	—	—
vapor	T57.3X1	T57.3X2	T57.3X3	T57.3X4	—	—
Pseudoephedrine	T44.991	T44.992	T44.993	T44.994	T44.995	T44.996
Psilocin	T40.991	T40.992	T40.993	T40.994	—	—
Psilocybin	T40.991	T40.992	T40.993	T40.994	—	—
Psilocybine	T40.991	T40.992	T40.993	T40.994	—	—
Psoralene (nonmedicinal)	T65.891	T65.892	T65.893	T65.894	—	—
Psoralens (medicinal)	T50.991	T50.992	T50.993	T50.994	T50.995	T50.996
PSP (phenolsulfonphthalein)	T50.8X1	T50.8X2	T50.8X3	T50.8X4	T50.8X5	T50.8X6
Psychodysleptic drug NEC	T40.901	T40.902	T40.903	T40.904	T40.905	T40.906
Psychostimulant	T43.601	T43.602	T43.603	T43.604	T43.605	T43.606
amphetamine	T43.621	T43.622	T43.623	T43.624	T43.625	T43.626
caffeine	T43.611	T43.612	T43.613	T43.614	T43.615	T43.616
methylphenidate	T43.631	T43.632	T43.633	T43.634	T43.635	T43.636
specified NEC	T43.691	T43.692	T43.693	T43.694	T43.695	T43.696
Psychotherapeutic drug NEC	T43.91	T43.92	T43.93	T43.94	T43.95	T43.96
antidepressants — see also Antidepressant	T43.201	T43.202	T43.203	T43.204	T43.205	T43.206
specified NEC	T43.8X1	T43.8X2	T43.8X3	T43.8X4	T43.8X5	T43.8X6
tranquilizers NEC	T43.501	T43.502	T43.503	T43.504	T43.505	T43.506
Psychotomimetic agents	T40.901	T40.902	T40.903	T40.904	T40.905	T40.906
Psychotropic drug NEC	T43.91	T43.92	T43.93	T43.94	T43.95	T43.96
specified NEC	T43.8X1	T43.8X2	T43.8X3	T43.8X4	T43.8X5	T43.8X6
Psyllium hydrophilic mucilloid	T47.4X1	T47.4X2	T47.4X3	T47.4X4	T47.4X5	T47.4X6
Pteroylglutamic acid	T45.8X1	T45.8X2	T45.8X3	T45.8X4	T45.8X5	T45.8X6
Pteroyltriglutamate	T45.1X1	T45.1X2	T45.1X3	T45.1X4	T45.1X5	T45.1X6
PTFE — see Polytetrafluoroethylene						
Pulp						
devitalizing paste	T49.7X1	T49.7X2	T49.7X3	T49.7X4	T49.7X5	T49.7X6
dressing	T49.7X1	T49.7X2	T49.7X3	T49.7X4	T49.7X5	T49.7X6
Pulsatilla	T62.2X1	T62.2X2	T62.2X3	T62.2X4	—	—
Pumpkin seed extract	T37.4X1	T37.4X2	T37.4X3	T37.4X4	T37.4X5	T37.4X6
Purex (bleach)	T54.91	T54.92	T54.93	T54.94	—	—
Purgative NEC — see also Cathartic	T47.4X1	T47.4X2	T47.4X3	T47.4X4	T47.4X5	T47.4X6
Purine analogue (antineoplastic)	T45.1X1	T45.1X2	T45.1X3	T45.1X4	T45.1X5	T45.1X6
Purine diuretics	T50.2X1	T50.2X2	T50.2X3	T50.2X4	T50.2X5	T50.2X6
Purinethol	T45.1X1	T45.1X2	T45.1X3	T45.1X4	T45.1X5	T45.1X6
PVP	T45.8X1	T45.8X2	T45.8X3	T45.8X4	T45.8X5	T45.8X6
Pyrabital	T39.8X1	T39.8X2	T39.8X3	T39.8X4	T39.8X5	T39.8X6
Pyramidon	T39.2X1	T39.2X2	T39.2X3	T39.2X4	T39.2X5	T39.2X6
Pyrantel	T37.4X1	T37.4X2	T37.4X3	T37.4X4	T37.4X5	T37.4X6

Substance	Poisoning, Accidental (Unintentional)	Poisoning, Intentional Self-Harm	Poisoning, Assault	Poisoning, Undetermined	Adverse Effect	Underdosing
Pyrathiazine	T45.0X1	T45.0X2	T45.0X3	T45.0X4	T45.0X5	T45.0X6
Pyrazinamide	T37.1X1	T37.1X2	T37.1X3	T37.1X4	T37.1X5	T37.1X6
Pyrazinoic acid (amide)	T37.1X1	T37.1X2	T37.1X3	T37.1X4	T37.1X5	T37.1X6
Pyrazole (derivatives)	T39.2X1	T39.2X2	T39.2X3	T39.2X4	T39.2X5	T39.2X6
Pyrazolone analgesic NEC	T39.2X1	T39.2X2	T39.2X3	T39.2X4	T39.2X5	T39.2X6
Pyrethrin, pyrethrum (nonmedicinal)	T60.2X1	T60.2X2	T60.2X3	T60.2X4	—	—
Pyrethrum extract	T49.0X1	T49.0X2	T49.0X3	T49.0X4	T49.0X5	T49.0X6
Pyribenzamine	T45.0X1	T45.0X2	T45.0X3	T45.0X4	T45.0X5	T45.0X6
Pyridine	T52.8X1	T52.8X2	T52.8X3	T52.8X4	—	—
aldoxime methiodide	T50.6X1	T50.6X2	T50.6X3	T50.6X4	T50.6X5	T50.6X6
aldoxime methyl chloride	T50.6X1	T50.6X2	T50.6X3	T50.6X4	T50.6X5	T50.6X6
vapor	T59.891	T59.892	T59.893	T59.894	—	—
Pyridium	T39.8X1	T39.8X2	T39.8X3	T39.8X4	T39.8X5	T39.8X6
Pyridostigmine bromide	T44.0X1	T44.0X2	T44.0X3	T44.0X4	T44.0X5	T44.0X6
Pyridoxal phosphate	T45.2X1	T45.2X2	T45.2X3	T45.2X4	T45.2X5	T45.2X6
Pyridoxine	T45.2X1	T45.2X2	T45.2X3	T45.2X4	T45.2X5	T45.2X6
Pyrilamine	T45.0X1	T45.0X2	T45.0X3	T45.0X4	T45.0X5	T45.0X6
Pyrimethamine	T37.2X1	T37.2X2	T37.2X3	T37.2X4	T37.2X5	T37.2X6
with sulfadoxine	T37.2X1	T37.2X2	T37.2X3	T37.2X4	T37.2X5	T37.2X6
Pyrimidine antagonist	T45.1X1	T45.1X2	T45.1X3	T45.1X4	T45.1X5	T45.1X6
Pyriminil	T60.4X1	T60.4X2	T60.4X3	T60.4X4	—	—
Pyrithione zinc	T49.4X1	T49.4X2	T49.4X3	T49.4X4	T49.4X5	T49.4X6
Pyrithyldione	T42.6X1	T42.6X2	T42.6X3	T42.6X4	T42.6X5	T42.6X6
Pyrogallic acid	T49.0X1	T49.0X2	T49.0X3	T49.0X4	T49.0X5	T49.0X6
Pyrogallol	T49.0X1	T49.0X2	T49.0X3	T49.0X4	T49.0X5	T49.0X6
Pyroxylin	T49.3X1	T49.3X2	T49.3X3	T49.3X4	T49.3X5	T49.3X6
Pyrrobutamine	T45.0X1	T45.0X2	T45.0X3	T45.0X4	T45.0X5	T45.0X6
Pyrrolizidine alkaloids	T62.8X1	T62.8X2	T62.8X3	T62.8X4	—	—
Pyrvinium chloride	T37.4X1	T37.4X2	T37.4X3	T37.4X4	T37.4X5	T37.4X6
PZI	T38.3X1	T38.3X2	T38.3X3	T38.3X4	T38.3X5	T38.3X6
Q						
Quaalude	T42.6X1	T42.6X2	T42.6X3	T42.6X4	T42.6X5	T42.6X6
Quarternary ammonium						
anti-infective	T49.0X1	T49.0X2	T49.0X3	T49.0X4	T49.0X5	T49.0X6
ganglion blocking	T44.2X1	T44.2X2	T44.2X3	T44.2X4	T44.2X5	T44.2X6
parasympatholytic	T44.3X1	T44.3X2	T44.3X3	T44.3X4	T44.3X5	T44.3X6
Quazepam	T42.4X1	T42.4X2	T42.4X3	T42.4X4	T42.4X5	T42.4X6
Quicklime	T54.3X1	T54.3X2	T54.3X3	T54.3X4	—	—
Quillaja extract	T48.4X1	T48.4X2	T48.4X3	T48.4X4	T48.4X5	T48.4X6

Substance	External Cause (T-Code)					
	Poisoning, Accidental (Unintentional)	Poisoning, Intentional Self-Harm	Poisoning, Assault	Poisoning, Undetermined	Adverse Effect	Underdosing
Quinacrine	T37.2X1	T37.2X2	T37.2X3	T37.2X4	T37.2X5	T37.2X6
Quinaglute	T46.2X1	T46.2X2	T46.2X3	T46.2X4	T46.2X5	T46.2X6
Quinalbarbital	T42.3X1	T42.3X2	T42.3X3	T42.3X4	T42.3X5	T42.3X6
Quinalbarbitone sodium	T42.3X1	T42.3X2	T42.3X3	T42.3X4	T42.3X5	T42.3X6
Quinalphos	T60.0X1	T60.0X2	T60.0X3	T60.0X4	—	—
Quinapril	T46.4X1	T46.4X2	T46.4X3	T46.4X4	T46.4X5	T46.4X6
Quinestradiol	T38.5X1	T38.5X2	T38.5X3	T38.5X4	T38.5X5	T38.5X6
Quinestradol	T38.5X1	T38.5X2	T38.5X3	T38.5X4	T38.5X5	T38.5X6
Quinestrol	T38.5X1	T38.5X2	T38.5X3	T38.5X4	T38.5X5	T38.5X6
Quinethazone	T50.2X1	T50.2X2	T50.2X3	T50.2X4	T50.2X5	T50.2X6
Quingestanol	T38.4X1	T38.4X2	T38.4X3	T38.4X4	T38.4X5	T38.4X6
Quinidine	T46.2X1	T46.2X2	T46.2X3	T46.2X4	T46.2X5	T46.2X6
Quinine	T37.2X1	T37.2X2	T37.2X3	T37.2X4	T37.2X5	T37.2X6
Quiniobine	T37.8X1	T37.8X2	T37.8X3	T37.8X4	T37.8X5	T37.8X6
Quinisocaine	T49.1X1	T49.1X2	T49.1X3	T49.1X4	T49.1X5	T49.1X6
Quinocide	T37.2X1	T37.2X2	T37.2X3	T37.2X4	T37.2X5	T37.2X6
Quinoline (derivatives) NEC	T37.8X1	T37.8X2	T37.8X3	T37.8X4	T37.8X5	T37.8X6
Quinupramine	T43.011	T43.012	T43.013	T43.014	T43.015	T43.016
Quotane	T41.3X1	T41.3X2	T41.3X3	T41.3X4	T41.3X5	T41.3X6
R						
Rabies						
immune globulin (human)	T50.Z11	T50.Z12	T50.Z13	T50.Z14	T50.Z15	T50.Z16
vaccine	T50.B91	T50.B92	T50.B93	T50.B94	T50.B95	T50.B96
Racemoramide	T40.2X1	T40.2X2	T40.2X3	T40.2X4	—	—
Racemorphan	T40.2X1	T40.2X2	T40.2X3	T40.2X4	T40.2X5	T40.2X6
Racepinefrin	T44.5X1	T44.5X2	T44.5X3	T44.5X4	T44.5X5	T44.5X6
Raclopride	T43.591	T43.592	T43.593	T43.594	T43.595	T43.596
Radiator alcohol	T51.1X1	T51.1X2	T51.1X3	T51.1X4	—	—
Radioactive drug NEC	T50.8X1	T50.8X2	T50.8X3	T50.8X4	T50.8X5	T50.8X6
Radio-opaque (drugs) (materials)	T50.8X1	T50.8X2	T50.8X3	T50.8X4	T50.8X5	T50.8X6
Ramifenazone	T39.2X1	T39.2X2	T39.2X3	T39.2X4	T39.2X5	T39.2X6
Ramipril	T46.4X1	T46.4X2	T46.4X3	T46.4X4	T46.4X5	T46.4X6
Ranitidine	T47.0X1	T47.0X2	T47.0X3	T47.0X4	T47.0X5	T47.0X6
Ranunculus	T62.2X1	T62.2X2	T62.2X3	T62.2X4	—	—
Rat poison NEC	T60.4X1	T60.4X2	T60.4X3	T60.4X4	—	—
Rattlesnake (venom)	T63.011	T63.012	T63.013	T63.014	—	—
Raubasine	T46.7X1	T46.7X2	T46.7X3	T46.7X4	T46.7X5	T46.7X6
Raudixin	T46.5X1	T46.5X2	T46.5X3	T46.5X4	T46.5X5	T46.5X6
Rautensin	T46.5X1	T46.5X2	T46.5X3	T46.5X4	T46.5X5	T46.5X6

Substance	External Cause (T-Code)					
	Poisoning, Accidental (Unintentional)	Poisoning, Intentional Self-Harm	Poisoning, Assault	Poisoning, Undetermined	Adverse Effect	Underdosing
Rautina	T46.5X1	T46.5X2	T46.5X3	T46.5X4	T46.5X5	T46.5X6
Rautotal	T46.5X1	T46.5X2	T46.5X3	T46.5X4	T46.5X5	T46.5X6
Rauwiloid	T46.5X1	T46.5X2	T46.5X3	T46.5X4	T46.5X5	T46.5X6
Rauwoldin	T46.5X1	T46.5X2	T46.5X3	T46.5X4	T46.5X5	T46.5X6
Rauwolfia (alkaloids)	T46.5X1	T46.5X2	T46.5X3	T46.5X4	T46.5X5	T46.5X6
Razoxane	T45.1X1	T45.1X2	T45.1X3	T45.1X4	T45.1X5	T45.1X6
Realgar	T57.0X1	T57.0X2	T57.0X3	T57.0X4	—	—
Recombinant (R) — *see specific protein*						
Red blood cells, packed	T45.8X1	T45.8X2	T45.8X3	T45.8X4	T45.8X5	T45.8X6
Red squill (scilliroside)	T60.4X1	T60.4X2	T60.4X3	T60.4X4	—	—
Reducing agent, industrial NEC	T65.891	T65.892	T65.893	T65.894	—	—
Refrigerant gas (chlorofluoro-carbon)	T53.5X1	T53.5X2	T53.5X3	T53.5X4	—	—
not chlorofluoro-carbon	T59.891	T59.892	T59.893	T59.894	—	—
Regroton	T50.2X1	T50.2X2	T50.2X3	T50.2X4	T50.2X5	T50.2X6
Rehydration salts (oral)	T50.3X1	T50.3X2	T50.3X3	T50.3X4	T50.3X5	T50.3X6
Rela	T42.8X1	T42.8X2	T42.8X3	T42.8X4	T42.8X5	T42.8X6
Relaxant, muscle						
anesthetic	T48.1X1	T48.1X2	T48.1X3	T48.1X4	T48.1X5	T48.1X6
central nervous system	T42.8X1	T42.8X2	T42.8X3	T42.8X4	T42.8X5	T42.8X6
skeletal NEC	T48.1X1	T48.1X2	T48.1X3	T48.1X4	T48.1X5	T48.1X6
smooth NEC	T44.3X1	T44.3X2	T44.3X3	T44.3X4	T44.3X5	T44.3X6
Remoxipride	T43.591	T43.592	T43.593	T43.594	T43.595	T43.596
Renese	T50.2X1	T50.2X2	T50.2X3	T50.2X4	T50.2X5	T50.2X6
Renografin	T50.8X1	T50.8X2	T50.8X3	T50.8X4	T50.8X5	T50.8X6
Replacement solution	T50.3X1	T50.3X2	T50.3X3	T50.3X4	T50.3X5	T50.3X6
Reproterol	T48.6X1	T48.6X2	T48.6X3	T48.6X4	T48.6X5	T48.6X6
Rescinnamine	T46.5X1	T46.5X2	T46.5X3	T46.5X4	T46.5X5	T46.5X6
Reserpin(e)	T46.5X1	T46.5X2	T46.5X3	T46.5X4	T46.5X5	T46.5X6
Resorcin, resorcinol (nonmedicinal)	T65.891	T65.892	T65.893	T65.894	—	—
medicinal	T49.4X1	T49.4X2	T49.4X3	T49.4X4	T49.4X5	T49.4X6
Respaire	T48.4X1	T48.4X2	T48.4X3	T48.4X4	T48.4X5	T48.4X6
Respiratory drug NEC	T48.901	T48.902	T48.903	T48.904	T48.905	T48.906
antiasthmatic NEC	T48.6X1	T48.6X2	T48.6X3	T48.6X4	T48.6X5	T48.6X6
anti-common-cold NEC	T48.5X1	T48.5X2	T48.5X3	T48.5X4	T48.5X5	T48.5X6
expectorant NEC	T48.4X1	T48.4X2	T48.4X3	T48.4X4	T48.4X5	T48.4X6
stimulant	T48.901	T48.902	T48.903	T48.904	T48.905	T48.906
Retinoic acid	T49.0X1	T49.0X2	T49.0X3	T49.0X4	T49.0X5	T49.0X6
Retinol	T45.2X1	T45.2X2	T45.2X3	T45.2X4	T45.2X5	T45.2X6
Rh (D) immune globulin (human)	T50.Z11	T50.Z12	T50.Z13	T50.Z14	T50.Z15	T50.Z16
Rhodine	T39.011	T39.012	T39.013	T39.014	T39.015	T39.016

TABLE OF DRUGS AND CHEMICALS

Substance	External Cause (T-Code)					
	Poisoning, Accidental (Unintentional)	Poisoning, Intentional Self-Harm	Poisoning, Assault	Poisoning, Undetermined	Adverse Effect	Underdosing
RhoGAM	T50.Z11	T50.Z12	T50.Z13	T50.Z14	T50.Z15	T50.Z16
Rhubarb						
dry extract	T47.2X1	T47.2X2	T47.2X3	T47.2X4	T47.2X5	T47.2X6
tincture, compound	T47.2X1	T47.2X2	T47.2X3	T47.2X4	T47.2X5	T47.2X6
Ribavirin	T37.5X1	T37.5X2	T37.5X3	T37.5X4	T37.5X5	T37.5X6
Riboflavin	T45.2X1	T45.2X2	T45.2X3	T45.2X4	T45.2X5	T45.2X6
Ribostamycin	T36.5X1	T36.5X2	T36.5X3	T36.5X4	T36.5X5	T36.5X6
Ricin	T62.2X1	T62.2X2	T62.2X3	T62.2X4	—	—
Ricinus communis	T62.2X1	T62.2X2	T62.2X3	T62.2X4	—	—
Rickettsial vaccine NEC	T50.A91	T50.A92	T50.A93	T50.A94	T50.A95	T50.A96
Rifabutin	T36.6X1	T36.6X2	T36.6X3	T36.6X4	T36.6X5	T36.6X6
Rifamide	T36.6X1	T36.6X2	T36.6X3	T36.6X4	T36.6X5	T36.6X6
Rifampicin	T36.6X1	T36.6X2	T36.6X3	T36.6X4	T36.6X5	T36.6X6
with isoniazid	T37.1X1	T37.1X2	T37.1X3	T37.1X4	T37.1X5	T37.1X6
Rifampin	T36.6X1	T36.6X2	T36.6X3	T36.6X4	T36.6X5	T36.6X6
Rifamycin	T36.6X1	T36.6X2	T36.6X3	T36.6X4	T36.6X5	T36.6X6
Rifaximin	T36.6X1	T36.6X2	T36.6X3	T36.6X4	T36.6X5	T36.6X6
Rimantadine	T37.5X1	T37.5X2	T37.5X3	T37.5X4	T37.5X5	T37.5X6
Rimazolium metilsulfate	T39.8X1	T39.8X2	T39.8X3	T39.8X4	T39.8X5	T39.8X6
Rimifon	T37.1X1	T37.1X2	T37.1X3	T37.1X4	T37.1X5	T37.1X6
Rimiterol	T48.6X1	T48.6X2	T48.6X3	T48.6X4	T48.6X5	T48.6X6
Ringer (lactate) solution	T50.3X1	T50.3X2	T50.3X3	T50.3X4	T50.3X5	T50.3X6
Ristocetin	T36.8X1	T36.8X2	T36.8X3	T36.8X4	T36.8X5	T36.8X6
Ritalin	T43.631	T43.632	T43.633	T43.634	T43.635	T43.636
Ritodrine	T44.5X1	T44.5X2	T44.5X3	T44.5X4	T44.5X5	T44.5X6
Roach killer — see Insecticide						
Rociverine	T44.3X1	T44.3X2	T44.3X3	T44.3X4	T44.3X5	T44.3X6
Rocky Mountain spotted fever vaccine	T50.A91	T50.A92	T50.A93	T50.A94	T50.A95	T50.A96
Rodenticide NEC	T60.4X1	T60.4X2	T60.4X3	T60.4X4	—	—
Rohypnol	T42.4X1	T42.4X2	T42.4X3	T42.4X4	T42.4X5	T42.4X6
Rokitamycin	T36.3X1	T36.3X2	T36.3X3	T36.3X4	T36.3X5	T36.3X6
Rolaids	T47.1X1	T47.1X2	T47.1X3	T47.1X4	T47.1X5	T47.1X6
Rolitetracycline	T36.4X1	T36.4X2 ·	T36.4X3	T36.4X4	T36.4X5	T36.4X6
Romilar	T48.3X1	T48.3X2	T48.3X3	T48.3X4	T48.3X5	T48.3X6
Ronifibrate	T46.6X1	T46.6X2	T46.6X3	T46.6X4	T46.6X5	T46.6X6
Rosaprostol	T47.1X1	T47.1X2	T47.1X3	T47.1X4	T47.1X5	T47.1X6
Rose bengal sodium (131I)	T50.8X1	T50.8X2	T50.8X3	T50.8X4	T50.8X5	T50.8X6
Rose water ointment	T49.3X1	T49.3X2	T49.3X3	T49.3X4	T49.3X5	T49.3X6
Rosoxacin	T37.8X1	T37.8X2	T37.8X3	T37.8X4	T37.8X5	T37.8X6
Rotenone	T60.2X1	T60.2X2	T60.2X3	T60.2X4	—	—

Substance	External Cause (T-Code)					
	Poisoning, Accidental (Unintentional)	Poisoning, Intentional Self-Harm	Poisoning, Assault	Poisoning, Undetermined	Adverse Effect	Underdosing
Rotoxamine	T45.0X1	T45.0X2	T45.0X3	T45.0X4	T45.0X5	T45.0X6
Rough-on-rats	T60.4X1	T60.4X2	T60.4X3	T60.4X4	—	—
Roxatidine	T47.0X1	T47.0X2	T47.0X3	T47.0X4	T47.0X5	T47.0X6
Roxithromycin	T36.3X1	T36.3X2	T36.3X3	T36.3X4	T36.3X5	T36.3X6
Rt-PA	T45.611	T45.612	T45.613	T45.614	T45.615	T45.616
Rubbing alcohol	T51.2X1	T51.2X2	T51.2X3	T51.2X4	—	—
Rubefacient	T49.4X1	T49.4X2	T49.4X3	T49.4X4	T49.4X5	T49.4X6
Rubella vaccine	T50.B91	T50.B92	T50.B93	T50.B94	T50.B95	T50.B96
Rubelogen	T50.B91	T50.B92	T50.B93	T50.B94	T50.B95	T50.B96
Rubeovax	T50.991	T50.992	T50.993	T50.994	T50.995	T50.996
Rubidium chloride Rb82	T50.8X1	T50.8X2	T50.8X3	T50.8X4	T50.8X5	T50.8X6
Rubidomycin	T45.1X1	T45.1X2	T45.1X3	T45.1X4	T45.1X5	T45.1X6
Rue	T62.2X1	T62.2X2	T62.2X3	T62.2X4	—	—
Rufocromomycin	T45.1X1	T45.1X2	T45.1X3	T45.1X4	T45.1X5	T45.1X6
Russel's viper venin	T45.7X1	T45.7X2	T45.7X3	T45.7X4	T45.7X5	T45.7X6
Ruta (graveolens)	T62.2X1	T62.2X2	T62.2X3	T62.2X4	—	—
Rutinum	T46.991	T46.992	T46.993	T46.994	T46.995	T46.996
Rutoside	T46.991	T46.992	T46.993	T46.994	T46.995	T46.996
S						
Sabadilla (plant)	T62.2X1	T62.2X2	T62.2X3	T62.2X4	—	—
pesticide	T60.2X1	T60.2X2	T60.2X3	T60.2X4	—	—
Saccharated iron oxide	T45.8X1	T45.8X2	T45.8X3	T45.8X4	T45.8X5	T45.8X6
Saccharin	T50.901	T50.902	T50.903	T50.904	T50.905	T50.906
Saccharomyces boulardii	T47.6X1	T47.6X2	T47.6X3	T47.6X4	T47.6X5	T47.6X6
Safflower oil	T46.6X1	T46.6X2	T46.6X3	T46.6X4	T46.6X5	T46.6X6
Safrazine	T43.1X1	T43.1X2	T43.1X3	T43.1X4	T43.1X5	T43.1X6
Salazosulfapyridine	T37.0X1	T37.0X2	T37.0X3	T37.0X4	T37.0X5	T37.0X6
Salbutamol	T48.6X1	T48.6X2	T48.6X3	T48.6X4	T48.6X5	T48.6X6
Salicylamide	T39.091	T39.092	T39.093	T39.094	T39.095	T39.096
Salicylate NEC	T39.091	T39.092	T39.093	T39.094	T39.095	T39.096
methyl	T49.3X1	T49.3X2	T49.3X3	T49.3X4	T49.3X5	T49.3X6
theobromine calcium	T50.2X1	T50.2X2	T50.2X3	T50.2X4	T50.2X5	T50.2X6
Salicylazosulfapyridine	T37.0X1	T37.0X2	T37.0X3	T37.0X4	T37.0X5	T37.0X6
Salicylhydroxamic acid	T49.0X1	T49.0X2	T49.0X3	T49.0X4	T49.0X5	T49.0X6
Salicylic acid	T49.4X1	T49.4X2	T49.4X3	T49.4X4	T49.4X5	T49.4X6
with benzoic acid	T49.4X1	T49.4X2	T49.4X3	T49.4X4	T49.4X5	T49.4X6
congeners	T39.091	T39.092	T39.093	T39.094	T39.095	T39.096
derivative	T39.091	T39.092	T39.093	T39.094	T39.095	T39.096
salts	T39.091	T39.092	T39.093	T39.094	T39.095	T39.096

TABLE OF DRUGS AND CHEMICALS

Substance	Poisoning, Accidental (Unintentional)	Poisoning, Intentional Self-Harm	Poisoning, Assault	Poisoning, Undetermined	Adverse Effect	Underdosing
	External Cause (T-Code)					
Salinazid	T37.1X1	T37.1X2	T37.1X3	T37.1X4	T37.1X5	T37.1X6
Salmeterol	T48.6X1	T48.6X2	T48.6X3	T48.6X4	T48.6X5	T48.6X6
Salol	T49.3X1	T49.3X2	T49.3X3	T49.3X4	T49.3X5	T49.3X6
Salsalate	T39.091	T39.092	T39.093	T39.094	T39.095	T39.096
Salt substitute	T50.901	T50.902	T50.903	T50.904	T50.905	T50.906
Salt-replacing drug	T50.901	T50.902	T50.903	T50.904	T50.905	T50.906
Salt-retaining mineralocorticoid	T50.0X1	T50.0X2	T50.0X3	T50.0X4	T50.0X5	T50.0X6
Saluretic NEC	T50.2X1	T50.2X2	T50.2X3	T50.2X4	T50.2X5	T50.2X6
Saluron	T50.2X1	T50.2X2	T50.2X3	T50.2X4	T50.2X5	T50.2X6
Salvarsan 606 (neosilver) (silver)	T37.8X1	T37.8X2	T37.8X3	T37.8X4	T37.8X5	T37.8X6
Sambucus canadensis	T62.2X1	T62.2X2	T62.2X3	T62.2X4	—	—
berry	T62.1X1	T62.1X2	T62.1X3	T62.1X4	—	—
Sandril	T46.5X1	T46.5X2	T46.5X3	T46.5X4	T46.5X5	T46.5X6
Sanguinaria canadensis	T62.2X1	T62.2X2	T62.2X3	T62.2X4	—	—
Saniflush (cleaner)	T54.2X1	T54.2X2	T54.2X3	T54.2X4	—	—
Santonin	T37.4X1	T37.4X2	T37.4X3	T37.4X4	T37.4X5	T37.4X6
Santyl	T49.8X1	T49.8X2	T49.8X3	T49.8X4	T49.8X5	T49.8X6
Saralasin	T46.5X1	T46.5X2	T46.5X3	T46.5X4	T46.5X5	T46.5X6
Sarcolysin	T45.1X1	T45.1X2	T45.1X3	T45.1X4	T45.1X5	T45.1X6
Sarkomycin	T45.1X1	T45.1X2	T45.1X3	T45.1X4	T45.1X5	T45.1X6
Saroten	T43.011	T43.012	T43.013	T43.014	T43.015	T43.016
Saturnine — *see Lead*						
Savin (oil)	T49.4X1	T49.4X2	T49.4X3	T49.4X4	T49.4X5	T49.4X6
Scammony	T47.2X1	T47.2X2	T47.2X3	T47.2X4	T47.2X5	T47.2X6
Scarlet red	T49.8X1	T49.8X2	T49.8X3	T49.8X4	T49.8X5	T49.8X6
Scheele's green	T57.0X1	T57.0X2	T57.0X3	T57.0X4	—	—
insecticide	T57.0X1	T57.0X2	T57.0X3	T57.0X4	—	—
Schizontozide (blood) (tissue)	T37.2X1	T37.2X2	T37.2X3	T37.2X4	T37.2X5	T37.2X6
Schradan	T60.0X1	T60.0X2	T60.0X3	T60.0X4	—	—
Schweinfurth green	T57.0X1	T57.0X2	T57.0X3	T57.0X4	—	—
insecticide	T57.0X1	T57.0X2	T57.0X3	T57.0X4	—	—
Scilla, rat poison	T60.4X1	T60.4X2	T60.4X3	T60.4X4	—	—
Scillaren	T60.4X1	T60.4X2	T60.4X3	T60.4X4	—	—
Sclerosing agent	T46.8X1	T46.8X2	T46.8X3	T46.8X4	T46.8X5	T46.8X6
Scombrotoxin	T61.11	T61.12	T61.13	T61.14	—	—
Scopolamine	T44.3X1	T44.3X2	T44.3X3	T44.3X4	T44.3X5	T44.3X6
Scopolia extract	T44.3X1	T44.3X2	T44.3X3	T44.3X4	T44.3X5	T44.3X6
Scouring powder	T65.891	T65.892	T65.893	T65.894	—	—

Substance	External Cause (T-Code)					
	Poisoning, Accidental (Unintentional)	Poisoning, Intentional Self-Harm	Poisoning, Assault	Poisoning, Undetermined	Adverse Effect	Underdosing
Sea						
anemone (sting)	T63.631	T63.632	T63.633	T63.634	—	—
cucumber (sting)	T63.691	T63.692	T63.693	T63.694	—	—
snake (bite) (venom)	T63.091	T63.092	T63.093	T63.094	—	—
urchin spine (puncture)	T63.691	T63.692	T63.693	T63.694	—	—
Seafood	T61.91	T61.92	T61.93	T61.94	—	—
specified NEC	T61.8X1	T61.8X2	T61.8X3	T61.8X4	—	—
Secbutabarbital	T42.3X1	T42.3X2	T42.3X3	T42.3X4	T42.3X5	T42.3X6
Secbutabarbitone	T42.3X1	T42.3X2	T42.3X3	T42.3X4	T42.3X5	T42.3X6
Secnidazole	T37.3X1	T37.3X2	T37.3X3	T37.3X4	T37.3X5	T37.3X6
Secobarbital	T42.3X1	T42.3X2	T42.3X3	T42.3X4	T42.3X5	T42.3X6
Seconal	T42.3X1	T42.3X2	T42.3X3	T42.3X4	T42.3X5	T42.3X6
Secretin	T50.8X1	T50.8X2	T50.8X3	T50.8X4	T50.8X5	T50.8X6
Sedative NEC	T42.71	T42.72	T42.73	T42.74	T42.75	T42.76
mixed NEC	T42.6X1	T42.6X2	T42.6X3	T42.6X4	T42.6X5	T42.6X6
Sedormid	T42.6X1	T42.6X2	T42.6X3	T42.6X4	T42.6X5	T42.6X6
Seed disinfectant or dressing	T60.8X1	T60.8X2	T60.8X3	T60.8X4	—	—
Seeds (poisonous)	T62.2X1	T62.2X2	T62.2X3	T62.2X4	—	—
Selegiline	T42.8X1	T42.8X2	T42.8X3	T42.8X4	T42.8X5	T42.8X6
Selenium NEC	T56.891	T56.892	T56.893	T56.894	—	—
disulfide or sulfide	T49.4X1	T49.4X2	T49.4X3	T49.4X4	T49.4X5	T49.4X6
fumes	T59.891	T59.892	T59.893	T59.894	—	—
sulfide	T49.4X1	T49.4X2	T49.4X3	T49.4X4	T49.4X5	T49.4X6
Selenomethionine (75Se)	T50.8X1	T50.8X2	T50.8X3	T50.8X4	T50.8X5	T50.8X6
Selsun	T49.4X1	T49.4X2	T49.4X3	T49.4X4	T49.4X5	T49.4X6
Semustine	T45.1X1	T45.1X2	T45.1X3	T45.1X4	T45.1X5	T45.1X6
Senega syrup	T48.4X1	T48.4X2	T48.4X3	T48.4X4	T48.4X5	T48.4X6
Senna	T47.2X1	T47.2X2	T47.2X3	T47.2X4	T47.2X5	T47.2X6
Sennoside A+B	T47.2X1	T47.2X2	T47.2X3	T47.2X4	T47.2X5	T47.2X6
Septisol	T49.2X1	T49.2X2	T49.2X3	T49.2X4	T49.2X5	T49.2X6
Seractide	T38.811	T38.812	T38.813	T38.814	T38.815	T38.816
Serax	T42.4X1	T42.4X2	T42.4X3	T42.4X4	T42.4X5	T42.4X6
Serenesil	T42.6X1	T42.6X2	T42.6X3	T42.6X4	T42.6X5	T42.6X6
Serenium (hydrochloride)	T37.91	T37.92	T37.93	T37.94	T37.95	T37.96
Serepax — see Oxazepam						
Sermorelin	T38.891	T38.892	T38.893	T38.894	T38.895	T38.896
Sernyl	T41.1X1	T41.1X2	T41.1X3	T41.1X4	T41.1X5	T41.1X6
Serotonin	T50.991	T50.992	T50.993	T50.994	T50.995	T50.996

TABLE OF DRUGS AND CHEMICALS

Substance	External Cause (T-Code)					
	Poisoning, Accidental (Unintentional)	Poisoning, Intentional Self-Harm	Poisoning, Assault	Poisoning, Undetermined	Adverse Effect	Underdosing
Serpasil	T46.5X1	T46.5X2	T46.5X3	T46.5X4	T46.5X5	T46.5X6
Serrapeptase	T45.3X1	T45.3X2	T45.3X3	T45.3X4	T45.3X5	T45.3X6
Serum						
antibotulinus	T50.Z11	T50.Z12	T50.Z13	T50.Z14	T50.Z15	T50.Z16
anticytotoxic	T50.Z11	T50.Z12	T50.Z13	T50.Z14	T50.Z15	T50.Z16
antidiphtheria	T50.Z11	T50.Z12	T50.Z13	T50.Z14	T50.Z15	T50.Z16
antimeningococcus	T50.Z11	T50.Z12	T50.Z13	T50.Z14	T50.Z15	T50.Z16
anti-Rh	T50.Z11	T50.Z12	T50.Z13	T50.Z14	T50.Z15	T50.Z16
anti-snake-bite	T50.Z11	T50.Z12	T50.Z13	T50.Z14	T50.Z15	T50.Z16
antitetanic	T50.Z11	T50.Z12	T50.Z13	T50.Z14	T50.Z15	T50.Z16
antitoxic	T50.Z11	T50.Z12	T50.Z13	T50.Z14	T50.Z15	T50.Z16
complement (inhibitor)	T45.8X1	T45.8X2	T45.8X3	T45.8X4	T45.8X5	T45.8X6
convalescent	T50.Z11	T50.Z12	T50.Z13	T50.Z14	T50.Z15	T50.Z16
hemolytic complement	T45.8X1	T45.8X2	T45.8X3	T45.8X4	T45.8X5	T45.8X6
immune (human)	T50.Z11	T50.Z12	T50.Z13	T50.Z14	T50.Z15	T50.Z16
protective NEC	T50.Z11	T50.Z12	T50.Z13	T50.Z14	T50.Z15	T50.Z16
Setastine	T45.0X1	T45.0X2	T45.0X3	T45.0X4	T45.0X5	T45.0X6
Setoperone	T43.591	T43.592	T43.593	T43.594	T43.595	T43.596
Sewer gas	T59.91	T59.92	T59.93	T59.94	—	—
Shampoo	T55.0X1	T55.0X2	T55.0X3	T55.0X4		
Shellfish, noxious, nonbacterial	T61.781	T61.782	T61.783	T61.784	—	—
Sildenafil	T46.7X1	T46.7X2	T46.7X3	T46.7X4	T46.7X5	T46.7X6
Silibinin	T50.991	T50.992	T50.993	T50.994	T50.995	T50.996
Silicone NEC	T65.891	T65.892	T65.893	T65.894	—	—
medicinal	T49.3X1	T49.3X2	T49.3X3	T49.3X4	T49.3X5	T49.3X6
Silvadene	T49.0X1	T49.0X2	T49.0X3	T49.0X4	T49.0X5	T49.0X6
Silver	T49.0X1	T49.0X2	T49.0X3	T49.0X4	T49.0X5	T49.0X6
anti-infectives	T49.0X1	T49.0X2	T49.0X3	T49.0X4	T49.0X5	T49.0X6
arsphenamine	T37.8X1	T37.8X2	T37.8X3	T37.8X4	T37.8X5	T37.8X6
colloidal	T49.0X1	T49.0X2	T49.0X3	T49.0X4	T49.0X5	T49.0X6
nitrate	T49.0X1	T49.0X2	T49.0X3	T49.0X4	T49.0X5	T49.0X6
ophthalmic preparation	T49.5X1	T49.5X2	T49.5X3	T49.5X4	T49.5X5	T49.5X6
toughened (keratolytic)	T49.4X1	T49.4X2	T49.4X3	T49.4X4	T49.4X5	T49.4X6
nonmedicinal (dust)	T56.891	T56.892	T56.893	T56.894	—	—
protein	T49.5X1	T49.5X2	T49.5X3	T49.5X4	T49.5X5	T49.5X6
salvarsan	T37.8X1	T37.8X2	T37.8X3	T37.8X4	T37.8X5	T37.8X6
sulfadiazine	T49.4X1	T49.4X2	T49.4X3	T49.4X4	T49.4X5	T49.4X6
Silymarin	T50.991	T50.992	T50.993	T50.994	T50.995	T50.996
Simaldrate	T47.1X1	T47.1X2	T47.1X3	T47.1X4	T47.1X5	T47.1X6
Simazine	T60.3X1	T60.3X2	T60.3X3	T60.3X4	—	—

Substance	External Cause (T-Code)					
	Poisoning, Accidental (Unintentional)	Poisoning, Intentional Self-Harm	Poisoning, Assault	Poisoning, Undetermined	Adverse Effect	Underdosing
Simethicone	T47.1X1	T47.1X2	T47.1X3	T47.1X4	T47.1X5	T47.1X6
Simfibrate	T46.6X1	T46.6X2	T46.6X3	T46.6X4	T46.6X5	T46.6X6
Simvastatin	T46.6X1	T46.6X2	T46.6X3	T46.6X4	T46.6X5	T46.6X6
Sincalide	T50.8X1	T50.8X2	T50.8X3	T50.8X4	T50.8X5	T50.8X6
Sinequan	T43.011	T43.012	T43.013	T43.014	T43.015	T43.016
Singoserp	T46.5X1	T46.5X2	T46.5X3	T46.5X4	T46.5X5	T46.5X6
Sintrom	T45.511	T45.512	T45.513	T45.514	T45.515	T45.516
Sisomicin	T36.5X1	T36.5X2	T36.5X3	T36.5X4	T36.5X5	T36.5X6
Sitosterols	T46.6X1	T46.6X2	T46.6X3	T46.6X4	T46.6X5	T46.6X6
Skeletal muscle relaxants	T48.1X1	T48.1X2	T48.1X3	T48.1X4	T48.1X5	T48.1X6
Skin						
agents (external)	T49.91	T49.92	T49.93	T49.94	T49.95	T49.96
specified NEC	T49.8X1	T49.8X2	T49.8X3	T49.8X4	T49.8X5	T49.8X6
test antigen	T50.8X1	T50.8X2	T50.8X3	T50.8X4	T50.8X5	T50.8X6
Sleep-eze	T45.0X1	T45.0X2	T45.0X3	T45.0X4	T45.0X5	T45.0X6
Sleeping draught, pill	T42.71	T42.72	T42.73	T42.74	T42.75	T42.76
Smallpox vaccine	T50.B11	T50.B12	T50.B13	T50.B14	T50.B15	T50.B16
Smelter fumes NEC	T56.91	T56.92	T56.93	T56.94	—	—
Smog	T59.1X1	T59.1X2	T59.1X3	T59.1X4	—	—
Smoke NEC	T59.811	T59.812	T59.813	T59.814	—	—
Smooth muscle relaxant	T44.3X1	T44.3X2	T44.3X3	T44.3X4	T44.3X5	T44.3X6
Snail killer NEC	T60.8X1	T60.8X2	T60.8X3	T60.8X4	—	—
Snake venom or bite	T63.001	T63.002	T63.003	T63.004	—	—
hemocoagulase	T45.7X1	T45.7X2	T45.7X3	T45.7X4	T45.7X5	T45.7X6
Snuff	T65.211	T65.212	T65.213	T65.214	—	—
Soap (powder) (product)	T55.0X1	T55.0X2	T55.0X3	T55.0X4	—	—
enema	T47.4X1	T47.4X2	T47.4X3	T47.4X4	T47.4X5	T47.4X6
medicinal, soft	T49.2X1	T49.2X2	T49.2X3	T49.2X4	T49.2X5	T49.2X6
superfatted	T49.2X1	T49.2X2	T49.2X3	T49.2X4	T49.2X5	T49.2X6
Sobrerol	T48.4X1	T48.4X2	T48.4X3	T48.4X4	T48.4X5	T48.4X6
Soda (caustic)	T54.3X1	T54.3X2	T54.3X3	T54.3X4	—	—
bicarb	T47.1X1	T47.1X2	T47.1X3	T47.1X4	T47.1X5	T47.1X6
chlorinated — see Sodium, hypochlorite						
Sodium						
acetosulfone	T37.1X1	T37.1X2	T37.1X3	T37.1X4	T37.1X5	T37.1X6
acetrizoate	T50.8X1	T50.8X2	T50.8X3	T50.8X4	T50.8X5	T50.8X6
acid phosphate	T50.3X1	T50.3X2	T50.3X3	T50.3X4	T50.3X5	T50.3X6
alginate	T47.8X1	T47.8X2	T47.8X3	T47.8X4	T47.8X5	T47.8X6
amidotrizoate	T50.8X1	T50.8X2	T50.8X3	T50.8X4	T50.8X5	T50.8X6
aminopterin	T45.1X1	T45.1X2	T45.1X3	T45.1X4	T45.1X5	T45.1X6

Substance	External Cause (T-Code)					
	Poisoning, Accidental (Unintentional)	Poisoning, Intentional Self-Harm	Poisoning, Assault	Poisoning, Undetermined	Adverse Effect	Underdosing
Sodium *(Continued)*						
amylosulfate	T47.8X1	T47.8X2	T47.8X3	T47.8X4	T47.8X5	T47.8X6
amytal	T42.3X1	T42.3X2	T42.3X3	T42.3X4	T42.3X5	T42.3X6
antimony gluconate	T37.3X1	T37.3X2	T37.3X3	T37.3X4	T37.3X5	T37.3X6
arsenate	T57.0X1	T57.0X2	T57.0X3	T57.0X4	—	—
aurothiomalate	T39.4X1	T39.4X2	T39.4X3	T39.4X4	T39.4X5	T39.4X6
aurothiosulfate	T39.4X1	T39.4X2	T39.4X3	T39.4X4	T39.4X5	T39.4X6
barbiturate	T42.3X1	T42.3X2	T42.3X3	T42.3X4	T42.3X5	T42.3X6
basic phosphate	T47.4X1	T47.4X2	T47.4X3	T47.4X4	T47.4X5	T47.4X6
bicarbonate	T47.1X1	T47.1X2	T47.1X3	T47.1X4	T47.1X5	T47.1X6
bichromate	T57.8X1	T57.8X2	T57.8X3	T57.8X4	—	—
biphosphate	T50.3X1	T50.3X2	T50.3X3	T50.3X4	T50.3X5	T50.3X6
bisulfate	T65.891	T65.892	T65.893	T65.894	—	—
borate						
cleanser	T57.8X1	T57.8X2	T57.8X3	T57.8X4	—	—
eye	T49.5X1	T49.5X2	T49.5X3	T49.5X4	T49.5X5	T49.5X6
therapeutic	T49.8X1	T49.8X2	T49.8X3	T49.8X4	T49.8X5	T49.8X6
bromide	T42.6X1	T42.6X2	T42.6X3	T42.6X4	T42.6X5	T42.6X6
cacodylate (nonmedicinal) NEC	T50.8X1	T50.8X2	T50.8X3	T50.8X4	T50.8X5	T50.8X6
anti-infective	T37.8X1	T37.8X2	T37.8X3	T37.8X4	T37.8X5	T37.8X6
herbicide	T60.3X1	T60.3X2	T60.3X3	T60.3X4	—	—
calcium edetate	T45.8X1	T45.8X2	T45.8X3	T45.8X4	T45.8X5	T45.8X6
carbonate NEC	T54.3X1	T54.3X2	T54.3X3	T54.3X4	—	—
chlorate NEC	T65.891	T65.892	T65.893	T65.894	—	—
herbicide	T54.91	T54.92	T54.93	T54.94	—	—
chloride	T50.3X1	T50.3X2	T50.3X3	T50.3X4	T50.3X5	T50.3X6
with glucose	T50.3X1	T50.3X2	T50.3X3	T50.3X4	T50.3X5	T50.3X6
chromate	T65.891	T65.892	T65.893	T65.894	—	—
citrate	T50.991	T50.992	T50.993	T50.994	T50.995	T50.996
cromoglicate	T48.6X1	T48.6X2	T48.6X3	T48.6X4	T48.6X5	T48.6X6
cyanide	T65.0X1	T65.0X2	T65.0X3	T65.0X4	—	—
cyclamate	T50.3X1	T50.3X2	T50.3X3	T50.3X4	T50.3X5	T50.3X6
dehydrocholate	T45.8X1	T45.8X2	T45.8X3	T45.8X4	T45.8X5	T45.8X6
diatrizoate	T50.8X1	T50.8X2	T50.8X3	T50.8X4	T50.8X5	T50.8X6
dibunate	T48.4X1	T48.4X2	T48.4X3	T48.4X4	T48.4X5	T48.4X6
dioctyl sulfosuccinate	T47.4X1	T47.4X2	T47.4X3	T47.4X4	T47.4X5	T47.4X6
dipantoyl ferrate	T45.8X1	T45.8X2	T45.8X3	T45.8X4	T45.8X5	T45.8X6
edetate	T45.8X1	T45.8X2	T45.8X3	T45.8X4	T45.8X5	T45.8X6
ethacrynate	T50.1X1	T50.1X2	T50.1X3	T50.1X4	T50.1X5	T50.1X6
feredetate	T45.8X1	T45.8X2	T45.8X3	T45.8X4	T45.8X5	T45.8X6

Substance	External Cause (T-Code)					
	Poisoning, Accidental (Unintentional)	Poisoning, Intentional Self-Harm	Poisoning, Assault	Poisoning, Undetermined	Adverse Effect	Underdosing
Sodium *(Continued)*						
Fluoride—*see Fluoride*						
fluoroacetate (dust) (pesticide)	T60.4X1	T60.4X2	T60.4X3	T60.4X4	—	—
free salt	T50.3X1	T50.3X2	T50.3X3	T50.3X4	T50.3X5	T50.3X6
fusidate	T36.8X1	T36.8X2	T36.8X3	T36.8X4	T36.8X5	T36.8X6
glucaldrate	T47.1X1	T47.1X2	T47.1X3	T47.1X4	T47.1X5	T47.1X6
glucosulfone	T37.1X1	T37.1X2	T37.1X3	T37.1X4	T37.1X5	T37.1X6
glutamate	T45.8X1	T45.8X2	T45.8X3	T45.8X4	T45.8X5	T45.8X6
hydrogen carbonate	T50.3X1	T50.3X2	T50.3X3	T50.3X4	T50.3X5	T50.3X6
hydroxide	T54.3X1	T54.3X2	T54.3X3	T54.3X4	—	—
hypochlorite (bleach) NEC	T54.3X1	T54.3X2	T54.3X3	T54.3X4	—	—
disinfectant	T54.3X1	T54.3X2	T54.3X3	T54.3X4	—	—
medicinal (anti-infective) (external)	T49.0X1	T49.0X2	T49.0X3	T49.0X4	T49.0X5	T49.0X6
vapor	T54.3X1	T54.3X2	T54.3X3	T54.3X4	—	—
hyposulfite	T49.0X1	T49.0X2	T49.0X3	T49.0X4	T49.0X5	T49.0X6
indigotin disulfonate	T50.8X1	T50.8X2	T50.8X3	T50.8X4	T50.8X5	T50.8X6
iodide	T50.991	T50.992	T50.993	T50.994	T50.995	T50.996
I-131	T50.8X1	T50.8X2	T50.8X3	T50.8X4	T50.8X5	T50.8X6
therapeutic	T38.2X1	T38.2X2	T38.2X3	T38.2X4	T38.2X5	T38.2X6
iodohippurate (131I)	T50.8X1	T50.8X2	T50.8X3	T50.8X4	T50.8X5	T50.8X6
iopodate	T50.8X1	T50.8X2	T50.8X3	T50.8X4	T50.8X5	T50.8X6
iothalamate	T50.8X1	T50.8X2	T50.8X3	T50.8X4	T50.8X5	T50.8X6
iron edetate	T45.4X1	T45.4X2	T45.4X3	T45.4X4	T45.4X5	T45.4X6
lactate (compound solution)	T45.8X1	T45.8X2	T45.8X3	T45.8X4	T45.8X5	T45.8X6
lauryl (sulfate)	T49.2X1	T49.2X2	T49.2X3	T49.2X4	T49.2X5	T49.2X6
(L)-triiodothyronine	T38.1X1	T38.1X2	T38.1X3	T38.1X4	T38.1X5	T38.1X6
magnesium citrate	T50.991	T50.992	T50.993	T50.994	T50.995	T50.996
mersalate	T50.2X1	T50.2X2	T50.2X3	T50.2X4	T50.2X5	T50.2X6
metasilicate	T65.891	T65.892	T65.893	T65.894	—	—
metrizoate	T50.8X1	T50.8X2	T50.8X3	T50.8X4	T50.8X5	T50.8X6
monofluoroacetate (pesticide)	T60.1X1	T60.1X2	T60.1X3	T60.1X4	—	—
morrhuate	T46.8X1	T46.8X2	T46.8X3	T46.8X4	T46.8X5	T46.8X6
nafcillin	T36.0X1	T36.0X2	T36.0X3	T36.0X4	T36.0X5	T36.0X6
nitrate (oxidizing agent)	T65.891	T65.892	T65.893	T65.894	—	—
nitrite	T50.6X1	T50.6X2	T50.6X3	T50.6X4	T50.6X5	T50.6X6
nitroferricyanide	T46.5X1	T46.5X2	T46.5X3	T46.5X4	T46.5X5	T46.5X6
nitroprusside	T46.5X1	T46.5X2	T46.5X3	T46.5X4	T46.5X5	T46.5X6
oxalate	T65.891	T65.892	T65.893	T65.894	—	—
oxide/peroxide	T65.891	T65.892	T65.893	T65.894	—	—
oxybate	T41.291	T41.292	T41.293	T41.294	T41.295	T41.296

Substance	External Cause (T-Code)					
	Poisoning, Accidental (Unintentional)	Poisoning, Intentional Self-Harm	Poisoning, Assault	Poisoning, Undetermined	Adverse Effect	Underdosing
Sodium *(Continued)*						
para-aminohippurate	T50.8X1	T50.8X2	T50.8X3	T50.8X4	T50.8X5	T50.8X6
perborate (nonmedicinal) NEC	T65.891	T65.892	T65.893	T65.894	—	—
medicinal	T49.0X1	T49.0X2	T49.0X3	T49.0X4	T49.0X5	T49.0X6
soap	T55.0X1	T55.0X2	T55.0X3	T55.0X4	—	—
percarbonate — *see Sodium, perborate*						
pertechnetate Tc99m	T50.8X1	T50.8X2	T50.8X3	T50.8X4	T50.8X5	T50.8X6
phosphate						
cellulose	T45.8X1	T45.8X2	T45.8X3	T45.8X4	T45.8X5	T45.8X6
dibasic	T47.2X1	T47.2X2	T47.2X3	T47.2X4	T47.2X5	T47.2X6
monobasic	T47.2X1	T47.2X2	T47.2X3	T47.2X4	T47.2X5	T47.2X6
phytate	T50.6X1	T50.6X2	T50.6X3	T50.6X4	T50.6X5	T50.6X6
picosulfate	T47.2X1	T47.2X2	T47.2X3	T47.2X4	T47.2X5	T47.2X6
polyhydroxyaluminium monocarbonate	T47.1X1	T47.1X2	T47.1X3	T47.1X4	T47.1X5	T47.1X6
polystyrene sulfonate	T50.3X1	T50.3X2	T50.3X3	T50.3X4	T50.3X5	T50.3X6
propionate	T49.0X1	T49.0X2	T49.0X3	T49.0X4	T49.0X5	T49.0X6
propyl hydroxybenzoate	T50.991	T50.992	T50.993	T50.994	T50.995	T50.996
psylliate	T46.8X1	T46.8X2	T46.8X3	T46.8X4	T46.8X5	T46.8X6
removing resins	T50.3X1	T50.3X2	T50.3X3	T50.3X4	T50.3X5	T50.3X6
salicylate	T39.091	T39.092	T39.093	T39.094	T39.095	T39.096
salt NEC	T50.3X1	T50.3X2	T50.3X3	T50.3X4	T50.3X5	T50.3X6
selenate	T60.2X1	T60.2X2	T60.2X3	T60.2X4	—	—
stibogluconate	T37.3X1	T37.3X2	T37.3X3	T37.3X4	T37.3X5	T37.3X6
sulfate	T47.4X1	T47.4X2	T47.4X3	T47.4X4	T47.4X5	T47.4X6
sulfoxone	T37.1X1	T37.1X2	T37.1X3	T37.1X4	T37.1X5	T37.1X6
tetradecyl sulfate	T46.8X1	T46.8X2	T46.8X3	T46.8X4	T46.8X5	T46.8X6
thiopental	T41.1X1	T41.1X2	T41.1X3	T41.1X4	T41.1X5	T41.1X6
thiosalicylate	T39.091	T39.092	T39.093	T39.094	T39.095	T39.096
thiosulfate	T50.6X1	T50.6X2	T50.6X3	T50.6X4	T50.6X5	T50.6X6
tolbutamide	T38.3X1	T38.3X2	T38.3X3	T38.3X4	T38.3X5	T38.3X6
l-triiodothyronine	T38.1X1	T38.1X2	T38.1X3	T38.1X4	T38.1X5	T38.1X6
tyropanoate	T50.8X1	T50.8X2	T50.8X3	T50.8X4	T50.8X5	T50.8X6
valproate	T42.6X1	T42.6X2	T42.6X3	T42.6X4	T42.6X5	T42.6X6
versenate	T50.6X1	T50.6X2	T50.6X3	T50.6X4	T50.6X5	T50.6X6
Sodium-free salt	T50.901	T50.902	T50.903	T50.904	T50.905	T50.906
Sodium-removing resin	T50.3X1	T50.3X2	T50.3X3	T50.3X4	T50.3X5	T50.3X6
Soft soap	T55.0X1	T55.0X2	T55.0X3	T55.0X4	—	—
Solanine	T62.2X1	T62.2X2	T62.2X3	T62.2X4	—	—
berries	T62.1X1	T62.1X2	T62.1X3	T62.1X4	—	—

Substance	Poisoning, Accidental (Unintentional)	Poisoning, Intentional Self-Harm	Poisoning, Assault	Poisoning, Undetermined	Adverse Effect	Underdosing
Solanum dulcamara	T62.2X1	T62.2X2	T62.2X3	T62.2X4	—	—
berries	T62.1X1	T62.1X2	T62.1X3	T62.1X4	—	—
Solapsone	T37.1X1	T37.1X2	T37.1X3	T37.1X4	T37.1X5	T37.1X6
Solar lotion	T49.3X1	T49.3X2	T49.3X3	T49.3X4	T49.3X5	T49.3X6
Solasulfone	T37.1X1	T37.1X2	T37.1X3	T37.1X4	T37.1X5	T37.1X6
Soldering fluid	T65.891	T65.892	T65.893	T65.894	—	—
Solid substance	T65.91	T65.92	T65.93	T65.94	—	—
specified NEC	T65.891	T65.892	T65.893	T65.894	—	—
Solvent, industrial NEC	T52.91	T52.92	T52.93	T52.94	—	—
naphtha	T52.0X1	T52.0X2	T52.0X3	T52.0X4	—	—
petroleum	T52.0X1	T52.0X2	T52.0X3	T52.0X4	—	—
specified NEC	T52.8X1	T52.8X2	T52.8X3	T52.8X4	—	—
Soma	T42.8X1	T42.8X2	T42.8X3	T42.8X4	T42.8X5	T42.8X6
Somatorelin	T38.891	T38.892	T38.893	T38.894	T38.895	T38.896
Somatostatin	T38.991	T38.992	T38.993	T38.994	T38.995	T38.996
Somatotropin	T38.811	T38.812	T38.813	T38.814	T38.815	T38.816
Somatrem	T38.811	T38.812	T38.813	T38.814	T38.815	T38.816
Somatropin	T38.811	T38.812	T38.813	T38.814	T38.815	T38.816
Sominex	T45.0X1	T45.0X2	T45.0X3	T45.0X4	T45.0X5	T45.0X6
Somnos	T42.6X1	T42.6X2	T42.6X3	T42.6X4	T42.6X5	T42.6X6
Somonal	T42.3X1	T42.3X2	T42.3X3	T42.3X4	T42.3X5	T42.3X6
Soneryl	T42.3X1	T42.3X2	T42.3X3	T42.3X4	T42.3X5	T42.3X6
Soothing syrup	T50.901	T50.902	T50.903	T50.904	T50.905	T50.906
Sopor	T42.6X1	T42.6X2	T42.6X3	T42.6X4	T42.6X5	T42.6X6
Soporific	T42.71	T42.72	T42.73	T42.74	T42.75	T42.76
Soporific drug	T42.71	T42.72	T42.73	T42.74	T42.75	T42.76
specified type NEC	T42.6X1	T42.6X2	T42.6X3	T42.6X4	T42.6X5	T42.6X6
Sorbide nitrate	T46.3X1	T46.3X2	T46.3X3	T46.3X4	T46.3X5	T46.3X6
Sorbitol	T47.4X1	T47.4X2	T47.4X3	T47.4X4	T47.4X5	T47.4X6
Sotalol	T44.7X1	T44.7X2	T44.7X3	T44.7X4	T44.7X5	T44.7X6
Sotradecol	T46.8X1	T46.8X2	T46.8X3	T46.8X4	T46.8X5	T46.8X6
Soysterol	T46.6X1	T46.6X2	T46.6X3	T46.6X4	T46.6X5	T46.6X6
Spacoline	T44.3X1	T44.3X2	T44.3X3	T44.3X4	T44.3X5	T44.3X6
Spanish fly	T49.8X1	T49.8X2	T49.8X3	T49.8X4	T49.8X5	T49.8X6
Sparine	T43.3X1	T43.3X2	T43.3X3	T43.3X4	T43.3X5	T43.3X6
Sparteine	T48.0X1	T48.0X2	T48.0X3	T48.0X4	T48.0X5	T48.0X6
Spasmolytic						
anticholinergics	T44.3X1	T44.3X2	T44.3X3	T44.3X4	T44.3X5	T44.3X6
autonomic	T44.3X1	T44.3X2	T44.3X3	T44.3X4	T44.3X5	T44.3X6

	External Cause (T-Code)					
Substance	Poisoning, Accidental (Unintentional)	Poisoning, Intentional Self-Harm	Poisoning, Assault	Poisoning, Undetermined	Adverse Effect	Underdosing
Spasmolytic *(Continued)*						
bronchial NEC	T48.6X1	T48.6X2	T48.6X3	T48.6X4	T48.6X5	T48.6X6
quaternary ammonium	T44.3X1	T44.3X2	T44.3X3	T44.3X4	T44.3X5	T44.3X6
skeletal muscle NEC	T48.1X1	T48.1X2	T48.1X3	T48.1X4	T48.1X5	T48.1X6
Spectinomycin	T36.5X1	T36.5X2	T36.5X3	T36.5X4	T36.5X5	T36.5X6
Speed	T43.621	T43.622	T43.623	T43.624	T43.625	T43.626
Spermicide	T49.8X1	T49.8X2	T49.8X3	T49.8X4	T49.8X5	T49.8X6
Spider (bite) (venom)	T63.391	T63.392	T63.393	T63.394	—	—
antivenin	T50.Z11	T50.Z12	T50.Z13	T50.Z14	T50.Z15	T50.Z16
Spigelia (root)	T37.4X1	T37.4X2	T37.4X3	T37.4X4	T37.4X5	T37.4X6
Spindle inactivator	T50.4X1	T50.4X2	T50.4X3	T50.4X4	T50.4X5	T50.4X6
Spiperone	T43.4X1	T43.4X2	T43.4X3	T43.4X4	T43.4X5	T43.4X6
Spiramycin	T36.3X1	T36.3X2	T36.3X3	T36.3X4	T36.3X5	T36.3X6
Spirapril	T46.4X1	T46.4X2	T46.4X3	T46.4X4	T46.4X5	T46.4X6
Spirilene	T43.591	T43.592	T43.593	T43.594	T43.595	T43.596
Spirit(s) (neutral) NEC	T51.0X1	T51.0X2	T51.0X3	T51.0X4	—	—
beverage	T51.0X1	T51.0X2	T51.0X3	T51.0X4	—	—
industrial	T51.0X1	T51.0X2	T51.0X3	T51.0X4	—	—
mineral	T52.0X1	T52.0X2	T52.0X3	T52.0X4	—	—
of salt — *see Hydrochloric acid*						
surgical	T51.0X1	T51.0X2	T51.0X3	T51.0X4	—	—
Spironolactone	T50.0X1	T50.0X2	T50.0X3	T50.0X4	T50.0X5	T50.0X6
Spiroperidol	T43.4X1	T43.4X2	T43.4X3	T43.4X4	T43.4X5	T43.4X6
Sponge, absorbable (gelatin)	T45.7X1	T45.7X2	T45.7X3	T45.7X4	T45.7X5	T45.7X6
Sporostacin	T49.0X1	T49.0X2	T49.0X3	T49.0X4	T49.0X5	T49.0X6
Spray (aerosol)	T65.91	T65.92	T65.93	T65.94	—	—
cosmetic	T65.891	T65.892	T65.893	T65.894	—	—
medicinal NEC	T50.901	T50.902	T50.903	T50.904	T50.905	T50.906
pesticides — *see Pesticides*						
specified content — *see specific substance*						
Spurge flax	T62.2X1	T62.2X2	T62.2X3	T62.2X4	—	—
Spurges	T62.2X1	T62.2X2	T62.2X3	T62.2X4	—	—
Sputum viscosity-lowering drug	T48.4X1	T48.4X2	T48.4X3	T48.4X4	T48.4X5	T48.4X6
Squill	T46.0X1	T46.0X2	T46.0X3	T46.0X4	T46.0X5	T46.0X6
rat poison	T60.4X1	T60.4X2	T60.4X3	T60.4X4	—	—
Squirting cucumber (cathartic)	T47.2X1	T47.2X2	T47.2X3	T47.2X4	T47.2X5	T47.2X6
Stains	T65.6X1	T65.6X2	T65.6X3	T65.6X4	—	—
Stannous fluoride	T49.7X1	T49.7X2	T49.7X3	T49.7X4	T49.7X5	T49.7X6
Stanolone	T38.7X1	T38.7X2	T38.7X3	T38.7X4	T38.7X5	T38.7X6
Stanozolol	T38.7X1	T38.7X2	T38.7X3	T38.7X4	T38.7X5	T38.7X6

	External Cause (T-Code)					
Substance	**Poisoning, Accidental (Unintentional)**	**Poisoning, Intentional Self-Harm**	**Poisoning, Assault**	**Poisoning, Undetermined**	**Adverse Effect**	**Underdosing**
Staphisagria or stavesacre (pediculicide)	T49.0X1	T49.0X2	T49.0X3	T49.0X4	T49.0X5	T49.0X6
Starch	T50.901	T50.902	T50.903	T50.904	T50.905	T50.906
Stelazine	T43.3X1	T43.3X2	T43.3X3	T43.3X4	T43.3X5	T43.3X6
Stemetil	T43.3X1	T43.3X2	T43.3X3	T43.3X4	T43.3X5	T43.3X6
Stepronin	T48.4X1	T48.4X2	T48.4X3	T48.4X4	T48.4X5	T48.4X6
Sterculia	T47.4X1	T47.4X2	T47.4X3	T47.4X4	T47.4X5	T47.4X6
Sternutator gas	T59.891	T59.892	T59.893	T59.894	—	—
Steroid	T38.0X1	T38.0X2	T38.0X3	T38.0X4	T38.0X5	T38.0X6
anabolic	T38.7X1	T38.7X2	T38.7X3	T38.7X4	T38.7X5	T38.7X6
androgenic	T38.7X1	T38.7X2	T38.7X3	T38.7X4	T38.7X5	T38.7X6
antineoplastic, hormone	T38.7X1	T38.7X2	T38.7X3	T38.7X4	T38.7X5	T38.7X6
estrogen	T38.5X1	T38.5X2	T38.5X3	T38.5X4	T38.5X5	T38.5X6
ENT agent	T49.6X1	T49.6X2	T49.6X3	T49.6X4	T49.6X5	T49.6X6
ophthalmic preparation	T49.5X1	T49.5X2	T49.5X3	T49.5X4	T49.5X5	T49.5X6
topical NEC	T49.0X1	T49.0X2	T49.0X3	T49.0X4	T49.0X5	T49.0X6
Stibine	T56.891	T56.892	T56.893	T56.894	—	—
Stibogluconate	T37.3X1	T37.3X2	T37.3X3	T37.3X4	T37.3X5	T37.3X6
Stibophen	T37.4X1	T37.4X2	T37.4X3	T37.4X4	T37.4X5	T37.4X6
Stilbamidine (isetionate)	T37.3X1	T37.3X2	T37.3X3	T37.3X4	T37.3X5	T37.3X6
Stilbestrol	T38.5X1	T38.5X2	T38.5X3	T38.5X4	T38.5X5	T38.5X6
Stilboestrol	T38.5X1	T38.5X2	T38.5X3	T38.5X4	T38.5X5	T38.5X6
Stimulant						
central nervous system — see also Psychostimulant	T43.601	T43.602	T43.603	T43.604	T43.605	T43.606
analeptics	T50.7X1	T50.7X2	T50.7X3	T50.7X4	T50.7X5	T50.7X6
opiate antagonist	T50.7X1	T50.7X2	T50.7X3	T50.7X4	T50.7X5	T50.7X6
psychotherapeutic NEC — see also Psychotherapeutic drug	T43.601	T43.602	T43.603	T43.604	T43.605	T43.606
specified NEC	T43.691	T43.692	T43.693	T43.694	T43.695	T43.696
respiratory	T48.901	T48.902	T48.903	T48.904	T48.905	T48.906
Stone-dissolving drug	T50.901	T50.902	T50.903	T50.904	T50.905	T50.906
Storage battery (cells) (acid)	T54.2X1	T54.2X2	T54.2X3	T54.2X4	—	—
Stovaine	T41.3X1	T41.3X2	T41.3X3	T41.3X4	T41.3X5	T41.3X6
infiltration (subcutaneous)	T41.3X1	T41.3X2	T41.3X3	T41.3X4	T41.3X5	T41.3X6
nerve block (peripheral) (plexus)	T41.3X1	T41.3X2	T41.3X3	T41.3X4	T41.3X5	T41.3X6
spinal	T41.3X1	T41.3X2	T41.3X3	T41.3X4	T41.3X5	T41.3X6
topical (surface)	T41.3X1	T41.3X2	T41.3X3	T41.3X4	T41.3X5	T41.3X6
Stovarsal	T37.8X1	T37.8X2	T37.8X3	T37.8X4	T37.8X5	T37.8X6
Stove gas — see Gas, stove	T57.91	T57.92	T57.93	T57.94	—	—
Stoxil	T49.5X1	T49.5X2	T49.5X3	T49.5X4	T49.5X5	T49.5X6
Stramonium	T48.6X1	T48.6X2	T48.6X3	T48.6X4	T48.6X5	T48.6X6
natural state	T62.2X1	T62.2X2	T62.2X3	T62.2X4	—	—

Substance	External Cause (T-Code)					
	Poisoning, Accidental (Unintentional)	Poisoning, Intentional Self-Harm	Poisoning, Assault	Poisoning, Undetermined	Adverse Effect	Underdosing
Streptodornase	T45.3X1	T45.3X2	T45.3X3	T45.3X4	T45.3X5	T45.3X6
Streptoduocin	T36.5X1	T36.5X2	T36.5X3	T36.5X4	T36.5X5	T36.5X6
Streptokinase	T45.611	T45.612	T45.613	T45.614	T45.615	T45.616
Streptomycin (derivative)	T36.5X1	T36.5X2	T36.5X3	T36.5X4	T36.5X5	T36.5X6
Streptonivicin	T36.5X1	T36.5X2	T36.5X3	T36.5X4	T36.5X5	T36.5X6
Streptovarycin	T36.5X1	T36.5X2	T36.5X3	T36.5X4	T36.5X5	T36.5X6
Streptozocin	T45.1X1	T45.1X2	T45.1X3	T45.1X4	T45.1X5	T45.1X6
Streptozotocin	T45.1X1	T45.1X2	T45.1X3	T45.1X4	T45.1X5	T45.1X6
Stripper (paint) (solvent)	T52.8X1	T52.8X2	T52.8X3	T52.8X4	—	—
Strobane	T60.1X1	T60.1X2	T60.1X3	T60.1X4	—	—
Strofantina	T46.0X1	T46.0X2	T46.0X3	T46.0X4	T46.0X5	T46.0X6
Strophanthin (g) (k)	T46.0X1	T46.0X2	T46.0X3	T46.0X4	T46.0X5	T46.0X6
Strophanthus	T46.0X1	T46.0X2	T46.0X3	T46.0X4	T46.0X5	T46.0X6
Strophantin	T46.0X1	T46.0X2	T46.0X3	T46.0X4	T46.0X5	T46.0X6
Strophantin-g	T46.0X1	T46.0X2	T46.0X3	T46.0X4	T46.0X5	T46.0X6
Strychnine (nonmedicinal) (pesticide) (salts)	T65.1X1	T65.1X2	T65.1X3	T65.1X4	—	—
medicinal	T48.291	T48.292	T48.293	T48.294	T48.295	T48.296
Strychnos (ignatii) — see Strychnine						
Styramate	T42.8X1	T42.8X2	T42.8X3	T42.8X4	T42.8X5	T42.8X6
Styrene	T65.891	T65.892	T65.893	T65.894	—	—
Succinimide, antiepileptic or anticonvulsant	T42.2X1	T42.2X2	T42.2X3	T42.2X4	T42.2X5	T42.2X6
mercuric — see Mercury						
Succinylcholine	T48.1X1	T48.1X2	T48.1X3	T48.1X4	T48.1X5	T48.1X6
Succinylsulfathiazole	T37.0X1	T37.0X2	T37.0X3	T37.0X4	T37.0X5	T37.0X6
Sucralfate	T47.1X1	T47.1X2	T47.1X3	T47.1X4	T47.1X5	T47.1X6
Sucrose	T50.3X1	T50.3X2	T50.3X3	T50.3X4	T50.3X5	T50.3X6
Sufentanil	T40.4X1	T40.4X2	T40.4X3	T40.4X4	T40.4X5	T40.4X6
Sulbactam	T36.0X1	T36.0X2	T36.0X3	T36.0X4	T36.0X5	T36.0X6
Sulbenicillin	T36.0X1	T36.0X2	T36.0X3	T36.0X4	T36.0X5	T36.0X6
Sulbentine	T49.0X1	T49.0X2	T49.0X3	T49.0X4	T49.0X5	T49.0X6
Sulfacetamide	T49.0X1	T49.0X2	T49.0X3	T49.0X4	T49.0X5	T49.0X6
ophthalmic preparation	T49.5X1	T49.5X2	T49.5X3	T49.5X4	T49.5X5	T49.5X6
Sulfachlorpyridazine	T37.0X1	T37.0X2	T37.0X3	T37.0X4	T37.0X5	T37.0X6
Sulfacitine	T37.0X1	T37.0X2	T37.0X3	T37.0X4	T37.0X5	T37.0X6
Sulfadiasulfone sodium	T37.0X1	T37.0X2	T37.0X3	T37.0X4	T37.0X5	T37.0X6
Sulfadiazine	T37.0X1	T37.0X2	T37.0X3	T37.0X4	T37.0X5	T37.0X6
silver (topical)	T49.0X1	T49.0X2	T49.0X3	T49.0X4	T49.0X5	T49.0X6
Sulfadimethoxine	T37.0X1	T37.0X2	T37.0X3	T37.0X4	T37.0X5	T37.0X6
Sulfadimidine	T37.0X1	T37.0X2	T37.0X3	T37.0X4	T37.0X5	T37.0X6

Substance	Poisoning, Accidental (Unintentional)	Poisoning, Intentional Self-Harm	Poisoning, Assault	Poisoning, Undetermined	Adverse Effect	Underdosing
			External Cause (T-Code)			
Sulfadoxine	T37.0X1	T37.0X2	T37.0X3	T37.0X4	T37.0X5	T37.0X6
with pyrimethamine	T37.2X1	T37.2X2	T37.2X3	T37.2X4	T37.2X5	T37.2X6
Sulfaethidole	T37.0X1	T37.0X2	T37.0X3	T37.0X4	T37.0X5	T37.0X6
Sulfafurazole	T37.0X1	T37.0X2	T37.0X3	T37.0X4	T37.0X5	T37.0X6
Sulfaguanidine	T37.0X1	T37.0X2	T37.0X3	T37.0X4	T37.0X5	T37.0X6
Sulfalene	T37.0X1	T37.0X2	T37.0X3	T37.0X4	T37.0X5	T37.0X6
Sulfaloxate	T37.0X1	T37.0X2	T37.0X3	T37.0X4	T37.0X5	T37.0X6
Sulfaloxic acid	T37.0X1	T37.0X2	T37.0X3	T37.0X4	T37.0X5	T37.0X6
Sulfamazone	T39.2X1	T39.2X2	T39.2X3	T39.2X4	T39.2X5	T39.2X6
Sulfamerazine	T37.0X1	T37.0X2	T37.0X3	T37.0X4	T37.0X5	T37.0X6
Sulfameter	T37.0X1	T37.0X2	T37.0X3	T37.0X4	T37.0X5	T37.0X6
Sulfamethazine	T37.0X1	T37.0X2	T37.0X3	T37.0X4	T37.0X5	T37.0X6
Sulfamethizole	T37.0X1	T37.0X2	T37.0X3	T37.0X4	T37.0X5	T37.0X6
Sulfamethoxazole	T37.0X1	T37.0X2	T37.0X3	T37.0X4	T37.0X5	T37.0X6
with trimethoprim	T36.8X1	T36.8X2	T36.8X3	T36.8X4	T36.8X5	T36.8X6
Sulfamethoxydiazine	T37.0X1	T37.0X2	T37.0X3	T37.0X4	T37.0X5	T37.0X6
Sulfamethoxypyridazine	T37.0X1	T37.0X2	T37.0X3	T37.0X4	T37.0X5	T37.0X6
Sulfamethylthiazole	T37.0X1	T37.0X2	T37.0X3	T37.0X4	T37.0X5	T37.0X6
Sulfametoxydiazine	T37.0X1	T37.0X2	T37.0X3	T37.0X4	T37.0X5	T37.0X6
Sulfamidopyrine	T39.2X1	T39.2X2	T39.2X3	T39.2X4	T39.2X5	T39.2X6
Sulfamonomethoxine	T37.0X1	T37.0X2	T37.0X3	T37.0X4	T37.0X5	T37.0X6
Sulfamoxole	T37.0X1	T37.0X2	T37.0X3	T37.0X4	T37.0X5	T37.0X6
Sulfamylon	T49.0X1	T49.0X2	T49.0X3	T49.0X4	T49.0X5	T49.0X6
Sulfan blue (diagnostic dye)	T50.8X1	T50.8X2	T50.8X3	T50.8X4	T50.8X5	T50.8X6
Sulfanilamide	T37.0X1	T37.0X2	T37.0X3	T37.0X4	T37.0X5	T37.0X6
Sulfanilylguanidine	T37.0X1	T37.0X2	T37.0X3	T37.0X4	T37.0X5	T37.0X6
Sulfaperin	T37.0X1	T37.0X2	T37.0X3	T37.0X4	T37.0X5	T37.0X6
Sulfaphenazole	T37.0X1	T37.0X2	T37.0X3	T37.0X4	T37.0X5	T37.0X6
Sulfaphenylthiazole	T37.0X1	T37.0X2	T37.0X3	T37.0X4	T37.0X5	T37.0X6
Sulfaproxyline	T37.0X1	T37.0X2	T37.0X3	T37.0X4	T37.0X5	T37.0X6
Sulfapyridine	T37.0X1	T37.0X2	T37.0X3	T37.0X4	T37.0X5	T37.0X6
Sulfapyrimidine	T37.0X1	T37.0X2	T37.0X3	T37.0X4	T37.0X5	T37.0X6
Sulfarsphenamine	T37.8X1	T37.8X2	T37.8X3	T37.8X4	T37.8X5	T37.8X6
Sulfasalazine	T37.0X1	T37.0X2	T37.0X3	T37.0X4	T37.0X5	T37.0X6
Sulfasuxidine	T37.0X1	T37.0X2	T37.0X3	T37.0X4	T37.0X5	T37.0X6
Sulfasymazine	T37.0X1	T37.0X2	T37.0X3	T37.0X4	T37.0X5	T37.0X6
Sulfated amylopectin	T47.8X1	T47.8X2	T47.8X3	T47.8X4	T47.8X5	T47.8X6
Sulfathiazole	T37.0X1	T37.0X2	T37.0X3	T37.0X4	T37.0X5	T37.0X6
Sulfatostearate	T49.2X1	T49.2X2	T49.2X3	T49.2X4	T49.2X5	T49.2X6

Substance	External Cause (T-Code)					
	Poisoning, Accidental (Unintentional)	Poisoning, Intentional Self-Harm	Poisoning, Assault	Poisoning, Undetermined	Adverse Effect	Underdosing
Sulfinpyrazone	T50.4X1	T50.4X2	T50.4X3	T50.4X4	T50.4X5	T50.4X6
Sulfiram	T49.0X1	T49.0X2	T49.0X3	T49.0X4	T49.0X5	T49.0X6
Sulfisomidine	T37.0X1	T37.0X2	T37.0X3	T37.0X4	T37.0X5	T37.0X6
Sulfisoxazole	T37.0X1	T37.0X2	T37.0X3	T37.0X4	T37.0X5	T37.0X6
ophthalmic preparation	T49.5X1	T49.5X2	T49.5X3	T49.5X4	T49.5X5	T49.5X6
Sulfobromophthalein (sodium)	T50.8X1	T50.8X2	T50.8X3	T50.8X4	T50.8X5	T50.8X6
Sulfobromphthalein	T50.8X1	T50.8X2	T50.8X3	T50.8X4	T50.8X5	T50.8X6
Sulfogaiacol	T48.4X1	T48.4X2	T48.4X3	T48.4X4	T48.4X5	T48.4X6
Sulfomyxin	T36.8X1	T36.8X2	T36.8X3	T36.8X4	T36.8X5	T36.8X6
Sulfonal	T42.6X1	T42.6X2	T42.6X3	T42.6X4	T42.6X5	T42.6X6
Sulfonamide NEC	T37.0X1	T37.0X2	T37.0X3	T37.0X4	T37.0X5	T37.0X6
eye	T49.5X1	T49.5X2	T49.5X3	T49.5X4	T49.5X5	T49.5X6
Sulfonazide	T37.1X1	T37.1X2	T37.1X3	T37.1X4	T37.1X5	T37.1X6
Sulfones	T37.1X1	T37.1X2	T37.1X3	T37.1X4	T37.1X5	T37.1X6
Sulfonethylmethane	T42.6X1	T42.6X2	T42.6X3	T42.6X4	T42.6X5	T42.6X6
Sulfonmethane	T42.6X1	T42.6X2	T42.6X3	T42.6X4	T42.6X5	T42.6X6
Sulfonphthal, sulfonphthol	T50.8X1	T50.8X2	T50.8X3	T50.8X4	T50.8X5	T50.8X6
Sulfonylurea derivatives, oral	T38.3X1	T38.3X2	T38.3X3	T38.3X4	T38.3X5	T38.3X6
Sulforidazine	T43.3X1	T43.3X2	T43.3X3	T43.3X4	T43.3X5	T43.3X6
Sulfoxone	T37.1X1	T37.1X2	T37.1X3	T37.1X4	T37.1X5	T37.1X6
Sulfur, sulfurated, sulfuric, sulfurous, sulfuryl (compounds NEC) (medicinal)	T49.4X1	T49.4X2	T49.4X3	T49.4X4	T49.4X5	T49.4X6
acid	T54.2X1	T54.2X2	T54.2X3	T54.2X4	—	—
dioxide (gas)	T59.1X1	T59.1X2	T59.1X3	T59.1X4	—	—
ether — see Ether(s)						
hydrogen	T59.6X1	T59.6X2	T59.6X3	T59.6X4	—	—
medicinal (keratolytic) (ointment) NEC	T49.4X1	T49.4X2	T49.4X3	T49.4X4	T49.4X5	T49.4X6
ointment	T49.0X1	T49.0X2	T49.0X3	T49.0X4	T49.0X5	T49.0X6
pesticide (vapor)	T60.91	T60.92	T60.93	T60.94	—	—
vapor NEC	T59.891	T59.892	T59.893	T59.894	—	—
Sulfuric acid	T54.2X1	T54.2X2	T54.2X3	T54.2X4	—	—
Sulglicotide	T47.1X1	T47.1X2	T47.1X3	T47.1X4	T47.1X5	T47.1X6
Sulindac	T39.391	T39.392	T39.393	T39.394	T39.395	T39.396
Sulisatin	T47.2X1	T47.2X2	T47.2X3	T47.2X4	T47.2X5	T47.2X6
Sulisobenzone	T49.3X1	T49.3X2	T49.3X3	T49.3X4	T49.3X5	T49.3X6
Sulkowitch's reagent	T50.8X1	T50.8X2	T50.8X3	T50.8X4	T50.8X5	T50.8X6
Sulmetozine	T44.3X1	T44.3X2	T44.3X3	T44.3X4	T44.3X5	T44.3X6
Suloctidil	T46.7X1	T46.7X2	T46.7X3	T46.7X4	T46.7X5	T46.7X6
Sulph — see also Sulf-						
Sulphadiazine	T37.0X1	T37.0X2	T37.0X3	T37.0X4	T37.0X5	T37.0X6
Sulphadimethoxine	T37.0X1	T37.0X2	T37.0X3	T37.0X4	T37.0X5	T37.0X6

Substance	External Cause (T-Code)					
	Poisoning, Accidental (Unintentional)	Poisoning, Intentional Self-Harm	Poisoning, Assault	Poisoning, Undetermined	Adverse Effect	Underdosing
Sulphadimidine	T37.0X1	T37.0X2	T37.0X3	T37.0X4	T37.0X5	T37.0X6
Sulphadione	T37.1X1	T37.1X2	T37.1X3	T37.1X4	T37.1X5	T37.1X6
Sulphafurazole	T37.0X1	T37.0X2	T37.0X3	T37.0X4	T37.0X5	T37.0X6
Sulphamethizole	T37.0X1	T37.0X2	T37.0X3	T37.0X4	T37.0X5	T37.0X6
Sulphamethoxazole	T37.0X1	T37.0X2	T37.0X3	T37.0X4	T37.0X5	T37.0X6
Sulphan blue	T50.8X1	T50.8X2	T50.8X3	T50.8X4	T50.8X5	T50.8X6
Sulphaphenazole	T37.0X1	T37.0X2	T37.0X3	T37.0X4	T37.0X5	T37.0X6
Sulphapyridine	T37.0X1	T37.0X2	T37.0X3	T37.0X4	T37.0X5	T37.0X6
Sulphasalazine	T37.0X1	T37.0X2	T37.0X3	T37.0X4	T37.0X5	T37.0X6
Sulphinpyrazone	T50.4X1	T50.4X2	T50.4X3	T50.4X4	T50.4X5	T50.4X6
Sulpiride	T43.591	T43.592	T43.593	T43.594	T43.595	T43.596
Sulprostone	T48.0X1	T48.0X2	T48.0X3	T48.0X4	T48.0X5	T48.0X6
Sulpyrine	T39.2X1	T39.2X2	T39.2X3	T39.2X4	T39.2X5	T39.2X6
Sultamicillin	T36.0X1	T36.0X2	T36.0X3	T36.0X4	T36.0X5	T36.0X6
Sulthiame	T42.6X1	T42.6X2	T42.6X3	T42.6X4	T42.6X5	T42.6X6
Sultiame	T42.6X1	T42.6X2	T42.6X3	T42.6X4	T42.6X5	T42.6X6
Sultopride	T43.591	T43.592	T43.593	T43.594	T43.595	T43.596
Sumatriptan	T39.8X1	T39.8X2	T39.8X3	T39.8X4	T39.8X5	T39.8X6
Sunflower seed oil	T46.6X1	T46.6X2	T46.6X3	T46.6X4	T46.6X5	T46.6X6
Superinone	T48.4X1	T48.4X2	T48.4X3	T48.4X4	T48.4X5	T48.4X6
Suprofen	T39.311	T39.312	T39.313	T39.314	T39.315	T39.316
Suramin (sodium)	T37.4X1	T37.4X2	T37.4X3	T37.4X4	T37.4X5	T37.4X6
Surfacaine	T41.3X1	T41.3X2	T41.3X3	T41.3X4	T41.3X5	T41.3X6
Surital	T41.1X1	T41.1X2	T41.1X3	T41.1X4	T41.1X5	T41.1X6
Sutilains	T45.3X1	T45.3X2	T45.3X3	T45.3X4	T45.3X5	T45.3X6
Suxamethonium (chloride)	T48.1X1	T48.1X2	T48.1X3	T48.1X4	T48.1X5	T48.1X6
Suxethonium (chloride)	T48.1X1	T48.1X2	T48.1X3	T48.1X4	T48.1X5	T48.1X6
Suxibuzone	T39.2X1	T39.2X2	T39.2X3	T39.2X4	T39.2X5	T39.2X6
Sweet oil (birch)	T49.3X1	T49.3X2	T49.3X3	T49.3X4	T49.3X5	T49.3X6
Sweet niter spirit	T46.3X1	T46.3X2	T46.3X3	T46.3X4	T46.3X5	T46.3X6
Sweetener	T50.901	T50.902	T50.903	T50.904	T50.905	T50.906
Sym-dichloroethyl ether	T53.6X1	T53.6X2	T53.6X3	T53.6X4	—	—
Sympatholytic NEC	T44.8X1	T44.8X2	T44.8X3	T44.8X4	T44.8X5	T44.8X6
haloalkylamine	T44.8X1	T44.8X2	T44.8X3	T44.8X4	T44.8X5	T44.8X6
Sympathomimetic NEC	T44.901	T44.902	T44.903	T44.904	T44.905	T44.906
anti-common-cold	T48.5X1	T48.5X2	T48.5X3	T48.5X4	T48.5X5	T48.5X6
bronchodilator	T48.6X1	T48.6X2	T48.6X3	T48.6X4	T48.6X5	T48.6X6
specified NEC	T44.991	T44.992	T44.993	T44.994	T44.995	T44.996
Synagis	T50.B91	T50.B92	T50.B93	T50.B94	T50.B95	T50.B96
Synalar	T49.0X1	T49.0X2	T49.0X3	T49.0X4	T49.0X5	T49.0X6

717

Substance	External Cause (T-Code)					
	Poisoning, Accidental (Unintentional)	Poisoning, Intentional Self-Harm	Poisoning, Assault	Poisoning, Undetermined	Adverse Effect	Underdosing
Synthroid	T38.1X1	T38.1X2	T38.1X3	T38.1X4	T38.1X5	T38.1X6
Syntocinon	T48.0X1	T48.0X2	T48.0X3	T48.0X4	T48.0X5	T48.0X6
Syrosingopine	T46.5X1	T46.5X2	T46.5X3	T46.5X4	T46.5X5	T46.5X6
Systemic drug	T45.91	T45.92	T45.93	T45.94	T45.95	T45.96
specified NEC	T45.8X1	T45.8X2	T45.8X3	T45.8X4	T45.8X5	T45.8X6
2,4,5-T	T60.3X1	T60.3X2	T60.3X3	T60.3X4	—	—
T						
Tablets — *see also specified substance*	T50.901	T50.902	T50.903	T50.904	T50.905	T50.906
Tace	T38.5X1	T38.5X2	T38.5X3	T38.5X4	T38.5X5	T38.5X6
Tacrine	T44.0X1	T44.0X2	T44.0X3	T44.0X4	T44.0X5	T44.0X6
Tadalafil	T46.7X1	T46.7X2	T46.7X3	T46.7X4	T46.7X5	T46.7X6
Talampicillin	T36.0X1	T36.0X2	T36.0X3	T36.0X4	T36.0X5	T36.0X6
Talbutal	T42.3X1	T42.3X2	T42.3X3	T42.3X4	T42.3X5	T42.3X6
Talc powder	T49.3X1	T49.3X2	T49.3X3	T49.3X4	T49.3X5	T49.3X6
Talcum	T49.3X1	T49.3X2	T49.3X3	T49.3X4	T49.3X5	T49.3X6
Taleranol	T38.6X1	T38.6X2	T38.6X3	T38.6X4	T38.6X5	T38.6X6
Tamoxifen	T38.6X1	T38.6X2	T38.6X3	T38.6X4	T38.6X5	T38.6X6
Tamsulosin	T44.6X1	T44.6X2	T44.6X3	T44.6X4	T44.6X5	T44.6X6
Tandearil, tanderil	T39.2X1	T39.2X2	T39.2X3	T39.2X4	T39.2X5	T39.2X6
Tannic acid	T49.2X1	T49.2X2	T49.2X3	T49.2X4	T49.2X5	T49.2X6
medicinal (astringent)	T49.2X1	T49.2X2	T49.2X3	T49.2X4	T49.2X5	T49.2X6
Tannin — *see Tannic acid*						
Tansy	T62.2X1	T62.2X2	T62.2X3	T62.2X4	—	—
TAO	T36.3X1	T36.3X2	T36.3X3	T36.3X4	T36.3X5	T36.3X6
Tapazole	T38.2X1	T38.2X2	T38.2X3	T38.2X4	T38.2X5	T38.2X6
Tar NEC	T52.0X1	T52.0X2	T52.0X3	T52.0X4	—	—
camphor	T60.1X1	T60.1X2	T60.1X3	T60.1X4	—	—
distillate	T49.1X1	T49.1X2	T49.1X3	T49.1X4	T49.1X5	T49.1X6
fumes	T59.891	T59.892	T59.893	T59.894	—	—
medicinal	T49.1X1	T49.1X2	T49.1X3	T49.1X4	T49.1X5	T49.1X6
ointment	T49.1X1	T49.1X2	T49.1X3	T49.1X4	T49.1X5	T49.1X6
Taractan	T43.591	T43.592	T43.593	T43.594	T43.595	T43.596
Tarantula (venomous)	T63.321	T63.322	T63.323	T63.324	—	—
Tartar emetic	T37.8X1	T37.8X2	T37.8X3	T37.8X4	T37.8X5	T37.8X6
Tartaric acid	T65.891	T65.892	T65.893	T65.894	—	—
Tartrated antimony (anti-infective)	T37.8X1	T37.8X2	T37.8X3	T37.8X4	T37.8X5	T37.8X6
Tartrate, laxative	T47.4X1	T47.4X2	T47.4X3	T47.4X4	T47.4X5	T47.4X6
Tauromustine	T45.1X1	T45.1X2	T45.1X3	T45.1X4	T45.1X5	T45.1X6
TCA — *see Trichloroacetic acid*						

Substance	External Cause (T-Code)					
	Poisoning, Accidental (Unintentional)	Poisoning, Intentional Self-Harm	Poisoning, Assault	Poisoning, Undetermined	Adverse Effect	Underdosing
TCDD	T53.7X1	T53.7X2	T53.7X3	T53.7X4	—	—
TDI (vapor)	T65.0X1	T65.0X2	T65.0X3	T65.0X4	—	—
Tear						
gas	T59.3X1	T59.3X2	T59.3X3	T59.3X4	—	—
solution	T49.5X1	T49.5X2	T49.5X3	T49.5X4	T49.5X5	T49.5X6
Teclothiazide	T50.2X1	T50.2X2	T50.2X3	T50.2X4	T50.2X5	T50.2X6
Teclozan	T37.3X1	T37.3X2	T37.3X3	T37.3X4	T37.3X5	T37.3X6
Tegafur	T45.1X1	T45.1X2	T45.1X3	T45.1X4	T45.1X5	T45.1X6
Tegretol	T42.1X1	T42.1X2	T42.1X3	T42.1X4	T42.1X5	T42.1X6
Teicoplanin	T36.8X1	T36.8X2	T36.8X3	T36.8X4	T36.8X5	T36.8X6
Telepaque	T50.8X1	T50.8X2	T50.8X3	T50.8X4	T50.8X5	T50.8X6
Tellurium	T56.891	T56.892	T56.893	T56.894	—	—
fumes	T56.891	T56.892	T56.893	T56.894	—	—
TEM	T45.1X1	T45.1X2	T45.1X3	T45.1X4	T45.1X5	T45.1X6
Temazepam	T42.4X1	T42.4X2	T42.4X3	T42.4X4	T42.4X5	T42.4X6
Temocillin	T36.0X1	T36.0X2	T36.0X3	T36.0X4	T36.0X5	T36.0X6
Tenamfetamine	T43.621	T43.622	T43.623	T43.624	T43.625	T43.626
Teniposide	T45.1X1	T45.1X2	T45.1X3	T45.1X4	T45.1X5	T45.1X6
Tenitramine	T46.3X1	T46.3X2	T46.3X3	T46.3X4	T46.3X5	T46.3X6
Tenoglicin	T48.4X1	T48.4X2	T48.4X3	T48.4X4	T48.4X5	T48.4X6
Tenonitrozole	T37.3X1	T37.3X2	T37.3X3	T37.3X4	T37.3X5	T37.3X6
Tenoxicam	T39.391	T39.392	T39.393	T39.394	T39.395	T39.396
TEPA	T45.1X1	T45.1X2	T45.1X3	T45.1X4	T45.1X5	T45.1X6
TEPP	T60.0X1	T60.0X2	T60.0X3	T60.0X4	—	—
Teprotide	T46.5X1	T46.5X2	T46.5X3	T46.5X4	T46.5X5	T46.5X6
Terazosin	T44.6X1	T44.6X2	T44.6X3	T44.6X4	T44.6X5	T44.6X6
Terbufos	T60.0X1	T60.0X2	T60.0X3	T60.0X4	—	—
Terbutaline	T48.6X1	T48.6X2	T48.6X3	T48.6X4	T48.6X5	T48.6X6
Terconazole	T49.0X1	T49.0X2	T49.0X3	T49.0X4	T49.0X5	T49.0X6
Terfenadine	T45.0X1	T45.0X2	T45.0X3	T45.0X4	T45.0X5	T45.0X6
Teriparatide (acetate)	T50.991	T50.992	T50.993	T50.994	T50.995	T50.996
Terizidone	T37.1X1	T37.1X2	T37.1X3	T37.1X4	T37.1X5	T37.1X6
Terlipressin	T38.891	T38.892	T38.893	T38.894	T38.895	T38.896
Terodiline	T46.3X1	T46.3X2	T46.3X3	T46.3X4	T46.3X5	T46.3X6
Teroxalene	T37.4X1	T37.4X2	T37.4X3	T37.4X4	T37.4X5	T37.4X6
Terpin(cis) hydrate	T48.4X1	T48.4X2	T48.4X3	T48.4X4	T48.4X5	T48.4X6
Terramycin	T36.4X1	T36.4X2	T36.4X3	T36.4X4	T36.4X5	T36.4X6
Tertatolol	T44.7X1	T44.7X2	T44.7X3	T44.7X4	T44.7X5	T44.7X6
Tessalon	T48.3X1	T48.3X2	T48.3X3	T48.3X4	T48.3X5	T48.3X6
Testolactone	T38.7X1	T38.7X2	T38.7X3	T38.7X4	T38.7X5	T38.7X6

Substance	External Cause (T-Code)					
	Poisoning, Accidental (Unintentional)	Poisoning, Intentional Self-Harm	Poisoning, Assault	Poisoning, Undetermined	Adverse Effect	Underdosing
Testosterone	T38.7X1	T38.7X2	T38.7X3	T38.7X4	T38.7X5	T38.7X6
Tetanus toxoid or vaccine	T50.A91	T50.A92	T50.A93	T50.A94	T50.A95	T50.A96
antitoxin	T50.Z11	T50.Z12	T50.Z13	T50.Z14	T50.Z15	T50.Z16
immune globulin (human)	T50.Z11	T50.Z12	T50.Z13	T50.Z14	T50.Z15	T50.Z16
toxoid	T50.A91	T50.A92	T50.A93	T50.A94	T50.A95	T50.A96
with diphtheria toxoid	T50.A21	T50.A22	T50.A23	T50.A24	T50.A25	T50.A26
with pertussis	T50.A11	T50.A12	T50.A13	T50.A14	T50.A15	T50.A16
Tetrabenazine	T43.591	T43.592	T43.593	T43.594	T43.595	T43.596
Tetracaine	T41.3X1	T41.3X2	T41.3X3	T41.3X4	T41.3X5	T41.3X6
nerve block (peripheral) (plexus)	T41.3X1	T41.3X2	T41.3X3	T41.3X4	T41.3X5	T41.3X6
regional	T41.3X1	T41.3X2	T41.3X3	T41.3X4	T41.3X5	T41.3X6
spinal	T41.3X1	T41.3X2	T41.3X3	T41.3X4	T41.3X5	T41.3X6
Tetrachlorethylene — see Tetrachloroethylene						
Tetrachlormethiazide	T50.2X1	T50.2X2	T50.2X3	T50.2X4	T50.2X5	T50.2X6
2,3,7,8-Tetrachlorodibenzo-p-dioxin	T53.7X1	T53.7X2	T53.7X3	T53.7X4	—	—
Tetrachloroethane	T53.6X1	T53.6X2	T53.6X3	T53.6X4	—	—
vapor	T53.6X1	T53.6X2	T53.6X3	T53.6X4	—	—
paint or varnish	T53.6X1	T53.6X2	T53.6X3	T53.6X4	—	—
Tetrachloroethylene (liquid)	T53.3X1	T53.3X2	T53.3X3	T53.3X4	—	—
medicinal	T37.4X1	T37.4X2	T37.4X3	T37.4X4	T37.4X5	T37.4X6
vapor	T53.3X1	T53.3X2	T53.3X3	T53.3X4	—	—
Tetrachloromethane — see Carbon tetrachloride						
Tetracosactide	T38.811	T38.812	T38.813	T38.814	T38.815	T38.816
Tetracosactrin	T38.811	T38.812	T38.813	T38.814	T38.815	T38.816
Tetracycline	T36.4X1	T36.4X2	T36.4X3	T36.4X4	T36.4X5	T36.4X6
ophthalmic preparation	T49.5X1	T49.5X2	T49.5X3	T49.5X4	T49.5X5	T49.5X6
topical NEC	T49.0X1	T49.0X2	T49.0X3	T49.0X4	T49.0X5	T49.0X6
Tetradifon	T60.8X1	T60.8X2	T60.8X3	T60.8X4	—	—
Tetradotoxin	T61.771	T61.772	T61.773	T61.774	—	—
Tetraethyl						
lead	T56.0X1	T56.0X2	T56.0X3	T56.0X4	—	—
pyrophosphate	T60.0X1	T60.0X2	T60.0X3	T60.0X4	—	—
Tetraethylammonium chloride	T44.2X1	T44.2X2	T44.2X3	T44.2X4	T44.2X5	T44.2X6
Tetraethylthiuram disulfide	T50.6X1	T50.6X2	T50.6X3	T50.6X4	T50.6X5	T50.6X6
Tetrahydroaminoacridine	T44.0X1	T44.0X2	T44.0X3	T44.0X4	T44.0X5	T44.0X6
Tetrahydrocannabinol	T40.7X1	T40.7X2	T40.7X3	T40.7X4	T40.7X5	T40.7X6
Tetrahydrofuran	T52.8X1	T52.8X2	T52.8X3	T52.8X4	—	—
Tetrahydronaphthalene	T52.8X1	T52.8X2	T52.8X3	T52.8X4	—	—
Tetrahydrozoline	T49.5X1	T49.5X2	T49.5X3	T49.5X4	T49.5X5	T49.5X6
Tetralin	T52.8X1	T52.8X2	T52.8X3	T52.8X4	—	—

Substance	External Cause (T-Code)					
	Poisoning, Accidental (Unintentional)	Poisoning, Intentional Self-Harm	Poisoning, Assault	Poisoning, Undetermined	Adverse Effect	Underdosing
Tetramethrin	T60.2X1	T60.2X2	T60.2X3	T60.2X4	—	—
Tetramethylthiuram (disulfide) NEC	T60.3X1	T60.3X2	T60.3X3	T60.3X4	—	—
medicinal	T49.0X1	T49.0X2	T49.0X3	T49.0X4	T49.0X5	T49.0X6
Tetramisole	T37.4X1	T37.4X2	T37.4X3	T37.4X4	T37.4X5	T37.4X6
Tetranicotinoyl fructose	T46.7X1	T46.7X2	T46.7X3	T46.7X4	T46.7X5	T46.7X6
Tetronal	T42.6X1	T42.6X2	T42.6X3	T42.6X4	T42.6X5	T42.6X6
Tetrazepam	T42.4X1	T42.4X2	T42.4X3	T42.4X4	T42.4X5	T42.4X6
Tetryl	T65.3X1	T65.3X2	T65.3X3	T65.3X4	—	—
Tetrylammonium chloride	T44.2X1	T44.2X2	T44.2X3	T44.2X4	T44.2X5	T44.2X6
Tetryzoline	T49.5X1	T49.5X2	T49.5X3	T49.5X4	T49.5X5	T49.5X6
Thalidomide	T45.1X1	T45.1X2	T45.1X3	T45.1X4	T45.1X5	T45.1X6
Thallium (compounds) (dust) NEC	T56.811	T56.812	T56.813	T56.814	—	—
pesticide	T60.4X1	T60.4X2	T60.4X3	T60.4X4	—	—
THC	T40.7X1	T40.7X2	T40.7X3	T40.7X4	T40.7X5	T40.7X6
Thebacon	T48.3X1	T48.3X2	T48.3X3	T48.3X4	T48.3X5	T48.3X6
Thebaine	T40.2X1	T40.2X2	T40.2X3	T40.2X4	T40.2X5	T40.2X6
Thenoic acid	T49.6X1	T49.6X2	T49.6X3	T49.6X4	T49.6X5	T49.6X6
Thenyldiamine	T45.0X1	T45.0X2	T45.0X3	T45.0X4	T45.0X5	T45.0X6
Theobromine (calcium salicylate)	T48.6X1	T48.6X2	T48.6X3	T48.6X4	T48.6X5	T48.6X6
sodium salicylate	T48.6X1	T48.6X2	T48.6X3	T48.6X4	T48.6X5	T48.6X6
Theophyllamine	T48.6X1	T48.6X2	T48.6X3	T48.6X4	T48.6X5	T48.6X6
Theophylline	T48.6X1	T48.6X2	T48.6X3	T48.6X4	T48.6X5	T48.6X6
aminobenzoic acid	T48.6X1	T48.6X2	T48.6X3	T48.6X4	T48.6X5	T48.6X6
ethylenediamine	T48.6X1	T48.6X2	T48.6X3	T48.6X4	T48.6X5	T48.6X6
piperazine p-amino-benzoate	T48.6X1	T48.6X2	T48.6X3	T48.6X4	T48.6X5	T48.6X6
Thiabendazole	T37.4X1	T37.4X2	T37.4X3	T37.4X4	T37.4X5	T37.4X6
Thialbarbital	T41.1X1	T41.1X2	T41.1X3	T41.1X4	T41.1X5	T41.1X6
Thiamazole	T38.2X1	T38.2X2	T38.2X3	T38.2X4	T38.2X5	T38.2X6
Thiambutosine	T37.1X1	T37.1X2	T37.1X3	T37.1X4	T37.1X5	T37.1X6
Thiamine	T45.2X1	T45.2X2	T45.2X3	T45.2X4	T45.2X5	T45.2X6
Thiamphenicol	T36.2X1	T36.2X2	T36.2X3	T36.2X4	T36.2X5	T36.2X6
Thiamylal	T41.1X1	T41.1X2	T41.1X3	T41.1X4	T41.1X5	T41.1X6
sodium	T41.1X1	T41.1X2	T41.1X3	T41.1X4	T41.1X5	T41.1X6
Thiazesim	T43.291	T43.292	T43.293	T43.294	T43.295	T43.296
Thiazides (diuretics)	T50.2X1	T50.2X2	T50.2X3	T50.2X4	T50.2X5	T50.2X6
Thiazinamium metilsulfate	T43.3X1	T43.3X2	T43.3X3	T43.3X4	T43.3X5	T43.3X6
Thiethylperazine	T43.3X1	T43.3X2	T43.3X3	T43.3X4	T43.3X5	T43.3X6
Thimerosal	T49.0X1	T49.0X2	T49.0X3	T49.0X4	T49.0X5	T49.0X6
ophthalmic preparation	T49.5X1	T49.5X2	T49.5X3	T49.5X4	T49.5X5	T49.5X6

Substance	External Cause (T-Code)					
	Poisoning, Accidental (Unintentional)	Poisoning, Intentional Self-Harm	Poisoning, Assault	Poisoning, Undetermined	Adverse Effect	Underdosing
Thioacetazone	T37.1X1	T37.1X2	T37.1X3	T37.1X4	T37.1X5	T37.1X6
with isoniazid	T37.1X1	T37.1X2	T37.1X3	T37.1X4	T37.1X5	T37.1X6
Thiobarbital sodium	T41.1X1	T41.1X2	T41.1X3	T41.1X4	T41.1X5	T41.1X6
Thiobarbiturate anesthetic	T41.1X1	T41.1X2	T41.1X3	T41.1X4	T41.1X5	T41.1X6
Thiobismol	T37.8X1	T37.8X2	T37.8X3	T37.8X4	T37.8X5	T37.8X6
Thiobutabarbital sodium	T41.1X1	T41.1X2	T41.1X3	T41.1X4	T41.1X5	T41.1X6
Thiocarbamate (insecticide)	T60.0X1	T60.0X2	T60.0X3	T60.0X4	—	—
Thiocarbamide	T38.2X1	T38.2X2	T38.2X3	T38.2X4	T38.2X5	T38.2X6
Thiocarbarsone	T37.8X1	T37.8X2	T37.8X3	T37.8X4	T37.8X5	T37.8X6
Thiocarlide	T37.1X1	T37.1X2	T37.1X3	T37.1X4	T37.1X5	T37.1X6
Thioctamide	T50.991	T50.992	T50.993	T50.994	T50.995	T50.996
Thioctic acid	T50.991	T50.992	T50.993	T50.994	T50.995	T50.996
Thiofos	T60.0X1	T60.0X2	T60.0X3	T60.0X4	—	—
Thioglycolate	T49.4X1	T49.4X2	T49.4X3	T49.4X4	T49.4X5	T49.4X6
Thioglycolic acid	T65.891	T65.892	T65.893	T65.894	—	—
Thioguanine	T45.1X1	T45.1X2	T45.1X3	T45.1X4	T45.1X5	T45.1X6
Thiomercaptomerin	T50.2X1	T50.2X2	T50.2X3	T50.2X4	T50.2X5	T50.2X6
Thiomerin	T50.2X1	T50.2X2	T50.2X3	T50.2X4	T50.2X5	T50.2X6
Thiomersal	T49.0X1	T49.0X2	T49.0X3	T49.0X4	T49.0X5	T49.0X6
Thionazin	T60.0X1	T60.0X2	T60.0X3	T60.0X4	—	—
Thiopental (sodium)	T41.1X1	T41.1X2	T41.1X3	T41.1X4	T41.1X5	T41.1X6
Thiopentone (sodium)	T41.1X1	T41.1X2	T41.1X3	T41.1X4	T41.1X5	T41.1X6
Thiopropazate	T43.3X1	T43.3X2	T43.3X3	T43.3X4	T43.3X5	T43.3X6
Thioproperazine	T43.3X1	T43.3X2	T43.3X3	T43.3X4	T43.3X5	T43.3X6
Thioridazine	T43.3X1	T43.3X2	T43.3X3	T43.3X4	T43.3X5	T43.3X6
Thiosinamine	T49.3X1	T49.3X2	T49.3X3	T49.3X4	T49.3X5	T49.3X6
Thiotepa	T45.1X1	T45.1X2	T45.1X3	T45.1X4	T45.1X5	T45.1X6
Thiothixene	T43.4X1	T43.4X2	T43.4X3	T43.4X4	T43.4X5	T43.4X6
Thiouracil (benzyl) (methyl) (propyl)	T38.2X1	T38.2X2	T38.2X3	T38.2X4	T38.2X5	T38.2X6
Thiourea	T38.2X1	T38.2X2	T38.2X3	T38.2X4	T38.2X5	T38.2X6
Thiphenamil	T44.3X1	T44.3X2	T44.3X3	T44.3X4	T44.3X5	T44.3X6
Thiram	T60.3X1	T60.3X2	T60.3X3	T60.3X4	—	—
medicinal	T49.2X1	T49.2X2	T49.2X3	T49.2X4	T49.2X5	T49.2X6
Thonzylamine (systemic)	T45.0X1	T45.0X2	T45.0X3	T45.0X4	T45.0X5	T45.0X6
mucosal decongestant	T48.5X1	T48.5X2	T48.5X3	T48.5X4	T48.5X5	T48.5X6
Thorazine	T43.3X1	T43.3X2	T43.3X3	T43.3X4	T43.3X5	T43.3X6
Thorium dioxide suspension	T50.8X1	T50.8X2	T50.8X3	T50.8X4	T50.8X5	T50.8X6
Thornapple	T62.2X1	T62.2X2	T62.2X3	T62.2X4	—	—
Throat drug NEC	T49.6X1	T49.6X2	T49.6X3	T49.6X4	T49.6X5	T49.6X6
Thrombin	T45.7X1	T45.7X2	T45.7X3	T45.7X4	T45.7X5	T45.7X6

	External Cause (T-Code)					
Substance	Poisoning, Accidental (Unintentional)	Poisoning, Intentional Self-Harm	Poisoning, Assault	Poisoning, Undetermined	Adverse Effect	Underdosing
Thrombolysin	T45.611	T45.612	T45.613	T45.614	T45.615	T45.616
Thromboplastin	T45.7X1	T45.7X2	T45.7X3	T45.7X4	T45.7X5	T45.7X6
Thurfyl nicotinate	T46.7X1	T46.7X2	T46.7X3	T46.7X4	T46.7X5	T46.7X6
Thymol	T49.0X1	T49.0X2	T49.0X3	T49.0X4	T49.0X5	T49.0X6
Thymopentin	T37.5X1	T37.5X2	T37.5X3	T37.5X4	T37.5X5	T37.5X6
Thymoxamine	T46.7X1	T46.7X2	T46.7X3	T46.7X4	T46.7X5	T46.7X6
Thymus extract	T38.891	T38.892	T38.893	T38.894	T38.895	T38.896
Thyreotrophic hormone	T38.811	T38.812	T38.813	T38.814	T38.815	T38.816
Thyroglobulin	T38.1X1	T38.1X2	T38.1X3	T38.1X4	T38.1X5	T38.1X6
Thyroid (hormone)	T38.1X1	T38.1X2	T38.1X3	T38.1X4	T38.1X5	T38.1X6
Thyrolar	T38.1X1	T38.1X2	T38.1X3	T38.1X4	T38.1X5	T38.1X6
Thyrotrophin	T38.811	T38.812	T38.813	T38.814	T38.815	T38.816
Thyrotropic hormone	T38.811	T38.812	T38.813	T38.814	T38.815	T38.816
Thyroxine	T38.1X1	T38.1X2	T38.1X3	T38.1X4	T38.1X5	T38.1X6
Tiabendazole	T37.4X1	T37.4X2	T37.4X3	T37.4X4	T37.4X5	T37.4X6
Tiamizide	T50.2X1	T50.2X2	T50.2X3	T50.2X4	T50.2X5	T50.2X6
Tianeptine	T43.291	T43.292	T43.293	T43.294	T43.295	T43.296
Tiapamil	T46.1X1	T46.1X2	T46.1X3	T46.1X4	T46.1X5	T46.1X6
Tiapride	T43.591	T43.592	T43.593	T43.594	T43.595	T43.596
Tiaprofenic acid	T39.311	T39.312	T39.313	T39.314	T39.315	T39.316
Tiaramide	T39.8X1	T39.8X2	T39.8X3	T39.8X4	T39.8X5	T39.8X6
Ticarcillin	T36.0X1	T36.0X2	T36.0X3	T36.0X4	T36.0X5	T36.0X6
Ticlatone	T49.0X1	T49.0X2	T49.0X3	T49.0X4	T49.0X5	T49.0X6
Ticlopidine	T45.521	T45.522	T45.523	T45.524	T45.525	T45.526
Ticrynafen	T50.1X1	T50.1X2	T50.1X3	T50.1X4	T50.1X5	T50.1X6
Tidiacic	T50.991	T50.992	T50.993	T50.994	T50.995	T50.996
Tiemonium	T44.3X1	T44.3X2	T44.3X3	T44.3X4	T44.3X5	T44.3X6
iodide	T44.3X1	T44.3X2	T44.3X3	T44.3X4	T44.3X5	T44.3X6
Tienilic acid	T50.1X1	T50.1X2	T50.1X3	T50.1X4	T50.1X5	T50.1X6
Tifenamil	T44.3X1	T44.3X2	T44.3X3	T44.3X4	T44.3X5	T44.3X6
Tigan	T45.0X1	T45.0X2	T45.0X3	T45.0X4	T45.0X5	T45.0X6
Tigloidine	T44.3X1	T44.3X2	T44.3X3	T44.3X4	T44.3X5	T44.3X6
Tilactase	T47.5X1	T47.5X2	T47.5X3	T47.5X4	T47.5X5	T47.5X6
Tiletamine	T41.291	T41.292	T41.293	T41.294	T41.295	T41.296
Tilidine	T40.4X1	T40.4X2	T40.4X3	T40.4X4	—	—
Timepidium bromide	T44.3X1	T44.3X2	T44.3X3	T44.3X4	T44.3X5	T44.3X6
Timiperone	T43.4X1	T43.4X2	T43.4X3	T43.4X4	T43.4X5	T43.4X6
Timolol	T44.7X1	T44.7X2	T44.7X3	T44.7X4	T44.7X5	T44.7X6
Tin (chloride) (dust) (oxide) NEC	T56.6X1	T56.6X2	T56.6X3	T56.6X4	—	—
anti-infectives	T37.8X1	T37.8X2	T37.8X3	T37.8X4	T37.8X5	T37.8X6

Substance	External Cause (T-Code)					
	Poisoning, Accidental (Unintentional)	Poisoning, Intentional Self-Harm	Poisoning, Assault	Poisoning, Undetermined	Adverse Effect	Underdosing
Tincture, iodine — see Iodine						
Tindal	T43.3X1	T43.3X2	T43.3X3	T43.3X4	T43.3X5	T43.3X6
Tinidazole	T37.3X1	T37.3X2	T37.3X3	T37.3X4	T37.3X5	T37.3X6
Tinoridine	T39.8X1	T39.8X2	T39.8X3	T39.8X4	T39.8X5	T39.8X6
Tiocarlide	T37.1X1	T37.1X2	T37.1X3	T37.1X4	T37.1X5	T37.1X6
Tioclomarol	T45.511	T45.512	T45.513	T45.514	T45.515	T45.516
Tioconazole	T49.0X1	T49.0X2	T49.0X3	T49.0X4	T49.0X5	T49.0X6
Tioguanine	T45.1X1	T45.1X2	T45.1X3	T45.1X4	T45.1X5	T45.1X6
Tiopronin	T50.991	T50.992	T50.993	T50.994	T50.995	T50.996
Tiotixene	T43.4X1	T43.4X2	T43.4X3	T43.4X4	T43.4X5	T43.4X6
Tioxolone	T49.4X1	T49.4X2	T49.4X3	T49.4X4	T49.4X5	T49.4X6
Tipepidine	T48.3X1	T48.3X2	T48.3X3	T48.3X4	T48.3X5	T48.3X6
Tiquizium bromide	T44.3X1	T44.3X2	T44.3X3	T44.3X4	T44.3X5	T44.3X6
Tiratricol	T38.1X1	T38.1X2	T38.1X3	T38.1X4	T38.1X5	T38.1X6
Tisopurine	T50.4X1	T50.4X2	T50.4X3	T50.4X4	T50.4X5	T50.4X6
Titanium (compounds) (vapor)	T56.891	T56.892	T56.893	T56.894	—	—
dioxide	T49.3X1	T49.3X2	T49.3X3	T49.3X4	T49.3X5	T49.3X6
ointment	T49.3X1	T49.3X2	T49.3X3	T49.3X4	T49.3X5	T49.3X6
oxide	T49.3X1	T49.3X2	T49.3X3	T49.3X4	T49.3X5	T49.3X6
tetrachloride	T56.891	T56.892	T56.893	T56.894	—	—
Titanocene	T56.891	T56.892	T56.893	T56.894	—	—
Titroid	T38.1X1	T38.1X2	T38.1X3	T38.1X4	T38.1X5	T38.1X6
Tizanidine	T42.8X1	T42.8X2	T42.8X3	T42.8X4	T42.8X5	T42.8X6
TMTD	T60.3X1	T60.3X2	T60.3X3	T60.3X4	—	—
TNT (fumes)	T65.3X1	T65.3X2	T65.3X3	T65.3X4	—	—
Toadstool	T62.0X1	T62.0X2	T62.0X3	T62.0X4	—	—
Tobacco NEC	T65.291	T65.292	T65.293	T65.294	—	—
cigarettes	T65.221	T65.222	T65.223	T65.224	—	—
Indian	T62.291	T62.292	T62.293	T62.294	—	—
smoke, second-hand	T65.221	T65.222	T65.223	T65.224	—	—
Tobramycin	T36.5X1	T36.5X2	T36.5X3	T36.5X4	T36.5X5	T36.5X6
Tocainide	T46.2X1	T46.2X2	T46.2X3	T46.2X4	T46.2X5	T46.2X6
Tocoferol	T45.2X1	T45.2X2	T45.2X3	T45.2X4	T45.2X5	T45.2X6
Tocopherol	T45.2X1	T45.2X2	T45.2X3	T45.2X4	T45.2X5	T45.2X6
acetate	T45.2X1	T45.2X2	T45.2X3	T45.2X4	T45.2X5	T45.2X6
Tocosamine	T48.0X1	T48.0X2	T48.0X3	T48.0X4	T48.0X5	T48.0X6
Todralazine	T46.5X1	T46.5X2	T46.5X3	T46.5X4	T46.5X5	T46.5X6
Tofisopam	T42.4X1	T42.4X2	T42.4X3	T42.4X4	T42.4X5	T42.4X6
Tofranil	T43.011	T43.012	T43.013	T43.014	T43.015	T43.016
Toilet deodorizer	T65.891	T65.892	T65.893	T65.894	—	—

Substance	Poisoning, Accidental (Unintentional)	Poisoning, Intentional Self-Harm	Poisoning, Assault	Poisoning, Undetermined	Adverse Effect	Underdosing
	External Cause (T-Code)					
Tolamolol	T44.7X1	T44.7X2	T44.7X3	T44.7X4	T44.7X5	T44.7X6
Tolazamide	T38.3X1	T38.3X2	T38.3X3	T38.3X4	T38.3X5	T38.3X6
Tolazoline	T46.7X1	T46.7X2	T46.7X3	T46.7X4	T46.7X5	T46.7X6
Tolbutamide (sodium)	T38.3X1	T38.3X2	T38.3X3	T38.3X4	T38.3X5	T38.3X6
Tolciclate	T49.0X1	T49.0X2	T49.0X3	T49.0X4	T49.0X5	T49.0X6
Tolmetin	T39.391	T39.392	T39.393	T39.394	T39.395	T39.396
Tolnaftate	T49.0X1	T49.0X2	T49.0X3	T49.0X4	T49.0X5	T49.0X6
Tolonidine	T46.5X1	T46.5X2	T46.5X3	T46.5X4	T46.5X5	T46.5X6
Toloxatone	T42.6X1	T42.6X2	T42.6X3	T42.6X4	T42.6X5	T42.6X6
Tolperisone	T44.3X1	T44.3X2	T44.3X3	T44.3X4	T44.3X5	T44.3X6
Tolserol	T42.8X1	T42.8X2	T42.8X3	T42.8X4	T42.8X5	T42.8X6
Toluene (liquid)	T52.2X1	T52.2X2	T52.2X3	T52.2X4	—	—
diisocyanate	T65.0X1	T65.0X2	T65.0X3	T65.0X4	—	—
Toluidine	T65.891	T65.892	T65.893	T65.894	—	—
vapor	T59.891	T59.892	T59.893	T59.894	—	—
Toluol (liquid)	T52.2X1	T52.2X2	T52.2X3	T52.2X4	—	—
vapor	T52.2X1	T52.2X2	T52.2X3	T52.2X4	—	—
Toluylenediamine	T65.3X1	T65.3X2	T65.3X3	T65.3X4	—	—
Tolylene-2,4-diisocyanate	T65.0X1	T65.0X2	T65.0X3	T65.0X4	—	—
Tonic NEC	T50.901	T50.902	T50.903	T50.904	T50.905	T50.906
Topical action drug NEC	T49.91	T49.92	T49.93	T49.94	T49.95	T49.96
ear, nose or throat	T49.6X1	T49.6X2	T49.6X3	T49.6X4	T49.6X5	T49.6X6
eye	T49.5X1	T49.5X2	T49.5X3	T49.5X4	T49.5X5	T49.5X6
skin	T49.91	T49.92	T49.93	T49.94	T49.95	T49.96
specified NEC	T49.8X1	T49.8X2	T49.8X3	T49.8X4	T49.8X5	T49.8X6
Toquizine	T44.3X1	T44.3X2	T44.3X3	T44.3X4	T44.3X5	T44.3X6
Toremifene	T38.6X1	T38.6X2	T38.6X3	T38.6X4	T38.6X5	T38.6X6
Tosylchloramide sodium	T49.8X1	T49.8X2	T49.8X3	T49.8X4	T49.8X5	T49.8X6
Toxaphene (dust) (spray)	T60.1X1	T60.1X2	T60.1X3	T60.1X4	—	—
Toxin, diphtheria (Schick Test)	T50.8X1	T50.8X2	T50.8X3	T50.8X4	T50.8X5	T50.8X6
Toxoid						
combined	T50.A21	T50.A22	T50.A23	T50.A24	T50.A25	T50.A26
diphtheria	T50.A91	T50.A92	T50.A93	T50.A94	T50.A95	T50.A96
tetanus	T50.A91	T50.A92	T50.A93	T50.A94	T50.A95	T50.A96
Trace element NEC	T45.8X1	T45.8X2	T45.8X3	T45.8X4	T45.8X5	T45.8X6
Tractor fuel NEC	T52.0X1	T52.0X2	T52.0X3	T52.0X4	—	—
Tragacanth	T50.991	T50.992	T50.993	T50.994	T50.995	T50.996
Tramadol	T40.4X1	T40.4X2	T40.4X3	T40.4X4	T40.4X5	T40.4X6
Tramazoline	T48.5X1	T48.5X2	T48.5X3	T48.5X4	T48.5X5	T48.5X6
Tranexamic acid	T45.621	T45.622	T45.623	T45.624	T45.625	T45.626

Substance	Poisoning, Accidental (Unintentional)	Poisoning, Intentional Self-Harm	Poisoning, Assault	Poisoning, Undetermined	Adverse Effect	Underdosing
Tranilast	T45.0X1	T45.0X2	T45.0X3	T45.0X4	T45.0X5	T45.0X6
Tranquilizer NEC	T43.501	T43.502	T43.503	T43.504	T43.505	T43.506
with hypnotic or sedative	T42.6X1	T42.6X2	T42.6X3	T42.6X4	T42.6X5	T42.6X6
benzodiazepine NEC	T42.4X1	T42.4X2	T42.4X3	T42.4X4	T42.4X5	T42.4X6
butyrophenone NEC	T43.4X1	T43.4X2	T43.4X3	T43.4X4	T43.4X5	T43.4X6
carbamate	T43.591	T43.592	T43.593	T43.594	T43.595	T43.596
dimethylamine	T43.3X1	T43.3X2	T43.3X3	T43.3X4	T43.3X5	T43.3X6
ethylamine	T43.3X1	T43.3X2	T43.3X3	T43.3X4	T43.3X5	T43.3X6
hydroxyzine	T43.591	T43.592	T43.593	T43.594	T43.595	T43.596
major NEC	T43.501	T43.502	T43.503	T43.504	T43.505	T43.506
penothiazine NEC	T43.3X1	T43.3X2	T43.3X3	T43.3X4	T43.3X5	T43.3X6
phenothiazine-based	T43.3X1	T43.3X2	T43.3X3	T43.3X4	T43.3X5	T43.3X6
piperazine NEC	T43.3X1	T43.3X2	T43.3X3	T43.3X4	T43.3X5	T43.3X6
piperidine	T43.3X1	T43.3X2	T43.3X3	T43.3X4	T43.3X5	T43.3X6
propylamine	T43.3X1	T43.3X2	T43.3X3	T43.3X4	T43.3X5	T43.3X6
specified NEC	T43.591	T43.592	T43.593	T43.594	T43.595	T43.596
thioxanthene NEC	T43.591	T43.592	T43.593	T43.594	T43.595	T43.596
Tranxene	T42.4X1	T42.4X2	T42.4X3	T42.4X4	T42.4X5	T42.4X6
Tranylcypromine	T43.1X1	T43.1X2	T43.1X3	T43.1X4	T43.1X5	T43.1X6
Trapidil	T46.3X1	T46.3X2	T46.3X3	T46.3X4	T46.3X5	T46.3X6
Trasentine	T44.3X1	T44.3X2	T44.3X3	T44.3X4	T44.3X5	T44.3X6
Travert	T50.3X1	T50.3X2	T50.3X3	T50.3X4	T50.3X5	T50.3X6
Trazodone	T43.211	T43.212	T43.213	T43.214	T43.215	T43.216
Trecator	T37.1X1	T37.1X2	T37.1X3	T37.1X4	T37.1X5	T37.1X6
Treosulfan	T45.1X1	T45.1X2	T45.1X3	T45.1X4	T45.1X5	T45.1X6
Tretamine	T45.1X1	T45.1X2	T45.1X3	T45.1X4	T45.1X5	T45.1X6
Tretinoin	T49.0X1	T49.0X2	T49.0X3	T49.0X4	T49.0X5	T49.0X6
Tretoquinol	T48.6X1	T48.6X2	T48.6X3	T48.6X4	T48.6X5	T48.6X6
Triacetin	T49.0X1	T49.0X2	T49.0X3	T49.0X4	T49.0X5	T49.0X6
Triacetoxyanthracene	T49.4X1	T49.4X2	T49.4X3	T49.4X4	T49.4X5	T49.4X6
Triacetyloleandomycin	T36.3X1	T36.3X2	T36.3X3	T36.3X4	T36.3X5	T36.3X6
Triamcinolone	T49.0X1	T49.0X2	T49.0X3	T49.0X4	T49.0X5	T49.0X6
ENT agent	T49.6X1	T49.6X2	T49.6X3	T49.6X4	T49.6X5	T49.6X6
hexacetonide	T49.0X1	T49.0X2	T49.0X3	T49.0X4	T49.0X5	T49.0X6
ophthalmic preparation	T49.5X1	T49.5X2	T49.5X3	T49.5X4	T49.5X5	T49.5X6
topical NEC	T49.0X1	T49.0X2	T49.0X3	T49.0X4	T49.0X5	T49.0X6
Triampyzine	T44.3X1	T44.3X2	T44.3X3	T44.3X4	T44.3X5	T44.3X6
Triamterene	T50.2X1	T50.2X2	T50.2X3	T50.2X4	T50.2X5	T50.2X6
Triazine (herbicide)	T60.3X1	T60.3X2	T60.3X3	T60.3X4	—	—
Triaziquone	T45.1X1	T45.1X2	T45.1X3	T45.1X4	T45.1X5	T45.1X6

Substance	External Cause (T-Code)					
	Poisoning, Accidental (Unintentional)	Poisoning, Intentional Self-Harm	Poisoning, Assault	Poisoning, Undetermined	Adverse Effect	Underdosing
Triazolam	T42.4X1	T42.4X2	T42.4X3	T42.4X4	T42.4X5	T42.4X6
Triazole (herbicide)	T60.3X1	T60.3X2	T60.3X3	T60.3X4	—	—
Tribenoside	T46.991	T46.992	T46.993	T46.994	T46.995	T46.996
Tribromacetaldehyde	T42.6X1	T42.6X2	T42.6X3	T42.6X4	T42.6X5	T42.6X6
Tribromoethanol, rectal	T41.291	T41.292	T41.293	T41.294	T41.295	T41.296
Tribromomethane	T42.6X1	T42.6X2	T42.6X3	T42.6X4	T42.6X5	T42.6X6
Trichlorethane	T53.2X1	T53.2X2	T53.2X3	T53.2X4	—	—
Trichlorethylene	T53.2X1	T53.2X2	T53.2X3	T53.2X4	—	—
Trichlorfon	T60.0X1	T60.0X2	T60.0X3	T60.0X4	—	—
Trichlormethiazide	T50.2X1	T50.2X2	T50.2X3	T50.2X4	T50.2X5	T50.2X6
Trichlormethine	T45.1X1	T45.1X2	T45.1X3	T45.1X4	T45.1X5	T45.1X6
Trichloroacetic acid, Trichloracetic acid	T54.2X1	T54.2X2	T54.2X3	T54.2X4	—	—
medicinal	T49.4X1	T49.4X2	T49.4X3	T49.4X4	T49.4X5	T49.4X6
Trichloroethane	T53.2X1	T53.2X2	T53.2X3	T53.2X4	—	—
Trichloroethanol	T42.6X1	T42.6X2	T42.6X3	T42.6X4	T42.6X5	T42.6X6
Trichloroethylene (liquid) (vapor)	T53.2X1	T53.2X2	T53.2X3	T53.2X4	—	—
anesthetic (gas)	T41.0X1	T41.0X2	T41.0X3	T41.0X4	T41.0X5	T41.0X6
vapor NEC	T53.2X1	T53.2X2	T53.2X3	T53.2X4	—	—
Trichloroethyl phosphate	T42.6X1	T42.6X2	T42.6X3	T42.6X4	T42.6X5	T42.6X6
Trichlorofluoromethane NEC	T53.5X1	T53.5X2	T53.5X3	T53.5X4	—	—
Trichloronate	T60.0X1	T60.0X2	T60.0X3	T60.0X4	—	—
2,4,5-Trichlorophen-oxyacetic acid	T60.3X1	T60.3X2	T60.3X3	T60.3X4	—	—
Trichloropropane	T53.6X1	T53.6X2	T53.6X3	T53.6X4	—	—
Trichlorotriethylamine	T45.1X1	T45.1X2	T45.1X3	T45.1X4	T45.1X5	T45.1X6
Trichomonacides NEC	T37.3X1	T37.3X2	T37.3X3	T37.3X4	T37.3X5	T37.3X6
Trichomycin	T36.7X1	T36.7X2	T36.7X3	T36.7X4	T36.7X5	T36.7X6
Triclobisonium chloride	T49.0X1	T49.0X2	T49.0X3	T49.0X4	T49.0X5	T49.0X6
Triclocarban	T49.0X1	T49.0X2	T49.0X3	T49.0X4	T49.0X5	T49.0X6
Triclofos	T42.6X1	T42.6X2	T42.6X3	T42.6X4	T42.6X5	T42.6X6
Triclosan	T49.0X1	T49.0X2	T49.0X3	T49.0X4	T49.0X5	T49.0X6
Tricresyl phosphate	T65.891	T65.892	T65.893	T65.894	—	—
solvent	T52.91	T52.92	T52.93	T52.94	—	—
Tricyclamol chloride	T44.3X1	T44.3X2	T44.3X3	T44.3X4	T44.3X5	T44.3X6
Tridesilon	T49.0X1	T49.0X2	T49.0X3	T49.0X4	T49.0X5	T49.0X6
Tridihexethyl iodide	T44.3X1	T44.3X2	T44.3X3	T44.3X4	T44.3X5	T44.3X6
Tridione	T42.2X1	T42.2X2	T42.2X3	T42.2X4	T42.2X5	T42.2X6
Trientine	T45.8X1	T45.8X2	T45.8X3	T45.8X4	T45.8X5	T45.8X6
Triethanolamine NEC	T54.3X1	T54.3X2	T54.3X3	T54.3X4	—	—
detergent	T54.3X1	T54.3X2	T54.3X3	T54.3X4	—	—
trinitrate (biphosphate)	T46.3X1	T46.3X2	T46.3X3	T46.3X4	T46.3X5	T46.3X6

Substance	External Cause (T-Code)					
	Poisoning, Accidental (Unintentional)	Poisoning, Intentional Self-Harm	Poisoning, Assault	Poisoning, Undetermined	Adverse Effect	Underdosing
Triethanomelamine	T45.1X1	T45.1X2	T45.1X3	T45.1X4	T45.1X5	T45.1X6
Triethylenemelamine	T45.1X1	T45.1X2	T45.1X3	T45.1X4	T45.1X5	T45.1X6
Triethylenephosphoramide	T45.1X1	T45.1X2	T45.1X3	T45.1X4	T45.1X5	T45.1X6
Triethylenethiophosphoramide	T45.1X1	T45.1X2	T45.1X3	T45.1X4	T45.1X5	T45.1X6
Trifluoperazine	T43.3X1	T43.3X2	T43.3X3	T43.3X4	T43.3X5	T43.3X6
Trifluoroethyl vinyl ether	T41.0X1	T41.0X2	T41.0X3	T41.0X4	T41.0X5	T41.0X6
Trifluperidol	T43.4X1	T43.4X2	T43.4X3	T43.4X4	T43.4X5	T43.4X6
Triflupromazine	T43.3X1	T43.3X2	T43.3X3	T43.3X4	T43.3X5	T43.3X6
Trifluridine	T37.5X1	T37.5X2	T37.5X3	T37.5X4	T37.5X5	T37.5X6
Triflusal	T45.521	T45.522	T45.523	T45.524	T45.525	T45.526
Trihexyphenidyl	T44.3X1	T44.3X2	T44.3X3	T44.3X4	T44.3X5	T44.3X6
Triiodothyronine	T38.1X1	T38.1X2	T38.1X3	T38.1X4	T38.1X5	T38.1X6
Trilene	T41.0X1	T41.0X2	T41.0X3	T41.0X4	T41.0X5	T41.0X6
Trilostane	T38.991	T38.992	T38.993	T38.994	T38.995	T38.996
Trimebutine	T44.3X1	T44.3X2	T44.3X3	T44.3X4	T44.3X5	T44.3X6
Trimecaine	T41.3X1	T41.3X2	T41.3X3	T41.3X4	T41.3X5	T41.3X6
Trimeprazine (tartrate)	T44.3X1	T44.3X2	T44.3X3	T44.3X4	T44.3X5	T44.3X6
Trimetaphan camsilate	T44.2X1	T44.2X2	T44.2X3	T44.2X4	T44.2X5	T44.2X6
Trimetazidine	T46.7X1	T46.7X2	T46.7X3	T46.7X4	T46.7X5	T46.7X6
Trimethadione	T42.2X1	T42.2X2	T42.2X3	T42.2X4	T42.2X5	T42.2X6
Trimethaphan	T44.2X1	T44.2X2	T44.2X3	T44.2X4	T44.2X5	T44.2X6
Trimethidinium	T44.2X1	T44.2X2	T44.2X3	T44.2X4	T44.2X5	T44.2X6
Trimethobenzamide	T45.0X1	T45.0X2	T45.0X3	T45.0X4	T45.0X5	T45.0X6
Trimethoprim	T37.8X1	T37.8X2	T37.8X3	T37.8X4	T37.8X5	T37.8X6
with sulfamethoxazole	T36.8X1	T36.8X2	T36.8X3	T36.8X4	T36.8X5	T36.8X6
Trimethylcarbinol	T51.3X1	T51.3X2	T51.3X3	T51.3X4	—	—
Trimethylpsoralen	T49.3X1	T49.3X2	T49.3X3	T49.3X4	T49.3X5	T49.3X6
Trimeton	T45.0X1	T45.0X2	T45.0X3	T45.0X4	T45.0X5	T45.0X6
Trimetrexate	T45.1X1	T45.1X2	T45.1X3	T45.1X4	T45.1X5	T45.1X6
Trimipramine	T43.011	T43.012	T43.013	T43.014	T43.015	T43.016
Trimustine	T45.1X1	T45.1X2	T45.1X3	T45.1X4	T45.1X5	T45.1X6
Trinitrine	T46.3X1	T46.3X2	T46.3X3	T46.3X4	T46.3X5	T46.3X6
Trinitrobenzol	T65.3X1	T65.3X2	T65.3X3	T65.3X4	—	—
Trinitrophenol	T65.3X1	T65.3X2	T65.3X3	T65.3X4	—	—
Trinitrotoluene (fumes)	T65.3X1	T65.3X2	T65.3X3	T65.3X4	—	—
Trional	T42.6X1	T42.6X2	T42.6X3	T42.6X4	T42.6X5	T42.6X6
Triorthocresyl phosphate	T65.891	T65.892	T65.893	T65.894	—	—
Trioxide of arsenic	T57.0X1	T57.0X2	T57.0X3	T57.0X4	—	—
Trioxysalen	T49.4X1	T49.4X2	T49.4X3	T49.4X4	T49.4X5	T49.4X6
Tripamide	T50.2X1	T50.2X2	T50.2X3	T50.2X4	T50.2X5	T50.2X6

Substance	External Cause (T-Code)					
	Poisoning, Accidental (Unintentional)	Poisoning, Intentional Self-Harm	Poisoning, Assault	Poisoning, Undetermined	Adverse Effect	Underdosing
Triparanol	T46.6X1	T46.6X2	T46.6X3	T46.6X4	T46.6X5	T46.6X6
Tripelennamine	T45.0X1	T45.0X2	T45.0X3	T45.0X4	T45.0X5	T45.0X6
Triperiden	T44.3X1	T44.3X2	T44.3X3	T44.3X4	T44.3X5	T44.3X6
Triperidol	T43.4X1	T43.4X2	T43.4X3	T43.4X4	T43.4X5	T43.4X6
Triphenylphosphate	T65.891	T65.892	T65.893	T65.894	—	—
Triple						
bromides	T42.6X1	T42.6X2	T42.6X3	T42.6X4	T42.6X5	T42.6X6
carbonate	T47.1X1	T47.1X2	T47.1X3	T47.1X4	T47.1X5	T47.1X6
vaccine						
DPT	T50.A11	T50.A12	T50.A13	T50.A14	T50.A15	T50.A16
including pertussis	T50.A11	T50.A12	T50.A13	T50.A14	T50.A15	T50.A16
MMR	T50.B91	T50.B92	—	—	—	—
Triprolidine	T45.0X1	T45.0X2	T45.0X3	T45.0X4	T45.0X5	T45.0X6
Trisodium hydrogen edetate	T50.6X1	T50.6X2	T50.6X3	T50.6X4	T50.6X5	T50.6X6
Trisoralen	T49.3X1	T49.3X2	T49.3X3	T49.3X4	T49.3X5	T49.3X6
Trisulfapyrimidines	T37.0X1	T37.0X2	T37.0X3	T37.0X4	T37.0X5	T37.0X6
Trithiozine	T44.3X1	T44.3X2	T44.3X3	T44.3X4	T44.3X5	T44.3X6
Tritiozine	T44.3X1	T44.3X2	T44.3X3	T44.3X4	T44.3X5	T44.3X6
Tritoqualine	T45.0X1	T45.0X2	T45.0X3	T45.0X4	T45.0X5	T45.0X6
Trofosfamide	T45.1X1	T45.1X2	T45.1X3	T45.1X4	T45.1X5	T45.1X6
Troleandomycin	T36.3X1	T36.3X2	T36.3X3	T36.3X4	T36.3X5	T36.3X6
Trolnitrate (phosphate)	T46.3X1	T46.3X2	T46.3X3	T46.3X4	T46.3X5	T46.3X6
Tromantadine	T37.5X1	T37.5X2	T37.5X3	T37.5X4	T37.5X5	T37.5X6
Trometamol	T50.2X1	T50.2X2	T50.2X3	T50.2X4	T50.2X5	T50.2X6
Tromethamine	T50.2X1	T50.2X2	T50.2X3	T50.2X4	T50.2X5	T50.2X6
Tronothane	T41.3X1	T41.3X2	T41.3X3	T41.3X4	T41.3X5	T41.3X6
Tropacine	T44.3X1	T44.3X2	T44.3X3	T44.3X4	T44.3X5	T44.3X6
Tropatepine	T44.3X1	T44.3X2	T44.3X3	T44.3X4	T44.3X5	T44.3X6
Tropicamide	T44.3X1	T44.3X2	T44.3X3	T44.3X4	T44.3X5	T44.3X6
Trospium chloride	T44.3X1	T44.3X2	T44.3X3	T44.3X4	T44.3X5	T44.3X6
Troxerutin	T46.991	T46.992	T46.993	T46.994	T46.995	T46.996
Troxidone	T42.2X1	T42.2X2	T42.2X3	T42.2X4	T42.2X5	T42.2X6
Tryparsamide	T37.3X1	T37.3X2	T37.3X3	T37.3X4	T37.3X5	T37.3X6
Trypsin	T45.3X1	T45.3X2	T45.3X3	T45.3X4	T45.3X5	T45.3X6
Tryptizol	T43.011	T43.012	T43.013	T43.014	T43.015	T43.016
TSH	T38.811	T38.812	T38.813	T38.814	T38.815	T38.816
Tuaminoheptane	T48.5X1	T48.5X2	T48.5X3	T48.5X4	T48.5X5	T48.5X6
Tuberculin, purified protein derivative (PPD)	T50.8X1	T50.8X2	T50.8X3	T50.8X4	T50.8X5	T50.8X6
Tubocurare	T48.1X1	T48.1X2	T48.1X3	T48.1X4	T48.1X5	T48.1X6
Tubocurarine (chloride)	T48.1X1	T48.1X2	T48.1X3	T48.1X4	T48.1X5	T48.1X6

Substance	Poisoning, Accidental (Unintentional)	External Cause (T-Code) Poisoning, Intentional Self-Harm	Poisoning, Assault	Poisoning, Undetermined	Adverse Effect	Underdosing
Tulobuterol	T48.6X1	T48.6X2	T48.6X3	T48.6X4	T48.6X5	T48.6X6
Turpentine (spirits of)	T52.8X1	T52.8X2	T52.8X3	T52.8X4	—	—
vapor	T52.8X1	T52.8X2	T52.8X3	T52.8X4	—	—
Tybamate	T43.591	T43.592	T43.593	T43.594	T43.595	T43.596
Tyloxapol	T48.4X1	T48.4X2	T48.4X3	T48.4X4	T48.4X5	T48.4X6
Tymazoline	T48.5X1	T48.5X2	T48.5X3	T48.5X4	T48.5X5	T48.5X6
Typhoid-paratyphoid vaccine	T50.A91	T50.A92	T50.A93	T50.A94	T50.A95	T50.A96
Typhus vaccine	T50.A91	T50.A92	T50.A93	T50.A94	T50.A95	T50.A96
Tyropanoate	T50.8X1	T50.8X2	T50.8X4	T50.8X4	T50.8X5	T50.8X6
Tyrothricin	T49.6X1	T49.6X2	T49.6X3	T49.6X4	T49.6X5	T49.6X6
ENT agent	T49.6X1	T49.6X2	T49.6X3	T49.6X4	T49.6X5	T49.6X6
ophthalmic preparation	T49.5X1	T49.5X2	T49.5X3	T49.5X4	T49.5X5	T49.5X6
U						
Ufenamate	T39.391	T39.392	T39.393	T39.394	T39.395	T39.396
Ultraviolet light protectant	T49.3X1	T49.3X2	T49.3X3	T49.3X4	T49.3X5	T49.3X6
Undecenoic acid	T49.0X1	T49.0X2	T49.0X3	T49.0X4	T49.0X5	T49.0X6
Undecoylium	T49.0X1	T49.0X2	T49.0X3	T49.0X4	T49.0X5	T49.0X6
Undecylenic acid (derivatives)	T49.0X1	T49.0X2	T49.0X3	T49.0X4	T49.0X5	T49.0X6
Unna's boot	T49.3X1	T49.3X2	T49.3X3	T49.3X4	T49.3X5	T49.3X6
Unsaturated fatty acid	T46.6X1	T46.6X2	T46.6X3	T46.6X4	T46.6X5	T46.6X6
Uracil mustard	T45.1X1	T45.1X2	T45.1X3	T45.1X4	T45.1X5	T45.1X6
Uramustine	T45.1X1	T45.1X2	T45.1X3	T45.1X4	T45.1X5	T45.1X6
Urapidil	T46.5X1	T46.5X2	T46.5X3	T46.5X4	T46.5X5	T46.5X6
Urari	T48.1X1	T48.1X2	T48.1X3	T48.1X4	T48.1X5	T48.1X6
Urate oxidase	T50.4X1	T50.4X2	T50.4X3	T50.4X4	T50.4X5	T50.4X6
Urea	T47.3X1	T47.3X2	T47.3X3	T47.3X4	T47.3X5	T47.3X6
peroxide	T49.0X1	T49.0X2	T49.0X3	T49.0X4	T49.0X5	T49.0X6
stibamine	T37.4X1	T37.4X2	T37.4X3	T37.4X4	T37.4X5	T37.4X6
topical	T49.8X1	T49.8X2	T49.8X3	T49.8X4	T49.8X5	T49.8X6
Urethane	T45.1X1	T45.1X2	T45.1X3	T45.1X4	T45.1X5	T45.1X6
Urginea (maritima) (scilla) — see Squill						
Uric acid metabolism drug NEC	T50.4X1	T50.4X2	T50.4X3	T50.4X4	T50.4X5	T50.4X6
Uricosuric agent	T50.4X1	T50.4X2	T50.4X3	T50.4X4	T50.4X5	T50.4X6
Urinary anti-infective	T37.8X1	T37.8X2	T37.8X3	T37.8X4	T37.8X5	T37.8X6
Urofollitropin	T38.811	T38.812	T38.813	T38.814	T38.815	T38.816
Urokinase	T45.611	T45.612	T45.613	T45.614	T45.615	T45.616
Urokon	T50.8X1	T50.8X2	T50.8X3	T50.8X4	T50.8X5	T50.8X6
Ursodeoxycholic acid	T50.991	T50.992	T50.993	T50.994	T50.995	T50.996
Ursodiol	T50.991	T50.992	T50.993	T50.994	T50.995	T50.996

TABLE OF DRUGS AND CHEMICALS

Substance	External Cause (T-Code)					
	Poisoning, Accidental (Unintentional)	Poisoning, Intentional Self-Harm	Poisoning, Assault	Poisoning, Undetermined	Adverse Effect	Underdosing
Urtica	T62.2X1	T62.2X2	T62.2X3	T62.2X4	—	—
Utility gas—see Gas, utility						
V						
Vaccine NEC	T50.Z91	T50.Z92	T50.Z93	T50.Z94	T50.Z95	T50.Z96
antineoplastic	T50.Z91	T50.Z92	T50.Z93	T50.Z94	T50.Z95	T50.Z96
bacterial NEC	T50.A91	T50.A92	T50.A93	T50.A94	T50.A95	T50.A96
with						
other bacterial component	T50.A91	T50.A92	T50.A93	T50.A94	T50.A95	T50.A96
pertussis component	T50.A91	T50.A92	T50.A93	T50.A94	T50.A95	T50.A96
viral-rickettsial component	T50.A91	T50.A92	T50.A93	T50.A94	T50.A95	T50.A96
mixed NEC	T50.A91	T50.A92	T50.A93	T50.A94	T50.A95	T50.A96
BCG	T50.A91	T50.A92	T50.A93	T50.A94	T50.A95	T50.A96
cholera	T50.A91	T50.A92	T50.A93	T50.A94	T50.A95	T50.A96
diphtheria	T50.A91	T50.A92	T50.A93	T50.A94	T50.A95	T50.A96
with tetanus	T50.A21	T50.A22	T50.A23	T50.A24	T50.A25	T50.A26
and pertussis	T50.A11	T50.A12	T50.A13	T50.A14	T50.A15	T50.A16
influenza	T50.B91	T50.B92	T50.B93	T50.B94	T50.B95	T50.B96
measles	T50.B91	T50.B92	T50.B93	T50.B94	T50.B95	T50.B96
with mumps and rubella	T50.B91	T50.B92	T50.B93	T50.B94	T50.B95	T50.B96
meningococcal	T50.A91	T50.A92	T50.A93	T50.A94	T50.A95	T50.A96
mumps	T50.B91	T50.B92	T50.B93	T50.B94	T50.B95	T50.B96
paratyphoid	T50.A91	T50.A92	T50.A93	T50.A94	T50.A95	T50.A96
pertussis	T50.A11	T50.A12	T50.A13	T50.A14	T50.A15	T50.A16
with diphtheria	T50.A11	T50.A12	T50.A13	T50.A14	T50.A15	T50.A16
and tetanus	T50.A11	T50.A12	T50.A13	T50.A14	T50.A15	T50.A16
plague	T50.A91	T50.A92	T50.A93	T50.A94	T50.A95	T50.A96
poliomyelitis	T50.B91	T50.B92	T50.B93	T50.B94	T50.B95	T50.B96
poliovirus	T50.B91	T50.B92	T50.B93	T50.B94	T50.B95	T50.B96
rabies	T50.B91	T50.B92	T50.B93	T50.B94	T50.B95	T50.B96
respiratory syncytial virus	T50.B91	T50.B92	T50.B93	T50.B94	T50.B95	T50.B96
rickettsial NEC	T50.A91	T50.A92	T50.A93	T50.A94	T50.A95	T50.A96
with						
bacterial component	T50.A21	T50.A22	T50.A23	T50.A24	T50.A25	T50.A26
Rocky Mountain spotted fever	T50.A91	T50.A92	T50.A93	T50.A94	T50.A95	T50.A96
rubella	T50.B91	T50.B92	T50.B93	T50.B94	T50.B95	T50.B96
sabin oral	T50.B91	T50.B92	T50.B93	T50.B94	T50.B95	T50.B96
smallpox	T50.B11	T50.B12	T50.B13	T50.B14	T50.B15	T50.B16
TAB	T50.A91	T50.A92	T50.A93	T50.A94	T50.A95	T50.A96
tetanus	T50.A91	T50.A92	T50.A93	T50.A94	T50.A95	T50.A96

TABLE OF DRUGS AND CHEMICALS

TABLE OF DRUGS AND CHEMICALS

Substance	External Cause (T-Code)					
	Poisoning, Accidental (Unintentional)	Poisoning, Intentional Self-Harm	Poisoning, Assault	Poisoning, Undetermined	Adverse Effect	Underdosing
Vaccine NEC *(Continued)*						
typhoid	T50.A91	T50.A92	T50.A93	T50.A94	T50.A95	T50.A96
typhus	T50.A91	T50.A92	T50.A93	T50.A94	T50.A95	T50.A96
viral NEC	T50.B91	T50.B92	T50.B93	T50.B94	T50.B95	T50.B96
yellow fever	T50.B91	T50.B92	T50.B93	T50.B94	T50.B95	T50.B96
Vaccinia immune globulin	T50.Z11	T50.Z12	T50.Z13	T50.Z14	T50.Z15	T50.Z16
Vaginal contraceptives	T49.8X1	T49.8X2	T49.8X3	T49.8X4	T49.8X5	T49.8X6
Valerian						
root	T42.6X1	T42.6X2	T42.6X3	T42.6X4	T42.6X5	T42.6X6
tincture	T42.6X1	T42.6X2	T42.6X3	T42.6X4	T42.6X5	T42.6X6
Valethamate bromide	T44.3X1	T44.3X2	T44.3X3	T44.3X4	T44.3X5	T44.3X6
Valisone	T49.0X1	T49.0X2	T49.0X3	T49.0X4	T49.0X5	T49.0X6
Valium	T42.4X1	T42.4X2	T42.4X3	T42.4X4	T42.4X5	T42.4X6
Valmid	T42.6X1	T42.6X2	T42.6X3	T42.6X4	T42.6X5	T42.6X6
Valnoctamide	T42.6X1	T42.6X2	T42.6X3	T42.6X4	T42.6X5	T42.6X6
Valproate (sodium)	T42.6X1	T42.6X2	T42.6X3	T42.6X4	T42.6X5	T42.6X6
Valproic acid	T42.6X1	T42.6X2	T42.6X3	T42.6X4	T42.6X5	T42.6X6
Valpromide	T42.6X1	T42.6X2	T42.6X3	T42.6X4	T42.6X5	T42.6X6
Vanadium	T56.891	T56.892	T56.893	T56.894	—	—
Vancomycin	T36.8X1	T36.8X2	T36.8X3	T36.8X4	T36.8X5	T36.8X6
Vapor — *see also Gas*	T59.91	T59.92	T59.93	T59.94	—	—
kiln (carbon monoxide)	T58.8X1	T58.8X2	T58.8X3	T58.8X4	—	—
lead — *see lead*						
specified source NEC	T59.891	T59.892	T59.893	T59.894	—	—
Vardenafil	T46.7X1	T46.7X2	T46.7X3	T46.7X4	T46.7X5	T46.7X6
Varicose reduction drug	T46.8X1	T46.8X2	T46.8X3	T46.8X4	T46.8X5	T46.8X6
Varnish	T65.4X1	T65.4X2	T65.4X3	T65.4X4	—	—
cleaner	T52.91	T52.92	T52.93	T52.94	—	—
Vaseline	T49.3X1	T49.3X2	T49.3X3	T49.3X4	T49.3X5	T49.3X6
Vasodilan	T46.7X1	T46.7X2	T46.7X3	T46.7X4	T46.7X5	T46.7X6
Vasodilator						
coronary NEC	T46.3X1	T46.3X2	T46.3X3	T46.3X4	T46.3X5	T46.3X6
peripheral NEC	T46.7X1	T46.7X2	T46.7X3	T46.7X4	T46.7X5	T46.7X6
Vasopressin	T38.891	T38.892	T38.893	T38.894	T38.895	T38.896
Vasopressor drugs	T38.891	T38.892	T38.893	T38.894	T38.895	T38.896
Vecuronium bromide	T48.1X1	T48.1X2	T48.1X3	T48.1X4	T48.1X5	T48.1X6
Vegetable extract, astringent	T49.2X1	T49.2X2	T49.2X3	T49.2X4	T49.2X5	T49.2X6
Venlafaxine	T43.211	T43.212	T43.213	T43.214	T43.215	T43.216

Substance	External Cause (T-Code)					
	Poisoning, Accidental (Unintentional)	Poisoning, Intentional Self-Harm	Poisoning, Assault	Poisoning, Undetermined	Adverse Effect	Underdosing
Venom, venomous (bite) (sting)	T63.91	T63.92	T63.93	T63.94	—	—
amphibian NEC	T63.831	T63.832	T63.833	T63.834	—	—
animal NEC	T63.891	T63.892	T63.893	T63.894	—	—
ant	T63.421	T63.422	T63.423	T63.424	—	—
arthropod NEC	T63.481	T63.482	T63.483	T63.484	—	—
bee	T63.441	T63.442	T63.443	T63.444	—	—
centipede	T63.411	T63.412	T63.413	T63.414	—	—
fish	T63.591	T63.592	T63.593	T63.594	—	—
frog	T63.811	T63.812	T63.813	T63.814	—	—
hornet	T63.451	T63.452	T63.453	T63.454	—	—
insect NEC	T63.481	T63.482	T63.483	T63.484	—	—
lizard	T63.121	T63.122	T63.123	T63.124	—	—
marine						
animals	T63.691	T63.692	T63.693	T63.694	—	—
bluebottle	T63.611	T63.612	T63.613	T63.614	—	—
jellyfish NEC	T63.621	T63.622	T63.623	T63.624	—	—
Portugese Man-o-war	T63.611	T63.612	T63.613	T63.614	—	—
sea anemone	T63.631	T63.632	T63.633	T63.634	—	—
specified NEC	T63.691	T63.692	T63.693	T63.694	—	—
fish	T63.591	T63.592	T63.593	T63.594	—	—
plants	T63.711	T63.712	T63.713	T63.714	—	—
sting ray	T63.511	T63.512	T63.513	T63.514	—	—
millipede (tropical)	T63.411	T63.412	T63.413	T63.414	—	—
plant NEC	T63.791	T63.792	T63.793	T63.794	—	—
marine	T63.711	T63.712	T63.713	T63.714	—	—
reptile	T63.191	T63.192	T63.193	T63.194	—	—
gila monster	T63.111	T63.112	T63.113	T63.114	—	—
lizard NEC	T63.121	T63.122	T63.123	T63.124	—	—
scorpion	T63.2X1	T63.2X2	T63.2X3	T63.2X4	—	—
snake	T63.001	T63.002	T63.003	T63.004	—	—
African NEC	T63.081	T63.082	T63.083	T63.084	—	—
American (North) (South) NEC	T63.061	T63.062	T63.063	T63.064	—	—
Asian	T63.081	T63.082	T63.083	T63.084	—	—
Australian	T63.071	T63.072	T63.073	T63.074	—	—
cobra	T63.041	T63.042	T63.043	T63.044	—	—
coral snake	T63.021	T63.022	T63.023	T63.024	—	—
rattlesnake	T63.011	T63.012	T63.013	T63.014	—	—
specified NEC	T63.091	T63.092	T63.093	T63.094	—	—
taipan	T63.031	T63.032	T63.033	T63.034	—	—

Substance	Poisoning, Accidental (Unintentional)	External Cause (T-Code)				
		Poisoning, Intentional Self-Harm	Poisoning, Assault	Poisoning, Undetermined	Adverse Effect	Underdosing
Venom, venomous *(Continued)*						
specified NEC	T63.891	T63.892	T63.893	T63.894	—	—
spider	T63.301	T63.302	T63.303	T63.304	—	—
black widow	T63.311	T63.312	T63.313	T63.314	—	—
brown recluse	T63.331	T63.332	T63.333	T63.334	—	—
specified NEC	T63.391	T63.392	T63.393	T63.394	—	—
tarantula	T63.321	T63.322	T63.323	T63.324	—	—
sting ray	T63.511	T63.512	T63.513	T63.514	—	—
toad	T63.821	T63.822	T63.823	T63.824	—	—
wasp	T63.461	T63.462	T63.463	T63.464	—	—
Venous sclerosing drug NEC	T46.8X1	T46.8X2	T46.8X3	T46.8X4	T46.8X5	T46.8X6
Ventolin—*see Albuterol*						
Verapamil	T46.1X1	T46.1X2	T46.1X3	T46.1X4	T46.1X5	T46.1X6
Veramon	T42.3X1	T42.3X2	T42.3X3	T42.3X4	T42.3X5	T42.3X6
Veratrine	T46.5X1	T46.5X2	T46.5X3	T46.5X4	T46.5X5	T46.5X6
Veratrum						
album	T62.2X1	T62.2X2	T62.2X3	T62.2X4	—	—
alkaloids	T46.5X1	T46.5X2	T46.5X3	T46.5X4	T46.5X5	T46.5X6
viride	T62.2X1	T62.2X2	T62.2X3	T62.2X4	—	—
Verdigris	T60.3X1	T60.3X2	T60.3X3	T60.3X4	—	—
Veronal	T42.3X1	T42.3X2	T42.3X3	T42.3X4	T42.3X5	T42.3X6
Veroxil	T37.4X1	T37.4X2	T37.4X3	T37.4X4	T37.4X5	T37.4X6
Versenate	T50.6X1	T50.6X2	T50.6X3	T50.6X4	T50.6X5	T50.6X6
Versidyne	T39.8X1	T39.8X2	T39.8X3	T39.8X4	T39.8X5	T39.8X6
Vetrabutine	T48.0X1	T48.0X2	T48.0X3	T48.0X4	T48.0X5	T48.0X6
Vidarabine	T37.5X1	T37.5X2	T37.5X3	T37.5X4	T37.5X5	T37.5X6
Vienna						
green	T57.0X1	T57.0X2	T57.0X3	T57.0X4	—	—
insecticide	T60.2X1	T60.2X2	T60.2X3	T60.2X4	—	—
red	T57.0X1	T57.0X2	T57.0X3	T57.0X4	—	—
pharmaceutical dye	T50.991	T50.992	T50.993	T50.994	T50.995	T50.996
Vigabatrin	T42.6X1	T42.6X2	T42.6X3	T42.6X4	T42.6X5	T42.6X6
Viloxazine	T43.291	T43.292	T43.293	T43.294	T43.295	T43.296
Viminol	T39.8X1	T39.8X2	T39.8X3	T39.8X4	T39.8X5	T39.8X6
Vinbarbital, vinbarbitone	T42.3X1	T42.3X2	T42.3X3	T42.3X4	T42.3X5	T42.3X6
Vinblastine	T45.1X1	T45.1X2	T45.1X3	T45.1X4	T45.1X5	T45.1X6
Vinburnine	T46.7X1	T46.7X2	T46.7X3	T46.7X4	T46.7X5	T46.7X6
Vincamine	T45.1X1	T45.1X2	T45.1X3	T45.1X4	T45.1X5	T45.1X6
Vincristine	T45.1X1	T45.1X2	T45.1X3	T45.1X4	T45.1X5	T45.1X6
Vindesine	T45.1X1	T45.1X2	T45.1X3	T45.1X4	T45.1X5	T45.1X6

Substance	Poisoning, Accidental (Unintentional)	Poisoning, Intentional Self-Harm	Poisoning, Assault	Poisoning, Undetermined	Adverse Effect	Underdosing
	External Cause (T-Code)					
Vinesthene, vinethene	T41.0X1	T41.0X2	T41.0X3	T41.0X4	T41.0X5	T41.0X6
Vinorelbine tartrate	T45.1X1	T45.1X2	T45.1X3	T45.1X4	T45.1X5	T45.1X6
Vinpocetine	T46.7X1	T46.7X2	T46.7X3	T46.7X4	T46.7X5	T46.7X6
Vinyl						
acetate	T65.891	T65.892	T65.893	T65.894	—	—
bital	T42.3X1	T42.3X2	T42.3X3	T42.3X4	T42.3X5	T42.3X6
bromide	T65.891	T65.892	T65.893	T65.894	—	—
chloride	T59.891	T59.892	T59.893	T59.894	—	—
ether	T41.0X1	T41.0X2	T41.0X3	T41.0X4	T41.0X5	T41.0X6
Vinylbital	T42.3X1	T42.3X2	T42.3X3	T42.3X4	T42.3X5	T42.3X6
Vinylidene chloride	T65.891	T65.892	T65.893	T65.894	—	—
Vioform	T37.8X1	T37.8X2	T37.8X3	T37.8X4	T37.8X5	T37.8X6
topical	T49.0X1	T49.0X2	T49.0X3	T49.0X4	T49.0X5	T49.0X6
Viomycin	T36.8X1	T36.8X2	T36.8X3	T36.8X4	T36.8X5	T36.8X6
Viosterol	T45.2X1	T45.2X2	T45.2X3	T45.2X4	T45.2X5	T45.2X6
Viper (venom)	T63.091	T63.092	T63.093	T63.094	—	—
Viprynium	T37.4X1	T37.4X2	T37.4X3	T37.4X4	T37.4X5	T37.4X6
Viquidil	T46.7X1	T46.7X2	T46.7X3	T46.7X4	T46.7X5	T46.7X6
Viral vaccine NEC	T50.B91	T50.B92	T50.B93	T50.B94	T50.B95	T50.B96
Virginiamycin	T36.8X1	T36.8X2	T36.8X3	T36.8X4	T36.8X5	T36.8X6
Virugon	T37.5X1	T37.5X2	T37.5X3	T37.5X4	T37.5X5	T37.5X6
Viscous agent	T50.901	T50.902	T50.903	T50.904	T50.905	T50.906
Visine	T49.5X1	T49.5X2	T49.5X3	T49.5X4	T49.5X5	T49.5X6
Visnadine	T46.3X1	T46.3X2	T46.3X3	T46.3X4	T46.3X5	T46.3X6
Vitamin NEC	T45.2X1	T45.2X2	T45.2X3	T45.2X4	T45.2X5	T45.2X6
A	T45.2X1	T45.2X2	T45.2X3	T45.2X4	T45.2X5	T45.2X6
B NEC	T45.2X1	T45.2X2	T45.2X3	T45.2X4	T45.2X5	T45.2X6
nicotinic acid	T46.7X1	T46.7X2	T46.7X3	T46.7X4	T46.7X5	T46.7X6
B1	T45.2X1	T45.2X2	T45.2X3	T45.2X4	T45.2X5	T45.2X6
B2	T45.2X1	T45.2X2	T45.2X3	T45.2X4	T45.2X5	T45.2X6
B6	T45.2X1	T45.2X2	T45.2X3	T45.2X4	T45.2X5	T45.2X6
B12	T45.2X1	T45.2X2	T45.2X3	T45.2X4	T45.2X5	T45.2X6
B15	T45.2X1	T45.2X2	T45.2X3	T45.2X4	T45.2X5	T45.2X6
C	T45.2X1	T45.2X2	T45.2X3	T45.2X4	T45.2X5	T45.2X6
D	T45.2X1	T45.2X2	T45.2X3	T45.2X4	T45.2X5	T45.2X6
D2	T45.2X1	T45.2X2	T45.2X3	T45.2X4	T45.2X5	T45.2X6
D3	T45.2X1	T45.2X2	T45.2X3	T45.2X4	T45.2X5	T45.2X6
E	T45.2X1	T45.2X2	T45.2X3	T45.2X4	T45.2X5	T45.2X6
E acetate	T45.2X1	T45.2X2	T45.2X3	T45.2X4	T45.2X5	T45.2X6
hematopoietic	T45.8X1	T45.8X2	T45.8X3	T45.8X4	T45.8X5	T45.8X6

Substance	External Cause (T-Code)					
	Poisoning, Accidental (Unintentional)	Poisoning, Intentional Self-Harm	Poisoning, Assault	Poisoning, Undetermined	Adverse Effect	Underdosing
Vitamin NEC *(Continued)*						
K NEC	T45.7X1	T45.7X2	T45.7X3	T45.7X4	T45.7X5	T45.7X6
K1	T45.7X1	T45.7X2	T45.7X3	T45.7X4	T45.7X5	T45.7X6
K2	T45.7X1	T45.7X2	T45.7X3	T45.7X4	T45.7X5	T45.7X6
PP	T45.2X1	T45.2X2	T45.2X3	T45.2X4	T45.2X5	T45.2X6
ulceroprotectant	T47.1X1	T47.1X2	T47.1X3	T47.1X4	T47.1X5	T47.1X6
Vleminckx's solution	T49.4X1	T49.4X2	T49.4X3	T49.4X4	T49.4X5	T49.4X6
Voltaren — *see Diclofenac sodium*						
W						
Warfarin	T45.511	T45.512	T45.513	T45.514	T45.515	T45.516
rodenticide	T60.4X1	T60.4X2	T60.4X3	T60.4X4	—	—
sodium	T60.4X1	T60.4X2	T60.4X3	T60.4X4	—	—
Wasp (sting)	T63.461	T63.462	T63.463	T63.464	—	—
Water						
balance drug	T50.3X1	T50.3X2	T50.3X3	T50.3X4	T50.3X5	T50.3X6
distilled	T50.3X1	T50.3X2	T50.3X3	T50.3X4	T50.3X5	T50.3X6
gas — *see Gas, water*						
incomplete combustion of — *see Carbon, monoxide, fuel, utility*						
hemlock	T62.2X1	T62.2X2	T62.2X3	T62.2X4	—	—
moccasin (venom)	T63.061	T63.062	T63.063	T63.064	—	—
purified	T50.3X1	T50.3X2	T50.3X3	T50.3X4	T50.3X5	T50.3X6
Wax (paraffin) (petroleum)	T52.0X1	T52.0X2	T52.0X3	T52.0X4	—	—
automobile	T65.891	T65.892	T65.893	T65.894	—	—
floor	T52.0X1	T52.0X2	T52.0X3	T52.0X4	—	—
Weed killers NEC	T60.3X1	T60.3X2	T60.3X3	T60.3X4	—	—
Welldorm	T42.6X1	T42.6X2	T42.6X3	T42.6X4	T42.6X5	T42.6X6
White						
arsenic	T57.0X1	T57.0X2	T57.0X3	T57.0X4	—	—
hellebore	T62.2X1	T62.2X2	T62.2X3	T62.2X4	—	—
lotion (keratolytic)	T49.4X1	T49.4X2	T49.4X3	T49.4X4	T49.4X5	T49.4X6
spirit	T52.0X1	T52.0X2	T52.0X3	T52.0X4	—	—
Whitewash	T65.891	T65.892	T65.893	T65.894	—	—
Whole blood (human)	T45.8X1	T45.8X2	T45.8X3	T45.8X4	T45.8X5	T45.8X6
Wild						
black cherry	T62.2X1	T62.2X2	T62.2X3	T62.2X4	—	—
poisonous plants NEC	T62.2X1	T62.2X2	T62.2X3	T62.2X4	—	—
Window cleaning fluid	T65.891	T65.892	T65.893	T65.894	—	—
Wintergreen (oil)	T49.3X1	T49.3X2	T49.3X3	T49.3X4	T49.3X5	T49.3X6

Substance	Poisoning, Accidental (Unintentional)	Poisoning, Intentional Self-Harm	Poisoning, Assault	Poisoning, Undetermined	Adverse Effect	Underdosing
		External Cause (T-Code)				
Wisterine	T62.2X1	T62.2X2	T62.2X3	T62.2X4	—	—
Witch hazel	T49.2X1	T49.2X2	T49.2X3	T49.2X4	T49.2X5	T49.2X6
Wood alcohol or spirit	T51.1X1	T51.1X2	T51.1X3	T51.1X4	—	—
Wool fat (hydrous)	T49.3X1	T49.3X2	T49.3X3	T49.3X4	T49.3X5	T49.3X6
Woorali	T48.1X1	T48.1X2	T48.1X3	T48.1X4	T48.1X5	T48.1X6
Wormseed, American	T37.4X1	T37.4X2	T37.4X3	T37.4X4	T37.4X5	T37.4X6
X						
Xamoterol	T44.5X1	T44.5X2	T44.5X3	T44.5X4	T44.5X5	T44.5X6
Xanthine diuretics	T50.2X1	T50.2X2	T50.2X3	T50.2X4	T50.2X5	T50.2X6
Xanthinol nicotinate	T46.7X1	T46.7X2	T46.7X3	T46.7X4	T46.7X5	T46.7X6
Xanthotoxin	T49.3X1	T49.3X2	T49.3X3	T49.3X4	T49.3X5	T49.3X6
Xantinol nicotinate	T46.7X1	T46.7X2	T46.7X3	T46.7X4	T46.7X5	T46.7X6
Xantocillin	T36.0X1	T36.0X2	T36.0X3	T36.0X4	T36.0X5	T36.0X6
Xenon (127Xe) (133Xe)	T50.8X1	T50.8X2	T50.8X3	T50.8X4	T50.8X5	T50.8X6
Xenysalate	T49.4X1	T49.4X2	T49.4X3	T49.4X4	T49.4X5	T49.4X6
Xibornol	T37.8X1	T37.8X2	T37.8X3	T37.8X4	T37.8X5	T37.8X6
Xigris	T45.511	T45.512	T45.513	T45.514	T45.515	T45.516
Xipamide	T50.2X1	T50.2X2	T50.2X3	T50.2X4	T50.2X5	T50.2X6
Xylene (vapor)	T52.2X1	T52.2X2	T52.2X3	T52.2X4	—	—
Xylocaine (infiltration) (topical)	T41.3X1	T41.3X2	T41.3X3	T41.3X4	T41.3X5	T41.3X6
nerve block (peripheral) (plexus)	T41.3X1	T41.3X2	T41.3X3	T41.3X4	T41.3X5	T41.3X6
spinal	T41.3X1	T41.3X2	T41.3X3	T41.3X4	T41.3X5	T41.3X6
Xylol (vapor)	T52.2X1	T52.2X2	T52.2X3	T52.2X4	—	—
Xylometazoline	T48.5X1	T48.5X2	T48.5X3	T48.5X4	T48.5X5	T48.5X6
Y						
Yeast	T45.2X1	T45.2X2	T45.2X3	T45.2X4	T45.2X5	T45.2X6
dried	T45.2X1	T45.2X2	T45.2X3	T45.2X4	T45.2X5	T45.2X6
Yellow						
fever vaccine	T50.B91	T50.B92	T50.B93	T50.B94	T50.B95	T50.B96
jasmine	T62.2X1	T62.2X2	T62.2X3	T62.2X4	—	—
phenolphthalein	T47.2X1	T47.2X2	T47.2X3	T47.2X4	T47.2X5	T47.2X6
Yew	T62.2X1	T62.2X2	T62.2X3	T62.2X4	—	—
Yohimbic acid	T40.991	T40.992	T40.993	T40.994	T40.995	T40.996
Z						
Zactane	T39.8X1	T39.8X2	T39.8X3	T39.8X4	T39.8X5	T39.8X6
Zalcitabine	T37.5X1	T37.5X2	T37.5X3	T37.5X4	T37.5X5	T37.5X6
Zaroxolyn	T50.2X1	T50.2X2	T50.2X3	T50.2X4	T50.2X5	T50.2X6

TABLE OF DRUGS AND CHEMICALS

Substance	Poisoning, Accidental (Unintentional)	Poisoning, Intentional Self-Harm	Poisoning, Assault	Poisoning, Undetermined	Adverse Effect	Underdosing
Zephiran (topical)	T49.0X1	T49.0X2	T49.0X3	T49.0X4	T49.0X5	T49.0X6
ophthalmic preparation	T49.5X1	T49.5X2	T49.5X3	T49.5X4	T49.5X5	T49.5X6
Zeranol	T38.7X1	T38.7X2	T38.7X3	T38.7X4	T38.7X5	T38.7X6
Zerone	T51.1X1	T51.1X2	T51.1X3	T51.1X4	—	—
Zidovudine	T37.5X1	T37.5X2	T37.5X3	T37.5X4	T37.5X5	T37.5X6
Zimeldine	T43.221	T43.222	T43.223	T43.224	T43.225	T43.226
Zinc (compounds) (fumes) (vapor) NEC	T56.5X1	T56.5X2	T56.5X3	T56.5X4	—	—
anti-infectives	T49.0X1	T49.0X2	T49.0X3	T49.0X4	T49.0X5	T49.0X6
antivaricose	T46.8X1	T46.8X2	T46.8X3	T46.8X4	T46.8X5	T46.8X6
bacitracin	T49.0X1	T49.0X2	T49.0X3	T49.0X4	T49.0X5	T49.0X6
chloride (mouthwash)	T49.6X1	T49.6X2	T49.6X3	T49.6X4	T49.6X5	T49.6X6
chromate	T56.5X1	T56.5X2	T56.5X3	T56.5X4	—	—
gelatin	T49.3X1	T49.3X2	T49.3X3	T49.3X4	T49.3X5	T49.3X6
oxide	T49.3X1	T49.3X2	T49.3X3	T49.3X4	T49.3X5	T49.3X6
plaster	T49.3X1	T49.3X2	T49.3X3	T49.3X4	T49.3X5	T49.3X6
peroxide	T49.0X1	T49.0X2	T49.0X3	T49.0X4	T49.0X5	T49.0X6
pesticides	T56.5X1	T56.5X2	T56.5X3	T56.5X4	—	—
phosphide	T60.4X1	T60.4X2	T60.4X3	T60.4X4	—	—
pyrithionate	T49.4X1	T49.4X2	T49.4X3	T49.4X4	T49.4X5	T49.4X6
stearate	T49.3X1	T49.3X2	T49.3X3	T49.3X4	T49.3X5	T49.3X6
sulfate	T49.5X1	T49.5X2	T49.5X3	T49.5X4	T49.5X5	T49.5X6
ENT agent	T49.6X1	T49.6X2	T49.6X3	T49.6X4	T49.6X5	T49.6X6
ophthalmic solution	T49.5X1	T49.5X2	T49.5X3	T49.5X4	T49.5X5	T49.5X6
topical NEC	T49.0X1	T49.0X2	T49.0X3	T49.0X4	T49.0X5	T49.0X6
undecylenate	T49.0X1	T49.0X2	T49.0X3	T49.0X4	T49.0X5	T49.0X6
Zineb	T60.0X1	T60.0X2	T60.0X3	T60.0X4	—	—
Zinostatin	T45.1X1	T45.1X2	T45.1X3	T45.1X4	T45.1X5	T45.1X6
Zipeprol	T48.3X1	T48.3X2	T48.3X3	T48.3X4	T48.3X5	T48.3X6
Zofenopril	T46.4X1	T46.4X2	T46.4X3	T46.4X4	T46.4X5	T46.4X6
Zolpidem	T42.6X1	T42.6X2	T42.6X3	T42.6X4	T42.6X5	T42.6X6
Zomepirac	T39.391	T39.392	T39.393	T39.394	T39.395	T39.396
Zopiclone	T42.6X1	T42.6X2	T42.6X3	T42.6X4	T42.6X5	T42.6X6
Zorubicin	T45.1X1	T45.1X2	T45.1X3	T45.1X4	T45.1X5	T45.1X6
Zotepine	T43.591	T43.592	T43.593	T43.594	T43.595	T43.596
Zovant	T45.511	T45.512	T45.513	T45.514	T45.515	T45.516
Zoxazolamine	T42.8X1	T42.8X2	T42.8X3	T42.8X4	T42.8X5	T42.8X6
Zuclopenthixol	T43.4X1	T43.4X2	T43.4X3	T43.4X4	T43.4X5	T43.4X6
Zygadenus (venenosus)	T62.2X1	T62.2X2	T62.2X3	T62.2X4	—	—
Zyprexa	T43.591	T43.592	T43.593	T43.594	T43.595	T43.596

External Cause
of Injuries Index

A

Abandonment (causing exposure to weather conditions) (with intent to injure or kill) NEC X58

Abuse (adult) (child) (mental) (physical) (sexual) X58

Accident (to) X58

  aircraft (in transit) (powered) —see also Accident, transport, aircraft

    due to, caused by cataclysm —see Forces of nature, by type

  animal-drawn vehicle —see Accident, transport, animal-drawn vehicle occupant

  animal-rider —see Accident, transport, animal-rider

  automobile —see Accident, transport, car occupant

  bare foot water skiier V94.4

  boat, boating —see also Accident, watercraft

    striking swimmer

      powered V94.11

      unpowered V94.12

  bus —see Accident, transport, bus occupant

  cable car, not on rails V98.0

    on rails —see Accident, transport, streetcar occupant

  car —see Accident, transport, car occupant

  caused by, due to

    animal NEC W64

    chain hoist W24.0

    cold (excessive) —see Exposure, cold

    corrosive liquid, substance —see Table of drugs and chemicals

    cutting or piercing instrument — see Contact, with, by type of instrument

    drive belt W24.0

    electric

      current —see Exposure, electric current

      motor (see also Contact, with, by type of machine) W31.3

      current (of) W86.8

    environmental factor NEC X58

    explosive material —see Explosion

    fire, flames —see Exposure, fire

    firearm missile —see Discharge, firearm by type

    heat (excessive) —see Heat

    hot —see Contact, with, hot

    ignition —see Ignition

    lifting device W24.0

    lightning —see subcategory T75.0

      causing fire —see Exposure, fire

    machine, machinery —see Contact, with, by type of machine

    natural factor NEC X58

    pulley (block) W24.0

    radiation —see Radiation

    steam X13.1

      inhalation X13.0

      pipe X16

    thunderbolt —see subcategory T75.0

      causing fire —see Exposure, fire

    transmission device W24.1

  coach —see Accident, transport, bus occupant

Accident (Continued)

  coal car —see Accident, transport, industrial vehicle occupant

  diving —see also Fall, into, water

    with

      drowning or submersion —see Drowning

  forklift —see Accident, transport, industrial vehicle occupant

  heavy transport vehicle NOS —see Accident, transport, truck occupant

  ice yacht V98.2

  in

    medical, surgical procedure

      as, or due to misadventure —see Misadventure

      causing an abnormal reaction or later complication without mention of misadventure (see also Complication of or following, by type of procedure) Y84.9

  land yacht V98.1

  late effect of —see W00-X58 with 7th character S

  logging car —see Accident, transport, industrial vehicle occupant

  machine, machinery —see also Contact, with, by type of machine

    on board watercraft V93.69

      explosion —see Explosion, in, watercraft

      fire —see Burn, on board watercraft

      powered craft V93.63

        ferry boat V93.61

        fishing boat V93.62

        jetskis V93.63

        liner V93.61

        merchant ship V93.60

        passenger ship V93.61

        sailboat V93.64

  mine tram —see Accident, transport, industrial vehicle occupant

  mobility scooter (motorized) —see Accident, transport, pedestrian, conveyance, specified type NEC

  motor scooter —see Accident, transport, motorcyclist

  motor vehicle NOS (traffic) (see also Accident, transport) V89.2

    nontraffic V89.0

    three-wheeled NOS —see Accident, transport, three-wheeled motor vehicle occupant

  motorcycle NOS —see Accident, transport, motorcyclist

  nonmotor vehicle NOS (nontraffic) (see also Accident, transport) V89.1

    traffic NOS V89.3

  nontraffic (victim's mode of transport NOS) V88.9

    collision (between) V88.7

      bus and truck V88.5

      car and:

        bus V88.3

        pickup V88.2

        three-wheeled motor vehicle V88.0

        train V88.6

        truck V88.4

        two-wheeled motor vehicle V88.0

        van V88.2

      specified vehicle NEC and:

        three-wheeled motor vehicle V88.1

        two-wheeled motor vehicle V88.1

Accident (Continued)

  nontraffic (Continued)

    known mode of transport —see Accident, transport, by type of vehicle

    noncollision V88.8

  on board watercraft V93.89

    powered craft V93.83

      ferry boat V93.81

      fishing boat V93.82

      jetskis V93.83

      liner V93.81

      merchant ship V93.80

      passenger ship V93.81

    unpowered craft V93.88

      canoe V93.85

      inflatable V93.86

        in tow

          recreational V94.31

          specified NEC V94.32

      kayak V93.85

      sailboat V93.84

      surf-board V93.88

      water skis V93.87

      windsurfer V93.88

  parachutist V97.29

    entangled in object V97.21

    injured on landing V97.22

  pedal cycle —see Accident, transport, pedal cyclist

  pedestrian (on foot)

    with

      another pedestrian W51

        with fall W03

          due to ice or snow W00.0

        on pedestrian conveyance NEC V00.09

      roller skater (in-line) V00.01

      skate boarder V00.02

      transport vehicle —see Accident, transport

    on pedestrian conveyance —see Accident, transport, pedestrian, conveyance

  pick-up truck or van —see Accident, transport, pickup truck occupant

  quarry truck —see Accident, transport, industrial vehicle occupant

  railway vehicle (any) (in motion) — see Accident, transport, railway vehicle occupant

    due to cataclysm —see Forces of nature, by type

  scooter (non-motorized) —see Accident, transport, pedestrian, conveyance, scooter

  sequelae of —see W00-X58 with 7th character S

  skateboard —see Accident, transport, pedestrian, conveyance, skateboard

  ski (ing) —see Accident, transport, pedestrian, conveyance

    lift V98.3

  specified cause NEC X58

  streetcar —see Accident, transport, streetcar occupant

  traffic (victim's mode of transport NOS) V87.9

    collision (between) V87.7

      bus and truck V87.5

      car and:

        bus V87.3

Accident *(Continued)*
 traffic *(Continued)*
  collision *(Continued)*
   car and: *(Continued)*
    pickup V87.2
    three-wheeled motor vehicle V87.0
    train V87.6
    truck V87.4
    two-wheeled motor vehicle V87.0
    van V87.2
    specified vehicle NEC and:
     three-wheeled motor vehicle
      V87.1
     two-wheeled motor vehicle V87.1
   known mode of transport —*see*
    Accident, transport, by type of
    vehicle
  noncollision V87.8
 transport (involving injury to) V99
  18 wheeler —*see* Accident, transport,
   truck occupant
  agricultural vehicle occupant
   (nontraffic) V84.9
   driver V84.5
   hanger-on V84.7
   passenger V84.6
   traffic V84.3
    driver V84.0
    hanger-on V84.2
    passenger V84.1
   while boarding or alighting V84.4
  aircraft NEC V97.89
   military NEC V97.818
    with civilian aircraft V97.810
    civilian injured by V97.811
   occupant injured (in)
    nonpowered craft accident V96.9
     balloon V96.00
      collision V96.03
      crash V96.01
      explosion V96.05
      fire V96.04
      forced landing V96.02
      specified type NEC V96.09
     glider V96.20
      collision V96.23
      crash V96.21
      explosion V96.25
      fire V96.24
      forced landing V96.22
      specified type NEC V96.29
     hang glider V96.10
      collision V96.13
      crash V96.11
      explosion V96.15
      fire V96.14
      forced landing V96.12
      specified type NEC V96.19
     specified craft NEC V96.8
    powered craft accident V95.9
     fixed wing NEC
      commercial V95.30
       collision V95.33
       crash V95.31
       explosion V95.35
       fire V95.34
       forced landing V95.32
       specified type NEC V95.39
      private V95.20
       collision V95.23
       crash V95.21
       explosion V95.25
       fire V95.24
       forced landing V95.22
       specified type NEC V95.29

Accident *(Continued)*
 transport *(Continued)*
  aircraft NEC *(Continued)*
   occupant injured *(Continued)*
    powered craft accident
     (Continued)
     glider V95.10
      collision V95.13
      crash V95.11
      explosion V95.15
      fire V95.14
      forced landing V95.12
      specified type NEC V95.19
     helicopter V95.00
      collision V95.03
      crash V95.01
      explosion V95.05
      fire V95.04
      forced landing V95.02
      specified type NEC V95.09
     spacecraft V95.40
      collision V95.43
      crash V95.41
      explosion V95.45
      fire V95.44
      forced landing V95.42
      specified type NEC V95.49
     specified craft NEC V95.8
     ultralight V95.10
      collision V95.13
      crash V95.11
      explosion V95.15
      fire V95.14
      forced landing V95.12
      specified type NEC V95.19
    specified accident NEC V97.0
    while boarding or alighting
     V97.1
   person (injured by)
    falling from, in or on aircraft
     V97.0
    machinery on aircraft V97.89
    on ground with aircraft
     involvement V97.39
    rotating propeller V97.32
    struck by object falling from
     aircraft V97.31
    sucked into aircraft jet V97.33
    while boarding or alighting
     aircraft V97.1
  airport (battery-powered) passenger
   vehicle —*see* Accident, transport,
   industrial vehicle occupant
  all-terrain vehicle occupant
   (nontraffic) V86.99
   driver V86.59
   dune buggy —*see* Accident,
    transport, dune buggy
    occupant
   hanger-on V86.79
   passenger V86.69
   snowmobile —*see* Accident,
    transport, snowmobile
    occupant
   traffic V86.39
    driver V86.09
    hanger-on V86.29
    passenger V86.19
   while boarding or alighting
    V86.49
  ambulance occupant (traffic) V86.31
   driver V86.01
   hanger-on V86.21
   nontraffic V86.91
    driver V86.51

Accident *(Continued)*
 transport *(Continued)*
  ambulance occupant *(Continued)*
    passenger V86.11
   while boarding or alighting
    V86.41
  animal-drawn vehicle occupant (in)
   V80.929
   collision (with)
    animal V80.12
     being ridden V80.711
    animal-drawn vehicle
     V80.721
    bus V80.42
    car V80.42
    fixed or stationary object
     V80.82
    military vehicle V80.920
    nonmotor vehicle V80.791
    pedal cycle V80.22
    pedestrian V80.12
    pickup V80.42
    railway train or vehicle V80.62
    specified motor vehicle NEC
     V80.52
    streetcar V80.731
    truck V80.42
    two-or three-wheeled motor
     vehicle V80.32
    van V80.42
   noncollision V80.02
   specified circumstance NEC V80. 928
  animal-rider V80.919
   collision (with)
    animal V80.11
     being ridden V80.710
    animal-drawn vehicle V80.720
    bus V80.41
    car V80.41
    fixed or stationary object V80.81
    military vehicle V80.910
    nonmotor vehicle V80.790
    pedal cycle V80.21
    pedestrian V80.11
    pickup V80.41
    railway train or vehicle V80.61
    specified motor vehicle NEC
     V80.51
    streetcar V80.730
    truck V80.41
    two- or three-wheeled motor
     vehicle V80.31
    van V80.41
   noncollision V80.018
    specified as horse rider V80.010
   specified circumstance NEC V80.918
  armored car —*see* Accident,
   transport, truck occupant
  battery-powered truck (baggage)
   (mail) —*see* Accident, transport,
   industrial vehicle occupant
  bus occupant V79.9
   collision (with)
    animal (traffic) V70.9
     being ridden (traffic) V76.9
      nontraffic V76.3
       while boarding or alighting
        V76.4
     nontraffic V70.3
      while boarding or alighting
       V70.4
    animal-drawn vehicle (traffic)
     V76.9
     nontraffic V76.3
      while boarding or alighting V76.4

Accident *(Continued)*
  transport *(Continued)*
    bus occupant *(Continued)*
      collision *(Continued)*
        bus (traffic) V74.9
          nontraffic V74.3
            while boarding or alighting
              V74.4
        car (traffic) V73.9
          nontraffic V73.3
            while boarding or alighting
              V73.4
        motor vehicle NOS (traffic)
          V79.60
          nontraffic V79.20
            specified type NEC (traffic)
              V79.69
              nontraffic V79.29
        pedal cycle (traffic) V71.9
          nontraffic V71.3
            while boarding or alighting
              V71.4
        pickup truck (traffic) V73.9
          nontraffic V73.3
            while boarding or alighting
              V73.4
        railway vehicle (traffic) V75.9
          nontraffic V75.3
            while boarding or alighting
              V75.4
        specified vehicle NEC (traffic)
          V76.9
          nontraffic V76.3
            while boarding or alighting
              V76.4
        stationary object (traffic) V77.9
          nontraffic V77.3
            while boarding or alighting
              V77.4
        streetcar (traffic) V76.9
          nontraffic V76.3
            while boarding or alighting
              V76.4
        three wheeled motor vehicle
          (traffic) V72.9
          nontraffic V72.3
            while boarding or alighting
              V72.4
        truck (traffic) V74.9
          nontraffic V74.3
            while boarding or alighting
              V74.4
        two wheeled motor vehicle
          (traffic) V72.9
          nontraffic V72.3
            while boarding or alighting
              V72.4
        van (traffic) V73.9
          nontraffic V73.3
            while boarding or alighting V73.4
      driver
        collision (with)
          animal (traffic) V70.5
            being ridden (traffic) V76.5
              nontraffic V76.0
            nontraffic V70.0
          animal-drawn vehicle (traffic)
            V76.5
            nontraffic V76.0
          bus (traffic) V74.5
            nontraffic V74.0
          car (traffic) V73.5
            nontraffic V73.0
          motor vehicle NOS (traffic)
            V79.40

Accident *(Continued)*
  transport *(Continued)*
    bus occupant *(Continued)*
      driver *(Continued)*
        collision *(Continued)*
          motor vehicle NOS *(Continued)*
            nontraffic V79.00
            specified type NEC (traffic)
              V79.49
              nontraffic V79.09
          pedal cycle (traffic) V71.5
            nontraffic V71.0
          pickup truck (traffic) V73.5
            nontraffic V73.0
          railway vehicle (traffic) V75.5
            nontraffic V75.0
          specified vehicle NEC (traffic)
            V76.5
            nontraffic V76.0
          stationary object (traffic) V77.5
            nontraffic V77.0
          streetcar (traffic) V76.5
            nontraffic V76.0
          three wheeled motor vehicle
            (traffic) V72.5
            nontraffic V72.0
          truck (traffic) V74.5
            nontraffic V74.0
          two wheeled motor vehicle
            (traffic) V72.5
            nontraffic V72.0
          van (traffic) V73.5
            nontraffic V73.0
        noncollision accident (traffic)
          V78.5
          nontraffic V78.0
      hanger-on
        collision (with)
          animal (traffic) V70.7
            being ridden (traffic) V76.7
              nontraffic V76.2
            nontraffic V70.2
          animal-drawn vehicle (traffic)
            V76.7
            nontraffic V76.2
          bus (traffic) V74.7
            nontraffic V74.2
          car (traffic) V73.7
            nontraffic V73.2
          pedal cycle (traffic) V71.7
            nontraffic V71.2
          pickup truck (traffic) V73.7
            nontraffic V73.2
          railway vehicle (traffic) V75.7
            nontraffic V75.2
          specified vehicle NEC (traffic)
            V76.7
            nontraffic V76.2
          stationary object (traffic) V77.7
            nontraffic V77.2
          streetcar (traffic) V76.7
            nontraffic V76.2
          three wheeled motor vehicle
            (traffic) V72.7
            nontraffic V72.2
          truck (traffic) V74.7
            nontraffic V74.2
          two wheeled motor vehicle
            (traffic) V72.7
            nontraffic V72.2
          van (traffic) V73.7
            nontraffic V73.2
        noncollision accident (traffic)
          V78.7
          nontraffic V78.2

Accident *(Continued)*
  transport *(Continued)*
    bus occupant *(Continued)*
      noncollision accident (traffic) V78.9
        nontraffic V78.3
          while boarding or alighting V78.4
      nontraffic V79.3
      passenger
        collision (with)
          animal (traffic) V70.6
            being ridden (traffic) V76.6
              nontraffic V76.1
            nontraffic V70.1
          animal-drawn vehicle (traffic)
            V76.6
            nontraffic V76.1
          bus (traffic) V74.6
            nontraffic V74.1
          car (traffic) V73.6
            nontraffic V73.1
          motor vehicle NOS (traffic)
            V79.50
            nontraffic V79.10
            specified type NEC (traffic)
              V79.59
              nontraffic V79.19
          pedal cycle (traffic) V71.6
            nontraffic V71.1
          pickup truck (traffic) V73.6
            nontraffic V73.1
          railway vehicle (traffic) V75.6
            nontraffic V75.1
          specified vehicle NEC (traffic)
            V76.6
            nontraffic V76.1
          stationary object (traffic) V77.6
            nontraffic V77.1
          streetcar (traffic) V76.6
            nontraffic V76.1
          three wheeled motor vehicle
            (traffic) V72.6
            nontraffic V72.1
          truck (traffic) V74.6
            nontraffic V74.1
          two wheeled motor vehicle
            (traffic) V72.6
            nontraffic V72.1
          van (traffic) V73.6
            nontraffic V73.1
        noncollision accident (traffic)
          V78.6
          nontraffic V78.1
      specified type NEC V79.88
        military vehicle V79.81
    cable car, not on rails V98.0
      on rails —*see* Accident, transport,
        streetcar occupant
    car occupant V49.9
      ambulance occupant —*see*
        Accident, transport,
        ambulance occupant
      collision (with)
        animal (traffic) V40.9
          being ridden (traffic) V46.9
            nontraffic V46.3
              while boarding or alighting
                V46.4
          nontraffic V40.3
            while boarding or alighting
              V40.4
        animal-drawn vehicle (traffic)
          V46.9
          nontraffic V46.3
            while boarding or alighting
              V46.4

Accident (Continued)
  transport (Continued)
    coal car —see Accident, transport,
      industrial vehicle occupant
    construction vehicle occupant
      (nontraffic) V85.9
      driver V85.5
      hanger-on V85.7
      passenger V85.6
      traffic V85.3
        driver V85.0
        hanger-on V85.2
        passenger V85.1
      while boarding or alighting V85.4
    dirt bike rider —see Accident, transport,
      all-terrain vehicle occupant
    due to cataclysm —see Forces of
      nature, by type
    dune buggy occupant (nontraffic)
      V86.93
      driver V86.53
      hanger-on V86.73
      passenger V86.63
      traffic V86.33
        driver V86.03
        hanger-on V86.23
        passenger V86.13
      while boarding or alighting
        V86.43
    forklift —see Accident, transport,
      industrial vehicle occupant
    go cart —see Accident, transport,
      all-terrain vehicle occupant
    golf cart —see Accident, transport,
      all-terrain vehicle occupant
    heavy transport vehicle occupant —
      see Accident, transport, truck
      occupant
    ice yacht V98.2
    industrial vehicle occupant
      (nontraffic) V83.9
      driver V83.5
      hanger-on V83.7
      passenger V83.6
      traffic V83.3
        driver V83.0
        hanger-on V83.2
        passenger V83.1
      while boarding or alighting V83.4
    interurban electric car —see Accident,
      transport, streetcar
    land yacht V98.1
    logging car —see Accident, transport,
      industrial vehicle occupant
    military vehicle occupant (traffic)
      V86.34
      driver V86.04
      hanger-on V86.24
      nontraffic V86.94
        driver V86.54
        hanger-on V86.74
        passenger V86.64
      passenger V86.14
      while boarding or alighting
        V86.44
    mine tram —see Accident, transport,
      industrial vehicle occupant
    motor vehicle NEC occupant (traffic)
      V86.39
      driver V86.09
      hanger-on V86.29
      nontraffic V86.99
        driver V86.59
        hanger-on V86.79
        passenger V86.69

Accident (Continued)
  transport (Continued)
    motor vehicle NEC occupant
      (Continued)
      passenger V86.19
      while boarding or alighting V86.49
    motorcoach —see Accident, transport,
      bus occupant
    motorcyclist V29.9
      collision (with)
        animal (traffic) V20.9
          being ridden (traffic) V26.9
            nontraffic V26.2
            while boarding or alighting
              V26.3
          nontraffic V20.2
          while boarding or alighting
            V20.3
        animal-drawn vehicle (traffic)
          V26.9
          nontraffic V26.2
          while boarding or alighting
            V26.3
        bus (traffic) V24.9
          nontraffic V24.2
          while boarding or alighting
            V24.3
        car (traffic) V23.9
          nontraffic V23.2
          while boarding or alighting
            V23.3
        motor vehicle NOS (traffic)
          V29.60
          nontraffic V29.20
          specified type NEC (traffic)
            V29.69
            nontraffic V29.29
        pedal cycle (traffic) V21.9
          nontraffic V21.2
          while boarding or alighting
            V21.3
        pickup truck (traffic) V23.9
          nontraffic V23.2
          while boarding or alighting
            V23.3
        railway vehicle (traffic) V25.9
          nontraffic V25.2
          while boarding or alighting
            V25.3
        specified vehicle NEC (traffic)
          V26.9
          nontraffic V26.2
          while boarding or alighting
            V26.3
        stationary object (traffic) V27.9
          nontraffic V27.2
          while boarding or alighting
            V27.3
        streetcar (traffic) V26.9
          nontraffic V26.2
          while boarding or alighting
            V26.3
        three wheeled motor vehicle
          (traffic) V22.9
          nontraffic V22.2
          while boarding or alighting
            V22.3
        truck (traffic) V24.9
          nontraffic V24.2
          while boarding or alighting V24.3
        two wheeled motor vehicle
          (traffic) V22.9
          nontraffic V22.2
          while boarding or alighting
            V22.3

Accident (Continued)
  transport (Continued)
    motorcyclist (Continued)
      collision (Continued)
        van (traffic) V23.9
          nontraffic V23.2
          while boarding or alighting V23.3
      driver
        collision (with)
          animal (traffic) V20.4
            being ridden (traffic) V26.4
              nontraffic V26.0
            nontraffic V20.0
          animal-drawn vehicle (traffic)
            V26.4
            nontraffic V26.0
          bus (traffic) V24.4
            nontraffic V24.0
          car (traffic) V23.4
            nontraffic V23.0
          motor vehicle NOS (traffic)
            V29.40
            nontraffic V29.00
            specified type NEC (traffic)
              V29.49
              nontraffic V29.09
          pedal cycle (traffic) V21.4
            nontraffic V21.0
          pickup truck (traffic) V23.4
            nontraffic V23.0
          railway vehicle (traffic) V25.4
            nontraffic V25.0
          specified vehicle NEC (traffic)
            V26.4
            nontraffic V26.0
          stationary object (traffic) V27.4
            nontraffic V27.0
          streetcar (traffic) V26.4
            nontraffic V26.0
          three wheeled motor vehicle
            (traffic) V22.4
            nontraffic V22.0
          truck (traffic) V24.4
            nontraffic V24.0
          two wheeled motor vehicle
            (traffic) V22.4
            nontraffic V22.0
          van (traffic) V23.4
            nontraffic V23.0
          noncollision accident (traffic)
            V28.4
            nontraffic V28.0
      noncollision accident (traffic) V28.9
        nontraffic V28.2
        while boarding or alighting V28.3
      nontraffic V29.3
      passenger
        collision (with)
          animal (traffic) V20.5
            being ridden (traffic) V26.5
              nontraffic V26.1
            nontraffic V20.1
          animal-drawn vehicle (traffic)
            V26.5
            nontraffic V26.1
          bus (traffic) V24.5
            nontraffic V24.1
          car (traffic) V23.5
            nontraffic V23.1
          motor vehicle NOS (traffic)
            V29.50
            nontraffic V29.10
            specified type NEC (traffic)
              V29.59
              nontraffic V29.19

Accident *(Continued)*
  transport *(Continued)*
    pedal cyclist *(Continued)*
      collision *(Continued)*
        animal *(Continued)*
          nontraffic V10.2
          while boarding or alighting
            V10.3
        animal-drawn vehicle (traffic) V16.9
          nontraffic V16.2
          while boarding or alighting
            V16.3
        bus (traffic) V14.9
          nontraffic V14.2
          while boarding or alighting
            V14.3
        car (traffic) V13.9
          nontraffic V13.2
          while boarding or alighting
            V13.3
        motor vehicle NOS (traffic)
          V19.60
          nontraffic V19.20
          specified type NEC (traffic)
          V19.69
          nontraffic V19.29
        pedal cycle (traffic) V11.9
          nontraffic V11.2
          while boarding or alighting
            V11.3
        pickup truck (traffic) V13.9
          nontraffic V13.2
          while boarding or alighting
            V13.3
        railway vehicle (traffic) V15.9
          nontraffic V15.2
          while boarding or alighting
            V15.3
        specified vehicle NEC (traffic)
          V16.9
          nontraffic V16.2
          while boarding or alighting
            V16.3
        stationary object (traffic) V17.9
          nontraffic V17.2
          while boarding or alighting
            V17.3
        streetcar (traffic) V16.9
          nontraffic V16.2
          while boarding or alighting
            V16.3
        three wheeled motor vehicle
          (traffic) V12.9
          nontraffic V12.2
          while boarding or alighting
            V12.3
        truck (traffic) V14.9
          nontraffic V14.2
          while boarding or alighting
            V14.3
        two wheeled motor vehicle
          (traffic) V12.9
          nontraffic V12.2
          while boarding or alighting
            V12.3
        van (traffic) V13.9
          nontraffic V13.2
          while boarding or alighting
            V13.3
      driver
        collision (with)
          animal (traffic) V10.4
            being ridden (traffic) V16.4
              nontraffic V16.0
            nontraffic V10.0

Accident *(Continued)*
  transport *(Continued)*
    pedal cyclist *(Continued)*
      driver *(Continued)*
        collision *(Continued)*
          animal-drawn vehicle (traffic)
          V16.4
          nontraffic V16.0
        bus (traffic) V14.4
          nontraffic V14.0
        car (traffic) V13.4
          nontraffic V13.0
        motor vehicle NOS (traffic)
          V19.40
          nontraffic V19.00
          specified type NEC (traffic)
          V19.49
          nontraffic V19.09
        pedal cycle (traffic) V11.4
          nontraffic V11.0
        pickup truck (traffic) V13.4
          nontraffic V13.0
        railway vehicle (traffic) V15.4
          nontraffic V15.0
        specified vehicle NEC (traffic)
          V16.4
          nontraffic V16.0
        stationary object (traffic) V17.4
          nontraffic V17.0
        streetcar (traffic) V16.4
          nontraffic V16.0
        three wheeled motor vehicle
          (traffic) V12.4
          nontraffic V12.0
        truck (traffic) V14.4
          nontraffic V14.0
        two wheeled motor vehicle
          (traffic) V12.4
          nontraffic V12.0
        van (traffic) V13.4
          nontraffic V13.0
        noncollision accident (traffic)
          V18.4
          nontraffic V18.0
      noncollision accident (traffic) V18.9
        nontraffic V18.2
        while boarding or alighting
          V18.3
      nontraffic V19.3
      passenger
        collision (with)
          animal (traffic) V10.5
            being ridden (traffic)
              V16.5
              nontraffic V16.1
            nontraffic V10.1
          animal-drawn vehicle (traffic)
          V16.5
          nontraffic V16.1
        bus (traffic) V14.5
          nontraffic V14.1
        car (traffic) V13.5
          nontraffic V13.1
        motor vehicle NOS (traffic)
          V19.50
          nontraffic V19.10
          specified type NEC (traffic)
          V19.59
          nontraffic V19.19
        pedal cycle (traffic) V11.5
          nontraffic V11.1
        pickup truck (traffic) V13.5
          nontraffic V13.1
        railway vehicle (traffic) V15.5
          nontraffic V15.1

Accident *(Continued)*
  transport *(Continued)*
    pedal cyclist *(Continued)*
      passenger *(Continued)*
        collision *(Continued)*
          specified vehicle NEC (traffic)
          V16.5
          nontraffic V16.1
        stationary object (traffic)
          V17.5
          nontraffic V17.1
        streetcar (traffic) V16.5
          nontraffic V16.1
        three wheeled motor vehicle
          (traffic) V12.5
          nontraffic V12.1
        truck (traffic) V14.5
          nontraffic V14.1
        two wheeled motor vehicle
          (traffic) V12.5
          nontraffic V12.1
        van (traffic) V13.5
          nontraffic V13.1
        noncollision accident (traffic)
          V18.5
          nontraffic V18.1
      specified type NEC V19.88
      military vehicle V19.81
    pedestrian
      conveyance (occupant) V09.9
        babystroller V00.828
        collision (with) V09.9
          animal being ridden or animal
            drawn vehicle V06.99
            nontraffic V06.09
            traffic V06.19
          bus or heavy transport
            V04.99
            nontraffic V04.09
            traffic V04.19
          car V03.99
            nontraffic V03.09
            traffic V03.19
          pedal cycle V01.99
            nontraffic V01.09
            traffic V01.19
          pick-up truck or van V03.99
            nontraffic V03.09
            traffic V03.19
          railway (train) (vehicle)
            V05.99
            nontraffic V05.09
            traffic V05.19
          stationary object V00.822
          streetcar V06.99
            nontraffic V06.09
            traffic V06.19
          two- or three-wheeled motor
            vehicle V02.99
            nontraffic V02.09
            traffic V02.19
          vehicle V09.9
            animal-drawn V06.99
             nontraffic V06.09
             traffic V06.19
            motor
             nontraffic V09.00
             traffic V09.20
        fall V00.821
        nontraffic V09.1
          involving motor vehicle
            NEC V09.00
        traffic V09.3
          involving motor vehicle
            NEC V09.20

Accident *(Continued)*
  transport *(Continued)*
    pedestrian *(Continued)*
      conveyance *(Continued)*
        flat-bottomed NEC V00.388
          collision (with) V09.9
            animal being ridden or
              animal drawn vehicle
              V06.99
              nontraffic V06.09
              traffic V06.19
            bus or heavy transport
              V04.99
              nontraffic V04.09
              traffic V04.19
            car V03.99
              nontraffic V03.09
              traffic V03.19
            pedal cycle V01.99
              nontraffic V01.09
              traffic V01.19
            pick-up truck or van V03.99
              nontraffic V03.09
              traffic V03.19
            railway (train) (vehicle)
              V05.99
              nontraffic V05.09
              traffic V05.19
            stationary object V00.382
            streetcar V06.99
              nontraffic V06.09
              traffic V06.19
            two-or three-wheeled motor
              vehicle V02.99
              nontraffic V02.09
              traffic V02.19
            vehicle V09.9
              animal-drawn V06.99
                nontraffic V06.09
                traffic V06.19
              motor
                nontraffic V09.00
                traffic V09.20
          fall V00.381
          nontraffic V09.1
            involving motor vehicle
              NEC V09.00
        snow
          board —*see* Accident,
            transport, pedestrian,
            conveyance, snow board
          ski —*see* Accident, transport,
            pedestrian, conveyance,
            skis (snow)
        traffic V09.3
          involving motor vehicle
            NEC V09.20
        gliding type NEC V00.288
          collision (with) V09.9
            animal being ridden or animal
              drawn vehicle V06.99
              nontraffic V06.09
              traffic V06.19
            bus or heavy transport V04.99
              nontraffic V04.09
              traffic V04.19
            car V03.99
              nontraffic V03.09
              traffic V03.19
            pedal cycle V01.99
              nontraffic V01.09
              traffic V01.19
            pick-up truck or van V03.99
              nontraffic V03.09
              traffic V03.19

Accident *(Continued)*
  transport *(Continued)*
    pedestrian *(Continued)*
      conveyance *(Continued)*
        gliding type NEC *(Continued)*
          collision *(Continued)*
            railway (train) (vehicle)
              V05.99
              nontraffic V05.09
              traffic V05.19
            stationary object V00.282
            streetcar V06.99
              nontraffic V06.09
              traffic V06.19
            two- or three-wheeled motor
              vehicle V02.99
              nontraffic V02.09
              traffic V02.19
            vehicle V09.9
              animal-drawn V06.99
                nontraffic V06.09
                traffic V06.19
              motor
                nontraffic V09.00
                traffic V09.20
          fall V00.281
          heelies —*see* Accident,
            transport, pedestrian,
            conveyance, heelies
          ice skate —*see* Accident,
            transport, pedestrian,
            conveyance, ice skate
          nontraffic V09.1
            involving motor vehicle
              NEC V09.00
          sled —*see* Accident, transport,
            pedestrian, conveyance,
            sled
          traffic V09.3
            involving motor vehicle
              NEC V09.20
            wheelies —*see* Accident,
             transport, pedestrian,
             conveyance, heelies
        heelies V00.158
          colliding with stationary object
            V00.152
          fall V00.151
        ice skates V00.218
          collision (with) V09.9
            animal being ridden or
              animal drawn vehicle
               V06.99
              nontraffic V06.09
              traffic V06.19
            bus or heavy transport
              V04.99
              nontraffic V04.09
              traffic V04.19
            car V03.99
              nontraffic V03.09
              traffic V03.19
            pedal cycle V01.99
              nontraffic V01.09
              traffic V01.19
            pick-up truck or van
              V03.99
              nontraffic V03.09
              traffic V03.19
            railway (train) (vehicle)
              V05.99
              nontraffic V05.09
              traffic V05.19
            stationary object
              V00.212

Accident *(Continued)*
  transport *(Continued)*
    pedestrian *(Continued)*
      conveyance *(Continued)*
        ice skates *(Continued)*
          collision *(Continued)*
            streetcar V06.99
              nontraffic V06.09
              traffic V06.19
            two- or three-wheeled motor
              vehicle V02.99
              nontraffic V02.09
              traffic V02.19
            vehicle V09.9
              animal-drawn V06.99
                nontraffic V06.09
                traffic V06.19
              motor
                nontraffic V09.00
                traffic V09.20
          fall V00.211
          nontraffic V09.1
            involving motor vehicle
              NEC V09.00
          traffic V09.3
            involving motor vehicle
              NEC V09.20
        motorized mobility scooter
          V00.838
          collision with stationary object
            V00.832
          fall from V00.831
          nontraffic V09.1
            involving motor vehicle V09.00
              military V09.01
              specified type NEC V09.09
        roller skates (non in-line) V00.128
          collision (with) V09.9
            animal being ridden or
              animal drawn vehicle
               V06.91
              nontraffic V06.01
              traffic V06.11
            bus or heavy transport
              V04.91
              nontraffic V04.01
              traffic V04.11
            car V03.91
              nontraffic V03.01
              traffic V03.11
            pedal cycle V01.91
              nontraffic V01.01
              traffic V01.11
            pick-up truck or van V03.91
              nontraffic V03.01
              traffic V03.11
            railway (train) (vehicle)
              V05.91
              nontraffic V05.01
              traffic V05.11
            stationary object V00.122
            streetcar V06.91
              nontraffic V06.01
              traffic V06.11
            two- or three-wheeled motor
              vehicle V02.91
              nontraffic V02.01
              traffic V02.11
            vehicle V09.9
              animal-drawn V06.91
                nontraffic V06.01
                traffic V06.11
              motor
                nontraffic V09.00
                traffic V09.20

Accident (Continued)
  transport (Continued)
    pedestrian (Continued)
      conveyance (Continued)
        roller skates (Continued)
          fall V00.121
          in-line V00.118
            collision —see also Accident,
              transport, pedestrian,
              conveyance occupant,
              roller skates, collision
              with stationary object
              V00.112
            fall V00.111
            nontraffic V09.1
              involving motor vehicle
                NEC V09.00
            traffic V09.3
              involving motor vehicle
                NEC V09.20
        rolling shoes V00.158
          colliding with stationary object
            V00.152
          fall V00.151
        rolling type NEC V00.188
          collision (with) V09.9
            animal being ridden or
              animal drawn vehicle
              V06.99
              nontraffic V06.09
              traffic V06.19
            bus or heavy transport
              V04.99
              nontraffic V04.09
              traffic V04.19
            car V03.99
              nontraffic V03.09
              traffic V03.19
            pedal cycle V01.99
              nontraffic V01.09
              traffic V01.19
            pick-up truck or van
              V03.99
              nontraffic V03.09
              traffic V03.19
            railway (train) (vehicle)
              V05.99
              nontraffic V05.09
              traffic V05.19
            stationary object V00.182
            streetcar V06.99
              nontraffic V06.09
              traffic V06.19
            two- or three-wheeled motor
              vehicle V02.99
              nontraffic V02.09
              traffic V02.19
            vehicle V09.9
              animal-drawn V06.99
                nontraffic V06.09
                traffic V06.19
              motor
                nontraffic V09.00
                traffic V09.20
          fall V00.181
          in-line roller skate —see
            Accident, transport,
            pedestrian, conveyance,
            roller skate, in-line
          nontraffic V09.1
            involving motor vehicle
              NEC V09.00
          roller skate —see Accident,
            transport, pedestrian,
            conveyance, roller skate

Accident (Continued)
  transport (Continued)
    pedestrian (Continued)
      conveyance (Continued)
        rolling type NEC (Continued)
          scooter (non-motorized) —see
            Accident, transport,
            pedestrian, conveyance,
            scooter
          skateboard —see Accident,
            transport, pedestrian,
            conveyance, skateboard
          traffic V09.3
            involving motor vehicle
              NEC V09.20
        scooter (non-motorized) V00.148
          collision (with) V09.9
            animal being ridden or
              animal drawn vehicle
              V06.99
              nontraffic V06.09
              traffic V06.19
            bus or heavy transport
              V04.99
              nontraffic V04.09
              traffic V04.19
            car V03.99
              nontraffic V03.09
              traffic V03.19
            pedal cycle V01.99
              nontraffic V01.09
              traffic V01.19
            pick-up truck or van V03.99
              nontraffic V03.09
              traffic V03.19
            railway (train) (vehicle)
              V05.99
              nontraffic V05.09
              traffic V05.19
            stationary object V00.142
            streetcar V06.99
              nontraffic V06.09
              traffic V06.19
            two- or three-wheeled motor
              vehicle V02.99
              nontraffic V02.09
              traffic V02.19
            vehicle V09.9
              animal-drawn V06.99
                nontraffic V06.09
                traffic V06.19
              motor
                nontraffic V09.00
                traffic V09.20
          fall V00.141
          nontraffic V09.1
            involving motor vehicle
              NEC V09.00
          traffic V09.3
            involving motor vehicle
              NEC V09.20
        skate board V00.138
          collision (with) V09.9
            animal being ridden or
              animal drawn vehicle
              V06.92
              nontraffic V06.02
              traffic V06.12
            bus or heavy transport
              V04.92
              nontraffic V04.02
              traffic V04.12
            car V03.92
              nontraffic V03.02
              traffic V03.12

Accident (Continued)
  transport (Continued)
    pedestrian (Continued)
      conveyance (Continued)
        skate board (Continued)
          collision (Continued)
            pedal cycle V01.92
              nontraffic V01.02
              traffic V01.12
            pick-up truck or van V03.92
              nontraffic V03.02
              traffic V03.12
            railway (train) (vehicle)
              V05.92
              nontraffic V05.02
              traffic V05.12
            stationary object V00.132
            streetcar V06.92
              nontraffic V06.02
              traffic V06.12
            two- or three-wheeled motor
              vehicle V02.92
              nontraffic V02.02
              traffic V02.12
            vehicle V09.9
              animal-drawn V06.92
                nontraffic V06.02
                traffic V06.12
              motor
                nontraffic V09.00
                traffic V09.20
          fall V00.131
          nontraffic V09.1
            involving motor vehicle
              NEC V09.00
          traffic V09.3
            involving motor vehicle
              NEC V09.20
        skis (snow) V00.328
          collision (with) V09.9
            animal being ridden or
              animal drawn vehicle
              V06.99
              nontraffic V06.09
              traffic V06.19
            bus or heavy transport V04.99
              nontraffic V04.09
              traffic V04.19
            car V03.99
              nontraffic V03.09
              traffic V03.19
            pedal cycle V01.99
              nontraffic V01.09
              traffic V01.19
            pick-up truck or van V03.99
              nontraffic V03.09
              traffic V03.19
            railway (train) (vehicle)
              V05.99
              nontraffic V05.09
              traffic V05.19
            stationary object V00.322
            streetcar V06.99
              nontraffic V06.09
              traffic V06.19
            two- or three-wheeled motor
              vehicle V02.99
              nontraffic V02.09
              traffic V02.19
            vehicle V09.9
              animal-drawn V06.99
                nontraffic V06.09
                traffic V06.19
              motor
                nontraffic V09.00
                traffic V09.20

Accident *(Continued)*
transport *(Continued)*
pedestrian *(Continued)*
conveyance *(Continued)*
skis *(Continued)*
fall V00.321
nontraffic V09.1
involving motor vehicle
NEC V09.00
traffic V09.3
involving motor vehicle
NEC V09.20
sled V00.228
collision (with) V09.9
animal being ridden or
animal drawn vehicle
V06.99
nontraffic V06.09
traffic V06.19
bus or heavy transport
V04.99
nontraffic V04.09
traffic V04.19
car V03.99
nontraffic V03.09
traffic V03.19
pedal cycle V01.99
nontraffic V01.09
traffic V01.19
pick-up truck or van V03.99
nontraffic V03.09
traffic V03.19
railway (train) (vehicle)
V05.99
nontraffic V05.09
traffic V05.19
stationary object V00.222
streetcar V06.99
nontraffic V06.09
traffic V06.19
two- or three-wheeled
motor vehicle V02.99
nontraffic V02.09
traffic V02.19
vehicle V09.9
animal-drawn V06.99
nontraffic V06.09
traffic V06.19
motor
nontraffic V09.00
traffic V09.20
fall V00.221
nontraffic V09.1
involving motor vehicle
NEC V09.00
traffic V09.3
involving motor vehicle
NEC V09.20
snow board V00.318
collision (with) V09.9
animal being ridden or
animal drawn vehicle
V06.99
nontraffic V06.09
traffic V06.19
bus or heavy transport
V04.99
nontraffic V04.09
traffic V04.19
car V03.99
nontraffic V03.09
traffic V03.19
pedal cycle V01.99
nontraffic V01.09
traffic V01.19

Accident *(Continued)*
transport *(Continued)*
pedestrian *(Continued)*
conveyance *(Continued)*
snow board *(Continued)*
collision *(Continued)*
pick-up truck or van V03.99
nontraffic V03.09
traffic V03.19
railway (train) (vehicle)
V05.99
nontraffic V05.09
traffic V05.19
stationary object V00.312
streetcar V06.99
nontraffic V06.09
traffic V06.19
two- or three-wheeled motor
vehicle V02.99
nontraffic V02.09
traffic V02.19
vehicle V09.9
animal-drawn V06.99
nontraffic V06.09
traffic V06.19
motor
nontraffic V09.00
traffic V09.20
fall V00.311
nontraffic V09.1
involving motor vehicle
NEC V09.00
traffic V09.3
involving motor vehicle
NEC V09.20
specified type NEC V00.898
collision (with) V09.9
animal being ridden or
animal drawn vehicle
V06.99
nontraffic V06.09
traffic V06.19
bus or heavy transport
V04.99
nontraffic V04.09
traffic V04.19
car V03.99
nontraffic V03.09
traffic V03.19
pedal cycle V01.99
nontraffic V01.09
traffic V01.19
pick-up truck or van V03.99
nontraffic V03.09
traffic V03.19
railway (train) (vehicle)
V05.99
nontraffic V05.09
traffic V05.19
stationary object V00.892
streetcar V06.99
nontraffic V06.09
traffic V06.19
two- or three-wheeled motor
vehicle V02.99
nontraffic V02.09
traffic V02.19
vehicle V09.9
animal-drawn V06.99
nontraffic V06.09
traffic V06.19
motor
nontraffic V09.00
traffic V09.20
fall V00.891

Accident *(Continued)*
transport *(Continued)*
pedestrian *(Continued)*
conveyance *(Continued)*
specified type NEC *(Continued)*
nontraffic V09.1
involving motor vehicle
NEC V09.00
traffic V09.3
involving motor vehicle
NEC V09.20
traffic V09.3
involving motor vehicle
V09.20
military V09.21
specified type NEC
V09.29
wheelchair (powered) V00.818
collision (with) V09.9
animal being ridden or
animal drawn vehicle
V06.99
nontraffic V06.09
traffic V06.19
bus or heavy transport
V04.99
nontraffic V04.09
traffic V04.19
car V03.99
nontraffic V03.09
traffic V03.19
pedal cycle V01.99
nontraffic V01.09
traffic V01.19
pick-up truck or van
V03.99
nontraffic V03.09
traffic V03.19
railway (train) (vehicle)
V05.99
nontraffic V05.09
traffic V05.19
stationary object V00.812
streetcar V06.99
nontraffic V06.09
traffic V06.19
two- or three-wheeled motor
vehicle V02.99
nontraffic V02.09
traffic V02.19
vehicle V09.9
animal-drawn V06.99
nontraffic V06.09
traffic V06.19
motor
nontraffic V09.00
traffic V09.20
fall V00.811
nontraffic V09.1
involving motor vehicle
NEC V09.00
traffic V09.3
involving motor vehicle
NEC V09.20
wheeled shoe V00.158
colliding with stationary object
V00.152
fall V00.151
on foot —*see also* Accident,
pedestrian
collision (with)
animal being ridden or animal
drawn vehicle V06.90
nontraffic V06.00
traffic V06.10

Accident *(Continued)*
  transport *(Continued)*
    pedestrian *(Continued)*
      on foot *(Continued)*
        collision *(Continued)*
          bus or heavy transport V04.90
            nontraffic V04.00
            traffic V04.10
          car V03.90
            nontraffic V03.00
            traffic V03.10
          pedal cycle V01.90
            nontraffic V01.00
            traffic V01.10
          pick-up truck or van V03.90
            nontraffic V03.00
            traffic V03.10
          railway (train) (vehicle) V05.90
            nontraffic V05.00
            traffic V05.10
          streetcar V06.90
            nontraffic V06.00
            traffic V06.10
          two- or three-wheeled motor vehicle V02.90
            nontraffic V02.00
            traffic V02.10
          vehicle V09.9
            animal-drawn V06.90
              nontraffic V06.00
              traffic V06.10
            motor
              nontraffic V09.00
              traffic V09.20
         nontraffic V09.1
          involving motor vehicle V09.00
            military V09.01
            specified type NEC V09.09
        traffic V09.3
          involving motor vehicle V09.20
            military V09.21
            specified type NEC V09.29
      person NEC (unknown way or transportation) V99
    collision (between)
      bus (with)
        heavy transport vehicle (traffic) V87.5
          nontraffic V88.5
      car (with)
        nontraffic V88.5
        bus (traffic) V87.3
          nontraffic V88.3
        heavy transport vehicle (traffic) V87.4
          nontraffic V88.4
        pick-up truck or van (traffic) V87.2
          nontraffic V88.2
        train or railway vehicle (traffic) V87.6
          nontraffic V88.6
        two- or three-wheeled motor vehicle (traffic) V87.0
          nontraffic V88.0
        motor vehicle (traffic) NEC V87.7
          nontraffic V88.7
        two- or three-wheeled vehicle (with) (traffic)
          motor vehicle NEC V87.1
          nontraffic V88.1
      nonmotor vehicle (collision) (noncollision) (traffic) V87.9
        nontraffic V88.9

Accident *(Continued)*
  transport *(Continued)*
    pickup truck occupant V59.9
      collision (with)
        animal (traffic) V50.9
          being ridden (traffic) V56.9
            nontraffic V56.3
            while boarding or alighting V56.4
          nontraffic V50.3
          while boarding or alighting V50.4
        animal-drawn vehicle (traffic) V56.9
          nontraffic V56.3
          while boarding or alighting V56.4
        bus (traffic) V54.9
          nontraffic V54.3
          while boarding or alighting V54.4
        car (traffic) V53.9
          nontraffic V53.3
          while boarding or alighting V53.4
        motor vehicle NOS (traffic) V59.60
          nontraffic V59.20
          specified type NEC (traffic) V59.69
            nontraffic V59.29
        pedal cycle (traffic) V51.9
          nontraffic V51.3
          while boarding or alighting V51.4
        pickup truck (traffic) V53.9
          nontraffic V53.3
          while boarding or alighting V53.4
        railway vehicle (traffic) V55.9
          nontraffic V55.3
          while boarding or alighting V55.4
        specified vehicle NEC (traffic) V56.9
          nontraffic V56.3
          while boarding or alighting V56.4
        stationary object (traffic) V57.9
          nontraffic V57.3
          while boarding or alighting V57.4
        streetcar (traffic) V56.9
          nontraffic V56.3
          while boarding or alighting V56.4
        three wheeled motor vehicle (traffic) V52.9
          nontraffic V52.3
          while boarding or alighting V52.4
        truck (traffic) V54.9
          nontraffic V54.3
          while boarding or alighting V54.4
        two wheeled motor vehicle (traffic) V52.9
          nontraffic V52.3
          while boarding or alighting V52.4
        van (traffic) V53.9
          nontraffic V53.3
          while boarding or alighting V53.4

Accident *(Continued)*
  transport *(Continued)*
    pickup truck occupant *(Continued)*
      driver
        collision (with)
          animal (traffic) V50.5
            being ridden (traffic) V56.5
              nontraffic V56.0
            nontraffic V50.0
          animal-drawn vehicle (traffic) V56.5
            nontraffic V56.0
          bus (traffic) V54.5
            nontraffic V54.0
          car (traffic) V53.5
            nontraffic V53.0
          motor vehicle NOS (traffic) V59.40
            nontraffic V59.00
            specified type NEC (traffic) V59.49
              nontraffic V59.09
          pedal cycle (traffic) V51.5
            nontraffic V51.0
          pickup truck (traffic) V53.5
            nontraffic V53.0
          railway vehicle (traffic) V55.5
            nontraffic V55.0
          specified vehicle NEC (traffic) V56.5
            nontraffic V56.0
          stationary object (traffic) V57.5
            nontraffic V57.0
          streetcar (traffic) V56.5
            nontraffic V56.0
          three wheeled motor vehicle (traffic) V52.5
            nontraffic V52.0
          truck (traffic) V54.5
            nontraffic V54.0
          two wheeled motor vehicle (traffic) V52.5
            nontraffic V52.0
          van (traffic) V53.5
            nontraffic V53.0
        noncollision accident (traffic) V58.5
          nontraffic V58.0
      hanger-on
        collision (with)
          animal (traffic) V50.7
            being ridden (traffic) V56.7
              nontraffic V56.2
            nontraffic V50.2
          animal-drawn vehicle (traffic) V56.7
            nontraffic V56.2
          bus (traffic) V54.7
            nontraffic V54.2
          car (traffic) V53.7
            nontraffic V53.2
          pedal cycle (traffic) V51.7
            nontraffic V51.2
          pickup truck (traffic) V53.7
            nontraffic V53.2
          railway vehicle (traffic) V55.7
            nontraffic V55.2
          specified vehicle NEC (traffic) V56.7
            nontraffic V56.2
          stationary object (traffic) V57.7
            nontraffic V57.2
          streetcar (traffic) V56.7
            nontraffic V56.2

A

Accident *(Continued)*
  transport *(Continued)*
    three-wheeled motor vehicle
      occupant *(Continued)*
        collision *(Continued)*
          three wheeled motor vehicle
            (traffic) V32.9
            nontraffic V32.3
            while boarding or alighting
              V32.4
          truck (traffic) V34.9
            nontraffic V34.3
            while boarding or alighting
              V34.4
          two wheeled motor vehicle
            (traffic) V32.9
            nontraffic V32.3
            while boarding or alighting
              V32.4
          van (traffic) V33.9
            nontraffic V33.3
            while boarding or alighting
              V33.4
        driver
          collision (with)
            animal (traffic) V30.5
              being ridden (traffic) V36.5
                nontraffic V36.0
              nontraffic V30.0
            animal-drawn vehicle (traffic)
              V36.5
              nontraffic V36.0
            bus (traffic) V34.5
              nontraffic V34.0
            car (traffic) V33.5
              nontraffic V33.0
            motor vehicle NOS (traffic)
              V39.40
              nontraffic V39.00
              specified type NEC (traffic)
                V39.49
                nontraffic V39.09
            pedal cycle (traffic) V31.5
              nontraffic V31.0
            pickup truck (traffic) V33.5
              nontraffic V33.0
            railway vehicle (traffic) V35.5
              nontraffic V35.0
            specified vehicle NEC (traffic)
              V36.5
              nontraffic V36.0
            stationary object (traffic) V37.5
              nontraffic V37.0
            streetcar (traffic) V36.5
              nontraffic V36.0
            three wheeled motor vehicle
              (traffic) V32.5
              nontraffic V32.0
            truck (traffic) V34.5
              nontraffic V34.0
            two wheeled motor vehicle
              (traffic) V32.5
              nontraffic V32.0
            van (traffic) V33.5
              nontraffic V33.0
          noncollision accident (traffic)
            V38.5
            nontraffic V38.0
        hanger-on
          collision (with)
            animal (traffic) V30.7
              being ridden (traffic)
                V36.7
                nontraffic V36.2
              nontraffic V30.2

Accident *(Continued)*
  transport *(Continued)*
    three-wheeled motor vehicle
      occupant *(Continued)*
        hanger-on *(Continued)*
          collision *(Continued)*
            animal-drawn vehicle (traffic)
              V36.7
              nontraffic V36.2
            bus (traffic) V34.7
              nontraffic V34.2
            car (traffic) V33.7
              nontraffic V33.2
            pedal cycle (traffic) V31.7
              nontraffic V31.2
            pickup truck (traffic) V33.7
              nontraffic V33.2
            railway vehicle (traffic) V35.7
              nontraffic V35.2
            specified vehicle NEC (traffic)
              V36.7
              nontraffic V36.2
            stationary object (traffic) V37.7
              nontraffic V37.2
            streetcar (traffic) V36.7
              nontraffic V36.2
            three wheeled motor vehicle
              (traffic) V32.7
              nontraffic V32.2
            truck (traffic) V34.7
              nontraffic V34.2
            two wheeled motor vehicle
              (traffic) V32.7
              nontraffic V32.2
            van (traffic) V33.7
              nontraffic V33.2
          noncollision accident (traffic)
            V38.7
            nontraffic V38.2
        noncollision accident (traffic)
          V38.9
          nontraffic V38.3
          while boarding or alighting
            V38.4
        nontraffic V39.3
        passenger
          collision (with)
            animal (traffic) V30.6
              being ridden (traffic) V36.6
                nontraffic V36.1
              nontraffic V30.1
            animal-drawn vehicle (traffic)
              V36.6
              nontraffic V36.1
            bus (traffic) V34.6
              nontraffic V34.1
            car (traffic) V33.6
              nontraffic V33.1
            motor vehicle NOS (traffic)
              V39.50
              nontraffic V39.10
              specified type NEC (traffic)
                V39.59
                nontraffic V39.19
            pedal cycle (traffic) V31.6
              nontraffic V31.1
            pickup truck (traffic) V33.6
              nontraffic V33.1
            railway vehicle (traffic) V35.6
              nontraffic V35.1
            specified vehicle NEC (traffic)
              V36.6
              nontraffic V36.1
            stationary object (traffic) V37.6
              nontraffic V37.1

Accident *(Continued)*
  transport *(Continued)*
    three-wheeled motor vehicle
      occupant *(Continued)*
        passenger *(Continued)*
          collision *(Continued)*
            streetcar (traffic) V36.6
              nontraffic V36.1
            three wheeled motor vehicle
              (traffic) V32.6
              nontraffic V32.1
            truck (traffic) V34.6
              nontraffic V34.1
            two wheeled motor vehicle
              (traffic) V32.6
              nontraffic V32.1
            van (traffic) V33.6
              nontraffic V33.1
          noncollision accident (traffic)
            V38.6
            nontraffic V38.1
        specified type NEC V39.89
        military vehicle V39.81
    tractor (farm) (and trailer) —*see*
      Accident, transport, agricultural
      vehicle occupant
    tram —*see* Accident, transport,
      streetcar
      in mine or quarry —*see* Accident,
        transport, industrial vehicle
        occupant
    trolley —*see* Accident, transport,
      streetcar
      in mine or quarry —*see* Accident,
        transport, industrial vehicle
        occupant
    truck (heavy) occupant V69.9
      collision (with)
        animal (traffic) V60.9
          being ridden (traffic) V66.9
            nontraffic V66.3
            while boarding or alighting
              V66.4
          nontraffic V60.3
          while boarding or alighting
            V60.4
        animal-drawn vehicle (traffic)
          V66.9
          nontraffic V66.3
          while boarding or alighting
            V66.4
        bus (traffic) V64.9
          nontraffic V64.3
          while boarding or alighting V64.4
        car (traffic) V63.9
          nontraffic V63.3
          while boarding or alighting
            V63.4
        motor vehicle NOS (traffic) V69.60
          nontraffic V69.20
          specified type NEC (traffic)
            V69.69
            nontraffic V69.29
        pedal cycle (traffic) V61.9
          nontraffic V61.3
          while boarding or alighting
            V61.4
        pickup truck (traffic) V63.9
          nontraffic V63.3
          while boarding or alighting
            V63.4
        railway vehicle (traffic) V65.9
          nontraffic V65.3
          while boarding or alighting
            V65.4

Accident *(Continued)*
 transport *(Continued)*
  truck occupant *(Continued)*
   collision *(Continued)*
    specified vehicle NEC (traffic) V66.9
     nontraffic V66.3
     while boarding or alighting V66.4
    stationary object (traffic) V67.9
     nontraffic V67.3
     while boarding or alighting V67.4
    streetcar (traffic) V66.9
     nontraffic V66.3
     while boarding or alighting V66.4
    three wheeled motor vehicle (traffic) V62.9
     nontraffic V62.3
     while boarding or alighting V62.4
    truck (traffic) V64.9
     nontraffic V64.3
     while boarding or alighting V64.4
    two wheeled motor vehicle (traffic) V62.9
     nontraffic V62.3
     while boarding or alighting V62.4
    van (traffic) V63.9
     nontraffic V63.3
     while boarding or alighting V63.4
   driver
    collision (with)
     animal (traffic) V60.5
      being ridden (traffic) V66.5
       nontraffic V66.0
      nontraffic V60.0
     animal-drawn vehicle (traffic) V66.5
      nontraffic V66.0
     bus (traffic) V64.5
      nontraffic V64.0
     car (traffic) V63.5
      nontraffic V63.0
     motor vehicle NOS (traffic) V69.40
      nontraffic V69.00
      specified type NEC (traffic) V69.49
       nontraffic V69.09
     pedal cycle (traffic) V61.5
      nontraffic V61.0
     pickup truck (traffic) V63.5
      nontraffic V63.0
     railway vehicle (traffic) V65.5
      nontraffic V65.0
     specified vehicle NEC (traffic) V66.5
      nontraffic V66.0
     stationary object (traffic) V67.5
      nontraffic V67.0
     streetcar (traffic) V66.5
      nontraffic V66.0
     three wheeled motor vehicle (traffic) V62.5
      nontraffic V62.0
     truck (traffic) V64.5
      nontraffic V64.0
     two wheeled motor vehicle (traffic) V62.5
      nontraffic V62.0

Accident *(Continued)*
 transport *(Continued)*
  truck occupant *(Continued)*
   driver *(Continued)*
    collision *(Continued)*
     van (traffic) V63.5
      nontraffic V63.0
    noncollision accident (traffic) V68.5
     nontraffic V68.0
   dump —*see* Accident, transport, construction vehicle occupant
   hanger-on
    collision (with)
     animal (traffic) V60.7
      being ridden (traffic) V66.7
       nontraffic V66.2
      nontraffic V60.2
     animal-drawn vehicle (traffic) V66.7
      nontraffic V66.2
     bus (traffic) V64.7
      nontraffic V64.2
     car (traffic) V63.7
      nontraffic V63.2
     pedal cycle (traffic) V61.7
      nontraffic V61.2
     pickup truck (traffic) V63.7
      nontraffic V63.2
     railway vehicle (traffic) V65.7
      nontraffic V65.2
     specified vehicle NEC (traffic) V66.7
      nontraffic V66.2
     stationary object (traffic) V67.7
      nontraffic V67.2
     streetcar (traffic) V66.7
      nontraffic V66.2
     three wheeled motor vehicle (traffic) V62.7
      nontraffic V62.2
     truck (traffic) V64.7
      nontraffic V64.2
     two wheeled motor vehicle (traffic) V62.7
      nontraffic V62.2
     van (traffic) V63.7
      nontraffic V63.2
    noncollision accident (traffic) V68.7
     nontraffic V68.2
   noncollision accident (traffic) V68.9
    nontraffic V68.3
    while boarding or alighting V68.4
   nontraffic V69.3
   passenger
    collision (with)
     animal (traffic) V60.6
      being ridden (traffic) V66.6
       nontraffic V66.1
      nontraffic V60.1
     animal-drawn vehicle (traffic) V66.6
      nontraffic V66.1
     bus (traffic) V64.6
      nontraffic V64.1
     car (traffic) V63.6
      nontraffic V63.1
     motor vehicle NOS (traffic) V69.50
      nontraffic V69.10
      specified type NEC (traffic) V69.59
       nontraffic V69.19

Accident *(Continued)*
 transport *(Continued)*
  truck occupant *(Continued)*
   passenger *(Continued)*
    collision *(Continued)*
     pedal cycle (traffic) V61.6
      nontraffic V61.1
     pickup truck (traffic) V63.6
      nontraffic V63.1
     railway vehicle (traffic) V65.6
      nontraffic V65.1
     specified vehicle NEC (traffic) V66.6
      nontraffic V66.1
     stationary object (traffic) V67.6
      nontraffic V67.1
     streetcar (traffic) V66.6
      nontraffic V66.1
     three wheeled motor vehicle (traffic) V62.6
      nontraffic V62.1
     truck (traffic) V64.6
      nontraffic V64.1
     two wheeled motor vehicle (traffic) V62.6
      nontraffic V62.1
     van (traffic) V63.6
      nontraffic V63.1
    noncollision accident (traffic) V68.6
     nontraffic V68.1
   pickup —*see* Accident, transport, pickup truck occupant
   specified type NEC V69.88
    military vehicle V69.81
  van occupant V59.9
   collision (with)
    animal (traffic) V50.9
     being ridden (traffic) V56.9
      nontraffic V56.3
      while boarding or alighting V56.4
     nontraffic V50.3
     while boarding or alighting V50.4
    animal-drawn vehicle (traffic) V56.9
     nontraffic V56.3
     while boarding or alighting V56.4
    bus (traffic) V54.9
     nontraffic V54.3
     while boarding or alighting V54.4
    car (traffic) V53.9
     nontraffic V53.3
     while boarding or alighting V53.4
    motor vehicle NOS (traffic) V59.60
     nontraffic V59.20
     specified type NEC (traffic) V59.69
      nontraffic V59.29
    pedal cycle (traffic) V51.9
     nontraffic V51.3
     while boarding or alighting V51.4
    pickup truck (traffic) V53.9
     nontraffic V53.3
     while boarding or alighting V53.4
    railway vehicle (traffic) V55.9
     nontraffic V55.3
     while boarding or alighting V55.4

Accident *(Continued)*
  transport *(Continued)*
    van occupant *(Continued)*
      collision *(Continued)*
        specified vehicle NEC (traffic)
          V56.9
          nontraffic V56.3
          while boarding or alighting
            V56.4
        stationary object (traffic) V57.9
          nontraffic V57.3
          while boarding or alighting
            V57.4
        streetcar (traffic) V56.9
          nontraffic V56.3
          while boarding or alighting
            V56.4
        three wheeled motor vehicle
          (traffic) V52.9
          nontraffic V52.3
          while boarding or alighting
            V52.4
        truck (traffic) V54.9
          nontraffic V54.3
          while boarding or alighting
            V54.4
        two wheeled motor vehicle
          (traffic) V52.9
          nontraffic V52.3
          while boarding or alighting
            V52.4
        van (traffic) V53.9
          nontraffic V53.3
          while boarding or alighting
            V53.4
      driver
        collision (with)
          animal (traffic) V50.5
            being ridden (traffic) V56.5
              nontraffic V56.0
            nontraffic V50.0
          animal-drawn vehicle (traffic)
            V56.5
            nontraffic V56.0
          bus (traffic) V54.5
            nontraffic V54.0
          car (traffic) V53.5
            nontraffic V53.0
          motor vehicle NOS (traffic)
            V59.40
            nontraffic V59.00
            specified type NEC (traffic)
              V59.49
              nontraffic V59.09
          pedal cycle (traffic) V51.5
            nontraffic V51.0
          pickup truck (traffic) V53.5
            nontraffic V53.0
          railway vehicle (traffic) V55.5
            nontraffic V55.0
          specified vehicle NEC (traffic)
            V56.5
            nontraffic V56.0
          stationary object (traffic) V57.5
            nontraffic V57.0
          streetcar (traffic) V56.5
            nontraffic V56.0
          three wheeled motor vehicle
            (traffic) V52.5
            nontraffic V52.0
          truck (traffic) V54.5
            nontraffic V54.0
          two wheeled motor vehicle
            (traffic) V52.5
            nontraffic V52.0

Accident *(Continued)*
  transport *(Continued)*
    van occupant *(Continued)*
      driver *(Continued)*
        collision *(Continued)*
          van (traffic) V53.5
            nontraffic V53.0
        noncollision accident (traffic)
          V58.5
          nontraffic V58.0
      hanger-on
        collision (with)
          animal (traffic) V50.7
            being ridden (traffic) V56.7
              nontraffic V56.2
            nontraffic V50.2
          animal-drawn vehicle (traffic)
            V56.7
            nontraffic V56.2
          bus (traffic) V54.7
            nontraffic V54.2
          car (traffic) V53.7
            nontraffic V53.2
          pedal cycle (traffic) V51.7
            nontraffic V51.2
          pickup truck (traffic) V53.7
            nontraffic V53.2
          railway vehicle (traffic) V55.7
            nontraffic V55.2
          specified vehicle NEC (traffic)
            V56.7
            nontraffic V56.2
          stationary object (traffic) V57.7
            nontraffic V57.2
          streetcar (traffic) V56.7
            nontraffic V56.2
          three wheeled motor vehicle
            (traffic) V52.7
            nontraffic V52.2
          truck (traffic) V54.7
            nontraffic V54.2
          two wheeled motor vehicle
            (traffic) V52.7
            nontraffic V52.2
          van (traffic) V53.7
            nontraffic V53.2
        noncollision accident (traffic)
          V58.7
          nontraffic V58.2
      noncollision accident (traffic) V58.9
        nontraffic V58.3
        while boarding or alighting
          V58.4
      nontraffic V59.3
      passenger
        collision (with)
          animal (traffic) V50.6
            being ridden (traffic) V56.6
              nontraffic V56.1
            nontraffic V50.1
          animal-drawn vehicle (traffic)
            V56.6
            nontraffic V56.1
          bus (traffic) V54.6
            nontraffic V54.1
          car (traffic) V53.6
            nontraffic V53.1
          motor vehicle NOS (traffic)
            V59.50
            nontraffic V59.10
            specified type NEC (traffic)
              V59.59
              nontraffic V59.19
          pedal cycle (traffic) V51.6
            nontraffic V51.1

Accident *(Continued)*
  transport *(Continued)*
    van occupant *(Continued)*
      passenger *(Continued)*
        collision *(Continued)*
          pickup truck (traffic)
            V53.6
            nontraffic V53.1
          railway vehicle (traffic)
            V55.6
            nontraffic V55.1
          specified vehicle NEC (traffic)
            V56.6
            nontraffic V56.1
          stationary object (traffic)
            V57.6
            nontraffic V57.1
          streetcar (traffic) V56.6
            nontraffic V56.1
          three wheeled motor vehicle
            (traffic) V52.6
            nontraffic V52.1
          truck (traffic) V54.6
            nontraffic V54.1
          two wheeled motor vehicle
            (traffic) V52.6
            nontraffic V52.1
          van (traffic) V53.6
            nontraffic V53.1
        noncollision accident (traffic)
          V58.6
          nontraffic V58.1
      specified type NEC V59.88
        military vehicle V59.81
      watercraft occupant —*see* Accident,
        watercraft
    vehicle NEC V89.9
      animal-drawn NEC —*see* Accident,
        transport, animal-drawn vehicle
        occupant
      special
        agricultural —*see* Accident,
          transport, agricultural vehicle
          occupant
        construction —*see* Accident,
          transport, construction vehicle
          occupant
        industrial —*see* Accident,
          transport, industrial
          vehicle occupant
        three-wheeled NEC (motorized) —
          see Accident, transport,
          three-wheeled motor vehicle
          occupant
    watercraft V94.9
      causing
        drowning B —*see* Drowning, due
          to, accident to, watercraft
        injury NEC V91.89
          crushed between craft and object
            V91.19
          powered craft V91.13
            ferry boat V91.11
            fishing boat V91.12
            jetskis V91.13
            liner V91.11
            merchant ship V91.10
            passenger ship V91.11
          unpowered craft V91.18
            canoe V91.15
            inflatable V91.16
            kayak V91.15
            sailboat V91.14
            surf-board V91.18
            windsurfer V91.18

Accident (*Continued*)
 watercraft (*Continued*)
  causing (*Continued*)
   injury NEC (*Continued*)
    fall on board V91.29
     powered craft V91.23
      ferry boat V91.21
      fishing boat V91.22
      jetskis V91.23
      liner V91.21
      merchant ship V91.20
      passenger ship V91.21
     unpowered craft
      canoe V91.25
      inflatable V91.26
      kayak V91.25
      sailboat V91.24
    fire on board causing burn
      V91.09
     powered craft V91.03
      ferry boat V91.01
      fishing boat V91.02
      jetskis V91.03
      liner V91.01
      merchant ship V91.00
      passenger ship V91.01
     unpowered craft V91.08
      canoe V91.05
      inflatable V91.06
      kayak V91.05
      sailboat V91.04
      surf-board V91.08
      water skis V91.07
      windsurfer V91.08
    hit by falling object V91.39
     powered craft V91.33
      ferry boat V91.31
      fishing boat V91.32
      jetskis V91.33
      liner V91.31
      merchant ship V91.30
      passenger ship V91.31
     unpowered craft V91.38
      canoe V91.35
      inflatable V91.36
      kayak V91.35
      sailboat V91.34
      surf-board V91.38
      water skis V91.37
      windsurfer V91.38
    specified type NEC V91.89
     powered craft V91.83
      ferry boat V91.81
      fishing boat V91.82
      jetskis V91.83
      liner V91.81
      merchant ship V91.80
      passenger ship V91.81
     unpowered craft V91.88
      canoe V91.85
      inflatable V91.86
      kayak V91.85
      sailboat V91.84
      surf-board V91.88
      water skis V91.87
      windsurfer V91.88
  due to, caused by cataclysm —*see*
   Forces of nature, by type
  military NEC V94.818
   with civilian watercraft V94.810
   civilian in water injured by
    V94.811
  nonpowered, struck by
   nonpowered vessel V94.22
   powered vessel V94.21

Accident (*Continued*)
 watercraft (*Continued*)
  specified type NEC V94.89
  striking swimmer
   powered V94.11
   unpowered V94.12
Acid throwing (assault) Y08.89
Activity (involving) (of victim at time of
  event) Y93.9
 aerobic and step exercise (class)
  Y93.A3
 alpine skiing Y93.23
 animal care NEC Y93.K9
 arts and handcrafts NEC Y93.D9
 athletics NEC Y93.79
 athletics played as a team or group
  NEC Y93.69
 athletics played individually NEC
  Y93.59
 baking Y93.G3
 ballet Y93.41
 barbells Y93.B3
 BASE (Building, Antenna, Span, Earth)
  jumping Y93.33
 baseball Y93.64
 basketball Y93.67
 bathing (personal) Y93.E1
 beach volleyball Y93.68
 bike riding Y93.55
 boogie boarding Y93.18
 bowling Y93.54
 boxing Y93.71
 brass instrument playing Y93.J4
 building construction Y93.H3
 bungee jumping Y93.34
 calisthenics Y93.A2
 canoeing (in calm and turbulent water)
  Y93.16
 capture the flag Y93.6A
 cardiorespiratory exercise NEC
  Y93.A9
 caregiving (providing) NEC
  Y93.F9
  bathing Y93.F1
  lifting Y93.F2
 cellular
  communication device Y93.C2
  telephone Y93.C2
 challenge course Y93.A5
 cheerleading Y93.45
 circuit training Y93.A4
 cleaning
  floor Y93.E5
 climbing NEC Y93.39
  mountain Y93.31
  rock Y93.31
  wall Y93.31
 clothing care and maintenance NEC
  Y93.E9
 combatives Y93.75
 computer
  keyboarding Y93.C1
  technology NEC Y93.C9
 confidence course Y93.A5
 construction (building) Y93.H3
 cooking and baking Y93.G3
 cool down exercises Y93.A2
 cricket Y93.69
 crocheting Y93.D1
 cross country skiing Y93.24
 dancing (all types) Y93.41
 digging
  dirt Y93.H1
 dirt digging Y93.H1
 dishwashing Y93.G1

Activity (*Continued*)
 diving (platform) (springboard)
  Y93.12
  underwater Y93.15
 dodge ball Y93.6A
 downhill skiing Y93.23
 drum playing Y93.J2
 dumbbells Y93.B3
 electronic
  devices NEC Y93.C9
   hand held interactive Y93.C2
  game playing (using) (with)
   interactive device Y93.C2
   keyboard or other stationary device
    Y93.C1
 elliptical machine Y93.A1
 exercise (s)
  machines ((primarily) for)
   cardiorespiratory conditioning
    Y93.A1
   muscle strengthening Y93.B1
  muscle strengthening (non-machine)
   NEC Y93.B9
 external motion NEC Y93.I9
  rollercoaster Y93.I1
 field hockey Y93.65
 figure skating (pairs) (singles)
  Y93.21
 flag football Y93.62
 floor mopping and cleaning
  Y93.E5
 food preparation and clean up
  Y93.G1
 football (American) NOS Y93.61
  flag Y93.62
  tackle Y93.61
  touch Y93.62
 four square Y93.6A
 free weights Y93.B3
 frisbee (ultimate) Y93.74
 furniture
  building Y93.D3
  finishing Y93.D3
  repair Y93.D3
 game playing (electronic)
  using interactive device Y93.C2
  using keyboard or other stationary
   device Y93.C1
 gardening Y93.H2
 golf Y93.53
 grass drills Y93.A6
 grilling and smoking food Y93.G2
 grooming and shearing an animal
  Y93.K3
 guerilla drills Y93.A6
 gymnastics (rhythmic) Y93.43
 hand held interactive electronic device
  Y93.C2
 handball Y93.73
 handcrafts NEC Y93.D9
 hang gliding Y93.35
 hiking (on level or elevated terrain)
  Y93.01
 hockey (ice) Y93.22
  field Y93.65
 horseback riding Y93.52
 household (interior) maintenance NEC
  Y93.E9
 ice NEC Y93.29
  dancing Y93.21
  hockey Y93.22
  skating Y93.21
 inline roller skating Y93.51
 ironing Y93.E4
 judo Y93.75

Activity *(Continued)*
jumping (off) NEC Y93.39
BASE (Building, Antenna, Span, Earth) Y93.33
bungee Y93.34
jacks Y93.A2
rope Y93.56
jumping jacks Y93.A2
jumping rope Y93.56
karate Y93.75
kayaking (in calm and turbulent water) Y93.16
keyboarding (computer) Y93.C1
kickball Y93.6A
knitting Y93.D1
lacrosse Y93.65
land maintenance NEC Y93.H9
landscaping Y93.H2
laundry Y93.E2
machines (exercise)
primarily for cardiorespiratory conditioning Y93.A1
primarily for muscle strengthening Y93.B1
maintenance
exterior building NEC Y93.H9
household (interior) NEC Y93.E9
land Y93.H9
property Y93.H9
marching (on level or elevated terrain) Y93.01
martial arts Y93.75
microwave oven Y93.G3
milking an animal Y93.K2
mopping (floor) Y93.E5
mountain climbing Y93.31
muscle strengthening
exercises (non-machine) NEC Y93.B9
machines Y93.B1
musical keyboard (electronic) playing Y93.J1
nordic skiing Y93.24
obstacle course Y93.A5
oven (microwave) Y93.G3
packing up and unpacking in moving to a new residence Y93.E6
parasailing Y93.19
percussion instrument playing NEC Y93.J2
personal
bathing and showering Y93.E1
hygiene NEC Y93.E8
showering Y93.E1
physical games generally associated with school recess, summer camp and children Y93.6A
physical training NEC Y93.A9
piano playing Y93.J1
pilates Y93.B4
platform diving Y93.12
playing musical instrument
brass instrument Y93.J4
drum Y93.J2
musical keyboard (electronic) Y93.J1
percussion instrument NEC Y93.J2
piano Y93.J1
string instrument Y93.J3
winds instrument Y93.J4
property maintenance
exterior NEC Y93.H9
interior NEC Y93.E9
pruning (garden and lawn) Y93.H2
pull-ups Y93.B2
push-ups Y93.B2
racquetball Y93.73

Activity *(Continued)*
rafting (in calm and turbulent water) Y93.16
raking (leaves) Y93.H1
rappelling Y93.32
refereeing a sports activity Y93.81
residential relocation Y93.E6
rhythmic gymnastics Y93.43
rhythmic movement NEC Y93.49
riding
horseback Y93.52
rollercoaster Y93.I1
rock climbing Y93.31
roller skating (inline) Y93.51
rollercoaster riding Y93.I1
rough housing and horseplay Y93.83
rowing (in calm and turbulent water) Y93.16
rugby Y93.63
SCUBA diving Y93.15
sewing Y93.D2
shoveling Y93.H1
dirt Y93.H1
snow Y93.H1
showering (personal) Y93.E1
sit-ups Y93.B2
skateboarding Y93.51
skating (ice) Y93.21
roller Y93.51
skiing (alpine) (downhill) Y93.23
cross country Y93.24
nordic Y93.24
water Y93.17
sledding (snow) Y93.23
sleeping (sleep) Y93.84
smoking and grilling food Y93.G2
snorkeling Y93.15
snow NEC Y93.29
boarding Y93.23
shoveling Y93.H1
sledding Y93.23
tubing Y93.23
soccer Y93.66
softball Y93.64
specified NEC Y93.89
spectator at an event Y93.82
sports NEC Y93.79
sports played as a team or group NEC Y93.69
sports played individually NEC Y93.59
springboard diving Y93.12
squash Y93.73
stationary bike Y93.A1
step (stepping) exercise (class) Y93.A3
stepper machine Y93.A1
stove Y93.G3
string instrument playing Y93.J3
surfing Y93.18
wind Y93.18
swimming Y93.11
tackle football Y93.61
tap dancing Y93.41
tennis Y93.73
tobogganing Y93.23
touch football Y93.62
track and field events (non-running) Y93.57
running Y93.02
trampoline Y93.44
treadmill Y93.A1
trimming shrubs Y93.H2
tubing (in calm and turbulent water) Y93.16
snow Y93.23

Activity *(Continued)*
ultimate frisbee Y93.74
underwater diving Y93.15
unpacking in moving to a new residence Y93.E6
use of stove, oven and microwave oven Y93.G3
vacuuming Y93.E3
volleyball (beach) (court) Y93.68
wake boarding Y93.17
walking (on level or elevated terrain) Y93.01
an animal Y93.K1
walking an animal Y93.K1
wall climbing Y93.31
warm up and cool down exercises Y93.A2
water NEC Y93.19
aerobics Y93.14
craft NEC Y93.19
exercise Y93.14
polo Y93.13
skiing Y93.17
sliding Y93.18
survival training and testing Y93.19
weeding (garden and lawn) Y93.H2
wind instrument playing Y93.J4
windsurfing Y93.18
wrestling Y93.72
yoga Y93.42
Adverse effect of drugs —*see* Table of Drugs and Chemicals
Aerosinusitis —*see* Air, pressure
After-effect, late —*see* Sequelae
Air
blast in war operations —*see* War operations, air blast
pressure
change, rapid
during
ascent W94.29
while (in) (surfacing from)
aircraft W94.23
deep water diving W94.21
underground W94.22
descent W94.39
in
aircraft W94.31
water W94.32
high, prolonged W94.0
low, prolonged W94.12
due to residence or long visit at high altitude W94.11
Alpine sickness W94.11
Altitude sickness W94.11
Anaphylactic shock, anaphylaxis —*see* Table of drugs and chemicals
Andes disease W94.11
Arachnidism, arachnoidism X58
Arson (with intent to injure or kill) X97
Asphyxia, asphyxiation
by
food (bone) (seed) —*see* categories T17 and T18
gas —*see also* Table of drugs and chemicals
legal
execution —*see* Legal, intervention, gas
intervention —*see* Legal, intervention, gas

Asphyxia, asphyxiation (Continued)
from
fire —see also Exposure, fire
in war operations —see War
operations, fire
ignition —see Ignition
vomitus T17.81
in war operations —see War operations,
restriction of airway
Aspiration
food (any type) (into respiratory
tract) (with asphyxia, obstruction
respiratory tract, suffocation) —see
categories T17 and T18
foreign body —see Foreign body,
aspiration
vomitus (with asphyxia,
obstruction respiratory tract,
suffocation) T17.81
Assassination (attempt) —see Assault
Assault (homicidal) (by) (in) Y09
arson X97
bite (of human being) Y04.1
bodily force Y04.8
bite Y04.1
bumping into Y04.2
sexual —see subcategories T74.0,
T76.0
unarmed fight Y04.0
bomb X96.9
antipersonnel X96.0
fertilizer X96.3
gasoline X96.1
letter X96.2
petrol X96.1
pipe X96.3
specified NEC X96.8
brawl (hand) (fists) (foot) (unarmed)
Y04.0
burning, burns (by fire) NEC X97
acid Y08.89
caustic, corrosive substance Y08.89
chemical from swallowing caustic,
corrosive substance —see Table
of drugs and chemicals
cigarette (s) X97
hot object X98.9
fluid NEC X98.2
household appliance X98.3
specified NEC X98.8
steam X98.0
tap water X98.1
vapors X98.0

Assault (Continued)
burning, burns NEC (Continued)
scalding —see Assault, burning
steam X98.0
vitriol Y08.89
caustic, corrosive substance (gas)
Y08.89
crashing of
aircraft Y08.81
motor vehicle Y03.8
pushed in front of Y02.0
run over Y03.0
specified NEC Y03.8
cutting or piercing instrument
X99.9
dagger X99.2
glass X99.0
knife X99.1
specified NEC X99.8
sword X99.2
dagger X99.2
drowning (in) X92.9
bathtub X92.0
natural water X92.3
specified NEC X92.8
swimming pool X92.1
following fall X92.2
dynamite X96.8
explosive (s) (material) X96.9
fight (hand) (fists) (foot) (unarmed)
Y04.0
with weapon —see Assault, by type
of weapon
fire X97
firearm X95.9
airgun X95.01
handgun X93
hunting rifle X94.1
larger X94.9
specified NEC X94.8
machine gun X94.2
shotgun X94.0
specified NEC X95.8
from high place Y01
gunshot (wound) NEC —see Assault,
firearm, by type
incendiary device X97
injury Y09
to child due to criminal abortion
attempt NEC Y08.89
knife X99.1
late effect of —see X92-Y08 with 7th
character S

Assault (Continued)
placing before moving object NEC Y02.8
motor vehicle Y02.0
poisoning —see categories T36-T65 with
7th character S
puncture, any part of body —see
Assault, cutting or piercing
instrument
pushing
before moving object NEC Y02.8
motor vehicle Y02.0
subway train Y02.1
train Y02.1
rape T74.2-
scalding —see Assault, burning
sequelae of —see X92-Y08 with 7th
character S
sexual (by bodily force) T74.2-
shooting —see Assault, firearm
specified means NEC Y08.89
stab, any part of body —see Assault,
cutting or piercing instrument
steam X98.0
striking against
other person Y04.2
sports equipment Y08.09
baseball bat Y08.02
hockey stick Y08.01
struck by
sports equipment Y08.09
baseball bat Y08.02
hockey stick Y08.01
submersion —see Assault, drowning
violence Y09
weapon Y09
blunt Y00
cutting or piercing —see Assault,
cutting or piercing instrument
firearm —see Assault, firearm
wound Y09
cutting —see Assault, cutting or
piercing instrument
gunshot —see Assault, firearm
knife X99.1
piercing —see Assault, cutting or
piercing instrument
puncture —see Assault, cutting or
piercing instrument
stab —see Assault, cutting or piercing
instrument
Attack by mammals NEC W55.89
Avalanche —see Landslide
Aviator's disease —see Air, pressure

A

B

Barotitis, barodontalgia, barosinusitis, barotrauma (otitic) (sinus) —see Air, pressure
Battered (baby) (child) (person) (syndrome) X58
Bayonet wound W26.1
  in
    legal intervention —see Legal, intervention, sharp object, bayonet
    war operations —see War operations, combat
  stated as undetermined whether accidental or intentional Y28.8
  suicide (attempt) X78.2
Bean in nose —see categories T17 and T18
Bed set on fire NEC —see Exposure, fire, uncontrolled, building, bed
Beheading (by guillotine)
  homicide X99.9
  legal execution —see Legal, intervention
Bending, injury in —see Overexertion
Bends —see Air, pressure, change
Bite, bitten by
  alligator W58.01
  arthropod (nonvenomous) NEC W57
  bull W55.21
  cat W55.01
  cow W55.21
  crocodile W58.11
  dog W54.0
  goat W55.31
  hoof stock NEC W55.31
  horse W55.11
  human being (accidentally) W50.3
    with intent to injure or kill Y04.1
    as, or caused by, a crowd or human stampede (with fall) W52
    assault Y04.1
    homicide (attempt) Y04.1
    in
      fight Y04.1
  insect (nonvenomous) W57
  lizard (nonvenomous) W59.01
  mammal NEC W55.81
    marine W56.31
  marine animal (nonvenomous) W56.81
  millipede W57
  moray eel W56.51
  mouse W53.01
  person (s) (accidentally) W50.3
    with intent to injure or kill Y04.1
    as, or caused by, a crowd or human stampede (with fall) W52
    assault Y04.1
    homicide (attempt) Y04.1
    in
      fight Y04.1
  pig W55.41
  raccoon W55.51
  rat W53.11
  reptile W59.81
    lizard W59.01
    snake W59.11
    turtle W59.21
      terrestrial W59.81
  rodent W53.81
    mouse W53.01
    rat W53.11
    specified NEC W53.81
    squirrel W53.21

Bite, bitten by (Continued)
  shark W56.41
  sheep W55.31
  snake (nonvenomous) W59.11
  spider (nonvenomous) W57
  squirrel W53.21
Blast (air) **in war operations** —see War operations, blast
Blizzard X37.2
Blood alcohol level Y90.9
  20-39mg/100ml Y90.1
  200-239mg/100ml Y90.7
  40-59mg/100ml Y90.2
  60-79mg/100ml Y90.3
  80-99mg/100ml Y90.4
  100-119mg/100ml Y90.5
  120-199mg/100ml Y90.6
  less than 20mg/100ml Y90.0
  presence in blood, level not specified Y90.9
Blow X58
  by law-enforcing agent, police (on duty) —see Legal, intervention, manhandling
    blunt object —see Legal, intervention, blunt object
Blowing up —see Explosion
Brawl (hand) (fists) (foot) Y04.0
Breakage (accidental) (part of)
  ladder (causing fall) W11
  scaffolding (causing fall) W12
Broken
  glass, contact with —see Contact, with, glass
  power line (causing electric shock) W85
Bumping against, into (accidentally)
  object NEC W22.8
    with fall —see Fall, due to, bumping against, object
    caused by crowd or human stampede (with fall) W52
    sports equipment W21.9
  person (s) W51
    with fall W03
      due to ice or snow W00.0
    assault Y04.2
    caused by, a crowd or human stampede (with fall) W52
    homicide (attempt) Y04.2
  sports equipment W21.9
Burn, burned, burning (accidental) (by) (from) (on)
  acid NEC —see Table of drugs and chemicals
  bed linen —see Exposure, fire, uncontrolled, in building, bed
  blowtorch X08.8
    with ignition of clothing NEC X06.2
      nightwear X05
  bonfire, campfire (controlled) —see also Exposure, fire, controlled, not in building
    uncontrolled —see Exposure, fire, uncontrolled, not in building
  candle X08.8
    with ignition of clothing NEC X06.2
      nightwear X05
  caustic liquid, substance (external) (internal) NEC —see Table of drugs and chemicals
  chemical (external) (internal) —see also Table of drugs and chemicals
    in war operations —see War operations, fire

Burn, burned, burning (Continued)
  cigar (s) or cigarette (s) X08.8
    with ignition of clothing NEC X06.2
      nightwear X05
  clothes, clothing NEC (from controlled fire) X06.2
    with conflagration —see Exposure, fire, uncontrolled, building
    not in building or structure —see Exposure, fire, uncontrolled, not in building
  cooker (hot) X15.8
    stated as undetermined whether accidental or intentional Y27.3
    suicide (attempt) X77.3
  electric blanket X16
  engine (hot) X17
  fire, flames —see Exposure, fire
  flare, Very pistol —see Discharge, firearm NEC
  heat
    from appliance (electrical) (household) X15.8
      cooker X15.8
      hotplate X15.2
      kettle X15.8
      light bulb X15.8
      saucepan X15.3
      skillet X15.3
      stated as undetermined whether accidental or intentional Y27.3
      stove X15.0
      suicide (attempt) X77.3
      toaster X15.1
    in local application or packing during medical or surgical procedure Y63.5
  heating
    appliance, radiator or pipe X16
  homicide (attempt) —see Assault, burning
  hot
    air X14.1
    cooker X15.8
    drink X10.0
    engine X17
    fat X10.2
    fluid NEC X12
    food X10.1
    gases X14.1
    heating appliance X16
    household appliance NEC X15.8
    kettle X15.8
    liquid NEC X12
    machinery X17
    metal (molten) (liquid) NEC X18
    object (not producing fire or flames) NEC X19
    oil (cooking) X10.2
    pipe (s) X16
    radiator X16
    saucepan (glass) (metal) X15.3
    stove (kitchen) X15.0
    substance NEC X19
      caustic or corrosive NEC —see Table of drugs and chemicals
    toaster X15.1
    tool X17
    vapor X13.1
    water (tap) —see Contact, with, hot, tap water
  hotplate X15.2
    suicide (attempt) X77.3
  ignition —see Ignition

Burn, burned, burning (*Continued*)
  in war operations —*see* War operations,
    fire
  inflicted by other person X97
    by hot objects, hot vapor, and steam —
      see Assault, burning, hot object
  internal, from swallowed caustic,
    corrosive liquid, substance —*see*
    Table of drugs and chemicals
  iron (hot) X15.8
    stated as undetermined whether
      accidental or intentional Y27.3
    suicide (attempt) X77.3
  kettle (hot) X15.8
    stated as undetermined whether
      accidental or intentional Y27.3
    suicide (attempt) X77.3
  lamp (flame) X08.8
    with ignition of clothing NEC X06.2
      nightwear X05
  lighter (cigar) (cigarette) X08.8
    with ignition of clothing NEC X06.2
      nightwear X05
  lightning —*see* subcategory T75.0
    causing fire —*see* Exposure, fire
  liquid (boiling) (hot) NEC X12
    stated as undetermined whether
      accidental or intentional Y27.2
    suicide (attempt) X77.2
  local application of externally applied
    substance in medical or surgical
    care Y63.5
  machinery (hot) X17
  matches X08.8
    with ignition of clothing NEC X06.2
      nightwear X05
  mattress —*see* Exposure, fire,
    uncontrolled, building, bed
  medicament, externally applied Y63.5
  metal (hot) (liquid) (molten) NEC X18
  nightwear (nightclothes, nightdress,
    gown, pajamas, robe) X05
  object (hot) NEC X19
  on board watercraft
    due to
      accident to watercraft V91.09
        powered craft V91.03
          ferry boat V91.01
          fishing boat V91.02
          jetskis V91.03
          liner V91.01
          merchant ship V91.00
          passenger ship V91.01

Burn, burned, burning (*Continued*)
  on board watercraft (*Continued*)
    due to (*Continued*)
      accident to watercraft (*Continued*)
        unpowered craft V91.08
          canoe V91.05
          inflatable V91.06
          kayak V91.05
          sailboat V91.04
          surf-board V91.08
          water skis V91.07
          windsurfer V91.08
      fire on board V93.09
        ferry boat V93.01
        fishing boat V93.02
        jetskis V93.03
        liner V93.01
        merchant ship V93.00
        passenger ship V93.01
        powered craft NEC V93.03
        sailboat V93.04
      specified heat source NEC on
        board V93.19
        ferry boat V93.11
        fishing boat V93.12
        jetskis V93.13
        liner V93.11
        merchant ship V93.10
        passenger ship V93.11
        powered craft NEC V93.13
        sailboat V93.14
  pipe (hot) X16
    smoking X08.8
      with ignition of clothing NEC
        X06.2
      nightwear X05
  powder —*see* Powder burn
  radiator (hot) X16
  saucepan (hot) (glass) (metal) X15.3
    stated as undetermined whether
      accidental or intentional
      Y27.3
    suicide (attempt) X77.3
  self-inflicted X76
    stated as undetermined whether
      accidental or intentional Y26
  stated as undetermined whether
    accidental or intentional Y27.0
  steam X13.1
    pipe X16
      stated as undetermined whether
        accidental or intentional
        Y27.8

Burn, burned, burning (*Continued*)
  steam (*Continued*)
    stated as undetermined whether
      accidental or intentional Y27.0
    suicide (attempt) X77.0
  stove (hot) (kitchen) X15.0
    stated as undetermined whether
      accidental or intentional Y27.3
    suicide (attempt) X77.3
  substance (hot) NEC X19
    boiling X12
      stated as undetermined whether
        accidental or intentional
        Y27.2
      suicide (attempt) X77.2
    molten (metal) X18
  suicide (attempt) NEC X76
    hot
      household appliance X77.3
      object X77.9
  stated as undetermined whether
    accidental or intentional Y27.0
  therapeutic misadventure
    heat in local application or packing
      during medical or surgical
      procedure Y63.5
    overdose of radiation Y63.2
  toaster (hot) X15.1
    stated as undetermined whether
      accidental or intentional Y27.3
    suicide (attempt) X77.3
  tool (hot) X17
  torch, welding X08.8
    with ignition of clothing NEC
      X06.2
    nightwear X05
  trash fire (controlled) —*see* Exposure,
    fire, controlled, not in building
    uncontrolled —*see* Exposure, fire,
      uncontrolled, not in building
  vapor (hot) X13.1
    stated as undetermined whether
      accidental or intentional Y27.0
    suicide (attempt) X77.0
  Very pistol —*see* Discharge, firearm
    NEC
Butted by animal W55.82
  bull W55.22
  cow W55.22
  goat W55.32
  horse W55.12
  pig W55.42
  sheep W55.32

C

Caisson disease —*see* Air, pressure, change
Campfire (exposure to) (controlled) —*see* also Exposure, fire, controlled, not in building
uncontrolled —*see* Exposure, fire, uncontrolled, not in building
Capital punishment (any means) —*see* Legal, intervention
Car sickness T75.3
Casualty (not due to war) NEC X58
war —*see* War operations
Cat
bite W55.01
scratch W55.03
Cataclysm, cataclysmic (any injury) NEC —*see* Forces of nature
Catching fire —*see* Exposure, fire
Caught
between
folding object W23.0
objects (moving) (stationary and moving) W23.0
and machinery —*see* Contact, with, by type of machine
stationary W23.1
sliding door and door frame W23.0
by, in
machinery (moving parts of) — *see* Contact, with, by type of machine
washing-machine wringer W23.0
under packing crate (due to losing grip) W23.1
Cave-in caused by cataclysmic earth surface movement or eruption —*see* Landslide
Change (s) **in air pressure** —*see* Air, pressure, change
Choked, choking (on) (any object except food or vomitus)
food (bone) (seed) —*see* categories T17 and T18
vomitus T17.81-
Civil insurrection —*see* War operations
Cloudburst (any injury) X37.8
Cold, exposure to (accidental) (excessive) (extreme) (natural) (place) **NEC** —*see* Exposure, cold
Collapse
building W20.1
burning (uncontrolled fire) X00.2
dam or man-made structure (causing earth movement) X36.0
machinery —*see* Contact, with, by type of machine
structure W20.1
burning (uncontrolled fire) X00.2
Collision (accidental) **NEC** (*see* also Accident, transport) V89.9
pedestrian W51
with fall W03
due to ice or snow W00.0
involving pedestrian conveyance — *see* Accident, transport, pedestrian, conveyance
and
crowd or human stampede (with fall) W52
object W22.8
with fall —*see* Fall, due to, bumping against, object
person (s) —*see* Collision, pedestrian

Collision (Continued)
transport vehicle NEC V89.9
and
avalanche, fallen or not moving — *see* Accident, transport
falling or moving B —*see* Landslide
landslide, fallen or not moving — *see* Accident, transport
falling or moving B —*see* Landslide
due to cataclysm —*see* Forces of nature, by type
intentional, purposeful suicide (attempt) —*see* Suicide, collision
Combustion, spontaneous —*see* Ignition
Complication (delayed) **of or following** (medical or surgical procedure) Y84.9
with misadventure —*see* Misadventure
amputation of limb (s) Y83.5
anastomosis (arteriovenous) (blood vessel) (gastrojejunal) (tendon) (natural or artificial material) Y83.2
aspiration (of fluid) Y84.4
tissue Y84.8
biopsy Y84.8
blood
sampling Y84.7
transfusion
procedure Y84.8
bypass Y83.2
catheterization (urinary) Y84.6
cardiac Y84.0
colostomy Y83.3
cystostomy Y83.3
dialysis (kidney) Y84.1
drug —*see* Table of drugs and chemicals
due to misadventure —*see* Misadventure
duodenostomy Y83.3
electroshock therapy Y84.3
external stoma, creation of Y83.3
formation of external stoma Y83.3
gastrostomy Y83.3
graft Y83.2
hypothermia (medically-induced) Y84.8
implant, implantation (of)
artificial
internal device (cardiac pacemaker) (electrodes in brain) (heart valve prosthesis) (orthopedic) Y83.1
material or tissue (for anastomosis or bypass) Y83.2
with creation of external stoma Y83.3
natural tissues (for anastomosis or bypass) Y83.2
with creation of external stoma Y83.3
infusion
procedure Y84.8
injection —*see* Table of drugs and chemicals
procedure Y84.8
insertion of gastric or duodenal sound Y84.5
insulin-shock therapy Y84.3
paracentesis (abdominal) (thoracic) (aspirative) Y84.4
procedures other than surgical operation —*see* Complication of or following, by type of procedure
radiological procedure or therapy Y84.2
removal of organ (partial) (total) NEC Y83.6

Complication (Continued)
sampling
blood Y84.7
fluid NEC Y84.4
tissue Y84.8
shock therapy Y84.3
surgical operation NEC (*see* also Complication of or following, by type of operation) Y83.9
reconstructive NEC Y83.4
with
anastomosis, bypass or graft Y83.2
formation of external stoma Y83.3
specified NEC Y83.8
transfusion —*see* also Table of drugs and chemicals
procedure Y84.8
transplant, transplantation (heart) (kidney) (liver) (whole organ, any) Y83.0
partial organ Y83.4
ureterostomy Y83.3
vaccination —*see* also Table of drugs and chemicals
procedure Y84.8
Compression
divers' squeeze —*see* Air, pressure, change
trachea by
food (lodged in esophagus) —*see* categories T17 and T18
vomitus (lodged in esophagus) T17.81-
Conflagration —*see* Exposure, fire, uncontrolled
Constriction (external)
hair W49.01
jewelry W49.04
ring W49.04
rubber band W49.03
specified item NEC W49.09
string W49.02
thread W49.02
Contact (accidental)
with
abrasive wheel (metalworking) W31.1
alligator W58.09
bite W58.01
crushing W58.03
strike W58.02
amphibian W62.9
frog W62.0
toad W62.1
animal (nonvenomous) NEC W64
marine W56.89
bite W56.81
dolphin —*see* Contact, with, dolphin
fish NEC —*see* Contact, with, fish
mammal —*see* Contact, with, mammal, marine
orca —*see* Contact, with, orca
sea lion —*see* Contact, with, sea lion
shark —*see* Contact, with, shark
strike W56.82
animate mechanical force NEC W64
arrow W21.89
not thrown, projected or falling W45.8
arthropods (nonvenomous) W57
axe W27.0
band-saw (industrial) W31.2
bayonet —*see* Bayonet wound
bee (s) X58

Contact *(Continued)*
  with *(Continued)*
    bench-saw (industrial) W31.2
    bird W61.99
      bite W61.91
      chicken —*see* Contact, with, chicken
      duck —*see* Contact, with, duck
      goose —*see* Contact, with, goose
      macaw —*see* Contact, with, macaw
      parrot —*see* Contact, with, parrot
      psittacine —*see* Contact, with, psittacine
      strike W61.92
      turkey —*see* Contact, with, turkey
    blender W29.0
    boiling water X12
      stated as undetermined whether accidental or intentional Y27.2
      suicide (attempt) X77.2
    bore, earth-drilling or mining (land) (seabed) W31.0
    buffalo —*see* Contact, with, hoof stock NEC
    bull W55.29
      bite W55.21
      gored W55.22
      strike W55.22
    bumper cars W31.81
    camel —*see* Contact, with, hoof stock NEC
    can
      lid W45.2
      opener W27.4
        powered W29.0
    cat W55.09
      bite W55.01
      scratch W55.03
    caterpillar (venomous) X58
    centipede (venomous) X58
    chain
      hoist W24.0
        agricultural operations W30.89
      saw W29.3
    chicken W61.39
      peck W61.33
      strike W61.32
    chisel W27.0
    circular saw W31.2
    cobra X58
    combine (harvester) W30.0
    conveyer belt W24.1
    cooker (hot) X15.8
      stated as undetermined whether accidental or intentional Y27.3
      suicide (attempt) X77.3
    coral X58
    cotton gin W31.82
    cow W55.29
      bite W55.21
      strike W55.22
    crane W24.0
      agricultural operations W30.89
    crocodile W58.19
      bite W58.11
      crushing W58.13
      strike W58.12
    dagger W26.1
      stated as undetermined whether accidental or intentional Y28.2
      suicide (attempt) X78.2
    dairy equipment W31.82
    dart W21.89
      not thrown, projected or falling W45.8

Contact *(Continued)*
  with *(Continued)*
    deer —*see* Contact, with, hoof stock NEC
    derrick W24.0
      agricultural operations W30.89
      hay W30.2
    dog W54.8
      bite W54.0
      strike W54.1
    dolphin W56.09
      bite W56.01
      strike W56.02
    donkey —*see* Contact, with, hoof stock NEC
    drill (powered) W29.8
      earth (land) (seabed) W31.0
      nonpowered W27.8
    drive belt W24.0
      agricultural operations W30.89
    dry ice —*see* Exposure, cold, man-made
    dryer (clothes) (powered) (spin) W29.2
    duck W61.69
      bite W61.61
      strike W61.62
    earth(-)
      drilling machine (industrial) W31.0
      scraping machine in stationary use W31.83
    edge of stiff paper W45.1
    electric
      beater W29.0
      blanket X16
      fan W29.2
        commercial W31.82
      knife W29.1
      mixer W29.0
    elevator (building) W24.0
      agricultural operations W30.89
      grain W30.3
    engine (s), hot NEC X17
    excavating machine W31.0
    farm machine W30.9
    feces —*see* Contact, with, by type of animal
    fer de lance X58
    fish W56.59
      bite W56.51
      shark —*see* Contact, with, shark
      strike W56.52
    flying horses W31.81
    forging (metalworking) machine W31.1
    fork W27.4
    forklift (truck) W24.0
      agricultural operations W30.89
    frog W62.0
    garden
      cultivator (powered) W29.3
        riding W30.89
      fork W27.1
    gas turbine W31.3
    Gila monster X58
    giraffe —*see* Contact, with, hoof stock NEC
    glass (sharp) (broken) W25
      with subsequent fall W18.02
      assault X99.0
      due to fall —*see* Fall, by type
      stated as undetermined whether accidental or intentional Y28. 0
      suicide (attempt) X78.0

Contact *(Continued)*
  with *(Continued)*
    goat W55.39
      bite W55.31
      strike W55.32
    goose W61.59
      bite W61.51
      strike W61.52
    hand
      saw W27.0
      tool (not powered) NEC W27.8
        powered W29.8
    harvester W30.0
    hay-derrick W30.2
    heat NEC X19
      from appliance (electrical) (household) —*see* Contact, with, hot, household appliance
      heating appliance X16
    heating
      appliance (hot) X16
      pad (electric) X16
    hedge-trimmer (powered) W29.3
    hoe W27.1
    hoist (chain) (shaft) NEC W24.0
      agricultural W30.89
    hoof stock NEC W55.39
      bite W55.31
      strike W55.32
    hornet (s) X58
    horse W55.19
      bite W55.11
      strike W55.12
    hot
      air X14.1
        inhalation X14.0
      cooker X15.8
      drinks X10.0
      engine X17
      fats X10.2
      fluids NEC X12
        assault X98.2
        suicide (attempt) X77.2
        undetermined whether accidental or intentional Y27.2
      food X10.1
      gases X14.1
        inhalation X14.0
      heating appliance X16
      household appliance X15.8
        assault X98.3
        cooker X15.8
        hotplate X15.2
        kettle X15.8
        light bulb X15.8
        object NEC X19
          assault X98.8
          stated as undetermined whether accidental or intentional Y27.9
          suicide (attempt) X77.8
        saucepan X15.3
        skillet X15.3
        stated as undetermined whether accidental or intentional Y27.3
        stove X15.0
        suicide (attempt) X77.3
        toaster X15.1
      kettle X15.8
      light bulb X15.8

Contact *(Continued)*
  with *(Continued)*
    hot *(Continued)*
      liquid NEC *(see also* Burning) X12
        drinks X10.0
        stated as undetermined whether
          accidental or intentional Y27.2
        suicide (attempt) X77.2
        tap water X11.8
          stated as undetermined
            whether accidental or
            intentional Y27.1
          suicide (attempt) X77.1
      machinery X17
      metal (molten) (liquid) NEC X18
      object (not producing fire or
        flames) NEC X19
      oil (cooking) X10.2
      pipe X16
      plate X15.2
      radiator X16
      saucepan (glass) (metal) X15.3
      skillet X15.3
      stove (kitchen) X15.0
      substance NEC X19
      tap-water X11.8
        assault X98.1
        heated on stove X12
          stated as undetermined
            whether accidental or
            intentional Y27.2
          suicide (attempt) X77.2
        in bathtub X11.0
        running X11.1
        stated as undetermined whether
          accidental or intentional Y27.1
        suicide (attempt) X77.1
      toaster X15.1
      tool X17
      vapors X13.1
        inhalation X13.0
      water (tap) X11.8
        boiling X12
          stated as undetermined
            whether accidental or
            intentional Y27.2
          suicide (attempt) X77.2
        heated on stove X12
          stated as undetermined
            whether accidental or
            intentional Y27.2
          suicide (attempt) X77.2
        in bathtub X11.0
        running X11.1
        stated as undetermined whether
          accidental or intentional
          Y27.1
        suicide (attempt) X77.1
      hotplate X15.2
      ice-pick W27.4
      insect (nonvenomous) NEC W57
      kettle (hot) X15.8
      knife W26.0
        assault X99.1
        electric W29.1
        stated as undetermined whether
          accidental or intentional Y28.1
        suicide (attempt) X78.1
      lathe (metalworking) W31.1
        turnings W45.8
        woodworking W31.2
      lawnmower (powered) (ridden) W28
        causing electrocution W86.8
          suicide (attempt) X83.1
        unpowered W27.1

Contact *(Continued)*
  with *(Continued)*
    lift, lifting (devices) W24.0
      agricultural operations W30.89
      shaft W24.0
    liquefied gas —*see* Exposure, cold,
      man-made
    liquid air, hydrogen, nitrogen —*see*
      Exposure, cold, man-made
    lizard (nonvenomous) W59.09
      bite W59.01
      strike W59.02
    llama —*see* Contact, with, hoof stock
      NEC
    macaw W61.19
      bite W61.11
      strike W61.12
    machine, machinery W31.9
      abrasive wheel W31.1
      agricultural including
          animal-powered W30.9
        combine harvester W30.0
        grain storage elevator W30.3
        hay derrick W30.2
        power take-off device W30.1
        reaper W30.0
        specified NEC W30.89
        thresher W30.0
        transport vehicle, stationary
          W30.81
      band saw W31.2
      bench saw W31.2
      circular saw W31.2
      commercial NEC W31.82
      drilling, metal (industrial)
        W31.1
      earth-drilling W31.0
      earthmoving or scraping
        W31.89
      excavating W31.89
      forging machine W31.1
      gas turbine W31.3
      hot X17
      internal combustion engine
        W31.3
      land drill W31.0
      lathe W31.1
      lifting (devices) W24.0
      metal drill W31.1
      metalworking (industrial) W31.1
      milling, metal W31.1
      mining W31.0
      molding W31.2
      overhead plane W31.2
      power press, metal W31.1
      prime mover W31.3
      printing W31.89
      radial saw W31.2
      recreational W31.81
      roller-coaster W31.81
      rolling mill, metal W31.1
      sander W31.2
      seabed drill W31.0
      shaft
        hoist W31.0
        lift W31.0
      specified NEC W31.89
      spinning W31.89
      steam engine W31.3
      transmission W24.1
      undercutter W31.0
      water driven turbine W31.3
      weaving W31.89
      woodworking or forming
        (industrial) W31.2

Contact *(Continued)*
  with *(Continued)*
    mammal (feces) (urine) W55.89
      bull —*see* Contact, with, bull
      cat —*see* Contact, with, cat
      cow —*see* Contact, with, cow
      goat —*see* Contact, with, goat
      hoof stock —*see* Contact, with, hoof
        stock
      horse —*see* Contact, with, horse
      marine W56.39
        dolphin —*see* Contact, with,
          dolphin
        orca —*see* Contact, with, orca
        sea lion —*see* Contact, with, sea
          lion
        specified NEC W56.39
          bite W56.31
          strike W56.32
      pig —*see* Contact, with, pig
      raccoon —*see* Contact, with, raccoon
      rodent —*see* Contact, with, rodent
      sheep —*see* Contact, with, sheep
      specified NEC W55.89
        bite W55.81
        strike W55.82
    marine
      animal W56.89
        bite W56.81
        dolphin —*see* Contact, with,
          dolphin
        fish NEC —*see* Contact, with, fish
        mammal —*see* Contact, with,
          mammal, marine
        orca —*see* Contact, with, orca
        sea lion —*see* Contact, with, sea
          lion
        shark —*see* Contact, with, shark
        strike W56.82
    meat
      grinder (domestic) W29.0
        industrial W31.82
        nonpowered W27.4
      slicer (domestic) W29.0
        industrial W31.82
    merry go round W31.81
    metal, (hot) (liquid) (molten) NEC
      X18
    millipede W57
    nail W45.0
      gun W29.4
    needle (sewing) W27.3
      hypodermic W46.0
        contaminated W46.1
    object (blunt) NEC
      hot NEC X19
      legal intervention —*see* Legal,
        intervention, blunt object
      sharp NEC W45.8
        inflicted by other person NEC
          W45.8
        stated as
          intentional homicide
            (attempt) —*see* Assault,
            cutting or piercing
            instrument
        legal intervention —*see* Legal,
          intervention, sharp object
        self-inflicted X78.9
    orca W56.29
      bite W56.21
      strike W56.22
    overhead plane W31.2
    paper (as sharp object) W45.1
    paper-cutter W27.5

Contact *(Continued)*
  with *(Continued)*
    parrot W61.09
      bite W61.01
      strike W61.02
    pig W55.49
      bite W55.41
      strike W55.42
    pipe, hot X16
    pitchfork W27.1
    plane (metal) (wood) W27.0
      overhead W31.2
    plant thorns, spines, sharp leaves or
        other mechanisms W60
    powered
      garden cultivator W29.3
      household appliance, implement,
          or machine W29.8
      saw (industrial) W31.2
        hand W29.8
    printing machine W31.89
    psittacine bird W61.29
      bite W61.21
      macaw —*see* Contace, with, macaw
      parrot —*see* Contact, with, parrot
      strike W61.22
    pulley (block) (transmission) W24.0
      agricultural operations W30.89
    raccoon W55.59
      bite W55.51
      strike W55.52
    radial-saw (industrial) W31.2
    radiator (hot) X16
    rake W27.1
    rattlesnake X58
    reaper W30.0
    reptile W59.89
      lizard —*see* Contact, with, lizard
      snake —*see* Contact, with, snake
      specified NEC W59.89
        bite W59.81
        crushing W59.83
        strike W59.82
      turtle —*see* Contact, with, turtle
    rivet gun (powered) W29.4
    road scraper —*see* Accident,
        transport, construction vehicle
    rodent (feces) (urine) W53.89
      bite W53.81
      mouse W53.09
        bite W53.01
      rat W53.19
        bite W53.11
      specified NEC W53.89
        bite W53.81
      squirrel W53.29
        bite W53.21
    roller coaster W31.81
    rope NEC W24.0
      agricultural operations W30.89
    saliva —*see* Contact, with, by type of
        animal
    sander W29.8
      industrial W31.2
    saucepan (hot) (glass) (metal) X15.3
    saw W27.0
      band (industrial) W31.2
      bench (industrial) W31.2
      chain W29.3
      hand W27.0
    sawing machine, metal W31.1
    scissors W27.2
    scorpion X58
    screwdriver W27.0
      powered W29.8

Contact *(Continued)*
  with *(Continued)*
    sea
      anemone, cucumber or urchin
          (spine) X58
      lion W56.19
        bite W56.11
        strike W56.12
    serpent —*see* Contact, with, snake,
        by type
    sewing-machine (electric) (powered)
        W29.2
      not powered W27.8
    shaft (hoist) (lift) (transmission) NEC
        W24.0
      agricultural W30.89
    shark W56.49
      bite W56.41
      strike W56.42
    shears (hand) W27.2
      powered (industrial) W31.1
      domestic W29.2
    sheep W55.39
      bite W55.31
      strike W55.32
    shovel W27.8
      steam —*see* Accident, transport,
          construction vehicle
    snake (nonvenomous) W59.19
      bite W59.11
      crushing W59.13
      strike W59.12
    spade W27.1
    spider (venomous) X58
    spin-drier W29.2
    spinning machine W31.89
    splinter W45.8
    sports equipment W21.9
    staple gun (powered) W29.8
    steam X13.1
      engine W31.3
      inhalation X13.0
      pipe X16
      shovel W31.89
    stove (hot) (kitchen) X15.0
    substance, hot NEC X19
      molten (metal) X18
    sword W26.1
      assault X99.2
      stated as undetermined whether
          accidental or intentional Y28.2
      suicide (attempt) X78.2
    tarantula X58
    thresher W30.0
    tin can lid W45.2
    toad W62.1
    toaster (hot) X15.1
    tool W27.8
      hand (not powered) W27.8
        auger W27.0
        axe W27.0
        can opener W27.4
        chisel W27.0
        fork W27.4
        garden W27.1
        handsaw W27.0
        hoe W27.1
        ice-pick W27.4
        kitchen utensil W27.4
        manual
          lawn mower W27.1
          sewing machine W27.8
        meat grinder W27.4
        needle (sewing) W27.3
          hypodermic W46.0
            contaminated W46.1

Contact *(Continued)*
  with *(Continued)*
    tool *(Continued)*
      hand *(Continued)*
        paper cutter W27.5
        pitchfork W27.1
        rake W27.1
        scissors W27.2
        screwdriver W27.0
        specified NEC W27.8
        workbench W27.0
      hot X17
      powered W29.8
        blender W29.0
          commercial W31.82
        can opener W29.0
          commercial W31.82
        chainsaw W29.3
        clothes dryer W29.2
          commercial W31.82
        dishwasher W29.2
          commercial W31.82
        edger W29.3
        electric fan W29.2
          commercial W31.82
        electric knife W29.1
        food processor W29.0
          commercial W31.82
        garbage disposal W29.0
          commercial W31.82
        garden tool W29.3
        hedge trimmer W29.3
        ice maker W29.0
          commercial W31.82
        kitchen appliance W29.0
          commercial W31.82
        lawn mower W28
        meat grinder W29.0
          commercial W31.82
        mixer W29.0
          commercial W31.82
        rototiller W29.3
        sewing machine W29.2
          commercial W31.82
        washing machine W29.2
          commercial W31.82
    transmission device (belt, cable,
        chain, gear, pinion, shaft)
        W24.1
      agricultural operations
          W30.89
    turbine (gas) (water-driven)
        W31.3
    turkey W61.49
      peck W61.43
      strike W61.42
    turtle (nonvenomous) W59.29
      bite W59.21
      strike W59.22
      terrestrial W59.89
        bite W59.81
        crushing W59.83
        strike W59.82
    under-cutter W31.0
    urine —*see* Contact, with, by type of
        animal
    vehicle
      agricultural use (transport) —
          see Accident, transport,
          agricultural vehicle
        not on public highway W30.81
      industrial use (transport) —*see*
          Accident, transport, industrial
          vehicle
        not on public highway W31.83

Contact (Continued)
  with (Continued)
    vehicle (Continued)
      off-road use (transport) —see
        Accident, transport, all-terrain
        or off-road vehicle
        not on public highway W31.83
      special construction use
        (transport) —see Accident,
        transport, construction vehicle
        not on public highway W31.83
    venomous
      animal X58
      arthropods X58
      lizard X58
      marine animal NEC X58
      marine plant NEC X58
      millipedes (tropical) X58
      plant (s) X58
      snake X58
      spider X58
      viper X58
      washing-machine (powered) W29.2
      wasp X58
      weaving-machine W31.89
      winch W24.0
        agricultural operations W30.89
      wire NEC W24.0
        agricultural operations W30.89
      wood slivers W45.8
      yellow jacket X58
      zebra —see Contact, with, hoof stock
        NEC
Coup de soleil X32
Crash
  aircraft (in transit) (powered) V95.9
    balloon V96.01
    fixed wing NEC (private) V95.21
      commercial V95.31
    glider V96.21
      hang V96.11
      powered V95.11

Crash (Continued)
  aircraft (Continued)
    helicopter V95.01
    in war operations —see War
      operations, destruction of
      aircraft
    microlight V95.11
    nonpowered V96.9
      specified NEC V96.8
    powered NEC V95.8
    stated as
      homicide (attempt) Y08.81
      suicide (attempt) X83.0
    ultralight V95.11
  spacecraft V95.41
  transport vehicle NEC (see also
    Accident, transport) V89.9
    homicide (attempt) Y03.8
    motor NEC (traffic) V89.2
      homicide (attempt) Y03.8
      suicide (attempt) —see Suicide,
        collision
Cruelty (mental) (physical) (sexual)
  X58
Crushed (accidentally) X58
  between objects (moving) (stationary
    and moving) W23.0
    stationary W23.1
  by
    alligator W58.03
    avalanche NEC B —see Landslide
    cave-in W20.0
      caused by cataclysmic earth
        surface movement B —see
        Landslide
    crocodile W58.13
    crowd or human stampede W52
    falling
      aircraft V97.39
        in war operations —see War
          operations, destruction of
          aircraft

Crushed (Continued)
  by (Continued)
    falling (Continued)
      earth, material W20.0
        caused by cataclysmic earth
          surface movement —see
          Landslide
      object NEC W20.8
    landslide NEC —see Landslide
    lizard (nonvenomous) W59.09
    machinery —see Contact, with, by
      type of machine
    reptile NEC W59.89
    snake (nonvenomous) W59.13
  in
    machinery —see Contact, with, by
      type of machine
Cut, cutting (any part of body)
  (accidental) —see also Contact, with,
    by object or machine
  during medical or surgical
    treatment as misadventure —see
    Misadventure, cut, by
    type of procedure
  homicide (attempt) —see Assault,
    cutting or piercing instrument
  inflicted by other person —see Assault,
    cutting or piercing instrument
  legal
    execution —see Legal, intervention
    intervention —see Legal, intervention,
      sharp object
  machine NEC (see also Contact,
    with, by type of machine)
    W31.9
  self-inflicted —see Suicide, cutting or
    piercing instrument
  suicide (attempt) —see Suicide, cutting
    or piercing instrument
Cyclone (any injury) X37.1

D

Drowning *(Continued)*
  in *(Continued)*
    natural water *(Continued)*
      stated as undetermined whether
        accidental or intentional
        Y21.4
      suicide (attempt) X71.3
    quarry —*see* Drowning, in, specified
      place NEC
    quenching tank —*see* Drowning, in,
      specified place NEC
    reservoir —*see* Drowning, in,
      specified place NEC
    river —*see* Drowning, in, natural
      water
    sea —*see* Drowning, in, natural water
    specified place NEC W73
      assault X92.8
      following
        dive or jump W16.811
          striking
            bottom W16.821
            wall W16.831

Drowning *(Continued)*
  in *(Continued)*
    specified place *(Continued)*
      following *(Continued)*
        fall W16.311
          striking
            bottom W16.321
            wall W16.331
      stated as undetermined whether
        accidental or intentional
        Y21.8
      suicide (attempt) X71.8
    stream —*see* Drowning, in, natural
      water
    swimming-pool W67
      assault X92.1
        following fall X92.2
      following
        dive or jump W16.511
          striking
            bottom W16.521
            wall W16.531

Drowning *(Continued)*
  in *(Continued)*
    swimming-pool *(Continued)*
      following *(Continued)*
        fall W16.011
          striking
            bottom W16.021
            wall W16.031
      stated as undetermined whether
        accidental or intentional Y21.2
        following fall Y21.3
      suicide (attempt) X71.1
        following fall X71.2
    war operations —*see* War operations,
      restriction of airway
    resulting from accident to watercraft —
      see Drowning, due to, accident,
      watercraft
  self-inflicted X71.9
  stated as undetermined whether
    accidental or intentional Y21.9
  suicide (attempt) X71.9

E

Earth (surface) movement NEC B —*see*
Forces of nature, earth movement
Earth falling (on) W20.0
caused by cataclysmic earth surface
movement or eruption B —*see*
Landslide
Earthquake (any injury) X34
Effect (s) (adverse) of
air pressure (any) —*see* Air, pressure
cold, excessive (exposure to) —*see*
Exposure, cold
heat (excessive) —*see* Heat
hot place (weather) B —*see* Heat
insolation X30
late —*see* Sequelae
motion —*see* Motion
nuclear explosion or weapon in war
operations —*see* War operations,
nuclear weapon
radiation —*see* Radiation
travel —*see* Travel
Electric shock (accidental) (by) (in) —*see*
Exposure, electric current
Electrocution (accidental) —*see* Exposure,
electric current
Endotracheal tube wrongly placed
during anesthetic procedure Y65.3
Entanglement
in
bed linen, causing suffocation —*see*
category T71
wheel of pedal cycle V19.88
Entry of foreign body or material —*see*
Foreign body
Environmental pollution related
condition —*see* Z57
Execution, legal (any method) —*see*
Legal, intervention
Exhaustion
cold —*see* Exposure, cold
due to excessive exertion —*see*
Overexertion
heat —*see* Heat
Explosion (accidental) (of) (with
secondary fire) W40.9
acetylene W40.1
aerosol can W36.1
air tank (compressed) (in machinery)
W36.2
aircraft (in transit) (powered) NEC
V95.9
balloon V96.05
fixed wing NEC (private) V95.25
commercial V95.35
glider V96.25
hang V96.15
powered V95.15
helicopter V95.05
in war operations —*see* War operations,
destruction of aircraft
microlight V95.15
nonpowered V96.9
specified NEC V96.8
powered NEC V95.8
stated as
homicide (attempt) Y03.8
suicide (attempt) X83.0
ultralight V95.15
anesthetic gas in operating room W40.1
antipersonnel bomb W40.8
assault X96.0
homicide (attempt) X96.0
suicide (attempt) X75

Explosion (Continued)
assault X96.9
bicycle tire W37.0
blasting (cap) (materials) W40.0
boiler (machinery), not on transport
vehicle W35
on watercraft —*see* Explosion, in,
watercraft
butane W40.1
caused by other person X96.9
coal gas W40.1
detonator W40.0
dump (munitions) W40.8
dynamite W40.0
in
assault X96.8
homicide (attempt) X96.8
legal intervention
injuring
bystander Y35.112
law enforcement personnel
Y35.111
suspect Y35.113
suicide (attempt) X75
explosive (material) W40.9
gas W40.1
in blasting operation W40.0
specified NEC W40.8
in
assault X96.8
homicide (attempt) X96.8
legal intervention
injuring
bystander Y35.192
law enforcement personnel
Y35.191
suspect Y35.193
suicide (attempt) X75
factory (munitions) W40.8
fertilizer bomb W40.8
assault X96.3
homicide (attempt) X96.3
suicide (attempt) X75
fire-damp W40.1
firearm (parts) NEC W34.19
airgun W34.110
BB gun W34.110
gas, air or spring-operated gun NEC
W34.118
handgun W32.1
hunting rifle W33.12
larger firearm W33.10
specified NEC W33.19
machine gun W33.13
paintball gun W34.111
pellet gun W34.110
shotgun W33.11
Very pistol [flare] W34.19
fireworks W39
gas (coal) (explosive) W40.1
cylinder W36.9
aerosol can W36.1
air tank W36.2
pressurized W36.3
specified NEC W36.8
gasoline (fumes) (tank) not in moving
motor vehicle W40.1
bomb W40.8
assault X96.1
homicide (attempt) X96.1
suicide (attempt) X75
in motor vehicle —*see* Accident,
transport, by type of
vehicle
grain store W40.8

Explosion (Continued)
grenade W40.8
in
assault X96.8
homicide (attempt) X96.8
legal intervention
injuring
bystander Y35.192
law enforcement personnel
Y35.191
suspect Y35.193
suicide (attempt) X75
handgun (parts) —*see* Explosion,
firearm, handgun (parts)
homicide (attempt) X96.9
antipersonnel bomb —*see* Explosion,
antipersonnel bomb
fertilizer bomb —*see* Explosion,
fertilizer bomb
gasoline bomb —*see* Explosion,
gasoline bomb
letter bomb —*see* Explosion, letter
bomb
pipe bomb —*see* Explosion, pipe
bomb
specified NEC X96.8
hose, pressurized W37.8
hot water heater, tank (in machinery)
W35
on watercraft —*see* Explosion, in,
watercraft
in, on
dump W40.8
factory W40.8
mine (of explosive gases) NEC
W40.1
watercraft V93.59
powered craft V93.53
ferry boat V93.51
fishing boat V93.52
jetskis V93.53
liner V93.51
merchant ship V93.50
passenger ship V93.51
sailboat V93.54
letter bomb W40.8
assault X96.2
homicide (attempt) X96.2
suicide (attempt) X75
machinery —*see also* Contact, with, by
type of machine
on board watercraft —*see* Explosion,
in, watercraft
pressure vessel —*see* Explosion, by
type of vessel
methane W40.1
mine W40.1
missile NEC W40.8
mortar bomb W40.8
in
assault X96.8
homicide (attempt) X96.8
legal intervention
injuring
bystander Y35.192
law enforcement personnel
Y35.191
suspect Y35.193
suicide (attempt) X75
munitions (dump) (factory) W40.8
pipe, pressurized W37.8
bomb W40.8
assault X96.4
homicide (attempt) X96.4
suicide (attempt) X75

Explosion (Continued)
pressure, pressurized
  cooker W38
  gas tank (in machinery) W36.3
  hose W37.8
  pipe W37.8
  specified device NEC W38
  tire W37.8
    bicycle W37.0
  vessel (in machinery) W38
propane W40.1
self-inflicted X75
shell (artillery) NEC W40.8
  during war operations —see War
    operations, explosion
  in
    legal intervention
      injuring
        bystander Y35.122
        law enforcement personnel
          Y35.121
        suspect Y35.123
    war —see War operations, explosion
spacecraft V95.45
stated as undetermined whether
  accidental or intentional Y25
steam or water lines (in machinery)
  W37.8
stove W40.9
suicide (attempt) X75
tire, pressurized W37.8
  bicycle W37.0
undetermined whether accidental or
  intentional Y25
vehicle tire NEC W37.8
  bicycle W37.0
war operations —see War operations,
  explosion
Exposure (to) X58
air pressure change —see Air, pressure
cold (accidental) (excessive) (extreme)
  (natural) (place) X31
  assault Y08.89
  due to
    man-made conditions W93.8
      dry ice (contact) W93.01
        inhalation W93.02
      liquid air (contact) (hydrogen)
        (nitrogen) W93.11
        inhalation W93.12
      refrigeration unit (deep freeze)
        W93.2
      suicide (attempt) X83.2
      weather (conditions) X31
  homicide (attempt) Y08.89
  self-inflicted X83.2
due to abandonment or neglect X58
electric current W86.8
  appliance (faulty) W86.8
    domestic W86.0
  caused by other person Y08.89
  conductor (faulty) W86.1
  control apparatus (faulty) W86.1
  electric power generating plant,
    distribution station W86.1
  electroshock gun —see Exposure,
    electric current, taser
  high-voltage cable W85
  homicide (attempt) Y08.89
  legal execution —see Legal,
    intervention, specified means NEC
  lightning —see subcategory T75.0
  live rail W86.8
  misadventure in medical or surgical
    procedure in electroshock
    therapy Y63.4

Exposure (Continued)
electric current (Continued)
  motor (electric) (faulty) W86.8
    domestic W86.0
  self-inflicted X83.1
  specified NEC W86.8
    domestic W86.0
  stun gun —see Exposure, electric
    current, taser
  suicide (attempt) X83.1
  taser W86.8
    assault Y08.89
    legal intervention —see category Y35
    self-harm (intentional) X83.8
    undetermined intent Y33
  third rail W86.8
  transformer (faulty) W86.1
  transmission lines W85
environmental tobacco smoke X58
excessive
  cold —see Exposure, cold
  heat (natural) NEC X30
    man-made W92
factor (s) NOS X58
  environmental NEC X58
    man-made NEC W99
    natural NEC B —see Forces of
      nature
  specified NEC X58
fire, flames (accidental) X08.8
  assault X97
  campfire —see Exposure, fire,
    controlled, not in building
  controlled (in)
    with ignition (of) clothing (see also
      Ignition, clothes) X06.2
      nightwear X05
    bonfire —see Exposure, fire,
      controlled, not in building
    brazier (in building or structure) —
      see also Exposure, fire,
      controlled, building
    not in building or structure —see
      Exposure, fire, controlled,
      not in building
    building or structure X02.0
      with
        fall from building X02.3
        from building X02.5
        injury due to building collapse
          X02.2
        smoke inhalation X02.1
      hit by object from building X02.4
      specified mode of injury NEC
        X02.8
    fireplace, furnace or stove —see
      Exposure, fire, controlled,
      building
    not in building or structure X03.0
      with
        fall X03.3
        smoke inhalation X03.1
      hit by object X03.4
      specified mode of injury NEC
        X03.8
    trash —see Exposure, fire,
      controlled, not in building
  fireplace —see Exposure, fire,
    controlled, building
  fittings or furniture (in building or
    structure) (uncontrolled) —see
    Exposure, fire, uncontrolled,
    building
  forest (uncontrolled) —see Exposure,
    fire, uncontrolled, not in building

Exposure (Continued)
fire, flames (Continued)
  grass (uncontrolled) —see Exposure,
    fire, uncontrolled, not in building
  hay (uncontrolled) —see Exposure,
    fire, uncontrolled, not in
    building
  homicide (attempt) X97
  ignition of highly flammable material
    X04
  in, of, on, starting in
    machinery —see Contact, with, by
      type of machine
    motor vehicle (in motion) (see also
      Accident, transport, occupant
      by type of vehicle) V87.8
      with collision —see Collision
    railway rolling stock, train, vehicle
      V81.81
      with collision —see Accident,
        transport, railway vehicle
        occupant
    street car (in motion) V82.8
      with collision —see Accident,
        transport, streetcar
        occupant
    transport vehicle NEC —see also
      Accident, transport
      with collision —see Collision
  war operations —see also War
    operations, fire
    from nuclear explosion —see War
      operations, nuclear weapons
  watercraft (in transit) (not in
    transit) V91.09
    localized —see Burn, on board
      watercraft, due to, fire on
      board
    powered craft V91.03
      ferry boat V91.01
      fishing boat V91.02
      jet skis V91.03
      liner V91.01
      merchant ship V91.00
      passenger ship V91.01
    unpowered craft V91.08
      canoe V91.05
      inflatable V91.06
      kayak V91.05
      sailboat V91.04
      surf-board V91.08
      waterskis V91.07
      windsurfer V91.08
  lumber (uncontrolled) —see
    Exposure, fire, uncontrolled, not
    in building
  mine (uncontrolled) —see Exposure,
    fire, uncontrolled, not in building
  prairie (uncontrolled) —see
    Exposure, fire, uncontrolled, not
    in building
  resulting from
    explosion —see Explosion
    lightning X08.8
  self-inflicted X76
  specified NEC X08.8
  started by other person X97
  stated as undetermined whether
    accidental or intentional Y26
  stove —see Exposure, fire, controlled,
    building
  suicide (attempt) X76
  tunnel (uncontrolled) —see
    Exposure, fire, uncontrolled, not
    in building

Exposure (*Continued*)
  fire, flames (*Continued*)
    uncontrolled
      in building or structure
        X00.0
        with
          fall from building X00.3
          injury due to building collapse
            X00.2
          jump from building X00.5
          smoke inhalation X00.1
        bed X08.00
          due to
            cigarette X08.01
            specified material NEC
              X08.09
        furniture NEC X08.20
          due to
            cigarette X08.21
            specified material NEC
              X08.29
        hit by object from building
          X00.4
        sofa X08.10
          due to
            cigarette X08.11
            specified material NEC
              X08.19
        specified mode of injury NEC
          X00.8
      not in building or structure (any)
        X01.0
        with
          fall X01.3
          smoke inhalation X01.1

Exposure (*Continued*)
  fire, flames (*Continued*)
    uncontrolled (*Continued*)
      not in building or structure
        (*Continued*)
        hit by object X01.4
        specified mode of injury NEC
          X01.8
      undetermined whether accidental or
        intentional Y26
  forces of nature NEC B —*see* Forces of
    nature
  G-forces (abnormal) W49.9
  gravitational forces (abnormal)
    W49.9
  heat (natural) NEC —*see* Heat
  high-pressure jet (hydraulic)
    (pneumatic) W49.9
  hydraulic jet W49.9
  inanimate mechanical force W49.9
  jet, high-pressure (hydraulic)
    (pneumatic) W49.9
  lightning —*see* subcategory T75.0
    causing fire —*see* Exposure, fire
  mechanical forces NEC W49.9
    animate NEC W64
    inanimate NEC W49.9
  noise W42.9
    supersonic W42.0
  noxious substance —*see* Table of drugs
    and chemical
  pneumatic jet W49.9
  prolonged in deep-freeze unit or
    refrigerator W93.2
  radiation —*see* Radiation

Exposure (*Continued*)
  smoke —*see* also Exposure, fire
    tobacco, second hand Z77.22
  specified factors NEC X58
  sunlight X32
    man-made (sun lamp) W89.8
      tanning bed W89.1
  supersonic waves W42.0
  transmission line (s), electric W85
  vibration W49.9
  waves
    infrasound W49.9
    sound W42.9
    supersonic W42.0
  weather NEC B —*see* Forces of nature
External cause status Y99.9
  child assisting in compensated work for
    family Y99.8
  civilian activity done for financial or
    other compensation Y99.0
  civilian activity done for income or pay
    Y99.0
  family member assisting in
    compensated work for other family
    member Y99.8
  hobby not done for income Y99.8
  leisure activity Y99.8
  military activity Y99.1
  off-duty activity of military personnel
    Y99.8
  recreation or sport not for income or
    while a student Y99.8
  specified NEC Y99.8
  student activity Y99.8
  volunteer activity Y99.2

F

Factors, supplemental
  alcohol
    blood level
      less than 20mg/100ml Y90.0
      presence in blood, level not
        specified Y90.9
      20-39mg/100ml Y90.1
      40-59mg/100ml Y90.2
      60-79mg/100ml Y90.3
      80-99mg/100ml Y90.4
      100-119mg/100ml Y90.5
      120-199mg/100ml Y90.6
      200-239mg/100ml Y90.7
      240mg/100ml or more Y90.8
      presence in blood, but level not
        specified Y90.9
  environmental-pollution-related
    condition —*see* Z57
  nosocomial condition Y95
  work-related condition Y99.0
Failure
  in suture or ligature during surgical
    procedure Y65.2
  mechanical, of instrument or apparatus
    (any) (during any medical or
    surgical procedure) Y65.8
  sterile precautions (during medical and
    surgical care) —*see* Misadventure,
    failure, sterile precautions, by type
    of procedure
  to
    introduce tube or instrument Y65.4
    endotracheal tube during
      anesthesia Y65.3
    make curve (transport vehicle)
      NEC —*see* Accident, transport
    remove tube or instrument Y65.4
Fall, falling (accidental) W19
  building W20.1
    burning (uncontrolled fire) X00.3
  down
    embankment W17.81
    escalator W10.0
    hill W17.81
    ladder W11
    ramp W10.2
    stairs, steps W10.9
  due to
    bumping against
      object W18.00
        sharp glass W18.02
        specified NEC W18.09
        sports equipment W18.01
      person W03
        due to ice or snow W00.0
        on pedestrian conveyance —
          see Accident, transport,
          pedestrian, conveyance
    collision with another person W03
      due to ice or snow W00.0
      involving pedestrian conveyance —
        see Accident, transport,
        pedestrian, conveyance
    grocery cart tipping over W17.82
    ice or snow W00.9
      from one level to another W00.2
      on stairs or steps W00.1
      involving pedestrian
        conveyance —*see* Accident,
        transport, pedestrian,
        conveyance
      on same level W00.0
    slipping (on moving sidewalk) W01.0

Fall, falling (Continued)
  due to (Continued)
    slipping (Continued)
      with subsequent striking against
        object W01.10
        furniture W01.190
        sharp object W01.119
          glass W01.110
          power tool or machine W01.111
          specified NEC W01.118
        specified NEC W01.198
    striking against
      object W18.00
        sharp glass W18.02
        specified NEC W18.09
        sports equipment W18.01
      person W03
        due to ice or snow W00.0
        on pedestrian conveyance —
          see Accident, transport,
          pedestrian, conveyance
  earth (with asphyxia or suffocation (by
    pressure)) —*see* Earth, falling
  from, off, out of
    aircraft NEC (with accident to aircraft
      NEC) V97.0
      while boarding or alighting V97.1
    balcony W13.0
    bed W06
    boat, ship, watercraft NEC (with
      drowning or submersion) —*see*
      Drowning, due to, fall overboard
      with hitting bottom or object V94.0
    bridge W13.1
    building W13.9
      burning (uncontrolled fire) X00.3
    cavity W17.2
    chair W07
    cherry picker W17.89
    cliff W15
    dock W17.4
    embankment W17.81
    escalator W10.0
    flagpole W13.8
    furniture NEC W08
    grocery cart W17.82
    haystack W17.89
    high place NEC W17.89
      stated as undetermined whether
        accidental or intentional Y30
    hole W17.2
    incline W10.2
    ladder W11
    lifting device W17.89
    machine, machinery —*see* also
      Contact, with, by type of machine
      not in operation W17.89
    manhole W17.1
    mobile elevated work platform
      [MEWP] W17.89
    motorized mobility scooter W05.2
    one level to another NEC W17.89
      intentional, purposeful, suicide
        (attempt) X80
      stated as undetermined whether
        accidental or intentional Y30
    pit W17.2
    playground equipment W09.8
      jungle gym W09.2
      slide W09.0
      swing W09.1
    quarry W17.89
    railing W13.9
    ramp W10.2
    roof W13.2

Fall, falling (Continued)
  from, off, out of (Continued)
    scaffolding W12
    scooter (nonmotorized) W05.1
      motorized mobility W05.2
    sky lift W17.89
    stairs, steps W10.9
      curb W10.1
      due to ice or snow W00.1
      escalator W10.0
      incline W10.2
      ramp W10.2
      sidewalk curb W10.1
      specified NEC W10.8
    stepladder W11
    storm drain W17.1
    streetcar NEC V82.6
      with antecedent collision —*see*
        Accident, transport, streetcar
        occupant
      while boarding or alighting V82.4
    structure NEC W13.8
      burning (uncontrolled fire) X00.3
    table W08
    toilet W18.11
      with subsequent striking against
        object W18.12
    train NEC V81.6
      during derailment (without
        antecedent collision) V81.7
      with antecedent collision —*see*
        Accident, transport, railway
        vehicle occupant
      while boarding or alighting V81.4
    transport vehicle after collision —*see*
      Accident, transport, by type of
      vehicle, collision
    tree W14
    vehicle (in motion) NEC (*see also*
      Accident, transport) V89.9
      motor NEC (*see also* Accident,
        transport, occupant, by type of
        vehicle) V87.8
      stationary W17.89
        while boarding or alighting
          B —*see* Accident, transport,
          by type of vehicle, while
          boarding or alighting
    viaduct W13.8
    wall W13.8
    watercraft —*see also* Drowning, due
      to, fall overboard
      with hitting bottom or object
        V94.0
    well W17.0
    wheelchair, non-moving W05.0
      powered —*see* Accident, transport,
        pedestrian, conveyance
        occupant, specified type NEC
    window W13.4
  in, on
    aircraft NEC V97.0
      with accident to aircraft V97.0
      while boarding or alighting
        V97.1
    bathtub (empty) W18.2
      filled W16.212
        causing drowning W16.211
    escalator W10.0
    incline W10.2
    ladder W11
    machine, machinery —*see* Contact,
      with, by type of machine
    object, edged, pointed or sharp (with
      cut) —*see* Fall, by type

Fall, falling (Continued)
  in, on (Continued)
    playground equipment W09.8
      jungle gym W09.2
      slide W09.0
      swing W09.1
    ramp W10.2
    scaffolding W12
    shower W18.2
      causing drowning W16.211
    staircase, stairs, steps W10.9
      curb W10.1
      due to ice or snow W00.1
      escalator W10.0
      incline W10.2
      specified NEC W10.8
    streetcar (without antecedent collision) V82.5
      with antecedent collision —see Accident, transport, streetcar occupant
      while boarding or alighting V82.4
    train (without antecedent collision) V81.5
      with antecedent collision —see Accident, transport, railway vehicle occupant
      during derailment (without antecedent collision) V81.7
        with antecedent collision —see Accident, transport, railway vehicle occupant
      while boarding or alighting V81.4
    transport vehicle after collision —see Accident, transport, by type of vehicle, collision
    watercraft V93.39
      due to
        accident to craft V91.29
          powered craft V91.23
            ferry boat V91.21
            fishing boat V91.22
            jetskis V91.23
            liner V91.21
            merchant ship V91.20
            passenger ship V91.21
          unpowered craft
            canoe V91.25
            inflatable V91.26
            kayak V91.25
            sailboat V91.24
        powered craft V93.33
          ferry boat V93.31
          fishing boat V93.32
          jetskis V93.33
          liner V93.31
          merchant ship V93.30
          passenger ship V93.31
        unpowered craft V93.38
          canoe V93.35
          inflatable V93.36
          kayak V93.35
          sailboat V93.34
          surf-board V93.38
          windsurfer V93.38
  into
    cavity W17.2
    dock W17.4
    fire —see Exposure, fire, by type
    haystack W17.89
    hole W17.2
    lake —see Fall, into, water
    manhole W17.1
    moving part of machinery —see Contact, with, by type of machine

Fall, falling (Continued)
  into (Continued)
    ocean —see Fall, into, water
    opening in surface NEC W17.89
    pit W17.2
    pond —see Fall, into, water
    quarry W17.89
    river —see Fall, into, water
    shaft W17.89
    storm drain W17.1
    stream —see Fall, into, water
    swimming pool —see also Fall, into, water, in, swimming pool
      empty W17.3
    tank W17.89
    water W16.42
      causing drowning W16.41
      from watercraft —see Drowning, due to, fall overboard
      hitting diving board W21.4
      in
        bathtub W16.212
          causing drowning W16.211
        bucket W16.222
          causing drowning W16.221
        natural body of water W16.112
          causing drowning W16.111
          striking
            bottom W16.122
              causing drowning W16.121
            side W16.132
              causing drowning W16.131
        specified water NEC W16.312
          causing drowning W16.311
          striking
            bottom W16.322
              causing drowning W16.321
            wall W16.332
              causing drowning W16.331
        swimming pool W16.012
          causing drowning W16.011
          striking
            bottom W16.022
              causing drowning W16.021
            wall W16.032
              causing drowning W16.031
        utility bucket W16.222
          causing drowning W16.221
    well W17.0
  involving
    bed W06
    chair W07
    furniture NEC W08
    glass —see Fall, by type
    playground equipment W09.8
      jungle gym W09.2
      slide W09.0
      swing W09.1
    roller blades —see Accident, transport, pedestrian, conveyance
    skateboard (s) —see Accident, transport, pedestrian, conveyance
    skates (ice) (in line) (roller) —see Accident, transport, pedestrian, conveyance
    skis —see Accident, transport, pedestrian, conveyance
    table W08
    wheelchair, non-moving W05.0
      powered —see Accident, transport, pedestrian, conveyance, specified type NEC

Fall, falling (Continued)
  object —see Struck by, object, falling
  off
    toilet W18.11
      with subsequent striking against object W18.12
  on same level W18.30
    due to
      specified NEC W18.39
      stepping on an object W18.31
  out of
    bed W06
    building NEC W13.8
    chair W07
    furniture NEC W08
    wheelchair, non-moving W05.0
      powered —see Accident, transport, pedestrian, conveyance, specified type NEC
    window W13.4
  over
    animal W01.0
    cliff W15
    embankment W17.81
    small object W01.0
  rock W20.8
  same level W18.30
    from
      being crushed, pushed, or stepped on by a crowd or human stampede W52
      collision, pushing, shoving, by or with other person W03
      slipping, stumbling, tripping W01.0
    involving ice or snow W00.0
      involving skates (ice) (roller), skateboard, skis —see Accident, transport, pedestrian, conveyance
  snowslide (avalanche) B —see Landslide
  stone W20.8
  structure W20.1
    burning (uncontrolled fire) X00.3
  through
    bridge W13.1
    floor W13.3
    roof W13.2
    wall W13.8
    window W13.4
  timber W20.8
  tree (caused by lightning) W20.8
  while being carried or supported by other person (s) W04
Fallen on by
  animal (not being ridden) NEC W55.89
Felo-de-se —see Suicide
Fight (hand) (fists) (foot) —see Assault, fight
Fire (accidental) —see Exposure, fire
Firearm discharge —see Discharge, firearm
Fireball effects from nuclear explosion in war operations —see War operations, nuclear weapons
Fireworks (explosion) W39
Flash burns from explosion —see Explosion
Flood (any injury) (caused by) X38
  collapse of man-made structure causing earth movement X36.0
  tidal wave —see Forces of nature, tidal wave
Food (any type) in
  air passages (with asphyxia, obstruction, or suffocation) —see categories T17 and T18

Food *(Continued)*
  alimentary tract causing asphyxia (due to compression of trachea) —*see* categories T17 and T18
Forces of nature X39.8
  avalanche X36.1
    causing transport accident —*see* Accident, transport, by type of vehicle
  blizzard X37.2
  cataclysmic storm X37.9
    with flood X38
    blizzard X37.2
    cloudburst X37.8
    cyclone X37.1
    dust storm X37.3
    hurricane X37.0
    specified storm NEC X37.8
    storm surge X37.0
    tornado X37.1
    twister X37.1
    typhoon X37.0
  cloudburst X37.8
  cold (natural) X31
  cyclone X37.1
  dam collapse causing earth movement X36.0
  dust storm X37.3
  earth movement X36.1
    caused by dam or structure collapse X36.0
    earthquake X34

Forces of nature *(Continued)*
  earthquake X34
  flood (caused by) X38
    dam collapse X36.0
    tidal wave B —*see* Forces of nature, tidal wave
  heat (natural) X30
  hurricane X37.0
  landslide X36.1
    causing transport accident —*see* Accident, transport, by type of vehicle
  lightning —*see* subcategory T75.0
    causing fire —*see* Exposure, fire
  mudslide X36.1
    causing transport accident —*see* Accident, transport, by type of vehicle
  radiation (natural) X39.08
    radon X39.01
  radon X39.01
  specified force NEC X39.8
  storm surge X37.0
  structure collapse causing earth movement X36.0
  sunlight X32
  tidal wave X37.41
    due to
      earthquake X37.41
      landslide X37.43
      storm X37.42
      volcanic eruption X37.41

Forces of nature *(Continued)*
  tornado X37.1
  tsunami X37.41
  twister X37.1
  typhoon X37.0
  volcanic eruption X35
Foreign body entering through skin W45.8
  can lid W45.2
  nail W45.0
  paper W45.1
  specified NEC W45.8
  splinter W45.8
Forest fire (exposure to) —*see* Exposure, fire, uncontrolled, not in building
Found injured X58
  from exposure (to) —*see* Exposure
  on
    highway, road(way), street V89.9
    railway right of way V81.9
Fracture (circumstances unknown or unspecified) X58
  due to specified cause NEC X58
Freezing —*see* Exposure, cold
Frostbite X31
  due to man-made conditions —*see* Exposure, cold, man-made
Frozen —*see* Exposure, cold

G

Gored by bull W55.22
Gunshot wound W34.00

H

Hailstones, injured by X39.8
Hanged herself or himself —*see* Hanging, self-inflicted
Hanging (accidental) (*see also* category T71)
  legal execution —*see* Legal, intervention, specified means NEC
Heat (effects of) (excessive) X30
  due to
    man-made conditions W92
      on board watercraft V93.29
        fishing boat V93.22
        merchant ship V93.20
        passenger ship V93.21
        sailboat V93.24
        specified powered craft NEC V93.23
    weather (conditions) X30

Heat *(Continued)*
  from
    electric heating apparatus causing burning X16
    nuclear explosion in war operations —*see* War operations, nuclear weapons
    inappropriate in local application or packing in medical or surgical procedure Y63.5
Hemorrhage
  delayed following medical or surgical treatment without mention of misadventure —*see* Complication of or following, by type of procedure
  during medical or surgical treatment as misadventure —*see* Misadventure, cut, by type of procedure

High
  altitude (effects) —*see* Air, pressure, low
  level of radioactivity, effects —*see* Radiation
  pressure (effects) —*see* Air, pressure, high
  temperature, effects —*see* Heat
Hit, hitting (accidental) by —*see* Struck by
Hitting against —*see* Striking against
Homicide (attempt) (justifiable) —*see* Assault
Hot
  place, effects —*see also* Heat
  weather, effects X30
House fire (uncontrolled) —*see* Exposure, fire, uncontrolled, building
Humidity, causing problem X39.8
Hunger X58
Hurricane (any injury) X37.0
Hypobarism, hypobaropathy —*see* Air, pressure, low

I

Ictus
caloris —*see also* Heat
solaris X30
Ignition (accidental) (*see also* Exposure, fire) X08.8
anesthetic gas in operating room W40.1
apparel X06.2
from highly flammable material X04
nightwear X05
bed linen (sheets) (spreads) (pillows) (mattress) —*see* Exposure, fire, uncontrolled, building, bed
benzine X04
clothes, clothing NEC (from controlled fire) X06.2
from
highly flammable material X04
ether X04
in operating room W40.1
explosive material —*see* Explosion
gasoline X04
jewelry (plastic) (any) X06.0
kerosene X04
material
explosive —*see* Explosion
highly flammable with secondary explosion X04
nightwear X05
paraffin X04
petrol X04
Immersion (accidental) —*see also* Drowning
hand or foot due to cold (excessive) X31
Implantation of quills of porcupine W55.89
Inanition (from) (hunger) X58
thirst X58.8
Inappropriate operation performed
correct operation on wrong side or body part (wrong side) (wrong site) Y65.53
operation intended for another patient done on wrong patient Y65.52
wrong operation performed on correct patient Y65.51
Inattention after, at birth (homicidal intent) (infanticidal intent) X58
Incident, adverse
device
anesthesiology Y70.8
accessory Y70.2
diagnostic Y70.0
miscellaneous Y70.8
monitoring Y70.0
prosthetic Y70.2
rehabilitative Y70.1
surgical Y70.3
therapeutic Y70.1
cardiovascular Y71.8
accessory Y71.2
diagnostic Y71.0
miscellaneous Y71.8
monitoring Y71.0
prosthetic Y71.2
rehabilitative Y71.1
surgical Y71.3
therapeutic Y71.1

Incident, adverse (*Continued*)
device (*Continued*)
gastroenterology Y73.8
accessory Y73.2
diagnostic Y73.0
miscellaneous Y73.8
monitoring Y73.0
prosthetic Y73.2
rehabilitative Y73.1
surgical Y73.3
therapeutic Y73.1
general
hospital Y74.8
accessory Y74.2
diagnostic Y74.0
miscellaneous Y74.8
monitoring Y74.0
prosthetic Y74.2
rehabilitative Y74.1
surgical Y74.3
therapeutic Y74.1
surgical Y81.8
accessory Y81.2
diagnostic Y81.0
miscellaneous Y81.8
monitoring Y81.0
prosthetic Y81.2
rehabilitative Y81.1
surgical Y81.3
therapeutic Y81.1
gynecological Y76.8
accessory Y76.2
diagnostic Y76.0
miscellaneous Y76.8
monitoring Y76.0
prosthetic Y76.2
rehabilitative Y76.1
surgical Y76.3
therapeutic Y76.1
medical Y82.9
specified type NEC Y82.8
neurological Y75.8
accessory Y75.2
diagnostic Y75.0
miscellaneous Y75.8
monitoring Y75.0
prosthetic Y75.2
rehabilitative Y75.1
surgical Y75.3
therapeutic Y75.1
obstetrical Y76.8
accessory Y76.2
diagnostic Y76.0
miscellaneous Y76.8
monitoring Y76.0
prosthetic Y76.2
rehabilitative Y76.1
surgical Y76.3
therapeutic Y76.1
ophthalmic Y77.8
accessory Y77.2
diagnostic Y77.0
miscellaneous Y77.8
monitoring Y77.0
prosthetic Y77.2
rehabilitative Y77.1
surgical Y77.3
therapeutic Y77.1
orthopedic Y79.8
accessory Y79.2
diagnostic Y79.0
miscellaneous Y79.8
monitoring Y79.0
prosthetic Y79.2

Incident, adverse (*Continued*)
device (*Continued*)
orthopedic (*Continued*)
rehabilitative Y79.1
surgical Y79.3
therapeutic Y79.1
otorhinolaryngological Y72.8
accessory Y72.2
diagnostic Y72.0
miscellaneous Y72.8
monitoring Y72.0
prosthetic Y72.2
rehabilitative Y72.1
surgical Y72.3
therapeutic Y72.1
personal use Y74.8
accessory Y74.2
diagnostic Y74.0
miscellaneous Y74.8
monitoring Y74.0
prosthetic Y74.2
rehabilitative Y74.1
surgical Y74.3
therapeutic Y74.1
physical medicine Y80.8
accessory Y80.2
diagnostic Y80.0
miscellaneous Y80.8
monitoring Y80.0
prosthetic Y80.2
rehabilitative Y80.1
surgical Y80.3
therapeutic Y80.1
plastic surgical Y81.8
accessory Y81.2
diagnostic Y81.0
miscellaneous Y81.8
monitoring Y81.0
prosthetic Y81.2
rehabilitative Y81.1
surgical Y81.3
therapeutic Y81.1
radiological Y78.8
accessory Y78.2
diagnostic Y78.0
miscellaneous Y78.8
monitoring Y78.0
prosthetic Y78.2
rehabilitative Y78.1
surgical Y78.3
therapeutic Y78.1
urology Y73.8
accessory Y73.2
diagnostic Y73.0
miscellaneous Y73.8
monitoring Y73.0
prosthetic Y73.2
rehabilitative Y73.1
surgical Y73.3
therapeutic Y73.1
Incineration (accidental) —*see* Exposure, fire
Infanticide —*see* Assault
Infrasound waves (causing injury) W49.9
Ingestion
foreign body (causing injury) (with obstruction) —*see* Foreign body, alimentary canal
poisonous
plant (s) X58
substance NEC —*see* Table of drugs and chemicals

Inhalation
excessively cold substance, man-
made —*see* Exposure, cold,
man-made
food (any type) (into respiratory
tract) (with asphyxia, obstruction
respiratory tract, suffocation) —*see*
categories T17 and T18
foreign body —*see* Foreign body,
aspiration
gastric contents (with asphyxia,
obstruction respiratory passage,
suffocation) T17.81-
hot air or gases X14.0
liquid air, hydrogen, nitrogen W93.12
suicide (attempt) X83.2
steam X13.0
assault X98.0
stated as undetermined whether
accidental or intentional Y27.0
suicide (attempt) X77.0
toxic gas —*see* Table of drugs and
chemicals
vomitus (with asphyxia, obstruction
respiratory passage, suffocation)
T17.81-

Injury, injured (accidental(ly)) NOS X58
by, caused by, from
assault —*see* Assault
law-enforcing agent, police, in course
of legal intervention —*see* Legal
intervention
suicide (attempt) X83.8
due to, in
civil insurrection —*see* War
operations
fight (*see also* Assault, fight) Y04.0
war operations —*see* War operations
homicide (*see also* Assault) Y09
inflicted (by)
in course of arrest (attempted),
suppression of disturbance,
maintenance of order, by
law-enforcing agents —*see* Legal
intervention
other person
stated as
accidental X58
intentional, homicide
(attempt) —*see* Assault
undetermined whether
accidental or intentional Y33

Injury, injured (*Continued*)
purposely (inflicted) by other
person (s) —*see* Assault
self-inflicted X83.8
stated as accidental X58
specified cause NEC X58
undetermined whether accidental
or intentional Y33
Insolation, effects X30
Insufficient nourishment X58
Interruption of respiration (by)
food (lodged in esophagus) —*see*
categories T17 and T18
vomitus (lodged in esophagus) T17.81-
Intervention, legal —*see* Legal
intervention
Intoxication
drug —*see* Table of drugs and
chemicals
poison —*see* Table of drugs and
chemicals

J

Jammed (accidentally)
between objects (moving) (stationary
and moving) W23.0
stationary W23.1
Jumped, jumping
before moving object NEC X81.8
motor vehicle X81.0
subway train X81.1
train X81.1
undetermined whether accidental or
intentional Y31
from
boat (into water) voluntarily, without
accident (to or on boat) W16.712
with
accident to or on boat —*see*
Accident, watercraft
drowning or submersion W16.711
suicide (attempt) X71.3
striking bottom W16.722
causing drowning W16.721

Jumped, jumping (*Continued*)
from (*Continued*)
building (*see also* Jumped, from, high
place) W13.9
burning (uncontrolled fire)
X00.5
high place NEC W17.89
suicide (attempt) X80
undetermined whether
accidental or intentional
Y30
structure (*see also* Jumped, from,
high place) W13.9
burning (uncontrolled fire)
X00.5
into water W16.92
causing drowning W16.91
from, off watercraft —*see* Jumped,
from, boat
in
natural body W16.612
causing drowning W16.611

Jumped, jumping (*Continued*)
into water (*Continued*)
in (*Continued*)
natural body (*Continued*)
striking bottom W16.622
causing drowning
W16.621
specified place NEC W16.812
causing drowning W16.811
striking
bottom W16.822
causing drowning W16.821
wall W16.832
causing drowning W16.831
swimming pool W16.512
causing drowning W16.511
striking
bottom W16.522
causing drowning W16.521
wall W16.532
causing drowning W16.531
suicide (attempt) X71.3

K

Kicked by
animal NEC W55.82
person (s) (accidentally) W50.1
with intent to injure or kill Y04.0
as, or caused by, a crowd or human
stampede (with fall) W52
assault Y04.0
homicide (attempt) Y04.0
in
fight Y04.0
legal intervention
injuring
bystander Y35.812
law enforcement personnel
Y35.811
suspect Y35.813

Kicking against
object W22.8
sports equipment W21.9
stationary W22.09
sports equipment W21.89
person —*see* Striking against, person
sports equipment W21.9
Killed, killing (accidentally) NOS (*see
also* Injury) X58
in
action —*see* War operations
brawl, fight (hand) (fists) (foot)
Y04.0
by weapon —*see also* Assault
cutting, piercing —*see* Assault,
cutting or piercing instrument
firearm —*see* Discharge, firearm, by
type, homicide

Killed, killing NOS (*Continued*)
self
stated as
accident NOS X58
suicide —*see* Suicide
undetermined whether accidental
or intentional Y33
Knocked down (accidentally) (by) NOS
X58
animal (not being ridden) NEC —*see
also* Struck by, by type of animal
crowd or human stampede W52
person W51
in brawl, fight Y04.0
transport vehicle NEC (*see also*
Accident, transport) V09.9

L

Laceration NEC —*see* Injury
Lack of
care (helpless person) (infant)
(newborn) X58
food except as result of abandonment
or neglect X58
due to abandonment or neglect
X58
water except as result of transport
accident X58
due to transport accident B —*see*
Accident, transport, by type
helpless person, infant, newborn
X58
Landslide (falling on transport vehicle)
X36.1
caused by collapse of man-made
structure X36.0
Late effect —*see* Sequelae
Legal
execution (any method) —*see* Legal,
intervention
intervention (by)
baton —*see* Legal, intervention, blunt
object, baton
bayonet —*see* Legal, intervention,
sharp object, bayonet
blow —*see* Legal, intervention,
manhandling
blunt object
baton
injuring
bystander Y35.312
law enforcement personnel
Y35.311
suspect Y35.313
injuring
bystander Y35.302
law enforcement personnel
Y35.301
suspect Y35.303
specified NEC
injuring
bystander Y35.392
law enforcement personnel
Y35.391
suspect Y35.393
stave
injuring
bystander Y35.392
law enforcement personnel
Y35.391
suspect Y35.393
bomb —*see* Legal, intervention,
explosive
cutting or piercing instrument —
see Legal, intervention, sharp
object
dynamite —*see* Legal, intervention,
explosive, dynamite
explosive (s)
dynamite
injuring
bystander Y35.112
law enforcement personnel
Y35.111
suspect Y35.113
grenade
injuring
bystander Y35.192
law enforcement personnel
Y35.191
suspect Y35.193

Legal *(Continued)*
intervention *(Continued)*
explosive *(Continued)*
injuring
bystander Y35.102
law enforcement personnel
Y35.101
suspect Y35.103
mortar bomb
injuring
bystander Y35.192
law enforcement personnel
Y35.191
suspect Y35.193
shell
injuring
bystander Y35.122
law enforcement personnel
Y35.121
suspect Y35.123
specified NEC
injuring
bystander Y35.192
law enforcement personnel
Y35.191
suspect Y35.193
firearm (s) (discharge)
handgun
injuring
bystander Y35.022
law enforcement personnel
Y35.021
suspect Y35.023
injuring
bystander Y35.002
law enforcement personnel Y35.001
suspect Y35.003
machine gun
injuring
bystander Y35.012
law enforcement personnel
Y35.011
suspect Y35.013
rifle pellet
injuring
bystander Y35.032
law enforcement personnel
Y35.031
suspect Y35.033
rubber bullet
injuring
bystander Y35.042
law enforcement personnel
Y35.041
suspect Y35.043
shotgun —*see* Legal, intervention,
firearm, specified NEC
specified NEC
injuring
bystander Y35.092
law enforcement personnel
Y35.091
suspect Y35.093
gas (asphyxiation) (poisoning)
injuring
bystander Y35.202
law enforcement personnel
Y35.201
suspect Y35.203
specified NEC
injuring
bystander Y35.292
law enforcement personnel
Y35.291
suspect Y35.293

Legal *(Continued)*
intervention *(Continued)*
gas *(Continued)*
tear gas
injuring
bystander Y35.212
law enforcement personnel
Y35.211
suspect Y35.213
grenade —*see* Legal, intervention,
explosive, grenade
injuring
bystander Y35.92
law enforcement personnel Y35.91
suspect Y35.93
late effect (of) (*see* with 7th character
S) Y35
manhandling
injuring
bystander Y35.812
law enforcement personnel
Y35.811
suspect Y35.813
sequelae (of) (*see* with 7th character
S) Y35
sharp objects
bayonet
injuring
bystander Y35.412
law enforcement personnel
Y35.411
suspect Y35.413
injuring
bystander Y35.402
law enforcement personnel
Y35.401
suspect Y35.403
specified NEC
injuring
bystander Y35.492
law enforcement personnel
Y35.491
suspect Y35.493
specified means NEC
injuring
bystander Y35.892
law enforcement personnel
Y35.891
suspect Y35.893
stabbing —*see* Legal, intervention,
sharp object
stave —*see* Legal, intervention, blunt
object, stave
tear gas —*see* Legal, intervention, gas,
tear gas
truncheon —*see* Legal, intervention,
blunt object, stave
Lightning (shock) (stroke) (struck by) —
see subcategory T75.0
causing fire —*see* Exposure, fire
Loss of control (transport vehicle) **NEC** —
see Accident, transport
Lost at sea NOS —*see* Drowning, due to,
fall overboard
Low
pressure (effects) —*see* Air, pressure, low
temperature (effects) —*see* Exposure,
cold
**Lying before train, vehicle or other
moving object** X81.8
subway train X81.1
train X81.1
undetermined whether accidental or
intentional Y31
Lynching —*see* Assault

M

Malfunction (mechanism or component) (of)
  firearm
    airgun W34.10
    BB gun W34.110
    gas, air or spring-operated gun NEC W34.118
    handgun W32.1
    hunting rifle W33.12
    larger firearm W33.10
      specified NEC W33.19
    machine gun W33.13
    paintball gun W34.111
    pellet gun W34.110
    shotgun W33.11
    specified NEC W34.19
    Very pistol [flare] W34.19
  handgun —see Malfunction, firearm, handgun
Maltreatment —see Perpetrator
Mangled (accidentally) NOS X58
Manhandling (in brawl, fight) Y04.0
  legal intervention —see Legal, intervention, manhandling
Manslaughter (nonaccidental) —see Assault
Mauled by animal NEC W55.89
Medical procedure, complication of (delayed or as an abnormal reaction without mention of misadventure) —see Complication of or following, by specified type of procedure
  due to or as a result of misadventure — see Misadventure
Melting (due to fire) —see also Exposure, fire
  apparel NEC X06.3
  clothes, clothing NEC X06.3
    nightwear X05
  fittings or furniture (burning building) (uncontrolled fire) X00.8
  nightwear X05
  plastic jewelry X06.1
Mental cruelty X58
Military operations (injuries to military and civilians occuring during peacetime on military property and during routine military exercises and operations) (by) (from) (involving) Y37.90-
  air blast Y37.20-
  aircraft
    destruction —see Military operations, destruction of aircraft
  airway restriction —see Military operations, restriction of airways
  asphyxiation —see Military operations, restriction of airways
  biological weapons Y37.6X-
  blast Y37.20-
  blast fragments Y37.20-
  blast wave Y37.20-
  blast wind Y37.20-
  bomb Y37.20-
    dirty Y37.50-
    gasoline Y37.31-
    incendiary Y37.31-
    petrol Y37.31-
  bullet Y37.43-
    incendiary Y37.32-
    rubber Y37.41-
  chemical weapons Y37.7X-

Military operations (Continued)
  combat
    hand to hand (unarmed) combat Y37.44-
    using blunt or piercing object Y37.45-
  conflagration —see Military operations, fire
  conventional warfare NEC Y37.49-
  depth-charge Y37.01-
  destruction of aircraft Y37.10-
    due to
      air to air missile Y37.11-
      collision with other aircraft Y37.12-
      detonation (accidental) of onboard munitions and explosives Y37.14-
      enemy fire or explosives Y37.11-
      explosive placed on aircraft Y37.11-
      onboard fire Y37.13-
      rocket propelled grenade [RPG] Y37.11-
      small arms fire Y37.11-
      surface to air missile Y37.11-
    specified NEC Y37.19-
  detonation (accidental) of
    onboard marine weapons Y37.05-
    own munitions or munitions launch device Y37.24-
  dirty bomb Y37.50-
  explosion (of) Y37.20-
    aerial bomb Y37.21-
    bomb NOS (see also Military operations, bomb (s)) Y37.20-
    fragments Y37.20-
    grenade Y37.29-
    guided missile Y37.22-
    improvised explosive device [IED] (person-borne) (roadside) (vehicle-borne) Y37.23-
    land mine Y37.29-
    marine mine (at sea) (in harbor) Y37.02-
    marine weapon Y37.00-
      specified NEC Y37.09-
    own munitions or munitions launch device (accidental) Y37.24-
    sea-based artillery shell Y37.03-
    specified NEC Y37.29-
    torpedo Y37.04-
  fire Y37.30-
    specified NEC Y37.39-
  firearms
    discharge Y37.43-
    pellets Y37.42-
  flamethrower Y37.33-
  fragments (from) (of)
    improvised explosive device [IED] (person-borne) (roadside) (vehicle-borne) Y37.26-
    munitions Y37.25-
    specified NEC Y37.29-
    weapons Y37.27-
  friendly fire Y37.92-
  hand to hand (unarmed) combat Y37.44-
  hot substances —see Military operations, fire
  incendiary bullet Y37.32-
  nuclear weapon (effects of) Y37.50-
    acute radiation exposure Y37.54-
    blast pressure Y37.51-
    direct blast Y37.51-
    direct heat Y37.53-
    fallout exposure Y37.54-
    fireball Y37.53-

Military operations (Continued)
  nuclear weapon (effects of) (Continued)
    indirect blast (struck or crushed by blast debris) (being thrown by blast) Y37.52-
    ionizing radiation (immediate exposure) Y37.54-
    nuclear radiation Y37.54-
    radiation
      ionizing (immediate exposure) Y37.54-
      nuclear Y37.54-
      thermal Y37.53-
    secondary effects Y37.54-
    specified NEC Y37.59-
    thermal radiation Y37.53-
  restriction of air (airway)
    intentional Y37.46-
    unintentional Y37.47-
  rubber bullets Y37.41-
  shrapnel NOS Y37.29-
  suffocation —see Military operations, restriction of airways
  unconventional warfare NEC Y37.7X-
  underwater blast NOS Y37.00-
  warfare
    conventional NEC Y37.49-
    unconventional NEC Y37.7X-
  weapon of mass destruction [WMD] Y37.91-
  weapons
    biological weapons Y37.6X-
    chemical Y37.7X-
    nuclear (effects of) Y37.50-
      acute radiation exposure Y37.54-
      blast pressure Y37.51-
      direct blast Y37.51-
      direct heat Y37.53-
      fallout exposure Y37.54-
      fireball Y37.53-
      indirect blast (struck or crushed by blast debris) (being thrown by blast) Y37.52-
      radiation
        ionizing (immediate exposure) Y37.54-
        nuclear Y37.54-
        thermal Y37.53-
      secondary effects Y37.54-
      specified NEC Y37.59-
    of mass destruction [WMD] Y37.91-
Misadventure (s) to patient (s) during surgical or medical care Y69
  contaminated medical or biological substance (blood, drug, fluid) Y64.9
    administered (by) NEC Y64.9
      immunization Y64.1
      infusion Y64.0
      injection Y64.1
      specified means NEC Y64.8
      transfusion Y64.0
      vaccination Y64.1
  excessive amount of blood or other fluid during transfusion or infusion Y63.0
  failure
    in dosage Y63.9
      electroshock therapy Y63.4
      inappropriate temperature (too hot or too cold) in local application and packing Y63.5

Misadventure (s) to patient (s) during surgical or medical care *(Continued)*
failure *(Continued)*
  in dosage *(Continued)*
    infusion
      excessive amount of fluid Y63.0
      incorrect dilution of fluid Y63.1
    insulin-shock therapy Y63.4
    nonadministration of necessary drug or biological substance Y63.62
    overdose —*see* Table of drugs and chemicals
    radiation, in therapy Y63.2
    radiation
      overdose Y63.2
    specified procedure NEC Y63.8
    transfusion
      excessive amount of blood Y63.0
  mechanical, of instrument or apparatus (any) (during any procedure) Y65.8
  sterile precautions (during procedure) Y62.9
    aspiration of fluid or tissue (by puncture or catheterization, except heart) Y62.6
    biopsy (except needle aspiration) Y62.8
      needle (aspirating) Y62.6
    blood sampling Y62.6
    catheterization Y62.6
      heart Y62.5
    dialysis (kidney) Y62.2
    endoscopic examination Y62.4
    enema Y62.8
    immunization Y62.3
    infusion Y62.1
    injection Y62.3

Misadventure (s) to patient (s) during surgical or medical care *(Continued)*
failure *(Continued)*
  sterile precautions *(Continued)*
    needle biopsy Y62.6
    paracentesis (abdominal) (thoracic) Y62.6
    perfusion Y62.2
    puncture (lumbar) Y62.6
    removal of catheter or packing Y62.8
    specified procedure NEC Y62.8
    surgical operation Y62.0
    transfusion Y62.1
    vaccination Y62.3
  suture or ligature during surgical procedure Y65.2
  to introduce or to remove tube or instrument B —*see* Failure, to
  hemorrhage —*see* Misadventure, cut, by type of procedure
  inadvertent exposure of patient to radiation Y63.3
  inappropriate
    operation performed —*see* Inappropriate operation performed
    temperature (too hot or too cold) in local application or packing Y63.5
  infusion (*see also* Misadventure, by type, infusion) Y69
    excessive amount of fluid Y63.0
    incorrect dilution of fluid Y63.1
    wrong fluid Y65.1
  mismatched blood in transfusion Y65.0
  nonadministration of necessary drug or biological substance Y63.62
  overdose —*see* Table of drugs and chemicals
    radiation (in therapy) Y63.2
  perforation —*see* Misadventure, cut, by type of procedure

Misadventure (s) to patient (s) during surgical or medical care *(Continued)*
performance of inappropriate operation —*see* Inappropriate operation performed
puncture —*see* Misadventure, cut, by type of procedure
specified type NEC Y65.8
  failure
    suture or ligature during surgical operation Y65.2
    to introduce or to remove tube or instrument B —*see* Failure, to
  infusion of wrong fluid Y65.1
  performance of inappropriate operation —*see* Inappropriate operation performed
  transfusion of mismatched blood Y65.0
  wrong
    fluid in infusion Y65.1
    placement of endotracheal tube during anesthetic procedure Y65.3
transfusion —*see* Misadventure, by type, transfusion
  excessive amount of blood Y63.0
  mismatched blood Y65.0
wrong
  drug given in error —*see* Table of drugs and chemicals
  fluid in infusion Y65.1
  placement of endotracheal tube during anesthetic procedure Y65.3
Mismatched blood in transfusion Y65.0
Motion sickness T75.3
Mountain sickness W94.11
Mudslide (of cataclysmic nature) —*see* Landslide
Murder (attempt) —*see* Assault

N

Nail, contact with W45.0
  gun W29.4
Neglect (criminal) (homicidal intent) X58
Noise (causing injury) (pollution) W42.9
  supersonic W42.0

Nonadministration (of)
  drug or biological substance (necessary) Y63.62
  surgical and medical care Y66
Nosocomial condition Y95

O

Object
  falling
    from, in, on, hitting
      machinery —*see* Contact, with, by type of machine
  set in motion by
    accidental explosion or rupture of pressure vessel W38
    firearm —*see* Discharge, firearm, by type
    machine (ry) —*see* Contact, with, by type of machine

Overdose (drug) —*see* Table of drugs and chemicals
  radiation Y63.2
Overexertion —*see* category Y93
Overexposure (accidental) (to)
  cold (*see also* Exposure, cold) X31
    due to man-made conditions —*see* Exposure, cold, man-made
  heat (*see also* Heat) X30
  radiation —*see* Radiation
  radioactivity W88.0
  sun (sunburn) X32
  weather NEC B —*see* Forces of nature
  wind NEC B —*see* Forces of nature

Overheated —*see* Heat
Overturning (accidental)
  machinery —*see* Contact, with, by type of machine
  transport vehicle NEC (*see also* Accident, transport) V89.9
  watercraft (causing drowning, submersion) —*see also* Drowning, due to, accident to, watercraft, overturning
    causing injury except drowning or submersion B —*see* Accident, watercraft, causing, injury NEC

M, N, & O

P

Parachute descent (voluntary) (without accident to aircraft) V97.29
 due to accident to aircraft —*see*
  Accident, transport, aircraft
Pecked by bird W61.99
Perforation during medical or surgical treatment as misadventure —*see*
 Misadventure, cut, by type of procedure
Perpetrator, perpetration, of assault, maltreatment and neglect (by) Y07.9
 boyfriend Y07.03
 brother Y07.410
  stepbrother Y07.435
 coach Y07.53
 cousin
  female Y07.491
  male Y07.490
 daycare provider Y07.519
  at-home
   adult care Y07.512
   childcare Y07.510
  care center
   adult care Y07.513
   childcare Y07.511
 family member NEC Y07.499
 father Y07.11
  adoptive Y07.13
  foster Y07.420
  stepfather Y07.430
 foster father Y07.420
 foster mother Y07.421
 girl friend Y07.04
 healthcare provider Y07.529
  mental health Y07.521
  specified NEC Y07.528
 husband Y07.01
 instructor Y07.53
 mother Y07.12
  adoptive Y07.14
  foster Y07.421
  stepmother Y07.433
 nonfamily member Y07.50
  specified NEC Y07.59
 nurse Y07.528
 occupational therapist Y07.528
 partner of parent
  female Y07.434
  male Y07.432
 physical therapist Y07.528
 sister Y07.411
 speech therapist Y07.528
 stepbrother Y07.435
 stepfather Y07.430
 stepmother Y07.433
 stepsister Y07.436
 teacher Y07.53
 wife Y07.02
Piercing —*see* Contact, with, by type of object or machine
Pinched
 between objects (moving) (stationary and moving) W23.0
  stationary W23.1
Pinned under machine (ry) —*see* Contact, with, by type of machine
Place of occurrence Y92.9
 abandoned house Y92.89
 airplane Y92.813
 airport Y92.520
 ambulatory health services establishment NEC Y92.538
 ambulatory surgery center Y92.530

Place of occurrence (*Continued*)
 amusement park Y92.831
 apartment (co-op) —*see* Place of occurrence, residence, apartment
 assembly hall Y92.29
 bank Y92.510
 barn Y92.71
 baseball field Y92.320
 basketball court Y92.310
 beach Y92.832
 boarding house —*see* Place of occurrence, residence, boarding house
 boat Y92.814
 bowling alley Y92.39
 bridge Y92.89
 building under construction Y92.61
 bus Y92.811
  station Y92.521
 cafe Y92.511
 campsite Y92.833
 campus —*see* Place of occurrence, school
 canal Y92.89
 car Y92.810
 casino Y92.59
 children's home —*see* Place of occurrence, residence, institutional, orphanage
 church Y92.22
 cinema Y92.26
 clubhouse Y92.29
 coal pit Y92.64
 college (community) Y92.214
 condominium —*see* Place of occurrence, residence, apartment
 construction area —*see* Place of occurrence, industrial and construction area
 convalescent home —*see* Place of occurrence, residence, institutional, nursing home
 court-house Y92.240
 cricket ground Y92.328
 cultural building Y92.258
  art gallery Y92.250
  museum Y92.251
  music hall Y92.252
  opera house Y92.253
  specified NEC Y92.258
  theater Y92.254
 dancehall Y92.252
 day nursery Y92.210
 dentist office Y92.531
 derelict house Y92.89
 desert Y92.820
 dock NOS Y92.89
 dockyard Y92.62
 doctor's office Y92.531
 dormitory —*see* Place of occurrence, residence, institutional, school dormitory
 dry dock Y92.62
 factory (building) (premises) Y92.63
 farm (land under cultivation) (outbuildings) Y92.79
  barn Y92.71
  chicken coop Y92.72
  field Y92.73
  hen house Y92.72
  house —*see* Place of occurrence, residence, house
  orchard Y92.74
  specified NEC Y92.79
 football field Y92.321
 forest Y92.821
 freeway Y92.411
 gallery Y92.250

Place of occurrence (*Continued*)
 garage (commercial) Y92.59
  boarding house Y92.044
  military base Y92.135
  mobile home Y92.025
  nursing home Y92.124
  orphanage Y92.114
  private house Y92.015
  reform school Y92.155
 gas station Y92.524
 gasworks Y92.69
 golf course Y92.39
 gravel pit Y92.64
 grocery Y92.512
 gymnasium Y92.39
 handball court Y92.318
 harbor Y92.89
 harness racing course Y92.39
 healthcare provider office Y92.531
 highway (interstate) Y92.411
 hill Y92.828
 hockey rink Y92.330
 home —*see* Place of occurrence, residence
 hospice —*see* Place of occurrence, residence, institutional, nursing home
 hospital Y92.239
  cafeteria Y92.233
  corridor Y92.232
  operating room Y92.234
  patient
   bathroom Y92.231
   room Y92.230
  specified NEC Y92.238
 hotel Y92.59
 house —*see also* Place of occurrence, residence
  abandoned Y92.89
  under construction Y92.61
 industrial and construction area (yard) Y92.69
  building under construction Y92.61
  dock Y92.62
  dry dock Y92.62
  factory Y92.63
  gasworks Y92.69
  mine Y92.64
  oil rig Y92.65
  pit Y92.64
  power station Y92.69
  shipyard Y92.62
  specified NEC Y92.69
  tunnel under construction Y92.69
  workshop Y92.69
 kindergarten Y92.211
 lacrosse field Y92.328
 lake Y92.828
 library Y92.241
 mall Y92.59
 market Y92.512
 marsh Y92.828
 military
  base —*see* Place of occurrence, residence, institutional, military base
  training ground Y92.84
 mine Y92.64
 mosque Y92.22
 motel Y92.59
 motorway (interstate) Y92.411
 mountain Y92.828
 movie-house Y92.26
 museum Y92.251
 music-hall Y92.252
 not applicable Y92.9
 nuclear power station Y92.69

Place of occurrence (*Continued*)
  nursing home —*see* Place of occurrence, residence, institutional, nursing home
  office building Y92.59
  offshore installation Y92.65
  oil rig Y92.65
  old people's home —*see* Place of occurrence, residence, institutional, specified NEC
  opera-house Y92.253
  orphanage —*see* Place of occurrence, residence, institutional, orphanage
  outpatient surgery center Y92.530
  park (public) Y92.830
    amusement Y92.831
  parking garage Y92.89
    lot Y92.481
  pavement Y92.480
  physician office Y92.531
  polo field Y92.328
  pond Y92.828
  post office Y92.242
  power station Y92.69
  prairie Y92.828
  prison —*see* Place of occurrence, residence, institutional, prison
  public
    administration building Y92.248
      city hall Y92.243
      courthouse Y92.240
      library Y92.241
      post office Y92.242
      specified NEC Y92.248
    building NEC Y92.29
    hall Y92.29
    place NOS Y92.89
  race course Y92.39
  radio station Y92.59
  railway line (bridge) Y92.85
  ranch (outbuildings) —*see* Place of occurrence, farm
  recreation area Y92.838
    amusement park Y92.831
    beach Y92.832
    campsite Y92.833
    park (public) Y92.830
    seashore Y92.832
    specified NEC Y92.838
  reform school —*see* Place of occurrence, residence, institutional, reform school
  religious institution Y92.22
  residence (non-institutional) (private) Y92.009
    apartment Y92.039
      bathroom Y92.031
      bedroom Y92.032
      kitchen Y92.030
      specified NEC Y92.038
    bathroom Y92.002
    bedroom Y92.003
    boarding house Y92.049
      bathroom Y92.041
      bedroom Y92.042
      driveway Y92.043
      garage Y92.044
      garden Y92.046
      kitchen Y92.040
      specified NEC Y92.048
      swimming pool Y92.045
      yard Y92.046
    dining room Y92.001
    garden Y92.007
    home Y92.009
    house, single family Y92.019
      bathroom Y92.012
      bedroom Y92.013
      dining room Y92.011
      driveway Y92.014

Place of occurrence (*Continued*)
  residence (*Continued*)
    house, single family (*Continued*)
      garage Y92.015
      garden Y92.017
      kitchen Y92.010
      specified NEC Y92.018
      swimming pool Y92.016
      yard Y92.017
    institutional Y92.10
      children's home —*see* Place of occurrence, residence, institutional, orphanage
      hospice —*see* Place of occurrence, residence, institutional, nursing home
      military base Y92.139
        barracks Y92.133
        garage Y92.135
        garden Y92.137
        kitchen Y92.130
        mess hall Y92.131
        specified NEC Y92.138
        swimming pool Y92.136
        yard Y92.137
      nursing home Y92.129
        bathroom Y92.121
        bedroom Y92.122
        driveway Y92.123
        garage Y92.124
        garden Y92.126
        kitchen Y92.120
        specified NEC Y92.128
        swimming pool Y92.125
        yard Y92.126
      orphanage Y92.119
        bathroom Y92.111
        bedroom Y92.112
        driveway Y92.113
        garage Y92.114
        garden Y92.116
        kitchen Y92.110
        specified NEC Y92.118
        swimming pool Y92.115
        yard Y92.116
      prison Y92.149
        bathroom Y92.142
        cell Y92.143
        courtyard Y92.147
        dining room Y92.141
        kitchen Y92.140
        specified NEC Y92.148
        swimming pool Y92.146
      reform school Y92.159
        bathroom Y92.152
        bedroom Y92.153
        dining room Y92.151
        driveway Y92.154
        garage Y92.155
        garden Y92.157
        kitchen Y92.150
        specified NEC Y92.158
        swimming pool Y92.156
        yard Y92.157
      school dormitory Y92.169
        bathroom Y92.162
        bedroom Y92.163
        dining room Y92.161
        kitchen Y92.160
        specified NEC Y92.168
      specified NEC Y92.199
        bathroom Y92.192
        bedroom Y92.193
        dining room Y92.191
        driveway Y92.194
        garage Y92.195
        garden Y92.197
        kitchen Y92.190
        specified NEC Y92.198

Place of occurrence (*Continued*)
  residence (*Continued*)
    institutional (*Continued*)
      specified NEC (*Continued*)
        swimming pool Y92.196
        yard Y92.197
    kitchen Y92.000
    mobile home Y92.029
      bathroom Y92.022
      bedroom Y92.023
      dining room Y92.021
      driveway Y92.024
      garage Y92.025
      garden Y92.027
      kitchen Y92.020
      specified NEC Y92.028
      swimming pool Y92.026
      yard Y92.027
    specified place in residence NEC Y92.009
    specified residence type NEC Y92.099
      bathroom Y92.091
      bedroom Y92.092
      driveway Y92.093
      garage Y92.094
      garden Y92.096
      kitchen Y92.090
      specified NEC Y92.098
      swimming pool Y92.095
      yard Y92.096
  restaurant Y92.511
  riding school Y92.39
  river Y92.828
  road Y92.488
  rodeo ring Y92.39
  rugby field Y92.328
  same day surgery center Y92.530
  sand pit Y92.64
  school (private) (public) (state) Y92.219
    college Y92.214
    daycare center Y92.210
    elementary school Y92.211
    high school Y92.213
    kindergarten Y92.211
    middle school Y92.212
    specified NEC Y92.218
    trace school Y92.215
    university Y92.214
    vocational school Y92.215
  sea (shore) Y92.832
  senior citizen center Y92.29
  service area
    airport Y92.520
    bus station Y92.521
    gas station Y92.524
    highway rest stop Y92.523
    railway station Y92.522
  shipyard Y92.62
  shop(commercial) Y92.513
  sidewalk Y92.480
  silo Y92.79
  skating rink (roller) Y92.331
    ice Y92.330
  slaughter house Y92.86
  soccer field Y92.322
  specified place NEC Y92.89
  sports area Y92.39
    athletic
      court Y92.318
        basketball Y92.310
        specified NEC Y92.318
        squash Y92.311
        tennis Y92.312
      field Y92.328
        baseball Y92.320
        cricket ground Y92.328
        football Y92.321
        hockey Y92.328

Place of occurrence *(Continued)*
  sports area *(Continued)*
    athletic *(Continued)*
      field *(Continued)*
        soccer Y92.322
        specified NEC Y92.328
    golf course Y92.39
    gymnasium Y92.39
    riding school Y92.39
    skating rink (roller) Y92.331
      ice Y92.330
    stadium Y92.39
    swimming pool Y92.34
  squash court Y92.311
  stadium Y92.39
  steeplechasing course Y92.39
  store Y92.512
  stream Y92.828
  street and highway Y92.410
    bike path Y92.482
    freeway Y92.411
    highway ramp Y92.415
    interstate highway Y92.411
    local residential or business street
      Y92.414
    motorway Y92.411
    parking lot Y92.481
    parkway Y92.412
    sidewalk Y92.480
    specified NEC Y92.488
    state road Y92.413
  subway car Y92.816
  supermarket Y92.512
  swamp Y92.828
  swimming pool (public) Y92.34
    private (at) Y92.095
      boarding house Y92.045
      military base Y92.136
      mobile home Y92.026
      nursing home Y92.125
      orphanage Y92.115
      prison Y92.146
      reform school Y92.156
      single family residence
        Y92.016
  synagogue Y92.22
  television station Y92.59
  tennis court Y92.312
  theater Y92.254
  trade area Y92.59
    bank Y92.510
    cafe Y92.511
    casino Y92.59
    garage Y92.59
    hotel Y92.59
    market Y92.512
    office building Y92.59
    radio station Y92.59
    restaurant Y92.511
    shop Y92.513
    shopping mall Y92.59
    store Y92.512
    supermarket Y92.512
    television station Y92.59
    warehouse Y92.59
  trailer park, residential —*see* Place of
    occurrence, residence, mobile
    home
  trailer site NOS Y92.89
  train Y92.815
    station Y92.522
  truck Y92.812
  tunnel under construction Y92. 69
  university Y92.214
  urgent (health) care center Y92.532
  vehicle (transport) Y92.818
    airplane Y92.813
    boat Y92.814
    bus Y92.811

Place of occurrence *(Continued)*
  vehicle *(Continued)*
    car Y92.810
    specified NEC Y92.818
    subway car Y92.816
    train Y92.815
    truck Y92.812
  warehouse Y92.59
  water reservoir Y92.89
  wilderness area Y92.828
    desert Y92.820
    forest Y92.821
    marsh Y92.828
    mountain Y92.828
    prairie Y92.828
    specified NEC Y92.828
    swamp Y92.828
  workshop Y92.69
  yard, private Y92.096
    boarding house Y92.046
    mobile home Y92.027
    single family house Y92.017
  youth center Y92.29
  zoo (zoological garden) Y92.834
Plumbism —*see* Table of drugs and
  chemicals, lead
Poisoning (accidental) (by) —*see* also
  Table of drugs and chemicals
  by plant, thorns, spines, sharp leaves or
    other mechanisms NEC X58
  carbon monoxide
    generated by
      motor vehicle —*see* Accident,
        transport
      watercraft (in transit) (not in
        transit) V93.89
        ferry boat V93.81
        fishing boat V93.82
        jet skis V93.83
        liner V93.81
        merchant ship V93.80
        passenger ship V93.81
        powered craft NEC V93.83
  caused by injection of poisons into
    skin by plant thorns, spines, sharp
    leaves X58
  marine or sea plants (venomous)
    X58
  exhaust gas
    generated by
      motor vehicle —*see* Accident,
        transport
      watercraft (in transit) (not in
        transit) V93.89
        ferry boat V93.81
        fishing boat V93.82
        jet skis V93.83
        liner V93.81
        merchant ship V93.80
        passenger ship V93.81
        powered craft NEC V93.83
  fumes or smoke due to
    explosion (see also Explosion) W40.9
    fire —*see* Exposure, fire
    ignition —*see* Ignition
  gas
    in legal intervention —*see* Legal,
      intervention, gas
    legal execution —*see* Legal,
      intervention, gas
    in war operations —*see* War operations
  legal
    execution —*see* Legal, intervention, gas
    intervention
      by gas —*see* Legal, intervention,
        gas
      other specified means —*see* Legal,
        intervention, specified means
        NEC

Powder burn (by) (from)
  airgun W34.110
  BB gun W34.110
  firearm NEC W34.19
  gas, air or spring-operated gun NEC
    W34.118
  handgun W32.1
  hunting rifle W33.12
  larger firearm W33.10
    specified NEC W33.19
  machine gun W33.13
  paintball gun W34.111
  pellet gun W34.110
  shotgun W33.11
  Very pistol [flare] W34.19
Premature cessation (of) surgical and
    medical care Y66
Privation (food) (water) X58
Procedure (operation)
  correct, on wrong side or body part
    (wrong side) (wrong site)
    Y65.53
  intended for another patient done on
    wrong patient Y65.52
  performed on patient not scheduled for
    surgery Y65.52
  performed on wrong patient
    Y65.52
  wrong, performed on correct patient
    Y65.51
Prolonged
  sitting in transport vehicle —*see* Travel,
    by type of vehicle
  stay in
    high altitude as cause of anoxia,
      barodontalgia, barotitis or
      hypoxia W94.11
    weightless environment X52
Pulling, excessive —*see* Overexertion
Puncture, puncturing —*see* also
    Contact, with, by type of object or
    machine
  by
    plant thorns, spines, sharp
      leaves or other mechanisms
      NEC W60
  during medical or surgical treatment
    as misadventure —*see*
    Misadventure, cut, by type
    of procedure
Pushed, pushing (accidental) (injury in)
    (overexertion) —*see* also Overexertion
  by other person (s) (accidental) W51
    with fall W03
      due to ice or snow W00.0
    as, or caused by, a crowd or human
      stampede (with fall) W52
    before moving object NEC Y02.8
      motor vehicle Y02.0
      subway train Y02.1
      train Y02.1
    from
      high place NEC
        in accidental circumstances
          W17.89
        stated as
          intentional, homicide (attempt)
            Y01
          undetermined whether
            accidental or intentional
            Y30
      transport vehicle NEC (see also
        Accident, transport) V89.9
        stated as
          intentional, homicide (attempt)
            Y08.89

R

Radiation (exposure to)
arc lamps W89.0
atomic power plant (malfunction) NEC W88.1
complication of or abnormal reaction to medical radiotherapy Y84.2
electromagnetic, ionizing W88.0
gamma rays W88.1
in
    war operations (from or following nuclear explosion) —*see also* War operations
inadvertent exposure of patient (receiving test or therapy) Y63.3
infrared (heaters and lamps) W90.1
    excessive heat from W92
ionized, ionizing (particles, artificially accelerated)
    radioisotopes W88.1
    specified NEC W88.8
    x-rays W88.0
isotopes, radioactive —*see* Radiation, radioactive isotopes
laser (s) W90.2
    in war operations —*see* War operations
    misadventure in medical care Y63.2
light sources (man-made visible and ultraviolet) W89.9
    natural X32
    specified NEC W89.8
    tanning bed W89.1
    welding light W89.0
man-made visible light W89.9
    specified NEC W89.8
    tanning bed W89.1
    welding light W89.0
microwave W90.8
misadventure in medical or surgical procedure Y63.2

Radiation *(Continued)*
natural NEC X39.08
    radon X39.01
overdose (in medical or surgical procedure) Y63.2
radar W90.0
radioactive isotopes (any) W88.1
    atomic power plant malfunction W88.1
    misadventure in medical or surgical treatment Y63.2
radiofrequency W90.0
radium NEC W88.1
sun X32
ultraviolet (light) (man-made) W89.9
    natural X32
    specified NEC W89.8
    tanning bed W89.1
    welding light W89.0
welding arc, torch, or light W89.0
    excessive heat from W92
x-rays (hard) (soft) W88.0
Range disease W94.11
Rape (attempted) T74.2-
Rat bite W53.11
Reaction, abnormal to medical procedure (*see also* Complication of or following, by type of procedure) Y84.9
with misadventure —*see* Misadventure
biologicals —*see* Table of drugs and chemicals
drugs —*see* Table of drugs and chemicals
vaccine —*see* Table of drugs and chemicals
Recoil
airgun W34.110
BB gun W34.110
firearm NEC W34.19
gas, air or spring-operated gun NEC W34.118

Recoil *(Continued)*
handgun W32.1
hunting rifle W33.12
larger firearm W33.10
    specified NEC W33.19
machine gun W33.13
paintball gun W34.111
pellet W34.110
shotgun W33.11
Very pistol [flare] W34.19
Reduction in
atmospheric pressure —*see* Air, pressure, change
Rock falling on or hitting (accidentally) (person) W20.8
in cave-in W20.0
Run over (accidentally) (by)
animal (not being ridden) NEC W55.89
machinery —*see* Contact, with, by specified type of machine
transport vehicle NEC (*see also* Accident, transport) V09.9
    intentional homicide (attempt) Y03.0
    motor NEC V09.20
        intentional homicide (attempt) Y03.0
Running
before moving object X81.8
    motor vehicle X81.0
Running off, away
animal (being ridden) (*see also* Accident, transport) V80.918
    not being ridden W55.89
animal-drawn vehicle NEC (*see also* Accident, transport) V80.928
highway, road(way), street
    transport vehicle NEC (*see also* Accident, transport) V89.9
Rupture pressurized devices —*see* Explosion, by type of device

S

Saturnism —see Table of drugs and chemicals, lead
Scald, scalding (accidental) (by) (from) (in) X19
air (hot) X14.1
gases (hot) X14.1
homicide (attempt) —see Assault, burning, hot object
inflicted by other person
stated as intentional, homicide (attempt) —see Assault, burning, hot object
liquid (boiling) (hot) NEC X12
stated as undetermined whether accidental or intentional Y27.2
suicide (attempt) X77.2
local application of externally applied substance in medical or surgical care Y63.5
metal (molten) (liquid) (hot) NEC X18
self-inflicted X77.9
stated as undetermined whether accidental or intentional Y27.8
steam X13.1
assault X98.0
stated as undetermined whether accidental or intentional Y27.0
suicide (attempt) X77.0
suicide (attempt) X77.9
vapor (hot) X13.1
assault X98.0
stated as undetermined whether accidental or intentional Y27.0
suicide (attempt) X77.0
Scratched by
cat W55.03
person (s) (accidentally) W50.4
with intent to injure or kill Y04.0
as, or caused by, a crowd or human stampede (with fall) W52
assault Y04.0
homicide (attempt) Y04.0
in
fight Y04.0
legal intervention
injuring
bystander Y35.892
law enforcement personnel Y35.891
suspect Y35.893
Seasickness T75.3
Self-harm NEC —see also External cause by type, undetermined whether accidental or intentional
intentional —see Suicide
poisoning NEC —see Table of drugs and biologicals, accident
Self-inflicted (injury) NEC —see also External cause by type, undetermined whether accidental or intentional
intentional —see Suicide
poisoning NEC —see Table of drugs and biologicals, accident
Sequelae (of)
accident NEC —see W00-X58 with 7th character S
assault (homicidal) (any means) —see X92-Y08 with 7th character S
homicide, attempt (any means) —see X92-Y08 with 7th character S
injury undetermined whether accidentally or purposely inflicted —see Y21-Y33 with 7th character S

Sequelae (Continued)
intentional self-harm (classifiable to X71-X83) —see X71-X83 with 7th character S
legal intervention (see with 7th character S Y35)
motor vehicle accident —see V00-V99 with 7th character S
suicide, attempt (any means) —see X71-X83 with 7th character S
transport accident —see V00-V99 with 7th character S
war operations —see War operations
Shock
electric —see Exposure, electric current
from electric appliance (any) (faulty) W86.8
domestic W86.0
suicide (attempt) X83.1
Shooting, shot (accidental (ly)) —see also Discharge, firearm, by type
herself or himself —see Discharge, firearm by type, self-inflicted
homicide (attempt) —see Discharge, firearm by type, homicide
in war operations —see War operations
inflicted by other person —see Discharge, firearm by type, homicide
accidental —see Discharge, firearm, by type of firearm
legal
execution —see Legal, intervention, firearm
intervention —see Legal, intervention, firearm
self-inflicted —see Discharge, firearm by type, suicide
accidental —see Discharge, firearm, by type of firearm
suicide (attempt) —see Discharge, firearm by type, suicide
Shoving (accidentally) by other person — see Pushing, by other person
Sickness
alpine W94.11
motion —see Motion
mountain W94.11
Sinking (accidental)
watercraft (causing drowning, submersion) B —see also Drowning, due to, accident to, watercraft, sinking
causing injury except drowning or submersion —see Accident, watercraft, causing, injury NEC
Siriasis X32
Slashed wrists —see Cut, self-inflicted
Slipping (accidental) (on same level) (with fall) W01.0
without fall W18.40
due to
specified NEC W18.49
stepping from one level to another W18.43
stepping into hole or opening W18.42
stepping on object W18.41
on
ice W00.0
with skates —see Accident, transport, pedestrian, conveyance
mud W01.0
oil W01.0

Slipping (Continued)
on (Continued)
snow W00.0
with skis —see Accident, transport, pedestrian, conveyance
surface (slippery) (wet) NEC W01.0
Sliver, wood, contact with W45.8
Smoldering (due to fire) —see Exposure, fire
Sodomy (attempted) by force T74.2-
Sound waves (causing injury) W42.9
supersonic W42.0
Splinter, contact with W45.8
Stab, stabbing B —see Cut
Starvation X58
Status of external cause Y99.9
child assisting in compensated work for family Y99.8
civilian activity done for financial or other compensation Y99.0
civilian activity done for income or pay Y99.0
family member assisting in compensated work for other family member Y99.8
hobby not done for income Y99.8
leisure activity Y99.8
military activity Y99.1
off-duty activity of military personnel Y99.8
recreation or sport not for income or while a student Y99.8
specified NEC Y99.8
student activity Y99.8
volunteer activity Y99.2
Stepped on
by
animal (not being ridden) NEC W55.89
crowd or human stampede W52
person W50.0
Stepping on
object W22.8
with fall W18.31
sports equipment W21.9
stationary W22.09
sports equipment W21.89
person W51
by crowd or human stampede W52
sports equipment W21.9
Sting
arthropod, nonvenomous W57
insect, nonvenomous W57
Storm (cataclysmic) B —see Forces of nature, cataclysmic storm
Straining, excessive —see Overexertion
Strangling —see Strangulation
Strangulation (accidental) —see category T71
Strenuous movements —see Repetitive movements
Striking against
airbag (automobile) W22.10
driver side W22.11
front passenger side W22.12
specified NEC W22.19
bottom when
diving or jumping into water (in) W16.822
causing drowning W16.821
from boat W16.722
causing drowning W16.721
natural body W16.622
causing drowning W16.821
swimming pool W16.522
causing drowning W16.521

Striking against *(Continued)*
bottom when *(Continued)*
falling into water (in) W16.322
causing drowning W16.321
fountain —*see* Striking against,
bottom when, falling into
water, specified NEC
natural body W16.122
causing drowning W16.121
reservoir —*see* Striking against,
bottom when, falling into
water, specified NEC
specified NEC W16.322
causing drowning W16.321
swimming pool W16.022
causing drowning W16.021
diving board (swimming-pool)
W21.4
object W22.8
with
drowning or submersion —*see*
Drowning
fall —*see* Fall, due to, bumping
against, object
caused by crowd or human stampede
(with fall) W52
furniture W22.03
lamppost W22.02
sports equipment W21.9
stationary W22.09
sports equipment W21.89
wall W22.01
person (s) W51
with fall W03
due to ice or snow W00.0
as, or caused by, a crowd or human
stampede (with fall) W52
assault Y04.2
homicide (attempt) Y04.2
sports equipment W21.9
wall (when) W22.01
diving or jumping into water (in)
W16.832
causing drowning W16.831
swimming pool W16.532
causing drowning W16.531
falling into water (in) W16.332
causing drowning W16.331
fountain —*see* Striking against,
wall when, falling into water,
specified NEC
natural body W16.132
causing drowning W16.131
reservoir —*see* Striking against,
wall when, falling into water,
specified NEC
specified NEC W16.332
causing drowning W16.331
swimming pool W16.032
causing drowning W16.031
swimming pool (when) W22.042
causing drowning W22.041
diving or jumping into water
W16.532
causing drowning W16.531
falling into water W16.032
causing drowning W16.031
Struck (accidentally) by
airbag (automobile) W22.10
driver side W22.11
front passenger side W22.12
specified NEC W22.19
alligator W58.02
animal (not being ridden) NEC W55.89
avalanche B —*see* Landslide

Struck by *(Continued)*
ball (hit) (thrown) W21.00
assault Y08.09
baseball W21.03
basketball W21.05
football W21.01
golf ball W21.04
football W21.01
soccer W21.02
softball W21.07
specified NEC W21.09
volleyball W21.06
bat or racquet
baseball bat W21.11
assault Y08.02
golf club W21.13
assault Y08.09
specified NEC W21.19
assault Y08.09
tennis racquet W21.12
assault Y08.09
bullet —*see also* Discharge, firearm by type
in war operations —*see* War
operations
crocodile W58.12
dog W54.1
flare, Very pistol —*see* Discharge,
firearm NEC
hailstones X39.8
hockey (ice)
field
puck W21.221
stick W21.211
puck W21.220
stick W21.210
assault Y08.01
landslide B —*see* Landslide
law-enforcement agent (on duty) —*see*
Legal, intervention, manhandling
with blunt object —*see* Legal,
intervention, blunt object
lightning —*see* subcategory T75.0
causing fire —*see* Exposure, fire
machine —*see* Contact, with, by type of
machine
mammal NEC W55.89
marine W56.32
marine animal W56.82
missile
firearm —*see* Discharge, firearm by type
in war operations —*see* War
operations, missile
object W22.8
blunt W22.8
assault Y00
suicide (attempt) X79
undetermined whether accidental
or intentional Y29
falling W20.8
from, in, on
building W20.1
burning (uncontrolled fire) X00.4
cataclysmic
earth surface movement NEC
B —*see* Landslide
storm B —*see* Forces of nature,
cataclysmic storm
cave-in W20.0
earthquake X34
machine (in operation) —*see*
Contact, with, by type of
machine
structure W20.1
burning X00.4
transport vehicle (in motion) —
see Accident, transport, by
type of vehicle

Struck by *(Continued)*
object *(Continued)*
falling *(Continued)*
from, in, on *(Continued)*
watercraft V93.49
due to
accident to craft V91.39
powered craft V91.33
ferry boat V91.31
fishing boat V91.32
jetskis V91.33
liner V91.31
merchant ship V91.30
passenger ship V91.31
unpowered craft V91.38
canoe V91.35
inflatable V91.36
kayak V91.35
sailboat V91.34
surf-board V91.38
windsurfer V91.38
powered craft V93.43
ferry boat V93.41
fishing boat V93.42
jetskis V93.43
liner V93.41
merchant ship V93.40
passenger ship V93.41
unpowered craft V93.48
sailboat V93.44
surf-board V93.48
windsurfer V93.48
moving NEC W20.8
projected W20.8
assault Y00
in sports W21.9
assault Y08.09
ball W21.00
baseball W21.03
basketball W21.05
football W21.01
golf ball W21.04
soccer W21.02
softball W21.07
specified NEC W21.09
volleyball W21.06
bat or racquet
baseball bat W21.11
assault Y08.02
golf club W21.13
assault Y08.09-
specified NEC W21.19
assault Y08.09
tennis racquet W21.12
assault Y08.09
hockey (ice)
field
puck W21.221
stick W21.211
puck W21.220
stick W21.210
assault Y08.01
specified NEC W21.89
set in motion by explosion —*see*
Explosion
thrown W20.8
assault Y00
in sports W21.9
assault Y08.09
ball W21.00
baseball W21.03
basketball W21.05
football W21.01
golf ball W21.04
soccer W21.02

Struck by (*Continued*)
object (*Continued*)
thrown (*Continued*)
in sports (*Continued*)
ball (*Continued*)
soft ball W21.07
specified NEC W21.09
volleyball W21.06
bat or racquet
baseball bat W21.11
assault Y08.02
golf club W21.13
assault Y08.09
specified NEC W21.19
assault Y08.09
tennis racquet W21.12
assault Y08.09
hockey (ice)
field
puck W21.221
stick W21.211
puck W21.220
stick W21.210
assault Y08.01
specified NEC W21.89
other person (s) W50.0
with
blunt object W22.8
intentional, homicide (attempt) Y00
sports equipment W21.9
undetermined whether accidental or intentional Y29
fall W03
due to ice or snow W00.0
as, or caused by, a crowd or human stampede (with fall) W52
assault Y04.2
homicide (attempt) Y04.2
in legal intervention
injuring
bystander Y35.812
law enforcement personnel Y35.811
suspect Y35.813
sports equipment W21.9
police (on duty) —*see* Legal, intervention, manhandling
with blunt object —*see* Legal, intervention, blunt object
sports equipment W21.9
assault Y08.09
ball W21.00
baseball W21.03
basketball W21.05
football W21.01
golf ball W21.04
soccer W21.02
soft ball W21.07
specified NEC W21.09
volleyball W21.06
bat or racquet
baseball bat W21.11
assault Y08.02
golf club W21.13
assault Y08.09
specified NEC W21.19
tennis racquet W21.12
assault Y08.09
cleats (shoe) W21.31
foot wear NEC W21.39
football helmet W21.81
hockey (ice)
field
puck W21.221
stick W21.211

Struck by (*Continued*)
sports equipment (*Continued*)
hockey (*Continued*)
puck W21.220
stick W21.210
assault Y08.01
skate blades W21.32
specified NEC W21.89
assault Y08.09
thunderbolt —*see* subcategory T75.0
causing fire —*see* Exposure, fire
transport vehicle NEC (*see also* Accident, transport) V09.9
intentional, homicide (attempt) Y03.0
motor NEC (*see also* Accident, transport) V09.20
homicide Y03.0
vehicle (transport) NEC —*see* Accident, transport, by type of vehicle
stationary (falling from jack, hydraulic lift, ramp) W20.8
Stumbling
without fall W18.40
due to
specified NEC W18.49
stepping from one level to another W18.43
stepping into hole or opening W18.42
stepping on object W18.41
over
animal NEC W01.0
with fall W18.09
carpet, rug or (small) object W22.8
with fall W18.09
person W51
with fall W03
due to ice or snow W00.0
Submersion (accidental) —*see* Drowning
Suffocation (accidental) (by external means) (by pressure) (mechanical) —*see also* category T71
due to, by
avalanche —*see* Landslide
explosion —*see* Explosion
fire —*see* Exposure, fire
food, any type (aspiration) (ingestion) (inhalation) —*see* categories T17 and T18
ignition —*see* Ignition
landslide —*see* Landslide
machine (ry) —*see* Contact, with, by type of machine
vomitus (aspiration) (inhalation) T17.81-
in
burning building X00.8
Suicide, suicidal (attempted) (by) X83.8
blunt object X79
burning, burns X76
hot object X77.9
fluid NEC X77.2
household appliance X77.3
specified NEC X77.8
steam X77.0
tap water X77.1
vapors X77.0
caustic substance —*see* Table of drugs and chemicals
cold, extreme X83.2
collision of motor vehicle with
motor vehicle X82.0
specified NEC X82.8
train X82.1
tree X82.2
crashing of aircraft X83.0

Suicide, suicidal (*Continued*)
cut (any part of body) X78.9
cutting or piercing instrument X78.9
dagger X78.2
glass X78.0
knife X78.1
specified NEC X78.8
sword X78.2
drowning (in) X71.9
bathtub X71.0
natural water X71.3
specified NEC X71.8
swimming pool X71.1
following fall X71.2
electrocution X83.1
explosive (s) (material) X75
fire, flames X76
firearm X74.9
airgun X74.01
handgun X72
hunting rifle X73.1
larger X73.9
specified NEC X73.8
machine gun X73.2
shotgun X73.0
specified NEC X74.8
hanging X83.8
hot object —*see* Suicide, burning, hot object
jumping
before moving object X81.8
motor vehicle X81.0
subway train X81.1
train X81.1
from high place X80
late effect of attempt —*see* X71-X83 with 7th character S
lying before moving object, train, vehicle X81.8
poisoning —*see* Table of drugs and chemicals
puncture (any part of body) —*see* Suicide, cutting or piercing instrument
scald —*see* Suicide, burning, hot object
sequelae of attempt —*see* X71-X83 with 7th character S
sharp object (any) —*see* Suicide, cutting or piercing instrument
shooting —*see* Suicide, firearm
specified means NEC X83.8
stab (any part of body) —*see* Suicide, cutting or piercing instrument
steam, hot vapors X77.0
strangulation X83.8
submersion —*see* Suicide, drowning
suffocation X83.8
wound NEC X83.8
Sunstroke X32
Supersonic waves (causing injury) W42.0
Surgical procedure, complication of (delayed or as an abnormal reaction without mention of misadventure) —*see also* Complication of or following, by type of procedure
due to or as a result of misadventure —*see* Misadventure
Swallowed, swallowing
foreign body —*see* Foreign body, alimentary canal
poison —*see* Table of drugs and chemicals
substance
caustic or corrosive —*see* Table of drugs and chemicals
poisonous —*see* Table of drugs and chemicals

T

Tackle in sport W03
Terrorism (involving) Y38.80
  biological weapons Y38.6X-
  chemical weapons Y38.7X-
  conflagration Y38.3X-
  explosion Y38.2X-
    destruction of aircraft Y38.1X-
    marine weapons Y38.0X-
  fire Y38.3X-
  firearms Y38.4X-
  hot substances Y38.5X-
  nuclear weapons Y38.5X-
  specified method NEC Y38.8X-
Thirst X58
Threat to breathing
  aspiration —*see* Aspiration
  due to cave-in, falling earth or
    substance NEC —*see* category T71
Thrown (accidentally)
  against part (any) of or object in
    transport vehicle (in motion) NEC
    (*see also* Accident, transport)
  from
    high place, homicide (attempt) Y01
    machinery —*see* Contact, with, by
      type of machine
    transport vehicle NEC (*see also*
      Accident, transport) V89.9
  off —*see* Thrown, from

Thunderbolt —*see* subcategory
  T75.0
  causing fire —*see* Exposure, fire
Tidal wave (any injury) NEC B —*see*
  Forces of nature, tidal wave
Took
  overdose (drug) —*see* Table of drugs
    and chemicals
  poison —*see* Table of drugs and
    chemicals
Tornado (any injury) X37.1
Torrential rain (any injury) X37.8
Torture X58
Trampled by animal NEC W55.89
Trapped (accidentally)
  between objects (moving) (stationary
    and moving) —*see* Caught
  by part (any) of
    motorcycle V29.88
    pedal cycle V19.88
    transport vehicle NEC (*see also*
      Accident, transport) V89.9
Travel (effects) (sickness) T75.3
Tree falling on or hitting (accidentally)
  (person) W20.8
Tripping
  without fall W18.40
    due to
      specified NEC W18.49
      stepping from one level to another
        W18.43

Tripping (Continued)
  without fall (Continued)
    due to (Continued)
      stepping into hole or opening
        W18.42
      stepping on object W18.41
  over
    animal W01.0
      with fall W01.0
    carpet, rug or (small) object
      W22.8
      with fall W18.09
    person W51
      with fall W03
        due to ice or snow W00.0
Twisted by person (s) (accidentally)
  W50.2
  with intent to injure or kill
    Y04.0
  as, or caused by, a crowd or
    human stampede (with fall)
    W52
  assault Y04.0
  homicide (attempt) Y04.0
  in
    fight Y04.0
    legal intervention —*see* Legal,
      intervention, manhandling
Twisting, excessive —*see*
  Overexertion

U

Underdosing of necessary drugs,
  medicaments or biological
  substances Y63.61
Undetermined intent (contact)
  (exposure)
  automobile collision Y32
  blunt object Y29
  drowning (submersion) (in) Y21.9
    bathtub Y21.0
      after fall Y21.1
    natural water (lake) (ocean) (pond)
      (river) (stream) Y21.4
    specified place NEC Y21.8
    swimming pool Y21.2
      after fall Y21.3
  explosive material Y25
  fall, jump or push from high place Y30
  falling, lying or running before moving
    object Y31
  fire Y26

Undetermined intent (Continued)
  firearm discharge Y24.9
    airgun (BB) (pellet) Y24.0
    handgun (pistol) (revolver)
      Y22
    hunting rifle Y23.1
    larger Y23.9
      hunting rifle Y23.1
      machine gun Y23.3
      military Y23.2
      shotgun Y23.0
      specified type NEC Y23.8
    machine gun Y23.3
    military Y23.2
    shotgun Y23.0
    specified type NEC Y24.8
    Very pistol Y24.8
  hot object Y27.9
    fluid NEC Y27.2
    household appliance Y27.3
    specified object NEC Y27.8
    steam Y27.0

Undetermined intent (Continued)
  hot object (Continued)
    tap water Y27.1
    vapor Y27.0
  jump, fall or push from high
    place Y30
  lying, falling or running before
    moving object Y31
  motor vehicle crash Y32
  push, fall or jump from high
    place Y30
  running, falling or lying before
    moving object Y31
  sharp object Y28.9
    dagger Y28.2
    glass Y28.0
    knife Y28.1
    specified object NEC
      Y28.8
    sword Y28.2
  smoke Y26
  specified event NEC Y33

V

Vibration (causing injury) W49.9
Victim (of)
  avalanche B —*see* Landslide
  earth movements NEC B —*see* Forces of
    nature, earth movement
  earthquake X34

Victim (Continued)
  flood B —*see* Flood
  landslide B —*see* Landslide
  lightning —*see* subcategory T75.0
    causing fire —*see* Exposure, fire
  storm (cataclysmic) NEC B —*see* Forces
    of nature, cataclysmic storm
  volcanic eruption X35

Volcanic eruption (any injury) X35
Vomitus, gastric contents in air passages
  (with asphyxia, obstruction or
  suffocation) T17.81-

W

Walked into stationary object (any) W22.09
  furniture W22.03
  lamppost W22.02
  wall W22.01
War operations (injuries to military
    personnel and civilians during war,
    civil insurrection and peacekeeping
    missions) (by) (from) (involving) Y36.90-
  after cessation of hostilities Y36.89-
    explosion (of)
      bomb placed during war
        operations Y36.82-
      mine placed during war operations
        Y36.81-
    specified NEC Y36.88-
  air blast Y36.20-
  aircraft
    destruction —see War operations,
      destruction of aircraft
    airway restriction —see War operations,
      restriction of airways
    asphyxiation —see War operations,
      restriction of airways
  biological weapons Y36.6X-
  blast Y36.20-
  blast fragments Y36.20-
  blast wave Y36.20-
  blast wind Y36.20-
  bomb Y36.20-
    dirty Y36.50-
    gasoline Y36.31-
    incendiary Y36.31-
    petrol Y36.31-
  bullet Y36.43-
    incendiary Y36.32-
    rubber Y36.41-
  chemical weapons Y36.7X-
  combat
    hand to hand (unarmed) combat
      Y36.44-
    using blunt or piercing object Y36.45-
  conflagration —see War operations, fire
  conventional warfare NEC Y36.49-
  depth-charge Y36.01-
  destruction of aircraft Y36.10-
    due to
      air to air missile Y36.11-
      collision with other aircraft Y36.12-
      detonation (accidental) of onboard
        munitions and explosives
        Y36.14-
      enemy fire or explosives Y36.11-
      explosive placed on aircraft Y36.11-
      onboard fire Y36.13-
      rocket propelled grenade [RPG]
        Y36.11-
      small arms fire Y36.11-
      surface to air missile Y36.11-
    specified NEC Y36.19-
  detonation (accidental) of
    onboard marine weapons Y36.05-
    own munitions or munitions launch
      device Y36.24-

War operations (Continued)
  dirty bomb Y36.50-
  explosion (of) Y36.20-
    aerial bomb Y36.21-
    after cessation of hostilities
      bomb placed during war operations
        Y36.82-
      mine placed during war operations
        Y36.81-
    bomb NOS (see also War operations,
      bomb (s)) Y36.20-
    fragments Y36.20-
    grenade Y36.29-
    guided missile Y36.22-
    improvised explosive device [IED]
      (person-borne) (roadside)
      (vehicle-borne) Y36.23-
    land mine Y36.29-
    marine mine (at sea) (in harbor)
      Y36.02-
    marine weapon Y36.00-
      specified NEC Y36.09-
    own munitions or munitions launch
      device (accidental) Y36.24-
    sea-based artillery shell Y36.03-
    specified NEC Y36.29-
    torpedo Y36.04-
  fire Y36.30-
    specified NEC Y36.39-
  firearms
    discharge Y36.43-
    pellets Y36.42-
  flamethrower Y36.33-
  fragments (from) (of)
    improvised explosive device [IED]
      (person-borne) (roadside)
      (vehicle-borne) Y36.26-
    munitions Y36.25-
    specified NEC Y36.29-
    weapons Y36.27-
  friendly fire Y36.92
  hand to hand (unarmed) combat
    Y36.44-
  hot substances —see War operations,
    fire
  incendiary bullet Y36.32-
  nuclear weapon (effects of) Y36.50-
    acute radiation exposure Y36.54-
    blast pressure Y36.51-
    direct blast Y36.51-
    direct heat Y36.53-
    fallout exposure Y36.54-
    fireball Y36.53-
    indirect blast (struck or crushed by
      blast debris) (being thrown by
      blast) Y36.52-
    ionizing radiation (immediate
      exposure) Y36.54-
    nuclear radiation Y36.54-
    radiation
      ionizing (immediate exposure)
        Y36.54-
      nuclear Y36.54-
      thermal Y36.53-
    secondary effects Y36.54-

War operations (Continued)
  nuclear weapon (Continued)
    specified NEC Y36.59-
    thermal radiation Y36.53-
  restriction of air (airway)
    intentional Y36.46-
    unintentional Y36.47-
  rubber bullets Y36.41-
  shrapnel NOS Y36.29-
  suffocation —see War operations,
    restriction of airways
  unconventional warfare NEC Y36.7X-
  underwater blast NOS Y36.00-
  warfare
    conventional NEC Y36.49-
    unconventional NEC Y36.7X-
  weapon of mass destruction [WMD]
    Y36.91
  weapons
    biological weapons Y36.6X-
    chemical Y36.7X-
    nuclear (effects of) Y36.50-
      acute radiation exposure Y36.54-
      blast pressure Y36.51-
      direct blast Y36.51-
      direct heat Y36.53-
      fallout exposure Y36.54-
      fireball Y36.53-
      indirect blast (struck or crushed by
        blast debris) (being thrown by
        blast) Y36.52-
      radiation
        ionizing (immediate exposure)
          Y36.54-
        nuclear Y36.54-
        thermal Y36.53-
      secondary effects Y36.54-
      specified NEC Y36.59-
    of mass destruction [WMD] Y36.91-
Washed
  away by flood —see Flood
  off road by storm (transport vehicle) —
    see Forces of nature, cataclysmic
    storm
Weather exposure NEC —see Forces of
    nature
Weightlessness (causing injury) (effects
    of) (in spacecraft, real or simulated)
    X52
Work related condition Y99.0
Wound (accidental) NEC (see also Injury)
    X58
  battle (see also War operations) Y36.90
  gunshot —see Discharge, firearm by
    type
Wreck transport vehicle NEC (see also
    Accident, transport) V89.9
Wrong
  device implanted into correct surgical
    site Y65.51
  fluid in infusion Y65.1
  patient, procedure performed on
    Y65.52
  procedure (operation) on correct
    patient Y65.51

PART III

ICD-10-CM Tabular List of Diseases and Injuries

C1 *communicable / transmissable*

Instructional Notations

Includes:

The word 'Includes' appears immediately under certain categories to further define, or give examples of, the content of the category.

Excludes Notes

The ICD-10-CM has two types of excludes notes. Each note has a different definition for use but they are both similar in that they indicate that codes excluded from each other are independent of each other.

Excludes1

A type 1 Excludes note is a pure excludes. It means 'NOT CODED HERE!' An Excludes1 note indicates that the code excluded should never be used at the same time as the code above the Excludes1 note. An Excludes1 is used when two conditions cannot occur together, such as a congenital form versus an acquired form of the same condition.

Excludes2

A type 2 excludes note represents 'Not included here'. An excludes2 note indicates that the condition excluded is not part of the condition it is excluded from but a patient may have both conditions at the same time. When an Excludes2 note appears under a code it is acceptable to use both the code and the excluded code together.

Code First/Use Additional Code notes (etiology/ manifestation paired codes)

Certain conditions have both an underlying etiology and multiple body system manifestations due to the underlying etiology. For such conditions the ICD-10-CM has a coding convention that requires the underlying condition be sequenced first followed by the manifestation. Wherever such a combination exists there is a 'use additional code' note at the etiology code, and a 'code first' note at the manifestation code. These instructional notes indicate the proper sequencing order of the codes, etiology followed by manifestation.

In most cases the manifestation codes will have in the code title, 'in diseases classified elsewhere.' Codes with this title are a component of the etiology/ manifestation convention. The code title indicates that it is a manifestation code. 'In diseases classified elsewhere' codes are never permitted to be used as first listed or principal diagnosis codes. They must be used in conjunction with an underlying condition code and they must be listed following the underlying condition.

Code Also

A code also note instructs that 2 codes may be required to fully describe a condition but the sequencing of the two codes is discretionary, depending on the severity of the conditions and the reason for the encounter.

7th characters and placeholder X

For codes less than 6 characters that require a 7th character a placeholder X should be assigned for all characters less than 6.
The 7th character must always be the 7th character of a code.

CHAPTER 1

CERTAIN INFECTIOUS AND PARASITIC DISEASES (A00-B99)

Includes   diseases generally recognized as communicable or transmissible

Use additional code to identify resistance to antimicrobial drugs (Z16-)

Excludes1   certain localized infections - see body system-related chapters
infectious and parasitic diseases complicating pregnancy, childbirth and the puerperium (O98.-)
influenza and other acute respiratory infections (J00-J22)

Excludes2   carrier or suspected carrier of infectious disease (Z22.-)
infectious and parasitic diseases specific to the perinatal period (P35-P39)

This chapter contains the following blocks:

A00-A09	Intestinal infectious diseases
A15-A19	Tuberculosis
A20-A28	Certain zoonotic bacterial diseases
A30-A49	Other bacterial diseases
A50-A64	Infections with a predominantly sexual mode of transmission
A65-A69	Other spirochetal diseases
A70-A74	Other diseases caused by chlamydiae
A75-A79	Rickettsioses
A80-A89	Viral and prion infections of the central nervous system
A90-A99	Arthropod-borne viral fevers and viral hemorrhagic fevers
B00-B09	Viral infections characterized by skin and mucous membrane lesions
B10	Other human herpesviruses
B15-B19	Viral hepatitis
B20	Human immunodeficiency virus [HIV] disease
B25-B34	Other viral diseases
B35-B49	Mycoses
B50-B64	Protozoal diseases
B65-B83	Helminthiases
B85-B89	Pediculosis, acariasis and other infestations
B90-B94	Sequelae of infectious and parasitic diseases
B95-B97	Bacterial and viral infectious agents
B99	Other infectious diseases

INTESTINAL INFECTIOUS DISEASES (A00-A09)

● **A00   Cholera**
     A serious, often deadly, infectious disease of the small intestine

    A00.0   Cholera due to Vibrio cholerae 01, biovar cholerae 🔊
       Classical cholera

    A00.1   Cholera due to Vibrio cholerae 01, biovar eltor 🔊
       Cholera eltor

    ■ **A00.9   Cholera, unspecified** 🔊

● **A01   Typhoid and paratyphoid fevers**
     Caused by Salmonella typhi and Salmonella paratyphi A, B, and C bacteria

    ● **A01.0   Typhoid fever**
       Infection due to Salmonella typhi

      ■ **A01.00   Typhoid fever, unspecified** 🔊

      A01.01   Typhoid meningitis 🔊

● Unacceptable Principal Diagnosis   ● Use Additional Character(s)   ■ Unspecified   ▶ Manifestation Code

  OGCR   Official Guidelines for Coding and Reporting | Excludes 1 | | Excludes 2 | | Includes | | Use additional | | Code first | | Code also |

A01.02 **Typhoid fever with heart involvement** 🦠
Typhoid endocarditis
Typhoid myocarditis

A01.03 **Typhoid pneumonia** 🦠

A01.04 **Typhoid arthritis** 🦠

A01.05 **Typhoid osteomyelitis** 🦠

A01.09 **Typhoid fever with other complications** 🦠

A01.1 **Paratyphoid fever A** 🦠

A01.2 **Paratyphoid fever B** 🦠

A01.3 **Paratyphoid fever C** 🦠

A01.4 **Paratyphoid fever, unspecified** 🦠
Infection due to Salmonella paratyphi NOS

● A02 **Other salmonella infections**

> **Includes**   infection or foodborne intoxication due to any Salmonella species other than S. typhi and S. paratyphi

A02.0 **Salmonella enteritis** 🦠
Salmonellosis

A02.1 **Salmonella sepsis** 🦠

● A02.2 **Localized salmonella infections**

A02.20 **Localized salmonella infection, unspecified** 🦠
Specified in the documentation as localized, but unspecified as to type

A02.21 **Salmonella meningitis** 🦠
Specified as localized in the meninges

A02.22 **Salmonella pneumonia** 🦠
Specified as localized in the lungs

A02.23 **Salmonella arthritis** 🦠
Specified as localized in the joints

A02.24 **Salmonella osteomyelitis** 🦠
Specified as localized in bone

A02.25 **Salmonella pyelonephritis** 🦠
Salmonella tubulo-interstitial nephropathy

A02.29 **Salmonella with other localized infection** 🦠
Specified as localized (because it is still under localized heading) but does not assign into any of the above codes

A02.8 **Other specified salmonella infections** 🦠
Any specified salmonella infection which does NOT assign into any of the above codes (not specified as localized)

A02.9 **Salmonella infection, unspecified** 🦠
Unspecified in the documentation as to specific type of salmonella

Item 1-1 Salmonella is a bacterium that lives in the intestines of fowl and mammals and can spread to humans through improper food preparation and cooking. Salmonellosis is an infection with the bacterium. Symptoms include diarrhea, fever, and abdominal cramps 12 to 72 hours after infection. The illness usually lasts 4 to 7 days, and most persons recover without treatment. The diarrhea may be so severe that the patient needs to be hospitalized. Patients with immunocompromised systems in chronic, ill health are more likely to have the infection invade their bloodstream with life-threatening results. For example, patients with sickle cell disease are more prone to salmonella osteomyelitis than others.

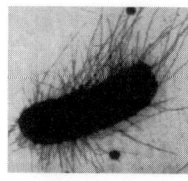

Figure 1-1   Electron micrograh of escherichia coli *(E. coli)* expressing P fimbriae. (From Mandell, Bennett, & Dolin: Principles and Practice of Infectious Diseases, 6th ed. 2005, Churchill Livingstone, An Imprint of Elsevier.)

Item 1-2 Escherichia coli [E. coli] is a gram-negative bacterium found in the intestinal tracts of humans and animals and is usually nonpathogenic. Pathogenic strains can cause diarrhea or pyogenic (pus-producing) infections. Can be a threat to food safety.

● A03 **Shigellosis**
An infectious disease caused by bacteria (Shigella)

A03.0 **Shigellosis due to Shigella dysenteriae** 🦠
Group A shigellosis [Shiga-Kruse dysentery]

A03.1 **Shigellosis due to Shigella flexneri**
Group B shigellosis

A03.2 **Shigellosis due to Shigella boydii**
Group C shigellosis

A03.3 **Shigellosis due to Shigella sonnei**
Group D shigellosis

A03.8 **Other shigellosis**

A03.9 **Shigellosis, unspecified**
Bacillary dysentery NOS

● A04 **Other bacterial intestinal infections**

> **Excludes1**   bacterial foodborne intoxications, NEC (A05.-) tuberculous enteritis (A18.32)

A04.0 **Enteropathogenic Escherichia coli infection** 🦠
Pertaining to or producing intestinal disease

A04.1 **Enterotoxigenic Escherichia coli infection** 🦠
Producing or containing intestinal toxin

A04.2 **Enteroinvasive Escherichia coli infection** 🦠
Capable of penetrating and spreading through intestinal mucosal epithelium

A04.3 **Enterohemorrhagic Escherichia coli infection** 🦠
Causing bloody diarrhea, resulting from microorganisms

A04.4 **Other intestinal Escherichia coli infections** 🦠
Escherichia coli enteritis NOS

A04.5 **Campylobacter enteritis** 🦠
Spiral shaped bacterium

A04.6 **Enteritis due to Yersinia enterocolitica** 🦠

> **Excludes1**   extraintestinal yersiniosis (A28.2)

Transmitted by infected food /water and person-to-person contact, affecting intestinal tract

A04.7 **Enterocolitis due to Clostridium difficile** 🦠
Foodborne intoxication by Clostridium difficile
Pseudomembraneous colitis
Marked by fibrinous deposit (false membrane) with enmeshed necrotic cells

A04.8 **Other specified bacterial intestinal infections** 🦠

A04.9 **Bacterial intestinal infection, unspecified** 🦠
Bacterial enteritis NOS

N Newborn Age: 0   **P** Pediatric Age: 0–17   **M** Maternity DX: 12–55   **A** Adult Age: 15–124   ♀ Females Only   ♂ Males Only

🦠 Complication\Comorbidity   🦠 Major C\C   🦠 Present on Admission Requirement   🦠 Hospital-Acquired Condition

791

CHAPTER 1 (A00-B99)

CHAPTER 1 (A00-B99)

● **A05 Other bacterial foodborne intoxications, not elsewhere classified**

> **Excludes1**   Clostridium difficile foodborne intoxication and infection (A04.7)
> Escherichia coli infection (A04.0-A04.4)
> listeriosis (A32.-)
> salmonella foodborne intoxication and infection (A02.-)
> toxic effect of noxious foodstuffs (T61-T62)

A05.0 Foodborne staphylococcal intoxication 🦠

A05.1 Botulism food poisoning 🦠
> Botulism NOS
> Classical foodborne intoxication due to Clostridium botulinum
>> **Excludes1**   infant botulism (A48.51)
>> wound botulism (A48.52)

A05.2 Foodborne Clostridium perfringens [Clostridium welchii] intoxication 🦠
> *Type A causes gas gangrene and necrotizing colitis; major cause of food poisoning in humans*
> Enteritis necroticans
> Pig-bel

A05.3 Foodborne Vibrio parahaemolyticus intoxication 🦠
> *Organism that survives only in high salt environment (halophilic), major cause of gastroenteritis due to consumption of raw or improperly cooked fish/seafood*

A05.4 Foodborne Bacillus cereus intoxication 🦠
> *Spore-forming species commonly found in soil, causes food poisoning from formation of intestinal toxins in contaminated foods*

A05.5 Foodborne Vibrio vulnificus intoxication 🦠
> *Species that survives in high salt environment (halophilic) with infection by eating raw seafood causes septicemia and cellulitis*

A05.8 Other specified bacterial foodborne intoxications 🦠

■ **A05.9 Bacterial foodborne intoxication, unspecified**

● **A06 Amebiasis**
> *An intestinal illness caused by the microscopic parasite Entamoeba histolytica*
> **Includes**   infection due to Entamoeba histolytica
> **Excludes1**   other protozoal intestinal diseases (A07.-)
> **Excludes2**   acanthamebiasis (B60.1-)
> Naegleriasis (B60.2)

A06.0 Acute amebic dysentery 🦠
> Acute amebiasis
> Intestinal amebiasis NOS

A06.1 Chronic intestinal amebiasis 🦠

A06.2 Amebic nondysenteric colitis 🦠
> *Pertaining to single cell microorganism*

A06.3 Ameboma of intestine 🦠
> *Tumorlike mass produced by localized inflammation often in intestine*
> Ameboma NOS

A06.4 Amebic liver abscess 🦠
> Hepatic amebiasis

A06.5 Amebic lung abscess 🦠
> Amebic abscess of lung (and liver)

A06.6 Amebic brain abscess 🦠
> Amebic abscess of brain (and liver) (and lung)

A06.7 Cutaneous amebiasis

● **A06.8 Amebic infection of other sites**

A06.81 Amebic cystitis 🦠

A06.82 Other amebic genitourinary infections 🦠
> Amebic balanitis
> Amebic vesiculitis
> Amebic vulvovaginitis

A06.89 Other amebic infections 🦠
> Amebic appendicitis
> Amebic splenic abscess

■ **A06.9 Amebiasis, unspecified**

● **A07 Other protozoal intestinal diseases**

A07.0 Balantidiasis
> Balantidial dysentery
> *Infection by protozoa that may cause diarrhea and dysentery, with ulceration of colonic mucous membranes*

A07.1 Giardiasis [lambliasis] 🦠
> *Common infection in small intestine spread by contaminated food, water, or direct person-to-person contact*

A07.2 Cryptosporidiosis 🦠
> *Human infection with protozoa usually seen as self-limited diarrhea in those who work with cattle*

A07.3 Isosporiasis 🦠
> *Human intestinal disease caused by protozoa*
> Infection due to Isospora belli and Isospora hominis
> Intestinal coccidiosis
> Isosporosis

A07.4 Cyclosporiasis 🦠
> *Infection by protozoa with most common species infecting humans being C cayetanensis*

A07.8 Other specified protozoal intestinal diseases 🦠
> Intestinal microsporidiosis
> Intestinal trichomoniasis
> Sarcocystosis
> Sarcosporidiosis

■ **A07.9 Protozoal intestinal disease, unspecified** 🦠
> Flagellate diarrhea
> Protozoal colitis
> Protozoal diarrhea
> Protozoal dysentery

● **A08 Viral and other specified intestinal infections**
> **Excludes1**   influenza with involvement of gastrointestinal tract (J09.X3, J10.2, J11.2)

A08.0 Rotaviral enteritis 🦠

● **A08.1 Acute gastroenteropathy due to Norwalk agent and other small round viruses**

A08.11 Acute gastroenteropathy due to Norwalk agent 🦠
> Acute gastroenteropathy due to Norovirus
> Acute gastroenteropathy due to Norwalk-like agent

A08.19 Acute gastroenteropathy due to other small round viruses 🦠
> Acute gastroenteropathy due to small round virus [SRV] NOS

A08.2 Adenoviral enteritis 🦠

● **A08.3 Other viral enteritis**

A08.31 Calicivirus enteritis 🦠

A08.32 Astrovirus enteritis 🦠

A08.39 Other viral enteritis 🦠
> Coxsackie virus enteritis
> Echovirus enteritis
> Enterovirus enteritis NEC
> Torovirus enteritis

● Unacceptable Principal Diagnosis   ● Use Additional Character(s)   ■ Unspecified   ▶ Manifestation Code
OGCR Official Guidelines for Coding and Reporting   Excludes 1   Excludes 2   Includes   Use additional   Code first   Code also
792

◼ **A08.4   Viral intestinal infection, unspecified**
     Viral enteritis NOS
     Viral gastroenteritis NOS
     Viral gastroenteropathy NOS

A08.8   Other specified intestinal infections

◼**A09   Infectious gastroenteritis and colitis, unspecified** 🦠
     Infectious colitis NOS
     Infectious enteritis NOS
     Infectious gastroenteritis NOS

     Excludes1   colitis NOS (K52.9)
              diarrhea NOS (R19.7)
              enteritis NOS (K52.9)
              gastroenteritis NOS (K52.9)
              noninfective gastroenteritis and colitis,
                 unspecified (K52.9)

TUBERCULOSIS (A15-A19)

Includes   infections due to Mycobacterium
           tuberculosis and Mycobacterium bovis

Excludes1   congenital tuberculosis (P37.0)
        nonspecific reaction to test for tuberculosis
           without active tuberculosis (R76.1-)
        pneumoconiosis associated with
           tuberculosis, any type in A15 (J65)
        positive PPD (R76.11)
        positive tuberculin skin test without active
           tuberculosis (R76.11)
        sequelae of tuberculosis (B90.-)
        silicotuberculosis (J65)

● **A15   Respiratory tuberculosis**

     A15.0   Tuberculosis of lung 🦠
           Tuberculous bronchiectasis
           Chronic dilatation of bronchi
           Tuberculous fibrosis of lung
           Tuberculous pneumonia
           Tuberculous pneumothorax

     A15.4   Tuberculosis of intrathoracic lymph nodes 🦠
           Tuberculosis of hilar lymph nodes
           Tuberculosis of mediastinal lymph nodes
           Tuberculosis of tracheobronchial lymph nodes

         Excludes1   tuberculosis specified as primary
                    (A15.7)

     A15.5   Tuberculosis of larynx, trachea and bronchus 🦠
           Tuberculosis of bronchus
           Tuberculosis of glottis
           Tuberculosis of larynx
           Tuberculosis of trachea

Figure 1-2   Far advanced bilteral pulmonary tuberculosis before and after 8 months of treatment with streptomycin, PAS, and isoniazid. (From Hinshaw HC, Garland LH: Diseases of the Chest, 2nd ed. Philadelphia, WB Saunders, 1963, p. 538.)

Item 1-3   Tuberculosis is a common and deadly infectious disease caused by the Mycobacterium tuberculosis organism. The first tuberculosis infection is called the **primary infection** and most commonly attacks the lungs but can affect the central nervous system, lymphatic system, circulatory system, genitourinary system, bones, joints, and even the skin. A **Ghon** lesion is the **initial lesion.** A **secondary lesion** occurs when the tubercle bacilli are carried to other areas.

Item 1-4   Although it primarily affects the lungs, the bacteria *Mycobacterium tuberculosis* can travel from the pulmonary circulation to virtually any organ in the body, much as a cancer metastasizes to a secondary site. If the immune system becomes compromised by age or disease, what would otherwise be a self-limiting primary tuberculosis in the lungs will develop in other organs. These are known as extrapulmonary sites.

     A15.6   Tuberculous pleurisy 🦠
           Tuberculosis of pleura
           Tuberculous empyema

         Excludes1   primary respiratory tuberculosis
                    (A15.7)

     A15.7   Primary respiratory tuberculosis 🦠

     A15.8   Other respiratory tuberculosis 🦠
           Mediastinal tuberculosis
           Nasopharyngeal tuberculosis
           Tuberculosis of nose
           Tuberculosis of sinus [any nasal]

◼ **A15.9   Respiratory tuberculosis unspecified** 🦠

● **A17   Tuberculosis of nervous system**

     A17.0   Tuberculous meningitis 🦠
           Tuberculosis of meninges (cerebral) (spinal)
           Tuberculous leptomeningitis

         Excludes1   tuberculous meningoencephalitis
                    (A17.82)

     A17.1   Meningeal tuberculoma 🦠
           Tuberculoma of meninges (cerebral) (spinal)

         Excludes2   tuberculoma of brain and spinal cord
                    (A17.81)

    ● **A17.8   Other tuberculosis of nervous system**

         A17.81   Tuberculoma of brain and spinal cord 🦠
              Tuberculous abscess of brain and spinal cord

         A17.82   Tuberculous meningoencephalitis 🦠
              Inflammation of brain and meninges;
                AKA cerebromeningitis and
                encephalomeningitis
              Tuberculous myelitis

         A17.83   Tuberculous neuritis 🦠
              Tuberculous mononeuropathy

         A17.89   Other tuberculosis of nervous system 🦠
              Tuberculous polyneuropathy

   ◼ **A17.9   Tuberculosis of nervous system, unspecified** 🦠

● **A18   Tuberculosis of other organs**

    ● **A18.0   Tuberculosis of bones and joints**

         A18.01   Tuberculosis of spine 🦠
              Pott's disease or curvature of spine
              Tuberculous arthritis
              Tuberculous osteomyelitis of spine
              Tuberculous spondylitis

         A18.02   Tuberculous arthritis of other joints 🦠
              Tuberculosis of hip (joint)
              Tuberculosis of knee (joint)

         A18.03   Tuberculosis of other bones 🦠
              Tuberculous mastoiditis
              Tuberculous osteomyelitis

CHAPTER 1 (A00-B99)

N   Newborn Age: 0   **P**   Pediatric Age: 0–17   **M**   Maternity DX: 12–55   **A**   Adult Age: 15–124   ♀   Females Only   ♂   Males Only

🦠   Complication\Comorbidity   🦠   Major C\C   🦠   Present on Admission Requirement   🦠   Hospital-Acquired Condition

A18.09 Other musculoskeletal tuberculosis
Tuberculous myositis
Tuberculous synovitis
Tuberculous tenosynovitis

● **A18.1 Tuberculosis of genitourinary system**

■ **A18.10 Tuberculosis of genitourinary system, unspecified**

A18.11 Tuberculosis of kidney and ureter

A18.12 Tuberculosis of bladder

A18.13 Tuberculosis of other urinary organs
Tuberculous urethritis

A18.14 Tuberculosis of prostate ♂   A

A18.15 Tuberculosis of other male genital organs ♂

A18.16 Tuberculosis of cervix ♀

A18.17 Tuberculous female pelvic inflammatory disease ♀
Tuberculous endometritis
Tuberculous oophoritis and salpingitis
Oophoritis = inflammation of ovary
Salpingitis = inflammation of fallopian tube

A18.18 Tuberculosis of other female genital organs ♀
Tuberculous ulceration of vulva

A18.2 Tuberculous peripheral lymphadenopathy
Tuberculous adenitis
Excludes2 tuberculosis of bronchial and mediastinal lymph nodes (A15.4)
tuberculosis of mesenteric and retroperitoneal lymph nodes (A18.39)
tuberculous tracheobronchial adenopathy (A15.4)

● **A18.3 Tuberculosis of intestines, peritoneum and mesenteric glands**

A18.31 Tuberculous peritonitis
Tuberculous ascites

A18.32 Tuberculous enteritis
Tuberculosis of anus and rectum
Tuberculosis of intestine (large) (small)

A18.39 Retroperitoneal tuberculosis
Tuberculosis of mesenteric glands
Tuberculosis of retroperitoneal (lymph glands)

A18.4 Tuberculosis of skin and subcutaneous tissue
Erythema induratum, tuberculous
Lupus excedens
Lupus vulgaris NOS
Lupus vulgaris of eyelid
Cutaneous tuberculosis characterized by reddish brown plaque on skin surrounded by papules and nodules
Scrofuloderma
Type of cutaneous tuberculosis, with direct extension of tuberculosis into skin from underlying structures; AKA tuberculosis colliquativa
Tuberculosis of external ear
Excludes2 lupus erythematosus (L93.-)
lupus NOS (M32.9)
systemic (M32.-)

● **A18.5 Tuberculosis of eye**
Excludes2 lupus vulgaris of eyelid (A18.4)

■ **A18.50 Tuberculosis of eye, unspecified**

A18.51 Tuberculous episcleritis
Inflammation of episclera and adjacent tissues

A18.52 Tuberculous keratitis
Tuberculous interstitial keratitis
Tuberculous keratoconjunctivitis (interstitial) (phlyctenular)
Inflammation of cornea and conjunctiva

A18.53 Tuberculous chorioretinitis
Inflammation of choroid and retina; retinochoroiditis

A18.54 Tuberculous iridocyclitis
Inflammation of iris and ciliary body

A18.59 Other tuberculosis of eye
Tuberculous conjunctivitis

A18.6 Tuberculosis of (inner) (middle) ear
Tuberculous otitis media
Excludes2 tuberculosis of external ear (A18.4)
tuberculous mastoiditis (A18.03)

A18.7 Tuberculosis of adrenal glands
Tuberculous Addison's disease

● **A18.8 Tuberculosis of other specified organs**

A18.81 Tuberculosis of thyroid gland

A18.82 Tuberculosis of other endocrine glands
Tuberculosis of pituitary gland
Tuberculosis of thymus gland

A18.83 Tuberculosis of digestive tract organs, not elsewhere classified
Excludes1 tuberculosis of intestine (A18.32)

A18.84 Tuberculosis of heart
Tuberculous cardiomyopathy
Tuberculous endocarditis
Tuberculous myocarditis
Tuberculous pericarditis

A18.85 Tuberculosis of spleen

A18.89 Tuberculosis of other sites
Tuberculosis of muscle
Tuberculous cerebral arteritis

● **A19 Miliary tuberculosis**
Includes disseminated tuberculosis
generalized tuberculosis
tuberculous polyserositis

A19.0 Acute miliary tuberculosis of a single specified site

A19.1 Acute miliary tuberculosis of multiple sites

■ **A19.2 Acute miliary tuberculosis, unspecified**

A19.8 Other miliary tuberculosis

■ **A19.9 Miliary tuberculosis, unspecified**

CERTAIN ZOONOTIC BACTERIAL DISEASES (A20-A28)

● **A20 Plague**
Infectious disease caused by a Yersinia pestis bacterium, transmitted by a rodent flea bite or handling of infected animal
Includes infection due to Yersinia pestis

A20.0 Bubonic plague

A20.1 Cellulocutaneous plague
Skin and subcutaneous tissue plague

Item 1–5 Miliary tuberculosis can be a life-threatening condition. If a tuberculous lesion enters a blood vessel, immense dissemination of tuberculous organisms can occur if the immune system is weak. High-risk populations—children under 4 years of age, the elderly, or the immunocompromised—are particularly prone to this type of infection. The lesions will have a millet seedlike appearance on chest x-ray. Bronchial washings and biopsy may aid in diagnosis.

● Unacceptable Principal Diagnosis   ● Use Additional Character(s)   ■ Unspecified   ▶ Manifestation Code
OGCR Official Guidelines for Coding and Reporting   Excludes 1   Excludes 2   Includes   Use additional   Code first   Code also

A20.2 Pneumonic plague 🦠
A20.3 Plague meningitis 🦠
A20.7 Septicemic plague 🦠
A20.8 Other forms of plague 🦠
    Abortive plague
    Asymptomatic plague
    Pestis minor
     Systemic bacterial disease
■ **A20.9 Plague, unspecified** 🦠
● **A21 Tularemia**
Caused by Francisella tularensis bacterium found in rodents, rabbits, and hares and transmitted to humans by contact with infected animal tissues or by ticks, biting flies, or mosquitoes

   Includes   deer-fly fever
                infection due to Francisella tularensis
                rabbit fever

A21.0 Ulceroglandular tularemia 🦠
Most common form of tularemia in humans is painful, swollen, erythematous papule at point of inoculation that ruptures to form shallow ulcer
A21.1 Oculoglandular tularemia 🦠
Primary site of entry is conjunctival sac, results in granulomatous corneal lesions
    Ophthalmic tularemia
A21.2 Pulmonary tularemia 🦠
A21.3 Gastrointestinal tularemia 🦠
    Abdominal tularemia
A21.7 Generalized tularemia 🦠
A21.8 Other forms of tularemia 🦠
■ **A21.9 Tularemia, unspecified** 🦠
● **A22 Anthrax**
An acute infectious disease caused by the spore-forming Bacillus anthracis; occurs in humans exposed to infected animals or tissue from infected animals

   Includes   infection due to Bacillus anthracis

A22.0 Cutaneous anthrax 🦠
    Malignant carbuncle
    Malignant pustule
A22.1 Pulmonary anthrax 🦠
    Inhalation anthrax
    Ragpicker's disease
    Woolsorter's disease
A22.2 Gastrointestinal anthrax 🦠
A22.7 Anthrax sepsis 🦠
    Infectious bacterial disease
    MCC: Only when the principal diagnosis is designated as an MCC
A22.8 Other forms of anthrax 🦠
    Anthrax meningitis
■ **A22.9 Anthrax, unspecified** 🦠

Item 1-6 Brucellosis: An infectious disease caused by the bacterium Brucella. Humans are infected by contact with contaminated animals or animal products. In humans brucellosis symptoms that are similar to the flu include fever, sweats, headaches, back pains, and physical weakness. Severe infections of the central nervous system or lining of the heart may occur. Brucellosis can also cause chronic symptoms that include recurrent fevers, joint pain, and fatigue.

● **A23 Brucellosis**
   Includes   Malta fever
                Mediterranean fever
                undulant fever

A23.0 Brucellosis due to Brucella melitensis
Resulting in flu-like symptoms that may lead to chronic symptoms that include recurrent fevers, joint pain, and fatigue
A23.1 Brucellosis due to Brucella abortus
Most common cause of brucellosis in humans; AKA Bang bacillus
A23.2 Brucellosis due to Brucella suis
Species found primarily in pigs, rabbits, and reindeer
A23.3 Brucellosis due to Brucella canis
Species that causes respiratory tract infection in humans
A23.8 Other brucellosis 🦠
■ **A23.9 Brucellosis, unspecified** 🦠
● **A24 Glanders and melioidosis**
Infection, usually of rodents, which spreads to other animals and humans, caused by Burkholderia pseudomallei through break in skin contaminated with infested soil or water

A24.0 Glanders 🦠
    Infection due to Pseudomonas mallei
    Malleus
A24.1 Acute and fulminating melioidosis 🦠
    Melioidosis pneumonia
    Melioidosis sepsis
A24.2 Subacute and chronic melioidosis 🦠
A24.3 Other melioidosis 🦠
■ **A24.9 Melioidosis, unspecified** 🦠
    Infection due to Pseudomonas pseudomallei NOS
    Whitmore's disease
● **A25 Rat-bite fevers**
RBF, infectious disease caused by Streptobacillus moniliformis or Spirillum minus.
A25.0 Spirillosis 🦠
Any disease condition caused by spirilla
    Sodoku
A25.1 Streptobacillosis 🦠
Acute, febrile human illness caused by bacteria transmitted by rats in most cases, passed from rodent to human via rodent's urine or mucous secretions; AKA rat fever
    Epidemic arthritic erythema
    Haverhill fever
    Streptobacillary rat-bite fever
■ **A25.9 Rat-bite fever, unspecified** 🦠
● **A26 Erysipeloid**
Infection with Erysipelothrix rhusiopathiae, occurring often as occupational disease resulting from handling infected fish, shellfish, meat, or poultry

A26.0 Cutaneous erysipeloid
    Erythema migrans
A26.7 Erysipelothrix sepsis 🦠
    MCC: Only when the principal diagnosis is designated as an MCC
A26.8 Other forms of erysipeloid
■ **A26.9 Erysipeloid, unspecified**
● **A27 Leptospirosis**
Occurs most commonly in the tropics
A27.0 Leptospirosis icterohemorrhagica 🦠
    Leptospiral or spirochetal jaundice (hemorrhagic)
    Weil's disease

N Newborn Age: 0   **P** Pediatric Age: 0–17   **M** Maternity DX: 12–55   **A** Adult Age: 15–124   ♀ Females Only   ♂ Males Only
🦠 Complication\Comorbidity   🦠 Major C\C   🦠 Present on Admission Requirement   🦠 Hospital-Acquired Condition

795

CHAPTER 1 (A00-B99)

● A27.8   Other forms of leptospirosis
    A27.81   Aseptic meningitis in leptospirosis 🦠
    A27.89   Other forms of leptospirosis 🦠
◻ A27.9   Leptospirosis, unspecified 🦠

● A28   Other zoonotic bacterial diseases, not elsewhere classified
    A28.0   Pasteurellosis 🦠
       Infection of humans or other animals by species of Pasteurella
    A28.1   Cat-scratch disease 🦠
       Cat-scratch fever
    A28.2   Extraintestinal yersiniosis 🦠
       Infection from Yersinia enterocolitica; AKA enteric yersiniosis, intestinal yersiniosis, Yersinia enteritis

       | Excludes1 | enteritis due to Yersinia enterocolitica (A04.6) |
       | | plague (A20.-) |

    A28.8   Other specified zoonotic bacterial diseases, not elsewhere classified 🦠
◻ A28.9   Zoonotic bacterial disease, unspecified 🦠

OTHER BACTERIAL DISEASES (A30-A49)

● A30   Leprosy [Hansen's disease]
    Chronic infectious disease attacking the skin, peripheral nerves, and mucous membranes

    | Includes | infection due to Mycobacterium leprae |
    | Excludes1 | sequelae of leprosy (B92) |

    A30.0   Indeterminate leprosy 🦠
       I leprosy
    A30.1   Tuberculoid leprosy 🦠
       TT leprosy
    A30.2   Borderline tuberculoid leprosy 🦠
       BT leprosy
    A30.3   Borderline leprosy 🦠
       BB leprosy
    A30.4   Borderline lepromatous leprosy 🦠
       BL leprosy
    A30.5   Lepromatous leprosy 🦠
       LL leprosy
    A30.8   Other forms of leprosy 🦠
◻ A30.9   Leprosy, unspecified 🦠

● A31   Infection due to other mycobacteria
    | Excludes2 | leprosy (A30.-) |
    | | tuberculosis (A15-A19) |

    A31.0   Pulmonary mycobacterial infection 🦠
       Infection due to Mycobacterium avium
       Infection due to Mycobacterium intracellulare [Battey bacillus]
       Infection due to Mycobacterium kansasii
    A31.1   Cutaneous mycobacterial infection 🦠
       Buruli ulcer
       Infection due to Mycobacterium marinum
       Infection due to Mycobacterium ulcerans
    A31.2   Disseminated mycobacterium avium-intracellulare complex (DMAC) 🦠
       MAC sepsis
    A31.8   Other mycobacterial infections 🦠
◻ A31.9   Mycobacterial infection, unspecified 🦠
       Atypical mycobacterial infection NOS
       Mycobacteriosis NOS

● A32   Listeriosis
    Infection caused by Listeria monocytogenes
    | Includes | listerial foodborne infection |
    | Excludes1 | neonatal (disseminated) listeriosis (P37.2) |
    A32.0   Cutaneous listeriosis 🦠
    A32.1   Listerial meningitis and meningoencephalitis
       A32.11   Listerial meningitis 🦠
       A32.12   Listerial meningoencephalitis 🦠
    A32.7   Listerial sepsis 🦠
       MCC: Only when the principal diagnosis is designated as an MCC
    A32.8   Other forms of listeriosis
       A32.81   Oculoglandular listeriosis 🦠
          Primary infection site is conjunctival sac, which if untreated may result in perforation of cornea and optic atrophy
       A32.82   Listerial endocarditis 🦠
          Exudative and proliferative inflammatory condition of endocardium caused by listeria bacteria
       A32.89   Other forms of listeriosis 🦠
          Listerial cerebral arteritis
◻ A32.9   Listeriosis, unspecified 🦠

A33   Tetanus neonatorum 🦠   N
    Neonate = newborn

A34   Obstetrical tetanus ♀ 🦠   M

A35   Other tetanus 🦠
    Tetanus NOS
    | Excludes1 | tetanus neonatorum (A33) |
    | | obstetrical tetanus (A34) |

● A36   Diphtheria
    A36.0   Pharyngeal diphtheria 🦠
       Diphtheritic membranous angina
       Tonsillar diphtheria
    A36.1   Nasopharyngeal diphtheria 🦠
    A36.2   Laryngeal diphtheria 🦠
       Diphtheritic laryngotracheitis
    A36.3   Cutaneous diphtheria 🦠
       | Excludes2 | erythrasma (L08.1) |
    A36.8   Other diphtheria
       A36.81   Diphtheritic cardiomyopathy 🦠
          Diphtheritic myocarditis
       A36.82   Diphtheritic radiculomyelitis 🦠
       A36.83   Diphtheritic polyneuritis 🦠
       A36.84   Diphtheritic tubulo-interstitial nephropathy 🦠
       A36.85   Diphtheritic cystitis 🦠
       A36.86   Diphtheritic conjunctivitis 🦠
       A36.89   Other diphtheritic complications 🦠
          Diphtheritic peritonitis
◻ A36.9   Diphtheria, unspecified 🦠

● A37   Whooping cough
    Pertussis is a highly contagious disease caused by the bacterium Bordetella pertussis and results in a whooping sounding cough.

Item 1-7 Diptheria: A highly contagious bacterial disease that results in the formation of an adherent membrane in the throat that may lead to suffocation. In its most poisonous form, it attacks the heart and lungs. It is spread by direct physical contact or breathing the aerosolized secretions of infected individuals. The exact location is specified in the codes.

● Unacceptable Principal Diagnosis   ● Use Additional Character(s)   ◻ Unspecified   ▶ Manifestation Code

OGCR Official Guidelines for Coding and Reporting   Excludes 1   Excludes 2   Includes   Use additional   Code first   Code also

● **A37.0 Whooping cough due to Bordetella pertussis**

     A37.00 Whooping cough due to Bordetella pertussis without pneumonia 🦠

     A37.01 Whooping cough due to Bordetella pertussis with pneumonia 🦠

         MCC: Only when the principal diagnosis is designated as an MCC

● **A37.1 Whooping cough due to Bordetella parapertussis**

     A37.10 Whooping cough due to Bordetella parapertussis without pneumonia 🦠

     A37.11 Whooping cough due to Bordetella parapertussis with pneumonia 🦠

         MCC: Only when the principal diagnosis is designated as an MCC

● **A37.8 Whooping cough due to other Bordetella species**

     A37.80 Whooping cough due to other Bordetella species without pneumonia 🦠

     A37.81 Whooping cough due to other Bordetella species with pneumonia 🦠

         MCC: Only when the principal diagnosis is designated as an MCC

● **A37.9 Whooping cough, unspecified species**

     ▪ **A37.90 Whooping cough, unspecified species without pneumonia** 🦠

     ▪ **A37.91 Whooping cough, unspecified species with pneumonia** 🦠

         MCC: Only when the principal diagnosis is designated as an MCC

● **A38 Scarlet fever**

     Most commonly caused by the bacteria Streptococcus pneumoniae and Neisseria meningitides

     Includes   scarlatina

     Excludes2   streptococcal sore throat (J02.0)

     A38.0 Scarlet fever with otitis media 🦠

     A38.1 Scarlet fever with myocarditis 🦠

     A38.8 Scarlet fever with other complications 🦠

     A38.9 Scarlet fever, uncomplicated 🦠
         Scarlet fever, NOS

● **A39 Meningococcal infection**

     Most commonly caused by the bacteria Streptococcus pneumoniae and Neisseria meningitides

     A39.0 Meningococcal meningitis 🦠

     A39.1 Waterhouse-Friderichsen syndrome 🦠
         Fulminating complication of meningococcemia
         Meningococcal hemorrhagic adrenalitis
         Meningococcic adrenal syndrome

     A39.2 Acute meningococcemia 🦠

     A39.3 Chronic meningococcemia 🦠

     ▪ **A39.4 Meningococcemia, unspecified** 🦠

     ● **A39.5 Meningococcal heart disease**

     ▪ **A39.50 Meningococcal carditis, unspecified** 🦠

     A39.51 Meningococcal endocarditis 🦠

     A39.52 Meningococcal myocarditis 🦠

     A39.53 Meningococcal pericarditis 🦠

     ● **A39.8 Other meningococcal infections**

     A39.81 Meningococcal encephalitis 🦠

     A39.82 Meningococcal retrobulbar neuritis 🦠
         Optic neuritis in portion of optic nerve posterior to eyeball; AKA postocular optic neuritis

     A39.83 Meningococcal arthritis 🦠

     A39.84 Postmeningococcal arthritis 🦠

     A39.89 Other meningococcal infections 🦠
         Meningococcal conjunctivitis

▪ **A39.9 Meningococcal infection, unspecified** 🦠
     Meningococcal disease NOS

● **A40 Streptococcal sepsis**

     Code first
     postprocedural streptococcal sepsis (T81.4)
     streptococcal sepsis during labor (O75.3)
     streptococcal sepsis following abortion or ectopic or molar pregnancy (O03-O07, O08.0)
     streptococcal sepsis following immunization (T88.0)
     streptococcal sepsis following infusion, transfusion or therapeutic injection (T80.2-)

     Excludes1   neonatal (P36.0-P36.1)
         puerperal sepsis (O85)
         sepsis due to Streptococcus, group D (A41.81)

     A40.0 Sepsis due to streptococcus, group A 🦠

     A40.1 Sepsis due to streptococcus, group B 🦠

     A40.3 Sepsis due to Streptococcus pneumoniae 🦠
         Pneumococcal sepsis

     A40.8 Other streptococcal sepsis 🦠

     ▪ **A40.9 Streptococcal sepsis, unspecified** 🦠

● **A41 Other sepsis**

     Code first
     postprocedural sepsis (T81.4)
     sepsis during labor (O75.3)
     sepsis following abortion, ectopic or molar pregnancy (O03-O07, O08.0)
     sepsis following immunization (T88.0)
     sepsis following infusion, transfusion or therapeutic injection (T80.2-)

     Excludes1   bacteremia NOS (R78.81)
         neonatal (P36.-)
         puerperal sepsis (O85)
         sepsis NOS (A41.9)
         streptococcal sepsis (A40.-)

     Excludes2   sepsis (due to) (in) actinomycotic (A42.7)
         sepsis (due to) (in) anthrax (A22.7)
         sepsis (due to) (in) candidal (B37.7)
         sepsis (due to) (in) Erysipelothrix (A26.7)
         sepsis (due to) (in) extraintestinal yersiniosis (A28.2)
         sepsis (due to) (in) gonococcal (A54.86)
         sepsis (due to) (in) herpesviral (B00.7)
         sepsis (due to) (in) listerial (A32.7)
         sepsis (due to) (in) melioidosis (A24.1)
         sepsis (due to) (in) meningococcal (A39.2-A39.4)
         sepsis (due to) (in) plague (A20.7)
         sepsis (due to) (in) tularemia (A21.7)
         toxic shock syndrome (A48.3)

     ● **A41.0 Sepsis due to Staphylococcus aureus**

     A41.01 Sepsis due to Methicillin susceptible Staphylococcus aureus 🦠
         MSSA sepsis
         Staphylococcus aureus sepsis NOS

     A41.02 Sepsis due to Methicillin resistant Staphylococcus aureus 🦠

     A41.1 Sepsis due to other specified staphylococcus 🦠
         Coagulase negative staphylococcus sepsis

     ▪ **A41.2 Sepsis due to unspecified staphylococcus** 🦠

     A41.3 Sepsis due to Hemophilus influenzae 🦠

     A41.4 Sepsis due to anaerobes 🦠

     Excludes1   gas gangrene (A48.0)

CHAPTER 1 (A00-B99)

● **A41.5 Sepsis due to other Gram-negative organisms**
  ■ **A41.50 Gram-negative sepsis, unspecified**
    Gram-negative sepsis NOS
  A41.51 Sepsis due to Escherichia coli [E. coli]
  A41.52 Sepsis due to Pseudomonas
    Pseudomonas aeroginosa
  A41.53 Sepsis due to Serratia
  A41.59 Other Gram-negative sepsis
● **A41.8 Other specified sepsis**
  A41.81 Sepsis due to Enterococcus
  A41.89 Other specified sepsis
■ **A41.9 Sepsis, unspecified organism**
  Septicemia NOS

● **A42 Actinomycosis**
  Excludes1 actinomycetoma (B47.1)
  A42.0 Pulmonary actinomycosis
  A42.1 Abdominal actinomycosis
  A42.2 Cervicofacial actinomycosis
  A42.7 Actinomycotic sepsis
  ● **A42.8 Other forms of actinomycosis**
    A42.81 Actinomycotic meningitis
    A42.82 Actinomycotic encephalitis
    A42.89 Other forms of actinomycosis
  ■ **A42.9 Actinomycosis, unspecified**

● **A43 Nocardiosis**
  A43.0 Pulmonary nocardiosis
  A43.1 Cutaneous nocardiosis
  A43.8 Other forms of nocardiosis
  ■ **A43.9 Nocardiosis, unspecified**

● **A44 Bartonellosis**
  A44.0 Systemic bartonellosis
    Oroya fever
  A44.1 Cutaneous and mucocutaneous bartonellosis
    Verruga peruana
  A44.8 Other forms of bartonellosis
  ■ **A44.9 Bartonellosis, unspecified**

A46 Erysipelas
  Excludes1 postpartum or puerperal erysipelas (O86.89)

● **A48 Other bacterial diseases, not elsewhere classified**
  Excludes1 actinomycetoma (B47.1)
  A48.0 Gas gangrene
    Clostridial cellulitis
    Clostridial myonecrosis
  A48.1 Legionnaires' disease
  A48.2 Nonpneumonic Legionnaires' disease [Pontiac fever]
  A48.3 Toxic shock syndrome
    Use additional code to identify the organism (B95, B96)
    Excludes1 endotoxic shock NOS (R57.8)
      sepsis NOS (A41.9)
  A48.4 Brazilian purpuric fever
    Systemic Hemophilus aegyptius infection

Item 1-8 Gas gangrene is a necrotizing subcutaneous infection that will cause tissue death. Patients with poor circulation (e.g., diabetes, peripheral nephropathy) will have low oxygen content in their tissues (hypoxia), which allows the Clostridium bacteria to flourish. Gas gangrene often occurs at the site of a surgical wound or trauma. Onset is sudden and dramatic. Treatment can include debridement, amputation, and/or hyperbaric oxygen treatments.

● **A48.5 Other specified botulism**
  Non-foodborne intoxication due to toxins of Clostridium botulinum [C. botulinum]
  Excludes1 food poisoning due to toxins of Clostridium botulinum (A05.1)
  A48.51 Infant botulism   P
  A48.52 Wound botulism
    Non-foodborne botulism NOS
    Use additional code for associated wound
  A48.8 Other specified bacterial diseases

● **A49 Bacterial infection of unspecified site**
  Excludes1 bacterial agents as the cause of diseases classified elsewhere (B95-B96)
    chlamydial infection NOS (A74.9)
    meningococcal infection NOS (A39.9)
    rickettsial infection NOS (A79.9)
    spirochetal infection NOS (A69.9)
  ● **A49.0 Staphylococcal infection, unspecified site**
    ■ **A49.01 Methicillin susceptible Staphylococcus aureus infection, unspecified site**
      Methicillin susceptible Staphylococcus aureus (MSSA) infection
      Staphylococcus aureus infection NOS
    ■ **A49.02 Methicillin resistant Staphylococcus aureus infection, unspecified site**
      Methicillin resistant Staphylococcus aureus (MRSA) infection
  ■ **A49.1 Streptococcal infection, unspecified site**
  ■ **A49.2 Hemophilus influenzae infection, unspecified site**
    Any of seven bacterium of genus Haemophilus
  ■ **A49.3 Mycoplasma infection, unspecified site**
    Bacterium of class Mollicutes, unusual group of bacteria distinguished by absence of cell wall
  ■ **A49.8 Other bacterial infections of unspecified site**
  ■ **A49.9 Bacterial infection, unspecified**
    Excludes1 bacteremia NOS (R78.81)

INFECTIONS WITH A PREDOMINANTLY SEXUAL MODE OF TRANSMISSION (A50-A64)

  Excludes1 human immunodeficiency virus [HIV] disease (B20)
    nonspecific and nongonococcal urethritis (N34.1)
    Reiter's disease (M02.3-)

● **A50 Congenital syphilis**
  ● **A50.0 Early congenital syphilis, symptomatic**
    Any congenital syphilitic condition specified as early or manifest less than two years after birth
    A50.01 Early congenital syphilitic oculopathy
    A50.02 Early congenital syphilitic osteochondropathy
    A50.03 Early congenital syphilitic pharyngitis
      Early congenital syphilitic laryngitis
    A50.04 Early congenital syphilitic pneumonia
    A50.05 Early congenital syphilitic rhinitis
    A50.06 Early cutaneous congenital syphilis
    A50.07 Early mucocutaneous congenital syphilis

Figure 1-3 Chancre of primary syphilis. (From Mandell, Bennrtt, & Dolin: Principles and Practice of Infectious Diseases, 6th ed. 2005, Churchill Livingstone, An Imprint of Elsevier.)

Item 1-9 Syphilis, also known as lues, is the most serious of the venereal diseases caused by *Treponema pallidum.* The **primary** stage is characterized by an ulceration known as **chancre,** which usually appears on the genitals but can also develop on the anus, lips, tonsils, breasts, or fingers. Syphilis is easy to cure in its early stages. A single intramuscular injection of penicillin will usually cure a person who has had syphilis for less than a year.

The **secondary** stage is characterized by a rash that can affect any area of the body. **Latent** syphilis is divided into **early,** which is diagnosed within two years of infection, and **late,** which is diagnosed two years or more after infection. Additional doses of penicillin or another antibiotic are needed to treat someone who has had syphilis for longer than a year. For those allergic to penicillin, there are other antibiotic treatments. **Congenital** syphilis is also labeled **early** or **late** based on the time of diagnosis.

A50.08   **Early visceral congenital syphilis** 🅒

A50.09   **Other early congenital syphilis, symptomatic** 🅒

A50.1   **Early congenital syphilis, latent**
      Congenital syphilis without clinical manifestations, with positive serological reaction and negative spinal fluid test, less than two years after birth

🔲A50.2   **Early congenital syphilis, unspecified** 🅒
      Congenital syphilis NOS less than two years after birth

⬤A50.3   **Late congenital syphilitic oculopathy**
      Excludes1   Hutchinson's triad (A50.53)

     🔲A50.30   **Late congenital syphilitic oculopathy, unspecified** 🅒

     A50.31   **Late congenital syphilitic interstitial keratitis** 🅒

     A50.32   **Late congenital syphilitic chorioretinitis** 🅒

     A50.39   **Other late congenital syphilitic oculopathy** 🅒

⬤A50.4   **Late congenital neurosyphilis [juvenile neurosyphilis]**
      Use additional code to identify any associated mental disorder
      Excludes1   Hutchinson's triad (A50.53)

     🔲A50.40   **Late congenital neurosyphilis, unspecified** 🅒
        Juvenile neurosyphilis NOS

     A50.41   **Late congenital syphilitic meningitis** 🅜

     A50.42   **Late congenital syphilitic encephalitis** 🅜

     A50.43   **Late congenital syphilitic polyneuropathy** 🅒

     A50.44   **Late congenital syphilitic optic nerve atrophy** 🅒

     A50.45   **Juvenile general paresis** 🅒
        Dementia paralytica juvenilis
        Juvenile tabetoparetic neurosyphilis

     A50.49   **Other late congenital neurosyphilis** 🅒
        Juvenile tabes dorsalis

⬤A50.5   **Other late congenital syphilis, symptomatic**
      Any congenital syphilitic condition specified as late or manifest two years or more after birth

     A50.51   **Clutton's joints** 🅒

     A50.52   **Hutchinson's teeth** 🅒

     A50.53   **Hutchinson's triad** 🅒

     A50.54   **Late congenital cardiovascular syphilis** 🅒

     A50.55   **Late congenital syphilitic arthropathy** 🅒

     A50.56   **Late congenital syphilitic osteochondropathy** 🅒

     A50.57   **Syphilitic saddle nose** 🅒

     A50.59   **Other late congenital syphilis, symptomatic** 🅒

A50.6   **Late congenital syphilis, latent**
      Congenital syphilis without clinical manifestations, with positive serological reaction and negative spinal fluid test, two years or more after birth.

🔲A50.7   **Late congenital syphilis, unspecified**
      Congenital syphilis NOS two years or more after birth.

🔲A50.9   **Congenital syphilis, unspecified**

⬤A51   **Early syphilis**

    A51.0   **Primary genital syphilis**
        Syphilitic chancre NOS

    A51.1   **Primary anal syphilis**

    A51.2   **Primary syphilis of other sites**

  ⬤A51.3   **Secondary syphilis of skin and mucous membranes**

     A51.31   **Condyloma latum** 🅒

     A51.32   **Syphilitic alopecia** 🅒

     A51.39   **Other secondary syphilis of skin** 🅒
        Syphilitic leukoderma
        Syphilitic mucous patch
        Excludes1 late syphilitic leukoderma (A52.79)

  ⬤A51.4   **Other secondary syphilis**

     A51.41   **Secondary syphilitic meningitis** 🅜

     A51.42   **Secondary syphilitic female pelvic disease** ♀ 🅒

     A51.43   **Secondary syphilitic oculopathy** 🅒
        Secondary syphilitic chorioretinitis
        Secondary syphilitic iridocyclitis, iritis
        Secondary syphilitic uveitis

     A51.44   **Secondary syphilitic nephritis** 🅒

     A51.45   **Secondary syphilitic hepatitis** 🅒

     A51.46   **Secondary syphilitic osteopathy** 🅒

     A51.49   **Other secondary syphilitic conditions** 🅒
        Secondary syphilitic lymphadenopathy
        Secondary syphilitic myositis

    A51.5   **Early syphilis, latent**
      Syphilis (acquired) without clinical manifestations, with positive serological reaction and negative spinal fluid test, less than two years after infection.

🔲A51.9   **Early syphilis, unspecified**

⬤A52   **Late syphilis**

  ⬤A52.0   **Cardiovascular and cerebrovascular syphilis**

     🔲A52.00   **Cardiovascular syphilis, unspecified** 🅒

     A52.01   **Syphilitic aneurysm of aorta** 🅒

     A52.02   **Syphilitic aortitis** 🅒

CHAPTER 1 (A00-B99)

N   Newborn Age: 0   **P**   Pediatric Age: 0–17   **M**   Maternity DX: 12–55   **A**   Adult Age: 15–124   ♀   Females Only   ♂   Males Only

🅒 Complication\Comorbidity   🅜 Major C\C   🔲 Present on Admission Requirement   🅗 Hospital-Acquired Condition

CHAPTER 1 (A00-B99)

A52.03 Syphilitic endocarditis 🦠
  Syphilitic aortic valve incompetence or stenosis
  Syphilitic mitral valve stenosis
  Syphilitic pulmonary valve regurgitation

A52.04 Syphilitic cerebral arteritis 🦠

A52.05 Other cerebrovascular syphilis 🦠
  Syphilitic cerebral aneurysm (ruptured) (non-ruptured)
  Syphilitic cerebral thrombosis

A52.06 Other syphilitic heart involvement 🦠
  Syphilitic coronary artery disease
  Syphilitic myocarditis
  Syphilitic pericarditis

A52.09 Other cardiovascular syphilis 🦠

● **A52.1 Symptomatic neurosyphilis**

■ **A52.10 Symptomatic neurosyphilis, unspecified** 🦠

A52.11 Tabes dorsalis 🦠
  Cognitive decline with progressive degeneration of posterior columns, roots, and ganglia of spinal cord, occur 15-20 years after initial infection of syphilis; AKA Duchenne disease
  Locomotor ataxia (progressive)
  Tabetic neurosyphilis

A52.12 Other cerebrospinal syphilis 🦠

A52.13 Late syphilitic meningitis 🦠

A52.14 Late syphilitic encephalitis 🦠

A52.15 Late syphilitic neuropathy 🦠
  Late syphilitic acoustic neuritis
  Late syphilitic optic (nerve) atrophy
  Late syphilitic polyneuropathy
  Late syphilitic retrobulbar neuritis

A52.16 Charcôt's arthropathy (tabetic) 🦠
  Progressive musculoskeletal condition characterized by joint dislocation, fractures, and deformities, results in progressive destruction of bone and soft tissue of weight-bearing joints

A52.17 General paresis 🦠
  Chronic meningoencephalitis results in loss of cortical function, or progressive dementia and generalized paralysis, occurring 10-20 years after initial infection of syphilis; AKA Bayle disease, dementia paralytica, paralytic dementiaparetic neurosyphilis, syphilitic meningoencephalitis
  Dementia paralytica

A52.19 Other symptomatic neurosyphilis 🦠
  Syphilitic parkinsonism

A52.2 Asymptomatic neurosyphilis 🦠

■ **A52.3 Neurosyphilis, unspecified** 🦠
  Gumma (syphilitic)
  Destructive lesions of syphilis
  Syphilis (late)
  Syphiloma

● **A52.7 Other symptomatic late syphilis**

A52.71 Late syphilitic oculopathy 🦠
  Late syphilitic chorioretinitis
  Late syphilitic episcleritis

A52.72 Syphilis of lung and bronchus 🦠

A52.73 Symptomatic late syphilis of other respiratory organs 🦠

A52.74 Syphilis of liver and other viscera 🦠
  Late syphilitic peritonitis

A52.75 Syphilis of kidney and ureter 🦠
  Syphilitic glomerular disease

A52.76 Other genitourinary symptomatic late syphilis 🦠
  Late syphilitic female pelvic inflammatory disease

A52.77 Syphilis of bone and joint 🦠

A52.78 Syphilis of other musculoskeletal tissue 🦠
  Late syphilitic bursitis
  Syphilis [stage unspecified] of bursa
  Syphilis [stage unspecified] of muscle
  Syphilis [stage unspecified] of synovium
  Syphilis [stage unspecified] of tendon

A52.79 Other symptomatic late syphilis 🦠
  Late syphilitic leukoderma
  Syphilis of adrenal gland
  Syphilis of pituitary gland
  Syphilis of thyroid gland
  Syphilitic splenomegaly
  | Excludes1 | syphilitic leukoderma (secondary) (A51.39) |

A52.8 Late syphilis, latent
  Syphilis (acquired) without clinical manifestations, with positive serological reaction and negative spinal fluid test, two years or more after infection

■ **A52.9 Late syphilis, unspecified**

● **A53 Other and unspecified syphilis**

■ **A53.0 Latent syphilis, unspecified as early or late**
  Latent syphilis NOS
  Positive serological reaction for syphilis

■ **A53.9 Syphilis, unspecified**
  Infection due to Treponema pallidum NOS
  Syphilis (acquired) NOS
  | Excludes1 | syphilis NOS under two years of age (A50.2) |

● **A54 Gonococcal infection**

● **A54.0 Gonococcal infection of lower genitourinary tract without periurethral or accessory gland abscess**
  | Excludes1 | gonococcal infection with genitourinary gland abscess (A54.1) gonococcal infection with periurethral abscess (A54.1) |

■ **A54.00 Gonococcal infection of lower genitourinary tract, unspecified** 🦠

■ **A54.01 Gonococcal cystitis and urethritis, unspecified** 🦠

■ **A54.02 Gonococcal vulvovaginitis, unspecified** ♀ 🦠

■ **A54.03 Gonococcal cervicitis, unspecified** ♀ 🦠

A54.09 Other gonococcal infection of lower genitourinary tract 🦠

A54.1 Gonococcal infection of lower genitourinary tract with periurethral and accessory gland abscess 🦠
  Gonococcal Bartholin's gland abscess

● **A54.2 Gonococcal pelviperitonitis and other gonococcal genitourinary infection**

A54.21 Gonococcal infection of kidney and ureter 🦠

A54.22 Gonococcal prostatitis ♂ 🦠

A54.23 Gonococcal infection of other male genital organs ♂ 🦠
  Gonococcal epididymitis
  Gonococcal orchitis

A54.24 Gonococcal female pelvic inflammatory disease ♀ 🦠
  Gonococcal pelviperitonitis
  | Excludes1 | gonococcal peritonitis (A54.85) |

A54.29 Other gonococcal genitourinary infections 🦠

● Unacceptable Principal Diagnosis   ● Use Additional Character(s)   ■ Unspecified   ▶ Manifestation Code
OGCR Official Guidelines for Coding and Reporting   Excludes 1   Excludes 2   Includes   Use additional   Code first   Code also

Item 1-10 An STD (sexually transmitted disease) caused by **Neisseria gonorrhoeae** that flourishes in the warm, moist areas of the reproductive tract. Untreated gonorrhea spreads to other parts of the body, causing inflammation of the testes or prostate or pelvic inflammatory disease (PID).

● **A54.3 Gonococcal infection of eye**

■ **A54.30 Gonococcal infection of eye, unspecified** 🦠

A54.31 Gonococcal conjunctivitis 🦠
> *Form of bacterial conjunctivitis contracted by newborns during delivery; AKA neonatal conjunctivitis*
Ophthalmia neonatorum due to gonococcus

A54.32 Gonococcal iridocyclitis 🦠
> *Inflammation of iris and of ciliary body due to gonococcal infection*

A54.33 Gonococcal keratitis 🦠
> *Inflammation of cornea due to gonococcal infection; AKA keratoconjunctivitis, keratopathy*

A54.39 Other gonococcal eye infection 🦠
Gonococcal endophthalmia

● **A54.4 Gonococcal infection of musculoskeletal system**

■ **A54.40 Gonococcal infection of musculoskeletal system, unspecified** 🦠

A54.41 Gonococcal spondylopathy 🦠
> *Disorder of vertebrae due to gonococcal infection; AKA rachiopathy*

A54.42 Gonococcal arthritis 🦠
> **Excludes2**   gonococcal infection of spine (A54.41)

A54.43 Gonococcal osteomyelitis 🦠
> **Excludes2**   gonococcal infection of spine (A54.41)

A54.49 Gonococcal infection of other musculoskeletal tissue 🦠
Gonococcal bursitis
Gonococcal myositis
Gonococcal synovitis
Gonococcal tenosynovitis

A54.5 Gonococcal pharyngitis

A54.6 Gonococcal infection of anus and rectum

● **A54.8 Other gonococcal infections**

A54.81 Gonococcal meningitis 🦠

A54.82 Gonococcal brain abscess 🦠

A54.83 Gonococcal heart infection 🦠
Gonococcal endocarditis
Gonococcal myocarditis
Gonococcal pericarditis

A54.84 Gonococcal pneumonia 🦠

A54.85 Gonococcal peritonitis 🦠
> **Excludes1**   gonococcal pelviperitonitis (A54.24)

A54.86 Gonococcal sepsis 🦠

A54.89 Other gonococcal infections 🦠
Gonococcal keratoderma
Gonococcal lymphadenitis

■ **A54.9 Gonococcal infection, unspecified** 🦠

A55 Chlamydial lymphogranuloma (venereum)
Climatic or tropical bubo
Durand-Nicolas-Favre disease
Esthiomene
Lymphogranuloma inguinale

● **A56 Other sexually transmitted chlamydial diseases**

> **Includes**   sexually transmitted diseases due to Chlamydia trachomatis

> **Excludes1**   neonatal chlamydial conjunctivitis (P39.1)
neonatal chlamydial pneumonia (P23.1)

> **Excludes2**   chlamydial lymphogranuloma (A55)
conditions classified to A74.-

● **A56.0 Chlamydial infection of lower genitourinary tract**

■ **A56.00 Chlamydial infection of lower genitourinary tract, unspecified**

A56.01 Chlamydial cystitis and urethritis

A56.02 Chlamydial vulvovaginitis ♀

A56.09 Other chlamydial infection of lower genitourinary tract
Chlamydial cervicitis

● **A56.1 Chlamydial infection of pelviperitoneum and other genitourinary organs**

A56.11 Chlamydial female pelvic inflammatory disease ♀

A56.19 Other chlamydial genitourinary infection
Chlamydial epididymitis
Chlamydial orchitis

■ **A56.2 Chlamydial infection of genitourinary tract, unspecified**

A56.3 Chlamydial infection of anus and rectum

A56.4 Chlamydial infection of pharynx

A56.8 Sexually transmitted chlamydial infection of other sites

A57 Chancroid
Ulcus molle
> *Sexually transmitted infection caused by bacteria, Haemophilus ducreyi*

A58 Granuloma inguinale
> *Chronic, progressive, ulcerative granulomatous disease*
Donovanosis

● **A59 Trichomoniasis**
> **Excludes2**   intestinal trichomoniasis (A07.8)
> *A common STD caused by a parasite, Trichomonas vaginalis*

● **A59.0 Urogenital trichomoniasis**

■ **A59.00 Urogenital trichomoniasis, unspecified**
Fluor (vaginalis) due to Trichomonas
Leukorrhea (vaginalis) due to Trichomonas

A59.01 Trichomonal vulvovaginitis ♀

A59.02 Trichomonal prostatitis ♂

A59.03 Trichomonal cystitis and urethritis

A59.09 Other urogenital trichomoniasis
> *Common sexually transmitted disease (STD) caused by single-celled protozoan parasite; AKA trich*
Trichomonas cervicitis

A59.8 Trichomoniasis of other sites

■ **A59.9 Trichomoniasis, unspecified**

● **A60 Anogenital herpesviral [herpes simplex] infections**

● **A60.0 Herpesviral infection of genitalia and urogenital tract**

■ **A60.00 Herpesviral infection of urogenital system, unspecified**

A60.01 Herpesviral infection of penis ♂

A60.02 Herpesviral infection of other male genital organs ♂

N Newborn Age: 0   **P** Pediatric Age: 0–17   **M** Maternity DX: 12–55   **A** Adult Age: 15–124   ♀ Females Only   ♂ Males Only

 Complication\Comorbidity   🦠 Major C\C   Present on Admission Requirement   Hospital-Acquired Condition

801

CHAPTER 1 (A00-B99)

CHAPTER 1 (A00-B99)

A60.03   **Herpesviral cervicitis ♀**

A60.04   **Herpesviral vulvovaginitis ♀**
Herpesviral [herpes simplex] ulceration
Herpesviral [herpes simplex] vaginitis
Herpesviral [herpes simplex] vulvitis

A60.09   **Herpesviral infection of other urogenital tract**

A60.1   **Herpesviral infection of perianal skin and rectum**

■ A60.9   **Anogenital herpesviral infection, unspecified**

● A63   **Other predominantly sexually transmitted diseases, not elsewhere classified**

Excludes2	molluscum contagiosum (B08.1)
	papilloma of cervix (D26.0)

A63.0   **Anogenital (venereal) warts**
Anogenital warts due to (human) papillomavirus [HPV]
Condyloma acuminatum

A63.8   **Other specified predominantly sexually transmitted diseases**

■ A64   **Unspecified sexually transmitted disease**

OTHER SPIROCHETAL DISEASES (A65-A69)

Excludes2	leptospirosis (A27.-)
	syphilis (A50-A53)

A65   **Nonvenereal syphilis**
Bejel
Endemic syphilis
Njovera

● A66   **Yaws**
Endemic, infectious, tropical disease caused by spirochete, spread by direct contact; AKA frambesia, framboesia, frambesia tropica

Includes	bouba
	frambesia (tropica)
	pian

A66.0   **Initial lesions of yaws**
Chancre of yaws
Frambesia, initial or primary
Initial frambesial ulcer
Mother yaw

A66.1   **Multiple papillomata and wet crab yaws**
Frambesioma
Pianoma
Plantar or palmar papilloma of yaws

A66.2   **Other early skin lesions of yaws**
Cutaneous yaws, less than five years after infection
Early yaws (cutaneous)(macular)(maculopapular) (micropapular)(papular)
Frambeside of early yaws

A66.3   **Hyperkeratosis of yaws**
Hypertrophy of stratum corneum of skin in which there are small, hard, verrucous scales
Ghoul hand
Hyperkeratosis, palmar or plantar (early) (late) due to yaws
Worm-eaten soles

A66.4   **Gummata and ulcers of yaws**
Small, rubbery granuloma with necrotic center and inflamed characteristic of advanced stage of syphilis; AKA syphiloma
Gummatous frambeside
Nodular late yaws (ulcerated)

A66.5   **Gangosa**
Manifestation of yaws that develops in the soft palate and spreads eroding bone, cartilage, and soft tissue
Rhinopharyngitis mutilans

A66.6   **Bone and joint lesions of yaws**
Yaws ganglion
Yaws goundou
Yaws gumma, bone
Yaws gummatous osteitis or periostitis
Yaws hydrarthrosis
Yaws osteitis
Yaws periostitis (hypertrophic)

A66.7   **Other manifestations of yaws**
Juxta-articular nodules of yaws
Mucosal yaws

A66.8   **Latent yaws**
Yaws without clinical manifestations, with positive serology

■ A66.9   **Yaws, unspecified**

● A67   **Pinta [carate]**
Group of nonvenereal diseases caused by Treponema species

A67.0   **Primary lesions of pinta**
Chancre (primary) of pinta
Papule (primary) of pinta

A67.1   **Intermediate lesions of pinta**
Erythematous plaques of pinta
Hyperchromic lesions of pinta
Hyperkeratosis of pinta
Pintids

A67.2   **Late lesions of pinta**
Achromic skin lesions of pinta
Cicatricial skin lesions of pinta
Dyschromic skin lesions of pinta

A67.3   **Mixed lesions of pinta**
Achromic with hyperchromic skin lesions of pinta [carate]

■ A67.9   **Pinta, unspecified**

● A68   **Relapsing fevers**

Includes	recurrent fever

Excludes2	Lyme disease (A69.2-)

A68.0   **Louse-borne relapsing fever** 🕭
Relapsing fever due to Borrelia recurrentis

A68.1   **Tick-borne relapsing fever** 🕭
Relapsing fever due to any Borrelia species other than Borrelia recurrentis

■ A68.9   **Relapsing fever, unspecified** 🕭

● A69   **Other spirochetal infections**

A69.0   **Necrotizing ulcerative stomatitis**
Cancrum oris
Fusospirochetal gangrene
Noma
Stomatitis gangrenosa

A69.1   **Other Vincent's infections** 🕭
Fusospirochetal pharyngitis
Necrotizing ulcerative (acute) gingivitis
Necrotizing ulcerative (acute) gingivostomatitis
Spirochetal stomatitis
Trench mouth
Vincent's angina
Vincent's gingivitis

● A69.2   **Lyme disease**
Erythema chronicum migrans due to Borrelia burgdorferi

■ A69.20   **Lyme disease, unspecified** 🕭

A69.21   **Meningitis due to Lyme disease** 🕭

A69.22   **Other neurologic disorders in Lyme disease** 🕭
Cranial neuritis
Meningoencephalitis
Polyneuropathy

● Unacceptable Principal Diagnosis   ● Use Additional Character(s)   ■ Unspecified   ▶ Manifestation Code

OGCR   Official Guidelines for Coding and Reporting | Excludes 1 | | Excludes 2 | Includes   Use additional   Code first   Code also

Item 1-11 Cancrum oris, also known as **noma** or **gangrenous stomatitis,** begins as an ulcer of the gingiva and results in a progressive gangrenous process.

    A69.23   **Arthritis due to Lyme disease** 🦠

    A69.29   **Other conditions associated with Lyme disease** 🦠
         Myopericarditis due to Lyme disease

   A69.8   **Other specified spirochetal infections**

   ▪ A69.9   **Spirochetal infection, unspecified**

OTHER DISEASES CAUSED BY CHLAMYDIAE (A70-A74)

   | Excludes1 | sexually transmitted chlamydial diseases (A55-A56)

  A70   **Chlamydia psittaci infections** 🦠
     Ornithosis
     Parrot fever
     Psittacosis

● A71   **Trachoma**
    | Excludes1 | sequelae of trachoma (B94.0)

   A71.0   **Initial stage of trachoma**
     Trachoma dubium

   A71.1   **Active stage of trachoma**
     Granular conjunctivitis (trachomatous)
     Trachomatous follicular conjunctivitis
     Trachomatous pannus

   ▪ A71.9   **Trachoma, unspecified**

● A74   **Other diseases caused by chlamydiae**
    | Excludes1 | neonatal chlamydial conjunctivitis (P39.1)
        neonatal chlamydial pneumonia (P23.1)
        Reiter's disease (M02.3-)
        sexually transmitted chlamydial diseases (A55-A56)

    | Excludes2 | chlamydial pneumonia (J16.0)

   A74.0   **Chlamydial conjunctivitis**
     Paratrachoma

   ● A74.8   **Other chlamydial diseases**

     A74.81   **Chlamydial peritonitis**

     A74.89   **Other chlamydial diseases**

   ▪ A74.9   **Chlamydial infection, unspecified**
     Chlamydiosis NOS

RICKETTSIOSES (A75-A79)

● A75   **Typhus fever**
    | Excludes1 | rickettsiosis due to Ehrlichia sennetsu (A79.2)

   A75.0   **Epidemic louse-borne typhus fever due to Rickettsia prowazekii** 🦠
     Organisms transmitted between humans via louse
     Classical typhus (fever)
     Epidemic (louse-borne) typhus

   A75.1   **Recrudescent typhus [Brill's disease]** 🦠
     Brill-Zinsser disease

   A75.2   **Typhus fever due to Rickettsia typhi** 🦠
     Murine (flea-borne) typhus

   A75.3   **Typhus fever due to Rickettsia tsutsugamushi** 🦠
     Scrub (mite-borne) typhus
     Tsutsugamushi fever

   ▪ A75.9   **Typhus fever, unspecified** 🦠
     Typhus (fever) NOS

● A77   **Spotted fever [tick-borne rickettsioses]**

   A77.0   **Spotted fever due to Rickettsia rickettsii** 🦠
     Rocky Mountain spotted fever
     Sao Paulo fever

Item 1–12 Rickettsioses are diseases spread from ticks, lice, fleas, or mites to humans.
   Typhus is spread to humans chiefly by the fleas of rats.
   Endemic identifies a disease as being present in low numbers of humans at all times, whereas **epidemic** identifies a disease as being present in high numbers of humans at a specific time. Morbidity (death) is higher in epidemic diseases.
   Brill's disease, also known as **Brill-Zinsser disease,** is spread from human to human by body lice and also from the lice of flying squirrels. **Scrub typhus** is spread in the same ways as Brill's disease.
   Malaria is spread to humans by mosquitoes.

   A77.1   **Spotted fever due to Rickettsia conorii** 🦠
     African tick typhus
     Boutonneuse fever
     India tick typhus
     Kenya tick typhus
     Marseilles fever
     Mediterranean tick fever

   A77.2   **Spotted fever due to Rickettsia siberica** 🦠
     North Asian tick fever
     Siberian tick typhus

   A77.3   **Spotted fever due to Rickettsia australis** 🦠
     Queensland tick typhus

   ● A77.4   **Ehrlichiosis**
     Type of tick-borne fever caused by bacteria infection
     | Excludes1 | Rickettsiosis due to Ehrlichia sennetsu (A79.81)

     ▪ A77.40   **Ehrlichiosis, unspecified** 🦠

     A77.41   **Ehrlichiosis chafeensis [E. chafeensis]** 🦠

     A77.49   **Other ehrlichiosis** 🦠

   A77.8   **Other spotted fevers** 🦠

   ▪ A77.9   **Spotted fever, unspecified** 🦠
     Tick-borne typhus NOS

  A78   **Q fever** 🦠
     Infection due to Coxiella burnetii
     Nine Mile fever
     Quadrilateral fever

● A79   **Other rickettsioses**

   A79.0   **Trench fever** 🦠
     Quintan fever
     Wolhynian fever

   A79.1   **Rickettsialpox due to Rickettsia akari** 🦠
     Kew Garden fever
     Vesicular rickettsiosis

   ● A79.8   **Other specified rickettsioses**

     A79.81   **Rickettsiosis due to Ehrlichia sennetsu** 🦠

     A79.89   **Other specified rickettsioses** 🦠

   ▪ A79.9   **Rickettsiosis, unspecified** 🦠
     Rickettsial infection NOS

VIRAL AND PRION INFECTIONS OF THE CENTRAL NERVOUS SYSTEM (A80-A89)

    | Excludes1 | postpolio syndrome (G14)
        sequelae of poliomyelitis (B91)
        sequelae of viral encephalitis (B94.1)

● A80   **Acute poliomyelitis**

   A80.0   **Acute paralytic poliomyelitis, vaccine-associated** 🦠

   A80.1   **Acute paralytic poliomyelitis, wild virus, imported** 🦠

   A80.2   **Acute paralytic poliomyelitis, wild virus, indigenous** 🦠

N Newborn Age: 0   **P** Pediatric Age: 0–17   **M** Maternity DX: 12–55   **A** Adult Age: 15–124   ♀ Females Only   ♂ Males Only

🦠 Complication\Comorbidity   🦠 Major C\C   🦠 Present on Admission Requirement   🦠 Hospital-Acquired Condition

CHAPTER 1 (A00-B99)

Item 1-13   Acute Poliomyelitis: Also called infantile paralysis and is caused by the poliovirus, which enters the body orally and infects the intestinal wall and then enters the blood stream and central nervous system, causing muscle weakness and paralysis. This disease has been nearly eradicated with the polio vaccine.

- ● **A80.3   Acute paralytic poliomyelitis, other and unspecified**
  - ■ **A80.30   Acute paralytic poliomyelitis, unspecified** 🔍
  - **A80.39   Other acute paralytic poliomyelitis** 🔍
  - **A80.4   Acute nonparalytic poliomyelitis**
- ■ **A80.9   Acute poliomyelitis, unspecified**

- ● **A81   Atypical virus infections of central nervous system**

  > **Includes**   diseases of the central nervous system caused by prions

  > Use additional code to identify:
  > dementia with behavioral disturbance (F02.81)
  > dementia without behavioral disturbance (F02.80)

  - ● **A81.0   Creutzfeldt-Jakob disease**
    - ■ **A81.00   Creutzfeldt-Jakob disease, unspecified** 🔍
      Jakob-Creutzfeldt disease, unspecified
    - **A81.01   Variant Creutzfeldt-Jakob disease** 🔍
      vCJD
    - **A81.09   Other Creutzfeldt-Jakob disease** 🔍
      CJD
      Familial Creutzfeldt-Jakob disease
      Iatrogenic Creutzfeldt-Jakob disease
      Sporadic Creutzfeldt-Jakob disease
      Subacute spongiform encephalopathy (with dementia)

  - **A81.1   Subacute sclerosing panencephalitis** 🔍
    Type of viral encephalitis that causes parenchymatous lesions in gray and white matter of brain
    Dawson's inclusion body encephalitis
    Van Bogaert's sclerosing leukoencephalopathy

  - **A81.2   Progressive multifocal leukoencephalopathy** 🔍
    Group of diseases affecting white matter of brain
    Multifocal leukoencephalopathy NOS

  - ● **A81.8   Other atypical virus infections of central nervous system**
    - **A81.81   Kuru** 🔍
    - **A81.82   Gerstmann-Sträussler-Scheinker syndrome** 🔍
      GSS syndrome
    - **A81.83   Fatal familial insomnia** 🔍
      FFI
    - **A81.89   Other atypical virus infections of central nervous system** 🔍

  - ■ **A81.9   Atypical virus infection of central nervous system, unspecified** 🔍
    Prion diseases of the central nervous system NOS

- ● **A82   Rabies**
  Viral disease affecting the central nervous system and transmitted from infected mammals to man.
  - **A82.0   Sylvatic rabies** 🔍
  - **A82.1   Urban rabies** 🔍
  - ■ **A82.9   Rabies, unspecified** 🔍

- ● **A83   Mosquito-borne viral encephalitis**
  Inflammation of the brain caused most commonly by Herpes Simplex virus.

  > **Includes**   mosquito-borne viral meningoencephalitis
  > **Excludes2**   Venezuelan equine encephalitis (A92.2)
  > West Nile fever (A92.3-)
  > West Nile virus (A92.3-)

  - **A83.0   Japanese encephalitis** 🔍
  - **A83.1   Western equine encephalitis** 🔍
  - **A83.2   Eastern equine encephalitis** 🔍
  - **A83.3   St. Louis encephalitis** 🔍

- **A83.4   Australian encephalitis** 🔍
  Kunjin virus disease
- **A83.5   California encephalitis** 🔍
  California meningoencephalitis
  La Crosse encephalitis
- **A83.6   Rocio virus disease** 🔍
  Mosquito-borne virus
- **A83.8   Other mosquito-borne viral encephalitis** 🔍
- ■ **A83.9   Mosquito-borne viral encephalitis, unspecified** 🔍

- ● **A84   Tick-borne viral encephalitis**

  > **Includes**   tick-borne viral meningoencephalitis

  - **A84.0   Far Eastern tick-borne encephalitis [Russian spring-summer encephalitis]** 🔍
  - **A84.1   Central European tick-borne encephalitis** 🔍
  - **A84.8   Other tick-borne viral encephalitis** 🔍
    Louping ill
    Powassan virus disease
  - ■ **A84.9   Tick-borne viral encephalitis, unspecified** 🔍

- ● **A85   Other viral encephalitis, not elsewhere classified**

  > **Includes**   specified viral encephalomyelitis NEC
  > specified viral meningoencephalitis NEC

  > **Excludes1**   benign myalgic encephalomyelitis (G93.3)
  > encephalitis due to:
  >   cytomegalovirus (B25.8)
  >   herpesvirus NEC (B10.0-)
  >   herpesvirus [herpes simplex] (B00.4)
  >   measles virus (B05.0)
  >   mumps virus (B26.2)
  >   poliomyelitis virus (A80.-)
  >   zoster (B02.0)
  > lymphocytic choriomeningitis (A87.2)

  - **A85.0   Enteroviral encephalitis** 🔍
    Enteroviral encephalomyelitis
  - **A85.1   Adenoviral encephalitis** 🔍
    Adenoviral meningoencephalitis
  - ■ **A85.2   Arthropod-borne viral encephalitis, unspecified** 🔍

    > **Excludes1**   West nile virus with encephalitis (A92.31)

  - **A85.8   Other specified viral encephalitis** 🔍
    Encephalitis lethargica
    Von Economo-Cruchet disease

- ■ **A86   Unspecified viral encephalitis** 🔍
  Viral encephalomyelitis NOS
  Viral meningoencephalitis NOS

- ● **A87   Viral meningitis**

  > **Excludes1**   meningitis due to herpesvirus [herpes simplex] (B00.3)
  > meningitis due to measles virus (B05.1)
  > meningitis due to mumps virus (B26.1)
  > meningitis due to poliomyelitis virus (A80.-)
  > meningitis due to zoster (B02.1)

  - **A87.0   Enteroviral meningitis** 🔍
    Group of common viruses responsible for the majority of viral meningitis
    Coxsackievirus meningitis
    Echovirus meningitis

Item 1-14   Encephalitis is an inflammation of the brain most often caused by a virus but may also be caused by a bacteria and most commonly transmitted by a mosquito. **Myelitis** is an inflammation of the spinal cord that may disrupt CNS function. Untreated myelitis may rapidly lead to permanent damage to the spinal cord. **Encephalomyelitis** is a general term for an inflammation of the brain and spinal cord.

● Unacceptable Principal Diagnosis   ● Use Additional Character(s)   ■ Unspecified   ▶ Manifestation Code

804   **OGCR** Official Guidelines for Coding and Reporting | Excludes 1 | | Excludes 2 | | Includes | | Use additional | | Code first | | Code also |

A87.1   **Adenoviral meningitis** 🦠

A87.2   **Lymphocytic choriomeningitis** 🦠
     Lymphocytic meningoencephalitis

A87.8   **Other viral meningitis** 🦠

A87.9   **Viral meningitis, unspecified** 🦠

● **A88**   **Other viral infections of central nervous system, not elsewhere classified**

> **Excludes1**   viral encephalitis NOS (A86)
>   viral meningitis NOS (A87.9)

A88.0   **Enteroviral exanthematous fever [Boston exanthem]** 🦠
     Infectious skin eruption

A88.1   **Epidemic vertigo**

A88.8   **Other specified viral infections of central nervous system** 🦠

■ **A89**   **Unspecified viral infection of central nervous system** 🦠

ARTHROPOD-BORNE VIRAL FEVERS AND VIRAL HEMORRHAGIC FEVERS (A90-A99)

A90   **Dengue fever [classical dengue]** 🦠
     Acute, self-limited disease, characterized by fever, prostration, severe muscle pains, headache, rash, lymphadenopathy, and leukopenia, caused by dengue virus; AKA breakbone, dandy

> **Excludes1**   dengue hemorrhagic fever (A91)

A91   **Dengue hemorrhagic fever** 🦠
     Serious follow-up to regular dengue, with symptoms of hemorrhage

● **A92**   **Other mosquito-borne viral fevers**

> **Excludes1**   Ross River disease (B33.1)

A92.0   **Chikungunya virus disease** 🦠
     Transmitted by mosquitoes
     Chikungunya (hemorrhagic) fever

A92.1   **O'nyong-nyong fever** 🦠
     Acute, nonfatal febrile disease transmitted by mosquitoes, which clinically resembles dengue and chikungunya

A92.2   **Venezuelan equine fever** 🦠
     Venezuelan equine encephalitis
     Venezuelan equine encephalomyelitis virus disease

● A92.3   **West Nile virus infection**
     West Nile fever

■ A92.30   **West Nile virus infection, unspecified** 🦠
     West Nile fever NOS
     West Nile fever without complications
     West Nile virus NOS

A92.31   **West Nile virus infection with encephalitis** 🦠
     West Nile encephalitis
     West Nile encephalomyelitis

A92.32   **West Nile virus infection with other neurologic manifestation** 🦠

> Use additional code to specify the neurologic manifestation

A92.39   **West Nile virus infection with other complications** 🦠

> Use additional code to specify the other conditions

A92.4   **Rift Valley fever** 🦠

A92.8   **Other specified mosquito-borne viral fevers** 🦠

■ A92.9   **Mosquito-borne viral fever, unspecified** 🦠

● **A93**   **Other arthropod-borne viral fevers, not elsewhere classified**

A93.0   **Oropouche virus disease** 🦠
     Tropical viral infection
     Oropouche fever

A93.1   **Sandfly fever** 🦠
     Pappataci fever
     Phlebotomus fever

A93.2   **Colorado tick fever** 🦠

A93.8   **Other specified arthropod-borne viral fevers** 🦠
     Piry virus disease
     Vesicular stomatitis virus disease [Indiana fever]

■ **A94**   **Unspecified arthropod-borne viral fever** 🦠
     Arboviral fever NOS
     Arbovirus infection NOS

● **A95**   **Yellow fever**
     Acute infectious disease transmitted by mosquitoes

A95.0   **Sylvatic yellow fever** 🦠
     Jungle yellow fever

A95.1   **Urban yellow fever** 🦠

■ A95.9   **Yellow fever, unspecified** 🦠

● **A96**   **Arenaviral hemorrhagic fever**
     Virus that causes various hemorrhagic fevers

A96.0   **Junin hemorrhagic fever** 🦠
     Argentinian hemorrhagic fever

A96.1   **Machupo hemorrhagic fever** 🦠
     Transmitted by contact with infected rodents
     Bolivian hemorrhagic fever

A96.2   **Lassa fever**
     Acute type of hemorrhagic fever caused by contact with disease carrying mouse or person

A96.8   **Other arenaviral hemorrhagic fevers** 🦠

■ A96.9   **Arenaviral hemorrhagic fever, unspecified** 🦠

● **A98**   **Other viral hemorrhagic fevers, not elsewhere classified**

> **Excludes1**   chikungunya hemorrhagic fever (A92.0)
>   dengue hemorrhagic fever (A91)

A98.0   **Crimean-Congo hemorrhagic fever** 🦠
     Virus transmitted by ticks and contact with blood, secretions, or fluids from infected humans or animals
     Central Asian hemorrhagic fever

A98.1   **Omsk hemorrhagic fever** 🦠
     Transmitted to humans by bites of infected ticks or contact with infected muskrats

A98.2   **Kyasanur Forest disease** 🦠
     Transmitted via infected monkeys, voles, ticks

A98.3   **Marburg virus disease**
     Rare, acute, often fatal type of hemorrhagic fever

A98.4   **Ebola virus disease**

A98.5   **Hemorrhagic fever with renal syndrome** 🦠
     Epidemic hemorrhagic fever
     Korean hemorrhagic fever
     Russian hemorrhagic fever
     Hantaan virus disease
     Hantavirus disease with renal manifestations
     Nephropathia epidemica
     Songo fever

> **Excludes1**   hantavirus (cardio)-pulmonary syndrome (B33.4)

A98.8   **Other specified viral hemorrhagic fevers** 🦠

■ **A99**   **Unspecified viral hemorrhagic fever** 🦠

CHAPTER 1 (A00-B99)

**VIRAL INFECTIONS CHARACTERIZED BY SKIN
AND MUCOUS MEMBRANE LESIONS (B00-B09)**

● **B00   Herpesviral [herpes simplex] infections**

> **Excludes1**   congenital herpesviral infections (P35.2)
>
> **Excludes2**   anogenital herpesviral infection (A60.-)
> gammaherpesviral mononucleosis (B27.0-)
> herpangina (B08.5)

B00.0   Eczema herpeticum
> *Cutaneous eruption caused by herpes simplex virus
> (HSV) type 1, HSV-2, coxsackievirus A16, or
> vaccinia virus*
> Kaposi's varicelliform eruption

B00.1   Herpesviral vesicular dermatitis
> *Vesicle formation; characteristics include formation of
> blisters and scabs on feet and legs*
> Herpes simplex facialis
> Herpes simplex labialis
> Herpes simplex otitis externa
> Vesicular dermatitis of ear
> Vesicular dermatitis of lip

**B00.2   Herpesviral gingivostomatitis and
pharyngotonsillitis** 🔖
> *Inflammation involving both gingivae and oral mucosa*
> Herpesviral pharyngitis
> *Inflammation of pharynx and tonsils; AKA
> tonsillopharyngitis*

B00.3   Herpesviral meningitis 🔖

B00.4   Herpesviral encephalitis 🔖
> Herpesviral meningoencephalitis
> Simian B disease

> **Excludes1**   herpesviral encephalitis due to
> herpesvirus 6 and 7 (B10.01, B10.09)
> non-simplex herpesviral encephalitis
> (B10.0-)

● **B00.5   Herpesviral ocular disease**

■ **B00.50   Herpesviral ocular disease, unspecified** 🔖

B00.51   Herpesviral iridocyclitis 🔖
> Herpesviral iritis
> Herpesviral uveitis, anterior

B00.52   Herpesviral keratitis 🔖
> Herpesviral keratoconjunctivitis

B00.53   Herpesviral conjunctivitis 🔖

B00.59   Other herpesviral disease of eye 🔖
> Herpesviral dermatitis of eyelid

B00.7   Disseminated herpesviral disease 🔖
> Herpesviral sepsis

● **B00.8   Other forms of herpesviral infections**

B00.81   Herpesviral hepatitis 🔖

B00.82   Herpes simplex myelitis 🔖

B00.89   Other herpesviral infection 🔖
> Herpesviral whitlow

■ **B00.9   Herpesviral infection, unspecified**
> Herpes simplex infection NOS

Item 1–15   Herpes is a viral disease for which there is no cure. There are two types of the herpes simplex virus: **Type I** causes **cold sores** or **fever blisters,** and **Type II** causes **genital herpes.** The virus can be spread from a sore on the lips to the genitals or from the genitals to the lips.

● **B01   Varicella [chickenpox]**
> *Very contagious disease caused by the varicella zoster virus
> that results in an itchy outbreak of skin blisters (varicella).
> The same virus causes shingles (zoster).*

B01.0   Varicella meningitis 🔖

● **B01.1   Varicella encephalitis, myelitis and
encephalomyelitis**
> Postchickenpox encephalitis, myelitis and
> encephalomyelitis

**B01.11   Varicella encephalitis and
encephalomyelitis** 🔖
> Postchickenpox encephalitis and
> encephalomyelitis

B01.12   Varicella myelitis 🔖
> Postchickenpox myelitis

B01.2   Varicella pneumonia 🔖

● **B01.8   Varicella with other complications**

B01.81   Varicella keratitis 🔖

B01.89   Other varicella complications 🔖

B01.9   Varicella without complication 🔖
> Varicella NOS

● **B02   Zoster [herpes zoster]**

> **Includes**   shingles
> zona

B02.0   Zoster encephalitis 🔖
> Zoster meningoencephalitis

B02.1   Zoster meningitis 🔖

● **B02.2   Zoster with other nervous system involvement**

B02.21   Postherpetic geniculate ganglionitis 🔖

B02.22   Postherpetic trigeminal neuralgia 🔖

B02.23   Postherpetic polyneuropathy 🔖

B02.24   Postherpetic myelitis 🔖
> Herpes zoster myelitis

**B02.29   Other postherpetic nervous system
involvement** 🔖
> Postherpetic radiculopathy

● **B02.3   Zoster ocular disease**

■ **B02.30   Zoster ocular disease, unspecified** 🔖

B02.31   Zoster conjunctivitis 🔖

B02.32   Zoster iridocyclitis 🔖

B02.33   Zoster keratitis 🔖
> Herpes zoster keratoconjunctivitis

B02.34   Zoster scleritis 🔖

B02.39   Other herpes zoster eye disease 🔖
> Zoster blepharitis

Figure 1-4   Primary herpes simplex in and around the mouth. The infection is usually acquired from siblings or parents and is readily transmitted to other direct contacts. (From Forbes, Jackson: Colour Atlas and Text of Clinical Medicine, International Edition. 2002, Mosby.)

Item 1-16 Zoster: Also known as ***shingles*** and is caused by the same virus as chickenpox. After exposure, the virus lies dormant in nerve tissue and is activated by factors including aging, stress, suppression of the immune system, and certain medication. It begins as a unilateral rash that leads to blisters and sores on the skin. It may involve the nerve pathways of the eye, forehead, nose, and eyelids and may be very painful with long term systemic effects.

● Unacceptable Principal Diagnosis   ● Use Additional Character(s)   ■ Unspecified   ▶ Manifestation Code

OGCR   Official Guidelines for Coding and Reporting | Excludes 1 | | Excludes 2 | | Includes | | Use additional | | Code first | | Code also |

Figure 1-5 Photograph of eyelids with marginal blepharitis. (From Mandell, Bennett, & Dolin: Principles and Practice of Infectious Diseases, 6th ed. 2005, Churchill Livingstone, An Imprint of Elsevier.)

Item 1-17 Blepharitis is a common condition in which the eyelid is swollen and yellow scaling and conjunctivitis develop. Usually the hair on the scalp and brow is involved.

B02.7 **Disseminated zoster**

B02.8 **Zoster with other complications**
Herpes zoster otitis externa

B02.9 **Zoster without complications**
Zoster NOS

B03 Smallpox
Note: In 1980 the 33rd World Health Assembly declared that smallpox had been eradicated. The classification is maintained for surveillance purposes.

B04 Monkeypox
Disease occurring in captive monkeys and other mammals that may be transmitted to humans, clinically similar to smallpox

B05 Measles

> **Includes**   morbilli

> **Excludes1**   subacute sclerosing panencephalitis (A81.1)

B05.0 **Measles complicated by encephalitis**
Postmeasles encephalitis

B05.1 **Measles complicated by meningitis**
Postmeasles meningitis

B05.2 **Measles complicated by pneumonia**
Postmeasles pneumonia

B05.3 **Measles complicated by otitis media**
Postmeasles otitis media

B05.4 **Measles with intestinal complications**

B05.8 **Measles with other complications**

    B05.81 **Measles keratitis and keratoconjunctivitis**

    B05.89 **Other measles complications**

B05.9 **Measles without complication**
Measles NOS

B06 Rubella [German measles]

> **Excludes1**   congenital rubella (P35.0)

B06.0 **Rubella with neurological complications**

    B06.00 **Rubella with neurological complication, unspecified**

    B06.01 **Rubella encephalitis**
      Rubella meningoencephalitis

    B06.02 **Rubella meningitis**

    B06.09 **Other neurological complications of rubella**

B06.8 **Rubella with other complications**

    B06.81 **Rubella pneumonia**

    B06.82 **Rubella arthritis**

    B06.89 **Other rubella complications**

B06.9 **Rubella without complication**
Rubella NOS

B07 Viral warts

> **Includes**   verruca simplex
> verruca vulgaris
> viral warts due to human papillomavirus

> **Excludes2**   anogenital (venereal) warts (A63.0)
> papilloma of bladder (D41.4)
> papilloma of cervix (D26.0)
> papilloma larynx (D14.1)

B07.0 **Plantar wart**
Verruca plantaris

B07.8 **Other viral warts**
Common wart
Flat wart
Verruca plana

B07.9 **Viral wart, unspecified**

B08 Other viral infections characterized by skin and mucous membrane lesions, not elsewhere classified

> **Excludes1**   vesicular stomatitis virus disease (A93.8)

B08.0 **Other orthopoxvirus infections**

> **Excludes2**   monkeypox (B04)

    B08.01 **Cowpox and vaccinia not from vaccine**

      B08.010 **Cowpox**

      B08.011 **Vaccinia not from vaccine**

>   **Excludes1**   vaccinia (from vaccination) (generalized) (T88.1)

    B08.02 **Orf virus disease**
      Contagious pustular dermatitis
      Ecthyma contagiosum

    B08.03 **Pseudocowpox [milker's node]**

    B08.04 **Paravaccinia, unspecified**

    B08.09 **Other orthopoxvirus infections**
      Orthopoxvirus infection NOS

B08.1 **Molluscum contagiosum**
Various skin diseases characterized by soft, rounded, cutaneous lesions

B08.2 **Exanthema subitum [sixth disease] Roseola infantum**
Acute, short-lived high fever in infants and young children followed by a rash mainly on the trunk, caused by human herpesvirus 6

    B08.20 **Exanthema subitum [sixth disease], unspecified Roseola infantum, unspecified**   P

    B08.21 **Exanthema subitum [sixth disease] due to human herpesvirus 6 Roseola infantum due to human herpesvirus 6**   P
      Virus results in sudden rash; infection results in lifelong persistence

    B08.22 **Exanthema subitum [sixth disease] due to human herpesvirus 7 Roseola infantum due to human herpesvirus 7**   P

B08.3 **Erythema infectiosum [fifth disease]**
Moderately contagious, epidemic disease in children caused by B19 virus; onset of rash that begins as redness of cheeks, later there is rash on trunk and limbs; when this fades, there may be central clearing that leaves lacelike pattern

B08.4 **Enteroviral vesicular stomatitis with exanthem**
Hand, foot and mouth disease
Check your documentation—this code is HAND, foot, and mouth disease. Code B08.8 is foot and mouth disease.

B08.5 **Enteroviral vesicular pharyngitis**
Herpangina

CHAPTER 1 (A00-B99)

N Newborn Age: 0   **P** Pediatric Age: 0–17   **M** Maternity DX: 12–55   **A** Adult Age: 15–124   ♀ Females Only   ♂ Males Only

Complication\Comorbidity   Major C\C   Present on Admission Requirement   Hospital-Acquired Condition

807

CHAPTER 1 (A00-B99)

- B08.6   **Parapoxvirus infections**
  - B08.60   **Parapoxvirus infection, unspecified**
  - B08.61   **Bovine stomatitis**
  - B08.62   **Sealpox**
  - B08.69   **Other parapoxvirus infections**
- B08.7   **Yatapoxvirus infections**
  - B08.70   **Yatapoxvirus infection, unspecified**
  - B08.71   **Tanapox virus disease** 🔧
  - B08.72   **Yaba pox virus disease**
            Yaba monkey tumor disease
  - B08.79   **Other yatapoxvirus infections**
- B08.8   **Other specified viral infections characterized by skin and mucous membrane lesions**
          Enteroviral lymphonodular pharyngitis
          Foot-and-mouth disease
          Check your documentation. Code B08.4 is for HAND, foot, and mouth disease.
          Poxvirus NEC

- B09   **Unspecified viral infection characterized by skin and mucous membrane lesions**
        Viral enanthema NOS
        Viral exanthema NOS

OTHER HUMAN HERPESVIRUSES (B10)

- B10   **Other human herpesviruses**
  - Excludes2   cytomegalovirus (B25.9)
              Epstein-Barr virus (B27.0-)
              herpes NOS (B00.9)
              herpes simplex (B00.-)
              herpes zoster (B02.-)
              human herpesvirus NOS (B00.-)
              human herpesvirus 1 and 2 (B00.-)
              human herpesvirus 3 (B01.-, B02-)
              human herpesvirus 4 (B27.0-)
              human herpesvirus 5 (B25.-)
              varicella (B01.-)
              zoster (B02.-)

  - B10.0   **Other human herpesvirus encephalitis**
    - Excludes2   herpes encephalitis NOS (B00.4)
                herpes simplex encephalitis (B00.4)
                human herpesvirus encephalitis (B00.4)
                simian B herpes virus encephalitis (B00.4)
    - B10.01   **Human herpesvirus 6 encephalitis** 🔧
              Sudden rash or roseola
    - B10.09   **Other human herpesvirus encephalitis** 🔧
              Human herpesvirus 7 encephalitis
              Virus closely related to human herpesvirus 6, but not known to cause any disease
  - B10.8   **Other human herpesvirus infection**
    - B10.81   **Human herpesvirus 6 infection**
              Causative agent of exanthema subitum that results in sudden rash
    - B10.82   **Human herpesvirus 7 infection**
              Closely related to human herpesvirus 6, but not known cause any disease
    - B10.89   **Other human herpesvirus infection**
              Human herpesvirus 8 infection
              May be the cause of Kaposi sarcoma, a malignant tumor
              Kaposi's sarcoma-associated herpesvirus infection

Figure 1-6   Hepatitis B viral infection. **A.** Liver parenchyma showing hepatocytes with diffuse granular cytoplasm, so-called ground glass hepatocytes (H&E). **B.** Immunoperoxidase stains from the same case, showing cytoplasmic inclusions of viral particles. (From Kumar: Robbins and Cotran: Pathologic Basis of Disease, 7th ed. 2005, Saunders, An Imprint of Elsevier.)

Item 1–18   Hepatitis A (HAV) was formerly called epidemic, infectious, short-incubation, or acute catarrhal jaundice hepatitis. The primary transmission mode is the oral–fecal route. **Hepatitis B (HBV)** was formerly called long-incubation period, serum, or homologous serum hepatitis. Transmission modes are through blood from infected persons and from body fluids of infected mother to neonate. **Hepatitis C (HCV),** caused by the hepatitis C virus, is primarily transfusion associated. **Hepatitis D (HDV),** also called delta hepatitis, is caused by the hepatitis D virus in patients formerly or currently infected with hepatitis B. **Hepatitis E (HEV)** is also called enterically transmitted non-A, non-B hepatitis. The primary transmission mode is the oral–fecal route, usually through contaminated water.

VIRAL HEPATITIS (B15-B19)

- Excludes1   sequelae of viral hepatitis (B94.2)
- Excludes2   cytomegaloviral hepatitis (B25.1)
            herpesviral [herpes simplex] hepatitis (B00.81)

- B15   **Acute hepatitis A**
  - B15.0   **Hepatitis A with hepatic coma** 🔧
  - B15.9   **Hepatitis A without hepatic coma** 🔧
            Hepatitis A (acute) (viral) NOS

- B16   **Acute hepatitis B**
  - B16.0   **Acute hepatitis B with delta-agent with hepatic coma** 🔧
  - B16.1   **Acute hepatitis B with delta-agent without hepatic coma** 🔧
  - B16.2   **Acute hepatitis B without delta-agent with hepatic coma** 🔧
  - B16.9   **Acute hepatitis B without delta-agent and without hepatic coma** 🔧
            Hepatitis B (acute) (viral) NOS

- B17   **Other acute viral hepatitis**
  - B17.0   **Acute delta-(super) infection of hepatitis B carrier** 🔧
  - B17.1   **Acute hepatitis C**
    - B17.10   **Acute hepatitis C without hepatic coma** 🔧
              Acute hepatitis C NOS
    - B17.11   **Acute hepatitis C with hepatic coma** 🔧
  - B17.2   **Acute hepatitis E** 🔧
  - B17.8   **Other specified acute viral hepatitis** 🔧
            Hepatitis non-A non-B (acute) (viral) NEC
  - B17.9   **Acute viral hepatitis, unspecified** 🔧
            Acute hepatitis NOS

- B18   **Chronic viral hepatitis**
  - B18.0   **Chronic viral hepatitis B with delta-agent** 🔧
  - B18.1   **Chronic viral hepatitis B without delta-agent** 🔧
            Chronic (viral) hepatitis B

● Unacceptable Principal Diagnosis   ● Use Additional Character(s)   ■ Unspecified   ▶ Manifestation Code

OGCR Official Guidelines for Coding and Reporting   Excludes 1   Excludes 2   Includes   Use additional   Code first   Code also

Figure 1-7 Kaposi's sarcoma. There are large confluent hyperpigmented patch-stage lesions with lymphedema. (From Cahen & Powderly: Infectious Disease, 2nd ed. 2004, Mosby, An imprint of Elsevier.)

Item 1-19 AIDS (acquired immune deficiency syndrome) is caused by **HIV** (human immunodeficiency virus). HIV affects certain white blood cells (T-4 lymphocytes) and destroys the ability of the cells to fight infections, making patients susceptible to a host of infectious diseases (e.g., *Pneumocystis carinii pneumonia (PCP)*, *Kaposi's sarcoma,* and *lymphoma*). *AIDS-related complex (ARC)* is an early stage of AIDS in which tests for HIV are positive but the symptoms are mild.

     B18.2   **Chronic viral hepatitis C**

     B18.8   **Other chronic viral hepatitis** 🏷

     B18.9   **Chronic viral hepatitis, unspecified** 🏷

● B19   **Unspecified viral hepatitis**

     B19.0   **Unspecified viral hepatitis with hepatic coma** 🏷

  ● B19.1   **Unspecified viral hepatitis B**

       B19.10   **Unspecified viral hepatitis B without hepatic coma** 🏷
         Unspecified viral hepatitis B NOS

       B19.11   **Unspecified viral hepatitis B with hepatic coma** 🏷

  ● B19.2   **Unspecified viral hepatitis C**

       B19.20   **Unspecified viral hepatitis C without hepatic coma**
         Viral hepatitis C NOS

       B19.21   **Unspecified viral hepatitis C with hepatic coma** 🏷

     B19.9   **Unspecified viral hepatitis without hepatic coma** 🏷
         Viral hepatitis NOS

     OGCR Section I. C.1.a

> Certain Infectious and Parasitic Diseases (A00-B99)
> a. Human Immunodeficiency Virus (HIV) Infections
>   1) Code only confirmed cases
>
>   Code only confirmed cases of HIV infection illness. This is an exception to the hospital inpatient guideline Section II, H.
>
>   In this context, "confirmation" does not require documentation of positive serology or culture for HIV; the provider's diagnostic statement that the patient is HIV positive, or has an HIV-related illness is sufficient.

HUMAN IMMUNODEFICIENCY VIRUS [HIV] DISEASE (B20)

B20   **Human immunodeficiency virus [HIV] disease** 🏷

   Includes   acquired immune deficiency syndrome [AIDS]
         AIDS-related complex [ARC]
         HIV infection, symptomatic

   Code first Human immunodeficiency virus [HIV] disease complicating pregnancy, childbirth and the puerperium, if applicable (O98.7-)

   Use additional code(s) to identify all manifestations of HIV infection

   Excludes1   asymptomatic human immunodeficiency virus [HIV] infection status (Z21)
         exposure to HIV virus (Z20.6)
         inconclusive serologic evidence of HIV (R75)

OTHER VIRAL DISEASES (B25-B34)

● B25   **Cytomegaloviral disease**
     AKA: HCMV or Human Herpesvirus 5 (HHV-5)

   Excludes1   congenital cytomegalovirus infection (P35.1)
         cytomegaloviral mononucleosis (B27.1-)

     B25.0   **Cytomegaloviral pneumonitis** 🏷
         MCC: Only when the principal diagnosis is designated as an MCC

     B25.1   **Cytomegaloviral hepatitis** 🏷
         MCC: Only when the principal diagnosis is designated as a CC

     B25.2   **Cytomegaloviral pancreatitis** 🏷
         MCC: Only when the principal diagnosis is designated as an MCC

     B25.8   **Other cytomegaloviral diseases** 🏷
         Cytomegaloviral encephalitis

     B25.9   **Cytomegaloviral disease, unspecified** 🏷

● B26   **Mumps**

   Includes   epidemic parotitis
         infectious parotitis
   Acute, contagious, viral disease

     B26.0   **Mumps orchitis** ♂ 🏷

     B26.1   **Mumps meningitis** 🏷

     B26.2   **Mumps encephalitis** 🏷

     B26.3   **Mumps pancreatitis** 🏷

  ● B26.8   **Mumps with other complications**

       B26.81   **Mumps hepatitis** 🏷

       B26.82   **Mumps myocarditis** 🏷

       B26.83   **Mumps nephritis** 🏷

       B26.84   **Mumps polyneuropathy** 🏷

       B26.85   **Mumps arthritis** 🏷

       B26.89   **Other mumps complications** 🏷

     B26.9   **Mumps without complication**
         Mumps NOS
         Mumps parotitis NOS

● B27   **Infectious mononucleosis**

   Includes   glandular fever
         monocytic angina
         Pfeiffer's disease

  ● B27.0   **Gammaherpesviral mononucleosis**
     AKA: Pfeiffer's disease, infective mononucleosis
     Mononucleosis due to Epstein-Barr virus

       B27.00   **Gammaherpesviral mononucleosis without complication**
         Infective mononucleosis

       B27.01   **Gammaherpesviral mononucleosis with polyneuropathy**

       B27.02   **Gammaherpesviral mononucleosis with meningitis**

       B27.09   **Gammaherpesviral mononucleosis with other complications**
         Hepatomegaly in gammaherpesviral mononucleosis

CHAPTER 1 (A00-B99)

N Newborn Age: 0   **P** Pediatric Age: 0–17   **M** Maternity DX: 12–55   **A** Adult Age: 15–124   ♀ Females Only   ♂ Males Only

🏷 Complication\Comorbidity   Major C\C   Present on Admission Requirement   Hospital-Acquired Condition

809

CHAPTER 1 (A00-B99)

- **B27.1   Cytomegaloviral mononucleosis**
  Infectious disease resembling infectious mononucleosis
  - **B27.10   Cytomegaloviral mononucleosis without complications**
  - **B27.11   Cytomegaloviral mononucleosis with polyneuropathy**
  - **B27.12   Cytomegaloviral mononucleosis with meningitis**
  - **B27.19   Cytomegaloviral mononucleosis with other complication**
    Hepatomegaly in cytomegaloviral mononucleosis

- **B27.8   Other infectious mononucleosis**
  - **B27.80   Other infectious mononucleosis without complication**
  - **B27.81   Other infectious mononucleosis with polyneuropathy**
  - **B27.82   Other infectious mononucleosis with meningitis**
  - **B27.89   Other infectious mononucleosis with other complication**
    Hepatomegaly in other infectious mononucleosis

- **B27.9   Infectious mononucleosis, unspecified**
  - **B27.90   Infectious mononucleosis, unspecified without complication**
  - **B27.91   Infectious mononucleosis, unspecified with polyneuropathy**
  - **B27.92   Infectious mononucleosis, unspecified with meningitis**
  - **B27.99   Infectious mononucleosis, unspecified with other complication**
    Hepatomegaly in unspecified infectious mononucleosis

- **B30   Viral conjunctivitis**
  > **Excludes1**   herpesviral [herpes simplex] ocular disease (B00.5)
  > ocular zoster (B02.3)
  - **B30.0   Keratoconjunctivitis due to adenovirus**
    Epidemic keratoconjunctivitis
    Shipyard eye
  - **B30.1   Conjunctivitis due to adenovirus**
    Acute adenoviral follicular conjunctivitis
    Swimming-pool conjunctivitis
  - **B30.2   Viral pharyngoconjunctivitis**
  - **B30.3   Acute epidemic hemorrhagic conjunctivitis (enteroviral)**
    Conjunctivitis due to coxsackievirus 24
    Conjunctivitis due to enterovirus 70
    Hemorrhagic conjunctivitis (acute)(epidemic)
  - **B30.8   Other viral conjunctivitis**
    Newcastle conjunctivitis
  - **B30.9   Viral conjunctivitis, unspecified**

- **B33   Other viral diseases, not elsewhere classified**
  - **B33.0   Epidemic myalgia**
    Acute infectious disease, caused by group A coxsackie viruses or other enteroviruses with symptoms that include sudden pain in chest or upper abdomen with fever
    Bornholm disease
  - **B33.1   Ross River disease** 🦠
    Epidemic polyarthritis and exanthema
    Ross River fever

- **B33.2   Viral carditis**
  Coxsackie (virus) carditis
  - **B33.20   Viral carditis, unspecified** 🦠
  - **B33.21   Viral endocarditis** 🦠
  - **B33.22   Viral myocarditis** 🦠
  - **B33.23   Viral pericarditis** 🦠
  - **B33.24   Viral cardiomyopathy**
- **B33.3   Retrovirus infections, not elsewhere classified**
  Retrovirus infection NOS
- **B33.4   Hantavirus (cardio)-pulmonary syndrome [HPS] [HCPS]** 🦠
  Hantavirus disease with pulmonary manifestations
  Sin nombre virus disease
  Use additional code to identify any associated acute kidney failure (N17.9)
  > **Excludes1**   hantavirus disease with renal manifestations (A98.5)
  > hemorrhagic fever with renal manifestations (A98.5)
- **B33.8   Other specified viral diseases**
  > **Excludes1**   anogenital human papillomavirus infection (A63.0)
  > viral warts due to human papillomavirus infection (B07)

- **B34   Viral infection of unspecified site**
  > **Excludes1**   anogenital human papillomavirus infection (A63.0)
  > cytomegaloviral disease NOS (B25.9)
  > herpesvirus [herpes simplex] infection NOS (B00.9)
  > retrovirus infection NOS (B33.3)
  > viral agents as the cause of diseases classified elsewhere (B97.-)
  > viral warts due to human papillomavirus infection (B07)
  - **B34.0   Adenovirus infection, unspecified**
  - **B34.1   Enterovirus infection, unspecified**
    Intestinal tract infection
    Coxsackievirus infection NOS
    Echovirus infection NOS
  - **B34.2   Coronavirus infection, unspecified**
    > **Excludes1**   pneumonia due to SARS-associated coronavirus (J12.81)
  - **B34.3   Parvovirus infection, unspecified** 🦠
  - **B34.4   Papovavirus infection, unspecified**
  - **B34.8   Other viral infections of unspecified site**
  - **B34.9   Viral infection, unspecified**
    Viremia NOS

MYCOSES (B35-B49)

> **Excludes2**   hypersensitivity pneumonitis due to organic dust (J67.-)
> mycosis fungoides (C84.0-)

- **B35   Dermatophytosis**
  AKA tinea or ringworm
  > **Includes**   favus
  > infections due to species of Epidermophyton, Micro-sporum and Trichophyton
  > tinea, any type except those in B36.-
  - **B35.0   Tinea barbae and tinea capitis**
    Beard ringworm
    Kerion
    Scalp ringworm
    Sycosis, mycotic

● Unacceptable Principal Diagnosis   ● Use Additional Character(s)   ■ Unspecified   ▶ Manifestation Code

OGCR   Official Guidelines for Coding and Reporting | Excludes 1 | | Excludes 2 | | Includes | | Use additional | | Code first | | Code also |

B35.1 **Tinea unguium**
White patches or pits on surface or edges of nails, followed by infection under nail plate
Dermatophytic onychia
Dermatophytosis of nail
Onychomycosis
Ringworm of nails

B35.2 **Tinea manuum**
Tinea of hands
Dermatophytosis of hand
Hand ringworm

B35.3 **Tinea pedis**
Tinea affecting feet
Athlete's foot
Dermatophytosis of foot
Foot ringworm

B35.4 **Tinea corporis**
Infecting skin areas other than hands
Ringworm of the body

B35.5 **Tinea imbricata**
Chronic tropical tinea corporis; AKA Oriental ringworm, tinea inguinalis, tinea cruris
Tokelau

B35.6 **Tinea cruris**
In groin or perineal area, spreading to adjacent regions; AKA jock itch, eczema marginatum, ringworm of groin, or t inguinalis
Dhobi itch
Groin ringworm
Jock itch

B35.8 **Other dermatophytoses**
Disseminated dermatophytosis
Granulomatous dermatophytosis

■ B35.9 **Dermatophytosis, unspecified**
Ringworm NOS

● B36 **Other superficial mycoses**

B36.0 **Pityriasis versicolor**
Common, chronic, symptomless disorder that includes macular patches of various sizes and shapes; AKA liver spots
Tinea flava
Tinea versicolor

B36.1 **Tinea nigra**
Minor fungal infection, with dark lesions, usually on skin of hands
Keratomycosis nigricans palmaris
Microsporosis nigra
Pityriasis nigra

B36.2 **White piedra**
White to light brown nodules on hair of beard, axilla, or groin; AKA trichosporosis
Tinea blanca

B36.3 **Black piedra**
Characterized by small black or brown nodules on shafts of scalp hair

B36.8 **Other specified superficial mycoses**

■ B36.9 **Superficial mycosis, unspecified**

● B37 **Candidiasis**
Includes	candidosis
	moniliasis
Excludes1	neonatal candidiasis (P37.5)

B37.0 **Candidal stomatitis** 🦠
Oral thrush

B37.1 **Pulmonary candidiasis** 🦠
Candidal bronchitis
Candidal pneumonia

Figure 1-8 Oral candidiasis (thrush). *(Courtesy of Stephen Raffanti, MD, MPH).* (From Mandell, Bennett, & Dolin: Principles and Practice of Infectious Diseases, 6th ed, 2005, Churchill Livingstone, An Imprint of Elsevier.)

Item 1–20 Candidiasis, also called oidiomycosis or moniliasis, is a fungal infection. It most often appears on moist cutaneous areas of the body but can also be responsible for a variety of systemic infections such as endocarditis, meningitis, arthritis, and myositis. Antifungal medications cure most yeast infections.

B37.2 **Candidiasis of skin and nail**
Candidal onychia
Candidal paronychia
Excludes2 diaper dermatitis (L22)

B37.3 **Candidiasis of vulva and vagina** ♀
Candidal vulvovaginitis
Monilial vulvovaginitis
Vaginal thrush

● B37.4 **Candidiasis of other urogenital sites**

B37.41 **Candidal cystitis and urethritis** 🦠 🦠

B37.42 **Candidal balanitis**
Male condition only

B37.49 **Other urogenital candidiasis** 🦠 🦠
Candidal pyelonephritis

B37.5 **Candidal meningitis** 🦠

B37.6 **Candidal endocarditis** 🦠

B37.7 **Candidal sepsis** 🦠
Disseminated candidiasis systemic candidiasis
MCC: Only when the principal diagnosis is designated as an MCC

● B37.8 **Candidiasis of other sites**

B37.81 **Candidal esophagitis** 🦠

B37.82 **Candidal enteritis** 🦠
Candidal proctitis

B37.83 **Candidal cheilitis** 🦠
Inflammation affecting lip

B37.84 **Candidal otitis externa** 🦠
Inflammation of external auditory canal

B37.89 **Other sites of candidiasis** 🦠
Infection manifested by invasive candidiasis
Candidal osteomyelitis

■ B37.9 **Candidiasis, unspecified**
Thrush NOS

● B38 **Coccidioidomycosis**
Fungal disease; AKA coccidioidosis, coccidioidal granuloma, Posadas, or Posadas-Wernicke disease

B38.0 **Acute pulmonary coccidioidomycosis** 🦠

B38.1 **Chronic pulmonary coccidioidomycosis** 🦠

■ B38.2 **Pulmonary coccidioidomycosis, unspecified** 🦠

B38.3 **Cutaneous coccidioidomycosis** 🦠

B38.4 **Coccidioidomycosis meningitis** 🦠

B38.7 **Disseminated coccidioidomycosis** 🦠
Generalized coccidioidomycosis

● B38.8 **Other forms of coccidioidomycosis**

B38.81 **Prostatic coccidioidomycosis** ♂ 🦠

B38.89 **Other forms of coccidioidomycosis** 🦠

■ B38.9 **Coccidioidomycosis, unspecified** 🦠

N Newborn Age: 0   **P** Pediatric Age: 0–17   **M** Maternity DX: 12–55   **A** Adult Age: 15–124   ♀ Females Only   ♂ Males Only

🦠 Complication\Comorbidity   🦠 Major C\C   🦠 Present on Admission Requirement   🦠 Hospital-Acquired Condition

811

CHAPTER 1 (A00-B99)

Item 1-21 Bird and bat droppings that fall into the soil give rise to a fungus that can spread airborne spores. When inhaled into the lungs, these spores divide and multiply into lesions. Histoplasmosis capsulatum takes three forms: primary (lodged in the lungs only), chronic (resembles TB), and disseminated (infection has moved to other organs). This is an opportunistic infection in immunosuppressed patients.

● **B39　Histoplasmosis**
　　Infection resulting from inhalation or ingestion of spores; AKA Darling disease

　　Code first *associated AIDS (B20)*

　　Use additional *code for any associated manifestations, such as:*
　　　endocarditis (I39)
　　　meningitis (G02)
　　　pericarditis (I32)
　　　retinitits (H32)

　　B39.0　Acute pulmonary histoplasmosis capsulati 🗫
　　B39.1　Chronic pulmonary histoplasmosis capsulati 🗫
■ **B39.2　Pulmonary histoplasmosis capsulati, unspecified** 🗫
　　B39.3　Disseminated histoplasmosis capsulati 🗫
　　　　Generalized histoplasmosis capsulati
■ **B39.4　Histoplasmosis capsulati, unspecified**
　　　　American histoplasmosis
　　B39.5　Histoplasmosis duboisii
　　　　African histoplasmosis
■ **B39.9　Histoplasmosis, unspecified**

● **B40　Blastomycosis**
　　Rare and potentially fatal infection caused by inhaling fungus found in moist soil in temperate climates.

　　Excludes1　Brazilian blastomycosis (B41.-)
　　　　keloidal blastomycosis (B48.0)

　　B40.0　Acute pulmonary blastomycosis 🗫
　　B40.1　Chronic pulmonary blastomycosis 🗫
■ **B40.2　Pulmonary blastomycosis, unspecified** 🗫
　　B40.3　Cutaneous blastomycosis 🗫
　　B40.7　Disseminated blastomycosis 🗫
　　　　Generalized blastomycosis
● **B40.8　Other forms of blastomycosis**
　　　B40.81　Blastomycotic meningoencephalitis 🗫
　　　　　Meningomyelitis due to blastomycosis
　　　B40.89　Other forms of blastomycosis 🗫
■ **B40.9　Blastomycosis, unspecified** 🗫

● **B41　Paracoccidioidomycosis**
　　Fungal infection usually chronic that begins in lungs, spreads to mucocutaneous areas which may extend to skin, tonsils, gastrointestinal lymphatics, liver, and spleen; AKA Almeida or Lutz-Splendore-Almeida disease, Brazilian or South American blastomycosis, or paracoccidioidal granuloma

　　Includes　Brazilian blastomycosis
　　　　Lutz' disease

　　B41.0　Pulmonary paracoccidioidomycosis 🗫
　　B41.7　Disseminated paracoccidioidomycosis 🗫
　　　　Generalized paracoccidioidomycosis
　　B41.8　Other forms of paracoccidioidomycosis 🗫
■ **B41.9　Paracoccidioidomycosis, unspecified** 🗫

● **B42　Sporotrichosis**
　　Chronic fungal infection with nodular lesions

　　B42.0　Pulmonary sporotrichosis
　　B42.1　Lymphocutaneous sporotrichosis
　　B42.7　Disseminated sporotrichosis
　　　　Generalized sporotrichosis

● **B42.8　Other forms of sporotrichosis**
　　　B42.81　Cerebral sporotrichosis
　　　　　Meningitis due to sporotrichosis
　　　B42.82　Sporotrichosis arthritis
　　　B42.89　Other forms of sporotrichosis
■ **B42.9　Sporotrichosis, unspecified**

● **B43　Chromomycosis and pheomycotic abscess**
　　Chronic fungal infection of skin, initiated at site of puncture affecting lower limb or foot (mossy foot)

　　B43.0　Cutaneous chromomycosis
　　　　Dermatitis verrucosa
　　B43.1　Pheomycotic brain abscess
　　　　Cerebral chromomycosis
　　B43.2　Subcutaneous pheomycotic abscess and cyst
　　B43.8　Other forms of chromomycosis
■ **B43.9　Chromomycosis, unspecified**

● **B44　Aspergillosis**
　　Infection marked by inflammatory lesions in skin, ear, orbit, nasal sinuses, lungs, and occasionally bones and meninges

　　Includes　aspergilloma

　　B44.0　Invasive pulmonary aspergillosis 🗫
　　　　MCC: Only when the principal diagnosis is designated as an MCC
　　B44.1　Other pulmonary aspergillosis 🗫
　　B44.2　Tonsillar aspergillosis 🗫
　　B44.7　Disseminated aspergillosis 🗫
　　　　Generalized aspergillosis
● **B44.8　Other forms of aspergillosis**
　　　B44.81　Allergic bronchopulmonary aspergillosis 🗫
　　　B44.89　Other forms of aspergillosis 🗫
■ **B44.9　Aspergillosis, unspecified** 🗫

● **B45　Cryptococcosis**
　　Infection in the immunocompromised and fatal if left untreated; AKA torulosis, Buschke, or Busse-Buschke disease

　　B45.0　Pulmonary cryptococcosis 🗫
　　B45.1　Cerebral cryptococcosis 🗫
　　　　Cryptococcal meningitis
　　　　Cryptococcosis meningocerebralis
　　　　MCC: Only when the principal diagnosis is designated as an MCC
　　B45.2　Cutaneous cryptococcosis 🗫
　　B45.3　Osseous cryptococcosis 🗫
　　B45.7　Disseminated cryptococcosis 🗫
　　　　Generalized cryptococcosis
　　B45.8　Other forms of cryptococcosis 🗫
■ **B45.9　Cryptococcosis, unspecified** 🗫

● **B46　Zygomycosis**
　　Fungal infections including subcutaneous lesions and infection of sinuses, brain, or lungs

　　B46.0　Pulmonary mucormycosis 🗫
　　　　Fungal infection affecting lung
　　B46.1　Rhinocerebral mucormycosis 🗫
　　B46.2　Gastrointestinal mucormycosis 🗫
　　B46.3　Cutaneous mucormycosis 🗫
　　　　Subcutaneous mucormycosis
　　B46.4　Disseminated mucormycosis 🗫
　　　　Generalized mucormycosis
■ **B46.5　Mucormycosis, unspecified** 🗫
　　B46.8　Other zygomycoses 🗫
　　　　Entomophthoromycosis
■ **B46.9　Zygomycosis, unspecified** 🗫
　　　　Phycomycosis NOS

● Unacceptable Principal Diagnosis　　● Use Additional Character(s)　　■ Unspecified　　▶ Manifestation Code

　OGCR　Official Guidelines for Coding and Reporting　　Excludes 1　　Excludes 2　　Includes　　Use additional　　Code first　　Code also

● **B47   Mycetoma**
Slow progressive, destructive fungal infection of cutaneous and subcutaneous tissues, fascia, and bone, primarily seen in foot (Madura foot) or leg

   B47.0   Eumycetoma 🕷
   Madura foot, mycotic Maduromycosis

   B47.1   Actinomycetoma 🕷

   ▪ **B47.9   Mycetoma, unspecified** 🕷
   Madura foot NOS

● **B48   Other mycoses, not elsewhere classified**

   B48.0   Lobomycosis
   Infection with symptoms of red, smooth, hard cutaneous nodules resembling keloids
   Keloidal blastomycosis
   Lobo's disease

   B48.1   Rhinosporidiosis
   Chronic, localized granulomatous fungal infection, affecting mucocutaneous tissues, usually of nose characterized by polyps, papillomas, and wartlike lesions

   B48.2   Allescheriasis 🕷
   Fungal infection
   Infection due to Pseudallescheria boydii
   | **Excludes1** | eumycetoma (B47.0) |

   B48.3   Geotrichosis 🕷
   Fungal infection usually of bronchi, lungs, mouth, or intestinal tract
   Geotrichum stomatitis

   B48.4   Penicillosis 🕷
   Fungal infection

   B48.8   Other specified mycoses 🕷
   Adiaspiromycosis
   Infection of tissue and organs by Alternaria
   Infection of tissue and organs by Drechslera
   Infection of tissue and organs by Fusarium
   Infection of tissue and organs by saprophytic fungi NEC

▪ **B49   Unspecified mycosis** 🕷
   Fungemia NOS

PROTOZOAL DISEASES (B50-B64)

| **Excludes1** | amebiasis (A06.-) |
| | other protozoal intestinal diseases (A07.-) |

● **B50   Plasmodium falciparum malaria**
Severe form of malaria that can be fatal
   | **Includes** | mixed infections of Plasmodium falciparum with any other Plasmodium species |

   B50.0   Plasmodium falciparum malaria with cerebral complications 🕷
   Cerebral malaria NOS

   B50.8   Other severe and complicated Plasmodium falciparum malaria 🕷
   Severe or complicated Plasmodium falciparum malaria NOS

   ▪ **B50.9   Plasmodium falciparum malaria, unspecified** 🕷

● **B51   Plasmodium vivax malaria**
   | **Includes** | mixed infections of Plasmodium vivax with other Plasmodium species, except Plasmodium falciparum |
   | **Excludes1** | plasmodium vivav with Plasmodium falciparum (B50.-) |

   B51.0   Plasmodium vivax malaria with rupture of spleen 🕷

   B51.8   Plasmodium vivax malaria with other complications 🕷

   B51.9   Plasmodium vivax malaria without complication 🕷
   Plasmodium vivax malaria NOS

● **B52   Plasmodium malariae malaria**
Causes fever that recurs at approximately three-day intervals (quartan fever), longer than two-day (tertian) intervals of other malarial parasites
Includes	mixed infections of Plasmodium malariae with other Plasmodium species, except Plasmodium falciparum and Plasmodium vivax
Excludes1	plasmodium falciparum (B50.-)
	plasmodium vivax (B51.-)

   B52.0   Plasmodium malariae malaria with nephropathy 🕷
   MCC: Only when the principal diagnosis is designated as a CC

   B52.8   Plasmodium malariae malaria with other complications 🕷

   B52.9   Plasmodium malariae malaria without complication 🕷
   Plasmodium malariae malaria NOS

● **B53   Other specified malaria**

   B53.0   Plasmodium ovale malaria 🕷
   Least diagnosed type of malaria spread by female mosquitoes of rare species
Excludes1	plasmodium ovale with Plasmodium falciparum (B50.-)
	plasmodium ovale with Plasmodium malariae (B52.-)
	plasmodium ovale with Plasmodium vivax (B51.-)

   B53.1   Malaria due to simian plasmodia 🕷
   Malaria-like disease (parasite infection)
Excludes1	malaria due to simian plasmodia with Plasmodium falciparum (B50.-)
	malaria due to simian plasmodia with Plasmodium malariae (B52.-)
	malaria due to simian plasmodia with Plasmodium ovale (B53.0)
	malaria due to simian plasmodia with Plasmodium vivax (B51.-)

   B53.8   Other malaria, not elsewhere classified 🕷

▪ **B54   Unspecified malaria** 🕷

● **B55   Leishmaniasis**
Protozoal infection

   B55.0   Visceral leishmaniasis 🕷
   Kala-azar
   Post-kala-azar dermal leishmaniasis

   B55.1   Cutaneous leishmaniasis 🕷

   B55.2   Mucocutaneous leishmaniasis 🕷

   ▪ **B55.9   Leishmaniasis, unspecified** 🕷

● **B56   African trypanosomiasis**
Human African trypanosomiasis (HAT) is transmitted by fly bites

   B56.0   Gambiense trypanosomiasis 🕷
   Infection due to Trypanosoma brucei gambiense
   West African sleeping sickness

   B56.1   Rhodesiense trypanosomiasis 🕷
   East African sleeping sickness
   Infection due to Trypanosoma brucei rhodesiense

   ▪ **B56.9   African trypanosomiasis, unspecified** 🕷
   Sleeping sickness NOS

CHAPTER 1 (A00-B99)

N Newborn Age: 0   **P** Pediatric Age: 0–17   **M** Maternity DX: 12–55   **A** Adult Age: 15–124   ♀ Females Only   ♂ Males Only
🕷 Complication\Comorbidity   🕷 Major C\C   🕷 Present on Admission Requirement   🕷 Hospital-Acquired Condition

CHAPTER 1 (A00-B99)

Item 1–22 Toxoplasmosis is caused by the protozoa **Toxoplasma gondii,** of which the house cat can be a host. Human infection occurs when contact is made with materials containing the pathogen, such as feces, contaminated soil, or ingestion of infected lamb, goat, or pork. Of the infected, very few have symptoms because a healthy person's immune system keeps the parasite from causing illness. When the immune system is compromised, symptoms may occur. Clinical symptoms include flu-like symptoms, but the disease progresses to include the eyes and the brain in babies.

● **B57 Chagas' disease**
    Tropical parasitic disease

    Includes   American trypanosomiasis
                infection due to Trypanosoma cruzi

    B57.0 Acute Chagas' disease with heart involvement 🦠
        Acute Chagas' disease with myocarditis

    B57.1 Acute Chagas' disease without heart involvement 🦠
        Acute Chagas' disease NOS

    B57.2 Chagas' disease (chronic) with heart involvement 🦠
        American trypanosomiasis NOS
        Chagas' disease (chronic) NOS
        Chagas' disease (chronic) with myocarditis
        Trypanosomiasis NOS

 ● **B57.3 Chagas' disease (chronic) with digestive system involvement**

      ◼ **B57.30 Chagas' disease with digestive system involvement, unspecified** 🦠

      B57.31 Megaesophagus in Chagas' disease 🦠

      B57.32 Megacolon in Chagas' disease 🦠

      B57.39 Other digestive system involvement in Chagas' disease 🦠

 ● **B57.4 Chagas' disease (chronic) with nervous system involvement**

      ◼ **B57.40 Chagas' disease with nervous system involvement, unspecified** 🦠

      B57.41 Meningitis in Chagas' disease 🦠

      B57.42 Meningoencephalitis in Chagas' disease 🦠

      B57.49 Other nervous system involvement in Chagas' disease 🦠

    B57.5 Chagas' disease (chronic) with other organ involvement 🦠

● **B58 Toxoplasmosis**
    Infection by protozoon transmitted in cysts in feces of cats

    Includes   infection due to Toxoplasma gondii

    Excludes1   congenital toxoplasmosis (P37.1)

 ● **B58.0 Toxoplasma oculopathy**

      ◼ **B58.00 Toxoplasma oculopathy, unspecified** 🦠

      B58.01 Toxoplasma chorioretinitis 🦠

      B58.09 Other toxoplasma oculopathy 🦠
              Toxoplasma uveitis

    B58.1 Toxoplasma hepatitis 🦠

    B58.2 Toxoplasma meningoencephalitis 🦠

    B58.3 Pulmonary toxoplasmosis 🦠

 ● **B58.8 Toxoplasmosis with other organ involvement**

      B58.81 Toxoplasma myocarditis 🦠

      B58.82 Toxoplasma myositis 🦠

      B58.83 Toxoplasma tubulo-interstitial nephropathy 🦠
              Toxoplasma pyelonephritis

      B58.89 Toxoplasmosis with other organ involvement 🦠

 ◼ **B58.9 Toxoplasmosis, unspecified** 🦠

B59 Pneumocystosis 🦠
    Caused by fungus
    Pneumonia due to Pneumocystis carinii
    Pneumonia due to Pneumocystis jiroveci

● **B60 Other protozoal diseases, not elsewhere classified**

    Excludes1   cryptosporidiosis (A07.2)
                 intestinal microsporidiosis (A07.8)
                 isosporiasis (A07.3)

    B60.0 Babesiosis 🦠
        Tickborne disease caused by microscopic organisms
        Piroplasmosis

 ● **B60.1 Acanthamebiasis**

      ◼ **B60.10 Acanthamebiasis, unspecified** 🦠

      B60.11 Meningoencephalitis due to Acanthamoeba (culbertsoni)

      B60.12 Conjunctivitis due to Acanthamoeba

      ● **B60.13 Keratoconjunctivitis due to Acanthamoeba**

      B60.19 Other acanthamebic disease 🦠

    B60.2 Naegleriasis 🦠
        Infection with microscopic organisms
        Primary amebic meningoencephalitis

    B60.8 Other specified protozoal diseases
        Microsporidiosis

◼ **B64 Unspecified protozoal disease**

HELMINTHIASES (B65-B83)

Diseases or infestations caused by parasitic worms

● **B65 Schistosomiasis [bilharziasis]**
    Infection with flukes (flat parasitic worms)

    Includes   snail fever

    B65.0 Schistosomiasis due to Schistosoma haematobium [urinary schistosomiasis] 🦠

    B65.1 Schistosomiasis due to Schistosoma mansoni [intestinal schistosomiasis] 🦠

    B65.2 Schistosomiasis due to Schistosoma japonicum 🦠
        Asiatic schistosomiasis

    B65.3 Cercarial dermatitis 🦠
        Swimmer's itch

    B65.8 Other schistosomiasis 🦠
        Infection due to Schistosoma intercalatum
        Infection due to Schistosoma mattheei
        Infection due to Schistosoma mekongi

 ◼ **B65.9 Schistosomiasis, unspecified** 🦠

● **B66 Other fluke infections**
    Trematode (parasitic worms)

    B66.0 Opisthorchiasis 🦠
        Infection due to cat liver fluke
        Infection due to Opisthorchis (felineus)(viverrini)

    B66.1 Clonorchiasis 🦠
        Chinese liver fluke disease
        Infection due to Clonorchis sinensis
        Oriental liver fluke disease

    B66.2 Dicroceliasis 🦠
        Liver fluke
        Infection due to Dicrocoelium dendriticum
        Lancet fluke infection

    B66.3 Fascioliasis 🦠
        Infection due to Fasciola gigantica
        Infection due to Fasciola hepatica
        Infection due to Fasciola indica
        Sheep liver fluke disease

● Unacceptable Principal Diagnosis   ● Use Additional Character(s)   ◼ Unspecified   ▶ Manifestation Code

814   **OGCR** Official Guidelines for Coding and Reporting   Excludes 1   Excludes 2   Includes   Use additional   Code first   Code also

Item 1-23 Echinococcosis: Also known as hydatid disease; is caused by Echinococcus granulosus, E. multilocularis, and E. vogeli tapeworms; and is contracted from infected food. Found in southern South America, the Mediterranean, the Middle East, central Asia, and Africa and uncommon in the United States but has been reported in California, New Mexico, Arizona and Utah. The disease is treated with medication over a long course as it is resistive.

- **B66.4   Paragonimiasis** 🦠
  Infection due to Paragonimus species
  Lung fluke disease
  Pulmonary distomiasis

- **B66.5   Fasciolopsiasis** 🦠
  Largest intestinal fluke in humans
  Infection due to Fasciolopsis buski
  Intestinal distomiasis

- **B66.8   Other specified fluke infections** 🦠
  Echinostomiasis
  Heterophyiasis
  Metagonimiasis
  Nanophyetiasis
  Watsoniasis

- **B66.9   Fluke infection, unspecified**

● **B67   Echinococcosis**
  Larval forms of tapeworms usually of liver or lungs

  Includes   hydatidosis

- **B67.0   Echinococcus granulosus infection of liver** 🦠
- **B67.1   Echinococcus granulosus infection of lung** 🦠
- **B67.2   Echinococcus granulosus infection of bone** 🦠
- ● **B67.3   Echinococcus granulosus infection, other and multiple sites**
  - **B67.31   Echinococcus granulosus infection, thyroid gland** 🦠
  - **B67.32   Echinococcus granulosus infection, multiple sites** 🦠
  - **B67.39   Echinococcus granulosus infection, other sites** 🦠
- **B67.4   Echinococcus granulosus infection, unspecified** 🦠
  Dog tapeworm (infection)
- **B67.5   Echinococcus multilocularis infection of liver** 🦠
- ● **B67.6   Echinococcus multilocularis infection, other and multiple sites**
  - **B67.61   Echinococcus multilocularis infection, multiple sites** 🦠
  - **B67.69   Echinococcus multilocularis infection, other sites** 🦠
- **B67.7   Echinococcus multilocularis infection, unspecified** 🦠
- **B67.8   Echinococcosis, unspecified, of liver** 🦠
- ● **B67.9   Echinococcosis, other and unspecified**
  - **B67.90   Echinococcosis, unspecified** 🦠
    Echinococcosis NOS
  - **B67.99   Other echinococcosis** 🦠

● **B68   Taeniasis**
  Intestinal tapeworm (cestode) infection from raw or undercooked meat of infected animal

  Excludes1   cysticercosis (B69.-)

- **B68.0   Taenia solium taeniasis** 🦠
  Pork tapeworm (infection)
- **B68.1   Taenia saginata taeniasis** 🦠
  Beef tapeworm (infection)
  Infection due to adult tapeworm Taenia saginata
- **B68.9   Taeniasis, unspecified** 🦠

● **B69   Cysticercosis**
  Systemic illness caused by the larvae of pork tapeworm

  Includes   cysticerciasis infection due to larval form of Taenia solium

- **B69.0   Cysticercosis of central nervous system** 🦠
- **B69.1   Cysticercosis of eye** 🦠
- ● **B69.8   Cysticercosis of other sites**
  - **B69.81   Myositis in cysticercosis** 🦠
  - **B69.89   Cysticercosis of other sites** 🦠
- **B69.9   Cysticercosis, unspecified** 🦠

● **B70   Diphyllobothriasis and sparganosis**
  Infection with tapeworms seen most often from inadequately cooked fish

- **B70.0   Diphyllobothriasis** 🦠
  Diphyllobothrium (adult) (latum) (pacificum) infection
  Fish tapeworm (infection)

  Excludes2   larval diphyllobothriasis (B70.1)

- **B70.1   Sparganosis** 🦠
  Infection with migrating tapeworm larvae, which invade subcutaneous tissues, causing inflammation and fibrosis that resembles cellulitis
  Infection due to Sparganum (mansoni) (proliferum)
  Infection due to Spirometra larva
  Larval diphyllobothriasis
  Spirometrosis

● **B71   Other cestode infections**
- **B71.0   Hymenolepiasis** 🦠
  Intestinal infestation with tapeworms
  Dwarf tapeworm infection
  Rat tapeworm (infection)
- **B71.1   Dipylidiasis** 🦠
  Infection with tapeworm common to dogs and cats and seen in children having close contact with infected pets
- **B71.8   Other specified cestode infections** 🦠
  Infection by the larval stage of a tapeworm, usually through fruit or vegetables
  Coenurosis
- **B71.9   Cestode infection, unspecified**
  Tapeworm (infection) NOS

B72   Dracunculiasis 🦠
  Infection with roundworms

  Includes   guinea worm infection
  infection due to Dracunculus medinensis

● **B73   Onchocerciasis**
  Infection with parasitic worm

  Includes   onchocerca volvulus infection
  onchocercosis
  river blindness

- ● **B73.0   Onchocerciasis with eye disease**
  - **B73.00   Onchocerciasis with eye involvement, unspecified** 🦠
  - **B73.01   Onchocerciasis with endophthalmitis** 🦠
  - **B73.02   Onchocerciasis with glaucoma** 🦠
  - **B73.09   Onchocerciasis with other eye involvement** 🦠
    Infestation of eyelid due to onchocerciasis
- **B73.1   Onchocerciasis without eye disease** 🦠

N Newborn Age: 0   **P** Pediatric Age: 0–17   **M** Maternity DX: 12–55   **A** Adult Age: 15–124   ♀ Females Only   ♂ Males Only

🦠 Complication\Comorbidity   🦠 Major C\C   🦠 Present on Admission Requirement   🦠 Hospital-Acquired Condition

815

● **B74 Filariasis** 🐛
Infestation with slender threadlike worms
> **Excludes2**   onchocerciasis (B73)
> tropical (pulmonary) eosinophilia NOS (J82)

    B74.0 Filariasis due to Wuchereria bancrofti 🐛
      Bancroftian elephantiasis
      Bancroftian filariasis

    B74.1 Filariasis due to Brugia malayi 🐛

    B74.2 Filariasis due to Brugia timori 🐛

    B74.3 Loiasis 🐛
      Infection with round worms growing in subcutaneous
        connective tissue
      Calabar swelling
      Eyeworm disease of Africa
      Loa loa infection

    B74.4 Mansonelliasis 🐛
      Infection with filarial parasite
      Infection due to Mansonella ozzardi
      Infection due to Mansonella perstans
      Infection due to Mansonella streptocerca

    B74.8 Other filariases 🐛
      Dirofilariasis

    ■ **B74.9 Filariasis, unspecified** 🐛

● **B75 Trichinellosis** 🐛
Infestation with parasitic roundworms ingested in undercooked
contaminated meat
> **Includes**   infection due to Trichinella species
> trichiniasis

● **B76 Hookworm diseases**
Occurs in hot, humid parts of world where larvae are soil
borne, enter digestive tract through skin of feet/legs or in
contaminated food/water; AKA ground itch
> **Includes**   uncinariasis

    B76.0 Ancylostomiasis 🐛
      Infection due to Ancylostoma species

    B76.1 Necatoriasis 🐛
      Infection due to Necator americanus

    B76.8 Other hookworm diseases 🐛

    ■ **B76.9 Hookworm disease, unspecified** 🐛
      Cutaneous larva migrans NOS

● **B77 Ascariasis**
Infection by roundworm in small intestine
> **Includes**   ascaridiasis
> roundworm infection

    B77.0 Ascariasis with intestinal complications 🐛

    ● **B77.8 Ascariasis with other complications**

      B77.81 Ascariasis pneumonia 🐛
        MCC: Only when the principal diagnosis
          is designated as an MCC

      B77.89 Ascariasis with other complications 🐛

    ■ **B77.9 Ascariasis, unspecified** 🐛

● **B78 Strongyloidiasis**
Infection with adult female roundworms
> **Excludes1**   trichostrongyliasis (B81.2)

    B78.0 Intestinal strongyloidiasis 🐛

    B78.1 Cutaneous strongyloidiasis

    B78.7 Disseminated strongyloidiasis 🐛

    ■ **B78.9 Strongyloidiasis, unspecified** 🐛

   B79 Trichuriasis 🐛
Intestinal infection with roundworms
> **Includes**   trichocephaliasis
> whipworm (disease)(infection)

   B80 Enterobiasis 🐛
Intestinal infection with pinworms
> **Includes**   oxyuriasis
> pinworm infection
> threadworm infection

● **B81 Other intestinal helminthiases, not elsewhere classified**
Diseases or infestations caused by parasitic worms
> **Excludes1**   angiostrongyliasis due to Parastrongylus
> cantonensis (B83.2)

    B81.0 Anisakiasis 🐛
      Roundworm infection via contaminated undercooked
        infected fish or marine mammals
      Infection due to Anisakis larva

    B81.1 Intestinal capillariasis 🐛
      Infestation with of parasites (nematodes)
      Capillariasis NOS
      Infection due to Capillaria philippinensis
> **Excludes2**   hepatic capillariasis (B83.8)

    B81.2 Trichostrongyliasis 🐛

    B81.3 Intestinal angiostrongyliasis 🐛
      Angiostrongyliasis due to Parastrongylus
        costaricensis

    B81.4 Mixed intestinal helminthiases 🐛
      Infection due to intestinal helminths classified to
        more than one of the categories B65.0-B81.3
        and B81.8
      Mixed helminthiasis NOS

    B81.8 Other specified intestinal helminthiases 🐛
      Infection due to Oesophagostomum species
        [esophagostomiasis]
      Infection due to Ternidens diminutus
        [ternidensiasis]

● **B82 Unspecified intestinal parasitism**

    ■ **B82.0 Intestinal helminthiasis, unspecified** 🐛
      Infected with worms

    ■ **B82.9 Intestinal parasitism, unspecified**

● **B83 Other helminthiases**
Caused by parasitic worms
> **Excludes1**   capillariasis NOS (B81.1)
> **Excludes2**   intestinal capillariasis (B81.1)

    B83.0 Visceral larva migrans
      Prolonged migration of nematode larvae
      Toxocariasis

    B83.1 Gnathostomiasis
      Infection with nematode occurring from ingested
        undercooked fish contaminated with larvae; larvae
        migrate to subcutaneous tissue or deeper tissues,
        results are abscesses
      Wandering swelling

    B83.2 Angiostrongyliasis due to Parastrongylus
    cantonensis
      Nematode infection caused by eating contaminated raw
        snails, slugs, or paratenic hosts such as prawns
        or crabs; larval worms migrate to central nervous
        system resulting in eosinophilic meningitis
      Eosinophilic meningoencephalitis due to
        Parastrongylus cantonensis
> **Excludes2**   intestinal angiostrongyliasis (B81.3)

    B83.3 Syngamiasis
      Infestation with gapeworm from turkey, pheasant,
        guinea fowl, goose, and wild birds
      Syngamosis

    B83.4 Internal hirudiniasis
      Infestation by leeches
> **Excludes2**   external hirudiniasis (B88.3)

● Unacceptable Principal Diagnosis   ● Use Additional Character(s)   ■ Unspecified   ▶ Manifestation Code

OGCR Official Guidelines for Coding and Reporting   [Excludes 1]   [Excludes 2]   Includes   Use additional   Code first   Code also

B83.8 Other specified helminthiases
Parasitic worm infestation
Acanthocephaliasis
Gongylonemiasis
Hepatic capillariasis
Metastrongyliasis
Thelaziasis

■ **B83.9 Helminthiasis, unspecified**
Worms NOS

> **Excludes1**   intestinal helminthiasis NOS (B82.0)

PEDICULOSIS, ACARIASIS AND OTHER INFESTATIONS (B85-B89)

Infestation of lice

● **B85 Pediculosis and phthiriasis**

B85.0 Pediculosis due to Pediculus humanus capitis
Head-louse infestation

B85.1 Pediculosis due to Pediculus humanus corporis
Body-louse infestation

■ **B85.2 Pediculosis, unspecified**

B85.3 Phthiriasis
Crab or pubic lice
Infestation by crab-louse
Infestation by Phthirus pubis

B85.4 Mixed pediculosis and phthiriasis
Infestation classifiable to more than one of the categories B85.0-B85.3

B86 Scabies
Sarcoptic itch
Contagious dermatitis caused by mites

● **B87 Myiasis**
Infestation by fly maggots

> **Includes**   infestation by larva of flies

B87.0 Cutaneous myiasis
Creeping myiasis

B87.1 Wound myiasis
Traumatic myiasis

B87.2 Ocular myiasis

B87.3 Nasopharyngeal myiasis
Laryngeal myiasis

B87.4 Aural myiasis

● **B87.8 Myiasis of other sites**

B87.81 Genitourinary myiasis

B87.82 Intestinal myiasis

B87.89 Myiasis of other sites

■ **B87.9 Myiasis, unspecified**

● **B88 Other infestations**

B88.0 Other acariasis
Acarine dermatitis
Dermatitis due to Demodex species
Dermatitis due to Dermanyssus gallinae
Dermatitis due to Liponyssoides sanguineus
Trombiculosis

> **Excludes2**   scabies (B86)

B88.1 Tungiasis [sandflea infestation]
Inflammatory skin disease caused by infestation of fleas

B88.2 Other arthropod infestations
Scarabiasis

B88.3 External hirudiniasis
Leech infestation NOS

> **Excludes2**   internal hirudiniasis (B83.4)

B88.8 Other specified infestations
Infection of topical fresh water fish parasite
Ichthyoparasitism due to Vandellia cirrhosa
Linguatulosis
Porocephaliasis

■ **B88.9 Infestation, unspecified**
Infestation (skin) NOS
Infestation by mites NOS
Skin parasites NOS

■ **B89 Unspecified parasitic disease**

SEQUELAE OF INFECTIOUS AND PARASITIC DISEASES (B90-B94)

Note: Categories B90-B94 are to be used to indicate conditions in categories A00-B89 as the cause of sequelae, which are themselves classified elsewhere. The 'sequelae' include conditions specified as such; they also include residuals of diseases classifiable to the above categories if there is evidence that the disease itself is no longer present. Codes from these categories are not to be used for chronic infections. Code chronic current infections to active infectious disease as appropriate.

Code first condition resulting from (sequela) the infectious or parasitic disease

● **B90 Sequelae of tuberculosis**
Condition resulting from tuberculosis

B90.0 Sequelae of central nervous system tuberculosis 🔒

B90.1 Sequelae of genitourinary tuberculosis 🔒

B90.2 Sequelae of tuberculosis of bones and joints 🔒

B90.8 Sequelae of tuberculosis of other organs 🔒

> **Excludes2**   sequelae of respiratory tuberculosis (B90.9)

B90.9 Sequelae of respiratory and unspecified tuberculosis 🔒
Sequelae of tuberculosis NOS

B91 Sequelae of poliomyelitis 🔒

> **Excludes1**   postpolio syndrome (G14)

B92 Sequelae of leprosy 🔒

● **B94 Sequelae of other and unspecified infectious and parasitic diseases**

B94.0 Sequelae of trachoma 🔒

B94.1 Sequelae of viral encephalitis 🔒

B94.2 Sequelae of viral hepatitis 🔒

B94.8 Sequelae of other specified infectious and parasitic diseases 🔒

■ **B94.9 Sequelae of unspecified infectious and parasitic disease** 🔒

OGCR   Section I.C.1.b

Certain infectious and parasitic diseases

Infectious agents as the cause of diseases classified to other chapters

Certain infections are classified in chapters other than Chapter 1 and no organism is identified as part of the infection code. In these instances, it is necessary to use an additional code from Chapter 1 to identify the organism. A code from category B95, Streptococcus, Staphylococcus, and Enterococcus as the cause of diseases classified to other chapters, B96, Other bacterial agents as the cause of diseases classified to other chapters, or B97, Viral agents as the cause of diseases classified to other chapters, is to be used as an additional code to identify the organism. An instructional note will be found at the infection code advising that an additional organism code is required.

N Newborn Age: 0   **P** Pediatric Age: 0–17   **M** Maternity DX: 12–55   **A** Adult Age: 15–124   ♀ Females Only   ♂ Males Only

🔒 Complication\Comorbidity   🔒 Major C\C   🔒 Present on Admission Requirement   🔒 Hospital-Acquired Condition

817

CHAPTER 1 (A00-B99)

BACTERIAL AND VIRAL INFECTIOUS AGENTS (B95-B97)

Note: These categories are provided for use as supplementary or additional codes to identify the infectious agent(s) in diseases classified elsewhere.
Code the disease first, then the bacterium.

● **B95** **Streptococcus, Staphylococcus, and Enterococcus as the cause of diseases classified elsewhere**

● *B95.0* *Streptococcus, group A, as the cause of diseases classified elsewhere*

● *B95.1* *Streptococcus, group B, as the cause of diseases classified elsewhere*

● *B95.2* *Enterococcus as the cause of diseases classified elsewhere*

● *B95.3* *Streptococcus pneumoniae as the cause of diseases classified elsewhere*

● *B95.4* *Other streptococcus as the cause of diseases classified elsewhere*

●■ *B95.5* *Unspecified streptococcus as the cause of diseases classified elsewhere*

● **B95.6** **Staphylococcus aureus as the cause of diseases classified elsewhere**

● *B95.61* *Methicillin susceptible Staphylococcus aureus infection as the cause of diseases classified elsewhere*
Methicillin susceptible Staphylococcus aureus (MSSA) infection as the cause of diseases classified elsewhere
Staphylococcus aureus infection NOS as the cause of diseases classified elsewhere

● *B95.62* *Methicillin resistant Staphylococcus aureus infection as the cause of diseases classified elsewhere*
Methicillin resistant staphylococcus aureus (MRSA) infection as the cause of diseases classified elsewhere

● *B95.7* *Other staphylococcus as the cause of diseases classified elsewhere*

●■ *B95.8* *Unspecified staphylococcus as the cause of diseases classified elsewhere*

● **B96** **Other bacterial agents as the cause of diseases classified elsewhere**

● *B96.0* *Mycoplasma pneumoniae [M. pneumoniae] as the cause of diseases classified elsewhere*
Pleuro-pneumonia-like-organism [PPLO]

● *B96.1* *Klebsiella pneumoniae [K. pneumoniae] as the cause of diseases classified elsewhere*

● *B96.2* **Escherichia coli [E. coli] as the cause of diseases classified elsewhere**

●■ *B96.20* *Unspecified Escherichia coli [E. coli] as the cause of diseases classified elsewhere*
Escherichia coli [E. coli] NOS

● *B96.21* *Shiga toxin-producing Escherichia coli [E. coli] (STEC) O157 as the cause of diseases classified elsewhere*
E. coli O157:H- (nonmotile) with confirmation of Shiga toxin
E. coli O157 with confirmation of Shiga toxin when H antigen is unknown, or is not H7
O157:H7 Escherichia coli [E.coli] with or without confirmation of Shiga toxin-production
Shiga toxin-producing Escherichia coli [E.coli] O157:H7 with or without confirmation of Shiga toxin-production
STEC O157:H7 with or without confirmation of Shiga toxin-production

● *B96.22* *Other specified Shiga toxin-producing Escherichia coli [E. coli] (STEC) as the cause of diseases classified elsewhere*
Non-O157 Shiga toxin-producing Escherichia coli [E.coli]
Non-O157 Shiga toxin-producing Escherichia coli [E.coli] with known O group

●■ *B96.23* *Unspecified Shiga toxin-producing Escherichia coli [E. coli] (STEC) as the cause of diseases classified elsewhere*
Shiga toxin-producing Escherichia coli [E. coli] with unspecified O group
STEC NOS

● *B96.29* *Other Escherichia coli [E. coli] as the cause of diseases classified elsewhere*
Non-Shiga toxin-producing E. coli

● *B96.3* *Hemophilus influenzae [H. influenzae] as the cause of diseases classified elsewhere*

● *B96.4* *Proteus (mirabilis) (morganii) as the cause of diseases classified elsewhere*

● *B96.5* *Pseudomonas (aeruginosa) (mallei) (pseudomallei) as the cause of diseases classified elsewhere*

● *B96.6* *Bacteroides fragilis [B. fragilis] as the cause of diseases classified elsewhere*

● *B96.7* *Clostridium perfringens [C. perfringens] as the cause of diseases classified elsewhere*

● **B96.8** **Other specified bacterial agents as the cause of diseases classified elsewhere**

● *B96.81* *Helicobacter pylori [H. pylori] as the cause of diseases classified elsewhere*

● *B96.82* *Vibrio vulnificus as the cause of diseases classified elsewhere*

● *B96.89* *Other specified bacterial agents as the cause of diseases classified elsewhere*

● **B97** **Viral agents as the cause of diseases classified elsewhere**

● *B97.0* *Adenovirus as the cause of diseases classified elsewhere*

● **B97.1** **Enterovirus as the cause of diseases classified elsewhere**

●■ *B97.10* *Unspecified enterovirus as the cause of diseases classified elsewhere*

● *B97.11* *Coxsackievirus as the cause of diseases classified elsewhere*

● *B97.12* *Echovirus as the cause of diseases classified elsewhere*

● *B97.19* *Other enterovirus as the cause of diseases classified elsewhere*

Item 1–24 Retrovirus develops by copying its RNA, genetic materials, into the DNA, which then produces new virus particles. It is from the Retroviridae virus family. **Human T-cell lymphotropic virus, Type I (HTLV-I)** is also called human T-cell leukemia virus, Type I, and is a retrovirus thought to cause T-cell leukemia/lymphoma. **Human T-cell lymphotropic virus, Type II (HTLV-II),** is also called human T-cell leukemia virus, Type II, and is a retrovirus associated with hematologic disorders.

HIV-2 is one of the serotypes of HIV and is usually confined to West Africa, whereas HIV-1 is found worldwide.

● B97.2   **Coronavirus as the cause of diseases classified elsewhere**
  ● B97.21   *SARS-associated coronavirus as the cause of diseases classified elsewhere* 🦠
      Excludes1   pneumonia due to SARS-associated coronavirus (J12.81)
  ● B97.29   *Other coronavirus as the cause of diseases classified elsewhere*

● B97.3   **Retrovirus as the cause of diseases classified elsewhere**
      Excludes1   human immunodeficiency virus [HIV] disease (B20)
  ● ■ B97.30   *Unspecified retrovirus as the cause of diseases classified elsewhere*
  ● B97.31   *Lentivirus as the cause of diseases classified elsewhere*
  ● B97.32   *Oncovirus as the cause of diseases classified elsewhere*
  ● B97.33   *Human T-cell lymphotrophic virus, type I [HTLV-I] as the cause of diseases classified elsewhere* 🦠
  ● B97.34   *Human T-cell lymphotrophic virus, type II [HTLV-II] as the cause of diseases classified elsewhere* 🦠
  ● B97.35   *Human immunodeficiency virus, type 2 [HIV 2] as the cause of diseases classified elsewhere* 🦠
  ● B97.39   *Other retrovirus as the cause of diseases classified elsewhere*

● B97.4   *Respiratory syncytial virus as the cause of diseases classified elsewhere*
● B97.5   *Reovirus as the cause of diseases classified elsewhere*
● B97.6   *Parvovirus as the cause of diseases classified elsewhere*
● B97.7   *Papillomavirus as the cause of diseases classified elsewhere*
● B97.8   **Other viral agents as the cause of diseases classified elsewhere**
  ● B97.81   *Human metapneumovirus as the cause of diseases classified elsewhere*
  ● B97.89   *Other viral agents as the cause of diseases classified elsewhere*

OTHER INFECTIOUS DISEASES (B99)

● B99   **Other and unspecified infectious diseases**
    B99.8   **Other infectious disease**
  ■ B99.9   **Unspecified infectious disease**

N Newborn Age: 0   P Pediatric Age: 0–17   M Maternity DX: 12–55   A Adult Age: 15–124   ♀ Females Only   ♂ Males Only   🦠 Complication\Comorbidity   🦠 Major C\C   Present on Admission Requirement   🦠 Hospital-Acquired Condition   819

CHAPTER 1 (A00-B99)

Item 2–1 Neoplasm: Neo = new, plasm = growth, development, formation. This new growth (mass, tumor) can be malignant or benign, which is confirmed by the pathology report. Do not assign a code to a neoplasm until you review the pathology report. Certain CPT codes will specify benign or malignant lesion, so be certain the diagnosis code supports the procedure code.

OGCR Section I.C.2

General Guidelines

Chapter 2 of the ICD-10-CM contains the codes for the most benign and all malignant neoplasms. Certain benign neoplasms, such as prostatic adenomas, may be found in the specific body system chapters. To properly code a neoplasm, it is necessary to determine from the record if the neoplasm is benign, in-situ, malignant, or, of uncertain histologic behavior. If malignant, any secondary (metastatic) sites should also be determined.

CHAPTER 2

NEOPLASMS (C00-D49)

This chapter contains the following blocks:

C00-C14	Malignant neoplasms of lip, oral cavity and pharynx
C15-C26	Malignant neoplasms of digestive organs
C30-C39	Malignant neoplasms of respiratory and intrathoracic organs
C40-C41	Malignant neoplasms of bone and articular cartilage
C43-C44	Melanoma and other malignant neoplasms of skin
C45-C49	Malignant neoplasms of mesothelial and soft tissue
C50	Malignant neoplasms of breast
C51-C58	Malignant neoplasms of female genital organs
C60-C63	Malignant neoplasms of male genital organs
C64-C68	Malignant neoplasms of urinary tract
C69-C72	Malignant neoplasms of eye, brain and other parts of central nervous system
C73-C75	Malignant neoplasms of thyroid and other endocrine glands
C7A	Malignant neuroendocrine tumors
C7B	Secondary neuroendocrine tumors
C76-C80	Malignant neoplasms of ill-defined, other secondary and unspecified sites
C81-C96	Malignant neoplasms of lymphoid, hematopoietic and related tissue
D00-D09	In situ neoplasms
D10-D36	Benign neoplasms, except benign neuroendocrine tumors
D3A	Benign neuroendocrine tumors
D37-D48	Neoplasms of uncertain behavior, polycythemia vera and myelodysplastic syndromes
D49	Neoplasms of unspecified behavior

Notes: Functional activity

All neoplasms are classified in this chapter, whether they are functionally active or not. An additional code from Chapter 4 may be used, to identify functional activity associated with any neoplasm.

Morphology [Histology]

Chapter 2 classifies neoplasms primarily by site (topography), with broad groupings for behavior, malignant, in situ, benign, etc. The Table of Neoplasms should be used to identify the correct topography code. In a few cases, such as for malignant melanoma and certain neuroendocrine tumors, the morphology (histologic type) is included in the category and codes.

Primary malignant neoplasms overlapping site boundaries

A primary malignant neoplasm that overlaps two or more contiguous (next to each other) sites should be classified to the subcategory/code .8 ('overlapping lesion'), unless the combination is specifically indexed elsewhere. For multiple neoplasms of the same site that are not contiguous, such as tumors in different quadrants of the same breast, codes for each site should be assigned.

Malignant neoplasm of ectopic tissue

Malignant neoplasms of ectopic tissue are to be coded to the site mentioned, e.g., ectopic pancreatic malignant neoplasms are coded to pancreas, unspecified (C25.9).

MALIGNANT NEOPLASMS (C00-C96)

MALIGNANT NEOPLASMS, STATED OR PRESUMED TO BE PRIMARY (OF SPECIFIED SITES), AND CERTAIN SPECIFIED HISTOLOGIES, EXCEPT NEUROENDOCRINE, AND OF LYMPHOID, HEMATOPOIETIC AND RELATED TISSUE (C00-C75)

MALIGNANT NEOPLASMS OF LIP, ORAL CAVITY AND PHARYNX (C00-C14)

● **C00　Malignant neoplasm of lip**

Use additional code to identify:
　　alcohol abuse and dependence (F10.-)
　　history of tobacco use (Z87.891)
　　tobacco dependence (F17.-)
　　tobacco use (Z72.0)

Excludes1	malignant melanoma of lip (C43.0)
	Merkel cell carcinoma of lip (C4A.0)
	other and unspecified malignant neoplasm of skin of lip (C44.0-)

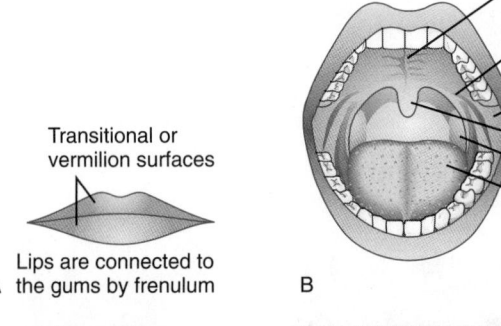

Figure 2-1 Anatomical structures of the mouth and lips. **A.** Transitional or vermilion borders. Lips are connected to the gums by frenulum. **B.** Dorsal surface. **C.** Ventral surface.

● Unacceptable Principal Diagnosis　　● Use Additional Character(s)　　■ Unspecified　　▶ Manifestation Code

820　　**OGCR** Official Guidelines for Coding and Reporting　　Excludes 1　　Excludes 2　　Includes　　Use additional　　Code first　　Code also

C00.0 Malignant neoplasm of external upper lip
Malignant neoplasm of lipstick area of upper lip
Malignant neoplasm of upper lip NOS
Malignant neoplasm of vermilion border of upper lip

C00.1 Malignant neoplasm of external lower lip
Malignant neoplasm of lower lip NOS
Malignant neoplasm of lipstick area of lower lip
Malignant neoplasm of vermilion border of lower lip

■ **C00.2 Malignant neoplasm of external lip, unspecified**
Malignant neoplasm of vermilion border of lip NOS

C00.3 Malignant neoplasm of upper lip, inner aspect
Malignant neoplasm of buccal aspect of upper lip
Malignant neoplasm of frenulum of upper lip
Malignant neoplasm of mucosa of upper lip
Malignant neoplasm of oral aspect of upper lip

C00.4 Malignant neoplasm of lower lip, inner aspect
Malignant neoplasm of buccal aspect of lower lip
Malignant neoplasm of frenulum of lower lip
Malignant neoplasm of mucosa of lower lip
Malignant neoplasm of oral aspect of lower lip

■ **C00.5 Malignant neoplasm of lip, unspecified, inner aspect**
Malignant neoplasm of buccal aspect of lip, unspecified
Malignant neoplasm of frenulum of lip, unspecified
Malignant neoplasm of mucosa of lip, unspecified
Malignant neoplasm of oral aspect of lip, unspecified

■ **C00.6 Malignant neoplasm of commissure of lip, unspecified**
Commissure: Site of union of corresponding parts

C00.8 Malignant neoplasm of overlapping sites of lip

■ **C00.9 Malignant neoplasm of lip, unspecified**

C01 Malignant neoplasm of base of tongue
Malignant neoplasm of dorsal surface of base of tongue
Malignant neoplasm of fixed part of tongue NOS
Malignant neoplasm of posterior third of tongue

Use additional code to identify:
alcohol abuse and dependence (F10.-)
history of tobacco use (Z87.891)
tobacco dependence (F17.-)
tobacco use (Z72.0)

● **C02 Malignant neoplasm of other and unspecified parts of tongue**

Use additional code to identify:
alcohol abuse and dependence (F10.-)
history of tobacco use (Z87.891)
tobacco dependence (F17.-)
tobacco use (Z72.0)

C02.0 Malignant neoplasm of dorsal surface of tongue
Malignant neoplasm of anterior two-thirds of tongue, dorsal surface

| Excludes2 | malignant neoplasm of dorsal surface of base of tongue (C01) |

C02.1 Malignant neoplasm of border of tongue
Malignant neoplasm of tip of tongue

C02.2 Malignant neoplasm of ventral surface of tongue
Malignant neoplasm of anterior two-thirds of tongue, ventral surface
Malignant neoplasm of frenulum linguae

■ **C02.3 Malignant neoplasm of anterior two-thirds of tongue, part unspecified**
Malignant neoplasm of middle third of tongue NOS
Malignant neoplasm of mobile part of tongue NOS

C02.4 Malignant neoplasm of lingual tonsil
Lingual tonsil: Aggregation of lymph follicles at root of tongue

| Excludes2 | malignant neoplasm of tonsil NOS (C09.9) |

C02.8 Malignant neoplasm of overlapping sites of tongue
Malignant neoplasm of two or more contiguous sites of tongue

■ **C02.9 Malignant neoplasm of tongue, unspecified**

● **C03 Malignant neoplasm of gum**

| Includes | malignant neoplasm of alveolar (ridge) mucosa
malignant neoplasm of gingiva |

Use additional code to identify:
alcohol abuse and dependence (F10.-)
history of tobacco use (Z87.891)
tobacco dependence (F17.-)
tobacco use (Z72.0)

| Excludes2 | malignant odontogenic neoplasms (C41.0-C41.1) |

C03.0 Malignant neoplasm of upper gum

C03.1 Malignant neoplasm of lower gum

■ **C03.9 Malignant neoplasm of gum, unspecified**

● **C04 Malignant neoplasm of floor of mouth**

Use additional code to identify:
alcohol abuse and dependence (F10.-)
history of tobacco use (Z87.891)
tobacco dependence (F17.-)
tobacco use (Z72.0)

C04.0 Malignant neoplasm of anterior floor of mouth
Malignant neoplasm of anterior to the premolar-canine junction

C04.1 Malignant neoplasm of lateral floor of mouth

C04.8 Malignant neoplasm of overlapping sites of floor of mouth

■ **C04.9 Malignant neoplasm of floor of mouth, unspecified**

● **C05 Malignant neoplasm of palate**

Use additional code to identify:
alcohol abuse and dependence (F10.-)
history of tobacco use (Z87.891)
tobacco dependence (F17.-)
tobacco use (Z72.0)

| Excludes1 | Kaposi's sarcoma of palate (C46.2) |

C05.0 Malignant neoplasm of hard palate

C05.1 Malignant neoplasm of soft palate

| Excludes2 | malignant neoplasm of nasopharyngeal surface of soft palate (C11.3) |

C05.2 Malignant neoplasm of uvula

C05.8 Malignant neoplasm of overlapping sites of palate

■ **C05.9 Malignant neoplasm of palate, unspecified**
Malignant neoplasm of roof of mouth

● **C06 Malignant neoplasm of other and unspecified parts of mouth**

Use additional code to identify:
alcohol abuse and dependence (F10.-)
history of tobacco use (Z87.891)
tobacco dependence (F17.-)
tobacco use (Z72.0)

C06.0 Malignant neoplasm of cheek mucosa
Malignant neoplasm of buccal mucosa NOS
Malignant neoplasm of internal cheek

CHAPTER 2 (C00-D49)

N Newborn Age: 0   P Pediatric Age: 0–17   M Maternity DX: 12–55   A Adult Age: 15–124   ♀ Females Only   ♂ Males Only

C06.1 Malignant neoplasm of vestibule of mouth
    Malignant neoplasm of buccal sulcus (upper) (lower)
    Malignant neoplasm of labial sulcus (upper) (lower)

C06.2 Malignant neoplasm of retromolar area

● **C06.8 Malignant neoplasm of overlapping sites of other and unspecified parts of mouth**

■ **C06.80 Malignant neoplasm of overlapping sites of unspecified parts of mouth**

C06.89 Malignant neoplasm of overlapping sites of other parts of mouth 'book leaf' neoplasm [ventral surface of tongue and floor of mouth]

■ **C06.9 Malignant neoplasm of mouth, unspecified**
    Malignant neoplasm of minor salivary gland, unspecified site
    Malignant neoplasm of oral cavity NOS

C07 Malignant neoplasm of parotid gland
    Use additional code to identify:
        alcohol abuse and dependence (F10.-)
        exposure to environmental tobacco smoke (Z77.22)
        exposure to tobacco smoke in the perinatal period (P96.81)
        history of tobacco use (Z87.891)
        occupational exposure to environmental tobacco smoke (Z57.31)
        tobacco dependence (F17.-)
        tobacco use (Z72.0)

● **C08 Malignant neoplasm of other and unspecified major salivary glands**
    Includes   malignant neoplasm of salivary ducts
    Use additional code to identify:
        alcohol abuse and dependence (F10.-)
        exposure to environmental tobacco smoke (Z77.22)
        exposure to tobacco smoke in the perinatal period (P96.81)
        history of tobacco use (Z87.891)
        occupational exposure to environmental tobacco smoke (Z57.31)
        tobacco dependence (F17.-)
        tobacco use (Z72.0)

    Excludes1   malignant neoplasms of specified minor salivary glands which are classified according to their anatomical location

    Excludes2   malignant neoplasms of minor salivary glands NOS (C06.9)
        malignant neoplasm of parotid gland (C07)

C08.0 Malignant neoplasm of submandibular gland
    Malignant neoplasm of submaxillary gland

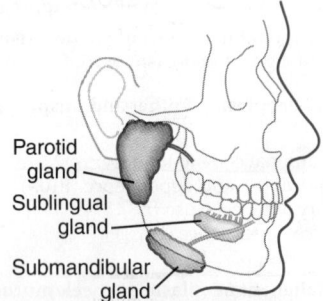

Figure 2-2 Major salivary glands.

Parotid gland
Sublingual gland
Submandibular gland

C08.1 Malignant neoplasm of sublingual gland

■ **C08.9 Malignant neoplasm of major salivary gland, unspecified**
    Malignant neoplasm of salivary gland (major) NOS

(See Plate 61 on page NAP-25.)

● **C09 Malignant neoplasm of tonsil**
    Use additional code to identify:
        alcohol abuse and dependence (F10.-)
        exposure to environmental tobacco smoke (Z77.22)
        exposure to tobacco smoke in the perinatal period (P96.81)
        history of tobacco use (Z87.891)
        occupational exposure to environmental tobacco smoke (Z57.31)
        tobacco dependence (F17.-)
        tobacco use (Z72.0)

    Excludes2   malignant neoplasm of lingual tonsil (C02.4)
        malignant neoplasm of pharyngeal tonsil (C11.1)

C09.0 Malignant neoplasm of tonsillar fossa
    Surface of palatine (two masses of lymphatic tissue on sides of throat) tonsils

C09.1 Malignant neoplasm of tonsillar pillar (anterior) (posterior)
    Extension from palatine (two masses of lymphatic tissue on sides of throat) tonsils

C09.8 Malignant neoplasm of overlapping sites of tonsil

■ **C09.9 Malignant neoplasm of tonsil, unspecified**
    Malignant neoplasm of tonsil NOS
    Malignant neoplasm of faucial tonsils
    Malignant neoplasm of palatine tonsils

● **C10 Malignant neoplasm of oropharynx**
    Area of throat at back of mouth
    Use additional code to identify:
        alcohol abuse and dependence (F10.-)
        exposure to environmental tobacco smoke (Z77.22)
        exposure to tobacco smoke in the perinatal period (P96.81)
        history of tobacco use (Z87.891)
        occupational exposure to environmental tobacco smoke (Z57.31)
        tobacco dependence (F17.-)
        tobacco use (Z72.0)

    Excludes2   malignant neoplasm of tonsil (C09.-)

C10.0 Malignant neoplasm of vallecula
    Vallecula, depression or furrow

C10.1 Malignant neoplasm of anterior surface of epiglottis
    Malignant neoplasm of epiglottis, free border [margin]
    Malignant neoplasm of glossoepiglottic fold(s)
    Excludes2   malignant neoplasm of epiglottis (suprahyoid portion) NOS (C32.1)

C10.2 Malignant neoplasm of lateral wall of oropharynx

C10.3 Malignant neoplasm of posterior wall of oropharynx

C10.4 Malignant neoplasm of branchial cleft
    Congenital slitlike openings formed between branchial arches pharyngeal groove
    Malignant neoplasm of branchial cyst [site of neoplasm]

C10.8 Malignant neoplasm of overlapping sites of oropharynx
    Malignant neoplasm of junctional region of oropharynx

■ **C10.9 Malignant neoplasm of oropharynx, unspecified**

● Unacceptable Principal Diagnosis   ● Use Additional Character(s)   ■ Unspecified   ▶ Manifestation Code
OGCR Official Guidelines for Coding and Reporting   Excludes 1   Excludes 2   Includes   Use additional   Code first   Code also

●**C11 Malignant neoplasm of nasopharynx**

Use additional code to identify:
    exposure to environmental tobacco smoke (Z77.22)
    exposure to tobacco smoke in the perinatal period (P96.81)
    history of tobacco use (Z87.891)
    occupational exposure to environmental tobacco smoke (Z57.31)
    tobacco dependence (F17.-)
    tobacco use (Z72.0)

C11.0 Malignant neoplasm of superior wall of nasopharynx
Part of pharynx that lies above soft palate
Malignant neoplasm of roof of nasopharynx

C11.1 Malignant neoplasm of posterior wall of nasopharynx
Malignant neoplasm of adenoid
Malignant neoplasm of pharyngeal tonsil

C11.2 Malignant neoplasm of lateral wall of nasopharynx
Malignant neoplasm of fossa of Rosenmüller
Malignant neoplasm of opening of auditory tube
Malignant neoplasm of pharyngeal recess

C11.3 Malignant neoplasm of anterior wall of nasopharynx
Malignant neoplasm of floor of nasopharynx
Malignant neoplasm of nasopharyngeal (anterior) (posterior) surface of soft palate
Malignant neoplasm of posterior margin of nasal choana
Malignant neoplasm of posterior margin of nasal septum

C11.8 Malignant neoplasm of overlapping sites of nasopharynx

■**C11.9 Malignant neoplasm of nasopharynx, unspecified**
Malignant neoplasm of nasopharyngeal wall NOS

C12 Malignant neoplasm of pyriform sinus
Malignant neoplasm of pyriform fossa

Use additional code to identify:
    exposure to environmental tobacco smoke (Z77.22)
    exposure to tobacco smoke in the perinatal period (P96.81)
    history of tobacco use (Z87.891)
    occupational exposure to environmental tobacco smoke (Z57.31)
    tobacco dependence (F17.-)
    tobacco use (Z72.0)

●**C13 Malignant neoplasm of hypopharynx**

Use additional code to identify:
    exposure to environmental tobacco smoke (Z77.22)
    exposure to tobacco smoke in the perinatal period (P96.81)
    history of tobacco use (Z87.891)
    occupational exposure to environmental tobacco smoke (Z57.31)
    tobacco dependence (F17.-)
    tobacco use (Z72.0)

Excludes2   malignant neoplasm of pyriform sinus (C12)

C13.0 Malignant neoplasm of postcricoid region
Behind the cricoid cartilage of neck

C13.1 Malignant neoplasm of aryepiglottic fold, hypopharyngeal aspect
Arytenoepiglottic fold, triangular opening between side of epiglottis and apex of arytenoid cartilage
Malignant neoplasm of aryepiglottic fold NOS
Malignant neoplasm of interarytenoid fold NOS
Malignant neoplasm of aryepiglottic fold marginal zone
Malignant neoplasm of interarytenoid fold marginal zone

Excludes2   malignant neoplasm of aryepiglottic fold or interarytenoid fold, laryngeal aspect (C32.1)

C13.2 Malignant neoplasm of posterior wall of hypopharynx

C13.8 Malignant neoplasm of overlapping sites of hypopharynx

■**C13.9 Malignant neoplasm of hypopharynx, unspecified**
Malignant neoplasm of hypopharyngeal wall NOS

●**C14 Malignant neoplasm of other and ill-defined sites in the lip, oral cavity and pharynx**

Use additional code to identify:
    alcohol abuse and dependence (F10.-)
    exposure to environmental tobacco smoke (Z77.22)
    exposure to tobacco smoke in the perinatal period (P96.81)
    history of tobacco use (Z87.891)
    occupational exposure to environmental tobacco smoke (Z57.31)
    tobacco dependence (F17.-)
    tobacco use (Z72.0)

Excludes1   malignant neoplasm of oral cavity NOS (C06.9)

■**C14.0 Malignant neoplasm of pharynx, unspecified**

C14.2 Malignant neoplasm of Waldeyer's ring

CHAPTER 2 (C00-D49)

Figure 2-3 The esophagus is the muscular tube that connects the pharynx and the stomach. The 10 inch (25 cm) long esophagus is divided into three parts: **cervical, thoracic,** and **abdominal.**

N Newborn Age: 0   **P** Pediatric Age: 0–17   **M** Maternity DX: 12–55   **A** Adult Age: 15–124   ♀ Females Only   ♂ Males Only

🖝 Complication\Comorbidity   🖝 Major C\C   🖝 Present on Admission Requirement   🖝 Hospital-Acquired Condition

823

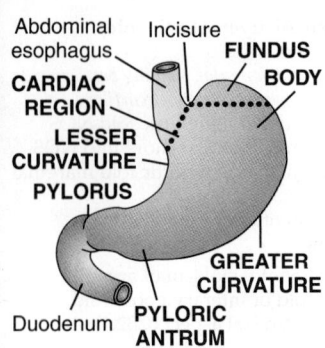

Figure 2-4 Parts of the stomach.

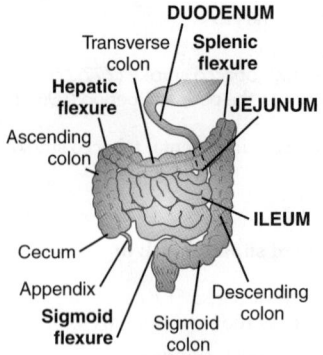

Figure 2-5 Small intestine and colon.

Item 2–2 The esophagus opens into the stomach through the **cardiac orifice**, also called the **cardioesophageal junction**. The **cardia** is adjacent to the cardiac orifice. The stomach widens into the **greater** and **lesser curvatures**. The **pyloric antrum** precedes the **pylorus**, which opens to the duodenum.

C14.8   **Malignant neoplasm of overlapping sites of lip, oral cavity and pharynx**
        Primary malignant neoplasm of two or more contiguous sites of lip, oral cavity and pharynx
        | Excludes 1 | 'book leaf' neoplasm [ventral surface of tongue and floor of mouth] (C06.89)

MALIGNANT NEOPLASM OF DIGESTIVE ORGANS (C15-C26)

| Excludes 1 | Kaposi's sarcoma of gastrointestinal sites (C46.4)

● **C15   Malignant neoplasms of esophagus**
        Use additional code to identify:
        alcohol abuse and dependence (F10.-)

C15.3   **Malignant neoplasm of upper third of esophagus** 🔧

C15.4   **Malignant neoplasm of middle third of esophagus** 🔧

C15.5   **Malignant neoplasm of lower third of esophagus** 🔧
        | Excludes 1 | malignant neoplasm of cardio-esophageal junction (C16.0)

C15.8   **Malignant neoplasm of overlapping sites of esophagus** 🔧

■ C15.9   **Malignant neoplasm of esophagus, unspecified** 🔧

● **C16   Malignant neoplasm of stomach**
        Use additional code to identify:
        alcohol abuse and dependence (F10.-)
        | Excludes 2 | malignant carcinoid tumor of the stomach (C7A.092)

C16.0   **Malignant neoplasm of cardia** 🔧
        Malignant neoplasm of cardiac orifice
        Malignant neoplasm of cardio-esophageal junction
        Malignant neoplasm of esophagus and stomach
        Malignant neoplasm of gastro-esophageal junction

C16.1   **Malignant neoplasm of fundus of stomach** 🔧

C16.2   **Malignant neoplasm of body of stomach** 🔧

C16.3   **Malignant neoplasm of pyloric antrum** 🔧
        Malignant neoplasm of gastric antrum

C16.4   **Malignant neoplasm of pylorus** 🔧
        Malignant neoplasm of prepylorus
        Malignant neoplasm of pyloric canal

■ C16.5   **Malignant neoplasm of lesser curvature of stomach, unspecified** 🔧
        Malignant neoplasm of lesser curvature of stomach, not classifiable to C16.1-C16.4

■ C16.6   **Malignant neoplasm of greater curvature of stomach, unspecified** 🔧
        Malignant neoplasm of greater curvature of stomach, not classifiable to C16.0-C16.4

C16.8   **Malignant neoplasm of overlapping sites of stomach** 🔧

■ C16.9   **Malignant neoplasm of stomach, unspecified** 🔧
        Gastric cancer NOS

● **C17   Malignant neoplasm of small intestine**
        | Excludes 1 | malignant carcinoid tumor of the small intestine (C7A.01)

C17.0   **Malignant neoplasm of duodenum** 🔧
        First or proximal portion of small intestine, extending from pylorus to jejunum

C17.1   **Malignant neoplasm of jejunum** 🔧
        Second section of small intestine, extending from duodenum to ileum

C17.2   **Malignant neoplasm of ileum** 🔧
        Distal and longest portion of small intestine, extending from jejunum to cecum
        | Excludes 1 | malignant neoplasm of ileocecal valve (C18.0)

C17.3   **Meckel's diverticulum, malignant** 🔧
        Appendage of ileum
        | Excludes 1 | Meckel's diverticulum, congenital (Q43.0)

C17.8   **Malignant neoplasm of overlapping sites of small intestine** 🔧

■ C17.9   **Malignant neoplasm of small intestine, unspecified** 🔧

● **C18   Malignant neoplasm of colon**
        | Excludes 1 | malignant carcinoid tumors of the colon (C7A.02)

C18.0   **Malignant neoplasm of cecum** 🔧
        First section of large intestine
        Malignant neoplasm of ileocecal valve

C18.1   **Malignant neoplasm of appendix** 🔧
        Blind ended tube connected to the cecum; AKA vermiform appendix

C18.2   **Malignant neoplasm of ascending colon** 🔧
        Ascending colon is between cecum and right colic flexure

C18.3   **Malignant neoplasm of hepatic flexure** 🔧
        A flexure is a bending in a structure or organ. Note the three flexures illustrated in Figure 2–5.

C18.4   **Malignant neoplasm of transverse colon** 🔧
        Portion of colon that runs transversely across upper part of abdomen, between right and left colic flexures

C18.5   **Malignant neoplasm of splenic flexure** 🔧
        Bend at junction of transverse and descending colon

● Unacceptable Principal Diagnosis   ● Use Additional Character(s)   ■ Unspecified   ▶ Manifestation Code

824   OGCR Official Guidelines for Coding and Reporting | Excludes 1 | | Excludes 2 | Includes   Use additional   Code first   Code also

CHAPTER 2 (C00-D49)

C18.6   Malignant neoplasm of descending colon
Portion between left colic flexure and sigmoid colon at pelvic brim; AKA iliac colon

C18.7   Malignant neoplasm of sigmoid colon
S-shaped part of colon extending from pelvic brim to third segment of sacrum
Malignant neoplasm of sigmoid (flexure)

> **Excludes1**   malignant neoplasm of rectosigmoid junction (C19)

C18.8   Malignant neoplasm of overlapping sites of colon

C18.9   Malignant neoplasm of colon, unspecified
Malignant neoplasm of large intestine NOS

C19   Malignant neoplasm of rectosigmoid junction
Malignant neoplasm of colon with rectum
Malignant neoplasm of rectosigmoid (colon)

> **Excludes1**   malignant carcinoid tumors of the colon (C7A.02-)

C20   Malignant neoplasm of rectum
Malignant neoplasm of rectal ampulla

> **Excludes1**   malignant carcinoid tumor of the rectum (C7A.026)

● C21   Malignant neoplasm of anus and anal canal

> **Excludes2**   malignant carcinoid tumors of the colon (C7A.02-)
> malignant melanoma of anal margin (C43.51)
> malignant melanoma of anal skin (C43.51)
> malignant melanoma of perianal skin (C43.51)
> other and unspecified malignant neoplasm of anal margin (C44.500, C44.510, C44.520, C44.590)
> other and unspecified malignant neoplasm of anal skin (C44.500, C44.510, C44.520, C44.590)
> other and unspecified malignant neoplasm of perianal skin (C44.500, C44.510, C44.520, C44.590)

C21.0   Malignant neoplasm of anus, unspecified

C21.1   Malignant neoplasm of anal canal
Terminal part of large intestine
Malignant neoplasm of anal sphincter

C21.2   Malignant neoplasm of cloacogenic zone

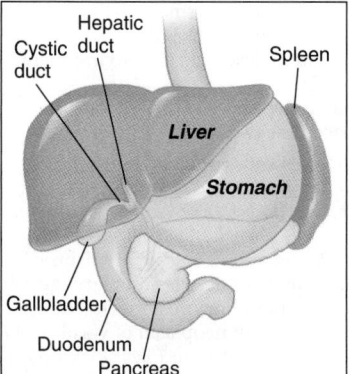

Figure 2-6 Diagram of liver, gallbladder, hepatic duct, pancreas, and spleen. (From Thibodeau and Patton: Anatomy and Physiology, 6th ed. 2007, Mosby.)

C21.8   Malignant neoplasm of overlapping sites of rectum, anus and anal canal
Malignant neoplasm of anorectal junction
Malignant neoplasm of anorectum
Primary malignant neoplasm of two or more contiguous sites of rectum, anus and anal canal

● C22   Malignant neoplasm of liver and intrahepatic bile ducts
Intrahepatic: Within liver

Use additional code to identify:
alcohol abuse and dependence (F10.-)
hepatitis B (B16.-, B18.0-B18.1) hepatitis C (B17.1-, B18.2)

> **Excludes1**   malignant neoplasm of biliary tract NOS (C24.9)
> secondary malignant neoplasm of liver and intrahepatic bile duct (C78.7)

C22.0   Liver cell carcinoma
Hepatocellular carcinoma
Hepatoma

C22.1   Intrahepatic bile duct carcinoma
Cholangiocarcinoma
Adenocarcinoma (cancer that originates in glandular tissue) arising from epithelium of intrahepatic bile ducts

> **Excludes1**   malignant neoplasm of hepatic duct (C24.0)

C22.2   Hepatoblastoma
Malignant intrahepatic tumor

C22.3   Angiosarcoma of liver
Kupffer cell sarcoma

C22.4   Other sarcomas of liver

C22.7   Other specified carcinomas of liver

C22.8   Malignant neoplasm of liver, primary, unspecified as to type

C22.9   Malignant neoplasm of liver, not specified as primary or secondary

C23   Malignant neoplasm of gallbladder

● C24   Malignant neoplasm of other and unspecified parts of biliary tract

> **Excludes1**   malignant neoplasm of intrahepatic bile duct (C22.1)

C24.0   Malignant neoplasm of extrahepatic bile duct
Extrahepatic = outside the liver
Malignant neoplasm of biliary duct or passage NOS
Malignant neoplasm of common bile duct
Malignant neoplasm of cystic duct
Malignant neoplasm of hepatic duct

C24.1   Malignant neoplasm of ampulla of Vater
Union of pancreatic duct and common bile duct

C24.8   Malignant neoplasm of overlapping sites of biliary tract
Malignant neoplasm involving both intrahepatic and extrahepatic bile ducts
Primary malignant neoplasm of two or more contiguous sites of biliary tract

C24.9   Malignant neoplasm of biliary tract, unspecified

● C25   Malignant neoplasm of pancreas
Check documentation for specific site.

Use additional code to identify:
alcohol abuse and dependence (F10.-)

C25.0   Malignant neoplasm of head of pancreas

C25.1   Malignant neoplasm of body of pancreas

C25.2   Malignant neoplasm of tail of pancreas

C25.3   Malignant neoplasm of pancreatic duct

CHAPTER 2 (C00-D49)

N Newborn Age: 0   **P** Pediatric Age: 0–17   **M** Maternity DX: 12–55   **A** Adult Age: 15–124   ♀ Females Only   ♂ Males Only

Complication\Comorbidity   Major C\C   Present on Admission Requirement   Hospital-Acquired Condition

CHAPTER 2 (C00-D49)

Item 2–3   **Islets** of Langerhans (endocrine producing cells comprising 1% to 2% of the pancreatic mass) make and secrete hormones that regulate the body's production of insulin, glucagon, and stomach acid. Breakdown of the insulin-producing cells can cause diabetes mellitus. Islet cell tumors can be benign or malignant and include glucagonomas, insulinomas, gastrinomas, and neuroendocrine tumor. The neoplasm table must be consulted for the correct neoplasm code.

C25.4   Malignant neoplasm of endocrine pancreas 🔹
     Malignant neoplasm of islets of Langerhans
     That part of the pancreas that acts as endocrine gland and consists of islets of Langerhans

     Use additional code to identify any functional activity.

C25.7   Malignant neoplasm of other parts of pancreas 🔹
     Malignant neoplasm of neck of pancreas

C25.8   Malignant neoplasm of overlapping sites of pancreas 🔹

C25.9   Malignant neoplasm of pancreas, unspecified 🔹

● **C26   Malignant neoplasm of other and ill-defined digestive organs**
     Excludes1   malignant neoplasm of peritoneum and retroperitoneum (C48.-)

C26.0   Malignant neoplasm of intestinal tract, part unspecified
     Malignant neoplasm of intestine NOS

C26.1   Malignant neoplasm of spleen
     Excludes1   Hodgkin lymphoma (C81.-)
                 non-Hodgkin lymphoma (C82-C85)

C26.9   Malignant neoplasm of ill-defined sites within the digestive system
     Malignant neoplasm of alimentary canal or tract NOS
     Malignant neoplasm of gastrointestinal tract NOS
     Excludes1   malignant neoplasm of abdominal NOS (C76.2)
                 malignant neoplasm of intra-abdominal NOS (C76.2)

MALIGNANT NEOPLASMS OF RESPIRATORY AND INTRATHORACIC ORGANS (C30-C39)

     Includes   malignant neoplasm of middle ear
     Excludes1   mesothelioma (C45.-)

● **C30   Malignant neoplasm of nasal cavity and middle ear**

C30.0   Malignant neoplasm of nasal cavity
     Malignant neoplasm of cartilage of nose
     Malignant neoplasm of nasal concha
     Malignant neoplasm of internal nose
     Malignant neoplasm of septum of nose
     Malignant neoplasm of vestibule of nose
     Anterior part of nasal cavity
     Excludes1   malignant neoplasm of nasal bone (C41.0)
                 malignant neoplasm of nose NOS (C76.0)
                 malignant neoplasm of olfactory bulb (C72.2-)
                 malignant neoplasm of posterior margin of nasal septum and choana (C11.3)
                 malignant melanoma of skin of nose (C43.31)
                 malignant neoplasm of turbinates (C41.0)
                 other and unspecified malignant neoplasm of skin of nose C44.301, C44.311, C44.321, C44.391)

Figure 2-7 Paranasal sinuses. (From Buck CJ: Step-by-Step Medical Coding, 2006 ed. Philadelphia, WB Saunders, 2006.)

C30.1   Malignant neoplasm of middle ear
     Malignant neoplasm of antrum tympanicum
     Boney cavity or chamber
     Malignant neoplasm of auditory tube
     Malignant neoplasm of eustachian tube
     Malignant neoplasm of inner ear
     Malignant neoplasm of mastoid air cells
     Malignant neoplasm of tympanic cavity
     Excludes1   malignant neoplasm of auricular canal (external) (C43.2-, C44.2-)
                 malignant neoplasm of bone of ear (meatus) (C41.0)
                 malignant neoplasm of cartilage of ear (C49.0)
                 malignant melanoma of skin of (external) ear (C43.2-)
                 other and unspecified malignant neoplasm of skin of (external) ear (C44.2-)

● **C31   Malignant neoplasm of accessory sinuses**
     Paired sinuses in bones of face

C31.0   Malignant neoplasm of maxillary sinus
     Malignant neoplasm of antrum (Highmore) (maxillary)

C31.1   Malignant neoplasm of ethmoidal sinus

C31.2   Malignant neoplasm of frontal sinus

C31.3   Malignant neoplasm of sphenoid sinus

C31.8   Malignant neoplasm of overlapping sites of accessory sinuses

C31.9   Malignant neoplasm of accessory sinus, unspecified

● **C32   Malignant neoplasm of larynx**
     Use additional code to identify:
     alcohol abuse and dependence (F10.-)
     exposure to environmental tobacco smoke (Z77.22)
     exposure to tobacco smoke in the perinatal period (P96.81)
     history of tobacco use (Z87.891)
     occupational exposure to environmental tobacco smoke (Z57.31)
     tobacco dependence (F17.-)
     tobacco use (Z72.0)

C32.0   Malignant neoplasm of glottis
     Vocal apparatus of larynx, consisting of true vocal cords (plicae vocales) and opening between them (rima glottidis)
     Malignant neoplasm of intrinsic larynx
     Malignant neoplasm of laryngeal commissure (anterior)(posterior)
     Malignant neoplasm of vocal cord (true) NOS
     True *vocal cords ("lower vocal folds") produce vocalization when air from the lungs passes between them. Check your documentation. Code C32.1 is for malignant neoplasm of the **false** vocal cords.*

● Unacceptable Principal Diagnosis   ● Use Additional Character(s)   ■ Unspecified   ▶ Manifestation Code

OGCR Official Guidelines for Coding and Reporting   Excludes 1   Excludes 2   Includes   Use additional   Code first   Code also

C32.1   **Malignant neoplasm of supraglottis**
Area of pharynx above glottis
Malignant neoplasm of aryepiglottic fold or
interarytenoid fold, laryngeal aspect
Malignant neoplasm of epiglottis (suprahyoid
portion) NOS
Malignant neoplasm of extrinsic larynx
Malignant neoplasm of false vocal cord
*False vocal cords ("upper vocal folds") are not involved
in vocalization. Check your documentation. Code
C32.0 is for true vocal cords.*
Malignant neoplasm of posterior (laryngeal)
surface of epiglottis
Malignant neoplasm of ventricular bands

> **Excludes2**   malignant neoplasm of anterior
> surface of epiglottis (C10.1)
> malignant neoplasm of aryepiglottic
> fold or interarytenoid fold:
> NOS (C13.1)
> hypopharyngeal aspect (C13.1)
> marginal zone (C13.1)

C32.2   **Malignant neoplasm of subglottis**
*Lowest part of larynx from just below vocal cords down
to top of trachea*

C32.3   **Malignant neoplasm of laryngeal cartilage**
*Cartilages of larynx, including cricoid, thyroid, and
epiglottic, and two each of arytenoid, corniculate,
and cuneiform*

C32.8   **Malignant neoplasm of overlapping sites of larynx**

C32.9   **Malignant neoplasm of larynx, unspecified**

C33   **Malignant neoplasm of trachea** 🅒
Use additional code to identify:
exposure to environmental tobacco smoke (Z77.22)
exposure to tobacco smoke in the perinatal period (P96.81)
history of tobacco use (Z87.891)
occupational exposure to environmental tobacco smoke
(Z57.31)
tobacco dependence (F17.-)
tobacco use (Z72.0)

C34   **Malignant neoplasm of bronchus and lung**
Use additional code to identify:
exposure to environmental tobacco smoke (Z77.22)
exposure to tobacco smoke in the perinatal period (P96.81)
history of tobacco use (Z87.891)
occupational exposure to environmental tobacco smoke
(Z57.31)
tobacco dependence (F17.-)
tobacco use (Z72.0)

> **Excludes1**   Kaposi's sarcoma of lung (C46.5-)
> malignant carcinoid tumor of the bronchus
> and lung (C7A.090)

C34.0   **Malignant neoplasm of main bronchus**
Malignant neoplasm of carina
Ridgelike structure
Malignant neoplasm of hilus (of lung)
Anatomic depression or pit

    C34.00   **Malignant neoplasm of unspecified main
bronchus** 🅒

    C34.01   **Malignant neoplasm of right main bronchus** 🅒

    C34.02   **Malignant neoplasm of left main
bronchus** 🅒

C34.1   **Malignant neoplasm of upper lobe, bronchus or
lung**

    C34.10   **Malignant neoplasm of unspecified
bronchus or lung** 🅒

    C34.11   **Malignant neoplasm of upper lobe, right
bronchus or lung** 🅒

    C34.12   **Malignant neoplasm of upper lobe, left
bronchus or lung** 🅒

C34.2   **Malignant neoplasm of middle lobe, bronchus or
lung** 🅒

C34.3   **Malignant neoplasm of lower lobe, bronchus or
lung**

    C34.30   **Malignant neoplasm of lower lobe,
unspecified bronchus or lung** 🅒

    C34.31   **Malignant neoplasm of lower lobe, right
bronchus or lung** 🅒

    C34.32   **Malignant neoplasm of lower lobe, left
bronchus or lung** 🅒

C34.8   **Malignant neoplasm of overlapping sites of
bronchus and lung**

    C34.80   **Malignant neoplasm of overlapping sites
of unspecified bronchus and lung** 🅒

    C34.81   **Malignant neoplasm of overlapping sites
of right bronchus and lung** 🅒

    C34.82   **Malignant neoplasm of overlapping sites
of left bronchus and lung** 🅒

C34.9   **Malignant neoplasm of unspecified part of bronchus
or lung**

    C34.90   **Malignant neoplasm of unspecified part of
unspecified bronchus or lung** 🅒
Lung cancer NOS

    C34.91   **Malignant neoplasm of unspecified part of
right bronchus or lung** 🅒

    C34.92   **Malignant neoplasm of unspecified part of
left bronchus or lung** 🅒

C37   **Malignant neoplasm of thymus** 🅒

> **Excludes1**   malignant carcinoid tumor of the thymus
> (C7A.091)

C38   **Malignant neoplasm of heart, mediastinum and pleura**

> **Excludes1**   mesothelioma (C45.-)

C38.0   **Malignant neoplasm of heart** 🅒
Malignant neoplasm of pericardium

> **Excludes1**   malignant neoplasm of great vessels
> (C49.3)

C38.1   **Malignant neoplasm of anterior mediastinum** 🅒

C38.2   **Malignant neoplasm of posterior mediastinum** 🅒

C38.3   **Malignant neoplasm of mediastinum, part
unspecified** 🅒

C38.4   **Malignant neoplasm of pleura** 🅒

C38.8   **Malignant neoplasm of overlapping sites of heart,
mediastinum and pleura** 🅒
*Pleura are comprised of serous membrane that lines
the thoracic cavity (parietal) and covers the lungs
(visceral).*

C39   **Malignant neoplasm of other and ill-defined sites in the
respiratory system and intrathoracic organs**
Intrathoracic: within thorax/chest

Use additional code to identify:
exposure to environmental tobacco smoke (Z77.22)
exposure to tobacco smoke in the perinatal period (P96.81)
history of tobacco use (Z87.891)
occupational exposure to environmental tobacco smoke
(Z57.31)
tobacco dependence (F17.-)
tobacco use (Z72.0)

> **Excludes1**   intrathoracic malignant neoplasm NOS (C76.1)
> thoracic malignant neoplasm NOS (C76.1)

C39.0   **Malignant neoplasm of upper respiratory tract,
part unspecified**

C39.9   **Malignant neoplasm of lower respiratory tract, part
unspecified**
Malignant neoplasm of respiratory tract NOS

N Newborn Age: 0   **P** Pediatric Age: 0–17   **M** Maternity DX: 12–55   **A** Adult Age: 15–124   ♀ Females Only   ♂ Males Only

🅒 Complication\Comorbidity   Major C\C   Present on Admission Requirement   Hospital-Acquired Condition

827

CHAPTER 2 (C00-D49)

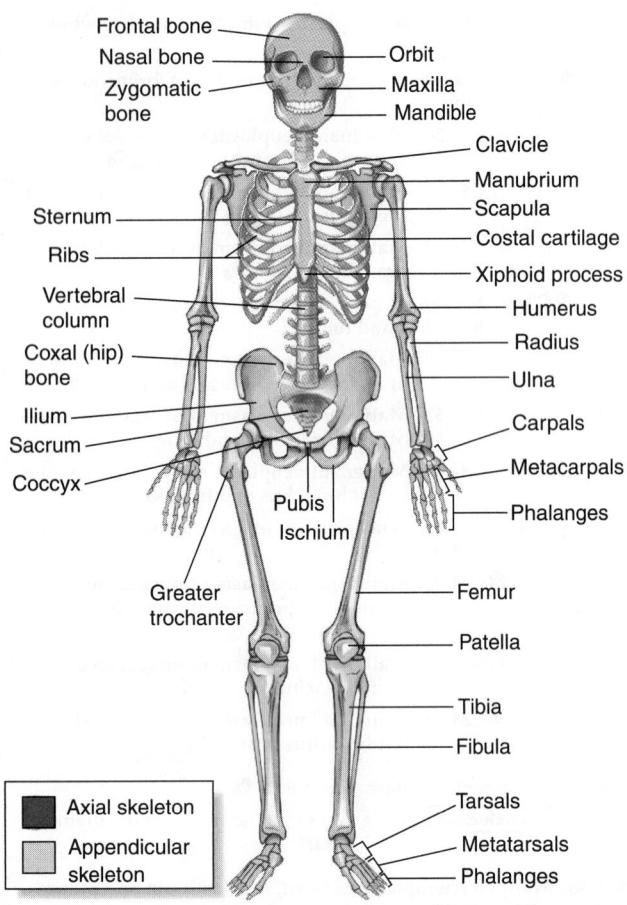

Frontal bone — Nasal bone — Orbit
Zygomatic bone — Maxilla — Mandible
Sternum — Clavicle — Manubrium — Scapula — Costal cartilage
Ribs — Xiphoid process
Vertebral column — Humerus — Radius
Coxal (hip) bone — Ulna
Ilium — Carpals
Sacrum — Metacarpals
Coccyx — Phalanges
Pubis — Ischium
Greater trochanter — Femur — Patella
Tibia — Fibula
Tarsals — Metatarsals — Phalanges

■ Axial skeleton
□ Appendicular skeleton

Figure 2-8 Diagram of skeleton of trunk and limbs with bones labled. (From Thibodeau and Patton: Anatomy and Physiology, 6th ed. 2007, Mosby.)

MALIGNANT NEOPLASMS OF BONE AND ARTICULAR CARTILAGE (C40-C41)

Includes   malignant neoplasm of cartilage (articular) (joint)
         malignant neoplasm of periosteum

Excludes1   malignant neoplasm of bone marrow NOS (C96.9)
         malignant neoplasm of synovia (C49.-)

● C40   **Malignant neoplasm of bone and articular cartilage of limbs**

Use additional code to identify major osseous defect, if applicable (M89.7-)

● C40.0   **Malignant neoplasm of scapula and long bones of upper limb**

■ C40.00   Malignant neoplasm of scapula and long bones of unspecified upper limb ●

C40.01   Malignant neoplasm of scapula and long bones of right upper limb ●

C40.02   Malignant neoplasm of scapula and long bones of left upper limb ●

● C40.1   **Malignant neoplasm of short bones of upper limb**

■ C40.10   Malignant neoplasm of short bones of unspecified upper limb ●

C40.11   Malignant neoplasm of short bones of right upper limb ●

C40.12   Malignant neoplasm of short bones of left upper limb ●

● C40.2   **Malignant neoplasm of long bones of lower limb**

■ C40.20   Malignant neoplasm of long bones of unspecified lower limb ●

C40.21   Malignant neoplasm of long bones of right lower limb ●

C40.22   Malignant neoplasm of long bones of left lower limb ●

● C40.3   **Malignant neoplasm of short bones of lower limb**

■ C40.30   Malignant neoplasm of short bones of unspecified lower limb ●

C40.31   Malignant neoplasm of short bones of right lower limb ●

C40.32   Malignant neoplasm of short bones of left lower limb ●

● C40.8   **Malignant neoplasm of overlapping sites of bone and articular cartilage of limb**

■ C40.80   Malignant neoplasm of overlapping sites of bone and articular cartilage of unspecified limb ●

C40.81   Malignant neoplasm of overlapping sites of bone and articular cartilage of right limb ●

C40.82   Malignant neoplasm of overlapping sites of bone and articular cartilage of left limb ●

● C40.9   **Malignant neoplasm of unspecified bones and articular cartilage of limb**

■ C40.90   Malignant neoplasm of unspecified bones and articular cartilage of unspecified limb ●

■ C40.91   Malignant neoplasm of unspecified bones and articular cartilage of right limb ●

■ C40.92   Malignant neoplasm of unspecified bones and articular cartilage of left limb ●

● C41   **Malignant neoplasm of bone and articular cartilage of other and unspecified sites**

Excludes1   malignant neoplasm of bones of limbs (C40.-)
         malignant neoplasm of cartilage of:
           ear (C49.0)
           eyelid (C49.0)
           larynx (C32.3)
           limbs (C40.-)
           nose (C30.0)

C41.0   **Malignant neoplasm of bones of skull and face** ●
Malignant neoplasm of maxilla (superior)
Malignant neoplasm of orbital bone

Excludes2   carcinoma, any type except intraosseous or odontogenic of:
         maxillary sinus (C31.0)
         upper jaw (C03.0)
         malignant neoplasm of jaw bone (lower) (C41.1)

C41.1   **Malignant neoplasm of mandible** ●
Malignant neoplasm of inferior maxilla
Malignant neoplasm of lower jaw bone

Excludes2   carcinoma, any type except intraosseous or odontogenic of:
         jaw NOS (C03.9)
         lower (C03.1)
         malignant neoplasm of upper jaw bone (C41.0)

C41.2   **Malignant neoplasm of vertebral column** ●

Excludes1   malignant neoplasm of sacrum and coccyx (C41.4)

C41.3   **Malignant neoplasm of ribs, sternum and clavicle** ●

C41.4   **Malignant neoplasm of pelvic bones, sacrum and coccyx** ●

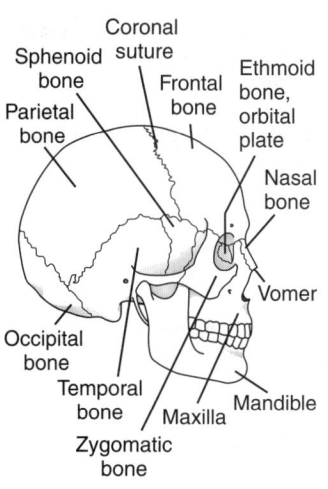

Figure 2-9 Bones of the skull.

- ■ C41.9 **Malignant neoplasm of bone and articular cartilage, unspecified** 🔧

MELANOMA AND OTHER MALIGNANT NEOPLASMS OF SKIN (C43-C44)

- ● C43 **Malignant melanoma of skin**
  - | Excludes1 | melanoma in situ (D03.-)
  - | Excludes2 | malignant melanoma of skin of genital organs (C51-C52, C60.-, C63.-)
    Merkel cell carcinoma (C4A.-)
    sites other than skin-code to malignant neoplasm of the site
  - C43.0 **Malignant melanoma of lip**
    - | Excludes1 | malignant neoplasm of vermilion border of lip (C00.0-C00.2)
  - ● C43.1 **Malignant melanoma of eyelid, including canthus**
    Canthus: Either corner of eye where upper and lower eyelids meet
    - ■ C43.10 **Malignant melanoma of unspecified eyelid, including canthus**
    - C43.11 **Malignant melanoma of right eyelid, including canthus**
    - C43.12 **Malignant melanoma of left eyelid, including canthus**

Figure 2-10 Malignant melanoma of skin. (From Goldman: Cecil Textbook of Medicine, 22nd ed. 2004, Saunders.)

Item 2–4 Malignant melanoma is a serious form of skin cancer that affects the melanocytes (pigment-forming cells) and is caused by ultraviolet (UV) rays from the sun that damage skin. It is most commonly seen in the 40- to 60-year-olds with fair skin, blue or green eyes, and red or blond hair who sunburn easily.

Melanoma can spread very rapidly and is the most deadly form of skin cancer. It is less common than other types of skin cancer. The rate of melanoma is increasing and currently is the leading cause of death from skin disease.

- ● C43.2 **Malignant melanoma of ear and external auricular canal**
  - ■ C43.20 **Malignant melanoma of unspecified ear and external auricular canal**
  - C43.21 **Malignant melanoma of right ear and external auricular canal**
  - C43.22 **Malignant melanoma of left ear and external auricular canal**
- ● C43.3 **Malignant melanoma of other and unspecified parts of face**
  - ■ C43.30 **Malignant melanoma of unspecified part of face**
  - C43.31 **Malignant melanoma of nose**
  - C43.39 **Malignant melanoma of other parts of face**
- C43.4 **Malignant melanoma of scalp and neck**
- ● C43.5 **Malignant melanoma of trunk**
  - | Excludes2 | malignant neoplasm of anus NOS (C21.0)
    malignant neoplasm of scrotum (C63.2)
  - C43.51 **Malignant melanoma of anal skin**
    Malignant melanoma of anal margin
    Malignant melanoma of perianal skin
  - C43.52 **Malignant melanoma of skin of breast**
  - C43.59 **Malignant melanoma of other part of trunk**
- ● C43.6 **Malignant melanoma of upper limb, including shoulder**
  - ■ C43.60 **Malignant melanoma of upper limb, including shoulder, unspecified side**
  - C43.61 **Malignant melanoma of right upper limb, including shoulder**
  - C43.62 **Malignant melanoma of left upper limb, including shoulder**
- ● C43.7 **Malignant melanoma of lower limb, including hip**
  - ■ C43.70 **Malignant melanoma of unspecified lower limb, including hip**
  - C43.71 **Malignant melanoma of right lower limb, including hip**
  - C43.72 **Malignant melanoma of left lower limb, including hip**
- C43.8 **Malignant melanoma of overlapping sites of skin**
- ■ C43.9 **Malignant melanoma of skin, unspecified**
  Malignant melanoma of unspecified site of skin
  Melanoma (malignant) NOS

- C4A **Merkel cell carcinoma**
  - C4A.0 **Merkel cell carcinoma of lip**
    - | Excludes1 | malignant neoplasm of vermilion border of lip (C00.0-C00.2)
  - ● C4A.1 **Merkel cell carcinoma of eyelid, including canthus**
    - ■ C4A.10 **Merkel cell carcinoma of unspecified eyelid, including canthus**
    - C4A.11 **Merkel cell carcinoma of right eyelid, including canthus**
    - C4A.12 **Merkel cell carcinoma of left eyelid, including canthus**
  - ● C4A.2 **Merkel cell carcinoma of ear and external auricular canal**
    - ■ C4A.20 **Merkel cell carcinoma of unspecified ear and external auricular canal**
    - C4A.21 **Merkel cell carcinoma of right ear and external auricular canal**
    - C4A.22 **Merkel cell carcinoma of left ear and external auricular canal**

CHAPTER 2 (C00-D49)

N Newborn Age: 0 **P** Pediatric Age: 0–17 **M** Maternity DX: 12–55 **A** Adult Age: 15–124 ♀ Females Only ♂ Males Only

🔧 Complication\Comorbidity 🔧 Major C\C 🔧 Present on Admission Requirement 🔧 Hospital-Acquired Condition

829

- ● C4A.3 Merkel cell carcinoma of other and unspecified parts of face
  - 🔲 C4A.30 Merkel cell carcinoma of unspecified part of face
  - C4A.31 Merkel cell carcinoma of nose
  - C4A.39 Merkel cell carcinoma of other parts of face
- C4A.4 Merkel cell carcinoma of scalp and neck
- ● C4A.5 Merkel cell carcinoma of trunk
  - **Excludes2** malignant neoplasm of anus NOS (C21.0)
    malignant neoplasm of scrotum (C63.2)
  - C4A.51 Merkel cell carcinoma of anal skin
    Merkel cell carcinoma of anal margin
    Merkel cell carcinoma of perianal skin
  - C4A.52 Merkel cell carcinoma of skin of breast
  - C4A.59 Merkel cell carcinoma of other part of trunk
- ● C4A.6 Merkel cell carcinoma of upper limb, including shoulder
  - 🔲 C4A.60 Merkel cell carcinoma of unspecified upper limb, including shoulder
  - C4A.61 Merkel cell carcinoma of right upper limb, including shoulder
  - C4A.62 Merkel cell carcinoma of left upper limb, including shoulder
- ● C4A.7 Merkel cell carcinoma of lower limb, including hip
  - 🔲 C4A.70 Merkel cell carcinoma of unspecified lower limb, including hip
  - C4A.71 Merkel cell carcinoma of right lower limb, including hip
  - C4A.72 Merkel cell carcinoma of left lower limb, including hip
- C4A.8 Merkel cell carcinoma of overlapping sites
- 🔲 C4A.9 Merkel cell carcinoma, unspecified
  Merkel cell carcinoma of unspecified site
  Merkel cell carcinoma NOS

- ● C44 Other and unspecified malignant neoplasm of skin
  - **Includes** malignant neoplasm of sebaceous glands
    malignant neoplasm of sweat glands
  - **Excludes1** Kaposi's sarcoma of skin (C46.0)
    malignant melanoma of skin (C43.-)
    malignant neoplasm of skin of genital organs (C51-C52, C60.-, C63.2)
    Merkel cell carcinoma (C4A.-)
  - ● C44.0 Other and unspecified malignant neoplasm of skin of lip
    - **Excludes1** malignant neoplasm of lip (C00.-)
    - 🔲 C44.00 Unspecified malignant neoplasm of skin of lip
    - C44.01 Basal cell carcinoma of skin of lip
    - C44.02 Squamous cell carcinoma of skin of lip
    - C44.09 Other specified malignant neoplasm of skin of lip
  - ● C44.1 Other and unspecified malignant neoplasm of skin of eyelid, including canthus
    - **Excludes1** connective tissue of eyelid (C49.0)
    - ● C44.10 Unspecified malignant neoplasm of skin of eyelid, including canthus
      - 🔲 C44.101 Unspecified malignant neoplasm of skin of unspecified eyelid, including canthus

- 🔲 C44.102 Unspecified malignant neoplasm of skin of right eyelid, including canthus
- 🔲 C44.109 Unspecified malignant neoplasm of skin of left eyelid, including canthus
- ● C44.11 Basal cell carcinoma of skin of eyelid, including canthus
  - 🔲 C44.111 Basal cell carcinoma of skin of unspecified eyelid, including canthus
  - C44.112 Basal cell carcinoma of skin of right eyelid, including canthus
  - C44.119 Basal cell carcinoma of skin of left eyelid, including canthus
- ● C44.12 Squamous cell carcinoma of skin of eyelid, including canthus
  - 🔲 C44.121 Squamous cell carcinoma of skin of unspecified eyelid, including canthus
  - C44.122 Squamous cell carcinoma of skin of right eyelid, including canthus
  - C44.129 Squamous cell carcinoma of skin of left eyelid, including canthus
- ● C44.19 Other specified malignant neoplasm of skin of eyelid, including canthus
  - 🔲 C44.191 Other specified malignant neoplasm of skin of unspecified eyelid, including canthus
  - C44.192 Other specified malignant neoplasm of skin of right eyelid, including canthus
  - C44.199 Other specified malignant neoplasm of skin of left eyelid, including canthus
- ● C44.2 Other and unspecified malignant neoplasm of skin of ear and external auricular canal
  - **Excludes1** connective tissue of ear (C49.0)
  - ● C44.20 Unspecified malignant neoplasm of skin of ear and external auricular canal
    - 🔲 C44.201 Unspecified malignant neoplasm of skin of unspecified ear and external auricular canal
    - C44.202 Unspecified malignant neoplasm of skin of right ear and external auricular canal
    - C44.209 Unspecified malignant neoplasm of skin of left ear and external auricular canal
  - ● C44.21 Basal cell carcinoma of skin of ear and external auricular canal
    - 🔲 C44.211 Basal cell carcinoma of skin of unspecified ear and external auricular canal
    - C44.212 Basal cell carcinoma of skin of right ear and external auricular canal
    - C44.219 Basal cell carcinoma of skin of left ear and external auricular canal

● C44.22 Squamous cell carcinoma of skin of ear and external auricular canal

   ■ C44.221 Squamous cell carcinoma of skin of unspecified ear and external auricular canal

   C44.222 Squamous cell carcinoma of skin of right ear and external auricular canal

   C44.229 Squamous cell carcinoma of skin of left ear and external auricular canal

● C44.29 Other specified malignant neoplasm of skin of ear and external auricular canal

   ■ C44.291 Other specified malignant neoplasm of skin of unspecified ear and external auricular canal

   C44.292 Other specified malignant neoplasm of skin of right ear and external auricular canal

   C44.299 Other specified malignant neoplasm of skin of left ear and external auricular canal

● C44.3 Other and unspecified malignant neoplasm of skin of other and unspecified parts of face

● C44.30 Unspecified malignant neoplasm of skin of other and unspecified parts of face

   ■ C44.300 Unspecified malignant neoplasm of skin of unspecified part of face

   ■ C44.301 Unspecified malignant neoplasm of skin of nose

   ■ C44.309 Unspecified malignant neoplasm of skin of other parts of face

● C44.31 Basal cell carcinoma of skin of other and unspecified parts of face

   ■ C44.310 Basal cell carcinoma of skin of unspecified parts of face

   C44.311 Basal cell carcinoma of skin of nose

   C44.319 Basal cell carcinoma of skin of other parts of face

● C44.32 Squamous cell carcinoma of skin of other and unspecified parts of face

   ■ C44.320 Squamous cell carcinoma of skin of unspecified parts of face

   C44.321 Squamous cell carcinoma of skin of nose

   C44.329 Squamous cell carcinoma of skin of other parts of face

● C44.39 Other specified malignant neoplasm of skin of other and unspecified parts of face

   ■ C44.390 Other specified malignant neoplasm of skin of unspecified parts of face

   C44.391 Other specified malignant neoplasm of skin of nose

   C44.399 Other specified malignant neoplasm of skin of other parts of face

● C44.4 Other and unspecified malignant neoplasm of skin of scalp and neck

   ■ C44.40 Unspecified malignant neoplasm of skin of scalp and neck

   C44.41 Basal cell carcinoma of skin of scalp and neck

   C44.42 Squamous cell carcinoma of skin of scalp and neck

   C44.49 Other specified malignant neoplasm of skin of scalp and neck

● C44.5 Other and unspecified malignant neoplasm of skin of trunk

   | Excludes1 | anus NOS (C21.0)
                  scrotum (C63.2)

● C44.50 Unspecified malignant neoplasm of skin of trunk

   ■ C44.500 Unspecified malignant neoplasm of anal skin
              Unspecified malignant neoplasm of anal margin
              Unspecified malignant neoplasm of perianal skin

   ■ C44.501 Unspecified malignant neoplasm of skin of breast

   ■ C44.509 Unspecified malignant neoplasm of skin of other part of trunk

● C44.51 Basal cell carcinoma of skin of trunk

   C44.510 Basal cell carcinoma of anal skin
            Basal cell carcinoma of anal margin
            Basal cell carcinoma of perianal skin

   C44.511 Basal cell carcinoma of skin of breast

   C44.519 Basal cell carcinoma of skin of other part of trunk

● C44.52 Squamous cell carcinoma of skin of trunk

   C44.520 Squamous cell carcinoma of anal skin
            Squamous cell carcinoma of anal margin
            Squamous cell carcinoma of perianal skin

   C44.521 Squamous cell carcinoma of skin of breast

   C44.529 Squamous cell carcinoma of skin of other part of trunk

● C44.59 Other specified malignant neoplasm of skin of trunk

   C44.590 Other specified malignant neoplasm of anal skin
            Other specified malignant neoplasm of anal margin
            Other specified malignant neoplasm of perianal skin

   C44.591 Other specified malignant neoplasm of skin of breast

   C44.599 Other specified malignant neoplasm of skin of other part of trunk

● **C44.6　Other and unspecified malignant neoplasm of skin of upper limb, including shoulder**

  ● **C44.60　Unspecified malignant neoplasm of skin of upper limb, including shoulder**

    ■ C44.601　Unspecified malignant neoplasm of skin of unspecified upper limb, including shoulder

    ■ C44.602　Unspecified malignant neoplasm of skin of right upper limb, including shoulder

    ■ C44.609　Unspecified malignant neoplasm of skin of left upper limb, including shoulder

  ● **C44.61　Basal cell carcinoma of skin of upper limb, including shoulder**

    ■ C44.611　Basal cell carcinoma of skin of unspecified upper limb, including shoulder

    C44.612　Basal cell carcinoma of skin of right upper limb, including shoulder

    C44.619　Basal cell carcinoma of skin of left upper limb, including shoulder

  ● **C44.62　Squamous cell carcinoma of skin of upper limb, including shoulder**

    ■ C44.621　Squamous cell carcinoma of skin of unspecified upper limb, including shoulder

    C44.622　Squamous cell carcinoma of skin of right upper limb, including shoulder

    C44.629　Squamous cell carcinoma of skin of left upper limb, including shoulder

  ● **C44.69　Other specified malignant neoplasm of skin of upper limb, including shoulder**

    ■ C44.691　Other specified malignant neoplasm of skin of unspecified upper limb, including shoulder

    C44.692　Other specified malignant neoplasm of skin of right upper limb, including shoulder

    C44.699　Other specified malignant neoplasm of skin of left upper limb, including shoulder

● **C44.7　Other and unspecified malignant neoplasm of skin of lower limb, including hip**

  ● **C44.70　Unspecified malignant neoplasm of skin of lower limb, including hip**

    ■ C44.701　Unspecified malignant neoplasm of skin of unspecified lower limb, including hip

    ■ C44.702　Unspecified malignant neoplasm of skin of right lower limb, including hip

    ■ C44.709　Unspecified malignant neoplasm of skin of left lower limb, including hip

  ● **C44.71　Basal cell carcinoma of skin of lower limb, including hip**

    ■ C44.711　Basal cell carcinoma of skin of unspecified lower limb, including hip

    C44.712　Basal cell carcinoma of skin of right lower limb, including hip

    C44.719　Basal cell carcinoma of skin of left lower limb, including hip

  ● **C44.72　Squamous cell carcinoma of skin of lower limb, including hip**

    ■ C44.721　Squamous cell carcinoma of skin of unspecified lower limb, including hip

    C44.722　Squamous cell carcinoma of skin of right lower limb, including hip

    C44.729　Squamous cell carcinoma of skin of left lower limb, including hip

  ● **C44.79　Other specified malignant neoplasm of skin of lower limb, including hip**

    ■ C44.791　Other specified malignant neoplasm of skin of unspecified lower limb, including hip

    C44.792　Other specified malignant neoplasm of skin of right lower limb, including hip

    C44.799　Other specified malignant neoplasm of skin of left lower limb, including hip

● **C44.8　Other and unspecified malignant neoplasm of overlapping sites of skin**

  ■ C44.80　Unspecified malignant neoplasm of overlapping sites of skin

  C44.81　Basal cell carcinoma of overlapping sites of skin

  C44.82　Squamous cell carcinoma of overlapping sites of skin

  C44.89　Other specified malignant neoplasm of overlapping sites of skin

● **C44.9　Other and unspecified malignant neoplasm of skin, unspecified**

  ■ C44.90　Unspecified malignant neoplasm of skin, unspecified
    Malignant neoplasm of unspecified site of skin

  ■ C44.91　Basal cell carcinoma of skin, unspecified

  ■ C44.92　Squamous cell carcinoma of skin, unspecified

  ■ C44.99　Other specified malignant neoplasm of skin, unspecified

---

MALIGNANT NEOPLASMS OF MESOTHELIAL AND SOFT TISSUE (C45-C49)

● **C45　Mesothelioma**
Malignant cells develop in protective lining that covers internal organs (mesothelium) caused by exposure to asbestos

  C45.0　Mesothelioma of pleura 🔗
    | Excludes1 | other malignant neoplasm of pleura (C38.4)

  C45.1　Mesothelioma of peritoneum 🔗
    Mesothelioma of cul-de-sac
    Mesothelioma of mesentery
    Mesothelioma of mesocolon
    Mesothelioma of omentum
    Mesothelioma of peritoneum (parietal) (pelvic)
    | Excludes1 | other malignant neoplasm of soft tissue of peritoneum (C48.-)

  C45.2　Mesothelioma of pericardium 🔗
    | Excludes1 | other malignant neoplasm of pericardium (C38.0)

  C45.7　Mesothelioma of other sites

  ■ **C45.9　Mesothelioma, unspecified**

● Unacceptable Principal Diagnosis　　● Use Additional Character(s)　　■ Unspecified　　▶ Manifestation Code

832　　**OGCR** Official Guidelines for Coding and Reporting　| Excludes 1 |　| Excludes 2 |　Includes　Use additional　Code first　Code also

CHAPTER 2 (C00-D49)

● **C46   Kaposi's sarcoma**

> *Code first* any human immunodeficiency virus [HIV]
> disease (B20)

     C46.0   Kaposi's sarcoma of skin 🔹

     C46.1   Kaposi's sarcoma of soft tissue 🔹
         Kaposi's sarcoma of blood vessel
         Kaposi's sarcoma of connective tissue
         Kaposi's sarcoma of fascia
         Kaposi's sarcoma of ligament
         Kaposi's sarcoma of lymphatic(s) NEC
         Kaposi's sarcoma of muscle

         | Excludes2 | Kaposi's sarcoma of lymph glands and nodes (C46.3) |

     C46.2   Kaposi's sarcoma of palate 🔹

     C46.3   Kaposi's sarcoma of lymph nodes 🔹

     C46.4   Kaposi's sarcoma of gastrointestinal sites 🔹

● **C46.5   Kaposi's sarcoma of lung**

    ◾ **C46.50   Kaposi's sarcoma of unspecified lung** 🔹

     C46.51   Kaposi's sarcoma of right lung 🔹

     C46.52   Kaposi's sarcoma of left lung 🔹

     C46.7   Kaposi's sarcoma of other sites 🔹

◾ **C46.9   Kaposi's sarcoma, unspecified** 🔹
         Kaposi's sarcoma of unspecified site

● **C47   Malignant neoplasm of peripheral nerves and autonomic nervous system**

     | Includes | malignant neoplasm of sympathetic and parasympathetic nerves and ganglia |

     | Excludes1 | Kaposi's sarcoma of soft tissue (C46.1) |

     C47.0   Malignant neoplasm of peripheral nerves of head, face and neck 🔹

         | Excludes1 | malignant neoplasm of peripheral nerves of orbit (C69.6-) |

● **C47.1   Malignant neoplasm of peripheral nerves of upper limb, including shoulder**

    ◾ **C47.10   Malignant neoplasm of peripheral nerves of unspecified upper limb, including shoulder** 🔹

     C47.11   Malignant neoplasm of peripheral nerves of right upper limb, including shoulder 🔹

     C47.12   Malignant neoplasm of peripheral nerves of left upper limb, including shoulder 🔹

● **C47.2   Malignant neoplasm of peripheral nerves of lower limb, including hip**

    ◾ **C47.20   Malignant neoplasm of peripheral nerves of unspecified lower limb, including hip** 🔹

     C47.21   Malignant neoplasm of peripheral nerves of right lower limb, including hip 🔹

     C47.22   Malignant neoplasm of peripheral nerves of left lower limb, including hip 🔹

     C47.3   Malignant neoplasm of peripheral nerves of thorax 🔹

     C47.4   Malignant neoplasm of peripheral nerves of abdomen 🔹

     C47.5   Malignant neoplasm of peripheral nerves of pelvis 🔹

◾ **C47.6   Malignant neoplasm of peripheral nerves of trunk, unspecified** 🔹
         Malignant neoplasm of peripheral nerves of unspecified part of trunk

     C47.8   Malignant neoplasm of overlapping sites of peripheral nerves and autonomic nervous system 🔹

◾ **C47.9   Malignant neoplasm of peripheral nerves and autonomic nervous system, unspecified** 🔹
         Malignant neoplasm of unspecified site of peripheral nerves and autonomic nervous system

● **C48   Malignant neoplasm of retroperitoneum and peritoneum**

     | Excludes1 | Kaposi's sarcoma of connective tissue (C46.1)
 mesothelioma (C45.-) |

     C48.0   Malignant neoplasm of retroperitoneum 🔹
         Behind/outside of peritoneum

     C48.1   Malignant neoplasm of specified parts of peritoneum 🔹
         Serous membrane lining abdominopelvic walls and covering viscera
         Malignant neoplasm of cul-de-sac
         Malignant neoplasm of mesentery
         Malignant neoplasm of mesocolon
         Malignant neoplasm of omentum
         Malignant neoplasm of parietal peritoneum
         Malignant neoplasm of pelvic peritoneum

◾ **C48.2   Malignant neoplasm of peritoneum, unspecified** 🔹

     C48.8   Malignant neoplasm of overlapping sites of retroperitoneum and peritoneum 🔹

CHAPTER 2 (C00-D49)

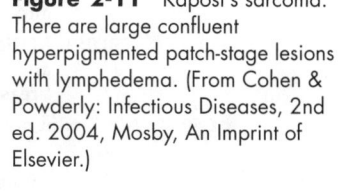

Figure 2-11   Kaposi's sarcoma. There are large confluent hyperpigmented patch-stage lesions with lymphedema. (From Cohen & Powderly: Infectious Diseases, 2nd ed. 2004, Mosby, An Imprint of Elsevier.)

Item 2–5   Kaposi's sarcoma is a cancer that causes patches of abnormal tissue to grow under the skin; in the lining of the mouth, nose, and throat; or in other organs, often beginning and spreading to other organs. Patients who have had organ transplants or patients with AIDS are at high risk for this malignancy.

CHAPTER 2 (C00-D49)

● **C49   Malignant neoplasm of other connective and soft tissue**

> **Includes**   malignant neoplasm of blood vessel
> malignant neoplasm of bursa
> malignant neoplasm of cartilage
> malignant neoplasm of fascia
> malignant neoplasm of fat
> malignant neoplasm of ligament, except uterine
> malignant neoplasm of lymphatic vessel
> malignant neoplasm of muscle
> malignant neoplasm of synovia
> malignant neoplasm of tendon (sheath)

> **Excludes1**   malignant neoplasm of cartilage (of):
> articular (C40-C41)
> larynx (C32.3)
> nose (C30.0)
> malignant neoplasm of connective tissue of breast (C50-)

> **Excludes2**   Kaposi's sarcoma of soft tissue (C46.1)
> malignant neoplasm of heart (C38.0)
> malignant neoplasm of peripheral nerves and autonomic nervous system (C47.-)
> malignant neoplasm of peritoneum (C48.2)
> malignant neoplasm of retroperitoneum (C48.0)
> malignant neoplasm of uterine ligament (C57.3)
> mesothelioma (C45.-)

C49.0   **Malignant neoplasm of connective and soft tissue of head, face and neck** 🔊
> Malignant neoplasm of connective tissue of ear
> Malignant neoplasm of connective tissue of eyelid
> **Excludes1**   connective tissue of orbit (C69.6-)

● **C49.1**   **Malignant neoplasm of connective and soft tissue of upper limb, including shoulder**

   ■ **C49.10**   Malignant neoplasm of connective and soft tissue of unspecified upper limb, including shoulder 🔊

   C49.11   Malignant neoplasm of connective and soft tissue of right upper limb, including shoulder 🔊

   C49.12   Malignant neoplasm of connective and soft tissue of left upper limb, including shoulder 🔊

● **C49.2**   **Malignant neoplasm of connective and soft tissue of lower limb, including hip**

   ■ **C49.20**   Malignant neoplasm of connective and soft tissue of unspecified lower limb, including hip 🔊

   C49.21   Malignant neoplasm of connective and soft tissue of right lower limb, including hip 🔊

   C49.22   Malignant neoplasm of connective and soft tissue of left lower limb, including hip 🔊

C49.3   **Malignant neoplasm of connective and soft tissue of thorax** 🔊
> Malignant neoplasm of axilla
> Malignant neoplasm of diaphragm
> Malignant neoplasm of great vessels
> **Excludes1**   malignant neoplasm of breast (C50.-)
> malignant neoplasm of heart (C38.0)
> malignant neoplasm of mediastinum (C38.1-C38.3)
> malignant neoplasm of thymus (C37)

C49.4   **Malignant neoplasm of connective and soft tissue of abdomen** 🔊
> Malignant neoplasm of abdominal wall
> Malignant neoplasm of hypochondrium

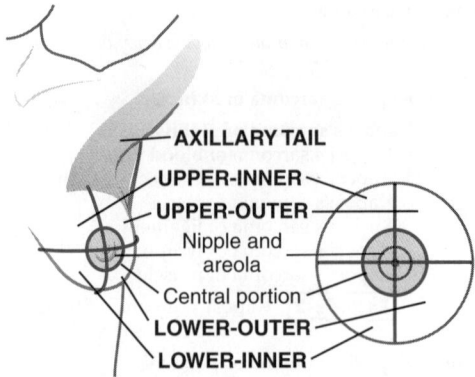

Figure 2-12   Femal breast quadrants and axillary tail.

C49.5   **Malignant neoplasm of connective and soft tissue of pelvis** 🔊
> Malignant neoplasm of buttock
> Malignant neoplasm of groin
> Malignant neoplasm of perineum

■ **C49.6**   **Malignant neoplasm of connective and soft tissue of trunk, unspecified** 🔊
> Malignant neoplasm of back NOS

C49.8   **Malignant neoplasm of overlapping sites of connective and soft tissue** 🔊
> Primary malignant neoplasm of two or more contiguous sites of connective and soft tissue

■ **C49.9**   **Malignant neoplasm of connective and soft tissue, unspecified** 🔊

MALIGNANT NEOPLASMS OF BREAST (C50)

● **C50   Malignant neoplasm of breast**

> **Includes**   connective tissue of breast
> Paget's disease of breast
> Paget's disease of nipple
> *Intraductal carcinoma of breast characterized by eczema-like inflammatory skin changes*

> **Use additional** code to identify estrogen receptor status (Z17.0, Z17.1)
> **Excludes1**   skin of breast (C44.501, C44.511, C44.521, C44.591)

● **C50.0**   **Malignant neoplasm of nipple and areola**

   ● **C50.01**   Malignant neoplasm of nipple and areola, female

     C50.011   Malignant neoplasm of nipple and areola, right female breast ♀

     C50.012   Malignant neoplasm of nipple and areola, left female breast ♀

     ■ **C50.019**   Malignant neoplasm of nipple and areola, unspecified female breast ♀

   ● **C50.02**   Malignant neoplasm of nipple and areola, male

     C50.021   Malignant neoplasm of nipple and areola, right male breast ♂

     C50.022   Malignant neoplasm of nipple and areola, left male breast ♂

     ■ **C50.029**   Malignant neoplasm of nipple and areola, unspecified male breast ♂

● Unacceptable Principal Diagnosis   ● Use Additional Character(s)   ■ Unspecified   ▶ Manifestation Code
OGCR Official Guidelines for Coding and Reporting | Excludes 1 | Excludes 2 | Includes | Use additional | Code first | Code also |

● **C50.1**   Malignant neoplasm of central portion of breast
  ● **C50.11**   Malignant neoplasm of central portion of breast, female
    C50.111   Malignant neoplasm of central portion of right female breast ♀
    C50.112   Malignant neoplasm of central portion of left female breast ♀
    ■ **C50.119**   Malignant neoplasm of central portion of unspecified female breast ♀
  ● **C50.12**   Malignant neoplasm of central portion of breast, male
    C50.121   Malignant neoplasm of central portion of right male breast ♂
    C50.122   Malignant neoplasm of central portion of left male breast ♂
    ■ **C50.129**   Malignant neoplasm of central portion of unspecified male breast ♂
● **C50.2**   Malignant neoplasm of upper-inner quadrant of breast
  ● **C50.21**   Malignant neoplasm of upper-inner quadrant of breast, female
    C50.211   Malignant neoplasm of upper-inner quadrant of right female breast ♀
    C50.212   Malignant neoplasm of upper-inner quadrant of left female breast ♀
    ■ **C50.219**   Malignant neoplasm of upper-inner quadrant of unspecified female breast ♀
  ● **C50.22**   Malignant neoplasm of upper-inner quadrant of breast, male
    C50.221   Malignant neoplasm of upper-inner quadrant of right male breast ♂
    C50.222   Malignant neoplasm of upper-inner quadrant of left male breast ♂
    ■ **C50.229**   Malignant neoplasm of upper-inner quadrant of unspecified male breast ♂
● **C50.3**   Malignant neoplasm of lower-inner quadrant of breast
  ● **C50.31**   Malignant neoplasm of lower-inner quadrant of breast, female
    C50.311   Malignant neoplasm of lower-inner quadrant of right female breast ♀
    C50.312   Malignant neoplasm of lower-inner quadrant of left female breast ♀
    ■ **C50.319**   Malignant neoplasm of lower-inner quadrant of unspecified female breast ♀
  ● **C50.32**   Malignant neoplasm of lower-inner quadrant of breast, male
    C50.321   Malignant neoplasm of lower-inner quadrant of right male breast ♂
    C50.322   Malignant neoplasm of lower-inner quadrant of left male breast ♂
    ■ **C50.329**   Malignant neoplasm of lower-inner quadrant of unspecified male breast ♂

● **C50.4**   Malignant neoplasm of upper-outer quadrant of breast
  ● **C50.41**   Malignant neoplasm of upper-outer quadrant of breast, female
    C50.411   Malignant neoplasm of upper-outer quadrant of right female breast ♀
    C50.412   Malignant neoplasm of upper-outer quadrant of left female breast ♀
    ■ **C50.419**   Malignant neoplasm of upper-outer quadrant of unspecified female breast ♀
  ● **C50.42**   Malignant neoplasm of upper-outer quadrant of breast, male
    C50.421   Malignant neoplasm of upper-outer quadrant of right male breast ♂
    C50.422   Malignant neoplasm of upper-outer quadrant of left male breast ♂
    ■ **C50.429**   Malignant neoplasm of upper-outer quadrant of unspecified male breast ♂
● **C50.5**   Malignant neoplasm of lower-outer quadrant of breast
  ● **C50.51**   Malignant neoplasm of lower-outer quadrant of breast, female
    C50.511   Malignant neoplasm of lower-outer quadrant of right female breast ♀
    C50.512   Malignant neoplasm of lower-outer quadrant of left female breast ♀
    ■ **C50.519**   Malignant neoplasm of lower-outer quadrant of unspecified female breast ♀
  ● **C50.52**   Malignant neoplasm of lower-outer quadrant of breast, male
    C50.521   Malignant neoplasm of lower-outer quadrant of right male breast ♂
    C50.522   Malignant neoplasm of lower-outer quadrant of left male breast ♂
    ■ **C50.529**   Malignant neoplasm of lower-outer quadrant of unspecified male breast ♂
● **C50.6**   Malignant neoplasm of axillary tail of breast
  ● **C50.61**   Malignant neoplasm of axillary tail of breast, female
    C50.611   Malignant neoplasm of axillary tail of right female breast ♀
    C50.612   Malignant neoplasm of axillary tail of left female breast ♀
    ■ **C50.619**   Malignant neoplasm of axillary tail of unspecified female breast ♀
  ● **C50.62**   Malignant neoplasm of axillary tail of breast, male
    C50.621   Malignant neoplasm of axillary tail of right male breast ♂
    C50.622   Malignant neoplasm of axillary tail of left male breast ♂
    ■ **C50.629**   Malignant neoplasm of axillary tail of unspecified male breast ♂

CHAPTER 2 (C00-D49)

N Newborn Age: 0   **P** Pediatric Age: 0–17   **M** Maternity DX: 12–55   **A** Adult Age: 15–124   ♀ Females Only   ♂ Males Only
Complication\Comorbidity   Major C\C   Present on Admission Requirement   Hospital-Acquired Condition
835

CHAPTER 2 (C00-D49)

- ● C50.8   Malignant neoplasm of overlapping sites of breast
  - ● C50.81   Malignant neoplasm of overlapping sites of breast, female
    - C50.811   Malignant neoplasm of overlapping sites of right female breast ♀
    - C50.812   Malignant neoplasm of overlapping sites of left female breast ♀
    - ■ C50.819   Malignant neoplasm of overlapping sites of unspecified female breast ♀
  - ● C50.82   Malignant neoplasm of overlapping sites of breast, male
    - C50.821   Malignant neoplasm of overlapping sites of right male breast ♂
    - C50.822   Malignant neoplasm of overlapping sites of left male breast ♂
    - ■ C50.829   Malignant neoplasm of overlapping sites of unspecified male breast ♂
- ● C50.9   Malignant neoplasm of breast of unspecified site
  - ● C50.91   Malignant neoplasm of breast of unspecified site, female
    - ■ C50.911   Malignant neoplasm of unspecified site of right female breast ♀
    - ■ C50.912   Malignant neoplasm of unspecified site of left female breast ♀
    - ■ C50.919   Malignant neoplasm of unspecified site of unspecified female breast ♀
  - ● C50.92   Malignant neoplasm of breast of unspecified site, male
    - ■ C50.921   Malignant neoplasm of unspecified site of right male breast ♂
    - ■ C50.922   Malignant neoplasm of unspecified site of left male breast ♂
    - ■ C50.929   Malignant neoplasm of unspecified site of unspecified male breast ♂

MALIGNANT NEOPLASMS OF FEMALE GENITAL ORGANS (C51-C58)

> **Includes**   malignant neoplasm of skin of female genital organs

- ● C51   Malignant neoplasm of vulva
  > **Excludes1**   carcinoma in situ of vulva (D07.1)
  - C51.0   Malignant neoplasm of labium majus ♀
    Outer folds of skin external female genitalia
    Malignant neoplasm of Bartholin's [greater vestibular] gland
  - C51.1   Malignant neoplasm of labium minus ♀
    Two inner folds surrounding vulva in female genitalia
  - C51.2   Malignant neoplasm of clitoris ♀
  - C51.8   Malignant neoplasm of overlapping sites of vulva ♀
  - ■ C51.9   Malignant neoplasm of vulva, unspecified ♀
    Malignant neoplasm of external female genitalia NOS
    Malignant neoplasm of pudendum

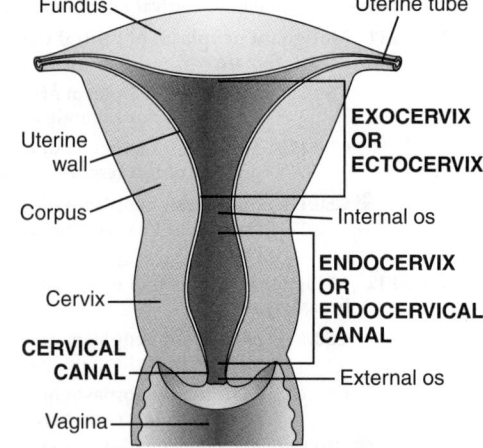

Figure 2-13   Cervix uteri.

- C52   Malignant neoplasm of vagina ♀
  > **Excludes1**   carcinoma in situ of vagina (D07.2)
- ● C53   Malignant neoplasm of cervix uteri
  > **Excludes1**   carcinoma in situ of cervix uteri (D06.-)
  - C53.0   Malignant neoplasm of endocervix ♀
    Inside the cervix
  - C53.1   Malignant neoplasm of exocervix ♀
    Outside the cervix
  - C53.8   Malignant neoplasm of overlapping sites of cervix uteri ♀
  - ■ C53.9   Malignant neoplasm of cervix uteri, unspecified ♀
- ● C54   Malignant neoplasm of corpus uteri
  - C54.0   Malignant neoplasm of isthmus uteri ♀
    Constricted part of uterus between cervix and body
    Malignant neoplasm of lower uterine segment
  - C54.1   Malignant neoplasm of endometrium ♀
    Lining of uterus
  - C54.2   Malignant neoplasm of myometrium ♀
    Middle layer of uterine wall consisting of smooth muscle supporting stromal and vascular tissue
  - C54.3   Malignant neoplasm of fundus uteri ♀
    Top rounded portion of uterus
  - C54.8   Malignant neoplasm of overlapping sites of corpus uteri ♀
    Main body of uterus
  - ■ C54.9   Malignant neoplasm of corpus uteri, unspecified ♀
- ■ C55   Malignant neoplasm of uterus, part unspecified ♀
- ● C56   Malignant neoplasm of ovary
  > Use additional code to identify any functional activity
  - C56.1   Malignant neoplasm of right ovary ♀
  - C56.2   Malignant neoplasm of left ovary ♀
  - ■ C56.9   Malignant neoplasm of unspecified ovary ♀
- ● C57   Malignant neoplasm of other and unspecified female genital organs
  - ● C57.0   Malignant neoplasm of fallopian tube
    Malignant neoplasm of oviduct
    Malignant neoplasm of uterine tube
    - ■ C57.00   Malignant neoplasm of unspecified fallopian tube ♀
    - C57.01   Malignant neoplasm of right fallopian tube ♀
    - C57.02   Malignant neoplasm of left fallopian tube ♀

● Unacceptable Principal Diagnosis   ● Use Additional Character(s)   ■ Unspecified   ▶ Manifestation Code

OGCR Official Guidelines for Coding and Reporting   Excludes 1   Excludes 2   Includes   Use additional   Code first   Code also

● C57.1　Malignant neoplasm of broad ligament

　　■ C57.10　Malignant neoplasm of unspecified broad ligament ♀

　　　C57.11　Malignant neoplasm of right broad ligament ♀

　　　C57.12　Malignant neoplasm of left broad ligament ♀

● C57.2　Malignant neoplasm of round ligament

　　■ C57.20　Malignant neoplasm of unspecified round ligament ♀

　　　C57.21　Malignant neoplasm of right round ligament ♀

　　　C57.22　Malignant neoplasm of left round ligament ♀

　C57.3　Malignant neoplasm of parametrium ♀
　　　　Malignant neoplasm of uterine ligament NOS

■ C57.4　Malignant neoplasm of uterine adnexa, unspecified ♀

　C57.7　Malignant neoplasm of other specified female genital organs ♀
　　　　Malignant neoplasm of wolffian body or duct

　C57.8　Malignant neoplasm of overlapping sites of female genital organs ♀
　　　　Primary malignant neoplasm of two or more contiguous sites of the female genital organs whose point of origin cannot be determined
　　　　Primary tubo-ovarian malignant neoplasm whose point of origin cannot be determined
　　　　Primary utero-ovarian malignant neoplasm whose point of origin cannot be determined

■ C57.9　Malignant neoplasm of female genital organ, unspecified ♀
　　　　Malignant neoplasm of female genitourinary tract NOS

C58　Malignant neoplasm of placenta ♀

　　| **Includes** | choriocarcinoma NOS |
　　| | chorionepithelioma NOS |

Excludes1	chorioadenoma (destruens) (D39.2)
	hydatidiform mole NOS (O01.9)
	invasive hydatidiform mole (D39.2)
	male choriocarcinoma NOS (C62.9-)
	malignant hydatidiform mole (D39.2)

MALIGNANT NEOPLASMS OF MALE GENITAL ORGANS (C60-C63)

　　| **Includes** | malignant neoplasm of skin of male genital organs |

● C60　Malignant neoplasm of penis

　C60.0　Malignant neoplasm of prepuce ♂
　　　　Malignant neoplasm of foreskin

　C60.1　Malignant neoplasm of glans penis ♂

　C60.2　Malignant neoplasm of body of penis ♂
　　　　Malignant neoplasm of corpus cavernosum

　C60.8　Malignant neoplasm of overlapping sites of penis ♂

■ C60.9　Malignant neoplasm of penis, unspecified ♂
　　　　Malignant neoplasm of skin of penis NOS

C61　Malignant neoplasm of prostate ♂

　　| **Excludes1** | malignant neoplasm of seminal vesicle (C63.7) |

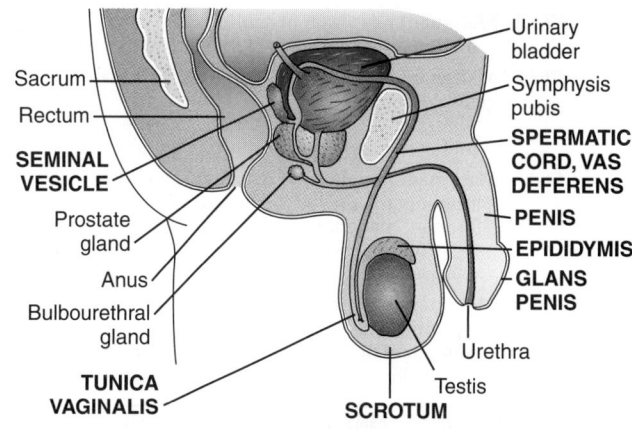

Figure 2-14　Penis and other male genital organs.

● C62　Malignant neoplasm of testis

　　Use additional code to identify any functional activity.

　● C62.0　Malignant neoplasm of undescended testis
　　　　Malignant neoplasm of ectopic testis
　　　　Malignant neoplasm of retained testis

　　■ C62.00　Malignant neoplasm of unspecified undescended testis ♂

　　　C62.01　Malignant neoplasm of undescended right testis ♂

　　　C62.02　Malignant neoplasm of undescended left testis ♂

　● C62.1　Malignant neoplasm of descended testis
　　　　Malignant neoplasm of scrotal testis

　　■ C62.10　Malignant neoplasm of unspecified descended testis, unspecified side ♂

　　　C62.11　Malignant neoplasm of descended right testis ♂

　　　C62.12　Malignant neoplasm of descended left testis ♂

　● C62.9　Malignant neoplasm of testis, unspecified whether descended or undescended

　　■ C62.90　Malignant neoplasm of unspecified testis, unspecified whether descended or undescended ♂
　　　　Malignant neoplasm of testis NOS

　　■ C62.91　Malignant neoplasm of right testis, unspecified whether descended or undescended ♂

　　■ C62.92　Malignant neoplasm of left testis, unspecified whether descended or undescended ♂

● C63　Malignant neoplasm of other and unspecified male genital organs

　● C63.0　Malignant neoplasm of epididymis

　　■ C63.00　Malignant neoplasm of unspecified epididymis ♂

　　　C63.01　Malignant neoplasm of right epididymis ♂

　　　C63.02　Malignant neoplasm of left epididymis ♂

　● C63.1　Malignant neoplasm of spermatic cord

　　■ C63.10　Malignant neoplasm of unspecified spermatic cord ♂

　　　C63.11　Malignant neoplasm of right spermatic cord ♂

　　　C63.12　Malignant neoplasm of left spermatic cord ♂

CHAPTER 2 (C00-D49)

C63.2 **Malignant neoplasm of scrotum ♂**
Malignant neoplasm of skin of scrotum

C63.7 **Malignant neoplasm of other specified male genital organs ♂**
Malignant neoplasm of seminal vesicle
Malignant neoplasm of tunica vaginalis

C63.8 **Malignant neoplasm of overlapping sites of male genital organs ♂**
Primary malignant neoplasm of two or more contiguous sites of male genital organs whose point of origin cannot be determined

■ C63.9 **Malignant neoplasm of male genital organ, unspecified ♂**
Malignant neoplasm of male genitourinary tract NOS

MALIGNANT NEOPLASMS OF URINARY TRACT (C64-C68)

● C64 **Malignant neoplasm of kidney, except renal pelvis**
| Excludes1 | malignant carcinoid tumor of the kidney (C7A.093) |
malignant neoplasm of renal calyces (C65.-)
malignant neoplasm of renal pelvis (C65.-)

C64.1 **Malignant neoplasm of right kidney, except renal pelvis 🔊**

C64.2 **Malignant neoplasm of left kidney, except renal pelvis 🔊**

■ C64.9 **Malignant neoplasm of unspecified kidney, except renal pelvis 🔊**

● C65 **Malignant neoplasm of renal pelvis**
| Includes | malignant neoplasm of pelviureteric junction |
malignant neoplasm of renal calyces

C65.1 **Malignant neoplasm of right renal pelvis 🔊**

C65.2 **Malignant neoplasm of left renal pelvis 🔊**

■ C65.9 **Malignant neoplasm of unspecified renal pelvis 🔊**

● C66 **Malignant neoplasm of ureter**
| Excludes1 | malignant neoplasm of ureteric orifice of bladder (C67.6) |

C66.1 **Malignant neoplasm of right ureter 🔊**

C66.2 **Malignant neoplasm of left ureter 🔊**

■ C66.9 **Malignant neoplasm of unspecified ureter 🔊**

● C67 **Malignant neoplasm of bladder**

C67.0 **Malignant neoplasm of trigone of bladder**
Triangular area formed by three openings in the floor of urinary bladder

C67.1 **Malignant neoplasm of dome of bladder**
Vaulted roof

C67.2 **Malignant neoplasm of lateral wall of bladder**
Side walls

C67.3 **Malignant neoplasm of anterior wall of bladder**
Front wall

C67.4 **Malignant neoplasm of posterior wall of bladder**
Back wall

C67.5 **Malignant neoplasm of bladder neck**
Joining of bladder and urethra
Malignant neoplasm of internal urethral orifice

C67.6 **Malignant neoplasm of ureteric orifice**
Opening from bladder to ureters

C67.7 **Malignant neoplasm of urachus**
Embryonic canal that connects the urinary bladder with the structure that forms the umbilical cord (allantois)

C67.8 **Malignant neoplasm of overlapping sites of bladder**

■ C67.9 **Malignant neoplasm of bladder, unspecified**

Figure 2-15 The brain.

● C68 **Malignant neoplasm of other and unspecified urinary organs**
| Excludes1 | malignant neoplasm of female genitourinary tract NOS (C57.9) |
malignant neoplasm of male genitourinary tract NOS (C63.9)

C68.0 **Malignant neoplasm of urethra 🔊**
| Excludes1 | malignant neoplasm of urethral orifice of bladder (C67.5) |

C68.1 **Malignant neoplasm of paraurethral glands 🔊**
Group of glands of female urethra drained by paraurethral ducts; AKA Skene glands, female prostate

C68.8 **Malignant neoplasm of overlapping sites of urinary organs 🔊**
Primary malignant neoplasm of two or more contiguous sites of urinary organs whose point of origin cannot be determined

■ C68.9 **Malignant neoplasm of urinary organ, unspecified 🔊**
Malignant neoplasm of urinary system NOS

MALIGNANT NEOPLASMS OF EYE, BRAIN AND OTHER PARTS OF CENTRAL NERVOUS SYSTEM (C69-C72)

● C69 **Malignant neoplasm of eye and adnexa**
| Excludes1 | malignant neoplasm of connective tissue of eyelid (C49.0) |
malignant neoplasm of eyelid (skin) (C43.1-, C44.1-)
malignant neoplasm of optic nerve (C72.3-)

● C69.0 **Malignant neoplasm of conjunctiva**

■ C69.00 **Malignant neoplasm of unspecified conjunctiva**

C69.01 **Malignant neoplasm of right conjunctiva**

C69.02 **Malignant neoplasm of left conjunctiva**

● C69.1 **Malignant neoplasm of cornea**

■ C69.10 **Malignant neoplasm of unspecified cornea**

C69.11 **Malignant neoplasm of right cornea**

C69.12 **Malignant neoplasm of left cornea**

● C69.2 **Malignant neoplasm of retina**
| Excludes1 | dark area on retina (D49.81) |
neoplasm of unspecified behavior of retina and choroid (D49.81)
retinal freckle (D49.81)

■ C69.20 **Malignant neoplasm of unspecified retina**

C69.21 **Malignant neoplasm of right retina**

C69.22 **Malignant neoplasm of left retina**

● Unacceptable Principal Diagnosis   ● Use Additional Character(s)   ■ Unspecified   ▶ Manifestation Code

838   **OGCR** Official Guidelines for Coding and Reporting | Excludes 1 | | Excludes 2 | | Includes | | Use additional | | Code first | | Code also |

CHAPTER 2 (C00-D49)

● **C69.3 Malignant neoplasm of choroid**
  ■ C69.30 Malignant neoplasm of unspecified choroid
  C69.31 Malignant neoplasm of right choroid
  C69.32 Malignant neoplasm of left choroid
● **C69.4 Malignant neoplasm of ciliary body**
  Malignant neoplasm of eyeball
  ■ C69.40 Malignant neoplasm of unspecified ciliary body
  C69.41 Malignant neoplasm of right ciliary body
  C69.42 Malignant neoplasm of left ciliary body
● **C69.5 Malignant neoplasm of lacrimal gland and duct**
  Malignant neoplasm of lacrimal sac
  Malignant neoplasm of nasolacrimal duct
  ■ C69.50 Malignant neoplasm of unspecified lacrimal gland and duct
  C69.51 Malignant neoplasm of right lacrimal gland and duct
  C69.52 Malignant neoplasm of left lacrimal gland and duct
● **C69.6 Malignant neoplasm of orbit**
  Malignant neoplasm of connective tissue of orbit
  Malignant neoplasm of extraocular muscle
  Malignant neoplasm of peripheral nerves of orbit
  Malignant neoplasm of retrobulbar tissue
  Malignant neoplasm of retro-ocular tissue
  Excludes1 malignant neoplasm of orbital bone (C41.0)
  ■ C69.60 Malignant neoplasm of unspecified orbit
  C69.61 Malignant neoplasm of right orbit
  C69.62 Malignant neoplasm of left orbit
● **C69.8 Malignant neoplasm of overlapping sites of eye and adnexa**
  ■ C69.80 Malignant neoplasm of overlapping sites of unspecified eye and adnexa
  C69.81 Malignant neoplasm of overlapping sites of right eye and adnexa
  C69.82 Malignant neoplasm of overlapping sites of left eye and adnexa
● **C69.9 Malignant neoplasm of unspecified site of eye**
  ■ C69.90 Malignant neoplasm of unspecified site of unspecified eye
  ■ C69.91 Malignant neoplasm of unspecified site of right eye
  ■ C69.92 Malignant neoplasm of unspecified site of left eye
● **C70 Malignant neoplasm of meninges**
  C70.0 Malignant neoplasm of cerebral meninges 🦠
  C70.1 Malignant neoplasm of spinal meninges 🦠
  ■ C70.9 Malignant neoplasm of meninges, unspecified 🦠
● **C71 Malignant neoplasm of brain**
  Excludes1 malignant neoplasm of cranial nerves (C72.2-C72.5)
  retrobulbar malignant neoplasm (C69.6-)
  C71.0 Malignant neoplasm of cerebrum, except lobes and ventricles 🦠
  Malignant neoplasm of supratentorial NOS
  C71.1 Malignant neoplasm of frontal lobe 🦠
  C71.2 Malignant neoplasm of temporal lobe 🦠
  C71.3 Malignant neoplasm of parietal lobe 🦠
  C71.4 Malignant neoplasm of occipital lobe 🦠

C71.5 Malignant neoplasm of cerebral ventricle 🦠
  Excludes1 malignant neoplasm of fourth cerebral ventricle (C71.7)
C71.6 Malignant neoplasm of cerebellum 🦠
C71.7 Malignant neoplasm of brain stem 🦠
  Malignant neoplasm of fourth cerebral ventricle
  Infratentorial malignant neoplasm NOS
C71.8 Malignant neoplasm of overlapping sites of brain 🦠
■ C71.9 Malignant neoplasm of brain, unspecified 🦠
● **C72 Malignant neoplasm of spinal cord, cranial nerves and other parts of central nervous system**
  Excludes1 malignant neoplasm of meninges (C70.-)
  malignant neoplasm of peripheral nerves and autonomic nervous system (C47.-)
  C72.0 Malignant neoplasm of spinal cord 🦠
  C72.1 Malignant neoplasm of cauda equina 🦠
  Lower end of spinal column
● C72.2 Malignant neoplasm of olfactory nerve
  Malignant neoplasm of olfactory bulb
  ■ C72.20 Malignant neoplasm of unspecified olfactory nerve 🦠
  C72.21 Malignant neoplasm of right olfactory nerve 🦠
  C72.22 Malignant neoplasm of left olfactory nerve 🦠
● C72.3 Malignant neoplasm of optic nerve
  ■ C72.30 Malignant neoplasm of unspecified optic nerve 🦠
  C72.31 Malignant neoplasm of right optic nerve 🦠
  C72.32 Malignant neoplasm of left optic nerve 🦠
● C72.4 Malignant neoplasm of acoustic nerve
  ■ C72.40 Malignant neoplasm of unspecified acoustic nerve 🦠
  C72.41 Malignant neoplasm of right acoustic nerve 🦠
  C72.42 Malignant neoplasm of left acoustic nerve 🦠
● C72.5 Malignant neoplasm of other and unspecified cranial nerves
  ■ C72.50 Malignant neoplasm of unspecified cranial nerve 🦠
  Malignant neoplasm of cranial nerve NOS
  C72.59 Malignant neoplasm of other cranial nerves 🦠
■ C72.9 Malignant neoplasm of central nervous system, unspecified 🦠
  Malignant neoplasm of unspecified site of central nervous system
  Malignant neoplasm of nervous system NOS

MALIGNANT NEOPLASMS OF THYROID AND OTHER ENDOCRINE GLANDS (C73-C75)

C73 **Malignant neoplasm of thyroid gland**
  Use additional code to identify any functional activity
● C74 **Malignant neoplasm of adrenal gland**
  ● C74.0 Malignant neoplasm of cortex of adrenal gland
    ■ C74.00 Malignant neoplasm of cortex of unspecified adrenal gland 🦠
    C74.01 Malignant neoplasm of cortex of right adrenal gland 🦠
    C74.02 Malignant neoplasm of cortex of left adrenal gland 🦠

N Newborn Age: 0 **P** Pediatric Age: 0–17 **M** Maternity DX: 12–55 **A** Adult Age: 15–124 ♀ Females Only ♂ Males Only

🦠 Complication\Comorbidity Major C\C Present on Admission Requirement Hospital-Acquired Condition

839

CHAPTER 2 (C00-D49)

CHAPTER 2 (C00-D49)

- C74.1 **Malignant neoplasm of medulla of adrenal gland**
  Pair of glands situated on top of or above each kidney ("suprarenal")

  - C74.10 **Malignant neoplasm of medulla of unspecified adrenal gland** 🞱

  - C74.11 **Malignant neoplasm of medulla of right adrenal gland** 🞱

  - C74.12 **Malignant neoplasm of medulla of left adrenal gland** 🞱

- C74.9 **Malignant neoplasm of unspecified part of adrenal gland**

  - C74.90 **Malignant neoplasm of unspecified part of unspecified adrenal gland** 🞱

  - C74.91 **Malignant neoplasm of unspecified part of right adrenal gland** 🞱

  - C74.92 **Malignant neoplasm of unspecified part of left adrenal gland** 🞱

- C75 **Malignant neoplasm of other endocrine glands and related structures**

  > **Excludes1** malignant carcinoid tumors (C7A.0-)
  > malignant neoplasm of adrenal gland (C74.-)
  > malignant neoplasm of endocrine pancreas (C25.4)
  > malignant neoplasm of islets of Langerhans (C25.4)
  > malignant neoplasm of ovary (C56-)
  > malignant neoplasm of testis (C62.-)
  > malignant neoplasm of thymus (C37)
  > malignant neoplasm of thyroid gland (C73)
  > malignant neuroendocrine tumors (C7A.-)

  - C75.0 **Malignant neoplasm of parathyroid gland** 🞱
  - C75.1 **Malignant neoplasm of pituitary gland** 🞱
  - C75.2 **Malignant neoplasm of craniopharyngeal duct** 🞱
  - C75.3 **Malignant neoplasm of pineal gland** 🞱
  - C75.4 **Malignant neoplasm of carotid body** 🞱
  - C75.5 **Malignant neoplasm of aortic body and other paraganglia** 🞱
  - C75.8 **Malignant neoplasm with pluriglandular involvement, unspecified** 🞱
  - C75.9 **Malignant neoplasm of endocrine gland, unspecified** 🞱

MALIGNANT NEUROENDOCRINE TUMORS (C7A)

- C7A **Malignant neuroendocrine tumors**

  > **Code also** any associated multiple endocrine neoplasia [MEN] syndromes (E31.2-)

  > **Use additional** code to identify any associated endocrine syndrome, such as:
  > carcinoid syndrome (E34.0)

  > **Excludes2** malignant pancreatic islet cell tumors (C25.4)
  > Merkel cell carcinoma (C4A.-)

  - C7A.0 **Malignant carcinoid tumors**

    - C7A.00 **Malignant carcinoid tumor of unspecified site** 🞱

    - C7A.01 **Malignant carcinoid tumors of the small intestine**

      - C7A.010 **Malignant carcinoid tumor of the duodenum** 🞱

      - C7A.011 **Malignant carcinoid tumor of the jejunum** 🞱

      - C7A.012 **Malignant carcinoid tumor of the ileum** 🞱

      - C7A.019 **Malignant carcinoid tumor of the small intestine, unspecified portion** 🞱

- C7A.02 **Malignant carcinoid tumors of the appendix, large intestine, and rectum**

  - C7A.020 **Malignant carcinoid tumor of the appendix** 🞱

  - C7A.021 **Malignant carcinoid tumor of the cecum** 🞱

  - C7A.022 **Malignant carcinoid tumor of the ascending colon** 🞱

  - C7A.023 **Malignant carcinoid tumor of the transverse colon** 🞱

  - C7A.024 **Malignant carcinoid tumor of the descending colon** 🞱

  - C7A.025 **Malignant carcinoid tumor of the sigmoid colon** 🞱

  - C7A.026 **Malignant carcinoid tumor of the rectum** 🞱

  - C7A.029 **Malignant carcinoid tumor of the large intestine, unspecified portion** 🞱
    Malignant carcinoid tumor of the colon NOS

- C7A.09 **Malignant carcinoid tumors of other sites**

  - C7A.090 **Malignant carcinoid tumor of the bronchus and lung** 🞱

  - C7A.091 **Malignant carcinoid tumor of the thymus** 🞱

  - C7A.092 **Malignant carcinoid tumor of the stomach** 🞱

  - C7A.093 **Malignant carcinoid tumor of the kidney** 🞱

  - C7A.094 **Malignant carcinoid tumor of the foregut NOS** 🞱

  - C7A.095 **Malignant carcinoid tumor of the midgut NOS** 🞱

  - C7A.096 **Malignant carcinoid tumor of the hindgut NOS** 🞱

  - C7A.098 **Malignant carcinoid tumors of other sites** 🞱

- C7A.1 **Malignant poorly differentiated neuroendocrine tumors** 🞱
  Malignant poorly differentiated neuroendocrine tumor NOS
  Malignant poorly differentiated neuroendocrine carcinoma, any site
  High grade neuroendocrine carcinoma, any site

- C7A.8 **Other malignant neuroendocrine tumors** 🞱
  Secondary neuroendocrine tumors (C7B)

- C7B **Secondary neuroendocrine tumors**

  > **Use additional** code to identify any functional activity

  - C7B.0 **Secondary carcinoid tumors**

    - C7B.00 **Secondary carcinoid tumors, unspecified site**

    - C7B.01 **Secondary carcinoid tumors of distant lymph nodes** 🞱

    - C7B.02 **Secondary carcinoid tumors of liver** 🞱

    - C7B.03 **Secondary carcinoid tumors of bone** 🞱

    - C7B.04 **Secondary carcinoid tumors of peritoneum** 🞱
      Mesentary metastasis of carcinoid tumor

    - C7B.09 **Secondary carcinoid tumors of other sites** 🞱

● Unacceptable Principal Diagnosis ● Use Additional Character(s) ■ Unspecified ▶ Manifestation Code

840   **OGCR** Official Guidelines for Coding and Reporting | Excludes 1 | | Excludes 2 | | Includes | | Use additional | | Code first | | Code also |

C7B.1 Secondary Merkel cell carcinoma
Merkel cell carcinoma nodal presentation
Merkel cell carcinoma visceral metastatic presentation

C7B.8 Other secondary neuroendocrine tumors 🔴

MALIGNANT NEOPLASMS OF ILL-DEFINED, OTHER SECONDARY AND UNSPECIFIED SITES (C76-C80)

● **C76 Malignant neoplasm of other and ill-defined sites**

  | Excludes1 | malignant neoplasm of female genitourinary tract NOS (C57.9)
      malignant neoplasm of male genitourinary tract NOS (C63.9)
      malignant neoplasm of lymphoid, hematopoietic and related tissue (C81-C96)
      malignant neoplasm of skin (C44.-)
      malignant neoplasm of unspecified site NOS (C80.1)

  C76.0 Malignant neoplasm of head, face and neck
      Malignant neoplasm of cheek NOS
      Malignant neoplasm of nose NOS

  C76.1 Malignant neoplasm of thorax
      Intrathoracic malignant neoplasm NOS
      Malignant neoplasm of axilla NOS
      Thoracic malignant neoplasm NOS

  C76.2 Malignant neoplasm of abdomen

  C76.3 Malignant neoplasm of pelvis
      Malignant neoplasm of groin NOS
      Malignant neoplasm of sites overlapping systems within the pelvis
      Rectovaginal (septum) malignant neoplasm
         Between rectum and vagina
      Rectovesical (septum) malignant neoplasm
         Between rectum and urinary bladder; AKA vesicorectal

● **C76.4 Malignant neoplasm of upper limb**

  ■ **C76.40 Malignant neoplasm of unspecified upper limb**

  C76.41 Malignant neoplasm of right upper limb

  C76.42 Malignant neoplasm of left upper limb

● **C76.5 Malignant neoplasm of lower limb**

  ■ **C76.50 Malignant neoplasm of unspecified lower limb**

  C76.51 Malignant neoplasm of right lower limb

  C76.52 Malignant neoplasm of left lower limb

  C76.8 Malignant neoplasm of other specified ill-defined sites
      Malignant neoplasm of overlapping ill-defined sites

● **C77 Secondary and unspecified malignant neoplasm of lymph nodes**

  | Excludes1 | malignant neoplasm of lymph nodes, specified as primary (C81-C88, C96.-)
      mesentary metastasis of carcinoid tumor (C7B.04)
      secondary carcinoid tumors of distant lymph nodes (C7B.01)

  ■ **C77.0 Secondary and unspecified malignant neoplasm of lymph nodes of head, face and neck** 🔴
      Secondary and unspecified malignant neoplasm of supraclavicular lymph nodes

  ■ **C77.1 Secondary and unspecified malignant neoplasm of intrathoracic lymph nodes** 🔴

  ■ **C77.2 Secondary and unspecified malignant neoplasm of intra-abdominal lymph nodes** 🔴

  ■ **C77.3 Secondary and unspecified malignant neoplasm of axilla and upper limb lymph nodes** 🔴
      Secondary and unspecified malignant neoplasm of pectoral lymph nodes

  ■ **C77.4 Secondary and unspecified malignant neoplasm of inguinal and lower limb lymph nodes** 🔴

  ■ **C77.5 Secondary and unspecified malignant neoplasm of intrapelvic lymph nodes** 🔴

  ■ **C77.8 Secondary and unspecified malignant neoplasm of lymph nodes of multiple regions** 🔴

  ■ **C77.9 Secondary and unspecified malignant neoplasm of lymph node, unspecified** 🔴

● **C78 Secondary malignant neoplasm of respiratory and digestive organs**

  | Excludes1 | lymph node metastases (C77.0)
      secondary carcinoid tumors of liver (C7B.02)
      secondary carcinoid tumors of peritoneum (C7B.04)

● **C78.0 Secondary malignant neoplasm of lung**

  ■ **C78.00 Secondary malignant neoplasm of unspecified lung** 🔴

  C78.01 Secondary malignant neoplasm of right lung 🔴

  C78.02 Secondary malignant neoplasm of left lung 🔴

  C78.1 Secondary malignant neoplasm of mediastinum 🔴
      Thoracic cavity between pleural cavities

  C78.2 Secondary malignant neoplasm of pleura 🔴
      Serous membrane covering lungs and lining thoracic cavity

● **C78.3 Secondary malignant neoplasm of other and unspecified respiratory organs**

  ■ **C78.30 Secondary malignant neoplasm of unspecified respiratory organ** 🔴

  C78.39 Secondary malignant neoplasm of other respiratory organs 🔴

  C78.4 Secondary malignant neoplasm of small intestine 🔴

  C78.5 Secondary malignant neoplasm of large intestine and rectum 🔴

  C78.6 Secondary malignant neoplasm of retroperitoneum and peritoneum 🔴

  C78.7 Secondary malignant neoplasm of liver and intrahepatic bile duct 🔴

● **C78.8 Secondary malignant neoplasm of other and unspecified digestive organs**

  ■ **C78.80 Secondary malignant neoplasm of unspecified digestive organ** 🔴

  C78.89 Secondary malignant neoplasm of other digestive organs 🔴

● **C79 Secondary malignant neoplasm of other and unspecified sites**

  | Excludes1 | lymph node metastases (C77.0)
      secondary carcinoid tumors (C7B.-)
      secondary neuroendocrine tumors (C7B.-)

● **C79.0 Secondary malignant neoplasm of kidney and renal pelvis**

  ■ **C79.00 Secondary malignant neoplasm of unspecified kidney and renal pelvis** 🔴

  C79.01 Secondary malignant neoplasm of right kidney and renal pelvis 🔴

  C79.02 Secondary malignant neoplasm of left kidney and renal pelvis 🔴

N Newborn Age: 0   **P** Pediatric Age: 0–17   **M** Maternity DX: 12–55   **A** Adult Age: 15–124   ♀ Females Only   ♂ Males Only

🔴 Complication\Comorbidity   🔴 Major C\C   🔴 Present on Admission Requirement   🔴 Hospital-Acquired Condition

841

CHAPTER 2 (C00-D49)

Item 2-6 The adrenal glands are a pair of glands situated on top of or above each kidney ("suprarenal") and chiefly responsible for regulating the stress response through the synthesis of corticosteroids and catecholamines, including cortisol and adrenaline.

● C79.1 **Secondary malignant neoplasm of bladder and other and unspecified urinary organs**

■ C79.10 **Secondary malignant neoplasm of unspecified urinary organs** 🕭

C79.11 **Secondary malignant neoplasm of bladder** 🕭

C79.19 **Secondary malignant neoplasm of other urinary organs** 🕭

● C79.2 **Secondary malignant neoplasm of skin** 🕭

> **Excludes1** secondary Merkel cell carcinoma (C7B.1)

● C79.3 **Secondary malignant neoplasm of brain and cerebral meninges**

C79.31 **Secondary malignant neoplasm of brain** 🕭

C79.32 **Secondary malignant neoplasm of cerebral meninges** 🕭

● C79.4 **Secondary malignant neoplasm of other and unspecified parts of nervous system**

■ C79.40 **Secondary malignant neoplasm of unspecified part of nervous system** 🕭

C79.49 **Secondary malignant neoplasm of other parts of nervous system** 🕭

● C79.5 **Secondary malignant neoplasm of bone and bone marrow**

> **Excludes1** secondary carcinoid tumors of bone (C7B.03)

C79.51 **Secondary malignant neoplasm of bone** 🕭

C79.52 **Secondary malignant neoplasm of bone marrow** 🕭

● C79.6 **Secondary malignant neoplasm of ovary**

■ C79.60 **Secondary malignant neoplasm of unspecified ovary** ♀ 🕭

C79.61 **Secondary malignant neoplasm of right ovary** ♀ 🕭

C79.62 **Secondary malignant neoplasm of left ovary** ♀ 🕭

● C79.7 **Secondary malignant neoplasm of adrenal gland**

■ C79.70 **Secondary malignant neoplasm of unspecified adrenal gland** 🕭

C79.71 **Secondary malignant neoplasm of right adrenal gland** 🕭

C79.72 **Secondary malignant neoplasm of left adrenal gland** 🕭

● C79.8 **Secondary malignant neoplasm of other specified sites**

C79.81 **Secondary malignant neoplasm of breast** 🕭

C79.82 **Secondary malignant neoplasm of genital organs** 🕭

C79.89 **Secondary malignant neoplasm of other specified sites** 🕭

■ C79.9 **Secondary malignant neoplasm of unspecified site** 🕭
Metastatic cancer NOS
Metastatic disease NOS

> **Excludes1** carcinomatosis NOS (C80.0)
> generalized cancer NOS (C80.0)
> malignant (primary) neoplasm of unspecified site (C80.1)

OGCR Section I.C.2.j and k

Disseminated malignant neoplasm, unspecified

j. Code C80.0, Disseminated malignant neoplasm, unspecified, is for use only in those cases where the patient has advanced metastatic disease and no known primary or secondary sites are specified. It should not be used in place of assigning codes for the primary site and all known secondary sites.

Malignant neoplasm without specification of site

k. Code C80.1, Malignant (primary) neoplasm, unspecified, equates to Cancer, unspecified. This code should only be used when no determination can be made as to the primary site of a malignancy. This code should rarely be used in the inpatient setting.

● C80 **Malignant neoplasm without specification of site**

> **Excludes1** malignant carcinoid tumor of unspecified site (C7A.00)
> malignant neoplasm of specified multiple sites-code to each site

■ C80.0 **Disseminated malignant neoplasm, unspecified** 🕭
Carcinomatosis NOS
Generalized cancer, unspecified site (primary) (secondary)
Generalized malignancy, unspecified site (primary) (secondary)

■ C80.1 **Malignant (primary) neoplasm, unspecified**
Cancer NOS
Cancer unspecified site (primary)
Carcinoma unspecified site (primary)
Malignancy unspecified site (primary)

> **Excludes1** secondary malignant neoplasm of unspecified site (C79.9)

● C80.2 **Malignant neoplasm associated with transplanted organ** 🕭

> *Code first* complication of transplanted organ (T86.-)
> Use additional code to identify the specific malignancy

(See Plate 315 on page NAP-1.)

MALIGNANT NEOPLASMS OF LYMPHOID, HEMATOPOIETIC AND RELATED TISSUE (C81-C96)

> **Excludes2** Kaposi's sarcoma of lymph nodes (C46.3)
> secondary and unspecified neoplasm of lymph nodes (C77.-)
> secondary neoplasm of bone marrow (C79.52)
> secondary neoplasm of spleen (C78.89)

● C81 **Hodgkin lymphoma**
Form of malignant lymphoma with four types, nodular sclerosis, mixed cellularity, lymphocyte depleted, and lymphocyte predominant

> **Excludes1** personal history of Hodgkin lymphoma (Z85.71)

● C81.0 **Nodular lymphocyte predominant Hodgkin lymphoma**
Least aggressive, least common, typically no symptoms
Lymphocytic-histiocytic predominance Hodgkin's disease

■ C81.00 **Nodular lymphocyte predominant Hodgkin lymphoma, unspecified site** 🕭

C81.01 **Nodular lymphocyte predominant Hodgkin lymphoma, lymph nodes of head, face, and neck** 🕭

C81.02 **Nodular lymphocyte predominant Hodgkin lymphoma, intrathoracic lymph nodes** 🕭

● Unacceptable Principal Diagnosis ● Use Additional Character(s) ■ Unspecified ▶ Manifestation Code

842 OGCR Official Guidelines for Coding and Reporting | Excludes 1 | Excludes 2 | Includes | Use additional | Code first | Code also

C81.03   Nodular lymphocyte predominant Hodgkin lymphoma, intra-abdominal lymph nodes 🅒

C81.04   Nodular lymphocyte predominant Hodgkin lymphoma, lymph nodes of axilla and upper limb 🅒

C81.05   Nodular lymphocyte predominant Hodgkin lymphoma, lymph nodes of inguinal region and lower limb 🅒

C81.06   Nodular lymphocyte predominant Hodgkin lymphoma, intrapelvic lymph nodes 🅒

C81.07   Nodular lymphocyte predominant Hodgkin lymphoma, spleen 🅒

C81.08   Nodular lymphocyte predominant Hodgkin lymphoma, lymph nodes of multiple sites 🅒

C81.09   Nodular lymphocyte predominant Hodgkin lymphoma, extranodal and solid organ sites 🅒

● C81.1   Nodular sclerosis classical Hodgkin lymphoma
Moderately aggressive; most common in young adults

■ C81.10   Nodular sclerosis classical Hodgkin lymphoma, unspecified site 🅒

C81.11   Nodular sclerosis classical Hodgkin lymphoma, lymph nodes of head, face, and neck 🅒

C81.12   Nodular sclerosis classical Hodgkin lymphoma, intrathoracic lymph nodes 🅒

C81.13   Nodular sclerosis classical Hodgkin lymphoma, intra-abdominal lymph nodes 🅒

C81.14   Nodular sclerosis classical Hodgkin lymphoma, lymph nodes of axilla and upper limb 🅒

C81.15   Nodular sclerosis classical Hodgkin lymphoma, lymph nodes of inguinal region and lower limb 🅒

C81.16   Nodular sclerosis classical Hodgkin lymphoma, intrapelvic lymph nodes 🅒

C81.17   Nodular sclerosis classical Hodgkin lymphoma, spleen 🅒

C81.18   Nodular sclerosis classical Hodgkin lymphoma, lymph nodes of multiple sites 🅒

C81.19   Nodular sclerosis classical Hodgkin lymphoma, extranodal and solid organ sites 🅒

● C81.2   Mixed cellularity classical Hodgkin lymphoma
A type of Hodgkin's that is moderately aggressive with mixed cell types

■ C81.20   Mixed cellularity classical Hodgkin lymphoma, unspecified site 🅒

C81.21   Mixed cellularity classical Hodgkin lymphoma, lymph nodes of head, face, and neck 🅒

C81.22   Mixed cellularity classical Hodgkin lymphoma, intrathoracic lymph nodes 🅒

C81.23   Mixed cellularity classical Hodgkin lymphoma, intra-abdominal lymph nodes 🅒

C81.24   Mixed cellularity classical Hodgkin lymphoma, lymph nodes of axilla and upper limb 🅒

C81.25   Mixed cellularity classical Hodgkin lymphoma, lymph nodes of inguinal region and lower limb 🅒

C81.26   Mixed cellularity classical Hodgkin lymphoma, intrapelvic lymph nodes 🅒

C81.27   Mixed cellularity classical Hodgkin lymphoma, spleen 🅒

C81.28   Mixed cellularity classical Hodgkin lymphoma, lymph nodes of multiple sites 🅒

C81.29   Mixed cellularity classical Hodgkin lymphoma, extranodal and solid organ sites 🅒

● C81.3   Lymphocyte depleted classical Hodgkin lymphoma
Most aggressive type with poor prognosis

■ C81.30   Lymphocyte depleted classical Hodgkin lymphoma, unspecified site 🅒

C81.31   Lymphocyte depleted classical Hodgkin lymphoma, lymph nodes of head, face, and neck 🅒

C81.32   Lymphocyte depleted classical Hodgkin lymphoma, intrathoracic lymph nodes 🅒

C81.33   Lymphocyte depleted classical Hodgkin lymphoma, intra-abdominal lymph nodes 🅒

C81.34   Lymphocyte depleted classical Hodgkin lymphoma, lymph nodes of axilla and upper limb 🅒

C81.35   Lymphocyte depleted classical Hodgkin lymphoma, lymph nodes of inguinal region and lower limb 🅒

C81.36   Lymphocyte depleted classical Hodgkin lymphoma, intrapelvic lymph nodes 🅒

C81.37   Lymphocyte depleted classical Hodgkin lymphoma, spleen 🅒

C81.38   Lymphocyte depleted classical Hodgkin lymphoma, lymph nodes of multiple sites 🅒

C81.39   Lymphocyte depleted classical Hodgkin lymphoma, extranodal and solid organ sites 🅒

● C81.4   Lymphocyte-rich classical Hodgkin lymphoma

Excludes1   nodular lymphocyte predominant Hodgkin lymphoma (C81.0-)

■ C81.40   Lymphocyte-rich classical Hodgkin lymphoma, unspecified site 🅒

C81.41   Lymphocyte-rich classical Hodgkin lymphoma, lymph nodes of head, face, and neck 🅒

C81.42   Lymphocyte-rich classical Hodgkin lymphoma, intrathoracic lymph nodes 🅒

C81.43   Lymphocyte-rich classical Hodgkin lymphoma, intra-abdominal lymph nodes 🅒

C81.44   Lymphocyte-rich classical Hodgkin lymphoma, lymph nodes of axilla and upper limb 🅒

C81.45   Lymphocyte-rich classical Hodgkin lymphoma, lymph nodes of inguinal region and lower limb 🅒

C81.46   Lymphocyte-rich classical Hodgkin lymphoma, intrapelvic lymph nodes 🅒

C81.47   Lymphocyte-rich classical Hodgkin lymphoma, spleen 🅒

C81.48   Lymphocyte-rich classical Hodgkin lymphoma, lymph nodes of multiple sites 🅒

C81.49   Lymphocyte-rich classical Hodgkin lymphoma, extranodal and solid organ sites 🅒

N Newborn Age: 0   **P** Pediatric Age: 0–17   **M** Maternity DX: 12–55   **A** Adult Age: 15–124   ♀ Females Only   ♂ Males Only

🅒 Complication\Comorbidity   🅒 Major C\C   🅒 Present on Admission Requirement   🅒 Hospital-Acquired Condition

843

● **C81.7** **Other classical Hodgkin lymphoma**
Classical Hodgkin lymphoma NOS

◻ **C81.70** Other classical Hodgkin lymphoma, unspecified site 🕭

C81.71 Other classical Hodgkin lymphoma, lymph nodes of head, face, and neck 🕭

C81.72 Other classical Hodgkin lymphoma, intrathoracic lymph nodes 🕭

C81.73 Other classical Hodgkin lymphoma, intra-abdominal lymph nodes 🕭

C81.74 Other classical Hodgkin lymphoma, lymph nodes of axilla and upper limb 🕭

C81.75 Other classical Hodgkin lymphoma, lymph nodes of inguinal region and lower limb 🕭

C81.76 Other classical Hodgkin lymphoma, intrapelvic lymph nodes 🕭

C81.77 Other classical Hodgkin lymphoma, spleen 🕭

C81.78 Other classical Hodgkin lymphoma, lymph nodes of multiple sites 🕭

C81.79 Other classical Hodgkin lymphoma, extranodal and solid organ sites 🕭

● **C81.9** **Hodgkin lymphoma, unspecified**

◻ **C81.90** Hodgkin lymphoma, unspecified, unspecified site 🕭

◻ **C81.91** Hodgkin lymphoma, unspecified, lymph nodes of head, face, and neck 🕭

◻ **C81.92** Hodgkin lymphoma, unspecified, intrathoracic lymph nodes 🕭

◻ **C81.93** Hodgkin lymphoma, unspecified, intra-abdominal lymph nodes 🕭

◻ **C81.94** Hodgkin lymphoma, unspecified, lymph nodes of axilla and upper limb 🕭

◻ **C81.95** Hodgkin lymphoma, unspecified, lymph nodes of inguinal region and lower limb 🕭

◻ **C81.96** Hodgkin lymphoma, unspecified, intrapelvic lymph nodes 🕭

◻ **C81.97** Hodgkin lymphoma, unspecified, spleen 🕭

◻ **C81.98** Hodgkin lymphoma, unspecified, lymph nodes of multiple sites 🕭

◻ **C81.99** Hodgkin lymphoma, unspecified, extranodal and solid organ sites 🕭

● **C82** **Follicular lymphoma**
Group of malignant lymphomas

Includes   follicular lymphoma with or without diffuse areas

Excludes1   mature T/NK-cell lymphomas (C84.-)
personal history of non-Hodgkin lymphoma (Z85.72)

● **C82.0** **Follicular lymphoma grade I**

◻ **C82.00** Follicular lymphoma grade I, unspecified site 🕭

C82.01 Follicular lymphoma grade I, lymph nodes of head, face, and neck 🕭

C82.02 Follicular lymphoma grade I, intrathoracic lymph nodes 🕭

C82.03 Follicular lymphoma grade I, intra-abdominal lymph nodes 🕭

C82.04 Follicular lymphoma grade I, lymph nodes of axilla and upper limb 🕭

C82.05 Follicular lymphoma grade I, lymph nodes of inguinal region and lower limb 🕭

C82.06 Follicular lymphoma grade I, intrapelvic lymph nodes 🕭

C82.07 Follicular lymphoma grade I, spleen 🕭

C82.08 Follicular lymphoma grade I, lymph nodes of multiple sites 🕭

C82.09 Follicular lymphoma grade I, extranodal and solid organ sites 🕭

● **C82.1** **Follicular lymphoma grade II**

◻ **C82.10** Follicular lymphoma grade II, unspecified site 🕭

C82.11 Follicular lymphoma grade II, lymph nodes of head, face, and neck 🕭

C82.12 Follicular lymphoma grade II, intrathoracic lymph nodes 🕭

C82.13 Follicular lymphoma grade II, intra-abdominal lymph nodes 🕭

C82.14 Follicular lymphoma grade II, lymph nodes of axilla and upper limb 🕭

C82.15 Follicular lymphoma grade II, lymph nodes of inguinal region and lower limb 🕭

C82.16 Follicular lymphoma grade II, intrapelvic lymph nodes 🕭

C82.17 Follicular lymphoma grade II, spleen 🕭

C82.18 Follicular lymphoma grade II, lymph nodes of multiple sites 🕭

C82.19 Follicular lymphoma grade II, extranodal and solid organ sites 🕭

● **C82.2** **Follicular lymphoma grade III, unspecified**

◻ **C82.20** Follicular lymphoma grade III, unspecified, unspecified site 🕭

◻ **C82.21** Follicular lymphoma grade III, unspecified, lymph nodes of head, face, and neck 🕭

◻ **C82.22** Follicular lymphoma grade III, unspecified, intrathoracic lymph nodes 🕭

◻ **C82.23** Follicular lymphoma grade III, unspecified, intra-abdominal lymph nodes 🕭

◻ **C82.24** Follicular lymphoma grade III, unspecified, lymph nodes of axilla and upper limb 🕭

◻ **C82.25** Follicular lymphoma grade III, unspecified, lymph nodes of inguinal region and lower limb 🕭

◻ **C82.26** Follicular lymphoma grade III, unspecified, intrapelvic lymph nodes 🕭

◻ **C82.27** Follicular lymphoma grade III, unspecified, spleen 🕭

◻ **C82.28** Follicular lymphoma grade III, unspecified, lymph nodes of multiple sites 🕭

◻ **C82.29** Follicular lymphoma grade III, unspecified, extranodal and solid organ sites 🕭

● **C82.3** **Follicular lymphoma grade IIIa**

◻ **C82.30** Follicular lymphoma grade IIIa, unspecified site 🕭

C82.31 Follicular lymphoma grade IIIa, lymph nodes of head, face, and neck 🕭

C82.32 Follicular lymphoma grade IIIa, intrathoracic lymph nodes 🕭

C82.33 Follicular lymphoma grade IIIa, intra-abdominal lymph nodes 🕭

CHAPTER 2 (C00-D49)

C82.34   Follicular lymphoma grade IIIa, lymph nodes of axilla and upper limb

C82.35   Follicular lymphoma grade IIIa, lymph nodes of inguinal region and lower limb

C82.36   Follicular lymphoma grade IIIa, intrapelvic lymph nodes

C82.37   Follicular lymphoma grade IIIa, spleen

C82.38   Follicular lymphoma grade IIIa, lymph nodes of multiple sites

C82.39   Follicular lymphoma grade IIIa, extranodal and solid organ sites

● C82.4   Follicular lymphoma grade IIIb

■ C82.40   Follicular lymphoma grade IIIb, unspecified site

C82.41   Follicular lymphoma grade IIIb, lymph nodes of head, face, and neck

C82.42   Follicular lymphoma grade IIIb, intrathoracic lymph nodes

C82.43   Follicular lymphoma grade IIIb, intra-abdominal lymph nodes

C82.44   Follicular lymphoma grade IIIb, lymph nodes of axilla and upper limb

C82.45   Follicular lymphoma grade IIIb, lymph nodes of inguinal region and lower limb

C82.46   Follicular lymphoma grade IIIb, intrapelvic lymph nodes

C82.47   Follicular lymphoma grade IIIb, spleen

C82.48   Follicular lymphoma grade IIIb, lymph nodes of multiple sites

C82.49   Follicular lymphoma grade IIIb, extranodal and solid organ sites

● C82.5   Diffuse follicle center lymphoma

■ C82.50   Diffuse follicle center lymphoma, unspecified site

C82.51   Diffuse follicle center lymphoma, lymph nodes of head, face, and neck

C82.52   Diffuse follicle center lymphoma, intrathoracic lymph nodes

C82.53   Diffuse follicle center lymphoma, intra-abdominal lymph nodes

C82.54   Diffuse follicle center lymphoma, lymph nodes of axilla and upper limb

C82.55   Diffuse follicle center lymphoma, lymph nodes of inguinal region and lower limb

C82.56   Diffuse follicle center lymphoma, intrapelvic lymph nodes

C82.57   Diffuse follicle center lymphoma, spleen

C82.58   Diffuse follicle center lymphoma, lymph nodes of multiple sites

C82.59   Diffuse follicle center lymphoma, extranodal and solid organ sites

● C82.6   Cutaneous follicle center lymphoma

■ C82.60   Cutaneous follicle center lymphoma, unspecified site

C82.61   Cutaneous follicle center lymphoma, lymph nodes of head, face, and neck

C82.62   Cutaneous follicle center lymphoma, intrathoracic lymph nodes

C82.63   Cutaneous follicle center lymphoma, intra-abdominal lymph nodes

C82.64   Cutaneous follicle center lymphoma, lymph nodes of axilla and upper limb

C82.65   Cutaneous follicle center lymphoma, lymph nodes of inguinal region and lower limb

C82.66   Cutaneous follicle center lymphoma, intrapelvic lymph nodes

C82.67   Cutaneous follicle center lymphoma, spleen

C82.68   Cutaneous follicle center lymphoma, lymph nodes of multiple sites

C82.69   Cutaneous follicle center lymphoma, extranodal and solid organ sites

● C82.8   Other types of follicular lymphoma

■ C82.80   Other types of follicular lymphoma, unspecified site

C82.81   Other types of follicular lymphoma, lymph nodes of head, face, and neck

C82.82   Other types of follicular lymphoma, intrathoracic lymph nodes

C82.83   Other types of follicular lymphoma, intra-abdominal lymph nodes

C82.84   Other types of follicular lymphoma, lymph nodes of axilla and upper limb

C82.85   Other types of follicular lymphoma, lymph nodes of inguinal region and lower limb

C82.86   Other types of follicular lymphoma, intrapelvic lymph nodes

C82.87   Other types of follicular lymphoma, spleen

C82.88   Other types of follicular lymphoma, lymph nodes of multiple sites

C82.89   Other types of follicular lymphoma, extranodal and solid organ sites

● C82.9   Follicular lymphoma, unspecified

■ C82.90   Follicular lymphoma, unspecified, unspecified site

■ C82.91   Follicular lymphoma, unspecified, lymph nodes of head, face, and neck

■ C82.92   Follicular lymphoma, unspecified, intrathoracic lymph nodes

■ C82.93   Follicular lymphoma, unspecified, intra-abdominal lymph nodes

■ C82.94   Follicular lymphoma, unspecified, lymph nodes of axilla and upper limb

■ C82.95   Follicular lymphoma, unspecified, lymph nodes of inguinal region and lower limb

■ C82.96   Follicular lymphoma, unspecified, intrapelvic lymph nodes

■ C82.97   Follicular lymphoma, unspecified, spleen

■ C82.98   Follicular lymphoma, unspecified, lymph nodes of multiple sites

■ C82.99   Follicular lymphoma, unspecified, extranodal and solid organ sites

● C83   Non-follicular lymphoma

Excludes1   personal history of non-Hodgkin lymphoma (Z85.72)

● C83.0   Small cell B-cell lymphoma
Lymphoplasmacytic lymphoma
Nodal marginal zone lymphoma
Non-leukemic variant of B-CLL
Splenic marginal zone lymphoma

Excludes1   chronic lymphocytic leukemia (C91.1)
mature T/NK-cell lymphomas (C84.-)
Waldenström macroglobulinemia (C88.0)

 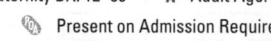

CHAPTER 2 (C00-D49)

■ C83.00   Small cell B-cell lymphoma, unspecified site 🦠

C83.01   Small cell B-cell lymphoma, lymph nodes of head, face, and neck 🦠

C83.02   Small cell B-cell lymphoma, intrathoracic lymph nodes 🦠

C83.03   Small cell B-cell lymphoma, intra-abdominal lymph nodes 🦠

C83.04   Small cell B-cell lymphoma, lymph nodes of axilla and upper limb 🦠

C83.05   Small cell B-cell lymphoma, lymph nodes of inguinal region and lower limb 🦠

C83.06   Small cell B-cell lymphoma, intrapelvic lymph nodes 🦠

C83.07   Small cell B-cell lymphoma, spleen 🦠

C83.08   Small cell B-cell lymphoma, lymph nodes of multiple sites 🦠

C83.09   Small cell B-cell lymphoma, extranodal and solid organ sites 🦠

● C83.1   Mantle cell lymphoma
     Centrocytic lymphoma
     Malignant lymphomatous polyposis

■ C83.10   Mantle cell lymphoma, unspecified site 🦠

C83.11   Mantle cell lymphoma, lymph nodes of head, face, and neck 🦠

C83.12   Mantle cell lymphoma, intrathoracic lymph nodes 🦠

C83.13   Mantle cell lymphoma, intra-abdominal lymph nodes 🦠

C83.14   Mantle cell lymphoma, lymph nodes of axilla and upper limb 🦠

C83.15   Mantle cell lymphoma, lymph nodes of inguinal region and lower limb 🦠

C83.16   Mantle cell lymphoma, intrapelvic lymph nodes 🦠

C83.17   Mantle cell lymphoma, spleen 🦠

C83.18   Mantle cell lymphoma, lymph nodes of multiple sites 🦠

C83.19   Mantle cell lymphoma, extranodal and solid organ sites 🦠

● C83.3   Diffuse large B-cell lymphoma
     Anaplastic diffuse large B-cell lymphoma
     CD30-positive diffuse large B-cell lymphoma
     Centroblastic diffuse large B-cell lymphoma
     Diffuse large B-cell lymphoma, subtype not specified
     Immunoblastic diffuse large B-cell lymphoma
     Plasmablastic diffuse large B-cell lymphoma
     Diffuse large B-cell lymphoma, subtype not specified
     T-cell rich diffuse large B-cell lymphoma

     | Excludes1 | mediastinal (thymic) large B-cell lymphoma (C85.2-)
                      mature T/NK-cell lymphomas (C84.-)

■ C83.30   Diffuse large B-cell lymphoma, unspecified site 🦠

C83.31   Diffuse large B-cell lymphoma, lymph nodes of head, face, and neck 🦠

C83.32   Diffuse large B-cell lymphoma, intrathoracic lymph nodes 🦠

C83.33   Diffuse large B-cell lymphoma, intra-abdominal lymph nodes 🦠

C83.34   Diffuse large B-cell lymphoma, lymph nodes of axilla and upper limb 🦠

C83.35   Diffuse large B-cell lymphoma, lymph nodes of inguinal region and lower limb 🦠

C83.36   Diffuse large B-cell lymphoma, intrapelvic lymph nodes 🦠

C83.37   Diffuse large B-cell lymphoma, spleen 🦠

C83.38   Diffuse large B-cell lymphoma, lymph nodes of multiple sites 🦠

C83.39   Diffuse large B-cell lymphoma, extranodal and solid organ sites 🦠

● C83.5   Lymphoblastic (diffuse) lymphoma
     Highly malignant type of non-Hodgkin lymphoma with diffuse infiltration
     B-precursor lymphoma
     Lymphoblastic B-cell lymphoma
     Lymphoblastic lymphoma NOS
     Lymphoblastic T-cell lymphoma
     T-precursor lymphoma

■ C83.50   Lymphoblastic (diffuse) lymphoma, unspecified site 🦠

C83.51   Lymphoblastic (diffuse) lymphoma, lymph nodes of head, face, and neck 🦠

C83.52   Lymphoblastic (diffuse) lymphoma, intrathoracic lymph nodes 🦠

C83.53   Lymphoblastic (diffuse) lymphoma, intra-abdominal lymph nodes 🦠

C83.54   Lymphoblastic (diffuse) lymphoma, lymph nodes of axilla and upper limb 🦠

C83.55   Lymphoblastic (diffuse) lymphoma, lymph nodes of inguinal region and lower limb 🦠

C83.56   Lymphoblastic (diffuse) lymphoma, intrapelvic lymph nodes 🦠

C83.57   Lymphoblastic (diffuse) lymphoma, spleen 🦠

C83.58   Lymphoblastic (diffuse) lymphoma, lymph nodes of multiple sites 🦠

C83.59   Lymphoblastic (diffuse) lymphoma, extranodal and solid organ sites 🦠

● C83.7   Burkitt lymphoma
     Form of small cell lymphoma
     Atypical Burkitt lymphoma
     Burkitt-like lymphoma

     | Excludes1 | mature B-cell leukemia Burkitt type (C91.A-)

■ C83.70   Burkitt lymphoma, unspecified site 🦠

C83.71   Burkitt lymphoma, lymph nodes of head, face, and neck 🦠

C83.72   Burkitt lymphoma, intrathoracic lymph nodes 🦠

C83.73   Burkitt lymphoma, intra-abdominal lymph nodes 🦠

C83.74   Burkitt lymphoma, lymph nodes of axilla and upper limb 🦠

C83.75   Burkitt lymphoma, lymph nodes of inguinal region and lower limb 🦠

C83.76   Burkitt lymphoma, intrapelvic lymph nodes 🦠

C83.77   Burkitt lymphoma, spleen 🦠

C83.78   Burkitt lymphoma, lymph nodes of multiple sites 🦠

C83.79   Burkitt lymphoma, extranodal and solid organ sites 🦠

● Unacceptable Principal Diagnosis   ● Use Additional Character(s)   ■ Unspecified   ▶ Manifestation Code

846   **OGCR** Official Guidelines for Coding and Reporting   Excludes 1   Excludes 2   Includes   Use additional   Code first   Code also

● C83.8 Other non-follicular lymphoma
  Intravascular large B-cell lymphoma
  Lymphoid granulomatosis
  Primary effusion B-cell lymphoma

  Excludes1   mediastinal (thymic) large B-cell
              lymphoma (C85.2-)
              T-cell rich B-cell lymphoma (C83.3-)

  ◼ C83.80 Other non-follicular lymphoma,
            unspecified site 🅒

  C83.81 Other non-follicular lymphoma, lymph
         nodes of head, face, and neck 🅒

  C83.82 Other non-follicular lymphoma,
         intrathoracic lymph nodes 🅒

  C83.83 Other non-follicular lymphoma, intra-
         abdominal lymph nodes 🅒

  C83.84 Other non-follicular lymphoma, lymph
         nodes of axilla and upper limb 🅒

  C83.85 Other non-follicular lymphoma, lymph
         nodes of inguinal region and lower limb 🅒

  C83.86 Other non-follicular lymphoma,
         intrapelvic lymph nodes 🅒

  C83.87 Other non-follicular lymphoma, spleen 🅒

  C83.88 Other non-follicular lymphoma, lymph
         nodes of multiple sites 🅒

  C83.89 Other non-follicular lymphoma,
         extranodal and solid organ sites 🅒

● C83.9 Non-follicular (diffuse) lymphoma, unspecified

  ◼ C83.90 Non-follicular (diffuse) lymphoma,
            unspecified, unspecified site 🅒

  ◼ C83.91 Non-follicular (diffuse) lymphoma,
            unspecified, lymph nodes of head, face,
            and neck 🅒

  ◼ C83.92 Non-follicular (diffuse) lymphoma,
            unspecified, intrathoracic lymph nodes 🅒

  ◼ C83.93 Non-follicular (diffuse) lymphoma,
            unspecified, intra-abdominal lymph
            nodes 🅒

  ◼ C83.94 Non-follicular (diffuse) lymphoma,
            unspecified, lymph nodes of axilla and
            upper limb 🅒

  ◼ C83.95 Non-follicular (diffuse) lymphoma,
            unspecified, lymph nodes of inguinal
            region and lower limb 🅒

  ◼ C83.96 Non-follicular (diffuse) lymphoma,
            unspecified, intrapelvic lymph nodes 🅒

  ◼ C83.97 Non-follicular (diffuse) lymphoma,
            unspecified, spleen 🅒

  ◼ C83.98 Non-follicular (diffuse) lymphoma,
            unspecified, lymph nodes of multiple
            sites 🅒

  ◼ C83.99 Non-follicular (diffuse) lymphoma,
            unspecified, extranodal and solid organ
            sites 🅒

● C84 Mature T/NK-cell lymphomas

  Excludes1   personal history of non-Hodgkin lymphoma
              (Z85.72)

● C84.0 Mycosis fungoides
  Chronic or rapidly progressive form of cutaneous
  T-cell lymphoma; AKA granuloma fungoides

  Excludes1   peripheral T-cell lymphoma, not
              classified (C84.4-)

  ◼ C84.00 Mycosis fungoides, unspecified site 🅒

  C84.01 Mycosis fungoides, lymph nodes of head,
         face, and neck 🅒

  C84.02 Mycosis fungoides, intrathoracic lymph
         nodes 🅒

C84.03 Mycosis fungoides, intra-abdominal
       lymph nodes 🅒

C84.04 Mycosis fungoides, lymph nodes of axilla
       and upper limb 🅒

C84.05 Mycosis fungoides, lymph nodes of
       inguinal region and lower limb 🅒

C84.06 Mycosis fungoides, intrapelvic lymph
       nodes 🅒

C84.07 Mycosis fungoides, spleen 🅒

C84.08 Mycosis fungoides, lymph nodes of
       multiple sites 🅒

C84.09 Mycosis fungoides, extranodal and solid
       organ sites 🅒

● C84.1 Sézary disease
  Type of cutaneous lymphoma affecting T-cells

  ◼ C84.10 Sézary disease, unspecified site 🅒

  C84.11 Sézary disease, lymph nodes of head, face,
         and neck 🅒

  C84.12 Sézary disease, intrathoracic lymph
         nodes 🅒

  C84.13 Sézary disease, intra-abdominal lymph
         nodes 🅒

  C84.14 Sézary disease, lymph nodes of axilla and
         upper limb 🅒

  C84.15 Sézary disease, lymph nodes of inguinal
         region and lower limb 🅒

  C84.16 Sézary disease, intrapelvic lymph nodes 🅒

  C84.17 Sézary disease, spleen 🅒

  C84.18 Sézary disease, lymph nodes of multiple
         sites 🅒

  C84.19 Sézary disease, extranodal and solid organ
         sites 🅒

● C84.4 Peripheral T-cell lymphoma, not classified
  Diverse group of blood carcinomas originating from
  T-cells, requiring aggressive chemotherapy
  Lennert's lymphoma
  Lymphoepithelioid lymphoma
  Mature T-cell lymphoma, not elsewhere classified

  ◼ C84.40 Peripheral T-cell lymphoma, not classified,
            unspecified site 🅒

  C84.41 Peripheral T-cell lymphoma, not classified,
         lymph nodes of head, face, and neck 🅒

  C84.42 Peripheral T-cell lymphoma, not classified,
         intrathoracic lymph nodes 🅒

  C84.43 Peripheral T-cell lymphoma, not classified,
         intra-abdominal lymph nodes 🅒

  C84.44 Peripheral T-cell lymphoma, not classified,
         lymph nodes of axilla and upper limb 🅒

  C84.45 Peripheral T-cell lymphoma, not classified,
         lymph nodes of inguinal region and lower
         limb 🅒

  C84.46 Peripheral T-cell lymphoma, not classified,
         intrapelvic lymph nodes 🅒

  C84.47 Peripheral T-cell lymphoma, not classified,
         spleen 🅒

  C84.48 Peripheral T-cell lymphoma, not classified,
         lymph nodes of multiple sites 🅒

  C84.49 Peripheral T-cell lymphoma, not classified,
         extranodal and solid organ sites 🅒

Item 2–7   Lymphosarcoma, also known as malignant lymphoma,
is a cancer of the lymph system exhibiting abnormal cells encompassing
an entire lymph node creating a diffuse pattern without any definite
organization. Diffuse pattern lymphoma has a more unfavorable survival
outlook than those with a follicular or nodular pattern. Reticulosarcoma is
the most common aggressive form of non-Hodgkin's lymphoma.

CHAPTER 2 (C00-D49)

● **C84.6**   **Anaplastic large cell lymphoma, ALK-positive**
Anaplastic large cell lymphoma, CD30-positive

▪ C84.60   Anaplastic large cell lymphoma, ALK-positive, unspecified site 🦠

C84.61   Anaplastic large cell lymphoma, ALK-positive, lymph nodes of head, face, and neck 🦠

C84.62   Anaplastic large cell lymphoma, ALK-positive, intrathoracic lymph nodes 🦠

C84.63   Anaplastic large cell lymphoma, ALK-positive, intra-abdominal lymph nodes 🦠

C84.64   Anaplastic large cell lymphoma, ALK-positive, lymph nodes of axilla and upper limb 🦠

C84.65   Anaplastic large cell lymphoma, ALK-positive, lymph nodes of inguinal region and lower limb 🦠

C84.66   Anaplastic large cell lymphoma, ALK-positive, intrapelvic lymph nodes 🦠

C84.67   Anaplastic large cell lymphoma, ALK-positive, spleen 🦠

C84.68   Anaplastic large cell lymphoma, ALK-positive, lymph nodes of multiple sites 🦠

C84.69   Anaplastic large cell lymphoma, ALK-positive, extranodal and solid organ sites 🦠

● **C84.7**   **Anaplastic large cell lymphoma, ALK-negative**

Excludes1   primary cutaneous CD30-positive T-cell proliferations (C86.6-)

▪ C84.70   Anaplastic large cell lymphoma, ALK-negative, unspecified site 🦠

C84.71   Anaplastic large cell lymphoma, ALK-negative, lymph nodes of head, face, and neck 🦠

C84.72   Anaplastic large cell lymphoma, ALK-negative, intrathoracic lymph nodes 🦠

C84.73   Anaplastic large cell lymphoma, ALK-negative, intra-abdominal lymph nodes 🦠

C84.74   Anaplastic large cell lymphoma, ALK-negative, lymph nodes of axilla and upper limb 🦠

C84.75   Anaplastic large cell lymphoma, ALK-negative, lymph nodes of inguinal region and lower limb 🦠

C84.76   Anaplastic large cell lymphoma, ALK-negative, intrapelvic lymph nodes 🦠

C84.77   Anaplastic large cell lymphoma, ALK-negative, spleen 🦠

C84.78   Anaplastic large cell lymphoma, ALK-negative, lymph nodes of multiple sites 🦠

C84.79   Anaplastic large cell lymphoma, ALK-negative, extranodal and solid organ sites 🦠

● **C84.A**   **Cutaneous T-cell lymphoma, unspecified**

▪ C84.A0   Cutaneous T-cell lymphoma, unspecified, unspecified site 🦠

▪ C84.A1   Cutaneous T-cell lymphoma, unspecified, lymph nodes of head, face, and neck 🦠

▪ C84.A2   Cutaneous T-cell lymphoma, unspecified, intrathoracic lymph nodes 🦠

▪ C84.A3   Cutaneous T-cell lymphoma, unspecified, intra-abdominal lymph nodes 🦠

▪ C84.A4   Cutaneous T-cell lymphoma, unspecified, lymph nodes of axilla and upper limb 🦠

▪ C84.A5   Cutaneous T-cell lymphoma, unspecified, lymph nodes of inguinal region and lower limb 🦠

▪ C84.A6   Cutaneous T-cell lymphoma, unspecified, intrapelvic lymph nodes 🦠

▪ C84.A7   Cutaneous T-cell lymphoma, unspecified, spleen 🦠

▪ C84.A8   Cutaneous T-cell lymphoma, unspecified, lymph nodes of multiple sites 🦠

▪ C84.A9   Cutaneous T-cell lymphoma, unspecified, extranodal and solid organ sites 🦠

● **C84.Z**   **Other mature T/NK-cell lymphomas**

Note: If T-cell lineage or involvement is mentioned in conjunction with a specific lymphoma, code to the more specific description.

Excludes1   angioimmunoblastic T-cell lymphoma (C86.5)
blastic NK-cell lymphoma (C86.4)
enteropathy-type T-cell lymphoma (C86.2)
extranodal NK-cell lymphoma, nasal type (C86.0)
hepatosplenic T-cell lymphoma (C86.1)
primary cutaneous CD30-positive T-cell proliferations (C86.6)
subcutaneous panniculitis-like T-cell lymphoma (C86.3)
T-cell leukemia (C91.1-)

▪ C84.Z0   Other mature T/NK-cell lymphomas, unspecified site 🦠

C84.Z1   Other mature T/NK-cell lymphomas, lymph nodes of head, face, and neck 🦠

C84.Z2   Other mature T/NK-cell lymphomas, intrathoracic lymph nodes 🦠

C84.Z3   Other mature T/NK-cell lymphomas, intra-abdominal lymph nodes 🦠

C84.Z4   Other mature T/NK-cell lymphomas, lymph nodes of axilla and upper limb 🦠

C84.Z5   Other mature T/NK-cell lymphomas, lymph nodes of inguinal region and lower limb 🦠

C84.Z6   Other mature T/NK-cell lymphomas, intrapelvic lymph nodes 🦠

C84.Z7   Other mature T/NK-cell lymphomas, spleen 🦠

C84.Z8   Other mature T/NK-cell lymphomas, lymph nodes of multiple sites 🦠

C84.Z9   Other mature T/NK-cell lymphomas, extranodal and solid organ sites 🦠

● **C84.9**   **Mature T/NK-cell lymphomas, unspecified**
NK/T cell lymphoma NOS

Excludes1   mature T-cell lymphoma, not elsewhere classified (C84.4-)

▪ C84.90   Mature T/NK-cell lymphomas, unspecified, unspecified site 🦠

▪ C84.91   Mature T/NK-cell lymphomas, unspecified, lymph nodes of head, face, and neck 🦠

▪ C84.92   Mature T/NK-cell lymphomas, unspecified, intrathoracic lymph nodes 🦠

▪ C84.93   Mature T/NK-cell lymphomas, unspecified, intra-abdominal lymph nodes 🦠

▪ C84.94   Mature T/NK-cell lymphomas, unspecified, lymph nodes of axilla and upper limb 🦠

● Unacceptable Principal Diagnosis   ● Use Additional Character(s)   ▪ Unspecified   ▶ Manifestation Code

OGCR Official Guidelines for Coding and Reporting   Excludes 1   Excludes 2   Includes   Use additional   Code first   Code also

CHAPTER 2 (C00-D49)

■ **C84.95**   Mature T/NK-cell lymphomas, unspecified, lymph nodes of inguinal region and lower limb 🝔

■ **C84.96**   Mature T/NK-cell lymphomas, unspecified, intrapelvic lymph nodes 🝔

■ **C84.97**   Mature T/NK-cell lymphomas, unspecified, spleen 🝔

■ **C84.98**   Mature T/NK-cell lymphomas, unspecified, lymph nodes of multiple sites 🝔

■ **C84.99**   Mature T/NK-cell lymphomas, unspecified, extranodal and solid organ sites 🝔

● **C85**   **Other specified and unspecified types of non-Hodgkin lymphoma**

> **Excludes1**   other specified types of T/NK-cell lymphoma (C86.-)
>
> personal history of non-Hodgkin lymphoma (Z85.72)

● **C85.1**   **Unspecified B-cell lymphoma**

> **Note:** If B-cell lineage or involvement is mentioned in conjunction with a specific lymphoma, code to the more specific description.

■ **C85.10**   Unspecified B-cell lymphoma, unspecified site 🝔

■ **C85.11**   Unspecified B-cell lymphoma, lymph nodes of head, face, and neck 🝔

■ **C85.12**   Unspecified B-cell lymphoma, intrathoracic lymph nodes 🝔

■ **C85.13**   Unspecified B-cell lymphoma, intra-abdominal lymph nodes 🝔

■ **C85.14**   Unspecified B-cell lymphoma, lymph nodes of axilla and upper limb 🝔

■ **C85.15**   Unspecified B-cell lymphoma, lymph nodes of inguinal region and lower limb 🝔

■ **C85.16**   Unspecified B-cell lymphoma, intrapelvic lymph nodes 🝔

■ **C85.17**   Unspecified B-cell lymphoma, spleen 🝔

■ **C85.18**   Unspecified B-cell lymphoma, lymph nodes of multiple sites 🝔

■ **C85.19**   Unspecified B-cell lymphoma, extranodal and solid organ sites 🝔

● **C85.2**   **Mediastinal (thymic) large B-cell lymphoma**

■ **C85.20**   Mediastinal (thymic) large B-cell lymphoma, unspecified site 🝔

C85.21   Mediastinal (thymic) large B-cell lymphoma, lymph nodes of head, face, and neck 🝔

C85.22   Mediastinal (thymic) large B-cell lymphoma, intrathoracic lymph nodes 🝔

C85.23   Mediastinal (thymic) large B-cell lymphoma, intra-abdominal lymph nodes 🝔

C85.24   Mediastinal (thymic) large B-cell lymphoma, lymph nodes of axilla and upper limb 🝔

C85.25   Mediastinal (thymic) large B-cell lymphoma, lymph nodes of inguinal region and lower limb 🝔

C85.26   Mediastinal (thymic) large B-cell lymphoma, intrapelvic lymph nodes 🝔

C85.27   Mediastinal (thymic) large B-cell lymphoma, spleen 🝔

C85.28   Mediastinal (thymic) large B-cell lymphoma, lymph nodes of multiple sites 🝔

C85.29   Mediastinal (thymic) large B-cell lymphoma, extranodal and solid organ sites 🝔

● **C85.8**   **Other specified types of non-Hodgkin lymphoma**

■ **C85.80**   Other specified types of non-Hodgkin lymphoma, unspecified site 🝔

C85.81   Other specified types of non-Hodgkin lymphoma, lymph nodes of head, face, and neck 🝔

C85.82   Other specified types of non-Hodgkin lymphoma, intrathoracic lymph nodes 🝔

C85.83   Other specified types of non-Hodgkin lymphoma, intra-abdominal lymph nodes 🝔

C85.84   Other specified types of non-Hodgkin lymphoma, lymph nodes of axilla and upper limb 🝔

C85.85   Other specified types of non-Hodgkin lymphoma, lymph nodes of inguinal region and lower limb 🝔

C85.86   Other specified types of non-Hodgkin lymphoma, intrapelvic lymph nodes 🝔

C85.87   Other specified types of non-Hodgkin lymphoma, spleen 🝔

C85.88   Other specified types of non-Hodgkin lymphoma, lymph nodes of multiple sites 🝔

C85.89   Other specified types of non-Hodgkin lymphoma, extranodal and solid organ sites 🝔

● **C85.9**   **Non-Hodgkin lymphoma, unspecified**

Lymphoma NOS

Malignant lymphoma NOS

Non-Hodgkin lymphoma NOS

■ **C85.90**   Non-Hodgkin lymphoma, unspecified, unspecified site 🝔

■ **C85.91**   Non-Hodgkin lymphoma, unspecified, lymph nodes of head, face, and neck 🝔

■ **C85.92**   Non-Hodgkin lymphoma, unspecified, intrathoracic lymph nodes 🝔

■ **C85.93**   Non-Hodgkin lymphoma, unspecified, intra-abdominal lymph nodes 🝔

■ **C85.94**   Non-Hodgkin lymphoma, unspecified, lymph nodes of axilla and upper limb 🝔

■ **C85.95**   Non-Hodgkin lymphoma, unspecified, lymph nodes of inguinal region and lower limb 🝔

■ **C85.96**   Non-Hodgkin lymphoma, unspecified, intrapelvic lymph nodes 🝔

■ **C85.97**   Non-Hodgkin lymphoma, unspecified, spleen 🝔

■ **C85.98**   Non-Hodgkin lymphoma, unspecified, lymph nodes of multiple sites 🝔

■ **C85.99**   Non-Hodgkin lymphoma, unspecified, extranodal and solid organ sites 🝔

N Newborn Age: 0   **P** Pediatric Age: 0–17   **M** Maternity DX: 12–55   **A** Adult Age: 15–124   ♀ Females Only   ♂ Males Only

🝔 Complication\Comorbidity   🝔 Major C\C   🝔 Present on Admission Requirement   🝔 Hospital-Acquired Condition

849

C86 Other specified types of T/NK-cell lymphoma
> **Excludes1** anaplastic large cell lymphoma, ALK
> negative (C84.7-)
> anaplastic large cell lymphoma, ALK
> positive (C84.6-)
> mature T/NK-cell lymphomas (C84.-)
> other specified types of non-Hodgkin
> lymphoma (C85.8-)

C86.0 Extranodal NK/T-cell lymphoma, nasal type 🖝

C86.1 Hepatosplenic T-cell lymphoma 🖝
  Alpha-beta and gamma delta types

C86.2 Enteropathy-type (intestinal) T-cell lymphoma 🖝
  Enteropathy associated T-cell lymphoma

C86.3 Subcutaneous panniculitis-like T-cell lymphoma 🖝

C86.4 Blastic NK-cell lymphoma 🖝

C86.5 Angioimmunoblastic T-cell lymphoma 🖝
  Angioimmunoblastic lymphadenopathy with
  dysproteinemia (AILD)

C86.6 Primary cutaneous CD30-positive T-cell
  proliferations 🖝
  Lymphomatoid papulosis
  Primary cutaneous anaplastic large cell lymphoma
  Primary cutaneous CD30-positive large T-cell
  lymphoma

● C88 Malignant immunoproliferative diseases and certain
  other B-cell lymphomas
  Diseases involving immune system
> **Excludes1** B-cell lymphoma, unspecified C85.1-
> personal history of other malignant
> neoplasms of lymphoid, hematopoietic
> and related tissues (Z85.79)

C88.0 Waldenström's macroglobulinemia
  Lymphoplasmacytic lymphoma with
  IgM-production
  Macroglobulinemia (idiopathic) (primary)
> **Excludes1** small cell B-cell lymphoma (C83.0)

C88.2 Heavy chain disease 🖝
  Franklin disease
  Gamma heavy chain disease
  Mu heavy chain disease

C88.3 Immunoproliferative small intestinal disease 🖝
  Alpha heavy chain disease
  Mediterranean lymphoma

C88.4 Extranodal marginal zone B-cell lymphoma of
  mucosa-associated lymphoid tissue [MALT-
  lymphoma] 🖝
  Lymphoma of skin-associated lymphoid tissue
  [SALT-lymphoma]
  Lymphoma of bronchial-associated lymphoid
  tissue [BALT-lymphoma]
> **Excludes1** high malignant (diffuse large B-cell)
> lymphoma (C83.3-)

C88.8 Other malignant immunoproliferative diseases 🖝

C88.9 Malignant immunoproliferative disease,
  unspecified 🖝
  Immunoproliferative disease NOS

● C90 Multiple myeloma and malignant plasma cell neoplasms
> **Excludes1** personal history of other malignant
> neoplasms of lymphoid, hematopoietic
> and related tissues (Z85.79)

● C90.0 Multiple myeloma
  Kahler's disease
  Medullary plasmacytoma
  Myelomatosis
  Plasma cell myeloma
> **Excludes1** solitary myeloma (C90.3-)
> solitary plasmacytoma (C90.3-)

C90.00 Multiple myeloma not having achieved
  remission 🖝
  Multiple myeloma with failed remission
  Multiple myeloma NOS

C90.01 Multiple myeloma in remission 🖝

C90.02 Multiple myeloma in relapse 🖝

● C90.1 Plasma cell leukemia
  Rare type of acute leukemia
  Plasmacytic leukemia

C90.10 Plasma cell leukemia not having achieved
  remission 🖝
  Plasma cell leukemia with failed remission
  Plasma cell leukemia NOS

C90.11 Plasma cell leukemia in remission 🖝

C90.12 Plasma cell leukemia in relapse 🖝

● C90.2 Extramedullary plasmacytoma
  *Malignant monoclonal plasma cell tumor growing in
  soft tissue; AKA plasma cell dyscrasias*

C90.20 Extramedullary plasmacytoma not having
  achieved remission 🖝
  Extramedullary plasmacytoma with failed
  remission
  Extramedullary plasmacytoma NOS

C90.21 Extramedullary plasmacytoma in
  remission 🖝

C90.22 Extramedullary plasmacytoma in relapse 🖝

C90.3 Solitary plasmacytoma
  Localized malignant plasma cell tumor NOS
  Plasmacytoma NOS
  Solitary myeloma

C90.30 Solitary plasmacytoma not having
  achieved remission 🖝
  Solitary plasmacytoma with failed
  remission
  Solitary plasmacytoma NOS

C90.31 Solitary plasmacytoma in remission 🖝

C90.32 Solitary plasmacytoma in relapse 🖝

● C91 Lymphoid leukemia
  Type of leukemia affecting circulating cells of lymphoid origin
> **Excludes1** personal history of leukemia (Z85.6)

● C91.0 Acute lymphoblastic leukemia [ALL]
  Note: Code C91.0 should only be used for T-cell
  and B-cell precusor leukemia

C91.00 Acute lymphoblastic leukemia not having
  achieved remission 🖝
  Acute lymphoblastic leukemia with failed
  remission
  Acute lymphoblastic leukemia NOS

C91.01 Acute lymphoblastic leukemia, in
  remission 🖝

C91.02 Acute lymphoblastic leukemia,
  in relapse 🖝

Item 2–8 Multiple myeloma is a cancer of a plasma cell (a type of white blood cell) and is an incurable but treatable disease. Immunoproliferative neoplasm is a term for diseases (mostly cancers) in which the immune system cells proliferate.

Item 2–9 Leukemia is a cancer (acute or chronic) of the blood-forming tissues of the bone marrow. Blood cells all start out as stem cells. They mature and become red cells, white cells, or platelets. There are three main types of leukocytes (white cells that fight infection): monocytes, lymphocytes, and granulocytes. **Acute monocytic leukemia** (AML) affects monocytes. **Acute lymphoid leukemia** (ALL) affects lymphocytes, and **acute myeloid leukemia** (AML) affects cells that typically develop into white blood cells (not lymphocytes), though it may develop in other blood cells.

● **C91.1** **Chronic lymphocytic leukemia of B-cell type**
Lymphoplasmacytic leukemia
Richter syndrome

> **Excludes1**   lymphoplasmacytic lymphoma (C83.0-)

C91.10 **Chronic lymphocytic leukemia of B-cell type not having achieved remission** 🗝
Chronic lymphocytic leukemia of B-cell type with failed remission
Chronic lymphocytic leukemia of B-cell type NOS

C91.11 **Chronic lymphocytic leukemia of B-cell type in remission** 🗝

C91.12 **Chronic lymphocytic leukemia of B-cell type in relapse** 🗝

● **C91.3** **Prolymphocytic leukemia of B-cell type**
Chronic leukemia with symptoms of large number of circulating lymphocytes

C91.30 **Prolymphocytic leukemia of B-cell type not having achieved remission** 🗝
Prolymphocytic leukemia of B-cell type with failed remission
Prolymphocytic leukemia of B-cell type NOS

C91.31 **Prolymphocytic leukemia of B-cell type, in remission** 🗝

C91.32 **Prolymphocytic leukemia of B-cell type, in relapse** 🗝

● **C91.4** **Hairy cell leukemia**
Chronic leukemia with splenomegaly and excessive number of abnormal large mononuclear cells covered by hairlike villi
Leukemic reticuloendotheliosis

C91.40 **Hairy cell leukemia not having achieved remission** 🗝
Hairy cell leukemia with failed remission
Hairy cell leukemia NOS

C91.41 **Hairy cell leukemia, in remission** 🗝

C91.42 **Hairy cell leukemia, in relapse** 🗝

● **C91.5** **Adult T-cell lymphoma/leukemia (HTLV-1-associated)**
Acute variant of adult T-cell lymphoma/leukemia (HTLV-1-associated)
Chronic variant of adult T-cell lymphoma/leukemia (HTLV-1-associated)
Lymphomatoid variant of adult T-cell lymphoma/leukemia (HTLV-1-associated)
Smouldering variant of adult T-cell lymphoma/leukemia (HTLV-1-associated)

C91.50 **Adult T-cell lymphoma/leukemia (HTLV-1-associated) not having achieved remission** 🗝   **A**
Adult T-cell lymphoma/leukemia (HTLV-1-associated) with failed remission
Adult T-cell lymphoma/leukemia (HTLV-1-associated) NOS

C91.51 **Adult T-cell lymphoma/leukemia (HTLV-1-associated), in remission** 🗝   **A**

C91.52 **Adult T-cell lymphoma/leukemia (HTLV-1-associated), in relapse** 🗝   **A**

● **C91.6** **Prolymphocytic leukemia of T-cell type**

C91.60 **Prolymphocytic leukemia of T-cell type not having achieved remission** 🗝
Prolymphocytic leukemia of T-cell type with failed remission
Prolymphocytic leukemia of T-cell type NOS

C91.61 **Prolymphocytic leukemia of T-cell type, in remission** 🗝

C91.62 **Prolymphocytic leukemia of T-cell type, in relapse** 🗝

● **C91.A** **Mature B-cell leukemia Burkitt-type**

> **Excludes1**   Burkitt lymphoma (C83.7-)

C91.A0 **Mature B-cell leukemia Burkitt-type not having achieved remission** 🗝
Mature B-cell leukemia Burkitt-type with failed remission
Mature B-cell leukemia Burkitt-type NOS

C91.A1 **Mature B-cell leukemia Burkitt-type, in remission** 🗝

C91.A2 **Mature B-cell leukemia Burkitt-type, in relapse** 🗝

● **C91.Z** **Other lymphoid leukemia**
T-cell large granular lymphocytic leukemia (associated with rheumatoid arthritis)

C91.Z0 **Other lymphoid leukemia not having achieved remission** 🗝
Other lymphoid leukemia with failed remission
Other lymphoid leukemia NOS

C91.Z1 **Other lymphoid leukemia, in remission** 🗝

C91.Z2 **Other lymphoid leukemia, in relapse** 🗝

● **C91.9** **Lymphoid leukemia, unspecified**

■ **C91.90** **Lymphoid leukemia, unspecified not having achieved remission** 🗝
Lymphoid leukemia with failed remission
Lymphoid leukemia NOS

■ **C91.91** **Lymphoid leukemia, unspecified, in remission** 🗝

■ **C91.92** **Lymphoid leukemia, unspecified, in relapse** 🗝

N Newborn Age: 0   **P** Pediatric Age: 0–17   **M** Maternity DX: 12–55   **A** Adult Age: 15–124   ♀ Females Only   ♂ Males Only
🗝 Complication\Comorbidity   🗝 Major C\C   🗝 Present on Admission Requirement   🗝 Hospital-Acquired Condition

851

CHAPTER 2 (C00-D49)

● **C92   Myeloid leukemia**

> **Includes**   granulocytic leukemia
>   myelogenous leukemia
>
> **Excludes1**   personal history of leukemia (Z85.6)

  ● **C92.0 Acute myeloblastic leukemia**

> Acute myeloblastic leukemia, minimal differentiation
> Acute myeloblastic leukemia (with maturation)
> Acute myeloblastic leukemia 1/ETO
> Acute myeloblastic leukemia M0
> Acute myeloblastic leukemia M1
> Acute myeloblastic leukemia M2
> Acute myeloblastic leukemia with t(8;21)
> Acute myeloblastic leukemia (without a FAB classification) NOS
> Refractory anemia with excess blasts in transformation [RAEB T]
>
> **Excludes1**   acute exacerbation of chronic myeloid leukemia (C92.10)
>   refractory anemia with excess of blasts not in transformation (D46.2-)

    C92.00 Acute myeloblastic leukemia, not having achieved remission 🔍

> Acute myeloblastic leukemia with failed remission
> Acute myeloblastic leukemia NOS

    C92.01 Acute myeloblastic leukemia, in remission 🔍

    C92.02 Acute myeloblastic leukemia, in relapse 🔍

  ● **C92.1 Chronic myeloid leukemia, BCR/ABL-positive**

> Chronic myelogenous leukemia, Philadelphia chromosome (Ph1) positive
> Chronic myelogenous leukemia, t(9;22) (q34;q11)
> Chronic myelogenous leukemia with crisis of blast cells
>
> **Excludes1**   atypical chronic myeloid leukemia BCR/ABL-negative (C92.2-)
>   chronic myelomonocytic leukemia (C93.1-)
>   chronic myeloproliferative disease (D47.1)

    C92.10 Chronic myeloid leukemia, BCR/ABL-positive, not having achieved remission 🔍

> Chronic myeloid leukemia, BCR/ABL-positive with failed remission
> Chronic myeloid leukemia, BCR/ABL-positive NOS

    C92.11 Chronic myeloid leukemia, BCR/ABL-positive, in remission 🔍

    C92.12 Chronic myeloid leukemia, BCR/ABL-positive, in relapse 🔍

  ● **C92.2 Atypical chronic myeloid leukemia, BCR/ABL-negative**

    C92.20 Atypical chronic myeloid leukemia, BCR/ABL-negative, not having achieved remission 🔍

> Atypical chronic myeloid leukemia, BCR/ABL-negative with failed remission
> Atypical chronic myeloid leukemia, BCR/ABL-negative NOS

    C92.21 Atypical chronic myeloid leukemia, BCR/ABL-negative, in remission 🔍

    C92.22 Atypical chronic myeloid leukemia, BCR/ABL-negative, in relapse 🔍

  ● **C92.3 Myeloid sarcoma**

> A malignant tumor of immature myeloid cells
> Chloroma
> Granulocytic sarcoma

    C92.30 Myeloid sarcoma, not having achieved remission 🔍

> Myeloid sarcoma with failed remission
> Myeloid sarcoma NOS

    C92.31 Myeloid sarcoma, in remission 🔍

    C92.32 Myeloid sarcoma, in relapse 🔍

  ● **C92.4 Acute promyelocytic leukemia**

> AML M3
> AML Me with t(15;17) and variants

    C92.40 Acute promyelocytic leukemia, not having achieved remission 🔍

> Acute promyelocytic leukemia with failed remission
> Acute promyelocytic leukemia NOS

    C92.41 Acute promyelocytic leukemia, in remission 🔍

    C92.42 Acute promyelocytic leukemia, in relapse 🔍

  ● **C92.5 Acute myelomonocytic leukemia**

> AML M4
> AML M4 Eo with inv(16) or t(16;16)

    C92.50 Acute myelomonocytic leukemia, not having achieved remission 🔍

> Acute myelomonocytic leukemia with failed remission
> Acute myelomonocytic leukemia NOS

    C92.51 Acute myelomonocytic leukemia, in remission 🔍

    C92.52 Acute myelomonocytic leukemia, in relapse 🔍

  ● **C92.6 Acute myeloid leukemia with 11q23-abnormality**

> Acute myeloid leukemia with variation of MLL-gene

    C92.60 Acute myeloid leukemia with 11q23-abnormality not having achieved remission 🔍

> Acute myeloid leukemia with 11q23-abnormality with failed remission
> Acute myeloid leukemia with 11q23-abnormality NOS

    C92.61 Acute myeloid leukemia with 11q23-abnormality in remission 🔍

    C92.62 Acute myeloid leukemia with 11q23-abnormality in relapse 🔍

  ● **C92.A Acute myeloid leukemia with multilineage dysplasia**

> Acute myeloid leukemia with dysplasia of remaining hematopoesis and/or myelodysplastic disease in its history

    C92.A0 Acute myeloid leukemia with multilineage dysplasia, not having achieved remission 🔍

> Acute myeloid leukemia with multilineage dysplasia with failed remission
> Acute myeloid leukemia with multilineage dysplasia NOS

    C92.A1 Acute myeloid leukemia with multilineage dysplasia, in remission 🔍

    C92.A2 Acute myeloid leukemia with multilineage dysplasia, in relapse 🔍

● Unacceptable Principal Diagnosis   ● Use Additional Character(s)   ■ Unspecified   ▶ Manifestation Code

OGCR Official Guidelines for Coding and Reporting   Excludes 1   Excludes 2   Includes   Use additional   Code first   Code also

● **C92.Z   Other myeloid leukemia**

     C92.Z0   Other myeloid leukemia not having achieved remission 🔹
         Myeloid leukemia NEC with failed remission
         Myeloid leukemia NEC

     C92.Z1   Other myeloid leukemia, in remission 🔹

     C92.Z2   Other myeloid leukemia, in relapse 🔹

● **C92.9   Myeloid leukemia, unspecified**

     ▪ **C92.90   Myeloid leukemia, unspecified, not having achieved remission** 🔹
         Myeloid leukemia, unspecified with failed remission
         Myeloid leukemia, unspecified NOS

     ▪ **C92.91   Myeloid leukemia, unspecified in remission** 🔹

     ▪ **C92.92   Myeloid leukemia, unspecified in relapse** 🔹

● **C93   Monocytic leukemia**

     Includes   monocytoid leukemia
     Excludes1   personal history of leukemia (Z85.6)

● **C93.0   Acute monoblastic/monocytic leukemia**
     AML M5
     AML M5a
     AML M5b

     C93.00   Acute monoblastic/monocytic leukemia, not having achieved remission 🔹
         Acute monoblastic/monocytic leukemia with failed remission
         Acute monoblastic/monocytic leukemia NOS

     C93.01   Acute monoblastic/monocytic leukemia, in remission 🔹

     C93.02   Acute monoblastic/monocytic leukemia, in relapse 🔹

● **C93.1   Chronic myelomonocytic leukemia**
     Chronic monocytic leukemia
     CMML-1
     CMML-2
     CMML with eosinophilia

     C93.10   Chronic myelomonocytic leukemia not having achieved remission 🔹
         Chronic myelomonocytic leukemia with failed remission
         Chronic myelomonocytic leukemia NOS

     C93.11   Chronic myelomonocytic leukemia, in remission 🔹

     C93.12   Chronic myelomonocytic leukemia, in relapse 🔹

● **C93.3   Juvenile myelomonocytic leukemia**

     C93.30   Juvenile myelomonocytic leukemia, not having achieved remission 🔹
         Juvenile myelomonocytic leukemia with failed remission
         Juvenile myelomonocytic leukemia NOS

     C93.31   Juvenile myelomonocytic leukemia, in remission 🔹

     C93.32   Juvenile myelomonocytic leukemia, in relapse 🔹

● **C93.Z   Other monocytic leukemia**

     C93.Z0   Other monocytic leukemia, not having achieved remission 🔹
         Other monocytic leukemia NOS

     C93.Z1   Other monocytic leukemia, in remission 🔹

     C93.Z2   Other monocytic leukemia, in relapse

● **C93.9   Monocytic leukemia, unspecified**

     ▪ **C93.90   Monocytic leukemia, unspecified, not having achieved remission** 🔹
         Monocytic leukemia, unspecified with failed remission
         Monocytic leukemia, unspecified NOS

     ▪ **C93.91   Monocytic leukemia, unspecified in remission** 🔹

     ▪ **C93.92   Monocytic leukemia, unspecified in relapse** 🔹

● **C94   Other leukemias of specified cell type**

     Excludes1   leukemic reticuloendotheliosis (C91.4-)
         myelodysplastic syndromes (D46.-)
         personal history of leukemia (Z85.6)
         plasma cell leukemia (C90.1-)

● **C94.0   Acute erythroid leukemia**
     Acute myeloid leukemia M6(a)(b)
     Erythroleukemia

     C94.00   Acute erythroid leukemia, not having achieved remission 🔹
         Acute erythroid leukemia with failed remission
         Acute erythroid leukemia NOS

     C94.01   Acute erythroid leukemia, in remission 🔹

     C94.02   Acute erythroid leukemia, in relapse 🔹

● **C94.2   Acute megakaryoblastic leukemia**
     Acute myeloid leukemia M7
     Acute megakaryocytic leukemia

     C94.20   Acute megakaryoblastic leukemia not having achieved remission 🔹
         Acute megakaryoblastic leukemia with failed remission
         Acute megakaryoblastic leukemia NOS

     C94.21   Acute megakaryoblastic leukemia, in remission 🔹

     C94.22   Acute megakaryoblastic leukemia, in relapse 🔹

● **C94.3   Mast cell leukemia**

     C94.30   Mast cell leukemia not having achieved remission 🔹
         Mast cell leukemia with failed remission
         Mast cell leukemia NOS

     C94.31   Mast cell leukemia, in remission 🔹

     C94.32   Mast cell leukemia, in relapse 🔹

● **C94.4   Acute panmyelosis with myelofibrosis**
     Acute myelofibrosis

     Excludes1   myelofibrosis NOS (D75.81)
         secondary myelofibrosis NOS (D75.81)

     C94.40   Acute panmyelosis with myelofibrosis not having achieved remission 🔹
         Acute myelofibrosis NOS
         Acute panmyelosis with myelofibrosis with failed remission
         Acute panmyelosis NOS

     C94.41   Acute panmyelosis with myelofibrosis, in remission 🔹

     C94.42   Acute panmyelosis with myelofibrosis, in relapse 🔹

C94.6   Myelodysplastic disease, not classified 🔹
     Myeloproliferative disease, not classified

N Newborn Age: 0   **P** Pediatric Age: 0–17   **M** Maternity DX: 12–55   **A** Adult Age: 15–124   ♀ Females Only   ♂ Males Only

🔹 Complication\Comorbidity   🔹 Major C\C   🔹 Present on Admission Requirement   🔹 Hospital-Acquired Condition

853

CHAPTER 2 (C00-D49)

● **C94.8   Other specified leukemias**
     Aggressive NK-cell leukemia
     Acute basophilic leukemia

     C94.80   Other specified leukemias not having achieved remission 🗅
         Other specified leukemia with failed remission
         Other specified leukemias NOS

     C94.81   Other specified leukemias, in remission 🗅

     C94.82   Other specified leukemias, in relapse 🗅

● **C95   Leukemia of unspecified cell type**
     | Excludes 1 | personal history of leukemia (Z85.6)

   ● **C95.0   Acute leukemia of unspecified cell type**
     Acute bilineal leukemia
     Acute mixed lineage leukemia
     Biphenotypic acute leukemia
     Stem cell leukemia of unclear lineage

     | Excludes 1 | acute exacerbation of unspecified chronic leukemia (C95.10)

     ■ **C95.00   Acute leukemia of unspecified cell type not having achieved remission** 🗅
         Acute leukemia of unspecified cell type with failed remission
         Acute leukemia NOS

     ■ **C95.01   Acute leukemia of unspecified cell type, in remission** 🗅

     ■ **C95.02   Acute leukemia of unspecified cell type, in relapse** 🗅

   ● **C95.1   Chronic leukemia of unspecified cell type**
     ■ **C95.10   Chronic leukemia of unspecified cell type not having achieved remission** 🗅
         Chronic leukemia of unspecified cell type with failed remission
         Chronic leukemia NOS

     ■ **C95.11   Chronic leukemia of unspecified cell type, in remission** 🗅

     ■ **C95.12   Chronic leukemia of unspecified cell type, in relapse** 🗅

   ● **C95.9   Leukemia, unspecified**
     ■ **C95.90   Leukemia, unspecified not having achieved remission** 🗅
         Leukemia, unspecified with failed remission
         Leukemia NOS

     ■ **C95.91   Leukemia, unspecified, in remission** 🗅

     ■ **C95.92   Leukemia, unspecified, in relapse** 🗅

● **C96   Other and unspecified malignant neoplasms of lymphoid, hematopoietic and related tissue**
     | Excludes 1 | personal history of other malignant neoplasms of lymphoid, hematopoietic and related tissues (Z85.79)

   C96.0   Multifocal and multisystemic (disseminated) Langerhans-cell histiocytosis 🗅
     Histiocytosis X, multisystemic
     Letterer-Siwe disease

     | Excludes 1 | adult pulmonary Langerhans cell histiocytosis (J84.82)
         multifocal and unisystemic Langerhans-cell histiocytosis (C96.5)
         unifocal Langerhans-cell histiocytosis (C96.6)

   C96.2   Malignant mast cell tumor 🗅
     Aggressive systemic mastocytosis
     Mast cell sarcoma

     | Excludes 1 | indolent mastocytosis (D47.0)
         mast cell leukemia (C94.30)
         mastocytosis (congenital) (cutaneous) (Q82.2)

   C96.4   Sarcoma of dendritic cells (accessory cells) 🗅
     Follicular dendritic cell sarcoma
     Interdigitating dendritic cell sarcoma
     Langerhans cell sarcoma

   C96.5   Multifocal and unisystemic Langerhans-cell histiocytosis 🗅
     Hand-Schüller-Christian disease
     Histiocytosis X, multifocal

     | Excludes 1 | multifocal and multisystemic (disseminated) Langerhans-cell histiocytosis (C96.0)
         unifocal Langerhans-cell histiocytosis (C96.6)

   C96.6   Unifocal Langerhans-cell histiocytosis 🗅
     Eosinophilic granuloma
     Histiocytosis X, unifocal
     Histiocytosis X NOS
     Langerhans-cell histiocytosis NOS

     | Excludes 1 | multifocal and multisysemic (disseminated) Langerhans-cell histiocytosis (C96.0)
         multifocal and unisystemic Langerhans-cell histiocytosis (C96.5)

   C96.A   Histiocytic sarcoma 🗅
     Malignant histiocytosis

   C96.Z   Other specified malignant neoplasms of lymphoid, hematopoietic and related tissue 🗅

   ■ **C96.9   Malignant neoplasm of lymphoid, hematopoietic and related tissue, unspecified** 🗅

●   Unacceptable Principal Diagnosis   ●   Use Additional Character(s)   ■   Unspecified   ▶   Manifestation Code

854

OGCR   Official Guidelines for Coding and Reporting | Excludes 1 | | Excludes 2 | Includes   Use additional   Code first   Code also

CHAPTER 2 (C00-D49)

In situ is carcinoma involving cells in localized tissues that has not spread to nearby tissues

IN SITU NEOPLASMS (D00-D09)

Includes   Bowen's disease
           erythroplasia
           grade III intraepithelial neoplasia
           Queyrat's erythroplasia

● **D00 Carcinoma in situ of oral cavity, esophagus and stomach**
     Excludes1   melanoma in situ (D03.-)

● **D00.0 Carcinoma in situ of lip, oral cavity and pharynx**
     Use additional code to identify:
     exposure to environmental tobacco smoke (Z77.22)
     exposure to tobacco smoke in the perinatal period
        (P96.81)
     history of tobacco use (Z87.891)
     occupational exposure to environmental tobacco
        smoke (Z57.31)
     tobacco dependence (F17.-)
     tobacco use (Z72.0)

     Excludes1   carcinoma in situ of aryepiglottic
                  fold or interarytenoid fold,
                  laryngeal aspect (D02.0)
                  carcinoma in situ of epiglottis NOS
                  (D02.0)
                  carcinoma in situ of epiglottis
                  suprahyoid portion (D02.0)
                  carcinoma in situ of skin of lip
                  (D03.0, D04.0)

  ■ **D00.00 Carcinoma in situ of oral cavity,
           unspecified site**

   **D00.01 Carcinoma in situ of labial mucosa and
           vermilion border**

   D00.02 Carcinoma in situ of buccal mucosa

   **D00.03 Carcinoma in situ of gingiva and
           edentulous alveolar ridge**

   D00.04 Carcinoma in situ of soft palate

   D00.05 Carcinoma in situ of hard palate

   D00.06 Carcinoma in situ of floor of mouth

   D00.07 Carcinoma in situ of tongue

   D00.08 Carcinoma in situ of pharynx
           Carcinoma in situ of aryepiglottic fold
              NOS
           Carcinoma in situ of hypopharyngeal
              aspect of aryepiglottic fold
           Carcinoma in situ of marginal zone of
              aryepiglottic fold

   D00.1 Carcinoma in situ of esophagus

   D00.2 Carcinoma in situ of stomach

● **D01 Carcinoma in situ of other and unspecified digestive
     organs**
     Excludes1   melanoma in situ (D03.-)

   D01.0 Carcinoma in situ of colon
     Excludes1   carcinoma in situ of rectosigmoid
                  junction (D01.1)

   D01.1 Carcinoma in situ of rectosigmoid junction

   D01.2 Carcinoma in situ of rectum

   D01.3 Carcinoma in situ of anus and anal canal
     Excludes1   carcinoma in situ of anal margin
                  (D04.5)
                  carcinoma in situ of anal skin (D04.5)
                  carcinoma in situ of perianal skin
                  (D04.5)

● **D01.4 Carcinoma in situ of other and unspecified parts of
     intestine**
     Excludes1   carcinoma in situ of ampulla of Vater
                  (D01.5)

   **D01.40 Carcinoma in situ of unspecified part of
           intestine**

   D01.49 Carcinoma in situ of other parts of intestine

   D01.5 Carcinoma in situ of liver, gallbladder and bile ducts
           Carcinoma in situ of ampulla of Vater

   **D01.7 Carcinoma in situ of other specified digestive
     organs**
           Carcinoma in situ of pancreas

  ■ **D01.9 Carcinoma in situ of digestive organ, unspecified**

● **D02 Carcinoma in situ of middle ear and respiratory system**
     Use additional code to identify:
     exposure to environmental tobacco smoke (Z77.22)
     exposure to tobacco smoke in the perinatal period (P96.81)
     history of tobacco use (Z87.891)
     occupational exposure to environmental tobacco smoke
        (Z57.31)
     tobacco dependence (F17.-)
     tobacco use (Z72.0)

     Excludes1   melanoma in situ (D03.-)

   D02.0 Carcinoma in situ of larynx
           Carcinoma in situ of aryepiglottic fold or
              interarytenoid fold, laryngeal aspect
           Carcinoma in situ of epiglottis (suprahyoid
              portion)
     Excludes1   carcinoma in situ of aryepiglottic
                  fold or interarytenoid fold NOS
                  (D00.08)
                  carcinoma in situ of hypopharyngeal
                  aspect (D00.08)
                  carcinoma in situ of marginal zone
                  (D00.08)

   D02.1 Carcinoma in situ of trachea

● **D02.2 Carcinoma in situ of bronchus and lung**

  ■ **D02.20 Carcinoma in situ of unspecified bronchus
           and lung**

   D02.21 Carcinoma in situ of right bronchus and lung

   **D02.22 Carcinoma in situ of left bronchus and
           lung**

   **D02.3 Carcinoma in situ of other parts of respiratory
     system**
           Carcinoma in situ of accessory sinuses
           Carcinoma in situ of middle ear
           Carcinoma in situ of nasal cavities
     Excludes1   carcinoma in situ of ear (external)
                  (skin) (D04.2-)
                  carcinoma in situ of nose NOS (D09.8)
                  carcinoma in situ of skin of nose
                  (D04.3)

  ■ **D02.4 Carcinoma in situ of respiratory system,
           unspecified**

● **D03 Melanoma in situ**

   D03.0 Melanoma in situ of lip

● **D03.1 Melanoma in situ of eyelid, including canthus**

  ■ **D03.10 Melanoma in situ of unspecified eyelid,
           including canthus**

   **D03.11 Melanoma in situ of right eyelid,
           including canthus**

   **D03.12 Melanoma in situ of left eyelid, including
           canthus**

● D03.2 **Melanoma in situ of ear and external auricular canal**

■ D03.20 Melanoma in situ of unspecified ear and external auricular canal

D03.21 Melanoma in situ of right ear and external auricular canal

D03.22 Melanoma in situ of left ear and external auricular canal

● D03.3 **Melanoma in situ of other and unspecified parts of face**

■ D03.30 Melanoma in situ of unspecified part of face

D03.39 Melanoma in situ of other parts of face

D03.4 **Melanoma in situ of scalp and neck**

● D03.5 **Melanoma in situ of trunk**

D03.51 Melanoma in situ of anal skin
Melanoma in situ of anal margin
Melanoma in situ of perianal skin

D03.52 Melanoma in situ of breast (skin) (soft tissue)

D03.59 Melanoma in situ of other part of trunk

● D03.6 **Melanoma in situ of upper limb, including shoulder**

■ D03.60 Melanoma in situ of unspecified upper limb, including shoulder

D03.61 Melanoma in situ of right upper limb, including shoulder

D03.62 Melanoma in situ of left upper limb, including shoulder

● D03.7 **Melanoma in situ of lower limb, including hip**

■ D03.70 Melanoma in situ of unspecified lower limb, including hip

D03.71 Melanoma in situ of right lower limb, including hip

D03.72 Melanoma in situ of left lower limb, including hip

D03.8 **Melanoma in situ of other sites**
Melanoma in situ of scrotum

> **Excludes1** carcinoma in situ of scrotum (D07.61)

■ D03.9 **Melanoma in situ, unspecified**

● D04 **Carcinoma in situ of skin**

> **Excludes1** erythroplasia of Queyrat (penis) NOS (D07.4)
> melanoma in situ (D03.-)

D04.0 **Carcinoma in situ of skin of lip**

> **Excludes1** carcinoma in situ of vermilion border of lip (D00.01)

● D04.1 **Carcinoma in situ of skin of eyelid, including canthus**

■ D04.10 Carcinoma in situ of skin of unspecified eyelid, including canthus

D04.11 Carcinoma in situ of skin of right eyelid, including canthus

D04.12 Carcinoma in situ of skin of left eyelid, including canthus

● D04.2 **Carcinoma in situ of skin of ear and external auricular canal**

■ D04.20 Carcinoma in situ of skin of unspecified ear and external auricular canal

D04.21 Carcinoma in situ of skin of right ear and external auricular canal

D04.22 Carcinoma in situ of skin of left ear and external auricular canal

● D04.3 **Carcinoma in situ of skin of other and unspecified parts of face**

■ D04.30 Carcinoma in situ of skin of unspecified part of face

D04.39 Carcinoma in situ of skin of other parts of face

D04.4 **Carcinoma in situ of skin of scalp and neck**

D04.5 **Carcinoma in situ of skin of trunk**
Carcinoma in situ of anal margin
Carcinoma in situ of anal skin
Carcinoma in situ of perianal skin
Carcinoma in situ of skin of breast

> **Excludes1** carcinoma in situ of anus NOS (D01.3)
> carcinoma in situ of scrotum (D07.61)
> carcinoma in situ of skin of genital organs (D07.-)

● D04.6 **Carcinoma in situ of skin of upper limb, including shoulder**

■ D04.60 Carcinoma in situ of skin of unspecified upper limb, including shoulder

D04.61 Carcinoma in situ of skin of right upper limb, including shoulder

D04.62 Carcinoma in situ of skin of left upper limb, including shoulder

● D04.7 **Carcinoma in situ of skin of lower limb, including hip**

■ D04.70 Carcinoma in situ of skin of unspecified lower limb, including hip

D04.71 Carcinoma in situ of skin of right lower limb, including hip

D04.72 Carcinoma in situ of skin of left lower limb, including hip

D04.8 **Carcinoma in situ of skin of other sites**

■ D04.9 **Carcinoma in situ of skin, unspecified**

● D05 **Carcinoma in situ of breast**

> **Excludes1** carcinoma in situ of skin of breast (D04.5)
> melanoma in situ of breast (skin) (D03.5)
> Paget's disease of breast or nipple (C50.-)

● D05.0 **Lobular carcinoma in situ of breast**

■ D05.00 Lobular carcinoma in situ of unspecified breast

D05.01 Lobular carcinoma in situ of right breast

D05.02 Lobular carcinoma in situ of left breast

● D05.1 **Intraductal carcinoma in situ of breast**

■ D05.10 Intraductal carcinoma in situ of unspecified breast

D05.11 Intraductal carcinoma in situ of right breast

D05.12 Intraductal carcinoma in situ of left breast

● D05.8 **Other specified type of carcinoma in situ of breast**

■ D05.80 Other specified type of carcinoma in situ of unspecified breast

D05.81 Other specified type of carcinoma in situ of right breast

D05.82 Other specified type of carcinoma in situ of left breast

● D05.9 **Unspecified type of carcinoma in situ of breast**

■ D05.90 Unspecified type of carcinoma in situ of unspecified breast

■ D05.91 Unspecified type of carcinoma in situ of right breast

■ D05.92 Unspecified type of carcinoma in situ of left breast

● Unacceptable Principal Diagnosis ● Use Additional Character(s) ■ Unspecified ▶ Manifestation Code

OGCR Official Guidelines for Coding and Reporting Excludes 1 Excludes 2 Includes Use additional Code first Code also

● **D06   Carcinoma in situ of cervix uteri**

     Includes   cervical adenocarcinoma in situ

              cervical intraepithelial glandular neoplasia

              cervical intraepithelial neoplasia III [CIN III]

              severe dysplasia of cervix uteri

     Excludes1   cervical intraepithelial neoplasia II [CIN II] (N87.1)

              cytologic evidence of malignancy of cervix without histologic confirmation (R87.614)

              high grade squamous intraepithelial lesion (HGSIL) of cervix (R87.613)

              melanoma in situ of cervix (D03.5)

              moderate cervical dysplasia (N87.1)

   D06.0   Carcinoma in situ of endocervix ♀

   D06.1   Carcinoma in situ of exocervix ♀

   D06.7   Carcinoma in situ of other parts of cervix ♀

   ■ **D06.9   Carcinoma in situ of cervix, unspecified** ♀

● **D07   Carcinoma in situ of other and unspecified genital organs**

     Excludes1   melanoma in situ of trunk (D03.5)

   D07.0   Carcinoma in situ of endometrium ♀

   D07.1   Carcinoma in situ of vulva ♀

     Severe dysplasia of vulva

     Vulvar intraepithelial neoplasia III [VIN III]

     Excludes1   moderate dysplasia of vulva (N90.1)

              vulvar intraepithelial neoplasia II [VIN II] (N90.1)

   D07.2   Carcinoma in situ of vagina ♀

     Severe dysplasia of vagina

     Vaginal intraepithelial neoplasia III [VIN III]

     Excludes1   moderate dysplasia of vagina (N89.1)

              vaginal intraepithelial neoplasia II [VIN II] (N89.1)

   ● **D07.3   Carcinoma in situ of other and unspecified female genital organs**

     ■ **D07.30   Carcinoma in situ of unspecified female genital organs** ♀

     D07.39   Carcinoma in situ of other female genital organs ♀

   D07.4   Carcinoma in situ of penis ♂

     Erythroplasia of Queyrat NOS

   D07.5   Carcinoma in situ of prostate ♂

     Prostatic intraepithelial neoplasia III (PIN III)

     Severe dysplasia of prostate

     Excludes1   dysplasia (mild) (moderate) of prostate (N42.3)

   ● **D07.6   Carcinoma in situ of other and unspecified male genital organs**

     ■ **D07.60   Carcinoma in situ of unspecified male genital organs** ♂

     D07.61   Carcinoma in situ of scrotum ♂

     D07.69   Carcinoma in situ of other male genital organs ♂

● **D09   Carcinoma in situ of other and unspecified sites**

     Excludes1   melanoma in situ (D03.-)

   D09.0   Carcinoma in situ of bladder

   ● **D09.1   Carcinoma in situ of other and unspecified urinary organs**

     ■ **D09.10   Carcinoma in situ of unspecified urinary organ**

     D09.19   Carcinoma in situ of other urinary organs

   ● **D09.2   Carcinoma in situ of eye**

     Excludes1   carcinoma in situ of skin of eyelid (D04.1-)

     ■ **D09.20   Carcinoma in situ of unspecified eye**

     D09.21   Carcinoma in situ of right eye

     D09.22   Carcinoma in situ of left eye

   D09.3   Carcinoma in situ of thyroid and other endocrine glands

     Excludes1   carcinoma in situ of endocrine pancreas (D01.7)

              carcinoma in situ of ovary (D07.39)

              carcinoma in situ of testis (D07.69)

   D09.8   Carcinoma in situ of other specified sites

   ■ **D09.9   Carcinoma in situ, unspecified**

BENIGN NEOPLASMS, EXCEPT BENIGN NEUROENDOCRINE TUMORS (D10-D36)

● **D10   Benign neoplasm of mouth and pharynx**

   D10.0   Benign neoplasm of lip

     Benign neoplasm of lip (frenulum) (inner aspect) (mucosa) (vermilion border)

     Excludes1   benign neoplasm of skin of lip (D22.0, D23.0)

   D10.1   Benign neoplasm of tongue

     Benign neoplasm of lingual tonsil

   D10.2   Benign neoplasm of floor of mouth

   ● **D10.3   Other and unspecified parts of mouth**

     ■ **D10.30   Benign neoplasm of unspecified part of mouth**

     D10.39   Benign neoplasm of other parts of mouth

       Benign neoplasm of minor salivary gland NOS

       Excludes1   benign odontogenic neoplasms (D16.4-D16.5)

              benign neoplasm of mucosa of lip (D10.0)

              benign neoplasm of nasopharyngeal surface of soft palate (D10.6)

   D10.4   Benign neoplasm of tonsil

     Benign neoplasm of tonsil (faucial) (palatine)

     Excludes1   benign neoplasm of lingual tonsil (D10.1)

              benign neoplasm of pharyngeal tonsil (D10.6)

              benign neoplasm of tonsillar fossa (D10.5)

              benign neoplasm of tonsillar pillars (D10.5)

   D10.5   Benign neoplasm of other parts of oropharynx

     Division of pharynx lying between soft palate and upper edge of epiglottis

     Benign neoplasm of epiglottis, anterior aspect

     Benign neoplasm of tonsillar fossa

     Benign neoplasm of tonsillar pillars

     Benign neoplasm of vallecula

     Excludes1   benign neoplasm of epiglottis NOS (D14.1)

              benign neoplasm of epiglottis, suprahyoid portion (D14.1)

   D10.6   Benign neoplasm of nasopharynx

     Segment of pharynx that lies above soft palate

     Benign neoplasm of pharyngeal tonsil

     Benign neoplasm of posterior margin of septum and choanae

CHAPTER 2 (C00-D49)

Figure 2-16   The esophagus is the muscular tube that connects the pharynx and the tomach. The 10 inch (25 cm) long esophagus is divided into three parts: **cervical, thoracic,** and **abdominal.**

D10.7   Benign neoplasm of hypopharynx
    Segment of pharynx that lies below upper edge of epiglottis and opens into larynx and esophagus

■ **D10.9   Benign neoplasm of pharynx, unspecified**

● **D11   Benign neoplasm of major salivary glands**
     Excludes1   benign neoplasms of specified minor salivary glands which are classified according to their anatomical location benign neoplasms of minor salivary glands NOS (D10.39)

D11.0   Benign neoplasm of parotid gland

D11.7   Benign neoplasm of other major salivary glands
     Benign neoplasm of sublingual salivary gland
     Benign neoplasm of submandibular salivary gland

■ **D11.9   Benign neoplasm of major salivary gland, unspecified**

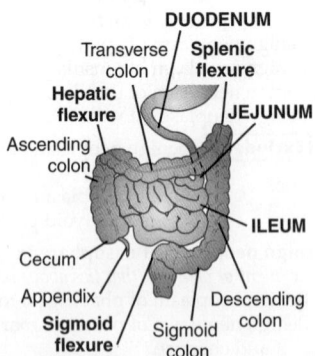

Figure 2-17   Small intestine and colon.

● **D12   Benign neoplasm of colon, rectum, anus and anal canal**
     Excludes1   benign carcinoid tumors of the large intestine, and rectum (D3A.02-)

D12.0   Benign neoplasm of cecum
     Benign neoplasm of ileocecal valve

D12.1   Benign neoplasm of appendix
     Excludes1   benign carcinoid tumor of the appendix (D3A.020)

D12.2   Benign neoplasm of ascending colon

D12.3   Benign neoplasm of transverse colon
     Benign neoplasm of hepatic flexure
     Benign neoplasm of splenic flexure
     Flexure is a bending in a structure or organ. Note the three flexures illustrated in Figure 2–17. Hepatic = liver, sigmoid = colon, splenic = spleen.

D12.4   Benign neoplasm of descending colon

D12.5   Benign neoplasm of sigmoid colon

■ **D12.6   Benign neoplasm of colon, unspecified**
     Adenomatosis of colon
     Benign neoplasm of large intestine NOS
     Polyposis (hereditary) of colon
     Excludes1   inflammatory polyp of colon (K51.4-)
          polyp of colon NOS (K63.5)

D12.7   Benign neoplasm of rectosigmoid junction
     Angle where sigmoid colon becomes rectum

D12.8   Benign neoplasm of rectum
     Excludes1   benign carcinoid tumor of the rectum (D3A.026)

D12.9   Benign neoplasm of anus and anal canal
     Benign neoplasm of anus NOS
     Excludes1   benign neoplasm of anal margin (D22.5, D23.5)
          benign neoplasm of anal skin (D22.5, D23.5)
          benign neoplasm of perianal skin (D22.5, D23.5)

● **D13   Benign neoplasm of other and ill-defined parts of digestive system**
     Excludes1   benign stromal tumors of digestive system (D21.4)

D13.0   Benign neoplasm of esophagus

D13.1   Benign neoplasm of stomach
     Excludes1   benign carcinoid tumor of the stomach (D3A.092)

D13.2   Benign neoplasm of duodenum
     Excludes1   benign carcinoid tumor of the duodenum (D3A.010)

● **D13.3   Benign neoplasm of other and unspecified parts of small intestine**
     Excludes1   benign carcinoid tumors of the small intestine (D3A.01-)
          benign neoplasm of ileocecal valve (D12.0)

■ **D13.30   Benign neoplasm of unspecified part of small intestine**

D13.39   Benign neoplasm of other parts of small intestine

D13.4   Benign neoplasm of liver
     Benign neoplasm of intrahepatic bile ducts

D13.5   Benign neoplasm of extrahepatic bile ducts
     Extensions of common hepatic bile duct (tube that collects bile from liver)

● Unacceptable Principal Diagnosis   ● Use Additional Character(s)   ■ Unspecified   ▶ Manifestation Code

858   **OGCR**   Official Guidelines for Coding and Reporting | Excludes 1 | | Excludes 2 | Includes   Use additional   Code first   Code also

CHAPTER 2 (C00-D49)

D13.6 Benign neoplasm of pancreas
> **Excludes1**   benign neoplasm of endocrine pancreas (D13.7)

D13.7 Benign neoplasm of endocrine pancreas
> *Pancreatic islets: Cells scattered throughout pancreas*
> Islet cell tumor
> Benign neoplasm of islets of Langerhans
> Use additional code to identify any functional activity.

D13.9 Benign neoplasm of ill-defined sites within the digestive system
> Benign neoplasm of digestive system NOS
> Benign neoplasm of intestine NOS
> Benign neoplasm of spleen

● **D14 Benign neoplasm of middle ear and respiratory system**

D14.0 Benign neoplasm of middle ear, nasal cavity and accessory sinuses
> Benign neoplasm of cartilage of nose
> **Excludes1**   benign neoplasm of auricular canal (external) (D22.2-, D23.2-)
> benign neoplasm of bone of ear (D16.4)
> benign neoplasm of bone of nose (D16.4)
> benign neoplasm of cartilage of ear (D21.0)
> benign neoplasm of ear (external) (skin) (D22.2-, D23.2-)
> benign neoplasm of nose NOS (D36.7)
> benign neoplasm of skin of nose (D22.39, D23.39)
> benign neoplasm of olfactory bulb (D33.3)
> benign neoplasm of posterior margin of septum and choanae (D10.6)
> polyp of accessory sinus (J33.8)
> polyp of ear (middle) (H74.4)
> polyp of nasal (cavity) (J33.-)

D14.1 Benign neoplasm of larynx
> Adenomatous polyp of larynx
> Benign neoplasm of epiglottis (suprahyoid portion)
> *Horseshoe shaped bone in anterior midline of neck between chin and thyroid cartilage*
> **Excludes1**   benign neoplasm of epiglottis, anterior aspect (D10.5)
> polyp (nonadenomatous) of vocal cord or larynx (J38.1)

D14.2 Benign neoplasm of trachea

● **D14.3 Benign neoplasm of bronchus and lung**
> **Excludes1**   benign carcinoid tumor of the bronchus and lung (D3A.090)

■ **D14.30 Benign neoplasm of unspecified bronchus and lung**

D14.31 Benign neoplasm of right bronchus and lung

D14.32 Benign neoplasm of left bronchus and lung

■ **D14.4 Benign neoplasm of respiratory system, unspecified**

● **D15 Benign neoplasm of other and unspecified intrathoracic organs**
> **Excludes1**   benign neoplasm of mesothelial tissue (D19.-)

D15.0 Benign neoplasm of thymus
> **Excludes1**   benign carcinoid tumor of the thymus (D3A.091)

D15.1 Benign neoplasm of heart
> **Excludes1**   benign neoplasm of great vessels (D21.3)

D15.2 Benign neoplasm of mediastinum

D15.7 Benign neoplasm of other specified intrathoracic organs

■ **D15.9 Benign neoplasm of intrathoracic organ, unspecified**

● **D16 Benign neoplasm of bone and articular cartilage**
> **Excludes1**   benign neoplasm of connective tissue of ear (D21.0)
> benign neoplasm of connective tissue of eyelid (D21.0)
> benign neoplasm of connective tissue of larynx (D14.1)
> benign neoplasm of connective tissue of nose (D14.0)
> benign neoplasm of synovia (D21.-)

● **D16.0 Benign neoplasm of scapula and long bones of upper limb**

■ **D16.00 Benign neoplasm of scapula and long bones of unspecified upper limb**

D16.01 Benign neoplasm of scapula and long bones of right upper limb

D16.02 Benign neoplasm of scapula and long bones of left upper limb

● **D16.1 Benign neoplasm of short bones of upper limb**

■ **D16.10 Benign neoplasm of short bones of unspecified upper limb**

D16.11 Benign neoplasm of short bones of right upper limb

D16.12 Benign neoplasm of short bones of left upper limb

● **D16.2 Benign neoplasm of long bones of lower limb**

■ **D16.20 Benign neoplasm of long bones of unspecified lower limb**

D16.21 Benign neoplasm of long bones of right lower limb

D16.22 Benign neoplasm of long bones of left lower limb

● **D16.3 Benign neoplasm of short bones of lower limb**

■ **D16.30 Benign neoplasm of short bones of unspecified lower limb**

D16.31 Benign neoplasm of short bones of right lower limb

D16.32 Benign neoplasm of short bones of left lower limb

CHAPTER 2 (C00-D49)

D16.4 Benign neoplasm of bones of skull and face
Benign neoplasm of maxilla (superior)
Benign neoplasm of orbital bone
Cavity or socket of skull in which eye and its appendages are located
Keratocyst of maxilla
Keratocystic odontogenic tumor of maxilla
Excludes1 benign neoplasm of lower jaw bone (D16.5)

D16.5 Benign neoplasm of lower jaw bone
Keratocyst of mandible
Keratocystic odontogenic tumor of mandible

D16.6 Benign neoplasm of vertebral column
Excludes1 benign neoplasm of sacrum and coccyx (D16.8)

D16.7 Benign neoplasm of ribs, sternum and clavicle

D16.8 Benign neoplasm of pelvic bones, sacrum and coccyx

D16.9 Benign neoplasm of bone and articular cartilage, unspecified

●D17 Benign lipomatous neoplasm
Slow growing benign tumors (rubbery masses) of mature fat cells enclosed in a thin fibrous capsule

D17.0 Benign lipomatous neoplasm of skin and subcutaneous tissue of head, face and neck

D17.1 Benign lipomatous neoplasm of skin and subcutaneous tissue of trunk

●D17.2 Benign lipomatous neoplasm of skin and subcutaneous tissue of limb
D17.20 Benign lipomatous neoplasm of skin and subcutaneous tissue of unspecified limb
D17.21 Benign lipomatous neoplasm of skin and subcutaneous tissue of right arm
D17.22 Benign lipomatous neoplasm of skin and subcutaneous tissue of left arm
D17.23 Benign lipomatous neoplasm of skin and subcutaneous tissue of right leg
D17.24 Benign lipomatous neoplasm of skin and subcutaneous tissue of left leg

●D17.3 Benign lipomatous neoplasm of skin and subcutaneous tissue of other and unspecified sites
D17.30 Benign lipomatous neoplasm of skin and subcutaneous tissue of unspecified sites
D17.39 Benign lipomatous neoplasm of skin and subcutaneous tissue of other sites

D17.4 Benign lipomatous neoplasm of intrathoracic organs

D17.5 Benign lipomatous neoplasm of intra-abdominal organs
Excludes1 benign lipomatous neoplasm of peritoneum and retroperitoneum (D17.79)

D17.6 Benign lipomatous neoplasm of spermatic cord ♂

●D17.7 Benign lipomatous neoplasm of other sites
D17.71 Benign lipomatous neoplasm of kidney
D17.72 Benign lipomatous neoplasm of other genitourinary organ
D17.79 Benign lipomatous neoplasm of other sites
Benign lipomatous neoplasm of peritoneum
Benign lipomatous neoplasm of retroperitoneum

D17.9 Benign lipomatous neoplasm, unspecified
Lipoma NOS

Figure 2-18 Hemangioma of skin and subcutaneous tissue. (From Yanoff: Ophthalmology, 2nd ed. 2004, Mosby, Inc.)

Item 2–10 Hemangiomas are abnormally dense collections of dilated capillaries that occur on the skin or in internal organs. Hemangiomas are both deep and superficial and undergo a rapid growth phase when the size increases rapidly, followed by a rest phase, in which the tumor changes very little, followed by an involutional phase in which the tumor begins to and can disappear altogether. **Lymphangiomas** or cystic hygroma are benign collections of overgrown lymph vessels and, although rare, may occur anywhere but most commonly on the head and neck of children and infants. Visceral organs, lungs, and gastrointestinal tract may also be involved.

●D18 Hemangioma and lymphangioma, any site
Excludes1 benign neoplasm of glomus jugulare (D35.6)
blue or pigmented nevus (D22.-)
nevus NOS (D22.-)
vascular nevus (Q82.5)

●D18.0 Hemangioma
Common type of vascular malformation
Angioma NOS
Cavernous nevus
D18.00 Hemangioma unspecified site
D18.01 Hemangioma of skin and subcutaneous tissue
D18.02 Hemangioma of intracranial structures
D18.03 Hemangioma of intra-abdominal structures
D18.09 Hemangioma of other sites

D18.1 Lymphangioma, any site

●D19 Benign neoplasm of mesothelial tissue
Mesothelial tissue is the membrane lining several body cavities
D19.0 Benign neoplasm of mesothelial tissue of pleura
D19.1 Benign neoplasm of mesothelial tissue of peritoneum
D19.7 Benign neoplasm of mesothelial tissue of other sites
D19.9 Benign neoplasm of mesothelial tissue, unspecified
Benign mesothelioma NOS

●D20 Benign neoplasm of soft tissue of retroperitoneum and peritoneum
Excludes1 benign lipomatous neoplasm of peritoneum and retroperitoneum (D17.79)
benign neoplasm of mesothelial tissue (D19.-)

D20.0 Benign neoplasm of soft tissue of retroperitoneum
D20.1 Benign neoplasm of soft tissue of peritoneum

● Unacceptable Principal Diagnosis   ● Use Additional Character(s)   ■ Unspecified   ▶ Manifestation Code
OGCR Official Guidelines for Coding and Reporting   Excludes 1   Excludes 2   Includes   Use additional   Code first   Code also

● **D21　Other benign neoplasms of connective and other soft tissue**

> **Includes**　　benign neoplasm of blood vessel
> benign neoplasm of bursa
> benign neoplasm of cartilage
> benign neoplasm of fascia
> benign neoplasm of fat
> benign neoplasm of ligament, except uterine
> benign neoplasm of lymphatic channel
> benign neoplasm of muscle
> benign neoplasm of synovia
> benign neoplasm of tendon (sheath)
> benign stromal tumors

> **Excludes1**　　benign neoplasm of articular cartilage (D16.-)
> benign neoplasm of cartilage of larynx (D14.1)
> benign neoplasm of cartilage of nose (D14.0)
> benign neoplasm of connective tissue of breast (D24.-)
> benign neoplasm of peripheral nerves and autonomic nervous system (D36.1-)
> benign neoplasm of peritoneum (D20.1)
> benign neoplasm of retroperitoneum (D20.0)
> benign neoplasm of uterine ligament, any (D28.2)
> benign neoplasm of vascular tissue (D18.-)
> hemangioma (D18.0-)
> lipomatous neoplasm (D17.-)
> lymphangioma (D18.1)
> uterine leiomyoma (D25.-)

D21.0　Benign neoplasm of connective and other soft tissue of head, face and neck
> Benign neoplasm of connective tissue of ear
> Benign neoplasm of connective tissue of eyelid

> **Excludes1**　　benign neoplasm of connective tissue of orbit (D31.6-)

● **D21.1　Benign neoplasm of connective and other soft tissue of upper limb, including shoulder**

　■ **D21.10　Benign neoplasm of connective and other soft tissue of unspecified upper limb, including shoulder**

　　D21.11　Benign neoplasm of connective and other soft tissue of right upper limb, including shoulder

　　D21.12　Benign neoplasm of connective and other soft tissue of left upper limb, including shoulder

● **D21.2　Benign neoplasm of connective and other soft tissue of lower limb, including hip**

　■ **D21.20　Benign neoplasm of connective and other soft tissue of unspecified lower limb, including hip**

　　D21.21　Benign neoplasm of connective and other soft tissue of right lower limb, including hip

　　D21.22　Benign neoplasm of connective and other soft tissue of left lower limb, including hip

D21.3　Benign neoplasm of connective and other soft tissue of thorax
> Benign neoplasm of axilla
> Benign neoplasm of diaphragm
> Benign neoplasm of great vessels

> **Excludes1**　　benign neoplasm of heart (D15.1)
> benign neoplasm of mediastinum (D15.2)
> benign neoplasm of thymus (D15.0)

D21.4　Benign neoplasm of connective and other soft tissue of abdomen Benign stromal tumors of abdomen

D21.5　Benign neoplasm of connective and other soft tissue of pelvis

> **Excludes1**　　benign neoplasm of any uterine ligament (D28.2)
> uterine leiomyoma (D25.-)

■ **D21.6　Benign neoplasm of connective and other soft tissue of trunk, unspecified**
> Benign neoplasm of back NOS

■ **D21.9　Benign neoplasm of connective and other soft tissue, unspecified**

● **D22　Melanocytic nevi**

> **Includes**　　atypical nevus
> blue hairy pigmented nevus
> nevus NOS

D22.0　Melanocytic nevi of lip
> *Skin lesions composed of nests of nevus cells with macules/papules*

● **D22.1　Melanocytic nevi of eyelid, including canthus**

　■ **D22.10　Melanocytic nevi of unspecified eyelid, including canthus**

　　D22.11　Melanocytic nevi of right eyelid, including canthus

　　D22.12　Melanocytic nevi of left eyelid, including canthus

● **D22.2　Melanocytic nevi of ear and external auricular canal**

　■ **D22.20　Melanocytic nevi of unspecified ear and external auricular canal**

　　D22.21　Melanocytic nevi of right ear and external auricular canal

　　D22.22　Melanocytic nevi of left ear and external auricular canal

● **D22.3　Melanocytic nevi of other and unspecified parts of face**

　■ **D22.30　Melanocytic nevi of unspecified part of face**

　　D22.39　Melanocytic nevi of other parts of face

D22.4　Melanocytic nevi of scalp and neck

D22.5　Melanocytic nevi of trunk
> Melanocytic nevi of anal margin
> Melanocytic nevi of anal skin
> Melanocytic nevi of perianal skin
> Melanocytic nevi of skin of breast

● **D22.6　Melanocytic nevi of upper limb, including shoulder**

　■ **D22.60　Melanocytic nevi of unspecified upper limb, including shoulder**

　　D22.61　Melanocytic nevi of right upper limb, including shoulder

　　D22.62　Melanocytic nevi of left upper limb, including shoulder

● **D22.7　Melanocytic nevi of lower limb, including hip**

　■ **D22.70　Melanocytic nevi of unspecified lower limb, including hip**

　　D22.71　Melanocytic nevi of right lower limb, including hip

　　D22.72　Melanocytic nevi of left lower limb, including hip

■ **D22.9　Melanocytic nevi, unspecified**

CHAPTER 2 (C00-D49)

N　Newborn Age: 0　　　**P**　Pediatric Age: 0–17　　　**M**　Maternity DX: 12–55　　　**A**　Adult Age: 15–124　　　♀　Females Only　　　♂　Males Only

　　Complication\Comorbidity　　　　Major C\C　　　Present on Admission Requirement　　　Hospital-Acquired Condition

861

● **D23   Other benign neoplasms of skin**

   Includes   benign neoplasm of hair follicles
               benign neoplasm of sebaceous glands
               benign neoplasm of sweat glands

   Excludes1   benign lipomatous neoplasms of skin (D17.0-D17.3)
               melanocytic nevi (D22.-)

D23.0   Other benign neoplasm of skin of lip

   Excludes1   benign neoplasm of vermilion border of lip (D10.0)

● **D23.1   Other benign neoplasm of skin of eyelid, including canthus**

■ **D23.10   Other benign neoplasm of skin unspecified of eyelid, including canthus**

D23.11   Other benign neoplasm of skin of right eyelid, including canthus

D23.12   Other benign neoplasm of skin of left eyelid, including canthus

● **D23.2   Other benign neoplasm of skin of ear and external auricular canal**

■ **D23.20   Other benign neoplasm of skin of unspecified ear and external auricular canal**

D23.21   Other benign neoplasm of skin of right ear and external auricular canal

D23.22   Other benign neoplasm of skin of left ear and external auricular canal

● **D23.3   Other benign neoplasm of skin of other and unspecified parts of face**

■ **D23.30   Other benign neoplasm of skin of unspecified part of face**

D23.39   Other benign neoplasm of skin of other parts of face

D23.4   Other benign neoplasm of skin of scalp and neck

D23.5   Other benign neoplasm of skin of trunk
   Other benign neoplasm of anal margin
   Other benign neoplasm of anal skin
   Other benign neoplasm of perianal skin
   Other benign neoplasm of skin of breast

   Excludes1   benign neoplasm of anus NOS (D12.9)

● **D23.6   Other benign neoplasm of skin of upper limb, including shoulder**

■ **D23.60   Other benign neoplasm of skin of unspecified upper limb, including shoulder**

D23.61   Other benign neoplasm of skin of right upper limb, including shoulder

D23.62   Other benign neoplasm of skin of left upper limb, including shoulder

● **D23.7   Other benign neoplasm of skin of lower limb, including hip**

■ **D23.70   Other benign neoplasm of skin of unspecified lower limb, including hip**

D23.71   Other benign neoplasm of skin of right lower limb, including hip

D23.72   Other benign neoplasm of skin of left lower limb, including hip

■ **D23.9   Other benign neoplasm of skin, unspecified**

● **D24   Benign neoplasm of breast**

   Includes   benign neoplasm of connective tissue of breast
            benign neoplasm of soft parts of breast
            fibroadenoma of breast

   Excludes2   adenofibrosis of breast (N60.2)
            benign cyst of breast (N60.-)
            benign mammary dysplasia (N60.-)
            benign neoplasm of skin of breast (D22.5, D23.5)
            fibrocystic disease of breast (N60.-)

D24.1   Benign neoplasm of right breast

D24.2   Benign neoplasm of left breast

■ **D24.9   Benign neoplasm of unspecified breast**

● **D25   Leiomyoma of uterus**
   Benign tumors or nodules of the uterine wall

   Includes   uterine fibroid
            uterine fibromyoma
            uterine myoma

D25.0   Submucous leiomyoma of uterus ♀

D25.1   Intramural leiomyoma of uterus ♀
   Interstitial leiomyoma of uterus

D25.2   Subserosal leiomyoma of uterus ♀
   Subperitoneal leiomyoma of uterus

■ **D25.9   Leiomyoma of uterus, unspecified ♀**

● **D26   Other benign neoplasms of uterus**

D26.0   Other benign neoplasm of cervix uteri ♀

D26.1   Other benign neoplasm of corpus uteri ♀

D26.7   Other benign neoplasm of other parts of uterus ♀

■ **D26.9   Other benign neoplasm of uterus, unspecified ♀**

● **D27   Benign neoplasm of ovary**

   Use additional code to identify any functional activity.

   Excludes2   corpus albicans cyst (N83.2)
            corpus luteum cyst (N83.1)
            endometrial cyst (N80.1)
            follicular (atretic) cyst (N83.0)
            graafian follicle cyst (N83.0)
            ovarian cyst NEC (N83.2)
            ovarian retention cyst (N83.2)

D27.0   Benign neoplasm of right ovary ♀

D27.1   Benign neoplasm of left ovary ♀

■ **D27.9   Benign neoplasm of unspecified ovary ♀**

● **D28   Benign neoplasm of other and unspecified female genital organs**

   Includes   adenomatous polyp
            benign neoplasm of skin of female genital organs
            benign teratoma

   Excludes1   epoophoron cyst (Q50.5)
            fimbrial cyst (Q50.4)
            Gartner's duct cyst (Q52.4)
            parovarian cyst (Q50.5)

D28.0   Benign neoplasm of vulva ♀

D28.1   Benign neoplasm of vagina ♀

Item 2–11 Teratoma: terat = monster, oma = mass, tumor. Alternate terms: dermoid cyst of the ovary, ovarian teratoma. Teratomas are neoplasms and arise from germ cells (ovaries in female and testes in male) and can be benign or malignant. Teratomas have been known to contain hair, nails, and teeth, giving them a bizarre ("monster") appearance.

● Unacceptable Principal Diagnosis   ● Use Additional Character(s)   ■ Unspecified   ▶ Manifestation Code
OGCR Official Guidelines for Coding and Reporting   Excludes 1   Excludes 2   Includes   Use additional   Code first   Code also

D28.2 **Benign neoplasm of uterine tubes and ligaments** ♀
Benign neoplasm of fallopian tube
Benign neoplasm of uterine ligament (broad)
(round)

D28.7 **Benign neoplasm of other specified female genital organs** ♀

▢ **D28.9** **Benign neoplasm of female genital organ, unspecified** ♀

● **D29** **Benign neoplasm of male genital organs**
     Includes   benign neoplasm of skin of male genital organs

D29.0 **Benign neoplasm of penis** ♂

D29.1 **Benign neoplasm of prostate** ♂
     Excludes1   enlarged prostate (N40.-)

● **D29.2** **Benign neoplasm of testis**
     Use additional code to identify any functional activity.

  ▢ **D29.20** **Benign neoplasm of unspecified testis** ♂
     D29.21 **Benign neoplasm of right testis** ♂
     D29.22 **Benign neoplasm of left testis** ♂

● **D29.3** **Benign neoplasm of epididymis**
  ▢ **D29.30** **Benign neoplasm of unspecified epididymis** ♂
     D29.31 **Benign neoplasm of right epididymis** ♂
     D29.32 **Benign neoplasm of left epididymis** ♂

D29.4 **Benign neoplasm of scrotum** ♂
Benign neoplasm of skin of scrotum

D29.8 **Benign neoplasm of other specified male genital organs** ♂
Benign neoplasm of seminal vesicle
Benign neoplasm of spermatic cord
Benign neoplasm of tunica vaginalis

▢ **D29.9** **Benign neoplasm of male genital organ, unspecified** ♂

● **D30** **Benign neoplasm of urinary organs**
● **D30.0** **Benign neoplasm of kidney**
     Excludes1   benign carcinoid tumor of the kidney (D3A.093)
       benign neoplasm of renal calyces (D30.1-)
       benign neoplasm of renal pelvis (D30.1-)

  ▢ **D30.00** **Benign neoplasm of unspecified kidney**
     D30.01 **Benign neoplasm of right kidney**
     D30.02 **Benign neoplasm of left kidney**

● **D30.1** **Benign neoplasm of renal pelvis**
  ▢ **D30.10** **Benign neoplasm of unspecified renal pelvis**
     D30.11 **Benign neoplasm of right renal pelvis**
     D30.12 **Benign neoplasm of left renal pelvis**

● **D30.2** **Benign neoplasm of ureter**
     Excludes1   benign neoplasm of ureteric orifice of bladder (D30.3)

  ▢ **D30.20** **Benign neoplasm of unspecified ureter**
     D30.21 **Benign neoplasm of right ureter**
     D30.22 **Benign neoplasm of left ureter**

D30.3 **Benign neoplasm of bladder**
Benign neoplasm of ureteric orifice of bladder
Benign neoplasm of urethral orifice of bladder

D30.4 **Benign neoplasm of urethra**
     Excludes1   benign neoplasm of urethral orifice of bladder (D30.3)

D30.8 **Benign neoplasm of other specified urinary organs**
Benign neoplasm of paraurethral glands

▢ **D30.9** **Benign neoplasm of urinary organ, unspecified**
Benign neoplasm of urinary system NOS

● **D31** **Benign neoplasm of eye and adnexa**
     Excludes1   benign neoplasm of connective tissue of eyelid (D21.0)
       benign neoplasm of optic nerve (D33.3)
       benign neoplasm of skin of eyelid (D22.1-, D23.1-)

● **D31.0** **Benign neoplasm of conjunctiva**
  ▢ **D31.00** **Benign neoplasm of unspecified conjunctiva**
     D31.01 **Benign neoplasm of right conjunctiva**
     D31.02 **Benign neoplasm of left conjunctiva**

● **D31.1** **Benign neoplasm of cornea**
  ▢ **D31.10** **Benign neoplasm of unspecified cornea**
     D31.11 **Benign neoplasm of right cornea**
     D31.12 **Benign neoplasm of left cornea**

● **D31.2** **Benign neoplasm of retina**
     Excludes1   dark area on retina (D49.81)
       hemangioma of retina (D49.81)
       neoplasm of unspecified behavior of retina and choroid (D49.81)
       retinal freckle (D49.81)

  ▢ **D31.20** **Benign neoplasm of unspecified retina**
     D31.21 **Benign neoplasm of right retina**
     D31.22 **Benign neoplasm of left retina**

● **D31.3** **Benign neoplasm of choroid**
     D31.30 **Benign neoplasm of unspecified choroid**
     D31.31 **Benign neoplasm of right choroid**
     D31.32 **Benign neoplasm of left choroid**

● **D31.4** **Benign neoplasm of ciliary body**
  ▢ **D31.40** **Benign neoplasm of unspecified ciliary body**
     D31.41 **Benign neoplasm of right ciliary body**
     D31.42 **Benign neoplasm of left ciliary body**

● **D31.5** **Benign neoplasm of lacrimal gland and duct**
Benign neoplasm of lacrimal sac
Benign neoplasm of nasolacrimal duct

  ▢ **D31.50** **Benign neoplasm of unspecified lacrimal gland and duct**
     D31.51 **Benign neoplasm of right lacrimal gland and duct**
     D31.52 **Benign neoplasm of left lacrimal gland and duct**

CHAPTER 2 (C00-D49)

- **D31.6 Benign neoplasm of unspecified site of orbit**
  Benign neoplasm of connective tissue of orbit
  Benign neoplasm of extraocular muscle
  Benign neoplasm of peripheral nerves of orbit
  Benign neoplasm of retrobulbar tissue
  Benign neoplasm of retro-ocular tissue

  Excludes1 benign neoplasm of orbital bone (D16.4)

  - **D31.60 Benign neoplasm of unspecified site of unspecified orbit**
  - **D31.61 Benign neoplasm of unspecified site of right orbit**
  - **D31.62 Benign neoplasm of unspecified site of left orbit**

- **D31.9 Benign neoplasm of unspecified part of eye**
  - **D31.90 Benign neoplasm of unspecified part of unspecified eye**
  - **D31.91 Benign neoplasm of unspecified part of right eye**
  - **D31.92 Benign neoplasm of unspecified part of left eye**

- **D32 Benign neoplasm of meninges**
  - **D32.0 Benign neoplasm of cerebral meninges**
  - **D32.1 Benign neoplasm of spinal meninges**
  - **D32.9 Benign neoplasm of meninges, unspecified**
    Meningioma NOS

- **D33 Benign neoplasm of brain and other parts of central nervous system**

  Excludes1 angioma (D18.0-)
  benign neoplasm of meninges (D32.-)
  benign neoplasm of peripheral nerves and autonomic nervous system (D36.1-)
  hemangioma (D18.0-)
  neurofibromatosis (Q85.0-)
  retro-ocular benign neoplasm (D31.6-)

  - **D33.0 Benign neoplasm of brain, supratentorial**
    Benign neoplasm of cerebral ventricle
    Benign neoplasm of cerebrum
    Benign neoplasm of frontal lobe
    Benign neoplasm of occipital lobe
    Benign neoplasm of parietal lobe
    Benign neoplasm of temporal lobe

    Excludes1 benign neoplasm of fourth ventricle (D33.1)

  - **D33.1 Benign neoplasm of brain, infratentorial**
    Benign neoplasm of brain stem
    Benign neoplasm of cerebellum
    Benign neoplasm of fourth ventricle

  - **D33.2 Benign neoplasm of brain, unspecified**
  - **D33.3 Benign neoplasm of cranial nerves**
    Benign neoplasm of olfactory bulb
  - **D33.4 Benign neoplasm of spinal cord**
  - **D33.7 Benign neoplasm of other specified parts of central nervous system**
  - **D33.9 Benign neoplasm of central nervous system, unspecified**
    Benign neoplasm of nervous system (central) NOS

- **D34 Benign neoplasm of thyroid gland**
  Use additional code to identify any functional activity.

- **D35 Benign neoplasm of other and unspecified endocrine glands**

  Use additional code to identify any functional activity.

  Excludes1 benign neoplasm of endocrine pancreas (D13.7)
  benign neoplasm of ovary (D27.-)
  benign neoplasm of testis (D29.2.-)
  benign neoplasm of thymus (D15.0)

  - **D35.0 Benign neoplasm of adrenal gland**
    - **D35.00 Benign neoplasm of unspecified adrenal gland**
    - **D35.01 Benign neoplasm of right adrenal gland**
    - **D35.02 Benign neoplasm of left adrenal gland**
  - **D35.1 Benign neoplasm of parathyroid gland**
  - **D35.2 Benign neoplasm of pituitary gland**
  - **D35.3 Benign neoplasm of craniopharyngeal duct**
  - **D35.4 Benign neoplasm of pineal gland**
  - **D35.5 Benign neoplasm of carotid body**
  - **D35.6 Benign neoplasm of aortic body and other paraganglia**
    Benign tumor of glomus jugulare
  - **D35.7 Benign neoplasm of other specified endocrine glands**
  - **D35.9 Benign neoplasm of endocrine gland, unspecified**
    Benign neoplasm of unspecified endocrine gland

- **D36 Benign neoplasm of other and unspecified sites**
  - **D36.0 Benign neoplasm of lymph nodes**
    Excludes1 lymphangioma (D18.1)
  - **D36.1 Benign neoplasm of peripheral nerves and autonomic nervous system**

    Excludes1 benign neoplasm of peripheral nerves of orbit (D31.6-)
    neurofibromatosis (Q85.0-)

    - **D36.10 Benign neoplasm of peripheral nerves and autonomic nervous system, unspecified**
    - **D36.11 Benign neoplasm of peripheral nerves and autonomic nervous system of face, head, and neck**
    - **D36.12 Benign neoplasm of peripheral nerves and autonomic nervous system, upper limb, including shoulder**
    - **D36.13 Benign neoplasm of peripheral nerves and autonomic nervous system of lower limb, including hip**
    - **D36.14 Benign neoplasm of peripheral nerves and autonomic nervous system of thorax**
    - **D36.15 Benign neoplasm of peripheral nerves and autonomic nervous system of abdomen**
    - **D36.16 Benign neoplasm of peripheral nerves and autonomic nervous system of pelvis**
    - **D36.17 Benign neoplasm of peripheral nerves and autonomic nervous system of trunk, unspecified**
  - **D36.7 Benign neoplasm of other specified sites**
    Benign neoplasm of nose NOS
  - **D36.9 Benign neoplasm, unspecified site**

CHAPTER 2 (C00-D49)

● Unacceptable Principal Diagnosis   ● Use Additional Character(s)   ■ Unspecified   ▶ Manifestation Code

OGCR Official Guidelines for Coding and Reporting   Excludes 1   Excludes 2   Includes   Use additional   Code first   Code also

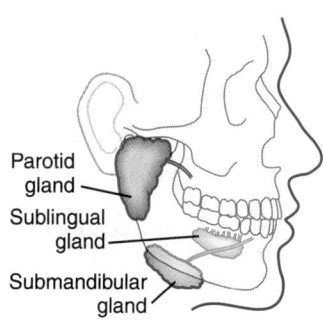

Figure 2-19 Major salivary glands.

Parotid gland
Sublingual gland
Submandibular gland

BENIGN NEUROENDOCRINE TUMORS (D3A)

● **D3A Benign neuroendocrine tumors**

Code also any associated multiple endocrine neoplasia [MEN] syndromes (E31.2-)

Use additional code to identify any associated endocrine syndrome, such as:
carcinoid syndrome (E34.0)

Excludes2   benign pancreatic islet cell tumors (D13.7)

● **D3A.0 Benign carcinoid tumors**

■ **D3A.00 Benign carcinoid tumor of unspecified site**
Carcinoid tumor NOS

● **D3A.01 Benign carcinoid tumors of the small intestine**

D3A.010 Benign carcinoid tumor of the duodenum

D3A.011 Benign carcinoid tumor of the jejunum

D3A.012 Benign carcinoid tumor of the ileum

■ **D3A.019 Benign carcinoid tumor of the small intestine, unspecified portion**

● **D3A.02 Benign carcinoid tumors of the appendix, large intestine, and rectum**

D3A.020 Benign carcinoid tumor of the appendix

D3A.021 Benign carcinoid tumor of the cecum

D3A.022 Benign carcinoid tumor of the ascending colon

D3A.023 Benign carcinoid tumor of the transverse colon

D3A.024 Benign carcinoid tumor of the descending colon

D3A.025 Benign carcinoid tumor of the sigmoid colon

D3A.026 Benign carcinoid tumor of the rectum

■ **D3A.029 Benign carcinoid tumor of the large intestine, unspecified portion**
Benign carcinoid tumor of the colon NOS

● **D3A.09 Benign carcinoid tumors of other sites**

D3A.090 Benign carcinoid tumor of the bronchus and lung

D3A.091 Benign carcinoid tumor of the thymus

D3A.092 Benign carcinoid tumor of the stomach

D3A.093 Benign carcinoid tumor of the kidney

D3A.094 Benign carcinoid tumor of the foregut NOS

D3A.095 Benign carcinoid tumor of the midgut NOS

D3A.096 Benign carcinoid tumor of the hindgut NOS

D3A.098 Benign carcinoid tumors of other sites

● **D3A.8 Other benign neuroendocrine tumors**
Neuroendocrine tumor NOS

NEOPLASMS OF UNCERTAIN BEHAVIOR, POLYCYTHEMIA VERA AND MYELODYSPLASTIC SYNDROMES (D37-D48)

Note: Categories D37-D44, and D48 classify by site neoplasms of uncertain behavior, i.e., histologic confirmation whether the neoplasm is malignant or benign cannot be made.

Excludes1   neoplasms of unspecified behavior (D49-)

● **D37 Neoplasm of uncertain behavior of oral cavity and digestive organs**

Excludes1   stromal tumors of uncertain behavior of digestive system (D48.1)

● **D37.0 Neoplasm of uncertain behavior of lip, oral cavity and pharynx**

Excludes1   neoplasm of uncertain behavior of aryepiglottic fold or interarytenoid fold, laryngeal aspect (D38.0)
neoplasm of uncertain behavior of epiglottis NOS (D38.0)
neoplasm of uncertain behavior of skin of lip (D48.5)
neoplasm of uncertain behavior of suprahyoid portion of epiglottis (D38.0)

D37.01 Neoplasm of uncertain behavior of lip
Neoplasm of uncertain behavior of vermilion border of lip

D37.02 Neoplasm of uncertain behavior of tongue

● **D37.03 Neoplasm of uncertain behavior of the major salivary glands**

D37.030 Neoplasm of uncertain behavior of the parotid salivary glands

D37.031 Neoplasm of uncertain behavior of the sublingual salivary glands

D37.032 Neoplasm of uncertain behavior of the submandibular salivary glands

■ **D37.039 Neoplasm of uncertain behavior of the major salivary glands, unspecified**

D37.04 Neoplasm of uncertain behavior of the minor salivary glands
Neoplasm of uncertain behavior of submucosal salivary glands of lip
Neoplasm of uncertain behavior of submucosal salivary glands of cheek
Neoplasm of uncertain behavior of submucosal salivary glands of hard palate
Neoplasm of uncertain behavior of submucosal salivary glands of soft palate

CHAPTER 2 (C00-D49)

N Newborn Age: 0   **P** Pediatric Age: 0–17   **M** Maternity DX: 12–55   **A** Adult Age: 15–124   ♀ Females Only   ♂ Males Only

Complication\Comorbidity   Major C\C   Present on Admission Requirement   Hospital-Acquired Condition   865

D37.05   Neoplasm of uncertain behavior of pharynx
> Neoplasm of uncertain behavior of aryepiglottic fold of pharynx NOS
> Neoplasm of uncertain behavior of hypopharyngeal aspect of aryepiglottic fold of pharynx
> Neoplasm of uncertain behavior of marginal zone of aryepiglottic fold of pharynx

■ **D37.09   Neoplasm of uncertain behavior of other specified sites of the oral cavity**

D37.1   Neoplasm of uncertain behavior of stomach

D37.2   Neoplasm of uncertain behavior of small intestine

D37.3   Neoplasm of uncertain behavior of appendix

D37.4   Neoplasm of uncertain behavior of colon

D37.5   Neoplasm of uncertain behavior of rectum
> Neoplasm of uncertain behavior of rectosigmoid junction
> *Rectosigmoid junction: Angle where sigmoid colon becomes rectum*

■ **D37.6   Neoplasm of uncertain behavior of liver, gallbladder and bile ducts**
> Neoplasm of uncertain behavior of ampulla of Vater
> *Ampulla of Vater: Enlarged segment of ducts from liver and pancreas at entry point to small intestine*

D37.8   Neoplasm of uncertain behavior of other specified digestive organs
> Neoplasm of uncertain behavior of anal canal
> Neoplasm of uncertain behavior of anal sphincter
> Neoplasm of uncertain behavior of anus NOS
> Neoplasm of uncertain behavior of esophagus
> Neoplasm of uncertain behavior of intestine NOS
> Neoplasm of uncertain behavior of pancreas
>
> | Excludes1 | neoplasm of uncertain behavior of anal margin (D48.5) |
> | --- | --- |
> | | neoplasm of uncertain behavior of anal skin (D48.5) |
> | | neoplasm of uncertain behavior of perianal skin (D48.5) |

D37.9   Neoplasm of uncertain behavior of digestive organ, unspecified

● **D38   Neoplasm of uncertain behavior of middle ear and respiratory and intrathoracic organs**

Excludes1	neoplasm of uncertain behavior of heart (D48.7)

D38.0   Neoplasm of uncertain behavior of larynx
> Neoplasm of uncertain behavior of aryepiglottic fold or interarytenoid fold, laryngeal aspect
> Neoplasm of uncertain behavior of epiglottis (suprahyoid portion)
>
> | Excludes1 | neoplasm of uncertain behavior of aryepiglottic fold or interarytenoid fold NOS (D37.05) |
> | --- | --- |
> | | neoplasm of uncertain behavior of hypopharyngeal aspect of aryepiglottic fold (D37.05) |
> | | neoplasm of uncertain behavior of marginal zone of aryepiglottic fold (D37.05) |

D38.1   Neoplasm of uncertain behavior of trachea, bronchus and lung

D38.2   Neoplasm of uncertain behavior of pleura

D38.3   Neoplasm of uncertain behavior of mediastinum

D38.4   Neoplasm of uncertain behavior of thymus

D38.5   Neoplasm of uncertain behavior of other respiratory organs
> Neoplasm of uncertain behavior of accessory sinuses
> Neoplasm of uncertain behavior of cartilage of nose
> Neoplasm of uncertain behavior of middle ear
> Neoplasm of uncertain behavior of nasal cavities
>
> | Excludes1 | neoplasm of uncertain behavior of ear (external) (skin) (D48.5) |
> | --- | --- |
> | | neoplasm of uncertain behavior of nose NOS (D48.7) |
> | | neoplasm of uncertain behavior of skin of nose (D48.5) |

D38.6   Neoplasm of uncertain behavior of respiratory organ, unspecified

● **D39   Neoplasm of uncertain behavior of female genital organs**

D39.0   Neoplasm of uncertain behavior of uterus ♀

● **D39.1   Neoplasm of uncertain behavior of ovary**
> Use additional code to identify any functional activity.

■ **D39.10   Neoplasm of uncertain behavior of unspecified ovary ♀**

D39.11   Neoplasm of uncertain behavior of right ovary ♀

D39.12   Neoplasm of uncertain behavior of left ovary ♀

D39.2   Neoplasm of uncertain behavior of placenta ♀
> Chorioadenoma destruens
> Invasive hydatidiform mole
> Malignant hydatidiform mole
>
> | Excludes1 | hydatidiform mole NOS (O01.9) |
> | --- | --- |

D39.8   Neoplasm of uncertain behavior of other specified female genital organs ♀
> Neoplasm of uncertain behavior of skin of female genital organs

■ **D39.9   Neoplasm of uncertain behavior of female genital organ, unspecified ♀**

● **D40   Neoplasm of uncertain behavior of male genital organs**

D40.0   Neoplasm of uncertain behavior of prostate ♂

● **D40.1   Neoplasm of uncertain behavior of testis**

■ **D40.10   Neoplasm of uncertain behavior of unspecified testis ♂**

D40.11   Neoplasm of uncertain behavior of right testis ♂

D40.12   Neoplasm of uncertain behavior of left testis ♂

D40.8   Neoplasm of uncertain behavior of other specified male genital organs ♂
> Neoplasm of uncertain behavior of skin of male genital organs

■ **D40.9   Neoplasm of uncertain behavior of male genital organ, unspecified ♂**

● **D41   Neoplasm of uncertain behavior of urinary organs**

● **D41.0   Neoplasm of uncertain behavior of kidney**

Excludes1	neoplasm of uncertain behavior of renal pelvis (D41.1-)

■ **D41.00   Neoplasm of uncertain behavior of unspecified kidney**

D41.01   Neoplasm of uncertain behavior of right kidney

D41.02   Neoplasm of uncertain behavior of left kidney

CHAPTER 2 (C00-D49)

● Unacceptable Principal Diagnosis   ● Use Additional Character(s)   ■ Unspecified   ▶ Manifestation Code

OGCR Official Guidelines for Coding and Reporting   Excludes 1   Excludes 2   Includes   Use additional   Code first   Code also

● **D41.1**   Neoplasm of uncertain behavior of renal pelvis

    ■ **D41.10**   Neoplasm of uncertain behavior of unspecified renal pelvis

     D41.11   Neoplasm of uncertain behavior of right renal pelvis

     D41.12   Neoplasm of uncertain behavior of left renal pelvis

● **D41.2**   Neoplasm of uncertain behavior of ureter

    ■ **D41.20**   Neoplasm of uncertain behavior of unspecified ureter

     D41.21   Neoplasm of uncertain behavior of right ureter

     D41.22   Neoplasm of uncertain behavior of left ureter

D41.3   Neoplasm of uncertain behavior of urethra

D41.4   Neoplasm of uncertain behavior of bladder

D41.8   Neoplasm of uncertain behavior of other specified urinary organs

■ **D41.9**   Neoplasm of uncertain behavior of unspecified urinary organ

● **D42**   Neoplasm of uncertain behavior of meninges

D42.0   Neoplasm of uncertain behavior of cerebral meninges

D42.1   Neoplasm of uncertain behavior of spinal meninges

■ **D42.9**   Neoplasm of uncertain behavior of meninges, unspecified

● **D43**   Neoplasm of uncertain behavior of brain and central nervous system

     Excludes1   neoplasm of uncertain behavior of peripheral nerves and autonomic nervous system (D48.2)

D43.0   Neoplasm of uncertain behavior of brain, supratentorial

     Superior to tentorium of cerebellum

     Neoplasm of uncertain behavior of cerebral ventricle

     Neoplasm of uncertain behavior of cerebrum

     Neoplasm of uncertain behavior of frontal lobe

     Neoplasm of uncertain behavior of occipital lobe

     Neoplasm of uncertain behavior of parietal lobe

     Neoplasm of uncertain behavior of temporal lobe

     Excludes1   neoplasm of uncertain behavior of fourth ventricle (D43.1)

D43.1   Neoplasm of uncertain behavior of brain, infratentorial

     Beneath the tentorium of cerebellum

     Neoplasm of uncertain behavior of brain stem

     Neoplasm of uncertain behavior of cerebellum

     Neoplasm of uncertain behavior of fourth ventricle

■ **D43.2**   Neoplasm of uncertain behavior of brain, unspecified

D43.3   Neoplasm of uncertain behavior of cranial nerves

D43.4   Neoplasm of uncertain behavior of spinal cord

D43.8   Neoplasm of uncertain behavior of other specified parts of central nervous system

■ **D43.9**   Neoplasm of uncertain behavior of central nervous system, unspecified

     Neoplasm of uncertain behavior of nervous system (central) NOS

● **D44**   Neoplasm of uncertain behavior of endocrine glands

     Excludes1   multiple endocrine adenomatosis (E31.2-)

         multiple endocrine neoplasia (E31.2-)

         neoplasm of uncertain behavior of endocrine pancreas (D37.8)

         neoplasm of uncertain behavior of ovary (D39.1-)

         neoplasm of uncertain behavior of testis (D40.1-)

         neoplasm of uncertain behavior of thymus (D38.4)

D44.0   Neoplasm of uncertain behavior of thyroid gland

● **D44.1**   Neoplasm of uncertain behavior of adrenal gland

     Use additional code to identify any functional activity.

    ■ **D44.10**   Neoplasm of uncertain behavior of unspecified adrenal gland

     D44.11   Neoplasm of uncertain behavior of right adrenal gland

     D44.12   Neoplasm of uncertain behavior of left adrenal gland

D44.2   Neoplasm of uncertain behavior of parathyroid gland

D44.3   Neoplasm of uncertain behavior of pituitary gland

     Use additional code to identify any functional activity.

D44.4   Neoplasm of uncertain behavior of craniopharyngeal duct

D44.5   Neoplasm of uncertain behavior of pineal gland

D44.6   Neoplasm of uncertain behavior of carotid body

D44.7   Neoplasm of uncertain behavior of aortic body and other paraganglia

■ **D44.9**   Neoplasm of uncertain behavior of unspecified endocrine gland

D45   Polycythemia vera

     Excludes1   familial polycythemia (D75.0)

         secondary polycythemia (D75.1)

     Primary polycythemia is D75.1. Check your documentation. Secondary polycythemia is D75.1. Check your documentation. Polycythemia is caused by too many red blood cells, which increase the thickness of blood (viscosity). This can cause engorgement of the spleen (splenomegaly) with extra RBCs and potential clot formation.

● **D46**   Myelodysplastic syndromes

     Use additional code for adverse effect, if applicable, to identify drug (T36-T50 with fifth or sixth character 5)

     Excludes2   drug-induced aplastic anemia (D61.1)

D46.0   Refractory anemia without ring sideroblasts, so stated

     Refractory anemia without sideroblasts, without excess of blasts

D46.1   Refractory anemia with ring sideroblasts RARS

● **D46.2**   Refractory anemia with excess of blasts

     Form of myelodysplasia with increased immature white blood cells (blasts) in bone marrow

    ■ **D46.20**   Refractory anemia with excess of blasts, unspecified RAEB NOS

     D46.21   Refractory anemia with excess of blasts 1 RAEB 1

         Bone marrow disease which results in insufficient RBCs (anemia) in which level of blasts is less than 10%

     D46.22   Refractory anemia with excess of blasts 2 RAEB 2 🦠

         Bone marrow disease manifested by insufficient numbers of RBCs (anemia) with level of blasts 10-20%

N Newborn Age: 0   **P** Pediatric Age: 0–17   **M** Maternity DX: 12–55   **A** Adult Age: 15–124   ♀ Females Only   ♂ Males Only

🦠 Complication\Comorbidity   🦠 Major C\C   🦠 Present on Admission Requirement   🦠 Hospital-Acquired Condition

867

CHAPTER 2 (C00-D49)

CHAPTER 2 (C00-D49)

D46.A **Refractory cytopenia with multilineage dysplasia**

D46.B **Refractory cytopenia with multilineage dysplasia and ring sideroblasts**
RCMD RS

D46.C **Myelodysplastic syndrome with isolated del(5q) chromosomal abnormality** 🔊
Myelodysplastic syndrome with 5q deletion
5q minus syndrome NOS

◼ **D46.4** **Refractory anemia, unspecified**

D46.Z **Other myelodysplastic syndromes**
> **Excludes1**   chronic myelomonocytic leukemia (C93.1-)

◼ **D46.9** **Myelodysplastic syndrome, unspecified**
Myelodysplasia NOS

● **D47** **Other neoplasms of uncertain behavior of lymphoid, hematopoietic and related tissue**

D47.0 **Histiocytic and mast cell tumors of uncertain behavior** 🔊
Indolent systemic mastocytosis
Mast cell tumor NOS
Mastocytoma NOS
> **Excludes1**   malignant mast cell tumor (C96.2)
> mastocytosis (congenital) (cutaneous) (Q82.2)

D47.1 **Chronic myeloproliferative disease** 🔊
Chronic neutrophilic leukemia
Myeloproliferative disease, unspecified
> **Excludes1**   atypical chronic myeloid leukemia BCR/ABL-negative (C92.2-)
> chronic myeloid leukemia BCR/ABL-positive (C92.1-)
> myelofibrosis NOS (D75.81)
> myelophthisic anemia (D61.82)
> myelophthisis (D61.82)
> secondary myelofibrosis NOS (D75.81)

D47.2 **Monoclonal gammopathy**
Monoclonal gammopathy of undetermined significance [MGUS]

D47.3 **Essential (hemorrhagic) thrombocythemia**
Essential thrombocytosis
Idiopathic hemorrhagic thrombocythemia

D47.4 **Osteomyelofibrosis**
Chronic idiopathic myelofibrosis
Myelofibrosis (idiopathic) (with myeloid metaplasia)
Myelosclerosis (megakaryocytic) with myeloid metaplasia
Secondary myelofibrosis in myeloproliferative disease
> **Excludes1**   acute myelofibrosis (C94.4-)

● **D47.Z** **Other specified neoplasms of uncertain behavior of lymphoid, hematopoietic and related tissue**

● **D47.Z1** **Post-transplant lymphoproliferative disorder (PTLD)** 🔊
> *Code first* complications of transplanted organs and tissue (T86.-)

D47.Z9 **Other specified neoplasms of uncertain behavior of lymphoid, hematopoietic and related tissue** 🔊
Histiocytic tumors of uncertain behavior

◼ **D47.9** **Neoplasm of uncertain behavior of lymphoid, hematopoietic and related tissue, unspecified** 🔊
Lymphoproliferative disease NOS

● **D48** **Neoplasm of uncertain behavior of other and unspecified sites**
> **Excludes1**   neurofibromatosis (nonmalignant) (Q85.0-)

D48.0 **Neoplasm of uncertain behavior of bone and articular cartilage**
> **Excludes1**   neoplasm of uncertain behavior of cartilage of ear (D48.1)
> neoplasm of uncertain behavior of cartilage of larynx (D38.0)
> neoplasm of uncertain behavior of cartilage of nose (D38.5)
> neoplasm of uncertain behavior of connective tissue of eyelid (D48.1)
> neoplasm of uncertain behavior of synovia (D48.1)

D48.1 **Neoplasm of uncertain behavior of connective and other soft tissue**
Neoplasm of uncertain behavior of connective tissue of ear
Neoplasm of uncertain behavior of connective tissue of eyelid
Stromal tumors of uncertain behavior of digestive system
> **Excludes1**   neoplasm of uncertain behavior of articular cartilage (D48.0)
> neoplasm of uncertain behavior of cartilage of larynx (D38.0)
> neoplasm of uncertain behavior of cartilage of nose (D38.5)
> neoplasm of uncertain behavior of connective tissue of breast (D48.6-)

D48.2 **Neoplasm of uncertain behavior of peripheral nerves and autonomic nervous system**
> **Excludes1**   neoplasm of uncertain behavior of peripheral nerves of orbit (D48.7)

D48.3 **Neoplasm of uncertain behavior of retroperitoneum**

D48.4 **Neoplasm of uncertain behavior of peritoneum**

D48.5 **Neoplasm of uncertain behavior of skin**
Neoplasm of uncertain behavior of anal margin
Neoplasm of uncertain behavior of anal skin
Neoplasm of uncertain behavior of perianal skin
Neoplasm of uncertain behavior of skin of breast
> **Excludes1**   neoplasm of uncertain behavior of anus NOS (D37.8)
> neoplasm of uncertain behavior of skin of genital organs (D39.8, D40.7)
> neoplasm of uncertain behavior of vermilion border of lip (D37.0)

● **D48.6** **Neoplasm of uncertain behavior of breast**
Neoplasm of uncertain behavior of connective tissue of breast
Cystosarcoma phyllodes
> **Excludes1**   neoplasm of uncertain behavior of skin of breast (D48.5)

◼ **D48.60** **Neoplasm of uncertain behavior of unspecified breast**

D48.61 **Neoplasm of uncertain behavior of right breast**

D48.62 **Neoplasm of uncertain behavior of left breast**

● Unacceptable Principal Diagnosis   ● Use Additional Character(s)   ◼ Unspecified   ▶ Manifestation Code
OGCR Official Guidelines for Coding and Reporting | Excludes 1 | | Excludes 2 | | Includes | | Use additional | | Code first | | Code also |

D48.7　**Neoplasm of uncertain behavior of other specified sites**
　　　Neoplasm of uncertain behavior of eye
　　　Neoplasm of uncertain behavior of heart
　　　Neoplasm of uncertain behavior of peripheral nerves of orbit

　　　Excludes1　neoplasm of uncertain behavior of connective tissue (D48.1)
　　　　　　　　neoplasm of uncertain behavior of skin of eyelid (D48.5)

■ D48.9　**Neoplasm of uncertain behavior, unspecified**

● **D49　Neoplasms of unspecified behavior**

　　　Note: Category D49 classifies by site neoplasms of unspecified morphology and behavior. The term 'mass', unless otherwise stated, is not to be regarded as a neoplastic growth.

　　　Includes　'growth' NOS
　　　　　　　neoplasm NOS
　　　　　　　new growth NOS
　　　　　　　tumor NOS

　　　Excludes1　neoplasms of uncertain behavior (D37-D44, D48)

■ D49.0　**Neoplasm of unspecified behavior of digestive system**

　　　Excludes1　neoplasm of unspecified behavior of margin of anus (D49.2)
　　　　　　　　neoplasm of unspecified behavior of perianal skin (D49.2)
　　　　　　　　neoplasm of unspecified behavior of skin of anus (D49.2)

■ D49.1　**Neoplasm of unspecified behavior of respiratory system**

■ D49.2　**Neoplasm of unspecified behavior of bone, soft tissue, and skin**

　　　Excludes1　neoplasm of unspecified behavior of anal canal (D49.0)
　　　　　　　　neoplasm of unspecified behavior of anus NOS (D49.0)
　　　　　　　　neoplasm of unspecified behavior of bone marrow (D49.9)
　　　　　　　　neoplasm of unspecified behavior of cartilage of larynx (D49.1)
　　　　　　　　neoplasm of unspecified behavior of cartilage of nose (D49.1)
　　　　　　　　neoplasm of unspecified behavior of connective tissue of breast (D49.3)
　　　　　　　　neoplasm of unspecified behavior of skin of genital organs (D49.5)
　　　　　　　　neoplasm of unspecified behavior of vermilion border of lip (D49.0)

■ D49.3　**Neoplasm of unspecified behavior of breast**

　　　Excludes1　neoplasm of unspecified behavior of skin of breast (D49.2)

■ D49.4　**Neoplasm of unspecified behavior of bladder**

■ D49.5　**Neoplasm of unspecified behavior of other genitourinary organs**

■ D49.6　**Neoplasm of unspecified behavior of brain**

　　　Excludes1　neoplasm of unspecified behavior of cerebral meninges (D49.7)
　　　　　　　　neoplasm of unspecified behavior of cranial nerves (D49.7)

● D49.7　**Neoplasm of unspecified behavior of endocrine glands and other parts of nervous system**

　　　Excludes1　neoplasm of unspecified behavior of peripheral, sympathetic, and parasympathetic nerves and ganglia (D49.2)

● D49.8　**Neoplasm of unspecified behavior of other specified sites**

　　　Excludes1　neoplasm of unspecified behavior of eyelid (skin) (D49.2)
　　　　　　　　neoplasm of unspecified behavior of eyelid cartilage (D49.2)
　　　　　　　　neoplasm of unspecified behavior of great vessels (D49.2)
　　　　　　　　neoplasm of unspecified behavior of optic nerve (D49.7)

　　■ D49.81　**Neoplasm of unspecified behavior of retina and choroid**
　　　　　Dark area on retina
　　　　　Retinal freckle

　　■ D49.89　**Neoplasm of unspecified behavior of other specified sites**

■ D49.9　**Neoplasm of unspecified behavior of unspecified site**

CHAPTER 3

DISEASES OF THE BLOOD AND BLOOD-FORMING ORGANS AND CERTAIN DISORDERS INVOLVING THE IMMUNE MECHANISM (D50-D89)

Excludes2   autoimmune disease (systemic) NOS (M35.9)
certain conditions originating in the perinatal period (P00-P96)
complications of pregnancy, childbirth and the puerperium (O00-O9A)
congenital malformations, deformations and chromosomal abnormalities (Q00-Q99)
endocrine, nutritional and metabolic diseases (E00-E88)
human immunodeficiency virus [HIV] disease (B20)
injury, poisoning and certain other consequences of external causes (S00-T88)
neoplasms (C00-D49)
symptoms, signs and abnormal clinical and laboratory findings, not elsewhere classified (R00-R94)

This chapter contains the following blocks:

D50-D53	Nutritional anemias
D55-D59	Hemolytic anemias
D60-D64	Aplastic and other anemias and other bone marrow failure syndromes
D65-D69	Coagulation defects, purpura and other hemorrhagic conditions
D70-D77	Other disorders of blood and blood-forming organs
D78	Intraoperative and postprocedural complications of the spleen
D80-D89	Certain disorders involving the immune mechanism

NUTRITIONAL ANEMIAS (D50-D53)

● **D50   Iron deficiency anemia**
A disease characterized by a decrease in the number of red cells (hemoglobin) in the blood.

Includes   asiderotic anemia
hypochromic anemia

D50.0   Iron deficiency anemia secondary to blood loss (chronic)
Posthemorrhagic anemia (chronic)

Excludes1   acute posthemorrhagic anemia (D62)
congenital anemia from fetal blood loss (P61.3)

D50.1   Sideropenic dysphagia
Web-like growth of membranes in throat that makes swallowing difficult
Kelly-Paterson syndrome
Plummer-Vinson syndrome

D50.8   Other iron deficiency anemias
Iron deficiency anemia due to inadequate dietary iron intake

■ **D50.9   Iron deficiency anemia, unspecified**

● **D51   Vitamin B12 deficiency anemia**

Excludes1   vitamin B12 deficiency (E53.8)

D51.0   Vitamin B12 deficiency anemia due to intrinsic factor deficiency
Addison anemia
Biermer anemia
Pernicious (congenital) anemia
Congenital intrinsic factor deficiency

D51.1   Vitamin B12 deficiency anemia due to selective vitamin B12 malabsorption with proteinuria
Imerslund (Gräsbeck) syndrome
Megaloblastic hereditary anemia

D51.2   Transcobalamin II deficiency

D51.3   Other dietary vitamin B12 deficiency anemia
Vegan anemia

D51.8   Other vitamin B12 deficiency anemias

■ **D51.9   Vitamin B12 deficiency anemia, unspecified**

● **D52   Folate deficiency anemia**

Excludes1   folate deficiency without anemia (E53.8)

D52.0   Dietary folate deficiency anemia
Nutritional megaloblastic anemia

● **D52.1   Drug-induced folate deficiency anemia**

Use additional code for adverse effect, if applicable, to identify drug (T36-T50 with fifth or sixth character 5)

D52.8   Other folate deficiency anemias

■ **D52.9   Folate deficiency anemia, unspecified**
Folic acid deficiency anemia NOS

● **D53   Other nutritional anemias**

Includes   megaloblastic anemia unresponsive to vitamin B12 or folate therapy

D53.0   Protein deficiency anemia
Amino-acid deficiency anemia
Orotaciduric anemia

Excludes1   Lesch-Nyhan syndrome (E79.1)

D53.1   Other megaloblastic anemias, not elsewhere classified
Megaloblastic anemia NOS

Excludes1   Di Guglielmo's disease (C94.0)

D53.2   Scorbutic anemia
Anemia resulting from deficiency of ascorbic acid (vitamin C)

Excludes1   scurvy (E54)

D53.8   Other specified nutritional anemias
Anemia associated with deficiency of copper
Anemia associated with deficiency of molybdenum
Anemia associated with deficiency of zinc

Excludes1   nutritional deficiencies without anemia, such as:
copper deficiency NOS (E61.0)
molybdenum deficiency NOS (E61.5)
zinc deficiency NOS (E60)

■ **D53.9   Nutritional anemia, unspecified**
Simple chronic anemia

Excludes1   anemia NOS (D64.9)

● Unacceptable Principal Diagnosis   ● Use Additional Character(s)   ■ Unspecified   ▶ Manifestation Code
OGCR   Official Guidelines for Coding and Reporting   Excludes 1   Excludes 2   Includes   Use additional   Code first   Code also

CHAPTER 3 (D50-D89)

HEMOLYTIC ANEMIAS (D55-D59)

● **D55 Anemia due to enzyme disorders**

     | Excludes1 | drug-induced enzyme deficiency anemia (D59.2)

     D55.0 Anemia due to glucose-6-phosphate dehydrogenase [G6PD] deficiency
         Favism
         G6PD deficiency anemia

     D55.1 Anemia due to other disorders of glutathione metabolism
         Anemia (due to) enzyme deficiencies, except G6PD, related to the hexose monophosphate [HMP] shunt pathway
         Anemia (due to) hemolytic nonspherocytic (hereditary), type I

     D55.2 Anemia due to disorders of glycolytic enzymes
         Hemolytic nonspherocytic (hereditary) anemia, type II
         Hexokinase deficiency anemia
         Pyruvate kinase [PK] deficiency anemia
         Triose-phosphate isomerase deficiency anemia

         | Excludes1 | disorders of glycolysis not associated with anemia (E74.8)

     D55.3 Anemia due to disorders of nucleotide metabolism

     D55.8 Other anemias due to enzyme disorders

     ■ **D55.9 Anemia due to enzyme disorder, unspecified**

● **D56 Thalassemia**
     Hereditary disorders characterized by low production of hemoglobin or excessive destruction of red blood cells

     | Excludes1 | sickle-cell thalassemia (D57.4-)

     D56.0 Alpha thalassemia
         Alpha thalassemia major
         Hemoglobin H Constant Spring
         Hemoglobin H disease
         Hydrops fetalis due to alpha thalassemia
         Severe alpha thalassemia
         Triple gene defect alpha thalassemia

         Use additional code, if applicable, for hydrops fetalis due to alpha thalassemia (P56.99)

         | Excludes1 | alpha thalassemia trait or minor (D56.3)
                 asymptomatic alpha thalassemia (D56.3)
                 hydrops fetalis due to isoimmunization (P56.0)
                 hydrops fetalis not due to immune hemolysis (P83.2)

     D56.1 Beta thalassemia
         Beta thalassemia major
         Cooley's anemia
         Homozygous beta thalassemia
         Severe beta thalassemia
         Thalassemia intermedia
         Thalassemia major

         | Excludes1 | beta thalassemia minor (D56.3)
                 beta thalassemia trait (D56.3)
                 delta-beta thalassemia (D56.2)
                 hemoglobin E-beta thalassemia (D56.5)
                 sickle-cell beta thalassemia (D57.4-)

     D56.2 Delta-beta thalassemia
         Homozygous delta-beta thalassemia

         | Excludes1 | delta-beta thalassemia minor (D56.3)
                 delta-beta thalassemia trait (D56.3)

     D56.3 Thalassemia minor
     Genetic disorders that have in common defective production of hemoglobin
         Alpha thalassemia minor
         Alpha thalassemia silent carrier
         Alpha thalassemia trait
         Beta thalassemia minor
         Beta thalassemia trait
         Delta-beta thalassemia minor
         Delta-beta thalassemia trait
         Thalassemia trait NOS

         | Excludes1 | alpha thalassemia (D56.0)
                 beta thalassemia (D56.1)
                 delta-beta thalassemia (D56.2)
                 hemoglobin E-beta thalassemia (D56.5)
                 sickle-cell trait (D57.3)

     D56.4 Hereditary persistence of fetal hemoglobin [HPFH]
     Persistent production of hemoglobin

     D56.5 Hemoglobin E-beta thalassemia

         | Excludes1 | beta thalassemia (D56.1)
                 beta thalassemia minor (D56.3)
                 beta thalassemia trait (D56.3)
                 delta-beta thalassemia (D56.2)
                 delta-beta thalassemia trait (D56.3)
                 hemoglobin E disease (D58.2)
                 other hemoglobinopathies (D58.2)
                 sickle-cell beta thalassemia (D57.4-)

     D56.8 Other thalassemias
         Dominant thalassemia
         Hemoglobin C thalassemia
         Mixed thalassemia
         Thalassemia with other hemoglobinopathy

         | Excludes1 | hemoglobin C disease (D58.2)
                 hemoglobin E disease (D58.2)
                 other hemoglobinopathies (D58.2)
                 sickle cell anemia (D57.-)
                 sickle-cell thalassemia (D57.4)

     ■ **D56.9 Thalassemia, unspecified**
         Mediterranean anemia (with other hemoglobinopathy)

● **D57 Sickle-cell disorders**
     Inherited disease in which red blood cells, normally disc-shaped, become crescent shaped.

     Use additional code for any associated fever (R50.81)

     | Excludes1 | other hemoglobinopathies (D58.-)

● **D57.0 Hb-SS disease with crisis**
         Sickle-cell disease NOS with crisis
         Hb-SS disease with vasoocclusive pain

     ■ **D57.00 Hb-SS disease with crisis, unspecified** 🐾

     D57.01 Hb-SS disease with acute chest syndrome 🐾

     D57.02 Hb-SS disease with splenic sequestration 🐾

     D57.1 Sickle-cell disease without crisis Hb-SS disease without crisis
         Sickle-cell anemia NOS
         Sickle-cell disease NOS
         Sickle-cell disorder NOS

CHAPTER 3 (D50-D89)

N Newborn Age: 0   **P** Pediatric Age: 0–17   **M** Maternity DX: 12–55   **A** Adult Age: 15–124   ♀ Females Only   ♂ Males Only

🐾 Complication\Comorbidity   🐾 Major C\C   🐾 Present on Admission Requirement   🐾 Hospital-Acquired Condition

871

● **D57.2   Sickle-cell/Hb-C disease**
     Hb-SC disease
     Hb-S/Hb-C disease

   D57.20   Sickle-cell/Hb-C disease without crisis

● **D57.21   Sickle-cell/Hb-C disease with crisis**

     D57.211   Sickle-cell/Hb-C disease with acute chest syndrome 🔖
       MCC: Only when the principal diagnosis is designated as a CC

     D57.212   Sickle-cell/Hb-C disease with splenic sequestration 🔖

■ **D57.219   Sickle-cell/Hb-C disease with crisis, unspecified** 🔖
       Sickle-cell/Hb-C disease with crisis NOS

   D57.3   Sickle-cell trait
     Hb-S trait
     Heterozygous hemoglobin S

● **D57.4   Sickle-cell thalassemia**
     Sickle-cell beta thalassemia
     Thalassemia Hb-S disease

   D57.40   Sickle-cell thalassemia without crisis
     Microdrepanocytosis
     Sickle-cell thalassemia NOS

● **D57.41   Sickle-cell thalassemia with crisis**
     Sickle-cell "crisis" is precipitated when abnormally crescent-shaped red blood cells form clots and interrupt blood flow to major organs, causing severe pain and organ damage.
     Sickle-cell thalassemia with vasoocclusive pain

     D57.411   Sickle-cell thalassemia with acute chest syndrome 🔖
       MCC: Only when the principal diagnosis is designated as a CC

     D57.412   Sickle-cell thalassemia with splenic sequestration 🔖

■ **D57.419   Sickle-cell thalassemia with crisis, unspecified** 🔖
       Sickle-cell thalassemia with crisis NOS

● **D57.8   Other sickle-cell disorders**
     Hb-SD disease
     Hb-SE disease

   D57.80   Other sickle-cell disorders without crisis

● **D57.81   Other sickle-cell disorders with crisis**

     D57.811   Other sickle-cell disorders with acute chest syndrome 🔖

     D57.812   Other sickle-cell disorders with splenic sequestration 🔖

■ **D57.819   Other sickle-cell disorders with crisis, unspecified** 🔖
       Other sickle-cell disorders with crisis NOS

● **D58   Other hereditary hemolytic anemias**
     Genetic condition in which bone marrow is unable to compensate for premature destruction of red blood cells

   Excludes1   hemolytic anemia of the newborn (P55.-)

   D58.0   Hereditary spherocytosis
     Presence of spherocytes (spherically shaped red blood cells)
     Acholuric (familial) jaundice
     Congenital (spherocytic) hemolytic icterus
     Minkowski-Chauffard syndrome

   D58.1   Hereditary elliptocytosis
     Presence of large numbers of elliptocytes in blood
     Elliptocytosis (congenital)
     Ovalocytosis (congenital) (hereditary)

   D58.2   Other hemoglobinopathies
     Abnormal hemoglobin NOS
     Congenital Heinz body anemia
     Hb-C disease
     Hb-D disease
     Hb-E disease
     Hemoglobinopathy NOS
     Unstable hemoglobin hemolytic disease

     Excludes1   familial polycythemia (D75.0)
       Hb-M disease (D74.0)
       hemoglobin E-beta thalassemia (D56.5)
       hereditary persistence of fetal hemoglobin [HPFH] (D56.4)
       high-altitude polycythemia (D75.1)
       methemoglobinemia (D74.-)
       other hemoglobinopathies with thalassemia (D56.8)

   D58.8   Other specified hereditary hemolytic anemias 🔖
     Stomatocytosis

■ **D58.9   Hereditary hemolytic anemia, unspecified** 🔖

● **D59   Acquired hemolytic anemia**

● **D59.0   Drug-induced autoimmune hemolytic anemia** 🔖
     Use additional code for adverse effect, if applicable, to identify drug (T36-T50 with fifth or sixth character 5)

   D59.1   Other autoimmune hemolytic anemias 🔖
     Autoimmune hemolytic disease (cold type) (warm type)
     Chronic cold hemagglutinin disease
     Cold agglutinin disease
     Cold agglutinin hemoglobinuria
     Cold type (secondary) (symptomatic) hemolytic anemia
     Warm type (secondary) (symptomatic) hemolytic anemia

     Excludes1   Evans syndrome (D69.41)
       hemolytic disease of newborn (P55.-)
       paroxysmal cold hemoglobinuria (D59.6)

● **D59.2   Drug-induced nonautoimmune hemolytic anemia** 🔖
     Drug-induced enzyme deficiency anemia
     Use additional code for adverse effect, if applicable, to identify drug (T36-T50 with fifth or sixth character 5)

   D59.3   Hemolytic-uremic syndrome 🔖
     Use additional code to identify associated:
     E. coli infection (B96.2-)
     Pneumococcal pneumonia (J13)
     Shigella dysenteriae (A03.9)

   D59.4   Other nonautoimmune hemolytic anemias 🔖
     Mechanical hemolytic anemia
     Microangiopathic hemolytic anemia
     Toxic hemolytic anemia

   D59.5   Paroxysmal nocturnal hemoglobinuria [Marchiafava-Micheli]

     Excludes1   hemoglobinuria NOS (R82.3)

●   Unacceptable Principal Diagnosis   ●   Use Additional Character(s)   ■   Unspecified   ▶   Manifestation Code

OGCR   Official Guidelines for Coding and Reporting   Excludes 1   Excludes 2   Includes   Use additional   Code first   Code also

D59.6 Hemoglobinuria due to hemolysis from other external causes
    Hemoglobinuria from exertion
    March hemoglobinuria
    Paroxysmal cold hemoglobinuria
    Use additional code (Chapter 20) to identify external cause
    Excludes1   hemoglobinuria NOS (R82.3)

D59.8 Other acquired hemolytic anemias

D59.9 Acquired hemolytic anemia, unspecified 🕭
    Idiopathic hemolytic anemia, chronic

APLASTIC AND OTHER ANEMIAS AND OTHER BONE MARROW FAILURE SYNDROMES (D60-D64)

D60 Acquired pure red cell aplasia [erythroblastopenia]
    Deficiency of erythroblasts
    Includes   red cell aplasia (acquired) (adult) (with thymoma)
    Excludes1   congenital red cell aplasia (D61.01)

D60.0 Chronic acquired pure red cell aplasia 🕭
    Lack of development of blood cell

D60.1 Transient acquired pure red cell aplasia 🕭

D60.8 Other acquired pure red cell aplasias 🕭

D60.9 Acquired pure red cell aplasia, unspecified 🕭

D61 Other aplastic anemias and other bone marrow failure syndromes
    Excludes1   neutropenia (D70.-)

D61.0 Constitutional aplastic anemia
    Condition where bone marrow is unable to produce blood cells

    D61.01 Constitutional (pure) red blood cell aplasia 🕭
        Blackfan-Diamond syndrome
        Congenital (pure) red cell aplasia
        Familial hypoplastic anemia
        Primary (pure) red cell aplasia
        Red cell (pure) aplasia of infants
        Excludes1   acquired red cell aplasia (D60.9)

    D61.09 Other constitutional aplastic anemia 🕭
        Fanconi's anemia
        Pancytopenia with malformations

D61.1 Drug-induced aplastic anemia 🕭
    Use additional code for adverse effect, if applicable, to identify drug (T36-T50 with fifth or sixth character 5)

D61.2 Aplastic anemia due to other external agents 🕭
    Code first , if applicable, toxic effects of substances chiefly nonmedicinal as to source (T51-T65)

D61.3 Idiopathic aplastic anemia 🕭

D61.8 Other specified aplastic anemias and other bone marrow failure syndromes

D61.81 Pancytopenia
    Marked deficiency of all the blood elements: Red blood cells (erythrocytes), white blood cells (leukocytes), and platelets (thrombocytes). Check laboratory results.
    Excludes1   pancytopenia (due to) (with) aplastic anemia (D61.9)
        pancytopenia (due to) (with) bone marrow infiltration (D61.82)
        pancytopenia (due to) (with) congenital (pure) red cell aplasia (D61.01)
        pancytopenia (due to) (with) hairy cell leukemia (C91.4-)
        pancytopenia (due to) (with) human immunodeficiency virus disease (B20.-)
        pancytopenia (due to) (with) leukoerythroblastic anemia (D61.82)
        pancytopenia (due to) (with) myelodysplastic syndromes (D46.-)
        pancytopenia (due to) (with) myeloproliferative disease (D47.1)

    D61.810 Antineoplastic chemotherapy induced pancytopenia 🕭
        Excludes2   aplastic anemia due to antineoplastic chemotherapy (D61.1)

    D61.811 Other drug-induced pancytopenia 🕭
        Excludes2   aplastic anemia due to drugs (D61.1)

    D61.818 Other pancytopenia 🕭

    D61.82 Myelophthisis 🕭
        Leukoerythroblastic anemia
        Myelophthisic anemia
        Panmyelophthisis
        Code also the underlying disorder, such as: malignant neoplasm of breast (C50.-) tuberculosis (A15.-)
        Excludes1   idiopathic myelofibrosis (D47.1)
            myelofibrosis NOS (D75.81)
            myelofibrosis with myeloid metaplasia (D47.4)
            primary myelofibrosis (D47.1)
            secondary myelofibrosis (D75.81)

    D61.89 Other specified aplastic anemias and other bone marrow failure syndromes 🕭

N Newborn Age: 0   **P** Pediatric Age: 0–17   **M** Maternity DX: 12–55   **A** Adult Age: 15–124   ♀ Females Only   ♂ Males Only

 Complication\Comorbidity   Major C\C   Present on Admission Requirement   🕭 Hospital-Acquired Condition

873

CHAPTER 3 (D50-D89)

CHAPTER 3 (D50-D89)

■ **D61.9 Aplastic anemia, unspecified** 🦴
   Hypoplastic anemia NOS
   Medullary hypoplasia

D62 Acute posthemorrhagic anemia 🦴
   | **Excludes1** | anemia due to chronic blood loss (D50.0)
   blood loss anemia NOS (D50.0)
   congenital anemia from fetal blood loss (P61.3) |

● **D63 Anemia in chronic diseases classified elsewhere**
   ● *D63.0 Anemia in neoplastic disease*
      Code first neoplasm (C00-D49)
      | **Excludes1** | anemia due to antineoplastic chemotherapy (D64.81)
      aplastic anemia due to antineoplastic chemotherapy (D61.1) |

      OGCR Section I.C.2.e.2.

      2) Anemia associated with chemotherapy, immunotherapy and radiation therapy

      When the admission/encounter is for management of an anemia associated with an adverse effect of the administration of chemotherapy or immunotherapy and the only treatment is for the anemia, the anemia code is sequenced first followed by the appropriate codes for the neoplasm and the adverse effect (T45.1X5, Adverse effect of antineoplastic and immunosuppressive drugs).

   ● *D63.1 Anemia in chronic kidney disease*
      Erythropoietin resistant anemia (EPO resistant anemia)
      Code first underlying chronic kidney disease (CKD) (N18.-)

   ● *D63.8 Anemia in other chronic diseases classified elsewhere*
      Code first underlying disease, such as:
         diphyllobothriasis (B70.0)
         hookworm disease (B76.0-B76.9)
         hypothyroidism (E00.0-E03.9)
         malaria (B50.0-B54)
         symptomatic late syphilis (A52.79)
         tuberculosis (A18.89)

● **D64 Other anemias**
   | **Excludes1** | refractory anemia (D46.-)
   refractory anemia with excess blasts in transformation [RAEB T] (C92.0-) |

   D64.0 Hereditary sideroblastic anemia
      Abnormal production RBCs (erythrocytes)
      Sex-linked hypochromic sideroblastic anemia

   ● **D64.1 Secondary sideroblastic anemia due to disease**
      Code first underlying disease

   ● **D64.2 Secondary sideroblastic anemia due to drugs and toxins**
      Code first poisoning due to drug or toxin, if applicable (T36-T65 with fifth or sixth character 1-4 or 6)
      Use additional code for adverse effect, if applicable, to identify drug (T36-T50 with fifth or sixth character 5)

   D64.3 Other sideroblastic anemias
      Sideroblastic anemia NOS
      Pyridoxine-responsive sideroblastic anemia NEC

   D64.4 Congenital dyserythropoietic anemia
      Any of several rare hereditary anemias, mostly types of macrocytic anemia
      Dyshematopoietic anemia (congenital)
      | **Excludes1** | Blackfan-Diamond syndrome (D61.01)
      Di Guglielmo's disease (C94.0) |

● **D64.8 Other specified anemias**
   D64.81 Anemia due to antineoplastic chemotherapy
      Antineoplastic chemotherapy induced anemia
      | **Excludes1** | anemia in neoplastic disease (D63.0)
      aplastic anemia due to antineoplastic chemotherapy (D61.1) |

   D64.89 Other specified anemias
      Infantile pseudoleukemia

■ **D64.9 Anemia, unspecified**

COAGULATION DEFECTS, PURPURA AND OTHER HEMORRHAGIC CONDITIONS (D65-D69)

D65 Disseminated intravascular coagulation [defibrination syndrome] 🦴
   Blood clots form and consume all coagulation proteins and platelets and disrupt normal coagulation, resulting in abnormal bleeding
   Afibrinogenemia, acquired
   Consumption coagulopathy
   Diffuse or disseminated intravascular coagulation [DIC]
   Fibrinolytic hemorrhage, acquired
   Fibrinolytic purpura
   Purpura fulminans
   | **Excludes1** | disseminated intravascular coagulation (complicating):
   abortion or ectopic or molar pregnancy (O00-O07, O08.1)
   in newborn (P60)
   pregnancy, childbirth and the puerperium (O45.0, O46.0, O67.0, O72.3) |

D66 Hereditary factor VIII deficiency 🦴
   Inherited coagulation disorder carried by females but most often affecting males
   Classical hemophilia
   Deficiency factor VIII (with functional defect)
   Hemophilia NOS
   Hemophilia A
   | **Excludes1** | factor VIII deficiency with vascular defect (D68.0) |

D67 Hereditary factor IX deficiency 🦴
   Christmas disease
   Factor IX deficiency (with functional defect)
   Hemophilia B
   Plasma thromboplastin component [PTC] deficiency

● **D68 Other coagulation defects**
   | **Excludes1** | abnormal coagulation profile (R79.1)
   coagulation defects complicating:
   abortion or ectopic or molar pregnancy (O00-O07, O08.1)
   pregnancy, childbirth and the puerperium (O45.0, O46.0, O67.0, O72.3) |

   D68.0 Von Willebrand's disease 🦴
      Congenital bleeding disorder
      Angiohemophilia
      Factor VIII deficiency with vascular defect
      Vascular hemophilia
      | **Excludes1** | capillary fragility (hereditary) (D69.8)
      factor VIII deficiency NOS (D66)
      factor VIII deficiency with functional defect (D66) |

   D68.1 Hereditary factor XI deficiency 🦴
      Deficiency of blood coagulation resulting in systemic blood-clotting defect
      Hemophilia C
      Plasma thromboplastin antecedent [PTA] deficiency
      Rosenthal's disease

● Unacceptable Principal Diagnosis   ● Use Additional Character(s)   ■ Unspecified   ▶ Manifestation Code
OGCR Official Guidelines for Coding and Reporting   Excludes 1   Excludes 2   Includes   Use additional   Code first   Code also

D68.2 Hereditary deficiency of other clotting factors 🔹
Blood clotting disorders caused by hereditary deficiencies of one or more clotting factors
AC globulin deficiency
Congenital afibrinogenemia
Deficiency of factor I [fibrinogen]
Deficiency of factor II [prothrombin]
Deficiency of factor V [labile]
Deficiency of factor VII [stable]
Deficiency of factor X [Stuart-Prower]
Deficiency of factor XII [Hageman]
Deficiency of factor XIII [fibrin stabilizing]
Dysfibrinogenemia (congenital)
Hypoproconvertinemia
Owren's disease
Proaccelerin deficiency

● **D68.3 Hemorrhagic disorder due to circulating anticoagulants**
Blood clotting disorders caused by anticoagulants (warfarin and heparin)

● **D68.31 Hemorrhagic disorder due to intrinsic circulating anticoagulants, antibodies, or inhibitors**

  D68.311 Acquired hemophilia 🔹
  Autoimmune hemophilia
  Autoimmune inhibitors to clotting factors
  Secondary hemophilia

  D68.312 Antiphospholipid antibody with hemorrhagic disorder 🔹
  Lupus anticoagulant (LAC) with hemorrhagic disorder
  Systemic lupus erythematosus [SLE] inhibitor with hemorrhagic disorder

Excludes1	antiphospholipid antibody, finding without diagnosis (R76.0)

  antiphospholipid antibody syndrome (D68.61)
  antiphospholipid antibody with hypercoagulable state (D68.61)
  lupus anticoagulant (LAC) finding without diagnosis (R76.0)
  lupus anticoagulant (LAC) with hypercoagulable state (D68.62)
  systemic lupus erythematosus [SLE] inhibitor finding without diagnosis (R76.0)
  systemic lupus erythematosus [SLE] inhibitor with hypercoagulable state (D68.62)

  D68.318 Other hemorrhagic disorder due to intrinsic circulating anticoagulants, antibodies, or inhibitors 🔹
  Antithromboplastinemia
  Antithromboplastinogenemia
  Hemorrhagic disorder due to intrinsic increase in antithrombin
  Hemorrhagic disorder due to intrinsic increase in anti-VIIIa
  Hemorrhagic disorder due to intrinsic increase in anti-IXa
  Hemorrhagic disorder due to intrinsic increase in anti-XIa

● **D68.32 Hemorrhagic disorder due to extrinsic circulating anticoagulants 🔹**
  Drug-induced hemorrhagic disorder
  Hemorrhagic disorder due to increase in anti-IIa
  Hemorrhagic disorder due to increase in anti-Xa
  Hyperheparinemia

  Use additional code for adverse effect, if applicable, to identify drug (T45.515, T45.525)

D68.4 Acquired coagulation factor deficiency 🔹
Deficiency of coagulation factor due to liver disease
Deficiency of coagulation factor due to vitamin K deficiency

Excludes1	vitamin K deficiency of newborn (P53)

● **D68.5 Primary thrombophilia**
AKA idiopathic thrombocytopenia, may be acquired or congenital and is a common cause of coagulation disorders.
Primary hypercoagulable states

Excludes1	antiphospholipid syndrome (D68.61)

  lupus anticoagulant (D68.62)
  secondary activated protein C resistance (D68.69)
  secondary antiphospholipid antibody syndrome (D68.69)
  secondary lupus anticoagulant with hypercoagulable state (D68.69)
  secondary systemic lupus erythematosus [SLE] inhibitor with hypercoagulable state (D68.69)
  systemic lupus erythematosus [SLE] inhibitor finding without diagnosis (R76.0)
  systemic lupus erythematosus [SLE] inhibitor with hemorrhagic disorder (D68.312)
  thrombotic thrombocytopenic purpura (M31.1)

  D68.51 Activated protein C resistance 🔹
  Factor V Leiden mutation

  D68.52 Prothrombin gene mutation 🔹

  D68.59 Other primary thrombophilia 🔹
  Antithrombin III deficiency
  Hypercoagulable state NOS
  Primary hypercoagulable state NEC
  Primary thrombophilia NEC
  Protein C deficiency
  Protein S deficiency
  Thrombophilia NOS

CHAPTER 3 (D50-D89)

● **D68.6 Other thrombophilia**
Other hypercoagulable states
> **Excludes1** diffuse or disseminated intravascular coagulation [DIC] (D65)
> heparin induced thrombocytopenia (HIT) (D75.82)
> hyperhomocysteinemia (E72.11)

  D68.61 Antiphospholipid syndrome 🔧
Anticardiolipin syndrome
Antiphospholipid antibody syndrome
> **Excludes1** anti-phospholipid antibody, finding without diagnosis (R76.0)
> anti-phospholipid antibody with hemorrhagic disorder (D68.312)
> lupus anticoagulant syndrome (D68.62)

  D68.62 Lupus anticoagulant syndrome 🔧
Lupus anticoagulant
Presence of systemic lupus erythematosus [SLE] inhibitor
> **Excludes1** anticardiolipin syndrome (D68.61)
> antiphospholipid syndrome (D68.61)
> lupus anticoagulant (LAC) finding without diagnosis (R79.0)
> lupus anticoagulant (LAC) with hemorrhagic disorder (D68.312)

  D68.69 Other thrombophilia 🔧
Hypercoagulable states NEC
Secondary hypercoagulable state NOS

 D68.8 Other specified coagulation defects 🔧
> **Excludes1** hemorrhagic disease of newborn (P53)

■ **D68.9 Coagulation defect, unspecified** 🔧

● **D69 Purpura and other hemorrhagic conditions**
Group of conditions characterized by small hemorrhages in skin, mucous membranes, or serosal surfaces
> **Excludes1** benign hypergammaglobulinemic purpura (D89.0)
> cryoglobulinemic purpura (D89.1)
> essential (hemorrhagic) thrombocythemia (D47.3)
> hemorrhagic thrombocythemia (D47.3)
> purpura fulminans (D65)
> thrombotic thrombocytopenic purpura (M31.1)
> Waldenström hypergammaglobulinemic purpura (D89.0)

 D69.0 Allergic purpura 🔧
Allergic vasculitis
Nonthrombocytopenic hemorrhagic purpura
Nonthrombocytopenic idiopathic purpura
Purpura anaphylactoid
Purpura Henoch(-Schönlein)
Purpura rheumatica
Vascular purpura
> **Excludes1** thrombocytopenic hemorrhagic purpura (D69.3)

 D69.1 Qualitative platelet defects
Bernard-Soulier [giant platelet] syndrome
Glanzmann's disease
Grey platelet syndrome
Thromboasthenia (hemorrhagic) (hereditary)
Thrombocytopathy
> **Excludes1** von Willebrand's disease (D68.0)

 D69.2 Other nonthrombocytopenic purpura
Purpura NOS
Purpura simplex
Senile purpura

 D69.3 Immune thrombocytopenic purpura 🔧
Hemorrhagic (thrombocytopenic) purpura
Idiopathic thrombocytopenic purpura
Tidal platelet dysgenesis

● **D69.4 Other primary thrombocytopenia**
> **Excludes1** transient neonatal thrombocytopenia (P61.0)
> Wiskott-Aldrich syndrome (D82.0)

  D69.41 Evans syndrome 🔧
Acquired hemolytic anemia and thrombocytopenia

  ● **D69.42 Congenital and hereditary thrombocytopenia purpura** 🔧
Congenital thrombocytopenia
Hereditary thrombocytopenia
Code first congenital or hereditary disorder, such as:
thrombocytopenia with absent radius (TAR syndrome) (Q87.2)

  D69.49 Other primary thrombocytopenia
Megakaryocytic hypoplasia
Primary thrombocytopenia NOS

● **D69.5 Secondary thrombocytopenia**
Acquired reduction of number of platelets required for blood clotting
> **Excludes1** heparin induced thrombocytopenia (HIT) (D75.82)
> transient thrombocytopenia of newborn (P61.0)

  D69.51 Posttransfusion purpura
Posttransfusion purpura from whole blood (fresh) or blood products PTP

  D69.59 Other secondary thrombocytopenia

■ **D69.6 Thrombocytopenia, unspecified**

 D69.8 Other specified hemorrhagic conditions
Capillary fragility (hereditary)
Vascular pseudohemophilia

■ **D69.9 Hemorrhagic condition, unspecified**

OTHER DISORDERS OF BLOOD AND BLOOD-FORMING ORGANS (D70-D77)

● **D70 Neutropenia**
Decrease in number of neutrophils (type of white blood cell)
> **Includes** agranulocytosis
> decreased absolute neurophile count (ANC)

> **Use additional** code for any associated:
> fever (R50.81)
> mucositis (J34.81, K12.3-, K92.81, N76.81)
> **Excludes1** neutropenic splenomegaly (D73.81)
> transient neonatal neutropenia (P61.5)

 D70.0 Congenital agranulocytosis
Reduced numbers of neutrophils (type of white blood cell)
Congenital neutropenia
Infantile genetic agranulocytosis
Kostmann's disease

● Unacceptable Principal Diagnosis   ● Use Additional Character(s)   ■ Unspecified   ▶ Manifestation Code
OGCR Official Guidelines for Coding and Reporting   Excludes 1   Excludes 2   Includes   Use additional   Code first   Code also

● **D70.1 Agranulocytosis secondary to cancer chemotherapy**
Decreased numbers of granulocytes (type of white blood cell)

Code also *underlying neoplasm*

Use additional code for adverse effect, if applicable, to identify drug (T45.1X5)

● **D70.2 Other drug-induced agranulocytosis**

Use additional code for adverse effect, if applicable, to identify drug (T36-T50 with fifth or sixth character 5)

D70.3 Neutropenia due to infection

D70.4 Cyclic neutropenia
Chronic neutropenia (low number of type of white blood cell)
Cyclic hematopoiesis
Periodic neutropenia

D70.8 Other neutropenia

■ **D70.9 Neutropenia, unspecified**

D71 Functional disorders of polymorphonuclear neutrophils
Polymorphonuclear: varying shapes of nucleus; AKA PMNs
Cell membrane receptor complex [CR3] defect
Chronic (childhood) granulomatous disease
Congenital dysphagocytosis
Progressive septic granulomatosis

● **D72 Other disorders of white blood cells**

Excludes1   basophilia (D72.824)
immunity disorders (D80-D89)
neutropenia (D70)
preleukemia (syndrome) (D46.9)

D72.0 Genetic anomalies of leukocytes
Alder (granulation) (granulocyte) anomaly
Alder syndrome
Hereditary leukocytic hypersegmentation
Hereditary leukocytic hyposegmentation
Hereditary leukomelanopathy
May-Hegglin (granulation) (granulocyte) anomaly
May-Hegglin syndrome
Pelger-Huët (granulation) (granulocyte) anomaly
Pelger-Huët syndrome

Excludes1   Chédiak (-Steinbrinck)-Higashi syndrome (E70.330)

D72.1 Eosinophilia
Formation and accumulation of high number of white cells in blood/tissue
Allergic eosinophilia
Hereditary eosinophilia

Excludes1   Löffler's syndrome (J82)
pulmonary eosinophilia (J82)

● **D72.8 Other specified disorders of white blood cells**

Excludes1   leukemia (C91-C95)

● **D72.81 Decreased white blood cell count**

Excludes1   neutropenia (D70.-)

D72.810 Lymphocytopenia
Decreased lymphocytes
Reduction in number of lympho cytes in blood

D72.818 Other decreased white blood cell count
Basophilic leukopenia
Eosinophilic leukopenia
Monocytopenia
Other decreased leukocytes
Plasmacytopenia

■ **D72.819 Decreased white blood cell count, unspecified**
Decreased leukocytes, unspecified
Leukocytopenia, unspecified
Leukopenia

Excludes1   malignant leukopenia (D70.9)

● **D72.82 Elevated white blood cell count**

Excludes1   eosinophilia (D72.1)

D72.820 Lymphocytosis (symptomatic)
Elevated lymphocytes
Excess of normal lymphocytes

D72.821 Monocytosis (symptomatic)

Excludes1   infectious mononucleosis (B27.-)

D72.822 Plasmacytosis
Presence of excess plasma cells

D72.823 Leukemoid reaction
Basophilic leukemoid reaction
Leukemoid reaction NOS
Lymphocytic leukemoid reaction
Monocytic leukemoid reaction
Myelocytic leukemoid reaction
Neutrophilic leukemoid reaction

D72.824 Basophilia
Increase of basophils in blood

D72.825 Bandemia
Bandemia without diagnosis of specific infection
Excess number of band cells (immature white blood cells) released by bone marrow

Excludes1   confirmed infection -code to infection leukemia (C91.-, C92.-, C93.-, C94.-, C95.-)

D72.828 Other elevated white blood cell count

■ **D72.829 Elevated white blood cell count, unspecified**
Elevated leukocytes, unspecified
Leukocytosis, unspecified

D72.89 Other specified disorders of white blood cells
Abnormality of white blood cells NEC

■ **D72.9 Disorder of white blood cells, unspecified**
Abnormal leukocyte differential NOS

● **D73 Diseases of spleen**

D73.0 Hyposplenism
Diminished functioning of spleen
Atrophy of spleen

Excludes1   asplenia (congenital) (Q89.01)
postsurgical absence of spleen (Z90.81)

CHAPTER 3 (D50-D89)

D73.1 Hypersplenism
Accelerated function of spleen

> **Excludes1**   neutropenic splenomegaly (D73.81)
> primary splenic neutropenia (D73.81)
> splenitis, splenomegaly in late
>   syphilis (A52.79)
> splenitis, splenomegaly in
>   tuberculosis (A18.85)
> splenomegaly NOS (R16.1)
> splenomegaly congenital (Q89.0)

D73.2 Chronic congestive splenomegaly
Enlargement of spleen

D73.3 Abscess of spleen

D73.4 Cyst of spleen

D73.5 Infarction of spleen
Splenic rupture, nontraumatic
Torsion of spleen

> **Excludes1**   rupture of spleen due to Plasmodium
> vivax malaria (B51.0)
> traumatic rupture of spleen (S36.03-)

● **D73.8 Other diseases of spleen**

D73.81 Neutropenic splenomegaly
Werner-Schultz disease
*Enlarged spleen responding to inadequate
number of neutrophils*

D73.89 Other diseases of spleen
Fibrosis of spleen NOS
Perisplenitis
Splenitis NOS

■ **D73.9 Disease of spleen, unspecified**

● **D74 Methemoglobinemia**
Excessive methemoglobin (form of hemoglobin)

D74.0 Congenital methemoglobinemia 🜛
Congenital NADH-methemoglobin reductase
deficiency
Hemoglobin-M [Hb-M] disease
Methemoglobinemia, hereditary

D74.8 Other methemoglobinemias 🜛
Acquired methemoglobinemia (with
sulfhemoglobinemia)
Toxic methemoglobinemia

■ **D74.9 Methemoglobinemia, unspecified** 🜛

● **D75 Other and unspecified diseases of blood and blood-
forming organs**

> **Excludes2**   acute lymphadenitis (L04.-)
> chronic lymphadenitis (I88.1)
> enlarged lymph nodes (R59.-)
> hypergammaglobulinemia NOS (D89.2)
> lymphadenitis NOS (I88.9)
> mesenteric lymphadenitis (acute) (chronic)
>   (I88.0)

D75.0 Familial erythrocytosis
*Genetic mutation of gene that results in increased
circulating RBCs*
Benign polycythemia
Familial polycythemia

> **Excludes1**   hereditary ovalocytosis (D58.1)

D75.1 Secondary polycythemia
Increase in total red cell mass
Acquired polycythemia
Emotional polycythemia
Erythrocytosis NOS
Hypoxemic polycythemia
Nephrogenous polycythemia
Polycythemia due to erythropoietin
Polycythemia due to fall in plasma volume
Polycythemia due to high altitude
Polycythemia due to stress
Polycythemia NOS
Relative polycythemia

> **Excludes1**   polycythemia neonatorum (P61.1)
> polycythemia vera (D45)

● **D75.8 Other specified diseases of blood and blood-
forming organs**

D75.81 Myelofibrosis 🜛
Replacing bone marrow by fibrous tissue
Myelofibrosis NOS
Secondary myelofibrosis NOS

Code first the underlying disorder, such as:
malignant neoplasm of breast (C50.-)

Use additional code, if applicable,
for associated therapy-related
myelodysplastic syndrome (D46.-)

Use additional code for adverse effect,
if applicable, to identify drug
(T45.1X5)

> **Excludes1**   acute myelofibrosis (C94.4-)
> idiopathic myelofibrosis
>   (D47.1)
> leukoerythroblastic anemia
>   (D61.82)
> myelofibrosis with myeloid
>   metaplasia (D47.4)
> myelophthisic anemia
>   (D61.82)
> myelophthisis (D61.82)
> primary myelofibrosis
>   (D47.1)

D75.82 Heparin induced thrombocytopenia (HIT)

**D75.89 Other specified diseases of blood and
blood-forming organs**

■ **D75.9 Disease of blood and blood-forming organs,
unspecified**

● **D76 Other specified diseases with participation of
lymphoreticular and reticulohistiocytic tissue**

> **Excludes1**   (Abt-) Letterer-Siwe disease (C96.0)
> eosinophilic granuloma (C96.6)
> Hand-Schüller-Christian disease (C96.5)
> histiocytic sarcoma (C96.A)
> histiocytosis X, multifocal (C96.5)
> histiocytosis X, unifocal (C96.6)
> malignant histiocytosis (C96.A)
> Langerhans-cell histiocytosis, multifocal
>   (C96.5)
> Langerhans-cell histiocytosis NOS (C96.6)
> Langerhans-cell histiocytosis, unifocal
>   (C96.6)

> **Excludes1**   leukemic reticuloendotheliosis or reticulosis
>   (C91.4-)
> lipomelanotic reticuloendotheliosis or
>   reticulosis (I89.8)

CHAPTER 3 (D50-D89)

● Unacceptable Principal Diagnosis   ● Use Additional Character(s)   ■ Unspecified   ▶ Manifestation Code
OGCR Official Guidelines for Coding and Reporting | Excludes 1 | | Excludes 2 | | Includes | | Use additional | | Code first | | Code also |

D76.1 Hemophagocytic lymphohistiocytosis 🗲
    Familial hemophagocytic reticulosis
    Histiocytoses of mononuclear phagocytes

D76.2 Hemophagocytic syndrome, infection-associated 🗲
    Use additional code to identify infectious agent or disease.

D76.3 Other histiocytosis syndromes 🗲
    Reticulohistiocytoma (giant-cell)
    Sinus histiocytosis with massive lymphadenopathy
    Xanthogranuloma

D77 Other disorders of blood and blood-forming organs in diseases classified elsewhere
    Code first underlying disease, such as:
    amyloidosis (E85-)
    congenital early syphilis (A50.0)
    echinococcosis (B67.0-B67.9)
    malaria (B50.0-B54)
    schistosomiasis [bilharziasis] (B65.0-B65.9)
    vitamin C deficiency (E54)
    Excludes1 rupture of spleen due to Plasmodium vivax malaria (B51.0)
    splenitis, splenomegaly in:
    late syphilis (A52.79)
    tuberculosis (A18.85)

INTRAOPERATIVE AND POSTPROCEDURAL COMPLICATIONS OF THE SPLEEN (D78)

D78 Intraoperative and postprocedural complications of the spleen

D78.0 Intraoperative hemorrhage and hematoma of the spleen complicating a procedure
    Excludes1 intraoperative hemorrhage and hematoma of the spleen due to accidental puncture or laceration during a procedure (D78.1-)

D78.01 Intraoperative hemorrhage and hematoma of the spleen complicating a procedure on the spleen 🗲

D78.02 Intraoperative hemorrhage and hematoma of the spleen complicating other procedure 🗲

D78.1 Accidental puncture and laceration of the spleen during a procedure

D78.11 Accidental puncture and laceration of the spleen during a procedure on the spleen 🗲

D78.12 Accidental puncture and laceration of the spleen during other procedure 🗲

D78.2 Postprocedural hemorrhage and hematoma of the spleen following a procedure

D78.21 Postprocedural hemorrhage and hematoma of the spleen following a procedure on the spleen 🗲

D78.22 Postprocedural hemorrhage and hematoma of the spleen following other procedure 🗲

D78.8 Other intraoperative and postprocedural complications of the spleen
    Use additional code, if applicable, to further specify disorder

D78.81 Other intraoperative complications of the spleen 🗲

D78.89 Other postprocedural complications of the spleen 🗲

CERTAIN DISORDERS INVOLVING THE IMMUNE MECHANISM (D80-D89)

Includes defects in the complement system
immunodeficiency disorders, except human immunodeficiency virus [HIV] disease
sarcoidosis

Excludes1 autoimmune disease (systemic) NOS (M35.9)
functional disorders of polymorphonuclear neutrophils (D71)
human immunodeficiency virus [HIV] disease (B20)

D80 Immunodeficiency with predominantly antibody defects

D80.0 Hereditary hypogammaglobulinemia 🗲
    Autosomal recessive agammaglobulinemia (Swiss type)
    X-linked agammaglobulinemia [Bruton] (with growth hormone deficiency)

D80.1 Nonfamilial hypogammaglobulinemia 🗲
    Abnormally low levels of all classes of immunoglobulins
    Agammaglobulinemia with immunoglobulin-bearing B-lymphocytes
    Common variable agammaglobulinemia [CVAgamma]
    Hypogammaglobulinemia NOS

D80.2 Selective deficiency of immunoglobulin A [IgA] 🗲

D80.3 Selective deficiency of immunoglobulin G [IgG] subclasses 🗲

D80.4 Selective deficiency of immunoglobulin M [IgM] 🗲

D80.5 Immunodeficiency with increased immunoglobulin M [IgM] 🗲

D80.6 Antibody deficiency with near-normal immunoglobulins or with hyperimmunoglobulinemia 🗲
    Abnormally high levels of immunoglobulins in serum

D80.7 Transient hypogammaglobulinemia of infancy 🗲 **N**

D80.8 Other immunodeficiencies with predominantly antibody defects 🗲
    Kappa light chain deficiency

D80.9 Immunodeficiency with predominantly antibody defects, unspecified 🗲

D81 Combined immunodeficiencies
    Excludes1 autosomal recessive agammaglobulinemia (Swiss type) (D80.0)

D81.0 Severe combined immunodeficiency [SCID] with reticular dysgenesis 🗲

D81.1 Severe combined immunodeficiency [SCID] with low T- and B-cell numbers 🗲

D81.2 Severe combined immunodeficiency [SCID] with low or normal B-cell numbers 🗲

D81.3 Adenosine deaminase [ADA] deficiency 🗲

D81.4 Nezelof's syndrome 🗲

D81.5 Purine nucleoside phosphorylase [PNP] deficiency 🗲

D81.6 Major histocompatibility complex class I deficiency 🗲
    Bare lymphocyte syndrome

D81.7 Major histocompatibility complex class II deficiency 🗲

CHAPTER 3 (D50-D89)

N Newborn Age: 0   P Pediatric Age: 0–17   M Maternity DX: 12–55   A Adult Age: 15–124   ♀ Females Only   ♂ Males Only
🗲 Complication\Comorbidity   Major C\C   Present on Admission Requirement   Hospital-Acquired Condition

879

CHAPTER 3 (D50-D89)

● **D81.8 Other combined immunodeficiencies**

　● **D81.81 Biotin-dependent carboxylase deficiency**
　　　Multiple carboxylase deficiency

　　　　| Excludes1 | biotin-dependent carboxylase deficiency due to dietary deficiency of biotin (E53.8) |

　　　D81.810 Biotinidase deficiency

　　　D81.818 Other biotin-dependent carboxylase deficiency
　　　　　Holocarboxylase synthetase deficiency
　　　　　Other multiple carboxylase deficiency

　　■ **D81.819 Biotin-dependent carboxylase deficiency, unspecified**
　　　　　Multiple carboxylase deficiency, unspecified

　　D81.89 Other combined immunodeficiencies 🕭

■ **D81.9 Combined immunodeficiency, unspecified** 🕭
　　Severe combined immunodeficiency disorder [SCID] NOS

● **D82 Immunodeficiency associated with other major defects**

　| Excludes1 | ataxia telangiectasia [Louis-Bar] (G11.3) |

　D82.0 Wiskott-Aldrich syndrome 🕭
　　X-linked immunodeficiency
　　Immunodeficiency with thrombocytopenia and eczema

　D82.1 Di George's syndrome 🕭
　　Congenital disorder with defective development of third and fourth pharyngeal pouches
　　Pharyngeal pouch syndrome
　　Thymic alymphoplasia
　　Thymic aplasia or hypoplasia with immunodeficiency

　D82.2 Immunodeficiency with short-limbed stature

　D82.3 Immunodeficiency following hereditary defective response to Epstein-Barr virus
　　X-linked lymphoproliferative disease

　D82.4 Hyperimmunoglobulin E [IgE] syndrome
　　Suspected genetic defect that produces high levels of antibody immunoglobulin (IgE) that causes skin and lung infections and eczema

　D82.8 Immunodeficiency associated with other specified major defects

■ **D82.9 Immunodeficiency associated with major defect, unspecified**

● **D83 Common variable immunodeficiency**

　D83.0 Common variable immunodeficiency with predominant abnormalities of B-cell numbers and function 🕭

　D83.1 Common variable immunodeficiency with predominant immunoregulatory T-cell disorders 🕭

　D83.2 Common variable immunodeficiency with autoantibodies to B- or T-cells 🕭

　D83.8 Other common variable immunodeficiencies 🕭

■ **D83.9 Common variable immunodeficiency, unspecified** 🕭

● **D84 Other immunodeficiencies**

　D84.0 Lymphocyte function antigen-1 [LFA-1] defect

　D84.1 Defects in the complement system
　　C1 esterase inhibitor [C1-INH] deficiency

　D84.8 Other specified immunodeficiencies 🕭

■ **D84.9 Immunodeficiency, unspecified** 🕭

● **D86 Sarcoidosis**

　D86.0 Sarcoidosis of lung

　D86.1 Sarcoidosis of lymph nodes

　D86.2 Sarcoidosis of lung with sarcoidosis of lymph nodes

　D86.3 Sarcoidosis of skin

　● **D86.8 Sarcoidosis of other sites**

　　D86.81 Sarcoid meningitis

　　D86.82 Multiple cranial nerve palsies in sarcoidosis

　　D86.83 Sarcoid iridocyclitis
　　　Rare large tumor with irregular surface of iris

　　D86.84 Sarcoid pyelonephritis
　　　Systemic disease of unknown etiology characterized by chronic granulomatous inflammation with tissue destruction of pelvis kidney
　　　Tubulo-interstitial nephropathy in sarcoidosis

　　D86.85 Sarcoid myocarditis

　　D86.86 Sarcoid arthropathy
　　　Polyarthritis in sarcoidosis

　　D86.87 Sarcoid myositis
　　　Granumloma of muscle

　　D86.89 Sarcoidosis of other sites
　　　Hepatic granuloma
　　　Uveoparotid fever [Heerfordt]

■ **D86.9 Sarcoidosis, unspecified**

● **D89 Other disorders involving the immune mechanism, not elsewhere classified**

　| Excludes1 | hyperglobulinemia NOS (R77.1) monoclonal gammopathy (of undetermined significance) (D47.2) |

　| Excludes2 | transplant failure and rejection (T86.-) |

　D89.0 Polyclonal hypergammaglobulinemia
　　Benign hypergammaglobulinemic purpura
　　Polyclonal gammopathy NOS

　D89.1 Cryoglobulinemia
　　Cryoglobulin (proteins) in blood that precipitate temperatures below 98.6° F; usually symptomatic of underlying disease
　　Cryoglobulinemic purpura
　　Cryoglobulinemic vasculitis
　　Essential cryoglobulinemia
　　Idiopathic cryoglobulinemia
　　Mixed cryoglobulinemia
　　Primary cryoglobulinemia
　　Secondary cryoglobulinemia

■ **D89.2 Hypergammaglobulinemia, unspecified**

　D89.3 Immune reconstitution syndrome
　　Immune reconstitution inflammatory syndrome [IRIS]

　　Use additional code for adverse effect, if applicable, to identify drug (T36-T50 with fifth or sixth character 5)

Item 3-1 Sarcoidosis: A symptom of an inflammation producing tiny lumps of cells (granulomas) in various organs, most commonly the lungs and lymph nodes, that affect organ function. Cause is unknown occurring primarily in 20- to 40-year-olds, African-American, especially women, and those of Asian, German, Irish Scandinavian, and Puerto Rican heritage.

● Unacceptable Principal Diagnosis   ● Use Additional Character(s)   ■ Unspecified   ▶ Manifestation Code
OGCR Official Guidelines for Coding and Reporting | Excludes 1 | | Excludes 2 | Includes Use additional Code first Code also

● **D89.8 Other specified disorders involving the immune mechanism, not elsewhere classified**

● **D89.81 Graft-versus-host disease**

Code first underlying cause, such as:
complications of transplanted organs and tissue (T86.-)
complications of blood transfusion (T80.89)

Use additional code to identify associated manifestations, such as:
desquamative dermatitis (L30.8)
diarrhea (R19.7)
elevated bilirubin (R17)
hair loss (L65.9)

● **D89.810 Acute graft-versus-host disease** 🅜

● **D89.811 Chronic graft-versus-host disease** 🅜

● **D89.812 Acute on chronic graft-versus-host disease** 🅜

●▪ **D89.813 Graft-versus-host disease, unspecified** 🅜

D89.82 Autoimmune lymphoproliferative syndrome [ALPS]

D89.89 Other specified disorders involving the immune mechanism, not elsewhere classified

| Excludes1 | human immunodeficiency virus disease (B20) |

▪ **D89.9 Disorder involving the immune mechanism, unspecified**

Immune disease NOS

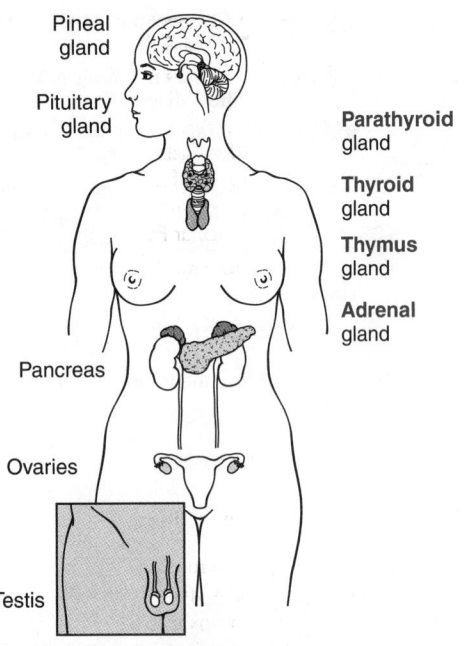

Figure 4-1   The endocrine system. (From Buck CJ: Step-by-Step Medical Coding, 2010 ed. Philadelphia, WB Saunders, 2010.)

CHAPTER 4

ENDOCRINE, NUTRITIONAL AND METABOLIC DISEASES (E00-E89)

All neoplasms, whether functionally active or not, are classified in Chapter 2. Appropriate codes in this chapter (i.e., E05.8, E07.0, E16-E31, E34.-) may be used as additional codes to indicate either functional activity by neoplasms and ectopic endocrine tissue or hyperfunction and hypofunction of endocrine glands associated with neoplasms and other conditions classified elsewhere.

> **Excludes1**   transitory endocrine and metabolic disorders specific to newborn (P70-P74)

This chapter contains the following blocks:

E00-E07	Disorders of thyroid gland
E08-E13	Diabetes mellitus
E15-E16	Other disorders of glucose regulation and pancreatic internal secretion
E20-E35	Disorders of other endocrine glands
E36	Intraoperative complications of endocrine system
E40-E46	Malnutrition
E50-E64	Other nutritional deficiencies
E65-E68	Overweight, obesity and other hyperalimentation
E70-E88	Metabolic disorders
E89	Postprocedural endocrine and metabolic complications and disorders, not elsewhere classified

DISORDERS OF THYROID GLAND (E00-E07)

● **E00**   **Congenital iodine-deficiency syndrome**

> Use additional code (F70-F79) to identify associated intellectual disabilities.
>
> **Excludes1**   subclinical iodine-deficiency hypothyroidism (E02)

E00.0   **Congenital iodine-deficiency syndrome, neurological type**
Endemic cretinism, neurological type

E00.1   **Congenital iodine-deficiency syndrome, myxedematous type**
Dry, waxy type of swelling (nonpitting edema) with abnormal deposits of mucin in skin (mucinosis) and other tissues
Endemic hypothyroid cretinism
Endemic cretinism, myxedematous type

E00.2   **Congenital iodine-deficiency syndrome, mixed type**
Endemic cretinism, mixed type

◧ **E00.9**   **Congenital iodine-deficiency syndrome, unspecified**
Congenital iodine-deficiency hypothyroidism NOS
Endemic cretinism NOS

● **E01**   **Iodine-deficiency related thyroid disorders and allied conditions**

> **Excludes1**   congenital iodine-deficiency syndrome (E00.-)
> subclinical iodine-deficiency hypothyroidism (E02)

E01.0   **Iodine-deficiency related diffuse (endemic) goiter**
Thyroid gland is enlarged

E01.1   **Iodine-deficiency related multinodular (endemic) goiter**
Iodine-deficiency related nodular goiter

◧ **E01.2**   **Iodine-deficiency related (endemic) goiter, unspecified**
Endemic goiter NOS

E01.8   **Other iodine-deficiency related thyroid disorders and allied conditions**
Acquired iodine-deficiency hypothyroidism NOS

Figure 4-2   **Goiter** is an enlargement of the thyroid gland.

Item 4–1   **Simple** goiter indicates no nodules are present. The most common type of goiter is a **diffuse colloidal**, also called a **nontoxic** or **endemic** goiter.

Item 4–2   **Hypothyroidism** is a condition in which there are insufficient levels of thyroxine. **Cretinism** is congenital hypothyroidism, which can result in mental and physical retardation.

● Unacceptable Principal Diagnosis   ● Use Additional Character(s)   ▨ Unspecified   ▶ Manifestation Code

OGCR   Official Guidelines for Coding and Reporting   Excludes 1   Excludes 2   Includes   Use additional   Code first   Code also

Figure 4-3 Typical appearance of patients with moderately severe primary hypothyroidism or myxedema. (From Larsen: Williams Textbook of Endocrinology, 10th ed. 2003, Saunders, An Imprint of Elsevier.)

Figure 4-4 Graves' disease. In Graves' disease, exophthalmos often looks more pronounced than it actually is because of the extreme lid retraction that may occur. This patient, for instance, had minimal proptosis of the left eye but marked lid retraction. (Courtesy Dr. HG Scheie. From Yanoff M, Fine BS: Ocular Pathology, ed 5. St. Louis, Mosby, 2002.)

Item 4–3 Thyrotoxicosis is a condition caused by excessive amounts of the thyroid hormone thyroxine production or hyperthyroidism. **Graves' disease is associated with hyperthyroidism** (known as **Basedow's disease** in Europe).

E02 Subclinical iodine-deficiency hypothyroidism

● **E03 Other hypothyroidism**
Excludes1 iodine-deficiency related hypothyroidism (E00-E02)
postprocedural hypothyroidism (E89.0)

E03.0 Congenital hypothyroidism with diffuse goiter
Congenital parenchymatous goiter (nontoxic)
Congenital goiter (nontoxic) NOS
Excludes1 transitory congenital goiter with normal function (P72.0)

E03.1 Congenital hypothyroidism without goiter
Aplasia of thyroid (with myxedema)
Congenital atrophy of thyroid
Congenital hypothyroidism NOS

E03.2 Hypothyroidism due to medicaments and other exogenous substances
Code first poisoning due to drug or toxin, if applicable (T36-T65 with fifth or sixth character 1-4 or 6)
Use additional code for adverse effect, if applicable, to identify drug (T36-T50 with fifth or sixth character 5)

E03.3 Postinfectious hypothyroidism
E03.4 Atrophy of thyroid (acquired)
Excludes1 congenital atrophy of thyroid (E03.1)

E03.5 Myxedema coma 🔖
Often fatal complication of long-term hypothyroidism

E03.8 Other specified hypothyroidism
■ **E03.9 Hypothyroidism, unspecified**
Myxedema NOS

● **E04 Other nontoxic goiter**
Excludes1 congenital goiter (NOS) (diffuse) (parenchymatous) (E03.0)
iodine-deficiency related goiter (E00-E02)

E04.0 Nontoxic diffuse goiter
Thyroid gland is enlarged
Diffuse (colloid) nontoxic goiter
Simple nontoxic goiter

E04.1 Nontoxic single thyroid nodule
Colloid nodule (cystic) (thyroid)
Nontoxic uninodular goiter
Thyroid (cystic) nodule NOS

E04.2 Nontoxic multinodular goiter
Enlarged thyroid gland with multiple nodules
Cystic goiter NOS
Multinodular (cystic) goiter NOS

E04.8 Other specified nontoxic goiter
■ **E04.9 Nontoxic goiter, unspecified**
Goiter NOS
Nodular goiter (nontoxic) NOS

● **E05 Thyrotoxicosis [hyperthyroidism]**
Enlarged thyroid gland with multiple nodules
Excludes1 chronic thyroiditis with transient thyrotoxicosis (E06.2)
neonatal thyrotoxicosis (P72.1)

● **E05.0 Thyrotoxicosis with diffuse goiter**
Exophthalmic or toxic goiter NOS
Graves' disease
Toxic diffuse goiter
E05.00 Thyrotoxicosis with diffuse goiter without thyrotoxic crisis or storm
E05.01 Thyrotoxicosis with diffuse goiter with thyrotoxic crisis or storm 🔖

● **E05.1 Thyrotoxicosis with toxic single thyroid nodule**
Thyrotoxicosis with toxic uninodular goiter
E05.10 Thyrotoxicosis with toxic single thyroid nodule without thyrotoxic crisis or storm
E05.11 Thyrotoxicosis with toxic single thyroid nodule with thyrotoxic crisis or storm 🔖

● **E05.2 Thyrotoxicosis with toxic multinodular goiter**
Toxic nodular goiter NOS
E05.20 Thyrotoxicosis with toxic multinodular goiter without thyrotoxic crisis or storm
E05.21 Thyrotoxicosis with toxic multinodular goiter with thyrotoxic crisis or storm 🔖

● **E05.3 Thyrotoxicosis from ectopic thyroid tissue**
E05.30 Thyrotoxicosis from ectopic thyroid tissue without thyrotoxic crisis or storm
E05.31 Thyrotoxicosis from ectopic thyroid tissue with thyrotoxic crisis or storm 🔖

● **E05.4 Thyrotoxicosis factitia**
E05.40 Thyrotoxicosis factitia without thyrotoxic crisis or storm
E05.41 Thyrotoxicosis factitia with thyrotoxic crisis or storm 🔖

● **E05.8 Other thyrotoxicosis**
Overproduction of thyroid-stimulating hormone
E05.80 Other thyrotoxicosis without thyrotoxic crisis or storm
E05.81 Other thyrotoxicosis with thyrotoxic crisis or storm 🔖

● **E05.9 Thyrotoxicosis, unspecified**
Hyperthyroidism NOS
■ **E05.90 Thyrotoxicosis, unspecified without thyrotoxic crisis or storm**
■ **E05.91 Thyrotoxicosis, unspecified with thyrotoxic crisis or storm** 🔖

N Newborn Age: 0   **P** Pediatric Age: 0–17   **M** Maternity DX: 12–55   **A** Adult Age: 15–124   ♀ Females Only   ♂ Males Only
🔖 Complication\Comorbidity   🔖 Major C\C   Present on Admission Requirement   Hospital-Acquired Condition
883

CHAPTER 4 (E00-E90)

● **E06   Thyroiditis**
An inflammation of the thyroid gland which results in an inability to convert iodine into thyroid hormone

Excludes1   postpartum thyroiditis (O90.5)

E06.0   Acute thyroiditis 🔗
Abscess of thyroid
Pyogenic thyroiditis
Suppurative thyroiditis

Use additional code (B95-B97) to identify infectious agent.

E06.1   Subacute thyroiditis
Inflammation of thyroid gland following viral upper respiratory infection
de Quervain thyroiditis
Giant-cell thyroiditis
Granulomatous thyroiditis
Nonsuppurative thyroiditis
Viral thyroiditis

Excludes1   autoimmune thyroiditis (E06.3)

E06.2   Chronic thyroiditis with transient thyrotoxicosis
Chronic inflammation of thyroid gland with intermittent overproduction of thyroid hormone

Excludes1   autoimmune thyroiditis (E06.3)

E06.3   Autoimmune thyroiditis
Hashimoto's thyroiditis
Hashitoxicosis (transient)
Lymphadenoid goiter
Lymphocytic thyroiditis
Struma lymphomatosa

● **E06.4   Drug-induced thyroiditis**
Use additional code for adverse effect, if applicable, to identify drug (T36-T50 with fifth or sixth character 5)

E06.5   Other chronic thyroiditis
Chronic fibrous thyroiditis
Chronic thyroiditis NOS
Ligneous thyroiditis
Riedel thyroiditis

■ **E06.9   Thyroiditis, unspecified**

● **E07   Other disorders of thyroid**

E07.0   Hypersecretion of calcitonin
C-cell hyperplasia of thyroid
Hypersecretion of thyrocalcitonin

E07.1   Dyshormogenetic goiter
Group of several types of goiter resulting from enzyme defects in hormone synthesis
Familial dyshormogenetic goiter
Pendred's syndrome

Excludes1   transitory congenital goiter with normal function (P72.0)

● **E07.8   Other specified disorders of thyroid**

E07.81   Sick-euthyroid syndrome
Euthyroid sick-syndrome

E07.89   Other specified disorders of thyroid
Abnormality of thyroid-binding globulin
Hemorrhage of thyroid
Infarction of thyroid

■ **E07.9   Disorder of thyroid, unspecified**

OGCR Section I.C.4.a

4.1 Diabetes mellitus
The diabetes mellitus codes are combination codes that include the type of diabetes mellitus, body system affected, and the complications affecting that body system. As many codes within a particular category as are necessary to describe all of the complications of the disease may be used. They should be sequenced based on the reason for a particular visit. Assign as many codes from categories E08–E13 as needed to identify all of the associated conditions that the patient has.

A metabolic disease that results in persistent hyperglycemia.

● **E08   Diabetes mellitus due to underlying condition**
Code first the underlying condition, such as:
congenital rubella (P35.0)
Cushing's syndrome (E24.-)
cystic fibrosis (E84.-)
malignant neoplasm (C00-C96)
malnutrition (E40-E46)
pancreatitis and other diseases of the pancreas (K85-K86.-)

Use additional code to identify any insulin use (Z79.4)

Excludes1   drug or chemical induced diabetes mellitus (E09.-)
gestational diabetes (O24.4-)
neonatal diabetes mellitus (P70.2)
postpancreatectomy diabetes mellitus (E13.-)
postprocedural diabetes mellitus (E13.-)
secondary diabetes mellitus NEC (E13.-)
type 1 diabetes mellitus (E10.-)
type 2 diabetes mellitus (E11.-)

● **E08.0   Diabetes mellitus due to underlying condition with hyperosmolarity**

● **E08.00   Diabetes mellitus due to underlying condition with hyperosmolarity without nonketotic hyperglycemic-hyperosmolar coma (NKHHC)** 🔗🔗

● **E08.01   Diabetes mellitus due to underlying condition with hyperosmolarity with coma** 🔗🔗

● **E08.1   Diabetes mellitus due to underlying condition with ketoacidosis**

● **E08.10   Diabetes mellitus due to underlying condition with ketoacidosis without coma** 🔗🔗

● **E08.11   Diabetes mellitus due to underlying condition with ketoacidosis with coma** 🔗

● **E08.2   Diabetes mellitus due to underlying condition with kidney complications**

● **E08.21   Diabetes mellitus due to underlying condition with diabetic nephropathy**
Diabetes mellitus due to underlying condition with intercapillary glomerulosclerosis
Diabetes mellitus due to underlying condition with intracapillary glomerulonephrosis
Diabetes mellitus due to underlying condition with Kimmelstiel-Wilson disease

● **E08.22   Diabetes mellitus due to underlying condition with diabetic chronic kidney disease**
Diabetes mellitus due to underlying condition with chronic kidney disease due to conditions classified to .21 and .22

Use additional code to identify stage of chronic kidney disease (N18.1-N18.6)

● **E08.29   Diabetes mellitus due to underlying condition with other diabetic kidney complication**
Renal tubular degeneration in diabetes mellitus due to underlying condition

● Unacceptable Principal Diagnosis   ● Use Additional Character(s)   ■ Unspecified   ▶ Manifestation Code
OGCR Official Guidelines for Coding and Reporting   Excludes 1   Excludes 2   Includes   Use additional   Code first   Code also

● **E08.3 Diabetes mellitus due to underlying condition with ophthalmic complications**

Changes in blood vessels of retina in which blood vessels swell and leak fluid into retinal surface.

● **E08.31 Diabetes mellitus due to underlying condition with unspecified diabetic retinopathy**

● ■ **E08.311 Diabetes mellitus due to underlying condition with unspecified diabetic retinopathy with macular edema**

● ■ **E08.319 Diabetes mellitus due to underlying condition with unspecified diabetic retinopathy without macular edema**

● **E08.32 Diabetes mellitus due to underlying condition with mild nonproliferative diabetic retinopathy**

Diabetes mellitus due to underlying condition with nonproliferative diabetic retinopathy NOS

● **E08.321 Diabetes mellitus due to underlying condition with mild nonproliferative diabetic retinopathy with macular edema**

● **E08.329 Diabetes mellitus due to underlying condition with mild nonproliferative diabetic retinopathy without macular edema**

● **E08.33 Diabetes mellitus due to underlying condition with moderate nonproliferative diabetic retinopathy**

● **E08.331 Diabetes mellitus due to underlying condition with moderate nonproliferative diabetic retinopathy with macular edema**

● **E08.339 Diabetes mellitus due to underlying condition with moderate nonproliferative diabetic retinopathy without macular edema**

● **E08.34 Diabetes mellitus due to underlying condition with severe nonproliferative diabetic retinopathy**

● **E08.341 Diabetes mellitus due to underlying condition with severe nonproliferative diabetic retinopathy with macular edema**

● **E08.349 Diabetes mellitus due to underlying condition with severe nonproliferative diabetic retinopathy without macular edema**

● **E08.35 Diabetes mellitus due to underlying condition with proliferative diabetic retinopathy**

● **E08.351 Diabetes mellitus due to underlying condition with proliferative diabetic retinopathy with macular edema**

● **E08.359 Diabetes mellitus due to underlying condition with proliferative diabetic retinopathy without macular edema**

● **E08.36 Diabetes mellitus due to underlying condition with diabetic cataract**

● **E08.39 Diabetes mellitus due to underlying condition with other diabetic ophthalmic complication**

● **E08.4 Diabetes mellitus due to underlying condition with neurological complications**

● ■ **E08.40 Diabetes mellitus due to underlying condition with diabetic neuropathy, unspecified**

● **E08.41 Diabetes mellitus due to underlying condition with diabetic mononeuropathy**

● **E08.42 Diabetes mellitus due to underlying condition with diabetic polyneuropathy**

Diabetes mellitus due to underlying condition with diabetic neuralgia

● **E08.43 Diabetes mellitus due to underlying condition with diabetic autonomic (poly) neuropathy**

Diabetes mellitus due to underlying condition with diabetic gastroparesis

● **E08.44 Diabetes mellitus due to underlying condition with diabetic amyotrophy**

● **E08.49 Diabetes mellitus due to underlying condition with other diabetic neurological complication**

● **E08.5 Diabetes mellitus due to underlying condition with circulatory complications**

● **E08.51 Diabetes mellitus due to underlying condition with diabetic peripheral angiopathy without gangrene**

● **E08.52 Diabetes mellitus due to underlying condition with diabetic peripheral angiopathy with gangrene** 🔖

Diabetes mellitus due to underlying condition with diabetic gangrene

MCC: Only when the principal diagnosis is designated as a CC

● **E08.59 Diabetes mellitus due to underlying condition with other circulatory complications**

● **E08.6 Diabetes mellitus due to underlying condition with other specified complications**

● **E08.61 Diabetes mellitus due to underlying condition with diabetic arthropathy**

● **E08.610 Diabetes mellitus due to underlying condition with diabetic neuropathic arthropathy**

Diabetes mellitus due to underlying condition with Charcôt's joints

● **E08.618 Diabetes mellitus due to underlying condition with other diabetic arthropathy**

● **E08.62 Diabetes mellitus due to underlying condition with skin complications**

● **E08.620 Diabetes mellitus due to underlying condition with diabetic dermatitis**

Diabetes mellitus due to underlying condition with diabetic necrobiosis lipoidica

● **E08.621 Diabetes mellitus due to underlying condition with foot ulcer**

Use additional code to identify site of ulcer (L97.4-, L97.5-)

 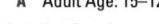
CHAPTER 4 (E00–E90)

CHAPTER 4 (E00-E90)

● **E08.622** **Diabetes mellitus due to underlying condition with other skin ulcer**
  > Use additional code to identify site of ulcer (L97.1-L97.9, L98.41-L98.49)

● **E08.628** **Diabetes mellitus due to underlying condition with other skin complications**

● **E08.63** **Diabetes mellitus due to underlying condition with oral complications**

● **E08.630** **Diabetes mellitus due to underlying condition with periodontal disease**

● **E08.638** **Diabetes mellitus due to underlying condition with other oral complications**

● **E08.64** **Diabetes mellitus due to underlying condition with hypoglycemia**

● **E08.641** **Diabetes mellitus due to underlying condition with hypoglycemia with coma** 🔖

● **E08.649** **Diabetes mellitus due to underlying condition with hypoglycemia without coma**

● **E08.65** **Diabetes mellitus due to underlying condition with hyperglycemia** 🔖

● **E08.69** **Diabetes mellitus due to underlying condition with other specified complication**
  > Use additional code to identify complication

● ■ **E08.8** **Diabetes mellitus due to underlying condition with unspecified complications**

● **E08.9** **Diabetes mellitus due to underlying condition without complications**

● **E09** **Drug or chemical induced diabetes mellitus**
  > Code first poisoning due to drug or toxin, if applicable (T36-T65 with fifth or sixth character 1-4 or 6)
  > Use additional code for adverse effect, if applicable, to identify drug (T36-T50 with fifth or sixth character 5)
  > Use additional code to identify any insulin use (Z79.4)

  | **Excludes1** | diabetes mellitus due to underlying condition (E08.-)
  gestational diabetes (O24.4-)
  neonatal diabetes mellitus (P70.2)
  postpancreatectomy diabetes mellitus (E13.-)
  postprocedural diabetes mellitus (E13.-)
  secondary diabetes mellitus NEC (E13.-)
  type 1 diabetes mellitus (E10.-)
  type 2 diabetes mellitus (E11.-)

● **E09.0** **Drug or chemical induced diabetes mellitus with hyperosmolarity**

● **E09.00** **Drug or chemical induced diabetes mellitus with hyperosmolarity without nonketotic hyperglycemic-hyperosmolar coma (NKHHC)** 🔖 🔖

● **E09.01** **Drug or chemical induced diabetes mellitus with hyperosmolarity with coma** 🔖 🔖

● **E09.1** **Drug or chemical induced diabetes mellitus with ketoacidosis**

● **E09.10** **Drug or chemical induced diabetes mellitus with ketoacidosis without coma** 🔖 🔖

● **E09.11** **Drug or chemical induced diabetes mellitus with ketoacidosis with coma** 🔖

● **E09.2** **Drug or chemical induced diabetes mellitus with kidney complications**

● **E09.21** **Drug or chemical induced diabetes mellitus with diabetic nephropathy**
  Drug or chemical induced diabetes mellitus with intercapillary glomerulosclerosis
  Drug or chemical induced diabetes mellitus with intracapillary glomerulonephrosis
  Drug or chemical induced diabetes mellitus with Kimmelstiel-Wilson disease

● **E09.22** **Drug or chemical induced diabetes mellitus with diabetic chronic kidney disease**
  Drug or chemical induced diabetes mellitus with chronic kidney disease due to conditions classified to .21 and .22
  > Use additional code to identify stage of chronic kidney disease (N18.1-N18.6)

● **E09.29** **Drug or chemical induced diabetes mellitus with other diabetic kidney complication**
  Drug or chemical induced diabetes mellitus with renal tubular degeneration

● **E09.3** **Drug or chemical induced diabetes mellitus with ophthalmic complications**

● **E09.31** **Drug or chemical induced diabetes mellitus with unspecified diabetic retinopathy**

● ■ **E09.311** **Drug or chemical induced diabetes mellitus with unspecified diabetic retinopathy with macular edema**

● ■ **E09.319** **Drug or chemical induced diabetes mellitus with unspecified diabetic retinopathy without macular edema**

● **E09.32** **Drug or chemical induced diabetes mellitus with mild nonproliferative diabetic retinopathy**
  Drug or chemical induced diabetes mellitus with nonproliferative diabetic retinopathy NOS

● **E09.321** **Drug or chemical induced diabetes mellitus with mild nonproliferative diabetic retinopathy with macular edema**

● **E09.329** **Drug or chemical induced diabetes mellitus with mild nonproliferative diabetic retinopathy without macular edema**

● **E09.33** **Drug or chemical induced diabetes mellitus with moderate nonproliferative diabetic retinopathy**

● **E09.331** **Drug or chemical induced diabetes mellitus with moderate nonproliferative diabetic retinopathy with macular edema**

● **E09.339** **Drug or chemical induced diabetes mellitus with moderate nonproliferative diabetic retinopathy without macular edema**

● Unacceptable Principal Diagnosis   ● Use Additional Character(s)   ■ Unspecified   ▶ Manifestation Code

OGCR Official Guidelines for Coding and Reporting   Excludes 1   Excludes 2   Includes   Use additional   Code first   Code also

● **E09.34**	**Drug or chemical induced diabetes mellitus with severe nonproliferative diabetic retinopathy**

   ● **E09.341**	**Drug or chemical induced diabetes mellitus with severe nonproliferative diabetic retinopathy with macular edema**

   ● **E09.349**	**Drug or chemical induced diabetes mellitus with severe nonproliferative diabetic retinopathy without macular edema**

● **E09.35**	**Drug or chemical induced diabetes mellitus with proliferative diabetic retinopathy**

   ● **E09.351**	**Drug or chemical induced diabetes mellitus with proliferative diabetic retinopathy with macular edema**

   ● **E09.359**	**Drug or chemical induced diabetes mellitus with proliferative diabetic retinopathy without macular edema**

● **E09.36**	**Drug or chemical induced diabetes mellitus with diabetic cataract**

● **E09.39**	**Drug or chemical induced diabetes mellitus with other diabetic ophthalmic complication**

● **E09.4**	**Drug or chemical induced diabetes mellitus with neurological complications**

   ●◼ **E09.40**	**Drug or chemical induced diabetes mellitus with neurological complications with diabetic neuropathy, unspecified**

   ● **E09.41**	**Drug or chemical induced diabetes mellitus with neurological complications with diabetic mononeuropathy**

   ● **E09.42**	**Drug or chemical induced diabetes mellitus with neurological complications with diabetic polyneuropathy**
     Drug or chemical induced diabetes mellitus with diabetic neuralgia

   ● **E09.43**	**Drug or chemical induced diabetes mellitus with neurological complications with diabetic autonomic (poly)neuropathy**
     Drug or chemical induced diabetes mellitus with diabetic gastroparesis

   ● **E09.44**	**Drug or chemical induced diabetes mellitus with neurological complications with diabetic amyotrophy**

   ● **E09.49**	**Drug or chemical induced diabetes mellitus with neurological complications with other diabetic neurological complication**

● **E09.5**	**Drug or chemical induced diabetes mellitus with circulatory complications**

   ● **E09.51**	**Drug or chemical induced diabetes mellitus with diabetic peripheral angiopathy without gangrene**

   ● **E09.52**	**Drug or chemical induced diabetes mellitus with diabetic peripheral angiopathy with gangrene** 🦠
     Drug or chemical induced diabetes mellitus with diabetic gangrene
     MCC: Only when the principal diagnosis is designated as a CC

   ● **E09.59**	**Drug or chemical induced diabetes mellitus with other circulatory complications**

● **E09.6**	**Drug or chemical induced diabetes mellitus with other specified complications**

   ● **E09.61**	**Drug or chemical induced diabetes mellitus with diabetic arthropathy**

      ● **E09.610**	**Drug or chemical induced diabetes mellitus with diabetic neuropathic arthropathy**
       Drug or chemical induced diabetes mellitus with Charcôt's joints
       Progressive degeneration of weight bearing joint

      ● **E09.618**	**Drug or chemical induced diabetes mellitus with other diabetic arthropathy**

   ● **E09.62**	**Drug or chemical induced diabetes mellitus with skin complications**

      ● **E09.620**	**Drug or chemical induced diabetes mellitus with diabetic dermatitis**
       Drug or chemical induced diabetes mellitus with diabetic necrobiosis lipoidica
       Necrotizing skin condition

      ● **E09.621**	**Drug or chemical induced diabetes mellitus with foot ulcer**
       Use additional code to identify site of ulcer (L97.4-, L97.5-)

      ● **E09.622**	**Drug or chemical induced diabetes mellitus with other skin ulcer**
       Use additional code to identify site of ulcer (L97.1-L97.9, L98.41-L98.49)

      ● **E09.628**	**Drug or chemical induced diabetes mellitus with other skin complications**

   ● **E09.63**	**Drug or chemical induced diabetes mellitus with oral complications**

      ● **E09.630**	**Drug or chemical induced diabetes mellitus with periodontal disease**

      ● **E09.638**	**Drug or chemical induced diabetes mellitus with other oral complications**

   ● **E09.64**	**Drug or chemical induced diabetes mellitus with hypoglycemia**

      ● **E09.641**	**Drug or chemical induced diabetes mellitus with hypoglycemia with coma** 🦠

      ● **E09.649**	**Drug or chemical induced diabetes mellitus with hypoglycemia without coma**

   ● **E09.65**	**Drug or chemical induced diabetes mellitus with hyperglycemia** 🦠

   ● **E09.69**	**Drug or chemical induced diabetes mellitus with other specified complication**
     Use additional code to identify complication

●◼ **E09.8**	**Drug or chemical induced diabetes mellitus with unspecified complications**

● **E09.9**	**Drug or chemical induced diabetes mellitus without complications**

CHAPTER 4 (E00-E90)

● **E10   Type 1 diabetes mellitus**

Includes   brittle diabetes (mellitus)
diabetes (mellitus) due to autoimmune
process
diabetes (mellitus) due to immune mediated
pancreatic islet beta-cell destruction
idiopathic diabetes (mellitus)
juvenile onset diabetes (mellitus)
ketosis-prone diabetes (mellitus)

Excludes1   diabetes mellitus due to underlying
condition (E08.-)
drug or chemical induced diabetes mellitus
(E09.-)
gestational diabetes (O24.4-)
hyperglycemia NOS (R73.9)
neonatal diabetes mellitus (P70.2)
postpancreatectomy diabetes mellitus
(E13.-)
postprocedural diabetes mellitus (E13.-)
secondary diabetes mellitus NEC (E13.-)
type 2 diabetes mellitus (E11.-)

● **E10.1   Type 1 diabetes mellitus with ketoacidosis**
*Acidosis accompanied by accumulation of ketone
bodies (ketosis) in body tissues and fluids*

　E10.10   Type 1 diabetes mellitus with ketoacidosis
without coma 🔖 🔖

　E10.11   Type 1 diabetes mellitus with ketoacidosis
with coma 🔖

● **E10.2   Type 1 diabetes mellitus with kidney complications**

　E10.21   Type 1 diabetes mellitus with diabetic
nephropathy
Type 1 diabetes mellitus with
intercapillary glomerulosclerosis
Type 1 diabetes mellitus with
intracapillary glomerulonephrosis
Type 1 diabetes mellitus with
Kimmelstiel-Wilson disease

　E10.22   Type 1 diabetes mellitus with diabetic
chronic kidney disease
Type 1 diabetes mellitus with chronic
kidney disease due to conditions
classified to .21 and .22

　　Use additional code to identify
stage of chronic kidney disease
(N18.1-N18.6)

　E10.29   Type 1 diabetes mellitus with other
diabetic kidney complication
Type 1 diabetes mellitus with renal
tubular degeneration

● **E10.3   Type 1 diabetes mellitus with ophthalmic
complications**

● **E10.31**   Type 1 diabetes mellitus with unspecified
diabetic retinopathy

　■ **E10.311**   Type 1 diabetes mellitus with
unspecified diabetic retinopathy
with macular edema

　■ **E10.319**   Type 1 diabetes mellitus with
unspecified diabetic retinopathy
without macular edema

● **E10.32**   Type 1 diabetes mellitus with mild
nonproliferative diabetic retinopathy
Type 1 diabetes mellitus with
nonproliferative diabetic retinopathy
NOS

　E10.321   Type 1 diabetes mellitus with
mild nonproliferative diabetic
retinopathy with macular edema

　E10.329   Type 1 diabetes mellitus with
mild nonproliferative diabetic
retinopathy without macular
edema

● **E10.33**   Type 1 diabetes mellitus with moderate
nonproliferative diabetic retinopathy

　E10.331   Type 1 diabetes mellitus with
moderate nonproliferative
diabetic retinopathy with
macular edema

　E10.339   Type 1 diabetes mellitus with
moderate nonproliferative
diabetic retinopathy without
macular edema

● **E10.34**   Type 1 diabetes mellitus with severe
nonproliferative diabetic retinopathy

　E10.341   Type 1 diabetes mellitus with
severe nonproliferative diabetic
retinopathy with macular edema

　E10.349   Type 1 diabetes mellitus with
severe nonproliferative diabetic
retinopathy without macular
edema

● **E10.35**   Type 1 diabetes mellitus with proliferative
diabetic retinopathy

　E10.351   Type 1 diabetes mellitus with
proliferative diabetic retinopathy
with macular edema

　E10.359   Type 1 diabetes mellitus with
proliferative diabetic retinopathy
without macular edema

　E10.36   Type 1 diabetes mellitus with diabetic
cataract

　E10.39   Type 1 diabetes mellitus with other
diabetic ophthalmic complication

● **E10.4   Type 1 diabetes mellitus with neurological
complications**

■ **E10.40**   Type 1 diabetes mellitus with diabetic
neuropathy, unspecified

　E10.41   Type 1 diabetes mellitus with diabetic
mononeuropathy

　E10.42   Type 1 diabetes mellitus with diabetic
polyneuropathy
Type 1 diabetes mellitus with diabetic
neuralgia

　E10.43   Type 1 diabetes mellitus with diabetic
autonomic (poly)neuropathy
Type 1 diabetes mellitus with diabetic
gastroparesis

　E10.44   Type 1 diabetes mellitus with diabetic
amyotrophy

　E10.49   Type 1 diabetes mellitus with other
diabetic neurological complication

● **E10.5   Type 1 diabetes mellitus with circulatory
complications**

　E10.51   Type 1 diabetes mellitus with diabetic
peripheral angiopathy without gangrene

　E10.52   Type 1 diabetes mellitus with diabetic
peripheral angiopathy with gangrene
Type 1 diabetes mellitus with diabetic
gangrene 🔖

　E10.59   Type 1 diabetes mellitus with other
circulatory complications

● **E10.6　Type 1 diabetes mellitus with other specified complications**

　● **E10.61　Type 1 diabetes mellitus with diabetic arthropathy**

　　E10.610　Type 1 diabetes mellitus with diabetic neuropathic arthropathy
　　　　　　Type 1 diabetes mellitus with Charcôt's joints

　　E10.618　Type 1 diabetes mellitus with other diabetic arthropathy

　● **E10.62　Type 1 diabetes mellitus with skin complications**

　　E10.620　Type 1 diabetes mellitus with diabetic dermatitis
　　　　　　Type 1 diabetes mellitus with diabetic necrobiosis lipoidica

　　E10.621　Type 1 diabetes mellitus with foot ulcer
　　　　　　Use additional code to identify site of ulcer (L97.4-, L97.5-)

　　E10.622　Type 1 diabetes mellitus with other skin ulcer
　　　　　　Use additional code to identify site of ulcer (L97.1-L97.9, L98.41-L98.49)

　　E10.628　Type 1 diabetes mellitus with other skin complications

　● **E10.63　Type 1 diabetes mellitus with oral complications**

　　E10.630　Type 1 diabetes mellitus with periodontal disease

　　E10.638　Type 1 diabetes mellitus with other oral complications

　● **E10.64　Type 1 diabetes mellitus with hypoglycemia**

　　E10.641　Type 1 diabetes mellitus with hypoglycemia with coma 🦠

　　E10.649　Type 1 diabetes mellitus with hypoglycemia without coma

　　E10.65　Type 1 diabetes mellitus with hyperglycemia 🦠

　　E10.69　Type 1 diabetes mellitus with other specified complication
　　　　　　Use additional code to identify complication

■ **E10.8　Type 1 diabetes mellitus with unspecified complications**

　E10.9　Type 1 diabetes mellitus without complications

● **E11　Type 2 diabetes mellitus**

　Includes　diabetes (mellitus) due to insulin secretory defect
　　　　　　diabetes NOS
　　　　　　insulin resistant diabetes (mellitus)

　Use additional code to identify any insulin use (Z79.4)

　Excludes1　diabetes mellitus due to underlying condition (E08.-)
　　　　　　drug or chemical induced diabetes mellitus (E09.-)
　　　　　　gestational diabetes (O24.4-)
　　　　　　neonatal diabetes mellitus (P70.2)
　　　　　　postpancreatectomy diabetes mellitus (E13.-)
　　　　　　postprocedural diabetes mellitus (E13.-)
　　　　　　secondary diabetes mellitus NEC (E13.-)
　　　　　　type 1 diabetes mellitus (E10.-)

● **E11.0　Type 2 diabetes mellitus with hyperosmolarity**

　E11.00　Type 2 diabetes mellitus with hyperosmolarity without nonketotic hyperglycemic-hyperosmolar coma (NKHHC) 🦠 🦠

　E11.01　Type 2 diabetes mellitus with hyperosmolarity with coma 🦠 🦠

● **E11.2　Type 2 diabetes mellitus with kidney complications**

　E11.21　Type 2 diabetes mellitus with diabetic nephropathy
　　　　Type 2 diabetes mellitus with intercapillary glomerulosclerosis
　　　　Type 2 diabetes mellitus with intracapillary glomerulonephrosis
　　　　Type 2 diabetes mellitus with Kimmelstiel-Wilson disease

　E11.22　Type 2 diabetes mellitus with diabetic chronic kidney disease
　　　　Type 2 diabetes mellitus with chronic kidney disease due to conditions classified to .21 and .22
　　　　Use additional code to identify stage of chronic kidney disease (N18.1-N18.6)

　E11.29　Type 2 diabetes mellitus with other diabetic kidney complication
　　　　Type 2 diabetes mellitus with renal tubular degeneration

● **E11.3　Type 2 diabetes mellitus with ophthalmic complications**

　● **E11.31　Type 2 diabetes mellitus with unspecified diabetic retinopathy**

　　■ **E11.311　Type 2 diabetes mellitus with unspecified diabetic retinopathy with macular edema**

　　■ **E11.319　Type 2 diabetes mellitus with unspecified diabetic retinopathy without macular edema**

　● **E11.32　Type 2 diabetes mellitus with mild nonproliferative diabetic retinopathy**
　　　　Type 2 diabetes mellitus with nonproliferative diabetic retinopathy NOS

　　E11.321　Type 2 diabetes mellitus with mild nonproliferative diabetic retinopathy with macular edema

　　E11.329　Type 2 diabetes mellitus with mild nonproliferative diabetic retinopathy without macular edema

　● **E11.33　Type 2 diabetes mellitus with moderate nonproliferative diabetic retinopathy**

　　E11.331　Type 2 diabetes mellitus with moderate nonproliferative diabetic retinopathy with macular edema

　　E11.339　Type 2 diabetes mellitus with moderate nonproliferative diabetic retinopathy without macular edema

　● **E11.34　Type 2 diabetes mellitus with severe nonproliferative diabetic retinopathy**

　　E11.341　Type 2 diabetes mellitus with severe nonproliferative diabetic retinopathy with macular edema

N Newborn Age: 0　　**P** Pediatric Age: 0–17　　**M** Maternity DX: 12–55　　**A** Adult Age: 15–124　　♀ Females Only　　♂ Males Only

🦠 Complication\Comorbidity　　🦠 Major C\C　　🦠 Present on Admission Requirement　　🦠 Hospital-Acquired Condition

889

CHAPTER 4 (E00-E90)

E11.349 Type 2 diabetes mellitus with severe nonproliferative diabetic retinopathy without macular edema

● E11.35 Type 2 diabetes mellitus with proliferative diabetic retinopathy

E11.351 Type 2 diabetes mellitus with proliferative diabetic retinopathy with macular edema

E11.359 Type 2 diabetes mellitus with proliferative diabetic retinopathy without macular edema

E11.36 Type 2 diabetes mellitus with diabetic cataract

E11.39 Type 2 diabetes mellitus with other diabetic ophthalmic complication

● E11.4 Type 2 diabetes mellitus with neurological complications

■ E11.40 Type 2 diabetes mellitus with diabetic neuropathy, unspecified

E11.41 Type 2 diabetes mellitus with diabetic mononeuropathy

E11.42 Type 2 diabetes mellitus with diabetic polyneuropathy
Type 2 diabetes mellitus with diabetic neuralgia

E11.43 Type 2 diabetes mellitus with diabetic autonomic (poly)neuropathy
Type 2 diabetes mellitus with diabetic gastroparesis

E11.44 Type 2 diabetes mellitus with diabetic amyotrophy

E11.49 Type 2 diabetes mellitus with other diabetic neurological complication

● E11.5 Type 2 diabetes mellitus with circulatory complications

E11.51 Type 2 diabetes mellitus with diabetic peripheral angiopathy without gangrene

E11.52 Type 2 diabetes mellitus with diabetic peripheral angiopathy with gangrene
Type 2 diabetes mellitus with diabetic gangrene 🐾

E11.59 Type 2 diabetes mellitus with other circulatory complications

● E11.6 Type 2 diabetes mellitus with other specified complications

● E11.61 Type 2 diabetes mellitus with diabetic arthropathy

E11.610 Type 2 diabetes mellitus with diabetic neuropathic arthropathy
Type 2 diabetes mellitus with Charcôt's joints

E11.618 Type 2 diabetes mellitus with other diabetic arthropathy

● E11.62 Type 2 diabetes mellitus with skin complications

E11.620 Type 2 diabetes mellitus with diabetic dermatitis
Type 2 diabetes mellitus with diabetic necrobiosis lipoidica

E11.621 Type 2 diabetes mellitus with foot ulcer
Use additional code to identify site of ulcer (L97.4-, L97.5-)

E11.622 Type 2 diabetes mellitus with other skin ulcer
Use additional code to identify site of ulcer (L97.1-L97.9, L98.41-L98.49)

E11.628 Type 2 diabetes mellitus with other skin complications

● E11.63 Type 2 diabetes mellitus with oral complications

E11.630 Type 2 diabetes mellitus with periodontal disease

E11.638 Type 2 diabetes mellitus with other oral complications

● E11.64 Type 2 diabetes mellitus with hypoglycemia

E11.641 Type 2 diabetes mellitus with hypoglycemia with coma 🐾

E11.649 Type 2 diabetes mellitus with hypoglycemia without coma

E11.65 Type 2 diabetes mellitus with hyperglycemia 🐾

E11.69 Type 2 diabetes mellitus with other specified complication
Use additional code to identify complication

■ E11.8 Type 2 diabetes mellitus with unspecified complications

E11.9 Type 2 diabetes mellitus without complications
MCE: Questionable admission when principal dx

● E13 Other specified diabetes mellitus

Includes diabetes mellitus due to genetic defects of beta-cell function
diabetes mellitus due to genetic defects in insulin action
postpancreatectomy diabetes mellitus
postprocedural diabetes mellitus
secondary diabetes mellitus NEC

Use additional code to identify any insulin use (Z79.4)

Excludes1 diabetes (mellitus) due to autoimmune process (E10.-)
diabetes (mellitus) due to immune mediated pancreatic islet beta-cell destruction (E10.-)
diabetes mellitus due to underlying condition (E08.-)
drug or chemical induced diabetes mellitus (E09.-)
gestational diabetes (O24.4-)
neonatal diabetes mellitus (P70.2)
type 2 diabetes mellitus (E11.-)

● E13.0 Other specified diabetes mellitus with hyperosmolarity

E13.00 Other specified diabetes mellitus with hyperosmolarity without nonketotic hyperglycemic-hyperosmolar coma (NKHHC) 🐾 🐾

E13.01 Other specified diabetes mellitus with hyperosmolarity with coma 🐾 🐾

● E13.1 Other specified diabetes mellitus with ketoacidosis

E13.10 Other specified diabetes mellitus with ketoacidosis without coma 🐾 🐾

E13.11 Other specified diabetes mellitus with ketoacidosis with coma 🐾

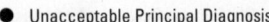

● Unacceptable Principal Diagnosis   ● Use Additional Character(s)   ■ Unspecified   ▶ Manifestation Code

OGCR Official Guidelines for Coding and Reporting   Excludes 1   Excludes 2   Includes   Use additional   Code first   Code also

● **E13.2 Other specified diabetes mellitus with kidney complications**

   E13.21 Other specified diabetes mellitus with diabetic nephropathy
      Other specified diabetes mellitus with intercapillary glomerulosclerosis
      Other specified diabetes mellitus with intracapillary glomerulonephrosis
      Other specified diabetes mellitus with Kimmelstiel-Wilson disease

   E13.22 Other specified diabetes mellitus with diabetic chronic kidney disease
      Other specified diabetes mellitus with chronic kidney disease due to conditions classified to .21 and .22
      Use additional code to identify stage of chronic kidney disease (N18.1-N18.6)

   E13.29 Other specified diabetes mellitus with other diabetic kidney complication
      Other specified diabetes mellitus with renal tubular degeneration

● **E13.3 Other specified diabetes mellitus with ophthalmic complications**

   ● **E13.31 Other specified diabetes mellitus with unspecified diabetic retinopathy**

      ■ **E13.311 Other specified diabetes mellitus with unspecified diabetic retinopathy with macular edema**

      ■ **E13.319 Other specified diabetes mellitus with unspecified diabetic retinopathy without macular edema**

   E13.32 Other specified diabetes mellitus with mild nonproliferative diabetic retinopathy
      Other specified diabetes mellitus with nonproliferative diabetic retinopathy NOS

      E13.321 Other specified diabetes mellitus with mild nonproliferative diabetic retinopathy with macular edema

      E13.329 Other specified diabetes mellitus with mild nonproliferative diabetic retinopathy without macular edema

   E13.33 Other specified diabetes mellitus with moderate nonproliferative diabetic retinopathy

      E13.331 Other specified diabetes mellitus with moderate nonproliferative diabetic retinopathy with macular edema

      E13.339 Other specified diabetes mellitus with moderate nonproliferative diabetic retinopathy without macular edema

   ● **E13.34 Other specified diabetes mellitus with severe nonproliferative diabetic retinopathy**

      E13.341 Other specified diabetes mellitus with severe nonproliferative diabetic retinopathy with macular edema

      E13.349 Other specified diabetes mellitus with severe nonproliferative diabetic retinopathy without macular edema

● **E13.35 Other specified diabetes mellitus with proliferative diabetic retinopathy**

      E13.351 Other specified diabetes mellitus with proliferative diabetic retinopathy with macular edema

      E13.359 Other specified diabetes mellitus with proliferative diabetic retinopathy without macular edema

   E13.36 Other specified diabetes mellitus with diabetic cataract

   E13.39 Other specified diabetes mellitus with other diabetic ophthalmic complication

● **E13.4 Other specified diabetes mellitus with neurological complications**

   ■ **E13.40 Other specified diabetes mellitus with diabetic neuropathy, unspecified**

   E13.41 Other specified diabetes mellitus with diabetic mononeuropathy

   E13.42 Other specified diabetes mellitus with diabetic polyneuropathy
      Other specified diabetes mellitus with diabetic neuralgia

   E13.43 Other specified diabetes mellitus with diabetic autonomic (poly)neuropathy
      Other specified diabetes mellitus with diabetic gastroparesis

   E13.44 Other specified diabetes mellitus with diabetic amyotrophy

   E13.49 Other specified diabetes mellitus with other diabetic neurological complication

● **E13.5 Other specified diabetes mellitus with circulatory complications**

   E13.51 Other specified diabetes mellitus with diabetic peripheral angiopathy without gangrene

   E13.52 Other specified diabetes mellitus with diabetic peripheral angiopathy with gangrene
      Other specified diabetes mellitus with diabetic gangrene
      MCC: Only when the principal diagnosis is designated as a CC

   E13.59 Other specified diabetes mellitus with other circulatory complications

● **E13.6 Other specified diabetes mellitus with other specified complications**

   ● **E13.61 Other specified diabetes mellitus with diabetic arthropathy**

      E13.610 Other specified diabetes mellitus with diabetic neuropathic arthropathy
         Other specified diabetes mellitus with Charcôt's joints

      E13.618 Other specified diabetes mellitus with other diabetic arthropathy

   ● **E13.62 Other specified diabetes mellitus with skin complications**

      E13.620 Other specified diabetes mellitus with diabetic dermatitis
         Other specified diabetes mellitus with diabetic necrobiosis lipoidica

N Newborn Age: 0   **P** Pediatric Age: 0–17   **M** Maternity DX: 12–55   **A** Adult Age: 15–124   ♀ Females Only   ♂ Males Only

Complication\Comorbidity   Major C\C   Present on Admission Requirement   Hospital-Acquired Condition

891

E13.621 Other specified diabetes mellitus with foot ulcer

> Use additional code to identify site of ulcer (L97.4-, L97.5-)

E13.622 Other specified diabetes mellitus with other skin ulcer

> Use additional code to identify site of ulcer (L97.1-L97.9, L98.41-L98.49)

E13.628 Other specified diabetes mellitus with other skin complications

● **E13.63 Other specified diabetes mellitus with oral complications**

E13.630 Other specified diabetes mellitus with periodontal disease

E13.638 Other specified diabetes mellitus with other oral complications

● **E13.64 Other specified diabetes mellitus with hypoglycemia**

E13.641 Other specified diabetes mellitus with hypoglycemia with coma 🔖

E13.649 Other specified diabetes mellitus with hypoglycemia without coma

E13.65 Other specified diabetes mellitus with hyperglycemia 🔖

E13.69 Other specified diabetes mellitus with other specified complication

> Use additional code to identify complication

◼ **E13.8 Other specified diabetes mellitus with unspecified complications**

E13.9 Other specified diabetes mellitus without complications

> MCE: Questionable admission when principal dx

OTHER DISORDERS OF GLUCOSE REGULATION AND PANCREATIC INTERNAL SECRETION (E15-E16)

E15 Nondiabetic hypoglycemic coma 🔖🔖

> **Includes** drug-induced insulin coma in nondiabetic
> hyperinsulinism with hypoglycemic coma
> hypoglycemic coma NOS

● **E16 Other disorders of pancreatic internal secretion**

● **E16.0 Drug-induced hypoglycemia without coma**

> Use additional code for adverse effect, if applicable, to identify drug (T36-T50 with fifth or sixth character 5)

E16.1 Other hypoglycemia

> Functional hyperinsulinism
> Functional nonhyperinsulinemic hypoglycemia
> Hyperinsulinism NOS
> Hyperplasia of pancreatic islet beta cells NOS

> **Excludes1** hypoglycemia in infant of diabetic mother (P70.1)
> neonatal hypoglycemia (P70.4)

◼ **E16.2 Hypoglycemia, unspecified**

E16.3 Increased secretion of glucagon

> Hyperplasia of pancreatic endocrine cells with glucagon excess

E16.4 Increased secretion of gastrin

> Hypergastrinemia
> Hyperplasia of pancreatic endocrine cells with gastrin excess
> Zollinger-Ellison syndrome

E16.8 Other specified disorders of pancreatic internal secretion

> Increased secretion from endocrine pancreas of growth hormone-releasing hormone
> Increased secretion from endocrine pancreas of pancreatic polypeptide
> Increased secretion from endocrine pancreas of somatostatin
> Increased secretion from endocrine pancreas of vasoactive-intestinal polypeptide

◼ **E16.9 Disorder of pancreatic internal secretion, unspecified**

> Islet-cell hyperplasia NOS
> Pancreatic endocrine cell hyperplasia NOS

DISORDERS OF OTHER ENDOCRINE GLANDS (E20-E35)

> **Excludes1** galactorrhea (N64.3)
> gynecomastia (N62)

● **E20 Hypoparathyroidism**

> *Greatly reduced function of parathyroid glands; AKA parathyroid insufficiency*

> **Excludes1** Di George's syndrome (D82.1)
> postprocedural hypoparathyroidism (E89.2)
> tetany NOS (R29.0)
> transitory neonatal hypoparathyroidism (P71.4)

E20.0 Idiopathic hypoparathyroidism

> *Rare condition, unknown cause; short dwarf-like with round face*

E20.1 Pseudohypoparathyroidism

> *Hereditary condition resembling hypoparathyroidism, but caused by inability to respond to parathyroid hormone*

E20.8 Other hypoparathyroidism

◼ **E20.9 Hypoparathyroidism, unspecified**

> Parathyroid tetany

● **E21 Hyperparathyroidism and other disorders of parathyroid gland**

> **Excludes1** adult osteomalacia (M83.-)
> ectopic hyperparathyroidism (E34.2)
> familial hypocalciuric hypercalcemia (E83.52)
> hungry bone syndrome (E83.81)
> infantile and juvenile osteomalacia (E55.0)

E21.0 Primary hyperparathyroidism

> Hyperplasia of parathyroid
> Osteitis fibrosa cystica generalisata [von Recklinghausen's disease of bone]

E21.1 Secondary hyperparathyroidism, not elsewhere classified

> **Excludes1** secondary hyperparathyroidism of renal origin (N25.81)

Item 4–4 Hyperparathyroidism is an overactive parathyroid gland that secretes excessive parathormone, causing increased levels of circulating calcium. This results in a loss of calcium in the bone (osteoporosis).

Hypoparathyroidism is an underactive parathyroid gland that results in decreased levels of circulating calcium. The primary manifestation is **tetany,** a continuous muscle spasm.

Figure 4-5 Tetany caused by hypoparathyroidism.

● Unacceptable Principal Diagnosis   ● Use Additional Character(s)   ◼ Unspecified   ▶ Manifestation Code

OGCR Official Guidelines for Coding and Reporting   Excludes 1   Excludes 2   Includes   Use additional   Code first   Code also

Item 4–5   Hyperadrenalism is overactivity of the adrenal cortex, which secretes corticosteroid hormones. Excessive glucocorticoid hormone results in hyperglycemia **(Cushing's syndrome),** and excessive aldosterone results in **Conn's syndrome. Adrenogenital syndrome** is the result of excessive secretion of androgens, male hormones, which stimulates premature sexual development. **Hypoadrenalism, Addison's disease,** is a condition in which the adrenal glands atrophy.

Figure 4-6   Centripetal and generalized obesity and dorsal kyphosis in a 30-year-old woman with Cushing's disease. (From Larsen: Williams Textbook of Endocrinology, 10th ed. 2003, Saunders, An Imprint of Elsevier.)

     E21.2   Other hyperparathyroidism
         Tertiary hyperparathyroidism
         Excludes1   familial hypocalciuric hypercalcemia (E83.52)

     ▪ **E21.3   Hyperparathyroidism, unspecified**

     E21.4   Other specified disorders of parathyroid gland

     ▪ **E21.5   Disorder of parathyroid gland, unspecified**

● **E22   Hyperfunction of pituitary gland**
         Excludes1   Cushing's syndrome (E24.-)
                Nelson's syndrome (E24.1)
                overproduction of ACTH not associated with Cushing's disease (E27.0)
                overproduction of pituitary ACTH (E24.0)
                overproduction of thyroid-stimulating hormone (E05.8-)

     E22.0   Acromegaly and pituitary gigantism
         Chronic disease caused by hypersecretion of growth hormone
         Overproduction of growth hormone
         Excludes1   constitutional gigantism (E34.4)
                constitutional tall stature (E34.4)
                increased secretion from endocrine pancreas of growth hormone-releasing hormone (E16.8)

     E22.1   Hyperprolactinemia 🦠
         Increased levels of prolactin
         Use additional code for adverse effect, if applicable, to identify drug (T36-T50 with fifth or sixth character 5)

     E22.2   Syndrome of inappropriate secretion of antidiuretic hormone 🦠

     E22.8   Other hyperfunction of pituitary gland 🦠
         Central precocious puberty

     ▪ **E22.9   Hyperfunction of pituitary gland, unspecified** 🦠

● **E23   Hypofunction and other disorders of the pituitary gland**
         Includes   the listed conditions whether the disorder is in the pituitary or the hypothalamus
         Excludes1   postprocedural hypopituitarism (E89.3)

     E23.0   Hypopituitarism 🦠
         Fertile eunuch syndrome
         Hypogonadotropic hypogonadism
         Idiopathic growth hormone deficiency
         Isolated deficiency of gonadotropin
         Isolated deficiency of growth hormone
         Isolated deficiency of pituitary hormone
         Kallmann's syndrome
         Lorain-Levi short stature
         Necrosis of pituitary gland (postpartum)
         Panhypopituitarism
         Pituitary cachexia
         Pituitary insufficiency NOS
         Pituitary short stature
         Sheehan's syndrome
         Simmonds' disease

● **E23.1   Drug-induced hypopituitarism**
         Use additional code for adverse effect, if applicable, to identify drug (T36-T50 with fifth or sixth character 5)

     E23.2   Diabetes insipidus 🦠
         Excludes1   nephrogenic diabetes insipidus (N25.1)

     E23.3   Hypothalamic dysfunction, not elsewhere classified
         Excludes1   Prader-Willi syndrome (Q87.1)
                Russell-Silver syndrome (Q87.1)

     E23.6   Other disorders of pituitary gland
         Abscess of pituitary
         Adiposogenital dystrophy

     ▪ **E23.7   Disorder of pituitary gland, unspecified**

● **E24   Cushing's syndrome**
         Excludes1   congenital adrenal hyperplasia (E25.0)

     E24.0   Pituitary-dependent Cushing's disease 🦠
         Overproduction of pituitary ACTH
         Pituitary-dependent hypercorticalism

     E24.1   Nelson's syndrome

     ● **E24.2   Drug-induced Cushing's syndrome** 🦠
         Use additional code for adverse effect, if applicable, to identify drug (T36-T50 with fifth or sixth character 5)

     E24.3   Ectopic ACTH syndrome 🦠

     E24.4   Alcohol-induced pseudo-Cushing's syndrome 🦠

     E24.8   Other Cushing's syndrome 🦠

     ▪ **E24.9   Cushing's syndrome, unspecified** 🦠

● **E25   Adrenogenital disorders**
         Disorder of production of steroid hormone in adrenal gland
         Includes   adrenogenital syndromes, virilizing or feminizing, whether acquired or due to adrenal hyperplasia consequent on inborn enzyme defects in hormone synthesis
                female adrenal pseudohermaphroditism
                female heterosexual precocious pseudopuberty
                male isosexual precocious pseudopuberty
                male macrogenitosomia praecox
                male sexual precocity with adrenal hyperplasia
                male virilization (female)
         Excludes1   indeterminate sex and pseudohermaphroditism (Q56)
                chromosomal abnormalities (Q90-Q99)

     E25.0   Congenital adrenogenital disorders associated with enzyme deficiency
         Congenital adrenal hyperplasia
         21-Hydroxylase deficiency
         Salt-losing congenital adrenal hyperplasia

N   Newborn Age: 0   **P**   Pediatric Age: 0–17   **M**   Maternity DX: 12–55   **A**   Adult Age: 15–124   ♀   Females Only   ♂   Males Only

🦠   Complication\Comorbidity   🦠   Major C\C   Present on Admission Requirement   Hospital-Acquired Condition

893

CHAPTER 4 (E00-E90)

E25.8 Other adrenogenital disorders
    Idiopathic adrenogenital disorder
> **Use additional** code for adverse effect, if
> applicable, to identify drug (T36-T50 with
> fifth or sixth character 5)

■ **E25.9 Adrenogenital disorder, unspecified**
    Adrenogenital syndrome NOS

● **E26 Hyperaldosteronism**
    Abnormality of electrolyte metabolism caused by excessive
    secretion of aldosterone

  ● **E26.0 Primary hyperaldosteronism**

    E26.01 Conn's syndrome
> **Code also** adrenal adenoma (D35.0)

    E26.02 Glucocorticoid-remediable aldosteronism
        Familial aldosteronism type I

    E26.09 Other primary hyperaldosteronism
        Primary aldosteronism due to adrenal
          hyperplasia (bilateral)

  E26.1 Secondary hyperaldosteronism

  ● **E26.8 Other hyperaldosteronism**

    E26.81 Bartter's syndrome

    E26.89 Other hyperaldosteronism

  ■ **E26.9 Hyperaldosteronism, unspecified**
    Aldosteronism NOS
    Hyperaldosteronism NOS

● **E27 Other disorders of adrenal gland**

  E27.0 Other adrenocortical overactivity ◐
    Overproduction of ACTH, not associated with
      Cushing's disease
    Premature adrenarche
> **Excludes1** Cushing's syndrome (E24.-)

  E27.1 Primary adrenocortical insufficiency ◐
    Addison's disease
    Autoimmune adrenalitis
> **Excludes1** Addison only phenotype
>   adrenoleukodystrophy (E71.528)
>   amyloidosis (E85-)
>   tuberculous Addison's disease (A18.7)
>   Waterhouse-Friderichsen syndrome
>   (A39.1)

  E27.2 Addisonian crisis ◐
    Acute onset of adrenocortical insufficiency
    Adrenal crisis
    Adrenocortical crisis

  ● **E27.3 Drug-induced adrenocortical insufficiency** ◐
> **Use additional** code for adverse effect, if
> applicable, to identify drug (T36-T50 with
> fifth or sixth character 5)

  ● **E27.4 Other and unspecified adrenocortical insufficiency**
> **Excludes1** adrenoleukodystrophy [Addison-
>   Schilder] (E71.528)
>   Waterhouse-Friderichsen syndrome
>   (A39.1)

    ■ **E27.40 Unspecified adrenocortical insufficiency** ◐
        Adrenocortical insufficiency NOS
        Hypoaldosteronism

    E27.49 Other adrenocortical insufficiency ◐
        Adrenal hemorrhage
        Adrenal infarction

  E27.5 Adrenomedullary hyperfunction ◐
    Adrenomedullary hyperplasia
    Catecholamine hypersecretion

  E27.8 Other specified disorders of adrenal gland
    Abnormality of cortisol-binding globulin

  ■ **E27.9 Disorder of adrenal gland, unspecified**

● **E28 Ovarian dysfunction**
> **Excludes1** isolated gonadotropin deficiency (E23.0)
>   postprocedural ovarian failure (E89.4-)

  E28.0 Estrogen excess ♀
> **Use additional** code for adverse effect, if
> applicable, to identify drug (T36-T50 with
> fifth or sixth character 5)

  E28.1 Androgen excess ♀
    Hypersecretion of ovarian androgens
> **Use additional** code for adverse effect, if
> applicable, to identify drug (T36-T50 with
> fifth or sixth character 5)

  E28.2 Polycystic ovarian syndrome ♀
    Sclerocystic ovary syndrome
    Stein-Leventhal syndrome

  ● **E28.3 Primary ovarian failure**
> **Excludes1** pure gonadal dysgenesis (Q99.1)
>   Turner's syndrome (Q96.-)

    ● **E28.31 Premature menopause**

      **E28.310 Symptomatic premature
            menopause** ♀   A
          Symptoms such as flushing,
            sleeplessness, headache,
            lack of concentration,
            associated with premature
            menopause

      **E28.319 Asymptomatic premature
            menopause** ♀   A
          Premature menopause NOS

    E28.39 Other primary ovarian failure ♀
        Decreased estrogen
        Resistant ovary syndrome

  E28.8 Other ovarian dysfunction ♀
    Ovarian hyperfunction NOS
> **Excludes1** postprocedural ovarian failure
>   (E89.4-)

  ■ **E28.9 Ovarian dysfunction, unspecified** ♀

● **E29 Testicular dysfunction**
> **Excludes1** androgen insensitivity syndrome (E34.5-)
>   azoospermia or oligospermia NOS
>   (N46.0-N46.1)
>   isolated gonadotropin deficiency (E23.0)
>   Klinefelter's syndrome (Q98.0-Q98.2, Q98.4)

  E29.0 Testicular hyperfunction ♂
    Hypersecretion of testicular hormones

  E29.1 Testicular hypofunction ♂
    Defective biosynthesis of testicular androgen NOS
    5-delta-Reductase deficiency (with male
      pseudohermaphroditism)
    Testicular hypogonadism NOS
> **Use additional** code for adverse effect, if
> applicable, to identify drug (T36-T50 with
> fifth or sixth character 5)
> **Excludes1** postprocedural testicular
>   hypofunction (E89.5)

  E29.8 Other testicular dysfunction ♂

  ■ **E29.9 Testicular dysfunction, unspecified** ♂

  ● Unacceptable Principal Diagnosis   ● Use Additional Character(s)   ■ Unspecified   ▶ Manifestation Code
OGCR Official Guidelines for Coding and Reporting   Excludes 1   Excludes 2   Includes   Use additional   Code first   Code also

CHAPTER 4 (E00-E90)

● **E30 Disorders of puberty, not elsewhere classified**

E30.0 Delayed puberty
Constitutional delay of puberty
Delayed sexual development

E30.1 Precocious puberty   P
Sexual maturation at earlier age than normal, or before age 8 in girls and 9 in boys, usually hormonal; AKA sexual precocity or pubertas praecox
Precocious menstruation

> Excludes1   Albright (-McCune) (-Sternberg) syndrome (Q78.1)
> central precocious puberty (E22.8)
> congenital adrenal hyperplasia (E25.0)
> female heterosexual precocious pseudopuberty (E25.-)
> male isosexual precocious pseudopuberty (E25.-)

E30.8 Other disorders of puberty   P
Premature thelarche

E30.9 Disorder of puberty, unspecified

● **E31 Polyglandular dysfunction**

> Excludes1   ataxia telangiectasia [Louis-Bar] (G11.3)
> dystrophia myotonica [Steinert] (G71.11)
> pseudohypoparathyroidism (E20.1)

E31.0 Autoimmune polyglandular failure
Schmidt's syndrome

E31.1 Polyglandular hyperfunction

> Excludes1   multiple endocrine adenomatosis (E31.2-)
> multiple endocrine neoplasia (E31.2-)

● **E31.2 Multiple endocrine neoplasia [MEN] syndromes**
Adenomatous hyperplasia and malignant tumors in endocrine glands
Multiple endocrine adenomatosis

> Code also any associated malignancies and other conditions associated with the syndromes

E31.20 Multiple endocrine neoplasia [MEN] syndrome, unspecified
Multiple endocrine adenomatosis NOS
Multiple endocrine neoplasia [MEN] syndrome NOS

E31.21 Multiple endocrine neoplasia [MEN] type I
Wermer's syndrome

E31.22 Multiple endocrine neoplasia [MEN] type IIA
Sipple's syndrome

E31.23 Multiple endocrine neoplasia [MEN] type IIB

E31.8 Other polyglandular dysfunction

E31.9 Polyglandular dysfunction, unspecified

● **E32 Diseases of thymus**

> Excludes1   aplasia or hypoplasia of thymus with immunodeficiency (D82.1)
> myasthenia gravis (G70.0)

E32.0 Persistent hyperplasia of thymus
Hypertrophy of thymus

E32.1 Abscess of thymus 🔹

E32.8 Other diseases of thymus

> Excludes1   aplasia or hypoplasia with immunodeficiency (D82.1)
> thymoma (D15.0)

E32.9 Disease of thymus, unspecified

● **E34 Other endocrine disorders**

> Excludes1   pseudohypoparathyroidism (E20.1)

E34.0 Carcinoid syndrome 🔹

> **Note:** May be used as an additional code to identify functional activity associated with a carcinoid tumor.

E34.1 Other hypersecretion of intestinal hormones

E34.2 Ectopic hormone secretion, not elsewhere classified

> Excludes1   ectopic ACTH syndrome (E24.3)

E34.3 Short stature due to endocrine disorder
Constitutional short stature
Laron-type short stature

> Excludes1   achondroplastic short stature (Q77.4)
> hypochondroplastic short stature (Q77.4)
> nutritional short stature (E45)
> pituitary short stature (E23.0)
> progeria (E34.8)
> renal short stature (N25.0)
> Russell-Silver syndrome (Q87.1)
> short-limbed stature with immunodeficiency (D82.2)
> short stature in specific dysmorphic syndromes - code to syndrome - see Alphabetical Index
> short stature NOS (R62.52)

E34.4 Constitutional tall stature
Constitutional gigantism

● **E34.5 Androgen insensitivity syndrome**

E34.50 Androgen insensitivity syndrome, unspecified
Androgen insensitivity NOS

E34.51 Complete androgen insensitivity syndrome
Complete androgen insensitivity
de Quervain syndrome
Goldberg-Maxwell syndrome

E34.52 Partial androgen insensitivity syndrome
Partial androgen insensitivity
Reifenstein syndrome

E34.8 Other specified endocrine disorders
Pineal gland dysfunction
Progeria

> Excludes2   pseudohypoparathyroidism (E20.1)

E34.9 Endocrine disorder, unspecified
Endocrine disturbance NOS
Hormone disturbance NOS

●◗ **E35 Disorders of endocrine glands in diseases classified elsewhere**

> Code first underlying disease, such as:
> late congenital syphilis of thymus gland [Dubois disease] (A50.5)
> tuberculous calcification of adrenal gland (B90.8)

> Excludes1   Echinococcus granulosus infection of thyroid gland (B67.3)
> meningococcal hemorrhagic adrenalitis (A39.1)
> syphilis of endocrine gland (A52.79)
> tuberculosis of adrenal gland, except calcification (A18.7)
> tuberculosis of endocrine gland NEC (A18.82)
> tuberculosis of thyroid gland (A18.81)
> Waterhouse-Friderichsen syndrome (A39.1)

CHAPTER 4 (E00-E90)

INTRAOPERATIVE COMPLICATIONS OF ENDOCRINE SYSTEM (E36)

● **E36**   **Intraoperative complications of endocrine system**

> **Excludes2**   postprocedural endocrine and metabolic complications and disorders, not elsewhere classified (E89.-)

   ● **E36.0**   **Intraoperative hemorrhage and hematoma of an endocrine system organ or structure complicating a procedure**

> **Excludes1**   intraoperative hemorrhage and hematoma of an endocrine system organ or structure due to accidental puncture or laceration during a procedure (E36.1-)

     E36.01   **Intraoperative hemorrhage and hematoma of an endocrine system organ or structure complicating an endocrine system procedure** 🔾

     E36.02   **Intraoperative hemorrhage and hematoma of an endocrine system organ or structure complicating other procedure** 🔾

   ● **E36.1**   **Accidental puncture and laceration of an endocrine system organ or structure during a procedure**

     E36.11   **Accidental puncture and laceration of an endocrine system organ or structure during an endocrine system procedure** 🔾

     E36.12   **Accidental puncture and laceration of an endocrine system organ or structure during other procedure** 🔾

     E36.8   **Other intraoperative complications of endocrine system**

> Use additional code, if applicable, to further specify disorder

MALNUTRITION (E40-E46)

> **Excludes1**   intestinal malabsorption (K90.-)
> sequelae of protein-calorie malnutrition (E64.0)

> **Excludes2**   nutritional anemias (D50-D53)
> starvation (T73.0)

E40   **Kwashiorkor** 🔾
Malnutrition produced by severe protein deficiency
Severe malnutrition with nutritional edema with dyspigmentation of skin and hair

> **Excludes1**   marasmic kwashiorkor (E42)

E41   **Nutritional marasmus** 🔾
Severe malnutrition with marasmus

> **Excludes1**   marasmic kwashiorkor (E42)

E42   **Marasmic kwashiorkor** 🔾
Severe protein malnutrition
Intermediate form severe protein-calorie malnutrition
Severe protein-calorie malnutrition with signs of both kwashiorkor and marasmus

■ **E43**   **Unspecified severe protein-calorie malnutrition** 🔾
Starvation edema

● **E44**   **Protein-calorie malnutrition of moderate and mild degree**

     E44.0   **Moderate protein-calorie malnutrition**

     E44.1   **Mild protein-calorie malnutrition**

E45   **Retarded development following protein-calorie malnutrition** 🔾
Nutritional short stature
Nutritional stunting
Physical retardation due to malnutrition

Item 4–6   **Bitot's spots** are the result of a buildup of keratin debris found on the superficial surface the conjunctiva; oval, triangular, or irregular in shape; and a sign of vitamin A deficiency and associated with night blindness. The disease may progress to **keratomalacia,** which can result in eventual prolapse of the iris and loss of the lens.

Figure 4-7   Bitot's spot on the conjunctiva.

■ **E46**   **Unspecified protein-calorie malnutrition** 🔾
Malnutrition NOS
Protein-calorie imbalance NOS

> **Excludes1**   nutritional deficiency NOS (E63.9)

OTHER NUTRITIONAL DEFICIENCIES (E50-E64)

> **Excludes2**   nutritional anemias (D50-D53)

● **E50**   **Vitamin A deficiency**

> **Excludes1**   sequelae of vitamin A deficiency (E64.1)

     E50.0   **Vitamin A deficiency with conjunctival xerosis**

     E50.1   **Vitamin A deficiency with Bitot's spot and conjunctival xerosis**
Bitot's spot in the young child

     E50.2   **Vitamin A deficiency with corneal xerosis**

     E50.3   **Vitamin A deficiency with corneal ulceration and xerosis**

     E50.4   **Vitamin A deficiency with keratomalacia**
Eye disorder that results in dry cornea caused by vitamin A deficiency

     E50.5   **Vitamin A deficiency with night blindness**

     E50.6   **Vitamin A deficiency with xerophthalmic scars of cornea**
Abnormal dryness and thickening of conjunctiva and cornea due to vitamin A deficiency

     E50.7   **Other ocular manifestations of vitamin A deficiency**
Xerophthalmia NOS

     E50.8   **Other manifestations of vitamin A deficiency**
Follicular keratosis
Xeroderma

   ■ **E50.9**   **Vitamin A deficiency, unspecified**
Hypovitaminosis A NOS

● **E51**   **Thiamine deficiency**

> **Excludes1**   sequelae of thiamine deficiency (E64.8)

   ● **E51.1**   **Beriberi**

     E51.11   **Dry beriberi** 🔾
Thiamine deficiency with nervous system manifestation most often caused by excessive alcohol consumption
Beriberi NOS
Beriberi with polyneuropathy

     E51.12   **Wet beriberi** 🔾
Thiamine deficiency with cardiovascular manifestation most often caused by excessive alcohol consumption
Beriberi with cardiovascular manifestations
Cardiovascular beriberi
Shoshin disease

     E51.2   **Wernicke's encephalopathy** 🔾
Acute disease of brain due to thiamine deficiency most often associated with excessive alcohol consumption

---

● Unacceptable Principal Diagnosis   ● Use Additional Character(s)   ■ Unspecified   ▶ Manifestation Code

OGCR   Official Guidelines for Coding and Reporting   Excludes 1   Excludes 2   Includes   Use additional   Code first   Code also

Figure 4-8 The sharply demarcated, characterstic scaling dermatitis of pellagra. (From Kumar: Robbins and Cotran: Pathologic Basis of Disease, 7th ed. 2005, Saunders, An Imprint of Elsevier.)

Item 4–7 Pellagra is associated with a deficiency of niacin and its precursor, **tryptophan.** Characteristics of the condition include diarrhea, dermatitis on exposed skin surfaces, dementia, and death. It is prevalent in developing countries where nutrition is inadequate. **Beriberi** is associated with thiamine deficiency.

E51.8   Other manifestations of thiamine deficiency 🔷

🔲 **E51.9   Thiamine deficiency, unspecified** 🔷

E52   Niacin deficiency [pellagra]
     Niacin (-tryptophan) deficiency
     Nicotinamide deficiency
     Pellagra (alcoholic)
     Excludes1   sequelae of niacin deficiency (E64.8)

⚫ **E53   Deficiency of other B group vitamins**
     Excludes1   sequelae of vitamin B deficiency (E64.8)

E53.0   Riboflavin deficiency 🔷
     Ariboflavinosis
     Vitamin B2 deficiency

E53.1   Pyridoxine deficiency
     Vitamin B6 deficiency
     Excludes1   pyridoxine-responsive sideroblastic anemia (D64.3)

E53.8   Deficiency of other specified B group vitamins
     Biotin deficiency
     Cyanocobalamin deficiency
     Folate deficiency
     Folic acid deficiency
     Pantothenic acid deficiency
     Vitamin B12 deficiency
     Excludes1   folate deficiency anemia (D52.-)
                   vitamin B12 deficiency anemia (D51.-)

🔲 **E53.9   Vitamin B deficiency, unspecified**

E54   Ascorbic acid deficiency
     Deficiency of vitamin C
     Scurvy
     Excludes1   scorbutic anemia (D53.2)
                   sequelae of vitamin C deficiency (E64.2)

⚫ **E55   Vitamin D deficiency**
     Excludes1   adult osteomalacia (M83.-)
                   osteoporosis (M80-)
                   sequelae of rickets (E64.3)

E55.0   Rickets, active 🔷
     Infantile osteomalacia
     Juvenile osteomalacia
     Softening of bone
     Excludes1   celiac rickets (K90.0)
                   Crohn's rickets (K50.-)
                   hereditary vitamin D-dependent rickets (E83.32)
                   inactive rickets (E64.3)
                   renal rickets (N25.0)
                   sequelae of rickets (E64.3)
                   vitamin D-resistant rickets (E83.31)

🔲 **E55.9   Vitamin D deficiency, unspecified**
     Avitaminosis D

⚫ **E56   Other vitamin deficiencies**
     Excludes1   sequelae of other vitamin deficiencies (E64.8)

E56.0   Deficiency of vitamin E

E56.1   Deficiency of vitamin K
     Excludes1   deficiency of coagulation factor due to vitamin K deficiency (D68.4)
                   vitamin K deficiency of newborn (P53)

E56.8   Deficiency of other vitamins

🔲 **E56.9   Vitamin deficiency, unspecified**

E58   Dietary calcium deficiency
     Excludes1   disorders of calcium metabolism (E83.5-)
                   sequelae of calcium deficiency (E64.8)

E59   Dietary selenium deficiency
     Keshan disease
     Excludes1   sequelae of selenium deficiency (E64.8)

E60   Dietary zinc deficiency

⚫ **E61   Deficiency of other nutrient elements**
     Use additional code for adverse effect, if applicable, to identify drug (T36-T50 with fifth or sixth character 5)
     Excludes1   disorders of mineral metabolism (E83.-)
                   iodine deficiency related thyroid disorders (E00-E02)
                   sequelae of malnutrition and other nutritional deficiencies (E64.-)

E61.0   Copper deficiency

E61.1   Iron deficiency
     Excludes1   iron deficiency anemia (D50.-)

E61.2   Magnesium deficiency

E61.3   Manganese deficiency

E61.4   Chromium deficiency

E61.5   Molybdenum deficiency

E61.6   Vanadium deficiency

E61.7   Deficiency of multiple nutrient elements

E61.8   Deficiency of other specified nutrient elements

🔲 **E61.9   Deficiency of nutrient element, unspecified**

⚫ **E63   Other nutritional deficiencies**
     Excludes1   dehydration (E86.0)
                   failure to thrive, adult (R62.7)
                   failure to thrive, child (R62.51)
                   feeding problems in newborn (P92.-)
                   sequelae of malnutrition and other nutritional deficiencies (E64.-)

E63.0   Essential fatty acid [EFA] deficiency

E63.1   Imbalance of constituents of food intake

E63.8   Other specified nutritional deficiencies

🔲 **E63.9   Nutritional deficiency, unspecified**

⚫ **E64   Sequelae of malnutrition and other nutritional deficiencies**
     Pathological condition resulting from disease, injury, or other trauma

     Note: This category is to be used to indicate conditions in categories E43, E44, E46, E50-E63 as the cause of sequelae, which are themselves classified elsewhere. The 'sequelae' include conditions specified as such; they also include the late effects of diseases classifiable to the above categories if the disease itself is no longer present

     Code first condition resulting from (sequela) of malnutrition and other nutritional deficiencies

⚫ **E64.0   Sequelae of protein-calorie malnutrition** 🔷
     Excludes2   retarded development following protein-calorie malnutrition (E45)

N   Newborn Age: 0   **P**   Pediatric Age: 0–17   **M**   Maternity DX: 12–55   **A**   Adult Age: 15–124   ♀   Females Only   ♂   Males Only

🔷   Complication\Comorbidity   🔷   Major C\C   🔷   Present on Admission Requirement   🔷   Hospital-Acquired Condition

*(right margin, vertical)* CHAPTER 4 (E00-E90)

- **E64.1** Sequelae of vitamin A deficiency
- **E64.2** Sequelae of vitamin C deficiency
- **E64.3** Sequelae of rickets
- **E64.8** Sequelae of other nutritional deficiencies
- **E64.9** Sequelae of unspecified nutritional deficiency

OVERWEIGHT, OBESITY AND OTHER HYPERALIMENTATION (E65-E68)

E65 Localized adiposity
Fat pad

E66 Overweight and obesity
Code first obesity complicating pregnancy, childbirth and the puerperium, if applicable (O99.21-)
Use additional code to identify body mass index (BMI), if known (Z68.-)
Excludes1 adiposogenital dystrophy (E23.6)
lipomatosis NOS (E88.2)
lipomatosis dolorosa [Dercum] (E88.2)
Prader-Willi syndrome (Q87.1)

E66.0 Obesity due to excess calories
E66.01 Morbid (severe) obesity due to excess calories
Excludes1 morbid (severe) obesity with alveolar hypoventilation (E66.2)
E66.09 Other obesity due to excess calories
MCE: Questionable admission when principal dx

E66.1 Drug-induced obesity
MCE: Questionable admission when principal dx
Use additional code for adverse effect, if applicable, to identify drug (T36-T50 with fifth or sixth character 5)

E66.2 Morbid (severe) obesity with alveolar hypoventilation
Uncommon condition of unknown cause leading to inadequate ventilation in lungs, even though lungs and airways are normal
Pickwickian syndrome

E66.3 Overweight
E66.8 Other obesity
MCE: Questionable admission when principal dx
E66.9 Obesity, unspecified
Obesity NOS
MCE: Questionable admission when principal dx

E67 Other hyperalimentation
Ingestion of more than optimal amount of nutrients
Excludes1 hyperalimentation NOS (R63.2)
sequelae of hyperalimentation (E68)
E67.0 Hypervitaminosis A
E67.1 Hypercarotinemia
E67.2 Megavitamin-B6 syndrome
E67.3 Hypervitaminosis D
E67.8 Other specified hyperalimentation

E68 Sequelae of hyperalimentation
Code first condition resulting from (sequela) of hyperalimentation

METABOLIC DISORDERS (E70-E88)

Excludes1 androgen insensitivity syndrome (E34.5-)
congenital adrenal hyperplasia (E25.0)
Ehlers-Danlos syndrome (Q79.6)
hemolytic anemias attributable to enzyme disorders (D55.-)
Marfan's syndrome (Q87.4)
5-alpha-reductase deficiency (E29.1)

E70 Disorders of aromatic amino-acid metabolism
E70.0 Classical phenylketonuria
Inherited disorder that increases to harmful levels amino acid phenylalanine
E70.1 Other hyperphenylalaninemias
E70.2 Disorders of tyrosine metabolism
Excludes1 transitory tyrosinemia of newborn (P74.5)
E70.20 Disorder of tyrosine metabolism, unspecified
Tyrosine: Nonessential amino acid occurring in most proteins
E70.21 Tyrosinemia
Congenital amino acid metabolism
Hypertyrosinemia
E70.29 Other disorders of tyrosine metabolism
Alkaptonuria
Ochronosis

E70.3 Albinism
Congenital condition of reduced or absent pigment in eyes, skin, and hair
E70.30 Albinism, unspecified
E70.31 Ocular albinism
E70.310 X-linked ocular albinism
E70.311 Autosomal recessive ocular albinism
E70.318 Other ocular albinism
E70.319 Ocular albinism, unspecified
E70.32 Oculocutaneous albinism
Partial or total lack of melanin pigment in eyes
Excludes1 Chediak-Higashi syndrome (E70.330)
Hermansky-Pudlak syndrome (E70.331)
E70.320 Tyrosinase negative oculocutaneous albinism
Albinism I
Oculocutaneous albinism ty-neg
E70.321 Tyrosinase positive oculocutaneous albinism
Albinism II
Oculocutaneous albinism ty-pos
E70.328 Other oculocutaneous albinism
Cross syndrome
E70.329 Oculocutaneous albinism, unspecified
E70.33 Albinism with hematologic abnormality
E70.330 Chediak-Higashi syndrome
E70.331 Hermansky-Pudlak syndrome
E70.338 Other albinism with hematologic abnormality
E70.339 Albinism with hematologic abnormality, unspecified
E70.39 Other specified albinism
Piebaldism

● **E70.4　Disorders of histidine metabolism**
◼ **E70.40　Disorders of histidine metabolism, unspecified** 🗗
　　E70.41　Histidinemia 🗗
　　E70.49　Other disorders of histidine metabolism 🗗
E70.5　Disorders of tryptophan metabolism 🗗
E70.8　Other disorders of aromatic amino-acid metabolism 🗗
◼ **E70.9　Disorder of aromatic amino-acid metabolism, unspecified** 🗗

● **E71　Disorders of branched-chain amino-acid metabolism and fatty-acid metabolism**

　E71.0　Maple-syrup-urine disease 🗗
　　Due to defect in amino acid catabolism, causing severe ketoacidosis with smell of maple syrup in urine and on body

● **E71.1　Other disorders of branched-chain amino-acid metabolism**
　● **E71.11　Branched-chain organic acidurias**
　　　E71.110　Isovaleric acidemia 🗗
　　　E71.111　3-methylglutaconic aciduria 🗗
　　　E71.118　Other branched-chain organic acidurias 🗗
　● **E71.12　Disorders of propionate metabolism**
　　　E71.120　Methylmalonic acidemia 🗗
　　　E71.121　Propionic acidemia 🗗
　　　E71.128　Other disorders of propionate metabolism 🗗
　　E71.19　Other disorders of branched-chain amino-acid metabolism 🗗
　　　　Hyperleucine-isoleucinemia
　　　　Hypervalinemia

◼ **E71.2　Disorder of branched-chain amino-acid metabolism, unspecified** 🗗

● **E71.3　Disorders of fatty-acid metabolism**
　┌─────────┐
　│ **Excludes1** │　peroxisomal disorders (E71.5)
　└─────────┘　　Refsum's disease (G60.1)
　　　　　　　　　Schilder's disease (G37.0)
　┌─────────┐
　│ **Excludes2** │　carnitine deficiency due to inborn error of metabolism (E71.42)
　└─────────┘

◼ **E71.30　Disorder of fatty-acid metabolism, unspecified**
　● **E71.31　Disorders of fatty-acid oxidation**
　　　E71.310　Long chain/very long chain acyl CoA dehydrogenase deficiency 🗗
　　　　　LCAD
　　　　　VLCAD
　　　E71.311　Medium chain acyl CoA dehydrogenase deficiency 🗗
　　　　　MCAD
　　　E71.312　Short chain acyl CoA dehydrogenase deficiency 🗗
　　　　　SCAD
　　　E71.313　Glutaric aciduria type II 🗗
　　　　　Glutaric aciduria type II A
　　　　　Glutaric aciduria type II B
　　　　　Glutaric aciduria type II C
　　　　┌─────────┐
　　　　│ **Excludes1** │　glutaric aciduria (type 1) NOS (E72.3)
　　　　└─────────┘

　　　E71.314　Muscle carnitine palmitoyltransferase deficiency 🗗
　　　E71.318　Other disorders of fatty-acid oxidation 🗗
　　E71.32　Disorders of ketone metabolism 🗗
　　E71.39　Other disorders of fatty-acid metabolism 🗗

● **E71.4　Disorders of carnitine metabolism**
　┌─────────┐
　│ **Excludes1** │　muscle carnitine palmitoyltransferase deficiency (E71.314)
　└─────────┘
◼ **E71.40　Disorder of carnitine metabolism, unspecified**
　　E71.41　Primary carnitine deficiency
　　E71.42　Carnitine deficiency due to inborn errors of metabolism
　　　　Code also associated inborn error or metabolism
　　E71.43　Iatrogenic carnitine deficiency
　　　　Iatrogenic: Outcomes from activity of physicians
　　　　Carnitine deficiency due to:
　　　　　hemodialysis
　　　　　Valproic acid therapy
● **E71.44　Other secondary carnitine deficiency**
　　　E71.440　Ruvalcaba-Myhre-Smith syndrome
　　　E71.448　Other secondary carnitine deficiency

● **E71.5　Peroxisomal disorders**
　　Class of conditions which lead to disorders of lipid metabolism
　┌─────────┐
　│ **Excludes1** │　Schilder's disease (G37.0)
　└─────────┘
◼ **E71.50　Peroxisomal disorder, unspecified** 🗗
　● **E71.51　Disorders of peroxisome biogenesis**
　　　　Group 1 peroxisomal disorders
　　　┌─────────┐
　　　│ **Excludes1** │　Refsum's disease (G60.1)
　　　└─────────┘
　　　E71.510　Zellweger syndrome 🗗
　　　E71.511　Neonatal adrenoleukodystrophy 🗗　　　**N**
　　　　┌─────────┐
　　　　│ **Excludes1** │　X-linked adreno-leukodystro-phy (E71.42-)
　　　　└─────────┘
　　　E71.518　Other disorders of peroxisome biogenesis 🗗
　● **E71.52　X-linked adrenoleukodystrophy**
　　　E71.520　Childhood cerebral X-linked adrenoleukodystrophy 🗗
　　　E71.521　Adolescent X-linked adrenoleukodystrophy 🗗
　　　E71.522　Adrenomyeloneuropathy 🗗
　　　E71.528　Other X-linked adrenoleukodystrophy 🗗
　　　　Addison only phenotype adrenoleukodystrophy
　　　　Addison-Schilder adrenoleukodystrophy
　◼ **E71.529　X-linked adrenoleukodystrophy, unspecified type** 🗗
　　E71.53　Other group 2 peroxisomal disorders 🗗

N Newborn Age: 0　　**P** Pediatric Age: 0–17　　**M** Maternity DX: 12–55　　**A** Adult Age: 15–124　　♀ Females Only　　♂ Males Only
🗗 Complication\Comorbidity　　🗗 Major C\C　　🗗 Present on Admission Requirement　　🗗 Hospital-Acquired Condition

899

CHAPTER 4 (E00-E90)

● **E71.54 Other peroxisomal disorders**

E71.540 **Rhizomelic chondrodysplasia punctata** 🕮
Rare, severe, inherited disorder with limb shortening, bone and cartilage abnormalities, abnormal facial appearance, severe mental retardation, psychomotor retardation, and cataracts

Excludes1 chondrodysplasia punctata NOS (Q77.3)

E71.541 **Zellweger-like syndrome** 🕮

E71.542 **Other group 3 peroxisomal disorders** 🕮

E71.548 **Other peroxisomal disorders** 🕮

● **E72 Other disorders of amino-acid metabolism**

Excludes1 disorders of:
aromatic amino-acid metabolism (E70.-)
branched-chain amino-acid metabolism (E71.0-E71.2)
fatty-acid metabolism (E71.3)
purine and pyrimidine metabolism (E79.-)
gout (M1A-, M10.-)

● **E72.0 Disorders of amino-acid transport**

Excludes1 disorders of tryptophan metabolism (E70.5)

■ E72.00 **Disorders of amino-acid transport, unspecified** 🕮

E72.01 **Cystinuria** 🕮
Hereditary aminoaciduria due to impairment of renal transport with predominant symptom of urinary cystine calculi

E72.02 **Hartnup's disease** 🕮
Inborn error of metabolism

E72.03 **Lowe's syndrome** 🕮
X-linked disorder with rickets, hydrophthalmia, congenital glaucoma, cataracts, mental retardation, and renal tubule dysfunction

Use additional code for associated glaucoma (H42)

E72.04 **Cystinosis** 🕮
Genetic disease with excessive depostits of amino acid cystine in cells
Fanconi (-de Toni) (-Debré) syndrome with cystinosis

Excludes1 Fanconi (-de Toni) (-Debré) syndrome without cystinosis (E72.09)

E72.09 **Other disorders of amino-acid transport** 🕮
Fanconi (-de Toni) (-Debré) syndrome, unspecified

● **E72.1 Disorders of sulfur-bearing amino-acid metabolism**

Excludes1 cystinosis (E72.04)
cystinuria (E72.01)
transcobalamin II deficiency (D51.2)

■ E72.10 **Disorders of sulfur-bearing amino-acid metabolism, unspecified** 🕮

E72.11 **Homocystinuria** 🕮
Cystathionine synthase deficiency

E72.12 **Methylenetetrahydrofolate reductase deficiency** 🕮

E72.19 **Other disorders of sulfur-bearing amino-acid metabolism** 🕮
Cystathioninuria
Methioninemia
Sulfite oxidase deficiency

● **E72.2 Disorders of urea cycle metabolism**

Excludes1 disorders of ornithine metabolism (E72.4)

■ E72.20 **Disorder of urea cycle metabolism, unspecified** 🕮
Hyperammonemia
Elevated levels of ammonia

Excludes1 hyperammonemia-hyperornithinemia-homocitrullinemia syndrome E72.4
transient hyperammonemia of newborn (P74.6)

E72.21 **Argininemia** 🕮
Disorder in which deficiency of enzyme arginase causes build up of arginine and ammonia in blood

E72.22 **Arginosuccinic aciduria** 🕮
Gene disorder of urea cycle resulting accumulation of ammonia

E72.23 **Citrullinemia** 🕮
Urea cycle disorder that causes ammonia and other toxic substances to accumulate in blood

E72.29 **Other disorders of urea cycle metabolism** 🕮

E72.3 Disorders of lysine and hydroxylysine metabolism 🕮
Glutaric aciduria NOS
Glutaric aciduria (type I)
Hydroxylysinemia
Hyperlysinemia

Excludes1 glutaric aciduria type II (E71.313)
Refsum's disease (G60.1)
Zellweger syndrome (E71.510)

E72.4 Disorders of ornithine metabolism 🕮
Hyperammonemia-Hyperornithinemia-Homocitrullinemia syndrome
Ornithinemia (types I, II)
Ornithine transcarbamylase deficiency

Excludes1 hereditary choroidal dystrophy (H31.2-)

● **E72.5 Disorders of glycine metabolism**

■ E72.50 **Disorder of glycine metabolism, unspecified** 🕮

E72.51 **Non-ketotic hyperglycinemia** 🕮

E72.52 **Trimethylaminuria** 🕮

E72.53 **Hyperoxaluria** 🕮
Oxalosis
Oxaluria

E72.59 **Other disorders of glycine metabolism** 🕮
D-glycericacidemia
Hyperhydroxyprolinemia
Hyperprolinemia (types I, II)
Sarcosinemia

E72.8 Other specified disorders of amino-acid metabolism 🕮
Disorders of beta-amino-acid metabolism
Disorders of gamma-glutamyl cycle

■ **E72.9 Disorder of amino-acid metabolism, unspecified** 🕮

● Unacceptable Principal Diagnosis   ● Use Additional Character(s)   ■ Unspecified   ▶ Manifestation Code
OGCR Official Guidelines for Coding and Reporting   Excludes 1   Excludes 2   Includes   Use additional   Code first   Code also

● **E73**   **Lactose intolerance**
     Intolerance for lactose, due to inherited deficiency of lactase
     activity in intestinal mucosa

   E73.0   **Congenital lactase deficiency**

   E73.1   **Secondary lactase deficiency**

   E73.8   **Other lactose intolerance**

   ▪ **E73.9**   **Lactose intolerance, unspecified**

● **E74**   **Other disorders of carbohydrate metabolism**
    | **Excludes1** | diabetes mellitus (E08-E13)
                   hypoglycemia NOS (E16.2)
                   increased secretion of glucagon (E16.3)
                   mucopolysaccharidosis (E76.0-E76.3)

● **E74.0**   **Glycogen storage disease**

   ▪ **E74.00**   **Glycogen storage disease, unspecified** 🔹

   E74.01   **von Gierke's disease** 🔹
         Type I glycogen storage disease

   E74.02   **Pompe disease** 🔹
         Cardiac glycogenosis
         Type II glycogen storage disease

   E74.03   **Cori disease** 🔹
         Forbes' disease
         Type III glycogen storage disease

   E74.04   **McArdle disease** 🔹
         Type V glycogen storage disease

   E74.09   **Other glycogen storage disease** 🔹
         Andersen disease
         Hers disease
         Tauri disease
         Glycogen storage disease, types 0, IV, VI-XI
         Liver phosphorylase deficiency
         Muscle phosphofructokinase deficiency

● **E74.1**   **Disorders of fructose metabolism**
    | **Excludes1** | muscle phosphofructokinase
                   deficiency (E74.09)

   ▪ **E74.10**   **Disorder of fructose metabolism,**
              unspecified

   E74.11   **Essential fructosuria**
         Fructokinase deficiency

   E74.12   **Hereditary fructose intolerance**
         Fructosemia

   E74.19   **Other disorders of fructose metabolism**
         Fructose-1, 6-diphosphatase deficiency

● **E74.2**   **Disorders of galactose metabolism**

   ▪ **E74.20**   **Disorders of galactose metabolism,**
              unspecified 🔹

   E74.21   **Galactosemia** 🔹
         Genetic disorders resulting from defective
         simple sugar (galactose) metabolism

   E74.29   **Other disorders of galactose metabolism** 🔹
         Galactokinase deficiency

● **E74.3**   **Other disorders of intestinal carbohydrate**
      absorption
    | **Excludes2** | lactose intolerance (E73.-)

   E74.31   **Sucrase-isomaltase deficiency**
         Deficiency in metabolism in intestinal mucosa
         results in malabsorption of sucrose and
         starch

   E74.39   **Other disorders of intestinal carbohydrate**
              absorption
         Disorder of intestinal carbohydrate
            absorption NOS
         Glucose-galactose malabsorption
         Sucrase deficiency

E74.4   **Disorders of pyruvate metabolism and**
      gluconeogenesis 🔹
         Deficiency of phosphoenolpyruvate
            carboxykinase
         Deficiency of pyruvate carboxylase
         Deficiency of pyruvate dehydrogenase
    | **Excludes1** | disorders of pyruvate metabolism
                   and gluconeogenesis with
                   anemia (D55.-)
                   Leigh's syndrome (G31.82)

E74.8   **Other specified disorders of carbohydrate**
      metabolism 🔹
         Essential pentosuria
         Renal glycosuria

▪ **E74.9**   **Disorder of carbohydrate metabolism, unspecif**

● **E75**   **Disorders of sphingolipid metabolism and other lipid**
     storage disorders
    | **Excludes1** | mucolipidosis, types I-III (E77.0-E77.1)
                   Refsum's disease (G60.1)

● **E75.0**   **GM2 gangliosidosis**
      Rare metabolic disorder that causes destruction of
      nerve cells of brain and spinal cord

   ▪ **E75.00**   **GM2 gangliosidosis, unspecified** 🔹

   E75.01   **Sandhoff disease** 🔹

   E75.02   **Tay-Sachs disease** 🔹

   E75.09   **Other GM2 gangliosidosis** 🔹
         Adult GM2 gangliosidosis
         Juvenile GM2 gangliosidosis

● **E75.1**   **Other and unspecified gangliosidosis**

   ▪ **E75.10**   **Unspecified gangliosidosis** 🔹
           Gangliosidosis NOS

   E75.11   **Mucolipidosis IV** 🔹
         Disorder with symptoms of psychomotor
         retardation and severe visual impairment

   E75.19   **Other gangliosidosis** 🔹
         GM1 gangliosidosis
         GM3 gangliosidosis

● **E75.2**   **Other sphingolipidosis**
      Lysosomal (a particle in a cytoplasm cell that contains
      digestive enzymes) storage diseases with
      symptoms of abnormal storage of amino acids
    | **Excludes1** | adrenoleukodystrophy [Addison-
                   Schilder] (E71.528)

   E75.21   **Fabry (-Anderson) disease**

   E75.22   **Gaucher disease**

   E75.23   **Krabbe disease** 🔹

   ● **E75.24**   **Niemann-Pick disease**

     E75.240   **Niemann-Pick disease type A**

     E75.241   **Niemann-Pick disease type B**

     E75.242   **Niemann-Pick disease type C**

     E75.243   **Niemann-Pick disease type D**

     E75.248   **Other Niemann-Pick disease**

     ▪ **E75.249**   **Niemann-Pick disease,**
                unspecified

   E75.25   **Metachromatic leukodystrophy** 🔹

   E75.29   **Other sphingolipidosis** 🔹
         Farber's syndrome
         Sulfatase deficiency
         Sulfatide lipidosis

▪ **E75.3**   **Sphingolipidosis, unspecified**

N   Newborn Age: 0   **P**   Pediatric Age: 0–17   **M**   Maternity DX: 12–55   **A**   Adult Age: 15–124   ♀   Females Only   ♂   Males Only

🔹   Complication\Comorbidity   🔹   Major C\C   🔹   Present on Admission Requirement   🔹   Hospital-Acquired Condition

901

Item 48 Leukodystrophy is characterized by degeneration and/or failure of the myelin formation of the central nervous system and sometimes of the peripheral nervous system. The disease is inherited and progressive.

E75.4 Neuronal ceroid lipofuscinosis 🔵
     Batten disease
     Bielschowsky-Jansky disease
     Kufs disease
     Spielmeyer-Vogt disease

E75.5 Other lipid storage disorders
     Cerebrotendinous cholesterosis [van Bogaert-
         Scherer-Epstein]
     Wolman's disease

E75.6 Lipid storage disorder, unspecified

● E76 Disorders of glycosaminoglycan metabolism

   ● E76.0 Mucopolysaccharidosis, type I
       Inborn metabolic disorder of enzymes that break down
         carbohydrates

     E76.01 Hurler's syndrome 🔵

     E76.02 Hurler-Scheie syndrome 🔵

     E76.03 Scheie's syndrome 🔵

   E76.1 Mucopolysaccharidosis, type II 🔵
       Inborn metabolic disorder of enzymes that break down
         carbohydrates occurs in 2-4 year old males
       Hunter's syndrome

   ● E76.2 Other mucopolysaccharidoses

     ● E76.21 Morquio mucopolysaccharidoses

       E76.210 Morquio A
           mucopolysaccharidoses 🔵
           Classic Morquio syndrome
           Morquio syndrome A
           Mucopolysaccharidosis, type IVA

       E76.211 Morquio B
           mucopolysaccharidoses 🔵
           Morquio-like
             mucopolysaccharidoses
           Morquio-like syndrome
           Morquio syndrome B
           Mucopolysaccharidosis, type IVB

       ■ E76.219 Morquio mucopolysaccharidoses,
           unspecified 🔵
           Morquio syndrome
           Mucopolysaccharidosis, type IV

     E76.22 Sanfilippo mucopolysaccharidoses 🔵
       Mucopolysaccharidosis, type III (A) (B)
         (C) (D)
       Sanfilippo A syndrome
       Sanfilippo B syndrome
       Sanfilippo C syndrome
       Sanfilippo D syndrome

     ■ E76.29 Other mucopolysaccharidoses 🔵
       beta-Glucuronidase deficiency
       Maroteaux-Lamy (mild) (severe)
         syndrome
       Mucopolysaccharidosis, types VI, VII

   E76.3 Mucopolysaccharidosis, unspecified 🔵

   E76.8 Other disorders of glycosaminoglycan
      metabolism 🔵

   ■ E76.9 Glucosaminoglycan metabolism disorder,
      unspecified 🔵

● E77 Disorders of glycoprotein metabolism

   E77.0 Defects in post-translational modification of
      lysosomal enzymes
      Mucolipidosis II [I-cell disease]
      Mucolipidosis III [pseudo-Hurler polydystrophy]

   E77.1 Defects in glycoprotein degradation 🔵
      Aspartylglucosaminuria
      Fucosidosis
      Mannosidosis
      Sialidosis [mucolipidosis I]

   E77.8 Other disorders of glycoprotein metabolism

   ■ E77.9 Disorder of glycoprotein metabolism, unspecified

● E78 Disorders of lipoprotein metabolism and other lipidemias
   | Excludes1 | sphingolipidosis (E75.0-E75.3)

   E78.0 Pure hypercholesterolemia
      Familial hypercholesterolemia
      Fredrickson's hyperlipoproteinemia, type IIa
      Hyperbetalipoproteinemia
      Hyperlipidemia, Group A
      Low-density-lipoprotein-type [LDL]
        hyperlipoproteinemia

   E78.1 Pure hyperglyceridemia
      Elevated fasting triglycerides
      Endogenous hyperglyceridemia
      Fredrickson's hyperlipoproteinemia, type IV
      Hyperlipidemia, group B
      Hyperprebetalipoproteinemia
      Very-low-density-lipoprotein-type [VLDL]
        hyperlipoproteinemia

   E78.2 Mixed hyperlipidemia
      Broad- or floating-betalipoproteinemia
      Combined hyperlipidemia NOS
      Elevated cholesterol with elevated triglycerides NEC
      Fredrickson's hyperlipoproteinemia, type IIb or III
      Hyperbetalipoproteinemia with
        prebetalipoproteinemia
      Hypercholesteremia with endogenous
        hyperglyceridemia
      Hyperlipidemia, group C
      Tubo-eruptive xanthoma
      Xanthoma tuberosum

     | Excludes1 | cerebrotendinous cholesterosis [van
           Bogaert-Scherer-Epstein] (E75.5)
           familial combined hyperlipidemia
           (E78.4)

   E78.3 Hyperchylomicronemia
      Chylomicron retention disease
      Fredrickson's hyperlipoproteinemia, type I or V
      Hyperlipidemia, group D
      Mixed hyperglyceridemia

   E78.4 Other hyperlipidemia
      Familial combined hyperlipidemia

   ■ E78.5 Hyperlipidemia, unspecified

   E78.6 Lipoprotein deficiency
      Abetalipoproteinemia
      Depressed HDL cholesterol
      High-density lipoprotein deficiency
      Hypoalphalipoproteinemia
      Hypobetalipoproteinemia (familial)
      Lecithin cholesterol acyltransferase deficiency
      Tangier disease

CHAPTER 4 (E00-E90)

● Unacceptable Principal Diagnosis   ● Use Additional Character(s)   ■ Unspecified   ▶ Manifestation Code

902   **OGCR** Official Guidelines for Coding and Reporting | Excludes 1 | | Excludes 2 | Includes   Use additional   Code first   Code also

- E78.7　**Disorders of bile acid and cholesterol metabolism**
  - **Excludes1**　Niemann-Pick disease type C (E75.242)
  - ■ E78.70　**Disorder of bile acid and cholesterol metabolism, unspecified**
  - E78.71　**Barth syndrome** 🦠 ⬡
  - E78.72　**Smith-Lemli-Opitz syndrome** 🦠 ⬡
  - E78.79　**Other disorders of bile acid and cholesterol metabolism**
- E78.8　**Other disorders of lipoprotein metabolism**
  - E78.81　**Lipoid dermatoarthritis**
  - ■ E78.89　**Other lipoprotein metabolism disorders**
- E78.9　**Disorder of lipoprotein metabolism, unspecified**

- E79　**Disorders of purine and pyrimidine metabolism**
  Purines, along with pyrimidines, signal RNA and DNA production
  - **Excludes1**　Ataxia-telangiectasia (Q87.1)
    Bloom's syndrome (Q82.8)
    Cockayne's syndrome (Q87.1)
    calculus of kidney (N20.0)
    combined immunodeficiency disorders (D81.-)
    Fanconi's anemia (D61.09)
    gout (M1A-M10.-)
    orotaciduric anemia (D53.0)
    progeria (E34.8)
    Werner's syndrome (E34.8)
    xeroderma pigmentosum (Q82.1)
  - E79.0　**Hyperuricemia without signs of inflammatory arthritis and tophaceous disease**
    Asymptomatic hyperuricemia
  - E79.1　**Lesch-Nyhan syndrome** 🦠
    HGPRT deficiency
  - E79.2　**Myoadenylate deaminase deficiency** 🦠
  - E79.8　**Other disorders of purine and pyrimidine metabolism** 🦠
    Hereditary xanthinuria
  - ■ E79.9　**Disorder of purine and pyrimidine metabolism, unspecified** 🦠

- E80　**Disorders of porphyrin and bilirubin metabolism**
  Group of chemical compounds in RBC's that combine with iron to form heme
  - **Includes**　defects of catalase and peroxidase
  - E80.0　**Hereditary erythropoietic porphyria** 🦠
    Congenital erythropoietic porphyria
    Erythropoietic protoporphyria
  - E80.1　**Porphyria cutanea tarda** 🦠
  - E80.2　**Other and unspecified porphyria**
    - ■ E80.20　**Unspecified porphyria** 🦠
      Porphyria NOS
    - E80.21　**Acute intermittent (hepatic) porphyria** 🦠
    - E80.29　**Other porphyria** 🦠
      Hereditary coproporphyria
  - E80.3　**Defects of catalase and peroxidase** 🦠
    Acatalasia [Takahara]
  - E80.4　**Gilbert syndrome**
  - E80.5　**Crigler-Najjar syndrome**
  - E80.6　**Other disorders of bilirubin metabolism**
    Dubin-Johnson syndrome
    Rotor's syndrome
  - ■ E80.7　**Disorder of bilirubin metabolism, unspecified**

- E83　**Disorders of mineral metabolism**
  - **Excludes1**　dietary mineral deficiency (E58-E61)
    parathyroid disorders (E20-E21)
    vitamin D deficiency (E55.-)
  - E83.0　**Disorders of copper metabolism**
    - ■ E83.00　**Disorder of copper metabolism, unspecified**
    - E83.01　**Wilson's disease**
      Code also associated Kayser Fleischer ring (H18.04-)
    - E83.09　**Other disorders of copper metabolism**
      Menkes' (kinky hair) (steely hair) disease
  - E83.1　**Disorders of iron metabolism**
    - **Excludes1**　iron deficiency anemia (D50.-)
      sideroblastic anemia (D64.0-D64.3)
    - ■ E83.10　**Disorder of iron metabolism, unspecified**
    - E83.11　**Hemochromatosis**
      - E83.110　**Hereditary hemochromatosis**
        Bronzed diabetes
        Pigmentary cirrhosis (of liver)
        Primary (hereditary) hemochromatosis
      - E83.111　**Hemochromatosis due to repeated red blood cell transfusions**
        Iron overload due to repeated red blood cell transfusions
        Transfusion (red blood cell) associated hemochromatosis
      - E83.118　**Other hemochromatosis**
      - ■ E83.119　**Hemochromatosis, unspecified**
    - E83.19　**Other disorders of iron metabolism**
      Use additional code, if applicable, for idiopathic pulmonary hemosiderosis (J84.03)
  - E83.2　**Disorders of zinc metabolism**
    Acrodermatitis enteropathica
  - E83.3　**Disorders of phosphorus metabolism and phosphatases**
    - **Excludes1**　adult osteomalacia (M83.-)
      osteoporosis (M80-)
    - ■ E83.30　**Disorder of phosphorus metabolism, unspecified**
    - E83.31　**Familial hypophosphatemia**
      Vitamin D-resistant osteomalacia
      Vitamin D-resistant rickets
      - **Excludes1**　vitamin D-deficiency rickets (E55.0)
    - E83.32　**Hereditary vitamin D-dependent rickets (type 1) (type 2)**
      25-hydroxyvitamin D 1-alpha-hydroxylase deficiency
      Pseudovitamin D deficiency
      Vitamin D receptor defect
    - E83.39　**Other disorders of phosphorus metabolism**
      Acid phosphatase deficiency
      Hypophosphatasia

N Newborn Age: 0　**P** Pediatric Age: 0–17　**M** Maternity DX: 12–55　**A** Adult Age: 15–124　♀ Females Only　♂ Males Only

🦠 Complication\Comorbidity　🦠 Major C\C　⬡ Present on Admission Requirement　⬡ Hospital-Acquired Condition

903

CHAPTER 4 (E00-E90)

E83.4 **Disorders of magnesium metabolism**

E83.40 **Disorders of magnesium metabolism, unspecified**

E83.41 **Hypermagnesemia**

E83.42 **Hypomagnesemia**

E83.49 **Other disorders of magnesium metabolism**

E83.5 **Disorders of calcium metabolism**

Excludes1   chondrocalcinosis (M11.1-M11.2)
hungry bone syndrome (E83.81)
hyperparathyroidism (E21.0-E21.3)

E83.50 **Unspecified disorder of calcium metabolism**

E83.51 **Hypocalcemia**

E83.52 **Hypercalcemia**
Familial hypocalciuric hypercalcemia

E83.59 **Other disorders of calcium metabolism**
Idiopathic hypercalciuria

E83.8 **Other disorders of mineral metabolism**

E83.81 **Hungry bone syndrome**

E83.89 **Other disorders of mineral metabolism**

E83.9 **Disorder of mineral metabolism, unspecified**

E84 **Cystic fibrosis**

Includes   mucoviscidosis

E84.0 **Cystic fibrosis with pulmonary manifestations** 🔖

Use additional code to identify any infectious organism present, such as:
Pseudomonas (B96.5)

E84.1 **Cystic fibrosis with intestinal manifestations**

E84.11 **Meconium ileus in cystic fibrosis** 🔖   N

Excludes1   meconium ileus not due to cystic fibrosis (P76.0)

E84.19 **Cystic fibrosis with other intestinal manifestations** 🔖
Distal intestinal obstruction syndrome

E84.8 **Cystic fibrosis with other manifestations** 🔖

E84.9 **Cystic fibrosis, unspecified** 🔖

E85 **Amyloidosis**
A disorder resulting from the abnormal deposition of a particular protein (amyloid) into tissues of the body.

Excludes1   Alzheimer's disease (G30.0-)

E85.0 **Non-neuropathic heredofamilial amyloidosis** 🔖
Familial Mediterranean fever
Hereditary amyloid nephropathy

E85.1 **Neuropathic heredofamilial amyloidosis** 🔖
Amyloid polyneuropathy (Portuguese)

E85.2 **Heredofamilial amyloidosis, unspecified** 🔖

E85.3 **Secondary systemic amyloidosis** 🔖
Hemodialysis-associated amyloidosis

E85.4 **Organ-limited amyloidosis** 🔖
Localized amyloidosis

E85.8 **Other amyloidosis** 🔖

E85.9 **Amyloidosis, unspecified** 🔖

Item 4-9 Circulating fluid volume is regulated by the amount of water and sodium ingested, excreted by the kidneys into the urine, and lost through the gastrointestinal tract, lungs, and skin. To maintain blood volume within a normal range, the kidneys regulate the amount of water and sodium lost into the urine. Too much (**fluid overload**) or too little fluid volume (**volume depletion**) will affect blood pressure. Severe cases of vomiting, diarrhea, bleeding, and burns (fluid loss through exposed burn surface area) can contribute to fluid loss. Internal body environment must maintain a precise balance (homeostasis) between too much fluid and too little fluid. This complex balancing mechanism is critical to good health.

E86 **Volume depletion**

Excludes1   dehydration of newborn (P74.1)
hypovolemic shock NOS (R57.1)
postprocedural hypovolemic shock (T81.11)
traumatic hypovolemic shock (T79.4)

E86.0 **Dehydration**
Excessive loss of body water

E86.1 **Hypovolemia**
Diminished volume of circulating blood
Depletion of volume of plasma

E86.9 **Volume depletion, unspecified**

E87 **Other disorders of fluid, electrolyte and acid-base balance**

Excludes1   diabetes insipidus (E23.2)
electrolyte imbalance associated with hyperemesis gravidarum (O21.1)
electrolyte imbalance following ectopic or molar pregnancy (O08.5)
familial periodic paralysis (G72.3)

E87.0 **Hyperosmolality and hypernatremia** 🔖
Sodium [Na] excess
Sodium [Na] overload

E87.1 **Hypo-osmolality and hyponatremia** 🔖
Sodium [Na] deficiency

Excludes1   syndrome of inappropriate secretion of antidiuretic hormone (E22.2)

E87.2 **Acidosis** 🔖
Acidosis NOS
Lactic acidosis
Metabolic acidosis
Respiratory acidosis

Excludes1   diabetic acidosis - see categories E08-E13 with ketoacidosis

E87.3 **Alkalosis** 🔖
Alkalosis NOS
Metabolic alkalosis
Respiratory alkalosis

E87.4 **Mixed disorder of acid-base balance** 🔖

E87.5 **Hyperkalemia**
Potassium [K] excess
Potassium [K] overload

E87.6 **Hypokalemia**
Potassium [K] deficiency

E87.7 **Fluid overload**

Excludes1   edema NOS (R60.9)
fluid retention (R60.9)

E87.70 **Fluid overload, unspecified**

E87.71 **Transfusion associated circulatory overload**
Fluid overload due to transfusion (blood) (blood components) TACO

E87.79 **Other fluid overload**

E87.8 **Other disorders of electrolyte and fluid balance, not elsewhere classified**
Electrolyte imbalance NOS
Hyperchloremia
Hypochloremia

● Unacceptable Principal Diagnosis   ● Use Additional Character(s)   ■ Unspecified   ▶ Manifestation Code
OGCR Official Guidelines for Coding and Reporting   Excludes 1   Excludes 2   Includes   Use additional   Code first   Code also

● **E88   Other and unspecified metabolic disorders**

Use additional codes for associated conditions

| Excludes1 | histiocytosis X (chronic) (C96.6) |

● **E88.0   Disorders of plasma-protein metabolism, not elsewhere classified**

Excludes1	disorder of lipoprotein metabolism (E78.-)
	monoclonal gammopathy (of undetermined significance) (D47.2)
	polyclonal hypergammaglobulinemia (D89.0)
	Waldenström macroglobulinemia (C88.0)

  E88.01   Alpha-1-antitrypsin deficiency AAT deficiency

  E88.09   Other disorders of plasma-protein metabolism, not elsewhere classified
  Bisalbuminemia

E88.1   Lipodystrophy, not elsewhere classified
Defective fat metabolism resulting in absence of subcutaneous fat
Lipodystrophy NOS

| Excludes1 | Whipple's disease (K90.81) |

E88.2   Lipomatosis, not elsewhere classified
Abnormal tumorlike accumulations of fat in tissue
Lipomatosis NOS
Lipomatosis (Check) dolorosa [Dercum]

E88.3   Tumor lysis syndrome 🅲
Tumor lysis syndrome (spontaneous)
Tumor lysis syndrome following antineoplastic drug chemotherapy

Use additional code for adverse effect, if applicable, to identify drug (T45.1X5)

● **E88.4   Mitochondrial metabolism disorders**
Congenital disorder of metabolism

Excludes1	disorders of pyruvate metabolism (E74.4)
	Kearns-Sayre syndrome (H49.81)
	Leber's disease (H47.22)
	Leigh's encephalopathy (G31.82)
	Mitochondrial myopathy, NEC (G71.3)
	Reye's syndrome (G93.7)

  ▪ **E88.40   Mitochondrial metabolism disorder, unspecified** 🅲

  E88.41   MELAS syndrome 🅲
  Mitochondrial myopathy, encephalopathy, lactic acidosis and stroke-like episodes

  E88.42   MERRF syndrome 🅲
  Myoclonic epilepsy associated with ragged-red fibers

  Code also myoclonic epilepsy (G40.3-)

  E88.49   Other mitochondrial metabolism disorders 🅲

● **E88.8   Other specified metabolic disorders**

  E88.81   Metabolic syndrome
  Dysmetabolic syndrome X

  Use additional codes for associated manifestations, such as:
  obesity (E66.-)

  E88.89   Other specified metabolic disorders
  Launois-Bensaude adenolipomatosis

  | Excludes1 | adult pulmonary Langerhans cell histiocytosis (J84.82) |

▪ **E88.9   Metabolic disorder, unspecified** 🅲

POSTPROCEDURAL ENDOCRINE AND METABOLIC COMPLICATIONS AND DISORDERS, NOT ELSEWHERE CLASSIFIED (E89)

● **E89   Postprocedural endocrine and metabolic complications and disorders, not elsewhere classified**

| Excludes2 | intraoperative complications of endocrine system organ or structure (E36.0-, E36.1-, E36.8) |

E89.0   Postprocedural hypothyroidism
Postirradiation hypothyroidism
Postsurgical hypothyroidism

E89.1   Postprocedural hypoinsulinemia 🅲
Postpancreatectomy hyperglycemia
Postsurgical hypoinsulinemia

Use additional code, if applicable, to identify:
acquired absence of pancreas (Z90.41-)
diabetes mellitus (postpancreatectomy) (postprocedural) (E13.-)
insulin use (Z79.4)

| Excludes1 | transient postprocedural hyperglycemia (R73.9) |
| | transient postprocedural hypoglycemia (E16.2) |

E89.2   Postprocedural hypoparathyroidism
Parathyroprival tetany

E89.3   Postprocedural hypopituitarism
Postirradiation hypopituitarism

● **E89.4   Postprocedural ovarian failure**

  E89.40   Asymptomatic postprocedural ovarian failure ♀
  Postprocedural ovarian failure NOS

  E89.41   Symptomatic postprocedural ovarian failure ♀
  Symptoms such as flushing, sleeplessness, headache, lack of concentration, associated with postprocedural menopause

E89.5   Postprocedural testicular hypofunction ♂

E89.6   Postprocedural adrenocortical (-medullary) hypofunction 🅲

● **E89.8   Other postprocedural endocrine and metabolic complications and disorders**

  ● **E89.81   Postprocedural hemorrhage and hematoma of an endocrine system organ or structure following a procedure**

    E89.810   Postprocedural hemorrhage and hematoma of an endocrine system organ or structure following an endocrine system procedure 🅲

    E89.811   Postprocedural hemorrhage and hematoma of an endocrine system organ or structure following other procedure 🅲

  E89.89   Other postprocedural endocrine and metabolic complications and disorders 🅲

  Use additional code, if applicable, to further specify disorder

CHAPTER 4 (E00-E90)

CHAPTER 5

MENTAL, BEHAVIORAL AND NEURODEVELOPMENTAL DISORDERS (F01-F99)

Includes   disorders of psychological development

Excludes2   symptoms, signs and abnormal clinical laboratory findings, not elsewhere classified (R00-R99)

This chapter contains the following blocks:

F01-F09	Mental disorders due to known physiological conditions
F10-F19	Mental and behavioral disorders due to psychoactive substance use
F20-F29	Schizophrenia, schizotypal, delusional, and other non-mood psychotic disorders
F30-F39	Mood [affective] disorders
F40-F48	Anxiety, dissociative, stress-related, somatoform and other nonpsychotic mental disorders
F50-F59	Behavioral syndromes associated with physiological disturbances and physical factors
F60-F69	Disorders of adult personality and behavior
F70-F79	Intellectual disabilities
F80-F89	Pervasive and specific developmental disorders
F90-F98	Behavioral and emotional disorders with onset usually occurring in childhood and adolescence
F99	Unspecified mental disorder

MENTAL DISORDERS DUE TO KNOWN PHYSIOLOGICAL CONDITIONS (F01-F09)

This block comprises a range of mental disorders grouped together on the basis of their having in common a demonstrable etiology in cerebral disease, brain injury, or other insult leading to cerebral dysfunction. The dysfunction may be primary, as in diseases, injuries, and insults that affect the brain directly and selectively; or secondary, as in systemic diseases and disorders that attack the brain only as one of the multiple organs or systems of the body that are involved.

● **F01**   **Vascular dementia**

Vascular dementia as a result of infarction of the brain due to vascular disease, including hypertensive cerebrovascular disease.

Includes   arteriosclerotic dementia

Code first the underlying physiological condition or sequelae of cerebrovascular disease.

● **F01.5**   **Vascular dementia**

    ● **F01.50**   **Vascular dementia without behavioral disturbance**   A

    ● **F01.51**   **Vascular dementia with behavioral disturbance** 🐾   A

        Vascular dementia with aggressive behavior

        Vascular dementia with combative behavior

        Vascular dementia with violent behavior

        Use additional code, if applicable, to identify wandering in vascular dementia (Z91.83)

● **F02**   **Dementia in other diseases classified elsewhere**

Code first the underlying physiological condition, such as:
   Alzheimer's (G30.-)
   cerebral lipidosis (E75.4)
   Creutzfeldt-Jakob disease (A81.0-)
   dementia with Lewy bodies (G31.83)
   epilepsy and recurrent seizures (G40.-)
   frontotemporal dementia (G31.09)
   hepatolenticular degeneration (E83.0)
   human immunodeficiency virus [HIV] disease (B20)
   hypercalcemia (E83.52)
   hypothyroidism, acquired (E00-E03.-)
   intoxications (T36-T65)
   Jakob-Creutzfeldt disease (A81.0-)
   multiple sclerosis (G35)
   neurosyphilis (A52.17)
   niacin deficiency [pellagra] (E52)
   Parkinson's disease (G20)
   Pick's disease (G31.01)
   polyarteritis nodosa (M30.0)
   systemic lupus erythematosus (M32.-)
   trypanosomiasis (B56.-, B57.-)
   vitamin B deficiency (E53.8)

Excludes1   dementia with Parkinsonism (G31.83)

Excludes2   dementia in alcohol and psychoactive substance disorders (F10-F19, with .17, .27, .97)
        vascular dementia (F01.5-)

● **F02.8**   **Dementia in other diseases classified elsewhere**

    ●▶ **F02.80**   *Dementia in other diseases classified elsewhere without behavioral disturbance*
        Dementia in other diseases classified elsewhere NOS

    ●▶ **F02.81**   *Dementia in other diseases classified elsewhere with behavioral disturbance* 🐾
        Dementia in other diseases classified elsewhere with aggressive behavior
        Dementia in other diseases classified elsewhere with combative behavior
        Dementia in other diseases classified elsewhere with violent behavior

        Use additional code, if applicable, to identify wandering in dementia in conditions classified elsewhere (Z91.83)

● **F03**   **Unspecified dementia**   A
   Presenile dementia NOS
   Presenile psychosis NOS
   Primary degenerative dementia NOS
   Senile dementia NOS
   Senile dementia depressed or paranoid type
   Senile psychosis NOS

Excludes1   senility NOS (R41.81)

Excludes2   mild memory disturbance due to known physiological condition (F06.8)
        senile dementia with delirium or acute confusional state (F05)

● **F03.9**   **Unspecified dementia**

    ■ **F03.90**   **Unspecified dementia without behavioral disturbance**
        Dementia NOS

Item 5-1 Psychosis was a term formerly applied to any mental disorder but is now restricted to disturbances of a great magnitude in which there is a personality disintegration and loss of contact with reality.

● Unacceptable Principal Diagnosis   ● Use Additional Character(s)   ■ Unspecified   ▶ Manifestation Code

OGCR Official Guidelines for Coding and Reporting   Excludes 1   Excludes 2   Includes   Use additional   Code first   Code also

CHAPTER 5 (F01-F99)

■ **F03.91 Unspecified dementia with behavioral disturbance**
Unspecified dementia with aggressive behavior
Unspecified dementia with combative behavior
Unspecified dementia with violent behavior
Use additional code, if applicable, to identify wandering in unspecified dementia (Z91.83)

F04 Amnestic disorder due to known physiological condition
Korsakov's psychosis or syndrome, nonalcoholic
Code first the underlying physiological condition

| Excludes1 | amnesia NOS (R41.3)
anterograde amnesia (R41.1)
dissociative amnesia (F44.0)
retrograde amnesia (R41.2) |

| Excludes2 | alcohol-induced or unspecified Korsakov's syndrome (F10.26, F10.96)
Korsakov's syndrome induced by other psychoactive substances (F13.26, F13.96, F19.16, F19.26, F19.96) |

F05 Delirium due to known physiological condition 🔹
Acute or subacute brain syndrome
Acute or subacute confusional state (nonalcoholic)
Acute or subacute infective psychosis
Acute or subacute organic reaction
Acute or subacute psycho-organic syndrome
Delirium of mixed etiology
Delirium superimposed on dementia
Sundowning
Code first the underlying physiological condition

| Excludes1 | delirium NOS (R41.0) |
| Excludes2 | delirium tremens alcohol-induced or unspecified (F10.231, F10.921) |

● **F06 Other mental disorders due to known physiological condition**

| Includes | mental disorders due to endocrine disorder
mental disorders due to exogenous hormone
mental disorders due to exogenous toxic substance
mental disorders due to primary cerebral disease
mental disorders due to somatic illness
mental disorders due to systemic disease affecting the brain |

Code first the underlying physiological condition

| Excludes1 | unspecified dementia (F03) |
| Excludes2 | delirium due to known physiological condition (F05)
dementia as classified in F01-F02
other mental disorders associated with alcohol and other psychoactive substances (F10-F19) |

F06.0 Psychotic disorder with hallucinations due to known physiological condition 🔹
Organic hallucinatory state (nonalcoholic)

| Excludes2 | hallucinations and perceptual disturbance induced by alcohol and other psychoactive substances (F10-F19 with .151, .251, .951)
schizophrenia (F20.-) |

F06.1 Catatonic disorder due to known physiological condition

| Excludes1 | catatonic stupor (R40.1)
stupor NOS (R40.1) |

| Excludes2 | catatonic schizophrenia (F20.2)
dissociative stupor (F44.2) |

F06.2 Psychotic disorder with delusions due to known physiological condition 🔹
Paranoid and paranoid-hallucinatory organic states
Schizophrenia-like psychosis in epilepsy

| Excludes2 | alcohol and drug-induced psychotic disorder (F10-F19 with .150, .250, .950)
brief psychotic disorder (F23)
delusional disorder (F22)
schizophrenia (F20.-) |

● **F06.3 Mood disorder due to known physiological condition**

| Excludes2 | mood disorders due to alcohol and other psychoactive substances (F10-F19 with .14, .24, .94)
mood disorders, not due to known physiological condition or unspecified (F30-F39) |

■ **F06.30 Mood disorder due to known physiological condition, unspecified**

F06.31 Mood disorder due to known physiological condition with depressive features

F06.32 Mood disorder due to known physiological condition with major depressive-like episode

F06.33 Mood disorder due to known physiological condition with manic features

F06.34 Mood disorder due to known physiological condition with mixed features

F06.4 Anxiety disorder due to known physiological condition

| Excludes2 | anxiety disorders due to alcohol and other psychoactive substances (F10-F19 with .180, .280, .980)
anxiety disorders, not due to known physiological condition or unspecified (F40.-, F41.-) |

F06.8 Other specified mental disorders due to known physiological condition
Epileptic psychosis NOS
Organic dissociative disorder
Organic emotionally labile [asthenic] disorder

● **F07 Personality and behavioral disorders due to known physiological condition**
Code first the underlying physiological condition

F07.0 Personality change due to known physiological condition
Frontal lobe syndrome
Limbic epilepsy personality syndrome
Lobotomy syndrome
Organic personality disorder
Organic pseudopsychopathic personality
Organic pseudoretarded personality
Postleucotomy syndrome
Code first underlying physiological condition

| Excludes1 | mild cognitive impairment (G31.84)
postconcussional syndrome (F07.81)
postencephalitic syndrome (F07.89)
signs and symptoms involving emotional state (R45.-) |

| Excludes2 | specific personality disorder (F60.-) |

N   Newborn Age: 0   P   Pediatric Age: 0–17   M   Maternity DX: 12–55   A   Adult Age: 15–124   ♀   Females Only   ♂   Males Only
🔹 Complication\Comorbidity   Major C\C   Present on Admission Requirement   Hospital-Acquired Condition
907

CHAPTER 5 (F01-F99)

07.8 **Other personality and behavioral disorders due to known physiological condition**

    F07.81 **Postconcussional syndrome**
        Postcontusional syndrome (encephalopathy)
        Post-traumatic brain syndrome, nonpsychotic

        Use additional code to identify associated post-traumatic headache, if applicable (G44.3-)

        Excludes1   current concussion (brain) (S06.0-)
                  postencephalitic syndrome (F07.89)

    F07.89 **Other personality and behavioral disorders due to known physiological condition**
        Postencephalitic syndrome
        Damage to temporal brain lobes with memory loss and abnormal behavior
        Right hemispheric organic affective disorder

● ■ **F07.9 Unspecified personality and behavioral disorder due to known physiological condition**
        Organic psychosyndrome
        Due to exposure to organic solvents

● **F09 Unspecified mental disorder due to known physiological condition**
    Mental disorder NOS due to known physiological condition
    Organic brain syndrome NOS
    Organic mental disorder NOS
    Organic psychosis NOS
    Symptomatic psychosis NOS

    Code first the underlying physiological condition
    Excludes1   psychosis NOS (F29)

MENTAL AND BEHAVIORAL DISORDERS DUE TO PSYCHOACTIVE SUBSTANCE USE (F10-F19)

● **F10 Alcohol related disorders**
    Use additional code for blood alcohol level, if applicable (Y90.-)

  ● **F10.1 Alcohol abuse**
    Excludes1   alcohol dependence (F10.2-)
                  alcohol use, unspecified (F10.9-)

    F10.10 **Alcohol abuse, uncomplicated**

  ● F10.12 **Alcohol abuse with intoxication**
        F10.120 **Alcohol abuse with intoxication, uncomplicated**
        F10.121 **Alcohol abuse with intoxication, delirium** 🔖
        ■ F10.129 **Alcohol abuse with intoxication, unspecified**

    F10.14 **Alcohol abuse with alcohol-induced mood disorder**

  ● F10.15 **Alcohol abuse with alcohol-induced psychotic disorder**
        F10.150 **Alcohol abuse with alcohol-induced psychotic disorder with delusions**
        F10.151 **Alcohol abuse with alcohol-induced psychotic disorder with hallucinations** 🔖
        ■ F10.159 **Alcohol abuse with alcohol-induced psychotic disorder, unspecified**

● **F10.18 Alcohol abuse with other alcohol-induced disorders**
    F10.180 **Alcohol abuse with alcohol-induced anxiety disorder**
    F10.181 **Alcohol abuse with alcohol-induced sexual dysfunction**
    F10.182 **Alcohol abuse with alcohol-induced sleep disorder**
    F10.188 **Alcohol abuse with other alcohol-induced disorder**

■ **F10.19 Alcohol abuse with unspecified alcohol-induced disorder**

● **F10.2 Alcohol dependence**
    Excludes1   alcohol abuse (F10.1-)
                  alcohol use, unspecified (F10.9-)
    Excludes2   toxic effect of alcohol (T51.0-)

    F10.20 **Alcohol dependence, uncomplicated**
    F10.21 **Alcohol dependence, in remission**

  ● F10.22 **Alcohol dependence with intoxication**
        Acute drunkenness (in alcoholism)
        Excludes1   alcohol dependence with withdrawal (F10.23-)

        F10.220 **Alcohol dependence with intoxication, uncomplicated**
        F10.221 **Alcohol dependence with intoxication delirium** 🔖
        ■ F10.229 **Alcohol dependence with intoxication, unspecified**

  ● F10.23 **Alcohol dependence with withdrawal**
        Excludes1   alcohol dependence with intoxication (F10.22-)

        F10.230 **Alcohol dependence with withdrawal, uncomplicated** 🔖
        F10.231 **Alcohol dependence with withdrawal delirium** 🔖
        F10.232 **Alcohol dependence with withdrawal with perceptual disturbance** 🔖
        ■ F10.239 **Alcohol dependence with withdrawal, unspecified** 🔖

    F10.24 **Alcohol dependence with alcohol-induced mood disorder**

  ● F10.25 **Alcohol dependence with alcohol-induced psychotic disorder**
        F10.250 **Alcohol dependence with alcohol-induced psychotic disorder with delusions**
        F10.251 **Alcohol dependence with alcohol-induced psychotic disorder with hallucinations** 🔖
        ■ F10.259 **Alcohol dependence with alcohol-induced psychotic disorder, unspecified**

    F10.26 **Alcohol dependence with alcohol-induced persisting amnestic disorder**

    F10.27 **Alcohol dependence with alcohol-induced persisting dementia** 🔖

● Unaccceptable Principal Diagnosis   ● Use Additional Character(s)   ■ Unspecified   ▶ Manifestation Code

OGCR Official Guidelines for Coding and Reporting   Excludes 1   Excludes 2   Includes   Use additional   Code first   Code also

● F10.28 Alcohol dependence with other alcohol-induced disorders

    F10.280 Alcohol dependence with alcohol-induced anxiety disorder

    F10.281 Alcohol dependence with alcohol-induced sexual dysfunction

    F10.282 Alcohol dependence with alcohol-induced sleep disorder

    F10.288 Alcohol dependence with other alcohol-induced disorder

■ F10.29 Alcohol dependence with unspecified alcohol-induced disorder

● F10.9 Alcohol use, unspecified

    | Excludes1 | alcohol abuse (F10.1-) |
    alcohol dependence (F10.2-)

● F10.92 Alcohol use, unspecified with intoxication

    ■ F10.920 Alcohol use, unspecified with intoxication, uncomplicated

    ■ F10.921 Alcohol use, unspecified with intoxication delirium 🦠

    ■ F10.929 Alcohol use, unspecified with intoxication, unspecified

    F10.94 Alcohol use, unspecified with alcohol-induced mood disorder 🦠

● F10.95 Alcohol use, unspecified with alcohol-induced psychotic disorder

    ■ F10.950 Alcohol use, unspecified with alcohol-induced psychotic disorder with delusions

    ■ F10.951 Alcohol use, unspecified with alcohol-induced psychotic disorder with hallucinations 🦠

    ■ F10.959 Alcohol use, unspecified with alcohol-induced psychotic disorder, unspecified

■ F10.96 Alcohol use, unspecified with alcohol-induced persisting amnestic disorder

■ F10.97 Alcohol use, unspecified with alcohol-induced persisting dementia 🦠

● F10.98 Alcohol use, unspecified with other alcohol-induced disorders

    ■ F10.980 Alcohol use, unspecified with alcohol-induced anxiety disorder 🦠

    ■ F10.981 Alcohol use, unspecified with alcohol-induced sexual dysfunction 🦠

    ■ F10.982 Alcohol use, unspecified with alcohol-induced sleep disorder

    ■ F10.988 Alcohol use, unspecified with other alcohol-induced disorder 🦠

■ F10.99 Alcohol use, unspecified with unspecified alcohol-induced disorder 🦠

● F11 Opioid related disorders

● F11.1 Opioid abuse

    | Excludes1 | opioid dependence (F11.2-) |
    opioid use, unspecified (F11.9-)

    F11.10 Opioid abuse, uncomplicated

● F11.12 Opioid abuse with intoxication

    F11.120 Opioid abuse with intoxication, uncomplicated

    F11.121 Opioid abuse with intoxication delirium 🦠

    F11.122 Opioid abuse with intoxication with perceptual disturbance 🦠

    ■ F11.129 Opioid abuse with intoxication, unspecified

    F11.14 Opioid abuse with opioid-induced mood disorder

● F11.15 Opioid abuse with opioid-induced psychotic disorder

    F11.150 Opioid abuse with opioid-induced psychotic disorder with delusions 🦠

    F11.151 Opioid abuse with opioid-induced psychotic disorder with hallucinations 🦠

    ■ F11.159 Opioid abuse with opioid-induced psychotic disorder, unspecified

● F11.18 Opioid abuse with other opioid-induced disorder

    F11.181 Opioid abuse with opioid-induced sexual dysfunction

    F11.182 Opioid abuse with opioid-induced sleep disorder

    F11.188 Opioid abuse with other opioid-induced disorder

■ F11.19 Opioid abuse with unspecified opioid-induced disorder

● F11.2 Opioid dependence

    | Excludes1 | opioid abuse (F11.1-) |
    opioid use, unspecified (F11.9-)

    | Excludes2 | opioid poisoning (T40.0--T40.2-) |

    F11.20 Opioid dependence, uncomplicated 🦠

    F11.21 Opioid dependence, in remission

● F11.22 Opioid dependence with intoxication

    | Excludes1 | opioid dependence with withdrawal (F11.23) |

    F11.220 Opioid dependence with intoxication, uncomplicated 🦠

    F11.221 Opioid dependence with intoxication delirium 🦠

    F11.222 Opioid dependence with intoxication with perceptual disturbance 🦠

    ■ F11.229 Opioid dependence with intoxication, unspecified 🦠

    F11.23 Opioid dependence with withdrawal 🦠

    | Excludes1 | opioid dependence with intoxication (F11.22-) |

    F11.24 Opioid dependence with opioid-induced mood disorder

● F11.25 Opioid dependence with opioid-induced psychotic disorder

    F11.250 Opioid dependence with opioid-induced psychotic disorder with delusions 🦠

    F11.251 Opioid dependence with opioid-induced psychotic disorder with hallucinations 🦠

    ■ F11.259 Opioid dependence with opioid-induced psychotic disorder, unspecified 🦠

CHAPTER 5 (F01-F99)

● **F11.28** Opioid dependence with other opioid-induced disorder

    F11.281 Opioid dependence with opioid-induced sexual dysfunction 🔖

    F11.282 Opioid dependence with opioid-induced sleep disorder 🔖

    F11.288 Opioid dependence with other opioid-induced disorder 🔖

◼ **F11.29** Opioid dependence with unspecified opioid-induced disorder 🔖

● **F11.9** Opioid use, unspecified

    Excludes1 opioid abuse (F11.1-)
                opioid dependence (F11.2-)

◼ **F11.90** Opioid use, unspecified, uncomplicated

● **F11.92** Opioid use, unspecified with intoxication

    Excludes1 opioid use, unspecified with withdrawal (F11.93)

    ◼ **F11.920** Opioid use, unspecified with intoxication, uncomplicated

    ◼ **F11.921** Opioid use, unspecified with intoxication delirium 🔖

    ◼ **F11.922** Opioid use, unspecified with intoxication with perceptual disturbance

    ◼ **F11.929** Opioid use, unspecified with intoxication, unspecified

◼ **F11.93** Opioid use, unspecified with withdrawal 🔖

    Excludes1 opioid use, unspecified with intoxication (F11.92-)

◼ **F11.94** Opioid use, unspecified with opioid-induced mood disorder

● **F11.95** Opioid use, unspecified with opioid-induced psychotic disorder

    ◼ **F11.950** Opioid use, unspecified with opioid-induced psychotic disorder with delusions 🔖

    ◼ **F11.951** Opioid use, unspecified with opioid-induced psychotic disorder with hallucinations 🔖

    ◼ **F11.959** Opioid use, unspecified with opioid-induced psychotic disorder, unspecified

● **F11.98** Opioid use, unspecified with other specified opioid-induced disorder

    ◼ **F11.981** Opioid use, unspecified with opioid-induced sexual dysfunction

    ◼ **F11.982** Opioid use, unspecified with opioid-induced sleep disorder

    ◼ **F11.988** Opioid use, unspecified with other opioid-induced disorder

◼ **F11.99** Opioid use, unspecified with unspecified opioid-induced disorder

● **F12** Cannabis related disorders

    Includes marijuana

● **F12.1** Cannabis abuse

    Excludes1 cannabis dependence (F12.2-)
                cannabis use, unspecified (F12.9-)

F12.10 Cannabis abuse, uncomplicated

● **F12.12** Cannabis abuse with intoxication

    F12.120 Cannabis abuse with intoxication, uncomplicated

    F12.121 Cannabis abuse with intoxication delirium 🔖

    F12.122 Cannabis abuse with intoxication with perceptual disturbance

    ◼ **F12.129** Cannabis abuse with intoxication, unspecified

● **F12.15** Cannabis abuse with psychotic disorder

    F12.150 Cannabis abuse with psychotic disorder with delusions 🔖

    F12.151 Cannabis abuse with psychotic disorder with hallucinations 🔖

    ◼ **F12.159** Cannabis abuse with psychotic disorder, unspecified

● **F12.18** Cannabis abuse with other cannabis-induced disorder

    F12.180 Cannabis abuse with cannabis-induced anxiety disorder

    F12.188 Cannabis abuse with other cannabis-induced disorder

◼ **F12.19** Cannabis abuse with unspecified cannabis-induced disorder

● **F12.2** Cannabis dependence

    Excludes1 cannabis abuse (F12.1-)
                cannabis use, unspecified (F12.9-)

    Excludes2 cannabis poisoning (T40.7-)

F12.20 Cannabis dependence, uncomplicated

F12.21 Cannabis dependence, in remission

● **F12.22** Cannabis dependence with intoxication

    F12.220 Cannabis dependence with intoxication, uncomplicated

    F12.221 Cannabis dependence with intoxication delirium 🔖

    F12.222 Cannabis dependence with intoxication with perceptual disturbance

    ◼ **F12.229** Cannabis dependence with intoxication, unspecified

● **F12.25** Cannabis dependence with psychotic disorder

    F12.250 Cannabis dependence with psychotic disorder with delusions 🔖

    F12.251 Cannabis dependence with psychotic disorder with hallucinations 🔖

    ◼ **F12.259** Cannabis dependence with psychotic disorder, unspecified

● Unacceptable Principal Diagnosis   ● Use Additional Character(s)   ◼ Unspecified   ▶ Manifestation Code

OGCR Official Guidelines for Coding and Reporting   Excludes 1   Excludes 2   Includes   Use additional   Code first   Code also

● **F12.28** Cannabis dependence with other cannabis-induced disorder

    F12.280 Cannabis dependence with cannabis-induced anxiety disorder

    F12.288 Cannabis dependence with other cannabis-induced disorder

■ **F12.29** Cannabis dependence with unspecified cannabis-induced disorder

● **F12.9** Cannabis use, unspecified

    | Excludes1 | cannabis abuse (F12.1-)
    cannabis dependence (F12.2-)

■ **F12.90** Cannabis use, unspecified, uncomplicated

● **F12.92** Cannabis use, unspecified with intoxication

    ■ F12.920 Cannabis use, unspecified with intoxication, uncomplicated

    ■ F12.921 Cannabis use, unspecified with intoxication delirium

    ■ F12.922 Cannabis use, unspecified with intoxication with perceptual disturbance

    ■ F12.929 Cannabis use, unspecified with intoxication, unspecified

● **F12.95** Cannabis use, unspecified with psychotic disorder

    ■ F12.950 Cannabis use, unspecified with psychotic disorder with delusions

    ■ F12.951 Cannabis use, unspecified with psychotic disorder with hallucinations

    ■ F12.959 Cannabis use, unspecified with psychotic disorder, unspecified

● **F12.98** Cannabis use, unspecified with other cannabis-induced disorder

    ■ F12.980 Cannabis use, unspecified with anxiety disorder

    ■ F12.988 Cannabis use, unspecified with other cannabis-induced disorder

■ **F12.99** Cannabis use, unspecified with unspecified cannabis-induced disorder

● **F13** Sedative, hypnotic, or anxiolytic related disorders

● **F13.1** Sedative, hypnotic or anxiolytic-related abuse

    | Excludes1 | sedative, hypnotic or anxiolytic-related dependence (F13.2-)
    sedative, hypnotic, or anxiolytic use, unspecified (F13.9-)

    F13.10 Sedative, hypnotic or anxiolytic abuse, uncomplicated

● **F13.12** Sedative, hypnotic or anxiolytic abuse with intoxication

    F13.120 Sedative, hypnotic or anxiolytic abuse with intoxication, uncomplicated

    F13.121 Sedative, hypnotic or anxiolytic abuse with intoxication delirium

    ■ F13.129 Sedative, hypnotic or anxiolytic abuse with intoxication, unspecified

    F13.14 Sedative, hypnotic or anxiolytic abuse with sedative, hypnotic or anxiolytic-induced mood disorder

● **F13.15** Sedative, hypnotic or anxiolytic abuse with sedative, hypnotic or anxiolyticinduced psychotic disorder

    F13.150 Sedative, hypnotic or anxiolytic abuse with sedative, hypnotic or anxiolytic-induced psychotic disorder with delusions

    F13.151 Sedative, hypnotic or anxiolytic abuse with sedative, hypnotic or anxiolytic-induced psychotic disorder with hallucinations

    ■ F13.159 Sedative, hypnotic or anxiolytic abuse with sedative, hypnotic or anxiolytic-induced psychotic disorder, unspecified

● **F13.18** Sedative, hypnotic or anxiolytic abuse with other sedative, hypnotic or anxiolytic-induced disorders

    F13.180 Sedative, hypnotic or anxiolytic abuse with sedative, hypnotic or anxiolytic-induced anxiety disorder

    F13.181 Sedative, hypnotic or anxiolytic abuse with sedative, hypnotic or anxiolytic-induced sexual dysfunction

    F13.182 Sedative, hypnotic or anxiolytic abuse with sedative, hypnotic or anxiolytic-induced sleep disorder

    F13.188 Sedative, hypnotic or anxiolytic abuse with other sedative, hypnotic or anxiolytic-induced disorder

■ **F13.19** Sedative, hypnotic or anxiolytic abuse with unspecified sedative, hypnotic or anxiolytic-induced disorder

● **F13.2** Sedative, hypnotic or anxiolytic-related dependence

    | Excludes1 | sedative, hypnotic or anxiolytic-related abuse (F13.1-)
    sedative, hypnotic, or anxiolytic use, unspecified (F13.9-)

    | Excludes2 | sedative, hypnotic, or anxiolytic poisoning (T42.-)

    F13.20 Sedative, hypnotic or anxiolytic dependence, uncomplicated

    F13.21 Sedative, hypnotic or anxiolytic dependence, in remission

● **F13.22** Sedative, hypnotic or anxiolytic dependence with intoxication

    | Excludes1 | sedative, hypnotic or anxiolytic dependence with withdrawal (F13.23-)

    F13.220 Sedative, hypnotic or anxiolytic dependence with intoxication, uncomplicated

    F13.221 Sedative, hypnotic or anxiolytic dependence with intoxication delirium

    ■ F13.229 Sedative, hypnotic or anxiolytic dependence with intoxication, unspecified

CHAPTER 5 (F01-F99)

● **F13.23 Sedative, hypnotic or anxiolytic dependence with withdrawal**

> **Excludes1** sedative, hypnotic or anxiolytic dependence with intoxication (F13.22-)

     F13.230 Sedative, hypnotic or anxiolytic dependence with withdrawal, uncomplicated

     F13.231 Sedative, hypnotic or anxiolytic dependence with withdrawal delirium

     F13.232 Sedative, hypnotic or anxiolytic dependence with withdrawal with perceptual disturbance

     F13.239 Sedative, hypnotic or anxiolytic dependence with withdrawal, unspecified

F13.24 Sedative, hypnotic or anxiolytic dependence with sedative, hypnotic or anxiolytic-induced mood disorder

● F13.25 Sedative, hypnotic or anxiolytic dependence with sedative, hypnotic or anxiolytic-induced psychotic disorder

     F13.250 Sedative, hypnotic or anxiolytic dependence with sedative, hypnotic or anxiolytic-induced psychotic disorder with delusions

     F13.251 Sedative, hypnotic or anxiolytic dependence with sedative, hypnotic or anxiolytic-induced psychotic disorder with hallucinations

     F13.259 Sedative, hypnotic or anxiolytic dependence with sedative, hypnotic or anxiolytic-induced psychotic disorder, unspecified

F13.26 Sedative, hypnotic or anxiolytic dependence with sedative, hypnotic or anxiolytic-induced persisting amnestic disorder

F13.27 Sedative, hypnotic or anxiolytic dependence with sedative, hypnotic or anxiolytic-induced persisting dementia

● F13.28 Sedative, hypnotic or anxiolytic dependence with other sedative, hypnotic or anxiolytic-induced disorders

     F13.280 Sedative, hypnotic or anxiolytic dependence with sedative, hypnotic or anxiolytic-induced anxiety disorder

     F13.281 Sedative, hypnotic or anxiolytic dependence with sedative, hypnotic or anxiolytic-induced sexual dysfunction

     F13.282 Sedative, hypnotic or anxiolytic dependence with sedative, hypnotic or anxiolytic-induced sleep disorder

     F13.288 Sedative, hypnotic or anxiolytic dependence with other sedative, hypnotic or anxiolytic-induced disorder

F13.29 Sedative, hypnotic or anxiolytic dependence with unspecified sedative, hypnotic or anxiolytic-induced disorder

● **F13.9 Sedative, hypnotic or anxiolytic-related use, unspecified**

> **Excludes1** sedative, hypnotic or anxiolytic-related abuse (F13.1-)
> sedative, hypnotic or anxiolytic-related dependence (F13.2-)

F13.90 Sedative, hypnotic, or anxiolytic use, unspecified, uncomplicated

● F13.92 Sedative, hypnotic or anxiolytic use, unspecified with intoxication

> **Excludes1** sedative, hypnotic or anxiolytic use, unspecified with withdrawal (F13.93-)

     F13.920 Sedative, hypnotic or anxiolytic use, unspecified with intoxication, uncomplicated

     F13.921 Sedative, hypnotic or anxiolytic use, unspecified with intoxication delirium

     F13.929 Sedative, hypnotic or anxiolytic use, unspecified with intoxication, unspecified

● F13.93 Sedative, hypnotic or anxiolytic use, unspecified with withdrawal

> **Excludes1** sedative, hypnotic or anxiolytic use, unspecified with intoxication (F13.92-)

     F13.930 Sedative, hypnotic or anxiolytic use, unspecified with withdrawal, uncomplicated

     F13.931 Sedative, hypnotic or anxiolytic use, unspecified with withdrawal delirium

     F13.932 Sedative, hypnotic or anxiolytic use, unspecified with withdrawal with perceptual disturbances

     F13.939 Sedative, hypnotic or anxiolytic use, unspecified with withdrawal, unspecified

F13.94 Sedative, hypnotic or anxiolytic use, unspecified with sedative, hypnotic or anxiolytic-induced mood disorder

● F13.95 Sedative, hypnotic or anxiolytic use, unspecified with sedative, hypnotic or anxiolytic-induced psychotic disorder

     F13.950 Sedative, hypnotic or anxiolytic use, unspecified with sedative, hypnotic or anxiolytic-induced psychotic disorder with delusions

     F13.951 Sedative, hypnotic or anxiolytic use, unspecified with sedative, hypnotic or anxiolytic-induced psychotic disorder with hallucinations

     F13.959 Sedative, hypnotic or anxiolytic use, unspecified with sedative, hypnotic or anxiolytic-induced psychotic disorder, unspecified

F13.96 Sedative, hypnotic or anxiolytic use, unspecified with sedative, hypnotic or anxiolytic-induced persisting amnestic disorder

■ **F13.97** Sedative, hypnotic or anxiolytic use, unspecified with sedative, hypnotic or anxiolytic-induced persisting dementia ℚ

● **F13.98** Sedative, hypnotic or anxiolytic use, unspecified with other sedative, hypnotic or anxiolytic-induced disorders

   ■ **F13.980** Sedative, hypnotic or anxiolytic use, unspecified with sedative, hypnotic or anxiolytic-induced anxiety disorder

   ■ **F13.981** Sedative, hypnotic or anxiolytic use, unspecified with sedative, hypnotic or anxiolytic-induced sexual dysfunction

   ■ **F13.982** Sedative, hypnotic or anxiolytic use, unspecified with sedative, hypnotic or anxiolytic-induced sleep disorder

   ■ **F13.988** Sedative, hypnotic or anxiolytic use, unspecified with other sedative, hypnotic or anxiolytic-induced disorder

■ **F13.99** Sedative, hypnotic or anxiolytic use, unspecified with unspecified sedative, hypnotic or anxiolytic-induced disorder

● **F14** **Cocaine related disorders**

   Excludes2   other stimulant-related disorders (F15.-)

● **F14.1** Cocaine abuse

   Excludes1   cocaine dependence (F14.2-)
                  cocaine use, unspecified (F14.9-)

   F14.10 Cocaine abuse, uncomplicated

● **F14.12** Cocaine abuse with intoxication

   F14.120 Cocaine abuse with intoxication, uncomplicated

   F14.121 Cocaine abuse with intoxication with delirium ℚ

   F14.122 Cocaine abuse with intoxication with perceptual disturbance

   ■ **F14.129** Cocaine abuse with intoxication, unspecified

   F14.14 Cocaine abuse with cocaine-induced mood disorder

● **F14.15** Cocaine abuse with cocaine-induced psychotic disorder

   F14.150 Cocaine abuse with cocaine-induced psychotic disorder with delusions ℚ

   F14.151 Cocaine abuse with cocaine-induced psychotic disorder with hallucinations ℚ

   ■ **F14.159** Cocaine abuse with cocaine-induced psychotic disorder, unspecified

● **F14.18** Cocaine abuse with other cocaine-induced disorder

   F14.180 Cocaine abuse with cocaine-induced anxiety disorder

   F14.181 Cocaine abuse with cocaine-induced sexual dysfunction

   F14.182 Cocaine abuse with cocaine-induced sleep disorder

   F14.188 Cocaine abuse with other cocaine-induced disorder

   ■ **F14.19** Cocaine abuse with unspecified cocaine-induced disorder

● **F14.2** Cocaine dependence

   Excludes1   cocaine abuse (F14.1-)
                  cocaine use, unspecified (F14.9-)

   Excludes2   cocaine poisoning (T40.5-)

   F14.20 Cocaine dependence, uncomplicated ℚ

   F14.21 Cocaine dependence, in remission

● **F14.22** Cocaine dependence with intoxication

   Excludes1   cocaine dependence with withdrawal (F14.23)

   F14.220 Cocaine dependence with intoxication, uncomplicated ℚ

   F14.221 Cocaine dependence with intoxication delirium ℚ

   F14.222 Cocaine dependence with intoxication with perceptual disturbance ℚ

   ■ **F14.229** Cocaine dependence with intoxication, unspecified

   F14.23 Cocaine dependence with withdrawal ℚ

   Excludes1   cocaine dependence with intoxication (F14.22-)

   F14.24 Cocaine dependence with cocaine-induced mood disorder

● **F14.25** Cocaine dependence with cocaine-induced psychotic disorder

   F14.250 Cocaine dependence with cocaine-induced psychotic disorder with delusions ℚ

   F14.251 Cocaine dependence with cocaine-induced psychotic disorder with hallucinations ℚ

   ■ **F14.259** Cocaine dependence with cocaine-induced psychotic disorder, unspecified ℚ

● **F14.28** Cocaine dependence with other cocaine-induced disorder

   F14.280 Cocaine dependence with cocaine-induced anxiety disorder ℚ

   F14.281 Cocaine dependence with cocaine-induced sexual dysfunction ℚ

   F14.282 Cocaine dependence with cocaine-induced sleep disorder ℚ

   F14.288 Cocaine dependence with other cocaine-induced disorder ℚ

   ■ **F14.29** Cocaine dependence with unspecified cocaine-induced disorder ℚ

● **F14.9** Cocaine use, unspecified

   Excludes1   cocaine abuse (F14.1-)
                  cocaine dependence (F14.2-)

   ■ **F14.90** Cocaine use, unspecified, uncomplicated

● **F14.92** Cocaine use, unspecified with intoxication

   ■ **F14.920** Cocaine use, unspecified with intoxication, uncomplicated

   ■ **F14.921** Cocaine use, unspecified with intoxication delirium ℚ

   ■ **F14.922** Cocaine use, unspecified with intoxication with perceptual disturbance

   ■ **F14.929** Cocaine use, unspecified with intoxication, unspecified

CHAPTER 5 (F01-F99)

N Newborn Age: 0   P Pediatric Age: 0–17   M Maternity DX: 12–55   A Adult Age: 15–124   ♀ Females Only   ♂ Males Only

ℚ Complication\Comorbidity   ℚ Major C\C   ℚ Present on Admission Requirement   ℚ Hospital-Acquired Condition

CHAPTER 5 (F01-F99)

● F14.94   Cocaine use, unspecified with cocaine-induced mood disorder

● F14.95   Cocaine use, unspecified with cocaine-induced psychotic disorder

     ■ F14.950   Cocaine use, unspecified with cocaine-induced psychotic disorder with delusions 🔎

     ■ F14.951   Cocaine use, unspecified with cocaine-induced psychotic disorder with hallucinations 🔎

     ■ F14.959   Cocaine use, unspecified with cocaine-induced psychotic disorder, unspecified

● F14.98   Cocaine use, unspecified with other specified cocaine-induced disorder

     ■ F14.980   Cocaine use, unspecified with cocaine-induced anxiety disorder

     ■ F14.981   Cocaine use, unspecified with cocaine-induced sexual dysfunction

     ■ F14.982   Cocaine use, unspecified with cocaine-induced sleep disorder

     ■ F14.988   Cocaine use, unspecified with other cocaine-induced disorder

     ■ F14.99   Cocaine use, unspecified with unspecified cocaine-induced disorder

● F15   Other stimulant related disorders

     Includes   amphetamine-related disorders
                  caffeine

     Excludes2   cocaine-related disorders (F14.-)

● F15.1   Other stimulant abuse

     Excludes1   other stimulant dependence (F15.2-)
                   other stimulant use, unspecified (F15.9-)

     F15.10   Other stimulant abuse, uncomplicated

● F15.12   Other stimulant abuse with intoxication

     F15.120   Other stimulant abuse with intoxication, uncomplicated

     F15.121   Other stimulant abuse with intoxication delirium 🔎

     F15.122   Other stimulant abuse with intoxication with perceptual disturbance

     ■ F15.129   Other stimulant abuse with intoxication, unspecified

     F15.14   Other stimulant abuse with stimulant-induced mood disorder

● F15.15   Other stimulant abuse with stimulant-induced psychotic disorder

     F15.150   Other stimulant abuse with stimulant-induced psychotic disorder with delusions 🔎

     F15.151   Other stimulant abuse with stimulant-induced psychotic disorder with hallucinations 🔎

     ■ F15.159   Other stimulant abuse with stimulant-induced psychotic disorder, unspecified

● F15.18   Other stimulant abuse with other stimulant-induced disorder

     F15.180   Other stimulant abuse with stimulant-induced anxiety disorder

     F15.181   Other stimulant abuse with stimulant-induced sexual dysfunction

     F15.182   Other stimulant abuse with stimulant-induced sleep disorder

     F15.188   Other stimulant abuse with other stimulant-induced disorder

     ■ F15.19   Other stimulant abuse with unspecified stimulant-induced disorder

● F15.2   Other stimulant dependence

     Excludes1   other stimulant abuse (F15.1-)
                   other stimulant use, unspecified (F15.9-)

     F15.20   Other stimulant dependence, uncomplicated 🔎

     F15.21   Other stimulant dependence, in remission

● F15.22   Other stimulant dependence with intoxication

     Excludes1   other stimulant dependence with withdrawal (F15.23)

     F15.220   Other stimulant dependence with intoxication, uncomplicated 🔎

     F15.221   Other stimulant dependence with intoxication delirium 🔎

     F15.222   Other stimulant dependence with intoxication with perceptual disturbance 🔎

     ■ F15.229   Other stimulant dependence with intoxication, unspecified 🔎

     F15.23   Other stimulant dependence with withdrawal 🔎

     Excludes1   other stimulant dependence with intoxication (F15.22-)

     F15.24   Other stimulant dependence with stimulant-induced mood disorder

● F15.25   Other stimulant dependence with stimulant-induced psychotic disorder

     F15.250   Other stimulant dependence with stimulant-induced psychotic disorder with delusions 🔎

     F15.251   Other stimulant dependence with stimulant-induced psychotic disorder with hallucinations 🔎

     ■ F15.259   Other stimulant dependence with stimulant-induced psychotic disorder, unspecified 🔎

● F15.28   Other stimulant dependence with other stimulant-induced disorder

     F15.280   Other stimulant dependence with stimulant-induced anxiety disorder 🔎

     F15.281   Other stimulant dependence with stimulant-induced sexual dysfunction 🔎

F15.282　Other stimulant dependence with stimulant-induced sleep disorder 🅒

F15.288　Other stimulant dependence with other stimulant-induced disorder 🅒

■ F15.29　Other stimulant dependence with unspecified stimulant-induced disorder 🅒

● F15.9　Other stimulant use, unspecified

Excludes1　other stimulant abuse (F15.1-)
other stimulant dependence (F15.2-)

■ F15.90　Other stimulant use, unspecified, uncomplicated

● F15.92　Other stimulant use, unspecified with intoxication

Excludes1　other stimulant use, unspecified with withdrawal (F15.93)

■ F15.920　Other stimulant use, unspecified with intoxication, uncomplicated

■ F15.921　Other stimulant use, unspecified with intoxication delirium 🅒

■ F15.922　Other stimulant use, unspecified with intoxication with perceptual disturbance

■ F15.929　Other stimulant use, unspecified with intoxication, unspecified

■ F15.93　Other stimulant use, unspecified with withdrawal 🅒

Excludes1　other stimulant use, unspecified with intoxication (F15.92-)

■ F15.94　Other stimulant use, unspecified with stimulant-induced mood disorder

● F15.95　Other stimulant use, unspecified with stimulant-induced psychotic disorder

■ F15.950　Other stimulant use, unspecified with stimulant-induced psychotic disorder with delusions 🅒

■ F15.951　Other stimulant use, unspecified with stimulant-induced psychotic disorder with hallucinations 🅒

■ F15.959　Other stimulant use, unspecified with stimulant-induced psychotic disorder, unspecified

● F15.98　Other stimulant use, unspecified with other stimulant-induced disorder

■ F15.980　Other stimulant use, unspecified with stimulant-induced anxiety disorder

■ F15.981　Other stimulant use, unspecified with stimulant-induced sexual dysfunction

■ F15.982　Other stimulant use, unspecified with stimulant-induced sleep disorder

■ F15.988　Other stimulant use, unspecified with other stimulant-induced disorder

■ F15.99　Other stimulant use, unspecified with unspecified stimulant-induced disorder

● F16　Hallucinogen related disorders

Includes　ecstasy
PCP
phencyclidine

● F16.1　Hallucinogen abuse

Excludes1　hallucinogen dependence (F16.2-)
hallucinogen use, unspecified (F16.9-)

F16.10　Hallucinogen abuse, uncomplicated

● F16.12　Hallucinogen abuse with intoxication

F16.120　Hallucinogen abuse with intoxication, uncomplicated

F16.121　Hallucinogen abuse with intoxication with delirium 🅒

F16.122　Hallucinogen abuse with intoxication with perceptual disturbance

■ F16.129　Hallucinogen abuse with intoxication, unspecified

F16.14　Hallucinogen abuse with hallucinogen-induced mood disorder

● F16.15　Hallucinogen abuse with hallucinogen-induced psychotic disorder

F16.150　Hallucinogen abuse with hallucinogen-induced psychotic disorder with delusions 🅒

F16.151　Hallucinogen abuse with hallucinogen-induced psychotic disorder with hallucinations 🅒

■ F16.159　Hallucinogen abuse with hallucinogen-induced psychotic disorder, unspecified

● F16.18　Hallucinogen abuse with other hallucinogen-induced disorder

F16.180　Hallucinogen abuse with hallucinogen-induced anxiety disorder

F16.183　Hallucinogen abuse with hallucinogen persisting perception disorder (flashbacks)

F16.188　Hallucinogen abuse with other hallucinogen-induced disorder

■ F16.19　Hallucinogen abuse with unspecified hallucinogen-induced disorder

● F16.2　Hallucinogen dependence

Excludes1　hallucinogen abuse (F16.1-)
hallucinogen use, unspecified (F16.9-)

F16.20　Hallucinogen dependence, uncomplicated 🅒

F16.21　Hallucinogen dependence, in remission

● F16.22　Hallucinogen dependence with intoxication

F16.220　Hallucinogen dependence with intoxication, uncomplicated 🅒

F16.221　Hallucinogen dependence with intoxication with delirium 🅒

■ F16.229　Hallucinogen dependence with intoxication, unspecified 🅒

F16.24　Hallucinogen dependence with hallucinogen-induced mood disorder

CHAPTER 5 (F01-F99)

● F16.25   Hallucinogen dependence with hallucinogen-induced psychotic disorder

    F16.250   Hallucinogen dependence with hallucinogen-induced psychotic disorder with delusions 🦠

    F16.251   Hallucinogen dependence with hallucinogen-induced psychotic disorder with hallucinations 🦠

    ▢ F16.259   Hallucinogen dependence with hallucinogen-induced psychotic disorder, unspecified 🦠

● F16.28   Hallucinogen dependence with other hallucinogen-induced disorder

    F16.280   Hallucinogen dependence with hallucinogen-induced anxiety disorder 🦠

    F16.283   Hallucinogen dependence with hallucinogen persisting perception disorder (flashbacks) 🦠

    F16.288   Hallucinogen dependence with other hallucinogen-induced disorder 🦠

▢ F16.29   Hallucinogen dependence with unspecified hallucinogen-induced disorder 🦠

● F16.9   Hallucinogen use, unspecified

   Excludes1   hallucinogen abuse (F16.1-)
               hallucinogen dependence (F16.2-)

▢ F16.90   Hallucinogen use, unspecified, uncomplicated

● F16.92   Hallucinogen use, unspecified with intoxication

    ▢ F16.920   Hallucinogen use, unspecified with intoxication, uncomplicated

    ▢ F16.921   Hallucinogen use, unspecified with intoxication with delirium 🦠

    ▢ F16.929   Hallucinogen use, unspecified with intoxication, unspecified

▢ F16.94   Hallucinogen use, unspecified with hallucinogen-induced mood disorder

● F16.95   Hallucinogen use, unspecified with hallucinogen-induced psychotic disorder

    ▢ F16.950   Hallucinogen use, unspecified with hallucinogen-induced psychotic disorder with delusions 🦠

    ▢ F16.951   Hallucinogen use, unspecified with hallucinogen-induced psychotic disorder with hallucinations 🦠

    ▢ F16.959   Hallucinogen use, unspecified with hallucinogen-induced psychotic disorder, unspecified

● F16.98   Hallucinogen use, unspecified with other specified hallucinogen-induced disorder

    ▢ F16.980   Hallucinogen use, unspecified with hallucinogen-induced anxiety disorder

    ▢ F16.983   Hallucinogen use, unspecified with hallucinogen persisting perception disorder (flashbacks)

    ▢ F16.988   Hallucinogen use, unspecified with other hallucinogen-induced disorder

▢ F16.99   Hallucinogen use, unspecified with unspecified hallucinogen-induced disorder

● F17   Nicotine dependence

   Excludes1   history of tobacco dependence (Z87.891)
               tobacco use NOS (Z72.0)

   Excludes2   tobacco use (smoking) during pregnancy, childbirth and the puerperium (O99.33-)
               toxic effect of nicotine (T65.2-)

● F17.2   Nicotine dependence

   ● F17.20   Nicotine dependence, unspecified

     ● ▢ F17.200   Nicotine dependence, unspecified, uncomplicated

     ● ▢ F17.201   Nicotine dependence, unspecified, in remission

     ▢ F17.203   Nicotine dependence unspecified, with withdrawal 🦠

     ▢ F17.208   Nicotine dependence, unspecified, with other nicotine-induced disorders

     ▢ F17.209   Nicotine dependence, unspecified, with unspecified nicotine-induced disorders

   ● F17.21   Nicotine dependence, cigarettes

     ● F17.210   Nicotine dependence, cigarettes, uncomplicated

     ● F17.211   Nicotine dependence, cigarettes, in remission

     F17.213   Nicotine dependence, cigarettes, with withdrawal 🦠

     F17.218   Nicotine dependence, cigarettes, with other nicotine-induced disorders

     ▢ F17.219   Nicotine dependence, cigarettes, with unspecified nicotine-induced disorders

   ● F17.22   Nicotine dependence, chewing tobacco

     ● F17.220   Nicotine dependence, chewing tobacco, uncomplicated

     ● F17.221   Nicotine dependence, chewing tobacco, in remission

     F17.223   Nicotine dependence, chewing tobacco, with withdrawal 🦠

     F17.228   Nicotine dependence, chewing tobacco, with other nicotine-induced disorders

     ▢ F17.229   Nicotine dependence, chewing tobacco, with unspecified nicotine-induced disorders

   ● F17.29   Nicotine dependence, other tobacco product

     ● F17.290   Nicotine dependence, other tobacco product, uncomplicated

     ● F17.291   Nicotine dependence, other tobacco product, in remission

     F17.293   Nicotine dependence, other tobacco product, with withdrawal 🦠

     F17.298   Nicotine dependence, other tobacco product, with other nicotine-induced disorders

     ▢ F17.299   Nicotine dependence, other tobacco product, with unspecified nicotine-induced disorders

CHAPTER 5 (F01-F99)

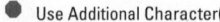

● Unacceptable Principal Diagnosis   ● Use Additional Character(s)   ▢ Unspecified   ▶ Manifestation Code

OGCR Official Guidelines for Coding and Reporting   Excludes 1   Excludes 2   Includes   Use additional   Code first   Code also

916

● **F18**   **Inhalant related disorders**

     Includes   volatile solvents

● **F18.1**   **Inhalant abuse**

     Excludes1   inhalant dependence (F18.2-)
                   inhalant use, unspecified (F18.9-)

     F18.10   Inhalant abuse, uncomplicated

●   F18.12   Inhalant abuse with intoxication

         F18.120   Inhalant abuse with intoxication, uncomplicated

         F18.121   Inhalant abuse with intoxication delirium 🝳

         ◼ F18.129   Inhalant abuse with intoxication, unspecified

     F18.14   Inhalant abuse with inhalant-induced mood disorder

●   F18.15   Inhalant abuse with inhalant-induced psychotic disorder

         F18.150   Inhalant abuse with inhalant-induced psychotic disorder with delusions 🝳

         F18.151   Inhalant abuse with inhalant-induced psychotic disorder with hallucinations 🝳

         ◼ F18.159   Inhalant abuse with inhalant-induced psychotic disorder, unspecified

     F18.17   Inhalant abuse with inhalant-induced dementia 🝳

●   F18.18   Inhalant abuse with other inhalant-induced disorders

         F18.180   Inhalant abuse with inhalant-induced anxiety disorder

         F18.188   Inhalant abuse with other inhalant-induced disorder

     ◼ F18.19   Inhalant abuse with unspecified inhalant-induced disorder

● **F18.2**   **Inhalant dependence**

     Excludes1   inhalant abuse (F18.1-)
                   inhalant use, unspecified (F18.9-)

     F18.20   Inhalant dependence, uncomplicated 🝳

     F18.21   Inhalant dependence, in remission

●   F18.22   Inhalant dependence with intoxication

         F18.220   Inhalant dependence with intoxication, uncomplicated 🝳

         F18.221   Inhalant dependence with intoxication delirium 🝳

         ◼ F18.229   Inhalant dependence with intoxication, unspecified 🝳

     F18.24   Inhalant dependence with inhalant-induced mood disorder

●   F18.25   Inhalant dependence with inhalant-induced psychotic disorder

         F18.250   Inhalant dependence with inhalant-induced psychotic disorder with delusions 🝳

         F18.251   Inhalant dependence with inhalant-induced psychotic disorder with hallucinations 🝳

         ◼ F18.259   Inhalant dependence with inhalant-induced psychotic disorder, unspecified 🝳

     F18.27   Inhalant dependence with inhalant-induced dementia 🝳

●   F18.28   Inhalant dependence with other inhalant-induced disorders

         F18.280   Inhalant dependence with inhalant-induced anxiety disorder 🝳

         F18.288   Inhalant dependence with other inhalant-induced disorder 🝳

     ◼ F18.29   Inhalant dependence with unspecified inhalant-induced disorder 🝳

● **F18.9**   **Inhalant use, unspecified**

     Excludes1   inhalant abuse (F18.1-)
                   inhalant dependence (F18.2-)

     ◼ F18.90   Inhalant use, unspecified, uncomplicated

●   F18.92   Inhalant use, unspecified with intoxication

         ◼ F18.920   Inhalant use, unspecified with intoxication, uncomplicated

         ◼ F18.921   Inhalant use, unspecified with intoxication with delirium 🝳

         ◼ F18.929   Inhalant use, unspecified with intoxication, unspecified

     ◼ F18.94   Inhalant use, unspecified with inhalant-induced mood disorder

●   F18.95   Inhalant use, unspecified with inhalant-induced psychotic disorder

         ◼ F18.950   Inhalant use, unspecified with inhalant-induced psychotic disorder with delusions 🝳

         ◼ F18.951   Inhalant use, unspecified with inhalant-induced psychotic disorder with hallucinations 🝳

         ◼ F18.959   Inhalant use, unspecified with inhalant-induced psychotic disorder, unspecified

     ◼ F18.97   Inhalant use, unspecified with inhalant-induced persisting dementia 🝳

●   F18.98   Inhalant use, unspecified with other inhalant-induced disorders

         ◼ F18.980   Inhalant use, unspecified with inhalant-induced anxiety disorder

         ◼ F18.988   Inhalant use, unspecified with other inhalant-induced disorder

     ◼ F18.99   Inhalant use, unspecified with unspecified inhalant-induced disorder

● **F19**   **Other psychoactive substance related disorders**

     Includes   polysubstance drug use (indiscriminate drug use)

● **F19.1**   **Other psychoactive substance abuse**

     Excludes1   other psychoactive substance dependence (F19.2-)
                   other psychoactive substance use, unspecified (F19.9-)

     F19.10   Other psychoactive substance abuse, uncomplicated

● F19.12   Other psychoactive substance abuse with intoxication

    F19.120   Other psychoactive substance abuse with intoxication, uncomplicated

    F19.121   Other psychoactive substance abuse with intoxication delirium 🐾

    F19.122   Other psychoactive substance abuse with intoxication with perceptual disturbances

    ■ F19.129   Other psychoactive substance abuse with intoxication, unspecified

F19.14   Other psychoactive substance abuse with psychoactive substance-induced mood disorder

● F19.15   Other psychoactive substance abuse with psychoactive substance-induced psychotic disorder

    F19.150   Other psychoactive substance abuse with psychoactive substance-induced psychotic disorder with delusions 🐾

    F19.151   Other psychoactive substance abuse with psychoactive substance-induced psychotic disorder with hallucinations 🐾

    ■ F19.159   Other psychoactive substance abuse with psychoactive substance-induced psychotic disorder, unspecified

F19.16   Other psychoactive substance abuse with psychoactive substance-induced persisting amnestic disorder

F19.17   Other psychoactive substance abuse with psychoactive substance-induced persisting dementia 🐾

● F19.18   Other psychoactive substance abuse with other psychoactive substance-induced disorders

    F19.180   Other psychoactive substance abuse with psychoactive substance-induced anxiety disorder

    F19.181   Other psychoactive substance abuse with psychoactive substance-induced sexual dysfunction

    F19.182   Other psychoactive substance abuse with psychoactive substance-induced sleep disorder

    F19.188   Other psychoactive substance abuse with other psychoactive substance-induced disorder

■ F19.19   Other psychoactive substance abuse with unspecified psychoactive substance-induced disorder

● F19.2   Other psychoactive substance dependence

    Excludes1   other psychoactive substance abuse (F19.1-)
          other psychoactive substance use, unspecified (F19.9-)

F19.20   Other psychoactive substance dependence, uncomplicated 🐾

F19.21   Other psychoactive substance dependence, in remission

● F19.22   Other psychoactive substance dependence with intoxication

    Excludes1   other psychoactive substance dependence with withdrawal (F19.23-)

    F19.220   Other psychoactive substance dependence with intoxication, uncomplicated 🐾

    F19.221   Other psychoactive substance dependence with intoxication delirium 🐾

    F19.222   Other psychoactive substance dependence with intoxication with perceptual disturbance 🐾

    ■ F19.229   Other psychoactive substance dependence with intoxication, unspecified 🐾

● F19.23   Other psychoactive substance dependence with withdrawal

    Excludes1   other psychoactive substance dependence with intoxication (F19.22-)

    F19.230   Other psychoactive substance dependence with withdrawal, uncomplicated 🐾

    F19.231   Other psychoactive substance dependence with withdrawal delirium 🐾

    F19.232   Other psychoactive substance dependence with withdrawal with perceptual disturbance 🐾

    ■ F19.239   Other psychoactive substance dependence with withdrawal, unspecified 🐾

F19.24   Other psychoactive substance dependence with psychoactive substance-induced mood disorder

● F19.25   Other psychoactive substance dependence with psychoactive substance-induced psychotic disorder

    F19.250   Other psychoactive substance dependence with psychoactive substance-induced psychotic disorder with delusions 🐾

    F19.251   Other psychoactive substance dependence with psychoactive substance-induced psychotic disorder with hallucinations 🐾

    ■ F19.259   Other psychoactive substance dependence with psychoactive substance-induced psychotic disorder, unspecified 🐾

F19.26   Other psychoactive substance dependence with psychoactive substance-induced persisting amnestic disorder 🐾

F19.27   Other psychoactive substance dependence with psychoactive substance-induced persisting dementia 🐾

● F19.28   Other psychoactive substance dependence with other psychoactive substance-induced disorders

    F19.280   Other psychoactive substance dependence with psychoactive substance-induced anxiety disorder 🐾

● Unacceptable Principal Diagnosis   ● Use Additional Character(s)   ■ Unspecified   ▶ Manifestation Code

OGCR Official Guidelines for Coding and Reporting   Excludes 1   Excludes 2   Includes   Use additional   Code first   Code also

CHAPTER 5 (F01-F99)

F19.281   Other psychoactive substance dependence with psychoactive substance-induced sexual dysfunction 🝐

F19.282   Other psychoactive substance dependence with psychoactive substance-induced sleep disorder 🝐

F19.288   Other psychoactive substance dependence with other psychoactive substance-induced disorder 🝐

● F19.29   Other psychoactive substance dependence with unspecified psychoactive substance-induced disorder 🝐

● **F19.9**   Other psychoactive substance use, unspecified

    Excludes1   other psychoactive substance abuse (F19.1-)
          other psychoactive substance dependence (F19.2-)

F19.90   Other psychoactive substance use, unspecified, uncomplicated

● F19.92   Other psychoactive substance use, unspecified with intoxication

    Excludes1   other psychoactive substance use, unspecified with withdrawal (F19.93)

F19.920   Other psychoactive substance use, unspecified with intoxication, uncomplicated

F19.921   Other psychoactive substance use, unspecified with intoxication with delirium 🝐

F19.922   Other psychoactive substance use, unspecified with intoxication with perceptual disturbance

F19.929   Other psychoactive substance use, unspecified with intoxication, unspecified

● F19.93   Other psychoactive substance use, unspecified with withdrawal

    Excludes1   other psychoactive substance use, unspecified with intoxication (F19.92-)

F19.930   Other psychoactive substance use, unspecified with withdrawal, uncomplicated 🝐

F19.931   Other psychoactive substance use, unspecified with withdrawal delirium 🝐

F19.932   Other psychoactive substance use, unspecified with withdrawal with perceptual disturbance 🝐

F19.939   Other psychoactive substance use, unspecified with withdrawal, unspecified 🝐

F19.94   Other psychoactive substance use, unspecified with psychoactive substance-induced mood disorder

● F19.95   Other psychoactive substance use, unspecified with psychoactive substance-induced psychotic disorder

F19.950   Other psychoactive substance use, unspecified with psychoactive substance-induced psychotic disorder with delusions 🝐

F19.951   Other psychoactive substance use, unspecified with psychoactive substance-induced psychotic disorder with hallucinations 🝐

F19.959   Other psychoactive substance use, unspecified with psychoactive substance-induced psychotic disorder, unspecified

F19.96   Other psychoactive substance use, unspecified with psychoactive substance-induced persisting amnestic disorder

F19.97   Other psychoactive substance use, unspecified with psychoactive substance-induced persisting dementia 🝐

● F19.98   Other psychoactive substance use, unspecified with other psychoactive substance-induced disorders

F19.980   Other psychoactive substance use, unspecified with psychoactive substance-induced anxiety disorder

F19.981   Other psychoactive substance use, unspecified with psychoactive substance-induced sexual dysfunction

F19.982   Other psychoactive substance use, unspecified with psychoactive substance-induced sleep disorder

F19.988   Other psychoactive substance use, unspecified with other psychoactive substance-induced disorder

F19.99   Other psychoactive substance use, unspecified with unspecified psychoactive substance-induced disorder

---

SCHIZOPHRENIA, SCHIZOTYPAL, DELUSIONAL, AND OTHER NON-MOOD PSYCHOTIC DISORDERS (F20-F29)

● **F20**   **Schizophrenia**
Personality disorders characterized by multiple mental and behavioral irregularities (may exhibit disorganized thinking, delusions, and auditory hallucinations.)

    Excludes1   brief psychotic disorder (F23)
          cyclic schizophrenia (F25.0)
          mood [affective] disorders with psychotic symptoms (F30.2, F31.2, F31.5, F31.64, F32.3, F33.3)
          schizoaffective disorder (F25.-)
          schizophrenic reaction NOS (F23)

    Excludes2   schizophrenic reaction in:
          alcoholism (F10.15-, F10.25-, F10.95-)
          brain disease (F06.2)
          epilepsy (F06.2)
          psychoactive drug use (F11-F19 with .15, .25, .95)
          schizotypal disorder (F21)

F20.0   **Paranoid schizophrenia** 🝐
     Paraphrenic schizophrenia

    Excludes1   involutional paranoid state (F22)
          paranoia (F22)

F20.1   **Disorganized schizophrenia** 🝐
     Hebephrenic schizophrenia
     Hebephrenia

N Newborn Age: 0   **P** Pediatric Age: 0–17   **M** Maternity DX: 12–55   **A** Adult Age: 15–124   ♀ Females Only   ♂ Males Only

🝐 Complication\Comorbidity   🝐 Major C\C   Present on Admission Requirement   🝐 Hospital-Acquired Condition

919

CHAPTER 5 (F01-F99)

F20.2 Catatonic schizophrenia
Schizophrenic catalepsy
Schizophrenic catatonia
Schizophrenic flexibilitas cerea
Excludes1 catatonic stupor (R40.1)

F20.3 Undifferentiated schizophrenia
Atypical schizophrenia
Excludes1 acute schizophrenia-like psychotic disorder (F23)
Excludes2 post-schizophrenic depression (F32.8)

F20.5 Residual schizophrenia
Restzustand (schizophrenic)
Schizophrenic residual state

F20.8 Other schizophrenia
F20.81 Schizophreniform disorder
Schizophreniform psychosis NOS
F20.89 Other schizophrenia
Cenesthopathic schizophrenia
Simple schizophrenia

F20.9 Schizophrenia, unspecified

F21 Schizotypal disorder
Personality disorder characterized by need for social isolation, odd behavior and thinking, and often unconventional beliefs
Borderline schizophrenia
Latent schizophrenia
Latent schizophrenic reaction
Prepsychotic schizophrenia
Prodromal schizophrenia
Pseudoneurotic schizophrenia
Pseudopsychopathic schizophrenia
Schizotypal personality disorder
Excludes2 Asperger's syndrome (F84.5)
schizoid personality disorder (F60.1)

F22 Delusional disorders
Delusional dysmorphophobia
Involutional paranoid state
Paranoia
Paranoia querulans
Paranoid psychosis
Paranoid state
Paraphrenia (late)
Sensitiver Beziehungswahn
Excludes1 mood [affective] disorders with psychotic symptoms (F30.2, F31.2, F31.5, F31.64, F32.3, F33.3)
paranoid schizophrenia (F20.0)
Excludes2 paranoid personality disorder (F60.0)
paranoid psychosis, psychogenic (F23)
paranoid reaction (F23)

F23 Brief psychotic disorder
Paranoid reaction
Psychogenic paranoid psychosis
Excludes2 mood [affective] disorders with psychotic symptoms (F30.2, F31.2, F31.5, F31.64, F32.3, F33.3)

F24 Shared psychotic disorder
Folie à deux
Induced paranoid disorder
Induced psychotic disorder

F25 Schizoaffective disorders
Mental disorder exhibiting major depressive episode, manic episode, or mixed episode occurs with symptoms of schizophrenia, and mood disorder
Excludes1 mood [affective] disorders with psychotic symptoms (F30.2, F31.2, F31.5, F31.64, F32.3, F33.3)
schizophrenia (F20.-)

F25.0 Schizoaffective disorder, bipolar type
Cyclic schizophrenia
Schizoaffective disorder, manic type
Schizoaffective disorder, mixed type
Schizoaffective psychosis, bipolar type
Schizophreniform psychosis, manic type

F25.1 Schizoaffective disorder, depressive type
Schizoaffective psychosis, depressive type
Schizophreniform psychosis, depressive type

F25.8 Other schizoaffective disorders

F25.9 Schizoaffective disorder, unspecified
Schizoaffective psychosis NOS

F28 Other psychotic disorder not due to a substance or known physiological condition
Chronic hallucinatory psychosis

F29 Unspecified psychosis not due to a substance or known physiological condition
Psychosis NOS
Excludes1 mental disorder NOS (F99)
unspecified mental disorder due to known physiological condition (F09)

MOOD [AFFECTIVE] DISORDERS (F30-F39)

F30 Manic episode
Elevated, expansive, or irritable mood
Includes bipolar disorder, single manic episode
mixed affective episode
Excludes1 bipolar disorder (F31.-)
major depressive disorder, single episode (F32.-)
major depressive disorder, recurrent (F33.-)

F30.1 Manic episode without psychotic symptoms
F30.10 Manic episode without psychotic symptoms, unspecified
F30.11 Manic episode without psychotic symptoms, mild
F30.12 Manic episode without psychotic symptoms, moderate
F30.13 Manic episode, severe, without psychotic symptoms

F30.2 Manic episode, severe with psychotic symptoms
Manic stupor
Mania with mood-congruent psychotic symptoms
Mania with mood-incongruent psychotic symptoms

F30.3 Manic episode in partial remission

F30.4 Manic episode in full remission

F30.8 Other manic episodes
Abnormality of mood resembling mania but less intense
Hypomania

F30.9 Manic episode, unspecified
Mania NOS

● **F31   Bipolar disorder**
   Mood disorders with history of manic, mixed, or hypomanic episodes

   Includes   manic-depressive illness
   manic-depressive psychosis
   manic-depressive reaction

   Excludes1   bipolar disorder, single manic episode (F30.-)
   major depressive disorder, single episode (F32.-)
   major depressive disorder, recurrent (F33.-)

   Excludes2   cyclothymia (F34.0)

   F31.0   Bipolar disorder, current episode hypomanic 🏵

● **F31.1   Bipolar disorder, current episode manic without psychotic features**

   ▪ **F31.10   Bipolar disorder, current episode manic without psychotic features, unspecified** 🏵

   F31.11   Bipolar disorder, current episode manic without psychotic features, mild 🏵

   F31.12   Bipolar disorder, current episode manic without psychotic features, moderate 🏵

   F31.13   Bipolar disorder, current episode manic without psychotic features, severe 🏵

   F31.2   Bipolar disorder, current episode manic severe with psychotic features 🏵
   Bipolar disorder, current episode manic with mood-congruent psychotic symptoms
   Bipolar disorder, current episode manic with mood-incongruent psychotic symptoms

● **F31.3   Bipolar disorder, current episode depressed, mild or moderate severity**

   ▪ **F31.30   Bipolar disorder, current episode depressed, mild or moderate severity, unspecified** 🏵

   F31.31   Bipolar disorder, current episode depressed, mild 🏵

   F31.32   Bipolar disorder, current episode depressed, moderate 🏵

   F31.4   Bipolar disorder, current episode depressed, severe, without psychotic features 🏵

   F31.5   Bipolar disorder, current episode depressed, severe, with psychotic features 🏵
   Bipolar disorder, current episode depressed with mood-incongruent psychotic symptoms
   Bipolar disorder, current episode depressed with mood-congruent psychotic symptoms

● **F31.6   Bipolar disorder, current episode mixed**

   ▪ **F31.60   Bipolar disorder, current episode mixed, unspecified** 🏵

   F31.61   Bipolar disorder, current episode mixed, mild 🏵

   F31.62   Bipolar disorder, current episode mixed, moderate 🏵

   F31.63   Bipolar disorder, current episode mixed, severe, without psychotic features 🏵

   F31.64   Bipolar disorder, current episode mixed, severe, with psychotic features 🏵
   Bipolar disorder, current episode mixed with mood-congruent psychotic symptoms
   Bipolar disorder, current episode mixed with mood-incongruent psychotic symptoms

● **F31.7   Bipolar disorder, currently in remission**

   ▪ **F31.70   Bipolar disorder, currently in remission, most recent episode unspecified**

   F31.71   Bipolar disorder, in partial remission, most recent episode hypomanic

   F31.72   Bipolar disorder, in full remission, most recent episode hypomanic

   F31.73   Bipolar disorder, in partial remission, most recent episode manic

   F31.74   Bipolar disorder, in full remission, most recent episode manic

   F31.75   Bipolar disorder, in partial remission, most recent episode depressed

   F31.76   Bipolar disorder, in full remission, most recent episode depressed

   F31.77   Bipolar disorder, in partial remission, most recent episode mixed

   F31.78   Bipolar disorder, in full remission, most recent episode mixed

● **F31.8   Other bipolar disorders**

   F31.81   Bipolar II disorder 🏵

   F31.89   Other bipolar disorder 🏵
   Recurrent manic episodes NOS

   ▪ **F31.9   Bipolar disorder, unspecified**

● **F32   Major depressive disorder, single episode**

   Includes   single episode of agitated depression
   single episode of depressive reaction
   single episode of major depression
   single episode of psychogenic depression
   single episode of reactive depression
   single episode of vital depression

   Excludes1   bipolar disorder (F31-)
   manic episode (F30-)
   recurrent depressive disorder (F33.-)

   Excludes2   adjustment disorder (F43.2)

   F32.0   Major depressive disorder, single episode, mild 🏵

   F32.1   Major depressive disorder, single episode, moderate 🏵

   F32.2   Major depressive disorder, single episode, severe without psychotic features 🏵

   F32.3   Major depressive disorder, single episode, severe with psychotic features 🏵
   Single episode of major depression with mood-congruent psychotic symptoms
   Single episode of major depression with mood-incongruent psychotic symptoms
   Single episode of major depression with psychotic symptoms
   Single episode of psychogenic depressive psychosis
   Single episode of psychotic depression
   Single episode of reactive depressive psychosis

   F32.4   Major depressive disorder, single episode, in partial remission

   F32.5   Major depressive disorder, single episode, in full remission

   F32.8   Other depressive episodes
   Atypical depression
   Post-schizophrenic depression
   Single episode of 'masked' depression NOS

   ▪ **F32.9   Major depressive disorder, single episode, unspecified**
   Depression NOS
   Depressive disorder NOS
   Major depression NOS

CHAPTER 5 (F01-F99)

N   Newborn Age: 0   P   Pediatric Age: 0–17   M   Maternity DX: 12–55   A   Adult Age: 15–124   ♀   Females Only   ♂   Males Only

🏵   Complication\Comorbidity   Major C\C   Present on Admission Requirement   Hospital-Acquired Condition

CHAPTER 5 (F01-F99)

● **F33   Major depressive disorder, recurrent**

Includes   recurrent episodes of depressive reaction
recurrent episodes of endogenous
  depression
recurrent episodes of major depression
recurrent episodes of psychogenic
  depression
recurrent episodes of reactive depression
recurrent episodes of seasonal depressive
  disorder
recurrent episodes of vital depression

Excludes1   bipolar disorder (F31.-)
manic episode (F30.-)

F33.0   Major depressive disorder, recurrent, mild 🜲

F33.1   Major depressive disorder, recurrent, moderate 🜲

**F33.2   Major depressive disorder, recurrent severe
without psychotic features** 🜲

**F33.3   Major depressive disorder, recurrent, severe with
psychotic symptoms** 🜲
Endogenous depression with psychotic
  symptoms
Recurrent severe episodes of major depression
  with mood-congruent psychotic symptoms
Recurrent severe episodes of major depression
  with mood-incongruent psychotic
  symptoms
Recurrent severe episodes of major depression
  with psychotic symptoms
Recurrent severe episodes of psychogenic
  depressive psychosis
Recurrent severe episodes of psychotic
  depression
Recurrent severe episodes of reactive depressive
  psychosis

● **F33.4   Major depressive disorder, recurrent, in remission**

■ **F33.40   Major depressive disorder, recurrent, in
remission, unspecified** 🜲

**F33.41   Major depressive disorder, recurrent, in
partial remission**

**F33.42   Major depressive disorder, recurrent, in
full remission**

F33.8   Other recurrent depressive disorders 🜲
Recurrent brief depressive episodes

■ **F33.9   Major depressive disorder, recurrent, unspecified** 🜲
Monopolar depression NOS

● **F34   Persistent mood [affective] disorders**

F34.0   Cyclothymic disorder
Affective personality disorder
Cycloid personality
Cyclothymia
Cyclothymic personality

F34.1   Dysthymic disorder
Depressive neurosis
Depressive personality disorder
Dysthymia
Neurotic depression
Persistent anxiety depression

Excludes2   anxiety depression (mild or not
persistent) (F41.8)

F34.8   Other persistent mood [affective] disorders 🜲

■ **F34.9   Persistent mood [affective] disorder, unspecified** 🜲

■ **F39   Unspecified mood [affective] disorder**
Affective psychosis NOS

ANXIETY, DISSOCIATIVE, STRESS-RELATED, SOMATOFORM AND OTHER NONPSYCHOTIC MENTAL DISORDERS (F40-F48)

● **F40   Phobic anxiety disorders**
*Irrational fear with avoidance of the feared subject, activity,
or situation even though the individual knows that the
reaction is excessive.*

● **F40.0   Agoraphobia**
Intense, irrational fear of open spaces

■ **F40.00   Agoraphobia, unspecified**

F40.01   Agoraphobia with panic disorder
Panic disorder with agoraphobia

Excludes1   panic disorder without
agoraphobia (F41.0)

F40.02   Agoraphobia without panic disorder

● **F40.1   Social phobias**
Anthropophobia
Social anxiety disorder of childhood
Social neurosis

■ **F40.10   Social phobia, unspecified**

F40.11   Social phobia, generalized

● **F40.2   Specific (isolated) phobias**

Excludes2   dysmorphophobia (nondelusional)
(F45.22)
nosophobia (F45.22)

● **F40.21   Animal type phobia**

F40.210   Arachnophobia
Fear of spiders

F40.218   Other animal type phobia

● **F40.22   Natural environment type phobia**

F40.220   Fear of thunderstorms

**F40.228   Other natural environment type
phobia**

● **F40.23   Blood, injection, injury type phobia**

F40.230   Fear of blood

F40.231   Fear of injections and transfusions

F40.232   Fear of other medical care

F40.233   Fear of injury

● **F40.24   Situational type phobia**

F40.240   Claustrophobia
Fear of closed spaces

F40.241   Acrophobia
Fear of heights

F40.242   Fear of bridges

F40.243   Fear of flying

F40.248   Other situational type phobia

● **F40.29   Other specified phobia**

F40.290   Androphobia
Fear of men

F40.291   Gynephobia
Fear of women

F40.298   Other specified phobia

F40.8   Other phobic anxiety disorders
Phobic anxiety disorder of childhood

■ **F40.9   Phobic anxiety disorder, unspecified**
Phobia NOS
Phobic state NOS

● Unacceptable Principal Diagnosis   ● Use Additional Character(s)   ■ Unspecified   ▶ Manifestation Code

922   **OGCR** Official Guidelines for Coding and Reporting   [Excludes 1] [Excludes 2] [Includes] [Use additional] [Code first] [Code also]

● **F41   Other anxiety disorders**

> | Excludes2 | anxiety in:
> acute stress reaction (F43.0)
> transient adjustment reaction (F43.2)
> neurasthenia (F48.8)
> psychophysiologic disorders (F45.-)
> separation anxiety (F93.0)

     F41.0   Panic disorder [episodic paroxysmal anxiety] without agoraphobia
         Panic attack
         Panic state

> | Excludes1 | panic disorder with agoraphobia (F40.01)

     F41.1   Generalized anxiety disorder
         Anxiety neurosis
         Anxiety reaction
         Anxiety state
         Overanxious disorder

> | Excludes2 | neurasthenia (F48.8)

     F41.3   Other mixed anxiety disorders

     F41.8   Other specified anxiety disorders
         Anxiety depression (mild or not persistent)
         Anxiety hysteria
         Mixed anxiety and depressive disorder

     ◼ **F41.9   Anxiety disorder, unspecified**
         Anxiety NOS

F42   Obsessive-compulsive disorder
     Anxiety disorder with recurrent obsessions or compulsions
     Anancastic neurosis
     Obsessive-compulsive neurosis

> | Excludes2 | obsessive-compulsive personality (disorder) (F60.5)
> obsessive-compulsive symptoms occurring in:
> depression (F32-F33)
> schizophrenia (F20.-)

● **F43   Reaction to severe stress and adjustment disorders**

     F43.0   Acute stress reaction
         Acute crisis reaction
         Acute reaction to stress
         Combat and operational stress reaction
         Combat fatigue
         Crisis state
         Psychic shock

     ● **F43.1   Post-traumatic stress disorder (PTSD)**
         Traumatic neurosis

         ◼ **F43.10   Post-traumatic stress disorder, unspecified**

         F43.11   Post-traumatic stress disorder, acute

         F43.12   Post-traumatic stress disorder, chronic

     ● **F43.2   Adjustment disorders**
         Culture shock
         Grief reaction
         Hospitalism in children

> | Excludes2 | separation anxiety disorder of childhood (F93.0)

         ◼ **F43.20   Adjustment disorder, unspecified**

         F43.21   Adjustment disorder with depressed mood

         F43.22   Adjustment disorder with anxiety

         F43.23   Adjustment disorder with mixed anxiety and depressed mood

         F43.24   Adjustment disorder with disturbance of conduct

         F43.25   Adjustment disorder with mixed disturbance of emotions and conduct

         F43.29   Adjustment disorder with other symptoms

     F43.8   Other reactions to severe stress

     ◼ **F43.9   Reaction to severe stress, unspecified**

● **F44   Dissociative and conversion disorders**

> | Includes | conversion hysteria
> conversion reaction
> hysteria
> hysterical psychosis

> | Excludes2 | malingering [conscious simulation] (Z76.5)

     F44.0   Dissociative amnesia
     Sudden loss of memory for personal information

> | Excludes1 | amnesia NOS (R41.3)
> anterograde amnesia (R41.1)
> retrograde amnesia (R41.2)

> | Excludes2 | alcohol-or other psychoactive substance-induced amnestic disorder (F10, F13, F19 with .26, .96)
> amnestic disorder due to known physiological condition (F04)
> postictal amnesia in epilepsy (G40.-)

     F44.1   Dissociative fugue
     Characterized by episode of sudden, unexpected travel with amnesia for past and partial to total confusion about identity or assumption of new identity

> | Excludes2 | postictal fugue in epilepsy (G40.-)

     F44.2   Dissociative stupor
     Profound diminution or absence of voluntary movement and responsiveness to external stimuli

> | Excludes1 | catatonic stupor (R40.1)
> stupor NOS (R40.1)

> | Excludes2 | catatonic disorder due to known physiological condition (F06.1)
> depressive stupor (F32, F33)
> manic stupor (F30, F31)

     F44.4   Conversion disorder with motor symptom or deficit
         Dissociative motor disorders
         Psychogenic aphonia
         Psychogenic dysphonia

     F44.5   Conversion disorder with seizures or convulsions
         Dissociative convulsions

     F44.6   Conversion disorder with sensory symptom or deficit
         Dissociative anesthesia and sensory loss
         Psychogenic deafness

     F44.7   Conversion disorder with mixed symptom presentation

     ● **F44.8   Other dissociative and conversion disorders**

         F44.81   Dissociative identity disorder
              Multiple personality disorder

         F44.89   Other dissociative and conversion disorders
              Ganser's syndrome
              Psychogenic confusion
              Psychogenic twilight state
              Trance and possession disorders

     ◼ **F44.9   Dissociative and conversion disorder, unspecified**
         Dissociative disorder NOS

CHAPTER 5 (F01-F99)

CHAPTER 5 (F01-F99)

OGCR Section I.C.5.a

Pain disorders related to psychological factors

Assign code F45.41, for pain that is exclusively psychological. Code F45.41, Pain disorder exclusively related to psychological factors, should be used following the appropriate code from category G89, Pain, not elsewhere classified, if there is documentation of a psychological component for a patient with acute or chronic pain.

See Section I.C.6. Pain

● **F45   Somatoform disorders**
Mental disorders characterized by symptoms suggesting general medical condition

    Excludes2   dissociative and conversion disorders (F44.-)
                 factitious disorders (F68.1-)
                 hair-plucking (F63.3)
                 lalling (F80.0)
                 lisping (F80.0)
                 malingering [conscious simulation] (Z76.5)
                 nail-biting (F98.8)
                 psychological or behavioral factors associated with disorders or diseases classified elsewhere (F54)
                 sexual dysfunction, not due to a substance or known physiological condition (F52.-)
                 thumb-sucking (F98.8)
                 tic disorders (in childhood and adolescence) (F95.-)
                 Tourette's syndrome (F95.2)
                 trichotillomania (F63.3)

   F45.0   Somatization disorder
         Briquet's disorder
         Multiple psychosomatic disorder

   F45.1   Undifferentiated somatoform disorder
         Undifferentiated psychosomatic disorder

● **F45.2   Hypochondriacal disorders**
Persistent, unrealistic preoccupation with possibility of having serious disease

    Excludes2   delusional dysmorphophobia (F22)
                 fixed delusions about bodily functions or shape (F22)

    ▪ **F45.20   Hypochondriacal disorder, unspecified**

    F45.21   Hypochondriasis
           Hypochondriacal neurosis

    F45.22   Body dysmorphic disorder
           Dysmorphophobia (nondelusional)
           Nosophobia

    F45.29   Other hypochondriacal disorders

● **F45.4   Pain disorders related to psychological factors**
    Excludes1   pain NOS (R52)

    F45.41   Pain disorder exclusively related to psychological factors
           Somatoform pain disorder (persistent)

    F45.42   Pain disorder with related psychological factors
           Code also associated acute or chronic pain (G89.-)

F45.8   Other somatoform disorders
     Psychogenic dysmenorrhea
     Psychogenic dysphagia, including 'globus hystericus'
     Psychogenic pruritus
     Psychogenic torticollis
     Somatoform autonomic dysfunction
     Teeth grinding
    Excludes1   sleep related teeth grinding (G47.63)

▪ **F45.9   Somatoform disorder, unspecified**
     Psychosomatic disorder NOS

● **F48   Other nonpsychotic mental disorders**

   F48.1   Depersonalization-derealization syndrome

   F48.2   Pseudobulbar affect
      Involuntary emotional expression disorder
      Code first underlying cause, if known, such as:
         amyotrophic lateral sclerosis (G12.21)
         multiple sclerosis (G35)
         sequelae of cerebrovascular disease (I69.-)
         sequelae of traumatic intracranial injury (S06.-)

   F48.8   Other specified nonpsychotic mental disorders
      Dhat syndrome
      Neurasthenia
      Occupational neurosis, including writer's cramp
      Psychasthenia
      Psychasthenic neurosis
      Psychogenic syncope

▪ **F48.9   Nonpsychotic mental disorder, unspecified**
     Neurosis NOS

BEHAVIORAL SYNDROMES ASSOCIATED WITH PHYSIOLOGICAL DISTURBANCES AND PHYSICAL FACTORS (F50-F59)

● **F50   Eating disorders**

    Excludes1   anorexia NOS (R63.0)
                 feeding difficulties (R63.3)
                 polyphagia (R63.2)

    Excludes2   feeding disorder in infancy or childhood (F98.2-)

● **F50.0   Anorexia nervosa**
    Excludes1   loss of appetite (R63.0)
                 psychogenic loss of appetite (F50.8)

    ▪ **F50.00   Anorexia nervosa, unspecified** 🔖

    F50.01   Anorexia nervosa, restricting type 🔖

    F50.02   Anorexia nervosa, binge eating/purging type 🔖
       Excludes1   bulimia nervosa (F50.2)

   F50.2   Bulimia nervosa 🔖
      Bulimia NOS
      Hyperorexia nervosa
    Excludes1   anorexia nervosa, binge eating/purging type (F50.02)

   F50.8   Other eating disorders
      Pica in adults
      Psychogenic loss of appetite
    Excludes2   pica of infancy and childhood (F98.3)

▪ **F50.9   Eating disorder, unspecified**
     Atypical anorexia nervosa
     Atypical bulimia nervosa

● Unacceptable Principal Diagnosis   ● Use Additional Character(s)   ▪ Unspecified   ▶ Manifestation Code

OGCR Official Guidelines for Coding and Reporting   Excludes 1   Excludes 2   Includes   Use additional   Code first   Code also

● **F51 Sleep disorders not due to a substance or known physiological condition**

> **Excludes2**   organic sleep disorders (G47.-)

● **F51.0 Insomnia not due to a substance or known physiological condition**

> **Excludes2**   alcohol related insomnia (F10.182, F10.282, F10.982)
> drug related insomnia (F11.182, F11.282, F11.982, F13.182, F13.282, F13.982, F14.182, F14.282, F14.982, F15.182, F15.282, F15.982, F19.182, F19.282, F19.982)
> insomnia NOS (G47.0-)
> insomnia due to known physiological condition (G47.0-)
> organic insomnia (G47.0-)
> sleep deprivation (Z72.820)

     F51.01 Primary insomnia
        Idiopathic insomnia

     F51.02 Adjustment insomnia

     F51.03 Paradoxical insomnia

     F51.04 Psychophysiologic insomnia

     F51.05 Insomnia due to other mental disorder
        Code also associated mental disorder

     F51.09 Other insomnia not due to a substance or known physiological condition

● **F51.1 Hypersomnia not due to a substance or known physiological condition**
        Hypersomnia: Excessive sleeping/sleepiness

> **Excludes2**   alcohol related hypersomnia (F10.182, F10.282, F10.982)
> drug related hypersomnia (F11.182, F11.282, F11.982, F13.182, F13.282, F13.982, F14.182, F14.282, F14.982, F15.182, F15.282, F15.982, F19.182, F19.282, F19.982)
> hypersomnia NOS (G47.10)
> hypersomnia due to known physiological condition (G47.10)
> idiopathic hypersomnia (G47.11, G47.12)
> narcolepsy (G47.4-)

     F51.11 Primary hypersomnia

     F51.12 Insufficient sleep syndrome

> **Excludes1**   sleep deprivation (Z72.820)

     F51.13 Hypersomnia due to other mental disorder
        Code also associated mental disorder

     F51.19 Other hypersomnia not due to a substance or known physiological condition

F51.3 Sleepwalking [somnambulism]

F51.4 Sleep terrors [night terrors]

F51.5 Nightmare disorder
     Dream anxiety disorder

F51.8 Other sleep disorders not due to a substance or known physiological condition

■ **F51.9 Sleep disorder not due to a substance or known physiological condition, unspecified**
     Emotional sleep disorder NOS

● **F52 Sexual dysfunction not due to a substance or known physiological condition**

> **Excludes2**   Dhat syndrome (F48.8)

F52.0 Hypoactive sexual desire disorder
     Anhedonia (sexual)
     Total loss of feeling of sexual pleasure
     Lack or loss of sexual desire

> **Excludes1**   decreased libido (R68.82)

F52.1 Sexual aversion disorder
     Sexual aversion and lack of sexual enjoyment

● **F52.2 Sexual arousal disorders**
     Failure of genital response

     F52.21 Male erectile disorder ♂
        Psychogenic impotence

> **Excludes1**   impotence of organic origin (N52.-)
> impotence NOS (N52.-)

     F52.22 Female sexual arousal disorder ♀
        Frigidity

● **F52.3 Orgasmic disorder**
     Inhibited orgasm
     Psychogenic anorgasmy

     F52.31 Female orgasmic disorder ♀

     F52.32 Male orgasmic disorder ♂

F52.4 Premature ejaculation ♂

F52.5 Vaginismus not due to a substance or known physiological condition ♀
     Psychogenic vaginismus

> **Excludes2**   vaginismus (due to a known physiological condition) (N94.2)

F52.6 Dyspareunia not due to a substance or known physiological condition ♀
     Dyspareunia: Difficult or painful sexual intercourse
     Psychogenic dyspareunia

> **Excludes2**   dyspareunia (due to a known physiological condition) (N94.1)

F52.8 Other sexual dysfunction not due to a substance or known physiological condition
     Excessive sexual drive
     Nymphomania
     Satyriasis

●■ **F52.9 Unspecified sexual dysfunction not due to a substance or known physiological condition**
     Sexual dysfunction NOS

F53 Puerperal psychosis ♀
     Postpartum depression
     Acute mental illness with sudden onset following childbirth with symptoms of affective psychosis, disorientation, and confusion are prevalent

> **Excludes1**   mood disorders with psychotic features (F30.2, F31.2, F31.5, F31.64, F32.3, F33.3)
> postpartum dysphoria (O90.6)
> psychosis in schizophrenia, schizotypal, delusional, and other psychotic disorders (F20-F29)

CHAPTER 5 (F01-F99)

CHAPTER 5 (F01-F99)

● ▶ **F54** *Psychological and behavioral factors associated with disorders or diseases classified elsewhere*
Psychological factors affecting physical conditions

Code first *the associated physical disorder, such as:*
asthma (J45.-)
dermatitis (L23-L25)
gastric ulcer (K25.-)
mucous colitis (K58.-)
ulcerative colitis (K51.-)
urticaria (L50.-)

Excludes2 tension-type headache (G44.2)

● **F55** **Abuse of non-psychoactive substances**
Excludes2 abuse of psychoactive substances (F10-F19)

F55.0 **Abuse of antacids**

F55.1 **Abuse of herbal or folk remedies**

F55.2 **Abuse of laxatives**

F55.3 **Abuse of steroids or hormones**

F55.4 **Abuse of vitamins**

F55.8 **Abuse of other non-psychoactive substances**

■ **F59** **Unspecified behavioral syndromes associated with physiological disturbances and physical factors**
Psychogenic physiological dysfunction NOS

DISORDERS OF ADULT PERSONALITY AND BEHAVIOR (F60-F69)

● **F60** **Specific personality disorders**
Long-term patterns of thoughts and behaviors causing serious problems with relationships and work.

F60.0 **Paranoid personality disorder**
Hostile, devious, and combative response to disappointments
Expansive paranoid personality (disorder)
Fanatic personality (disorder)
Querulant personality (disorder)
Paranoid personality (disorder)
Sensitive paranoid personality (disorder)

Excludes2 paranoia (F22)
paranoia querulans (F22)
paranoid psychosis (F22)
paranoid schizophrenia (F20.0)
paranoid state (F22)

F60.1 **Schizoid personality disorder**
Detachment from social relationships with minimal emotional experiences and expressions

Excludes2 Asperger's syndrome (F84.5)
delusional disorder (F22)
schizoid disorder of childhood (F84.5)
schizophrenia (F20.-)
schizotypal disorder (F21)

F60.2 **Antisocial personality disorder**
Continuous and chronic antisocial behavior
Amoral personality (disorder)
Asocial personality (disorder)
Dissocial personality disorder
Psychopathic personality (disorder)
Sociopathic personality (disorder)

Excludes1 conduct disorders (F91.-)
Excludes2 borderline personality disorder (F60.3)

F60.3 **Borderline personality disorder**
Instability of mood, self-image or sense of self, and interpersonal relationships
Aggressive personality (disorder)
Emotionally unstable personality disorder
Explosive personality (disorder)

Excludes2 antisocial personality disorder (F60.2)

F60.4 **Histrionic personality disorder**
Personality disorder with excessive emotional and attention-seeking behavior
Hysterical personality (disorder)
Psychoinfantile personality (disorder)

F60.5 **Obsessive-compulsive personality disorder**
Anankastic personality (disorder)
Compulsive personality (disorder)
Obsessional personality (disorder)

Excludes2 obsessive-compulsive disorder (F42)

F60.6 **Avoidant personality disorder**
Anxious personality disorder

F60.7 **Dependent personality disorder**
Asthenic personality (disorder)
Inadequate personality (disorder)
Passive personality (disorder)

● **F60.8** **Other specific personality disorders**

F60.81 **Narcissistic personality disorder**
Vanity, conceit, egotism or indifference to plight of others

F60.89 **Other specific personality disorders**
Eccentric personality disorder
'Haltlose' type personality disorder
Immature personality disorder
Passive-aggressive personality disorder
Psychoneurotic personality disorder
Self-defeating personality disorder

■ **F60.9** **Personality disorder, unspecified**
Character disorder NOS
Character neurosis NOS
Pathological personality NOS

● **F63** **Impulse disorders**
Excludes2 habitual excessive use of alcohol or psychoactive substances (F10-F19)
impulse disorders involving sexual behavior (F65.-)

F63.0 **Pathological gambling**
Compulsive gambling
Excludes1 gambling and betting NOS (Z72.6)
Excludes2 excessive gambling by manic patients (F30, F31)
gambling in antisocial personality disorder (F60.2)

F63.1 **Pyromania**
Pathological fire-setting
Excludes2 fire-setting (by) (in):
adult with antisocial personality disorder (F60.2)
alcohol or psychoactive substance intoxication (F10-F19)
conduct disorders (F91.-)
mental disorders due to known physiological condition (F01-F09)
schizophrenia (F20.-)

● Unacceptable Principal Diagnosis ● Use Additional Character(s) ■ Unspecified ▶ Manifestation Code
OGCR Official Guidelines for Coding and Reporting Excludes 1 Excludes 2 Includes Use additional Code first Code also

F63.2   Kleptomania
Pathological stealing
> **Excludes1**   shoplifting as the reason for observation for suspected mental disorder (Z03.8)
> **Excludes2**   depressive disorder with stealing (F31-F33)
> stealing due to underlying mental condition-code to mental condition
> stealing in mental disorders due to known physiological condition (F01-F09)

F63.3   Trichotillomania
Hair plucking
> **Excludes2**   other stereotyped movement disorder (F98.4)

● **F63.8   Other impulse disorders**
    F63.81   Intermittent explosive disorder
    F63.89   Other impulse disorders

■ **F63.9   Impulse disorder, unspecified**
Impulse control disorder NOS

● **F64 Gender identity disorders**
    F64.1   Gender identity disorder in adolescence and adulthood
     Dual role transvestism
     Transsexualism
> Use additional code to identify sex reassignment status (Z87.890)
> **Excludes1**   gender identity disorder in childhood (F64.2)
> **Excludes2**   fetishistic transvestism (F65.1)

    F64.2   Gender identity disorder of childhood   **P**
> **Excludes1**   gender identity disorder in adolescence and adulthood (F64.1)
> **Excludes2**   sexual maturation disorder (F66)

    F64.8   Other gender identity disorders
■ **F64.9   Gender identity disorder, unspecified**
Gender-role disorder NOS

● **F65   Paraphilias**
    F65.0   Fetishism
Intense sexual urges and arousing fantasies using inanimate objects

    F65.1   Transvestic fetishism
Intense sexual urges, arousal, or orgasm associated with fantasized/actual cross-dressing
Fetishistic transvestism

    F65.2   Exhibitionism
    F65.3   Voyeurism
Sexual urges or arousal involving real or fantasized observation of unsuspecting people who are naked, disrobing, or engaging in sexual activity

    F65.4   Pedophilia
● **F65.5   Sadomasochism**
    ■ **F65.50   Sadomasochism, unspecified**
    F65.51   Sexual masochism
    F65.52   Sexual sadism

● **F65.8   Other paraphilias**
    F65.81   Frotteurism
Sexual arousal or orgasm is achieved by rubbing up against another person (or fantasies of), in crowded place with unsuspecting victim

    F65.89   Other paraphilias
Necrophilia

■ **F65.9   Paraphilia, unspecified**
Sexual deviation NOS

F66   Other sexual disorders
Sexual maturation disorder
Sexual relationship disorder

● **F68   Other disorders of adult personality and behavior**
● **F68.1   Factitious disorder**
Compensation neurosis
Elaboration of physical symptoms for psychological reasons
Hospital hopper syndrome
Münchhausen's syndrome
Peregrinating patient
> **Excludes2**   factitial dermatitis (L98.1)
> person feigning illness (with obvious motivation) (Z76.5)

    ■ **F68.10   Factitious disorder, unspecified** 🅒
    F68.11   Factitious disorder with predominantly psychological signs and symptoms
    F68.12   Factitious disorder with predominantly physical signs and symptoms 🅒
    F68.13   Factitious disorder with combined psychological and physical signs and symptoms

    F68.8   Other specified disorders of adult personality and behavior

■ **F69   Unspecified disorder of adult personality and behavior**   **A**

INTELLECTUAL DISABILITIES (F70-F79)

Code first any associated physical or developmental disorders
> **Excludes1**   borderline intellectual functioning, IQ above 70 to 84 (R41.83)

F70   Mild intellectual disabilities
IQ level 50-55 to approximately 70
Mild mental subnormality

F71   Moderate intellectual disabilities
IQ level 35-40 to 50-55
Moderate mental subnormality

F72   Severe intellectual disabilities 🅒
IQ 20-25 to 35-40
Severe mental subnormality

F73   Profound intellectual disabilities 🅒
IQ level below 20-25
Profound mental subnormality

F78   Other intellectual disabilities

■ **F79   Unspecified intellectual disabilities**
Mental deficiency NOS
Mental subnormality NOS

N Newborn Age: 0   **P** Pediatric Age: 0–17   **M** Maternity DX: 12–55   **A** Adult Age: 15–124   ♀ Females Only   ♂ Males Only
🅒 Complication\Comorbidity   🅒 Major C\C   Present on Admission Requirement   Hospital-Acquired Condition
927

PERVASIVE AND SPECIFIC DEVELOPMENTAL DISORDERS (F80-F89)

● **F80   Specific developmental disorders of speech and language**

    F80.0   Phonological disorder
        Communication disorder of unknown cause,
          characterized by failure to use age-appropriate
          sounds
        Dyslalia
        Functional speech articulation disorder
        Lalling
        Lisping
        Phonological developmental disorder
        Speech articulation developmental disorder

        Excludes1   speech articulation impairment due to aphasia NOS (R47.01)
             speech articulation impairment due to apraxia (R48.2)

        Excludes2   speech articulation impairment due to hearing loss (F80.4)
             speech articulation impairment due to intellectual disabilities (F70-F79)
             speech articulation impairment with expressive language developmental disorder (F80.1)
             speech articulation impairment with mixed receptive expressive language developmental disorder (F80.2)

    F80.1   Expressive language disorder
        Developmental dysphasia or aphasia, expressive type

        Excludes1   mixed receptive-expressive language disorder (F80.2)
             dysphasia and aphasia NOS (R47.-)

        Excludes2   acquired aphasia with epilepsy [Landau-Kleffner] (G40.80-)
             intellectual disabilities (F70-F79)
             pervasive developmental disorders (F84.-)
             selective mutism (F94.0)

    F80.2   Mixed receptive-expressive language disorder
        Developmental dysphasia or aphasia, receptive type
        Developmental Wernicke's aphasia

        Excludes1   central auditory processing disorder (H93.25)
             dysphasia or aphasia NOS (R47.-)
             expressive language disorder (F80.1)
             expressive type dysphasia or aphasia (F80.1)
             word deafness (H93.25)

        Excludes2   acquired aphasia with epilepsy [Landau-Kleffner] (G40.80-)
             intellectual disabilities (F70-F79)
             pervasive developmental disorders (F84.-)
             selective mutism (F94.0)

    F80.4   Speech and language development delay due to hearing loss
        Code also type of hearing loss (H90.-, H91.-)

    ● **F80.8   Other developmental disorders of speech or language**

        F80.81   Childhood onset fluency disorder
            Cluttering NOS
            Stuttering NOS

            Excludes1   adult onset fluency disorder (F98.5)
                fluency disorder in conditions classified elsewhere (R47.82)
                fluency disorder (stuttering) following cerebrovascular disease (I69. with final characters -23)

        F80.89   Other developmental disorders of speech and language

    ■ **F80.9   Developmental disorder of speech and language, unspecified**
        Communication disorder NOS
        Language disorder NOS

● **F81   Specific developmental disorders of scholastic skills**

    F81.0   Specific reading disorder
        'Backward reading'
        Developmental dyslexia
        Specific reading retardation

        Excludes1   alexia NOS (R48.0)
             dyslexia NOS (R48.0)

    F81.2   Mathematics disorder
        Developmental acalculia
        Developmental arithmetical disorder
        Developmental Gerstmann's syndrome

        Excludes1   acalculia NOS (R48.8)

        Excludes2   arithmetical difficulties associated with a reading disorder (F81.0)
             arithmetical difficulties associated with a spelling disorder (F81.81)
             arithmetical difficulties due to inadequate teaching (Z55.8)

    ● **F81.8   Other developmental disorders of scholastic skills**

        F81.81   Disorder of written expression
            Specific spelling disorder

        F81.89   Other developmental disorders of scholastic skills

    ● ■ **F81.9   Developmental disorder of scholastic skills, unspecified**
        Knowledge acquisition disability NOS
        Learning disability NOS
        Learning disorder NOS

   F82   Specific developmental disorder of motor function
        Clumsy child syndrome
        Developmental coordination disorder
        Developmental dyspraxia

    Excludes1   abnormalities of gait and mobility (R26.-)
         lack of coordination (R27.-)

    Excludes2   lack of coordination secondary to intellectual disabilities (F70-F79)

● **F84   Pervasive developmental disorders**
    Use additional code to identify any associated medical condition and intellectual disabilities.

    F84.0   Autistic disorder ✆
        Infantile autism
        Infantile psychosis
        Kanner's syndrome

        Excludes1   Asperger's syndrome (F84.5)

● Unacceptable Principal Diagnosis   ● Use Additional Character(s)   ■ Unspecified   ▶ Manifestation Code
OGCR Official Guidelines for Coding and Reporting   Excludes 1   Excludes 2   Includes   Use additional   Code first   Code also

F84.2   Rett's syndrome 🦠
Neurodevelopmental disorder

> **Excludes1**   Asperger's syndrome (F84.5)
> Autistic disorder (F84.0)
> other childhood disintegrative
> disorder (F84.3)

F84.3   Other childhood disintegrative disorder 🦠   P
Dementia infantilis
*At least two years of normal development followed
by significant loss of language abilities, social
skills, bowel/bladder control, motor skills*
Disintegrative psychosis
Heller's syndrome
*At least two years of normal development followed
by significant loss of language abilities, social
skills, bowel/bladder control, motor skills*
Symbiotic psychosis
*Abnormal relationship to mothering figure,
characterized by intense separation anxiety,
severe regression, giving up of useful speech,
and autism*

> Use additional code to identify any associated
> neurological condition.

> **Excludes1**   Asperger's syndrome (F84.5)
> Autistic disorder (F84.0)
> Rett's syndrome (F84.2)

F84.5   Asperger's syndrome 🦠
Developmental disorder
Asperger's disorder
Autistic psychopathy
Schizoid disorder of childhood

F84.8   Other pervasive developmental disorders 🦠
Overactive disorder associated with intellectual
disabilities and stereotyped movements

F84.9   Pervasive developmental disorder, unspecified 🦠
Atypical autism

F88   Other disorders of psychological development
Developmental agnosia

F89   Unspecified disorder of psychological development
Developmental disorder NOS

BEHAVIORAL AND EMOTIONAL DISORDERS WITH ONSET USUALLY OCCURRING IN CHILDHOOD AND ADOLESCENCE (F90-F98)

Note: Codes within categories F90-F98 may be used
regardless of the age of a patient. These disorders
generally have onset within the childhood or adolescent
years, but may continue throughout life or not be
diagnosed until adulthood.

F90   Attention-deficit hyperactivity disorders

> **Includes**   attention deficit disorder with hyperactivity
> attention deficit syndrome with hyperactivity

> **Excludes2**   anxiety disorders (F40.-, F41.-)
> mood [affective] disorders (F30-F39)
> pervasive developmental disorders (F84.-)
> schizophrenia (F20.-)

Attention deficit disorder with hyperactivity=ADHD

**F90.0   Attention-deficit hyperactivity disorder,
predominantly inattentive type**

**F90.1   Attention-deficit hyperactivity disorder,
predominantly hyperactive type**

**F90.2   Attention-deficit hyperactivity disorder, combined
type**

F90.8   Attention-deficit hyperactivity disorder, other type

**F90.9   Attention-deficit hyperactivity disorder,
unspecified type**
Attention-deficit hyperactivity disorder of
childhood or adolescence NOS
Attention-deficit hyperactivity disorder NOS

F91   Conduct disorders
Childhood/adolescence disruptive behavior disorder

> **Excludes1**   antisocial behavior (Z72.81-)
> antisocial personality disorder (F60.2)

> **Excludes2**   conduct problems associated with attention-
> deficit hyperactivity disorder (F90.-)
> mood [affective] disorders (F30-F39)
> pervasive developmental disorders (F84.-)
> schizophrenia (F20.-)

F91.0   Conduct disorder confined to family context

F91.1   Conduct disorder, childhood-onset type
Unsocialized conduct disorder
Conduct disorder, solitary aggressive type
Unsocialized aggressive disorder

F91.2   Conduct disorder, adolescent-onset type
Socialized conduct disorder
Conduct disorder, group type

F91.3   Oppositional defiant disorder

F91.8   Other conduct disorders

F91.9   Conduct disorder, unspecified
Behavioral disorder NOS
Conduct disorder NOS
Disruptive behavior disorder NOS

F93   Emotional disorders with onset specific to childhood

F93.0   Separation anxiety disorder of childhood   P

> **Excludes2**   mood [affective] disorders (F30-F39)
> nonpsychotic mental disorders
> (F40-F48)
> phobic anxiety disorder of childhood
> (F40.8)
> social phobia (F40.1)

F93.8   Other childhood emotional disorders   P
Identity disorder

> **Excludes2**   gender identity disorder of
> childhood (F64.2)

F93.9   Childhood emotional disorder, unspecified   P

**F94   Disorders of social functioning with onset specific to
childhood and adolescence**

F94.0   Selective mutism
Elective mutism

> **Excludes2**   pervasive developmental disorders
> (F84.-)
> schizophrenia (F20.-)
> specific developmental disorders of
> speech and language (F80.-)
> transient mutism as part of
> separation anxiety in young
> children (F93.0)

F94.1   Reactive attachment disorder of childhood   P

> Use additional code to identify any associated
> failure to thrive or growth retardation

> **Excludes1**   disinhibited attachment disorder of
> childhood (F94.2)
> normal variation in pattern of
> selective attachment

> **Excludes2**   Asperger's syndrome (F84.5)
> maltreatment syndromes (T74.-)
> sexual or physical abuse in childhood,
> resulting in psychosocial
> problems (Z62.81-)

N Newborn Age: 0   **P** Pediatric Age: 0–17   **M** Maternity DX: 12–55   **A** Adult Age: 15–124   ♀ Females Only   ♂ Males Only

🦠 Complication\Comorbidity   🦠 Major C\C   🦠 Present on Admission Requirement   🦠 Hospital-Acquired Condition

929

Item 5–2 Enuresis: Bed wetting by children at night. Causes can be either psychological or medical (diabetes, urinary tract infections, or abnormalities). **Encopresis:** Overflow incontinence of bowels sometimes resulting from chronic constipation or fecal impaction. Check the documentation for additional diagnoses.

F94.2　Disinhibited attachment disorder of childhood　P
　　Affectionless psychopathy
　　Institutional syndrome

> **Excludes1**　reactive attachment disorder of childhood (F94.l)

> **Excludes2**　Asperger's syndrome (F84.5)
> 　　attention-deficit hyperactivity disorders (F90.-)
> 　　hospitalism in children (F43.2-)

F94.8　Other childhood disorders of social functioning　P

F94.9　Childhood disorder of social functioning, unspecified　P

● **F95　Tic disorder**
　　Involuntary twitch

F95.0　Transient tic disorder

F95.1　Chronic motor or vocal tic disorder

F95.2　Tourette's disorder
　　Combined vocal and multiple motor tic disorder [de la Tourette]
　　Tourette's syndrome

F95.8　Other tic disorders

F95.9　Tic disorder, unspecified
　　Tic NOS

● **F98　Other behavioral and emotional disorders with onset usually occurring in childhood and adolescence**

> **Excludes2**　breath-holding spells (R06.89)
> 　　gender identity disorder of childhood (F64.2)
> 　　Kleine-Levin syndrome (G47.13)
> 　　obsessive-compulsive disorder (F42)
> 　　sleep disorders not due to a substance or known physiological condition (F51.-)

F98.0　Enuresis not due to a substance or known physiological condition
　　Enuresis: Urinary incontinence
　　Enuresis (primary) (secondary) of nonorganic origin
　　Functional enuresis
　　Psychogenic enuresis
　　Urinary incontinence of nonorganic origin

> **Excludes1**　enuresis NOS (R32)

F98.1　Encopresis not due to a substance or known physiological condition
　　Encopresis: Fecal incontinence
　　Functional encopresis
　　Incontinence of feces of nonorganic origin
　　Psychogenic encopresis

　　Use additional code to identify the cause of any coexisting constipation.

> **Excludes1**　encopresis NOS (R15-)

● **F98.2　Other feeding disorders of infancy and childhood**

> **Excludes1**　feeding difficulties (R63.3)

> **Excludes2**　anorexia nervosa and other eating disorders (F50.-)
> 　　feeding problems of newborn (P92.-)
> 　　pica of infancy or childhood (F98.3)

F98.21　Rumination disorder of infancy　P

F98.29　Other feeding disorders of infancy and early childhood　P

F98.3　Pica of infancy and childhood　P
　　Craving and eating substances such as paint, clay, or dirt to replace a nutritional deficit in the body.

F98.4　Stereotyped movement disorders
　　Stereotype/habit disorder

> **Excludes1**　abnormal involuntary movements (R25.-)

> **Excludes2**　compulsions in obsessive-compulsive disorder (F42)
> 　　hair plucking (F63.3)
> 　　movement disorders of organic origin (G20-G25)
> 　　nail-biting (F98.8)
> 　　nose-picking (F98.8)
> 　　stereotypies that are part of a broader psychiatric condition (F01-F95)
> 　　thumb-sucking (F98.8)
> 　　tic disorders (F95.-)
> 　　trichotillomania (F63.3)

F98.5　Adult onset fluency disorder

> **Excludes1**　childhood onset fluency disorder (F80.81)
> 　　dysphasia (R47.02)
> 　　fluency disorder in conditions classified elsewhere (R47.82)
> 　　fluency disorder (stuttering) following cerebrovascular disease (I69. with final characters -23)
> 　　tic disorders (F95.-)

F98.8　Other specified behavioral and emotional disorders with onset usually occurring in childhood and adolescence　P
　　Excessive masturbation
　　Nail-biting
　　Nose-picking
　　Thumb-sucking

F98.9　Unspecified behavioral and emotional disorders with onset usually occurring in childhood and adolescence　P

UNSPECIFIED MENTAL DISORDER (F99)

F99　Mental disorder, not otherwise specified
　　Mental illness NOS

> **Excludes1**　unspecified mental disorder due to known physiological condition (F09)

● Unacceptable Principal Diagnosis　　● Use Additional Character(s)　　■ Unspecified　　▶ Manifestation Code
OGCR Official Guidelines for Coding and Reporting　　Excludes 1　　Excludes 2　　Includes　　Use additional　　Code first　　Code also

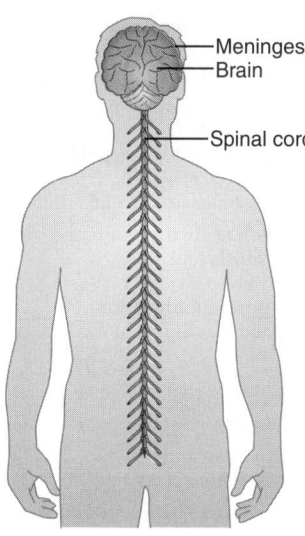

—Meninges
—Brain

—Spinal cord

Figure 6-1 The brain and spinal cord make up the central nervous system.

Item 6–1 The two major classifications of the nervous system are the peripheral nervous system and the central nervous system (CNS). The central nervous system is comprised of the brain and the spinal cord. The peripheral nervous system is comprised of the parasympathetic and sympathetic systems. **Encephalitis** is the swelling of the brain. **Meningitis** is swelling of the covering of the brain, the meninges. Types and causes of brain infections are:

Type Cause
purulent bacterial
aseptic/abacterial viral
chronic meningitis mycobacterial and fungal

CHAPTER 6

DISEASES OF THE NERVOUS SYSTEM
(G00-G99)

Excludes2	certain conditions originating in the perinatal period (P04-P96)
	certain infectious and parasitic diseases (A00-B99)
	complications of pregnancy, childbirth and the puerperium (O00-O9A)
	congenital malformations, deformations, and chromosomal abnormalities (Q00-Q99)
	endocrine, nutritional and metabolic diseases (E00-E88)
	injury, poisoning and certain other consequences of external causes (S00-T88)
	neoplasms (C00-D49)
	symptoms, signs and abnormal clinical and laboratory findings, not elsewhere classified (R00-R94)

This chapter contains the following blocks:

G00-G09	Inflammatory diseases of the central nervous system
G10-G14	Systemic atrophies primarily affecting the central nervous system
G20-G26	Extrapyramidal and movement disorders
G30-G32	Other degenerative diseases of the nervous system
G35-G37	Demyelinating diseases of the central nervous system
G40-G47	Episodic and paroxysmal disorders
G50-G59	Nerve, nerve root and plexus disorders
G60-G65	Polyneuropathies and other disorders of the peripheral nervous system
G70-G73	Diseases of myoneural junction and muscle
G80-G83	Cerebral palsy and other paralytic syndromes
G89-G99	Other disorders of the nervous system

INFLAMMATORY DISEASES OF THE CENTRAL NERVOUS SYSTEM (G00-G09)

● **G00   Bacterial meningitis, not elsewhere classified**
An infection of the cerebrospinal fluid surrounding the spinal cord and brain.

Includes	bacterial arachnoiditis
	bacterial leptomeningitis
	bacterial meningitis
	bacterial pachymeningitis

Excludes1	bacterial:
	meningoencephalitis (G04.2)
	meningomyelitis (G04.2)

G00.0   Hemophilus meningitis 🦠
     Meningitis due to Hemophilus influenzae

G00.1   Pneumococcal meningitis 🦠

G00.2   Streptococcal meningitis 🦠
     Use additional code to further identify organism (B95.0-B95.5)

G00.3   Staphylococcal meningitis 🦠
     Use additional code to further identify organism (B95.61-B95.8)

G00.8   Other bacterial meningitis 🦠
     Meningitis due to Escherichia coli
     Meningitis due to Friedländer bacillus
     Meningitis due to Klebsiella
     Use additional code to further identify organism (B96.-)

▪ **G00.9   Bacterial meningitis, unspecified** 🦠
     Meningitis due to gram-negative bacteria, unspecified
     Purulent meningitis NOS
     Pyogenic meningitis NOS
     Suppurative meningitis NOS

● ▶ *G01   Meningitis in bacterial diseases classified elsewhere* 🦠
Code first underlying disease

Excludes1	meningitis (in):
	gonococcal (A54.81)
	leptospirosis (A27.81)
	listeriosis (A32.11)
	Lyme disease (A69.21)
	meningococcal (A39.0)
	neurosyphilis (A52.13)
	tuberculosis (A17.0)
	meningoencephalitis and meningomyelitis in bacterial diseases classified elsewhere (G05)

N Newborn Age: 0   **P** Pediatric Age: 0–17   **M** Maternity DX: 12–55   **A** Adult Age: 15–124   ♀ Females Only   ♂ Males Only

🦠 Complication\Comorbidity   🦠 Major C\C   🦠 Present on Admission Requirement   🦠 Hospital-Acquired Condition

931

CHAPTER 6 (G00-G99)

CHAPTER 6 (G00-G99)

● ▶ **G02**   *Meningitis in other infectious and parasitic diseases classified elsewhere* 🦠

     Code first underlying disease, such as:
        African trypanosomiasis (B56.-)
        poliovirus infection (A80.-)

     | Excludes1 | candidal meningitis (B37.5)
                    coccidioidomycosis meningitis (B38.4)
                    cryptococcal meningitis (B45.1)
                    herpesviral [herpes simplex] meningitis
                       (B00.3)
                    infectious mononucleosis complicated
                       by meningitis (B27.- with fourth
                       character 2)
                    measles complicated by meningitis (B05.1)
                    meningoencephalitis and meningomyelitis
                       in other infectious and parasitic diseases
                       classified elsewhere (G05)
                    mumps meningitis (B26.1)
                    rubella meningitis (B06.02)
                    varicella [chickenpox] meningitis (B01.0)
                    zoster meningitis (B02.1)

● **G03**   **Meningitis due to other and unspecified causes**

     | Includes | arachnoiditis NOS
                   leptomeningitis NOS
                   meningitis NOS
                   pachymeningitis NOS

     | Excludes1 | meningoencephalitis (G04.-)
                    meningomyelitis (G04.-)

    G03.0   **Nonpyogenic meningitis** 🦠
           Aseptic meningitis
           Nonbacterial meningitis

    G03.1   **Chronic meningitis** 🦠

    G03.2   **Benign recurrent meningitis [Mollaret]** 🦠

    G03.8   **Meningitis due to other specified causes** 🦠

    ◻ **G03.9**   **Meningitis, unspecified** 🦠
           Arachnoiditis (spinal) NOS

● **G04**   **Encephalitis, myelitis and encephalomyelitis**

     | Includes | acute ascending myelitis
                   meningoencephalitis
                   meningomyelitis

     | Excludes1 | encephalopathy NOS (G93.40)
                    other noninfectious acute disseminated
                       encephalomyelitis (noninfectious
                       ADEM) (G04.81)

     | Excludes2 | acute transverse myelitis (G37.3-)
                    alcoholic encephalopathy (G31.2)
                    benign myalgic encephalomyelitis (G93.3)
                    multiple sclerosis (G35)
                    subacute necrotizing myelitis (G37.4)
                    toxic encephalitis (G92)
                    toxic encephalopathy (G92)

    ● **G04.0**   **Acute disseminated encephalitis and encephalomyelitis (ADEM)**

        | Excludes1 | acute necrotizing hemorrhagic
                        encephalopathy (G04.3-)

      G04.00   **Acute disseminated encephalitis and encephalomyelitis, unspecified** 🦠

      G04.01   **Postinfectious acute disseminated encephalitis and encephalomyelitis (postinfectious ADEM)** 🦠

         | Excludes1 | post chickenpox encephalitis
                         (B01.1)
                      post measles encephalitis
                         (B05.0)
                      post measles myelitis (B05.1)

      G04.02   **Postimmunization acute disseminated encephalitis, myelitis and encephalomyelitis**
          Encephalitis, post immunization
          Encephalomyelitis, post immunization

        | Use additional | code to identify the
               vaccine (T50.A-, T50.B-, T50.Z-)

    G04.1   **Tropical spastic paraplegia** 🦠

    G04.2   **Bacterial meningoencephalitis and meningomyelitis, not elsewhere classified** 🦠

● **G04.3**   **Acute necrotizing hemorrhagic encephalopathy**
         Sudden and severe CNS disease with pathology of hemorrhages and necrosis of white matter

     | Excludes1 | acute disseminated encephalitis and
                        encephalomyelitis (G04.0-)

      G04.30   **Acute necrotizing hemorrhagic encephalopathy, unspecified** 🦠

      G04.31   **Postinfectious acute necrotizing hemorrhagic encephalopathy** 🦠

      G04.32   **Postimmunization acute necrotizing hemorrhagic encephalopathy**

        | Use additional | code to identify vaccine
              (T50.A-, T50.B-, T50.Z-)

      G04.39   **Other acute necrotizing hemorrhagic encephalopathy**

        | Code also | underlying etiology, if
              applicable

● **G04.8**   **Other encephalitis, myelitis and encephalomyelitis**
        | Code also | any associated seizure (G40.-, R56.9)

      G04.81   **Other encephalitis and encephalomyelitis** 🦠
          Noninfectious acute disseminated
             encephalomyelitis (noninfectious
             ADEM)

      G04.89   **Other myelitis** 🦠

● **G04.9**   **Encephalitis, myelitis and encephalomyelitis, unspecified**

    ◻ **G04.90**   **Encephalitis and encephalomyelitis, unspecified** 🦠
          Ventriculitis (cerebral) NOS

    ◻ **G04.91**   **Myelitis, unspecified** 🦠

● G05　Encephalitis, myelitis and encephalomyelitis in diseases classified elsewhere

    Code first underlying disease, such as:
      human immunodeficiency virus [HIV] disease (B20)
      poliovirus (A80.-)
      suppurative otitis media (H66.01-H66.4)
      trichinellosis (B75)

    | Excludes1 | adenoviral encephalitis, myelitis and encephalomyelitis (A85.1)
      congenital toxoplasmosis encephalitis, myelitis and encephalomyelitis (P37.1)
      cytomegaloviral encephalitis, myelitis and encephalomyelitis (B25.8)
      encephalitis, myelitis and encephalomyelitis (in) measles (B05.0)
      encephalitis, myelitis and encephalomyelitis (in) systemic lupus erythematosus (M32.19)
      enteroviral encephalitis, myelitis and encephalomyelitis (A85.0)
      herpesviral [herpes simplex] encephalitis, myelitis and encephalomyelitis (B00.4)
      listerial encephalitis, myelitis and encephalomyelitis (A32.12)
      meningococcal encephalitis, myelitis and encephalomyelitis (A39.81)
      mumps encephalitis, myelitis and encephalomyelitis (B26.2)
      postchickenpox encephalitis, myelitis and encephalomyelitis (B01.1-)
      rubella encephalitis, myelitis and encephalomyelitis (B06.01)
      toxoplasmosis encephalitis, myelitis and encephalomyelitis (B58.2)
      zoster encephalitis, myelitis and encephalomyelitis (B02.0)

● ▶ **G05.3　Encephalitis and encephalomyelitis in diseases classified elsewhere** 🦠
    Meningoencephalitis in diseases classified elsewhere

● ▶ **G05.4　Myelitis in diseases classified elsewhere** 🦠
    Meningomyelitis in diseases classified elsewhere

● G06　Intracranial and intraspinal abscess and granuloma
    An accumulation of pus in either the brain or spinal cord

    | Use additional | code (B95-B97) to identify infectious agent.

    G06.0　Intracranial abscess and granuloma 🦠
      Brain [any part] abscess (embolic)
      Cerebellar abscess (embolic)
      Cerebral abscess (embolic)
      Intracranial epidural abscess or granuloma
      Intracranial extradural abscess or granuloma
      Intracranial subdural abscess or granuloma
      Otogenic abscess (embolic)

      | Excludes1 | tuberculous intracranial abscess and granuloma (A17.81)

    G06.1　Intraspinal abscess and granuloma 🦠
      Abscess (embolic) of spinal cord [any part]
      Intraspinal epidural abscess or granuloma
      Intraspinal extradural abscess or granuloma
      Intraspinal subdural abscess or granuloma

      | Excludes1 | tuberculous intraspinal abscess and granuloma (A17.81)

    ■ **G06.2　Extradural and subdural abscess, unspecified** 🦠

● ▶ G07　*Intracranial and intraspinal abscess and granuloma in diseases classified elsewhere* 🦠

    Code first underlying disease, such as:
      schistosomiasis granuloma of brain (B65.-)

    | Excludes1 | abscess of brain:
      amebic (A06.6)
      chromomycotic (B43.1)
      gonococcal (A54.82)
      tuberculous (A17.81)
      tuberculoma of meninges (A17.1)

G08　Intracranial and intraspinal phlebitis and thrombophlebitis 🦠
    Septic embolism of intracranial or intraspinal venous sinuses and veins
    Septic endophlebitis of intracranial or intraspinal venous sinuses and veins
    Septic phlebitis of intracranial or intraspinal venous sinuses and veins
    Septic thrombophlebitis of intracranial or intraspinal venous sinuses and veins
    Septic thrombosis of intracranial or intraspinal venous sinuses and veins

    | Excludes1 | intracranial phlebitis and thrombophlebitis complicating:
      abortion, ectopic or molar pregnancy (O00-O07, O08.7)
      pregnancy, childbirth and the puerperium (O22.5, O87.3)
      nonpyogenic intracranial phlebitis and thrombophlebitis (I67.6)
      nonpyogenic intraspinal phlebitis and thrombophlebitis (G95.1)

● G09　Sequelae of inflammatory diseases of central nervous system 🦠

    Note: Category G09 is to be used to indicate conditions whose primary classification is to G00-G08 as the cause of sequelae, themselves classifiable elsewhere. The 'sequelae' include conditions specified as residuals.

    Code first condition resulting from (sequela) of inflammatory diseases of central nervous system

---

SYSTEMIC ATROPHIES PRIMARILY AFFECTING THE CENTRAL NERVOUS SYSTEM (G10-G14)

G10　Huntington's disease 🦠
    Genetic disease with degeneration of cells of the nervous system, including brain
    Huntington's chorea
    Huntington's dementia

● G11　Hereditary ataxia
    Genetic neurological disorder affecting coordination

    | Excludes2 | cerebral palsy (G80.-)
      hereditary and idiopathic neuropathy (G60.-)
      metabolic disorders (E70-E88)

    G11.0　Congenital nonprogressive ataxia 🦠

    G11.1　Early-onset cerebellar ataxia 🦠
      Early-onset cerebellar ataxia with essential tremor
      Early-onset cerebellar ataxia with myoclonus [Hunt's ataxia]
      Early-onset cerebellar ataxia with retained tendon reflexes
      Friedreich's ataxia (autosomal recessive)
      X-linked recessive spinocerebellar ataxia

Item 6–2 Huntington's chorea is an inherited degenerative disorder of the central nervous system and is characterized by ceaseless, jerky movements and progressive cognitive and behavioral deterioration.

CHAPTER 6 (G00-G99)

G11.2   Late-onset cerebellar ataxia 🖐   A

G11.3   Cerebellar ataxia with defective DNA repair 🖐
Ataxia telangiectasia [Louis-Bar]

> | Excludes2 | Cockayne's syndrome (Q87.1) |

> other disorders of purine and
> pyrimidine metabolism (E79.-)
> xeroderma pigmentosum (Q82.1)

G11.4   Hereditary spastic paraplegia 🖐

G11.8   Other hereditary ataxias 🖐

◼ **G11.9   Hereditary ataxia, unspecified** 🖐
Hereditary cerebellar ataxia NOS
Hereditary cerebellar degeneration
Hereditary cerebellar disease
Hereditary cerebellar syndrome

● **G12   Spinal muscular atrophy and related syndromes**

**G12.0   Infantile spinal muscular atrophy, type I
[Werdnig-Hoffman]** 🖐

G12.1   Other inherited spinal muscular atrophy 🖐
Adult form spinal muscular atrophy
Childhood form, type II spinal muscular atrophy
Distal spinal muscular atrophy
Juvenile form, type III spinal muscular atrophy
[Kugelberg-Welander]
Progressive bulbar palsy of childhood [Fazio-
Londe]
Scapuloperoneal form spinal muscular atrophy

● **G12.2   Motor neuron disease**
*Progressive disease of motor neurons that carry
impluses to muscles to move*

◼ **G12.20   Motor neuron disease, unspecified** 🖐

G12.21   Amyotrophic lateral sclerosis 🖐   A
Lou Gehrig's disease (ALS)
Progressive spinal muscle atrophy

G12.22   Progressive bulbar palsy 🖐

G12.29   Other motor neuron disease 🖐
Familial motor neuron disease
Primary lateral sclerosis

**G12.8   Other spinal muscular atrophies and related
syndromes** 🖐

◼ **G12.9   Spinal muscular atrophy, unspecified** 🖐

● **G13   Systemic atrophies primarily affecting central nervous
system in diseases classified elsewhere**

● ▶ *G13.0   Paraneoplastic neuromyopathy and neuropathy*
Carcinomatous neuromyopathy
Sensorial paraneoplastic neuropathy [Denny Brown]

> *Code first underlying neoplasm (C00-D49)*

● ▶ *G13.1   Other systemic atrophy primarily affecting central
nervous system in neoplastic disease*
Paraneoplastic limbic encephalopathy

> *Code first underlying neoplasm (C00-D49)*

● ▶ *G13.2   Systemic atrophy primarily affecting the central
nervous system in myxedema*

> *Code first underlying disease, such as:*
> hypothyroidism (E03.-)
> myxedematous congenital iodine deficiency
> (E00.1)

● ▶ *G13.8   Systemic atrophy primarily affecting central
nervous system in other diseases classified
elsewhere*

> *Code first underlying disease*

G14   Postpolio syndrome 🖐

> | Includes | Postpolio myelitic syndrome |
> | Excludes1 | sequelae of poliomyelitis (B91) |

EXTRAPYRAMIDAL AND MOVEMENT DISORDERS (G20-G26)

G20   Parkinson's disease
*Progressive disease of the nervous system that affects muscle
coordination*
Hemiparkinsonism
Idiopathic Parkinsonism or Parkinson's disease
Paralysis agitans
Parkinsonism or Parkinson's disease NOS
Primary Parkinsonism or Parkinson's disease

> | Excludes1 | dementia with Parkinsonism (G31.83) |

● **G21   Secondary parkinsonism**
*Symptoms of Parkinson's caused by medicines, illness, or other
nervous system disorder*

> | Excludes1 | dementia with Parkinsonism (G31.83) |

> Huntington's disease (G10)
> Shy-Drager syndrome (G90.3)
> syphilitic Parkinsonism (A52.19)

● **G21.0   Malignant neuroleptic syndrome** 🖐

> Use additional code for adverse effect, if
> applicable, to identify drug (T43.3X5,
> T43.4X5, T43.505, T43.595)

> | Excludes1 | neuroleptic induced parkinsonism |

> (G21.11)

● **G21.1   Other drug-induced secondary parkinsonism**

● **G21.11   Neuroleptic induced parkinsonism** 🖐

> Use additional code for adverse effect,
> if applicable, to identify drug
> (T43.3X5, T43.4X5, T43.505, T43.595)

> | Excludes1 | malignant neuroleptic |

> syndrome (G21.0)

● **G21.19   Other drug induced secondary
parkinsonism** 🖐

> Use additional code for adverse effect, if
> applicable, to identify drug (T36-T50
> with fifth or sixth character 5)

● **G21.2   Secondary parkinsonism due to other external
agents** 🖐

> *Code first (T51-T65) to identify external agent*

G21.3   Postencephalitic parkinsonism 🖐

G21.4   Vascular parkinsonism

G21.8   Other secondary parkinsonism 🖐

◼ **G21.9   Secondary parkinsonism, unspecified** 🖐

● **G23   Other degenerative diseases of basal ganglia**

> | Excludes2 | multi-system degeneration of the autonomic |

> nervous system (G90.3)

G23.0   Hallervorden-Spatz disease 🖐
Pigmentary pallidal degeneration

**G23.1   Progressive supranuclear ophthalmoplegia
[Steele-Richardson-Olszewski]** 🖐
Progressive supranuclear palsy

G23.2   Striatonigral degeneration 🖐

**G23.8   Other specified degenerative diseases of basal
ganglia** 🖐
Calcification of basal ganglia

◼ **G23.9   Degenerative disease of basal ganglia,
unspecified** 🖐

●   Unacceptable Principal Diagnosis   ●   Use Additional Character(s)   ◼   Unspecified   ▶   Manifestation Code
OGCR   Official Guidelines for Coding and Reporting | Excludes 1 | | Excludes 2 | Includes   Use additional   Code first   Code also

● **G24 Dystonia**
Involuntary movements
   Includes dyskinesia
   Excludes2 athetoid cerebral palsy (G80.3)

● **G24.0 Drug induced dystonia**
   Use additional code for adverse effect, if applicable, to identify drug (T36-T50 with fifth or sixth character 5)

   ● **G24.01 Drug induced subacute dyskinesia**
     Drug induced blepharospasm
     Drug induced orofacial dyskinesia
     Neuroleptic induced tardive dyskinesia
     Tardive dyskinesia

   ● **G24.02 Drug induced acute dystonia** 🌑
     Acute dystonic reaction to drugs
     Neuroleptic induced acute dystonia

   ● **G24.09 Other drug induced dystonia** 🌑

G24.1 Genetic torsion dystonia
   Dystonia deformans progressiva
   Dystonia musculorum deformans
   Familial torsion dystonia
   Idiopathic familial dystonia
   Idiopathic (torsion) dystonia NOS
   (Schwalbe-) Ziehen-Oppenheim disease

G24.2 Idiopathic nonfamilial dystonia 🌑

G24.3 Spasmodic torticollis
Head tilts toward one side and chin is elevated and turned toward opposite side (wry neck)
   Excludes1 congenital torticollis (Q68.0)
     hysterical torticollis (F44.4)
     ocular torticollis (R29.891)
     psychogenic torticollis (F45.8)
     torticollis NOS (M43.6)
     traumatic recurrent torticollis (S13.4)

G24.4 Idiopathic orofacial dystonia
   Orofacial dyskinesia
   Excludes1 drug induced orofacial dyskinesia (G24.01)

G24.5 Blepharospasm
Tonic spasm of orbicularis oculi muscle, producing closure of eyelids
   Excludes1 drug induced blepharospasm (G24.01)

G24.8 Other dystonia 🌑
   Acquired torsion dystonia NOS

◼ **G24.9 Dystonia, unspecified**
   Dyskinesia NOS

● **G25 Other extrapyramidal and movement disorders**
Extrapyramidal: Other than pyramidal tracts
   Excludes2 sleep related movement disorders (G47.6-)

G25.0 Essential tremor
   Familial tremor
   Excludes1 tremor NOS (R25.1)

● **G25.1 Drug-induced tremor**
   Use additional code for adverse effect, if applicable, to identify drug (T36-T50 with fifth or sixth character 5)

G25.2 Other specified forms of tremor
   Intention tremor

G25.3 Myoclonus
Shocklike contractions muscle(s)
   Drug-induced myoclonus
   Palatal myoclonus
   Use additional code for adverse effect, if applicable, to identify drug (T36-T50 with fifth or sixth character 5)
   Excludes1 facial myokymia (G51.4)
     myoclonic epilepsy (G40.-)

● **G25.4 Drug-induced chorea**
   Use additional code for adverse effect, if applicable, to identify drug (T36-T50 with fifth or sixth character 5)

G25.5 Other chorea
Continual, involuntary, jerky, movements
   Chorea NOS
   Excludes1 chorea NOS with heart involvement (I02.0)
     Huntington's chorea (G10)
     rheumatic chorea (I02.-)
     Sydenham's chorea (I02.-)

● **G25.6 Drug induced tics and other tics of organic origin**

   ● **G25.61 Drug induced tics**
     Use additional code for adverse effect, if applicable, to identify drug (T36-T50 with fifth or sixth character 5)

   G25.69 Other tics of organic origin
     Excludes1 habit spasm (F95.9)
     tic NOS (F95.9)
     Tourette's syndrome (F95.2)

● **G25.7 Other and unspecified drug induced movement disorders**
   Use additional code for adverse effect, if applicable, to identify drug (T36-T50 with fifth or sixth character 5)

   ● ◼ **G25.70 Drug induced movement disorder, unspecified**

   ● **G25.71 Drug induced akathisia**
     Drug induced acathisia
     Neuroleptic induced acute akathisia

   ● **G25.79 Other drug induced movement disorders**

● **G25.8 Other specified extrapyramidal and movement disorders**
   G25.81 Restless legs syndrome
   G25.82 Stiff-man syndrome 🌑
   G25.83 Benign shuddering attacks
   G25.89 Other specified extrapyramidal and movement disorders

◼ **G25.9 Extrapyramidal and movement disorder, unspecified** 🌑

● ◗ **G26 Extrapyramidal and movement disorders in diseases classified elsewhere**
   Code first underlying disease

CHAPTER 6 (G00-G99)

CHAPTER 6 (G00-G99)

OTHER DEGENERATIVE DISEASES OF THE NERVOUS SYSTEM (G30-G32)

● **G30   Alzheimer's disease**
  Progressive central neurodegenerative disorder

  Includes   Alzheimer's dementia senile and presenile
                 forms

  Use additional code to identify:
    delirium, if applicable (F05)
    dementia with behavioral disturbance (F02.81)
    dementia without behavioral disturbance (F02.80)

  Excludes1   senile degeneration of brain NEC (G31.1)
                  senile dementia NOS (F03)
                  senility NOS (R41.81)

  G30.0   Alzheimer's disease with early onset

  G30.1   Alzheimer's disease with late onset   A

  G30.8   Other Alzheimer's disease

  ▪ **G30.9   Alzheimer's disease, unspecified**

● **G31   Other degenerative diseases of nervous system, not
          elsewhere classified**

  Use additional code to identify:
    dementia with behavioral disturbance (F02.81)
    dementia without behavioral disturbance (F02.80)

  Excludes2   Reye's syndrome (G93.7)

  ● **G31.0   Frontotemporal dementia**

    G31.01   Pick's disease
             Primary progressive aphasia
             Progressive isolated aphasia

    G31.09   Other frontotemporal dementia
             Frontal dementia

  **G31.1   Senile degeneration of brain, not elsewhere
            classified**

    Excludes1   Alzheimer's disease (G30.-)
                    senility NOS (R41.81)

  G31.2   Degeneration of nervous system due to alcohol
          Alcoholic cerebellar ataxia
          Alcoholic cerebellar degeneration
          Alcoholic cerebral degeneration
          Alcoholic encephalopathy
          Dysfunction of the autonomic nervous system due
            to alcohol

    Code also associated alcoholism (F10.-)

  ● **G31.8   Other specified degenerative diseases of nervous
             system**

    G31.81   Alpers' disease 🕮
             *Rare neuronal degeneration of cerebral
               cortex disease of young children*
             Grey-matter degeneration

    G31.82   Leigh's disease 🕮
             *Rare neurometabolic disorder that affects
               central nervous system*
             Subacute necrotizing encephalopathy

    G31.83   Dementia with Lewy bodies
             Closely allied to Parkinson's Disease
             Dementia with Parkinsonism
             Lewy body dementia
             Lewy body disease

  G31.84   Mild cognitive impairment, so stated

    Excludes1   age related cognitive decline
                      (R41.81)
                    altered mental status (R41.82)
                    cerebral degeneration (G31.9)
                    change in mental status
                      (R41.82)
                    cognitive deficits following
                      (sequelae of) cerebral
                      hemorrhage or infarction
                      (I69.01, I69.11, I69.21,
                      I69.31, I69.81, I69.91)
                    cognitive impairment due
                      to intracranial or head
                      injury (S06.-)
                    dementia (F01.-, F02.-, F03)
                    mild memory disturbance
                      (F06.8)
                    neurologic neglect syndrome
                      (R41.4)
                    personality change,
                      nonpsychotic (F68.8)

  G31.85   Corticobasal degeneration

  **G31.89   Other specified degenerative diseases of
             nervous system**

  ▪ **G31.9   Degenerative disease of nervous system, unspecified**

● **G32   Other degenerative disorders of nervous system in
          diseases classified elsewhere**

  ●▶ *G32.0   Subacute combined degeneration of spinal cord in
             diseases classified elsewhere* 🕮
           Dana-Putnam syndrome
           Sclerosis of spinal cord (combined) (dorsolateral)
             (posterolateral)

    Code first underlying disease, such as:
      vitamin B12 deficiency (E53.8)
      anemia (D51.9)
      dietary (D51.3)
      pernicious (D51.0)

    Excludes1   syphilitic combined degeneration of
                    spinal cord (A52.11)

  ● **G32.8   Other specified degenerative disorders of nervous
             system in diseases classified elsewhere**

    Code first underlying disease, such as:
      amyloidosis cerebral degeneration (E85-)
      cerebral degeneration (due to) hypothyroidism
        (E00.0-E03.9)
      cerebral degeneration (due to) neoplasm
        (C00-D49)
      cerebral degeneration (due to) vitamin B
        deficiency, except thiamine (E52-E53.-)

    Excludes1   superior hemorrhagic
                    polioencephalitis [Wernicke's
                    encephalopathy] (E51.2)

  ●▶ *G32.81   Cerebellar ataxia in diseases classified
             elsewhere*

    Code first underlying disease, such as:
      cerebellar ataxia (in) neoplastic
        disease (paraneoplastic cerebellar
        degeneration) (C00-D49)

    Excludes1   systemic atrophy primarily
                    affecting the central
                    nervous system in
                    alcoholic cerebellar
                    ataxia (G31.2)
                    systemic atrophy primarily
                    affecting the central
                    nervous system in
                    myxedema (G13.2)

● Unacceptable Principal Diagnosis   ● Use Additional Character(s)   ▪ Unspecified   ▶ Manifestation Code
OGCR Official Guidelines for Coding and Reporting   Excludes 1   Excludes 2   Includes   Use additional   Code first   Code also

● ▸ *G32.89*   *Other specified degenerative disorders of nervous system in diseases classified elsewhere*
     Degenerative encephalopathy in diseases classified elsewhere

---

DEMYELINATING DISEASES OF THE CENTRAL NERVOUS SYSTEM (G35-G37)

G35   Multiple sclerosis
Destruction of central nervous system; four types: relapsing remitting, secondary progressive, primary progressive, and progressive relapsing
     Disseminated multiple sclerosis
     Generalized multiple sclerosis
     Multiple sclerosis NOS
     Multiple sclerosis of brain stem
     Multiple sclerosis of cord

● **G36   Other acute disseminated demyelination**
     Excludes1   postinfectious encephalitis and encephalomyelitis NOS (G04.01)

   G36.0   Neuromyelitis optica [Devic] 🦠
Inflammatory disorder in which immune system attacks optic nerves and spinal cord producing inflammation of optic nerve (optic neuritis) and spinal cord (myelitis)
     Demyelination in optic neuritis
     Excludes1   optic neuritis NOS (H46)

   G36.1   Acute and subacute hemorrhagic leukoencephalitis [Hurst] 🦠

   G36.8   Other specified acute disseminated demyelination 🦠

   ▪ **G36.9   Acute disseminated demyelination, unspecified** 🦠

● **G37   Other demyelinating diseases of central nervous system**
Destruction of central nervous system

   G37.0   Diffuse sclerosis of central nervous system 🦠
     Periaxial encephalitis
     Schilder's disease
     Excludes1   X linked adrenoleukodystrophy (E71.52-)

   G37.1   Central demyelination of corpus callosum 🦠

   G37.2   Central pontine myelinolysis 🦠

   G37.3   Acute transverse myelitis in demyelinating disease of central nervous system 🦠
     Acute transverse myelitis NOS
     Acute transverse myelopathy
     Excludes1   multiple sclerosis (G35)
         neuromyelitis optica [Devic] (G36.0)

   G37.4   Subacute necrotizing myelitis of central nervous system 🦠

   G37.5   Concentric sclerosis [Baló] of central nervous system 🦠

   G37.8   Other specified demyelinating diseases of central nervous system 🦠

   ▪ **G37.9   Demyelinating disease of central nervous system, unspecified** 🦠

EPISODIC AND PAROXYSMAL DISORDERS (G40-G47)

● **G40   Epilepsy and recurrent seizures**
Note: The following terms are to be considered equivalent to intractable: pharmacoresistant (pharmacologically resistant), treatment resistant, refractory (medically) and poorly controlled
     Excludes1   conversion disorder with seizures (F44.5)
         convulsions NOS (R56.9)
         hippocampal sclerosis (G93.81)
         mesial temporal sclerosis (G93.81)
         post traumatic seizures (R56.1)
         seizure (convulsive) NOS (R56.9)
         seizure of newborn (P90)
         temporal sclerosis (G93.81)
         Todd's paralysis (G83.8)

● **G40.0   Localization-related (focal) (partial) idiopathic epilepsy and epileptic syndromes with seizures of localized onset**
     Benign childhood epilepsy with centrotemporal EEG spikes
     Childhood epilepsy with occipital EEG paroxysms
     Excludes1   adult onset localization-related epilepsy (G40.1-, G40.2-)

   ● **G40.00   Localization-related (focal) (partial) idiopathic epilepsy and epileptic syndromes with seizures of localized onset, not intractable**
     Localization-related (focal) (partial) idiopathic epilepsy and epileptic syndromes with seizures of localized onset without intractability

     G40.001   Localization-related (focal) (partial) idiopathic epilepsy and epileptic syndromes with seizures of localized onset, not intractable, with status epilepticus 🦠

     G40.009   Localization-related (focal) (partial) idiopathic epilepsy and epileptic syndromes with seizures of localized onset, not intractable, without status epilepticus 🦠
       Localization-related (focal) (partial) idiopathic epilepsy and epileptic syndromes with seizures of localized onset NOS

   ● **G40.01   Localization-related (focal) (partial) idiopathic epilepsy and epileptic syndromes with seizures of localized onset, intractable**

     G40.011   Localization-related (focal) (partial) idiopathic epilepsy and epileptic syndromes with seizures of localized onset, intractable, with status epilepticus 🦠

     G40.019   Localization-related (focal) (partial) idiopathic epilepsy and epileptic syndromes with seizures of localized onset, intractable, without status epilepticus 🦠

Item 6-3   Multiple sclerosis (MS) is a nervous system disease affecting the brain and spinal cord by damaging the myelin sheath surrounding and protecting nerve cells. The damage slows down/ blocks messages between the brain and body. Symptoms are: visual disturbances, muscle weakness, coordination and balance issues, numbness, prickling, thinking and memory problems. The cause is unknown, though it is thought that it may be an autoimmune disease. It affects women more than men, between 20 and 40 years of age. MS can be mild, but it may cause the loss of ability to write, walk, and speak. There is no cure, but medication may slow or control symptoms.

N Newborn Age: 0   **P** Pediatric Age: 0–17   **M** Maternity DX: 12–55   **A** Adult Age: 15–124   ♀ Females Only   ♂ Males Only
🦠 Complication\Comorbidity   🦠 Major C\C   🦠 Present on Admission Requirement   🦠 Hospital-Acquired Condition

CHAPTER 6 (G00-G99)

● **G40.1 Localization-related (focal) (partial) symptomatic epilepsy and epileptic syndromes with simple partial seizures**
    Attacks without alteration of consciousness
    Epilepsia partialis continua [Kozhevnikof]
    Simple partial seizures developing into secondarily generalized seizures

  ● **G40.10 Localization-related (focal) (partial) symptomatic epilepsy and epileptic syndromes with simple partial seizures, not intractable**
      Localization-related (focal) (partial) symptomatic epilepsy and epileptic syndromes with simple partial seizures without intractability

      G40.101 Localization-related (focal) (partial) symptomatic epilepsy and epileptic syndromes with simple partial seizures, not intractable, with status epilepticus 🦠

      G40.109 Localization-related (focal) (partial) symptomatic epilepsy and epileptic syndromes with simple partial seizures, not intractable, without status epilepticus 🦠
          Localization-related (focal) (partial) symptomatic epilepsy and epileptic syndromes with simple partial seizures NOS

  ● **G40.11 Localization-related (focal) (partial) symptomatic epilepsy and epileptic syndromes with simple partial seizures, intractable**

      G40.111 Localization-related (focal) (partial) symptomatic epilepsy and epileptic syndromes with simple partial seizures, intractable, with status epilepticus 🦠

      G40.119 Localization-related (focal) (partial) symptomatic epilepsy and epileptic syndromes with simple partial seizures, intractable, without status epilepticus 🦠

● **G40.2 Localization-related (focal) (partial) symptomatic epilepsy and epileptic syndromes with complex partial seizures**
    Attacks with alteration of consciousness, often with automatisms
    Complex partial seizures developing into secondarily generalized seizures

  ● **G40.20 Localization-related (focal) (partial) symptomatic epilepsy and epileptic syndromes with complex partial seizures, not intractable**
      Localization-related (focal) (partial) symptomatic epilepsy and epileptic syndromes with complex partial seizures without intractability

      G40.201 Localization-related (focal) (partial) symptomatic epilepsy and epileptic syndromes with complex partial seizures, not intractable, with status epilepticus 🦠

      G40.209 Localization-related (focal) (partial) symptomatic epilepsy and epileptic syndromes with complex partial seizures, not intractable, without status epilepticus 🦠
          Localization-related (focal) (partial) symptomatic epilepsy and epileptic syndromes with complex partial seizures NOS

  ● **G40.21 Localization-related (focal) (partial) symptomatic epilepsy and epileptic syndromes with complex partial seizures, intractable**

      G40.211 Localization-related (focal) (partial) symptomatic epilepsy and epileptic syndromes with complex partial seizures, intractable, with status epilepticus 🦠

      G40.219 Localization-related (focal) (partial) symptomatic epilepsy and epileptic syndromes with complex partial seizures, intractable, without status epilepticus 🦠

● **G40.3 Generalized idiopathic epilepsy and epileptic syndromes**
    Code also MERRF syndrome, if applicable (E88.42)

  ● **G40.30 Generalized idiopathic epilepsy and epileptic syndromes, not intractable**
      Generalized idiopathic epilepsy and epileptic syndromes without intractability

      G40.301 Generalized idiopathic epilepsy and epileptic syndromes, not intractable, with status epilepticus 🦠

      G40.309 Generalized idiopathic epilepsy and epileptic syndromes, not intractable, without status epilepticus
          Generalized idiopathic epilepsy and epileptic syndromes NOS

  ● **G40.31 Generalized idiopathic epilepsy and epileptic syndromes, intractable**

      G40.311 Generalized idiopathic epilepsy and epileptic syndromes, intractable, with status epilepticus 🦠

      G40.319 Generalized idiopathic epilepsy and epileptic syndromes, intractable, without status epilepticus 🦠

● **G40.A Absence epileptic syndrome**
    Childhood absence epilepsy [pyknolepsy]
    Juvenile absence epilepsy
    Absence epileptic syndrome, NOS

  ● **G40.A0 Absence epileptic syndrome, not intractable**

      G40.A01 Absence epileptic syndrome, not intractable, with status epilepticus

      G40.A09 Absence epileptic syndrome, not intractable, without status epilepticus

CHAPTER 6 (G00-G99)

● Unacceptable Principal Diagnosis   ● Use Additional Character(s)   ■ Unspecified   ▶ Manifestation Code
OGCR Official Guidelines for Coding and Reporting   Excludes 1   Excludes 2   Includes   Use additional   Code first   Code also

●G40.A1 **Absence epileptic syndrome, intractable**

    G40.A11 **Absence epileptic syndrome, intractable, with status epilepticus**

    G40.A19 **Absence epileptic syndrome, intractable, without status epilepticus**

●G40.B **Juvenile myoclonic epilepsy [impulsive petit mal]**

 ●G40.B0 **Juvenile myoclonic epilepsy, not intractable**

    G40.B01 **Juvenile myoclonic epilepsy, not intractable, with status epilepticus**

    G40.B09 **Juvenile myoclonic epilepsy, not intractable, without status epilepticus**

 ●G40.B1 **Juvenile myoclonic epilepsy, intractable**

    G40.B11 **Juvenile myoclonic epilepsy, intractable, with status epilepticus**

    G40.B19 **Juvenile myoclonic epilepsy, intractable, without status epilepticus**

●G40.4 **Other generalized epilepsy and epileptic syndromes**
    Epilepsy with grand mal seizures on awakening
    Epilepsy with myoclonic absences
    Epilepsy with myoclonic-astatic seizures
    Grand mal seizure NOS
    Nonspecific atonic epileptic seizures
    Nonspecific clonic epileptic seizures
    Nonspecific myoclonic epileptic seizures
    Nonspecific tonic epileptic seizures
    Nonspecific tonic-clonic epileptic seizures
    Symptomatic early myoclonic encephalopathy

 ●G40.40 **Other generalized epilepsy and epileptic syndromes, not intractable**
    Other generalized epilepsy and epileptic syndromes without intractability
    Other generalized epilepsy and epileptic syndromes NOS

    G40.401 **Other generalized epilepsy and epileptic syndromes, not intractable, with status epilepticus**

    G40.409 **Other generalized epilepsy and epileptic syndromes, not intractable, without status epilepticus**

 ●G40.41 **Other generalized epilepsy and epileptic syndromes, intractable**

    G40.411 **Other generalized epilepsy and epileptic syndromes, intractable, with status epilepticus**

    G40.419 **Other generalized epilepsy and epileptic syndromes, intractable, without status epilepticus**

●G40.5 **Epileptic seizures related to external causes**
    Epileptic seizures related to alcohol
    Epileptic seizures related to drugs
    Epileptic seizures related to hormonal changes
    Epileptic seizures related to sleep deprivation
    Epileptic seizures related to stress

    Code also, if applicable, associated epilepsy and recurrent seizures (G40.-)

    Use additional code for adverse effect, if applicable, to identify drug (T36-T50 with fifth or sixth character 5)

 ●G40.50 **Epileptic seizures related to external causes, not intractable**

    G40.501 **Epileptic seizures related to external causes, not intractable, with status epilepticus**

    G40.509 **Epileptic seizures related to external causes, not intractable, without status epilepticus**
    Epileptic seizures related to external causes, NOS

●G40.8 **Other epilepsy and recurrent seizures**
    Epilepsies and epileptic syndromes undetermined as to whether they are focal or generalized
    Landau-Kleffner syndrome

 ●G40.80 **Other epilepsy**

    G40.801 **Other epilepsy, not intractable, with status epilepticus**
    Other epilepsy without intractability with status epilepticus

    G40.802 **Other epilepsy, not intractable, without status epilepticus**
    Other epilepsy NOS
    Other epilepsy without intractability without status epilepticus

    G40.803 **Other epilepsy, intractable, with status epilepticus**

    G40.804 **Other epilepsy, intractable, without status epilepticus**

 ●G40.81 **Lennox-Gastaut syndrome**

    G40.811 **Lennox-Gastaut syndrome, not intractable, with status epilepticus**

    G40.812 **Lennox-Gastaut syndrome, not intractable, without status epilepticus**

    G40.813 **Lennox-Gastaut syndrome, intractable, with status epilepticus**

    G40.814 **Lennox-Gastaut syndrome, intractable, without status epilepticus**

 ●G40.82 **Epileptic spasms**
    Infantile spasms
    Salaam attacks
    West's syndrome

    G40.821 **Epileptic spasms, not intractable, with status epilepticus**

    G40.822 **Epileptic spasms, not intractable, without status epilepticus**

    G40.823 **Epileptic spasms, intractable, with status epilepticus**

    G40.824 **Epileptic spasms, intractable, without status epilepticus**

CHAPTER 6 (G00-G99)

G40.89 **Other seizures** 🔖
  | Excludes1 | post traumatic seizures (R56.1)
  recurrent seizures NOS (G40.909)
  seizure NOS (R56.9)

● **G40.9 Epilepsy, unspecified**
  ● G40.90 **Epilepsy, unspecified, not intractable**
    Epilepsy, unspecified, without intractability
    ■ G40.901 **Epilepsy, unspecified, not intractable, with status epilepticus**
    ■ G40.909 **Epilepsy, unspecified, not intractable, without status epilepticus**
      Epilepsy NOS
      Epileptic convulsions NOS
      Epileptic fits NOS
      Epileptic seizures NOS
      Recurrent seizures NOS
      Seizure disorder NOS

  ● G40.91 **Epilepsy, unspecified, intractable**
    Intractable seizure disorder NOS
    ■ G40.911 **Epilepsy, unspecified, intractable, with status epilepticus** 🔖
    ■ G40.919 **Epilepsy, unspecified, intractable, without status epilepticus** 🔖

● **G43 Migraine**
  Note: The following terms are to be considered equivalent to intractable: pharmacoresistant (pharmacologically resistant), treatment resistant, refractory (medically) and poorly controlled
  Use additional code for adverse effect, if applicable, to identify drug (T36-T50 with fifth or sixth character 5)
  | Excludes1 | headache NOS (R51)
  headache syndromes (G44.-)
  lower half migraine (G44.00)

  ● **G43.0 Migraine without aura**
    Neurological disorder, generally recurring headaches without early symptom (aura)
    Common migraine
    | Excludes1 | chronic migraine without aura (G43.7-)

    ● G43.00 **Migraine without aura, not intractable**
      Migraine without aura without mention of refractory migraine
      Neurological disorder, generally recurring headaches without early symptom (aura); resistant to cure, relief, or control
      G43.001 **Migraine without aura, not intractable, with status migrainosus**
      G43.009 **Migraine without aura, not intractable, without status migrainosus**
        Migraine without aura NOS

    ● G43.01 **Migraine without aura, intractable**
      Migraine without aura with refractory migraine
      Intractable migraine: Not easily cured or managed; relentless pain from a migraine
      G43.011 **Migraine without aura, intractable, with status migrainosus**
      G43.019 **Migraine without aura, intractable, without status migrainosus**

Item 6–4 Migraine headache is described as an intense pulsing or throbbing pain in one area of the head. It can be accompanied by extreme sensitivity to light (photophobic) and sound and is three times more common in women than in men. Symptoms include nausea and vomiting. Research indicates migraine headaches are caused by inherited abnormalities in genes that control the activities of certain cell populations in the brain.

  ● G43.1 **Migraine with aura**
    Basilar migraine
    Classical migraine
    Migraine equivalents
    Migraine preceded or accompanied by transient focal neurological phenomena
    Migraine triggered seizures
    Migraine with acute-onset aura
    Migraine with aura without headache (migraine equivalents)
    Migraine with prolonged aura
    Migraine with typical aura
    Retinal migraine
    Code also any associated seizure (G40.-, R56.9)
    | Excludes1 | persistent migraine aura (G43.5-, G43.6-)

    ● G43.10 **Migraine with aura, not intractable**
      Migraine with aura without mention of refractory migraine
      G43.101 **Migraine with aura, not intractable, with status migrainosus**
      G43.109 **Migraine with aura, not intractable, without status migrainosus**
        Migraine with aura NOS

    ● G43.11 **Migraine with aura, intractable**
      Migraine with aura with refractory migraine
      G43.111 **Migraine with aura, intractable, with status migrainosus**
      G43.119 **Migraine with aura, intractable, without status migrainosus**

  ● G43.4 **Hemiplegic migraine**
    Familial migraine
    Sporadic migraine
    Inherited migraine disorder causing temporary paralysis of one side of body followed by severe headache and nausea

    ● G43.40 **Hemiplegic migraine, not intractable**
      Hemiplegic migraine without refractory migraine
      G43.401 **Hemiplegic migraine, not intractable, with status migrainosus**
      G43.409 **Hemiplegic migraine, not intractable, without status migrainosus**
        Hemiplegic migraine NOS

    ● G43.41 **Hemiplegic migraine, intractable**
      Hemiplegic migraine with refractory migraine
      G43.411 **Hemiplegic migraine, intractable, with status migrainosus**
      G43.419 **Hemiplegic migraine, intractable, without status migrainosus**

● Unacceptable Principal Diagnosis   ● Use Additional Character(s)   ■ Unspecified   ▶ Manifestation Code

940   **OGCR** Official Guidelines for Coding and Reporting | Excludes 1 | | Excludes 2 | Includes   Use additional   Code first   Code also

● **G43.5 Persistent migraine aura without cerebral infarction**

● **G43.50 Persistent migraine aura without cerebral infarction, not intractable**
Persistent migraine aura without cerebral infarction, without refractory migraine

G43.501 Persistent migraine aura without cerebral infarction, not intractable, with status migrainosus

G43.509 Persistent migraine aura without cerebral infarction, not intractable, without status migrainosus
Persistent migraine aura NOS

● **G43.51 Persistent migraine aura without cerebral infarction, intractable**
Persistent migraine aura without cerebral infarction, with refractory migraine

G43.511 Persistent migraine aura without cerebral infarction, intractable, with status migrainosus

G43.519 Persistent migraine aura without cerebral infarction, intractable, without status migrainosus

● **G43.6 Persistent migraine aura with cerebral infarction**
Visual, motor, or psychic disturbances, paresthesias, and related neurologic abnormalities accompanying migraine

Code also the type of cerebral infarction (I63.-)

● **G43.60 Persistent migraine aura with cerebral infarction, not intractable**
Persistent migraine aura with cerebral infarction, without refractory migraine

G43.601 Persistent migraine aura with cerebral infarction, not intractable, with status migrainosus 🅒

G43.609 Persistent migraine aura with cerebral infarction, not intractable, without status migrainosus 🅒

● **G43.61 Persistent migraine aura with cerebral infarction, intractable**
Persistent migraine aura with cerebral infarction, with refractory migraine

G43.611 Persistent migraine aura with cerebral infarction, intractable, with status migrainosus 🅒

G43.619 Persistent migraine aura with cerebral infarction, intractable, without status migrainosus 🅒

● **G43.7 Chronic migraine without aura**
Transformed migraine

Excludes1   migraine without aura (G43.0-)

● **G43.70 Chronic migraine without aura, not intractable**
Chronic migraine without aura, without refractory migraine

G43.701 Chronic migraine without aura, not intractable, with status migrainosus

G43.709 Chronic migraine without aura, not intractable, without status migrainosus
Chronic migraine without aura NOS

● **G43.71 Chronic migraine without aura, intractable**
Chronic migraine without aura, with refractory migraine

G43.711 Chronic migraine without aura, intractable, with status migrainosus

G43.719 Chronic migraine without aura, intractable, without status migrainosus

● **G43.A Cyclical vomiting**

● **G43.A0 Cyclical vomiting, not intractable**
Cyclical vomiting, without refractory migraine

● **G43.A1 Cyclical vomiting, intractable**
Cyclical vomiting, with refractory migraine

● **G43.B Ophthalmoplegic migraine**

● **G43.B0 Ophthalmoplegic migraine, not intractable**
Ophthalmoplegic migraine, without refractory migraine

● **G43.B1 Ophthalmoplegic migraine, intractable**
Ophthalmoplegic migraine, with refractory migraine

● **G43.C Periodic headache syndromes in child or adult**

● **G43.C0 Periodic headache syndromes in child or adult, not intractable**
Periodic headache syndromes in child or adult, without refractory migraine

● **G43.C1 Periodic headache syndromes in child or adult, intractable**
Periodic headache syndromes in child or adult, with refractory migraine

● **G43.D Abdominal migraine**

● **G43.D0 Abdominal migraine, not intractable**
Abdominal migraine, without refractory migraine

● **G43.D1 Abdominal migraine, intractable**
Abdominal migraine, with refractory migraine

● **G43.8 Other migraine**

● **G43.80 Other migraine, not intractable**
Other migraine, without refractory migraine

G43.801 Other migraine, not intractable, with status migrainosus

G43.809 Other migraine, not intractable, without status migrainosus

● **G43.81 Other migraine, intractable**
Other migraine, with refractory migraine

G43.811 Other migraine, intractable, with status migrainosus

G43.819 Other migraine, intractable, without status migrainosus

● **G43.82 Menstrual migraine, not intractable**
Menstrual headache, not intractable
Menstrual migraine, without refractory migraine
Menstrually related migraine, not intractable
Pre-menstrual headache, not intractable
Pre-menstrual migraine, not intractable
Pure menstrual migraine, not intractable

Code also associated premenstrual tension syndrome (N94.3)

G43.821 Menstrual migraine, not intractable, with status migrainosus ♀

G43.829 Menstrual migraine, not intractable, without status migrainosus ♀
　　Menstrual migraine NOS

● **G43.83** Menstrual migraine, intractable
　　Menstrual headache, intractable
　　Menstrual migraine, with refractory migraine
　　Menstrually related migraine, intractable
　　Pre-menstrual headache, intractable
　　Pre-menstrual migraine, intractable
　　Pure menstrual migraine, intractable

　　Code also associated premenstrual tension syndrome (N94.3)

　　G43.831 Menstrual migraine, intractable, with status migrainosus ♀

　　G43.839 Menstrual migraine, intractable, without status migrainosus ♀

● **G43.9** Migraine, unspecified

　● **G43.90** Migraine, unspecified, not intractable
　　Migraine, unspecified, without refractory migraine

　　■ **G43.901** Migraine, unspecified, not intractable, with status migrainosus
　　　Status migrainosus NOS

　　■ **G43.909** Migraine, unspecified, not intractable, without status migrainosus
　　　Migraine NOS

　● **G43.91** Migraine, unspecified, intractable
　　Migraine, unspecified, with refractory migraine

　　■ **G43.911** Migraine, unspecified, intractable, with status migrainosus

　　■ **G43.919** Migraine, unspecified, intractable, without status migrainosus

● **G44** Other headache syndromes

　Excludes1 headache NOS (R51)
　Excludes2 atypical facial pain (G50.1)
　　headache due to lumbar puncture (G97.1)
　　migraines (G43.-)
　　trigeminal neuralgia (G50.0)

● **G44.0** Cluster headaches and other trigeminal autonomic cephalgias (TAC)

　● **G44.00** Cluster headache syndrome, unspecified
　　Ciliary neuralgia
　　Cluster headache NOS
　　Histamine cephalgia
　　Lower half migraine
　　Migrainous neuralgia

　　■ **G44.001** Cluster headache syndrome, unspecified, intractable

　　■ **G44.009** Cluster headache syndrome, unspecified, not intractable
　　　Cluster headache syndrome NOS

　● **G44.01** Episodic cluster headache

　　G44.011 Episodic cluster headache, intractable

　　G44.019 Episodic cluster headache, not intractable
　　　Episodic cluster headache NOS

● **G44.02** Chronic cluster headache

　　■ **G44.021** Chronic cluster headache, intractable

　　G44.029 Chronic cluster headache, not intractable
　　　Chronic cluster headache NOS

● **G44.03** Episodic paroxysmal hemicrania
　　Paroxysmal hemicrania NOS

　　G44.031 Episodic paroxysmal hemicrania, intractable

　　G44.039 Episodic paroxysmal hemicrania, not intractable
　　　Episodic paroxysmal hemicrania NOS

● **G44.04** Chronic paroxysmal hemicrania
　　Unilateral headache

　　G44.041 Chronic paroxysmal hemicrania, intractable

　　G44.049 Chronic paroxysmal hemicrania, not intractable
　　　Chronic paroxysmal hemicrania NOS

● **G44.05** Short lasting unilateral neuralgiform headache with conjunctival injection and tearing (SUNCT)

　　G44.051 Short lasting unilateral neuralgiform headache with conjunctival injection and tearing (SUNCT), intractable

　　G44.059 Short lasting unilateral neuralgiform headache with conjunctival injection and tearing (SUNCT), not intractable
　　　Short lasting unilateral neuralgiform headache with conjunctival injection and tearing (SUNCT) NOS

● **G44.09** Other trigeminal autonomic cephalgias (TAC)
　　Cluster headaches

　　G44.091 Other trigeminal autonomic cephalgias (TAC), intractable

　　G44.099 Other trigeminal autonomic cephalgias (TAC), not intractable

G44.1 Vascular headache, not elsewhere classified

　Excludes2 cluster headache (G44.0)
　　complicated headache syndromes (G44.5-)
　　drug-induced headache (G44.4-)
　　migraine (G43.-)
　　other specified headache syndromes (G44.8-)
　　post-traumatic headache (G44.3-)
　　tension-type headache (G44.2-)

● **G44.2** Tension-type headache

　● **G44.20** Tension-type headache, unspecified

　　G44.201 Tension-type headache, unspecified, intractable

　　■ **G44.209** Tension-type headache, unspecified, not intractable
　　　Tension headache NOS

　● **G44.21** Episodic tension-type headache

　　G44.211 Episodic tension-type headache, intractable

　　G44.219 Episodic tension-type headache, not intractable
　　　Episodic tension-type headache NOS

● **G44.22**   **Chronic tension-type headache**

    G44.221   **Chronic tension-type headache, intractable**

    G44.229   **Chronic tension-type headache, not intractable**
         Chronic tension-type headache NOS

● **G44.3**   **Post-traumatic headache**

   ● **G44.30**   **Post-traumatic headache, unspecified**

     ●■ **G44.301**   **Post-traumatic headache, unspecified, intractable**

     ●■ **G44.309**   **Post-traumatic headache, unspecified, not intractable**
         Post-traumatic headache NOS

   ● **G44.31**   **Acute post-traumatic headache**

     ● **G44.311**   **Acute post-traumatic headache, intractable**

     ● **G44.319**   **Acute post-traumatic headache, not intractable**
         Acute post-traumatic headache NOS

   ● **G44.32**   **Chronic post-traumatic headache**

     ● **G44.321**   **Chronic post-traumatic headache, intractable**

     ● **G44.329**   **Chronic post-traumatic headache, not intractable**
         Chronic post-traumatic headache NOS

● **G44.4**   **Drug-induced headache, not elsewhere classified**
     Medication overuse headache

     Use additional code for adverse effect, if applicable, to identify drug (T36-T50 with fifth or sixth character 5)

   ● **G44.40**   **Drug-induced headache, not elsewhere classified, not intractable**

   ● **G44.41**   **Drug-induced headache, not elsewhere classified, intractable**

● **G44.5**   **Complicated headache syndromes**

    G44.51   **Hemicrania continua**
       Persistent unilateral headache

    G44.52   **New daily persistent headache (NDPH)**

    G44.53   **Primary thunderclap headache**

    G44.59   **Other complicated headache syndrome**

● **G44.8**   **Other specified headache syndromes**

    G44.81   **Hypnic headache**
       Benign primary headaches

    G44.82   **Headache associated with sexual activity**
       Orgasmic headache
       Preorgasmic headache

    G44.83   **Primary cough headache**

    G44.84   **Primary exertional headache**

    G44.85   **Primary stabbing headache**

    G44.89   **Other headache syndrome**

● **G45**   **Transient cerebral ischemic attacks and related syndromes**

    Excludes1   neonatal cerebral ischemia (P91.0)
                transient retinal artery occlusion (H34.0-)

    G45.0   **Vertebro-basilar artery syndrome** 🗲

    G45.1   **Carotid artery syndrome (hemispheric)** 🗲

    G45.2   **Multiple and bilateral precerebral artery syndromes** 🗲

    G45.3   **Amaurosis fugax** 🗲
       Transient visual loss in one eye

    G45.4   **Transient global amnesia**
       Episode of short-term memory loss, nonrecurrent, lasting few hours

     Excludes1   amnesia NOS (R41.3)

    G45.8   **Other transient cerebral ischemic attacks and related syndromes** 🗲

  ■ G45.9   **Transient cerebral ischemic attack, unspecified** 🗲
       Spasm of cerebral artery
       TIA
       Transient cerebral ischemia NOS

● **G46**   **Vascular syndromes of brain in cerebrovascular diseases**

    Code first underlying cerebrovascular disease (I60-I69)

   ● **G46.0**   **Middle cerebral artery syndrome** 🗲

   ● **G46.1**   **Anterior cerebral artery syndrome** 🗲

   ● **G46.2**   **Posterior cerebral artery syndrome** 🗲

   ● **G46.3**   **Brain stem stroke syndrome**
       Benedikt syndrome
       Claude syndrome
       Foville syndrome
       Millard-Gubler syndrome
       Wallenberg syndrome
       Weber syndrome

   ● **G46.4**   **Cerebellar stroke syndrome**

   ● **G46.5**   **Pure motor lacunar syndrome**
       Occlusion of single deep penetrating artery

   ● **G46.6**   **Pure sensory lacunar syndrome**

   ● **G46.7**   **Other lacunar syndromes**

   ● **G46.8**   **Other vascular syndromes of brain in cerebrovascular diseases**

● **G47**   **Sleep disorders**

    Excludes2   nightmares (F51.5)
               nonorganic sleep disorders (F51.-)
               sleep terrors (F51.4)
               sleepwalking (F51.3)

   ● **G47.0**   **Insomnia**

     Excludes2   alcohol related insomnia (F10.182, F10.282, F10.982)
               drug related insomnia F11.182, F11.282, F11.982, F13.182, F13.282, F13.982, F14.182, F14.282, F14.982, F15.182, F15.282, F15.982, F19.182, F19.282, F19.982
               idiopathic insomnia (F51.01)
               insomnia due to a mental disorder (F51.05)
               insomnia not due to a substance or known physiological condition (F51.0-)
               nonorganic insomnia (F51.0-)
               primary insomnia (F51.01)
               sleep apnea (G47.3-)

    ■ G47.00   **Insomnia, unspecified**
       Insomnia NOS

    G47.01   **Insomnia due to medical condition**

       Code also associated medical condition

    G47.09   **Other insomnia**

CHAPTER 6 (G00-G99)

- G47.1 **Hypersomnia**
  - **Excludes2** alcohol-related hypersomnia (F10.182, F10.282, F10.982)
    drug-related hypersomnia F11.182, F11.282, F11.982, F13.182, F13.282, F13.982, F14.182, F14.282, F14.982, F15.182, F15.282, F15.982, F19.182, F19.282, F19.982
    hypersomnia due to a mental disorder (F51.13)
    hypersomnia not due to a substance or known physiological condition (F51.1-)
    primary hypersomnia (F51.11)
    sleep apnea (G47.3-)
  - G47.10 **Hypersomnia, unspecified**
    Hypersomnia NOS
  - G47.11 **Idiopathic hypersomnia with long sleep time**
    Idiopathic hypersomnia NOS
  - G47.12 **Idiopathic hypersomnia without long sleep time**
  - G47.13 **Recurrent hypersomnia**
    Kleine-Levin syndrome
    Menstrual related hypersomnia
  - G47.14 **Hypersomnia due to medical condition**
    Code also associated medical condition
  - G47.19 **Other hypersomnia**
- G47.2 **Circadian rhythm sleep disorders**
  Disorders of the sleep wake schedule
  Inversion of nyctohemeral rhythm
  Inversion of sleep rhythm
  - G47.20 **Circadian rhythm sleep disorder, unspecified type**
    Sleep wake schedule disorder NOS
  - G47.21 **Circadian rhythm sleep disorder, delayed sleep phase type**
    Delayed sleep phase syndrome
  - G47.22 **Circadian rhythm sleep disorder, advanced sleep phase type**
  - G47.23 **Circadian rhythm sleep disorder, irregular sleep wake type**
    Irregular sleep-wake pattern
  - G47.24 **Circadian rhythm sleep disorder, free running type**
  - G47.25 **Circadian rhythm sleep disorder, jet lag type**
  - G47.26 **Circadian rhythm sleep disorder, shift work type**
  - G47.27 *Circadian rhythm sleep disorder in conditions classified elsewhere*
    Code first underlying condition
  - G47.29 **Other circadian rhythm sleep disorder**
- G47.3 **Sleep apnea**
  Characterized by episodes in which breathing stops during sleep
  Code also any associated underlying condition
  - **Excludes1** apnea NOS R06.81
    Cheyne-Stokes breathing (R06.3)
    pickwickian syndrome (E66.2)
    sleep apnea of newborn (P28.3)
  - G47.30 **Sleep apnea, unspecified**
    Sleep apnea NOS
  - G47.31 **Primary central sleep apnea**
  - G47.32 **High altitude periodic breathing**

- G47.33 **Obstructive sleep apnea (adult) (pediatric)**
  - **Excludes1** obstructive sleep apnea of newborn (P28.3)
- G47.34 **Idiopathic sleep related nonobstructive alveolar hypoventilation**
  Sleep related hypoxia
- G47.35 **Congenital central alveolar hypoventilation syndrome**
- G47.36 *Sleep related hypoventilation in conditions classified elsewhere*
  Sleep related hypoxemia in conditions classified elsewhere
  Code first underlying condition
- G47.37 *Central sleep apnea in conditions classified elsewhere*
  Code first underlying condition
- G47.39 **Other sleep apnea**
- G47.4 **Narcolepsy and cataplexy**
  *Cataplexy is a disorder evidenced by seizures including minor slacking of the facial muscles to complete collapse and often affects people who have **narcolepsy**, a disorder in which there is great difficulty remaining awake during the daytime.*
  - G47.41 **Narcolepsy**
    - G47.411 **Narcolepsy with cataplexy**
    - G47.419 **Narcolepsy without cataplexy**
      Narcolepsy NOS
  - G47.42 **Narcolepsy in conditions classified elsewhere**
    - G47.421 *Narcolepsy in conditions classified elsewhere with cataplexy*
    - G47.429 *Narcolepsy in conditions classified elsewhere without cataplexy*
- G47.5 **Parasomnia**
  - **Excludes1** alcohol induced parasomnia (F10.182, F10.282, F10.982)
    drug induced parasomnia (F11.182, F11.282, F11.982, F13.182, F13.282, F13.982, F14.182, F14.982, F15.182, F15.282, F15.982, F19.182, F19.282, F19.982)
    parasomnia not due to a substance or known physiological condition (F51.8)
  - G47.50 **Parasomnia, unspecified**
    Parasomnia NOS
  - G47.51 **Confusional arousals**
  - G47.52 **REM sleep behavior disorder**
  - G47.53 **Recurrent isolated sleep paralysis**
  - G47.54 *Parasomnia in conditions classified elsewhere*
    Code first underlying condition
  - G47.59 **Other parasomnia**
- G47.6 **Sleep related movement disorders**
  - **Excludes2** restless legs syndrome (G25.81)
  - G47.61 **Periodic limb movement disorder**
    Periodic limb movement disorder
  - G47.62 **Sleep related leg cramps**
  - G47.63 **Sleep related bruxism**
    - **Excludes1** psychogenic bruxism (F45.8)
  - G47.69 **Other sleep related movement disorders**

● Unacceptable Principal Diagnosis   ● Use Additional Character(s)   ■ Unspecified   ▶ Manifestation Code

OGCR Official Guidelines for Coding and Reporting | Excludes 1 | | Excludes 2 | | Includes | | Use additional | | Code first | | Code also |

G47.8   Other sleep disorders

■ G47.9   Sleep disorder, unspecified
      Sleep disorder NOS

(See Plate 118 on page NAP-6.)

NERVE, NERVE ROOT AND PLEXUS DISORDERS (G50-G59)

Excludes1	current traumatic nerve, nerve root and plexus disorders - see Injury, nerve by body region
	neuralgia NOS (M79.2)
	neuritis NOS (M79.2)
	peripheral neuritis in pregnancy (O26.82-)
	radiculitis NOS (M54.1-)

● G50   Disorders of trigeminal nerve

    Includes   disorders of 5th cranial nerve

   G50.0   Trigeminal neuralgia
       Syndrome of paroxysmal facial pain
       Tic douloureux

   G50.1   Atypical facial pain

   G50.8   Other disorders of trigeminal nerve

■ G50.9   Disorder of trigeminal nerve, unspecified

● G51   Facial nerve disorders

    Includes   disorders of 7th cranial nerve

   G51.0   Bell's palsy
       Facial palsy

   G51.1   Geniculate ganglionitis
       Rare disorder with symptoms of severe pain deep in ear, spreading to ear canal, outer ear, mastoid or eye regions

Excludes1	postherpetic geniculate ganglionitis (B02.21)

   G51.2   Melkersson's syndrome
       Melkersson-Rosenthal syndrome

   G51.3   Clonic hemifacial spasm

   G51.4   Facial myokymia
       Involuntary facial muscle movement

   G51.8   Other disorders of facial nerve

■ G51.9   Disorder of facial nerve, unspecified

● G52   Disorders of other cranial nerves

Excludes2	disorders of acoustic [8th] nerve (H93.3)
	disorders of optic [2nd] nerve (H46, H47.0)
	paralytic strabismus due to nerve palsy (H49.0-H49.2)

   G52.0   Disorders of olfactory nerve
       Disorders of 1st cranial nerve

   G52.1   Disorders of glossopharyngeal nerve
       Disorder of 9th cranial nerve
       Glossopharyngeal neuralgia

   G52.2   Disorders of vagus nerve
       Disorders of pneumogastric [10th] nerve

   G52.3   Disorders of hypoglossal nerve
       Disorders of 12th cranial nerve

   G52.7   Disorders of multiple cranial nerves
       Polyneuritis cranialis

   G52.8   Disorders of other specified cranial nerves

■ G52.9   Cranial nerve disorder, unspecified

Item 6-5 Trigeminal neuralgia, tic douloureux, is a pain syndrome diagnosed from the patient's history alone. The condition is characterized by pain and a brief facial spasm or tic. Pain is unilateral and follows the sensory distribution of cranial nerve V, typically radiating to the maxillary (V2) or mandibular (V3) area.

Item 6-6   The most common facial nerve disorder is **Bell's Palsy,** which occurs suddenly and results in facial drooping unilaterally. This disorder is the result of a reaction to a virus that causes the facial nerve in the ear to swell resulting in pressure in the bony canal.

●▶ G53   *Cranial nerve disorders in diseases classified elsewhere*

      Code first underlying disease, such as:
       neoplasm (C00-D49)

Excludes1	multiple cranial nerve palsy in sarcoidosis (D86.82)
	multiple cranial nerve palsy in syphilis (A52.15)
	postherpetic geniculate ganglionitis (B02.21)
	postherpetic trigeminal neuralgia (B02.22)

● G54   Nerve root and plexus disorders
     Raiculopathy (nerve root disorder) caused by pressure on nerve root, most common cause is herniation of intervertebral disk. Plexus disorders (plexopathies) are due to compression or injury.

Excludes1	current traumatic nerve root and plexus disorders - see nerve injury by body region
	intervertebral disc disorders (M50-M51)
	neuralgia or neuritis NOS (M79.2)
	neuritis or radiculitis:
	brachial NOS (M54.13)
	lumbar NOS (M54.16)
	lumbosacral NOS (M54.17)
	thoracic NOS (M54.14)
	radiculitis NOS (M54.10)
	radiculopathy NOS (M54.10)
	spondylosis (M47.-)

   G54.0   Brachial plexus disorders
       Thoracic outlet syndrome

   G54.1   Lumbosacral plexus disorders

   G54.2   Cervical root disorders, not elsewhere classified

● G54.3   Thoracic root disorders, not elsewhere classified

   G54.4   Lumbosacral root disorders, not elsewhere classified

   G54.5   Neuralgic amyotrophy
       Parsonage-Aldren-Turner syndrome
       Shoulder-girdle neuritis

Excludes1	neuralgic amyotrophy in diabetes mellitus (E08-E13 with .44)

   G54.6   Phantom limb syndrome with pain
       Sensations (cramping, itching) in a limb that no longer exists.

   G54.7   Phantom limb syndrome without pain
       Phantom limb syndrome NOS

   G54.8   Other nerve root and plexus disorders

■ G54.9   Nerve root and plexus disorder, unspecified

●▶ G55   *Nerve root and plexus compressions in diseases classified elsewhere*

      Code first underlying disease, such as:
       neoplasm (C00-D49)

Excludes1	nerve root compression (due to) (in) ankylosing spondylitis (M45.-)
	nerve root compression (due to) (in) dorsopathies (M53.-, M54.-)
	nerve root compression (due to) (in) intervertebral disc disorders (M50.1-, M51.1-)
	nerve root compression (due to) (in) spondylopathies (M46.-, M48.-)
	nerve root compression (due to) (in) spondylosis (M47.0-M47.2.-)

CHAPTER 6 (G00-G99)

N Newborn Age: 0   **P** Pediatric Age: 0–17   **M** Maternity DX: 12–55   **A** Adult Age: 15–124   ♀ Females Only   ♂ Males Only

🔖 Complication\Comorbidity   🔖 Major C\C   🔖 Present on Admission Requirement   🔖 Hospital-Acquired Condition

945

(See Plates 472 and 473 on pages NAP-8 and NAP-9.)

- **G56   Mononeuropathies of upper limb**
  - Excludes1   current traumatic nerve disorder - see nerve injury by body region
  - **G56.0   Carpal tunnel syndrome**
    - G56.00   Carpal tunnel syndrome, unspecified upper limb
    - G56.01   Carpal tunnel syndrome, right upper limb
    - G56.02   Carpal tunnel syndrome, left upper limb
  - **G56.1   Other lesions of median nerve**
    - G56.10   Other lesions of median nerve, unspecified side
    - G56.11   Other lesions of median nerve, right upper limb
    - G56.12   Other lesions of median nerve, left upper limb
  - **G56.2   Lesion of ulnar nerve**
    Tardy ulnar nerve palsy
    - G56.20   Lesion of ulnar nerve, unspecified upper limb
    - G56.21   Lesion of ulnar nerve, right upper limb
    - G56.22   Lesion of ulnar nerve, left upper limb
  - **G56.3   Lesion of radial nerve**
    - G56.30   Lesion of radial nerve, unspecified upper limb
    - G56.31   Lesion of radial nerve, right upper limb
    - G56.32   Lesion of radial nerve, left upper limb
  - **G56.4   Causalgia of upper limb**
    Intense burning pain and sensitivity to slight touch
    Complex regional pain syndrome II of upper limb
    - Excludes1   complex regional pain syndrome I of lower limb (G90.52-)
      complex regional pain syndrome I of upper limb (G90.51-)
      complex regional pain syndrome II of lower limb (G57.7-)
      reflex sympathetic dystrophy of lower limb (G90.52-)
      reflex sympathetic dystrophy (G90.51-)
    - G56.40   Causalgia of unspecified upper limb
    - G56.41   Causalgia of right upper limb
    - G56.42   Causalgia of left upper limb
  - **G56.8   Other specified mononeuropathies of upper limb**
    Disease of a single nerve
    Interdigital neuroma of upper limb
    - G56.80   Other specified mononeuropathies of unspecified upper limb
    - G56.81   Other specified mononeuropathies of right upper limb
    - G56.82   Other specified mononeuropathies of left upper limb
  - **G56.9   Unspecified mononeuropathy of upper limb**
    Disease of a single nerve
    - G56.90   Unspecified mononeuropathy of unspecified upper limb
    - G56.91   Unspecified mononeuropathy of right upper limb
    - G56.92   Unspecified mononeuropathy of left upper limb

- **G57   Mononeuropathies of lower limb**
  - Excludes1   current traumatic nerve disorder - see nerve injury by body region

(See Plates 544 and 545 on pages NAP-10 and NAP-11.)

  - **G57.0   Lesion of sciatic nerve**
    - Excludes1   sciatica NOS (M54.3-)
    - Excludes2   sciatica attributed to intervertebral disc disorder (M51.1-)
    - G57.00   Lesion of sciatic nerve, unspecified lower limb
    - G57.01   Lesion of sciatic nerve, right lower limb
    - G57.02   Lesion of sciatic nerve, left lower limb
  - **G57.1   Meralgia paresthetica**
    Numbness or pain in outer thigh caused by injury to nerve
    Lateral cutaneous nerve of thigh syndrome
    - G57.10   Meralgia paresthetica, unspecified lower limb
    - G57.11   Meralgia paresthetica, right lower limb
    - G57.12   Meralgia paresthetica, left lower limb
  - **G57.2   Lesion of femoral nerve**
    - G57.20   Lesion of femoral nerve, unspecified lower limb
    - G57.21   Lesion of femoral nerve, right lower limb
    - G57.22   Lesion of femoral nerve, left lower limb
  - **G57.3   Lesion of lateral popliteal nerve**
    Peroneal nerve palsy
    - G57.30   Lesion of lateral popliteal nerve, unspecified lower limb
    - G57.31   Lesion of lateral popliteal nerve, right lower limb
    - G57.32   Lesion of lateral popliteal nerve, left lower limb
  - **G57.4   Lesion of medial popliteal nerve**
    - G57.40   Lesion of medial popliteal nerve, unspecified lower limb
    - G57.41   Lesion of medial popliteal nerve, right lower limb
    - G57.42   Lesion of medial popliteal nerve, left lower limb
  - **G57.5   Tarsal tunnel syndrome**
    - G57.50   Tarsal tunnel syndrome, unspecified lower limb
    - G57.51   Tarsal tunnel syndrome, right lower limb
    - G57.52   Tarsal tunnel syndrome, left lower limb
  - **G57.6   Lesion of plantar nerve**
    Morton's metatarsalgia
    - G57.60   Lesion of plantar nerve, unspecified lower limb
    - G57.61   Lesion of plantar nerve, right lower limb
    - G57.62   Lesion of plantar nerve, left lower limb

● Unacceptable Principal Diagnosis   ● Use Additional Character(s)   ■ Unspecified   ▶ Manifestation Code
OGCR Official Guidelines for Coding and Reporting   Excludes 1   Excludes 2   Includes   Use additional   Code first   Code also

● **G57.7 Causalgia of lower limb**
Complex regional pain syndrome II of lower limb

> **Excludes1**   complex regional pain syndrome I of lower limb (G90.52-)
> complex regional pain syndrome I of upper limb (G90.51-)
> complex regional pain syndrome II of upper limb (G56.4-)
> reflex sympathetic dystrophy of lower limb (G90.52-)
> reflex sympathetic dystrophy of upper limb (G90.51-)

■ **G57.70 Causalgia of unspecified lower limb**

G57.71 Causalgia of right lower limb

G57.72 Causalgia of left lower limb

● **G57.8 Other specified mononeuropathies of lower limb**
Interdigital neuroma of lower limb

■ **G57.80 Other specified mononeuropathies of unspecified lower limb**

G57.81 Other specified mononeuropathies of right lower limb

G57.82 Other specified mononeuropathies of left lower limb

● **G57.9 Unspecified mononeuropathy of lower limb**

■ **G57.90 Unspecified mononeuropathy of unspecified lower limb**

■ **G57.91 Unspecified mononeuropathy of right lower limb**

■ **G57.92 Unspecified mononeuropathy of left lower limb**

● **G58 Other mononeuropathies**

G58.0 Intercostal neuropathy

G58.7 Mononeuritis multiplex

G58.8 Other specified mononeuropathies

■ **G58.9 Mononeuropathy, unspecified**

●◗ *G59 Mononeuropathy in diseases classified elsewhere*

> *Code first underlying disease*

> **Excludes1**   diabetic mononeuropathy (E09-E14 with .41)
> syphilitic nerve paralysis (A52.19)
> syphilitic neuritis (A52.15)
> tuberculous mononeuropathy (A17.83)

POLYNEUROPATHIES AND OTHER DISORDERS OF THE PERIPHERAL NERVOUS SYSTEM (G60-G65)

> **Excludes1**   neuralgia NOS (M79.2)
> neuritis NOS (M79.2)
> peripheral neuritis in pregnancy (O26.82-)
> radiculitis NOS (M54.10)

● **G60 Hereditary and idiopathic neuropathy**

G60.0 Hereditary motor and sensory neuropathy
Charcot-Marie-Tooth disease
Déjerine-Sottas disease
Hereditary motor and sensory neuropathy, types I-IV
Hypertrophic neuropathy of infancy
Peroneal muscular atrophy (axonal type) (hypertrophic type)
Roussy-Lévy syndrome

G60.1 Refsum's disease 🅒
Genetic disorder affecting fatty acid metabolism
Infantile Refsum disease

G60.2 Neuropathy in association with hereditary ataxia

G60.3 Idiopathic progressive neuropathy

Item 6–7   The **peripheral nervous system** consists of 31 pairs of spinal nerves, 12 pairs of cranial nerves, and the autonomic nerves, which are divided into the parasympathetic and sympathetic nerves. The cranial nerves are: olfactory (I), optic (II), oculomotor (III), trochlear (IV), trigeminal (V), abducens (VI), facial (VII), vestibulocochlear (VIII), glossopharyngeal (IX), vagus (X), accessory (XI), and hypoglossal (XII).

G60.8 Other hereditary and idiopathic neuropathies
Dominantly inherited sensory neuropathy
Morvan's disease
Nelaton's syndrome
Recessively inherited sensory neuropathy

■ **G60.9 Hereditary and idiopathic neuropathy, unspecified**

● **G61 Inflammatory polyneuropathy**

G61.0 Guillain-Barré syndrome 🅒
Autoimmune disease affecting peripheral nervous system
Acute (post-)infective polyneuritis
Miller Fisher Syndrome

● **G61.1 Serum neuropathy**

> Use additional code for adverse effect, if applicable, to identify serum (T50.-)

● **G61.8 Other inflammatory polyneuropathies**

G61.81 Chronic inflammatory demyelinating polyneuritis 🅒

G61.89 Other inflammatory polyneuropathies

■ **G61.9 Inflammatory polyneuropathy, unspecified**

● **G62 Other and unspecified polyneuropathies**

● **G62.0 Drug-induced polyneuropathy**

> Use additional code for adverse effect, if applicable, to identify drug (T36-T50 with fifth or sixth character 5)

G62.1 Alcoholic polyneuropathy
Malfunction of many peripheral nerves throughout the body

● **G62.2 Polyneuropathy due to other toxic agents**

> Code first (T51-T65) to identify toxic agent

● **G62.8 Other specified polyneuropathies**

G62.81 Critical illness polyneuropathy 🅒
Acute motor neuropathy

G62.82 Radiation-induced polyneuropathy

> Use additional external cause code (W88-W90, X39.0-) to identify cause

G62.89 Other specified polyneuropathies

■ **G62.9 Polyneuropathy, unspecified**
Neuropathy NOS

CHAPTER 6 (G00-G99)

●▶ **G63   Polyneuropathy in diseases classified elsewhere**

Code first underlying disease, such as:
   amyloidosis (E85-)
   endocrine disease, except diabetes (E00-E07, E15-E16,
      E20-E34)
   metabolic diseases (E70-E88)
   neoplasm (C00-D49)
   nutritional deficiency (E40-E64)

   | Excludes1 | polyneuropathy (in):

   polyneuropathy (in):
      diabetes mellitus (E08-E13 with .42)
      diphtheria (A36.83)
      infectious mononucleosis (B27.0-B27.9
         with 1)
      Lyme disease (A69.22)
      mumps (B26.84)
      postherpetic (B02.23)
      rheumatoid arthritis (M05.33)
      scleroderma (M34.83)
      systemic lupus erythematosus (M32.19)

G64   Other disorders of peripheral nervous system
   Disorder of peripheral nervous system NOS

● **G65   Sequelae of inflammatory and toxic polyneuropathies**

   Code first condition resulting from (sequela) of inflammatory
      and toxic polyneuropathies

   ● **G65.0   Sequelae of Guillain-Barré syndrome**

   ● **G65.1   Sequelae of other inflammatory polyneuropathy**

   ● **G65.2   Sequelae of toxic polyneuropathy**

DISEASES OF MYONEURAL JUNCTION AND MUSCLE (G70-G73)

● **G70   Myasthenia gravis and other myoneural disorders**

   | Excludes1 | botulism (A05.1, A48.51-A48.52)
                    transient neonatal myasthenia gravis (P94.0)

● **G70.0   Myasthenia gravis**
   *Acquired and results in fatigable muscle weakness
   exacerbated by activity and improved with rest.*

   **G70.00   Myasthenia gravis without (acute)
      exacerbation**
      Myasthenia gravis NOS

   G70.01   Myasthenia gravis with (acute) exacerbation 🔗
      Myasthenia gravis in crisis

● **G70.1   Toxic myoneural disorders**
   *Dysfunction at junction of muscle and motor nerve
   (myoneural junction)*

   Code first (T51-T65) to identify toxic agent

Item 6–8   Muscular dystrophies (MD) are a group of rare inherited muscle diseases. Voluntary muscles become progressively weaker. In the late stages of MD, fat and connective tissue replace muscle fibers. In some types of muscular dystrophy, heart muscles, other involuntary muscles, and other organs are affected. **Myopathies** is a general term for neuromuscular diseases in which the muscle fibers dysfunction for any one of many reasons, resulting in muscular weakness.

Figure 6-2   A. Parasympathetic nervous system. **B.** Sympathetic nervous system. (From Buck CJ: Step-by-Step Medical Coding, 2nd ed. Philadelphia, WB Saunders, 1998, pp 186 and 187.)

● Unacceptable Principal Diagnosis   ● Use Additional Character(s)   ■ Unspecified   ▶ Manifestation Code

OGCR   Official Guidelines for Coding and Reporting | Excludes 1 | | Excludes 2 | | Includes | | Use additional | | Code first | | Code also |

G70.2   **Congenital and developmental myasthenia**

● **G70.8**   **Other specified myoneural disorders**

■   G70.80   **Lambert-Eaton syndrome, unspecified**
     Lambert-Eaton syndrome NOS

G70.81   *Lambert-Eaton syndrome in disease classified elsewhere*

     Code first underlying disease

     | Excludes1 | Lambert-Eaton syndrome in neoplastic disease (G73.1)

G70.89   **Other specified myoneural disorders**

■ **G70.9**   **Myoneural disorder, unspecified**

● **G71**   **Primary disorders of muscles**

     | Excludes2 | arthrogryposis multiplex congenita (Q74.3)
     metabolic disorders (E70-E88)
     myositis (M60.-)

G71.0   **Muscular dystrophy** 🔖
     Autosomal recessive, childhood type, muscular dystrophy resembling Duchenne or Becker muscular dystrophy
     Benign [Becker] muscular dystrophy
     Benign scapuloperoneal muscular dystrophy with early contractures [Emery-Dreifuss]
     Congenital muscular dystrophy NOS
     Congenital muscular dystrophy with specific morphological abnormalities of the muscle fiber
     Distal muscular dystrophy
     Facioscapulohumeral muscular dystrophy
     Limb-girdle muscular dystrophy
     Ocular muscular dystrophy
     Oculopharyngeal muscular dystrophy
     Scapuloperoneal muscular dystrophy
     Severe [Duchenne] muscular dystrophy

● **G71.1**   **Myotonic disorders**
     Inherited disorder that affects muscles tone

G71.11   **Myotonic muscular dystrophy**
     Dystrophia myotonica [Steinert]
     Myotonia atrophica
     Myotonic dystrophy
     Proximal myotonic myopathy (PROMM)
     Steinert disease

G71.12   **Myotonia congenita**
     Acetazolamide responsive myotonia congenita
     Dominant myotonia congenita [Thomsen disease]
     Myotonia levior
     Recessive myotonia congenita [Becker disease]

G71.13   **Myotonic chondrodystrophy**
     Chondrodystrophic myotonia
     Congenital myotonic chondrodystrophy
     Schwartz-Jampel disease

● G71.14   **Drug induced myotonia**

     Use additional code for adverse effect, if applicable, to identify drug (T36-T50 with fifth or sixth character 5)

G71.19   **Other specified myotonic disorders**
     Myotonia fluctuans
     Myotonia permanens
     Neuromyotonia [Isaacs]
     Paramyotonia congenita (of von Eulenburg)
     Pseudomyotonia
     Symptomatic myotonia

G71.2   **Congenital myopathies** 🔖
     Central core disease
     Fiber-type disproportion
     Minicore disease
     Multicore disease
     Myotubular (centronuclear) myopathy
     Nemaline myopathy

     | Excludes1 | arthrogryposis multiplex congenita (Q74.3)

G71.3   **Mitochondrial myopathy, not elsewhere classified**
     Myopathies associated with increased number of enlarged, often abnormal, mitochondria in muscle fibers

     | Excludes1 | Kearns-Sayre syndrome (H49.81)
     Leber's disease (H47.21)
     Leigh's encephalopathy (G31.82)
     mitochondrial metabolism disorders (E88.4.-)
     Reye's syndrome (G93.7)

G71.8   **Other primary disorders of muscles**

■ **G71.9**   **Primary disorder of muscle, unspecified**
     Hereditary myopathy NOS

● **G72**   **Other and unspecified myopathies**

     | Excludes1 | arthrogryposis multiplex congenita (Q74.3)
     dermatopolymyositis (M33.-)
     ischemic infarction of muscle (M62.2-)
     myositis (M60.-)
     polymyositis (M33.2.-)

● **G72.0**   **Drug-induced myopathy** 🔖

     Use additional code for adverse effect, if applicable, to identify drug (T36-T50 with fifth or sixth character 5)

G72.1   **Alcoholic myopathy** 🔖

     Use additional code to identify alcoholism (F10.-)

● **G72.2**   **Myopathy due to other toxic agents** 🔖

     Code first (T51-T65) to identify toxic agent

G72.3   **Periodic paralysis**
     Familial periodic paralysis
     Hyperkalemic periodic paralysis (familial)
     Hypokalemic periodic paralysis (familial)
     Myotonic periodic paralysis (familial)
     Normokalemic paralysis (familial)
     Potassium sensitive periodic paralysis

     | Excludes1 | paramyotonia congenita (of von Eulenburg) (G71.19)

● **G72.4**   **Inflammatory and immune myopathies, not elsewhere classified**

G72.41   **Inclusion body myositis [IBM]**

G72.49   **Other inflammatory and immune myopathies, not elsewhere classified**
     Inflammatory myopathy NOS

● **G72.8**   **Other specified myopathies**

G72.81   **Critical illness myopathy** 🔖
     Acute necrotizing myopathy
     Acute quadriplegic myopathy
     Intensive care (ICU) myopathy
     Myopathy of critical illness

G72.89   **Other specified myopathies**

■ **G72.9**   **Myopathy, unspecified**

N   Newborn Age: 0   **P**   Pediatric Age: 0–17   **M**   Maternity DX: 12–55   **A**   Adult Age: 15–124   ♀   Females Only   ♂   Males Only

🔖   Complication\Comorbidity   🔖   Major C\C   🔖   Present on Admission Requirement   🔖   Hospital-Acquired Condition

949

CHAPTER 6 (G00-G99)

CHAPTER 6 (G00-G99)

● **G73   Disorders of myoneural junction and muscle in diseases classified elsewhere**

  ● *G73.1 Lambert-Eaton syndrome in neoplastic disease*
     Rare autoimmune disorder affecting calcium channels of nerve-muscle (neuromuscular) junction

     Code first *underlying neoplasm (C00-D49)*

       Excludes1 Lambert-Eaton syndrome not associated with neoplasm (G70.80-G70.81)

  ●▶ *G73.3 Myasthenic syndromes in other diseases classified elsewhere* 🔎

     Code first *underlying disease, such as:*
      neoplasm (C00-D49)
      thyrotoxicosis (E05.-)

  ●▶ *G73.7 Myopathy in diseases classified elsewhere*

     Code first *underlying disease, such as:*
      hyperparathyroidism (E21.0, E21.3)
      hypoparathyroidism (E20.-)
      glycogen storage disease (E74.0)
      lipid storage disorders (E75.-)

       Excludes1 myopathy in:
           rheumatoid arthritis (M05.32)
           sarcoidosis (D86.87)
           scleroderma (M34.82)
           sicca syndrome [Sjögren] (M35.03)
           systemic lupus erythematosus (M32.19)

CEREBRAL PALSY AND OTHER PARALYTIC SYNDROMES (G80-G83)

● **G80 Cerebral palsy**

    Excludes1 hereditary spastic paraplegia (G11.4)

  G80.0 **Spastic quadriplegic cerebral palsy** 🔎
     Congenital spastic paralysis (cerebral)

  G80.1 **Spastic diplegic cerebral palsy** 🔎
     Spastic cerebral palsy NOS

  G80.2 **Spastic hemiplegic cerebral palsy** 🔎

  G80.3 **Athetoid cerebral palsy** 🔎
     Result of damage to cerebellum or basal ganglia responsible for processing neuromuscular signals
     Double athetosis (syndrome)
     Dyskinetic cerebral palsy
     Dystonic cerebral palsy
     Vogt disease

  G80.4 **Ataxic cerebral palsy**
     Poor muscle tone and coordination

  G80.8 **Other cerebral palsy**
     Mixed cerebral palsy syndromes

  ◼ G80.9 **Cerebral palsy, unspecified**
     Cerebral palsy NOS

OGCR Section I.C.6.a.

Dominant/nondominant side

Codes from category G81, Hemiplegia and hemiparesis, and subcategories, G83.1, Monoplegia of lower limb, G83.2, Monoplegia of upper limb, and G83.3, Monoplegia, unspecified, identify whether the dominant and nondominant side is affected. Should the affected side be documented, but not specified as dominant or nondominant, and the classification system does not indicate a default, code selection is as follows:

• For ambidextrous patients, the default should be dominant.

• If the left side is affected, the default is non-dominant.

• If the right side is affected, the default is dominant.

Item 6–9 Hemiplegia is complete paralysis of one side of the body—arm, leg, and trunk. **Hemiparesis** is a generalized weakness or incomplete paralysis of one side of the body. If most activities (eating, writing) are performed with the right hand, the right is the dominant side, and the left is the nondominant side. **Quadriplegia,** also called tetraplegia, is the complete paralysis of all four limbs. **Quadriparesis** is the incomplete paralysis of all four limbs. Nerve damage in C1–C4 is associated with lower limb paralysis, and C5–C7 damage is associated with upper limb paralysis. **Diplegia** is the paralysis of the upper limbs. **Monoplegia** is the complete paralysis of one limb.

● **G81 Hemiplegia and hemiparesis**

  Note: This category is to be used only when hemiplegia (complete)(incomplete) is reported without further specification, or is stated to be old or longstanding but of unspecified cause. The category is also for use in multiple coding to identify these types of hemiplegia resulting from any cause.

    Excludes1 congenital cerebral palsy (G80.-)
      hemiplegia and hemiparesis due to sequela of cerebrovascular disease (I69.05-, I69.15-, I69.25-, I69.35-, I69.85-, I69.95-)

  ● **G81.0 Flaccid hemiplegia**
    Paralysis of half of body with loss of tone of muscles of paralyzed part and absence of tendon reflexes

    ◼ G81.00 **Flaccid hemiplegia affecting unspecified side** 🔎

      G81.01 **Flaccid hemiplegia affecting right dominant side** 🔎

      G81.02 **Flaccid hemiplegia affecting left dominant side** 🔎

      G81.03 **Flaccid hemiplegia affecting right nondominant side** 🔎

      G81.04 **Flaccid hemiplegia affecting left nondominant side** 🔎

  ● **G81.1 Spastic hemiplegia**
    Paralysis of half of body with spasticity of muscles of paralyzed part and increased tendon reflexes

    ◼ G81.10 **Spastic hemiplegia affecting unspecified side** 🔎

      G81.11 **Spastic hemiplegia affecting right dominant side** 🔎

      G81.12 **Spastic hemiplegia affecting left dominant side** 🔎

      G81.13 **Spastic hemiplegia affecting right nondominant side** 🔎

      G81.14 **Spastic hemiplegia affecting left nondominant side** 🔎

  ● **G81.9 Hemiplegia, unspecified**

    ◼ G81.90 **Hemiplegia, unspecified affecting unspecified side** 🔎

    ◼ G81.91 **Hemiplegia, unspecified affecting right dominant side** 🔎

    ◼ G81.92 **Hemiplegia, unspecified affecting left dominant side** 🔎

    ◼ G81.93 **Hemiplegia, unspecified affecting right nondominant side** 🔎

    ◼ G81.94 **Hemiplegia, unspecified affecting left nondominant side** 🔎

  ● Unacceptable Principal Diagnosis   ● Use Additional Character(s)   ◼ Unspecified   ▶ Manifestation Code

OGCR Official Guidelines for Coding and Reporting | Excludes 1 | | Excludes 2 | | Includes | | Use additional | | Code first | | Code also |

- **G82 Paraplegia (paraparesis) and quadriplegia (quadriparesis)**

    Note: This category is to be used only when the listed conditions are reported without further specification, or are stated to be old or longstanding but of unspecified cause. The category is also for use in multiple coding to identify these conditions resulting from any cause.

    Excludes1   congenital cerebral palsy (G80.-)
    functional quadriplegia (R53.2)
    hysterical paralysis (F44.4)

- **G82.2 Paraplegia**
    Paralysis of both lower limbs NOS
    Paraparesis (lower) NOS
    Paraplegia (lower) NOS

    - **G82.20 Paraplegia, unspecified**
    - **G82.21 Paraplegia, complete**
    - **G82.22 Paraplegia, incomplete**

- **G82.5 Quadriplegia**
    Paralysis of all limbs; AKA tetraplegia

    - **G82.50 Quadriplegia, unspecified**
    - **G82.51 Quadriplegia, C1-C4 complete**
    - **G82.52 Quadriplegia, C1-C4 incomplete**
    - **G82.53 Quadriplegia, C5-C7 complete**
    - **G82.54 Quadriplegia, C5-C7 incomplete**

- **G83 Other paralytic syndromes**

    Note: This category is to be used only when the listed conditions are reported without further specification, or are stated to be old or longstanding but of unspecified cause. The category is also for use in multiple coding to identify these conditions resulting from any cause.

    Includes   paralysis (complete) (incomplete), except as in G80-G82

- **G83.0 Diplegia of upper limbs**
    Paralysis affecting limbs on both sides; AKA bilateral paralysis
    Diplegia (upper)
    Paralysis of both upper limbs

- **G83.1 Monoplegia of lower limb**
    Paralysis of limb on one side
    Paralysis of lower limb

    Excludes1   monoplegia of lower limbs due to sequela of cerebrovascular disease (I69.04-, I69.14-, I69.24-, I69.34-, I69.84-, I69.94-)

    - **G83.10 Monoplegia of lower limb affecting unspecified side**
    - **G83.11 Monoplegia of lower limb affecting right dominant side**
    - **G83.12 Monoplegia of lower limb affecting left dominant side**
    - **G83.13 Monoplegia of lower limb affecting right nondominant side**
    - **G83.14 Monoplegia of lower limb affecting left nondominant side**

- **G83.2 Monoplegia of upper limb**
    Paralysis of upper limb

    Excludes1   monoplegia of upper limbs due to sequela of cerebrovascular disease (I69.03-, I69.13-, I69.23-, I69.33-, I69.83-, I69.93-)

    - **G83.20 Monoplegia of upper limb affecting unspecified side**
    - **G83.21 Monoplegia of upper limb affecting right dominant side**
    - **G83.22 Monoplegia of upper limb affecting left dominant side**
    - **G83.23 Monoplegia of upper limb affecting right nondominant side**
    - **G83.24 Monoplegia of upper limb affecting left nondominant side**

- **G83.3 Monoplegia, unspecified**
    - **G83.30 Monoplegia, unspecified affecting unspecified side**
    - **G83.31 Monoplegia, unspecified affecting right dominant side**
    - **G83.32 Monoplegia, unspecified affecting left dominant side**
    - **G83.33 Monoplegia, unspecified affecting right nondominant side**
    - **G83.34 Monoplegia, unspecified affecting left nondominant side**

- **G83.4 Cauda equina syndrome**
    Aching pain due to compression of spinal nerve roots
    Neurogenic bladder due to cauda equina syndrome
    Excludes1   cord bladder NOS (G95.89)
    neurogenic bladder NOS (N31.9)

- **G83.5 Locked-in state**

- **G83.8 Other specified paralytic syndromes**
    Excludes1   paralytic syndromes due to current spinal cord injury-code to spinal cord injury (S14, S24, S34)

    - **G83.81 Brown-Séquard syndrome**
    - **G83.82 Anterior cord syndrome**
    - **G83.83 Posterior cord syndrome**
    - **G83.84 Todd's paralysis (postepileptic)**
    - **G83.89 Other specified paralytic syndromes**

- **G83.9 Paralytic syndrome, unspecified**

CHAPTER 6 (G00-G99)

N Newborn Age: 0   **P** Pediatric Age: 0–17   **M** Maternity DX: 12–55   **A** Adult Age: 15–124   ♀ Females Only   ♂ Males Only
 Complication\Comorbidity   Major C\C   Present on Admission Requirement   Hospital-Acquired Condition

951

CHAPTER 6 (G00-G99)

OTHER DISORDERS OF THE NERVOUS SYSTEM (G89-G99)

● **G89   Pain, not elsewhere classified**

Code also related psychological factors associated with pain (F45.42)

Excludes1   generalized pain NOS (R52)
pain disorders exclusively related to psychological factors (F45.41)
pain NOS (R52)

Excludes2   atypical face pain (G50.1)
headache syndromes (G44.-)
localized pain, unspecified type - code to pain by site, such as:
    abdomen pain (R10.-)
    back pain (M54.9)
    breast pain (N64.4)
    chest pain (R07.1-R07.9)
    ear pain (H92.0-)
    eye pain (H57.1)
    headache (R51)
    joint pain (M25.5-)
    limb pain (M79.6-)
    lumbar region pain (M54.5)
    painful urination (R30.9)
    pelvic and perineal pain (R10.2)
    shoulder pain (M25.51-)
    spine pain (M54.-)
    throat pain (R07.0)
    tongue pain (K14.6)
    tooth pain (K08.8)
renal colic (N23)
migraines (G43.-)
myalgia (M79.1)
pain from prosthetic devices, implants, and grafts (T82.84, T83.84, T84.84, T85.84)
phantom limb syndrome with pain (G54.6)
vulvar vestibulitis (N94.810)
vulvodynia (N94.81-)

G89.0   Central pain syndrome
Neurological condition causing intractable pain resulting from damage to CNS
Déjérine-Roussy syndrome
Myelopathic pain syndrome
Thalamic pain syndrome (hyperesthetic)

● **G89.1   Acute pain, not elsewhere classified**

G89.11   Acute pain due to trauma

G89.12   Acute post-thoracotomy pain
Post-thoracotomy pain NOS

G89.18   Other acute postprocedural pain
Postoperative pain NOS
Postprocedural pain NOS

● **G89.2   Chronic pain, not elsewhere classified**

Excludes1   causalgia, lower limb (G57.7-)
causalgia, upper limb (G56.4-)
central pain syndrome (G89.0)
chronic pain syndrome (G89.4)
complex regional pain syndrome II, lower limb (G57.7-)
complex regional pain syndrome II, upper limb (G56.4-)
neoplasm related chronic pain (G89.3)
reflex sympathetic dystrophy (G90.5-)

G89.21   Chronic pain due to trauma

G89.22   Chronic post-thoracotomy pain

G89.28   Other chronic postprocedural pain
Other chronic postoperative pain

G89.29   Other chronic pain

G89.3   Neoplasm related pain (acute) (chronic)
Cancer associated pain
Pain due to malignancy (primary) (secondary)
Tumor associated pain

G89.4   Chronic pain syndrome
Chronic pain associated with significant psychosocial dysfunction

● **G90   Disorders of autonomic nervous system**

Excludes1   dysfunction of the autonomic nervous system due to alcohol (G31.2)

● **G90.0   Idiopathic peripheral autonomic neuropathy**

G90.01   Carotid sinus syncope
Carotid sinus syndrome

G90.09   Other idiopathic peripheral autonomic neuropathy
Idiopathic peripheral autonomic neuropathy NOS

G90.1   Familial dysautonomia [Riley-Day] 🔎
Inherited disorder that affects nerve function

G90.2   Horner's syndrome
Due to damage of the sympathetic nervous system
Bernard(-Horner) syndrome
Cervical sympathetic dystrophy or paralysis

G90.3   Multi-system degeneration of the autonomic nervous system 🐾
Neurogenic orthostatic hypotension [Shy-Drager]
Excludes1   orthostatic hypotension NOS (I95.1)

G90.4   Autonomic dysreflexia
Syndrome resulting from lesions of spinal cord
Use additional code to identify the cause, such as:
fecal impaction (K56.41)
pressure ulcer (pressure area) (L89.-)
urinary tract infection (N39.0)

● **G90.5   Complex regional pain syndrome I (CRPS I)**
Reflex sympathetic dystrophy
Excludes1   causalgia of lower limb (G57.7-)
causalgia of upper limb (G56.4-)
complex regional pain syndrome II of lower limb (G57.7-)
complex regional pain syndrome II of upper limb (G56.4-)

G90.50   Complex regional pain syndrome I, unspecified 🐾

● **G90.51   Complex regional pain syndrome I of upper limb**

G90.511   Complex regional pain syndrome I of right upper limb 🐾

G90.512   Complex regional pain syndrome I of left upper limb 🐾

G90.513   Complex regional pain syndrome I of upper limb, bilateral 🐾

◼ **G90.519   Complex regional pain syndrome I of unspecified upper limb** 🐾

● **G90.52   Complex regional pain syndrome I of lower limb**

G90.521   Complex regional pain syndrome I of right lower limb 🐾

G90.522   Complex regional pain syndrome I of left lower limb 🐾

G90.523   Complex regional pain syndrome I of lower limb, bilateral 🐾

◼ **G90.529   Complex regional pain syndrome I of unspecified lower limb** 🐾

G90.59   Complex regional pain syndrome I of other specified site 🐾

● Unacceptable Principal Diagnosis   ● Use Additional Character(s)   ◼ Unspecified   ▶ Manifestation Code

952   **OGCR** Official Guidelines for Coding and Reporting   Excludes 1   Excludes 2   Includes   Use additional   Code first   Code also

G90.8 Other disorders of autonomic nervous system

G90.9 Disorder of the autonomic nervous system, unspecified

● **G91 Hydrocephalus**

Dilatation of cerebral ventricles, accompanied by accumulation of cerebrospinal fluid

Includes   acquired hydrocephalus

Excludes1   Arnold-Chiari syndrome with hydrocephalus (Q07.-)
congenital hydrocephalus (Q03.-)
spina bifida with hydrocephalus (Q05.-)

G91.0 Communicating hydrocephalus ⚕
Secondary normal pressure hydrocephalus

G91.1 Obstructive hydrocephalus ⚕

G91.2 (Idiopathic) normal pressure hydrocephalus ⚕
Normal pressure hydrocephalus NOS

G91.3 Post-traumatic hydrocephalus, unspecified ⚕

● ▶ **G91.4 *Hydrocephalus in diseases classified elsewhere***

Code first underlying condition, such as:
congenital syphilis (A50.4-)
neoplasm (C00-D49)

Excludes1   hydrocephalus due to congenital toxoplasmosis (P37.1)

G91.8 Other hydrocephalus ⚕

G91.9 Hydrocephalus, unspecified ⚕

G92 Toxic encephalopathy ⚕
Disorder or disease of brain caused by chemicals
Toxic encephalitis
Toxic metabolic encephalopathy
Code first (T51-T65) to identify toxic agent

● **G93 Other disorders of brain**

G93.0 Cerebral cysts
Arachnoid cyst
Porencephalic cyst, acquired

Excludes1   acquired periventricular cysts of newborn (P91.1)
congenital cerebral cysts (Q04.6)

G93.1 Anoxic brain damage, not elsewhere classified ⚕
Permanent brain damage by lack of oxygen perfusion through brain tissues.

Excludes1   cerebral anoxia due to anesthesia during labor and delivery (O74.3)
cerebral anoxia due to anesthesia during the puerperium (O89.2)
neonatal anoxia (P84)

G93.2 Benign intracranial hypertension

Excludes1   hypertensive encephalopathy (I67.4)

G93.3 Postviral fatigue syndrome
Benign myalgic encephalomyelitis

Excludes1   chronic fatigue syndrome NOS (R53.82)

● **G93.4 Other and unspecified encephalopathy**

Excludes1   alcoholic encephalopathy (G31.2)
encephalopathy in diseases classified elsewhere (G94)
hypertensive encephalopathy (I67.4)
toxic (metabolic) encephalopathy (G92)

G93.40 Encephalopathy, unspecified ⚕

G93.41 Metabolic encephalopathy ⚕
Septic encephalopathy

G93.49 Other encephalopathy ⚕
Encephalopathy NEC

G93.5 Compression of brain ⚕
Arnold-Chiari type 1 compression of brain
Compression of brain (stem)
Herniation of brain (stem)

Excludes1   diffuse traumatic compression of brain (S06.2-)
focal traumatic compression of brain (S06.3-)

G93.6 Cerebral edema ⚕

Excludes1   cerebral edema due to birth injury (P11.0)
traumatic cerebral edema (S06.1-)

G93.7 Reye's syndrome ⚕   **P**
Life-threatening neurological condition, usually follows viral illness
Code first (T39.0-), if salicylates-induced

● **G93.8 Other specified disorders of brain**

G93.81 Temporal sclerosis
Hippocampal sclerosis
Mesial temporal sclerosis

G93.82 Brain death

G93.89 Other specified disorders of brain
Postradiation encephalopathy

G93.9 Disorder of brain, unspecified

● ▶ **G94 *Other disorders of brain in diseases classified elsewhere***
Code first underlying disease

Excludes1   encephalopathy in congenital syphilis (A50.49)
encephalopathy in influenza (J09.X9, J10.81, J11.81)
encephalopathy in syphilis (A52.19)
hydrocephalus in diseases classified elsewhere (G91.4)

● **G95 Other and unspecified diseases of spinal cord**

Excludes2   myelitis (G04.-)

G95.0 Syringomyelia and syringobulbia ⚕

● **G95.1 Vascular myelopathies**

Excludes2   intraspinal phlebitis and thrombophlebitis, except non-pyogenic (G08)

G95.11 Acute infarction of spinal cord (embolic) (nonembolic) ⚕
Anoxia of spinal cord
Arterial thrombosis of spinal cord

G95.19 Other vascular myelopathies ⚕
Edema of spinal cord
Hematomyelia
Nonpyogenic intraspinal phlebitis and thrombophlebitis
Subacute necrotic myelopathy

● **G95.2 Other and unspecified cord compression**

G95.20 Unspecified cord compression ⚕

G95.29 Other cord compression ⚕

● **G95.8 Other specified diseases of spinal cord**

Excludes1   neurogenic bladder NOS (N31.9)
neurogenic bladder due to cauda equina syndrome (G83.4)
neuromuscular dysfunction of bladder without spinal cord lesion (N31.-)

G95.81 Conus medullaris syndrome ⚕
Damage to gray matter and/or nerve roots in lower end of spinal cord

CHAPTER 6 (G00-G99)

N Newborn Age: 0   **P** Pediatric Age: 0–17   **M** Maternity DX: 12–55   **A** Adult Age: 15–124   ♀ Females Only   ♂ Males Only

 Complication\Comorbidity   Major C\C   Present on Admission Requirement   Hospital-Acquired Condition

953

CHAPTER 6 (G00-G99)

G95.89 Other specified diseases of spinal cord 🔊
Cord bladder NOS
Drug-induced myelopathy
Radiation-induced myelopathy
Excludes1 myelopathy NOS (G95.9)

G95.9 Disease of spinal cord, unspecified 🔊
Myelopathy NOS

● **G96** Other disorders of central nervous system

G96.0 Cerebrospinal fluid leak 🔊
Excludes1 cerebrospinal fluid leak from spinal puncture (G97.0)

● **G96.1** Disorders of meninges, not elsewhere classified

G96.11 Dural tear 🔊
Excludes1 accidental puncture or laceration of dura during a procedure (G97.41)

G96.12 Meningeal adhesions (cerebral) (spinal)

G96.19 Other disorders of meninges, not elsewhere classified

G96.8 Other specified disorders of central nervous system

G96.9 Disorder of central nervous system, unspecified

● **G97** Intraoperative and postprocedural complications and disorders of nervous system, not elsewhere classified
Excludes2 intraoperative and postprocedural cerebrovascular infarction (I97.81-, I97.82-)

G97.0 Cerebrospinal fluid leak from spinal puncture 🔊

G97.1 Other reaction to spinal and lumbar puncture
Headache due to lumbar puncture

G97.2 Intracranial hypotension following ventricular shunting 🔊

● **G97.3** Intraoperative hemorrhage and hematoma of a nervous system organ or structure complicating a procedure
Excludes1 intraoperative hemorrhage and hematoma of a nervous system organ or structure due to accidental puncture and laceration during a procedure (G97.4-)

G97.31 Intraoperative hemorrhage and hematoma of a nervous system organ or structure complicating a nervous system procedure 🔊

G97.32 Intraoperative hemorrhage and hematoma of a nervous system organ or structure complicating other procedure 🔊

● **G97.4** Accidental puncture and laceration of a nervous system organ or structure during a procedure

G97.41 Accidental puncture or laceration of dura during a procedure 🔊
Incidental (inadvertent) durotomy

G97.48 Accidental puncture and laceration of other nervous system organ or structure during a nervous system procedure 🔊

G97.49 Accidental puncture and laceration of other nervous system organ or structure during other procedure 🔊

● **G97.5** Postprocedural hemorrhage and hematoma of a nervous system organ or structure following a procedure

G97.51 Postprocedural hemorrhage and hematoma of a nervous system organ or structure following a nervous system procedure 🔊

G97.52 Postprocedural hemorrhage and hematoma of a nervous system organ or structure following other procedure 🔊

● **G97.8** Other intraoperative and postprocedural complications and disorders of nervous system
Use additional code to further specify disorder

G97.81 Other intraoperative complications of nervous system 🔊

G97.82 Other postprocedural complications and disorders of nervous system 🔊

● **G98** Other disorders of nervous system not elsewhere classified
Includes nervous system disorder NOS

G98.0 Neurogenic arthritis, not elsewhere classified
Nonsyphilitic neurogenic arthropathy NEC
Nonsyphilitic neurogenic spondylopathy NEC
Excludes1 spondylopathy (in):
syringomyelia and syringobulbia (G95.0)
tabes dorsalis (A52.11)

G98.8 Other disorders of nervous system
Nervous system disorder NOS

● **G99** Other disorders of nervous system in diseases classified elsewhere

●) **G99.0** *Autonomic neuropathy in diseases classified elsewhere* 🔊
Code first underlying disease, such as:
amyloidosis (E85-)
gout (M1A-, M10.-)
hyperthyroidism (E05.-)
Excludes1 diabetic autonomic neuropathy (E09-14 with .43)

●) **G99.2** *Myelopathy in diseases classified elsewhere* 🔊
Code first underlying disease, such as:
neoplasm (C00-D49)
Excludes1 myelopathy in:
intervertebral disease (M50.0-, M51.0-)
spondylosis (M47.0-, M47.1-)

●) **G99.8** *Other specified disorders of nervous system in diseases classified elsewhere*
Code first underlying disorder, such as:
amyloidosis (E85-)
avitaminosis (E56.9)
Excludes1 nervous system involvement in:
cysticercosis (B69.0)
rubella (B06.0-)
syphilis (A52.1-)

● Unacceptable Principal Diagnosis ● Use Additional Character(s) ■ Unspecified ▶ Manifestation Code
OGCR Official Guidelines for Coding and Reporting Excludes 1 Excludes 2 Includes Use additional Code first Code also

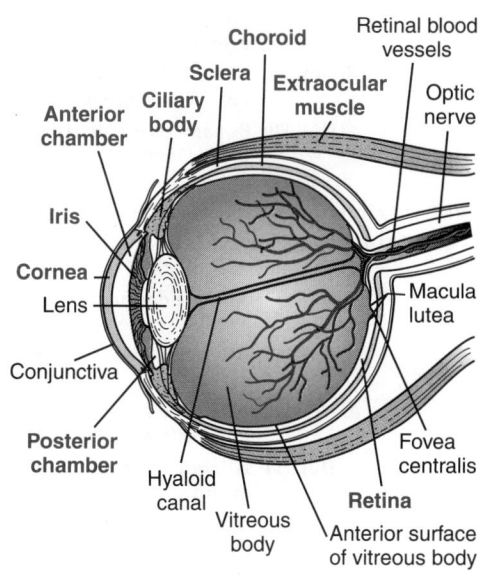

Retinal blood vessels
Choroid
Sclera
Extraocular muscle
Ciliary body
Optic nerve
Anterior chamber
Iris
Cornea
Lens
Conjunctiva
Macula lutea
Posterior chamber
Hyaloid canal
Vitreous body
Fovea centralis
Retina
Anterior surface of vitreous body

Figure 7–1 Eye and ocular adnexa. (From Buck CJ: Step-by-Step Medical Coding, 2010 ed. Philadelphia, WB Saunders, 2010.)

(See Plate 87 on page NAP-15.)

CHAPTER 7

DISEASES OF THE EYE AND ADNEXA (H00-H59)

Note: Use an external cause code following the code for the eye condition, if applicable, to identify the cause of the eye condition

Excludes2   certain conditions originating in the perinatal period (P04-P96)
certain infectious and parasitic diseases (A00-B99)
complications of pregnancy, childbirth and the puerperium (O00-O9A)
congenital malformations, deformations, and chromosomal abnormalities (Q00-Q99)
diabetes mellitus related eye conditions (E09.3-, E10.3-, E11.3-, E13.3-)
endocrine, nutritional and metabolic diseases (E00-E88)
injury (trauma) of eye and orbit (S05.-)
injury, poisoning and certain other consequences of external causes (S00-T88)
neoplasms (C00-D49)
symptoms, signs and abnormal clinical and laboratory findings, not elsewhere classified (R00-R94)
syphilis related eye disorders (A50.01, A50.3-, A51.43, A52.71)

This chapter contains the following blocks:

H00-H05	Disorders of eyelid, lacrimal system and orbit
H10-H11	Disorders of conjunctiva
H15-H22	Disorders of sclera, cornea, iris and ciliary body
H25-H28	Disorders of lens
H30-H36	Disorders of choroid and retina
H40-H42	Glaucoma
H43-H44	Disorders of vitreous body and globe

H46-H47	Disorders of optic nerve and visual pathways
H49-H52	Disorders of ocular muscles, binocular movement, accommodation and refraction
H53-H54	Visual disturbances and blindness
H55-H57	Other disorders of eye and adnexa
H59	Intraoperative and postprocedural complications and disorders of eye and adnexa, not elsewhere classified

DISORDERS OF EYELID, LACRIMAL SYSTEM AND ORBIT (H00-H05)

Excludes2   open wound of eyelid (S01.1-)
superficial injury of eyelid (S00.1-, S00.2-)

● **H00 Hordeolum and chalazion**
Hordeolum: inflammatory staphylococcal infection of sebaceous glands of eyelids; AKA stye. Chalazion: eyelid mass

  ● **H00.0 Hordeolum (externum) (internum) of eyelid**
  Bacterial infection (staphylococcus) of the sebaceous gland of the eyelid (stye)

    ● **H00.01 Hordeolum externum**
    Hordeolum NOS
    Stye

      H00.011 Hordeolum externum right upper eyelid

      H00.012 Hordeolum externum right lower eyelid

      H00.013 Hordeolum externum right eye, unspecified eyelid

      H00.014 Hordeolum externum left upper eyelid

      H00.015 Hordeolum externum left lower eyelid

      H00.016 Hordeolum externum left eye, unspecified eyelid

      H00.019 Hordeolum externum unspecified eye, unspecified eyelid

    ● **H00.02 Hordeolum internum**
    Infection of meibomian gland

      H00.021 Hordeolum internum right upper eyelid

      H00.022 Hordeolum internum right lower eyelid

      H00.023 Hordeolum internum right eye, unspecified eyelid

      H00.024 Hordeolum internum left upper eyelid

      H00.025 Hordeolum internum left lower eyelid

      H00.026 Hordeolum internum left eye, unspecified eyelid

      H00.029 Hordeolum internum unspecified eye, unspecified eyelid

    ● **H00.03 Abscess of eyelid**
    Furuncle of eyelid

      H00.031 Abscess of right upper eyelid

      H00.032 Abscess of right lower eyelid

      H00.033 Abscess of eyelid right eye, unspecified eyelid

N Newborn Age: 0   **P** Pediatric Age: 0–17   **M** Maternity DX: 12–55   **A** Adult Age: 15–124   ♀ Females Only   ♂ Males Only

🅒 Complication\Comorbidity   Major C\C   Present on Admission Requirement   Hospital-Acquired Condition

955

H00.034   Abscess of left upper eyelid

H00.035   Abscess of left lower eyelid

■ H00.036   Abscess of eyelid left eye, unspecified eyelid

■ H00.039   Abscess of eyelid unspecified eye, unspecified eyelid

● **H00.1 Chalazion**

Often caused by accumulation of meibomian gland secretions resulting from a blockage of duct.

Meibomian (gland) cyst

Excludes2   infected meibomian gland (H00.02-)

H00.11   Chalazion right upper eyelid

H00.12   Chalazion right lower eyelid

■ H00.13   Chalazion right eye, unspecified eyelid

H00.14   Chalazion left upper eyelid

H00.15   Chalazion left lower eyelid

■ H00.16   Chalazion left eye, unspecified eyelid

■ H00.19   Chalazion unspecified eye, unspecified eyelid

● **H01 Other inflammation of eyelid**

● **H01.0 Blepharitis**

Inflammation of eyelids

Excludes1   blepharoconjunctivitis (H10.5-)

● H01.00   Unspecified blepharitis

■ H01.001   Unspecified blepharitis right upper eyelid

■ H01.002   Unspecified blepharitis right lower eyelid

■ H01.003   Unspecified blepharitis right eye, unspecified eyelid

■ H01.004   Unspecified blepharitis left upper eyelid

■ H01.005   Unspecified blepharitis left lower eyelid

■ H01.006   Unspecified blepharitis left eye, unspecified eyelid

■ H01.009   Unspecified blepharitis unspecified eye, unspecified eyelid

● H01.01   Ulcerative blepharitis

H01.011   Ulcerative blepharitis right upper eyelid

H01.012   Ulcerative blepharitis right lower eyelid

■ H01.013   Ulcerative blepharitis right eye, unspecified eyelid

H01.014   Ulcerative blepharitis left upper eyelid

H01.015   Ulcerative blepharitis left lower eyelid

■ H01.016   Ulcerative blepharitis left eye, unspecified eyelid

■ H01.019   Ulcerative blepharitis unspecified eye, unspecified eyelid

● H01.02   Squamous blepharitis

H01.021   Squamous blepharitis right upper eyelid

H01.022   Squamous blepharitis right lower eyelid

■ H01.023   Squamous blepharitis right eye, unspecified eyelid

H01.024   Squamous blepharitis left upper eyelid

H01.025   Squamous blepharitis left lower eyelid

■ H01.026   Squamous blepharitis left eye, unspecified eyelid

■ H01.029   Squamous blepharitis unspecified eye, unspecified eyelid

● **H01.1 Noninfectious dermatoses of eyelid**

● H01.11   Allergic dermatitis of eyelid

Contact dermatitis of eyelid

H01.111   Allergic dermatitis of right upper eyelid

H01.112   Allergic dermatitis of right lower eyelid

■ H01.113   Allergic dermatitis of right eye, unspecified eyelid

H01.114   Allergic dermatitis of left upper eyelid

H01.115   Allergic dermatitis of left lower eyelid

■ H01.116   Allergic dermatitis of left eye, unspecified eyelid

■ H01.119   Allergic dermatitis of unspecified eye, unspecified eyelid

● H01.12   Discoid lupus erythematosus of eyelid

H01.121   Discoid lupus erythematosus of right upper eyelid

H01.122   Discoid lupus erythematosus of right lower eyelid

■ H01.123   Discoid lupus erythematosus of right eye, unspecified eyelid

H01.124   Discoid lupus erythematosus of left upper eyelid

H01.125   Discoid lupus erythematosus of left lower eyelid

■ H01.126   Discoid lupus erythematosus of left eye, unspecified eyelid

■ H01.129   Discoid lupus erythematosus of unspecified eye, unspecified eyelid

● H01.13   Eczematous dermatitis of eyelid

H01.131   Eczematous dermatitis of right upper eyelid

H01.132   Eczematous dermatitis of right lower eyelid

■ H01.133   Eczematous dermatitis of right eye, unspecified eyelid

H01.134   Eczematous dermatitis of left upper eyelid

H01.135   Eczematous dermatitis of left lower eyelid

■ H01.136   Eczematous dermatitis of left eye, unspecified eyelid

■ H01.139   Eczematous dermatitis of unspecified eye, unspecified eyelid

● H01.14   Xeroderma of eyelid

Abnormally dry

H01.141   Xeroderma of right upper eyelid

H01.142   Xeroderma of right lower eyelid

■ H01.143   Xeroderma of right eye, unspecified eyelid

● Unacceptable Principal Diagnosis   ● Use Additional Character(s)   ■ Unspecified   ▶ Manifestation Code

956   OGCR Official Guidelines for Coding and Reporting   Excludes 1   Excludes 2   Includes   Use additional   Code first   Code also

Figure 7-2 Right lower eyelid entropion. Note the inward rotation of the tarsal plate about the horizontal axis and the resultant contact between the mucocutaneous junction and ocular surface. (From Yanoff: Ophthalmology, 2nd ed. 2004, Mosby, Inc.)

     H01.144   Xeroderma of left upper eyelid

     H01.145   Xeroderma of left lower eyelid

     H01.146   Xeroderma of left eye, unspecified eyelid

     H01.149   Xeroderma of unspecified eye, unspecified eyelid

H01.8   Other specified inflammations of eyelid

H01.9   Unspecified inflammation of eyelid
     Inflammation of eyelid NOS

● H02   **Other disorders of eyelid**
     Turning inward (inversion) of eyelid margin and ingrowing eyelashes

     Excludes1   congenital malformations of eyelid (Q10.0-Q10.3)

● H02.0   **Entropion and trichiasis of eyelid**

   ● H02.00   **Unspecified entropion of eyelid**

     H02.001   Unspecified entropion of right upper eyelid

     H02.002   Unspecified entropion of right lower eyelid

     H02.003   Unspecified entropion of right eye, unspecified eyelid

     H02.004   Unspecified entropion of left upper eyelid

     H02.005   Unspecified entropion of left lower eyelid

     H02.006   Unspecified entropion of left eye, unspecified eyelid

     H02.009   Unspecified entropion of unspecified eye, unspecified eyelid

   ● H02.01   **Cicatricial entropion of eyelid**
     Scar

     H02.011   Cicatricial entropion of right upper eyelid

     H02.012   Cicatricial entropion of right lower eyelid

     H02.013   Cicatricial entropion of right eye, unspecified eyelid

     H02.014   Cicatricial entropion of left upper eyelid

     H02.015   Cicatricial entropion of left lower eyelid

     H02.016   Cicatricial entropion of left eye, unspecified eyelid

     H02.019   Cicatricial entropion of unspecified eye, unspecified eyelid

   ● H02.02   **Mechanical entropion of eyelid**
     Turning inward (inversion) of eyelid margin due to lack of support

     H02.021   Mechanical entropion of right upper eyelid

     H02.022   Mechanical entropion of right lower eyelid

     H02.023   Mechanical entropion of right eye, unspecified eyelid

     H02.024   Mechanical entropion of left upper eyelid

     H02.025   Mechanical entropion of left lower eyelid

     H02.026   Mechanical entropion of left eye, unspecified eyelid

     H02.029   Mechanical entropion of unspecified eye, unspecified eyelid

   ● H02.03   **Senile entropion of eyelid**
     Turning inward (inversion) of eyelid margin due to aging

     H02.031   Senile entropion of right upper eyelid   **A**

     H02.032   Senile entropion of right lower eyelid   **A**

     H02.033   Senile entropion of right eye, unspecified eyelid   **A**

     H02.034   Senile entropion of left upper eyelid   **A**

     H02.035   Senile entropion of left lower eyelid   **A**

     H02.036   Senile entropion of left eye, unspecified eyelid   **A**

     H02.039   Senile entropion of unspecified eye, unspecified eyelid   **A**

   ● H02.04   **Spastic entropion of eyelid**
     Turning inward (inversion) of eyelid margin caused by spasm of muscle

     H02.041   Spastic entropion of right upper eyelid

     H02.042   Spastic entropion of right lower eyelid

     H02.043   Spastic entropion of right eye, unspecified eyelid

     H02.044   Spastic entropion of left upper eyelid

     H02.045   Spastic entropion of left lower eyelid

     H02.046   Spastic entropion of left eye, unspecified eyelid

     H02.049   Spastic entropion of unspecified eye, unspecified eyelid

   ● H02.05   **Trichiasis without entropian**
     Ingrowing hairs of eyelashes

     H02.051   Trichiasis without entropian right upper eyelid

     H02.052   Trichiasis without entropian right lower eyelid

     H02.053   Trichiasis without entropian right eye, unspecified eyelid

     H02.054   Trichiasis without entropian left upper eyelid

     H02.055   Trichiasis without entropian left lower eyelid

     H02.056   Trichiasis without entropian left eye, unspecified eyelid

     H02.059   Trichiasis without entropian unspecified eye, unspecified eyelid

CHAPTER 7 (H00-H59)

CHAPTER 7 (H00-H59)

● **H02.1   Ectropion of eyelid**
Eversion (pulling away) of eyelid

  ● **H02.10   Unspecified ectropion of eyelid**

    ■ H02.101   Unspecified ectropion of right upper eyelid

    ■ H02.102   Unspecified ectropion of right lower eyelid

    ■ H02.103   Unspecified ectropion of right eye, unspecified eyelid

    ■ H02.104   Unspecified ectropion of left upper eyelid

    ■ H02.105   Unspecified ectropion of left lower eyelid

    ■ H02.106   Unspecified ectropion of left eye, unspecified eyelid

    ■ H02.109   Unspecified ectropion of unspecified eye, unspecified eyelid

  ● **H02.11   Cicatricial ectropion of eyelid**
Pulling of eyelid down and away from eye due to scar or tightening

    H02.111   Cicatricial ectropion of right upper eyelid

    H02.112   Cicatricial ectropion of right lower eyelid

    ■ H02.113   Cicatricial ectropion of right eye, unspecified eyelid

    H02.114   Cicatricial ectropion of left upper eyelid

    H02.115   Cicatricial ectropion of left lower eyelid

    ■ H02.116   Cicatricial ectropion of left eye, unspecified eyelid

    ■ H02.119   Cicatricial ectropion of unspecified eye, unspecified eyelid

  ● **H02.12   Mechanical ectropion of eyelid**
Eversion (pulling away) of eyelid due to lack of support

    H02.121   Mechanical ectropion of right upper eyelid

    H02.122   Mechanical ectropion of right lower eyelid

    ■ H02.123   Mechanical ectropion of right eye, unspecified eyelid

    H02.124   Mechanical ectropion of left upper eyelid

    H02.125   Mechanical ectropion of left lower eyelid

    ■ H02.126   Mechanical ectropion of left eye, unspecified eyelid

    ■ H02.129   Mechanical ectropion of unspecified eye, unspecified eyelid

  ● **H02.13   Senile ectropion of eyelid**
Eversion (pulling away) of eyelid due to age

    H02.131   Senile ectropion of right upper eyelid   A

    H02.132   Senile ectropion of right lower eyelid   A

    ■ H02.133   Senile ectropion of right eye, unspecified eyelid   A

    H02.134   Senile ectropion of left upper eyelid   A

    H02.135   Senile ectropion of left lower eyelid   A

    ■ H02.136   Senile ectropion of left eye, unspecified eyelid   A

    ■ H02.139   Senile ectropion of unspecified eye, unspecified eyelid   A

  ● **H02.14   Spastic ectropion of eyelid**
Eversion (pulling away) of eyelid due to tonic muscle spasm

    H02.141   Spastic ectropion of right upper eyelid

    H02.142   Spastic ectropion of right lower eyelid

    ■ H02.143   Spastic ectropion of right eye, unspecified eyelid

    H02.144   Spastic ectropion of left upper eyelid

    H02.145   Spastic ectropion of left lower eyelid

    ■ H02.146   Spastic ectropion of left eye, unspecified eyelid

    ■ H02.149   Spastic ectropion of unspecified eye, unspecified eyelid

● **H02.2   Lagophthalmos**
Condition in which eye cannot completely close

  ● **H02.20   Unspecified lagophthalmos**

    ■ H02.201   Unspecified lagophthalmos right upper eyelid

    ■ H02.202   Unspecified lagophthalmos right lower eyelid

    ■ H02.203   Unspecified lagophthalmos right eye, unspecified eyelid

    ■ H02.204   Unspecified lagophthalmos left upper eyelid

    ■ H02.205   Unspecified lagophthalmos left lower eyelid

    ■ H02.206   Unspecified lagophthalmos left eye, unspecified eyelid

    ■ H02.209   Unspecified lagophthalmos unspecified eye, unspecified eyelid

  ● **H02.21   Cicatricial lagophthalmos**
Upper or lower eyelid does not close due to scar or tightening

    H02.211   Cicatricial lagophthalmos right upper eyelid

    H02.212   Cicatricial lagophthalmos right lower eyelid

    ■ H02.213   Cicatricial lagophthalmos right eye, unspecified eyelid

    H02.214   Cicatricial lagophthalmos left upper eyelid

    H02.215   Cicatricial lagophthalmos left lower eyelid

    ■ H02.216   Cicatricial lagophthalmos left eye, unspecified eyelid

    ■ H02.219   Cicatricial lagophthalmos unspecified eye, unspecified eyelid

  ● **H02.22   Mechanical lagophthalmos**
Inability to close lids due to structural disorder

    H02.221   Mechanical lagophthalmos right upper eyelid

    H02.222   Mechanical lagophthalmos right lower eyelid

    ■ H02.223   Mechanical lagophthalmos right eye, unspecified eyelid

● Unacceptable Principal Diagnosis   ● Use Additional Character(s)   ■ Unspecified   ▶ Manifestation Code

OGCR   Official Guidelines for Coding and Reporting | Excludes 1 | | Excludes 2 | | Includes | | Use additional | | Code first | | Code also |

Figure 7-3   Piosis of eyelid. (From Yanoff: Ophthalmology, 2nd ed. 2004, Mosby, Inc.)

Item 7–1   Ptosis of eyelid is drooping of the upper eyelid over the pupil when the eyes are fully opened resulting from nerve or muscle damage, which may require surgical correction.

H02.224   **Mechanical lagophthalmos left upper eyelid**

H02.225   **Mechanical lagophthalmos left lower eyelid**

H02.226   **Mechanical lagophthalmos left eye, unspecified eyelid**

H02.229   **Mechanical lagophthalmos unspecified eye, unspecified eyelid**

● H02.23   **Paralytic lagophthalmos**
     Eyelids do not close due to paralysis

H02.231   **Paralytic lagophthalmos right upper eyelid**

H02.232   **Paralytic lagophthalmos right lower eyelid**

H02.233   **Paralytic lagophthalmos right eye, unspecified eyelid**

H02.234   **Paralytic lagophthalmos left upper eyelid**

H02.235   **Paralytic lagophthalmos left lower eyelid**

H02.236   **Paralytic lagophthalmos left eye, unspecified eyelid**

H02.239   **Paralytic lagophthalmos unspecified eye, unspecified eyelid**

(See Plate 81, middle, on page NAP-17.)

● H02.3   **Blepharochalasis**
     Relaxation of skin of eyelid, due to atrophy of intercellular tissue
     Pseudoptosis

H02.30   **Blepharochalasis unspecified eye, unspecified eyelid**

H02.31   **Blepharochalasis right upper eyelid**

H02.32   **Blepharochalasis right lower eyelid**

H02.33   **Blepharochalasis right eye, unspecified eyelid**

H02.34   **Blepharochalasis left upper eyelid**

H02.35   **Blepharochalasis left lower eyelid**

H02.36   **Blepharochalasis left eye, unspecified eyelid**

● H02.4   **Ptosis of eyelid**
     Falling forward, drooping, sagging of eyelid

● H02.40   **Unspecified ptosis of eyelid**

H02.401   **Unspecified ptosis of right eyelid**

H02.402   **Unspecified ptosis of left eyelid**

H02.403   **Unspecified ptosis of bilateral eyelids**

H02.409   **Unspecified ptosis of unspecified eyelid**

● H02.41   **Mechanical ptosis of eyelid**

H02.411   **Mechanical ptosis of right eyelid**

H02.412   **Mechanical ptosis of left eyelid**

H02.413   **Mechanical ptosis of bilateral eyelids**

H02.419   **Mechanical ptosis of unspecified eyelid**

● H02.42   **Myogenic ptosis of eyelid**

H02.421   **Myogenic ptosis of right eyelid**

H02.422   **Myogenic ptosis of left eyelid**

H02.423   **Myogenic ptosis of bilateral eyelids**

H02.429   **Myogenic ptosis of unspecified eyelid**

● H02.43   **Paralytic ptosis of eyelid**
     Neurogenic ptosis of eyelid

H02.431   **Paralytic ptosis of right eyelid**

H02.432   **Paralytic ptosis of left eyelid**

H02.433   **Paralytic ptosis of bilateral eyelids**

H02.439   **Paralytic ptosis unspecified eyelid**

● H02.5   **Other disorders affecting eyelid function**
     Excludes2   blepharospasm (G24.5)
           organic tic (G25.69)
           psychogenic tic (F95.-)

● H02.51   **Abnormal innervation syndrome**

H02.511   **Abnormal innervation syndrome right upper eyelid**

H02.512   **Abnormal innervation syndrome right lower eyelid**

H02.513   **Abnormal innervation syndrome right eye, unspecified eyelid**

H02.514   **Abnormal innervation syndrome left upper eyelid**

H02.515   **Abnormal innervation syndrome left lower eyelid**

H02.516   **Abnormal innervation syndrome left eye, unspecified eyelid**

H02.519   **Abnormal innervation syndrome unspecified eye, unspecified eyelid**

● H02.52   **Blepharophimosis**
     Drooping of eyelid with reduced lid size
     Ankyloblepharon

H02.521   **Blepharophimosis right upper eyelid**

H02.522   **Blepharophimosis right lower eyelid**

H02.523   **Blepharophimosis right eye, unspecified eyelid**

H02.524   **Blepharophimosis left upper eyelid**

H02.525   **Blepharophimosis left lower eyelid**

H02.526   **Blepharophimosis left eye, unspecified eyelid**

H02.529   **Blepharophimosis unspecified eye, unspecified lid**

CHAPTER 7 (H00-H59)

N   Newborn Age: 0   **P**   Pediatric Age: 0–17   **M**   Maternity DX: 12–55   **A**   Adult Age: 15–124   ♀   Females Only   ♂   Males Only

   Complication\Comorbidity   Major C\C   Present on Admission Requirement   Hospital-Acquired Condition

959

● **H02.53   Eyelid retraction**
Eyelid lag

    H02.531   Eyelid retraction right upper eyelid

    H02.532   Eyelid retraction right lower eyelid

    ■ **H02.533   Eyelid retraction right eye, unspecified eyelid**

    H02.534   Eyelid retraction left upper eyelid

    H02.535   Eyelid retraction left lower eyelid

    ■ **H02.536   Eyelid retraction left eye, unspecified eyelid**

    ■ **H02.539   Eyelid retraction unspecified eye, unspecified lid**

H02.59   Other disorders affecting eyelid function
Deficient blink reflex
Sensory disorders

● **H02.6   Xanthelasma of eyelid**
Yellow-to-orange patches or pimples clustered together on eyelid

    ■ **H02.60   Xanthelasma of unspecified eye, unspecified eyelid**

    H02.61   Xanthelasma of right upper eyelid

    H02.62   Xanthelasma of right lower eyelid

    ■ **H02.63   Xanthelasma of right eye, unspecified eyelid**

    H02.64   Xanthelasma of left upper eyelid

    H02.65   Xanthelasma of left lower eyelid

    ■ **H02.66   Xanthelasma of left eye, unspecified eyelid**

● **H02.7   Other and unspecified degenerative disorders of eyelid and periocular area**

    ■ **H02.70   Unspecified degenerative disorders of eyelid and periocular area**

    ● **H02.71   Chloasma of eyelid and periocular area**
Dyspigmentation of eyelid
Hyperpigmentation of eyelid

        H02.711   Chloasma of right upper eyelid and periocular area

        H02.712   Chloasma of right lower eyelid and periocular area

        ■ **H02.713   Chloasma of right eye, unspecified eyelid and periocular area**

        H02.714   Chloasma of left upper eyelid and periocular area

        H02.715   Chloasma of left lower eyelid and periocular area

        ■ **H02.716   Chloasma of left eye, unspecified eyelid and periocular area**

        ■ **H02.719   Chloasma of unspecified eye, unspecified eyelid and periocular area**

    ● **H02.72   Madarosis of eyelid and periocular area**
Loss of eyelashes and/or eyebrows
Hypotrichosis of eyelid

        H02.721   Madarosis of right upper eyelid and periocular area

        H02.722   Madarosis of right lower eyelid and periocular area

        ■ **H02.723   Madarosis of right eye, unspecified eyelid and periocular area**

        H02.724   Madarosis of left upper eyelid and periocular area

        H02.725   Madarosis of left lower eyelid and periocular area

        ■ **H02.726   Madarosis of left eye, unspecified eyelid and periocular area**

        ■ **H02.729   Madarosis of unspecified eye, unspecified eyelid and periocular area**

    ● **H02.73   Vitiligo of eyelid and periocular area**
Skin pigmentation disease characterized by white patches
Hypopigmentation of eyelid

        H02.731   Vitiligo of right upper eyelid and periocular area

        H02.732   Vitiligo of right lower eyelid and periocular area

        ■ **H02.733   Vitiligo of right eye, unspecified eyelid and periocular area**

        H02.734   Vitiligo of left upper eyelid and periocular area

        H02.735   Vitiligo of left lower eyelid and periocular area

        ■ **H02.736   Vitiligo of left eye, unspecified eyelid and periocular area**

        ■ **H02.739   Vitiligo of unspecified eye, unspecified eyelid and periocular area**

● **H02.79   Other degenerative disorders of eyelid and periocular area**

● **H02.8   Other specified disorders of eyelid**

    ● **H02.81   Retained foreign body in eyelid**

        Use additional code to identify the type of retained foreign body (Z18.-)

        Excludes1   laceration of eyelid with foreign body (S01.12-)
retained intraocular foreign body (H44.6-, H44.7-)
superficial foreign body of eyelid and periocular area (S00.25-)

        H02.811   Retained foreign body in right upper eyelid

        H02.812   Retained foreign body in right lower eyelid

        ■ **H02.813   Retained foreign body in right eye, unspecified eyelid**

        H02.814   Retained foreign body in left upper eyelid

        H02.815   Retained foreign body in left lower eyelid

        ■ **H02.816   Retained foreign body in left eye, unspecified eyelid**

        ■ **H02.819   Retained foreign body in unspecified eye, unspecified eyelid**

    ● **H02.82   Cysts of eyelid**
Sebaceous cyst of eyelid

        H02.821   Cysts of right upper eyelid

        H02.822   Cysts of right lower eyelid

        ■ **H02.823   Cysts of right eye, unspecified eyelid**

        H02.824   Cysts of left upper eyelid

        H02.825   Cysts of left lower eyelid

        ■ **H02.826   Cysts of left eye, unspecified eyelid**

        ■ **H02.829   Cysts of unspecified eye, unspecified eyelid**

● Unacceptable Principal Diagnosis   ● Use Additional Character(s)   ■ Unspecified   ▶ Manifestation Code

OGCR Official Guidelines for Coding and Reporting   Excludes 1   Excludes 2   Includes   Use additional   Code first   Code also

● **H02.83 Dermatochalasis of eyelid**
   Skin is inelastic and hangs loosely in folds

   H02.831 Dermatochalasis of right upper eyelid

   H02.832 Dermatochalasis of right lower eyelid

   ■ **H02.833 Dermatochalasis of right eye, unspecified eyelid**

   H02.834 Dermatochalasis of left upper eyelid

   H02.835 Dermatochalasis of left lower eyelid

   ■ **H02.836 Dermatochalasis of left eye, unspecified eyelid**

   ■ **H02.839 Dermatochalasis of unspecified eye, unspecified eyelid**

● **H02.84 Edema of eyelid**
   Hyperemia of eyelid

   H02.841 Edema of right upper eyelid

   H02.842 Edema of right lower eyelid

   ■ **H02.843 Edema of right eye, unspecified eyelid**

   H02.844 Edema of left upper eyelid

   H02.845 Edema of left lower eyelid

   ■ **H02.846 Edema of left eye, unspecified eyelid**

   ■ **H02.849 Edema of unspecified eye, unspecified eyelid**

● **H02.85 Elephantiasis of eyelid**
   Massive secondary lymphedema with hypertrophy of skin and subcutaneous tissues (pachyderma)

   H02.851 Elephantiasis of right upper eyelid

   H02.852 Elephantiasis of right lower eyelid

   ■ **H02.853 Elephantiasis of right eye, unspecified eyelid**

   H02.854 Elephantiasis of left upper eyelid

   H02.855 Elephantiasis of left lower eyelid

   ■ **H02.856 Elephantiasis of left eye, unspecified eyelid**

   ■ **H02.859 Elephantiasis of unspecified eye, unspecified eyelid**

● **H02.86 Hypertrichosis of eyelid**
   Excessive growth of hair

   H02.861 Hypertrichosis of right upper eyelid

   H02.862 Hypertrichosis of right lower eyelid

   ■ **H02.863 Hypertrichosis of right eye, unspecified eyelid**

   H02.864 Hypertrichosis of left upper eyelid

   H02.865 Hypertrichosis of left lower eyelid

   ■ **H02.866 Hypertrichosis of left eye, unspecified eyelid**

   ■ **H02.869 Hypertrichosis of unspecified eye, unspecified eyelid**

● **H02.87 Vascular anomalies of eyelid**

   H02.871 Vascular anomalies of right upper eyelid

   H02.872 Vascular anomalies of right lower eyelid

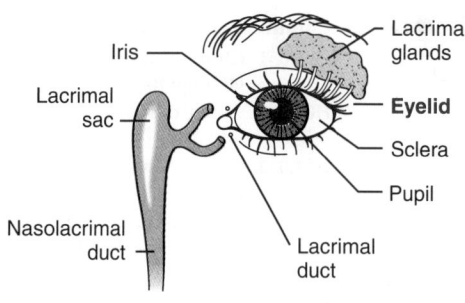

Figure 7-4 Lacrimal apparatus. (From Buck CJ: Step-by-Step Medical Coding, St. Louis, WB Saunders, 2010, p 645.)

(See Plate 82 on page NAP-19.)

   ■ **H02.873 Vascular anomalies of right eye, unspecified eyelid**

   H02.874 Vascular anomalies of left upper eyelid

   H02.875 Vascular anomalies of left lower eyelid

   ■ **H02.876 Vascular anomalies of left eye, unspecified eyelid**

   ■ **H02.879 Vascular anomalies of unspecified eye, unspecified eyelid**

   H02.89 Other specified disorders of eyelid
   Hemorrhage of eyelid

■ **H02.9 Unspecified disorder of eyelid**
   Disorder of eyelid NOS

● **H04 Disorders of lacrimal system**

   Excludes1   congenital malformations of lacrimal system (Q10.4-Q10.6)

   ● **H04.0 Dacryoadenitis**
      Inflammation of lacrimal gland

      ● **H04.00 Unspecified dacryoadenitis**

         ■ **H04.001 Unspecified dacryoadenitis, right lacrimal gland**

         ■ **H04.002 Unspecified dacryoadenitis, left lacrimal gland**

         ■ **H04.003 Unspecified dacryoadenitis, bilateral lacrimal glands**

         ■ **H04.009 Unspecified dacryoadenitis, unspecified lacrimal gland**

      ● **H04.01 Acute dacryoadenitis**

         H04.011 Acute dacryoadenitis, right lacrimal gland

         H04.012 Acute dacryoadenitis, left lacrimal gland

         H04.013 Acute dacryoadenitis, bilateral lacrimal glands

         ■ **H04.019 Acute dacryoadenitis, unspecified lacrimal gland**

      ● **H04.02 Chronic dacryoadenitis**

         H04.021 Chronic dacryoadenitis, right lacrimal gland

         H04.022 Chronic dacryoadenitis, left lacrimal gland

         H04.023 Chronic dacryoadenitis, bilateral lacrimal glands

         ■ **H04.029 Chronic dacryoadenitis, unspecified lacrimal gland**

N Newborn Age: 0   **P** Pediatric Age: 0–17   **M** Maternity DX: 12–55   **A** Adult Age: 15–124   ♀ Females Only   ♂ Males Only

 Complication\Comorbidity   Major C\C   Present on Admission Requirement   Hospital-Acquired Condition

961

CHAPTER 7 (H00-H59)

- ● H04.03 Chronic enlargement of lacrimal gland
  - H04.031 Chronic enlargement of right lacrimal gland
  - H04.032 Chronic enlargement of left lacrimal gland
  - H04.033 Chronic enlargement of bilateral lacrimal glands
  - ■ H04.039 Chronic enlargement of unspecified lacrimal gland
- ● H04.1 Other disorders of lacrimal gland
  - ● H04.11 Dacryops
    Watery eye or distention of lacrimal duct due to fluid
    - H04.111 Dacryops of right lacrimal gland
    - H04.112 Dacryops of left lacrimal gland
    - H04.113 Dacryops of bilateral lacrimal glands
    - ■ H04.119 Dacryops of unspecified lacrimal gland
  - ● H04.12 Dry eye syndrome
    Tear film insufficiency, NOS
    - H04.121 Dry eye syndrome of right lacrimal gland
    - H04.122 Dry eye syndrome of left lacrimal gland
    - H04.123 Dry eye syndrome of bilateral lacrimal glands
    - ■ H04.129 Dry eye syndrome of unspecified lacrimal gland
  - ● H04.13 Lacrimal cyst
    Lacrimal cystic degeneration
    - H04.131 Lacrimal cyst right lacrimal gland
    - H04.132 Lacrimal cyst left lacrimal gland
    - H04.133 Lacrimal cyst bilateral lacrimal glands
    - ■ H04.139 Lacrimal cyst unspecified lacrimal gland
  - ● H04.14 Primary lacrimal gland atrophy
    - H04.141 Primary lacrimal gland atrophy, right lacrimal gland
    - H04.142 Primary lacrimal gland atrophy, left lacrimal gland
    - H04.143 Primary lacrimal gland atrophy, bilateral lacrimal glands
    - ■ H04.149 Primary lacrimal gland atrophy, unspecified lacrimal gland
  - ● H04.15 Secondary lacrimal gland atrophy
    - H04.151 Secondary lacrimal gland atrophy, right lacrimal gland
    - H04.152 Secondary lacrimal gland atrophy, left lacrimal gland
    - H04.153 Secondary lacrimal gland atrophy, bilateral lacrimal glands
    - ■ H04.159 Secondary lacrimal gland atrophy, unspecified lacrimal gland
  - ● H04.16 Lacrimal gland dislocation
    - H04.161 Lacrimal gland dislocation, right lacrimal gland
    - H04.162 Lacrimal gland dislocation, left lacrimal gland
    - H04.163 Lacrimal gland dislocation, bilateral lacrimal glands
    - ■ H04.169 Lacrimal gland dislocation, unspecified lacrimal gland
  - H04.19 Other specified disorders of lacrimal gland
- ● H04.2 Epiphora
  Overflow of tears due to stricture of lacrimal passages; AKA lacrimation
  - ● H04.20 Unspecified epiphora
    - ■ H04.201 Unspecified epiphora, right lacrimal gland
    - ■ H04.202 Unspecified epiphora, left lacrimal gland
    - ■ H04.203 Unspecified epiphora, bilateral lacrimal glands
    - ■ H04.209 Unspecified epiphora, unspecified lacrimal gland
  - ● H04.21 Epiphora due to excess lacrimation
    - H04.211 Epiphora due to excess lacrimation, right lacrimal gland
    - H04.212 Epiphora due to excess lacrimation, left lacrimal gland
    - H04.213 Epiphora due to excess lacrimation, bilateral lacrimal glands
    - ■ H04.219 Epiphora due to excess lacrimation, unspecified lacrimal gland
  - ● H04.22 Epiphora due to insufficient drainage
    - H04.221 Epiphora due to insufficient drainage, right lacrimal gland
    - H04.222 Epiphora due to insufficient drainage, left lacrimal gland
    - H04.223 Epiphora due to insufficient drainage, bilateral lacrimal glands
    - ■ H04.229 Epiphora due to insufficient drainage, unspecified lacrimal gland
- ● H04.3 Acute and unspecified inflammation of lacrimal passages
  - **Excludes1** neonatal dacryocystitis (P39.1)
  - ● H04.30 Unspecified dacryocystitis
    - ■ H04.301 Unspecified dacryocystitis of right lacrimal passage
    - ■ H04.302 Unspecified dacryocystitis of left lacrimal passage
    - ■ H04.303 Unspecified dacryocystitis of bilateral lacrimal passages
    - ■ H04.309 Unspecified dacryocystitis of unspecified lacrimal passage
  - ● H04.31 Phlegmonous dacryocystitis
    Cellulitis of lacrimal sac
    - H04.311 Phlegmonous dacryocystitis of right lacrimal passage
    - H04.312 Phlegmonous dacryocystitis of left lacrimal passage
    - H04.313 Phlegmonous dacryocystitis of bilateral lacrimal passages
    - ■ H04.319 Phlegmonous dacryocystitis of unspecified lacrimal passage
  - ● H04.32 Acute dacryocystitis
    Acute dacryopericystitis
    - H04.321 Acute dacryocystitis of right lacrimal passage
    - H04.322 Acute dacryocystitis of left lacrimal passage
    - H04.323 Acute dacryocystitis of bilateral lacrimal passages
    - ■ H04.329 Acute dacryocystitis of unspecified lacrimal passage

● Unacceptable Principal Diagnosis   ● Use Additional Character(s)   ■ Unspecified   ▶ Manifestation Code
OGCR Official Guidelines for Coding and Reporting   Excludes 1   Excludes 2   Includes   Use additional   Code first   Code also

● **H04.33   Acute lacrimal canaliculitis**

  H04.331   Acute lacrimal canaliculitis of right lacrimal passage

  H04.332   Acute lacrimal canaliculitis of left lacrimal passage

  H04.333   Acute lacrimal canaliculitis of bilateral lacrimal passages

  ■ **H04.339   Acute lacrimal canaliculitis of unspecified lacrimal passage**

● **H04.4   Chronic inflammation of lacrimal passages**

  ● **H04.41   Chronic dacryocystitis**
    Inflammation of lacrimal sac

    H04.411   Chronic dacryocystitis of right lacrimal passage

    H04.412   Chronic dacryocystitis of left lacrimal passage

    H04.413   Chronic dacryocystitis of bilateral lacrimal passages

    ■ **H04.419   Chronic dacryocystitis of unspecified lacrimal passage**

  ● **H04.42   Chronic lacrimal canaliculitis**
    Inflammation of lacrimal ducts

    H04.421   Chronic lacrimal canaliculitis of right lacrimal passage

    H04.422   Chronic lacrimal canaliculitis of left lacrimal passage

    H04.423   Chronic lacrimal canaliculitis of bilateral lacrimal passages

    ■ **H04.429   Chronic lacrimal canaliculitis of unspecified lacrimal passage**

  ● **H04.43   Chronic lacrimal mucocele**
    Accumulation of mucous secretion

    H04.431   Chronic lacrimal mucocele of right lacrimal passage

    H04.432   Chronic lacrimal mucocele of left lacrimal passage

    H04.433   Chronic lacrimal mucocele of bilateral lacrimal passages

    ■ **H04.439   Chronic lacrimal mucocele of unspecified lacrimal passage**

● **H04.5   Stenosis and insufficiency of lacrimal passages**

  ● **H04.51   Dacryolith**
    Concretion in lacrimal sac/duct; AKA lacrimal calculus

    H04.511   Dacryolith of right lacrimal passage

    H04.512   Dacryolith of left lacrimal passage

    H04.513   Dacryolith of bilateral lacrimal passages

    ■ **H04.519   Dacryolith of unspecified lacrimal passage**

  ● **H04.52   Eversion of lacrimal punctum**
    Turning out of lacrimal drainage opening

    H04.521   Eversion of right lacrimal punctum

    H04.522   Eversion of left lacrimal punctum

    H04.523   Eversion of bilateral lacrimal punctum

    ■ **H04.529   Eversion of unspecified lacrimal punctum**

● **H04.53   Neonatal obstruction of nasolacrimal duct**

  | **Excludes1** | congenital stenosis and stricture of lacrimal duct (Q10.5) |

  H04.531   Neonatal obstruction of right nasolacrimal duct   N

  H04.532   Neonatal obstruction of left nasolacrimal duct   N

  H04.533   Neonatal obstruction of bilateral nasolacrimal duct   N

  ■ **H04.539   Neonatal obstruction of unspecified nasolacrimal duct**   N

● **H04.54   Stenosis of lacrimal canaliculi**

  H04.541   Stenosis of right lacrimal canaliculi

  H04.542   Stenosis of left lacrimal canaliculi

  H04.543   Stenosis of bilateral lacrimal canaliculi

  ■ **H04.549   Stenosis of unspecified lacrimal canaliculi**

● **H04.55   Acquired stenosis of nasolacrimal duct**

  H04.551   Acquired stenosis of right nasolacrimal duct

  H04.552   Acquired stenosis of left nasolacrimal duct

  H04.553   Acquired stenosis of bilateral nasolacrimal duct

  ■ **H04.559   Acquired stenosis of unspecified nasolacrimal duct**

● **H04.56   Stenosis of lacrimal punctum**

  H04.561   Stenosis of right lacrimal punctum

  H04.562   Stenosis of left lacrimal punctum

  H04.563   Stenosis of bilateral lacrimal punctum

  ■ **H04.569   Stenosis of unspecified lacrimal punctum**

● **H04.57   Stenosis of lacrimal sac**

  H04.571   Stenosis of right lacrimal sac

  H04.572   Stenosis of left lacrimal sac

  H04.573   Stenosis of bilateral lacrimal sac

  ■ **H04.579   Stenosis of unspecified lacrimal sac**

● **H04.6   Other changes of lacrimal passages**

  ● **H04.61   Lacrimal fistula**

    H04.611   Lacrimal fistula right lacrimal passage

    H04.612   Lacrimal fistula left lacrimal passage

    H04.613   Lacrimal fistula bilateral lacrimal passages

    ■ **H04.619   Lacrimal fistula unspecified lacrimal passage**

  H04.69   Other changes of lacrimal passages

● **H04.8   Other disorders of lacrimal system**

  ● **H04.81   Granuloma of lacrimal passages**
    Inflammatory response due to infectious or noninfectious agents

    H04.811   Granuloma of right lacrimal passage

    H04.812   Granuloma of left lacrimal passage

H04.813 Granuloma of bilateral lacrimal
passages

■ H04.819 Granuloma of unspecified
lacrimal passage

H04.89 Other disorders of lacrimal system

■ H04.9 Disorder of lacrimal system, unspecified

● H05 Disorders of orbit

> **Excludes1**   congenital malformation of orbit (Q10.7)

● H05.0 Acute inflammation of orbit

H05.00 Unspecified acute inflammation of orbit

● H05.01 Cellulitis of orbit
Infection of soft tissue of orbit
Abscess of orbit

H05.011 Cellulitis of right orbit 🦟

H05.012 Cellulitis of left orbit 🦟

H05.013 Cellulitis of bilateral orbits 🦟

■ H05.019 Cellulitis of unspecified orbit 🦟

● H05.02 Osteomyelitis of orbit
Infection of boney orbit of eye

H05.021 Osteomyelitis of right orbit 🦟

H05.022 Osteomyelitis of left orbit 🦟

H05.023 Osteomyelitis of bilateral
orbits 🦟

■ H05.029 Osteomyelitis of unspecified
orbit 🦟

● H05.03 Periostitis of orbit
*Inflammation of periosteum (membrane
covering bone surface)*

H05.031 Periostitis of right orbit 🦟

H05.032 Periostitis of left orbit 🦟

H05.033 Periostitis of bilateral orbits 🦟

■ H05.039 Periostitis of unspecified orbit 🦟

● H05.04 Tenonitis of orbit
*Inflammation of tenon capsule (space
enclosing fascia of Tenon between
eyeball and fat of orbit)*

H05.041 Tenonitis of right orbit

H05.042 Tenonitis of left orbit

H05.043 Tenonitis of bilateral orbits

■ H05.049 Tenonitis of unspecified orbit

● H05.1 Chronic inflammatory disorders of orbit

■ H05.10 Unspecified chronic inflammatory
disorders of orbit

● H05.11 Granuloma of orbit
Pseudotumor (inflammatory) of orbit

H05.111 Granuloma of right orbit

H05.112 Granuloma of left orbit

H05.113 Granuloma of bilateral orbits

■ H05.119 Granuloma of unspecified orbit

● H05.12 Orbital myositis
*Inflammation of extraocular muscles of
orbit*

H05.121 Orbital myositis, right orbit

H05.122 Orbital myositis, left orbit

H05.123 Orbital myositis, bilateral

■ H05.129 Orbital myositis, unspecified
orbit

● H05.2 Exophthalmic conditions
Bulging eyes

■ H05.20 Unspecified exophthalmos

● H05.21 Displacement (lateral) of globe

H05.211 Displacement (lateral) of globe,
right eye

H05.212 Displacement (lateral) of globe,
left eye

H05.213 Displacement (lateral) of globe,
bilateral

■ H05.219 Displacement (lateral) of globe,
unspecified eye

● H05.22 Edema of orbit
Orbital congestion

H05.221 Edema of right orbit

H05.222 Edema of left orbit

H05.223 Edema of bilateral orbit

■ H05.229 Edema of unspecified orbit

● H05.23 Hemorrhage of orbit

H05.231 Hemorrhage of right orbit

H05.232 Hemorrhage of left orbit

H05.233 Hemorrhage of bilateral orbit

■ H05.239 Hemorrhage of unspecified orbit

● H05.24 Constant exophthalmos
*Constant bulging eyes, often symptom of
Graves disease*

H05.241 Constant exophthalmos, right eye

H05.242 Constant exophthalmos, left eye

H05.243 Constant exophthalmos, bilateral

■ H05.249 Constant exophthalmos,
unspecified eye

● H05.25 Intermittent exophthalmos
*Intermittent bulging eye occurring with
bending forward or sharp turning
of head*

H05.251 Intermittent exophthalmos, right
eye

H05.252 Intermittent exophthalmos, left
eye

H05.253 Intermittent exophthalmos,
bilateral

■ H05.259 Intermittent exophthalmos,
unspecified eye

● H05.26 Pulsating exophthalmos
*Bulging eyes with pulsation and bruit, often
due to aneurysm pushing eye forward*

H05.261 Pulsating exophthalmos, right eye

H05.262 Pulsating exophthalmos, left eye

H05.263 Pulsating exophthalmos, bilateral

■ H05.269 Pulsating exophthalmos,
unspecified eye

● H05.3 Deformity of orbit

> **Excludes1**   congenital deformity of orbit (Q10.7)
> hypertelorism (Q75.2)

■ H05.30 Unspecified deformity of orbit

● H05.31 Atrophy of orbit

H05.311 Atrophy of right orbit

H05.312 Atrophy of left orbit

H05.313 Atrophy of bilateral orbit

■ H05.319 Atrophy of unspecified orbit

CHAPTER 7 (H00-H59)

● Unacceptable Principal Diagnosis   ● Use Additional Character(s)   ■ Unspecified   ▶ Manifestation Code

OGCR Official Guidelines for Coding and Reporting   Excludes 1   Excludes 2   Includes   Use additional   Code first   Code also

● **H05.32 Deformity of orbit due to bone disease**
> [Code also] associated bone disease

   H05.321 Deformity of right orbit due to bone disease

   H05.322 Deformity of left orbit due to bone disease

   H05.323 Deformity of bilateral orbits due to bone disease

   ■ **H05.329 Deformity of unspecified orbit due to bone disease**

● **H05.33 Deformity of orbit due to trauma or surgery**

   H05.331 Deformity of right orbit due to trauma or surgery

   H05.332 Deformity of left orbit due to trauma or surgery

   H05.333 Deformity of bilateral orbits due to trauma or surgery

   ■ **H05.339 Deformity of unspecified orbit due to trauma or surgery**

● **H05.34 Enlargement of orbit**

   H05.341 Enlargement of right orbit

   H05.342 Enlargement of left orbit

   H05.343 Enlargement of bilateral orbits

   ■ **H05.349 Enlargement of unspecified orbit**

● **H05.35 Exostosis of orbit**

   H05.351 Exostosis of right orbit

   H05.352 Exostosis of left orbit

   H05.353 Exostosis of bilateral orbits

   ■ **H05.359 Exostosis of unspecified orbit**

● **H05.4 Enophthalmos**
> *Recessed eyeball into orbit*

   ● **H05.40 Unspecified enophthalmos**

    ■ **H05.401 Unspecified enophthalmos, right eye**

    ■ **H05.402 Unspecified enophthalmos, left eye**

    ■ **H05.403 Unspecified enophthalmos, bilateral**

    ■ **H05.409 Unspecified enophthalmos, unspecified eye**

   ● **H05.41 Enophthalmos due to atrophy of orbital tissue**

    H05.411 Enophthalmos due to atrophy of orbital tissue, right eye

    H05.412 Enophthalmos due to atrophy of orbital tissue, left eye

    H05.413 Enophthalmos due to atrophy of orbital tissue, bilateral

    ■ **H05.419 Enophthalmos due to atrophy of orbital tissue, unspecified eye**

   ● **H05.42 Enophthalmos due to trauma or surgery**

    H05.421 Enophthalmos due to trauma or surgery, right eye

    H05.422 Enophthalmos due to trauma or surgery, left eye

    H05.423 Enophthalmos due to trauma or surgery, bilateral

    ■ **H05.429 Enophthalmos due to trauma or surgery, unspecified eye**

● **H05.5 Retained (old) foreign body following penetrating wound of orbit**
> Retrobulbar foreign body
>
> [Use additional] code to identify the type of retained foreign body (Z18.-)
>
> [Excludes1]   current penetrating wound of orbit (S05.4-)
>
> [Excludes2]   retained foreign body of eyelid (H02.81-)
> retained intraocular foreign body (H44.6-, H44.7-)

   ■ **H05.50 Retained (old) foreign body following penetrating wound of unspecified orbit**

   H05.51 Retained (old) foreign body following penetrating wound of right orbit

   H05.52 Retained (old) foreign body following penetrating wound of left orbit

   H05.53 Retained (old) foreign body following penetrating wound of bilateral orbits

● **H05.8 Other disorders of orbit**

   ● **H05.81 Cyst of orbit**
> Encephalocele of orbit

    H05.811 Cyst of right orbit

    H05.812 Cyst of left orbit

    H05.813 Cyst of bilateral orbits

    ■ **H05.819 Cyst of unspecified orbit**

   ● **H05.82 Myopathy of extraocular muscles**
> *Weakness of muscles of eye*

    H05.821 Myopathy of extraocular muscles, right orbit

    H05.822 Myopathy of extraocular muscles, left orbit

    H05.823 Myopathy of extraocular muscles, bilateral

    ■ **H05.829 Myopathy of extraocular muscles, unspecified orbit**

   H05.89 Other disorders of orbit

   ■ **H05.9 Unspecified disorder of orbit**

DISORDERS OF CONJUNCTIVA (H10-H11)

(See Plate 81, upper, on page NAP-18.)

● **H10 Conjunctivitis**
> *Inflammation of membrane of the inside of the eyelid or on surface of eye (conjunctiva)*
>
> [Excludes1]   keratoconjunctivitis (H16.2-)

   ● **H10.0 Mucopurulent conjunctivitis**

    ● **H10.01 Acute follicular conjunctivitis**

     H10.011 Acute follicular conjunctivitis, right eye

     H10.012 Acute follicular conjunctivitis, left eye

     H10.013 Acute follicular conjunctivitis, bilateral

     ■ **H10.019 Acute follicular conjunctivitis, unspecified eye**

    ● **H10.02 Other mucopurulent conjunctivitis**

     H10.021 Other mucopurulent conjunctivitis, right eye

     H10.022 Other mucopurulent conjunctivitis, left eye

     H10.023 Other mucopurulent conjunctivitis, bilateral

     ■ **H10.029 Other mucopurulent conjunctivitis, unspecified eye**

CHAPTER 7 (H00-H59)

● H10.1 Acute atopic conjunctivitis
　　　　Acute papillary conjunctivitis
　■ H10.10 Acute atopic conjunctivitis, unspecified eye
　　H10.11 Acute atopic conjunctivitis, right eye
　　H10.12 Acute atopic conjunctivitis, left eye
　　H10.13 Acute atopic conjunctivitis, bilateral
● H10.2 Other acute conjunctivitis
　● H10.21 Acute toxic conjunctivitis
　　　　Acute chemical conjunctivitis
　　　　Code first (T51-T65) *to identify chemical and intent*
　　　　　| Excludes1 | burn and corrosion of eye and adnexa (T26.-)
　　H10.211 Acute toxic conjunctivitis, right eye
　　H10.212 Acute toxic conjunctivitis, left eye
　　H10.213 Acute toxic conjunctivitis, bilateral
　■ H10.219 Acute toxic conjunctivitis, unspecified eye
　● H10.22 Pseudomembranous conjunctivitis
　　H10.221 Pseudomembranous conjunctivitis, right eye
　　H10.222 Pseudomembranous conjunctivitis, left eye
　　H10.223 Pseudomembranous conjunctivitis, bilateral
　■ H10.229 Pseudomembranous conjunctivitis, unspecified eye
　● H10.23 Serous conjunctivitis, except viral
　　　　| Excludes1 | viral conjunctivitis (B30.-)
　　H10.231 Serous conjunctivitis, except viral, right eye
　　H10.232 Serous conjunctivitis, except viral, left eye
　　H10.233 Serous conjunctivitis, except viral, bilateral
　■ H10.239 Serous conjunctivitis, except viral, unspecified eye
● H10.3 Unspecified acute conjunctivitis
　　　　| Excludes1 | ophthalmia neonatorum NOS (P39.1)
　■ H10.30 Unspecified acute conjunctivitis, unspecified eye
　■ H10.31 Unspecified acute conjunctivitis, right eye
　■ H10.32 Unspecified acute conjunctivitis, left eye
　■ H10.33 Unspecified acute conjunctivitis, bilateral
● H10.4 Chronic conjunctivitis
　● H10.40 Unspecified chronic conjunctivitis
　　■ H10.401 Unspecified chronic conjunctivitis, right eye
　　■ H10.402 Unspecified chronic conjunctivitis, left eye
　　■ H10.403 Unspecified chronic conjunctivitis, bilateral
　　■ H10.409 Unspecified chronic conjunctivitis, unspecified eye
　● H10.41 Chronic giant papillary conjunctivitis
　　　　Inflammation of membrane of the inside of the eyelid or on surface of eye often associated with contact lens wear
　　H10.411 Chronic giant papillary conjunctivitis, right eye

　　H10.412 Chronic giant papillary conjunctivitis, left eye
　　H10.413 Chronic giant papillary conjunctivitis, bilateral
　■ H10.419 Chronic giant papillary conjunctivitis, unspecified eye
● H10.42 Simple chronic conjunctivitis
　　H10.421 Simple chronic conjunctivitis, right eye
　　H10.422 Simple chronic conjunctivitis, left eye
　　H10.423 Simple chronic conjunctivitis, bilateral
　■ H10.429 Simple chronic conjunctivitis, unspecified eye
● H10.43 Chronic follicular conjunctivitis
　　　　Inflammation of membrane of the inside of the eyelid or on surface of eye due to topical medications or infection
　　H10.431 Chronic follicular conjunctivitis, right eye
　　H10.432 Chronic follicular conjunctivitis, left eye
　　H10.433 Chronic follicular conjunctivitis, bilateral
　■ H10.439 Chronic follicular conjunctivitis, unspecified eye
　H10.44 Vernal conjunctivitis
　　　　Affecting children, especially boys in which there are flattened papules with thick, gelatinous exudate on conjunctivae on inside of upper lid
　　　　| Excludes1 | vernal keratoconjunctivitis with limbar and corneal involvement (H16.26-)
　H10.45 Other chronic allergic conjunctivitis
● H10.5 Blepharoconjunctivitis
　　　　Inflammation of eyelids and conjunctiva
　● H10.50 Unspecified blepharoconjunctivitis
　　■ H10.501 Unspecified blepharoconjunctivitis, right eye
　　■ H10.502 Unspecified blepharoconjunctivitis, left eye
　　■ H10.503 Unspecified blepharoconjunctivitis, bilateral
　　■ H10.509 Unspecified blepharoconjunctivitis, unspecified eye
　● H10.51 Ligneous conjunctivitis
　　H10.511 Ligneous conjunctivitis, right eye
　　H10.512 Ligneous conjunctivitis, left eye
　　H10.513 Ligneous conjunctivitis, bilateral
　　■ H10.519 Ligneous conjunctivitis, unspecified eye
　● H10.52 Angular blepharoconjunctivitis
　　H10.521 Angular blepharoconjunctivitis, right eye
　　H10.522 Angular blepharoconjunctivitis, left eye
　　H10.523 Angular blepharoconjunctivitis, bilateral
　　■ H10.529 Angular blepharoconjunctivitis, unspecified eye

● Unacceptable Principal Diagnosis　　● Use Additional Character(s)　　■ Unspecified　　▶ Manifestation Code
OGCR Official Guidelines for Coding and Reporting　| Excludes 1 |　| Excludes 2 |　Includes　Use additional　Code first　Code also

● H10.53   **Contact blepharoconjunctivitis**

    H10.531   **Contact blepharoconjunctivitis, right eye**

    H10.532   **Contact blepharoconjunctivitis, left eye**

    H10.533   **Contact blepharoconjunctivitis, bilateral**

    ■ H10.539   **Contact blepharoconjunctivitis, unspecified eye**

● H10.8   **Other conjunctivitis**

  ● H10.81   **Pingueculitis**

    Inflammation of a yellow, raised thickening on the white of the eye associated with chronic dry eyes

    Excludes1   pinguecula (H11.15-)

    H10.811   **Pingueculitis, right eye**

    H10.812   **Pingueculitis, left eye**

    H10.813   **Pingueculitis, bilateral**

    ■ H10.819   **Pingueculitis, unspecified eye**

  H10.89   **Other conjunctivitis**

■ H10.9   **Unspecified conjunctivitis**

● H11   **Other disorders of conjunctiva**

  Excludes1   keratoconjunctivitis (H16.2-)

 ● H11.0   **Pterygium of eye**

    Excludes1   pseudopterygium (H11.81-)

  ● H11.00   **Unspecified pterygium of eye**

    ■ H11.001   **Unspecified pterygium of right eye**

    ■ H11.002   **Unspecified pterygium of left eye**

    ■ H11.003   **Unspecified pterygium of eye, bilateral**

    ■ H11.009   **Unspecified pterygium of unspecified eye**

  ● H11.01   **Amyloid pterygium**

    H11.011   **Amyloid pterygium of right eye**

    H11.012   **Amyloid pterygium of left eye**

    H11.013   **Amyloid pterygium of eye, bilateral**

    ■ H11.019   **Amyloid pterygium of unspecified eye**

  ● H11.02   **Central pterygium of eye**

    H11.021   **Central pterygium of right eye**

    H11.022   **Central pterygium of left eye**

    H11.023   **Central pterygium of eye, bilateral**

    ■ H11.029   **Central pterygium of unspecified eye**

  ● H11.03   **Double pterygium of eye**

    H11.031   **Double pterygium of right eye**

    H11.032   **Double pterygium of left eye**

    H11.033   **Double pterygium of eye, bilateral**

    ■ H11.039   **Double pterygium of unspecified eye**

  ● H11.04   **Peripheral pterygium of eye, stationary**

    H11.041   **Peripheral pterygium, stationary, right eye**

    H11.042   **Peripheral pterygium, stationary, left eye**

    H11.043   **Peripheral pterygium, stationary, bilateral**

    ■ H11.049   **Peripheral pterygium, stationary, unspecified eye**

  ● H11.05   **Peripheral pterygium of eye, progressive**

    H11.051   **Peripheral pterygium, progressive, right eye**

    H11.052   **Peripheral pterygium, progressive, left eye**

    H11.053   **Peripheral pterygium, progressive, bilateral**

    ■ H11.059   **Peripheral pterygium, progressive, unspecified eye**

  ● H11.06   **Recurrent pterygium of eye**

    H11.061   **Recurrent pterygium of right eye**

    H11.062   **Recurrent pterygium of left eye**

    H11.063   **Recurrent pterygium of eye, bilateral**

    ■ H11.069   **Recurrent pterygium of unspecified eye**

● H11.1   **Conjunctival degenerations and deposits**

  Excludes2   pseudopterygium (H11.81)

 ■ H11.10   **Unspecified conjunctival degenerations**

 ● H11.11   **Conjunctival deposits**

    H11.111   **Conjunctival deposits, right eye**

    H11.112   **Conjunctival deposits, left eye**

    H11.113   **Conjunctival deposits, bilateral**

    ■ H11.119   **Conjunctival deposits, unspecified eye**

 ● H11.12   **Conjunctival concretions**

    White to yellow nodules within or beneath conjunctiva

    H11.121   **Conjunctival concretions, right eye**

    H11.122   **Conjunctival concretions, left eye**

    H11.123   **Conjunctival concretions, bilateral**

    ■ H11.129   **Conjunctival concretions, unspecified eye**

 ● H11.13   **Conjunctival pigmentations**

    Conjunctival argyrosis [argyria]

    H11.131   **Conjunctival pigmentations, right eye**

    H11.132   **Conjunctival pigmentations, left eye**

    H11.133   **Conjunctival pigmentations, bilateral**

    ■ H11.139   **Conjunctival pigmentations, unspecified eye**

 ● H11.14   **Conjunctival xerosis, unspecified**

    Excludes1   xerosis of conjunctiva due to vitamin A deficiency (E50.0, E50.1)

    H11.141   **Conjunctival xerosis, unspecified, right eye**

    H11.142   **Conjunctival xerosis, unspecified, left eye**

Figure 7-5   Double pterygium. Not both nasal and temporal pterygia in a 57-year-old farmer. (From Yanoff: Ophthalmology, 2nd ed. 2004, Mosby, Inc.)

Item 7–2 Pterygium is Greek for batlike. The condition is characterized by a membrane that extends from the limbus to the center of the cornea and resembles a wing.

N Newborn Age: 0   **P** Pediatric Age: 0–17   **M** Maternity DX: 12–55   **A** Adult Age: 15–124   ♀ Females Only   ♂ Males Only

🝆 Complication\Comorbidity   Major C\C   Present on Admission Requirement   Hospital-Acquired Condition

H11.143   Conjunctival xerosis, unspecified, bilateral

■ H11.149   Conjunctival xerosis, unspecified, unspecified eye

● H11.15   Pinguecula
Yellowish spot near sclerocorneal junction, usually on nasal side; associated with aging

   Excludes1   pingueculitis (H10.81-)

H11.151   Pinguecula, right eye

H11.152   Pinguecula, left eye

H11.153   Pinguecula, bilateral

■ H11.159   Pinguecula, unspecified eye

● H11.2   Conjunctival scars

  ● H11.21   Conjunctival adhesions and strands (localized)

H11.211   Conjunctival adhesions and strands (localized), right eye

H11.212   Conjunctival adhesions and strands (localized), left eye

H11.213   Conjunctival adhesions and strands (localized), bilateral

■ H11.219   Conjunctival adhesions and strands (localized), unspecified eye

  ● H11.22   Conjunctival granuloma

H11.221   Conjunctival granuloma, right eye

H11.222   Conjunctival granuloma, left eye

H11.223   Conjunctival granuloma, bilateral

■ H11.229   Conjunctival granuloma, unspecified

  ● H11.23   Symblepharon
Adhesion between tarsal conjunctiva and bulbar conjunctiva

H11.231   Symblepharon, right eye

H11.232   Symblepharon, left eye

H11.233   Symblepharon, bilateral

■ H11.239   Symblepharon, unspecified eye

  ● H11.24   Scarring of conjunctiva

H11.241   Scarring of conjunctiva, right eye

H11.242   Scarring of conjunctiva, left eye

H11.243   Scarring of conjunctiva, bilateral

■ H11.249   Scarring of conjunctiva, unspecified eye

● H11.3   Conjunctival hemorrhage
Subconjunctival hemorrhage

■ H11.30   Conjunctival hemorrhage, unspecified eye

H11.31   Conjunctival hemorrhage, right eye

H11.32   Conjunctival hemorrhage, left eye

H11.33   Conjunctival hemorrhage, bilateral

● H11.4   Other conjunctival vascular disorders and cysts

  ● H11.41   Vascular abnormalities of conjunctiva
Conjunctival aneurysm

H11.411   Vascular abnormalities of conjunctiva, right eye

H11.412   Vascular abnormalities of conjunctiva, left eye

H11.413   Vascular abnormalities of conjunctiva, bilateral

■ H11.419   Vascular abnormalities of conjunctiva, unspecified eye

● H11.42   Conjunctival edema

H11.421   Conjunctival edema, right eye

H11.422   Conjunctival edema, left eye

H11.423   Conjunctival edema, bilateral

■ H11.429   Conjunctival edema, unspecified eye

● H11.43   Conjunctival hyperemia

H11.431   Conjunctival hyperemia, right eye

H11.432   Conjunctival hyperemia, left eye

H11.433   Conjunctival hyperemia, bilateral

■ H11.439   Conjunctival hyperemia, unspecified eye

● H11.44   Conjunctival cysts

H11.441   Conjunctival cysts, right eye

H11.442   Conjunctival cysts, left eye

H11.443   Conjunctival cysts, bilateral

■ H11.449   Conjunctival cysts, unspecified eye

● H11.8   Other specified disorders of conjunctiva

  ● H11.81   Pseudopterygium of conjunctiva
Conjunctival scar attached to cornea

H11.811   Pseudopterygium of conjunctiva, right eye

H11.812   Pseudopterygium of conjunctiva, left eye

H11.813   Pseudopterygium of conjunctiva, bilateral

■ H11.819   Pseudopterygium of conjunctiva, unspecified eye

  ● H11.82   Conjunctivochalasis
Conjunctiva bulges over eyelid margin or covers lower punctum

H11.821   Conjunctivochalasis, right eye

H11.822   Conjunctivochalasis, left eye

H11.823   Conjunctivochalasis, bilateral

■ H11.829   Conjunctivochalasis, unspecified eye

H11.89   Other specified disorders of conjunctiva

■ H11.9   Unspecified disorder of conjunctiva

DISORDERS OF SCLERA, CORNEA, IRIS AND CILIARY BODY (H15-H22)

● H15   Disorders of sclera

  ● H15.0   Scleritis
Inflammation of the white (sclera and episclera) of the eye.

  ● H15.00   Unspecified scleritis

■ H15.001   Unspecified scleritis, right eye

■ H15.002   Unspecified scleritis, left eye

■ H15.003   Unspecified scleritis, bilateral

■ H15.009   Unspecified scleritis, unspecified eye

  ● H15.01   Anterior scleritis

H15.011   Anterior scleritis, right eye

H15.012   Anterior scleritis, left eye

H15.013   Anterior scleritis, bilateral

■ H15.019   Anterior scleritis, unspecified eye

● Unacceptable Principal Diagnosis   ● Use Additional Character(s)   ■ Unspecified   ▶ Manifestation Code

OGCR   Official Guidelines for Coding and Reporting   Excludes 1   Excludes 2   Includes   Use additional   Code first   Code also

● **H15.02 Brawny scleritis**
Swelling around the cornea that is gelantinous in appearance
   H15.021 Brawny scleritis, right eye
   H15.022 Brawny scleritis, left eye
   H15.023 Brawny scleritis, bilateral
   ■ H15.029 Brawny scleritis, unspecified eye

● **H15.03 Posterior scleritis**
Sclerotenonitis
   H15.031 Posterior scleritis, right eye
   H15.032 Posterior scleritis, left eye
   H15.033 Posterior scleritis, bilateral
   ■ H15.039 Posterior scleritis, unspecified eye

● **H15.04 Scleritis with corneal involvement**
   H15.041 Scleritis with corneal involvement, right eye
   H15.042 Scleritis with corneal involvement, left eye
   H15.043 Scleritis with corneal involvement, bilateral
   ■ H15.049 Scleritis with corneal involvement, unspecified eye

● **H15.05 Scleromalacia perforans**
Necrotic without inflammation; usually associated with rheumatoid arthritis
   H15.051 Scleromalacia perforans, right eye
   H15.052 Scleromalacia perforans, left eye
   H15.053 Scleromalacia perforans, bilateral
   ■ H15.059 Scleromalacia perforans, unspecified eye

● **H15.09 Other scleritis**
Scleral abscess
   H15.091 Other scleritis, right eye
   H15.092 Other scleritis, left eye
   H15.093 Other scleritis, bilateral
   ■ H15.099 Other scleritis, unspecified eye

● **H15.1 Episcleritis**
Inflammation of the white (sclera and episclera) of the eye.

● **H15.10 Unspecified episcleritis**
   ■ H15.101 Unspecified episcleritis, right eye
   ■ H15.102 Unspecified episcleritis, left eye
   ■ H15.103 Unspecified episcleritis, bilateral
   ■ H15.109 Unspecified episcleritis, unspecified eye

● **H15.11 Episcleritis periodica fugax**
Transient, recurrent inflammation of portion of episclera (connective tissue on the surface of the sclera)
   H15.111 Episcleritis periodica fugax, right eye
   H15.112 Episcleritis periodica fugax, left eye
   H15.113 Episcleritis periodica fugax, bilateral
   ■ H15.119 Episcleritis periodica fugax, unspecified eye

● **H15.12 Nodular episcleritis**
Characterized by tender, localized, moveable nodule within inflamed area
   H15.121 Nodular episcleritis, right eye
   H15.122 Nodular episcleritis, left eye

   H15.123 Nodular episcleritis, bilateral
   ■ H15.129 Nodular episcleritis, unspecified eye

● **H15.8 Other disorders of sclera**
   Excludes2   blue sclera (Q13.5)
     degenerative myopia (H44.2-)

● **H15.81 Equatorial staphyloma**
   H15.811 Equatorial staphyloma, right eye
   H15.812 Equatorial staphyloma, left eye
   H15.813 Equatorial staphyloma, bilateral
   ■ H15.819 Equatorial staphyloma, unspecified eye

● **H15.82 Localized anterior staphyloma**
   H15.821 Localized anterior staphyloma, right eye
   H15.822 Localized anterior staphyloma, left eye
   H15.823 Localized anterior staphyloma, bilateral
   ■ H15.829 Localized anterior staphyloma, unspecified eye

● **H15.83 Staphyloma posticum**
   H15.831 Staphyloma posticum, right eye
   H15.832 Staphyloma posticum, left eye
   H15.833 Staphyloma posticum, bilateral
   ■ H15.839 Staphyloma posticum, unspecified eye

● **H15.84 Scleral ectasia**
   H15.841 Scleral ectasia, right eye
   H15.842 Scleral ectasia, left eye
   H15.843 Scleral ectasia, bilateral
   ■ H15.849 Scleral ectasia, unspecified eye

● **H15.85 Ring staphyloma**
   H15.851 Ring staphyloma, right eye
   H15.852 Ring staphyloma, left eye
   H15.853 Ring staphyloma, bilateral
   ■ H15.859 Ring staphyloma, unspecified eye

   H15.89 Other disorders of sclera
■ **H15.9 Unspecified disorder of sclera**

● **H16 Keratitis**
● **H16.0 Corneal ulcer**
● **H16.00 Unspecified corneal ulcer**
   ■ H16.001 Unspecified corneal ulcer, right eye
   ■ H16.002 Unspecified corneal ulcer, left eye
   ■ H16.003 Unspecified corneal ulcer, bilateral
   ■ H16.009 Unspecified corneal ulcer, unspecified eye

● **H16.01 Central corneal ulcer**
   H16.011 Central corneal ulcer, right eye
   H16.012 Central corneal ulcer, left eye
   H16.013 Central corneal ulcer, bilateral
   ■ H16.019 Central corneal ulcer, unspecified eye

N Newborn Age: 0   P Pediatric Age: 0–17   M Maternity DX: 12–55   A Adult Age: 15–124   ♀ Females Only   ♂ Males Only
Complication\Comorbidity   Major C\C   Present on Admission Requirement   Hospital-Acquired Condition   969
CHAPTER 7 (H00-H59)

CHAPTER 7 (H00–H59)

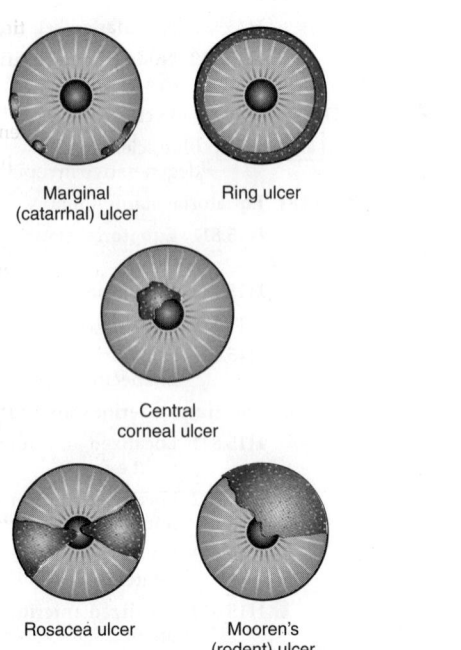

Figure 7-6   Corneal ulcers: marginal, ring, central corneal, rosacea, and Mooren's.

Item 7–3 An infected ulcer is usually called a **serpiginous** or **hypopyon** ulcer which is a pus sac in the anterior chamber of the eye. **Marginal** ulcers are usually asymptomatic, not primary, and are often superficial and simple. More severe marginal ulcers spread to form a ring ulcer. **Ring** ulcers can extend around the entire corneal periphery. **Central corneal** ulcers develop when there is an abrasion to the epithelium and an infection develops in the eroded area. The **pyocyaneal** ulcer is the most serious corneal infection, which, if left untreated, can lead to loss of the eye.

- ● H16.02   Ring corneal ulcer
  -     H16.021   Ring corneal ulcer, right eye
  -     H16.022   Ring corneal ulcer, left eye
  -     H16.023   Ring corneal ulcer, bilateral
  - ▪ H16.029   Ring corneal ulcer, unspecified eye
- ● H16.03   Corneal ulcer with hypopyon
  -     H16.031   Corneal ulcer with hypopyon, right eye
  -     H16.032   Corneal ulcer with hypopyon, left eye
  -     H16.033   Corneal ulcer with hypopyon, bilateral
  - ▪ H16.039   Corneal ulcer with hypopyon, unspecified eye
- ● H16.04   Marginal corneal ulcer
  -     H16.041   Marginal corneal ulcer, right eye
  -     H16.042   Marginal corneal ulcer, left eye
  -     H16.043   Marginal corneal ulcer, bilateral
  - ▪ H16.049   Marginal corneal ulcer, unspecified eye

- ● H16.05   Mooren's corneal ulcer
  -     H16.051   Mooren's corneal ulcer, right eye
  -     H16.052   Mooren's corneal ulcer, left eye
  -     H16.053   Mooren's corneal ulcer, bilateral
  - ▪ H16.059   Mooren's corneal ulcer, unspecified eye
- ● H16.06   Mycotic corneal ulcer
  -     H16.061   Mycotic corneal ulcer, right eye
  -     H16.062   Mycotic corneal ulcer, left eye
  -     H16.063   Mycotic corneal ulcer, bilateral
  - ▪ H16.069   Mycotic corneal ulcer, unspecified eye
- ● H16.07   Perforated corneal ulcer
  -     H16.071   Perforated corneal ulcer, right eye
  -     H16.072   Perforated corneal ulcer, left eye
  -     H16.073   Perforated corneal ulcer, bilateral
  - ▪ H16.079   Perforated corneal ulcer, unspecified eye
- ● H16.1   Other and unspecified superficial keratitis without conjunctivitis
  - ● H16.10   Unspecified superficial keratitis
    - ▪ H16.101   Unspecified superficial keratitis, right eye
    - ▪ H16.102   Unspecified superficial keratitis, left eye
    - ▪ H16.103   Unspecified superficial keratitis, bilateral
    - ▪ H16.109   Unspecified superficial keratitis, unspecified eye
  - ● H16.11   Macular keratitis
    Areolar keratitis
    Nummular keratitis
    Stellate keratitis
    Striate keratitis
    -     H16.111   Macular keratitis, right eye
    -     H16.112   Macular keratitis, left eye
    -     H16.113   Macular keratitis, bilateral
    - ▪ H16.119   Macular keratitis, unspecified eye
  - ● H16.12   Filamentary keratitis
    -     H16.121   Filamentary keratitis, right eye
    -     H16.122   Filamentary keratitis, left eye
    -     H16.123   Filamentary keratitis, bilateral
    - ▪ H16.129   Filamentary keratitis, unspecified eye
  - ● H16.13   Photokeratitis
    Snow blindness
    Welders' keratitis
    -     H16.131   Photokeratitis, right eye
    -     H16.132   Photokeratitis, left eye
    -     H16.133   Photokeratitis, bilateral
    - ▪ H16.139   Photokeratitis, unspecified eye
  - ● H16.14   Punctate keratitis
    -     H16.141   Punctate keratitis, right eye
    -     H16.142   Punctate keratitis, left eye
    -     H16.143   Punctate keratitis, bilateral
    - ▪ H16.149   Punctate keratitis, unspecified eye

● Unacceptable Principal Diagnosis   ● Use Additional Character(s)   ▪ Unspecified   ▶ Manifestation Code

OGCR   Official Guidelines for Coding and Reporting   Excludes 1   Excludes 2   Includes   Use additional   Code first   Code also

● **H16.2   Keratoconjunctivitis**

  ● **H16.20   Unspecified keratoconjunctivitis**
      Superficial keratitis with conjunctivitis
      NOS

    ■ **H16.201   Unspecified keratoconjunctivitis, right eye**

    ■ **H16.202   Unspecified keratoconjunctivitis, left eye**

    ■ **H16.203   Unspecified keratoconjunctivitis, bilateral**

    ■ **H16.209   Unspecified keratoconjunctivitis, unspecified eye**

  ● **H16.21   Exposure keratoconjunctivitis**

     H16.211   Exposure keratoconjunctivitis, right eye

     H16.212   Exposure keratoconjunctivitis, left eye

     H16.213   Exposure keratoconjunctivitis, bilateral

    ■ **H16.219   Exposure keratoconjunctivitis, unspecified eye**

  ● **H16.22   Keratoconjunctivitis sicca, not specified as Sjögren's**

     Excludes1   Sjogren's syndrome (M35.01)

     H16.221   Keratoconjunctivitis sicca, not specified as Sjögren's, right eye

     H16.222   Keratoconjunctivitis sicca, not specified as Sjögren's, left eye

     H16.223   Keratoconjunctivitis sicca, not specified as Sjögren's, bilateral

    ■ **H16.229   Keratoconjunctivitis sicca, not specified as Sjögren's, unspecified eye**

  ● **H16.23   Neurotrophic keratoconjunctivitis**

     H16.231   Neurotrophic keratoconjunctivitis, right eye

     H16.232   Neurotrophic keratoconjunctivitis, left eye

     H16.233   Neurotrophic keratoconjunctivitis, bilateral

    ■ **H16.239   Neurotrophic keratoconjunctivitis, unspecified eye**

  ● **H16.24   Ophthalmia nodosa**

     H16.241   Ophthalmia nodosa, right eye

     H16.242   Ophthalmia nodosa, left eye

     H16.243   Ophthalmia nodosa, bilateral

    ■ **H16.249   Ophthalmia nodosa, unspecified eye**

  ● **H16.25   Phlyctenular keratoconjunctivitis**

     H16.251   Phlyctenular keratoconjunctivitis, right eye

     H16.252   Phlyctenular keratoconjunctivitis, left eye

     H16.253   Phlyctenular keratoconjunctivitis, bilateral

    ■ **H16.259   Phlyctenular keratoconjunctivitis, unspecified eye**

  ● **H16.26   Vernal keratoconjunctivitis, with limbar and corneal involvement**

     Excludes1   vernal conjunctivitis without limbar and corneal involvement (H10.44)

     H16.261   Vernal keratoconjunctivitis, with limbar and corneal involvement, right eye

     H16.262   Vernal keratoconjunctivitis, with limbar and corneal involvement, left eye

     H16.263   Vernal keratoconjunctivitis, with limbar and corneal involvement, bilateral

    ■ **H16.269   Vernal keratoconjunctivitis, with limbar and corneal involvement, unspecified eye**

  ● **H16.29   Other keratoconjunctivitis**

     H16.291   Other keratoconjunctivitis, right eye

     H16.292   Other keratoconjunctivitis, left eye

     H16.293   Other keratoconjunctivitis, bilateral

    ■ **H16.299   Other keratoconjunctivitis, unspecified eye**

● **H16.3   Interstitial and deep keratitis**

  ● **H16.30   Unspecified interstitial keratitis**

    ■ **H16.301   Unspecified interstitial keratitis, right eye**

    ■ **H16.302   Unspecified interstitial keratitis, left eye**

    ■ **H16.303   Unspecified interstitial keratitis, bilateral**

    ■ **H16.309   Unspecified interstitial keratitis, unspecified eye**

  ● **H16.31   Corneal abscess**

     H16.311   Corneal abscess, right eye

     H16.312   Corneal abscess, left eye

     H16.313   Corneal abscess, bilateral

    ■ **H16.319   Corneal abscess, unspecified eye**

  ● **H16.32   Diffuse interstitial keratitis**
      Cogan's syndrome

     H16.321   Diffuse interstitial keratitis, right eye

     H16.322   Diffuse interstitial keratitis, left eye

     H16.323   Diffuse interstitial keratitis, bilateral

    ■ **H16.329   Diffuse interstitial keratitis, unspecified eye**

  ● **H16.33   Sclerosing keratitis**

     H16.331   Sclerosing keratitis, right eye

     H16.332   Sclerosing keratitis, left eye

     H16.333   Sclerosing keratitis, bilateral

    ■ **H16.339   Sclerosing keratitis, unspecified eye**

  ● **H16.39   Other interstitial and deep keratitis**

     H16.391   Other interstitial and deep keratitis, right eye

     H16.392   Other interstitial and deep keratitis, left eye

CHAPTER 7 (H00-H59)

N   Newborn Age: 0   **P**   Pediatric Age: 0–17   **M**   Maternity DX: 12–55   **A**   Adult Age: 15–124   ♀   Females Only   ♂   Males Only

   Complication\Comorbidity   Major C\C   Present on Admission Requirement   Hospital-Acquired Condition

971

       H16.393   Other interstitial and deep keratitis, bilateral

       ■ H16.399   Other interstitial and deep keratitis, unspecified eye

● H16.4   Corneal neovascularization

   ● H16.40   Unspecified corneal neovascularization

     ■ H16.401   Unspecified corneal neovascularization, right eye

     ■ H16.402   Unspecified corneal neovascularization, left eye

     ■ H16.403   Unspecified corneal neovascularization, bilateral

     ■ H16.409   Unspecified corneal neovascularization, unspecified eye

   ● H16.41   Ghost vessels (corneal)

     H16.411   Ghost vessels (corneal), right eye

     H16.412   Ghost vessels (corneal), left eye

     H16.413   Ghost vessels (corneal), bilateral

     ■ H16.419   Ghost vessels (corneal), unspecified eye

   ● H16.42   Pannus (corneal)

     H16.421   Pannus (corneal), right eye

     H16.422   Pannus (corneal), left eye

     H16.423   Pannus (corneal), bilateral

     ■ H16.429   Pannus (corneal), unspecified eye

   ● H16.43   Localized vascularization of cornea

     H16.431   Localized vascularization of cornea, right eye

     H16.432   Localized vascularization of cornea, left eye

     H16.433   Localized vascularization of cornea, bilateral

     ■ H16.439   Localized vascularization of cornea, unspecified eye

   ● H16.44   Deep vascularization of cornea

     H16.441   Deep vascularization of cornea, right eye

     H16.442   Deep vascularization of cornea, left eye

     H16.443   Deep vascularization of cornea, bilateral

     ■ H16.449   Deep vascularization of cornea, unspecified eye

● H16.8   Other keratitis

■ H16.9   Unspecified keratitis

● H17   Corneal scars and opacities

   ● H17.0   Adherent leukoma

     ■ H17.00   Adherent leukoma, unspecified eye

     H17.01   Adherent leukoma, right eye

     H17.02   Adherent leukoma, left eye

     H17.03   Adherent leukoma, bilateral

   ● H17.1   Central corneal opacity

     ■ H17.10   Central corneal opacity, unspecified eye

     H17.11   Central corneal opacity, right eye

     H17.12   Central corneal opacity, left eye

     H17.13   Central corneal opacity, bilateral

● H17.8   Other corneal scars and opacities

   ● H17.81   Minor opacity of cornea
      Corneal nebula

     H17.811   Minor opacity of cornea, right eye

     H17.812   Minor opacity of cornea, left eye

     H17.813   Minor opacity of cornea, bilateral

     ■ H17.819   Minor opacity of cornea, unspecified eye

   ● H17.82   Peripheral opacity of cornea

     H17.821   Peripheral opacity of cornea, right eye

     H17.822   Peripheral opacity of cornea, left eye

     H17.823   Peripheral opacity of cornea, bilateral

     ■ H17.829   Peripheral opacity of cornea, unspecified eye

   H17.89   Other corneal scars and opacities

■ H17.9   Unspecified corneal scar and opacity

● H18   Other disorders of cornea

   ● H18.0   Corneal pigmentations and deposits

     ● H18.00   Unspecified corneal deposit

       ■ H18.001   Unspecified corneal deposit, right eye

       ■ H18.002   Unspecified corneal deposit, left eye

       ■ H18.003   Unspecified corneal deposit, bilateral

       ■ H18.009   Unspecified corneal deposit, unspecified eye

     ● H18.01   Anterior corneal pigmentations
       Staehli's line

       H18.011   Anterior corneal pigmentations, right eye

       H18.012   Anterior corneal pigmentations, left eye

       H18.013   Anterior corneal pigmentations, bilateral

       ■ H18.019   Anterior corneal pigmentations, unspecified eye

     ● H18.02   Argentous corneal deposits

       H18.021   Argentous corneal deposits, right eye

       H18.022   Argentous corneal deposits, left eye

       H18.023   Argentous corneal deposits, bilateral

       ■ H18.029   Argentous corneal deposits, unspecified eye

     ● H18.03   Corneal deposits in metabolic disorders

       Code also associated metabolic disorder

       H18.031   Corneal deposits in metabolic disorders, right eye

       H18.032   Corneal deposits in metabolic disorders, left eye

       H18.033   Corneal deposits in metabolic disorders, bilateral

       ■ H18.039   Corneal deposits in metabolic disorders, unspecified eye

---

● Unacceptable Principal Diagnosis   ● Use Additional Character(s)   ■ Unspecified   ▶ Manifestation Code

OGCR Official Guidelines for Coding and Reporting   Excludes 1   Excludes 2   Includes   Use additional   Code first   Code also

972

● **H18.04 Kayser-Fleischer ring**
     Code also associated Wilson's disease (E83.01)

     H18.041 Kayser-Fleischer ring, right eye

     H18.042 Kayser-Fleischer ring, left eye

     H18.043 Kayser-Fleischer ring, bilateral

     ■ H18.049 Kayser-Fleischer ring, unspecified eye

● **H18.05 Posterior corneal pigmentations**
     Krukenberg's spindle

     H18.051 Posterior corneal pigmentations, right eye

     H18.052 Posterior corneal pigmentations, left eye

     H18.053 Posterior corneal pigmentations, bilateral

     ■ H18.059 Posterior corneal pigmentations, unspecified eye

● **H18.06 Stromal corneal pigmentations**
     Hematocornea

     H18.061 Stromal corneal pigmentations, right eye

     H18.062 Stromal corneal pigmentations, left eye

     H18.063 Stromal corneal pigmentations, bilateral

     ■ H18.069 Stromal corneal pigmentations, unspecified eye

● **H18.1 Bullous keratopathy**

     ■ H18.10 Bullous keratopathy, unspecified eye

     H18.11 Bullous keratopathy, right eye

     H18.12 Bullous keratopathy, left eye

     H18.13 Bullous keratopathy, bilateral

● **H18.2 Other and unspecified corneal edema**

     ■ H18.20 Unspecified corneal edema

     ● H18.21 Corneal edema secondary to contact lens

       Excludes2 / other corneal disorders due to contact lens (H18.82-)

     H18.211 Corneal edema secondary to contact lens, right eye

     H18.212 Corneal edema secondary to contact lens, left eye

     H18.213 Corneal edema secondary to contact lens, bilateral

     ■ H18.219 Corneal edema secondary to contact lens, unspecified eye

     ● H18.22 Idiopathic corneal edema

     H18.221 Idiopathic corneal edema, right eye

     H18.222 Idiopathic corneal edema, left eye

     H18.223 Idiopathic corneal edema, bilateral

     ■ H18.229 Idiopathic corneal edema, unspecified eye

     ● H18.23 Secondary corneal edema

     H18.231 Secondary corneal edema, right eye

     H18.232 Secondary corneal edema, left eye

     H18.233 Secondary corneal edema, bilateral

     ■ H18.239 Secondary corneal edema, unspecified eye

● **H18.3 Changes of corneal membranes**

     ■ H18.30 Unspecified corneal membrane change

     ● H18.31 Folds and rupture in Bowman's membrane

     H18.311 Folds and rupture in Bowman's membrane, right eye

     H18.312 Folds and rupture in Bowman's membrane, left eye

     H18.313 Folds and rupture in Bowman's membrane, bilateral

     ■ H18.319 Folds and rupture in Bowman's membrane, unspecified eye

     ● H18.32 Folds in Descemet's membrane

     H18.321 Folds in Descemet's membrane, right eye

     H18.322 Folds in Descemet's membrane, left eye

     H18.323 Folds in Descemet's membrane, bilateral

     ■ H18.329 Folds in Descemet's membrane, unspecified eye

     ● H18.33 Rupture in Descemet's membrane

     H18.331 Rupture in Descemet's membrane, right eye

     H18.332 Rupture in Descemet's membrane, left eye

     H18.333 Rupture in Descemet's membrane, bilateral

     ■ H18.339 Rupture in Descemet's membrane, unspecified eye

● **H18.4 Corneal degeneration**

     Excludes1   Mooren's ulcer (H16.0-)
                 recurrent erosion of cornea (H18.83-)

     ■ H18.40 Unspecified corneal degeneration

     ● H18.41 Arcus senilis
       Senile corneal changes

     H18.411 Arcus senilis, right eye

     H18.412 Arcus senilis, left eye

     H18.413 Arcus senilis, bilateral

     ■ H18.419 Arcus senilis, unspecified eye

     ● H18.42 Band keratopathy

     H18.421 Band keratopathy, right eye

     H18.422 Band keratopathy, left eye

     H18.423 Band keratopathy, bilateral

     ■ H18.429 Band keratopathy, unspecified eye

     H18.43 Other calcerous corneal degeneration

     ● H18.44 Keratomalacia

       Excludes1   keratomalacia due to vitamin A deficiency (E50.4)

     H18.441 Keratomalacia, right eye

     H18.442 Keratomalacia, left eye

     H18.443 Keratomalacia, bilateral

     ■ H18.449 Keratomalacia, unspecified eye

     ● H18.45 Nodular corneal degeneration

     H18.451 Nodular corneal degeneration, right eye

     H18.452 Nodular corneal degeneration, left eye

     H18.453 Nodular corneal degeneration, bilateral

     ■ H18.459 Nodular corneal degeneration, unspecified eye

CHAPTER 7 (H00-H59)

N Newborn Age: 0   **P** Pediatric Age: 0–17   **M** Maternity DX: 12–55   **A** Adult Age: 15–124   ♀ Females Only   ♂ Males Only

Complication\Comorbidity   Major C\C   Present on Admission Requirement   Hospital-Acquired Condition

973

● **H18.46 Peripheral corneal degeneration**

    H18.461 Peripheral corneal degeneration, right eye

    H18.462 Peripheral corneal degeneration, left eye

    H18.463 Peripheral corneal degeneration, bilateral

    ■ H18.469 Peripheral corneal degeneration, unspecified eye

    H18.49 Other corneal degeneration

● **H18.5 Hereditary corneal dystrophies**

    ■ H18.50 Unspecified hereditary corneal dystrophies

    H18.51 Endothelial corneal dystrophy
          Fuchs' dystrophy

    H18.52 Epithelial (juvenile) corneal dystrophy

    H18.53 Granular corneal dystrophy

    H18.54 Lattice corneal dystrophy

    H18.55 Macular corneal dystrophy

    H18.59 Other hereditary corneal dystrophies

● **H18.6 Keratoconus**

    ● H18.60 Keratoconus, unspecified

        ■ H18.601 Keratoconus, unspecified, right eye

        ■ H18.602 Keratoconus, unspecified, left eye

        ■ H18.603 Keratoconus, unspecified, bilateral

        ■ H18.609 Keratoconus, unspecified, unspecified eye

    ● H18.61 Keratoconus, stable

        H18.611 Keratoconus, stable, right eye

        H18.612 Keratoconus, stable, left eye

        H18.613 Keratoconus, stable, bilateral

        ■ H18.619 Keratoconus, stable, unspecified eye

    ● H18.62 Keratoconus, unstable
            Acute hydrops

        H18.621 Keratoconus, unstable, right eye

        H18.622 Keratoconus, unstable, left eye

        H18.623 Keratoconus, unstable, bilateral

        ■ H18.629 Keratoconus, unstable, unspecified eye

● **H18.7 Other and unspecified corneal deformities**

    | Excludes1 | congenital malformations of cornea (Q13.3-Q13.4) |

    ■ H18.70 Unspecified corneal deformity

    ● H18.71 Corneal ectasia

        H18.711 Corneal ectasia, right eye

        H18.712 Corneal ectasia, left eye

        H18.713 Corneal ectasia, bilateral

        ■ H18.719 Corneal ectasia, unspecified eye

    ● H18.72 Corneal staphyloma

        H18.721 Corneal staphyloma, right eye

        H18.722 Corneal staphyloma, left eye

        H18.723 Corneal staphyloma, bilateral

        ■ H18.729 Corneal staphyloma, unspecified eye

    ● H18.73 Descemetocele

        H18.731 Descemetocele, right eye

        H18.732 Descemetocele, left eye

        H18.733 Descemetocele, bilateral

        ■ H18.739 Descemetocele, unspecified eye

    ● H18.79 Other corneal deformities

        H18.791 Other corneal deformities, right eye

        H18.792 Other corneal deformities, left eye

        H18.793 Other corneal deformities, bilateral

        ■ H18.799 Other corneal deformities, unspecified eye

● **H18.8 Other specified disorders of cornea**

    ● H18.81 Anesthesia and hypoesthesia of cornea

        H18.811 Anesthesia and hypoesthesia of cornea, right eye

        H18.812 Anesthesia and hypoesthesia of cornea, left eye

        H18.813 Anesthesia and hypoesthesia of cornea, bilateral

        ■ H18.819 Anesthesia and hypoesthesia of cornea, unspecified eye

    ● H18.82 Corneal disorder due to contact lens

    | Excludes2 | corneal edema due to contact lens (H18.21-) |

        H18.821 Corneal disorder due to contact lens, right eye

        H18.822 Corneal disorder due to contact lens, left eye

        H18.823 Corneal disorder due to contact lens, bilateral

        ■ H18.829 Corneal disorder due to contact lens, unspecified eye

    ● H18.83 Recurrent erosion of cornea

        H18.831 Recurrent erosion of cornea, right eye

        H18.832 Recurrent erosion of cornea, left eye

        H18.833 Recurrent erosion of cornea, bilateral

        ■ H18.839 Recurrent erosion of cornea, unspecified eye

Figure 7-7 Lateral view of the displacement of the cone apex in keratoconus. (From Yanoff: Ophthalmology, 2nd ed. 2004, Mosby, Inc.)

Item 7-4 Keratoconus results in corneal degeneration that begins in childhood, gradually changes the cornea from a round to cone shape, decreasing visual acuity. Treatment includes contact lenses. In severe cases the need for corneal transplant may be the treatment of choice; however, newer technologies may use high frequency radio energy to shrink the edges of the cornea, pulling the central area back to a more normal shape. It can help delay or avoid the need for a corneal transplantation.

● Unacceptable Principal Diagnosis   ● Use Additional Character(s)   ■ Unspecified   ▶ Manifestation Code

OGCR Official Guidelines for Coding and Reporting   Excludes 1   Excludes 2   Includes   Use additional   Code first   Code also

CHAPTER 7 (H00-H59)

● **H18.89 Other specified disorders of cornea**

     H18.891   Other specified disorders of cornea, right eye

     H18.892   Other specified disorders of cornea, left eye

     H18.893   Other specified disorders of cornea, bilateral

     ■ H18.899   Other specified disorders of cornea, unspecified eye

■ **H18.9 Unspecified disorder of cornea**

● **H20 Iridocyclitis**

   ● **H20.0 Acute and subacute iridocyclitis**

     Acute anterior uveitis
     Acute cyclitis
     Acute iritis
     Subacute anterior uveitis
     Subacute cyclitis
     Subacute iritis

     Excludes1   iridocyclitis, iritis, uveitis (due to) (in) diabetes mellitus (E08-E13 with .39)
     iridocyclitis, iritis, uveitis (due to) (in) diphtheria (A36.89)
     iridocyclitis, iritis, uveitis (due to) (in) gonococcal (A54.32)
     iridocyclitis, iritis, uveitis (due to) (in) herpes (simplex) (B00.51)
     iridocyclitis, iritis, uveitis (due to) (in) herpes zoster (B02.32)
     iridocyclitis, iritis, uveitis (due to) (in) late congenital syphilis (A50.39)
     iridocyclitis, iritis, uveitis (due to) (in) late syphilis (A52.71)
     iridocyclitis, iritis, uveitis (due to) (in) sarcoidosis (D86.83)
     iridocyclitis, iritis, uveitis (due to) (in) syphilis (A51.43)
     iridocyclitis, iritis, uveitis (due to) (in) toxoplasmosis (B58.09)
     iridocyclitis, iritis, uveitis (due to) (in) tuberculosis (A18.54)

     ■ **H20.00 Unspecified acute and subacute iridocyclitis** 🔷

   ● **H20.01 Primary iridocyclitis**

     H20.011   **Primary iridocyclitis, right eye** 🔷

     H20.012   **Primary iridocyclitis, left eye** 🔷

     H20.013   **Primary iridocyclitis, bilateral** 🔷

     ■ H20.019   **Primary iridocyclitis, unspecified eye** 🔷

   ● **H20.02 Recurrent acute iridocyclitis**

     H20.021   **Recurrent acute iridocyclitis, right eye** 🔷

     H20.022   **Recurrent acute iridocyclitis, left eye** 🔷

     H20.023   **Recurrent acute iridocyclitis, bilateral** 🔷

     ■ H20.029   **Recurrent acute iridocyclitis, unspecified eye** 🔷

   ● **H20.03 Secondary infectious iridocyclitis**

     H20.031   **Secondary infectious iridocyclitis, right eye** 🔷

     H20.032   **Secondary infectious iridocyclitis, left eye** 🔷

     H20.033   **Secondary infectious iridocyclitis, bilateral** 🔷

     ■ H20.039   **Secondary infectious iridocyclitis, unspecified eye** 🔷

   ● **H20.04 Secondary noninfectious iridocyclitis**

     H20.041   **Secondary noninfectious iridocyclitis, right eye**

     H20.042   **Secondary noninfectious iridocyclitis, left eye**

     H20.043   **Secondary noninfectious iridocyclitis, bilateral**

     ■ H20.049   **Secondary noninfectious iridocyclitis, unspecified eye**

   ● **H20.05 Hypopyon**

     H20.051   **Hypopyon, right eye**

     H20.052   **Hypopyon, left eye**

     H20.053   **Hypopyon, bilateral**

     ■ H20.059   **Hypopyon, unspecified eye**

● **H20.1 Chronic iridocyclitis**

     Use additional code for any associated cataract (H26.21-)

     Excludes2   posterior cyclitis (H30.2-)

   ■ **H20.10 Chronic iridocyclitis, unspecified eye**

   H20.11 Chronic iridocyclitis, right eye

   H20.12 Chronic iridocyclitis, left eye

   H20.13 Chronic iridocyclitis, bilateral

● **H20.2 Lens-induced iridocyclitis**

   ■ **H20.20 Lens-induced iridocyclitis, unspecified eye**

   H20.21 Lens-induced iridocyclitis, right eye

   H20.22 Lens-induced iridocyclitis, left eye

   H20.23 Lens-induced iridocyclitis, bilateral

● **H20.8 Other iridocyclitis**

     Excludes2   glaucomatocyclitis crises (H40.4-)
     posterior cyclitis (H30.2-)
     sympathetic uveitis (H44.13-)

   ● **H20.81 Fuchs' heterochromic cyclitis**

     H20.811   **Fuchs' heterochromic cyclitis, right eye**

     H20.812   **Fuchs' heterochromic cyclitis, left eye**

     H20.813   **Fuchs' heterochromic cyclitis, bilateral**

     ■ H20.819   **Fuchs' heterochromic cyclitis, unspecified eye**

   ● **H20.82 Vogt-Koyanagi syndrome**

     H20.821   **Vogt-Koyanagi syndrome, right eye**

     H20.822   **Vogt-Koyanagi syndrome, left eye**

     H20.823   **Vogt-Koyanagi syndrome, bilateral**

     ■ H20.829   **Vogt-Koyanagi syndrome, unspecified eye**

■ **H20.9 Unspecified iridocyclitis** 🔷
     Uveitis NOS

● **H21 Other disorders of iris and ciliary body**

     Excludes2   sympathetic uveitis (H44.1-)

   ● **H21.0 Hyphema**

     Excludes1   traumatic hyphema (S05.1-)

   ■ **H21.00 Hyphema, unspecified eye**

   H21.01 Hyphema, right eye

   H21.02 Hyphema, left eye

   H21.03 Hyphema, bilateral

N Newborn Age: 0   **P** Pediatric Age: 0–17   **M** Maternity DX: 12–55   **A** Adult Age: 15–124   ♀ Females Only   ♂ Males Only

🔷 Complication\Comorbidity   🔷 Major C\C   🔷 Present on Admission Requirement   🔷 Hospital-Acquired Condition

● **H21.1 Other vascular disorders of iris and ciliary body**
     Neovascularization of iris or ciliary body
     Rubeosis iridis
     Rubeosis of iris

  ● **H21.1X Other vascular disorders of iris and ciliary body**

     H21.1X1 Other vascular disorders of iris and ciliary body, right eye

     H21.1X2 Other vascular disorders of iris and ciliary body, left eye

     H21.1X3 Other vascular disorders of iris and ciliary body, bilateral

     ▪ **H21.1X9 Other vascular disorders of iris and ciliary body, unspecified eye**

● **H21.2 Degeneration of iris and ciliary body**

  ● **H21.21 Degeneration of chamber angle**

     H21.211 Degeneration of chamber angle, right eye

     H21.212 Degeneration of chamber angle, left eye

     H21.213 Degeneration of chamber angle, bilateral

     ▪ **H21.219 Degeneration of chamber angle, unspecified eye**

  ● **H21.22 Degeneration of ciliary body**

     H21.221 Degeneration of ciliary body, right eye

     H21.222 Degeneration of ciliary body, left eye

     H21.223 Degeneration of ciliary body, bilateral

     ▪ **H21.229 Degeneration of ciliary body, unspecified eye**

  ● **H21.23 Degeneration of iris (pigmentary)**
     Translucency of iris

     H21.231 Degeneration of iris (pigmentary), right eye

     H21.232 Degeneration of iris (pigmentary), left eye

     H21.233 Degeneration of iris (pigmentary), bilateral

     ▪ **H21.239 Degeneration of iris (pigmentary), unspecified eye**

  ● **H21.24 Degeneration of pupillary margin**

     H21.241 Degeneration of pupillary margin, right eye

     H21.242 Degeneration of pupillary margin, left eye

     H21.243 Degeneration of pupillary margin, bilateral

     ▪ **H21.249 Degeneration of pupillary margin, unspecified eye**

  ● **H21.25 Iridoschisis**

     H21.251 Iridoschisis, right eye

     H21.252 Iridoschisis, left eye

     H21.253 Iridoschisis, bilateral

     ▪ **H21.259 Iridoschisis, unspecified eye**

  ● **H21.26 Iris atrophy (essential) (progressive)**

     H21.261 Iris atrophy (essential) (progressive), right eye

     H21.262 Iris atrophy (essential) (progressive), left eye

     H21.263 Iris atrophy (essential) (progressive), bilateral

     ▪ **H21.269 Iris atrophy (essential) (progressive), unspecified eye**

  ● **H21.27 Miotic pupillary cyst**

     H21.271 Miotic pupillary cyst, right eye

     H21.272 Miotic pupillary cyst, left eye

     H21.273 Miotic pupillary cyst, bilateral

     ▪ **H21.279 Miotic pupillary cyst, unspecified eye**

   H21.29 Other iris atrophy

● **H21.3 Cyst of iris, ciliary body and anterior chamber**
     Excludes2   miotic pupillary cyst (H21.27-)

  ● **H21.30 Idiopathic cysts of iris, ciliary body or anterior chamber**
     Cyst of iris, ciliary body or anterior chamber NOS

     H21.301 Idiopathic cysts of iris, ciliary body or anterior chamber, right eye

     H21.302 Idiopathic cysts of iris, ciliary body or anterior chamber, left eye

     H21.303 Idiopathic cysts of iris, ciliary body or anterior chamber, bilateral

     ▪ **H21.309 Idiopathic cysts of iris, ciliary body or anterior chamber, unspecified eye**

  ● **H21.31 Exudative cysts of iris or anterior chamber**

     H21.311 Exudative cysts of iris or anterior chamber, right eye

     H21.312 Exudative cysts of iris or anterior chamber, left eye

     H21.313 Exudative cysts of iris or anterior chamber, bilateral

     ▪ **H21.319 Exudative cysts of iris or anterior chamber, unspecified eye**

  ● **H21.32 Implantation cysts of iris, ciliary body or anterior chamber**

     H21.321 Implantation cysts of iris, ciliary body or anterior chamber, right eye

     H21.322 Implantation cysts of iris, ciliary body or anterior chamber, left eye

     H21.323 Implantation cysts of iris, ciliary body or anterior chamber, bilateral

     ▪ **H21.329 Implantation cysts of iris, ciliary body or anterior chamber, unspecified eye**

  ● **H21.33 Parasitic cyst of iris, ciliary body or anterior chamber**

     H21.331 Parasitic cyst of iris, ciliary body or anterior chamber, right eye ▸

     H21.332 Parasitic cyst of iris, ciliary body or anterior chamber, left eye ▸

     H21.333 Parasitic cyst of iris, ciliary body or anterior chamber, bilateral ▸

     ▪ **H21.339 Parasitic cyst of iris, ciliary body or anterior chamber, unspecified eye** ▸

● **H21.34 Primary cyst of pars plana**

    H21.341 Primary cyst of pars plana, right eye

    H21.342 Primary cyst of pars plana, left eye

    H21.343 Primary cyst of pars plana, bilateral

    ■ H21.349 Primary cyst of pars plana, unspecified eye

● **H21.35 Exudative cyst of pars plana**

    H21.351 Exudative cyst of pars plana, right eye

    H21.352 Exudative cyst of pars plana, left eye

    H21.353 Exudative cyst of pars plana, bilateral

    ■ H21.359 Exudative cyst of pars plana, unspecified eye

● **H21.4 Pupillary membranes**
    Iris bombé
    Pupillary occlusion
    Pupillary seclusion

    | Excludes1 | congenital pupillary membranes (Q13.8) |

    ■ H21.40 Pupillary membranes, unspecified eye

    H21.41 Pupillary membranes, right eye

    H21.42 Pupillary membranes, left eye

    H21.43 Pupillary membranes, bilateral

● **H21.5 Other and unspecified adhesions and disruptions of iris and ciliary body**

    | Excludes1 | corectopia (Q13.2) |

    ● H21.50 Unspecified adhesions of iris
        Synechia (iris) NOS

        ■ H21.501 Unspecified adhesions of iris, right eye

        ■ H21.502 Unspecified adhesions of iris, left eye

        ■ H21.503 Unspecified adhesions of iris, bilateral

        ■ H21.509 Unspecified adhesions of iris and ciliary body, unspecified eye

    ● H21.51 Anterior synechiae (iris)

        H21.511 Anterior synechiae (iris), right eye

        H21.512 Anterior synechiae (iris), left eye

        H21.513 Anterior synechiae (iris), bilateral

        ■ H21.519 Anterior synechiae (iris), unspecified eye

    ● H21.52 Goniosynechiae

        H21.521 Goniosynechiae, right eye

        H21.522 Goniosynechiae, left eye

        H21.523 Goniosynechiae, bilateral

        ■ H21.529 Goniosynechiae, unspecified eye

    ● H21.53 Iridodialysis

        H21.531 Iridodialysis, right eye

        H21.532 Iridodialysis, left eye

        H21.533 Iridodialysis, bilateral

        ■ H21.539 Iridodialysis, unspecified eye

    ● H21.54 Posterior synechiae (iris)

        H21.541 Posterior synechiae (iris), right eye

        H21.542 Posterior synechiae (iris), left eye

        H21.543 Posterior synechiae (iris), bilateral

        ■ H21.549 Posterior synechiae (iris), unspecified eye

● **H21.55 Recession of chamber angle**

    H21.551 Recession of chamber angle, right eye

    H21.552 Recession of chamber angle, left eye

    H21.553 Recession of chamber angle, bilateral

    ■ H21.559 Recession of chamber angle, unspecified eye

● **H21.56 Pupillary abnormalities**
    Deformed pupil
    Ectopic pupil
    Rupture of sphincter, pupil

    | Excludes1 | congenital deformity of pupil (Q13.2-) |

    H21.561 Pupillary abnormality, right eye

    H21.562 Pupillary abnormality, left eye

    H21.563 Pupillary abnormality, bilateral

    ■ H21.569 Pupillary abnormality, unspecified eye

● **H21.8 Other specified disorders of iris and ciliary body**

    ● H21.81 Floppy iris syndrome
        Intraoperative floppy iris syndrome (IFIS)

        Use additional code for adverse effect, if applicable, to identify drug (T36-T50 with fifth or sixth character 5)

    H21.82 Plateau iris syndrome (post-iridectomy) (postprocedural)

    H21.89 Other specified disorders of iris and ciliary body

    ■ H21.9 Unspecified disorder of iris and ciliary body

▶ *H22 Disorders of iris and ciliary body in diseases classified elsewhere*

    Code first underlying disease, such as:
    gout (M1A-, M10.-)

DISORDERS OF LENS (H25-H28)

● **H25 Age-related cataract**
    Senile cataract

    | Excludes2 | capsular glaucoma with pseudoexfoliation of lens (H40.1-) |

    ● H25.0 Age-related incipient cataract

        ● H25.01 Cortical age-related cataract

            H25.011 Cortical age-related cataract, right eye   **A**

            H25.012 Cortical age-related cataract, left eye   **A**

            H25.013 Cortical age-related cataract, bilateral   **A**

            ■ H25.019 Cortical age-related cataract, unspecified eye   **A**

        ● H25.03 Anterior subcapsular polar age-related cataract

            H25.031 Anterior subcapsular polar age-related cataract, right eye   **A**

            H25.032 Anterior subcapsular polar age-related cataract, left eye   **A**

            H25.033 Anterior subcapsular polar age-related cataract, bilateral   **A**

            ■ H25.039 Anterior subcapsular polar age-related cataract, unspecified eye   **A**

N Newborn Age: 0   **P** Pediatric Age: 0–17   **M** Maternity DX: 12–55   **A** Adult Age: 15–124   ♀ Females Only   ♂ Males Only

🅒 Complication\Comorbidity   🅜 Major C\C   🅟 Present on Admission Requirement   🅗 Hospital-Acquired Condition

977

CHAPTER 7 (H00-H59)

Figure 7-8   Age-related cataract. Nuclear sclerosis and cortical lens opacities are present. (From Yanoff: Ophthalmology, 2nd ed. 2004, Mosby, Inc.)

Item 7–5 **Senile** cataracts are linked to the aging process. The most common area for the formation of a cataract is the cortical area of the lens. **Polar cataracts** can be either anterior or posterior. **Anterior polar cataracts** are more common and are small, white, capsular cataracts located on the anterior portion of the lens. **Total cataracts,** also called **complete** or **mature,** cause an opacity of all fibers of the lens. **Hypermature** describes a mature cataract with a swollen, milky cortex that covers the entire lens. **Immature,** also called **incipient,** cataracts have a clear cortex and are only slightly opaque. Treatment for all cataracts is the removal of the lens.

● H25.04   **Posterior subcapsular polar age-related cataract**

     H25.041   **Posterior subcapsular polar age-related cataract, right eye**   A

     H25.042   **Posterior subcapsular polar age-related cataract, left eye**   A

     H25.043   **Posterior subcapsular polar age-related cataract, bilateral**   A

     ■ H25.049   **Posterior subcapsular polar age-related cataract, unspecified eye**   A

● H25.09   **Other age-related incipient cataract**
     Coronary age-related cataract
     Punctate age-related cataract
     Water clefts

     H25.091   **Other age-related incipient cataract, right eye**   A

     H25.092   **Other age-related incipient cataract, left eye**   A

     H25.093   **Other age-related incipient cataract, bilateral**   A

     ■ H25.099   **Other age-related incipient cataract, unspecified eye**   A

● H25.1   **Age-related nuclear cataract**
     Cataracta brunescens
     Nuclear sclerosis cataract

     ■ H25.10   **Age-related nuclear cataract, unspecified eye**   A

     H25.11   **Age-related nuclear cataract, right eye**   A

     H25.12   **Age-related nuclear cataract, left eye**   A

     H25.13   **Age-related nuclear cataract, bilateral**   A

● H25.2   **Age-related cataract, morgagnian type**
     Age-related hypermature cataract

     ■ H25.20   **Age-related cataract, morgagnian type, unspecified eye**   A

     H25.21   **Age-related cataract, morgagnian type, right eye**   A

     H25.22   **Age-related cataract, morgagnian type, left eye**   A

     H25.23   **Age-related cataract, morgagnian type, bilateral**   A

● H25.8   **Other age-related cataract**

     ● H25.81   **Combined forms of age-related cataract**

        H25.811   **Combined forms of age-related cataract, right eye**   A

        H25.812   **Combined forms of age-related cataract, left eye**   A

        H25.813   **Combined forms of age-related cataract, bilateral**   A

        ■ H25.819   **Combined forms of age-related cataract, unspecified eye**   A

     H25.89   **Other age-related cataract**   A

■ H25.9   **Unspecified age-related cataract**   A

● H26   **Other cataract**

     | Excludes1 | congenital cataract (Q12.0)

     ● H26.0   **Infantile and juvenile cataract**

        ● H26.00   **Unspecified infantile and juvenile cataract**

          ■ H26.001   **Unspecified infantile and juvenile cataract, right eye**   P

          ■ H26.002   **Unspecified infantile and juvenile cataract, left eye**   P

          ■ H26.003   **Unspecified infantile and juvenile cataract, bilateral**   P

          ■ H26.009   **Unspecified infantile and juvenile cataract, unspecified eye**   P

        ● H26.01   **Infantile and juvenile cortical, lamellar, or zonular cataract**

          H26.011   **Infantile and juvenile cortical, lamellar, or zonular cataract, right eye**   P

          H26.012   **Infantile and juvenile cortical, lamellar, or zonular cataract, left eye**   P

          H26.013   **Infantile and juvenile cortical, lamellar, or zonular cataract, bilateral**   P

          ■ H26.019   **Infantile and juvenile cortical, lamellar, or zonular cataract, unspecified eye**   P

        ● H26.03   **Infantile and juvenile nuclear cataract**

          H26.031   **Infantile and juvenile nuclear cataract, right eye**   P

          H26.032   **Infantile and juvenile nuclear cataract, left eye**   P

          H26.033   **Infantile and juvenile nuclear cataract, bilateral**   P

          ■ H26.039   **Infantile and juvenile nuclear cataract, unspecified eye**   P

        ● H26.04   **Anterior subcapsular polar infantile and juvenile cataract**

          H26.041   **Anterior subcapsular polar infantile and juvenile cataract, right eye**   P

          H26.042   **Anterior subcapsular polar infantile and juvenile cataract, left eye**   P

          H26.043   **Anterior subcapsular polar infantile and juvenile cataract, bilateral**   P

          ■ H26.049   **Anterior subcapsular polar infantile and juvenile cataract, unspecified eye**   P

●   Unacceptable Principal Diagnosis   ●   Use Additional Character(s)   ■   Unspecified   ▶   Manifestation Code

OGCR   Official Guidelines for Coding and Reporting | Excludes 1 | | Excludes 2 | | Includes | | Use additional | | Code first | | Code also |

● **H26.05** **Posterior subcapsular polar infantile and juvenile cataract**

     H26.051 **Posterior subcapsular polar infantile and juvenile cataract, right eye**   P

     H26.052 **Posterior subcapsular polar infantile and juvenile cataract, left eye**   P

     H26.053 **Posterior subcapsular polar infantile and juvenile cataract, bilateral**   P

     ■ **H26.059** **Posterior subcapsular polar infantile and juvenile cataract, unspecified eye**   P

● **H26.06** **Combined forms of infantile and juvenile cataract**

     H26.061 **Combined forms of infantile and juvenile cataract, right eye**   P

     H26.062 **Combined forms of infantile and juvenile cataract, left eye**   P

     H26.063 **Combined forms of infantile and juvenile cataract bilateral**   P

     ■ **H26.069** **Combined forms of infantile and juvenile cataract, unspecified eye**   P

     H26.09 **Other infantile and juvenile cataract**   P

● **H26.1** **Traumatic cataract**

     Use additional code (Chapter 20) to identify external cause

● **H26.10** **Unspecified traumatic cataract**

     ■ **H26.101** **Unspecified traumatic cataract, right eye**

     ■ **H26.102** **Unspecified traumatic cataract, left eye**

     ■ **H26.103** **Unspecified traumatic cataract, bilateral**

     ■ **H26.109** **Unspecified traumatic cataract, unspecified eye**

● **H26.11** **Localized traumatic opacities**

     H26.111 **Localized traumatic opacities, right eye**

     H26.112 **Localized traumatic opacities, left eye**

     H26.113 **Localized traumatic opacities, bilateral**

     ■ **H26.119** **Localized traumatic opacities, unspecified eye**

● **H26.12** **Partially resolved traumatic cataract**

     H26.121 **Partially resolved traumatic cataract, right eye**

     H26.122 **Partially resolved traumatic cataract, left eye**

     H26.123 **Partially resolved traumatic cataract, bilateral**

     ■ **H26.129** **Partially resolved traumatic cataract, unspecified eye**

● **H26.13** **Total traumatic cataract**

     H26.131 **Total traumatic cataract, right eye**

     H26.132 **Total traumatic cataract, left eye**

     H26.133 **Total traumatic cataract, bilateral**

     ■ **H26.139** **Total traumatic cataract, unspecified eye**

● **H26.2** **Complicated cataract**

     ■ **H26.20** **Unspecified complicated cataract**
     Cataracta complicata NOS

     ● **H26.21** **Cataract with neovascularization**

         Code also associated condition, such as: chronic iridocyclitis (H20.1-)

         H26.211 **Cataract with neovascularization, right eye**

         H26.212 **Cataract with neovascularization, left eye**

         H26.213 **Cataract with neovascularization, bilateral**

         ■ **H26.219** **Cataract with neovascularization, unspecified eye**

     ● **H26.22** **Cataract secondary to ocular disorders (degenerative) (inflammatory)**

         Code also associated ocular disorder

         H26.221 **Cataract secondary to ocular disorders (degenerative) (inflammatory), right eye**

         H26.222 **Cataract secondary to ocular disorders (degenerative) (inflammatory), left eye**

         H26.223 **Cataract secondary to ocular disorders (degenerative) (inflammatory), bilateral**

         ■ **H26.229** **Cataract secondary to ocular disorders (degenerative) (inflammatory), unspecified eye**

     ● **H26.23** **Glaucomatous flecks (subcapsular)**

         Code first underlying glaucoma (H40-H42)

         ● **H26.231** **Glaucomatous flecks (subcapsular), right eye**

         ● **H26.232** **Glaucomatous flecks (subcapsular), left eye**

         ● **H26.233** **Glaucomatous flecks (subcapsular), bilateral**

         ● ■ **H26.239** **Glaucomatous flecks (subcapsular), unspecified eye**

● **H26.3** **Drug-induced cataract**
     Toxic cataract

     Use additional code for adverse effect, if applicable, to identify drug (T36-T50 with fifth or sixth character 5)

     ● ■ **H26.30** **Drug-induced cataract, unspecified eye**

     ● **H26.31** **Drug-induced cataract, right eye**

     ● **H26.32** **Drug-induced cataract, left eye**

     ● **H26.33** **Drug-induced cataract, bilateral**

● **H26.4** **Secondary cataract**

     ■ **H26.40** **Unspecified secondary cataract**

     ● **H26.41** **Soemmering's ring**

         H26.411 **Soemmering's ring, right eye**

         H26.412 **Soemmering's ring, left eye**

         H26.413 **Soemmering's ring, bilateral**

         ■ **H26.419** **Soemmering's ring, unspecified eye**

     ● **H26.49** **Other secondary cataract**

         H26.491 **Other secondary cataract, right eye**

         H26.492 **Other secondary cataract, left eye**

         H26.493 **Other secondary cataract, bilateral**

         ■ **H26.499** **Other secondary cataract, unspecified eye**

CHAPTER 7 (H00-H59)

N Newborn Age: 0   **P** Pediatric Age: 0–17   **M** Maternity DX: 12–55   **A** Adult Age: 15–124   ♀ Females Only   ♂ Males Only

     Complication\Comorbidity   Major C\C   Present on Admission Requirement   Hospital-Acquired Condition

CHAPTER 7 (H00-H59)

H26.8   Other specified cataract

■ H26.9   Unspecified cataract

● H27   Other disorders of lens

> **Excludes1**   congenital lens malformations (Q12.-)
> mechanical complications of intraocular lens implant (T85.2)
> pseudophakia (Z96.1)

● H27.0   Aphakia

> Acquired absence of lens
> Acquired aphakia
> Aphakia due to trauma

> **Excludes1**   cataract extraction status (Z98.4-)
> congenital absence of lens (Q12.3)
> congenital aphakia (Q12.3)

■ H27.00   Aphakia, unspecified eye

H27.01   Aphakia, right eye

H27.02   Aphakia, left eye

H27.03   Aphakia, bilateral

● H27.1   Dislocation of lens

■ H27.10   Unspecified dislocation of lens

● H27.11   Subluxation of lens

> H27.111   Subluxation of lens, right eye

> H27.112   Subluxation of lens, left eye

> H27.113   Subluxation of lens, bilateral

> ■ H27.119   Subluxation of lens, unspecified eye

● H27.12   Anterior dislocation of lens

> H27.121   Anterior dislocation of lens, right eye

> H27.122   Anterior dislocation of lens, left eye

> H27.123   Anterior dislocation of lens, bilateral

> ■ H27.129   Anterior dislocation of lens, unspecified eye

● H27.13   Posterior dislocation of lens

> H27.131   Posterior dislocation of lens, right eye

> H27.132   Posterior dislocation of lens, left eye

> H27.133   Posterior dislocation of lens, bilateral

> ■ H27.139   Posterior dislocation of lens, unspecified eye

H27.8   Other specified disorders of lens

■ H27.9   Unspecified disorder of lens

● ▶ *H28   Cataract in diseases classified elsewhere*

> *Code first underlying disease, such as:*
> hypoparathyroidism (E20.-)
> myotonia (G71.1-)
> myxedema (E03.-)
> protein-calorie malnutrition (E40-E46)

> **Excludes1**   cataract in diabetes mellitus (E08.33, E09.33, E10.33, E11.33, E13.33)

DISORDERS OF CHOROID AND RETINA (H30-H36)

(See Plate 90 on page NAP-16.)

● H30   Chorioretinal inflammation

● H30.0   Focal chorioretinal inflammation

> Focal chorioretinitis
> Focal choroiditis
> Focal retinitis
> Focal retinochoroiditis

● H30.00   Unspecified focal chorioretinal inflammation

> Focal chorioretinitis NOS
> Focal choroiditis NOS
> Focal retinitis NOS
> Focal retinochoroiditis NOS

> ■ H30.001   Unspecified focal chorioretinal inflammation, right eye

> ■ H30.002   Unspecified focal chorioretinal inflammation, left eye

> ■ H30.003   Unspecified focal chorioretinal inflammation, bilateral

> ■ H30.009   Unspecified focal chorioretinal inflammation, unspecified eye

● H30.01   Focal chorioretinal inflammation, juxtapapillary

> H30.011   Focal chorioretinal inflammation, juxtapapillary, right eye

> H30.012   Focal chorioretinal inflammation, juxtapapillary, left eye

> H30.013   Focal chorioretinal inflammation, juxtapapillary, bilateral

> ■ H30.019   Focal chorioretinal inflammation, juxtapapillary, unspecified eye

● H30.02   Focal chorioretinal inflammation of posterior pole

> H30.021   Focal chorioretinal inflammation of posterior pole, right eye

> H30.022   Focal chorioretinal inflammation of posterior pole, left eye

> H30.023   Focal chorioretinal inflammation of posterior pole, bilateral

> ■ H30.029   Focal chorioretinal inflammation of posterior pole, unspecified eye

● H30.03   Focal chorioretinal inflammation, peripheral

> H30.031   Focal chorioretinal inflammation, peripheral, right eye

> H30.032   Focal chorioretinal inflammation, peripheral, left eye

> H30.033   Focal chorioretinal inflammation, peripheral, bilateral

> ■ H30.039   Focal chorioretinal inflammation, peripheral, unspecified eye

● H30.04   Focal chorioretinal inflammation, macular or paramacular

> H30.041   Focal chorioretinal inflammation, macular or paramacular, right eye

> H30.042   Focal chorioretinal inflammation, macular or paramacular, left eye

> H30.043   Focal chorioretinal inflammation, macular or paramacular, bilateral

> ■ H30.049   Focal chorioretinal inflammation, macular or paramacular, unspecified eye

● Unacceptable Principal Diagnosis   ● Use Additional Character(s)   ■ Unspecified   ▶ Manifestation Code

OGCR Official Guidelines for Coding and Reporting   Excludes 1   Excludes 2   Includes   Use additional   Code first   Code also

● **H30.1 Disseminated chorioretinal inflammation**
Disseminated chorioretinitis
Disseminated choroiditis
Disseminated retinitis
Disseminated retinochoroiditis
> Excludes2   exudative retinopathy (H35.02-)

● **H30.10 Unspecified disseminated chorioretinal inflammation**
Disseminated chorioretinitis NOS
Disseminated choroiditis NOS
Disseminated retinitis NOS
Disseminated retinochoroiditis NOS

    ■ **H30.101** Unspecified disseminated chorioretinal inflammation, right eye 🐾

    ■ **H30.102** Unspecified disseminated chorioretinal inflammation, left eye 🐾

    ■ **H30.103** Unspecified disseminated chorioretinal inflammation, bilateral 🐾

    ■ **H30.109** Unspecified disseminated chorioretinal inflammation, unspecified eye 🐾

● **H30.11 Disseminated chorioretinal inflammation of posterior pole**

    H30.111 Disseminated chorioretinal inflammation of posterior pole, right eye 🐾

    H30.112 Disseminated chorioretinal inflammation of posterior pole, left eye 🐾

    H30.113 Disseminated chorioretinal inflammation of posterior pole, bilateral 🐾

    ■ **H30.119** Disseminated chorioretinal inflammation of posterior pole, unspecified eye 🐾

● **H30.12 Disseminated chorioretinal inflammation, peripheral**

    H30.121 Disseminated chorioretinal inflammation, peripheral right eye 🐾

    H30.122 Disseminated chorioretinal inflammation, peripheral, left eye 🐾

    H30.123 Disseminated chorioretinal inflammation, peripheral, bilateral 🐾

    ■ **H30.129** Disseminated chorioretinal inflammation, peripheral, unspecified eye 🐾

● **H30.13 Disseminated chorioretinal inflammation, generalized**

    H30.131 Disseminated chorioretinal inflammation, generalized, right eye 🐾

    H30.132 Disseminated chorioretinal inflammation, generalized, left eye 🐾

    H30.133 Disseminated chorioretinal inflammation, generalized, bilateral 🐾

    ■ **H30.139** Disseminated chorioretinal inflammation, generalized, unspecified eye 🐾

● **H30.14 Acute posterior multifocal placoid pigment epitheliopathy**

    H30.141 Acute posterior multifocal placoid pigment epitheliopathy, right eye 🐾

    H30.142 Acute posterior multifocal placoid pigment epitheliopathy, left eye 🐾

    H30.143 Acute posterior multifocal placoid pigment epitheliopathy, bilateral 🐾

    ■ **H30.149** Acute posterior multifocal placoid pigment epitheliopathy, unspecified eye 🐾

● **H30.2 Posterior cyclitis**
Pars planitis

    ■ **H30.20** Posterior cyclitis, unspecified eye

    H30.21 Posterior cyclitis, right eye

    H30.22 Posterior cyclitis, left eye

    H30.23 Posterior cyclitis, bilateral

● **H30.8 Other chorioretinal inflammations**

● **H30.81 Harada's disease**

    H30.811 Harada's disease, right eye

    H30.812 Harada's disease, left eye

    H30.813 Harada's disease, bilateral

    ■ **H30.819** Harada's disease, unspecified eye

● **H30.89 Other chorioretinal inflammations**

    H30.891 Other chorioretinal inflammations, right eye 🐾

    H30.892 Other chorioretinal inflammations, left eye 🐾

    H30.893 Other chorioretinal inflammations, bilateral 🐾

    ■ **H30.899** Other chorioretinal inflammations, unspecified eye 🐾

● **H30.9 Unspecified chorioretinal inflammation**
Chorioretinitis NOS
Choroiditis NOS
Neuroretinitis NOS
Retinitis NOS
Retinochoroiditis NOS

    ■ **H30.90** Unspecified chorioretinal inflammation, unspecified eye 🐾

    ■ **H30.91** Unspecified chorioretinal inflammation, right eye 🐾

    ■ **H30.92** Unspecified chorioretinal inflammation, left eye 🐾

    ■ **H30.93** Unspecified chorioretinal inflammation, bilateral 🐾

● **H31 Other disorders of choroid**

● **H31.0 Chorioretinal scars**
> Excludes2   postsurgical chorioretinal scars (H59.81-)

● **H31.00 Unspecified chorioretinal scars**

    ■ **H31.001** Unspecified chorioretinal scars, right eye

    ■ **H31.002** Unspecified chorioretinal scars, left eye

    ■ **H31.003** Unspecified chorioretinal scars, bilateral

    ■ **H31.009** Unspecified chorioretinal scars, unspecified eye

CHAPTER 7 (H00-H59)

● H31.01 Macula scars of posterior pole (postinflammatory) (post-traumatic)

> Excludes1 postprocedural choriorentinal scar (H59.81-)

H31.011 Macula scars of posterior pole (postinflammatory) (post-traumatic), right eye

H31.012 Macula scars of posterior pole (postinflammatory) (post-traumatic), left eye

H31.013 Macula scars of posterior pole (postinflammatory) (post-traumatic), bilateral

■ H31.019 Macula scars of posterior pole (postinflammatory) (post-traumatic), unspecified eye

● H31.02 Solar retinopathy

H31.021 Solar retinopathy, right eye

H31.022 Solar retinopathy, left eye

H31.023 Solar retinopathy, bilateral

■ H31.029 Solar retinopathy, unspecified eye

● H31.09 Other chorioretinal scars

H31.091 Other chorioretinal scars, right eye

H31.092 Other chorioretinal scars, left eye

H31.093 Other chorioretinal scars, bilateral

■ H31.099 Other chorioretinal scars, unspecified eye

● H31.1 Choroidal degeneration

> Excludes2 angioid streaks of macula (H35.33)

● H31.10 Unspecified choroidal degeneration
Choroidal sclerosis NOS

■ H31.101 Choroidal degeneration, unspecified, right eye

■ H31.102 Choroidal degeneration, unspecified, left eye

■ H31.103 Choroidal degeneration, unspecified, bilateral

■ H31.109 Choroidal degeneration, unspecified, unspecified eye

● H31.11 Age-related choroidal atrophy

H31.111 Age-related choroidal atrophy, right eye   A

H31.112 Age-related choroidal atrophy, left eye   A

H31.113 Age-related choroidal atrophy, bilateral   A

■ H31.119 Age-related choroidal atrophy, unspecified eye   A

● H31.12 Diffuse secondary atrophy of choroid

H31.121 Diffuse secondary atrophy of choroid, right eye

H31.122 Diffuse secondary atrophy of choroid, left eye

H31.123 Diffuse secondary atrophy of choroid, bilateral

■ H31.129 Diffuse secondary atrophy of choroid, unspecified eye

● H31.2 Hereditary choroidal dystrophy

> Excludes2 hyperornithinemia (E72.4)
> ornithinemia (E72.4)

■ H31.20 Hereditary choroidal dystrophy, unspecified

H31.21 Choroideremia

H31.22 Choroidal dystrophy (central areolar) (generalized) (peripapillary)

H31.23 Gyrate atrophy, choroid

H31.29 Other hereditary choroidal dystrophy

● H31.3 Choroidal hemorrhage and rupture

● H31.30 Unspecified choroidal hemorrhage

■ H31.301 Unspecified choroidal hemorrhage, right eye

■ H31.302 Unspecified choroidal hemorrhage, left eye

■ H31.303 Unspecified choroidal hemorrhage, bilateral

■ H31.309 Unspecified choroidal hemorrhage, unspecified eye

● H31.31 Expulsive choroidal hemorrhage

H31.311 Expulsive choroidal hemorrhage, right eye

H31.312 Expulsive choroidal hemorrhage, left eye

H31.313 Expulsive choroidal hemorrhage, bilateral

■ H31.319 Expulsive choroidal hemorrhage, unspecified eye

● H31.32 Choroidal rupture

H31.321 Choroidal rupture, right eye ☾

H31.322 Choroidal rupture, left eye ☾

H31.323 Choroidal rupture, bilateral ☾

■ H31.329 Choroidal rupture, unspecified eye ☾

● H31.4 Choroidal detachment

● H31.40 Unspecified choroidal detachment

■ H31.401 Unspecified choroidal detachment, right eye ☾

■ H31.402 Unspecified choroidal detachment, left eye ☾

■ H31.403 Unspecified choroidal detachment, bilateral ☾

■ H31.409 Unspecified choroidal detachment, unspecified eye ☾

● H31.41 Hemorrhagic choroidal detachment

H31.411 Hemorrhagic choroidal detachment, right eye ☾

H31.412 Hemorrhagic choroidal detachment, left eye ☾

H31.413 Hemorrhagic choroidal detachment, bilateral ☾

■ H31.419 Hemorrhagic choroidal detachment, unspecified eye ☾

● H31.42 Serous choroidal detachment

H31.421 Serous choroidal detachment, right eye ☾

H31.422 Serous choroidal detachment, left eye ☾

H31.423 Serous choroidal detachment, bilateral ☾

■ H31.429 Serous choroidal detachment, unspecified eye ☾

● Unacceptable Principal Diagnosis   ● Use Additional Character(s)   ■ Unspecified   ▶ Manifestation Code

OGCR Official Guidelines for Coding and Reporting   Excludes 1   Excludes 2   Includes   Use additional   Code first   Code also

NON-RHEGMATOGENOUS
RETINAL DETACHMENT

- Vitreous
- Retina
- Protein-rich fluid in sub-retinal space
- Retinal pigment epithelium

VITREOUS DETACHMENT

- Vitreous
- Posterior hyaloid
- Internal limiting membrane

RHEGMATOGENOUS RETINAL DETACHMENT

Blood
- Vitreous
- Posterior hyaloid
- Retina
- Retinal tear
- Liquified vitreous
- Retinal pigment epithelium

Figure 7-9   Rential detachment. (From Kumar: Robbins and Cotran: Pathologic Basis of Disease, 7th ed. 2005, Saunders.)

H31.8 Other specified disorders of choroid

H31.9 Unspecified disorder of choroid

● ◗ **H32 *Chorioretinal disorders in diseases classified elsewhere***

  Code first underlying disease, such as:
    congenital toxoplasmosis (P37.1)
    histoplasmosis (B39.-)
    leprosy (A30.-)

  Excludes1 chorioretinitis (in):
      toxoplasmosis (acquired) (B58.01)
      tuberculosis (A18.53)

● **H33 Retinal detachments and breaks**

  Excludes1 detachment of retinal pigment epithelium (H35.72-, H35.73-)

● **H33.0 Retinal detachment with retinal break**
    Rhegmatogenous retinal detachment

  Excludes1 serous retinal detachment (without retinal break) (H33.2-)

  ● **H33.00 Unspecified retinal detachment with retinal break**

      H33.001 Unspecified retinal detachment with retinal break, right eye

      H33.002 Unspecified retinal detachment with retinal break, left eye

Item 7–6   Retinal detachments and defects are conditions of the eye in which the retina separates from the underlying tissue. Initial detachment may be localized, requiring rapid treatment (medical emergency) to avoid the entire retina from detaching which leads to vision loss and blindness.

      H33.003 Unspecified retinal detachment with retinal break, bilateral

      H33.009 Unspecified retinal detachment with retinal break, unspecified eye

  ● **H33.01 Retinal detachment with single break**

      H33.011 Retinal detachment with single break, right eye

      H33.012 Retinal detachment with single break, left eye

      H33.013 Retinal detachment with single break, bilateral

      H33.019 Retinal detachment with single break, unspecified eye

  ● **H33.02 Retinal detachment with multiple breaks**

      H33.021 Retinal detachment with multiple breaks, right eye

      H33.022 Retinal detachment with multiple breaks, left eye

      H33.023 Retinal detachment with multiple breaks, bilateral

      H33.029 Retinal detachment with multiple breaks, unspecified eye

  ● **H33.03 Retinal detachment with giant retinal tear**

      H33.031 Retinal detachment with giant retinal tear, right eye

      H33.032 Retinal detachment with giant retinal tear, left eye

      H33.033 Retinal detachment with giant retinal tear, bilateral

      H33.039 Retinal detachment with giant retinal tear, unspecified eye

  ● **H33.04 Retinal detachment with retinal dialysis**

      H33.041 Retinal detachment with retinal dialysis, right eye

      H33.042 Retinal detachment with retinal dialysis, left eye

      H33.043 Retinal detachment with retinal dialysis, bilateral

      H33.049 Retinal detachment with retinal dialysis, unspecified eye

  ● **H33.05 Total retinal detachment**

      H33.051 Total retinal detachment, right eye

      H33.052 Total retinal detachment, left eye

      H33.053 Total retinal detachment, bilateral

      H33.059 Total retinal detachment, unspecified eye

● **H33.1 Retinoschisis and retinal cysts**

  Excludes1 congenital retinoschisis (Q14.1)
      microcystoid degeneration of retina (H35.42-)

  ● **H33.10 Unspecified retinoschisis**

      H33.101 Unspecified retinoschisis, right eye

      H33.102 Unspecified retinoschisis, left eye

      H33.103 Unspecified retinoschisis, bilateral

      H33.109 Unspecified retinoschisis, unspecified eye

N Newborn Age: 0   **P** Pediatric Age: 0–17   **M** Maternity DX: 12–55   **A** Adult Age: 15–124   ♀ Females Only   ♂ Males Only

🅒 Complication\Comorbidity   🅜 Major C\C   🅟 Present on Admission Requirement   🅗 Hospital-Acquired Condition

983

CHAPTER 7 (H00-H59)

● **H33.11   Cyst of ora serrata**
     H33.111   Cyst of ora serrata, right eye
     H33.112   Cyst of ora serrata, left eye
     H33.113   Cyst of ora serrata, bilateral
     ■ H33.119   Cyst of ora serrata, unspecified eye

● **H33.12   Parasitic cyst of retina**
     H33.121   Parasitic cyst of retina, right eye 🕮
     H33.122   Parasitic cyst of retina, left eye 🕮
     H33.123   Parasitic cyst of retina, bilateral 🕮
     ■ H33.129   Parasitic cyst of retina, unspecified eye 🕮

● **H33.19   Other retinoschisis and retinal cysts**
     Pseudocyst of retina
     H33.191   Other retinoschisis and retinal cysts, right eye
     H33.192   Other retinoschisis and retinal cysts, left eye
     H33.193   Other retinoschisis and retinal cysts, bilateral
     ■ H33.199   Other retinoschisis and retinal cysts, unspecified eye

● **H33.2   Serous retinal detachment**
     Retinal detachment NOS
     Retinal detachment without retinal break
     | Excludes1 | central serous chorioretinopathy (H35.71-)
     ■ H33.20   Serous retinal detachment, unspecified eye 🕮
     H33.21   Serous retinal detachment, right eye 🕮
     H33.22   Serous retinal detachment, left eye 🕮
     H33.23   Serous retinal detachment, bilateral 🕮

● **H33.3   Retinal breaks without detachment**
     | Excludes1 | chorioretinal scars after surgery for detachment (H59.81-)
                     peripheral retinal degeneration without break (H35.4-)
     ● H33.30   Unspecified retinal break
         ■ H33.301   Unspecified retinal break, right eye
         ■ H33.302   Unspecified retinal break, left eye
         ■ H33.303   Unspecified retinal break, bilateral
         ■ H33.309   Unspecified retinal break, unspecified eye

     ● H33.31   Horseshoe tear of retina without detachment
         Operculum of retina without detachment
         H33.311   Horseshoe tear of retina without detachment, right eye
         H33.312   Horseshoe tear of retina without detachment, left eye
         H33.313   Horseshoe tear of retina without detachment, bilateral
         ■ H33.319   Horseshoe tear of retina without detachment, unspecified eye

     ● H33.32   Round hole of retina without detachment
         H33.321   Round hole, right eye
         H33.322   Round hole, left eye
         H33.323   Round hole, bilateral
         ■ H33.329   Round hole, unspecified eye

● **H33.33   Multiple defects of retina without detachment**
     H33.331   Multiple defects of retina without detachment, right eye
     H33.332   Multiple defects of retina without detachment, left eye
     H33.333   Multiple defects of retina without detachment, bilateral
     ■ H33.339   Multiple defects of retina without detachment, unspecified eye

● **H33.4   Traction detachment of retina**
     Proliferative vitreo-retinopathy with retinal detachment
     ■ H33.40   Traction detachment of retina, unspecified eye 🕮
     H33.41   Traction detachment of retina, right eye 🕮
     H33.42   Traction detachment of retina, left eye 🕮
     H33.43   Traction detachment of retina, bilateral 🕮

   H33.8   Other retinal detachments 🕮

● **H34   Retinal vascular occlusions**
     Blockage in vessel of the retina
     | Excludes1 | amaurosis fugax (G45.3)
   ● **H34.0   Transient retinal artery occlusion**
     ■ H34.00   Transient retinal artery occlusion, unspecified eye 🕮
     H34.01   Transient retinal artery occlusion, right eye 🕮
     H34.02   Transient retinal artery occlusion, left eye 🕮
     H34.03   Transient retinal artery occlusion, bilateral 🕮

   ● **H34.1   Central retinal artery occlusion**
     ■ H34.10   Central retinal artery occlusion, unspecified eye 🕮
     H34.11   Central retinal artery occlusion, right eye 🕮
     H34.12   Central retinal artery occlusion, left eye 🕮
     H34.13   Central retinal artery occlusion, bilateral 🕮

   ● **H34.2   Other retinal artery occlusions**
     ● H34.21   Partial retinal artery occlusion
         Hollenhorst's plaque
         Retinal microembolism
         H34.211   Partial retinal artery occlusion, right eye 🕮
         H34.212   Partial retinal artery occlusion, left eye 🕮
         H34.213   Partial retinal artery occlusion, bilateral 🕮
         ■ H34.219   Partial retinal artery occlusion, unspecified eye 🕮

     ● H34.23   Retinal artery branch occlusion
         H34.231   Retinal artery branch occlusion, right eye 🕮
         H34.232   Retinal artery branch occlusion, left eye 🕮
         H34.233   Retinal artery branch occlusion, bilateral 🕮
         ■ H34.239   Retinal artery branch occlusion, unspecified eye 🕮

● Unacceptable Principal Diagnosis   ● Use Additional Character(s)   ■ Unspecified   ▶ Manifestation Code
OGCR Official Guidelines for Coding and Reporting | Excludes 1 | | Excludes 2 | | Includes | | Use additional | | Code first | | Code also |

● **H34.8 Other retinal vascular occlusions**
  ● **H34.81 Central retinal vein occlusion**
    H34.811 **Central retinal vein occlusion, right eye** 🔧
    H34.812 **Central retinal vein occlusion, left eye** 🔧
    H34.813 **Central retinal vein occlusion, bilateral** 🔧
    ◩ H34.819 **Central retinal vein occlusion, unspecified eye** 🔧
  ● **H34.82 Venous engorgement**
    Incipient retinal vein occlusion
    Partial retinal vein occlusion
    H34.821 **Venous engorgement, right eye**
    H34.822 **Venous engorgement, left eye**
    H34.823 **Venous engorgement, bilateral**
    ◩ H34.829 **Venous engorgement, unspecified eye**
  ● **H34.83 Tributary (branch) retinal vein occlusion**
    H34.831 **Tributary (branch) retinal vein occlusion, right eye**
    H34.832 **Tributary (branch) retinal vein occlusion, left eye**
    H34.833 **Tributary (branch) retinal vein occlusion, bilateral**
    ◩ H34.839 **Tributary (branch) retinal vein occlusion, unspecified eye**
◩ **H34.9 Unspecified retinal vascular occlusion** 🔧

  OGCR Section I. C.9.a.5.

> Hypertensive Retinopathy
>
> Subcategory H35.0, Background retinopathy and retinal vascular changes, should be used with a code from category I10–I15, Hypertensive disease to include the systemic hypertension. The sequencing is based on the reason for the encounter.

● **H35 Other retinal disorders**
  Excludes2   diabetic retinal disorders (E08.311- E08.359, E09.311- E09.359, E10.311- E10.359, E11.311- E11.359, E13.311- E13.359)
● **H35.0 Background retinopathy and retinal vascular changes**
  Code also any associated hypertension (I10-)
  ◩ **H35.00 Unspecified background retinopathy**
  ● **H35.01 Changes in retinal vascular appearance**
    Retinal vascular sheathing
    H35.011 **Changes in retinal vascular appearance, right eye**
    H35.012 **Changes in retinal vascular appearance, left eye**
    H35.013 **Changes in retinal vascular appearance, bilateral**
    ◩ H35.019 **Changes in retinal vascular appearance, unspecified eye**
  ● **H35.02 Exudative retinopathy**
    Coats retinopathy
    H35.021 **Exudative retinopathy, right eye**
    H35.022 **Exudative retinopathy, left eye**
    H35.023 **Exudative retinopathy, bilateral**
    ◩ H35.029 **Exudative retinopathy, unspecified eye**

● **H35.03 Hypertensive retinopathy**
    H35.031 **Hypertensive retinopathy, right eye**
    H35.032 **Hypertensive retinopathy, left eye**
    H35.033 **Hypertensive retinopathy, bilateral**
    ◩ H35.039 **Hypertensive retinopathy, unspecified eye**
● **H35.04 Retinal micro-aneurysms, unspecified**
    H35.041 **Retinal micro-aneurysms, unspecified, right eye**
    H35.042 **Retinal micro-aneurysms, unspecified, left eye**
    H35.043 **Retinal micro-aneurysms, unspecified, bilateral**
    ◩ H35.049 **Retinal micro-aneurysms, unspecified, unspecified eye**
● **H35.05 Retinal neovascularization, unspecified**
    H35.051 **Retinal neovascularization, unspecified, right eye**
    H35.052 **Retinal neovascularization, unspecified, left eye**
    H35.053 **Retinal neovascularization, unspecified, bilateral**
    ◩ H35.059 **Retinal neovascularization, unspecified, unspecified eye**
● **H35.06 Retinal vasculitis**
    Eales disease
    Retinal perivasculitis
    H35.061 **Retinal vasculitis, right eye**
    H35.062 **Retinal vasculitis, left eye**
    H35.063 **Retinal vasculitis, bilateral**
    ◩ H35.069 **Retinal vasculitis, unspecified eye**
● **H35.07 Retinal telangiectasis**
    H35.071 **Retinal telangiectasis, right eye**
    H35.072 **Retinal telangiectasis, left eye**
    H35.073 **Retinal telangiectasis, bilateral**
    ◩ H35.079 **Retinal telangiectasis, unspecified eye**
    H35.09 **Other intraretinal microvascular abnormalities**
    Retinal varices
H35.1 **Retinopathy of prematurity**
  ● **H35.10 Retinopathy of prematurity, unspecified**
    Retinopathy of prematurity NOS
    ◩ H35.101 **Retinopathy of prematurity, unspecified, right eye**
    ◩ H35.102 **Retinopathy of prematurity, unspecified, left eye**
    ◩ H35.103 **Retinopathy of prematurity, unspecified, bilateral**
    ◩ H35.109 **Retinopathy of prematurity, unspecified, unspecified eye**
  ● **H35.11 Retinopathy of prematurity, stage 0**
    H35.111 **Retinopathy of prematurity, stage 0, right eye**
    H35.112 **Retinopathy of prematurity, stage 0, left eye**
    H35.113 **Retinopathy of prematurity, stage 0, bilateral**
    ◩ H35.119 **Retinopathy of prematurity, stage 0, unspecified eye**

N Newborn Age: 0   **P** Pediatric Age: 0–17   **M** Maternity DX: 12–55   **A** Adult Age: 15–124   ♀ Females Only   ♂ Males Only

🔧 Complication\Comorbidity   🔧 Major C\C   🔧 Present on Admission Requirement   🔧 Hospital-Acquired Condition

985

CHAPTER 7 (H00-H59)

● H35.12   Retinopathy of prematurity, stage 1

    H35.121   Retinopathy of prematurity, stage 1, right eye

    H35.122   Retinopathy of prematurity, stage 1, left eye

    H35.123   Retinopathy of prematurity, stage 1, bilateral

    ■ H35.129   Retinopathy of prematurity, stage 1, unspecified eye

● H35.13   Retinopathy of prematurity, stage 2

    H35.131   Retinopathy of prematurity, stage 2, right eye

    H35.132   Retinopathy of prematurity, stage 2, left eye

    H35.133   Retinopathy of prematurity, stage 2, bilateral

    ■ H35.139   Retinopathy of prematurity, stage 2, unspecified eye

● H35.14   Retinopathy of prematurity, stage 3

    H35.141   Retinopathy of prematurity, stage 3, right eye

    H35.142   Retinopathy of prematurity, stage 3, left eye

    H35.143   Retinopathy of prematurity, stage 3, bilateral

    ■ H35.149   Retinopathy of prematurity, stage 3, unspecified eye

● H35.15   Retinopathy of prematurity, stage 4

    H35.151   Retinopathy of prematurity, stage 4, right eye

    H35.152   Retinopathy of prematurity, stage 4, left eye

    H35.153   Retinopathy of prematurity, stage 4, bilateral

    ■ H35.159   Retinopathy of prematurity, stage 4, unspecified eye

● H35.16   Retinopathy of prematurity, stage 5

    H35.161   Retinopathy of prematurity, stage 5, right eye

    H35.162   Retinopathy of prematurity, stage 5, left eye

    H35.163   Retinopathy of prematurity, stage 5, bilateral

    ■ H35.169   Retinopathy of prematurity, stage 5, unspecified eye

● H35.17   Retrolental fibroplasia

    H35.171   Retrolental fibroplasia, right eye

    H35.172   Retrolental fibroplasia, left eye

    H35.173   Retrolental fibroplasia, bilateral

    ■ H35.179   Retrolental fibroplasia, unspecified eye

● H35.2   Other non-diabetic proliferative retinopathy

    Proliferative vitreo-retinopathy

    Excludes1   proliferative vitreo-retinopathy with retinal detachment (H33.4-)

    ■ H35.20   Other non-diabetic proliferative retinopathy, unspecified eye

    H35.21   Other non-diabetic proliferative retinopathy, right eye

    H35.22   Other non-diabetic proliferative retinopathy, left eye

    H35.23   Other non-diabetic proliferative retinopathy, bilateral

Item 7-7   Macular degeneration is typically age-related, chronic, and is evidenced by deterioration of the macula (the part of the retina that provides for central field vision), resulting in blurred vision or a blind spot in the center of visual field while not affecting peripheral vision.

● H35.3   Degeneration of macula and posterior pole

    ■ H35.30   Unspecified macular degeneration   **A**

       Age-related macular degeneration

    H35.31   Nonexudative age-related macular degeneration   **A**

       Atrophic age-related macular degeneration

    H35.32   Exudative age-related macular degeneration   **A**

    H35.33   Angioid streaks of macula

    ● H35.34   Macular cyst, hole, or pseudohole

       H35.341   Macular cyst, hole, or pseudohole, right eye

       H35.342   Macular cyst, hole, or pseudohole, left eye

       H35.343   Macular cyst, hole, or pseudohole, bilateral

       ■ H35.349   Macular cyst, hole, or pseudohole, unspecified eye

    ● H35.35   Cystoid macular degeneration

       Excludes1   cystoid macular edema following cataract surgery (H59.03-)

       H35.351   Cystoid macular degeneration, right eye

       H35.352   Cystoid macular degeneration, left eye

       H35.353   Cystoid macular degeneration, bilateral

       ■ H35.359   Cystoid macular degeneration, unspecified eye

    ● H35.36   Drusen (degenerative) of macula

       H35.361   Drusen (degenerative) of macula, right eye

       H35.362   Drusen (degenerative) of macula, left eye

       H35.363   Drusen (degenerative) of macula, bilateral

       ■ H35.369   Drusen (degenerative) of macula, unspecified eye

    ● H35.37   Puckering of macula

       H35.371   Puckering of macula, right eye

       H35.372   Puckering of macula, left eye

       H35.373   Puckering of macula, bilateral

       ■ H35.379   Puckering of macula, unspecified eye

    ● H35.38   Toxic maculopathy

       Code first poisoning due to drug or toxin, if applicable (T36-T65 with fifth or sixth character 1-4 or 6)

       Use additional code for adverse effect, if applicable, to identify drug (T36-T50 with fifth or sixth character 5)

       H35.381   Toxic maculopathy, right eye

       H35.382   Toxic maculopathy, left eye

       H35.383   Toxic maculopathy, bilateral

       ■ H35.389   Toxic maculopathy, unspecified eye

● Unacceptable Principal Diagnosis   ● Use Additional Character(s)   ■ Unspecified   ▶ Manifestation Code

OGCR Official Guidelines for Coding and Reporting   Excludes 1   Excludes 2   Includes   Use additional   Code first   Code also

● **H35.4   Peripheral retinal degeneration**

> **Excludes1**   hereditary retinal degeneration
> (dystrophy) (H35.5-)
> peripheral retinal degeneration with
> retinal break (H33.3-)

■ **H35.40   Unspecified peripheral retinal
degeneration**

● **H35.41   Lattice degeneration of retina**
> Palisade degeneration of retina

    **H35.411   Lattice degeneration of retina,
right eye**

    **H35.412   Lattice degeneration of retina,
left eye**

    **H35.413   Lattice degeneration of retina,
bilateral**

    ■ **H35.419   Lattice degeneration of retina,
unspecified eye**

● **H35.42   Microcystoid degeneration of retina**

    **H35.421   Microcystoid degeneration of
retina, right eye**

    **H35.422   Microcystoid degeneration of
retina, left eye**

    **H35.423   Microcystoid degeneration of
retina, bilateral**

    ■ **H35.429   Microcystoid degeneration of
retina, unspecified eye**

● **H35.43   Paving stone degeneration of retina**

    **H35.431   Paving stone degeneration of
retina, right eye**

    **H35.432   Paving stone degeneration of
retina, left eye**

    **H35.433   Paving stone degeneration of
retina, bilateral**

    ■ **H35.439   Paving stone degeneration of
retina, unspecified eye**

● **H35.44   Age-related reticular degeneration of retina**

    **H35.441   Age-related reticular
degeneration of retina, right eye A**

    **H35.442   Age-related reticular
degeneration of retina, left eye   A**

    **H35.443   Age-related reticular
degeneration of retina, bilateral A**

    ■ **H35.449   Age-related reticular
degeneration of retina,
unspecified eye   A**

● **H35.45   Secondary pigmentary degeneration**

    **H35.451   Secondary pigmentary
degeneration, right eye**

    **H35.452   Secondary pigmentary
degeneration, left eye**

    **H35.453   Secondary pigmentary
degeneration, bilateral**

    ■ **H35.459   Secondary pigmentary
degeneration, unspecified eye**

● **H35.46   Secondary vitreoretinal degeneration**

    **H35.461   Secondary vitreoretinal
degeneration, right eye**

    **H35.462   Secondary vitreoretinal
degeneration, left eye**

    **H35.463   Secondary vitreoretinal
degeneration, bilateral**

    ■ **H35.469   Secondary vitreoretinal
degeneration, unspecified eye**

● **H35.5   Hereditary retinal dystrophy**

> **Excludes1**   dystrophies primarily involving
> Bruch's membrane (H31.1-)

■ **H35.50   Unspecified hereditary retinal dystrophy**

H35.51   Vitreoretinal dystrophy

H35.52   Pigmentary retinal dystrophy
> Albipunctate retinal dystrophy
> Retinitis pigmentosa
> Tapetoretinal dystrophy

**H35.53   Other dystrophies primarily involving the
sensory retina**
> Stargardt's disease

**H35.54   Dystrophies primarily involving the
retinal pigment epithelium**
> Vitelliform retinal dystrophy

● **H35.6   Retinal hemorrhage**

■ **H35.60   Retinal hemorrhage, unspecified eye**

H35.61   Retinal hemorrhage, right eye

H35.62   Retinal hemorrhage, left eye

H35.63   Retinal hemorrhage, bilateral

● **H35.7   Separation of retinal layers**

> **Excludes1**   retinal detachment (serous) (H33.2-)
> rhegmatogenous retinal detachment
> (H33.0-)

■ **H35.70   Unspecified separation of retinal layers** 🔹

● **H35.71   Central serous chorioretinopathy**

    **H35.711   Central serous chorioretinopathy,
right eye**

    **H35.712   Central serous chorioretinopathy,
left eye**

    **H35.713   Central serous chorioretinopathy,
bilateral**

    ■ **H35.719   Central serous chorioretinopathy,
unspecified eye**

● **H35.72   Serous detachment of retinal pigment
epithelium**

    **H35.721   Serous detachment of retinal
pigment epithelium, right eye** 🔹

    **H35.722   Serous detachment of retinal
pigment epithelium, left eye** 🔹

    **H35.723   Serous detachment of retinal
pigment epithelium, bilateral** 🔹

    ■ **H35.729   Serous detachment of retinal
pigment epithelium, unspecified
eye** 🔹

● **H35.73   Hemorrhagic detachment of retinal
pigment epithelium**

    **H35.731   Hemorrhagic detachment of retinal
pigment epithelium, right eye** 🔹

    **H35.732   Hemorrhagic detachment of retinal
pigment epithelium, left eye** 🔹

    **H35.733   Hemorrhagic detachment of
retinal pigment epithelium,
bilateral** 🔹

    ■ **H35.739   Hemorrhagic detachment of
retinal pigment epithelium,
unspecified eye** 🔹

N Newborn Age: 0   **P** Pediatric Age: 0–17   **M** Maternity DX: 12–55   **A** Adult Age: 15–124   ♀ Females Only   ♂ Males Only

🔹 Complication\Comorbidity   🔹 Major C\C   🔹 Present on Admission Requirement   🔹 Hospital-Acquired Condition

987

CHAPTER 7 (H00-H59)

- **H35.8 Other specified retinal disorders**
  - Excludes2   retinal hemorrhage (H35.6-)
  - **H35.81 Retinal edema**
    - Retinal cotton wool spots
  - **H35.82 Retinal ischemia** 🏷
  - **H35.89 Other specified retinal disorders**
- **H35.9 Unspecified retinal disorder**

- **H36 *Retinal disorders in diseases classified elsewhere***
  - *Code first* underlying disease, such as:
    - lipid storage disorders (E75.-)
    - sickle-cell disorders (D57.-)
  - Excludes1   arteriosclerotic retinopathy (H35.0-)
    - diabetic retinopathy (E08.3-, E09.3-, E10.3-, E11.3-, E13.3-)

GLAUCOMA (H40-H42)

- **H40 Glaucoma**
  - *Intraocular pressure (IOP) that is too high results from too much aqueous humor and because of excess production or inadequate drainage, optic nerve damage and vision loss may occur.*
  - Excludes1   absolute glaucoma (H44.51-)
    - congenital glaucoma (Q15.0)
    - traumatic glaucoma due to birth injury (P15.3)
  - **H40.0 Glaucoma suspect**
    - **H40.00 Preglaucoma, unspecified**
      - H40.001 Preglaucoma, unspecified, right eye
      - H40.002 Preglaucoma, unspecified, left eye
      - H40.003 Preglaucoma, unspecified, bilateral
      - H40.009 Preglaucoma, unspecified, unspecified eye
    - **H40.01 Open angle with borderline findings, low risk**
      - Open angle, low risk
      - H40.011 Open angle with borderline findings, low risk, right eye
      - H40.012 Open angle with borderline findings, low risk, left eye
      - H40.013 Open angle with borderline findings, low risk, bilateral
      - H40.019 Open angle with borderline findings, low risk, unspecified eye
    - **H40.02 Open angle with borderline findings, high risk**
      - Open angle, high risk
      - H40.021 Open angle with borderline findings, high risk, right eye
      - H40.022 Open angle with borderline findings, high risk, left eye
      - H40.023 Open angle with borderline findings, high risk, bilateral
      - H40.029 Open angle with borderline findings, high risk, unspecified eye
    - **H40.03 Anatomical narrow angle**
      - Primary angle closure suspect
      - H40.031 Anatomical narrow angle, right eye
      - H40.032 Anatomical narrow angle, left eye
      - H40.033 Anatomical narrow angle, bilateral
      - H40.039 Anatomical narrow angle, unspecified eye
    - **H40.04 Steroid responder**
      - H40.041 Steroid responder, right eye
      - H40.042 Steroid responder, left eye
      - H40.043 Steroid responder, bilateral
      - H40.049 Steroid responder, unspecified eye
    - **H40.05 Ocular hypertension**
      - H40.051 Ocular hypertension, right eye
      - H40.052 Ocular hypertension, left eye
      - H40.053 Ocular hypertension, bilateral
      - H40.059 Ocular hypertension, unspecified eye
    - **H40.06 Primary angle closure without glaucoma damage**
      - H40.061 Primary angle closure without glaucoma damage, right eye
      - H40.062 Primary angle closure without glaucoma damage, left eye
      - H40.063 Primary angle closure without glaucoma damage, bilateral
      - H40.069 Primary angle closure without glaucoma damage, unspecified eye
  - **H40.1 Open-angle glaucoma**
    - **H40.10 Unspecified open-angle glaucoma**
      - One of the following 7th characters is to be assigned to code H40.10 to designate the stage of glaucoma

0	stage unspecified
1	mild stage
2	moderate stage
3	severe stage
4	indeterminate stage
    - **H40.11 Primary open-angle glaucoma**
      - Chronic simple glaucoma
      - One of the following 7th characters is to be assigned to code H40.11 to designate the stage of glaucoma

0	stage unspecified
1	mild stage
2	moderate stage
3	severe stage
4	indeterminate stage
    - **H40.12 Low-tension glaucoma**
      - One of the following 7th characters is to be assigned to each code in subcategory H40.12 to designate the stage of glaucoma

0	stage unspecified
1	mild stage
2	moderate stage
3	severe stage
4	indeterminate stage

      - **H40.121 Low-tension glaucoma, right eye**
      - **H40.122 Low-tension glaucoma, left eye**
      - **H40.123 Low-tension glaucoma, bilateral**
      - **H40.129 Low-tension glaucoma, unspecified eye**

● Unacceptable Principal Diagnosis   ● Use Additional Character(s)   ■ Unspecified   ▶ Manifestation Code
OGCR Official Guidelines for Coding and Reporting   Excludes 1   Excludes 2   Includes   Use additional   Code first   Code also

CHAPTER 7 (H00-H59)

● **H40.13** **Pigmentary glaucoma**

One of the following 7th characters is to be assigned to each code in subcategory H40.13 to designate the stage of glaucoma

0	stage unspecified
1	mild stage
2	moderate stage
3	severe stage
4	indeterminate stage

● **H40.131** **Pigmentary glaucoma, right eye**

● **H40.132** **Pigmentary glaucoma, left eye**

● **H40.133** **Pigmentary glaucoma, bilateral**

●■ **H40.139** **Pigmentary glaucoma, unspecified eye**

● **H40.14** **Capsular glaucoma with pseudoexfoliation of lens**

One of the following 7th characters is to be assigned to each code in subcategory H40.15 to designate the stage of glaucoma

0	stage unspecified
1	mild stage
2	moderate stage
3	severe stage
4	indeterminate stage

● **H40.141** **Capsular glaucoma with pseudoexfoliation of lens, right eye**

● **H40.142** **Capsular glaucoma with pseudoexfoliation of lens, left eye**

● **H40.143** **Capsular glaucoma with pseudoexfoliation of lens, bilateral**

●■ **H40.149** **Capsular glaucoma with pseudoexfoliation of lens, unspecified eye**

● **H40.15** **Residual stage of open-angle glaucoma**

    H40.151 **Residual stage of open-angle glaucoma, right eye**

    H40.152 **Residual stage of open-angle glaucoma, left eye**

    H40.153 **Residual stage of open-angle glaucoma, bilateral**

■ **H40.159** **Residual stage of open-angle glaucoma, unspecified eye**

● **H40.2** **Primary angle-closure glaucoma**

    Excludes1   aqueous misdirection (H40.83-)
                malignant glaucoma (H40.83-)

●■ **H40.20** **Unspecified primary angle-closure glaucoma**

One of the following 7th characters is to be assigned to code H40.20 to designate the stage of glaucoma

0	stage unspecified
1	mild stage
2	moderate stage
3	severe stage
4	indeterminate stage

● **H40.21** **Acute angle-closure glaucoma**

    Acute angle-closure glaucoma attack
    Acute angle-closure glaucoma crisis

    H40.211 **Acute angle-closure glaucoma, right eye** 🔵

    H40.212 **Acute angle-closure glaucoma, left eye** 🔵

    H40.213 **Acute angle-closure glaucoma, bilateral** 🔵

■ **H40.219** **Acute angle-closure glaucoma, unspecified eye** 🔵

● **H40.22** **Chronic angle-closure glaucoma**

    Chronic primary angle closure glaucoma

One of the following 7th characters is to be assigned to each code in subcategory H40.22 to designate the stage of glaucoma

0	stage unspecified
1	mild stage
2	moderate stage
3	severe stage
4	indeterminate stage

● **H40.221** **Chronic angle-closure glaucoma, right eye**

● **H40.222** **Chronic angle-closure glaucoma, left eye**

● **H40.223** **Chronic angle-closure glaucoma, bilateral**

●■ **H40.229** **Chronic angle-closure glaucoma, unspecified eye**

● **H40.23** **Intermittent angle-closure glaucoma**

    H40.231 **Intermittent angle-closure glaucoma, right eye**

    H40.232 **Intermittent angle-closure glaucoma, left eye**

    H40.233 **Intermittent angle-closure glaucoma, bilateral**

■ **H40.239** **Intermittent angle-closure glaucoma, unspecified eye**

● **H40.24** **Residual stage of angle-closure glaucoma**

    H40.241 **Residual stage of angle-closure glaucoma, right eye**

    H40.242 **Residual stage of angle-closure glaucoma, left eye**

    H40.243 **Residual stage of angle-closure glaucoma, bilateral**

■ **H40.249** **Residual stage of angle-closure glaucoma, unspecified eye**

● **H40.3** **Glaucoma secondary to eye trauma**

    Code also underlying condition

One of the following 7th characters is to be assigned to each code in subcategory H40.3 to designate the stage of glaucoma

0	stage unspecified
1	mild stage
2	moderate stage
3	severe stage
4	indeterminate stage

●■ **H40.30** **Glaucoma secondary to eye trauma, unspecified eye**

● **H40.31** **Glaucoma secondary to eye trauma, right eye**

N Newborn Age: 0   **P** Pediatric Age: 0–17   **M** Maternity DX: 12–55   **A** Adult Age: 15–124   ♀ Females Only   ♂ Males Only

🔵 Complication\Comorbidity   🔵 Major C\C   🔵 Present on Admission Requirement   🔵 Hospital-Acquired Condition

989

● H40.32   Glaucoma secondary to eye trauma, left eye

● H40.33   Glaucoma secondary to eye trauma, bilateral

● **H40.4   Glaucoma secondary to eye inflammation**

Code also underlying condition

One of the following 7th characters is to be assigned to each code in subcategory H40.4 to designate the stage of glaucoma

0   stage unspecified
1   mild stage
2   moderate stage
3   severe stage
4   indeterminate stage

● ■ H40.40   Glaucoma secondary to eye inflammation, unspecified eye

● H40.41   Glaucoma secondary to eye inflammation, right eye

● H40.42   Glaucoma secondary to eye inflammation, left eye

● H40.43   Glaucoma secondary to eye inflammation, bilateral

● **H40.5   Glaucoma secondary to other eye disorders**

Code also underlying eye disorder

One of the following 7th characters is to be assigned to each code in subcategory H40.5 to designate the stage of glaucoma

0   stage unspecified
1   mild stage
2   moderate stage
3   severe stage
4   indeterminate stage

● ■ H40.50   Glaucoma secondary to other eye disorders, unspecified eye

● H40.51   Glaucoma secondary to other eye disorders, right eye

● H40.52   Glaucoma secondary to other eye disorders, left eye

● H40.53   Glaucoma secondary to other eye disorders, bilateral

● **H40.6   Glaucoma secondary to drugs**

Use additional code for adverse effect, if applicable, to identify drug (T36-T50 with fifth or sixth character 5)

One of the following 7th characters is to be assigned to each code in subcategory H40.6 to designate the stage of glaucoma

0   stage unspecified
1   mild stage
2   moderate stage
3   severe stage
4   indeterminate stage

● ● ■ H40.60   Glaucoma secondary to drugs, unspecified eye

● ● H40.61   Glaucoma secondary to drugs, right eye

● ● H40.62   Glaucoma secondary to drugs, left eye

● ● H40.63   Glaucoma secondary to drugs, bilateral

● **H40.8   Other glaucoma**

● H40.81   Glaucoma with increased episcleral venous pressure

H40.811   Glaucoma with increased episcleral venous pressure, right eye

H40.812   Glaucoma with increased episcleral venous pressure, left eye

H40.813   Glaucoma with increased episcleral venous pressure, bilateral

■ H40.819   Glaucoma with increased episcleral venous pressure, unspecified eye

● H40.82   Hypersecretion glaucoma

H40.821   Hypersecretion glaucoma, right eye

H40.822   Hypersecretion glaucoma, left eye

H40.823   Hypersecretion glaucoma, bilateral

■ H40.829   Hypersecretion glaucoma, unspecified eye

● H40.83   Aqueous misdirection
Malignant glaucoma

H40.831   Aqueous misdirection, right eye

H40.832   Aqueous misdirection, left eye

H40.833   Aqueous misdirection, bilateral

■ H40.839   Aqueous misdirection, unspecified eye

H40.89   Other specified glaucoma

■ **H40.9   Unspecified glaucoma**

● ▶ **H42   *Glaucoma in diseases classified elsewhere***

Code first underlying condition, such as:
amyloidosis (E85-)
aniridia (Q13.1)
Lowe's syndrome (E72.03)
Reiger's anomaly (Q13.81)
specified metabolic disorder (E70-E88)

Excludes1   glaucoma (in):
diabetes mellitus (E08.39, E09.39, E10.39, E11.39, E13.39)
onchocerciasis (B73.02)
syphilis (A52.71)
tuberculous (A18.59)

DISORDERS OF VITREOUS BODY AND GLOBE (H43-H44)

● **H43   Disorders of vitreous body**

● **H43.0   Vitreous prolapse**

Excludes1   vitreous syndrome following cataract surgery (H59.0-)
traumatic vitreous prolapse (S05.2-)

■ H43.00   Vitreous prolapse, unspecified eye

H43.01   Vitreous prolapse, right eye

H43.02   Vitreous prolapse, left eye

H43.03   Vitreous prolapse, bilateral

● Unacceptable Principal Diagnosis   ● Use Additional Character(s)   ■ Unspecified   ▶ Manifestation Code

OGCR   Official Guidelines for Coding and Reporting   Excludes 1   Excludes 2   Includes   Use additional   Code first   Code also

● H43.1 Vitreous hemorrhage
  ■ H43.10 Vitreous hemorrhage, unspecified eye
    H43.11 Vitreous hemorrhage, right eye
    H43.12 Vitreous hemorrhage, left eye
    H43.13 Vitreous hemorrhage, bilateral
● H43.2 Crystalline deposits in vitreous body
  ■ H43.20 Crystalline deposits in vitreous body, unspecified eye
    H43.21 Crystalline deposits in vitreous body, right eye
    H43.22 Crystalline deposits in vitreous body, left eye
    H43.23 Crystalline deposits in vitreous body, bilateral
● H43.3 Other vitreous opacities
  ● H43.31 Vitreous membranes and strands
    H43.311 Vitreous membranes and strands, right eye
    H43.312 Vitreous membranes and strands, left eye
    H43.313 Vitreous membranes and strands, bilateral
  ■ H43.319 Vitreous membranes and strands, unspecified eye
  ● H43.39 Other vitreous opacities
    Vitreous floaters
    Small clumps of cells that float in the vitreous of the eye, appearing as black specks or dots in the field of vision and common in the aging eye.
    H43.391 Other vitreous opacities, right eye
    H43.392 Other vitreous opacities, left eye
    H43.393 Other vitreous opacities, bilateral
  ■ H43.399 Other vitreous opacities, unspecified eye
● H43.8 Other disorders of vitreous body
    Excludes1 proliferative vitreo-retinopathy with retinal detachment (H33.4)
    Excludes2 vitreous abscess (H44.02-)
  ● H43.81 Vitreous degeneration
    Vitreous detachment
    H43.811 Vitreous degeneration, right eye
    H43.812 Vitreous degeneration, left eye
    H43.813 Vitreous degeneration, bilateral
  ■ H43.819 Vitreous degeneration, unspecified eye
  ● H43.82 Vitreomacular adhesion
    Vitreomacular traction
    H43.821 Vitreomacular adhesion, right eye
    H43.822 Vitreomacular adhesion, left eye
    H43.823 Vitreomacular adhesion, bilateral
  ■ H43.829 Vitreomacular adhesion, unspecified eye
    H43.89 Other disorders of vitreous body
■ H43.9 Unspecified disorder of vitreous body

● H44 Disorders of globe
    Includes disorders affecting multiple structures of eye
● H44.0 Purulent endophthalmitis
    Use additional code to identify organism
    Excludes1 bleb associated endophthalmitis (H59.4-)
  ● H44.00 Unspecified purulent endophthalmitis
    ■ H44.001 Unspecified purulent endophthalmitis, right eye 🦟
    ■ H44.002 Unspecified purulent endophthalmitis, left eye 🦟
    ■ H44.003 Unspecified purulent endophthalmitis, bilateral 🦟
    ■ H44.009 Unspecified purulent endophthalmitis, unspecified eye 🦟
  ● H44.01 Panophthalmitis (acute)
    H44.011 Panophthalmitis (acute), right eye 🦟
    H44.012 Panophthalmitis (acute), left eye 🦟
    H44.013 Panophthalmitis (acute), bilateral 🦟
    ■ H44.019 Panophthalmitis (acute), unspecified eye 🦟
  ● H44.02 Vitreous abscess (chronic)
    H44.021 Vitreous abscess (chronic), right eye 🦟
    H44.022 Vitreous abscess (chronic), left eye 🦟
    H44.023 Vitreous abscess (chronic), bilateral 🦟
    ■ H44.029 Vitreous abscess (chronic), unspecified eye 🦟
● H44.1 Other endophthalmitis
    Excludes1 bleb associated endophthalmitis (H59.4-)
    Excludes2 ophthalmia nodosa (H16.2-)
  ● H44.11 Panuveitis
    H44.111 Panuveitis, right eye 🦟
    H44.112 Panuveitis, left eye 🦟
    H44.113 Panuveitis, bilateral 🦟
    ■ H44.119 Panuveitis, unspecified eye 🦟
  ● H44.12 Parasitic endophthalmitis, unspecified
    H44.121 Parasitic endophthalmitis, unspecified, right eye 🦟
    H44.122 Parasitic endophthalmitis, unspecified, left eye 🦟
    H44.123 Parasitic endophthalmitis, unspecified, bilateral 🦟
    ■ H44.129 Parasitic endophthalmitis, unspecified, unspecified eye 🦟
  ● H44.13 Sympathetic uveitis
    H44.131 Sympathetic uveitis, right eye 🦟
    H44.132 Sympathetic uveitis, left eye 🦟
    H44.133 Sympathetic uveitis, bilateral 🦟
    ■ H44.139 Sympathetic uveitis, unspecified eye 🦟
    H44.19 Other endophthalmitis 🦟

CHAPTER 7 (H00-H59)

N Newborn Age: 0   **P** Pediatric Age: 0–17   **M** Maternity DX: 12–55   **A** Adult Age: 15–124   ♀ Females Only   ♂ Males Only

🦟 Complication\Comorbidity   🦟 Major C\C   🦟 Present on Admission Requirement   🦟 Hospital-Acquired Condition

991

● H44.2   Degenerative myopia
     Malignant myopia
  ■ H44.20   Degenerative myopia, unspecified eye
     H44.21   Degenerative myopia, right eye
     H44.22   Degenerative myopia, left eye
     H44.23   Degenerative myopia, bilateral

● H44.3   Other and unspecified degenerative disorders of globe
  ■ H44.30   Unspecified degenerative disorder of globe
  ● H44.31   Chalcosis
     H44.311   Chalcosis, right eye
     H44.312   Chalcosis, left eye
     H44.313   Chalcosis, bilateral
    ■ H44.319   Chalcosis, unspecified eye
  ● H44.32   Siderosis of eye
     H44.321   Siderosis of eye, right eye
     H44.322   Siderosis of eye, left eye
     H44.323   Siderosis of eye, bilateral
    ■ H44.329   Siderosis of eye, unspecified eye
  ● H44.39   Other degenerative disorders of globe
     H44.391   Other degenerative disorders of globe, right eye
     H44.392   Other degenerative disorders of globe, left eye
     H44.393   Other degenerative disorders of globe, bilateral
    ■ H44.399   Other degenerative disorders of globe, unspecified eye

● H44.4   Hypotony of eye
  ■ H44.40   Unspecified hypotony of eye
  ● H44.41   Flat anterior chamber hypotony of eye
     H44.411   Flat anterior chamber hypotony of right eye
     H44.412   Flat anterior chamber hypotony of left eye
     H44.413   Flat anterior chamber hypotony of eye, bilateral
    ■ H44.419   Flat anterior chamber hypotony of unspecified eye
  ● H44.42   Hypotony of eye due to ocular fistula
     H44.421   Hypotony of right eye due to ocular fistula
     H44.422   Hypotony of left eye due to ocular fistula
     H44.423   Hypotony of eye due to ocular fistula, bilateral
    ■ H44.429   Hypotony of unspecified eye due to ocular fistula
  ● H44.43   Hypotony of eye due to other ocular disorders
     H44.431   Hypotony of eye due to other ocular disorders, right eye
     H44.432   Hypotony of eye due to other ocular disorders, left eye
     H44.433   Hypotony of eye due to other ocular disorders, bilateral
    ■ H44.439   Hypotony of eye due to other ocular disorders, unspecified eye

● H44.44   Primary hypotony of eye
     H44.441   Primary hypotony of right eye
     H44.442   Primary hypotony of left eye
     H44.443   Primary hypotony of eye, bilateral
    ■ H44.449   Primary hypotony of unspecified eye

● H44.5   Degenerated conditions of globe
  ■ H44.50   Unspecified degenerated conditions of globe
  ● H44.51   Absolute glaucoma
     H44.511   Absolute glaucoma, right eye
     H44.512   Absolute glaucoma, left eye
     H44.513   Absolute glaucoma, bilateral
    ■ H44.519   Absolute glaucoma, unspecified eye
  ● H44.52   Atrophy of globe
     Phthisis bulbi
     H44.521   Atrophy of globe, right eye
     H44.522   Atrophy of globe, left eye
     H44.523   Atrophy of globe, bilateral
    ■ H44.529   Atrophy of globe, unspecified eye
  ● H44.53   Leucocoria
     H44.531   Leucocoria, right eye
     H44.532   Leucocoria, left eye
     H44.533   Leucocoria, bilateral
    ■ H44.539   Leucocoria, unspecified eye

● H44.6   Retained (old) intraocular foreign body, magnetic
     Use additional code to identify magnetic foreign body (Z18.11)
     Excludes1   current intraocular foreign body (S05.-)
     Excludes2   retained foreign body in eyelid (H02.81-)
                 retained (old) foreign body following penetrating wound of orbit (H05.5-)
                 retained (old) intraocular foreign body, nonmagnetic (H44.7-)
  ● H44.60   Unspecified retained (old) intraocular foreign body, magnetic
    ■ H44.601   Unspecified retained (old) intraocular foreign body, magnetic, right eye
    ■ H44.602   Unspecified retained (old) intraocular foreign body, magnetic, left eye
    ■ H44.603   Unspecified retained (old) intraocular foreign body, magnetic, bilateral
    ■ H44.609   Unspecified retained (old) intraocular foreign body, magnetic, unspecified eye
  ● H44.61   Retained (old) magnetic foreign body in anterior chamber
     H44.611   Retained (old) magnetic foreign body in anterior chamber, right eye
     H44.612   Retained (old) magnetic foreign body in anterior chamber, left eye
     H44.613   Retained (old) magnetic foreign body in anterior chamber, bilateral

● Unacceptable Principal Diagnosis   ● Use Additional Character(s)   ■ Unspecified   ▶ Manifestation Code
OGCR Official Guidelines for Coding and Reporting   Excludes 1   Excludes 2   Includes   Use additional   Code first   Code also

H44.619 Retained (old) magnetic foreign body in anterior chamber, unspecified eye

● H44.62 Retained (old) magnetic foreign body in iris or ciliary body

H44.621 Retained (old) magnetic foreign body in iris or ciliary body, right eye

H44.622 Retained (old) magnetic foreign body in iris or ciliary body, left eye

H44.623 Retained (old) magnetic foreign body in iris or ciliary body, bilateral

H44.629 Retained (old) magnetic foreign body in iris or ciliary body, unspecified eye

● H44.63 Retained (old) magnetic foreign body in lens

H44.631 Retained (old) magnetic foreign body in lens, right eye

H44.632 Retained (old) magnetic foreign body in lens, left eye

H44.633 Retained (old) magnetic foreign body in lens, bilateral

H44.639 Retained (old) magnetic foreign body in lens, unspecified eye

● H44.64 Retained (old) magnetic foreign body in posterior wall of globe

H44.641 Retained (old) magnetic foreign body in posterior wall of globe, right eye

H44.642 Retained (old) magnetic foreign body in posterior wall of globe, left eye

H44.643 Retained (old) magnetic foreign body in posterior wall of globe, bilateral

H44.649 Retained (old) magnetic foreign body in posterior wall of globe, unspecified eye

● H44.65 Retained (old) magnetic foreign body in vitreous body

H44.651 Retained (old) magnetic foreign body in vitreous body, right eye

H44.652 Retained (old) magnetic foreign body in vitreous body, left eye

H44.653 Retained (old) magnetic foreign body in vitreous body, bilateral

H44.659 Retained (old) magnetic foreign body in vitreous body, unspecified eye

● H44.69 Retained (old) intraocular foreign body, magnetic, in other or multiple sites

H44.691 Retained (old) intraocular foreign body, magnetic, in other or multiple sites, right eye

H44.692 Retained (old) intraocular foreign body, magnetic, in other or multiple sites, left eye

H44.693 Retained (old) intraocular foreign body, magnetic, in other or multiple sites, bilateral

H44.699 Retained (old) intraocular foreign body, magnetic, in other or multiple sites, unspecified eye

● H44.7 Retained (old) intraocular foreign body, nonmagnetic

Use additional code to identify nonmagnetic foreign body (Z18.01-Z18.10, Z18.12, Z18.2-Z18.9)

Excludes1 current intraocular foreign body (S05.-)

Excludes2 retained foreign body in eyelid (H02.81-)
retained (old) foreign body following penetrating wound of orbit (H05.5-)
retained (old) intraocular foreign body, magnetic (H44.6-)

● H44.70 Unspecified retained (old) intraocular foreign body, nonmagnetic

H44.701 Unspecified retained (old) intraocular foreign body, nonmagnetic, right eye

H44.702 Unspecified retained (old) intraocular foreign body, nonmagnetic, left eye

H44.703 Unspecified retained (old) intraocular foreign body, nonmagnetic, bilateral

H44.709 Unspecified retained (old) intraocular foreign body, nonmagnetic, unspecified eye
Retained (old) intraocular foreign body NOS

● H44.71 Retained (nonmagnetic) (old) foreign body in anterior chamber

H44.711 Retained (nonmagnetic) (old) foreign body in anterior chamber, right eye

H44.712 Retained (nonmagnetic) (old) foreign body in anterior chamber, left eye

H44.713 Retained (nonmagnetic) (old) foreign body in anterior chamber, bilateral

H44.719 Retained (nonmagnetic) (old) foreign body in anterior chamber, unspecified eye

● H44.72 Retained (nonmagnetic) (old) foreign body in iris or ciliary body

H44.721 Retained (nonmagnetic) (old) foreign body in iris or ciliary body, right eye

H44.722 Retained (nonmagnetic) (old) foreign body in iris or ciliary body, left eye

H44.723 Retained (nonmagnetic) (old) foreign body in iris or ciliary body, bilateral

H44.729 Retained (nonmagnetic) (old) foreign body in iris or ciliary body, unspecified eye

● H44.73 Retained (nonmagnetic) (old) foreign body in lens

H44.731 Retained (nonmagnetic) (old) foreign body in lens, right eye

H44.732 Retained (nonmagnetic) (old) foreign body in lens, left eye

H44.733 Retained (nonmagnetic) (old) foreign body in lens, bilateral

■ H44.739 Retained (nonmagnetic) (old) foreign body in lens, unspecified eye

● H44.74 Retained (nonmagnetic) (old) foreign body in posterior wall of globe

H44.741 Retained (nonmagnetic) (old) foreign body in posterior wall of globe, right eye

H44.742 Retained (nonmagnetic) (old) foreign body in posterior wall of globe, left eye

H44.743 Retained (nonmagnetic) (old) foreign body in posterior wall of globe, bilateral

■ H44.749 Retained (nonmagnetic) (old) foreign body in posterior wall of globe, unspecified eye

● H44.75 Retained (nonmagnetic) (old) foreign body in vitreous body

H44.751 Retained (nonmagnetic) (old) foreign body in vitreous body, right eye

H44.752 Retained (nonmagnetic) (old) foreign body in vitreous body, left eye

H44.753 Retained (nonmagnetic) (old) foreign body in vitreous body, bilateral

■ H44.759 Retained (nonmagnetic) (old) foreign body in vitreous body, unspecified eye

● H44.79 Retained (old) intraocular foreign body, nonmagnetic, in other or multiple sites

H44.791 Retained (old) intraocular foreign body, nonmagnetic, in other or multiple sites, right eye

H44.792 Retained (old) intraocular foreign body, nonmagnetic, in other or multiple sites, left eye

H44.793 Retained (old) intraocular foreign body, nonmagnetic, in other or multiple sites, bilateral

■ H44.799 Retained (old) intraocular foreign body, nonmagnetic, in other or multiple sites, unspecified eye

● H44.8 Other disorders of globe

● H44.81 Hemophthalmos

H44.811 Hemophthalmos, right eye

H44.812 Hemophthalmos, left eye

H44.813 Hemophthalmos, bilateral

■ H44.819 Hemophthalmos, unspecified eye

● H44.82 Luxation of globe

H44.821 Luxation of globe, right eye

H44.822 Luxation of globe, left eye

H44.823 Luxation of globe, bilateral

■ H44.829 Luxation of globe, unspecified eye

H44.89 Other disorders of globe

■ H44.9 Unspecified disorder of globe

(See Plate 86 on page NAP-7.)

DISORDERS OF OPTIC NERVE AND VISUAL PATHWAYS (H46-H47)

● H46 Optic neuritis

Excludes2 ischemic optic neuropathy (H47.01-)
neuromyelitis optica [Devic] (G36.0)

● H46.0 Optic papillitis

■ H46.00 Optic papillitis, unspecified eye 🔒

H46.01 Optic papillitis, right eye 🔒

H46.02 Optic papillitis, left eye 🔒

H46.03 Optic papillitis, bilateral 🔒

● H46.1 Retrobulbar neuritis
Retrobulbar neuritis NOS

Excludes1 syphilitic retrobulbar neuritis (A52.15)

■ H46.10 Retrobulbar neuritis, unspecified eye 🔒

H46.11 Retrobulbar neuritis, right eye 🔒

H46.12 Retrobulbar neuritis, left eye 🔒

H46.13 Retrobulbar neuritis, bilateral 🔒

H46.2 Nutritional optic neuropathy

● H46.3 Toxic optic neuropathy
Code first (T51-T65) *to identify cause*

H46.8 Other optic neuritis 🔒

■ H46.9 Unspecified optic neuritis 🔒

● H47 Other disorders of optic [2nd] nerve and visual pathways

● H47.0 Disorders of optic nerve, not elsewhere classified

● H47.01 Ischemic optic neuropathy

H47.011 Ischemic optic neuropathy, right eye

H47.012 Ischemic optic neuropathy, left eye

H47.013 Ischemic optic neuropathy, bilateral

■ H47.019 Ischemic optic neuropathy, unspecified eye

● H47.02 Hemorrhage in optic nerve sheath

H47.021 Hemorrhage in optic nerve sheath, right eye

H47.022 Hemorrhage in optic nerve sheath, left eye

H47.023 Hemorrhage in optic nerve sheath, bilateral

■ H47.029 Hemorrhage in optic nerve sheath, unspecified eye

● H47.03 Optic nerve hypoplasia

H47.031 Optic nerve hypoplasia, right eye

H47.032 Optic nerve hypoplasia, left eye

H47.033 Optic nerve hypoplasia, bilateral

■ H47.039 Optic nerve hypoplasia, unspecified eye

● H47.09 Other disorders of optic nerve, not elsewhere classified
Compression of optic nerve

H47.091 Other disorders of optic nerve, not elsewhere classified, right eye

H47.092 Other disorders of optic nerve, not elsewhere classified, left eye

H47.093 Other disorders of optic nerve, not elsewhere classified, bilateral

■ H47.099 Other disorders of optic nerve, not elsewhere classified, unspecified eye

● Unacceptable Principal Diagnosis   ● Use Additional Character(s)   ■ Unspecified   ▶ Manifestation Code

OGCR Official Guidelines for Coding and Reporting   Excludes 1   Excludes 2   Includes   Use additional   Code first   Code also

Figure 7-10   Papilledema. (From Behrma: Nelson Textbook of Pediatrics, 17th ed. 2004, Saunders.)

Item 7-8   Papilledema is swelling of the optic disc caused by increased intracranial pressure. It is most often bilateral and occurs quickly (hours) or over weeks of time. It is a common symptom of a brain tumor. The term should not be used to describe optic disc swelling with underlying infectious, infiltrative, or inflammatory etiologies.

- **H47.1   Papilledema**
  - **H47.10   Unspecified papilledema** 🦠
  - H47.11   Papilledema associated with increased intracranial pressure 🦠
  - H47.12   Papilledema associated with decreased ocular pressure
  - H47.13   Papilledema associated with retinal disorder
  - **H47.14   Foster-Kennedy syndrome**
    - H47.141   Foster-Kennedy syndrome, right eye
    - H47.142   Foster-Kennedy syndrome, left eye
    - H47.143   Foster-Kennedy syndrome, bilateral
    - **H47.149   Foster-Kennedy syndrome, unspecified eye**
- **H47.2   Optic atrophy**
  - **H47.20   Unspecified optic atrophy**
  - **H47.21   Primary optic atrophy**
    - H47.211   Primary optic atrophy, right eye
    - H47.212   Primary optic atrophy, left eye
    - H47.213   Primary optic atrophy, bilateral
    - **H47.219   Primary optic atrophy, unspecified eye**
  - H47.22   Hereditary optic atrophy
    Leber's optic atrophy

- **H47.23   Glaucomatous optic atrophy**
  - H47.231   Glaucomatous optic atrophy, right eye
  - H47.232   Glaucomatous optic atrophy, left eye
  - H47.233   Glaucomatous optic atrophy, bilateral
  - **H47.239   Glaucomatous optic atrophy, unspecified eye**
- **H47.29   Other optic atrophy**
  Temporal pallor of optic disc
  - H47.291   Other optic atrophy, right eye
  - H47.292   Other optic atrophy, left eye
  - H47.293   Other optic atrophy, bilateral
  - **H47.299   Other optic atrophy, unspecified eye**
- **H47.3   Other disorders of optic disc**
  - **H47.31   Coloboma of optic disc**
    - H47.311   Coloboma of optic disc, right eye
    - H47.312   Coloboma of optic disc, left eye
    - H47.313   Coloboma of optic disc, bilateral
    - **H47.319   Coloboma of optic disc, unspecified eye**
  - **H47.32   Drusen of optic disc**
    - H47.321   Drusen of optic disc, right eye
    - H47.322   Drusen of optic disc, left eye
    - H47.323   Drusen of optic disc, bilateral
    - **H47.329   Drusen of optic disc, unspecified eye**
  - **H47.33   Pseudopapilledema of optic disc**
    - H47.331   Pseudopapilledema of optic disc, right eye
    - H47.332   Pseudopapilledema of optic disc, left eye
    - H47.333   Pseudopapilledema of optic disc, bilateral
    - **H47.339   Pseudopapilledema of optic disc, unspecified eye**
  - **H47.39   Other disorders of optic disc**
    - H47.391   Other disorders of optic disc, right eye
    - H47.392   Other disorders of optic disc, left eye
    - H47.393   Other disorders of optic disc, bilateral
    - **H47.399   Other disorders of optic disc, unspecified eye**
- **H47.4   Disorders of optic chiasm**
  Code also underlying condition
  - H47.41   Disorders of optic chiasm in (due to) inflammatory disorders 🦠
  - H47.42   Disorders of optic chiasm in (due to) neoplasm 🦠
  - H47.43   Disorders of optic chiasm in (due to) vascular disorders 🦠
  - H47.49   Disorders of optic chiasm in (due to) other disorders 🦠

N   Newborn Age: 0   **P**   Pediatric Age: 0–17   **M**   Maternity DX: 12–55   **A**   Adult Age: 15–124   ♀   Females Only   ♂   Males Only

🦠 Complication\Comorbidity   🦠 Major C\C   🦠 Present on Admission Requirement   🦠 Hospital-Acquired Condition

995

CHAPTER 7 (H00-H59)

CHAPTER 7 (H00-H59)

● **H47.5 Disorders of other visual pathways**
Disorders of optic tracts, geniculate nuclei and
optic radiations
Code also underlying condition

● H47.51 **Disorders of visual pathways in (due to) inflammatory disorders**

H47.511 **Disorders of visual pathways in (due to) inflammatory disorders, right side** ●

H47.512 **Disorders of visual pathways in (due to) inflammatory disorders, left side** ●

■ H47.519 **Disorders of visual pathways in (due to) inflammatory disorders, unspecified side** ●

● H47.52 **Disorders of visual pathways in (due to) neoplasm**

H47.521 **Disorders of visual pathways in (due to) neoplasm, right side** ●

H47.522 **Disorders of visual pathways in (due to) neoplasm, left side** ●

■ H47.529 **Disorders of visual pathways in (due to) neoplasm, unspecified side** ●

● H47.53 **Disorders of visual pathways in (due to) vascular disorders**

H47.531 **Disorders of visual pathways in (due to) vascular disorders, right side** ●

H47.532 **Disorders of visual pathways in (due to) vascular disorders, left side** ●

■ H47.539 **Disorders of visual pathways in (due to) vascular disorders, unspecified side** ●

● **H47.6 Disorders of visual cortex**
Code also underlying condition
Excludes1 injury to visual cortex S04.04

● H47.61 **Cortical blindness**

H47.611 **Cortical blindness, right side of brain**

H47.612 **Cortical blindness, left side of brain**

■ H47.619 **Cortical blindness, unspecified side of brain**

● H47.62 **Disorders of visual cortex in (due to) inflammatory disorders**

H47.621 **Disorders of visual cortex in (due to) inflammatory disorders, right side of brain** ●

H47.622 **Disorders of visual cortex in (due to) inflammatory disorders, left side of brain** ●

■ H47.629 **Disorders of visual cortex in (due to) inflammatory disorders, unspecified side of brain** ●

● H47.63 **Disorders of visual cortex in (due to) neoplasm**

H47.631 **Disorders of visual cortex in (due to) neoplasm, right side of brain** ●

H47.632 **Disorders of visual cortex in (due to) neoplasm, left side of brain** ●

■ H47.639 **Disorders of visual cortex in (due to) neoplasm, unspecified side of brain** ●

Item 7–9 Strabismus or esotropia (crossed eyes) is a condition of the extraocular eye muscles, resulting in an inability of the eyes to focus and also affects depth perception.

Figure 7-11 A. Image of strabismus. **B.** Exotropia. (**A** from Yanoff: Ophthalmology, 2nd ed. 2004, Mosby, Inc. **B** from Rakel: Textbook of Family Practice, 7th ed. 2007, Saunders.)

● H47.64 **Disorders of visual cortex in (due to) vascular disorders**

H47.641 **Disorders of visual cortex in (due to) vascular disorders, right side of brain** ●

H47.642 **Disorders of visual cortex in (due to) vascular disorders, left side of brain** ●

■ H47.649 **Disorders of visual cortex in (due to) vascular disorders, unspecified side of brain** ●

■ H47.9 **Unspecified disorder of visual pathways**

DISORDERS OF OCULAR MUSCLES, BINOCULAR MOVEMENT, ACCOMMODATION AND REFRACTION (H49-H52)

Excludes2 nystagmus and other irregular eye movements (H55)

● H49 **Paralytic strabismus**

Excludes2 internal ophthalmoplegia (H52.51-)
internuclear ophthalmoplegia (H51.2-)
progressive supranuclear ophthalmoplegia (G23.1)

● H49.0 **Third [oculomotor] nerve palsy**

■ H49.00 **Third [oculomotor] nerve palsy, unspecified eye**

H49.01 **Third [oculomotor] nerve palsy, right eye**

H49.02 **Third [oculomotor] nerve palsy, left eye**

H49.03 **Third [oculomotor] nerve palsy, bilateral**

● H49.1 **Fourth [trochlear] nerve palsy**

■ H49.10 **Fourth [trochlear] nerve palsy, unspecified eye**

H49.11 **Fourth [trochlear] nerve palsy, right eye**

H49.12 **Fourth [trochlear] nerve palsy, left eye**

H49.13 **Fourth [trochlear] nerve palsy, bilateral**

● H49.2 **Sixth [abducent] nerve palsy**

■ H49.20 **Sixth [abducent] nerve palsy, unspecified eye**

H49.21 **Sixth [abducent] nerve palsy, right eye**

H49.22 **Sixth [abducent] nerve palsy, left eye**

H49.23 **Sixth [abducent] nerve palsy, bilateral**

● Unacceptable Principal Diagnosis   ● Use Additional Character(s)   ■ Unspecified   ▶ Manifestation Code
OGCR Official Guidelines for Coding and Reporting   Excludes 1   Excludes 2   Includes   Use additional   Code first   Code also

● H49.3 Total (external) ophthalmoplegia

◻ H49.30 Total (external) ophthalmoplegia, unspecified eye

H49.31 Total (external) ophthalmoplegia, right eye

H49.32 Total (external) ophthalmoplegia, left eye

H49.33 Total (external) ophthalmoplegia, bilateral

● H49.4 Progressive external ophthalmoplegia

Excludes1   Kearns-Sayre syndrome (H49.81-)

◻ H49.40 Progressive external ophthalmoplegia, unspecified eye

H49.41 Progressive external ophthalmoplegia, right eye

H49.42 Progressive external ophthalmoplegia, left eye

H49.43 Progressive external ophthalmoplegia, bilateral

● H49.8 Other paralytic strabismus

● H49.81 Kearns-Sayre syndrome
Progressive external ophthalmoplegia with pigmentary retinopathy

Use additional code for other manifestation, such as:
heart block (I45.9)

H49.811 Kearns-Sayre syndrome, right eye 🐾

H49.812 Kearns-Sayre syndrome, left eye 🐾

H49.813 Kearns-Sayre syndrome, bilateral 🐾

◻ H49.819 Kearns-Sayre syndrome, unspecified eye 🐾

● H49.88 Other paralytic strabismus
External ophthalmoplegia NOS

H49.881 Other paralytic strabismus, right eye

H49.882 Other paralytic strabismus, left eye

H49.883 Other paralytic strabismus, bilateral

◻ H49.889 Other paralytic strabismus, unspecified eye

◻ H49.9 Unspecified paralytic strabismus

● H50 Other strabismus

● H50.0 Esotropia
Convergent concomitant strabismus

Excludes1   intermittent esotropia (H50.31-, H50.32)

◻ H50.00 Unspecified esotropia

● H50.01 Monocular esotropia

H50.011 Monocular esotropia, right eye

H50.012 Monocular esotropia, left eye

● H50.02 Monocular esotropia with A pattern

H50.021 Monocular esotropia with A pattern, right eye

H50.022 Monocular esotropia with A pattern, left eye

● H50.03 Monocular esotropia with V pattern

H50.031 Monocular esotropia with V pattern, right eye

H50.032 Monocular esotropia with V pattern, left eye

● H50.04 Monocular esotropia with other noncomitancies

H50.041 Monocular esotropia with other noncomitancies, right eye

H50.042 Monocular esotropia with other noncomitancies, left eye

H50.05 Alternating esotropia

H50.06 Alternating esotropia with A pattern

H50.07 Alternating esotropia with V pattern

H50.08 Alternating esotropia with other noncomitancies

● H50.1 Exotropia
Misalignment in which one eye deviates outward (away from nose) while the other fixates normally
Divergent concomitant strabismus

Excludes1   intermittent exotropia (H50.33-, H50.34)

◻ H50.10 Unspecified exotropia

● H50.11 Monocular exotropia

H50.111 Monocular exotropia, right eye

H50.112 Monocular exotropia, left eye

● H50.12 Monocular exotropia with A pattern

H50.121 Monocular exotropia with A pattern, right eye

H50.122 Monocular exotropia with A pattern, left eye

● H50.13 Monocular exotropia with V pattern

H50.131 Monocular exotropia with V pattern, right eye

H50.132 Monocular exotropia with V pattern, left eye

● H50.14 Monocular exotropia with other noncomitancies

H50.141 Monocular exotropia with other noncomitancies, right eye

H50.142 Monocular exotropia with other noncomitancies, left eye

H50.15 Alternating exotropia

H50.16 Alternating exotropia with A pattern

H50.17 Alternating exotropia with V pattern

H50.18 Alternating exotropia with other noncomitancies

● H50.2 Vertical strabismus
Hypertropia

H50.21 Vertical strabismus, right eye

H50.22 Vertical strabismus, left eye

● H50.3 Intermittent heterotropia
Displacement of an organ or part of an organ from its normal position

◻ H50.30 Unspecified intermittent heterotropia

● H50.31 Intermittent monocular esotropia

H50.311 Intermittent monocular esotropia, right eye

H50.312 Intermittent monocular esotropia, left eye

H50.32 Intermittent alternating esotropia

N Newborn Age: 0   **P** Pediatric Age: 0–17   **M** Maternity DX: 12–55   **A** Adult Age: 15–124   ♀ Females Only   ♂ Males Only

🐾 Complication\Comorbidity   Major C\C   Present on Admission Requirement   Hospital-Acquired Condition

997

CHAPTER 7 (H00–H59)

- H50.33 Intermittent monocular exotropia
  - H50.331 Intermittent monocular exotropia, right eye
  - H50.332 Intermittent monocular exotropia, left eye
  - H50.34 Intermittent alternating exotropia
- H50.4 Other and unspecified heterotropia
  - H50.40 Unspecified heterotropia
  - H50.41 Cyclotropia
    - H50.411 Cyclotropia, right eye
    - H50.412 Cyclotropia, left eye
  - H50.42 Monofixation syndrome
  - H50.43 Accommodative component in esotropia
- H50.5 Heterophoria
  One or both eyes wander away from the position where both eyes are looking together in the same direction
  - H50.50 Unspecified heterophoria
  - H50.51 Esophoria
    Eye deviates inward (toward the nose)
  - H50.52 Exophoria
    Eye deviates outward (toward the ear)
  - H50.53 Vertical heterophoria
  - H50.54 Cyclophoria
  - H50.55 Alternating heterophoria
- H50.6 Mechanical strabismus
  - H50.60 Mechanical strabismus, unspecified
  - H50.61 Brown's sheath syndrome
    - H50.611 Brown's sheath syndrome, right eye
    - H50.612 Brown's sheath syndrome, left eye
  - H50.69 Other mechanical strabismus
    Strabismus due to adhesions
    Traumatic limitation of duction of eye muscle
- H50.8 Other specified strabismus
  - H50.81 Duane's syndrome
    - H50.811 Duane's syndrome, right eye
    - H50.812 Duane's syndrome, left eye
  - H50.89 Other specified strabismus
- H50.9 Unspecified strabismus

- H51 Other disorders of binocular movement
  - H51.0 Palsy (spasm) of conjugate gaze
  - H51.1 Convergence insufficiency and excess
    - H51.11 Convergence insufficiency
    - H51.12 Convergence excess
  - H51.2 Internuclear ophthalmoplegia
    - H51.20 Internuclear ophthalmoplegia, unspecified eye
    - H51.21 Internuclear ophthalmoplegia, right eye
    - H51.22 Internuclear ophthalmoplegia, left eye
    - H51.23 Internuclear ophthalmoplegia, bilateral
  - H51.8 Other specified disorders of binocular movement
  - H51.9 Unspecified disorder of binocular movement

Item 7–10 Disorders of refraction: **Hypermetropia,** or farsightedness, means focus at a distance is adequate but not on close objects. **Myopia** is near-sightedness or short-sightedness and means the focus on nearby objects is clear but distant objects appear blurred. **Astigmatism** is warping of the curvature of the cornea so light rays entering do not meet a single focal point, resulting in a distorted image. **Anisometropia** is unequal refractive power in which one eye may be myopic (near-sighted) and the other hyperopic (far-sighted). **Presbyopia** is the loss of focus on near objects, which occurs with age because the lens loses elasticity.

- H52 Disorders of refraction and accommodation
  - H52.0 Hypermetropia
    - H52.00 Hypermetropia, unspecified eye
    - H52.01 Hypermetropia, right eye
    - H52.02 Hypermetropia, left eye
    - H52.03 Hypermetropia, bilateral
  - H52.1 Myopia
    Excludes1   degenerative myopia (H44.2-)
    - H52.10 Myopia, unspecified eye
    - H52.11 Myopia, right eye
    - H52.12 Myopia, left eye
    - H52.13 Myopia, bilateral
  - H52.2 Astigmatism
    - H52.20 Unspecified astigmatism
      - H52.201 Unspecified astigmatism, right eye
      - H52.202 Unspecified astigmatism, left eye
      - H52.203 Unspecified astigmatism, bilateral
      - H52.209 Unspecified astigmatism, unspecified eye
    - H52.21 Irregular astigmatism
      - H52.211 Irregular astigmatism, right eye
      - H52.212 Irregular astigmatism, left eye
      - H52.213 Irregular astigmatism, bilateral
      - H52.219 Irregular astigmatism, unspecified eye
    - H52.22 Regular astigmatism
      - H52.221 Regular astigmatism, right eye
      - H52.222 Regular astigmatism, left eye
      - H52.223 Regular astigmatism, bilateral
      - H52.229 Regular astigmatism, unspecified eye
  - H52.3 Anisometropia and aniseikonia
    - H52.31 Anisometropia
    - H52.32 Aniseikonia
  - H52.4 Presbyopia
  - H52.5 Disorders of accommodation
    - H52.51 Internal ophthalmoplegia (complete) (total)
      - H52.511 Internal ophthalmoplegia (complete) (total), right eye
      - H52.512 Internal ophthalmoplegia (complete) (total), left eye
      - H52.513 Internal ophthalmoplegia (complete) (total), bilateral
      - H52.519 Internal ophthalmoplegia (complete) (total), unspecified eye

● H52.52 Paresis of accommodation

    H52.521 Paresis of accommodation, right eye

    H52.522 Paresis of accommodation, left eye

    H52.523 Paresis of accommodation, bilateral

    ■ H52.529 Paresis of accommodation, unspecified eye

● H52.53 Spasm of accommodation

    H52.531 Spasm of accommodation, right eye

    H52.532 Spasm of accommodation, left eye

    H52.533 Spasm of accommodation, bilateral

    ■ H52.539 Spasm of accommodation, unspecified eye

H52.6 Other disorders of refraction

■ H52.7 Unspecified disorder of refraction

VISUAL DISTURBANCES AND BLINDNESS (H53-H54)

● H53 Visual disturbances

  ● H53.0 Amblyopia ex anopsia

    Excludes1 amblyopia due to vitamin A deficiency (E50.5)

    ● H53.00 Unspecified amblyopia

      ■ H53.001 Unspecified amblyopia, right eye

      ■ H53.002 Unspecified amblyopia, left eye

      ■ H53.003 Unspecified amblyopia, bilateral

      ■ H53.009 Unspecified amblyopia, unspecified eye

    ● H53.01 Deprivation amblyopia

      H53.011 Deprivation amblyopia, right eye

      H53.012 Deprivation amblyopia, left eye

      H53.013 Deprivation amblyopia, bilateral

      ■ H53.019 Deprivation amblyopia, unspecified eye

    ● H53.02 Refractive amblyopia

      H53.021 Refractive amblyopia, right eye

      H53.022 Refractive amblyopia, left eye

      H53.023 Refractive amblyopia, bilateral

      ■ H53.029 Refractive amblyopia, unspecified eye

    ● H53.03 Strabismic amblyopia

      Excludes1 strabismus (H50.-)

      H53.031 Strabismic amblyopia, right eye

      H53.032 Strabismic amblyopia, left eye

      H53.033 Strabismic amblyopia, bilateral

      ■ H53.039 Strabismic amblyopia, unspecified eye

  ● H53.1 Subjective visual disturbances

    Excludes1 subjective visual disturbances due to vitamin A deficiency (E50.5)
               visual hallucinations (R44.1)

    ■ H53.10 Unspecified subjective visual disturbances

    H53.11 Day blindness
      Hemeralopia

    ● H53.12 Transient visual loss
      Scintillating scotoma

      Excludes1 amaurosis fugax (G45.3-)
             transient retinal artery occlusion (H34.0-)

      H53.121 Transient visual loss, right eye 🔖

      H53.122 Transient visual loss, left eye 🔖

      H53.123 Transient visual loss, bilateral 🔖

      ■ H53.129 Transient visual loss, unspecified eye 🔖

    ● H53.13 Sudden visual loss

      H53.131 Sudden visual loss, right eye 🔖

      H53.132 Sudden visual loss, left eye 🔖

      H53.133 Sudden visual loss, bilateral 🔖

      ■ H53.139 Sudden visual loss, unspecified eye 🔖

  ● H53.14 Visual discomfort
    Asthenopia
    Photophobia

    H53.141 Visual discomfort, right eye

    H53.142 Visual discomfort, left eye

    H53.143 Visual discomfort, bilateral

    ■ H53.149 Visual discomfort, unspecified

  H53.15 Visual distortions of shape and size
    Metamorphopsia

  H53.16 Psychophysical visual disturbances

  H53.19 Other subjective visual disturbances
    Visual halos

H53.2 Diplopia
  Double vision

● H53.3 Other and unspecified disorders of binocular vision

  ■ H53.30 Unspecified disorder of binocular vision

  H53.31 Abnormal retinal correspondence

  H53.32 Fusion with defective stereopsis

  H53.33 Simultaneous visual perception without fusion

  H53.34 Suppression of binocular vision

● H53.4 Visual field defects

  ■ H53.40 Unspecified visual field defects

  ● H53.41 Scotoma involving central area
    Central scotoma

    H53.411 Scotoma involving central area, right eye

    H53.412 Scotoma involving central area, left eye

    H53.413 Scotoma involving central area, bilateral

    ■ H53.419 Scotoma involving central area, unspecified eye

  ● H53.42 Scotoma of blind spot area
    Enlarged blind spot

    H53.421 Scotoma of blind spot area, right eye

    H53.422 Scotoma of blind spot area, left eye

    H53.423 Scotoma of blind spot area, bilateral

    ■ H53.429 Scotoma of blind spot area, unspecified eye

CHAPTER 7 (H00-H59)

N Newborn Age: 0   **P** Pediatric Age: 0–17   **M** Maternity DX: 12–55   **A** Adult Age: 15–124   ♀ Females Only   ♂ Males Only

🔖 Complication\Comorbidity   🔖 Major C\C   🔖 Present on Admission Requirement   🔖 Hospital-Acquired Condition

999

● H53.43 Sector or arcuate defects
Arcuate scotoma
Bjerrum scotoma

    H53.431 Sector or arcuate defects, right eye

    H53.432 Sector or arcuate defects, left eye

    H53.433 Sector or arcuate defects, bilateral

    ■ H53.439 Sector or arcuate defects, unspecified eye

● H53.45 Other localized visual field defect
Peripheral visual field defect
Ring scotoma NOS
Scotoma NOS

    H53.451 Other localized visual field defect, right eye

    H53.452 Other localized visual field defect, left eye

    H53.453 Other localized visual field defect, bilateral

    ■ H53.459 Other localized visual field defect, unspecified eye

● H53.46 Homonymous bilateral field defects
Homonymous hemianop(s)ia
Quadrant anop(s)ia

    H53.461 Homonymous bilateral field defects, right side

    H53.462 Homonymous bilateral field defects, left side

    ■ H53.469 Homonymous bilateral field defects, unspecified side
        Homonymous bilateral field defects NOS

    H53.47 Heteronymous bilateral field defects
    Heteronymous hemianop(s)ia

● H53.48 Generalized contraction of visual field

    H53.481 Generalized contraction of visual field, right eye

    H53.482 Generalized contraction of visual field, left eye

    H53.483 Generalized contraction of visual field, bilateral

    ■ H53.489 Generalized contraction of visual field, unspecified eye

● H53.5 Color vision deficiencies
Color blindness

    Excludes2 day blindness (H53.11)

    ■ **H53.50 Unspecified color vision deficiencies**
    Color blindness NOS

    H53.51 Achromatopsia

    H53.52 Acquired color vision deficiency

    H53.53 Deuteranomaly
    Deuteranopia

    H53.54 Protanomaly
    Protanopia

    H53.55 Tritanomaly
    Tritanopia

    H53.59 Other color vision deficiencies

● H53.6 Night blindness
    Excludes1 night blindness due to vitamin A deficiency (E50.5)

    ■ **H53.60 Unspecified night blindness**

    H53.61 Abnormal dark adaptation curve

    H53.62 Acquired night blindness

    H53.63 Congenital night blindness

    H53.69 Other night blindness

H53.7 Vision sensitivity deficiencies

    H53.71 Glare sensitivity

    H53.72 Impaired contrast sensitivity

H53.8 Other visual disturbances

■ **H53.9 Unspecified visual disturbance**

● H54 Blindness and low vision
    Note: For definition of visual impairment categories see table below.

    Code first any associated underlying cause of the blindness

    Excludes1 amaurosis fugax (G45.3)

    H54.0 Blindness, both eyes
    Visual impairment categories 3, 4, 5 in both eyes.

    ● H54.1 Blindness, one eye, low vision other eye
    Visual impairment categories 3, 4, 5 in one eye, with categories 1 or 2 in the other eye.

       ■ **H54.10 Blindness, one eye, low vision other eye, unspecified eyes**

       H54.11 Blindness, right eye, low vision left eye

       H54.12 Blindness, left eye, low vision right eye

    H54.2 Low vision, both eyes
    Visual impairment categories 1 or 2 in both eyes.

    H54.3 Unqualified visual loss, both eyes
    Visual impairment category 9 in both eyes.

    ● H54.4 Blindness, one eye
    Visual impairment categories 3, 4, 5 in one eye [normal vision in other eye]

       ■ **H54.40 Blindness, one eye, unspecified eye**

       H54.41 Blindness, right eye, normal vision left eye

       H54.42 Blindness, left eye, normal vision right eye

    ● H54.5 Low vision, one eye
    Visual impairment categories 1 or 2 in one eye [normal vision in other eye].

       ■ **H54.50 Low vision, one eye, unspecified eye**

       H54.51 Low vision, right eye, normal vision left eye

       H54.52 Low vision, left eye, normal vision right eye

    ● H54.6 Unqualified visual loss, one eye
    Visual impairment category 9 in one eye [normal vision in other eye].

       ■ **H54.60 Unqualified visual loss, one eye, unspecified**

       H54.61 Unqualified visual loss, right eye, normal vision left eye

       H54.62 Unqualified visual loss, left eye, normal vision right eye

● Unacceptable Principal Diagnosis   ● Use Additional Character(s)   ■ Unspecified   ▶ Manifestation Code

OGCR Official Guidelines for Coding and Reporting   Excludes 1   Excludes 2   Includes   Use additional   Code first   Code also

● ■ **H54.7 Unspecified visual loss**
Visual impairment category 9 NOS

H54.8 Legal blindness, as defined in USA
Blindness NOS according to USA definition

> **Excludes1**   legal blindness with specification of impairment level (H54.0-H54.7)

> **Note:** The table below gives a classification of severity of visual impairment recommended by a WHO Study Group on the Prevention of Blindness, Geneva, 6-10 November 1972.

> The term 'low vision' in category H54 comprises categories 1 and 2 of the table, the term 'blindness' categories 3, 4 and 5, and the term 'unqualified visual loss' category 9.

> If the extent of the visual field is taken into account, patients with a field no greater than 10 but greater than 5 around central fixation should be placed in category 3 and patients with a field no greater than 5 around central fixation should be placed in category 4, even if the central acuity is not impaired.

Category of visual impairment	Visual acuity with best possible correction	
	Maximum less than:	**Minimum equal to or better than:**
	6/18	6/60
3/10 (0.3)	1/10 (0.1)	
20/70	20/200	
	6/60	3/60
1/10 (0.1)	1/20 (0.05)	
20/200	20/400	
	3/60	1/60 (finger counting at one meter)
1/20 (0.05)	1/50 (0.02)	
20/400	5/300 (20/1200)	
	1/60 (finger counting at one meter)	Light perception
1/50 (0.02)		
5/300		
	No light perception	
	Undetermined or unspecified	

OTHER DISORDERS OF EYE AND ADNEXA (H55-H57)

● **H55 Nystagmus and other irregular eye movements**
  ● **H55.0 Nystagmus**
     Rapid, involuntary movements of the eyes in the horizontal or vertical direction.

    ■ **H55.00 Unspecified nystagmus**
    H55.01 Congenital nystagmus
    H55.02 Latent nystagmus
    H55.03 Visual deprivation nystagmus
    H55.04 Dissociated nystagmus
    H55.09 Other forms of nystagmus
  ● **H55.8 Other irregular eye movements**
    H55.81 Saccadic eye movements
    H55.89 Other irregular eye movements

● **H57 Other disorders of eye and adnexa**
  ● **H57.0 Anomalies of pupillary function**
    ■ **H57.00 Unspecified anomaly of pupillary function**
    H57.01 Argyll Robertson pupil, atypical

> **Excludes1**   syphilitic Argyll Robertson pupil (A52.19)

    H57.02 Anisocoria
    H57.03 Miosis
    H57.04 Mydriasis
    ● **H57.05 Tonic pupil**
      H57.051 Tonic pupil, right eye
      H57.052 Tonic pupil, left eye
      H57.053 Tonic pupil, bilateral
      ■ **H57.059 Tonic pupil, unspecified eye**
    H57.09 Other anomalies of pupillary function
  ● **H57.1 Ocular pain**
    ■ **H57.10 Ocular pain, unspecified eye**
    H57.11 Ocular pain, right eye
    H57.12 Ocular pain, left eye
    H57.13 Ocular pain, bilateral
  H57.8 Other specified disorders of eye and adnexa
  ● ■ **H57.9 Unspecified disorder of eye and adnexa**

INTRAOPERATIVE AND POSTPROCEDURAL COMPLICATIONS AND DISORDERS OF EYE AND ADNEXA, NOT ELSEWHERE CLASSIFIED (H59)

● **H59 Intraoperative and postprocedural complications and disorders of eye and adnexa, not elsewhere classified**

> **Excludes1**   mechanical complication of intraocular lens (T85.2)
> mechanical complication of other ocular prosthetic devices, implants and grafts (T85.3)
> pseudophakia (Z96.1)
> secondary cataracts (H26.4-)

  ● **H59.0 Disorders of the eye following cataract surgery**
    ● **H59.01 Keratopathy (bullous aphakic) following cataract surgery**
      Vitreal corneal syndrome
      Vitreous (touch) syndrome

      H59.011 Keratopathy (bullous aphakic) following cataract surgery, right eye 🅲
      H59.012 Keratopathy (bullous aphakic) following cataract surgery, left eye 🅲
      H59.013 Keratopathy (bullous aphakic) following cataract surgery, bilateral 🅲
      ■ **H59.019 Keratopathy (bullous aphakic) following cataract surgery, unspecified eye** 🅲
    ● **H59.02 Cataract (lens) fragments in eye following cataract surgery**
      H59.021 Cataract (lens) fragments in eye following cataract surgery, right eye
      H59.022 Cataract (lens) fragments in eye following cataract surgery, left eye
      H59.023 Cataract (lens) fragments in eye following cataract surgery, bilateral

N Newborn Age: 0   **P** Pediatric Age: 0–17   **M** Maternity DX: 12–55   **A** Adult Age: 15–124   ♀ Females Only   ♂ Males Only

🅲 Complication\Comorbidity   🅲 Major C\C   Present on Admission Requirement   Hospital-Acquired Condition

1001

CHAPTER 7 (H00-H59)

CHAPTER 7 (H00–H59)

◼ H59.029   Cataract (lens) fragments in eye following cataract surgery, unspecified eye

● H59.03   Cystoid macular edema following cataract surgery

H59.031   Cystoid macular edema following cataract surgery, right eye 🖉

H59.032   Cystoid macular edema following cataract surgery, left eye 🖉

H59.033   Cystoid macular edema following cataract surgery, bilateral 🖉

◼ H59.039   Cystoid macular edema following cataract surgery, unspecified eye 🖉

● H59.09   Other disorders of the eye following cataract surgery

H59.091   Other disorders of the right eye following cataract surgery 🖉

H59.092   Other disorders of the left eye following cataract surgery 🖉

H59.093   Other disorders of the eye following cataract surgery, bilateral 🖉

◼ H59.099   Other disorders of unspecified eye following cataract surgery 🖉

● H59.1   Intraoperative hemorrhage and hematoma of eye and adnexa complicating a procedure

> **Excludes1**   intraoperative hemorrhage and hematoma of eye and adnexa due to accidental puncture or laceration during a procedure (H59.2-)

● H59.11   Intraoperative hemorrhage and hematoma of eye and adnexa complicating an ophthalmic procedure

H59.111   Intraoperative hemorrhage and hematoma of right eye and adnexa complicating an ophthalmic procedure 🖉

H59.112   Intraoperative hemorrhage and hematoma of left eye and adnexa complicating an ophthalmic procedure 🖉

H59.113   Intraoperative hemorrhage and hematoma of eye and adnexa complicating an ophthalmic procedure, bilateral 🖉

◼ H59.119   Intraoperative hemorrhage and hematoma of unspecified eye and adnexa complicating an ophthalmic procedure 🖉

● H59.12   Intraoperative hemorrhage and hematoma of eye and adnexa complicating other procedure

H59.121   Intraoperative hemorrhage and hematoma of right eye and adnexa complicating other procedure 🖉

H59.122   Intraoperative hemorrhage and hematoma of left eye and adnexa complicating other procedure 🖉

H59.123   Intraoperative hemorrhage and hematoma of eye and adnexa complicating other procedure, bilateral 🖉

◼ H59.129   Intraoperative hemorrhage and hematoma of unspecified eye and adnexa complicating other procedure 🖉

● H59.2   Accidental puncture and laceration of eye and adnexa during a procedure

● H59.21   Accidental puncture and laceration of eye and adnexa during an ophthalmic procedure

H59.211   Accidental puncture and laceration of right eye and adnexa during an ophthalmic procedure 🖉

H59.212   Accidental puncture and laceration of left eye and adnexa during an ophthalmic procedure 🖉

H59.213   Accidental puncture and laceration of eye and adnexa during an ophthalmic procedure, bilateral 🖉

◼ H59.219   Accidental puncture and laceration of unspecified eye and adnexa during an ophthalmic procedure 🖉

● H59.22   Accidental puncture and laceration of eye and adnexa during other procedure

H59.221   Accidental puncture and laceration of right eye and adnexa during other procedure 🖉

H59.222   Accidental puncture and laceration of left eye and adnexa during other procedure 🖉

H59.223   Accidental puncture and laceration of eye and adnexa during other procedure, bilateral 🖉

◼ H59.229   Accidental puncture and laceration of unspecified eye and adnexa during other procedure 🖉

● H59.3   Postprocedural hemorrhage and hematoma of eye and adnexa following a procedure

● H59.31   Postprocedural hemorrhage and hematoma of eye and adnexa following an ophthalmic procedure

H59.311   Postprocedural hemorrhage and hematoma of right eye and avdnexa following an ophthalmic procedure 🖉

H59.312   Postprocedural hemorrhage and hematoma of left eye and adnexa following an ophthalmic procedure 🖉

H59.313   Postprocedural hemorrhage and hematoma of eye and adnexa following an ophthalmic procedure, bilateral 🖉

◼ H59.319   Postprocedural hemorrhage and hematoma of unspecified eye and adnexa following an ophthalmic procedure 🖉

● H59.32   Postprocedural hemorrhage and hematoma of eye and adnexa following other procedure

H59.321   Postprocedural hemorrhage and hematoma of right eye and adnexa following other procedure 🖉

H59.322   Postprocedural hemorrhage and hematoma of left eye and adnexa following other procedure 🖉

● Unacceptable Principal Diagnosis	● Use Additional Character(s)	◼ Unspecified	▶ Manifestation Code

OGCR   Official Guidelines for Coding and Reporting   Excludes 1   Excludes 2   Includes   Use additional   Code first   Code also

H59.323   Postprocedural hemorrhage and hematoma of eye and adnexa following other procedure, bilateral 🏥

■ H59.329   Postprocedural hemorrhage and hematoma of unspecified eye and adnexa following other procedure 🏥

● H59.4   **Inflammation (infection) of postprocedural bleb**
Postprocedural blebitis

     Excludes1   filtering (vitreous) bleb after glaucoma surgery status (Z98.83)

■ H59.40   Inflammation (infection) of postprocedural bleb, unspecified

H59.41   Inflammation (infection) of postprocedural bleb, stage 1

H59.42   Inflammation (infection) of postprocedural bleb, stage 2

H59.43   Inflammation (infection) of postprocedural bleb, stage 3
Bleb endophthalmitis

● H59.8   **Other intraoperative and postprocedural complications and disorders of eye and adnexa, not elsewhere classified**

● H59.81   Chorioretinal scars after surgery for detachment

H59.811   Chorioretinal scars after surgery for detachment, right eye 🏥

H59.812   Chorioretinal scars after surgery for detachment, left eye 🏥

H59.813   Chorioretinal scars after surgery for detachment, bilateral 🏥

■ H59.819   Chorioretinal scars after surgery for detachment, unspecified eye 🏥

H59.88   Other intraoperative complications of eye and adnexa, not elsewhere classified 🏥

H59.89   Other postprocedural complications and disorders of eye and adnexa, not elsewhere classified 🏥

N   Newborn Age: 0   **P**   Pediatric Age: 0–17   **M**   Maternity DX: 12–55   **A**   Adult Age: 15–124   ♀   Females Only   ♂   Males Only

 Complication\Comorbidity   Major C\C   🏥 Present on Admission Requirement   🏥 Hospital-Acquired Condition

1003

CHAPTER 7 (H00-H59)

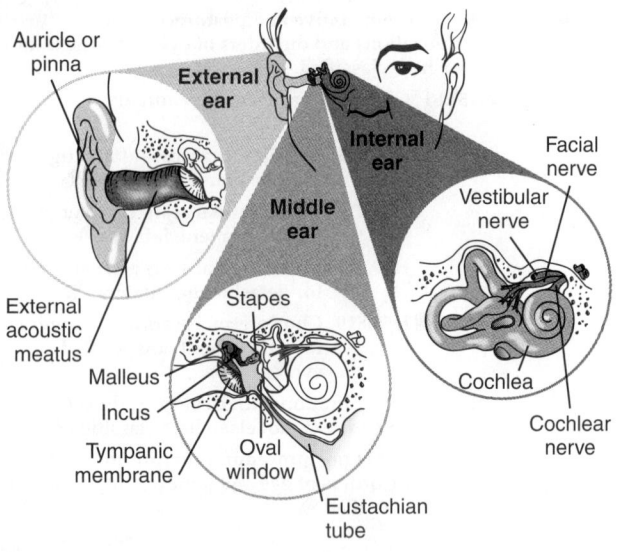

Figure 8-1 Auditory system. (From Buck CJ: Step-by-Step Medical Coding, 2010 ed. Philadelphia, WB Saunders, 2010.)

(See Plate 92 on page NAP-20.)

CHAPTER 8

DISEASES OF THE EAR AND MASTOID PROCESS (H60-H95)

Note: Use an external cause code following the code for the ear condition, if applicable, to identify the cause of the ear condition

Excludes2   certain conditions originating in the perinatal period (P04-P96)
certain infectious and parasitic diseases (A00-B99)
complications of pregnancy, childbirth and the puerperium (O00-O9A)
congenital malformations, deformations and chromosomal abnormalities (Q00-Q99)
endocrine, nutritional and metabolic diseases (E00-E88)
injury, poisoning and certain other consequences of external causes (S00-T88)
neoplasms (C00-D49)
symptoms, signs and abnormal clinical and laboratory findings, not elsewhere classified (R00-R94)

This chapter contains the following blocks:

H60-H62	Diseases of external ear
H65-H75	Diseases of middle ear and mastoid
H80-H83	Diseases of inner ear
H90-H94	Other disorders of ear
H95	Intraoperative and postprocedural complications and disorders of ear and mastoid process, not elsewhere classified

DISEASES OF EXTERNAL EAR (H60-H62)

● **H60 Otitis externa**
  ● **H60.0 Abscess of external ear**
    Boil of external ear
    Carbuncle of auricle or external auditory canal
    Furuncle of external ear
    ■ H60.00 Abscess of external ear, unspecified ear
    H60.01 Abscess of right external ear
    H60.02 Abscess of left external ear
    H60.03 Abscess of external ear, bilateral
  ● **H60.1 Cellulitis of external ear**
    Cellulitis of auricle
    Cellulitis of external auditory canal
    ■ H60.10 Cellulitis of external ear, unspecified ear
    H60.11 Cellulitis of right external ear
    H60.12 Cellulitis of left external ear
    H60.13 Cellulitis of external ear, bilateral
  ● **H60.2 Malignant otitis externa**
    ■ H60.20 Malignant otitis externa, unspecified ear 🔊
    H60.21 Malignant otitis externa, right ear 🔊
    H60.22 Malignant otitis externa, left ear 🔊
    H60.23 Malignant otitis externa, bilateral 🔊
  ● **H60.3 Other infective otitis externa**
    ● H60.31 Diffuse otitis externa
      H60.311 Diffuse otitis externa, right ear
      H60.312 Diffuse otitis externa, left ear
      H60.313 Diffuse otitis externa, bilateral
      ■ H60.319 Diffuse otitis externa, unspecified ear
    ● H60.32 Hemorrhagic otitis externa
      H60.321 Hemorrhagic otitis externa, right ear
      H60.322 Hemorrhagic otitis externa, left ear
      H60.323 Hemorrhagic otitis externa, bilateral
      ■ H60.329 Hemorrhagic otitis externa, unspecified ear
    ● H60.33 Swimmer's ear
      H60.331 Swimmer's ear, right ear
      H60.332 Swimmer's ear, left ear
      H60.333 Swimmer's ear, bilateral
      ■ H60.339 Swimmer's ear, unspecified ear
    ● H60.39 Other infective otitis externa
      H60.391 Other infective otitis externa, right ear
      H60.392 Other infective otitis externa, left ear
      H60.393 Other infective otitis externa, bilateral
      ■ H60.399 Other infective otitis externa, unspecified ear

● Unacceptable Principal Diagnosis   ● Use Additional Character(s)   ■ Unspecified   ▶ Manifestation Code
OGCR Official Guidelines for Coding and Reporting   Excludes 1   Excludes 2   Includes   Use additional   Code first   Code also

CHAPTER 8 (H60-H95)

● **H60.4   Cholesteatoma of external ear**
     Keratosis obturans of external ear (canal)
     Excludes2   cholesteatoma of middle ear
               (H71.-)
               recurrent cholesteatoma of
                 postmastoidectomy cavity
                 (H95.0-)
   ■ **H60.40   Cholesteatoma of external ear, unspecified ear**
     H60.41   Cholesteatoma of right external ear
     H60.42   Cholesteatoma of left external ear
     H60.43   Cholesteatoma of external ear, bilateral

● **H60.5   Acute noninfective otitis externa**
   ● **H60.50   Unspecified acute noninfective otitis externa**
       Acute otitis externa NOS
     ■ **H60.501   Unspecified acute noninfective otitis externa, right ear**
     ■ **H60.502   Unspecified acute noninfective otitis externa, left ear**
     ■ **H60.503   Unspecified acute noninfective otitis externa, bilateral**
     ■ **H60.509   Unspecified acute noninfective otitis externa, unspecified ear**
   ● **H60.51   Acute actinic otitis externa**
     H60.511   Acute actinic otitis externa, right ear
     H60.512   Acute actinic otitis externa, left ear
     H60.513   Acute actinic otitis externa, bilateral
     ■ **H60.519   Acute actinic otitis externa, unspecified ear**
   ● **H60.52   Acute chemical otitis externa**
     H60.521   Acute chemical otitis externa, right ear
     H60.522   Acute chemical otitis externa, left ear
     H60.523   Acute chemical otitis externa, bilateral
     ■ **H60.529   Acute chemical otitis externa, unspecified ear**
   ● **H60.53   Acute contact otitis externa**
     H60.531   Acute contact otitis externa, right ear
     H60.532   Acute contact otitis externa, left ear
     H60.533   Acute contact otitis externa, bilateral
     ■ **H60.539   Acute contact otitis externa, unspecified ear**
   ● **H60.54   Acute eczematoid otitis externa**
     H60.541   Acute eczematoid otitis externa, right ear
     H60.542   Acute eczematoid otitis externa, left ear
     H60.543   Acute eczematoid otitis externa, bilateral
     ■ **H60.549   Acute eczematoid otitis externa, unspecified ear**

● **H60.55   Acute reactive otitis externa**
     H60.551   Acute reactive otitis externa, right ear
     H60.552   Acute reactive otitis externa, left ear
     H60.553   Acute reactive otitis externa, bilateral
     ■ **H60.559   Acute reactive otitis externa, unspecified ear**
● **H60.59   Other noninfective acute otitis externa**
     H60.591   Other noninfective acute otitis externa, right ear
     H60.592   Other noninfective acute otitis externa, left ear
     H60.593   Other noninfective acute otitis externa, bilateral
     ■ **H60.599   Other noninfective acute otitis externa, unspecified ear**
● **H60.6   Unspecified chronic otitis externa**
   ■ **H60.60   Unspecified chronic otitis externa, unspecified ear**
   ■ **H60.61   Unspecified chronic otitis externa, right ear**
   ■ **H60.62   Unspecified chronic otitis externa, left ear**
   ■ **H60.63   Unspecified chronic otitis externa, bilateral**
● **H60.8   Other otitis externa**
   ● **H60.8X   Other otitis externa**
     H60.8X1   Other otitis externa, right ear
     H60.8X2   Other otitis externa, left ear
     H60.8X3   Other otitis externa, bilateral
     ■ **H60.8X9   Other otitis externa, unspecified ear**
● **H60.9   Unspecified otitis externa**
   ■ **H60.90   Unspecified otitis externa, unspecified ear**
   ■ **H60.91   Unspecified otitis externa, right ear**
   ■ **H60.92   Unspecified otitis externa, left ear**
   ■ **H60.93   Unspecified otitis externa, bilateral**

● **H61   Other disorders of external ear**
   ● **H61.0   Chondritis and perichondritis of external ear**
       Chondrodermatitis nodularis chronica helicis
       Perichondritis of auricle
       Perichondritis of pinna
   ● **H61.00   Unspecified perichondritis of external ear**
     ■ **H61.001   Unspecified perichondritis of right external ear**
     ■ **H61.002   Unspecified perichondritis of left external ear**
     ■ **H61.003   Unspecified perichondritis of external ear, bilateral**
     ■ **H61.009   Unspecified perichondritis of external ear, unspecified ear**
   ● **H61.01   Acute perichondritis of external ear**
     H61.011   Acute perichondritis of right external ear
     H61.012   Acute perichondritis of left external ear
     H61.013   Acute perichondritis of external ear, bilateral
     ■ **H61.019   Acute perichondritis of external ear, unspecified ear**

CHAPTER 8 (H60-H95)

N Newborn Age: 0   **P** Pediatric Age: 0–17   **M** Maternity DX: 12–55   **A** Adult Age: 15–124   ♀ Females Only   ♂ Males Only
🔗 Complication\Comorbidity   🔗 Major C\C   🔗 Present on Admission Requirement   🔗 Hospital-Acquired Condition

1005

● **H61.02 Chronic perichondritis of external ear**

    H61.021 Chronic perichondritis of right external ear

    H61.022 Chronic perichondritis of left external ear

    H61.023 Chronic perichondritis of external ear, bilateral

    ■ **H61.029 Chronic perichondritis of external ear, unspecified ear**

● **H61.03 Chondritis of external ear**
Chondritis of auricle
Chondritis of pinna

    H61.031 Chondritis of right external ear

    H61.032 Chondritis of left external ear

    H61.033 Chondritis of external ear, bilateral

    ■ **H61.039 Chondritis of external ear, unspecified ear**

● **H61.1 Noninfective disorders of pinna**

    Excludes2   cauliflower ear (M95.1-)
                gouty tophi of ear (M1A-, M10.-)

● **H61.10 Unspecified noninfective disorders of pinna**
Disorder of pinna NOS

    ■ **H61.101 Unspecified noninfective disorders of pinna, right ear**

    ■ **H61.102 Unspecified noninfective disorders of pinna, left ear**

    ■ **H61.103 Unspecified noninfective disorders of pinna, bilateral**

    ■ **H61.109 Unspecified noninfective disorders of pinna, unspecified ear**

● **H61.11 Acquired deformity of pinna**
Acquired deformity of auricle

    Excludes2   cauliflower ear (M95.1-)

    H61.111 Acquired deformity of pinna, right ear

    H61.112 Acquired deformity of pinna, left ear

    H61.113 Acquired deformity of pinna, bilateral

    ■ **H61.119 Acquired deformity of pinna, unspecified ear**

● **H61.12 Hematoma of pinna**
Hematoma of auricle

    H61.121 Hematoma of pinna, right ear

    H61.122 Hematoma of pinna, left ear

    H61.123 Hematoma of pinna, bilateral

    ■ **H61.129 Hematoma of pinna, unspecified ear**

● **H61.19 Other noninfective disorders of pinna**

    H61.191 Noninfective disorders of pinna, right ear

    H61.192 Noninfective disorders of pinna, left ear

    H61.193 Noninfective disorders of pinna, bilateral

    ■ **H61.199 Noninfective disorders of pinna, unspecified ear**

● **H61.2 Impacted cerumen**
Wax in ear

    ■ **H61.20 Impacted cerumen, unspecified ear**
MCE: Questionable admission when principal dx

    H61.21 Impacted cerumen, right ear
MCE: Questionable admission when principal dx

    H61.22 Impacted cerumen, left ear
MCE: Questionable admission when principal dx

    H61.23 Impacted cerumen, bilateral
MCE: Questionable admission when principal dx

● **H61.3 Acquired stenosis of external ear canal**
Collapse of external ear canal

    Excludes1   postprocedural stenosis of external ear canal (H95.81-)

● **H61.30 Acquired stenosis of external ear canal, unspecified**

    ■ **H61.301 Acquired stenosis of right external ear canal, unspecified**

    ■ **H61.302 Acquired stenosis of left external ear canal, unspecified**

    ■ **H61.303 Acquired stenosis of external ear canal, unspecified, bilateral**

    ■ **H61.309 Acquired stenosis of external ear canal, unspecified, unspecified ear**

● **H61.31 Acquired stenosis of external ear canal secondary to trauma**

    H61.311 Acquired stenosis of right external ear canal secondary to trauma

    H61.312 Acquired stenosis of left external ear canal secondary to trauma

    H61.313 Acquired stenosis of external ear canal secondary to trauma, bilateral

    ■ **H61.319 Acquired stenosis of external ear canal secondary to trauma, unspecified ear**

● **H61.32 Acquired stenosis of external ear canal secondary to inflammation and infection**

    H61.321 Acquired stenosis of right external ear canal secondary to inflammation and infection

    H61.322 Acquired stenosis of left external ear canal secondary to inflammation and infection

    H61.323 Acquired stenosis of external ear canal secondary to inflammation and infection, bilateral

    ■ **H61.329 Acquired stenosis of external ear canal secondary to inflammation and infection, unspecified ear**

● **H61.39 Other acquired stenosis of external ear canal**

    H61.391 Other acquired stenosis of right external ear canal

    H61.392 Other acquired stenosis of left external ear canal

    H61.393 Other acquired stenosis of external ear canal, bilateral

    ■ **H61.399 Other acquired stenosis of external ear canal, unspecified ear**

● **H61.8 Other specified disorders of external ear**

  ● **H61.81 Exostosis of external canal**

     H61.811 Exostosis of right external canal

     H61.812 Exostosis of left external canal

     H61.813 Exostosis of external canal, bilateral

     ■ **H61.819 Exostosis of external canal, unspecified ear**

  ● **H61.89 Other specified disorders of external ear**

     H61.891 Other specified disorders of right external ear

     H61.892 Other specified disorders of left external ear

     H61.893 Other specified disorders of external ear, bilateral

     ■ **H61.899 Other specified disorders of external ear, unspecified ear**

● **H61.9 Disorder of external ear, unspecified**

  ■ **H61.90 Disorder of external ear, unspecified, unspecified ear**

  ■ **H61.91 Disorder of right external ear, unspecified**

  ■ **H61.92 Disorder of left external ear, unspecified**

  ■ **H61.93 Disorder of external ear, unspecified, bilateral**

● **H62 Disorders of external ear in diseases classified elsewhere**

  ● **H62.4 Otitis externa in other diseases classified elsewhere**

    Code first underlying disease, such as:
     erysipelas (A46)
     impetigo (L01.0)

    Excludes1   otitis externa (in):
      candidiasis (B37.84)
      herpes viral [herpes simplex]
       (B00.1)
      herpes zoster (B02.8)

   ● ■▶ *H62.40 Otitis externa in other diseases classified elsewhere, unspecified ear*

   ● ▶ *H62.41 Otitis externa in other diseases classified elsewhere, right ear*

   ● ▶ *H62.42 Otitis externa in other diseases classified elsewhere, left ear*

   ● ▶ *H62.43 Otitis externa in other diseases classified elsewhere, bilateral*

  ● **H62.8 Other disorders of external ear in diseases classified elsewhere**

    Code first underlying disease, such as:
     gout (M1A-, M10.-)

   ● **H62.8X Other disorders of external ear in diseases classified elsewhere**

     ● ▶ *H62.8X1 Other disorders of right external ear in diseases classified elsewhere*

     ● ▶ *H62.8X2 Other disorders of left external ear in diseases classified elsewhere*

     ● ▶ *H62.8X3 Other disorders of external ear in diseases classified elsewhere, bilateral*

     ● ■▶ *H62.8X9 Other disorders of external ear in diseases classified elsewhere, unspecified ear*

DISEASES OF MIDDLE EAR AND MASTOID (H65-H75)

(See Plate 94 on page NAP-21.)

● **H65 Nonsuppurative otitis media**

  Bacterial or viral infection or inflammation of the middle ear; may result in fluid accumulation with pain and temporary hearing loss.

  Includes   nonsuppurative otitis media with myringitis

  Use additional code for any associated perforated tympanic membrane (H72.-)

  Use additional code to identify:
   exposure to environmental tobacco smoke (Z77.22)
   exposure to tobacco smoke in the perinatal period (P96.81)
   history of tobacco use (Z87.891)
   occupational exposure to environmental tobacco smoke (Z57.31)
   tobacco dependence (F17.-)
   tobacco use (Z72.0)

  ● **H65.0 Acute serous otitis media**

    Acute and subacute secretory otitis

   ■ **H65.00 Acute serous otitis media, unspecified ear**

   H65.01 Acute serous otitis media, right ear

   H65.02 Acute serous otitis media, left ear

   H65.03 Acute serous otitis media, bilateral

   H65.04 Acute serous otitis media, recurrent, right ear

   H65.05 Acute serous otitis media, recurrent, left ear

   H65.06 Acute serous otitis media, recurrent, bilateral

   ■ **H65.07 Acute serous otitis media, recurrent, unspecified ear**

  ● **H65.1 Other acute nonsuppurative otitis media**

    Excludes1   otitic barotrauma (T70.0)
      otitis media (acute) NOS (H66.9)

   ● **H65.11 Acute and subacute allergic otitis media (mucoid) (sanguinous) (serous)**

    H65.111 Acute and subacute allergic otitis media (mucoid) (sanguinous) (serous), right ear

    H65.112 Acute and subacute allergic otitis media (mucoid) (sanguinous) (serous), left ear

    H65.113 Acute and subacute allergic otitis media (mucoid) (sanguinous) (serous), bilateral

    H65.114 Acute and subacute allergic otitis media (mucoid) (sanguinous) (serous), recurrent, right ear

    H65.115 Acute and subacute allergic otitis media (mucoid) (sanguinous) (serous), recurrent, left ear

    H65.116 Acute and subacute allergic otitis media (mucoid) (sanguinous) (serous), recurrent, bilateral

    ■ **H65.117 Acute and subacute allergic otitis media (mucoid) (sanguinous) (serous), recurrent, unspecified ear**

    ■ **H65.119 Acute and subacute allergic otitis media (mucoid) (sanguinous) (serous), unspecified ear**

CHAPTER 8 (H60-H95)

● **H65.19 Other acute nonsuppurative otitis media**
Acute and subacute mucoid otitis media
Acute and subacute nonsuppurative otitis media NOS
Acute and subacute sanguinous otitis media
Acute and subacute seromucinous otitis media

     H65.191 Other acute nonsuppurative otitis media, right ear

     H65.192 Other acute nonsuppurative otitis media, left ear

     H65.193 Other acute nonsuppurative otitis media, bilateral

     H65.194 Other acute nonsuppurative otitis media, recurrent, right ear

     H65.195 Other acute nonsuppurative otitis media, recurrent, left ear

     H65.196 Other acute nonsuppurative otitis media, recurrent, bilateral

     ■ **H65.197 Other acute nonsuppurative otitis media recurrent, unspecified ear**

     ■ **H65.199 Other acute nonsuppurative otitis media, unspecified ear**

● **H65.2 Chronic serous otitis media**
Chronic tubotympanal catarrh

     ■ **H65.20 Chronic serous otitis media, unspecified ear**

     H65.21 Chronic serous otitis media, right ear

     H65.22 Chronic serous otitis media, left ear

     H65.23 Chronic serous otitis media, bilateral

● **H65.3 Chronic mucoid otitis media**
Chronic mucinous otitis media
Chronic secretory otitis media
Chronic transudative otitis media
Glue ear

     Excludes1   adhesive middle ear disease (H74.1)

     ■ **H65.30 Chronic mucoid otitis media, unspecified ear**

     H65.31 Chronic mucoid otitis media, right ear

     H65.32 Chronic mucoid otitis media, left ear

     H65.33 Chronic mucoid otitis media, bilateral

● **H65.4 Other chronic nonsuppurative otitis media**

     ● **H65.41 Chronic allergic otitis media**

         H65.411 Chronic allergic otitis media, right ear

         H65.412 Chronic allergic otitis media, left ear

         H65.413 Chronic allergic otitis media, bilateral

         ■ **H65.419 Chronic allergic otitis media, unspecified ear**

     ● **H65.49 Other chronic nonsuppurative otitis media**
Chronic exudative otitis media
Chronic nonsuppurative otitis media NOS
Chronic otitis media with effusion (nonpurulent)
Chronic seromucinous otitis media

         H65.491 Other chronic nonsuppurative otitis media, right ear

         H65.492 Other chronic nonsuppurative otitis media, left ear

         H65.493 Other chronic nonsuppurative otitis media, bilateral

         ■ **H65.499 Other chronic nonsuppurative otitis media, unspecified ear**

● **H65.9 Unspecified nonsuppurative otitis media**
Allergic otitis media NOS
Catarrhal otitis media NOS
Exudative otitis media NOS
Mucoid otitis media NOS
Otitis media with effusion (nonpurulent) NOS
Secretory otitis media NOS
Seromucinous otitis media NOS
Serous otitis media NOS
Transudative otitis media NOS

     ■ **H65.90 Unspecified nonsuppurative otitis media, unspecified ear**

     ■ **H65.91 Unspecified nonsuppurative otitis media, right ear**

     ■ **H65.92 Unspecified nonsuppurative otitis media, left ear**

     ■ **H65.93 Unspecified nonsuppurative otitis media, bilateral**

● **H66 Suppurative and unspecified otitis media**
Suppurative: Discharging pus

     Includes   suppurative and unspecified otitis media with myringitis

     Use additional code for any associated perforated tympanic membrane (H72.-)

     Use additional code to identify:
exposure to environmental tobacco smoke (Z77.22)
exposure to tobacco smoke in the perinatal period (P96.81)
history of tobacco use (Z87.891)
occupational exposure to environmental tobacco smoke (Z57.31)
tobacco dependence (F17.-)
tobacco use (Z72.0)

● **H66.0 Acute suppurative otitis media**

     ● **H66.00 Acute suppurative otitis media without spontaneous rupture of ear drum**

         H66.001 Acute suppurative otitis media without spontaneous rupture of ear drum, right ear

         H66.002 Acute suppurative otitis media without spontaneous rupture of ear drum, left ear

         H66.003 Acute suppurative otitis media without spontaneous rupture of ear drum, bilateral

         H66.004 Acute suppurative otitis media without spontaneous rupture of ear drum, recurrent, right ear

         H66.005 Acute suppurative otitis media without spontaneous rupture of ear drum, recurrent, left ear

         H66.006 Acute suppurative otitis media without spontaneous rupture of ear drum, recurrent, bilateral

         ■ **H66.007 Acute suppurative otitis media without spontaneous rupture of ear drum, recurrent, unspecified ear**

         ■ **H66.009 Acute suppurative otitis media without spontaneous rupture of ear drum, unspecified ear**

● **H66.01 Acute suppurative otitis media with spontaneous rupture of ear drum**

 H66.011 Acute suppurative otitis media with spontaneous rupture of ear drum, right ear

 H66.012 Acute suppurative otitis media with spontaneous rupture of ear drum, left ear

 H66.013 Acute suppurative otitis media with spontaneous rupture of ear drum, bilateral

 H66.014 Acute suppurative otitis media with spontaneous rupture of ear drum, recurrent, right ear

 H66.015 Acute suppurative otitis media with spontaneous rupture of ear drum, recurrent, left ear

 H66.016 Acute suppurative otitis media with spontaneous rupture of ear drum, recurrent, bilateral

 H66.017 Acute suppurative otitis media with spontaneous rupture of ear drum, recurrent, unspecified ear

 H66.019 Acute suppurative otitis media with spontaneous rupture of ear drum, unspecified ear

● **H66.1 Chronic tubotympanic suppurative otitis media**
Benign chronic suppurative otitis media
Chronic tubotympanic disease

 H66.10 Chronic tubotympanic suppurative otitis media, unspecified

 H66.11 Chronic tubotympanic suppurative otitis media, right ear

 H66.12 Chronic tubotympanic suppurative otitis media, left ear

 H66.13 Chronic tubotympanic suppurative otitis media, bilateral

● **H66.2 Chronic atticoantral suppurative otitis media**
Chronic atticoantral disease

 H66.20 Chronic atticoantral suppurative otitis media, unspecified ear

 H66.21 Chronic atticoantral suppurative otitis media, right ear

 H66.22 Chronic atticoantral suppurative otitis media, left ear

 H66.23 Chronic atticoantral suppurative otitis media, bilateral

● **H66.3 Other chronic suppurative otitis media**
Chronic suppurative otitis media NOS
Excludes1 tuberculous otitis media (A18.6)

● **H66.3X Other chronic suppurative otitis media**

 H66.3X1 Other chronic suppurative otitis media, right ear

 H66.3X2 Other chronic suppurative otitis media, left ear

 H66.3X3 Other chronic suppurative otitis media, bilateral

 H66.3X9 Other chronic suppurative otitis media, unspecified ear

● **H66.4 Suppurative otitis media, unspecified**
Purulent otitis media NOS

 H66.40 Suppurative otitis media, unspecified, unspecified ear

 H66.41 Suppurative otitis media, unspecified, right ear

 H66.42 Suppurative otitis media, unspecified, left ear

 H66.43 Suppurative otitis media, unspecified, bilateral

● **H66.9 Otitis media, unspecified**
Otitis media NOS
Acute otitis media NOS
Chronic otitis media NOS

 H66.90 Otitis media, unspecified, unspecified ear

 H66.91 Otitis media, unspecified, right ear

 H66.92 Otitis media, unspecified, left ear

 H66.93 Otitis media, unspecified, bilateral

● **H67 Otitis media in diseases classified elsewhere**
Code first underlying disease, such as:
viral disease NEC (B00-B34)
Use additional code for any associated perforated tympanic membrane (H72.-)
Excludes1 otitis media in:
influenza (J09.X9, J10.83, J11.83)
measles (B05.3)
scarlet fever (A38.0)
tuberculosis (A18.6)

 H67.1 Otitis media in diseases classified elsewhere, right ear

 H67.2 Otitis media in diseases classified elsewhere, left ear

 H67.3 Otitis media in diseases classified elsewhere, bilateral

 H67.9 Otitis media in diseases classified elsewhere, unspecified ear

● **H68 Eustachian salpingitis and obstruction**

● **H68.0 Eustachian salpingitis**

● **H68.00 Unspecified Eustachian salpingitis**

 H68.001 Unspecified Eustachian salpingitis, right ear

 H68.002 Unspecified Eustachian salpingitis, left ear

 H68.003 Unspecified Eustachian salpingitis, bilateral

 H68.009 Unspecified Eustachian salpingitis, unspecified ear

● **H68.01 Acute Eustachian salpingitis**

 H68.011 Acute Eustachian salpingitis, right ear

 H68.012 Acute Eustachian salpingitis, left ear

 H68.013 Acute Eustachian salpingitis, bilateral

 H68.019 Acute Eustachian salpingitis, unspecified ear

● **H68.02 Chronic Eustachian salpingitis**

 H68.021 Chronic Eustachian salpingitis, right ear

 H68.022 Chronic Eustachian salpingitis, left ear

 H68.023 Chronic Eustachian salpingitis, bilateral

 H68.029 Chronic Eustachian salpingitis, unspecified ear

CHAPTER 8 (H60-H95)

● **H68.1   Obstruction of Eustachian tube**
    Stenosis of Eustachian tube
    Stricture of Eustachian tube

  ● **H68.10   Unspecified obstruction of Eustachian tube**

    ■ H68.101   Unspecified obstruction of Eustachian tube, right ear

    ■ H68.102   Unspecified obstruction of Eustachian tube, left ear

    ■ H68.103   Unspecified obstruction of Eustachian tube, bilateral

    ■ H68.109   Unspecified obstruction of Eustachian tube, unspecified ear

  ● **H68.11   Osseous obstruction of Eustachian tube**

    H68.111   Osseous obstruction of Eustachian tube, right ear

    H68.112   Osseous obstruction of Eustachian tube, left ear

    H68.113   Osseous obstruction of Eustachian tube, bilateral

    ■ H68.119   Osseous obstruction of Eustachian tube, unspecified ear

  ● **H68.12   Intrinsic cartilagenous obstruction of Eustachian tube**

    H68.121   Intrinsic cartilagenous obstruction of Eustachian tube, right ear

    H68.122   Intrinsic cartilagenous obstruction of Eustachian tube, left ear

    H68.123   Intrinsic cartilagenous obstruction of Eustachian tube, bilateral

    ■ H68.129   Intrinsic cartilagenous obstruction of Eustachian tube, unspecified ear

  ● **H68.13   Extrinsic cartilagenous obstruction of Eustachian tube**
    Compression of Eustachian tube

    H68.131   Extrinsic cartilagenous obstruction of Eustachian tube, right ear

    H68.132   Extrinsic cartilagenous obstruction of Eustachian tube, left ear

    H68.133   Extrinsic cartilagenous obstruction of Eustachian tube, bilateral

    ■ H68.139   Extrinsic cartilagenous obstruction of Eustachian tube, unspecified ear

● **H69   Other and unspecified disorders of Eustachian tube**

  ● **H69.0   Patulous Eustachian tube**

    ■ H69.00   Patulous Eustachian tube, unspecified ear

    H69.01   Patulous Eustachian tube, right ear

    H69.02   Patulous Eustachian tube, left ear

    H69.03   Patulous Eustachian tube, bilateral

  ● **H69.8   Other specified disorders of Eustachian tube**

    ■ H69.80   Other specified disorders of Eustachian tube, unspecified ear

    H69.81   Other specified disorders of Eustachian tube, right ear

    H69.82   Other specified disorders of Eustachian tube, left ear

    H69.83   Other specified disorders of Eustachian tube, bilateral

  ● **H69.9   Unspecified Eustachian tube disorder**

    ■ H69.90   Unspecified Eustachian tube disorder, unspecified ear

    ■ H69.91   Unspecified Eustachian tube disorder, right ear

    ■ H69.92   Unspecified Eustachian tube disorder, left ear

    ■ H69.93   Unspecified Eustachian tube disorder, bilateral

● **H70   Mastoiditis and related conditions**

  ● **H70.0   Acute mastoiditis**
    Abscess of mastoid
    Empyema of mastoid

  ● **H70.00   Acute mastoiditis without complications**

    H70.001   Acute mastoiditis without complications, right ear ✇

    H70.002   Acute mastoiditis without complications, left ear ✇

    H70.003   Acute mastoiditis without complications, bilateral ✇

    ■ H70.009   Acute mastoiditis without complications, unspecified ear ✇

  ● **H70.01   Subperiosteal abscess of mastoid**

    H70.011   Subperiosteal abscess of mastoid, right ear ✇

    H70.012   Subperiosteal abscess of mastoid, left ear ✇

    H70.013   Subperiosteal abscess of mastoid, bilateral ✇

    ■ H70.019   Subperiosteal abscess of mastoid, unspecified ear ✇

  ● **H70.09   Acute mastoiditis with other complications**

    H70.091   Acute mastoiditis with other complications, right ear ✇

    H70.092   Acute mastoiditis with other complications, left ear ✇

    H70.093   Acute mastoiditis with other complications, bilateral ✇

    ■ H70.099   Acute mastoiditis with other complications, unspecified ear ✇

  ● **H70.1   Chronic mastoiditis**
    Caries of mastoid
    Fistula of mastoid

    | Excludes1 | tuberculous mastoiditis (A18.03) |

    ■ H70.10   Chronic mastoiditis, unspecified ear

    H70.11   Chronic mastoiditis, right ear

    H70.12   Chronic mastoiditis, left ear

    H70.13   Chronic mastoiditis, bilateral

Item 8–1   Mastoiditis is an infection of the portion of the temporal bone of the skull that is behind the ear (mastoid process) caused by an untreated otitis media, leading to an infection of the surrounding structures which may include the brain.

●   Unacceptable Principal Diagnosis   ●   Use Additional Character(s)   ■   Unspecified   ▶   Manifestation Code

OGCR   Official Guidelines for Coding and Reporting | Excludes 1 | | Excludes 2 | | Includes | | Use additional | | Code first | | Code also |

● **H70.2**   **Petrositis**
     Inflammation of petrous bone
   ● **H70.20**   Unspecified petrositis
      ■ H70.201   Unspecified petrositis, right ear
      ■ H70.202   Unspecified petrositis, left ear
      ■ H70.203   Unspecified petrositis, bilateral
      ■ H70.209   Unspecified petrositis, unspecified ear
   ● **H70.21**   Acute petrositis
      H70.211   Acute petrositis, right ear
      H70.212   Acute petrositis, left ear
      H70.213   Acute petrositis, bilateral
      ■ H70.219   Acute petrositis, unspecified ear
   ● **H70.22**   Chronic petrositis
      H70.221   Chronic petrositis, right ear
      H70.222   Chronic petrositis, left ear
      H70.223   Chronic petrositis, bilateral
      ■ H70.229   Chronic petrositis, unspecified ear
● **H70.8**   **Other mastoiditis and related conditions**
     Excludes1   preauricular sinus and cyst (Q18.1)
                  sinus, fistula, and cyst of branchial cleft (Q18.0)
   ● **H70.81**   Postauricular fistula
      H70.811   Postauricular fistula, right ear
      H70.812   Postauricular fistula, left ear
      H70.813   Postauricular fistula, bilateral
      ■ H70.819   Postauricular fistula, unspecified ear
   ● **H70.89**   Other mastoiditis and related conditions
      H70.891   Other mastoiditis and related conditions, right ear
      H70.892   Other mastoiditis and related conditions, left ear
      H70.893   Other mastoiditis and related conditions, bilateral
      ■ H70.899   Other mastoiditis and related conditions, unspecified ear
● **H70.9**   **Unspecified mastoiditis**
     ■ H70.90   Unspecified mastoiditis, unspecified ear
     ■ H70.91   Unspecified mastoiditis, right ear
     ■ H70.92   Unspecified mastoiditis, left ear
     ■ H70.93   Unspecified mastoiditis, bilateral

● **H71**   **Cholesteatoma of middle ear**
     Excludes2   cholesteatoma of external ear (H60.4-)
                  recurrent cholesteatoma of postmastoidectomy cavity (H95.0-)
   ● **H71.0**   **Cholesteatoma of attic**
      ■ H71.00   Cholesteatoma of attic, unspecified ear
      H71.01   Cholesteatoma of attic, right ear
      H71.02   Cholesteatoma of attic, left ear
      H71.03   Cholesteatoma of attic, bilateral
   ● **H71.1**   **Cholesteatoma of tympanum**
      ■ H71.10   Cholesteatoma of tympanum, unspecified ear
      H71.11   Cholesteatoma of tympanum, right ear
      H71.12   Cholesteatoma of tympanum, left ear
      H71.13   Cholesteatoma of tympanum, bilateral

● **H71.2**   **Cholesteatoma of mastoid**
     ■ H71.20   Cholesteatoma of mastoid, unspecified ear
     H71.21   Cholesteatoma of mastoid, right ear
     H71.22   Cholesteatoma of mastoid, left ear
     H71.23   Cholesteatoma of mastoid, bilateral
● **H71.3**   **Diffuse cholesteatosis**
     ■ H71.30   Diffuse cholesteatosis, unspecified ear
     H71.31   Diffuse cholesteatosis, right ear
     H71.32   Diffuse cholesteatosis, left ear
     H71.33   Diffuse cholesteatosis, bilateral
● **H71.9**   **Unspecified cholesteatoma**
     ■ H71.90   Unspecified cholesteatoma, unspecified ear
     ■ H71.91   Unspecified cholesteatoma, right ear
     ■ H71.92   Unspecified cholesteatoma, left ear
     ■ H71.93   Unspecified cholesteatoma, bilateral

(See Plate 93 on page NAP-21.)

● **H72**   **Perforation of tympanic membrane**
     Hole or rupture in ear drum
     Includes   persistent post-traumatic perforation of ear drum
                    postinflammatory perforation of ear drum
     Code first any associated otitis media (H65.-, H66.1-, H66.2-, H66.3-, H66.4-, H66.9-, H67.-)
     Excludes1   acute suppurative otitis media with rupture of the tympanic membrane (H66.01-)
                  traumatic rupture of ear drum (S09.2-)
   ● **H72.0**   **Central perforation of tympanic membrane**
      ■ H72.00   Central perforation of tympanic membrane, unspecified ear
      H72.01   Central perforation of tympanic membrane, right ear
      H72.02   Central perforation of tympanic membrane, left ear
      H72.03   Central perforation of tympanic membrane, bilateral
   ● **H72.1**   **Attic perforation of tympanic membrane**
      Perforation of pars flaccida
      ■ H72.10   Attic perforation of tympanic membrane, unspecified ear
      H72.11   Attic perforation of tympanic membrane, right ear
      H72.12   Attic perforation of tympanic membrane, left ear
      H72.13   Attic perforation of tympanic membrane, bilateral
   ● **H72.2**   **Other marginal perforations of tympanic membrane**
     ● **H72.2X**   Other marginal perforations of tympanic membrane
       H72.2X1   Other marginal perforations of tympanic membrane, right ear
       H72.2X2   Other marginal perforations of tympanic membrane, left ear
       H72.2X3   Other marginal perforations of tympanic membrane, bilateral
       ■ H72.2X9   Other marginal perforations of tympanic membrane, unspecified ear

CHAPTER 8 (H60-H95)

● H72.8   **Other perforations of tympanic membrane**

   ● H72.81   **Multiple perforations of tympanic membrane**

       H72.811   **Multiple perforations of tympanic membrane, right ear**

       H72.812   **Multiple perforations of tympanic membrane, left ear**

       H72.813   **Multiple perforations of tympanic membrane, bilateral**

      ■ H72.819   **Multiple perforations of tympanic membrane, unspecified ear**

   ● H72.82   **Total perforations of tympanic membrane**

       H72.821   **Total perforations of tympanic membrane, right ear**

       H72.822   **Total perforations of tympanic membrane, left ear**

       H72.823   **Total perforations of tympanic membrane, bilateral**

      ■ H72.829   **Total perforations of tympanic membrane, unspecified ear**

  ● H72.9   **Unspecified perforation of tympanic membrane**

   ■ H72.90   **Unspecified perforation of tympanic membrane, unspecified ear**

   ■ H72.91   **Unspecified perforation of tympanic membrane, right ear**

   ■ H72.92   **Unspecified perforation of tympanic membrane, left ear**

   ■ H72.93   **Unspecified perforation of tympanic membrane, bilateral**

● H73   **Other disorders of tympanic membrane**

  ● H73.0   **Acute myringitis**

      Excludes1   acute myringitis with otitis media (H65, H66)

   ● H73.00   **Unspecified acute myringitis**
       Acute tympanitis NOS

       H73.001   **Acute myringitis, right ear**

       H73.002   **Acute myringitis, left ear**

       H73.003   **Acute myringitis, bilateral**

      ■ H73.009   **Acute myringitis, unspecified ear**

   ● H73.01   **Bullous myringitis**

       H73.011   **Bullous myringitis, right ear**

       H73.012   **Bullous myringitis, left ear**

       H73.013   **Bullous myringitis, bilateral**

      ■ H73.019   **Bullous myringitis, unspecified ear**

   ● H73.09   **Other acute myringitis**

       H73.091   **Other acute myringitis, right ear**

       H73.092   **Other acute myringitis, left ear**

       H73.093   **Other acute myringitis, bilateral**

      ■ H73.099   **Other acute myringitis, unspecified ear**

  ● H73.1   **Chronic myringitis**
      Chronic tympanitis

      Excludes1   chronic myringitis with otitis media (H65, H66)

   ■ H73.10   **Chronic myringitis, unspecified ear**

    H73.11   **Chronic myringitis, right ear**

    H73.12   **Chronic myringitis, left ear**

    H73.13   **Chronic myringitis, bilateral**

● H73.2   **Unspecified myringitis**

   ■ H73.20   **Unspecified myringitis, unspecified ear**

   ■ H73.21   **Unspecified myringitis, right ear**

   ■ H73.22   **Unspecified myringitis, left ear**

   ■ H73.23   **Unspecified myringitis, bilateral**

● H73.8   **Other specified disorders of tympanic membrane**

  ● H73.81   **Atrophic flaccid tympanic membrane**

       H73.811   **Atrophic flaccid tympanic membrane, right ear**

       H73.812   **Atrophic flaccid tympanic membrane, left ear**

       H73.813   **Atrophic flaccid tympanic membrane, bilateral**

      ■ H73.819   **Atrophic flaccid tympanic membrane, unspecified ear**

  ● H73.82   **Atrophic nonflaccid tympanic membrane**

       H73.821   **Atrophic nonflaccid tympanic membrane, right ear**

       H73.822   **Atrophic nonflaccid tympanic membrane, left ear**

       H73.823   **Atrophic nonflaccid tympanic membrane, bilateral**

      ■ H73.829   **Atrophic nonflaccid tympanic membrane, unspecified ear**

  ● H73.89   **Other specified disorders of tympanic membrane**

       H73.891   **Other specified disorders of tympanic membrane, right ear**

       H73.892   **Other specified disorders of tympanic membrane, left ear**

       H73.893   **Other specified disorders of tympanic membrane, bilateral**

      ■ H73.899   **Other specified disorders of tympanic membrane, unspecified ear**

● H73.9   **Unspecified disorder of tympanic membrane**

   ■ H73.90   **Unspecified disorder of tympanic membrane, unspecified ear**

   ■ H73.91   **Unspecified disorder of tympanic membrane, right ear**

   ■ H73.92   **Unspecified disorder of tympanic membrane, left ear**

   ■ H73.93   **Unspecified disorder of tympanic membrane, bilateral**

● H74   **Other disorders of middle ear mastoid**

      Excludes2   mastoiditis (H70.-)

  ● H74.0   **Tympanosclerosis**

    H74.01   **Tympanosclerosis, right ear**

    H74.02   **Tympanosclerosis, left ear**

    H74.03   **Tympanosclerosis, bilateral**

   ■ H74.09   **Tympanosclerosis, unspecified ear**

  ● H74.1   **Adhesive middle ear disease**
      Adhesive otitis

      Excludes1   glue ear (H65.3-)

    H74.11   **Adhesive right middle ear disease**

    H74.12   **Adhesive left middle ear disease**

    H74.13   **Adhesive middle ear disease, bilateral**

   ■ H74.19   **Adhesive middle ear disease, unspecified ear**

CHAPTER 8 (H60-H95)

● Unacceptable Principal Diagnosis   ● Use Additional Character(s)   ■ Unspecified   ▶ Manifestation Code

OGCR Official Guidelines for Coding and Reporting   Excludes 1   Excludes 2   Includes   Use additional   Code first   Code also

● H74.2 Discontinuity and dislocation of ear ossicles

  ▪ H74.20 Discontinuity and dislocation of ear ossicles, unspecified ear

    H74.21 Discontinuity and dislocation of right ear ossicles

    H74.22 Discontinuity and dislocation of left ear ossicles

    H74.23 Discontinuity and dislocation of ear ossicles, bilateral

● H74.3 Other acquired abnormalities of ear ossicles

  ● H74.31 Ankylosis of ear ossicles

      H74.311 Ankylosis of ear ossicles, right ear

      H74.312 Ankylosis of ear ossicles, left ear

      H74.313 Ankylosis of ear ossicles, bilateral

    ▪ H74.319 Ankylosis of ear ossicles, unspecified ear

  ● H74.32 Partial loss of ear ossicles

      H74.321 Partial loss of ear ossicles, right ear

      H74.322 Partial loss of ear ossicles, left ear

      H74.323 Partial loss of ear ossicles, bilateral

    ▪ H74.329 Partial loss of ear ossicles, unspecified ear

  ● H74.39 Other acquired abnormalities of ear ossicles

      H74.391 Other acquired abnormalities of right ear ossicles

      H74.392 Other acquired abnormalities of left ear ossicles

      H74.393 Other acquired abnormalities of ear ossicles, bilateral

    ▪ H74.399 Other acquired abnormalities of ear ossicles, unspecified ear

● H74.4 Polyp of middle ear

  ▪ H74.40 Polyp of middle ear, unspecified ear

    H74.41 Polyp of right middle ear

    H74.42 Polyp of left middle ear

    H74.43 Polyp of middle ear, bilateral

● H74.8 Other specified disorders of middle ear and mastoid

  ● H74.8X Other specified disorders of middle ear and mastoid

      H74.8X1 Other specified disorders of right middle ear and mastoid

      H74.8X2 Other specified disorders of left middle ear and mastoid

      H74.8X3 Other specified disorders of middle ear and mastoid, bilateral

    ▪ H74.8X9 Other specified disorders of middle ear and mastoid, unspecified ear

● H74.9 Unspecified disorder of middle ear and mastoid

  ▪ H74.90 Unspecified disorder of middle ear and mastoid, unspecified ear

  ▪ H74.91 Unspecified disorder of right middle ear and mastoid

  ▪ H74.92 Unspecified disorder of left middle ear and mastoid

  ▪ H74.93 Unspecified disorder of middle ear and mastoid, bilateral

● H75 Other disorders of middle ear and mastoid in diseases classified elsewhere

  Code first underlying disease

● H75.0 Mastoiditis in infectious and parasitic diseases classified elsewhere

  | Excludes1 | mastoiditis (in):
              syphilis (A52.77)
              tuberculosis (A18.03)

  ● ▪ ▸ *H75.00 Mastoiditis in infectious and parasitic diseases classified elsewhere, unspecified ear*

  ● ▸ *H75.01 Mastoiditis in infectious and parasitic diseases classified elsewhere, right ear*

  ● ▸ *H75.02 Mastoiditis in infectious and parasitic diseases classified elsewhere, left ear*

  ● ▸ *H75.03 Mastoiditis in infectious and parasitic diseases classified elsewhere, bilateral*

● H75.8 Other specified disorders of middle ear and mastoid in diseases classified elsewhere

  ● ▪ ▸ *H75.80 Other specified disorders of middle ear and mastoid in diseases classified elsewhere, unspecified ear*

  ● ▸ *H75.81 Other specified disorders of right middle ear and mastoid in diseases classified elsewhere*

  ● ▸ *H75.82 Other specified disorders of left middle ear and mastoid in diseases classified elsewhere*

  ● ▸ *H75.83 Other specified disorders of middle ear and mastoid in diseases classified elsewhere, bilateral*

DISEASES OF INNER EAR (H80-H83)

(See Plate 95 on page NAP-21.)

● H80 Otosclerosis

  Inherited middle ear spongelike bone growth causing hearing loss

  | Includes | Otospongiosis

● H80.0 Otosclerosis involving oval window, nonobliterative

  ▪ H80.00 Otosclerosis involving oval window, nonobliterative, unspecified ear

    H80.01 Otosclerosis involving oval window, nonobliterative, right ear

    H80.02 Otosclerosis involving oval window, nonobliterative, left ear

    H80.03 Otosclerosis involving oval window, nonobliterative, bilateral

N Newborn Age: 0   **P** Pediatric Age: 0–17   **M** Maternity DX: 12–55   **A** Adult Age: 15–124   ♀ Females Only   ♂ Males Only

🔖 Complication\Comorbidity   🔖 Major C\C   🔖 Present on Admission Requirement   🔖 Hospital-Acquired Condition

1013

● **H80.1 Otosclerosis involving oval window, obliterative**

◻ **H80.10 Otosclerosis involving oval window, obliterative, unspecified ear**

H80.11 Otosclerosis involving oval window, obliterative, right ear

H80.12 Otosclerosis involving oval window, obliterative, left ear

H80.13 Otosclerosis involving oval window, obliterative, bilateral

● **H80.2 Cochlear otosclerosis**
Otosclerosis involving otic capsule
Otosclerosis involving round window

◻ **H80.20 Cochlear otosclerosis, unspecified ear**

H80.21 Cochlear otosclerosis, right ear

H80.22 Cochlear otosclerosis, left ear

H80.23 Cochlear otosclerosis, bilateral

● **H80.8 Other otosclerosis**

◻ **H80.80 Other otosclerosis, unspecified ear**

H80.81 Other otosclerosis, right ear

H80.82 Other otosclerosis, left ear

H80.83 Other otosclerosis, bilateral

● **H80.9 Unspecified otosclerosis**

◻ **H80.90 Unspecified otosclerosis, unspecified ear**

◻ **H80.91 Unspecified otosclerosis, right ear**

◻ **H80.92 Unspecified otosclerosis, left ear**

◻ **H80.93 Unspecified otosclerosis, bilateral**

● **H81 Disorders of vestibular function**

> **Excludes1**   epidemic vertigo (A88.1)
> vertigo NOS (R42)

● **H81.0 Ménière's disease**
Vestibular disorder that produces recurring symptoms including severe and intermittent hearing loss including the feeling of ear pressure or pain.
Labyrinthine hydrops
Ménière's syndrome or vertigo

H81.01 Ménière's disease, right ear

H81.02 Ménière's disease, left ear

H81.03 Ménière's disease, bilateral

◻ **H81.09 Ménière's disease, unspecified ear**

● **H81.1 Benign paroxysmal vertigo**

◻ **H81.10 Benign paroxysmal vertigo, unspecified ear**

H81.11 Benign paroxysmal vertigo, right ear

H81.12 Benign paroxysmal vertigo, left ear

H81.13 Benign paroxysmal vertigo, bilateral

● **H81.2 Vestibular neuronitis**

◻ **H81.20 Vestibular neuronitis, unspecified ear**

H81.21 Vestibular neuronitis, right ear

H81.22 Vestibular neuronitis, left ear

H81.23 Vestibular neuronitis, bilateral

● **H81.3 Other peripheral vertigo**

● **H81.31 Aural vertigo**

H81.311 Aural vertigo, right ear

H81.312 Aural vertigo, left ear

H81.313 Aural vertigo, bilateral

◻ **H81.319 Aural vertigo, unspecified ear**

● **H81.39 Other peripheral vertigo**
Lermoyez' syndrome
Otogenic vertigo
Peripheral vertigo NOS

H81.391 Other peripheral vertigo, right ear

H81.392 Other peripheral vertigo, left ear

H81.393 Other peripheral vertigo, bilateral

◻ **H81.399 Other peripheral vertigo, unspecified ear**

● **H81.4 Vertigo of central origin**
Central positional nystagmus

H81.41 Vertigo of central origin, right ear

H81.42 Vertigo of central origin, left ear

H81.43 Vertigo of central origin, bilateral

◻ **H81.49 Vertigo of central origin, unspecified ear**

● **H81.8 Other disorders of vestibular function**

● **H81.8X Other disorders of vestibular function**

H81.8X1 Other disorders of vestibular function, right ear

H81.8X2 Other disorders of vestibular function, left ear

H81.8X3 Other disorders of vestibular function, bilateral

◻ **H81.8X9 Other disorders of vestibular function, unspecified ear**

● **H81.9 Unspecified disorder of vestibular function**
Vertiginous syndrome NOS

◻ **H81.90 Unspecified disorder of vestibular function, unspecified ear**

◻ **H81.91 Unspecified disorder of vestibular function, right ear**

◻ **H81.92 Unspecified disorder of vestibular function, left ear**

◻ **H81.93 Unspecified disorder of vestibular function, bilateral**

● **H82 Vertiginous syndromes in diseases classified elsewhere**
Code first underlying disease

> **Excludes1**   epidemic vertigo (A88.1)

●▶ *H82.1 Vertiginous syndromes in diseases classified elsewhere, right ear*

●▶ *H82.2 Vertiginous syndromes in diseases classified elsewhere, left ear*

●▶ *H82.3 Vertiginous syndromes in diseases classified elsewhere, bilateral*

●◻▶ *H82.9 Vertiginous syndromes in diseases classified elsewhere, unspecified ear*

● **H83 Other diseases of inner ear**

● **H83.0 Labyrinthitis**
Balance disorder that follows URI or head injury.

H83.01 Labyrinthitis, right ear

H83.02 Labyrinthitis, left ear

H83.03 Labyrinthitis, bilateral

◻ **H83.09 Labyrinthitis, unspecified ear**

● **H83.1 Labyrinthine fistula**

H83.11 Labyrinthine fistula, right ear

H83.12 Labyrinthine fistula, left ear

H83.13 Labyrinthine fistula, bilateral

◻ **H83.19 Labyrinthine fistula, unspecified ear**

● Unacceptable Principal Diagnosis   ● Use Additional Character(s)   ◻ Unspecified   ▶ Manifestation Code
OGCR Official Guidelines for Coding and Reporting | Excludes 1 | | Excludes 2 | Includes   Use additional   Code first   Code also

● **H83.2 Labyrinthine dysfunction**
Labyrinthine hypersensitivity
Labyrinthine hypofunction
Labyrinthine loss of function

  ● **H83.2X Labyrinthine dysfunction**

    H83.2X1 Labyrinthine dysfunction, right ear

    H83.2X2 Labyrinthine dysfunction, left ear

    H83.2X3 Labyrinthine dysfunction, bilateral

    ■ **H83.2X9 Labyrinthine dysfunction, unspecified ear**

● **H83.3 Noise effects on inner ear**
Acoustic trauma of inner ear
Noise-induced hearing loss of inner ear

  ● **H83.3X Noise effects on inner ear**

    H83.3X1 Noise effects on right inner ear

    H83.3X2 Noise effects on left inner ear

    H83.3X3 Noise effects on inner ear, bilateral

    ■ **H83.3X9 Noise effects on inner ear, unspecified ear**

● **H83.8 Other specified diseases of inner ear**

  ● **H83.8X Other specified diseases of inner ear**

    H83.8X1 Other specified diseases of right inner ear

    H83.8X2 Other specified diseases of left inner ear

    H83.8X3 Other specified diseases of inner ear, bilateral

    ■ **H83.8X9 Other specified diseases of inner ear, unspecified ear**

● **H83.9 Unspecified disease of inner ear**

  ■ **H83.90 Unspecified disease of inner ear, unspecified ear**

  ■ **H83.91 Unspecified disease of right inner ear**

  ■ **H83.92 Unspecified disease of left inner ear**

  ■ **H83.93 Unspecified disease of inner ear, bilateral**

OTHER DISORDERS OF EAR (H90-H94)

● **H90 Conductive and sensorineural hearing loss**

  | **Excludes1** | deaf nonspeaking NEC (H91.3)
deafness NOS (H91.9-)
hearing loss NOS (H91.9-)
noise-induced hearing loss (H83.3-)
ototoxic hearing loss (H91.0-)
sudden (idiopathic) hearing loss (H91.2-) |

  H90.0 Conductive hearing loss, bilateral

● **H90.1 Conductive hearing loss, unilateral with unrestricted hearing on the contralateral side**

  H90.11 Conductive hearing loss, unilateral, right ear, with unrestricted hearing on the contralateral side

  H90.12 Conductive hearing loss, unilateral, left ear, with unrestricted hearing on the contralateral side

■ **H90.2 Conductive hearing loss, unspecified**
Conductive deafness NOS

  H90.3 Sensorineural hearing loss, bilateral

● **H90.4 Sensorineural hearing loss, unilateral with unrestricted hearing on the contralateral side**

  H90.41 Sensorineural hearing loss, unilateral, right ear, with unrestricted hearing on the contralateral side

  H90.42 Sensorineural hearing loss, unilateral, left ear, with unrestricted hearing on the contralateral side

■ **H90.5 Unspecified sensorineural hearing loss**
Central hearing loss NOS
Congenital deafness NOS
Neural hearing loss NOS
Perceptive hearing loss NOS
Sensorineural deafness NOS
Sensory hearing loss NOS

  | **Excludes1** | abnormal auditory perception (H93.2-)
psychogenic deafness (F44.6) |

  H90.6 Mixed conductive and sensorineural hearing loss, bilateral

● **H90.7 Mixed conductive and sensorineural hearing loss, unilateral with unrestricted hearing on the contralateral side**

  H90.71 Mixed conductive and sensorineural hearing loss, unilateral, right ear, with unrestricted hearing on the contralateral side

  H90.72 Mixed conductive and sensorineural hearing loss, unilateral, left ear, with unrestricted hearing on the contralateral side

■ **H90.8 Mixed conductive and sensorineural hearing loss, unspecified**

● **H91 Other and unspecified hearing loss**

  | **Excludes1** | abnormal auditory perception (H93.2-)
hearing loss as classified in H90.-
impacted cerumen (H61.2-)
noise-induced hearing loss (H83.3-)
psychogenic deafness (F44.6)
transient ischemic deafness (H93.01-) |

● **H91.0 Ototoxic hearing loss**

  Code first poisoning due to drug or toxin, if applicable (T36-T65 with fifth or sixth character 1-4 or 6)

  Use additional code for adverse effect, if applicable, to identify drug (T36-T50 with fifth or sixth character 5)

  ● **H91.01 Ototoxic hearing loss, right ear**

  ● **H91.02 Ototoxic hearing loss, left ear**

  ● **H91.03 Ototoxic hearing loss, bilateral**

  ●■ **H91.09 Ototoxic hearing loss, unspecified ear**

● **H91.1 Presbycusis**
Presbyacusia

  ■ **H91.10 Presbycusis, unspecified ear**

  H91.11 Presbycusis, right ear

  H91.12 Presbycusis, left ear

  H91.13 Presbycusis, bilateral

● **H91.2 Sudden idiopathic hearing loss**
Sudden hearing loss NOS

  ■ **H91.20 Sudden idiopathic hearing loss, unspecified ear**

  H91.21 Sudden idiopathic hearing loss, right ear

  H91.22 Sudden idiopathic hearing loss, left ear

  H91.23 Sudden idiopathic hearing loss, bilateral

CHAPTER 8 (H60-H95)

N Newborn Age: 0   **P** Pediatric Age: 0–17   **M** Maternity DX: 12–55   **A** Adult Age: 15–124   ♀ Females Only   ♂ Males Only

🅒 Complication\Comorbidity   Major C\C   Present on Admission Requirement   Hospital-Acquired Condition

1015

CHAPTER 8 (H60-H95)

H91.3 Deaf nonspeaking, not elsewhere classified

● H91.8 Other specified hearing loss

  ● H91.8X Other specified hearing loss

    H91.8X1 Other specified hearing loss, right ear

    H91.8X2 Other specified hearing loss, left ear

    H91.8X3 Other specified hearing loss, bilateral

    H91.8X9 Other specified hearing loss, unspecified ear

● H91.9 Unspecified hearing loss
Deafness NOS
High frequency deafness
Low frequency deafness

  H91.90 Unspecified hearing loss, unspecified ear

  H91.91 Unspecified hearing loss, right ear

  H91.92 Unspecified hearing loss, left ear

  H91.93 Unspecified hearing loss, bilateral

● H92 Otalgia and effusion of ear

  ● H92.0 Otalgia

    H92.01 Otalgia, right ear

    H92.02 Otalgia, left ear

    H92.03 Otalgia, bilateral

    H92.09 Otalgia, unspecified ear

  ● H92.1 Otorrhea

    Excludes1 leakage of cerebrospinal fluid through ear (G96.0)

    H92.10 Otorrhea, unspecified ear

    H92.11 Otorrhea, right ear

    H92.12 Otorrhea, left ear

    H92.13 Otorrhea, bilateral

  ● H92.2 Otorrhagia

    Excludes1 traumatic otorrhagia - code to injury

    H92.20 Otorrhagia, unspecified ear

    H92.21 Otorrhagia, right ear

    H92.22 Otorrhagia, left ear

    H92.23 Otorrhagia, bilateral

● H93 Other disorders of ear, not elsewhere classified

  ● H93.0 Degenerative and vascular disorders of ear

    Excludes1 presbycusis (H91.1)

    ● H93.01 Transient ischemic deafness

      H93.011 Transient ischemic deafness, right ear

      H93.012 Transient ischemic deafness, left ear

      H93.013 Transient ischemic deafness, bilateral

      H93.019 Transient ischemic deafness, unspecified ear

    ● H93.09 Unspecified degenerative and vascular disorders of ear

      H93.091 Unspecified degenerative and vascular disorders of right ear

      H93.092 Unspecified degenerative and vascular disorders of left ear

      H93.093 Unspecified degenerative and vascular disorders of ear, bilateral

      H93.099 Unspecified degenerative and vascular disorders of unspecified ear

  ● H93.1 Tinnitus
Perception of sound (ringing, buzzing, humming, whistling tunes, or singing)

    H93.11 Tinnitus, right ear

    H93.12 Tinnitus, left ear

    H93.13 Tinnitus, bilateral

    H93.19 Tinnitus, unspecified ear

  ● H93.2 Other abnormal auditory perceptions

    Excludes2 auditory hallucinations (R44.0)

    ● H93.21 Auditory recruitment

      H93.211 Auditory recruitment, right ear

      H93.212 Auditory recruitment, left ear

      H93.213 Auditory recruitment, bilateral

      H93.219 Auditory recruitment, unspecified ear

    ● H93.22 Diplacusis

      H93.221 Diplacusis, right ear

      H93.222 Diplacusis, left ear

      H93.223 Diplacusis, bilateral

      H93.229 Diplacusis, unspecified ear

    ● H93.23 Hyperacusis

      H93.231 Hyperacusis, right ear

      H93.232 Hyperacusis, left ear

      H93.233 Hyperacusis, bilateral

      H93.239 Hyperacusis, unspecified ear

    ● H93.24 Temporary auditory threshold shift

      H93.241 Temporary auditory threshold shift, right ear

      H93.242 Temporary auditory threshold shift, left ear

      H93.243 Temporary auditory threshold shift, bilateral

      H93.249 Temporary auditory threshold shift, unspecified ear

    H93.25 Central auditory processing disorder
Congenital auditory imperception
Word deafness

      Excludes1 mixed receptive-expressive language disorder (F80.2)

    ● H93.29 Other abnormal auditory perceptions

      H93.291 Other abnormal auditory perceptions, right ear

      H93.292 Other abnormal auditory perceptions, left ear

      H93.293 Other abnormal auditory perceptions, bilateral

      H93.299 Other abnormal auditory perceptions, unspecified ear

● Unacceptable Principal Diagnosis   ● Use Additional Character(s)   ■ Unspecified   ▶ Manifestation Code

OGCR Official Guidelines for Coding and Reporting   Excludes 1   Excludes 2   Includes   Use additional   Code first   Code also

● **H93.3   Disorders of acoustic nerve**
     Disorder of 8th cranial nerve
     Excludes1   acoustic neuroma (D33.3)
                  syphilitic acoustic neuritis (A52.15)

   ● **H93.3X   Disorders of acoustic nerve**
       H93.3X1   Disorders of right acoustic nerve
       H93.3X2   Disorders of left acoustic nerve
       H93.3X3   Disorders of bilateral acoustic nerves
       ■ **H93.3X9   Disorders of unspecified acoustic nerve**

● **H93.8   Other specified disorders of ear**
   ● **H93.8X   Other specified disorders of ear**
       H93.8X1   Other specified disorders of right ear
       H93.8X2   Other specified disorders of left ear
       H93.8X3   Other specified disorders of ear, bilateral
       ■ **H93.8X9   Other specified disorders of ear, unspecified ear**

● **H93.9   Unspecified disorder of ear**
   ● **H93.90   Unspecified disorder of ear, unspecified ear**
   ●■ **H93.91   Unspecified disorder of right ear**
   ●■ **H93.92   Unspecified disorder of left ear**
   ●■ **H93.93   Unspecified disorder of ear, bilateral**

● **H94   Other disorders of ear in diseases classified elsewhere**
   ● **H94.0   Acoustic neuritis in infectious and parasitic diseases classified elsewhere**
     Code first *underlying disease, such as:*
     parasitic disease (B65-B89)
     Excludes1   acoustic neuritis (in):
                  herpes zoster (B02.29)
                  syphilis (A52.15)

   ●■▶ *H94.00   Acoustic neuritis in infectious and parasitic diseases classified elsewhere, unspecified ear*
   ●▶ *H94.01   Acoustic neuritis in infectious and parasitic diseases classified elsewhere, right ear*
   ●▶ *H94.02   Acoustic neuritis in infectious and parasitic diseases classified elsewhere, left ear*
   ●▶ *H94.03   Acoustic neuritis in infectious and parasitic diseases classified elsewhere, bilateral*

   ● **H94.8   Other specified disorders of ear in diseases classified elsewhere**
     Code first *underlying disease, such as:*
     congenital syphilis (A50.0)
     Excludes1   aural myiasis (B87.4)
                  syphilitic labyrinthitis (A52.79)

   ●■▶ *H94.80   Other specified disorders of ear in diseases classified elsewhere, unspecified ear*
   ●▶ *H94.81   Other specified disorders of right ear in diseases classified elsewhere*
   ●▶ *H94.82   Other specified disorders of left ear in diseases classified elsewhere*
   ●▶ *H94.83   Other specified disorders of ear in diseases classified elsewhere, bilateral*

● **H95   Intraoperative and postprocedural complications and disorders of ear and mastoid process, not elsewhere classified**
   ● **H95.0   Recurrent cholesteatoma of postmastoidectomy cavity**
     ■ **H95.00   Recurrent cholesteatoma of postmastoidectomy cavity, unspecified ear**
     H95.01   Recurrent cholesteatoma of postmastoidectomy cavity, right ear
     H95.02   Recurrent cholesteatoma of postmastoidectomy cavity, left ear
     H95.03   Recurrent cholesteatoma of postmastoidectomy cavity, bilateral ears

   ● **H95.1   Other disorders of ear and mastoid process following mastoidectomy**
     ● **H95.11   Chronic inflammation of postmastoidectomy cavity**
       H95.111   Chronic inflammation of postmastoidectomy cavity, right ear
       H95.112   Chronic inflammation of postmastoidectomy cavity, left ear
       H95.113   Chronic inflammation of postmastoidectomy cavity, bilateral ears
       ■ **H95.119   Chronic inflammation of postmastoidectomy cavity, unspecified ear**

     ● **H95.12   Granulation of postmastoidectomy cavity**
       H95.121   Granulation of postmastoidectomy cavity, right ear
       H95.122   Granulation of postmastoidectomy cavity, left ear
       H95.123   Granulation of postmastoidectomy cavity, bilateral ears
       ■ **H95.129   Granulation of postmastoidectomy cavity, unspecified ear**

     ● **H95.13   Mucosal cyst of postmastoidectomy cavity**
       H95.131   Mucosal cyst of postmastoidectomy cavity, right ear
       H95.132   Mucosal cyst of postmastoidectomy cavity, left ear
       H95.133   Mucosal cyst of postmastoidectomy cavity, bilateral ears
       ■ **H95.139   Mucosal cyst of postmastoidectomy cavity, unspecified ear**

CHAPTER 8 (H60-H95)

CHAPTER 8 (H60-H95)

● H95.19   Other disorders following mastoidectomy

    H95.191   Other disorders following mastoidectomy, right ear

    H95.192   Other disorders following mastoidectomy, left ear

    H95.193   Other disorders following mastoidectomy, bilateral ears

    ■ H95.199   Other disorders following mastoidectomy, unspecified ear

● H95.2   Intraoperative hemorrhage and hematoma of ear and mastoid process complicating a procedure

    Excludes1   intraoperative hemorrhage and hematoma of ear and mastoid process due to accidental puncture or laceration during a procedure (H95.3-)

    H95.21   Intraoperative hemorrhage and hematoma of ear and mastoid process complicating a procedure on the ear and mastoid process

    H95.22   Intraoperative hemorrhage and hematoma of ear and mastoid process complicating other procedure

● H95.3   Accidental puncture and laceration of ear and mastoid process during a procedure

    H95.31   Accidental puncture and laceration of the ear and mastoid process during a procedure on the ear and mastoid process

    H95.32   Accidental puncture and laceration of the ear and mastoid process during other procedure

● H95.4   Postprocedural hemorrhage and hematoma of ear and mastoid process following a procedure

    H95.41   Postprocedural hemorrhage and hematoma of ear and mastoid process following a procedure on the ear and mastoid process

    H95.42   Postprocedural hemorrhage and hematoma of ear and mastoid process following other procedure

● H95.8   Other intraoperative and postprocedural complications and disorders of the ear and mastoid process, not elsewhere classified

    Excludes2   postprocedural complications and disorders following mastoidectomy (H95.0-, H95.1-)

    ● H95.81   Postprocedural stenosis of external ear canal

      H95.811   Postprocedural stenosis of right external ear canal

      H95.812   Postprocedural stenosis of left external ear canal

      H95.813   Postprocedural stenosis of external ear canal, bilateral

      ■ H95.819   Postprocedural stenosis of unspecified external ear canal

    H95.88   Other intraoperative complications and disorders of the ear and mastoid process, not elsewhere classified

      Use additional code, if applicable, to further specify disorder

    H95.89   Other postprocedural complications and disorders of the ear and mastoid process, not elsewhere classified

      Use additional code, if applicable, to further specify disorder

● Unacceptable Principal Diagnosis   ● Use Additional Character(s)   ■ Unspecified   ▶ Manifestation Code
OGCR Official Guidelines for Coding and Reporting   Excludes 1   Excludes 2   Includes   Use additional   Code first   Code also

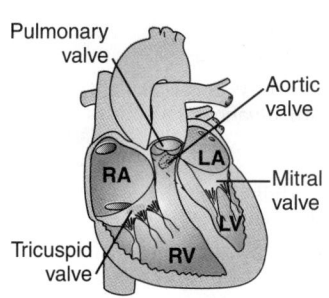

Figure 9-1 Cardiovascular valves.

Item 9–1 Rheumatic fever is the inflammation of the valve(s) of the heart, usually the mitral or aortic, which leads to valve damage. Rheumatic heart inflammations are usually **pericarditis** (sac surrounding heart), **endocarditis** (heart cavity), or **myocarditis** (heart muscle).

CHAPTER 9 DISEASES OF THE CIRCULATORY SYSTEM (I00-I99)

Excludes2 certain conditions originating in the perinatal period (P04-P96)
certain infectious and parasitic diseases (A00-B99)
complications of pregnancy, childbirth and the puerperium (O00-O9A)
congenital malformations, deformations, and chromosomal abnormalities (Q00-Q99)
endocrine, nutritional and metabolic diseases (E00-E88)
injury, poisoning and certain other consequences of external causes (S00-T88)
neoplasms (C00-D49)
symptoms, signs and abnormal clinical and laboratory findings, not elsewhere classified (R00-R94)
systemic connective tissue disorders (M30-M36)
transient cerebral ischemic attacks and related syndromes (G45.-)

This chapter contains the following blocks:

I00-I02	Acute rheumatic fever
I05-I09	Chronic rheumatic heart diseases
I10-I15	Hypertensive diseases
I20-I25	Ischemic heart diseases
I26-I28	Pulmonary heart disease and diseases of pulmonary circulation
I30-I52	Other forms of heart disease
I60-I69	Cerebrovascular diseases
I70-I79	Diseases of arteries, arterioles and capillaries
I80-I89	Diseases of veins, lymphatic vessels and lymph nodes, not elsewhere classified
I95-I99	Other and unspecified disorders of the circulatory system

ACUTE RHEUMATIC FEVER (I00-I02)

I00 Rheumatic fever without heart involvement
Includes arthritis, rheumatic, acute or subacute
Excludes1 rheumatic fever with heart involvement (I01.0 - I01.9)

Item 9–2 Rheumatic chorea, also called Sydenham's, juvenile, minor, simple, or St. Vitus' dance, is a major symptom of rheumatic fever and is characterized by ceaseless, involuntary, jerky, purposeless movements.

● I01 Rheumatic fever with heart involvement
Excludes1 chronic diseases of rheumatic origin (I05-I09) unless rheumatic fever is also present or there is evidence of reactivation or activity of the rheumatic process.

I01.0 **Acute rheumatic pericarditis** 🍊
Any condition in I00 with pericarditis
Rheumatic pericarditis (acute)
Excludes1 acute pericarditis not specified as rheumatic (I30.-)

I01.1 **Acute rheumatic endocarditis** 🍊
Any condition in I00 with endocarditis or valvulitis
Acute rheumatic valvulitis

I01.2 **Acute rheumatic myocarditis** 🍊
Any condition in I00 with myocarditis

I01.8 **Other acute rheumatic heart disease** 🍊
Any condition in I00 with other or multiple types of heart involvement
Acute rheumatic pancarditis

■ I01.9 **Acute rheumatic heart disease, unspecified** 🍊
Any condition in I00 with unspecified type of heart involvement
Rheumatic carditis, acute
Rheumatic heart disease, active or acute

● I02 Rheumatic chorea
Includes Sydenham's chorea
Excludes1 chorea NOS (G25.5)
Huntington's chorea (G10)

I02.0 **Rheumatic chorea with heart involvement** 🍊
Chorea NOS with heart involvement
Rheumatic chorea with heart involvement of any type classifiable under I01.-

I02.9 **Rheumatic chorea without heart involvement** 🍊
Rheumatic chorea NOS

CHRONIC RHEUMATIC HEART DISEASES (I05-I09)

● I05 Rheumatic mitral valve diseases
Includes conditions classifiable to both I05.0 and I05.2-I05.9, whether specified as rheumatic or not
Excludes1 mitral valve disease specified as nonrheumatic (I34.-)
mitral valve disease with aortic and/or tricuspid valve involvement (I08.-)

I05.0 **Rheumatic mitral stenosis**
Mitral (valve) obstruction (rheumatic)

I05.1 **Rheumatic mitral insufficiency**
Rheumatic mitral incompetence
Rheumatic mitral regurgitation
Excludes1 mitral insufficiency not specified as rheumatic (I34.0)

(See Plate 244 on page NAP-30.)

Item 9–3 Mitral stenosis is the narrowing of the mitral valve separating the left atrium from the left ventricle. **Mitral insufficiency** is the improper closure of the mitral valve which may lead to enlargement (hypertrophy) of the left atrium.

N Newborn Age: 0 P Pediatric Age: 0–17 M Maternity DX: 12–55 A Adult Age: 15-124 ♀ Females Only ♂ Males Only
🍊 Complication\Comorbidity Major C\C Present on Admission Requirement Hospital-Acquired Condition
1019

CHAPTER 9 (I00-I99)

Item 9–4 Aortic stenosis is the narrowing of the aortic valve located between the left ventricle and the aorta. **Aortic insufficiency** is the improper closure of the aortic valve which may lead to enlargement (hypertrophy) of the left ventricle.

I05.8   **Other rheumatic mitral valve diseases**
Rheumatic mitral (valve) failure

I05.9   **Rheumatic mitral valve disease, unspecified**
Rheumatic mitral (valve) disorder (chronic) NOS

● **I06**   **Rheumatic aortic valve diseases**

> Excludes1   aortic valve disease not specified as rheumatic (I35.-)
> aortic valve disease with mitral and/or tricuspid valve involvement (I08.-)

I06.0   **Rheumatic aortic stenosis**
Rheumatic aortic (valve) obstruction

I06.1   **Rheumatic aortic insufficiency**
Rheumatic aortic incompetence
Rheumatic aortic regurgitation

I06.2   **Rheumatic aortic stenosis with insufficiency**
Rheumatic aortic stenosis with incompetence or regurgitation

I06.8   **Other rheumatic aortic valve diseases**

I06.9   **Rheumatic aortic valve disease, unspecified**
Rheumatic aortic (valve) disease NOS

● **I07**   **Rheumatic tricuspid valve diseases**

> Includes   rheumatic tricuspid valve diseases specified as rheumatic or unspecified

> Excludes1   tricuspid valve disease specified as nonrheumatic (I36.-)
> tricuspid valve disease with aortic and/or mitral valve involvement (I08.-)

I07.0   **Rheumatic tricuspid stenosis**
Tricuspid (valve) stenosis (rheumatic)

I07.1   **Rheumatic tricuspid insufficiency**
Tricuspid (valve) insufficiency (rheumatic)

I07.2   **Rheumatic tricuspid stenosis and insufficiency**

I07.8   **Other rheumatic tricuspid valve diseases**

I07.9   **Rheumatic tricuspid valve disease, unspecified**
Rheumatic tricuspid valve disorder NOS

● **I08**   **Multiple valve diseases**

> Includes   multiple valve diseases specified as rheumatic or unspecified

> Excludes1   endocarditis, valve unspecified (I38)
> multiple valve disease specified a nonrheumatic (I34.-, I35.-, I36.-, I37.-, I38.-, Q22.-, Q23.-, Q24.8-)
> rheumatic valve disease NOS (I09.1)

I08.0   **Rheumatic disorders of both mitral and aortic valves**
Involvement of both mitral and aortic valves specified as rheumatic or unspecified

I08.1   **Rheumatic disorders of both mitral and tricuspid valves**

I08.2   **Rheumatic disorders of both aortic and tricuspid valves**

I08.3   **Combined rheumatic disorders of mitral, aortic and tricuspid valves**

I08.8   **Other rheumatic multiple valve diseases**

I08.9   **Rheumatic multiple valve disease, unspecified**

● **I09**   **Other rheumatic heart diseases**

I09.0   **Rheumatic myocarditis** 🔗

> Excludes1   myocarditis not specified as rheumatic (I51.4)

I09.1   **Rheumatic diseases of endocardium, valve unspecified**
Rheumatic endocarditis (chronic)
Rheumatic valvulitis (chronic)

> Excludes1   endocarditis, valve unspecified (I38)

I09.2   **Chronic rheumatic pericarditis** 🔗
Adherent pericardium, rheumatic
Chronic rheumatic mediastinopericarditis
Chronic rheumatic myopericarditis

> Excludes1   chronic pericarditis not specified as rheumatic (I31.-)

● **I09.8**   **Other specified rheumatic heart diseases**

I09.81   **Rheumatic heart failure** 🔗

> Use additional code to identify type of heart failure (I50.-)

I09.89   **Other specified rheumatic heart diseases**
Rheumatic disease of pulmonary valve

I09.9   **Rheumatic heart disease, unspecified**
Rheumatic carditis

> Excludes1   rheumatoid carditis (M05.31)

HYPERTENSIVE DISEASES (I10-I15)

> Use additional code to identify:
> exposure to environmental tobacco smoke (Z77.22)
> history of tobacco use (Z87.891)
> occupational exposure to environmental tobacco smoke (Z57.31)
> tobacco dependence (F17.-)
> tobacco use (Z72.0)

> Excludes1   hypertensive disease complicating pregnancy, childbirth and the puerperium (O10-O11, O13-O16)
> neonatal hypertension (P29.2)
> primary pulmonary hypertension (I27.0)

I10   **Essential (primary) hypertension**

> Includes   high blood pressure
> hypertension (arterial) (benign) (essential) (malignant) (primary) (systemic)

> Excludes1   hypertensive disease complicating pregnancy, childbirth and the puerperium (O10-O11, O13-O16)

> Excludes2   essential (primary) hypertension involving vessels of brain (I60-I69)
> essential (primary) hypertension involving vessels of eye (H35.0-)

MCE: Questionable admission when principal dx

● **I11**   **Hypertensive heart disease**

> Includes   any condition in I51.4-I51.9 due to hypertension

I11.0   **Hypertensive heart disease with heart failure**
Hypertensive heart failure

> Use additional code to identify type of heart failure (I50.-)

I11.9   **Hypertensive heart disease without heart failure**
Hypertensive heart disease NOS

Item 9–5 Hypertension is caused by high arterial blood pressure in the arteries. **Essential, primary,** or **idiopathic** hypertension occurs without identifiable organic cause. **Secondary** hypertension is that which has an organic cause. **Malignant** hypertension is severely elevated blood pressure. **Benign** hypertension is mildly elevated blood pressure.

● Unacceptable Principal Diagnosis   ● Use Additional Character(s)   ■ Unspecified   ▶ Manifestation Code

OGCR Official Guidelines for Coding and Reporting   Excludes 1   Excludes 2   Includes   Use additional   Code first   Code also

OGCR Section I.C.9.a.2

Hypertensive Chronic Kidney Disease

Assign codes from category I12, Hypertensive chronic kidney disease, when both hypertension and a condition classifiable to category N18, Chronic kidney disease (CKD), are present. Unlike hypertension with heart disease, ICD-10-CM presumes a cause-and-effect relationship and classifies chronic kidney disease with hypertension as hypertensive chronic kidney disease.

The appropriate code from category N18 should be used as a secondary code with a code from category I12 to identify the stage of chronic kidney disease.

See Section I.C.14. Chronic kidney disease.

If a patient has hypertensive chronic kidney disease and acute renal failure, an additional code for the acute renal failure is required.

● **I12**   **Hypertensive chronic kidney disease**

     Includes   any condition in N18 and N26 - due to
              hypertension
              arteriosclerosis of kidney
              arteriosclerotic nephritis (chronic)
                (interstitial)
              hypertensive nephropathy
              nephrosclerosis

     Excludes1   hypertension due to kidney disease (I15.0,
              I15.1)
              renovascular hypertension (I15.0)
              secondary hypertension (I15.-)

     Excludes2   acute kidney failure (N17.-)

   I12.0   **Hypertensive chronic kidney disease with stage 5 chronic kidney disease or end stage renal disease** 🔵

       Use additional code to identify the stage of chronic kidney disease (N18.5, N18.6)

   ■ **I12.9**   **Hypertensive chronic kidney disease with stage 1 through stage 4 chronic kidney disease, or unspecified chronic kidney disease**
       Hypertensive chronic kidney disease NOS
       Hypertensive renal disease NOS

       Use additional code to identify the stage of chronic kidney disease (N18.1-N18.4, N18.9)

OGCR Section I.c.9.a.6

Hypertensive Heart and Chronic Kidney Disease

Assign codes from combination category I13, Hypertensive heart and chronic kidney disease, when both hypertensive kidney disease and hypertensive heart disease are stated in the diagnosis. Assume a relationship between the hypertension and the chronic kidney disease, whether or not the condition is so designated. If heart failure is present, assign an additional code from category I50 to identify the type of heart failure.

The appropriate code from category N18, Chronic kidney disease, should be used as a secondary code with a code from category I13 to identify the stage of chronic kidney disease.

See Section I.C.14. Chronic kidney disease.

The codes in category I13, Hypertensive heart and chronic kidney disease, are combination codes that include hypertension, heart disease and chronic kidney disease. The Includes note at I13 specifies that the conditions included at I11 and I12 are included together in I13. If a patient has hypertension, heart disease and chronic kidney disease then a code from I13 should be used, not individual codes for hypertension, heart disease and chronic kidney disease, or codes from I11 or I12.

For patients with both acute renal failure and chronic kidney disease an additional code for acute renal failure is required.

● **I13**   **Hypertensive heart and chronic kidney disease**

     Includes   any condition in I11.- with any condition in
              I12.- cardiorenal disease
              cardiovascular renal disease

   ■ **I13.0**   **Hypertensive heart and chronic kidney disease with heart failure and stage 1 through stage 4 chronic kidney disease, or unspecified chronic kidney disease** 🔵

       Use additional code to identify type of heart failure (I50.-)

       Use additional code to identify stage of chronic kidney disease (N18.1-N18.4, N18.9)

   ● **I13.1**   **Hypertensive heart and chronic kidney disease without heart failure**

     ■ **I13.10**   **Hypertensive heart and chronic kidney disease without heart failure, with stage 1 through stage 4 chronic kidney disease, or unspecified chronic kidney disease**
         Hypertensive heart disease and hypertensive chronic kidney disease NOS

         Use additional code to identify the stage of chronic kidney disease (N18.1-N18.4, N18.9)

     I13.11   **Hypertensive heart and chronic kidney disease without heart failure, with stage 5 chronic kidney disease, or end stage renal disease** 🔵

         Use additional code to identify the stage of chronic kidney disease (N18.5, N18.6)

   I13.2   **Hypertensive heart and chronic kidney disease with heart failure and with stage 5 chronic kidney disease, or end stage renal disease** 🔵

       Use additional code to identify type of heart failure (I50.-)

       Use additional code to identify the stage of chronic kidney disease (N18.5, N18.6)

OGCR Section I.9.a.6

Hypertension, Secondary

Secondary hypertension is due to an underlying condition. Two codes are required: one to identify the underlying etiology and one from category I15 to identify the hypertension. Sequencing of codes is determined by the reason for admission/encounter.

● **I15**   **Secondary hypertension**

     Code also underlying condition

     Excludes1   postprocedural hypertension (I97.3)

     Excludes2   secondary hypertension involving vessels of
              brain (I60-I69)
              secondary hypertension involving vessels of
              eye (H35.0-)

   I15.0   **Renovascular hypertension**

   I15.1   **Hypertension secondary to other renal disorders**

   I15.2   **Hypertension secondary to endocrine disorders**

   I15.8   **Other secondary hypertension**

   ■ **I15.9**   **Secondary hypertension, unspecified**

CHAPTER 9 (I00-I99)

N Newborn Age: 0   **P** Pediatric Age: 0–17   **M** Maternity DX: 12–55   **A** Adult Age: 15–124   ♀ Females Only   ♂ Males Only

🔵 Complication\Comorbidity   🔵 Major C\C   🔵 Present on Admission Requirement   🔵 Hospital-Acquired Condition   **1021**

ISCHEMIC HEART DISEASES (I20-I25)

Use additional code to identify presence of hypertension (I10-I15)

● **I20**   **Angina pectoris**

Chest pain/discomfort due to lack of oxygen to the heart muscle. Principal symptom of myocardial infarction.

Use additional code to identify:
exposure to environmental tobacco smoke (Z77.22)
history of tobacco use (Z87.891)
occupational exposure to environmental tobacco smoke (Z57.31)
tobacco dependence (F17.-)
tobacco use (Z72.0)

Excludes1   angina pectoris with atherosclerotic heart disease of native coronary arteries (I25.1-)
atherosclerosis of coronary artery bypass graft(s) and coronary artery of transplanted heart with angina pectoris (I25.7-)
postinfarction angina (I23.7)

   I20.0   **Unstable angina** 🔹
Accelerated angina
Crescendo angina
De novo effort angina
Intermediate coronary syndrome
Preinfarction syndrome
Worsening effort angina

   I20.1   **Angina pectoris with documented spasm** 🔹
Angiospastic angina
Prinzmetal angina
Spasm-induced angina
Variant angina

   I20.8   **Other forms of angina pectoris**
Angina equivalent
Angina of effort
Coronary slow flow syndrome
Stenocardia

Use additional code(s) for symptoms associated with angina equivalent

   ■ **I20.9**   **Angina pectoris, unspecified**
Angina NOS
Anginal syndrome
Cardiac angina
Ischemic chest pain

I21   **ST elevation (STEMI) and non-ST elevation (NSTEMI) myocardial infarction**

Includes   cardiac infarction
coronary (artery) embolism
coronary (artery) occlusion
coronary (artery) rupture
coronary (artery) thrombosis
infarction of heart, myocardium, or ventricle
myocardial infarction specified as acute or with a stated duration of 4 weeks (28 days) or less from onset

Use additional code, if applicable, to identify:
exposure to environmental tobacco smoke (Z77.22)
history of tobacco use (Z87.891)
occupational exposure to environmental tobacco smoke (Z57.31)
status post administration of tPA (rtPA) in a different facility within the last 24 hours prior to admission to current facility (Z92.82)
tobacco dependence (F17.-)
tobacco use (Z72.0)

Excludes2   old myocardial infarction (I25.2)
postmyocardial infarction syndrome (I24.1)
subsequent myocardial infarction (I22.-)

● **I21.0**   **ST elevation (STEMI) myocardial infarction of anterior wall**

   I21.01   **ST elevation (STEMI) myocardial infarction involving left main coronary artery** 🔹

   I21.02   **ST elevation (STEMI) myocardial infarction involving left anterior descending coronary artery** 🔹
ST elevation (STEMI) myocardial infarction involving diagonal coronary artery

   I21.09   **ST elevation (STEMI) myocardial infarction involving other coronary artery of anterior wall** 🔹
Acute transmural myocardial infarction of anterior wall
Anteroapical transmural (Q wave) infarction (acute)
Anterolateral transmural (Q wave) infarction (acute)
Anteroseptal transmural (Q wave) infarction (acute)
Transmural (Q wave) infarction (acute) (of) anterior (wall) NOS

● **I21.1**   **ST elevation (STEMI) myocardial infarction of inferior wall**

   I21.11   **ST elevation (STEMI) myocardial infarction involving right coronary artery** 🔹
Inferoposterior transmural (Q wave) infarction (acute)

   I21.19   **ST elevation (STEMI) myocardial infarction involving other coronary artery of inferior wall** 🔹
Acute transmural myocardial infarction of inferior wall
Inferolateral transmural (Q wave) infarction (acute)
Transmural (Q wave) infarction (acute) (of) diaphragmatic wall
Transmural (Q wave) infarction (acute) (of) inferior (wall) NOS

Excludes2   ST elevation (STEMI) myocardial infarction involving left circumflex coronary artery (I21.21)

OGCR   See Section I.c.9.e.3

Acute myocardial infarction, unspecified

Code I21.3, ST elevation (STEMI) myocardial infarction of unspecified site, is the default for unspecified acute myocardial infarction. If only STEMI or transmural MI without the site is documented, assign I21.3.

● Unacceptable Principal Diagnosis   ● Use Additional Character(s)   ■ Unspecified   ▶ Manifestation Code
OGCR Official Guidelines for Coding and Reporting   Excludes 1   Excludes 2   Includes   Use additional   Code first   Code also

CHAPTER 9 (I00-I99)

● **I21.2** **ST elevation (STEMI) myocardial infarction of other sites**

     I21.21 **ST elevation (STEMI) myocardial infarction involving left circumflex coronary artery** 🔖
         ST elevation (STEMI) myocardial infarction involving oblique marginal coronary artery

     I21.29 **ST elevation (STEMI) myocardial infarction involving other sites** 🔖
         Acute transmural myocardial infarction of other sites
         Apical-lateral transmural (Q wave) infarction (acute)
         Basal-lateral transmural (Q wave) infarction (acute)
         High lateral transmural (Q wave) infarction (acute)
         Lateral (wall) NOS transmural (Q wave) infarction (acute)
         Posterior (true) transmural (Q wave) infarction (acute)
         Posterobasal transmural (Q wave) infarction (acute)
         Posterolateral transmural (Q wave) infarction (acute)
         Posteroseptal transmural (Q wave) infarction (acute)
         Septal transmural (Q wave) infarction (acute) NOS

■ **I21.3** **ST elevation (STEMI) myocardial infarction of unspecified site** 🔖
     Acute transmural myocardial infarction of unspecified site
     Myocardial infarction (acute) NOS
     Transmural (Q wave) myocardial infarction NOS

I21.4 **Non-ST elevation (NSTEMI) myocardial infarction** 🔖
     Acute subendocardial myocardial infarction
     Non-Q wave myocardial infarction NOS
     Nontransmural myocardial infarction NOS

● **I22** **Subsequent ST elevation (STEMI) and non-ST elevation (NSTEMI) myocardial infarction**

     Includes   acute myocardial infarction occurring within four weeks (28 days) of a previous acute myocardial infarction, regardless of site
         cardiac infarction
         coronary (artery) embolism
         coronary (artery) occlusion
         coronary (artery) rupture
         coronary (artery) thrombosis
         infarction of heart, myocardium, or ventricle
         recurrent myocardial infarction
         reinfarction of myocardium
         rupture of heart, myocardium, or ventricle

     Use additional code, if applicable, to identify:
     exposure to environmental tobacco smoke (Z77.22)
     history of tobacco use (Z87.891)
     occupational exposure to environmental tobacco smoke (Z57.31)
     status post administration of tPA (rtPA) in a different facility within the last 24 hours prior to admission to current facility (Z92.82)
     tobacco dependence (F17.-)
     tobacco use (Z72.0)

I22.0 **Subsequent ST elevation (STEMI) myocardial infarction of anterior wall** 🔖
     Subsequent acute transmural myocardial infarction of anterior wall
     Subsequent transmural (Q wave) infarction (acute)(of) anterior (wall) NOS
     Subsequent anteroapical transmural (Q wave) infarction (acute)
     Subsequent anterolateral transmural (Q wave) infarction (acute)
     Subsequent anteroseptal transmural (Q wave) infarction (acute)

I22.1 **Subsequent ST elevation (STEMI) myocardial infarction of inferior wall** 🔖
     Subsequent acute transmural myocardial infarction of inferior wall
     Subsequent transmural (Q wave) infarction (acute)(of) diaphragmatic wall
     Subsequent transmural (Q wave) infarction (acute)(of) inferior (wall) NOS
     Subsequent inferolateral transmural (Q wave) infarction (acute)
     Subsequent inferoposterior transmural (Q wave) infarction (acute)

I22.2 **Subsequent non-ST elevation (NSTEMI) myocardial infarction** 🔖
     Subsequent acute subendocardial myocardial infarction
     Subsequent non-Q wave myocardial infarction NOS
     Subsequent nontransmural myocardial infarction NOS

I22.8 **Subsequent ST elevation (STEMI) myocardial infarction of other sites** 🔖
     Subsequent acute transmural myocardial infarction of other sites
     Subsequent apical-lateral transmural (Q wave) myocardial infarction (acute)
     Subsequent basal-lateral transmural (Q wave) myocardial infarction (acute)
     Subsequent high lateral transmural (Q wave) myocardial infarction (acute)
     Subsequent transmural (Q wave) myocardial infarction (acute)(of) lateral (wall) NOS
     Subsequent posterior (true) transmural (Q wave) myocardial infarction (acute)
     Subsequent posterobasal transmural (Q wave) myocardial infarction (acute)
     Subsequent posterolateral transmural (Q wave) myocardial infarction (acute)
     Subsequent posteroseptal transmural (Q wave) myocardial infarction (acute)
     Subsequent septal NOS transmural (Q wave) myocardial infarction (acute)

■ **I22.9** **Subsequent ST elevation (STEMI) myocardial infarction of unspecified site** 🔖
     Subsequent acute myocardial infarction of unspecified site
     Subsequent myocardial infarction (acute) NOS

N Newborn Age: 0   **P** Pediatric Age: 0–17   **M** Maternity DX: 12–55   **A** Adult Age: 15–124   ♀ Females Only   ♂ Males Only
🔖 Complication\Comorbidity   🔖 Major C\C   🔖 Present on Admission Requirement   🔖 Hospital-Acquired Condition
1023

CHAPTER 9 (I00-I99)

● **I23 Certain current complications following ST elevation (STEMI) and non-ST elevation (NSTEMI) myocardial infarction (within the 28 day period)**

> **Note:** A code from category I23 must be used in conjunction with a code from category I21 or category I22. The I23 code should be sequenced first, if it is the reason for encounter, or, it should be sequenced after the I21 or I22 code if the complication of the MI occurs during the encounter for the MI.

I23.0 Hemopericardium as current complication following acute myocardial infarction 🖥 **A**

> **Excludes1** hemopericardium not specified as current complication following acute myocardial infarction (I31.2)

I23.1 Atrial septal defect as current complication following acute myocardial infarction 🖥 **A**

> **Excludes1** acquired atrial septal defect not specified as current complication following acute myocardial infarction (I51.0)

I23.2 Ventricular septal defect as current complication following acute myocardial infarction 🖥 **A**

> **Excludes1** acquired ventricular septal defect not specified as current complication following acute myocardial infarction (I51.0)

I23.3 Rupture of cardiac wall without hemopericardium as current complication following acute myocardial infarction 🖥 **A**

I23.4 Rupture of chordae tendineae as current complication following acute myocardial infarction 🖥

> **Excludes1** rupture of chordae tendineae not specified as current complication following acute myocardial infarction (I51.1)

I23.5 Rupture of papillary muscle as current complication following acute myocardial infarction 🖥

> **Excludes1** rupture of papillary muscle not specified as current complication following acute myocardial infarction (I51.2)

I23.6 Thrombosis of atrium, auricular appendage, and ventricle as current complications following acute myocardial infarction 🖥 **A**

> **Excludes1** thrombosis of atrium, auricular appendage, and ventricle not specified as current complication following acute myocardial infarction (I51.3)

I23.7 Postinfarction angina 🖥 **A**

I23.8 Other current complications following acute myocardial infarction 🖥 **A**

● **I24 Other acute ischemic heart diseases**

> **Excludes1** angina pectoris (I20.-)
> transient myocardial ischemia in newborn (P29.4)

I24.0 Acute coronary thrombosis not resulting in myocardial infarction 🖥
Acute coronary (artery) (vein) embolism not resulting in myocardial infarction
Acute coronary (artery) (vein) occlusion not resulting in myocardial infarction
Acute coronary (artery) (vein) thromboembolism not resulting in myocardial infarction

> **Excludes1** atherosclerotic heart disease (I25.1-)

Item 9–6 Classification is based on the location of the atherosclerosis. **"Of native coronary artery"** indicates the atherosclerosis is within an original heart artery. **"Of autologous vein bypass graft"** indicates that the atherosclerosis is within a vein graft that was taken from within the patient. **"Of nonautologous biological bypass graft"** indicates the atherosclerosis is within a vessel grafted from other than the patient. **"Of artery bypass graft"** indicates the atherosclerosis is within an artery that was grafted from within the patient.

I24.1 Dressler's syndrome 🖥
Postmyocardial infarction syndrome

> **Excludes1** postinfarction angina (I23.7)

I24.8 Other forms of acute ischemic heart disease 🖥

■ **I24.9 Acute ischemic heart disease, unspecified** 🖥

> **Excludes1** ischemic heart disease (chronic) NOS (I25.9)

● **I25 Chronic ischemic heart disease**

> Use additional code to identify:
> chronic total occlusion of coronary artery (I25.82)
> exposure to environmental tobacco smoke (Z77.22)
> history of tobacco use (Z87.891)
> occupational exposure to environmental tobacco smoke (Z57.31)
> tobacco dependence (F17.-)
> tobacco use (Z72.0)

OGCR See Section I.9.b.

Atherosclerotic Coronary Artery Disease and Angina

ICD-10-CM has combination codes for atherosclerotic heart disease with angina pectoris. The subcategories for these codes are I25.11, Atherosclerotic heart disease of native coronary artery with angina pectoris and I25.7, Atherosclerosis of coronary artery bypass graft(s) and coronary artery of transplanted heart with angina pectoris.

When using one of these combination codes it is not necessary to use an additional code for angina pectoris. A causal relationship can be assumed in a patient with both atherosclerosis and angina pectoris, unless the documentation indicates the angina is due to something other than the atherosclerosis.

If a patient with coronary artery disease is admitted due to an acute myocardial infarction (AMI), the AMI should be sequenced before the coronary artery disease.

See Section I.C.9. Acute myocardial infarction (AMI)

(See Plates 218 and 219 on pages NAP-26 and NAP-27.)

● **I25.1 Atherosclerotic heart disease of native coronary artery**
Disease in which fatty deposits form on the walls of arteries
Atherosclerotic cardiovascular disease
Coronary (artery) atheroma
Coronary (artery) atherosclerosis
Coronary (artery) disease
Coronary (artery) sclerosis

> Use additional code, if applicable, to identify:
> coronary atherosclerosis due to calcified coronary lesion (I25.84)
> coronary atherosclerosis due to lipid rich plaque (I25.83)

> **Excludes2** atheroembolism (I75.-)
> atherosclerosis of coronary artery bypass graft(s) and transplanted heart (I25.7-)

I25.10 Atherosclerotic heart disease of native coronary artery without angina pectoris A
Atherosclerotic heart disease NOS

● Unacceptable Principal Diagnosis ● Use Additional Character(s) ■ Unspecified ▶ Manifestation Code
OGCR Official Guidelines for Coding and Reporting | Excludes 1 | Excludes 2 | Includes | Use additional | Code first | Code also

Figure 9-2 Atherosclerotic plaque.

Atherosclerotic plaque (atheromas)

● **I25.11**   **Atherosclerotic heart disease of native coronary artery with angina pectoris**

    I25.110   **Atherosclerotic heart disease of native coronary artery with unstable angina pectoris** 🖜   **A**

       Excludes1   unstable angina without atherosclerotic heart disease (I20.0)

    I25.111   **Atherosclerotic heart disease of native coronary artery with angina pectoris with documented spasm**   **A**

       Excludes1   angina pectoris with documented spasm without atherosclerotic heart disease (I20.1)

    I25.118   **Atherosclerotic heart disease of native coronary artery with other forms of angina pectoris**   **A**

       Excludes1   other forms of angina pectoris without atherosclerotic heart disease (I20.8)

    ▢ **I25.119**   **Atherosclerotic heart disease of native coronary artery with unspecified angina pectoris**   **A**
       Atherosclerotic heart disease with angina NOS
       Atherosclerotic heart disease with ischemic chest pain

       Excludes1   unspecified angina pectoris without atherosclerotic heart disease (I20.9)

I25.2   **Old myocardial infarction** 🖜
    Healed myocardial infarction
    Past myocardial infarction diagnosed by ECG or other investigation, but currently presenting no symptoms

I25.3   **Aneurysm of heart** 🖜
    Mural aneurysm
    Ventricular aneurysm

● **I25.4**   **Coronary artery aneurysm and dissection**

    I25.41   **Coronary artery aneurysm**
       Coronary arteriovenous fistula, acquired

       Excludes1   congenital coronary (artery) aneurysm (Q24.5)

    I25.42   **Coronary artery dissection** 🖜

I25.5   **Ischemic cardiomyopathy**
    Excludes2   coronary atherosclerosis (I25.1-, I25.7-)

I25.6   **Silent myocardial ischemia**

● **I25.7**   **Atherosclerosis of coronary artery bypass graft(s) and coronary artery of transplanted heart with angina pectoris**

    Use additional code, if applicable, to identify:
    coronary atherosclerosis due to calcified coronary lesion (I25.84)
    coronary atherosclerosis due to lipid rich plaque (I25.83)

    Excludes1   atherosclerosis of bypass graft(s) of transplanted heart without angina pectoris (I25.812)
       atherosclerosis of coronary artery bypass graft(s) without angina pectoris (I25.810)
       atherosclerosis of native coronary artery of transplanted heart without angina pectoris (I25.811)
       embolism or thrombus of coronary artery bypass graft(s) (T82.8-)

● **I25.70**   **Atherosclerosis of coronary artery bypass graft(s), unspecified, with angina pectoris**

    ▢ **I25.700**   **Atherosclerosis of coronary artery bypass graft(s), unspecified, with unstable angina pectoris** 🖜   **A**

       Excludes1   unstable angina pectoris without atherosclerosis of coronary artery bypass graft (I20.0)

    ▢ **I25.701**   **Atherosclerosis of coronary artery bypass graft(s), unspecified, with angina pectoris with documented spasm**   **A**

       Excludes1   angina pectoris with documented spasm without atherosclerosis of coronary artery bypass graft (I20.1)

    ▢ **I25.708**   **Atherosclerosis of coronary artery bypass graft(s), unspecified, with other forms of angina pectoris**   **A**

       Excludes1   other forms of angina pectoris without atherosclerosis of coronary artery bypass graft (I20.8)

    ▢ **I25.709**   **Atherosclerosis of coronary artery bypass graft(s), unspecified, with unspecified angina pectoris**   **A**

       Excludes1   unspecified angina pectoris without atherosclerosis of coronary artery bypass graft (I20.9)

CHAPTER 9 (I00-I99)

N Newborn Age: 0   **P** Pediatric Age: 0–17   **M** Maternity DX: 12–55   **A** Adult Age: 15–124   ♀ Females Only   ♂ Males Only

🖜 Complication\Comorbidity   🖜 Major C\C   🖜 Present on Admission Requirement   🖜 Hospital-Acquired Condition

1025

● **I25.71**   **Atherosclerosis of autologous vein coronary artery bypass graft(s) with angina pectoris**

    I25.710   **Atherosclerosis of autologous vein coronary artery bypass graft(s) with unstable angina pectoris** ✪ **A**

       | Excludes 1 | unstable angina without atherosclerosis of autologous vein coronary artery bypass graft(s) (I20.0)

    I25.711   **Atherosclerosis of autologous vein coronary artery bypass graft(s) with angina pectoris with documented spasm** ✪ **A**

       | Excludes 1 | angina pectoris with documented spasm without atherosclerosis of autologous vein coronary artery bypass graft(s) (I20.1)

    I25.718   **Atherosclerosis of autologous vein coronary artery bypass graft(s) with other forms of angina pectoris** ✪ **A**

       | Excludes 1 | other forms of angina pectoris without atherosclerosis of autologous vein coronary artery bypass graft(s) (I20.8)

    ■ **I25.719**   **Atherosclerosis of autologous vein coronary artery bypass graft(s) with unspecified angina pectoris** ✪ **A**

       | Excludes 1 | unspecified angina pectoris without atherosclerosis of autologous vein coronary artery bypass graft(s) (I20.9)

● **I25.72**   **Atherosclerosis of autologous artery coronary artery bypass graft(s) with angina pectoris**

    Atherosclerosis of internal mammary artery graft with angina pectoris

    I25.720   **Atherosclerosis of autologous artery coronary artery bypass graft(s) with unstable angina pectoris** ✪ **A**

       | Excludes 1 | unstable angina without atherosclerosis of autologous artery coronary artery bypass graft(s) (I20.0)

    I25.721   **Atherosclerosis of autologous artery coronary artery bypass graft(s) with angina pectoris with documented spasm** ✪ **A**

       | Excludes 1 | angina pectoris with documented spasm without atherosclerosis of autologous artery coronary artery bypass graft(s) (I20.1)

    I25.728   **Atherosclerosis of autologous artery coronary artery bypass graft(s) with other forms of angina pectoris** ✪ **A**

       | Excludes 1 | other forms of angina pectoris without atherosclerosis of autologous artery coronary artery bypass graft(s) (I20.8)

    ■ **I25.729**   **Atherosclerosis of autologous artery coronary artery bypass graft(s) with unspecified angina pectoris** ✪ **A**

       | Excludes 1 | unspecified angina pectoris without atherosclerosis of autologous artery coronary artery bypass graft(s) (I20.9)

● **I25.73**   **Atherosclerosis of nonautologous biological coronary artery bypass graft(s) with angina pectoris**

    I25.730   **Atherosclerosis of nonautologous biological coronary artery bypass graft(s) with unstable angina pectoris** ✪ **A**

       | Excludes 1 | unstable angina without atherosclerosis of non-autologous biological coronary artery bypass graft(s) (I20.0)

    I25.731   **Atherosclerosis of nonautologous biological coronary artery bypass graft(s) with angina pectoris with documented spasm** ✪ **A**

       | Excludes 1 | angina pectoris with documented spasm without atherosclerosis of non-autologous biological coronary artery bypass graft(s) (I20.1)

● Unacceptable Principal Diagnosis   ● Use Additional Character(s)   ■ Unspecified   ▶ Manifestation Code

OGCR Official Guidelines for Coding and Reporting | Excludes 1 | | Excludes 2 | Includes   Use additional   Code first   Code also

I25.738 **Atherosclerosis of nonautologous biological coronary artery bypass graft(s) with other forms of angina pectoris** 🔹   A

> Excludes1   other forms of angina pectoris without atherosclerosis of nonautologous biological coronary artery bypass graft(s) (I20.8)

I25.739 **Atherosclerosis of nonautologous biological coronary artery bypass graft(s) with unspecified angina pectoris** 🔹   A

> Excludes1   unspecified angina pectoris without atherosclerosis of nonautologous biological coronary artery bypass graft(s) (I20.9)

● I25.75 **Atherosclerosis of native coronary artery of transplanted heart with angina pectoris**

> Excludes1   atherosclerosis of native coronary artery of transplanted heart without angina pectoris (I25.811)

I25.750 **Atherosclerosis of native coronary artery of transplanted heart with unstable angina** 🔹

I25.751 **Atherosclerosis of native coronary artery of transplanted heart with angina pectoris with documented spasm** 🔹

I25.758 **Atherosclerosis of native coronary artery of transplanted heart with other forms of angina pectoris** 🔹

I25.759 **Atherosclerosis of native coronary artery of transplanted heart with unspecified angina pectoris** 🔹

● I25.76 **Atherosclerosis of bypass graft of coronary artery of transplanted heart with angina pectoris**

> Excludes1   atherosclerosis of bypass graft of coronary artery of transplanted heart without angina pectoris (I25.812)

I25.760 **Atherosclerosis of bypass graft of coronary artery of transplanted heart with unstable angina** 🔹   A

I25.761 **Atherosclerosis of bypass graft of coronary artery of transplanted heart with angina pectoris with documented spasm** 🔹   A

I25.768 **Atherosclerosis of bypass graft of coronary artery of transplanted heart with other forms of angina pectoris** 🔹   A

I25.769 **Atherosclerosis of bypass graft of coronary artery of transplanted heart with unspecified angina pectoris** 🔹   A

● I25.79 **Atherosclerosis of other coronary artery bypass graft(s) with angina pectoris**   A

I25.790 **Atherosclerosis of other coronary artery bypass graft(s) with unstable angina pectoris** 🔹

> Excludes1   unstable angina without atherosclerosis of other coronary artery bypass graft(s) (I20.0)

I25.791 **Atherosclerosis of other coronary artery bypass graft(s) with angina pectoris with documented spasm** 🔹   A

> Excludes1   angina pectoris with documented spasm without atherosclerosis of other coronary artery bypass graft(s) (I20.1)

I25.798 **Atherosclerosis of other coronary artery bypass graft(s) with other forms of angina pectoris** 🔹   A

> Excludes1   other forms of angina pectoris without atherosclerosis of other coronary artery bypass graft(s) (I20.8)

I25.799 **Atherosclerosis of other coronary artery bypass graft(s) with unspecified angina pectoris** 🔹   A

> Excludes1   unspecified angina pectoris without atherosclerosis of other coronary artery bypass graft(s) (I20.9)

● I25.8 **Other forms of chronic ischemic heart disease**

● I25.81 **Atherosclerosis of other coronary vessels without angina pectoris**

Use additional code, if applicable, to identify:
coronary atherosclerosis due to calcified coronary lesion (I25.84)
coronary atherosclerosis due to lipid rich plaque (I25.83)

> Excludes1   atherosclerotic heart disease of native coronary artery without angina pectoris (I25.10)

CHAPTER 9 (I00-I99)

I25.810   Atherosclerosis of coronary artery bypass graft(s) without angina pectoris 🔒   A

Atherosclerosis of coronary artery bypass graft NOS

> **Excludes1**   atherosclerosis of coronary bypass graft(s) with angina pectoris (I25.70--I25.73-, I25.79-)

I25.811   Atherosclerosis of native coronary artery of transplanted heart without angina pectoris 🔒

Atherosclerosis of native coronary artery of transplanted heart NOS

> **Excludes1**   atherosclerosis of native coronary artery of transplanted heart with angina pectoris (I25.75-)

I25.812   Atherosclerosis of bypass graft of coronary artery of transplanted heart without angina pectoris 🔒 A

Atherosclerosis of bypass graft of transplanted heart NOS

> **Excludes1**   atherosclerosis of bypass graft of transplanted heart with angina pectoris (I25.76)

● **I25.82   Chronic total occlusion of coronary artery**

Complete occlusion of coronary artery
Total occlusion of coronary artery

Code first coronary atherosclerosis (I25.1-, I25.7-, I25.81-)

> **Excludes1**   acute coronary occlusion with myocardial infarction (I21.-, I22.-)
> acute coronary occlusion without myocardial infarction (I24.0)

● **I25.83   Coronary atherosclerosis due to lipid rich plaque   A**

Code first coronary atherosclerosis (I25.1-, I25.7-, I25.81-)

I25.84   Coronary atherosclerosis due to calcified coronary lesion

Coronary atherosclerosis due to severely calcified coronary lesion

Code first coronary atherosclerosis (I25.1-, I25.7-, I25.81-)

I25.89   Other forms of chronic ischemic heart disease

▪ **I25.9   Chronic ischemic heart disease, unspecified**

Ischemic heart disease (chronic) NOS

Item 9-7 Pulmonary heart disease or **cor pulmonale** is right ventricle hypertrophy or RVH as a result of a respiratory disorder increasing back flow pressure to the right ventricle. Left untreated, cor pulmonale leads to right-heart failure and death.

PULMONARY HEART DISEASE AND DISEASES OF PULMONARY CIRCULATION (I26-I28)

● **I26   Pulmonary embolism**

> **Includes**   pulmonary (acute)(artery)(vein) infarction
> pulmonary (acute)(artery)(vein) thromboembolism
> pulmonary (acute)(artery)(vein) thrombosis

> **Excludes2**   chronic pulmonary embolism (I27.82)
> personal history of pulmonary embolism (Z86.711)
> pulmonary embolism due to trauma (T79.0, T79.1)
> pulmonary embolism due to complications of surgical and medical care (T80.0, T81.7-, T82.8-)
> pulmonary embolism complicating:
>   abortion, ectopic or molar pregnancy (O00-O07, O08.2)
>   pregnancy, childbirth and the puerperium (O88.-)
> septic (non-pulmonary) arterial embolism (I76)

● **I26.0   Pulmonary embolism with acute cor pulmonale**

● **I26.01   Septic pulmonary embolism with acute cor pulmonale 🔒**

> *Code first* underlying infection

MCC: Only when the principal diagnosis is designated as an MCC

I26.02   Saddle embolus of pulmonary artery with acute cor pulmonale

I26.09   Other pulmonary embolism with acute cor pulmonale 🔒 🔒

Acute cor pulmonale NOS

MCC: Only when the principal diagnosis is designated as an MCC

● **I26.9   Pulmonary embolism without acute cor pulmonale**

● **I26.90   Septic pulmonary embolism without acute cor pulmonale 🔒**

> *Code first* underlying infection

I26.92   Saddle embolus of pulmonary artery without acute cor pulmonale

I26.99   Other pulmonary embolism without acute cor pulmonale 🔒 🔒

Acute pulmonary embolism NOS
Pulmonary embolism NOS

● **I27   Other pulmonary heart diseases**

I27.0   Primary pulmonary hypertension 🔒

> **Excludes1**   pulmonary hypertension NOS (I27.2)
> secondary pulmonary hypertension (I27.2)

I27.1   Kyphoscoliotic heart disease 🔒

I27.2   Other secondary pulmonary hypertension

Pulmonary hypertension NOS

Code also associated underlying condition

● **I27.8   Other specified pulmonary heart diseases**

I27.81   Cor pulmonale (chronic)

Cor pulmonale NOS

> **Excludes1**   acute cor pulmonale (I26.0-)

I27.82   Chronic pulmonary embolism 🔒

> Use additional code, if applicable, for associated long-term (current) use of anticoagulants (Z79.01)

> **Excludes1**   personal history of pulmonary embolism (Z86.711)

● Unacceptable Principal Diagnosis   ● Use Additional Character(s)   ▪ Unspecified   ▶ Manifestation Code

OGCR Official Guidelines for Coding and Reporting   Excludes 1   Excludes 2   Includes   Use additional   Code first   Code also

I27.89 **Other specified pulmonary heart diseases**
Eisenmenger's complex
Eisenmenger's syndrome
Excludes1 Eisenmenger's defect (Q21.8)

■ I27.9 **Pulmonary heart disease, unspecified**
Chronic cardiopulmonary disease

● I28 **Other diseases of pulmonary vessels**

I28.0 **Arteriovenous fistula of pulmonary vessels** 🗫
Excludes1 congenital arteriovenous fistula
(Q25.72)

I28.1 **Aneurysm of pulmonary artery** 🗫
Excludes1 congenital aneurysm (Q25.79)
congenital arteriovenous aneurysm
(Q25.72)

I28.8 **Other diseases of pulmonary vessels**
Pulmonary arteritis
Pulmonary endarteritis
Rupture of pulmonary vessels
Stenosis of pulmonary vessels
Stricture of pulmonary vessels

■ I28.9 **Disease of pulmonary vessels, unspecified**

OTHER FORMS OF HEART DISEASE (I30-I52)

● I30 **Acute pericarditis**
Inflammation of pericardium (sac surrounding the heart)
caused by an infection.

Includes acute mediastinopericarditis
acute myopericarditis
acute pericardial effusion
acute pleuropericarditis
acute pneumopericarditis

Excludes1 Dressler's syndrome (I24.1)
rheumatic pericarditis (acute) (I01.0)

I30.0 **Acute nonspecific idiopathic pericarditis** 🗫

I30.1 **Infective pericarditis** 🗫
Pneumococcal pericarditis
Pneumopyopericardium
Purulent pericarditis
Pyopericarditis
Pyopericardium
Pyopneumopericardium
Staphylococcal pericarditis
Streptococcal pericarditis
Suppurative pericarditis
Viral pericarditis
Use additional code (B95-B97) to identify
infectious agent

I30.8 **Other forms of acute pericarditis** 🗫

■ I30.9 **Acute pericarditis, unspecified** 🗫

● I31 **Other diseases of pericardium**
Excludes1 diseases of pericardium specified as
rheumatic (I09.2)
postcardiotomy syndrome (I97.0)
traumatic injury to pericardium (S26.-)

I31.0 **Chronic adhesive pericarditis** 🗫
Accretio cordis
Adherent pericardium
Adhesive mediastinopericarditis

I31.1 **Chronic constrictive pericarditis** 🗫
Concretio cordis
Pericardial calcification

I31.2 **Hemopericardium, not elsewhere classified** 🗫
Excludes1 hemopericardium as current
complication following acute
myocardial infarction (I23.0)

I31.3 **Pericardial effusion (noninflammatory)** 🗫
Chylopericardium
Excludes1 acute pericardial effusion (I30.9)

● I31.4 **Cardiac tamponade** 🗫
Code first underlying cause

I31.8 **Other specified diseases of pericardium** 🗫
Epicardial plaques
Focal pericardial adhesions

■ I31.9 **Disease of pericardium, unspecified** 🗫
Pericarditis (chronic) NOS

● ◗ I32 *Pericarditis in diseases classified elsewhere* 🗫
Code first underlying disease
Excludes1 pericarditis (in):
coxsackie (virus) (B33.23)
gonococcal (A54.83)
meningococcal (A39.53)
rheumatoid (arthritis) (M05.31)
syphilitic (A52.06)
systemic lupus erythematosus (M32.12)
tuberculosis (A18.84)

● I33 **Acute and subacute endocarditis**
Inflammation/infection of lining of heart, affecting heart valves
including replacement valves and is usually caused by a
bacterial infection
Excludes1 acute rheumatic endocarditis (I01.1)
endocarditis NOS (I38)

I33.0 **Acute and subacute infective endocarditis** 🗫
Bacterial endocarditis (acute) (subacute)
Infective endocarditis (acute) (subacute) NOS
Endocarditis lenta (acute) (subacute)
Malignant endocarditis (acute) (subacute)
Purulent endocarditis (acute) (subacute)
Septic endocarditis (acute) (subacute)
Ulcerative endocarditis (acute) (subacute)
Vegetative endocarditis (acute) (subacute)
Use additional code (B95-B97) to identify
infectious agent

■ I33.9 **Acute and subacute endocarditis, unspecified** 🗫
Acute endocarditis NOS
Acute myoendocarditis NOS
Acute periendocarditis NOS
Subacute endocarditis NOS
Subacute myoendocarditis NOS
Subacute periendocarditis NOS

● I34 **Nonrheumatic mitral valve disorders**
Excludes1 mitral valve disease (I05.9)
mitral valve failure (I05.8)
mitral valve stenosis (I05.0)
mitral valve disorder of unspecified cause
with diseases of aortic and/or tricuspid
valve(s) (I08.-)
mitral valve disorder of unspecified cause
with mitral stenosis or obstruction (I05.0)
mitral valve disorder specified as congenital
(Q23.2, Q23.3)
mitral valve disorder specified as rheumatic
(I05.-)

I34.0 **Nonrheumatic mitral (valve) insufficiency**
Nonrheumatic mitral (valve) incompetence NOS
Nonrheumatic mitral (valve) regurgitation NOS

I34.1 **Nonrheumatic mitral (valve) prolapse**
Floppy nonrheumatic mitral valve syndrome
Excludes1 Marfan's syndrome (Q87.4-)

I34.2 **Nonrheumatic mitral (valve) stenosis**

I34.8 **Other nonrheumatic mitral valve disorders**

■ I34.9 **Nonrheumatic mitral valve disorder, unspecified**

N Newborn Age: 0 P Pediatric Age: 0–17 M Maternity DX: 12–55 A Adult Age: 15–124 ♀ Females Only ♂ Males Only
🗫 Complication\Comorbidity 🗫 Major C\C Present on Admission Requirement 🗫 Hospital-Acquired Condition

1029

CHAPTER 9 (I00-I99)

● **I35   Nonrheumatic aortic valve disorders**

> **Excludes1**   aortic valve disorder of unspecified cause but with diseases of mitral and/or tricuspid valve(s) (I08.-)
> aortic valve disorder specified as congenital (Q23.0, Q23.1)
> aortic valve disorder specified as rheumatic (I06.-)
> hypertrophic subaortic stenosis (I42.1)

I35.0   Nonrheumatic aortic (valve) stenosis

I35.1   Nonrheumatic aortic (valve) insufficiency
> Nonrheumatic aortic (valve) incompetence NOS
> Nonrheumatic aortic (valve) regurgitation NOS

I35.2   Nonrheumatic aortic (valve) stenosis with insufficiency

I35.8   Other nonrheumatic aortic valve disorders

■ **I35.9   Nonrheumatic aortic valve disorder, unspecified**

● **I36   Nonrheumatic tricuspid valve disorders**

> **Excludes1**   tricuspid valve disorders of unspecified cause (I07.-)
> tricuspid valve disorders specified as congenital (Q22.4, Q22.8, Q22.9)
> tricuspid valve disorders specified as rheumatic (I07.-)
> tricuspid valve disorders with aortic and/or mitral valve involvement (I08.-)

I36.0   Nonrheumatic tricuspid (valve) stenosis

I36.1   Nonrheumatic tricuspid (valve) insufficiency
> Nonrheumatic tricuspid (valve) incompetence
> Nonrheumatic tricuspid (valve) regurgitation

I36.2   Nonrheumatic tricuspid (valve) stenosis with insufficiency

I36.8   Other nonrheumatic tricuspid valve disorders

■ **I36.9   Nonrheumatic tricuspid valve disorder, unspecified**

● **I37   Nonrheumatic pulmonary valve disorders**

> **Excludes1**   pulmonary valve disorder specified as congenital (Q22.1, Q22.2, Q22.3)
> pulmonary valve disorder specified as rheumatic (I09.89)

I37.0   Nonrheumatic pulmonary valve stenosis

I37.1   Nonrheumatic pulmonary valve insufficiency
> Nonrheumatic pulmonary valve incompetence
> Nonrheumatic pulmonary valve regurgitation

I37.2   Nonrheumatic pulmonary valve stenosis with insufficiency

I37.8   Other nonrheumatic pulmonary valve disorders

■ **I37.9   Nonrheumatic pulmonary valve disorder, unspecified**

■ **I38   Endocarditis, valve unspecified** 🦠

> **Includes**   endocarditis (chronic) NOS
> valvular incompetence NOS
> valvular insufficiency NOS
> valvular regurgitation NOS
> valvular stenosis NOS
> valvulitis (chronic) NOS

> **Excludes1**   congenital insufficiency of cardiac valve NOS (Q24.8)
> congenital stenosis of cardiac valve NOS (Q24.8)
> endocardial fibroelastosis (I42.4)
> endocarditis specified as rheumatic (I09.1)

● ▶ **I39   *Endocarditis and heart valve disorders in diseases classified elsewhere*** 🦠

> *Code first* underlying disease, such as:
> Q fever (A78)

> **Excludes1**   endocardial involvement in:
> candidiasis (B37.6)
> gonococcal infection (A54.83)
> Libman-Sacks disease (M32.11)
> listerosis (A32.82)
> meningococcal infection (A39.51)
> rheumatoid arthritis (M05.31)
> syphilis (A52.03)
> tuberculosis (A18.84)
> typhoid fever (A01.02)

● **I40   Acute myocarditis**

> *Inflammation of heart muscle due to infection (viral/bacterial).*

> **Includes**   subacute myocarditis

> **Excludes1**   acute rheumatic myocarditis (I01.2)

I40.0   Infective myocarditis 🦠
> Septic myocarditis

> **Use additional** code (B95-B97) to identify infectious agent

I40.1   Isolated myocarditis 🦠
> Fiedler's myocarditis
> Giant cell myocarditis
> Idiopathic myocarditis

I40.8   Other acute myocarditis 🦠

■ **I40.9   Acute myocarditis, unspecified** 🦠

● ▶ **I41   *Myocarditis in diseases classified elsewhere*** 🦠

> *Code first* underlying disease, such as:
> typhus (A75.0-A75.9)

> **Excludes1**   myocarditis (in):
> Chagas' disease (chronic) (B57.2)
> acute (B57.0)
> coxsackie (virus) infection (B33.22)
> diphtheritic (A36.81)
> gonococcal (A54.83)
> influenzal (J09.X9, J10.82, J11.82)
> meningococcal (A39.52)
> mumps (B26.82)
> rheumatoid arthritis (M05.31)
> sarcoid (D86.85)
> syphilis (A52.06)
> toxoplasmosis (B58.81)
> tuberculous (A18.84)

● **I42   Cardiomyopathy**

> *Disease of the heart muscle resulting in an abnormally enlarged, weakened, thickened, and/or stiffened muscles*

> **Includes**   myocardiopathy

> *Code first* cardiomyopathy complicating pregnancy and puerperium (O99.4)

> **Excludes1**   ischemic cardiomyopathy (I25.5)
> peripartum cardiomyopathy (O90.3)

> **Excludes2**   ventricular hypertrophy (I51.7)

I42.0   Dilated cardiomyopathy 🦠
> Congestive cardiomyopathy

I42.1   Obstructive hypertrophic cardiomyopathy 🦠
> Hypertrophic subaortic stenosis (idiopathic)

I42.2   Other hypertrophic cardiomyopathy 🦠
> Nonobstructive hypertrophic cardiomyopathy

I42.3   Endomyocardial (eosinophilic) disease 🦠
> Endomyocardial (tropical) fibrosis
> Löffler's endocarditis

● Unacceptable Principal Diagnosis   ● Use Additional Character(s)   ■ Unspecified   ▶ Manifestation Code

1030   **OGCR**   Official Guidelines for Coding and Reporting   Excludes 1   Excludes 2   Includes   Use additional   Code first   Code also

I42.4   **Endocardial fibroelastosis** 🅒
         Congenital cardiomyopathy
         Elastomyofibrosis

I42.5   **Other restrictive cardiomyopathy** 🅒
         Constrictive cardiomyopathy NOS

I42.6   **Alcoholic cardiomyopathy** 🅒
         Code also presence of alcoholism (F10.-)

I42.7   **Cardiomyopathy due to drug and external agent** 🅒
         Code first poisoning due to drug or toxin, if applicable
         (T36-T65 with fifth or sixth character 1-4 or 6)

         Use additional code for adverse effect, if
         applicable, to identify drug (T36-T50 with
         fifth or sixth character 5)

I42.8   **Other cardiomyopathies** 🅒

I42.9   **Cardiomyopathy, unspecified** 🅒
         Cardiomyopathy (primary) (secondary) NOS

●▶ I43   *Cardiomyopathy in diseases classified elsewhere* 🅒
         Code first underlying disease, such as:
             amyloidosis (E85-)
             glycogen storage disease (E74.0)
             gout (M10.0-)
             thyrotoxicosis (E05.0-E05.9-)
         Excludes1   cardiomyopathy (in):
                         coxsackie (virus) (B33.24)
                         diphtheria (A36.81)
                         sarcoidosis (D86.85)
                         tuberculosis (A18.84)

● I44   **Atrioventricular and left bundle-branch block**
         *Conduction problem resulting in arrhythmias/dysrhythmias
         due to a lack of electrical impulses being transmitted
         normally through the heart.*

I44.0   **Atrioventricular block, first degree**

I44.1   **Atrioventricular block, second degree**
         Atrioventricular block, type I and II
         Möbitz block, type I and II
         Second degree block, type I and II
         Wenckebach's block

I44.2   **Atrioventricular block, complete** 🅒
         Complete heart block NOS
         Third degree block

● I44.3 **Other and unspecified atrioventricular block**
         Atrioventricular block NOS

         I44.30   **Unspecified atrioventricular block**

         I44.39   **Other atrioventricular block**

I44.4   **Left anterior fascicular block**
         MCE: Questionable admission when principal dx

I44.5   **Left posterior fascicular block**
         MCE: Questionable admission when principal dx

● I44.6 **Other and unspecified fascicular block**

         I44.60   **Unspecified fascicular block**
                   Left bundle-branch hemiblock NOS
                   MCE: Questionable admission when
                   principal dx

         I44.69   **Other fascicular block**
                   MCE: Questionable admission when
                   principal dx

I44.7   **Left bundle-branch block, unspecified**
         MCE: Questionable admission when principal dx

● I45   **Other conduction disorders**

I45.0   **Right fascicular block**
         MCE: Questionable admission when principal dx

● I45.1 **Other and unspecified right bundle-branch block**

         I45.10   **Unspecified right bundle-branch block**
                   Right bundle-branch block NOS
                   MCE: Questionable admission when
                   principal dx

         I45.19   **Other right bundle-branch block**
                   MCE: Questionable admission when
                   principal dx

I45.2   **Bifascicular block** 🅒

I45.3   **Trifascicular block** 🅒

I45.4   **Nonspecific intraventricular block**
         Bundle-branch block NOS

I45.5   **Other specified heart block**
         Sinoatrial block
         Sinoauricular block
         Excludes1   heart block NOS (I45.9)

I45.6   **Pre-excitation syndrome**
         Accelerated atrioventricular conduction
         Accessory atrioventricular conduction
         Anomalous atrioventricular excitation
         Lown-Ganong-Levine syndrome
         Pre-excitation atrioventricular conduction
         Wolff-Parkinson-White syndrome

● I45.8 **Other specified conduction disorders**

         I45.81   **Long QT syndrome**

         I45.89   **Other specified conduction disorders** 🅒
                   Atrioventricular [AV] dissociation
                   Interference dissociation
                   Isorhythmic dissociation
                   Nonparoxysmal AV nodal tachycardia

I45.9   **Conduction disorder, unspecified**
         Heart block NOS
         Stokes-Adams syndrome

● I46   **Cardiac arrest**
         Excludes1   cardiogenic shock (R57.0)

● I46.2 **Cardiac arrest due to underlying cardiac condition** 🅒
         Code first underlying cardiac condition
         MCC: Only if patient discharged alive

● I46.8 **Cardiac arrest due to other underlying condition** 🅒
         Code first underlying condition
         MCC: Only if patient discharged alive

I46.9   **Cardiac arrest, cause unspecified** 🅒
         MCC: Only if patient discharged alive

● I47   **Paroxysmal tachycardia**
         Code first tachycardia complicating:
             abortion or ectopic or molar pregnancy (O00-O07, O08.8)
             obstetric surgery and procedures (O75.4)
         Excludes1   tachycardia:
                         NOS (R00.0)
                         sinoauricular NOS (R00.0)
                         sinus [sinusal] NOS (R00.0)

I47.0   **Re-entry ventricular arrhythmia** 🅒

I47.1   **Supraventricular tachycardia** 🅒
         Atrial (paroxysmal) tachycardia
         Atrioventricular [AV] (paroxysmal) tachycardia
         Atrioventricular re-entrant (nodal) tachycardia
             [AVNRT] [AVRT]
         Junctional (paroxysmal) tachycardia
         Nodal (paroxysmal) tachycardia

I47.2   **Ventricular tachycardia** 🅒

I47.9   **Paroxysmal tachycardia, unspecified**
         Bouveret (-Hoffman) syndrome

N Newborn Age: 0   **P** Pediatric Age: 0–17   **M** Maternity DX: 12–55   **A** Adult Age: 15–124   ♀ Females Only   ♂ Males Only

🅒 Complication\Comorbidity   🅒 Major C\C   🅒 Present on Admission Requirement   🅒 Hospital-Acquired Condition

1031

CHAPTER 9 (I00-I99)

CHAPTER 9 (I00-I99)

● **I48   Atrial fibrillation and flutter**
*Most common abnormal heart rhythm (arrhythmia) presenting
as irregular, rapid beating (tachycardia) of the heart's
upper chamber.*

   I48.0   Paroxysmal atrial fibrillation

   I48.1   Persistent atrial fibrillation 🦠
Rapid contractions of the upper heart chamber

   I48.2   Chronic atrial fibrillation
Permanent atrial fibrillation

   I48.3   Typical atrial flutter
Type I atrial flutter

   I48.4   Atypical atrial flutter
Type II atrial flutter

  ● **I48.9   Unspecified atrial fibrillation and atrial flutter**

     ■ **I48.91   Unspecified atrial fibrillation**

     ■ **I48.92   Unspecified atrial flutter**

● **I49   Other cardiac arrhythmias**
Code first cardiac arrhythmia complicating:
  abortion or ectopic or molar pregnancy (O00-O07,
   O08.8)
  obstetric surgery and procedures (O75.4)

   | Excludes1 | bradycardia:
        NOS (R00.1)
        sinoatrial (R00.1)
        sinus (R00.1)
        vagal (R00.1)
       neonatal dysrhythmia (P29.1-)

  ● **I49.0   Ventricular fibrillation and flutter**

     I49.01   Ventricular fibrillation 🦠
       MCC: Only if patient discharged alive

     I49.02   Ventricular flutter 🦠

   I49.1   Atrial premature depolarization
Atrial premature beats

   I49.2   Junctional premature depolarization 🦠

   I49.3   Ventricular premature depolarization

  ● **I49.4   Other and unspecified premature depolarization**

     ■ **I49.40   Unspecified premature depolarization**
       Premature beats NOS

     I49.49   Other premature depolarization
       Ectopic beats
       Extrasystoles
       Extrasystolic arrhythmias
       Premature contractions

   I49.5   Sick sinus syndrome
Tachycardia-bradycardia syndrome

   I49.8   Other specified cardiac arrhythmias
Coronary sinus rhythm disorder
Ectopic rhythm disorder
Nodal rhythm disorder

  ■ **I49.9   Cardiac arrhythmia, unspecified**
Arrhythmia (cardiac) NOS

● **I50   Heart failure**
Code first heart failure complicating abortion or ectopic or
  molar pregnancy (O00-O07, O08.8)
heart failure following surgery (I97.13-)
heart failure due to hypertension (I11.0)
heart failure due to hypertension with chronic kidney
  disease (I13.-)
obstetric surgery and procedures (O75.4)
rheumatic heart failure (I09.81)

   | Excludes1 | cardiac arrest (I46.-)
        neonatal cardiac failure (P29.0)

   I50.1   Left ventricular failure 🦠
Cardiac asthma
Edema of lung with heart disease NOS
Edema of lung with heart failure
Left heart failure
Pulmonary edema with heart disease NOS
Pulmonary edema with heart failure

    | Excludes1 | edema of lung without heart disease
        or heart failure (J81.-)
       pulmonary edema without heart
        disease or failure (J81.-)

  ● **I50.2   Systolic (congestive) heart failure**

    | Excludes1 | combined systolic (congestive) and
        diastolic (congestive) heart
        failure (I50.4-)

    ■ **I50.20   Unspecified systolic (congestive) heart
       failure** 🦠

    I50.21   Acute systolic (congestive) heart failure 🦠
       Presenting a short and relatively severe episode

    I50.22   Chronic systolic (congestive) heart failure 🦠
       Long-lasting, presenting over time

    **I50.23   Acute on chronic systolic (congestive)
       heart failure** 🦠
       *Combination code. What was a chronic
       condition now has an acute exacerbation
       (to make more severe).*

  ● **I50.3   Diastolic (congestive) heart failure**

    | Excludes1 | combined systolic (congestive) and
        diastolic (congestive) heart
        failure (I50.4-)

    ■ **I50.30   Unspecified diastolic (congestive) heart
       failure** 🦠

    I50.31   Acute diastolic (congestive) heart failure 🦠

    **I50.32   Chronic diastolic (congestive) heart
       failure** 🦠

    **I50.33   Acute on chronic diastolic (congestive)
       heart failure** 🦠

  ● **I50.4   Combined systolic (congestive) and diastolic
     (congestive) heart failure**

    ■ **I50.40   Unspecified combined systolic
       (congestive) and diastolic (congestive)
       heart failure** 🦠

    **I50.41   Acute combined systolic (congestive) and
       diastolic (congestive) heart failure** 🦠

    **I50.42   Chronic combined systolic (congestive)
       and diastolic (congestive) heart failure** 🦠

    **I50.43   Acute on chronic combined systolic
       (congestive) and diastolic (congestive)
       heart failure** 🦠

Item 9-8 Congestive heart failure (CHF) is a condition in which
the left ventricle of the heart cannot pump enough blood to the body. The
blood flow from the heart slows or returns to the heart from the venous
system back flow resulting in congestion (fluid accumulation) particularly
in the abdomen. Most commonly, fluid collects in the lungs and results in
shortness of breath, especially when in a reclining position.

● Unacceptable Principal Diagnosis   ● Use Additional Character(s)   ■ Unspecified   ▶ Manifestation Code
OGCR Official Guidelines for Coding and Reporting | Excludes 1 | | Excludes 2 | | Includes | | Use additional | | Code first | | Code also |

◼ **I50.9**   **Heart failure, unspecified**
Biventricular (heart) failure NOS
Cardiac, heart or myocardial failure NOS
Congestive heart disease
Congestive heart failure NOS
Right ventricular failure (secondary to left heart failure)
Excludes1   fluid overload (E87.70)

● **I51**   **Complications and ill-defined descriptions of heart disease**
Excludes1   any condition in I51.4-I51.9 due to hypertension (I11.-)
any condition in I51.4-I51.9 due to hypertension and chronic kidney disease (I13.-)
heart disease specified as rheumatic (I00-I09)

I51.0   **Cardiac septal defect, acquired** 🪙   A
Acquired septal atrial defect (old)
Acquired septal auricular defect (old)
Acquired septal ventricular defect (old)
Excludes1   cardiac septal defect as current complication following acute myocardial infarction (I23.1, I23.2)

I51.1   **Rupture of chordae tendineae, not elsewhere classified** 🪙
Excludes1   rupture of chordae tendineae as current complication following acute myocardial infarction (I23.4)

I51.2   **Rupture of papillary muscle, not elsewhere classified** 🪙
Excludes1   rupture of papillary muscle as current complication following acute myocardial infarction (I23.5)

I51.3   **Intracardiac thrombosis, not elsewhere classified** 🪙   A
Apical thrombosis (old)
Atrial thrombosis (old)
Auricular thrombosis (old)
Mural thrombosis (old)
Ventricular thrombosis (old)
Excludes1   intracardiac thrombosis as current complication following acute myocardial infarction (I23.6)

◼ **I51.4**   **Myocarditis, unspecified**
Chronic (interstitial) myocarditis
Myocardial fibrosis
Myocarditis NOS
Excludes1   acute or subacute myocarditis (I40.-)

I51.5   **Myocardial degeneration**
Fatty degeneration of heart or myocardium
Myocardial disease
Senile degeneration of heart or myocardium

I51.7   **Cardiomegaly**
Cardiac dilatation
Cardiac hypertrophy
Ventricular dilatation

● **I51.8**   **Other ill-defined heart diseases**
I51.81   **Takotsubo syndrome** 🪙
Reversible left ventricular dysfunction following sudden emotional stress
Stress induced cardiomyopathy
Takotsubo cardiomyopathy
Transient left ventricular apical ballooning syndrome

I51.89   **Other ill-defined heart diseases**
Carditis (acute)(chronic)
Pancarditis (acute)(chronic)

◼ **I51.9**   **Heart disease, unspecified**

● ▸ *I52*   *Other heart disorders in diseases classified elsewhere*
Code first underlying disease, such as:
congenital syphilis (A50.5)
mucopolysaccharidosis (E76.3)
schistosomiasis (B65.0-B65.9)
Excludes1   heart disease (in):
gonococcal infection (A54.83)
meningococcal infection (A39.50)
rheumatoid arthritis (M05.31)
syphilis (A52.06)

CEREBROVASCULAR DISEASES (I60-I69)

Use additional code to identify presence of:
alcohol abuse and dependence (F10.-)
exposure to environmental tobacco smoke (Z77.22)
history of tobacco use (Z87.891)
hypertension (I10-I15)
occupational exposure to environmental tobacco smoke (Z57.31)
tobacco dependence (F17.-)
tobacco use (Z72.0)
Excludes1   transient cerebral ischemic attacks and related syndromes (G45.-)
traumatic intracranial hemorrhage (S06.-)

● **I60**   **Nontraumatic subarachnoid hemorrhage**
Includes   ruptured cerebral aneurysm
Excludes1   sequelae of subarachnoid hemorrhage (I69.0-)
syphilitic ruptured cerebral aneurysm (A52.05)

● **I60.0**   **Nontraumatic subarachnoid hemorrhage from carotid siphon and bifurcation**
◼ **I60.00**   **Nontraumatic subarachnoid hemorrhage from unspecified carotid siphon and bifurcation** 🪙
I60.01   **Nontraumatic subarachnoid hemorrhage from right carotid siphon and bifurcation** 🪙
I60.02   **Nontraumatic subarachnoid hemorrhage from left carotid siphon and bifurcation** 🪙

● **I60.1**   **Nontraumatic subarachnoid hemorrhage from middle cerebral artery**
◼ **I60.10**   **Nontraumatic subarachnoid hemorrhage from unspecified middle cerebral artery** 🪙
I60.11   **Nontraumatic subarachnoid hemorrhage from right middle cerebral artery** 🪙
I60.12   **Nontraumatic subarachnoid hemorrhage from left middle cerebral artery** 🪙

N Newborn Age: 0   P Pediatric Age: 0–17   M Maternity DX: 12–55   A Adult Age: 15–124   ♀ Females Only   ♂ Males Only
🪙 Complication\Comorbidity   🪙 Major C\C   Present on Admission Requirement   Hospital-Acquired Condition
1033

- **I60.2 Nontraumatic subarachnoid hemorrhage from anterior communicating artery**
  - ▪ **I60.20 Nontraumatic subarachnoid hemorrhage from unspecified anterior communicating artery**
  - **I60.21 Nontraumatic subarachnoid hemorrhage from right anterior communicating artery**
  - **I60.22 Nontraumatic subarachnoid hemorrhage from left anterior communicating artery**
- **I60.3 Nontraumatic subarachnoid hemorrhage from posterior communicating artery**
  - ▪ **I60.30 Nontraumatic subarachnoid hemorrhage from unspecified posterior communicating artery**
  - **I60.31 Nontraumatic subarachnoid hemorrhage from right posterior communicating artery**
  - **I60.32 Nontraumatic subarachnoid hemorrhage from left posterior communicating artery**
- **I60.4 Nontraumatic subarachnoid hemorrhage from basilar artery**
- **I60.5 Nontraumatic subarachnoid hemorrhage from vertebral artery**
  - ▪ **I60.50 Nontraumatic subarachnoid hemorrhage from unspecified vertebral artery**
  - **I60.51 Nontraumatic subarachnoid hemorrhage from right vertebral artery**
  - **I60.52 Nontraumatic subarachnoid hemorrhage from left vertebral artery**
- **I60.6 Nontraumatic subarachnoid hemorrhage from other intracranial arteries**
- ▪ **I60.7 Nontraumatic subarachnoid hemorrhage from unspecified intracranial artery**
  - Ruptured (congenital) berry aneurysm
  - Ruptured (congenital) cerebral aneurysm
  - Subarachnoid hemorrhage (nontraumatic) from cerebral artery NOS
  - Subarachnoid hemorrhage (nontraumatic) from communicating artery NOS
  - **Excludes1** berry aneurysm, nonruptured (I67.1)
- **I60.8 Other nontraumatic subarachnoid hemorrhage**
  - Meningeal hemorrhage
  - Rupture of cerebral arteriovenous malformation
- ▪ **I60.9 Nontraumatic subarachnoid hemorrhage, unspecified**

- ● **I61 Nontraumatic intracerebral hemorrhage**
  - **Excludes1** sequelae of intracerebral hemorrhage (I69.1-)
  - **I61.0 Nontraumatic intracerebral hemorrhage in hemisphere, subcortical**
    - Deep intracerebral hemorrhage (nontraumatic)
  - **I61.1 Nontraumatic intracerebral hemorrhage in hemisphere, cortical**
    - Cerebral lobe hemorrhage (nontraumatic)
    - Superficial intracerebral hemorrhage (nontraumatic)
  - ▪ **I61.2 Nontraumatic intracerebral hemorrhage in hemisphere, unspecified**
  - **I61.3 Nontraumatic intracerebral hemorrhage in brain stem**
  - **I61.4 Nontraumatic intracerebral hemorrhage in cerebellum**
  - **I61.5 Nontraumatic intracerebral hemorrhage, intraventricular**

- **I61.6 Nontraumatic intracerebral hemorrhage, multiple localized**
- **I61.8 Other nontraumatic intracerebral hemorrhage**
- ▪ **I61.9 Nontraumatic intracerebral hemorrhage, unspecified**

- ● **I62 Other and unspecified nontraumatic intracranial hemorrhage**
  - **Excludes1** sequelae of intracranial hemorrhage (I69.2)
  - ● **I62.0 Nontraumatic subdural hemorrhage**
    - ▪ **I62.00 Nontraumatic subdural hemorrhage, unspecified**
    - **I62.01 Nontraumatic acute subdural hemorrhage**
    - **I62.02 Nontraumatic subacute subdural hemorrhage**
    - **I62.03 Nontraumatic chronic subdural hemorrhage**
  - **I62.1 Nontraumatic extradural hemorrhage**
    - Nontraumatic epidural hemorrhage
  - ▪ **I62.9 Nontraumatic intracranial hemorrhage, unspecified**

(See Plate 141 on page NAP-28.)

- ● **I63 Cerebral infarction**
  - **Includes** occlusion and stenosis of cerebral and precerebral arteries, resulting in cerebral infarction
  - **Use additional** code, if applicable, to identify status post administration of tPA (rtPA) in a different facility within the last 24 hours prior to admission to current facility (Z92.82)
  - **Excludes1** sequelae of cerebral infarction (I69.3-)
  - ● **I63.0 Cerebral infarction due to thrombosis of precerebral arteries**
    - ▪ **I63.00 Cerebral infarction due to thrombosis of unspecified precerebral artery**
    - ● **I63.01 Cerebral infarction due to thrombosis of vertebral artery**
      - **I63.011 Cerebral infarction due to thrombosis of right vertebral artery**
      - **I63.012 Cerebral infarction due to thrombosis of left vertebral artery**
      - ▪ **I63.019 Cerebral infarction due to thrombosis of unspecified vertebral artery**
    - **I63.02 Cerebral infarction due to thrombosis of basilar artery**
    - ● **I63.03 Cerebral infarction due to thrombosis of carotid artery**
      - **I63.031 Cerebral infarction due to thrombosis of right carotid artery**
      - **I63.032 Cerebral infarction due to thrombosis of left carotid artery**
      - ▪ **I63.039 Cerebral infarction due to thrombosis of unspecified carotid artery**
    - **I63.09 Cerebral infarction due to thrombosis of other precerebral artery**

● Unacceptable Principal Diagnosis ● Use Additional Character(s) ▪ Unspecified ▶ Manifestation Code
OGCR Official Guidelines for Coding and Reporting | Excludes 1 | Excludes 2 | Includes | Use additional | Code first | Code also

CHAPTER 9 (I00-I99)

● **I63.1**   **Cerebral infarction due to embolism of precerebral arteries**

   ■ **I63.10**   Cerebral infarction due to embolism of unspecified precerebral artery 🔒

   ● **I63.11**   Cerebral infarction due to embolism of vertebral artery

     I63.111   Cerebral infarction due to embolism of right vertebral artery 🔒

     I63.112   Cerebral infarction due to embolism of left vertebral artery 🔒

     ■ **I63.119**   Cerebral infarction due to embolism of unspecified vertebral artery 🔒

   I63.12   Cerebral infarction due to embolism of basilar artery 🔒

   ● **I63.13**   Cerebral infarction due to embolism of carotid artery

     I63.131   Cerebral infarction due to embolism of right carotid artery 🔒

     I63.132   Cerebral infarction due to embolism of left carotid artery 🔒

     ■ **I63.139**   Cerebral infarction due to embolism of unspecified carotid artery 🔒

   I63.19   Cerebral infarction due to embolism of other precerebral artery 🔒

● **I63.2**   **Cerebral infarction due to unspecified occlusion or stenosis of precerebral arteries**

   ■ **I63.20**   Cerebral infarction due to unspecified occlusion or stenosis of unspecified precerebral arteries 🔒

   ● **I63.21**   Cerebral infarction due to unspecified occlusion or stenosis of vertebral arteries

     ■ **I63.211**   Cerebral infarction due to unspecified occlusion or stenosis of right vertebral arteries 🔒

     ■ **I63.212**   Cerebral infarction due to unspecified occlusion or stenosis of left vertebral arteries 🔒

     ■ **I63.219**   Cerebral infarction due to unspecified occlusion or stenosis of unspecified vertebral arteries 🔒

   ■ **I63.22**   Cerebral infarction due to unspecified occlusion or stenosis of basilar arteries 🔒

   ● **I63.23**   Cerebral infarction due to unspecified occlusion or stenosis of carotid arteries

     ■ **I63.231**   Cerebral infarction due to unspecified occlusion or stenosis of right carotid arteries 🔒

     ■ **I63.232**   Cerebral infarction due to unspecified occlusion or stenosis of left carotid arteries 🔒

     ■ **I63.239**   Cerebral infarction due to unspecified occlusion or stenosis of unspecified carotid arteries 🔒

   ■ **I63.29**   Cerebral infarction due to unspecified occlusion or stenosis of other precerebral arteries 🔒

● **I63.3**   **Cerebral infarction due to thrombosis of cerebral arteries**

   ■ **I63.30**   Cerebral infarction due to thrombosis of unspecified cerebral artery 🔒

   ● **I63.31**   Cerebral infarction due to thrombosis of middle cerebral artery

     I63.311   Cerebral infarction due to thrombosis of right middle cerebral artery 🔒

     I63.312   Cerebral infarction due to thrombosis of left middle cerebral artery 🔒

     ■ **I63.319**   Cerebral infarction due to thrombosis of unspecified middle cerebral artery 🔒

   ● **I63.32**   Cerebral infarction due to thrombosis of anterior cerebral artery

     I63.321   Cerebral infarction due to thrombosis of right anterior cerebral artery 🔒

     I63.322   Cerebral infarction due to thrombosis of left anterior cerebral artery 🔒

     ■ **I63.329**   Cerebral infarction due to thrombosis of unspecified anterior cerebral artery 🔒

   ● **I63.33**   Cerebral infarction due to thrombosis of posterior cerebral artery

     I63.331   Cerebral infarction due to thrombosis of right posterior cerebral artery 🔒

     I63.332   Cerebral infarction due to thrombosis of left posterior cerebral artery 🔒

     ■ **I63.339**   Cerebral infarction due to thrombosis of unspecified posterior cerebral artery 🔒

   ● **I63.34**   Cerebral infarction due to thrombosis of cerebellar artery

     I63.341   Cerebral infarction due to thrombosis of right cerebellar artery 🔒

     I63.342   Cerebral infarction due to thrombosis of left cerebellar artery 🔒

     ■ **I63.349**   Cerebral infarction due to thrombosis of unspecified cerebellar artery 🔒

   I63.39   Cerebral infarction due to thrombosis of other cerebral artery 🔒

● **I63.4**   **Cerebral infarction due to embolism of cerebral arteries**

   ■ **I63.40**   Cerebral infarction due to embolism of unspecified cerebral artery 🔒

   ● **I63.41**   Cerebral infarction due to embolism of middle cerebral artery

     I63.411   Cerebral infarction due to embolism of right middle cerebral artery 🔒

     I63.412   Cerebral infarction due to embolism of left middle cerebral artery 🔒

     ■ **I63.419**   Cerebral infarction due to embolism of unspecified middle cerebral artery 🔒

N Newborn Age: 0   **P** Pediatric Age: 0–17   **M** Maternity DX: 12–55   **A** Adult Age: 15–124   ♀ Females Only   ♂ Males Only

🔒 Complication\Comorbidity   🔒 Major C\C   🔒 Present on Admission Requirement   🔒 Hospital-Acquired Condition

CHAPTER 9 (I00-I99)

1035

CHAPTER 9 (I00-I99)

● **I63.42**   Cerebral infarction due to embolism of anterior cerebral artery

     I63.421   Cerebral infarction due to embolism of right anterior cerebral artery 🔾

     I63.422   Cerebral infarction due to embolism of left anterior cerebral artery 🔾

     ■ **I63.429**   Cerebral infarction due to embolism of unspecified anterior cerebral artery 🔾

● **I63.43**   Cerebral infarction due to embolism of posterior cerebral artery

     I63.431   Cerebral infarction due to embolism of right posterior cerebral artery 🔾

     I63.432   Cerebral infarction due to embolism of left posterior cerebral artery 🔾

     ■ **I63.439**   Cerebral infarction due to embolism of unspecified posterior cerebral artery 🔾

● **I63.44**   Cerebral infarction due to embolism of cerebellar artery

     I63.441   Cerebral infarction due to embolism of right cerebellar artery 🔾

     I63.442   Cerebral infarction due to embolism of left cerebellar artery 🔾

     ■ **I63.449**   Cerebral infarction due to embolism of unspecified cerebellar artery 🔾

     I63.49   Cerebral infarction due to embolism of other cerebral artery 🔾

● **I63.5**   Cerebral infarction due to unspecified occlusion or stenosis of cerebral arteries

     ■ **I63.50**   Cerebral infarction due to unspecified occlusion or stenosis of unspecified cerebral artery 🔾

     ● **I63.51**   Cerebral infarction due to unspecified occlusion or stenosis of middle cerebral artery

         ■ **I63.511**   Cerebral infarction due to unspecified occlusion or stenosis of right middle cerebral artery 🔾

         ■ **I63.512**   Cerebral infarction due to unspecified occlusion or stenosis of left middle cerebral artery 🔾

         ■ **I63.519**   Cerebral infarction due to unspecified occlusion or stenosis of unspecified middle cerebral artery 🔾

     ● **I63.52**   Cerebral infarction due to unspecified occlusion or stenosis of anterior cerebral artery

         ■ **I63.521**   Cerebral infarction due to unspecified occlusion or stenosis of right anterior cerebral artery 🔾

         ■ **I63.522**   Cerebral infarction due to unspecified occlusion or stenosis of left anterior cerebral artery 🔾

         ■ **I63.529**   Cerebral infarction due to unspecified occlusion or stenosis of unspecified anterior cerebral artery 🔾

● **I63.53**   Cerebral infarction due to unspecified occlusion or stenosis of posterior cerebral artery

     ■ **I63.531**   Cerebral infarction due to unspecified occlusion or stenosis of right posterior cerebral artery 🔾

     ■ **I63.532**   Cerebral infarction due to unspecified occlusion or stenosis of left posterior cerebral artery 🔾

     ■ **I63.539**   Cerebral infarction due to unspecified occlusion or stenosis of unspecified posterior cerebral artery 🔾

● **I63.54**   Cerebral infarction due to unspecified occlusion or stenosis of cerebellar artery

     ■ **I63.541**   Cerebral infarction due to unspecified occlusion or stenosis of right cerebellar artery 🔾

     ■ **I63.542**   Cerebral infarction due to unspecified occlusion or stenosis of left cerebellar artery 🔾

     ■ **I63.549**   Cerebral infarction due to unspecified occlusion or stenosis of unspecified cerebellar artery 🔾

     ■ **I63.59**   Cerebral infarction due to unspecified occlusion or stenosis of other cerebral artery 🔾

     I63.6   Cerebral infarction due to cerebral venous thrombosis, nonpyogenic 🔾

     I63.8   Other cerebral infarction 🔾

     ■ **I63.9**   Cerebral infarction, unspecified 🔾
              Stroke NOS

● **I65**   Occlusion and stenosis of precerebral arteries, not resulting in cerebral infarction

     Includes   embolism of precerebral artery
            narrowing of precerebral artery
            obstruction (complete) (partial) of precerebral artery
            thrombosis of precerebral artery

     Excludes 1   insufficiency, NOS, of precerebral artery (G45.-)
            insufficiency of precerebral arteries causing cerebral infarction (I63.0-I63.2)

● **I65.0**   Occlusion and stenosis of vertebral artery

     I65.01   Occlusion and stenosis of right vertebral artery

     I65.02   Occlusion and stenosis of left vertebral artery

     I65.03   Occlusion and stenosis of bilateral vertebral arteries

     ■ **I65.09**   Occlusion and stenosis of unspecified vertebral artery

     I65.1   Occlusion and stenosis of basilar artery

● **I65.2**   Occlusion and stenosis of carotid artery

     I65.21   Occlusion and stenosis of right carotid artery

     I65.22   Occlusion and stenosis of left carotid artery

     I65.23   Occlusion and stenosis of bilateral carotid arteries

     ■ **I65.29**   Occlusion and stenosis of unspecified carotid artery

---

● Unacceptable Principal Diagnosis   ● Use Additional Character(s)   ■ Unspecified   ▶ Manifestation Code

OGCR Official Guidelines for Coding and Reporting   Excludes 1   Excludes 2   Includes   Use additional   Code first   Code also

1036

I65.8   **Occlusion and stenosis of other precerebral arteries**

■ I65.9   **Occlusion and stenosis of unspecified precerebral artery**
       Occlusion and stenosis of precerebral artery NOS

● **I66**   **Occlusion and stenosis of cerebral arteries, not resulting in cerebral infarction**

     Includes   embolism of cerebral artery
                 narrowing of cerebral artery
                 obstruction (complete) (partial) of cerebral artery
                 thrombosis of cerebral artery

     Excludes1   occlusion and stenosis of cerebral artery causing cerebral infarction (I63.3-I63.5)

● I66.0   **Occlusion and stenosis of middle cerebral artery**

     I66.01   **Occlusion and stenosis of right middle cerebral artery**

     I66.02   **Occlusion and stenosis of left middle cerebral artery**

     I66.03   **Occlusion and stenosis of bilateral middle cerebral arteries**

     ■ I66.09   **Occlusion and stenosis of unspecified middle cerebral artery**

● I66.1   **Occlusion and stenosis of anterior cerebral artery**

     I66.11   **Occlusion and stenosis of right anterior cerebral artery**

     I66.12   **Occlusion and stenosis of left anterior cerebral artery**

     I66.13   **Occlusion and stenosis of bilateral anterior cerebral arteries**

     ■ I66.19   **Occlusion and stenosis of unspecified anterior cerebral artery**

● I66.2   **Occlusion and stenosis of posterior cerebral artery**

     I66.21   **Occlusion and stenosis of right posterior cerebral artery**

     I66.22   **Occlusion and stenosis of left posterior cerebral artery**

     I66.23   **Occlusion and stenosis of bilateral posterior cerebral arteries**

     ■ I66.29   **Occlusion and stenosis of unspecified posterior cerebral artery**

I66.3   **Occlusion and stenosis of cerebellar arteries**

I66.8   **Occlusion and stenosis of other cerebral arteries**
       Occlusion and stenosis of perforating arteries

■ I66.9   **Occlusion and stenosis of unspecified cerebral artery**

● **I67**   **Other cerebrovascular diseases**

     Excludes1   sequelae of the listed conditions (I69.8)

I67.0   **Dissection of cerebral arteries, nonruptured** 🔹

     Excludes1   ruptured cerebral arteries (I60.7)

I67.1   **Cerebral aneurysm, nonruptured**
       Cerebral aneurysm NOS
       Cerebral arteriovenous fistula, acquired
       Internal carotid artery aneurysm, intracranial portion
       Internal carotid artery aneurysm, NOS

     Excludes1   congenital cerebral aneurysm, nonruptured (Q28.-)
                ruptured cerebral aneurysm (I60.7)

I67.2   **Cerebral atherosclerosis**   **A**
       Atheroma of cerebral and precerebral arteries

I67.3   **Progressive vascular leukoencephalopathy** 🔹
       Binswanger's disease

I67.4   **Hypertensive encephalopathy** 🔹

I67.5   **Moyamoya disease** 🔹

I67.6   **Nonpyogenic thrombosis of intracranial venous system** 🔹
       Nonpyogenic thrombosis of cerebral vein
       Nonpyogenic thrombosis of intracranial venous sinus

     Excludes1   nonpyogenic thrombosis of intracranial venous system causing infarction (I63.6)

I67.7   **Cerebral arteritis, not elsewhere classified** 🔹
       Granulomatous angiitis of the nervous system

     Excludes1   allergic granulomatous angiitis (M30.1)

● I67.8   **Other specified cerebrovascular diseases**

     I67.81   **Acute cerebrovascular insufficiency** 🔹
         Acute cerebrovascular insufficiency unspecified as to location or reversibility

     I67.82   **Cerebral ischemia** 🔹
         Chronic cerebral ischemia

     I67.83   **Posterior reversible encephalopathy syndrome** 🔹
         PRES

     ● I67.84   **Cerebral vasospasm and vasoconstriction**

         I67.841   **Reversible cerebrovascular vasoconstriction syndrome** 🔹
            Call-Fleming syndrome

            Code first underlying condition, if applicable, such as eclampsia (O15.00-O15.9)

         I67.848   **Other cerebrovascular vasospasm and vasoconstriction** 🔹

     I67.89   **Other cerebrovascular disease** 🔹

■ I67.9   **Cerebrovascular disease, unspecified**

● **I68**   **Cerebrovascular disorders in diseases classified elsewhere**

     ●▶ *I68.0*   *Cerebral amyloid angiopathy*
         Code first underlying amyloidosis (E85-)

     ●▶ *I68.2*   *Cerebral arteritis in other diseases classified elsewhere* 🔹
         Code first underlying disease

     Excludes1   cerebral arteritis (in):
                 listerosis (A32.89)
                 systemic lupus erythematosus (M32.19)
                 syphilis (A52.04)
                 tuberculosis (A18.89)

     ●▶ *I68.8*   *Other cerebrovascular disorders in diseases classified elsewhere*
         Code first underlying disease

     Excludes1   syphilitic cerebral aneurysm (A52.05)

N   Newborn Age: 0   **P**   Pediatric Age: 0–17   **M**   Maternity DX: 12–55   **A**   Adult Age: 15–124   ♀   Females Only   ♂   Males Only

🔹 Complication\Comorbidity   🔹 Major C\C   🔹 Present on Admission Requirement   🔹 Hospital-Acquired Condition   **1037**

OGCR Section I.c.9.d.

Sequelae of Cerebrovascular Disease

1) Category I69, Sequelae of Cerebrovascular disease

Category I69 is used to indicate conditions classifiable to categories I60-I67 as the causes of sequela (neurologic deficits), themselves classified elsewhere. These "late effects" include neurologic deficits that persist after initial onset of conditions classifiable to categories I60-I67. The neurologic deficits caused by cerebrovascular disease may be present from the onset of may arise at any time after the onset of the condition classifiable to categories I60-I67.

2) Codes from category I69 with codes from I60-I67

Codes from category I69 may be assigned on a health care record with codes from I60-I67, if the patient has a current cerebrovascular disease and deficits from an old cerebrovascular disease.

● **I69**   **Sequelae of cerebrovascular disease**

    Note: Category I69 is to be used to indicate conditions in I60-I67 as the cause of sequelae. The 'sequelae' include conditions specified as such or as residuals which may occur at any time after the onset of the causal condition.

    Excludes1   personal history of cerebral infarction without residual deficit (Z86.73)

           personal history of prolonged reversible ischemic neurologic deficit (PRIND) (Z86.73)

           personal history of reversible ischemic neurologcial deficit (RIND) (Z86.73)

           sequelae of traumatic intracranial injury (S06.-)

           transient ischemic attack (TIA) (G45.9)

● **I69.0**   **Sequelae of nontraumatic subarachnoid hemorrhage**

  ■ **I69.00**   Unspecified sequelae of nontraumatic subarachnoid hemorrhage

    I69.01   Cognitive deficits following nontraumatic subarachnoid hemorrhage

  ● **I69.02**   Speech and language deficits following nontraumatic subarachnoid hemorrhage

      I69.020   Aphasia following nontraumatic subarachnoid hemorrhage

      I69.021   Dysphasia following nontraumatic subarachnoid hemorrhage

      I69.022   Dysarthria following nontraumatic subarachnoid hemorrhage

      I69.023   Fluency disorder following nontraumatic subarachnoid hemorrhage

          Stuttering following nontraumatic subarachnoid hemorrhage

      I69.028   Other speech and language deficits following nontraumatic subarachnoid hemorrhage

  ● **I69.03**   Monoplegia of upper limb following nontraumatic subarachnoid hemorrhage

      I69.031   Monoplegia of upper limb following nontraumatic subarachnoid hemorrhage affecting right dominant side

      I69.032   Monoplegia of upper limb following nontraumatic subarachnoid hemorrhage affecting left dominant side

      I69.033   Monoplegia of upper limb following nontraumatic subarachnoid hemorrhage affecting right non-dominant side

      I69.034   Monoplegia of upper limb following nontraumatic subarachnoid hemorrhage affecting left non-dominant side

  ■ **I69.039**   Monoplegia of upper limb following nontraumatic subarachnoid hemorrhage affecting unspecified side

  ● **I69.04**   Monoplegia of lower limb following nontraumatic subarachnoid hemorrhage

      I69.041   Monoplegia of lower limb following nontraumatic subarachnoid hemorrhage affecting right dominant side

      I69.042   Monoplegia of lower limb following nontraumatic subarachnoid hemorrhage affecting left dominant side

      I69.043   Monoplegia of lower limb following nontraumatic subarachnoid hemorrhage affecting right non-dominant side

      I69.044   Monoplegia of lower limb following nontraumatic subarachnoid hemorrhage affecting left non-dominant side

  ■ **I69.049**   Monoplegia of lower limb following nontraumatic subarachnoid hemorrhage affecting unspecified side

  ● **I69.05**   Hemiplegia and hemiparesis following nontraumatic subarachnoid hemorrhage

      I69.051   Hemiplegia and hemiparesis following nontraumatic subarachnoid hemorrhage affecting right dominant side

      I69.052   Hemiplegia and hemiparesis following nontraumatic subarachnoid hemorrhage affecting left dominant side

      I69.053   Hemiplegia and hemiparesis following nontraumatic subarachnoid hemorrhage affecting right non-dominant side

      I69.054   Hemiplegia and hemiparesis following nontraumatic subarachnoid hemorrhage affecting left non-dominant side

  ■ **I69.059**   Hemiplegia and hemiparesis following nontraumatic subarachnoid hemorrhage affecting unspecified side

● Unacceptable Principal Diagnosis   ● Use Additional Character(s)   ■ Unspecified   ▶ Manifestation Code

OGCR Official Guidelines for Coding and Reporting   Excludes 1   Excludes 2   Includes   Use additional   Code first   Code also

● **I69.06** **Other paralytic syndrome following nontraumatic subarachnoid hemorrhage**

     Use additional code to identify type of paralytic syndrome, such as:
     locked-in state (G83.5)
     quadriplegia (G82.5-)

     Excludes1 hemiplegia/hemiparesis following nontraumatic subarachnoid hemorrhage (I69.05-)
       monoplegia of lower limb following nontraumatic subarachnoid hemorrhage (I69.04-)
       monoplegia of upper limb following nontraumatic subarachnoid hemorrhage (I69.03-)

     I69.061 **Other paralytic syndrome following nontraumatic subarachnoid hemorrhage affecting right dominant side**

     I69.062 **Other paralytic syndrome following nontraumatic subarachnoid hemorrhage affecting left dominant side**

     I69.063 **Other paralytic syndrome following nontraumatic subarachnoid hemorrhage affecting right non-dominant side**

     I69.064 **Other paralytic syndrome following nontraumatic subarachnoid hemorrhage affecting left non-dominant side**

     I69.065 **Other paralytic syndrome following nontraumatic subarachnoid hemorrhage, bilateral**

     ■ **I69.069** **Other paralytic syndrome following nontraumatic subarachnoid hemorrhage affecting unspecified side**

● **I69.09** **Other sequelae of nontraumatic subarachnoid hemorrhage**

     I69.090 **Apraxia following nontraumatic subarachnoid hemorrhage**

     I69.091 **Dysphagia following nontraumatic subarachnoid hemorrhage**

       Use additional code to identify the type of dysphagia, if known (R13.1-)

     I69.092 **Facial weakness following nontraumatic subarachnoid hemorrhage**
       Facial droop following nontraumatic subarachnoid hemorrhage

     I69.093 **Ataxia following nontraumatic subarachnoid hemorrhage**

I69.098 **Other sequelae following nontraumatic subarachnoid hemorrhage**
     Alterations of sensation following nontraumatic subarachnoid hemorrhage
     Disturbance of vision following nontraumatic subarachnoid hemorrhage

     Use additional code to identify the sequelae

● **I69.1** **Sequelae of nontraumatic intracerebral hemorrhage**

     ■ **I69.10** **Unspecified sequelae of nontraumatic intracerebral hemorrhage**

     I69.11 **Cognitive deficits following nontraumatic intracerebral hemorrhage**

     ● **I69.12** **Speech and language deficits following nontraumatic intracerebral hemorrhage**

       I69.120 **Aphasia following nontraumatic intracerebral hemorrhage**

       I69.121 **Dysphasia following nontraumatic intracerebral hemorrhage**

       I69.122 **Dysarthria following nontraumatic intracerebral hemorrhage**

       I69.123 **Fluency disorder following nontraumatic intracerebral hemorrhage**
       Stuttering following nontraumatic subarachnoid hemorrhage

       I69.128 **Other speech and language deficits following nontraumatic intracerebral hemorrhage**

     ● **I69.13** **Monoplegia of upper limb following nontraumatic intracerebral hemorrhage**

       I69.131 **Monoplegia of upper limb following nontraumatic intracerebral hemorrhage affecting right dominant side**

       I69.132 **Monoplegia of upper limb following nontraumatic intracerebral hemorrhage affecting left dominant side**

       I69.133 **Monoplegia of upper limb following nontraumatic intracerebral hemorrhage affecting right non-dominant side**

       I69.134 **Monoplegia of upper limb following nontraumatic intracerebral hemorrhage affecting left non-dominant side**

       ■ **I69.139** **Monoplegia of upper limb following nontraumatic intracerebral hemorrhage affecting unspecified side**

     ● **I69.14** **Monoplegia of lower limb following nontraumatic intracerebral hemorrhage**

       I69.141 **Monoplegia of lower limb following nontraumatic intracerebral hemorrhage affecting right dominant side**

CHAPTER 9 (I00-I99)

CHAPTER 9 (I00-I99)

I69.142 Monoplegia of lower limb following nontraumatic intracerebral hemorrhage affecting left dominant side

I69.143 Monoplegia of lower limb following nontraumatic intracerebral hemorrhage affecting right non-dominant side

I69.144 Monoplegia of lower limb following nontraumatic intracerebral hemorrhage affecting left non-dominant side

I69.149 Monoplegia of lower limb following nontraumatic intracerebral hemorrhage affecting unspecified side

● **I69.15** Hemiplegia and hemiparesis following nontraumatic intracerebral hemorrhage

I69.151 Hemiplegia and hemiparesis following nontraumatic intracerebral hemorrhage affecting right dominant side

I69.152 Hemiplegia and hemiparesis following nontraumatic intracerebral hemorrhage affecting left dominant side

I69.153 Hemiplegia and hemiparesis following nontraumatic intracerebral hemorrhage affecting right non-dominant side

I69.154 Hemiplegia and hemiparesis following nontraumatic intracerebral hemorrhage affecting left non-dominant side

I69.159 Hemiplegia and hemiparesis following nontraumatic intracerebral hemorrhage affecting unspecified side

● **I69.16** Other paralytic syndrome following nontraumatic intracerebral hemorrhage

Use additional code to identify type of paralytic syndrome, such as:
locked-in state (G83.5)
quadriplegia (G82.5-)

Excludes1 hemiplegia/hemiparesis following nontraumatic intracerebral hemorrhage (I69.15-)
monoplegia of lower limb following nontraumatic intracerebral hemorrhage (I69.14-)
monoplegia of upper limb following nontraumatic intracerebral hemorrhage (I69.13-)

I69.161 Other paralytic syndrome following nontraumatic intracerebral hemorrhage affecting right dominant side

I69.162 Other paralytic syndrome following nontraumatic intracerebral hemorrhage affecting left dominant side

I69.163 Other paralytic syndrome following nontraumatic intracerebral hemorrhage affecting right non-dominant side

I69.164 Other paralytic syndrome following nontraumatic intracerebral hemorrhage affecting left non-dominant side

I69.165 Other paralytic syndrome following nontraumatic intracerebral hemorrhage, bilateral

I69.169 Other paralytic syndrome following nontraumatic intracerebral hemorrhage affecting unspecified side

● **I69.19** Other sequelae of nontraumatic intracerebral hemorrhage

I69.190 Apraxia following nontraumatic intracerebral hemorrhage

I69.191 Dysphagia following nontraumatic intracerebral hemorrhage

Use additional code to identify the type of dysphagia, if known (R13.1-)

I69.192 Facial weakness following nontraumatic intracerebral hemorrhage
Facial droop following nontraumatic intracerebral hemorrhage

I69.193 Ataxia following nontraumatic intracerebral hemorrhage

I69.198 Other sequelae of nontraumatic intracerebral hemorrhage
Alteration of sensations following nontraumatic intracerebral hemorrhage
Disturbance of vision following nontraumatic intracerebral hemorrhage

Use additional code to identify the sequelae

● **I69.2** Sequelae of other nontraumatic intracranial hemorrhage

I69.20 Unspecified sequelae of other nontraumatic intracranial hemorrhage

I69.21 Cognitive deficits following other nontraumatic intracranial hemorrhage

● **I69.22** Speech and language deficits following other nontraumatic intracranial hemorrhage

I69.220 Aphasia following other nontraumatic intracranial hemorrhage

I69.221 Dysphasia following other nontraumatic intracranial hemorrhage

I69.222 Dysarthria following other nontraumatic intracranial hemorrhage

I69.223   **Fluency disorder following other nontraumatic intracranial hemorrhage** 🔖
              Stuttering following nontraumatic subarachnoid hemorrhage

I69.228   **Other speech and language deficits following other nontraumatic intracranial hemorrhage** 🔖

● I69.23   **Monoplegia of upper limb following other nontraumatic intracranial hemorrhage**

I69.231   **Monoplegia of upper limb following other nontraumatic intracranial hemorrhage affecting right dominant side** 🔖

I69.232   **Monoplegia of upper limb following other nontraumatic intracranial hemorrhage affecting left dominant side** 🔖

I69.233   **Monoplegia of upper limb following other nontraumatic intracranial hemorrhage affecting right non-dominant side** 🔖

I69.234   **Monoplegia of upper limb following other nontraumatic intracranial hemorrhage affecting left non-dominant side** 🔖

■ I69.239 **Monoplegia of upper limb following other nontraumatic intracranial hemorrhage affecting unspecified side** 🔖

● I69.24   **Monoplegia of lower limb following other nontraumatic intracranial hemorrhage**

I69.241   **Monoplegia of lower limb following other nontraumatic intracranial hemorrhage affecting right dominant side** 🔖

I69.242   **Monoplegia of lower limb following other nontraumatic intracranial hemorrhage affecting left dominant side** 🔖

I69.243   **Monoplegia of lower limb following other nontraumatic intracranial hemorrhage affecting right non-dominant side** 🔖

I69.244   **Monoplegia of lower limb following other nontraumatic intracranial hemorrhage affecting left non-dominant side** 🔖

■ I69.249 **Monoplegia of lower limb following other nontraumatic intracranial hemorrhage affecting unspecified side** 🔖

● I69.25   **Hemiplegia and hemiparesis following other nontraumatic intracranial hemorrhage**

I69.251   **Hemiplegia and hemiparesis following other nontraumatic intracranial hemorrhage affecting right dominant side** 🔖🔖

I69.252   **Hemiplegia and hemiparesis following other nontraumatic intracranial hemorrhage affecting left dominant side** 🔖🔖

I69.253   **Hemiplegia and hemiparesis following other nontraumatic intracranial hemorrhage affecting right non-dominant side** 🔖🔖

I69.254   **Hemiplegia and hemiparesis following other nontraumatic intracranial hemorrhage affecting left non-dominant side** 🔖🔖

■ I69.259 **Hemiplegia and hemiparesis following other nontraumatic intracranial hemorrhage affecting unspecified side** 🔖🔖

● I69.26   **Other paralytic syndrome following other nontraumatic intracranial hemorrhage**

   Use additional code to identify type of paralytic syndrome, such as:
   locked-in state (G83.5)
   quadriplegia (G82.5-)

   Excludes1 hemiplegia/hemiparesis following other nontraumatic intracranial hemorrhage (I69.25-)
   monoplegia of lower limb following other nontraumatic intracranial hemorrhage (I69.24-)
   monoplegia of upper limb following other nontraumatic intracranial hemorrhage (I69.23-)

I69.261   **Other paralytic syndrome following other nontraumatic intracranial hemorrhage affecting right dominant side** 🔖

I69.262   **Other paralytic syndrome following other nontraumatic intracranial hemorrhage affecting left dominant side** 🔖

I69.263   **Other paralytic syndrome following other nontraumatic intracranial hemorrhage affecting right non-dominant side** 🔖

I69.264   **Other paralytic syndrome following other nontraumatic intracranial hemorrhage affecting left non-dominant side** 🔖

I69.265   **Other paralytic syndrome following other nontraumatic intracranial hemorrhage, bilateral** 🔖

■ I69.269 **Other paralytic syndrome following other nontraumatic intracranial hemorrhage affecting unspecified side** 🔖

● I69.29   **Other sequelae of other nontraumatic intracranial hemorrhage**

I69.290   **Apraxia following other nontraumatic intracranial hemorrhage** 🔖

I69.291   **Dysphagia following other nontraumatic intracranial hemorrhage** 🔖

   Use additional code to identify the type of dysphagia, if known (R13.1-)

N Newborn Age: 0   **P** Pediatric Age: 0–17   **M** Maternity DX: 12–55   **A** Adult Age: 15–124   ♀ Females Only   ♂ Males Only

🔖 Complication\Comorbidity   🔖 Major C\C   🔖 Present on Admission Requirement   🔖 Hospital-Acquired Condition

CHAPTER 9 (I00-I99)

1041

I69.292 **Facial weakness following other nontraumatic intracranial hemorrhage** 🔍

    Facial droop following other nontraumatic intracranial hemorrhage

I69.293 **Ataxia following other nontraumatic intracranial hemorrhage** 🔍

I69.298 **Other sequelae of other nontraumatic intracranial hemorrhage** 🔍

    Alteration of sensation following other nontraumatic intracranial hemorrhage

    Disturbance of vision following other nontraumatic intracranial hemorrhage

    Use additional code to identify the sequelae

● **I69.3** **Sequelae of cerebral infarction**
Sequelae of stroke NOS

■ **I69.30** **Unspecified sequelae of cerebral infarction** 🔍

I69.31 **Cognitive deficits following cerebral infarction** 🔍

● **I69.32** **Speech and language deficits following cerebral infarction**

I69.320 **Aphasia following cerebral infarction** 🔍

I69.321 **Dysphasia following cerebral infarction** 🔍

I69.322 **Dysarthria following cerebral infarction** 🔍

I69.323 **Fluency disorder following cerebral infarction** 🔍

    Stuttering following nontraumatic subarachnoid hemorrhage

I69.328 **Other speech and language deficits following cerebral infarction** 🔍

● **I69.33** **Monoplegia of upper limb following cerebral infarction**

I69.331 **Monoplegia of upper limb following cerebral infarction affecting right dominant side** 🔍

I69.332 **Monoplegia of upper limb following cerebral infarction affecting left dominant side** 🔍

I69.333 **Monoplegia of upper limb following cerebral infarction affecting right non-dominant side** 🔍

I69.334 **Monoplegia of upper limb following cerebral infarction affecting left non-dominant side** 🔍

■ **I69.339** **Monoplegia of upper limb following cerebral infarction affecting unspecified side** 🔍

● **I69.34** **Monoplegia of lower limb following cerebral infarction**

I69.341 **Monoplegia of lower limb following cerebral infarction affecting right dominant side** 🔍

I69.342 **Monoplegia of lower limb following cerebral infarction affecting left dominant side** 🔍

I69.343 **Monoplegia of lower limb following cerebral infarction affecting right non-dominant side** 🔍

I69.344 **Monoplegia of lower limb following cerebral infarction affecting left non-dominant side** 🔍

■ **I69.349** **Monoplegia of lower limb following cerebral infarction affecting unspecified side** 🔍

● **I69.35** **Hemiplegia and hemiparesis following cerebral infarction**

I69.351 **Hemiplegia and hemiparesis following cerebral infarction affecting right dominant side** 🔍🔍

I69.352 **Hemiplegia and hemiparesis following cerebral infarction affecting left dominant side** 🔍🔍

I69.353 **Hemiplegia and hemiparesis following cerebral infarction affecting right non-dominant side** 🔍🔍

I69.354 **Hemiplegia and hemiparesis following cerebral infarction affecting left non-dominant side** 🔍🔍

■ **I69.359** **Hemiplegia and hemiparesis following cerebral infarction affecting unspecified side** 🔍🔍

● **I69.36** **Other paralytic syndrome following cerebral infarction**

Use additional code to identify type of paralytic syndrome, such as:
locked-in state (G83.5)
quadriplegia (G82.5-)

    Excludes1 hemiplegia/hemiparesis following cerebral infarction (I69.35-)
monoplegia of lower limb following cerebral infarction (I69.34-)
monoplegia of upper limb following cerebral infarction (I69.33-)

I69.361 **Other paralytic syndrome following cerebral infarction affecting right dominant side** 🔍

I69.362 **Other paralytic syndrome following cerebral infarction affecting left dominant side** 🔍

I69.363 **Other paralytic syndrome following cerebral infarction affecting right non-dominant side** 🔍

I69.364 **Other paralytic syndrome following cerebral infarction affecting left non-dominant side** 🔍

I69.365 **Other paralytic syndrome following cerebral infarction, bilateral** 🔍

■ **I69.369** **Other paralytic syndrome following cerebral infarction affecting unspecified side** 🔍

● Unacceptable Principal Diagnosis   ● Use Additional Character(s)   ■ Unspecified   ▶ Manifestation Code

OGCR Official Guidelines for Coding and Reporting   Excludes 1   Excludes 2   Includes   Use additional   Code first   Code also

CHAPTER 9 (I00-I99)

● **I69.39   Other sequelae of cerebral infarction**

    I69.390   Apraxia following cerebral infarction 🔍

    I69.391   Dysphagia following cerebral infarction 🔍

       Use additional code to identify the type of dysphagia, if known (R13.1-)

    I69.392   Facial weakness following cerebral infarction 🔍

       Facial droop following cerebral infarction

    I69.393   Ataxia following cerebral infarction 🔍

    I69.398   Other sequelae of cerebral infarction 🔍

       Alteration of sensation following cerebral infarction

       Disturbance of vision following cerebral infarction

       Use additional code to identify the sequelae

● **I69.8   Sequelae of other cerebrovascular diseases**

    Excludes1   sequelae of traumatic intracranial injury (S06.-)

■ **I69.80   Unspecified sequelae of other cerebrovascular disease** 🔍

   I69.81   Cognitive deficits following other cerebrovascular disease 🔍

● **I69.82   Speech and language deficits following other cerebrovascular disease**

    ■ **I69.820   Aphasia following other cerebrovascular disease** 🔍

    I69.821   Dysphasia following other cerebrovascular disease 🔍

    I69.822   Dysarthria following other cerebrovascular disease 🔍

    I69.823   Fluency disorder following other cerebrovascular disease 🔍

       Stuttering following nontraumatic subarachnoid hemorrhage

    I69.828   Other speech and language deficits following other cerebrovascular disease 🔍

● **I69.83   Monoplegia of upper limb following other cerebrovascular disease**

    I69.831   Monoplegia of upper limb following other cerebrovascular disease affecting right dominant side 🔍

    I69.832   Monoplegia of upper limb following other cerebrovascular disease affecting left dominant side 🔍

    I69.833   Monoplegia of upper limb following other cerebrovascular disease affecting right non-dominant side 🔍

    I69.834   Monoplegia of upper limb following other cerebrovascular disease affecting left non-dominant side 🔍

    ■ **I69.839   Monoplegia of upper limb following other cerebrovascular disease affecting unspecified side** 🔍

● **I69.84   Monoplegia of lower limb following other cerebrovascular disease**

    I69.841   Monoplegia of lower limb following other cerebrovascular disease affecting right dominant side 🔍

    I69.842   Monoplegia of lower limb following other cerebrovascular disease affecting left dominant side 🔍

    I69.843   Monoplegia of lower limb following other cerebrovascular disease affecting right non-dominant side 🔍

    I69.844   Monoplegia of lower limb following other cerebrovascular disease affecting left non-dominant side 🔍

    ■ **I69.849   Monoplegia of lower limb following other cerebrovascular disease affecting unspecified side** 🔍

● **I69.85   Hemiplegia and hemiparesis following other cerebrovascular disease**

    I69.851   Hemiplegia and hemiparesis following other cerebrovascular disease affecting right dominant side 🔍🔍

    I69.852   Hemiplegia and hemiparesis following other cerebrovascular disease affecting left dominant side 🔍🔍

    I69.853   Hemiplegia and hemiparesis following other cerebrovascular disease affecting right non-dominant side 🔍🔍

    I69.854   Hemiplegia and hemiparesis following other cerebrovascular disease affecting left non-dominant side 🔍🔍

    ■ **I69.859   Hemiplegia and hemiparesis following other cerebrovascular disease affecting unspecified side** 🔍🔍

● **I69.86   Other paralytic syndrome following other cerebrovascular disease**

       Use additional code to identify type of paralytic syndrome, such as:
       locked-in state (G83.5)
       quadriplegia (G82.5-)

    Excludes1   hemiplegia/hemiparesis following other cerebrovascular disease (I69.85-)

       monoplegia of lower limb following other cerebrovascular disease (I69.84-)

       monoplegia of upper limb following other cerebrovascular disease (I69.83-)

    I69.861   Other paralytic syndrome following other cerebrovascular disease affecting right dominant side 🔍

N   Newborn Age: 0   **P**   Pediatric Age: 0–17   **M**   Maternity DX: 12–55   **A**   Adult Age: 15–124   ♀   Females Only   ♂   Males Only

🔍 Complication\Comorbidity   🔍 Major C\C   Present on Admission Requirement   🔍 Hospital-Acquired Condition

1043

CHAPTER 9 (I00-I99)

I69.862   Other paralytic syndrome following other cerebrovascular disease affecting left dominant side 🔍

I69.863   Other paralytic syndrome following other cerebrovascular disease affecting right non-dominant side 🔍

I69.864   Other paralytic syndrome following other cerebrovascular disease affecting left non-dominant side 🔍

I69.865   Other paralytic syndrome following other cerebrovascular disease, bilateral 🔍

■ I69.869   Other paralytic syndrome following other cerebrovascular disease affecting unspecified side 🔍

● I69.89   Other sequelae of other cerebrovascular disease

I69.890   Apraxia following other cerebrovascular disease 🔍

I69.891   Dysphagia following other cerebrovascular disease 🔍

> Use additional code to identify the type of dysphagia, if known (R13.1-)

I69.892   Facial weakness following other cerebrovascular disease 🔍
> Facial droop following other cerebrovascular disease

I69.893   Ataxia following other cerebrovascular disease 🔍

I69.898   Other sequelae of other cerebrovascular disease 🔍
> Alteration of sensation following other cerebrovascular disease
> Disturbance of vision following other cerebrovascular disease

> Use additional code to identify the sequelae

● I69.9   Sequelae of unspecified cerebrovascular diseases

Excludes1   sequelae of stroke (I69.3)
sequelae of traumatic intracranial injury (S06.-)

■ I69.90   Unspecified sequelae of unspecified cerebrovascular disease 🔍

■ I69.91   Cognitive deficits following unspecified cerebrovascular disease 🔍

● I69.92   Speech and language deficits following unspecified cerebrovascular disease

■ I69.920   Aphasia following unspecified cerebrovascular disease 🔍

■ I69.921   Dysphasia following unspecified cerebrovascular disease 🔍

■ I69.922   Dysarthria following unspecified cerebrovascular disease 🔍

■ I69.923   Fluency disorder following unspecified cerebrovascular disease 🔍
> Stuttering following nontraumatic subarachnoid hemorrhage

■ I69.928   Other speech and language deficits following unspecified cerebrovascular disease 🔍

● I69.93   Monoplegia of upper limb following unspecified cerebrovascular disease

■ I69.931   Monoplegia of upper limb following unspecified cerebrovascular disease affecting right dominant side 🔍

■ I69.932   Monoplegia of upper limb following unspecified cerebrovascular disease affecting left dominant side 🔍

■ I69.933   Monoplegia of upper limb following unspecified cerebrovascular disease affecting right non-dominant side 🔍

■ I69.934   Monoplegia of upper limb following unspecified cerebrovascular disease affecting left non-dominant side 🔍

■ I69.939   Monoplegia of upper limb following unspecified cerebrovascular disease affecting unspecified side 🔍

● I69.94   Monoplegia of lower limb following unspecified cerebrovascular disease

■ I69.941   Monoplegia of lower limb following unspecified cerebrovascular disease affecting right dominant side 🔍

■ I69.942   Monoplegia of lower limb following unspecified cerebrovascular disease affecting left dominant side 🔍

■ I69.943   Monoplegia of lower limb following unspecified cerebrovascular disease affecting right non-dominant side 🔍

■ I69.944   Monoplegia of lower limb following unspecified cerebrovascular disease affecting left non-dominant side 🔍

■ I69.949   Monoplegia of lower limb following unspecified cerebrovascular disease affecting unspecified side 🔍

● I69.95   Hemiplegia and hemiparesis following unspecified cerebrovascular disease

■ I69.951   Hemiplegia and hemiparesis following unspecified cerebrovascular disease affecting right dominant side 🔹🔍

■ I69.952   Hemiplegia and hemiparesis following unspecified cerebrovascular disease affecting left dominant side 🔹🔍

■ I69.953   Hemiplegia and hemiparesis following unspecified cerebrovascular disease affecting right non-dominant side 🔹🔍

■ I69.954   Hemiplegia and hemiparesis following unspecified cerebrovascular disease affecting left non-dominant side 🔹🔍

■ I69.959   Hemiplegia and hemiparesis following unspecified cerebrovascular disease affecting unspecified side 🔹🔍

● Unacceptable Principal Diagnosis   ● Use Additional Character(s)   ■ Unspecified   ▶ Manifestation Code

OGCR Official Guidelines for Coding and Reporting   Excludes 1   Excludes 2   Includes   Use additional   Code first   Code also

● **I69.96** **Other paralytic syndrome following unspecified cerebrovascular disease**

Use additional code to identify type of paralytic syndrome, such as:
locked-in state (G83.5)
quadriplegia (G82.5-)

Excludes1 | hemiplegia/hemiparesis following unspecified cerebrovascular disease (I69.95-)
monoplegia of lower limb following unspecified cerebrovascular disease (I69.94-)
monoplegia of upper limb following unspecified cerebrovascular disease (I69.93-)

■ I69.961 **Other paralytic syndrome following unspecified cerebrovascular disease affecting right dominant side** 🖐

■ I69.962 **Other paralytic syndrome following unspecified cerebrovascular disease affecting left dominant side** 🖐

■ I69.963 **Other paralytic syndrome following unspecified cerebrovascular disease affecting right non-dominant side** 🖐

■ I69.964 **Other paralytic syndrome following unspecified cerebrovascular disease affecting left non-dominant side** 🖐

■ I69.965 **Other paralytic syndrome following unspecified cerebrovascular disease, bilateral** 🖐

■ I69.969 **Other paralytic syndrome following unspecified cerebrovascular disease affecting unspecified side** 🖐

● **I69.99** **Other sequelae of unspecified cerebrovascular disease**

■ I69.990 **Apraxia following unspecified cerebrovascular disease** 🖐

■ I69.991 **Dysphagia following unspecified cerebrovascular disease**

Use additional code to identify the type of dysphagia, if known (R13.1-)

■ I69.992 **Facial weakness following unspecified cerebrovascular disease** 🖐
Facial droop following unspecified cerebrovascular disease

■ I69.993 **Ataxia following unspecified cerebrovascular disease** 🖐

■ I69.998 **Other sequelae following unspecified cerebrovascular disease** 🖐
Alteration in sensation following unspecified cerebrovascular disease
Disturbance of vision following unspecified cerebrovascular disease

Use additional code to identify the sequelae

DISEASES OF ARTERIES, ARTERIOLES AND CAPILLARIES (I70-I79)

● **I70** **Atherosclerosis**

Includes | arteriolosclerosis
arterial degeneration
arteriosclerosis
arteriosclerotic vascular disease
arteriovascular degeneration
atheroma
endarteritis deformans or obliterans
senile arteritis
senile endarteritis
vascular degeneration

Use additional code to identify:
exposure to environmental tobacco smoke (Z77.22)
history of tobacco use (Z87.891)
occupational exposure to environmental tobacco smoke (Z57.31)
tobacco dependence (F17.-)
tobacco use (Z72.0)

Excludes2 | arteriosclerotic cardiovascular disease (I25.1-)
arteriosclerotic heart disease (I25.1-)
atheroembolism (I75.-)
cerebral atherosclerosis (I67.2)
coronary atherosclerosis (I25.1-)
mesenteric atherosclerosis (K55.1)
precerebral atherosclerosis (I67.2)
primary pulmonary atherosclerosis (I27.0)

I70.0 **Atherosclerosis of aorta** A

I70.1 **Atherosclerosis of renal artery** A
Goldblatt's kidney

Excludes2 | atherosclerosis of renal arterioles (I12.-)

(See Plates 500, 501, and 502 on pages NAP-12 – NAP-14.)

● **I70.2** **Atherosclerosis of native arteries of the extremities**
Mönckeberg's (medial) sclerosis

Use additional code, if applicable, to identify chronic total occlusion of artery of extremity (I70.92)

Excludes2 | atherosclerosis of bypass graft of extremities (I70.30-I70.79)

● **I70.20** **Unspecified atherosclerosis of native arteries of extremities**

■ I70.201 **Unspecified atherosclerosis of native arteries of extremities, right leg** A

■ I70.202 **Unspecified atherosclerosis of native arteries of extremities, left leg** A

■ I70.203 **Unspecified atherosclerosis of native arteries of extremities, bilateral legs** A

■ I70.208 **Unspecified atherosclerosis of native arteries of extremities, other extremity** A

■ I70.209 **Unspecified atherosclerosis of native arteries of extremities, unspecified extremity** A

● **I70.21** **Atherosclerosis of native arteries of extremities with intermittent claudication**

I70.211 **Atherosclerosis of native arteries of extremities with intermittent claudication, right leg** A

I70.212   Atherosclerosis of native arteries of extremities with intermittent claudication, left leg   A

I70.213   Atherosclerosis of native arteries of extremities with intermittent claudication, bilateral legs   A

I70.218   Atherosclerosis of native arteries of extremities with intermittent claudication, other extremity   A

I70.219   Atherosclerosis of native arteries of extremities with intermittent claudication, unspecified extremity   A

I70.22   Atherosclerosis of native arteries of extremities with rest pain

> **Includes**   any condition classifiable to I70.21-

I70.221   Atherosclerosis of native arteries of extremities with rest pain, right leg   A

I70.222   Atherosclerosis of native arteries of extremities with rest pain, left leg   A

I70.223   Atherosclerosis of native arteries of extremities with rest pain, bilateral legs   A

I70.228   Atherosclerosis of native arteries of extremities with rest pain, other extremity   A

I70.229   Atherosclerosis of native arteries of extremities with rest pain, unspecified extremity   A

I70.23   Atherosclerosis of native arteries of right leg with ulceration

> **Includes**   any condition classifiable to I70.211 and I70.221

> **Use additional** code to identify severity of ulcer (L97.- with fifth character 1)

I70.231   Atherosclerosis of native arteries of right leg with ulceration of thigh   A

I70.232   Atherosclerosis of native arteries of right leg with ulceration of calf   A

I70.233   Atherosclerosis of native arteries of right leg with ulceration of ankle   A

I70.234   Atherosclerosis of native arteries of right leg with ulceration of heel and midfoot   A
> Atherosclerosis of native arteries of right leg with ulceration of plantar surface of midfoot

I70.235   Atherosclerosis of native arteries of right leg with ulceration of other part of foot   A
> Atherosclerosis of native arteries of right leg extremities with ulceration of toe

I70.238   Atherosclerosis of native arteries of right leg with ulceration of other part of lower right leg   A

I70.239   Atherosclerosis of native arteries of right leg with ulceration of unspecified site   A

I70.24   Atherosclerosis of native arteries of left leg with ulceration

> **Includes**   any condition classifiable to I70.212 and I70.222

> **Use additional** code to identify severity of ulcer (L97.- with fifth character 2)

I70.241   Atherosclerosis of native arteries of left leg with ulceration of thigh   A

I70.242   Atherosclerosis of native arteries of left leg with ulceration of calf   A

I70.243   Atherosclerosis of native arteries of left leg with ulceration of ankle   A

I70.244   Atherosclerosis of native arteries of left leg with ulceration of heel and midfoot   A
> Atherosclerosis of native arteries of left leg with ulceration of plantar surface of midfoot

I70.245   Atherosclerosis of native arteries of left leg with ulceration of other part of foot   A
> Atherosclerosis of native arteries of left leg extremities with ulceration of toe

I70.248   Atherosclerosis of native arteries of left leg with ulceration of other part of lower left leg   A

I70.249   Atherosclerosis of native arteries of left leg with ulceration of unspecified site   A

I70.25   Atherosclerosis of native arteries of other extremities with ulceration   A

> **Includes**   any condition classifiable to I70.218 and I70.228

> **Use additional** code to identify the severity of the ulcer (L98.49-)

I70.26   Atherosclerosis of native arteries of extremities with gangrene

> **Includes**   any condition classifiable to I70.21-, I70.22-, I70.23-, I70.24-, and I70.25-

> **Use additional** code to identify the severity of any ulcer (L98.49-), if applicable

I70.261   Atherosclerosis of native arteries of extremities with gangrene, right leg   A

I70.262   Atherosclerosis of native arteries of extremities with gangrene, left leg   A

I70.263   Atherosclerosis of native arteries of extremities with gangrene, bilateral legs   A

I70.268   Atherosclerosis of native arteries of extremities with gangrene, other extremity   A

I70.269   Atherosclerosis of native arteries of extremities with gangrene, unspecified extremity   A

● **I70.29   Other atherosclerosis of native arteries of extremities**

I70.291   Other atherosclerosis of native arteries of extremities, right leg **A**

I70.292   Other atherosclerosis of native arteries of extremities, left leg **A**

I70.293   Other atherosclerosis of native arteries of extremities, bilateral legs **A**

I70.298   Other atherosclerosis of native arteries of extremities, other extremity **A**

◻ I70.299   Other atherosclerosis of native arteries of extremities, unspecified extremity **A**

● **I70.3   Atherosclerosis of unspecified type of bypass graft(s) of the extremities**

Use additional code, if applicable, to identify chronic total occlusion of artery of extremity (I70.92)

Excludes1   embolism or thrombus of bypass graft(s) of extremities (T82.8-)

● **I70.30   Unspecified atherosclerosis of unspecified type of bypass graft(s) of the extremities**

◻ 70.301   Unspecified atherosclerosis of unspecified type of bypass graft(s) of the extremities, right leg **A**

◻ I70.302   Unspecified atherosclerosis of unspecified type of bypass graft(s) of the extremities, left leg **A**

◻ I70.303   Unspecified atherosclerosis of unspecified type of bypass graft(s) of the extremities, bilateral legs **A**

◻ I70.308   Unspecified atherosclerosis of unspecified type of bypass graft(s) of the extremities, other extremity **A**

◻ I70.309   Unspecified atherosclerosis of unspecified type of bypass graft(s) of the extremities, unspecified extremity **A**

● **I70.31   Atherosclerosis of unspecified type of bypass graft(s) of the extremities with intermittent claudication**

◻ I70.311   Atherosclerosis of unspecified type of bypass graft(s) of the extremities with intermittent claudication, right leg **A**

◻ I70.312   Atherosclerosis of unspecified type of bypass graft(s) of the extremities with intermittent claudication, left leg **A**

◻ I70.313   Atherosclerosis of unspecified type of bypass graft(s) of the extremities with intermittent claudication, bilateral legs **A**

◻ I70.318   Atherosclerosis of unspecified type of bypass graft(s) of the extremities with intermittent claudication, other extremity **A**

◻ I70.319   Atherosclerosis of unspecified type of bypass graft(s) of the extremities with intermittent claudication, unspecified extremity **A**

● **I70.32   Atherosclerosis of unspecified type of bypass graft(s) of the extremities with rest pain**

Includes   any condition classifiable to I70.31-

◻ I70.321   Atherosclerosis of unspecified type of bypass graft(s) of the extremities with rest pain, right leg **A**

◻ I70.322   Atherosclerosis of unspecified type of bypass graft(s) of the extremities with rest pain, left leg **A**

◻ I70.323   Atherosclerosis of unspecified type of bypass graft(s) of the extremities with rest pain, bilateral legs **A**

◻ I70.328   Atherosclerosis of unspecified type of bypass graft(s) of the extremities with rest pain, other extremity **A**

◻ I70.329   Atherosclerosis of unspecified type of bypass graft(s) of the extremities with rest pain, unspecified extremity **A**

● **I70.33   Atherosclerosis of unspecified type of bypass graft(s) of the right leg with ulceration**

Includes   any condition classifiable to I70.311 and I70.321

Use additional code to identify severity of ulcer (L97.- with fifth character 1)

◻ I70.331   Atherosclerosis of unspecified type of bypass graft(s) of the right leg with ulceration of thigh ◔ **A**
  MCC: Only when the principal diagnosis is designated as a CC

◻ I70.332   Atherosclerosis of unspecified type of bypass graft(s) of the right leg with ulceration of calf ◔ **A**
  MCC: Only when the principal diagnosis is designated as a CC

◻ I70.333   Atherosclerosis of unspecified type of bypass graft(s) of the right leg with ulceration of ankle ◔ **A**
  MCC: Only when the principal diagnosis is designated as a CC

◻ I70.334   Atherosclerosis of unspecified type of bypass graft(s) of the right leg with ulceration of heel and midfoot ◔ **A**
  Atherosclerosis of unspecified type of bypass graft(s) of right leg with ulceration of plantar surface of midfoot
  MCC: Only when the principal diagnosis is designated as a CC

◻ I70.335   Atherosclerosis of unspecified type of bypass graft(s) of the right leg with ulceration of other part of foot **A**
  Atherosclerosis of unspecified type of bypass graft(s) of the right leg with ulceration of toe

CHAPTER 9 (I00-I99)

■ I70.338   Atherosclerosis of unspecified
type of bypass graft(s) of the
right leg with ulceration of other
part of lower leg 🦠   A
> MCC: Only when the principal
> diagnosis is designated as
> a CC

■ I70.339   Atherosclerosis of unspecified
type of bypass graft(s) of the
right leg with ulceration of
unspecified site 🦠   A
> MCC: Only when the principal
> diagnosis is designated as
> a CC

● I70.34   Atherosclerosis of unspecified type
of bypass graft(s) of the left leg with
ulceration

> **Includes**   any condition classifiable to
> I70.312 and I70.322

> Use additional code to identify severity
> of ulcer (L97.- with fifth character 2)

■ I70.341   Atherosclerosis of unspecified
type of bypass graft(s) of the left
leg with ulceration of thigh 🦠   A
> MCC: Only when the principal
> diagnosis is designated as
> a CC

■ I70.342   Atherosclerosis of unspecified
type of bypass graft(s) of the left
leg with ulceration of calf 🦠   A
> MCC: Only when the principal
> diagnosis is designated as
> a CC

■ I70.343   Atherosclerosis of unspecified
type of bypass graft(s) of the left
leg with ulceration of ankle 🦠   A
> MCC: Only when the principal
> diagnosis is designated as
> a CC

■ I70.344   Atherosclerosis of unspecified
type of bypass graft(s) of the left
leg with ulceration of heel and
midfoot 🦠   A
> Atherosclerosis of unspecified
> type of bypass graft(s) of
> left leg with ulceration of
> plantar surface of midfoot
> MCC: Only when the principal
> diagnosis is designated as
> a CC

■ I70.345   Atherosclerosis of unspecified
type of bypass graft(s) of the left
leg with ulceration of other part
of foot   A
> Atherosclerosis of unspecified
> type of bypass graft(s) of
> the left leg with ulceration
> of toe

■ I70.348   Atherosclerosis of unspecified
type of bypass graft(s) of the left
leg with ulceration of other part
of lower leg 🦠   A
> MCC: Only when the principal
> diagnosis is designated as
> a CC

■ I70.349   Atherosclerosis of unspecified
type of bypass graft(s) of the left
leg with ulceration of unspecified
site 🦠   A
> MCC: Only when the principal
> diagnosis is designated as
> a CC

■ I70.35   Atherosclerosis of unspecified type of
bypass graft(s) of other extremity with
ulceration   A

> **Includes**   any condition classifiable to
> I70.318 and I70.328

> Use additional code to identify severity
> of ulcer (L98.49-)

● I70.36   Atherosclerosis of unspecified type of
bypass graft(s) of the extremities with
gangrene

> **Includes**   any condition classifiable to
> I70.31-, I70.32-, I70.33-,
> I70.34-, I70.35

> Use additional code to identify the
> severity of any ulcer (L98.49-), if
> applicable

■ I70.361   Atherosclerosis of unspecified
type of bypass graft(s) of the
extremities with gangrene, right
leg 🦠   A
> MCC: Only when the principal
> diagnosis is designated as
> a CC

■ I70.362   Atherosclerosis of unspecified type
of bypass graft(s) of the extremities
with gangrene, left leg 🦠   A
> MCC: Only when the principal
> diagnosis is designated as
> a CC

■ I70.363   Atherosclerosis of unspecified
type of bypass graft(s) of the
extremities with gangrene,
bilateral legs 🦠   A
> MCC: Only when the principal
> diagnosis is designated as
> a CC

■ I70.368   Atherosclerosis of unspecified
type of bypass graft(s) of the
extremities with gangrene, other
extremity 🦠   A
> MCC: Only when the principal
> diagnosis is designated as
> a CC

■ I70.369   Atherosclerosis of unspecified
type of bypass graft(s) of the
extremities with gangrene,
unspecified extremity 🦠   A
> MCC: Only when the principal
> diagnosis is designated as
> a CC

● I70.39   Other atherosclerosis of unspecified type
of bypass graft(s) of the extremities

■ I70.391   Other atherosclerosis of
unspecified type of bypass graft(s)
of the extremities, right leg   A

■ I70.392   Other atherosclerosis of
unspecified type of bypass graft(s)
of the extremities, left leg   A

■ I70.393   Other atherosclerosis of
unspecified type of bypass
graft(s) of the extremities,
bilateral legs   A

■ I70.398   Other atherosclerosis of
unspecified type of bypass
graft(s) of the extremities, other
extremity   A

■ I70.399   Other atherosclerosis of
unspecified type of bypass
graft(s) of the extremities,
unspecified extremity   A

CHAPTER 9 (I00-I99)

● **I70.4**   **Atherosclerosis of autologous vein bypass graft(s) of the extremities**

> **Use additional** code, if applicable, to identify chronic total occlusion of artery of extremity (I70.92)

■ **I70.40**   **Unspecified atherosclerosis of autologous vein bypass graft(s) of the extremities**

   ■ **I70.401**   Unspecified atherosclerosis of autologous vein bypass graft(s) of the extremities, right leg   **A**

   ■ **I70.402**   Unspecified atherosclerosis of autologous vein bypass graft(s) of the extremities, left leg   **A**

   ■ **I70.403**   Unspecified atherosclerosis of autologous vein bypass graft(s) of the extremities, bilateral legs   **A**

   ■ **I70.408**   Unspecified atherosclerosis of autologous vein bypass graft(s) of the extremities, other extremity   **A**

   ■ **I70.409**   Unspecified atherosclerosis of autologous vein bypass graft(s) of the extremities, unspecified extremity   **A**

● **I70.41**   **Atherosclerosis of autologous vein bypass graft(s) of the extremities with intermittent claudication**

   I70.411   Atherosclerosis of autologous vein bypass graft(s) of the extremities with intermittent claudication, right leg   **A**

   I70.412   Atherosclerosis of autologous vein bypass graft(s) of the extremities with intermittent claudication, left leg   **A**

   I70.413   Atherosclerosis of autologous vein bypass graft(s) of the extremities with intermittent claudication, bilateral legs   **A**

   I70.418   Atherosclerosis of autologous vein bypass graft(s) of the extremities with intermittent claudication, other extremity   **A**

   ■ **I70.419**   Atherosclerosis of autologous vein bypass graft(s) of the extremities with intermittent claudication, unspecified extremity   **A**

● **I70.42**   **Atherosclerosis of autologous vein bypass graft(s) of the extremities with rest pain**

> **Includes**   any condition classifiable to I70.41-

   I70.421   Atherosclerosis of autologous vein bypass graft(s) of the extremities with rest pain, right leg   **A**

   I70.422   Atherosclerosis of autologous vein bypass graft(s) of the extremities with rest pain, left leg   **A**

   I70.423   Atherosclerosis of autologous vein bypass graft(s) of the extremities with rest pain, bilateral legs   **A**

   I70.428   Atherosclerosis of autologous vein bypass graft(s) of the extremities with rest pain, other extremity   **A**

   ■ **I70.429**   Atherosclerosis of autologous vein bypass graft(s) of the extremities with rest pain, unspecified extremity   **A**

● **I70.43**   **Atherosclerosis of autologous vein bypass graft(s) of the right leg with ulceration**

> **Includes**   any condition classifiable to I70.411 and I70.421

> **Use additional** code to identify severity of ulcer (L97.- with fifth character 1)

   I70.431   Atherosclerosis of autologous vein bypass graft(s) of the right leg with ulceration of thigh 🔗   **A**
     MCC: Only when the principal diagnosis is designated as a CC

   I70.432   Atherosclerosis of autologous vein bypass graft(s) of the right leg with ulceration of calf 🔗   **A**
     MCC: Only when the principal diagnosis is designated as a CC

   I70.433   Atherosclerosis of autologous vein bypass graft(s) of the right leg with ulceration of ankle 🔗   **A**
     MCC: Only when the principal diagnosis is designated as a CC

   I70.434   Atherosclerosis of autologous vein bypass graft(s) of the right leg with ulceration of heel and midfoot 🔗   **A**
     Atherosclerosis of autologous vein bypass graft(s) of right leg with ulceration of plantar surface of midfoot
     MCC: Only when the principal diagnosis is designated as a CC

   I70.435   Atherosclerosis of autologous vein bypass graft(s) of the right leg with ulceration of other part of foot
     Atherosclerosis of autologous vein bypass graft(s) of right leg with ulceration of toe

   I70.438   Atherosclerosis of autologous vein bypass graft(s) of the right leg with ulceration of other part of lower leg 🔗   **A**
     MCC: Only when the principal diagnosis is designated as a CC

   ■ **I70.439**   Atherosclerosis of autologous vein bypass graft(s) of the right leg with ulceration of unspecified site 🔗   **A**
     MCC: Only when the principal diagnosis is designated as a CC

● **I70.44**   **Atherosclerosis of autologous vein bypass graft(s) of the left leg with ulceration**

> **Includes**   any condition classifiable to I70.412 and I70.422

> **Use additional** code to identify severity of ulcer (L97.- with fifth character 2)

   I70.441   Atherosclerosis of autologous vein bypass graft(s) of the left leg with ulceration of thigh 🔗   **A**
     MCC: Only when the principal diagnosis is designated as a CC

N Newborn Age: 0   **P** Pediatric Age: 0–17   **M** Maternity DX: 12–55   **A** Adult Age: 15–124   ♀ Females Only   ♂ Males Only
🔗 Complication\Comorbidity   Major C\C   Present on Admission Requirement   Hospital-Acquired Condition

CHAPTER 9 (I00-I99)

1049

I70.442 Atherosclerosis of autologous vein bypass graft(s) of the left leg with ulceration of calf 🔊   **A**
    MCC: Only when the principal diagnosis is designated as a CC

I70.443 Atherosclerosis of autologous vein bypass graft(s) of the left leg with ulceration of ankle 🔊   **A**

I70.444 Atherosclerosis of autologous vein bypass graft(s) of the left leg with ulceration of heel and midfoot 🔊   **A**
    Atherosclerosis of autologous vein bypass graft(s) of left leg with ulceration of plantar surface of midfoot
    MCC: Only when the principal diagnosis is designated as a CC

I70.445 Atherosclerosis of autologous vein bypass graft(s) of the left leg with ulceration of other part of foot   **A**
    Atherosclerosis of autologous vein bypass graft(s) of left leg with ulceration of toe

I70.448 Atherosclerosis of autologous vein bypass graft(s) of the left leg with ulceration of other part of lower leg 🔊   **A**
    MCC: Only when the principal diagnosis is designated as a CC

■ **I70.449** Atherosclerosis of autologous vein bypass graft(s) of the left leg with ulceration of unspecified site 🔊   **A**
    MCC: Only when the principal diagnosis is designated as a CC

I70.45 Atherosclerosis of autologous vein bypass graft(s) of other extremity with ulceration   **A**
    Includes any condition classifiable to I70.418, I70.428, and I70.438

    Use additional code to identify severity of ulcer (L98.49-)

● **I70.46** Atherosclerosis of autologous vein bypass graft(s) of the extremities with gangrene
    Includes any condition classifiable to I70.41-, I70.42-, and I70.43-, I70.44-, I70.45

    Use additional code to identify the severity of any ulcer (L98.49-), if applicable

I70.461 Atherosclerosis of autologous vein bypass graft(s) of the extremities with gangrene, right leg 🔊   **A**
    MCC: Only when the principal diagnosis is designated as a CC

I70.462 Atherosclerosis of autologous vein bypass graft(s) of the extremities with gangrene, left leg 🔊   **A**
    MCC: Only when the principal diagnosis is designated as a CC

I70.463 Atherosclerosis of autologous vein bypass graft(s) of the extremities with gangrene, bilateral legs 🔊   **A**
    MCC: Only when the principal diagnosis is designated as a CC

I70.468 Atherosclerosis of autologous vein bypass graft(s) of the extremities with gangrene, other extremity 🔊   **A**
    MCC: Only when the principal diagnosis is designated as a CC

■ **I70.469** Atherosclerosis of autologous vein bypass graft(s) of the extremities with gangrene, unspecified extremity 🔊   **A**
    MCC: Only when the principal diagnosis is designated as a CC

● **I70.49** Other atherosclerosis of autologous vein bypass graft(s) of the extremities

I70.491 Other atherosclerosis of autologous vein bypass graft(s) of the extremities, right leg   **A**

I70.492 Other atherosclerosis of autologous vein bypass graft(s) of the extremities, left leg   **A**

I70.493 Other atherosclerosis of autologous vein bypass graft(s) of the extremities, bilateral legs **A**

I70.498 Other atherosclerosis of autologous vein bypass graft(s) of the extremities, other extremity   **A**

■ **I70.499** Other atherosclerosis of autologous vein bypass graft(s) of the extremities, unspecified extremity   **A**

● **I70.5** Atherosclerosis of nonautologous biological bypass graft(s) of the extremities
    Use additional code, if applicable, to identify chronic total occlusion of artery of extremity (I70.92)

■ **I70.50** Unspecified atherosclerosis of nonautologous biological bypass graft(s) of the extremities

■ **I70.501** Unspecified atherosclerosis of nonautologous biological bypass graft(s) of the extremities, right leg   **A**

■ **I70.502** Unspecified atherosclerosis of nonautologous biological bypass graft(s) of the extremities, left leg   **A**

■ **I70.503** Unspecified atherosclerosis of nonautologous biological bypass graft(s) of the extremities, bilateral legs   **A**

■ **I70.508** Unspecified atherosclerosis of nonautologous biological bypass graft(s) of the extremities, other extremity   **A**

■ **I70.509** Unspecified atherosclerosis of nonautologous biological bypass graft(s) of the extremities, unspecified extremity   **A**

● Unacceptable Principal Diagnosis   ● Use Additional Character(s)   ■ Unspecified   ▶ Manifestation Code
OGCR Official Guidelines for Coding and Reporting   Excludes 1   Excludes 2   Includes   Use additional   Code first   Code also

CHAPTER 9 (I00-I99)

● **I70.51   Atherosclerosis of nonautologous biological bypass graft(s) of the extremities intermittent claudication**

　I70.511   Atherosclerosis of nonautologous biological bypass graft(s) of the extremities with intermittent claudication, right leg   **A**

　I70.512   Atherosclerosis of nonautologous biological bypass graft(s) of the extremities with intermittent claudication, left leg   **A**

　I70.513   Atherosclerosis of nonautologous biological bypass graft(s) of the extremities with intermittent claudication, bilateral legs   **A**

　I70.518   Atherosclerosis of nonautologous biological bypass graft(s) of the extremities with intermittent claudication, other extremity   **A**

　■ I70.519   Atherosclerosis of nonautologous biological bypass graft(s) of the extremities with intermittent claudication, unspecified extremity   **A**

● **I70.52   Atherosclerosis of nonautologous biological bypass graft(s) of the extremities with rest pain**

Includes   any condition classifiable to I70.51-

　I70.521   Atherosclerosis of nonautologous biological bypass graft(s) of the extremities with rest pain, right leg   **A**

　I70.522   Atherosclerosis of nonautologous biological bypass graft(s) of the extremities with rest pain, left leg   **A**

　I70.523   Atherosclerosis of nonautologous biological bypass graft(s) of the extremities with rest pain, bilateral legs   **A**

　I70.528   Atherosclerosis of nonautologous biological bypass graft(s) of the extremities with rest pain, other extremity   **A**

　■ I70.529   Atherosclerosis of nonautologous biological bypass graft(s) of the extremities with rest pain, unspecified extremity   **A**

● **I70.53   Atherosclerosis of nonautologous biological bypass graft(s) of the right leg with ulceration**

Includes   any condition classifiable to I70.511 and I70.521

Use additional code to identify severity of ulcer (L97.- with fifth character 1)

　I70.531   Atherosclerosis of nonautologous biological bypass graft(s) of the right leg with ulceration of thigh 🦠   **A**
　　MCC: Only when the principal diagnosis is designated as a CC

　I70.532   Atherosclerosis of nonautologous biological bypass graft(s) of the right leg with ulceration of calf 🦠   **A**
　　MCC: Only when the principal diagnosis is designated as a CC

　I70.533   Atherosclerosis of nonautologous biological bypass graft(s) of the right leg with ulceration of ankle 🦠   **A**
　　MCC: Only when the principal diagnosis is designated as a CC

　I70.534   Atherosclerosis of nonautologous biological bypass graft(s) of the right leg with ulceration of heel and midfoot 🦠   **A**
　　Atherosclerosis of nonautologous biological bypass graft(s) of right leg with ulceration of plantar surface of midfoot
　　MCC: Only when the principal diagnosis is designated as a CC

　I70.535   Atherosclerosis of nonautologous biological bypass graft(s) of the right leg with ulceration of other part of foot   **A**
　　Atherosclerosis of nonautologous biological bypass graft(s) of the right leg with ulceration of toe

　I70.538   Atherosclerosis of nonautologous biological bypass graft(s) of the right leg with ulceration of other part of lower leg 🦠   **A**
　　MCC: Only when the principal diagnosis is designated as a CC

　■ I70.539   Atherosclerosis of nonautologous biological bypass graft(s) of the right leg with ulceration of unspecified site 🦠   **A**
　　MCC: Only when the principal diagnosis is designated as a CC

● **I70.54   Atherosclerosis of nonautologous biological bypass graft(s) of the left leg with ulceration**

Includes   any condition classifiable to I70.512 and I70.522

Use additional code to identify severity of ulcer (L97.- with fifth character 2)

　I70.541   Atherosclerosis of nonautologous biological bypass graft(s) of the left leg with ulceration of thigh 🦠   **A**
　　MCC: Only when the principal diagnosis is designated as a CC

　I70.542   Atherosclerosis of nonautologous biological bypass graft(s) of the left leg with ulceration of calf 🦠 **A**
　　MCC: Only when the principal diagnosis is designated as a CC

I70.543   Atherosclerosis of nonautologous biological bypass graft(s) of the left leg with ulceration of ankle 🔒   A
> MCC: Only when the principal diagnosis is designated as a CC

I70.544   Atherosclerosis of nonautologous biological bypass graft(s) of the left leg with ulceration of heel and midfoot 🔒   A
> Atherosclerosis of nonautologous biological bypass graft(s) of left leg with ulceration of plantar surface of midfoot
> MCC: Only when the principal diagnosis is designated as a CC

I70.545   Atherosclerosis of nonautologous biological bypass graft(s) of the left leg with ulceration of other part of foot   A
> Atherosclerosis of nonautologous biological bypass graft(s) of the left leg with ulceration of toe

I70.548   Atherosclerosis of nonautologous biological bypass graft(s) of the left leg with ulceration of other part of lower leg 🔒   A
> MCC: Only when the principal diagnosis is designated as a CC

■ I70.549   Atherosclerosis of nonautologous biological bypass graft(s) of the left leg with ulceration of unspecified site 🔒   A
> MCC: Only when the principal diagnosis is designated as a CC

I70.55   Atherosclerosis of nonautologous biological bypass graft(s) of other extremity with ulceration   A
> **Includes** any condition classifiable to I70.518, I70.528, and I70.538
>
> **Use additional** code to identify severity of ulcer (L98.49)

● I70.56   Atherosclerosis of nonautologous biological bypass graft(s) of the extremities with gangrene
> **Includes** any condition classifiable to I70.51-, I70.52-, and I70.53-, I70.54-, I70.55
>
> **Use additional** code to identify the severity of any ulcer (L98.49-), if applicable

I70.561   Atherosclerosis of nonautologous biological bypass graft(s) of the extremities with gangrene, right leg 🔒   A
> MCC: Only when the principal diagnosis is designated as a CC

I70.562   Atherosclerosis of nonautologous biological bypass graft(s) of the extremities with gangrene, left leg 🔒   A
> MCC: Only when the principal diagnosis is designated as a CC

I70.563   Atherosclerosis of nonautologous biological bypass graft(s) of the extremities with gangrene, bilateral legs 🔒   A
> MCC: Only when the principal diagnosis is designated as a CC

I70.568   Atherosclerosis of nonautologous biological bypass graft(s) of the extremities with gangrene, other extremity 🔒   A
> MCC: Only when the principal diagnosis is designated as a CC

■ I70.569   Atherosclerosis of nonautologous biological bypass graft(s) of the extremities with gangrene, unspecified extremity 🔒   A
> MCC: Only when the principal diagnosis is designated as a CC

● I70.59   Other atherosclerosis of nonautologous biological bypass graft(s) of the extremities

I70.591   Other atherosclerosis of nonautologous biological bypass graft(s) of the extremities, right leg   A

I70.592   Other atherosclerosis of nonautologous biological bypass graft(s) of the extremities, left leg   A

I70.593   Other atherosclerosis of nonautologous biological bypass graft(s) of the extremities, bilateral legs   A

I70.598   Other atherosclerosis of nonautologous biological bypass graft(s) of the extremities, other extremity   A

■ I70.599   Other atherosclerosis of nonautologous biological bypass graft(s) of the extremities, unspecified extremity   A

● I70.6   Atherosclerosis of nonbiological bypass graft(s) of the extremities
> **Use additional** code, if applicable, to identify chronic total occlusion of artery of extremity (I70.92)

● I70.60   Unspecified atherosclerosis of nonbiological bypass graft(s) of the extremities

■ I70.601   Unspecified atherosclerosis of nonbiological bypass graft(s) of the extremities, right leg   A

■ I70.602   Unspecified atherosclerosis of nonbiological bypass graft(s) of the extremities, left leg   A

■ I70.603   Unspecified atherosclerosis of nonbiological bypass graft(s) of the extremities, bilateral legs   A

■ I70.608 Unspecified atherosclerosis of nonbiological bypass graft(s) of the extremities, other extremity **A**

■ I70.609 Unspecified atherosclerosis of nonbiological bypass graft(s) of the extremities, unspecified extremity **A**

● I70.61 Atherosclerosis of nonbiological bypass graft(s) of the extremities with intermittent claudication

  I70.611 Atherosclerosis of nonbiological bypass graft(s) of the extremities with intermittent claudication, right leg **A**

  I70.612 Atherosclerosis of nonbiological bypass graft(s) of the extremities with intermittent claudication, left leg **A**

  I70.613 Atherosclerosis of nonbiological bypass graft(s) of the extremities with intermittent claudication, bilateral legs **A**

  I70.618 Atherosclerosis of nonbiological bypass graft(s) of the extremities with intermittent claudication, other extremity **A**

■ I70.619 Atherosclerosis of nonbiological bypass graft(s) of the extremities with intermittent claudication, unspecified extremity **A**

● I70.62 Atherosclerosis of nonbiological bypass graft(s) of the extremities with rest pain

  Includes any condition classifiable to I70.61-

  I70.621 Atherosclerosis of nonbiological bypass graft(s) of the extremities with rest pain, right leg **A**

  I70.622 Atherosclerosis of nonbiological bypass graft(s) of the extremities with rest pain, left leg **A**

  I70.623 Atherosclerosis of nonbiological bypass graft(s) of the extremities with rest pain, bilateral legs **A**

  I70.628 Atherosclerosis of nonbiological bypass graft(s) of the extremities with rest pain, other extremity **A**

■ I70.629 Atherosclerosis of nonbiological bypass graft(s) of the extremities with rest pain, unspecified extremity **A**

● I70.63 Atherosclerosis of nonbiological bypass graft(s) of the right leg with ulceration

  Includes any condition classifiable to I70.611 and I70.621

  Use additional code to identify severity of ulcer (L97.- with fifth character 1)

  I70.631 Atherosclerosis of nonbiological bypass graft(s) of the right leg with ulceration of thigh 🦴 **A**
      MCC: Only when the principal diagnosis is designated as a CC

  I70.632 Atherosclerosis of nonbiological bypass graft(s) of the right leg with ulceration of calf 🦴 **A**
      MCC: Only when the principal diagnosis is designated as a CC

I70.633 Atherosclerosis of nonbiological bypass graft(s) of the right leg with ulceration of ankle 🦴 **A**
    MCC: Only when the principal diagnosis is designated as a CC

I70.634 Atherosclerosis of nonbiological bypass graft(s) of the right leg with ulceration of heel and midfoot 🦴 **A**
    Atherosclerosis of nonbiological bypass graft(s) of right leg with ulceration of plantar surface of midfoot
    MCC: Only when the principal diagnosis is designated as a CC

I70.635 Atherosclerosis of nonbiological bypass graft(s) of the right leg with ulceration of other part of foot **A**
    Atherosclerosis of nonbiological bypass graft(s) of the right leg with ulceration of toe

I70.638 Atherosclerosis of nonbiological bypass graft(s) of the right leg with ulceration of other part of lower leg 🦴 **A**
    MCC: Only when the principal diagnosis is designated as a CC

■ I70.639 Atherosclerosis of nonbiological bypass graft(s) of the right leg with ulceration of unspecified site 🦴 **A**
    MCC: Only when the principal diagnosis is designated as a CC

● I70.64 Atherosclerosis of nonbiological bypass graft(s) of the left leg with ulceration

  Includes any condition classifiable to I70.612 and I70.622

  Use additional code to identify severity of ulcer (L97.- with fifth character 2)

  I70.641 Atherosclerosis of nonbiological bypass graft(s) of the left leg with ulceration of thigh 🦴 **A**
      MCC: Only when the principal diagnosis is designated as a CC

  I70.642 Atherosclerosis of nonbiological bypass graft(s) of the left leg with ulceration of calf 🦴 **A**
      MCC: Only when the principal diagnosis is designated as a CC

  I70.643 Atherosclerosis of nonbiological bypass graft(s) of the left leg with ulceration of ankle 🦴 **A**
      MCC: Only when the principal diagnosis is designated as a CC

CHAPTER 9 (I00-I99)

I70.644   **Atherosclerosis of nonbiological bypass graft(s) of the left leg with ulceration of heel and midfoot** 🦠   A
     Atherosclerosis of nonbiological bypass graft(s) of left leg with ulceration of plantar surface of midfoot
     MCC: Only when the principal diagnosis is designated as a CC

I70.645   **Atherosclerosis of nonbiological bypass graft(s) of the left leg with ulceration of other part of foot**   A
     Atherosclerosis of nonbiological bypass graft(s) of the left leg with ulceration of toe

I70.648   **Atherosclerosis of nonbiological bypass graft(s) of the left leg with ulceration of other part of lower leg** 🦠   A
     MCC: Only when the principal diagnosis is designated as a CC

■ I70.649   **Atherosclerosis of nonbiological bypass graft(s) of the left leg with ulceration of unspecified site** 🦠 A
     MCC: Only when the principal diagnosis is designated as a CC

I70.65   **Atherosclerosis of nonbiological bypass graft(s) of other extremity with ulceration** A
     Includes   any condition classifiable to I70.618 and I70.628
     Use additional code to identify severity of ulcer (L98.49-)

● I70.66   **Atherosclerosis of nonbiological bypass graft(s) of the extremities with gangrene**
     Includes   any condition classifiable to I70.61-, I70.62-, I70.63-, I70.64-, I70.65
     Use additional code to identify the severity of any ulcer (L98.49-), if applicable

I70.661   **Atherosclerosis of nonbiological bypass graft(s) of the extremities with gangrene, right leg** 🦠   A
     MCC: Only when the principal diagnosis is designated as a CC

I70.662   **Atherosclerosis of nonbiological bypass graft(s) of the extremities with gangrene, left leg** 🦠   A
     MCC: Only when the principal diagnosis is designated as a CC

I70.663   **Atherosclerosis of nonbiological bypass graft(s) of the extremities with gangrene, bilateral legs** 🦠   A
     MCC: Only when the principal diagnosis is designated as a CC

I70.668   **Atherosclerosis of nonbiological bypass graft(s) of the extremities with gangrene, other extremity** 🦠   A
     MCC: Only when the principal diagnosis is designated as a CC

■ I70.669   **Atherosclerosis of nonbiological bypass graft(s) of the extremities with gangrene, unspecified extremity** 🦠   A
     MCC: Only when the principal diagnosis is designated as a CC

● I70.69   **Other atherosclerosis of nonbiological bypass graft(s) of the extremities**

I70.691   **Other atherosclerosis of nonbiological bypass graft(s) of the extremities, right leg**   A

I70.692   **Other atherosclerosis of nonbiological bypass graft(s) of the extremities, left leg**   A

I70.693   **Other atherosclerosis of nonbiological bypass graft(s) of the extremities, bilateral legs**   A

I70.698   **Other atherosclerosis of nonbiological bypass graft(s) of the extremities, other extremity** A

■ I70.699   **Other atherosclerosis of nonbiological bypass graft(s) of the extremities, unspecified extremity**   A

● I70.7   **Atherosclerosis of other type of bypass graft(s) of the extremities**
     Use additional code, if applicable, to identify chronic total occlusion of artery of extremity (I70.92)

● I70.70   **Unspecified atherosclerosis of other type of bypass graft(s) of the extremities**

■ I70.701   **Unspecified atherosclerosis of other type of bypass graft(s) of the extremities, right leg**   A

■ I70.702   **Unspecified atherosclerosis of other type of bypass graft(s) of the extremities, left leg**   A

■ I70.703   **Unspecified atherosclerosis of other type of bypass graft(s) of the extremities, bilateral legs**   A

■ I70.708   **Unspecified atherosclerosis of other type of bypass graft(s) of the extremities, other extremity** A

■ I70.709   **Unspecified atherosclerosis of other type of bypass graft(s) of the extremities, unspecified extremity**   A

● I70.71   **Atherosclerosis of other type of bypass graft(s) of the extremities with intermittent claudication**

I70.711   **Atherosclerosis of other type of bypass graft(s) of the extremities with intermittent claudication, right leg**   A

I70.712   **Atherosclerosis of other type of bypass graft(s) of the extremities with intermittent claudication, left leg**   A

I70.713   **Atherosclerosis of other type of bypass graft(s) of the extremities with intermittent claudication, bilateral legs**   A

I70.718   **Atherosclerosis of other type of bypass graft(s) of the extremities with intermittent claudication, other extremity**   A

■ **I70.719** **Atherosclerosis of other type of bypass graft(s) of the extremities with intermittent claudication, unspecified extremity**   **A**

● **I70.72** **Atherosclerosis of other type of bypass graft(s) of the extremities with rest pain**

> **Includes**   any condition classifiable to I70.71-

I70.721 **Atherosclerosis of other type of bypass graft(s) of the extremities with rest pain, right leg**   **A**

I70.722 **Atherosclerosis of other type of bypass graft(s) of the extremities with rest pain, left leg**   **A**

I70.723 **Atherosclerosis of other type of bypass graft(s) of the extremities with rest pain, bilateral legs**   **A**

I70.728 **Atherosclerosis of other type of bypass graft(s) of the extremities with rest pain, other extremity**   **A**

■ **I70.729** **Atherosclerosis of other type of bypass graft(s) of the extremities with rest pain, unspecified extremity**   **A**

● **I70.73** **Atherosclerosis of other type of bypass graft(s) of the right leg with ulceration**

> **Includes**   any condition classifiable to I70.711 and I70.721

> **Use additional** code to identify severity of ulcer (L97.- with fifth character 1)

I70.731 **Atherosclerosis of other type of bypass graft(s) of the right leg with ulceration of thigh** 🔵   **A**
> MCC: Only when the principal diagnosis is designated as a CC

I70.732 **Atherosclerosis of other type of bypass graft(s) of the right leg with ulceration of calf** 🔵   **A**
> MCC: Only when the principal diagnosis is designated as a CC

I70.733 **Atherosclerosis of other type of bypass graft(s) of the right leg with ulceration of ankle** 🔵   **A**
> MCC: Only when the principal diagnosis is designated as a CC

I70.734 **Atherosclerosis of other type of bypass graft(s) of the right leg with ulceration of heel and midfoot** 🔵   **A**
> Atherosclerosis of other type of bypass graft(s) of right leg with ulceration of plantar surface of midfoot
> MCC: Only when the principal diagnosis is designated as a CC

I70.735 **Atherosclerosis of other type of bypass graft(s) of the right leg with ulceration of other part of foot**   **A**
> Atherosclerosis of other type of bypass graft(s) of right leg with ulceration of toe

I70.738 **Atherosclerosis of other type of bypass graft(s) of the right leg with ulceration of other part of lower leg** 🔵   **A**
> MCC: Only when the principal diagnosis is designated as a CC

■ **I70.739** **Atherosclerosis of other type of bypass graft(s) of the right leg with ulceration of unspecified site** 🔵   **A**
> MCC: Only when the principal diagnosis is designated as a CC

● **I70.74** **Atherosclerosis of other type of bypass graft(s) of the left leg with ulceration**

> **Includes**   any condition classifiable to I70.712 and I70.722

> **Use additional** code to identify severity of ulcer (L97.- with fifth character 2)

I70.741 **Atherosclerosis of other type of bypass graft(s) of the left leg with ulceration of thigh** 🔵   **A**
> MCC: Only when the principal diagnosis is designated as a CC

I70.742 **Atherosclerosis of other type of bypass graft(s) of the left leg with ulceration of calf** 🔵   **A**
> MCC: Only when the principal diagnosis is designated as a CC

I70.743 **Atherosclerosis of other type of bypass graft(s) of the left leg with ulceration of ankle** 🔵   **A**
> MCC: Only when the principal diagnosis is designated as a CC

I70.744 **Atherosclerosis of other type of bypass graft(s) of the left leg with ulceration of heel and midfoot** 🔵   **A**
> Atherosclerosis of other type of bypass graft(s) of left leg with ulceration of plantar surface of midfoot
> MCC: Only when the principal diagnosis is designated as a CC

I70.745 **Atherosclerosis of other type of bypass graft(s) of the left leg with ulceration of other part of foot**   **A**
> Atherosclerosis of other type of bypass graft(s) of left leg with ulceration of toe

I70.748 **Atherosclerosis of other type of bypass graft(s) of the left leg with ulceration of other part of lower leg** 🔵   **A**
> MCC: Only when the principal diagnosis is designated as a CC

■ **I70.749** **Atherosclerosis of other type of bypass graft(s) of the left leg with ulceration of unspecified site** 🔵 **A**
> MCC: Only when the principal diagnosis is designated as a CC

N Newborn Age: 0   **P** Pediatric Age: 0–17   **M** Maternity DX: 12–55   **A** Adult Age: 15–124   ♀ Females Only   ♂ Males Only
🔵 Complication\Comorbidity   🔵 Major C\C   🔵 Present on Admission Requirement   🔵 Hospital-Acquired Condition

CHAPTER 9 (I00-I99)

1055

● **I70.75** **Atherosclerosis of other type of bypass graft(s) of other extremity with ulceration** A

> **Includes**   any condition classifiable to I70.718 and I70.728

> **Use additional** code to identify severity of ulcer (L98.49)

● **I70.76** **Atherosclerosis of other type of bypass graft(s) of the extremities with gangrene**

> **Includes**   any condition classifiable to I70.71-, I70.72-, I70.73-, I70.74-, I70.75

> **Use additional** code to identify the severity of any ulcer (L98.49-), if applicable

     I70.761 **Atherosclerosis of other type of bypass graft(s) of the extremities with gangrene, right leg** 🝆   A
> MCC: Only when the principal diagnosis is designated as a CC

     I70.762 **Atherosclerosis of other type of bypass graft(s) of the extremities with gangrene, left leg** 🝆   A
> MCC: Only when the principal diagnosis is designated as a CC

     I70.763 **Atherosclerosis of other type of bypass graft(s) of the extremities with gangrene, bilateral legs** 🝆 A
> MCC: Only when the principal diagnosis is designated as a CC

     I70.768 **Atherosclerosis of other type of bypass graft(s) of the extremities with gangrene, other extremity** 🝆A
> MCC: Only when the principal diagnosis is designated as a CC

     I70.769 **Atherosclerosis of other type of bypass graft(s) of the extremities with gangrene, unspecified extremity** 🝆   A
> MCC: Only when the principal diagnosis is designated as a CC

● **I70.79** **Other atherosclerosis of other type of bypass graft(s) of the extremities**

     I70.791 **Other atherosclerosis of other type of bypass graft(s) of the extremities, right leg**   A

     I70.792 **Other atherosclerosis of other type of bypass graft(s) of the extremities, left leg**   A

     I70.793 **Other atherosclerosis of other type of bypass graft(s) of the extremities, bilateral legs**   A

     I70.798 **Other atherosclerosis of other type of bypass graft(s) of the extremities, other extremity**   A

     I70.799 **Other atherosclerosis of other type of bypass graft(s) of the extremities, unspecified extremity**   A

I70.8 **Atherosclerosis of other arteries**   A

● **I70.9** **Other and unspecified atherosclerosis**

     I70.90 **Unspecified atherosclerosis**   A

     I70.91 **Generalized atherosclerosis**   A

● **I70.92** **Chronic total occlusion of artery of the extremities**   A

> Complete occlusion of artery of the extremities
> Total occlusion of artery of the extremities

> *Code first* atherosclerosis of arteries of the extremities (I70.2-, I70.3-, I70.4-, I70.5-, I70.6-, I70.7-)

> **Excludes1**   acute occlusion of artery of the extremity (I70.2-, I70.3-, I70.4-)

● **I71** **Aortic aneurysm and dissection**

> **Excludes1**   aortic ectasia (I77.81-)
> syphilitic aortic aneurysm (A52.01)
> traumatic aortic aneurysm (S25.09, S35.09)

● **I71.0** **Dissection of aorta**

     ■ **I71.00** **Dissection of unspecified site of aorta** 🝆

     I71.01 **Dissection of thoracic aorta** 🝆

     I71.02 **Dissection of abdominal aorta** 🝆

     I71.03 **Dissection of thoracoabdominal aorta** 🝆

I71.1 **Thoracic aortic aneurysm, ruptured** 🝆

I71.2 **Thoracic aortic aneurysm, without rupture**

I71.3 **Abdominal aortic aneurysm, ruptured** 🝆

I71.4 **Abdominal aortic aneurysm, without rupture**

I71.5 **Thoracoabdominal aortic aneurysm, ruptured** 🝆

I71.6 **Thoracoabdominal aortic aneurysm, without rupture**

■ **I71.8** **Aortic aneurysm of unspecified site, ruptured** 🝆
> Rupture of aorta NOS

■ **I71.9** **Aortic aneurysm of unspecified site, without rupture**
> Aneurysm of aorta
> Dilatation of aorta
> Hyaline necrosis of aorta

● **I72** **Other aneurysm**

> **Includes**   aneurysm (cirsoid) (false) (ruptured)

> **Excludes2**   acquired aneurysm (I77.0)
> aneurysm (of) aorta (I71.-)
> aneurysm (of) arteriovenous NOS (Q27.3-)
> carotid artery dissection (I77.71)
> cerebral (nonruptured) aneurysm (I67.1)
> coronary aneurysm (I25.4)
> coronary artery dissection (I25.42)
> dissection of artery NEC (I77.79)
> heart aneurysm (I25.3)
> iliac artery dissection (I77.72)
> pulmonary artery aneurysm (I28.1)
> renal artery dissection (I77.73)
> retinal aneurysm (H35.0)
> ruptured cerebral aneurysm (I60.7)
> varicose aneurysm (I77.0)
> vertebral artery dissection (I77.74)

I72.0 **Aneurysm of carotid artery**
> Aneurysm of common carotid artery
> Aneurysm of external carotid artery
> Aneurysm of internal carotid artery, extracranial portion

> **Excludes1**   aneurysm of internal carotid artery, intracranial portion (I67.1)
> aneurysm of internal carotid artery NOS (I67.1)

I72.1 **Aneurysm of artery of upper extremity**

I72.2 **Aneurysm of renal artery**

I72.3 **Aneurysm of iliac artery**

I72.4 **Aneurysm of artery of lower extremity**

I72.8 **Aneurysm of other specified arteries**

■ **I72.9** **Aneurysm of unspecified site**

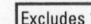

● Unacceptable Principal Diagnosis   ● Use Additional Character(s)   ■ Unspecified   ▶ Manifestation Code

   OGCR Official Guidelines for Coding and Reporting   [Excludes 1]   [Excludes 2]   Includes   Use additional   Code first   Code also

● **I73   Other peripheral vascular diseases**
  Excludes2 chilblains (T69.1)
    frostbite (T33- T34)
    immersion hand or foot (T69.0-)
    spasm of cerebral artery (G45.9)

● **I73.0   Raynaud's syndrome**
  Diminishing oxygen supply to fingers, toes, nose, and ears when exposed to temperature changes or stress
  Raynaud's disease
  Raynaud's phenomenon (secondary)

  I73.00   Raynaud's syndrome without gangrene

  I73.01   Raynaud's syndrome with gangrene 🔴
    MCC: Only when the principal diagnosis is designated as a CC

I73.1   Thromboangiitis obliterans [Buerger's disease]
  Inflammatory occlusive disease resulting in poor circulation to the legs, feet, and sometimes the hands due to progressive inflammatory narrowing and eventually obliteration of the small arteries

● **I73.8   Other specified peripheral vascular diseases**
  Excludes1 diabetic (peripheral) angiopathy (E08-E13 with .51-.52)

  I73.81   Erythromelalgia

  I73.89   Other specified peripheral vascular diseases
    Acrocyanosis
    Erythrocyanosis
    Simple acroparesthesia [Schultze's type]
    Vasomotor acroparesthesia [Nothnagel's type]

■ **I73.9   Peripheral vascular disease, unspecified**
    Intermittent claudication
    Peripheral angiopathy NOS
    Spasm of artery
    Excludes1 atherosclerosis of the extremities (I70.2--I70.7-)

● **I74   Arterial embolism and thrombosis**
  Includes embolic infarction
    embolic occlusion
    thrombotic infarction
    thrombotic occlusion

  Code first embolism and thrombosis complicating abortion or ectopic or molar pregnancy (O00-O07, O08.2)
    embolism and thrombosis complicating pregnancy, childbirth and the puerperium (O88.-)
  Excludes2 atheroembolism (I75.-)
    basilar embolism and thrombosis (I63.0-I63.2, I65.1)
    carotid embolism and thrombosis (I63.0-I63.2, I65.2)
    cerebral embolism and thrombosis (I63.3-I63.5, I66.-)
    coronary embolism and thrombosis (I21-I25)
    mesenteric embolism and thrombosis (K55.0)
    ophthalmic embolism and thrombosis (H34.-)
    precerebral embolism and thrombosis NOS (I63.0-I63.2, I65.9)
    pulmonary embolism and thrombosis (I26.-)
    renal embolism and thrombosis (N28.0)
    retinal embolism and thrombosis (H34.-)
    septic embolism and thrombosis (I76)
    vertebral embolism and thrombosis (I63.0-I63.2, I65.0)

Item 9–9 An **embolus** is a mass of undissolved matter present in the blood that is transported by the blood current. A **thrombus** is a blood clot that occludes or shuts off a vessel. When a thrombus is dislodged, it becomes an embolus.

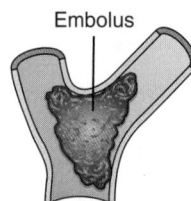

Embolus

Figure 9-3 An arterial embolus.

● **I74.0   Embolism and thrombosis of abdominal aorta**

  I74.01   Saddle embolus of abdominal aorta

  I74.09   Other arterial embolism and thrombosis of abdominal aorta
    Aortic bifurcation syndrome
    Aortoiliac obstruction
    Leriche's syndrome

● **I74.1   Embolism and thrombosis of other and unspecified parts of aorta**

  ■ **I74.10   Embolism and thrombosis of unspecified parts of aorta** 🔴

  I74.11   Embolism and thrombosis of thoracic aorta 🔴

  I74.19   Embolism and thrombosis of other parts of aorta 🔴

  I74.2   Embolism and thrombosis of arteries of the upper extremities 🔴

  I74.3   Embolism and thrombosis of arteries of the lower extremities 🔴

■ **I74.4   Embolism and thrombosis of arteries of extremities, unspecified** 🔴
    Peripheral arterial embolism NOS

  I74.5   Embolism and thrombosis of iliac artery 🔴

  I74.8   Embolism and thrombosis of other arteries 🔴

■ **I74.9   Embolism and thrombosis of unspecified artery** 🔴

● **I75   Atheroembolism**
  Includes atherothrombotic microembolism
    cholesterol embolism

● **I75.0   Atheroembolism of extremities**

  ● **I75.01   Atheroembolism of upper extremity**

    I75.011   Atheroembolism of right upper extremity 🔴

    I75.012   Atheroembolism of left upper extremity 🔴

    I75.013   Atheroembolism of bilateral upper extremities 🔴

    ■ **I75.019   Atheroembolism of unspecified upper extremity** 🔴

  ● **I75.02   Atheroembolism of lower extremity**

    I75.021   Atheroembolism of right lower extremity 🔴

    I75.022   Atheroembolism of left lower extremity 🔴

    I75.023   Atheroembolism of bilateral lower extremities 🔴

    I75.029   Atheroembolism of unspecified lower extremity 🔴

CHAPTER 9 (I00-I99)

● **I75.8   Atheroembolism of other sites**

    I75.81   **Atheroembolism of kidney** 🔖

       Use additional code for any associated acute kidney failure and chronic kidney disease (N17.-, N18.-)

    I75.89   **Atheroembolism of other site** 🔖

● **I76   Septic arterial embolism** 🔖

   Code first underlying infection, such as:
     infective endocarditis (I33.0)
     lung abscess (J85.-)

   Use additional code to identify the site of the embolism (I74.-)

   | **Excludes2** | septic pulmonary embolism (I26.01, I26.90)

● **I77   Other disorders of arteries and arterioles**

   | **Excludes2** | collagen (vascular) diseases (M30-M36)
                 hypersensitivity angiitis (M31.0)
                 pulmonary artery (I28.-)

  I77.0   Arteriovenous fistula, acquired
    Aneurysmal varix
    Arteriovenous aneurysm, acquired

    | **Excludes1** | arteriovenous aneurysm NOS (Q27.3-)
               presence of arteriovenous shunt (fistula) for dialysis (Z99.2)
               traumatic - see injury of blood vessel by body region

    | **Excludes2** | cerebral (I67.1)
               coronary (I25.4)

  I77.1   Stricture of artery
    Narrowing of artery

  I77.2   Rupture of artery 🔖
    Erosion of artery
    Fistula of artery
    Ulcer of artery

    | **Excludes1** | traumatic rupture of artery - see injury of blood vessel by body region

  I77.3   Arterial fibromuscular dysplasia
    Fibromuscular hyperplasia (of) carotid artery
    Fibromuscular hyperplasia (of) renal artery

  I77.4   Celiac artery compression syndrome 🔖

  I77.5   Necrosis of artery 🔖

◼ **I77.6   Arteritis, unspecified**
    Aortitis NOS
    Endarteritis NOS

    | **Excludes1** | arteritis or endarteritis:
               aortic arch (M31.4)
               cerebral NEC (I67.7)
               coronary (I25.89)
               deformans (I70.-)
               giant cell (M31.5., M31.6)
               obliterans (I70.-)
               senile (I70.-)

● **I77.7   Other arterial dissection**

    | **Excludes2** | dissection of aorta (I71.0-)
               dissection of coronary artery (I25.42)

    I77.71   **Dissection of carotid artery** 🔖

    I77.72   **Dissection of iliac artery** 🔖

    I77.73   **Dissection of renal artery** 🔖

    I77.74   **Dissection of vertebral artery** 🔖

    I77.79   **Dissection of other artery** 🔖

● **I77.8   Other specified disorders of arteries and arterioles**

    I77.81   **Aortic ectasia**
       Ectasis aorta

       | **Excludes1** | aortic aneurysm and dissection (I71.0-)

      I77.810   **Thoracic aortic ectasia**

      I77.811   **Abdominal aortic ectasia**

      I77.812   **Thoracoabdominal aortic ectasia**

     ◼ I77.819   **Aortic ectasia, unspecified site**

    I77.89   **Other specified disorders of arteries and arterioles**

◼ **I77.9   Disorder of arteries and arterioles, unspecified**

● **I78   Diseases of capillaries**

  I78.0   Hereditary hemorrhagic telangiectasia
    Rendu-Osler-Weber disease

  I78.1   Nevus, non-neoplastic
    Araneus nevus
    Senile nevus
    Spider nevus
    Stellar nevus

    | **Excludes1** | nevus NOS (D22.-)
               vascular NOS (Q82.5)

    | **Excludes2** | blue nevus (D22.-)
               flammeus nevus (Q82.5)
               hairy nevus (D22.-)
               melanocytic nevus (D22.-)
               pigmented nevus (D22.-)
               portwine nevus (Q82.5)
               sanguineous nevus (Q82.5)
               strawberry nevus (Q82.5)
               verrucous nevus (Q82.5)

◼ **I78.8   Other diseases of capillaries**

◼ **I78.9   Disease of capillaries, unspecified**

● **I79   Disorders of arteries, arterioles and capillaries in diseases classified elsewhere**

  ●▶ *I79.0   Aneurysm of aorta in diseases classified elsewhere*

    Code first underlying disease

    | **Excludes1** | syphilitic aneurysm (A52.01)

  ●▶ *I79.1   Aortitis in diseases classified elsewhere*

    Code first underlying disease

    | **Excludes1** | syphilitic aortitis (A52.02)

  ●▶ *I79.8   Other disorders of arteries, arterioles and capillaries in diseases classified elsewhere*

    Code first underlying disease, such as:
      amyloidosis (E85-)

    | **Excludes1** | diabetic (peripheral) angiopathy (E08-E13 with .51-.52) endarteritis:
               syphilitic (A52.09)
               tuberculous (A18.89)

● Unacceptable Principal Diagnosis   ● Use Additional Character(s)   ◼ Unspecified   ▶ Manifestation Code

OGCR Official Guidelines for Coding and Reporting | Excludes 1 | | Excludes 2 | Includes   Use additional   Code first   Code also

DISEASES OF VEINS, LYMPHATIC VESSELS AND LYMPH NODES, NOT ELSEWHERE CLASSIFIED (I80-I89)

● **I80   Phlebitis and thrombophlebitis**
Inflammation of a vein with infiltration of walls (phlebitis).

> **Includes** endophlebitis
>   inflammation, vein
>   periphlebitis
>   suppurative phlebitis

> *Code first* phlebitis and thrombophlebitis complicating abortion, ectopic or molar pregnancy (O00-O07, O08.7)
> phlebitis and thrombophlebitis complicating pregnancy, childbirth and the puerperium (O22.-, O87.-)

> **Excludes1** venous embolism and thrombosis of lower extremities (I82.4-, I82.5-, I82.81-)

● **I80.0   Phlebitis and thrombophlebitis of superficial vessels of lower extremities**
      Phlebitis and thrombophlebitis of femoropopliteal vein

■ **I80.00   Phlebitis and thrombophlebitis of superficial vessels of unspecified lower extremity**

I80.01   Phlebitis and thrombophlebitis of superficial vessels of right lower extremity

I80.02   Phlebitis and thrombophlebitis of superficial vessels of left lower extremity

I80.03   Phlebitis and thrombophlebitis of superficial vessels of lower extremities, bilateral

● **I80.1   Phlebitis and thrombophlebitis of femoral vein**

■ **I80.10   Phlebitis and thrombophlebitis of unspecified femoral vein** 🚫

I80.11   Phlebitis and thrombophlebitis of right femoral vein 🚫

I80.12   Phlebitis and thrombophlebitis of left femoral vein 🚫

I80.13   Phlebitis and thrombophlebitis of femoral vein, bilateral 🚫

● **I80.2   Phlebitis and thrombophlebitis of other and unspecified deep vessels of lower extremities**

● **I80.20   Phlebitis and thrombophlebitis of unspecified deep vessels of lower extremities**

■ **I80.201   Phlebitis and thrombophlebitis of unspecified deep vessels of right lower extremity** 🚫

■ **I80.202   Phlebitis and thrombophlebitis of unspecified deep vessels of left lower extremity** 🚫

■ **I80.203   Phlebitis and thrombophlebitis of unspecified deep vessels of lower extremities, bilateral** 🚫

■ **I80.209   Phlebitis and thrombophlebitis of unspecified deep vessels of unspecified lower extremity** 🚫

● **I80.21   Phlebitis and thrombophlebitis of iliac vein**

I80.211   Phlebitis and thrombophlebitis of right iliac vein 🚫

I80.212   Phlebitis and thrombophlebitis of left iliac vein 🚫

I80.213   Phlebitis and thrombophlebitis of iliac vein, bilateral 🚫

■ **I80.219   Phlebitis and thrombophlebitis of unspecified iliac vein** 🚫

● **I80.22   Phlebitis and thrombophlebitis of popliteal vein**

I80.221   Phlebitis and thrombophlebitis of right popliteal vein 🚫

I80.222   Phlebitis and thrombophlebitis of left popliteal vein 🚫

I80.223   Phlebitis and thrombophlebitis of popliteal vein, bilateral 🚫

■ **I80.229   Phlebitis and thrombophlebitis of unspecified popliteal vein** 🚫

● **I80.23   Phlebitis and thrombophlebitis of tibial vein**

I80.231   Phlebitis and thrombophlebitis of right tibial vein 🚫

I80.232   Phlebitis and thrombophlebitis of left tibial vein 🚫

I80.233   Phlebitis and thrombophlebitis of tibial vein, bilateral 🚫

■ **I80.239   Phlebitis and thrombophlebitis of unspecified tibial vein** 🚫

● **I80.29   Phlebitis and thrombophlebitis of other deep vessels of lower extremities**

I80.291   Phlebitis and thrombophlebitis of other deep vessels of right lower extremity 🚫

I80.292   Phlebitis and thrombophlebitis of other deep vessels of left lower extremity 🚫

I80.293   Phlebitis and thrombophlebitis of other deep vessels of lower extremity, bilateral 🚫

■ **I80.299   Phlebitis and thrombophlebitis of other deep vessels of unspecified lower extremity** 🚫

■ **I80.3   Phlebitis and thrombophlebitis of lower extremities, unspecified**

I80.8   Phlebitis and thrombophlebitis of other sites

■ **I80.9   Phlebitis and thrombophlebitis of unspecified site**

I81   Portal vein thrombosis 🚫
Portal (vein) obstruction

> **Excludes2** hepatic vein thrombosis (I82.0)
> phlebitis of portal vein (K75.1)

● **I82   Other venous embolism and thrombosis**

> *Code first* *venous embolism and thrombosis complicating:*
> abortion, ectopic or molar pregnancy (O00-O07, O08.7)
> pregnancy, childbirth and the puerperium (O22.-, O87.-)

> **Excludes2** venous embolism and thrombosis (of):
> cerebral (I63.6, I67.6)
> coronary (I21-I25)
> intracranial and intraspinal, septic or NOS (G08)
> intracranial, nonpyogenic (I67.6)
> intraspinal, nonpyogenic (G95.1)
> mesenteric (K55.0)
> portal (I81)
> pulmonary (I26.-)

I82.0   Budd-Chiari syndrome 🚫
Hepatic vein thrombosis

I82.1   Thrombophlebitis migrans 🚫
"White leg" is the other term to describe a migrating thrombus.

N Newborn Age: 0   **P** Pediatric Age: 0–17   **M** Maternity DX: 12–55   **A** Adult Age: 15–124   ♀ Females Only   ♂ Males Only

🚫 Complication\Comorbidity   🚫 Major C\C   🚫 Present on Admission Requirement   🚫 Hospital-Acquired Condition

1059

CHAPTER 9 (I00-I99)

● **I82.2**   **Embolism and thrombosis of vena cava and other thoracic veins**

  ● **I82.21**   **Embolism and thrombosis of superior vena cava**

    I82.210   **Acute embolism and thrombosis of superior vena cava** 🦴
          Embolism and thrombosis of superior vena cava NOS

    I82.211   **Chronic embolism and thrombosis of superior vena cava** 🦴

  ● **I82.22**   **Embolism and thrombosis of inferior vena cava**

    I82.220   **Acute embolism and thrombosis of inferior vena cava** 🦴
          Embolism and thrombosis of inferior vena cava NOS

    I82.221   **Chronic embolism and thrombosis of inferior vena cava** 🦴

  ● **I82.29**   **Embolism and thrombosis of other thoracic veins**
      Embolism and thrombosis of brachiocephalic (innominate) vein

    I82.290   **Acute embolism and thrombosis of other thoracic veins** 🦴

    I82.291   **Chronic embolism and thrombosis of other thoracic veins** 🦴

I82.3   **Embolism and thrombosis of renal vein** 🦴

● **I82.4**   **Acute embolism and thrombosis of deep veins of lower extremity**

  ● **I82.40**   **Acute embolism and thrombosis of unspecified deep veins of lower extremity**
      Deep vein thrombosis NOS
      DVT NOS

    | Excludes1 | acute embolism and thrombosis of unspecified deep veins of distal lower extremity (I82.4b-)
          acute embolism and thrombosis of unspecified deep veins of proximal lower extremity (I82.4a-)

    ▪ **I82.401**   **Acute embolism and thrombosis of unspecified deep veins of right lower extremity** 🦴

    ▪ **I82.402**   **Acute embolism and thrombosis of unspecified deep veins of left lower extremity** 🦴

    ▪ **I82.403**   **Acute embolism and thrombosis of unspecified deep veins of lower extremity, bilateral** 🦴

    ▪ **I82.409**   **Acute embolism and thrombosis of unspecified deep veins of unspecified lower extremity** 🦴

  ● **I82.41**   **Acute embolism and thrombosis of femoral vein**

    I82.411   **Acute embolism and thrombosis of right femoral vein** 🦴

    I82.412   **Acute embolism and thrombosis of left femoral vein** 🦴

    I82.413   **Acute embolism and thrombosis of femoral vein, bilateral** 🦴

    ▪ **I82.419**   **Acute embolism and thrombosis of unspecified femoral vein** 🦴

● **I82.42**   **Acute embolism and thrombosis of iliac vein**

    I82.421   **Acute embolism and thrombosis of right iliac vein** 🦴

    I82.422   **Acute embolism and thrombosis of left iliac vein** 🦴

    I82.423   **Acute embolism and thrombosis of iliac vein, bilateral** 🦴

    ▪ **I82.429**   **Acute embolism and thrombosis of unspecified iliac vein** 🦴

● **I82.43**   **Acute embolism and thrombosis of popliteal vein**

    I82.431   **Acute embolism and thrombosis of right popliteal vein** 🦴

    I82.432   **Acute embolism and thrombosis of left popliteal vein** 🦴

    I82.433   **Acute embolism and thrombosis of popliteal vein, bilateral** 🦴

    ▪ **I82.439**   **Acute embolism and thrombosis of unspecified popliteal vein** 🦴

● **I82.44**   **Acute embolism and thrombosis of tibial vein**

    I82.441   **Acute embolism and thrombosis of right tibial vein** 🦴

    I82.442   **Acute embolism and thrombosis of left tibial vein** 🦴

    I82.443   **Acute embolism and thrombosis of tibial vein, bilateral** 🦴

    ▪ **I82.449**   **Acute embolism and thrombosis of unspecified tibial vein** 🦴

● **I82.49**   **Acute embolism and thrombosis of other specified deep vein of lower extremity**

    I82.491   **Acute embolism and thrombosis of other specified deep vein of right lower extremity** 🦴

    I82.492   **Acute embolism and thrombosis of other specified deep vein of left lower extremity** 🦴

    I82.493   **Acute embolism and thrombosis of other specified deep vein of lower extremity, bilateral** 🦴

    ▪ **I82.499**   **Acute embolism and thrombosis of other specified deep vein of unspecified lower extremity** 🦴

● **I82.4Y**   **Acute embolism and thrombosis of unspecified deep veins of proximal lower extremity**
      Acute embolism and thrombosis of deep vein of thigh NOS
      Acute embolism and thrombosis of deep vein of upper leg NOS

    I82.4Y1   **Acute embolism and thrombosis of unspecified deep veins of right proximal lower extremity** 🦴

    I82.4Y2   **Acute embolism and thrombosis of unspecified deep veins of left proximal lower extremity** 🦴

    ▪ **I82.4Y3**   **Acute embolism and thrombosis of unspecified deep veins of proximal lower extremity, bilateral** 🦴

    ▪ **I82.4Y9**   **Acute embolism and thrombosis of unspecified deep veins of unspecified proximal lower extremity** 🦴

● Unacceptable Principal Diagnosis   ● Use Additional Character(s)   ▪ Unspecified   ▸ Manifestation Code

OGCR Official Guidelines for Coding and Reporting | Excludes 1 | | Excludes 2 | Includes   Use additional   Code first   Code also

● **I82.4Z**   **Acute embolism and thrombosis of unspecified deep veins of distal lower extremity**

Acute embolism and thrombosis of deep vein of calf NOS

Acute embolism and thrombosis of deep vein of lower leg NOS

▨ **I82.4Z1**   Acute embolism and thrombosis of unspecified deep veins of right distal lower extremity 🔧 🔧

▨ **I82.4Z2**   Acute embolism and thrombosis of unspecified deep veins of left distal lower extremity 🔧 🔧

▨ **I82.4Z3**   Acute embolism and thrombosis of unspecified deep veins of distal lower extremity, bilateral 🔧 🔧

▨ **I82.4Z9**   Acute embolism and thrombosis of unspecified deep veins of unspecified distal lower extremity 🔧 🔧

● **I82.5**   **Chronic embolism and thrombosis of deep veins of lower extremity**

Use additional code, if applicable, for associated long-term (current) use of anticoagulants (Z79.01)

Excludes1   personal history of venous embolism and thrombosis (Z86.718)

● **I82.50**   **Chronic embolism and thrombosis of unspecified deep veins of lower extremity**

Excludes1   chronic embolism and thrombosis of unspecified deep veins of distal lower extremity (I82.5b-)
chronic embolism and thrombosis of unspecified deep veins of proximal lower extremity (I82.5a-)

▨ **I82.501**   Chronic embolism and thrombosis of unspecified deep veins of right lower extremity 🔧

▨ **I82.502**   Chronic embolism and thrombosis of unspecified deep veins of left lower extremity 🔧

▨ **I82.503**   Chronic embolism and thrombosis of unspecified deep veins of lower extremity, bilateral 🔧

▨ **I82.509**   Chronic embolism and thrombosis of unspecified deep veins of unspecified lower extremity 🔧

● **I82.51**   **Chronic embolism and thrombosis of femoral vein**

I82.511   Chronic embolism and thrombosis of right femoral vein 🔧

I82.512   Chronic embolism and thrombosis of left femoral vein 🔧

I82.513   Chronic embolism and thrombosis of femoral vein, bilateral 🔧

▨ **I82.519**   Chronic embolism and thrombosis of unspecified femoral vein 🔧

Item 9–10   Varicose/Varicosities (varix = singular, varices = plural): Enlarged, engorged, tortuous, twisted vascular vessels (veins, arteries, lymphatics). As such, the condition can present in various parts of the body, although the most familiar locations are the lower extremities. A common complication of varices is thrombophlebitis. Varicosities of the anus and rectum are called hemorrhoids.

Figure 9-4   Varicose veins of the legs. (From Goldman: *Cecil Medicine*, 23rd ed. 2008, Saunders.)

● **I82.52**   **Chronic embolism and thrombosis of iliac vein**

I82.521   Chronic embolism and thrombosis of right iliac vein 🔧

I82.522   Chronic embolism and thrombosis of left iliac vein 🔧

I82.523   Chronic embolism and thrombosis of iliac vein, bilateral 🔧

▨ **I82.529**   Chronic embolism and thrombosis of unspecified iliac vein 🔧

● **I82.53**   **Chronic embolism and thrombosis of popliteal vein**

I82.531   Chronic embolism and thrombosis of right popliteal vein 🔧

I82.532   Chronic embolism and thrombosis of left popliteal vein 🔧

I82.533   Chronic embolism and thrombosis of popliteal vein, bilateral 🔧

▨ **I82.539**   Chronic embolism and thrombosis of unspecified popliteal vein 🔧

● **I82.54**   **Chronic embolism and thrombosis of tibial vein**

I82.541   Chronic embolism and thrombosis of right tibial vein 🔧

I82.542   Chronic embolism and thrombosis of left tibial vein 🔧

I82.543   Chronic embolism and thrombosis of tibial vein, bilateral 🔧

▨ **I82.549**   Chronic embolism and thrombosis of unspecified tibial vein 🔧

N Newborn Age: 0   **P** Pediatric Age: 0–17   **M** Maternity DX: 12–55   **A** Adult Age: 15–124   ♀ Females Only   ♂ Males Only

🔧 Complication\Comorbidity   🔧 Major C\C   🔧 Present on Admission Requirement   🔧 Hospital-Acquired Condition

1061

CHAPTER 9 (I00-I99)

● **I82.59**   **Chronic embolism and thrombosis of other specified deep vein of lower extremity**

     I82.591   Chronic embolism and thrombosis of other specified deep vein of right lower extremity ✎

     I82.592   Chronic embolism and thrombosis of other specified deep vein of left lower extremity ✎

     I82.593   Chronic embolism and thrombosis of other specified deep vein of lower extremity, bilateral ✎

     ■ **I82.599**   Chronic embolism and thrombosis of other specified deep vein of unspecified lower extremity ✎

● **I82.5Y**   **Chronic embolism and thrombosis of unspecified deep veins of proximal lower extremity**
     Chronic embolism and thrombosis of deep veins of thigh NOS
     Chronic embolism and thrombosis of deep veins of upper leg NOS

     ■ **I82.5Y1**   Chronic embolism and thrombosis of unspecified deep veins of right proximal lower extremity ✎

     ■ **I82.5Y2**   Chronic embolism and thrombosis of unspecified deep veins of left proximal lower extremity ✎

     ■ **I82.5Y3**   Chronic embolism and thrombosis of unspecified deep veins of proximal lower extremity, bilateral ✎

     ■ **I82.5Y9**   Chronic embolism and thrombosis of unspecified deep veins of unspecified proximal lower extremity ✎

● **I82.5Z**   **Chronic embolism and thrombosis of unspecified deep veins of distal lower extremity**
     Chronic embolism and thrombosis of deep veins of calf NOS
     Chronic embolism and thrombosis of deep veins of lower leg NOS

     ■ **I82.5Z1**   Chronic embolism and thrombosis of unspecified deep veins of right distal lower extremity ✎

     ■ **I82.5Z2**   Chronic embolism and thrombosis of unspecified deep veins of left distal lower extremity ✎

     ■ **I82.5Z3**   Chronic embolism and thrombosis of unspecified deep veins of distal lower extremity, bilateral ✎

     ■ **I82.5Z9**   Chronic embolism and thrombosis of unspecified deep veins of unspecified distal lower extremity ✎

● **I82.6**   **Acute embolism and thrombosis of veins of upper extremity**

   ● **I82.60**   **Acute embolism and thrombosis of unspecified veins of upper extremity**

     ■ **I82.601**   Acute embolism and thrombosis of unspecified veins of right upper extremity ✎

     ■ **I82.602**   Acute embolism and thrombosis of unspecified veins of left upper extremity ✎

     ■ **I82.603**   Acute embolism and thrombosis of unspecified veins of upper extremity, bilateral ✎

     ■ **I82.609**   Acute embolism and thrombosis of unspecified veins of unspecified upper extremity ✎

   ● **I82.61**   **Acute embolism and thrombosis of superficial veins of upper extremity**
     Acute embolism and thrombosis of antecubital vein
     Acute embolism and thrombosis of basilic vein
     Acute embolism and thrombosis of cephalic vein

     I82.611   Acute embolism and thrombosis of superficial veins of right upper extremity ✎

     I82.612   Acute embolism and thrombosis of superficial veins of left upper extremity ✎

     I82.613   Acute embolism and thrombosis of superficial veins of upper extremity, bilateral ✎

     ■ **I82.619**   Acute embolism and thrombosis of superficial veins of unspecified upper extremity ✎

   ● **I82.62**   **Acute embolism and thrombosis of deep veins of upper extremity**
     Acute embolism and thrombosis of brachial vein
     Acute embolism and thrombosis of radial vein
     Acute embolism and thrombosis of ulnar vein

     I82.621   Acute embolism and thrombosis of deep veins of right upper extremity ✎

     I82.622   Acute embolism and thrombosis of deep veins of left upper extremity ✎

     I82.623   Acute embolism and thrombosis of deep veins of upper extremity, bilateral ✎

     ■ **I82.629**   Acute embolism and thrombosis of deep veins of unspecified upper extremity ✎

● **I82.7**   **Chronic embolism and thrombosis of veins of upper extremity**

     Use additional code, if applicable, for associated long-term (current) use of anticoagulants (Z79.01)

     Excludes1   personal history of venous embolism and thrombosis (Z86.718)

   ● **I82.70**   **Chronic embolism and thrombosis of unspecified veins of upper extremity**

● Unacceptable Principal Diagnosis   ● Use Additional Character(s)   ■ Unspecified   ▶ Manifestation Code

1062

OGCR   Official Guidelines for Coding and Reporting   Excludes 1   Excludes 2   Includes   Use additional   Code first   Code also

■ I82.701 Chronic embolism and thrombosis of unspecified veins of right upper extremity 🌣

■ I82.702 Chronic embolism and thrombosis of unspecified veins of left upper extremity 🌣

■ I82.703 Chronic embolism and thrombosis of unspecified veins of upper extremity, bilateral 🌣

■ I82.709 Chronic embolism and thrombosis of unspecified veins of unspecified upper extremity 🌣

● I82.71 Chronic embolism and thrombosis of superficial veins of upper extremity
Chronic embolism and thrombosis of antecubital vein
Chronic embolism and thrombosis of basilic vein
Chronic embolism and thrombosis of cephalic vein

I82.711 Chronic embolism and thrombosis of superficial veins of right upper extremity 🌣

I82.712 Chronic embolism and thrombosis of superficial veins of left upper extremity 🌣

I82.713 Chronic embolism and thrombosis of superficial veins of upper extremity, bilateral 🌣

■ I82.719 Chronic embolism and thrombosis of superficial veins of unspecified upper extremity 🌣

● I82.72 Chronic embolism and thrombosis of deep veins of upper extremity
Chronic embolism and thrombosis of brachial vein
Chronic embolism and thrombosis of radial vein
Chronic embolism and thrombosis of ulnar vein

I82.721 Chronic embolism and thrombosis of deep veins of right upper extremity 🌣

I82.722 Chronic embolism and thrombosis of deep veins of left upper extremity 🌣

I82.723 Chronic embolism and thrombosis of deep veins of upper extremity, bilateral 🌣

■ I82.729 Chronic embolism and thrombosis of deep veins of unspecified upper extremity 🌣

● I82.A Embolism and thrombosis of axillary vein

● I82.A1 Acute embolism and thrombosis of axillary vein

I82.A11 Acute embolism and thrombosis of right axillary vein 🌣

I82.A12 Acute embolism and thrombosis of left axillary vein 🌣

I82.A13 Acute embolism and thrombosis of axillary vein, bilateral 🌣

■ I82.A19 Acute embolism and thrombosis of unspecified axillary vein 🌣

● I82.A2 Chronic embolism and thrombosis of axillary vein

I82.A21 Chronic embolism and thrombosis of right axillary vein 🌣

I82.A22 Chronic embolism and thrombosis of left axillary vein 🌣

I82.A23 Chronic embolism and thrombosis of axillary vein, bilateral 🌣

■ I82.A29 Chronic embolism and thrombosis of unspecified axillary vein 🌣

● I82.B Embolism and thrombosis of subclavian vein

● I82.B1 Acute embolism and thrombosis of subclavian vein

I82.B11 Acute embolism and thrombosis of right subclavian vein 🌣

I82.B12 Acute embolism and thrombosis of left subclavian vein 🌣

I82.B13 Acute embolism and thrombosis of subclavian vein, bilateral 🌣

■ I82.B19 Acute embolism and thrombosis of unspecified subclavian vein 🌣

● I82.B2 Chronic embolism and thrombosis of subclavian vein

I82.B21 Chronic embolism and thrombosis of right subclavian vein 🌣

I82.B22 Chronic embolism and thrombosis of left subclavian vein 🌣

I82.B23 Chronic embolism and thrombosis of subclavian vein, bilateral 🌣

■ I82.B29 Chronic embolism and thrombosis of unspecified subclavian vein 🌣

● I82.C Embolism and thrombosis of internal jugular vein

● I82.C1 Acute embolism and thrombosis of internal jugular vein

I82.C11 Acute embolism and thrombosis of right internal jugular vein 🌣

I82.C12 Acute embolism and thrombosis of left internal jugular vein 🌣

I82.C13 Acute embolism and thrombosis of internal jugular vein, bilateral 🌣

■ I82.C19 Acute embolism and thrombosis of unspecified internal jugular vein 🌣

● I82.C2 Chronic embolism and thrombosis of internal jugular vein

I82.C21 Chronic embolism and thrombosis of right internal jugular vein 🌣

I82.C22 Chronic embolism and thrombosis of left internal jugular vein 🌣

I82.C23 Chronic embolism and thrombosis of internal jugular vein, bilateral 🌣

■ I82.C29 Chronic embolism and thrombosis of unspecified internal jugular vein 🌣

CHAPTER 9 (I00-I99)

N Newborn Age: 0   **P** Pediatric Age: 0–17   **M** Maternity DX: 12–55   **A** Adult Age: 15–124   ♀ Females Only   ♂ Males Only

🌣 Complication\Comorbidity   🌣 Major C\C   🌣 Present on Admission Requirement   🌣 Hospital-Acquired Condition

1063

CHAPTER 9 (I00-I99)

● **I82.8**   **Embolism and thrombosis of other specified veins**

Use additional code, if applicable, for associated long-term (current) use of anticoagulants (Z79.01)

● **I82.81**   **Embolism and thrombosis of superficial veins of lower extremities**

Embolism and thrombosis of saphenous vein (greater) (lesser)

I82.811   **Embolism and thrombosis of superficial veins of right lower extremities** ✪

I82.812   **Embolism and thrombosis of superficial veins of left lower extremities** ✪

I82.813   **Embolism and thrombosis of superficial veins of lower extremities, bilateral** ✪

◼ **I82.819**   **Embolism and thrombosis of superficial veins of unspecified lower extremities** ✪

● **I82.89**   **Embolism and thrombosis of other specified veins**

I82.890   **Acute embolism and thrombosis of other specified veins** ✪

I82.891   **Chronic embolism and thrombosis of other specified veins** ✪

● **I82.9**   **Embolism and thrombosis of unspecified vein**

◼ **I82.90**   **Acute embolism and thrombosis of unspecified vein** ✪

Embolism of vein NOS
Thrombosis (vein) NOS

◼ **I82.91**   **Chronic embolism and thrombosis of unspecified vein** ✪

● **I83**   **Varicose veins of lower extremities**

| Excludes1 | varicose veins complicating pregnancy (O22.0-) |

varicose veins complicating the puerperium (O87.4)

● **I83.0**   **Varicose veins of lower extremities with ulcer**

Use additional code to identify severity of ulcer (L97.-)

● **I83.00**   **Varicose veins of unspecified lower extremity with ulcer**

◼ **I83.001**   **Varicose veins of unspecified lower extremity with ulcer of thigh**   A

◼ **I83.002**   **Varicose veins of unspecified lower extremity with ulcer of calf**   A

◼ **I83.003**   **Varicose veins of unspecified lower extremity with ulcer of ankle**   A

◼ **I83.004**   **Varicose veins of unspecified lower extremity with ulcer of heel and midfoot**   A

Varicose veins of unspecified lower extremity with ulcer of plantar surface of midfoot

◼ **I83.005**   **Varicose veins of unspecified lower extremity with ulcer other part of foot**   A

Varicose veins of unspecified lower extremity with ulcer of toe

◼ **I83.008**   **Varicose veins of unspecified lower extremity with ulcer other part of lower leg**   A

◼ **I83.009**   **Varicose veins of unspecified lower extremity with ulcer of unspecified site**   A

● **I83.01**   **Varicose veins of right lower extremity with ulcer**

I83.011   **Varicose veins of right lower extremity with ulcer of thigh**   A

I83.012   **Varicose veins of right lower extremity with ulcer of calf**   A

I83.013   **Varicose veins of right lower extremity with ulcer of ankle**   A

I83.014   **Varicose veins of right lower extremity with ulcer of heel and midfoot**   A

Varicose veins of right lower extremity with ulcer of plantar surface of midfoot

I83.015   **Varicose veins of right lower extremity with ulcer other part of foot**   A

Varicose veins of right lower extremity with ulcer of toe

I83.018   **Varicose veins of right lower extremity with ulcer other part of lower leg**   A

◼ **I83.019**   **Varicose veins of right lower extremity with ulcer of unspecified site**   A

● **I83.02**   **Varicose veins of left lower extremity with ulcer**

I83.021   **Varicose veins of left lower extremity with ulcer of thigh**   A

I83.022   **Varicose veins of left lower extremity with ulcer of calf**   A

I83.023   **Varicose veins of left lower extremity with ulcer of ankle**   A

I83.024   **Varicose veins of left lower extremity with ulcer of heel and midfoot**   A

Varicose veins of left lower extremity with ulcer of plantar surface of midfoot

I83.025   **Varicose veins of left lower extremity with ulcer other part of foot**   A

Varicose veins of left lower extremity with ulcer of toe

I83.028   **Varicose veins of left lower extremity with ulcer other part of lower leg**   A

◼ **I83.029**   **Varicose veins of left lower extremity with ulcer of unspecified site**   A

● **I83.1**   **Varicose veins of lower extremities with inflammation**

Stasis dermatitis

◼ **I83.10**   **Varicose veins of unspecified lower extremity with inflammation**   A

I83.11   **Varicose veins of right lower extremity with inflammation**   A

I83.12   **Varicose veins of left lower extremity with inflammation**   A

● **I83.2   Varicose veins of lower extremities with both ulcer and inflammation**

> Use additional code to identify severity of ulcer (L97.-)

  ● **I83.20   Varicose veins of unspecified lower extremity with both ulcer and inflammation**

    ■ **I83.201   Varicose veins of unspecified lower extremity with both ulcer of thigh and inflammation 🦠   A**

    ■ **I83.202   Varicose veins of unspecified lower extremity with both ulcer of calf and inflammation 🦠   A**

    ■ **I83.203   Varicose veins of unspecified lower extremity with both ulcer of ankle and inflammation 🦠   A**

    ■ **I83.204   Varicose veins of unspecified lower extremity with both ulcer of heel and midfoot and inflammation 🦠   A**

> Varicose veins of unspecified lower extremity with both ulcer of plantar surface of midfoot and inflammation

    ■ **I83.205   Varicose veins of unspecified lower extremity with both ulcer other part of foot and inflammation 🦠   A**

> Varicose veins of unspecified lower extremity with both ulcer of toe and inflammation

    ■ **I83.208   Varicose veins of unspecified lower extremity with both ulcer of other part of lower extremity and inflammation 🦠   A**

    ■ **I83.209   Varicose veins of unspecified lower extremity with both ulcer of unspecified site and inflammation 🦠   A**

  ● **I83.21   Varicose veins of right lower extremity with both ulcer and inflammation**

    I83.211   Varicose veins of right lower extremity with both ulcer of thigh and inflammation 🦠   A

    I83.212   Varicose veins of right lower extremity with both ulcer of calf and inflammation 🦠   A

    I83.213   Varicose veins of right lower extremity with both ulcer of ankle and inflammation 🦠   A

    I83.214   Varicose veins of right lower extremity with both ulcer of heel and midfoot and inflammation 🦠   A

> Varicose veins of right lower extremity with both ulcer of plantar surface of midfoot and inflammation

    I83.215   Varicose veins of right lower extremity with both ulcer other part of foot and inflammation 🦠 A

> Varicose veins of right lower extremity with both ulcer of toe and inflammation

    I83.218   Varicose veins of right lower extremity with both ulcer of other part of lower extremity and inflammation 🦠   A

    ■ **I83.219   Varicose veins of right lower extremity with both ulcer of unspecified site and inflammation 🦠   A**

  ● **I83.22   Varicose veins of left lower extremity with both ulcer and inflammation**

    I83.221   Varicose veins of left lower extremity with both ulcer of thigh and inflammation 🦠   A

    I83.222   Varicose veins of left lower extremity with both ulcer of calf and inflammation 🦠   A

    I83.223   Varicose veins of left lower extremity with both ulcer of ankle and inflammation 🦠   A

    I83.224   Varicose veins of left lower extremity with both ulcer of heel and midfoot and inflammation 🦠   A

> Varicose veins of left lower extremity with both ulcer of plantar surface of midfoot and inflammation

    I83.225   Varicose veins of left lower extremity with both ulcer other part of foot and inflammation 🦠 A

> Varicose veins of left lower extremity with both ulcer of toe and inflammation

    I83.228   Varicose veins of left lower extremity with both ulcer of other part of lower extremity and inflammation 🦠   A

    ■ **I83.229   Varicose veins of left lower extremity with both ulcer of unspecified site and inflammation 🦠   A**

● **I83.8   Varicose veins of lower extremities with other complications**

  ● **I83.81   Varicose veins of lower extremities with pain**

    I83.811   Varicose veins of right lower extremities with pain   A

    I83.812   Varicose veins of left lower extremities with pain   A

    I83.813   Varicose veins of bilateral lower extremities with pain   A

    ■ **I83.819   Varicose veins of unspecified lower extremities with pain   A**

  ● **I83.89   Varicose veins of lower extremities with other complications**

> Varicose veins of lower extremities with edema
>
> Varicose veins of lower extremities with swelling

    I83.891   Varicose veins of right lower extremities with other complications   A

    I83.892   Varicose veins of left lower extremities with other complications   A

    I83.893   Varicose veins of bilateral lower extremities with other complications   A

    ■ **I83.899   Varicose veins of unspecified lower extremities with other complications   A**

N Newborn Age: 0   **P** Pediatric Age: 0–17   **M** Maternity DX: 12–55   **A** Adult Age: 15–124   ♀ Females Only   ♂ Males Only

🦠 Complication\Comorbidity   🦠 Major C\C   🦠 Present on Admission Requirement   🦠 Hospital-Acquired Condition

1065

CHAPTER 9 (I00-I99)

● **I83.9   Asymptomatic varicose veins of lower extremities**
Phlebectasia of lower extremities
Varicose veins of lower extremities
Varix of lower extremities

■ **I83.90   Asymptomatic varicose veins of unspecified lower extremity**   A
Varicose veins NOS

I83.91   Asymptomatic varicose veins of right lower extremity   A

I83.92   Asymptomatic varicose veins of left lower extremity   A

I83.93   Asymptomatic varicose veins of bilateral lower extremities   A

● **I85   Esophageal varices**
Use additional code to identify:
alcohol abuse and dependence (F10.-)

● **I85.0   Esophageal varices**
Idiopathic esophageal varices
Primary esophageal varices

I85.00   Esophageal varices without bleeding 🕭
Esophageal varices NOS

I85.01   Esophageal varices with bleeding 🕭

● **I85.1   Secondary esophageal varices**
Esophageal varices secondary to alcoholic liver disease
Esophageal varices secondary to cirrhosis of liver
Esophageal varices secondary to schistosomiasis
Esophageal varices secondary to toxic liver disease

Code first underlying disease

● **I85.10   Secondary esophageal varices without bleeding** 🕭

● **I85.11   Secondary esophageal varices with bleeding** 🕭

● **I86   Varicose veins of other sites**

   Excludes1   varicose veins of unspecified site (I83.9-)
   Excludes2   retinal varices (H35.0-)

I86.0   Sublingual varices

I86.1   Scrotal varices ♂
Varicocele

I86.2   Pelvic varices

I86.3   Vulval varices ♀

   Excludes1   vulval varices complicating childbirth and the puerperium (O87.8)
vulval varices complicating pregnancy (O22.1-)

I86.4   Gastric varices

I86.8   Varicose veins of other specified sites   A
Varicose ulcer of nasal septum

● **I87   Other disorders of veins**

● **I87.0   Postthrombotic syndrome**
Chronic venous hypertension due to deep vein thrombosis
Postphlebitic syndrome

   Excludes1   chronic venous hypertension without deep vein thrombosis (I87.3-)

● **I87.00   Postthrombotic syndrome without complications**
Asymptomatic Postthrombotic syndrome

I87.001   Postthrombotic syndrome without complications of right lower extremity

I87.002   Postthrombotic syndrome without complications of left lower extremity

I87.003   Postthrombotic syndrome without complications of bilateral lower extremity

■ **I87.009   Postthrombotic syndrome without complications of unspecified extremity**
Postthrombotic syndrome NOS

● **I87.01   Postthrombotic syndrome with ulcer**

   Use additional code to specify site and severity of ulcer (L97.-)

I87.011   Postthrombotic syndrome with ulcer of right lower extremity 🕭

I87.012   Postthrombotic syndrome with ulcer of left lower extremity 🕭

I87.013   Postthrombotic syndrome with ulcer of bilateral lower extremity 🕭

■ **I87.019   Postthrombotic syndrome with ulcer of unspecified lower extremity** 🕭

● **I87.02   Postthrombotic syndrome with inflammation**

I87.021   Postthrombotic syndrome with inflammation of right lower extremity

I87.022   Postthrombotic syndrome with inflammation of left lower extremity

I87.023   Postthrombotic syndrome with inflammation of bilateral lower extremity

■ **I87.029   Postthrombotic syndrome with inflammation of unspecified lower extremity**

● **I87.03   Postthrombotic syndrome with ulcer and inflammation**

   Use additional code to specify site and severity of ulcer (L97.-)

I87.031   Postthrombotic syndrome with ulcer and inflammation of right lower extremity 🕭

I87.032   Postthrombotic syndrome with ulcer and inflammation of left lower extremity 🕭

I87.033   Postthrombotic syndrome with ulcer and inflammation of bilateral lower extremity 🕭

■ **I87.039   Postthrombotic syndrome with ulcer and inflammation of unspecified lower extremity** 🕭

● **I87.09   Postthrombotic syndrome with other complications**

I87.091   Postthrombotic syndrome with other complications of right lower extremity

I87.092   Postthrombotic syndrome with other complications of left lower extremity

I87.093   Postthrombotic syndrome with other complications of bilateral lower extremity

■ **I87.099   Postthrombotic syndrome with other complications of unspecified lower extremity**

●   Unacceptable Principal Diagnosis   ●   Use Additional Character(s)   ■   Unspecified   ▶   Manifestation Code
OGCR   Official Guidelines for Coding and Reporting   Excludes 1   Excludes 2   Includes   Use additional   Code first   Code also

I87.1　Compression of vein 🔷
　　Stricture of vein
　　Vena cava syndrome (inferior) (superior)
　　Excludes2 compression of pulmonary vein
　　　　　(I28.8)

I87.2　Venous insufficiency (chronic) (peripheral)

● **I87.3　Chronic venous hypertension (idiopathic)**
　　Stasis edema
　　Excludes1 chronic venous hypertension due to
　　　　　deep vein thrombosis (I87.0-)
　　　　　varicose veins of lower extremities
　　　　　(I83.-)

● **I87.30　Chronic venous hypertension (idiopathic) without complications**
　　Asymptomatic chronic venous hypertension (idiopathic)

　I87.301　Chronic venous hypertension (idiopathic) without complications of right lower extremity

　I87.302　Chronic venous hypertension (idiopathic) without complications of left lower extremity

　I87.303　Chronic venous hypertension (idiopathic) without complications of bilateral lower extremity

　■ **I87.309　Chronic venous hypertension (idiopathic) without complications of unspecified lower extremity**
　　　Chronic venous hypertension NOS

● **I87.31　Chronic venous hypertension (idiopathic) with ulcer**
　　Use additional code to specify site and severity of ulcer (L97.-)

　I87.311　Chronic venous hypertension (idiopathic) with ulcer of right lower extremity 🔷

　I87.312　Chronic venous hypertension (idiopathic) with ulcer of left lower extremity 🔷

　I87.313　Chronic venous hypertension (idiopathic) with ulcer of bilateral lower extremity 🔷

　■ **I87.319　Chronic venous hypertension (idiopathic) with ulcer of unspecified lower extremity** 🔷

● **I87.32　Chronic venous hypertension (idiopathic) with inflammation**

　I87.321　Chronic venous hypertension (idiopathic) with inflammation of right lower extremity

　I87.322　Chronic venous hypertension (idiopathic) with inflammation of left lower extremity

　I87.323　Chronic venous hypertension (idiopathic) with inflammation of bilateral lower extremity

　■ **I87.329　Chronic venous hypertension (idiopathic) with inflammation of unspecified lower extremity**

● **I87.33　Chronic venous hypertension (idiopathic) with ulcer and inflammation**
　　Use additional code to specify site and severity of ulcer (L97.-)

　I87.331　Chronic venous hypertension (idiopathic) with ulcer and inflammation of right lower extremity 🔷

　I87.332　Chronic venous hypertension (idiopathic) with ulcer and inflammation of left lower extremity 🔷

　I87.333　Chronic venous hypertension (idiopathic) with ulcer and inflammation of bilateral lower extremity 🔷

　■ **I87.339　Chronic venous hypertension (idiopathic) with ulcer and inflammation of unspecified lower extremity** 🔷

● **I87.39　Chronic venous hypertension (idiopathic) with other complications**

　I87.391　Chronic venous hypertension (idiopathic) with other complications of right lower extremity

　I87.392　Chronic venous hypertension (idiopathic) with other complications of left lower extremity

　I87.393　Chronic venous hypertension (idiopathic) with other complications of bilateral lower extremity

　■ **I87.399　Chronic venous hypertension (idiopathic) with other complications of unspecified lower extremity**

I87.8　Other specified disorders of veins
　　Phlebosclerosis
　　Venofibrosis

■ **I87.9　Disorder of vein, unspecified**

● **I88　Nonspecific lymphadenitis**
　　Excludes1 acute lymphadenitis, except mesenteric
　　　　　(L04.-)
　　　　　enlarged lymph nodes NOS (R59.-)
　　　　　human immunodeficiency virus [HIV]
　　　　　disease resulting in generalized
　　　　　lymphadenopathy (B20)

I88.0　Nonspecific mesenteric lymphadenitis
　　Mesenteric lymphadenitis (acute)(chronic)

I88.1　Chronic lymphadenitis, except mesenteric
　　Adenitis
　　Lymphadenitis

I88.8　Other nonspecific lymphadenitis

■ **I88.9　Nonspecific lymphadenitis, unspecified**
　　Lymphadenitis NOS

● **I89**   **Other noninfective disorders of lymphatic vessels and lymph nodes**

> **Excludes1**   chylocele, tunica vaginalis (nonfilarial) NOS (N50.8)
> enlarged lymph nodes NOS (R59.-)
> filarial chylocele (B74.-)
> hereditary lymphedema (Q82.0)

I89.0   **Lymphedema, not elsewhere classified**
Elephantiasis (nonfilarial) NOS
Lymphangiectasis
Obliteration, lymphatic vessel
Praecox lymphedema
Secondary lymphedema

> **Excludes1**   postmastectomy lymphedema (I97.2)

I89.1   **Lymphangitis**
Chronic lymphangitis
Lymphangitis NOS
Subacute lymphangitis

> **Excludes1**   acute lymphangitis (L03.-)

I89.8   **Other specified noninfective disorders of lymphatic vessels and lymph nodes**
Chylocele (nonfilarial)
Chylous ascites
Chylous cyst
Lipomelanotic reticulosis
Lymph node or vessel fistula
Lymph node or vessel infarction
Lymph node or vessel rupture

■ **I89.9**   **Noninfective disorder of lymphatic vessels and lymph nodes, unspecified**
Disease of lymphatic vessels NOS

OTHER AND UNSPECIFIED DISORDERS OF THE CIRCULATORY SYSTEM (I95-I99)

● **I95**   **Hypotension**
Subnormal arterial blood pressure

> **Excludes1**   cardiovascular collapse (R57.9)
> maternal hypotension syndrome (O26.5-)
> nonspecific low blood pressure reading NOS (R03.1)

I95.0   **Idiopathic hypotension**

I95.1   **Orthostatic hypotension**
Hypotension, postural
Moving from a sitting or reclining position to a standing position precipitates a sudden drop in blood pressure (hypotension).

> **Excludes1**   neurogenic orthostatic hypotension [Shy-Drager] (G90.3)
> orthostatic hypotension due to drugs (I95.2)

I95.2   **Hypotension due to drugs**
Orthostatic hypotension due to drugs
Use additional code for adverse effect, if applicable, to identify drug (T36-T50 with fifth or sixth character 5)

I95.3   **Hypotension of hemodialysis**
Intra-dialytic hypotension

● **I95.8**   **Other hypotension**

I95.81   **Postprocedural hypotension**

I95.89   **Other hypotension**
Chronic hypotension

■ **I95.9**   **Hypotension, unspecified**

I96   **Gangrene, not elsewhere classified** 🔧
Gangrenous cellulitis

> **Excludes1**   gangrene in atherosclerosis of native arteries of the extremities (I70.26)
> gangrene of certain specified sites - *see* Alphabetical Index
> gangrene in diabetes mellitus (E08-E13)
> gangrene in hernia (K40.1, K40.4, K41.1, K41.4, K42.1, K43.1-, K44.1, K45.1, K46.1)
> gangrene in other peripheral vascular diseases (I73.-)
> gas gangrene (A48.0)
> pyoderma gangrenosum (L88)

● **I97**   **Intraoperative and postprocedural complications and disorders of circulatory system, not elsewhere classified**

> **Excludes2**   postprocedural shock (T81.1-)

I97.0   **Postcardiotomy syndrome**

● **I97.1**   **Other postprocedural cardiac functional disturbances**

> **Excludes2**   acute pulmonary insufficiency following thoracic surgery (J95.1)
> intraoperative cardiac functional disturbances (I97.7-)

● **I97.11**   **Postprocedural cardiac insufficiency**

I97.110   **Postprocedural cardiac insufficiency following cardiac surgery**

I97.111   **Postprocedural cardiac insufficiency following other surgery**

● **I97.12**   **Postprocedural cardiac arrest**

I97.120   **Postprocedural cardiac arrest following cardiac surgery**

I97.121   **Postprocedural cardiac arrest following other surgery**

● **I97.13**   **Postprocedural heart failure**
Use additional code to identify the heart failure (I50.-)

I97.130   **Postprocedural heart failure following cardiac surgery**

I97.131   **Postprocedural heart failure following other surgery**

● **I97.19**   **Other postprocedural cardiac functional disturbances**
Use additional code, if applicable, to further specify disorder

I97.190   **Other postprocedural cardiac functional disturbances following cardiac surgery**

I97.191   **Other postprocedural cardiac functional disturbances following other surgery**

I97.2   **Postmastectomy lymphedema syndrome**   A
Elephantiasis due to mastectomy
Obliteration of lymphatic vessels

I97.3   **Postprocedural hypertension**

● **I97.4**   **Intraoperative hemorrhage and hematoma of a circulatory system organ or structure complicating a procedure**

     Excludes1   intraoperative hemorrhage and hematoma of a circulatory system organ or structure due to accidental puncture and laceration during a procedure (I97.5-)

     Excludes2   intraoperative cerebrovascular hemorrhage complicating a procedure (G97.3-)

    ● **I97.41**   **Intraoperative hemorrhage and hematoma of a circulatory system organ or structure complicating a circulatory system procedure**

       I97.410   **Intraoperative hemorrhage and hematoma of a circulatory system organ or structure complicating a cardiac catheterization** 🔹

       I97.411   **Intraoperative hemorrhage and hematoma of a circulatory system organ or structure complicating a cardiac bypass** 🔹

       I97.418   **Intraoperative hemorrhage and hematoma of a circulatory system organ or structure complicating other circulatory system procedure** 🔹

    I97.42   **Intraoperative hemorrhage and hematoma of a circulatory system organ or structure complicating other procedure** 🔹

● **I97.5**   **Accidental puncture and laceration of a circulatory system organ or structure during a procedure**

     Excludes2   accidental puncture and laceration of brain during a procedure (G97.4-)

    I97.51   **Accidental puncture and laceration of a circulatory system organ or structure during a circulatory system procedure** 🔹

    I97.52   **Accidental puncture and laceration of a circulatory system organ or structure during other procedure** 🔹

● **I97.6**   **Postprocedural hemorrhage and hematoma of a circulatory system organ or structure following a procedure**

     Excludes2   postprocedural cerebrovascular hemorrhage complicating a procedure (G97.5-)

    ● **I97.61**   **Postprocedural hemorrhage and hematoma of a circulatory system organ or structure following a circulatory system procedure**

       I97.610   **Postprocedural hemorrhage and hematoma of a circulatory system organ or structure following a cardiac catheterization** 🔹

       I97.611   **Postprocedural hemorrhage and hematoma of a circulatory system organ or structure following cardiac bypass** 🔹

       I97.618   **Postprocedural hemorrhage and hematoma of a circulatory system organ or structure following other circulatory system procedure** 🔹

    I97.62   **Postprocedural hemorrhage and hematoma of a circulatory system organ or structure following other procedure** 🔹

● **I97.7**   **Intraoperative cardiac functional disturbances**

     Excludes2   acute pulmonary insufficiency following thoracic surgery (J95.1)
            postprocedural cardiac functional disturbances (I97.1-)

    ● **I97.71**   **Intraoperative cardiac arrest**

       I97.710   **Intraoperative cardiac arrest during cardiac surgery** 🔹

       I97.711   **Intraoperative cardiac arrest during other surgery** 🔹

    ● **I97.79**   **Other intraoperative cardiac functional disturbances**

      Use additional code, if applicable, to further specify disorder

       I97.790   **Other intraoperative cardiac functional disturbances during cardiac surgery** 🔹

       I97.791   **Other intraoperative cardiac functional disturbances during other surgery** 🔹

● **I97.8**   **Other intraoperative and postprocedural complications and disorders of the circulatory system, not elsewhere classified**

      Use additional code, if applicable, to further specify disorder

    ● **I97.81**   **Intraoperative cerebrovascular infarction**

       I97.810   **Intraoperative cerebrovascular infarction during cardiac surgery** 🔹

       I97.811   **Intraoperative cerebrovascular infarction during other surgery** 🔹

    ● **I97.82**   **Postprocedural cerebrovascular infarction**

       I97.820   **Postprocedural cerebrovascular infarction during cardiac surgery** 🔹

       I97.821   **Postprocedural cerebrovascular infarction during other surgery** 🔹

    I97.88   **Other intraoperative complications of the circulatory system, not elsewhere classified** 🔹

    I97.89   **Other postprocedural complications and disorders of the circulatory system, not elsewhere classified** 🔹

● **I99**   **Other and unspecified disorders of circulatory system**

    I99.8   **Other disorder of circulatory system**

    ■ **I99.9**   **Unspecified disorder of circulatory system**

N   Newborn Age: 0   **P**   Pediatric Age: 0–17   **M**   Maternity DX: 12–55   **A**   Adult Age: 15–124   ♀   Females Only   ♂   Males Only

🔹 Complication\Comorbidity   🔹 Major C\C   🔹 Present on Admission Requirement   🔹 Hospital-Acquired Condition   **1069**

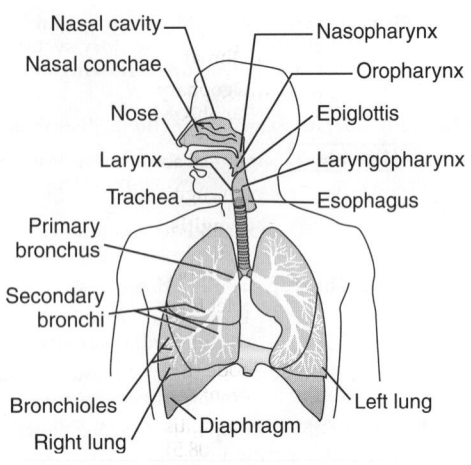

Figure 10-1 Respiratory system. (From Buck CJ: Step-by-Step Medical Coding, 2006 ed. Philadelphia, WB Saunders, 2006.)

Figure 10-2 Paranasal sinuses. (From Buck CJ: Step-by-Step Medical Coding. 2006 ed. Philadelphia, WB Saunders, 2006.)

Item 10-1 Pharyngitis is painful inflammation of the pharynx (sore throat). Ninety percent of the infections are caused by a virus with the remaining being bacterial and rarely a fungus (candidiasis). Other irritants such as pollutants, chemicals, or smoke may cause similar symptoms.

OGCR Section I.C.10.a.1

10.1 Chronic Obstructive Pulmonary Disease (COPD) and Asthma

CHAPTER 10

DISEASES OF THE RESPIRATORY SYSTEM (J00-J99)

Note: When a respiratory condition is described as occurring in more than one site and is not specifically indexed, it should be classified to the lower anatomic site (e.g. tracheobronchitis to bronchitis in J40).

Use additional code, where applicable, to identify:
exposure to environmental tobacco smoke (Z77.22)
exposure to tobacco smoke in the perinatal period (P96.81)
history of tobacco use (Z87.891)
occupational exposure to environmental tobacco smoke (Z57.31)
tobacco dependence (F17.-)
tobacco use (Z72.0)

Excludes2
certain conditions originating in the perinatal period (P04-P96)
certain infectious and parasitic diseases (A00-B99)
complications of pregnancy, childbirth and the puerperium (O00-O99A)
congenital malformations, deformations and chromosomal abnormalities (Q00-Q99)
endocrine, nutritional and metabolic diseases (E00-E88)
injury, poisoning and certain other consequences of external causes (S00-T88)
neoplasms (C00-D49)
smoke inhalation (T59.81-)
symptoms, signs and abnormal clinical and laboratory findings, not elsewhere classified (R00-R94)

This chapter contains the following blocks:

J00-J06	Acute upper respiratory infections
J09-J18	Influenza and pneumonia
J20-J22	Other acute lower respiratory infections
J30-J39	Other diseases of upper respiratory tract
J40-J47	Chronic lower respiratory diseases
J60-J70	Lung diseases due to external agents
J80-J84	Other respiratory diseases principally affecting the interstitium
J85-J86	Suppurative and necrotic conditions of the lower respiratory tract
J90-J94	Other diseases of the pleura
J95	Intraoperative and postprocedural complications and disorders of respiratory system, not elsewhere classified
J96-J99	Other diseases of the respiratory system

ACUTE UPPER RESPIRATORY INFECTIONS (J00-J06)

Excludes1	chronic obstructive pulmonary disease with acute lower respiratory infection (J44.0)
	influenza virus with other respiratory manifestations (J09.X2, J10.1, J11.1)

J00   Acute nasopharyngitis [common cold]
     Acute rhinitis
     Coryza (acute)
     Infective nasopharyngitis NOS
     Infective rhinitis
     Nasal catarrh, acute
     Nasopharyngitis NOS

Excludes1	acute pharyngitis (J02.-)
	acute sore throat NOS (J02.9)
	pharyngitis NOS (J02.9)
	rhinitis NOS (J31.0)
	sore throat NOS (J02.9)

Excludes2	allergic rhinitis (J30.1-J30.9)
	chronic pharyngitis (J31.2)
	chronic rhinitis (J31.0)
	chronic sore throat (J31.2)
	nasopharyngitis, chronic (J31.1)
	vasomotor rhinitis (J30.0)

(See Plate 49 on page NAP-24.)

● **J01   Acute sinusitis**

Includes	acute abscess of sinus
	acute empyema of sinus
	acute infection of sinus
	acute inflammation of sinus
	acute suppuration of sinus

     Use additional code (B95-B97) to identify infectious agent.

Excludes1	sinusitis NOS (J32.9)
Excludes2	chronic sinusitis (J32.0-J32.8)

● **J01.0   Acute maxillary sinusitis**
     Acute antritis

     ■ **J01.00   Acute maxillary sinusitis, unspecified**

     J01.01   Acute recurrent maxillary sinusitis

● **J01.1   Acute frontal sinusitis**

     ■ **J01.10   Acute frontal sinusitis, unspecified**

     J01.11   Acute recurrent frontal sinusitis

● **J01.2   Acute ethmoidal sinusitis**

     ■ **J01.20   Acute ethmoidal sinusitis, unspecified**

     J01.21   Acute recurrent ethmoidal sinusitis

● **J01.3   Acute sphenoidal sinusitis**

     ■ **J01.30   Acute sphenoidal sinusitis, unspecified**

     J01.31   Acute recurrent sphenoidal sinusitis

● **J01.4   Acute pansinusitis**

     ■ **J01.40   Acute pansinusitis, unspecified**

     J01.41   Acute recurrent pansinusitis

● **J01.8   Other acute sinusitis**

     J01.80   Other acute sinusitis
         Acute sinusitis involving more than one sinus but not pansinusitis

     J01.81   Other acute recurrent sinusitis
         Acute recurrent sinusitis involving more than one sinus but not pansinusitis

● **J01.9   Acute sinusitis, unspecified**

     ■ **J01.90   Acute sinusitis, unspecified**

     ■ **J01.91   Acute recurrent sinusitis, unspecified**

● **J02   Acute pharyngitis**

Includes	acute sore throat

Excludes1	acute laryngopharyngitis (J06.0)
	peritonsillar abscess (J36)
	pharyngeal abscess (J39.1)
	retropharyngeal abscess (J39.0)

Excludes2	chronic pharyngitis (J31.2)

J02.0   Streptococcal pharyngitis
     Septic pharyngitis
     Streptococcal sore throat

Excludes2	scarlet fever (A38.-)

J02.8   Acute pharyngitis due to other specified organisms

     Use additional code (B95-B97) to identify infectious agent

Excludes1	pharyngitis due to coxsackie virus (B08.5)
	pharyngitis due to gonococcus (A54.5)
	acute pharyngitis due to herpes [simplex] virus (B00.2)
	acute pharyngitis due to infectious mononucleosis (B27.-)
	enteroviral vesicular pharyngitis (B08.5)

■ **J02.9   Acute pharyngitis, unspecified**
     Gangrenous pharyngitis (acute)
     Infective pharyngitis (acute) NOS
     Pharyngitis (acute) NOS
     Sore throat (acute) NOS
     Suppurative pharyngitis (acute)
     Ulcerative pharyngitis (acute)

● **J03   Acute tonsillitis**
     Inflammation of pharyngeal tonsils caused by virus or bacteria

Excludes1	acute sore throat (J02.-)
	hypertrophy of tonsils (J35.1)
	peritonsillar abscess (J36)
	sore throat NOS (J02.9)
	streptococcal sore throat (J02.0)

Excludes2	chronic tonsillitis (J35.0)

● **J03.0   Streptococcal tonsillitis**

     ■ **J03.00   Acute streptococcal tonsillitis, unspecified**

     J03.01   Acute recurrent streptococcal tonsillitis

● **J03.8   Acute tonsillitis due to other specified organisms**

     Use additional code (B95-B97) to identify infectious agent.

Excludes1	diphtheritic tonsillitis (A36.0)
	herpesviral pharyngotonsillitis (B00.2)
	streptococcal tonsillitis (J03.0)
	tuberculous tonsillitis (A15.8)
	Vincent's tonsillitis (A69.1)

     J03.80   Acute tonsillitis due to other specified organisms

     J03.81   Acute recurrent tonsillitis due to other specified organisms

● **J03.9   Acute tonsillitis, unspecified**
     Follicular tonsillitis (acute)
     Gangrenous tonsillitis (acute)
     Infective tonsillitis (acute)
     Tonsillitis (acute) NOS
     Ulcerative tonsillitis (acute)

     ■ **J03.90   Acute tonsillitis, unspecified**

     ■ **J03.91   Acute recurrent tonsillitis, unspecified**

CHAPTER 10 (J00-J99)

Item 10–2 **Laryngitis** is an inflammation of the larynx (voice box) resulting in hoarse voice or the complete loss of the voice. **Tracheitis** is an inflammation of the trachea (often following a URI) commonly caused by *staphylococcus aureus* resulting in inspiratory stridor (crowing sound on inspiration) and a croup like cough.

● **J04   Acute laryngitis and tracheitis**

  Use additional code (B95-B97) to identify infectious agent.

  Excludes1 acute obstructive laryngitis [croup] and epiglottitis (J05.-)

  Excludes2 laryngismus (stridulus) (J38.5)

  J04.0   Acute laryngitis
  Edematous laryngitis (acute)
  Laryngitis (acute) NOS
  Subglottic laryngitis (acute)
  Suppurative laryngitis (acute)
  Ulcerative laryngitis (acute)

    Excludes1 acute obstructive laryngitis (J05.0)
    Excludes2 chronic laryngitis (J37.0)

  ● **J04.1   Acute tracheitis**
  Acute viral tracheitis
  Catarrhal tracheitis (acute)
  Tracheitis (acute) NOS

    Excludes2 chronic tracheitis (J42)

    J04.10   Acute tracheitis without obstruction

    J04.11   Acute tracheitis with obstruction 🔾

  J04.2   Acute laryngotracheitis
  Laryngotracheitis NOS
  Tracheitis (acute) with laryngitis (acute)

    Excludes1 acute obstructive laryngotracheitis (J05.0)
    Excludes2 chronic laryngotracheitis (J37.1)

  ● **J04.3   Supraglottitis, unspecified**

    ▪ **J04.30   Supraglottitis, unspecified, without obstruction**

    ▪ **J04.31   Supraglottitis, unspecified, with obstruction** 🔾

● **J05   Acute obstructive laryngitis [croup] and epiglottitis**

  Use additional code (B95-B97) to identify infectious agent.

  J05.0   Acute obstructive laryngitis [croup]
  Obstructive laryngitis (acute) NOS
  Obstructive laryngotracheitis NOS

  J05.1   Acute epiglottitis

    Excludes2 epiglottitis, chronic (J37.0)

    J05.10   Acute epiglottitis without obstruction 🔾
    Epiglottitis NOS

    J05.11   Acute epiglottitis with obstruction 🔾

● **J06   Acute upper respiratory infections of multiple and unspecified sites**

  Excludes1 acute respiratory infection NOS (J22)
  streptococcal pharyngitis (J02.0)

  J06.0   Acute laryngopharyngitis

  ▪ **J06.9   Acute upper respiratory infection, unspecified**
  Upper respiratory disease, acute
  Upper respiratory infection NOS

INFLUENZA AND PNEUMONIA (J09-J18)

  Excludes2 allergic or eosinophilic pneumonia (J82)
  aspiration pneumonia NOS (J69.0)
  meconium pneumonia (P24.01)
  neonatal aspiration pneumonia (P24.-)
  pneumonia due to solids and liquids (J69-)
  congenital pneumonia (P23.9)
  lipid pneumonia (J69.1)
  rheumatic pneumonia (I00)
  ventilator associated pneumonia (J95.851)

● **J09   Influenza due to certain identified influenza viruses**

  Excludes1 influenza due to other influenza viruses (J10.-)
  influenza due to unidentified influenza virus (J11.-)
  seasonal influenza due to other identified influenza virus (J10.-)
  seasonal influenza due to unidentified influenza virus (J11.-)

● **J09.X   Influenza due to identified novel influenza A virus**
  Avian influenza
  Bird influenza
  Influenza A/H5N1
  Influenza of other animal origin, not bird or swine
  Swine influenza virus (viruses that normally cause infections in pigs)

  J09.X1   Influenza due to identified novel influenza A virus with pneumonia

    Code also , if applicable, associated:
    lung abscess (J85.1)
    other specified type of pneumonia

  J09.X2   Influenza due to identified novel influenza A virus with other respiratory manifestations
  Influenza due to identified novel influenza A virus NOS
  Influenza due to identified novel influenza A virus with laryngitis
  Influenza due to identified novel influenza A virus with pharyngitis
  Influenza due to identified novel influenza A virus with upper respiratory symptoms

    Use additional code, if applicable, for associated:
    pleural effusion (J91.8)
    sinusitis (J01.-)

  J09.X3   Influenza due to identified novel influenza A virus with gastrointestinal manifestations
  Influenza due to identified novel influenza A virus gastroenteritis

    Excludes1 'intestinal flu' [viral gastroenteritis] (A08.-)

  J09.X9   Influenza due to identified novel influenza A virus with other manifestations
  Influenza due to identified novel influenza A virus with encephalopathy
  Influenza due to identified novel influenza A virus with myocarditis
  Influenza due to identified novel influenza A virus with otitis media

    Use additional code to identify manifestation

● Unacceptable Principal Diagnosis   ● Use Additional Character(s)   ▪ Unspecified   ▶ Manifestation Code

OGCR Official Guidelines for Coding and Reporting   Excludes 1   Excludes 2   Includes   Use additional   Code first   Code also

● J10   Influenza due to other identified influenza virus

Use additional code to identify the virus (B97.-)

Excludes1   influenza due to avian influenza virus
(J09.X-)
influenza due to swine flu (J09.X-)
influenza due to unidentified influenza
virus (J11.-)

● J10.0   Influenza due to other identified influenza virus
with pneumonia

Code also associated lung abscess, if applicable
(J85.1)

■ J10.00   Influenza due to other identified influenza
virus with unspecified type of
pneumonia

J10.01   Influenza due to other identified influenza
virus with the same other identified
influenza virus pneumonia

J10.08   Influenza due to other identified influenza
virus with other specified pneumonia

Code also other specified type of
pneumonia

J10.1   Influenza due to other identified influenza virus
with other respiratory manifestations
Influenza due to other identified influenza virus
NOS
Influenza due to other identified influenza virus
with laryngitis
Influenza due to other identified influenza virus
with pharyngitis
Influenza due to other identified influenza virus
with upper respiratory symptoms

Use additional code for associated pleural
effusion, if applicable (J91.8)

Use additional code for associated sinusitis, if
applicable (J01.-)

J10.2   Influenza due to other identified influenza virus
with gastrointestinal manifestations
Influenza due to other identified influenza virus
gastroenteritis

Excludes1   'intestinal flu' [viral gastroenteritis]
(A08.-)

● J10.8   Influenza due to other identified influenza virus
with other manifestations

J10.81   Influenza due to other identified influenza
virus with encephalopathy

J10.82   Influenza due to other identified influenza
virus with myocarditis

J10.83   Influenza due to other identified influenza
virus with otitis media

Use additional code for any associated
perforated tympanic membrane
(H72.-)

J10.89   Influenza due to other identified influenza
virus with other manifestations

Use additional codes to identify the
manifestations

● J11   Influenza due to unidentified influenza virus

● J11.0   Influenza due to unidentified influenza virus with
pneumonia

Code also associated lung abscess, if applicable
(J85.1)

J11.00   Influenza due to unidentified influenza
virus with unspecified type of
pneumonia
Influenza with pneumonia NOS

J11.08   Influenza due to unidentified influenza
virus with specified pneumonia

Code also other specified type of
pneumonia

■ J11.1   Influenza due to unidentified influenza virus with
other respiratory manifestations
Influenza NOS
Influenzal laryngitis NOS
Influenzal pharyngitis NOS
Influenza with upper respiratory symptoms NOS

Use additional code for associated pleural
effusion, if applicable (J91.8)

Use additional code for associated sinusitis, if
applicable (J01.-)

■ J11.2   Influenza due to unidentified influenza virus with
gastrointestinal manifestations
Influenza gastroenteritis NOS

Excludes1   'intestinal flu' [viral gastroenteritis]
(A08.-)

● J11.8   Influenza due to unidentified influenza virus with
other manifestations

■ J11.81   Influenza due to unidentified influenza
virus with encephalopathy
Influenzal encephalopathy NOS

■ J11.82   Influenza due to unidentified influenza
virus with myocarditis
Influenzal myocarditis NOS

■ J11.83   Influenza due to unidentified influenza
virus with otitis media
Influenzal otitis media NOS

Use additional code for any associated
perforated tympanic membrane
(H72.-)

J11.89   Influenza due to unidentified influenza
virus with other manifestations

Use additional codes to identify the
manifestations

● J12   Viral pneumonia, not elsewhere classified

Includes   bronchopneumonia due to viruses other
than influenza viruses

Code first associated influenza, if applicable (J09.X1, J10.0-,
J11.0-)

Code also associated abscess, if applicable (J85.1)

Excludes1   aspiration pneumonia due to anesthesia
during labor and delivery (O74.0)
aspiration pneumonia due to anesthesia
during pregnancy (O29)
aspiration pneumonia due to anesthesia
during puerperium (O89.0)
aspiration pneumonia due to solids and
liquids (J69.-)
aspiration pneumonia NOS (J69.0)
congenital pneumonia (P23.0)
congenital rubella pneumonitis (P35.0)
interstitial pneumonia NOS (J84.9)
lipid pneumonia (J69.1)
neonatal aspiration pneumonia (P24.-)

J12.0   Adenoviral pneumonia

J12.1   Respiratory syncytial virus pneumonia

J12.2   Parainfluenza virus pneumonia

J12.3   Human metapneumovirus pneumonia

Item 10–3 Pneumonia is an infection of the lungs, caused by a variety
of microorganisms, including viruses, most commonly the *Streptococcus
pneumoniae* (pneumococcus) bacteria, fungi, and parasites. Pneumonia
occurs when the immune system is weakened, often by a URI or influenza.

CHAPTER 10 (J00-J99)

● **J12.8   Other viral pneumonia**

    J12.81   Pneumonia due to SARS-associated coronavirus 🦠

        Severe acute respiratory syndrome NOS

    J12.89   Other viral pneumonia 🦠

■ **J12.9   Viral pneumonia, unspecified** 🦠

■ **J13   Pneumonia due to Streptococcus pneumoniae** 🦠

    Bronchopneumonia due to S. pneumoniae

    Code first associated influenza, if applicable (J09.X1, J10.0-, J11.0-)

    Code also associated abscess, if applicable (J85.1)

    Excludes1   congenital pneumonia due to S. pneumoniae (P23.6)

        lobar pneumonia, unspecified organism (J18.1)

        pneumonia due to other streptococci (J15.3-J15.4)

J14   Pneumonia due to Hemophilus influenzae 🦠

    Bronchopneumonia due to H. influenzae

    Code first associated influenza, if applicable (J09.X1, J10.0-, J11.0-)

    Code also associated abscess, if applicable (J85.1)

    Excludes1   congenital pneumonia due to H. influenzae (P23.6)

● **J15   Bacterial pneumonia, not elsewhere classified**

    Includes   bronchopneumonia due to bacteria other than S. pneumoniae and H. influenzae

    Code first associated influenza, if applicable (J09.X1, J10.0-, J11.0-)

    Code also associated abscess, if applicable (J85.1)

    Excludes1   chlamydial pneumonia (J16.0)

        congenital pneumonia (P23.-)

        Legionnaires' disease (A48.1)

        spirochetal pneumonia (A69.8)

    J15.0   Pneumonia due to Klebsiella pneumoniae 🦠

    J15.1   Pneumonia due to Pseudomonas 🦠

●   **J15.2   Pneumonia due to staphylococcus**

      ■ **J15.20   Pneumonia due to staphylococcus, unspecified** 🦠

      ● **J15.21   Pneumonia due to staphylococcus aureus**

        J15.211   Pneumonia due to Methicillin susceptible Staphylococcus aureus 🦠

          MSSA pneumonia

          Pneumonia due to Staphylococcus aureus NOS

        J15.212   Pneumonia due to Methicillin resistant Staphylococcus aureus 🦠

        J15.29   Pneumonia due to other staphylococcus 🦠

    J15.3   Pneumonia due to streptococcus, group B 🦠

    J15.4   Pneumonia due to other streptococci 🦠

      Excludes1   pneumonia due to streptococcus, group B (J15.3)

        pneumonia due to Streptococcus pneumoniae (J13)

    J15.5   Pneumonia due to Escherichia coli 🦠

    J15.6   Pneumonia due to other aerobic Gram-negative bacteria 🦠

      Pneumonia due to Serratia marcescens

    J15.7   Pneumonia due to Mycoplasma pneumoniae 🦠

    J15.8   Pneumonia due to other specified bacteria 🦠

    ■ **J15.9   Unspecified bacterial pneumonia** 🦠

      Pneumonia due to gram-positive bacteria

● **J16   Pneumonia due to other infectious organisms, not elsewhere classified**

    Code first associated influenza, if applicable (J09.X1, J10.0-, J11.0-)

    Code also associated abscess, if applicable (J85.1)

    Excludes1   congenital pneumonia (P23.-)

        ornithosis (A70)

        pneumocystosis (B59)

        pneumonia NOS (J18.9)

    J16.0   Chlamydial pneumonia 🦠

    J16.8   Pneumonia due to other specified infectious organisms 🦠

●▶ **J17   *Pneumonia in diseases classified elsewhere*** 🦠

    Code first underlying disease, such as:

      Q fever (A78)

      rheumatic fever (I00)

      schistosomiasis (B65.0-B65.9)

    Excludes1   candidial pneumonia (B37.1)

        chlamydial pneumonia (J16.0)

        gonorrheal pneumonia (A54.84)

        histoplasmosis pneumonia (B39.0-B39.2)

        measles pneumonia (B05.2)

        nocardiosis pneumonia (A43.0)

        pneumocystosis (B59)

        pneumonia due to Pneumocystis carinii (B59)

        pneumonia due to Pneumocystis jiroveci (B59)

        pneumonia in actinomycosis (A42.0)

        pneumonia in anthrax (A22.1)

        pneumonia in ascariasis (B77.81)

        pneumonia in aspergillosis (B44.0-B44.1)

        pneumonia in coccidioidomycosis (B38.0-B38.2)

        pneumonia in cytomegalovirus disease (B25.0)

        pneumonia in toxoplasmosis (B58.3)

        rubella pneumonia (B06.81)

        salmonella pneumonia (A02.22)

        spirochetal infection NEC with pneumonia (A69.8)

        tularemia pneumonia (A21.2)

        typhoid fever with pneumonia (A01.03)

        varicella pneumonia (B01.2)

        whooping cough with pneumonia (A37 with fifth-character 1)

● **J18   Pneumonia, unspecified organism**

    Code first associated influenza, if applicable (J09.X1, J10.0-, J11.0-)

    Excludes1   abscess of lung with pneumonia (J85.1)

        aspiration pneumonia due to anesthesia during labor and delivery (O74.0)

        aspiration pneumonia due to anesthesia during pregnancy (O29)

        aspiration pneumonia due to anesthesia during puerperium (O89.0)

        aspiration pneumonia due to solids and liquids (J69.-)

        aspiration pneumonia NOS (J69.0)

        congenital pneumonia (P23.0)

        drug-induced interstitial lung disorder (J70.2-J70.4)

        interstitial pneumonia NOS (J84.9)

        lipid pneumonia (J69.1)

        neonatal aspiration pneumonia (P24.-)

        pneumonitis due to external agents (J67-J70)

        pneumonitis due to fumes and vapors (J68.0)

        usual interstitial pneumonia (J84.17)

● Unacceptable Principal Diagnosis   ● Use Additional Character(s)   ■ Unspecified   ▶ Manifestation Code

OGCR Official Guidelines for Coding and Reporting   Excludes 1   Excludes 2   Includes   Use additional   Code first   Code also

■ **J18.0   Bronchopneumonia, unspecified organism** 🦠

     Excludes1   hypostatic bronchopneumonia (J18.2)

                    lipid pneumonia (J69.1)

     Excludes2   acute bronchiolitis (J21.-)

                    chronic bronchiolitis (J44.9)

■ **J18.1   Lobar pneumonia, unspecified organism** 🦠

■ **J18.2   Hypostatic pneumonia, unspecified organism** 🦠

     Hypostatic bronchopneumonia

     Passive pneumonia

■ **J18.8   Other pneumonia, unspecified organism** 🦠

■ **J18.9   Pneumonia, unspecified organism** 🦠

OTHER ACUTE LOWER RESPIRATORY INFECTIONS (J20-J22)

     Excludes1   chronic obstructive pulmonary disease with acute lower respiratory infection (J44.0)

● **J20   Acute bronchitis**

Inflammation/irritation of the bronchial tubes lasting 2-3 weeks, most commonly caused by a virus.

     Includes   acute and subacute bronchitis (with) bronchospasm

                   acute and subacute bronchitis (with) tracheitis

                   acute and subacute bronchitis (with) tracheobronchitis, acute

                   acute and subacute fibrinous bronchitis

                   acute and subacute membranous bronchitis

                   acute and subacute purulent bronchitis

                   acute and subacute septic bronchitis

     Excludes2   acute bronchitis with bronchiectasis (J47.0)

                   acute bronchitis with chronic obstructive asthma (J44.0)

                   acute bronchitis with chronic obstructive pulmonary disease (J44.0)

                   allergic bronchitis NOS (J45.909-)

                   bronchitis due to chemicals, fumes and vapors (J68.0)

                   bronchitis NOS (J40)

                   chronic bronchitis NOS (J42)

                   chronic mucopurulent bronchitis (J41.1)

                   chronic obstructive bronchitis (J44.-)

                   chronic obstructive tracheobronchitis (J44.-)

                   chronic simple bronchitis (J41.0)

                   chronic tracheobronchitis (J42)

                   tracheobronchitis NOS (J40)

     J20.0   Acute bronchitis due to Mycoplasma pneumoniae

     J20.1   Acute bronchitis due to Hemophilus influenzae

     J20.2   Acute bronchitis due to streptococcus

     J20.3   Acute bronchitis due to coxsackievirus

     J20.4   Acute bronchitis due to parainfluenza virus

     J20.5   Acute bronchitis due to respiratory syncytial virus

     J20.6   Acute bronchitis due to rhinovirus

     J20.7   Acute bronchitis due to echovirus

     J20.8   Acute bronchitis due to other specified organisms

■   **J20.9   Acute bronchitis, unspecified**

● **J21   Acute bronchiolitis**

Bronchiolitis obliterans with organizing pneumonia (BOOP) inflammation of bronchioles and surrounding tissue in lung.

     Includes   acute bronchiolitis with bronchospasm

     Excludes2   respiratory bronchiolitis interstitial lung disease (J84.115)

     J21.0   Acute bronchiolitis due to respiratory syncytial virus 🦠

     J21.1   Acute bronchiolitis due to human metapneumovirus 🦠

     J21.8   Acute bronchiolitis due to other specified organisms 🦠

■ **J21.9   Acute bronchiolitis, unspecified** 🦠

     Bronchiolitis (acute)

     Excludes1   chronic bronchiolitis (J44.-)

■ **J22   Unspecified acute lower respiratory infection**

     Acute (lower) respiratory (tract) infection NOS

     Excludes1   upper respiratory infection (acute) (J06.9)

OTHER DISEASES OF UPPER RESPIRATORY TRACT (J30-J39)

● **J30   Vasomotor and allergic rhinitis**

     Includes   spasmodic rhinorrhea

     Excludes1   allergic rhinitis with asthma (bronchial) (J45.909)

                   rhinitis NOS (J31.0)

     J30.0   Vasomotor rhinitis

     J30.1   Allergic rhinitis due to pollen

         Allergy NOS due to pollen

         Hay fever

         Pollinosis

     J30.2   Other seasonal allergic rhinitis

     J30.5   Allergic rhinitis due to food

●   **J30.8   Other allergic rhinitis**

         J30.81   Allergic rhinitis due to animal (cat) (dog) hair and dander

         J30.89   Other allergic rhinitis

                 Perennial allergic rhinitis

■   **J30.9   Allergic rhinitis, unspecified**

● **J31   Chronic rhinitis, nasopharyngitis and pharyngitis**

     Use additional code to identify:

         exposure to environmental tobacco smoke (Z77.22)

         exposure to tobacco smoke in the perinatal period (P96.81)

         history of tobacco use (Z87.891)

         occupational exposure to environmental tobacco smoke (Z57.31)

         tobacco dependence (F17.-)

         tobacco use (Z72.0)

     J31.0   Chronic rhinitis

         Atrophic rhinitis (chronic)

         Granulomatous rhinitis (chronic)

         Hypertrophic rhinitis (chronic)

         Obstructive rhinitis (chronic)

         Ozena

         Purulent rhinitis (chronic)

         Rhinitis (chronic) NOS

         Ulcerative rhinitis (chronic)

         Excludes1   allergic rhinitis (J30.1-J30.9)

                       vasomotor rhinitis (J30.0)

     J31.1   Chronic nasopharyngitis

         Excludes2   acute nasopharyngitis (J00)

     J31.2   Chronic pharyngitis

         Chronic sore throat

         Atrophic pharyngitis (chronic)

         Granular pharyngitis (chronic)

         Hypertrophic pharyngitis (chronic)

         Excludes2   acute pharyngitis (J02.9)

N Newborn Age: 0   **P** Pediatric Age: 0–17   **M** Maternity DX: 12–55   **A** Adult Age: 15–124   ♀ Females Only   ♂ Males Only

🦠 Complication\C   🦠 Major C\C   🦠 Present on Admission Requirement   🦠 Hospital-Acquired Condition

1075

Item 10–4   Nasal polyps are an abnormal growth of tissue (tumor) projecting from a mucous membrane and attached to the surface by a narrow elongated stalk (pedunculated). Nasal polyps usually originate in the ethmoid sinus but also may occur in the maxillary sinus. Symptoms are nasal block, sinusitis, anosmia, and secondary infections.

● **J32   Chronic sinusitis**

> **Includes**   sinus abscess
> sinus empyema
> sinus infection
> sinus suppuration

> **Use additional** code to identify:
> exposure to environmental tobacco smoke (Z77.22)
> exposure to tobacco smoke in the perinatal period (P96.81)
> history of tobacco use (Z87.891)
> infectious agent (B95-B97)
> occupational exposure to environmental tobacco smoke (Z57.31)
> tobacco dependence (F17.-)
> tobacco use (Z72.0)

> **Excludes2**   acute sinusitis (J01.-)

J32.0   Chronic maxillary sinusitis
Antritis (chronic)
Maxillary sinusitis NOS

J32.1   Chronic frontal sinusitis
Frontal sinusitis NOS

J32.2   Chronic ethmoidal sinusitis
Ethmoidal sinusitis NOS

> **Excludes1**   Woakes' ethmoiditis (J33.1)

J32.3   Chronic sphenoidal sinusitis
Sphenoidal sinusitis NOS

J32.4   Chronic pansinusitis
Pansinusitis NOS

J32.8   Other chronic sinusitis
Sinusitis (chronic) involving more than one sinus but not pansinusitis

■ **J32.9   Chronic sinusitis, unspecified**
Sinusitis (chronic) NOS

● **J33   Nasal polyp**

> **Use additional** code to identify:
> exposure to environmental tobacco smoke (Z77.22)
> exposure to tobacco smoke in the perinatal period (P96.81)
> history of tobacco use (Z87.891)
> occupational exposure to environmental tobacco smoke (Z57.31)
> tobacco dependence (F17.-)
> tobacco use (Z72.0)

> **Excludes1**   adenomatous polyps (D14.0)

J33.0   Polyp of nasal cavity
Choanal polyp
Nasopharyngeal polyp

J33.1   Polypoid sinus degeneration
Woakes' syndrome or ethmoiditis

J33.8   Other polyp of sinus
Accessory polyp of sinus
Ethmoidal polyp of sinus
Maxillary polyp of sinus
Sphenoidal polyp of sinus

■ **J33.9   Nasal polyp, unspecified**

● **J34   Other and unspecified disorders of nose and nasal sinuses**

> **Excludes2**   varicose ulcer of nasal septum (I86.8)

J34.0   Abscess, furuncle and carbuncle of nose
Cellulitis of nose
Necrosis of nose
Ulceration of nose

─ Deviated septal cartilage

Figure 10-3   Deviated nasal septum.

Item 10–5   A **deviated nasal septum** is the displacement of the septal cartilage that separates the nares. This displacement causes obstructed air flow through the nasal passages. A child can be born with this displacement (congenital), or the condition may be acquired through trauma, such as a sports injury. Symptoms include nasal block, sinusitis, and related secondary infections. Septoplasty is surgical repair of this condition.

J34.1   Cyst and mucocele of nose and nasal sinus

J34.2   Deviated nasal septum
Deflection or deviation of septum (nasal) (acquired)

> **Excludes1**   congenital deviated nasal septum (Q67.4)

J34.3   Hypertrophy of nasal turbinates

● **J34.8   Other specified disorders of nose and nasal sinuses**

J34.81   Nasal mucositis (ulcerative)

> **Code also** type of associated therapy, such as:
> antineoplastic and immunosuppressive drugs (T45.1x-)
> radiological procedure and radiotherapy (Y84.2)

> **Excludes2**   gastrointestinal mucositis (ulcerative) (K92.81)
> mucositis (ulcerative) of vagina and vulva (N76.81)
> oral mucositis (ulcerative) (K12.3-)

J34.89   Other specified disorders of nose and nasal sinuses
Perforation of nasal septum NOS
Rhinolith

■ **J34.9   Unspecified disorder of nose and nasal sinuses**

● **J35   Chronic diseases of tonsils and adenoids**

> **Use additional** code to identify:
> exposure to environmental tobacco smoke (Z77.22)
> exposure to tobacco smoke in the perinatal period (P96.81)
> history of tobacco use (Z87.891)
> occupational exposure to environmental tobacco smoke (Z57.31)
> tobacco dependence (F17.-)
> tobacco use (Z72.0)

● **J35.0   Chronic tonsillitis and adenoiditis**

> **Excludes2**   acute tonsillitis (J03.-)

J35.01   Chronic tonsillitis

J35.02   Chronic adenoiditis

J35.03   Chronic tonsillitis and adenoiditis

J35.1   Hypertrophy of tonsils
Enlargement of tonsils

> **Excludes1**   hypertrophy of tonsils with tonsillitis (J35.0-)

J35.2   Hypertrophy of adenoids
Enlargement of adenoids

> **Excludes1**   hypertrophy of adenoids with adenoiditis (J35.0-)

● Unacceptable Principal Diagnosis   ● Use Additional Character(s)   ■ Unspecified   ▶ Manifestation Code

1076   **OGCR**   Official Guidelines for Coding and Reporting   [Excludes 1] [Excludes 2] Includes Use additional Code first Code also

J35.3   **Hypertrophy of tonsils with hypertrophy of adenoids**

> **Excludes1**   hypertrophy of tonsils and adenoids with tonsillitis and adenoiditis (J35.03)

J35.8   **Other chronic diseases of tonsils and adenoids**
Adenoid vegetations
Amygdalolith
Calculus, tonsil
Cicatrix of tonsil (and adenoid)
Tonsillar tag
Ulcer of tonsil

■ **J35.9**   **Chronic disease of tonsils and adenoids, unspecified**
Disease (chronic) of tonsils and adenoids NOS

J36   **Peritonsillar abscess** 🗲

> **Includes**   abscess of tonsil
> peritonsillar cellulitis
> quinsy

Use additional code (B95-B97) to identify infectious agent.

> **Excludes1**   acute tonsillitis (J03.-)
> chronic tonsillitis (J35.0)
> retropharyngeal abscess (J39.0)
> tonsillitis NOS (J03.9-)

● **J37**   **Chronic laryngitis and laryngotracheitis**
Use additional code to identify:
exposure to environmental tobacco smoke (Z77.22)
exposure to tobacco smoke in the perinatal period (P96.81)
history of tobacco use (Z87.891)
infectious agent (B95-B97)
occupational exposure to environmental tobacco smoke (Z57.31)
tobacco dependence (F17.-)
tobacco use (Z72.0)

J37.0   **Chronic laryngitis**
Catarrhal laryngitis
Hypertrophic laryngitis
Sicca laryngitis

> **Excludes2**   acute laryngitis (J04.0)
> obstructive (acute) laryngitis (J05.0)

J37.1   **Chronic laryngotracheitis**
Laryngitis, chronic, with tracheitis (chronic)
Tracheitis, chronic, with laryngitis

> **Excludes1**   chronic tracheitis (J42)
> **Excludes2**   acute laryngotracheitis (J04.2)
> acute tracheitis (J04.1)

● **J38**   **Diseases of vocal cords and larynx, not elsewhere classified**
Use additional code to identify:
exposure to environmental tobacco smoke (Z77.22)
exposure to tobacco smoke in the perinatal period (P96.81)
history of tobacco use (Z87.891)
occupational exposure to environmental tobacco smoke (Z57.31)
tobacco dependence (F17.-)
tobacco use (Z72.0)

> **Excludes1**   congenital laryngeal stridor (P28.89)
> obstructive laryngitis (acute) (J05.0)
> postprocedural subglottic stenosis (J95.5)
> stridor (R06.1)
> ulcerative laryngitis (J04.0)

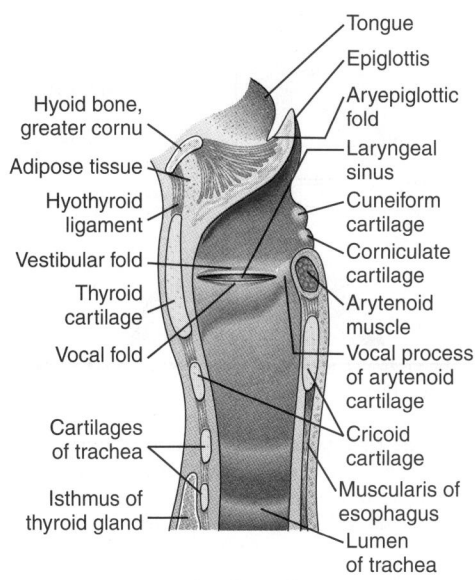

Figure 10-4   Coronal section of the larynx.

Item 10-6   The **larynx** extends from the tongue to the trachea and is divided into an upper and lower portion separated by folds. The framework of the larynx is cartilage composed of the single cricoid, thyroid, and epiglottic cartilages, and the paired arytenoid, cuneiform, and corniculate cartilages.

● **J38.0**   **Paralysis of vocal cords and larynx**
Laryngoplegia
Paralysis of glottis

■ **J38.00**   **Paralysis of vocal cords and larynx, unspecified**

J38.01   **Paralysis of vocal cords and larynx, unilateral**

J38.02   **Paralysis of vocal cords and larynx, bilateral**

J38.1   **Polyp of vocal cord and larynx**

> **Excludes1**   adenomatous polyps (D14.1)

J38.2   **Nodules of vocal cords**
Chorditis (fibrinous)(nodosa)(tuberosa)
Singer's nodes
Teacher's nodes

J38.3   **Other diseases of vocal cords**
Abscess of vocal cords
Cellulitis of vocal cords
Granuloma of vocal cords
Leukokeratosis of vocal cords
Leukoplakia of vocal cords

J38.4   **Edema of larynx**
Edema (of) glottis
Subglottic edema
Supraglottic edema

> **Excludes1**   acute obstructive laryngitis [croup] (J05.0)
> edematous laryngitis (J04.0)

J38.5   **Laryngeal spasm**
Laryngismus (stridulus)

J38.6   **Stenosis of larynx**

N   Newborn Age: 0   **P**   Pediatric Age: 0–17   **M**   Maternity DX: 12–55   **A**   Adult Age: 15–124   ♀ Females Only   ♂ Males Only

🗲 Complication\Comorbidity   🗲 Major C\C   ◉ Present on Admission Requirement   ◉ Hospital-Acquired Condition   1077

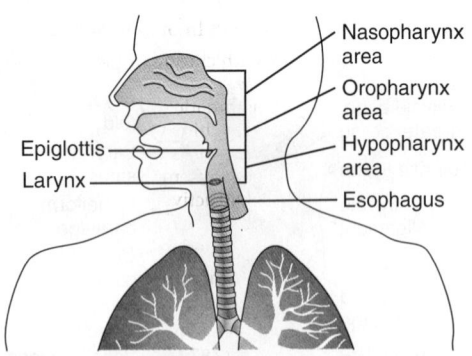

Figure 10-5 The pharynx.

Item 10–7 The **pharynx** is the passage for both food and air between the mouth and the esophagus and is divided into three areas: nasopharynx, oropharynx, and hypopharynx. The hypopharynx branches into the esophagus and the voice box.

J38.7 Other diseases of larynx
Abscess of larynx
Cellulitis of larynx
Disease of larynx NOS
Necrosis of larynx
Pachyderma of larynx
Perichondritis of larynx
Ulcer of larynx

● **J39 Other diseases of upper respiratory tract**
Excludes1 acute respiratory infection NOS (J22)
acute upper respiratory infection (J06.9)
upper respiratory inflammation due to chemicals, gases, fumes or vapors (J68.2)

J39.0 Retropharyngeal and parapharyngeal abscess 🔗
Peripharyngeal abscess
Excludes1 peritonsillar abscess (J36)

J39.1 Other abscess of pharynx 🔗
Cellulitis of pharynx
Nasopharyngeal abscess

J39.2 Other diseases of pharynx
Cyst of pharynx
Edema of pharynx
Excludes2 chronic pharyngitis (J31.2)
ulcerative pharyngitis (J02.9)

■ **J39.3 Upper respiratory tract hypersensitivity reaction, site unspecified**
Excludes1 hypersensitivity reaction of upper respiratory tract, such as:
extrinsic allergic alveolitis (J67.9)
pneumoconiosis (J60-J67.9)

J39.8 Other specified diseases of upper respiratory tract
■ **J39.9 Disease of upper respiratory tract, unspecified**

CHRONIC LOWER RESPIRATORY DISEASES (J40-J47)
Excludes1 bronchitis due to chemicals, gases, fumes and vapors (J68.0)
Excludes2 cystic fibrosis (E84.-)

J40 Bronchitis, not specified as acute or chronic
Bronchitis NOS
Catarrhal bronchitis
Bronchitis with tracheitis NOS
Tracheobronchitis NOS
Use additional code to identify:
exposure to environmental tobacco smoke (Z77.22)
exposure to tobacco smoke in the perinatal period (P96.81)
history of tobacco use (Z87.891)
occupational exposure to environmental tobacco smoke (Z57.31)
tobacco dependence (F17.-)
tobacco use (Z72.0)
Excludes1 allergic bronchitis NOS (J45.909-)
asthmatic bronchitis NOS (J45.9-)
bronchitis due to chemicals, gases, fumes and vapors (J68.0)

● **J41 Simple and mucopurulent chronic bronchitis**
Use additional code to identify:
exposure to environmental tobacco smoke (Z77.22)
exposure to tobacco smoke in the perinatal period (P96.81)
history of tobacco use (Z87.891)
occupational exposure to environmental tobacco smoke (Z57.31)
tobacco dependence (F17.-)
tobacco use (Z72.0)
Excludes1 chronic bronchitis NOS (J42)
chronic obstructive bronchitis (J44.-)

J41.0 Simple chronic bronchitis
J41.1 Mucopurulent chronic bronchitis
J41.8 Mixed simple and mucopurulent chronic bronchitis

■ **J42 Unspecified chronic bronchitis**
Chronic bronchitis NOS
Chronic tracheitis
Chronic tracheobronchitis
Use additional code to identify:
exposure to environmental tobacco smoke (Z77.22)
exposure to tobacco smoke in the perinatal period (P96.81)
history of tobacco use (Z87.891)
occupational exposure to environmental tobacco smoke (Z57.31)
tobacco dependence (F17.-)
tobacco use (Z72.0)
Excludes1 chronic asthmatic bronchitis (J44.-)
chronic bronchitis with airways obstruction (J44.-)
chronic emphysematous bronchitis (J44.-)
chronic obstructive pulmonary disease NOS (J44.9)
simple and mucopurulent chronic bronchitis (J41.-)

CHAPTER 10 (J00-J99)

● Unacceptable Principal Diagnosis ● Use Additional Character(s) ■ Unspecified ▶ Manifestation Code
OGCR Official Guidelines for Coding and Reporting | Excludes 1 | Excludes 2 | Includes | Use additional | Code first | Code also

Item 10–8 Chronic bronchitis is usually defined as being present in any patient who has persistent cough with sputum production for at least three months in at least two consecutive years. **Simple chronic bronchitis** is marked by a productive cough but no pathological airflow obstruction. **Chronic obstructive pulmonary disease (COPD)** is a group of conditions—bronchitis, emphysema, asthma, bronchiectasis, allergic alveolitis—marked by dyspnea. **Catarrhal** bronchitis is an acute form of bronchitis marked by profuse mucus and pus production (**mucopurulent** discharge). **Croupous** bronchitis, also known as pseudomembranous, fibrinous, plastic, exudative, or membranous, is marked by a violent cough and dyspnea.

● **J43   Emphysema**

Use additional code to identify:
    exposure to environmental tobacco smoke (Z77.22)
    history of tobacco use (Z87.891)
    occupational exposure to environmental tobacco smoke (Z57.31)
    tobacco dependence (F17.-)
    tobacco use (Z72.0)

Excludes1
    compensatory emphysema (J98.3)
    emphysema due to inhalation of chemicals, gases, fumes or vapors (J68.4)
    emphysema with chronic (obstructive) bronchitis (J44.-)
    emphysematous (obstructive) bronchitis (J44.-)
    interstitial emphysema (J98.2)
    mediastinal emphysema (J98.2)
    neonatal interstitial emphysema (P25.0)
    surgical (subcutaneous) emphysema (T81.82)
    traumatic subcutaneous emphysema (T79.7)

J43.0 Unilateral pulmonary emphysema [MacLeod's syndrome]
    Swyer-James syndrome
    Unilateral emphysema
    Unilateral hyperlucent lung
    Unilateral pulmonary artery functional hypoplasia
    Unilateral transparency of lung

J43.1 Panlobular emphysema
    Panacinar emphysema

J43.2 Centrilobular emphysema

J43.8 Other emphysema

■ **J43.9 Emphysema, unspecified**
    Bullous emphysema (lung)(pulmonary)
    Emphysema (lung)(pulmonary) NOS
    Emphysematous bleb
    Vesicular emphysema (lung)(pulmonary)

Item 10–9 Asthma is a bronchial condition marked by airway obstruction, hyper-responsiveness, and inflammation. **Extrinsic** asthma, also known as allergic asthma, is characterized by the same symptoms that occur with exposure to allergens and is divided into the following types: **atopic, occupational, and allergic bronchopulmonary aspergillosis. Intrinsic** asthma occurs in patients who have no history of allergy or sensitivities to allergens and is divided into the following types: **nonreaginic and pharmacologic. Status asthmaticus** is the most severe form of asthma attack and can last for days or weeks.

● **J44   Other chronic obstructive pulmonary disease**

Includes
    asthma with chronic obstructive pulmonary disease
    chronic asthmatic (obstructive) bronchitis
    chronic bronchitis with airways obstruction
    chronic bronchitis with emphysema
    chronic emphysematous bronchitis
    chronic obstructive asthma
    chronic obstructive bronchitis
    chronic obstructive tracheobronchitis

Code also type of asthma, if applicable (J45.-)
Use additional code to identify:
    exposure to environmental tobacco smoke (Z77.22)
    history of tobacco use (Z87.891)
    occupational exposure to environmental tobacco smoke (Z57.31)
    tobacco dependence (F17.-)
    tobacco use (Z72.0)

Excludes1
    bronchiectasis (J47.-)
    chronic bronchitis NOS (J42)
    chronic simple and mucopurulent bronchitis (J41.-)
    chronic tracheitis (J42)
    chronic tracheobronchitis (J42)
    emphysema without chronic bronchitis (J43.-)
    lung diseases due to external agents (J60-J70)

J44.0 Chronic obstructive pulmonary disease with acute lower respiratory infection 🕭
    Use additional code to identify the infection

J44.1 Chronic obstructive pulmonary disease with (acute) exacerbation 🕭
    Decompensated COPD
    Decompensated COPD with (acute) exacerbation

Excludes2
    chronic obstructive pulmonary disease [COPD] with acute bronchitis (J44.0)

■ **J44.9 Chronic obstructive pulmonary disease, unspecified**
    Chronic obstructive airway disease NOS
    Chronic obstructive lung disease NOS

● **J45   Asthma**
    Allergic (predominantly) asthma
    Allergic bronchitis NOS
    Allergic rhinitis with asthma
    Atopic asthma
    Extrinsic allergic asthma
    Hay fever with asthma
    Idiosyncratic asthma
    Intrinsic nonallergic asthma
    Nonallergic asthma

Use additional code to identify:
    exposure to environmental tobacco smoke (Z77.22)
    exposure to tobacco smoke in the perinatal period (P96.81)
    history of tobacco use (Z87.891)
    occupational exposure to environmental tobacco smoke (Z57.31)
    tobacco dependence (F17.-)
    tobacco use (Z72.0)

Excludes1
    detergent asthma (J69.8)
    eosinophilic asthma (J82)
    lung diseases due to external agents (J60-J70)
    miner's asthma (J60)
    wheezing NOS (R06.2)
    wood asthma (J67.8)

Excludes2
    asthma with chronic obstructive pulmonary disease (J44.9)
    chronic asthmatic (obstructive) bronchitis (J44.9)
    chronic obstructive asthma (J44.9)

CHAPTER 10 (J00-J99)

N Newborn Age: 0   **P** Pediatric Age: 0–17   **M** Maternity DX: 12–55   **A** Adult Age: 15–124   ♀ Females Only   ♂ Males Only
🕭 Complication\Comorbidity   🕭 Major C\C   Present on Admission Requirement   Hospital-Acquired Condition

1079

CHAPTER 10 (J00-J99)

● **J45.2 Mild intermittent asthma**

    J45.20   **Mild intermittent asthma, uncomplicated**
           Mild intermittent asthma NOS

    J45.21   **Mild intermittent asthma with (acute) exacerbation** 🔍

    J45.22   **Mild intermittent asthma with status asthmaticus** 🔍

● **J45.3 Mild persistent asthma**

    J45.30   **Mild persistent asthma, uncomplicated**
           Mild persistent asthma NOS

    J45.31   **Mild persistent asthma with (acute) exacerbation** 🔍

    J45.32   **Mild persistent asthma with status asthmaticus** 🔍

● **J45.4 Moderate persistent asthma**

    J45.40   **Moderate persistent asthma, uncomplicated**
           Moderate persistent asthma NOS

    J45.41   **Moderate persistent asthma with (acute) exacerbation** 🔍

    J45.42   **Moderate persistent asthma with status asthmaticus** 🔍

● **J45.5 Severe persistent asthma**

    J45.50   **Severe persistent asthma, uncomplicated**
           Severe persistent asthma NOS

    J45.51   **Severe persistent asthma with (acute) exacerbation** 🔍

    J45.52   **Severe persistent asthma with status asthmaticus** 🔍

● **J45.9 Other and unspecified asthma**

  ● **J45.90 Unspecified asthma**
           Asthmatic bronchitis NOS
           Childhood asthma NOS
           Late onset asthma

     ■ J45.901   **Unspecified asthma with (acute) exacerbation** 🔍

     ■ J45.902   **Unspecified asthma with status asthmaticus** 🔍

     ■ J45.909   **Unspecified asthma, uncomplicated**
              Asthma NOS

  ● **J45.99 Other asthma**

    J45.990   **Exercise induced bronchospasm**

    J45.991   **Cough variant asthma**

    J45.998   **Other asthma**

● **J47 Bronchiectasis**

   Includes bronchiolectasis

   Use additional code to identify:
     exposure to environmental tobacco smoke (Z77.22)
     exposure to tobacco smoke in the perinatal period (P96.81)
     history of tobacco use (Z87.891)
     occupational exposure to environmental tobacco smoke (Z57.31)
     tobacco dependence (F17.-)
     tobacco use (Z72.0)

   Excludes1 congenital bronchiectasis (Q33.4)
              tuberculous bronchiectasis (current disease) (A15.0)

    J47.0   **Bronchiectasis with acute lower respiratory infection** 🔍
           Bronchiectasis with acute bronchitis

    J47.1   **Bronchiectasis with (acute) exacerbation** 🔍

    J47.9   **Bronchiectasis, uncomplicated**
           Bronchiectasis NOS

Figure 10-6 Progressive massive fibrosis superimposed on coal workers' pneumoconiosis. The large, blackened scars are located principally in the upper lobe. (From Cotran R, Kumar V, Collins T: Robbins Pathologic Basis of Disease, 6th ed. Philadelphia, WB Saunders, 1999, p 730. Courtesy of Dr. Warner Laquer, Dr. Jerome Kleinerman, and the National Institute of Occupational Safety and Health, Morgantown, WV.)

Item 10–10 **Pneumoconiosis** refers to a lung condition resulting from exposure to inorganic or organic airborne particles, such as coal dust or moldy hay, as well as chemical fumes and vapors, such as insecticides. In this condition, the lungs retain the airborne particles.

LUNG DISEASES DUE TO EXTERNAL AGENTS (J60-J70)

   Excludes2 asthma (J45.-)
          malignant neoplasm of bronchus and lung (C34.-)

J60 Coalworker's pneumoconiosis   **A**
   Anthracosilicosis
   Anthracosis
   Black lung disease
   Coalworker's lung
   Excludes1 coalworker pneumoconiosis with tuberculosis, any type in A15 (J65)

J61 Pneumoconiosis due to asbestos and other mineral fibers **A**
   Asbestosis
   Excludes1 pleural plaque with asbestosis (J92.0)
         pneumoconiosis with tuberculosis, any type in A15 (J65)

● **J62 Pneumoconiosis due to dust containing silica**
   Includes silicotic fibrosis (massive) of lung
   Excludes1 pneumoconiosis with tuberculosis, any type in A15 (J65)

    J62.0   **Pneumoconiosis due to talc dust**

    J62.8   **Pneumoconiosis due to other dust containing silica**
           Silicosis NOS

● **J63 Pneumoconiosis due to other inorganic dusts**
   Excludes1 pneumoconiosis with tuberculosis, any type in A15 (J65)

    J63.0   **Aluminosis (of lung)**

    J63.1   **Bauxite fibrosis (of lung)**

    J63.2   **Berylliosis**

    J63.3   **Graphite fibrosis (of lung)**

    J63.4   **Siderosis**

    J63.5   **Stannosis**

    J63.6   **Pneumoconiosis due to other specified inorganic dusts**

■ **J64 Unspecified pneumoconiosis**
   Excludes1 pneumonoconiosis with tuberculosis, any type in A15 (J65)

J65 Pneumoconiosis associated with tuberculosis
   Any condition in J60-J64 with tuberculosis, any type in A15
   Silicotuberculosis

● Unacceptable Principal Diagnosis   ● Use Additional Character(s)   ■ Unspecified   ▶ Manifestation Code

OGCR Official Guidelines for Coding and Reporting | Excludes 1 | | Excludes 2 | | Includes | | Use additional | | Code first | | Code also |

● **J66** **Airway disease due to specific organic dust**

Excludes2 allergic alveolitis (J67.-)
asbestosis (J61)
bagassosis (J67.1)
farmer's lung (J67.0)
hypersensitivity pneumonitis due to organic
dust (J67.-)
reactive airways dysfunction syndrome
(J68.3)

J66.0 **Byssinosis**
Airway disease due to cotton dust

J66.1 **Flax-dressers' disease**

J66.2 **Cannabinosis**

J66.8 **Airway disease due to other specific organic dusts**

● **J67** **Hypersensitivity pneumonitis due to organic dust**

Includes allergic alveolitis and pneumonitis due to
inhaled organic dust and particles of
fungal, actinomycetic or other origin

Excludes1 pneumonitis due to inhalation of chemicals,
gases, fumes or vapors (J68.0)

J67.0 **Farmer's lung**
Harvester's lung
Haymaker's lung
Moldy hay disease

J67.1 **Bagassosis**
Bagasse disease
Bagasse pneumonitis

J67.2 **Bird fancier's lung**
Budgerigar fancier's disease or lung
Pigeon fancier's disease or lung

J67.3 **Suberosis**
Corkhandler's disease or lung
Corkworker's disease or lung

J67.4 **Maltworker's lung**
Alveolitis due to Aspergillus clavatus

J67.5 **Mushroom-worker's lung**

J67.6 **Maple-bark-stripper's lung**
Alveolitis due to Cryptostroma corticale
Cryptostromosis

J67.7 **Air conditioner and humidifier lung** 🦠
Allergic alveolitis due to fungal, thermophilic
actinomycetes and other organisms growing
in ventilation [air conditioning] systems

J67.8 **Hypersensitivity pneumonitis due to other organic
dusts** 🦠
Cheese-washer's lung
Coffee-worker's lung
Fish-meal worker's lung
Furrier's lung
Sequoiosis

▪ J67.9 **Hypersensitivity pneumonitis due to unspecified
organic dust** 🦠
Allergic alveolitis (extrinsic) NOS
Hypersensitivity pneumonitis NOS

● **J68** **Respiratory conditions due to inhalation of chemicals,
gases, fumes and vapors**

Code first (T51-T65) *to identify cause*

Use additional code to identify associated respiratory
conditions, such as:
acute respiratory failure (J96.0-)

● J68.0 **Bronchitis and pneumonitis due to chemicals,
gases, fumes and vapors** 🦠
Chemical bronchitis (acute)

● J68.1 **Pulmonary edema due to chemicals, gases, fumes
and vapors** 🦠
Chemical pulmonary edema (acute) (chronic)

Excludes1 pulmonary edema (acute) (chronic)
NOS (J81.-)

● J68.2 **Upper respiratory inflammation due to chemicals,
gases, fumes and vapors, not elsewhere classified**

● J68.3 **Other acute and subacute respiratory conditions
due to chemicals, gases, fumes and vapors**
Reactive airways dysfunction syndrome

J68.4 **Chronic respiratory conditions due to chemicals,
gases, fumes and vapors**
Emphysema (diffuse) (chronic) due to inhalation
of chemicals, gases, fumes and vapors
Obliterative bronchiolitis (chronic) (subacute) due
to inhalation of chemicals, gases, fumes and
vapors
Pulmonary fibrosis (chronic) due to inhalation of
chemicals, gases, fumes and vapors

Excludes1 chronic pulmonary edema due to
chemicals, gases, fumes and
vapors (J68.1)

● J68.8 **Other respiratory conditions due to chemicals,
gases, fumes and vapors**

● ▪ J68.9 **Unspecified respiratory condition due to
chemicals, gases, fumes and vapors**

● **J69** **Pneumonitis due to solids and liquids**

Excludes1 neonatal aspiration syndromes (P24.-)
postprocedural pneumonitis (J95.4)

J69.0 **Pneumonitis due to inhalation of food and
vomit** 🦠
Aspiration pneumonia NOS
Aspiration pneumonia (due to) food
(regurgitated)
Aspiration pneumonia (due to) gastric secretions
Aspiration pneumonia (due to) milk
Aspiration pneumonia (due to) vomit

Code also any associated foreign body in
respiratory tract (T17.-)

Excludes1 chemical pneumonitis due to
anesthesia (J95.4)
obstetric aspiration pneumonitis
(O74.0)

● J69.1 **Pneumonitis due to inhalation of oils and
essences** 🦠
Exogenous lipoid pneumonia
Lipid pneumonia NOS

Code first (T51-T65) *to identify substance*

Excludes1 endogenous lipoid pneumonia
(J84.89)

● J69.8 **Pneumonitis due to inhalation of other solids and
liquids** 🦠
Pneumonitis due to aspiration of blood
Pneumonitis due to aspiration of detergent

Code first (T51-T65) *to identify substance*

● **J70** **Respiratory conditions due to other external agents**

J70.0 **Acute pulmonary manifestations due to
radiation** 🦠
Radiation pneumonitis

Use additional code (W88-W90, X39.0-) to identify
the external cause

J70.1 **Chronic and other pulmonary manifestations due
to radiation** 🦠
Fibrosis of lung following radiation

Use additional code (W88-W90, X39.0-) to identify
the external cause

N Newborn Age: 0   **P** Pediatric Age: 0–17   **M** Maternity DX: 12–55   **A** Adult Age: 15–124   ♀ Females Only   ♂ Males Only

🦠 Complication\Comorbidity   🦠 Major C\C   Present on Admission Requirement   🦠 Hospital-Acquired Condition

1081

● J70.2   **Acute drug-induced interstitial lung disorders**

Use additional code for adverse effect, if applicable, to identify drug (T36-T50 with fifth or sixth character 5)

Excludes1   interstitial pneumonia NOS (J84.9)
lymphoid interstitial pneumonia (J84.2)

● J70.3   **Chronic drug-induced interstitial lung disorders**

Use additional code for adverse effect, if applicable, to identify drug (T36-T50 with fifth or sixth character 5)

Excludes1   interstitial pneumonia NOS (J84.9)
lymphoid interstitial pneumonia (J84.2)

● ■ J70.4   **Drug-induced interstitial lung disorders, unspecified**

Use additional code for adverse effect, if applicable, to identify drug (T36-T50 with fifth or sixth character 5)

Excludes1   interstitial pneumonia NOS (J84.9)
lymphoid interstitial pneumonia (J84.2)

J70.5   **Respiratory conditions due to smoke inhalation**
Smoke inhalation NOS

Excludes1   smoke inhalation due to chemicals, gases, fumes and vapors (J68.9)

● J70.8   **Respiratory conditions due to other specified external agents**

Code first (T51-T65) to identify the external agent

● ■ J70.9   **Respiratory conditions due to unspecified external agent**

Code first (T51-T65) to identify the external agent

OTHER RESPIRATORY DISEASES PRINCIPALLY AFFECTING THE INTERSTITIUM (J80-J84)

J80   **Acute respiratory distress syndrome** 🔎
Acute respiratory distress syndrome in adult or child
Adult hyaline membrane disease

Excludes1   respiratory distress syndrome in newborn (perinatal) (P22.0)

● J81   **Pulmonary edema**

Use additional code to identify:
exposure to environmental tobacco smoke (Z77.22)
history of tobacco use (Z87.891)
occupational exposure to environmental tobacco smoke (Z57.31)
tobacco dependence (F17.-)
tobacco use (Z72.0)

Excludes1   chemical (acute) pulmonary edema (J68.1)
hypostatic pneumonia (J18.2)
passive pneumonia (J18.2)
pulmonary edema due to external agents (J60-J70)
pulmonary edema with heart disease NOS (I50.1)
pulmonary edema with heart failure (I50.1)

J81.0   **Acute pulmonary edema** 🔎
Acute edema of lung

J81.1   **Chronic pulmonary edema** 🔎
Pulmonary congestion (chronic) (passive)
Pulmonary edema NOS

J82   **Pulmonary eosinophilia, not elsewhere classified** 🔎
Allergic pneumonia
Eosinophilic asthma
Eosinophilic pneumonia
Löffler's pneumonia
Tropical (pulmonary) eosinophilia NOS

Excludes1   pulmonary eosinophilia due to aspergillosis (B44.-)
pulmonary eosinophilia due to drugs (J70.2-J70.4)
pulmonary eosinophilia due to specified parasitic infection (B50-B83)
pulmonary eosinophilia due to systemic connective tissue disorders (M30-M36)
pulmonary infiltrate NOS (R91.8)

● J84   **Other interstitial pulmonary diseases**

Excludes1   drug-induced interstitial lung disorders (J70.2-J70.4)
interstitial emphysema (J98.2)
lung diseases due to external agents (J60-J70)

● J84.0   **Alveolar and parieto-alveolar conditions**

J84.01   **Alveolar proteinosis** 🔎

J84.02   **Pulmonary alveolar microlithiasis** 🔎

J84.03   **Idiopathic pulmonary hemosiderosis** 🔎
Essential brown induration of lung

Code first underlying disease, such as:
disorders of iron metabolism (E83.1-)

Excludes1   acute idiopathic pulmonary hemorrhage in infants [AIPHI] (R04.81)

J84.09   **Other alveolar and parieto-alveolar conditions** 🔎

● J84.1   **Other interstitial pulmonary diseases with fibrosis**

Excludes1   pulmonary fibrosis (chronic) due to inhalation of chemicals, gases, fumes or vapors (J68.4)
pulmonary fibrosis (chronic) following radiation (J70.1)

■ J84.10   **Pulmonary fibrosis, unspecified**
Capillary fibrosis of lung
Cirrhosis of lung (chronic) NOS
Fibrosis of lung (atrophic) (chronic) (confluent) (massive) (perialveolar) (peribronchial) NOS
Induration of lung (chronic) NOS
Postinflammatory pulmonary fibrosis

● J84.11   **Idiopathic interstitial pneumonia**

Excludes1   lymphoid interstitial pneumonia (J84.2)
pneumocystis pneumonia (B59)

J84.111   **Idiopathic interstitial pneumonia, not otherwise specified**

● Unacceptable Principal Diagnosis   ● Use Additional Character(s)   ■ Unspecified   ▶ Manifestation Code
OGCR Official Guidelines for Coding and Reporting   Excludes 1   Excludes 2   Includes   Use additional   Code first   Code also

J84.112   Idiopathic pulmonary fibrosis
Cryptogenic fibrosing alveolitis
Idiopathic fibrosing alveolitis

J84.113   Idiopathic non-specific interstitial pneumonitis

Excludes1	non-specific interstitial pneumonia NOS, or due to known underlying cause (J84.89)

J84.114   Acute interstitial pneumonitis
Hamman-Rich syndrome

Excludes1	pneumocystis pneumonia (B59)

J84.115   Respiratory bronchiolitis interstitial lung disease

J84.116   Cryptogenic organizing pneumonia

Excludes1	organizing pneumonia NOS, or due to known underlying cause (J84.89)

J84.117   Desquamative interstitial pneumonia

J84.17   Other interstitial pulmonary diseases with fibrosis in diseases classified elsewhere
Interstitial pneumonia (nonspecific) (usual) due to collagen vascular disease
Interstitial pneumonia (nonspecific) (usual) in diseases classified elsewhere
Organizing pneumonia due to collagen vascular disease
Organizing pneumonia in diseases classified elsewhere

Code first underlying disease, such as:
progressive systemic sclerosis (M34.0)
rheumatoid arthritis (M05.00-M06.9)
systemic lupus erythematosis (M32.0-M32.9)

J84.2   Lymphoid interstitial pneumonia 🕭
Lymphoid interstitial pneumonitis

● **J84.8   Other specified interstitial pulmonary diseases**

Excludes1	exogenous lipoid pneumonia (J69.1) unspecified lipoid pneumonia (J69.1)

J84.81   Lymphangioleiomyomatosis 🕭
Lymphangiomyomatosis

J84.82   Adult pulmonary Langerhans cell histiocytosis 🕭
Adult PLCH

J84.83   Surfactant mutations of the lung 🕭

● **J84.84   Other interstitial lung diseases of childhood**

J84.841   Neuroendocrine cell hyperplasia of infancy 🕭

J84.842   Pulmonary interstitial glycogenosis 🕭

J84.843   Alveolar capillary dysplasia with vein misalignment 🕭

J84.848   Other interstitial lung diseases of childhood 🕭

J84.89   Other specified interstitial pulmonary diseases 🕭
Endogenous lipoid pneumonia
Interstitial pneumonitis
Non-specific interstitial pneumonitis NOS
Organizing pneumonia due to known underlying cause
Organizing pneumonia NOS

Code first, *if applicable:*
poisoning due to drug or toxin (T51-T65 with fifth or sixth character to indicate intent), for toxic pneumonopathy underlying cause of pneumonopathy, if known

Use additional code, for adverse effect, to identify drug (T36-T50 with fifth or sixth character 5), if drug-induced

Excludes1	cryptogenic organizing pneumonia (J84.846) idiopathic non-specific interstitial pneumonitis (J84.843) lipoid pneumonia, exogenous or unspecified (J69.1) lymphoid interstitial pneumonia (J84.2)

■ **J84.9   Interstitial pulmonary disease, unspecified** 🕭
Interstitial pneumonia NOS

SUPPURATIVE AND NECROTIC CONDITIONS OF THE LOWER RESPIRATORY TRACT (J85-J86)

● **J85   Abscess of lung and mediastinum**
Use additional code (B95-B97) to identify infectious agent.

J85.0   Gangrene and necrosis of lung 🕭

J85.1   Abscess of lung with pneumonia 🕭
Code also the type of pneumonia

J85.2   Abscess of lung without pneumonia 🕭
Abscess of lung NOS

J85.3   Abscess of mediastinum 🕭

CHAPTER 10 (J00-J99)

Item 10–11 Empyema is a condition in which pus accumulates in a body cavity. Empyema **with fistula** occurs when the pus passes from one cavity to another organ or structure.

● **J86 Pyothorax**

Use additional code (B95-B97) to identify infectious agent.

Excludes1   abscess of lung (J85.-)
pyothorax due to tuberculosis (A15.6)

J86.0 Pyothorax with fistula 🖊
Bronchocutaneous fistula
Bronchopleural fistula
Hepatopleural fistula
Mediastinal fistula
Pleural fistula
Thoracic fistula
Any condition classifiable to J86.9 with fistula

J86.9 Pyothorax without fistula 🖊
Abscess of pleura
Abscess of thorax
Empyema (chest) (lung) (pleura)
Fibrinopurulent pleurisy
Purulent pleurisy
Pyopneumothorax
Septic pleurisy
Seropurulent pleurisy
Suppurative pleurisy

OTHER DISEASES OF THE PLEURA (J90-J94)

J90 **Pleural effusion, not elsewhere classified** 🖊
Encysted pleurisy
Pleural effusion NOS
Pleurisy with effusion (exudative) (serous)

Excludes1   chylous (pleural) effusion (J94.0)
malignant pleural effusion (J91.0))
pleurisy NOS (R09.1)
tuberculous pleural effusion (A15.6)

● J91 **Pleural effusion in conditions classified elsewhere**

Excludes2   pleural effusion in heart failure (I50.-)
pleural effusion in systemic lupus erythematosus (M32.13)

●▶ *J91.0   Malignant pleural effusion* 🖊

Code first underlying neoplasm

●▶ *J91.8   Pleural effusion in other conditions classified elsewhere* 🖊

Code first underlying disease, such as:
filariasis (B74.0-B74.9)
influenza (J09.X2, J10.1, J11.1)

● J92 **Pleural plaque**

Includes   pleural thickening

J92.0 Pleural plaque with presence of asbestos

J92.9 Pleural plaque without asbestos
Pleural plaque NOS

● J93 **Pneumothorax and air leak**
Collapsed lung

Excludes1   congenital or perinatal pneumothorax (P25.1)
postprocedural air leak (J95.812)
postprocedural pneumothorax (J95.811)
traumatic pneumothorax (S27.0)
tuberculous (current disease) pneumothorax (A15.-)
pyopneumothorax (J86.-)

J93.0 **Spontaneous tension pneumothorax** 🖊
Tension pneumothorax (most serious type) occurs when air (positive pressure) collects in the pleural space

● J93.1 **Other spontaneous pneumothorax**

J93.11   Primary spontaneous pneumothorax 🖊

J93.12   Secondary spontaneous pneumothorax 🖊

Code first underlying condition, such as:
catamenial pneumothorax due to endometriosis (N80.8)
cystic fibrosis (E84.-)
eosinophilic pneumonia (J82)
lymphangioleiomyomatosis (J84.81)
malignant neoplasm of bronchus and lung (C34.-)
Marfan's syndrome (Q87.4)
pneumonia due to Pneumocystis carinii (B59)
secondary malignant neoplasm of lung (C78.0-)
spontaneous rupture of the esophagus (K22.3)

● J93.8 **Other pneumothorax and air leak**

J93.81   Chronic pneumothorax 🖊

J93.82   Other air leak 🖊
Persistent air leak

J93.83   Other pneumothorax 🖊
Acute pneumothorax
Spontaneous pneumothorax NOS

◼ J93.9 **Pneumothorax, unspecified** 🖊
Pneumothorax NOS

● J94 **Other pleural conditions**

Excludes1   pleurisy NOS (R09.1)
traumatic hemopneumothorax (S27.2)
traumatic hemothorax (S27.1)
tuberculous pleural conditions (current disease) (A15.-)

J94.0 Chylous effusion 🖊
Chyliform effusion

J94.1 Fibrothorax

J94.2 Hemothorax 🖊
Hemopneumothorax

J94.8 Other specified pleural conditions
Hydropneumothorax
Hydrothorax

◼ **J94.9 Pleural condition, unspecified**

● Unacceptable Principal Diagnosis   ● Use Additional Character(s)   ◼ Unspecified   ▶ Manifestation Code
OGCR Official Guidelines for Coding and Reporting | Excludes 1 | | Excludes 2 | Includes   Use additional   Code first   Code also

INTRAOPERATIVE AND POSTPROCEDURAL COMPLICATIONS AND DISORDERS OF RESPIRATORY SYSTEM, NOT ELSEWHERE CLASSIFIED (J95)

● **J95**   Intraoperative and postprocedural complications and disorders of respiratory system, not elsewhere classified

Excludes2   aspiration pneumonia (J69.-)
emphysema (subcutaneous) resulting from a procedure (T81.82)
hypostatic pneumonia (J18.2)
pulmonary manifestations due to radiation (J70.0- J70.1)

● **J95.0**   Tracheostomy complications

■ **J95.00**   Unspecified tracheostomy complication

J95.01   Hemorrhage from tracheostomy stoma

J95.02   Infection of tracheostomy stoma
Use additional code to identify type of infection, such as:
cellulitis of neck (L03.8)
sepsis (A40, A41.-)

J95.03   Malfunction of tracheostomy stoma
Mechanical complication of tracheostomy stoma
Obstruction of tracheostomy airway
Tracheal stenosis due to tracheostomy

J95.04   Tracheo-esophageal fistula following tracheostomy

J95.09   Other tracheostomy complication

J95.1   Acute pulmonary insufficiency following thoracic surgery
Excludes2   functional disturbances following cardiac surgery (I97.0, I97.1-)

J95.2   Acute pulmonary insufficiency following nonthoracic surgery
Excludes2   functional disturbances following cardiac surgery (I97.0, I97.1-)

J95.3   Chronic pulmonary insufficiency following surgery
Excludes2   functional disturbances following cardiac surgery (I97.0, I97.1-)

● **J95.4**   Chemical pneumonitis due to anesthesia
Mendelson's syndrome
Postprocedural aspiration pneumonia
Use additional code for adverse effect, if applicable, to identify drug (T41.- with fifth or sixth character 5)
Excludes1   aspiration pneumonitis due to anesthesia complicating labor and delivery (O74.0)
aspiration pneumonitis due to anesthesia complicating pregnancy (O29)
aspiration pneumonitis due to anesthesia complicating the puerperium (O89.01)

J95.5   Postprocedural subglottic stenosis

● **J95.6**   Intraoperative hemorrhage and hematoma of a respiratory system organ or structure complicating a procedure
Excludes1   intraoperative hemorrhage and hematoma of a respiratory system organ or structure due to accidental puncture and laceration during procedure (J95.7-)

J95.61   Intraoperative hemorrhage and hematoma of a respiratory system organ or structure complicating a respiratory system procedure

J95.62   Intraoperative hemorrhage and hematoma of a respiratory system organ or structure complicating other procedure

● **J95.7**   Accidental puncture and laceration of a respiratory system organ or structure during a procedure
Excludes2   postprocedural pneumothorax (J95.8)

J95.71   Accidental puncture and laceration of a respiratory system organ or structure during a respiratory system procedure

J95.72   Accidental puncture and laceration of a respiratory system organ or structure during other procedure

● **J95.8**   Other intraoperative and postprocedural complications and disorders of respiratory system, not elsewhere classified

● **J95.81**   Postprocedural pneumothorax and air leak

J95.811   Postprocedural pneumothorax

J95.812   Postprocedural air leak

● **J95.82**   Postprocedural respiratory failure
Excludes1   Respiratory failure in other conditions (J96.-)

J95.821   Acute postprocedural respiratory failure
Postprocedural respiratory failure NOS

J95.822   Acute and chronic postprocedural respiratory failure

● **J95.83**   Postprocedural hemorrhage and hematoma of a respiratory system organ or structure following a procedure

J95.830   Postprocedural hemorrhage and hematoma of a respiratory system organ or structure following a respiratory system procedure

J95.831   Postprocedural hemorrhage and hematoma of a respiratory system organ or structure following other procedure

J95.84   Transfusion-related acute lung injury (TRALI)

● **J95.85**   Complication of respirator [ventilator]

J95.850   Mechanical complication of respirator
Excludes1   encounter for respirator [ventilator] dependence during power failure (Z99.12)

J95.851   Ventilator associated pneumonia
Ventilator associated pneumonitis
Use additional code to identify the organism, if known (B95.-, B96.-, B97.-)
Excludes1   ventilator lung in newborn (P27.8)

J95.859   Other complication of respirator [ventilator]

N Newborn Age: 0   **P** Pediatric Age: 0–17   **M** Maternity DX: 12–55   **A** Adult Age: 15–124   ♀ Females Only   ♂ Males Only
Complication\Comorbidity   Major C\C   Present on Admission Requirement   Hospital-Acquired Condition

CHAPTER 10 (J00-J99)

1085

J95.88   **Other intraoperative complications of respiratory system, not elsewhere classified** 🦠

J95.89   **Other postprocedural complications and disorders of respiratory system, not elsewhere classified** 🦠

> Use additional code to identify disorder, such as:
> aspiration pneumonia (J69.-)
> bacterial or viral pneumonia (J12-J18)
>
> | Excludes2 | acute pulmonary insufficiency following thoracic surgery (J95.1)
> postprocedural subglottic stenosis (J95.5)

OTHER DISEASES OF THE RESPIRATORY SYSTEM (J96-J99)

● **J96   Respiratory failure, not elsewhere classified**

> | Excludes1 | acute respiratory distress syndrome (J80)
> cardiorespiratory failure (R09.2)
> newborn respiratory distress syndrome (P22.0)
> postprocedural respiratory failure (J95.82-)
> respiratory arrest (R09.2)
> respiratory arrest of newborn (P28.81)
> respiratory failure of newborn (P28.5)

● **J96.0   Acute respiratory failure**

■ J96.00   **Acute respiratory failure, unspecified whether with hypoxia or hypercapnia** 🦠

J96.01   **Acute respiratory failure with hypoxia** 🦠

J96.02   **Acute respiratory failure with hypercapnia** 🦠

● **J96.1   Chronic respiratory failure**

■ J96.10   **Chronic respiratory failure, unspecified whether with hypoxia or hypercapnia** 🦠

J96.11   **Chronic respiratory failure with hypoxia** 🦠

J96.12   **Chronic respiratory failure with hypercapnia** 🦠

● **J96.2   Acute and chronic respiratory failure**
Acute on chronic respiratory failure

■ J96.20   **Acute and chronic respiratory failure, unspecified whether with hypoxia or hypercapnia** 🦠

J96.21   **Acute and chronic respiratory failure with hypoxia** 🦠

J96.22   **Acute and chronic respiratory failure with hypercapnia** 🦠

● **J96.9   Respiratory failure, unspecified**

■ J96.90   **Respiratory failure, unspecified, unspecified whether with hypoxia or hypercapnia** 🦠

■ J96.91   **Respiratory failure, unspecified with hypoxia** 🦠

■ J96.92   **Respiratory failure, unspecified with hypercapnia** 🦠

● **J98   Other respiratory disorders**

> Use additional code to identify:
> exposure to environmental tobacco smoke (Z77.22)
> exposure to tobacco smoke in the perinatal period (P96.81)
> history of tobacco use (Z87.891)
> occupational exposure to environmental tobacco smoke (Z57.31)
> tobacco dependence (F17.-)
> tobacco use (Z72.0)
>
> | Excludes1 | newborn apnea (P28.4)
> newborn sleep apnea (P28.3)
>
> | Excludes2 | apnea NOS (R06.81)
> sleep apnea (G47.3-)

● **J98.0   Diseases of bronchus, not elsewhere classified**

J98.01   **Acute bronchospasm**

> | Excludes1 | acute bronchiolitis with bronchospasm (J21.-)
> acute bronchitis with bronchospasm (J20.-)
> asthma (J45.-)
> exercise induced bronchospasm (J45.990)

J98.09   **Other diseases of bronchus, not elsewhere classified**
Broncholithiasis
Calcification of bronchus
Stenosis of bronchus
Tracheobronchial collapse
Tracheobronchial dyskinesia
Ulcer of bronchus

● **J98.1   Pulmonary collapse**

> | Excludes1 | therapeutic collapse of lung status (Z98.3)

J98.11   **Atelectasis** 🦠

> | Excludes1 | newborn atelectasis
> tuberculous atelectasis (current disease) (A15)

J98.19   **Other pulmonary collapse** 🦠

J98.2   **Interstitial emphysema**
Mediastinal emphysema

> | Excludes1 | emphysema NOS (J43.9)
> emphysema in newborn (P25.0)
> surgical emphysema (subcutaneous) (T81.82)
> traumatic subcutaneous emphysema (T79.7)

J98.3   **Compensatory emphysema**

J98.4   **Other disorders of lung**
Calcification of lung
Cystic lung disease (acquired)
Lung disease NOS
Pulmolithiasis

> | Excludes1 | acute interstitial pneumonitis (J84.114)
> pulmonary insufficiency following surgery (J95.1-J95.2)

● Unacceptable Principal Diagnosis   ● Use Additional Character(s)   ■ Unspecified   ▶ Manifestation Code

OGCR   Official Guidelines for Coding and Reporting | Excludes 1 | | Excludes 2 | Includes   Use additional   Code first   Code also

J98.5 **Diseases of mediastinum, not elsewhere classified** 🕙🕙
     Fibrosis of mediastinum
     Hernia of mediastinum
     Retraction of mediastinum
     Mediastinitis
     Excludes2   abscess of mediastinum (J85.3)

J98.6 **Disorders of diaphragm**
     Diaphragmatitis
     Paralysis of diaphragm
     Relaxation of diaphragm
     Excludes1   congenital malformation of
                 diaphragm NEC (Q79.1)
                 congenital diaphragmatic hernia
                 (Q79.0)
     Excludes2   diaphragmatic hernia (K44.-)

J98.8 **Other specified respiratory disorders**

■ **J98.9** **Respiratory disorder, unspecified**
     Respiratory disease (chronic) NOS

● ▶ **J99** *Respiratory disorders in diseases classified elsewhere*
     Code first underlying disease, such as:
         amyloidosis (E85-)
         ankylosing spondylitis (M45)
         congenital syphilis (A50.5)
         cryoglobulinemia (D89.1)
         early congenital syphilis (A50.0)
         schistosomiasis (B65.0-B65.9)
     Excludes1   respiratory disorders in:
         amebiasis (A06.5)
         blastomycosis (B40.0-B40.2)
         candidiasis (B37.1)
         coccidioidomycosis (B38.0-B38.2)
         cystic fibrosis with pulmonary
             manifestations (E84.0)
         dermatomyositis (M33.01, M33.11)
         histoplasmosis (B39.0-B39.2)
         late syphilis (A52.72, A52.73)
         polymyositis (M33.21)
         sicca syndrome (M35.02)
         systemic lupus erythematosus (M32.13)
         systemic sclerosis (M34.81)
         Wegener's granulomatosis
            (M31.30-M31.31)

N Newborn Age: 0   **P** Pediatric Age: 0–17   **M** Maternity DX: 12–55   **A** Adult Age: 15–124   ♀ Females Only   ♂ Males Only

🕙 Complication\Comorbidity   🕙 Major C\C   🕙 Present on Admission Requirement   🕙 Hospital-Acquired Condition   **1087**

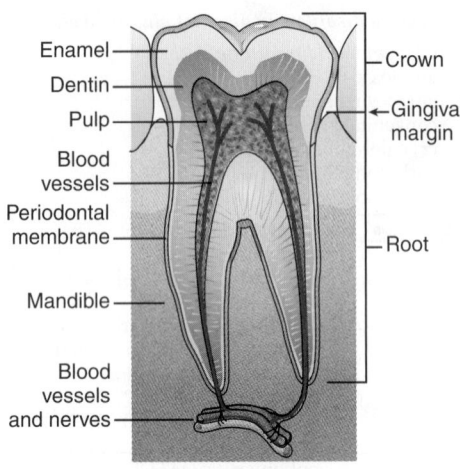

Figure 11-1 Anatomy of a tooth.

Item 11-1 Anodontia is the congenital absence of teeth. **Hypodontia** is partial anodontia. **Oligodontia** is the congenital absence of some teeth, whereas **supernumerary** is having more teeth than the normal number. **Mesiodens** are small extra teeth that often appear in pairs, although single small teeth are not uncommon.

CHAPTER 11

DISEASES OF THE DIGESTIVE SYSTEM (K00-K95)

| Excludes2 | certain conditions originating in the perinatal period (P04-P96)
certain infectious and parasitic diseases (A00-B99)
complications of pregnancy, childbirth and the puerperium (O00-O9A)
congenital malformations, deformations and chromosomal abnormalities (Q00-Q99)
endocrine, nutritional and metabolic diseases (E00-E88)
injury, poisoning and certain other consequences of external causes (S00-T88)
neoplasms (C00-D49)
symptoms, signs and abnormal clinical and laboratory findings, not elsewhere classified (R00-R94)

This chapter contains the following blocks:

K00-K14	Diseases of oral cavity and salivary glands
K20-K31	Diseases of esophagus, stomach and duodenum
K35-K38	Diseases of appendix
K40-K46	Hernia
K50-K52	Noninfective enteritis and colitis
K55-K64	Other diseases of intestines
K65-K68	Diseases of peritoneum and retroperitoneum
K70-K77	Diseases of liver
K80-K87	Disorders of gallbladder, biliary tract and pancreas
K90-K95	Other diseases of the digestive system

DISEASES OF ORAL CAVITY AND SALIVARY GLANDS (K00-K14)

● **K00**   **Disorders of tooth development and eruption**
    | Excludes2 | embedded and impacted teeth (K01.-)

   K00.0   **Anodontia**
       Hypodontia
       Oligodontia
       | Excludes1 | acquired absence of teeth (K08.1-)

   K00.1   **Supernumerary teeth**
       Distomolar
       Fourth molar
       Mesiodens
       Paramolar
       Supplementary teeth
       | Excludes2 | supernumerary roots (K00.2)

   K00.2   **Abnormalities of size and form of teeth**
       Concrescence of teeth
       Fusion of teeth
       Gemination of teeth
       Dens evaginatus
       Dens in dente
       Dens invaginatus
       Enamel pearls
       Macrodontia
       Microdontia
       Peg-shaped [conical] teeth
       Supernumerary roots
       Taurodontism
       Tuberculum paramolare
       | Excludes1 | abnormalities of teeth due to congenital syphilis (A50.5)
               tuberculum Carabelli, which is regarded as a normal variation and should not be coded

   K00.3   **Mottled teeth**
       Dental fluorosis
       Mottling of enamel
       Nonfluoride enamel opacities
       | Excludes2 | deposits [accretions] on teeth (K03.6)

   K00.4   **Disturbances in tooth formation**
       Aplasia and hypoplasia of cementum
       Dilaceration of tooth
       Enamel hypoplasia (neonatal) (postnatal) (prenatal)
       Regional odontodysplasia
       Turner's tooth
       | Excludes1 | Hutchinson's teeth and mulberry molars in congenital syphilis (A50.5)
       | Excludes2 | mottled teeth (K00.3)

   K00.5   **Hereditary disturbances in tooth structure, not elsewhere classified**
       Amelogenesis imperfecta
       Dentinogenesis imperfecta
       Odontogenesis imperfecta
       Dentinal dysplasia
       Shell teeth

   K00.6   **Disturbances in tooth eruption**
       Dentia praecox
       Natal tooth
       Neonatal tooth
       Premature eruption of tooth
       Premature shedding of primary [deciduous] tooth
       Prenatal teeth
       Retained [persistent] primary tooth
       | Excludes2 | embedded and impacted teeth (K01.-)

● Unacceptable Principal Diagnosis   ◐ Use Additional Character(s)   ■ Unspecified   ▶ Manifestation Code
OGCR Official Guidelines for Coding and Reporting | Excludes 1 | | Excludes 2 | Includes   Use additional   Code first   Code also

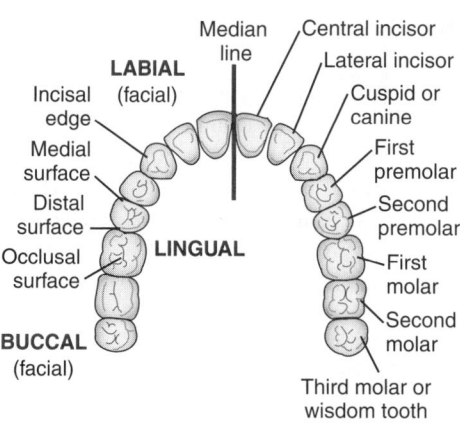

Figure 11-2   The permanent teeth within the dental arch.

Item 11–2 Each dental arch (jaw) normally contains 16 teeth. Tooth decay or **dental caries** is a disease of the enamel, dentin, and cementum of the tooth and can result in a cavity.

K00.7   Teething syndrome

K00.8   Other disorders of tooth development
Color changes during tooth formation
Intrinsic staining of teeth NOS
> **Excludes2**   posteruptive color changes (K03.7)

K00.9   Disorder of tooth development, unspecified
Disorder of odontogenesis NOS

● **K01   Embedded and impacted teeth**
> **Excludes1**   abnormal position of fully erupted teeth (M26.3-)

K01.0   Embedded teeth

K01.1   Impacted teeth

● **K02   Dental caries**
> **Includes**   dental cavities
>   tooth decay

K02.3   Arrested dental caries
Arrested coronal and root caries

● **K02.5   Dental caries on pit and fissure surface**
Dental caries on chewing surface of tooth

    K02.51   Dental caries on pit and fissure surface limited to enamel
       White spot lesions [initial caries] on pit and fissure surface of tooth

    K02.52   Dental caries on pit and fissure surface penetrating into dentin

    K02.53   Dental caries on pit and fissure surface penetrating into pulp

● **K02.6   Dental caries on smooth surface**

    K02.61   Dental caries on smooth surface limited to enamel
       White spot lesions [initial caries] on smooth surface of tooth

    K02.62   Dental caries on smooth surface penetrating into dentin

    K02.63   Dental caries on smooth surface penetrating into pulp

K02.7   Dental root caries

K02.9   Dental caries, unspecified

● **K03   Other diseases of hard tissues of teeth**
> **Excludes2**   bruxism (F45.8)
>   dental caries (K02.-)
>   teeth-grinding NOS (F45.8)

K03.0   Excessive attrition of teeth
Approximal wear of teeth
Occlusal wear of teeth

K03.1   Abrasion of teeth
Dentifrice abrasion of teeth
Habitual abrasion of teeth
Occupational abrasion of teeth
Ritual abrasion of teeth
Traditional abrasion of teeth
Wedge defect NOS

K03.2   Erosion of teeth
Erosion of teeth due to diet
Erosion of teeth due to drugs and medicaments
Erosion of teeth due to persistent vomiting
Erosion of teeth NOS
Idiopathic erosion of teeth
Occupational erosion of teeth

K03.3   Pathological resorption of teeth
Internal granuloma of pulp
Resorption of teeth (external)

K03.4   Hypercementosis
Cementation hyperplasia

K03.5   Ankylosis of teeth

K03.6   Deposits [accretions] on teeth
Betel deposits [accretions] on teeth
Black deposits [accretions] on teeth
Extrinsic staining of teeth NOS
Green deposits [accretions] on teeth
Materia alba deposits [accretions] on teeth
Orange deposits [accretions] on teeth
Staining of teeth NOS
Subgingival dental calculus
Supragingival dental calculus
Tobacco deposits [accretions] on teeth

K03.7   Posteruptive color changes of dental hard tissues
> **Excludes2**   deposits [accretions] on teeth (K03.6)

● **K03.8   Other specified diseases of hard tissues of teeth**

    K03.81   Cracked tooth
>   **Excludes1**   asymptomatic craze lines in enamel - omit code
>   broken or fractured tooth due to trauma (S02.5)

    K03.89   Other specified diseases of hard tissues of teeth

K03.9   Disease of hard tissues of teeth, unspecified

K04   Diseases of pulp and periapical tissues

K04.0   Pulpitis 🦷
Acute pulpitis
Chronic (hyperplastic) (ulcerative) pulpitis
Irreversible pulpitis
Reversible pulpitis

K04.1   Necrosis of pulp
Pulpal gangrene

K04.2   Pulp degeneration
Denticles
Pulpal calcifications
Pulpal stones

K04.3   Abnormal hard tissue formation in pulp
Secondary or irregular dentine

K04.4   Acute apical periodontitis of pulpal origin 🦷
Acute apical periodontitis NOS
> **Excludes1**   acute periodontitis (K05.2-)

CHAPTER 11 (K00-K95)

N Newborn Age: 0   **P** Pediatric Age: 0–17   **M** Maternity DX: 12–55   **A** Adult Age: 15–124   ♀ Females Only   ♂ Males Only
🦷 Complication\Comorbidity   🦷 Major C\C   🦷 Present on Admission Requirement   🦷 Hospital-Acquired Condition

Item 11–3   **Acute gingivitis,** also known as orilitis or ulitis, is the short-term, severe inflammation of the gums (gingiva) caused by bacteria. **Chronic gingivitis** is persistent inflammation of the gums. When the gingivitis moves into the periodontium it is called periodontitis, also known as paradentitis.

K04.5   **Chronic apical periodontitis**
     Apical or periapical granuloma
     Apical periodontitis NOS
     Excludes1   chronic periodontitis (K05.3-)

K04.6   **Periapical abscess with sinus**
     Dental abscess with sinus
     Dentoalveolar abscess with sinus

K04.7   **Periapical abscess without sinus**
     Dental abscess without sinus
     Dentoalveolar abscess without sinus
     Periapical abscess without sinus

K04.8   **Radicular cyst**
     Apical (periodontal) cyst
     Periapical cyst
     Residual radicular cyst
     Excludes2   lateral periodontal cyst (K09.0)

● K04.9   **Other and unspecified diseases of pulp and periapical tissues**
     ◼ K04.90   **Unspecified diseases of pulp and periapical tissues**
        K04.99   **Other diseases of pulp and periapical tissues**

● K05   **Gingivitis and periodontal diseases**
     Use additional code to identify:
     alcohol abuse and dependence (F10.-)
     exposure to environmental tobacco smoke (Z77.22)
     exposure to tobacco smoke in the perinatal period (P96.81)
     history of tobacco use (Z87.891)
     occupational exposure to environmental tobacco smoke (Z57.31)
     tobacco dependence (F17.-)
     tobacco use (Z72.0)

● K05.0   **Acute gingivitis**
     Excludes1   acute necrotizing ulcerative gingivitis (A69.1)
        herpesviral [herpes simplex] gingivostomatitis (B00.2)
     K05.00   **Acute gingivitis, plaque induced**
        Acute gingivitis NOS
     K05.01   **Acute gingivitis, non-plaque induced**

● K05.1   **Chronic gingivitis**
     Desquamative gingivitis (chronic)
     Gingivitis (chronic) NOS
     Hyperplastic gingivitis (chronic)
     Simple marginal gingivitis (chronic)
     Ulcerative gingivitis (chronic)
     K05.10   **Chronic gingivitis, plaque induced**
        Chronic gingivitis NOS
        Gingivitis NOS
     K05.11   **Chronic gingivitis, non-plaque induced**

● K05.2   **Aggressive periodontitis**
     Acute pericoronitis
     Excludes1   acute apical periodontitis (K04.4)
        periapical abscess (K04.7)
        periapical abscess with sinus (K04.6)
     ◼ K05.20   **Aggressive periodontitis, unspecified**
     K05.21   **Aggressive periodontitis, localized**
        Periodontal abscess
     K05.22   **Aggressive periodontitis, generalized**

● K05.3   **Chronic periodontitis**
     Chronic pericoronitis
     Complex periodontitis
     Periodontitis NOS
     Simplex periodontitis
     Excludes1   chronic apical periodontitis (K04.5)
     ◼ K05.30   **Chronic periodontitis, unspecified**
     K05.31   **Chronic periodontitis, localized**
     K05.32   **Chronic periodontitis, generalized**

K05.4   **Periodontosis**
     Juvenile periodontosis

K05.5   **Other periodontal diseases**
     Excludes2   leukoplakia of gingiva (K13.21)

◼ K05.6   **Periodontal disease, unspecified**

● K06   **Other disorders of gingiva and edentulous alveolar ridge**
     Excludes2   acute gingivitis (K05.0)
        atrophy of edentulous alveolar ridge (K08.2)
        chronic gingivitis (K05.1)
        gingivitis NOS (K05.1)

K06.0   **Gingival recession**
     Gingival recession (generalized) (localized) (postinfective) (postprocedural)

K06.1   **Gingival enlargement**
     Gingival fibromatosis

K06.2   **Gingival and edentulous alveolar ridge lesions associated with trauma**
     Irritative hyperplasia of edentulous ridge [denture hyperplasia]
     Use additional code (Chapter 20) to identify external cause or denture status (Z97.2)

K06.8   **Other specified disorders of gingiva and edentulous alveolar ridge**
     Fibrous epulis
     Flabby alveolar ridge
     Giant cell epulis
     Peripheral giant cell granuloma of gingiva
     Pyogenic granuloma of gingiva
     Excludes2   gingival cyst (K09.0)

◼ K06.9   **Disorder of gingiva and edentulous alveolar ridge, unspecified**

● K08   **Other disorders of teeth and supporting structures**
     Excludes2   dentofacial anomalies [including malocclusion] (M26.-)
        disorders of jaw (M27.-)

K08.0   **Exfoliation of teeth due to systemic causes**
     Code also underlying systemic condition

● K08.1   **Complete loss of teeth**
     Acquired loss of teeth, complete
     Excludes1   congenital absence of teeth (K00.0)
        exfoliation of teeth due to systemic causes (K08.0)
        partial loss of teeth (K08.4-)
     ● K08.10   **Complete loss of teeth, unspecified cause**
        ◼ K08.101   **Complete loss of teeth, unspecified cause, class I**
        ◼ K08.102   **Complete loss of teeth, unspecified cause, class II**
        ◼ K08.103   **Complete loss of teeth, unspecified cause, class III**
        ◼ K08.104   **Complete loss of teeth, unspecified cause, class IV**
        ◼ K08.109   **Complete loss of teeth, unspecified cause, unspecified class**
          Edentulism NOS

CHAPTER 11 (K00-K95)

● Unacceptable Principal Diagnosis   ● Use Additional Character(s)   ◼ Unspecified   ▶ Manifestation Code

1090   **OGCR** Official Guidelines for Coding and Reporting | Excludes 1 | | Excludes 2 | | Includes | | Use additional | | Code first | | Code also |

● K08.11 **Complete loss of teeth due to trauma**

    K08.111 **Complete loss of teeth due to trauma, class I**

    K08.112 **Complete loss of teeth due to trauma, class II**

    K08.113 **Complete loss of teeth due to trauma, class III**

    K08.114 **Complete loss of teeth due to trauma, class IV**

    ■ K08.119 **Complete loss of teeth due to trauma, unspecified class**

● K08.12 **Complete loss of teeth due to periodontal diseases**

    K08.121 **Complete loss of teeth due to periodontal diseases, class I**

    K08.122 **Complete loss of teeth due to periodontal diseases, class II**

    K08.123 **Complete loss of teeth due to periodontal diseases, class III**

    K08.124 **Complete loss of teeth due to periodontal diseases, class IV**

    ■ K08.129 **Complete loss of teeth due to periodontal diseases, unspecified class**

● K08.13 **Complete loss of teeth due to caries**

    K08.131 **Complete loss of teeth due to caries, class I**

    K08.132 **Complete loss of teeth due to caries, class II**

    K08.133 **Complete loss of teeth due to caries, class III**

    K08.134 **Complete loss of teeth due to caries, class IV**

    ■ K08.139 **Complete loss of teeth due to caries, unspecified class**

● K08.19 **Complete loss of teeth due to other specified cause**

    K08.191 **Complete loss of teeth due to other specified cause, class I**

    K08.192 **Complete loss of teeth due to other specified cause, class II**

    K08.193 **Complete loss of teeth due to other specified cause, class III**

    K08.194 **Complete loss of teeth due to other specified cause, class IV**

    ■ K08.199 **Complete loss of teeth due to other specified cause, unspecified class**

● K08.2 **Atrophy of edentulous alveolar ridge**

    ■ K08.20 **Unspecified atrophy of edentulous alveolar ridge**
        Atrophy of the mandible NOS
        Atrophy of the maxilla NOS

    K08.21 **Minimal atrophy of the mandible**
        Minimal atrophy of the edentulous mandible

    K08.22 **Moderate atrophy of the mandible**
        Moderate atrophy of the edentulous mandible

    K08.23 **Severe atrophy of the mandible**
        Severe atrophy of the edentulous mandible

    K08.24 **Minimal atrophy of maxilla**
        Minimal atrophy of the edentulous maxilla

    K08.25 **Moderate atrophy of the maxilla**
        Moderate atrophy of the edentulous maxilla

    K08.26 **Severe atrophy of the maxilla**
        Severe atrophy of the edentulous maxilla

K08.3 **Retained dental root**

● K08.4 **Partial loss of teeth**
    Acquired loss of teeth, partial

    | Excludes1 | complete loss of teeth (K08.1-) congenital absence of teeth (K00.0) |
    | Excludes2 | exfoliation of teeth due to systemic causes (K08.0) |

    ● K08.40 **Partial loss of teeth, unspecified cause**

       ■ K08.401 **Partial loss of teeth, unspecified cause, class I**

       ■ K08.402 **Partial loss of teeth, unspecified cause, class II**

       ■ K08.403 **Partial loss of teeth, unspecified cause, class III**

       ■ K08.404 **Partial loss of teeth, unspecified cause, class IV**

       ■ K08.409 **Partial loss of teeth, unspecified cause, unspecified class**
           Tooth extraction status NOS

    ● K08.41 **Partial loss of teeth due to trauma**

       K08.411 **Partial loss of teeth due to trauma, class I**

       K08.412 **Partial loss of teeth due to trauma, class II**

       K08.413 **Partial loss of teeth due to trauma, class III**

       K08.414 **Partial loss of teeth due to trauma, class IV**

       ■ K08.419 **Partial loss of teeth due to trauma, unspecified class**

    ● K08.42 **Partial loss of teeth due to periodontal diseases**

       K08.421 **Partial loss of teeth due to periodontal diseases, class I**

       K08.422 **Partial loss of teeth due to periodontal diseases, class II**

       K08.423 **Partial loss of teeth due to periodontal diseases, class III**

       K08.424 **Partial loss of teeth due to periodontal diseases, class IV**

       ■ K08.429 **Partial loss of teeth due to periodontal diseases, unspecified class**

    ● K08.43 **Partial loss of teeth due to caries**

       K08.431 **Partial loss of teeth due to caries, class I**

       K08.432 **Partial loss of teeth due to caries, class II**

       K08.433 **Partial loss of teeth due to caries, class III**

       K08.434 **Partial loss of teeth due to caries, class IV**

       ■ K08.439 **Partial loss of teeth due to caries, unspecified class**

CHAPTER 11 (K00–K95)

● **K08.49 Partial loss of teeth due to other specified cause**

    K08.491 Partial loss of teeth due to other specified cause, class I

    K08.492 Partial loss of teeth due to other specified cause, class II

    K08.493 Partial loss of teeth due to other specified cause, class III

    K08.494 Partial loss of teeth due to other specified cause, class IV

    ■ **K08.499 Partial loss of teeth due to other specified cause, unspecified class**

● **K08.5 Unsatisfactory restoration of tooth**
    Defective bridge, crown, filling
    Defective dental restoration

    Excludes1 dental restoration status (Z98.811)

    Excludes2 endosseous dental implant failure (M27.6-)
        unsatisfactory endodontic treatment (M27.5-)

■ **K08.50 Unsatisfactory restoration of tooth, unspecified**
    Defective dental restoration NOS

K08.51 Open restoration margins of tooth
    Dental restoration failure of marginal integrity
    Open margin on tooth restoration
    Poor gingival margin to tooth restoration

K08.52 Unrepairable overhanging of dental restorative materials
    Overhanging of tooth restoration

● **K08.53 Fractured dental restorative material**

    Excludes1 cracked tooth (K03.81)
        traumatic fracture of tooth (S02.5)

    K08.530 Fractured dental restorative material without loss of material

    K08.531 Fractured dental restorative material with loss of material

    ■ **K08.539 Fractured dental restorative material, unspecified**

K08.54 Contour of existing restoration of tooth biologically incompatible with oral health
    Dental restoration failure of periodontal anatomical integrity
    Unacceptable contours of existing restoration of tooth
    Unacceptable morphology of existing restoration of tooth

K08.55 Allergy to existing dental restorative material

    Use additional code to identify the specific type of allergy

K08.56 Poor aesthetic of existing restoration of tooth
    Dental restoration aesthetically inadequate or displeasing

K08.59 Other unsatisfactory restoration of tooth
    Other defective dental restoration

K08.8 Other specified disorders of teeth and supporting structures
    Enlargement of alveolar ridge NOS
    Irregular alveolar process
    Toothache NOS

■ **K08.9 Disorder of teeth and supporting structures, unspecified**

● **K09 Cysts of oral region, not elsewhere classified**

    Includes lesions showing histological features both of aneurysmal cyst and of another fibro-osseous lesion

    Excludes2 cysts of jaw (M27.0-, M27.4-)
        radicular cyst (K04.8)

K09.0 Developmental odontogenic cysts
    Dentigerous cyst
    Eruption cyst
    Follicular cyst
    Gingival cyst
    Lateral periodontal cyst
    Primordial cyst

    Excludes2 keratocysts D16.4, D16.5
        odontogenic keratocystic tumors D16.4, D16.5

K09.1 Developmental (nonodontogenic) cysts of oral region
    Cyst (of) incisive canal
    Cyst (of) palatine of papilla
    Globulomaxillary cyst
    Median palatal cyst
    Nasoalveolar cyst
    Nasolabial cyst
    Nasopalatine duct cyst

K09.8 Other cysts of oral region, not elsewhere classified
    Dermoid cyst
    Epidermoid cyst
    Lymphoepithelial cyst
    Epstein's pearl

■ **K09.9 Cyst of oral region, unspecified**

● **K11 Diseases of salivary glands**

    Use additional code to identify:
    alcohol abuse and dependence (F10.-)
    exposure to environmental tobacco smoke (Z77.22)
    exposure to tobacco smoke in the perinatal period (P96.81)
    history of tobacco use (Z87.891)
    occupational exposure to environmental tobacco smoke (Z57.31)
    tobacco dependence (F17.-)
    tobacco use (Z72.0)

K11.0 Atrophy of salivary gland

K11.1 Hypertrophy of salivary gland

● **K11.2 Sialoadenitis**
    Parotitis

    Excludes1 epidemic parotitis (B26.-)
        mumps (B26.-)
        uveoparotid fever [Heerfordt] (D86.89)

    ■ **K11.20 Sialoadenitis, unspecified**

    K11.21 Acute sialoadenitis

        Excludes1 acute recurrent sialoadenitis (K11.22)

    K11.22 Acute recurrent sialoadenitis

    K11.23 Chronic sialoadenitis

K11.3 Abscess of salivary gland 🔾

K11.4 Fistula of salivary gland 🔾

    Excludes1 congenital fistula of salivary gland (Q38.4)

Item 11-4 Atrophy is wasting away of a tissue or organ, whereas **hypertrophy** is overdevelopment or enlargement of a tissue or organ. **Sialoadenitis** is salivary gland inflammation. **Parotitis** is the inflammation of the parotid gland. In the epidemic form, parotitis is also known as mumps. **Sialolithiasis** is the formation of calculus within a salivary gland. **Mucocele** is a polyp composed of mucus.

● Unacceptable Principal Diagnosis   ● Use Additional Character(s)   ■ Unspecified   ▶ Manifestation Code

OGCR Official Guidelines for Coding and Reporting   Excludes 1   Excludes 2   Includes   Use additional   Code first   Code also

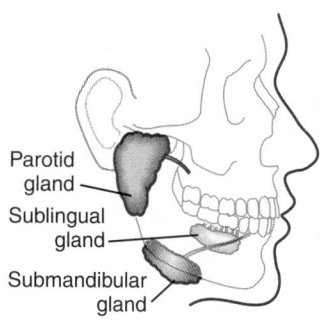

Figure 11-3   Major salivary glands.

(See Plate 61 on page NAP-25.)

K11.5   Sialolithiasis
    Calculus of salivary gland or duct
    Stone of salivary gland or duct

K11.6   Mucocele of salivary gland
    Mucous extravasation cyst of salivary gland
    Mucous retention cyst of salivary gland
    Ranula

K11.7   Disturbances of salivary secretion
    Hypoptyalism
    Ptyalism
    Xerostomia
    Excludes2   dry mouth NOS (R68.2)

K11.8   Other diseases of salivary glands
    Benign lymphoepithelial lesion of salivary gland
    Mikulicz' disease
    Necrotizing sialometaplasia
    Sialectasia
    Stenosis of salivary duct
    Stricture of salivary duct
    Excludes1   sicca syndrome [Sjögren] (M35.0-)

K11.9   Disease of salivary gland, unspecified
    Sialoadenopathy NOS

● **K12   Stomatitis and related lesions**
    Use additional code to identify:
    alcohol abuse and dependence (F10.-)
    exposure to environmental tobacco smoke (Z77.22)
    exposure to tobacco smoke in the perinatal period (P96.81)
    history of tobacco use (Z87.891)
    occupational exposure to environmental tobacco smoke (Z57.31)
    tobacco dependence (F17.-)
    tobacco use (Z72.0)
    Excludes1   cancrum oris (A69.0)
                cheilitis (K13.0)
                gangrenous stomatitis (A69.0)
                herpesviral [herpes simplex] gingivostomatitis (B00.2)
                noma (A69.0)

K12.0   Recurrent oral aphthae
    Aphthous stomatitis (major) (minor)
    Bednar's aphthae
    Periadenitis mucosa necrotica recurrens
    Recurrent aphthous ulcer
    Stomatitis herpetiformis

Item 11-5   Stomatitis is the inflammation of the oral mucosa. **Mucositis** is the inflammation of the mucous membranes lining the digestive tract from the mouth to the anus. It is a common side effect of chemotherapy and of radiotherapy that involves any part of the digestive tract.

K12.1   Other forms of stomatitis
    Stomatitis NOS
    Denture stomatitis
    Ulcerative stomatitis
    Vesicular stomatitis
    Excludes1   acute necrotizing ulcerative stomatitis (A69.1)
                Vincent's stomatitis (A69.1)

K12.2   Cellulitis and abscess of mouth ⊗
    Cellulitis of mouth (floor)
    Submandibular abscess
    Excludes2   abscess of salivary gland (K11.3)
                abscess of tongue (K14.0)
                periapical abscess (K04.6-K04.7)
                periodontal abscess (K05.21)
                peritonsillar abscess (J36)

● **K12.3   Oral mucositis (ulcerative)**
    Mucositis (oral) (oropharyneal)
    Excludes2   gastrointestinal mucositis (ulcerative) (K92.81)
                mucositis (ulcerative) of vagina and vulva (N76.81)
                nasal mucositis (ulcerative) (J34.81)

■ **K12.30   Oral mucositis (ulcerative), unspecified**

K12.31   Oral mucositis (ulcerative) due to antineoplastic therapy
    Use additional code for adverse effect, if applicable, to identify antineoplastic and immunosuppressive drugs (T45.1x5)
    Use additional code for other antineoplastic therapy, such as: radiological procedure and radiotherapy (Y84.2)

K12.32   Oral mucositis (ulcerative) due to other drugs
    Use additional code for adverse effect, if applicable, to identify drug (T36-T50 with fifth or sixth character 5)

K12.33   Oral mucositis (ulcerative) due to radiation
    Use additional external cause code (W88-W90, X39.0-) to identify cause

K12.39   Other oral mucositis (ulcerative)
    Viral oral mucositis (ulcerative)

● **K13   Other diseases of lip and oral mucosa**
    Includes   epithelial disturbances of tongue
    Use additional code to identify:
    alcohol abuse and dependence (F10.-)
    exposure to environmental tobacco smoke (Z77.22)
    exposure to tobacco smoke in the perinatal period (P96.81)
    history of tobacco use (Z87.891)
    occupational exposure to environmental tobacco smoke (Z57.31)
    tobacco dependence (F17.-)
    tobacco use (Z72.0)
    Excludes2   certain disorders of gingiva and edentulous alveolar ridge (K05-K06)
                cysts of oral region (K09.-)
                diseases of tongue (K14.-)
                stomatitis and related lesions (K12.-)

CHAPTER 11 (K00-K95)

N Newborn Age: 0   **P** Pediatric Age: 0-17   **M** Maternity DX: 12-55   **A** Adult Age: 15-124   ♀ Females Only   ♂ Males Only

 Complication\Comorbidity   Major C\C   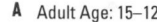 Present on Admission Requirement   ⊗ Hospital-Acquired Condition

1093

K13.0 Diseases of lips
Abscess of lips
Angular cheilitis
Cellulitis of lips
Cheilitis NOS
Cheilodynia
Cheilosis
Exfoliative cheilitis
Fistula of lips
Glandular cheilitis
Hypertrophy of lips
Perlèche NEC

Excludes1 ariboflavinosis (E53.0)
cheilitis due to radiation-related disorders (L55-L59)
congenital fistula of lips (Q38.0)
congenital hypertrophy of lips (Q18.6)
Perlèche due to candidiasis (B37.83)
Perlèche due to riboflavin deficiency (E53.0)

K13.1 Cheek and lip biting

● **K13.2 Leukoplakia and other disturbances of oral epithelium, including tongue**

Excludes1 carcinoma in situ of oral epithelium (D00.0-)
hairy leukoplakia (K13.3)

K13.21 Leukoplakia of oral mucosa, including tongue
Considered precancerous and evidenced by thickened white patches of epithelium on mucous membranes
Leukokeratosis of oral mucosa
Leukoplakia of gingiva, lips, tongue

Excludes1 hairy leukoplakia (K13.3)
leukokeratosis nicotina palati (K13.24)

K13.22 Minimal keratinized residual ridge mucosa
Minimal keratinization of alveolar ridge mucosa

K13.23 Excessive keratinized residual ridge mucosa
Excessive keratinization of alveolar ridge mucosa

K13.24 Leukokeratosis nicotina palati
Smoker's palate

K13.29 Other disturbances of oral epithelium, including tongue
Erythroplakia of mouth or tongue
Focal epithelial hyperplasia of mouth or tongue
Leukoedema of mouth or tongue
Other oral epithelium disturbances

K13.3 Hairy leukoplakia

K13.4 Granuloma and granuloma-like lesions of oral mucosa
Eosinophilic granuloma
Granuloma pyogenicum
Verrucous xanthoma

K13.5 Oral submucous fibrosis
Submucous fibrosis of tongue

Figure 11-4 Oral leukoplakia and associated squamous carcinoma. (From Feldman: Sleisenger & Fordtran's Gastrointestinal and Liver Disease, 8th ed. 2006, Saunders, An Imprint of Elsevier.)

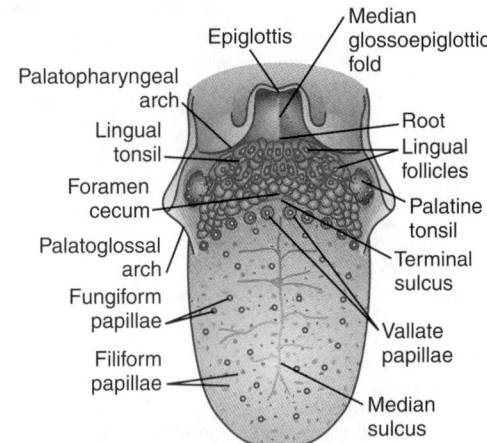
Figure 11-5 Structure of the tongue.

K13.6 Irritative hyperplasia of oral mucosa
Excludes2 irritative hyperplasia of edentulous ridge [denture hyperplasia] (K06.2)

● **K13.7 Other and unspecified lesions of oral mucosa**
(See Plate 58 on page NAP-23.)
■ **K13.70 Unspecified lesions of oral mucosa**
K13.79 Other lesions of oral mucosa
Focal oral mucinosis

● **K14 Diseases of tongue**
Use additional code to identify:
alcohol abuse and dependence (F10.-)
exposure to environmental tobacco smoke (Z77.22)
history of tobacco use (Z87.891)
occupational exposure to environmental tobacco smoke (Z57.31)
tobacco dependence (F17.-)
tobacco use (Z72.0)

Excludes2 erythroplakia (K13.29)
focal epithelial hyperplasia (K13.29)
leukedema of tongue (K13.29)
leukoplakia of tongue (K13.21)
hairy leukoplakia (K13.3)
macroglossia (congenital) (Q38.2)
submucous fibrosis of tongue (K13.5)

K14.0 Glossitis
Abscess of tongue
Ulceration (traumatic) of tongue
Excludes1 atrophic glossitis (K14.4)

K14.1 Geographic tongue
Benign migratory glossitis
Glossitis areata exfoliativa

K14.2 Median rhomboid glossitis

K14.3 Hypertrophy of tongue papillae
Black hairy tongue
Coated tongue
Hypertrophy of foliate papillae
Lingua villosa nigra

K14.4 Atrophy of tongue papillae
Atrophic glossitis

K14.5 Plicated tongue
Fissured tongue
Furrowed tongue
Scrotal tongue
Excludes1 fissured tongue, congenital (Q38.3)

● Unacceptable Principal Diagnosis   ● Use Additional Character(s)   ■ Unspecified   ▶ Manifestation Code
OGCR Official Guidelines for Coding and Reporting   Excludes 1   Excludes 2   Includes   Use additional   Code first   Code also

K14.6 Glossodynia
　　Glossopyrosis
　　Painful tongue

K14.8 Other diseases of tongue
　　Atrophy of tongue
　　Crenated tongue
　　Enlargement of tongue
　　Glossocele
　　Glossoptosis
　　Hypertrophy of tongue

K14.9 Disease of tongue, unspecified
　　Glossopathy NOS

DISEASES OF ESOPHAGUS, STOMACH AND DUODENUM (K20-K31)

> **Excludes2**　hiatus hernia (K44.-)

K20 Esophagitis
> Use additional code to identify:
> alcohol abuse and dependence (F10.-)
>
> **Excludes1**　erosion of esophagus (K22.1-)
> esophagitis with gastro-esophageal reflux
>   disease (K21.0)
> reflux esophagitis (K21.0)
> ulcerative esophagitis (K22.1-)
>
> **Excludes2**　eosinophilic gastritis or gastroenteritis
>   (K52.81)

K20.0 Eosinophilic esophagitis

K20.8 Other esophagitis
　　Abscess of esophagus

K20.9 Esophagitis, unspecified
　　Esophagitis NOS

K21 Gastro-esophageal reflux disease
> **Excludes1**　newborn esophageal reflux (P78.83)

K21.0 Gastro-esophageal reflux disease with esophagitis
　　Reflux esophagitis

K21.9 Gastro-esophageal reflux disease without esophagitis
　　Esophageal reflux NOS

K22 Other diseases of esophagus
> **Excludes2**　esophageal varices (I85.-)

K22.0 Achalasia of cardia
　　Achalasia NOS
　　Cardiospasm
> **Excludes1**　congenital cardiospasm (Q39.5)

K22.1 Ulcer of esophagus
　　Barrett's ulcer
　　Erosion of esophagus
　　Fungal ulcer of esophagus
　　Peptic ulcer of esophagus
　　Ulcer of esophagus due to ingestion of chemicals
　　Ulcer of esophagus due to ingestion of drugs and
　　　medicaments
　　Ulcerative esophagitis
> *Code first* poisoning due to drug or toxin, if applicable
>   (T36-T65 with fifth or sixth character 1-4 or 6)
> Use additional code for adverse effect, if
>   applicable, to identify drug (T36-T50 with
>   fifth or sixth character 5)
> **Excludes1**　Barrett's esophagus (K22.87-)

K22.10 Ulcer of esophagus without bleeding 🦠
　　Ulcer of esophagus NOS

K22.11 Ulcer of esophagus with bleeding 🦠
> **Excludes2**　bleeding esophageal varices
>   (I85.01, I85.11)

Item 11-6 Esophageal reflux is the return flow of the contents of the stomach to the esophagus and is referred to as GERD and/or "heartburn." **Gastroesophageal reflux** is the return flow of the contents of the stomach and duodenum to the esophagus. **Esophageal leukoplakia** are white areas on the mucous membrane of the esophagus for which no specific cause can be identified.

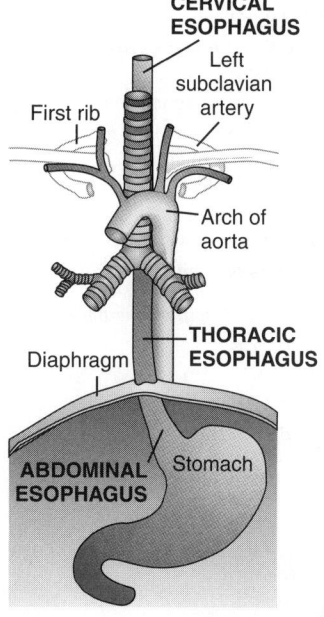

Figure 11-6 The esophagus is the muscular tube that connects the pharynx and the stomach. The 10 inch (25 cm) long esophagus is divided into three parts: cervical, thoracic, and abdominal.

K22.2 Esophageal obstruction
　　Compression of esophagus
　　Constriction of esophagus
　　Stenosis of esophagus
　　Stricture of esophagus
> **Excludes1**　congenital stenosis or stricture of
>   esophagus (Q39.3)

K22.3 Perforation of esophagus 🦠
　　Rupture of esophagus
> **Excludes1**　traumatic perforation of (thoracic)
>   esophagus (S27.8-)

K22.4 Dyskinesia of esophagus
　　Difficulty in moving
　　Corkscrew esophagus
　　Diffuse esophageal spasm
　　Spasm of esophagus
> **Excludes1**　cardiospasm (K22.0)

K22.5 Diverticulum of esophagus, acquired
　　Esophageal pouch, acquired
> **Excludes1**　diverticulum of esophagus
>   (congenital) (Q39.6)

K22.6 Gastro-esophageal laceration-hemorrhage syndrome 🦠
　　Mallory-Weiss syndrome

K22.7 Barrett's esophagus
　　Barrett's disease
　　Barrett's syndrome
> **Excludes1**　Barrett's ulcer (K22.1)
>   malignant neoplasm of esophagus
>   (C15.-)

K22.70 Barrett's esophagus without dysplasia
　　Barrett's esophagus NOS

CHAPTER 11 (K00-K95)

N Newborn Age: 0   **P** Pediatric Age: 0–17   **M** Maternity DX: 12–55   **A** Adult Age: 15–124   ♀ Females Only   ♂ Males Only
🦠 Complication\Comorbidity   🦠 Major C\C   🦠 Present on Admission Requirement   🦠 Hospital-Acquired Condition

1095

Item 11-7 Achalasia is a condition in which the smooth muscle fibers of the esophagus do not relax. Most frequently, this condition occurs at the esophagogastric sphincter. **Cardiospasm,** also known as **megaesophagus,** is achalasia of the thoracic esophagus.

- **K22.71 Barrett's esophagus with dysplasia**
  - K22.710 Barrett's esophagus with low grade dysplasia
  - K22.711 Barrett's esophagus with high grade dysplasia
  - K22.719 Barrett's esophagus with dysplasia, unspecified
- **K22.8 Other specified diseases of esophagus**
  Hemorrhage of esophagus NOS
  - **Excludes2** esophageal varices (I85.-)
  Paterson-Kelly syndrome (D50.1)
- **K22.9 Disease of esophagus, unspecified**

- **K23 Disorders of esophagus in diseases classified elsewhere**
  Code first underlying disease, such as:
  congenital syphilis (A50.5)
  - **Excludes1** late syphilis (A52.79)
  megaesophagus due to Chagas' disease (B57.31)
  tuberculosis (A18.83)

- **K25 Gastric ulcer**
  - **Includes** erosion (acute) of stomach
  pylorus ulcer (peptic)
  stomach ulcer (peptic)
  - **Use additional** code to identify:
  alcohol abuse and dependence (F10.-)
  - **Excludes1** acute gastritis (K29.0-)
  peptic ulcer NOS (K27.-)
  - K25.0 Acute gastric ulcer with hemorrhage
  - K25.1 Acute gastric ulcer with perforation
  - K25.2 Acute gastric ulcer with both hemorrhage and perforation
  - K25.3 Acute gastric ulcer without hemorrhage or perforation
  - K25.4 Chronic or unspecified gastric ulcer with hemorrhage
  - K25.5 Chronic or unspecified gastric ulcer with perforation
  - K25.6 Chronic or unspecified gastric ulcer with both hemorrhage and perforation
  - K25.7 Chronic gastric ulcer without hemorrhage or perforation
  - K25.9 Gastric ulcer, unspecified as acute or chronic, without hemorrhage or perforation

- **K26 Duodenal ulcer**
  - **Includes** erosion (acute) of duodenum
  duodenum ulcer (peptic)
  postpyloric ulcer (peptic)
  - **Use additional** code to identify:
  alcohol abuse and dependence (F10.-)
  - **Excludes1** peptic ulcer NOS (K27.-)
  - K26.0 Acute duodenal ulcer with hemorrhage
  - K26.1 Acute duodenal ulcer with perforation
  - K26.2 Acute duodenal ulcer with both hemorrhage and perforation
  - K26.3 Acute duodenal ulcer without hemorrhage or perforation

Figure 11-7 A. Ulcer. **B.** Perforated ulcer. **C.** Laparoscopic view of a perforated duodenal ulcer *(arrow)* with fibrinous exudate on the adjacent peritoneum. (**C** from Feldman: Sleisenger & Fordtran's Gastrointestinal and Liver Disease, 8th ed. 2006, Saunders, An Imprint of Elsevier.)

Item 11-8 Gastric ulcers are lesions of the stomach that result in the death of the tissue and a defect of the surface. **Perforated ulcers** are those in which the lesion penetrates the gastric wall, leaving a hole. **Peptic ulcers** are lesions of the stomach or the duodenum. **Peptic** refers to the gastric juice, pepsin.

- K26.4 Chronic or unspecified duodenal ulcer with hemorrhage
- K26.5 Chronic or unspecified duodenal ulcer with perforation
- K26.6 Chronic or unspecified duodenal ulcer with both hemorrhage and perforation
- K26.7 Chronic duodenal ulcer without hemorrhage or perforation
- K26.9 Duodenal ulcer, unspecified as acute or chronic, without hemorrhage or perforation

- **K27 Peptic ulcer, site unspecified**
  - **Includes** gastroduodenal ulcer NOS
  peptic ulcer NOS
  - **Use additional** code to identify:
  alcohol abuse and dependence (F10.-)
  - **Excludes1** peptic ulcer of newborn (P78.82)
  - K27.0 Acute peptic ulcer, site unspecified, with hemorrhage
  - K27.1 Acute peptic ulcer, site unspecified, with perforation
  - K27.2 Acute peptic ulcer, site unspecified, with both hemorrhage and perforation
  - K27.3 Acute peptic ulcer, site unspecified, without hemorrhage or perforation
  - K27.4 Chronic or unspecified peptic ulcer, site unspecified, with hemorrhage
  - K27.5 Chronic or unspecified peptic ulcer, site unspecified, with perforation
  - K27.6 Chronic or unspecified peptic ulcer, site unspecified, with both hemorrhage and perforation
  - K27.7 Chronic peptic ulcer, site unspecified, without hemorrhage or perforation
  - K27.9 Peptic ulcer, site unspecified, unspecified as acute or chronic, without hemorrhage or perforation

● Unacceptable Principal Diagnosis   ● Use Additional Character(s)   ■ Unspecified   ▶ Manifestation Code
OGCR Official Guidelines for Coding and Reporting   Excludes 1   Excludes 2   Includes   Use additional   Code first   Code also

● **K28   Gastrojejunal ulcer**

     Includes   anastomotic ulcer (peptic) or erosion
                     gastrocolic ulcer (peptic) or erosion
                     gastrointestinal ulcer (peptic) or erosion
                     gastrojejunal ulcer (peptic) or erosion
                     jejunal ulcer (peptic) or erosion
                     marginal ulcer (peptic) or erosion
                     stomal ulcer (peptic) or erosion

     Use additional code to identify:
         alcohol abuse and dependence (F10.-)

     Excludes1   primary ulcer of small intestine (K63.3)

     K28.0   Acute gastrojejunal ulcer with hemorrhage 🦠

     K28.1   Acute gastrojejunal ulcer with perforation 🦠

     K28.2   Acute gastrojejunal ulcer with both hemorrhage and perforation 🦠

     ■ **K28.3   Acute gastrojejunal ulcer without hemorrhage or perforation** 🦠

     ■ **K28.4   Chronic or unspecified gastrojejunal ulcer with hemorrhage** 🦠

     ■ **K28.5   Chronic or unspecified gastrojejunal ulcer with perforation** 🦠

     K28.6   Chronic or unspecified gastrojejunal ulcer with both hemorrhage and perforation 🦠

     K28.7   Chronic gastrojejunal ulcer without hemorrhage or perforation

     ■ **K28.9   Gastrojejunal ulcer, unspecified as acute or chronic, without hemorrhage or perforation**

● **K29   Gastritis and duodenitis**

     Excludes1   eosinophilic gastritis or gastroenteritis (K52.81)
                    Zollinger-Ellison syndrome (E16.4)

     ● **K29.0   Acute gastritis**

         Use additional code to identify:
             alcohol abuse and dependence (F10.-)

         Excludes1   erosion (acute) of stomach (K25.-)

         K29.00   Acute gastritis without bleeding

         K29.01   Acute gastritis with bleeding 🦠

     ● **K29.2   Alcoholic gastritis**

         Use additional code to identify:
             alcohol abuse and dependence (F10.-)

         K29.20   Alcoholic gastritis without bleeding

         K29.21   Alcoholic gastritis with bleeding 🦠

     ● **K29.3   Chronic superficial gastritis**

         K29.30   Chronic superficial gastritis without bleeding

         K29.31   Chronic superficial gastritis with bleeding 🦠

     ● **K29.4   Chronic atrophic gastritis**
         Gastric atrophy

         K29.40   Chronic atrophic gastritis without bleeding

         K29.41   Chronic atrophic gastritis with bleeding 🦠

     ● **K29.5   Unspecified chronic gastritis**
         Chronic antral gastritis
         Chronic fundal gastritis

         ■ **K29.50   Unspecified chronic gastritis without bleeding**

         ■ **K29.51   Unspecified chronic gastritis with bleeding** 🦠

Item 11–9   Gastritis is a severe inflammation of the stomach. **Atrophic gastritis** is a chronic inflammation of the stomach that results in destruction of the cells of the mucosa of the stomach. Duodenitis is an inflammation of the duodenum, the first section of the small intestine.

     ● **K29.6   Other gastritis**
         Giant hypertrophic gastritis
         Granulomatous gastritis
         Ménétrier's disease

         K29.60   Other gastritis without bleeding

         K29.61   Other gastritis with bleeding 🦠

     ● **K29.7   Gastritis, unspecified**

         ■ **K29.70   Gastritis, unspecified, without bleeding**

         ■ **K29.71   Gastritis, unspecified, with bleeding** 🦠

     ● **K29.8   Duodenitis**

         K29.80   Duodenitis without bleeding

         K29.81   Duodenitis with bleeding 🦠

     ● **K29.9   Gastroduodenitis, unspecified**

         ■ **K29.90   Gastroduodenitis, unspecified, without bleeding**

         ■ **K29.91   Gastroduodenitis, unspecified, with bleeding** 🦠

K30   Functional dyspepsia
     Indigestion

     Excludes1   dyspepsia NOS (R10.13)
                heartburn (R12)
                nervous dyspepsia (F45.8)
                neurotic dyspepsia (F45.8)
                psychogenic dyspepsia (F45.8)

● **K31   Other diseases of stomach and duodenum**
     Includes   functional disorders of stomach

     Excludes2   diabetic gastroparesis (E08.43, E09.43, E10.43, E11.43, E13.43)
                diverticulum of duodenum (K57.00-K57.13)

     K31.0   Acute dilatation of stomach 🦠
         Acute distention of stomach

     K31.1   Adult hypertrophic pyloric stenosis 🦠   **A**
         Pyloric stenosis NOS

         Excludes1   congenital or infantile pyloric stenosis (Q40.0)

     K31.2   Hourglass stricture and stenosis of stomach

         Excludes1   congenital hourglass stomach (Q40.2)
                hourglass contraction of stomach (K31.89)

     K31.3   Pylorospasm, not elsewhere classified

         Excludes1   congenital or infantile pylorospasm (Q40.0)
                neurotic pylorospasm (F45.8)
                psychogenic pylorospasm (F45.8)

     K31.4   Gastric diverticulum

         Excludes1   congenital diverticulum of stomach (Q40.2)

     K31.5   Obstruction of duodenum 🦠
         Constriction of duodenum
         Duodenal ileus (chronic)
         Stenosis of duodenum
           Narrowing
         Stricture of duodenum
           Narrowing
         Volvulus of duodenum
           Twisting/knotting

         Excludes1   congenital stenosis of duodenum (Q41.0)

N Newborn Age: 0   **P** Pediatric Age: 0–17   **M** Maternity DX: 12–55   **A** Adult Age: 15–124   ♀ Females Only   ♂ Males Only
🦠 Complication\Comorbidity   🦠 Major C\C   🦠 Present on Admission Requirement   🦠 Hospital-Acquired Condition
1097

Item 11–10 **Achlorhydria,** also known as gastric anacidity, is the absence of gastric acid.

K31.6 **Fistula of stomach and duodenum** 🔗
    Gastrocolic fistula
    Gastrojejunocolic fistula

K31.7 **Polyp of stomach and duodenum**
    Excludes1   adenomatous polyp of stomach (D13.1)

● **K31.8** **Other specified diseases of stomach and duodenum**

  ● **K31.81** **Angiodysplasia of stomach and duodenum**

    K31.811 **Angiodysplasia of stomach and duodenum with bleeding** 🔗

    K31.819 **Angiodysplasia of stomach and duodenum without bleeding**
        Angiodysplasia of stomach and duodenum NOS

  K31.82 **Dieulafoy lesion (hemorrhagic) of stomach and duodenum** 🔗
    Excludes2   Dieulafoy lesion of intestine (K63.81)

  K31.83 **Achlorhydria**

  K31.84 **Gastroparesis**
    Gastroparalysis
    Code first underlying disease, if known, such as:
      anorexia nervosa (F50.0-)
      diabetes mellitus (E08.43, E09.43, E10.43, E11.43, E13.43)
      scleroderma (M34.-)

  K31.89 **Other diseases of stomach and duodenum**

■ **K31.9** **Disease of stomach and duodenum, unspecified**

DISEASES OF APPENDIX (K35-K38)

● **K35** **Acute appendicitis**

  K35.2 **Acute appendicitis with generalized peritonitis** 🔗
    Appendicitis (acute) with generalized (diffuse) peritonitis following rupture or perforation of appendix
    Appendicitis with peritonitis NOS
    Perforated appendix NOS
    Ruptured appendix NOS

  K35.3 **Acute appendicitis with localized peritonitis** 🔗
    Acute appendicitis with localized peritonitis with or without rupture or perforation of appendix
    Acute appendicitis with peritoneal abscess

  ● **K35.8** **Other and unspecified acute appendicitis**

    ■ **K35.80** **Unspecified acute appendicitis** 🔗
      Acute appendicitis NOS
      Acute appendicitis without (localized) (generalized) peritonitis

    K35.89 **Other acute appendicitis** 🔗

K36 **Other appendicitis**
  Chronic appendicitis
  Recurrent appendicitis

■ **K37** **Unspecified appendicitis**
  Excludes1 -unspecified appendicitis with peritonitis (K35.2-K35.3)

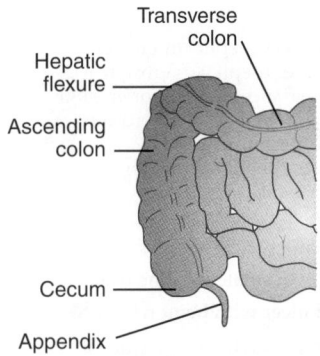

Figure 11-8 Acute appendicitis is the inflammation of the appendix, usually associated with obstruction. Most often this is a disease of adolescents and young adults.

Transverse colon
Hepatic flexure
Ascending colon
Cecum
Appendix

● **K38** **Other diseases of appendix**

  K38.0 **Hyperplasia of appendix**

  K38.1 **Appendicular concretions**
    Fecalith of appendix
    Stercolith of appendix

  K38.2 **Diverticulum of appendix**

  K38.3 **Fistula of appendix**

  K38.8 **Other specified diseases of appendix**
    Intussusception of appendix

■ **K38.9** **Disease of appendix, unspecified**

HERNIA (K40-K46)

Note: Hernia with both gangrene and obstruction is classified to hernia with gangrene.

  Includes acquired hernia
    congenital [except diaphragmatic or hiatus] hernia
    recurrent hernia

● **K40** **Inguinal hernia**
  Includes bubonocele
    direct inguinal hernia
    double inguinal hernia
    indirect inguinal hernia
    inguinal hernia NOS
    oblique inguinal hernia
    scrotal hernia

● **K40.0** **Bilateral inguinal hernia, with obstruction, without gangrene**
  Inguinal hernia (bilateral) causing obstruction without gangrene
  Incarcerated inguinal hernia (bilateral) without gangrene
  Irreducible inguinal hernia (bilateral) without gangrene
  Strangulated inguinal hernia (bilateral) without gangrene

  K40.00 **Bilateral inguinal hernia, with obstruction, without gangrene, not specified as recurrent** 🔗
    Bilateral inguinal hernia, with obstruction, without gangrene NOS

  K40.01 **Bilateral inguinal hernia, with obstruction, without gangrene, recurrent** 🔗

● **K40.1** **Bilateral inguinal hernia, with gangrene**

  K40.10 **Bilateral inguinal hernia, with gangrene, not specified as recurrent** 🔗
    Bilateral inguinal hernia, with gangrene NOS

  K40.11 **Bilateral inguinal hernia, with gangrene, recurrent** 🔗

● Unacceptable Principal Diagnosis   ● Use Additional Character(s)   ■ Unspecified   ▶ Manifestation Code

1098   **OGCR** Official Guidelines for Coding and Reporting   Excludes 1 Excludes 2 Includes Use additional Code first Code also

Item 11-11 Hernias of the groin are the most common type, accounting for 80 percent of all hernias. There are two major types of inguinal hernias: indirect (oblique) affecting men only and direct. **Indirect inguinal hernias** result when the intestines emerge through the abdominal wall in an indirect fashion through the inguinal canal. **Direct inguinal hernias** penetrate through the abdominal wall in a direct fashion. **Femoral hernias** occur at the femoral ring where the femoral vessels enter the thigh and is most common in women. An abdominal wall hernia is also called a ventral or epigastric hernia and occurs in both sexes. Classification is based on location of the hernia and whether there is obstruction or gangrene.

Ventral, epigastric, or incisional hernia occurs on the abdominal surface caused by musculature weakness or a tear at a previous surgical site and is evidenced by a bulge that changes in size, becoming larger with exertion. An **incarcerated** hernia is one in which the intestines become trapped in the hernia. A **strangulated** hernia is one in which the blood supply to the intestines is lost. Hiatal hernia occurs when a loop of the stomach protrudes upward through the small opening in the diaphragm through which the esophagus passes, leaving the abdominal cavity and entering the chest. It occurs in both sexes.

- **K40.2 Bilateral inguinal hernia, without obstruction or gangrene**
    - **K40.20 Bilateral inguinal hernia, without obstruction or gangrene, not specified as recurrent**
        Bilateral inguinal hernia NOS
    - **K40.21 Bilateral inguinal hernia, without obstruction or gangrene, recurrent**
- **K40.3 Unilateral inguinal hernia, with obstruction, without gangrene**
    Inguinal hernia (unilateral) causing obstruction without gangrene
    Incarcerated inguinal hernia (unilateral) without gangrene
    Irreducible inguinal hernia (unilateral) without gangrene
    Strangulated inguinal hernia (unilateral) without gangrene
    - **K40.30 Unilateral inguinal hernia, with obstruction, without gangrene, not specified as recurrent**
        Inguinal hernia, with obstruction NOS
        Unilateral inguinal hernia, with obstruction, without gangrene NOS
    - **K40.31 Unilateral inguinal hernia, with obstruction, without gangrene, recurrent**
- **K40.4 Unilateral inguinal hernia, with gangrene**
    - **K40.40 Unilateral inguinal hernia, with gangrene, not specified as recurrent**
        Inguinal hernia with gangrene NOS
        Unilateral inguinal hernia with gangrene NOS
    - **K40.41 Unilateral inguinal hernia, with gangrene, recurrent**
- **K40.9 Unilateral inguinal hernia, without obstruction or gangrene**
    - **K40.90 Unilateral inguinal hernia, without obstruction or gangrene, not specified as recurrent**
        Inguinal hernia NOS
        Unilateral inguinal hernia NOS
    - **K40.91 Unilateral inguinal hernia, without obstruction or gangrene, recurrent**

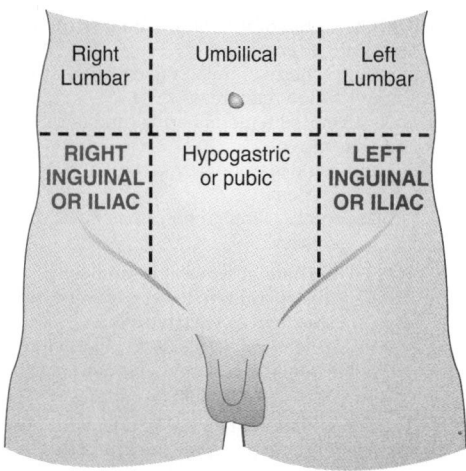

Figure 11-9 Inguinal hernias are those are located in the inguinal or iliac areas of the abdomen.

- **K41 Femoral hernia**
    - **K41.0 Bilateral femoral hernia, with obstruction, without gangrene**
        Femoral hernia (bilateral) causing obstruction, without gangrene
        Incarcerated femoral hernia (bilateral), without gangrene
        Irreducible femoral hernia (bilateral), without gangrene
        Strangulated femoral hernia (bilateral), without gangrene
        - **K41.00 Bilateral femoral hernia, with obstruction, without gangrene, not specified as recurrent**
            Bilateral femoral hernia, with obstruction, without gangrene NOS
        - **K41.01 Bilateral femoral hernia, with obstruction, without gangrene, recurrent**
    - **K41.1 Bilateral femoral hernia, with gangrene**
        - **K41.10 Bilateral femoral hernia, with gangrene, not specified as recurrent**
            Bilateral femoral hernia, with gangrene NOS
        - **K41.11 Bilateral femoral hernia, with gangrene, recurrent**
    - **K41.2 Bilateral femoral hernia, without obstruction or gangrene**
        - **K41.20 Bilateral femoral hernia, without obstruction or gangrene, not specified as recurrent**
            Bilateral femoral hernia NOS
        - **K41.21 Bilateral femoral hernia, without obstruction or gangrene, recurrent**

CHAPTER 11 (K00-K95)

● **K41.3 Unilateral femoral hernia, with obstruction, without gangrene**
Femoral hernia (unilateral) causing obstruction, without gangrene
Incarcerated femoral hernia (unilateral), without gangrene
Irreducible femoral hernia (unilateral), without gangrene
Strangulated femoral hernia (unilateral), without gangrene

  K41.30 Unilateral femoral hernia, with obstruction, without gangrene, not specified as recurrent 🔊
Femoral hernia, with obstruction NOS
Unilateral femoral hernia, with obstruction NOS

  K41.31 Unilateral femoral hernia, with obstruction, without gangrene, recurrent 🔊

● **K41.4 Unilateral femoral hernia, with gangrene**

  K41.40 Unilateral femoral hernia, with gangrene, not specified as recurrent 🔊
Femoral hernia, with gangrene NOS
Unilateral femoral hernia, with gangrene NOS

  K41.41 Unilateral femoral hernia, with gangrene, recurrent 🔊

● **K41.9 Unilateral femoral hernia, without obstruction or gangrene**

  K41.90 Unilateral femoral hernia, without obstruction or gangrene, not specified as recurrent
Femoral hernia NOS
Unilateral femoral hernia NOS

  K41.91 Unilateral femoral hernia, without obstruction or gangrene, recurrent

● **K42 Umbilical hernia**
| **Includes** | paraumbilical hernia |

| **Excludes1** | omphalocele (Q79.2) |

  K42.0 Umbilical hernia with obstruction, without gangrene 🔊
Umbilical hernia causing obstruction, without gangrene
Incarcerated umbilical hernia, without gangrene
Irreducible umbilical hernia, without gangrene
Strangulated umbilical hernia, without gangrene

  K42.1 Umbilical hernia with gangrene 🔊
Gangrenous umbilical hernia

  K42.9 Umbilical hernia without obstruction or gangrene
Umbilical hernia NOS

● **K43 Ventral hernia**

  K43.0 Incisional hernia with obstruction, without gangrene 🔊
Incisional hernia causing obstruction, without gangrene
Incarcerated incisional hernia, without gangrene
Irreducible incisional hernia, without gangrene
Strangulated incisional hernia, without gangrene

  K43.1 Incisional hernia with gangrene 🔊
Gangrenous incisional hernia

  K43.2 Incisional hernia without obstruction or gangrene
Incisional hernia NOS

K43.3 Parastomal hernia with obstruction, without gangrene
Incarcerated parastomal hernia, without gangrene
Irreducible parastomal hernia, without gangrene
Parastomal hernia causing obstruction, without gangrene
Strangulated parastomal hernia, without gangrene

K43.4 Parastomal hernia with gangrene
Gangrenous parastomal hernia

K43.5 Parastomal hernia without obstruction or gangrene
Parastomal hernia NOS

K43.6 Other and unspecified ventral hernia with obstruction, without gangrene
Epigastric hernia causing obstruction, without gangrene
Hypogastric hernia causing obstruction, without gangrene
Incarcerated epigastric hernia without gangrene
Incarcerated hypogastric hernia without gangrene
Incarcerated midline hernia without gangrene
Incarcerated spigelian hernia without gangrene
Incarcerated subxiphoid hernia without gangrene
Irreducible epigastric hernia without gangrene
Irreducible hypogastric hernia without gangrene
Irreducible midline hernia without gangrene
Irreducible spigelian hernia without gangrene
Irreducible subxiphoid hernia without gangrene
Midline hernia causing obstruction, without gangrene
Spigelian hernia causing obstruction, without gangrene
Strangulated epigastric hernia without gangrene
Strangulated hypogastric hernia without gangrene
Strangulated midline hernia without gangrene
Strangulated spigelian hernia without gangrene
Strangulated subxiphoid hernia without gangrene
Subxiphoid hernia causing obstruction, without gangrene

K43.7 Other and unspecified ventral hernia with gangrene
Any condition listed under K43.6 specified as gangrenous

K43.9 Ventral hernia without obstruction or gangrene
Epigastric hernia
Ventral hernia NOS

● **K44 Diaphragmatic hernia**
| **Includes** | hiatus hernia (esophageal) (sliding) paraesophageal hernia |

| **Excludes1** | congenital diaphragmatic hernia (Q79.0) congenital hiatus hernia (Q40.1) |

K44.0 Diaphragmatic hernia with obstruction, without gangrene 🔊
Diaphragmatic hernia causing obstruction
Incarcerated diaphragmatic hernia
Irreducible diaphragmatic hernia
Strangulated diaphragmatic hernia

K44.1 Diaphragmatic hernia with gangrene 🔊
Gangrenous diaphragmatic hernia

K44.9 Diaphragmatic hernia without obstruction or gangrene
Diaphragmatic hernia NOS

● Unacceptable Principal Diagnosis   ● Use Additional Character(s)   ■ Unspecified   ▶ Manifestation Code
OGCR Official Guidelines for Coding and Reporting   Excludes 1   Excludes 2   Includes   Use additional   Code first   Code also

CHAPTER 11 (K00-K95)

● **K45** **Other abdominal hernia**

> **Includes** abdominal hernia, specified site NEC
> lumbar hernia
> obturator hernia
> pudendal hernia
> retroperitoneal hernia
> sciatic hernia

  K45.0 **Other specified abdominal hernia with obstruction, without gangrene** 🦠
> Other specified abdominal hernia causing obstruction
> Other specified incarcerated abdominal hernia
> Other specified irreducible abdominal hernia
> Other specified strangulated abdominal hernia

  K45.1 **Other specified abdominal hernia with gangrene** 🦠
> Any condition listed under K45 specified as gangrenous

  K45.8 **Other specified abdominal hernia without obstruction or gangrene**

● **K46** **Unspecified abdominal hernia**

> **Includes** enterocele
> epiplocele
> hernia NOS
> interstitial hernia
> intestinal hernia
> intra-abdominal hernia

> **Excludes1** vaginal enterocele (N81.5)

  ■ **K46.0** **Unspecified abdominal hernia with obstruction, without gangrene** 🦠
> Unspecified abdominal hernia causing obstruction
> Unspecified incarcerated abdominal hernia
> Unspecified irreducible abdominal hernia
> Unspecified strangulated abdominal hernia

  ■ **K46.1** **Unspecified abdominal hernia with gangrene** 🦠
> Any condition listed under K46 specified as gangrenous

  ■ **K46.9** **Unspecified abdominal hernia without obstruction or gangrene**
> Abdominal hernia NOS

(See Plate 284 on page NAP-29.)

NONINFECTIVE ENTERITIS AND COLITIS (K50-K52)

> **Includes** noninfective inflammatory bowel disease
> **Excludes1** irritable bowel syndrome (K58.-)
> megacolon (K59.3)

● **K50** **Crohn's disease [regional enteritis]**

> **Includes** granulomatous enteritis

> **Use additional** code to identify manifestations, such as:
> pyoderma gangrenosum (L88)

> **Excludes1** ulcerative colitis (K51.-)

  ● **K50.0** **Crohn's disease of small intestine**
> Crohn's disease [regional enteritis] of duodenum
> Crohn's disease [regional enteritis] of ileum
> Crohn's disease [regional enteritis] of jejunum
> Regional ileitis
> Terminal ileitis

> > **Excludes1** Crohn's disease of both small and large intestine (K50.8-)

    K50.00 **Crohn's disease of small intestine without complications** 🦠

Item 11–12 **Crohn's disease,** also known as **regional enteritis,** is a chronic inflammatory disease of the intestines. Classification is based on location in the small (duodenum, ileum, jejunum) or large (cecum, colon, rectum, anal canal) intestine.

  ● **K50.01** **Crohn's disease of small intestine with complications**

    K50.011 **Crohn's disease of small intestine with rectal bleeding** 🦠

    K50.012 **Crohn's disease of small intestine with intestinal obstruction** 🦠
> MCC: Only when the principal diagnosis is designated as a CC

    K50.013 **Crohn's disease of small intestine with fistula** 🦠
> MCC: Only when the principal diagnosis is designated as a CC

    K50.014 **Crohn's disease of small intestine with abscess** 🦠
> MCC: Only when the principal diagnosis is designated as a CC

    K50.018 **Crohn's disease of small intestine with other complication** 🦠

    ■ **K50.019** **Crohn's disease of small intestine with unspecified complications** 🦠

  ● **K50.1** **Crohn's disease of large intestine**
> Crohn's disease [regional enteritis] of colon
> Crohn's disease [regional enteritis] of large bowel
> Crohn's disease [regional enteritis] of rectum
> Granulomatous colitis
> Regional colitis

> > **Excludes1** Crohn's disease of both small and large intestine (K50.8)

    K50.10 **Crohn's disease of large intestine without complications** 🦠

  ● **K50.11** **Crohn's disease of large intestine with complications**

    K50.111 **Crohn's disease of large intestine with rectal bleeding** 🦠

    K50.112 **Crohn's disease of large intestine with intestinal obstruction** 🦠
> MCC: Only when the principal diagnosis is designated as a CC

    K50.113 **Crohn's disease of large intestine with fistula** 🦠
> MCC: Only when the principal diagnosis is designated as a CC

    K50.114 **Crohn's disease of large intestine with abscess** 🦠
> MCC: Only when the principal diagnosis is designated as a CC

    K50.118 **Crohn's disease of large intestine with other complication** 🦠

    ■ **K50.119** **Crohn's disease of large intestine with unspecified complications** 🦠

CHAPTER 11 (K00-K95)

CHAPTER 11 (K00-K95)

● **K50.8**   Crohn's disease of both small and large intestine

    K50.80   Crohn's disease of both small and large intestine without complications ✪

● **K50.81**   Crohn's disease of both small and large intestine with complications

        K50.811 Crohn's disease of both small and large intestine with rectal bleeding ✪

        K50.812 Crohn's disease of both small and large intestine with intestinal obstruction ✪
            MCC: Only when the principal diagnosis is designated as a CC

        K50.813 Crohn's disease of both small and large intestine with fistula ✪
            MCC: Only when the principal diagnosis is designated as a CC

        K50.814 Crohn's disease of both small and large intestine with abscess ✪
            MCC: Only when the principal diagnosis is designated as a CC

        K50.818 Crohn's disease of both small and large intestine with other complication ✪

       ■ **K50.819** Crohn's disease of both small and large intestine with unspecified complications ✪

● **K50.9**   Crohn's disease, unspecified

  ■ **K50.90**   Crohn's disease, unspecified, without complications ✪
        Crohn's disease NOS
        Regional enteritis NOS

● **K50.91**   Crohn's disease, unspecified, with complications

    ■ **K50.911** Crohn's disease, unspecified, with rectal bleeding ✪
            MCC: Only when the principal diagnosis is designated as a CC

    ■ **K50.912** Crohn's disease, unspecified, with intestinal obstruction ✪
            MCC: Only when the principal diagnosis is designated as a CC

    ■ **K50.913** Crohn's disease, unspecified, with fistula ✪
            MCC: Only when the principal diagnosis is designated as a CC

■ **K50.914** Crohn's disease, unspecified, with abscess ✪

■ **K50.918** Crohn's disease, unspecified, with other complication ✪

■ **K50.919** Crohn's disease, unspecified, with unspecified complications ✪

● **K51**   Ulcerative colitis

  Use additional code to identify manifestations, such as: pyoderma gangrenosum (L88)

  Excludes1   Crohn's disease [regional enteritis] (K50.-)

● **K51.0**   Ulcerative (chronic) pancolitis
    Backwash ileitis

    K51.00   Ulcerative (chronic) pancolitis without complications ✪
        Ulcerative (chronic) pancolitis NOS

● **K51.01**   Ulcerative (chronic) pancolitis with complications

        K51.011 Ulcerative (chronic) pancolitis with rectal bleeding ✪

        K51.012 Ulcerative (chronic) pancolitis with intestinal obstruction ✪
            MCC: Only when the principal diagnosis is designated as a CC

        K51.013 Ulcerative (chronic) pancolitis with fistula ✪
            MCC: Only when the principal diagnosis is designated as a CC

        K51.014 Ulcerative (chronic) pancolitis with abscess ✪
            MCC: Only when the principal diagnosis is designated as a CC

        K51.018 Ulcerative (chronic) pancolitis with other complication ✪

       ■ **K51.019** Ulcerative (chronic) pancolitis with unspecified complications ✪

● **K51.2**   Ulcerative (chronic) proctitis

    K51.20   Ulcerative (chronic) proctitis without complications ✪
        Ulcerative (chronic) proctitis NOS

● **K51.21**   Ulcerative (chronic) proctitis with complications

        K51.211 Ulcerative (chronic) proctitis with rectal bleeding ✪

        K51.212 Ulcerative (chronic) proctitis with intestinal obstruction ✪
            MCC: Only when the principal diagnosis is designated as a CC

        K51.213 Ulcerative (chronic) proctitis with fistula ✪
            MCC: Only when the principal diagnosis is designated as a CC

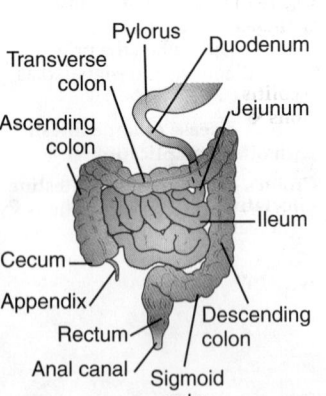

Figure 11-10 Small and large intestines.

Item 11–13 Ulcerative colitis attacks the colonic mucosa and forms abscesses. The disease involves the intestines. Classification is based on the location:

- Enterocolitis: large and small intestine
- Ileocolitis: ileum and colon
- Proctitis: rectum
- Proctosigmoiditis: sigmoid colon and rectum

  ● Unacceptable Principal Diagnosis   ● Use Additional Character(s)   ■ Unspecified   ▶ Manifestation Code

OGCR Official Guidelines for Coding and Reporting   Excludes 1   Excludes 2   Includes   Use additional   Code first   Code also

K51.214 **Ulcerative (chronic) proctitis with abstract abscess** 🦠
    MCC: Only when the principal diagnosis is designated as a CC

K51.218 **Ulcerative (chronic) proctitis with other complication** 🦠

▪ K51.219 **Ulcerative (chronic) proctitis with unspecified complications** 🦠

● K51.3 **Ulcerative (chronic) rectosigmoiditis**

K51.30 **Ulcerative (chronic) rectosigmoiditis without complications** 🦠
    Ulcerative (chronic) rectosigmoiditis NOS

● K51.31 **Ulcerative (chronic) rectosigmoiditis with complications**

K51.311 **Ulcerative (chronic) rectosigmoiditis with rectal bleeding** 🦠

K51.312 **Ulcerative (chronic) rectosigmoiditis with intestinal obstruction** 🦠
    MCC: Only when the principal diagnosis is designated as a CC

K51.313 **Ulcerative (chronic) rectosigmoiditis with fistula** 🦠
    MCC: Only when the principal diagnosis is designated as a CC

K51.314 **Ulcerative (chronic) rectosigmoiditis with abscess** 🦠
    MCC: Only when the principal diagnosis is designated as a CC

K51.318 **Ulcerative (chronic) rectosigmoiditis with other complication** 🦠

▪ K51.319 **Ulcerative (chronic) rectosigmoiditis with unspecified complications** 🦠

● K51.4 **Inflammatory polyps of colon**
    | Excludes1 | adenomatous polyp of colon (D12.6)
    polyposis of colon (D12.6)
    polyps of colon NOS (K63.5)

K51.40 **Inflammatory polyps of colon without complications** 🦠
    Inflammatory polyps of colon NOS

● K51.41 **Inflammatory polyps of colon with complications**

K51.411 **Inflammatory polyps of colon with rectal bleeding** 🦠

K51.412 **Inflammatory polyps of colon with intestinal obstruction** 🦠
    MCC: Only when the principal diagnosis is designated as a CC

K51.413 **Inflammatory polyps of colon with fistula** 🦠
    MCC: Only when the principal diagnosis is designated as a CC

K51.414 **Inflammatory polyps of colon with abscess** 🦠
    MCC: Only when the principal diagnosis is designated as a CC

K51.418 **Inflammatory polyps of colon with other complication** 🦠

▪ K51.419 **Inflammatory polyps of colon with unspecified complications** 🦠

● K51.5 **Left sided colitis**
    Left hemicolitis

K51.50 **Left sided colitis without complications** 🦠
    Left sided colitis NOS

● K51.51 **Left sided colitis with complications**

K51.511 **Left sided colitis with rectal bleeding** 🦠

K51.512 **Left sided colitis with intestinal obstruction** 🦠
    MCC: Only when the principal diagnosis is designated as a CC

K51.513 **Left sided colitis with fistula** 🦠
    MCC: Only when the principal diagnosis is designated as a CC

K51.514 **Left sided colitis with abscess** 🦠
    MCC: Only when the principal diagnosis is designated as a CC

K51.518 **Left sided colitis with other complication** 🦠

▪ K51.519 **Left sided colitis with unspecified complications** 🦠

● K51.8 **Other ulcerative colitis**

K51.80 **Other ulcerative colitis without complications** 🦠

● K51.81 **Other ulcerative colitis with complications**

K51.811 **Other ulcerative colitis with rectal bleeding** 🦠

K51.812 **Other ulcerative colitis with intestinal obstruction** 🦠
    MCC: Only when the principal diagnosis is designated as a CC

K51.813 **Other ulcerative colitis with fistula** 🦠
    MCC: Only when the principal diagnosis is designated as a CC

K51.814 **Other ulcerative colitis with abscess** 🦠
    MCC: Only when the principal diagnosis is designated as a CC

K51.818 **Other ulcerative colitis with other complication** 🦠

▪ K51.819 **Other ulcerative colitis with unspecified complications** 🦠

● K51.9 **Ulcerative colitis, unspecified**

▪ K51.90 **Ulcerative colitis, unspecified, without complications** 🦠

● K51.91 **Ulcerative colitis, unspecified, with complications**

▪ K51.911 **Ulcerative colitis, unspecified with rectal bleeding** 🦠

▪ K51.912 **Ulcerative colitis, unspecified with intestinal obstruction** 🦠
    MCC: Only when the principal diagnosis is designated as a CC

CHAPTER 11 (K00-K95)

N Newborn Age: 0   **P** Pediatric Age: 0–17   **M** Maternity DX: 12–55   **A** Adult Age: 15–124   ♀ Females Only   ♂ Males Only

🦠 Complication\Comorbidity   🦠 Major C\C   🦠 Present on Admission Requirement   🦠 Hospital-Acquired Condition

1103

■ **K51.913 Ulcerative colitis, unspecified with fistula** 🔗
     MCC: Only when the principal diagnosis is designated as a CC

■ **K51.914 Ulcerative colitis, unspecified with abscess** 🔗
     MCC: Only when the principal diagnosis is designated as a CC

■ **K51.918 Ulcerative colitis, unspecified with other complication** 🔗

■ **K51.919 Ulcerative colitis, unspecified with unspecified complications** 🔗

● **K52 Other and unspecified noninfective gastroenteritis and colitis**

   K52.0 Gastroenteritis and colitis due to radiation 🔗

● **K52.1 Toxic gastroenteritis and colitis** 🔗
     Drug-induced gastroenteritis and colitis
     Code first (T51-T65) *to identify toxic agent*
     Use additional code for adverse effect, if applicable, to identify drug (T36-T50 with fifth or sixth character 5)

   K52.2 Allergic and dietetic gastroenteritis and colitis
     Food hypersensitivity gastroenteritis or colitis
     Use additional code to identify type of food allergy (Z91.01-, Z91.02-)

● **K52.8 Other specified noninfective gastroenteritis and colitis**

   K52.81 Eosinophilic gastritis or gastroenteritis
     Eosinophilic enteritis
     | Excludes1 | eosinophilic esophagitis (K20.0)

   K52.82 Eosinophilic colitis

   K52.89 Other specified noninfective gastroenteritis and colitis
     Collagenous colitis
     Lymphocytic colitis
     Microscopic colitis (collagenous or lymphocytic)

■ **K52.9 Noninfective gastroenteritis and colitis, unspecified**
     Colitis NOS
     Enteritis NOS
     Gastroenteritis NOS
     Ileitis NOS
     Jejunitis NOS
     Sigmoiditis NOS
     | Excludes1 | diarrhea NOS (R19.7)
                   functional diarrhea (K59.1)
                    infectious gastroenteritis and colitis NOS (A09)
                    neonatal diarrhea (noninfective) (P78.3)
                    psychogenic diarrhea (F45.8)

OTHER DISEASES OF INTESTINES (K55-K64)

● **K55 Vascular disorders of intestine**
   | Excludes1 | necrotizing enterocolitis of newborn (P77.-)

   K55.0 Acute vascular disorders of intestine 🔗
     Acute fulminant ischemic colitis
     Acute intestinal infarction
     Acute small intestine ischemia
     Infarction of appendices epiploicae
     Mesenteric (artery) (vein) embolism
     Mesenteric (artery) (vein) infarction
     Mesenteric (artery) (vein) thrombosis
     Necrosis of intestine
     Subacute ischemic colitis

   K55.1 Chronic vascular disorders of intestine 🔗
     Chronic ischemic colitis
     Chronic ischemic enteritis
     Chronic ischemic enterocolitis
     Ischemic stricture of intestine
     Mesenteric atherosclerosis
     Mesenteric vascular insufficiency

● **K55.2 Angiodysplasia of colon**

   K55.20 Angiodysplasia of colon without hemorrhage

   K55.21 Angiodysplasia of colon with hemorrhage 🔗

   K55.8 Other vascular disorders of intestine 🔗

■ **K55.9 Vascular disorder of intestine, unspecified** 🔗
     Ischemic colitis
     Ischemic enteritis
     Ischemic enterocolitis

● **K56 Paralytic ileus and intestinal obstruction without hernia**
   | Excludes1 | congenital stricture or stenosis of intestine (Q41-Q42)
                cystic fibrosis with meconium ileus (E84.11)
                ischemic stricture of intestine (K55.1)
                meconium ileus NOS (P76.0)
                neonatal intestinal obstructions classifiable to P76.-
                obstruction of duodenum (K31.5)
                postprocedural intestinal obstruction (K91.3)
                stenosis of anus or rectum (K62.4)
                intestinal obstruction with hernia (K40-K46)

   K56.0 Paralytic ileus 🔗
     Paralysis of bowel
     Paralysis of colon
     Paralysis of intestine
     | Excludes1 | gallstone ileus (K56.3)
                 ileus NOS (K56.7)
                 obstructive ileus NOS (K56.69)

   K56.1 Intussusception 🔗
     Intussusception or invagination of bowel
     Intussusception or invagination of colon
     Intussusception or invagination of intestine
     Intussusception or invagination of rectum
     | Excludes2 | intussusception of appendix (K38.8)

   K56.2 Volvulus 🔗
     Strangulation of colon or intestine
     Torsion of colon or intestine
     Twist of colon or intestine
     | Excludes2 | volvulus of duodenum (K31.5)

Item 11–14 Intussusception is the prolapse (telescoping) of a part of the intestine into another adjacent part of the intestine. Intussusception may be enteric (ileoileal, jejunoileal, jejunojejunal), colic (colocolic), or intracolic (ileocecal, ileocolic).

● Unacceptable Principal Diagnosis   ● Use Additional Character(s)   ■ Unspecified   ▶ Manifestation Code
OGCR Official Guidelines for Coding and Reporting | Excludes 1 | | Excludes 2 | Includes   Use additional   Code first   Code also

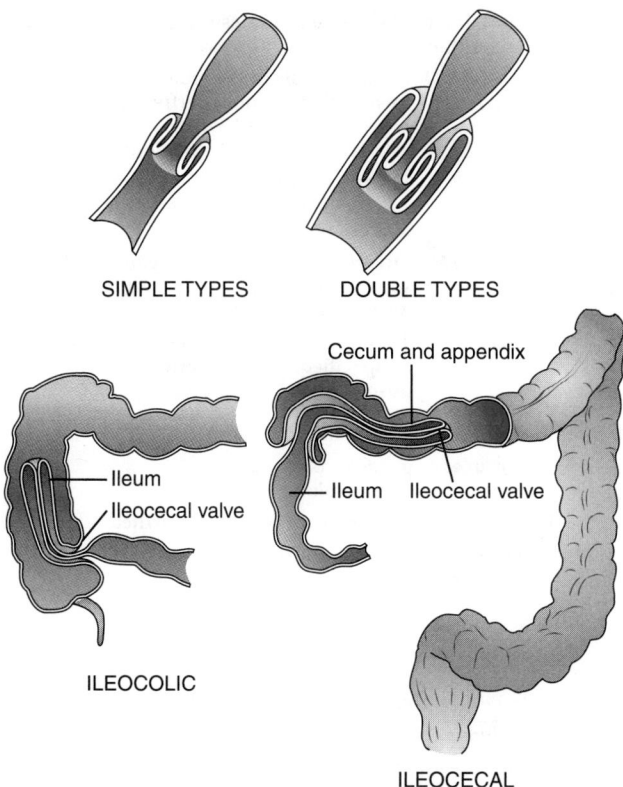

SIMPLE TYPES   DOUBLE TYPES

Cecum and appendix

Ileum
Ileocecal valve   Ileum   Ileocecal valve

ILEOCOLIC   ILEOCECAL

Figure 11-11 Types of intussusception.

Item 11–15 Volvulus is the twisting of a segment of the intestine, resulting in obstruction. Paralytic ileus is paralysis of the intestine. It need not be a complete paralysis, but it must prohibit the passage of food through the intestine and lead to intestinal blockage. It is a common aftermath of some types of surgery.

K56.3 Gallstone ileus 🦠
  Obstruction of intestine by gallstone

● **K56.4 Other impaction of intestine**

  K56.41 Fecal impaction
    Excludes1 constipation (K59.0-)
      incomplete defecation (R15.0)

  K56.49 Other impaction of intestine 🦠

K56.5 Intestinal adhesions [bands] with obstruction (postprocedural) (postinfection) 🦠
  Abdominal hernia due to adhesions with obstruction
  Peritoneal adhesions [bands] with intestinal obstruction (postprocedural) (postinfection)

● **K56.6 Other and unspecified intestinal obstruction**

  ◾ **K56.60 Unspecified intestinal obstruction**
    Intestinal obstruction NOS 🦠
    Excludes1 intestinal obstruction due to specified condition-code to condition

    K56.69 Other intestinal obstruction 🦠
      Enterostenosis NOS
      Obstructive ileus NOS
      Occlusion of colon or intestine NOS
      Stenosis of colon or intestine NOS
      Stricture of colon or intestine NOS
      Excludes1 intestinal obstruction due to specified condition-code to condition

  ◾ **K56.7 Ileus, unspecified** 🦠
    Excludes1 obstructive ileus (K56.69)

● **K57 Diverticular disease of intestine**
  Excludes1 congenital diverticulum of intestine (Q43.8)
    Meckel's diverticulum (Q43.0)
  Excludes2 diverticulum of appendix (K38.2)

● **K57.0 Diverticulitis of small intestine with perforation and abscess**
  Diverticulitis of small intestine with peritonitis
  Excludes1 diverticulitis of both small and large intestine with perforation and abscess (K57.4-)

  K57.00 Diverticulitis of small intestine with perforation and abscess without bleeding 🦠
    MCC: Only when the principal diagnosis is designated as a CC

  K57.01 Diverticulitis of small intestine with perforation and abscess with bleeding 🦠
    MCC: Only when the principal diagnosis is designated as a CC

● **K57.1 Diverticular disease of small intestine without perforation or abscess**
  Excludes1 diverticular disease of both small and large intestine without perforation or abscess (K57.5-)

  K57.10 Diverticulosis of small intestine without perforation or abscess without bleeding
    Diverticular disease of small intestine NOS

  K57.11 Diverticulosis of small intestine without perforation or abscess with bleeding 🦠

  K57.12 Diverticulitis of small intestine without perforation or abscess without bleeding 🦠

  K57.13 Diverticulitis of small intestine without perforation or abscess with bleeding 🦠

● **K57.2 Diverticulitis of large intestine with perforation and abscess**
  Diverticulitis of colon with peritonitis
  Excludes1 diverticulitis of both small and large intestine with perforation and abscess (K57.4-)

  K57.20 Diverticulitis of large intestine with perforation and abscess without bleeding 🦠
    MCC: Only when the principal diagnosis is designated as a CC

  K57.21 Diverticulitis of large intestine with perforation and abscess with bleeding 🦠
    MCC: Only when the principal diagnosis is designated as a CC

Item 11–16 Diverticula of the intestines are acquired herniations of the mucosa. Diverticulum (singular): Pocket or pouch that bulges outward through a weak spot (herniation) in the colon. Diverticula (plural). **Diverticulosis** is the condition of having diverticula. **Diverticulitis** is inflammation of these pouches or herniations. Classification is based on location (small intestine or colon) and whether it occurs with or without hemorrhage.

CHAPTER 11 (K00-K95)

● **K57.3** **Diverticular disease of large intestine without perforation or abscess**

> **Excludes1**   diverticular disease of both small and large intestine without perforation or abscess (K57.5-)

     K57.30 **Diverticulosis of large intestine without perforation or abscess without bleeding**
         Diverticular disease of colon NOS

     K57.31 **Diverticulosis of large intestine without perforation or abscess with bleeding** 🔍

     K57.32 **Diverticulitis of large intestine without perforation or abscess without bleeding** 🔍

     K57.33 **Diverticulitis of large intestine without perforation or abscess with bleeding** 🔍

● **K57.4** **Diverticulitis of both small and large intestine with perforation and abscess**
     Diverticulitis of both small and large intestine with peritonitis

     K57.40 **Diverticulitis of both small and large intestine with perforation and abscess without bleeding** 🔍
         MCC: Only when the principal diagnosis is designated as a CC

     K57.41 **Diverticulitis of both small and large intestine with perforation and abscess with bleeding** 🔍
         MCC: Only when the principal diagnosis is designated as a CC

● **K57.5** **Diverticular disease of both small and large intestine without perforation or abscess**

     K57.50 **Diverticulosis of both small and large intestine without perforation or abscess without bleeding**
         Diverticular disease of both small and large intestine NOS

     K57.51 **Diverticulosis of both small and large intestine without perforation or abscess with bleeding** 🔍

     K57.52 **Diverticulitis of both small and large intestine without perforation or abscess without bleeding** 🔍
         MCC: Only when the principal diagnosis is designated as a CC

     K57.53 **Diverticulitis of both small and large intestine without perforation or abscess with bleeding** 🔍

● **K57.8** **Diverticulitis of intestine, part unspecified, with perforation and abscess**
     Diverticulitis of intestine NOS with peritonitis

     ▪ K57.80 **Diverticulitis of intestine, part unspecified, with perforation and abscess without bleeding** 🔍
         MCC: Only when the principal diagnosis is designated as a CC

     ▪ K57.81 **Diverticulitis of intestine, part unspecified, with perforation and abscess with bleeding** 🔍
         MCC: Only when the principal diagnosis is designated as a CC

● **K57.9** **Diverticular disease of intestine, part unspecified, without perforation or abscess**

     ▪ K57.90 **Diverticulosis of intestine, part unspecified, without perforation or abscess without bleeding**
         Diverticular disease of intestine NOS

     ▪ K57.91 **Diverticulosis of intestine, part unspecified, without perforation or abscess with bleeding** 🔍

     ▪ K57.92 **Diverticulitis of intestine, part unspecified, without perforation or abscess without bleeding** 🔍

     ▪ K57.93 **Diverticulitis of intestine, part unspecified, without perforation or abscess with bleeding** 🔍

● **K58** **Irritable bowel syndrome**

> **Includes**   irritable colon
>   spastic colon

     K58.0 **Irritable bowel syndrome with diarrhea**

     K58.9 **Irritable bowel syndrome without diarrhea**
         Irritable bowel syndrome NOS

● **K59** **Other functional intestinal disorders**

> **Excludes1**   change in bowel habit NOS (R19.4)
>   intestinal malabsorption (K90.-)
>   psychogenic intestinal disorders (F45.8)

> **Excludes2**   functional disorders of stomach (K31.-)

● **K59.0** **Constipation**

> **Excludes1**   fecal impaction (K56.41)
>   incomplete defecation (R15.0)

     ▪ K59.00 **Constipation, unspecified**

     K59.01 **Slow transit constipation**

     K59.02 **Outlet dysfunction constipation**

     K59.09 **Other constipation**

     K59.1 **Functional diarrhea**

> **Excludes1**   diarrhea NOS (R19.7)
>   irritable bowel syndrome with diarrhea (K58.0)

     K59.2 **Neurogenic bowel, not elsewhere classified** 🔍

     K59.3 **Megacolon, not elsewhere classified** 🔍
         Dilatation of colon
         Toxic megacolon

> *Code first* (T51-T65) *to identify toxic agent*

> **Excludes1**   congenital megacolon (aganglionic) (Q43.1)
>   megacolon (due to) (in) Chagas' disease (B57.32)
>   megacolon (due to) (in) Clostridium difficile (A04.7)
>   megacolon (due to) (in) Hirschsprung's disease (Q43.1)

     K59.4 **Anal spasm**
         Proctalgia fugax

     K59.8 **Other specified functional intestinal disorders**
         Atony of colon Pseudo-obstruction (acute) (chronic) of intestine

     ▪ K59.9 **Functional intestinal disorder, unspecified**

CHAPTER 11 (K00-K95)

● Unacceptable Principal Diagnosis   ● Use Additional Character(s)   ▪ Unspecified   ▶ Manifestation Code

1106   **OGCR** Official Guidelines for Coding and Reporting   Excludes 1   Excludes 2   Includes   Use additional   Code first   Code also

Item 11-17 A **fissure** is a groove in the surface, whereas a **fistula** is an abnormal passage. An **abscess** is an accumulation of pus in a tissue cavity resulting from a bacterial or parasitic infection.

● **K60 Fissure and fistula of anal and rectal regions**

> **Excludes1** fissure and fistula of anal and rectal regions with abscess or cellulitis (K61.-)

> **Excludes2** anal sphincter tear (healed) (nontraumatic) (old) (K62.81)

K60.0 Acute anal fissure

K60.1 Chronic anal fissure

■ **K60.2 Anal fissure, unspecified**

K60.3 Anal fistula

K60.4 Rectal fistula
> Fistula of rectum to skin
>> **Excludes1** rectovaginal fistula (N82.3)
>> vesicorectal fistula (N32.1)

K60.5 Anorectal fistula

● **K61 Abscess of anal and rectal regions**

> **Includes** abscess of anal and rectal regions
> cellulitis of anal and rectal regions

K61.0 Anal abscess 🦠
> Perianal abscess
>> **Excludes1** intrasphincteric abscess (K61.4)

K61.1 Rectal abscess 🦠
> Perirectal abscess
>> **Excludes1** ischiorectal abscess (K61.3)

K61.2 Anorectal abscess 🦠

K61.3 Ischiorectal abscess 🦠
> Abscess of ischiorectal fossa

K61.4 Intrasphincteric abscess 🦠

● **K62 Other diseases of anus and rectum**

> **Includes** anal canal

> **Excludes2** colostomy and enterostomy malfunction (K94.0-, K91.4-)
> fecal incontinence (R15)
> hemorrhoids (K64.-)

K62.0 Anal polyp

K62.1 Rectal polyp
>> **Excludes1** adenomatous polyp (D12.8)

K62.2 Anal prolapse
> Prolapse of anal canal

K62.3 Rectal prolapse
> Prolapse of rectal mucosa

K62.4 Stenosis of anus and rectum
> Stricture of anus (sphincter)

K62.5 Hemorrhage of anus and rectum 🦠
>> **Excludes1** gastrointestinal bleeding NOS (K92.2)
>> melena (K92.1)
>> neonatal rectal hemorrhage (P54.2)

K62.6 Ulcer of anus and rectum 🦠
> Solitary ulcer of anus and rectum
> Stercoral ulcer of anus and rectum
>> **Excludes1** fissure and fistula of anus and rectum (K60.-)
>> ulcerative colitis (K51.-)

K62.7 Radiation proctitis
> Use additional code to identify the type of radiation (W90.-)

● **K62.8 Other specified diseases of anus and rectum**
> **Excludes2** ulcerative proctitis (K51.2)

K62.81 Anal sphincter tear (healed) (nontraumatic) (old)
> Tear of anus, nontraumatic
> Use additional code for any associated fecal incontinence (R15-)
>> **Excludes2** anal fissure (K60.-)
>> anal sphincter tear (healed) (old) complicating delivery (O34.7-)
>> traumatic tear of anal sphincter (S31.831)

K62.82 Dysplasia of anus
> Anal intraepithelial neoplasia I and II (AIN I and II) (histologically confirmed)
> Dysplasia of anus NOS
> Mild and moderate dysplasia of anus (histologically confirmed)
>> **Excludes1** abnormal results from anal cytologic examination without histologic confirmation (R85.61-)
>> anal intraepithelial neoplasia III (D01.3)
>> carcinoma in situ of anus (D01.3)
>> HGSIL of anus (R85.613)
>> severe dysplasia of anus (D01.3)

K62.89 Other specified diseases of anus and rectum
> Proctitis NOS
> Use additional code for any associated fecal incontinence (R15-)

■ **K62.9 Disease of anus and rectum, unspecified**

● **K63 Other diseases of intestine**

K63.0 Abscess of intestine 🦠
>> **Excludes1** abscess of intestine with Crohn's disease (K50.014, K50.114, K50.814, K50.914)
>> abscess of intestine with diverticular disease (K57.0, K57.2, K57.4, K57.8)
>> abscess of intestine with ulcerative colitis (K51.014, K51.114, K51.214, K51.314, K51.414, K51.514, K51.814, K51.914)
>> **Excludes2** abscess of anal and rectal regions (K61.-)
>> abscess of appendix (K35.3)

K63.1 Perforation of intestine (nontraumatic) 🦠
> Perforation (nontraumatic) of rectum
>> **Excludes1** perforation (nontraumatic) of duodenum (K26.-)
>> perforation (nontraumatic) of intestine with diverticular disease (K57.0, K57.2, K57.4, K57.8)
>> **Excludes2** perforation (nontraumatic) of appendix (K35.2, K35.3)

CHAPTER 11 (K00-K95)

K63.2 Fistula of intestine 🔹

> **Excludes1**   fistula of duodenum (K31.6)
> fistula of intestine with Crohn's
>   disease (K50.013, K50.113,
>   K50.813, K50.913)
> fistula of intestine with ulcerative
>   colitis (K51.013, K51.113,
>   K51.213, K51.313, K51.413,
>   K51.513, K51.813, K51.913)

> **Excludes2**   fistula of anal and rectal regions
>   (K60.-)
> fistula of appendix (K38.3)
> intestinal-genital fistula, female
>   (N82.2-N82.4)
> vesicointestinal fistula (N32.1)

K63.3 Ulcer of intestine 🔹
     Primary ulcer of small intestine

> **Excludes1**   duodenal ulcer (K26.-)
> gastrointestinal ulcer (K28.-)
> gastrojejunal ulcer (K28.-)
> jejunal ulcer (K28.-)
> peptic ulcer, site unspecified (K27.-)
> ulcer of intestine with perforation
>   (K63.1)
> ulcer of anus or rectum (K62.6)
> ulcerative colitis (K51.-)

K63.4 Enteroptosis

K63.5 Polyp of colon

> **Excludes1**   adenomatous polyp of colon (D12.6)
> inflammatory polyp of colon (K51.4-)
> polyposis of colon (D12.6)

● **K63.8 Other specified diseases of intestine**

     K63.81 Dieulafoy lesion of intestine 🔹

>   **Excludes2**   Dieulafoy lesion of stomach
>   and duodenum (K31.82)

     K63.89 Other specified diseases of intestine

■ **K63.9 Disease of intestine, unspecified**

● **K64 Hemorrhoids and perianal venous thrombosis**

> **Includes**   piles
> **Excludes1**   hemorrhoids complicating childbirth and
>   the puerperium (O87.2)
> hemorrhoids complicating pregnancy
>   (O22.4)

K64.0 First degree hemorrhoids
     Grade/stage I hemorrhoids
     Hemorrhoids (bleeding) without prolapse outside
        of anal canal

K64.1 Second degree hemorrhoids
     Grade/stage II hemorrhoids
     Hemorrhoids (bleeding) that prolapse with
        straining, but retract spontaneously

K64.2 Third degree hemorrhoids
     Grade/stage III hemorrhoids
     Hemorrhoids (bleeding) that prolapse with
        straining and require manual replacement
        back inside anal canal

K64.3 Fourth degree hemorrhoids
     Grade/stage IV hemorrhoids
     Hemorrhoids (bleeding) with prolapsed tissue
        that cannot be manually replaced

K64.4 Residual hemorrhoidal skin tags
     External hemorrhoids, NOS
     Skin tags of anus

K64.5 Perianal venous thrombosis
     External hemorrhoids with thrombosis
     Perianal hematoma
     Thrombosed hemorrhoids NOS

Item 11-18   Peritonitis is an inflammation of the lining (peritoneum) of the abdominal cavity and surface of the intestines.

     K64.8 Other hemorrhoids
        Internal hemorrhoids, without mention of degree
        Prolapsed hemorrhoids, degree not specified

■ **K64.9 Unspecified hemorrhoids**
        Hemorrhoids (bleeding) NOS
        Hemorrhoids (bleeding) without mention of
           degree

DISEASES OF PERITONEUM AND RETROPERITONEUM (K65-K68)

● **K65 Peritonitis**

> **Use additional** code (B95-B97), to identify infectious
> agent

> **Excludes1**   acute appendicitis with generalized
>   peritonitis (K35.2)
> aseptic peritonitis (T81.6)
> benign paroxysmal peritonitis (E85.0)
> chemical peritonitis (T81.6)
> diverticulitis of both small and large
>   intestine with peritonitis (K57.4-)
> diverticulitis of colon with peritonitis
>   (K57.2-)
> diverticulitis of intestine, NOS, with
>   peritonitis (K57.8-)
> diverticulitis of small intestine with
>   peritonitis (K57.0-)
> gonococcal peritonitis (A54.85)
> neonatal peritonitis (P78.0-P78.1)
> pelvic peritonitis, female (N73.3-N73.5)
> periodic familial peritonitis (E85.0)
> peritonitis due to talc or other foreign
>   substance (T81.6)
> peritonitis in chlamydia (A74.81)
> peritonitis in diphtheria (A36.89)
> peritonitis in syphilis (late) (A52.74)
> peritonitis in tuberculosis (A18.31)
> peritonitis with or following abortion or
>   ectopic or molar pregnancy (O00-O07,
>   O08.0)
> peritonitis with or following appendicitis
>   (K35.-)
> peritonitis with or following diverticular
>   disease of intestine (K57.-)
> puerperal peritonitis (O85)
> retroperitoneal infections (K68.-)

K65.0 Generalized (acute) peritonitis 🔹
     Pelvic peritonitis (acute), male
     Subphrenic peritonitis (acute)
     Suppurative peritonitis (acute)

K65.1 Peritoneal abscess 🔹
     Abdominopelvic abscess
     Abscess (of) omentum
     Abscess (of) peritoneum
     Mesenteric abscess
     Retrocecal abscess
     Subdiaphragmatic abscess
     Subhepatic abscess
     Subphrenic abscess

K65.2 Spontaneous bacterial peritonitis 🔹

> **Excludes1**   bacterial peritonitis NOS K65.9

K65.3 Choleperitonitis 🔹
     Peritonitis due to bile

K65.4 Sclerosing mesenteritis 🔹
     Fat necrosis of peritoneum
     (Idiopathic) sclerosing mesenteric fibrosis
     Mesenteric lipodystrophy
     Mesenteric panniculitis
     Retractile mesenteritis

●   Unacceptable Principal Diagnosis   ●   Use Additional Character(s)   ■   Unspecified   ▶   Manifestation Code

OGCR   Official Guidelines for Coding and Reporting   Excludes 1   Excludes 2   Includes   Use additional   Code first   Code also

1108

Item 11-19 Retroperitoneal infections occur between the posterior parietal peritoneum and posterior abdominal wall where the kidneys, adrenal glands, ureters, duodenum, ascending colon, descending colon, pancreas, and the large vessels and nerves are located.

K65.8   Other peritonitis
     Chronic proliferative peritonitis
     Peritonitis due to urine

■ **K65.9   Peritonitis, unspecified**
     Bacterial peritonitis NOS

● **K66   Other disorders of peritoneum**
     Excludes2   ascites (R18.-)
                 peritoneal effusion (chronic) (R18.8)

   K66.0   Peritoneal adhesions (postprocedural) (postinfection)
     Adhesions (of) abdominal (wall)
     Adhesions (of) diaphragm
     Adhesions (of) intestine
     Adhesions (of) male pelvis
     Adhesions (of) omentum
     Adhesions (of) stomach
     Adhesive bands
     Mesenteric adhesions
     Excludes1   female pelvic adhesions [bands] (N73.6)
                 peritoneal adhesions with intestinal obstruction (K56.5)

   K66.1   Hemoperitoneum
     Excludes1   traumatic hemoperitoneum (S36.8-)

   K66.8   Other specified disorders of peritoneum

■   **K66.9   Disorder of peritoneum, unspecified**

●) **K67   *Disorders of peritoneum in infectious diseases classified elsewhere***
     Code first underlying disease, such as:
     congenital syphilis (A50.0)
     helminthiasis (B65.0 - B83.9)
     Excludes1   peritonitis in chlamydia (A74.81)
                 peritonitis in diphtheria (A36.89)
                 peritonitis in gonococcal (A54.85)
                 peritonitis in syphilis (late) (A52.74)
                 peritonitis in tuberculosis (A18.31)

● **K68   Disorders of retroperitoneum**
   ● **K68.1   Retroperitoneal abscess**
     K68.11   Postprocedural retroperitoneal abscess
     K68.12   Psoas muscle abscess
     K68.19   Other retroperitoneal abscess

   K68.9   Other disorders of retroperitoneum

DISEASES OF LIVER (K70-K77)

Excludes1   jaundice NOS (R17)
Excludes2   hemochromatosis (E83.11-)
                Reye's syndrome (G93.7)
                viral hepatitis (B15-B19)
                Wilson's disease (E83.0)

● **K70   Alcoholic liver disease**
     Use additional code to identify:
     alcohol abuse and dependence (F10.-)

   K70.0   Alcoholic fatty liver   **A**

●   **K70.1   Alcoholic hepatitis**
     K70.10   Alcoholic hepatitis without ascites   **A**
     K70.11   Alcoholic hepatitis with ascites   **A**

   K70.2   Alcoholic fibrosis and sclerosis of liver   **A**

Item 11-20 Cirrhosis is the progressive fibrosis of the liver resulting in loss of liver function. The main causes of cirrhosis of the liver are alcohol abuse, chronic hepatitis (inflammation of the liver), biliary disease, and excessive amounts of iron. **Alcoholic cirrhosis of the liver** is also called portal, Laënnec's, or fatty nutritional cirrhosis.

● **K70.3   Alcoholic cirrhosis of liver**
     Alcoholic cirrhosis NOS

     K70.30   Alcoholic cirrhosis of liver without ascites   **A**

     K70.31   Alcoholic cirrhosis of liver with ascites   **A**

● **K70.4   Alcoholic hepatic failure**
     Acute alcoholic hepatic failure
     Alcoholic hepatic failure NOS
     Chronic alcoholic hepatic failure
     Subacute alcoholic hepatic failure

     K70.40   Alcoholic hepatic failure without coma   **A**

     K70.41   Alcoholic hepatic failure with coma   **A**
           MCC: Only when the principal diagnosis is designated as an MCC

■   **K70.9   Alcoholic liver disease, unspecified**   **A**

● **K71   Toxic liver disease**
     Includes   drug-induced idiosyncratic (unpredictable) liver disease
              drug-induced toxic (predictable) liver disease

     Code first poisoning due to drug or toxin, if applicable (T36-T65 with fifth or sixth character 1-4 or 6)

     Use additional code for adverse effect, if applicable, to identify drug (T36-T50 with fifth or sixth character 5)

     Excludes2   alcoholic liver disease (K70.-)
                 Budd-Chiari syndrome (I82.0)

● **K71.0   Toxic liver disease with cholestasis**
     Cholestasis with hepatocyte injury
     'Pure' cholestasis

● **K71.1   Toxic liver disease with hepatic necrosis**
     Hepatic failure (acute) (chronic) due to drugs

     ● **K71.10   Toxic liver disease with hepatic necrosis, without coma**

     ● **K71.11   Toxic liver disease with hepatic necrosis, with coma**
           MCC: Only when the principal diagnosis is designated as an MCC

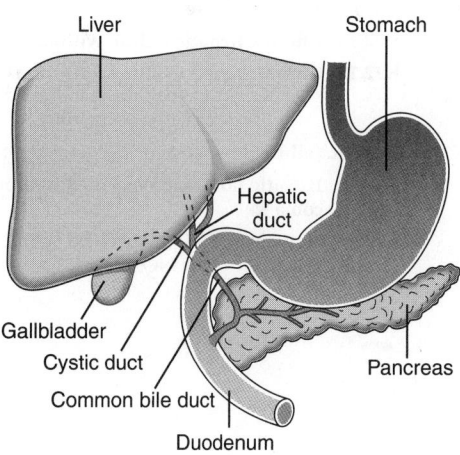

Figure 11-12   Liver and bile ducts.

N Newborn Age: 0   **P** Pediatric Age: 0–17   **M** Maternity DX: 12–55   **A** Adult Age: 15–124   ♀ Females Only   ♂ Males Only

Complication\Comorbidity   Major C\C   Present on Admission Requirement   Hospital-Acquired Condition

1109

CHAPTER 11 (K00-K95)

CHAPTER 11 (K00-K95)

● K71.2 Toxic liver disease with acute hepatitis

● K71.3 Toxic liver disease with chronic persistent hepatitis

● K71.4 Toxic liver disease with chronic lobular hepatitis

● K71.5 Toxic liver disease with chronic active hepatitis
  Toxic liver disease with lupoid hepatitis

  ● K71.50 Toxic liver disease with chronic active hepatitis without ascites

  ● K71.51 Toxic liver disease with chronic active hepatitis with ascites

● K71.6 Toxic liver disease with hepatitis, not elsewhere classified

● K71.7 Toxic liver disease with fibrosis and cirrhosis of liver

● K71.8 Toxic liver disease with other disorders of liver
  Toxic liver disease with focal nodular hyperplasia
  Toxic liver disease with hepatic granulomas
  Toxic liver disease with peliosis hepatis
  Toxic liver disease with veno-occlusive disease of liver

● ■ K71.9 Toxic liver disease, unspecified

● K72 Hepatic failure, not elsewhere classified

  Includes acute hepatitis NEC, with hepatic failure
  fulminant hepatitis NEC, with hepatic failure
  hepatic encephalopathy NOS
  liver (cell) necrosis with hepatic failure
  malignant hepatitis NEC, with hepatic failure
  yellow liver atrophy or dystrophy

  Excludes1 alcoholic hepatic failure (K70.4)
  hepatic failure complicating abortion or ectopic or molar pregnancy (O00-O07, O08.8)
  hepatic failure complicating pregnancy, childbirth and the puerperium (O26.6-)
  hepatic failure with toxic liver disease (K71.1-)
  icterus of newborn (P55-P59)
  postprocedural hepatic failure (K91.82)
  viral hepatitis with hepatic coma (B15-B19)

  ● K72.0 Acute and subacute hepatic failure

    K72.00 Acute and subacute hepatic failure without coma 🦟

    K72.01 Acute and subacute hepatic failure with coma 🦟
      MCC: Only when the principal diagnosis is designated as an MCC

  ● K72.1 Chronic hepatic failure

    K72.10 Chronic hepatic failure without coma

    K72.11 Chronic hepatic failure with coma
      MCC: Only when the principal diagnosis is designated as an MCC

  ● K72.9 Hepatic failure, unspecified

    ■ K72.90 Hepatic failure, unspecified without coma 🦟

    ■ K72.91 Hepatic failure, unspecified with coma 🦟
      Hepatic coma NOS

● K73 Chronic hepatitis, not elsewhere classified

  Excludes1 alcoholic hepatitis (chronic) (K70.1-)
  drug-induced hepatitis (chronic) (K71.-)
  granulomatous hepatitis (chronic) NEC (K75.3)
  reactive, nonspecific hepatitis (chronic) (K75.2)
  viral hepatitis (chronic) (B15-B19)

  K73.0 Chronic persistent hepatitis, not elsewhere classified

  K73.1 Chronic lobular hepatitis, not elsewhere classified

  K73.2 Chronic active hepatitis, not elsewhere classified

  K73.8 Other chronic hepatitis, not elsewhere classified

  ■ K73.9 Chronic hepatitis, unspecified

● K74 Fibrosis and cirrhosis of liver

  Code also, if applicable, viral hepatitis (acute) (chronic) (B15-B19)

  Excludes1 alcoholic cirrhosis (of liver) (K70.3)
  alcoholic fibrosis of liver (K70.2)
  cardiac sclerosis of liver (K76.1)
  cirrhosis (of liver) with toxic liver disease (K71.7)
  congenital cirrhosis (of liver) (P78.81)
  pigmentary cirrhosis (of liver) (E83.110)

  K74.0 Hepatic fibrosis

  K74.1 Hepatic sclerosis

  K74.2 Hepatic fibrosis with hepatic sclerosis

  K74.3 Primary biliary cirrhosis
    Chronic nonsuppurative destructive cholangitis

  K74.4 Secondary biliary cirrhosis

  ■ K74.5 Biliary cirrhosis, unspecified

  ● K74.6 Other and unspecified cirrhosis of liver

    ■ K74.60 Unspecified cirrhosis of liver
      Cirrhosis (of liver) NOS

    K74.69 Other cirrhosis of liver
      Cryptogenic cirrhosis (of liver)
      Macronodular cirrhosis (of liver)
      Micronodular cirrhosis (of liver)
      Mixed type cirrhosis (of liver)
      Portal cirrhosis (of liver)
      Postnecrotic cirrhosis (of liver)

● K75 Other inflammatory liver diseases

  Excludes2 toxic liver disease (K71.-)

  K75.0 Abscess of liver 🦟
    Cholangitic hepatic abscess
    Hematogenic hepatic abscess
    Hepatic abscess NOS
    Lymphogenic hepatic abscess
    Pylephlebitic hepatic abscess

    Excludes1 amebic liver abscess (A06.4)
    cholangitis without liver abscess (K83.0)
    pylephlebitis without liver abscess (K75.1)

  K75.1 Phlebitis of portal vein 🦟
    Pylephlebitis

    Excludes1 pylephlebitic liver abscess (K75.0)

  K75.2 Nonspecific reactive hepatitis

    Excludes1 acute or subacute hepatitis (K72.0-)
    chronic hepatitis NEC (K73.-)
    viral hepatitis (B15-B19)

● Unacceptable Principal Diagnosis   ● Use Additional Character(s)   ■ Unspecified   ▶ Manifestation Code

K75.3   Granulomatous hepatitis, not elsewhere classified

> Excludes1   acute or subacute hepatitis (K72.0-)
> chronic hepatitis NEC (K73.-)
> viral hepatitis (B15-B19)

K75.4   Autoimmune hepatitis
> Lupoid hepatitis NEC

● **K75.8**   Other specified inflammatory liver diseases

     K75.81   Nonalcoholic steatohepatitis (NASH)

     K75.89   Other specified inflammatory liver diseases

■ **K75.9**   Inflammatory liver disease, unspecified
> Hepatitis NOS

> Excludes1   acute or subacute hepatitis (K72.0-)
> chronic hepatitis NEC (K73.-)
> viral hepatitis (B15-B19)

● **K76**   Other diseases of liver

> Excludes2   alcoholic liver disease (K70.-)
> amyloid degeneration of liver (E85-)
> cystic disease of liver (congenital) (Q44.6)
> hepatic vein thrombosis (I82.0)
> hepatomegaly NOS (R16.0)
> pigmentary cirrhosis (of liver) (E83.110)
> portal vein thrombosis (I81)
> toxic liver disease (K71.-)

K76.0   Fatty (change of) liver, not elsewhere classified
> Nonalcoholic fatty liver disease (NAFLD)

> Excludes1   nonalcoholic steatohepatitis (NASH) (K75.81)

K76.1   Chronic passive congestion of liver
> Cardiac cirrhosis
> Cardiac sclerosis

K76.2   Central hemorrhagic necrosis of liver 🦠

> Excludes1   liver necrosis with hepatic failure (K72.-)

K76.3   Infarction of liver 🦠

K76.4   Peliosis hepatis
> Hepatic angiomatosis

K76.5   Hepatic veno-occlusive disease

> Excludes1   Budd-Chiari syndrome (I82.0)

K76.6   Portal hypertension 🦠

> Use additional code for any associated complications, such as:
> portal hypertensive gastropathy (K31.89)

K76.7   Hepatorenal syndrome 🦠

> Excludes1   hepatorenal syndrome following labor and delivery (O90.4)
> postprocedural hepatorenal syndrome (K91.82)

● **K76.8**   Other specified diseases of liver

     K76.81   Hepatopulmonary syndrome

> Code first underlying liver disease, such as:
> alcoholic cirrhosis of liver (K70.3-)
> cirrhosis of liver without mention of alcohol (K74.6-)

     K76.89   Other specified diseases of liver
> Cyst (simple) of liver
> Focal nodular hyperplasia of liver
> Hepatoptosis

■ **K76.9**   Liver disease, unspecified

● ◗ **K77**   *Liver disorders in diseases classified elsewhere* 🦠

> *Code first* underlying disease, such as:
> amyloidosis (E85-)
> congenital syphilis (A50.0, A50.5)
> congenital toxoplasmosis (P37.1)
> schistosomiasis (B65.0-B65.9)

> Excludes1   alcoholic hepatitis (K70.1-)
> alcoholic liver disease (K70.-)
> cytomegaloviral hepatitis (B25.1)
> herpesviral [herpes simplex] hepatitis (B00.81)
> infectious mononucleosis with liver disease (B27.0-B27.9 with .9)
> mumps hepatitis (B26.81)
> sarcoidosis with liver disease (D86.89)
> secondary syphilis with liver disease (A51.45)
> syphilis (late) with liver disease (A52.74)
> toxoplasmosis (acquired) hepatitis (B58.1)
> tuberculosis with liver disease (A18.83)

DISORDERS OF GALLBLADDER, BILIARY TRACT AND PANCREAS (K80–K87)

● **K80**   Cholelithiasis
> *Presence or formation of gallstones*

> Excludes1   retained cholelithiasis following cholecystectomy (K91.86)

● **K80.0**   Calculus of gallbladder with acute cholecystitis
> Any condition listed in K80.2 with acute cholecystitis
> *Check documentation for acute/chronic gallbladder/ common bile duct either with or without obstruction.*

     K80.00   Calculus of gallbladder with acute cholecystitis without obstruction 🦠

     K80.01   Calculus of gallbladder with acute cholecystitis with obstruction 🦠

● **K80.1**   Calculus of gallbladder with other cholecystitis

     K80.10   Calculus of gallbladder with chronic cholecystitis without obstruction 🦠
> Cholelithiasis with cholecystitis NOS

     K80.11   Calculus of gallbladder with chronic cholecystitis with obstruction 🦠

     K80.12   Calculus of gallbladder with acute and chronic cholecystitis without obstruction 🦠

     K80.13   Calculus of gallbladder with acute and chronic cholecystitis with obstruction 🦠

     K80.18   Calculus of gallbladder with other cholecystitis without obstruction 🦠

     K80.19   Calculus of gallbladder with other cholecystitis with obstruction 🦠

● **K80.2**   Calculus of gallbladder without cholecystitis
> Cholecystolithiasis without cholecystitis
> Cholelithiasis (without cholecystitis)
> Colic (recurrent) of gallbladder (without cholecystitis)
> Gallstone (impacted) of cystic duct (without cholecystitis)
> Gallstone (impacted) of gallbladder (without cholecystitis)

     K80.20   Calculus of gallbladder without cholecystitis without obstruction

     K80.21   Calculus of gallbladder without cholecystitis with obstruction 🦠

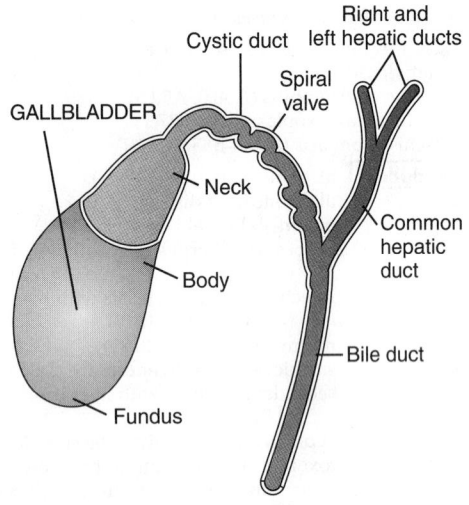

Figure 11-13   *Gallbladder and bile ducts.*

● **K80.3**   **Calculus of bile duct with cholangitis**
     Any condition listed in K80.5 with cholangitis

  ■ **K80.30**   **Calculus of bile duct with cholangitis, unspecified, without obstruction**

  ■ **K80.31**   **Calculus of bile duct with cholangitis, unspecified, with obstruction** 🦠

     K80.32   **Calculus of bile duct with acute cholangitis without obstruction**

     K80.33   **Calculus of bile duct with acute cholangitis with obstruction** 🦠

     K80.34   **Calculus of bile duct with chronic cholangitis without obstruction**

     K80.35   **Calculus of bile duct with chronic cholangitis with obstruction** 🦠

     K80.36   **Calculus of bile duct with acute and chronic cholangitis without obstruction**

     K80.37   **Calculus of bile duct with acute and chronic cholangitis with obstruction** 🦠

● **K80.4**   **Calculus of bile duct with cholecystitis**
     Any condition listed in K80.5 with cholecystitis (with cholangitis)

  ■ **K80.40**   **Calculus of bile duct with cholecystitis, unspecified, without obstruction** 🦠

  ■ **K80.41**   **Calculus of bile duct with cholecystitis, unspecified, with obstruction** 🦠

     K80.42   **Calculus of bile duct with acute cholecystitis without obstruction** 🦠

     K80.43   **Calculus of bile duct with acute cholecystitis with obstruction** 🦠

     K80.44   **Calculus of bile duct with chronic cholecystitis without obstruction** 🦠

     K80.45   **Calculus of bile duct with chronic cholecystitis with obstruction** 🦠

     K80.46   **Calculus of bile duct with acute and chronic cholecystitis without obstruction** 🦠

     K80.47   **Calculus of bile duct with acute and chronic cholecystitis with obstruction** 🦠

● **K80.5**   **Calculus of bile duct without cholangitis or cholecystitis**
     Choledocholithiasis (without cholangitis or cholecystitis)
     Gallstone (impacted) of bile duct NOS (without cholangitis or cholecystitis)
     Gallstone (impacted) of common duct (without cholangitis or cholecystitis)
     Gallstone (impacted) of hepatic duct (without cholangitis or cholecystitis)
     Hepatic cholelithiasis (without cholangitis or cholecystitis)
     Hepatic colic (recurrent) (without cholangitis or cholecystitis)

     K80.50   **Calculus of bile duct without cholangitis or cholecystitis without obstruction**

     K80.51   **Calculus of bile duct without cholangitis or cholecystitis with obstruction** 🦠

● **K80.6**   **Calculus of gallbladder and bile duct with cholecystitis**

  ■ **K80.60**   **Calculus of gallbladder and bile duct with cholecystitis, unspecified, without obstruction** 🦠

  ■ **K80.61**   **Calculus of gallbladder and bile duct with cholecystitis, unspecified, with obstruction** 🦠

     K80.62   **Calculus of gallbladder and bile duct with acute cholecystitis without obstruction** 🦠

     K80.63   **Calculus of gallbladder and bile duct with acute cholecystitis with obstruction** 🦠

     K80.64   **Calculus of gallbladder and bile duct with chronic cholecystitis without obstruction** 🦠

     K80.65   **Calculus of gallbladder and bile duct with chronic cholecystitis with obstruction** 🦠

     K80.66   **Calculus of gallbladder and bile duct with acute and chronic cholecystitis without obstruction** 🦠

     K80.67   **Calculus of gallbladder and bile duct with acute and chronic cholecystitis with obstruction** 🦠

● **K80.7**   **Calculus of gallbladder and bile duct without cholecystitis**

     K80.70   **Calculus of gallbladder and bile duct without cholecystitis without obstruction**

     K80.71   **Calculus of gallbladder and bile duct without cholecystitis with obstruction** 🦠

● **K80.8**   **Other cholelithiasis**

     K80.80   **Other cholelithiasis without obstruction**

     K80.81   **Other cholelithiasis with obstruction** 🦠

● **K81**   **Cholecystitis**
     Chronic or acute inflammation of the gallbladder.

     Excludes1   cholecystitis with cholelithiasis (K80.-)

     K81.0   **Acute cholecystitis** 🦠
       Abscess of gallbladder
       Angiocholecystitis
       Emphysematous (acute) cholecystitis
       Empyema of gallbladder
       Gangrene of gallbladder
       Gangrenous cholecystitis
       Suppurative cholecystitis

     K81.1   **Chronic cholecystitis**

     K81.2   **Acute cholecystitis with chronic cholecystitis** 🦠

  ■ **K81.9**   **Cholecystitis, unspecified**

●   Unacceptable Principal Diagnosis   ●   Use Additional Character(s)   ■   Unspecified   ▶   Manifestation Code

OGCR   Official Guidelines for Coding and Reporting   Excludes 1   Excludes 2   Includes   Use additional   Code first   Code also

● **K82   Other diseases of gallbladder**

     Excludes1   nonvisualization of gallbladder (R93.2)
                postcholecystectomy syndrome (K91.5)

   K82.0   Obstruction of gallbladder 🕮
       Occlusion of cystic duct or gallbladder without
          cholelithiasis
       Stenosis of cystic duct or gallbladder without
          cholelithiasis
       Stricture of cystic duct or gallbladder without
          cholelithiasis

       Excludes1   obstruction of gallbladder with
                   cholelithiasis (K80.-)

   K82.1   Hydrops of gallbladder 🕮
       Mucocele of gallbladder

   K82.2   Perforation of gallbladder 🕮
       Rupture of cystic duct or gallbladder

   K82.3   Fistula of gallbladder 🕮
       Cholecystocolic fistula
       Cholecystoduodenal fistula

   K82.4   Cholesterolosis of gallbladder
       Strawberry gallbladder

       Excludes1   cholesterolosis of gallbladder with
                   cholecystitis (K81.-)
                cholesterolosis of gallbladder with
                   cholelithiasis (K80.-)

   K82.8   Other specified diseases of gallbladder
       Adhesions of cystic duct or gallbladder
       Atrophy of cystic duct or gallbladder
       Cyst of cystic duct or gallbladder
       Dyskinesia of cystic duct or gallbladder
       Hypertrophy of cystic duct or gallbladder
       Nonfunctioning of cystic duct or gallbladder
       Ulcer of cystic duct or gallbladder

 ◼ **K82.9   Disease of gallbladder, unspecified**

● **K83   Other diseases of biliary tract**

     Excludes1   postcholecystectomy syndrome (K91.5)
     Excludes2   conditions involving the gallbladder
                (K81-K82)
              conditions involving the cystic duct
                (K81-K82)

   K83.0   Cholangitis 🕮
       Ascending cholangitis
       Cholangitis NOS
       Primary cholangitis
       Recurrent cholangitis
       Sclerosing cholangitis
       Secondary cholangitis
       Stenosing cholangitis
       Suppurative cholangitis

       Excludes1   cholangitic liver abscess (K75.0)
                cholangitis with choledocholithiasis
                   (K80.3-, K80.4-)
                chronic nonsuppurative destructive
                   cholangitis (K74.3)

   K83.1   Obstruction of bile duct 🕮
       Occlusion of bile duct without cholelithiasis
       Stenosis of bile duct without cholelithiasis
       Stricture of bile duct without cholelithiasis

       Excludes1   congenital obstruction of bile duct
                   (Q44.3)
                obstruction of bile duct with
                   cholelithiasis (K80.-)

   K83.2   Perforation of bile duct 🕮
       Rupture of bile duct

   K83.3   Fistula of bile duct 🕮
       Choledochoduodenal fistula

   K83.4   Spasm of sphincter of Oddi

   K83.5   Biliary cyst

   K83.8   Other specified diseases of biliary tract
       Adhesions of biliary tract
       Atrophy of biliary tract
       Hypertrophy of biliary tract
       Ulcer of biliary tract

 ◼ **K83.9   Disease of biliary tract, unspecified**

● **K85   Acute pancreatitis**
     *Inflammatory process in which pancreatic enzymes autodigest
     the gland.*

     Includes   abscess of pancreas
                acute necrosis of pancreas
                acute (recurrent) pancreatitis
                gangrene of (gangrenous) pancreas
                hemorrhagic pancreatitis
                infective necrosis of pancreas
                subacute pancreatitis
                suppurative pancreatitis

   K85.0   Idiopathic acute pancreatitis 🕮

   K85.1   Biliary acute pancreatitis 🕮
       Gallstone pancreatitis

   K85.2   Alcohol induced acute pancreatitis 🕮

       Excludes2   alcohol induced chronic pancreatitis
                   (K86.0)

   K85.3   Drug induced acute pancreatitis 🕮

       Use additional code for adverse effect, if
          applicable, to identify drug (T36-T50 with
          fifth or sixth character 5)

       Use additional code to identify drug abuse and
          dependence (F11.- F17.-)

   K85.8   Other acute pancreatitis 🕮

 ◼ **K85.9   Acute pancreatitis, unspecified** 🕮
       Pancreatitis NOS

● **K86   Other diseases of pancreas**

     Excludes2   fibrocystic disease of pancreas (E84.-)
              islet cell tumor (of pancreas) (D13.7)
              pancreatic steatorrhea (K90.3)

   K86.0   Alcohol-induced chronic pancreatitis 🕮

       Use additional code to identify:
          alcohol abuse and dependence (F10.-)

       Excludes2   alcohol induced acute pancreatitis
                   (K85.2)

   K86.1   Other chronic pancreatitis 🕮
       Chronic pancreatitis NOS
       Infectious chronic pancreatitis
       Recurrent chronic pancreatitis
       Relapsing chronic pancreatitis

   K86.2   Cyst of pancreas 🕮

   K86.3   Pseudocyst of pancreas 🕮

   K86.8   Other specified diseases of pancreas
       Aseptic pancreatic necrosis
       Atrophy of pancreas
       Calculus of pancreas
       Cirrhosis of pancreas
       Fibrosis of pancreas
       Pancreatic fat necrosis
       Pancreatic infantilism
       Pancreatic necrosis NOS

 ◼ **K86.9   Disease of pancreas, unspecified**

CHAPTER 11 (K00-K95)

N   Newborn Age: 0   **P**   Pediatric Age: 0–17   **M**   Maternity DX: 12–55   **A**   Adult Age: 15–124   ♀   Females Only   ♂   Males Only

🕮   Complication\Comorbidity   🕮   Major C\C   🕮   Present on Admission Requirement   🕮   Hospital-Acquired Condition   **1113**

CHAPTER 11 (K00-K95)

● ▶ **K87   Disorders of gallbladder, biliary tract and pancreas in diseases classified elsewhere**

　　　Code first underlying disease

　　　Excludes1   cytomegaloviral pancreatitis (B25.2)
　　　　　　　　mumps pancreatitis (B26.3)
　　　　　　　　syphilitic gallbladder (A52.74)
　　　　　　　　syphilitic pancreas (A52.74)
　　　　　　　　tuberculosis of gallbladder (A18.83)
　　　　　　　　tuberculosis of pancreas (A18.83)

OTHER DISEASES OF THE DIGESTIVE SYSTEM (K90-K95)

● **K90   Intestinal malabsorption**

　　　Excludes1   intestinal malabsorption following gastrointestinal surgery (K91.2)

K90.0   Celiac disease
　　　Gluten-sensitive enteropathy
　　　Idiopathic steatorrhea
　　　Nontropical sprue

K90.1   Tropical sprue 🕯
　　　Sprue NOS
　　　Tropical steatorrhea

K90.2   Blind loop syndrome, not elsewhere classified 🕯
　　　Blind loop syndrome NOS

　　　Excludes1   congenital blind loop syndrome (Q43.8)
　　　　　　　　postsurgical blind loop syndrome (K91.2)

K90.3   Pancreatic steatorrhea 🕯

K90.4   Malabsorption due to intolerance, not elsewhere classified 🕯
　　　Malabsorption due to intolerance to carbohydrate
　　　Malabsorption due to intolerance to fat
　　　Malabsorption due to intolerance to protein
　　　Malabsorption due to intolerance to starch

　　　Excludes2   gluten-sensitive enteropathy (K90.0)
　　　　　　　　lactose intolerance (E73.-)

● **K90.8   Other intestinal malabsorption**

　　K90.81   Whipple's disease 🕯

　　K90.89   Other intestinal malabsorption 🕯

■ **K90.9   Intestinal malabsorption, unspecified** 🕯

● **K91   Intraoperative and postprocedural complications and disorders of digestive system, not elsewhere classified**

　　　Excludes2   complications of artificial opening of digestive system (K94.-)
　　　　　　　　complications of bariatric procedures (K95.-)
　　　　　　　　gastrojejunal ulcer (K28.-)
　　　　　　　　postprocedural (radiation) retroperitoneal abscess (K68.11)
　　　　　　　　radiation colitis (K52.0)
　　　　　　　　radiation gastroenteritis (K52.0)
　　　　　　　　radiation proctitis (K62.7)

K91.0   Vomiting following gastrointestinal surgery

K91.1   Postgastric surgery syndromes
　　　Dumping syndrome
　　　Postgastrectomy syndrome
　　　Postvagotomy syndrome

■ **K91.2   Postsurgical malabsorption, not elsewhere classified** 🕯
　　　Postsurgical blind loop syndrome

　　　Excludes1   malabsorption osteomalacia in adults (M83.2)
　　　　　　　　malabsorption osteoporosis, postsurgical (M80.8-, M81.8)

K91.3   Postprocedural intestinal obstruction 🕯

K91.5   Postcholecystectomy syndrome

● **K91.6   Intraoperative hemorrhage and hematoma of a digestive system organ or structure complicating a procedure**

　　　Excludes1   intraoperative hemorrhage and hematoma of a digestive system organ or structure due to accidental puncture and laceration during a procedure (K91.7-)

　　K91.61   Intraoperative hemorrhage and hematoma of a digestive system organ or structure complicating a digestive sytem procedure 🕯

　　K91.62   Intraoperative hemorrhage and hematoma of a digestive system organ or structure complicating other procedure 🕯

● **K91.7   Accidental puncture and laceration of a digestive system organ or structure during a procedure**

　　K91.71   Accidental puncture and laceration of a digestive system organ or structure during a digestive system procedure 🕯

　　K91.72   Accidental puncture and laceration of a digestive system organ or structure during other procedure 🕯

● **K91.8   Other intraoperative and postprocedural complications and disorders of digestive system**

　　K91.81   Other intraoperative complications of digestive system 🕯

　　K91.82   Postprocedural hepatic failure 🕯

　　K91.83   Postprocedural hepatorenal syndrome 🕯

● **K91.84   Postprocedural hemorrhage and hematoma of a digestive system organ or structure following a procedure**

　　　K91.840   Postprocedural hemorrhage and hematoma of a digestive system organ or structure following a digestive system procedure 🕯

　　　K91.841   Postprocedural hemorrhage and hematoma of a digestive system organ or structure following other procedure 🕯

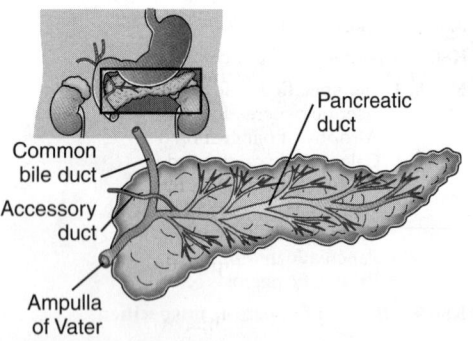

Figure 11-14   Pancreatic ductal system.

Pancreatic duct
Common bile duct
Accessory duct
Ampulla of Vater

● Unacceptable Principal Diagnosis　　● Use Additional Character(s)　　■ Unspecified　　▶ Manifestation Code

OGCR Official Guidelines for Coding and Reporting　　Excludes 1　　Excludes 2　　Includes　　Use additional　　Code first　　Code also

● **K91.85 Complications of intestinal pouch**

     K91.850   Pouchitis 🔴
         Inflammation of internal
         ileoanal pouch

     K91.858   Other complications of intestinal
         pouch 🔴

     K91.86   Retained cholelithiasis following
         cholecystectomy

     K91.89   Other postprocedural complications and
         disorders of digestive system 🔴

         Use additional code, if applicable, to
         further specify disorder

         | Excludes2 | postprocedural
         retroperitoneal abscess
         (K68.11)

● **K92 Other diseases of digestive system**

     | Excludes1 | neonatal gastrointestinal hemorrhage
     (P54.0-P54.3)

     K92.0   Hematemesis 🔴

     K92.1   Melena 🔴

         | Excludes1 | occult blood in feces (R19.5)

     K92.2   Gastrointestinal hemorrhage, unspecified 🔴
         Gastric hemorrhage NOS
         Intestinal hemorrhage NOS

         | Excludes1 | acute hemorrhagic gastritis (K29.01)
         hemorrhage of anus and rectum
         (K62.5)
         angiodysplasia of stomach with
         hemorrhage (K31.811)
         diverticular disease with
         hemorrhage (K57.-)
         gastritis and duodenitis with
         hemorrhage (K29.-)
         peptic ulcer with hemorrhage
         (K25-K28)

● **K92.8   Other specified diseases of the digestive system**

     K92.81   Gastrointestinal mucositis (ulcerative) 🔴

         Code also type of associated therapy,
         such as:
         antineoplastic and immunosuppressive
         drugs (T45.1x-)
         radiological procedure and
         radiotherapy (Y84.2)

         | Excludes2 | mucositis (ulcerative) of
         vagina and vulva
         (N76.81)
         nasal mucositis (ulcerative)
         (J34.81)
         oral mucositis (ulcerative)
         (K12.3-)

     K92.89   Other specified diseases of the digestive
         system

     ■ **K92.9   Disease of digestive system, unspecified**

● **K94 Complications of artificial openings of the digestive system**

● **K94.0   Colostomy complications**

     ■ **K94.00   Colostomy complication, unspecified**

     K94.01   Colostomy hemorrhage 🔴

     K94.02   Colostomy infection 🔴

         Use additional code to specify type of
         infection, such as:
         cellulitis of abdominal wall (L03.311)
         sepsis (A40.-, A41.-)

     K94.03   Colostomy malfunction 🔴
         Mechanical complication of colostomy

     K94.09   Other complications of colostomy 🔴

● **K94.1   Enterostomy complications**

     ■ **K94.10   Enterostomy complication, unspecified**

     K94.11   Enterostomy hemorrhage 🔴

     K94.12   Enterostomy infection 🔴

         Use additional code to specify type of
         infection, such as:
         cellulitis of abdominal wall (L03.311)
         sepsis (A40.-, A41.-)

     K94.13   Enterostomy malfunction 🔴
         Mechanical complication of enterostomy

     K94.19   Other complications of enterostomy 🔴

● **K94.2   Gastrostomy complications**

     ■ **K94.20   Gastrostomy complication, unspecified**

     K94.21   Gastrostomy hemorrhage

     K94.22   Gastrostomy infection 🔴

         Use additional code to specify type of
         infection, such as:
         cellulitis of abdominal wall (L03.311)
         sepsis (A40.-, A41.-)

     K94.23   Gastrostomy malfunction 🔴
         Mechanical complication of gastrostomy

     K94.29   Other complications of gastrostomy

● **K94.3   Esophagostomy complications**

     ■ **K94.30   Esophagostomy complications,
         unspecified** 🔴

     K94.31   Esophagostomy hemorrhage 🔴

     K94.32   Esophagostomy infection 🔴

         Use additional code to identify the
         infection

     K94.33   Esophagostomy malfunction 🔴
         Mechanical complication of
         esophagostomy

     K94.39   Other complications of esophagostomy 🔴

● **K95 Complications of bariatric procedures**

● **K95.0   Complications of gastric band procedure**

     K95.01   Infection due to gastric band procedure

         Use additional code to specify type of
         infection or organism, such as:
         bacterial and viral infectious agents
         (B95-, B96-)
         cellulitis of abdominal wall (L03.311)
         sepsis (A40.-, A41.-)

     **K95.09   Other complications of gastric band
         procedure**

         Use additional code, if applicable, to
         further specify complication

● **K95.8   Complications of other bariatric procedure**

     | Excludes1 | complications of gastric band
     surgery (K95.0-)

     K95.81   Infection due to other bariatric procedure

         Use additional code to specify type of
         infection or organism, such as:
         bacterial and viral infectious agents
         (B95-, B96-)
         cellulitis of abdominal wall (L03.311)
         sepsis (A40.-, A41.-)

     **K95.89   Other complications of other bariatric
         procedure**

         Use additional code, if applicable, to
         further specify complication

CHAPTER 11 (K00-K95)

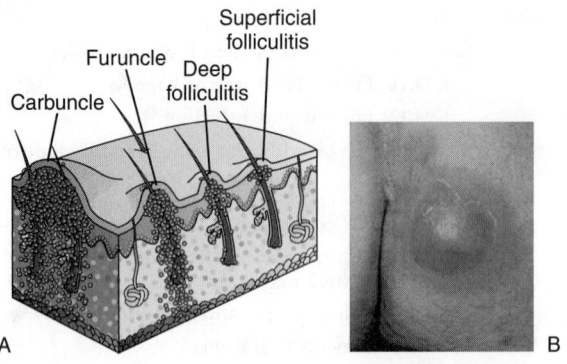

Figure 12-1 Furuncle, also known as a boil, is a staphylococcal infection. The organism enters the body through a hair follicle and so furuncles usually appear in hairy areas of the body. A cluster of furuncles is known as a carbuncle and involves infection into the deep subcutaneous fascia. These usually appear on the back and neck. (**B** from Habif: Clinical Dermatology, 4th ed. 2004, Mosby.)

CHAPTER 12

DISEASES OF THE SKIN AND SUBCUTANEOUS TISSUE (L00-L99)

Excludes2   certain conditions originating in the perinatal period (P04-P96)
certain infectious and parasitic diseases (A00-B99)
complications of pregnancy, childbirth and the puerperium (O00-O9A)
congenital malformations, deformations, and chromosomal abnormalities (Q00-Q99)
endocrine, nutritional and metabolic diseases (E00-E88)
lipomelanotic reticulosis (I89.8)
neoplasms (C00-D49)
symptoms, signs and abnormal clinical and laboratory findings, not elsewhere classified (R00-R94)
systemic connective tissue disorders (M30-M36)
viral warts (B07.-)

This chapter contains the following blocks:

L00-L08	Infections of the skin and subcutaneous tissue
L10-L14	Bullous disorders
L20-L30	Dermatitis and eczema
L40-L45	Papulosquamous disorders
L49-L54	Urticaria and erythema
L55-L59	Radiation-related disorders of the skin and subcutaneous tissue
L60-L75	Disorders of skin appendages
L76	Intraoperative and postprocedural complications of skin and subcutaneous tissue
L80-L99	Other disorders of the skin and subcutaneous tissue

INFECTIONS OF THE SKIN AND SUBCUTANEOUS TISSUE (L00-L08)

Use additional code (B95-B97) to identify infectious agent.

Excludes2   hordeolum (H00.0)
infective dermatitis (L30.3)
local infections of skin classified in Chapter 1
lupus panniculitis (L93.2)
panniculitis NOS (M79.3)
panniculitis of neck and back (M54.0-)
Perlèche NOS (K13.0)
Perlèche due to candidiasis (B37.0)
Perlèche due to riboflavin deficiency (E53.0)
pyogenic granuloma (L98.0)
relapsing panniculitis [Weber-Christian] (M35.6)
viral warts (B07.-)
zoster (B02.-)

L00   Staphylococcal scalded skin syndrome
Ritter's disease

Use additional code to identify percentage of skin exfoliation (L49-)

Excludes1   bullous impetigo (L01.03)
pemphigus neonatorum (L01.03)
toxic epidermal necrolysis [Lyell] (L51.2)

● **L01   Impetigo**
Contagious skin infection caused by a streptococcus or staphylococcus aureus, common skin infections among children.

Excludes1   impetigo herpetiformis (L40.1)

● **L01.0   Impetigo**
Impetigo contagiosa
Impetigo vulgaris

◾ **L01.00   Impetigo, unspecified**
Impetigo NOS

L01.01   Non-bullous impetigo

L01.02   Bockhart's impetigo
Impetigo follicularis
Perifolliculitis NOS
Superficial pustular perifolliculitis

L01.03   Bullous impetigo
Impetigo neonatorum
Pemphigus neonatorum
Neonate = newborn

L01.09   Other impetigo
Ulcerative impetigo

L01.1   Impetiginization of other dermatoses

● **L02   Cutaneous abscess, furuncle and carbuncle**

Use additional code to identify organism (B95-B96)

Excludes2   abscess of anus and rectal regions (K61.-)
abscess of female genital organs (external) (N76.4)
abscess of male genital organs (external) (N48.2, N49.-)

● **L02.0   Cutaneous abscess, furuncle and carbuncle of face**

Excludes2   abscess of ear, external (H60.0)
abscess of eyelid (H00.0)
abscess of head [any part, except face] (L02.8)
abscess of lacrimal gland (H04.0)
abscess of lacrimal passages (H04.3)
abscess of mouth (K12.2)
abscess of nose (J34.0)
abscess of orbit (H05.0)
submandibular abscess (K12.2)

L02.01   Cutaneous abscess of face 🖉

● Unacceptable Principal Diagnosis   ● Use Additional Character(s)   ◾ Unspecified   ▸ Manifestation Code

1116   OGCR Official Guidelines for Coding and Reporting   Excludes 1   Excludes 2   Includes   Use additional   Code first   Code also

L02.02   Furuncle of face
  Boil of face
  Folliculitis of face

L02.03   Carbuncle of face

● **L02.1   Cutaneous abscess, furuncle and carbuncle of neck**

 L02.11   Cutaneous abscess of neck 🦠

 L02.12   Furuncle of neck
  Boil of neck
  Folliculitis of neck

 L02.13   Carbuncle of neck

● **L02.2   Cutaneous abscess, furuncle and carbuncle of trunk**

 | **Excludes1** | non-newborn omphalitis (L08.82)
   omphalitis of newborn (P38.-)

 | **Excludes2** | abscess of breast (N61)
   abscess of buttocks (L02.3)
   abscess of female external genital
    organs (N76.4)
   abscess of male external genital
    organs (N48.2, N49.-)
   abscess of hip (L02.4)

 ● **L02.21   Cutaneous abscess of trunk**

  L02.211   Cutaneous abscess of abdominal wall 🦠

  L02.212   Cutaneous abscess of back [any part, except buttock] 🦠

  L02.213   Cutaneous abscess of chest wall 🦠

  L02.214   Cutaneous abscess of groin 🦠

  L02.215   Cutaneous abscess of perineum 🦠

  L02.216   Cutaneous abscess of umbilicus 🦠

  ■ **L02.219   Cutaneous abscess of trunk, unspecified** 🦠

 ● **L02.22   Furuncle of trunk**
  Boil of trunk
  Folliculitis of trunk

  L02.221   Furuncle of abdominal wall

  L02.222   Furuncle of back [any part, except buttock]

  L02.223   Furuncle of chest wall

  L02.224   Furuncle of groin

  L02.225   Furuncle of perineum

  L02.226   Furuncle of umbilicus

  ■ **L02.229   Furuncle of trunk, unspecified**

 ● **L02.23   Carbuncle of trunk**

  L02.231   Carbuncle of abdominal wall

  L02.232   Carbuncle of back [any part, except buttock]

  L02.233   Carbuncle of chest wall

  L02.234   Carbuncle of groin

  L02.235   Carbuncle of perineum

  L02.236   Carbuncle of umbilicus

  ■ **L02.239   Carbuncle of trunk, unspecified**

● **L02.3   Cutaneous abscess, furuncle and carbuncle of buttock**

 | **Excludes1** | pilonidal cyst with abscess (L05.01)

 L02.31   Cutaneous abscess of buttock 🦠
  Cutaneous abscess of gluteal region

 L02.32   Furuncle of buttock
  Boil of buttock
  Folliculitis of buttock
  Furuncle of gluteal region

 L02.33   Carbuncle of buttock
  Carbuncle of gluteal region

● **L02.4   Cutaneous abscess, furuncle and carbuncle of limb**

 | **Excludes2** | Cutaneous abscess, furuncle and
   carbuncle of groin (L02.214,
   L02.224, L02.234)
   Cutaneous abscess, furuncle and
   carbuncle of hand (L02.5-)
   Cutaneous abscess, furuncle and
   carbuncle of foot (L02.6-)

 ● **L02.41   Cutaneous abscess of limb**

  L02.411   Cutaneous abscess of right axilla 🦠

  L02.412   Cutaneous abscess of left axilla 🦠

  L02.413   Cutaneous abscess of right upper limb 🦠

  L02.414   Cutaneous abscess of left upper limb 🦠

  L02.415   Cutaneous abscess of right lower limb 🦠

  L02.416   Cutaneous abscess of left lower limb 🦠

  ■ **L02.419   Cutaneous abscess of limb, unspecified** 🦠

 ● **L02.42   Furuncle of limb**
  Boil of limb
  Folliculitis of limb

  L02.421   Furuncle of right axilla

  L02.422   Furuncle of left axilla

  L02.423   Furuncle of right upper limb

  L02.424   Furuncle of left upper limb

  L02.425   Furuncle of right lower limb

  L02.426   Furuncle of left lower limb

  ■ **L02.429   Furuncle of limb, unspecified**

 ● **L02.43   Carbuncle of limb**

  L02.431   Carbuncle of right axilla

  L02.432   Carbuncle of left axilla

  L02.433   Carbuncle of right upper limb

  L02.434   Carbuncle of left upper limb

  L02.435   Carbuncle of right lower limb

  L02.436   Carbuncle of left lower limb

  ■ **L02.439   Carbuncle of limb, unspecified**

● **L02.5   Cutaneous abscess, furuncle and carbuncle of hand**

 ● **L02.51   Cutaneous abscess of hand**

  L02.511   Cutaneous abscess of right hand 🦠

  L02.512   Cutaneous abscess of left hand 🦠

  ■ **L02.519   Cutaneous abscess of unspecified hand** 🦠

N Newborn Age: 0 **P** Pediatric Age: 0–17 **M** Maternity DX: 12–55 **A** Adult Age: 15–124 ♀ Females Only ♂ Males Only

🦠 Complication\Comorbidity 🦠 Major C\C 🦠 Present on Admission Requirement 🦠 Hospital-Acquired Condition

CHAPTER 12 (L00-L99)

1117

CHAPTER 12 (L00-L99)

● **L02.52**   **Furuncle hand**
     Boil of hand
     Folliculitis of hand

    L02.521   **Furuncle right hand**

    L02.522   **Furuncle left hand**

    ■ **L02.529**   **Furuncle unspecified hand**

● **L02.53**   **Carbuncle of hand**

    L02.531   **Carbuncle of right hand**

    L02.532   **Carbuncle of left hand**

    ■ **L02.539**   **Carbuncle of unspecified hand**

● **L02.6**   **Cutaneous abscess, furuncle and carbuncle of foot**

   ● **L02.61**   **Cutaneous abscess of foot**

     L02.611   **Cutaneous abscess of right foot** ✪

     L02.612   **Cutaneous abscess of left foot** ✪

     ■ **L02.619**   **Cutaneous abscess of unspecified foot** ✪

   ● **L02.62**   **Furuncle of foot**
       Boil of foot
       Folliculitis of foot

     L02.621   **Furuncle of right foot**

     L02.622   **Furuncle of left foot**

     ■ **L02.629**   **Furuncle of unspecified foot**

   ● **L02.63**   **Carbuncle of foot**

     L02.631   **Carbuncle of right foot**

     L02.632   **Carbuncle of left foot**

     ■ **L02.639**   **Carbuncle of unspecified foot**

● **L02.8**   **Cutaneous abscess, furuncle and carbuncle of other sites**

   ● **L02.81**   **Cutaneous abscess of other sites**

     L02.811   **Cutaneous abscess of head [any part, except face]** ✪

     L02.818   **Cutaneous abscess of other sites** ✪

   ● **L02.82**   **Furuncle of other sites**
       Boil of other sites
       Folliculitis of other sites

     L02.821   **Furuncle of head [any part, except face]**

     L02.828   **Furuncle of other sites**

   ● **L02.83**   **Carbuncle of other sites**

     L02.831   **Carbuncle of head [any part, except face]**

     L02.838   **Carbuncle of other sites**

● **L02.9**   **Cutaneous abscess, furuncle and carbuncle, unspecified**

   ■ **L02.91**   **Cutaneous abscess, unspecified** ✪

   ■ **L02.92**   **Furuncle, unspecified**
       Boil NOS
       Furunculosis NOS

   ■ **L02.93**   **Carbuncle, unspecified**

Item 12-1   **Onychia** is an inflammation of the tissue surrounding the nail with pus accumulation and loss of the nail, resulting from microscopic pathogens entering through small wounds. **Paronychia** is a nail disease also known as felon or whitlow and is a bacterial or fungal infection.

● **L03**   **Cellulitis and acute lymphangitis**

   | Excludes2 | cellulitis of anal and rectal region (K61.-)
                cellulitis of external auditory canal (H60.1)
                cellulitis of eyelid (H00.0)
                cellulitis of female external genital organs (N76.4)
                cellulitis of lacrimal apparatus (H04.3)
                cellulitis of male external genital organs (N48.2, N49.-)
                cellulitis of mouth (K12.2)
                cellulitis of nose (J34.0)
                eosinophilic cellulitis [Wells] (L98.3)
                febrile neutrophilic dermatosis [Sweet] (L98.2)
                lymphangitis (chronic) (subacute) (I89.1)

   ● **L03.0**   **Cellulitis and acute lymphangitis of finger and toe**
       Infection of nail
       Onychia
       Paronychia
       Perionychia

    ● **L03.01**   **Cellulitis of finger**
         Felon
         Whitlow

      | Excludes1 | herpetic whitlow (B00.89)

      L03.011   **Cellulitis of right finger**

      L03.012   **Cellulitis of left finger**

      ■ **L03.019**   **Cellulitis of unspecified finger**

    ● **L03.02**   **Acute lymphangitis of finger**
         Hangnail with lymphangitis of finger

      L03.021   **Acute lymphangitis of right finger**

      L03.022   **Acute lymphangitis of left finger**

      ■ **L03.029**   **Acute lymphangitis of unspecified finger**

    ● **L03.03**   **Cellulitis of toe**

      L03.031   **Cellulitis of right toe**

      L03.032   **Cellulitis of left toe**

      ■ **L03.039**   **Cellulitis of unspecified toe**

    ● **L03.04**   **Acute lymphangitis of toe**
         Hangnail with lymphangitis of toe

      L03.041   **Acute lymphangitis of right toe**

      L03.042   **Acute lymphangitis of left toe**

      ■ **L03.049**   **Acute lymphangitis of unspecified toe**

   ● **L03.1**   **Cellulitis and acute lymphangitis of other parts of limb**

    ● **L03.11**   **Cellulitis of other parts of limb**

      | Excludes2 | cellulitis of fingers (L03.01-)
                cellulitis of toes (L03.03-)
                groin (L03.314)

      L03.111   **Cellulitis of right axilla** ✪

      L03.112   **Cellulitis of left axilla** ✪

      L03.113   **Cellulitis of right upper limb** ✪

●   Unacceptable Principal Diagnosis   ●   Use Additional Character(s)   ■   Unspecified   ▸   Manifestation Code

OGCR   Official Guidelines for Coding and Reporting | Excludes 1 | | Excludes 2 | | Includes | | Use additional | | Code first | | Code also |

L03.114   Cellulitis of left upper limb 🦠

L03.115   Cellulitis of right lower limb 🦠

L03.116   Cellulitis of left lower limb 🦠

▢ L03.119   Cellulitis of unspecified part of limb 🦠

● L03.12   Acute lymphangitis of other parts of limb

　　| Excludes2 | acute lymphangitis of fingers (L03.2-) |
　　acute lymphangitis of toes (L03.4-)
　　acute lymphangitis of groin (L03.324)

L03.121   Acute lymphangitis of right axilla 🦠

L03.122   Acute lymphangitis of left axilla 🦠

L03.123   Acute lymphangitis of right upper limb 🦠

L03.124   Acute lymphangitis of left upper limb 🦠

L03.125   Acute lymphangitis of right lower limb 🦠

L03.126   Acute lymphangitis of left lower limb 🦠

▢ L03.129   Acute lymphangitis of unspecified part of limb 🦠

● L03.2   Cellulitis and acute lymphangitis of face and neck

● L03.21   Cellulitis and acute lymphangitis of face

L03.211   Cellulitis of face 🦠

　　| Excludes2 | cellulitis of ear (H60.1-) |
　　cellulitis of eyelid (H00.0-)
　　cellulitis of head (L03.81)
　　cellulitis of lacrimal apparatus (H04.3)
　　cellulitis of lip (K13.0)
　　cellulitis of mouth (K12.2)
　　cellulitis of nose (internal) (J34.0)
　　cellulitis of orbit (H05.0)
　　cellulitis of scalp (L03.81)

L03.212   Acute lymphangitis of face 🦠

● L03.22   Cellulitis and acute lymphangitis of neck

L03.221   Cellulitis of neck 🦠

L03.222   Acute lymphangitis of neck 🦠

Item 12-2   Cellulitis is an acute spreading bacterial infection below the surface of the skin characterized by redness (erythema), warmth, swelling, pain, fever, chills, and enlarged lymph nodes ("swollen glands").

● L03.3   Cellulitis and acute lymphangitis of trunk

● L03.31   Cellulitis of trunk

　　| Excludes2 | cellulitis of anal and rectal regions (K61.-) |
　　cellulitis of breast NOS (N61)
　　cellulitis of female external genital organs (N76.4)
　　cellulitis of male external genital organs (N48.2, N49.-)
　　omphalitis of newborn (P38.-)
　　puerperal cellulitis of breast (O91.2)

L03.311   Cellulitis of abdominal wall 🦠

　　| Excludes2 | cellulitis of umbilicus (L03.316) |
　　cellulitis of groin (L03.314)

L03.312   Cellulitis of back [any part except buttock] 🦠

L03.313   Cellulitis of chest wall 🦠

L03.314   Cellulitis of groin 🦠

L03.315   Cellulitis of perineum 🦠

L03.316   Cellulitis of umbilicus 🦠

L03.317   Cellulitis of buttock 🦠

▢ L03.319   Cellulitis of trunk, unspecified 🦠

● L03.32   Acute lymphangitis of trunk

L03.321   Acute lymphangitis of abdominal wall 🦠

L03.322   Acute lymphangitis of back [any part except buttock] 🦠

L03.323   Acute lymphangitis of chest wall 🦠

L03.324   Acute lymphangitis of groin 🦠

L03.325   Acute lymphangitis of perineum 🦠

L03.326   Acute lymphangitis of umbilicus 🦠

L03.327   Acute lymphangitis of buttock 🦠

▢ L03.329   Acute lymphangitis of trunk, unspecified 🦠

● L03.8   Cellulitis and acute lymphangitis of other sites

● L03.81   Cellulitis of other sites

L03.811   Cellulitis of head [any part, except face] 🦠
　　　Cellulitis of scalp
　　　| Excludes2 | cellulitis of face (L03.211) |

L03.818   Cellulitis of other sites 🦠

● L03.89   Acute lymphangitis of other sites

L03.891   Acute lymphangitis of head [any part, except face] 🦠

L03.898   Acute lymphangitis of other sites 🦠

CHAPTER 12 (L00-L99)

N Newborn Age: 0   **P** Pediatric Age: 0–17   **M** Maternity DX: 12–55   **A** Adult Age: 15–124   ♀ Females Only   ♂ Males Only

🦠 Complication\Comorbidity   🦠 Major C\C   🦠 Present on Admission Requirement   🦠 Hospital-Acquired Condition

1119

- L03.9 **Cellulitis and acute lymphangitis, unspecified**
  - ■ L03.90 **Cellulitis, unspecified** 🔊
  - ■ L03.91 **Acute lymphangitis, unspecified** 🔊
    - Excludes1 | lymphangitis NOS (I89.1)

- L04 **Acute lymphadenitis**
  - *Short-term inflammation of lymph nodes which can be regionalized to involve a given area of the lymph system or systemic involving much of the body*
    - Includes | abscess (acute) of lymph nodes, except mesenteric
      - acute lymphadenitis, except mesenteric
    - Excludes1 | chronic or subacute lymphadenitis, except mesenteric (I88.1)
      - enlarged lymph nodes (R59.-)
      - human immunodeficiency virus [HIV] disease resulting in generalized lymphadenopathy (B20)
      - lymphadenitis NOS (I88.9)
      - nonspecific mesenteric lymphadenitis (I88.0)
  - L04.0 **Acute lymphadenitis of face, head and neck**
  - L04.1 **Acute lymphadenitis of trunk**
  - L04.2 **Acute lymphadenitis of upper limb**
    - Acute lymphadenitis of axilla
    - Acute lymphadenitis of shoulder
  - L04.3 **Acute lymphadenitis of lower limb**
    - Acute lymphadenitis of hip
      - Excludes2 | acute lymphadenitis of groin (L04.1)
  - L04.8 **Acute lymphadenitis of other sites**
  - ■ L04.9 **Acute lymphadenitis, unspecified**

- L05 **Pilonidal cyst and sinus**
  - L05.0 **Pilonidal cyst and sinus with abscess**
    - L05.01 **Pilonidal cyst with abscess** 🔊
      - Parasacral dimple with abscess
      - Pilonidal abscess
      - Pilonidal dimple with abscess
      - Postanal dimple with abscess
    - L05.02 **Pilonidal sinus with abscess** 🔊
      - Coccygeal fistula with abscess
      - Coccygeal sinus with abscess
      - Pilonidal fistula with abscess
  - L05.9 **Pilonidal cyst and sinus without abscess**
    - L05.91 **Pilonidal cyst without abscess**
      - Parasacral dimple
      - Pilonidal dimple
      - Postanal dimple
      - Pilonidal cyst NOS
    - L05.92 **Pilonidal sinus without abscess**
      - Coccygeal fistula
      - Coccygeal sinus without abscess
      - Pilonidal fistula

- L08 **Other local infections of skin and subcutaneous tissue**
  - L08.0 **Pyoderma**
    - Dermatitis gangrenosa
    - Purulent dermatitis
    - Septic dermatitis
    - Suppurative dermatitis
      - Excludes1 | pyoderma gangrenosum (L88)
        - pyoderma vegetans (L08.81)
  - L08.1 **Erythrasma** 🔊
  - L08.8 **Other specified local infections of the skin and subcutaneous tissue**
    - L08.81 **Pyoderma vegetans**
      - Excludes1 | pyoderma gangrenosum (L88)
        - pyoderma NOS (L08.0)

Figure 12-2 Impetigo. A thick, honey-yellow adherent crust covers the entire eroded surface. (From Habif: Clinical Dermatology, 4th ed. 2004, Mosby, Inc.)

Item 12–3 Abscess is a localized collection of pus in tissues or organs and is a sign of infection resulting in swelling and inflammation.

Item 12–4 Pilonidal cyst, also called a coccygeal cyst, is the result of a disorder called pilonidal disease. The cyst usually contains hair and pus.

- L08.82 **Omphalitis not of newborn**
  - Excludes1 | omphalitis of newborn (P38.-)
- L08.89 **Other specified local infections of the skin and subcutaneous tissue**
- ■ L08.9 **Local infection of the skin and subcutaneous tissue, unspecified**

BULLOUS DISORDERS (L10-L14)

- Excludes1 | benign familial pemphigus [Hailey-Hailey] (Q82.8)
  - staphylococcal scalded skin syndrome (L00)
  - toxic epidermal necrolysis [Lyell] (L51.2)

- L10 **Pemphigus**
  - Excludes1 | pemphigus neonatorum (L01.03)
  - L10.0 **Pemphigus vulgaris** 🔊
  - L10.1 **Pemphigus vegetans** 🔊
  - L10.2 **Pemphigus foliaceous** 🔊
  - L10.3 **Brazilian pemphigus [fogo selvagem]** 🔊
  - L10.4 **Pemphigus erythematosus** 🔊
    - Senear-Usher syndrome
  - L10.5 **Drug-induced pemphigus** 🔊
    - Use additional code for adverse effect, if applicable, to identify drug (T36-T50 with fifth or sixth character 5)
  - L10.8 **Other pemphigus**
    - L10.81 **Paraneoplastic pemphigus** 🔊
    - L10.89 **Other pemphigus** 🔊
  - ■ L10.9 **Pemphigus, unspecified** 🔊

- L11 **Other acantholytic disorders**
  - L11.0 **Acquired keratosis follicularis**
    - Excludes1 | keratosis follicularis (congenital) [Darier-White] (Q82.8)
  - L11.1 **Transient acantholytic dermatosis [Grover]**
  - L11.8 **Other specified acantholytic disorders**
  - ■ L11.9 **Acantholytic disorder, unspecified**

- L12 **Pemphigoid**
  - Excludes1 | herpes gestationis (O26.4-)
    - impetigo herpetiformis (L40.1)
  - L12.0 **Bullous pemphigoid** 🔊
  - L12.1 **Cicatricial pemphigoid**
    - Benign mucous membrane pemphigoid
  - L12.2 **Chronic bullous disease of childhood**   P
    - Juvenile dermatitis herpetiformis

● Unacceptable Principal Diagnosis   ● Use Additional Character(s)   ■ Unspecified   ▶ Manifestation Code

1120   OGCR Official Guidelines for Coding and Reporting | Excludes 1 | | Excludes 2 | Includes   Use additional   Code first   Code also

● **L12.3   Acquired epidermolysis bullosa**
>   **Excludes1**   epidermolysis bullosa (congenital)
>   (Q81.-)

■ **L12.30   Acquired epidermolysis bullosa,
  unspecified** 🔗

● **L12.31   Epidermolysis bullosa due to drug** 🔗
>   Use additional code for adverse effect, if
>   applicable, to identify drug (T36-T50
>   with fifth or sixth character 5)

L12.35   Other acquired epidermolysis bullosa 🔗

L12.8   Other pemphigoid 🔗

■ **L12.9   Pemphigoid, unspecified** 🔗

● **L13   Other bullous disorders**

L13.0   Dermatitis herpetiformis
   Duhring's disease
   Hydroa herpetiformis
>   **Excludes1**   juvenile dermatitis herpetiformis
>   (L12.2)
>   senile dermatitis herpetiformis
>   (L12.0)

L13.1   Subcorneal pustular dermatitis
   Sneddon-Wilkinson disease

L13.8   Other specified bullous disorders

■ **L13.9   Bullous disorder, unspecified**

●▶ *L14   Bullous disorders in diseases classified elsewhere*
   Code first underlying disease

DERMATITIS AND ECZEMA (L20-L30)

Note: In this block the terms dermatitis and eczema are
used synonymously and interchangeably.
>   **Excludes2**   chronic (childhood) granulomatous disease
>   (D71)
>   dermatitis gangrenosa (L08.0)
>   dermatitis herpetiformis (L13.0)
>   dry skin dermatitis (L85.3)
>   factitial dermatitis (L98.1)
>   perioral dermatitis (L71.0)
>   radiation-related disorders of the skin and
>   subcutaneous tissue (L55-L59)
>   stasis dermatitis (I83.1-I83.2)

● **L20   Atopic dermatitis**

L20.0   Besnier's prurigo

● **L20.8   Other atopic dermatitis**
>   **Excludes2**   circumscribed neurodermatitis
>   (L28.0)

L20.81   Atopic neurodermatitis
   Diffuse neurodermatitis

L20.82   Flexural eczema

L20.83   Infantile (acute) (chronic) eczema   P

L20.84   Intrinsic (allergic) eczema

L20.89   Other atopic dermatitis

■ **L20.9   Atopic dermatitis, unspecified**

● **L21   Seborrheic dermatitis**
>   **Excludes2**   infective dermatitis (L30.3)
>   seborrheic keratosis (L82.-)

L21.0   Seborrhea capitis   P
   Cradle cap

L21.1   Seborrheic infantile dermatitis   P

L21.8   Other seborrheic dermatitis

■ **L21.9   Seborrheic dermatitis, unspecified**
   Seborrhea NOS

Item 12–5   Dermatitis herpetiformis, also known as Duhring's
disease, is a systemic disease characterized by small blisters (3 to 5 mm)
and occasionally large bullae (> 5 mm).

Figure 12-3   Dermatitis herpetiformis. (From Arnold HL, Odom
RB, James WD: Andrews' Diseases of the Skin, Clinical Dermatology,
8th ed. Philadelphia, WB Saunders, 1990, p 553.)

Item 12–6   Seborrheic dermatitis is characterized by greasy,
scaly, red patches and is associated with oily skin and scalp.

Figure 12-4   Seborrheic
dermatitis. (From Cohen BA: Atlas
of Pediatric Dermatology, St. Louis,
Mosby, 1993.)

Item 12–7   Atopic dermatitis, also known as atopic eczema,
infantile eczema, disseminated neuro dermatitis, flexural eczema, and
prurigo diathesique (Besnier), is characterized by intense itching and is
often hereditary.

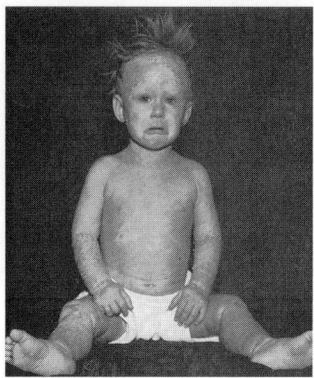

Figure 12-5   Atopic
dermatitis. (From Moschella
SL, Hurley HJ: Dermatology,
2nd ed. Philadelphia, WB
Saunders, 1985, p 336.)

CHAPTER 12 (L00-L99)

L22   Diaper dermatitis
     Diaper erythema
     Diaper rash
     Psoriasiform diaper rash

● **L23   Allergic contact dermatitis**

   Excludes1   allergy NOS (T78.40)
          contact dermatitis NOS (L25.9)
          dermatitis NOS (L30.9)

   Excludes2   dermatitis due to substances taken
            internally (L27.-)
          dermatitis of eyelid (H01.1-)
          diaper dermatitis (L22)
          eczema of external ear (H60.5-)
          irritant contact dermatitis (L24.-)
          perioral dermatitis (L71.0)
          radiation-related disorders of the skin and
            subcutaneous tissue (L55-L59)

● **L23.0   Allergic contact dermatitis due to metals**
     Allergic contact dermatitis due to chromium
     Allergic contact dermatitis due to nickel

● **L23.1   Allergic contact dermatitis due to adhesives**

● **L23.2   Allergic contact dermatitis due to cosmetics**

● **L23.3   Allergic contact dermatitis due to drugs in contact with skin**

   Use additional code for adverse effect, if
     applicable, to identify drug (T36-T50 with
     fifth or sixth character 5)

     Excludes2   dermatitis due to ingested drugs and
            medicaments (L27.0-L27.1)

● **L23.4   Allergic contact dermatitis due to dyes**

● **L23.5   Allergic contact dermatitis due to other chemical products**
     Allergic contact dermatitis due to cement
     Allergic contact dermatitis due to insecticide
     Allergic contact dermatitis due to plastic
     Allergic contact dermatitis due to rubber

● **L23.6   Allergic contact dermatitis due to food in contact with the skin**

     Excludes2   dermatitis due to ingested food
            (L27.2)

● **L23.7   Allergic contact dermatitis due to plants, except food**
     Excludes2   allergy NOS due to pollen (J30.1)

● **L23.8   Allergic contact dermatitis due to other agents**

● **L23.81   Allergic contact dermatitis due to animal (cat) (dog) dander**
     Allergic contact dermatitis due to animal (cat) (dog) hair

● **L23.89   Allergic contact dermatitis due to other agents**

● ■ **L23.9   Allergic contact dermatitis, unspecified cause**
     Allergic contact eczema NOS

● **L24   Irritant contact dermatitis**

   Excludes1   allergy NOS (T78.40)
          contact dermatitis NOS (L25.9)
          dermatitis NOS (L30.9)

   Excludes2   allergic contact dermatitis (L23.-)
          dermatitis due to substances taken
            internally (L27.-)
          dermatitis of eyelid (H01.1-)
          diaper dermatitis (L22)
          eczema of external ear (H60.5-)
          perioral dermatitis (L71.0)
          radiation-related disorders of the skin and
            subcutaneous tissue (L55-L59)

● **L24.0   Irritant contact dermatitis due to detergents**

● **L24.1   Irritant contact dermatitis due to oils and greases**

● **L24.2   Irritant contact dermatitis due to solvents**
     Irritant contact dermatitis due to chlorocompound
     Irritant contact dermatitis due to cyclohexane
     Irritant contact dermatitis due to ester
     Irritant contact dermatitis due to glycol
     Irritant contact dermatitis due to hydrocarbon
     Irritant contact dermatitis due to ketone

● **L24.3   Irritant contact dermatitis due to cosmetics**

● **L24.4   Irritant contact dermatitis due to drugs in contact with skin**

   Use additional code for adverse effect, if
     applicable, to identify drug (T36-T50 with
     fifth or sixth character 5)

● **L24.5   Irritant contact dermatitis due to other chemical products**
     Irritant contact dermatitis due to cement
     Irritant contact dermatitis due to insecticide
     Irritant contact dermatitis due to plastic
     Irritant contact dermatitis due to rubber

● **L24.6   Irritant contact dermatitis due to food in contact with skin**

     Excludes2   dermatitis due to ingested food
            (L27.2)

● **L24.7   Irritant contact dermatitis due to plants, except food**

     Excludes2   allergy NOS to pollen (J30.1)

● **L24.8   Irritant contact dermatitis due to other agents**

● **L24.81   Irritant contact dermatitis due to metals**
     Irritant contact dermatitis due to chromium
     Irritant contact dermatitis due to nickel

● **L24.89   Irritant contact dermatitis due to other agents**
     Irritant contact dermatitis due to dyes

● ■ **L24.9   Irritant contact dermatitis, unspecified cause**
     Irritant contact eczema NOS

● **L25   Unspecified contact dermatitis**

   Excludes1   allergic contact dermatitis (L23.-)
          allergy NOS (T78.40)
          dermatitis NOS (L30.9)
          irritant contact dermatitis (L24.-)

   Excludes2   dermatitis due to ingested substances (L27.-)
          dermatitis of eyelid (H01.1-)
          eczema of external ear (H60.5-)
          perioral dermatitis (L71.0)
          radiation-related disorders of the skin and
            subcutaneous tissue (L55-L59)

● ■ **L25.0   Unspecified contact dermatitis due to cosmetics**

● ■ **L25.1   Unspecified contact dermatitis due to drugs in contact with skin**

   Use additional code for adverse effect, if
     applicable, to identify drug (T36-T50 with
     fifth or sixth character 5)

     Excludes2   dermatitis due to ingested drugs and
            medicaments (L27.0-L27.1)

● ■ **L25.2   Unspecified contact dermatitis due to dyes**

● ■ **L25.3   Unspecified contact dermatitis due to other chemical products**
     Unspecified contact dermatitis due to cement
     Unspecified contact dermatitis due to insecticide

● ■ **L25.4   Unspecified contact dermatitis due to food in contact with skin**

     Excludes2   dermatitis due to ingested food
            (L27.2)

● ■ **L25.5 Unspecified contact dermatitis due to plants, except food**

| **Excludes1** | nettle rash (L50.9) |

| **Excludes2** | allergy NOS due to pollen (J30.1) |

● ■ **L25.8 Unspecified contact dermatitis due to other agents**

● ■ **L25.9 Unspecified contact dermatitis, unspecified cause**
Contact dermatitis (occupational) NOS
Contact eczema (occupational) NOS

L26 Exfoliative dermatitis
Hebra's pityriasis

| **Excludes1** | Ritter's disease (L00) |

● **L27 Dermatitis due to substances taken internally**

| **Excludes1** | allergy NOS (T78.40) |

Excludes2	adverse food reaction, except dermatitis (T78.0-T78.1)
	contact dermatitis (L23-L25)
	drug photoallergic response (L56.1)
	drug phototoxic response (L56.0)
	urticaria (L50.-)

● **L27.0 Generalized skin eruption due to drugs and medicaments taken internally**
Use additional code for adverse effect, if applicable, to identify drug (T36-T50 with fifth or sixth character 5)

● **L27.1 Localized skin eruption due to drugs and medicaments taken internally**
Use additional code for adverse effect, if applicable, to identify drug (T36-T50 with fifth or sixth character 5)

● **L27.2 Dermatitis due to ingested food**

| **Excludes2** | dermatitis due to food in contact with skin (L23.6, L24.6, L25.4) |

● **L27.8 Dermatitis due to other substances taken internally**

● ■ **L27.9 Dermatitis due to unspecified substance taken internally**

● **L28 Lichen simplex chronicus and prurigo**

L28.0 Lichen simplex chronicus
Circumscribed neurodermatitis
Lichen NOS

L28.1 Prurigo nodularis

L28.2 Other prurigo
Prurigo NOS   Prurigo mitis
Prurigo Hebra   Urticaria papulosa

● **L29 Pruritus**

| **Excludes1** | neurotic excoriation (L98.1) |
| | psychogenic pruritus (F45.8) |

L29.0 Pruritus ani

L29.1 Pruritus scroti ♂

L29.2 Pruritus vulvae ♀

■ **L29.3 Anogenital pruritus, unspecified**

L29.8 Other pruritus

■ **L29.9 Pruritus, unspecified**
Itch NOS

● **L30 Other and unspecified dermatitis**

Excludes2	contact dermatitis (L23-L25)
	dry skin dermatitis (L85.3)
	small plaque parapsoriasis (L41.3)
	stasis dermatitis (I83.1-.2)

L30.0 Nummular dermatitis

L30.1 Dyshidrosis [pompholyx]

L30.2 Cutaneous autosensitization
Candidid [levurid]   Eczematid
Dermatophytid

L30.3 Infective dermatitis
Infectious eczematoid dermatitis

L30.4 Erythema intertrigo

L30.5 Pityriasis alba

L30.8 Other specified dermatitis

■ **L30.9 Dermatitis, unspecified**
Eczema NOS

PAPULOSQUAMOUS DISORDERS (L40-L45)

● **L40 Psoriasis**

L40.0 Psoriasis vulgaris
Nummular psoriasis   Plaque psoriasis

L40.1 Generalized pustular psoriasis
Impetigo herpetiformis
Von Zumbusch's disease

L40.2 Acrodermatitis continua

L40.3 Pustulosis palmaris et plantaris

L40.4 Guttate psoriasis

● **L40.5 Arthropathic psoriasis**

■ **L40.50 Arthropathic psoriasis, unspecified**

L40.51 Distal interphalangeal psoriatic arthropathy

L40.52 Psoriatic arthritis mutilans

L40.53 Psoriatic spondylitis

L40.54 Psoriatic juvenile arthropathy

L40.59 Other psoriatic arthropathy

L40.8 Other psoriasis
Flexural psoriasis

■ **L40.9 Psoriasis, unspecified**

● **L41 Parapsoriasis**

| **Excludes1** | poikiloderma vasculare atrophicans (L94.5) |

L41.0 Pityriasis lichenoides et varioliformis acuta
Mucha-Habermann disease

L41.1 Pityriasis lichenoides chronica

L41.2 Lymphomatoid papulosis

L41.3 Small plaque parapsoriasis

L41.4 Large plaque parapsoriasis

L41.5 Retiform parapsoriasis

L41.8 Other parapsoriasis

■ **L41.9 Parapsoriasis, unspecified**

L42 Pityriasis rosea

Item 12–8 Psoriasis is a chronic, recurrent inflammatory skin disease characterized by small patches covered with thick silvery scales. **Parapsoriasis** is a treatment-resistant erythroderma. **Pityriasis rosea** is characterized by a herald patch that is a single large lesion and that usually appears on the trunk and is followed by scattered, smaller lesions.

CHAPTER 12 (L00-L99)

N Newborn Age: 0	**P** Pediatric Age: 0–17	**M** Maternity DX: 12–55	**A** Adult Age: 15–124	♀ Females Only	♂ Males Only

🅒 Complication\Comorbidity   🅜 Major C\C   Present on Admission Requirement   Hospital-Acquired Condition

● **L43 Lichen planus**

> Excludes1   lichen planopilaris (L66.1)

   L43.0 Hypertrophic lichen planus

   L43.1 Bullous lichen planus

● **L43.2 Lichenoid drug reaction**

> Use additional code for adverse effect, if
> applicable, to identify drug (T36-T50 with
> fifth or sixth character 5)

   L43.3 Subacute (active) lichen planus
      Lichen planus tropicus

   L43.8 Other lichen planus

■ **L43.9 Lichen planus, unspecified**

● **L44 Other papulosquamous disorders**

   L44.0 Pityriasis rubra pilaris

   L44.1 Lichen nitidus

   L44.2 Lichen striatus

   L44.3 Lichen ruber moniliformis

   L44.4 Infantile papular acrodermatitis [Gianotti-Crosti] P

   L44.8 Other specified papulosquamous disorders

■ **L44.9 Papulosquamous disorder, unspecified**

●◗ *L45 Papulosquamous disorders in diseases classified elsewhere*

> *Code first underlying disease*

URTICARIA AND ERYTHEMA (L49-L54)

> Excludes1   Lyme disease (A69.2-)
> rosacea (L71.-)

● **L49 Exfoliation due to erythematous conditions according to extent of body surface involved**

> Code first erythematous condition causing exfoliation,
> such as:
>   Ritter's disease (L00)
>   (Staphylococcal) scalded skin syndrome (L00)
>   Stevens-Johnson syndrome (L51.1)
>   Stevens-Johnson syndrome-toxic epidermal necrolysis
>   overlap syndrome (L51.3)
>   Toxic epidermal necrolysis (L51.2)

● **L49.0 Exfoliation due to erythematous condition involving less than 10 percent of body surface**
      Exfoliation due to erythematous condition NOS

● **L49.1 Exfoliation due to erythematous condition involving 10-19 percent of body surface**

● **L49.2 Exfoliation due to erythematous condition involving 20-29 percent of body surface**

● **L49.3 Exfoliation due to erythematous condition involving 30-39 percent of body surface** ✆

● **L49.4 Exfoliation due to erythematous condition involving 40-49 percent of body surface** ✆

● **L49.5 Exfoliation due to erythematous condition involving 50-59 percent of body surface** ✆

● **L49.6 Exfoliation due to erythematous condition involving 60-69 percent of body surface** ✆

● **L49.7 Exfoliation due to erythematous condition involving 70-79 percent of body surface** ✆

● **L49.8 Exfoliation due to erythematous condition involving 80-89 percent of body surface** ✆

● **L49.9 Exfoliation due to erythematous condition involving 90 or more percent of body surface** ✆

Figure 12-6 Erythematous plaques with silvery scales in a patient with psoriasis. (From Goldman: Cecil Textbook of Medicine, 22nd ed. 2004, Saunders.)

Figure 12-7 Urticaria (hives). *(Courtesy of Davis Effron, MD.)* (From Marx: Rosen's Emergency Medicine: Concepts and Clinical Practice, 6th ed. 2006, Mosby, Inc.)

Item 12–9 Urticaria is a vascular reaction in which wheals surrounded by a red halo appear and cause severe itching. The causes of urticaria or hives are extensive and varied (e.g., food, heat, cold, drugs, stress, infections).

● **L50 Urticaria**

> Excludes1   allergic contact dermatitis (L23.-)
> angioneurotic edema (T78.3)
> giant urticaria (T78.3)
> hereditary angio-edema (D84.1)
> Quincke's edema (T78.3)
> serum urticaria (T80.6-)
> solar urticaria (L56.3)
> urticaria neonatorum (P83.8)
> urticaria papulosa (L28.2)
> urticaria pigmentosa (Q82.2)

   L50.0 Allergic urticaria

   L50.1 Idiopathic urticaria

   L50.2 Urticaria due to cold and heat

   L50.3 Dermatographic urticaria

   L50.4 Vibratory urticaria

   L50.5 Cholinergic urticaria

   L50.6 Contact urticaria

   L50.8 Other urticaria
      Chronic urticaria
      Recurrent periodic urticaria

■ **L50.9 Urticaria, unspecified**

CHAPTER 12 (L00-L99)

1124

● Unacceptable Principal Diagnosis   ● Use Additional Character(s)   ■ Unspecified   ◗ Manifestation Code

OGCR Official Guidelines for Coding and Reporting | Excludes 1 | | Excludes 2 | Includes Use additional Code first Code also

● **L51   Erythema multiforme**

> Use additional code for adverse effect, if applicable, to identify drug (T36-T50 with fifth or sixth character 5)

> Use additional code to identify associated manifestations, such as:
> arthropathy associated with dermatological disorders (M14.8-)
> conjunctival edema (H11.42)
> conjunctivitis (H10.22-)
> corneal scars and opacities (H17.-)
> corneal ulcer (H16.0-)
> edema of eyelid (H02.84)
> inflammation of eyelid (H01.8)
> keratoconjunctivitis sicca (H16.22-)
> mechanical lagophthalmos (H02.22-)
> stomatitis (K12.-)
> symblepharon (H11.23-)

> Use additional code to identify percentage of skin exfoliation (L49-)

> **Excludes1**   staphylococcal scalded skin syndrome (L00)
> Ritter's disease (L00)

L51.0   **Nonbullous erythema multiforme**

L51.1   **Stevens-Johnson syndrome** 🔒

L51.2   **Toxic epidermal necrolysis [Lyell]** 🔒

L51.3   **Stevens-Johnson syndrome-toxic epidermal necrolysis overlap syndrome** 🔒
> SJS-TEN overlap syndrome

L51.8   **Other erythema multiforme**

◼ L51.9   **Erythema multiforme, unspecified**
> Erythema iris
> Erythema multiforme major NOS
> Erythema multiforme minor NOS
> Herpes iris

L52   **Erythema nodosum**

> **Excludes1**   tuberculous erythema nodosum (A18.4)

● **L53   Other erythematous conditions**

> **Excludes1**   erythema ab igne (L59.0)
> erythema due to external agents in contact with skin (L23-L25)
> erythema intertrigo (L30.4)

● L53.0   **Toxic erythema** 🔒

> *Code first* poisoning due to drug or toxin, if applicable (T36-T65 with fifth or sixth character 1-4 or 6)

> Use additional code for adverse effect, if applicable, to identify drug (T36-T50 with fifth or sixth character 5)

> **Excludes1**   neonatal erythema toxicum (P83.1)

L53.1   **Erythema annulare centrifugum** 🔒

L53.2   **Erythema marginatum** 🔒

L53.3   **Other chronic figurate erythema** 🔒

L53.8   **Other specified erythematous conditions**

◼ L53.9   **Erythematous condition, unspecified**
> Erythema NOS
> Erythroderma NOS

● ◗ *L54   Erythema in diseases classified elsewhere*
> *Code first* underlying disease

RADIATION-RELATED DISORDERS OF THE SKIN AND SUBCUTANEOUS TISSUE (L55-L59)

● **L55   Sunburn**

L55.0   **Sunburn of first degree**

L55.1   **Sunburn of second degree**

L55.2   **Sunburn of third degree**

◼ L55.9   **Sunburn, unspecified**

● **L56   Other acute skin changes due to ultraviolet radiation**

> Use additional code to identify the source of the ultraviolet radiation (W89, X32)

● L56.0   **Drug phototoxic response**

> Use additional code for adverse effect, if applicable, to identify drug (T36-T50 with fifth or sixth character 5)

● L56.1   **Drug photoallergic response**

> Use additional code for adverse effect, if applicable, to identify drug (T36-T50 with fifth or sixth character 5)

L56.2   **Photocontact dermatitis [berloque dermatitis]**

L56.3   **Solar urticaria**

L56.4   **Polymorphous light eruption**

L56.5   **Disseminated superficial actinic porokeratosis (DSAP)**

L56.8   **Other specified acute skin changes due to ultraviolet radiation**

◼ L56.9   **Acute skin change due to ultraviolet radiation, unspecified**

● **L57   Skin changes due to chronic exposure to nonionizing radiation**

> Use additional code to identify the source of the ultraviolet radiation (W89, X32)

L57.0   **Actinic keratosis**
> Keratosis NOS   Solar keratosis
> Senile keratosis

L57.1   **Actinic reticuloid**

L57.2   **Cutis rhomboidalis nuchae**

L57.3   **Poikiloderma of Civatte**

L57.4   **Cutis laxa senilis**
> Elastosis senilis

L57.5   **Actinic granuloma**

L57.8   **Other skin changes due to chronic exposure to nonionizing radiation**
> Farmer's skin   Solar dermatitis
> Sailor's skin

◼ L57.9   **Skin changes due to chronic exposure to nonionizing radiation, unspecified**

● **L58   Radiodermatitis**

> Use additional code to identify the source of the radiation (W88, W90)

L58.0   **Acute radiodermatitis**

L58.1   **Chronic radiodermatitis**

◼ L58.9   **Radiodermatitis, unspecified**

● **L59   Other disorders of skin and subcutaneous tissue related to radiation**

L59.0   **Erythema ab igne [dermatitis ab igne]**

L59.8   **Other specified disorders of the skin and subcutaneous tissue related to radiation**

◼ L59.9   **Disorder of the skin and subcutaneous tissue related to radiation, unspecified**

N Newborn Age: 0   **P** Pediatric Age: 0–17   **M** Maternity DX: 12–55   **A** Adult Age: 15–124   ♀ Females Only   ♂ Males Only

🔒 Complication\Comorbidity   🔒 Major C\C   🔒 Present on Admission Requirement   🔒 Hospital-Acquired Condition

1125

DISORDERS OF SKIN APPENDAGES (L60-L75)

| Excludes1 | congenital malformations of integument (Q84.-) |

● **L60 Nail disorders**

| Excludes2 | clubbing of nails (R68.3) |
| | onychia and paronychia (L03.0-) |

L60.0 Ingrowing nail

L60.1 Onycholysis

L60.2 Onychogryphosis

L60.3 Nail dystrophy

L60.4 Beau's lines

L60.5 Yellow nail syndrome

L60.8 Other nail disorders

■ L60.9 Nail disorder, unspecified

●▶ *L62 Nail disorders in diseases classified elsewhere*

Code first underlying disease, such as:
pachydermoperiostosis (M89.4-)

● **L63 Alopecia areata**

L63.0 Alopecia (capitis) totalis

L63.1 Alopecia universalis

L63.2 Ophiasis

L63.8 Other alopecia areata

■ L63.9 Alopecia areata, unspecified

● **L64 Androgenic alopecia**

| Includes | male-pattern baldness |

● **L64.0 Drug-induced androgenic alopecia**

Use additional code for adverse effect, if applicable, to identify drug (T36-T50 with fifth or sixth character 5)

L64.8 Other androgenic alopecia

■ L64.9 Androgenic alopecia, unspecified

Item 12-10 Alopecia is lack of hair and takes many forms. The most common is male pattern alopecia, also known as **androgenetic alopecia. Telogen effluvium** is early and excessive loss of hair resulting from a trauma to the hair follicle (fever, drugs, surgery, etc.).

Figure 12-8 Male pattern alopecia.

● **L65 Other nonscarring hair loss**

Use additional code for adverse effect, if applicable, to identify drug (T36-T50 with fifth or sixth character 5)

| Excludes1 | trichotillomania (F63.3) |

L65.0 Telogen effluvium

L65.1 Anagen effluvium

L65.2 Alopecia mucinosa

L65.8 Other specified nonscarring hair loss

■ L65.9 Nonscarring hair loss, unspecified
Alopecia NOS

● **L66 Cicatricial alopecia [scarring hair loss]**

L66.0 Pseudopelade

L66.1 Lichen planopilaris
Follicular lichen planus

L66.2 Folliculitis decalvans

L66.3 Perifolliculitis capitis abscedens

L66.4 Folliculitis ulerythematosa reticulata

L66.8 Other cicatricial alopecia

■ L66.9 Cicatricial alopecia, unspecified

● **L67 Hair color and hair shaft abnormalities**

Excludes1	monilethrix (Q84.1)
	pili annulati (Q84.1)
	telogen effluvium (L65.0)

L67.0 Trichorrhexis nodosa

L67.1 Variations in hair color
Canities
Greyness, hair (premature)
Heterochromia of hair
Poliosis circumscripta, acquired
Poliosis NOS

L67.8 Other hair color and hair shaft abnormalities
Fragilitas crinium

■ L67.9 Hair color and hair shaft abnormality, unspecified

● **L68 Hypertrichosis**

Includes	excess hair
Excludes1	congenital hypertrichosis (Q84.2)
	persistent lanugo (Q84.2)

L68.0 Hirsutism
Excessive growth of hair

L68.1 Acquired hypertrichosis lanuginosa

L68.2 Localized hypertrichosis

L68.3 Polytrichia

L68.8 Other hypertrichosis

■ L68.9 Hypertrichosis, unspecified

● **L70 Acne**

| Excludes2 | acne keloid (L73.0) |

L70.0 Acne vulgaris

L70.1 Acne conglobata

L70.2 Acne varioliformis
Acne necrotica miliaris

L70.3 Acne tropica

L70.4 Infantile acne   P

L70.5 Acné excoriée des jeunes filles
Picker's acne

L70.8 Other acne

■ L70.9 Acne, unspecified

● Unacceptable Principal Diagnosis   ● Use Additional Character(s)   ■ Unspecified   ▶ Manifestation Code

OGCR Official Guidelines for Coding and Reporting   Excludes 1   Excludes 2   Includes   Use additional   Code first   Code also

● **L71 Rosacea**
> Use additional code for adverse effect, if applicable, to identify drug (T36-T50 with fifth or sixth character 5)

     L71.0 Perioral dermatitis

     L71.1 Rhinophyma

     L71.8 Other rosacea

    ■ **L71.9 Rosacea, unspecified**

● **L72 Follicular cysts of skin and subcutaneous tissue**

     L72.0 Epidermal cyst

    ● **L72.1 Pilar and trichodermal cyst**

       L72.11 Pilar cyst

       L72.12 Trichodermal cyst
         Trichilemmal (proliferating) cyst

     L72.3 Sebaceous cyst
> **Excludes2**   pilar cyst (L72.11)
>   trichilemmal (proliferating) cyst (L72.12)

     L72.2 Steatocystoma multiplex

     L72.8 Other follicular cysts of the skin and subcutaneous tissue

    ■ **L72.9 Follicular cyst of the skin and subcutaneous tissue, unspecified**

● **L73 Other follicular disorders**

     L73.0 Acne keloid

     L73.1 Pseudofolliculitis barbae

     L73.2 Hidradenitis suppurativa

     L73.8 Other specified follicular disorders
       Sycosis barbae

    ■ **L73.9 Follicular disorder, unspecified**

● **L74 Eccrine sweat disorders**
> **Excludes2**   generalized hyperhidrosis (R61)

     L74.0 Miliaria rubra

     L74.1 Miliaria crystallina

     L74.2 Miliaria profunda
       Miliaria tropicalis

    ■ **L74.3 Miliaria, unspecified**

     L74.4 Anhidrosis
       Hypohidrosis

    ● **L74.5 Focal hyperhidrosis**

      ● **L74.51 Primary focal hyperhidrosis**

         L74.510 Primary focal hyperhidrosis, axilla

         L74.511 Primary focal hyperhidrosis, face

         L74.512 Primary focal hyperhidrosis, palms

         L74.513 Primary focal hyperhidrosis, soles

        ■ **L74.519 Primary focal hyperhidrosis, unspecified**

       L74.52 Secondary focal hyperhidrosis
         Frey's syndrome

     L74.8 Other eccrine sweat disorders

    ■ **L74.9 Eccrine sweat disorder, unspecified**
       Sweat gland disorder NOS

● **L75 Apocrine sweat disorders**
> **Excludes1**   dyshidrosis (L30.1)
>   hidradenitis suppurativa (L73.2)

     L75.0 Bromhidrosis

     L75.1 Chromhidrosis

     L75.2 Apocrine miliaria
       Fox-Fordyce disease

     L75.8 Other apocrine sweat disorders

    ■ **L75.9 Apocrine sweat disorder, unspecified**
       Intraoperative and postprocedural complications of skin and subcutaneous tissue (L76)

INTRAOPERATIVE AND POSTPROCEDURAL COMPLICATIONS OF SKIN AND SUBCUTANEOUS TISSUE (L76)

● **L76 Intraoperative and postprocedural complications of skin and subcutaneous tissue**

    ● **L76.0 Intraoperative hemorrhage and hematoma of skin and subcutaneous tissue complicating a procedure**
> **Excludes1**   intraoperative hemorrhage and hematoma of skin and subcutaneous tissue due to accidental puncture and laceration during a procedure (L76.1-)

       L76.01 Intraoperative hemorrhage and hematoma of skin and subcutaneous tissue complicating a dermatologic procedure 🔹

       L76.02 Intraoperative hemorrhage and hematoma of skin and subcutaneous tissue complicating other procedure 🔹

    ● **L76.1 Accidental puncture and laceration of skin and subcutaneous tissue during a procedure**

       L76.11 Accidental puncture and laceration of skin and subcutaneous tissue during a dermatologic procedure 🔹

       L76.12 Accidental puncture and laceration of skin and subcutaneous tissue during other procedure 🔹

    ● **L76.2 Postprocedural hemorrhage and hematoma of skin and subcutaneous tissue following a procedure**

       L76.21 Postprocedural hemorrhage and hematoma of skin and subcutaneous tissue following a dermatologic procedure 🔹

       L76.22 Postprocedural hemorrhage and hematoma of skin and subcutaneous tissue following other procedure 🔹

    ● **L76.8 Other intraoperative and postprocedural complications of skin and subcutaneous tissue**
> Use additional code, if applicable, to further specify disorder

       L76.81 Other intraoperative complications of skin and subcutaneous tissue

       L76.82 Other postprocedural complications of skin and subcutaneous tissue

OTHER DISORDERS OF THE SKIN AND SUBCUTANEOUS TISSUE (L80-L99)

L80 Vitiligo
> **Excludes2**   vitiligo of eyelids (H02.73-)
>   vitiligo of vulva (N90.89)

CHAPTER 12 (L00-L99)

N Newborn Age: 0   **P** Pediatric Age: 0–17   **M** Maternity DX: 12–55   **A** Adult Age: 15–124   ♀ Females Only   ♂ Males Only

🔹 Complication\Comorbidity   🔹 Major C\C   🔹 Present on Admission Requirement   🔹 Hospital-Acquired Condition

1127

CHAPTER 12 (L00–L99)

● **L81   Other disorders of pigmentation**

> Excludes1   birthmark NOS (Q82.5)
> Peutz-Jeghers syndrome (Q85.8)

> Excludes2   nevus - see Alphabetical Index

L81.0   Postinflammatory hyperpigmentation

L81.1   Chloasma

L81.2   Freckles

L81.3   Café au lait spots

L81.4   Other melanin hyperpigmentation
> Lentigo

L81.5   Leukoderma, not elsewhere classified

L81.6   Other disorders of diminished melanin formation

L81.7   Pigmented purpuric dermatosis
> Angioma serpiginosum

L81.8   Other specified disorders of pigmentation
> Iron pigmentation
> Tattoo pigmentation

■ **L81.9   Disorder of pigmentation, unspecified**

● **L82   Seborrheic keratosis**

> Includes   dermatosis papulosa nigra
> Leser-Trélat disease

> Excludes2   seborrheic dermatitis (L21.-)

L82.0   Inflamed seborrheic keratosis

L82.1   Other seborrheic keratosis
> Seborrheic keratosis NOS

L83   Acanthosis nigricans
> Confluent and reticulated papillomatosis

L84   Corns and callosities
> Callus
> Clavus

● **L85   Other epidermal thickening**

> Excludes2   hypertrophic disorders of the skin (L91.-)

L85.0   Acquired ichthyosis

> Excludes1   congenital ichthyosis (Q80.-)

L85.1   Acquired keratosis [keratoderma] palmaris et plantaris

> Excludes1   inherited keratosis palmaris et plantaris (Q82.8)

L85.2   Keratosis punctata (palmaris et plantaris) L85.3
> Xerosis cutis
> Dry skin dermatitis

L85.8   Other specified epidermal thickening
> Cutaneous horn

■ **L85.9   Epidermal thickening, unspecified**

●◗ *L86   Keratoderma in diseases classified elsewhere*
> *Firm horny papules that have a cobblestone appearance.*

> Code first *underlying disease, such as:*
> Reiter's disease (M02.3-)

> Excludes1   gonococcal keratoderma (A54.89)
> gonococcal keratosis (A54.89)
> keratoderma due to vitamin A deficiency (E50.8)
> keratosis due to vitamin A deficiency (E50.8)
> xeroderma due to vitamin A deficiency (E50.8)

● **L87   Transepidermal elimination disorders**

> Excludes1   granuloma annulare (perforating) (L92.0)

L87.0   Keratosis follicularis et parafollicularis in cutem penetrans
> Kyrle disease
> Hyperkeratosis follicularis penetrans

L87.1   Reactive perforating collagenosis

L87.2   Elastosis perforans serpiginosa

L87.8   Other transepidermal elimination disorders

■ **L87.9   Transepidermal elimination disorder, unspecified**

L88   Pyoderma gangrenosum 🔖
> Phagedenic pyoderma

> Excludes1   dermatitis gangrenosa (L08.0)

● **L89   Pressure ulcer**

> Includes   bed sore   pressure area
> decubitus ulcer   pressure sore
> plaster ulcer

> Code first *any associated gangrene (I96)*

> Excludes2   decubitus (trophic) ulcer of cervix (uteri) (N86)
> diabetic ulcers (E08.621, E08.622, E09.621, E09.622, E10.621, E10.622, E11.621, E11.622, E13.621, E13.622)
> non-pressure chronic ulcer of skin (L97.-)
> skin infections (L00-L08)
> varicose ulcer (I83.0, I83.2)

● **L89.0   Pressure ulcer of elbow**

> ● **L89.00   Pressure ulcer of unspecified elbow**

> > ■ **L89.000   Pressure ulcer of unspecified elbow, unstageable**

> > ■ **L89.001   Pressure ulcer of unspecified elbow, stage 1**
> > > Healing pressure ulcer of unspecified elbow, stage 1
> > > Pressure pre-ulcer skin changes limited to persistent focal edema, unspecified elbow

> > ■ **L89.002   Pressure ulcer of unspecified elbow, stage 2**
> > > Healing pressure ulcer of unspecified elbow, stage 2
> > > Pressure ulcer with abrasion, blister, partial thickness skin loss involving epidermis and/or dermis, unspecified elbow

> > ■ **L89.003   Pressure ulcer of unspecified elbow, stage 3** 🔖🔖   A
> > > Healing pressure ulcer of unspecified elbow, stage 3
> > > Pressure ulcer with full thickness skin loss involving damage or necrosis of subcutaneous tissue, unspecified elbow

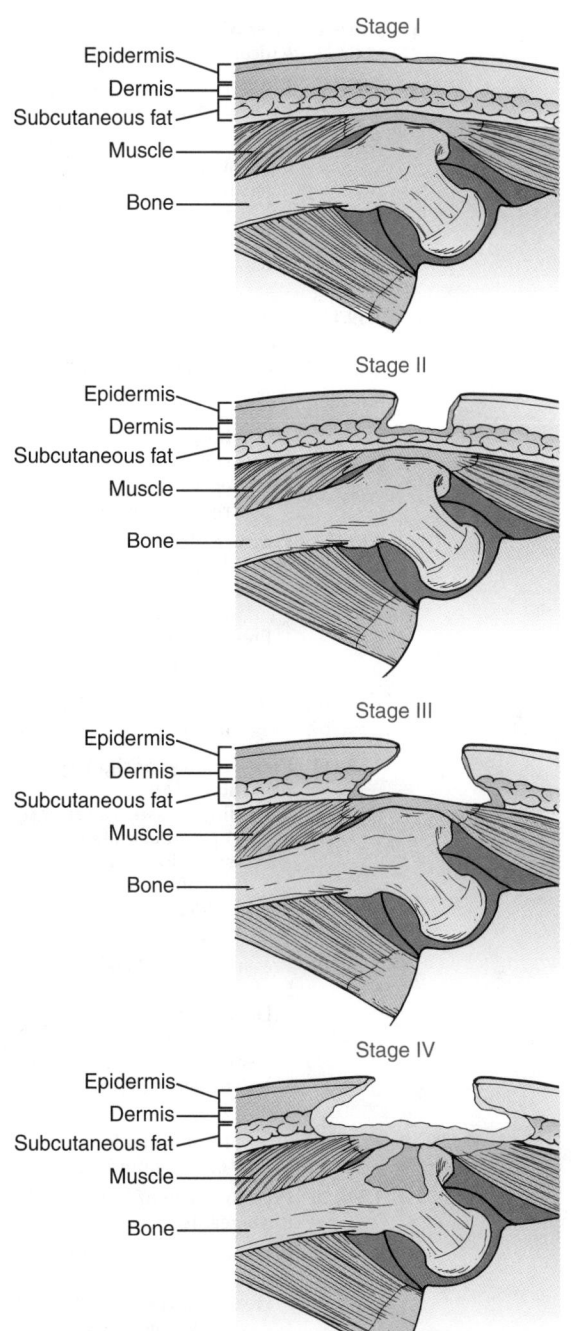

Stage I

Epidermis
Dermis
Subcutaneous fat
Muscle
Bone

Stage II

Epidermis
Dermis
Subcutaneous fat
Muscle
Bone

Stage III

Epidermis
Dermis
Subcutaneous fat
Muscle
Bone

Stage IV

Epidermis
Dermis
Subcutaneous fat
Muscle
Bone

Figure 12-9 Stage I, II, III, and IV of pressure ulcers.

■ **L89.004 Pressure ulcer of unspecified elbow, stage 4** 🏥🏥   **A**
    Healing pressure ulcer of unspecified elbow, stage 4
    Pressure ulcer with necrosis of soft tissues through to underlying muscle, tendon, or bone, unspecified elbow

■ **L89.009 Pressure ulcer of unspecified elbow, unspecified stage**
    Healing pressure ulcer of elbow NOS
    Healing pressure ulcer of unspecified elbow, unspecified stage

● **L89.01 Pressure ulcer of right elbow**

L89.010 Pressure ulcer of right elbow, unstageable

L89.011 Pressure ulcer of right elbow, stage 1
    Healing pressure ulcer of right elbow, stage 1
    Pressure pre-ulcer skin changes limited to persistent focal edema, right elbow

L89.012 Pressure ulcer of right elbow, stage 2
    Healing pressure ulcer of right elbow, stage 2
    Pressure ulcer with abrasion, blister, partial thickness skin loss involving epidermis and/or dermis, right elbow

L89.013 Pressure ulcer of right elbow, stage 3 🏥🏥   **A**
    Healing pressure ulcer of right elbow, stage 3
    Pressure ulcer with full thickness skin loss involving damage or necrosis of subcutaneous tissue, right elbow

L89.014 Pressure ulcer of right elbow, stage 4 🏥🏥   **A**
    Healing pressure ulcer of right elbow, stage 4
    Pressure ulcer with necrosis of soft tissues through to underlying muscle, tendon, or bone, right elbow

■ **L89.019 Pressure ulcer of right elbow, unspecified stage**
    Healing pressure right of elbow NOS
    Healing pressure ulcer of unspecified elbow, unspecified stage

● **L89.02 Pressure ulcer of left elbow**

L89.020 Pressure ulcer of left elbow, unstageable

L89.021 Pressure ulcer of left elbow, stage 1
    Healing pressure ulcer of left elbow, stage 1
    Pressure pre-ulcer skin changes limited to persistent focal edema, left elbow

L89.022 Pressure ulcer of left elbow, stage 2
    Healing pressure ulcer of left elbow, stage 2
    Pressure ulcer with abrasion, blister, partial thickness skin loss involving epidermis and/or dermis, left elbow

L89.023 Pressure ulcer of left elbow, stage 3 🏥🏥   **A**
    Healing pressure ulcer of left elbow, stage 3
    Pressure ulcer with full thickness skin loss involving damage or necrosis of subcutaneous tissue, left elbow

CHAPTER 12 (L00-L99)

L89.024   **Pressure ulcer of left elbow, stage 4** 🔲🔲   A
Healing pressure ulcer of left elbow, stage 4
Pressure ulcer with necrosis of soft tissues through to underlying muscle, tendon, or bone, left elbow

L89.029   **Pressure ulcer of left elbow, unspecified stage**
Healing pressure ulcer of left of elbow NOS
Healing pressure ulcer of unspecified elbow, unspecified stage

● **L89.1**   **Pressure ulcer of back**

  ● **L89.10**   **Pressure ulcer of unspecified part of back**

L89.100   **Pressure ulcer of unspecified part of back, unstageable**

L89.101   **Pressure ulcer of unspecified part of back, stage 1**
Healing pressure ulcer of unspecified part of back, stage 1
Pressure pre-ulcer skin changes limited to persistent focal edema, unspecified part of back

L89.102   **Pressure ulcer of unspecified part of back, stage 2**
Healing pressure ulcer of unspecified part of back, stage 2
Pressure ulcer with abrasion, blister, partial thickness skin loss involving epidermis and/or dermis, unspecified part of back

L89.103   **Pressure ulcer of unspecified part of back, stage 3** 🔲🔲   A
Healing pressure ulcer of unspecified part of back, stage 3
Pressure ulcer with full thickness skin loss involving damage or necrosis of subcutaneous tissue, unspecified part of back

L89.104   **Pressure ulcer of unspecified part of back, stage 4** 🔲🔲   A
Healing pressure ulcer of unspecified part of back, stage 4
Pressure ulcer with necrosis of soft tissues through to underlying muscle, tendon, or bone, unspecified part of back

L89.109   **Pressure ulcer of unspecified part of back, unspecified stage**
Healing pressure ulcer of unspecified part of back NOS
Healing pressure ulcer of unspecified part of back, unspecified stage

● **L89.11**   **Pressure ulcer of right upper back**
Pressure ulcer of right shoulder blade

L89.110   **Pressure ulcer of right upper back, unstageable**

L89.111   **Pressure ulcer of right upper back, stage 1**
Healing pressure ulcer of right upper back, stage 1
Pressure pre-ulcer skin changes limited to persistent focal edema, right upper back

L89.112   **Pressure ulcer of right upper back, stage 2**
Healing pressure ulcer of right upper back, stage 2
Pressure ulcer with abrasion, blister, partial thickness skin loss involving epidermis and/or dermis, right upper back

L89.113   **Pressure ulcer of right upper back, stage 3** 🔲🔲   A
Healing pressure ulcer of right upper back, stage 3
Pressure ulcer with full thickness skin loss involving damage or necrosis of subcutaneous tissue, right upper back

L89.114   **Pressure ulcer of right upper back, stage 4** 🔲🔲   A
Healing pressure ulcer of right upper back, stage 4
Pressure ulcer with necrosis of soft tissues through to underlying muscle, tendon, or bone, right upper back

L89.119   **Pressure ulcer of right upper back, unspecified stage**
Healing pressure ulcer of right upper back NOS
Healing pressure ulcer of right upper back, unspecified stage

● **L89.12**   **Pressure ulcer of left upper back**
Pressure ulcer of left shoulder blade

L89.120   **Pressure ulcer of left upper back, unstageable**

L89.121   **Pressure ulcer of left upper back, stage 1**
Healing pressure ulcer of left upper back, stage 1
Pressure pre-ulcer skin changes limited to persistent focal edema, left upper back

L89.122   **Pressure ulcer of left upper back, stage 2**
Healing pressure ulcer of left upper back, stage 2
Pressure ulcer with abrasion, blister, partial thickness skin loss involving epidermis and/or dermis, left upper back

L89.123   **Pressure ulcer of left upper back, stage 3** 🏷️🏷️   **A**
     Healing pressure ulcer of left upper back, stage 3
     Pressure ulcer with full thickness skin loss involving damage or necrosis of subcutaneous tissue, left upper back

L89.124   **Pressure ulcer of left upper back, stage 4** 🏷️🏷️   **A**
     Healing pressure ulcer of left upper back, stage 4
     Pressure ulcer with necrosis of soft tissues through to underlying muscle, tendon, or bone, left upper back

🔲 L89.129   **Pressure ulcer of left upper back, unspecified stage**
     Healing pressure ulcer of left upper back NOS
     Healing pressure ulcer of left upper back, unspecified stage

⬤ **L89.13 Pressure ulcer of right lower back**

L89.130   **Pressure ulcer of right lower back, unstageable**

L89.131   **Pressure ulcer of right lower back, stage 1**
     Healing pressure ulcer of right lower back, stage 1
     Pressure pre-ulcer skin changes limited to persistent focal edema, right lower back

L89.132   **Pressure ulcer of right lower back, stage 2**
     Healing pressure ulcer of right lower back, stage 2
     Pressure ulcer with abrasion, blister, partial thickness skin loss involving epidermis and/or dermis, right lower back

L89.133   **Pressure ulcer of right lower back, stage 3** 🏷️🏷️   **A**
     Healing pressure ulcer of right lower back, stage 3
     Pressure ulcer with full thickness skin loss involving damage or necrosis of subcutaneous tissue, right lower back

L89.134   **Pressure ulcer of right lower back, stage 4** 🏷️🏷️   **A**
     Healing pressure ulcer of right lower back, stage 4
     Pressure ulcer with necrosis of soft tissues through to underlying muscle, tendon, or bone, right lower back

🔲 L89.139   **Pressure ulcer of right lower back, unspecified stage**
     Healing pressure ulcer of right lower back NOS
     Healing pressure ulcer of right lower back, unspecified stage

⬤ **L89.14**   **Pressure ulcer of left lower back**

L89.140   **Pressure ulcer of left lower back, unstageable**

L89.141   **Pressure ulcer of left lower back, stage 1**
     Healing pressure ulcer of left lower back, stage 1
     Pressure pre-ulcer skin changes limited to persistent focal edema, left lower back

L89.142   **Pressure ulcer of left lower back, stage 2**
     Healing pressure ulcer of left lower back, stage 2
     Pressure ulcer with abrasion, blister, partial thickness skin loss involving epidermis and/or dermis, left lower back

L89.143   **Pressure ulcer of left lower back, stage 3** 🏷️🏷️   **A**
     Healing pressure ulcer of left lower back, stage 3
     Pressure ulcer with full thickness skin loss involving damage or necrosis of subcutaneous tissue, left lower back

L89.144   **Pressure ulcer of left lower back, stage 4** 🏷️🏷️   **A**
     Healing pressure ulcer of left lower back, stage 4
     Pressure ulcer with necrosis of soft tissues through to underlying muscle, tendon, or bone, left lower back

🔲 L89.149   **Pressure ulcer of left lower back, unspecified stage**
     Healing pressure ulcer of left lower back NOS
     Healing pressure ulcer of left lower back, unspecified stage

⬤ **L89.15**   **Pressure ulcer of sacral region**
     Pressure ulcer of coccyx
     Pressure ulcer of tailbone

L89.150   **Pressure ulcer of sacral region, unstageable**

L89.151   **Pressure ulcer of sacral region, stage 1**
     Healing pressure ulcer of sacral region, stage 1
     Pressure pre-ulcer skin changes limited to persistent focal edema, sacral region

L89.152   **Pressure ulcer of sacral region, stage 2**
     Healing pressure ulcer of sacral region, stage 2
     Pressure ulcer with abrasion, blister, partial thickness skin loss involving epidermis and/or dermis, sacral region

---

L89.153 **Pressure ulcer of sacral region, stage 3** 🦠🦠   A

     Healing pressure ulcer of sacral region, stage 3

     Pressure ulcer with full thickness skin loss involving damage or necrosis of subcutaneous tissue, sacral region

L89.154 **Pressure ulcer of sacral region, stage 4** 🦠🦠   A

     Healing pressure ulcer of sacral region, stage 4

     Pressure ulcer with necrosis of soft tissues through to underlying muscle, tendon, or bone, sacral region

■ L89.159 **Pressure ulcer of sacral region, unspecified stage**

     Healing pressure ulcer of sacral region NOS

     Healing pressure ulcer of sacral region, unspecified stage

● L89.2 **Pressure ulcer of hip**

  ● L89.20 **Pressure ulcer of unspecified hip**

    ■ L89.200 **Pressure ulcer of unspecified hip, unstageable**

    ■ L89.201 **Pressure ulcer of unspecified hip, stage 1**

       Healing pressure ulcer of unspecified hip back, stage 1

       Pressure pre-ulcer skin changes limited to persistent focal edema, unspecified hip

    ■ L89.202 **Pressure ulcer of unspecified hip, stage 2**

       Healing pressure ulcer of unspecified hip, stage 2

       Pressure ulcer with abrasion, blister, partial thickness skin loss involving epidermis and/or dermis, unspecified hip

    ■ L89.203 **Pressure ulcer of unspecified hip, stage 3** 🦠🦠   A

       Healing pressure ulcer of unspecified hip, stage 3

       Pressure ulcer with full thickness skin loss involving damage or necrosis of subcutaneous tissue, unspecified hip

    ■ L89.204 **Pressure ulcer of unspecified hip, stage 4** 🦠🦠   A

       Healing pressure ulcer of unspecified hip, stage 4

       Pressure ulcer with necrosis of soft tissues through to underlying muscle, tendon, or bone, unspecified hip

    ■ L89.209 **Pressure ulcer of unspecified hip, unspecified stage**

       Healing pressure ulcer of unspecified hip NOS

       Healing pressure ulcer of unspecified hip, unspecified stage

■ L89.21 **Pressure ulcer of right hip**

L89.210 **Pressure ulcer of right hip, unstageable**

L89.211 **Pressure ulcer of right hip, stage 1**

     Healing pressure ulcer of right hip back, stage 1

     Pressure pre-ulcer skin changes limited to persistent focal edema, right hip

L89.212 **Pressure ulcer of right hip, stage 2**

     Healing pressure ulcer of right hip, stage 2

     Pressure ulcer with abrasion, blister, partial thickness skin loss involving epidermis and/or dermis, right hip

L89.213 **Pressure ulcer of right hip, stage 3** 🦠🦠   A

     Healing pressure ulcer of right hip, stage 3

     Pressure ulcer with full thickness skin loss involving damage or necrosis of subcutaneous tissue, right hip

L89.214 **Pressure ulcer of right hip, stage 4** 🦠🦠

     Healing pressure ulcer of right hip, stage 4

     Pressure ulcer with necrosis of soft tissues through to underlying muscle, tendon, or bone, right hip

■ L89.219 **Pressure ulcer of right hip, unspecified stage**

     Healing pressure ulcer of right hip NOS

     Healing pressure ulcer of right hip, unspecified stage

● L89.22 **Pressure ulcer of left hip**

L89.220 **Pressure ulcer of left hip, unstageable**

L89.221 **Pressure ulcer of left hip, stage 1**

     Healing pressure ulcer of left hip back, stage 1

     Pressure pre-ulcer skin changes limited to persistent focal edema, left hip

L89.222 **Pressure ulcer of left hip, stage 2**

     Healing pressure ulcer of left hip, stage 2

     Pressure ulcer with abrasion, blister, partial thickness skin loss involving epidermis and/or dermis, left hip

L89.223 **Pressure ulcer of left hip, stage 3** 🦠🦠

     Healing pressure ulcer of left hip, stage 3

     Pressure ulcer with full thickness skin loss involving damage or necrosis of subcutaneous tissue, left hip

CHAPTER 12 (L00-L99)

L89.224 **Pressure ulcer of left hip, stage 4** 🔵🔵
Healing pressure ulcer of left hip, stage 4
Pressure ulcer with necrosis of soft tissues through to underlying muscle, tendon, or bone, left hip

◼ L89.229 **Pressure ulcer of left hip, unspecified stage**
Healing pressure ulcer of left hip NOS
Healing pressure ulcer of left hip, unspecified stage

● **L89.3 Pressure ulcer of buttock**

● **L89.30 Pressure ulcer of unspecified buttock**

◼ L89.300 **Pressure ulcer of unspecified buttock, unstageable**

◼ L89.301 **Pressure ulcer of unspecified buttock, stage 1**
Healing pressure ulcer of unspecified buttock, stage 1
Pressure pre-ulcer skin changes limited to persistent focal edema, unspecified buttock

◼ L89.302 **Pressure ulcer of unspecified buttock, stage 2**
Healing pressure ulcer of unspecified buttock, stage 2
Pressure ulcer with abrasion, blister, partial thickness skin loss involving epidermis and/or dermis, unspecified buttock

◼ L89.303 **Pressure ulcer of unspecified buttock, stage 3** 🔵🔵
Healing pressure ulcer of unspecified buttock, stage 3
Pressure ulcer with full thickness skin loss involving damage or necrosis of subcutaneous tissue, unspecified buttock

◼ L89.304 **Pressure ulcer of unspecified buttock, stage 4** 🔵🔵
Healing pressure ulcer of unspecified buttock, stage 4
Pressure ulcer with necrosis of soft tissues through to underlying muscle, tendon, or bone, unspecified buttock

◼ L89.309 **Pressure ulcer of unspecified buttock, unspecified stage**
Healing pressure ulcer of unspecified buttock NOS
Healing pressure ulcer of unspecified buttock, unspecified stage

● **L89.31 Pressure ulcer of right buttock**

L89.310 **Pressure ulcer of right buttock, unstageable**

L89.311 **Pressure ulcer of right buttock, stage 1**
Healing pressure ulcer of right buttock, stage 1
Pressure pre-ulcer skin changes limited to persistent focal edema, right buttock

L89.312 **Pressure ulcer of right buttock, stage 2**
Healing pressure ulcer of right buttock, stage 2
Pressure ulcer with abrasion, blister, partial thickness skin loss involving epidermis and/or dermis, right buttock

L89.313 **Pressure ulcer of right buttock, stage 3** 🔵🔵
Healing pressure ulcer of right buttock, stage 3
Pressure ulcer with full thickness skin loss involving damage or necrosis of subcutaneous tissue, right buttock

L89.314 **Pressure ulcer of right buttock, stage 4** 🔵🔵
Healing pressure ulcer of right buttock, stage 4
Pressure ulcer with necrosis of soft tissues through to underlying muscle, tendon, or bone, right buttock

◼ L89.319 **Pressure ulcer of right buttock, unspecified stage**
Healing pressure ulcer of right buttock NOS
Healing pressure ulcer of right buttock, unspecified stage

● **L89.32 Pressure ulcer of left buttock**

L89.320 **Pressure ulcer of left buttock, unstageable**

L89.321 **Pressure ulcer of left buttock, stage 1**
Healing pressure ulcer of left buttock, stage 1
Pressure pre-ulcer skin changes limited to persistent focal edema, left buttock

L89.322 **Pressure ulcer of left buttock, stage 2**
Healing pressure ulcer of left buttock, stage 2
Pressure ulcer with abrasion, blister, partial thickness skin loss involving epidermis and/or dermis, left buttock

L89.323 **Pressure ulcer of left buttock, stage 3** 🔵🔵
Healing pressure ulcer of left buttock, stage 3
Pressure ulcer with full thickness skin loss involving damage or necrosis of subcutaneous tissue, left buttock

L89.324 **Pressure ulcer of left buttock, stage 4** 🔵🔵
Healing pressure ulcer of left buttock, stage 4
Pressure ulcer with necrosis of soft tissues through to underlying muscle, tendon, or bone, left buttock

CHAPTER 12 (L00–L99)

■ L89.329 **Pressure ulcer of left buttock, unspecified stage**
    Healing pressure ulcer of left buttock NOS
    Healing pressure ulcer of left buttock, unspecified stage

● L89.4 **Pressure ulcer of contiguous site of back, buttock and hip**

  ■ L89.40 **Pressure ulcer of contiguous site of back, buttock and hip, unspecified stage**
    Healing pressure ulcer of contiguous site of back, buttock and hip NOS
    Healing pressure ulcer of contiguous site of back, buttock and hip, unspecified stage

  L89.41 **Pressure ulcer of contiguous site of back, buttock and hip, stage 1**
    Healing pressure ulcer of contiguous site of back, buttock and hip, stage 1
    Pressure pre-ulcer skin changes limited to persistent focal edema, contiguous site of back, buttock and hip

  L89.42 **Pressure ulcer of contiguous site of back, buttock and hip, stage 2**
    Healing pressure ulcer of contiguous site of back, buttock and hip, stage 2
    Pressure ulcer with abrasion, blister, partial thickness skin loss involving epidermis and/or dermis, contiguous site of back, buttock and hip

  L89.43 **Pressure ulcer of contiguous site of back, buttock and hip, stage 3** 🔖🔖
    Healing pressure ulcer of contiguous site of back, buttock and hip, stage 3
    Pressure ulcer with full thickness skin loss involving damage or necrosis of subcutaneous tissue, contiguous site of back, buttock and hip

  L89.44 **Pressure ulcer of contiguous site of back, buttock and hip, stage 4** 🔖🔖
    Healing pressure ulcer of contiguous site of back, buttock and hip, stage 4
    Pressure ulcer with necrosis of soft tissues through to underlying muscle, tendon, or bone, contiguous site of back, buttock and hip

  L89.45 **Pressure ulcer of contiguous site of back, buttock and hip, unstageable**

● L89.5 **Pressure ulcer of ankle**

  ● L89.50 **Pressure ulcer of unspecified ankle**

    ■ L89.500 **Pressure ulcer of unspecified ankle, unstageable**

    ■ L89.501 **Pressure ulcer of unspecified ankle, stage 1**
      Healing pressure ulcer of unspecified ankle, stage 1
      Pressure pre-ulcer skin changes limited to persistent focal edema, unspecified ankle

    ■ L89.502 **Pressure ulcer of unspecified ankle, stage 2**
      Healing pressure ulcer of unspecified ankle, stage 2
      Pressure ulcer with abrasion, blister, partial thickness skin loss involving epidermis and/or dermis, unspecified ankle

■ L89.503 **Pressure ulcer of unspecified ankle, stage 3** 🔖🔖
    Healing pressure ulcer of unspecified ankle, stage 3
    Pressure ulcer with full thickness skin loss involving damage or necrosis of subcutaneous tissue, unspecified ankle

■ L89.504 **Pressure ulcer of unspecified ankle, stage 4** 🔖🔖
    Healing pressure ulcer of unspecified ankle, stage 4
    Pressure ulcer with necrosis of soft tissues through to underlying muscle, tendon, or bone, unspecified ankle

■ L89.509 **Pressure ulcer of unspecified ankle, unspecified stage**
    Healing pressure ulcer of unspecified ankle NOS
    Healing pressure ulcer of unspecified ankle, unspecified stage

● L89.51 **Pressure ulcer of right ankle**

  L89.510 **Pressure ulcer of right ankle, unstageable**

  L89.511 **Pressure ulcer of right ankle, stage 1**
    Healing pressure ulcer of right ankle, stage 1
    Pressure pre-ulcer skin changes limited to persistent focal edema, right ankle

  L89.512 **Pressure ulcer of right ankle, stage 2**
    Healing pressure ulcer of right ankle, stage 2
    Pressure ulcer with abrasion, blister, partial thickness skin loss involving epidermis and/or dermis, right ankle

  L89.513 **Pressure ulcer of right ankle, stage 3** 🔖🔖
    Healing pressure ulcer of right ankle, stage 3
    Pressure ulcer with full thickness skin loss involving damage or necrosis of subcutaneous tissue, right ankle

  L89.514 **Pressure ulcer of right ankle, stage 4** 🔖🔖
    Healing pressure ulcer of right ankle, stage 4
    Pressure ulcer with necrosis of soft tissues through to underlying muscle, tendon, or bone, right ankle

■ L89.519 **Pressure ulcer of right ankle, unspecified stage**
    Healing pressure ulcer of right ankle NOS
    Healing pressure ulcer of right ankle, unspecified stage

● Unacceptable Principal Diagnosis   ● Use Additional Character(s)   ■ Unspecified   ▶ Manifestation Code
OGCR Official Guidelines for Coding and Reporting   Excludes 1   Excludes 2   Includes   Use additional   Code first   Code also

● **L89.52   Pressure ulcer of left ankle**

   L89.520   Pressure ulcer of left ankle, unstageable

   L89.521   Pressure ulcer of left ankle, stage 1
      Healing pressure ulcer of left ankle, stage 1
      Pressure pre-ulcer skin changes limited to persistent focal edema, left ankle

   L89.522   Pressure ulcer of left ankle, stage 2
      Healing pressure ulcer of left ankle, stage 2
      Pressure ulcer with abrasion, blister, partial thickness skin loss involving epidermis and/or dermis, left ankle

   L89.523   Pressure ulcer of left ankle, stage 3 🪙 🪙
      Healing pressure ulcer of left ankle, stage 3
      Pressure ulcer with full thickness skin loss involving damage or necrosis of subcutaneous tissue, left ankle

   L89.524   Pressure ulcer of left ankle, stage 4 🪙 🪙
      Healing pressure ulcer of left ankle, stage 4
      Pressure ulcer with necrosis of soft tissues through to underlying muscle, tendon, or bone, left ankle

   ■ **L89.529 Pressure ulcer of left ankle, unspecified stage**
      Healing pressure ulcer of left ankle NOS
      Healing pressure ulcer of left ankle, unspecified stage

● **L89.6   Pressure ulcer of heel**

  ● **L89.60   Pressure ulcer of unspecified heel**

   ■ **L89.600   Pressure ulcer of unspecified heel, unstageable**

   ■ **L89.601   Pressure ulcer of unspecified heel, stage 1**
      Healing pressure ulcer of unspecified heel, stage 1
      Pressure pre-ulcer skin changes limited to persistent focal edema, unspecified heel

   ■ **L89.602   Pressure ulcer of unspecified heel, stage 2**
      Healing pressure ulcer of unspecified heel, stage 2
      Pressure ulcer with abrasion, blister, partial thickness skin loss involving epidermis and/or dermis, unspecified heel

   ■ **L89.603   Pressure ulcer of unspecified heel, stage 3 🪙 🪙**
      Healing pressure ulcer of unspecified heel, stage 3
      Pressure ulcer with full thickness skin loss involving damage or necrosis of subcutaneous tissue, unspecified heel

   ■ **L89.604   Pressure ulcer of unspecified heel, stage 4 🪙 🪙**
      Healing pressure ulcer of unspecified heel, stage 4
      Pressure ulcer with necrosis of soft tissues through to underlying muscle, tendon, or bone, unspecified heel

   ■ **L89.609   Pressure ulcer of unspecified heel, unspecified stage**
      Healing pressure ulcer of unspecified heel NOS
      Healing pressure ulcer of unspecified heel, unspecified stage

● **L89.61   Pressure ulcer of right heel**

   L89.610   Pressure ulcer of right heel, unstageable

   L89.611   Pressure ulcer of right heel, stage 1
      Healing pressure ulcer of right heel, stage 1
      Pressure pre-ulcer skin changes limited to persistent focal edema, right heel

   L89.612   Pressure ulcer of right heel, stage 2
      Healing pressure ulcer of right heel, stage 2
      Pressure ulcer with abrasion, blister, partial thickness skin loss involving epidermis and/or dermis, right heel

   L89.613   Pressure ulcer of right heel, stage 3 🪙 🪙
      Healing pressure ulcer of right heel, stage 3
      Pressure ulcer with full thickness skin loss involving damage or necrosis of subcutaneous tissue, right heel

   L89.614   Pressure ulcer of right heel, stage 4 🪙 🪙
      Healing pressure ulcer of right heel, stage 4
      Pressure ulcer with necrosis of soft tissues through to underlying muscle, tendon, or bone, right heel

   ■ **L89.619   Pressure ulcer of right heel, unspecified stage**
      Healing pressure ulcer of right heel NOS
      Healing pressure ulcer of unspecified heel, right stage

●L89.62   Pressure ulcer of left heel

L89.620   Pressure ulcer of left heel, unstageable

L89.621   Pressure ulcer of left heel, stage 1
Healing pressure ulcer of left heel, stage 1
Pressure pre-ulcer skin changes limited to persistent focal edema, left heel

L89.622   Pressure ulcer of left heel, stage 2
Healing pressure ulcer of left heel, stage 2
Pressure ulcer with abrasion, blister, partial thickness skin loss involving epidermis and/or dermis, left heel

L89.623   Pressure ulcer of left heel, stage 3 🖢🖢
Healing pressure ulcer of left heel, stage 3
Pressure ulcer with full thickness skin loss involving damage or necrosis of subcutaneous tissue, left heel

L89.624   Pressure ulcer of left heel, stage 4 🖢🖢
Healing pressure ulcer of left heel, stage 4
Pressure ulcer with necrosis of soft tissues through to underlying muscle, tendon, or bone, left heel

◼L89.629   Pressure ulcer of left heel, unspecified stage
Healing pressure ulcer of left heel NOS
Healing pressure ulcer of left heel, unspecified stage

●L89.8   Pressure ulcer of other site

●L89.81   Pressure ulcer of head
Pressure ulcer of face

L89.810   Pressure ulcer of head, unstageable

L89.811   Pressure ulcer of head, stage 1
Healing pressure ulcer of head, stage 1
Pressure pre-ulcer skin changes limited to persistent focal edema, head

L89.812   Pressure ulcer of head, stage 2
Healing pressure ulcer of head, stage 2
Pressure ulcer with abrasion, blister, partial thickness skin loss involving epidermis and/or dermis, head

L89.813   Pressure ulcer of head, stage 3 🖢🖢
Healing pressure ulcer of head, stage 3
Pressure ulcer with full thickness skin loss involving damage or necrosis of subcutaneous tissue, head

L89.814   Pressure ulcer of head, stage 4 🖢🖢
Healing pressure ulcer of head, stage 4
Pressure ulcer with necrosis of soft tissues through to underlying muscle, tendon, or bone, head

◼L89.819   Pressure ulcer of head, unspecified stage
Healing pressure ulcer of head NOS
Healing pressure ulcer of head, unspecified stage

●L89.89   Pressure ulcer of other site

L89.890   Pressure ulcer of other site, unstageable

L89.891   Pressure ulcer of other site, stage 1
Healing pressure ulcer of other site, stage 1
Pressure pre-ulcer skin changes limited to persistent focal edema, other site

L89.892   Pressure ulcer of other site, stage 2
Healing pressure ulcer of other site, stage 2
Pressure ulcer with abrasion, blister, partial thickness skin loss involving epidermis and/or dermis, other site

L89.893   Pressure ulcer of other site, stage 3 🖢🖢
Healing pressure ulcer of other site, stage 3
Pressure ulcer with full thickness skin loss involving damage or necrosis of subcutaneous tissue, other site

L89.894   Pressure ulcer of other site, stage 4 🖢🖢
Healing pressure ulcer of other site, stage 4
Pressure ulcer with necrosis of soft tissues through to underlying muscle, tendon, or bone, other site

●L89.899   Pressure ulcer of other site, unspecified stage
Healing pressure ulcer of other site NOS
Healing pressure ulcer of other site, unspecified stage

●L89.9   Pressure ulcer of unspecified site

◼L89.90   Pressure ulcer of unspecified site, unspecified stage
Healing pressure ulcer of unspecified site NOS
Healing pressure ulcer of unspecified site, unspecified stage

◼L89.91   Pressure ulcer of unspecified site, stage 1
Healing pressure ulcer of unspecified site, stage 1
Pressure pre-ulcer skin changes limited to persistent focal edema, unspecified site

● Unacceptable Principal Diagnosis   ● Use Additional Character(s)   ◼ Unspecified   ▶ Manifestation Code

OGCR Official Guidelines for Coding and Reporting   Excludes 1   Excludes 2   Includes   Use additional   Code first   Code also

■ **L89.92　Pressure ulcer of unspecified site, stage 2**
　　　Healing pressure ulcer of unspecified site,
　　　　stage 2
　　　Pressure ulcer with abrasion, blister,
　　　　partial thickness skin loss involving
　　　　epidermis and/or dermis,
　　　　unspecified site

■ **L89.93　Pressure ulcer of unspecified site, stage 3** 🦠🦠
　　　Healing pressure ulcer of unspecified site,
　　　　stage 3
　　　Pressure ulcer with full thickness skin
　　　　loss involving damage or necrosis of
　　　　subcutaneous tissue, unspecified site

■ **L89.94　Pressure ulcer of unspecified site, stage 4** 🦠🦠
　　　Healing pressure ulcer of unspecified site,
　　　　stage 4
　　　Pressure ulcer with necrosis of soft tissues
　　　　through to underlying muscle,
　　　　tendon, or bone, unspecified site

● **L89.95　Pressure ulcer of unspecified site, unstageable**

● **L90　Atrophic disorders of skin**

L90.0　Lichen sclerosus et atrophicus
> **Excludes2**　lichen sclerosus of external female
> 　　　genital organs (N90.4)
> 　　　lichen sclerosus of external male
> 　　　genital organs (N48.0)

L90.1　Anetoderma of Schweninger-Buzzi

L90.2　Anetoderma of Jadassohn-Pellizzari

L90.3　Atrophoderma of Pasini and Pierini

L90.4　Acrodermatitis chronica atrophicans

L90.5　Scar conditions and fibrosis of skin
　　　Adherent scar (skin)
　　　Cicatrix
　　　Disfigurement of skin due to scar
　　　Fibrosis of skin NOS
　　　Scar NOS
> **Excludes2**　hypertrophic scar (L91.0)
> 　　　keloid scar (L91.0)

L90.6　Striae atrophicae

L90.8　Other atrophic disorders of skin

■ **L90.9　Atrophic disorder of skin, unspecified**

● **L91　Hypertrophic disorders of skin**

L91.0　Keloid scar
　　　Hypertrophic scar
　　　Keloid
> **Excludes2**　acne keloid (L73.0)
> 　　　scar NOS (L90.5)

L91.8　Other hypertrophic disorders of the skin

■ **L91.9　Hypertrophic disorder of the skin, unspecified**

● **L92　Granulomatous disorders of skin and subcutaneous tissue**
> **Excludes2**　actinic granuloma (L57.5)

L92.0　Granuloma annulare
　　　Perforating granuloma annulare

L92.1　Necrobiosis lipoidica, not elsewhere classified
> **Excludes1**　necrobiosis lipoidica associated with
> 　　　diabetes mellitus (E08-E13 with
> 　　　.620)

L92.2　Granuloma faciale [eosinophilic granuloma of skin]

Item 12-11　Scleroderma means hard skin. It is a group of diseases that causes abnormal growth of connective tissues that support the skin and organs. There are two types: localized scleroderma affecting the skin and systemic scleroderma affecting blood vessels and internal organs and the skin.

L92.3　Foreign body granuloma of the skin and subcutaneous tissue
> Use additional code to identify the type of
> 　　　retained foreign body (Z18.-)

L92.8　Other granulomatous disorders of the skin and subcutaneous tissue

■ **L92.9　Granulomatous disorder of the skin and subcutaneous tissue, unspecified**

● **L93　Lupus erythematosus**
> Use additional code for adverse effect, if applicable, to
> 　　　identify drug (T36-T50 with fifth or sixth character 5)
> **Excludes1**　lupus exedens (A18.4)
> 　　　lupus vulgaris (A18.4)
> 　　　scleroderma (M34.-)
> 　　　systemic lupus erythematosus (M32.-)

L93.0　Discoid lupus erythematosus
　　　Lupus erythematosus NOS

L93.1　Subacute cutaneous lupus erythematosus

L93.2　Other local lupus erythematosus
　　　Lupus erythematosus profundus
　　　Lupus panniculitis

● **L94　Other localized connective tissue disorders**
> **Excludes1**　systemic connective tissue disorders
> 　　　(M30-M36)

L94.0　Localized scleroderma [morphea]
　　　Circumscribed scleroderma

L94.1　Linear scleroderma
　　　En coup de sabre lesion

L94.2　Calcinosis cutis

L94.3　Sclerodactyly

L94.4　Gottron's papules

L94.5　Poikiloderma vasculare atrophicans

L94.6　Ainhum

L94.8　Other specified localized connective tissue disorders

■ **L94.9　Localized connective tissue disorder, unspecified**

● **L95　Vasculitis limited to skin, not elsewhere classified**
> **Excludes1**　angioma serpiginosum (L81.7)
> 　　　Henoch(-Schönlein) purpura (D69.0)
> 　　　hypersensitivity angiitis (M31.0)
> 　　　lupus panniculitis (L93.2)
> 　　　panniculitis NOS (M79.3)
> 　　　panniculitis of neck and back (M54.0-)
> 　　　polyarteritis nodosa (M30.0)
> 　　　relapsing panniculitis (M35.6)
> 　　　rheumatoid vasculitis (M05.2)
> 　　　serum sickness (T80.6-)
> 　　　urticaria (L50.-)
> 　　　Wegener's granulomatosis (M31.3-)

L95.0　Livedoid vasculitis
　　　Atrophie blanche (en plaque)

L95.1　Erythema elevatum diutinum

L95.8　Other vasculitis limited to the skin

■ **L95.9　Vasculitis limited to the skin, unspecified**

CHAPTER 12 (L00-L99)

● L97   Non-pressure chronic ulcer of lower limb, not elsewhere classified

> **Includes**   chronic ulcer of skin of lower limb NOS
> non-healing ulcer of skin
> non-infected sinus of skin
> trophic ulcer NOS
> tropical ulcer NOS
> ulcer of skin of lower limb NOS

> *Code first* any associated underlying condition, such as:
> any associated gangrene (I96)
> atherosclerosis of the lower extremities (I70.23-, I70.24-,
> I70.33-, I70.34-, I70.43-, I70.44-, I70.53-, I70.54-,
> I70.63-, I70.64-, I70.73-, I70.74-)
> chronic venous hypertension (I87.31-, I87.33-)
> diabetic ulcers (E08.621, E08.622, E09.621, E09.622,
> E10.621, E10.622, E11.621, E11.622, E13.621,
> E13.622)
> postphlebitic syndrome (I87.01-, I87.03-)
> postthrombotic syndrome (I87.01-, I87.03-)
> varicose ulcer (I83.0-, I83.2-)

> **Excludes2**   pressure ulcer (pressure area) (L89.-)
> skin infections (L00-L08)
> specific infections classified to A00-B99

● L97.1   Non-pressure chronic ulcer of thigh

    ● L97.10   Non-pressure chronic ulcer of unspecified thigh

       ▪ L97.101   Non-pressure chronic ulcer of unspecified thigh limited to breakdown of skin 🔍

       ▪ L97.102   Non-pressure chronic ulcer of unspecified thigh with fat layer exposed 🔍

       ▪ L97.103   Non-pressure chronic ulcer of unspecified thigh with necrosis of muscle 🔍

       ▪ L97.104   Non-pressure chronic ulcer of unspecified thigh with necrosis of bone 🔍

       ▪ L97.109   Non-pressure chronic ulcer of unspecified thigh with unspecified severity 🔍

    ● L97.11   Non-pressure chronic ulcer of right thigh

       L97.111   Non-pressure chronic ulcer of right thigh limited to breakdown of skin 🔍

       L97.112   Non-pressure chronic ulcer of right thigh with fat layer exposed 🔍

       L97.113   Non-pressure chronic ulcer of right thigh with necrosis of muscle 🔍

       L97.114   Non-pressure chronic ulcer of right thigh with necrosis of bone 🔍

       ▪ L97.119   Non-pressure chronic ulcer of right thigh with unspecified severity 🔍

    ● L97.12   Non-pressure chronic ulcer of left thigh

       L97.121   Non-pressure chronic ulcer of left thigh limited to breakdown of skin 🔍

       L97.122   Non-pressure chronic ulcer of left thigh with fat layer exposed 🔍

       L97.123   Non-pressure chronic ulcer of left thigh with necrosis of muscle 🔍

       L97.124   Non-pressure chronic ulcer of left thigh with necrosis of bone 🔍

       ▪ L97.129   Non-pressure chronic ulcer of left thigh with unspecified severity 🔍

● L97.2   Non-pressure chronic ulcer of calf

    ● L97.20   Non-pressure chronic ulcer of unspecified calf

       ▪ L97.201   Non-pressure chronic ulcer of unspecified calf limited to breakdown of skin 🔍

       ▪ L97.202   Non-pressure chronic ulcer of unspecified calf with fat layer exposed 🔍

       ▪ L97.203   Non-pressure chronic ulcer of unspecified calf with necrosis of muscle 🔍

       ▪ L97.204   Non-pressure chronic ulcer of unspecified calf with necrosis of bone 🔍

       ▪ L97.209   Non-pressure chronic ulcer of unspecified calf with unspecified severity 🔍

    ● L97.21   Non-pressure chronic ulcer of right calf

       L97.211   Non-pressure chronic ulcer of right calf limited to breakdown of skin 🔍

       L97.212   Non-pressure chronic ulcer of right calf with fat layer exposed 🔍

       L97.213   Non-pressure chronic ulcer of right calf with necrosis of muscle 🔍

       L97.214   Non-pressure chronic ulcer of right calf with necrosis of bone 🔍

       ▪ L97.219   Non-pressure chronic ulcer of right calf with unspecified severity 🔍

    ● L97.22   Non-pressure chronic ulcer of left calf

       L97.221   Non-pressure chronic ulcer of left calf limited to breakdown of skin 🔍

       L97.222   Non-pressure chronic ulcer of left calf with fat layer exposed 🔍

       L97.223   Non-pressure chronic ulcer of left calf with necrosis of muscle 🔍

       L97.224   Non-pressure chronic ulcer of left calf with necrosis of bone 🔍

       ▪ L97.229   Non-pressure chronic ulcer of left calf with unspecified severity 🔍

● L97.3   Non-pressure chronic ulcer of ankle

    ● L97.30   Non-pressure chronic ulcer of unspecified ankle

       ▪ L97.301   Non-pressure chronic ulcer of unspecified ankle limited to breakdown of skin 🔍

       ▪ L97.302   Non-pressure chronic ulcer of unspecified ankle with fat layer exposed 🔍

       ▪ L97.303   Non-pressure chronic ulcer of unspecified ankle with necrosis of muscle 🔍

● Unacceptable Principal Diagnosis   ● Use Additional Character(s)   ▪ Unspecified   ▶ Manifestation Code
OGCR Official Guidelines for Coding and Reporting   Excludes 1   Excludes 2   Includes   Use additional   Code first   Code also

L97.304　Non-pressure chronic ulcer of unspecified ankle with necrosis of bone 🦠

L97.309　Non-pressure chronic ulcer of unspecified ankle with unspecified severity 🦠

● L97.31　Non-pressure chronic ulcer of right ankle

L97.311　Non-pressure chronic ulcer of right ankle limited to breakdown of skin 🦠

L97.312　Non-pressure chronic ulcer of right ankle with fat layer exposed 🦠

L97.313　Non-pressure chronic ulcer of right ankle with necrosis of muscle 🦠

L97.314　Non-pressure chronic ulcer of right ankle with necrosis of bone 🦠

L97.319　Non-pressure chronic ulcer of right ankle with unspecified severity 🦠

● L97.32　Non-pressure chronic ulcer of left ankle

L97.321　Non-pressure chronic ulcer of left ankle limited to breakdown of skin 🦠

L97.322　Non-pressure chronic ulcer of left ankle with fat layer exposed 🦠

L97.323　Non-pressure chronic ulcer of left ankle with necrosis of muscle 🦠

L97.324　Non-pressure chronic ulcer of left ankle with necrosis of bone 🦠

L97.329　Non-pressure chronic ulcer of left ankle with unspecified severity 🦠

● L97.4　Non-pressure chronic ulcer of heel and midfoot
Non-pressure chronic ulcer of plantar surface of midfoot

● L97.40　Non-pressure chronic ulcer of unspecified heel and midfoot

L97.401　Non-pressure chronic ulcer of unspecified heel and midfoot limited to breakdown of skin 🦠

L97.402　Non-pressure chronic ulcer of unspecified heel and midfoot with fat layer exposed 🦠

L97.403　Non-pressure chronic ulcer of unspecified heel and midfoot with necrosis of muscle 🦠

L97.404　Non-pressure chronic ulcer of unspecified heel and midfoot with necrosis of bone 🦠

L97.409　Non-pressure chronic ulcer of unspecified heel and midfoot with unspecified severity 🦠

● L97.41　Non-pressure chronic ulcer of right heel and midfoot

L97.411　Non-pressure chronic ulcer of right heel and midfoot limited to breakdown of skin 🦠

L97.412　Non-pressure chronic ulcer of right heel and midfoot with fat layer exposed 🦠

L97.413　Non-pressure chronic ulcer of right heel and midfoot with necrosis of muscle 🦠

L97.414　Non-pressure chronic ulcer of right heel and midfoot with necrosis of bone 🦠

L97.419　Non-pressure chronic ulcer of right heel and midfoot with unspecified severity 🦠

● L97.42　Non-pressure chronic ulcer of left heel and midfoot

L97.421　Non-pressure chronic ulcer of left heel and midfoot limited to breakdown of skin 🦠

L97.422　Non-pressure chronic ulcer of left heel and midfoot with fat layer exposed 🦠

L97.423　Non-pressure chronic ulcer of left heel and midfoot with necrosis of muscle 🦠

L97.424　Non-pressure chronic ulcer of left heel and midfoot with necrosis of bone 🦠

L97.429　Non-pressure chronic ulcer of left heel and midfoot with unspecified severity 🦠

● L97.5　Non-pressure chronic ulcer of other part of foot
Non-pressure chronic ulcer of toe

● L97.50　Non-pressure chronic ulcer of other part of unspecified foot

L97.501　Non-pressure chronic ulcer of other part of unspecified foot limited to breakdown of skin

L97.502　Non-pressure chronic ulcer of other part of unspecified foot with fat layer exposed

L97.503　Non-pressure chronic ulcer of other part of unspecified foot with necrosis of muscle

L97.504　Non-pressure chronic ulcer of other part of unspecified foot with necrosis of bone

L97.509　Non-pressure chronic ulcer of other part of unspecified foot with unspecified severity

● L97.51　Non-pressure chronic ulcer of other part of right foot

L97.511　Non-pressure chronic ulcer of other part of right foot limited to breakdown of skin

L97.512　Non-pressure chronic ulcer of other part of right foot with fat layer exposed

L97.513　Non-pressure chronic ulcer of other part of right foot with necrosis of muscle

L97.514　Non-pressure chronic ulcer of other part of right foot with necrosis of bone

L97.519　Non-pressure chronic ulcer of other part of right foot with unspecified severity

N Newborn Age: 0　　**P** Pediatric Age: 0–17　　**M** Maternity DX: 12–55　　**A** Adult Age: 15–124　　♀ Females Only　　♂ Males Only

🦠 Complication\Comorbidity　　🦠 Major C\C　　◐ Present on Admission Requirement　　🦠 Hospital-Acquired Condition

CHAPTER 12 (L00-L99)

1139

● **L97.52** Non-pressure chronic ulcer of other part of left foot

  L97.521 Non-pressure chronic ulcer of other part of left foot limited to breakdown of skin

  L97.522 Non-pressure chronic ulcer of other part of left foot with fat layer exposed

  L97.523 Non-pressure chronic ulcer of other part of left foot with necrosis of muscle

  L97.524 Non-pressure chronic ulcer of other part of left foot with necrosis of bone

  L97.529 Non-pressure chronic ulcer of other part of left foot with unspecified severity

● **L97.8** Non-pressure chronic ulcer of other part of lower leg

● **L97.80** Non-pressure chronic ulcer of other part of unspecified lower leg

  L97.801 Non-pressure chronic ulcer of other part of unspecified lower leg limited to breakdown of skin

  L97.802 Non-pressure chronic ulcer of other part of unspecified lower leg with fat layer exposed

  L97.803 Non-pressure chronic ulcer of other part of unspecified lower leg with necrosis of muscle

  L97.804 Non-pressure chronic ulcer of other part of unspecified lower leg with necrosis of bone

  L97.809 Non-pressure chronic ulcer of other part of unspecified lower leg with unspecified severity

● **L97.81** Non-pressure chronic ulcer of other part of right lower leg

  L97.811 Non-pressure chronic ulcer of other part of right lower leg limited to breakdown of skin

  L97.812 Non-pressure chronic ulcer of other part of right lower leg with fat layer exposed

  L97.813 Non-pressure chronic ulcer of other part of right lower leg with necrosis of muscle

  L97.814 Non-pressure chronic ulcer of other part of right lower leg with necrosis of bone

  L97.819 Non-pressure chronic ulcer of other part of right lower leg with unspecified severity

● **L97.82** Non-pressure chronic ulcer of other part of left lower leg

  L97.821 Non-pressure chronic ulcer of other part of left lower leg limited to breakdown of skin

  L97.822 Non-pressure chronic ulcer of other part of left lower leg with fat layer exposed

  L97.823 Non-pressure chronic ulcer of other part of left lower leg with necrosis of muscle

  L97.824 Non-pressure chronic ulcer of other part of left lower leg with necrosis of bone

  L97.829 Non-pressure chronic ulcer of other part of left lower leg with unspecified severity

● **L97.9** Non-pressure chronic ulcer of unspecified part of lower leg

● **L97.90** Non-pressure chronic ulcer of unspecified part of unspecified lower leg

  L97.901 Non-pressure chronic ulcer of unspecified part of unspecified lower leg limited to breakdown of skin

  L97.902 Non-pressure chronic ulcer of unspecified part of unspecified lower leg with fat layer exposed

  L97.903 Non-pressure chronic ulcer of unspecified part of unspecified lower leg with necrosis of muscle

  L97.904 Non-pressure chronic ulcer of unspecified part of unspecified lower leg with necrosis of bone

  L97.909 Non-pressure chronic ulcer of unspecified part of unspecified lower leg with unspecified severity

● **L97.91** Non-pressure chronic ulcer of unspecified part of right lower leg

  L97.911 Non-pressure chronic ulcer of unspecified part of right lower leg limited to breakdown of skin

  L97.912 Non-pressure chronic ulcer of unspecified part of right lower leg with fat layer exposed

  L97.913 Non-pressure chronic ulcer of unspecified part of right lower leg with necrosis of muscle

  L97.914 Non-pressure chronic ulcer of unspecified part of right lower leg with necrosis of bone

  L97.919 Non-pressure chronic ulcer of unspecified part of right lower leg with unspecified severity

● **L97.92**   **Non-pressure chronic ulcer of unspecified part of left lower leg**
- ■ **L97.921**   Non-pressure chronic ulcer of unspecified part of left lower leg limited to breakdown of skin 🔗
- ■ **L97.922**   Non-pressure chronic ulcer of unspecified part of left lower leg with fat layer exposed 🔗
- ■ **L97.923**   Non-pressure chronic ulcer of unspecified part of left lower leg with necrosis of muscle 🔗
- ■ **L97.924**   Non-pressure chronic ulcer of unspecified part of left lower leg with necrosis of bone 🔗
- ■ **L97.929**   Non-pressure chronic ulcer of unspecified part of left lower leg with unspecified severity 🔗

● **L98**   **Other disorders of skin and subcutaneous tissue, not elsewhere classified**

L98.0   **Pyogenic granuloma**
> **Excludes2**   pyogenic granuloma of gingiva (K06.8)
> pyogenic granuloma of maxillary alveolar ridge (K04.5)
> pyogenic granuloma of oral mucosa (K13.4)

L98.1   **Factitial dermatitis**
Neurotic excoriation

L98.2   **Febrile neutrophilic dermatosis [Sweet]**

L98.3   **Eosinophilic cellulitis [Wells]** 🔗

● **L98.4**   **Non-pressure chronic ulcer of skin, not elsewhere classified**
Chronic ulcer of skin NOS
Tropical ulcer NOS
Ulcer of skin NOS
> **Excludes2**   pressure ulcer (pressure area) (L89.-)
> gangrene (I96)
> skin infections (L00-L08)
> specific infections classified to A00-B99
> ulcer of lower limb NEC (L97.-)
> varicose ulcer (I83.0-I82.2)

● **L98.41**   **Non-pressure chronic ulcer of buttock**
- **L98.411**   Non-pressure chronic ulcer of buttock limited to breakdown of skin
- **L98.412**   Non-pressure chronic ulcer of buttock with fat layer exposed
- **L98.413**   Non-pressure chronic ulcer of buttock with necrosis of muscle
- **L98.414**   Non-pressure chronic ulcer of buttock with necrosis of bone
- ■ **L98.419**   Non-pressure chronic ulcer of buttock with unspecified severity

● **L98.42**   **Non-pressure chronic ulcer of back**
- **L98.421**   Non-pressure chronic ulcer of back limited to breakdown of skin
- **L98.422**   Non-pressure chronic ulcer of back with fat layer exposed
- **L98.423**   Non-pressure chronic ulcer of back with necrosis of muscle
- **L98.424**   Non-pressure chronic ulcer of back with necrosis of bone
- ■ **L98.429**   Non-pressure chronic ulcer of back with unspecified severity

● **L98.49**   **Non-pressure chronic ulcer of skin of other sites**
Non-pressure chronic ulcer of skin NOS
- **L98.491**   Non-pressure chronic ulcer of skin of other sites limited to breakdown of skin
- **L98.492**   Non-pressure chronic ulcer of skin of other sites with fat layer exposed
- **L98.493**   Non-pressure chronic ulcer of skin of other sites with necrosis of muscle
- **L98.494**   Non-pressure chronic ulcer of skin of other sites with necrosis of bone
- ■ **L98.499**   Non-pressure chronic ulcer of skin of other sites with unspecified severity

L98.5   **Mucinosis of the skin**
Focal mucinosis
Lichen myxedematosus
> **Excludes1**   focal oral mucinosis (K13.79)
> myxedema (E03.9)

L98.6   **Other infiltrative disorders of the skin and subcutaneous tissue**
> **Excludes1**   hyalinosis cutis et mucosae (E78.89)

L98.8   **Other specified disorders of the skin and subcutaneous tissue**

■ **L98.9**   **Disorder of the skin and subcutaneous tissue, unspecified**

● ▷ *L99*   *Other disorders of skin and subcutaneous tissue in diseases classified elsewhere*
> *Code first* underlying disease, such as:
> amyloidosis (E85-)
> **Excludes1**   skin disorders in diabetes (E08-E13 with .62)
> skin disorders in gonorrhea (A54.89)
> skin disorders in syphilis (A51.31, A52.79)

CHAPTER 12 (L00-L99)

a. Site and laterality
Most of the codes within Chapter 13 have site and laterality designations. The site represents the bone, joint or the muscle involved. For some conditions where more than one bone, joint or muscle is usually involved, such as osteoarthritis, there is a "multiple sites" code available. For categories where no multiple site code is provided and more than one bone, joint or muscle is involved, multiple codes should be used to indicate the different sites involved.

1) Bone versus joint
For certain conditions, the bone may be affected at the upper or lower end, (e.g., avascular necrosis of bone, M87, Osteoporosis, M80, M81). Though the portion of the bone affected may be at the joint, the site designation will be the bone, not the joint.

b. Acute traumatic versus chronic or recurrent musculoskeletal conditions
Many musculoskeletal conditions are a result of previous injury or trauma to a site, or are recurrent conditions. Bone, joint or muscle conditions that are the result of a healed injury are usually found in chapter 13. Recurrent bone, joint or muscle conditions are also usually found in chapter 13. Any current, acute injury should be coded to the appropriate injury code from chapter 19. Chronic or recurrent conditions should generally be coded with a code from chapter 13. If it is difficult to determine from the documentation in the record which code is best to describe a condition, query the provider.

c. Coding of Pathologic Fractures
7th character A is for use as long as the patient is receiving active treatment for the fracture. Examples of active treatment are: surgical treatment, emergency department encounter, evaluation and treatment by a new physician. 7th character, D is to be used for encounters after the patient has completed active treatment. The other 7th characters, listed under each subcategory in the Tabular List, are to be used for subsequent encounters for treatment of problems associated with the healing, such as malunions and nonunions, and sequelae. Care for complications of surgical treatment for fracture repairs during the healing or recovery phase should be coded with the appropriate complication codes.

See Section I.C.19. Coding of traumatic fractures.

CHAPTER 13

DISEASES OF THE MUSCULOSKELETAL SYSTEM AND CONNECTIVE TISSUE (M00-M99)

Note: Use an external cause code following the code for the musculoskeletal condition, if applicable, to identify the cause of the musculoskeletal condition

Excludes2 arthropathic psoriasis (L40.5-)
certain conditions originating in the perinatal period (P04-P96)
certain infectious and parasitic diseases (A00-B99)
compartment syndrome (traumatic) (T79.A-)
complications of pregnancy, childbirth and the puerperium (O00-O9A)
congenital malformations, deformations, and chromosomal abnormalities (Q00-Q99)
endocrine, nutritional and metabolic diseases (E00-E88)
injury, poisoning and certain other consequences of external causes (S00-T88)
neoplasms (C00-D49)
symptoms, signs and abnormal clinical and laboratory findings, not elsewhere classified (R00-R94)

This chapter contains the following blocks:

M00-M02	Infectious arthropathies
M05-M14	Inflammatory polyarthropathies
M15-M19	Osteoarthritis
M20-M25	Other joint disorders
M26-M27	Dentofacial anomalies [including malocclusion] and other disorders of jaw
M30-M36	Systemic connective tissue disorders
M40-M43	Deforming dorsopathies
M45-M49	Spondylopathies
M50-M54	Other dorsopathies
M60-M63	Disorders of muscles
M65-M67	Disorders of synovium and tendon
M70-M79	Other soft tissue disorders
M80-M85	Disorders of bone density and structure
M86-M90	Other osteopathies
M91-M94	Chondropathies
M95	Other disorders of the musculoskeletal system and connective tissue
M96	Intraoperative and postprocedural complications and disorders of musculoskeletal system, not elsewhere classified
M99	Biomechanical lesions, not elsewhere classified

ARTHROPATHIES (M00-M25)

Includes Disorders affecting predominantly peripheral (limb) joints

INFECTIOUS ARTHROPATHIES (M00-M02)

Note: This block comprises arthropathies due to microbiological agents.

Distinction is made between the following types of etiological relationship:

a) direct infection of joint, where organisms invade synovial tissue and microbial antigen is present in the joint;

b) indirect infection, which may be of two types: a reactive arthropathy, where microbial infection of the body is established but neither organisms nor antigens can be identified in the joint, and a postinfective arthropathy, where microbial antigen is present but recovery of an organism is inconstant and evidence of local multiplication is lacking.

● M00 Pyogenic arthritis
● M00.0 Staphylococcal arthritis and polyarthritis
Use additional code (B95.61-B95.8) to identify bacterial agent
Excludes2 infection and inflammatory reaction due to internal joint prosthesis (T84.5-)
■ M00.00 Staphylococcal arthritis, unspecified joint
● M00.01 Staphylococcal arthritis, shoulder
M00.011 Staphylococcal arthritis, right shoulder
M00.012 Staphylococcal arthritis, left shoulder
■ M00.019 Staphylococcal arthritis, unspecified shoulder

● M00.02 Staphylococcal arthritis, elbow

    M00.021 Staphylococcal arthritis, right elbow 🕏

    M00.022 Staphylococcal arthritis, left elbow 🕏

    ▣ M00.029 Staphylococcal arthritis, unspecified elbow 🕏

● M00.03 Staphylococcal arthritis, wrist
    Staphylococcal arthritis of carpal bones

    M00.031 Staphylococcal arthritis, right wrist 🕏

    M00.032 Staphylococcal arthritis, left wrist 🕏

    ▣ M00.039 Staphylococcal arthritis, unspecified wrist 🕏

● M00.04 Staphylococcal arthritis, hand
    Staphylococcal arthritis of metacarpus and phalanges

    M00.041 Staphylococcal arthritis, right hand 🕏

    M00.042 Staphylococcal arthritis, left hand 🕏

    ▣ M00.049 Staphylococcal arthritis, unspecified hand 🕏

● M00.05 Staphylococcal arthritis, hip

    M00.051 Staphylococcal arthritis, right hip 🕏

    M00.052 Staphylococcal arthritis, left hip 🕏

    ▣ M00.059 Staphylococcal arthritis, unspecified hip 🕏

● M00.06 Staphylococcal arthritis, knee

    M00.061 Staphylococcal arthritis, right knee 🕏

    M00.062 Staphylococcal arthritis, left knee 🕏

    ▣ M00.069 Staphylococcal arthritis, unspecified knee 🕏

● M00.07 Staphylococcal arthritis, ankle and foot
    Staphylococcal arthritis, tarsus, metatarsus and phalanges

    M00.071 Staphylococcal arthritis, right ankle and foot 🕏

    M00.072 Staphylococcal arthritis, left ankle and foot 🕏

    ▣ M00.079 Staphylococcal arthritis, unspecified ankle and foot 🕏

    M00.08 Staphylococcal arthritis, vertebrae 🕏

    M00.09 Staphylococcal polyarthritis 🕏

● M00.1 Pneumococcal arthritis and polyarthritis

    ▣ M00.10 Pneumococcal arthritis, unspecified joint 🕏

● M00.11 Pneumococcal arthritis, shoulder

    M00.111 Pneumococcal arthritis, right shoulder 🕏

    M00.112 Pneumococcal arthritis, left shoulder 🕏

    ▣ M00.119 Pneumococcal arthritis, unspecified shoulder 🕏

● M00.12 Pneumococcal arthritis, elbow

    M00.121 Pneumococcal arthritis, right elbow 🕏

    M00.122 Pneumococcal arthritis, left elbow 🕏

    ▣ M00.129 Pneumococcal arthritis, unspecified elbow 🕏

● M00.13 Pneumococcal arthritis, wrist
    Pneumococcal arthritis of carpal bones

    M00.131 Pneumococcal arthritis, right wrist 🕏

    M00.132 Pneumococcal arthritis, left wrist 🕏

    ▣ M00.139 Pneumococcal arthritis, unspecified wrist 🕏

● M00.14 Pneumococcal arthritis, hand
    Pneumococcal arthritis of metacarpus and phalanges

    M00.141 Pneumococcal arthritis, right hand 🕏

    M00.142 Pneumococcal arthritis, left hand 🕏

    ▣ M00.149 Pneumococcal arthritis, unspecified hand 🕏

● M00.15 Pneumococcal arthritis, hip

    M00.151 Pneumococcal arthritis, right hip 🕏

    M00.152 Pneumococcal arthritis, left hip 🕏

    ▣ M00.159 Pneumococcal arthritis, unspecified hip 🕏

● M00.16 Pneumococcal arthritis, knee

    M00.161 Pneumococcal arthritis, right knee 🕏

    M00.162 Pneumococcal arthritis, left knee 🕏

    ▣ M00.169 Pneumococcal arthritis, unspecified knee 🕏

● M00.17 Pneumococcal arthritis, ankle and foot
    Pneumococcal arthritis, tarsus, metatarsus and phalanges

    M00.171 Pneumococcal arthritis, right ankle and foot 🕏

    M00.172 Pneumococcal arthritis, left ankle and foot 🕏

    ▣ M00.179 Pneumococcal arthritis, unspecified ankle and foot 🕏

    M00.18 Pneumococcal arthritis, vertebrae 🕏

    M00.19 Pneumococcal polyarthritis 🕏

● M00.2 Other streptococcal arthritis and polyarthritis

    Use additional code (B95.0-B95.2, B95.4-B95.5) to identify bacterial agent

    ▣ M00.20 Other streptococcal arthritis, unspecified joint 🕏

● M00.21 Other streptococcal arthritis, shoulder

    M00.211 Other streptococcal arthritis, right shoulder 🕏

    M00.212 Other streptococcal arthritis, left shoulder 🕏

    ▣ M00.219 Other streptococcal arthritis, unspecified shoulder 🕏

CHAPTER 13 (M00-M99)

CHAPTER 13 (M00-M99)

● M00.22   Other streptococcal arthritis, elbow
- M00.221   Other streptococcal arthritis, right elbow 🔎
- M00.222   Other streptococcal arthritis, left elbow 🔎
- ■ M00.229   Other streptococcal arthritis, unspecified elbow 🔎

● M00.23   Other streptococcal arthritis, wrist
     Other streptococcal arthritis of carpal bones
- M00.231   Other streptococcal arthritis, right wrist 🔎
- M00.232   Other streptococcal arthritis, left wrist 🔎
- ■ M00.239   Other streptococcal arthritis, unspecified wrist 🔎

● M00.24   Other streptococcal arthritis, hand
     Other streptococcal arthritis metacarpus and phalanges
- M00.241   Other streptococcal arthritis, right hand 🔎
- M00.242   Other streptococcal arthritis, left hand 🔎
- ■ M00.249   Other streptococcal arthritis, unspecified hand 🔎

● M00.25   Other streptococcal arthritis, hip
- M00.251   Other streptococcal arthritis, right hip 🔎
- M00.252   Other streptococcal arthritis, left hip 🔎
- ■ M00.259   Other streptococcal arthritis, unspecified hip 🔎

● M00.26   Other streptococcal arthritis, knee
- M00.261   Other streptococcal arthritis, right knee 🔎
- M00.262   Other streptococcal arthritis, left knee 🔎
- ■ M00.269   Other streptococcal arthritis, unspecified knee 🔎

● M00.27   Other streptococcal arthritis, ankle and foot
     Other streptococcal arthritis, tarsus, metatarsus and phalanges
- M00.271   Other streptococcal arthritis, right ankle and foot 🔎
- M00.272   Other streptococcal arthritis, left ankle and foot 🔎
- ■ M00.279   Other streptococcal arthritis, unspecified ankle and foot 🔎

M00.28   Other streptococcal arthritis, vertebrae 🔎

M00.29   Other streptococcal polyarthritis 🔎

● M00.8   Arthritis and polyarthritis due to other bacteria
     Use additional code (B96) to identify bacteria
- ■ M00.80   Arthritis due to other bacteria, unspecified joint 🔎
- ● M00.81   Arthritis due to other bacteria, shoulder
  - M00.811   Arthritis due to other bacteria, right shoulder 🔎
  - M00.812   Arthritis due to other bacteria, left shoulder 🔎
  - ■ M00.819   Arthritis due to other bacteria, unspecified shoulder 🔎

● M00.82   Arthritis due to other bacteria, elbow
- M00.821   Arthritis due to other bacteria, right elbow 🔎
- M00.822   Arthritis due to other bacteria, left elbow 🔎
- ■ M00.829   Arthritis due to other bacteria, unspecified elbow 🔎

● M00.83   Arthritis due to other bacteria, wrist
     Arthritis due to other bacteria, carpal bones
- M00.831   Arthritis due to other bacteria, right wrist 🔎
- M00.832   Arthritis due to other bacteria, left wrist 🔎
- ■ M00.839   Arthritis due to other bacteria, unspecified wrist 🔎

● M00.84   Arthritis due to other bacteria, hand
     Arthritis due to other bacteria, metacarpus and phalanges
- M00.841   Arthritis due to other bacteria, right hand 🔎
- M00.842   Arthritis due to other bacteria, left hand 🔎
- ■ M00.849   Arthritis due to other bacteria, unspecified hand 🔎

● M00.85   Arthritis due to other bacteria, hip
- M00.851   Arthritis due to other bacteria, right hip 🔎
- M00.852   Arthritis due to other bacteria, left hip 🔎
- ■ M00.859   Arthritis due to other bacteria, unspecified hip 🔎

● M00.86   Arthritis due to other bacteria, knee
- M00.861   Arthritis due to other bacteria, right knee 🔎
- M00.862   Arthritis due to other bacteria, left knee 🔎
- ■ M00.869   Arthritis due to other bacteria, unspecified knee 🔎

● M00.87   Arthritis due to other bacteria, ankle and foot
     Arthritis due to other bacteria, tarsus, metatarsus, and phalanges
- M00.871   Arthritis due to other bacteria, right ankle and foot 🔎
- M00.872   Arthritis due to other bacteria, left ankle and foot 🔎
- ■ M00.879   Arthritis due to other bacteria, unspecified ankle and foot 🔎

M00.88   Arthritis due to other bacteria, vertebrae 🔎

M00.89   Polyarthritis due to other bacteria 🔎

■ M00.9   Pyogenic arthritis, unspecified 🔎
     Infective arthritis NOS

● Unacceptable Principal Diagnosis   ● Use Additional Character(s)   ■ Unspecified   ▶ Manifestation Code

OGCR   Official Guidelines for Coding and Reporting   Excludes 1   Excludes 2   Includes   Use additional   Code first   Code also

● **M01 Direct infections of joint in infectious and parasitic diseases classified elsewhere**

> *Code first* underlying disease, such as:
> leprosy [Hansen's disease] (A30.-)
> mycoses (B35-B49)
> O'nyong-nyong fever (A92.1)
> paratyphoid fever (A01.1-A01.4)

Excludes1	arthritis, arthropathy (in):

gonococcal (A54.42)
Lyme disease (A69.23)
meningococcal (A39.83)
postmeningococcal (A39.84)
mumps (B26.85)
postinfective (M02.-)
reactive (M04.0-)
rubella (B06.82)
sarcoidosis (D86.86)
typhoid fever (A01.04)
tuberculosis (A18.02)
spine (A18.01)

● **M01.X Direct infection of joint in infectious and parasitic diseases classified elsewhere**

● ■▶ *M01.X0 Direct infection of unspecified joint in infectious and parasitic diseases classified elsewhere* 🦠

● *M01.X1 Direct infection of shoulder joint in infectious and parasitic diseases classified elsewhere*

● ▶ *M01.X11 Direct infection of right shoulder in infectious and parasitic diseases classified elsewhere* 🦠

● ▶ *M01.X12 Direct infection of left shoulder in infectious and parasitic diseases classified elsewhere* 🦠

● ■▶ *M01.X19 Direct infection of unspecified shoulder in infectious and parasitic diseases classified elsewhere* 🦠

● *M01.X2 Direct infection of elbow in infectious and parasitic diseases classified elsewhere*

● ▶ *M01.X21 Direct infection of right elbow in infectious and parasitic diseases classified elsewhere* 🦠

● ▶ *M01.X22 Direct infection of left elbow in infectious and parasitic diseases classified elsewhere* 🦠

● ■▶ *M01.X29 Direct infection of unspecified elbow in infectious and parasitic diseases classified elsewhere* 🦠

● *M01.X3 Direct infection of wrist in infectious and parasitic diseases classified elsewhere*
> Direct infection of carpal bones in infectious and parasitic diseases classified elsewhere

● ▶ *M01.X31 Direct infection of right wrist in infectious and parasitic diseases classified elsewhere* 🦠

● ▶ *M01.X32 Direct infection of left wrist in infectious and parasitic diseases classified elsewhere* 🦠

● ■▶ *M01.X39 Direct infection of unspecified wrist in infectious and parasitic diseases classified elsewhere* 🦠

● **M01.X4 Direct infection of hand in infectious and parasitic diseases classified elsewhere**
> Direct infection of metacarpus and phalanges in infectious and parasitic diseases classified elsewhere

● ▶ *M01.X41 Direct infection of right hand in infectious and parasitic diseases classified elsewhere* 🦠

● ▶ *M01.X42 Direct infection of left hand in infectious and parasitic diseases classified elsewhere* 🦠

● ■▶ *M01.X49 Direct infection of unspecified hand in infectious and parasitic diseases classified elsewhere* 🦠

● **M01.X5 Direct infection of hip in infectious and parasitic diseases classified elsewhere**

● ▶ *M01.X51 Direct infection of right hip in infectious and parasitic diseases classified elsewhere* 🦠

● ▶ *M01.X52 Direct infection of left hip in infectious and parasitic diseases classified elsewhere* 🦠

● ■▶ *M01.X59 Direct infection of unspecified hip in infectious and parasitic diseases classified elsewhere* 🦠

● **M01.X6 Direct infection of knee in infectious and parasitic diseases classified elsewhere**

● ▶ *M01.X61 Direct infection of right knee in infectious and parasitic diseases classified elsewhere* 🦠

● ▶ *M01.X62 Direct infection of left knee in infectious and parasitic diseases classified elsewhere* 🦠

● ■▶ *M01.X69 Direct infection of unspecified knee in infectious and parasitic diseases classified elsewhere* 🦠

● **M01.X7 Direct infection of ankle and foot in infectious and parasitic diseases classified elsewhere**
> Direct infection of tarsus, metatarsus and phalanges in infectious and parasitic diseases classified elsewhere

● ▶ *M01.X71 Direct infection of right ankle and foot in infectious and parasitic diseases classified elsewhere* 🦠

● ▶ *M01.X72 Direct infection of left ankle and foot in infectious and parasitic diseases classified elsewhere* 🦠

● ■▶ *M01.X79 Direct infection of unspecified ankle and foot in infectious and parasitic diseases classified elsewhere* 🦠

● ▶ *M01.X8 Direct infection of vertebrae in infectious and parasitic diseases classified elsewhere* 🦠

● ▶ *M01.X9 Direct infection of multiple joints in infectious and parasitic diseases classified elsewhere* 🦠

CHAPTER 13 (M00-M99)

N Newborn Age: 0   P Pediatric Age: 0–17   M Maternity DX: 12–55   A Adult Age: 15–124   ♀ Females Only   ♂ Males Only

🦠 Complication\Comorbidity   🦠 Major C\C   🦠 Present on Admission Requirement   🦠 Hospital-Acquired Condition

CHAPTER 13 (M00-M99)

● **M02   Postinfective and reactive arthropathies**

> *Code first* underlying disease, such as:
> congenital syphilis [Clutton's joints] (A50.5)
> enteritis due to Yersinia enterocolitica (A04.6)
> infective endocarditis (I33.0)
> viral hepatitis (B15-B19)

> **Excludes1**   Behçet's disease (M35.2)
> direct infections of joint in infectious and parasitic diseases classified elsewhere (M01.-)
> postinfectious arthritis (in):
>   meningococcal (A39.84)
>   mumps (B26.85)
>   rubella (B06.82)
>   syphilis (late) (A52.77)
> rheumatic fever (I00)
> tabetic arthropathy [Charcôt's] (A52.16)

● **M02.0   Arthropathy following intestinal bypass**

    ▪ **M02.00   Arthropathy following intestinal bypass, unspecified site**

    ● **M02.01   Arthropathy following intestinal bypass, shoulder**

       M02.011   Arthropathy following intestinal bypass, right shoulder

       M02.012   Arthropathy following intestinal bypass, left shoulder

       ▪ **M02.019   Arthropathy following intestinal bypass, unspecified shoulder**

    ● **M02.02   Arthropathy following intestinal bypass, elbow**

       M02.021   Arthropathy following intestinal bypass, right elbow

       M02.022   Arthropathy following intestinal bypass, left elbow

       ▪ **M02.029   Arthropathy following intestinal bypass, unspecified elbow**

    ● **M02.03   Arthropathy following intestinal bypass, wrist**
> Arthropathy following intestinal bypass, carpal bones

       M02.031   Arthropathy following intestinal bypass, right wrist

       M02.032   Arthropathy following intestinal bypass, left wrist

       ▪ **M02.039   Arthropathy following intestinal bypass, unspecified wrist**

    ● **M02.04   Arthropathy following intestinal bypass, hand**
> Arthropathy following intestinal bypass, metacarpals and phalanges

       M02.041   Arthropathy following intestinal bypass, right hand

       M02.042   Arthropathy following intestinal bypass, left hand

       ▪ **M02.049   Arthropathy following intestinal bypass, unspecified hand**

    ● **M02.05   Arthropathy following intestinal bypass, hip**

       M02.051   Arthropathy following intestinal bypass, right hip

       M02.052   Arthropathy following intestinal bypass, left hip

       ▪ **M02.059   Arthropathy following intestinal bypass, unspecified hip**

● **M02.06   Arthropathy following intestinal bypass, knee**

       M02.061   Arthropathy following intestinal bypass, right knee

       M02.062   Arthropathy following intestinal bypass, left knee

       ▪ **M02.069   Arthropathy following intestinal bypass, unspecified knee**

● **M02.07   Arthropathy following intestinal bypass, ankle and foot**
> Arthropathy following intestinal bypass, tarsus, metatarsus and phalanges

       M02.071   Arthropathy following intestinal bypass, right ankle and foot

       M02.072   Arthropathy following intestinal bypass, left ankle and foot

       ▪ **M02.079   Arthropathy following intestinal bypass, unspecified ankle and foot**

    M02.08   Arthropathy following intestinal bypass, vertebrae

    M02.09   Arthropathy following intestinal bypass, multiple sites

● **M02.1   Postdysenteric arthropathy**

    ▪ **M02.10   Postdysenteric arthropathy, unspecified site** 🦴

    ● **M02.11   Postdysenteric arthropathy, shoulder**

       M02.111   Postdysenteric arthropathy, right shoulder 🦴

       M02.112   Postdysenteric arthropathy, left shoulder 🦴

       ▪ **M02.119   Postdysenteric arthropathy, unspecified shoulder** 🦴

    ● **M02.12   Postdysenteric arthropathy, elbow**

       M02.121   Postdysenteric arthropathy, right elbow 🦴

       M02.122   Postdysenteric arthropathy, left elbow 🦴

       ▪ **M02.129   Postdysenteric arthropathy, unspecified elbow** 🦴

    ● **M02.13   Postdysenteric arthropathy, wrist**
> Postdysenteric arthropathy, carpal bones

       M02.131   Postdysenteric arthropathy, right wrist 🦴

       M02.132   Postdysenteric arthropathy, left wrist 🦴

       ▪ **M02.139   Postdysenteric arthropathy, unspecified wrist** 🦴

    ● **M02.14   Postdysenteric arthropathy, hand**
> Postdysenteric arthropathy, metacarpus and phalanges

       M02.141   Postdysenteric arthropathy, right hand 🦴

       M02.142   Postdysenteric arthropathy, left hand 🦴

       ▪ **M02.149   Postdysenteric arthropathy, unspecified hand** 🦴

●   Unacceptable Principal Diagnosis   ●   Use Additional Character(s)   ▪   Unspecified   ▸   Manifestation Code

OGCR   Official Guidelines for Coding and Reporting   Excludes 1   Excludes 2   Includes   Use additional   Code first   Code also

● M02.15   Postdysenteric arthropathy, hip

    M02.151   Postdysenteric arthropathy, right hip 🦴

    M02.152   Postdysenteric arthropathy, left hip 🦴

    M02.159   Postdysenteric arthropathy, unspecified hip 🦴

● M02.16   Postdysenteric arthropathy, knee

    M02.161   Postdysenteric arthropathy, right knee 🦴

    M02.162   Postdysenteric arthropathy, left knee 🦴

    M02.169   Postdysenteric arthropathy, unspecified knee 🦴

● M02.17   Postdysenteric arthropathy, ankle and foot
    Postdysenteric arthropathy, tarsus, metatarsus and phalanges

    M02.171   Postdysenteric arthropathy, right ankle and foot 🦴

    M02.172   Postdysenteric arthropathy, left ankle and foot 🦴

    M02.179   Postdysenteric arthropathy, unspecified ankle and foot 🦴

    M02.18   Postdysenteric arthropathy, vertebrae 🦴

    M02.19   Postdysenteric arthropathy, multiple sites 🦴

● M02.2   Postimmunization arthropathy

    M02.20   Postimmunization arthropathy, unspecified site

● M02.21   Postimmunization arthropathy, shoulder

    M02.211   Postimmunization arthropathy, right shoulder

    M02.212   Postimmunization arthropathy, left shoulder

    M02.219   Postimmunization arthropathy, unspecified shoulder

● M02.22   Postimmunization arthropathy, elbow

    M02.221   Postimmunization arthropathy, right elbow

    M02.222   Postimmunization arthropathy, left elbow

    M02.229   Postimmunization arthropathy, unspecified elbow

● M02.23   Postimmunization arthropathy, wrist
    Postimmunization arthropathy, carpal bones

    M02.231   Postimmunization arthropathy, right wrist

    M02.232   Postimmunization arthropathy, left wrist

    M02.239   Postimmunization arthropathy, unspecified wrist

● M02.24   Postimmunization arthropathy, hand
    Postimmunization arthropathy, metacarpus and phalanges

    M02.241   Postimmunization arthropathy, right hand

    M02.242   Postimmunization arthropathy, left hand

    M02.249   Postimmunization arthropathy, unspecified hand

● M02.25   Postimmunization arthropathy, hip

    M02.251   Postimmunization arthropathy, right hip

    M02.252   Postimmunization arthropathy, left hip

    M02.259   Postimmunization arthropathy, unspecified hip

● M02.26   Postimmunization arthropathy, knee

    M02.261   Postimmunization arthropathy, right knee

    M02.262   Postimmunization arthropathy, left knee

    M02.269   Postimmunization arthropathy, unspecified knee

● M02.27   Postimmunization arthropathy, ankle and foot
    Postimmunization arthropathy, tarsus, metatarsus and phalanges

    M02.271   Postimmunization arthropathy, right ankle and foot

    M02.272   Postimmunization arthropathy, left ankle and foot

    M02.279   Postimmunization arthropathy, unspecified ankle and foot

    M02.28   Postimmunization arthropathy, vertebrae

    M02.29   Postimmunization arthropathy, multiple sites

● M02.3   Reiter's disease
    Reactive arthritis

    M02.30   Reiter's disease, unspecified site 🦴
       MCC: Only when the principal diagnosis is designated as a CC

● M02.31   Reiter's disease, shoulder

    M02.311   Reiter's disease, right shoulder 🦴
       MCC: Only when the principal diagnosis is designated as a CC

    M02.312   Reiter's disease, left shoulder 🦴
       MCC: Only when the principal diagnosis is designated as a CC

    M02.319   Reiter's disease, unspecified shoulder 🦴
       MCC: Only when the principal diagnosis is designated as a CC

● M02.32   Reiter's disease, elbow

    M02.321   Reiter's disease, right elbow 🦴
       MCC: Only when the principal diagnosis is designated as a CC

    M02.322   Reiter's disease, left elbow 🦴
       MCC: Only when the principal diagnosis is designated as a CC

    M02.329   Reiter's disease, unspecified elbow 🦴
       MCC: Only when the principal diagnosis is designated as a CC

N Newborn Age: 0   **P** Pediatric Age: 0–17   **M** Maternity DX: 12–55   **A** Adult Age: 15–124   ♀ Females Only   ♂ Males Only

🦴 Complication\Comorbidity   🦴 Major C\C   Present on Admission Requirement   Hospital-Acquired Condition

1147

CHAPTER 13 (M00-M99)

● **M02.33 Reiter's disease, wrist**
Reiter's disease, carpal bones

   M02.331 Reiter's disease, right wrist 🐾
      MCC: Only when the principal diagnosis is designated as a CC

   M02.332 Reiter's disease, left wrist 🐾
      MCC: Only when the principal diagnosis is designated as a CC

   ■ **M02.339 Reiter's disease, unspecified wrist** 🐾
      MCC: Only when the principal diagnosis is designated as a CC

● **M02.34 Reiter's disease, hand**
Reiter's disease, metacarpus and phalanges

   M02.341 Reiter's disease, right hand 🐾
      MCC: Only when the principal diagnosis is designated as a CC

   M02.342 Reiter's disease, left hand 🐾
      MCC: Only when the principal diagnosis is designated as a CC

   ■ **M02.349 Reiter's disease, unspecified hand** 🐾
      MCC: Only when the principal diagnosis is designated as a CC

● **M02.35 Reiter's disease, hip**

   M02.351 Reiter's disease, right hip 🐾
      MCC: Only when the principal diagnosis is designated as a CC

   M02.352 Reiter's disease, left hip 🐾
      MCC: Only when the principal diagnosis is designated as a CC

   ■ **M02.359 Reiter's disease, unspecified hip** 🐾
      MCC: Only when the principal diagnosis is designated as a CC

● **M02.36 Reiter's disease, knee**

   M02.361 Reiter's disease, right knee 🐾
      MCC: Only when the principal diagnosis is designated as a CC

   M02.362 Reiter's disease, left knee 🐾
      MCC: Only when the principal diagnosis is designated as a CC

   ■ **M02.369 Reiter's disease, unspecified knee** 🐾
      MCC: Only when the principal diagnosis is designated as a CC

● **M02.37 Reiter's disease, ankle and foot**
Reiter's disease, tarsus, metatarsus and phalanges

   M02.371 Reiter's disease, right ankle and foot 🐾
      MCC: Only when the principal diagnosis is designated as a CC

   M02.372 Reiter's disease, left ankle and foot 🐾
      MCC: Only when the principal diagnosis is designated as a CC

   ■ **M02.379 Reiter's disease, unspecified ankle and foot** 🐾
      MCC: Only when the principal diagnosis is designated as a CC

● **M02.38 Reiter's disease, vertebrae** 🐾
      MCC: Only when the principal diagnosis is designated as a CC

● **M02.39 Reiter's disease, multiple sites** 🐾
      MCC: Only when the principal diagnosis is designated as a CC

● **M02.8 Other reactive arthropathies**

  ■ **M02.80 Other reactive arthropathies, unspecified site** 🐾

● **M02.81 Other reactive arthropathies, shoulder**

   M02.811 Other reactive arthropathies, right shoulder 🐾

   M02.812 Other reactive arthropathies, left shoulder 🐾

   ■ **M02.819 Other reactive arthropathies, unspecified shoulder** 🐾

● **M02.82 Other reactive arthropathies, elbow**

   M02.821 Other reactive arthropathies, right elbow 🐾

   M02.822 Other reactive arthropathies, left elbow 🐾

   ■ **M02.829 Other reactive arthropathies, unspecified elbow** 🐾

● **M02.83 Other reactive arthropathies, wrist**
Other reactive arthropathies, carpal bones

   M02.831 Other reactive arthropathies, right wrist 🐾

   M02.832 Other reactive arthropathies, left wrist 🐾

   ■ **M02.839 Other reactive arthropathies, unspecified wrist** 🐾

● **M02.84 Other reactive arthropathies, hand**
Other reactive arthropathies, metacarpus and phalanges

   M02.841 Other reactive arthropathies, right hand 🐾

   M02.842 Other reactive arthropathies, left hand 🐾

   ■ **M02.849 Other reactive arthropathies, unspecified hand** 🐾

● **M02.85 Other reactive arthropathies, hip**

   M02.851 Other reactive arthropathies, right hip 🐾

   M02.852 Other reactive arthropathies, left hip 🐾

   ■ **M02.859 Other reactive arthropathies, unspecified hip** 🐾

● **M02.86 Other reactive arthropathies, knee**

   M02.861 Other reactive arthropathies, right knee 🐾

   M02.862 Other reactive arthropathies, left knee 🐾

   ■ **M02.869 Other reactive arthropathies, unspecified knee** 🐾

● Unacceptable Principal Diagnosis   ● Use Additional Character(s)   ■ Unspecified   ▶ Manifestation Code
OGCR Official Guidelines for Coding and Reporting   Excludes 1   Excludes 2   Includes   Use additional   Code first   Code also

● **M02.87 Other reactive arthropathies, ankle and foot**
     Other reactive arthropathies, tarsus, metatarsus and phalanges

     M02.871 Other reactive arthropathies, right ankle and foot 🅒

     M02.872 Other reactive arthropathies, left ankle and foot 🅒

     ■ **M02.879 Other reactive arthropathies, unspecified ankle and foot** 🅒

◗ *M02.88 Other reactive arthropathies, vertebrae* 🅒

◗ *M02.89 Other reactive arthropathies, multiple sites* 🅒

■◗ *M02.9 Reactive arthropathy, unspecified*

INFLAMMATORY POLYARTHROPATHIES (M05-M14)

● **M05 Rheumatoid arthritis with rheumatoid factor**

     | Excludes1 | rheumatic fever (I00)
                  juvenile rheumatoid arthritis (M08.-)
                  rheumatoid arthritis of spine (M45.-)

● **M05.0 Felty's syndrome**
     Rheumatoid arthritis with splenoadenomegaly and leukopenia

     ■ **M05.00 Felty's syndrome, unspecified site**

     ● **M05.01 Felty's syndrome, shoulder**

         M05.011 Felty's syndrome, right shoulder

         M05.012 Felty's syndrome, left shoulder

         ■ **M05.019 Felty's syndrome, unspecified shoulder**

     ● **M05.02 Felty's syndrome, elbow**

         M05.021 Felty's syndrome, right elbow

         M05.022 Felty's syndrome, left elbow

         ■ **M05.029 Felty's syndrome, unspecified elbow**

     ● **M05.03 Felty's syndrome, wrist**
         Felty's syndrome, carpal bones

         M05.031 Felty's syndrome, right wrist

         M05.032 Felty's syndrome, left wrist

         ■ **M05.039 Felty's syndrome, unspecified wrist**

     ● **M05.04 Felty's syndrome, hand**
         Felty's syndrome, metacarpus and phalanges

         M05.041 Felty's syndrome, right hand

         M05.042 Felty's syndrome, left hand

         ■ **M05.049 Felty's syndrome, unspecified hand**

     ● **M05.05 Felty's syndrome, hip**

         M05.051 Felty's syndrome, right hip

         M05.052 Felty's syndrome, left hip

         ■ **M05.059 Felty's syndrome, unspecified hip**

● **M05.06 Felty's syndrome, knee**

     M05.061 Felty's syndrome, right knee

     M05.062 Felty's syndrome, left knee

     ■ **M05.069 Felty's syndrome, unspecified knee**

● **M05.07 Felty's syndrome, ankle and foot**
     Felty's syndrome, tarsus, metatarsus and phalanges

     M05.071 Felty's syndrome, right ankle and foot

     M05.072 Felty's syndrome, left ankle and foot

     ■ **M05.079 Felty's syndrome, unspecified ankle and foot**

     M05.09 Felty's syndrome, multiple sites

● **M05.1 Rheumatoid lung disease with rheumatoid arthritis**

     ■ **M05.10 Rheumatoid lung disease with rheumatoid arthritis of unspecified site**

     ● **M05.11 Rheumatoid lung disease with rheumatoid arthritis of shoulder**

         M05.111 Rheumatoid lung disease with rheumatoid arthritis of right shoulder

         M05.112 Rheumatoid lung disease with rheumatoid arthritis of left shoulder

         ■ **M05.119 Rheumatoid lung disease with rheumatoid arthritis of unspecified shoulder**

     ● **M05.12 Rheumatoid lung disease with rheumatoid arthritis of elbow**

         M05.121 Rheumatoid lung disease with rheumatoid arthritis of right elbow

         M05.122 Rheumatoid lung disease with rheumatoid arthritis of left elbow

         ■ **M05.129 Rheumatoid lung disease with rheumatoid arthritis of unspecified elbow**

     ● **M05.13 Rheumatoid lung disease with rheumatoid arthritis of wrist**
         Rheumatoid lung disease with rheumatoid arthritis, carpal bones

         M05.131 Rheumatoid lung disease with rheumatoid arthritis of right wrist

         M05.132 Rheumatoid lung disease with rheumatoid arthritis of left wrist

         ■ **M05.139 Rheumatoid lung disease with rheumatoid arthritis of unspecified wrist**

     ● **M05.14 Rheumatoid lung disease with rheumatoid arthritis of hand**
         Rheumatoid lung disease with rheumatoid arthritis, metacarpus and phalanges

         M05.141 Rheumatoid lung disease with rheumatoid arthritis of right hand

         M05.142 Rheumatoid lung disease with rheumatoid arthritis of left hand

         ■ **M05.149 Rheumatoid lung disease with rheumatoid arthritis of unspecified hand**

Item 13-1 Rheumatoid arthritis (RA) is a chronic systemic inflammatory disease of undetermined etiology involving primarily the synovial membranes and articular structures of multiple joints. The disease is often progressive and results in pain, stiffness, and swelling of joints. In late stages, deformity, ankylosis, and other **inflammatory polyarthropathies** develop.

N Newborn Age: 0   **P** Pediatric Age: 0–17   **M** Maternity DX: 12–55   **A** Adult Age: 15–124   ♀ Females Only   ♂ Males Only

🅒 Complication\Comorbidity   🅜 Major C\C   ■ Present on Admission Requirement   🅗 Hospital-Acquired Condition

1149

CHAPTER 13 (M00-M99)

CHAPTER 13 (M00-M99)

● **M05.15 Rheumatoid lung disease with rheumatoid arthritis of hip**

   M05.151 Rheumatoid lung disease with rheumatoid arthritis of right hip

   M05.152 Rheumatoid lung disease with rheumatoid arthritis of left hip

   ■ M05.159 Rheumatoid lung disease with rheumatoid arthritis of unspecified hip

● **M05.16 Rheumatoid lung disease with rheumatoid arthritis of knee**

   M05.161 Rheumatoid lung disease with rheumatoid arthritis of right knee

   M05.162 Rheumatoid lung disease with rheumatoid arthritis of left knee

   ■ M05.169 Rheumatoid lung disease with rheumatoid arthritis of unspecified knee

● **M05.17 Rheumatoid lung disease with rheumatoid arthritis of ankle and foot**

   Rheumatoid lung disease with rheumatoid arthritis, tarsus, metatarsus and phalanges

   M05.171 Rheumatoid lung disease with rheumatoid arthritis of right ankle and foot

   M05.172 Rheumatoid lung disease with rheumatoid arthritis of left ankle and foot

   ■ M05.179 Rheumatoid lung disease with rheumatoid arthritis of unspecified ankle and foot

   M05.19 Rheumatoid lung disease with rheumatoid arthritis of multiple sites

● **M05.2 Rheumatoid vasculitis with rheumatoid arthritis**

   ■ M05.20 Rheumatoid vasculitis with rheumatoid arthritis of unspecified site

● M05.21 Rheumatoid vasculitis with rheumatoid arthritis of shoulder

   M05.211 Rheumatoid vasculitis with rheumatoid arthritis of right shoulder

   M05.212 Rheumatoid vasculitis with rheumatoid arthritis of left shoulder

   ■ M05.219 Rheumatoid vasculitis with rheumatoid arthritis of unspecified shoulder

● M05.22 Rheumatoid vasculitis with rheumatoid arthritis of elbow

   M05.221 Rheumatoid vasculitis with rheumatoid arthritis of right elbow

   M05.222 Rheumatoid vasculitis with rheumatoid arthritis of left elbow

   ■ M05.229 Rheumatoid vasculitis with rheumatoid arthritis of unspecified elbow

● **M05.23 Rheumatoid vasculitis with rheumatoid arthritis of wrist**

   Rheumatoid vasculitis with rheumatoid arthritis, carpal bones

   M05.231 Rheumatoid vasculitis with rheumatoid arthritis of right wrist

   M05.232 Rheumatoid vasculitis with rheumatoid arthritis of left wrist

   ■ M05.239 Rheumatoid vasculitis with rheumatoid arthritis of unspecified wrist

● **M05.24 Rheumatoid vasculitis with rheumatoid arthritis of hand**

   Rheumatoid vasculitis with rheumatoid arthritis, metacarpus and phalanges

   M05.241 Rheumatoid vasculitis with rheumatoid arthritis of right hand

   M05.242 Rheumatoid vasculitis with rheumatoid arthritis of left hand

   ■ M05.249 Rheumatoid vasculitis with rheumatoid arthritis of unspecified hand

● M05.25 Rheumatoid vasculitis with rheumatoid arthritis of hip

   M05.251 Rheumatoid vasculitis with rheumatoid arthritis of right hip

   M05.252 Rheumatoid vasculitis with rheumatoid arthritis of left hip

   ■ M05.259 Rheumatoid vasculitis with rheumatoid arthritis of unspecified hip

● M05.26 Rheumatoid vasculitis with rheumatoid arthritis of knee

   M05.261 Rheumatoid vasculitis with rheumatoid arthritis of right knee

   M05.262 Rheumatoid vasculitis with rheumatoid arthritis of left knee

   ■ M05.269 Rheumatoid vasculitis with rheumatoid arthritis of unspecified knee

● M05.27 Rheumatoid vasculitis with rheumatoid arthritis of ankle and foot

   Rheumatoid vasculitis with rheumatoid arthritis, tarsus, metatarsus and phalanges

   M05.271 Rheumatoid vasculitis with rheumatoid arthritis of right ankle and foot

   M05.272 Rheumatoid vasculitis with rheumatoid arthritis of left ankle and foot

   ■ M05.279 Rheumatoid vasculitis with rheumatoid arthritis of unspecified ankle and foot

   M05.29 Rheumatoid vasculitis with rheumatoid arthritis of multiple sites

● Unacceptable Principal Diagnosis   ● Use Additional Character(s)   ■ Unspecified   ▶ Manifestation Code

OGCR Official Guidelines for Coding and Reporting   Excludes 1   Excludes 2   Includes   Use additional   Code first   Code also

● **M05.3** **Rheumatoid heart disease with rheumatoid arthritis**
  Rheumatoid carditis
  Rheumatoid endocarditis
  Rheumatoid myocarditis
  Rheumatoid pericarditis

■ **M05.30** Rheumatoid heart disease with rheumatoid arthritis of unspecified site

● **M05.31** Rheumatoid heart disease with rheumatoid arthritis of shoulder

     M05.311 Rheumatoid heart disease with rheumatoid arthritis of right shoulder

     M05.312 Rheumatoid heart disease with rheumatoid arthritis of left shoulder

     ■ **M05.319** Rheumatoid heart disease with rheumatoid arthritis of unspecified shoulder

● **M05.32** Rheumatoid heart disease with rheumatoid arthritis of elbow

     M05.321 Rheumatoid heart disease with rheumatoid arthritis of right elbow

     M05.322 Rheumatoid heart disease with rheumatoid arthritis of left elbow

     ■ **M05.329** Rheumatoid heart disease with rheumatoid arthritis of unspecified elbow

● **M05.33** Rheumatoid heart disease with rheumatoid arthritis of wrist
  Rheumatoid heart disease with rheumatoid arthritis, carpal bones

     M05.331 Rheumatoid heart disease with rheumatoid arthritis of right wrist

     M05.332 Rheumatoid heart disease with rheumatoid arthritis of left wrist

     ■ **M05.339** Rheumatoid heart disease with rheumatoid arthritis of unspecified wrist

● **M05.34** Rheumatoid heart disease with rheumatoid arthritis of hand
  Rheumatoid heart disease with rheumatoid arthritis, metacarpus and phalanges

     M05.341 Rheumatoid heart disease with rheumatoid arthritis of right hand

     M05.342 Rheumatoid heart disease with rheumatoid arthritis of left hand

     ■ **M05.349** Rheumatoid heart disease with rheumatoid arthritis of unspecified hand

● **M05.35** Rheumatoid heart disease with rheumatoid arthritis of hip

     M05.351 Rheumatoid heart disease with rheumatoid arthritis of right hip

     M05.352 Rheumatoid heart disease with rheumatoid arthritis of left hip

     ■ **M05.359** Rheumatoid heart disease with rheumatoid arthritis of unspecified hip

● **M05.36** Rheumatoid heart disease with rheumatoid arthritis of knee

     M05.361 Rheumatoid heart disease with rheumatoid arthritis of right knee

     M05.362 Rheumatoid heart disease with rheumatoid arthritis of left knee

     ■ **M05.369** Rheumatoid heart disease with rheumatoid arthritis of unspecified knee

● **M05.37** Rheumatoid heart disease with rheumatoid arthritis of ankle and foot
  Rheumatoid heart disease with rheumatoid arthritis, tarsus, metatarsus and phalanges

     M05.371 Rheumatoid heart disease with rheumatoid arthritis of right ankle and foot

     M05.372 Rheumatoid heart disease with rheumatoid arthritis of left ankle and foot

     ■ **M05.379** Rheumatoid heart disease with rheumatoid arthritis of unspecified ankle and foot

M05.39 Rheumatoid heart disease with rheumatoid arthritis of multiple sites

● **M05.4** **Rheumatoid myopathy with rheumatoid arthritis**

■ **M05.40** Rheumatoid myopathy with rheumatoid arthritis of unspecified site 🔖
  MCC: Only when the principal diagnosis is designated as a CC

● **M05.41** Rheumatoid myopathy with rheumatoid arthritis of shoulder

     M05.411 Rheumatoid myopathy with rheumatoid arthritis of right shoulder 🔖
       MCC: Only when the principal diagnosis is designated as a CC

     M05.412 Rheumatoid myopathy with rheumatoid arthritis of left shoulder 🔖
       MCC: Only when the principal diagnosis is designated as a CC

     ■ **M05.419** Rheumatoid myopathy with rheumatoid arthritis of unspecified shoulder 🔖
       MCC: Only when the principal diagnosis is designated as a CC

● **M05.42** Rheumatoid myopathy with rheumatoid arthritis of elbow

     M05.421 Rheumatoid myopathy with rheumatoid arthritis of right elbow 🔖
       MCC: Only when the principal diagnosis is designated as a CC

     M05.422 Rheumatoid myopathy with rheumatoid arthritis of left elbow 🔖
       MCC: Only when the principal diagnosis is designated as a CC

     ■ **M05.429** Rheumatoid myopathy with rheumatoid arthritis of unspecified elbow 🔖
       MCC: Only when the principal diagnosis is designated as a CC

CHAPTER 13 (M00-M99)

N Newborn Age: 0   **P** Pediatric Age: 0–17   **M** Maternity DX: 12–55   **A** Adult Age: 15–124   ♀ Females Only   ♂ Males Only

 Complication\Comorbidity   Major C\C   Present on Admission Requirement   Hospital-Acquired Condition

1151

CHAPTER 13 (M00-M99)

● **M05.43 Rheumatoid myopathy with rheumatoid arthritis of wrist**
Rheumatoid myopathy with rheumatoid arthritis, carpal bones

 M05.431 Rheumatoid myopathy with rheumatoid arthritis of right wrist 🔖
   MCC: Only when the principal diagnosis is designated as a CC

 M05.432 Rheumatoid myopathy with rheumatoid arthritis of left wrist 🔖
   MCC: Only when the principal diagnosis is designated as a CC

 ■ **M05.439 Rheumatoid myopathy with rheumatoid arthritis of unspecified wrist** 🔖
   MCC: Only when the principal diagnosis is designated as a CC

● **M05.44 Rheumatoid myopathy with rheumatoid arthritis of hand**
Rheumatoid myopathy with rheumatoid arthritis, metacarpus and phalanges

 M05.441 Rheumatoid myopathy with rheumatoid arthritis of right hand 🔖
   MCC: Only when the principal diagnosis is designated as a CC

 M05.442 Rheumatoid myopathy with rheumatoid arthritis of left hand 🔖
   MCC: Only when the principal diagnosis is designated as a CC

 ■ **M05.449 Rheumatoid myopathy with rheumatoid arthritis of unspecified hand** 🔖
   MCC: Only when the principal diagnosis is designated as a CC

● **M05.45 Rheumatoid myopathy with rheumatoid arthritis of hip**

 M05.451 Rheumatoid myopathy with rheumatoid arthritis of right hip 🔖
   MCC: Only when the principal diagnosis is designated as a CC

 M05.452 Rheumatoid myopathy with rheumatoid arthritis of left hip 🔖
   MCC: Only when the principal diagnosis is designated as a CC

 ■ **M05.459 Rheumatoid myopathy with rheumatoid arthritis of unspecified hip** 🔖
   MCC: Only when the principal diagnosis is designated as a CC

● **M05.46 Rheumatoid myopathy with rheumatoid arthritis of knee**

 M05.461 Rheumatoid myopathy with rheumatoid arthritis of right knee 🔖
   MCC: Only when the principal diagnosis is designated as a CC

 M05.462 Rheumatoid myopathy with rheumatoid arthritis of left knee 🔖
   MCC: Only when the principal diagnosis is designated as a CC

 ■ **M05.469 Rheumatoid myopathy with rheumatoid arthritis of unspecified knee** 🔖
   MCC: Only when the principal diagnosis is designated as a CC

● **M05.47 Rheumatoid myopathy with rheumatoid arthritis of ankle and foot**
Rheumatoid myopathy with rheumatoid arthritis, tarsus, metatarsus and phalanges

 M05.471 Rheumatoid myopathy with rheumatoid arthritis of right ankle and foot 🔖
   MCC: Only when the principal diagnosis is designated as a CC

 M05.472 Rheumatoid myopathy with rheumatoid arthritis of left ankle and foot 🔖
   MCC: Only when the principal diagnosis is designated as a CC

 ■ **M05.479 Rheumatoid myopathy with rheumatoid arthritis of unspecified ankle and foot** 🔖
   MCC: Only when the principal diagnosis is designated as a CC

 M05.49 Rheumatoid myopathy with rheumatoid arthritis of multiple sites 🔖
   MCC: Only when the principal diagnosis is designated as a CC

● **M05.5 Rheumatoid polyneuropathy with rheumatoid arthritis**

 ■ **M05.50 Rheumatoid polyneuropathy with rheumatoid arthritis of unspecified site**

 ● **M05.51 Rheumatoid polyneuropathy with rheumatoid arthritis of shoulder**

  M05.511 Rheumatoid polyneuropathy with rheumatoid arthritis of right shoulder

  M05.512 Rheumatoid polyneuropathy with rheumatoid arthritis of left shoulder

  ■ **M05.519 Rheumatoid polyneuropathy with rheumatoid arthritis of unspecified shoulder**

● Unacceptable Principal Diagnosis ● Use Additional Character(s) ■ Unspecified ▶ Manifestation Code
OGCR Official Guidelines for Coding and Reporting Excludes 1 Excludes 2 Includes Use additional Code first Code also

● **M05.52 Rheumatoid polyneuropathy with rheumatoid arthritis of elbow**

　M05.521 Rheumatoid polyneuropathy with rheumatoid arthritis of right elbow

　M05.522 Rheumatoid polyneuropathy with rheumatoid arthritis of left elbow

　■ **M05.529 Rheumatoid polyneuropathy with rheumatoid arthritis of unspecified elbow**

● **M05.53 Rheumatoid polyneuropathy with rheumatoid arthritis of wrist**
　　Rheumatoid polyneuropathy with rheumatoid arthritis, carpal bones

　M05.531 Rheumatoid polyneuropathy with rheumatoid arthritis of right wrist

　M05.532 Rheumatoid polyneuropathy with rheumatoid arthritis of left wrist

　■ **M05.539 Rheumatoid polyneuropathy with rheumatoid arthritis of unspecified wrist**

● **M05.54 Rheumatoid polyneuropathy with rheumatoid arthritis of hand**
　　Rheumatoid polyneuropathy with rheumatoid arthritis, metacarpus and phalanges

　M05.541 Rheumatoid polyneuropathy with rheumatoid arthritis of right hand

　M05.542 Rheumatoid polyneuropathy with rheumatoid arthritis of left hand

　■ **M05.549 Rheumatoid polyneuropathy with rheumatoid arthritis of unspecified hand**

● **M05.55 Rheumatoid polyneuropathy with rheumatoid arthritis of hip**

　M05.551 Rheumatoid polyneuropathy with rheumatoid arthritis of right hip

　M05.552 Rheumatoid polyneuropathy with rheumatoid arthritis of left hip

　■ **M05.559 Rheumatoid polyneuropathy with rheumatoid arthritis of unspecified hip**

● **M05.56 Rheumatoid polyneuropathy with rheumatoid arthritis of knee**

　M05.561 Rheumatoid polyneuropathy with rheumatoid arthritis of right knee

　M05.562 Rheumatoid polyneuropathy with rheumatoid arthritis of left knee

　■ **M05.569 Rheumatoid polyneuropathy with rheumatoid arthritis of unspecified knee**

● **M05.57 Rheumatoid polyneuropathy with rheumatoid arthritis of ankle and foot**
　　Rheumatoid polyneuropathy with rheumatoid arthritis, tarsus, metatarsus and phalanges

　M05.571 Rheumatoid polyneuropathy with rheumatoid arthritis of right ankle and foot

　M05.572 Rheumatoid polyneuropathy with rheumatoid arthritis of left ankle and foot

　■ **M05.579 Rheumatoid polyneuropathy with rheumatoid arthritis of unspecified ankle and foot**

　M05.59 Rheumatoid polyneuropathy with rheumatoid arthritis of multiple sites

● **M05.6 Rheumatoid arthritis with involvement of other organs and systems**

　■ **M05.60 Rheumatoid arthritis of unspecified site with involvement of other organs and systems**

　● **M05.61 Rheumatoid arthritis of shoulder with involvement of other organs and systems**

　　M05.611 Rheumatoid arthritis of right shoulder with involvement of other organs and systems

　　M05.612 Rheumatoid arthritis of left shoulder with involvement of other organs and systems

　　■ **M05.619 Rheumatoid arthritis of unspecified shoulder with involvement of other organs and systems**

　● **M05.62 Rheumatoid arthritis of elbow with involvement of other organs and systems**

　　M05.621 Rheumatoid arthritis of right elbow with involvement of other organs and systems

　　M05.622 Rheumatoid arthritis of left elbow with involvement of other organs and systems

　　■ **M05.629 Rheumatoid arthritis of unspecified elbow with involvement of other organs and systems**

　● **M05.63 Rheumatoid arthritis of wrist with involvement of other organs and systems**
　　　Rheumatoid arthritis of carpal bones with involvement of other organs and systems

　　M05.631 Rheumatoid arthritis of right wrist with involvement of other organs and systems

　　M05.632 Rheumatoid arthritis of left wrist with involvement of other organs and systems

　　■ **M05.639 Rheumatoid arthritis of unspecified wrist with involvement of other organs and systems**

● **M05.64 Rheumatoid arthritis of hand with involvement of other organs and systems**
   Rheumatoid arthritis of metacarpus and phalanges with involvement of other organs and systems

   M05.641 Rheumatoid arthritis of right hand with involvement of other organs and systems

   M05.642 Rheumatoid arthritis of left hand with involvement of other organs and systems

   ◾ **M05.649 Rheumatoid arthritis of unspecified hand with involvement of other organs and systems**

● **M05.65 Rheumatoid arthritis of hip with involvement of other organs and systems**

   M05.651 Rheumatoid arthritis of right hip with involvement of other organs and systems

   M05.652 Rheumatoid arthritis of left hip with involvement of other organs and systems

   ◾ **M05.659 Rheumatoid arthritis of unspecified hip with involvement of other organs and systems**

● **M05.66 Rheumatoid arthritis of knee with involvement of other organs and systems**

   M05.661 Rheumatoid arthritis of right knee with involvement of other organs and systems

   M05.662 Rheumatoid arthritis of left knee with involvement of other organs and systems

   ◾ **M05.669 Rheumatoid arthritis of unspecified knee with involvement of other organs and systems**

● **M05.67 Rheumatoid arthritis of ankle and foot with involvement of other organs and systems**
   Rheumatoid arthritis of tarsus, metatarsus and phalanges with involvement of other organs and systems

   M05.671 Rheumatoid arthritis of right ankle and foot with involvement of other organs and systems

   M05.672 Rheumatoid arthritis of left ankle and foot with involvement of other organs and systems

   ◾ **M05.679 Rheumatoid arthritis of unspecified ankle and foot with involvement of other organs and systems**

M05.69 Rheumatoid arthritis of multiple sites with involvement of other organs and systems

● **M05.7 Rheumatoid arthritis with rheumatoid factor without organ or systems involvement**

   ◾ **M05.70 Rheumatoid arthritis with rheumatoid factor of unspecified site without organ or systems involvement**

● **M05.71 Rheumatoid arthritis with rheumatoid factor of shoulder without organ or systems involvement**

   M05.711 Rheumatoid arthritis with rheumatoid factor of right shoulder without organ or systems involvement

   M05.712 Rheumatoid arthritis with rheumatoid factor of left shoulder without organ or systems involvement

   ◾ **M05.719 Rheumatoid arthritis with rheumatoid factor of unspecified shoulder without organ or systems involvement**

● **M05.72 Rheumatoid arthritis with rheumatoid factor of elbow without organ or systems involvement**

   M05.721 Rheumatoid arthritis with rheumatoid factor of right elbow without organ or systems involvement

   M05.722 Rheumatoid arthritis with rheumatoid factor of left elbow without organ or systems involvement

   ◾ **M05.729 Rheumatoid arthritis with rheumatoid factor of unspecified elbow without organ or systems involvement**

● **M05.73 Rheumatoid arthritis with rheumatoid factor of wrist without organ or systems involvement**

   M05.731 Rheumatoid arthritis with rheumatoid factor of right wrist without organ or systems involvement

   M05.732 Rheumatoid arthritis with rheumatoid factor of left wrist without organ or systems involvement

   ◾ **M05.739 Rheumatoid arthritis with rheumatoid factor of unspecified wrist without organ or systems involvement**

● **M05.74 Rheumatoid arthritis with rheumatoid factor of hand without organ or systems involvement**

   M05.741 Rheumatoid arthritis with rheumatoid factor of right hand without organ or systems involvement

   M05.742 Rheumatoid arthritis with rheumatoid factor of left hand without organ or systems involvement

   ◾ **M05.749 Rheumatoid arthritis with rheumatoid factor of unspecified hand without organ or systems involvement**

● **M05.75 Rheumatoid arthritis with rheumatoid factor of hip without organ or systems involvement**

   M05.751 Rheumatoid arthritis with rheumatoid factor of right hip without organ or systems involvement

● Unacceptable Principal Diagnosis   ● Use Additional Character(s)   ◾ Unspecified   ▶ Manifestation Code

OGCR Official Guidelines for Coding and Reporting | Excludes 1 | | Excludes 2 | | Includes | | Use additional | | Code first | | Code also |

     M05.752 Rheumatoid arthritis with rheumatoid factor of left hip without organ or systems involvement

     ■ M05.759 Rheumatoid arthritis with rheumatoid factor of unspecified hip without organ or systems involvement

● M05.76 Rheumatoid arthritis with rheumatoid factor of knee without organ or systems involvement

     M05.761 Rheumatoid arthritis with rheumatoid factor of right knee without organ or systems involvement

     M05.762 Rheumatoid arthritis with rheumatoid factor of left knee without organ or systems involvement

     ■ M05.769 Rheumatoid arthritis with rheumatoid factor of unspecified knee without organ or systems involvement

● M05.77 Rheumatoid arthritis with rheumatoid factor of ankle and foot without organ or systems involvement

     M05.771 Rheumatoid arthritis with rheumatoid factor of right ankle and foot without organ or systems involvement

     M05.772 Rheumatoid arthritis with rheumatoid factor of left ankle and foot without organ or systems involvement

     ■ M05.779 Rheumatoid arthritis with rheumatoid factor of unspecified ankle and foot without organ or systems involvement

M05.79 Rheumatoid arthritis with rheumatoid factor of multiple sites without organ or systems involvement

● M05.8 Other rheumatoid arthritis with rheumatoid factor

     ■ M05.80 Other rheumatoid arthritis with rheumatoid factor of unspecified site

● M05.81 Other rheumatoid arthritis with rheumatoid factor of shoulder

     M05.811 Other rheumatoid arthritis with rheumatoid factor of right shoulder

     M05.812 Other rheumatoid arthritis with rheumatoid factor of left shoulder

     ■ M05.819 Other rheumatoid arthritis with rheumatoid factor of unspecified shoulder

● M05.82 Other rheumatoid arthritis with rheumatoid factor of elbow

     M05.821 Other rheumatoid arthritis with rheumatoid factor of right elbow

     M05.822 Other rheumatoid arthritis with rheumatoid factor of left elbow

     ■ M05.829 Other rheumatoid arthritis with rheumatoid factor of unspecified elbow

● M05.83 Other rheumatoid arthritis with rheumatoid factor of wrist

     M05.831 Other rheumatoid arthritis with rheumatoid factor of right wrist

     M05.832 Other rheumatoid arthritis with rheumatoid factor of left wrist

     ■ M05.839 Other rheumatoid arthritis with rheumatoid factor of unspecified wrist

● M05.84 Other rheumatoid arthritis with rheumatoid factor of hand

     M05.841 Other rheumatoid arthritis with rheumatoid factor of right hand

     M05.842 Other rheumatoid arthritis with rheumatoid factor of left hand

     ■ M05.849 Other rheumatoid arthritis with rheumatoid factor of unspecified hand

● M05.85 Other rheumatoid arthritis with rheumatoid factor of hip

     M05.851 Other rheumatoid arthritis with rheumatoid factor of right hip

     M05.852 Other rheumatoid arthritis with rheumatoid factor of left hip

     ■ M05.859 Other rheumatoid arthritis with rheumatoid factor of unspecified hip

● M05.86 Other rheumatoid arthritis with rheumatoid factor of knee

     M05.861 Other rheumatoid arthritis with rheumatoid factor of right knee

     M05.862 Other rheumatoid arthritis with rheumatoid factor of left knee

     ■ M05.869 Other rheumatoid arthritis with rheumatoid factor of unspecified knee

● M05.87 Other rheumatoid arthritis with rheumatoid factor of ankle and foot

     M05.871 Other rheumatoid arthritis with rheumatoid factor of right ankle and foot

     M05.872 Other rheumatoid arthritis with rheumatoid factor of left ankle and foot

     ■ M05.879 Other rheumatoid arthritis with rheumatoid factor of unspecified ankle and foot

M05.89 Other rheumatoid arthritis with rheumatoid factor of multiple sites

■ M05.9 Rheumatoid arthritis with rheumatoid factor, unspecified

● M06 Other rheumatoid arthritis

     ● M06.0 Rheumatoid arthritis without rheumatoid factor

     ■ M06.00 Rheumatoid arthritis without rheumatoid factor, unspecified site

     ● M06.01 Rheumatoid arthritis without rheumatoid factor, shoulder

     M06.011 Rheumatoid arthritis without rheumatoid factor, right shoulder

     M06.012 Rheumatoid arthritis without rheumatoid factor, left shoulder

     ■ M06.019 Rheumatoid arthritis without rheumatoid factor, unspecified shoulder

CHAPTER 13 (M00-M99)

M06.02 Rheumatoid arthritis without rheumatoid factor, elbow

   M06.021 Rheumatoid arthritis without rheumatoid factor, right elbow

   M06.022 Rheumatoid arthritis without rheumatoid factor, left elbow

   M06.029 Rheumatoid arthritis without rheumatoid factor, unspecified elbow

M06.03 Rheumatoid arthritis without rheumatoid factor, wrist

   M06.031 Rheumatoid arthritis without rheumatoid factor, right wrist

   M06.032 Rheumatoid arthritis without rheumatoid factor, left wrist

   M06.039 Rheumatoid arthritis without rheumatoid factor, unspecified wrist

M06.04 Rheumatoid arthritis without rheumatoid factor, hand

   M06.041 Rheumatoid arthritis without rheumatoid factor, right hand

   M06.042 Rheumatoid arthritis without rheumatoid factor, left hand

   M06.049 Rheumatoid arthritis without rheumatoid factor, unspecified hand

M06.05 Rheumatoid arthritis without rheumatoid factor, hip

   M06.051 Rheumatoid arthritis without rheumatoid factor, right hip

   M06.052 Rheumatoid arthritis without rheumatoid factor, left hip

   M06.059 Rheumatoid arthritis without rheumatoid factor, unspecified hip

M06.06 Rheumatoid arthritis without rheumatoid factor, knee

   M06.061 Rheumatoid arthritis without rheumatoid factor, right knee

   M06.062 Rheumatoid arthritis without rheumatoid factor, left knee

   M06.069 Rheumatoid arthritis without rheumatoid factor, unspecified knee

M06.07 Rheumatoid arthritis without rheumatoid factor, ankle and foot

   M06.071 Rheumatoid arthritis without rheumatoid factor, right ankle and foot

   M06.072 Rheumatoid arthritis without rheumatoid factor, left ankle and foot

   M06.079 Rheumatoid arthritis without rheumatoid factor, unspecified ankle and foot

M06.08 Rheumatoid arthritis without rheumatoid factor, vertebrae

M06.09 Rheumatoid arthritis without rheumatoid factor, multiple sites

M06.1 Adult-onset Still's disease　　　　　A

  Excludes1 Still's disease NOS (M08.2-)

M06.2 Rheumatoid bursitis

  M06.20 Rheumatoid bursitis, unspecified site

  M06.21 Rheumatoid bursitis, shoulder

   M06.211 Rheumatoid bursitis, right shoulder

   M06.212 Rheumatoid bursitis, left shoulder

   M06.219 Rheumatoid bursitis, unspecified shoulder

  M06.22 Rheumatoid bursitis, elbow

   M06.221 Rheumatoid bursitis, right elbow

   M06.222 Rheumatoid bursitis, left elbow

   M06.229 Rheumatoid bursitis, unspecified elbow

  M06.23 Rheumatoid bursitis, wrist

   M06.231 Rheumatoid bursitis, right wrist

   M06.232 Rheumatoid bursitis, left wrist

   M06.239 Rheumatoid bursitis, unspecified wrist

  M06.24 Rheumatoid bursitis, hand

   M06.241 Rheumatoid bursitis, right hand

   M06.242 Rheumatoid bursitis, left hand

   M06.249 Rheumatoid bursitis, unspecified hand

  M06.25 Rheumatoid bursitis, hip

   M06.251 Rheumatoid bursitis, right hip

   M06.252 Rheumatoid bursitis, left hip

   M06.259 Rheumatoid bursitis, unspecified hip

  M06.26 Rheumatoid bursitis, knee

   M06.261 Rheumatoid bursitis, right knee

   M06.262 Rheumatoid bursitis, left knee

   M06.269 Rheumatoid bursitis, unspecified knee

  M06.27 Rheumatoid bursitis, ankle and foot

   M06.271 Rheumatoid bursitis, right ankle and foot

   M06.272 Rheumatoid bursitis, left ankle and foot

   M06.279 Rheumatoid bursitis, unspecified ankle and foot

  M06.28 Rheumatoid bursitis, vertebrae

  M06.29 Rheumatoid bursitis, multiple sites

M06.3 Rheumatoid nodule

  M06.30 Rheumatoid nodule, unspecified site

  M06.31 Rheumatoid nodule, shoulder

   M06.311 Rheumatoid nodule, right shoulder

   M06.312 Rheumatoid nodule, left shoulder

   M06.319 Rheumatoid nodule, unspecified shoulder

  M06.32 Rheumatoid nodule, elbow

   M06.321 Rheumatoid nodule, right elbow

   M06.322 Rheumatoid nodule, left elbow

   M06.329 Rheumatoid nodule, unspecified elbow

CHAPTER 13 (M00-M99)

● Unacceptable Principal Diagnosis　● Use Additional Character(s)　▪ Unspecified　▶ Manifestation Code
OGCR Official Guidelines for Coding and Reporting　Excludes 1　Excludes 2　Includes　Use additional　Code first　Code also

● **M06.33 Rheumatoid nodule, wrist**
   M06.331 Rheumatoid nodule, right wrist
   M06.332 Rheumatoid nodule, left wrist
   ■ **M06.339 Rheumatoid nodule, unspecified wrist**
● **M06.34 Rheumatoid nodule, hand**
   M06.341 Rheumatoid nodule, right hand
   M06.342 Rheumatoid nodule, left hand
   ■ **M06.349 Rheumatoid nodule, unspecified hand**
● **M06.35 Rheumatoid nodule, hip**
   M06.351 Rheumatoid nodule, right hip
   M06.352 Rheumatoid nodule, left hip
   ■ **M06.359 Rheumatoid nodule, unspecified hip**
● **M06.36 Rheumatoid nodule, knee**
   M06.361 Rheumatoid nodule, right knee
   M06.362 Rheumatoid nodule, left knee
   ■ **M06.369 Rheumatoid nodule, unspecified knee**
● **M06.37 Rheumatoid nodule, ankle and foot**
   M06.371 Rheumatoid nodule, right ankle and foot
   M06.372 Rheumatoid nodule, left ankle and foot
   ■ **M06.379 Rheumatoid nodule, unspecified ankle and foot**
M06.38 Rheumatoid nodule, vertebrae
M06.39 Rheumatoid nodule, multiple sites
M06.4 Inflammatory polyarthropathy
   Excludes1 polyarthritis NOS (M13.0)
● **M06.8 Other specified rheumatoid arthritis**
   ■ **M06.80 Other specified rheumatoid arthritis, unspecified site**
   ● **M06.81 Other specified rheumatoid arthritis, shoulder**
     M06.811 Other specified rheumatoid arthritis, right shoulder
     M06.812 Other specified rheumatoid arthritis, left shoulder
     ■ **M06.819 Other specified rheumatoid arthritis, unspecified shoulder**
   ● **M06.82 Other specified rheumatoid arthritis, elbow**
     M06.821 Other specified rheumatoid arthritis, right elbow
     M06.822 Other specified rheumatoid arthritis, left elbow
     ■ **M06.829 Other specified rheumatoid arthritis, unspecified elbow**
   ● **M06.83 Other specified rheumatoid arthritis, wrist**
     M06.831 Other specified rheumatoid arthritis, right wrist
     M06.832 Other specified rheumatoid arthritis, left wrist
     ■ **M06.839 Other specified rheumatoid arthritis, unspecified wrist**
   ● **M06.84 Other specified rheumatoid arthritis, hand**
     M06.841 Other specified rheumatoid arthritis, right hand

     M06.842 Other specified rheumatoid arthritis, left hand
     ■ **M06.849 Other specified rheumatoid arthritis, unspecified hand**
   ● **M06.85 Other specified rheumatoid arthritis, hip**
     M06.851 Other specified rheumatoid arthritis, right hip
     M06.852 Other specified rheumatoid arthritis, left hip
     ■ **M06.859 Other specified rheumatoid arthritis, unspecified hip**
   ● **M06.86 Other specified rheumatoid arthritis, knee**
     M06.861 Other specified rheumatoid arthritis, right knee
     M06.862 Other specified rheumatoid arthritis, left knee
     ■ **M06.869 Other specified rheumatoid arthritis, unspecified knee**
   ● **M06.87 Other specified rheumatoid arthritis, ankle and foot**
     M06.871 Other specified rheumatoid arthritis, right ankle and foot
     M06.872 Other specified rheumatoid arthritis, left ankle and foot
     ■ **M06.879 Other specified rheumatoid arthritis, unspecified ankle and foot**
   M06.88 Other specified rheumatoid arthritis, vertebrae
   M06.89 Other specified rheumatoid arthritis, multiple sites
■ **M06.9 Rheumatoid arthritis, unspecified**

● **M07 Enteropathic arthropathies**
   Code also associated enteropathy, such as:
   regional enteritis [Crohn's disease] (K50.-)
   ulcerative colitis (K51.-)
   Excludes1 psoriatic arthropathies (L40.5-)
   ● **M07.6 Enteropathic arthropathies**
     ■ **M07.60 Enteropathic arthropathies, unspecified site**
     ● **M07.61 Enteropathic arthropathies, shoulder**
       M07.611 Enteropathic arthropathies, right shoulder
       M07.612 Enteropathic arthropathies, left shoulder
       ■ **M07.619 Enteropathic arthropathies, unspecified shoulder**
     ● **M07.62 Enteropathic arthropathies, elbow**
       M07.621 Enteropathic arthropathies, right elbow
       M07.622 Enteropathic arthropathies, left elbow
       ■ **M07.629 Enteropathic arthropathies, unspecified elbow**
     ● **M07.63 Enteropathic arthropathies, wrist**
       M07.631 Enteropathic arthropathies, right wrist
       M07.632 Enteropathic arthropathies, left wrist
       ■ **M07.639 Enteropathic arthropathies, unspecified wrist**

N Newborn Age: 0   **P** Pediatric Age: 0–17   **M** Maternity DX: 12–55   **A** Adult Age: 15–124   ♀ Females Only   ♂ Males Only
Complication\Comorbidity   Major C\C   Present on Admission Requirement   Hospital-Acquired Condition
1157

CHAPTER 13 (M00-M99)

● M07.64 Enteropathic arthropathies, hand

    M07.641 Enteropathic arthropathies, right hand

    M07.642 Enteropathic arthropathies, left hand

    ■ M07.649 Enteropathic arthropathies, unspecified hand

● M07.65 Enteropathic arthropathies, hip

    M07.651 Enteropathic arthropathies, right hip

    M07.652 Enteropathic arthropathies, left hip

    ■ M07.659 Enteropathic arthropathies, unspecified hip

● M07.66 Enteropathic arthropathies, knee

    M07.661 Enteropathic arthropathies, right knee

    M07.662 Enteropathic arthropathies, left knee

    ■ M07.669 Enteropathic arthropathies, unspecified knee

● M07.67 Enteropathic arthropathies, ankle and foot

    M07.671 Enteropathic arthropathies, right ankle and foot

    M07.672 Enteropathic arthropathies, left ankle and foot

    ■ M07.679 Enteropathic arthropathies, unspecified ankle and foot

M07.68 Enteropathic arthropathies, vertebrae

M07.69 Enteropathic arthropathies, multiple sites

● **M08 Juvenile arthritis**

   Code also any associated underlying condition, such as:
   regional enteritis [Crohn's disease] (K50.-)
   ulcerative colitis (K51.-)

   Excludes1 arthropathy in Whipple's disease (M14.8)
                Felty's syndrome (M05.0)
                juvenile dermatomyositis (M33.0-)
                psoriatic juvenile arthropathy (L40.54)

● M08.0 Unspecified juvenile rheumatoid arthritis
    Juvenile rheumatoid arthritis with or without rheumatoid factor

    ■ M08.00 Unspecified juvenile rheumatoid arthritis of unspecified site

    ● M08.01 Unspecified juvenile rheumatoid arthritis, shoulder

       ■ M08.011 Unspecified juvenile rheumatoid arthritis, right shoulder

       ■ M08.012 Unspecified juvenile rheumatoid arthritis, left shoulder

       ■ M08.019 Unspecified juvenile rheumatoid arthritis, unspecified shoulder

    ● M08.02 Unspecified juvenile rheumatoid arthritis of elbow

       ■ M08.021 Unspecified juvenile rheumatoid arthritis, right elbow

       ■ M08.022 Unspecified juvenile rheumatoid arthritis, left elbow

       ■ M08.029 Unspecified juvenile rheumatoid arthritis, unspecified elbow

● M08.03 Unspecified juvenile rheumatoid arthritis, wrist

   ■ M08.031 Unspecified juvenile rheumatoid arthritis, right wrist

   ■ M08.032 Unspecified juvenile rheumatoid arthritis, left wrist

   ■ M08.039 Unspecified juvenile rheumatoid arthritis, unspecified wrist

● M08.04 Unspecified juvenile rheumatoid arthritis, hand

   ■ M08.041 Unspecified juvenile rheumatoid arthritis, right hand

   ■ M08.042 Unspecified juvenile rheumatoid arthritis, left hand

   ■ M08.049 Unspecified juvenile rheumatoid arthritis, unspecified hand

● M08.05 Unspecified juvenile rheumatoid arthritis, hip

   ■ M08.051 Unspecified juvenile rheumatoid arthritis, right hip

   ■ M08.052 Unspecified juvenile rheumatoid arthritis, left hip

   ■ M08.059 Unspecified juvenile rheumatoid arthritis, unspecified hip

● M08.06 Unspecified juvenile rheumatoid arthritis, knee

   ■ M08.061 Unspecified juvenile rheumatoid arthritis, right knee

   ■ M08.062 Unspecified juvenile rheumatoid arthritis, left knee

   ■ M08.069 Unspecified juvenile rheumatoid arthritis, unspecified knee

● M08.07 Unspecified juvenile rheumatoid arthritis, ankle and foot

   ■ M08.071 Unspecified juvenile rheumatoid arthritis, right ankle and foot

   ■ M08.072 Unspecified juvenile rheumatoid arthritis, left ankle and foot

   ■ M08.079 Unspecified juvenile rheumatoid arthritis, unspecified ankle and foot

■ M08.08 Unspecified juvenile rheumatoid arthritis, vertebrae

■ M08.09 Unspecified juvenile rheumatoid arthritis, multiple sites

M08.1 Juvenile ankylosing spondylitis

   Excludes1 ankylosing spondylitis in adults (M45.0-)

● M08.2 Juvenile rheumatoid arthritis with systemic onset
   Still's disease NOS

   Excludes1 adult-onset Still's disease (M06.1-)

■ M08.20 Juvenile rheumatoid arthritis with systemic onset, unspecified site

● M08.21 Juvenile rheumatoid arthritis with systemic onset, shoulder

   M08.211 Juvenile rheumatoid arthritis with systemic onset, right shoulder

   M08.212 Juvenile rheumatoid arthritis with systemic onset, left shoulder

   ■ M08.219 Juvenile rheumatoid arthritis with systemic onset, unspecified shoulder

● Unacceptable Principal Diagnosis   ● Use Additional Character(s)   ■ Unspecified   ▶ Manifestation Code

1158   **OGCR** Official Guidelines for Coding and Reporting   Excludes 1   Excludes 2   Includes   Use additional   Code first   Code also

● M08.22   Juvenile rheumatoid arthritis with systemic onset, elbow

     M08.221   Juvenile rheumatoid arthritis with systemic onset, right elbow

     M08.222   Juvenile rheumatoid arthritis with systemic onset, left elbow

     ▨ M08.229   Juvenile rheumatoid arthritis with systemic onset, unspecified elbow

● M08.23   Juvenile rheumatoid arthritis with systemic onset, wrist

     M08.231   Juvenile rheumatoid arthritis with systemic onset, right wrist

     M08.232   Juvenile rheumatoid arthritis with systemic onset, left wrist

     ▨ M08.239   Juvenile rheumatoid arthritis with systemic onset, unspecified wrist

● M08.24   Juvenile rheumatoid arthritis with systemic onset, hand

     M08.241   Juvenile rheumatoid arthritis with systemic onset, right hand

     M08.242   Juvenile rheumatoid arthritis with systemic onset, left hand

     ▨ M08.249   Juvenile rheumatoid arthritis with systemic onset, unspecified hand

● M08.25   Juvenile rheumatoid arthritis with systemic onset, hip

     M08.251   Juvenile rheumatoid arthritis with systemic onset, right hip

     M08.252   Juvenile rheumatoid arthritis with systemic onset, left hip

     ▨ M08.259   Juvenile rheumatoid arthritis with systemic onset, unspecified hip

● M08.26   Juvenile rheumatoid arthritis with systemic onset, knee

     M08.261   Juvenile rheumatoid arthritis with systemic onset, right knee

     M08.262   Juvenile rheumatoid arthritis with systemic onset, left knee

     ▨ M08.269   Juvenile rheumatoid arthritis with systemic onset, unspecified knee

● M08.27   Juvenile rheumatoid arthritis with systemic onset, ankle and foot

     M08.271   Juvenile rheumatoid arthritis with systemic onset, right ankle and foot

     M08.272   Juvenile rheumatoid arthritis with systemic onset, left ankle and foot

     ▨ M08.279   Juvenile rheumatoid arthritis with systemic onset, unspecified ankle and foot

     M08.28   Juvenile rheumatoid arthritis with systemic onset, vertebrae

     M08.29   Juvenile rheumatoid arthritis with systemic onset, multiple sites

M08.3   Juvenile rheumatoid polyarthritis (seronegative)

● M08.4   Pauciarticular juvenile rheumatoid arthritis

     ▨ M08.40   Pauciarticular juvenile rheumatoid arthritis, unspecified site

     ● M08.41   Pauciarticular juvenile rheumatoid arthritis, shoulder

         M08.411   Pauciarticular juvenile rheumatoid arthritis, right shoulder

         M08.412   Pauciarticular juvenile rheumatoid arthritis, left shoulder

         ▨ M08.419   Pauciarticular juvenile rheumatoid arthritis, unspecified shoulder

     ● M08.42   Pauciarticular juvenile rheumatoid arthritis, elbow

         M08.421   Pauciarticular juvenile rheumatoid arthritis, right elbow

         M08.422   Pauciarticular juvenile rheumatoid arthritis, left elbow

         ▨ M08.429   Pauciarticular juvenile rheumatoid arthritis, unspecified elbow

     ● M08.43   Pauciarticular juvenile rheumatoid arthritis, wrist

         M08.431   Pauciarticular juvenile rheumatoid arthritis, right wrist

         M08.432   Pauciarticular juvenile rheumatoid arthritis, left wrist

         ▨ M08.439   Pauciarticular juvenile rheumatoid arthritis, unspecified wrist

     ● M08.44   Pauciarticular juvenile rheumatoid arthritis, hand

         M08.441   Pauciarticular juvenile rheumatoid arthritis, right hand

         M08.442   Pauciarticular juvenile rheumatoid arthritis, left hand

         ▨ M08.449   Pauciarticular juvenile rheumatoid arthritis, unspecified hand

     ● M08.45   Pauciarticular juvenile rheumatoid arthritis, hip

         M08.451   Pauciarticular juvenile rheumatoid arthritis, right hip

         M08.452   Pauciarticular juvenile rheumatoid arthritis, left hip

         ▨ M08.459   Pauciarticular juvenile rheumatoid arthritis, unspecified hip

     ● M08.46   Pauciarticular juvenile rheumatoid arthritis, knee

         M08.461   Pauciarticular juvenile rheumatoid arthritis, right knee

         M08.462   Pauciarticular juvenile rheumatoid arthritis, left knee

         ▨ M08.469   Pauciarticular juvenile rheumatoid arthritis, unspecified knee

● **M08.47 Pauciarticular juvenile rheumatoid arthritis, ankle and foot**

    M08.471 Pauciarticular juvenile rheumatoid arthritis, right ankle and foot

    M08.472 Pauciarticular juvenile rheumatoid arthritis, left ankle and foot

    ■ **M08.479 Pauciarticular juvenile rheumatoid arthritis, unspecified ankle and foot**

    M08.48 Pauciarticular juvenile rheumatoid arthritis, vertebrae

● **M08.8 Other juvenile arthritis**

  ■ **M08.80 Other juvenile arthritis, unspecified site**

  ● **M08.81 Other juvenile arthritis, shoulder**

    M08.811 Other juvenile arthritis, right shoulder

    M08.812 Other juvenile arthritis, left shoulder

    ■ **M08.819 Other juvenile arthritis, unspecified shoulder**

  ● **M08.82 Other juvenile arthritis, elbow**

    M08.821 Other juvenile arthritis, right elbow

    M08.822 Other juvenile arthritis, left elbow

    ■ **M08.829 Other juvenile arthritis, unspecified elbow**

  ● **M08.83 Other juvenile arthritis, wrist**

    M08.831 Other juvenile arthritis, right wrist

    M08.832 Other juvenile arthritis, left wrist

    ■ **M08.839 Other juvenile arthritis, unspecified wrist**

  ● **M08.84 Other juvenile arthritis, hand**

    M08.841 Other juvenile arthritis, right hand

    M08.842 Other juvenile arthritis, left hand

    ■ **M08.849 Other juvenile arthritis, unspecified hand**

  ● **M08.85 Other juvenile arthritis, hip**

    M08.851 Other juvenile arthritis, right hip

    M08.852 Other juvenile arthritis, left hip

    ■ **M08.859 Other juvenile arthritis, unspecified hip**

  ● **M08.86 Other juvenile arthritis, knee**

    M08.861 Other juvenile arthritis, right knee

    M08.862 Other juvenile arthritis, left knee

    ■ **M08.869 Other juvenile arthritis, unspecified knee**

  ● **M08.87 Other juvenile arthritis, ankle and foot**

    M08.871 Other juvenile arthritis, right ankle and foot

    M08.872 Other juvenile arthritis, left ankle and foot

    ■ **M08.879 Other juvenile arthritis, unspecified ankle and foot**

  M08.88 Other juvenile arthritis, vertebrae

  M08.89 Other juvenile arthritis, multiple sites

● **M08.9 Juvenile arthritis, unspecified**

    | Excludes1 | juvenile rheumatoid arthritis, unspecified (M08.0-) |

  ■ **M08.90 Juvenile arthritis, unspecified, unspecified site**

  ● **M08.91 Juvenile arthritis, unspecified, shoulder**

    ■ **M08.911 Juvenile arthritis, unspecified, right shoulder**

    ■ **M08.912 Juvenile arthritis, unspecified, left shoulder**

    ■ **M08.919 Juvenile arthritis, unspecified, unspecified shoulder**

  ● **M08.92 Juvenile arthritis, unspecified, elbow**

    ■ **M08.921 Juvenile arthritis, unspecified, right elbow**

    ■ **M08.922 Juvenile arthritis, unspecified, left elbow**

    ■ **M08.929 Juvenile arthritis, unspecified, unspecified elbow**

  ● **M08.93 Juvenile arthritis, unspecified, wrist**

    ■ **M08.931 Juvenile arthritis, unspecified, right wrist**

    ■ **M08.932 Juvenile arthritis, unspecified, left wrist**

    ■ **M08.939 Juvenile arthritis, unspecified, unspecified wrist**

  ● **M08.94 Juvenile arthritis, unspecified, hand**

    ■ **M08.941 Juvenile arthritis, unspecified, right hand**

    ■ **M08.942 Juvenile arthritis, unspecified, left hand**

    ■ **M08.949 Juvenile arthritis, unspecified, unspecified hand**

  ● **M08.95 Juvenile arthritis, unspecified, hip**

    ■ **M08.951 Juvenile arthritis, unspecified, right hip**

    ■ **M08.952 Juvenile arthritis, unspecified, left hip**

    ■ **M08.959 Juvenile arthritis, unspecified, unspecified hip**

  ● **M08.96 Juvenile arthritis, unspecified, knee**

    ■ **M08.961 Juvenile arthritis, unspecified, right knee**

    ■ **M08.962 Juvenile arthritis, unspecified, left knee**

    ■ **M08.969 Juvenile arthritis, unspecified, unspecified knee**

  ● **M08.97 Juvenile arthritis, unspecified, ankle and foot**

    ■ **M08.971 Juvenile arthritis, unspecified, right ankle and foot**

    ■ **M08.972 Juvenile arthritis, unspecified, left ankle and foot**

    ■ **M08.979 Juvenile arthritis, unspecified, unspecified ankle and foot**

  ■ **M08.98 Juvenile arthritis, unspecified, vertebrae**

  ■ **M08.99 Juvenile arthritis, unspecified, multiple sites**

● Unacceptable Principal Diagnosis   ● Use Additional Character(s)   ■ Unspecified   ▶ Manifestation Code

OGCR Official Guidelines for Coding and Reporting   Excludes 1   Excludes 2   Includes   Use additional   Code first   Code also

● **M1A Chronic gout**

     Use additional code to identify:

         Autonomic neuropathy in diseases classified elsewhere (G99.0)

         Calculus of urinary tract in diseases classified elsewhere (N22)

         Cardiomyopathy in diseases classified elsewhere (I43)

         Disorders of external ear in diseases classified elsewhere (H61.1-, H62.8-)

         Disorders of iris and ciliary body in diseases classified elsewhere (H22)

         Glomerular disorders in diseases classified elsewhere (N08)

     Excludes1   acute gout (M10-)

                 gout NOS (M10.-)

     The appropriate 7th character is to be added to each code from category M1A

         0   without tophus (tophi)

         1   with tophus (tophi)

● **M1A.0 Idiopathic chronic gout**

     Chronic gouty bursitis

     Primary chronic gout

     ■ **M1A.00 Idiopathic chronic gout, unspecified site**

     ● **M1A.01 Idiopathic chronic gout, shoulder**

         M1A.011 Idiopathic chronic gout, right shoulder

         M1A.012 Idiopathic chronic gout, left shoulder

         ■ **M1A.019 Idiopathic chronic gout, unspecified shoulder**

     ● **M1A.02 Idiopathic chronic gout, elbow**

         M1A.021 Idiopathic chronic gout, right elbow

         M1A.022 Idiopathic chronic gout, left elbow

         ■ **M1A.029 Idiopathic chronic gout, unspecified elbow**

     ● **M1A.03 Idiopathic chronic gout, wrist**

         M1A.031 Idiopathic chronic gout, right wrist

         M1A.032 Idiopathic chronic gout, left wrist

         ■ **M1A.039 Idiopathic chronic gout, unspecified wrist**

     ● **M1A.04 Idiopathic chronic gout, hand**

         M1A.041 Idiopathic chronic gout, right hand

         M1A.042 Idiopathic chronic gout, left hand

         ■ **M1A.049 Idiopathic chronic gout, unspecified hand**

     ● **M1A.05 Idiopathic chronic gout, hip**

         M1A.051 Idiopathic chronic gout, right hip

         M1A.052 Idiopathic chronic gout, left hip

         ■ **M1A.059 Idiopathic chronic gout, unspecified hip**

     ● **M1A.06 Idiopathic chronic gout, knee**

         M1A.061 Idiopathic chronic gout, right knee

         M1A.062 Idiopathic chronic gout, left knee

         ■ **M1A.069 Idiopathic chronic gout, unspecified knee**

● **M1A.07 Idiopathic chronic gout, ankle and foot**

     M1A.071 Idiopathic chronic gout, right ankle and foot

     M1A.072 Idiopathic chronic gout, left ankle and foot

     ■ **M1A.079 Idiopathic chronic gout, unspecified ankle and foot**

     M1A.08 Idiopathic chronic gout, vertebrae

     M1A.09 Idiopathic chronic gout, multiple sites

M1A.1 Lead-induced chronic gout

     Code first toxic effects of lead and its compounds (T56.0-)

■ **M1A.10 Lead-induced chronic gout, unspecified site**

● **M1A.11 Lead-induced chronic gout, shoulder**

     M1A.111 Lead-induced chronic gout, right shoulder

     M1A.112 Lead-induced chronic gout, left shoulder

     ■ **M1A.119 Lead-induced chronic gout, unspecified shoulder**

● **M1A.12 Lead-induced chronic gout, elbow**

     M1A.121 Lead-induced chronic gout, right elbow

     M1A.122 Lead-induced chronic gout, left elbow

     ■ **M1A.129 Lead-induced chronic gout, unspecified elbow**

● **M1A.13 Lead-induced chronic gout, wrist**

     M1A.131 Lead-induced chronic gout, right wrist

     M1A.132 Lead-induced chronic gout, left wrist

     ■ **M1A.139 Lead-induced chronic gout, unspecified wrist**

● **M1A.14 Lead-induced chronic gout, hand**

     M1A.141 Lead-induced chronic gout, right hand

     M1A.142 Lead-induced chronic gout, left hand

     ■ **M1A.149 Lead-induced chronic gout, unspecified hand**

● **M1A.15 Lead-induced chronic gout, hip**

     M1A.151 Lead-induced chronic gout, right hip

     M1A.152 Lead-induced chronic gout, left hip

     ■ **M1A.159 Lead-induced chronic gout, unspecified hip**

● **M1A.16 Lead-induced chronic gout, knee**

     M1A.161 Lead-induced chronic gout, right knee

     M1A.162 Lead-induced chronic gout, left knee

     ■ **M1A.169 Lead-induced chronic gout, unspecified knee**

● **M1A.17 Lead-induced chronic gout, ankle and foot**

     M1A.171 Lead-induced chronic gout, right ankle and foot

     M1A.172 Lead-induced chronic gout, left ankle and foot

     ■ **M1A.179 Lead-induced chronic gout, unspecified ankle and foot**

CHAPTER 13 (M00-M99)

M1A.18 Lead-induced chronic gout, vertebrae

M1A.19 Lead-induced chronic gout, multiple sites

● M1A.2 Drug-induced chronic gout

> Use additional code for adverse effect, if applicable, to identify drug (T36-T50 with fifth or sixth character 5)

■ M1A.20 Drug-induced chronic gout, unspecified site

● M1A.21 Drug-induced chronic gout, shoulder

M1A.211 Drug-induced chronic gout, right shoulder

M1A.212 Drug-induced chronic gout, left shoulder

■ M1A.219 Drug-induced chronic gout, unspecified shoulder

● M1A.22 Drug-induced chronic gout, elbow

M1A.221 Drug-induced chronic gout, right elbow

M1A.222 Drug-induced chronic gout, left elbow

■ M1A.229 Drug-induced chronic gout, unspecified elbow

● M1A.23 Drug-induced chronic gout, wrist

M1A.231 Drug-induced chronic gout, right wrist

M1A.232 Drug-induced chronic gout, left wrist

■ M1A.239 Drug-induced chronic gout, unspecified wrist

● M1A.24 Drug-induced chronic gout, hand

M1A.241 Drug-induced chronic gout, right hand

M1A.242 Drug-induced chronic gout, left hand

■ M1A.249 Drug-induced chronic gout, unspecified hand

● M1A.25 Drug-induced chronic gout, hip

M1A.251 Drug-induced chronic gout, right hip

M1A.252 Drug-induced chronic gout, left hip

■ M1A.259 Drug-induced chronic gout, unspecified hip

● M1A.26 Drug-induced chronic gout, knee

M1A.261 Drug-induced chronic gout, right knee

M1A.262 Drug-induced chronic gout, left knee

■ M1A.269 Drug-induced chronic gout, unspecified knee

● M1A.27 Drug-induced chronic gout, ankle and foot

M1A.271 Drug-induced chronic gout, right ankle and foot

M1A.272 Drug-induced chronic gout, left ankle and foot

■ M1A.279 Drug-induced chronic gout, unspecified ankle and foot

M1A.28 Drug-induced chronic gout, vertebrae

M1A.29 Drug-induced chronic gout, multiple sites

● M1A.3 Chronic gout due to renal impairment

> Code first associated renal disease

■ M1A.30 Chronic gout due to renal impairment, unspecified site

● M1A.31 Chronic gout due to renal impairment, shoulder

M1A.311 Chronic gout due to renal impairment, right shoulder

M1A.312 Chronic gout due to renal impairment, left shoulder

■ M1A.319 Chronic gout due to renal impairment, unspecified shoulder

● M1A.32 Chronic gout due to renal impairment, elbow

M1A.321 Chronic gout due to renal impairment, right elbow

M1A.322 Chronic gout due to renal impairment, left elbow

■ M1A.329 Chronic gout due to renal impairment, unspecified elbow

■ M1A.33 Chronic gout due to renal impairment, wrist

M1A.331 Chronic gout due to renal impairment, right wrist

M1A.332 Chronic gout due to renal impairment, left wrist

■ M1A.339 Chronic gout due to renal impairment, unspecified wrist

● M1A.34 Chronic gout due to renal impairment, hand

M1A.341 Chronic gout due to renal impairment, right hand

M1A.342 Chronic gout due to renal impairment, left hand

■ M1A.349 Chronic gout due to renal impairment, unspecified hand

● M1A.35 Chronic gout due to renal impairment, hip

M1A.351 Chronic gout due to renal impairment, right hip

M1A.352 Chronic gout due to renal impairment, left hip

■ M1A.359 Chronic gout due to renal impairment, unspecified hip

● M1A.36 Chronic gout due to renal impairment, knee

M1A.361 Chronic gout due to renal impairment, right knee

M1A.362 Chronic gout due to renal impairment, left knee

■ M1A.369 Chronic gout due to renal impairment, unspecified knee

● M1A.37 Chronic gout due to renal impairment, ankle and foot

M1A.371 Chronic gout due to renal impairment, right ankle and foot

M1A.372 Chronic gout due to renal impairment, left ankle and foot

■ M1A.379 Chronic gout due to renal impairment, unspecified ankle and foot

M1A.38 Chronic gout due to renal impairment, vertebrae

M1A.39 Chronic gout due to renal impairment, multiple sites

● Unacceptable Principal Diagnosis ● Use Additional Character(s) ■ Unspecified ▶ Manifestation Code
OGCR Official Guidelines for Coding and Reporting Excludes 1 Excludes 2 Includes Use additional Code first Code also

CHAPTER 13 (M00-M99)

● M1A.4 Other secondary chronic gout
    Code first associated condition
    ■ M1A.40 Other secondary chronic gout, unspecified site
    ● M1A.41 Other secondary chronic gout, shoulder
        M1A.411 Other secondary chronic gout, right shoulder
        M1A.412 Other secondary chronic gout, left shoulder
        ■ M1A.419 Other secondary chronic gout, unspecified shoulder
    ● M1A.42 Other secondary chronic gout, elbow
        M1A.421 Other secondary chronic gout, right elbow
        M1A.422 Other secondary chronic gout, left elbow
        ■ M1A.429 Other secondary chronic gout, unspecified elbow
    ● M1A.43 Other secondary chronic gout, wrist
        M1A.431 Other secondary chronic gout, right wrist
        M1A.432 Other secondary chronic gout, left wrist
        ■ M1A.439 Other secondary chronic gout, unspecified wrist
    ● M1A.44 Other secondary chronic gout, hand
        M1A.441 Other secondary chronic gout, right hand
        M1A.442 Other secondary chronic gout, left hand
        ■ M1A.449 Other secondary chronic gout, unspecified hand
    ● M1A.45 Other secondary chronic gout, hip
        M1A.451 Other secondary chronic gout, right hip
        M1A.452 Other secondary chronic gout, left hip
        ■ M1A.459 Other secondary chronic gout, unspecified hip
    ● M1A.46 Other secondary chronic gout, knee
        M1A.461 Other secondary chronic gout, right knee
        M1A.462 Other secondary chronic gout, left knee
        ■ M1A.469 Other secondary chronic gout, unspecified knee
    ● M1A.47 Other secondary chronic gout, ankle and foot
        M1A.471 Other secondary chronic gout, right ankle and foot
        M1A.472 Other secondary chronic gout, left ankle and foot
        ■ M1A.479 Other secondary chronic gout, unspecified ankle and foot
    M1A.48 Other secondary chronic gout, vertebrae
    M1A.49 Other secondary chronic gout, multiple sites
● M1A.9 Chronic gout, unspecified

● M10 Gout
    Accumulation of uric acid that results in swollen, red, hot, painful, stiff joints.
    Acute gout
    Gout attack
    Gout flare
    Gout NOS
    Podagra
    Use additional code to identify:
      Autonomic neuropathy in diseases classified elsewhere (G99.0)
      Calculus of urinary tract in diseases classified elsewhere (N22)
      Cardiomyopathy in diseases classified elsewhere (I43)
      Disorders of external ear in diseases classified elsewhere (H61.1-, H62.8-)
      Disorders of iris and ciliary body in diseases classified elsewhere (H22)
      Glomerular disorders in diseases classified elsewhere (N08)
    Excludes1   chronic gout (M1A-)
    ● M10.0 Idiopathic gout
      Gouty bursitis
      Primary gout
      ■ M10.00 Idiopathic gout, unspecified site
      ● M10.01 Idiopathic gout, shoulder
          M10.011 Idiopathic gout, right shoulder
          M10.012 Idiopathic gout, left shoulder
          ■ M10.019 Idiopathic gout, unspecified shoulder
      ● M10.02 Idiopathic gout, elbow
          M10.021 Idiopathic gout, right elbow
          M10.022 Idiopathic gout, left elbow
          ■ M10.029 Idiopathic gout, unspecified elbow
      ● M10.03 Idiopathic gout, wrist
          M10.031 Idiopathic gout, right wrist
          M10.032 Idiopathic gout, left wrist
          ■ M10.039 Idiopathic gout, unspecified wrist
      ● M10.04 Idiopathic gout, hand
          M10.041 Idiopathic gout, right hand
          M10.042 Idiopathic gout, left hand
          ■ M10.049 Idiopathic gout, unspecified hand
      ● M10.05 Idiopathic gout, hip
          M10.051 Idiopathic gout, right hip
          M10.052 Idiopathic gout, left hip
          ■ M10.059 Idiopathic gout, unspecified hip
      ● M10.06 Idiopathic gout, knee
          M10.061 Idiopathic gout, right knee
          M10.062 Idiopathic gout, left knee
          ■ M10.069 Idiopathic gout, unspecified knee
      ● M10.07 Idiopathic gout, ankle and foot
          M10.071 Idiopathic gout, right ankle and foot
          M10.072 Idiopathic gout, left ankle and foot
          ■ M10.079 Idiopathic gout, unspecified ankle and foot
      M10.08 Idiopathic gout, vertebrae
      M10.09 Idiopathic gout, multiple sites

CHAPTER 13 (M00-M99)

● **M10.1 Lead-induced gout**

Code first *toxic effects of lead and its compounds (T56.0-)*

■ **M10.10 Lead-induced gout, unspecified site**

● **M10.11 Lead-induced gout, shoulder**

    M10.111 Lead-induced gout, right shoulder

    M10.112 Lead-induced gout, left shoulder

   ■ M10.119 Lead-induced gout, unspecified shoulder

● **M10.12 Lead-induced gout, elbow**

    M10.121 Lead-induced gout, right elbow

    M10.122 Lead-induced gout, left elbow

   ■ M10.129 Lead-induced gout, unspecified elbow

● **M10.13 Lead-induced gout, wrist**

    M10.131 Lead-induced gout, right wrist

    M10.132 Lead-induced gout, left wrist

   ■ M10.139 Lead-induced gout, unspecified wrist

● **M10.14 Lead-induced gout, hand**

    M10.141 Lead-induced gout, right hand

    M10.142 Lead-induced gout, left hand

   ■ M10.149 Lead-induced gout, unspecified hand

● **M10.15 Lead-induced gout, hip**

    M10.151 Lead-induced gout, right hip

    M10.152 Lead-induced gout, left hip

   ■ M10.159 Lead-induced gout, unspecified hip

● **M10.16 Lead-induced gout, knee**

    M10.161 Lead-induced gout, right knee

    M10.162 Lead-induced gout, left knee

   ■ M10.169 Lead-induced gout, unspecified knee

● **M10.17 Lead-induced gout, ankle and foot**

    M10.171 Lead-induced gout, right ankle and foot

    M10.172 Lead-induced gout, left ankle and foot

   ■ M10.179 Lead-induced gout, unspecified ankle and foot

    M10.18 Lead-induced gout, vertebrae

    M10.19 Lead-induced gout, multiple sites

● **M10.2 Drug-induced gout**

Use additional code for adverse effect, if applicable, to identify drug (T36-T50 with fifth or sixth character 5)

●■ **M10.20 Drug-induced gout, unspecified site**

● **M10.21 Drug-induced gout, shoulder**

   ● M10.211 Drug-induced gout, right shoulder

   ● M10.212 Drug-induced gout, left shoulder

  ●■ M10.219 Drug-induced gout, unspecified shoulder

● **M10.22 Drug-induced gout, elbow**

   ● M10.221 Drug-induced gout, right elbow

   ● M10.222 Drug-induced gout, left elbow

  ●■ M10.229 Drug-induced gout, unspecified elbow

● **M10.23 Drug-induced gout, wrist**

   ● M10.231 Drug-induced gout, right wrist

   ● M10.232 Drug-induced gout, left wrist

  ●■ M10.239 Drug-induced gout, unspecified wrist

● **M10.24 Drug-induced gout, hand**

   ● M10.241 Drug-induced gout, right hand

   ● M10.242 Drug-induced gout, left hand

  ●■ M10.249 Drug-induced gout, unspecified hand

● **M10.25 Drug-induced gout, hip**

   ● M10.251 Drug-induced gout, right hip

   ● M10.252 Drug-induced gout, left hip

  ●■ M10.259 Drug-induced gout, unspecified hip

● **M10.26 Drug-induced gout, knee**

   ● M10.261 Drug-induced gout, right knee

   ● M10.262 Drug-induced gout, left knee

  ●■ M10.269 Drug-induced gout, unspecified knee

● **M10.27 Drug-induced gout, ankle and foot**

   ● M10.271 Drug-induced gout, right ankle and foot

   ● M10.272 Drug-induced gout, left ankle and foot

  ●■ M10.279 Drug-induced gout, unspecified ankle and foot

● M10.28 Drug-induced gout, vertebrae

● M10.29 Drug-induced gout, multiple sites

● **M10.3 Gout due to renal impairment**

Code also *associated renal disease*

■ **M10.30 Gout due to renal impairment, unspecified site**

● **M10.31 Gout due to renal impairment, shoulder**

    M10.311 Gout due to renal impairment, right shoulder

    M10.312 Gout due to renal impairment, left shoulder

   ■ M10.319 Gout due to renal impairment, unspecified shoulder

● **M10.32 Gout due to renal impairment, elbow**

    M10.321 Gout due to renal impairment, right elbow

    M10.322 Gout due to renal impairment, left elbow

   ■ M10.329 Gout due to renal impairment, unspecified elbow

● **M10.33 Gout due to renal impairment, wrist**

    M10.331 Gout due to renal impairment, right wrist

    M10.332 Gout due to renal impairment, left wrist

   ■ M10.339 Gout due to renal impairment, unspecified wrist

● **M10.34 Gout due to renal impairment, hand**

    M10.341 Gout due to renal impairment, right hand

    M10.342 Gout due to renal impairment, left hand

   ■ M10.349 Gout due to renal impairment, unspecified hand

● Unacceptable Principal Diagnosis   ● Use Additional Character(s)   ■ Unspecified   ▶ Manifestation Code

OGCR Official Guidelines for Coding and Reporting   Excludes 1   Excludes 2   Includes   Use additional   Code first   Code also

- M10.35 Gout due to renal impairment, hip
  - M10.351 Gout due to renal impairment, right hip
  - M10.352 Gout due to renal impairment, left hip
  - M10.359 Gout due to renal impairment, unspecified hip
- M10.36 Gout due to renal impairment, knee
  - M10.361 Gout due to renal impairment, right knee
  - M10.362 Gout due to renal impairment, left knee
  - M10.369 Gout due to renal impairment, unspecified knee
- M10.37 Gout due to renal impairment, ankle and foot
  - M10.371 Gout due to renal impairment, right ankle and foot
  - M10.372 Gout due to renal impairment, left ankle and foot
  - M10.379 Gout due to renal impairment, unspecified ankle and foot
  - M10.38 Gout due to renal impairment, vertebrae
  - M10.39 Gout due to renal impairment, multiple sites
- M10.4 Other secondary gout
  - *Code first* associated condition
  - M10.40 Other secondary gout, unspecified site
- M10.41 Other secondary gout, shoulder
  - M10.411 Other secondary gout, right shoulder
  - M10.412 Other secondary gout, left shoulder
  - M10.419 Other secondary gout, unspecified shoulder
- M10.42 Other secondary gout, elbow
  - M10.421 Other secondary gout, right elbow
  - M10.422 Other secondary gout, left elbow
  - M10.429 Other secondary gout, unspecified elbow
- M10.43 Other secondary gout, wrist
  - M10.431 Other secondary gout, right wrist
  - M10.432 Other secondary gout, left wrist
  - M10.439 Other secondary gout, unspecified wrist
- M10.44 Other secondary gout, hand
  - M10.441 Other secondary gout, right hand
  - M10.442 Other secondary gout, left hand
  - M10.449 Other secondary gout, unspecified hand
- M10.45 Other secondary gout, hip
  - M10.451 Other secondary gout, right hip
  - M10.452 Other secondary gout, left hip
  - M10.459 Other secondary gout, unspecified hip

- M10.46 Other secondary gout, knee
  - M10.461 Other secondary gout, right knee
  - M10.462 Other secondary gout, left knee
  - M10.469 Other secondary gout, unspecified knee
- M10.47 Other secondary gout, ankle and foot
  - M10.471 Other secondary gout, right ankle and foot
  - M10.472 Other secondary gout, left ankle and foot
  - M10.479 Other secondary gout, unspecified ankle and foot
  - M10.48 Other secondary gout, vertebrae
  - M10.49 Other secondary gout, multiple sites
- M10.9 Gout, unspecified
  - Gout NOS

- M11 Other crystal arthropathies
  - M11.0 Hydroxyapatite deposition disease
    - M11.00 Hydroxyapatite deposition disease, unspecified site
    - M11.01 Hydroxyapatite deposition disease, shoulder
      - M11.011 Hydroxyapatite deposition disease, right shoulder
      - M11.012 Hydroxyapatite deposition disease, left shoulder
      - M11.019 Hydroxyapatite deposition disease, unspecified shoulder
    - M11.02 Hydroxyapatite deposition disease, elbow
      - M11.021 Hydroxyapatite deposition disease, right elbow
      - M11.022 Hydroxyapatite deposition disease, left elbow
      - M11.029 Hydroxyapatite deposition disease, unspecified elbow
    - M11.03 Hydroxyapatite deposition disease, wrist
      - M11.031 Hydroxyapatite deposition disease, right wrist
      - M11.032 Hydroxyapatite deposition disease, left wrist
      - M11.039 Hydroxyapatite deposition disease, unspecified wrist
    - M11.04 Hydroxyapatite deposition disease, hand
      - M11.041 Hydroxyapatite deposition disease, right hand
      - M11.042 Hydroxyapatite deposition disease, left hand
      - M11.049 Hydroxyapatite deposition disease, unspecified hand
    - M11.05 Hydroxyapatite deposition disease, hip
      - M11.051 Hydroxyapatite deposition disease, right hip
      - M11.052 Hydroxyapatite deposition disease, left hip
      - M11.059 Hydroxyapatite deposition disease, unspecified hip

CHAPTER 13 (M00-M99)

CHAPTER 13 (M00-M99)

● **M11.06** Hydroxyapatite deposition disease, knee

    M11.061 Hydroxyapatite deposition disease, right knee

    M11.062 Hydroxyapatite deposition disease, left knee

    ■ M11.069 Hydroxyapatite deposition disease, unspecified knee

● **M11.07** Hydroxyapatite deposition disease, ankle and foot

    M11.071 Hydroxyapatite deposition disease, right ankle and foot

    M11.072 Hydroxyapatite deposition disease, left ankle and foot

    ■ M11.079 Hydroxyapatite deposition disease, unspecified ankle and foot

    M11.08 Hydroxyapatite deposition disease, vertebrae

    M11.09 Hydroxyapatite deposition disease, multiple sites

● **M11.1** Familial chondrocalcinosis

    ■ M11.10 Familial chondrocalcinosis, unspecified site

● **M11.11** Familial chondrocalcinosis, shoulder

    M11.111 Familial chondrocalcinosis, right shoulder

    M11.112 Familial chondrocalcinosis, left shoulder

    ■ M11.119 Familial chondrocalcinosis, unspecified shoulder

● **M11.12** Familial chondrocalcinosis, elbow

    M11.121 Familial chondrocalcinosis, right elbow

    M11.122 Familial chondrocalcinosis, left elbow

    ■ M11.129 Familial chondrocalcinosis, unspecified elbow

● **M11.13** Familial chondrocalcinosis, wrist

    M11.131 Familial chondrocalcinosis, right wrist

    M11.132 Familial chondrocalcinosis, left wrist

    ■ M11.139 Familial chondrocalcinosis, unspecified wrist

● **M11.14** Familial chondrocalcinosis, hand

    M11.141 Familial chondrocalcinosis, right hand

    M11.142 Familial chondrocalcinosis, left hand

    ■ M11.149 Familial chondrocalcinosis, unspecified hand

● **M11.15** Familial chondrocalcinosis, hip

    M11.151 Familial chondrocalcinosis, right hip

    M11.152 Familial chondrocalcinosis, left hip

    ■ M11.159 Familial chondrocalcinosis, unspecified hip

● **M11.16** Familial chondrocalcinosis, knee

    M11.161 Familial chondrocalcinosis, right knee

    M11.162 Familial chondrocalcinosis, left knee

    ■ M11.169 Familial chondrocalcinosis, unspecified knee

● **M11.17** Familial chondrocalcinosis, ankle and foot

    M11.171 Familial chondrocalcinosis, right ankle and foot

    M11.172 Familial chondrocalcinosis, left ankle and foot

    ■ M11.179 Familial chondrocalcinosis, unspecified ankle and foot

    M11.18 Familial chondrocalcinosis, vertebrae

    M11.19 Familial chondrocalcinosis, multiple sites

● **M11.2** Other chondrocalcinosis
Chondrocalcinosis NOS

    ■ M11.20 Other chondrocalcinosis, unspecified site

● **M11.21** Other chondrocalcinosis, shoulder

    M11.211 Other chondrocalcinosis, right shoulder

    M11.212 Other chondrocalcinosis, left shoulder

    ■ M11.219 Other chondrocalcinosis, unspecified shoulder

● **M11.22** Other chondrocalcinosis, elbow

    M11.221 Other chondrocalcinosis, right elbow

    M11.222 Other chondrocalcinosis, left elbow

    ■ M11.229 Other chondrocalcinosis, unspecified elbow

● **M11.23** Other chondrocalcinosis, wrist

    M11.231 Other chondrocalcinosis, right wrist

    M11.232 Other chondrocalcinosis, left wrist

    ■ M11.239 Other chondrocalcinosis, unspecified wrist

● **M11.24** Other chondrocalcinosis, hand

    M11.241 Other chondrocalcinosis, right hand

    M11.242 Other chondrocalcinosis, left hand

    ■ M11.249 Other chondrocalcinosis, unspecified hand

● **M11.25** Other chondrocalcinosis, hip

    M11.251 Other chondrocalcinosis, right hip

    M11.252 Other chondrocalcinosis, left hip

    ■ M11.259 Other chondrocalcinosis, unspecified hip

● **M11.26** Other chondrocalcinosis, knee

    M11.261 Other chondrocalcinosis, right knee

    M11.262 Other chondrocalcinosis, left knee

    ■ M11.269 Other chondrocalcinosis, unspecified knee

● Unacceptable Principal Diagnosis   ● Use Additional Character(s)   ■ Unspecified   ▶ Manifestation Code

OGCR Official Guidelines for Coding and Reporting   Excludes 1   Excludes 2   Includes   Use additional   Code first   Code also

- ● M11.27 Other chondrocalcinosis, ankle and foot
  - M11.271 Other chondrocalcinosis, right ankle and foot
  - M11.272 Other chondrocalcinosis, left ankle and foot
  - ■ M11.279 Other chondrocalcinosis, unspecified ankle and foot
- M11.28 Other chondrocalcinosis, vertebrae
- M11.29 Other chondrocalcinosis, multiple sites
- ● M11.8 Other specified crystal arthropathies
  - ■ M11.80 Other specified crystal arthropathies, unspecified site
  - ● M11.81 Other specified crystal arthropathies, shoulder
    - M11.811 Other specified crystal arthropathies, right shoulder
    - M11.812 Other specified crystal arthropathies, left shoulder
    - ■ M11.819 Other specified crystal arthropathies, unspecified shoulder
  - ● M11.82 Other specified crystal arthropathies, elbow
    - M11.821 Other specified crystal arthropathies, right elbow
    - M11.822 Other specified crystal arthropathies, left elbow
    - ■ M11.829 Other specified crystal arthropathies, unspecified elbow
  - ● M11.83 Other specified crystal arthropathies, wrist
    - M11.831 Other specified crystal arthropathies, right wrist
    - M11.832 Other specified crystal arthropathies, left wrist
    - ■ M11.839 Other specified crystal arthropathies, unspecified wrist
  - ● M11.84 Other specified crystal arthropathies, hand
    - M11.841 Other specified crystal arthropathies, right hand
    - M11.842 Other specified crystal arthropathies, left hand
    - ■ M11.849 Other specified crystal arthropathies, unspecified hand
  - ● M11.85 Other specified crystal arthropathies, hip
    - M11.851 Other specified crystal arthropathies, right hip
    - M11.852 Other specified crystal arthropathies, left hip
    - ■ M11.859 Other specified crystal arthropathies, unspecified hip
  - ● M11.86 Other specified crystal arthropathies, knee
    - M11.861 Other specified crystal arthropathies, right knee
    - M11.862 Other specified crystal arthropathies, left knee
    - ■ M11.869 Other specified crystal arthropathies, unspecified knee
  - ● M11.87 Other specified crystal arthropathies, ankle and foot
    - M11.871 Other specified crystal arthropathies, right ankle and foot

- M11.872 Other specified crystal arthropathies, left ankle and foot
  - ■ M11.879 Other specified crystal arthropathies, unspecified ankle and foot
- M11.88 Other specified crystal arthropathies, vertebrae
- M11.89 Other specified crystal arthropathies, multiple sites
- ■ M11.9 Crystal arthropathy, unspecified
- ● M12 Other and unspecified arthropathy
  - **Excludes1**   arthrosis (M15-M19)
  - cricoarytenoid arthropathy (J38.7)
  - ● M12.0 Chronic postrheumatic arthropathy [Jaccoud]
    - ■ M12.00 Chronic postrheumatic arthropathy [Jaccoud], unspecified site
    - ● M12.01 Chronic postrheumatic arthropathy [Jaccoud], shoulder
      - M12.011 Chronic postrheumatic arthropathy [Jaccoud], right shoulder
      - M12.012 Chronic postrheumatic arthropathy [Jaccoud], left shoulder
      - ■ M12.019 Chronic postrheumatic arthropathy [Jaccoud], unspecified shoulder
    - ● M12.02 Chronic postrheumatic arthropathy [Jaccoud], elbow
      - M12.021 Chronic postrheumatic arthropathy [Jaccoud], right elbow
      - M12.022 Chronic postrheumatic arthropathy [Jaccoud], left elbow
      - ■ M12.029 Chronic postrheumatic arthropathy [Jaccoud], unspecified elbow
    - ● M12.03 Chronic postrheumatic arthropathy [Jaccoud], wrist
      - M12.031 Chronic postrheumatic arthropathy [Jaccoud], right wrist
      - M12.032 Chronic postrheumatic arthropathy [Jaccoud], left wrist
      - ■ M12.039 Chronic postrheumatic arthropathy [Jaccoud], unspecified wrist
    - ● M12.04 Chronic postrheumatic arthropathy [Jaccoud], hand
      - M12.041 Chronic postrheumatic arthropathy [Jaccoud], right hand
      - M12.042 Chronic postrheumatic arthropathy [Jaccoud], left hand
      - ■ M12.049 Chronic postrheumatic arthropathy [Jaccoud], unspecified hand
    - ● M12.05 Chronic postrheumatic arthropathy [Jaccoud], hip
      - M12.051 Chronic postrheumatic arthropathy [Jaccoud], right hip
      - M12.052 Chronic postrheumatic arthropathy [Jaccoud], left hip
      - ■ M12.059 Chronic postrheumatic arthropathy [Jaccoud], unspecified hip

N Newborn Age: 0   **P** Pediatric Age: 0–17   **M** Maternity DX: 12–55   **A** Adult Age: 15–124   ♀ Females Only   ♂ Males Only

 Complication\Comorbidity   Major C\C   Present on Admission Requirement   Hospital-Acquired Condition

1167

CHAPTER 13 (M00-M99)

CHAPTER 13 (M00-M99)

● M12.06   Chronic postrheumatic arthropathy [Jaccoud], knee

    M12.061   Chronic postrheumatic arthropathy [Jaccoud], right knee

    M12.062   Chronic postrheumatic arthropathy [Jaccoud], left knee

    ■ M12.069   Chronic postrheumatic arthropathy [Jaccoud], unspecified knee

● M12.07   Chronic postrheumatic arthropathy [Jaccoud], ankle and foot

    M12.071   Chronic postrheumatic arthropathy [Jaccoud], right ankle and foot

    M12.072   Chronic postrheumatic arthropathy [Jaccoud], left ankle and foot

    ■ M12.079   Chronic postrheumatic arthropathy [Jaccoud], unspecified ankle and foot

    M12.08   Chronic postrheumatic arthropathy [Jaccoud], vertebrae

    M12.09   Chronic postrheumatic arthropathy [Jaccoud], multiple sites

● M12.1   Kaschin-Beck disease
        Osteochondroarthrosis deformans endemica

    ■ M12.10   Kaschin-Beck disease, unspecified site

● M12.11   Kaschin-Beck disease, shoulder

    M12.111   Kaschin-Beck disease, right shoulder

    M12.112   Kaschin-Beck disease, left shoulder

    ■ M12.119   Kaschin-Beck disease, unspecified shoulder

● M12.12   Kaschin-Beck disease, elbow

    M12.121   Kaschin-Beck disease, right elbow

    M12.122   Kaschin-Beck disease, left elbow

    ■ M12.129   Kaschin-Beck disease, unspecified elbow

● M12.13   Kaschin-Beck disease, wrist

    M12.131   Kaschin-Beck disease, right wrist

    M12.132   Kaschin-Beck disease, left wrist

    ■ M12.139   Kaschin-Beck disease, unspecified wrist

● M12.14   Kaschin-Beck disease, hand

    M12.141   Kaschin-Beck disease, right hand

    M12.142   Kaschin-Beck disease, left hand

    ■ M12.149   Kaschin-Beck disease, unspecified hand

● M12.15   Kaschin-Beck disease, hip

    M12.151   Kaschin-Beck disease, right hip

    M12.152   Kaschin-Beck disease, left hip

    ■ M12.159   Kaschin-Beck disease, unspecified hip

● M12.16   Kaschin-Beck disease, knee

    M12.161   Kaschin-Beck disease, right knee

    M12.162   Kaschin-Beck disease, left knee

    ■ M12.169   Kaschin-Beck disease, unspecified knee

● M12.17   Kaschin-Beck disease, ankle and foot

    M12.171   Kaschin-Beck disease, right ankle and foot

    M12.172   Kaschin-Beck disease, left ankle and foot

    ■ M12.179   Kaschin-Beck disease, unspecified ankle and foot

    M12.18   Kaschin-Beck disease, vertebrae

    M12.19   Kaschin-Beck disease, multiple sites

● M12.2   Villonodular synovitis (pigmented)

    ■ M12.20   Villonodular synovitis (pigmented), unspecified site

● M12.21   Villonodular synovitis (pigmented), shoulder

    M12.211   Villonodular synovitis (pigmented), right shoulder

    M12.212   Villonodular synovitis (pigmented), left shoulder

    ■ M12.219   Villonodular synovitis (pigmented), unspecified shoulder

● M12.22   Villonodular synovitis (pigmented), elbow

    M12.221   Villonodular synovitis (pigmented), right elbow

    M12.222   Villonodular synovitis (pigmented), left elbow

    ■ M12.229   Villonodular synovitis (pigmented), unspecified elbow

● M12.23   Villonodular synovitis (pigmented), wrist

    M12.231   Villonodular synovitis (pigmented), right wrist

    M12.232   Villonodular synovitis (pigmented), left wrist

    ■ M12.239   Villonodular synovitis (pigmented), unspecified wrist

● M12.24   Villonodular synovitis (pigmented), hand

    M12.241   Villonodular synovitis (pigmented), right hand

    M12.242   Villonodular synovitis (pigmented), left hand

    ■ M12.249   Villonodular synovitis (pigmented), unspecified hand

● M12.25   Villonodular synovitis (pigmented), hip

    M12.251   Villonodular synovitis (pigmented), right hip

    M12.252   Villonodular synovitis (pigmented), left hip

    ■ M12.259   Villonodular synovitis (pigmented), unspecified hip

● M12.26   Villonodular synovitis (pigmented), knee

    M12.261   Villonodular synovitis (pigmented), right knee

    M12.262   Villonodular synovitis (pigmented), left knee

    ■ M12.269   Villonodular synovitis (pigmented), unspecified knee

● Unacceptable Principal Diagnosis   ● Use Additional Character(s)   ■ Unspecified   ▶ Manifestation Code

OGCR Official Guidelines for Coding and Reporting   Excludes 1   Excludes 2   Includes   Use additional   Code first   Code also

● M12.27 Villonodular synovitis (pigmented), ankle and foot

   M12.271 Villonodular synovitis (pigmented), right ankle and foot

   M12.272 Villonodular synovitis (pigmented), left ankle and foot

   ■ M12.279 Villonodular synovitis (pigmented), unspecified ankle and foot

  M12.28 Villonodular synovitis (pigmented), vertebrae

  M12.29 Villonodular synovitis (pigmented), multiple sites

● M12.3 Palindromic rheumatism

  ■ M12.30 Palindromic rheumatism, unspecified site

● M12.31 Palindromic rheumatism, shoulder

   M12.311 Palindromic rheumatism, right shoulder

   M12.312 Palindromic rheumatism, left shoulder

   ■ M12.319 Palindromic rheumatism, unspecified shoulder

● M12.32 Palindromic rheumatism, elbow

   M12.321 Palindromic rheumatism, right elbow

   M12.322 Palindromic rheumatism, left elbow

   ■ M12.329 Palindromic rheumatism, unspecified elbow

● M12.33 Palindromic rheumatism, wrist

   M12.331 Palindromic rheumatism, right wrist

   M12.332 Palindromic rheumatism, left wrist

   ■ M12.339 Palindromic rheumatism, unspecified wrist

● M12.34 Palindromic rheumatism, hand

   M12.341 Palindromic rheumatism, right hand

   M12.342 Palindromic rheumatism, left hand

   ■ M12.349 Palindromic rheumatism, unspecified hand

● M12.35 Palindromic rheumatism, hip

   M12.351 Palindromic rheumatism, right hip

   M12.352 Palindromic rheumatism, left hip

   ■ M12.359 Palindromic rheumatism, unspecified hip

● M12.36 Palindromic rheumatism, knee

   M12.361 Palindromic rheumatism, right knee

   M12.362 Palindromic rheumatism, left knee

   ■ M12.369 Palindromic rheumatism, unspecified knee

● M12.37 Palindromic rheumatism, ankle and foot

   M12.371 Palindromic rheumatism, right ankle and foot

   M12.372 Palindromic rheumatism, left ankle and foot

   ■ M12.379 Palindromic rheumatism, unspecified ankle and foot

  M12.38 Palindromic rheumatism, vertebrae

  M12.39 Palindromic rheumatism, multiple sites

● M12.4 Intermittent hydrarthrosis

  ■ M12.40 Intermittent hydrarthrosis, unspecified site

● M12.41 Intermittent hydrarthrosis, shoulder

   M12.411 Intermittent hydrarthrosis, right shoulder

   M12.412 Intermittent hydrarthrosis, left shoulder

   ■ M12.419 Intermittent hydrarthrosis, unspecified shoulder

● M12.42 Intermittent hydrarthrosis, elbow

   M12.421 Intermittent hydrarthrosis, right elbow

   M12.422 Intermittent hydrarthrosis, left elbow

   ■ M12.429 Intermittent hydrarthrosis, unspecified elbow

● M12.43 Intermittent hydrarthrosis, wrist

   M12.431 Intermittent hydrarthrosis, right wrist

   M12.432 Intermittent hydrarthrosis, left wrist

   ■ M12.439 Intermittent hydrarthrosis, unspecified wrist

● M12.44 Intermittent hydrarthrosis, hand

   M12.441 Intermittent hydrarthrosis, right hand

   M12.442 Intermittent hydrarthrosis, left hand

   ■ M12.449 Intermittent hydrarthrosis, unspecified hand

● M12.45 Intermittent hydrarthrosis, hip

   M12.451 Intermittent hydrarthrosis, right hip

   M12.452 Intermittent hydrarthrosis, left hip

   ■ M12.459 Intermittent hydrarthrosis, unspecified hip

● M12.46 Intermittent hydrarthrosis, knee

   M12.461 Intermittent hydrarthrosis, right knee

   M12.462 Intermittent hydrarthrosis, left knee

   ■ M12.469 Intermittent hydrarthrosis, unspecified knee

● M12.47 Intermittent hydrarthrosis, ankle and foot

   M12.471 Intermittent hydrarthrosis, right ankle and foot

   M12.472 Intermittent hydrarthrosis, left ankle and foot

   ■ M12.479 Intermittent hydrarthrosis, unspecified ankle and foot

  M12.48 Intermittent hydrarthrosis, other site

  M12.49 Intermittent hydrarthrosis, multiple sites

CHAPTER 13 (M00-M99)

● M12.5 **Traumatic arthropathy**

> | Excludes1 | current injury-see Alphabetic Index |
> |---|---|
> | | post-traumatic osteoarthritis (of): |
> | | NOS (M19.1-) |
> | | first carpometacarpal joint |
> | | (M18.2-M18.3) |
> | | hip (M16.4-M16.5) |
> | | knee (M17.2-M17.3) |
> | | other single joints (M19.1-) |

  ◾ M12.50 Traumatic arthropathy, unspecified site

  ● M12.51 Traumatic arthropathy, shoulder

       M12.511 Traumatic arthropathy, right shoulder

       M12.512 Traumatic arthropathy, left shoulder

       ◾ M12.519 Traumatic arthropathy, unspecified shoulder

  ● M12.52 Traumatic arthropathy, elbow

       M12.521 Traumatic arthropathy, right elbow

       M12.522 Traumatic arthropathy, left elbow

       ◾ M12.529 Traumatic arthropathy, unspecified elbow

  ● M12.53 Traumatic arthropathy, wrist

       M12.531 Traumatic arthropathy, right wrist

       M12.532 Traumatic arthropathy, left wrist

       ◾ M12.539 Traumatic arthropathy, unspecified wrist

  ● M12.54 Traumatic arthropathy, hand

       M12.541 Traumatic arthropathy, right hand

       M12.542 Traumatic arthropathy, left hand

       ◾ M12.549 Traumatic arthropathy, unspecified hand

  ● M12.55 Traumatic arthropathy, hip

       M12.551 Traumatic arthropathy, right hip

       M12.552 Traumatic arthropathy, left hip

       ◾ M12.559 Traumatic arthropathy, unspecified hip

  ● M12.56 Traumatic arthropathy, knee

       M12.561 Traumatic arthropathy, right knee

       M12.562 Traumatic arthropathy, left knee

       ◾ M12.569 Traumatic arthropathy, unspecified knee

  ● M12.57 Traumatic arthropathy, ankle and foot

       M12.571 Traumatic arthropathy, right ankle and foot

       M12.572 Traumatic arthropathy, left ankle and foot

       ◾ M12.579 Traumatic arthropathy, unspecified ankle and foot

     M12.58 Traumatic arthropathy, vertebrae

     M12.59 Traumatic arthropathy, multiple sites

● M12.8 **Other specific arthropathies, not elsewhere classified**
    Transient arthropathy

  ◾ M12.80 Other specific arthropathies, not elsewhere classified, unspecified site

  ● M12.81 Other specific arthropathies, not elsewhere classified, shoulder

       M12.811 Other specific arthropathies, not elsewhere classified, right shoulder

       M12.812 Other specific arthropathies, not elsewhere classified, left shoulder

       ◾ M12.819 Other specific arthropathies, not elsewhere classified, unspecified shoulder

  ● M12.82 Other specific arthropathies, not elsewhere classified, elbow

       M12.821 Other specific arthropathies, not elsewhere classified, right elbow

       M12.822 Other specific arthropathies, not elsewhere classified, left elbow

       ◾ M12.829 Other specific arthropathies, not elsewhere classified, unspecified elbow

  ● M12.83 Other specific arthropathies, not elsewhere classified, wrist

       M12.831 Other specific arthropathies, not elsewhere classified, right wrist

       M12.832 Other specific arthropathies, not elsewhere classified, left wrist

       ◾ M12.839 Other specific arthropathies, not elsewhere classified, unspecified wrist

  ● M12.84 Other specific arthropathies, not elsewhere classified, hand

       M12.841 Other specific arthropathies, not elsewhere classified, right hand

       M12.842 Other specific arthropathies, not elsewhere classified, left hand

       ◾ M12.849 Other specific arthropathies, not elsewhere classified, unspecified hand

  ● M12.85 Other specific arthropathies, not elsewhere classified, hip

       M12.851 Other specific arthropathies, not elsewhere classified, right hip

       M12.852 Other specific arthropathies, not elsewhere classified, left hip

       ◾ M12.859 Other specific arthropathies, not elsewhere classified, unspecified hip

  ● M12.86 Other specific arthropathies, not elsewhere classified, knee

       M12.861 Other specific arthropathies, not elsewhere classified, right knee

       M12.862 Other specific arthropathies, not elsewhere classified, left knee

       ◾ M12.869 Other specific arthropathies, not elsewhere classified, unspecified knee

  ● M12.87 Other specific arthropathies, not elsewhere classified, ankle and foot

       M12.871 Other specific arthropathies, not elsewhere classified, right ankle and foot

       M12.872 Other specific arthropathies, not elsewhere classified, left ankle and foot

       ◾ M12.879 Other specific arthropathies, not elsewhere classified, unspecified ankle and foot

     M12.88 Other specific arthropathies, not elsewhere classified, vertebrae

     M12.89 Other specific arthropathies, not elsewhere classified, multiple sites

◾ M12.9 **Arthropathy, unspecified**

● Unacceptable Principal Diagnosis   ● Use Additional Character(s)   ◾ Unspecified   ▶ Manifestation Code

OGCR Official Guidelines for Coding and Reporting   Excludes 1   Excludes 2   Includes   Use additional   Code first   Code also

● **M13 Other arthritis**

> **Excludes1**   arthrosis (M15-M19)
> osteoarthritis (M15-M19)

■ **M13.0 Polyarthritis, unspecified**

● **M13.1 Monoarthritis, not elsewhere classified**

> ■ **M13.10 Monoarthritis, not elsewhere classified, unspecified site**

> ● **M13.11 Monoarthritis, not elsewhere classified, shoulder**

>> **M13.111 Monoarthritis, not elsewhere classified, right shoulder**

>> **M13.112 Monoarthritis, not elsewhere classified, left shoulder**

>> ■ **M13.119 Monoarthritis, not elsewhere classified, unspecified shoulder**

> ● **M13.12 Monoarthritis, not elsewhere classified, elbow**

>> **M13.121 Monoarthritis, not elsewhere classified, right elbow**

>> **M13.122 Monoarthritis, not elsewhere classified, left elbow**

>> ■ **M13.129 Monoarthritis, not elsewhere classified, unspecified elbow**

> ● **M13.13 Monoarthritis, not elsewhere classified, wrist**

>> **M13.131 Monoarthritis, not elsewhere classified, right wrist**

>> **M13.132 Monoarthritis, not elsewhere classified, left wrist**

>> ■ **M13.139 Monoarthritis, not elsewhere classified, unspecified wrist**

> ● **M13.14 Monoarthritis, not elsewhere classified, hand**

>> **M13.141 Monoarthritis, not elsewhere classified, right hand**

>> **M13.142 Monoarthritis, not elsewhere classified, left hand**

>> ■ **M13.149 Monoarthritis, not elsewhere classified, unspecified hand**

> ● **M13.15 Monoarthritis, not elsewhere classified, hip**

>> **M13.151 Monoarthritis, not elsewhere classified, right hip**

>> **M13.152 Monoarthritis, not elsewhere classified, left hip**

>> ■ **M13.159 Monoarthritis, not elsewhere classified, unspecified hip**

> ● **M13.16 Monoarthritis, not elsewhere classified, knee**

>> **M13.161 Monoarthritis, not elsewhere classified, right knee**

>> **M13.162 Monoarthritis, not elsewhere classified, left knee**

>> ■ **M13.169 Monoarthritis, not elsewhere classified, unspecified knee**

> ● **M13.17 Monoarthritis, not elsewhere classified, ankle and foot**

>> **M13.171 Monoarthritis, not elsewhere classified, right ankle and foot**

>> **M13.172 Monoarthritis, not elsewhere classified, left ankle and foot**

>> ■ **M13.179 Monoarthritis, not elsewhere classified, unspecified ankle and foot**

● **M13.8 Other specified arthritis**
Allergic arthritis

> **Excludes1**   osteoarthritis (M15-M19)

> ■ **M13.80 Other specified arthritis, unspecified site**

> ● **M13.81 Other specified arthritis, shoulder**

>> **M13.811 Other specified arthritis, right shoulder**

>> **M13.812 Other specified arthritis, left shoulder**

>> ■ **M13.819 Other specified arthritis, unspecified shoulder**

> ● **M13.82 Other specified arthritis, elbow**

>> **M13.821 Other specified arthritis, right elbow**

>> **M13.822 Other specified arthritis, left elbow**

>> ■ **M13.829 Other specified arthritis, unspecified elbow**

> ● **M13.83 Other specified arthritis, wrist**

>> **M13.831 Other specified arthritis, right wrist**

>> **M13.832 Other specified arthritis, left wrist**

>> ■ **M13.839 Other specified arthritis, unspecified wrist**

> ● **M13.84 Other specified arthritis, hand**

>> **M13.841 Other specified arthritis, right hand**

>> **M13.842 Other specified arthritis, left hand**

>> ■ **M13.849 Other specified arthritis, unspecified hand**

> ● **M13.85 Other specified arthritis, hip**

>> **M13.851 Other specified arthritis, right hip**

>> **M13.852 Other specified arthritis, left hip**

>> ■ **M13.859 Other specified arthritis, unspecified hip**

> ● **M13.86 Other specified arthritis, knee**

>> **M13.861 Other specified arthritis, right knee**

>> **M13.862 Other specified arthritis, left knee**

>> ■ **M13.869 Other specified arthritis, unspecified knee**

> ● **M13.87 Other specified arthritis, ankle and foot**

>> **M13.871 Other specified arthritis, right ankle and foot**

>> **M13.872 Other specified arthritis, left ankle and foot**

>> ■ **M13.879 Other specified arthritis, unspecified ankle and foot**

> **M13.88 Other specified arthritis, other site**

> **M13.89 Other specified arthritis, multiple sites**

CHAPTER 13 (M00-M99)

N Newborn Age: 0   **P** Pediatric Age: 0–17   **M** Maternity DX: 12–55   **A** Adult Age: 15–124   ♀ Females Only   ♂ Males Only

🏷 Complication\Comorbidity   🏷 Major C\C   🏷 Present on Admission Requirement   🏷 Hospital-Acquired Condition

1171

CHAPTER 13 (M00-M99)

● **M14 Arthropathies in other diseases classified elsewhere**

> **Excludes1** arthropathy in:
>> diabetes mellitus (E08-E13 with 4th character 61)
>> hematological disorders (M36.2-M36.3)
>> hypersensitivity reactions (M36.4)
>> neoplastic disease (M36.1)
>> neurosyphillis (A52.16)
>> sarcoidosis (D86.86)
>
>> enteropathic arthropathies (M07.0-)
>> juvenile psoriatic arthropathy (L40.54)
>> lipoid dermatoarthritis (E78.81)

● **M14.6 Charcôt's joint**
> Neuropathic arthropathy
>
> **Excludes1** Charcôt's joint in diabetes mellitus (E08-E13 with final characters 610)
>> Charcôt's joint in tabes dorsalis (A52.16)

●■ **M14.60 Charcôt's joint, unspecified site**

● **M14.61 Charcôt's joint, shoulder**

> ● **M14.611 Charcôt's joint, right shoulder**
>
> ● **M14.612 Charcôt's joint, left shoulder**
>
> ●■ **M14.619 Charcôt's joint, unspecified shoulder**

● **M14.62 Charcôt's joint, elbow**

> ● **M14.621 Charcôt's joint, right elbow**
>
> ● **M14.622 Charcôt's joint, left elbow**
>
> ●■ **M14.629 Charcôt's joint, unspecified elbow**

● **M14.63 Charcôt's joint, wrist**

> ● **M14.631 Charcôt's joint, right wrist**
>
> ● **M14.632 Charcôt's joint, left wrist**
>
> ●■ **M14.639 Charcôt's joint, unspecified wrist**

● **M14.64 Charcôt's joint, hand**

> ● **M14.641 Charcôt's joint, right hand**
>
> ● **M14.642 Charcôt's joint, left hand**
>
> ●■ **M14.649 Charcôt's joint, unspecified hand**

● **M14.65 Charcôt's joint, hip**

> ● **M14.651 Charcôt's joint, right hip**
>
> ● **M14.652 Charcôt's joint, left hip**
>
> ●■ **M14.659 Charcôt's joint, unspecified hip**

● **M14.66 Charcôt's joint, knee**

> ● **M14.661 Charcôt's joint, right knee**
>
> ● **M14.662 Charcôt's joint, left knee**
>
> ●■ **M14.669 Charcôt's joint, unspecified knee**

● **M14.67 Charcôt's joint, ankle and foot**

> ● **M14.671 Charcôt's joint, right ankle and foot**
>
> ● **M14.672 Charcôt's joint, left ankle and foot**
>
> ●■ **M14.679 Charcôt's joint, unspecified ankle and foot**

● **M14.68 Charcôt's joint, vertebrae**

● **M14.69 Charcôt's joint, multiple sites**

● **M14.8 Arthropathies in other specified diseases classified elsewhere**

> *Code first* underlying disease, such as:
>> amyloidosis (E85-)
>> erythema multiforme (L51.-)
>> erythema nodosum (L52)
>> hemochromatosis (E83.11-)
>> hyperparathyroidism (E21.-)
>> hypothyroidism (E00-E03)
>> sickle-cell disorders (D57.-)
>> thyrotoxicosis [hyperthyroidism] (E05.-)
>> Whipple's disease (K90.81)

●■▶ *M14.80 Arthropathies in other specified diseases classified elsewhere, unspecified site*

● *M14.81 Arthropathies in other specified diseases classified elsewhere, shoulder*

> ●▶ *M14.811 Arthropathies in other specified diseases classified elsewhere, right shoulder*
>
> ●▶ *M14.812 Arthropathies in other specified diseases classified elsewhere, left shoulder*
>
> ●■▶ *M14.819 Arthropathies in other specified diseases classified elsewhere, unspecified shoulder*

● *M14.82 Arthropathies in other specified diseases classified elsewhere, elbow*

> ●▶ *M14.821 Arthropathies in other specified diseases classified elsewhere, right elbow*
>
> ●▶ *M14.822 Arthropathies in other specified diseases classified elsewhere, left elbow*
>
> ●■▶ *M14.829 Arthropathies in other specified diseases classified elsewhere, unspecified elbow*

● *M14.83 Arthropathies in other specified diseases classified elsewhere, wrist*

> ●▶ *M14.831 Arthropathies in other specified diseases classified elsewhere, right wrist*
>
> ●▶ *M14.832 Arthropathies in other specified diseases classified elsewhere, left wrist*
>
> ●■▶ *M14.839 Arthropathies in other specified diseases classified elsewhere, unspecified wrist*

● *M14.84 Arthropathies in other specified diseases classified elsewhere, hand*

> ●▶ *M14.841 Arthropathies in other specified diseases classified elsewhere, right hand*
>
> ●▶ *M14.842 Arthropathies in other specified diseases classified elsewhere, left hand*
>
> ●■▶ *M14.849 Arthropathies in other specified diseases classified elsewhere, unspecified hand*

● Unacceptable Principal Diagnosis   ● Use Additional Character(s)   ■ Unspecified   ▶ Manifestation Code

OGCR Official Guidelines for Coding and Reporting   Excludes 1   Excludes 2   Includes   Use additional   Code first   Code also

● **M14.85 Arthropathies in other specified diseases classified elsewhere, hip**

    ●❯ *M14.851 Arthropathies in other specified diseases classified elsewhere, right hip*

    ●❯ *M14.852 Arthropathies in other specified diseases classified elsewhere, left hip*

    ●■❯ *M14.859 Arthropathies in other specified diseases classified elsewhere, unspecified hip*

● **M14.86 Arthropathies in other specified diseases classified elsewhere, knee**

    ●❯ *M14.861 Arthropathies in other specified diseases classified elsewhere, right knee*

    ●❯ *M14.862 Arthropathies in other specified diseases classified elsewhere, left knee*

    ●■❯ *M14.869 Arthropathies in other specified diseases classified elsewhere, unspecified knee*

● **M14.87 Arthropathies in other specified diseases classified elsewhere, ankle and foot**

    ●❯ *M14.871 Arthropathies in other specified diseases classified elsewhere, right ankle and foot*

    ●❯ *M14.872 Arthropathies in other specified diseases classified elsewhere, left ankle and foot*

    ●■❯ *M14.879 Arthropathies in other specified diseases classified elsewhere, unspecified ankle and foot*

    ●❯ *M14.88 Arthropathies in other specified diseases classified elsewhere, vertebrae*

    ●❯ *M14.89 Arthropathies in other specified diseases classified elsewhere, multiple sites*

OSTEOARTHRITIS (M15-M19)

Osteoarthritis is the most common degenerative joint disease and form of arthritis that breaks down the cartilage causing pain, swelling, and reduced motion in the joints.

    Excludes2   osteoarthritis of spine (M47.-)

● **M15 Polyosteoarthritis**

    Includes   arthritis of multiple sites

    Excludes1   bilateral involvement of single joint (M16-M19)

    M15.0 Primary generalized (osteo)arthritis

    M15.1 Heberden's nodes (with arthropathy)
      Interphalangeal distal osteoarthritis

    M15.2 Bouchard's nodes (with arthropathy)
      Juxtaphalangeal distal osteoarthritis

    M15.3 Secondary multiple arthritis
      Post-traumatic polyosteoarthritis

    M15.4 Erosive (osteo)arthritis

    M15.8 Other polyosteoarthritis

    ■ **M15.9 Polyosteoarthritis, unspecified**
      Generalized osteoarthritis NOS

● **M16 Osteoarthritis of hip**

    M16.0 Bilateral primary osteoarthritis of hip

    ● **M16.1 Unilateral primary osteoarthritis of hip**
      Primary osteoarthritis of hip NOS

      ■ **M16.10 Unilateral primary osteoarthritis, unspecified hip**

      M16.11 Unilateral primary osteoarthritis, right hip

      M16.12 Unilateral primary osteoarthritis, left hip

    M16.2 Bilateral osteoarthritis resulting from hip dysplasia

    ● **M16.3 Unilateral osteoarthritis resulting from hip dysplasia**
      Dysplastic osteoarthritis of hip NOS

      ■ **M16.30 Unilateral osteoarthritis resulting from hip dysplasia, unspecified hip**

      M16.31 Unilateral osteoarthritis resulting from hip dysplasia, right hip

      M16.32 Unilateral osteoarthritis resulting from hip dysplasia, left hip

    M16.4 Bilateral post-traumatic osteoarthritis of hip

    ● **M16.5 Unilateral post-traumatic osteoarthritis of hip**
      Post-traumatic osteoarthritis of hip NOS

      ■ **M16.50 Unilateral post-traumatic osteoarthritis, unspecified hip**

      M16.51 Unilateral post-traumatic osteoarthritis, right hip

      M16.52 Unilateral post-traumatic osteoarthritis, left hip

    M16.6 Other bilateral secondary osteoarthritis of hip

    M16.7 Other unilateral secondary osteoarthritis of hip
      Secondary osteoarthritis of hip NOS

    ■ **M16.9 Osteoarthritis of hip, unspecified**

● **M17 Osteoarthritis of knee**

    M17.0 Bilateral primary osteoarthritis of knee

    ● **M17.1 Unilateral primary osteoarthritis of knee**
      Primary osteoarthritis of knee NOS

      ■ **M17.10 Unilateral primary osteoarthritis, unspecified knee**

      M17.11 Unilateral primary osteoarthritis, right knee

      M17.12 Unilateral primary osteoarthritis, left knee

    M17.2 Bilateral post-traumatic osteoarthritis of knee

    ● **M17.3 Unilateral post-traumatic osteoarthritis of knee**
      Post-traumatic osteoarthritis of knee NOS

      ■ **M17.30 Unilateral post-traumatic osteoarthritis, unspecified knee**

      M17.31 Unilateral post-traumatic osteoarthritis, right knee

      M17.32 Unilateral post-traumatic osteoarthritis, left knee

    M17.4 Other bilateral secondary osteoarthritis of knee

    M17.5 Other unilateral secondary osteoarthritis of knee
      Secondary osteoarthritis of knee NOS

    ■ **M17.9 Osteoarthritis of knee, unspecified**

● **M18 Osteoarthritis of first carpometacarpal joint**

    M18.0 Bilateral primary osteoarthritis of first carpometacarpal joints

    ● **M18.1 Unilateral primary osteoarthritis of first carpometacarpal joint**
      Primary osteoarthritis of first carpometacarpal joint NOS

      ■ **M18.10 Unilateral primary osteoarthritis of first carpometacarpal joint, unspecified hand**

      M18.11 Unilateral primary osteoarthritis of first carpometacarpal joint, right hand

      M18.12 Unilateral primary osteoarthritis of first carpometacarpal joint, left hand

CHAPTER 13 (M00-M99)

N Newborn Age: 0   **P** Pediatric Age: 0–17   **M** Maternity DX: 12–55   **A** Adult Age: 15–124   ♀ Females Only   ♂ Males Only

Complication\Comorbidity   Major C\C   Present on Admission Requirement   Hospital-Acquired Condition

1173

CHAPTER 13 (M00-M99)

M18.2 Bilateral post-traumatic osteoarthritis of first carpometacarpal joints

● **M18.3 Unilateral post-traumatic osteoarthritis of first carpometacarpal joint**
Post-traumatic osteoarthritis of first carpometacarpal joint NOS

■ **M18.30 Unilateral post-traumatic osteoarthritis of first carpometacarpal joint, unspecified hand**

M18.31 Unilateral post-traumatic osteoarthritis of first carpometacarpal joint, right hand

M18.32 Unilateral post-traumatic osteoarthritis of first carpometacarpal joint, left hand

M18.4 Other bilateral secondary osteoarthritis of first carpometacarpal joints

● **M18.5 Other unilateral secondary osteoarthritis of first carpometacarpal joint**
Secondary osteoarthritis of first carpometacarpal joint NOS

■ **M18.50 Other unilateral secondary osteoarthritis of first carpometacarpal joint, unspecified hand**

M18.51 Other unilateral secondary osteoarthritis of first carpometacarpal joint, right hand

M18.52 Other unilateral secondary osteoarthritis of first carpometacarpal joint, left hand

■ **M18.9 Osteoarthritis of first carpometacarpal joint, unspecified**

● **M19 Other and unspecified osteoarthritis**

Excludes1	polyarthritis (M15.-)
Excludes2	arthrosis of spine (M47.-)
	hallux rigidus (M20.2)
	osteoarthritis of spine (M47.-)

● **M19.0 Primary osteoarthritis of other joints**

● **M19.01 Primary osteoarthritis, shoulder**

M19.011 Primary osteoarthritis, right shoulder

M19.012 Primary osteoarthritis, left shoulder

■ **M19.019 Primary osteoarthritis, unspecified shoulder**

● **M19.02 Primary osteoarthritis, elbow**

M19.021 Primary osteoarthritis, right elbow

M19.022 Primary osteoarthritis, left elbow

■ **M19.029 Primary osteoarthritis, unspecified elbow**

● **M19.03 Primary osteoarthritis, wrist**

M19.031 Primary osteoarthritis, right wrist

M19.032 Primary osteoarthritis, left wrist

■ **M19.039 Primary osteoarthritis, unspecified wrist**

● **M19.04 Primary osteoarthritis, hand**

Excludes2	primary osteoarthritis of first carpometacarpal joint (M18.0-, M18.1-)

M19.041 Primary osteoarthritis, right hand

M19.042 Primary osteoarthritis, left hand

■ **M19.049 Primary osteoarthritis, unspecified hand**

● **M19.07 Primary osteoarthritis ankle and foot**

M19.071 Primary osteoarthritis, right ankle and foot

M19.072 Primary osteoarthritis, left ankle and foot

■ **M19.079 Primary osteoarthritis, unspecified ankle and foot**

● **M19.1 Post-traumatic osteoarthritis of other joints**

● **M19.11 Post-traumatic osteoarthritis, shoulder**

M19.111 Post-traumatic osteoarthritis, right shoulder

M19.112 Post-traumatic osteoarthritis, left shoulder

■ **M19.119 Post-traumatic osteoarthritis, unspecified shoulder**

● **M19.12 Post-traumatic osteoarthritis, elbow**

M19.121 Post-traumatic osteoarthritis, right elbow

M19.122 Post-traumatic osteoarthritis, left elbow

■ **M19.129 Post-traumatic osteoarthritis, unspecified elbow**

● **M19.13 Post-traumatic osteoarthritis, wrist**

M19.131 Post-traumatic osteoarthritis, right wrist

M19.132 Post-traumatic osteoarthritis, left wrist

■ **M19.139 Post-traumatic osteoarthritis, unspecified wrist**

● **M19.14 Post-traumatic osteoarthritis, hand**

Excludes2	post-traumatic osteoarthritis of first carpometacarpal joint (M18.2-, M18.3-)

M19.141 Post-traumatic osteoarthritis, right hand

M19.142 Post-traumatic osteoarthritis, left hand

■ **M19.149 Post-traumatic osteoarthritis, unspecified hand**

● **M19.17 Post-traumatic osteoarthritis, ankle and foot**

M19.171 Post-traumatic osteoarthritis, right ankle and foot

M19.172 Post-traumatic osteoarthritis, left ankle and foot

■ **M19.179 Post-traumatic osteoarthritis, unspecified ankle and foot**

● **M19.2 Secondary osteoarthritis of other joints**

● **M19.21 Secondary osteoarthritis, shoulder**

M19.211 Secondary osteoarthritis, right shoulder

M19.212 Secondary osteoarthritis, left shoulder

■ **M19.219 Secondary osteoarthritis, unspecified shoulder**

● **M19.22 Secondary osteoarthritis, elbow**

M19.221 Secondary osteoarthritis, right elbow

M19.222 Secondary osteoarthritis, left elbow

■ **M19.229 Secondary osteoarthritis, unspecified elbow**

● Unacceptable Principal Diagnosis   ● Use Additional Character(s)   ■ Unspecified   ▶ Manifestation Code
OGCR Official Guidelines for Coding and Reporting   Excludes 1   Excludes 2   Includes   Use additional   Code first   Code also

● M19.23 Secondary osteoarthritis, wrist

    M19.231 Secondary osteoarthritis, right wrist

    M19.232 Secondary osteoarthritis, left wrist

    ■ M19.239 Secondary osteoarthritis, unspecified wrist

● M19.24 Secondary osteoarthritis, hand

    M19.241 Secondary osteoarthritis, right hand

    M19.242 Secondary osteoarthritis, left hand

    ■ M19.249 Secondary osteoarthritis, unspecified hand

● M19.27 Secondary osteoarthritis, ankle and foot

    M19.271 Secondary osteoarthritis, right ankle and foot

    M19.272 Secondary osteoarthritis, left ankle and foot

    ■ M19.279 Secondary osteoarthritis, unspecified ankle and foot

● M19.9 Osteoarthritis, unspecified site

    ■ M19.90 Unspecified osteoarthritis, unspecified site
        Arthrosis NOS
        Arthritis NOS
        Osteoarthritis NOS

    ■ M19.91 Primary osteoarthritis, unspecified site
        Primary osteoarthritis NOS

    ■ M19.92 Post-traumatic osteoarthritis, unspecified site
        Post-traumatic osteoarthritis NOS

    ■ M19.93 Secondary osteoarthritis, unspecified site
        Secondary osteoarthritis NOS

OTHER JOINT DISORDERS (M20-M25)

> **Excludes2** joints of the spine (M40-M54)

● M20 Acquired deformities of fingers and toes

> **Excludes1** acquired absence of fingers and toes (Z89.-)
> congenital absence of fingers and toes (Q71.3-, Q72.3-)
> congenital deformities and malformations of fingers and toes (Q66.-, Q68-Q70, Q74.-)

● M20.0 Deformity of finger(s)

> **Excludes1** clubbing of fingers (R68.3)
> palmar fascial fibromatosis [Dupuytren] (M72.0)
> trigger finger (M65.3)

  ● M20.00 Unspecified deformity of finger(s)

    ■ M20.001 Unspecified deformity of right finger(s)

    ■ M20.002 Unspecified deformity of left finger(s)

    ■ M20.009 Unspecified deformity of unspecified finger(s)

  ● M20.01 Mallet finger

    M20.011 Mallet finger of right finger(s)

    M20.012 Mallet finger of left finger(s)

    ■ M20.019 Mallet finger of unspecified finger(s)

● M20.02 Boutonnière deformity

    M20.021 Boutonnière deformity of right finger(s)

    M20.022 Boutonnière deformity of left finger(s)

    ■ M20.029 Boutonnière deformity of unspecified finger(s)

● M20.03 Swan-neck deformity

    M20.031 Swan-neck deformity of right finger(s)

    M20.032 Swan-neck deformity of left finger(s)

    ■ M20.039 Swan-neck deformity of unspecified finger(s)

● M20.09 Other deformity of finger(s)

    M20.091 Other deformity of right finger(s)

    M20.092 Other deformity of left finger(s)

    ■ M20.099 Other deformity of finger(s), unspecified finger(s)

● M20.1 Hallux valgus (acquired)
    Bunion

    ■ M20.10 Hallux valgus (acquired), unspecified foot

    M20.11 Hallux valgus (acquired), right foot

    M20.12 Hallux valgus (acquired), left foot

● M20.2 Hallux rigidus

    ■ M20.20 Hallux rigidus, unspecified foot

    M20.21 Hallux rigidus, right foot

    M20.22 Hallux rigidus, left foot

● M20.3 Hallux varus (acquired)

    ■ M20.30 Hallux varus (acquired), unspecified foot

    M20.31 Hallux varus (acquired), right foot

    M20.32 Hallux varus (acquired), left foot

● M20.4 Other hammer toe(s) (acquired)

    ■ M20.40 Other hammer toe(s) (acquired), unspecified foot

    M20.41 Other hammer toe(s) (acquired), right foot

    M20.42 Other hammer toe(s) (acquired), left foot

Figure 13-1 Hallux valgus or bunion.

Item 13–2 Hallux valgus or bunion is a sometimes painful structural deformity caused by an inflammation of the bursal sac at the base of the metatarsophalangeal joint (big toe). **Hallus varus** is a deviation of the great toe to the inner side of the foot or away from the next toe.

CHAPTER 13 (M00-M99)

N Newborn Age: 0   **P** Pediatric Age: 0–17   **M** Maternity DX: 12–55   **A** Adult Age: 15–124   ♀ Females Only   ♂ Males Only

  Complication\Comorbidity   Major C\C   Present on Admission Requirement   Hospital-Acquired Condition

1175

Item 13-3 Cubitus valgus is a deformity of the elbow resulting in an increased carrying angle in which the arm extends at the side and the palm faces forward, which results in the forearm and hand extended at a greater than 15 degrees.

- M20.5 Other deformities of toe(s) (acquired)
  - M20.5X Other deformities of toe(s) (acquired)
    - M20.5X1 Other deformities of toe(s) (acquired), right foot
    - M20.5X2 Other deformities of toe(s) (acquired), left foot
    - M20.5X9 Other deformities of toe(s) (acquired), unspecified foot
- M20.6 Acquired deformities of toe(s), unspecified
  - M20.60 Acquired deformities of toe(s), unspecified, unspecified foot
  - M20.61 Acquired deformities of toe(s), unspecified, right foot
  - M20.62 Acquired deformities of toe(s), unspecified, left foot
- M21 Other acquired deformities of limbs
  - Excludes1 acquired absence of limb (Z89.-)
    congenital absence of limbs (Q71-Q73)
    congenital deformities and malformations of limbs (Q65-Q66, Q68-Q74)
  - Excludes2 acquired deformities of fingers or toes (M20.-)
    coxa plana (M91.2)
  - M21.0 Valgus deformity, not elsewhere classified
    - Excludes1 metatarsus valgus (Q66.6)
      talipes calcaneovalgus (Q66.4)
    - M21.00 Valgus deformity, not elsewhere classified, unspecified site
    - M21.02 Valgus deformity, not elsewhere classified, elbow
      Cubitus valgus
      - M21.021 Valgus deformity, not elsewhere classified, right elbow
      - M21.022 Valgus deformity, not elsewhere classified, left elbow
      - M21.029 Valgus deformity, not elsewhere classified, unspecified elbow
    - M21.05 Valgus deformity, not elsewhere classified, hip
      - M21.051 Valgus deformity, not elsewhere classified, right hip
      - M21.052 Valgus deformity, not elsewhere classified, left hip
      - M21.059 Valgus deformity, not elsewhere classified, unspecified hip
    - M21.06 Valgus deformity, not elsewhere classified, knee
      Genu valgum
      Knock knee
      - M21.061 Valgus deformity, not elsewhere classified, right knee
      - M21.062 Valgus deformity, not elsewhere classified, left knee
      - M21.069 Valgus deformity, not elsewhere classified, unspecified knee

Item 13-4 Cubitus varus is a deformity of the elbow resulting in the arm extended at the side and the palm facing forward so that the forearm and hand are held at less than 5 degrees, decreasing the carrying angle.

- M21.07 Valgus deformity, not elsewhere classified, ankle
  - M21.071 Valgus deformity, not elsewhere classified, right ankle
  - M21.072 Valgus deformity, not elsewhere classified, left ankle
  - M21.079 Valgus deformity, not elsewhere classified, unspecified ankle
- M21.1 Varus deformity, not elsewhere classified
  - Excludes1 metatarsus varus (Q66.2)
    tibia vara (M92.5)
  - M21.10 Varus deformity, not elsewhere classified, unspecified site
  - M21.12 Varus deformity, not elsewhere classified, elbow
    Cubitus varus, elbow
    - M21.121 Varus deformity, not elsewhere classified, right elbow
    - M21.122 Varus deformity, not elsewhere classified, left elbow
    - M21.129 Varus deformity, not elsewhere classified, unspecified elbow
  - M21.15 Varus deformity, not elsewhere classified, hip
    - M21.151 Varus deformity, not elsewhere classified, right hip
    - M21.152 Varus deformity, not elsewhere classified, left hip
    - M21.159 Varus deformity, not elsewhere classified, unspecified
  - M21.16 Varus deformity, not elsewhere classified, knee
    Bow leg
    Genu varum
    - M21.161 Varus deformity, not elsewhere classified, right knee
    - M21.162 Varus deformity, not elsewhere classified, left knee
    - M21.169 Varus deformity, not elsewhere classified, unspecified knee
  - M21.17 Varus deformity, not elsewhere classified, ankle
    - M21.171 Varus deformity, not elsewhere classified, right ankle
    - M21.172 Varus deformity, not elsewhere classified, left ankle
    - M21.179 Varus deformity, not elsewhere classified, unspecified ankle
- M21.2 Flexion deformity
  - M21.20 Flexion deformity, unspecified site
  - M21.21 Flexion deformity, shoulder
    - M21.211 Flexion deformity, right shoulder
    - M21.212 Flexion deformity, left shoulder
    - M21.219 Flexion deformity, unspecified shoulder

● Unacceptable Principal Diagnosis ● Use Additional Character(s) ■ Unspecified ▶ Manifestation Code
OGCR Official Guidelines for Coding and Reporting Excludes 1 Excludes 2 Includes Use additional Code first Code also

CHAPTER 13 (M00-M99)

● M21.22   Flexion deformity, elbow

 M21.221   Flexion deformity, right elbow

 M21.222   Flexion deformity, left elbow

 ■ M21.229   Flexion deformity, unspecified elbow

● M21.23   Flexion deformity, wrist

 M21.231   Flexion deformity, right wrist

 M21.232   Flexion deformity, left wrist

 ■ M21.239   Flexion deformity, unspecified wrist

● M21.24   Flexion deformity, finger joints

 M21.241   Flexion deformity, right finger joints

 M21.242   Flexion deformity, left finger joints

 ■ M21.249   Flexion deformity, unspecified finger joints

● M21.25   Flexion deformity, hip

 M21.251   Flexion deformity, right hip

 M21.252   Flexion deformity, left hip

 ■ M21.259   Flexion deformity, unspecified hip

● M21.26   Flexion deformity, knee

 M21.261   Flexion deformity, right knee

 M21.262   Flexion deformity, left knee

 ■ M21.269   Flexion deformity, unspecified knee

● M21.27   Flexion deformity, ankle and toes

 M21.271   Flexion deformity, right ankle and toes

 M21.272   Flexion deformity, left ankle and toes

 ■ M21.279   Flexion deformity, unspecified ankle and toes

● M21.3   Wrist or foot drop (acquired)

 ● M21.33   Wrist drop (acquired)

  M21.331   Wrist drop, right wrist

  M21.332   Wrist drop, left wrist

  ■ M21.339   Wrist drop, unspecified wrist

 ● M21.37   Foot drop (acquired)

  M21.371   Foot drop, right foot

  M21.372   Foot drop, left foot

  ■ M21.379   Foot drop, unspecified foot

● M21.4   Flat foot [pes planus] (acquired)

 Excludes1 congenital pes planus (Q66.5-)

 ■ M21.40   Flat foot [pes planus] (acquired), unspecified foot

 M21.41   Flat foot [pes planus] (acquired), right foot

 M21.42   Flat foot [pes planus] (acquired), left foot

● M21.5   Acquired clawhand, clubhand, clawfoot and clubfoot

 Excludes1 clubfoot, not specified as acquired (Q66.89)

 ● M21.51   Acquired clawhand

  M21.511   Acquired clawhand, right hand

  M21.512   Acquired clawhand, left hand

  ■ M21.519   Acquired clawhand, unspecified hand

● M21.52   Acquired clubhand

 M21.521   Acquired clubhand, right hand

 M21.522   Acquired clubhand, left hand

 ■ M21.529   Acquired clubhand, unspecified hand

● M21.53   Acquired clawfoot

 M21.531   Acquired clawfoot, right foot

 M21.532   Acquired clawfoot, left foot

 ■ M21.539   Acquired clawfoot, unspecified foot

● M21.54   Acquired clubfoot

 M21.541   Acquired clubfoot, right foot

 M21.542   Acquired clubfoot, left foot

 ■ M21.549   Acquired clubfoot, unspecified foot

● M21.6   Other acquired deformities of foot

 Excludes2 deformities of toe (acquired) (M20.1-(M20.6)

 ● M21.6X   Other acquired deformities of foot

  M21.6X1   Other acquired deformities of right foot

  M21.6X2   Other acquired deformities of left foot

  ■ M21.6X9   Other acquired deformities of unspecified foot

● M21.7   Unequal limb length (acquired)

 Note: The site used should correspond to the shorter limb.

 ■ M21.70   Unequal limb length (acquired), unspecified site

 ● M21.72   Unequal limb length (acquired), humerus

  M21.721   Unequal limb length (acquired), right humerus

  M21.722   Unequal limb length (acquired), left humerus

  ■ M21.729   Unequal limb length (acquired), unspecified humerus

 ● M21.73   Unequal limb length (acquired), ulna and radius

  M21.731   Unequal limb length (acquired), right ulna

  M21.732   Unequal limb length (acquired), left ulna

  M21.733   Unequal limb length (acquired), right radius

  M21.734   Unequal limb length (acquired), left radius

  ■ M21.739   Unequal limb length (acquired), unspecified ulna and radius

 ● M21.75   Unequal limb length (acquired), femur

  M21.751   Unequal limb length (acquired), right femur

  M21.752   Unequal limb length (acquired), left femur

  ■ M21.759   Unequal limb length (acquired), unspecified femur

 ● M21.76   Unequal limb length (acquired), tibia and fibula

  M21.761   Unequal limb length (acquired), right tibia

  M21.762   Unequal limb length (acquired), left tibia

N Newborn Age: 0 **P** Pediatric Age: 0–17 **M** Maternity DX: 12–55 **A** Adult Age: 15–124 ♀ Females Only ♂ Males Only

🔖 Complication\Comorbidity 🔖 Major C\C 🔖 Present on Admission Requirement 🔖 Hospital-Acquired Condition

1177

M21.763   Unequal limb length (acquired), right fibula

M21.764   Unequal limb length (acquired), left fibula

◼ M21.769   Unequal limb length (acquired), unspecified tibia and fibula

● M21.8   Other specified acquired deformities of limbs

> Excludes2   coxa plana (M91.2)

◼ M21.80   Other specified acquired deformities of unspecified limb

● M21.82   Other specified acquired deformities of upper arm

M21.821   Other specified acquired deformities of right upper arm

M21.822   Other specified acquired deformities of left upper arm

◼ M21.829   Other specified acquired deformities of unspecified upper arm

● M21.83   Other specified acquired deformities of forearm

M21.831   Other specified acquired deformities of right forearm

M21.832   Other specified acquired deformities of left forearm

◼ M21.839   Other specified acquired deformities of unspecified forearm

● M21.85   Other specified acquired deformities of thigh

M21.851   Other specified acquired deformities of right thigh

M21.852   Other specified acquired deformities of left thigh

◼ M21.859   Other specified acquired deformities of unspecified thigh

● M21.86   Other specified acquired deformities of lower leg

M21.861   Other specified acquired deformities of right lower leg

M21.862   Other specified acquired deformities of left lower leg

◼ M21.869   Other specified acquired deformities of unspecified lower leg

● M21.9   Unspecified acquired deformity of limb and hand

◼ M21.90   Unspecified acquired deformity of unspecified limb

● M21.92   Unspecified acquired deformity of upper arm

◼ M21.921   Unspecified acquired deformity of right upper arm

◼ M21.922   Unspecified acquired deformity of left upper arm

◼ M21.929   Unspecified acquired deformity of unspecified upper arm

● M21.93   Unspecified acquired deformity of forearm

◼ M21.931   Unspecified acquired deformity of right forearm

◼ M21.932   Unspecified acquired deformity of left forearm

◼ M21.939   Unspecified acquired deformity of unspecified forearm

● M21.94   Unspecified acquired deformity of hand

◼ M21.941   Unspecified acquired deformity of hand, right hand

◼ M21.942   Unspecified acquired deformity of hand, left hand

◼ M21.949   Unspecified acquired deformity of hand, unspecified hand

● M21.95   Unspecified acquired deformity of thigh

◼ M21.951   Unspecified acquired deformity of right thigh

◼ M21.952   Unspecified acquired deformity of left thigh

◼ M21.959   Unspecified acquired deformity of unspecified thigh

● M21.96   Unspecified acquired deformity of lower leg

◼ M21.961   Unspecified acquired deformity of right lower leg

◼ M21.962   Unspecified acquired deformity of left lower leg

◼ M21.969   Unspecified acquired deformity of unspecified lower leg

● M22   Disorder of patella

> Excludes1   traumatic dislocation of patella (S83.0-)

● M22.0   Recurrent dislocation of patella

◼ M22.00   Recurrent dislocation of patella, unspecified knee

M22.01   Recurrent dislocation of patella, right knee

M22.02   Recurrent dislocation of patella, left knee

● M22.1   Recurrent subluxation of patella
Incomplete dislocation of patella

◼ M22.10   Recurrent subluxation of patella, unspecified knee

M22.11   Recurrent subluxation of patella, right knee

M22.12   Recurrent subluxation of patella, left knee

● M22.2   Patellofemoral disorders

● M22.2X   Patellofemoral disorders

M22.2X1   Patellofemoral disorders, right knee

M22.2X2   Patellofemoral disorders, left knee

◼ M22.2X9   Patellofemoral disorders, unspecified knee

● M22.3   Other derangements of patella

● M22.3X   Other derangements of patella

M22.3X1   Other derangements of patella, right knee

M22.3X2   Other derangements of patella, left knee

◼ M22.3X9   Other derangements of patella, unspecified knee

● M22.4   Chondromalacia patellae

◼ M22.40   Chondromalacia patellae, unspecified knee

M22.41   Chondromalacia patellae, right knee

M22.42   Chondromalacia patellae, left knee

- M22.8 Other disorders of patella
  - M22.8X Other disorders of patella
    - M22.8X1 Other disorders of patella, right knee
    - M22.8X2 Other disorders of patella, left knee
    - M22.8X9 Other disorders of patella, unspecified knee
- M22.9 Unspecified disorder of patella
  - M22.90 Unspecified disorder of patella, unspecified knee
  - M22.91 Unspecified disorder of patella, right knee
  - M22.92 Unspecified disorder of patella, left knee

- M23 Internal derangement of knee
  - Excludes1 ankylosis (M24.66)
    current injury - see injury of knee and lower leg (S80-S89)
    deformity of knee (M21.-)
    osteochondritis dissecans (M93.2)
    recurrent dislocation or subluxation of joints (M24.4)
    recurrent dislocation or subluxation of patella (M22.0-M22.1)
  - M23.0 Cystic meniscus
    - M23.00 Cystic meniscus, unspecified meniscus
      Cystic meniscus, unspecified lateral meniscus
      Cystic meniscus, unspecified medial meniscus
      - M23.000 Cystic meniscus, unspecified lateral meniscus, right knee
      - M23.001 Cystic meniscus, unspecified lateral meniscus, left knee
      - M23.002 Cystic meniscus, unspecified lateral meniscus, unspecified knee
      - M23.003 Cystic meniscus, unspecified medial meniscus, right knee
      - M23.004 Cystic meniscus, unspecified medial meniscus, left knee
      - M23.005 Cystic meniscus, unspecified medial meniscus, unspecified knee
      - M23.006 Cystic meniscus, unspecified meniscus, right knee
      - M23.007 Cystic meniscus, unspecified meniscus, left knee
      - M23.009 Cystic meniscus, unspecified meniscus, unspecified knee
    - M23.01 Cystic meniscus, anterior horn of medial meniscus
      - M23.011 Cystic meniscus, anterior horn of medial meniscus, right knee
      - M23.012 Cystic meniscus, anterior horn of medial meniscus, left knee
      - M23.019 Cystic meniscus, anterior horn of medial meniscus, unspecified knee
    - M23.02 Cystic meniscus, posterior horn of medial meniscus
      - M23.021 Cystic meniscus, posterior horn of medial meniscus, right knee
      - M23.022 Cystic meniscus, posterior horn of medial meniscus, left knee
      - M23.029 Cystic meniscus, posterior horn of medial meniscus, unspecified knee
  - M23.03 Cystic meniscus, other medial meniscus
    - M23.031 Cystic meniscus, other medial meniscus, right knee
    - M23.032 Cystic meniscus, other medial meniscus, left knee
    - M23.039 Cystic meniscus, other medial meniscus, unspecified knee
  - M23.04 Cystic meniscus, anterior horn of lateral meniscus
    - M23.041 Cystic meniscus, anterior horn of lateral meniscus, right knee
    - M23.042 Cystic meniscus, anterior horn of lateral meniscus, left knee
    - M23.049 Cystic meniscus, anterior horn of lateral meniscus, unspecified knee
  - M23.05 Cystic meniscus, posterior horn of lateral meniscus
    - M23.051 Cystic meniscus, posterior horn of lateral meniscus, right knee
    - M23.052 Cystic meniscus, posterior horn of lateral meniscus, left knee
    - M23.059 Cystic meniscus, posterior horn of lateral meniscus, unspecified knee
  - M23.06 Cystic meniscus, other lateral meniscus
    - M23.061 Cystic meniscus, other lateral meniscus, right knee
    - M23.062 Cystic meniscus, other lateral meniscus, left knee
    - M23.069 Cystic meniscus, other lateral meniscus, unspecified knee

(See Plate 509 on page NAP-31.)

  - M23.2 Derangement of meniscus due to old tear or injury
    Old bucket-handle tear
    - M23.20 Derangement of unspecified meniscus due to old tear or injury
      Derangement of unspecified lateral meniscus due to old tear or injury
      Derangement of unspecified medial meniscus due to old tear or injury
      - M23.200 Derangement of unspecified lateral meniscus due to old tear or injury, right knee
      - M23.201 Derangement of unspecified lateral meniscus due to old tear or injury, left knee
      - M23.202 Derangement of unspecified lateral meniscus due to old tear or injury, unspecified knee
      - M23.203 Derangement of unspecified medial meniscus due to old tear or injury, right knee
      - M23.204 Derangement of unspecified medial meniscus due to old tear or injury, left knee
      - M23.205 Derangement of unspecified medial meniscus due to old tear or injury, unspecified knee
      - M23.206 Derangement of unspecified meniscus due to old tear or injury, right knee

CHAPTER 13 (M00-M99)

M23.207 Derangement of unspecified meniscus due to old tear or injury, left knee

M23.209 Derangement of unspecified meniscus due to old tear or injury, unspecified knee

● **M23.21 Derangement of anterior horn of medial meniscus due to old tear or injury**

M23.211 Derangement of anterior horn of medial meniscus due to old tear or injury, right knee

M23.212 Derangement of anterior horn of medial meniscus due to old tear or injury, left knee

M23.219 Derangement of anterior horn of medial meniscus due to old tear or injury, unspecified knee

● **M23.22 Derangement of posterior horn of medial meniscus due to old tear or injury**

M23.221 Derangement of posterior horn of medial meniscus due to old tear or injury, right knee

M23.222 Derangement of posterior horn of medial meniscus due to old tear or injury, left knee

M23.229 Derangement of posterior horn of medial meniscus due to old tear or injury, unspecified knee

● **M23.23 Derangement of other medial meniscus due to old tear or injury**

M23.231 Derangement of other medial meniscus due to old tear or injury, right knee

M23.232 Derangement of other medial meniscus due to old tear or injury, left knee

M23.239 Derangement of other medial meniscus due to old tear or injury, unspecified knee

● **M23.24 Derangement of anterior horn of lateral meniscus due to old tear or injury**

M23.241 Derangement of anterior horn of lateral meniscus due to old tear or injury, right knee

M23.242 Derangement of anterior horn of lateral meniscus due to old tear or injury, left knee

M23.249 Derangement of anterior horn of lateral meniscus due to old tear or injury, unspecified knee

● **M23.25 Derangement of posterior horn of lateral meniscus due to old tear or injury**

M23.251 Derangement of posterior horn of lateral meniscus due to old tear or injury, right knee

M23.252 Derangement of posterior horn of lateral meniscus due to old tear or injury, left knee

M23.259 Derangement of posterior horn of lateral meniscus due to old tear or injury, unspecified knee

● **M23.26 Derangement of other lateral meniscus due to old tear or injury**

M23.261 Derangement of other lateral meniscus due to old tear or injury, right knee

M23.262 Derangement of other lateral meniscus due to old tear or injury, left knee

M23.269 Derangement of other lateral meniscus due to old tear or injury, unspecified knee

● **M23.3 Other meniscus derangements**
Degenerate meniscus
Detached meniscus
Retained meniscus

● **M23.30 Other meniscus derangements, unspecified meniscus**
Other meniscus derangements, unspecified lateral meniscus
Other meniscus derangements, unspecified medial meniscus

M23.300 Other meniscus derangements, unspecified lateral meniscus, right knee

M23.301 Other meniscus derangements, unspecified lateral meniscus, left knee

M23.302 Other meniscus derangements, unspecified lateral meniscus, unspecified knee

M23.303 Other meniscus derangements, unspecified medial meniscus, right knee

M23.304 Other meniscus derangements, unspecified medial meniscus, left knee

M23.305 Other meniscus derangements, unspecified medial meniscus, unspecified knee

M23.306 Other meniscus derangements, unspecified meniscus, right knee

M23.307 Other meniscus derangements, unspecified meniscus, left knee

M23.309 Other meniscus derangements, unspecified meniscus, unspecified knee

● **M23.31 Other meniscus derangements, anterior horn of medial meniscus**

M23.311 Other meniscus derangements, anterior horn of medial meniscus, right knee

M23.312 Other meniscus derangements, anterior horn of medial meniscus, left knee

M23.319 Other meniscus derangements, anterior horn of medial meniscus, unspecified knee

● **M23.32 Other meniscus derangements, posterior horn of medial meniscus**

M23.321 Other meniscus derangements, posterior horn of medial meniscus, right knee

M23.322 Other meniscus derangements, posterior horn of medial meniscus, left knee

M23.329 Other meniscus derangements, posterior horn of medial meniscus, unspecified knee

● Unacceptable Principal Diagnosis   ● Use Additional Character(s)   ▪ Unspecified   ▶ Manifestation Code

OGCR Official Guidelines for Coding and Reporting   Excludes 1   Excludes 2   Includes   Use additional   Code first   Code also

CHAPTER 13 (M00-M99)

● M23.33 **Other meniscus derangements, other medial meniscus**

    M23.331 **Other meniscus derangements, other medial meniscus, right knee**

    M23.332 **Other meniscus derangements, other medial meniscus, left knee**

    M23.339 **Other meniscus derangements, other medial meniscus, unspecified knee**

● M23.34 **Other meniscus derangements, anterior horn of lateral meniscus**

    M23.341 **Other meniscus derangements, anterior horn of lateral meniscus, right knee**

    M23.342 **Other meniscus derangements, anterior horn of lateral meniscus, left knee**

    M23.349 **Other meniscus derangements, anterior horn of lateral meniscus, unspecified knee**

● M23.35 **Other meniscus derangements, posterior horn of lateral meniscus**

    M23.351 **Other meniscus derangements, posterior horn of lateral meniscus, right knee**

    M23.352 **Other meniscus derangements, posterior horn of lateral meniscus, left knee**

    M23.359 **Other meniscus derangements, posterior horn of lateral meniscus, unspecified knee**

● M23.36 **Other meniscus derangements, other lateral meniscus**

    M23.361 **Other meniscus derangements, other lateral meniscus, right knee**

    M23.362 **Other meniscus derangements, other lateral meniscus, left knee**

    M23.369 **Other meniscus derangements, other lateral meniscus, unspecified knee**

● M23.4 **Loose body in knee**

    M23.40 **Loose body in knee, unspecified knee**

    M23.41 **Loose body in knee, right knee**

    M23.42 **Loose body in knee, left knee**

● M23.5 **Chronic instability of knee**

    M23.50 **Chronic instability of knee, unspecified knee**

    M23.51 **Chronic instability of knee, right knee**

    M23.52 **Chronic instability of knee, left knee**

● M23.6 **Other spontaneous disruption of ligament(s) of knee**

    ● M23.60 **Other spontaneous disruption of unspecified ligament of knee**

        M23.601 **Other spontaneous disruption of unspecified ligament of right knee**

        M23.602 **Other spontaneous disruption of unspecified ligament of left knee**

        M23.609 **Other spontaneous disruption of unspecified ligament of unspecified knee**

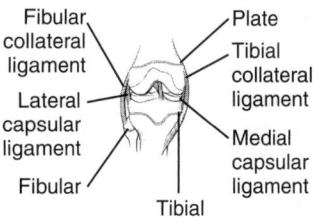

Figure 13-2 Collateral and cruciate ligament of knee. (From DeLee: DeLee and Drez's Orthopaedic Sports Medicine, 2nd ed. 2002, Saunders.)

● M23.61 **Other spontaneous disruption of anterior cruciate ligament of knee**

    M23.611 **Other spontaneous disruption of anterior cruciate ligament of right knee**

    M23.612 **Other spontaneous disruption of anterior cruciate ligament of left knee**

    M23.619 **Other spontaneous disruption of anterior cruciate ligament of unspecified knee**

● M23.62 **Other spontaneous disruption of posterior cruciate ligament of knee**

    M23.621 **Other spontaneous disruption of posterior cruciate ligament of right knee**

    M23.622 **Other spontaneous disruption of posterior cruciate ligament of left knee**

    M23.629 **Other spontaneous disruption of posterior cruciate ligament of unspecified knee**

● M23.63 **Other spontaneous disruption of medial collateral ligament of knee**

    M23.631 **Other spontaneous disruption of medial collateral ligament of right knee**

    M23.632 **Other spontaneous disruption of medial collateral ligament of left knee**

    M23.639 **Other spontaneous disruption of medial collateral ligament of unspecified knee**

● M23.64 **Other spontaneous disruption of lateral collateral ligament of knee**

    M23.641 **Other spontaneous disruption of lateral collateral ligament of right knee**

    M23.642 **Other spontaneous disruption of lateral collateral ligament of left knee**

    M23.649 **Other spontaneous disruption of lateral collateral ligament of unspecified knee**

● M23.67 **Other spontaneous disruption of capsular ligament of knee**

    M23.671 **Other spontaneous disruption of capsular ligament of right knee**

    M23.672 **Other spontaneous disruption of capsular ligament of left knee**

    M23.679 **Other spontaneous disruption of capsular ligament of unspecified knee**

CHAPTER 13 (M00-M99)

N Newborn Age: 0   **P** Pediatric Age: 0–17   **M** Maternity DX: 12–55   **A** Adult Age: 15–124   ♀ Females Only   ♂ Males Only

🗝 Complication\Comorbidity   🗝 Major C\C   ◑ Present on Admission Requirement   ◔ Hospital-Acquired Condition

1181

CHAPTER 13 (M00-M99)

● **M23.8 Other internal derangements of knee**
    Laxity of ligament of knee
    Snapping knee

  ● **M23.8X Other internal derangements of knee**

      M23.8X1 Other internal derangements of right knee

      M23.8X2 Other internal derangements of left knee

      ■ **M23.8X9 Other internal derangements of unspecified knee**

● **M23.9 Unspecified internal derangement of knee**

  ■ **M23.90 Unspecified internal derangement of unspecified knee**

  ■ **M23.91 Unspecified internal derangement of right knee**

  ■ **M23.92 Unspecified internal derangement of left knee**

● **M24 Other specific joint derangements**

  Excludes1   current injury - see injury of joint by body region

  Excludes2   ganglion (M67.4)
                snapping knee (M23.8-)
                temporomandibular joint disorders (M26.6-)

  ● **M24.0 Loose body in joint**

    Excludes2   loose body in knee (M23.4)

    ■ **M24.00 Loose body in unspecified joint**

    ● **M24.01 Loose body in shoulder**

      M24.011 Loose body in right shoulder

      M24.012 Loose body in left shoulder

      ■ **M24.019 Loose body in unspecified shoulder**

    ● **M24.02 Loose body in elbow**

      M24.021 Loose body in right elbow

      M24.022 Loose body in left elbow

      ■ **M24.029 Loose body in unspecified elbow**

    ● **M24.03 Loose body in wrist**

      M24.031 Loose body in right wrist

      M24.032 Loose body in left wrist

      ■ **M24.039 Loose body in unspecified wrist**

    ● **M24.04 Loose body in finger joints**

      M24.041 Loose body in right finger joint(s)

      M24.042 Loose body in left finger joint(s)

      ■ **M24.049 Loose body in unspecified finger joint(s)**

    ● **M24.05 Loose body in hip**

      M24.051 Loose body in right hip

      M24.052 Loose body in left hip

      ■ **M24.059 Loose body in unspecified hip**

    ● **M24.07 Loose body in ankle and toe joints**

      M24.071 Loose body in right ankle

      M24.072 Loose body in left ankle

      M24.073 Loose body in unspecified ankle

      M24.074 Loose body in right toe joint(s)

      M24.075 Loose body in left toe joint(s)

      ■ **M24.076 Loose body in unspecified toe joints**

    M24.08 Loose body, other site

● **M24.1 Other articular cartilage disorders**

  Excludes2   chondrocalcinosis (M11.1, M11.2-)
                internal derangement of knee (M23.-)
                metastatic calcification (E83.5)
                ochronosis (E70.2)

  ■ **M24.10 Other articular cartilage disorders, unspecified site**

  ● **M24.11 Other articular cartilage disorders, shoulder**

    M24.111 Other articular cartilage disorders, right shoulder

    M24.112 Other articular cartilage disorders, left shoulder

    ■ **M24.119 Other articular cartilage disorders, unspecified shoulder**

  ● **M24.12 Other articular cartilage disorders, elbow**

    M24.121 Other articular cartilage disorders, right elbow

    M24.122 Other articular cartilage disorders, left elbow

    ■ **M24.129 Other articular cartilage disorders, unspecified elbow**

  ● **M24.13 Other articular cartilage disorders, wrist**

    M24.131 Other articular cartilage disorders, right wrist

    M24.132 Other articular cartilage disorders, left wrist

    ■ **M24.139 Other articular cartilage disorders, unspecified wrist**

  ● **M24.14 Other articular cartilage disorders, hand**

    M24.141 Other articular cartilage disorders, right hand

    M24.142 Other articular cartilage disorders, left hand

    ■ **M24.149 Other articular cartilage disorders, unspecified hand**

  ● **M24.15 Other articular cartilage disorders, hip**

    M24.151 Other articular cartilage disorders, right hip

    M24.152 Other articular cartilage disorders, left hip

    ■ **M24.159 Other articular cartilage disorders, unspecified hip**

  ● **M24.17 Other articular cartilage disorders, ankle and foot**

    M24.171 Other articular cartilage disorders, right ankle

    M24.172 Other articular cartilage disorders, left ankle

    ■ **M24.173 Other articular cartilage disorders, unspecified ankle**

    M24.174 Other articular cartilage disorders, right foot

    M24.175 Other articular cartilage disorders, left foot

    ■ **M24.176 Other articular cartilage disorders, unspecified foot**

● Unacceptable Principal Diagnosis   ● Use Additional Character(s)   ■ Unspecified   ▶ Manifestation Code
OGCR Official Guidelines for Coding and Reporting   Excludes 1   Excludes 2   Includes   Use additional   Code first   Code also

- **M24.2 Disorder of ligament**
  Instability secondary to old ligament injury
  Ligamentous laxity NOS
  > **Excludes1**   familial ligamentous laxity (M35.7)
  > **Excludes2**   internal derangement of knee (M23.5-M23.89)
  - M24.20 Disorder of ligament, unspecified site
  - M24.21 Disorder of ligament, shoulder
    - M24.211 Disorder of ligament, right shoulder
    - M24.212 Disorder of ligament, left shoulder
    - M24.219 Disorder of ligament, unspecified shoulder
  - M24.22 Disorder of ligament, elbow
    - M24.221 Disorder of ligament, right elbow
    - M24.222 Disorder of ligament, left elbow
    - M24.229 Disorder of ligament, unspecified elbow
  - M24.23 Disorder of ligament, wrist
    - M24.231 Disorder of ligament, right wrist
    - M24.232 Disorder of ligament, left wrist
    - M24.239 Disorder of ligament, unspecified wrist
  - M24.24 Disorder of ligament, hand
    - M24.241 Disorder of ligament, right hand
    - M24.242 Disorder of ligament, left hand
    - M24.249 Disorder of ligament, unspecified hand
  - M24.25 Disorder of ligament, hip
    - M24.251 Disorder of ligament, right hip
    - M24.252 Disorder of ligament, left hip
    - M24.259 Disorder of ligament, unspecified hip
  - M24.27 Disorder of ligament, ankle and foot
    - M24.271 Disorder of ligament, right ankle
    - M24.272 Disorder of ligament, left ankle
    - M24.273 Disorder of ligament, unspecified ankle
    - M24.274 Disorder of ligament, right foot
    - M24.275 Disorder of ligament, left foot
    - M24.276 Disorder of ligament, unspecified foot
  - M24.28 Disorder of ligament, vertebrae
- **M24.3 Pathological dislocation of joint, not elsewhere classified**
  > **Excludes1**   congenital dislocation or displacement of joint - see congenital malformations and deformations of the musculoskeletal system (Q65-Q79)
  > current injury - see injury of joints and ligaments by body region
  > recurrent dislocation of joint (M24.4-)
  - M24.30 Pathological dislocation of unspecified joint, not elsewhere classified
  - M24.31 Pathological dislocation of shoulder, not elsewhere classified
    - M24.311 Pathological dislocation of right shoulder, not elsewhere classified
    - M24.312 Pathological dislocation of left shoulder, not elsewhere classified
  - M24.319 Pathological dislocation of unspecified shoulder, not elsewhere classified
- M24.32 Pathological dislocation of elbow, not elsewhere classified
    - M24.321 Pathological dislocation of right elbow, not elsewhere classified
    - M24.322 Pathological dislocation of left elbow, not elsewhere classified
    - M24.329 Pathological dislocation of unspecified elbow, not elsewhere classified
  - M24.33 Pathological dislocation of wrist, not elsewhere classified
    - M24.331 Pathological dislocation of right wrist, not elsewhere classified
    - M24.332 Pathological dislocation of left wrist, not elsewhere classified
    - M24.339 Pathological dislocation of unspecified wrist, not elsewhere classified
  - M24.34 Pathological dislocation of hand, not elsewhere classified
    - M24.341 Pathological dislocation of right hand, not elsewhere classified
    - M24.342 Pathological dislocation of left hand, not elsewhere classified
    - M24.349 Pathological dislocation of unspecified hand, not elsewhere classified
  - M24.35 Pathological dislocation of hip, not elsewhere classified
    - M24.351 Pathological dislocation of right hip, not elsewhere classified
    - M24.352 Pathological dislocation of left hip, not elsewhere classified
    - M24.359 Pathological dislocation of unspecified hip, not elsewhere classified
  - M24.36 Pathological dislocation of knee, not elsewhere classified
    - M24.361 Pathological dislocation of right knee, not elsewhere classified
    - M24.362 Pathological dislocation of left knee, not elsewhere classified
    - M24.369 Pathological dislocation of unspecified knee, not elsewhere classified
  - M24.37 Pathological dislocation of ankle and foot, not elsewhere classified
    - M24.371 Pathological dislocation of right ankle, not elsewhere classified
    - M24.372 Pathological dislocation of left ankle, not elsewhere classified
    - M24.373 Pathological dislocation of unspecified ankle, not elsewhere classified
    - M24.374 Pathological dislocation of right foot, not elsewhere classified
    - M24.375 Pathological dislocation of left foot, not elsewhere classified
    - M24.376 Pathological dislocation of unspecified foot, not elsewhere classified

N Newborn Age: 0   **P** Pediatric Age: 0–17   **M** Maternity DX: 12–55   **A** Adult Age: 15–124   ♀ Females Only   ♂ Males Only

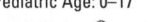 Complication\Comorbidity   Major C\C   Present on Admission Requirement   Hospital-Acquired Condition

1183

CHAPTER 13 (M00-M99)

● M24.4 **Recurrent dislocation of joint**
    Recurrent subluxation of joint

    | Excludes2 | recurrent dislocation of patella (M22.0-M22.1) |
                recurrent vertebral dislocation (M43.3-, M43.4, M43.5-)

■ M24.40 Recurrent dislocation, unspecified joint

● M24.41 Recurrent dislocation, shoulder
    M24.411 Recurrent dislocation, right shoulder
    M24.412 Recurrent dislocation, left shoulder
    ■ M24.419 Recurrent dislocation, unspecified shoulder

● M24.42 Recurrent dislocation, elbow
    M24.421 Recurrent dislocation, right elbow
    M24.422 Recurrent dislocation, left elbow
    ■ M24.429 Recurrent dislocation, unspecified elbow

● M24.43 Recurrent dislocation, wrist
    M24.431 Recurrent dislocation, right wrist
    M24.432 Recurrent dislocation, left wrist
    ■ M24.439 Recurrent dislocation, unspecified wrist

● M24.44 Recurrent dislocation, hand and finger(s)
    M24.441 Recurrent dislocation, right hand
    M24.442 Recurrent dislocation, left hand
    ■ M24.443 Recurrent dislocation, unspecified hand
    M24.444 Recurrent dislocation, right finger
    M24.445 Recurrent dislocation, left finger
    ■ M24.446 Recurrent dislocation, unspecified finger

● M24.45 Recurrent dislocation, hip
    M24.451 Recurrent dislocation, right hip
    M24.452 Recurrent dislocation, left hip
    ■ M24.459 Recurrent dislocation, unspecified hip

● M24.46 Recurrent dislocation, knee
    M24.461 Recurrent dislocation, right knee
    M24.462 Recurrent dislocation, left knee
    ■ M24.469 Recurrent dislocation, unspecified knee

● M24.47 Recurrent dislocation, ankle, foot and toes
    M24.471 Recurrent dislocation, right ankle
    M24.472 Recurrent dislocation, left ankle
    ■ M24.473 Recurrent dislocation, unspecified ankle
    M24.474 Recurrent dislocation, right foot
    M24.475 Recurrent dislocation, left foot
    M24.476 Recurrent dislocation, unspecified foot
    M24.477 Recurrent dislocation, right toe(s)
    M24.478 Recurrent dislocation, left toe(s)
    ■ M24.479 Recurrent dislocation, unspecified toe(s)

● M24.5 **Contracture of joint**

    | Excludes1 | contracture of muscle without contracture of joint (M62.4-) |
                contracture of tendon (sheath) without contracture of joint (M62.4-)
                Dupuytren's contracture (M72.0)

    | Excludes2 | acquired deformities of limbs (M20-M21) |

■ M24.50 Contracture, unspecified joint

● M24.51 Contracture, shoulder
    M24.511 Contracture, right shoulder
    M24.512 Contracture, left shoulder
    ■ M24.519 Contracture, unspecified shoulder

● M24.52 Contracture, elbow
    M24.521 Contracture, right elbow
    M24.522 Contracture, left elbow
    ■ M24.529 Contracture, unspecified elbow

● M24.53 Contracture, wrist
    M24.531 Contracture, right wrist
    M24.532 Contracture, left wrist
    ■ M24.539 Contracture, unspecified wrist

● M24.54 Contracture, hand
    M24.541 Contracture, right hand
    M24.542 Contracture, left hand
    ■ M24.549 Contracture, unspecified hand

● M24.55 Contracture, hip
    M24.551 Contracture, right hip
    M24.552 Contracture, left hip
    ■ M24.559 Contracture, unspecified hip

● M24.56 Contracture, knee
    M24.561 Contracture, right knee
    M24.562 Contracture, left knee
    ■ M24.569 Contracture, unspecified knee

● M24.57 Contracture, ankle and foot
    M24.571 Contracture, right ankle
    M24.572 Contracture, left ankle
    ■ M24.573 Contracture, unspecified ankle
    M24.574 Contracture, right foot
    M24.575 Contracture, left foot
    ■ M24.576 Contracture, unspecified foot

● M24.6 **Ankylosis of joint**

    | Excludes1 | stiffness of joint without ankylosis (M25.6-) |

    | Excludes2 | spine (M43.2-) |

■ M24.60 Ankylosis, unspecified joint

● M24.61 Ankylosis, shoulder
    M24.611 Ankylosis, right shoulder
    M24.612 Ankylosis, left shoulder
    ■ M24.619 Ankylosis, unspecified shoulder

● M24.62 Ankylosis, elbow
    M24.621 Ankylosis, right elbow
    M24.622 Ankylosis, left elbow
    ■ M24.629 Ankylosis, unspecified elbow

● Unacceptable Principal Diagnosis   ● Use Additional Character(s)   ■ Unspecified   ▶ Manifestation Code

OGCR Official Guidelines for Coding and Reporting   Excludes 1   Excludes 2   Includes   Use additional   Code first   Code also

1184

Item 13-5 Ankylosis or arthrokleisis is a consolidation of a joint due to disease, injury, or surgical procedure. Spondylosis is the degeneration of the vertebral processes and formation of osteophytes and commonly occurs with age. **Spondylitis** or ankylosing spondylitis is a type of arthritis that affects the spine or backbone causing back pain and stiffness.

● M24.63 Ankylosis, wrist
    M24.631 Ankylosis, right wrist
    M24.632 Ankylosis, left wrist
    ■ M24.639 Ankylosis, unspecified wrist
● M24.64 Ankylosis, hand
    M24.641 Ankylosis, right hand
    M24.642 Ankylosis, left hand
    ■ M24.649 Ankylosis, unspecified hand
● M24.65 Ankylosis, hip
    M24.651 Ankylosis, right hip
    M24.652 Ankylosis, left hip
    ■ M24.659 Ankylosis, unspecified hip
● M24.66 Ankylosis, knee
    M24.661 Ankylosis, right knee
    M24.662 Ankylosis, left knee
    ■ M24.669 Ankylosis, unspecified knee
● M24.67 Ankylosis, ankle and foot
    M24.671 Ankylosis, right ankle
    M24.672 Ankylosis, left ankle
    ■ M24.673 Ankylosis, unspecified ankle
    M24.674 Ankylosis, right foot
    M24.675 Ankylosis, left foot
    ■ M24.676 Ankylosis, unspecified foot
 M24.7 Protrusio acetabuli
● M24.8 Other specific joint derangements, not elsewhere classified
    Excludes2   iliotibial band syndrome (M76.3)
  ■ M24.80 Other specific joint derangements of unspecified joint, not elsewhere classified
● M24.81 Other specific joint derangements of shoulder, not elsewhere classified
    M24.811 Other specific joint derangements of right shoulder, not elsewhere classified
    M24.812 Other specific joint derangements of left shoulder, not elsewhere classified
    ■ M24.819 Other specific joint derangements of unspecified shoulder, not elsewhere classified
● M24.82 Other specific joint derangements of elbow, not elsewhere classified
    M24.821 Other specific joint derangements of right elbow, not elsewhere classified
    M24.822 Other specific joint derangements of left elbow, not elsewhere classified
    ■ M24.829 Other specific joint derangements of unspecified elbow, not elsewhere classified

● M24.83 Other specific joint derangements of wrist, not elsewhere classified
    M24.831 Other specific joint derangements of right wrist, not elsewhere classified
    M24.832 Other specific joint derangements of left wrist, not elsewhere classified
    ■ M24.839 Other specific joint derangements of unspecified wrist, not elsewhere classified
● M24.84 Other specific joint derangements of hand, not elsewhere classified
    M24.841 Other specific joint derangements of right hand, not elsewhere classified
    M24.842 Other specific joint derangements of left hand, not elsewhere classified
    ■ M24.849 Other specific joint derangements of unspecified hand, not elsewhere classified
● M24.85 Other specific joint derangements of hip, not elsewhere classified
    Irritable hip
    M24.851 Other specific joint derangements of right hip, not elsewhere classified
    M24.852 Other specific joint derangements of left hip, not elsewhere classified
    ■ M24.859 Other specific joint derangements of unspecified hip, not elsewhere classified
● M24.87 Other specific joint derangements of ankle and foot, not elsewhere classified
    M24.871 Other specific joint derangements of right ankle, not elsewhere classified
    M24.872 Other specific joint derangements of left ankle, not elsewhere classified
    ■ M24.873 Other specific joint derangements of unspecified ankle, not elsewhere classified
    M24.874 Other specific joint derangements of right foot, not elsewhere classified
    M24.875 Other specific joint derangements left foot, not elsewhere classified
    ■ M24.876 Other specific joint derangements of unspecified foot, not elsewhere classified
■ M24.9 Joint derangement, unspecified

CHAPTER 13 (M00-M99)

● **M25 Other joint disorder, not elsewhere classified**

    | Excludes2 | abnormality of gait and mobility (R26.-)
                     acquired deformities of limb (M20-M21)
                     calcification of bursa (M71.4-)
                     calcification of shoulder (joint) (M75.3)
                     calcification of tendon (M65.2-)
                     difficulty in walking (R26.2)
                     temporomandibular joint disorder (M26.6-)

  ● **M25.0 Hemarthrosis**

      | Excludes1 | current injury - see injury of joint by
                         body region
                       hemophilic arthropathy (M36.2)

    ■ M25.00 Hemarthrosis, unspecified joint 🦴

    ● M25.01 Hemarthrosis, shoulder

        M25.011 Hemarthrosis, right shoulder 🦴

        M25.012 Hemarthrosis, left shoulder 🦴

        ■ M25.019 Hemarthrosis, unspecified
                shoulder 🦴

    ● M25.02 Hemarthrosis, elbow

        M25.021 Hemarthrosis, right elbow 🦴

        M25.022 Hemarthrosis, left elbow 🦴

        ■ M25.029 Hemarthrosis, unspecified
                elbow 🦴

    ● M25.03 Hemarthrosis, wrist

        M25.031 Hemarthrosis, right wrist 🦴

        M25.032 Hemarthrosis, left wrist 🦴

        ■ M25.039 Hemarthrosis, unspecified
                wrist 🦴

    ● M25.04 Hemarthrosis, hand

        M25.041 Hemarthrosis, right hand 🦴

        M25.042 Hemarthrosis, left hand 🦴

        ■ M25.049 Hemarthrosis, unspecified
                hand 🦴

    ● M25.05 Hemarthrosis, hip

        M25.051 Hemarthrosis, right hip 🦴

        M25.052 Hemarthrosis, left hip 🦴

        ■ M25.059 Hemarthrosis, unspecified hip 🦴

    ● M25.06 Hemarthrosis, knee

        M25.061 Hemarthrosis, right knee 🦴

        M25.062 Hemarthrosis, left knee 🦴

        ■ M25.069 Hemarthrosis, unspecified
                knee 🦴

    ● M25.07 Hemarthrosis, ankle and foot

        M25.071 Hemarthrosis, right ankle 🦴

        M25.072 Hemarthrosis, left ankle 🦴

        ■ M25.073 Hemarthrosis, unspecified
                ankle 🦴

        M25.074 Hemarthrosis, right foot 🦴

        M25.075 Hemarthrosis, left foot 🦴

        ■ M25.076 Hemarthrosis, unspecified foot 🦴

    M25.08 Hemarthrosis, vertebrae 🦴

  ● **M25.1 Fistula of joint**

    ■ M25.10 Fistula, unspecified joint

    ● M25.11 Fistula, shoulder

        M25.111 Fistula, right shoulder

        M25.112 Fistula, left shoulder

        ■ M25.119 Fistula, unspecified shoulder

● M25.12 Fistula, elbow

    M25.121 Fistula, right elbow

    M25.122 Fistula, left elbow

    ■ M25.129 Fistula, unspecified elbow

● M25.13 Fistula, wrist

    M25.131 Fistula, right wrist

    M25.132 Fistula, left wrist

    ■ M25.139 Fistula, unspecified wrist

● M25.14 Fistula, hand

    M25.141 Fistula, right hand

    M25.142 Fistula, left hand

    ■ M25.149 Fistula, unspecified hand

● M25.15 Fistula, hip

    M25.151 Fistula, right hip

    M25.152 Fistula, left hip

    ■ M25.159 Fistula, unspecified hip

● M25.16 Fistula, knee

    M25.161 Fistula, right knee

    M25.162 Fistula, left knee

    ■ M25.169 Fistula, unspecified knee

● M25.17 Fistula, ankle and foot

    M25.171 Fistula, right ankle

    M25.172 Fistula, left ankle

    ■ M25.173 Fistula, unspecified ankle

    M25.174 Fistula, right foot

    M25.175 Fistula, left foot

    ■ M25.176 Fistula, unspecified foot

  M25.18 Fistula, vertebrae

● **M25.2 Flail joint**

  ■ M25.20 Flail joint, unspecified joint

  ● M25.21 Flail joint, shoulder

    M25.211 Flail joint, right shoulder

    M25.212 Flail joint, left shoulder

    ■ M25.219 Flail joint, unspecified shoulder

  ● M25.22 Flail joint, elbow

    M25.221 Flail joint, right elbow

    M25.222 Flail joint, left elbow

    ■ M25.229 Flail joint, unspecified elbow

  ● M25.23 Flail joint, wrist

    M25.231 Flail joint, right wrist

    M25.232 Flail joint, left wrist

    ■ M25.239 Flail joint, unspecified wrist

  ● M25.24 Flail joint, hand

    M25.241 Flail joint, right hand

    M25.242 Flail joint, left hand

    ■ M25.249 Flail joint, unspecified hand

  ● M25.25 Flail joint, hip

    M25.251 Flail joint, right hip

    M25.252 Flail joint, left hip

    ■ M25.259 Flail joint, unspecified hip

  ● M25.26 Flail joint, knee

    M25.261 Flail joint, right knee

    M25.262 Flail joint, left knee

    ■ M25.269 Flail joint, unspecified knee

● Unacceptable Principal Diagnosis   ● Use Additional Character(s)   ■ Unspecified   ▶ Manifestation Code

OGCR Official Guidelines for Coding and Reporting | Excludes 1 | | Excludes 2 | | Includes | | Use additional | | Code first | | Code also |

● M25.27 Flail joint, ankle and foot

    M25.271 Flail joint, right ankle and foot

    M25.272 Flail joint, left ankle and foot

    ■ M25.279 Flail joint, unspecified ankle and foot

    M25.28 Flail joint, other site

● M25.3 Other instability of joint

    Excludes1 instability of joint secondary to old ligament injury (M24.2-)
    instability of joint secondary to removal of joint prosthesis (M96.8-)

    Excludes2 spinal instabilities (M53.2-)

    ■ M25.30 Other instability, unspecified joint

● M25.31 Other instability, shoulder

    M25.311 Other instability, right shoulder

    M25.312 Other instability, left shoulder

    ■ M25.319 Other instability, unspecified shoulder

● M25.32 Other instability, elbow

    M25.321 Other instability, right elbow

    M25.322 Other instability, left elbow

    ■ M25.329 Other instability, unspecified elbow

● M25.33 Other instability, wrist

    M25.331 Other instability, right wrist

    M25.332 Other instability, left wrist

    ■ M25.339 Other instability, unspecified wrist

● M25.34 Other instability, hand

    M25.341 Other instability, right hand

    M25.342 Other instability, left hand

    ■ M25.349 Other instability, unspecified hand

● M25.35 Other instability, hip

    M25.351 Other instability, right hip

    M25.352 Other instability, left hip

    ■ M25.359 Other instability, unspecified hip

● M25.36 Other instability, knee

    M25.361 Other instability, right knee

    M25.362 Other instability, left knee

    ■ M25.369 Other instability, unspecified knee

● M25.37 Other instability, ankle and foot

    M25.371 Other instability, right ankle

    M25.372 Other instability, left ankle

    ■ M25.373 Other instability, unspecified ankle

    M25.374 Other instability, right foot

    M25.375 Other instability, left foot

    ■ M25.376 Other instability, unspecified foot

● M25.4 Effusion of joint

    Excludes1 hydrarthrosis in yaws (A66.6)
    intermittent hydrarthrosis (M12.4-)
    other infective (teno)synovitis (M65.1-)

    ■ M25.40 Effusion, unspecified joint

● M25.41 Effusion, shoulder

    M25.411 Effusion, right shoulder

    M25.412 Effusion, left shoulder

    ■ M25.419 Effusion, unspecified shoulder

● M25.42 Effusion, elbow

    M25.421 Effusion, right elbow

    M25.422 Effusion, left elbow

    ■ M25.429 Effusion, unspecified elbow

● M25.43 Effusion, wrist

    M25.431 Effusion, right wrist

    M25.432 Effusion, left wrist

    ■ M25.439 Effusion, unspecified wrist

● M25.44 Effusion, hand

    M25.441 Effusion, right hand

    M25.442 Effusion, left hand

    ■ M25.449 Effusion, unspecified hand

● M25.45 Effusion, hip

    M25.451 Effusion, right hip

    M25.452 Effusion, left hip

    ■ M25.459 Effusion, unspecified hip

● M25.46 Effusion, knee

    M25.461 Effusion, right knee

    M25.462 Effusion, left knee

    ■ M25.469 Effusion, unspecified knee

● M25.47 Effusion, ankle and foot

    M25.471 Effusion, right ankle

    M25.472 Effusion, left ankle

    ■ M25.473 Effusion, unspecified ankle

    M25.474 Effusion, right foot

    M25.475 Effusion, left foot

    ■ M25.476 Effusion, unspecified foot

    M25.48 Effusion, other site

● M25.5 Pain in joint

    Excludes2 pain in hand (M79.64-)
    pain in fingers (M79.64-)
    pain in foot (M79.67-)
    pain in limb (M79.6-)
    pain in toes (M79.67-)

    ■ M25.50 Pain in unspecified joint

● M25.51 Pain in shoulder

    M25.511 Pain in right shoulder

    M25.512 Pain in left shoulder

    ■ M25.519 Pain in unspecified shoulder

● M25.52 Pain in elbow

    M25.521 Pain in right elbow

    M25.522 Pain in left elbow

    ■ M25.529 Pain in unspecified elbow

● M25.53 Pain in wrist

    M25.531 Pain in right wrist

    M25.532 Pain in left wrist

    ■ M25.539 Pain in unspecified wrist

● M25.55 Pain in hip

    M25.551 Pain in right hip

    M25.552 Pain in left hip

    ■ M25.559 Pain in unspecified hip

CHAPTER 13 (M00-M99)

CHAPTER 13 (M00-M99)

● M25.56 Pain in knee

   M25.561 Pain in right knee

   M25.562 Pain in left knee

   ■ M25.569 Pain in unspecified knee

● M25.57 Pain in ankle

   M25.571 Pain in right ankle

   M25.572 Pain in left ankle

   ■ M25.579 Pain in unspecified ankle

● M25.6 Stiffness of joint, not elsewhere classified

   Excludes1   ankylosis of joint (M24.6-)
               contracture of joint (M24.5-)

   ■ M25.60 Stiffness of unspecified joint, not
             elsewhere classified

   ● M25.61 Stiffness of shoulder, not elsewhere
             classified

      M25.611 Stiffness of right shoulder, not
              elsewhere classified

      M25.612 Stiffness of left shoulder, not
              elsewhere classified

      ■ M25.619 Stiffness of unspecified shoulder,
               not elsewhere classified

   ● M25.62 Stiffness of elbow, not elsewhere classified

      M25.621 Stiffness of right elbow, not
              elsewhere classified

      M25.622 Stiffness of left elbow, not
              elsewhere classified

      ■ M25.629 Stiffness of unspecified elbow,
               not elsewhere classified

   ● M25.63 Stiffness of wrist, not elsewhere classified

      M25.631 Stiffness of right wrist, not
              elsewhere classified

      M25.632 Stiffness of left wrist, not
              elsewhere classified

      ■ M25.639 Stiffness of unspecified wrist, not
               elsewhere classified

   ● M25.64 Stiffness of hand, not elsewhere classified

      M25.641 Stiffness of right hand, not
              elsewhere classified

      M25.642 Stiffness of left hand, not
              elsewhere classified

      ■ M25.649 Stiffness of unspecified hand, not
               elsewhere classified

   ● M25.65 Stiffness of hip, not elsewhere classified

      M25.651 Stiffness of right hip, not
              elsewhere classified

      M25.652 Stiffness of left hip, not
              elsewhere classified

      ■ M25.659 Stiffness of unspecified hip, not
               elsewhere classified

   ● M25.66 Stiffness of knee, not elsewhere classified

      M25.661 Stiffness of right knee, not
              elsewhere classified

      M25.662 Stiffness of left knee, not
              elsewhere classified

      ■ M25.669 Stiffness of unspecified knee, not
               elsewhere classified

   ● M25.67 Stiffness of ankle and foot, not elsewhere
             classified

      M25.671 Stiffness of right ankle, not
              elsewhere classified

      M25.672 Stiffness of left ankle, not
              elsewhere classified

   ■ M25.673 Stiffness of unspecified ankle,
            not elsewhere classified

   M25.674 Stiffness of right foot, not
           elsewhere classified

   M25.675 Stiffness of left foot, not
           elsewhere classified

   ■ M25.676 Stiffness of unspecified foot, not
            elsewhere classified

● M25.7 Osteophyte

   ■ M25.70 Osteophyte, unspecified joint

   ● M25.71 Osteophyte, shoulder

      M25.711 Osteophyte, right shoulder

      M25.712 Osteophyte, left shoulder

      ■ M25.719 Osteophyte, unspecified shoulder

   ● M25.72 Osteophyte, elbow

      M25.721 Osteophyte, right elbow

      M25.722 Osteophyte, left elbow

      ■ M25.729 Osteophyte, unspecified elbow

   ● M25.73 Osteophyte, wrist

      M25.731 Osteophyte, right wrist

      M25.732 Osteophyte, left wrist

      ■ M25.739 Osteophyte, unspecified wrist

   ● M25.74 Osteophyte, hand

      M25.741 Osteophyte, right hand

      M25.742 Osteophyte, left hand

      ■ M25.749 Osteophyte, unspecified hand

   ● M25.75 Osteophyte, hip

      M25.751 Osteophyte, right hip

      M25.752 Osteophyte, left hip

      ■ M25.759 Osteophyte, unspecified hip

   ● M25.76 Osteophyte, knee

      M25.761 Osteophyte, right knee

      M25.762 Osteophyte, left knee

      ■ M25.769 Osteophyte, unspecified knee

   ● M25.77 Osteophyte, ankle and foot

      M25.771 Osteophyte, right ankle

      M25.772 Osteophyte, left ankle

      ■ M25.773 Osteophyte, unspecified ankle

      M25.774 Osteophyte, right foot

      M25.775 Osteophyte, left foot

      ■ M25.776 Osteophyte, unspecified foot

   M25.78 Osteophyte, vertebrae

● M25.8 Other specified joint disorders

   ■ M25.80 Other specified joint disorders,
            unspecified joint

   ● M25.81 Other specified joint disorders, shoulder

      M25.811 Other specified joint disorders,
              right shoulder

      M25.812 Other specified joint disorders,
              left shoulder

      ■ M25.819 Other specified joint disorders,
               unspecified shoulder

   ● M25.82 Other specified joint disorders, elbow

      M25.821 Other specified joint disorders,
              right elbow

      M25.822 Other specified joint disorders,
              left elbow

      ■ M25.829 Other specified joint disorders,
               unspecified elbow

● Unacceptable Principal Diagnosis   ● Use Additional Character(s)   ■ Unspecified   ▶ Manifestation Code

OGCR Official Guidelines for Coding and Reporting   Excludes 1   Excludes 2   Includes   Use additional   Code first   Code also

● **M25.83 Other specified joint disorders, wrist**

    M25.831 Other specified joint disorders, right wrist

    M25.832 Other specified joint disorders, left wrist

    ◻ **M25.839 Other specified joint disorders, unspecified wrist**

● **M25.84 Other specified joint disorders, hand**

    M25.841 Other specified joint disorders, right hand

    M25.842 Other specified joint disorders, left hand

    ◻ **M25.849 Other specified joint disorders, unspecified hand**

● **M25.85 Other specified joint disorders, hip**

    M25.851 Other specified joint disorders, right hip

    M25.852 Other specified joint disorders, left hip

    ◻ **M25.859 Other specified joint disorders, unspecified hip**

● **M25.86 Other specified joint disorders, knee**

    M25.861 Other specified joint disorders, right knee

    M25.862 Other specified joint disorders, left knee

    ◻ **M25.869 Other specified joint disorders, unspecified knee**

● **M25.87 Other specified joint disorders, ankle and foot**

    M25.871 Other specified joint disorders, right ankle and foot

    M25.872 Other specified joint disorders, left ankle and foot

    ◻ **M25.879 Other specified joint disorders, unspecified ankle and foot**

◻ **M25.9 Joint disorder, unspecified**

DENTOFACIAL ANOMALIES [INCLUDING MALOCCLUSION] AND OTHER DISORDERS OF JAW (M26-M27)

    Excludes1   hemifacial atrophy or hypertrophy (Q67.4)
                  unilateral condylar hyperplasia or hypoplasia (M27.8)

● **M26 Dentofacial anomalies [including malocclusion]**

   ● **M26.0 Major anomalies of jaw size**

     Excludes1   acromegaly (E22.0)
                   Robin's syndrome (Q87.0)

    ◻ **M26.00 Unspecified anomaly of jaw size**

    M26.01 Maxillary hyperplasia

    M26.02 Maxillary hypoplasia

    M26.03 Mandibular hyperplasia

    M26.04 Mandibular hypoplasia

    M26.05 Macrogenia

    M26.06 Microgenia

    M26.07 Excessive tuberosity of jaw
        Entire maxillary tuberosity

    M26.09 Other specified anomalies of jaw size

Figure 13-3   Dental malocclusion.

Item 13–6   **Hyperplasia** is a condition of overdevelopment, whereas **hypoplasia** is a condition of underdevelopment. **Macrogenia** is overdevelopment of the chin, whereas **microgenia** is underdevelopment of the chin.

● **M26.1 Anomalies of jaw-cranial base relationship**

    ◻ **M26.10 Unspecified anomaly of jaw-cranial base relationship**

    M26.11 Maxillary asymmetry

    M26.12 Other jaw asymmetry

    M26.19 Other specified anomalies of jaw-cranial base relationship

● **M26.2 Anomalies of dental arch relationship**

    ◻ **M26.20 Unspecified anomaly of dental arch relationship**

   ● **M26.21 Malocclusion, Angle's class**

     M26.211 Malocclusion, Angle's class I
        Neutro-occlusion

     M26.212 Malocclusion, Angle's class II
        Disto-occlusion Division I
        Disto-occlusion Division II

     M26.213 Malocclusion, Angle's class III
        Mesio-occlusion

     ◻ **M26.219 Malocclusion, Angle's class, unspecified**

   ● **M26.22 Open occlusal relationship**

     M26.220 Open anterior occlusal relationship
        Anterior openbite

     M26.221 Open posterior occlusal relationship
        Posterior openbite

    M26.23 Excessive horizontal overlap
        Excessive horizontal overjet

    M26.24 Reverse articulation
        Crossbite (anterior) (posterior)

    M26.25 Anomalies of interarch distance

    M26.29 Other anomalies of dental arch relationship
        Midline deviation of dental arch
        Overbite (excessive) deep
        Overbite (excessive) horizontal
        Overbite (excessive) vertical
        Posterior lingual occlusion of mandibular teeth

● **M26.3 Anomalies of tooth position of fully erupted tooth or teeth**

    Excludes2   embedded and impacted teeth (K01.-)

    ◻ **M26.30 Unspecified anomaly of tooth position of fully erupted tooth or teeth**
        Abnormal spacing of fully erupted tooth or teeth NOS
        Displacement of fully erupted tooth or teeth NOS
        Transposition of fully erupted tooth or teeth NOS

CHAPTER 13 (M00-M99)

CHAPTER 13 (M00-M99)

M26.31　Crowding of fully erupted teeth

M26.32　Excessive spacing of fully erupted teeth
　　　　Diastema of fully erupted tooth or teeth NOS

M26.33　Horizontal displacement of fully erupted tooth or teeth
　　　　Tipped tooth or teeth
　　　　Tipping of fully erupted tooth

M26.34　Vertical displacement of fully erupted tooth or teeth
　　　　Extruded tooth
　　　　Infraeruption of tooth or teeth
　　　　Supraeruption of tooth or teeth

M26.35　Rotation of fully erupted tooth or teeth

M26.36　Insufficient interocclusal distance of fully erupted teeth (ridge)
　　　　Lack of adequate intermaxillary vertical dimension of fully erupted teeth

M26.37　Excessive interocclusal distance of fully erupted teeth
　　　　Excessive intermaxillary vertical dimension of fully erupted teeth
　　　　Loss of occlusal vertical dimension of fully erupted teeth

M26.39　Other anomalies of tooth position of fully erupted tooth or teeth

■ M26.4　Malocclusion, unspecified

● M26.5　Dentofacial functional abnormalities
　　Excludes1　bruxism (F45.8)
　　　　　　　　teeth-grinding NOS (F45.8)

■ M26.50　Dentofacial functional abnormalities, unspecified

M26.51　Abnormal jaw closure

M26.52　Limited mandibular range of motion

M26.53　Deviation in opening and closing of the mandible

M26.54　Insufficient anterior guidance
　　　　Insufficient anterior occlusal guidance

M26.55　Centric occlusion maximum intercuspation discrepancy
　　　　Excludes1　centric occlusion NOS (M26.59)

M26.56　Non-working side interference
　　　　Balancing side interference

M26.57　Lack of posterior occlusal support

M26.59　Other dentofacial functional abnormalities
　　　　Centric occlusion (of teeth) NOS
　　　　Malocclusion due to abnormal swallowing
　　　　Malocclusion due to mouth breathing
　　　　Malocclusion due to tongue, lip or finger habits

● M26.6　Temporomandibular joint disorders
　　Excludes2　current temporomandibular joint dislocation (S03.0)
　　　　　　　　current temporomandibular joint sprain (S03.4)

■ M26.60　Temporomandibular joint disorder, unspecified

M26.61　Adhesions and ankylosis of temporomandibular joint

M26.62　Arthralgia of temporomandibular joint

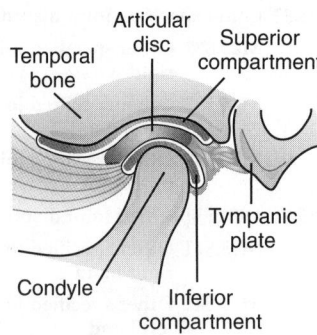

Figure 13-4　Temporomandibular joint.

Item 13-7　Dysfunction of the temporomandibular joint is termed **temporomandibular joint (TMJ) syndrome** and is characterized by pain and tenderness/spasm of the muscles of mastication, joint noise, and in the later stages, limited mandibular movement.

M26.63　Articular disc disorder of temporomandibular joint

M26.69　Other specified disorders of temporomandibular joint

● M26.7　Dental alveolar anomalies

■ M26.70　Unspecified alveolar anomaly

M26.71　Alveolar maxillary hyperplasia

M26.72　Alveolar mandibular hyperplasia

M26.73　Alveolar maxillary hypoplasia

M26.74　Alveolar mandibular hypoplasia

M26.79　Other specified alveolar anomalies

● M26.8　Other dentofacial anomalies

M26.81　Anterior soft tissue impingement
　　　　Anterior soft tissue impingement on teeth

M26.82　Posterior soft tissue impingement
　　　　Posterior soft tissue impingement on teeth

M26.89　Other dentofacial anomalies

■ M26.9　Dentofacial anomaly, unspecified

● M27　Other diseases of jaws

M27.0　Developmental disorders of jaws
　　　　Latent bone cyst of jaw
　　　　Stafne's cyst
　　　　Torus mandibularis
　　　　Torus palatinus

M27.1　Giant cell granuloma, central
　　　　Giant cell granuloma NOS
　　　　Excludes1　peripheral giant cell granuloma (K06.8)

M27.2　Inflammatory conditions of jaws
　　　　Osteitis of jaw(s)
　　　　Osteomyelitis (neonatal) jaw(s)
　　　　Osteoradionecrosis jaw(s)
　　　　Periostitis jaw(s)
　　　　Sequestrum of jaw bone
　　　　Use additional code (W88-W90, X39.0) to identify radiation, if radiation-induced
　　　　Excludes2　osteonecrosis of jaw due to drug (M87.180)

M27.3　Alveolitis of jaws
　　　　Alveolar osteitis
　　　　Dry socket

● **M27.4 Other and unspecified cysts of jaw**

> **Excludes1** cysts of oral region (K09.-)
> latent bone cyst of jaw (M27.0)
> Stafne's cyst (M27.0)

  ■ **M27.40 Unspecified cyst of jaw**
    Cyst of jaw NOS

  M27.49 Other cysts of jaw
    Aneurysmal cyst of jaw
    Hemorrhagic cyst of jaw
    Traumatic cyst of jaw

● **M27.5 Periradicular pathology associated with previous endodontic treatment**

  M27.51 Perforation of root canal space due to endodontic treatment

  M27.52 Endodontic overfill

  M27.53 Endodontic underfill

  M27.59 Other periradicular pathology associated with previous endodontic treatment

● **M27.6 Endosseous dental implant failure**

  M27.61 Osseointegration failure of dental implant
    Hemorrhagic complications of dental implant placement
    Iatrogenic osseointegration failure of dental implant
    Osseointegration failure of dental implant due to complications of systemic disease
    Osseointegration failure of dental implant due to poor bone quality
    Pre-integration failure of dental implant NOS
    Pre-osseointegration failure of dental implant

  M27.62 Post-osseointegration biological failure of dental implant
    Failure of dental implant due to lack of attached gingiva
    Failure of dental implant due to occlusal trauma (caused by poor prosthetic design)
    Failure of dental implant due to parafunctional habits
    Failure of dental implant due to periodontal infection (peri–implantitis)
    Failure of dental implant due to poor oral hygiene
    Iatrogenic post-osseointegration failure of dental implant
    Post-osseointegration failure of dental implant due to complications of systemic disease

  M27.63 Post-osseointegration mechanical failure of dental implant
    Failure of dental prosthesis causing loss of dental implant
    Fracture of dental implant

> **Excludes2** cracked tooth (K03.81)
> fractured dental restorative material with loss of material (K08.531)
> fractured dental restorative material without loss of material (K08.530)
> fractured tooth (S02.5)

  M27.69 Other endosseous dental implant failure
    Dental implant failure NOS

● **M27.8 Other specified diseases of jaws**
  Cherubism
  Exostosis
  Fibrous dysplasia
  Unilateral condylar hyperplasia
  Unilateral condylar hypoplasia

> **Excludes1** jaw pain (R68.84)

■ **M27.9 Disease of jaws, unspecified**

SYSTEMIC CONNECTIVE TISSUE DISORDERS (M30-M36)

> **Includes** autoimmune disease NOS
> collagen (vascular) disease NOS
> systemic autoimmune disease
> systemic collagen (vascular) disease

> **Excludes1** autoimmune disease, single organ or single cell-type - code to relevant condition category

● **M30 Polyarteritis nodosa and related conditions**

> **Excludes1** microscopic polyarteritis (M31.7)

  M30.0 Polyarteritis nodosa 🦠

  M30.1 Polyarteritis with lung involvement [Churg-Strauss] 🦠
    Allergic granulomatous angiitis

  M30.2 Juvenile polyarteritis 🦠

  M30.3 Mucocutaneous lymph node syndrome [Kawasaki] 🦠

  M30.8 Other conditions related to polyarteritis nodosa 🦠
    Polyangiitis overlap syndrome

● **M31 Other necrotizing vasculopathies**

  M31.0 Hypersensitivity angiitis 🦠
    Goodpasture's syndrome

  M31.1 Thrombotic microangiopathy 🦠
    Thrombotic thrombocytopenic purpura

  M31.2 Lethal midline granuloma 🦠

  M31.3 Wegener's granulomatosis
    Necrotizing respiratory granulomatosis

    M31.30 Wegener's granulomatosis without renal involvement 🦠
      Wegener's granulomatosis NOS

    M31.31 Wegener's granulomatosis with renal involvement 🦠

  M31.4 Aortic arch syndrome [Takayasu] 🦠

  M31.5 Giant cell arteritis with polymyalgia rheumatica

  M31.6 Other giant cell arteritis

  M31.7 Microscopic polyangiitis 🦠
    Microscopic polyarteritis

> **Excludes1** polyarteritis nodosa (M30.0)

  M31.8 Other specified necrotizing vasculopathies 🦠
    Hypocomplementemic vasculitis
    Septic vasculitis

■ **M31.9 Necrotizing vasculopathy, unspecified** 🦠

● **M32 Systemic lupus erythematosus (SLE)**
Autoimmune inflammatory connective tissue disease of unknown cause that occurs most often in women.

> **Excludes1** lupus erythematosus (discoid) (NOS) (L93.0)

● **M32.0 Drug-induced systemic lupus erythematosus**

> **Use additional** code for adverse effect, if applicable, to identify drug (T36-T50 with fifth or sixth character 5)

CHAPTER 13 (M00-M99)

● **M32.1 Systemic lupus erythematosus with organ or system involvement**

■ **M32.10 Systemic lupus erythematosus, organ or system involvement unspecified**

M32.11 Endocarditis in systemic lupus erythematosus 🔒
Libman-Sacks disease
MCC: Only when the principal diagnosis is designated as a CC

M32.12 Pericarditis in systemic lupus erythematosus 🔒
Lupus pericarditis
MCC: Only when the principal diagnosis is designated as a CC

M32.13 Lung involvement in systemic lupus erythematosus
Pleural effusion due to systemic lupus erythematosus

M32.14 Glomerular disease in systemic lupus erythematosus
Lupus renal disease NOS

M32.15 Tubulo-interstitial nephropathy in systemic lupus erythematosus

M32.19 Other organ or system involvement in systemic lupus erythematosus

M32.8 Other forms of systemic lupus erythematosus

■ **M32.9 Systemic lupus erythematosus, unspecified**
SLE NOS
Systemic lupus erythematosus NOS
Systemic lupus erythematosus without organ involvement

● **M33 Dermatopolymyositis**

● **M33.0 Juvenile dermatopolymyositis**

■ **M33.00 Juvenile dermatopolymyositis, organ involvement unspecified** 🔒

M33.01 Juvenile dermatopolymyositis with respiratory involvement 🔒

M33.02 Juvenile dermatopolymyositis with myopathy 🔒
MCC: Only when the principal diagnosis is designated as a CC

M33.09 Juvenile dermatopolymyositis with other organ involvement 🔒

● **M33.1 Other dermatopolymyositis**

■ **M33.10 Other dermatopolymyositis, organ involvement unspecified** 🔒

M33.11 Other dermatopolymyositis with respiratory involvement 🔒

M33.12 Other dermatopolymyositis with myopathy 🔒
MCC: Only when the principal diagnosis is designated as a CC

M33.19 Other dermatopolymyositis with other organ involvement 🔒

● **M33.2 Polymyositis**

■ **M33.20 Polymyositis, organ involvement unspecified** 🔒

M33.21 Polymyositis with respiratory involvement 🔒

M33.22 Polymyositis with myopathy 🔒
MCC: Only when the principal diagnosis is designated as a CC

M33.29 Polymyositis with other organ involvement 🔒

● **M33.9 Dermatopolymyositis, unspecified**

■ **M33.90 Dermatopolymyositis, unspecified, organ involvement unspecified** 🔒

■ **M33.91 Dermatopolymyositis, unspecified with respiratory involvement** 🔒

■ **M33.92 Dermatopolymyositis, unspecified with myopathy** 🔒
MCC: Only when the principal diagnosis is designated as a CC

■ **M33.99 Dermatopolymyositis, unspecified with other organ involvement** 🔒

● **M34 Systemic sclerosis [scleroderma]**

| **Excludes1** | circumscribed scleroderma (L94.0) neonatal scleroderma (P83.8) |

M34.0 Progressive systemic sclerosis

M34.1 CR(E)ST syndrome
Combination of calcinosis, Raynaud's phenomenon, esophageal dysfunction, sclerodactyly, telangiectasia

M34.2 Systemic sclerosis induced by drug and chemical

Code first poisoning due to drug or toxin, if applicable (T36-T65 with fifth or sixth character 1-4 or 6)

Use additional code for adverse effect, if applicable, to identify drug (T36-T50 with fifth or sixth character 5)

● **M34.8 Other forms of systemic sclerosis**

M34.81 Systemic sclerosis with lung involvement 🔒
MCC: Only when the principal diagnosis is designated as a CC

M34.82 Systemic sclerosis with myopathy 🔒
MCC: Only when the principal diagnosis is designated as a CC

M34.83 Systemic sclerosis with polyneuropathy

M34.89 Other systemic sclerosis

■ **M34.9 Systemic sclerosis, unspecified**

● **M35 Other systemic involvement of connective tissue**

| **Excludes1** | reactive perforating collagenosis (L87.1) |

● **M35.0 Sicca syndrome [Sjögren]**

■ **M35.00 Sicca syndrome, unspecified**

M35.01 Sicca syndrome with keratoconjunctivitis

M35.02 Sicca syndrome with lung involvement

M35.03 Sicca syndrome with myopathy 🔒
MCC: Only when the principal diagnosis is designated as a CC

M35.04 Sicca syndrome with tubulo-interstitial nephropathy
Renal tubular acidosis in sicca syndrome

M35.09 Sicca syndrome with other organ involvement

M35.1 Other overlap syndromes 🔒
Mixed connective tissue disease

| **Excludes1** | polyangiitis overlap syndrome (M30.8) |

M35.2 Behçet's disease 🔒

M35.3 Polymyalgia rheumatica

| **Excludes1** | polymyalgia rheumatica with giant cell arteritis (M31.5) |

Item 13-8 Polymyalgia rheumatica is a syndrome characterized by aching and morning stiffness and is related to aging and hereditary predisposition.

● Unacceptable Principal Diagnosis   ● Use Additional Character(s)   ■ Unspecified   ▶ Manifestation Code
OGCR Official Guidelines for Coding and Reporting | Excludes 1 | | Excludes 2 | Includes   Use additional   Code first   Code also

M35.4 **Diffuse (eosinophilic) fasciitis**

M35.5 **Multifocal fibrosclerosis** 🦠

M35.6 **Relapsing panniculitis [Weber-Christian]**
> **Excludes1**   lupus panniculitis (L93.2)
> panniculitis NOS (M79.3-)

M35.7 **Hypermobility syndrome**
Familial ligamentous laxity
> **Excludes1**   Ehlers-Danlos syndrome (Q79.6)
> ligamentous laxity, NOS (M24.2-)

M35.8 **Other specified systemic involvement of connective tissue** 🦠

☐ M35.9 **Systemic involvement of connective tissue, unspecified**
Autoimmune disease (systemic) NOS
Collagen (vascular) disease NOS

● **M36 Systemic disorders of connective tissue in diseases classified elsewhere**
> **Excludes2**   arthropathies in diseases classified elsewhere (M14.-)

●▶ *M36.0 Dermato(poly)myositis in neoplastic disease* 🦠
> *Code first underlying neoplasm (C00-D49)*

●▶ *M36.1 Arthropathy in neoplastic disease*
> *Code first underlying neoplasm, such as:*
> leukemia (C91-C95)
> malignant histiocytosis (C96.A)
> multiple myeloma (C90.0)

●▶ *M36.2 Hemophilic arthropathy*
Hemarthrosis in hemophilic arthropathy
> *Code first underlying disease, such as:*
> factor VIII deficiency (D66)
> with vascular defect (D68.0)
> factor IX deficiency (D67)
> hemophilia (classical) (D66)
> hemophilia B (D67)
> hemophilia C (D68.1)

●▶ *M36.3 Arthropathy in other blood disorders*

●▶ *M36.4 Arthropathy in hypersensitivity reactions classified elsewhere*
> *Code first underlying disease, such as:*
> Henoch (-Schönlein) purpura (D69.0)
> serum sickness (T80.6-)

●▶ *M36.8 Systemic disorders of connective tissue in other diseases classified elsewhere*
> *Code first underlying disease, such as:*
> alkaptonuria (E70.2)
> hypogammaglobulinemia (D80.-)
> ochronosis (E70.2)

DORSOPATHIES (M40-M54)

DEFORMING DORSOPATHIES (M40-M43)

● **M40 Kyphosis and lordosis**
> **Excludes1**   congenital kyphosis and lordosis (Q76.4)
> kyphoscoliosis (M41.-)
> postprocedural kyphosis and lordosis (M96.-)

● M40.0 **Postural kyphosis**
> **Excludes1**   osteochondrosis of spine (M42.-)
☐ M40.00 Postural kyphosis, site unspecified
M40.03 Postural kyphosis, cervicothoracic region
M40.04 Postural kyphosis, thoracic region
M40.05 Postural kyphosis, thoracolumbar region

Item 13–9 Kyphosis is an abnormal curvature of the spine. **Senile kyphosis** is a result of disc degeneration causing ossification (turning to bone). **Adolescent** or **juvenile** kyphosis is also known as **Scheuermann's disease,** a condition in which the discs of the lower thoracic spine herniate, causing the disc space to narrow and the spine to tilt forward. This condition is attributed to poor posture. Lordosis or swayback is an abnormal curvature of the spine resulting in an inward curve of the lumbar spine just above the buttocks. Scoliosis causes a sideways curve to the spine. The curves are S- or C-shaped, and it is most commonly acquired in late childhood and early teen years, when growth is fast.

● M40.1 **Other secondary kyphosis**
☐ M40.10 Other secondary kyphosis, site unspecified
M40.12 Other secondary kyphosis, cervical region
M40.13 Other secondary kyphosis, cervicothoracic region
M40.14 Other secondary kyphosis, thoracic region
M40.15 Other secondary kyphosis, thoracolumbar region

● M40.2 **Other and unspecified kyphosis**
● M40.20 **Unspecified kyphosis**
☐ M40.202 Unspecified kyphosis, cervical region
☐ M40.203 Unspecified kyphosis, cervicothoracic region
☐ M40.204 Unspecified kyphosis, thoracic region
☐ M40.205 Unspecified kyphosis, thoracolumbar region
☐ M40.209 Unspecified kyphosis, site unspecified
● M40.29 **Other kyphosis**
M40.292 Other kyphosis, cervical region
M40.293 Other kyphosis, cervicothoracic region
M40.294 Other kyphosis, thoracic region
M40.295 Other kyphosis, thoracolumbar region
☐ M40.299 Other kyphosis, site unspecified

● M40.3 **Flatback syndrome**
☐ M40.30 Flatback syndrome, site unspecified
M40.35 Flatback syndrome, thoracolumbar region
M40.36 Flatback syndrome, lumbar region
M40.37 Flatback syndrome, lumbosacral region

● M40.4 **Postural lordosis**
> *Abnormal increase in the normal curvature of the lumbar spine (sway back)*
Acquired lordosis
☐ M40.40 Postural lordosis, site unspecified
M40.45 Postural lordosis, thoracolumbar region
M40.46 Postural lordosis, lumbar region
M40.47 Postural lordosis, lumbosacral region

● M40.5 **Lordosis, unspecified**
☐ M40.50 Lordosis, unspecified, site unspecified
☐ M40.55 Lordosis, unspecified, thoracolumbar region
☐ M40.56 Lordosis, unspecified, lumbar region
☐ M40.57 Lordosis, unspecified, lumbosacral region

N Newborn Age: 0   P Pediatric Age: 0–17   M Maternity DX: 12–55   A Adult Age: 15–124   ♀ Females Only   ♂ Males Only
🦠 Complication\Comorbidity   Major C\C   Present on Admission Requirement   Hospital-Acquired Condition
1193

● M41 **Scoliosis**

> **Includes**   kyphoscoliosis
>
> **Excludes1**   congenital scoliosis NOS (Q67.5)
>   congenital scoliosis due to bony
>   malformation (Q76.3)
>   postural congenital scoliosis (Q67.5)
>   kyphoscoliotic heart disease (I27.1)
>   postprocedural scoliosis (M96.-)

● M41.0 **Infantile idiopathic scoliosis**

■ M41.00 **Infantile idiopathic scoliosis, site unspecified**

M41.02 **Infantile idiopathic scoliosis, cervical region**

M41.03 **Infantile idiopathic scoliosis, cervicothoracic region**

M41.04 **Infantile idiopathic scoliosis, thoracic region**

M41.05 **Infantile idiopathic scoliosis, thoracolumbar region**

M41.06 **Infantile idiopathic scoliosis, lumbar region**

M41.07 **Infantile idiopathic scoliosis, lumbosacral region**

M41.08 **Infantile idiopathic scoliosis, sacral and sacrococcygeal region**

● M41.1 **Juvenile and adolescent idiopathic scoliosis**

● M41.11 **Juvenile idiopathic scoliosis**

M41.112 **Juvenile idiopathic scoliosis, cervical region**

M41.113 **Juvenile idiopathic scoliosis, cervicothoracic region**

M41.114 **Juvenile idiopathic scoliosis, thoracic region**

M41.115 **Juvenile idiopathic scoliosis, thoracolumbar region**

M41.116 **Juvenile idiopathic scoliosis, lumbar region**

M41.117 **Juvenile idiopathic scoliosis, lumbosacral region**

■ M41.119 **Juvenile idiopathic scoliosis, site unspecified**

● M41.12 **Adolescent scoliosis**

M41.122 **Adolescent idiopathic scoliosis, cervical region**

M41.123 **Adolescent idiopathic scoliosis, cervicothoracic region**

M41.124 **Adolescent idiopathic scoliosis, thoracic region**

M41.125 **Adolescent idiopathic scoliosis, thoracolumbar region**

M41.126 **Adolescent idiopathic scoliosis, lumbar region**

M41.127 **Adolescent idiopathic scoliosis, lumbosacral region**

■ M41.129 **Adolescent idiopathic scoliosis, site unspecified**

● M41.2 **Other idiopathic scoliosis**

■ M41.20 **Other idiopathic scoliosis, site unspecified**

M41.22 **Other idiopathic scoliosis, cervical region**

M41.23 **Other idiopathic scoliosis, cervicothoracic region**

M41.24 **Other idiopathic scoliosis, thoracic region**

M41.25 **Other idiopathic scoliosis, thoracolumbar region**

M41.26 **Other idiopathic scoliosis, lumbar region**

M41.27 **Other idiopathic scoliosis, lumbosacral region**

● M41.3 **Thoracogenic scoliosis**

■ M41.30 **Thoracogenic scoliosis, site unspecified**

M41.34 **Thoracogenic scoliosis, thoracic region**

M41.35 **Thoracogenic scoliosis, thoracolumbar region**

● M41.4 **Neuromuscular scoliosis**

> Scoliosis secondary to cerebral palsy, Friedreich's ataxia, poliomyelitis and other neuromuscular disorders
>
> **Code also** underlying condition

■ M41.40 **Neuromuscular scoliosis, site unspecified**

M41.41 **Neuromuscular scoliosis, occipito-atlanto-axial region**

M41.42 **Neuromuscular scoliosis, cervical region**

M41.43 **Neuromuscular scoliosis, cervicothoracic region**

M41.44 **Neuromuscular scoliosis, thoracic region**

M41.45 **Neuromuscular scoliosis, thoracolumbar region**

M41.46 **Neuromuscular scoliosis, lumbar region**

M41.47 **Neuromuscular scoliosis, lumbosacral region**

● M41.5 **Other secondary scoliosis**

■ M41.50 **Other secondary scoliosis, site unspecified**

M41.52 **Other secondary scoliosis, cervical region**

M41.53 **Other secondary scoliosis, cervicothoracic region**

M41.54 **Other secondary scoliosis, thoracic region**

M41.55 **Other secondary scoliosis, thoracolumbar region**

M41.56 **Other secondary scoliosis, lumbar region**

M41.57 **Other secondary scoliosis, lumbosacral region**

● M41.8 **Other forms of scoliosis**

■ M41.80 **Other forms of scoliosis, site unspecified**

M41.82 **Other forms of scoliosis, cervical region**

M41.83 **Other forms of scoliosis, cervicothoracic region**

M41.84 **Other forms of scoliosis, thoracic region**

M41.85 **Other forms of scoliosis, thoracolumbar region**

M41.86 **Other forms of scoliosis, lumbar region**

M41.87 **Other forms of scoliosis, lumbosacral region**

■ M41.9 **Scoliosis, unspecified**

● **M42 Spinal osteochondrosis**
  ● **M42.0 Juvenile osteochondrosis of spine**
    Calvé's disease
    Scheuermann's disease
    Excludes1 postural kyphosis (M40.0)
    ■ **M42.00 Juvenile osteochondrosis of spine, site unspecified**
    M42.01 Juvenile osteochondrosis of spine, occipito-atlanto-axial region
    M42.02 Juvenile osteochondrosis of spine, cervical region
    M42.03 Juvenile osteochondrosis of spine, cervicothoracic region
    M42.04 Juvenile osteochondrosis of spine, thoracic region
    M42.05 Juvenile osteochondrosis of spine, thoracolumbar region
    M42.06 Juvenile osteochondrosis of spine, lumbar region
    M42.07 Juvenile osteochondrosis of spine, lumbosacral region
    M42.08 Juvenile osteochondrosis of spine, sacral and sacrococcygeal region
    M42.09 Juvenile osteochondrosis of spine, multiple sites in spine

  ● **M42.1 Adult osteochondrosis of spine**
    ■ **M42.10 Adult osteochondrosis of spine, site unspecified**   A
    M42.11 Adult osteochondrosis of spine, occipitoatlanto-axial region   A
    M42.12 Adult osteochondrosis of spine, cervical region   A
    M42.13 Adult osteochondrosis of spine, cervicothoracic region   A
    M42.14 Adult osteochondrosis of spine, thoracic region   A
    M42.15 Adult osteochondrosis of spine, thoracolumbar region   A
    M42.16 Adult osteochondrosis of spine, lumbar region   A
    M42.17 Adult osteochondrosis of spine, lumbosacral region   A
    M42.18 Adult osteochondrosis of spine, sacral and sacrococcygeal region   A
    M42.19 Adult osteochondrosis of spine, multiple sites in spine   A

  ■ **M42.9 Spinal osteochondrosis, unspecified**

● **M43 Other deforming dorsopathies**
  Excludes1 congenital spondylolysis and spondylolisthesis (Q76.2)
    hemivertebra (Q76.3-Q76.4)
    Klippel-Feil syndrome (Q76.1)
    lumbarization and sacralization (Q76.4)
    platyspondylisis (Q76.4)
    spina bifida occulta (Q76.0)
    spinal curvature in osteoporosis (M80-)
    spinal curvature in Paget's disease of bone [osteitis deformans] (M88.-)

  ● **M43.0 Spondylolysis**
    Excludes1 congenital spondylolysis (Q76.2)
    spondylolisthesis (M43.1)
    ■ **M43.00 Spondylolysis, site unspecified**
    M43.01 Spondylolysis, occipito-atlanto-axial region

Item 13–10 Spondylolisthesis is a condition caused by the slipping forward of one disc over another.

    M43.02 Spondylolysis, cervical region
    M43.03 Spondylolysis, cervicothoracic region
    M43.04 Spondylolysis, thoracic region
    M43.05 Spondylolysis, thoracolumbar region
    M43.06 Spondylolysis, lumbar region
    M43.07 Spondylolysis, lumbosacral region
    M43.08 Spondylolysis, sacral and sacrococcygeal region
    M43.09 Spondylolysis, multiple sites in spine

  ● **M43.1 Spondylolisthesis**
    Excludes1 acute traumatic of lumbosacral region (S33.1)
      acute traumatic of sites other than lumbosacral - code to Fracture, vertebra, by region
      congenital spondylolisthesis (Q76.2)
    ■ **M43.10 Spondylolisthesis, site unspecified**
    M43.11 Spondylolisthesis, occipito-atlanto-axial region
    M43.12 Spondylolisthesis, cervical region
    M43.13 Spondylolisthesis, cervicothoracic region
    M43.14 Spondylolisthesis, thoracic region
    M43.15 Spondylolisthesis, thoracolumbar region
    M43.16 Spondylolisthesis, lumbar region
    M43.17 Spondylolisthesis, lumbosacral region
    M43.18 Spondylolisthesis, sacral and sacrococcygeal region
    M43.19 Spondylolisthesis, multiple sites in spine

  ● **M43.2 Fusion of spine**
    Ankylosis of spinal joint
    Excludes1 ankylosing spondylitis (M45.0-)
      congenital fusion of spine (Q76.4)
    Excludes2 arthrodesis status (Z98.1)
      pseudoarthrosis after fusion or arthrodesis (M96.0)
    ■ **M43.20 Fusion of spine, site unspecified**
    M43.21 Fusion of spine, occipito-atlanto-axial region
    M43.22 Fusion of spine, cervical region
    M43.23 Fusion of spine, cervicothoracic region
    M43.24 Fusion of spine, thoracic region
    M43.25 Fusion of spine, thoracolumbar region
    M43.26 Fusion of spine, lumbar region
    M43.27 Fusion of spine, lumbosacral region
    M43.28 Fusion of spine, sacral and sacrococcygeal region

  M43.3 Recurrent atlantoaxial dislocation with myelopathy
  M43.4 Other recurrent atlantoaxial dislocation
  ● **M43.5 Other recurrent vertebral dislocation**
    Excludes1 biomechanical lesions NEC (M99.-)
    ● **M43.5X Other recurrent vertebral dislocation**
      M43.5X2 Other recurrent vertebral dislocation, cervical region
      M43.5X3 Other recurrent vertebral dislocation, cervicothoracic region

N Newborn Age: 0   **P** Pediatric Age: 0–17   **M** Maternity DX: 12–55   **A** Adult Age: 15–124   ♀ Females Only   ♂ Males Only

◐ Complication\Comorbidity   ◎ Major C\C   ◎ Present on Admission Requirement   ◎ Hospital-Acquired Condition

1195

CHAPTER 13 (M00-M99)

M43.5X4 Other recurrent vertebral
dislocation, thoracic region

M43.5X5 Other recurrent vertebral
dislocation, thoracolumbar
region

M43.5X6 Other recurrent vertebral
dislocation, lumbar region

M43.5X7 Other recurrent vertebral
dislocation, lumbosacral region

M43.5X8 Other recurrent vertebral
dislocation, sacral and
sacrococcygeal region

■ M43.5X9 Other recurrent vertebral
dislocation, site unspecified

M43.6 Torticollis
Excludes1 congenital (sternomastoid) torticollis
(Q68.0)
current injury - see Injury, of spine,
by body region ocular torticollis
(R29.891)
psychogenic torticollis (F45.8)
spasmodic torticollis (G24.3)
torticollis due to birth injury (P15.2)

● M43.8 Other specified deforming dorsopathies
Excludes2 kyphosis and lordosis (M40.-)
scoliosis (M41.-)

● M43.8X Other specified deforming dorsopathies
M43.8X1 Other specified deforming
dorsopathies, occipito-atlanto-
axial region

M43.8X2 Other specified deforming
dorsopathies, cervical region

M43.8X3 Other specified deforming
dorsopathies, cervicothoracic
region

M43.8X4 Other specified deforming
dorsopathies, thoracic region

M43.8X5 Other specified deforming
dorsopathies, thoracolumbar
region

M43.8X6 Other specified deforming
dorsopathies, lumbar region

M43.8X7 Other specified deforming
dorsopathies, lumbosacral region

M43.8X8 Other specified deforming
dorsopathies, sacral and
sacrococcygeal region

■ M43.8X9 Other specified deforming
dorsopathies, site unspecified

■ M43.9 Deforming dorsopathy, unspecified
Curvature of spine NOS

SPONDYLOPATHIES (M45-M49)

● M45 Ankylosing spondylitis
Rheumatoid arthritis of spine
Excludes1 arthropathy in Reiter's disease (M02.3-)
juvenile (ankylosing) spondylitis (M08.1)
Excludes2 Behçet's disease (M35.2)

M45.0 Ankylosing spondylitis of multiple sites in spine

M45.1 Ankylosing spondylitis of occipito-atlanto-axial
region

M45.2 Ankylosing spondylitis of cervical region

M45.3 Ankylosing spondylitis of cervicothoracic region

M45.4 Ankylosing spondylitis of thoracic region

M45.5 Ankylosing spondylitis of thoracolumbar region

M45.6 Ankylosing spondylitis lumbar region

M45.7 Ankylosing spondylitis of lumbosacral region

M45.8 Ankylosing spondylitis sacral and sacrococcygeal
region

■ M45.9 Ankylosing spondylitis of unspecified sites in
spine

● M46 Other inflammatory spondylopathies
● M46.0 Spinal enthesopathy
Disorder of ligamentous or muscular attachments
of spine

■ M46.00 Spinal enthesopathy, site unspecified

M46.01 Spinal enthesopathy, occipito-atlanto-axial
region

M46.02 Spinal enthesopathy, cervical region

M46.03 Spinal enthesopathy, cervicothoracic
region

M46.04 Spinal enthesopathy, thoracic region

M46.05 Spinal enthesopathy, thoracolumbar
region

M46.06 Spinal enthesopathy, lumbar region

M46.07 Spinal enthesopathy, lumbosacral region

M46.08 Spinal enthesopathy, sacral and
sacrococcygeal region

M46.09 Spinal enthesopathy, multiple sites in
spine

M46.1 Sacroiliitis, not elsewhere classified

● M46.2 Osteomyelitis of vertebra

■ M46.20 Osteomyelitis of vertebra, site
unspecified ◐

M46.21 Osteomyelitis of vertebra, occipito-atlanto-
axial region ◐

M46.22 Osteomyelitis of vertebra, cervical
region ◐

M46.23 Osteomyelitis of vertebra, cervicothoracic
region ◐

M46.24 Osteomyelitis of vertebra, thoracic
region ◐

M46.25 Osteomyelitis of vertebra, thoracolumbar
region ◐

M46.26 Osteomyelitis of vertebra, lumbar
region ◐

M46.27 Osteomyelitis of vertebra, lumbosacral
region ◐

M46.28 Osteomyelitis of vertebra, sacral and
sacrococcygeal region ◐

● M46.3 Infection of intervertebral disc (pyogenic)
Use additional code (B95-B97) to identify
infectious agent

■ M46.30 Infection of intervertebral disc (pyogenic),
site unspecified ◐

M46.31 Infection of intervertebral disc (pyogenic),
occipito-atlanto-axial region ◐

M46.32 Infection of intervertebral disc (pyogenic),
cervical region ◐

M46.33 Infection of intervertebral disc (pyogenic),
cervicothoracic region ◐

M46.34 Infection of intervertebral disc (pyogenic),
thoracic region ◐

● Unacceptable Principal Diagnosis   ● Use Additional Character(s)   ■ Unspecified   ▶ Manifestation Code
OGCR Official Guidelines for Coding and Reporting   Excludes 1   Excludes 2   Includes   Use additional   Code first   Code also

M46.35 Infection of intervertebral disc (pyogenic), thoracolumbar region 🦴

M46.36 Infection of intervertebral disc (pyogenic), lumbar region 🦴

M46.37 Infection of intervertebral disc (pyogenic), lumbosacral region 🦴

M46.38 Infection of intervertebral disc (pyogenic), sacral and sacrococcygeal region 🦴

M46.39 Infection of intervertebral disc (pyogenic), multiple sites in spine 🦴

● M46.4 Discitis, unspecified
  ◼ M46.40 Discitis, unspecified, site unspecified
  ◼ M46.41 Discitis, unspecified, occipito-atlanto-axial region
  ◼ M46.42 Discitis, unspecified, cervical region
  ◼ M46.43 Discitis, unspecified, cervicothoracic region
  ◼ M46.44 Discitis, unspecified, thoracic region
  ◼ M46.45 Discitis, unspecified, thoracolumbar region
  ◼ M46.46 Discitis, unspecified, lumbar region
  ◼ M46.47 Discitis, unspecified, lumbosacral region
  ◼ M46.48 Discitis, unspecified, sacral and sacrococcygeal region
  ◼ M46.49 Discitis, unspecified, multiple sites in spine

● M46.5 Other infective spondylopathies
  ◼ M46.50 Other infective spondylopathies, site unspecified
  M46.51 Other infective spondylopathies, occipitoatlanto-axial region
  M46.52 Other infective spondylopathies, cervical region
  M46.53 Other infective spondylopathies, cervicothoracic region
  M46.54 Other infective spondylopathies, thoracic region
  M46.55 Other infective spondylopathies, thoracolumbar region
  M46.56 Other infective spondylopathies, lumbar region
  M46.57 Other infective spondylopathies, lumbosacral region
  M46.58 Other infective spondylopathies, sacral and sacrococcygeal region
  M46.59 Other infective spondylopathies, multiple sites in spine

● M46.8 Other specified inflammatory spondylopathies
  ◼ M46.80 Other specified inflammatory spondylopathies, site unspecified
  M46.81 Other specified inflammatory spondylopathies, occipito-atlanto-axial region
  M46.82 Other specified inflammatory spondylopathies, cervical region
  M46.83 Other specified inflammatory spondylopathies, cervicothoracic region
  M46.84 Other specified inflammatory spondylopathies, thoracic region
  M46.85 Other specified inflammatory spondylopathies, thoracolumbar region
  M46.86 Other specified inflammatory spondylopathies, lumbar region

M46.87 Other specified inflammatory spondylopathies, lumbosacral region

M46.88 Other specified inflammatory spondylopathies, sacral and sacrococcygeal region

M46.89 Other specified inflammatory spondylopathies, multiple sites in spine

● M46.9 Unspecified inflammatory spondylopathy
  ◼ M46.90 Unspecified inflammatory spondylopathy, site unspecified
  ◼ M46.91 Unspecified inflammatory spondylopathy, occipito-atlanto-axial region
  ◼ M46.92 Unspecified inflammatory spondylopathy, cervical region
  ◼ M46.93 Unspecified inflammatory spondylopathy, cervicothoracic region
  ◼ M46.94 Unspecified inflammatory spondylopathy, thoracic region
  ◼ M46.95 Unspecified inflammatory spondylopathy, thoracolumbar region
  ◼ M46.96 Unspecified inflammatory spondylopathy, lumbar region
  ◼ M46.97 Unspecified inflammatory spondylopathy, lumbosacral region
  ◼ M46.98 Unspecified inflammatory spondylopathy, sacral and sacrococcygeal region
  ◼ M46.99 Unspecified inflammatory spondylopathy, multiple sites in spine

● M47 Spondylosis
  Includes arthrosis or osteoarthritis of spine
  degeneration of facet joints

● M47.0 Anterior spinal and vertebral artery compression syndromes
  ● M47.01 Anterior spinal artery compression syndromes
    M47.011 Anterior spinal artery compression syndromes, occipito-atlanto-axial region 🦴
    M47.012 Anterior spinal artery compression syndromes, cervical region 🦴
    M47.013 Anterior spinal artery compression syndromes, cervicothoracic region 🦴
    M47.014 Anterior spinal artery compression syndromes, thoracic region 🦴
    M47.015 Anterior spinal artery compression syndromes, thoracolumbar region 🦴
    M47.016 Anterior spinal artery compression syndromes, lumbar region 🦴
    ◼ M47.019 Anterior spinal artery compression syndromes, site unspecified 🦴
  ● M47.02 Vertebral artery compression syndromes
    M47.021 Vertebral artery compression syndromes, occipito-atlanto-axial region 🦴
    M47.022 Vertebral artery compression syndromes, cervical region 🦴
    ◼ M47.029 Vertebral artery compression syndromes, site unspecified 🦴

CHAPTER 13 (M00-M99)

● M47.1 Other spondylosis with myelopathy
Spondylogenic compression of spinal cord

Excludes1 vertebral subluxation
(M43.3-M43.59)

■ M47.10 Other spondylosis with myelopathy, site unspecified 🔊

M47.11 Other spondylosis with myelopathy, occipito-atlanto-axial region 🔊

M47.12 Other spondylosis with myelopathy, cervical region 🔊

M47.13 Other spondylosis with myelopathy, cervicothoracic region 🔊

M47.14 Other spondylosis with myelopathy, thoracic region 🔊

M47.15 Other spondylosis with myelopathy, thoracolumbar region 🔊

M47.16 Other spondylosis with myelopathy, lumbar region 🔊

M47.17 Other spondylosis with myelopathy, lumbosacral region 🔊

M47.18 Other spondylosis with myelopathy, sacral and sacrococcygeal region 🔊

● M47.2 Other spondylosis with radiculopathy

■ M47.20 Other spondylosis with radiculopathy, site unspecified

M47.21 Other spondylosis with radiculopathy, occipito-atlanto-axial region

M47.22 Other spondylosis with radiculopathy, cervical region

M47.23 Other spondylosis with radiculopathy, cervicothoracic region

M47.24 Other spondylosis with radiculopathy, thoracic region

M47.25 Other spondylosis with radiculopathy, thoracolumbar region

M47.26 Other spondylosis with radiculopathy, lumbar region

M47.27 Other spondylosis with radiculopathy, lumbosacral region

M47.28 Other spondylosis with radiculopathy, sacral and sacrococcygeal region

● M47.8 Other spondylosis

● M47.81 Spondylosis without myelopathy or radiculopathy

M47.811 Spondylosis without myelopathy or radiculopathy, occipito-atlanto-axial region

M47.812 Spondylosis without myelopathy or radiculopathy, cervical region

M47.813 Spondylosis without myelopathy or radiculopathy, cervicothoracic region

M47.814 Spondylosis without myelopathy or radiculopathy, thoracic region

M47.815 Spondylosis without myelopathy or radiculopathy, thoracolumbar region

M47.816 Spondylosis without myelopathy or radiculopathy, lumbar region

M47.817 Spondylosis without myelopathy or radiculopathy, lumbosacral region

M47.818 Spondylosis without myelopathy or radiculopathy, sacral and sacrococcygeal region

■ M47.819 Spondylosis without myelopathy or radiculopathy, site unspecified

● M47.89 Other spondylosis

M47.891 Other spondylosis, occipito-atlanto-axial region

M47.892 Other spondylosis, cervical region

M47.893 Other spondylosis, cervicothoracic region

M47.894 Other spondylosis, thoracic region

M47.895 Other spondylosis, thoracolumbar region

M47.896 Other spondylosis, lumbar region

M47.897 Other spondylosis, lumbosacral region

M47.898 Other spondylosis, sacral and sacrococcygeal region

■ M47.899 Other spondylosis, site unspecified

■ M47.9 Spondylosis, unspecified

● M48 Other spondylopathies

● M48.0 Spinal stenosis
Caudal stenosis

■ M48.00 Spinal stenosis, site unspecified

M48.01 Spinal stenosis, occipito-atlanto-axial region

M48.02 Spinal stenosis, cervical region

M48.03 Spinal stenosis, cervicothoracic region

M48.04 Spinal stenosis, thoracic region

M48.05 Spinal stenosis, thoracolumbar region

M48.06 Spinal stenosis, lumbar region

M48.07 Spinal stenosis, lumbosacral region

M48.08 Spinal stenosis, sacral and sacrococcygeal region

● M48.1 Ankylosing hyperostosis [Forestier]
Diffuse idiopathic skeletal hyperostosis [DISH]

■ M48.10 Ankylosing hyperostosis [Forestier], site unspecified

M48.11 Ankylosing hyperostosis [Forestier], occipito-atlanto-axial region

M48.12 Ankylosing hyperostosis [Forestier], cervical region

M48.13 Ankylosing hyperostosis [Forestier], cervicothoracic region

M48.14 Ankylosing hyperostosis [Forestier], thoracic region

M48.15 Ankylosing hyperostosis [Forestier], thoracolumbar region

M48.16 Ankylosing hyperostosis [Forestier], lumbar region

M48.17 Ankylosing hyperostosis [Forestier], lumbosacral region

M48.18 Ankylosing hyperostosis [Forestier], sacral and sacrococcygeal region

M48.19 Ankylosing hyperostosis [Forestier], multiple sites in spine

● Unacceptable Principal Diagnosis   ● Use Additional Character(s)   ■ Unspecified   ▶ Manifestation Code

OGCR Official Guidelines for Coding and Reporting   Excludes 1   Excludes 2   Includes   Use additional   Code first   Code also

CHAPTER 13 (M00-M99)

● M48.2   **Kissing spine**
    ■ **M48.20   Kissing spine, site unspecified**
      M48.21   Kissing spine, occipito-atlanto-axial region
      M48.22   Kissing spine, cervical region
      M48.23   Kissing spine, cervicothoracic region
      M48.24   Kissing spine, thoracic region
      M48.25   Kissing spine, thoracolumbar region
      M48.26   Kissing spine, lumbar region
      M48.27   Kissing spine, lumbosacral region

● M48.3   **Traumatic spondylopathy**
    ■ **M48.30   Traumatic spondylopathy, site unspecified** 🅒
      M48.31   Traumatic spondylopathy, occipito-atlanto-axial region 🅒
      M48.32   Traumatic spondylopathy, cervical region 🅒
      M48.33   Traumatic spondylopathy, cervicothoracic region 🅒
      M48.34   Traumatic spondylopathy, thoracic region 🅒
      M48.35   Traumatic spondylopathy, thoracolumbar region 🅒
      M48.36   Traumatic spondylopathy, lumbar region 🅒
      M48.37   Traumatic spondylopathy, lumbosacral region 🅒
      M48.38   Traumatic spondylopathy, sacral and sacrococcygeal region 🅒

● M48.4   **Fatigue fracture of vertebra**
    Stress fracture of vertebra

Excludes1	pathological fracture NOS (M84.4-)
	pathological fracture of vertebra due to neoplasm (M84.58)
	pathological fracture of vertebra due to other diagnosis (M84.68)
	pathological fracture of vertebra due to osteoporosis (M80.-)
	traumatic fracture of vertebrae (S12.0-S12.3-, S22.0-, S32.0-)

The appropriate 7th character is to be added to each code from subcategory M48.4:

A	initial encounter for fracture
D	subsequent encounter for fracture with routine healing
G	subsequent encounter for fracture with delayed healing
S	sequela of fracture

    ■ **M48.40   Fatigue fracture of vertebra, site unspecified** D, G, S 🅟
      M48.41   Fatigue fracture of vertebra, occipitoatlanto-axial region D, G, S 🅟
      M48.42   Fatigue fracture of vertebra, cervical region D, G, S 🅟
      M48.43   Fatigue fracture of vertebra, cervicothoracic region D, G, S 🅟
      M48.44   Fatigue fracture of vertebra, thoracic region D, G, S 🅟
      M48.45   Fatigue fracture of vertebra, thoracolumbar region D, G, S 🅟

      M48.46   Fatigue fracture of vertebra, lumbar region D, G, S 🅟
      M48.47   Fatigue fracture of vertebra, lumbosacral region D, G, S 🅟
      M48.48   Fatigue fracture of vertebra, sacral and sacrococcygeal region D, G, S 🅟

● M48.5   **Collapsed vertebra, not elsewhere classified**
    Collapsed vertebra NOS
    Wedging of vertebra NOS

Excludes1	current injury - see Injury of spine, by body region
	fatigue fracture of vertebra (M48.4)
	pathological fracture of vertebra due to neoplasm (M84.58)
	pathological fracture of vertebra due to other diagnosis (M84.68)
	pathological fracture of vertebra due to osteoporosis (M80.-)
	pathological fracture NOS (M84.4-)
	stress fracture of vertebra (M48.4-)
	traumatic fracture of vertebra (S12.-, S22.-, S32.-)

The appropriate 7th character is to be added to each code from subcategory M48.5:

A	initial encounter for fracture
D	subsequent encounter for fracture with routine healing
G	subsequent encounter for fracture with delayed healing
S	sequela of fracture

    ■ **M48.50   Collapsed vertebra, not elsewhere classified, site unspecified** A 🅒, D, G, S 🅟
      M48.51   Collapsed vertebra, not elsewhere classified, occipito-atlanto-axial region A 🅒, D, G, S 🅟
      M48.52   Collapsed vertebra, not elsewhere classified, cervical region A 🅒, D, G, S 🅟
      M48.53   Collapsed vertebra, not elsewhere classified, cervicothoracic region A 🅒, D, G, S 🅟
      M48.54   Collapsed vertebra, not elsewhere classified, thoracic region A 🅒, D, G, S 🅟
      M48.55   Collapsed vertebra, not elsewhere classified, thoracolumbar region A 🅒, D, G, S 🅟
      M48.56   Collapsed vertebra, not elsewhere classified, lumbar region A 🅒, D, G, S 🅟
      M48.57   Collapsed vertebra, not elsewhere classified, lumbosacral region A 🅒, D, G, S 🅟
      M48.58   Collapsed vertebra, not elsewhere classified, sacral and sacrococcygeal region A 🅒, D, G, S 🅟

● M48.8   **Other specified spondylopathies**
    Ossification of posterior longitudinal ligament
    ● **M48.8X   Other specified spondylopathies**
      M48.8X1   Other specified spondylopathies, occipito-atlanto-axial region
      M48.8X2   Other specified spondylopathies, cervical region
      M48.8X3   Other specified spondylopathies, cervicothoracic region

CHAPTER 13 (M00-M99)

N Newborn Age: 0   **P** Pediatric Age: 0–17   **M** Maternity DX: 12–55   **A** Adult Age: 15–124   ♀ Females Only   ♂ Males Only

🅒 Complication\Comorbidity   🅜 Major C\C   🅟 Present on Admission Requirement   🅗 Hospital-Acquired Condition

1199

M48.8X4 Other specified spondylopathies, thoracic region

M48.8X5 Other specified spondylopathies, thoracolumbar region

M48.8X6 Other specified spondylopathies, lumbar region

M48.8X7 Other specified spondylopathies, lumbosacral region

M48.8X8 Other specified spondylopathies, sacral and sacrococcygeal region

M48.8X9 Other specified spondylopathies, site unspecified

M48.9 Spondylopathy, unspecified

M49 Spondylopathies in diseases classified elsewhere

Includes　curvature of spine in diseases classified elsewhere
deformity of spine in diseases classified elsewhere
kyphosis in diseases classified elsewhere
scoliosis in diseases classified elsewhere
spondylopathy in diseases classified elsewhere

Code first underlying disease, such as:
brucellosis (A23.-)
Charcot-Marie-Tooth disease (G60.0)
enterobacterial infections (A01-A04)
osteitis fibrosa cystica (E21.0)

Excludes1　curvature of spine in tuberculosis [Pott's] (A18.01)
enteropathic arthropathies (M07.-)
neuropathic spondylopathy (in):
nonsyphilitic NEC (G98.0)
syringomyelia (G95.0)
tabes dorsalis (A52.11)
spondylitis (in):
gonococcal (A54.41)
syphilis (acquired) (A52.77)
neuropathic [tabes dorsalis] (A52.11)
tuberculosis (A18.01)
typhoid fever (A01.05)

M49.8 Spondylopathy in diseases classified elsewhere

M49.80 Spondylopathy in diseases classified elsewhere, site unspecified

M49.81 Spondylopathy in diseases classified elsewhere, occipito-atlanto-axial region

M49.82 Spondylopathy in diseases classified elsewhere, cervical region

M49.83 Spondylopathy in diseases classified elsewhere, cervicothoracic region

M49.84 Spondylopathy in diseases classified elsewhere, thoracic region

M49.85 Spondylopathy in diseases classified elsewhere, thoracolumbar region

M49.86 Spondylopathy in diseases classified elsewhere, lumbar region

M49.87 Spondylopathy in diseases classified elsewhere, lumbosacral region

M49.88 Spondylopathy in diseases classified elsewhere, sacral and sacrococcygeal region

M49.89 Spondylopathy in diseases classified elsewhere, multiple sites in spine

OTHER DORSOPATHIES (M50-M54)

Excludes1　current injury - see injury of spine by body region discitis NOS (M46.4-)

M50 Cervical disc disorders

Note: Code to the most superior level of disorder.

Includes　cervicothoracic disc disorders with cervicalgia
cervicothoracic disc disorders

M50.0 Cervical disc disorder with myelopathy

M50.00 Cervical disc disorder with myelopathy, unspecified cervical region

M50.01 Cervical disc disorder with myelopathy, occipito-atlanto-axial region

M50.02 Cervical disc disorder with myelopathy, mid-cervical region

M50.03 Cervical disc disorder with myelopathy, cervicothoracic region

M50.1 Cervical disc disorder with radiculopathy

Excludes2　brachial radiculitis NOS (M54.13)

M50.10 Cervical disc disorder with radiculopathy, unspecified cervical region

M50.11 Cervical disc disorder with radiculopathy, occipito-atlanto-axial region

M50.12 Cervical disc disorder with radiculopathy, mid-cervical region

M50.13 Cervical disc disorder with radiculopathy, cervicothoracic region

M50.2 Other cervical disc displacement

M50.20 Other cervical disc displacement, unspecified cervical region

M50.21 Other cervical disc displacement, occipitoatlanto-axial region

M50.22 Other cervical disc displacement, mid-cervical region

M50.23 Other cervical disc displacement, cervicothoracic region

M50.3 Other cervical disc degeneration

M50.30 Other cervical disc degeneration, unspecified cervical region

M50.31 Other cervical disc degeneration, occipitoatlanto-axial region

M50.32 Other cervical disc degeneration, mid-cervical region

M50.33 Other cervical disc degeneration, cervicothoracic region

M50.8 Other cervical disc disorders

M50.80 Other cervical disc disorders, unspecified cervical region

M50.81 Other cervical disc disorders, occipitoatlanto-axial region

M50.82 Other cervical disc disorders, mid-cervical region

M50.83 Other cervical disc disorders, cervicothoracic region

● M50.9 Cervical disc disorder, unspecified

    ■ M50.90 Cervical disc disorder, unspecified, unspecified cervical region

    ■ M50.91 Cervical disc disorder, unspecified, occipito-atlanto-axial region

    ■ M50.92 Cervical disc disorder, unspecified, mid-cervical region

    ■ M50.93 Cervical disc disorder, unspecified, cervicothoracic region

● M51 Thoracic, thoracolumbar, and lumbosacral intervertebral disc disorders

    Excludes2   cervical and cervicothoracic disc disorders (M50.-)

          sacral and sacrococcygeal disorders (M53.3)

● M51.0 Thoracic, thoracolumbar and lumbosacral intervertebral disc disorders with myelopathy

    M51.04 Intervertebral disc disorders with myelopathy, thoracic region 🌑

    M51.05 Intervertebral disc disorders with myelopathy, thoracolumbar region 🌑

    M51.06 Intervertebral disc disorders with myelopathy, lumbar region 🌑

    M51.07 Intervertebral disc disorders with myelopathy, lumbosacral region 🌑

● M51.1 Thoracic, thoracolumbar and lumbosacral intervertebral disc disorders with radiculopathy

    Sciatica due to intervertebral disc disorder

    Excludes1   lumbar radiculitis NOS (M54.16)

          sciatica NOS (M54.3)

    M51.14 Intervertebral disc disorders with radiculopathy, thoracic region

    M51.15 Intervertebral disc disorders with radiculopathy, thoracolumbar region

    M51.16 Intervertebral disc disorders with radiculopathy, lumbar region

    M51.17 Intervertebral disc disorders with radiculopathy, lumbosacral region

● M51.2 Other thoracic, thoracolumbar and lumbosacral intervertebral disc displacement

    Lumbago due to displacement of intervertebral disc

    M51.24 Other intervertebral disc displacement, thoracic region

    M51.25 Other intervertebral disc displacement, thoracolumbar region

    M51.26 Other intervertebral disc displacement, lumbar region

    M51.27 Other intervertebral disc displacement, lumbosacral region

● M51.3 Other thoracic, thoracolumbar and lumbosacral intervertebral disc degeneration

    M51.34 Other intervertebral disc degeneration, thoracic region

    M51.35 Other intervertebral disc degeneration, thoracolumbar region

    M51.36 Other intervertebral disc degeneration, lumbar region

    M51.37 Other intervertebral disc degeneration, lumbosacral region

● M51.4 Schmorl's nodes

    M51.44 Schmorl's nodes, thoracic region

    M51.45 Schmorl's nodes, thoracolumbar region

    M51.46 Schmorl's nodes, lumbar region

    M51.47 Schmorl's nodes, lumbosacral region

● M51.8 Other thoracic, thoracolumbar and lumbosacral intervertebral disc disorders

    M51.84 Other intervertebral disc disorders, thoracic region

    M51.85 Other intervertebral disc disorders, thoracolumbar region

    M51.86 Other intervertebral disc disorders, lumbar region

    M51.87 Other intervertebral disc disorders, lumbosacral region

■ M51.9 Unspecified thoracic, thoracolumbar and lumbosacral intervertebral disc disorder

● M53 Other and unspecified dorsopathies, not elsewhere classified

    M53.0 Cervicocranial syndrome

        Posterior cervical sympathetic syndrome

    M53.1 Cervicobrachial syndrome

        Excludes2   cervical disc disorder (M50.-)

              thoracic outlet syndrome (G54.0)

● M53.2 Spinal instabilities

    ● M53.2X Spinal instabilities

        M53.2X1 Spinal instabilities, occipito-atlanto-axial region

        M53.2X2 Spinal instabilities, cervical region

        M53.2X3 Spinal instabilities, cervicothoracic region

        M53.2X4 Spinal instabilities, thoracic region

        M53.2X5 Spinal instabilities, thoracolumbar region

        M53.2X6 Spinal instabilities, lumbar region

        M53.2X7 Spinal instabilities, lumbosacral region

        M53.2X8 Spinal instabilities, sacral and sacrococcygeal region

        ■ M53.2X9 Spinal instabilities, site unspecified

    M53.3 Sacrococcygeal disorders, not elsewhere classified

        Coccygodynia

● M53.8 Other specified dorsopathies

    ■ M53.80 Other specified dorsopathies, site unspecified

    M53.81 Other specified dorsopathies, occipito-atlanto-axial region

    M53.82 Other specified dorsopathies, cervical region

    M53.83 Other specified dorsopathies, cervicothoracic region

    M53.84 Other specified dorsopathies, thoracic region

    M53.85 Other specified dorsopathies, thoracolumbar region

CHAPTER 13 (M00-M99)

N Newborn Age: 0   **P** Pediatric Age: 0–17   **M** Maternity DX: 12–55   **A** Adult Age: 15–124   ♀ Females Only   ♂ Males Only

🌑 Complication\Comorbidity   🌑 Major C\C   🌑 Present on Admission Requirement   🌑 Hospital-Acquired Condition

1201

CHAPTER 13 (M00-M99)

M53.86 **Other specified dorsopathies, lumbar region**

M53.87 **Other specified dorsopathies, lumbosacral region**

M53.88 **Other specified dorsopathies, sacral and sacrococcygeal region**

■ M53.9 **Dorsopathy, unspecified**

● M54 **Dorsalgia**

> **Excludes1** psychogenic dorsalgia (F45.41)

● M54.0 **Panniculitis affecting regions of neck and back**

> **Excludes1** lupus panniculitis (L93.2)
> panniculitis NOS (M79.3)
> relapsing [Weber-Christian] panniculitis (M35.6)

■ M54.00 **Panniculitis affecting regions of neck and back, site unspecified**

M54.01 **Panniculitis affecting regions of neck and back, occipito-atlanto-axial region**

M54.02 **Panniculitis affecting regions of neck and back, cervical region**

M54.03 **Panniculitis affecting regions of neck and back, cervicothoracic region**

M54.04 **Panniculitis affecting regions of neck and back, thoracic region**

M54.05 **Panniculitis affecting regions of neck and back, thoracolumbar region**

M54.06 **Panniculitis affecting regions of neck and back, lumbar region**

M54.07 **Panniculitis affecting regions of neck and back, lumbosacral region**

M54.08 **Panniculitis affecting regions of neck and back, sacral and sacrococcygeal region**

M54.09 **Panniculitis affecting regions, neck and back, multiple sites in spine**

● M54.1 **Radiculopathy**
Brachial neuritis or radiculitis NOS
Lumbar neuritis or radiculitis NOS
Lumbosacral neuritis or radiculitis NOS
Thoracic neuritis or radiculitis NOS
Radiculitis NOS

> **Excludes1** neuralgia and neuritis NOS (M79.2)
> radiculopathy with cervical disc disorder (M50.1)
> radiculopathy with lumbar and other intervertebral disc disorder (M51.1-)
> radiculopathy with spondylosis (M47.2-)

■ M54.10 **Radiculopathy, site unspecified**

M54.11 **Radiculopathy, occipito-atlanto-axial region**

M54.12 **Radiculopathy, cervical region**

M54.13 **Radiculopathy, cervicothoracic region**

M54.14 **Radiculopathy, thoracic region**

M54.15 **Radiculopathy, thoracolumbar region**

M54.16 **Radiculopathy, lumbar region**

M54.17 **Radiculopathy, lumbosacral region**

M54.18 **Radiculopathy, sacral and sacrococcygeal region**

M54.2 **Cervicalgia**

> **Excludes1** cervicalgia due to intervertebral cervical disc disorder (M50.-)

● M54.3 **Sciatica**

> **Excludes1** lesion of sciatic nerve (G57.0)
> sciatica due to intervertebral disc disorder (M51.1-)
> sciatica with lumbago (M54.4-)

■ M54.30 **Sciatica, unspecified side**

M54.31 **Sciatica, right side**

M54.32 **Sciatica, left side**

● M54.4 **Lumbago with sciatica**

> **Excludes1** lumbago with sciatica due to intervertebral disc disorder (M51.1-)

■ M54.40 **Lumbago with sciatica, unspecified side**

M54.41 **Lumbago with sciatica, right side**

M54.42 **Lumbago with sciatica, left side**

M54.5 **Low back pain**
Loin pain
Lumbago NOS

> **Excludes1** low back strain S39.012
> lumbago due to intervertebral disc displacement (M51.2-)
> lumbago with sciatica (M54.4-)

M54.6 **Pain in thoracic spine**

> **Excludes1** pain in thoracic spine due to intervertebral disc disorder (M51.)

● M54.8 **Other dorsalgia**

> **Excludes1** dorsalgia in thoracic region (M54.6)
> low back pain (M54.5)

M54.81 **Occipital neuralgia**

M54.89 **Other dorsalgia**

■ M54.9 **Dorsalgia, unspecified**
Backache NOS
Back pain NOS

SOFT TISSUE DISORDERS (M60-M79)

DISORDERS OF MUSCLES (M60-M63)

> **Excludes1** dermatopolymyositis (M33.-)
> muscular dystrophies and myopathies (G71-G72)
> myopathy in:
> amyloidosis (E85-)
> polyarteritis nodosa (M30.0)
> rheumatoid arthritis (M05.32)
> scleroderma (M34.-)
> Sjögren's syndrome (M35.03)
> systemic lupus erythematosus (M32.-)

● M60 **Myositis**

> **Excludes2** inclusion body myositis [IBM] (G72.41)

● M60.0 **Infective myositis**
Tropical pyomyositis

> Use additional code (B95-B97) to identify infectious agent

● M60.00 **Infective myositis, unspecified site**

■ M60.000 **Infective myositis, unspecified right arm** ✆
Infective myositis, right upper limb NOS

● Unacceptable Principal Diagnosis   ● Use Additional Character(s)   ■ Unspecified   ▶ Manifestation Code
OGCR Official Guidelines for Coding and Reporting   Excludes 1   Excludes 2   Includes   Use additional   Code first   Code also

■ M60.001 Infective myositis, unspecified
left arm 🦠
    Infective myositis, left upper
limb NOS

■ M60.002 Infective myositis, unspecified
arm 🦠
    Infective myositis, upper limb
NOS

■ M60.003 Infective myositis, unspecified
right leg 🦠
    Infective myositis, right lower
limb NOS

■ M60.004 Infective myositis, unspecified
left leg 🦠
    Infective myositis, left lower
limb NOS

■ M60.005 Infective myositis, unspecified
leg 🦠
    Infective myositis, lower limb
NOS

■ M60.009 Infective myositis, unspecified
site 🦠

● M60.01 Infective myositis, shoulder
    M60.011 Infective myositis, right
shoulder 🦠
    M60.012 Infective myositis, left
shoulder 🦠
■ M60.019 Infective myositis, unspecified
shoulder 🦠

● M60.02 Infective myositis, upper arm
    M60.021 Infective myositis, right upper
arm 🦠
    M60.022 Infective myositis, left upper
arm 🦠
■ M60.029 Infective myositis, unspecified
upper arm 🦠

● M60.03 Infective myositis, forearm
    M60.031 Infective myositis, right
forearm 🦠
    M60.032 Infective myositis, left forearm 🦠
■ M60.039 Infective myositis, unspecified
forearm 🦠

● M60.04 Infective myositis, hand and fingers
    M60.041 Infective myositis, right hand 🦠
    M60.042 Infective myositis, left hand 🦠
■ M60.043 Infective myositis, unspecified
hand 🦠
    M60.044 Infective myositis, right
finger(s)🦠
    M60.045 Infective myositis, left finger(s)🦠
■ M60.046 Infective myositis, unspecified
finger(s)🦠

● M60.05 Infective myositis, thigh
    M60.051 Infective myositis, right thigh 🦠
    M60.052 Infective myositis, left thigh 🦠
■ M60.059 Infective myositis, unspecified
thigh 🦠

● M60.06 Infective myositis, lower leg
    M60.061 Infective myositis, right lower
leg 🦠
    M60.062 Infective myositis, left lower
leg 🦠
■ M60.069 Infective myositis, unspecified
lower leg 🦠

● M60.07 Infective myositis, ankle, foot and toes
    M60.070 Infective myositis, right ankle 🦠
    M60.071 Infective myositis, left ankle 🦠
■ M60.072 Infective myositis, unspecified
ankle 🦠
    M60.073 Infective myositis, right foot 🦠
    M60.074 Infective myositis, left foot 🦠
■ M60.075 Infective myositis, unspecified
foot 🦠
    M60.076 Infective myositis, right toe(s)🦠
    M60.077 Infective myositis, left toe(s)🦠
■ M60.078 Infective myositis, unspecified
toe(s)🦠

M60.08 Infective myositis, other site 🦠
M60.09 Infective myositis, multiple sites 🦠

● M60.1 Interstitial myositis
■ M60.10 Interstitial myositis of unspecified site
● M60.11 Interstitial myositis, shoulder
    M60.111 Interstitial myositis, right shoulder
    M60.112 Interstitial myositis, left shoulder
■ M60.119 Interstitial myositis, unspecified
shoulder

● M60.12 Interstitial myositis, upper arm
    M60.121 Interstitial myositis, right upper
arm
    M60.122 Interstitial myositis, left upper
arm
■ M60.129 Interstitial myositis, unspecified
upper arm

● M60.13 Interstitial myositis, forearm
    M60.131 Interstitial myositis, right
forearm
    M60.132 Interstitial myositis, left forearm
■ M60.139 Interstitial myositis, unspecified
forearm

● M60.14 Interstitial myositis, hand
    M60.141 Interstitial myositis, right hand
    M60.142 Interstitial myositis, left hand
■ M60.149 Interstitial myositis, unspecified
hand

● M60.15 Interstitial myositis, thigh
    M60.151 Interstitial myositis, right thigh
    M60.152 Interstitial myositis, left thigh
■ M60.159 Interstitial myositis, unspecified
thigh

● M60.16 Interstitial myositis, lower leg
    M60.161 Interstitial myositis, right lower
leg
    M60.162 Interstitial myositis, left lower leg
■ M60.169 Interstitial myositis, unspecified
lower leg

● M60.17 Interstitial myositis, ankle and foot
    M60.171 Interstitial myositis, right ankle
and foot
    M60.172 Interstitial myositis, left ankle
and foot
■ M60.179 Interstitial myositis, unspecified
ankle and foot

M60.18 Interstitial myositis, other site
M60.19 Interstitial myositis, multiple sites

CHAPTER 13 (M00-M99)

CHAPTER 13 (M00-M99)

● M60.2 Foreign body granuloma of soft tissue, not elsewhere classified

Use additional code to identify the type of retained foreign body (Z18.-)

Excludes1 foreign body granuloma of skin and subcutaneous tissue (L92.3)

■ M60.20 Foreign body granuloma of soft tissue, not elsewhere classified, unspecified site

● M60.21 Foreign body granuloma of soft tissue, not elsewhere classified, shoulder

M60.211 Foreign body granuloma of soft tissue, not elsewhere classified, right shoulder

M60.212 Foreign body granuloma of soft tissue, not elsewhere classified, left shoulder

■ M60.219 Foreign body granuloma of soft tissue, not elsewhere classified, unspecified shoulder

● M60.22 Foreign body granuloma of soft tissue, not elsewhere classified, upper arm

M60.221 Foreign body granuloma of soft tissue, not elsewhere classified, right upper arm

M60.222 Foreign body granuloma of soft tissue, not elsewhere classified, left upper arm

■ M60.229 Foreign body granuloma of soft tissue, not elsewhere classified, unspecified upper arm

● M60.23 Foreign body granuloma of soft tissue, not elsewhere classified, forearm

M60.231 Foreign body granuloma of soft tissue, not elsewhere classified, right forearm

M60.232 Foreign body granuloma of soft tissue, not elsewhere classified, left forearm

■ M60.239 Foreign body granuloma of soft tissue, not elsewhere classified, unspecified forearm

● M60.24 Foreign body granuloma of soft tissue, not elsewhere classified, hand

M60.241 Foreign body granuloma of soft tissue, not elsewhere classified, right hand

M60.242 Foreign body granuloma of soft tissue, not elsewhere classified, left hand

■ M60.249 Foreign body granuloma of soft tissue, not elsewhere classified, unspecified hand

● M60.25 Foreign body granuloma of soft tissue, not elsewhere classified, thigh

M60.251 Foreign body granuloma of soft tissue, not elsewhere classified, right thigh

M60.252 Foreign body granuloma of soft tissue, not elsewhere classified, left thigh

■ M60.259 Foreign body granuloma of soft tissue, not elsewhere classified, unspecified thigh

● M60.26 Foreign body granuloma of soft tissue, not elsewhere classified, lower leg

M60.261 Foreign body granuloma of soft tissue, not elsewhere classified, right lower leg

M60.262 Foreign body granuloma of soft tissue, not elsewhere classified, left lower leg

■ M60.269 Foreign body granuloma of soft tissue, not elsewhere classified, unspecified lower leg

● M60.27 Foreign body granuloma of soft tissue, not elsewhere classified, ankle and foot

M60.271 Foreign body granuloma of soft tissue, not elsewhere classified, right ankle and foot

M60.272 Foreign body granuloma of soft tissue, not elsewhere classified, left ankle and foot

■ M60.279 Foreign body granuloma of soft tissue, not elsewhere classified, unspecified ankle and foot

M60.28 Foreign body granuloma of soft tissue, not elsewhere classified, other site

● M60.8 Other myositis

■ M60.80 Other myositis, unspecified site

● M60.81 Other myositis shoulder

M60.811 Other myositis, right shoulder

M60.812 Other myositis, left shoulder

■ M60.819 Other myositis, unspecified shoulder

● M60.82 Other myositis, upper arm

M60.821 Other myositis, right upper arm

M60.822 Other myositis, left upper arm

■ M60.829 Other myositis, unspecified upper arm

● M60.83 Other myositis, forearm

M60.831 Other myositis, right forearm

M60.832 Other myositis, left forearm

■ M60.839 Other myositis, unspecified forearm

● M60.84 Other myositis, hand

M60.841 Other myositis, right hand

M60.842 Other myositis, left hand

■ M60.849 Other myositis, unspecified hand

● M60.85 Other myositis, thigh

M60.851 Other myositis, right thigh

M60.852 Other myositis, left thigh

■ M60.859 Other myositis, unspecified thigh

● M60.86 Other myositis, lower leg

M60.861 Other myositis, right lower leg

M60.862 Other myositis, left lower leg

■ M60.869 Other myositis, unspecified lower leg

● M60.87 Other myositis, ankle and foot

M60.871 Other myositis, right ankle and foot

M60.872 Other myositis, left ankle and foot

■ M60.879 Other myositis, unspecified ankle and foot

● Unacceptable Principal Diagnosis   ● Use Additional Character(s)   ■ Unspecified   ▶ Manifestation Code

OGCR Official Guidelines for Coding and Reporting   Excludes 1   Excludes 2   Includes   Use additional   Code first   Code also

M60.88 Other myositis, other site

M60.89 Other myositis, multiple sites

■ M60.9 Myositis, unspecified

● M61 Calcification and ossification of muscle

  ● M61.0 Myositis ossificans traumatica

    ■ M61.00 Myositis ossificans traumatica, unspecified site

    ● M61.01 Myositis ossificans traumatica, shoulder

      M61.011 Myositis ossificans traumatica, right shoulder

      M61.012 Myositis ossificans traumatica, left shoulder

      ■ M61.019 Myositis ossificans traumatica, unspecified shoulder

    ● M61.02 Myositis ossificans traumatica, upper arm

      M61.021 Myositis ossificans traumatica, right upper arm

      M61.022 Myositis ossificans traumatica, left upper arm

      ■ M61.029 Myositis ossificans traumatica, unspecified upper arm

    ● M61.03 Myositis ossificans traumatica, forearm

      M61.031 Myositis ossificans traumatica, right forearm

      M61.032 Myositis ossificans traumatica, left forearm

      ■ M61.039 Myositis ossificans traumatica, unspecified forearm

    ● M61.04 Myositis ossificans traumatica, hand

      M61.041 Myositis ossificans traumatica, right hand

      M61.042 Myositis ossificans traumatica, left hand

      ■ M61.049 Myositis ossificans traumatica, unspecified hand

    ● M61.05 Myositis ossificans traumatica, thigh

      M61.051 Myositis ossificans traumatica, right thigh

      M61.052 Myositis ossificans traumatica, left thigh

      ■ M61.059 Myositis ossificans traumatica, unspecified thigh

    ● M61.06 Myositis ossificans traumatica, lower leg

      M61.061 Myositis ossificans traumatica, right lower leg

      M61.062 Myositis ossificans traumatica, left lower leg

      ■ M61.069 Myositis ossificans traumatica, unspecified lower leg

    ● M61.07 Myositis ossificans traumatica, ankle and foot

      M61.071 Myositis ossificans traumatica, right ankle and foot

      M61.072 Myositis ossificans traumatica, left ankle and foot

      ■ M61.079 Myositis ossificans traumatica, unspecified ankle and foot

    M61.08 Myositis ossificans traumatica, other site

    M61.09 Myositis ossificans traumatica, multiple sites

● M61.1 Myositis ossificans progressiva
Fibrodysplasia ossificans progressiva

  ■ M61.10 Myositis ossificans progressiva, unspecified site

  ● M61.11 Myositis ossificans progressiva, shoulder

    M61.111 Myositis ossificans progressiva, right shoulder

    M61.112 Myositis ossificans progressiva, left shoulder

    ■ M61.119 Myositis ossificans progressiva, unspecified shoulder

  ● M61.12 Myositis ossificans progressiva, upper arm

    M61.121 Myositis ossificans progressiva, right upper arm

    M61.122 Myositis ossificans progressiva, left upper arm

    ■ M61.129 Myositis ossificans progressiva, unspecified arm

  ● M61.13 Myositis ossificans progressiva, forearm

    M61.131 Myositis ossificans progressiva, right forearm

    M61.132 Myositis ossificans progressiva, left forearm

    ■ M61.139 Myositis ossificans progressiva, unspecified forearm

  ● M61.14 Myositis ossificans progressiva, hand and finger(s)

    M61.141 Myositis ossificans progressiva, right hand

    M61.142 Myositis ossificans progressiva, left hand

    ■ M61.143 Myositis ossificans progressiva, unspecified hand

    M61.144 Myositis ossificans progressiva, right finger(s)

    M61.145 Myositis ossificans progressiva, left finger(s)

    ■ M61.146 Myositis ossificans progressiva, unspecified finger(s)

  ● M61.15 Myositis ossificans progressiva, thigh

    M61.151 Myositis ossificans progressiva, right thigh

    M61.152 Myositis ossificans progressiva, left thigh

    ■ M61.159 Myositis ossificans progressiva, unspecified thigh

  ● M61.16 Myositis ossificans progressiva, lower leg

    M61.161 Myositis ossificans progressiva, right lower leg

    M61.162 Myositis ossificans progressiva, left lower leg

    ■ M61.169 Myositis ossificans progressiva, unspecified lower leg

  ● M61.17 Myositis ossificans progressiva, ankle, foot and toe(s)

    M61.171 Myositis ossificans progressiva, right ankle

    M61.172 Myositis ossificans progressiva, left ankle

    ■ M61.173 Myositis ossificans progressiva, unspecified ankle

CHAPTER 13 (M00-M99)

N Newborn Age: 0   **P** Pediatric Age: 0–17   **M** Maternity DX: 12–55   **A** Adult Age: 15–124   ♀ Females Only   ♂ Males Only

Complication\Comorbidity   Major C\C   Present on Admission Requirement   Hospital-Acquired Condition

1205

M61.174 Myositis ossificans progressiva, right foot

M61.175 Myositis ossificans progressiva, left foot

■M61.176 Myositis ossificans progressiva, unspecified foot

M61.177 Myositis ossificans progressiva, right toe(s)

M61.178 Myositis ossificans progressiva, left toe(s)

■M61.179 Myositis ossificans progressiva, unspecified toe(s)

M61.18 Myositis ossificans progressiva, other site

M61.19 Myositis ossificans progressiva, multiple sites

●M61.2 Paralytic calcification and ossification of muscle
Myositis ossificans associated with quadriplegia or paraplegia

■M61.20 Paralytic calcification and ossification of muscle, unspecified site

●M61.21 Paralytic calcification and ossification of muscle, shoulder

M61.211 Paralytic calcification and ossification of muscle, right shoulder

M61.212 Paralytic calcification and ossification of muscle, left shoulder

■M61.219 Paralytic calcification and ossification of muscle, unspecified shoulder

●M61.22 Paralytic calcification and ossification of muscle, upper arm

M61.221 Paralytic calcification and ossification of muscle, right upper arm

M61.222 Paralytic calcification and ossification of muscle, left upper arm

■M61.229 Paralytic calcification and ossification of muscle, unspecified upper arm

●M61.23 Paralytic calcification and ossification of muscle, forearm

M61.231 Paralytic calcification and ossification of muscle, right forearm

M61.232 Paralytic calcification and ossification of muscle, left forearm

■M61.239 Paralytic calcification and ossification of muscle, unspecified forearm

●M61.24 Paralytic calcification and ossification of muscle, hand

M61.241 Paralytic calcification and ossification of muscle, right hand

M61.242 Paralytic calcification and ossification of muscle, left hand

■M61.249 Paralytic calcification and ossification of muscle, unspecified hand

●M61.25 Paralytic calcification and ossification of muscle, thigh

M61.251 Paralytic calcification and ossification of muscle, right thigh

M61.252 Paralytic calcification and ossification of muscle, left thigh

■M61.259 Paralytic calcification and ossification of muscle, unspecified thigh

●M61.26 Paralytic calcification and ossification of muscle, lower leg

M61.261 Paralytic calcification and ossification of muscle, right lower leg

M61.262 Paralytic calcification and ossification of muscle, left lower leg

■M61.269 Paralytic calcification and ossification of muscle, unspecified lower leg

●M61.27 Paralytic calcification and ossification of muscle, ankle and foot

M61.271 Paralytic calcification and ossification of muscle, right ankle and foot

M61.272 Paralytic calcification and ossification of muscle, left ankle and foot

■M61.279 Paralytic calcification and ossification of muscle, unspecified ankle and foot

M61.28 Paralytic calcification and ossification of muscle, other site

M61.29 Paralytic calcification and ossification of muscle, multiple sites

●M61.3 Calcification and ossification of muscles associated with burns
Myositis ossificans associated with burns

■M61.30 Calcification and ossification of muscles associated with burns, unspecified site

●M61.31 Calcification and ossification of muscles associated with burns, shoulder

M61.311 Calcification and ossification of muscles associated with burns, right shoulder

M61.312 Calcification and ossification of muscles associated with burns, left shoulder

■M61.319 Calcification and ossification of muscles associated with burns, unspecified shoulder

●M61.32 Calcification and ossification of muscles associated with burns, upper arm

M61.321 Calcification and ossification of muscles associated with burns, right upper arm

M61.322 Calcification and ossification of muscles associated with burns, left upper arm

■M61.329 Calcification and ossification of muscles associated with burns, unspecified upper arm

● Unacceptable Principal Diagnosis   ● Use Additional Character(s)   ■ Unspecified   ▶ Manifestation Code

OGCR Official Guidelines for Coding and Reporting   Excludes 1   Excludes 2   Includes   Use additional   Code first   Code also

● M61.33 Calcification and ossification of muscles associated with burns, forearm

    M61.331 Calcification and ossification of muscles associated with burns, right forearm

    M61.332 Calcification and ossification of muscles associated with burns, left forearm

    ■ M61.339 Calcification and ossification of muscles associated with burns, unspecified forearm

● M61.34 Calcification and ossification of muscles associated with burns, hand

    M61.341 Calcification and ossification of muscles associated with burns, right hand

    M61.342 Calcification and ossification of muscles associated with burns, left hand

    ■ M61.349 Calcification and ossification of muscles associated with burns, unspecified hand

● M61.35 Calcification and ossification of muscles associated with burns, thigh

    M61.351 Calcification and ossification of muscles associated with burns, right thigh

    M61.352 Calcification and ossification of muscles associated with burns, left thigh

    ■ M61.359 Calcification and ossification of muscles associated with burns, unspecified thigh

● M61.36 Calcification and ossification of muscles associated with burns, lower leg

    M61.361 Calcification and ossification of muscles associated with burns, right lower leg

    M61.362 Calcification and ossification of muscles associated with burns, left lower leg

    ■ M61.369 Calcification and ossification of muscles associated with burns, unspecified lower leg

● M61.37 Calcification and ossification of muscles associated with burns, ankle and foot

    M61.371 Calcification and ossification of muscles associated with burns, right ankle and foot

    M61.372 Calcification and ossification of muscles associated with burns, left ankle and foot

    ■ M61.379 Calcification and ossification of muscles associated with burns, unspecified ankle and foot

M61.38 Calcification and ossification of muscles associated with burns, other site

M61.39 Calcification and ossification of muscles associated with burns, multiple sites

● M61.4 Other calcification of muscle

    Excludes1   calcific tendinitis NOS (M65.2-)
                 calcific tendinitis of shoulder (M75.3)

    ■ M61.40 Other calcification of muscle, unspecified site

● M61.41 Other calcification of muscle, shoulder

    M61.411 Other calcification of muscle, right shoulder

    M61.412 Other calcification of muscle, left shoulder

    ■ M61.419 Other calcification of muscle, unspecified shoulder

● M61.42 Other calcification of muscle, upper arm

    M61.421 Other calcification of muscle, right upper arm

    M61.422 Other calcification of muscle, left upper arm

    ■ M61.429 Other calcification of muscle, unspecified upper arm

● M61.43 Other calcification of muscle, forearm

    M61.431 Other calcification of muscle, right forearm

    M61.432 Other calcification of muscle, left forearm

    ■ M61.439 Other calcification of muscle, unspecified forearm

● M61.44 Other calcification of muscle, hand

    M61.441 Other calcification of muscle, right hand

    M61.442 Other calcification of muscle, left hand

    ■ M61.449 Other calcification of muscle, unspecified hand

● M61.45 Other calcification of muscle, thigh

    M61.451 Other calcification of muscle, right thigh

    M61.452 Other calcification of muscle, left thigh

    ■ M61.459 Other calcification of muscle, unspecified thigh

● M61.46 Other calcification of muscle, lower leg

    M61.461 Other calcification of muscle, right lower leg

    M61.462 Other calcification of muscle, left lower leg

    ■ M61.469 Other calcification of muscle, unspecified lower leg

● M61.47 Other calcification of muscle, ankle and foot

    M61.471 Other calcification of muscle, right ankle and foot

    M61.472 Other calcification of muscle, left ankle and foot

    ■ M61.479 Other calcification of muscle, unspecified ankle and foot

M61.48 Other calcification of muscle, other site

M61.49 Other calcification of muscle, multiple sites

CHAPTER 13 (M00-M99)

- **M61.5 Other ossification of muscle**
  - **M61.50** Other ossification of muscle, unspecified site
  - **M61.51** Other ossification of muscle, shoulder
    - M61.511 Other ossification of muscle, right shoulder
    - M61.512 Other ossification of muscle, left shoulder
    - M61.519 Other ossification of muscle, unspecified shoulder
  - **M61.52** Other ossification of muscle, upper arm
    - M61.521 Other ossification of muscle, right upper arm
    - M61.522 Other ossification of muscle, left upper arm
    - M61.529 Other ossification of muscle, unspecified upper arm
  - **M61.53** Other ossification of muscle, forearm
    - M61.531 Other ossification of muscle, right forearm
    - M61.532 Other ossification of muscle, left forearm
    - M61.539 Other ossification of muscle, unspecified forearm
  - **M61.54** Other ossification of muscle, hand
    - M61.541 Other ossification of muscle, right hand
    - M61.542 Other ossification of muscle, left hand
    - M61.549 Other ossification of muscle, unspecified hand
  - **M61.55** Other ossification of muscle, thigh
    - M61.551 Other ossification of muscle, right thigh
    - M61.552 Other ossification of muscle, left thigh
    - M61.559 Other ossification of muscle, unspecified thigh
  - **M61.56** Other ossification of muscle, lower leg
    - M61.561 Other ossification of muscle, right lower leg
    - M61.562 Other ossification of muscle, left lower leg
    - M61.569 Other ossification of muscle, unspecified lower leg
  - **M61.57** Other ossification of muscle, ankle and foot
    - M61.571 Other ossification of muscle, right ankle and foot
    - M61.572 Other ossification of muscle, left ankle and foot
    - M61.579 Other ossification of muscle, unspecified ankle and foot
  - M61.58 Other ossification of muscle, other site
  - M61.59 Other ossification of muscle, multiple sites
- **M61.9 Calcification and ossification of muscle, unspecified**

- **M62 Other disorders of muscle**
  - **Excludes1** alcoholic myopathy (G72.1)
    cramp and spasm (R25.2)
    drug-induced myopathy (G72.0)
    myalgia (M79.1)
    stiff-man syndrome (G25.82)
  - **Excludes2** nontraumatic hematoma of muscle (M79.81)
  - **M62.0 Separation of muscle (nontraumatic)**
    Diastasis of muscle
    - **Excludes1** diastasis recti complicating pregnancy, labor and delivery (O71.8)
      traumatic separation of muscle - see strain of muscle by body region
    - **M62.00** Separation of muscle (nontraumatic), unspecified site
    - **M62.01** Separation of muscle (nontraumatic), shoulder
      - M62.011 Separation of muscle (nontraumatic), right shoulder
      - M62.012 Separation of muscle (nontraumatic), left shoulder
      - M62.019 Separation of muscle (nontraumatic), unspecified shoulder
    - **M62.02** Separation of muscle (nontraumatic), upper arm
      - M62.021 Separation of muscle (nontraumatic), right upper arm
      - M62.022 Separation of muscle (nontraumatic), left upper arm
      - M62.029 Separation of muscle (nontraumatic), unspecified upper arm
    - **M62.03** Separation of muscle (nontraumatic), forearm
      - M62.031 Separation of muscle (nontraumatic), right forearm
      - M62.032 Separation of muscle (nontraumatic), left forearm
      - M62.039 Separation of muscle (nontraumatic), unspecified forearm
    - **M62.04** Separation of muscle (nontraumatic), hand
      - M62.041 Separation of muscle (nontraumatic), right hand
      - M62.042 Separation of muscle (nontraumatic), left hand
      - M62.049 Separation of muscle (nontraumatic), unspecified hand
    - **M62.05** Separation of muscle (nontraumatic), thigh
      - M62.051 Separation of muscle (nontraumatic), right thigh
      - M62.052 Separation of muscle (nontraumatic), left thigh
      - M62.059 Separation of muscle (nontraumatic), unspecified thigh
    - **M62.06** Separation of muscle (nontraumatic), lower leg
      - M62.061 Separation of muscle (nontraumatic), right lower leg
      - M62.062 Separation of muscle (nontraumatic), left lower leg
      - M62.069 Separation of muscle (nontraumatic), unspecified lower leg

● Unacceptable Principal Diagnosis   ● Use Additional Character(s)   ■ Unspecified   ▶ Manifestation Code
OGCR Official Guidelines for Coding and Reporting   Excludes 1   Excludes 2   Includes   Use additional   Code first   Code also

● **M62.07 Separation of muscle (nontraumatic), ankle and foot**

　M62.071 Separation of muscle (nontraumatic), right ankle and foot

　M62.072 Separation of muscle (nontraumatic), left ankle and foot

　■ M62.079 Separation of muscle (nontraumatic), unspecified ankle and foot

　M62.08 Separation of muscle (nontraumatic), other site

● **M62.1 Other rupture of muscle (nontraumatic)**

　Excludes1　traumatic rupture of muscle - see strain of muscle by body region

　Excludes2　rupture of tendon (M66.-)

　■ M62.10 Other rupture of muscle (nontraumatic), unspecified site

● M62.11 Other rupture of muscle (nontraumatic), shoulder

　M62.111 Other rupture of muscle (nontraumatic), right shoulder

　M62.112 Other rupture of muscle (nontraumatic), left shoulder

　■ M62.119 Other rupture of muscle (nontraumatic), unspecified shoulder

● M62.12 Other rupture of muscle (nontraumatic), upper arm

　M62.121 Other rupture of muscle (nontraumatic), right upper arm

　M62.122 Other rupture of muscle (nontraumatic), left upper arm

　■ M62.129 Other rupture of muscle (nontraumatic), unspecified upper arm

● M62.13 Other rupture of muscle (nontraumatic), forearm

　M62.131 Other rupture of muscle (nontraumatic), right forearm

　M62.132 Other rupture of muscle (nontraumatic), left forearm

　■ M62.139 Other rupture of muscle (nontraumatic), unspecified forearm

● M62.14 Other rupture of muscle (nontraumatic), hand

　M62.141 Other rupture of muscle (nontraumatic), right hand

　M62.142 Other rupture of muscle (nontraumatic), left hand

　■ M62.149 Other rupture of muscle (nontraumatic), unspecified hand

● M62.15 Other rupture of muscle (nontraumatic), thigh

　M62.151 Other rupture of muscle (nontraumatic), right thigh

　M62.152 Other rupture of muscle (nontraumatic), left thigh

　■ M62.159 Other rupture of muscle (nontraumatic), unspecified thigh

● M62.16 Other rupture of muscle (nontraumatic), lower leg

　M62.161 Other rupture of muscle (nontraumatic), right lower leg

　M62.162 Other rupture of muscle (nontraumatic), left lower leg

　■ M62.169 Other rupture of muscle (nontraumatic), unspecified lower leg

● M62.17 Other rupture of muscle (nontraumatic), ankle and foot

　M62.171 Other rupture of muscle (nontraumatic), right ankle and foot

　M62.172 Other rupture of muscle (nontraumatic), left ankle and foot

　■ M62.179 Other rupture of muscle (nontraumatic), unspecified ankle and foot

　M62.18 Other rupture of muscle (nontraumatic), other site

● M62.2 Nontraumatic ischemic infarction of muscle

　Excludes1　compartment syndrome (traumatic) (T79.A-)
　　nontraumatic compartment syndrome (M79.A-)
　　traumatic ischemia of muscle (T79.6)
　　rhabdomyolysis (M62.82)
　　Volkmann's ischemic contracture (T79.6)

　■ M62.20 Nontraumatic ischemic infarction of muscle, unspecified site

● M62.21 Nontraumatic ischemic infarction of muscle, shoulder

　M62.211 Nontraumatic ischemic infarction of muscle, right shoulder

　M62.212 Nontraumatic ischemic infarction of muscle, left shoulder

　■ M62.219 Nontraumatic ischemic infarction of muscle, unspecified shoulder

● M62.22 Nontraumatic ischemic infarction of muscle, upper arm

　M62.221 Nontraumatic ischemic infarction of muscle, right upper arm

　M62.222 Nontraumatic ischemic infarction of muscle, left upper arm

　■ M62.229 Nontraumatic ischemic infarction of muscle, unspecified upper arm

● M62.23 Nontraumatic ischemic infarction of muscle, forearm

　M62.231 Nontraumatic ischemic infarction of muscle, right forearm

　M62.232 Nontraumatic ischemic infarction of muscle, left forearm

　■ M62.239 Nontraumatic ischemic infarction of muscle, unspecified forearm

● M62.24 Nontraumatic ischemic infarction of muscle, hand

　M62.241 Nontraumatic ischemic infarction of muscle, right hand

　M62.242 Nontraumatic ischemic infarction of muscle, left hand

　■ M62.249 Nontraumatic ischemic infarction of muscle, unspecified hand

● **M62.25 Nontraumatic ischemic infarction of muscle, thigh**

     M62.251 Nontraumatic ischemic infarction of muscle, right thigh

     M62.252 Nontraumatic ischemic infarction of muscle, left thigh

     ■ M62.259 Nontraumatic ischemic infarction of muscle, unspecified thigh

● **M62.26 Nontraumatic ischemic infarction of muscle, lower leg**

     M62.261 Nontraumatic ischemic infarction of muscle, right lower leg

     M62.262 Nontraumatic ischemic infarction of muscle, left lower leg

     ■ M62.269 Nontraumatic ischemic infarction of muscle, unspecified lower leg

● **M62.27 Nontraumatic ischemic infarction of muscle, ankle and foot**

     M62.271 Nontraumatic ischemic infarction of muscle, right ankle and foot

     M62.272 Nontraumatic ischemic infarction of muscle, left ankle and foot

     ■ M62.279 Nontraumatic ischemic infarction of muscle, unspecified ankle and foot

     M62.28 Nontraumatic ischemic infarction of muscle, other site

M62.3 Immobility syndrome (paraplegic)

M62.4 Contracture of muscle

CONTRACTURE OF TENDON (SHEATH)

Excludes1 contracture of joint (M24.5-)

■ M62.40 Contracture of muscle, unspecified site

● **M62.41 Contracture of muscle, shoulder**

     M62.411 Contracture of muscle, right shoulder

     M62.412 Contracture of muscle, left shoulder

     ■ M62.419 Contracture of muscle, unspecified shoulder

● **M62.42 Contracture of muscle, upper arm**

     M62.421 Contracture of muscle, right upper arm

     M62.422 Contracture of muscle, left upper arm

     ■ M62.429 Contracture of muscle, unspecified upper arm

● **M62.43 Contracture of muscle, forearm**

     M62.431 Contracture of muscle, right forearm

     M62.432 Contracture of muscle, left forearm

     ■ M62.439 Contracture of muscle, unspecified forearm

● **M62.44 Contracture of muscle, hand**

     M62.441 Contracture of muscle, right hand

     M62.442 Contracture of muscle, left hand

     ■ M62.449 Contracture of muscle, unspecified hand

● **M62.45 Contracture of muscle, thigh**

     M62.451 Contracture of muscle, right thigh

     M62.452 Contracture of muscle, left thigh

     ■ M62.459 Contracture of muscle, unspecified thigh

● **M62.46 Contracture of muscle, lower leg**

     M62.461 Contracture of muscle, right lower leg

     M62.462 Contracture of muscle, left lower leg

     ■ M62.469 Contracture of muscle, unspecified lower leg

● **M62.47 Contracture of muscle, ankle and foot**

     M62.471 Contracture of muscle, right ankle and foot

     M62.472 Contracture of muscle, left ankle and foot

     ■ M62.479 Contracture of muscle, unspecified ankle and foot

     M62.48 Contracture of muscle, other site

     M62.49 Contracture of muscle, multiple sites

● **M62.5 Muscle wasting and atrophy, not elsewhere classified**

     Disuse atrophy NEC

     Excludes1 neuralgic amyotrophy (G54.5) progressive muscular atrophy (G12.29)

     Excludes2 pelvic muscle wasting (N81.84)

■ M62.50 Muscle wasting and atrophy, not elsewhere classified, unspecified site

● **M62.51 Muscle wasting and atrophy, not elsewhere classified, shoulder**

     M62.511 Muscle wasting and atrophy, not elsewhere classified, right shoulder

     M62.512 Muscle wasting and atrophy, not elsewhere classified, left shoulder

     ■ M62.519 Muscle wasting and atrophy, not elsewhere classified, unspecified shoulder

● **M62.52 Muscle wasting and atrophy, not elsewhere classified, upper arm**

     M62.521 Muscle wasting and atrophy, not elsewhere classified, right upper arm

     M62.522 Muscle wasting and atrophy, not elsewhere classified, left upper arm

     ■ M62.529 Muscle wasting and atrophy, not elsewhere classified, unspecified upper arm

● **M62.53 Muscle wasting and atrophy, not elsewhere classified, forearm**

     M62.531 Muscle wasting and atrophy, not elsewhere classified, right forearm

     M62.532 Muscle wasting and atrophy, not elsewhere classified, left forearm

     ■ M62.539 Muscle wasting and atrophy, not elsewhere classified, unspecified forearm

● Unacceptable Principal Diagnosis   ● Use Additional Character(s)   ■ Unspecified   ▶ Manifestation Code

OGCR Official Guidelines for Coding and Reporting   Excludes 1   Excludes 2   Includes   Use additional   Code first   Code also

● **M62.54 Muscle wasting and atrophy, not elsewhere classified, hand**

     M62.541 Muscle wasting and atrophy, not elsewhere classified, right hand

     M62.542 Muscle wasting and atrophy, not elsewhere classified, left hand

     ■ **M62.549 Muscle wasting and atrophy, not elsewhere classified, unspecified hand**

● **M62.55 Muscle wasting and atrophy, not elsewhere classified, thigh**

     M62.551 Muscle wasting and atrophy, not elsewhere classified, right thigh

     M62.552 Muscle wasting and atrophy, not elsewhere classified, left thigh

     ■ **M62.559 Muscle wasting and atrophy, not elsewhere classified, unspecified thigh**

● **M62.56 Muscle wasting and atrophy, not elsewhere classified, lower leg**

     M62.561 Muscle wasting and atrophy, not elsewhere classified, right lower leg

     M62.562 Muscle wasting and atrophy, not elsewhere classified, left lower leg

     ■ **M62.569 Muscle wasting and atrophy, not elsewhere classified, unspecified lower leg**

● **M62.57 Muscle wasting and atrophy, not elsewhere classified, ankle and foot**

     M62.571 Muscle wasting and atrophy, not elsewhere classified, right ankle and foot

     M62.572 Muscle wasting and atrophy, not elsewhere classified, left ankle and foot

     ■ **M62.579 Muscle wasting and atrophy, not elsewhere classified, unspecified ankle and foot**

     M62.58 Muscle wasting and atrophy, not elsewhere classified, other site

     M62.59 Muscle wasting and atrophy, not elsewhere classified, multiple sites

● **M62.8 Other specified disorders of muscle**

     | Excludes2 | nontraumatic hematoma of muscle (M79.81)

     M62.81 Muscle weakness (generalized)

     M62.82 Rhabdomyolysis 🅼

         | Excludes1 | traumatic rhabdomyolysis (T79.6)

● **M62.83 Muscle spasm**

     M62.830 Muscle spasm of back

     M62.831 Muscle spasm of calf
         Charley-horse

     M62.838 Other muscle spasm

     M62.89 Other specified disorders of muscle
         Muscle (sheath) hernia

■ **M62.9 Disorder of muscle, unspecified**

● **M63 Disorders of muscle in diseases classified elsewhere**

     Code first underlying disease, such as:
         leprosy (A30.-)
         neoplasm (C49.-, C79.89, D21.-, D48.1)
         schistosomiasis (B65.-)
         trichinellosis (B75)

     | Excludes1 | myopathy in cysticercosis (B69.81)
         myopathy in endocrine diseases (G73.7)
         myopathy in metabolic diseases (G73.7)
         myopathy in sarcoidosis (D86.87)
         myopathy in secondary syphilis (A51.49)
         myopathy in syphilis (late) (A52.78)
         myopathy in toxoplasmosis (B58.82)
         myopathy in tuberculosis (A18.09)

● **M63.8 Disorders of muscle in diseases classified elsewhere**

     ● ■ ▶ *M63.80 Disorders of muscle in diseases classified elsewhere, unspecified site*

     ● **M63.81 Disorders of muscle in diseases classified elsewhere, shoulder**

         ● ▶ *M63.811 Disorders of muscle in diseases classified elsewhere, right shoulder*

         ● ▶ *M63.812 Disorders of muscle in diseases classified elsewhere, left shoulder*

         ● ■ ▶ *M63.819 Disorders of muscle in diseases classified elsewhere, unspecified shoulder*

     ● **M63.82 Disorders of muscle in diseases classified elsewhere, upper arm**

         ● ▶ *M63.821 Disorders of muscle in diseases classified elsewhere, right upper arm*

         ● ▶ *M63.822 Disorders of muscle in diseases classified elsewhere, left upper arm*

         ● ■ ▶ *M63.829 Disorders of muscle in diseases classified elsewhere, unspecified upper arm*

     ● **M63.83 Disorders of muscle in diseases classified elsewhere, forearm**

         ● ▶ *M63.831 Disorders of muscle in diseases classified elsewhere, right forearm*

         ● ▶ *M63.832 Disorders of muscle in diseases classified elsewhere, left forearm*

         ● ■ ▶ *M63.839 Disorders of muscle in diseases classified elsewhere, unspecified forearm*

     ● **M63.84 Disorders of muscle in diseases classified elsewhere, hand**

         ● ▶ *M63.841 Disorders of muscle in diseases classified elsewhere, right hand*

         ● ▶ *M63.842 Disorders of muscle in diseases classified elsewhere, left hand*

         ● ■ ▶ *M63.849 Disorders of muscle in diseases classified elsewhere, unspecified hand*

     ● **M63.85 Disorders of muscle in diseases classified elsewhere, thigh**

         ● ▶ *M63.851 Disorders of muscle in diseases classified elsewhere, right thigh*

         ● ▶ *M63.852 Disorders of muscle in diseases classified elsewhere, left thigh*

         ● ■ ▶ *M63.859 Disorders of muscle in diseases classified elsewhere, unspecified thigh*

CHAPTER 13 (M00-M99)

N Newborn Age: 0   **P** Pediatric Age: 0–17   **M** Maternity DX: 12–55   **A** Adult Age: 15–124   ♀ Females Only   ♂ Males Only

🅒 Complication\Comorbidity   🅜 Major C\C   🅟 Present on Admission Requirement   🅗 Hospital-Acquired Condition

1211

CHAPTER 13 (M00-M99)

● M63.86 Disorders of muscle in diseases classified elsewhere, lower leg
- ●▶ *M63.861 Disorders of muscle in diseases classified elsewhere, right lower leg*
- ●▶ *M63.862 Disorders of muscle in diseases classified elsewhere, left lower leg*
- ●■▶ *M63.869 Disorders of muscle in diseases classified elsewhere, unspecified lower leg*

● M63.87 Disorders of muscle in diseases classified elsewhere, ankle and foot
- ●▶ *M63.871 Disorders of muscle in diseases classified elsewhere, right ankle and foot*
- ●▶ *M63.872 Disorders of muscle in diseases classified elsewhere, left ankle and foot*
- ●■▶ *M63.879 Disorders of muscle in diseases classified elsewhere, unspecified ankle and foot*

●▶ *M63.88 Disorders of muscle in diseases classified elsewhere, other site*

●▶ *M63.89 Disorders of muscle in diseases classified elsewhere, multiple sites*

DISORDERS OF SYNOVIUM AND TENDON (M65-M67)

● M65 Synovitis and tenosynovitis

    Excludes1   chronic crepitant synovitis of hand and wrist (M70.0-)
                 current injury - see injury of ligament or tendon by body region
                 soft tissue disorders related to use, overuse and pressure (M70.-)

● M65.0 Abscess of tendon sheath

        Use additional code (B95-B96) to identify bacterial agent

- ■ M65.00 Abscess of tendon sheath, unspecified site
- ● M65.01 Abscess of tendon sheath, shoulder
  - M65.011 Abscess of tendon sheath, right shoulder
  - M65.012 Abscess of tendon sheath, left shoulder
  - ■ M65.019 Abscess of tendon sheath, unspecified shoulder
- ● M65.02 Abscess of tendon sheath, upper arm
  - M65.021 Abscess of tendon sheath, right upper arm
  - M65.022 Abscess of tendon sheath, left upper arm
  - ■ M65.029 Abscess of tendon sheath, unspecified upper arm

● M65.03 Abscess of tendon sheath, forearm
- M65.031 Abscess of tendon sheath, right forearm
- M65.032 Abscess of tendon sheath, left forearm
- ■ M65.039 Abscess of tendon sheath, unspecified forearm

● M65.04 Abscess of tendon sheath, hand
- M65.041 Abscess of tendon sheath, right hand
- M65.042 Abscess of tendon sheath, left hand
- ■ M65.049 Abscess of tendon sheath, unspecified hand

● M65.05 Abscess of tendon sheath, thigh
- M65.051 Abscess of tendon sheath, right thigh
- M65.052 Abscess of tendon sheath, left thigh
- ■ M65.059 Abscess of tendon sheath, unspecified thigh

● M65.06 Abscess of tendon sheath, lower leg
- M65.061 Abscess of tendon sheath, right lower leg
- M65.062 Abscess of tendon sheath, left lower leg
- ■ M65.069 Abscess of tendon sheath, unspecified lower leg

● M65.07 Abscess of tendon sheath, ankle and foot
- M65.071 Abscess of tendon sheath, right ankle and foot
- M65.072 Abscess of tendon sheath, left ankle and foot
- ■ M65.079 Abscess of tendon sheath, unspecified ankle and foot

M65.08 Abscess of tendon sheath, other site

● M65.1 Other infective (teno)synovitis
- ■ M65.10 Other infective (teno)synovitis, unspecified site
- ● M65.11 Other infective (teno)synovitis, shoulder
  - M65.111 Other infective (teno)synovitis, right shoulder
  - M65.112 Other infective (teno)synovitis, left shoulder
  - ■ M65.119 Other infective (teno)synovitis, unspecified shoulder
- ● M65.12 Other infective (teno)synovitis, elbow
  - M65.121 Other infective (teno)synovitis, right elbow
  - M65.122 Other infective (teno)synovitis, left elbow
  - ■ M65.129 Other infective (teno)synovitis, unspecified elbow
- ● M65.13 Other infective (teno)synovitis, wrist
  - M65.131 Other infective (teno)synovitis, right wrist
  - M65.132 Other infective (teno)synovitis, left wrist
  - ■ M65.139 Other infective (teno)synovitis, unspecified wrist

Item 13–11   **Synovitis** is an inflammation of a synovial membrane resulting in pain on motion and is characterized by fluctuating swelling due to effusion in a synovial sac. **Tenosynovitis** is an inflammation of a tendon sheath and occurs most commonly in the wrists, hands, and feet. Bursitis is inflammation of a bursa (fluid filled sac) caused by repetitive use, trauma, infection, or systemic inflammatory disease. Bursae act as protectors and facilitate movement between bones and overlapping muscles (deep bursae) or between bones and tendons/skin (superficial bursae).

●   Unacceptable Principal Diagnosis   ●   Use Additional Character(s)   ■   Unspecified   ▶   Manifestation Code

1212   **OGCR**   Official Guidelines for Coding and Reporting   Excludes 1   Excludes 2   Includes   Use additional   Code first   Code also

● M65.14 Other infective (teno)synovitis, hand

     M65.141 Other infective (teno)synovitis, right hand

     M65.142 Other infective (teno)synovitis, left hand

     ■ M65.149 Other infective (teno)synovitis, unspecified hand

● M65.15 Other infective (teno)synovitis, hip

     M65.151 Other infective (teno)synovitis, right hip

     M65.152 Other infective (teno)synovitis, left hip

     ■ M65.159 Other infective (teno)synovitis, unspecified hip

● M65.16 Other infective (teno)synovitis, knee

     M65.161 Other infective (teno)synovitis, right knee

     M65.162 Other infective (teno)synovitis, left knee

     ■ M65.169 Other infective (teno)synovitis, unspecified knee

● M65.17 Other infective (teno)synovitis, ankle and foot

     M65.171 Other infective (teno)synovitis, right ankle and foot

     M65.172 Other infective (teno)synovitis, left ankle and foot

     ■ M65.179 Other infective (teno)synovitis, unspecified ankle and foot

   M65.18 Other infective (teno)synovitis, other site

   M65.19 Other infective (teno)synovitis, multiple sites

● M65.2 Calcific tendinitis

     Excludes1   tendinitis as classified in M75-M77 calcified tendinitis of shoulder (M75.3)

■ M65.20 Calcific tendinitis, unspecified site

● M65.22 Calcific tendinitis, upper arm

     M65.221 Calcific tendinitis, right upper arm

     M65.222 Calcific tendinitis, left upper arm

     ■ M65.229 Calcific tendinitis, unspecified upper arm

● M65.23 Calcific tendinitis, forearm

     M65.231 Calcific tendinitis, right forearm

     M65.232 Calcific tendinitis, left forearm

     ■ M65.239 Calcific tendinitis, unspecified forearm

● M65.24 Calcific tendinitis, hand

     M65.241 Calcific tendinitis, right hand

     M65.242 Calcific tendinitis, left hand

     ■ M65.249 Calcific tendinitis, unspecified hand

● M65.25 Calcific tendinitis, thigh

     M65.251 Calcific tendinitis, right thigh

     M65.252 Calcific tendinitis, left thigh

     ■ M65.259 Calcific tendinitis, unspecified thigh

● M65.26 Calcific tendinitis, lower leg

     M65.261 Calcific tendinitis, right lower leg

     M65.262 Calcific tendinitis, left lower leg

     ■ M65.269 Calcific tendinitis, unspecified lower leg

● M65.27 Calcific tendinitis, ankle and foot

     M65.271 Calcific tendinitis, right ankle and foot

     M65.272 Calcific tendinitis, left ankle and foot

     ■ M65.279 Calcific tendinitis, unspecified ankle and foot

   M65.28 Calcific tendinitis, other site

   M65.29 Calcific tendinitis, multiple sites

● M65.3 Trigger finger

     Nodular tendinous disease

■ M65.30 Trigger finger, unspecified finger

● M65.31 Trigger thumb

     M65.311 Trigger thumb, right thumb

     M65.312 Trigger thumb, left thumb

     ■ M65.319 Trigger thumb, unspecified thumb

● M65.32 Trigger finger, index finger

     M65.321 Trigger finger, right index finger

     M65.322 Trigger finger, left index finger

     ■ M65.329 Trigger finger, unspecified index finger

● M65.33 Trigger finger, middle finger

     M65.331 Trigger finger, right middle finger

     M65.332 Trigger finger, left middle finger

     ■ M65.339 Trigger finger, unspecified middle finger

● M65.34 Trigger finger, ring finger

     M65.341 Trigger finger, right ring finger

     M65.342 Trigger finger, left ring finger

     ■ M65.349 Trigger finger, unspecified ring finger

● M65.35 Trigger finger, little finger

     M65.351 Trigger finger, right little finger

     M65.352 Trigger finger, left little finger

     ■ M65.359 Trigger finger, unspecified little finger

   M65.4 Radial styloid tenosynovitis [de Quervain]

● M65.8 Other synovitis and tenosynovitis

■ M65.80 Other synovitis and tenosynovitis, unspecified site

● M65.81 Other synovitis and tenosynovitis, shoulder

     M65.811 Other synovitis and tenosynovitis, right shoulder

     M65.812 Other synovitis and tenosynovitis, left shoulder

     ■ M65.819 Other synovitis and tenosynovitis, unspecified shoulder

CHAPTER 13 (M00-M99)

N Newborn Age: 0   **P** Pediatric Age: 0–17   **M** Maternity DX: 12–55   **A** Adult Age: 15–124   ♀ Females Only   ♂ Males Only

🝡 Complication\Comorbidity   🝡 Major C\C   🝡 Present on Admission Requirement   🝡 Hospital-Acquired Condition

1213

CHAPTER 13 (M00-M99)

● M65.82 Other synovitis and tenosynovitis, upper arm

    M65.821 Other synovitis and tenosynovitis, right upper arm

    M65.822 Other synovitis and tenosynovitis, left upper arm

    ■ M65.829 Other synovitis and tenosynovitis, unspecified upper arm

● M65.83 Other synovitis and tenosynovitis, forearm

    M65.831 Other synovitis and tenosynovitis, right forearm

    M65.832 Other synovitis and tenosynovitis, left forearm

    ■ M65.839 Other synovitis and tenosynovitis, unspecified forearm

● M65.84 Other synovitis and tenosynovitis, hand

    M65.841 Other synovitis and tenosynovitis, right hand

    M65.842 Other synovitis and tenosynovitis, left hand

    ■ M65.849 Other synovitis and tenosynovitis, unspecified hand

● M65.85 Other synovitis and tenosynovitis, thigh

    M65.851 Other synovitis and tenosynovitis, right thigh

    M65.852 Other synovitis and tenosynovitis, left thigh

    ■ M65.859 Other synovitis and tenosynovitis, unspecified thigh

● M65.86 Other synovitis and tenosynovitis, lower leg

    M65.861 Other synovitis and tenosynovitis, right lower leg

    M65.862 Other synovitis and tenosynovitis, left lower leg

    ■ M65.869 Other synovitis and tenosynovitis, unspecified lower leg

● M65.87 Other synovitis and tenosynovitis, ankle and foot

    M65.871 Other synovitis and tenosynovitis, right ankle and foot

    M65.872 Other synovitis and tenosynovitis, left ankle and foot

    ■ M65.879 Other synovitis and tenosynovitis, unspecified ankle and foot

    M65.88 Other synovitis and tenosynovitis, other site

    M65.89 Other synovitis and tenosynovitis, multiple sites

■ M65.9 Synovitis and tenosynovitis, unspecified

● M66 Spontaneous rupture of synovium and tendon

    Includes   rupture that occurs when a normal force is applied to tissues that are inferred to have less than normal strength

    Excludes2   rotator cuff syndrome (M75.1-)
rupture where an abnormal force is applied to normal tissue - see injury of tendon by body region

    M66.0 Rupture of popliteal cyst

● M66.1 Rupture of synovium
Rupture of synovial cyst

    Excludes2   rupture of popliteal cyst (M66.0)

    ■ M66.10 Rupture of synovium, unspecified joint

● M66.11 Rupture of synovium, shoulder

    M66.111 Rupture of synovium, right shoulder

    M66.112 Rupture of synovium, left shoulder

    ■ M66.119 Rupture of synovium, unspecified shoulder

● M66.12 Rupture of synovium, elbow

    M66.121 Rupture of synovium, right elbow

    M66.122 Rupture of synovium, left elbow

    ■ M66.129 Rupture of synovium, unspecified elbow

● M66.13 Rupture of synovium, wrist

    M66.131 Rupture of synovium, right wrist

    M66.132 Rupture of synovium, left wrist

    ■ M66.139 Rupture of synovium, unspecified wrist

● M66.14 Rupture of synovium, hand and fingers

    M66.141 Rupture of synovium, right hand

    M66.142 Rupture of synovium, left hand

    ■ M66.143 Rupture of synovium, unspecified hand

    M66.144 Rupture of synovium, right finger(s)

    M66.145 Rupture of synovium, left finger(s)

    ■ M66.146 Rupture of synovium, unspecified finger(s)

● M66.15 Rupture of synovium, hip

    M66.151 Rupture of synovium, right hip

    M66.152 Rupture of synovium, left hip

    ■ M66.159 Rupture of synovium, unspecified hip

● M66.17 Rupture of synovium, ankle, foot and toes

    M66.171 Rupture of synovium, right ankle

    M66.172 Rupture of synovium, left ankle

    ■ M66.173 Rupture of synovium, unspecified ankle

    M66.174 Rupture of synovium, right foot

    M66.175 Rupture of synovium, left foot

    ■ M66.176 Rupture of synovium, unspecified foot

    M66.177 Rupture of synovium, right toe(s)

    M66.178 Rupture of synovium, left toe(s)

    ■ M66.179 Rupture of synovium, unspecified toe(s)

    M66.18 Rupture of synovium, other site

● Unacceptable Principal Diagnosis   ● Use Additional Character(s)   ■ Unspecified   ▶ Manifestation Code

OGCR Official Guidelines for Coding and Reporting   Excludes 1   Excludes 2   Includes   Use additional   Code first   Code also

● M66.2 Spontaneous rupture of extensor tendons

■ M66.20 Spontaneous rupture of extensor tendons, unspecified site

● M66.21 Spontaneous rupture of extensor tendons, shoulder

   M66.211 Spontaneous rupture of extensor tendons, right shoulder

   M66.212 Spontaneous rupture of extensor tendons, left shoulder

   ■ M66.219 Spontaneous rupture of extensor tendons, unspecified shoulder

● M66.22 Spontaneous rupture of extensor tendons, upper arm

   M66.221 Spontaneous rupture of extensor tendons, right upper arm

   M66.222 Spontaneous rupture of extensor tendons, left upper arm

   ■ M66.229 Spontaneous rupture of extensor tendons, unspecified upper arm

● M66.23 Spontaneous rupture of extensor tendons, forearm

   M66.231 Spontaneous rupture of extensor tendons, right forearm

   M66.232 Spontaneous rupture of extensor tendons, left forearm

   ■ M66.239 Spontaneous rupture of extensor tendons, unspecified forearm

● M66.24 Spontaneous rupture of extensor tendons, hand

   M66.241 Spontaneous rupture of extensor tendons, right hand

   M66.242 Spontaneous rupture of extensor tendons, left hand

   ■ M66.249 Spontaneous rupture of extensor tendons, unspecified hand

● M66.25 Spontaneous rupture of extensor tendons, thigh

   M66.251 Spontaneous rupture of extensor tendons, right thigh

   M66.252 Spontaneous rupture of extensor tendons, left thigh

   ■ M66.259 Spontaneous rupture of extensor tendons, unspecified thigh

● M66.26 Spontaneous rupture of extensor tendons, lower leg

   M66.261 Spontaneous rupture of extensor tendons, right lower leg

   M66.262 Spontaneous rupture of extensor tendons, left lower leg

   ■ M66.269 Spontaneous rupture of extensor tendons, unspecified lower leg

● M66.27 Spontaneous rupture of extensor tendons, ankle and foot

   M66.271 Spontaneous rupture of extensor tendons, right ankle and foot

   M66.272 Spontaneous rupture of extensor tendons, left ankle and foot

   ■ M66.279 Spontaneous rupture of extensor tendons, unspecified ankle and foot

   M66.28 Spontaneous rupture of extensor tendons, other site

   M66.29 Spontaneous rupture of extensor tendons, multiple sites

● M66.3 Spontaneous rupture of flexor tendons

■ M66.30 Spontaneous rupture of flexor tendons, unspecified site

● M66.31 Spontaneous rupture of flexor tendons, shoulder

   M66.311 Spontaneous rupture of flexor tendons, right shoulder

   M66.312 Spontaneous rupture of flexor tendons, left shoulder

   ■ M66.319 Spontaneous rupture of flexor tendons, unspecified shoulder

● M66.32 Spontaneous rupture of flexor tendons, upper arm

   M66.321 Spontaneous rupture of flexor tendons, right upper arm

   M66.322 Spontaneous rupture of flexor tendons, left upper arm

   ■ M66.329 Spontaneous rupture of flexor tendons, unspecified upper arm

● M66.33 Spontaneous rupture of flexor tendons, forearm

   M66.331 Spontaneous rupture of flexor tendons, right forearm

   M66.332 Spontaneous rupture of flexor tendons, left forearm

   ■ M66.339 Spontaneous rupture of flexor tendons, unspecified forearm

● M66.34 Spontaneous rupture of flexor tendons, hand

   M66.341 Spontaneous rupture of flexor tendons, right hand

   M66.342 Spontaneous rupture of flexor tendons, left hand

   ■ M66.349 Spontaneous rupture of flexor tendons, unspecified hand

● M66.35 Spontaneous rupture of flexor tendons, thigh

   M66.351 Spontaneous rupture of flexor tendons, right thigh

   M66.352 Spontaneous rupture of flexor tendons, left thigh

   ■ M66.359 Spontaneous rupture of flexor tendons, unspecified thigh

● M66.36 Spontaneous rupture of flexor tendons, lower leg

   M66.361 Spontaneous rupture of flexor tendons, right lower leg

   M66.362 Spontaneous rupture of flexor tendons, left lower leg

   ■ M66.369 Spontaneous rupture of flexor tendons, unspecified lower leg

● M66.37 Spontaneous rupture of flexor tendons, ankle and foot

   M66.371 Spontaneous rupture of flexor tendons, right ankle and foot

   M66.372 Spontaneous rupture of flexor tendons, left ankle and foot

   ■ M66.379 Spontaneous rupture of flexor tendons, unspecified ankle and foot

   M66.38 Spontaneous rupture of flexor tendons, other site

   M66.39 Spontaneous rupture of flexor tendons, multiple sites

N Newborn Age: 0   **P** Pediatric Age: 0–17   **M** Maternity DX: 12–55   **A** Adult Age: 15–124   ♀ Females Only   ♂ Males Only

🔹 Complication\Comorbidity   🔹 Major C\C   🔹 Present on Admission Requirement   🔹 Hospital-Acquired Condition

CHAPTER 13 (M00-M99)

1215

● **M66.8**   **Spontaneous rupture of other tendons**

■ M66.80   Spontaneous rupture of other tendons, unspecified site

● M66.81   Spontaneous rupture of other tendons, shoulder

     M66.811   Spontaneous rupture of other tendons, right shoulder

     M66.812   Spontaneous rupture of other tendons, left shoulder

     ■ M66.819   Spontaneous rupture of other tendons, unspecified shoulder

● M66.82   Spontaneous rupture of other tendons, upper arm

     M66.821   Spontaneous rupture of other tendons, right upper arm

     M66.822   Spontaneous rupture of other tendons, left upper arm

     ■ M66.829   Spontaneous rupture of other tendons, unspecified upper arm

● M66.83   Spontaneous rupture of other tendons, forearm

     M66.831   Spontaneous rupture of other tendons, right forearm

     M66.832   Spontaneous rupture of other tendons, left forearm

     ■ M66.839   Spontaneous rupture of other tendons, unspecified forearm

● M66.84   Spontaneous rupture of other tendons, hand

     M66.841   Spontaneous rupture of other tendons, right hand

     M66.842   Spontaneous rupture of other tendons, left hand

     ■ M66.849   Spontaneous rupture of other tendons, unspecified hand

● M66.85   Spontaneous rupture of other tendons, thigh

     M66.851   Spontaneous rupture of other tendons, right thigh

     M66.852   Spontaneous rupture of other tendons, left thigh

     ■ M66.859   Spontaneous rupture of other tendons, unspecified thigh

● M66.86   Spontaneous rupture of other tendons, lower leg

     M66.861   Spontaneous rupture of other tendons, right lower leg

     M66.862   Spontaneous rupture of other tendons, left lower leg

     ■ M66.869   Spontaneous rupture of other tendons, unspecified lower leg

● M66.87   Spontaneous rupture of other tendons, ankle and foot

     M66.871   Spontaneous rupture of other tendons, right ankle and foot

     M66.872   Spontaneous rupture of other tendons, left ankle and foot

     ■ M66.879   Spontaneous rupture of other tendons, unspecified ankle and foot

M66.88   Spontaneous rupture of other tendons, other

M66.89   Spontaneous rupture of other tendons, multiple sites

■ **M66.9**   **Spontaneous rupture of unspecified tendon**
    Rupture at musculotendinous junction, nontraumatic

● **M67**   **Other disorders of synovium and tendon**

    Excludes1   palmar fascial fibromatosis [Dupuytren] (M72.0)
                tendinitis NOS (M77.9-)
                xanthomatosis localized to tendons (E78.2)

● **M67.0**   **Short Achilles tendon (acquired)**

■ M67.00   Short Achilles tendon (acquired), unspecified ankle

M67.01   Short Achilles tendon (acquired), right ankle

M67.02   Short Achilles tendon (acquired), left ankle

● **M67.2**   **Synovial hypertrophy, not elsewhere classified**

    Excludes1   villonodular synovitis (pigmented) (M12.2-)

■ M67.20   Synovial hypertrophy, not elsewhere classified, unspecified site

● M67.21   Synovial hypertrophy, not elsewhere classified, shoulder

     M67.211   Synovial hypertrophy, not elsewhere classified, right shoulder

     M67.212   Synovial hypertrophy, not elsewhere classified, left shoulder

     ■ M67.219   Synovial hypertrophy, not elsewhere classified, unspecified shoulder

● M67.22   Synovial hypertrophy, not elsewhere classified, upper arm

     M67.221   Synovial hypertrophy, not elsewhere classified, right upper arm

     M67.222   Synovial hypertrophy, not elsewhere classified, left upper arm

     ■ M67.229   Synovial hypertrophy, not elsewhere classified, unspecified upper arm

● M67.23   Synovial hypertrophy, not elsewhere classified, forearm

     M67.231   Synovial hypertrophy, not elsewhere classified, right forearm

     M67.232   Synovial hypertrophy, not elsewhere classified, left forearm

     ■ M67.239   Synovial hypertrophy, not elsewhere classified, unspecified forearm

● M67.24   Synovial hypertrophy, not elsewhere classified, hand

     M67.241   Synovial hypertrophy, not elsewhere classified, right hand

     M67.242   Synovial hypertrophy, not elsewhere classified, left hand

     ■ M67.249   Synovial hypertrophy, not elsewhere classified, unspecified hand

● Unacceptable Principal Diagnosis   ● Use Additional Character(s)   ■ Unspecified   ▶ Manifestation Code

OGCR Official Guidelines for Coding and Reporting   Excludes 1   Excludes 2   Includes   Use additional   Code first   Code also

● **M67.25** Synovial hypertrophy, not elsewhere classified, thigh
     M67.251 Synovial hypertrophy, not elsewhere classified, right thigh
     M67.252 Synovial hypertrophy, not elsewhere classified, left thigh
     ■ **M67.259** Synovial hypertrophy, not elsewhere classified, unspecified thigh

● **M67.26** Synovial hypertrophy, not elsewhere classified, lower leg
     M67.261 Synovial hypertrophy, not elsewhere classified, right lower leg
     M67.262 Synovial hypertrophy, not elsewhere classified, left lower leg
     ■ **M67.269** Synovial hypertrophy, not elsewhere classified, unspecified lower leg

● **M67.27** Synovial hypertrophy, not elsewhere classified, ankle and foot
     M67.271 Synovial hypertrophy, not elsewhere classified, right ankle and foot
     M67.272 Synovial hypertrophy, not elsewhere classified, left ankle and foot
     ■ **M67.279** Synovial hypertrophy, not elsewhere classified, unspecified ankle and foot

     M67.28 Synovial hypertrophy, not elsewhere classified, other site

     M67.29 Synovial hypertrophy, not elsewhere classified, multiple sites

● **M67.3** Transient synovitis
     Toxic synovitis
     Excludes1 palindromic rheumatism (M12.3-)

■ **M67.30** Transient synovitis, unspecified site

● **M67.31** Transient synovitis, shoulder
     M67.311 Transient synovitis, right shoulder
     M67.312 Transient synovitis, left shoulder
     ■ **M67.319** Transient synovitis, unspecified shoulder

● **M67.32** Transient synovitis, elbow
     M67.321 Transient synovitis, right elbow
     M67.322 Transient synovitis, left elbow
     ■ **M67.329** Transient synovitis, unspecified elbow

● **M67.33** Transient synovitis, wrist
     M67.331 Transient synovitis, right wrist
     M67.332 Transient synovitis, left wrist
     ■ **M67.339** Transient synovitis, unspecified wrist

● **M67.34** Transient synovitis, hand
     M67.341 Transient synovitis, right hand
     M67.342 Transient synovitis, left hand
     ■ **M67.349** Transient synovitis, unspecified hand

● **M67.35** Transient synovitis, hip
     M67.351 Transient synovitis, right hip
     M67.352 Transient synovitis, left hip
     ■ **M67.359** Transient synovitis, unspecified hip

● **M67.36** Transient synovitis, knee
     M67.361 Transient synovitis, right knee
     M67.362 Transient synovitis, left knee
     ■ **M67.369** Transient synovitis, unspecified knee

● **M67.37** Transient synovitis, ankle and foot
     M67.371 Transient synovitis, right ankle and foot
     M67.372 Transient synovitis, left ankle and foot
     ■ **M67.379** Transient synovitis, unspecified ankle and foot

     M67.38 Transient synovitis, other site

     M67.39 Transient synovitis, multiple sites

● **M67.4** Ganglion
     Ganglion of joint or tendon (sheath)
     Excludes1 ganglion in yaws (A66.6)
     Excludes2 cyst of bursa (M71.2-M71.3)
                 cyst of synovium (M71.2-M71.3)

■ **M67.40** Ganglion, unspecified site

● **M67.41** Ganglion, shoulder
     M67.411 Ganglion, right shoulder
     M67.412 Ganglion, left shoulder
     ■ **M67.419** Ganglion, unspecified shoulder

● **M67.42** Ganglion, elbow
     M67.421 Ganglion, right elbow
     M67.422 Ganglion, left elbow
     ■ **M67.429** Ganglion, unspecified elbow

● **M67.43** Ganglion, wrist
     M67.431 Ganglion, right wrist
     M67.432 Ganglion, left wrist
     ■ **M67.439** Ganglion, unspecified wrist

● **M67.44** Ganglion, hand
     M67.441 Ganglion, right hand
     M67.442 Ganglion, left hand
     ■ **M67.449** Ganglion, unspecified hand

● **M67.45** Ganglion, hip
     M67.451 Ganglion, right hip
     M67.452 Ganglion, left hip
     ■ **M67.459** Ganglion, unspecified hip

● **M67.46** Ganglion, knee
     M67.461 Ganglion, right knee
     M67.462 Ganglion, left knee
     ■ **M67.469** Ganglion, unspecified knee

● **M67.47** Ganglion, ankle and foot
     M67.471 Ganglion, right ankle and foot
     M67.472 Ganglion, left ankle and foot
     ■ **M67.479** Ganglion, unspecified ankle and foot

     M67.48 Ganglion, other site

     M67.49 Ganglion, multiple sites

CHAPTER 13 (M00-M99)

● M67.5 Plica syndrome
          Plica knee
  ■ M67.50 Plica syndrome, unspecified knee
    M67.51 Plica syndrome, right knee
    M67.52 Plica syndrome, left knee
● M67.8 Other specified disorders of synovium and tendon
  ■ M67.80 Other specified disorders of synovium and tendon, unspecified site
  ● M67.81 Other specified disorders of synovium and tendon, shoulder
    M67.811 Other specified disorders of synovium, right shoulder
    M67.812 Other specified disorders of synovium, left shoulder
    M67.813 Other specified disorders of tendon, right shoulder
    M67.814 Other specified disorders of tendon, left shoulder
  ■ M67.819 Other specified disorders of synovium and tendon, unspecified shoulder
  ● M67.82 Other specified disorders of synovium and tendon, elbow
    M67.821 Other specified disorders of synovium, right elbow
    M67.822 Other specified disorders of synovium, left elbow
    M67.823 Other specified disorders of tendon, right elbow
    M67.824 Other specified disorders of tendon, left elbow
  ■ M67.829 Other specified disorders of synovium and tendon, unspecified elbow
  ● M67.83 Other specified disorders of synovium and tendon, wrist
    M67.831 Other specified disorders of synovium, right wrist
    M67.832 Other specified disorders of synovium, left wrist
    M67.833 Other specified disorders of tendon, right wrist
    M67.834 Other specified disorders of tendon, left wrist
  ■ M67.839 Other specified disorders of synovium and tendon, unspecified forearm
  ● M67.84 Other specified disorders of synovium and tendon, hand
    M67.841 Other specified disorders of synovium, right hand
    M67.842 Other specified disorders of synovium, left hand
    M67.843 Other specified disorders of tendon, right hand
    M67.844 Other specified disorders of tendon, left hand
  ■ M67.849 Other specified disorders of synovium and tendon, unspecified hand

● M67.85 Other specified disorders of synovium and tendon, hip
    M67.851 Other specified disorders of synovium, right hip
    M67.852 Other specified disorders of synovium, left hip
    M67.853 Other specified disorders of tendon, right hip
    M67.854 Other specified disorders of tendon, left hip
  ■ M67.859 Other specified disorders of synovium and tendon, unspecified hip
● M67.86 Other specified disorders of synovium and tendon, knee
    M67.861 Other specified disorders of synovium, right knee
    M67.862 Other specified disorders of synovium, left knee
    M67.863 Other specified disorders of tendon, right knee
    M67.864 Other specified disorders of tendon, left knee
  ■ M67.869 Other specified disorders of synovium and tendon, unspecified knee
● M67.87 Other specified disorders of synovium and tendon, ankle and foot
    M67.871 Other specified disorders of synovium, right ankle and foot
    M67.872 Other specified disorders of synovium, left ankle and foot
    M67.873 Other specified disorders of tendon, right ankle and foot
    M67.874 Other specified disorders of tendon, left ankle and foot
  ■ M67.879 Other specified disorders of synovium and tendon, unspecified ankle and foot
    M67.88 Other specified disorders of synovium and tendon, other site
    M67.89 Other specified disorders of synovium and tendon, multiple sites
● M67.9 Unspecified disorder of synovium and tendon
  ■ M67.90 Unspecified disorder of synovium and tendon, unspecified site
  ● M67.91 Unspecified disorder of synovium and tendon, shoulder
    ■ M67.911 Unspecified disorder of synovium and tendon, right shoulder
    ■ M67.912 Unspecified disorder of synovium and tendon, left shoulder
    ■ M67.919 Unspecified disorder of synovium and tendon, unspecified shoulder

● Unacceptable Principal Diagnosis   ● Use Additional Character(s)   ■ Unspecified   ▶ Manifestation Code
OGCR Official Guidelines for Coding and Reporting   Excludes 1   Excludes 2   Includes   Use additional   Code first   Code also

● **M67.92** Unspecified disorder of synovium and tendon, upper arm

  ■ **M67.921** Unspecified disorder of synovium and tendon, right upper arm

  ■ **M67.922** Unspecified disorder of synovium and tendon, left upper arm

  ■ **M67.929** Unspecified disorder of synovium and tendon, unspecified upper arm

● **M67.93** Unspecified disorder of synovium and tendon, forearm

  ■ **M67.931** Unspecified disorder of synovium and tendon, right forearm

  ■ **M67.932** Unspecified disorder of synovium and tendon, left forearm

  ■ **M67.939** Unspecified disorder of synovium and tendon, unspecified forearm

● **M67.94** Unspecified disorder of synovium and tendon, hand

  ■ **M67.941** Unspecified disorder of synovium and tendon, right hand

  ■ **M67.942** Unspecified disorder of synovium and tendon, left hand

  ■ **M67.949** Unspecified disorder of synovium and tendon, unspecified hand

● **M67.95** Unspecified disorder of synovium and tendon, thigh

  ■ **M67.951** Unspecified disorder of synovium and tendon, right thigh

  ■ **M67.952** Unspecified disorder of synovium and tendon, left thigh

  ■ **M67.959** Unspecified disorder of synovium and tendon, unspecified thigh

● **M67.96** Unspecified disorder of synovium and tendon, lower leg

  ■ **M67.961** Unspecified disorder of synovium and tendon, right lower leg

  ■ **M67.962** Unspecified disorder of synovium and tendon, left lower leg

  ■ **M67.969** Unspecified disorder of synovium and tendon, unspecified lower leg

● **M67.97** Unspecified disorder of synovium and tendon, ankle and foot

  ■ **M67.971** Unspecified disorder of synovium and tendon, right ankle and foot

  ■ **M67.972** Unspecified disorder of synovium and tendon, left ankle and foot

  ■ **M67.979** Unspecified disorder of synovium and tendon, unspecified ankle and foot

■ **M67.98** Unspecified disorder of synovium and tendon, other site

■ **M67.99** Unspecified disorder of synovium and tendon, multiple sites

OTHER SOFT TISSUE DISORDERS (M70-M79)

● **M70** Soft tissue disorders related to use, overuse and pressure

  Includes soft tissue disorders of occupational origin

  Use additional external cause code to identify activity causing disorder (Y93.-)

  Excludes1 bursitis NOS (M71.9-)

  Excludes2 bursitis of shoulder (M75.5) enthesopathies (M76-M77) pressure ulcer (pressure area) (L89.-)

● **M70.0** Crepitant synovitis (acute) (chronic) of hand and wrist

  ● **M70.03** Crepitant synovitis (acute) (chronic), wrist

     M70.031 Crepitant synovitis (acute) (chronic), right wrist

     M70.032 Crepitant synovitis (acute) (chronic), left wrist

    ■ **M70.039** Crepitant synovitis (acute) (chronic), unspecified wrist

  ● **M70.04** Crepitant synovitis (acute) (chronic), hand

     M70.041 Crepitant synovitis (acute) (chronic), right hand

     M70.042 Crepitant synovitis (acute) (chronic), left hand

    ■ **M70.049** Crepitant synovitis (acute) (chronic), unspecified hand

● **M70.1** Bursitis of hand

  ■ **M70.10** Bursitis, unspecified hand

   M70.11 Bursitis, right hand

   M70.12 Bursitis, left hand

● **M70.2** Olecranon bursitis

  ■ **M70.20** Olecranon bursitis, unspecified elbow

   M70.21 Olecranon bursitis, right elbow

   M70.22 Olecranon bursitis, left elbow

● **M70.3** Other bursitis of elbow

  ■ **M70.30** Other bursitis of elbow, unspecified elbow

   M70.31 Other bursitis of elbow, right elbow

   M70.32 Other bursitis of elbow, left elbow

● **M70.4** Prepatellar bursitis

  ■ **M70.40** Prepatellar bursitis, unspecified knee

   M70.41 Prepatellar bursitis, right knee

   M70.42 Prepatellar bursitis, left knee

● **M70.5** Other bursitis of knee

  ■ **M70.50** Other bursitis of knee, unspecified knee

   M70.51 Other bursitis of knee, right knee

   M70.52 Other bursitis of knee, left knee

● **M70.6** Trochanteric bursitis

  Trochanteric tendinitis

  ■ **M70.60** Trochanteric bursitis, unspecified hip

   M70.61 Trochanteric bursitis, right hip

   M70.62 Trochanteric bursitis, left hip

● **M70.7** Other bursitis of hip

  Ischial bursitis

  ■ **M70.70** Other bursitis of hip, unspecified hip

   M70.71 Other bursitis of hip, right hip

   M70.72 Other bursitis of hip, left hip

CHAPTER 13 (M00-M99)

● **M70.8 Other soft tissue disorders related to use, overuse and pressure**

■ M70.80 Other soft tissue disorders related to use, overuse and pressure of unspecified site

● M70.81 Other soft tissue disorders related to use, overuse and pressure of shoulder

M70.811 Other soft tissue disorders related to use, overuse and pressure, right shoulder

M70.812 Other soft tissue disorders related to use, overuse and pressure, left shoulder

■ M70.819 Other soft tissue disorders related to use, overuse and pressure, unspecified shoulder

● M70.82 Other soft tissue disorders related to use, overuse and pressure of upper arm

M70.821 Other soft tissue disorders related to use, overuse and pressure, right upper arm

M70.822 Other soft tissue disorders related to use, overuse and pressure, left upper arm

■ M70.829 Other soft tissue disorders related to use, overuse and pressure, unspecified upper arms

● M70.83 Other soft tissue disorders related to use, overuse and pressure of forearm

M70.831 Other soft tissue disorders related to use, overuse and pressure, right forearm

M70.832 Other soft tissue disorders related to use, overuse and pressure, left forearm

■ M70.839 Other soft tissue disorders related to use, overuse and pressure, unspecified forearm

● M70.84 Other soft tissue disorders related to use, overuse and pressure of hand

M70.841 Other soft tissue disorders related to use, overuse and pressure, right hand

M70.842 Other soft tissue disorders related to use, overuse and pressure, left hand

■ M70.849 Other soft tissue disorders related to use, overuse and pressure, unspecified hand

● M70.85 Other soft tissue disorders related to use, overuse and pressure of thigh

M70.851 Other soft tissue disorders related to use, overuse and pressure, right thigh

M70.852 Other soft tissue disorders related to use, overuse and pressure, left thigh

■ M70.859 Other soft tissue disorders related to use, overuse and pressure, unspecified thigh

● M70.86 Other soft tissue disorders related to use, overuse and pressure lower leg

M70.861 Other soft tissue disorders related to use, overuse and pressure, right lower leg

M70.862 Other soft tissue disorders related to use, overuse and pressure, left lower leg

■ M70.869 Other soft tissue disorders related to use, overuse and pressure, unspecified leg

● M70.87 Other soft tissue disorders related to use, overuse and pressure of ankle and foot

M70.871 Other soft tissue disorders related to use, overuse and pressure, right ankle and foot

M70.872 Other soft tissue disorders related to use, overuse and pressure, left ankle and foot

■ M70.879 Other soft tissue disorders related to use, overuse and pressure, unspecified ankle and foot

M70.88 Other soft tissue disorders related to use, overuse and pressure other site

M70.89 Other soft tissue disorders related to use, overuse and pressure multiple sites

● **M70.9 Unspecified soft tissue disorder related to use, overuse and pressure**

■ M70.90 Unspecified soft tissue disorder related to use, overuse and pressure of unspecified site

● M70.91 Unspecified soft tissue disorder related to use, overuse and pressure of shoulder

■ M70.911 Unspecified soft tissue disorder related to use, overuse and pressure, right shoulder

■ M70.912 Unspecified soft tissue disorder related to use, overuse and pressure, left shoulder

■ M70.919 Unspecified soft tissue disorder related to use, overuse and pressure, unspecified shoulder

● M70.92 Unspecified soft tissue disorder related to use, overuse and pressure of upper arm

■ M70.921 Unspecified soft tissue disorder related to use, overuse and pressure, right upper arm

■ M70.922 Unspecified soft tissue disorder related to use, overuse and pressure, left upper arm

■ M70.929 Unspecified soft tissue disorder related to use, overuse and pressure, unspecified upper arm

● M70.93 Unspecified soft tissue disorder related to use, overuse and pressure of forearm

■ M70.931 Unspecified soft tissue disorder related to use, overuse and pressure, right forearm

■ M70.932 Unspecified soft tissue disorder related to use, overuse and pressure, left forearm

■ M70.939 Unspecified soft tissue disorder related to use, overuse and pressure, unspecified forearm

● Unacceptable Principal Diagnosis   ● Use Additional Character(s)   ■ Unspecified   ▶ Manifestation Code
OGCR Official Guidelines for Coding and Reporting   Excludes 1   Excludes 2   Includes   Use additional   Code first   Code also

● M70.94 Unspecified soft tissue disorder related to use, overuse and pressure of hand

■ M70.941 Unspecified soft tissue disorder related to use, overuse and pressure, right hand

■ M70.942 Unspecified soft tissue disorder related to use, overuse and pressure, left hand

■ M70.949 Unspecified soft tissue disorder related to use, overuse and pressure, unspecified hand

● M70.95 Unspecified soft tissue disorder related to use, overuse and pressure of thigh

■ M70.951 Unspecified soft tissue disorder related to use, overuse and pressure, right thigh

■ M70.952 Unspecified soft tissue disorder related to use, overuse and pressure, left thigh

■ M70.959 Unspecified soft tissue disorder related to use, overuse and pressure, unspecified thigh

● M70.96 Unspecified soft tissue disorder related to use, overuse and pressure lower leg

■ M70.961 Unspecified soft tissue disorder related to use, overuse and pressure, right lower leg

■ M70.962 Unspecified soft tissue disorder related to use, overuse and pressure, left lower leg

■ M70.969 Unspecified soft tissue disorder related to use, overuse and pressure, unspecified lower leg

● M70.97 Unspecified soft tissue disorder related to use, overuse and pressure of ankle and foot

■ M70.971 Unspecified soft tissue disorder related to use, overuse and pressure, right ankle and foot

■ M70.972 Unspecified soft tissue disorder related to use, overuse and pressure, left ankle and foot

M70.979 Unspecified soft tissue disorder related to use, overuse and pressure, unspecified ankle and foot

■ M70.98 Unspecified soft tissue disorder related to use, overuse and pressure other

■ M70.99 Unspecified soft tissue disorder related to use, overuse and pressure multiple sites

● M71 Other bursopathies

Excludes1   bunion (M20.1)
bursitis related to use, overuse or pressure (M70.-)
enthesopathies (M76-M77)

● M71.0 Abscess of bursa

Use additional code (B95.-, B96.-) to identify causative organism

■ M71.00 Abscess of bursa, unspecified site

● M71.01 Abscess of bursa, shoulder

M71.011 Abscess of bursa, right shoulder

M71.012 Abscess of bursa, left shoulder

■ M71.019 Abscess of bursa, unspecified shoulder

● M71.02 Abscess of bursa, elbow

M71.021 Abscess of bursa, right elbow

M71.022 Abscess of bursa, left elbow

■ M71.029 Abscess of bursa, unspecified elbow

● M71.03 Abscess of bursa, wrist

M71.031 Abscess of bursa, right wrist

M71.032 Abscess of bursa, left wrist

■ M71.039 Abscess of bursa, unspecified wrist

● M71.04 Abscess of bursa, hand

M71.041 Abscess of bursa, right hand

M71.042 Abscess of bursa, left hand

■ M71.049 Abscess of bursa, unspecified hand

● M71.05 Abscess of bursa, hip

M71.051 Abscess of bursa, right hip

M71.052 Abscess of bursa, left hip

■ M71.059 Abscess of bursa, unspecified hip

● M71.06 Abscess of bursa, knee

M71.061 Abscess of bursa, right knee

M71.062 Abscess of bursa, left knee

■ M71.069 Abscess of bursa, unspecified knee

● M71.07 Abscess of bursa, ankle and foot

M71.071 Abscess of bursa, right ankle and foot

M71.072 Abscess of bursa, left ankle and foot

■ M71.079 Abscess of bursa, unspecified ankle and foot

M71.08 Abscess of bursa, other site

M71.09 Abscess of bursa, multiple sites

● M71.1 Other infective bursitis

Use additional code (B95.-, B96.-) to identify causative organism

■ M71.10 Other infective bursitis, unspecified site

● M71.11 Other infective bursitis, shoulder

M71.111 Other infective bursitis, right shoulder

M71.112 Other infective bursitis, left shoulder

■ M71.119 Other infective bursitis, unspecified shoulder

● M71.12 Other infective bursitis, elbow

M71.121 Other infective bursitis, right elbow

M71.122 Other infective bursitis, left elbow

■ M71.129 Other infective bursitis, unspecified elbow

● M71.13 Other infective bursitis, wrist

M71.131 Other infective bursitis, right wrist

M71.132 Other infective bursitis, left wrist

■ M71.139 Other infective bursitis, unspecified wrist

CHAPTER 13 (M00-M99)

● M71.14   Other infective bursitis, hand
     M71.141   Other infective bursitis, right hand
     M71.142   Other infective bursitis, left hand
     ■ M71.149   Other infective bursitis, unspecified hand
● M71.15   Other infective bursitis, hip
     M71.151   Other infective bursitis, right hip
     M71.152   Other infective bursitis, left hip
     ■ M71.159   Other infective bursitis, unspecified hip
● M71.16   Other infective bursitis, knee
     M71.161   Other infective bursitis, right knee
     M71.162   Other infective bursitis, left knee
     ■ M71.169   Other infective bursitis, unspecified knee
● M71.17   Other infective bursitis, ankle and foot
     M71.171   Other infective bursitis, right ankle and foot
     M71.172   Other infective bursitis, left ankle and foot
     ■ M71.179   Other infective bursitis, unspecified ankle and foot
   M71.18   Other infective bursitis, other site
   M71.19   Other infective bursitis, multiple sites
● M71.2   Synovial cyst of popliteal space [Baker]
     Popliteal space = popliteal cavity, popliteal fossa. Depression in the posterior aspect of the knee (behind the knee).

     | Excludes1 | synovial cyst of popliteal space with rupture (M66.0)

   ■ M71.20   Synovial cyst of popliteal space [Baker], unspecified knee
   M71.21   Synovial cyst of popliteal space [Baker], right knee
   M71.22   Synovial cyst of popliteal space [Baker], left knee
● M71.3   Other bursal cyst
     Synovial cyst NOS

     | Excludes1 | synovial cyst with rupture (M66.1-)

   ■ M71.30   Other bursal cyst, unspecified site
   ● M71.31   Other bursal cyst, shoulder
     M71.311   Other bursal cyst, right shoulder
     M71.312   Other bursal cyst, left shoulder
     ■ M71.319   Other bursal cyst, unspecified shoulder
   ● M71.32   Other bursal cyst, elbow
     M71.321   Other bursal cyst, right elbow
     M71.322   Other bursal cyst, left elbow
     ■ M71.329   Other bursal cyst, unspecified elbow
   ● M71.33   Other bursal cyst, wrist
     M71.331   Other bursal cyst, right wrist
     M71.332   Other bursal cyst, left wrist
     ■ M71.339   Other bursal cyst, unspecified wrist

● M71.34   Other bursal cyst, hand
     M71.341   Other bursal cyst, right hand
     M71.342   Other bursal cyst, left hand
     ■ M71.349   Other bursal cyst, unspecified hand
● M71.35   Other bursal cyst, hip
     M71.351   Other bursal cyst, right hip
     M71.352   Other bursal cyst, left hip
     ■ M71.359   Other bursal cyst, unspecified hip
● M71.37   Other bursal cyst, ankle and foot
     M71.371   Other bursal cyst, right ankle and foot
     M71.372   Other bursal cyst, left ankle and foot
     ■ M71.379   Other bursal cyst, unspecified ankle and foot
   M71.38   Other bursal cyst, other site
   M71.39   Other bursal cyst, multiple sites
● M71.4   Calcium deposit in bursa

     | Excludes2 | calcium deposit in bursa of shoulder (M75.3)

   ■ M71.40   Calcium deposit in bursa, unspecified site
   ● M71.42   Calcium deposit in bursa, elbow
     M71.421   Calcium deposit in bursa, right elbow
     M71.422   Calcium deposit in bursa, left elbow
     ■ M71.429   Calcium deposit in bursa, unspecified elbow
   ● M71.43   Calcium deposit in bursa, wrist
     M71.431   Calcium deposit in bursa, right wrist
     M71.432   Calcium deposit in bursa, left wrist
     ■ M71.439   Calcium deposit in bursa, unspecified wrist
   ● M71.44   Calcium deposit in bursa, hand
     M71.441   Calcium deposit in bursa, right hand
     M71.442   Calcium deposit in bursa, left hand
     ■ M71.449   Calcium deposit in bursa, unspecified hand
   ● M71.45   Calcium deposit in bursa, hip
     M71.451   Calcium deposit in bursa, right hip
     M71.452   Calcium deposit in bursa, left hip
     ■ M71.459   Calcium deposit in bursa, unspecified hip
   ● M71.46   Calcium deposit in bursa, knee
     M71.461   Calcium deposit in bursa, right knee
     M71.462   Calcium deposit in bursa, left knee
     ■ M71.469   Calcium deposit in bursa, unspecified knee

●   Unacceptable Principal Diagnosis   ●   Use Additional Character(s)   ■   Unspecified   ▶   Manifestation Code

OGCR   Official Guidelines for Coding and Reporting | Excludes 1 | | Excludes 2 | Includes   Use additional   Code first   Code also

●M71.47 Calcium deposit in bursa, ankle and foot

    M71.471 Calcium deposit in bursa, right ankle and foot

    M71.472 Calcium deposit in bursa, left ankle and foot

    ■M71.479 Calcium deposit in bursa, unspecified ankle and foot

   M71.48 Calcium deposit in bursa, other site

   M71.49 Calcium deposit in bursa, multiple sites

●M71.5 Other bursitis, not elsewhere classified

> **Excludes1**   bursitis NOS (M71.9-)
>
> **Excludes2**   bursitis of shoulder (M75.5)
> bursitis of tibial collateral [Pellegrini-Stieda] (M76.4)

  ■M71.50 Other bursitis, not elsewhere classified, unspecified site

●M71.52 Other bursitis, not elsewhere classified, elbow

    M71.521 Other bursitis, not elsewhere classified, right elbow

    M71.522 Other bursitis, not elsewhere classified, left elbow

    ■M71.529 Other bursitis, not elsewhere classified, unspecified elbow

●M71.53 Other bursitis, not elsewhere classified, wrist

    M71.531 Other bursitis, not elsewhere classified, right wrist

    M71.532 Other bursitis, not elsewhere classified, left wrist

    ■M71.539 Other bursitis, not elsewhere classified, unspecified wrist

●M71.54 Other bursitis, not elsewhere classified, hand

    M71.541 Other bursitis, not elsewhere classified, right hand

    M71.542 Other bursitis, not elsewhere classified, left hand

    ■M71.549 Other bursitis, not elsewhere classified, unspecified hand

●M71.55 Other bursitis, not elsewhere classified, hip

    M71.551 Other bursitis, not elsewhere classified, right hip

    M71.552 Other bursitis, not elsewhere classified, left hip

    ■M71.559 Other bursitis, not elsewhere classified, unspecified hip

●M71.56 Other bursitis, not elsewhere classified, knee

    M71.561 Other bursitis, not elsewhere classified, right knee

    M71.562 Other bursitis, not elsewhere classified, left knee

    ■M71.569 Other bursitis, not elsewhere classified, unspecified knee

●M71.57 Other bursitis, not elsewhere classified, ankle and foot

    M71.571 Other bursitis, not elsewhere classified, right ankle and foot

    M71.572 Other bursitis, not elsewhere classified, left ankle and foot

    ■M71.579 Other bursitis, not elsewhere classified, unspecified ankle and foot

   M71.58 Other bursitis, not elsewhere classified, other site

●M71.8 Other specified bursopathies

  ■M71.80 Other specified bursopathies, unspecified site

●M71.81 Other specified bursopathies, shoulder

    M71.811 Other specified bursopathies, right shoulder

    M71.812 Other specified bursopathies, left shoulder

    ■M71.819 Other specified bursopathies, unspecified shoulder

●M71.82 Other specified bursopathies, elbow

    M71.821 Other specified bursopathies, right elbow

    M71.822 Other specified bursopathies, left elbow

    ■M71.829 Other specified bursopathies, unspecified elbow

●M71.83 Other specified bursopathies, wrist

    M71.831 Other specified bursopathies, right wrist

    M71.832 Other specified bursopathies, left wrist

    ■M71.839 Other specified bursopathies, unspecified wrist

●M71.84 Other specified bursopathies, hand

    M71.841 Other specified bursopathies, right hand

    M71.842 Other specified bursopathies, left hand

    ■M71.849 Other specified bursopathies, unspecified hand

●M71.85 Other specified bursopathies, hip

    M71.851 Other specified bursopathies, right hip

    M71.852 Other specified bursopathies, left hip

    ■M71.859 Other specified bursopathies, unspecified hip

●M71.86 Other specified bursopathies, knee

    M71.861 Other specified bursopathies, right knee

    M71.862 Other specified bursopathies, left knee

    ■M71.869 Other specified bursopathies, unspecified knee

●M71.87 Other specified bursopathies, ankle and foot

    M71.871 Other specified bursopathies, right ankle and foot

    M71.872 Other specified bursopathies, left ankle and foot

    ■M71.879 Other specified bursopathies, unspecified ankle and foot

   M71.88 Other specified bursopathies, other site

   M71.89 Other specified bursopathies, multiple sites

■M71.9 Bursopathy, unspecified
    Bursitis NOS

N Newborn Age: 0   **P** Pediatric Age: 0–17   **M** Maternity DX: 12–55   **A** Adult Age: 15–124   ♀ Females Only   ♂ Males Only

🏵 Complication\Comorbidity   🏵 Major C\C   🏵 Present on Admission Requirement   🏵 Hospital-Acquired Condition

1223

CHAPTER 13 (M00-M99)

● M72 Fibroblastic disorders

Excludes2   retroperitoneal fibromatosis (D48.3)

M72.0 Palmar fascial fibromatosis [Dupuytren]   A

M72.1 Knuckle pads

M72.2 Plantar fascial fibromatosis
Plantar fasciitis

M72.4 Pseudosarcomatous fibromatosis
Nodular fasciitis

M72.6 Necrotizing fasciitis 🔖
Use additional code (B95.-, B96.-) to identify
causative organism

M72.8 Other fibroblastic disorders
Abscess of fascia
Fasciitis NEC
Other infective fasciitis
Use additional code to (B95.-, B96.-) identify
causative organism

Excludes1   diffuse (eosinophilic) fasciitis (M35.4)
             necrotizing fasciitis (M72.6)
             nodular fasciitis (M72.4)
             perirenal fasciitis NOS (N13.5)
             perirenal fasciitis with infection
                (N13.6)
             plantar fasciitis (M72.2)

■ M72.9 Fibroblastic disorder, unspecified
Fasciitis NOS
Fibromatosis NOS

● M75 Shoulder lesions

Excludes2   shoulder-hand syndrome (M89.0-)

● M75.0 Adhesive capsulitis of shoulder
Frozen shoulder
Periarthritis of shoulder

■ M75.00 Adhesive capsulitis of unspecified shoulder

M75.01 Adhesive capsulitis of right shoulder

M75.02 Adhesive capsulitis of left shoulder

● M75.1 Rotator cuff tear or rupture, not specified as
traumatic
Rotator cuff syndrome
Supraspinatus syndrome
Supraspinatus tear or rupture, not specified as
traumatic

Excludes1   tear of rotator cuff, traumatic
             (S46.01-)

● M75.10 Unspecified rotator cuff tear or rupture,
not specified as traumatic

■ M75.100 Unspecified rotator cuff tear or
rupture of unspecified shoulder,
not specified as traumatic

■ M75.101 Unspecified rotator cuff tear or
rupture of right shoulder, not
specified as traumatic

■ M75.102 Unspecified rotator cuff tear or
rupture of left shoulder, not
specified as traumatic

● M75.11 Incomplete rotator cuff tear or rupture not
specified as traumatic

■ M75.110 Incomplete rotator cuff tear or
rupture of unspecified shoulder,
not specified as traumatic

M75.111 Incomplete rotator cuff tear or
rupture of right shoulder, not
specified as traumatic

M75.112 Incomplete rotator cuff tear or
rupture of left shoulder, not
specified as traumatic

● M75.12 Complete rotator cuff tear or rupture not
specified as traumatic

■ M75.120 Complete rotator cuff tear or
rupture of unspecified shoulder,
not specified as traumatic

M75.121 Complete rotator cuff tear or
rupture of right shoulder, not
specified as traumatic

M75.122 Complete rotator cuff tear or
rupture of left shoulder, not
specified as traumatic

● M75.2 Bicipital tendinitis

■ M75.20 Bicipital tendinitis, unspecified shoulder

M75.21 Bicipital tendinitis, right shoulder

M75.22 Bicipital tendinitis, left shoulder

● M75.3 Calcific tendinitis of shoulder
Calcified bursa of shoulder

■ M75.30 Calcific tendinitis of unspecified shoulder

M75.31 Calcific tendinitis of right shoulder

M75.32 Calcific tendinitis of left shoulder

● M75.4 Impingement syndrome of shoulder

■ M75.40 Impingement syndrome of unspecified
shoulder

M75.41 Impingement syndrome of right shoulder

M75.42 Impingement syndrome of left shoulder

● M75.5 Bursitis of shoulder

■ M75.50 Bursitis of unspecified shoulder

M75.51 Bursitis of right shoulder

M75.52 Bursitis of left shoulder

● M75.8 Other shoulder lesions

■ M75.80 Other shoulder lesions, unspecified
shoulder

M75.81 Other shoulder lesions, right shoulder

M75.82 Other shoulder lesions, left shoulder

● M75.9 Shoulder lesion, unspecified

■ M75.90 Shoulder lesion, unspecified, unspecified
shoulder

■ M75.91 Shoulder lesion, unspecified, right shoulder

■ M75.92 Shoulder lesion, unspecified, left shoulder

● M76 Enthesopathies, lower limb, excluding foot

Excludes2   bursitis due to use, overuse and pressure
             (M70.-)
             enthesopathies of ankle and foot (M77.5-)

● M76.0 Gluteal tendinitis

■ M76.00 Gluteal tendinitis, unspecified hip

M76.01 Gluteal tendinitis, right hip

M76.02 Gluteal tendinitis, left hip

● M76.1 Psoas tendinitis

■ M76.10 Psoas tendinitis, unspecified hip

M76.11 Psoas tendinitis, right hip

M76.12 Psoas tendinitis, left hip

● M76.2 Iliac crest spur

■ M76.20 Iliac crest spur, unspecified hip

M76.21 Iliac crest spur, right hip

M76.22 Iliac crest spur, left hip

● M76.3 Iliotibial band syndrome

■ M76.30 Iliotibial band syndrome, unspecified leg

M76.31 Iliotibial band syndrome, right leg

M76.32 Iliotibial band syndrome, left leg

● M76.4   Tibial collateral bursitis [Pellegrini-Stieda]
   ■ M76.40   Tibial collateral bursitis [Pellegrini-Stieda], unspecified leg
     M76.41   Tibial collateral bursitis [Pellegrini-Stieda], right leg
     M76.42   Tibial collateral bursitis [Pellegrini-Stieda], left leg

● M76.5   Patellar tendinitis
   ■ M76.50   Patellar tendinitis, unspecified knee
     M76.51   Patellar tendinitis, right knee
     M76.52   Patellar tendinitis, left knee

● M76.6   Achilles tendinitis
     Achilles bursitis
   ■ M76.60   Achilles tendinitis, unspecified leg
     M76.61   Achilles tendinitis, right leg
     M76.62   Achilles tendinitis, left leg

● M76.7   Peroneal tendinitis
   ■ M76.70   Peroneal tendinitis, unspecified leg
     M76.71   Peroneal tendinitis, right leg
     M76.72   Peroneal tendinitis, left leg

● M76.8   Other specified enthesopathies of lower limb, excluding foot
   ● M76.81   Anterior tibial syndrome
     M76.811   Anterior tibial syndrome, right leg
     M76.812   Anterior tibial syndrome, left leg
     ■ M76.819   Anterior tibial syndrome, unspecified leg
   ● M76.82   Posterior tibial tendinitis
     M76.821   Posterior tibial tendinitis, right leg
     M76.822   Posterior tibial tendinitis, left leg
     ■ M76.829   Posterior tibial tendinitis, unspecified leg
   ● M76.89   Other specified enthesopathies of lower limb, excluding foot
     M76.891   Other specified enthesopathies of right lower limb, excluding foot
     M76.892   Other specified enthesopathies of left lower limb, excluding foot
     ■ M76.899   Other specified enthesopathies of unspecified lower limb, excluding foot

■ M76.9   Unspecified enthesopathy, lower limb, excluding foot

● M77   Other enthesopathies
   Excludes1   bursitis NOS (M71.9-)
   Excludes2   bursitis due to use, overuse and pressure (M70.-)
     osteophyte (M25.7)
     spinal enthesopathy (M46.0-)

● M77.0   Medial epicondylitis
   ■ M77.00   Medial epicondylitis, unspecified elbow
     M77.01   Medial epicondylitis, right elbow
     M77.02   Medial epicondylitis, left elbow

● M77.1   Lateral epicondylitis
     Tennis elbow
   ■ M77.10   Lateral epicondylitis, unspecified elbow
     M77.11   Lateral epicondylitis, right elbow
     M77.12   Lateral epicondylitis, left elbow

● M77.2   Periarthritis of wrist
   ■ M77.20   Periarthritis, unspecified wrist
     M77.21   Periarthritis, right wrist
     M77.22   Periarthritis, left wrist

● M77.3   Calcaneal spur
   ■ M77.30   Calcaneal spur, unspecified foot
     M77.31   Calcaneal spur, right foot
     M77.32   Calcaneal spur, left foot

● M77.4   Metatarsalgia
   Excludes1   Morton's metatarsalgia (G57.6)
   ■ M77.40   Metatarsalgia, unspecified foot
     M77.41   Metatarsalgia, right foot
     M77.42   Metatarsalgia, left foot

● M77.5   Other enthesopathy of foot
   ■ M77.50   Other enthesopathy of unspecified foot
     M77.51   Other enthesopathy of right foot
     M77.52   Other enthesopathy of left foot

     M77.8   Other enthesopathies, not elsewhere classified

■ M77.9   Enthesopathy, unspecified
     Bone spur NOS
     Capsulitis NOS
     Periarthritis NOS
     Tendinitis NOS

● M79   Other and unspecified soft tissue disorders, not elsewhere classified
   Excludes1   psychogenic rheumatism (F45.8)
     soft tissue pain, psychogenic (F45.41)

■ M79.0   Rheumatism, unspecified
   Excludes1   fibromyalgia (M79.7)
     palindromic rheumatism (M12.3-)

     M79.1   Myalgia
     Myofascial pain syndrome
   Excludes1   fibromyalgia (M79.7)
     myositis (M60.-)

■ M79.2   Neuralgia and neuritis, unspecified
   Excludes1   brachial radiculitis NOS (M54.1)
     lumbosacral radiculitis NOS (M54.1)
     mononeuropathies (G56-G58)
     radiculitis NOS (M54.1)
     sciatica (M54.3-M54.4)

■ M79.3   Panniculitis, unspecified
   Excludes1   lupus panniculitis (L93.2)
     neck and back panniculitis (M54.0-)
     relapsing [Weber-Christian] panniculitis (M35.6)

     M79.4   Hypertrophy of (infrapatellar) fat pad

     M79.5   Residual foreign body in soft tissue
   Excludes1   foreign body granuloma of skin and subcutaneous tissue (L92.3)
     foreign body granuloma of soft tissue (M60.2-)

● M79.6   Pain in limb, hand, foot, fingers and toes
   Excludes2   pain in joint (M25.5-)
   ● M79.60   Pain in limb, unspecified
     M79.601   Pain in right arm
      Pain in right upper limb NOS
     M79.602   Pain in left arm
      Pain in left upper limb NOS
     ■ M79.603   Pain in arm, unspecified
      Pain in upper limb NOS

N Newborn Age: 0   **P** Pediatric Age: 0–17   **M** Maternity DX: 12–55   **A** Adult Age: 15–124   ♀ Females Only   ♂ Males Only

Complication\Comorbidity   Major C\C   Present on Admission Requirement   Hospital-Acquired Condition

CHAPTER 13 (M00-M99)

1225

M79.604 **Pain in right leg**
Pain in right lower limb NOS

M79.605 **Pain in left leg**
Pain in left lower limb NOS

■ M79.606 **Pain in leg, unspecified**
Pain in lower limb NOS

■ M79.609 **Pain in unspecified limb**
Pain in limb NOS

● M79.62 **Pain in upper arm**
Pain in axillary region

M79.621 **Pain in right upper arm**

M79.622 **Pain in left upper arm**

■ M79.629 **Pain in unspecified upper arm**

● M79.63 **Pain in forearm**

M79.631 **Pain in right forearm**

M79.632 **Pain in left forearm**

■ M79.639 **Pain in unspecified forearm**

● M79.64 **Pain in hand and fingers**

M79.641 **Pain in right hand**

M79.642 **Pain in left hand**

■ M79.643 **Pain in unspecified hand**

M79.644 **Pain in right finger(s)**

M79.645 **Pain in left finger(s)**

■ M79.646 **Pain in unspecified finger(s)**

● M79.65 **Pain in thigh**

M79.651 **Pain in right thigh**

M79.652 **Pain in left thigh**

■ M79.659 **Pain in unspecified thigh**

● M79.66 **Pain in lower leg**

M79.661 **Pain in right lower leg**

M79.662 **Pain in left lower leg**

■ M79.669 **Pain in unspecified lower leg**

● M79.67 **Pain in foot and toes**

M79.671 **Pain in right foot**

M79.672 **Pain in left foot**

■ M79.673 **Pain in unspecified foot**

M79.674 **Pain in right toe(s)**

M79.675 **Pain in left toe(s)**

■ M79.676 **Pain in unspecified toe(s)**

M79.7 **Fibromyalgia**
Fibromyositis
Fibrositis
Myofibrositis

● M79.A **Nontraumatic compartment syndrome**

Code first, if applicable, associated postprocedural complication

Excludes1 compartment syndrome NOS (T79.A-)
fibromyalgia (M79.7) nontraumatic ischemic infarction of muscle (M62.2-)
traumatic compartment syndrome (T79.A-)

● M79.A1 **Nontraumatic compartment syndrome of upper extremity**
Nontraumatic compartment syndrome of shoulder, arm, forearm, wrist, hand, and fingers

M79.A11 **Nontraumatic compartment syndrome of right upper extremity**

M79.A12 **Nontraumatic compartment syndrome of left upper extremity**

■ M79.A19 **Nontraumatic compartment syndrome of unspecified upper extremity**

● M79.A2 **Nontraumatic compartment syndrome of lower extremity**
Nontraumatic compartment syndrome of hip, buttock, thigh, leg, foot, and toes

M79.A21 **Nontraumatic compartment syndrome of right lower extremity**

M79.A22 **Nontraumatic compartment syndrome of left lower extremity**

■ M79.A29 **Nontraumatic compartment syndrome of unspecified lower extremity**

M79.A3 **Nontraumatic compartment syndrome of abdomen**

M79.A9 **Nontraumatic compartment syndrome of other sites**

● M79.8 **Other specified soft tissue disorders**

M79.81 **Nontraumatic hematoma of soft tissue**
Nontraumatic hematoma of muscle
Nontraumatic seroma of muscle and soft tissue

M79.89 **Other specified soft tissue disorders**
Polyalgia

■ M79.9 **Soft tissue disorder, unspecified**

OGCR See Section I.C., Chapter 13.d.

Osteoporosis

OSTEOPATHIES AND CHONDROPATHIES (M80-M94)

DISORDERS OF BONE DENSITY AND STRUCTURE (M80-M85)

M80 **Osteoporosis with current pathological fracture**
Excessive skeletal fragility (porous bone) resulting in bone fractures

Includes osteoporosis with current fragility fracture

Use additional code to identify major osseous defect, if applicable (M89.7-)

Excludes1 collapsed vertebra NOS (M48.5)
pathological fracture NOS (M84.4)
wedging of vertebra NOS (M48.5)

Excludes2 personal history of (healed) osteoporosis fracture (Z87.310)

The appropriate 7th character is to be added to each code from category M80:

A	initial encounter for fracture
D	subsequent encounter for fracture with routine healing
G	subsequent encounter for fracture with delayed healing
K	subsequent encounter for fracture with nonunion *Total failure of fracture healing*
P	subsequent encounter for fracture with malunion *Fracture ends do not heal together correctly.*
S	sequela

●M80.0 **Age-related osteoporosis with current pathological fracture**
    Involutional osteoporosis with current pathological fracture
    Osteoporosis NOS with current pathological fracture
    Postmenopausal osteoporosis with current pathological fracture
    Senile osteoporosis with current pathological fracture

■M80.00 **Age-related osteoporosis with current pathological fracture, unspecified site** A, K, P 🍥, D, G, S 🍥

●M80.01 **Age-related osteoporosis with current pathological fracture, shoulder**

M80.011 **Age-related osteoporosis with current pathological fracture, right shoulder** A, K, P 🍥, D, G, S 🍥

M80.012 **Age-related osteoporosis with current pathological fracture, left shoulder** A, K, P 🍥, D, G, S 🍥

■M80.019 **Age-related osteoporosis with current pathological fracture, unspecified shoulder** A, K, P 🍥, D, G, S 🍥

●M80.02 **Age-related osteoporosis with current pathological fracture, humerus**

M80.021 **Age-related osteoporosis with current pathological fracture, right humerus** A, K, P 🍥, D, G, S 🍥

M80.022 **Age-related osteoporosis with current pathological fracture, left humerus** A, K, P 🍥, D, G, S 🍥

■M80.029 **Age-related osteoporosis with current pathological fracture, unspecified humerus** A, K, P 🍥, D, G, S 🍥

●M80.03 **Age-related osteoporosis with current pathological fracture, forearm**
    Age-related osteoporosis with current pathological fracture of wrist

M80.031 **Age-related osteoporosis with current pathological fracture, right forearm** A, K, P 🍥, D, G, S 🍥

M80.032 **Age-related osteoporosis with current pathological fracture, left forearm** A, K, P 🍥, D, G, S 🍥

■M80.039 **Age-related osteoporosis with current pathological fracture, unspecified forearm** A, K, P 🍥, D, G, S 🍥

●M80.04 **Age-related osteoporosis with current pathological fracture, hand**

M80.041 **Age-related osteoporosis with current pathological fracture, right hand** A, K, P 🍥, D, G, S 🍥

M80.042 **Age-related osteoporosis with current pathological fracture, left hand** A, K, P 🍥, D, G, S 🍥

■M80.049 **Age-related osteoporosis with current pathological fracture, unspecified hand** A, K, P 🍥, D, G, S 🍥

●M80.05 **Age-related osteoporosis with current pathological fracture, femur**
    Age-related osteoporosis with current pathological fracture of hip

M80.051 **Age-related osteoporosis with current pathological fracture, right femur** A, K, P 🍥, D, G, S 🍥

M80.052 **Age-related osteoporosis with current pathological fracture, left femur** A, K, P 🍥, D, G, S 🍥

■M80.059 **Age-related osteoporosis with current pathological fracture, unspecified femur** A, K, P 🍥, D, G, S 🍥

●M80.06 **Age-related osteoporosis with current pathological fracture, lower leg**

M80.061 **Age-related osteoporosis with current pathological fracture, right lower leg** A, K, P 🍥, D, G, S 🍥

M80.062 **Age-related osteoporosis with current pathological fracture, left lower leg** A, K, P 🍥, D, G, S 🍥

■M80.069 **Age-related osteoporosis with current pathological fracture, unspecified lower leg** A, K, P 🍥, D, G, S 🍥

●M80.07 **Age-related osteoporosis with current pathological fracture, ankle and foot**

M80.071 **Age-related osteoporosis with current pathological fracture, right ankle and foot** A, K, P 🍥, D, G, S 🍥

M80.072 **Age-related osteoporosis with current pathological fracture, left ankle and foot** A, K, P 🍥, D, G, S 🍥

■M80.079 **Age-related osteoporosis with current pathological fracture, unspecified ankle and foot** A, K, P 🍥, D, G, S 🍥

M80.08 **Age-related osteoporosis with current pathological fracture, vertebra(e)** A, K, P 🍥, D, G, S 🍥

●M80.8 **Other osteoporosis with current pathological fracture**
    Drug-induced osteoporosis with current pathological fracture
    Idiopathic osteoporosis with current pathological fracture
    Osteoporosis of disuse with current pathological fracture
    Postoophorectomy osteoporosis with current pathological fracture
    Postsurgical malabsorption osteoporosis with current pathological fracture
    Post-traumatic osteoporosis with current pathological fracture

    Use additional code for adverse effect, if applicable, to identify drug (T36-T50 with fifth or sixth character 5)

■M80.80 **Other osteoporosis with current pathological fracture, unspecified site** A, K, P 🍥, D, G, S 🍥

CHAPTER 13 (M00-M99)

N Newborn Age: 0   **P** Pediatric Age: 0–17   **M** Maternity DX: 12–55   **A** Adult Age: 15–124   ♀ Females Only   ♂ Males Only

🍥 Complication\Comorbidity   🍥 Major C\C   🍥 Present on Admission Requirement   🍥 Hospital-Acquired Condition

1227

CHAPTER 13 (M00-M99)

● **M80.81 Other osteoporosis with pathological fracture, shoulder**

    M80.811 Other osteoporosis with current pathological fracture, right shoulder A, K, P 🖰, D, G, S 🖰

    M80.812 Other osteoporosis with current pathological fracture, left shoulder A, K, P 🖰, D, G, S 🖰

    ■ **M80.819** Other osteoporosis with current pathological fracture, unspecified shoulder A, K, P 🖰, D, G, S 🖰

● **M80.82 Other osteoporosis with current pathological fracture, humerus**

    M80.821 Other osteoporosis with current pathological fracture, right humerus A, K, P 🖰, D, G, S 🖰

    M80.822 Other osteoporosis with current pathological fracture, left humerus A, K, P 🖰, D, G, S 🖰

    ■ **M80.829** Other osteoporosis with current pathological fracture, unspecified humerus A, K, P 🖰, D, G, S 🖰

● **M80.83 Other osteoporosis with current pathological fracture, forearm**
    Other osteoporosis with current pathological fracture of wrist

    M80.831 Other osteoporosis with current pathological fracture, right forearm A, K, P 🖰, D, G, S 🖰

    M80.832 Other osteoporosis with current pathological fracture, left forearm A, K, P 🖰, D, G, S 🖰

    ■ **M80.839** Other osteoporosis with current pathological fracture, unspecified forearm A, K, P 🖰, D, G, S 🖰

● **M80.84 Other osteoporosis with current pathological fracture, hand**

    M80.841 Other osteoporosis with current pathological fracture, right hand A, K, P 🖰, D, G, S 🖰

    M80.842 Other osteoporosis with current pathological fracture, left hand A, K, P 🖰, D, G, S 🖰

    ■ **M80.849** Other osteoporosis with current pathological fracture, unspecified hand A, K, P 🖰, D, G, S 🖰

● **M80.85 Other osteoporosis with current pathological fracture, femur**
    Other osteoporosis with current pathological fracture of hip

    M80.851 Other osteoporosis with current pathological fracture, right femur A, K, P 🖰, D, G, S 🖰

    M80.852 Other osteoporosis with current pathological fracture, left femur A, K, P 🖰, D, G, S 🖰

    ■ **M80.859** Other osteoporosis with current pathological fracture, unspecified femur A, K, P 🖰, D, G, S 🖰

● **M80.86 Other osteoporosis with current pathological fracture, lower leg**

    M80.861 Other osteoporosis with current pathological fracture, right lower leg A, K, P 🖰, D, G, S 🖰

    M80.862 Other osteoporosis with current pathological fracture, left lower leg A, K, P 🖰, D, G, S 🖰

    ■ **M80.869** Other osteoporosis with current pathological fracture, unspecified lower leg A, K, P 🖰, D, G, S 🖰

● **M80.87 Other osteoporosis with current pathological fracture, ankle and foot**

    M80.871 Other osteoporosis with current pathological fracture, right ankle and foot A, K, P 🖰, D, G, S 🖰

    M80.872 Other osteoporosis with current pathological fracture, left ankle and foot A, K, P 🖰, D, G, S 🖰

    ■ **M80.879** Other osteoporosis with current pathological fracture, unspecified ankle and foot A, K, P 🖰, D, G, S 🖰

  M80.88 Other osteoporosis with current pathological fracture, vertebra(e) A, K, P 🖰, D, G, S 🖰

● **M81 Osteoporosis without current pathological fracture**

    Use additional code to identify:
    major osseous defect, if applicable (M89.7-)
    personal history of (healed) osteoporosis fracture, if applicable (Z87.310)

    Excludes1 osteoporosis with current pathological fracture (M80.-)
                Sudeck's atrophy (M89.0)

  M81.0 Age-related osteoporosis without current pathological fracture   A
    Involutional osteoporosis without current pathological fracture
    Osteoporosis NOS
    Postmenopausal osteoporosis without current pathological fracture
    Senile osteoporosis without current pathological fracture

  M81.6 Localized osteoporosis [Lequesne]
    Excludes1 Sudeck's atrophy (M89.0)

  M81.8 Other osteoporosis without current pathological fracture
    Drug-induced osteoporosis without current pathological fracture
    Idiopathic osteoporosis without current pathological fracture
    Osteoporosis of disuse without current pathological fracture
    Postoophorectomy osteoporosis without current pathological fracture
    Postsurgical malabsorption osteoporosis without current pathological fracture
    Post-traumatic osteoporosis without current pathological fracture

    Use additional code for adverse effect, if applicable, to identify drug (T36-T50 with fifth or sixth character 5)

● Unacceptable Principal Diagnosis   ● Use Additional Character(s)   ■ Unspecified   ▶ Manifestation Code

OGCR Official Guidelines for Coding and Reporting   Excludes 1   Excludes 2   Includes   Use additional   Code first   Code also

● **M83   Adult osteomalacia**

> **Excludes1**   infantile and juvenile osteomalacia (E55.0)
> renal osteodystrophy (N25.0)
> rickets (active) (E55.0)
> rickets (active) sequelae (E64.3)
> vitamin D-resistant osteomalacia (E83.3)
> vitamin D-resistant rickets (active) (E83.3)

M83.0   Puerperal osteomalacia ♀   **M**

M83.1   Senile osteomalacia   **A**

M83.2   Adult osteomalacia due to malabsorption   **A**
> Postsurgical malabsorption osteomalacia in adults

M83.3   Adult osteomalacia due to malnutrition   **A**

M83.4   Aluminum bone disease

● **M83.5   Other drug-induced osteomalacia in adults**   **A**
> Use additional code for adverse effect, if applicable, to identify drug (T36-T50 with fifth or sixth character 5)

M83.8   Other adult osteomalacia   **A**

■ **M83.9   Adult osteomalacia, unspecified**   **A**

● **M84   Disorder of continuity of bone**

> **Excludes2**   traumatic fracture of bone-see fracture, by site

● **M84.3   Stress fracture**
> Fatigue fracture
> March fracture
> Stress fracture NOS
> Stress reaction

> Use additional external cause code(s) to identify the cause of the stress fracture

> **Excludes1**   pathological fracture NOS (M84.4.-)
> pathological fracture due to osteoporosis (M80.-)
> traumatic fracture (S12.-, S22.-, S32.-, S42.-, S52.-, S62.-, S72.-, S82.-, S92.-)

> **Excludes2**   personal history of (healed) stress (fatigue) fracture (Z87.312)
> stress fracture of vertebra (M48.4-)

> The appropriate 7th character is to be added to each code from subcategory M84.3:

> | | |
> |---|---|
> | A | initial encounter for fracture |
> | D | subsequent encounter for fracture with routine healing |
> | G | subsequent encounter for fracture with delayed healing |
> | K | subsequent encounter for fracture with nonunion |
> | P | subsequent encounter for fracture with malunion |
> | S | sequela |

■ **M84.30   Stress fracture, unspecified site** K, P 🔵, D, G, S 🔵

● **M84.31   Stress fracture, shoulder**

> **M84.311   Stress fracture, right shoulder** K, P 🔵, D, G, S 🔵

> **M84.312   Stress fracture, left shoulder** K, P 🔵, D, G, S 🔵

> ■ **M84.319   Stress fracture, unspecified shoulder** K, P 🔵, D, G, S 🔵

● **M84.32   Stress fracture, humerus**

> **M84.321   Stress fracture, right humerus** K, P 🔵, D, G, S 🔵

> **M84.322   Stress fracture, left humerus** K, P 🔵, D, G, S 🔵

> ■ **M84.329   Stress fracture, unspecified humerus** K, P 🔵, D, G, S 🔵

● **M84.33   Stress fracture, ulna and radius**

> **M84.331   Stress fracture, right ulna** K, P 🔵, D, G, S 🔵

> **M84.332   Stress fracture, left ulna** K, P 🔵, D, G, S 🔵

> **M84.333   Stress fracture, right radius** K, P 🔵, D, G, S 🔵

> **M84.334   Stress fracture, left radius** K, P 🔵, D, G, S 🔵

> ■ **M84.339   Stress fracture, unspecified ulna and radius** K, P 🔵, D, G, S 🔵

● **M84.34   Stress fracture, hand and fingers**

> **M84.341   Stress fracture, right hand** K, P 🔵, D, G, S 🔵

> **M84.342   Stress fracture, left hand** K, P 🔵, D, G, S 🔵

> ■ **M84.343   Stress fracture, unspecified hand** K, P 🔵, D, G, S 🔵

> **M84.344   Stress fracture, right finger(s)** K, P 🔵, D, G, S 🔵

> **M84.345   Stress fracture, left finger(s)** K, P 🔵, D, G, S 🔵

> ■ **M84.346   Stress fracture, unspecified finger(s)** K, P 🔵, D, G, S 🔵

● **M84.35   Stress fracture, pelvis and femur**
> Stress fracture, hip

> **M84.350   Stress fracture, pelvis** K, P 🔵, D, G, S 🔵

> **M84.351   Stress fracture, right femur** K, P 🔵, D, G, S 🔵

> **M84.352   Stress fracture, left femur** K, P 🔵, D, G, S 🔵

> ■ **M84.353   Stress fracture, unspecified femur** K, P 🔵, D, G, S 🔵

> ■ **M84.359   Stress fracture, hip, unspecified** K, P 🔵, D, G, S 🔵

● **M84.36   Stress fracture, tibia and fibula**

> **M84.361   Stress fracture, right tibia** K, P 🔵, D, G, S 🔵

> **M84.362   Stress fracture, left tibia** K, P 🔵, D, G, S 🔵

> **M84.363   Stress fracture, right fibula** K, P 🔵, D, G, S 🔵

> **M84.364   Stress fracture, left fibula** K, P 🔵, D, G, S 🔵

> ■ **M84.369   Stress fracture, unspecified tibia and fibula** K, P 🔵, D, G, S 🔵

● **M84.37   Stress fracture, ankle, foot and toes**

> **M84.371   Stress fracture, right ankle** K, P 🔵, D, G, S 🔵

> **M84.372   Stress fracture, left ankle** K, P 🔵, D, G, S 🔵

> ■ **M84.373   Stress fracture, unspecified ankle** K, P 🔵, D, G, S 🔵

CHAPTER 13 (M00-M99)

N   Newborn Age: 0   **P**   Pediatric Age: 0–17   **M**   Maternity DX: 12–55   **A**   Adult Age: 15–124   ♀   Females Only   ♂   Males Only

 Complication\Comorbidity   Major C\C   Present on Admission Requirement   Hospital-Acquired Condition

1229

CHAPTER 13 (M00-M99)

M84.374   Stress fracture, right foot K, P ⬟, D, G, S ⬟

M84.375   Stress fracture, left foot K, P ⬟, D, G, S ⬟

■ M84.376   Stress fracture, unspecified foot K, P ⬟, D, G, S ⬟

M84.377   Stress fracture, right toe(s) K, P ⬟, D, G, S ⬟

M84.378   Stress fracture, left toe(s) K, P ⬟, D, G, S ⬟

■ M84.379   Stress fracture, unspecified toe(s) K, P ⬟, D, G, S ⬟

M84.38   Stress fracture, other site K, P ⬟, D, G, S ⬟

> **Excludes2**   stress fracture of vertebra (M48.4-)

● M84.4   **Pathological fracture, not elsewhere classified**
Chronic fracture
Pathological fracture NOS

> **Excludes1**   collapsed vertebra NEC (M48.5)
> pathological fracture in neoplastic disease (M84.5-)
> pathological fracture in osteoporosis (M80.-)
> pathological fracture in other disease (M84.6-)
> stress fracture (M84.3-)
> traumatic fracture (S12.-, S22.-, S32.-, S42.-, S52.-, S62.-, S72.-, S82.-, S92.-)

> **Excludes2**   personal history of (healed) pathological fracture (Z87.311)

The appropriate 7th character is to be added to each code from subcategory M84.4:

A	initial encounter for fracture
D	subsequent encounter for fracture with routine healing
G	subsequent encounter for fracture with delayed healing
K	subsequent encounter for fracture with nonunion
P	subsequent encounter for fracture with malunion
S	sequela

■ M84.40   Pathological fracture, unspecified site A, K, P ⬟, D, G, S ⬟

● M84.41   Pathological fracture, shoulder

    M84.411   Pathological fracture, right shoulder A, K, P ⬟, D, G, S ⬟

    M84.412   Pathological fracture, left shoulder A, K, P ⬟, D, G, S ⬟

    ■ M84.419   Pathological fracture, unspecified shoulder A, K, P ⬟, D, G, S ⬟

● M84.42   Pathological fracture, humerus

    M84.421   Pathological fracture, right humerus A, K, P ⬟, D, G, S ⬟

    M84.422   Pathological fracture, left humerus A, K, P ⬟, D, G, S ⬟

    ■ M84.429   Pathological fracture, unspecified humerus A, K, P ⬟, D, G, S ⬟

● M84.43   Pathological fracture, ulna and radius

    M84.431   Pathological fracture, right ulna A, K, P ⬟, D, G, S ⬟

    M84.432   Pathological fracture, left ulna A, K, P ⬟, D, G, S ⬟

    M84.433   Pathological fracture, right radius A, K, P ⬟, D, G, S ⬟

    M84.434   Pathological fracture, left radius A, K, P ⬟, D, G, S ⬟

    ■ M84.439   Pathological fracture, unspecified ulna and radius A, K, P ⬟, D, G, S ⬟

● M84.44   Pathological fracture, hand and fingers

    M84.441   Pathological fracture, right hand A, K, P ⬟, D, G, S ⬟

    M84.442   Pathological fracture, left hand A, K, P ⬟, D, G, S ⬟

    ■ M84.443   Pathological fracture, unspecified hand A, K, P ⬟, D, G, S ⬟

    M84.444   Pathological fracture, right finger(s) A, K, P ⬟, D, G, S ⬟

    M84.445   Pathological fracture, left finger(s) A, K, P ⬟, D, G, S ⬟

    ■ M84.446   Pathological fracture, unspecified finger(s) A, K, P ⬟, D, G, S ⬟

● M84.45   Pathological fracture, femur and pelvis

    M84.451   Pathological fracture, right femur A, K, P ⬟, D, G, S ⬟

    M84.452   Pathological fracture, left femur A, K, P ⬟, D, G, S ⬟

    ■ M84.453   Pathological fracture, unspecified femur A, K, P ⬟, D, G, S ⬟

    M84.454   Pathological fracture, pelvis A, K, P ⬟, D, G, S ⬟

    ■ M84.459   Pathological fracture, hip, unspecified A, K, P ⬟, D, G, S ⬟

● M84.46   Pathological fracture, tibia and fibula

    M84.461   Pathological fracture, right tibia A, K, P ⬟, D, G, S ⬟

    M84.462   Pathological fracture, left tibia A, K, P ⬟, D, G, S ⬟

    M84.463   Pathological fracture, right fibula A, K, P ⬟, D, G, S ⬟

    M84.464   Pathological fracture, left fibula A, K, P ⬟, D, G, S ⬟

    ■ M84.469   Pathological fracture, unspecified tibia and fibula A, K, P ⬟, D, G, S ⬟

● M84.47   Pathological fracture, ankle, foot and toes

    M84.471   Pathological fracture, right ankle A, K, P ⬟, D, G, S ⬟

    M84.472   Pathological fracture, left ankle A, K, P ⬟, D, G, S ⬟

    ■ M84.473   Pathological fracture, unspecified ankle A, K, P ⬟, D, G, S ⬟

    M84.474   Pathological fracture, right foot A, K, P ⬟, D, G, S ⬟

OGCR Section I.a, Chapter 13.C.

> Coding of Pathologic Fractures
>
> 7th character A is for use as long as the patient is receiving active treatment for the fracture. Examples of active treatment are: surgical treatment, emergency department encounter, evaluation and treatment by a new physician. 7th character, D is to be used for encounters after the patient has completed active treatment. The other 7th characters, listed under each subcategory in the Tabular List, are to be used for subsequent encounters for treatment of problems associated with the healing, such as malunions, nonunions, and sequelae.
>
> Care for complications of surgical treatment for fracture repairs during the healing or recovery phase should be coded with the appropriate complication codes.
>
> *See Section I.C.19. Coding of traumatic fractures.*

     M84.475 **Pathological fracture, left foot** A, K, P 🦠, D, G, S 🦠

     ■ M84.476 **Pathological fracture, unspecified foot** A, K, P 🦠, D, G, S 🦠

     M84.477 **Pathological fracture, right toe(s)** A, K, P 🦠, D, G, S 🦠

     M84.478 **Pathological fracture, left toe(s)** A, K, P 🦠, D, G, S 🦠

     ■ M84.479 **Pathological fracture, unspecified toe(s)** A, K, P 🦠, D, G, S 🦠

   M84.48 **Pathological fracture, other site** A, K, P 🦠

● M84.5 **Pathological fracture in neoplastic disease**

> Code also underlying neoplasm
>
> The appropriate 7th character is to be added to each code from subcategory M84.5:
>
> | | |
> |---|---|
> | A | initial encounter for fracture |
> | D | subsequent encounter for fracture with routine healing |
> | G | subsequent encounter for fracture with delayed healing |
> | K | subsequent encounter for fracture with nonunion |
> | P | subsequent encounter for fracture with malunion |
> | S | sequela |

   ■ M84.50 **Pathological fracture in neoplastic disease, unspecified site** A, K, P 🦠, D, G, S 🦠

● M84.51 **Pathological fracture in neoplastic disease, shoulder**

     M84.511 **Pathological fracture in neoplastic disease, right shoulder** A, K, P 🦠, D, G, S 🦠

     M84.512 **Pathological fracture in neoplastic disease, left shoulder** A, K, P 🦠, D, G, S 🦠

     ■ M84.519 **Pathological fracture in neoplastic disease, unspecified shoulder** A, K, P 🦠, D, G, S 🦠

● M84.52 **Pathological fracture in neoplastic disease, humerus**

     M84.521 **Pathological fracture in neoplastic disease, right humerus** A, K, P 🦠, D, G, S 🦠

     M84.522 **Pathological fracture in neoplastic disease, left humerus** A, K, P 🦠, D, G, S 🦠

     ■ M84.529 **Pathological fracture in neoplastic disease, unspecified humerus** A, K, P 🦠, D, G, S 🦠

● M84.53 **Pathological fracture in neoplastic disease, ulna and radius**

     M84.531 **Pathological fracture in neoplastic disease, right ulna** A, K, P 🦠, D, G, S 🦠

     M84.532 **Pathological fracture in neoplastic disease, left ulna** A, K, P 🦠, D, G, S 🦠

     M84.533 **Pathological fracture in neoplastic disease, right radius** A, K, P 🦠, D, G, S 🦠

     M84.534 **Pathological fracture in neoplastic disease, left radius** A, K, P 🦠, D, G, S 🦠

     ■ M84.539 **Pathological fracture in neoplastic disease, unspecified ulna and radius** A, K, P 🦠, D, G, S 🦠

● M84.54 **Pathological fracture in neoplastic disease, hand**

     M84.541 **Pathological fracture in neoplastic disease, right hand** A, K, P 🦠, D, G, S 🦠

     M84.542 **Pathological fracture in neoplastic disease, left hand** A, K, P 🦠, D, G, S 🦠

     ■ M84.549 **Pathological fracture in neoplastic disease, unspecified hand** A, K, P 🦠, D, G, S 🦠

● M84.55 **Pathological fracture in neoplastic disease, pelvis and femur**

     M84.550 **Pathological fracture in neoplastic disease, pelvis** A, K, P 🦠, D, G, S 🦠

     M84.551 **Pathological fracture in neoplastic disease, right femur** A, K, P 🦠, D, G, S 🦠

     M84.552 **Pathological fracture in neoplastic disease, left femur** A, K, P 🦠, D, G, S 🦠

     ■ M84.553 **Pathological fracture in neoplastic disease, unspecified femur** A, K, P 🦠, D, G, S 🦠

     ■ M84.559 **Pathological fracture in neoplastic disease, hip, unspecified** A, K, P 🦠, D, G, S 🦠

● M84.56 **Pathological fracture in neoplastic disease, tibia and fibula**

     M84.561 **Pathological fracture in neoplastic disease, right tibia** A, K, P 🦠, D, G, S 🦠

     M84.562 **Pathological fracture in neoplastic disease, left tibia** A, K, P 🦠, D, G, S 🦠

     M84.563 **Pathological fracture in neoplastic disease, right fibula** A, K, P 🦠, D, G, S 🦠

     M84.564 **Pathological fracture in neoplastic disease, left fibula** A, K, P 🦠, D, G, S 🦠

     ■ M84.569 **Pathological fracture in neoplastic disease, unspecified tibia and fibula** A, K, P 🦠, D, G, S 🦠

CHAPTER 13 (M00-M99)

N Newborn Age: 0	**P** Pediatric Age: 0–17	**M** Maternity DX: 12–55	**A** Adult Age: 15–124	♀ Females Only	♂ Males Only

🦠 Complication\Comorbidity   🦠 Major C\C   🦠 Present on Admission Requirement   🦠 Hospital-Acquired Condition

1231

CHAPTER 13 (M00-M99)

● M84.57   Pathological fracture in neoplastic disease, ankle and foot

     M84.571   Pathological fracture in neoplastic disease, right ankle A, K, P 🦴, D, G, S 🦴

     M84.572   Pathological fracture in neoplastic disease, left ankle A, K, P 🦴, D, G, S 🦴

     ■ M84.573   Pathological fracture in neoplastic disease, unspecified ankle A, K, P 🦴, D, G, S 🦴

     M84.574   Pathological fracture in neoplastic disease, right foot A, K, P 🦴, D, G, S 🦴

     M84.575   Pathological fracture in neoplastic disease, left foot A, K, P 🦴, D, G, S 🦴

     ■ M84.576   Pathological fracture in neoplastic disease, unspecified foot A, K, P 🦴, D, G, S 🦴

     M84.58   Pathological fracture in neoplastic disease, vertebrae A, K, P 🦴, D, G, S 🦴

● M84.6   Pathological fracture in other disease

     Code also underlying condition

     Excludes1   pathological fracture in osteoporosis (M80.-)

     The appropriate 7th character is to be added to each code from subcategory M84.6:

     A   initial encounter for fracture
     D   subsequent encounter for fracture with routine healing
     G   subsequent encounter for fracture with delayed healing
     K   subsequent encounter for fracture with nonunion
     P   subsequent encounter for fracture with malunion
     S   sequela

     ■ M84.60   Pathological fracture in other disease, unspecified site A, K, P 🦴, D, G, S 🦴

● M84.61   Pathological fracture in other disease, shoulder

     M84.611   Pathological fracture in other disease, right shoulder A, K, P 🦴, D, G, S 🦴

     M84.612   Pathological fracture in other disease, left shoulder A, K, P 🦴, D, G, S 🦴

     ■ M84.619   Pathological fracture in other disease, unspecified shoulder A, K, P 🦴, D, G, S 🦴

● M84.62   Pathological fracture in other disease, humerus

     M84.621   Pathological fracture in other disease, right humerus A, K, P 🦴, D, G, S 🦴

     M84.622   Pathological fracture in other disease, left humerus A, K, P 🦴, D, G, S 🦴

     ■ M84.629   Pathological fracture in other disease, unspecified humerus A, K, P 🦴, D, G, S 🦴

● M84.63   Pathological fracture in other disease, ulna and radius

     M84.631   Pathological fracture in other disease, right ulna A, K, P 🦴, D, G, S 🦴

     M84.632   Pathological fracture in other disease, left ulna A, K, P 🦴, D, G, S 🦴

     M84.633   Pathological fracture in other disease, right radius A, K, P 🦴, D, G, S 🦴

     M84.634   Pathological fracture in other disease, left radius A, K, P 🦴, D, G, S 🦴

     ■ M84.639   Pathological fracture in other disease, unspecified ulna and radius A, K, P 🦴, D, G, S 🦴

● M84.64   Pathological fracture in other disease, hand

     M84.641   Pathological fracture in other disease, right hand A, K, P 🦴, D, G, S 🦴

     M84.642   Pathological fracture in other disease, left hand A, K, P 🦴, D, G, S 🦴

     ■ M84.649   Pathological fracture in other disease, unspecified hand A, K, P 🦴, D, G, S 🦴

● M84.65   Pathological fracture in other disease, pelvis and femur

     M84.650   Pathological fracture in other disease, pelvis A, K, P 🦴, D, G, S 🦴

     M84.651   Pathological fracture in other disease, right femur A, K, P 🦴, D, G, S 🦴

     M84.652   Pathological fracture in other disease, left femur A, K, P 🦴, D, G, S 🦴

     ■ M84.653   Pathological fracture in other disease, unspecified femur A, K, P 🦴, D, G, S 🦴

     ■ M84.659   Pathological fracture in other disease, hip, unspecified A, K, P 🦴, D, G, S 🦴

● M84.66   Pathological fracture in other disease, tibia and fibula

     M84.661   Pathological fracture in other disease, right tibia A, K, P 🦴, D, G, S 🦴

     M84.662   Pathological fracture in other disease, left tibia A, K, P 🦴, D, G, S 🦴

     M84.663   Pathological fracture in other disease, right fibula A, K, P 🦴, D, G, S 🦴

     M84.664   Pathological fracture in other disease, left fibula A, K, P 🦴, D, G, S 🦴

     ■ M84.669   Pathological fracture in other disease, unspecified tibia and fibula A, K, P 🦴, D, G, S 🦴

● Unacceptable Principal Diagnosis   ● Use Additional Character(s)   ■ Unspecified   ▶ Manifestation Code

OGCR Official Guidelines for Coding and Reporting   Excludes 1   Excludes 2   Includes   Use additional   Code first   Code also

● **M84.67 Pathological fracture in other disease, ankle and foot**

    M84.671 Pathological fracture in other disease, right ankle A, K, P 🪙, D, G, S 🪙

    M84.672 Pathological fracture in other disease, left ankle A, K, P 🪙, D, G, S 🪙

    ■ **M84.673 Pathological fracture in other disease, unspecified ankle** A, K, P 🪙, D, G, S 🪙

    M84.674 Pathological fracture in other disease, right foot A, K, P 🪙, D, G, S 🪙

    M84.675 Pathological fracture in other disease, left foot A, K, P 🪙, D, G, S 🪙

    ■ **M84.676 Pathological fracture in other disease, unspecified foot** A, K, P 🪙, D, G, S 🪙

    M84.68 Pathological fracture in other disease, other site A, K, P 🪙, D, G, S 🪙

● **M84.8 Other disorders of continuity of bone**

    ■ **M84.80 Other disorders of continuity of bone, unspecified site**

    ● **M84.81 Other disorders of continuity of bone, shoulder**

      M84.811 Other disorders of continuity of bone, right shoulder

      M84.812 Other disorders of continuity of bone, left shoulder

      ■ **M84.819 Other disorders of continuity of bone, unspecified shoulder**

    ● **M84.82 Other disorders of continuity of bone, humerus**

      M84.821 Other disorders of continuity of bone, right humerus

      M84.822 Other disorders of continuity of bone, left humerus

      ■ **M84.829 Other disorders of continuity of bone, unspecified humerus**

    ● **M84.83 Other disorders of continuity of bone, ulna and radius**

      M84.831 Other disorders of continuity of bone, right ulna

      M84.832 Other disorders of continuity of bone, left ulna

      M84.833 Other disorders of continuity of bone, right radius

      M84.834 Other disorders of continuity of bone, left radius

      ■ **M84.839 Other disorders of continuity of bone, unspecified ulna and radius**

    ● **M84.84 Other disorders of continuity of bone, hand**

      M84.841 Other disorders of continuity of bone, right hand

      M84.842 Other disorders of continuity of bone, left hand

      ■ **M84.849 Other disorders of continuity of bone, unspecified hand**

● **M84.85 Other disorders of continuity of bone, pelvic region and thigh**

    M84.851 Other disorders of continuity of bone, right pelvic region and thigh

    M84.852 Other disorders of continuity of bone, left pelvic region and thigh

    ■ **M84.859 Other disorders of continuity of bone, unspecified pelvic region and thigh**

● **M84.86 Other disorders of continuity of bone, tibia and fibula**

    M84.861 Other disorders of continuity of bone, right tibia

    M84.862 Other disorders of continuity of bone, left tibia

    M84.863 Other disorders of continuity of bone, right fibula

    M84.864 Other disorders of continuity of bone, left fibula

    ■ **M84.869 Other disorders of continuity of bone, unspecified tibia and fibula**

● **M84.87 Other disorders of continuity of bone, ankle and foot**

    M84.871 Other disorders of continuity of bone, right ankle and foot

    M84.872 Other disorders of continuity of bone, left ankle and foot

    ■ **M84.879 Other disorders of continuity of bone, unspecified ankle and foot**

    M84.88 Other disorders of continuity of bone, other site

    ■ **M84.9 Disorder of continuity of bone, unspecified**

● **M85 Other disorders of bone density and structure**

    Excludes1   osteogenesis imperfecta (Q78.0)
      osteopetrosis (Q78.2)
      osteopoikilosis (Q78.8)
      polyostotic fibrous dysplasia (Q78.1)

   ● **M85.0 Fibrous dysplasia (monostotic)**

    Excludes2   fibrous dysplasia of jaw (M27.8)

    ■ **M85.00 Fibrous dysplasia (monostotic), unspecified site**

    ● **M85.01 Fibrous dysplasia (monostotic), shoulder**

      M85.011 Fibrous dysplasia (monostotic), right shoulder

      M85.012 Fibrous dysplasia (monostotic), left shoulder

      ■ **M85.019 Fibrous dysplasia (monostotic), unspecified shoulder**

    ● **M85.02 Fibrous dysplasia (monostotic), upper arm**

      M85.021 Fibrous dysplasia (monostotic), right upper arm

      M85.022 Fibrous dysplasia (monostotic), left upper arm

      ■ **M85.029 Fibrous dysplasia (monostotic), unspecified upper arm**

    ● **M85.03 Fibrous dysplasia (monostotic), forearm**

      M85.031 Fibrous dysplasia (monostotic), right forearm

      M85.032 Fibrous dysplasia (monostotic), left forearm

      ■ **M85.039 Fibrous dysplasia (monostotic), unspecified forearm**

CHAPTER 13 (M00-M99)

- M85.04   Fibrous dysplasia (monostotic), hand
  - M85.041   Fibrous dysplasia (monostotic), right hand
  - M85.042   Fibrous dysplasia (monostotic), left hand
  - M85.049   Fibrous dysplasia (monostotic), unspecified hand
- M85.05   Fibrous dysplasia (monostotic), thigh
  - M85.051   Fibrous dysplasia (monostotic), right thigh
  - M85.052   Fibrous dysplasia (monostotic), left thigh
  - M85.059   Fibrous dysplasia (monostotic), unspecified thigh
- M85.06   Fibrous dysplasia (monostotic), lower leg
  - M85.061   Fibrous dysplasia (monostotic), right lower leg
  - M85.062   Fibrous dysplasia (monostotic), left lower leg
  - M85.069   Fibrous dysplasia (monostotic), unspecified lower leg
- M85.07   Fibrous dysplasia (monostotic), ankle and foot
  - M85.071   Fibrous dysplasia (monostotic), right ankle and foot
  - M85.072   Fibrous dysplasia (monostotic), left ankle and foot
  - M85.079   Fibrous dysplasia (monostotic), unspecified ankle and foot
  - M85.08   Fibrous dysplasia (monostotic), other site
  - M85.09   Fibrous dysplasia (monostotic), multiple sites
- M85.1   Skeletal fluorosis
  - M85.10   Skeletal fluorosis, unspecified site
  - M85.11   Skeletal fluorosis, shoulder
    - M85.111   Skeletal fluorosis, right shoulder
    - M85.112   Skeletal fluorosis, left shoulder
    - M85.119   Skeletal fluorosis, unspecified shoulder
  - M85.12   Skeletal fluorosis, upper arm
    - M85.121   Skeletal fluorosis, right upper arm
    - M85.122   Skeletal fluorosis, left upper arm
    - M85.129   Skeletal fluorosis, unspecified upper arm
  - M85.13   Skeletal fluorosis, forearm
    - M85.131   Skeletal fluorosis, right forearm
    - M85.132   Skeletal fluorosis, left forearm
    - M85.139   Skeletal fluorosis, unspecified forearm
  - M85.14   Skeletal fluorosis, hand
    - M85.141   Skeletal fluorosis, right hand
    - M85.142   Skeletal fluorosis, left hand
    - M85.149   Skeletal fluorosis, unspecified hand
  - M85.15   Skeletal fluorosis, thigh
    - M85.151   Skeletal fluorosis, right thigh
    - M85.152   Skeletal fluorosis, left thigh
    - M85.159   Skeletal fluorosis, unspecified thigh
- M85.16   Skeletal fluorosis, lower leg
  - M85.161   Skeletal fluorosis, right lower leg
  - M85.162   Skeletal fluorosis, left lower leg
  - M85.169   Skeletal fluorosis, unspecified lower leg
- M85.17   Skeletal fluorosis, ankle and foot
  - M85.171   Skeletal fluorosis, right ankle and foot
  - M85.172   Skeletal fluorosis, left ankle and foot
  - M85.179   Skeletal fluorosis, unspecified ankle and foot
  - M85.18   Skeletal fluorosis, other site
  - M85.19   Skeletal fluorosis, multiple sites
- M85.2   Hyperostosis of skull
- M85.3   Osteitis condensans
  - M85.30   Osteitis condensans, unspecified site
  - M85.31   Osteitis condensans, shoulder
    - M85.311   Osteitis condensans, right shoulder
    - M85.312   Osteitis condensans, left shoulder
    - M85.319   Osteitis condensans, unspecified shoulder
  - M85.32   Osteitis condensans, upper arm
    - M85.321   Osteitis condensans, right upper arm
    - M85.322   Osteitis condensans, left upper arm
    - M85.329   Osteitis condensans, unspecified upper arm
  - M85.33   Osteitis condensans, forearm
    - M85.331   Osteitis condensans, right forearm
    - M85.332   Osteitis condensans, left forearm
    - M85.339   Osteitis condensans, unspecified forearm
  - M85.34   Osteitis condensans, hand
    - M85.341   Osteitis condensans, right hand
    - M85.342   Osteitis condensans, left hand
    - M85.349   Osteitis condensans, unspecified hand
  - M85.35   Osteitis condensans, thigh
    - M85.351   Osteitis condensans, right thigh
    - M85.352   Osteitis condensans, left thigh
    - M85.359   Osteitis condensans, unspecified thigh
  - M85.36   Osteitis condensans, lower leg
    - M85.361   Osteitis condensans, right lower leg
    - M85.362   Osteitis condensans, left lower leg
    - M85.369   Osteitis condensans, unspecified lower leg
  - M85.37   Osteitis condensans, ankle and foot
    - M85.371   Osteitis condensans, right ankle and foot
    - M85.372   Osteitis condensans, left ankle and foot
    - M85.379   Osteitis condensans, unspecified ankle and foot

● Unacceptable Principal Diagnosis   ● Use Additional Character(s)   ■ Unspecified   ▶ Manifestation Code

OGCR Official Guidelines for Coding and Reporting   Excludes 1   Excludes 2   Includes   Use additional   Code first   Code also

M85.38   Osteitis condensans, other site

M85.39   Osteitis condensans, multiple sites

● M85.4   Solitary bone cyst

> **Excludes2**   solitary cyst of jaw (M27.4)

■ M85.40   Solitary bone cyst, unspecified site

● M85.41   Solitary bone cyst, shoulder

    M85.411   Solitary bone cyst, right shoulder

    M85.412   Solitary bone cyst, left shoulder

    ■ M85.419   Solitary bone cyst, unspecified shoulder

● M85.42   Solitary bone cyst, humerus

    M85.421   Solitary bone cyst, right humerus

    M85.422   Solitary bone cyst, left humerus

    ■ M85.429   Solitary bone cyst, unspecified humerus

● M85.43   Solitary bone cyst, ulna and radius

    M85.431   Solitary bone cyst, right ulna and radius

    M85.432   Solitary bone cyst, left ulna and radius

    ■ M85.439   Solitary bone cyst, unspecified ulna and radius

● M85.44   Solitary bone cyst, hand

    M85.441   Solitary bone cyst, right hand

    M85.442   Solitary bone cyst, left hand

    ■ M85.449   Solitary bone cyst, unspecified hand

● M85.45   Solitary bone cyst, pelvis

    M85.451   Solitary bone cyst, right pelvis

    M85.452   Solitary bone cyst, left pelvis

    ■ M85.459   Solitary bone cyst, unspecified pelvis

● M85.46   Solitary bone cyst, tibia and fibula

    M85.461   Solitary bone cyst, right tibia and fibula

    M85.462   Solitary bone cyst, left tibia and fibula

    ■ M85.469   Solitary bone cyst, unspecified tibia and fibula

● M85.47   Solitary bone cyst, ankle and foot

    M85.471   Solitary bone cyst, right ankle and foot

    M85.472   Solitary bone cyst, left ankle and foot

    ■ M85.479   Solitary bone cyst, unspecified ankle and foot

M85.48   Solitary bone cyst, other site

● M85.5   Aneurysmal bone cyst

> **Excludes2**   aneurysmal cyst of jaw (M27.4)

■ M85.50   Aneurysmal bone cyst, unspecified site

● M85.51   Aneurysmal bone cyst, shoulder

    M85.511   Aneurysmal bone cyst, right shoulder

    M85.512   Aneurysmal bone cyst, left shoulder

    ■ M85.519   Aneurysmal bone cyst, unspecified shoulder

● M85.52   Aneurysmal bone cyst, upper arm

    M85.521   Aneurysmal bone cyst, right upper arm

    M85.522   Aneurysmal bone cyst, left upper arm

    ■ M85.529   Aneurysmal bone cyst, unspecified upper arm

● M85.53   Aneurysmal bone cyst, forearm

    M85.531   Aneurysmal bone cyst, right forearm

    M85.532   Aneurysmal bone cyst, left forearm

    ■ M85.539   Aneurysmal bone cyst, unspecified forearm

● M85.54   Aneurysmal bone cyst, hand

    M85.541   Aneurysmal bone cyst, right hand

    M85.542   Aneurysmal bone cyst, left hand

    ■ M85.549   Aneurysmal bone cyst, unspecified hand

● M85.55   Aneurysmal bone cyst, thigh

    M85.551   Aneurysmal bone cyst, right thigh

    M85.552   Aneurysmal bone cyst, left thigh

    ■ M85.559   Aneurysmal bone cyst, unspecified thigh

● M85.56   Aneurysmal bone cyst, lower leg

    M85.561   Aneurysmal bone cyst, right lower leg

    M85.562   Aneurysmal bone cyst, left lower leg

    ■ M85.569   Aneurysmal bone cyst, unspecified lower leg

● M85.57   Aneurysmal bone cyst, ankle and foot

    M85.571   Aneurysmal bone cyst, right ankle and foot

    M85.572   Aneurysmal bone cyst, left ankle and foot

    ■ M85.579   Aneurysmal bone cyst, unspecified ankle and foot

M85.58   Aneurysmal bone cyst, other site

M85.59   Aneurysmal bone cyst, multiple sites

● M85.6   Other cyst of bone

> **Excludes1**   cyst of jaw NEC (M27.4)
> osteitis fibrosa cystica generalisata [von Recklinghausen's disease of bone] (E21.0)

■ M85.60   Other cyst of bone, unspecified site

● M85.61   Other cyst of bone, shoulder

    M85.611   Other cyst of bone, right shoulder

    M85.612   Other cyst of bone, left shoulder

    ■ M85.619   Other cyst of bone, unspecified shoulder

● M85.62   Other cyst of bone, upper arm

    M85.621   Other cyst of bone, right upper arm

    M85.622   Other cyst of bone, left upper arm

    ■ M85.629   Other cyst of bone, unspecified upper arm

N Newborn Age: 0   **P** Pediatric Age: 0–17   **M** Maternity DX: 12–55   **A** Adult Age: 15–124   ♀ Females Only   ♂ Males Only

Complication\Comorbidity   Major C\C   Present on Admission Requirement   Hospital-Acquired Condition

1235

● M85.63   Other cyst of bone, forearm

     M85.631   Other cyst of bone, right forearm

     M85.632   Other cyst of bone, left forearm

     ■ M85.639   Other cyst of bone, unspecified forearm

● M85.64   Other cyst of bone, hand

     M85.641   Other cyst of bone, right hand

     M85.642   Other cyst of bone, left hand

     ■ M85.649   Other cyst of bone, unspecified hand

● M85.65   Other cyst of bone, thigh

     M85.651   Other cyst of bone, right thigh

     M85.652   Other cyst of bone, left thigh

     ■ M85.659   Other cyst of bone, unspecified thigh

● M85.66   Other cyst of bone, lower leg

     M85.661   Other cyst of bone, right lower leg

     M85.662   Other cyst of bone, left lower leg

     ■ M85.669   Other cyst of bone, unspecified lower leg

● M85.67   Other cyst of bone, ankle and foot

     M85.671   Other cyst of bone, right ankle and foot

     M85.672   Other cyst of bone, left ankle and foot

     ■ M85.679   Other cyst of bone, unspecified ankle and foot

     M85.68   Other cyst of bone, other site

     M85.69   Other cyst of bone, multiple sites

● M85.8   Other specified disorders of bone density and structure

     Hyperostosis of bones, except skull
     Osteosclerosis, acquired

Excludes1	diffuse idiopathic skeletal hyperostosis [DISH] (M48.1) osteosclerosis congenita (Q77.4) osteosclerosis fragilitas (generalista) (Q78.2) osteosclerosis myelofibrosis (D75.81)

     ■ M85.80   Other specified disorders of bone density and structure, unspecified site

● M85.81   Other specified disorders of bone density and structure, shoulder

     M85.811   Other specified disorders of bone density and structure, right shoulder

     M85.812   Other specified disorders of bone density and structure, left shoulder

     ■ M85.819   Other specified disorders of bone density and structure, unspecified shoulder

● M85.82   Other specified disorders of bone density and structure, upper arm

     M85.821   Other specified disorders of bone density and structure, right upper arm

     M85.822   Other specified disorders of bone density and structure, left upper arm

     ■ M85.829   Other specified disorders of bone density and structure, unspecified upper arm

● M85.83   Other specified disorders of bone density and structure, forearm

     M85.831   Other specified disorders of bone density and structure, right forearm

     M85.832   Other specified disorders of bone density and structure, left forearm

     ■ M85.839   Other specified disorders of bone density and structure, unspecified forearm

● M85.84   Other specified disorders of bone density and structure, hand

     M85.841   Other specified disorders of bone density and structure, right hand

     M85.842   Other specified disorders of bone density and structure, left hand

     ■ M85.849   Other specified disorders of bone density and structure, unspecified hand

● M85.85   Other specified disorders of bone density and structure, thigh

     M85.851   Other specified disorders of bone density and structure, right thigh

     M85.852   Other specified disorders of bone density and structure, left thigh

     ■ M85.859   Other specified disorders of bone density and structure, unspecified thigh

● M85.86   Other specified disorders of bone density and structure, lower leg

     M85.861   Other specified disorders of bone density and structure, right lower leg

     M85.862   Other specified disorders of bone density and structure, left lower leg

     ■ M85.869   Other specified disorders of bone density and structure, unspecified lower leg

● M85.87   Other specified disorders of bone density and structure, ankle and foot

     M85.871   Other specified disorders of bone density and structure, right ankle and foot

     M85.872   Other specified disorders of bone density and structure, left ankle and foot

     ■ M85.879   Other specified disorders of bone density and structure, unspecified ankle and foot

     M85.88   Other specified disorders of bone density and structure, other site

     M85.89   Other specified disorders of bone density and structure, multiple sites

■ M85.9   Disorder of bone density and structure, unspecified

● Unacceptable Principal Diagnosis   ● Use Additional Character(s)   ■ Unspecified   ▶ Manifestation Code

OGCR Official Guidelines for Coding and Reporting | Excludes 1 | | Excludes 2 | Includes   Use additional   Code first   Code also

Figure 13-5 Osteomyelitis of the spine. A lateral view of the lower thoracic spine demonstrates destruction of the disk space *(arrow)* as well as destruction of the adjoining vertebral bodies. (From Mettler: Essentials of Radiology, 2nd ed. 2005, Saunders, An Imprint of Elsevier.)

Item 13-12 Osteomyelitis is an inflammation of the bone. **Acute osteomyelitis** is a rapidly destructive, pus-producing infection capable of causing severe bone destruction. **Chronic osteomyelitis** can remain long after the initial acute episode has passed and may lead to a recurrence of the acute phase. **Brodie's abscess** is an encapsulated focal abscess that must be surgically drained. Periostitis is an inflammation of the periosteum, a dense membrane composed of fibrous connective tissue that closely wraps all bone, except those with articulating surfaces in joints, which are covered by synovial membranes.

OTHER OSTEOPATHIES (M86-M90)

> **Excludes1**   postprocedural osteopathies (M96.-)

● **M86 Osteomyelitis**

> Use additional code (B95-B97) to identify infectious agent

> Use additional code to identify major osseous defect, if applicable (M89.7-)

> **Excludes1**   osteomyelitis due to:
> echinococcus (B67.2)
> gonococcus (A54.43)
> salmonella (A02.24)

> **Excludes2**   ostemyelitis of:
> orbit (H05.0-)
> petrous bone (H70.2-)
> vertebra (M46.2-)

● **M86.0 Acute hematogenous osteomyelitis**

■ **M86.00 Acute hematogenous osteomyelitis, unspecified site** 🔧

● **M86.01 Acute hematogenous osteomyelitis, shoulder**

    M86.011 Acute hematogenous osteomyelitis, right shoulder 🔧

    M86.012 Acute hematogenous osteomyelitis, left shoulder 🔧

    ■ M86.019 Acute hematogenous osteomyelitis, unspecified shoulder 🔧

● **M86.02 Acute hematogenous osteomyelitis, humerus**

    M86.021 Acute hematogenous osteomyelitis, right humerus 🔧

    M86.022 Acute hematogenous osteomyelitis, left humerus 🔧

    ■ M86.029 Acute hematogenous osteomyelitis, unspecified humerus 🔧

● **M86.03 Acute hematogenous osteomyelitis, radius and ulna**

    M86.031 Acute hematogenous osteomyelitis, right radius and ulna 🔧

    M86.032 Acute hematogenous osteomyelitis, left radius and ulna 🔧

    ■ M86.039 Acute hematogenous osteomyelitis, unspecified radius and ulna 🔧

● **M86.04 Acute hematogenous osteomyelitis, hand**

    M86.041 Acute hematogenous osteomyelitis, right hand 🔧

    M86.042 Acute hematogenous osteomyelitis, left hand 🔧

    ■ M86.049 Acute hematogenous osteomyelitis, unspecified hand 🔧

● **M86.05 Acute hematogenous osteomyelitis, femur**

    M86.051 Acute hematogenous osteomyelitis, right femur 🔧

    M86.052 Acute hematogenous osteomyelitis, left femur 🔧

    ■ M86.059 Acute hematogenous osteomyelitis, unspecified femur 🔧

● **M86.06 Acute hematogenous osteomyelitis, tibia and fibula**

    M86.061 Acute hematogenous osteomyelitis, right tibia and fibula 🔧

    M86.062 Acute hematogenous osteomyelitis, left tibia and fibula 🔧

    ■ M86.069 Acute hematogenous osteomyelitis, unspecified tibia and fibula 🔧

● **M86.07 Acute hematogenous osteomyelitis, ankle and foot**

    M86.071 Acute hematogenous osteomyelitis, right ankle and foot 🔧

    M86.072 Acute hematogenous osteomyelitis, left ankle and foot 🔧

    ■ M86.079 Acute hematogenous osteomyelitis, unspecified ankle and foot 🔧

    M86.08 Acute hematogenous osteomyelitis, other sites 🔧

    M86.09 Acute hematogenous osteomyelitis, multiple sites 🔧

● **M86.1 Other acute osteomyelitis**

    ■ M86.10 Other acute osteomyelitis, unspecified site 🔧

● **M86.11 Other acute osteomyelitis, shoulder**

    M86.111 Other acute osteomyelitis, right shoulder 🔧

    M86.112 Other acute osteomyelitis, left shoulder 🔧

    ■ M86.119 Other acute osteomyelitis, unspecified shoulder 🔧

N Newborn Age: 0   **P** Pediatric Age: 0–17   **M** Maternity DX: 12–55   **A** Adult Age: 15–124   ♀ Females Only   ♂ Males Only

🔧 Complication\Comorbidity   🔧 Major C\C   🔧 Present on Admission Requirement   🔧 Hospital-Acquired Condition

1237

CHAPTER 13 (M00-M99)

● M86.12 Other acute osteomyelitis, humerus
   M86.121 Other acute osteomyelitis, right humerus 🦴
   M86.122 Other acute osteomyelitis, left humerus 🦴
   ■ M86.129 Other acute osteomyelitis, unspecified humerus 🦴
● M86.13 Other acute osteomyelitis, radius and ulna
   M86.131 Other acute osteomyelitis, right radius and ulna 🦴
   M86.132 Other acute osteomyelitis, left radius and ulna 🦴
   ■ M86.139 Other acute osteomyelitis, unspecified radius and ulna 🦴
● M86.14 Other acute osteomyelitis, hand
   M86.141 Other acute osteomyelitis, right hand 🦴
   M86.142 Other acute osteomyelitis, left hand 🦴
   ■ M86.149 Other acute osteomyelitis, unspecified hand 🦴
● M86.15 Other acute osteomyelitis, femur
   M86.151 Other acute osteomyelitis, right femur 🦴
   M86.152 Other acute osteomyelitis, left femur 🦴
   ■ M86.159 Other acute osteomyelitis, unspecified femur 🦴
● M86.16 Other acute osteomyelitis, tibia and fibula
   M86.161 Other acute osteomyelitis, right tibia and fibula 🦴
   M86.162 Other acute osteomyelitis, left tibia and fibula 🦴
   ■ M86.169 Other acute osteomyelitis, unspecified tibia and fibula 🦴
● M86.17 Other acute osteomyelitis, ankle and foot
   M86.171 Other acute osteomyelitis, right ankle and foot 🦴
   M86.172 Other acute osteomyelitis, left ankle and foot 🦴
   ■ M86.179 Other acute osteomyelitis, unspecified ankle and foot 🦴
   M86.18 Other acute osteomyelitis, other site 🦴
   M86.19 Other acute osteomyelitis, multiple sites 🦴
● M86.2 Subacute osteomyelitis
  ■ M86.20 Subacute osteomyelitis, unspecified site 🦴
● M86.21 Subacute osteomyelitis, shoulder
   M86.211 Subacute osteomyelitis, right shoulder 🦴
   M86.212 Subacute osteomyelitis, left shoulder 🦴
   ■ M86.219 Subacute osteomyelitis, unspecified shoulder 🦴
● M86.22 Subacute osteomyelitis, humerus
   M86.221 Subacute osteomyelitis, right humerus 🦴
   M86.222 Subacute osteomyelitis, left humerus 🦴
   ■ M86.229 Subacute osteomyelitis, unspecified humerus 🦴

● M86.23 Subacute osteomyelitis, radius and ulna
   M86.231 Subacute osteomyelitis, right radius and ulna 🦴
   M86.232 Subacute osteomyelitis, left radius and ulna 🦴
   ■ M86.239 Subacute osteomyelitis, unspecified radius and ulna 🦴
● M86.24 Subacute osteomyelitis, hand
   M86.241 Subacute osteomyelitis, right hand 🦴
   M86.242 Subacute osteomyelitis, left hand 🦴
   ■ M86.249 Subacute osteomyelitis, unspecified hand 🦴
● M86.25 Subacute osteomyelitis, femur
   M86.251 Subacute osteomyelitis, right femur 🦴
   M86.252 Subacute osteomyelitis, left femur 🦴
   ■ M86.259 Subacute osteomyelitis, unspecified femur 🦴
● M86.26 Subacute osteomyelitis, tibia and fibula
   M86.261 Subacute osteomyelitis, right tibia and fibula 🦴
   M86.262 Subacute osteomyelitis, left tibia and fibula 🦴
   ■ M86.269 Subacute osteomyelitis, unspecified tibia and fibula 🦴
● M86.27 Subacute osteomyelitis, ankle and foot
   M86.271 Subacute osteomyelitis, right ankle and foot 🦴
   M86.272 Subacute osteomyelitis, left ankle and foot 🦴
   ■ M86.279 Subacute osteomyelitis, unspecified ankle and foot 🦴
   M86.28 Subacute osteomyelitis, other site 🦴
   M86.29 Subacute osteomyelitis, multiple sites 🦴
● M86.3 Chronic multifocal osteomyelitis
  ■ M86.30 Chronic multifocal osteomyelitis, unspecified site 🦴
● M86.31 Chronic multifocal osteomyelitis, shoulder
   M86.311 Chronic multifocal osteomyelitis, right shoulder 🦴
   M86.312 Chronic multifocal osteomyelitis, left shoulder 🦴
   ■ M86.319 Chronic multifocal osteomyelitis, unspecified shoulder 🦴
● M86.32 Chronic multifocal osteomyelitis, humerus
   M86.321 Chronic multifocal osteomyelitis, right humerus 🦴
   M86.322 Chronic multifocal osteomyelitis, left humerus 🦴
   ■ M86.329 Chronic multifocal osteomyelitis, unspecified humerus 🦴
● M86.33 Chronic multifocal osteomyelitis, radius and ulna
   M86.331 Chronic multifocal osteomyelitis, right radius and ulna 🦴
   M86.332 Chronic multifocal osteomyelitis, left radius and ulna 🦴
   ■ M86.339 Chronic multifocal osteomyelitis, unspecified radius and ulna 🦴

● Unacceptable Principal Diagnosis   ● Use Additional Character(s)   ■ Unspecified   ▶ Manifestation Code
OGCR Official Guidelines for Coding and Reporting   Excludes 1   Excludes 2   Includes   Use additional   Code first   Code also

● M86.34 Chronic multifocal osteomyelitis, hand

     M86.341 Chronic multifocal osteomyelitis, right hand 🦠

     M86.342 Chronic multifocal osteomyelitis, left hand 🦠

     ■ M86.349 Chronic multifocal osteomyelitis, unspecified hand 🦠

● M86.35 Chronic multifocal osteomyelitis, femur

     M86.351 Chronic multifocal osteomyelitis, right femur 🦠

     M86.352 Chronic multifocal osteomyelitis, left femur 🦠

     ■ M86.359 Chronic multifocal osteomyelitis, unspecified femur 🦠

● M86.36 Chronic multifocal osteomyelitis, tibia and fibula

     M86.361 Chronic multifocal osteomyelitis, right tibia and fibula 🦠

     M86.362 Chronic multifocal osteomyelitis, left tibia and fibula 🦠

     ■ M86.369 Chronic multifocal osteomyelitis, unspecified tibia and fibula 🦠

● M86.37 Chronic multifocal osteomyelitis, ankle and foot

     M86.371 Chronic multifocal osteomyelitis, right ankle and foot 🦠

     M86.372 Chronic multifocal osteomyelitis, left ankle and foot 🦠

     ■ M86.379 Chronic multifocal osteomyelitis, unspecified ankle and foot 🦠

     M86.38 Chronic multifocal osteomyelitis, other site 🦠

     M86.39 Chronic multifocal osteomyelitis, multiple sites 🦠

● M86.4 Chronic osteomyelitis with draining sinus

     ■ M86.40 Chronic osteomyelitis with draining sinus, unspecified site 🦠

     ● M86.41 Chronic osteomyelitis with draining sinus, shoulder

         M86.411 Chronic osteomyelitis with draining sinus, right shoulder 🦠

         M86.412 Chronic osteomyelitis with draining sinus, left shoulder 🦠

         ■ M86.419 Chronic osteomyelitis with draining sinus, unspecified shoulder 🦠

     ● M86.42 Chronic osteomyelitis with draining sinus, humerus

         M86.421 Chronic osteomyelitis with draining sinus, right humerus 🦠

         M86.422 Chronic osteomyelitis with draining sinus, left humerus 🦠

         ■ M86.429 Chronic osteomyelitis with draining sinus, unspecified humerus 🦠

     ● M86.43 Chronic osteomyelitis with draining sinus, radius and ulna

         M86.431 Chronic osteomyelitis with draining sinus, right radius and ulna 🦠

         M86.432 Chronic osteomyelitis with draining sinus, left radius and ulna 🦠

         ■ M86.439 Chronic osteomyelitis with draining sinus, unspecified radius and ulna 🦠

● M86.44 Chronic osteomyelitis with draining sinus, hand

     M86.441 Chronic osteomyelitis with draining sinus, right hand 🦠

     M86.442 Chronic osteomyelitis with draining sinus, left hand 🦠

     ■ M86.449 Chronic osteomyelitis with draining sinus, unspecified hand 🦠

● M86.45 Chronic osteomyelitis with draining sinus, femur

     M86.451 Chronic osteomyelitis with draining sinus, right femur 🦠

     M86.452 Chronic osteomyelitis with draining sinus, left femur 🦠

     ■ M86.459 Chronic osteomyelitis with draining sinus, unspecified femur 🦠

● M86.46 Chronic osteomyelitis with draining sinus, tibia and fibula

     M86.461 Chronic osteomyelitis with draining sinus, right tibia and fibula 🦠

     M86.462 Chronic osteomyelitis with draining sinus, left tibia and fibula 🦠

     ■ M86.469 Chronic osteomyelitis with draining sinus, unspecified tibia and fibula 🦠

● M86.47 Chronic osteomyelitis with draining sinus, ankle and foot

     M86.471 Chronic osteomyelitis with draining sinus, right ankle and foot 🦠

     M86.472 Chronic osteomyelitis with draining sinus, left ankle and foot 🦠

     ■ M86.479 Chronic osteomyelitis with draining sinus, unspecified ankle and foot 🦠

     M86.48 Chronic osteomyelitis with draining sinus, other site 🦠

     M86.49 Chronic osteomyelitis with draining sinus, multiple sites 🦠

● M86.5 Other chronic hematogenous osteomyelitis

     ■ M86.50 Other chronic hematogenous osteomyelitis, unspecified site 🦠

     ● M86.51 Other chronic hematogenous osteomyelitis, shoulder

         M86.511 Other chronic hematogenous osteomyelitis, right shoulder 🦠

         M86.512 Other chronic hematogenous osteomyelitis, left shoulder 🦠

         ■ M86.519 Other chronic hematogenous osteomyelitis, unspecified shoulder 🦠

     ● M86.52 Other chronic hematogenous osteomyelitis, humerus

         M86.521 Other chronic hematogenous osteomyelitis, right humerus 🦠

         M86.522 Other chronic hematogenous osteomyelitis, left humerus 🦠

         ■ M86.529 Other chronic hematogenous osteomyelitis, unspecified humerus 🦠

N Newborn Age: 0   **P** Pediatric Age: 0–17   **M** Maternity DX: 12–55   **A** Adult Age: 15–124   ♀ Females Only   ♂ Males Only

🦠 Complication\Comorbidity   ■ Major C\C   Present on Admission Requirement   Hospital-Acquired Condition

1239

● M86.53 Other chronic hematogenous osteomyelitis, radius and ulna

    M86.531 Other chronic hematogenous osteomyelitis, right radius and ulna 🦴

    M86.532 Other chronic hematogenous osteomyelitis, left radius and ulna 🦴

    ■ M86.539 Other chronic hematogenous osteomyelitis, unspecified radius and ulna 🦴

● M86.54 Other chronic hematogenous osteomyelitis, hand

    M86.541 Other chronic hematogenous osteomyelitis, right hand 🦴

    M86.542 Other chronic hematogenous osteomyelitis, left hand 🦴

    ■ M86.549 Other chronic hematogenous osteomyelitis, unspecified hand 🦴

● M86.55 Other chronic hematogenous osteomyelitis, femur

    M86.551 Other chronic hematogenous osteomyelitis, right femur 🦴

    M86.552 Other chronic hematogenous osteomyelitis, left femur 🦴

    ■ M86.559 Other chronic hematogenous osteomyelitis, unspecified femur 🦴

● M86.56 Other chronic hematogenous osteomyelitis, tibia and fibula

    M86.561 Other chronic hematogenous osteomyelitis, right tibia and fibula 🦴

    M86.562 Other chronic hematogenous osteomyelitis, left tibia and fibula 🦴

    ■ M86.569 Other chronic hematogenous osteomyelitis, unspecified tibia and fibula 🦴

● M86.57 Other chronic hematogenous osteomyelitis, ankle and foot

    M86.571 Other chronic hematogenous osteomyelitis, right ankle and foot 🦴

    M86.572 Other chronic hematogenous osteomyelitis, left ankle and foot 🦴

    ■ M86.579 Other chronic hematogenous osteomyelitis, unspecified ankle and foot 🦴

M86.58 Other chronic hematogenous osteomyelitis, other site 🦴

M86.59 Other chronic hematogenous osteomyelitis, multiple sites 🦴

● M86.6 Other chronic osteomyelitis

    ■ M86.60 Other chronic osteomyelitis, unspecified site 🦴

● M86.61 Other chronic osteomyelitis, shoulder

    M86.611 Other chronic osteomyelitis, right shoulder 🦴

    M86.612 Other chronic osteomyelitis, left shoulder 🦴

    ■ M86.619 Other chronic osteomyelitis, unspecified shoulder 🦴

● M86.62 Other chronic osteomyelitis, humerus

    M86.621 Other chronic osteomyelitis, right humerus 🦴

    M86.622 Other chronic osteomyelitis, left humerus 🦴

    ■ M86.629 Other chronic osteomyelitis, unspecified humerus 🦴

● M86.63 Other chronic osteomyelitis, radius and ulna

    M86.631 Other chronic osteomyelitis, right radius and ulna 🦴

    M86.632 Other chronic osteomyelitis, left radius and ulna 🦴

    ■ M86.639 Other chronic osteomyelitis, unspecified radius and ulna 🦴

● M86.64 Other chronic osteomyelitis, hand

    M86.641 Other chronic osteomyelitis, right hand 🦴

    M86.642 Other chronic osteomyelitis, left hand 🦴

    ■ M86.649 Other chronic osteomyelitis, unspecified hand 🦴

● M86.65 Other chronic osteomyelitis, thigh

    M86.651 Other chronic osteomyelitis, right thigh 🦴

    M86.652 Other chronic osteomyelitis, left thigh 🦴

    ■ M86.659 Other chronic osteomyelitis, unspecified thigh 🦴

● M86.66 Other chronic osteomyelitis, tibia and fibula

    M86.661 Other chronic osteomyelitis, right tibia and fibula 🦴

    M86.662 Other chronic osteomyelitis, left tibia and fibula 🦴

    ■ M86.669 Other chronic osteomyelitis, unspecified tibia and fibula 🦴

● M86.67 Other chronic osteomyelitis, ankle and foot

    M86.671 Other chronic osteomyelitis, right ankle and foot 🦴

    M86.672 Other chronic osteomyelitis, left ankle and foot 🦴

    ■ M86.679 Other chronic osteomyelitis, unspecified ankle and foot 🦴

M86.68 Other chronic osteomyelitis, other site 🦴

M86.69 Other chronic osteomyelitis, multiple sites 🦴

● M86.8 Other osteomyelitis
Brodie's abscess

● M86.8X Other osteomyelitis

    M86.8X0 Other osteomyelitis, multiple sites 🦴

    M86.8X1 Other osteomyelitis, shoulder 🦴

    M86.8X2 Other osteomyelitis, upper arm 🦴

    M86.8X3 Other osteomyelitis, forearm 🦴

    M86.8X4 Other osteomyelitis, hand 🦴

    M86.8X5 Other osteomyelitis, thigh 🦴

    M86.8X6 Other osteomyelitis, lower leg 🦴

    M86.8X7 Other osteomyelitis, ankle and foot 🦴

    M86.8X8 Other osteomyelitis, other site 🦴

    ■ M86.8X9 Other osteomyelitis, unspecified sites 🦴

■ M86.9 Osteomyelitis, unspecified 🦴
Infection of bone NOS
Periostitis without osteomyelitis

● Unacceptable Principal Diagnosis   ● Use Additional Character(s)   ■ Unspecified   ▶ Manifestation Code

OGCR Official Guidelines for Coding and Reporting   Excludes 1   Excludes 2   Includes   Use additional   Code first   Code also

● **M87   Osteonecrosis**

    Includes   avascular necrosis of bone

    Use additional code to identify major osseous defect, if applicable (M89.7-)

    Excludes1   juvenile osteonecrosis (M91-M92)
                  osteochondropathies (M90-M93)

 ● **M87.0   Idiopathic aseptic necrosis of bone**

    ■ **M87.00   Idiopathic aseptic necrosis of unspecified bone** 🗇

    ● **M87.01   Idiopathic aseptic necrosis of shoulder**
         Idiopathic aseptic necrosis of clavicle and scapula

       M87.011   Idiopathic aseptic necrosis of right shoulder 🗇

       M87.012   Idiopathic aseptic necrosis of left shoulder 🗇

       ■ **M87.019   Idiopathic aseptic necrosis of unspecified shoulder** 🗇

    ● **M87.02   Idiopathic aseptic necrosis of humerus**

       M87.021   Idiopathic aseptic necrosis of right humerus 🗇

       M87.022   Idiopathic aseptic necrosis of left humerus 🗇

       ■ **M87.029   Idiopathic aseptic necrosis of unspecified humerus** 🗇

    ● **M87.03   Idiopathic aseptic necrosis of radius, ulna and carpus**

       M87.031   Idiopathic aseptic necrosis of right radius 🗇

       M87.032   Idiopathic aseptic necrosis of left radius 🗇

       ■ **M87.033   Idiopathic aseptic necrosis of unspecified radius** 🗇

       M87.034   Idiopathic aseptic necrosis of right ulna 🗇

       M87.035   Idiopathic aseptic necrosis of left ulna 🗇

       ■ **M87.036   Idiopathic aseptic necrosis of unspecified ulna** 🗇

       M87.037   Idiopathic aseptic necrosis of right carpus 🗇

       M87.038   Idiopathic aseptic necrosis of left carpus 🗇

       ■ **M87.039   Idiopathic aseptic necrosis of unspecified carpus** 🗇

    ● **M87.04   Idiopathic aseptic necrosis of hand and fingers**
         Idiopathic aseptic necrosis of metacarpals and phalanges of hands

       M87.041   Idiopathic aseptic necrosis of right hand 🗇

       M87.042   Idiopathic aseptic necrosis of left hand 🗇

       ■ **M87.043   Idiopathic aseptic necrosis of unspecified hand** 🗇

       M87.044   Idiopathic aseptic necrosis of right finger(s) 🗇

       M87.045   Idiopathic aseptic necrosis of left finger(s) 🗇

       ■ **M87.046   Idiopathic aseptic necrosis of unspecified finger(s)** 🗇

    ● **M87.05   Idiopathic aseptic necrosis of pelvis and femur**

       M87.050   Idiopathic aseptic necrosis of pelvis 🗇

       M87.051   Idiopathic aseptic necrosis of right femur 🗇

       M87.052   Idiopathic aseptic necrosis of left femur 🗇

       ■ **M87.059   Idiopathic aseptic necrosis of unspecified femur** 🗇
          Idiopathic aseptic necrosis of hip NOS

    ● **M87.06   Idiopathic aseptic necrosis of tibia and fibula**

       M87.061   Idiopathic aseptic necrosis of right tibia 🗇

       M87.062   Idiopathic aseptic necrosis of left tibia 🗇

       ■ **M87.063   Idiopathic aseptic necrosis of unspecified tibia** 🗇

       M87.064   Idiopathic aseptic necrosis of right fibula 🗇

       M87.065   Idiopathic aseptic necrosis of left fibula 🗇

       ■ **M87.066   Idiopathic aseptic necrosis of unspecified fibula** 🗇

    ● **M87.07   Idiopathic aseptic necrosis of ankle, foot and toes**
         Idiopathic aseptic necrosis of metatarsus, tarsus, and phalanges of toes

       M87.071   Idiopathic aseptic necrosis of right ankle 🗇

       M87.072   Idiopathic aseptic necrosis of left ankle 🗇

       ■ **M87.073   Idiopathic aseptic necrosis of unspecified ankle** 🗇

       M87.074   Idiopathic aseptic necrosis of right foot 🗇

       M87.075   Idiopathic aseptic necrosis of left foot 🗇

       ■ **M87.076   Idiopathic aseptic necrosis of unspecified foot** 🗇

       M87.077   Idiopathic aseptic necrosis of right toe(s) 🗇

       M87.078   Idiopathic aseptic necrosis of left toe(s) 🗇

       ■ **M87.079   Idiopathic aseptic necrosis of unspecified toe(s)** 🗇

    M87.08   Idiopathic aseptic necrosis of bone, other site 🗇

    M87.09   Idiopathic aseptic necrosis of bone, multiple sites 🗇

 ● **M87.1   Osteonecrosis due to drugs**

    Use additional code for adverse effect, if applicable, to identify drug (T36-T50 with fifth or sixth character 5)

    ●■ **M87.10   Osteonecrosis due to drugs, unspecified bone** 🗇

    ● **M87.11   Osteonecrosis due to drugs, shoulder**

       ● **M87.111   Osteonecrosis due to drugs, right shoulder** 🗇

       ● **M87.112   Osteonecrosis due to drugs, left shoulder** 🗇

       ●■ **M87.119   Osteonecrosis due to drugs, unspecified shoulder** 🗇

N Newborn Age: 0   **P** Pediatric Age: 0–17   **M** Maternity DX: 12–55   **A** Adult Age: 15–124   ♀ Females Only   ♂ Males Only

🗇 Complication\Comorbidity   🗇 Major C\C   🗇 Present on Admission Requirement   🗇 Hospital-Acquired Condition

1241

- M87.12 Osteonecrosis due to drugs, humerus
  - M87.121 Osteonecrosis due to drugs, right humerus
  - M87.122 Osteonecrosis due to drugs, left humerus
  - M87.129 Osteonecrosis due to drugs, unspecified humerus
- M87.13 Osteonecrosis due to drugs of radius, ulna and carpus
  - M87.131 Osteonecrosis due to drugs of right radius
  - M87.132 Osteonecrosis due to drugs of left radius
  - M87.133 Osteonecrosis due to drugs of unspecified radius
  - M87.134 Osteonecrosis due to drugs of right ulna
  - M87.135 Osteonecrosis due to drugs of left ulna
  - M87.136 Osteonecrosis due to drugs of unspecified ulna
  - M87.137 Osteonecrosis due to drugs of right carpus
  - M87.138 Osteonecrosis due to drugs of left carpus
  - M87.139 Osteonecrosis due to drugs of unspecified carpus
- M87.14 Osteonecrosis due to drugs, hand and fingers
  - M87.141 Osteonecrosis due to drugs, right hand
  - M87.142 Osteonecrosis due to drugs, left hand
  - M87.143 Osteonecrosis due to drugs, unspecified hand
  - M87.144 Osteonecrosis due to drugs, right finger(s)
  - M87.145 Osteonecrosis due to drugs, left finger(s)
  - M87.146 Osteonecrosis due to drugs, unspecified finger(s)
- M87.15 Osteonecrosis due to drugs, pelvis and femur
  - M87.150 Osteonecrosis due to drugs, pelvis
  - M87.151 Osteonecrosis due to drugs, right femur
  - M87.152 Osteonecrosis due to drugs, left femur
  - M87.159 Osteonecrosis due to drugs, unspecified femur
- M87.16 Osteonecrosis due to drugs, tibia and fibula
  - M87.161 Osteonecrosis due to drugs, right tibia
  - M87.162 Osteonecrosis due to drugs, left tibia
  - M87.163 Osteonecrosis due to drugs, unspecified tibia
  - M87.164 Osteonecrosis due to drugs, right fibula
  - M87.165 Osteonecrosis due to drugs, left fibula
  - M87.166 Osteonecrosis due to drugs, unspecified fibula

- M87.17 Osteonecrosis due to drugs, ankle, foot and toes
  - M87.171 Osteonecrosis due to drugs, right ankle
  - M87.172 Osteonecrosis due to drugs, left ankle
  - M87.173 Osteonecrosis due to drugs, unspecified ankle
  - M87.174 Osteonecrosis due to drugs, right foot
  - M87.175 Osteonecrosis due to drugs, left foot
  - M87.176 Osteonecrosis due to drugs, unspecified foot
  - M87.177 Osteonecrosis due to drugs, right toe(s)
  - M87.178 Osteonecrosis due to drugs, left toe(s)
  - M87.179 Osteonecrosis due to drugs, unspecified toe(s)
- M87.18 Osteonecrosis due to drugs, other site
  - M87.180 Osteonecrosis due to drugs, jaw
  - M87.188 Osteonecrosis due to drugs, other site
- M87.19 Osteonecrosis due to drugs, multiple sites
- M87.2 Osteonecrosis due to previous trauma
  - M87.20 Osteonecrosis due to previous trauma, unspecified bone
  - M87.21 Osteonecrosis due to previous trauma, shoulder
    - M87.211 Osteonecrosis due to previous trauma, right shoulder
    - M87.212 Osteonecrosis due to previous trauma, left shoulder
    - M87.219 Osteonecrosis due to previous trauma, unspecified shoulder
  - M87.22 Osteonecrosis due to previous trauma, humerus
    - M87.221 Osteonecrosis due to previous trauma, right humerus
    - M87.222 Osteonecrosis due to previous trauma, left humerus
    - M87.229 Osteonecrosis due to previous trauma, unspecified humerus
  - M87.23 Osteonecrosis due to previous trauma of radius, ulna and carpus
    - M87.231 Osteonecrosis due to previous trauma of right radius
    - M87.232 Osteonecrosis due to previous trauma of left radius
    - M87.233 Osteonecrosis due to previous trauma of unspecified radius
    - M87.234 Osteonecrosis due to previous trauma of right ulna
    - M87.235 Osteonecrosis due to previous trauma of left ulna
    - M87.236 Osteonecrosis due to previous trauma of unspecified ulna
    - M87.237 Osteonecrosis due to previous trauma of right carpus
    - M87.238 Osteonecrosis due to previous trauma of left carpus
    - M87.239 Osteonecrosis due to previous trauma of unspecified carpus

- Unacceptable Principal Diagnosis   Use Additional Character(s)   ◼ Unspecified   ▶ Manifestation Code
OGCR Official Guidelines for Coding and Reporting   Excludes 1   Excludes 2   Includes   Use additional   Code first   Code also

● M87.24 Osteonecrosis due to previous trauma, hand and fingers

   M87.241 Osteonecrosis due to previous trauma, right hand %

   M87.242 Osteonecrosis due to previous trauma, left hand %

   ■ M87.243 Osteonecrosis due to previous trauma, unspecified hand %

   M87.244 Osteonecrosis due to previous trauma, right finger(s) %

   M87.245 Osteonecrosis due to previous trauma, left finger(s) %

   ■ M87.246 Osteonecrosis due to previous trauma, unspecified finger(s) %

● M87.25 Osteonecrosis due to previous trauma, pelvis and femur

   M87.250 Osteonecrosis due to previous trauma, pelvis %

   M87.251 Osteonecrosis due to previous trauma, right femur %

   M87.252 Osteonecrosis due to previous trauma, left femur %

   ■ M87.256 Osteonecrosis due to previous trauma, unspecified femur %

● M87.26 Osteonecrosis due to previous trauma, tibia and fibula

   M87.261 Osteonecrosis due to previous trauma, right tibia %

   M87.262 Osteonecrosis due to previous trauma, left tibia %

   ■ M87.263 Osteonecrosis due to previous trauma, unspecified tibia %

   M87.264 Osteonecrosis due to previous trauma, right fibula %

   M87.265 Osteonecrosis due to previous trauma, left fibula %

   ■ M87.266 Osteonecrosis due to previous trauma, unspecified fibula %

● M87.27 Osteonecrosis due to previous trauma, ankle, foot and toes

   M87.271 Osteonecrosis due to previous trauma, right ankle %

   M87.272 Osteonecrosis due to previous trauma, left ankle %

   ■ M87.273 Osteonecrosis due to previous trauma, unspecified ankle %

   M87.274 Osteonecrosis due to previous trauma, right foot %

   M87.275 Osteonecrosis due to previous trauma, left foot %

   ■ M87.276 Osteonecrosis due to previous trauma, unspecified foot %

   M87.277 Osteonecrosis due to previous trauma, right toe(s) %

   M87.278 Osteonecrosis due to previous trauma, left toe(s) %

   ■ M87.279 Osteonecrosis due to previous trauma, unspecified toe(s) %

M87.28 Osteonecrosis due to previous trauma, other site %

M87.29 Osteonecrosis due to previous trauma, multiple sites %

● M87.3 Other secondary osteonecrosis

   ■ M87.30 Other secondary osteonecrosis, unspecified bone %

   ● M87.31 Other secondary osteonecrosis, shoulder

     M87.311 Other secondary osteonecrosis, right shoulder %

     M87.312 Other secondary osteonecrosis, left shoulder %

     ■ M87.319 Other secondary osteonecrosis, unspecified shoulder %

   ● M87.32 Other secondary osteonecrosis, humerus

     M87.321 Other secondary osteonecrosis, right humerus %

     M87.322 Other secondary osteonecrosis, left humerus %

     ■ M87.329 Other secondary osteonecrosis, unspecified humerus %

   ● M87.33 Other secondary osteonecrosis of radius, ulna and carpus

     M87.331 Other secondary osteonecrosis of right radius %

     M87.332 Other secondary osteonecrosis of left radius %

     ■ M87.333 Other secondary osteonecrosis of unspecified radius %

     M87.334 Other secondary osteonecrosis of right ulna %

     M87.335 Other secondary osteonecrosis of left ulna %

     ■ M87.336 Other secondary osteonecrosis of unspecified ulna %

     M87.337 Other secondary osteonecrosis of right carpus %

     M87.338 Other secondary osteonecrosis of left carpus %

     ■ M87.339 Other secondary osteonecrosis of unspecified carpus %

   ● M87.34 Other secondary osteonecrosis, hand and fingers

     M87.341 Other secondary osteonecrosis, right hand %

     M87.342 Other secondary osteonecrosis, left hand %

     ■ M87.343 Other secondary osteonecrosis, unspecified hand %

     M87.344 Other secondary osteonecrosis, right finger(s) %

     M87.345 Other secondary osteonecrosis, left finger(s) %

     ■ M87.346 Other secondary osteonecrosis, unspecified finger(s) %

   ● M87.35 Other secondary osteonecrosis, pelvis and femur

     M87.350 Other secondary osteonecrosis, pelvis %

     M87.351 Other secondary osteonecrosis, right femur %

     M87.352 Other secondary osteonecrosis, left femur %

     ■ M87.353 Other secondary osteonecrosis, unspecified femur %

CHAPTER 13 (M00-M99)

N Newborn Age: 0   **P** Pediatric Age: 0–17   **M** Maternity DX: 12–55   **A** Adult Age: 15–124   ♀ Females Only   ♂ Males Only

% Complication\Comorbidity   % Major C\C   Present on Admission Requirement   % Hospital-Acquired Condition

1243

CHAPTER 13 (M00-M99)

● M87.36 Other secondary osteonecrosis, tibia and fibula

    M87.361 Other secondary osteonecrosis, right tibia 🦴

    M87.362 Other secondary osteonecrosis, left tibia 🦴

    M87.363 Other secondary osteonecrosis, unspecified tibia 🦴

    M87.364 Other secondary osteonecrosis, right fibula 🦴

    M87.365 Other secondary osteonecrosis, left fibula 🦴

    M87.366 Other secondary osteonecrosis, unspecified fibula 🦴

● M87.37 Other secondary osteonecrosis, ankle and foot

    M87.371 Other secondary osteonecrosis, right ankle 🦴

    M87.372 Other secondary osteonecrosis, left ankle 🦴

    M87.373 Other secondary osteonecrosis, unspecified ankle 🦴

    M87.374 Other secondary osteonecrosis, right foot 🦴

    M87.375 Other secondary osteonecrosis, left foot 🦴

    M87.376 Other secondary osteonecrosis, unspecified foot 🦴

    M87.377 Other secondary osteonecrosis, right toe(s) 🦴

    M87.378 Other secondary osteonecrosis, left toe(s) 🦴

    M87.379 Other secondary osteonecrosis, unspecified toe(s) 🦴

    M87.38 Other secondary osteonecrosis, other site 🦴

    M87.39 Other secondary osteonecrosis, multiple sites 🦴

● M87.8 Other osteonecrosis

    M87.80 Other osteonecrosis, unspecified bone 🦴

●   M87.81 Other osteonecrosis, shoulder

    M87.811 Other osteonecrosis, right shoulder 🦴

    M87.812 Other osteonecrosis, left shoulder 🦴

    M87.819 Other osteonecrosis, unspecified shoulder 🦴

●   M87.82 Other osteonecrosis, humerus

    M87.821 Other osteonecrosis, right humerus 🦴

    M87.822 Other osteonecrosis, left humerus 🦴

    M87.829 Other osteonecrosis, unspecified humerus 🦴

●   M87.83 Other osteonecrosis of radius, ulna and carpus

    M87.831 Other osteonecrosis of right radius 🦴

    M87.832 Other osteonecrosis of left radius 🦴

    M87.833 Other osteonecrosis of unspecified radius 🦴

    M87.834 Other osteonecrosis of right ulna 🦴

    M87.835 Other osteonecrosis of left ulna 🦴

    M87.836 Other osteonecrosis of unspecified ulna 🦴

    M87.837 Other osteonecrosis of right carpus 🦴

    M87.838 Other osteonecrosis of left carpus 🦴

    M87.839 Other osteonecrosis of unspecified carpus 🦴

● M87.84 Other osteonecrosis, hand and fingers

    M87.841 Other osteonecrosis, right hand 🦴

    M87.842 Other osteonecrosis, left hand 🦴

    M87.843 Other osteonecrosis, unspecified hand 🦴

    M87.844 Other osteonecrosis, right finger(s) 🦴

    M87.845 Other osteonecrosis, left finger(s) 🦴

    M87.849 Other osteonecrosis, unspecified finger(s) 🦴

● M87.85 Other osteonecrosis, pelvis and femur

    M87.850 Other osteonecrosis, pelvis 🦴

    M87.851 Other osteonecrosis, right femur 🦴

    M87.852 Other osteonecrosis, left femur 🦴

    M87.859 Other osteonecrosis, unspecified femur 🦴

● M87.86 Other osteonecrosis, tibia and fibula

    M87.861 Other osteonecrosis, right tibia 🦴

    M87.862 Other osteonecrosis, left tibia 🦴

    M87.863 Other osteonecrosis, unspecified tibia 🦴

    M87.864 Other osteonecrosis, right fibula 🦴

    M87.865 Other osteonecrosis, left fibula 🦴

    M87.869 Other osteonecrosis, unspecified fibula 🦴

● M87.87 Other osteonecrosis, ankle, foot and toes

    M87.871 Other osteonecrosis, right ankle 🦴

    M87.872 Other osteonecrosis, left ankle 🦴

    M87.873 Other osteonecrosis, unspecified ankle 🦴

    M87.874 Other osteonecrosis, right foot 🦴

    M87.875 Other osteonecrosis, left foot 🦴

    M87.876 Other osteonecrosis, unspecified foot 🦴

    M87.877 Other osteonecrosis, right toe(s) 🦴

    M87.878 Other osteonecrosis, left toe(s) 🦴

    M87.879 Other osteonecrosis, unspecified toe(s) 🦴

    M87.88 Other osteonecrosis, other site 🦴

    M87.89 Other osteonecrosis, multiple sites 🦴

M87.9 Osteonecrosis, unspecified 🦴
    Necrosis of bone NOS

● Unacceptable Principal Diagnosis   ● Use Additional Character(s)   ■ Unspecified   ▶ Manifestation Code

OGCR Official Guidelines for Coding and Reporting   Excludes 1   Excludes 2   Includes   Use additional   Code first   Code also

● **M88 Osteitis deformans [Paget's disease of bone]**
Chronic disorder that results in enlarged and deformed bones. The excessive breakdown and formation of bone tissue causes bones to weaken and results in bone pain, arthritis, deformities, and fractures.

Excludes1   osteitis deformans in neoplastic disease (M90.6)

M88.0 Osteitis deformans of skull

M88.1 Osteitis deformans of vertebrae

● **M88.8 Osteitis deformans of other bones**

● **M88.81 Osteitis deformans of shoulder**

M88.811 Osteitis deformans of right shoulder

M88.812 Osteitis deformans of left shoulder

M88.819 Osteitis deformans of unspecified shoulder

● **M88.82 Osteitis deformans of upper arm**

M88.821 Osteitis deformans of right upper arm

M88.822 Osteitis deformans of left upper arm

M88.829 Osteitis deformans of unspecified upper arm

● **M88.83 Osteitis deformans of forearm**

M88.831 Osteitis deformans of right forearm

M88.832 Osteitis deformans of left forearm

M88.839 Osteitis deformans of unspecified forearm

● **M88.84 Osteitis deformans of hand**

M88.841 Osteitis deformans of right hand

M88.842 Osteitis deformans of left hand

M88.849 Osteitis deformans of unspecified hand

● **M88.85 Osteitis deformans of thigh**

M88.851 Osteitis deformans of right thigh

M88.852 Osteitis deformans of left thigh

M88.859 Osteitis deformans of unspecified thigh

● **M88.86 Osteitis deformans of lower leg**

M88.861 Osteitis deformans of right lower leg

M88.862 Osteitis deformans of left lower leg

M88.869 Osteitis deformans of unspecified lower leg

● **M88.87 Osteitis deformans of ankle and foot**

M88.871 Osteitis deformans of right ankle and foot

M88.872 Osteitis deformans of left ankle and foot

M88.879 Osteitis deformans of unspecified ankle and foot

M88.88 Osteitis deformans of other bones

Excludes2   osteitis deformans of skull (M88.0)
osteitis deformans of vertebrae (M88.1)

M88.89 Osteitis deformans of multiple sites

M88.9 Osteitis deformans of unspecified bone

● **M89 Other disorders of bone**

● **M89.0 Algoneurodystrophy**
Shoulder-hand syndrome
Sudeck's atrophy

Excludes1   causalgia, lower limb (G57.7-)
causalgia, upper limb (G56.4-)
complex regional pain syndrome II, lower limb (G57.7-)
complex regional pain syndrome II, upper limb (G56.4-)
reflex sympathetic dystrophy (G90.5-)

M89.00 Algoneurodystrophy, unspecified site

● **M89.01 Algoneurodystrophy, shoulder**

M89.011 Algoneurodystrophy, right shoulder

M89.012 Algoneurodystrophy, left shoulder

M89.019 Algoneurodystrophy, unspecified shoulder

● **M89.02 Algoneurodystrophy, upper arm**

M89.021 Algoneurodystrophy, right upper arm

M89.022 Algoneurodystrophy, left upper arm

M89.029 Algoneurodystrophy, unspecified upper arm

● **M89.03 Algoneurodystrophy, forearm**

M89.031 Algoneurodystrophy, right forearm

M89.032 Algoneurodystrophy, left forearm

M89.039 Algoneurodystrophy, unspecified forearm

● **M89.04 Algoneurodystrophy, hand**

M89.041 Algoneurodystrophy, right hand

M89.042 Algoneurodystrophy, left hand

M89.049 Algoneurodystrophy, unspecified hand

● **M89.05 Algoneurodystrophy, thigh**

M89.051 Algoneurodystrophy, right thigh

M89.052 Algoneurodystrophy, left thigh

M89.059 Algoneurodystrophy, unspecified thigh

● **M89.06 Algoneurodystrophy, lower leg**

M89.061 Algoneurodystrophy, right lower leg

M89.062 Algoneurodystrophy, left lower leg

M89.069 Algoneurodystrophy, unspecified lower leg

● **M89.07 Algoneurodystrophy, ankle and foot**

M89.071 Algoneurodystrophy, right ankle and foot

M89.072 Algoneurodystrophy, left ankle and foot

M89.079 Algoneurodystrophy, unspecified ankle and foot

M89.08 Algoneurodystrophy, other site

M89.09 Algoneurodystrophy, multiple sites

CHAPTER 13 (M00-M99)

● M89.1 Physeal arrest
    Arrest of growth plate
    Epiphyseal arrest
    Growth plate arrest

  ● M89.12 Physeal arrest, humerus

    M89.121 Complete physeal arrest, right proximal humerus

    M89.122 Complete physeal arrest, left proximal humerus

    M89.123 Partial physeal arrest, right proximal humerus

    M89.124 Partial physeal arrest, left proximal humerus

    M89.125 Complete physeal arrest, right distal humerus

    M89.126 Complete physeal arrest, left distal humerus

    M89.127 Partial physeal arrest, right distal humerus

    M89.128 Partial physeal arrest, left distal humerus

    ■ M89.129 Physeal arrest, humerus, unspecified

  ● M89.13 Physeal arrest, forearm

    M89.131 Complete physeal arrest, right distal radius

    M89.132 Complete physeal arrest, left distal radius

    M89.133 Partial physeal arrest, right distal radius

    M89.134 Partial physeal arrest, left distal radius

    M89.138 Other physeal arrest of forearm

    ■ M89.139 Physeal arrest, forearm, unspecified

  ● M89.15 Physeal arrest, femur

    M89.151 Complete physeal arrest, right proximal femur

    M89.152 Complete physeal arrest, left proximal femur

    M89.153 Partial physeal arrest, right proximal femur

    M89.154 Partial physeal arrest, left proximal femur

    M89.155 Complete physeal arrest, right distal femur

    M89.156 Complete physeal arrest, left distal femur

    M89.157 Partial physeal arrest, right distal femur

    M89.158 Partial physeal arrest, left distal femur

    ■ M89.159 Physeal arrest, femur, unspecified

● M89.16 Physeal arrest, lower leg

    M89.160 Complete physeal arrest, right proximal tibia

    M89.161 Complete physeal arrest, left proximal tibia

    M89.162 Partial physeal arrest, right proximal tibia

    M89.163 Partial physeal arrest, left proximal tibia

    M89.164 Complete physeal arrest, right distal tibia

    M89.165 Complete physeal arrest, left distal tibia

    M89.166 Partial physeal arrest, right distal tibia

    M89.167 Partial physeal arrest, left distal tibia

    M89.168 Other physeal arrest of lower leg

    ■ M89.169 Physeal arrest, lower leg, unspecified

  M89.18 Physeal arrest, other site

● M89.2 Other disorders of bone development and growth

  ■ M89.20 Other disorders of bone development and growth, unspecified site

  ● M89.21 Other disorders of bone development and growth, shoulder

    M89.211 Other disorders of bone development and growth, right shoulder

    M89.212 Other disorders of bone development and growth, left shoulder

    ■ M89.219 Other disorders of bone development and growth, unspecified shoulder

  ● M89.22 Other disorders of bone development and growth, humerus

    M89.221 Other disorders of bone development and growth, right humerus

    M89.222 Other disorders of bone development and growth, left humerus

    ■ M89.229 Other disorders of bone development and growth, unspecified humerus

  ● M89.23 Other disorders of bone development and growth, ulna and radius

    M89.231 Other disorders of bone development and growth, right ulna

    M89.232 Other disorders of bone development and growth, left ulna

    M89.233 Other disorders of bone development and growth, right radius

CHAPTER 13 (M00-M99)

● Unacceptable Principal Diagnosis   ● Use Additional Character(s)   ■ Unspecified   ▶ Manifestation Code
OGCR Official Guidelines for Coding and Reporting   Excludes 1   Excludes 2   Includes   Use additional   Code first   Code also

M89.234 Other disorders of bone development and growth, left radius

■ M89.239 Other disorders of bone development and growth, unspecified ulna and radius

● M89.24 Other disorders of bone development and growth, hand

M89.241 Other disorders of bone development and growth, right hand

M89.242 Other disorders of bone development and growth, left hand

■ M89.249 Other disorders of bone development and growth, unspecified hand

● M89.25 Other disorders of bone development and growth, femur

M89.251 Other disorders of bone development and growth, right femur

M89.252 Other disorders of bone development and growth, left femur

■ M89.259 Other disorders of bone development and growth, unspecified femur

● M89.26 Other disorders of bone development and growth, tibia and fibula

M89.261 Other disorders of bone development and growth, right tibia

M89.262 Other disorders of bone development and growth, left tibia

M89.263 Other disorders of bone development and growth, right fibula

M89.264 Other disorders of bone development and growth, left fibula

■ M89.269 Other disorders of bone development and growth, unspecified lower leg

● M89.27 Other disorders of bone development and growth, ankle and foot

M89.271 Other disorders of bone development and growth, right ankle and foot

M89.272 Other disorders of bone development and growth, left ankle and foot

■ M89.279 Other disorders of bone development and growth, unspecified ankle and foot

M89.28 Other disorders of bone development and growth, other site

M89.29 Other disorders of bone development and growth, multiple sites

● M89.3 Hypertrophy of bone

■ M89.30 Hypertrophy of bone, unspecified site

● M89.31 Hypertrophy of bone, shoulder

M89.311 Hypertrophy of bone, right shoulder

M89.312 Hypertrophy of bone, left shoulder

■ M89.319 Hypertrophy of bone, unspecified shoulder

● M89.32 Hypertrophy of bone, humerus

M89.321 Hypertrophy of bone, right humerus

M89.322 Hypertrophy of bone, left humerus

■ M89.329 Hypertrophy of bone, unspecified humerus

● M89.33 Hypertrophy of bone, ulna and radius

M89.331 Hypertrophy of bone, right ulna

M89.332 Hypertrophy of bone, left ulna

M89.333 Hypertrophy of bone, right radius

M89.334 Hypertrophy of bone, left radius

■ M89.339 Hypertrophy of bone, unspecified ulna and radius

● M89.34 Hypertrophy of bone, hand

M89.341 Hypertrophy of bone, right hand

M89.342 Hypertrophy of bone, left hand

■ M89.349 Hypertrophy of bone, unspecified hand

● M89.35 Hypertrophy of bone, femur

M89.351 Hypertrophy of bone, right femur

M89.352 Hypertrophy of bone, left femur

■ M89.359 Hypertrophy of bone, unspecified femur

● M89.36 Hypertrophy of bone, tibia and fibula

M89.361 Hypertrophy of bone, right tibia

M89.362 Hypertrophy of bone, left tibia

M89.363 Hypertrophy of bone, right fibula

M89.364 Hypertrophy of bone, left fibula

■ M89.369 Hypertrophy of bone, unspecified tibia and fibula

● M89.37 Hypertrophy of bone, ankle and foot

M89.371 Hypertrophy of bone, right ankle and foot

M89.372 Hypertrophy of bone, left ankle and foot

■ M89.379 Hypertrophy of bone, unspecified ankle and foot

M89.38 Hypertrophy of bone, other site

M89.39 Hypertrophy of bone, multiple sites

● M89.4 Other hypertrophic osteoarthropathy
Marie-Bamberger disease
Pachydermoperiostosis

■ M89.40 Other hypertrophic osteoarthropathy, unspecified site

● M89.41 Other hypertrophic osteoarthropathy, shoulder

M89.411 Other hypertrophic osteoarthropathy, right shoulder

M89.412 Other hypertrophic osteoarthropathy, left shoulder

N Newborn Age: 0   **P** Pediatric Age: 0–17   **M** Maternity DX: 12–55   **A** Adult Age: 15–124   ♀ Females Only   ♂ Males Only
Complication\Comorbidity   Major C\C   Present on Admission Requirement   Hospital-Acquired Condition

1247

M89.419 Other hypertrophic osteoarthropathy, unspecified shoulder

M89.42 Other hypertrophic osteoarthropathy, upper arm

M89.421 Other hypertrophic osteoarthropathy, right upper arm

M89.422 Other hypertrophic osteoarthropathy, left upper arm

M89.429 Other hypertrophic osteoarthropathy, unspecified upper arm

M89.43 Other hypertrophic osteoarthropathy, forearm

M89.431 Other hypertrophic osteoarthropathy, right forearm

M89.432 Other hypertrophic osteoarthropathy, left forearm

M89.439 Other hypertrophic osteoarthropathy, unspecified forearm

M89.44 Other hypertrophic osteoarthropathy, hand

M89.441 Other hypertrophic osteoarthropathy, right hand

M89.442 Other hypertrophic osteoarthropathy, left hand

M89.449 Other hypertrophic osteoarthropathy, unspecified hand

M89.45 Other hypertrophic osteoarthropathy, thigh

M89.451 Other hypertrophic osteoarthropathy, right thigh

M89.452 Other hypertrophic osteoarthropathy, left thigh

M89.459 Other hypertrophic osteoarthropathy, unspecified thigh

M89.46 Other hypertrophic osteoarthropathy, lower leg

M89.461 Other hypertrophic osteoarthropathy, right lower leg

M89.462 Other hypertrophic osteoarthropathy, left lower leg

M89.469 Other hypertrophic osteoarthropathy, unspecified lower leg

M89.47 Other hypertrophic osteoarthropathy, ankle and foot

M89.471 Other hypertrophic osteoarthropathy, right ankle and foot

M89.472 Other hypertrophic osteoarthropathy, left ankle and foot

M89.479 Other hypertrophic osteoarthropathy, unspecified ankle and foot

M89.48 Other hypertrophic osteoarthropathy, other site

M89.49 Other hypertrophic osteoarthropathy, multiple sites

M89.5 Osteolysis

Use additional code to identify major osseous defect, if applicable (M89.7-)

Excludes2 periprosthetic osteolysis of internal prosthetic joint (T84.05-)

M89.50 Osteolysis, unspecified site

M89.51 Osteolysis, shoulder

M89.511 Osteolysis, right shoulder

M89.512 Osteolysis, left shoulder

M89.519 Osteolysis, unspecified shoulder

M89.52 Osteolysis, upper arm

M89.521 Osteolysis, right upper arm

M89.522 Osteolysis, left upper arm

M89.529 Osteolysis, unspecified upper arm

M89.53 Osteolysis, forearm

M89.531 Osteolysis, right forearm

M89.532 Osteolysis, left forearm

M89.539 Osteolysis, unspecified forearm

M89.54 Osteolysis, hand

M89.541 Osteolysis, right hand

M89.542 Osteolysis, left hand

M89.549 Osteolysis, unspecified hand

M89.55 Osteolysis, thigh

M89.551 Osteolysis, right thigh

M89.552 Osteolysis, left thigh

M89.559 Osteolysis, unspecified thigh

M89.56 Osteolysis, lower leg

M89.561 Osteolysis, right lower leg

M89.562 Osteolysis, left lower leg

M89.569 Osteolysis, unspecified lower leg

M89.57 Osteolysis, ankle and foot

M89.571 Osteolysis, right ankle and foot

M89.572 Osteolysis, left ankle and foot

M89.579 Osteolysis, unspecified ankle and foot

M89.58 Osteolysis, other site

M89.59 Osteolysis, multiple sites

M89.6 Osteopathy after poliomyelitis

Use additional code (B91) to identify previous poliomyelitis

Excludes1 postpolio syndrome (G14)

M89.60 Osteopathy after poliomyelitis, unspecified site

M89.61 Osteopathy after poliomyelitis, shoulder

M89.611 Osteopathy after poliomyelitis, right shoulder

M89.612 Osteopathy after poliomyelitis, left shoulder

M89.619 Osteopathy after poliomyelitis, unspecified shoulder

M89.62 Osteopathy after poliomyelitis, upper arm

M89.621 Osteopathy after poliomyelitis, right upper arm

M89.622 Osteopathy after poliomyelitis, left upper arm

M89.629 Osteopathy after poliomyelitis, unspecified upper arm

● M89.63   Osteopathy after poliomyelitis, forearm

     M89.631   Osteopathy after poliomyelitis, right forearm

     M89.632   Osteopathy after poliomyelitis, left forearm

     ▪ M89.639   Osteopathy after poliomyelitis, unspecified forearm

● M89.64   Osteopathy after poliomyelitis, hand

     M89.641   Osteopathy after poliomyelitis, right hand

     M89.642   Osteopathy after poliomyelitis, left hand

     ▪ M89.649   Osteopathy after poliomyelitis, unspecified hand

● M89.65   Osteopathy after poliomyelitis, thigh

     M89.651   Osteopathy after poliomyelitis, right thigh

     M89.652   Osteopathy after poliomyelitis, left thigh

     ▪ M89.659   Osteopathy after poliomyelitis, unspecified thigh

● M89.66   Osteopathy after poliomyelitis, lower leg

     M89.661   Osteopathy after poliomyelitis, right lower leg

     M89.662   Osteopathy after poliomyelitis, left lower leg

     ▪ M89.669   Osteopathy after poliomyelitis, unspecified lower leg

● M89.67   Osteopathy after poliomyelitis, ankle and foot

     M89.671   Osteopathy after poliomyelitis, right ankle and foot

     M89.672   Osteopathy after poliomyelitis, left ankle and foot

     ▪ M89.679   Osteopathy after poliomyelitis, unspecified ankle and foot

     M89.68   Osteopathy after poliomyelitis, other site

     M89.69   Osteopathy after poliomyelitis, multiple sites

● M89.7   **Major osseous defect**

     Code first underlying disease, if known, such as:
     aseptic necrosis of bone (M87.-)
     malignant neoplasm of bone (C40.-)
     osteolysis (M89.5)
     osteomyelitis (M86.-)
     osteonecrosis (M87.-)
     osteoporosis (M80.-, M81.-)
     periprosthetic osteolysis (T84.05-)

     ▪ M89.70   Major osseous defect, unspecified site

● M89.71   Major osseous defect, shoulder region
     Major osseous defect clavicle or scapula

     M89.711   Major osseous defect, right shoulder region

     M89.712   Major osseous defect, left shoulder region

     ▪ M89.719   Major osseous defect, unspecified shoulder region

● M89.72   Major osseous defect, humerus

     M89.721   Major osseous defect, right humerus

     M89.722   Major osseous defect, left humerus

     ▪ M89.729   Major osseous defect, unspecified humerus

● M89.73   Major osseous defect, forearm
     Major osseous defect of radius and ulna

     M89.731   Major osseous defect, right forearm

     M89.732   Major osseous defect, left forearm

     ▪ M89.739   Major osseous defect, unspecified forearm

● M89.74   Major osseous defect, hand
     Major osseous defect of carpus, fingers, metacarpus

     M89.741   Major osseous defect, right hand

     M89.742   Major osseous defect, left hand

     ▪ M89.749   Major osseous defect, unspecified hand

● M89.75   Major osseous defect, pelvic region and thigh
     Major osseous defect of femur and pelvis

     M89.751   Major osseous defect, right pelvic region and thigh

     M89.752   Major osseous defect, left pelvic region and thigh

     ▪ M89.759   Major osseous defect, unspecified pelvic region and thigh

● M89.76   Major osseous defect, lower leg
     Major osseous defect of fibula and tibia

     M89.761   Major osseous defect, right lower leg

     M89.762   Major osseous defect, left lower leg

     ▪ M89.769   Major osseous defect, unspecified lower leg

● M89.77   Major osseous defect, ankle and foot
     Major osseous defect of metatarsus, tarsus, toes

     M89.771   Major osseous defect, right ankle and foot

     M89.772   Major osseous defect, left ankle and foot

     ▪ M89.779   Major osseous defect, unspecified ankle and foot

     M89.78   Major osseous defect, other site

     M89.79   Major osseous defect, multiple sites

● M89.8   **Other specified disorders of bone**
     Infantile cortical hyperostoses
     Post-traumatic subperiosteal ossification

● M89.8X   Other specified disorders of bone

     M89.8X0   Other specified disorders of bone, multiple sites

     M89.8X1   Other specified disorders of bone, shoulder

     M89.8X2   Other specified disorders of bone, upper arm

     M89.8X3   Other specified disorders of bone, forearm

     M89.8X4   Other specified disorders of bone, hand

     M89.8X5   Other specified disorders of bone, thigh

     M89.8X6   Other specified disorders of bone, lower leg

     M89.8X7   Other specified disorders of bone, ankle and foot

CHAPTER 13 (M00-M99)

CHAPTER 13 (M00-M99)

M89.8X8 Other specified disorders of
    bone, other site

■ M89.8X9 Other specified disorders of
    bone, unspecified site

■ **M89.9 Disorder of bone, unspecified**

● **M90 Osteopathies in diseases classified elsewhere**

> **Excludes1** osteochondritis, osteomyelitis, and
>   osteopathy (in):
>   cryptococcosis (B45.3)
>   diabetes mellitus (E08-E13 with 4th
>   character .61-)
>   gonococcal (A54.43)
>   neurogenic syphilis (A52.11)
>   renal osteodystrophy (N25.0)
>   salmonellosis (A02.24)
>   secondary syphilis (A51.46)
>   syphilis (late) (A52.77)

● **M90.5 Osteonecrosis in diseases classified elsewhere**

> *Code first* underlying disease, such as:
>   caisson disease (T70.3)
>   hemoglobinopathy (D50-D64)

●■▶ *M90.50 Osteonecrosis in diseases classified*
    elsewhere, unspecified site ℞
      MCC: Only when the principal diagnosis
      is designated as a CC

● **M90.51 Osteonecrosis in diseases classified**
    elsewhere, shoulder

●▶ *M90.511 Osteonecrosis in diseases*
    classified elsewhere, right
    shoulder ℞
      MCC: Only when the principal
      diagnosis is designated as
      a CC

●▶ *M90.512 Osteonecrosis in diseases*
    classified elsewhere, left
    shoulder ℞
      MCC: Only when the principal
      diagnosis is designated as
      a CC

●■▶ *M90.519 Osteonecrosis in diseases*
    classified elsewhere, unspecified
    shoulder ℞
      MCC: Only when the principal
      diagnosis is designated as
      a CC

● **M90.52 Osteonecrosis in diseases classified**
    elsewhere, upper arm

●▶ *M90.521 Osteonecrosis in diseases*
    classified elsewhere, right upper
    arm ℞
      MCC: Only when the principal
      diagnosis is designated as
      a CC

●▶ *M90.522 Osteonecrosis in diseases*
    classified elsewhere, left upper
    arm ℞
      MCC: Only when the principal
      diagnosis is designated as
      a CC

●■▶ *M90.529 Osteonecrosis in diseases*
    classified elsewhere, unspecified
    upper arm ℞
      MCC: Only when the principal
      diagnosis is designated as
      a CC

● **M90.53 Osteonecrosis in diseases classified**
    elsewhere, forearm

●▶ *M90.531 Osteonecrosis in diseases*
    classified elsewhere, right
    forearm ℞
      MCC: Only when the principal
      diagnosis is designated as
      a CC

●▶ *M90.532 Osteonecrosis in diseases*
    classified elsewhere, left
    forearm ℞
      MCC: Only when the principal
      diagnosis is designated as
      a CC

●■▶ *M90.539 Osteonecrosis in diseases*
    classified elsewhere, unspecified
    forearm ℞
      MCC: Only when the principal
      diagnosis is designated as
      a CC

● **M90.54 Osteonecrosis in diseases classified**
    elsewhere, hand

●▶ *M90.541 Osteonecrosis in diseases*
    classified elsewhere, right hand ℞
      MCC: Only when the principal
      diagnosis is designated as
      a CC

●▶ *M90.542 Osteonecrosis in diseases*
    classified elsewhere, left hand ℞
      MCC: Only when the principal
      diagnosis is designated as
      a CC

●■▶ *M90.549 Osteonecrosis in diseases*
    classified elsewhere, unspecified
    hand ℞
      MCC: Only when the principal
      diagnosis is designated as
      a CC

● **M90.55 Osteonecrosis in diseases classified**
    elsewhere, thigh

●▶ *M90.551 Osteonecrosis in diseases*
    classified elsewhere, right thigh ℞
      MCC: Only when the principal
      diagnosis is designated as
      a CC

●▶ *M90.552 Osteonecrosis in diseases*
    classified elsewhere, left thigh ℞
      MCC: Only when the principal
      diagnosis is designated as
      a CC

●■▶ *M90.559 Osteonecrosis in diseases*
    classified elsewhere, unspecified
    thigh ℞
      MCC: Only when the principal
      diagnosis is designated as
      a CC

● **M90.56 Osteonecrosis in diseases classified**
    elsewhere, lower leg

●▶ *M90.561 Osteonecrosis in diseases*
    classified elsewhere, right lower
    leg ℞
      MCC: Only when the principal
      diagnosis is designated as
      a CC

●▶ *M90.562 Osteonecrosis in diseases*
    classified elsewhere, left lower
    leg ℞
      MCC: Only when the principal
      diagnosis is designated as
      a CC

● Unacceptable Principal Diagnosis   ● Use Additional Character(s)   ■ Unspecified   ▶ Manifestation Code

OGCR Official Guidelines for Coding and Reporting   Excludes 1   Excludes 2   Includes   Use additional   Code first   Code also

● ■) *M90.569 Osteonecrosis in diseases classified elsewhere, unspecified lower leg* 🝖
     MCC: Only when the principal diagnosis is designated as a CC

● **M90.57 Osteonecrosis in diseases classified elsewhere, ankle and foot**

  ●) *M90.571 Osteonecrosis in diseases classified elsewhere, right ankle and foot* 🝖
       MCC: Only when the principal diagnosis is designated as a CC

  ●) *M90.572 Osteonecrosis in diseases classified elsewhere, left ankle and foot* 🝖
       MCC: Only when the principal diagnosis is designated as a CC

  ● ■) *M90.579 Osteonecrosis in diseases classified elsewhere, unspecified ankle and foot* 🝖
       MCC: Only when the principal diagnosis is designated as a CC

●) *M90.58 Osteonecrosis in diseases classified elsewhere, other site* 🝖
     MCC: Only when the principal diagnosis is designated as a CC

●) *M90.59 Osteonecrosis in diseases classified elsewhere, multiple sites* 🝖
     MCC: Only when the principal diagnosis is designated as a CC

● **M90.6 Osteitis deformans in neoplastic diseases**
     Osteitis deformans in malignant neoplasm of bone

     Code first the neoplasm (C40.-, C41.-)

     Excludes1   osteitis deformans [Paget's disease of bone] (M88.-)

● ■) *M90.60 Osteitis deformans in neoplastic diseases, unspecified site*

  ● **M90.61 Osteitis deformans in neoplastic diseases, shoulder**

    ●) *M90.611 Osteitis deformans in neoplastic diseases, right shoulder*

    ●) *M90.612 Osteitis deformans in neoplastic diseases, left shoulder*

    ■) *M90.619 Osteitis deformans in neoplastic diseases, unspecified shoulder*

  ● **M90.62 Osteitis deformans in neoplastic diseases, upper arm**

    ●) *M90.621 Osteitis deformans in neoplastic diseases, right upper arm*

    ●) *M90.622 Osteitis deformans in neoplastic diseases, left upper arm*

    ● ■) *M90.629 Osteitis deformans in neoplastic diseases, unspecified upper arm*

  ● **M90.63 Osteitis deformans in neoplastic diseases, forearm**

    ●) *M90.631 Osteitis deformans in neoplastic diseases, right forearm*

    ●) *M90.632 Osteitis deformans in neoplastic diseases, left forearm*

    ● ■) *M90.639 Osteitis deformans in neoplastic diseases, unspecified forearm*

● **M90.64 Osteitis deformans in neoplastic diseases, hand**

  ●) *M90.641 Osteitis deformans in neoplastic diseases, right hand*

  ●) *M90.642 Osteitis deformans in neoplastic diseases, left hand*

  ● ■) *M90.649 Osteitis deformans in neoplastic diseases, unspecified hand*

● **M90.65 Osteitis deformans in neoplastic diseases, thigh**

  ●) *M90.651 Osteitis deformans in neoplastic diseases, right thigh*

  ●) *M90.652 Osteitis deformans in neoplastic diseases, left thigh*

  ● ■) *M90.659 Osteitis deformans in neoplastic diseases, unspecified thigh*

● **M90.66 Osteitis deformans in neoplastic diseases, lower leg**

  ●) *M90.661 Osteitis deformans in neoplastic diseases, right lower leg*

  ●) *M90.662 Osteitis deformans in neoplastic diseases, left lower leg*

  ● ■) *M90.669 Osteitis deformans in neoplastic diseases, unspecified lower leg*

● **M90.67 Osteitis deformans in neoplastic diseases, ankle and foot**

  ●) *M90.671 Osteitis deformans in neoplastic diseases, right ankle and foot*

  ●) *M90.672 Osteitis deformans in neoplastic diseases, left ankle and foot*

  ● ■) *M90.679 Osteitis deformans in neoplastic diseases, unspecified ankle and foot*

●) *M90.68 Osteitis deformans in neoplastic diseases, other site*

●) *M90.69 Osteitis deformans in neoplastic diseases, multiple sites*

● **M90.8 Osteopathy in diseases classified elsewhere**

     Code first underlying disease, such as:
     rickets (E55.0)
     vitamin-D-resistant rickets (E83.3)

● ■) *M90.80 Osteopathy in diseases classified elsewhere, unspecified site*

  ● **M90.81 Osteopathy in diseases classified elsewhere, shoulder**

    ●) *M90.811 Osteopathy in diseases classified elsewhere, right shoulder*

    ●) *M90.812 Osteopathy in diseases classified elsewhere, left shoulder*

    ● ■) *M90.819 Osteopathy in diseases classified elsewhere, unspecified shoulder*

  ● **M90.82 Osteopathy in diseases classified elsewhere, upper arm**

    ●) *M90.821 Osteopathy in diseases classified elsewhere, right upper arm*

    ●) *M90.822 Osteopathy in diseases classified elsewhere, left upper arm*

    ● ■) *M90.829 Osteopathy in diseases classified elsewhere, unspecified upper arm*

CHAPTER 13 (M00-M99)

CHAPTER 13 (M00-M99)

● M90.83 Osteopathy in diseases classified elsewhere, forearm

  ● ▶ *M90.831 Osteopathy in diseases classified elsewhere, right forearm*

  ● ▶ *M90.832 Osteopathy in diseases classified elsewhere, left forearm*

  ● ■▶ *M90.839 Osteopathy in diseases classified elsewhere, unspecified forearm*

● M90.84 Osteopathy in diseases classified elsewhere, hand

  ● ▶ *M90.841 Osteopathy in diseases classified elsewhere, right hand*

  ● ▶ *M90.842 Osteopathy in diseases classified elsewhere, left hand*

  ● ■▶ *M90.849 Osteopathy in diseases classified elsewhere, unspecified hand*

● M90.85 Osteopathy in diseases classified elsewhere, thigh

  ● ▶ *M90.851 Osteopathy in diseases classified elsewhere, right thigh*

  ● ▶ *M90.852 Osteopathy in diseases classified elsewhere, left thigh*

  ● ■▶ *M90.859 Osteopathy in diseases classified elsewhere, unspecified thigh*

● M90.86 Osteopathy in diseases classified elsewhere, lower leg

  ● ▶ *M90.861 Osteopathy in diseases classified elsewhere, right lower leg*

  ● ▶ *M90.862 Osteopathy in diseases classified elsewhere, left lower leg*

  ● ■▶ *M90.869 Osteopathy in diseases classified elsewhere, unspecified lower leg*

● M90.87 Osteopathy in diseases classified elsewhere, ankle and foot

  ● ▶ *M90.871 Osteopathy in diseases classified elsewhere, right ankle and foot*

  ● ▶ *M90.872 Osteopathy in diseases classified elsewhere, left ankle and foot*

  ● ■▶ *M90.879 Osteopathy in diseases classified elsewhere, unspecified ankle and foot*

● ▶ *M90.88 Osteopathy in diseases classified elsewhere, other site*

● ▶ *M90.89 Osteopathy in diseases classified elsewhere, multiple sites*

CHONDROPATHIES (M91-M94)

Excludes1   postprocedural chondropathies (M96.-)

● M91 Juvenile osteochondrosis of hip and pelvis

Excludes1   slipped upper femoral epiphysis (nontraumatic) (M93.0)

M91.0 Juvenile osteochondrosis of pelvis
  Osteochondrosis (juvenile) of:
   acetabulum
   iliac crest [Buchanan]
   ischiopubic synchondrosis [van Neck]
   symphysis pubis [Pierson]

● M91.1 Juvenile osteochondrosis of head of femur [Legg-Calvé-Perthes]

  ■ M91.10 Juvenile osteochondrosis of head of femur [Legg-Calvé-Perthes], unspecified leg

  M91.11 Juvenile osteochondrosis of head of femur [Legg-Calvé-Perthes], right leg

  M91.12 Juvenile osteochondrosis of head of femur [Legg-Calvé-Perthes], left leg

● M91.2 Coxa plana
  Hip deformity due to previous juvenile osteochondrosis

  ■ M91.20 Coxa plana, unspecified hip
  M91.21 Coxa plana, right hip
  M91.22 Coxa plana, left hip

● M91.3 Pseudocoxalgia
  ■ M91.30 Pseudocoxalgia, unspecified hip
  M91.31 Pseudocoxalgia, right hip
  M91.32 Pseudocoxalgia, left hip

● M91.4 Coxa magna
  ■ M91.40 Coxa magna, unspecified hip
  M91.41 Coxa magna, right hip
  M91.42 Coxa magna, left hip

● M91.8 Other juvenile osteochondrosis of hip and pelvis
  Juvenile osteochondrosis after reduction of congenital dislocation of hip

  ■ M91.80 Other juvenile osteochondrosis of hip and pelvis, unspecified leg

  M91.81 Other juvenile osteochondrosis of hip and pelvis, right leg

  M91.82 Other juvenile osteochondrosis of hip and pelvis, left leg

● M91.9 Juvenile osteochondrosis of hip and pelvis, unspecified

  ■ M91.90 Juvenile osteochondrosis of hip and pelvis, unspecified, unspecified leg

  ■ M91.91 Juvenile osteochondrosis of hip and pelvis, unspecified, right leg

  ■ M91.92 Juvenile osteochondrosis of hip and pelvis, unspecified, left leg

● M92 Other juvenile osteochondrosis

● M92.0 Juvenile osteochondrosis of humerus
  Osteochondrosis (juvenile) of capitulum of humerus [Panner]
  Osteochondrosis (juvenile) of head of humerus [Haas]

  ■ M92.00 Juvenile osteochondrosis of humerus, unspecified arm

  M92.01 Juvenile osteochondrosis of humerus, right arm

  M92.02 Juvenile osteochondrosis of humerus, left arm

● M92.1 Juvenile osteochondrosis of radius and ulna
  Osteochondrosis (juvenile) of lower ulna [Burns]
  Osteochondrosis (juvenile) of radial head [Brailsford]

  ■ M92.10 Juvenile osteochondrosis of radius and ulna, unspecified arm

  M92.11 Juvenile osteochondrosis of radius and ulna, right arm

  M92.12 Juvenile osteochondrosis of radius and ulna, left arm

● Unacceptable Principal Diagnosis   ● Use Additional Character(s)   ■ Unspecified   ▶ Manifestation Code
OGCR Official Guidelines for Coding and Reporting   Excludes 1   Excludes 2   Includes   Use additional   Code first   Code also

● **M92.2 Juvenile osteochondrosis, hand**

  ● **M92.20 Unspecified juvenile osteochondrosis, hand**

    ■ **M92.201 Unspecified juvenile osteochondrosis, right hand**

    ■ **M92.202 Unspecified juvenile osteochondrosis, left hand**

    ■ **M92.209 Unspecified juvenile osteochondrosis, unspecified hand**

  ● **M92.21 Osteochondrosis (juvenile) of carpal lunate [Kienböck]**

    M92.211 Osteochondrosis (juvenile) of carpal lunate [Kienböck], right hand

    M92.212 Osteochondrosis (juvenile) of carpal lunate [Kienböck], left hand

    ■ **M92.219 Osteochondrosis (juvenile) of carpal lunate [Kienböck], unspecified hand**

  ● **M92.22 Osteochondrosis (juvenile) of metacarpal heads [Mauclaire]**

    M92.221 Osteochondrosis (juvenile) of metacarpal heads [Mauclaire], right hand

    M92.222 Osteochondrosis (juvenile) of metacarpal heads [Mauclaire], left hand

    ■ **M92.229 Osteochondrosis (juvenile) of metacarpal heads [Mauclaire], unspecified hand**

  ● **M92.29 Other juvenile osteochondrosis, hand**

    M92.291 Other juvenile osteochondrosis, right hand

    M92.292 Other juvenile osteochondrosis, left hand

    ■ **M92.299 Other juvenile osteochondrosis, unspecified hand**

● **M92.3 Other juvenile osteochondrosis, upper limb**

  ■ **M92.30 Other juvenile osteochondrosis, unspecified upper limb**

  M92.31 Other juvenile osteochondrosis, right upper limb

  M92.32 Other juvenile osteochondrosis, left upper limb

● **M92.4 Juvenile osteochondrosis of patella**

  Osteochondrosis (juvenile) of primary patellar center [Köhler]

  Osteochondrosis (juvenile) of secondary patellar center [Sinding Larsen]

  ■ **M92.40 Juvenile osteochondrosis of patella, unspecified knee**

  M92.41 Juvenile osteochondrosis of patella, right knee

  M92.42 Juvenile osteochondrosis of patella, left knee

● **M92.5 Juvenile osteochondrosis of tibia and fibula**

  Osteochondrosis (juvenile) of proximal tibia [Blount]

  Osteochondrosis (juvenile) of tibial tubercle [Osgood-Schlatter]

  Tibia vara

  ■ **M92.50 Juvenile osteochondrosis of tibia and fibula, unspecified leg**

  M92.51 Juvenile osteochondrosis of tibia and fibula, right leg

  M92.52 Juvenile osteochondrosis of tibia and fibula, left leg

● **M92.6 Juvenile osteochondrosis of tarsus**

  Osteochondrosis (juvenile) of calcaneum [Sever]

  Osteochondrosis (juvenile) of os tibiale externum [Haglund]

  Osteochondrosis (juvenile) of talus [Diaz]

  Osteochondrosis (juvenile) of tarsal navicular [Köhler]

  ■ **M92.60 Juvenile osteochondrosis of tarsus, unspecified ankle**

  M92.61 Juvenile osteochondrosis of tarsus, right ankle

  M92.62 Juvenile osteochondrosis of tarsus, left ankle

● **M92.7 Juvenile osteochondrosis of metatarsus**

  Osteochondrosis (juvenile) of fifth metatarsus [Iselin]

  Osteochondrosis (juvenile) of second metatarsus [Freiberg]

  ■ **M92.70 Juvenile osteochondrosis of metatarsus, unspecified foot**

  M92.71 Juvenile osteochondrosis of metatarsus, right foot

  M92.72 Juvenile osteochondrosis of metatarsus, left foot

M92.8 Other specified juvenile osteochondrosis

  Calcaneal apophysitis

■ **M92.9 Juvenile osteochondrosis, unspecified**

  Juvenile apophysitis NOS

  Juvenile epiphysitis NOS

  Juvenile osteochondritis NOS

  Juvenile osteochondrosis NOS

● **M93 Other osteochondropathies**

  Excludes2   osteochondrosis of spine (M42.-)

● **M93.0 Slipped upper femoral epiphysis (nontraumatic)**

  Use additional code for associated chondrolysis (M94.3)

  ● **M93.00 Unspecified slipped upper femoral epiphysis (nontraumatic)**

    ■ **M93.001 Unspecified slipped upper femoral epiphysis (nontraumatic), right hip**

    ■ **M93.002 Unspecified slipped upper femoral epiphysis (nontraumatic), left hip**

    ■ **M93.003 Unspecified slipped upper femoral epiphysis (nontraumatic), unspecified hip**

CHAPTER 13 (M00-M99)

N Newborn Age: 0   **P** Pediatric Age: 0–17   **M** Maternity DX: 12–55   **A** Adult Age: 15–124   ♀ Females Only   ♂ Males Only

🐾 Complication\Comorbidity   🐾 Major C\C   🐾 Present on Admission Requirement   🐾 Hospital-Acquired Condition

1253

● M93.01 Acute slipped upper femoral epiphysis (nontraumatic)

    M93.011 Acute slipped upper femoral epiphysis (nontraumatic), right hip

    M93.012 Acute slipped upper femoral epiphysis (nontraumatic), left hip

    ■ M93.013 Acute slipped upper femoral epiphysis (nontraumatic), unspecified hip

● M93.02 Chronic slipped upper femoral epiphysis (nontraumatic)

    M93.021 Chronic slipped upper femoral epiphysis (nontraumatic), right hip

    M93.022 Chronic slipped upper femoral epiphysis (nontraumatic), left hip

    ■ M93.023 Chronic slipped upper femoral epiphysis (nontraumatic), unspecified hip

● M93.03 Acute on chronic slipped upper femoral epiphysis (nontraumatic)

    M93.031 Acute on chronic slipped upper femoral epiphysis (nontraumatic), right hip

    M93.032 Acute on chronic slipped upper femoral epiphysis (nontraumatic), left hip

    ■ M93.033 Acute on chronic slipped upper femoral epiphysis (nontraumatic), unspecified hip

M93.1 Kienböck's disease of adults   **A**
    Adult osteochondrosis of carpal lunates

● M93.2 Osteochondritis dissecans

    ■ M93.20 Osteochondritis dissecans of unspecified site

    ● M93.21 Osteochondritis dissecans of shoulder

        M93.211 Osteochondritis dissecans, right shoulder

        M93.212 Osteochondritis dissecans, left shoulder

        ■ M93.219 Osteochondritis dissecans, unspecified shoulder

    ● M93.22 Osteochondritis dissecans of elbow

        M93.221 Osteochondritis dissecans, right elbow

        M93.222 Osteochondritis dissecans, left elbow

        ■ M93.229 Osteochondritis dissecans, unspecified elbow

    ● M93.23 Osteochondritis dissecans of wrist

        M93.231 Osteochondritis dissecans, right wrist

        M93.232 Osteochondritis dissecans, left wrist

        ■ M93.239 Osteochondritis dissecans, unspecified wrist

    ● M93.24 Osteochondritis dissecans of joints of hand

        M93.241 Osteochondritis dissecans, joints of right hand

        M93.242 Osteochondritis dissecans, joints of left hand

        ■ M93.249 Osteochondritis dissecans, joints of unspecified hand

● M93.25 Osteochondritis dissecans of hip

    M93.251 Osteochondritis dissecans, right hip

    M93.252 Osteochondritis dissecans, left hip

    ■ M93.259 Osteochondritis dissecans, unspecified hip

● M93.26 Osteochondritis dissecans knee

    M93.261 Osteochondritis dissecans, right knee

    M93.262 Osteochondritis dissecans, left knee

    ■ M93.269 Osteochondritis dissecans, unspecified knee

● M93.27 Osteochondritis dissecans of ankle and joints of foot

    M93.271 Osteochondritis dissecans, right ankle and joints of right foot

    M93.272 Osteochondritis dissecans, left ankle and joints of left foot

    ■ M93.279 Osteochondritis dissecans, unspecified ankle and joints of foot

    M93.28 Osteochondritis dissecans other site

    M93.29 Osteochondritis dissecans multiple sites

● M93.8 Other specified osteochondropathies

    ■ M93.80 Other specified osteochondropathies of unspecified site

    ● M93.81 Other specified osteochondropathies of shoulder

        M93.811 Other specified osteochondropathies, right shoulder

        M93.812 Other specified osteochondropathies, left shoulder

        ■ M93.819 Other specified osteochondropathies, unspecified shoulder

    ● M93.82 Other specified osteochondropathies of upper arm

        M93.821 Other specified osteochondropathies, right upper arm

        M93.822 Other specified osteochondropathies, left upper arm

        ■ M93.829 Other specified osteochondropathies, unspecified upper arm

    ● M93.83 Other specified osteochondropathies of forearm

        M93.831 Other specified osteochondropathies, right forearm

        M93.832 Other specified osteochondropathies, left forearm

        ■ M93.839 Other specified osteochondropathies, unspecified forearm

● Unacceptable Principal Diagnosis   ● Use Additional Character(s)   ■ Unspecified   ▶ Manifestation Code

OGCR Official Guidelines for Coding and Reporting   Excludes 1   Excludes 2   Includes   Use additional   Code first   Code also

● M93.84   Other specified osteochondropathies of hand

     M93.841   Other specified osteochondropathies, right hand

     M93.842   Other specified osteochondropathies, left hand

     ■ M93.849   Other specified osteochondropathies, unspecified hand

● M93.85   Other specified osteochondropathies of thigh

     M93.851   Other specified osteochondropathies, right thigh

     M93.852   Other specified osteochondropathies, left thigh

     ■ M93.859   Other specified osteochondropathies, unspecified thigh

● M93.86   Other specified osteochondropathies lower leg

     M93.861   Other specified osteochondropathies, right lower leg

     M93.862   Other specified osteochondropathies, left lower leg

     ■ M93.869   Other specified osteochondropathies, unspecified lower leg

● M93.87   Other specified osteochondropathies of ankle and foot

     M93.871   Other specified osteochondropathies, right ankle and foot

     M93.872   Other specified osteochondropathies, left ankle and foot

     ■ M93.879   Other specified osteochondropathies, unspecified ankle and foot

     M93.88   Other specified osteochondropathies other

     M93.89   Other specified osteochondropathies multiple sites

● M93.9   Osteochondropathy, unspecified

     Apophysitis NOS
     Epiphysitis NOS
     Osteochondritis NOS
     Osteochondrosis NOS

     ■ M93.90   Osteochondropathy, unspecified of unspecified site

● M93.91   Osteochondropathy, unspecified of shoulder

     ■ M93.911   Osteochondropathy, unspecified, right shoulder

     ■ M93.912   Osteochondropathy, unspecified, left shoulder

     ■ M93.919   Osteochondropathy, unspecified, unspecified shoulder

● M93.92   Osteochondropathy, unspecified of upper arm

     ■ M93.921   Osteochondropathy, unspecified, right upper arm

     ■ M93.922   Osteochondropathy, unspecified, left upper arm

     ■ M93.929   Osteochondropathy, unspecified, unspecified upper arm

● M93.93   Osteochondropathy, unspecified of forearm

     ■ M93.931   Osteochondropathy, unspecified, right forearm

     ■ M93.932   Osteochondropathy, unspecified, left forearm

     ■ M93.939   Osteochondropathy, unspecified, unspecified forearm

● M93.94   Osteochondropathy, unspecified of hand

     ■ M93.941   Osteochondropathy, unspecified, right hand

     ■ M93.942   Osteochondropathy, unspecified, left hand

     ■ M93.949   Osteochondropathy, unspecified, unspecified hand

● M93.95   Osteochondropathy, unspecified of thigh

     ■ M93.951   Osteochondropathy, unspecified, right thigh

     ■ M93.952   Osteochondropathy, unspecified, left thigh

     ■ M93.959   Osteochondropathy, unspecified, unspecified thigh

● M93.96   Osteochondropathy, unspecified lower leg

     ■ M93.961   Osteochondropathy, unspecified, right lower leg

     ■ M93.962   Osteochondropathy, unspecified, left lower leg

     ■ M93.969   Osteochondropathy, unspecified, unspecified lower leg

● M93.97   Osteochondropathy, unspecified of ankle and foot

     ■ M93.971   Osteochondropathy, unspecified, right ankle and foot

     ■ M93.972   Osteochondropathy, unspecified, left ankle and foot

     ■ M93.979   Osteochondropathy, unspecified, unspecified ankle and foot

     ■ M93.98   Osteochondropathy, unspecified other

     ■ M93.99   Osteochondropathy, unspecified multiple sites

● M94   Other disorders of cartilage

     M94.0   Chondrocostal junction syndrome [Tietze]
        Costochondritis

     M94.1   Relapsing polychondritis

● M94.2   Chondromalacia

     | Excludes1 | chondromalacia patellae (M22.4)

     ■ M94.20   Chondromalacia, unspecified site

● M94.21   Chondromalacia, shoulder

     M94.211   Chondromalacia, right shoulder

     M94.212   Chondromalacia, left shoulder

     ■ M94.219   Chondromalacia, unspecified shoulder

N Newborn Age: 0   **P** Pediatric Age: 0–17   **M** Maternity DX: 12–55   **A** Adult Age: 15–124   ♀ Females Only   ♂ Males Only

   Complication\Comorbidity   Major C\C   Present on Admission Requirement   Hospital-Acquired Condition

1255

CHAPTER 13 (M00-M99)

● M94.22 Chondromalacia, elbow

  M94.221 Chondromalacia, right elbow

  M94.222 Chondromalacia, left elbow

  ■ M94.229 Chondromalacia, unspecified elbow

● M94.23 Chondromalacia, wrist

  M94.231 Chondromalacia, right wrist

  M94.232 Chondromalacia, left wrist

  ■ M94.239 Chondromalacia, unspecified wrist

● M94.24 Chondromalacia, joints of hand

  M94.241 Chondromalacia, joints of right hand

  M94.242 Chondromalacia, joints of left hand

  ■ M94.249 Chondromalacia, joints of unspecified hand

● M94.25 Chondromalacia, hip

  M94.251 Chondromalacia, right hip

  M94.252 Chondromalacia, left hip

  ■ M94.259 Chondromalacia, unspecified hip

● M94.26 Chondromalacia, knee

  M94.261 Chondromalacia, right knee

  M94.262 Chondromalacia, left knee

  ■ M94.269 Chondromalacia, unspecified knee

● M94.27 Chondromalacia, ankle and joints of foot

  M94.271 Chondromalacia, right ankle and joints of right foot

  M94.272 Chondromalacia, left ankle and joints of left foot

  ■ M94.279 Chondromalacia, unspecified ankle and joints of foot

  M94.28 Chondromalacia, other site

  M94.29 Chondromalacia, multiple sites

● M94.3 Chondrolysis

  Code first any associated slipped upper femoral epiphysis (nontraumatic) (M93.0-)

● M94.35 Chondrolysis, hip

  M94.351 Chondrolysis, right hip

  M94.352 Chondrolysis, left hip

  ■ M94.359 Chondrolysis, unspecified hip

● M94.8 Other specified disorders of cartilage

  ● M94.8X Other specified disorders of cartilage

  M94.8X0 Other specified disorders of cartilage, multiple sites

  M94.8X1 Other specified disorders of cartilage, shoulder

  M94.8X2 Other specified disorders of cartilage, upper arm

  M94.8X3 Other specified disorders of cartilage, forearm

  M94.8X4 Other specified disorders of cartilage, hand

  M94.8X5 Other specified disorders of cartilage, thigh

  M94.8X6 Other specified disorders of cartilage, lower leg

  M94.8X7 Other specified disorders of cartilage, ankle and foot

  M94.8X8 Other specified disorders of cartilage, other site

  ■ M94.8X9 Other specified disorders of cartilage, unspecified sites

  ■ M94.9 Disorder of cartilage, unspecified

OTHER DISORDERS OF THE MUSCULOSKELETAL SYSTEM AND CONNECTIVE TISSUE (M95)

● M95 Other acquired deformities of musculoskeletal system and connective tissue

  Excludes2 acquired absence of limbs and organs (Z89-Z90)

  acquired deformities of limbs (M20-M21)

  congenital malformations and deformations of the musculoskeletal system (Q65-Q79)

  deforming dorsopathies (M40-M43)

  dentofacial anomalies [including malocclusion] (M26.-)

  postprocedural musculoskeletal disorders (M96.-)

  M95.0 Acquired deformity of nose

  Excludes2 deviated nasal septum (J34.2)

● M95.1 Cauliflower ear

  Excludes2 other acquired deformities of ear (H61.1)

  ■ M95.10 Cauliflower ear, unspecified ear

  M95.11 Cauliflower ear, right ear

  M95.12 Cauliflower ear, left ear

  M95.2 Other acquired deformity of head

  M95.3 Acquired deformity of neck

  M95.4 Acquired deformity of chest and rib

  M95.5 Acquired deformity of pelvis

  Excludes1 maternal care for known or suspected disproportion (O33.-)

  M95.8 Other specified acquired deformities of musculoskeletal system

  ■ M95.9 Acquired deformity of musculoskeletal system, unspecified

INTRAOPERATIVE AND POSTPROCEDURAL COMPLICATIONS AND DISORDERS OF MUSCULOSKELETAL SYSTEM, NOT ELSEWHERE CLASSIFIED (M96)

● M96 Intraoperative and postprocedural complications and disorders of musculoskeletal system, not elsewhere classified

  Excludes2 arthropathy following intestinal bypass (M02.0-)

  complications of internal orthopedic prosthetic devices, implants and grafts (T84.-)

  disorders associated with osteoporosis (M80)

  presence of functional implants and other devices (Z96-Z97)

● M96.0 Pseudarthrosis after fusion or arthrodesis ✑

  M96.1 Postlaminectomy syndrome, not elsewhere classified

  M96.2 Postradiation kyphosis

  M96.3 Postlaminectomy kyphosis

  M96.4 Postsurgical lordosis

  M96.5 Postradiation scoliosis

● Unacceptable Principal Diagnosis   ● Use Additional Character(s)   ■ Unspecified   ▶ Manifestation Code

OGCR Official Guidelines for Coding and Reporting   Excludes 1   Excludes 2   Includes   Use additional   Code first   Code also

● **M96.6** **Fracture of bone following insertion of orthopedic implant, joint prosthesis, or bone plate**

     Intraoperative fracture of bone during insertion of orthopedic implant, joint prosthesis, or bone plate

     | Excludes2 | complication of internal orthopedic devices, implants or grafts (T84.-)

● **M96.62** **Fracture of humerus following insertion of orthopedic implant, joint prosthesis, or bone plate**

     M96.621 Fracture of humerus following insertion of orthopedic implant, joint prosthesis, or bone plate, right arm 🦴

     M96.622 Fracture of humerus following insertion of orthopedic implant, joint prosthesis, or bone plate, left arm 🦴

     ■ **M96.629** Fracture of humerus following insertion of orthopedic implant, joint prosthesis, or bone plate, unspecified arm 🦴

● **M96.63** **Fracture of radius or ulna following insertion of orthopedic implant, joint prosthesis, or bone plate**

     M96.631 Fracture of radius or ulna following insertion of orthopedic implant, joint prosthesis, or bone plate, right arm 🦴

     M96.632 Fracture of radius or ulna following insertion of orthopedic implant, joint prosthesis, or bone plate, left arm 🦴

     ■ **M96.639** Fracture of radius or ulna following insertion of orthopedic implant, joint prosthesis, or bone plate, unspecified arm 🦴

M96.65 Fracture of pelvis following insertion of orthopedic implant, joint prosthesis, or bone plate 🦴

● **M96.66** **Fracture of femur following insertion of orthopedic implant, joint prosthesis, or bone plate**

     M96.661 Fracture of femur following insertion of orthopedic implant, joint prosthesis, or bone plate, right leg 🦴

     M96.662 Fracture of femur following insertion of orthopedic implant, joint prosthesis, or bone plate, left leg 🦴

     ■ **M96.669** Fracture of femur following insertion of orthopedic implant, joint prosthesis, or bone plate, unspecified leg 🦴

● **M96.67** **Fracture of tibia or fibula following insertion of orthopedic implant, joint prosthesis, or bone plate**

     M96.671 Fracture of tibia or fibula following insertion of orthopedic implant, joint prosthesis, or bone plate, right leg 🦴

     M96.672 Fracture of tibia or fibula following insertion of orthopedic implant, joint prosthesis, or bone plate, left leg 🦴

     ■ **M96.679** Fracture of tibia or fibula following insertion of orthopedic implant, joint prosthesis, or bone plate, unspecified leg 🦴

M96.69 Fracture of other bone following insertion of orthopedic implant, joint prosthesis, or bone plate 🦴

● **M96.8** **Other intraoperative and postprocedural complications and disorders of musculoskeletal system, not elsewhere classified**

● **M96.81** **Intraoperative hemorrhage and hematoma of a musculoskeletal structure complicating a procedure**

     | Excludes1 | intraoperative hemorrhage and hematoma of a musculoskeletal structure due to accidental puncture and laceration during a procedure (M98.82-)

     M96.810 Intraoperative hemorrhage and hematoma of a musculoskeletal structure complicating a musculoskeletal system procedure 🦴

     M96.811 Intraoperative hemorrhage and hematoma of a musculoskeletal structure complicating other procedure 🦴

● **M96.82** **Accidental puncture and laceration of a musculoskeletal structure during a procedure**

     M96.820 Accidental puncture and laceration of a musculoskeletal structure during a musculoskeletal system procedure 🦴

     M96.821 Accidental puncture and laceration of a musculoskeletal structure during other procedure 🦴

● **M96.83** **Postprocedural hemorrhage and hematoma of a musculoskeletal structure following a procedure**

     M96.830 Postprocedural hemorrhage and hematoma of a musculoskeletal structure following a musculoskeletal system procedure 🦴

     M96.831 Postprocedural hemorrhage and hematoma of a musculoskeletal structure following other procedure 🦴

M96.89 Other intraoperative and postprocedural complications and disorders of the musculoskeletal system 🦴

     Instability of joint secondary to removal of joint prosthesis

     Use additional code, if applicable, to further specify disorder

N Newborn Age: 0   **P** Pediatric Age: 0–17   **M** Maternity DX: 12–55   **A** Adult Age: 15–124   ♀ Females Only   ♂ Males Only

🦴 Complication\Comorbidity   🦴 Major C\C   🦴 Present on Admission Requirement   🦴 Hospital-Acquired Condition

1257

CHAPTER 13 (M00-M99)

BIOMECHANICAL LESIONS, NOT ELSEWHERE CLASSIFIED (M99)

● M99 Biomechanical lesions, not elsewhere classified

> **Note:** This category should not be used if the condition can be classified elsewhere.

● M99.0 Segmental and somatic dysfunction

M99.00 Segmental and somatic dysfunction of head region

M99.01 Segmental and somatic dysfunction of cervical region

M99.02 Segmental and somatic dysfunction of thoracic region

M99.03 Segmental and somatic dysfunction of lumbar region

M99.04 Segmental and somatic dysfunction of sacral region

M99.05 Segmental and somatic dysfunction of pelvic region

M99.06 Segmental and somatic dysfunction of lower extremity

M99.07 Segmental and somatic dysfunction of upper extremity

M99.08 Segmental and somatic dysfunction of rib cage

M99.09 Segmental and somatic dysfunction of abdomen and other regions

● M99.1 Subluxation complex (vertebral)

M99.10 Subluxation complex (vertebral) of head region

M99.11 Subluxation complex (vertebral) of cervical region

M99.12 Subluxation complex (vertebral) of thoracic region

M99.13 Subluxation complex (vertebral) of lumbar region

M99.14 Subluxation complex (vertebral) of sacral region

M99.15 Subluxation complex (vertebral) of pelvic region

M99.16 Subluxation complex (vertebral) of lower extremity

M99.17 Subluxation complex (vertebral) of upper extremity

M99.18 Subluxation complex (vertebral) of rib cage

M99.19 Subluxation complex (vertebral) of abdomen and other regions

● M99.2 Subluxation stenosis of neural canal

M99.20 Subluxation stenosis of neural canal of head region

M99.21 Subluxation stenosis of neural canal of cervical region

M99.22 Subluxation stenosis of neural canal of thoracic region

M99.23 Subluxation stenosis of neural canal of lumbar region

M99.24 Subluxation stenosis of neural canal of sacral region

M99.25 Subluxation stenosis of neural canal of pelvic region

M99.26 Subluxation stenosis of neural canal of lower extremity

M99.27 Subluxation stenosis of neural canal of upper extremity

M99.28 Subluxation stenosis of neural canal of rib cage

M99.29 Subluxation stenosis of neural canal of abdomen and other regions

● M99.3 Osseous stenosis of neural canal

M99.30 Osseous stenosis of neural canal of head region

M99.31 Osseous stenosis of neural canal of cervical region

M99.32 Osseous stenosis of neural canal of thoracic region

M99.33 Osseous stenosis of neural canal of lumbar region

M99.34 Osseous stenosis of neural canal of sacral region

M99.35 Osseous stenosis of neural canal of pelvic region

M99.36 Osseous stenosis of neural canal of lower extremity

M99.37 Osseous stenosis of neural canal of upper extremity

M99.38 Osseous stenosis of neural canal of rib cage

M99.39 Osseous stenosis of neural canal of abdomen and other regions

● M99.4 Connective tissue stenosis of neural canal

M99.40 Connective tissue stenosis of neural canal of head region

M99.41 Connective tissue stenosis of neural canal of cervical region

M99.42 Connective tissue stenosis of neural canal of thoracic region

M99.43 Connective tissue stenosis of neural canal of lumbar region

M99.44 Connective tissue stenosis of neural canal of sacral region

M99.45 Connective tissue stenosis of neural canal of pelvic region

M99.46 Connective tissue stenosis of neural canal of lower extremity

M99.47 Connective tissue stenosis of neural canal of upper extremity

M99.48 Connective tissue stenosis of neural canal of rib cage

M99.49 Connective tissue stenosis of neural canal of abdomen and other regions

● M99.5   Intervertebral disc stenosis of neural canal

     M99.50   Intervertebral disc stenosis of neural canal of head region

     M99.51   Intervertebral disc stenosis of neural canal of cervical region

     M99.52   Intervertebral disc stenosis of neural canal of thoracic region

     M99.53   Intervertebral disc stenosis of neural canal of lumbar region

     M99.54   Intervertebral disc stenosis of neural canal of sacral region

     M99.55   Intervertebral disc stenosis of neural canal of pelvic region

     M99.56   Intervertebral disc stenosis of neural canal of lower extremity

     M99.57   Intervertebral disc stenosis of neural canal of upper extremity

     M99.58   Intervertebral disc stenosis of neural canal of rib cage

     M99.59   Intervertebral disc stenosis of neural canal of abdomen and other regions

● M99.6   Osseous and subluxation stenosis of intervertebral foramina

     M99.60   Osseous and subluxation stenosis of intervertebral foramina of head region

     M99.61   Osseous and subluxation stenosis of intervertebral foramina of cervical region

     M99.62   Osseous and subluxation stenosis of intervertebral foramina of thoracic region

     M99.63   Osseous and subluxation stenosis of intervertebral foramina of lumbar region

     M99.64   Osseous and subluxation stenosis of intervertebral foramina of sacral region

     M99.65   Osseous and subluxation stenosis of intervertebral foramina of pelvic region

     M99.66   Osseous and subluxation stenosis of intervertebral foramina of lower extremity

     M99.67   Osseous and subluxation stenosis of intervertebral foramina of upper extremity

     M99.68   Osseous and subluxation stenosis of intervertebral foramina of rib cage

     M99.69   Osseous and subluxation stenosis of intervertebral foramina of abdomen and other regions

● M99.7   Connective tissue and disc stenosis of intervertebral foramina

     M99.70   Connective tissue and disc stenosis of intervertebral foramina of head region

     M99.71   Connective tissue and disc stenosis of intervertebral foramina of cervical region

     M99.72   Connective tissue and disc stenosis of intervertebral foramina of thoracic region

     M99.73   Connective tissue and disc stenosis of intervertebral foramina of lumbar region

     M99.74   Connective tissue and disc stenosis of intervertebral foramina of sacral region

     M99.75   Connective tissue and disc stenosis of intervertebral foramina of pelvic region

     M99.76   Connective tissue and disc stenosis of intervertebral foramina of lower extremity

     M99.77   Connective tissue and disc stenosis of intervertebral foramina of upper extremity

     M99.78   Connective tissue and disc stenosis of intervertebral foramina of rib cage

     M99.79   Connective tissue and disc stenosis of intervertebral foramina of abdomen and other regions

● M99.8   Other biomechanical lesions

     M99.80   Other biomechanical lesions of head region

     M99.81   Other biomechanical lesions of cervical region

     M99.82   Other biomechanical lesions of thoracic region

     M99.83   Other biomechanical lesions of lumbar region

     M99.84   Other biomechanical lesions of sacral region

     M99.85   Other biomechanical lesions of pelvic region

     M99.86   Other biomechanical lesions of lower extremity

     M99.87   Other biomechanical lesions of upper extremity

     M99.88   Other biomechanical lesions of rib cage

     M99.89   Other biomechanical lesions of abdomen and other regions

■ M99.9   Biomechanical lesion, unspecified

CHAPTER 13 (M00-M99)

Item 14–1 Nephritis (inflammation) or **nephropathy** (disease) **with lesion of proliferative glomerulonephritis** results from a streptococcal infection.

Nephritis (inflammation) or **nephropathy** (disease) **with lesion of membranous glomerulonephritis** is characterized by deposits along the epithelial side of the basement membrane.

Nephritis (inflammation) or **nephropathy** (disease) **with lesion of membranoproliferative glomerulonephritis** is characterized by alterations in the basement membranes of the kidney and the glomerular cells.

Nephritis (inflammation) or **nephropathy** (disease) **with lesion of rapidly progressive glomerulonephritis** is characterized by rapid and progressive decline in renal function.

Nephritis (inflammation) or **nephropathy** (disease) **with lesion of renal cortical necrosis** is characterized by death of the cortical tissues.

Nephritis (inflammation) or **nephropathy** (disease) **with lesion of renal medullary necrosis** is characterized by death of the tissues that collect urine.

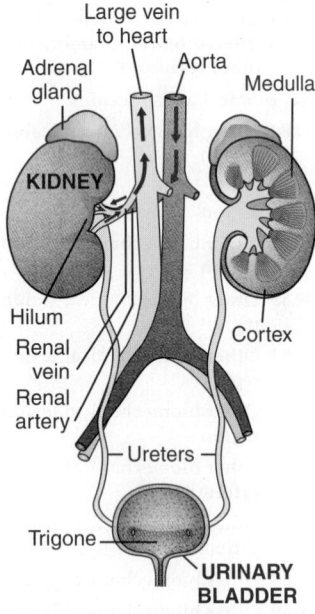

Figure 14-1   Kidneys within the urinary system.

Item 14–2 Glomerulonephritis is nephritis accompanied by inflammation of the glomeruli of the kidney, resulting in the degeneration of the glomeruli and the nephrons.

Acute glomerulonephritis primarily affects children and young adults and is usually a result of a streptococcal infection.

Proliferative glomerulonephritis is the acute form of the disease resulting from a streptococcal infection.

Rapidly progressive glomerulonephritis, also known as **crescentic** or **malignant glomerulonephritis**, is the acute form of the disease, which leads quickly to rapid and progressive decline in renal function.

CHAPTER 14

DISEASES OF THE GENITOURINARY SYSTEM (N00-N99)

Excludes2   certain conditions originating in the perinatal period (P04-P96)
certain infectious and parasitic diseases (A00-B99)
complications of pregnancy, childbirth and the puerperium (O00-O9A)
congenital malformations, deformations and chromosomal abnormalities (Q00-Q99)
endocrine, nutritional and metabolic diseases (E00-E88)
injury, poisoning and certain other consequences of external causes (S00-T88)
neoplasms (C00-D49)
symptoms, signs and abnormal clinical and laboratory findings, not elsewhere classified (R00-R94)

This chapter contains the following blocks:

N00-N08	Glomerular diseases
N10-N16	Renal tubulo-interstitial diseases
N17-N19	Acute kidney failure and chronic kidney disease
N20-N23	Urolithiasis
N25-N29	Other disorders of kidney and ureter
N30-N39	Other diseases of the urinary system
N40-N53	Diseases of male genital organs
N60-N65	Disorders of breast
N70-N77	Inflammatory diseases of female pelvic organs
N80-N98	Noninflammatory disorders of female genital tract
N99	Intraoperative and postprocedural complications and disorders of genitourinary system, not elsewhere classified

GLOMERULAR DISEASES (N00-N08)

Code also any associated kidney failure (N17-N19)

Excludes1   hypertensive chronic kidney disease (I12.-)

● **N00   Acute nephritic syndrome**

Includes   acute glomerular disease
acute glomerulonephritis
acute nephritis

Excludes1   acute tubulo-interstitial nephritis (N10)
nephritic syndrome NOS (N05.-)

N00.0   Acute nephritic syndrome with minor glomerular abnormality
Acute nephritic syndrome with minimal change lesion

N00.1   Acute nephritic syndrome with focal and segmental glomerular lesions
Acute nephritic syndrome with focal and segmental hyalinosis
Acute nephritic syndrome with focal and segmental sclerosis
Acute nephritic syndrome with focal glomerulonephritis

N00.2   Acute nephritic syndrome with diffuse membranous glomerulonephritis

N00.3   Acute nephritic syndrome with diffuse mesangial proliferative glomerulonephritis

● Unacceptable Principal Diagnosis   ● Use Additional Character(s)   ■ Unspecified   ▶ Manifestation Code
OGCR Official Guidelines for Coding and Reporting   Excludes 1   Excludes 2   Includes   Use additional   Code first   Code also

N00.4   **Acute nephritic syndrome with diffuse endocapillary proliferative glomerulonephritis** 🔵

N00.5   **Acute nephritic syndrome with diffuse mesangiocapillary glomerulonephritis** 🔵
> Acute nephritic syndrome with membranoproliferative glomerulonephritis, types 1 and 3, or NOS

N00.6   **Acute nephritic syndrome with dense deposit disease** 🔵
> Acute nephritic syndrome with membranoproliferative glomerulonephritis, type 2

N00.7   **Acute nephritic syndrome with diffuse crescentic glomerulonephritis** 🔵
> Acute nephritic syndrome with extracapillary glomerulonephritis

N00.8   **Acute nephritic syndrome with other morphologic changes** 🔵
> Acute nephritic syndrome with proliferative glomerulonephritis NOS

◾ **N00.9**   **Acute nephritic syndrome with unspecified morphologic changes** 🔵

● **N01**   **Rapidly progressive nephritic syndrome**

> **Includes**   rapidly progressive glomerular disease
> rapidly progressive glomerulonephritis
> rapidly progressive nephritis

> **Excludes1**   nephritic syndrome NOS (N05.-)

N01.0   **Rapidly progressive nephritic syndrome with minor glomerular abnormality** 🔵
> Rapidly progressive nephritic syndrome with minimal change lesion

N01.1   **Rapidly progressive nephritic syndrome with focal and segmental glomerular lesions** 🔵
> Rapidly progressive nephritic syndrome with focal and segmental hyalinosis
> Rapidly progressive nephritic syndrome with focal and segmental sclerosis
> Rapidly progressive nephritic syndrome with focal glomerulonephritis

N01.2   **Rapidly progressive nephritic syndrome with diffuse membranous glomerulonephritis** 🔵

N01.3   **Rapidly progressive nephritic syndrome with diffuse mesangial proliferative glomerulonephritis** 🔵

N01.4   **Rapidly progressive nephritic syndrome with diffuse endocapillary proliferative glomerulonephritis** 🔵

N01.5   **Rapidly progressive nephritic syndrome with diffuse mesangiocapillary glomerulonephritis** 🔵
> Rapidly progressive nephritic syndrome with membranoproliferative glomerulonephritis, types 1 and 3, or NOS

N01.6   **Rapidly progressive nephritic syndrome with dense deposit disease** 🔵
> Rapidly progressive nephritic syndrome with membranoproliferative glomerulonephritis, type 2

N01.7   **Rapidly progressive nephritic syndrome with diffuse crescentic glomerulonephritis** 🔵
> Rapidly progressive nephritic syndrome with extracapillary glomerulonephritis

N01.8   **Rapidly progressive nephritic syndrome with other morphologic changes** 🔵
> Rapidly progressive nephritic syndrome with proliferative glomerulonephritis NOS

◾ **N01.9**   **Rapidly progressive nephritic syndrome with unspecified morphologic changes** 🔵

● **N02**   **Recurrent and persistent hematuria**

> **Excludes1**   acute cystitis with hematuria (N30.01)
> acute prostatitis with hematuria (N41.01)
> chronic prostatitis with hematuria (N41.11)
> hematuria NOS (R31.9)
> hematuria not associated with specified morphologic lesions (R31.-)

N02.0   **Recurrent and persistent hematuria with minor glomerular abnormality** 🔵
> Recurrent and persistent hematuria with minimal change lesion

N02.1   **Recurrent and persistent hematuria with focal and segmental glomerular lesions** 🔵
> Recurrent and persistent hematuria with focal and segmental hyalinosis
> Recurrent and persistent hematuria with focal and segmental sclerosis
> Recurrent and persistent hematuria with focal glomerulonephritis

N02.2   **Recurrent and persistent hematuria with diffuse membranous glomerulonephritis** 🔵

N02.3   **Recurrent and persistent hematuria with diffuse mesangial proliferative glomerulonephritis** 🔵

N02.4   **Recurrent and persistent hematuria with diffuse endocapillary proliferative glomerulonephritis** 🔵

N02.5   **Recurrent and persistent hematuria with diffuse mesangiocapillary glomerulonephritis** 🔵
> Recurrent and persistent hematuria with membranoproliferative glomerulonephritis, types 1 and 3, or NOS

N02.6   **Recurrent and persistent hematuria with dense deposit disease** 🔵
> Recurrent and persistent hematuria with membranoproliferative glomerulonephritis, type 2

N02.7   **Recurrent and persistent hematuria with diffuse crescentic glomerulonephritis** 🔵
> Recurrent and persistent hematuria with extracapillary glomerulonephritis

N02.8   **Recurrent and persistent hematuria with other morphologic changes** 🔵
> Recurrent and persistent hematuria with proliferative glomerulonephritis NOS

◾ **N02.9**   **Recurrent and persistent hematuria with unspecified morphologic changes** 🔵

Item 14–3 Chronic glomerulonephritis (GN) persists over a period of years, with remissions and exacerbation.

Chronic GN with lesion of proliferative glomerulonephritis results from a streptococcal infection.

Chronic GN with lesion of membranous glomerulonephritis, also known as membranous nephropathy, is characterized by deposits along the epithelial side of the basement membrane.

Chronic GN with lesion of membrano-proliferative glomerulonephritis (MPGN) is a group of disorders characterized by alterations in the basement membranes of the kidney and the glomerular cells.

Chronic GN with lesion of rapidly progressive glomerulonephritis is characterized by necrosis, endothelial proliferation, and mesangial proliferation. The condition is marked by rapid and progressive decline in renal function.

CHAPTER 14 (N00–N99)

N Newborn Age: 0   **P** Pediatric Age: 0–17   **M** Maternity DX: 12–55   **A** Adult Age: 15–124   ♀ Females Only   ♂ Males Only

🔵 Complication\Comorbidity   🔵 Major C\C   🔵 Present on Admission Requirement   🔵 Hospital-Acquired Condition

1261

● **N03 Chronic nephritic syndrome**

> **Includes** chronic glomerular disease
> chronic glomerulonephritis
> chronic nephritis

> **Excludes1** chronic tubulo-interstitial nephritis (N11.-)
> diffuse sclerosing glomerulonephritis
> (N05.8-)
> nephritic syndrome NOS (N05.-)

N03.0 Chronic nephritic syndrome with minor glomerular abnormality ⚕
> Chronic nephritic syndrome with minimal change lesion

N03.1 Chronic nephritic syndrome with focal and segmental glomerular lesions ⚕
> Chronic nephritic syndrome with focal and segmental hyalinosis
> Chronic nephritic syndrome with focal and segmental sclerosis
> Chronic nephritic syndrome with focal glomerulonephritis

N03.2 Chronic nephritic syndrome with diffuse membranous glomerulonephritis ⚕

N03.3 Chronic nephritic syndrome with diffuse mesangial proliferative glomerulonephritis ⚕

N03.4 Chronic nephritic syndrome with diffuse endocapillary proliferative glomerulonephritis ⚕

N03.5 Chronic nephritic syndrome with diffuse mesangiocapillary glomerulonephritis ⚕
> Chronic nephritic syndrome with membranoproliferative glomerulonephritis, types 1 and 3, or NOS

N03.6 Chronic nephritic syndrome with dense deposit disease ⚕
> Chronic nephritic syndrome with membranoproliferative glomerulonephritis, type 2

N03.7 Chronic nephritic syndrome with diffuse crescentic glomerulonephritis ⚕
> Chronic nephritic syndrome with extracapillary glomerulonephritis

N03.8 Chronic nephritic syndrome with other morphologic changes ⚕
> Chronic nephritic syndrome with proliferative glomerulonephritis NOS

■ **N03.9 Chronic nephritic syndrome with unspecified morphologic changes** ⚕

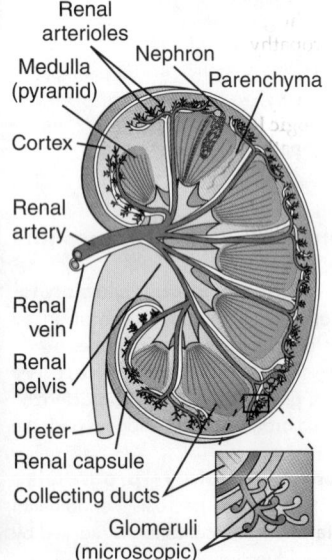

Renal arterioles
Nephron
Medulla (pyramid)
Parenchyma
Cortex
Renal artery
Renal vein
Renal pelvis
Ureter
Renal capsule
Collecting ducts
Glomeruli (microscopic)

Figure 14-2 Kidney cross section

Item 14-4 Nephrotic syndrome (NS) is marked by massive proteinuria (protein in the urine) and water retention. Patients with NS are particularly vulnerable to staphylococcal and pneumococcal infections. NS with lesion of proliferative glomerulonephritis results from a streptococcal infection. NS with lesion of membranous glomerulonephritis results in thickening of the capillary walls. NS with lesion of minimal change glomerulonephritis is usually a benign disorder that occurs mostly in children and requires electron microscopy (biopsy) to verify changes in the glomeruli.

● **N04 Nephrotic syndrome**

> **Includes** congenital nephrotic syndrome
> lipoid nephrosis

N04.0 Nephrotic syndrome with minor glomerular abnormality ⚕
> Nephrotic syndrome with minimal change lesion

N04.1 Nephrotic syndrome with focal and segmental glomerular lesions ⚕
> Nephrotic syndrome with focal and segmental hyalinosis
> Nephrotic syndrome with focal and segmental sclerosis
> Nephrotic syndrome with focal glomerulonephritis

N04.2 Nephrotic syndrome with diffuse membranous glomerulonephritis ⚕

N04.3 Nephrotic syndrome with diffuse mesangial proliferative glomerulonephritis ⚕

N04.4 Nephrotic syndrome with diffuse endocapillary proliferative glomerulonephritis ⚕

N04.5 Nephrotic syndrome with diffuse mesangiocapillary glomerulonephritis ⚕
> Nephrotic syndrome with membranoproliferative glomerulonephritis, types 1 and 3, or NOS

N04.6 Nephrotic syndrome with dense deposit disease ⚕
> Nephrotic syndrome with membranoproliferative glomerulonephritis, type 2

N04.7 Nephrotic syndrome with diffuse crescentic glomerulonephritis ⚕
> Nephrotic syndrome with extracapillary glomerulonephritis

N04.8 Nephrotic syndrome with other morphologic changes ⚕
> Nephrotic syndrome with proliferative glomerulonephritis NOS

■ **N04.9 Nephrotic syndrome with unspecified morphologic changes** ⚕

● **N05 Unspecified nephritic syndrome**

> **Includes** glomerular disease NOS
> glomerulonephritis NOS
> nephritis NOS
> nephropathy NOS and renal disease NOS with morphological lesion specified in .0-.8

> **Excludes1** nephropathy NOS with no stated morphological lesion (N28.9)
> renal disease NOS with no stated morphological lesion (N28.9)
> tubulo-interstitial nephritis NOS (N12)

■ **N05.0 Unspecified nephritic syndrome with minor glomerular abnormality**
> Unspecified nephritic syndrome with minimal change lesion

● Unacceptable Principal Diagnosis   ● Use Additional Character(s)   ■ Unspecified   ▶ Manifestation Code
OGCR Official Guidelines for Coding and Reporting   Excludes 1   Excludes 2   Includes   Use additional   Code first   Code also

CHAPTER 14 (N00-N99)

■ **N05.1** **Unspecified nephritic syndrome with focal and segmental glomerular lesions**
Unspecified nephritic syndrome with focal and segmental hyalinosis
Unspecified nephritic syndrome with focal and segmental sclerosis
Unspecified nephritic syndrome with focal glomerulonephritis

■ **N05.2** **Unspecified nephritic syndrome with diffuse membranous glomerulonephritis** 🔾

■ **N05.3** **Unspecified nephritic syndrome with diffuse mesangial proliferative glomerulonephritis** 🔾

■ **N05.4** **Unspecified nephritic syndrome with diffuse endocapillary proliferative glomerulonephritis** 🔾

■ **N05.5** **Unspecified nephritic syndrome with diffuse mesangiocapillary glomerulonephritis** 🔾
Unspecified nephritic syndrome with membranoproliferative glomerulonephritis, types 1 and 3, or NOS

■ **N05.6** **Unspecified nephritic syndrome with dense deposit disease**
Unspecified nephritic syndrome with membranoproliferative glomerulonephritis, type 2

■ **N05.7** **Unspecified nephritic syndrome with diffuse crescentic glomerulonephritis**
Unspecified nephritic syndrome with extracapillary glomerulonephritis

■ **N05.8** **Unspecified nephritic syndrome with other morphologic changes**
Unspecified nephritic syndrome with proliferative glomerulonephritis NOS

■ **N05.9** **Unspecified nephritic syndrome with unspecified morphologic changes**

● **N06** **Isolated proteinuria with specified morphological lesion**
⬛ **Excludes1** proteinuria not associated with specific morphologic lesions (R80.0)

N06.0 **Isolated proteinuria with minor glomerular abnormality**
Isolated proteinuria with minimal change lesion

N06.1 **Isolated proteinuria with focal and segmental glomerular lesions**
Isolated proteinuria with focal and segmental hyalinosis
Isolated proteinuria with focal and segmental sclerosis
Isolated proteinuria with focal glomerulonephritis

N06.2 **Isolated proteinuria with diffuse membranous glomerulonephritis** 🔾

N06.3 **Isolated proteinuria with diffuse mesangial proliferative glomerulonephritis** 🔾

N06.4 **Isolated proteinuria with diffuse endocapillary proliferative glomerulonephritis** 🔾

N06.5 **Isolated proteinuria with diffuse mesangiocapillary glomerulonephritis** 🔾
Isolated proteinuria with membranoproliferative glomerulonephritis, types 1 and 3, or NOS

N06.6 **Isolated proteinuria with dense deposit disease**
Isolated proteinuria with membranoproliferative glomerulonephritis, type 2

N06.7 **Isolated proteinuria with diffuse crescentic glomerulonephritis**
Isolated proteinuria with extracapillary glomerulonephritis

N06.8 **Isolated proteinuria with other morphologic lesion**
Isolated proteinuria with proliferative glomerulonephritis NOS

■ **N06.9** **Isolated proteinuria with unspecified morphologic lesion**

● **N07** **Hereditary nephropathy, not elsewhere classified**
⬛ **Excludes2** Alport's syndrome (Q87.81-)
hereditary amyloid nephropathy (E85-)
nail patella syndrome (Q87.2)
non-neuropathic heredofamilial amyloidosis (E85-)

N07.0 **Hereditary nephropathy, not elsewhere classified with minor glomerular abnormality**
Hereditary nephropathy, not elsewhere classified with minimal change lesion

N07.1 **Hereditary nephropathy, not elsewhere classified with focal and segmental glomerular lesions**
Hereditary nephropathy, not elsewhere classified with focal and segmental hyalinosis
Hereditary nephropathy, not elsewhere classified with focal and segmental sclerosis
Hereditary nephropathy, not elsewhere classified with focal glomerulonephritis

N07.2 **Hereditary nephropathy, not elsewhere classified with diffuse membranous glomerulonephritis** 🔾

N07.3 **Hereditary nephropathy, not elsewhere classified with diffuse mesangial proliferative glomerulonephritis** 🔾

N07.4 **Hereditary nephropathy, not elsewhere classified with diffuse endocapillary proliferative glomerulonephritis** 🔾

N07.5 **Hereditary nephropathy, not elsewhere classified with diffuse mesangiocapillary glomerulonephritis** 🔾
Hereditary nephropathy, not elsewhere classified with membranoproliferative glomerulonephritis, types 1 and 3, or NOS

N07.6 **Hereditary nephropathy, not elsewhere classified with dense deposit disease**
Hereditary nephropathy, not elsewhere classified with membranoproliferative glomerulonephritis, type 2

N07.7 **Hereditary nephropathy, not elsewhere classified with diffuse crescentic glomerulonephritis**
Hereditary nephropathy, not elsewhere classified with extracapillary glomerulonephritis

N07.8 **Hereditary nephropathy, not elsewhere classified with other morphologic lesions**
Hereditary nephropathy, not elsewhere classified with proliferative glomerulonephritis NOS

■ **N07.9** **Hereditary nephropathy, not elsewhere classified with unspecified morphologic lesions**

N Newborn Age: 0   **P** Pediatric Age: 0–17   **M** Maternity DX: 12–55   **A** Adult Age: 15–124   ♀ Females Only   ♂ Males Only

🔾 Complication\Comorbidity   🔾 Major C\C   🔾 Present on Admission Requirement   🔾 Hospital-Acquired Condition

● ▶ **N08** *Glomerular disorders in diseases classified elsewhere*
  Glomerulonephritis
  Nephritis
  Nephropathy

  Code first underlying disease, such as:
    amyloidosis (E85-)
    congenital syphilis (A50.5)
    cryoglobulinemia (D89.1)
    disseminated intravascular coagulation (D65)
    gout (M1A-, M10.-)
    microscopic polyangiitis (M31.7)
    multiple myeloma (C90.0-)
    sepsis (A40.0-A41.9)
    sickle-cell disease (D57.0-D57.8)

  | **Excludes1** | glomerulonephritis, nephritis and nephropathy (in): |

    antiglomerular basement membrane disease (M31.0)
    diabetes (E08-E13 with .21)
    gonococcal (A54.21)
    Goodpasture's syndrome (M31.0)
    hemolytic-uremic syndrome (D59.3)
    lupus (M32.14)
    mumps (B26.83)
    syphilis (A52.75)
    systemic lupus erythematosus (M32.14)
    Wegener's granulomatosis (M31.31)
  pyelonephritis in diseases classified elsewhere (N16)
  renal tubulo-interstitial disorders classified elsewhere (N16)

RENAL TUBULO-INTERSTITIAL DISEASES (N10-N16)

  | **Includes** | pyelonephritis |
  | **Excludes1** | pyeloureteritis cystica (N28.85) |

N10 **Acute tubulo-interstitial nephritis** 🕹🕹
  Acute infectious interstitial nephritis
  Acute pyelitis
  Acute pyelonephritis
  Hemoglobin nephrosis
  Myoglobin nephrosis

  Use additional code (B95-B97), to identify infectious agent

● **N11** **Chronic tubulo-interstitial nephritis**
Includes	chronic infectious interstitial nephritis
	chronic pyelitis
	chronic pyelonephritis

  Use additional code (B95-B97), to identify infectious agent

  N11.0 **Nonobstructive reflux-associated chronic pyelonephritis** 🕹
    Pyelonephritis (chronic) associated with (vesicoureteral) reflux

    | **Excludes1** | vesicoureteral reflux NOS (N13.70) |

Item 14–5 Pyelonephritis is an infection of the kidneys and ureters and may be chronic or acute in one or both kidneys.

  N11.1 **Chronic obstructive pyelonephritis** 🕹
    Pyelonephritis (chronic) associated with anomaly of pelviureteric junction
    Pyelonephritis (chronic) associated with anomaly of pyeloureteric junction
    Pyelonephritis (chronic) associated with crossing of vessel
    Pyelonephritis (chronic) associated with kinking of ureter
    Pyelonephritis (chronic) associated with obstruction of ureter
    Pyelonephritis (chronic) associated with stricture of pelviureteric junction
    Pyelonephritis (chronic) associated with stricture of ureter

    | **Excludes1** | calculous pyelonephritis (N20.9) |
    | | obstructive uropathy (N13.-) |

    MCC: Only when the principal diagnosis is designated as a CC

  N11.8 **Other chronic tubulo-interstitial nephritis** 🕹
    Nonobstructive chronic pyelonephritis NOS

  ▪ **N11.9** **Chronic tubulo-interstitial nephritis, unspecified** 🕹 🕹
    Chronic interstitial nephritis NOS
    Chronic pyelitis NOS
    Chronic pyelonephritis NOS

N12 **Tubulo-interstitial nephritis, not specified as acute or chronic** 🕹 🕹
  Interstitial nephritis NOS
  Pyelitis NOS
  Pyelonephritis NOS

  | **Excludes1** | calculous pyelonephritis (N20.9) |

● **N13** **Obstructive and reflux uropathy**
Excludes2	calculus of kidney and ureter without hydronephrosis (N20.-)
	congenital obstructive defects of renal pelvis and ureter (Q62.0-Q62.3)
	hydronephrosis with ureteropelvic junction obstruction (Q62.1)
	obstructive pyelonephritis (N11.1)

  N13.1 **Hydronephrosis with ureteral stricture, not elsewhere classified** 🕹
    | **Excludes1** | hydronephrosis with ureteral stricture with infection (N13.6) |

  N13.2 **Hydronephrosis with renal and ureteral calculous obstruction** 🕹
    | **Excludes1** | hydronephrosis with renal and ureteral calculous obstruction with infection (N13.6) |

Figure 14-3 Acute pyelonephritis. Cortical surface exhibits grayish white areas of inflammation and abscess formation. (From Kumar: Robbins and Cartan: Pathologic Basis of Disease, 7th ed. 2005, Saunders, An Imprint of Elsevier.)

Figure 14-4 Hydronephrosis of the kidney, with marked dilation of pelvis and calyces and thinning of renal parenchyma. (From Kumar: Robbins and Cartan: Pathologic Basis of Disease, 7th ed. 2005, Saunders, An Imprint of Elsevier.)

● Unacceptable Principal Diagnosis   ● Use Additional Character(s)   ▪ Unspecified   ▶ Manifestation Code
OGCR Official Guidelines for Coding and Reporting | Excludes 1 | | Excludes 2 | | Includes | | Use additional | | Code first | | Code also |

● **N13.3 Other and unspecified hydronephrosis**

> **Excludes1**   hydronephrosis with infection (N13.6)

■ **N13.30 Unspecified hydronephrosis** 🅒

N13.39 Other hydronephrosis 🅒

N13.4 Hydroureter 🅒

> **Excludes1**   congenital hydroureter (Q62.3-)
> hydroureter with infection (N13.6)
> vesicoureteral-reflux with
> hydroureter (N13.73-)

N13.5 Crossing vessel and stricture of ureter without hydronephrosis

> Kinking and stricture of ureter without hydronephrosis

> **Excludes1**   crossing vessel and stricture of ureter
> without hydronephrosis with
> infection (N13.6)

N13.6 Pyonephrosis 🅒 🅜

> Conditions in N13.1-N13.5 with infection
> Obstructive uropathy with infection

> **Use additional** code (B95-B97), to identify
> infectious agent

● **N13.7 Vesicoureteral-reflux**

> **Excludes1**   reflux-associated pyelonephritis
> (N11.0)

■ **N13.70 Vesicoureteral-reflux, unspecified**

> *Occurs when urine flows from bladder back
> into ureters*
> Vesicoureteral-reflux NOS

N13.71 Vesicoureteral-reflux without reflux nephropathy

● **N13.72 Vesicoureteral-reflux with reflux nephropathy without hydroureter**

N13.721 Vesicoureteral-reflux with reflux nephropathy without hydroureter, unilateral

N13.722 Vesicoureteral-reflux with reflux nephropathy without hydroureter, bilateral

■ **N13.729 Vesicoureteral-reflux with reflux nephropathy without hydroureter, unspecified**

● **N13.73 Vesicoureteral-reflux with reflux nephropathy with hydroureter**

N13.731 Vesicoureteral-reflux with reflux nephropathy with hydroureter, unilateral

N13.732 Vesicoureteral-reflux with reflux nephropathy with hydroureter, bilateral

■ **N13.739 Vesicoureteral-reflux with reflux nephropathy with hydroureter, unspecified**

N13.8 Other obstructive and reflux uropathy 🅒

> Urinary tract obstruction due to specified cause

> **Code first**, if applicable, any causal condition first,
> such as:
> enlarged prostate (N40.1)

■ **N13.9 Obstructive and reflux uropathy, unspecified**

> Urinary tract obstruction NOS

● **N14 Drug- and heavy-metal-induced tubulo-interstitial and tubular conditions**

> **Code first** *poisoning due to drug or toxin, if applicable
> (T36-T65 with fifth or sixth character 1-4 or 6)*

> **Use additional** code for adverse effect, if applicable, to
> identify drug (T36-T50 with fifth or sixth character 5)

● **N14.0 Analgesic nephropathy**

● **N14.1 Nephropathy induced by other drugs, medicaments and biological substances**

● ■ **N14.2 Nephropathy induced by unspecified drug, medicament or biological substance**

● **N14.3 Nephropathy induced by heavy metals**

● **N14.4 Toxic nephropathy, not elsewhere classified**

● **N15 Other renal tubulo-interstitial diseases**

N15.0 Balkan nephropathy

> Balkan endemic nephropathy

N15.1 Renal and perinephric abscess 🅜 🅜

N15.8 Other specified renal tubulo-interstitial diseases

■ **N15.9 Renal tubulo-interstitial disease, unspecified**

> Infection of kidney NOS

> **Excludes1**   urinary tract infection NOS (N39.0)

● ◗ **N16** *Renal tubulo-interstitial disorders in diseases classified elsewhere*

> Pyelonephritis
> Tubulo-interstitial nephritis

> **Code first** *underlying disease, such as:*
> brucellosis (A23.0-A23.9)
> cryoglobulinemia (D89.1)
> glycogen storage disease (E74.0)
> leukemia (C91-C95)
> lymphoma (C81.0-C85.9, C96.0-C96.9)
> multiple myeloma (C90.0-)
> sepsis (A40.0-A41.9)
> Wilson's disease (E83.0)

> **Excludes1**   diphtheritic pyelonephritis and tubulo-
> interstitial nephritis (A36.84)
> pyelonephritis and tubulo-interstitial
> nephritis in candidiasis (B37.49)
> pyelonephritis and tubulo-interstitial
> nephritis in cystinosis (E72.04)
> pyelonephritis and tubulo-interstitial
> nephritis in salmonella infection
> (A02.25)
> pyelonephritis and tubulo-interstitial
> nephritis in sarcoidosis (D86.84)
> pyelonephritis and tubulo-interstitial
> nephritis in sicca syndrome [Sjogren's]
> (M35.04)
> pyelonephritis and tubulo-interstitial
> nephritis in systemic lupus
> erythematosus (M32.15)
> pyelonephritis and tubulo-interstitial
> nephritis in toxoplasmosis (B58.83)
> renal tubular degeneration in diabetes
> (E08-E13 with .29)
> syphilitic pyelonephritis and tubulo-
> interstitial nephritis (A52.75)

CHAPTER 14 (N00-N99)

N   Newborn Age: 0   **P**   Pediatric Age: 0–17   **M**   Maternity DX: 12–55   **A**   Adult Age: 15–124   ♀   Females Only   ♂   Males Only

🅒   Complication\Comorbidity   🅜   Major C\C   🅟   Present on Admission Requirement   🅗   Hospital-Acquired Condition

1265

Item 14–6 Decreased blood flow is the usual cause of **acute renal failure** that offers a good prognosis for recovery.

    Chronic renal failure is usually the result of long-standing kidney disease and is a very serious condition that generally results in death.

ACUTE KIDNEY FAILURE AND CHRONIC KIDNEY DISEASE (N17-N19)

> **Excludes2**   congenital renal failure (P96.0)
>   drug- and heavy-metal-induced tubulo-
>   interstitial and tubular conditions (N14.-)
>   extrarenal uremia (R39.2)
>   hemolytic-uremic syndrome (D59.3)
>   hepatorenal syndrome (K76.7)
>   postpartum hepatorenal syndrome (O90.4)
>   posttraumatic renal failure (T79.5)
>   prerenal uremia (R39.2)
>   renal failure:
>   complicating abortion or ectopic or molar
>   pregnancy (O00-O07, O08.4)
>   following labor and delivery (O90.4)
>   postprocedural (N99.0)

● **N17 Acute kidney failure**

    Code also associated underlying condition

> **Excludes1**   posttraumatic renal failure (T79.5)

   N17.0 Acute kidney failure with tubular necrosis 🔹
      Acute tubular necrosis
      Renal tubular necrosis
      Tubular necrosis NOS

   N17.1 Acute kidney failure with acute cortical necrosis 🔹
      Acute cortical necrosis
      Cortical necrosis NOS
      Renal cortical necrosis

   N17.2 Acute kidney failure with medullary necrosis 🔹
      Medullary [papillary] necrosis NOS
      Acute medullary [papillary] necrosis
      Renal medullary [papillary] necrosis

   N17.8 Other acute kidney failure 🔹

■ **N17.9 Acute kidney failure, unspecified** 🔹
      Acute kidney injury (nontraumatic)

> **Excludes2**   traumatic kidney injury (S37.0-)

● **N18 Chronic kidney disease (CKD)**

    Code first any associated:
      diabetic chronic kidney disease (E08.22, E09.22, E10.22,
        E11.22, E13.22)
      hypertensive chronic kidney disease (I12.-, I13.-)

    Use additional code to identify kidney transplant status,
      if applicable, (Z94.0)

   N18.1 Chronic kidney disease, stage 1

   N18.2 Chronic kidney disease, stage 2 (mild)

   N18.3 Chronic kidney disease, stage 3 (moderate)

   N18.4 Chronic kidney disease, stage 4 (severe) 🔹

   N18.5 Chronic kidney disease, stage 5 🔹

> **Excludes1**   chronic kidney disease, stage 5
>   requiring chronic dialysis
>   (N18.6)

   N18.6 End stage renal disease 🔹
      Chronic kidney disease requiring chronic dialysis

     Use additional code to identify dialysis status
      (Z99.2)

■ **N18.9 Chronic kidney disease, unspecified**
      Chronic renal disease
      Chronic renal failure NOS
      Chronic renal insufficiency
      Chronic uremia
      Renal disease NOS

■ **N19 Unspecified kidney failure**
    Uremia NOS

> **Excludes1**   acute kidney failure (N17.-)
>   chronic kidney disease (N18.-)
>   chronic uremia (N18.9)
>   extrarenal uremia (R39.2)
>   prerenal uremia (R39.2)
>   renal insufficiency (acute) (N28.9)
>   uremia of newborn (P96.0)

UROLITHIASIS (N20-N23)

● **N20 Calculus of kidney and ureter**
    Calculous pyelonephritis

> **Excludes1**   nephrocalcinosis (E83.5)
>   that with hydronephrosis (N13.2)

   N20.0 Calculus of kidney
      Nephrolithiasis NOS   Staghorn calculus
      Renal calculus   Stone in kidney
      Renal stone

   N20.1 Calculus of ureter 🔹
      Ureteric stone

   N20.2 Calculus of kidney with calculus of ureter

■ **N20.9 Urinary calculus, unspecified**

● **N21 Calculus of lower urinary tract**

> **Includes**   calculus of lower urinary tract with cystitis
>   and urethritis

   N21.0 Calculus in bladder
      Calculus in diverticulum of bladder
      Urinary bladder stone

> **Excludes2**   staghorn calculus (N20.0)

   N21.1 Calculus in urethra

> **Excludes2**   calculus of prostate (N42.0)

   N21.8 Other lower urinary tract calculus

■ **N21.9 Calculus of lower urinary tract, unspecified**

> **Excludes1**   calculus of urinary tract NOS (N20.9)

● ▶ **N22 Calculus of urinary tract in diseases classified elsewhere**

    Code first underlying disease, such as:
      gout (M1A-, M10.-)
      schistosomiasis (B65.0-B65.9)

■ **N23 Unspecified renal colic**

Figure 14-5 Multiple urinary calculi.

Multiple calculi

● Unacceptable Principal Diagnosis   ● Use Additional Character(s)   ■ Unspecified   ▶ Manifestation Code

OGCR Official Guidelines for Coding and Reporting   Excludes 1   Excludes 2   Includes   Use additional   Code first   Code also

OTHER DISORDERS OF KIDNEY AND URETER (N25-N29)

> **Excludes2** disorders of kidney and ureter with urolithiasis (N20-N23)

● **N25 Disorders resulting from impaired renal tubular function**

> **Excludes1** metabolic disorders classifiable to E70-E88

    N25.0 **Renal osteodystrophy**
      Azotemic osteodystrophy
      Phosphate-losing tubular disorders
      Renal rickets
      Renal short stature

    N25.1 **Nephrogenic diabetes insipidus** 🦠

> **Excludes1** diabetes insipidus NOS (E23.2)

● N25.8 **Other disorders resulting from impaired renal tubular function**

      N25.81 **Secondary hyperparathyroidism of renal origin** 🦠

> **Excludes1** secondary hyperparathyroidism, non-renal (E21.1)

      N25.89 **Other disorders resulting from impaired renal tubular function**
        Hypokalemic nephropathy
        Lightwood-Albright syndrome
        Renal tubular acidosis NOS

■ N25.9 **Disorder resulting from impaired renal tubular function, unspecified**

● **N26 Unspecified contracted kidney**

> **Excludes1** contracted kidney due to hypertension (I12.-)
> diffuse sclerosing glomerulonephritis (N05.8.-)
> hypertensive nephrosclerosis (arteriolar) (arteriosclerotic) (I12.-)
> small kidney of unknown cause (N27.-)

    N26.1 **Atrophy of kidney (terminal)**

    N26.2 **Page kidney**

    N26.9 **Renal sclerosis, unspecified**

● **N27 Small kidney of unknown cause**

> **Includes** oligonephronia

    N27.0 **Small kidney, unilateral**

    N27.1 **Small kidney, bilateral**

■ N27.9 **Small kidney, unspecified**

● **N28 Other disorders of kidney and ureter, not elsewhere classified**

    N28.0 **Ischemia and infarction of kidney** 🦠
      Renal artery embolism
      Renal artery obstruction
      Renal artery occlusion
      Renal artery thrombosis
      Renal infarct

> **Excludes1** atherosclerosis of renal artery (extrarenal part) (I70.1)
> congenital stenosis of renal artery (Q27.1)
> Goldblatt's kidney (I70.1)

    N28.1 **Cyst of kidney, acquired**
      Cyst (multiple)(solitary) of kidney, acquired

> **Excludes1** cystic kidney disease (congenital) (Q61.-)

● N28.8 **Other specified disorders of kidney and ureter**

> **Excludes1** hydroureter (N13.4)
> ureteric stricture with hydronephrosis (N13.1)
> ureteric stricture without hydronephrosis (N13.5)

    N28.81 **Hypertrophy of kidney**

    N28.82 **Megaloureter**

    N28.83 **Nephroptosis**

    N28.84 **Pyelitis cystica** 🦠 🦠

    N28.85 **Pyeloureteritis cystica** 🦠 🦠

    N28.86 **Ureteritis cystica** 🦠 🦠

    N28.89 **Other specified disorders of kidney and ureter**

■ N28.9 **Disorder of kidney and ureter, unspecified**
      Nephropathy NOS
      Renal disease (acute) NOS
      Renal insufficiency (acute)

> **Excludes1** chronic renal insufficiency (N18.9)
> unspecified nephritic syndrome (N05-)

●▶ N29 *Other disorders of kidney and ureter in diseases classified elsewhere*

> *Code first* underlying disease, such as:
> amyloidosis (E85-)
> nephrocalcinosis (E83.5)
> schistosomiasis (B65.0-B65.9)

> **Excludes1** disorders of kidney and ureter in:
> cystinosis (E72.0)
> gonorrhea (A54.21)
> syphilis (A52.75)
> tuberculosis (A18.11)

OTHER DISEASES OF THE URINARY SYSTEM (N30-N39)

> **Excludes1** urinary infection (complicating):
> abortion or ectopic or molar pregnancy (O00-O07, O08.8)
> pregnancy, childbirth and the puerperium (O23.-, O75.3, O86.2-)

● N30 **Cystitis**

Infection of bladder and irritation in lower urinary tract

> **Use additional** code to identify infectious agent (B95-B97)

> **Excludes1** prostatocystitis (N41.3)

● N30.0 **Acute cystitis**

> **Excludes1** irradiation cystitis (N30.4-)
> trigonitis (N30.3-)

    N30.00 **Acute cystitis without hematuria** 🦠 🦠

    N30.01 **Acute cystitis with hematuria** 🦠 🦠

● N30.1 **Interstitial cystitis (chronic)**

Ongoing infection of kidney glomeruli and tubules

    N30.10 **Interstitial cystitis (chronic) without hematuria**

    N30.11 **Interstitial cystitis (chronic) with hematuria**

● N30.2 **Other chronic cystitis**

    N30.20 **Other chronic cystitis without hematuria**

    N30.21 **Other chronic cystitis with hematuria**

● N30.3 **Trigonitis**

Inflammation of triangular area of bladder (where the ureters and urethra come together)
    Urethrotrigonitis

    N30.30 **Trigonitis without hematuria**

    N30.31 **Trigonitis with hematuria**

N Newborn Age: 0   **P** Pediatric Age: 0–17   **M** Maternity DX: 12–55   **A** Adult Age: 15–124   ♀ Females Only   ♂ Males Only

 Complication\Comorbidity   Major C\C   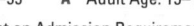 Present on Admission Requirement   Hospital-Acquired Condition

1267

CHAPTER 14 (N00-N99)

● N30.4 **Irradiation cystitis**

    N30.40 **Irradiation cystitis without hematuria** 🔖

    N30.41 **Irradiation cystitis with hematuria** 🔖

● N30.8 **Other cystitis**
    Abscess of bladder

    N30.80 **Other cystitis without hematuria**

    N30.81 **Other cystitis with hematuria**

● N30.9 **Cystitis, unspecified**

    ◻ N30.90 **Cystitis, unspecified without hematuria**

    ◻ N30.91 **Cystitis, unspecified with hematuria**

● N31 **Neuromuscular dysfunction of bladder, not elsewhere classified**

    Use additional code to identify any associated urinary incontinence (N39.3-N39.4-)

    | Excludes1 | cord bladder NOS (G95.89) |
    neurogenic bladder due to cauda equina syndrome (G83.4)
    neuromuscular dysfunction due to spinal cord lesion (G95.89)

    N31.0 **Uninhibited neuropathic bladder, not elsewhere classified**

    N31.1 **Reflex neuropathic bladder, not elsewhere classified**

    N31.2 **Flaccid neuropathic bladder, not elsewhere classified**
    Atonic (motor) (sensory) neuropathic bladder
    Diminished tone of bladder muscle
    Autonomous neuropathic bladder
    Nonreflex neuropathic bladder

    N31.8 **Other neuromuscular dysfunction of bladder**

    ◻ N31.9 **Neuromuscular dysfunction of bladder, unspecified**
    Neurogenic bladder dysfunction NOS

● N32 **Other disorders of bladder**

    | Excludes2 | calculus of bladder (N21.0) |
    cystocele (N81.1-)
    hernia or prolapse of bladder, female (N81.1-)

    N32.0 **Bladder-neck obstruction**
    Bladder-neck stenosis (acquired)

       | Excludes1 | congenital bladder-neck obstruction (Q64.3-) |

    N32.1 **Vesicointestinal fistula** 🔖
    Vesicorectal fistula

    N32.2 **Vesical fistula, not elsewhere classified** 🔖

       | Excludes1 | fistula between bladder and female genital tract (N82.0-N82.1) |

    N32.3 **Diverticulum of bladder**
    Formation of sac from a herniation of wall of bladder

       | Excludes1 | congenital diverticulum of bladder (Q64.6) |
    diverticulitis of bladder (N30.8-)

    ● N32.8 **Other specified disorders of bladder**

       N32.81 **Overactive bladder**
       Detrusor muscle hyperactivity

         | Excludes1 | frequent urination due to specified bladder condition- code to condition |

       N32.89 **Other specified disorders of bladder**
       Bladder hemorrhage
       Bladder hypertrophy
       Calcified bladder
       Contracted bladder

    ◻ N32.9 **Bladder disorder, unspecified**

● ▶ N33 *Bladder disorders in diseases classified elsewhere*
    Code first underlying disease, such as:
    schistosomiasis (B65.0-B65.9)

    | Excludes1 | bladder disorder in: |
    syphilis (A52.76)
    tuberculosis (A18.12)
    cystitis (in):
    candidal infection (B37.41)
    chlamydial (A56.01)
    diphtheritic (A36.85)
    gonorrhea (A54.01)
    syphilitic (A52.76)
    trichomonal infection (A59.03)
    neurogenic bladder (N31.-)

● N34 **Urethritis and urethral syndrome**
    Use additional code (B95-B97), to identify infectious agent

    | Excludes2 | Reiter's disease (M02.3-) |
    urethritis in diseases with a predominantly sexual mode of transmission (A50-A64)
    urethrotrigonitis (N30.3-)

    N34.0 **Urethral abscess** 🔖 🔖
    Abscess (of) Cowper's gland
    Abscess (of) Littré's gland
    Abscess (of) urethral (gland)
    Periurethral abscess

       | Excludes1 | urethral caruncle (N36.2) |

    N34.1 **Nonspecific urethritis**
    Nongonococcal urethritis
    Nonvenereal urethritis

    N34.2 **Other urethritis**
    Inflammation of urethra
    Meatitis, urethral
    Postmenopausal urethritis
    Ulcer of urethra (meatus)
    Urethritis NOS

    ◻ N34.3 **Urethral syndrome, unspecified**

● N35 **Urethral stricture**
    Narrowing of lumen of urethra caused by scarring due to infection or injury

    | Excludes1 | congenital urethral stricture (Q64.3-) |
    postprocedural urethral stricture (N99.1-)

    ● N35.0 **Post-traumatic urethral stricture**
    Urethral stricture due to injury

       | Excludes1 | postprocedural urethral stricture (N99.1-) |

       ● N35.01 **Post-traumatic urethral stricture, male**

          N35.010 **Post-traumatic urethral stricture, male, meatal** ♂

          N35.011 **Post-traumatic bulbous urethral stricture**

          N35.012 **Post-traumatic membranous urethral stricture**

          N35.013 **Post-traumatic anterior urethral stricture**

          ◻ N35.014 **Post-traumatic urethral stricture, male, unspecified** ♂

       ● N35.02 **Post-traumatic urethral stricture, female**

          N35.021 **Urethral stricture due to childbirth** ♀

          N35.028 **Other post-traumatic urethral stricture, female** ♀

● Unacceptable Principal Diagnosis   ● Use Additional Character(s)   ◻ Unspecified   ▶ Manifestation Code

1268   **OGCR** Official Guidelines for Coding and Reporting | Excludes 1 | | Excludes 2 | | Includes | | Use additional | | Code first | | Code also |

CHAPTER 14 (N00-N99)

● **N35.1** **Postinfective urethral stricture, not elsewhere classified**

     Excludes1   urethral stricture associated with schistosomiasis (B65.-, N29)
               gonococcal urethral stricture (A54.01)
               syphilitic urethral stricture (A52.76)

   ● **N35.11** **Postinfective urethral stricture, not elsewhere classified, male**

     N35.111 **Postinfective urethral stricture, not elsewhere classified, male, meatal** ♂

     N35.112 **Postinfective bulbous urethral stricture, not elsewhere classified**

     N35.113 **Postinfective membranous urethral stricture, not elsewhere classified**

     N35.114 **Postinfective anterior urethral stricture, not elsewhere classified**

     ▪ **N35.119** **Postinfective urethral stricture, not elsewhere classified, male, unspecified** ♂

   N35.12 **Postinfective urethral stricture, not elsewhere classified, female** ♀

  N35.8 **Other urethral stricture**

     Excludes1   postprocedural urethral stricture (N99.1-)

  ▪ **N35.9** **Urethral stricture, unspecified**

● **N36** **Other disorders of urethra**

  N36.0 **Urethral fistula** 🦠
     Urethroperineal fistula
     Urethrorectal fistula
     Urinary fistula NOS

     Excludes1   urethroscrotal fistula (N50.8)
               urethrovaginal fistula (N82.1)
               urethrovesicovaginal fistula (N82.1)

  N36.1 **Urethral diverticulum**

  N36.2 **Urethral caruncle**

  ● **N36.4** **Urethral functional and muscular disorders**

     Use additional code to identify associated urinary stress incontinence (N39.3)

     N36.41 **Hypermobility of urethra**

     N36.42 **Intrinsic sphincter deficiency (ISD)**

     N36.43 **Combined hypermobility of urethra and intrinsic sphincter deficiency**

     N36.44 **Muscular disorders of urethra**
          Bladder sphincter dyssynergy

  N36.5 **Urethral false passage**

  N36.8 **Other specified disorders of urethra**

  ▪ **N36.9** **Urethral disorder, unspecified**

● ◗ *N37* *Urethral disorders in diseases classified elsewhere*

     Code first underlying disease

     Excludes1   urethritis (in):
          candidal infection (B37.41)
          chlamydial (A56.01)
          gonorrhea (A54.01)
          syphilis (A52.76)
          trichomonal infection (A59.03)
          tuberculosis (A18.13)

● **N39** **Other disorders of urinary system**

     Excludes2   hematuria NOS (R31-)
               recurrent or persistent hematuria (N02.-)
               recurrent or persistent hematuria with specified morphological lesion (N02.-)
               proteinuria NOS (R80.-)

  N39.0 **Urinary tract infection, site not specified** 🦠 🦠

     Use additional code (B95-B97), to identify infectious agent

     Excludes1   candidiasis of urinary tract (B37.4-)
               neonatal urinary tract infection (P39.3)
               urinary tract infection of specified site, such as:
                 cystitis (N30.-)
                 urethritis (N34.-)

  N39.3 **Stress incontinence (female) (male)**

     Code also any associated overactive bladder (N32.81)

     Excludes1   mixed incontinence (N39.46)

  ● **N39.4** **Other specified urinary incontinence**

     Code also any associated overactive bladder (N32.81)

     Excludes1   enuresis NOS (R32)
               functional urinary incontinence (R39.81)
               urinary incontinence associated with cognitive impairment (R39.81)
               urinary incontinence NOS (R32)
               urinary incontinence of nonorganic origin (F98.0)

     N39.41 **Urge incontinence**

         Excludes1   mixed incontinence (N39.46)

     N39.42 **Incontinence without sensory awareness**

     N39.43 **Post-void dribbling**

     N39.44 **Nocturnal enuresis**

     N39.45 **Continuous leakage**

     N39.46 **Mixed incontinence**
          Urge and stress incontinence

   ● **N39.49** **Other specified urinary incontinence**

     N39.490 **Overflow incontinence**

     N39.498 **Other specified urinary incontinence**
          Reflex incontinence
          Total incontinence

  N39.8 **Other specified disorders of urinary system**

  ▪ **N39.9** **Disorder of urinary system, unspecified**

N Newborn Age: 0   **P** Pediatric Age: 0–17   **M** Maternity DX: 12–55   **A** Adult Age: 15–124   ♀ Females Only   ♂ Males Only

🦠 Complication\Comorbidity   🦠 Major C\C   🦠 Present on Admission Requirement   🦠 Hospital-Acquired Condition

1269

CHAPTER 14 (N00-N99)

DISEASES OF MALE GENITAL ORGANS (N40-N53)

(See Plate 387 on page NAP-5.)

● N40 **Enlarged prostate**

    Includes   adenofibromatous hypertrophy of prostate
        benign hypertrophy of the prostate
           Enlargement of prostate gland usually
              occurring with age and causing
              obstructed urine flow
        benign prostatic hyperplasia
        benign prostatic hypertrophy
        BPH
        nodular prostate
        polyp of prostate

    Excludes1 benign neoplasms of prostate (adenoma,
        benign) (fibroadenoma) (fibroma)
        (myoma) (D29.1)
        malignant neoplasm of prostate (C61)

  N40.0 **Enlarged prostate without lower urinary tract
    symptoms** ♂   A
      Enlarged prostate without LUTS
      Enlarged prostate NOS

  N40.1 **Enlarged prostate with lower urinary tract
    symptoms (LUTS)** ♂   A
      Enlarged prostate with LUTS

      Use additional code for associated symptoms,
        when specified:
        incomplete bladder emptying (R39.14)
        nocturia (R35.1)
        straining on urination (R39.16)
        urinary frequency (R35.0)
        urinary hesitancy (R39.11)
        urinary incontinence (N39.4-)
        urinary obstruction (N13.8)
        urinary retention (R33.8)
        urinary urgency (R39.15)
        weak urinary stream (R39.12)

  N40.2 **Nodular prostate without lower urinary tract
    symptoms** ♂
      Nodular prostate without LUTS

  N40.3 **Nodular prostate with lower urinary tract
    symptoms** ♂
      Use additional code for associated symptoms,
        when specified:
        incomplete bladder emptying (R39.14)
        nocturia (R35.1)
        straining on urination (R39.16)
        urinary frequency (R35.0)
        urinary hesitancy (R39.11)
        urinary incontinence (N39.4-)
        urinary obstruction (N13.8)
        urinary retention (R33.8)
        urinary urgency (R39.15)
        weak urinary stream (R39.12)

● N41 **Inflammatory diseases of prostate**

    Use additional code (B95-B97), to identify infectious
      agent

  N41.0 **Acute prostatitis** ♂ 🦠   A
  N41.1 **Chronic prostatitis** ♂   A
  N41.2 **Abscess of prostate** ♂ 🦠   A
  N41.3 **Prostatocystitis** ♂   A
  N41.4 **Granulomatous prostatitis** ♂   A
  N41.8 **Other inflammatory diseases of prostate** ♂ A
  ■ N41.9 **Inflammatory disease of prostate, unspecified** ♂ A
      Prostatitis NOS

● N42 **Other and unspecified disorders of prostate**

  N42.0 **Calculus of prostate** ♂   A
      Prostatic stone

  N42.1 **Congestion and hemorrhage of prostate** ♂ A
      Excludes1 enlarged prostate (N40.-)
           hematuria (R31.-)
           hyperplasia of prostate (N40.-)
           inflammatory diseases of prostate
             (N41.-)

  N42.3 **Dysplasia of prostate** ♂
      Prostatic intraepithelial neoplasia I (PIN I)
      Prostatic intraepithelial neoplasia II (PIN II)
      Excludes1 prostatic intraepithelial neoplasia III
           (PIN III) (D07.5)

● N42.8 **Other specified disorders of prostate**

  N42.81 **Prostatodynia syndrome** ♂   A
      Painful prostate syndrome
  N42.82 **Prostatosis syndrome** ♂   A
  N42.83 **Cyst of prostate** ♂
  N42.89 **Other specified disorders of prostate** ♂ A
■ N42.9 **Disorder of prostate, unspecified** ♂   A

● N43 **Hydrocele and spermatocele**

    Includes   hydrocele of spermatic cord, testis or tunica
        vaginalis
    Excludes1 congenital hydrocele (P83.5)

  N43.0 **Encysted hydrocele** ♂
  N43.1 **Infected hydrocele** ♂ 🦠
      Use additional code (B95-B97), to identify
        infectious agent

  N43.2 **Other hydrocele** ♂
■ N43.3 **Hydrocele, unspecified** ♂
● N43.4 **Spermatocele of epididymis**
      Spermatic cyst

  ■ N43.40 **Spermatocele of epididymis,
    unspecified** ♂
  N43.41 **Spermatocele of epididymis, single** ♂
  N43.42 **Spermatocele of epididymis, multiple** ♂

Item 14–7 **Hydrocele** is a sac of fluid accumulating in the testes membrane.

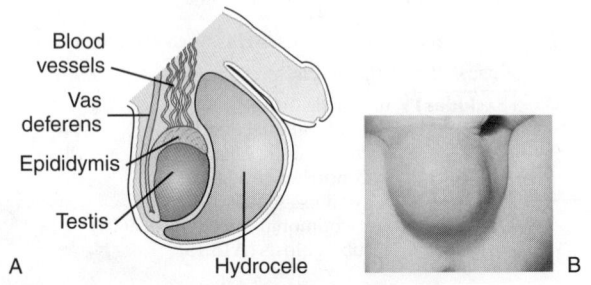

  Blood
  vessels
  Vas
  deferens
  Epididymis
  Testis
  A   Hydrocele   B

Figure 14-6 **A.** Hydrocele. **B.** Newborn with large right hydrocele. (**B** from Behrman: Nelson Textbook of Pediatrics, 17th ed. 2004, Saunders, An Imprint of Elsevier.)

● Unacceptable Principal Diagnosis   ● Use Additional Character(s)   ■ Unspecified   ▶ Manifestation Code
OGCR Official Guidelines for Coding and Reporting   Excludes 1   Excludes 2   Includes   Use additional   Code first   Code also

● **N44   Noninflammatory disorders of testis**
  ● **N44.0   Torsion of testis**
    ◼ **N44.00   Torsion of testis, unspecified** ♂ 🦠
       N44.01   Extravaginal torsion of spermatic cord ♂ 🦠
       N44.02   Intravaginal torsion of spermatic cord ♂ 🦠
         Torsion of spermatic cord NOS
       N44.03   Torsion of appendix testis ♂ 🦠
       N44.04   Torsion of appendix epididymis ♂ 🦠
   N44.1   Cyst of tunica albuginea testis ♂
   N44.2   Benign cyst of testis ♂
   N44.8   Other noninflammatory disorders of the testis ♂

● **N45   Orchitis and epididymitis**
     Orchitis is inflammation of one or both of the testes as a
     result of mumps or other infection, trauma, or metastasis.
     Epididymitis is inflammation of the tubular structure
     that connects the testicle with the vas deferens.
     Use additional code (B95-B97), to identify infectious
     agent
   N45.1   Epididymitis ♂
   N45.2   Orchitis ♂
   N45.3   Epididymo-orchitis ♂
   N45.4   Abscess of epididymis or testis ♂ 🦠

● **N46   Male infertility**
     Excludes1   vasectomy status (Z98.52)
  ● **N46.0   Azoospermia**
     Absolute male infertility
     Male infertility due to germinal (cell) aplasia
     Male infertility due to spermatogenic arrest
     (complete)
       N46.01   Organic azoospermia ♂   A
         Azoospermia NOS
    ● **N46.02   Azoospermia due to extratesticular causes**
       Code also associated cause
       N46.021   Azoospermia due to drug
         therapy ♂   A
       N46.022   Azoospermia due to infection ♂ A
       N46.023   Azoospermia due to obstruction
         of efferent ducts ♂   A
       N46.024   Azoospermia due to radiation ♂ A
       N46.025   Azoospermia due to systemic
         disease ♂   A
       N46.029   Azoospermia due to other
         extratesticular causes ♂   A
  ● **N46.1   Oligospermia**
     Male infertility due to germinal cell desquamation
     Male infertility due to hypospermatogenesis
     Male infertility due to incomplete spermatogenic
     arrest
       N46.11   Organic oligospermia ♂   A
         Oligospermia NOS

● **N46.12   Oligospermia due to extratesticular causes**
     Code also associated cause
       N46.121   Oligospermia due to drug
         therapy ♂   A
       N46.122   Oligospermia due to infection ♂ A
       N46.123   Oligospermia due to obstruction
         of efferent ducts ♂   A
       N46.124   Oligospermia due to radiation ♂ A
       N46.125   Oligospermia due to systemic
         disease ♂   A
       N46.129   Oligospermia due to other
         extratesticular causes ♂   A
   N46.8   Other male infertility ♂   A
  ◼ **N46.9   Male infertility, unspecified** ♂   A

● **N47   Disorders of prepuce**
   N47.0   Adherent prepuce, newborn   N
   N47.1   Phimosis ♂
   N47.2   Paraphimosis ♂
   N47.3   Deficient foreskin ♂
   N47.4   Benign cyst of prepuce ♂
   N47.5   Adhesions of prepuce and glans penis ♂
   N47.6   Balanoposthitis ♂
     Use additional code (B95-B97), to identify
     infectious agent
     Excludes1   balanitis (N48.1)
   N47.7   Other inflammatory diseases of prepuce ♂
     Use additional code (B95-B97), to identify
     infectious agent
   N47.8   Other disorders of prepuce ♂

● **N48   Other disorders of penis**
   N48.0   Leukoplakia of penis ♂
     Balanitis xerotica obliterans
     Kraurosis of penis
     Lichen sclerosus of external male genital organs
     Excludes1   carcinoma in situ of penis (D07.4)
   N48.1   Balanitis ♂
     Use additional code (B95-B97), to identify
     infectious agent
     Excludes1   amebic balanitis (A06.8)
       balanitis xerotica obliterans (N48.0)
       candidal balanitis (B37.42)
       gonococcal balanitis (A54.23)
       herpesviral [herpes simplex]
         balanitis (A60.01)
  ● **N48.2   Other inflammatory disorders of penis**
     Use additional code (B95-B97), to identify
     infectious agent
     Excludes1   balanitis (N48.1)
       balanitis xerotica obliterans (N48.0)
       balanoposthitis (N47.6)
       N48.21   Abscess of corpus cavernosum and penis ♂
       N48.22   Cellulitis of corpus cavernosum and
         penis ♂
       N48.29   Other inflammatory disorders of penis ♂

CHAPTER 14 (N00-N99)

Item 14-8 Male infertility is the inability of the female sex partner to conceive after one year of unprotected intercourse.

   Azoospermia is no sperm ejaculated and **oligospermia** is few sperm ejaculated—both resulting in infertility. Extratesticular causes such as injury, infections, radiation, and chemotherapy may also cause male infertility.

N   Newborn Age: 0   P   Pediatric Age: 0–17   M   Maternity DX: 12–55   A   Adult Age: 15–124   ♀   Females Only   ♂   Males Only

🦠 Complication\Comorbidity   🦠 Major C\C   ■ Present on Admission Requirement   🦠 Hospital-Acquired Condition

CHAPTER 14 (N00-N99)

● **N48.3 Priapism**
Painful erection
Code first underlying cause

▪ **N48.30 Priapism, unspecified** ♂ 🕭

N48.31 Priapism due to trauma ♂ 🕭

▸ **N48.32** *Priapism due to disease classified elsewhere* ♂ 🕭

N48.33 Priapism, drug-induced ♂ 🕭

N48.39 Other priapism ♂ 🕭

N48.5 Ulcer of penis ♂

N48.6 Induration penis plastica ♂
Peyronie's disease
Plastic induration of penis

● **N48.8 Other specified disorders of penis**

N48.81 Thrombosis of superficial vein of penis ♂

N48.82 Acquired torsion of penis ♂
Acquired torsion of penis NOS
> **Excludes1**   congenital torsion of penis (Q55.63)

N48.83 Acquired buried penis ♂
> **Excludes1**   congenital hidden penis (Q55.64)

N48.89 Other specified disorders of penis ♂

▪ **N48.9 Disorder of penis, unspecified** ♂

● **N49 Inflammatory disorders of male genital organs, not elsewhere classified**
Use additional code (B95-B97), to identify infectious agent
> **Excludes1**   inflammation of penis (N48.1, N48.2-)
> orchitis and epididymitis (N45.-)

N49.0 Inflammatory disorders of seminal vesicle ♂
Vesiculitis NOS

N49.1 Inflammatory disorders of spermatic cord, tunica vaginalis and vas deferens ♂
Vasitis

N49.2 Inflammatory disorders of scrotum ♂

N49.3 Fournier gangrene ♂

N49.8 Inflammatory disorders of other specified male genital organs ♂
Inflammation of multiple sites in male genital organs

▪ **N49.9 Inflammatory disorder of unspecified male genital organ** ♂
Abscess of unspecified male genital organ
Boil of unspecified male genital organ
Carbuncle of unspecified male genital organ
Cellulitis of unspecified male genital organ

Figure 14-7   **A.** Torsion of testis. **B.** Torsion of testis. (**B** from Kumar: Robbins and Catran: Pathologic Basis of Disease, 7th ed. 2005, Saunders, An Imprint of Elsevier.)

● **N50 Other and unspecified disorders of male genital organs**
> **Excludes2**   torsion of testis (N44.0-)

N50.0 Atrophy of testis ♂

N50.1 Vascular disorders of male genital organs ♂
Hematocele, NOS, of male genital organs
Hemorrhage of male genital organs
Thrombosis of male genital organs

N50.3 Cyst of epididymis ♂

N50.8 Other specified disorders of male genital organs ♂
Atrophy of scrotum, seminal vesicle, spermatic cord, tunica vaginalis and vas deferens
Edema of scrotum, seminal vesicle, spermatic cord, testis, tunica vaginalis and vas deferens
Hypertrophy of scrotum, seminal vesicle, spermatic cord, testis, tunica vaginalis and vas deferens
Ulcer of scrotum, seminal vesicle, spermatic cord, testis, tunica vaginalis and vas deferens
Chylocele, tunica vaginalis (nonfilarial) NOS
Urethroscrotal fistula
Stricture of spermatic cord, tunica vaginalis, and vas deferens

▪ **N50.9 Disorder of male genital organs, unspecified** ♂

● ▸ **N51** *Disorders of male genital organs in diseases classified elsewhere* ♂
Code first underlying disease, such as:
filariasis (B74.0-B74.9)
> **Excludes1**   amebic balanitis (A06.8)
> candidal balanitis (B37.42)
> gonococcal balanitis (A54.23)
> gonococcal prostatitis (A54.22)
> herpesviral [herpes simplex] balanitis (A60.01)
> trichomonal prostatitis (A59.02)
> tuberculous prostatitis (A18.14)

● **N52 Male erectile dysfunction**
> **Excludes1**   psychogenic impotence (F52.21)

● **N52.0 Vasculogenic erectile dysfunction**

N52.01 Erectile dysfunction due to arterial insufficiency ♂   A

N52.02 Corporo-venous occlusive erectile dysfunction ♂   A

N52.03 Combined arterial insufficiency and corporo-venous occlusive erectile dysfunction ♂   A

Item 14–9 Seminal vesiculitis is an inflammation of the seminal vesicle. Spermatocele is a benign cystic accumulation of sperm arising from the head of the epididymis. Torsion of the testis is a medical emergency occurring most commonly in boys 7 to 12 years of age and results from a congenital abnormality of the covering of the testis allowing the testis to twist within its sac and cutting off the blood supply to the testis.

● Unacceptable Principal Diagnosis   ● Use Additional Character(s)   ▪ Unspecified   ▸ Manifestation Code

1272   **OGCR** Official Guidelines for Coding and Reporting   Excludes 1   Excludes 2   Includes   Use additional   Code first   Code also

●▶N52.1 *Erectile dysfunction due to diseases classified elsewhere* ♂   A
      Code first underlying disease

N52.2 **Drug-induced erectile dysfunction** ♂   A

●N52.3 **Post-surgical erectile dysfunction**

    N52.31 **Erectile dysfunction following radical prostatectomy** ♂   A

    N52.32 **Erectile dysfunction following radical cystectomy** ♂   A

    N52.33 **Erectile dysfunction following urethral surgery** ♂   A

    N52.34 **Erectile dysfunction following simple prostatectomy** ♂   A

    N52.39 **Other post-surgical erectile dysfunction** ♂   A

N52.8 **Other male erectile dysfunction** ♂   A

▪N52.9 **Male erectile dysfunction, unspecified** ♂   A
      Impotence NOS

●N53 **Other male sexual dysfunction**
    Excludes1   psychogenic sexual dysfunction (F52.-)

●N53.1 **Ejaculatory dysfunction**
      Excludes1   premature ejaculation (F52.4)

    N53.11 **Retarded ejaculation** ♂

    N53.12 **Painful ejaculation** ♂

    N53.13 **Anejaculatory orgasm** ♂

    N53.14 **Retrograde ejaculation** ♂

    N53.19 **Other ejaculatory dysfunction** ♂
      Ejaculatory dysfunction NOS

N53.8 **Other male sexual dysfunction** ♂

▪N53.9 **Unspecified male sexual dysfunction** ♂

DISORDERS OF BREAST (N60-N65)

    Excludes1   disorders of breast associated with childbirth (O91-O92)

●N60 **Benign mammary dysplasia**
    Benign lumpiness of breast
    Includes   fibrocystic mastopathy

●N60.0 **Solitary cyst of breast**
    Cyst of breast

    N60.01 **Solitary cyst of right breast**

    N60.02 **Solitary cyst of left breast**

    ▪N60.09 **Solitary cyst of unspecified breast**

●N60.1 **Diffuse cystic mastopathy**
    Cystic breast
    Fibrocystic disease of breast
      Excludes1   diffuse cystic mastopathy with epithelial proliferation (N60.3-)

    N60.11 **Diffuse cystic mastopathy of right breast** A

    N60.12 **Diffuse cystic mastopathy of left breast** A

    ▪N60.19 **Diffuse cystic mastopathy of unspecified breast** A

●N60.2 **Fibroadenosis of breast**
    Adenofibrosis of breast
      Excludes2   fibroadenoma of breast (D24.-)

    N60.21 **Fibroadenosis of right breast**

    N60.22 **Fibroadenosis of left breast**

    ▪N60.29 **Fibroadenosis of unspecified breast**

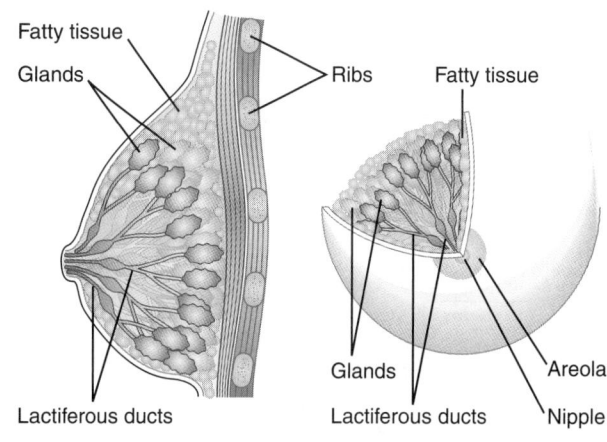

Figure 14-8   Breast.

●N60.3 **Fibrosclerosis of breast**
    Cystic mastopathy with epithelial proliferation

    N60.31 **Fibrosclerosis of right breast**

    N60.32 **Fibrosclerosis of left breast**

    ▪N60.39 **Fibrosclerosis of unspecified breast**

●N60.4 **Mammary duct ectasia**

    N60.41 **Mammary duct ectasia of right breast**

    N60.42 **Mammary duct ectasia of left breast**

    ▪N60.49 **Mammary duct ectasia of unspecified breast**

●N60.8 **Other benign mammary dysplasias**

    N60.81 **Other benign mammary dysplasias of right breast**

    N60.82 **Other benign mammary dysplasias of left breast**

    ▪N60.89 **Other benign mammary dysplasias of unspecified breast**

●N60.9 **Unspecified benign mammary dysplasia**

    ▪N60.91 **Unspecified benign mammary dysplasia of right breast**

    ▪N60.92 **Unspecified benign mammary dysplasia of left breast**

    ▪N60.99 **Unspecified benign mammary dysplasia of unspecified breast**

N61 **Inflammatory disorders of breast**
    Abscess (acute) (chronic) (nonpuerperal) of areola
    Abscess (acute) (chronic) (nonpuerperal) of breast
    Carbuncle of breast
    Infective mastitis (acute) (subacute) (nonpuerperal)
    Mastitis (acute) (subacute) (nonpuerperal) NOS
    Excludes1   inflammatory carcinoma of breast (C50.9)
      inflammatory disorder of breast associated with childbirth (O91.-)
      neonatal infective mastitis (P39.0)
      thrombophlebitis of breast [Mondor's disease] (I80.8)

N Newborn Age: 0   **P** Pediatric Age: 0–17   **M** Maternity DX: 12–55   **A** Adult Age: 15–124   ♀ Females Only   ♂ Males Only

🅒 Complication\Comorbidity   🅜 Major C\C   🄿 Present on Admission Requirement   🅗 Hospital-Acquired Condition

1273

CHAPTER 14 (N00-N99)

N62   Hypertrophy of breast
     Gynecomastia
     Hypertrophy of breast NOS
     Massive pubertal hypertrophy of breast

     Excludes1   breast engorgement of newborn (P83.4)
                 disproportion of reconstructed breast
                    (N65.1)

N63   Unspecified lump in breast
     Nodule(s) NOS in breast

N64   Other disorders of breast

     Excludes2   mechanical complication of breast prosthesis
                 and implant (T85.4-)

     N64.0   Fissure and fistula of nipple

     N64.1   Fat necrosis of breast
            Fat necrosis (segmental) of breast

            Code first breast necrosis due to breast graft (T85.89)

     N64.2   Atrophy of breast

     N64.3   Galactorrhea not associated with childbirth
            Excessive or spontaneous flow of milk

     N64.4   Mastodynia

     N64.5   Other signs and symptoms in breast

            Excludes2   abnormal findings on diagnostic
                       imaging of breast (R92.-)

            N64.51   Induration of breast

            N64.52   Nipple discharge

                 Excludes1   abnormal findings in nipple
                           discharge (R89.-)

            N64.53   Retraction of nipple

            N64.59   Other signs and symptoms in breast

     N64.8   Other specified disorders of breast

            N64.81   Ptosis of breast   A

                 Excludes1   ptosis of native breast in
                           relation to reconstructed
                           breast (N65.1)

            N64.82   Hypoplasia of breast   A
                 Micromastia

                 Excludes1   congenital absence of breast
                           (Q83.0)

                           hypoplasia of native
                           breast in relation to
                           reconstructed breast
                           (N65.1)

            N64.89   Other specified disorders of breast
                 Galactocele
                 Subinvolution of breast (postlactational)

     N64.9   Disorder of breast, unspecified

N65   Deformity and disproportion of reconstructed breast

     N65.0   Deformity of reconstructed breast   A
            Contour irregularity in reconstructed breast
            Excess tissue in reconstructed breast
            Misshapen reconstructed breast

     N65.1   Disproportion of reconstructed breast   A
            Breast asymmetry between native breast and
                 reconstructed breast
            Disproportion between native breast and
                 reconstructed breast

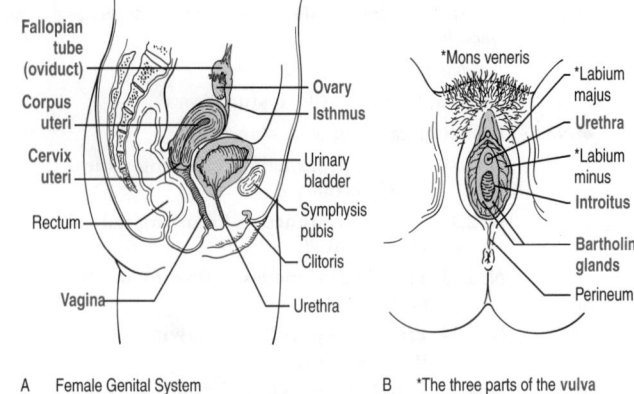

A   Female Genital System   B   *The three parts of the vulva

Figure 14-9   A. Female genital system. **B.** External female genital system. (From Buck CJ: Step-by-Step Medical Coding, 2010 ed. Philadelphia, WB Saunders, 2010.)

Item 14–10 Salpingitis is an infection of one or both fallopian tubes. **Oophoritis** is an infection of one or both ovaries.

INFLAMMATORY DISEASES OF FEMALE PELVIC ORGANS (N70-N77)

     Excludes1   inflammatory diseases of female pelvic
                 organs complicating:
                 abortion or ectopic or molar pregnancy
                     (O00-O07, O08.0)
                 pregnancy, childbirth and the puerperium
                     (O23.-, O75.3, O85, O86.-)

(See Plate 360 on page NAP-32.)

N70   Salpingitis and oophoritis
     Oophoritis = inflammation of ovary
     Salpingitis = inflammation of falloplan tube

     Includes   abscess (of) fallopian tube
               abscess (of) ovary
               pyosalpinx
               salpingo-oophoritis
               tubo-ovarian abscess
               tubo-ovarian inflammatory disease

     Use additional code (B95-B97), to identify infectious
            agent

     Excludes1   gonococcal infection (A54.24)
                 tuberculous infection (A18.17)

     N70.0   Acute salpingitis and oophoritis

            N70.01   Acute salpingitis ♀

            N70.02   Acute oophoritis ♀

            N70.03   Acute salpingitis and oophoritis ♀

     N70.1   Chronic salpingitis and oophoritis
            Hydrosalpinx

            N70.11   Chronic salpingitis ♀

            N70.12   Chronic oophoritis ♀

            N70.13   Chronic salpingitis and oophoritis ♀

     N70.9   Salpingitis and oophoritis, unspecified

            N70.91   Salpingitis, unspecified ♀

            N70.92   Oophoritis, unspecified ♀

            N70.93   Salpingitis and oophoritis, unspecified ♀

● Unacceptable Principal Diagnosis   ● Use Additional Character(s)   ▪ Unspecified   ▶ Manifestation Code

1274   **OGCR**   Official Guidelines for Coding and Reporting   Excludes 1   Excludes 2   Includes   Use additional   Code first   Code also

● N71   **Inflammatory disease of uterus, except cervix**

   Includes   endo (myo) metritis
                  metritis
                  myometritis
                  pyometra
                  uterine abscess

   Use additional code (B95-B97), to identify infectious
   agent

   Excludes1   hyperplastic endometritis (N85.0-)
                   infection of uterus following delivery (O85,
                   O86-)

   N71.0   **Acute inflammatory disease of uterus** ♀ 🎗
   N71.1   **Chronic inflammatory disease of uterus** ♀
   ■ N71.9   **Inflammatory disease of uterus, unspecified** ♀

N72   **Inflammatory disease of cervix uteri** ♀

   Includes   cervicitis (with or without erosion or
                  ectropion)
                  endocervicitis (with or without erosion or
                  ectropion)
                  exocervicitis (with or without erosion or
                  ectropion)

   Use additional code (B95-B97), to identify infectious
   agent

   Excludes1   erosion and ectropion of cervix without
                   cervicitis (N86)

● N73   **Other female pelvic inflammatory diseases**

   Use additional code (B95-B97), to identify infectious
   agent

   N73.0   **Acute parametritis and pelvic cellulitis** ♀ 🎗
           Abscess of broad ligament
           Abscess of parametrium
           Pelvic cellulitis, female

   N73.1   **Chronic parametritis and pelvic cellulitis** ♀
           Any condition in N73.0 specified as chronic

           Excludes1   tuberculous parametritis and pelvic
                           cellultis (A18.17)

   ■ N73.2   **Unspecified parametritis and pelvic cellulitis** ♀
           Any condition in N73.0 unspecified whether acute
           or chronic

   N73.3   **Female acute pelvic peritonitis** ♀ 🎗
   N73.4   **Female chronic pelvic peritonitis** ♀ 🎗

           Excludes1   tuberculous pelvic (female)
                           peritonitis (A18.17)

   ■ N73.5   **Female pelvic peritonitis, unspecified** ♀
   N73.6   **Female pelvic peritoneal adhesions
           (postinfective)** ♀

           Excludes2   postprocedural pelvic peritoneal
                           adhesions (N99.4)

   N73.8   **Other specified female pelvic inflammatory
           diseases** ♀

   ■ N73.9   **Female pelvic inflammatory disease, unspecified** ♀
           Female pelvic infection or inflammation NOS

●❱ N74   *Female pelvic inflammatory disorders in diseases classified
          elsewhere* ♀

   Code first underlying disease

   Excludes1   cervicitis:
                   chlamydial (A56.02)
                   gonococcal (A54.03)
                   herpesviral [herpes simplex] (A60.03)
                   syphilitic (A52.76)
                   trichomonal (A59.09)
                   tuberculous (A18.16)
                   pelvic inflammatory disease:
                   chlamydial (A56.11)
                   gonococcal (A54.24)
                   herpesviral [herpes simplex] (A60.09)
                   syphilitic (A52.76)
                   tuberculous (A18.17)

● N75   **Diseases of Bartholin's gland**

   N75.0   **Cyst of Bartholin's gland** ♀
           Cysts filled with liquid or semisolid material.

   N75.1   **Abscess of Bartholin's gland** ♀ 🎗
           Localized collection of pus

   N75.8   **Other diseases of Bartholin's gland** ♀
           Bartholinitis

   ■ N75.9   **Disease of Bartholin's gland, unspecified** ♀

● N76   **Other inflammation of vagina and vulva**

   Use additional code (B95-B97), to identify infectious
   agent

   Excludes2   senile (atrophic) vaginitis (N95.2)
                   vulvar vestibulitis (N94.810)

   N76.0   **Acute vaginitis** ♀
           Acute vulvovaginitis
           Vaginitis NOS
           Vulvovaginitis NOS

   N76.1   **Subacute and chronic vaginitis** ♀
           Chronic vulvovaginitis
           Subacute vulvovaginitis

   N76.2   **Acute vulvitis** ♀
           Vulvitis NOS

   N76.3   **Subacute and chronic vulvitis** ♀
   N76.4   **Abscess of vulva** ♀ 🎗
           Furuncle of vulva

   N76.5   **Ulceration of vagina** ♀
   N76.6   **Ulceration of vulva** ♀
   ● N76.8   **Other specified inflammation of vagina and vulva**

           N76.81   **Mucositis (ulcerative) of vagina and
                    vulva** ♀ 🎗

                    Code also type of associated therapy,
                    such as:
                    antineoplastic and immunosuppressive
                    drugs (T45.1x-)
                    radiological procedure and
                    radiotherapy (Y84.2)

                    Excludes2   gastrointestinal mucositis
                                    (ulcerative) (K92.81)
                                    nasal mucositis (ulcerative)
                                    (J34.81)
                                    oral mucositis (ulcerative)
                                    (K12.3-)

           N76.89   **Other specified inflammation of vagina
                    and vulva** ♀

N Newborn Age: 0   **P** Pediatric Age: 0–17   **M** Maternity DX: 12–55   **A** Adult Age: 15–124   ♀ Females Only   ♂ Males Only

🎗 Complication\Comorbidity   🎗 Major C\C   🎗 Present on Admission Requirement   🎗 Hospital-Acquired Condition

1275

CHAPTER 14 (N00-N99)

● N77   **Vulvovaginal ulceration and inflammation in diseases classified elsewhere**

   ● ◗ **N77.0**   *Ulceration of vulva in diseases classified elsewhere* ♀

       Code first underlying disease, such as:
         Behçet's disease (M35.2)

       | **Excludes1** | ulceration of vulva in gonococcal infection (A54.02)
           ulceration of vulva in herpesviral [herpes simplex] infection (A60.04)
           ulceration of vulva in syphilis (A51.0)
           ulceration of vulva in tuberculosis (A18.18)

   ● ◗ **N77.1**   *Vaginitis, vulvitis and vulvovaginitis in diseases classified elsewhere* ♀

       Code first underlying disease, such as:
         pinworm (B80)

       | **Excludes1** | vaginitis, vulvitis and vulvovaginitis (in):
           candidiasis (B37.3)
           chlamydial (A56.02)
           gonococcal infection (A54.02)
           herpesviral [herpes simplex] infection (A60.04)
           syphilitic, early (A51.0)
           syphilitic, late (A52.76)
           trichomonal (A59.01)
           tuberculous (A18.18)

NONINFLAMMATORY DISORDERS OF FEMALE GENITAL TRACT (N80-N98)

● **N80**   **Endometriosis**

   N80.0   **Endometriosis of uterus** ♀
      Adenomyosis
      | **Excludes1** | stromal endometriosis (D39.0)

   N80.1   **Endometriosis of ovary** ♀

   N80.2   **Endometriosis of fallopian tube** ♀

   N80.3   **Endometriosis of pelvic peritoneum** ♀

   N80.4   **Endometriosis of rectovaginal septum and vagina** ♀

   N80.5   **Endometriosis of intestine** ♀

   N80.6   **Endometriosis in cutaneous scar** ♀

   N80.8   **Other endometriosis** ♀

   ■ **N80.9**   **Endometriosis, unspecified** ♀

● **N81**   **Female genital prolapse**

   | **Excludes1** | genital prolapse complicating pregnancy, labor or delivery (O34.5-)
         prolapse and hernia of ovary and fallopian tube (N83.4)
         prolapse of vaginal vault after hysterectomy (N99.3)

   N81.0   **Urethrocele** ♀

      | **Excludes1** | urethrocele with cystocele (N81.1-)
         urethrocele with prolapse of uterus (N81.2-N81.4)

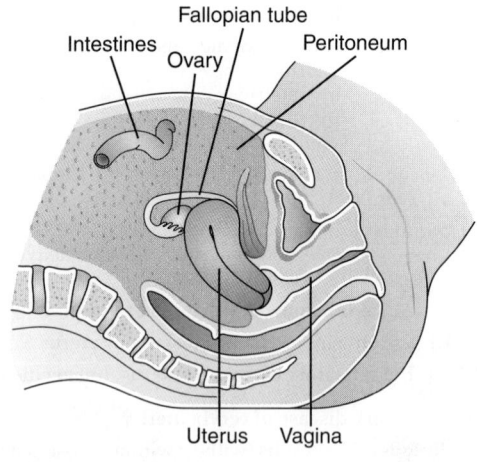

Figure 14-10   Sites of potential endometrial implants.

● **N81.1**   **Cystocele**
      Cystocele with urethrocele
      Cystourethrocele

      | **Excludes1** | cystocele with prolapse of uterus (N81.2-N81.4)

   ■ **N81.10**   **Cystocele, unspecified** ♀
      Prolapse of (anterior) vaginal wall NOS

   N81.11   **Cystocele, midline** ♀

   N81.12   **Cystocele, lateral** ♀
      Paravaginal cystocele

   N81.2   **Incomplete uterovaginal prolapse** ♀
      First degree uterine prolapse
      Prolapse of cervix NOS
      Second degree uterine prolapse
      | **Excludes1** | cervical stump prolaspe (N81.85)

   N81.3   **Complete uterovaginal prolapse** ♀
      Procidentia (uteri) NOS
      Third degree uterine prolapse

   ■ **N81.4**   **Uterovaginal prolapse, unspecified** ♀
      Prolapse of uterus NOS

   N81.5   **Vaginal enterocele** ♀
      | **Excludes1** | enterocele with prolapse of uterus (N81.2-N81.4)

   N81.6   **Rectocele** ♀
      Prolapse of posterior vaginal wall
      Use additional code for any associated fecal incontinence, if applicable (R15-)
      | **Excludes2** | perineocele N81.81
         rectal prolapse (K62.3)
         rectocele with prolapse of uterus (N81.2-N81.4)

● **N81.8**   **Other female genital prolapse**

   N81.81   **Perineocele** ♀

   N81.82   **Incompetence or weakening of pubocervical tissue** ♀

   N81.83   **Incompetence or weakening of rectovaginal tissue** ♀

   N81.84   **Pelvic muscle wasting** ♀
      Disuse atrophy of pelvic muscles and anal sphincter

   N81.85   **Cervical stump prolapse** ♀

   N81.89   **Other female genital prolapse** ♀
      Deficient perineum
      Old laceration of muscles of pelvic floor

■ **N81.9**   **Female genital prolapse, unspecified** ♀

Item 14–11 Endometriosis is a condition for which no clear cause has been identified. Endometrial tissue is expelled from the uterus into the abdominal cavity and can implant onto a variety of organs. Classification is based on the site of implant of the endometrial tissue.

● Unaccepptable Principal Diagnosis   ● Use Additional Character(s)   ■ Unspecified   ◗ Manifestation Code
OGCR Official Guidelines for Coding and Reporting | Excludes 1 | | Excludes 2 | Includes   Use additional   Code first   Code also

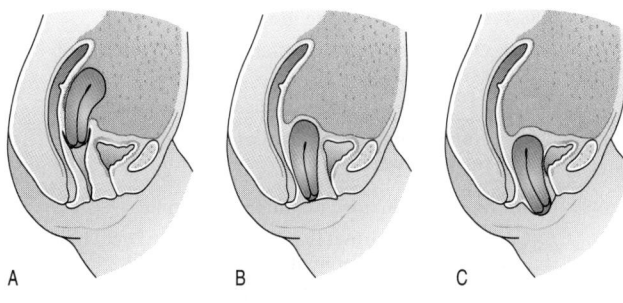

Figure 14-11 Three stages of uterine prolapse. **A.** Uterus is prolapsed. **B.** Vagina and uterus are prolapsed (incomplete uterovaginal prolapse). **C.** Vagina and uterus are completely prolapsed and are exposed through the external genitalia (complete uterovaginal prolapse).

● **N82 Fistulae involving female genital tract**
    | **Excludes1** | vesicointestinal fistulae (N32.1) |

  N82.0 Vesicovaginal fistula ♀ 🦠

  N82.1 Other female urinary-genital tract fistulae ♀ 🦠
       Cervicovesical fistula
       Ureterovaginal fistula
       Urethrovaginal fistula
       Uteroureteric fistula
       Uterovesical fistula

  N82.2 Fistula of vagina to small intestine ♀ 🦠

  N82.3 Fistula of vagina to large intestine ♀ 🦠
       Rectovaginal fistula

  N82.4 Other female intestinal-genital tract fistulae ♀ 🦠
       Intestinouterine fistula

  N82.5 Female genital tract-skin fistulae ♀ 🦠
       Uterus to abdominal wall fistula
       Vaginoperineal fistula

  N82.8 Other female genital tract fistulae ♀ 🦠

  🔲 **N82.9 Female genital tract fistula, unspecified** ♀ 🦠

● **N83 Noninflammatory disorders of ovary, fallopian tube and broad ligament**
    | **Excludes2** | hydrosalpinx (N70.1-) |

  N83.0 Follicular cyst of ovary ♀
       Cyst of graafian follicle
       Hemorrhagic follicular cyst (of ovary)

  N83.1 Corpus luteum cyst ♀
       Hemorrhagic corpus luteum cyst

● **N83.2 Other and unspecified ovarian cysts**
    | **Excludes1** | developmental ovarian cyst (Q50.1) |
    | | neoplastic ovarian cyst (D27.-) |
    | | polycystic ovarian syndrome (E28.2) |
    | | Stein-Leventhal syndrome (E28.2) |

    🔲 **N83.20 Unspecified ovarian cysts** ♀

    N83.29 Other ovarian cysts ♀
         Retention cyst of ovary
         Simple cyst of ovary

● **N83.3 Acquired atrophy of ovary and fallopian tube**

    N83.31 Acquired atrophy of ovary ♀

    N83.32 Acquired atrophy of fallopian tube ♀

    N83.33 Acquired atrophy of ovary and fallopian tube ♀

  N83.4 Prolapse and hernia of ovary and fallopian tube ♀

● **N83.5 Torsion of ovary, ovarian pedicle and fallopian tube**
       Torsion of accessory tube

    N83.51 Torsion of ovary and ovarian pedicle ♀ 🦠

    N83.52 Torsion of fallopian tube ♀ 🦠
         Torsion of hydatid of Morgagni

    N83.53 Torsion of ovary, ovarian pedicle and fallopian tube ♀ 🦠

  N83.6 Hematosalpinx ♀
    | **Excludes1** | hematosalpinx (with) (in): |
    | | hematocolpos (N89.7) |
    | | hematometra (N85.7) |
    | | tubal pregnancy (O00.1) |

  N83.7 Hematoma of broad ligament ♀

  N83.8 Other noninflammatory disorders of ovary, fallopian tube and broad ligament ♀
       Broad ligament laceration syndrome [Allen-Masters]

  🔲 **N83.9 Noninflammatory disorder of ovary, fallopian tube and broad ligament, unspecified** ♀

● **N84 Polyp of female genital tract**
    | **Excludes1** | adenomatous polyp (D28.-) |
    | | placental polyp (O90.89) |

  N84.0 Polyp of corpus uteri ♀
       Polyp of endometrium
       Polyp of uterus NOS
    | **Excludes1** | polypoid endometrial hyperplasia (N85.0-) |

  N84.1 Polyp of cervix uteri ♀
       Mucous polyp of cervix

  N84.2 Polyp of vagina ♀

  N84.3 Polyp of vulva ♀
       Polyp of labia

  N84.8 Polyp of other parts of female genital tract ♀

  🔲 **N84.9 Polyp of female genital tract, unspecified** ♀

● **N85 Other noninflammatory disorders of uterus, except cervix**
    | **Excludes1** | endometriosis (N80.-) |
    | | inflammatory diseases of uterus (N71.-) |
    | | noninflammatory disorders of cervix, except malposition (N86-N88) |
    | | polyp of corpus uteri (N84.0) |
    | | uterine prolapse (N81.-) |

● **N85.0 Endometrial hyperplasia**

    🔲 **N85.00 Endometrial hyperplasia, unspecified** ♀
         Hyperplasia (adenomatous) (cystic) (glandular) of endometrium
         Hyperplastic endometritis

    N85.01 Benign endometrial hyperplasia ♀
         Endometrial hyperplasia (complex) (simple) without atypia

    N85.02 Endometrial intraepithelial neoplasia [EIN] ♀
         Endometrial hyperplasia with atypia
      | **Excludes1** | malignant neoplasm of endometrium (with endometrial intraepithelial neoplasia [EIN]) (C54.1) |

  N85.2 Hypertrophy of uterus ♀
       Bulky or enlarged uterus
    | **Excludes1** | puerperal hypertrophy of uterus (O90.89) |

N Newborn Age: 0   **P** Pediatric Age: 0–17   **M** Maternity DX: 12–55   **A** Adult Age: 15–124   ♀ Females Only   ♂ Males Only
🦠 Complication\Comorbidity   🦠 Major C\C   Present on Admission Requirement   Hospital-Acquired Condition

CHAPTER 14 (N00-N99)

1277

CHAPTER 14 (N00-N99)

N85.3 Subinvolution of uterus ♀
> **Excludes1**   puerperal subinvolution of uterus (O90.89)

N85.4 Malposition of uterus ♀
Anteversion of uterus
Retroflexion of uterus
Retroversion of uterus
> **Excludes1**   malposition of uterus complicating pregnancy, labor or delivery (O34.5-, O65.5)

N85.5 Inversion of uterus ♀
> **Excludes1**   current obstetric trauma (O71.2) postpartum inversion of uterus (O71.2)

N85.6 Intrauterine synechiae ♀

N85.7 Hematometra ♀
Hematosalpinx with hematometra
> **Excludes1**   hematometra with hematocolpos (N89.7)

N85.8 Other specified noninflammatory disorders of uterus ♀
Atrophy of uterus, acquired
Fibrosis of uterus NOS

N85.9 Noninflammatory disorder of uterus, unspecified ♀
Disorder of uterus NOS

N86 Erosion and ectropion of cervix uteri ♀
Decubitus (trophic) ulcer of cervix
Eversion of cervix
> **Excludes1**   erosion and ectropion of cervix with cervicitis (N72)

● **N87 Dysplasia of cervix uteri**
> **Excludes1**   abnormal results from cervical cytologic examination without histologic confirmation (R87.61-)
> carcinoma in situ of cervix uteri (D06.-)
> cervical intraepithelial neoplasia III [CIN III] (D06.-)
> HGSIL of cervix (R87.613)
> severe dysplasia of cervix uteri (D06.-)

N87.0 Mild cervical dysplasia ♀
Cervical intraepithelial neoplasia I [CIN I]

N87.1 Moderate cervical dysplasia ♀
Cervical intraepithelial neoplasia II [CIN II]

N87.9 Dysplasia of cervix uteri, unspecified ♀
Anaplasia of cervix
Cervical atypism
Cervical dysplasia NOS

● **N88 Other noninflammatory disorders of cervix uteri**
> **Excludes2**   inflammatory disease of cervix (N72) polyp of cervix (N84.1)

N88.0 Leukoplakia of cervix uteri ♀

N88.1 Old laceration of cervix uteri ♀
Adhesions of cervix
> **Excludes1**   current obstetric trauma (O71.3)

N88.2 Stricture and stenosis of cervix uteri ♀
> **Excludes1**   stricture and stenosis of cervix uteri complicating labor (O65.5)

N88.3 Incompetence of cervix uteri ♀
Investigation and management of (suspected) cervical incompetence in a nonpregnant woman
> **Excludes1**   cervical incompetence complicating pregnancy (O34.3-)

N88.4 Hypertrophic elongation of cervix uteri ♀

N88.8 Other specified noninflammatory disorders of cervix uteri ♀
> **Excludes1**   current obstetric trauma (O71.3)

N88.9 Noninflammatory disorder of cervix uteri, unspecified ♀

● **N89 Other noninflammatory disorders of vagina**
> **Excludes1**   abnormal results from vaginal cytologic examination without histologic confirmation (R87.62-)
> carcinoma in situ of vagina (D07.2)
> HGSIL of vagina (R87.623)
> inflammation of vagina (N76.-)
> senile (atrophic) vaginitis (N95.2)
> severe dysplasia of vagina (D07.2)
> trichomonal leukorrhea (A59.00)
> vaginal intraepithelial neoplasia [VAIN], grade III (D07.2)

N89.0 Mild vaginal dysplasia ♀
Vaginal intraepithelial neoplasia [VAIN], grade I

N89.1 Moderate vaginal dysplasia ♀
Vaginal intraepithelial neoplasia [VAIN], grade II

N89.3 Dysplasia of vagina, unspecified ♀

N89.4 Leukoplakia of vagina ♀

N89.5 Stricture and atresia of vagina ♀
Vaginal adhesions　　　Vaginal stenosis
> **Excludes1**   congenital atresia or stricture (Q52.4) postprocedural adhesions of vagina (N99.2)

N89.6 Tight hymenal ring ♀
Rigid hymen　　　Tight introitus
> **Excludes1**   imperforate hymen (Q52.3)

N89.7 Hematocolpos ♀
Hematocolpos with hematometra or hematosalpinx

N89.8 Other specified noninflammatory disorders of vagina ♀
Leukorrhea NOS
Old vaginal laceration
Pessary ulcer of vagina
> **Excludes1**   current obstetric trauma (O70.-, O71.4, O71.7-O71.8)
> old laceration involving muscles of pelvic floor (N81.8)

N89.9 Noninflammatory disorder of vagina, unspecified ♀

● **N90 Other noninflammatory disorders of vulva and perineum**
> **Excludes1**   anogenital (venereal) warts (A63.0)
> carcinoma in situ of vulva (D07.1)
> condyloma acuminatum (A63.0)
> current obstetric trauma (O70.-, O71.7-O71.8)
> inflammation of vulva (N76.-)
> severe dysplasia of vulva (D07.1)
> vulvar intraepithelial neoplasm III [VIN III] (D07.1)

N90.0 Mild vulvar dysplasia ♀
Vulvar intraepithelial neoplasia [VIN], grade I

N90.1 Moderate vulvar dysplasia ♀
Vulvar intraepithelial neoplasia [VIN], grade II

N90.3 Dysplasia of vulva, unspecified ♀

N90.4 Leukoplakia of vulva ♀
Dystrophy of vulva
Kraurosis of vulva
Lichen sclerosus of external female genital organs

N90.5 Atrophy of vulva ♀
Stenosis of vulva

N90.6 Hypertrophy of vulva ♀
Hypertrophy of labia

N90.7 Vulvar cyst ♀

● **N90.8 Other specified noninflammatory disorders of vulva and perineum**

● **N90.81 Female genital mutilation status**
Female genital cutting status

◼ **N90.810 Female genital mutilation status, unspecified ♀**
Female genital cutting status, unspecified
Female genital mutilation status NOS

N90.811 Female genital mutilation Type I status ♀
Clitorectomy status
Female genital cutting Type I status

N90.812 Female genital mutilation Type II status ♀
Clitorectomy with excision of labia minora status
Female genital cutting Type II status

N90.813 Female genital mutilation Type III status ♀
Female genital cutting Type III status
Infibulation status

N90.818 Other female genital mutilation status ♀
Female genital cutting Type IV status
Female genital mutilation Type IV status
Other female genital cutting status

N90.89 Other specified noninflammatory disorders of vulva and perineum ♀
Adhesions of vulva
Hypertrophy of clitoris

◼ **N90.9 Noninflammatory disorder of vulva and perineum, unspecified ♀**

● **N91 Absent, scanty and rare menstruation**
Excludes1 ovarian dysfunction (E28.-)

N91.0 Primary amenorrhea ♀

N91.1 Secondary amenorrhea ♀

◼ **N91.2 Amenorrhea, unspecified ♀**

N91.3 Primary oligomenorrhea ♀

N91.4 Secondary oligomenorrhea ♀

◼ **N91.5 Oligomenorrhea, unspecified ♀**
Hypomenorrhea NOS

● **N92 Excessive, frequent and irregular menstruation**
Excludes1 postmenopausal bleeding (N95.0)
precocious puberty (menstruation) (E30.1)

N92.0 Excessive and frequent menstruation with regular cycle ♀
Heavy periods NOS   Polymenorrhea
Menorrhagia NOS

N92.1 Excessive and frequent menstruation with irregular cycle ♀
Irregular intermenstrual bleeding
Irregular, shortened intervals between menstrual bleeding
Menometrorrhagia
Metrorrhagia

N92.2 Excessive menstruation at puberty ♀   P
Excessive bleeding associated with onset of menstrual periods
Pubertal menorrhagia
Puberty bleeding

N92.3 Ovulation bleeding ♀
Regular intermenstrual bleeding

N92.4 Excessive bleeding in the premenopausal period ♀
Climacteric menorrhagia or metrorrhagia
Menopausal menorrhagia or metrorrhagia
Preclimacteric menorrhagia or metrorrhagia
Premenopausal menorrhagia or metrorrhagia

N92.5 Other specified irregular menstruation ♀

◼ **N92.6 Irregular menstruation, unspecified ♀**
Irregular bleeding NOS
Irregular periods NOS
Excludes1 irregular menstruation with:
lengthened intervals or scanty bleeding (N91.3-N91.5)
shortened intervals or excessive bleeding (N92.1)

● **N93 Other abnormal uterine and vaginal bleeding**
Excludes1 neonatal vaginal hemorrhage (P54.6)
precocious puberty (menstruation) (E30.1)
pseudomenses (P54.6)

N93.0 Postcoital and contact bleeding ♀

N93.8 Other specified abnormal uterine and vaginal bleeding ♀
Dysfunctional or functional uterine or vaginal bleeding NOS

◼ **N93.9 Abnormal uterine and vaginal bleeding, unspecified ♀**

● **N94 Pain and other conditions associated with female genital organs and menstrual cycle**

N94.0 Mittelschmerz ♀
Ovulation pain

N94.1 Dyspareunia ♀
Painful intercourse/coitus
Excludes1 psychogenic dyspareunia (F52.6)

N94.2 Vaginismus ♀
Vagina tightness
Excludes1 psychogenic vaginismus (F52.5)

N94.3 Premenstrual tension syndrome ♀
AKA: PMS
Premenstrual dysphoric disorder
Code also associated menstrual migraine (G43.82-, G43.83-)

N94.4 Primary dysmenorrhea ♀
Lifelong painful menstruation

N94.5 Secondary dysmenorrhea ♀
Later onset of painful menstruation

◼ **N94.6 Dysmenorrhea, unspecified ♀**
Excludes1 psychogenic dysmenorrhea (F45.8)

● **N94.8 Other specified conditions associated with female genital organs and menstrual cycle**

  ● **N94.81 Vulvodynia**

    N94.810 Vulvar vestibulitis ♀

    N94.818 Other vulvodynia ♀

    ■ **N94.819 Vulvodynia, unspecified ♀**
      Vulvodynia NOS

  N94.89 Other specified conditions associated with female genital organs and menstrual cycle ♀

■ **N94.9 Unspecified condition associated with female genital organs and menstrual cycle ♀**

● **N95 Menopausal and other perimenopausal disorders**
  Menopausal and other perimenopausal disorders due to naturally occurring (age-related) menopause and perimenopause

  | Excludes1 | excessive bleeding in the premenopausal period (N92.4)
  menopausal and perimenopausal disorders due to artificial or premature menopause (E89.4-, E28.31-)
  premature menopause (E28.31-) |

  | Excludes2 | postmenopausal osteoporosis (M81.0-)
  postmenopausal osteoporosis with current pathological fracture (M80.0-)
  postmenopausal urethritis (N34.2) |

  N95.0 Postmenopausal bleeding ♀

  N95.1 Menopausal and female climacteric states ♀
    Symptoms such as flushing, sleeplessness, headache, lack of concentration, associated with natural (age-related) menopause

    Use additional code for associated symptoms

    | Excludes1 | asymptomatic menopausal state (Z78.0)
    symptoms associated with artificial menopause (E89.41)
    symptoms associated with premature menopause (E28.310) |

  N95.2 Postmenopausal atrophic vaginitis ♀
    Senile (atrophic) vaginitis

  N95.8 Other specified menopausal and perimenopausal disorders ♀

  ■ **N95.9 Unspecified menopausal and perimenopausal disorder ♀**

N96 Recurrent pregnancy loss ♀
  Investigation or care in a nonpregnant woman with history of recurrent pregnancy loss

  | Excludes1 | recurrent pregnancy loss with current pregnancy (O26.2-) |

● **N97 Female infertility**

  | Includes | inability to achieve a pregnancy
  sterility, female NOS |

  | Excludes1 | female infertility associated with:
  hypopituitarism (E23.0)
  Stein-Leventhal syndrome (E28.2) |

  | Excludes2 | incompetence of cervix uteri (N88.3) |

  N97.0 Female infertility associated with anovulation ♀

N97.1 Female infertility of tubal origin ♀
  Female infertility associated with congenital anomaly of tube
  Female infertility due to tubal block
  Female infertility due to tubal occlusion
  Female infertility due to tubal stenosis

N97.2 Female infertility of uterine origin ♀
  Female infertility associated with congenital anomaly of uterus
  Female infertility due to nonimplantation of ovum

N97.8 Female infertility of other origin ♀

■ **N97.9 Female infertility, unspecified ♀**

● **N98 Complications associated with artificial fertilization**

  N98.0 Infection associated with artificial insemination ♀ 🦠

  N98.1 Hyperstimulation of ovaries ♀ 🦠
    Hyperstimulation of ovaries NOS
    Hyperstimulation of ovaries associated with induced ovulation

  N98.2 Complications of attempted introduction of fertilized ovum following in vitro fertilization ♀ 🦠

  N98.3 Complications of attempted introduction of embryo in embryo transfer ♀ 🦠

  N98.8 Other complications associated with artificial fertilization ♀ 🦠

  ■ **N98.9 Complication associated with artificial fertilization, unspecified ♀ 🦠**

INTRAOPERATIVE AND POSTPROCEDURAL COMPLICATIONS AND DISORDERS OF GENITOURINARY SYSTEM, NOT ELSEWHERE CLASSIFIED (N99)

● **N99 Intraoperative and postprocedural complications and disorders of genitourinary system, not elsewhere classified**

  | Excludes2 | irradiation cystitis (N30.4-)
  postoophorectomy osteoporosis with current pathological fracture (M80.8-)
  postoophorectomy osteoporosis without current pathological fracture (M81.8) |

  N99.0 Postprocedural (acute) (chronic) kidney failure

    Use additional code to type of kidney disease

  ● **N99.1 Postprocedural urethral stricture**
    Postcatheterization urethral stricture

    ● **N99.11 Postprocedural urethral stricture, male**

      N99.110 Postprocedural urethral stricture, male, meatal ♂

      N99.111 Postprocedural bulbous urethral stricture

      N99.112 Postprocedural membranous urethral stricture

      N99.113 Postprocedural anterior urethral stricture

      ■ **N99.114 Postprocedural urethral stricture, male, unspecified ♂**

    N99.12 Postprocedural urethral stricture, female ♀

  N99.2 Postprocedural adhesions of vagina ♀

  N99.3 Prolapse of vaginal vault after hysterectomy ♀

  N99.4 Postprocedural pelvic peritoneal adhesions

    | Excludes2 | pelvic peritoneal adhesions NOS (N73.6)
    postinfective pelvic peritoneal adhesions (N73.6) |

CHAPTER 14 (N00-N99)

1280

● Unacceptable Principal Diagnosis   ● Use Additional Character(s)   ■ Unspecified   ▶ Manifestation Code
OGCR Official Guidelines for Coding and Reporting | Excludes 1 | | Excludes 2 | Includes   Use additional   Code first   Code also

● **N99.5**   **Complications of stoma of urinary tract**

> **Excludes2**   mechanical complication of urinary (indwelling) catheter (T83.0-)

   ● **N99.51**   **Complication of cystostomy**

     N99.510   Cystostomy hemorrhage

     N99.511   Cystostomy infection

     N99.512   Cystostomy malfunction

     N99.518   Other cystostomy complication

   ● **N99.52**   **Complication of other external stoma of urinary tract**

     N99.520   Hemorrhage of other external stoma of urinary tract

     N99.521   Infection of other external stoma of urinary tract

     N99.522   Malfunction of other external stoma of urinary tract

     N99.528   Other complication of other external stoma of urinary tract

   ● **N99.53**   **Complication of other stoma of urinary tract**

     N99.530   Hemorrhage of other stoma of urinary tract

     N99.531   Infection of other stoma of urinary tract

     N99.532   Malfunction of other stoma of urinary tract

     N99.538   Other complication of other stoma of urinary tract

● **N99.6**   **Intraoperative hemorrhage and hematoma of a genitourinary system organ or structure complicating a procedure**

> **Excludes1**   intraoperative hemorrhage and hematoma of a genitourinary system organ or structure due to accidental puncture or laceration during a procedure (N99.7-)

   N99.61   Intraoperative hemorrhage and hematoma of a genitourinary system organ or structure complicating a genitourinary system procedure 🏥

   N99.62   Intraoperative hemorrhage and hematoma of a genitourinary system organ or structure complicating other procedure 🏥

● **N99.7**   **Accidental puncture and laceration of a genitourinary system organ or structure during a procedure**

   N99.71   Accidental puncture and laceration of a genitourinary system organ or structure during a genitourinary system procedure 🏥

   N99.72   Accidental puncture and laceration of a genitourinary system organ or structure during other procedure 🏥

● **N99.8**   **Other intraoperative and postprocedural complications and disorders of genitourinary system**

   N99.81   Other intraoperative complications of genitourinary system

   ● **N99.82**   **Postprocedural hemorrhage and hematoma of a genitourinary system organ or structure following a procedure**

     N99.820   Postprocedural hemorrhage and hematoma of a genitourinary system organ or structure following a genitourinary system procedure 🏥 ⬦

     N99.821   Postprocedural hemorrhage and hematoma of a genitourinary system organ or structure following other procedure 🏥

   N99.83   Residual ovary syndrome ♀

   N99.89   Other postprocedural complications and disorders of genitourinary system

N   Newborn Age: 0   **P**   Pediatric Age: 0–17   **M**   Maternity DX: 12–55   **A**   Adult Age: 15–124   ♀   Females Only   ♂   Males Only

🏥   Complication\Comorbidity   Major C\C   Present on Admission Requirement   Hospital-Acquired Condition

1281

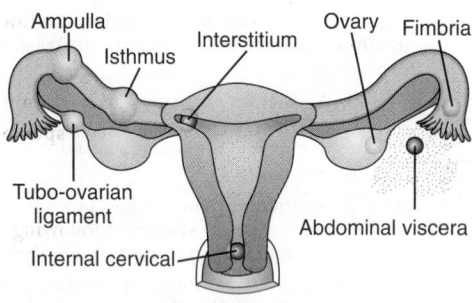

Ampulla — Isthmus — Interstitium — Ovary — Fimbria — Tubo-ovarian ligament — Abdominal viscera — Internal cervical

Figure 15-1 Implantation sites of ectopic pregnancy.

Item 15–1 Ectopic pregnancy most often occurs in the fallopian tube. Pregnancy outside the uterus may end in a lifethreatening rupture.

OGCR See Section I.C.15.

Chapter 15 Pregnancy, Childbirth, and the Puerperium

(See Plate 375 on page NAP-4.)

CHAPTER 15

PREGNANCY, CHILDBIRTH AND THE PUERPERIUM (O00-O9A)

Note: CODES FROM THIS CHAPTER ARE FOR USE ONLY ON MATERNAL RECORDS, NEVER ON NEWBORN RECORDS

Codes from this chapter are for use for conditions related to or aggravated by the pregnancy, childbirth, or by the puerperium (maternal causes or obstetric causes)

Trimesters are counted from the first day of the last menstrual period. They are defined as follows:

1st trimester - less than 14 weeks 0 days

2nd trimester - 14 weeks 0 days to less than 28 weeks 0 days

3rd trimester - 28 weeks 0 days until delivery

Use additional code from category Z3A, Weeks of gestation, to identify the specific week of the pregnancy

Excludes1 supervision of normal pregnancy (Z34.-)

Excludes2 mental and behavioral disorders associated with the puerperium (F53)
obstetrical tetanus (A34)
postpartum necrosis of pituitary gland (E23.0)
puerperal osteomalacia (M83.0)

This chapter contains the following blocks:

O00-O08	Pregnancy with abortive outcome
O09	Supervision of high risk pregnancy
O10-O16	Edema, proteinuria and hypertensive disorders in pregnancy, childbirth and the puerperium
O20-O29	Other maternal disorders predominantly related to pregnancy
O30-O48	Maternal care related to the fetus and amniotic cavity and possible delivery problems
O60-O77	Complications of labor and delivery
O80, O82	Encounter for delivery
O85-O92	Complications predominantly related to the puerperium
O94-O9A	Other obstetric conditions, not elsewhere classified

PREGNANCY WITH ABORTIVE OUTCOME (O00-O08)

Excludes1 continuing pregnancy in multiple gestation after abortion of one fetus or more (O31.1-, O31.3-)

● **O00 Ectopic pregnancy**

Includes　ruptured ectopic pregnancy

Use additional code from category O08 to identify any associated complication

O00.0 Abdominal pregnancy ♀ 🦠　　　　　　**M**

Excludes1 maternal care for viable fetus in abdominal pregnancy (O36.7-)

O00.1 Tubal pregnancy ♀ 🦠　　　　　　　**M**
Fallopian pregnancy
Rupture of (fallopian) tube due to pregnancy
Tubal abortion

O00.2 Ovarian pregnancy ♀ 🦠　　　　　　**M**

O00.8 Other ectopic pregnancy ♀ 🦠　　　**M**
Cervical pregnancy
Cornual pregnancy
Intraligamentous pregnancy
Mural pregnancy

■ **O00.9 Ectopic pregnancy, unspecified** ♀ 🦠　**M**

● **O01 Hydatidiform mole**

Use additional code from category O08 to identify any associated complication

Excludes1 chorioadenoma (destruens) (D39.2)
malignant hydatidiform mole (D39.2)

O01.0 Classical hydatidiform mole ♀　　　**M**
Complete hydatidiform mole

O01.1 Incomplete and partial hydatidiform mole ♀　**M**

■ **O01.9 Hydatidiform mole, unspecified** ♀　**M**
Trophoblastic disease NOS
Vesicular mole NOS

● **O02 Other abnormal products of conception**

Use additional code from category O08 to identify any associated complication

Excludes1 papyraceous fetus (O31.0-)

O02.0 Blighted ovum and nonhydatidiform mole ♀　**M**
Carneous mole　　　　Molar pregnancy NEC
Fleshy mole　　　　　Pathological ovum
Intrauterine mole NOS

O02.1 Missed abortion ♀　　　　　　　　**M**
Early fetal death, before completion of 20 weeks of gestation, with retention of dead fetus

Excludes1 failed induced abortion (O07.-)
fetal death (intrauterine) (late) (O36.4)
missed abortion with blighted ovum (O02.0)
missed abortion with hydatidiform mole (O01.-)
missed abortion with nonhydatidiform (O02.0)
missed abortion with other abnormal products of conception (O02.8-)
missed delivery (O36.4)
stillbirth (P95)

Item 15–2 A **hydatidiform** mole is a benign tumor of the placenta. The tumor secretes a hormone, chorionic gonadotropic hormone (CGH), that indicates a positive pregnancy test.

● Unacceptable Principal Diagnosis　　　● Use Additional Character(s)　　　■ Unspecified　　　▶ Manifestation Code

1282　　**OGCR** Official Guidelines for Coding and Reporting　　Excludes 1　Excludes 2　Includes　Use additional　Code first　Code also

● **O02.8 Other specified abnormal products of conception**

> | Excludes1 | abnormal products of conception with blighted ovum (O02.0)
> abnormal products of conception with hydatidiform mole (O01.-)
> abnormal products of conception with nonhydatidiform mole (O02.0)

> **O02.81 Inappropriate change in quantitative human chorionic gonadotropin (hCG) in early pregnancy** ♀   M
>> Biochemical pregnancy
>> Chemical pregnancy
>> Inappropriate level of quantitative human chorionic gonadotropin (hCG) for gestational age in early pregnancy

> **O02.89 Other abnormal products of conception** ♀   M

■ **O02.9 Abnormal product of conception, unspecified** ♀   M

● **O03 Spontaneous abortion**

> **Note:** Incomplete abortion includes retained products of conception following spontaneous abortion.

> | Includes | miscarriage

> **O03.0 Genital tract and pelvic infection following incomplete spontaneous abortion** ♀ 🦠   M
>> Endometritis following incomplete spontaneous abortion
>> Oophoritis following incomplete spontaneous abortion
>> Parametritis following incomplete spontaneous abortion
>> Pelvic peritonitis following incomplete spontaneous abortion
>> Salpingitis following incomplete spontaneous abortion
>> Salpingo-oophoritis following incomplete spontaneous abortion

>> | Excludes1 | sepsis following incomplete spontaneous abortion (O03.37)
>> urinary tract infection following incomplete spontaneous abortion (O03.38)

> **O03.1 Delayed or excessive hemorrhage following incomplete spontaneous abortion** ♀   M
>> Afibrinogenemia following incomplete spontaneous abortion
>> Defibrination syndrome following incomplete spontaneous abortion
>> Hemolysis following incomplete spontaneous abortion
>> Intravascular coagulation following incomplete spontaneous abortion

> **O03.2 Embolism following incomplete spontaneous abortion** ♀ 🦠   M
>> Air embolism following incomplete spontaneous abortion
>> Amniotic fluid embolism following incomplete spontaneous abortion
>> Blood-clot embolism following incomplete spontaneous abortion
>> Embolism NOS following incomplete spontaneous abortion
>> Fat embolism following incomplete spontaneous abortion
>> Pulmonary embolism following incomplete spontaneous abortion
>> Pyemic embolism following incomplete spontaneous abortion
>> Septic or septicopyemic embolism following incomplete spontaneous abortion
>> Soap embolism following incomplete spontaneous abortion

● **O03.3 Other and unspecified complications following incomplete spontaneous abortion**

> ■ **O03.30 Unspecified complication following incomplete spontaneous abortion** ♀ 🦠   M

> **O03.31 Shock following incomplete spontaneous abortion** ♀ 🦠   M
>> Circulatory collapse following incomplete spontaneous abortion
>> Shock (postprocedural) following incomplete spontaneous abortion

>> | Excludes1 | shock due to infection following incomplete spontaneous abortion (O03.37)

> **O03.32 Renal failure following incomplete spontaneous abortion** ♀ 🦠   M
>> Kidney failure (acute) following incomplete spontaneous abortion
>> Oliguria following incomplete spontaneous abortion
>> Renal shutdown following incomplete spontaneous abortion
>> Renal tubular necrosis following incomplete spontaneous abortion
>> Uremia following incomplete spontaneous abortion

> **O03.33 Metabolic disorder following incomplete spontaneous abortion** ♀ 🦠   M

> **O03.34 Damage to pelvic organs following incomplete spontaneous abortion** ♀ 🦠   M
>> Laceration, perforation, tear or chemical damage of bladder following incomplete spontaneous abortion
>> Laceration, perforation, tear or chemical damage of bowel following incomplete spontaneous abortion
>> Laceration, perforation, tear or chemical damage of broad ligament following incomplete spontaneous abortion
>> Laceration, perforation, tear or chemical damage of cervix following incomplete spontaneous abortion
>> Laceration, perforation, tear or chemical damage of periurethral tissue following incomplete spontaneous abortion
>> Laceration, perforation, tear or chemical damage of uterus following incomplete spontaneous abortion
>> Laceration, perforation, tear or chemical damage of vagina following incomplete spontaneous abortion

> **O03.35 Other venous complications following incomplete spontaneous abortion** ♀ 🦠   M

> **O03.36 Cardiac arrest following incomplete spontaneous abortion** ♀ 🦠   M

> **O03.37 Sepsis following incomplete spontaneous abortion** ♀ 🦠   M

>> | Use additional | code to identify infectious agent (B95-B97)

>> | Use additional | code to identify severe sepsis, if applicable (R65.2-)

>> | Excludes1 | septic or septicopyemic embolism following incomplete spontaneous abortion (O03.2)

CHAPTER 15 (O00-O9A)

O03.38 Urinary tract infection following incomplete spontaneous abortion ♀   M
     Cystitis following incomplete spontaneous abortion

O03.39 Incomplete spontaneous abortion with other complications ♀   M

O03.4 Incomplete spontaneous abortion without complication ♀   M

O03.5 Genital tract and pelvic infection following complete or unspecified spontaneous abortion ♀   M
     Endometritis following complete or unspecified spontaneous abortion
     Oophoritis following complete or unspecified spontaneous abortion
     Parametritis following complete or unspecified spontaneous abortion
     Pelvic peritonitis following complete or unspecified spontaneous abortion
     Salpingitis following complete or unspecified spontaneous abortion
     Salpingo-oophoritis following complete or unspecified spontaneous abortion

     Excludes1   sepsis following complete or unspecified spontaneous abortion (O03.87)
          urinary tract infection following complete or unspecified spontaneous abortion (O03.88)

O03.6 Delayed or excessive hemorrhage following complete or unspecified spontaneous abortion ♀ M
     Afibrinogenemia following complete or unspecified spontaneous abortion
     Defibrination syndrome following complete or unspecified spontaneous abortion
     Hemolysis following complete or unspecified spontaneous abortion
     Intravascular coagulation following complete or unspecified spontaneous abortion

O03.7 Embolism following complete or unspecified spontaneous abortion ♀   M
     Air embolism following complete or unspecified spontaneous abortion
     Amniotic fluid embolism following complete or unspecified spontaneous abortion
     Blood-clot embolism following complete or unspecified spontaneous abortion
     Embolism NOS following complete or unspecified spontaneous abortion
     Fat embolism following complete or unspecified spontaneous abortion
     Pulmonary embolism following complete or unspecified spontaneous abortion
     Pyemic embolism following complete or unspecified spontaneous abortion
     Septic or septicopyemic embolism following complete or unspecified spontaneous abortion
     Soap embolism following complete or unspecified spontaneous abortion

● **O03.8 Other and unspecified complications following complete or unspecified spontaneous abortion**

    O03.80 Unspecified complication following complete or unspecified spontaneous abortion ♀   M

O03.81 Shock following complete or unspecified spontaneous abortion ♀   M
     Circulatory collapse following complete or unspecified spontaneous abortion
     Shock (postprocedural) following complete or unspecified spontaneous abortion

     Excludes1   shock due to infection following complete or unspecified spontaneous abortion (O03.87)

O03.82 Renal failure following complete or unspecified spontaneous abortion ♀   M
     Kidney failure (acute) following complete or unspecified spontaneous abortion
     Oliguria following complete or unspecified spontaneous abortion
     Renal shutdown following complete or unspecified spontaneous abortion
     Renal tubular necrosis following complete or unspecified spontaneous abortion
     Uremia following complete or unspecified spontaneous abortion

O03.83 Metabolic disorder following complete or unspecified spontaneous abortion ♀   M

O03.84 Damage to pelvic organs following complete or unspecified spontaneous abortion ♀   M
     Laceration, perforation, tear or chemical damage of bladder following complete or unspecified spontaneous abortion
     Laceration, perforation, tear or chemical damage of bowel following complete or unspecified spontaneous abortion
     Laceration, perforation, tear or chemical damage of broad ligament following complete or unspecified spontaneous abortion
     Laceration, perforation, tear or chemical damage of cervix following complete or unspecified spontaneous abortion
     Laceration, perforation, tear or chemical damage of periurethral tissue following complete or unspecified spontaneous abortion
     Laceration, perforation, tear or chemical damage of uterus following complete or unspecified spontaneous abortion
     Laceration, perforation, tear or chemical damage of vagina following complete or unspecified spontaneous abortion

O03.85 Other venous complications following complete or unspecified spontaneous abortion ♀   M

O03.86 Cardiac arrest following complete or unspecified spontaneous abortion ♀   M

O03.87 Sepsis following complete or unspecified spontaneous abortion ♀   M

     Use additional code to identify infectious agent (B95-B97)

     Use additional code to identify severe sepsis, if applicable (R65.2-)

     Excludes1   septic or septicopyemic embolism following complete or unspecified spontaneous abortion (O03.7)

● Unacceptable Principal Diagnosis   ● Use Additional Character(s)   ▨ Unspecified   ▶ Manifestation Code
OGCR Official Guidelines for Coding and Reporting   Excludes 1   Excludes 2   Includes   Use additional   Code first   Code also

CHAPTER 15 (O00-O9A)

■ **O03.88 Urinary tract infection following complete or unspecified spontaneous abortion** ♀ 🦠 **M**
    Cystitis following complete or unspecified spontaneous abortion

■ **O03.89 Complete or unspecified spontaneous abortion with other complications** ♀ 🦠 **M**

■ **O03.9 Complete or unspecified spontaneous abortion without complication** ♀ **M**
    Miscarriage NOS
    Spontaneous abortion NOS

● **O04 Complications following (induced) termination of pregnancy**

> **Includes** complications following (induced) termination of pregnancy

> **Excludes1** encounter for elective termination of pregnancy, uncomplicated (Z33.2)
> failed attempted termination of pregnancy (O07.-)

O04.5 Genital tract and pelvic infection following (induced) termination of pregnancy ♀ 🦠 **M**
    Endometritis following (induced) termination of pregnancy
    Oophoritis following (induced) termination of pregnancy
    Parametritis following (induced) termination of pregnancy
    Pelvic peritonitis following (induced) termination of pregnancy
    Salpingitis following (induced) termination of pregnancy
    Salpingo-oophoritis following (induced) termination of pregnancy

> **Excludes1** sepsis following (induced) termination of pregnancy (O04.87)
> urinary tract infection following (induced) termination of pregnancy (O04.88)

O04.6 Delayed or excessive hemorrhage following (induced) termination of pregnancy ♀ **M**
    Afibrinogenemia following (induced) termination of pregnancy
    Defibrination syndrome following (induced) termination of pregnancy
    Hemolysis following (induced) termination of pregnancy
    Intravascular coagulation following (induced) termination of pregnancy

O04.7 Embolism following (induced) termination of pregnancy ♀ 🦠 **M**
    Air embolism following (induced) termination of pregnancy
    Amniotic fluid embolism following (induced) termination of pregnancy
    Blood-clot embolism following (induced) termination of pregnancy
    Embolism NOS following (induced) termination of pregnancy
    Fat embolism following (induced) termination of pregnancy
    Pulmonary embolism following (induced) termination of pregnancy
    Pyemic embolism following (induced) termination of pregnancy
    Septic or septicopyemic embolism following (induced) termination of pregnancy
    Soap embolism following (induced) termination of pregnancy

● **O04.8 (Induced) termination of pregnancy with other and unspecified complications**

■ **O04.80 (Induced) termination of pregnancy with unspecified complications** ♀ 🦠 **M**

O04.81 Shock following (induced) termination of pregnancy ♀ 🦠 **M**
    Circulatory collapse following (induced) termination of pregnancy
    Shock (postprocedural) following (induced) termination of pregnancy

> **Excludes1** shock due to infection following (induced) termination of pregnancy (O04.87)

O04.82 Renal failure following (induced) termination of pregnancy ♀ 🦠 **M**
    Kidney failure (acute) following (induced) termination of pregnancy
    Oliguria following (induced) termination of pregnancy
    Renal shutdown following (induced) termination of pregnancy
    Renal tubular necrosis following (induced) termination of pregnancy
    Uremia following (induced) termination of pregnancy

O04.83 Metabolic disorder following (induced) termination of pregnancy ♀ 🦠 **M**

O04.84 Damage to pelvic organs following (induced) termination of pregnancy ♀ 🦠 **M**
    Laceration, perforation, tear or chemical damage of bladder following (induced) termination of pregnancy
    Laceration, perforation, tear or chemical damage of bowel following (induced) termination of pregnancy
    Laceration, perforation, tear or chemical damage of broad ligament following (induced) termination of pregnancy
    Laceration, perforation, tear or chemical damage of cervix following (induced) termination of pregnancy
    Laceration, perforation, tear or chemical damage of periurethral tissue following (induced) termination of pregnancy
    Laceration, perforation, tear or chemical damage of uterus following (induced) termination of pregnancy
    Laceration, perforation, tear or chemical damage of vagina following (induced) termination of pregnancy

O04.85 Other venous complications following (induced) termination of pregnancy ♀ 🦠 **M**

O04.86 Cardiac arrest following (induced) termination of pregnancy ♀ 🦠 **M**

O04.87 Sepsis following (induced) termination of pregnancy ♀ 🦠 **M**

> **Use additional** code to identify infectious agent (B95-B97)

> **Use additional** code to identify severe sepsis, if applicable (R65.2-)

> **Excludes1** septic or septicopyemic embolism following (induced) termination of pregnancy (O04.7)

N Newborn Age: 0   **P** Pediatric Age: 0–17   **M** Maternity DX: 12–55   **A** Adult Age: 15–124   ♀ Females Only   ♂ Males Only

🦠 Complication\Comorbidity   🦠 Major C\C   🦠 Present on Admission Requirement   🦠 Hospital-Acquired Condition

1285

CHAPTER 15 (O00-O9A)

CHAPTER 15 (O00-O9A)

O04.88 Urinary tract infection following (induced) termination of pregnancy ♀ 🕭   M

Cystitis following (induced) termination of pregnancy

O04.89 (Induced) termination of pregnancy with other complications ♀ 🕭   M

● **O07 Failed attempted termination of pregnancy**

Includes   failure of attempted induction of termination of pregnancy
incomplete elective abortion

Excludes1   incomplete spontaneous abortion (O03.0-)

O07.0 Genital tract and pelvic infection following failed attempted termination of pregnancy ♀ 🕭   M

Endometritis following failed attempted termination of pregnancy
Oophoritis following failed attempted termination of pregnancy
Parametritis following failed attempted termination of pregnancy
Pelvic peritonitis following failed attempted termination of pregnancy
Salpingitis following failed attempted termination of pregnancy
Salpingo-oophoritis following failed attempted termination of pregnancy

Excludes1   sepsis following failed attempted termination of pregnancy (O07.37)
urinary tract infection following failed attempted termination of pregnancy (O07.38)

O07.1 Delayed or excessive hemorrhage following failed attempted termination of pregnancy ♀ 🕭   M

Afibrinogenemia following failed attempted termination of pregnancy
Defibrination syndrome following failed attempted termination of pregnancy
Hemolysis following failed attempted termination of pregnancy
Intravascular coagulation following failed attempted termination of pregnancy

O07.2 Embolism following failed attempted termination of pregnancy ♀ 🕭   M

Air embolism following failed attempted termination of pregnancy
Amniotic fluid embolism following failed attempted termination of pregnancy
Blood-clot embolism following failed attempted termination of pregnancy
Embolism NOS following failed attempted termination of pregnancy
Fat embolism following failed attempted termination of pregnancy
Pulmonary embolism following failed attempted termination of pregnancy
Pyemic embolism following failed attempted termination of pregnancy
Septic or septicopyemic embolism following failed attempted termination of pregnancy
Soap embolism following failed attempted termination of pregnancy

● **O07.3 Failed attempted termination of pregnancy with other and unspecified complications**

▪ **O07.30 Failed attempted termination of pregnancy with unspecified complications** ♀ 🕭   M

O07.31 Shock following failed attempted termination of pregnancy ♀ 🕭   M

Circulatory collapse following failed attempted termination of pregnancy
Shock (postprocedural) following failed attempted termination of pregnancy

Excludes1   shock due to infection following failed attempted termination of pregnancy (O07.37)

O07.32 Renal failure following failed attempted termination of pregnancy ♀ 🕭   M

Kidney failure (acute) following failed attempted termination of pregnancy
Oliguria following failed attempted termination of pregnancy
Renal shutdown following failed attempted termination of pregnancy
Renal tubular necrosis following failed attempted termination of pregnancy
Uremia following failed attempted termination of pregnancy

O07.33 Metabolic disorder following failed attempted termination of pregnancy ♀ 🕭 M

O07.34 Damage to pelvic organs following failed attempted termination of pregnancy ♀ 🕭 M

Laceration, perforation, tear or chemical damage of bladder following failed attempted termination of pregnancy
Laceration, perforation, tear or chemical damage of bowel following failed attempted termination of pregnancy
Laceration, perforation, tear or chemical damage of broad ligament following failed attempted termination of pregnancy
Laceration, perforation, tear or chemical damage of cervix following failed attempted termination of pregnancy
Laceration, perforation, tear or chemical damage of periurethral tissue following failed attempted termination of pregnancy
Laceration, perforation, tear or chemical damage of uterus following failed attempted termination of pregnancy
Laceration, perforation, tear or chemical damage of vagina following failed attempted termination of pregnancy

O07.35 Other venous complications following failed attempted termination of pregnancy ♀ 🕭   M

O07.36 Cardiac arrest following failed attempted termination of pregnancy ♀ 🕭   M

O07.37 Sepsis following failed attempted termination of pregnancy ♀ 🕭   M

Use additional code (B95-B97), to identify infectious agent

Use additional code (R65.2-) to identify severe sepsis, if applicable

Excludes1   septic or septicopyemic embolism following failed attempted termination of pregnancy (O07.2)

● Unacceptable Principal Diagnosis   ● Use Additional Character(s)   ▪ Unspecified   ▶ Manifestation Code

OGCR Official Guidelines for Coding and Reporting   Excludes 1   Excludes 2   Includes   Use additional   Code first   Code also

O07.38 **Urinary tract infection following failed attempted termination of pregnancy** ♀ 🔗 M
     Cystitis following failed attempted termination of pregnancy

O07.39 **Failed attempted termination of pregnancy with other complications** ♀ 🔗   M

O07.4 **Failed attempted termination of pregnancy without complication** ♀   M

● O08 **Complications following ectopic and molar pregnancy**
     This category is for use with categories O00-O02 to identify any associated complications.

O08.0 **Genital tract and pelvic infection following ectopic and molar pregnancy** ♀ 🔗   M
     Endometritis following ectopic and molar pregnancy
     Oophoritis following ectopic and molar pregnancy
     Parametritis following ectopic and molar pregnancy
     Pelvic peritonitis following ectopic and molar pregnancy
     Salpingitis following ectopic and molar pregnancy
     Salpingo-oophoritis following ectopic and molar pregnancy

     Excludes1   sepsis following ectopic and molar pregnancy (O08.82)
           urinary tract infection (O08.83)

O08.1 **Delayed or excessive hemorrhage following ectopic and molar pregnancy** ♀ 🔗   M
     Afibrinogenemia following ectopic and molar pregnancy
     Defibrination syndrome following ectopic and molar pregnancy
     Hemolysis following ectopic and molar pregnancy
     Intravascular coagulation following ectopic and molar pregnancy

     Excludes1   delayed or excessive hemorrhage due to incomplete abortion (O03.1)

O08.2 **Embolism following ectopic and molar pregnancy** ♀ 🔗   M
     Air embolism following ectopic and molar pregnancy
     Amniotic fluid embolism following ectopic and molar pregnancy
     Blood-clot embolism following ectopic and molar pregnancy
     Embolism NOS following ectopic and molar pregnancy
     Fat embolism following ectopic and molar pregnancy
     Pulmonary embolism following ectopic and molar pregnancy
     Pyemic embolism following ectopic and molar pregnancy
     Septic or septicopyemic embolism following ectopic and molar pregnancy
     Soap embolism following ectopic and molar pregnancy

O08.3 **Shock following ectopic and molar pregnancy** ♀ 🔗   M
     Circulatory collapse following ectopic and molar pregnancy
     Shock (postprocedural) following ectopic and molar pregnancy

     Excludes1   shock due to infection following ectopic and molar pregnancy (O08.82)

O08.4 **Renal failure following ectopic and molar pregnancy** ♀ 🔗   M
     Kidney failure (acute) following ectopic and molar pregnancy
     Oliguria following ectopic and molar pregnancy
     Renal shutdown following ectopic and molar pregnancy
     Renal tubular necrosis following ectopic and molar pregnancy
     Uremia following ectopic and molar pregnancy

O08.5 **Metabolic disorders following an ectopic and molar pregnancy** ♀ 🔗   M

O08.6 **Damage to pelvic organs and tissues following an ectopic and molar pregnancy** ♀ 🔗   M
     Laceration, perforation, tear or chemical damage of bladder following an ectopic and molar pregnancy
     Laceration, perforation, tear or chemical damage of bowel following an ectopic and molar pregnancy
     Laceration, perforation, tear or chemical damage of broad ligament following an ectopic and molar pregnancy
     Laceration, perforation, tear or chemical damage of cervix following an ectopic and molar pregnancy
     Laceration, perforation, tear or chemical damage of periurethral tissue following an ectopic and molar pregnancy
     Laceration, perforation, tear or chemical damage of uterus following an ectopic and molar pregnancy
     Laceration, perforation, tear or chemical damage of vagina following an ectopic and molar pregnancy

O08.7 **Other venous complications following an ectopic and molar pregnancy** ♀ 🔗   M

● O08.8 **Other complications following an ectopic and molar pregnancy**

O08.81 **Cardiac arrest following an ectopic and molar pregnancy** ♀ 🔗   M

O08.82 **Sepsis following ectopic and molar pregnancy** ♀ 🔗   M
     Use additional code (B95-B97), to identify infectious agent
     Use additional code (R65.2-) to identify severe sepsis, if applicable

     Excludes1   septic or septicopyemic embolism following ectopic and molar pregnancy (O08.2)

O08.83 **Urinary tract infection following an ectopic and molar pregnancy** ♀ 🔗   M
     Cystitis following an ectopic and molar pregnancy

O08.89 **Other complications following an ectopic and molar pregnancy** ♀ 🔗   M

■ O08.9 **Unspecified complication following an ectopic and molar pregnancy** ♀ 🔗   M

N Newborn Age: 0   **P** Pediatric Age: 0–17   **M** Maternity DX: 12–55   **A** Adult Age: 15–124   ♀ Females Only   ♂ Males Only
🔗 Complication\Comorbidity   🔗 Major C\C   Present on Admission Requirement   🔗 Hospital-Acquired Condition

1287

SUPERVISION OF HIGH RISK PREGNANCY (O09)

● **O09   Supervision of high risk pregnancy**

  ● **O09.0   Supervision of pregnancy with history of infertility**

    ■● **O09.00   Supervision of pregnancy with history of infertility, unspecified trimester** ♀ 🐾   **M**

    ● **O09.01   Supervision of pregnancy with history of infertility, first trimester** ♀ 🐾   **M**

    ● **O09.02   Supervision of pregnancy with history of infertility, second trimester** ♀ 🐾   **M**

    ● **O09.03   Supervision of pregnancy with history of infertility, third trimester** ♀ 🐾   **M**

  ● **O09.1   Supervision of pregnancy with history of ectopic or molar pregnancy**

    ■● **O09.10   Supervision of pregnancy with history of ectopic or molar pregnancy, unspecified trimester** ♀ 🐾   **M**

    ● **O09.11   Supervision of pregnancy with history of ectopic or molar pregnancy, first trimester** ♀ 🐾   **M**

    ● **O09.12   Supervision of pregnancy with history of ectopic or molar pregnancy, second trimester** ♀ 🐾   **M**

    ● **O09.13   Supervision of pregnancy with history of ectopic or molar pregnancy, third trimester** ♀ 🐾   **M**

  ● **O09.2   Supervision of pregnancy with other poor reproductive or obstetric history**

    Excludes2   pregnancy care for patient with history of recurrent pregnancy loss (O26.2-)

    ● **O09.21   Supervision of pregnancy with history of pre-term labor**

      ● **O09.211   Supervision of pregnancy with history of pre-term labor, first trimester** ♀ 🐾   **M**

      ● **O09.212   Supervision of pregnancy with history of pre-term labor, second trimester** ♀ 🐾   **M**

      ● **O09.213   Supervision of pregnancy with history of pre-term labor, third trimester** ♀ 🐾   **M**

      ■● **O09.219   Supervision of pregnancy with history of pre-term labor, unspecified trimester** ♀ 🐾   **M**

    ● **O09.29   Supervision of pregnancy with other poor reproductive or obstetric history**

      Supervision of pregnancy with history of neonatal death

      Supervision of pregnancy with history of stillbirth

      ● **O09.291   Supervision of pregnancy with other poor reproductive or obstetric history, first trimester** ♀ 🐾   **M**

      ● **O09.292   Supervision of pregnancy with other poor reproductive or obstetric history, second trimester** ♀ 🐾   **M**

      ● **O09.293   Supervision of pregnancy with other poor reproductive or obstetric history, third trimester** ♀ 🐾   **M**

      ■● **O09.299   Supervision of pregnancy with other poor reproductive or obstetric history, unspecified trimester** ♀ 🐾   **M**

  ● **O09.3   Supervision of pregnancy with insufficient antenatal care**

    Supervision of concealed pregnancy

    Supervision of hidden pregnancy

    ■● **O09.30   Supervision of pregnancy with insufficient antenatal care, unspecified trimester** ♀ 🐾   **M**

    ● **O09.31   Supervision of pregnancy with insufficient antenatal care, first trimester** ♀ 🐾   **M**

    ● **O09.32   Supervision of pregnancy with insufficient antenatal care, second trimester** ♀ 🐾   **M**

    ● **O09.33   Supervision of pregnancy with insufficient antenatal care, third trimester** ♀ 🐾   **M**

  ● **O09.4   Supervision of pregnancy with grand multiparity**

    ■● **O09.40   Supervision of pregnancy with grand multiparity, unspecified trimester** ♀ 🐾   **M**

    ● **O09.41   Supervision of pregnancy with grand multiparity, first trimester** ♀   **M**

    ● **O09.42   Supervision of pregnancy with grand multiparity, second trimester** ♀   **M**

    ● **O09.43   Supervision of pregnancy with grand multiparity, third trimester** ♀   **M**

  ● **O09.5   Supervision of elderly primigravida and multigravida**

    Pregnancy for a female 35 years and older at expected date of delivery

    ● **O09.51   Supervision of elderly primigravida**

      ● **O09.511   Supervision of elderly primigravida, first trimester** ♀ 🐾   **M**

      ● **O09.512   Supervision of elderly primigravida, second trimester** ♀ 🐾   **M**

      ● **O09.513   Supervision of elderly primigravida, third trimester** ♀ 🐾   **M**

      ■● **O09.519   Supervision of elderly primigravida, unspecified trimester** ♀ 🐾   **M**

    ● **O09.52   Supervision of elderly multigravida**

      ● **O09.521   Supervision of elderly multigravida, first trimester** ♀ 🐾   **M**

      ● **O09.522   Supervision of elderly multigravida, second trimester** ♀ 🐾   **M**

      ● **O09.523   Supervision of elderly multigravida, third trimester** ♀ 🐾   **M**

      ■● **O09.529   Supervision of elderly multigravida, unspecified trimester** ♀ 🐾   **M**

  ● **O09.6   Supervision of young primigravida and multigravida**

    Supervision of pregnancy for a female less than 16 years old at expected date of delivery

    ● **O09.61   Supervision of young primigravida**

      ● **O09.611   Supervision of young primigravida, first trimester** ♀ 🐾   **M**

      ● **O09.612   Supervision of young primigravida, second trimester** ♀ 🐾   **M**

      ● **O09.613   Supervision of young primigravida, third trimester** ♀ 🐾   **M**

● Unacceptable Principal Diagnosis   ● Use Additional Character(s)   ■ Unspecified   ▶ Manifestation Code

OGCR Official Guidelines for Coding and Reporting   Excludes 1   Excludes 2   Includes   Use additional   Code first   Code also

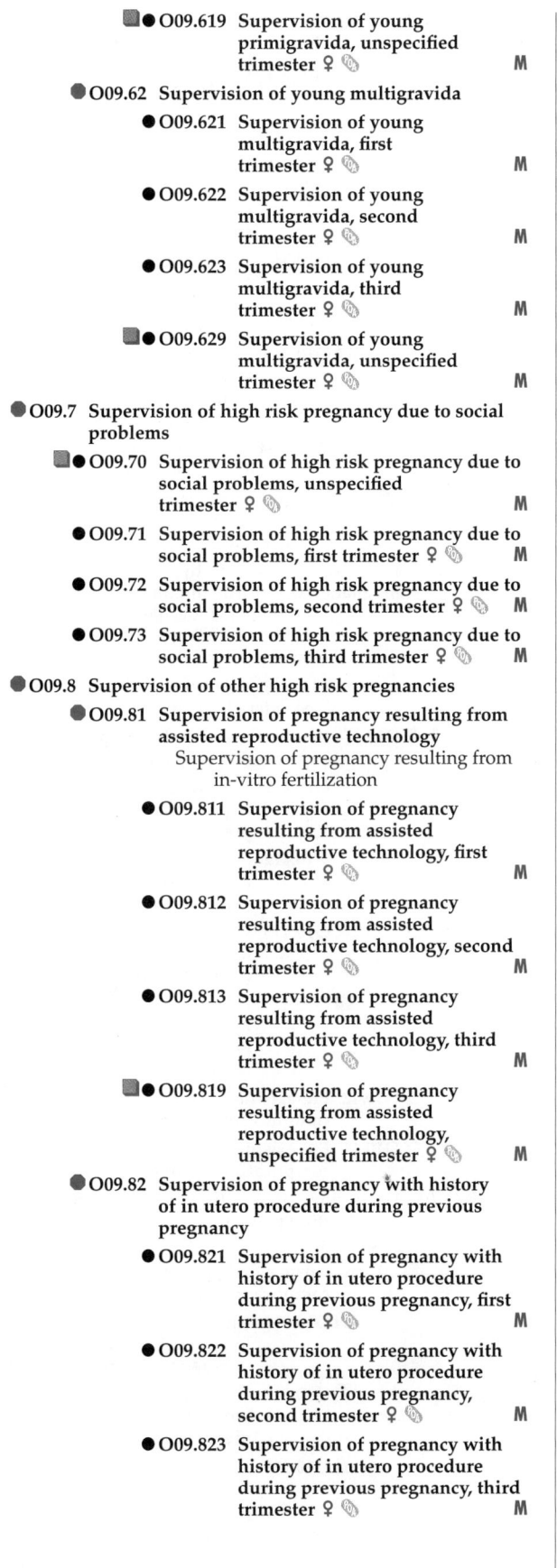

● O09.619 Supervision of young primigravida, unspecified trimester ♀ 🔍   M

● O09.62 Supervision of young multigravida

   ● O09.621 Supervision of young multigravida, first trimester ♀ 🔍   M

   ● O09.622 Supervision of young multigravida, second trimester ♀ 🔍   M

   ● O09.623 Supervision of young multigravida, third trimester ♀ 🔍   M

   ● O09.629 Supervision of young multigravida, unspecified trimester ♀ 🔍   M

● O09.7 Supervision of high risk pregnancy due to social problems

   ● O09.70 Supervision of high risk pregnancy due to social problems, unspecified trimester ♀ 🔍   M

   ● O09.71 Supervision of high risk pregnancy due to social problems, first trimester ♀ 🔍   M

   ● O09.72 Supervision of high risk pregnancy due to social problems, second trimester ♀ 🔍   M

   ● O09.73 Supervision of high risk pregnancy due to social problems, third trimester ♀ 🔍   M

● O09.8 Supervision of other high risk pregnancies

   ● O09.81 Supervision of pregnancy resulting from assisted reproductive technology
     Supervision of pregnancy resulting from in-vitro fertilization

     ● O09.811 Supervision of pregnancy resulting from assisted reproductive technology, first trimester ♀ 🔍   M

     ● O09.812 Supervision of pregnancy resulting from assisted reproductive technology, second trimester ♀ 🔍   M

     ● O09.813 Supervision of pregnancy resulting from assisted reproductive technology, third trimester ♀ 🔍   M

     ● O09.819 Supervision of pregnancy resulting from assisted reproductive technology, unspecified trimester ♀ 🔍   M

   ● O09.82 Supervision of pregnancy with history of in utero procedure during previous pregnancy

     ● O09.821 Supervision of pregnancy with history of in utero procedure during previous pregnancy, first trimester ♀ 🔍   M

     ● O09.822 Supervision of pregnancy with history of in utero procedure during previous pregnancy, second trimester ♀ 🔍   M

     ● O09.823 Supervision of pregnancy with history of in utero procedure during previous pregnancy, third trimester ♀ 🔍   M

● O09.829 Supervision of pregnancy with history of in utero procedure during previous pregnancy, unspecified trimester ♀ 🔍   M

     Excludes1   supervision of pregnancy affected by in utero procedure during current pregnancy (O35.7)

● O09.89 Supervision of other high risk pregnancies

   ● O09.891 Supervision of other high risk pregnancies, first trimester ♀ 🔍 M

   ● O09.892 Supervision of other high risk pregnancies, second trimester ♀ 🔍   M

   ● O09.893 Supervision of other high risk pregnancies, third trimester ♀ 🔍   M

   ● O09.899 Supervision of other high risk pregnancies, unspecified trimester ♀ 🔍   M

● O09.9 Supervision of high risk pregnancy, unspecified

   ● O09.90 Supervision of high risk pregnancy, unspecified, unspecified trimester ♀ 🔍   M

   ● O09.91 Supervision of high risk pregnancy, unspecified, first trimester ♀ 🔍   M

   ● O09.92 Supervision of high risk pregnancy, unspecified, second trimester ♀ 🔍   M

   ● O09.93 Supervision of high risk pregnancy, unspecified, third trimester ♀ 🔍   M

EDEMA, PROTEINURIA AND HYPERTENSIVE DISORDERS IN PREGNANCY, CHILDBIRTH AND THE PUERPERIUM (O10-O16)

● O10 Pre-existing hypertension complicating pregnancy, childbirth and the puerperium

   Includes   pre-existing hypertension with pre-existing proteinuria complicating pregnancy, childbirth and the puerperium

   Excludes2   pre-existing hypertension with superimposed pre-eclampsia complicating pregnancy, childbirth and the puerperium (O11.-)

● O10.0 Pre-existing essential hypertension complicating pregnancy, childbirth and the puerperium
     Any condition in I10 specified as a reason for obstetric care during pregnancy, childbirth or the puerperium

   ● O10.01 Pre-existing essential hypertension complicating pregnancy

     O10.011 Pre-existing essential hypertension complicating pregnancy, first trimester ♀ 🍴   M

     O10.012 Pre-existing essential hypertension complicating pregnancy, second trimester ♀ 🍴   M

     O10.013 Pre-existing essential hypertension complicating pregnancy, third trimester ♀ 🍴 M

     O10.019 Pre-existing essential hypertension complicating pregnancy, unspecified trimester ♀   M

O10.02   Pre-existing essential hypertension complicating childbirth ♀ 🐾   M

O10.03   Pre-existing essential hypertension complicating the puerperium ♀ 🐾   M

● **O10.1**   Pre-existing hypertensive heart disease complicating pregnancy, childbirth and the puerperium

> Any condition in I11 specified as a reason for obstetric care during pregnancy, childbirth or the puerperium

> Use additional code from I11 to identify the type of hypertensive heart disease

   ● **O10.11**   Pre-existing hypertensive heart disease complicating pregnancy

     O10.111   Pre-existing hypertensive heart disease complicating pregnancy, first trimester ♀   M

     O10.112   Pre-existing hypertensive heart disease complicating pregnancy, second trimester ♀   M

     O10.113   Pre-existing hypertensive heart disease complicating pregnancy, third trimester ♀   M

     ■ **O10.119**   Pre-existing hypertensive heart disease complicating pregnancy, unspecified trimester ♀   M

   O10.12   Pre-existing hypertensive heart disease complicating childbirth ♀   M

   O10.13   Pre-existing hypertensive heart disease complicating the puerperium ♀   M

● **O10.2**   Pre-existing hypertensive chronic kidney disease complicating pregnancy, childbirth and the puerperium

> Any condition in I12 specified as a reason for obstetric care during pregnancy, childbirth or the puerperium

> Use additional code from I12 to identify the type of hypertensive chronic kidney disease

   ● **O10.21**   Pre-existing hypertensive chronic kidney disease complicating pregnancy

     O10.211   Pre-existing hypertensive chronic kidney disease complicating pregnancy, first trimester ♀   M

     O10.212   Pre-existing hypertensive chronic kidney disease complicating pregnancy, second trimester ♀   M

     O10.213   Pre-existing hypertensive chronic kidney disease complicating pregnancy, third trimester ♀   M

     ■ **O10.219**   Pre-existing hypertensive chronic kidney disease complicating pregnancy, unspecified trimester ♀   M

   O10.22   Pre-existing hypertensive chronic kidney disease complicating childbirth ♀   M

   O10.23   Pre-existing hypertensive chronic kidney disease complicating the puerperium ♀   M

● **O10.3**   Pre-existing hypertensive heart and chronic kidney disease complicating pregnancy, childbirth and the puerperium

> Any condition in I13 specified as a reason for obstetric care during pregnancy, childbirth or the puerperium

> Use additional code from I13 to identify the type of hypertensive heart and chronic kidney disease

● **O10.31**   Pre-existing hypertensive heart and chronic kidney disease complicating pregnancy

     O10.311   Pre-existing hypertensive heart and chronic kidney disease complicating pregnancy, first trimester ♀   M

     O10.312   Pre-existing hypertensive heart and chronic kidney disease complicating pregnancy, second trimester ♀   M

     O10.313   Pre-existing hypertensive heart and chronic kidney disease complicating pregnancy, third trimester ♀   M

     ■ **O10.319**   Pre-existing hypertensive heart and chronic kidney disease complicating pregnancy, unspecified trimester ♀   M

   O10.32   Pre-existing hypertensive heart and chronic kidney disease complicating childbirth ♀ M

   O10.33   Pre-existing hypertensive heart and chronic kidney disease complicating the puerperium ♀   M

● **O10.4**   Pre-existing secondary hypertension complicating pregnancy, childbirth and the puerperium

> Any condition in I15 specified as a reason for obstetric care during pregnancy, childbirth or the puerperium

> Use additional code from I15 to identify the type of secondary hypertension

   ● **O10.41**   Pre-existing secondary hypertension complicating pregnancy

     O10.411   Pre-existing secondary hypertension complicating pregnancy, first trimester ♀ 🐾   M

     O10.412   Pre-existing secondary hypertension complicating pregnancy, second trimester ♀ 🐾 M

     O10.413   Pre-existing secondary hypertension complicating pregnancy, third trimester ♀ 🐾   M

     ■ **O10.419**   Pre-existing secondary hypertension complicating pregnancy, unspecified trimester ♀   M

   O10.42   Pre-existing secondary hypertension complicating childbirth ♀ 🐾   M

   O10.43   Pre-existing secondary hypertension complicating the puerperium ♀ 🐾   M

● **O10.9**   Unspecified pre-existing hypertension complicating pregnancy, childbirth and the puerperium

   ● **O10.91**   Unspecified pre-existing hypertension complicating pregnancy

     ■ **O10.911**   Unspecified pre-existing hypertension complicating pregnancy, first trimester ♀ 🐾   M

     ■ **O10.912**   Unspecified pre-existing hypertension complicating pregnancy, second trimester ♀ 🐾 M

     ■ **O10.913**   Unspecified pre-existing hypertension complicating pregnancy, third trimester ♀ 🐾   M

     ■ **O10.919**   Unspecified pre-existing hypertension complicating pregnancy, unspecified trimester ♀   M

●   Unacceptable Principal Diagnosis   ●   Use Additional Character(s)   ■   Unspecified   ▶   Manifestation Code

1290   **OGCR**   Official Guidelines for Coding and Reporting   Excludes 1   Excludes 2   Includes   Use additional   Code first   Code also

◼ O10.92   Unspecified pre-existing hypertension complicating childbirth ♀ 🐾   M

◼ O10.93   Unspecified pre-existing hypertension complicating the puerperium ♀ 🐾   M

● O11   Pre-existing hypertension with pre-eclampsia

> **Includes**   conditions in O10 complicated by pre-eclampsia
> pre-eclampsia superimposed pre-existing hypertension

> Use additional code from O10 to identify the type of hypertension

O11.1   Pre-existing hypertension with pre-eclampsia, first trimester ♀ 🐾   M

O11.2   Pre-existing hypertension with pre-eclampsia, second trimester ♀ 🐾   M

O11.3   Pre-existing hypertension with pre-eclampsia, third trimester ♀ 🐾   M

◼ O11.9   Pre-existing hypertension with pre-eclampsia, unspecified trimester ♀   M

● O12   Gestational [pregnancy-induced] edema and proteinuria without hypertension

   ● O12.0   Gestational edema

     ◼ O12.00   Gestational edema, unspecified trimester ♀   M

     O12.01   Gestational edema, first trimester ♀   M

     O12.02   Gestational edema, second trimester ♀   M

     O12.03   Gestational edema, third trimester ♀   M

   ● O12.1   Gestational proteinuria

     ◼ O12.10   Gestational proteinuria, unspecified trimester ♀   M

     O12.11   Gestational proteinuria, first trimester ♀ 🐾   M

     O12.12   Gestational proteinuria, second trimester ♀ 🐾   M

     O12.13   Gestational proteinuria, third trimester ♀ 🐾   M

   ● O12.2   Gestational edema with proteinuria

     ◼ O12.20   Gestational edema with proteinuria, unspecified trimester ♀   M

     O12.21   Gestational edema with proteinuria, first trimester ♀ 🐾   M

     O12.22   Gestational edema with proteinuria, second trimester ♀ 🐾   M

     O12.23   Gestational edema with proteinuria, third trimester ♀ 🐾   M

● O13   Gestational [pregnancy-induced] hypertension without significant proteinuria

> **Includes**   gestational hypertension NOS

O13.1   Gestational [pregnancy-induced] hypertension without significant proteinuria, first trimester ♀ 🐾   M

O13.2   Gestational [pregnancy-induced] hypertension without significant proteinuria, second trimester ♀ 🐾   M

O13.3   Gestational [pregnancy-induced] hypertension without significant proteinuria, third trimester ♀ 🐾   M

◼ O13.9   Gestational [pregnancy-induced] hypertension without significant proteinuria, unspecified trimester ♀   M

● O14   Pre-eclampsia

> **Excludes1**   pre-existing hypertension with pre-eclampsia (O11)

   ● O14.0   Mild to moderate pre-eclampsia

     ◼ O14.00   Mild to moderate pre-eclampsia, unspecified trimester ♀   M

     O14.02   Mild to moderate pre-eclampsia, second trimester ♀ 🐾   M

     O14.03   Mild to moderate pre-eclampsia, third trimester ♀ 🐾   M

   ● O14.1   Severe pre-eclampsia

> **Excludes1**   HELLP syndrome (O14.2-)
> *H=hemolysis, EL=elevated liver enzymes, LP=low platelet count*

     ◼ O14.10   Severe pre-eclampsia, unspecified trimester ♀   M

     O14.12   Severe pre-eclampsia, second trimester ♀ 🐾   M

     O14.13   Severe pre-eclampsia, third trimester ♀🐾M

   ● O14.2   HELLP syndrome

> Severe pre-eclampsia with hemolysis, elevated liver enzymes and low platelet count (HELLP)

     ◼ O14.20   HELLP syndrome (HELLP), unspecified trimester ♀   M

     O14.22   HELLP syndrome (HELLP), second trimester ♀ 🐾   M

     O14.23   HELLP syndrome (HELLP), third trimester ♀ 🐾   M

   ● O14.9   Unspecified pre-eclampsia

     ◼ O14.90   Unspecified pre-eclampsia, unspecified trimester ♀ 🐾   M

     ◼ O14.92   Unspecified pre-eclampsia, second trimester ♀ 🐾   M

     ◼ O14.93   Unspecified pre-eclampsia, third trimester ♀ 🐾   M

● O15   Eclampsia

> **Includes**   convulsions following conditions in O10-O14 and O16

   ● O15.0   Eclampsia in pregnancy

     ◼ O15.00   Eclampsia in pregnancy, unspecified trimester ♀   M

     O15.02   Eclampsia in pregnancy, second trimester ♀ 🐾   M

     O15.03   Eclampsia in pregnancy, third trimester ♀ 🐾   M

   O15.1   Eclampsia in labor ♀ 🐾   M

   O15.2   Eclampsia in the puerperium ♀ 🐾   M

   ◼ O15.9   Eclampsia, unspecified as to time period ♀   M
     Eclampsia NOS

● O16   Unspecified maternal hypertension

   ◼ O16.1   Unspecified maternal hypertension, first trimester ♀ 🐾   M

   ◼ O16.2   Unspecified maternal hypertension, second trimester ♀ 🐾   M

   ◼ O16.3   Unspecified maternal hypertension, third trimester ♀ 🐾   M

   ◼ O16.9   Unspecified maternal hypertension, unspecified trimester ♀ 🐾   M

CHAPTER 15 (O00-O9A)

OTHER MATERNAL DISORDERS PREDOMINANTLY RELATED TO PREGNANCY (O20-O29)

Excludes2   maternal care related to the fetus and amniotic cavity and possible delivery problems (O30-O48)
maternal diseases classifiable elsewhere but complicating pregnancy, labor and delivery, and the puerperium (O98-O99)

● **O20   Hemorrhage in early pregnancy**

Includes   hemorrhage before completion of 20 weeks gestation

Excludes1   pregnancy with abortive outcome (O00-O08)

O20.0   Threatened abortion ♀ 🐾   M
Hemorrhage specified as due to threatened abortion

O20.8   Other hemorrhage in early pregnancy ♀   M

▪ **O20.9   Hemorrhage in early pregnancy, unspecified** ♀ 🐾 M

● **O21   Excessive vomiting in pregnancy**

O21.0   Mild hyperemesis gravidarum ♀   M
Hyperemesis gravidarum, mild or unspecified, starting before the end of the 20th week of gestation

O21.1   Hyperemesis gravidarum with metabolic disturbance ♀   M
Hyperemesis gravidarum, starting before the end of the 20th week of gestation, with metabolic disturbance such as carbohydrate depletion
Hyperemesis gravidarum, starting before the end of the 20th week of gestation, with metabolic disturbance such as dehydration
Hyperemesis gravidarum, starting before the end of the 20th week of gestation, with metabolic disturbance such as electrolyte imbalance

O21.2   Late vomiting of pregnancy ♀   M
Excessive vomiting starting after 20 completed weeks of gestation

O21.8   Other vomiting complicating pregnancy ♀   M
Vomiting due to diseases classified elsewhere, complicating pregnancy
Use additional code, to identify cause

▪ **O21.9   Vomiting of pregnancy, unspecified** ♀   M

● **O22   Venous complications and hemorrhoids in pregnancy**

Excludes1   venous complications of:
abortion NOS (O03.9)
ectopic or molar pregnancy (O08.7)
failed attempted abortion (O07.35)
induced abortion (O04.85)
spontaneous abortion (O03.89)

Excludes2   obstetric pulmonary embolism (O88.-)
venous complications and hemorrhoids of childbirth and the puerperium (O87.-)

● **O22.0   Varicose veins of lower extremity in pregnancy**
Varicose veins NOS in pregnancy

▪ **O22.00   Varicose veins of lower extremity in pregnancy, unspecified trimester** ♀   M

O22.01   Varicose veins of lower extremity in pregnancy, first trimester ♀   M

O22.02   Varicose veins of lower extremity in pregnancy, second trimester ♀   M

O22.03   Varicose veins of lower extremity in pregnancy, third trimester ♀   M

● **O22.1   Genital varices in pregnancy**
Perineal varices in pregnancy
Vaginal varices in pregnancy
Vulval varices in pregnancy

▪ **O22.10   Genital varices in pregnancy, unspecified trimester** ♀   M

O22.11   Genital varices in pregnancy, first trimester ♀   M

O22.12   Genital varices in pregnancy, second trimester ♀   M

O22.13   Genital varices in pregnancy, third trimester ♀   M

● **O22.2   Superficial thrombophlebitis in pregnancy**
Phlebitis in pregnancy NOS
Thrombophlebitis of legs in pregnancy
Thrombosis in pregnancy NOS
Use additional code to identify the superficial thrombophlebitis (I80.0-)

▪ **O22.20   Superficial thrombophlebitis in pregnancy, unspecified trimester** ♀ 🐾   M

O22.21   Superficial thrombophlebitis in pregnancy, first trimester ♀ 🐾   M

O22.22   Superficial thrombophlebitis in pregnancy, second trimester ♀ 🐾   M

O22.23   Superficial thrombophlebitis in pregnancy, third trimester ♀ 🐾   M

● **O22.3   Deep phlebothrombosis in pregnancy**
Deep vein thrombosis, antepartum
Use additional code to identify the deep vein thrombosis (I82.4-, I82.5-, I82.62-. I82.72-)
Use additional code, if applicable, for associated long-term (current) use of anticoagulants (Z79.01)

▪ **O22.30   Deep phlebothrombosis in pregnancy, unspecified trimester** ♀ 🐾   M

O22.31   Deep phlebothrombosis in pregnancy, first trimester ♀ 🐾   M

O22.32   Deep phlebothrombosis in pregnancy, second trimester ♀ 🐾   M

O22.33   Deep phlebothrombosis in pregnancy, third trimester ♀ 🐾   M

● **O22.4   Hemorrhoids in pregnancy**

▪ **O22.40   Hemorrhoids in pregnancy, unspecified trimester** ♀ 🐾   M

O22.41   Hemorrhoids in pregnancy, first trimester ♀ 🐾   M

O22.42   Hemorrhoids in pregnancy, second trimester ♀ 🐾   M

O22.43   Hemorrhoids in pregnancy, third trimester ♀ 🐾   M

● **O22.5   Cerebral venous thrombosis in pregnancy**
Cerebrovenous sinus thrombosis in pregnancy

▪ **O22.50   Cerebral venous thrombosis in pregnancy, unspecified trimester** ♀ 🐾   M

O22.51   Cerebral venous thrombosis in pregnancy, first trimester ♀ 🐾   M

O22.52   Cerebral venous thrombosis in pregnancy, second trimester ♀ 🐾   M

O22.53   Cerebral venous thrombosis in pregnancy, third trimester ♀ 🐾   M

● **O22.8   Other venous complications in pregnancy**

● **O22.8X   Other venous complications in pregnancy**

O22.8X1   Other venous complications in pregnancy, first trimester ♀ 🐾   M

● Unacceptable Principal Diagnosis   ● Use Additional Character(s)   ▪ Unspecified   ▶ Manifestation Code

OGCR   Official Guidelines for Coding and Reporting   Excludes 1   Excludes 2   Includes   Use additional   Code first   Code also

O22.8X2 Other venous complications in pregnancy, second trimester ♀ M

O22.8X3 Other venous complications in pregnancy, third trimester ♀ M

O22.8X9 Other venous complications in pregnancy, unspecified trimester ♀ M

● **O22.9** Venous complication in pregnancy, unspecified
　　Gestational phlebitis NOS
　　Gestational phlebopathy NOS
　　Gestational thrombosis NOS

O22.90 Venous complication in pregnancy, unspecified, unspecified trimester ♀ M

O22.91 Venous complication in pregnancy, unspecified, first trimester ♀ M

O22.92 Venous complication in pregnancy, unspecified, second trimester ♀ M

O22.93 Venous complication in pregnancy, unspecified, third trimester ♀ M

● **O23** Infections of genitourinary tract in pregnancy
　Use additional code to identify organism (B95.-, B96.-)

　Excludes2　gonococcal infections complicating pregnancy, childbirth and the puerperium (O98.2)
　　　infections with a predominantly sexual mode of transmission NOS complicating pregnancy, childbirth and the puerperium (O98.3)
　　　syphilis complicating pregnancy, childbirth and the puerperium (O98.1)
　　　tuberculosis of genitourinary system complicating pregnancy, childbirth and the puerperium (O98.0)
　　　venereal disease NOS complicating pregnancy, childbirth and the puerperium (O98.3)

● **O23.0** Infections of kidney in pregnancy
　　Pyelonephritis in pregnancy

O23.00 Infections of kidney in pregnancy, unspecified trimester ♀ M

O23.01 Infections of kidney in pregnancy, first trimester ♀ M

O23.02 Infections of kidney in pregnancy, second trimester ♀ M

O23.03 Infections of kidney in pregnancy, third trimester ♀ M

● **O23.1** Infections of bladder in pregnancy

O23.10 Infections of bladder in pregnancy, unspecified trimester ♀ M

O23.11 Infections of bladder in pregnancy, first trimester ♀ M

O23.12 Infections of bladder in pregnancy, second trimester ♀ M

O23.13 Infections of bladder in pregnancy, third trimester ♀ M

● **O23.2** Infections of urethra in pregnancy

O23.20 Infections of urethra in pregnancy, unspecified trimester ♀ M

O23.21 Infections of urethra in pregnancy, first trimester ♀ M

O23.22 Infections of urethra in pregnancy, second trimester ♀ M

O23.23 Infections of urethra in pregnancy, third trimester ♀ M

● **O23.3** Infections of other parts of urinary tract in pregnancy

O23.30 Infections of other parts of urinary tract in pregnancy, unspecified trimester ♀ M

O23.31 Infections of other parts of urinary tract in pregnancy, first trimester ♀ M

O23.32 Infections of other parts of urinary tract in pregnancy, second trimester ♀ M

O23.33 Infections of other parts of urinary tract in pregnancy, third trimester ♀ M

● **O23.4** Unspecified infection of urinary tract in pregnancy

O23.40 Unspecified infection of urinary tract in pregnancy, unspecified trimester ♀ M

O23.41 Unspecified infection of urinary tract in pregnancy, first trimester ♀ M

O23.42 Unspecified infection of urinary tract in pregnancy, second trimester ♀ M

O23.43 Unspecified infection of urinary tract in pregnancy, third trimester ♀ M

● **O23.5** Infections of the genital tract in pregnancy

● **O23.51** Infection of cervix in pregnancy

O23.511 Infections of cervix in pregnancy, first trimester ♀ M

O23.512 Infections of cervix in pregnancy, second trimester ♀ M

O23.513 Infections of cervix in pregnancy, third trimester ♀ M

O23.519 Infections of cervix in pregnancy, unspecified trimester ♀ M

● **O23.52** Salpingo-oophoritis in pregnancy
　　Oophoritis = inflammation of ovary
　　Salpingitis = inflammation of fallopian tube
　　Oophoritis in pregnancy
　　Salpingitis in pregnancy

O23.521 Salpingo-oophoritis in pregnancy, first trimester ♀ M

O23.522 Salpingo-oophoritis in pregnancy, second trimester ♀ M

O23.523 Salpingo-oophoritis in pregnancy, third trimester ♀ M

O23.529 Salpingo-oophoritis in pregnancy, unspecified trimester ♀ M

● **O23.59** Infection of other part of genital tract in pregnancy

O23.591 Infection of other part of genital tract in pregnancy, first trimester ♀ M

O23.592 Infection of other part of genital tract in pregnancy, second trimester ♀ M

O23.593 Infection of other part of genital tract in pregnancy, third trimester ♀ M

O23.599 Infection of other part of genital tract in pregnancy, unspecified trimester ♀ M

N Newborn Age: 0　　**P** Pediatric Age: 0–17　　**M** Maternity DX: 12–55　　**A** Adult Age: 15–124　　♀ Females Only　　♂ Males Only

 Complication\Comorbidity　　 Major C\C　　 Present on Admission Requirement　　 Hospital-Acquired Condition

1293

CHAPTER 15 (O00-O9A)

● **O23.9 Unspecified genitourinary tract infection in pregnancy**
    Genitourinary tract infection in pregnancy NOS

    ■ **O23.90 Unspecified genitourinary tract infection in pregnancy, unspecified trimester** ♀   M

    ■ **O23.91 Unspecified genitourinary tract infection in pregnancy, first trimester** ♀ 🦠   M

    ■ **O23.92 Unspecified genitourinary tract infection in pregnancy, second trimester** ♀ 🦠   M

    ■ **O23.93 Unspecified genitourinary tract infection in pregnancy, third trimester** ♀ 🦠   M

OGCR Section I.C.15.g.

g. Diabetes mellitus in pregnancy

Diabetes mellitus is a significant complicating factor in pregnancy. Pregnant women who are diabetic should be assigned a code from category O24, Diabetes mellitus in pregnancy, childbirth, and the puerperium, first, followed by the appropriate diabetes code(s)(E08-E13) from Chapter 4.

OGCR Section I.C.15.i.

i. Gestational (pregnancy induced) diabetes

Gestational (pregnancy induced) diabetes can occur during the second and third trimester of pregnancy in women who were not diabetic prior to pregnancy. Gestational diabetes can cause complications in the pregnancy similar to those of pre-existing diabetes mellitus. It also puts the woman at greater risk of developing diabetes after the pregnancy. Codes for gestational diabetes are in subcategory O24.4, Gestational diabetes mellitus. No other code from category O24, Diabetes mellitus in pregnancy, childbirth, and the puerperium, should be used with a code from O24.4

The codes under subcategory O24.4 include diet controlled and insulin controlled. If a patient with gestational diabetes is treated with both diet and insulin, only the code for insulin-controlled is required. Code Z79.4, Long-term (current) use of insulin, should not be assigned with codes from subcategory O24.4.

An abnormal glucose tolerance in pregnancy is assigned a code from subcategory O99.81, Abnormal glucose complicating pregnancy, childbirth, and the puerperium.

● **O24 Diabetes mellitus in pregnancy, childbirth, and the puerperium**

  ● **O24.0 Pre-existing diabetes mellitus, type 1, in pregnancy, childbirth and the puerperium**
    Juvenile onset diabetes mellitus, in pregnancy, childbirth and the puerperium
    Ketosis-prone diabetes mellitus in pregnancy, childbirth and the puerperium

    Use additional code from category E10 to further identify any manifestations

    ● **O24.01 Pre-existing diabetes mellitus, type 1, in pregnancy**

      O24.011 Pre-existing diabetes mellitus, type 1, in pregnancy, first trimester ♀ 🦠   M

      O24.012 Pre-existing diabetes mellitus, type 1, in pregnancy, second trimester ♀ 🦠   M

      O24.013 Pre-existing diabetes mellitus, type 1, in pregnancy, third trimester ♀ 🦠   M

      ■ **O24.019 Pre-existing diabetes mellitus, type 1, in pregnancy, unspecified trimester** ♀ 🦠   M

    O24.02 Pre-existing diabetes mellitus, type 1, in childbirth ♀ 🦠   M

    O24.03 Pre-existing diabetes mellitus, type 1, in the puerperium ♀ 🦠   M

  ● **O24.1 Pre-existing diabetes mellitus, type 2, in pregnancy, childbirth and the puerperium**
    Insulin-resistant diabetes mellitus in pregnancy, childbirth and the puerperium

    Use additional code (for):
    from category E11 to further identify any manifestations
    long-term (current) use of insulin (Z79.4)

    ● **O24.11 Pre-existing diabetes mellitus, type 2, in pregnancy**

      O24.111 Pre-existing diabetes mellitus, type 2, in pregnancy, first trimester ♀ 🦠   M

      O24.112 Pre-existing diabetes mellitus, type 2, in pregnancy, second trimester ♀ 🦠   M

      O24.113 Pre-existing diabetes mellitus, type 2, in pregnancy, third trimester ♀ 🦠   M

      ■ **O24.119 Pre-existing diabetes mellitus, type 2, in pregnancy, unspecified trimester** ♀ 🦠   M

    O24.12 Pre-existing diabetes mellitus, type 2, in childbirth ♀ 🦠   M

    O24.13 Pre-existing diabetes mellitus, type 2, in the puerperium ♀ 🦠   M

  ● **O24.3 Unspecified pre-existing diabetes mellitus in pregnancy, childbirth and the puerperium**

    Use additional code (for):
    from category E11 to further identify any manifestation
    long-term (current) use of insulin (Z79.4)

    ● **O24.31 Unspecified pre-existing diabetes mellitus in pregnancy**

      ■ **O24.311 Unspecified pre-existing diabetes mellitus in pregnancy, first trimester** ♀ 🦠   M

      ■ **O24.312 Unspecified pre-existing diabetes mellitus in pregnancy, second trimester** ♀ 🦠   M

      ■ **O24.313 Unspecified pre-existing diabetes mellitus in pregnancy, third trimester** ♀ 🦠   M

      ■ **O24.319 Unspecified pre-existing diabetes mellitus in pregnancy, unspecified trimester** ♀ 🦠   M

    ■ **O24.32 Unspecified pre-existing diabetes mellitus in childbirth** ♀ 🦠   M

    ■ **O24.33 Unspecified pre-existing diabetes mellitus in the puerperium** ♀ 🦠   M

  ● **O24.4 Gestational diabetes mellitus**
    Diabetes mellitus arising in pregnancy
    Gestational diabetes mellitus NOS

    ● **O24.41 Gestational diabetes mellitus in pregnancy**

      O24.410 Gestational diabetes mellitus in pregnancy, diet controlled ♀   M

      O24.414 Gestational diabetes mellitus in pregnancy, insulin controlled ♀ M

      ■ **O24.419 Gestational diabetes mellitus in pregnancy, unspecified control** ♀   M

● Unacceptable Principal Diagnosis   ● Use Additional Character(s)   ■ Unspecified   ▶ Manifestation Code
OGCR Official Guidelines for Coding and Reporting   Excludes 1   Excludes 2   Includes   Use additional   Code first   Code also

● **O24.42 Gestational diabetes mellitus in childbirth**

    O24.420   Gestational diabetes mellitus in childbirth, diet controlled ♀   **M**

    O24.424   Gestational diabetes mellitus in childbirth, insulin controlled ♀ **M**

    ■ O24.429   Gestational diabetes mellitus in childbirth, unspecified control ♀   **M**

● **O24.43 Gestational diabetes mellitus in the puerperium**

    O24.430   Gestational diabetes mellitus in the puerperium, diet controlled ♀   **M**

    O24.434   Gestational diabetes mellitus in the puerperium, insulin controlled ♀   **M**

    ■ O24.439   Gestational diabetes mellitus in the puerperium, unspecified control ♀   **M**

● **O24.8 Other pre-existing diabetes mellitus in pregnancy, childbirth, and the puerperium**

    Use additional code (for):
    from categories E08, E09 and E13 to further identify any manifestation
    long-term (current) use of insulin (Z79.4)

  ● **O24.81 Other pre-existing diabetes mellitus in pregnancy**

    O24.811   Other pre-existing diabetes mellitus in pregnancy, first trimester ♀ 🝖   **M**

    O24.812   Other pre-existing diabetes mellitus in pregnancy, second trimester ♀ 🝖   **M**

    O24.813   Other pre-existing diabetes mellitus in pregnancy, third trimester ♀ 🝖   **M**

    ■ O24.819   Other pre-existing diabetes mellitus in pregnancy, unspecified trimester ♀ 🝖   **M**

  O24.82   Other pre-existing diabetes mellitus in childbirth ♀ 🝖   **M**

  O24.83   Other pre-existing diabetes mellitus in the puerperium ♀ 🝖   **M**

● **O24.9 Unspecified diabetes mellitus in pregnancy, childbirth and the puerperium**

    Use additional code for long-term (current) use of insulin (Z79.4)

  ● **O24.91 Unspecified diabetes mellitus in pregnancy**

    ■ O24.911   Unspecified diabetes mellitus in pregnancy, first trimester ♀ 🝖 **M**

    ■ O24.912   Unspecified diabetes mellitus in pregnancy, second trimester ♀ 🝖   **M**

    ■ O24.913   Unspecified diabetes mellitus in pregnancy, third trimester ♀ 🝖 **M**

    ■ O24.919   Unspecified diabetes mellitus in pregnancy, unspecified trimester ♀ 🝖   **M**

  ■ O24.92   Unspecified diabetes mellitus in childbirth ♀   **M**

  ■ O24.93   Unspecified diabetes mellitus in the puerperium ♀ 🝖   **M**

● **O25 Malnutrition in pregnancy, childbirth and the puerperium**

  ● **O25.1 Malnutrition in pregnancy**

    ■ O25.10   Malnutrition in pregnancy, unspecified trimester ♀   **M**

    O25.11   Malnutrition in pregnancy, first trimester ♀   **M**

    O25.12   Malnutrition in pregnancy, second trimester ♀   **M**

    O25.13   Malnutrition in pregnancy, third trimester ♀   **M**

  O25.2   Malnutrition in childbirth ♀   **M**

  O25.3   Malnutrition in the puerperium ♀   **M**

● **O26 Maternal care for other conditions predominantly related to pregnancy**

  ● **O26.0 Excessive weight gain in pregnancy**

    Excludes2   gestational edema (O12.0, O12.2)

    ■ O26.00   Excessive weight gain in pregnancy, unspecified trimester ♀   **M**

    O26.01   Excessive weight gain in pregnancy, first trimester ♀   **M**

    O26.02   Excessive weight gain in pregnancy, second trimester ♀   **M**

    O26.03   Excessive weight gain in pregnancy, third trimester ♀   **M**

  ● **O26.1 Low weight gain in pregnancy**

    ■ O26.10   Low weight gain in pregnancy, unspecified trimester ♀   **M**

    O26.11   Low weight gain in pregnancy, first trimester ♀   **M**

    O26.12   Low weight gain in pregnancy, second trimester ♀   **M**

    O26.13   Low weight gain in pregnancy, third trimester ♀   **M**

  ● **O26.2 Pregnancy care for patient with recurrent pregnancy loss**

    ■ O26.20   Pregnancy care for patient with recurrent pregnancy loss, unspecified trimester ♀ **M**

    O26.21   Pregnancy care for patient with recurrent pregnancy loss, first trimester ♀ 🝖   **M**

    O26.22   Pregnancy care for patient with recurrent pregnancy loss, second trimester ♀ 🝖   **M**

    O26.23   Pregnancy care for patient with recurrent pregnancy loss, third trimester ♀ 🝖   **M**

  ● **O26.3 Retained intrauterine contraceptive device in pregnancy**

    ■ O26.30   Retained intrauterine contraceptive device in pregnancy, unspecified trimester ♀   **M**

    O26.31   Retained intrauterine contraceptive device in pregnancy, first trimester ♀   **M**

    O26.32   Retained intrauterine contraceptive device in pregnancy, second trimester ♀   **M**

    O26.33   Retained intrauterine contraceptive device in pregnancy, third trimester ♀   **M**

  ● **O26.4 Herpes gestationis**

    ■ O26.40   Herpes gestationis, unspecified trimester ♀   **M**

    O26.41   Herpes gestationis, first trimester ♀   **M**

    O26.42   Herpes gestationis, second trimester ♀   **M**

    O26.43   Herpes gestationis, third trimester ♀   **M**

CHAPTER 15 (O00-O9A)

N Newborn Age: 0   **P** Pediatric Age: 0–17   **M** Maternity DX: 12–55   **A** Adult Age: 15–124   ♀ Females Only   ♂ Males Only

🝖 Complication\Comorbidity   🝖 Major C\C   🝖 Present on Admission Requirement   🝖 Hospital-Acquired Condition

1295

● **O26.5   Maternal hypotension syndrome**
Supine hypotensive syndrome

◻ **O26.50   Maternal hypotension syndrome, unspecified trimester** ♀   M

O26.51   Maternal hypotension syndrome, first trimester ♀ 🔗   M

O26.52   Maternal hypotension syndrome, second trimester ♀ 🔗   M

O26.53   Maternal hypotension syndrome, third trimester ♀ 🔗   M

● **O26.6   Liver and biliary tract disorders in pregnancy, childbirth and the puerperium**

Use additional code to identify the specific disorder

Excludes2   hepatorenal syndrome following labor and delivery (O90.4)

● **O26.61   Liver and biliary tract disorders in pregnancy**

O26.611   Liver and biliary tract disorders in pregnancy, first trimester ♀ 🔗   M

O26.612   Liver and biliary tract disorders in pregnancy, second trimester ♀ 🔗M

O26.613   Liver and biliary tract disorders in pregnancy, third trimester ♀ 🔗   M

◻ **O26.619   Liver and biliary tract disorders in pregnancy, unspecified trimester** ♀   M

O26.62   Liver and biliary tract disorders in childbirth ♀ 🔗   M

O26.63   Liver and biliary tract disorders in the puerperium ♀   M

● **O26.7   Subluxation of symphysis (pubis) in pregnancy, childbirth and the puerperium**

Excludes1   traumatic separation of symphysis (pubis) during childbirth (O71.6)

● **O26.71   Subluxation of symphysis (pubis) in pregnancy**

O26.711   Subluxation of symphysis (pubis) in pregnancy, first trimester ♀   M

O26.712   Subluxation of symphysis (pubis) in pregnancy, second trimester ♀   M

O26.713   Subluxation of symphysis (pubis) in pregnancy, third trimester ♀   M

◻ **O26.719   Subluxation of symphysis (pubis) in pregnancy, unspecified trimester** ♀   M

O26.72   Subluxation of symphysis (pubis) in childbirth ♀   M

O26.73   Subluxation of symphysis (pubis) in the puerperium ♀   M

● **O26.8   Other specified pregnancy related conditions**

● **O26.81   Pregnancy related exhaustion and fatigue**

O26.811   Pregnancy related exhaustion and fatigue, first trimester ♀   M

O26.812   Pregnancy related exhaustion and fatigue, second trimester ♀   M

O26.813   Pregnancy related exhaustion and fatigue, third trimester ♀   M

◻ **O26.819   Pregnancy related exhaustion and fatigue, unspecified trimester** ♀   M

● **O26.82   Pregnancy related peripheral neuritis**

O26.821   Pregnancy related peripheral neuritis, first trimester ♀   M

O26.822   Pregnancy related peripheral neuritis, second trimester ♀   M

O26.823   Pregnancy related peripheral neuritis, third trimester ♀   M

◻ **O26.829   Pregnancy related peripheral neuritis, unspecified trimester** ♀   M

● **O26.83   Pregnancy related renal disease**

Use additional code to identify the specific disorder

O26.831   Pregnancy related renal disease, first trimester ♀ 🔗   M

O26.832   Pregnancy related renal disease, second trimester ♀ 🔗   M

O26.833   Pregnancy related renal disease, third trimester ♀ 🔗   M

◻ **O26.839   Pregnancy related renal disease, unspecified trimester** ♀   M

● **O26.84   Uterine size-date discrepancy complicating pregnancy**

Excludes1   encounter for suspected problem with fetal growth ruled out (Z03.74)

O26.841   Uterine size-date discrepancy, first trimester ♀   M

O26.842   Uterine size-date discrepancy, second trimester ♀   M

O26.843   Uterine size-date discrepancy, third trimester ♀   M

◻ **O26.849   Uterine size-date discrepancy, unspecified trimester** ♀   M

● **O26.85   Spotting complicating pregnancy**

O26.851   Spotting complicating pregnancy, first trimester ♀   M

O26.852   Spotting complicating pregnancy, second trimester ♀   M

O26.853   Spotting complicating pregnancy, third trimester ♀   M

◻ **O26.859   Spotting complicating pregnancy, unspecified trimester** ♀   M

O26.86   Pruritic urticarial papules and plaques of pregnancy (PUPPP) ♀   M
Polymorphic eruption of pregnancy

● **O26.87   Cervical shortening**

Excludes1   encounter for suspected cervical shortening ruled out (Z03.75)

O26.872   Cervical shortening, second trimester ♀ 🔗   M

O26.873   Cervical shortening, third trimester ♀ 🔗   M

◻ **O26.879   Cervical shortening, unspecified trimester** ♀ 🔗   M

● Unacceptable Principal Diagnosis   ● Use Additional Character(s)   ◻ Unspecified   ▶ Manifestation Code

1296   **OGCR** Official Guidelines for Coding and Reporting | Excludes 1 | | Excludes 2 | | Includes | | Use additional | | Code first | | Code also |

● **O26.89 Other specified pregnancy related conditions**

    O26.891 Other specified pregnancy related conditions, first trimester ♀ M

    O26.892 Other specified pregnancy related conditions, second trimester ♀ M

    O26.893 Other specified pregnancy related conditions, third trimester ♀ M

    ■ **O26.899** Other specified pregnancy related conditions, unspecified trimester ♀ M

● **O26.9 Pregnancy related conditions, unspecified**

    ■ **O26.90** Pregnancy related conditions, unspecified, unspecified trimester ♀ M

    ■ **O26.91** Pregnancy related conditions, unspecified, first trimester ♀ M

    ■ **O26.92** Pregnancy related conditions, unspecified, second trimester ♀ M

    ■ **O26.93** Pregnancy related conditions, unspecified, third trimester ♀ M

● **O28 Abnormal findings on antenatal screening of mother**

    Excludes1   diagnostic findings classified elsewhere - see Alphabetical Index

    O28.0 Abnormal hematological finding on antenatal screening of mother ♀ M

    O28.1 Abnormal biochemical finding on antenatal screening of mother ♀ M

    O28.2 Abnormal cytological finding on antenatal screening of mother ♀ M

    O28.3 Abnormal ultrasonic finding on antenatal screening of mother ♀ M

    O28.4 Abnormal radiological finding on antenatal screening of mother ♀ M

    O28.5 Abnormal chromosomal and genetic finding on antenatal screening of mother ♀ M

    O28.8 Other abnormal findings on antenatal screening of mother ♀ M

    ■ **O28.9** Unspecified abnormal findings on antenatal screening of mother ♀ M

● **O29 Complications of anesthesia during pregnancy**

    Includes   maternal complications arising from the administration of a general, regional or local anesthetic, analgesic or other sedation during pregnancy

    Use additional code, if necessary, to identify the complication

    Excludes2   complications of anesthesia during labor and delivery (O74.-) complications of anesthesia during the puerperium (O89.-)

● **O29.0 Pulmonary complications of anesthesia during pregnancy**

    ● **O29.01 Aspiration pneumonitis due to anesthesia during pregnancy**

        Inhalation of stomach contents or secretions NOS due to anesthesia during pregnancy

        Mendelson's syndrome due to anesthesia during pregnancy

        O29.011 Aspiration pneumonitis due to anesthesia during pregnancy, first trimester ♀ M

        O29.012 Aspiration pneumonitis due to anesthesia during pregnancy, second trimester ♀ M

        O29.013 Aspiration pneumonitis due to anesthesia during pregnancy, third trimester ♀ M

        ■ **O29.019** Aspiration pneumonitis due to anesthesia during pregnancy, unspecified trimester ♀ M

    ● **O29.02 Pressure collapse of lung due to anesthesia during pregnancy**

        O29.021 Pressure collapse of lung due to anesthesia during pregnancy, first trimester ♀ M

        O29.022 Pressure collapse of lung due to anesthesia during pregnancy, second trimester ♀ M

        O29.023 Pressure collapse of lung due to anesthesia during pregnancy, third trimester ♀ M

        ■ **O29.029** Pressure collapse of lung due to anesthesia during pregnancy, unspecified trimester ♀ M

    ● **O29.09 Other pulmonary complications of anesthesia during pregnancy**

        O29.091 Other pulmonary complications of anesthesia during pregnancy, first trimester ♀ M

        O29.092 Other pulmonary complications of anesthesia during pregnancy, second trimester ♀ M

        O29.093 Other pulmonary complications of anesthesia during pregnancy, third trimester ♀ M

        ■ **O29.099** Other pulmonary complications of anesthesia during pregnancy, unspecified trimester ♀ M

● **O29.1 Cardiac complications of anesthesia during pregnancy**

    ● **O29.11 Cardiac arrest due to anesthesia during pregnancy**

        O29.111 Cardiac arrest due to anesthesia during pregnancy, first trimester ♀ M

        O29.112 Cardiac arrest due to anesthesia during pregnancy, second trimester ♀ M

        O29.113 Cardiac arrest due to anesthesia during pregnancy, third trimester ♀ M

        ■ **O29.119** Cardiac arrest due to anesthesia during pregnancy, unspecified trimester ♀ M

    ● **O29.12 Cardiac failure due to anesthesia during pregnancy**

        O29.121 Cardiac failure due to anesthesia during pregnancy, first trimester ♀ M

        O29.122 Cardiac failure due to anesthesia during pregnancy, second trimester ♀ M

        O29.123 Cardiac failure due to anesthesia during pregnancy, third trimester ♀ M

        ■ **O29.129** Cardiac failure due to anesthesia during pregnancy, unspecified trimester ♀ M

CHAPTER 15 (O00-O9A)

● O29.19   Other cardiac complications of anesthesia during pregnancy

    O29.191   Other cardiac complications of anesthesia during pregnancy, first trimester ♀   M

    O29.192   Other cardiac complications of anesthesia during pregnancy, second trimester ♀   M

    O29.193   Other cardiac complications of anesthesia during pregnancy, third trimester ♀   M

    ▪ O29.199   Other cardiac complications of anesthesia during pregnancy, unspecified trimester ♀   M

● O29.2   Central nervous system complications of anesthesia during pregnancy

 ● O29.21   Cerebral anoxia due to anesthesia during pregnancy

    O29.211   Cerebral anoxia due to anesthesia during pregnancy, first trimester ♀   M

    O29.212   Cerebral anoxia due to anesthesia during pregnancy, second trimester ♀   M

    O29.213   Cerebral anoxia due to anesthesia during pregnancy, third trimester ♀   M

    ▪ O29.219   Cerebral anoxia due to anesthesia during pregnancy, unspecified trimester ♀   M

 ● O29.29   Other central nervous system complications of anesthesia during pregnancy

    O29.291   Other central nervous system complications of anesthesia during pregnancy, first trimester ♀   M

    O29.292   Other central nervous system complications of anesthesia during pregnancy, second trimester ♀   M

    O29.293   Other central nervous system complications of anesthesia during pregnancy, third trimester ♀   M

    ▪ O29.299   Other central nervous system complications of anesthesia during pregnancy, unspecified trimester ♀   M

● O29.3   Toxic reaction to local anesthesia during pregnancy

 ● O29.3X   Toxic reaction to local anesthesia during pregnancy

    O29.3X1   Toxic reaction to local anesthesia during pregnancy, first trimester ♀   M

    O29.3X2   Toxic reaction to local anesthesia during pregnancy, second trimester ♀   M

    O29.3X3   Toxic reaction to local anesthesia during pregnancy, third trimester ♀   M

    ▪ O29.3X9   Toxic reaction to local anesthesia during pregnancy, unspecified trimester ♀   M

● O29.4   Spinal and epidural anesthesia induced headache during pregnancy

 ▪ O29.40   Spinal and epidural anesthesia induced headache during pregnancy, unspecified trimester ♀   M

    O29.41   Spinal and epidural anesthesia induced headache during pregnancy, first trimester ♀   M

    O29.42   Spinal and epidural anesthesia induced headache during pregnancy, second trimester ♀   M

    O29.43   Spinal and epidural anesthesia induced headache during pregnancy, third trimester ♀   M

● O29.5   Other complications of spinal and epidural anesthesia during pregnancy

 ● O29.5X   Other complications of spinal and epidural anesthesia during pregnancy

    O29.5X1   Other complications of spinal and epidural anesthesia during pregnancy, first trimester ♀   M

    O29.5X2   Other complications of spinal and epidural anesthesia during pregnancy, second trimester ♀   M

    O29.5X3   Other complications of spinal and epidural anesthesia during pregnancy, third trimester ♀   M

    ▪ O29.5X9   Other complications of spinal and epidural anesthesia during pregnancy, unspecified trimester ♀   M

● O29.6   Failed or difficult intubation for anesthesia during pregnancy

 ▪ O29.60   Failed or difficult intubation for anesthesia during pregnancy, unspecified trimester ♀   M

    O29.61   Failed or difficult intubation for anesthesia during pregnancy, first trimester ♀   M

    O29.62   Failed or difficult intubation for anesthesia during pregnancy, second trimester ♀   M

    O29.63   Failed or difficult intubation for anesthesia during pregnancy, third trimester ♀   M

● O29.8   Other complications of anesthesia during pregnancy

 ● O29.8X   Other complications of anesthesia during pregnancy

    O29.8X1   Other complications of anesthesia during pregnancy, first trimester ♀   M

    O29.8X2   Other complications of anesthesia during pregnancy, second trimester ♀   M

    O29.8X3   Other complications of anesthesia during pregnancy, third trimester ♀   M

    ▪ O29.8X9   Other complications of anesthesia during pregnancy, unspecified trimester ♀   M

● Unacceptable Principal Diagnosis   ● Use Additional Character(s)   ▪ Unspecified   ▶ Manifestation Code

OGCR Official Guidelines for Coding and Reporting | Excludes 1 | | Excludes 2 | Includes   Use additional   Code first   Code also

● **O29.9   Unspecified complication of anesthesia during pregnancy**

   ◼ O29.90   Unspecified complication of anesthesia during pregnancy, unspecified trimester ♀ M

   ◼ O29.91   Unspecified complication of anesthesia during pregnancy, first trimester ♀   M

   ◼ O29.92   Unspecified complication of anesthesia during pregnancy, second trimester ♀   M

   ◼ O29.93   Unspecified complication of anesthesia during pregnancy, third trimester ♀   M

MATERNAL CARE RELATED TO THE FETUS AND AMNIOTIC CAVITY AND POSSIBLE DELIVERY PROBLEMS (O30-O48)

● **O30   Multiple gestation**

> Code also any complications specific to multiple gestation

 ● **O30.0   Twin pregnancy**

  ● O30.00   Twin pregnancy, unspecified number of placenta and unspecified number of amniotic sacs

    ◼● O30.001   Twin pregnancy, unspecified number of placenta and unspecified number of amniotic sacs, first trimester ♀ 🪙   M

    ◼● O30.002   Twin pregnancy, unspecified number of placenta and unspecified number of amniotic sacs, second trimester ♀ 🪙   M

    ◼● O30.003   Twin pregnancy, unspecified number of placenta and unspecified number of amniotic sacs, third trimester ♀ 🪙   M

    ◼● O30.009   Twin pregnancy, unspecified number of placenta and unspecified number of amniotic sacs, unspecified trimester ♀   M

  ● O30.01   Twin pregnancy, monochorionic/monoamniotic

> Twin pregnancy, one placenta, one amniotic sac

> **Excludes1**   conjoined twins (O30.02-)

    ● O30.011   Twin pregnancy, monochorionic/monoamniotic, first trimester ♀ 🪙   M

    ● O30.012   Twin pregnancy, monochorionic/monoamniotic, second trimester ♀ 🪙   M

    ● O30.013   Twin pregnancy, monochorionic/monoamniotic, third trimester ♀ 🪙   M

    ◼● O30.019   Twin pregnancy, monochorionic/monoamniotic, unspecified trimester ♀   M

  ● O30.02   Conjoined twin pregnancy

    O30.021   Conjoined twin pregnancy, first trimester ♀   M

    O30.022   Conjoined twin pregnancy, second trimester ♀   M

    O30.023   Conjoined twin pregnancy, third trimester ♀   M

    ◼ O30.029   Conjoined twin pregnancy, unspecified trimester ♀

  ● O30.03   Twin pregnancy, monochorionic/diamniotic

> Twin pregnancy, one placenta, two amniotic sacs

    ● O30.031   Twin pregnancy, monochorionic/diamniotic, first trimester ♀ 🪙 M

    ● O30.032   Twin pregnancy, monochorionic/diamniotic, second trimester ♀ 🪙   M

    ● O30.033   Twin pregnancy, monochorionic/diamniotic, third trimester ♀ 🪙 M

    ◼● O30.039   Twin pregnancy, monochorionic/diamniotic, unspecified trimester ♀   M

  ● O30.04   Twin pregnancy, dichorionic/diamniotic

> Twin pregnancy, two placentae, two amniotic sacs

    ● O30.041   Twin pregnancy, dichorionic/diamniotic, first trimester ♀ 🪙   M

    ● O30.042   Twin pregnancy, dichorionic/diamniotic, second trimester ♀ 🪙   M

    ● O30.043   Twin pregnancy, dichorionic/diamniotic, third trimester ♀ 🪙 M

    ◼● O30.049   Twin pregnancy, dichorionic/diamniotic, unspecified trimester ♀   M

  ● O30.09   Twin pregnancy, unable to determine number of placenta and number of amniotic sacs

    ● O30.091   Twin pregnancy, unable to determine number of placenta and number of amniotic sacs, first trimester ♀ 🪙   M

    ● O30.092   Twin pregnancy, unable to determine number of placenta and number of amniotic sacs, second trimester ♀ 🪙   M

    ● O30.093   Twin pregnancy, unable to determine number of placenta and number of amniotic sacs, third trimester ♀ 🪙   M

    ◼● O30.099   Twin pregnancy, unable to determine number of placenta and number of amniotic sacs, unspecified trimester ♀   M

 ● **O30.1   Triplet pregnancy**

  ● O30.10   Triplet pregnancy, unspecified number of placenta and unspecified number of amniotic sacs

    ● O30.101   Triplet pregnancy, unspecified number of placenta and unspecified number of amniotic sacs, first trimester ♀ 🪙   M

    ● O30.102   Triplet pregnancy, unspecified number of placenta and unspecified number of amniotic sacs, second trimester ♀ 🪙   M

    ● O30.103   Triplet pregnancy, unspecified number of placenta and unspecified number of amniotic sacs, third trimester ♀ 🪙   M

    ◼● O30.109   Triplet pregnancy, unspecified number of placenta and unspecified number of amniotic sacs, unspecified trimester ♀   M

N Newborn Age: 0   **P** Pediatric Age: 0–17   **M** Maternity DX: 12–55   **A** Adult Age: 15–124   ♀ Females Only   ♂ Males Only

🪙 Complication\Comorbidity   🪙 Major C\C   Present on Admission Requirement   🪙 Hospital-Acquired Condition

1299

CHAPTER 15 (O00-O9A)

● O30.11   Triplet pregnancy with two or more monochorionic fetuses

   ● O30.111   Triplet pregnancy with two or more monochorionic fetuses, first trimester ♀ 🍼   M

   ● O30.112   Triplet pregnancy with two or more monochorionic fetuses, second trimester ♀ 🍼   M

   ● O30.113   Triplet pregnancy with two or more monochorionic fetuses, third trimester ♀ 🍼   M

   ■● O30.119   Triplet pregnancy with two or more monochorionic fetuses, unspecified trimester ♀   M

● O30.12   Triplet pregnancy with two or more monoamniotic fetuses

   ● O30.121   Triplet pregnancy with two or more monoamniotic fetuses, first trimester ♀ 🍼   M

   ● O30.122   Triplet pregnancy with two or more monoamniotic fetuses, second trimester ♀ 🍼   M

   ● O30.123   Triplet pregnancy with two or more monoamniotic fetuses, third trimester ♀ 🍼   M

   ■● O30.129   Triplet pregnancy with two or more monoamniotic fetuses, unspecified trimester ♀   M

● O30.19   Triplet pregnancy, unable to determine number of placenta and number of amniotic sacs

   ● O30.191   Triplet pregnancy, unable to determine number of placenta and number of amniotic sacs, first trimester ♀ 🍼   M

   ● O30.192   Triplet pregnancy, unable to determine number of placenta and number of amniotic sacs, second trimester ♀ 🍼   M

   ● O30.193   Triplet pregnancy, unable to determine number of placenta and number of amniotic sacs, third trimester ♀ 🍼   M

   ■● O30.199   Triplet pregnancy, unable to determine number of placenta and number of amniotic sacs, unspecified trimester ♀   M

● O30.2   Quadruplet pregnancy

 ● O30.20   Quadruplet pregnancy, unspecified number of placenta and unspecified number of amniotic sacs

   ● O30.201   Quadruplet pregnancy, unspecified number of placenta and unspecified number of amniotic sacs, first trimester ♀ 🍼   M

   ● O30.202   Quadruplet pregnancy, unspecified number of placenta and unspecified number of amniotic sacs, second trimester ♀ 🍼   M

   ● O30.203   Quadruplet pregnancy, unspecified number of placenta and unspecified number of amniotic sacs, third trimester ♀ 🍼   M

   ■● O30.209   Quadruplet pregnancy, unspecified number of placenta and unspecified number of amniotic sacs, unspecified trimester ♀   M

● O30.21   Quadruplet pregnancy with two or more monochorionic fetuses

   ● O30.211   Quadruplet pregnancy with two or more monochorionic fetuses, first trimester ♀ 🍼   M

   ● O30.212   Quadruplet pregnancy with two or more monochorionic fetuses, second trimester ♀ 🍼   M

   ● O30.213   Quadruplet pregnancy with two or more monochorionic fetuses, third trimester ♀ 🍼   M

   ■● O30.219   Quadruplet pregnancy with two or more monochorionic fetuses, unspecified trimester ♀   M

● O30.22   Quadruplet pregnancy with two or more monoamniotic fetuses

   ● O30.221   Quadruplet pregnancy with two or more monoamniotic fetuses, first trimester ♀ 🍼   M

   ● O30.222   Quadruplet pregnancy with two or more monoamniotic fetuses, second trimester ♀ 🍼   M

   ● O30.223   Quadruplet pregnancy with two or more monoamniotic fetuses, third trimester ♀ 🍼   M

   ■● O30.229   Quadruplet pregnancy with two or more monoamniotic fetuses, unspecified trimester ♀   M

● O30.29   Quadruplet pregnancy, unable to determine number of placenta and number of amniotic sacs

   ● O30.291   Quadruplet pregnancy, unable to determine number of placenta and number of amniotic sacs, first trimester ♀ 🍼   M

   ● O30.292   Quadruplet pregnancy, unable to determine number of placenta and number of amniotic sacs, second trimester ♀ 🍼   M

   ● O30.293   Quadruplet pregnancy, unable to determine number of placenta and number of amniotic sacs, third trimester ♀ 🍼   M

   ■● O30.299   Quadruplet pregnancy, unable to determine number of placenta and number of amniotic sacs, unspecified trimester ♀   M

● O30.8   Other specified multiple gestation
   Multiple gestation pregnancy greater then quadruplets

 ● O30.80   Other specified multiple gestation, unspecified number of placenta and unspecified number of amniotic sacs

   ● O30.801   Other specified multiple gestation, unspecified number of placenta and unspecified number of amniotic sacs, first trimester ♀ 🍼   M

   ● O30.802   Other specified multiple gestation, unspecified number of placenta and unspecified number of amniotic sacs, second trimester ♀ 🍼   M

● Unacceptable Principal Diagnosis   ● Use Additional Character(s)   ■ Unspecified   ▶ Manifestation Code

OGCR Official Guidelines for Coding and Reporting   Excludes 1   Excludes 2   Includes   Use additional   Code first   Code also

● O30.803   Other specified multiple gestation, unspecified number of placenta and unspecified number of amniotic sacs, third trimester ♀   M

● O30.809   Other specified multiple gestation, unspecified number of placenta and unspecified number of amniotic sacs, unspecified trimester ♀   M

● O30.81   Other specified multiple gestation with two or more monochorionic fetuses

     ● O30.811   Other specified multiple gestation with two or more monochorionic fetuses, first trimester ♀   M

     ● O30.812   Other specified multiple gestation with two or more monochorionic fetuses, second trimester ♀   M

     ● O30.813   Other specified multiple gestation with two or more monochorionic fetuses, third trimester ♀   M

     ● O30.819   Other specified multiple gestation with two or more monochorionic fetuses, unspecified trimester ♀   M

● O30.82   Other specified multiple gestation with two or more monoamniotic fetuses

     ● O30.821   Other specified multiple gestation with two or more monoamniotic fetuses, first trimester ♀   M

     ● O30.822   Other specified multiple gestation with two or more monoamniotic fetuses, second trimester ♀   M

     ● O30.823   Other specified multiple gestation with two or more monoamniotic fetuses, third trimester ♀   M

     ● O30.829   Other specified multiple gestation with two or more monoamniotic fetuses, unspecified trimester ♀   M

● O30.89   Other specified multiple gestation, unable to determine number of placenta and number of amniotic sacs

     ● O30.891   Other specified multiple gestation, unable to determine number of placenta and number of amniotic sacs, first trimester ♀   M

     ● O30.892   Other specified multiple gestation, unable to determine number of placenta and number of amniotic sacs, second trimester ♀   M

     ● O30.893   Other specified multiple gestation, unable to determine number of placenta and number of amniotic sacs, third trimester ♀   M

     ● O30.899   Other specified multiple gestation, unable to determine number of placenta and number of amniotic sacs, unspecified trimester ♀   M

● O30.9   Multiple gestation, unspecified
     Multiple pregnancy NOS

     ● O30.90   Multiple gestation, unspecified, unspecified trimester ♀   M

     ● O30.91   Multiple gestation, unspecified, first trimester ♀   M

     ● O30.92   Multiple gestation, unspecified, second trimester ♀   M

     ● O30.93   Multiple gestation, unspecified, third trimester ♀   M

● O31   Complications specific to multiple gestation

     | Excludes2 | delayed delivery of second twin, triplet, etc. (O63.2)
     malpresentation of one fetus or more (O32.5)
     placental transfusion syndromes (O43.0-)

     One of the following 7th characters is to be assigned to each code under category O31. 7th character 0 is for single gestations and multiple gestations where the fetus is unspecified. 7th characters 1 through 9 are for cases of multiple gestations to identify the fetus for which the code applies. The appropriate code from category O30, Multiple gestation, must also be assigned when assigning a code from category O31 that has a 7th character of 1 through 9.

     | 0 | not applicable or unspecified |
     | 1 | fetus 1 |
     | 2 | fetus 2 |
     | 3 | fetus 3 |
     | 4 | fetus 4 |
     | 5 | fetus 5 |
     | 9 | other fetus |

● O31.0   Papyraceous fetus
     Fetus compressus

     ● O31.00   Papyraceous fetus, unspecified trimester

     ● O31.01   Papyraceous fetus, first trimester

     ● O31.02   Papyraceous fetus, second trimester

     ● O31.03   Papyraceous fetus, third trimester

● O31.1   Continuing pregnancy after spontaneous abortion of one fetus or more

     ● O31.10   Continuing pregnancy after spontaneous abortion of one fetus or more, unspecified trimester

     ● O31.11   Continuing pregnancy after spontaneous abortion of one fetus or more, first trimester

     ● O31.12   Continuing pregnancy after spontaneous abortion of one fetus or more, second trimester

     ● O31.13   Continuing pregnancy after spontaneous abortion of one fetus or more, third trimester

● O31.2   Continuing pregnancy after intrauterine death of one fetus or more

     ● O31.20   Continuing pregnancy after intrauterine death of one fetus or more, unspecified trimester

     ● O31.21   Continuing pregnancy after intrauterine death of one fetus or more, first trimester

     ● O31.22   Continuing pregnancy after intrauterine death of one fetus or more, second trimester

     ● O31.23   Continuing pregnancy after intrauterine death of one fetus or more, third trimester

N   Newborn Age: 0   **P**   Pediatric Age: 0–17   **M**   Maternity DX: 12–55   **A**   Adult Age: 15–124   ♀   Females Only   ♂   Males Only

 Complication\Comorbidity   Major C\C   Present on Admission Requirement   Hospital-Acquired Condition

1301

CHAPTER 15 (O00-O9A)

● **O31.3 Continuing pregnancy after elective fetal reduction of one fetus or more**
Continuing pregnancy after selective termination of one fetus or more

●■ **O31.30 Continuing pregnancy after elective fetal reduction of one fetus or more, unspecified trimester**

● **O31.31 Continuing pregnancy after elective fetal reduction of one fetus or more, first trimester**

● **O31.32 Continuing pregnancy after elective fetal reduction of one fetus or more, second trimester**

● **O31.33 Continuing pregnancy after elective fetal reduction of one fetus or more, third trimester**

● **O31.8 Other complications specific to multiple gestation**

● **O31.8X Other complications specific to multiple gestation**

● **O31.8X1 Other complications specific to multiple gestation, first trimester** ✆

● **O31.8X2 Other complications specific to multiple gestation, second trimester** ✆

● **O31.8X3 Other complications specific to multiple gestation, third trimester** ✆

●■ **O31.8X9 Other complications specific to multiple gestation, unspecified trimester**

● **O32 Maternal care for malpresentation of fetus**

Includes the listed conditions as a reason for observation, hospitalization or other obstetric care of the mother, or for cesarean delivery before onset of labor

Excludes1 malpresentation of fetus with obstructed labor (O64.-)

One of the following 7th characters is to be assigned to each code under category O32. 7th character 0 is for single gestations and multiple gestations where the fetus is unspecified. 7th characters 1 through 9 are for cases of multiple gestations to identify the fetus for which the code applies. The appropriate code from category O30, Multiple gestation, must also be assigned when assigning a code from category O32 that has a 7th character of 1 through 9.

0	not applicable or unspecified
1	fetus 1
2	fetus 2
3	fetus 3
4	fetus 4
5	fetus 5
9	other fetus

● **O32.0 Maternal care for unstable lie**

● **O32.1 Maternal care for breech presentation**
Maternal care for buttocks presentation
Maternal care for complete breech
Maternal care for frank breech

Excludes1 footling presentation (O32.8)
incomplete breech (O32.8)

● **O32.2 Maternal care for transverse and oblique lie**
Maternal care for oblique presentation
Maternal care for transverse presentation

● **O32.3 Maternal care for face, brow and chin presentation**

● **O32.4 Maternal care for high head at term**
Maternal care for failure of head to enter pelvic brim

● **O32.6 Maternal care for compound presentation**

● **O32.8 Maternal care for other malpresentation of fetus**
Maternal care for footling presentation
Maternal care for incomplete breech

●■ **O32.9 Maternal care for malpresentation of fetus, unspecified**

● **O33 Maternal care for disproportion**

Includes the listed conditions as a reason for observation, hospitalization or other obstetric care of the mother, or for cesarean delivery before onset of labor

Excludes1 disproportion with obstructed labor (O65-O66)

O33.0 Maternal care for disproportion due to deformity of maternal pelvic bones ♀ ✆ **M**
Maternal care for disproportion due to pelvic deformity causing disproportion NOS

O33.1 Maternal care for disproportion due to generally contracted pelvis ♀ **M**
Maternal care for disproportion due to contracted pelvis NOS causing disproportion

O33.2 Maternal care for disproportion due to inlet contraction of pelvis ♀ **M**
Maternal care for disproportion due to inlet contraction (pelvis) causing disproportion

O33.3 Maternal care for disproportion due to outlet contraction of pelvis
Maternal care for disproportion due to mid-cavity contraction (pelvis)
Maternal care for disproportion due to outlet contraction (pelvis)

One of the following 7th characters is to be assigned to code O33.3. 7th character 0 is for single gestations and multiple gestations where the fetus is unspecified. 7th characters 1 through 9 are for cases of multiple gestations to identify the fetus for which the code applies. The appropriate code from category O30, Multiple gestation, must also be assigned when assigning code O33.3 with a 7th character of 1 through 9.

0	not applicable or unspecified
1	fetus 1
2	fetus 2
3	fetus 3
4	fetus 4
5	fetus 5
9	other fetus

● Unacceptable Principal Diagnosis   ● Use Additional Character(s)   ■ Unspecified   ▶ Manifestation Code
OGCR Official Guidelines for Coding and Reporting   Excludes 1   Excludes 2   Includes   Use additional   Code first   Code also

● **O33.4 Maternal care for disproportion of mixed maternal and fetal origin**

> One of the following 7th characters is to be assigned to code O33.4. 7th character 0 is for single gestations and multiple gestations where the fetus is unspecified. 7th characters 1 through 9 are for cases of multiple gestations to identify the fetus for which the code applies. The appropriate code from category O30, Multiple gestation, must also be assigned when assigning code O33.4 with a 7th character of 1 through 9.

0	not applicable or unspecified
1	fetus 1
2	fetus 2
3	fetus 3
4	fetus 4
5	fetus 5
9	other fetus

● **O33.5 Maternal care for disproportion due to unusually large fetus**

> Maternal care for disproportion due to disproportion of fetal origin with normally formed fetus
> Maternal care for disproportion due to fetal disproportion NOS

> One of the following 7th characters is to be assigned to code O33.5. 7th character 0 is for single gestations and multiple gestations where the fetus is unspecified. 7th characters 1 through 9 are for cases of multiple gestations to identify the fetus for which the code applies. The appropriate code from category O30, Multiple gestation, must also be assigned when assigning code O33.5 with a 7th character of 1 through 9.

0	not applicable or unspecified
1	fetus 1
2	fetus 2
3	fetus 3
4	fetus 4
5	fetus 5
9	other fetus

● **O33.6 Maternal care for disproportion due to hydrocephalic fetus**

> One of the following 7th characters is to be assigned to code O33.6. 7th character 0 is for single gestations and multiple gestations where the fetus is unspecified. 7th characters 1 through 9 are for cases of multiple gestations to identify the fetus for which the code applies. The appropriate code from category O30, Multiple gestation, must also be assigned when assigning code O33.6 with a 7th character of 1 through 9.

0	not applicable or unspecified
1	fetus 1
2	fetus 2
3	fetus 3
4	fetus 4
5	fetus 5
9	other fetus

● **O33.7 Maternal care for disproportion due to other fetal deformities** ♀ **M**

> Maternal care for disproportion due to fetal ascites
> Maternal care for disproportion due to fetal hydrops
> Maternal care for disproportion due to fetal meningomyelocele
> Maternal care for disproportion due to fetal sacral teratoma
> Maternal care for disproportion due to fetal tumor

> **Excludes1**   obstructed labor due to other fetal deformities (O66.3)

O33.8 Maternal care for disproportion of other origin ♀ **M**

■ **O33.9 Maternal care for disproportion, unspecified** ♀   **M**

> Maternal care for disproportion due to cephalopelvic disproportion NOS
> Maternal care for disproportion due to fetopelvic disproportion NOS

● **O34 Maternal care for abnormality of pelvic organs**

> **Includes**   the listed conditions as a reason for hospitalization or other obstetric care of the mother, or for cesarean delivery before onset of labor

> *Code first* any associated obstructed labor (O65.5)

> Use additional code for specific condition

● **O34.0 Maternal care for congenital malformation of uterus**

■ **O34.00 Maternal care for unspecified congenital malformation of uterus, unspecified trimester** ♀   **M**

■ **O34.01 Maternal care for unspecified congenital malformation of uterus, first trimester** ♀ **M**

■ **O34.02 Maternal care for unspecified congenital malformation of uterus, second trimester** ♀   **M**

■ **O34.03 Maternal care for unspecified congenital malformation of uterus, third trimester** ♀ **M**

● **O34.1 Maternal care for benign tumor of corpus uteri**

> **Excludes2**   maternal care for benign tumor of cervix (O34.4-)
> maternal care for malignant neoplasm of uterus (O9A.1-)

■ **O34.10 Maternal care for benign tumor of corpus uteri, unspecified trimester** ♀   **M**

O34.11 Maternal care for benign tumor of corpus uteri, first trimester ♀   **M**

O34.12 Maternal care for benign tumor of corpus uteri, second trimester ♀   **M**

O34.13 Maternal care for benign tumor of corpus uteri, third trimester ♀   **M**

● **O34.2 Maternal care due to uterine scar from previous surgery**

O34.21 Maternal care for scar from previous cesarean delivery ♀   **M**

O34.29 Maternal care due to uterine scar from other previous surgery ♀   **M**

N Newborn Age: 0   **P** Pediatric Age: 0–17   **M** Maternity DX: 12–55   **A** Adult Age: 15–124   ♀ Females Only   ♂ Males Only

🐾 Complication\Comorbidity   🐾 Major C\C   🐾 Present on Admission Requirement   🐾 Hospital-Acquired Condition

1303

● O34.3 **Maternal care for cervical incompetence**
    Maternal care for cerclage with or without cervical
        incompetence
    Maternal care for Shirodkar suture with or
        without cervical incompetence

■ O34.30 Maternal care for cervical incompetence,
            unspecified trimester ♀   M

  O34.31 Maternal care for cervical incompetence,
            first trimester ♀ 🐾   M

  O34.32 Maternal care for cervical incompetence,
            second trimester ♀ 🐾   M

  O34.33 Maternal care for cervical incompetence,
            third trimester ♀ 🐾   M

● O34.4 **Maternal care for other abnormalities of cervix**

■ O34.40 Maternal care for other abnormalities of
            cervix, unspecified trimester ♀   M

  O34.41 Maternal care for other abnormalities of
            cervix, first trimester ♀   M

  O34.42 Maternal care for other abnormalities of
            cervix, second trimester ♀   M

  O34.43 Maternal care for other abnormalities of
            cervix, third trimester ♀   M

● O34.5 **Maternal care for other abnormalities of gravid
         uterus**

  ● O34.51 Maternal care for incarceration of gravid
              uterus

    O34.511 Maternal care for incarceration of
              gravid uterus, first trimester ♀   M

    O34.512 Maternal care for incarceration
              of gravid uterus, second
              trimester ♀   M

    O34.513 Maternal care for incarceration of
              gravid uterus, third trimester ♀ M

  ■ O34.519 Maternal care for incarceration of
              gravid uterus, unspecified
              trimester ♀   M

  ● O34.52 Maternal care for prolapse of gravid uterus

    O34.521 Maternal care for prolapse of
              gravid uterus, first trimester ♀ M

    O34.522 Maternal care for prolapse
              of gravid uterus, second
              trimester ♀   M

    O34.523 Maternal care for prolapse of
              gravid uterus, third trimester ♀ M

  ■ O34.529 Maternal care for prolapse of
              gravid uterus, unspecified
              trimester ♀   M

  ● O34.53 Maternal care for retroversion of gravid
              uterus

    O34.531 Maternal care for retroversion of
              gravid uterus, first trimester ♀ M

    O34.532 Maternal care for retroversion
              of gravid uterus, second
              trimester ♀   M

    O34.533 Maternal care for retroversion of
              gravid uterus, third trimester ♀ M

  ■ O34.539 Maternal care for retroversion of
              gravid uterus, unspecified
              trimester ♀   M

● O34.59 **Maternal care for other abnormalities of
         gravid uterus**

  O34.591 Maternal care for other
            abnormalities of gravid uterus,
            first trimester ♀   M

  O34.592 Maternal care for other
            abnormalities of gravid uterus,
            second trimester ♀   M

  O34.593 Maternal care for other
            abnormalities of gravid uterus,
            third trimester ♀   M

■ O34.599 Maternal care for other
            abnormalities of gravid uterus,
            unspecified trimester ♀   M

● O34.6 **Maternal care for abnormality of vagina**
    Excludes2   maternal care for vaginal varices in
                     pregnancy (O22.1-)

■ O34.60 Maternal care for abnormality of vagina,
            unspecified trimester ♀   M

  O34.61 Maternal care for abnormality of vagina,
            first trimester ♀   M

  O34.62 Maternal care for abnormality of vagina,
            second trimester ♀   M

  O34.63 Maternal care for abnormality of vagina,
            third trimester ♀   M

● O34.7 **Maternal care for abnormality of vulva and
         perineum**
    Excludes2   maternal care for perineal and vulval
                     varices in pregnancy (O22.1-)

■ O34.70 Maternal care for abnormality of vulva
            and perineum, unspecified trimester ♀   M

  O34.71 Maternal care for abnormality of vulva
            and perineum, first trimester ♀   M

  O34.72 Maternal care for abnormality of vulva
            and perineum, second trimester ♀   M

  O34.73 Maternal care for abnormality of vulva
            and perineum, third trimester ♀   M

● O34.8 **Maternal care for other abnormalities of pelvic
         organs**

■ O34.80 Maternal care for other abnormalities of
            pelvic organs, unspecified trimester ♀   M

  O34.81 Maternal care for other abnormalities of
            pelvic organs, first trimester ♀   M

  O34.82 Maternal care for other abnormalities of
            pelvic organs, second trimester ♀   M

  O34.83 Maternal care for other abnormalities of
            pelvic organs, third trimester ♀   M

● O34.9 **Maternal care for abnormality of pelvic organ,
         unspecified**

■ O34.90 Maternal care for abnormality of pelvic
            organ, unspecified, unspecified
            trimester ♀   M

■ O34.91 Maternal care for abnormality of pelvic
            organ, unspecified, first trimester ♀   M

■ O34.92 Maternal care for abnormality of pelvic
            organ, unspecified, second trimester ♀   M

■ O34.93 Maternal care for abnormality of pelvic
            organ, unspecified, third trimester ♀   M

● Unacceptable Principal Diagnosis   ● Use Additional Character(s)   ■ Unspecified   ▶ Manifestation Code

OGCR Official Guidelines for Coding and Reporting | Excludes 1 | | Excludes 2 | | Includes | | Use additional | | Code first | | Code also |

OGCR Section I.C.15.e.l.

Fetal Conditions Affecting the Management of the Mother

1) Code from categories O35 and O36

Codes from categories O35, Maternal care for known or suspected fetal abnormality and damage, and O36, Maternal care for other fetal problems, are assigned only when the fetal condition is actually responsible for modifying the management of the mother, i.e., by requiring diagnostic studies, additional observation, special care, or termination of pregnancy. The fact that the fetal condition exists does not justify assigning a code from this series to the mother's record.

2) In utero surgery

In cases when surgery is performed on the fetus, a diagnosis code from category O35, Maternal care for known or suspected fetal abnormality and damage, should be assigned identifying the fetal condition. Assign the appropriate procedure code for the procedure performed.

No code from Chapter 16, the perinatal codes, should be used on the mother's record to identify fetal conditions. Surgery performed in utero on a fetus is still to be coded as an obstetric encounter.

● O35　Maternal care for known or suspected fetal abnormality and damage

Includes　the listed conditions in the fetus as a reason for hospitalization or other obstetric care to the mother, or for termination of pregnancy

Code also any associated maternal condition

Excludes1　encounter for suspected maternal and fetal conditions ruled out (Z03.7-)

One of the following 7th characters is to be assigned to each code under category O35. 7th character 0 is for single gestations and multiple gestations where the fetus is unspecified. 7th characters 1 through 9 are for cases of multiple gestations to identify the fetus for which the code applies. The appropriate code from category O30, Multiple gestation, must also be assigned when assigning a code from category O35 that has a 7th character of 1 through 9.

0	not applicable or unspecified
1	fetus 1
2	fetus 2
3	fetus 3
4	fetus 4
5	fetus 5
9	other fetus

● O35.0　Maternal care for (suspected) central nervous system malformation in fetus
　Maternal care for fetal anencephaly
　Maternal care for fetal hydrocephalus
　Maternal care for fetal spina bifida

Excludes2　chromosomal abnormality in fetus (O35.1)

● O35.1　Maternal care for (suspected) chromosomal abnormality in fetus

● O35.2　Maternal care for (suspected) hereditary disease in fetus

Excludes2　chromosomal abnormality in fetus (O35.1)

● O35.3　Maternal care for (suspected) damage to fetus from viral disease in mother
　Maternal care for damage to fetus from maternal cytomegalovirus infection
　Maternal care for damage to fetus from maternal rubella

● O35.4　Maternal care for (suspected) damage to fetus from alcohol

● O35.5　Maternal care for (suspected) damage to fetus by drugs
　Maternal care for damage to fetus from drug addiction

● O35.6　Maternal care for (suspected) damage to fetus by radiation

● O35.7　Maternal care for (suspected) damage to fetus by other medical procedures
　Maternal care for damage to fetus by amniocentesis
　Maternal care for damage to fetus by biopsy procedures
　Maternal care for damage to fetus by hematological investigation
　Maternal care for damage to fetus by intrauterine contraceptive device
　Maternal care for damage to fetus by intrauterine surgery

● O35.8　Maternal care for other (suspected) fetal abnormality and damage
　Maternal care for damage to fetus from maternal listeriosis
　Maternal care for damage to fetus from maternal toxoplasmosis

●■ O35.9　Maternal care for (suspected) fetal abnormality and damage, unspecified

● O36　Maternal care for other fetal problems

Includes　the listed conditions in the fetus as a reason for hospitalization or other obstetric care of the mother, or for termination of pregnancy

Excludes1　encounter for suspected maternal and fetal conditions ruled out (Z03.7-)
　placental transfusion syndromes (O43.0-)

Excludes2　labor and delivery complicated by fetal stress (O77.-)

One of the following 7th characters is to be assigned to each code under category O36. 7th character 0 is for single gestations and multiple gestations where the fetus is unspecified. 7th characters 1 through 9 are for cases of multiple gestations to identify the fetus for which the code applies. The appropriate code from category O30, Multiple gestation, must also be assigned when assigning a code from category O36 that has a 7th character of 1 through 9.

0	not applicable or unspecified
1	fetus 1
2	fetus 2
3	fetus 3
4	fetus 4
5	fetus 5
9	other fetus

● O36.0　Maternal care for rhesus isoimmunization
　Maternal care for Rh incompatibility (with hydrops fetalis)

● O36.01　Maternal care for anti-D [Rh] antibodies

● O36.011　Maternal care for anti-D [Rh] antibodies, first trimester ⚕

● O36.012　Maternal care for anti-D [Rh] antibodies, second trimester ⚕

● O36.013　Maternal care for anti-D [Rh] antibodies, third trimester ⚕

●■ O36.019　Maternal care for anti-D [Rh] antibodies, unspecified trimester

CHAPTER 15 (O00-O9A)

N Newborn Age: 0　P Pediatric Age: 0–17　M Maternity DX: 12–55　A Adult Age: 15–124　♀ Females Only　♂ Males Only

⚕ Complication\Comorbidity　⚕ Major C\C　⚕ Present on Admission Requirement　⚕ Hospital-Acquired Condition

● O36.09 **Maternal care for other rhesus isoimmunization**

  ● O36.091 **Maternal care for other rhesus isoimmunization, first trimester** 🔓

  ● O36.092 **Maternal care for other rhesus isoimmunization, second trimester** 🔓

  ● O36.093 **Maternal care for other rhesus isoimmunization, third trimester** 🔓

  ●■ O36.099 **Maternal care for other rhesus isoimmunization, unspecified trimester**

● O36.1 **Maternal care for other isoimmunization**
  Maternal care for ABO isoimmunization

  ● O36.11 **Maternal care for Anti-A sensitization**
    Maternal care for isoimmunization NOS (with hydrops fetalis)

    ● O36.111 **Maternal care for Anti-A sensitization, first trimester**

    ● O36.112 **Maternal care for Anti-A sensitization, second trimester**

    ● O36.113 **Maternal care for Anti-A sensitization, third trimester**

    ●■ O36.119 **Maternal care for Anti-A sensitization, unspecified trimester**

  ● O36.19 **Maternal care for other isoimmunization**
    Maternal care for Anti-B sensitization

    ● O36.191 **Maternal care for other isoimmunization, first trimester**

    ● O36.192 **Maternal care for other isoimmunization, second trimester**

    ● O36.193 **Maternal care for other isoimmunization, third trimester**

    ●■ O36.199 **Maternal care for other isoimmunization, unspecified trimester**

● O36.2 **Maternal care for hydrops fetalis**
  Maternal care for hydrops fetalis NOS
  Maternal care for hydrops fetalis not associated with isoimmunization

Excludes1	hydrops fetalis associated with ABO isoimmunization (O36.1-)
	hydrops fetalis associated with rhesus isoimmunization (O36.0-)

  ●■ O36.20 **Maternal care for hydrops fetalis, unspecified trimester**

  ● O36.21 **Maternal care for hydrops fetalis, first trimester**

  ● O36.22 **Maternal care for hydrops fetalis, second trimester**

  ● O36.23 **Maternal care for hydrops fetalis, third trimester**

● O36.4 **Maternal care for intrauterine death** 🔓
  Maternal care for intrauterine fetal death NOS
  Maternal care for intrauterine fetal death after completion of 20 weeks of gestation
  Maternal care for late fetal death
  Maternal care for missed delivery

Excludes1	missed abortion (O02.1)
	stillbirth (P95)

● O36.5 **Maternal care for known or suspected poor fetal growth**

  ● O36.51 **Maternal care for known or suspected placental insufficiency**

    ● O36.511 **Maternal care for known or suspected placental insufficiency, first trimester** 🔓

    ● O36.512 **Maternal care for known or suspected placental insufficiency, second trimester** 🔓

    ● O36.513 **Maternal care for known or suspected placental insufficiency, third trimester** 🔓

    ●■ O36.519 **Maternal care for known or suspected placental insufficiency, unspecified trimester**

  ● O36.59 **Maternal care for other known or suspected poor fetal growth**
    Maternal care for known or suspected light-for-dates NOS
    Maternal care for known or suspected small-for-dates NOS

    ● O36.591 **Maternal care for other known or suspected poor fetal growth, first trimester** 🔓

    ● O36.592 **Maternal care for other known or suspected poor fetal growth, second trimester** 🔓

    ● O36.593 **Maternal care for other known or suspected poor fetal growth, third trimester** 🔓

    ●■ O36.599 **Maternal care for other known or suspected poor fetal growth, unspecified trimester**

● O36.6 **Maternal care for excessive fetal growth**
  Maternal care for known or suspected large-for-dates

  ●■ O36.60 **Maternal care for excessive fetal growth, unspecified trimester**

  ● O36.61 **Maternal care for excessive fetal growth, first trimester**

  ● O36.62 **Maternal care for excessive fetal growth, second trimester**

  ● O36.63 **Maternal care for excessive fetal growth, third trimester**

● O36.7 **Maternal care for viable fetus in abdominal pregnancy**

  ●■ O36.70 **Maternal care for viable fetus in abdominal pregnancy, unspecified trimester**

  ● O36.71 **Maternal care for viable fetus in abdominal pregnancy, first trimester**

  ● O36.72 **Maternal care for viable fetus in abdominal pregnancy, second trimester**

  ● O36.73 **Maternal care for viable fetus in abdominal pregnancy, third trimester**

● O36.8 **Maternal care for other specified fetal problems**

  ● O36.80 **Pregnancy with inconclusive fetal viability**
    Encounter to determine fetal viability of pregnancy

● Unacceptable Principal Diagnosis   ● Use Additional Character(s)   ■ Unspecified   ▶ Manifestation Code

OGCR Official Guidelines for Coding and Reporting | Excludes 1 | | Excludes 2 | Includes   Use additional   Code first   Code also

1306

● O36.81   Decreased fetal movements
   ● O36.812   Decreased fetal movements, second trimester
   ● O36.813   Decreased fetal movements, third trimester
   ●■ O36.819   Decreased fetal movements, unspecified trimester
● O36.82   Fetal anemia and thrombocytopenia
   O36.821   Fetal anemia and thrombocytopenia, first trimester
   O36.822   Fetal anemia and thrombocytopenia, second trimester
   O36.823   Fetal anemia and thrombocytopenia, third trimester
   ■ O36.829   Fetal anemia and thrombocytopenia, unspecified trimester
● O36.89   Maternal care for other specified fetal problems
   ● O36.891   Maternal care for other specified fetal problems, first trimester
   ● O36.892   Maternal care for other specified fetal problems, second trimester
   ● O36.893   Maternal care for other specified fetal problems, third trimester
   ●■ O36.899   Maternal care for other specified fetal problems, unspecified trimester
● O36.9   Maternal care for fetal problem, unspecified
   ●■ O36.90   Maternal care for fetal problem, unspecified, unspecified trimester
   ●■ O36.91   Maternal care for fetal problem, unspecified, first trimester
   ●■ O36.92   Maternal care for fetal problem, unspecified, second trimester
   ●■ O36.93   Maternal care for fetal problem, unspecified, third trimester

● O40   **Polyhydramnios**
Overabundance of amniotic fluid

Includes	hydramnios
Excludes1	encounter for suspected maternal and fetal conditions ruled out (Z03.7-)

One of the following 7th characters is to be assigned to each code under category O40. 7th character 0 is for single gestations and multiple gestations where the fetus is unspecified. 7th characters 1 through 9 are for cases of multiple gestations to identify the fetus for which the code applies. The appropriate code from category O30, Multiple gestation, must also be assigned when assigning a code from category O40 that has a 7th character of 1 through 9.

0	not applicable or unspecified
1	fetus 1
2	fetus 2
3	fetus 3
4	fetus 4
5	fetus 5
9	other fetus

● O40.1   Polyhydramnios, first trimester 🦠
● O40.2   Polyhydramnios, second trimester 🦠
● O40.3   Polyhydramnios, third trimester 🦠
●■ O40.9   Polyhydramnios, unspecified trimester

● O41   **Other disorders of amniotic fluid and membranes**

Excludes1	encounter for suspected maternal and fetal conditions ruled out (Z03.7-)

One of the following 7th characters is to be assigned to each code under category O41. 7th character 0 is for single gestations and multiple gestations where the fetus is unspecified. 7th characters 1 through 9 are for cases of multiple gestations to identify the fetus for which the code applies. The appropriate code from category O30, Multiple gestation, must also be assigned when assigning a code from category O41 that has a 7th character of 1 through 9.

0	not applicable or unspecified
1	fetus 1
2	fetus 2
3	fetus 3
4	fetus 4
5	fetus 5
9	other fetus

● O41.0   Oligohydramnios
Scant volume of amniotic fluid
Oligohydramnios without rupture of membranes
   ●■ O41.00   Oligohydramnios, unspecified trimester
   ● O41.01   Oligohydramnios, first trimester 🦠
   ● O41.02   Oligohydramnios, second trimester 🦠
   ● O41.03   Oligohydramnios, third trimester 🦠
● O41.1   Infection of amniotic sac and membranes
   ● O41.10   Infection of amniotic sac and membranes, unspecified
     ●■ O41.101   Infection of amniotic sac and membranes, unspecified, first trimester 🦠
     ●■ O41.102   Infection of amniotic sac and membranes, unspecified, second trimester 🦠
     ●■ O41.103   Infection of amniotic sac and membranes, unspecified, third trimester 🦠
     ●■ O41.109   Infection of amniotic sac and membranes, unspecified, unspecified trimester
   ● O41.12   Chorioamnionitis
     ● O41.121   Chorioamnionitis, first trimester 🦠
     ● O41.122   Chorioamnionitis, second trimester 🦠
     ● O41.123   Chorioamnionitis, third trimester 🦠
     ●■ O41.129   Chorioamnionitis, unspecified trimester
   ● O41.14   Placentitis
     ● O41.141   Placentitis, first trimester 🦠
     ● O41.142   Placentitis, second trimester 🦠
     ● O41.143   Placentitis, third trimester 🦠
     ●■ O41.149   Placentitis, unspecified trimester

N   Newborn Age: 0   **P**   Pediatric Age: 0–17   **M**   Maternity DX: 12–55   **A**   Adult Age: 15–124   ♀   Females Only   ♂   Males Only

🦠 Complication\Comorbidity   🦠 Major C\C   🦠 Present on Admission Requirement   🦠 Hospital-Acquired Condition

1307

CHAPTER 15 (O00-O9A)

CHAPTER 15 (O00-O9A)

- ● O41.8   Other specified disorders of amniotic fluid and membranes
  - ● O41.8X   Other specified disorders of amniotic fluid and membranes
    - ● O41.8X1   Other specified disorders of amniotic fluid and membranes, first trimester 🔗
    - ● O41.8X2   Other specified disorders of amniotic fluid and membranes, second trimester 🔗
    - ● O41.8X3   Other specified disorders of amniotic fluid and membranes, third trimester 🔗
    - ●◻ O41.8X9   Other specified disorders of amniotic fluid and membranes, unspecified trimester
- ● O41.9   Disorder of amniotic fluid and membranes, unspecified
  - ●◻ O41.90   Disorder of amniotic fluid and membranes, unspecified, unspecified trimester
  - ●◻ O41.91   Disorder of amniotic fluid and membranes, unspecified, first trimester
  - ●◻ O41.92   Disorder of amniotic fluid and membranes, unspecified, second trimester
  - ●◻ O41.93   Disorder of amniotic fluid and membranes, unspecified, third trimester
- ● O42   Premature rupture of membranes
  - ● O42.0   Premature rupture of membranes, onset of labor within 24 hours of rupture
    - ◻ O42.00   Premature rupture of membranes, onset of labor within 24 hours of rupture, unspecified weeks of gestation ♀   M
    - ● O42.01   Preterm premature rupture of membranes, onset of labor within 24 hours of rupture
      Premature rupture of membranes before 37 completed weeks of gestation
      - O42.011   Preterm premature rupture of membranes, onset of labor within 24 hours of rupture, first trimester ♀   M
      - O42.012   Preterm premature rupture of membranes, onset of labor within 24 hours of rupture, second trimester ♀   M
      - O42.013   Preterm premature rupture of membranes, onset of labor within 24 hours of rupture, third trimester ♀   M
      - ◻ O42.019   Preterm premature rupture of membranes, onset of labor within 24 hours of rupture, unspecified trimester ♀   M
    - O42.02   Full-term premature rupture of membranes, onset of labor within 24 hours of rupture ♀   M
      Premature rupture of membranes after 37 completed weeks of gestation
- ● O42.1   Premature rupture of membranes, onset of labor more than 24 hours following rupture
  - ◻ O42.10   Premature rupture of membranes, onset of labor more than 24 hours following rupture, unspecified weeks of gestation ♀   M
  - ● O42.11   Preterm premature rupture of membranes, onset of labor more than 24 hours following rupture
    Premature rupture of membranes before 37 completed weeks of gestation
    - O42.111   Preterm premature rupture of membranes, onset of labor more than 24 hours following rupture, first trimester ♀   M
    - O42.112   Preterm premature rupture of membranes, onset of labor more than 24 hours following rupture, second trimester ♀   M
    - O42.113   Preterm premature rupture of membranes, onset of labor more than 24 hours following rupture, third trimester ♀   M
    - ◻ O42.119   Preterm premature rupture of membranes, onset of labor more than 24 hours following rupture, unspecified trimester ♀   M
  - O42.12   Full-term premature rupture of membranes, onset of labor more than 24 hours following rupture ♀   M
    Premature rupture of membranes after 37 completed weeks of gestation
- ● O42.9   Premature rupture of membranes, unspecified as to length of time between rupture and onset of labor
  - ◻ O42.90   Premature rupture of membranes, unspecified as to length of time between rupture and onset of labor, unspecified weeks of gestation ♀   M
  - ● O42.91   Preterm premature rupture of membranes, unspecified as to length of time between rupture and onset of labor
    Premature rupture of membranes before 37 completed weeks of gestation
    - ◻ O42.911   Preterm premature rupture of membranes, unspecified as to length of time between rupture and onset of labor, first trimester ♀   M
    - ◻ O42.912   Preterm premature rupture of membranes, unspecified as to length of time between rupture and onset of labor, second trimester ♀   M
    - ◻ O42.913   Preterm premature rupture of membranes, unspecified as to length of time between rupture and onset of labor, third trimester ♀   M
    - ◻ O42.919   Preterm premature rupture of membranes, unspecified as to length of time between rupture and onset of labor, unspecified trimester ♀   M
  - ◻ O42.92   Full-term premature rupture of membranes, unspecified as to length of time between rupture and onset of labor ♀   M
    Premature rupture of membranes after 37 completed weeks of gestation

● Unacceptable Principal Diagnosis   ● Use Additional Character(s)   ◻ Unspecified   ▶ Manifestation Code
OGCR Official Guidelines for Coding and Reporting   Excludes 1   Excludes 2   Includes   Use additional   Code first   Code also

● **O43　Placental disorders**

> **Excludes2**　maternal care for poor fetal growth due to placental insufficiency (O36.5-)
> placenta previa (O44.-)
> placental polyp (O90.89)
> placentitis (O41.14-)
> premature separation of placenta [abruptio placentae] (O45.-)

● **O43.0　Placental transfusion syndromes**

　● **O43.01　Fetomaternal placental transfusion syndrome**
　　　Maternofetal placental transfusion syndrome

　　　O43.011　Fetomaternal placental transfusion syndrome, first trimester ♀　　M

　　　O43.012　Fetomaternal placental transfusion syndrome, second trimester ♀　　M

　　　O43.013　Fetomaternal placental transfusion syndrome, third trimester ♀　　M

　　　O43.019　Fetomaternal placental transfusion syndrome, unspecified trimester ♀　　M

　● **O43.02　Fetus-to-fetus placental transfusion syndrome**

　　　O43.021　Fetus-to-fetus placental transfusion syndrome, first trimester ♀　　M

　　　O43.022　Fetus-to-fetus placental transfusion syndrome, second trimester ♀　　M

　　　O43.023　Fetus-to-fetus placental transfusion syndrome, third trimester ♀　　M

　　　O43.029　Fetus-to-fetus placental transfusion syndrome, unspecified trimester ♀　　M

● **O43.1　Malformation of placenta**

　● **O43.10　Malformation of placenta, unspecified**
　　　Abnormal placenta NOS

　　　O43.101　Malformation of placenta, unspecified, first trimester ♀　　M

　　　O43.102　Malformation of placenta, unspecified, second trimester ♀ M

　　　O43.103　Malformation of placenta, unspecified, third trimester ♀　　M

　　　O43.109　Malformation of placenta, unspecified, unspecified trimester ♀　　M

　● **O43.11　Circumvallate placenta**

　　　O43.111　Circumvallate placenta, first trimester ♀　　M

　　　O43.112　Circumvallate placenta, second trimester ♀　　M

　　　O43.113　Circumvallate placenta, third trimester ♀　　M

　　　O43.119　Circumvallate placenta, unspecified trimester ♀　　M

　● **O43.12　Velamentous insertion of umbilical cord**

　　　O43.121　Velamentous insertion of umbilical cord, first trimester ♀ M

　　　O43.122　Velamentous insertion of umbilical cord, second trimester ♀　　M

　　　O43.123　Velamentous insertion of umbilical cord, third trimester ♀　　M

　　　O43.129　Velamentous insertion of umbilical cord, unspecified trimester ♀　　M

　● **O43.19　Other malformation of placenta**

　　　O43.191　Other malformation of placenta, first trimester ♀　　M

　　　O43.192　Other malformation of placenta, second trimester ♀　　M

　　　O43.193　Other malformation of placenta, third trimester ♀　　M

　　　O43.199　Other malformation of placenta, unspecified trimester ♀　　M

● **O43.2　Morbidly adherent placenta**

> **Code also** associated third stage postpartum hemorrhage, if applicable (O72.0)
>
> **Excludes1**　retained placenta (O73.-)

　● **O43.21　Placenta accreta**

　　　O43.211　Placenta accreta, first trimester ♀　　M

　　　O43.212　Placenta accreta, second trimester ♀　　M

　　　O43.213　Placenta accreta, third trimester ♀　　M

　　　O43.219　Placenta accreta, unspecified trimester ♀　　M

　● **O43.22　Placenta increta**

　　　O43.221　Placenta increta, first trimester ♀　　M

　　　O43.222　Placenta increta, second trimester ♀　　M

　　　O43.223　Placenta increta, third trimester ♀　　M

　　　O43.229　Placenta increta, unspecified trimester ♀　　M

　● **O43.23　Placenta percreta**

　　　O43.231　Placenta percreta, first trimester ♀　　M

　　　O43.232　Placenta percreta, second trimester ♀　　M

　　　O43.233　Placenta percreta, third trimester ♀　　M

　　　O43.239　Placenta percreta, unspecified trimester ♀　　M

● **O43.8　Other placental disorders**

　● **O43.81　Placental infarction**

　　　O43.811　Placental infarction, first trimester ♀　　M

　　　O43.812　Placental infarction, second trimester ♀　　M

　　　O43.813　Placental infarction, third trimester ♀　　M

　　　O43.819　Placental infarction, unspecified trimester ♀　　M

　● **O43.89　Other placental disorders**
　　　Placental dysfunction

　　　O43.891　Other placental disorders, first trimester ♀　　M

　　　O43.892　Other placental disorders, second trimester ♀　　M

N Newborn Age: 0　　P Pediatric Age: 0–17　　M Maternity DX: 12–55　　A Adult Age: 15–124　　♀ Females Only　　♂ Males Only
🔴 Complication\Comorbidity　　🔷 Major C\C　　Present on Admission Requirement　　Hospital-Acquired Condition

1309

        O43.893 Other placental disorders, third
              trimester ♀   M

        O43.899 Other placental disorders,
              unspecified trimester ♀   M

● O43.9 Unspecified placental disorder

    O43.90 Unspecified placental disorder,
        unspecified trimester ♀   M

    O43.91 Unspecified placental disorder, first
        trimester ♀   M

    O43.92 Unspecified placental disorder, second
        trimester ♀   M

    O43.93 Unspecified placental disorder, third
        trimester ♀   M

● O44 Placenta previa

  ● O44.0 Placenta previa specified as without hemorrhage
      Low implantation of placenta specified as without
      hemorrhage

    O44.00 Placenta previa specified as without
        hemorrhage, unspecified trimester ♀   M

    O44.01 Placenta previa specified as without
        hemorrhage, first trimester ♀ 🐾   M

    O44.02 Placenta previa specified as without
        hemorrhage, second trimester ♀ 🐾   M

    O44.03 Placenta previa specified as without
        hemorrhage, third trimester ♀ 🐾   M

  ● O44.1 Placenta previa with hemorrhage
      Low implantation of placenta, NOS or with
      hemorrhage
      Marginal placenta previa, NOS or with
      hemorrhage
      Partial placenta previa, NOS or with hemorrhage
      Total placenta previa, NOS or with hemorrhage

    Excludes1   labor and delivery complicated by
             hemorrhage from vasa previa
             (O69.4)

    O44.10 Placenta previa with hemorrhage,
        unspecified trimester ♀   M

    O44.11 Placenta previa with hemorrhage, first
        trimester ♀ 🐾   M

    O44.12 Placenta previa with hemorrhage, second
        trimester ♀ 🐾   M

    O44.13 Placenta previa with hemorrhage, third
        trimester ♀ 🐾   M

● O45 Premature separation of placenta [abruptio placentae]

  ● O45.0 Premature separation of placenta with coagulation
    defect

  ● O45.00 Premature separation of placenta with
    coagulation defect, unspecified

    O45.001 Premature separation of placenta
        with coagulation defect,
        unspecified, first trimester ♀ 🐾 M

    O45.002 Premature separation of placenta
        with coagulation defect,
        unspecified, second
        trimester ♀ 🐾   M

    O45.003 Premature separation of
        placenta with coagulation
        defect, unspecified, third
        trimester ♀   M

    O45.009 Premature separation of placenta
        with coagulation defect,
        unspecified, unspecified
        trimester ♀   M

  ● O45.01 Premature separation of placenta with
    afibrinogenemia
      Premature separation of placenta with
      hypofibrinogenemia

    O45.011 Premature separation of placenta
        with afibrinogenemia, first
        trimester ♀ 🐾   M

    O45.012 Premature separation of placenta
        with afibrinogenemia, second
        trimester ♀ 🐾   M

    O45.013 Premature separation of placenta
        with afibrinogenemia, third
        trimester ♀ 🐾   M

    O45.019 Premature separation of placenta
        with afibrinogenemia,
        unspecified trimester ♀   M

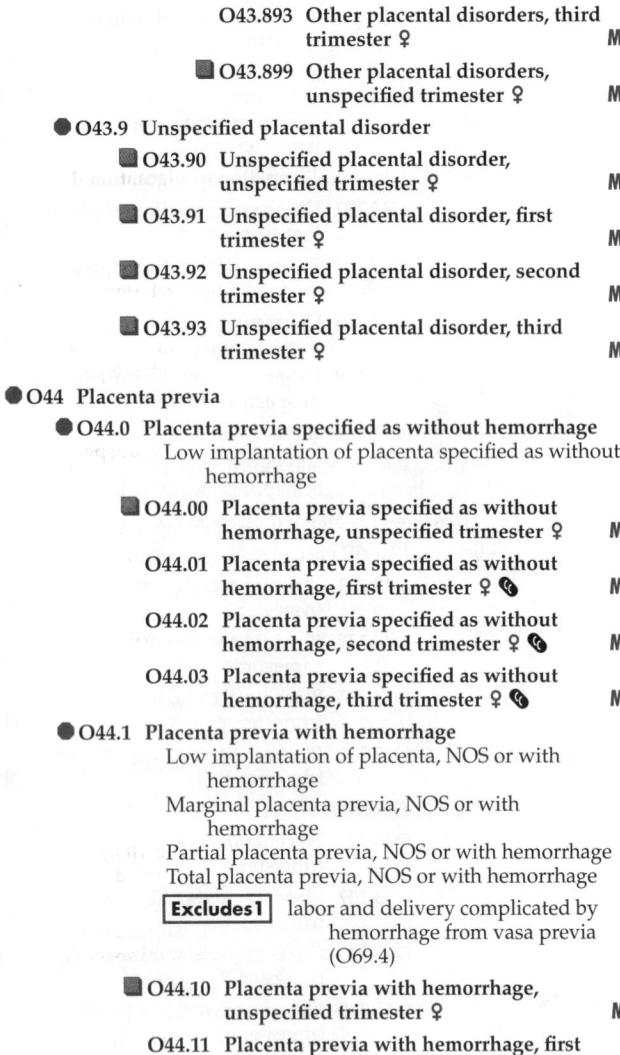

Figure 15-2   A. Marginal placento previa. **B.** Partial placenta previa. **C.** Total placento previa.

Item 15-3   Placenta previa is a condition in which the opening of the cervix is obstructed by the displaced placenta. The three types, marginal, partial, and total, are varying degrees of placenta displacement. Placenta abruption is the premature breaking away of the placenta from the site of the uterine implant before the delivery of the fetus.

Figure 15-3   Abruptio placentae is classified according to the grade of separation of the placenta from the uterine wall. **A.** Mild separation in which hemorrhage is internal. **B.** Moderate separation in which there is external hemorrhage. **C.** Severe separation in which there is external hemorrhage and extreme separation.

● Unacceptable Principal Diagnosis   ● Use Additional Character(s)   ▪ Unspecified   ▶ Manifestation Code

OGCR   Official Guidelines for Coding and Reporting   Excludes 1   Excludes 2   Includes   Use additional   Code first   Code also

● O45.02 Premature separation of placenta with disseminated intravascular coagulation

    O45.021 Premature separation of placenta with disseminated intravascular coagulation, first trimester ♀ 🍂 M

    O45.022 Premature separation of placenta with disseminated intravascular coagulation, second trimester ♀ 🍂 M

    O45.023 Premature separation of placenta with disseminated intravascular coagulation, third trimester ♀ 🍂M

    ◾O45.029 Premature separation of placenta with disseminated intravascular coagulation, unspecified trimester ♀ M

● O45.09 Premature separation of placenta with other coagulation defect

    O45.091 Premature separation of placenta with other coagulation defect, first trimester ♀ 🍂 M

    O45.092 Premature separation of placenta with other coagulation defect, second trimester ♀ 🍂 M

    O45.093 Premature separation of placenta with other coagulation defect, third trimester ♀ 🍂 M

    ◾O45.099 Premature separation of placenta with other coagulation defect, unspecified trimester ♀ M

● O45.8 Other premature separation of placenta

  ● O45.8X Other premature separation of placenta

    O45.8X1 Other premature separation of placenta, first trimester 🍂 ♀ M

    O45.8X2 Other premature separation of placenta, second trimester 🍂 ♀ M

    O45.8X3 Other premature separation of placenta, third trimester 🍂 ♀ M

    ◾O45.8X9 Other premature separation of placenta, unspecified trimester ♀M

● O45.9 Premature separation of placenta, unspecified
    Abruptio placentae NOS

  ◾O45.90 Premature separation of placenta, unspecified, unspecified trimester ♀ M

  ◾O45.91 Premature separation of placenta, unspecified, first trimester ♀ 🍂 M

  ◾O45.92 Premature separation of placenta, unspecified, second trimester ♀ 🍂 M

  ◾O45.93 Premature separation of placenta, unspecified, third trimester ♀ 🍂 M

● O46 Antepartum hemorrhage, not elsewhere classified

  [Excludes1] hemorrhage in early pregnancy (O20.-)
    intrapartum hemorrhage NEC (O67.-)
    placenta previa (O44.-)
    premature separation of placenta [abruptio placentae] (O45.-)

● O46.0 Antepartum hemorrhage with coagulation defect

  ● O46.00 Antepartum hemorrhage with coagulation defect, unspecified

    ◾O46.001 Antepartum hemorrhage with coagulation defect, unspecified, first trimester ♀ 🍂 M

    ◾O46.002 Antepartum hemorrhage with coagulation defect, unspecified, second trimester ♀ 🍂 M

    ◾O46.003 Antepartum hemorrhage with coagulation defect, unspecified, third trimester ♀ 🍂 M

    ◾O46.009 Antepartum hemorrhage with coagulation defect, unspecified, unspecified trimester ♀ M

  ● O46.01 Antepartum hemorrhage with afibrinogenemia
    Antepartum hemorrhage with hypofibrinogenemia

    O46.011 Antepartum hemorrhage with afibrinogenemia, first trimester ♀ 🍂 M

    O46.012 Antepartum hemorrhage with afibrinogenemia, second trimester ♀ 🍂 M

    O46.013 Antepartum hemorrhage with afibrinogenemia, third trimester ♀ 🍂 M

    ◾O46.019 Antepartum hemorrhage with afibrinogenemia, unspecified trimester ♀ M

  ● O46.02 Antepartum hemorrhage with disseminated intravascular coagulation

    O46.021 Antepartum hemorrhage with disseminated intravascular coagulation, first trimester ♀ 🍂 M

    O46.022 Antepartum hemorrhage with disseminated intravascular coagulation, second trimester ♀ 🍂 M

    O46.023 Antepartum hemorrhage with disseminated intravascular coagulation, third trimester ♀ 🍂 M

    ◾O46.029 Antepartum hemorrhage with disseminated intravascular coagulation, unspecified trimester ♀ M

  ● O46.09 Antepartum hemorrhage with other coagulation defect

    O46.091 Antepartum hemorrhage with other coagulation defect, first trimester ♀ 🍂 M

    O46.092 Antepartum hemorrhage with other coagulation defect, second trimester ♀ 🍂 M

    O46.093 Antepartum hemorrhage with other coagulation defect, third trimester ♀ 🍂 M

    ◾O46.099 Antepartum hemorrhage with other coagulation defect, unspecified trimester ♀ M

N Newborn Age: 0   **P** Pediatric Age: 0–17   **M** Maternity DX: 12–55   **A** Adult Age: 15–124   ♀ Females Only   ♂ Males Only

🍂 Complication\Comorbidity   🍂 Major C\C   🍂 Present on Admission Requirement   🍂 Hospital-Acquired Condition

1311

CHAPTER 15 (O00–O9A)

CHAPTER 15 (O00-O9A)

● **O46.8 Other antepartum hemorrhage**
  ● **O46.8x Other antepartum hemorrhage**
    O46.8x1 Other antepartum hemorrhage, first trimester ♀   M
    O46.8x2 Other antepartum hemorrhage, second trimester ♀   M
    O46.8x3 Other antepartum hemorrhage, third trimester ♀   M
    ■ O46.8x9 Other antepartum hemorrhage, unspecified trimester ♀   M

● **O46.9 Antepartum hemorrhage, unspecified**
  ■ O46.90 Antepartum hemorrhage, unspecified, unspecified trimester ♀   M
  ■ O46.91 Antepartum hemorrhage, unspecified, first trimester ♀   M
  ■ O46.92 Antepartum hemorrhage, unspecified, second trimester ♀   M
  ■ O46.93 Antepartum hemorrhage, unspecified, third trimester ♀   M

● **O47 False labor**
  Includes Braxton Hicks contractions
              threatened labor
  Excludes1 preterm labor (O60.-)
  ● **O47.0 False labor before 37 completed weeks of gestation**
    ■ O47.00 False labor before 37 completed weeks of gestation, unspecified trimester ♀   M
    O47.02 False labor before 37 completed weeks of gestation, second trimester ♀ 🦠   M
    O47.03 False labor before 37 completed weeks of gestation, third trimester ♀ 🦠   M
  O47.1 False labor at or after 37 completed weeks of gestation ♀ 🦠   M
  ■ O47.9 False labor, unspecified ♀   M

● **O48 Late pregnancy**
  O48.0 Post-term pregnancy ♀   M
    Pregnancy over 40 completed weeks to 42 completed weeks gestation
  O48.1 Prolonged pregnancy ♀   M
    Pregnancy which has advanced beyond 42 completed weeks gestation

COMPLICATIONS OF LABOR AND DELIVERY (O60-O77)

● **O60 Preterm labor**
  Includes onset (spontaneous) of labor before 37 completed weeks of gestation
  Excludes1 false labor (O47.0-)
            threatened labor NOS (O47.0-)
  ● **O60.0 Preterm labor without delivery**
    ■ O60.00 Preterm labor without delivery, unspecified trimester ♀   M
    O60.02 Preterm labor without delivery, second trimester ♀ 🦠   M
    O60.03 Preterm labor without delivery, third trimester ♀ 🦠   M

● **O60.1 Preterm labor with preterm delivery**
  One of the following 7th characters is to be assigned to each code under subcategory O60.1. 7th character 0 is for single gestations and multiple gestations where the fetus is unspecified. 7th characters 1 through 9 are for cases of multiple gestations to identify the fetus for which the code applies. The appropriate code from category O30, Multiple gestation, must also be assigned when assigning a code from subcategory O60.1 that has a 7th character of 1 through 9.

    0   not applicable or unspecified
    1   fetus 1
    2   fetus 2
    3   fetus 3
    4   fetus 4
    5   fetus 5
    9   other fetus

  ●■ O60.10 Preterm labor with preterm delivery, unspecified trimester 🦠
    Preterm labor with delivery NOS
  O60.12 Preterm labor second trimester with preterm delivery second trimester 🦠
  O60.13 Preterm labor second trimester with preterm delivery third trimester 🦠
  O60.14 Preterm labor third trimester with preterm delivery third trimester 🦠

● **O60.2 Term delivery with preterm labor**
  One of the following 7th characters is to be assigned to each code under subcategory O60.2. 7th character 0 is for single gestations and multiple gestations where the fetus is unspecified. 7th characters 1 through 9 are for cases of multiple gestations to identify the fetus for which the code applies. The appropriate code from category O30, Multiple gestation, must also be assigned when assigning a code from subcategory O60.2 that has a 7th character of 1 through 9.

    0   not applicable or unspecified
    1   fetus 1
    2   fetus 2
    3   fetus 3
    4   fetus 4
    5   fetus 5
    9   other fetus

  ●■ O60.20 Term delivery with preterm labor, unspecified trimester 🦠
  O60.22 Term delivery with preterm labor, second trimester 🦠
  O60.23 Term delivery with preterm labor, third trimester 🦠

● **O61 Failed induction of labor**
  O61.0 Failed medical induction of labor ♀   M
    Failed induction (of labor) by oxytocin
    Failed induction (of labor) by prostaglandins
  O61.1 Failed instrumental induction of labor ♀   M
    Failed mechanical induction (of labor)
    Failed surgical induction (of labor)
  O61.8 Other failed induction of labor ♀   M
  ■ O61.9 Failed induction of labor, unspecified ♀   M

● Unacceptable Principal Diagnosis   ● Use Additional Character(s)   ■ Unspecified   ▶ Manifestation Code
OGCR Official Guidelines for Coding and Reporting   Excludes 1   Excludes 2   Includes   Use additional   Code first   Code also

● **O62 Abnormalities of forces of labor**

    O62.0 Primary inadequate contractions ♀   M
          Failure of cervical dilatation
          Primary hypotonic uterine dysfunction
          Uterine inertia during latent phase of labor

    O62.1 Secondary uterine inertia ♀   M
          Arrested active phase of labor
          Secondary hypotonic uterine dysfunction

    O62.2 Other uterine inertia ♀   M
          Atony of uterus without hemorrhage
          Atony of uterus NOS
          Desultory labor
          Hypotonic uterine dysfunction NOS
          Irregular labor
          Poor contractions
          Slow slope active phase of labor
          Uterine inertia NOS

          Excludes1   atony of uterus with hemorrhage
                    (postpartum) (O72.1)
                  postpartum atony of uterus without
                    hemorrhage (O75.89)

    O62.3 Precipitate labor ♀   M

    **O62.4 Hypertonic, incoordinate, and prolonged uterine
           contractions** ♀   M
          Cervical spasm
          Contraction ring dystocia
          Dyscoordinate labor
          Hour-glass contraction of uterus
          Hypertonic uterine dysfunction
          Incoordinate uterine action
          Tetanic contractions
          Uterine dystocia NOS
          Uterine spasm

          Excludes1   dystocia (fetal) (maternal) NOS (O66.9)

    O62.8 Other abnormalities of forces of labor ♀   M

    ■ **O62.9 Abnormality of forces of labor, unspecified** ♀   M

● **O63 Long labor**

    O63.0 Prolonged first stage (of labor) ♀   M

    O63.1 Prolonged second stage (of labor) ♀   M

    O63.2 Delayed delivery of second twin, triplet, etc. ♀   M

    ■ **O63.9 Long labor, unspecified** ♀ 🩸   M
          Prolonged labor NOS

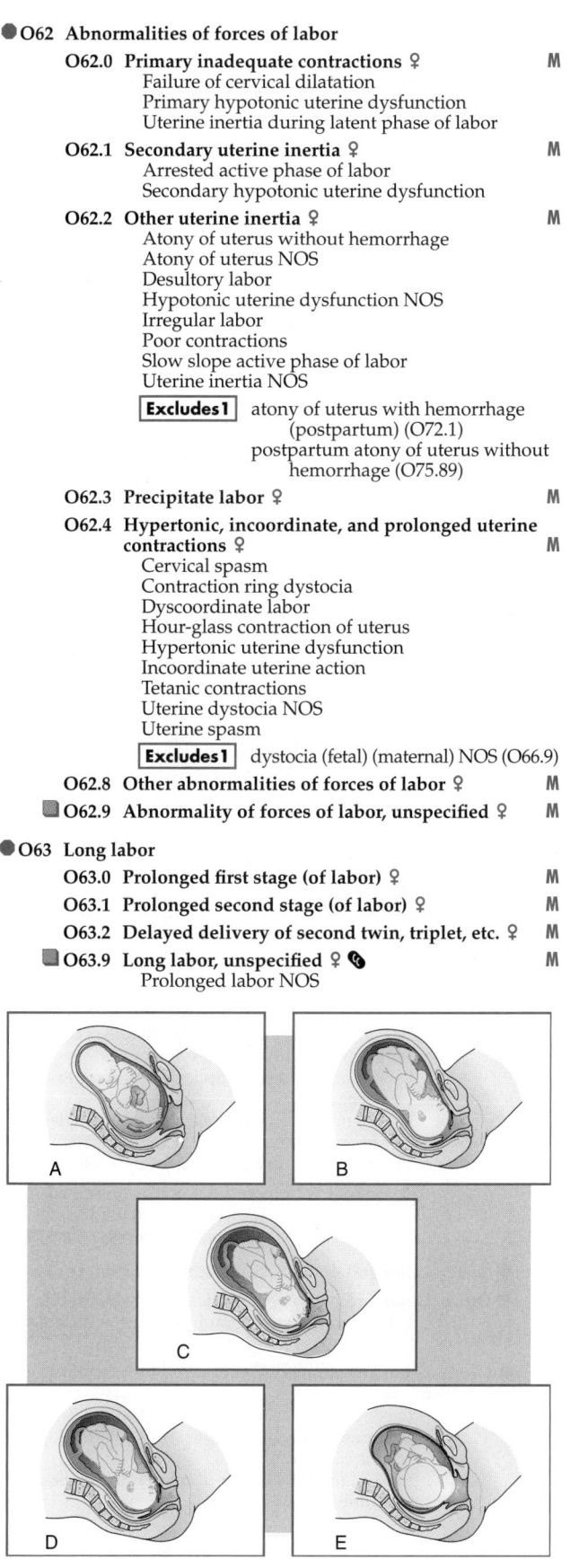

Figure 15-4   Five types of malposition and malpresentation of the fetus: **A.** Breech. **B.** Vertex. **C.** Face. **D.** Brow. **E.** Shoulder.

● **O64 Obstructed labor due to malposition and malpresentation
    of fetus**

    One of the following 7th characters is to be assigned to
    each code under category O64. 7th character 0 is for
    single gestations and multiple gestations where the
    fetus is unspecified. 7th characters 1 through 9 are
    for cases of multiple gestations to identify the fetus
    for which the code applies. The appropriate code
    from category O30, Multiple gestation, must also be
    assigned when assigning a code from category O64
    that has a 7th character of 1 through 9.

0	not applicable or unspecified
1	fetus 1
2	fetus 2
3	fetus 3
4	fetus 4
5	fetus 5
9	other fetus

    ● **O64.0 Obstructed labor due to incomplete rotation of
           fetal head**
          Deep transverse arrest
          Obstructed labor due to persistent occipitoiliac
            (position)
          Obstructed labor due to persistent
            occipitoposterior (position)
          Obstructed labor due to persistent occipitosacral
            (position)
          Obstructed labor due to persistent
            occipitotransverse (position)

    ● **O64.1 Obstructed labor due to breech presentation**
          Obstructed labor due to buttocks presentation
          Obstructed labor due to complete breech
            presentation
          Obstructed labor due to frank breech presentation

    ● **O64.2 Obstructed labor due to face presentation**
          Obstructed labor due to chin presentation

    ● **O64.3 Obstructed labor due to brow presentation**

    ● **O64.4 Obstructed labor due to shoulder presentation**
          Prolapsed arm

          Excludes1   impacted shoulders (O66.0)
                       shoulder dystocia (O66.0)

    ● **O64.5 Obstructed labor due to compound presentation**

    ● **O64.8 Obstructed labor due to other malposition and
           malpresentation**
          Obstructed labor due to footling presentation
          Obstructed labor due to incomplete breech
            presentation

    ● ■ **O64.9 Obstructed labor due to malposition and
           malpresentation, unspecified**

● **O65 Obstructed labor due to maternal pelvic abnormality**

    O65.0 Obstructed labor due to deformed pelvis ♀   M

    **O65.1 Obstructed labor due to generally contracted
           pelvis** ♀   M

    O65.2 Obstructed labor due to pelvic inlet contraction ♀M

    **O65.3 Obstructed labor due to pelvic outlet and mid-
           cavity contraction** ♀   M

    ■ **O65.4 Obstructed labor due to fetopelvic disproportion,
           unspecified** ♀   M

          Excludes1   dystocia due to abnormality of fetus
                       (O66.2-O66.3)

    **O65.5 Obstructed labor due to abnormality of maternal
           pelvic organs** ♀   M
          Obstructed labor due to conditions listed in O34.-
          Use additional code to identify abnormality of
            pelvic organs O34.-

    **O65.8 Obstructed labor due to other maternal pelvic
           abnormalities**   M

    ■ **O65.9 Obstructed labor due to maternal pelvic
           abnormality, unspecified** ♀   M

N Newborn Age: 0   **P** Pediatric Age: 0–17   **M** Maternity DX: 12–55   **A** Adult Age: 15–124   ♀ Females Only   ♂ Males Only

🩸 Complication\Comorbidity   🩸 Major C\C   🩸 Present on Admission Requirement   🩸 Hospital-Acquired Condition

1313

Figure 15-5 Hydrocephalic fetus causing disproportion.

CHAPTER 15 (O00-O9A)

● **O66 Other obstructed labor**

    O66.0 Obstructed labor due to shoulder dystocia ♀   **M**
         Impacted shoulders

    O66.1 Obstructed labor due to locked twins ♀   **M**

    O66.2 Obstructed labor due to unusually large fetus ♀   **M**

    O66.3 Obstructed labor due to other abnormalities of fetus ♀   **M**
         Dystocia due to fetal ascites
         Dystocia due to fetal hydrops
         Dystocia due to fetal meningomyelocele
         Dystocia due to fetal sacral teratoma
         Dystocia due to fetal tumor
         Dystocia due to hydrocephalic fetus
         Use additional code to identify cause of obstruction

  ● **O66.4 Failed trial of labor**

      ■ **O66.40 Failed trial of labor, unspecified ♀**   **M**

      O66.41 Failed attempted vaginal birth after previous cesarean delivery ♀   **M**
           Code first rupture of uterus, if applicable (O71.0-, O71.1)

    O66.5 Attempted application of vacuum extractor and forceps ♀   **M**
         Attempted application of vacuum or forceps, with subsequent delivery by forceps or cesarean delivery

    O66.6 Obstructed labor due to other multiple fetuses ♀   **M**

    O66.8 Other specified obstructed labor ♀   **M**
         Use additional code to identify cause of obstruction

  ■ **O66.9 Obstructed labor, unspecified ♀**   **M**
         Dystocia NOS
         Fetal dystocia NOS
         Maternal dystocia NOS

● **O67 Labor and delivery complicated by intrapartum hemorrhage, not elsewhere classified**

     Excludes1 antepartum hemorrhage NEC (O46.-)
                placenta previa (O44.-)
                premature separation of placenta [abruptio placentae] (O45.-)

     Excludes2 postpartum hemorrhage (O72.-)

    O67.0 Intrapartum hemorrhage with coagulation defect ♀   **M**
         Intrapartum hemorrhage (excessive) associated with afibrinogenemia
         Intrapartum hemorrhage (excessive) associated with disseminated intravascular coagulation
         Intrapartum hemorrhage (excessive) associated with hyperfibrinolysis
         Intrapartum hemorrhage (excessive) associated with hypofibrinogenemia

    O67.8 Other intrapartum hemorrhage ♀   **M**
         Excessive intrapartum hemorrhage

  ■ **O67.9 Intrapartum hemorrhage, unspecified ♀**   **M**

● **O68 Labor and delivery complicated by abnormality of fetal acid-base balance ♀ ⚲**   **M**
     Fetal acidemia complicating labor and delivery
     Fetal acidosis complicating labor and delivery
     Fetal alkalosis complicating labor and delivery
     Fetal metabolic acidemia complicating labor and delivery

     Excludes1 fetal stress NOS (O77.9)
                labor and delivery complicated by electrocardiographic evidence of fetal stress (O77.8)
                labor and delivery complicated by ultrasonic evidence of fetal stress (O77.8)

     Excludes2 abnormality in fetal heart rate or rhythm (O76)
                labor and delivery complicated by meconium in amniotic fluid (O77.0)

● **O69 Labor and delivery complicated by umbilical cord complications**

     One of the following 7th characters is to be assigned to each code under category O69. 7th character 0 is for single gestations and multiple gestations where the fetus is unspecified. 7th characters 1 through 9 are for cases of multiple gestations to identify the fetus for which the code applies. The appropriate code from category O30, Multiple gestation, must also be assigned when assigning a code from category O69 that has a 7th character of 1 through 9.

0	not applicable or unspecified
1	fetus 1
2	fetus 2
3	fetus 3
4	fetus 4
5	fetus 5
9	other fetus

● **O69.0 Labor and delivery complicated by prolapse of cord**

● **O69.1 Labor and delivery complicated by cord around neck, with compression**
     Excludes1 labor and delivery complicated by cord around neck, without compression (O69.81)

● **O69.2 Labor and delivery complicated by other cord entanglement, with compression**
     Labor and delivery complicated by compression of cord NOS
     Labor and delivery complicated by entanglement of cords of twins in monoamniotic sac
     Labor and delivery complicated by knot in cord
     Excludes1 labor and delivery complicated by other cord entanglement, without compression (O69.82)

● **O69.3 Labor and delivery complicated by short cord**

● **O69.4 Labor and delivery complicated by vasa previa**
     Labor and delivery complicated by hemorrhage from vasa previa

● **O69.5 Labor and delivery complicated by vascular lesion of cord**
     Labor and delivery complicated by cord bruising
     Labor and delivery complicated by cord hematoma
     Labor and delivery complicated by thrombosis of umbilical vessels

● Unacceptable Principal Diagnosis   ● Use Additional Character(s)   ■ Unspecified   ▸ Manifestation Code

OGCR Official Guidelines for Coding and Reporting   Excludes 1   Excludes 2   Includes   Use additional   Code first   Code also

● **O69.8 Labor and delivery complicated by other cord complications**

   ● **O69.81 Labor and delivery complicated by cord around neck, without compression**

   ● **O69.82 Labor and delivery complicated by other cord entanglement, without compression**

   ● **O69.89 Labor and delivery complicated by other cord complications**

●■ **O69.9 Labor and delivery complicated by cord complication, unspecified**

● **O70 Perineal laceration during delivery**

    | Includes | episiotomy extended by laceration |

    | Excludes1 | obstetric high vaginal laceration alone (O71.4) |

  O70.0 First degree perineal laceration during delivery ♀M
    Perineal laceration, rupture or tear involving fourchette during delivery
    Perineal laceration, rupture or tear involving labia during delivery
    Perineal laceration, rupture or tear involving skin during delivery
    Perineal laceration, rupture or tear involving vagina during delivery
    Perineal laceration, rupture or tear involving vulva during delivery
    Slight perineal laceration, rupture or tear during delivery

  O70.1 Second degree perineal laceration during delivery ♀   **M**
    Perineal laceration, rupture or tear during delivery as in O70.0, also involving pelvic floor
    Perineal laceration, rupture or tear during delivery as in O70.0, also involving perineal muscles
    Perineal laceration, rupture or tear during delivery as in O70.0, also involving vaginal muscles

    | Excludes1 | perineal laceration involving anal sphincter (O70.2) |

  O70.2 Third degree perineal laceration during delivery ♀ ⬤   **M**
    Perineal laceration, rupture or tear during delivery as in O70.1, also involving anal sphincter
    Perineal laceration, rupture or tear during delivery as in O70.1, also involving rectovaginal septum
    Perineal laceration, rupture or tear during delivery as in O70.1, also involving sphincter NOS

    | Excludes1 | anal sphincter tear during delivery without third degree perineal laceration (O70.4) |
    | | perineal laceration involving anal or rectal mucosa (O70.3) |

  O70.3 Fourth degree perineal laceration during delivery ♀ ⬤   **M**
    Perineal laceration, rupture or tear during delivery as in O70.2, also involving anal mucosa
    Perineal laceration, rupture or tear during delivery as in O70.2, also involving rectal mucosa

  O70.4 Anal sphincter tear complicating delivery, not associated with third degree laceration ♀ ⬤   **M**

    | Excludes1 | anal sphincter tear with third degree perineal laceration (O70.2) |

  ■ **O70.9 Perineal laceration during delivery, unspecified ♀M**

Vaginal opening   Urethral opening

       - - - - - A
       - - - - - B
       - - - - - C
       - - - - - D

Anus

Figure 15-6 Perineal lacerations: **A.** First-degree is laceration of superficial tissues. **B.** Second-degree is limited to the pelvic floor and may involve the perineal or vaginal muscles. **C.** Third-degree involves the anal sphincter. **D.** Fourth-degree involves anal or rectal muscosa.

● **O71 Other obstetric trauma**

    | Includes | obstetric damage from instruments |

  ● **O71.0 Rupture of uterus (spontaneous) before onset of labor**

    | Excludes1 | disruption of (current) cesarean delivery wound (O90.0) |
    | | laceration of uterus, NEC (O71.81) |

   ■ **O71.00 Rupture of uterus before onset of labor, unspecified trimester ♀**   **M**

   O71.02 Rupture of uterus before onset of labor, second trimester ♀ ⬤   **M**

   O71.03 Rupture of uterus before onset of labor, third trimester ♀ ⬤   **M**

  O71.1 Rupture of uterus during labor ♀ ⬤   **M**
    Rupture of uterus not stated as occurring before onset of labor

    | Excludes1 | disruption of cesarean delivery wound (O90.0) |
    | | laceration of uterus, NEC (O71.81) |

  O71.2 Postpartum inversion of uterus ♀ ⬤   **M**

  O71.3 Obstetric laceration of cervix ♀ ⬤   **M**
    Annular detachment of cervix

  O71.4 Obstetric high vaginal laceration alone ♀ ⬤   **M**
    Laceration of vaginal wall without perineal laceration

    | Excludes1 | obstetric high vaginal laceration with perineal laceration (O70.-) |

  O71.5 Other obstetric injury to pelvic organs ♀ ⬤   **M**
    Obstetric injury to bladder
    Obstetric injury to urethra

    | Excludes2 | obstetric periurethral trauma (O71.82) |

  O71.6 Obstetric damage to pelvic joints and ligaments ♀ ⬤   **M**
    Obstetric avulsion of inner symphyseal cartilage
    Obstetric damage to coccyx
    Obstetric traumatic separation of symphysis (pubis)

CHAPTER 15 (O00-O9A)

N Newborn Age: 0   P Pediatric Age: 0–17   M Maternity DX: 12–55   A Adult Age: 15–124   ♀ Females Only   ♂ Males Only

⬤ Complication\Comorbidity   ⬤ Major C\C   ⬤ Present on Admission Requirement   ⬤ Hospital-Acquired Condition

CHAPTER 15 (O00-O9A)

O71.7　**Obstetric hematoma of pelvis** ♀ 🔖　　M
　　　　Obstetric hematoma of perineum
　　　　Obstetric hematoma of vagina
　　　　Obstetric hematoma of vulva

● O71.8　**Other specified obstetric trauma**

　　O71.81　**Laceration of uterus, not elsewhere classified** ♀　　M

　　O71.82　**Other specified trauma to perineum and vulva** ♀　　M
　　　　　　Obstetric periurethral trauma

　　O71.89　**Other specified obstetric trauma** ♀　　M

▪ O71.9　**Obstetric trauma, unspecified** ♀　　M

● O72　**Postpartum hemorrhage**

　　Includes　hemorrhage after delivery of fetus or infant

　　O72.0　**Third-stage hemorrhage** ♀ 🔖　　M
　　　　　Hemorrhage associated with retained, trapped or adherent placenta
　　　　　Retained placenta NOS

　　　　　Code also type of adherent placenta (O43.2-)

　　O72.1　**Other immediate postpartum hemorrhage** ♀ 🔖　M
　　　　　Hemorrhage following delivery of placenta
　　　　　Postpartum hemorrhage (atonic) NOS
　　　　　Uterine atony with hemorrhage

　　　　　Excludes1　uterine atony NOS (O62.2)
　　　　　　　　　　uterine atony without hemorrhage (O62.2)
　　　　　　　　　　postpartum atony of uterus without hemorrhage (O75.89)

　　O72.2　**Delayed and secondary postpartum hemorrhage** ♀ 🔖　　M
　　　　　Hemorrhage associated with retained portions of placenta or membranes after the first 24 hours following delivery of placenta
　　　　　Retained products of conception NOS, following delivery

　　O72.3　**Postpartum coagulation defects** ♀　　M
　　　　　Postpartum afibrinogenemia
　　　　　Postpartum fibrinolysis

● O73　**Retained placenta and membranes, without hemorrhage**

　　Excludes1　placenta accreta (O43.21-)
　　　　　　　　placenta increta (O43.22-)
　　　　　　　　placenta percreta (O43.23-)

　　O73.0　**Retained placenta without hemorrhage** ♀　　M
　　　　　Adherent placenta, without hemorrhage
　　　　　Trapped placenta without hemorrhage

　　O73.1　**Retained portions of placenta and membranes, without hemorrhage** ♀　　M
　　　　　Retained products of conception following delivery, without hemorrhage

● O74　**Complications of anesthesia during labor and delivery**

　　Includes　maternal complications arising from the administration of a general, regional or local anesthetic, analgesic or other sedation during labor and delivery

　　Use additional code, if applicable, to identify specific complication

　　O74.0　**Aspiration pneumonitis due to anesthesia during labor and delivery** ♀　　M
　　　　　Inhalation of stomach contents or secretions NOS due to anesthesia during labor and delivery
　　　　　Mendelson's syndrome due to anesthesia during labor and delivery

O74.1　**Other pulmonary complications of anesthesia during labor and delivery** ♀　　M

O74.2　**Cardiac complications of anesthesia during labor and delivery** ♀　　M

O74.3　**Central nervous system complications of anesthesia during labor and delivery** ♀　　M

O74.4　**Toxic reaction to local anesthesia during labor and delivery** ♀　　M

O74.5　**Spinal and epidural anesthesia-induced headache during labor and delivery** ♀　　M

O74.6　**Other complications of spinal and epidural anesthesia during labor and delivery** ♀　　M

O74.7　**Failed or difficult intubation for anesthesia during labor and delivery** ♀　　M

O74.8　**Other complications of anesthesia during labor and delivery** ♀　　M

▪ O74.9　**Complication of anesthesia during labor and delivery, unspecified** ♀　　M

● O75　**Other complications of labor and delivery, not elsewhere classified**

　　Excludes2　puerperal (postpartum) infection (O86.-)
　　　　　　　　puerperal (postpartum) sepsis (O85)

　　O75.0　**Maternal distress during labor and delivery** ♀　　M

　　O75.1　**Shock during or following labor and delivery** ♀ 🔖　　M
　　　　　Obstetric shock following labor and delivery

　　O75.2　**Pyrexia during labor, not elsewhere classified** ♀ 🔖　　M

　　O75.3　**Other infection during labor** ♀ 🔖　　M
　　　　　Sepsis during labor

　　　　　Use additional code (B95-B97), to identify infectious agent

　　O75.4　**Other complications of obstetric surgery and procedures** ♀　　M
　　　　　Cardiac arrest following obstetric surgery or procedures
　　　　　Cardiac failure following obstetric surgery or procedures
　　　　　Cerebral anoxia following obstetric surgery or procedures
　　　　　Pulmonary edema following obstetric surgery or procedures

　　　　　Use additional code to identify specific complication

　　　　　Excludes2　complications of anesthesia during labor and delivery (O74.-)
　　　　　　　　　　disruption of obstetrical (surgical) wound (O90.0-O90.1)
　　　　　　　　　　hematoma of obstetrical (surgical) wound (O90.2)
　　　　　　　　　　infection of obstetrical (surgical) wound (O86.0)

　　O75.5　**Delayed delivery after artificial rupture of membranes** ♀　　M

● O75.8　**Other specified complications of labor and delivery**

　　O75.81　**Maternal exhaustion complicating labor and delivery** ♀　　M

● Unacceptable Principal Diagnosis　　　● Use Additional Character(s)　　　▪ Unspecified　　　▶ Manifestation Code

OGCR Official Guidelines for Coding and Reporting　　Excludes 1　　Excludes 2　　Includes　　Use additional　　Code first　　Code also

O75.82　**Onset (spontaneous) of labor after 37 completed weeks of gestation but before 39 completed weeks gestation, with delivery by (planned) cesarean section** ♀ M

Delivery by (planned) cesarean section occurring after 37 completed weeks of gestation but before 39 completed weeks gestation due to (spontaneous) onset of labor

Use additional code to specify reason for planned cesarean section such as:
cephalopelvic disproportion (normally formed fetus) (O33.9)
previous cesarean delivery (O34.21)

O75.89　**Other specified complications of labor and delivery** ♀　　　　　M

▢ O75.9　**Complication of labor and delivery, unspecified** ♀　　　　　M

O76　**Abnormality in fetal heart rate and rhythm complicating labor and delivery** ♀　　　　　M

Depressed fetal heart rate tones complicating labor and delivery
Fetal bradycardia complicating labor and delivery
Fetal heart rate decelerations complicating labor and delivery
Fetal heart rate irregularity complicating labor and delivery
Fetal heart rate abnormal variability complicating labor and delivery
Fetal tachycardia complicating labor and delivery
Non-reassuring fetal heart rate or rhythm complicating labor and delivery

Excludes1　fetal stress NOS (O77.9)
labor and delivery complicated by electrocardiographic evidence of fetal stress (O77.8)
labor and delivery complicated by ultrasonic evidence of fetal stress (O77.8)

Excludes2　fetal metabolic acidemia (O68)
other fetal stress (O77.0-O77.1)

● O77　**Other fetal stress complicating labor and delivery**

O77.0　**Labor and delivery complicated by meconium in amniotic fluid** ♀　　　　　M

O77.1　**Fetal stress in labor or delivery due to drug administration** ♀　　　　　M

O77.8　**Labor and delivery complicated by other evidence of fetal stress** ♀　　　　　M

Labor and delivery complicated by electrocardiographic evidence of fetal stress
Labor and delivery complicated by ultrasonic evidence of fetal stress

Excludes1　abnormality of fetal acid-base balance (O68)
abnormality in fetal heart rate or rhythm (O76)
fetal metabolic acidemia (O68)

▢ O77.9　**Labor and delivery complicated by fetal stress, unspecified** ♀　　　　　M

Excludes1　abnormality of fetal acid-base balance (O68)
abnormality in fetal heart rate or rhythm (O76)
fetal metabolic acidemia (O68)

Figure 15-7　The four stages of normal delivery: **I.** Lightening, which occurs 2 to 4 weeks before birth, at which time the fetus turns with head toward the vagina. **II.** Regular contractions begin, the amniotic sac ruptures, and dilation is complete. **III.** Delivery of the head and rotation. **IV.** Expulsion of placenta.

OGCR Section I.C., Chapter 15.m.

Normal Delivery, Code O80

1) Encounter for full term uncomplicated delivery

Code O80 should be assigned when a woman is admitted for a full-term normal delivery and delivers a single, healthy infant without any complications antepartum, during the delivery, or postpartum during the delivery episode. Code O80 is always a principal diagnosis. It is not to be used if any other code from chapter 15 is needed to describe a current complication of the antenatal, delivery, or perinatal period. Additional codes from other chapters may be used with code O80 if they are not related to or are in any way complicating the pregnancy.

2) Uncomplicated delivery with resolved antepartum complication

Code O80 may be used if the patient had a complication at some point during the pregnancy, but the complication is not present at the time of the admission for delivery.

3) Outcome of delivery for O80

Z37.0, Single live brith, is the only outcome of delivery code appropriate for use with O80.

ENCOUNTER FOR DELIVERY (O80-O82)

O80　**Encounter for full-term uncomplicated delivery** ♀ 🖐 M

Delivery requiring minimal or no assistance, with or without episiotomy, without fetal manipulation [e.g., rotation version] or instrumentation [forceps] of a spontaneous, cephalic, vaginal, full-term, single, live-born infant. This code is for use as a single diagnosis code and is not to be used with any other code from chapter 15. This code must be accompanied by a delivery code from the appropriate procedure classification.

Use additional code to indicate outcome of delivery (Z37.0)

O82　**Encounter for cesarean delivery without indication** ♀　　M

This code must be accompanied by a delivery code from the appropriate procedure classification.

Use additional code to indicate outcome of delivery (Z37.0)

CHAPTER 15 (O00-O9A)

COMPLICATIONS PREDOMINANTLY RELATED TO THE PUERPERIUM (O85-O92)

Excludes2	mental and behavioral disorders associated with the puerperium (F53)
	obstetrical tetanus (A34)
	puerperal osteomalacia (M83.0)

O85   Puerperal sepsis ♀ 🐾   **M**

Postpartum sepsis
Puerperal peritonitis
Puerperal pyemia

Use additional code (B95-B97), to identify infectious agent

Use additional code (R65.2-) to identify severe sepsis, if applicable

Excludes1	fever of unknown origin following delivery (O86.4)
	genital tract infection following delivery (O86.1-)
	obstetric pyemic and septic embolism (O88.3-)
	puerperal septic thrombophlebitis (O86.81)
	urinary tract infection following delivery (O86.2-)

| Excludes2 | sepsis during labor (O75.3) |

● **O86   Other puerperal infections**

Use additional code (B95-B97), to identify infectious agent

| Excludes2 | infection during labor (O75.3) |
| | obstetrical tetanus (A34) |

O86.0   Infection of obstetric surgical wound ♀   **M**

Infected cesarean delivery wound following delivery
Infected perineal repair following delivery

● **O86.1   Other infection of genital tract following delivery**

    O86.11   Cervicitis following delivery ♀ 🐾   **M**

    O86.12   Endometritis following delivery ♀ 🐾   **M**

    O86.13   Vaginitis following delivery ♀ 🐾   **M**

    O86.19   Other infection of genital tract following delivery ♀ 🐾   **M**

● **O86.2   Urinary tract infection following delivery**

    O86.20   Urinary tract infection following delivery, unspecified ♀ 🐾   **M**

       Puerperal urinary tract infection NOS

    O86.21   Infection of kidney following delivery ♀ 🐾   **M**

    O86.22   Infection of bladder following delivery ♀ 🐾   **M**

       Infection of urethra following delivery

    O86.29   Other urinary tract infection following delivery ♀ 🐾   **M**

O86.4   Pyrexia of unknown origin following delivery ♀ 🐾 M

Puerperal infection NOS following delivery
Puerperal pyrexia NOS following delivery

| Excludes2 | pyrexia during labor (O75.2) |

● **O86.8   Other specified puerperal infections**

    O86.81   Puerperal septic thrombophlebitis ♀ 🐾   M

    O86.89   Other specified puerperal infections ♀ 🐾M

● **O87   Venous complications and hemorrhoids in the puerperium**

| Includes | venous complications in labor, delivery and the puerperium |

Excludes2	obstetric embolism (O88.-)
	puerperal septic thrombophlebitis (O86.81)
	venous complications in pregnancy (O22.-)

O87.0   Superficial thrombophlebitis in the puerperium ♀ 🐾   **M**

Puerperal phlebitis NOS
Puerperal thrombosis NOS

O87.1   Deep phlebothrombosis in the puerperium ♀ 🐾 M

Deep vein thrombosis, postpartum
Pelvic thrombophlebitis, postpartum

Use additional code to identify the deep vein thrombosis (I82.4-, I82.5-, I82.62-. I82.72-)

Use additional code, if applicable, for associated long-term (current) use of anticoagulants (Z79.01)

O87.2   Hemorrhoids in the puerperium ♀ 🐾   **M**

O87.3   Cerebral venous thrombosis in the puerperium ♀ 🐾   **M**

Cerebrovenous sinus thrombosis in the puerperium

O87.4   Varicose veins of lower extremity in the puerperium ♀   **M**

O87.8   Other venous complications in the puerperium ♀ 🐾   **M**

Genital varices in the puerperium

■ **O87.9   Venous complication in the puerperium, unspecified ♀**   **M**

Puerperal phlebopathy NOS

O88   Obstetric embolism

Excludes1	embolism complicating abortion NOS (O03.2)
	embolism complicating ectopic or molar pregnancy (O08.2)
	embolism complicating failed attempted abortion (O07.2, O07.7)
	embolism complicating induced abortion (O04.7)
	embolism complicating spontaneous abortion (O03.2, O03.7)

● **O88.0   Obstetric air embolism**

    ● **O88.01   Obstetric air embolism in pregnancy**

       O88.011   Air embolism in pregnancy, first trimester ♀ 🐾   **M**

       O88.012   Air embolism in pregnancy, second trimester ♀ 🐾   **M**

       O88.013   Air embolism in pregnancy, third trimester ♀ 🐾   **M**

       ■ **O88.019   Air embolism in pregnancy, unspecified trimester ♀**   **M**

    O88.02   Air embolism in childbirth ♀ 🐾   **M**

    O88.03   Air embolism in the puerperium ♀ 🐾   **M**

● **O88.1 Amniotic fluid embolism**
Anaphylactoid syndrome in pregnancy

  ● **O88.11 Amniotic fluid embolism in pregnancy**

    O88.111 Amniotic fluid embolism in pregnancy, first trimester ♀ 🦠 M

    O88.112 Amniotic fluid embolism in pregnancy, second trimester ♀ 🦠 M

    O88.113 Amniotic fluid embolism in pregnancy, third trimester ♀ 🦠 M

    O88.119 Amniotic fluid embolism in pregnancy, unspecified trimester ♀   M

   O88.12 Amniotic fluid embolism in childbirth ♀ 🦠   M

   O88.13 Amniotic fluid embolism in the puerperium ♀ 🦠   M

● **O88.2 Obstetric thromboembolism**

  ● **O88.21 Thromboembolism in pregnancy**
Obstetric (pulmonary) embolism NOS

    O88.211 Thromboembolism in pregnancy, first trimester ♀ 🦠   M

    O88.212 Thromboembolism in pregnancy, second trimester ♀ 🦠   M

    O88.213 Thromboembolism in pregnancy, third trimester ♀ 🦠   M

    O88.219 Thromboembolism in pregnancy, unspecified trimester ♀   M

   O88.22 Thromboembolism in childbirth ♀ 🦠 M

   O88.23 Thromboembolism in the puerperium ♀ 🦠   M
Puerperal (pulmonary) embolism NOS

● **O88.3 Obstetric pyemic and septic embolism**

  ● **O88.31 Pyemic and septic embolism in pregnancy**

    O88.311 Pyemic and septic embolism in pregnancy, first trimester ♀ 🦠 M

    O88.312 Pyemic and septic embolism in pregnancy, second trimester ♀ 🦠 M

    O88.313 Pyemic and septic embolism in pregnancy, third trimester ♀ 🦠 M

    O88.319 Pyemic and septic embolism in pregnancy, unspecified trimester ♀ 🦠   M

   O88.32 Pyemic and septic embolism in childbirth ♀ 🦠   M

   O88.33 Pyemic and septic embolism in the puerperium ♀ 🦠   M

● **O88.8 Other obstetric embolism**
Obstetric fat embolism

  ● **O88.81 Other embolism in pregnancy**

    O88.811 Other embolism in pregnancy, first trimester ♀ 🦠   M

    O88.812 Other embolism in pregnancy, second trimester ♀ 🦠   M

    O88.813 Other embolism in pregnancy, third trimester ♀ 🦠   M

    O88.819 Other embolism in pregnancy, unspecified trimester ♀   M

   O88.82 Other embolism in childbirth ♀ 🦠   M

   O88.83 Other embolism in the puerperium ♀ 🦠 M

● **O89 Complications of anesthesia during the puerperium**

  Includes   maternal complications arising from the administration of a general, regional or local anesthetic, analgesic or other sedation during the puerperium

  Use additional code, if applicable, to identify specific complication

  ● **O89.0 Pulmonary complications of anesthesia during the puerperium**

    O89.01 Aspiration pneumonitis due to anesthesia during the puerperium ♀   M
Inhalation of stomach contents or secretions NOS due to anesthesia during the puerperium
Mendelson's syndrome due to anesthesia during the puerperium

    O89.09 Other pulmonary complications of anesthesia during the puerperium ♀   M

   O89.1 Cardiac complications of anesthesia during the puerperium ♀   M

   O89.2 Central nervous system complications of anesthesia during the puerperium ♀   M

   O89.3 Toxic reaction to local anesthesia during the puerperium ♀   M

   O89.4 Spinal and epidural anesthesia-induced headache during the puerperium ♀   M

   O89.5 Other complications of spinal and epidural anesthesia during the puerperium ♀   M

   O89.6 Failed or difficult intubation for anesthesia during the puerperium ♀   M

   O89.8 Other complications of anesthesia during the puerperium ♀   M

   O89.9 Complication of anesthesia during the puerperium, unspecified ♀   M

● **O90 Complications of the puerperium, not elsewhere classified**

  O90.0 Disruption of cesarean delivery wound ♀   M
Dehiscence of cesarean delivery wound

    Excludes1   rupture of uterus (spontaneous) before onset of labor (O71.0-)
rupture of uterus during labor (O71.1)

  O90.1 Disruption of perineal obstetric wound ♀   M
Disruption of wound of episiotomy
Disruption of wound of perineal laceration
Secondary perineal tear

  O90.2 Hematoma of obstetric wound ♀   M

  O90.3 Peripartum cardiomyopathy ♀ 🦠   M
Conditions in I42.- arising during pregnancy and the puerperium

    Excludes1   pre-existing heart disease complicating pregnancy and the puerperium (O99.4-)

  O90.4 Postpartum acute kidney failure ♀ 🦠   M
Hepatorenal syndrome following labor and delivery

  O90.5 Postpartum thyroiditis ♀   M

  O90.6 Postpartum mood disturbance ♀   M
Postpartum blues   Postpartum sadness
Postpartum dysphoria

    Excludes1   postpartum depression (F53)
puerperal psychosis (F53)

CHAPTER 15 (O00-O9A)

N Newborn Age: 0   **P** Pediatric Age: 0–17   **M** Maternity DX: 12–55   **A** Adult Age: 15–124   ♀ Females Only   ♂ Males Only

🦠 Complication\Comorbidity   🦠 Major C\C   🦠 Present on Admission Requirement   🦠 Hospital-Acquired Condition

1319

CHAPTER 15 (O00-O9A)

● O90.8　Other complications of the puerperium, not elsewhere classified

　　O90.81　Anemia of the puerperium ♀　　M
　　　　　Postpartum anemia NOS

　　　　　Excludes1　pre-existing anemia complicating the puerperium (O99.03)

　　■ O90.89　Other complications of the puerperium, not elsewhere classified ♀　　M
　　　　　Placental polyp

　　O90.9　Complication of the puerperium, unspecified ♀　　M

● O91　Infections of breast associated with pregnancy, the puerperium and lactation

　　Use additional code to identify infection

● O91.0　Infection of nipple associated with pregnancy, the puerperium and lactation

　　● O91.01　Infection of nipple associated with pregnancy
　　　　　Gestational abscess of nipple

　　　　O91.011　Infection of nipple associated with pregnancy, first trimester ♀　　M

　　　　O91.012　Infection of nipple associated with pregnancy, second trimester ♀　　M

　　　　O91.013　Infection of nipple associated with pregnancy, third trimester ♀　　M

　　　■ O91.019　Infection of nipple associated with pregnancy, unspecified trimester ♀　　M

　　O91.02　Infection of nipple associated with the puerperium ♀　　M
　　　　　Puerperal abscess of nipple

　　O91.03　Infection of nipple associated with lactation ♀　　M
　　　　　Abscess of nipple associated with lactation

● O91.1　Abscess of breast associated with pregnancy, the puerperium and lactation

　　● O91.11　Abscess of breast associated with pregnancy
　　　　　Gestational mammary abscess
　　　　　Gestational purulent mastitis
　　　　　Gestational subareolar abscess

　　　　O91.111　Abscess of breast associated with pregnancy, first trimester ♀ ⬤　　M

　　　　O91.112　Abscess of breast associated with pregnancy, second trimester ♀ ⬤　　M

　　　　O91.113　Abscess of breast associated with pregnancy, third trimester ♀ ⬤　M

　　　■ O91.119　Abscess of breast associated with pregnancy, unspecified trimester ♀　　M

　　O91.12　Abscess of breast associated with the puerperium ♀ ⬤　　M
　　　　　Puerperal mammary abscess
　　　　　Puerperal purulent mastitis
　　　　　Puerperal subareolar abscess

　　O91.13　Abscess of breast associated with lactation ♀　　M
　　　　　Mammary abscess associated with lactation
　　　　　Purulent mastitis associated with lactation
　　　　　Subareolar abscess associated with lactation

● O91.2　Nonpurulent mastitis associated with pregnancy, the puerperium and lactation

　　● O91.21　Nonpurulent mastitis associated with pregnancy
　　　　　Gestational interstitial mastitis
　　　　　Gestational lymphangitis of breast
　　　　　Gestational mastitis NOS
　　　　　Gestational parenchymatous mastitis

　　　　O91.211　Nonpurulent mastitis associated with pregnancy, first trimester ♀　　M

　　　　O91.212　Nonpurulent mastitis associated with pregnancy, second trimester ♀　　M

　　　　O91.213　Nonpurulent mastitis associated with pregnancy, third trimester ♀　　M

　　　■ O91.219　Nonpurulent mastitis associated with pregnancy, unspecified trimester ♀　　M

　　O91.22　Nonpurulent mastitis associated with the puerperium ♀　　M
　　　　　Puerperal interstitial mastitis
　　　　　Puerperal lymphangitis of breast
　　　　　Puerperal mastitis NOS
　　　　　Puerperal parenchymatous mastitis

　　O91.23　Nonpurulent mastitis associated with lactation ♀　　M
　　　　　Interstitial mastitis associated with lactation
　　　　　Lymphangitis of breast associated with lactation
　　　　　Mastitis NOS associated with lactation
　　　　　Parenchymatous mastitis associated with lactation

● O92　Other disorders of breast and disorders of lactation associated with pregnancy and the puerperium

● O92.0　Retracted nipple associated with pregnancy, the puerperium, and lactation

　　● O92.01　Retracted nipple associated with pregnancy

　　　　O92.011　Retracted nipple associated with pregnancy, first trimester ♀　　M

　　　　O92.012　Retracted nipple associated with pregnancy, second trimester ♀　M

　　　　O92.013　Retracted nipple associated with pregnancy, third trimester ♀　　M

　　　■ O92.019　Retracted nipple associated with pregnancy, unspecified trimester ♀　　M

　　O92.02　Retracted nipple associated with the puerperium ♀　　M

　　O92.03　Retracted nipple associated with lactation ♀　　M

● O92.1　Cracked nipple associated with pregnancy, the puerperium, and lactation
　　　　Fissure of nipple, gestational or puerperal

　　● O92.11　Cracked nipple associated with pregnancy

　　　　O92.111　Cracked nipple associated with pregnancy, first trimester ♀　　M

　　　　O92.112　Cracked nipple associated with pregnancy, second trimester ♀　　M

　　　　O92.113　Cracked nipple associated with pregnancy, third trimester ♀　　M

　　　■ O92.119　Cracked nipple associated with pregnancy, unspecified trimester ♀　　M

● Unacceptable Principal Diagnosis　　● Use Additional Character(s)　　■ Unspecified　　▶ Manifestation Code
OGCR Official Guidelines for Coding and Reporting　　Excludes 1　　Excludes 2　　Includes　　Use additional　　Code first　　Code also

O92.12   **Cracked nipple associated with the puerperium** ♀   M

O92.13   **Cracked nipple associated with lactation** ♀   M

● O92.2   **Other and unspecified disorders of breast associated with pregnancy and the puerperium**

◻ O92.20   **Unspecified disorder of breast associated with pregnancy and the puerperium** ♀   M

O92.29   **Other disorders of breast associated with pregnancy and the puerperium** ♀   M

O92.3   **Agalactia** ♀   M
Primary agalactia
> **Excludes1**   elective agalactia (O92.5)
> secondary agalactia (O92.5)
> therapeutic agalactia (O92.5)

O92.4   **Hypogalactia** ♀   M

O92.5   **Suppressed lactation** ♀   M
Elective agalactia   Therapeutic agalactia
Secondary agalactia
> **Excludes1**   primary agalactia (O92.3)

O92.6   **Galactorrhea** ♀   M

● O92.7   **Other and unspecified disorders of lactation**

◻ O92.70   **Unspecified disorders of lactation** ♀   M

O92.79   **Other disorders of lactation** ♀   M
Puerperal galactocele

OGCR Section I.C.2.l.3.

Malignant neoplasm in a pregnant patient

When a pregnant woman has a malignant neoplasm, a code from subcategory O9A.1-, Malignant neoplasm complicating pregnancy, childbirth, and the puerperium, should be sequenced first, followed by the appropriate code from Chapter 2 to indicate the type of neoplasm.

OTHER OBSTETRIC CONDITIONS, NOT ELSEWHERE CLASSIFIED (O94-O9A)

● O94   **Sequelae of complication of pregnancy, childbirth, and the puerperium** ♀ 🔾   M

Note: This category is to be used to indicate conditions in O00-O77.-, O85-O94 and O98-O9A.- as the cause of late effects. The 'sequelae' include conditions specified as such, or as late effects, which may occur at any time after the puerperium.

Code first condition resulting from (sequela) of complication of pregnancy, childbirth, and the puerperium

O98   **Maternal infectious and parasitic diseases classifiable elsewhere but complicating pregnancy, childbirth and the puerperium**

Includes   the listed conditions when complicating the pregnant state, when aggravated by the pregnancy, or as a reason for obstetric care

Use additional code (Chapter 1), to identify specific infectious or parasitic disease

> **Excludes2**   herpes gestationis (O26.4-)
> infectious carrier state (O99.82-, O99.83-)
> obstetrical tetanus (A34)
> puerperal infection (O86.-)
> puerperal sepsis (O85)
> when the reason for maternal care is that the disease is known or suspected to have affected the fetus (O35-O36)

● O98.0   **Tuberculosis complicating pregnancy, childbirth and the puerperium**
Conditions in A15-A19

● O98.01   **Tuberculosis complicating pregnancy**

O98.011   **Tuberculosis complicating pregnancy, first trimester** ♀ 🔾   M

O98.012   **Tuberculosis complicating pregnancy, second trimester** ♀ 🔾 M

O98.013   **Tuberculosis complicating pregnancy, third trimester** ♀ 🔾 M

◻ O98.019   **Tuberculosis complicating pregnancy, unspecified trimester** ♀   M

O98.02   **Tuberculosis complicating childbirth** ♀ 🔾 M

O98.03   **Tuberculosis complicating the puerperium** ♀ 🔾   M

● O98.1   **Syphilis complicating pregnancy, childbirth and the puerperium**
Conditions in A50-A53

● O98.11   **Syphilis complicating pregnancy**

O98.111   **Syphilis complicating pregnancy, first trimester** ♀ 🔾   M

O98.112   **Syphilis complicating pregnancy, second trimester** ♀ 🔾   M

O98.113   **Syphilis complicating pregnancy, third trimester** ♀ 🔾   M

◻ O98.119   **Syphilis complicating pregnancy, unspecified trimester** ♀   M

O98.12   **Syphilis complicating childbirth** ♀ 🔾   M

O98.13   **Syphilis complicating the puerperium** ♀ 🔾   M

● O98.2   **Gonorrhea complicating pregnancy, childbirth and the puerperium**
Conditions in A54.-

● O98.21   **Gonorrhea complicating pregnancy**

O98.211   **Gonorrhea complicating pregnancy, first trimester** ♀ 🔾   M

O98.212   **Gonorrhea complicating pregnancy, second trimester** ♀ 🔾   M

O98.213   **Gonorrhea complicating pregnancy, third trimester** ♀ 🔾   M

◻ O98.219   **Gonorrhea complicating pregnancy, unspecified trimester** ♀   M

O98.22   **Gonorrhea complicating childbirth** ♀ 🔾 M

O98.23   **Gonorrhea complicating the puerperium** ♀ 🔾   M

● O98.3   **Other infections with a predominantly sexual mode of transmission complicating pregnancy, childbirth and the puerperium**
Conditions in A55-A64

● O98.31   **Other infections with a predominantly sexual mode of transmission complicating pregnancy**

O98.311   **Other infections with a predominantly sexual mode of transmission complicating pregnancy, first trimester** ♀ 🔾   M

O98.312   **Other infections with a predominantly sexual mode of transmission complicating pregnancy, second trimester** ♀ 🔾M

O98.313   **Other infections with a predominantly sexual mode of transmission complicating pregnancy, third trimester** ♀ 🔾 M

O98.319 Other infections with a predominantly sexual mode of transmission complicating pregnancy, unspecified trimester ♀   M

O98.32 Other infections with a predominantly sexual mode of transmission complicating childbirth ♀ 🦠   M

O98.33 Other infections with a predominantly sexual mode of transmission complicating the puerperium ♀ 🦠   M

● **O98.4** Viral hepatitis complicating pregnancy, childbirth and the puerperium
Conditions in B15-B19

● **O98.41** Viral hepatitis complicating pregnancy

O98.411 Viral hepatitis complicating pregnancy, first trimester ♀ 🦠   M

O98.412 Viral hepatitis complicating pregnancy, second trimester ♀ 🦠 M

O98.413 Viral hepatitis complicating pregnancy, third trimester ♀ 🦠   M

O98.419 Viral hepatitis complicating pregnancy, unspecified trimester ♀   M

O98.42 Viral hepatitis complicating childbirth ♀ 🦠   M

O98.43 Viral hepatitis complicating the puerperium ♀ 🦠   M

● **O98.5** Other viral diseases complicating pregnancy, childbirth and the puerperium
Conditions in A80-B09, B25-B34, R87.81-, R87.82-

Excludes:1 human immunodeficiency virus [HIV] disease complicating pregnancy, childbirth and the puerperium (O98.7-)

● **O98.51** Other viral diseases complicating pregnancy

O98.511 Other viral diseases complicating pregnancy, first trimester ♀ 🦠   M

O98.512 Other viral diseases complicating pregnancy, second trimester ♀ 🦠 M

O98.513 Other viral diseases complicating pregnancy, third trimester ♀ 🦠   M

O98.519 Other viral diseases complicating pregnancy, unspecified trimester ♀   M

O98.52 Other viral diseases complicating childbirth ♀ 🦠   M

O98.53 Other viral diseases complicating the puerperium ♀ 🦠   M

● **O98.6** Protozoal diseases complicating pregnancy, childbirth and the puerperium
Conditions in B50-B64

● **O98.61** Protozoal diseases complicating pregnancy

O98.611 Protozoal diseases complicating pregnancy, first trimester ♀ 🦠   M

O98.612 Protozoal diseases complicating pregnancy, second trimester ♀ 🦠   M

O98.613 Protozoal diseases complicating pregnancy, third trimester ♀ 🦠 M

O98.619 Protozoal diseases complicating pregnancy, unspecified trimester ♀   M

O98.62 Protozoal diseases complicating childbirth ♀ 🦠   M

O98.63 Protozoal diseases complicating the puerperium ♀ 🦠   M

● **O98.7** Human immunodeficiency virus [HIV] disease complicating pregnancy, childbirth and the puerperium

Use additional code to identify the type of HIV disease:
Acquired immune deficiency syndrome (AIDS) (B20)
Asymptomatic HIV status (Z21)
HIV positive NOS (Z21)
Symptomatic HIV disease (B20)

OGCR Section I.C.15.f.

HIV Infection in Pregnancy, Childbirth and the Puerperium

During pregnancy, childbirth or the puerperium, a patient admitted because of an HIV-related illness should receive a principal diagnosis from subcategory O98.7-. Human immunodeficiency [HIV] disease complicating pregnancy, childbirth and the puerperium, followed by the code(s) for the HIV-related illness(es).

Patients with asymptomatic HIV infection status admitted during pregnancy, childbirth, or the puerperium should receive codes of O98.7- and Z21, Asymptomatic human immunodeficiency virus [HIV] infection status.

● **O98.71** Human immunodeficiency virus [HIV] disease complicating pregnancy

O98.711 Human immunodeficiency virus [HIV] disease complicating pregnancy, first trimester ♀ 🦠   M

O98.712 Human immunodeficiency virus [HIV] disease complicating pregnancy, second trimester ♀ 🦠   M

O98.713 Human immunodeficiency virus [HIV] disease complicating pregnancy, third trimester ♀ 🦠   M

O98.719 Human immunodeficiency virus [HIV] disease complicating pregnancy, unspecified trimester ♀   M

O98.72 Human immunodeficiency virus [HIV] disease complicating childbirth ♀ 🦠   M

O98.73 Human immunodeficiency virus [HIV] disease complicating the puerperium ♀ 🦠   M

● **O98.8** Other maternal infectious and parasitic diseases complicating pregnancy, childbirth and the puerperium

● **O98.81** Other maternal infectious and parasitic diseases complicating pregnancy

O98.811 Other maternal infectious and parasitic diseases complicating pregnancy, first trimester ♀ 🦠   M

O98.812 Other maternal infectious and parasitic diseases complicating pregnancy, second trimester ♀ 🦠   M

● Unacceptable Principal Diagnosis   ● Use Additional Character(s)   ■ Unspecified   ▶ Manifestation Code

OGCR Official Guidelines for Coding and Reporting | Excludes 1 | | Excludes 2 | | Includes | | Use additional | | Code first | | Code also |

O98.813   Other maternal infectious and parasitic diseases complicating pregnancy, third trimester ♀ 🐷 **M**

O98.819   Other maternal infectious and parasitic diseases complicating pregnancy, unspecified trimester ♀ **M**

O98.82   Other maternal infectious and parasitic diseases complicating childbirth ♀ 🐷 **M**

O98.83   Other maternal infectious and parasitic diseases complicating the puerperium ♀ 🐷 **M**

● O98.9   Unspecified maternal infectious and parasitic disease complicating pregnancy, childbirth and the puerperium

● O98.91   Unspecified maternal infectious and parasitic disease complicating pregnancy

O98.911   Unspecified maternal infectious and parasitic disease complicating pregnancy, first trimester ♀ 🐷 **M**

O98.912   Unspecified maternal infectious and parasitic disease complicating pregnancy, second trimester ♀ 🐷 **M**

O98.913   Unspecified maternal infectious and parasitic disease complicating pregnancy, third trimester ♀ 🐷 **M**

O98.919   Unspecified maternal infectious and parasitic disease complicating pregnancy, unspecified trimester ♀ **M**

O98.92   Unspecified maternal infectious and parasitic disease complicating childbirth ♀ 🐷 **M**

O98.93   Unspecified maternal infectious and parasitic disease complicating the puerperium ♀ 🐷 **M**

● O99   Other maternal diseases classifiable elsewhere but complicating pregnancy, childbirth and the puerperium

Includes: conditions which complicate the pregnant state, are aggravated by the pregnancy or are a main reason for obstetric care

Use additional code to identify specific condition

Excludes2   when the reason for maternal care is that the condition is known or suspected to have affected the fetus (O35-O36)

● O99.0   Anemia complicating pregnancy, childbirth and the puerperium
Conditions in D50-D64

Excludes1   anemia arising in the puerperium (O90.81)
postpartum anemia NOS (O90.81)

● O99.01   Anemia complicating pregnancy

O99.011   Anemia complicating pregnancy, first trimester ♀ **M**

O99.012   Anemia complicating pregnancy, second trimester ♀ **M**

O99.013   Anemia complicating pregnancy, third trimester ♀ **M**

O99.019   Anemia complicating pregnancy, unspecified trimester ♀ **M**

O99.02   Anemia complicating childbirth ♀ **M**

O99.03   Anemia complicating the puerperium ♀ **M**

Excludes1   postpartum anemia not pre-existing prior to delivery (O90-.81)

● O99.1   Other diseases of the blood and blood-forming organs and certain disorders involving the immune mechanism complicating pregnancy, childbirth and the puerperium
Conditions in D65-D89

Excludes2   hemorrhage with coagulation defects (O45.-, O46.0-, O67.0, O72.3)

● O99.11   Other diseases of the blood and blood-forming organs and certain disorders involving the immune mechanism complicating pregnancy

O99.111   Other diseases of the blood and blood-forming organs and certain disorders involving the immune mechanism complicating pregnancy, first trimester ♀ 🐷 **M**

O99.112   Other diseases of the blood and blood-forming organs and certain disorders involving the immune mechanism complicating pregnancy, second trimester ♀ 🐷 **M**

O99.113   Other diseases of the blood and blood-forming organs and certain disorders involving the immune mechanism complicating pregnancy, third trimester ♀ 🐷 **M**

O99.119   Other diseases of the blood and blood-forming organs and certain disorders involving the immune mechanism complicating pregnancy, unspecified trimester ♀ 🐷 **M**

O99.12   Other diseases of the blood and blood-forming organs and certain disorders involving the immune mechanism complicating childbirth ♀ 🐷 **M**

O99.13   Other diseases of the blood and blood-forming organs and certain disorders involving the immune mechanism complicating the puerperium ♀ 🐷 **M**

● O99.2   Endocrine, nutritional and metabolic diseases complicating pregnancy, childbirth and the puerperium
Conditions in E00-E88

Excludes2   diabetes mellitus (O24.-)
malnutrition (O25.-)
postpartum thyroiditis (O90.5)

● O99.21   Obesity complicating pregnancy, childbirth, and the puerperium

Use additional code to identify the type of obesity (E66.-)

O99.210   Obesity complicating pregnancy, unspecified trimester ♀ **M**

O99.211   Obesity complicating pregnancy, first trimester ♀ **M**

O99.212   Obesity complicating pregnancy, second trimester ♀ **M**

O99.213   Obesity complicating pregnancy, third trimester ♀ **M**

O99.214   Obesity complicating childbirth ♀ **M**

O99.215   Obesity complicating the puerperium ♀ **M**

N Newborn Age: 0   **P** Pediatric Age: 0–17   **M** Maternity DX: 12–55   **A** Adult Age: 15–124   ♀ Females Only   ♂ Males Only

 Complication\Comorbidity   🐷 Major C\C   Present on Admission Requirement   Hospital-Acquired Condition

1323

CHAPTER 15 (O00-O9A)

● **O99.28** **Other endocrine, nutritional and metabolic diseases complicating pregnancy, childbirth and the puerperium**

◾ O99.280 Endocrine, nutritional and metabolic diseases complicating pregnancy, unspecified trimester ♀   M

O99.281 Endocrine, nutritional and metabolic diseases complicating pregnancy, first trimester ♀   M

O99.282 Endocrine, nutritional and metabolic diseases complicating pregnancy, second trimester ♀   M

O99.283 Endocrine, nutritional and metabolic diseases complicating pregnancy, third trimester ♀   M

O99.284 Endocrine, nutritional and metabolic diseases complicating childbirth ♀   M

O99.285 Endocrine, nutritional and metabolic diseases complicating the puerperium ♀   M

● **O99.3** **Mental disorders and diseases of the nervous system complicating pregnancy, childbirth and the puerperium**

● **O99.31** **Alcohol use complicating pregnancy, childbirth, and the puerperium**

> Use additional code(s) from F10 to identify manifestations of the alcohol use

◾ O99.310 Alcohol use complicating pregnancy, unspecified trimester ♀   M

O99.311 Alcohol use complicating pregnancy, first trimester ♀   M

O99.312 Alcohol use complicating pregnancy, second trimester ♀   M

O99.313 Alcohol use complicating pregnancy, third trimester ♀   M

O99.314 Alcohol use complicating childbirth ♀   M

O99.315 Alcohol use complicating the puerperium ♀   M

● **O99.32** **Drug use complicating pregnancy, childbirth, and the puerperium**

> Use additional code(s) from F11-F16 and F18-F19 to identify manifestations of the drug use

◾ O99.320 Drug use complicating pregnancy, unspecified trimester ♀   M

O99.321 Drug use complicating pregnancy, first trimester ♀ 🕮   M

O99.322 Drug use complicating pregnancy, second trimester ♀ 🕮   M

O99.323 Drug use complicating pregnancy, third trimester ♀ 🕮   M

O99.324 Drug use complicating childbirth ♀ 🕮   M

O99.325 Drug use complicating the puerperium ♀ 🕮   M

● **O99.33** **Smoking (tobacco) complicating pregnancy, childbirth, and the puerperium**

> Use additional code from F17 to identify type of tobacco

◾ O99.330 Smoking (tobacco) complicating pregnancy, unspecified trimester ♀   M

O99.331 Smoking (tobacco) complicating pregnancy, first trimester ♀   M

O99.332 Smoking (tobacco) complicating pregnancy, second trimester ♀   M

O99.333 Smoking (tobacco) complicating pregnancy, third trimester ♀   M

O99.334 Smoking (tobacco) complicating childbirth ♀   M

O99.335 Smoking (tobacco) complicating the puerperium ♀   M

● **O99.34** **Other mental disorders complicating pregnancy, childbirth, and the puerperium**
Conditions in F01-F09 and F20-F99

> **Excludes2**   postpartum mood disturbance (O90.6)
> postnatal psychosis (F53)
> puerperal psychosis (F53)

◾ O99.340 Other mental disorders complicating pregnancy, unspecified trimester ♀   M

O99.341 Other mental disorders complicating pregnancy, first trimester ♀   M

O99.342 Other mental disorders complicating pregnancy, second trimester ♀   M

O99.343 Other mental disorders complicating pregnancy, third trimester ♀   M

O99.344 Other mental disorders complicating childbirth ♀   M

O99.345 Other mental disorders complicating the puerperium ♀ M

● **O99.35** **Diseases of the nervous system complicating pregnancy, childbirth, and the puerperium**
Conditions in G00-G99

> **Excludes2**   pregnancy related peripheral neuritis (O26.8-)

◾ O99.350 Diseases of the nervous system complicating pregnancy, unspecified trimester ♀   M

O99.351 Diseases of the nervous system complicating pregnancy, first trimester ♀   M

O99.352 Diseases of the nervous system complicating pregnancy, second trimester ♀   M

O99.353 Diseases of the nervous system complicating pregnancy, third trimester ♀   M

O99.354 Diseases of the nervous system complicating childbirth ♀ 🕮   M

O99.355 Diseases of the nervous system complicating the puerperium ♀ 🕮   M

● **O99.4 Diseases of the circulatory system complicating pregnancy, childbirth and the puerperium**
Conditions in I00-I99

    Excludes1   peripartum cardiomyopathy (O90.3)

    Excludes2   hypertensive disorders (O10-O16)
obstetric embolism (O88.-)
venous complications and cerebrovenous sinus thrombosis in labor, childbirth and the puerperium (O87.-)
venous complications and cerebrovenous sinus thrombosis in pregnancy (O22.-)

● **O99.41 Diseases of the circulatory system complicating pregnancy**

  O99.411 Diseases of the circulatory system complicating pregnancy, first trimester ♀ 🩸   M

  O99.412 Diseases of the circulatory system complicating pregnancy, second trimester ♀ 🩸   M

  O99.413 Diseases of the circulatory system complicating pregnancy, third trimester ♀ 🩸   M

  ■**O99.419 Diseases of the circulatory system complicating pregnancy, unspecified trimester** ♀   M

O99.42 Diseases of the circulatory system complicating childbirth ♀ 🩸   M

O99.43 Diseases of the circulatory system complicating the puerperium ♀ 🩸   M

● **O99.5 Diseases of the respiratory system complicating pregnancy, childbirth and the puerperium**
Conditions in J00-J99

● **O99.51 Diseases of the respiratory system complicating pregnancy**

  O99.511 Diseases of the respiratory system complicating pregnancy, first trimester ♀   M

  O99.512 Diseases of the respiratory system complicating pregnancy, second trimester ♀   M

  O99.513 Diseases of the respiratory system complicating pregnancy, third trimester ♀   M

  ■**O99.519 Diseases of the respiratory system complicating pregnancy, unspecified trimester** ♀   M

O99.52 Diseases of the respiratory system complicating childbirth ♀   M

O99.53 Diseases of the respiratory system complicating the puerperium ♀   M

● **O99.6 Diseases of the digestive system complicating pregnancy, childbirth and the puerperium**
Conditions in K00-K93

    Excludes2   liver and biliary tract disorders in pregnancy, childbirth and the puerperium (O26.6-)

● **O99.61 Diseases of the digestive system complicating pregnancy**

  O99.611 Diseases of the digestive system complicating pregnancy, first trimester ♀   M

  O99.612 Diseases of the digestive system complicating pregnancy, second trimester ♀   M

  O99.613 Diseases of the digestive system complicating pregnancy, third trimester ♀   M

  ■**O99.619 Diseases of the digestive system complicating pregnancy, unspecified trimester** ♀   M

O99.62 Diseases of the digestive system complicating childbirth ♀   M

O99.63 Diseases of the digestive system complicating the puerperium ♀   M

● **O99.7 Diseases of the skin and subcutaneous tissue complicating pregnancy, childbirth and the puerperium**
Conditions in L00-L99

    Excludes2   herpes gestationis (O26.4)
pruritic urticarial papules and plaques of pregnancy (PUPPP) (O26.86)

● **O99.71 Diseases of the skin and subcutaneous tissue complicating pregnancy**

  O99.711 Diseases of the skin and subcutaneous tissue complicating pregnancy, first trimester ♀   M

  O99.712 Diseases of the skin and subcutaneous tissue complicating pregnancy, second trimester ♀   M

  O99.713 Diseases of the skin and subcutaneous tissue complicating pregnancy, third trimester ♀   M

  ■**O99.719 Diseases of the skin and subcutaneous tissue complicating pregnancy, unspecified trimester** ♀   M

O99.72 Diseases of the skin and subcutaneous tissue complicating childbirth ♀   M

O99.73 Diseases of the skin and subcutaneous tissue complicating the puerperium ♀   M

● **O99.8 Other specified diseases and conditions complicating pregnancy, childbirth and the puerperium**
Conditions in D00-D48, H00-H95, M00-N99, and Q00-Q99

Use additional code to identify condition

    Excludes2   genitourinary infections in pregnancy (O23.-)
infection of genitourinary tract following delivery (O86.1-O86.3)
malignant neoplasm complicating pregnancy, childbirth and the puerperium (O9A.1-)
maternal care for known or suspected abnormality of maternal pelvic organs (O34.-)
postpartum acute kidney failure (O90.4)
traumatic injuries in pregnancy (O9A.2-)

● **O99.81 Abnormal glucose complicating pregnancy, childbirth and the puerperium**

    Excludes1   gestational diabetes (O24.4-)

  O99.810 Abnormal glucose complicating pregnancy ♀   M

  O99.814 Abnormal glucose complicating childbirth ♀   M

  O99.815 Abnormal glucose complicating the puerperium ♀   M

CHAPTER 15 (O00-O9A)

CHAPTER 15 (O00-O9A)

● **O99.82** **Streptococcus B carrier state complicating pregnancy, childbirth and the puerperium**

   ● **O99.820** **Streptococcus B carrier state complicating pregnancy** ♀   M

   O99.824 **Streptococcus B carrier state complicating childbirth** ♀   M

   ● **O99.825** **Streptococcus B carrier state complicating the puerperium** ♀ 🞷   M

● **O99.83** **Other infection carrier state complicating pregnancy, childbirth and the puerperium**

   Use additional code to identify the carrier state (Z22.-)

   O99.830 **Other infection carrier state complicating pregnancy** ♀ 🞷   M

   O99.834 **Other infection carrier state complicating childbirth** ♀ 🞷   M

   O99.835 **Other infection carrier state complicating the puerperium** ♀ 🞷   M

● **O99.84** **Bariatric surgery status complicating pregnancy, childbirth and the puerperium**

   Gastric banding status complicating pregnancy, childbirth and the puerperium

   Gastric bypass status for obesity complicating pregnancy, childbirth and the puerperium

   Obesity surgery status complicating pregnancy, childbirth and the puerperium

   ■ **O99.840** **Bariatric surgery status complicating pregnancy, unspecified trimester** ♀   M

   O99.841 **Bariatric surgery status complicating pregnancy, first trimester** ♀   M

   O99.842 **Bariatric surgery status complicating pregnancy, second trimester** ♀   M

   O99.843 **Bariatric surgery status complicating pregnancy, third trimester** ♀   M

   O99.844 **Bariatric surgery status complicating childbirth** ♀   M

   O99.845 **Bariatric surgery status complicating the puerperium** ♀ M

O99.89 **Other specified diseases and conditions complicating pregnancy, childbirth and the puerperium** ♀   M

● **O9A** **Maternal malignant neoplasms, traumatic injuries and abuse classifiable elsewhere but complicating pregnancy, childbirth and the puerperium**

● **O9A.1** **Malignant neoplasm complicating pregnancy, childbirth and the puerperium**

   Conditions in C00-C96

   Use additional code to identify neoplasm

   Excludes2 maternal care for benign tumor of corpus uteri (O34.1-)

         maternal care for benign tumor of cervix (O34.4-)

● **O9A.11** **Malignant neoplasm complicating pregnancy**

   O9A.111 **Malignant neoplasm complicating pregnancy, first trimester** ♀   M

   O9A.112 **Malignant neoplasm complicating pregnancy, second trimester** ♀   M

   O9A.113 **Malignant neoplasm complicating pregnancy, third trimester** ♀   M

   ■ **O9A.119** **Malignant neoplasm complicating pregnancy, unspecified trimester** ♀   M

O9A.12 **Malignant neoplasm complicating childbirth** ♀   M

O9A.13 **Malignant neoplasm complicating the puerperium** ♀   M

● **O9A.2** **Injury, poisoning and certain other consequences of external causes complicating pregnancy, childbirth and the puerperium**

   Conditions in S00-T88, except T74 and T76

   Use additional code(s) to identify the injury or poisoning

   Excludes2 physical, sexual and psychological abuse complicating pregnancy, childbirth and the puerperium (O9A.3-, O9A.4-, O9A.5-)

● **O9A.21** **Injury, poisoning and certain other consequences of external causes complicating pregnancy**

   O9A.211 **Injury, poisoning and certain other consequences of external causes complicating pregnancy, first trimester** ♀   M

   O9A.212 **Injury, poisoning and certain other consequences of external causes complicating pregnancy, second trimester** ♀   M

   O9A.213 **Injury, poisoning and certain other consequences of external causes complicating pregnancy, third trimester** ♀   M

   ■ **O9A.219** **Injury, poisoning and certain other consequences of external causes complicating pregnancy, unspecified trimester** ♀   M

O9A.22 **Injury, poisoning and certain other consequences of external causes complicating childbirth** ♀   M

O9A.23 **Injury, poisoning and certain other consequences of external causes complicating the puerperium** ♀   M

● **O9A.3** **Physical abuse complicating pregnancy, childbirth and the puerperium**

   Conditions in T74.11 or T76.11

   Use additional code (if applicable):

    to identify any associated current injury due to physical abuse

    to identify the perpetrator of abuse (Y07.-)

   Excludes2 sexual abuse complicating pregnancy, childbirth and the puerperium (O9A.4)

● **O9A.31** **Physical abuse complicating pregnancy**

   O9A.311 **Physical abuse complicating pregnancy, first trimester** ♀   M

   O9A.312 **Physical abuse complicating pregnancy, second trimester** ♀   M

   O9A.313 **Physical abuse complicating pregnancy, third trimester** ♀   M

   ■ **O9A.319** **Physical abuse complicating pregnancy, unspecified trimester** ♀   M

● Unacceptable Principal Diagnosis   ● Use Additional Character(s)   ■ Unspecified   ▶ Manifestation Code

OGCR Official Guidelines for Coding and Reporting   Excludes 1   Excludes 2   Includes   Use additional   Code first   Code also

O9A.32 **Physical abuse complicating childbirth** ♀ M

O9A.33 **Physical abuse complicating the puerperium** ♀   M

● O9A.4 **Sexual abuse complicating pregnancy, childbirth and the puerperium**
Conditions in T74.21 or T76.21

Use additional code (if applicable):
to identify any associated current injury due to sexual abuse
to identify the perpetrator of abuse (Y07.-)

● O9A.41 **Sexual abuse complicating pregnancy**

O9A.411 **Sexual abuse complicating pregnancy, first trimester** ♀   M

O9A.412 **Sexual abuse complicating pregnancy, second trimester** ♀   M

O9A.413 **Sexual abuse complicating pregnancy, third trimester** ♀   M

■ O9A.419 **Sexual abuse complicating pregnancy, unspecified trimester** ♀   M

O9A.42 **Sexual abuse complicating childbirth** ♀   M

O9A.43 **Sexual abuse complicating the puerperium** ♀   M

● O9A.5 **Psychological abuse complicating pregnancy, childbirth and the puerperium**
Conditions in T74.31 or T76.31

Use additional code to identify the perpetrator of abuse (Y07.-)

● O9A.51 **Psychological abuse complicating pregnancy**

O9A.511 **Psychological abuse complicating pregnancy, first trimester** ♀   M

O9A.512 **Psychological abuse complicating pregnancy, second trimester** ♀   M

O9A.513 **Psychological abuse complicating pregnancy, third trimester** ♀   M

■ O9A.519 **Psychological abuse complicating pregnancy, unspecified trimester** ♀   M

O9A.52 **Psychological abuse complicating childbirth** ♀   M

O9A.53 **Psychological abuse complicating the puerperium** ♀   M

N Newborn Age: 0   **P** Pediatric Age: 0–17   **M** Maternity DX: 12–55   **A** Adult Age: 15–124   ♀ Females Only   ♂ Males Only

 Complication\Comorbidity   Major C\C   Present on Admission Requirement   Hospital-Acquired Condition

1327

OGCR See Section I.C., Chapter 16
Newborn (Perinatal) Guidelines

CHAPTER 16

CERTAIN CONDITIONS ORIGINATING IN THE PERINATAL PERIOD (P00-P96)

Note: Codes from this chapter are for use on newborn records only, never on maternal records.

Includes conditions that have their origin in the fetal or perinatal period (before birth through the first 28 days after birth) even if morbidity occurs later

Excludes2 congenital malformations, deformations and chromosomal abnormalities (Q00-Q99)
endocrine, nutritional and metabolic diseases (E00-E88)
injury, poisoning and certain other consequences of external causes (S00-T88)
neoplasms (C00-D49)
tetanus neonatorum (A33)

This chapter contains the following blocks:

P00-P04	Newborn affected by maternal factors and by complications of pregnancy, labor, and delivery
P05-P08	Disorders of newborns related to length of gestation and fetal growth
P09	Abnormal findings on neonatal screening
P10-P15	Birth trauma
P19-P29	Respiratory and cardiovascular disorders specific to the perinatal period
P35-P39	Infections specific to the perinatal period
P50-P61	Hemorrhagic and hematological disorders of newborn
P70-P74	Transitory endocrine and metabolic disorders specific to newborn
P76-P78	Digestive system disorders of newborn
P80-P83	Conditions involving the integument and temperature regulation of newborn
P84	Other problems with newborn
P90-P96	Other disorders originating in the perinatal period

NEWBORN AFFECTED BY MATERNAL FACTORS AND BY COMPLICATIONS OF PREGNANCY, LABOR, AND DELIVERY (P00–P04)

Note: These codes are for use when the listed maternal conditions are specified as the cause of confirmed morbidity or potential morbidity which have their origin in the perinatal period (before birth through the first 28 days after birth). Codes from these categories are also for use for newborns who are suspected of having an abnormal condition resulting from exposure from the mother or the birth process, but without signs or symptoms, and, which after examination and observation, is found not to exist. These codes may be used even if treatment is begun for a suspected condition that is ruled out.

● **P00** **Newborn (suspected to be) affected by maternal conditions that may be unrelated to present pregnancy**

Code first any current condition in newborn

Excludes2 newborn (suspected to be) affected by maternal complications of pregnancy (P01.-)
newborn affected by maternal endocrine and metabolic disorders (P70–P74)
newborn affected by noxious substances transmitted via placenta or breast milk (P04.-)

P00.0 **Newborn (suspected to be) affected by maternal hypertensive disorders**   N
Newborn (suspected to be) affected by maternal conditions classifiable to O10-O11, O13-O16

P00.1 **Newborn (suspected to be) affected by maternal renal and urinary tract diseases**   N
Newborn (suspected to be) affected by maternal conditions classifiable to N00-N39

P00.2 **Newborn (suspected to be) affected by maternal infectious and parasitic diseases**   N
Newborn (suspected to be) affected by maternal infectious disease classifiable to A00-B99, J09 and J10

Excludes1 infections specific to the perinatal period (P35-P39)
maternal genital tract or other localized infections (P00.8)

P00.3 **Newborn (suspected to be) affected by other maternal circulatory and respiratory diseases**   N
Newborn (suspected to be) affected by maternal conditions classifiable to I00-I99, J00-J99, Q20-Q34 and not included in P00.0, P00.2

P00.4 **Newborn (suspected to be) affected by maternal nutritional disorders**   N
Newborn (suspected to be) affected by maternal disorders classifiable to E40-E64
Maternal malnutrition NOS

P00.5 **Newborn (suspected to be) affected by maternal injury**   N
Newborn (suspected to be) affected by maternal conditions classifiable to O9A.2-

P00.6 **Newborn (suspected to be) affected by surgical procedure on mother**   N
Newborn (suspected to be) affected by amniocentesis

Excludes1 Cesarean delivery for present delivery (P03.4)
damage to placenta from amniocentesis, cesarean delivery or surgical induction (P02.1)
previous surgery to uterus or pelvic organs (P03.89)

Excludes2 newborn affected by complication of (fetal) intrauterine procedure (P96.5)

P00.7 **Newborn (suspected to be) affected by other medical procedures on mother, not elsewhere classified**   N
Newborn (suspected to be) affected by radiation to mother

Excludes1 damage to placenta from amniocentesis, cesarean delivery or surgical induction (P02.1)
newborn affected by other complications of labor and delivery (P03.-)

● Unacceptable Principal Diagnosis   ● Use Additional Character(s)   ■ Unspecified   ▶ Manifestation Code
OGCR Official Guidelines for Coding and Reporting   Excludes 1   Excludes 2   Includes   Use additional   Code first   Code also

● **P00.8   Newborn (suspected to be) affected by other maternal conditions**

     P00.81   Newborn (suspected to be) affected by periodontal disease in mother   N

     P00.89   Newborn (suspected to be) affected by other maternal conditions 🔍   N

        Newborn (suspected to be) affected by conditions classifiable to T80-T88

        Newborn (suspected to be) affected by maternal genital tract or other localized infections

        Newborn (suspected to be) affected by maternal systemic lupus erythematosus

■ **P00.9   Newborn (suspected to be) affected by unspecified maternal condition**   N

● **P01   Newborn (suspected to be) affected by maternal complications of pregnancy**

     Code first any current condition in newborn

     P01.0   Newborn (suspected to be) affected by incompetent cervix   N

     P01.1   Newborn (suspected to be) affected by premature rupture of membranes   N

     P01.2   Newborn (suspected to be) affected by oligohydramnios   N

        Excludes1   oligohydramnios due to premature rupture of membranes (P01.1)

     P01.3   Newborn (suspected to be) affected by polyhydramnios   N

        Excess of amniotic fluid, usually > 2000 mL

        Newborn (suspected to be) affected by hydramnios

     P01.4   Newborn (suspected to be) affected by ectopic pregnancy   N

        Newborn (suspected to be) affected by abdominal pregnancy

     P01.5   Newborn (suspected to be) affected by multiple pregnancy   N

        Newborn (suspected to be) affected by triplet (pregnancy)

        Newborn (suspected to be) affected by twin (pregnancy)

     P01.6   Newborn (suspected to be) affected by maternal death   N

     P01.7   Newborn (suspected to be) affected by malpresentation before labor   N

        Newborn (suspected to be) affected by breech presentation before labor

        Newborn (suspected to be) affected by external version before labor

        Newborn (suspected to be) affected by face presentation before labor

        Newborn (suspected to be) affected by transverse lie before labor

        Newborn (suspected to be) affected by unstable lie before labor

     P01.8   Newborn (suspected to be) affected by other maternal complications of pregnancy   N

     ■ **P01.9   Newborn (suspected to be) affected by maternal complication of pregnancy, unspecified**   N

● **P02   Newborn (suspected to be) affected by complications of placenta, cord and membranes**

     Code first any current condition in newborn

     P02.0   Newborn (suspected to be) affected by placenta previa   N

P02.1   Newborn (suspected to be) affected by other forms of placental separation and hemorrhage   N

     Newborn (suspected to be) affected by abruptio placenta

     Newborn (suspected to be) affected by accidental hemorrhage

     Newborn (suspected to be) affected by antepartum hemorrhage

     Newborn (suspected to be) affected by damage to placenta from amniocentesis, cesarean delivery or surgical induction

     Newborn (suspected to be) affected by maternal blood loss

     Newborn (suspected to be) affected by premature separation of placenta

● **P02.2   Newborn (suspected to be) affected by other and unspecified morphological and functional abnormalities of placenta**

     ■ **P02.20   Newborn (suspected to be) affected by unspecified morphological and functional abnormalities of placenta**   N

     P02.29   Newborn (suspected to be) affected by other morphological and functional abnormalities of placenta   N

        Newborn (suspected to be) affected by placental dysfunction

        Newborn (suspected to be) affected by placental infarction

        Newborn (suspected to be) affected by placental insufficiency

P02.3   Newborn (suspected to be) affected by placental transfusion syndromes   N

     Newborn (suspected to be) affected by placental and cord abnormalities resulting in twin-to-twin or other transplacental transfusion

P02.4   Newborn (suspected to be) affected by prolapsed cord   N

P02.5   Newborn (suspected to be) affected by other compression of umbilical cord   N

     Newborn (suspected to be) affected by umbilical cord (tightly) around neck

     Newborn (suspected to be) affected by entanglement of umbilical cord

     Newborn (suspected to be) affected by knot in umbilical cord

● **P02.6   Newborn (suspected to be) affected by other and unspecified conditions of umbilical cord**

     ■ **P02.60   Newborn (suspected to be) affected by unspecified conditions of umbilical cord**   N

     P02.69   Newborn (suspected to be) affected by other conditions of umbilical cord   N

        Newborn (suspected to be) affected by short umbilical cord

        Newborn (suspected to be) affected by vasa previa

        Excludes1   newborn affected by single umbilical artery (Q27.0)

P02.7   Newborn (suspected to be) affected by chorioamnionitis   N

     Inflammation of chorion and amnion

     Newborn (suspected to be) affected by amnionitis

     Newborn (suspected to be) affected by membranitis

     Newborn (suspected to be) affected by placentitis

P02.8   Newborn (suspected to be) affected by other abnormalities of membranes   N

■ **P02.9   Newborn (suspected to be) affected by abnormality of membranes, unspecified**   N

CHAPTER 16 (P00-P96)

N Newborn Age: 0   **P** Pediatric Age: 0–17   **M** Maternity DX: 12–55   **A** Adult Age: 15–124   ♀ Females Only   ♂ Males Only

🔍 Complication\Comorbidity   🔍 Major C\C   🔍 Present on Admission Requirement   🔍 Hospital-Acquired Condition

CHAPTER 16 (P00-P96)

● **P03 Newborn (suspected to be) affected by other complications of labor and delivery**

Code first any current condition in newborn

P03.0 Newborn (suspected to be) affected by breech delivery and extraction   N

P03.1 Newborn (suspected to be) affected by other malpresentation, malposition and disproportion during labor and delivery   N

Newborn (suspected to be) affected by contracted pelvis

Newborn (suspected to be) affected by conditions classifiable to O64-O66

Newborn (suspected to be) affected by persistent occipitoposterior

Newborn (suspected to be) affected by transverse lie

P03.2 Newborn (suspected to be) affected by forceps delivery   N

P03.3 Newborn (suspected to be) affected by delivery by vacuum extractor [ventouse]   N

P03.4 Newborn (suspected to be) affected by Cesarean delivery   N

P03.5 Newborn (suspected to be) affected by precipitate delivery   N

Newborn (suspected to be) affected by rapid second stage

P03.6 Newborn (suspected to be) affected by abnormal uterine contractions   N

Newborn (suspected to be) affected by conditions classifiable to O62.-, except O62.3

Newborn (suspected to be) affected by hypertonic labor

Newborn (suspected to be) affected by uterine inertia

● **P03.8 Newborn (suspected to be) affected by other specified complications of labor and delivery**

● **P03.81 Newborn (suspected to be) affected by abnormality in fetal (intrauterine) heart rate or rhythm**

Excludes1   neonatal cardiac dysrhythmia (P29.1-)

P03.810 Newborn (suspected to be) affected by abnormality in fetal (intrauterine) heart rate or rhythm before the onset of labor   N

P03.811 Newborn (suspected to be) affected by abnormality in fetal (intrauterine) heart rate or rhythm during labor   N

P03.819 Newborn (suspected to be) affected by abnormality in fetal (intrauterine) heart rate or rhythm, unspecified as to time of onset   N

P03.82 Meconium passage during delivery   N

Excludes1   meconium aspiration (P24.00, P24.01)
meconium staining (P96.83)

P03.89 Newborn (suspected to be) affected by other specified complications of labor and delivery

Newborn (suspected to be) affected by abnormality of maternal soft tissues

Newborn (suspected to be) affected by conditions classifiable to O60-O75 and by procedures used in labor and delivery not included in P02.- and P03.0-P03.6

Newborn (suspected to be) affected by induction of labor

P03.9 Newborn (suspected to be) affected by complication of labor and delivery, unspecified   N

● **P04 Newborn (suspected to be) affected by noxious substances transmitted via placenta or breast milk**

Includes   nonteratogenic effects of substances transmitted via placenta

Excludes2   congenital malformations (Q00-Q99)
neonatal jaundice from excessive hemolysis due to drugs or toxins transmitted from mother (P58.4)
newborn in contact with and (suspected) exposures hazardous to health not transmitted via placenta or breast milk (Z77.-)

● **P04.0 Newborn (suspected to be) affected by maternal anesthesia and analgesia in pregnancy, labor and delivery**   N

Newborn (suspected to be) affected by reactions and intoxications from maternal opiates and tranquilizers administered during labor and delivery

P04.1 Newborn (suspected to be) affected by other maternal medication   N

Newborn (suspected to be) affected by cancer chemotherapy

Newborn (suspected to be) affected by cytotoxic drugs

Excludes1   dysmorphism due to warfarin (Q86.2)
fetal hydantoin syndrome (Q86.1)
maternal use of drugs of addiction (P04.4-)

P04.2 Newborn (suspected to be) affected by maternal use of tobacco   N

Newborn (suspected to be) affected by exposure in utero to tobacco smoke

Excludes2   newborn exposure to environmental tobacco smoke (P96.81)

P04.3 Newborn (suspected to be) affected by maternal use of alcohol   N

Excludes1   fetal alcohol syndrome (Q86.0)

● **P04.4 Newborn (suspected to be) affected by maternal use of drugs of addiction**

P04.41 Newborn (suspected to be) affected by maternal use of cocaine   N
'Crack baby'

P04.49 Newborn (suspected to be) affected by maternal use of other drugs of addiction   N

Excludes2   newborn (suspected to be) affected by maternal anesthesia and analgesia (P04.0)
withdrawal symptoms from maternal use of drugs of addiction (P96.1)

P04.5 Newborn (suspected to be) affected by maternal use of nutritional chemical substances   N

P04.6 Newborn (suspected to be) affected by maternal exposure to environmental chemical substances   N

P04.8 Newborn (suspected to be) affected by other maternal noxious substances   N

P04.9 Newborn (suspected to be) affected by maternal noxious substance, unspecified   N

● Unacceptable Principal Diagnosis   ● Use Additional Character(s)   ■ Unspecified   ▶ Manifestation Code

OGCR   Official Guidelines for Coding and Reporting   Excludes 1   Excludes 2   Includes   Use additional   Code first   Code also

OGCR Section I.C.16.d.

Prematurity and Fetal Growth Retardation

Providers utilize different criteria in determining prematurity. A code for prematurity should not be assigned unless it is documented. Assignment of codes in categories P05, Disorders of newborn related to slow fetal growth and fetal malnutrition, and P07, Disorders of newborn related to short gestation and low birth weight, not elsewhere classified, should be based on the recorded birth weight and estimated gestational age. Codes from category P05 should not be assigned with codes from category P07.

When both birth weight and gestational age are available, two codes from category P07 should be assigned, with the code for birth weight sequenced before the code for gestational age.

A code from P05 and codes from P07.2 and P07.3 may be used to specify weeks of gestation as documented by the provider in the record.

DISORDERS OF NEWBORN RELATED TO LENGTH OF GESTATION AND FETAL GROWTH (P05-P08)

● **P05**   **Disorders of newborn related to slow fetal growth and fetal malnutrition**

   ● **P05.0**   **Newborn light for gestational age**
      Newborn light-for-dates

     ■ **P05.00**   **Newborn light for gestational age, unspecified weight**   N

       P05.01   **Newborn light for gestational age, less than 500 grams**   N

       P05.02   **Newborn light for gestational age, 500-749 grams**   N

       P05.03   **Newborn light for gestational age, 750-999 grams**   N

       P05.04   **Newborn light for gestational age, 1000-1249 grams**   N

       P05.05   **Newborn light for gestational age, 1250-1499 grams**   N

       P05.06   **Newborn light for gestational age, 1500-1749 grams**   N

       P05.07   **Newborn light for gestational age, 1750-1999 grams**   N

       P05.08   **Newborn light for gestational age, 2000-2499 grams**   N

   ● **P05.1**   **Newborn small for gestational age**
      Newborn small-and-light-for-dates
      Newborn small-for-dates

     ■ **P05.10**   **Newborn small for gestational age, unspecified weight**   N

       P05.11   **Newborn small for gestational age, less than 500 grams**   N

       P05.12   **Newborn small for gestational age, 500-749 grams**   N

       P05.13   **Newborn small for gestational age, 750-999 grams**   N

       P05.14   **Newborn small for gestational age, 1000-1249 grams**   N

       P05.15   **Newborn small for gestational age, 1250-1499 grams**   N

       P05.16   **Newborn small for gestational age, 1500-1749 grams**   N

       P05.17   **Newborn small for gestational age, 1750-1999 grams**   N

       P05.18   **Newborn small for gestational age, 2000-2499 grams**   N

   P05.2   **Newborn affected by fetal (intrauterine) malnutrition not light or small for gestational age**   N
      Infant, not light or small for gestational age, showing signs of fetal malnutrition, such as dry, peeling skin and loss of subcutaneous tissue

     | Excludes1 | newborn affected by fetal malnutrition with light for gestational age (P05.0-)
           newborn affected by fetal malnutrition with small for gestational age (P05.1-)

   ■ **P05.9**   **Newborn affected by slow intrauterine growth, unspecified**   N
      Newborn affected by fetal growth retardation NOS

● **P07**   **Disorders of newborn related to short gestation and low birth weight, not elsewhere classified**

     Note: When both birth weight and gestational age of the newborn are available, both should be coded with birth weight sequenced before gestational age.

     | Includes | the listed conditions, without further specification, as the cause of morbidity or additional care, in newborn

     | Excludes1 | low birth weight due to slow fetal growth and fetal malnutrition (P05.-)

   ● **P07.0**   **Extremely low birth weight newborn**
      Newborn birth weight 999 g. or less

     ■ **P07.00**   **Extremely low birth weight newborn, unspecified weight**   N

       P07.01   **Extremely low birth weight newborn, less than 500 grams**   N

       P07.02   **Extremely low birth weight newborn, 500-749 grams**   N

       P07.03   **Extremely low birth weight newborn, 750-999 grams**   N

   ● **P07.1**   **Other low birth weight newborn**
      Newborn birth weight 1000-2499 g.

     ■ **P07.10**   **Other low birth weight newborn, unspecified weight**   N

       P07.14   **Other low birth weight newborn, 1000-1249 grams**   N

       P07.15   **Other low birth weight newborn, 1250-1499 grams**   N

       P07.16   **Other low birth weight newborn, 1500-1749 grams**   N

       P07.17   **Other low birth weight newborn, 1750-1999 grams**   N

       P07.18   **Other low birth weight newborn, 2000-2499 grams**   N

   ● **P07.2**   **Extreme immaturity of newborn**
      Less than 28 completed weeks (less than 196 completed days) of gestation

     ■ **P07.20**   **Extreme immaturity of newborn, unspecified weeks of gestation**   N
       Gestational age less than 28 completed weeks NOS

       P07.21   **Extreme immaturity of newborn, gestational age less than 23 completed weeks**   N
       Extreme immaturity of newborn, gestational age less than 23 weeks, 0 days

CHAPTER 16 (P00-P96)

P07.22   **Extreme immaturity of newborn, gestational age 23 completed weeks**   N
Extreme immaturity of newborn, gestational age 23 weeks, 0 days through 23 weeks, 6 days

P07.23   **Extreme immaturity of newborn, gestational age 24 completed weeks**   N
Extreme immaturity of newborn, gestational age 24 weeks, 0 days through 24 weeks, 6 days

P07.24   **Extreme immaturity of newborn, gestational age 25 completed weeks**   N
Extreme immaturity of newborn, gestational age 25 weeks, 0 days through 25 weeks, 6 days

P07.25   **Extreme immaturity of newborn, gestational age 26 completed weeks**   N
Extreme immaturity of newborn, gestational age 26 weeks, 0 days through 26 weeks, 6 days

P07.26   **Extreme immaturity of newborn, gestational age 27 completed weeks**   N
Extreme immaturity of newborn, gestational age 27 weeks, 0 days through 27 weeks, 6 days

● **P07.3**   **Preterm [premature] newborn [other]**
28 completed weeks or more but less than 37 completed weeks (196 completed days but less than 259 completed days) of gestation
Prematurity NOS

■ **P07.30**   **Preterm newborn, unspecified weeks of gestation**   N

P07.31   **Preterm newborn, gestational age 28 completed weeks**   N
Preterm newborn, gestational age 28 weeks, 0 days through 28 weeks, 6 days

P07.32   **Preterm newborn, gestational age 29 completed weeks**   N
Preterm newborn, gestational age 29 weeks, 0 days through 29 weeks, 6 days

P07.33   **Preterm newborn, gestational age 30 completed weeks**   N
Preterm newborn, gestational age 30 weeks, 0 days through 30 weeks, 6 days

P07.34   **Preterm newborn, gestational age 31 completed weeks**   N
Preterm newborn, gestational age 31 weeks, 0 days through 31 weeks, 6 days

P07.35   **Preterm newborn, gestational age 32 completed weeks**   N
Preterm newborn, gestational age 32 weeks, 0 days through 32 weeks, 6 days

P07.36   **Preterm newborn, gestational age 33 completed weeks**   N
Preterm newborn, gestational age 33 weeks, 0 days through 33 weeks, 6 days

P07.37   **Preterm newborn, gestational age 34 completed weeks**   N
Preterm newborn, gestational age 34 weeks, 0 days through 34 weeks, 6 days

P07.38   **Preterm newborn, gestational age 35 completed weeks**   N
Preterm newborn, gestational age 35 weeks, 0 days through 35 weeks, 6 days

P07.39   **Preterm newborn, gestational age 36 completed weeks**   N
Preterm newborn, gestational age 36 weeks, 0 days through 36 weeks, 6 days

● **P08**   **Disorders of newborn related to long gestation and high birth weight**

Note: When both birth weight and gestational age of the newborn are available, priority of assignment should be given to birth weight.

Includes   the listed conditions, without further specification, as causes of morbidity or additional care, in newborn

P08.0   **Exceptionally large newborn baby**   N
Usually implies a birth weight of 4500 g. or more
Excludes1   syndrome of infant of diabetic mother (P70.1)
syndrome of infant of mother with gestational diabetes (P70.0)

P08.1   **Other heavy for gestational age newborn**   N
Other newborn heavy- or large-for-dates regardless of period of gestation
Usually implies a birth weight of 4000 g. to 4499 g.
Excludes1   newborn with a birth weight of 4500 or more (P08.0)
syndrome of infant of diabetic mother (P70.1)
syndrome of infant of mother with gestational diabetes (P70.0)

● **P08.2**   **Late newborn, not heavy for gestational age**

P08.21   **Post-term newborn**   N
Newborn with gestation period over 40 completed weeks to 42 completed weeks

P08.22   **Prolonged gestation of newborn**   N
Newborn with gestation period over 42 completed weeks (294 days or more), not heavy- or large-for-dates
Postmaturity NOS

ABNORMAL FINDINGS ON NEONATAL SCREENING (P09)

P09   **Abnormal findings on neonatal screening**   N

Use additional code to identify signs, symptoms and conditions associated with the screening
Excludes2   nonspecific serologic evidence of human immunodeficiency virus [HIV] (R75)

● Unacceptable Principal Diagnosis   ● Use Additional Character(s)   ■ Unspecified   ▶ Manifestation Code
OGCR Official Guidelines for Coding and Reporting   Excludes 1   Excludes 2   Includes   Use additional   Code first   Code also

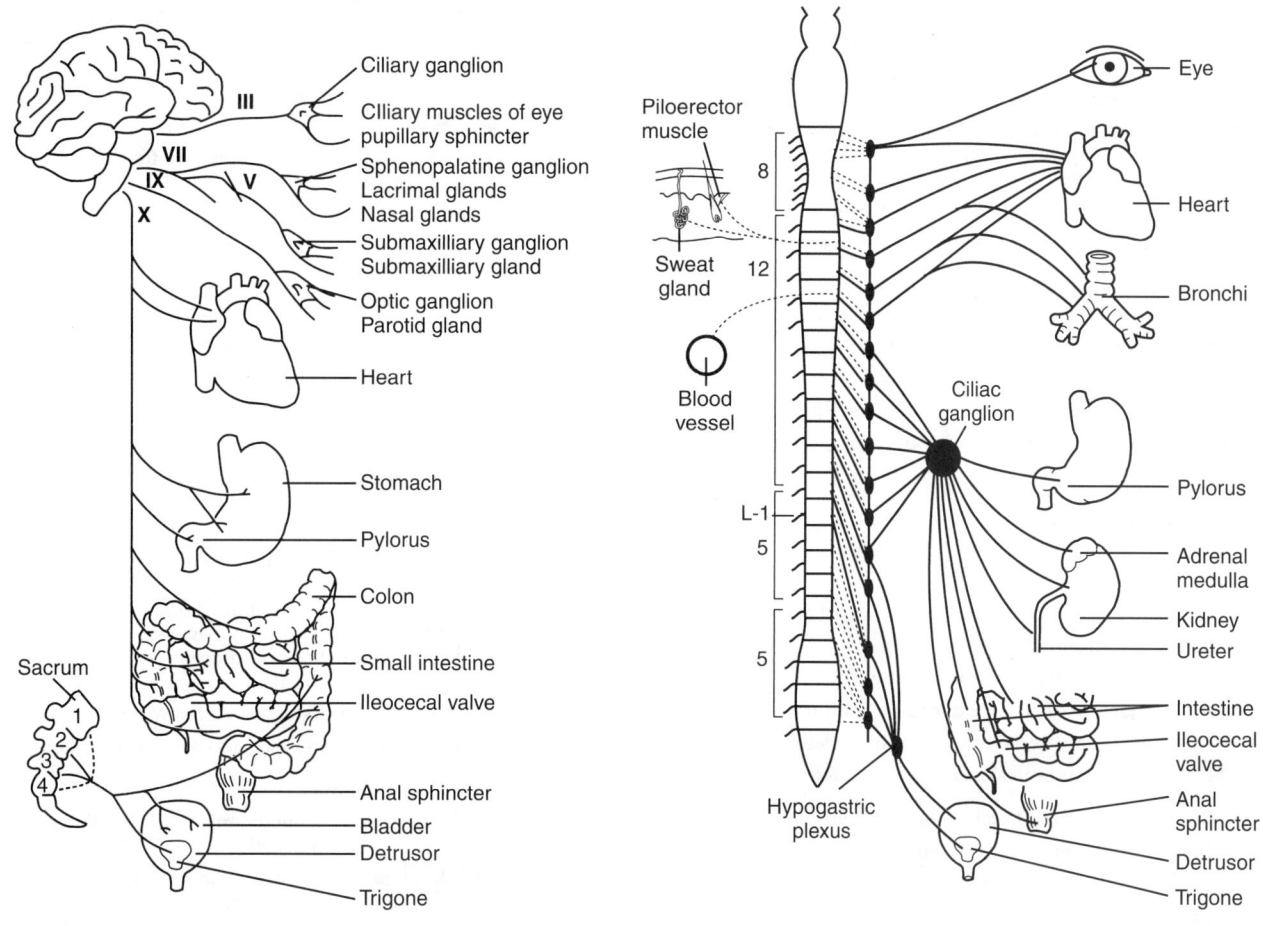

Figure 16-1 **A.** Parasympathetic nervous system. **B.** Sympathetic nervous system. (From Buck CJ: Step-by Step Medical Coding, Philadelphia, WB Saunders, 2010.)

Item 16–1 The **peripheral nervous system** consists of 31 pairs of spinal nerves, 12 pairs of cranial nerves, and the autonomic nerves, which are divided into the parasympathetic and sympathetic nerves. The cranial nerves are: olfactory (I), optic (II), oculomotor (III), trochlear (IV), trigeminal (V), abducens (VI), facial (VII), vestibulocochlear (VIII), glossopharyngeal (IX), vagus (X), accessory (XI), and hypoglossal (XII).

BIRTH TRAUMA (P10-P15)

● **P10** **Intracranial laceration and hemorrhage due to birth injury**
     Excludes1 intracranial hemorrhage of newborn NOS (P52.9)
                intracranial hemorrhage of newborn due to anoxia or hypoxia (P52.-)
                nontraumatic intracranial hemorrhage of newborn (P52.-)

   P10.0 **Subdural hemorrhage due to birth injury** 🚩 **N**
       Subdural hematoma (localized) due to birth injury
       Excludes1 subdural hemorrhage accompanying tentorial tear (P10.4)

   P10.1 **Cerebral hemorrhage due to birth injury** 🚩 **N**
   P10.2 **Intraventricular hemorrhage due to birth injury** 🚩 **N**

   P10.3 **Subarachnoid hemorrhage due to birth injury** 🚩 **N**
   P10.4 **Tentorial tear due to birth injury** 🚩 **N**
       Pertaining to tentorium of cerebellum (extension of dura mater that separates cerebellum from inferior portion of occipital lobes)

   P10.8 **Other intracranial lacerations and hemorrhages due to birth injury** 🚩 **N**
   ■ **P10.9** **Unspecified intracranial laceration and hemorrhage due to birth injury** 🚩 **N**

● **P11** **Other birth injuries to central nervous system**
   P11.0 **Cerebral edema due to birth injury** 🚩 **N**
   P11.1 **Other specified brain damage due to birth injury** **N**
   ■ **P11.2** **Unspecified brain damage due to birth injury** 🚩 **N**
   P11.3 **Birth injury to facial nerve** **N**
       Facial palsy due to birth injury
   P11.4 **Birth injury to other cranial nerves** **N**
   P11.5 **Birth injury to spine and spinal cord** **N**
       Fracture of spine due to birth injury
   ■ **P11.9** **Birth injury to central nervous system, unspecified** 🚩 **N**

N Newborn Age: 0 **P** Pediatric Age: 0–17 **M** Maternity DX: 12–55 **A** Adult Age: 15–124 ♀ Females Only ♂ Males Only
🚩 Complication\Comorbidity 🚩 Major C\C 🚩 Present on Admission Requirement 🚩 Hospital-Acquired Condition

1333

- **P12**   Birth injury to scalp
  - P12.0   Cephalhematoma due to birth injury   N
  - P12.1   Chignon (from vacuum extraction) due to birth injury   N
  - P12.2   Epicranial subaponeurotic hemorrhage due to birth injury 🔧   N
    - Subgaleal hemorrhage
  - P12.3   Bruising of scalp due to birth injury   N
  - P12.4   Injury of scalp of newborn due to monitoring equipment   N
    - Sampling incision of scalp of newborn
    - Scalp clip (electrode) injury of newborn
  - ● P12.8   Other birth injuries to scalp
    - P12.81   Caput succedaneum   N
    - P12.89   Other birth injuries to scalp   N
  - ■ P12.9   Birth injury to scalp, unspecified   N

- **P13**   Birth injury to skeleton
  - Excludes2   birth injury to spine (P11.5)
  - P13.0   Fracture of skull due to birth injury   N
  - P13.1   Other birth injuries to skull   N
    - Excludes1   cephalhematoma (P12.0)
  - P13.2   Birth injury to femur   N
  - P13.3   Birth injury to other long bones   N
  - P13.4   Fracture of clavicle due to birth injury   N
  - P13.8   Birth injuries to other parts of skeleton   N
  - ■ P13.9   Birth injury to skeleton, unspecified   N

- **P14**   Birth injury to peripheral nervous system
  - P14.0   Erb's paralysis due to birth injury   N
  - P14.1   Klumpke's paralysis due to birth injury   N
  - P14.2   Phrenic nerve paralysis due to birth injury   N
  - P14.3   Other brachial plexus birth injuries   N
  - P14.8   Birth injuries to other parts of peripheral nervous system   N
  - ■ P14.9   Birth injury to peripheral nervous system, unspecified   N

- **P15**   Other birth injuries
  - P15.0   Birth injury to liver   N
    - Rupture of liver due to birth injury
  - P15.1   Birth injury to spleen   N
    - Rupture of spleen due to birth injury
  - P15.2   Sternomastoid injury due to birth injury   N
  - P15.3   Birth injury to eye   N
    - Subconjunctival hemorrhage due to birth injury
    - Traumatic glaucoma due to birth injury
  - P15.4   Birth injury to face   N
    - Facial congestion due to birth injury
  - P15.5   Birth injury to external genitalia   N
  - P15.6   Subcutaneous fat necrosis due to birth injury   N
  - P15.8   Other specified birth injuries   N
  - ■ P15.9   Birth injury, unspecified   N

RESPIRATORY AND CARDIOVASCULAR DISORDERS SPECIFIC TO THE PERINATAL PERIOD (P19-P29)

- **P19**   Metabolic acidemia in newborn
  - Includes   metabolic acidemia in newborn
  - P19.0   Metabolic acidemia in newborn first noted before onset of labor   N
  - P19.1   Metabolic acidemia in newborn first noted during labor   N
  - P19.2   Metabolic acidemia noted at birth   N
  - ■ P19.9   Metabolic acidemia, unspecified   N

- **P22**   Respiratory distress of newborn
  - Excludes1   respiratory arrest of newborn (P28.81)
    - respiratory failure of newborn NOS (P28.5)
  - P22.0   Respiratory distress syndrome of newborn 🔧   N
    - Cardiorespiratory distress syndrome of newborn
    - Hyaline membrane disease
    - Idiopathic respiratory distress syndrome [IRDS or RDS] of newborn
    - Pulmonary hypoperfusion syndrome
    - Respiratory distress syndrome, type I
  - P22.1   Transient tachypnea of newborn   N
    - Idiopathic tachypnea of newborn
    - Respiratory distress syndrome, type II
    - Wet lung syndrome
  - P22.8   Other respiratory distress of newborn   N
  - ■ P22.9   Respiratory distress of newborn, unspecified   N

- **P23**   Congenital pneumonia
  - Includes   infective pneumonia acquired in utero or during birth
  - Excludes1   neonatal pneumonia resulting from aspiration (P24.-)
  - P23.0   Congenital pneumonia due to viral agent 🔧   N
    - Use additional code (B97) to identify organism
    - Excludes1   congenital rubella pneumonitis (P35.0)
  - P23.1   Congenital pneumonia due to Chlamydia 🔧   N
  - P23.2   Congenital pneumonia due to staphylococcus 🔧   N
  - P23.3   Congenital pneumonia due to streptococcus, group B 🔧   N
  - P23.4   Congenital pneumonia due to Escherichia coli 🔧   N
  - P23.5   Congenital pneumonia due to Pseudomonas 🔧   N
  - P23.6   Congenital pneumonia due to other bacterial agents 🔧   N
    - Congenital pneumonia due to Hemophilus influenzae
    - Congenital pneumonia due to Klebsiella pneumoniae
    - Congenital pneumonia due to Mycoplasma
    - Congenital pneumonia due to Streptococcus, except group B
    - Use additional code (B95-B96) to identify organism
  - P23.8   Congenital pneumonia due to other organisms 🔧   N
  - ■ P23.9   Congenital pneumonia, unspecified 🔧   N

● Unacceptable Principal Diagnosis   ● Use Additional Character(s)   ■ Unspecified   ▶ Manifestation Code

OGCR Official Guidelines for Coding and Reporting   Excludes 1   Excludes 2   Includes   Use additional   Code first   Code also

● **P24 Neonatal aspiration**

> **Includes**   aspiration in utero and during delivery

● **P24.0   Meconium aspiration**

> **Excludes1**   meconium passage (without aspiration) during delivery (P03.82)
>
> meconium staining (P96.83)

     P24.00   Meconium aspiration without respiratory symptoms   N
> Meconium aspiration NOS

     P24.01   Meconium aspiration with respiratory symptoms 🦠   N
> Meconium aspiration pneumonia
> Meconium aspiration pneumonitis
> Meconium aspiration syndrome NOS
>
> **Use additional** code to identify any secondary pulmonary hypertension, if applicable (I27.2)

● **P24.1   Neonatal aspiration of (clear) amniotic fluid and mucus**
> Neonatal aspiration of liquor (amnii)

     P24.10   Neonatal aspiration of (clear) amniotic fluid and mucus without respiratory symptoms   N
> Neonatal aspiration of amniotic fluid and mucus NOS

     P24.11   Neonatal aspiration of (clear) amniotic fluid and mucus with respiratory symptoms 🦠   N
> Neonatal aspiration of amniotic fluid and mucus with pneumonia
> Neonatal aspiration of amniotic fluid and mucus with pneumonitis
>
> **Use additional** code to identify any secondary pulmonary hypertension, if applicable (I27.2)

● **P24.2   Neonatal aspiration of blood**

     P24.20   Neonatal aspiration of blood without respiratory symptoms   N
> Neonatal aspiration of blood NOS

     P24.21   Neonatal aspiration of blood with respiratory symptoms 🦠   N
> Neonatal aspiration of blood with pneumonia
> Neonatal aspiration of blood with pneumonitis
>
> **Use additional** code to identify any secondary pulmonary hypertension, if applicable (I27.2)

● **P24.3   Neonatal aspiration of milk and regurgitated food**
> Neonatal aspiration of stomach contents

     P24.30   Neonatal aspiration of milk and regurgitated food without respiratory symptoms   N
> Neonatal aspiration of milk and regurgitated food NOS

     P24.31   Neonatal aspiration of milk and regurgitated food with respiratory symptoms 🦠   N
> Neonatal aspiration of milk and regurgitated food with pneumonia
> Neonatal aspiration of milk and regurgitated food with pneumonitis
>
> **Use additional** code to identify any secondary pulmonary hypertension, if applicable (I27.2)

● **P24.8   Other neonatal aspiration**

     P24.80   Other neonatal aspiration without respiratory symptoms   N
> Neonatal aspiration NEC

     P24.81   Other neonatal aspiration with respiratory symptoms 🦠   N
> Neonatal aspiration pneumonia NEC
> Neonatal aspiration with pneumonitis NEC
> Neonatal aspiration with pneumonia NOS
> Neonatal aspiration with pneumonitis NOS
>
> **Use additional** code to identify any secondary pulmonary hypertension, if applicable (I27.2)

■ **P24.9   Neonatal aspiration, unspecified**   N

● **P25   Interstitial emphysema and related conditions originating in the perinatal period**

     P25.0   Interstitial emphysema originating in the perinatal period 🦠   N

     P25.1   Pneumothorax originating in the perinatal period 🦠   N

     P25.2   Pneumomediastinum originating in the perinatal period 🦠   N

     P25.3   Pneumopericardium originating in the perinatal period 🦠   N

     P25.8   Other conditions related to interstitial emphysema originating in the perinatal period 🦠   N

● **P26   Pulmonary hemorrhage originating in the perinatal period**

> **Excludes1**   acute idiopathic hemorrhage in infants over 28 days old (R04.81)

     P26.0   Tracheobronchial hemorrhage originating in the perinatal period 🦠   N

     P26.1   Massive pulmonary hemorrhage originating in the perinatal period 🦠   N

     P26.8   Other pulmonary hemorrhages originating in the perinatal period 🦠   N

     ■ **P26.9   Unspecified pulmonary hemorrhage originating in the perinatal period** 🦠   N

● **P27   Chronic respiratory disease originating in the perinatal period**

> **Excludes1**   respiratory distress of newborn (P22.0-P22.9)

     P27.0   Wilson-Mikity syndrome 🦠
> Pulmonary dysmaturity

     P27.1   Bronchopulmonary dysplasia originating in the perinatal period 🦠

     P27.8   Other chronic respiratory diseases originating in the perinatal period 🦠
> Congenital pulmonary fibrosis
> Ventilator lung in newborn

     ■ **P27.9   Unspecified chronic respiratory disease originating in the perinatal period** 🦠

●P28   Other respiratory conditions originating in the perinatal period

> **Excludes1**   congenital malformations of the respiratory system (Q30-Q34)

P28.0   Primary atelectasis of newborn 🔾   N
> *Failure of lungs to expand properly at birth*
> Primary failure to expand terminal respiratory units
> Pulmonary hypoplasia associated with short gestation
> Pulmonary immaturity NOS

●P28.1   Other and unspecified atelectasis of newborn

▪P28.10   Unspecified atelectasis of newborn 🔾   N
> Atelectasis of newborn NOS

P28.11   Resorption atelectasis without respiratory distress syndrome 🔾   N
> **Excludes1**   resorption atelectasis with respiratory distress syndrome (P22.0)

P28.19   Other atelectasis of newborn 🔾   N
> Partial atelectasis of newborn
> Secondary atelectasis of newborn

P28.2   Cyanotic attacks of newborn 🔾   N
> **Excludes1**   apnea of newborn (P28.3-P28.4)

P28.3   Primary sleep apnea of newborn 🔾   N
> Central sleep apnea of newborn
> Obstructive sleep apnea of newborn
> Sleep apnea of newborn NOS

P28.4   Other apnea of newborn 🔾   N
> Apnea of prematurity
> Obstructive apnea of newborn
> **Excludes1**   obstructive sleep apnea of newborn (P28.3)

P28.5   Respiratory failure of newborn 🔾   N
> **Excludes1**   respiratory arrest of newborn (P28.81)
> respiratory distress of newborn (P22.0-)

●P28.8   Other specified respiratory conditions of newborn

P28.81   Respiratory arrest of newborn 🔾   N

P28.89   Other specified respiratory conditions of newborn   N
> Congenital laryngeal stridor
> Sniffles in newborn
> Snuffles in newborn
> **Excludes1**   early congenital syphilitic rhinitis (A50.0)

▪P28.9   Respiratory condition of newborn, unspecified   N
> Respiratory depression in newborn

●P29   Cardiovascular disorders originating in the perinatal period

> **Excludes1**   congenital malformations of the circulatory system (Q20-Q28)

P29.0   Neonatal cardiac failure   N

●P29.1   Neonatal cardiac dysrhythmia

P29.11   Neonatal tachycardia   N

P29.12   Neonatal bradycardia   N

P29.2   Neonatal hypertension   N

P29.3   Persistent fetal circulation 🔾🔾   N
> Delayed closure of ductus arteriosus
> (Persistent) pulmonary hypertension of newborn

P29.4   Transient myocardial ischemia in newborn   N

●P29.8   Other cardiovascular disorders originating in the perinatal period

P29.81   Cardiac arrest of newborn 🔾   N

P29.89   Other cardiovascular disorders originating in the perinatal period   N

▪P29.9   Cardiovascular disorder originating in the perinatal period, unspecified   N

INFECTIONS SPECIFIC TO THE PERINATAL PERIOD (P35-P39)

Infections acquired in utero, during birth via the umbilicus, or during the first 28 days after birth

> **Excludes2**   asymptomatic human immunodeficiency virus [HIV] infection status (Z21)
> congenital gonococcal infection (A54.-)
> congenital pneumonia (P23.-)
> congenital syphilis (A50.-)
> human immunodeficiency virus [HIV] disease (B20)
> infant botulism (A48.51)
> infectious diseases not specific to the perinatal period (A00-B99, J09, J10.-)
> intestinal infectious disease (A00-A09)
> laboratory evidence of human immunodeficiency virus [HIV] (R75)
> tetanus neonatorum (A33)

●P35   Congenital viral diseases

> **Includes**   infections acquired in utero or during birth

P35.0   Congenital rubella syndrome 🔾   N
> Congenital rubella pneumonitis

P35.1   Congenital cytomegalovirus infection 🔾   N
> *Viruses transmitted by multiple routes that cause mild/subclinical infection*

P35.2   Congenital herpesviral [herpes simplex] infection 🔾   N

P35.3   Congenital viral hepatitis 🔾   N

P35.8   Other congenital viral diseases 🔾   N
> Congenital varicella [chickenpox]

▪P35.9   Congenital viral disease, unspecified 🔾   N

●P36   Bacterial sepsis of newborn

> **Includes**   congenital sepsis

> Use additional code(s), if applicable, to identify severe sepsis (R65.2-) and associated acute organ dysfunction(s)

P36.0   Sepsis of newborn due to streptococcus, group B 🔾   N

●P36.1   Sepsis of newborn due to other and unspecified streptococci

▪P36.10   Sepsis of newborn due to unspecified streptococci 🔾   N

P36.19   Sepsis of newborn due to other streptococci 🔾   N

P36.2   Sepsis of newborn due to Staphylococcus aureus 🔾   N

●P36.3   Sepsis of newborn due to other and unspecified staphylococci

▪P36.30   Sepsis of newborn due to unspecified staphylococci 🔾   N

P36.39   Sepsis of newborn due to other staphylococci 🔾   N

P36.4   Sepsis of newborn due to Escherichia coli 🔾   N

P36.5   Sepsis of newborn due to anaerobes 🔾   N

● Unacceptable Principal Diagnosis   ● Use Additional Character(s)   ▪ Unspecified   ▶ Manifestation Code
OGCR Official Guidelines for Coding and Reporting   Excludes 1   Excludes 2   Includes   Use additional   Code first   Code also

P36.8   **Other bacterial sepsis of newborn** 🕸   N
> Use additional code from category B96 to identify organism

■ **P36.9**   **Bacterial sepsis of newborn, unspecified** 🕸   N

● **P37**   **Other congenital infectious and parasitic diseases**
> **Excludes2**   congenital syphilis (A50.-)
> infectious neonatal diarrhea (A00-A09)
> necrotizing enterocolitis in newborn (P77.-)
> noninfectious neonatal diarrhea (P78.3)
> ophthalmia neonatorum due to gonococcus (A54.31)
> tetanus neonatorum (A33)

P37.0   **Congenital tuberculosis** 🕸   N

P37.1   **Congenital toxoplasmosis** 🕸   N
> *Parasitic infection, often causing mild flu-like illness*
> Hydrocephalus due to congenital toxoplasmosis

P37.2   **Neonatal (disseminated) listeriosis** 🕸   N
> *Acquired transplacentally or during/after parturition in which symptoms are those of sepsis*

P37.3   **Congenital falciparum malaria** 🕸   N

P37.4   **Other congenital malaria** 🕸   N

P37.5   **Neonatal candidiasis**   N

P37.8   **Other specified congenital infectious and parasitic diseases** 🕸   N

■ **P37.9**   **Congenital infectious or parasitic disease, unspecified** 🕸   N

● **P38**   **Omphalitis of newborn**
> *Inflammation of umbilicus*
> **Excludes1**   omphalitis not of newborn (L08.82)
> tetanus omphalitis (A33)
> umbilical hemorrhage of newborn (P51.-)

P38.1   **Omphalitis with mild hemorrhage** 🕸   N

P38.9   **Omphalitis without hemorrhage** 🕸   N
> Omphalitis of newborn NOS

● **P39**   **Other infections specific to the perinatal period**
> Use additional code to identify organism or specific infection

P39.0   **Neonatal infective mastitis** 🕸   N
> **Excludes1**   breast engorgement of newborn (P83.4)
> noninfective mastitis of newborn (P83.4)

P39.1   **Neonatal conjunctivitis and dacryocystitis**   N
> Neonatal chlamydial conjunctivitis
> Ophthalmia neonatorum NOS
> *Neonate = newborn*
> **Excludes1**   gonococcal conjunctivitis (A54.31)

P39.2   **Intra-amniotic infection affecting newborn, not elsewhere classified** 🕸   N

P39.3   **Neonatal urinary tract infection** 🕸   N

P39.4   **Neonatal skin infection** 🕸   N
> Neonatal pyoderma
> **Excludes1**   pemphigus neonatorum (L00)
> staphylococcal scalded skin syndrome (L00)

P39.8   **Other specified infections specific to the perinatal period** 🕸   N

■ **P39.9**   **Infection specific to the perinatal period, unspecified** 🕸   N

HEMORRHAGIC AND HEMATOLOGICAL DISORDERS OF NEWBORN (P50-P61)

> **Excludes1**   congenital stenosis and stricture of bile ducts (Q44.3)
> Crigler-Najjar syndrome (E80.5)
> Dubin-Johnson syndrome (E80.6)
> Gilbert syndrome (E80.4)
> hereditary hemolytic anemias (D55-D58)

● **P50**   **Newborn affected by intrauterine (fetal) blood loss**
> **Excludes1**   congenital anemia from intrauterine (fetal) blood loss (P61.3)

P50.0   **Newborn affected by intrauterine (fetal) blood loss from vasa previa**   N

P50.1   **Newborn affected by intrauterine (fetal) blood loss from ruptured cord**   N

P50.2   **Newborn affected by intrauterine (fetal) blood loss from placenta**   N

P50.3   **Newborn affected by hemorrhage into co-twin**   N

P50.4   **Newborn affected by hemorrhage into maternal circulation**   N

P50.5   **Newborn affected by intrauterine (fetal) blood loss from cut end of co-twin's cord**   N

P50.8   **Newborn affected by other intrauterine (fetal) blood loss**   N

■ **P50.9**   **Newborn affected by intrauterine (fetal) blood loss, unspecified**   N
> Newborn affected by fetal hemorrhage NOS

● **P51**   **Umbilical hemorrhage of newborn**
> **Excludes1**   omphalitis with mild hemorrhage (P38.1)
> umbilical hemorrhage from cut end of co-twins cord (P50.5)

P51.0   **Massive umbilical hemorrhage of newborn**   N

P51.8   **Other umbilical hemorrhages of newborn**   N
> Slipped umbilical ligature NOS

■ **P51.9**   **Umbilical hemorrhage of newborn, unspecified**   N

● **P52**   **Intracranial nontraumatic hemorrhage of newborn**
> **Includes**   intracranial hemorrhage due to anoxia or hypoxia
> **Excludes1**   intracranial hemorrhage due to birth injury (P10.-)
> intracranial hemorrhage due to other injury (S06.-)

P52.0   **Intraventricular (nontraumatic) hemorrhage, grade 1, of newborn** 🕸   N
> Subependymal hemorrhage (without intraventricular extension)
> Bleeding into germinal matrix

P52.1   **Intraventricular (nontraumatic) hemorrhage, grade 2, of newborn** 🕸   N
> Subependymal hemorrhage with intraventricular extension
> Bleeding into ventricle

● **P52.2**   **Intraventricular (nontraumatic) hemorrhage, grade 3 and grade 4, of newborn**

P52.21   **Intraventricular (nontraumatic) hemorrhage, grade 3, of newborn** 🕸   N
> Subependymal hemorrhage with intraventricular extension with enlargement of ventricle

P52.22   **Intraventricular (nontraumatic) hemorrhage, grade 4, of newborn** 🕸   N
> Bleeding into cerebral cortex
> Subependymal hemorrhage with intracerebral extension

N Newborn Age: 0   **P** Pediatric Age: 0–17   **M** Maternity DX: 12–55   **A** Adult Age: 15–124   ♀ Females Only   ♂ Males Only
🕸 Complication\Comorbidity   🕸 Major C\C   Present on Admission Requirement   🕸 Hospital-Acquired Condition
1337

CHAPTER 16 (P00-P96)

P52.3 Unspecified intraventricular (nontraumatic) hemorrhage of newborn   N

P52.4 Intracerebral (nontraumatic) hemorrhage of newborn   N

P52.5 Subarachnoid (nontraumatic) hemorrhage of newborn   N

P52.6 Cerebellar (nontraumatic) and posterior fossa hemorrhage of newborn   N

P52.8 Other intracranial (nontraumatic) hemorrhages of newborn   N

P52.9 Intracranial (nontraumatic) hemorrhage of newborn, unspecified   N

P53 Hemorrhagic disease of newborn   N
Vitamin K deficiency of newborn

P54 Other neonatal hemorrhages
> Excludes1   newborn affected by (intrauterine) blood loss (P50.-)
> pulmonary hemorrhage originating in the perinatal period (P26.-)

P54.0 Neonatal hematemesis   N
Vomiting of blood
> Excludes1   neonatal hematemesis due to swallowed maternal blood (P78.2)

P54.1 Neonatal melena   N
Dark-colored feces stained with blood pigments
> Excludes1   neonatal melena due to swallowed maternal blood (P78.2)

P54.2 Neonatal rectal hemorrhage   N

P54.3 Other neonatal gastrointestinal hemorrhage   N

P54.4 Neonatal adrenal hemorrhage   N

P54.5 Neonatal cutaneous hemorrhage   N
Neonatal bruising
Neonatal ecchymoses
Neonatal petechiae
Neonatal superficial hematomata
> Excludes2   bruising of scalp due to birth injury (P12.3)
> cephalhematoma due to birth injury (P12.0)

P54.6 Neonatal vaginal hemorrhage ♀   N
Neonatal pseudomenses

P54.8 Other specified neonatal hemorrhages   N

P54.9 Neonatal hemorrhage, unspecified   N

P55 Hemolytic disease of newborn
AKA erythroblastosis fetalis and is due to Rh isoimmunization, result of Rh blood factor incompatibilities between mother (Rh negative) and fetus (Rh positive)

P55.0 Rh isoimmunization of newborn   N

P55.1 ABO isoimmunization of newborn   N

P55.8 Other hemolytic diseases of newborn   N

P55.9 Hemolytic disease of newborn, unspecified   N

P56 Hydrops fetalis due to hemolytic disease
Caused by maternal sensitization to fetal blood group antigen
> Excludes1   hydrops fetalis NOS (P83.2)

P56.0 Hydrops fetalis due to isoimmunization   N

P56.9 Hydrops fetalis due to other and unspecified hemolytic disease

P56.90 Hydrops fetalis due to unspecified hemolytic disease   N

P56.99 Hydrops fetalis due to other hemolytic disease   N

P57 Kernicterus
High levels of bilirubin in blood, with severe neural symptoms

P57.0 Kernicterus due to isoimmunization   N

P57.8 Other specified kernicterus   N
> Excludes1   Crigler-Najjar syndrome (E80.5)

P57.9 Kernicterus, unspecified   N

P58 Neonatal jaundice due to other excessive hemolysis
> Excludes1   jaundice due to isoimmunization (P55-P57)

P58.0 Neonatal jaundice due to bruising   N

P58.1 Neonatal jaundice due to bleeding   N

P58.2 Neonatal jaundice due to infection   N

P58.3 Neonatal jaundice due to polycythemia   N

P58.4 Neonatal jaundice due to drugs or toxins transmitted from mother or given to newborn
> Code first poisoning due to drug or toxin, if applicable (T36-T65 with fifth or sixth character 1-4 or 6)
> Use additional code for adverse effect, if applicable, to identify drug (T36-T50 with fifth or sixth character 5)

P58.41 Neonatal jaundice due to drugs or toxins transmitted from mother   N

P58.42 Neonatal jaundice due to drugs or toxins given to newborn   N

P58.5 Neonatal jaundice due to swallowed maternal blood   N

P58.8 Neonatal jaundice due to other specified excessive hemolysis   N

P58.9 Neonatal jaundice due to excessive hemolysis, unspecified   N

P59 Neonatal jaundice from other and unspecified causes
> Excludes1   jaundice due to inborn errors of metabolism (E70-E88)
> kernicterus (P57.-)

P59.0 Neonatal jaundice associated with preterm delivery   N
Hyperbilirubinemia of prematurity
Jaundice due to delayed conjugation associated with preterm delivery

P59.1 Inspissated bile syndrome   N

P59.2 Neonatal jaundice from other and unspecified hepatocellular damage
> Excludes1   congenital viral hepatitis (P35.3)

P59.20 Neonatal jaundice from unspecified hepatocellular damage   N

P59.29 Neonatal jaundice from other hepatocellular damage   N
Neonatal giant cell hepatitis
Neonatal (idiopathic) hepatitis

P59.3 Neonatal jaundice from breast milk inhibitor   N

P59.8 Neonatal jaundice from other specified causes   N

P59.9 Neonatal jaundice, unspecified   N
Neonatal physiological jaundice (intense) (prolonged) NOS

P60 Disseminated intravascular coagulation of newborn   N
Defibrination syndrome of newborn

● Unacceptable Principal Diagnosis   ● Use Additional Character(s)   ■ Unspecified   ▶ Manifestation Code

OGCR Official Guidelines for Coding and Reporting   Excludes 1   Excludes 2   Includes   Use additional   Code first   Code also

● **P61**   **Other perinatal hematological disorders**

> **Excludes1**   transient hypogammaglobulinemia of infancy (D80.7)

    P61.0   **Transient neonatal thrombocytopenia** 🦠   **N**
> *Lack of sufficient numbers of circulating thrombocytes (platelets)*
> Neonatal thrombocytopenia due to exchange transfusion
> Neonatal thrombocytopenia due to idiopathic maternal thrombocytopenia
> Neonatal thrombocytopenia due to isoimmunization

    P61.1   **Polycythemia neonatorum**   **N**
> *Neonate = newborn*

    P61.2   **Anemia of prematurity** 🦠   **N**

    P61.3   **Congenital anemia from fetal blood loss** 🦠   **N**

    P61.4   **Other congenital anemias, not elsewhere classified** 🦠   **N**
> Congenital anemia NOS

    P61.5   **Transient neonatal neutropenia** 🦠🦠   **N**
> *Low levels of granulocytic neutrophilic white blood cells*
> > **Excludes1**   congenital neutropenia (nontransient) (D70.0)

    P61.6   **Other transient neonatal disorders of coagulation** 🦠   **N**

    P61.8   **Other specified perinatal hematological disorders**   **N**

    ◼ **P61.9**   **Perinatal hematological disorder, unspecified**   **N**

TRANSITORY ENDOCRINE AND METABOLIC DISORDERS SPECIFIC TO NEWBORN (P70-P74)

> **Includes**   transitory endocrine and metabolic disturbances caused by the infant's response to maternal endocrine and metabolic factors, or its adjustment to extrauterine environment

● **P70**   **Transitory disorders of carbohydrate metabolism specific to newborn**

    P70.0   **Syndrome of infant of mother with gestational diabetes**   **N**
> Newborn (with hypoglycemia) affected by maternal gestational diabetes
> > **Excludes1**   newborn (with hypoglycemia) affected by maternal (pre-existing) diabetes mellitus (P70.1)
> > syndrome of infant of a diabetic mother (P70.1)

    P70.1   **Syndrome of infant of a diabetic mother**   **N**
> Newborn (with hypoglycemia) affected by maternal (pre-existing) diabetes mellitus
> > **Excludes1**   newborn (with hypoglycemia) affected by maternal gestational diabetes (P70.0)
> > syndrome of infant of mother with gestational diabetes (P70.0)

    P70.2   **Neonatal diabetes mellitus** 🦠   **N**

    P70.3   **Iatrogenic neonatal hypoglycemia**   **N**

    P70.4   **Other neonatal hypoglycemia**   **N**
> Transitory neonatal hypoglycemia

    P70.8   **Other transitory disorders of carbohydrate metabolism of newborn** 🦠   **N**

    ◼ **P70.9**   **Transitory disorder of carbohydrate metabolism of newborn, unspecified**   **N**

● **P71**   **Transitory neonatal disorders of calcium and magnesium metabolism**

    P71.0   **Cow's milk hypocalcemia in newborn** 🦠   **N**

    P71.1   **Other neonatal hypocalcemia** 🦠   **N**
> > **Excludes1**   neonatal hypoparathyroidism (P71.4)

    P71.2   **Neonatal hypomagnesemia** 🦠   **N**

    P71.3   **Neonatal tetany without calcium or magnesium deficiency** 🦠   **N**
> Neonatal tetany NOS

    P71.4   **Transitory neonatal hypoparathyroidism** 🦠   **N**

    P71.8   **Other transitory neonatal disorders of calcium and magnesium metabolism** 🦠   **N**

    ◼ **P71.9**   **Transitory neonatal disorder of calcium and magnesium metabolism, unspecified** 🦠   **N**

● **P72**   **Other transitory neonatal endocrine disorders**

> **Excludes1**   congenital hypothyroidism with or without goiter (E03.0-E03.1)
> dyshormogenetic goiter (E07.1)
> Pendred's syndrome (E07.1)

    P72.0   **Neonatal goiter, not elsewhere classified** 🦠   **N**
> Transitory congenital goiter with normal functioning

    P72.1   **Transitory neonatal hyperthyroidism** 🦠   **N**
> Neonatal thyrotoxicosis

    P72.2   **Other transitory neonatal disorders of thyroid function, not elsewhere classified** 🦠   **N**
> Transitory neonatal hypothyroidism

    P72.8   **Other specified transitory neonatal endocrine disorders** 🦠   **N**

    ◼ **P72.9**   **Transitory neonatal endocrine disorder, unspecified**   **N**

● **P74**   **Other transitory neonatal electrolyte and metabolic disturbances**

    P74.0   **Late metabolic acidosis of newborn** 🦠   **N**
> > **Excludes1**   (fetal) metabolic acidosis of newborn (P19)

    P74.1   **Dehydration of newborn**   **N**

    P74.2   **Disturbances of sodium balance of newborn**   **N**

    P74.3   **Disturbances of potassium balance of newborn**   **N**

    P74.4   **Other transitory electrolyte disturbances of newborn**   **N**

    P74.5   **Transitory tyrosinemia of newborn** 🦠   **N**

    P74.6   **Transitory hyperammonemia of newborn** 🦠   **N**

    P74.8   **Other transitory metabolic disturbances of newborn** 🦠   **N**
> Amino-acid metabolic disorders described as transitory

    ◼ **P74.9**   **Transitory metabolic disturbance of newborn, unspecified**   **N**

DIGESTIVE SYSTEM DISORDERS OF NEWBORN (P76-P78)

● **P76**   **Other intestinal obstruction of newborn**

    P76.0   **Meconium plug syndrome**   **N**
> *Intestinal obstruction; most often seen in premature infants*
> Meconium ileus NOS
> > **Excludes1**   meconium ileus in cystic fibrosis (E84.11)

    P76.1   **Transitory ileus of newborn** 🦠   **N**
> *Temporary obstruction of ileus (small intestine)*
> > **Excludes1**   Hirschsprung's disease (Q43.1)

N Newborn Age: 0   **P** Pediatric Age: 0–17   **M** Maternity DX: 12–55   **A** Adult Age: 15–124   ♀ Females Only   ♂ Males Only

🦠 Complication\Comorbidity   🦠 Major C\C   🦠 Present on Admission Requirement   🦠 Hospital-Acquired Condition

1339

P76.2 Intestinal obstruction due to inspissated milk   N
Being thickened, dried, or made less fluid

P76.8 Other specified intestinal obstruction of newborn   N
> Excludes1   intestinal obstruction classifiable to K56.-

P76.9 Intestinal obstruction of newborn, unspecified   N

P77 Necrotizing enterocolitis of newborn

P77.1 Stage 1 necrotizing enterocolitis in newborn   N
Necrotizing enterocolitis without pneumatosis, without perforation

P77.2 Stage 2 necrotizing enterocolitis in newborn   N
Necrotizing enterocolitis with pneumatosis, without perforation

P77.3 Stage 3 necrotizing enterocolitis in newborn   N
Necrotizing enterocolitis with perforation
Necrotizing enterocolitis with pneumatosis and perforation

P77.9 Necrotizing enterocolitis in newborn, unspecified   N
Necrotizing enterocolitis in newborn, NOS

P78 Other perinatal digestive system disorders
> Excludes1   cystic fibrosis (E84.0-E84.9)
> neonatal gastrointestinal hemorrhages (P54.0-P54.3)

P78.0 Perinatal intestinal perforation   N
Meconium peritonitis

P78.1 Other neonatal peritonitis   N
Neonatal peritonitis NOS

P78.2 Neonatal hematemesis and melena due to swallowed maternal blood   N

P78.3 Noninfective neonatal diarrhea   N
Neonatal diarrhea NOS

P78.8 Other specified perinatal digestive system disorders

  P78.81 Congenital cirrhosis (of liver)   N

  P78.82 Peptic ulcer of newborn   N

  P78.83 Newborn esophageal reflux   N
Neonatal esophageal reflux

  P78.89 Other specified perinatal digestive system disorders   N

P78.9 Perinatal digestive system disorder, unspecified   N

CONDITIONS INVOLVING THE INTEGUMENT AND TEMPERATURE REGULATION OF NEWBORN (P80-P83)

P80 Hypothermia of newborn

P80.0 Cold injury syndrome   N
Severe and usually chronic hypothermia associated with a pink flushed appearance, edema and neurological and biochemical abnormalities.
> Excludes1   mild hypothermia of newborn (P80.8)

P80.8 Other hypothermia of newborn   N
Mild hypothermia of newborn

P80.9 Hypothermia of newborn, unspecified   N

P81 Other disturbances of temperature regulation of newborn

P81.0 Environmental hyperthermia of newborn   N

P81.8 Other specified disturbances of temperature regulation of newborn   N

P81.9 Disturbance of temperature regulation of newborn, unspecified   N
Fever of newborn NOS

P83 Other conditions of integument specific to newborn
> Excludes1   congenital malformations of skin and integument (Q80-Q84)
> hydrops fetalis due to hemolytic disease (P56.-)
> neonatal skin infection (P39.4)
> staphylococcal scalded skin syndrome (L00)
> Excludes2   cradle cap (L21.0)
> diaper [napkin] dermatitis (L22)

P83.0 Sclerema neonatorum   N
Neonate = newborn

P83.1 Neonatal erythema toxicum   N
Benign, generalized, transient pustules that become firm vesicles

P83.2 Hydrops fetalis not due to hemolytic disease   N
Severe, life-threatening problem of severe edema (swelling) as result of too much fluid leaving blood and entering tissue
Hydrops fetalis NOS

P83.3 Other and unspecified edema specific to newborn

  P83.30 Unspecified edema specific to newborn   N

  P83.39 Other edema specific to newborn   N

P83.4 Breast engorgement of newborn   N
Noninfective mastitis of newborn

P83.5 Congenital hydrocele   N

P83.6 Umbilical polyp of newborn   N

P83.8 Other specified conditions of integument specific to newborn   N
Bronze baby syndrome
Neonatal scleroderma
Urticaria neonatorum

P83.9 Condition of the integument specific to newborn, unspecified   N

OTHER PROBLEMS WITH NEWBORN (P84)

P84 Other problems with newborn   N
Acidemia of newborn
Acidosis of newborn
Anoxia of newborn NOS
Asphyxia of newborn NOS
Hypercapnia of newborn
Hypoxemia of newborn
Hypoxia of newborn NOS
Mixed metabolic and respiratory acidosis of newborn
> Excludes1   intracranial hemorrhage due to anoxia or hypoxia (P52.-)
> hypoxic ischemic encephalopathy [HIE] (P91.6-)
> late metabolic acidosis of newborn (P74.0)

OTHER DISORDERS ORIGINATING IN THE PERINATAL PERIOD (P90-P96)

P90 Convulsions of newborn   N
> Excludes1   benign myoclonic epilepsy in infancy (G40.3-)
> benign neonatal convulsions (familial) (G40.3-)

P91 Other disturbances of cerebral status of newborn

P91.0 Neonatal cerebral ischemia   N

P91.1 Acquired periventricular cysts of newborn   N

P91.2 Neonatal cerebral leukomalacia   N
Degeneration of white matter adjacent to cerebral ventricles following cerebral hypoxia or brain ischemia in neonates
Periventricular leukomalacia

P91.3 Neonatal cerebral irritability   N

● Unacceptable Principal Diagnosis   ● Use Additional Character(s)   ■ Unspecified   ▶ Manifestation Code
OGCR Official Guidelines for Coding and Reporting   Excludes 1   Excludes 2   Includes   Use additional   Code first   Code also

P91.4 Neonatal cerebral depression 🔖   N

P91.5 Neonatal coma 🔖   N

● **P91.6 Hypoxic ischemic encephalopathy [HIE]**

   ■ **P91.60 Hypoxic ischemic encephalopathy [HIE], unspecified** 🔖   N

   P91.61 Mild hypoxic ischemic encephalopathy [HIE] 🔖   N

   P91.62 Moderate hypoxic ischemic encephalopathy [HIE] 🔖   N

   P91.63 Severe hypoxic ischemic encephalopathy [HIE] 🔖   N

P91.8 Other specified disturbances of cerebral status of newborn   N

■ **P91.9 Disturbance of cerebral status of newborn, unspecified**   N

● **P92 Feeding problems of newborn**

   Excludes1   feeding problems in child over 28 days old (R63.3)

   ● **P92.0 Vomiting of newborn**

     Excludes1   vomiting of child over 28 days old (R11.-)

     P92.01 Bilious vomiting of newborn 🔖   N

       Excludes1   bilious vomiting in child over 28 days old (R11.4)

     P92.09 Other vomiting of newborn   N

       Excludes1   regurgitation of food in newborn (P92.1)

   P92.1 Regurgitation and rumination of newborn   N

   P92.2 Slow feeding of newborn   N

   P92.3 Underfeeding of newborn   N

   P92.4 Overfeeding of newborn   N

   P92.5 Neonatal difficulty in feeding at breast   N

   P92.6 Failure to thrive in newborn   N

     Excludes1   failure to thrive in child over 28 days old (R62.51)

   P92.8 Other feeding problems of newborn   N

   ■ **P92.9 Feeding problem of newborn, unspecified**   N

● **P93 Reactions and intoxications due to drugs administered to newborn**

   Includes   reactions and intoxications due to drugs administered to fetus affecting newborn

   Excludes1   jaundice due to drugs or toxins transmitted from mother or given to newborn (P58.4-)

     reactions and intoxications from maternal opiates, tranquilizers and other medication (P04.0-P04.1, P04.4)

     withdrawal symptoms from maternal use of drugs of addiction (P96.1)

     withdrawal symptoms from therapeutic use of drugs in newborn (P96.2)

   P93.0 Grey baby syndrome 🔖   N

     Grey syndrome from chloramphenicol administration in newborn

   P93.8 Other reactions and intoxications due to drugs administered to newborn 🔖   N

     Use additional code for adverse effect, if applicable, to identify drug (T36-T50 with fifth or sixth character 5)

● **P94 Disorders of muscle tone of newborn**

   P94.0 Transient neonatal myasthenia gravis 🔖   N

     Excludes1   myasthenia gravis (G70.0)

P94.1 Congenital hypertonia   N

P94.2 Congenital hypotonia   N

   Floppy baby syndrome, unspecified

P94.8 Other disorders of muscle tone of newborn   N

■ **P94.9 Disorder of muscle tone of newborn, unspecified**   N

P95 Stillbirth   N

   Deadborn fetus NOS

   Fetal death of unspecified cause

   Stillbirth NOS

   Excludes1   maternal care for intrauterine death (O36.4)

     missed abortion (O02.1)

     outcome of delivery, stillbirth (Z37.1, Z37.3, Z37.4, Z37.7)

   OGCR Section I.C.16.g.

   Stillbirth

   Code P95, Stillbirth, is only for use for institutions that maintain separate records for stillbirths. No other code should be used with P95. Code P95 should not be used on the mother's record.

● **P96 Other conditions originating in the perinatal period**

   P96.0 Congenital renal failure   N

     Uremia of newborn

   P96.1 Neonatal withdrawal symptoms from maternal use of drugs of addiction 🔖   N

     Drug withdrawal syndrome in infant of dependent mother

     Neonatal abstinence syndrome

     Excludes1   reactions and intoxications from maternal opiates and tranquilizers administered during labor and delivery (P04.0)

   P96.2 Withdrawal symptoms from therapeutic use of drugs in newborn 🔖   N

   P96.3 Wide cranial sutures of newborn   N

     Neonatal craniotabes

   P96.5 Complication to newborn due to (fetal) intrauterine procedure   N

     Excludes2   newborn (suspected to be) affected by amniocentesis (P00.6)

   ● **P96.8 Other specified conditions originating in the perinatal period**

     P96.81 Exposure to (parental) (environmental) tobacco smoke in the perinatal period

       Excludes2   newborn affected by in utero exposure to tobacco (P04.2)

       exposure to environmental tobacco smoke after the perinatal period (Z77.22)

     P96.82 Delayed separation of umbilical cord   N

     P96.83 Meconium staining   N

       Excludes1   meconium aspiration (P24.00, P24.01)

       meconium passage during delivery (P03.82)

     P96.89 Other specified conditions originating in the perinatal period   N

       Use additional code to specify condition

   ■ **P96.9 Condition originating in the perinatal period, unspecified**   N

     Congenital debility NOS

N   Newborn Age: 0   P   Pediatric Age: 0–17   M   Maternity DX: 12–55   A   Adult Age: 15–124   ♀ Females Only   ♂ Males Only

🔖 Complication\Comorbidity   🔖 Major C\C   🔖 Present on Admission Requirement   🔖 Hospital-Acquired Condition

OGCR See Section III, Chapter 17

CHAPTER 17

CONGENITAL MALFORMATIONS, DEFORMATIONS AND CHROMOSOMAL ABNORMALITIES (Q00-Q99)

Note: Codes from this chapter are not for use on maternal or fetal records

Excludes1 inborn errors of metabolism (E70-E88)

This chapter contains the following blocks:

Q00-Q07	Congenital malformations of the nervous system
Q10-Q18	Congenital malformations of eye, ear, face and neck
Q20-Q28	Congenital malformations of the circulatory system
Q30-Q34	Congenital malformations of the respiratory system
Q35-Q37	Cleft lip and cleft palate
Q38-Q45	Other congenital malformations of the digestive system
Q50-Q56	Congenital malformations of genital organs
Q60-Q64	Congenital malformations of the urinary system
Q65-Q79	Congenital malformations and deformations of the musculoskeletal system
Q80-Q89	Other congenital malformations
Q90-Q99	Chromosomal abnormalities, not elsewhere classified

CONGENITAL MALFORMATIONS OF THE NERVOUS SYSTEM (Q00–Q07)

● **Q00 Anencephaly and similar malformations**

Q00.0 Anencephaly
Absence of skull with cerebral hemispheres missing or reduced to small masses attached to base of cranium
Acephaly
Acrania
Amyelencephaly
Hemianencephaly
Hemicephaly

Q00.1 Craniorachischisis
Developmental anomaly consisting of fissure of cranium and vertebral column

Q00.2 Iniencephaly
Developmental anomaly characterized by enlargement of foramen magnum and absence of laminae and spinous processes of cervical, dorsal

● **Q01 Encephalocele**
Sac-like protrusions of brain and membranes visible through an opening in skull

Includes Arnold-Chiari syndrome, type III
encephalocystocele
encephalomyelocele
hydroencephalocele
hydromeningocele, cranial
meningocele, cerebral
meningoencephalocele

Excludes1 Meckel-Gruber syndrome (Q61.9)

Q01.0 Frontal encephalocele

Q01.1 Nasofrontal encephalocele

Q01.2 Occipital encephalocele

Figure 17-1 An infant with a large occipital encephalocele. The large skin-covered encephalocele is visible. (From Townsend: Sabiston Textbook of Surgery, 17th ed. 2004, Sounders, An Imprint of Elsevier.)

Q01.8 Encephalocele of other sites

■ **Q01.9 Encephalocele, unspecified**

● **Q02 Microcephaly**
Head size measures significantly below normal based on standardized charts

Includes hydromicrocephaly
micrencephalon

Excludes1 Meckel-Gruber syndrome (Q61.9)

● **Q03 Congenital hydrocephalus**
Accumulation of cerebrospinal fluid in ventricles resulting in swelling and enlargement

Includes hydrocephalus in newborn

Excludes1 Arnold-Chiari syndrome, type II (Q07.0-)
acquired hydrocephalus (G91.-)
hydrocephalus due to congenital toxoplasmosis (P37.1)
hydrocephalus with spina bifida (Q05.0-Q05.4)

Q03.0 Malformations of aqueduct of Sylvius
Anomaly of aqueduct of Sylvius
Obstruction of aqueduct of Sylvius, congenital
Stenosis of aqueduct of Sylvius

Q03.1 Atresia of foramina of Magendie and Luschka
Dandy-Walker syndrome

Q03.8 Other congenital hydrocephalus

■ **Q03.9 Congenital hydrocephalus, unspecified**

● **Q04 Other congenital malformations of brain**
Excludes1 cyclopia (Q87.0)
macrocephaly (Q75.3)

Q04.0 Congenital malformations of corpus callosum
Agenesis of corpus callosum

Q04.1 Arhinencephaly
Congenital absence of olfactory bulbs, tract, or nerves

Q04.2 Holoprosencephaly
Failure of cleavage of forebrain (prosencephalon) resulting in incomplete or absent cortical separation and deficits in midline facial development

Q04.3 Other reduction deformities of brain
Absence of part of brain   Agyria
Agenesis of part of brain
Cerebral cortex are not fully formed, brain surface is smooth
Aplasia of part of brain
Hydranencephaly
Hypoplasia of part of brain
Lissencephaly
Congenital malformation or absence of convolutions of cerebral cortex
Microgyria
Malformation of brain characterized by excessive number of small convolutions (gyri) on surface
Pachygyria
Reduction in number of sulci of cerebrum

Excludes1 congenital malformations of corpus callosum (Q04.0)

● Unacceptable Principal Diagnosis   ● Use Additional Character(s)   ■ Unspecified   ▶ Manifestation Code
OGCR Official Guidelines for Coding and Reporting   Excludes 1   Excludes 2   Includes   Use additional   Code first   Code also

Q04.4 **Septo-optic dysplasia of brain** 🦠 🦠

Q04.5 **Megalencephaly** 🦠 🦠
    Abnormally large brain

Q04.6 **Congenital cerebral cysts** 🦠 🦠
    Porencephaly   Schizencephaly

    | Excludes1 | acquired porencephalic cyst (G93.0) |

Q04.8 **Other specified congenital malformations of brain** 🦠 🦠
    Arnold-Chiari syndrome, type IV
    Macrogyria

☐ Q04.9 **Congenital malformation of brain, unspecified** 🦠
    Congenital anomaly NOS of brain
    Congenital deformity NOS of brain
    Congenital disease or lesion NOS of brain
    Multiple anomalies NOS of brain, congenital

● Q05 **Spina bifida**
    Developmental anomaly characterized by defective closure of vertebral arch, through which spinal cord and meninges may protrude

    Includes hydromeningocele (spinal)
                 meningocele (spinal)
                 meningomyelocele
                 myelocele
                 myelomeningocele
                 rachischisis
                 spina bifida (aperta)(cystica)
                 syringomyelocele

    Use additional code for any associated paraplegia (paraparesis) (G82.2-)

    | Excludes1 | Arnold-Chiari syndrome, type II (Q07.0-) |
    | | spina bifida occulta (Q76.0) |

Q05.0 **Cervical spina bifida with hydrocephalus** 🦠 🦠

Q05.1 **Thoracic spina bifida with hydrocephalus** 🦠 🦠
    Dorsal spina bifida with hydrocephalus
    Thoracolumbar spina bifida with hydrocephalus

Q05.2 **Lumbar spina bifida with hydrocephalus** 🦠 🦠
    Lumbosacral spina bifida with hydrocephalus

Q05.3 **Sacral spina bifida with hydrocephalus** 🦠 🦠

☐ Q05.4 **Unspecified spina bifida with hydrocephalus** 🦠 🦠

Q05.5 **Cervical spina bifida without hydrocephalus**

Q05.6 **Thoracic spina bifida without hydrocephalus** 🦠
    Dorsal spina bifida NOS
    Thoracolumbar spina bifida NOS

Q05.7 **Lumbar spina bifida without hydrocephalus** 🦠
    Lumbosacral spina bifida NOS

Q05.8 **Sacral spina bifida without hydrocephalus** 🦠

☐ Q05.9 **Spina bifida, unspecified** 🦠 🦠

● Q06 **Other congenital malformations of spinal cord**

Q06.0 **Amyelia** 🦠
    Congenital absence of spinal cord

Q06.1 **Hypoplasia and dysplasia of spinal cord** 🦠
    Underdevelopment of spinal cord
    Atelomyelia
        Congenitally incomplete development of spinal cord
    Myelatelia
    Myelodysplasia of spinal cord
        Defective development of spinal cord, especially lower segments

Q06.2 **Diastematomyelia** 🦠
    Congenital anomaly, associated with spina bifida, in which spinal cord is split into halves and surrounded by dural sac

Q06.3 **Other congenital cauda equina malformations** 🦠

Q06.4 **Hydromyelia** 🦠
    Dilation of central canal of spinal cord with increased fluid accumulation
    Hydrorachis

Q06.8 **Other specified congenital malformations of spinal cord** 🦠

☐ Q06.9 **Congenital malformation of spinal cord, unspecified** 🦠
    Congenital anomaly NOS of spinal cord
    Congenital deformity NOS of spinal cord
    Congenital disease or lesion NOS of spinal cord

● Q07 **Other congenital malformations of nervous system**

    | Excludes2 | congenital central alveolar hypoventilation syndrome (G47.35) |
    | | familial dysautonomia [Riley-Day] (G90.1) |
    | | neurofibromatosis (nonmalignant) (Q85.0-) |

● Q07.0 **Arnold-Chiari syndrome**
    Herniation of cerebellar tonsils and vermis through foramen magnum into spinal canal
    Arnold-Chiari syndrome, type II

    | Excludes1 | Arnold-Chiari syndrome, type III (Q01.-) |
    | | Arnold-Chiari syndrome, type IV (Q04.8) |

    Q07.00 **Arnold-Chiari syndrome without spina bifida or hydrocephalus** 🦠

    Q07.01 **Arnold-Chiari syndrome with spina bifida** 🦠 🦠

    Q07.02 **Arnold-Chiari syndrome with hydrocephalus** 🦠 🦠

    Q07.03 **Arnold-Chiari syndrome with spina bifida and hydrocephalus** 🦠 🦠

Q07.8 **Other specified congenital malformations of nervous system** 🦠
    Agenesis of nerve
    Displacement of brachial plexus
    Jaw-winking syndrome
    Marcus Gunn's syndrome

☐ Q07.9 **Congenital malformation of nervous system, unspecified** 🦠
    Congenital anomaly NOS of nervous system
    Congenital deformity NOS of nervous system
    Congenital disease or lesion NOS of nervous system

CONGENITAL MALFORMATIONS OF EYE, EAR, FACE AND NECK (Q10-Q18)

    | Excludes2 | cleft lip and cleft palate (Q35-Q37) |
    | | congenital malformation of: |
    | | cervical spine (Q05.0, Q05.5, Q67.5, Q76.0-Q76.4) |
    | | larynx (Q31.-) |
    | | lip NEC (Q38.0) |
    | | nose (Q30.-) |
    | | parathyroid gland (Q89.2) |
    | | thyroid gland (Q89.2) |

● Q10 **Congenital malformations of eyelid, lacrimal apparatus and orbit**

    | Excludes1 | cryptophthalmos NOS (Q11.2) |
    | | cryptophthalmos syndrome (Q87.0) |

Q10.0 **Congenital ptosis** 🦠
    Prolapse or drooping of upper eyelid from paralysis of third nerve or from sympathetic innervations

Q10.1 **Congenital ectropion** 🦠
    Outward turning of eyelid

Q10.2 **Congenital entropion** 🦠
    Inward turning of eyelid

N Newborn Age: 0   **P** Pediatric Age: 0–17   **M** Maternity DX: 12–55   **A** Adult Age: 15–124   ♀ Females Only   ♂ Males Only

🦠 Complication\Comorbidity   🦠 Major C\C   🦠 Present on Admission Requirement   🦠 Hospital-Acquired Condition

1343

CHAPTER 17 (Q00-Q99)

Q10.3 **Other congenital malformations of eyelid**
Ablepharon
Blepharophimosis, congenital
Coloboma of eyelid
Congenital absence or agenesis of cilia
Congenital absence or agenesis of eyelid
Congenital accessory eyelid
Congenital accessory eye muscle
Congenital malformation of eyelid NOS

Q10.4 **Absence and agenesis of lacrimal apparatus**
Congenital absence of punctum lacrimale

Q10.5 **Congenital stenosis and stricture of lacrimal duct**

Q10.6 **Other congenital malformations of lacrimal apparatus**
Congenital malformation of lacrimal apparatus NOS

Q10.7 **Congenital malformation of orbit**

● **Q11** **Anophthalmos, microphthalmos and macrophthalmos**
Absence of eye and optic pit

Q11.0 **Cystic eyeball**

Q11.1 **Other anophthalmos**
Anophthalmos NOS
Agenesis of eye
Absence of eye
Aplasia of eye

Q11.2 **Microphthalmos**
Partial absence of eye and optic pit
Cryptophthalmos NOS
Dysplasia of eye
Hypoplasia of eye
Rudimentary eye
Excludes1 cryptophthalmos syndrome (Q87.0)

Q11.3 **Macrophthalmos**
Congenital enlargement of eyes
Excludes1 macrophthalmos in congenital glaucoma (Q15.0)

● **Q12** **Congenital lens malformations**

Q12.0 **Congenital cataract**

Q12.1 **Congenital displaced lens**

Q12.2 **Coloboma of lens**

Q12.3 **Congenital aphakia**

Q12.4 **Spherophakia**
Smaller, more spherical optic lens than normal

Q12.8 **Other congenital lens malformations**
Microphakia

■ **Q12.9** **Congenital lens malformation, unspecified**

Figure 17-2 Bilateral congenital **hydrophthalmia,** in which the eyes are very large in comparison to the other facial features due to glaucoma.

● **Q13** **Congenital malformations of anterior segment of eye**

Q13.0 **Coloboma of iris**
Coloboma NOS

Q13.1 **Absence of iris**
Aniridia
Use additional code for associated glaucoma (H42)

Q13.2 **Other congenital malformations of iris**
Anisocoria, congenital
Atresia of pupil
Congenital malformation of iris NOS
Corectopia

Q13.3 **Congenital corneal opacity**

Q13.4 **Other congenital corneal malformations**
Congenital malformation of cornea NOS
Microcornea
Peter's anomaly

Q13.5 **Blue sclera**
Condition of unusual blueness of sclera; not harmful

● **Q13.8** **Other congenital malformations of anterior segment of eye**

Q13.81 **Rieger's anomaly**
Use additional code for associated glaucoma (H42)

Q13.89 **Other congenital malformations of anterior segment of eye**

■ **Q13.9** **Congenital malformation of anterior segment of eye, unspecified**

● **Q14** **Congenital malformations of posterior segment of eye**
Excludes2 optic nerve hypoplasia (H47.03-)

Q14.0 **Congenital malformation of vitreous humor**
Congenital vitreous opacity

Q14.1 **Congenital malformation of retina**
Congenital retinal aneurysm

Q14.2 **Congenital malformation of optic disc**
Coloboma of optic disc

Q14.3 **Congenital malformation of choroid**

Q14.8 **Other congenital malformations of posterior segment of eye**
Coloboma of the fundus

■ **Q14.9** **Congenital malformation of posterior segment of eye, unspecified**

● **Q15** **Other congenital malformations of eye**
Excludes1 congenital nystagmus (H55.01)
ocular albinism (E70.31-)
optic nerve hypoplasia (H47.03-)
retinitis pigmentosa (H35.52)

Q15.0 **Congenital glaucoma**
Axenfeld's anomaly
Buphthalmos
Congenital syndrome characterized by port-wine nevus covering portions of face and cranium
Glaucoma of childhood
Glaucoma of newborn
Hydrophthalmos
Keratoglobus, congenital, with glaucoma
Macrocornea with glaucoma
Macrophthalmos in congenital glaucoma
Megalocornea with glaucoma

Q15.8 **Other specified congenital malformations of eye**

■ **Q15.9** **Congenital malformation of eye, unspecified**
Congenital anomaly of eye
Congenital deformity of eye

● Unacceptable Principal Diagnosis   ● Use Additional Character(s)   ■ Unspecified   ▶ Manifestation Code
OGCR Official Guidelines for Coding and Reporting   Excludes 1   Excludes 2   Includes   Use additional   Code first   Code also

● **Q16 Congenital malformations of ear causing impairment of hearing**

> **Excludes1**   congenital deafness (H90.-)

Q16.0 Congenital absence of (ear) auricle 🖾

Q16.1 Congenital absence, atresia and stricture of auditory canal (external) 🖾
>> Congenital atresia or stricture of osseous meatus

Q16.2 Absence of eustachian tube 🖾

Q16.3 Congenital malformation of ear ossicles 🖾
>> Congenital fusion of ear ossicles

Q16.4 Other congenital malformations of middle ear 🖾
>> Congenital malformation of middle ear NOS

Q16.5 Congenital malformation of inner ear 🖾
>> Congenital anomaly of membranous labyrinth
>> Congenital anomaly of organ of Corti

■ **Q16.9 Congenital malformation of ear causing impairment of hearing, unspecified** 🖾
>> Congenital absence of ear NOS

● **Q17 Other congenital malformations of ear**

> **Excludes1**   congenital malformations of ear with impairment of hearing (Q16.0-Q16.9)
> preauricular sinus (Q18.1)

Q17.0 Accessory auricle 🖾
>> Accessory tragus
>> Polyotia
>> Preauricular appendage or tag
>> Supernumerary ear
>> Supernumerary lobule

Q17.1 Macrotia 🖾
>> *Enlarged ears*

Q17.2 Microtia 🖾
>> *An abnormally small or underdeveloped external ear*

Q17.3 Other misshapen ear 🖾
>> Pointed ear

Q17.4 Misplaced ear 🖾
>> Low-set ears
>> **Excludes1**   cervical auricle (Q18.2)

Q17.5 Prominent ear 🖾
>> Bat ear

Q17.8 Other specified congenital malformations of ear 🖾
>> Congenital absence of lobe of ear

■ **Q17.9 Congenital malformation of ear, unspecified** 🖾
>> Congenital anomaly of ear NOS

● **Q18 Other congenital malformations of face and neck**

> **Excludes1**   cleft lip and cleft palate (Q35-Q37)
> conditions classified to Q67.0-Q67.4
> congenital malformations of skull and face bones (Q75.-)
> cyclopia (Q87.0)
> dentofacial anomalies [including malocclusion] (M26.-)
> malformation syndromes affecting facial appearance (Q87.0)
> persistent thyroglossal duct (Q89.2)

Q18.0 Sinus, fistula and cyst of branchial cleft 🖾
>> Branchial vestige
>> *Brachial remnants (cysts, fistula, skin tags) that are developmental anomalies*

Q18.1 Preauricular sinus and cyst 🖾
>> Fistula of auricle, congenital
>> Cervicoaural fistula
>> *Abnormal passage in neck originating from first branchial cleft*

Q18.2 Other branchial cleft malformations 🖾
>> Branchial cleft malformation NOS
>> Cervical auricle
>> Otocephaly

Q18.3 Webbing of neck 🖾
>> Pterygium colli
>> *Thick fold of skin on side of neck*

Q18.4 Macrostomia 🖾
>> *Results from failure of union of maxillary and mandibular processes, results in abnormally large mouth*

Q18.5 Microstomia 🖾

Q18.6 Macrocheilia 🖾
>> *Excessive size of lips*
>> Hypertrophy of lip, congenital

Q18.7 Microcheilia 🖾
>> *Abnormal smallness of lips*

Q18.8 Other specified congenital malformations of face and neck 🖾
>> Medial cyst of face and neck
>> Medial fistula of face and neck
>> Medial sinus of face and neck

■ **Q18.9 Congenital malformation of face and neck, unspecified** 🖾
>> Congenital anomaly NOS of face and neck

CONGENITAL MALFORMATIONS OF THE CIRCULATORY SYSTEM (Q20-Q28)

● **Q20 Congenital malformations of cardiac chambers and connections**

> **Excludes1**   dextrocardia with situs inversus (Q89.3)
> mirror-image atrial arrangement with situs inversus (Q89.3)

Q20.0 Common arterial trunk 🖾🖾
>> Persistent truncus arteriosus
>> **Excludes1**   aortic septal defect (Q21.4)

Q20.1 Double outlet right ventricle 🖾🖾
>> Taussig-Bing syndrome

Q20.2 Double outlet left ventricle 🖾🖾

Q20.3 Discordant ventriculoarterial connection 🖾🖾
>> Dextrotransposition of aorta
>> Transposition of great vessels (complete)

Q20.4 Double inlet ventricle 🖾🖾
>> Common ventricle
>> Cor triloculare biatriatum
>> Single ventricle

Q20.5 Discordant atrioventricular connection 🖾🖾
>> Corrected transposition
>> Levotransposition
>> Ventricular inversion

Q20.6 Isomerism of atrial appendages 🖾
>> Isomerism of atrial appendages with asplenia or polysplenia

Q20.8 Other congenital malformations of cardiac chambers and connections 🖾🖾
>> Cor binoculare

■ **Q20.9 Congenital malformation of cardiac chambers and connections, unspecified** 🖾

N Newborn Age: 0   **P** Pediatric Age: 0–17   **M** Maternity DX: 12–55   **A** Adult Age: 15–124   ♀ Females Only   ♂ Males Only

🖾 Complication\Comorbidity   🖾 Major C\C   🖾 Present on Admission Requirement   🖾 Hospital-Acquired Condition   **1345**

● **Q21 Congenital malformations of cardiac septa**
> **Excludes1** acquired cardiac septal defect (I51.0)

Q21.0 Ventricular septal defect 🦶🖐
> Roger's disease

Q21.1 Atrial septal defect 🦶🖐
> Coronary sinus defect
> Patent or persistent foramen ovale
> Patent or persistent ostium secundum defect (type II)
> Patent or persistent sinus venosus defect

Q21.2 Atrioventricular septal defect 🦶🖐
> Common atrioventricular canal
> Endocardial cushion defect
> Ostium primum atrial septal defect (type I)

Q21.3 Tetralogy of Fallot 🦶🖐
> Ventricular septal defect with pulmonary stenosis or atresia, dextroposition of aorta and hypertrophy of right ventricle.

Q21.4 Aortopulmonary septal defect 🖐
> Aortic septal defect
> Aortopulmonary window

Q21.8 Other congenital malformations of cardiac septa 🖐
> Eisenmenger's defect
> Pentalogy of Fallot
> > **Excludes1** Eisenmenger's complex (I27.8)
> > Eisenmenger's syndrome (I27.8)

▢ **Q21.9 Congenital malformation of cardiac septum, unspecified**
> Septal (heart) defect NOS

● **Q22 Congenital malformations of pulmonary and tricuspid valves**

Q22.0 Pulmonary valve atresia 🦶🖐

Q22.1 Congenital pulmonary valve stenosis 🦶🖐

Q22.2 Congenital pulmonary valve insufficiency 🦶🖐
> Congenital pulmonary valve regurgitation

Q22.3 Other congenital malformations of pulmonary valve 🦶🖐
> Congenital malformation of pulmonary valve NOS
> Supernumerary cusps of pulmonary valve

Q22.4 Congenital tricuspid stenosis 🦶🖐
> Congenital tricuspid atresia

Q22.5 Ebstein's anomaly 🦶🖐
> *Malformation of tricuspid valve*

Q22.6 Hypoplastic right heart syndrome 🦶🖐

Q22.8 Other congenital malformations of tricuspid valve 🦶🖐

▢ **Q22.9 Congenital malformation of tricuspid valve, unspecified** 🦶🖐

● **Q23 Congenital malformations of aortic and mitral valves**

Q23.0 Congenital stenosis of aortic valve 🦶🖐
> Congenital aortic atresia
> Congenital aortic stenosis NOS
> > **Excludes1** congenital stenosis of aortic valve in hypoplastic left heart syndrome (Q23.4)
> > congenital subaortic stenosis (Q24.4)
> > supravalvular aortic stenosis (congenital) (Q25.3)

Q23.1 Congenital insufficiency of aortic valve 🦶🖐
> Bicuspid aortic valve
> Congenital aortic insufficiency

Q23.2 Congenital mitral stenosis 🦶🖐
> Congenital mitral atresia

Q23.3 Congenital mitral insufficiency 🦶🖐

Q23.4 Hypoplastic left heart syndrome 🦶🖐

Q23.8 Other congenital malformations of aortic and mitral valves 🖐

▢ **Q23.9 Congenital malformation of aortic and mitral valves, unspecified** 🖐

● **Q24 Other congenital malformations of heart**
> **Excludes1** endocardial fibroelastosis (I42.4)

Q24.0 Dextrocardia 🦶🖐
> *Heart is located in right hemithorax*
> > **Excludes1** dextrocardia with situs inversus (Q89.3)
> > isomerism of atrial appendages (with asplenia or polysplenia) (Q20.6)
> > mirror-image atrial arrangement with situs inversus (Q89.3)

Q24.1 Levocardia 🦶🖐
> *Normal position of heart but related structures on wrong side*

Q24.2 Cor triatriatum 🦶🖐
> *Congenital heart defect; left atrium is subdivided*

Q24.3 Pulmonary infundibular stenosis 🦶🖐
> Subvalvular pulmonic stenosis

Q24.4 Congenital subaortic stenosis 🦶🖐

Q24.5 Malformation of coronary vessels 🦶🖐
> Congenital coronary (artery) aneurysm

Q24.6 Congenital heart block 🦶🖐

Q24.8 Other specified congenital malformations of heart 🖐
> Congenital diverticulum of left ventricle
> Congenital malformation of myocardium
> Congenital malformation of pericardium
> Malposition of heart
> Uhl's disease

▢ **Q24.9 Congenital malformation of heart, unspecified** 🖐
> Congenital anomaly of heart
> Congenital disease of heart

● **Q25 Congenital malformations of great arteries**

Q25.0 Patent ductus arteriosus 🦶🖐
> *Fetal blood vessel connecting left pulmonary artery directly to descending aorta*
> Patent ductus Botallo
> Persistent ductus arteriosus

Q25.1 Coarctation of aorta 🦶🖐
> Coarctation of aorta (preductal) (postductal)

Q25.2 Atresia of aorta 🦶🖐

Q25.3 Supravalvular aortic stenosis 🦶🖐
> > **Excludes1** congenital aortic stenosis NOS (Q23.0)
> > congenital stenosis of aortic valve (Q23.0)

Q25.4 Other congenital malformations of aorta 🦶🖐
> Absence of aorta
> Aneurysm of sinus of Valsalva (ruptured)
> Aplasia of aorta
> Congenital aneurysm of aorta
> Congenital malformations of aorta
> Congenital dilatation of aorta
> Double aortic arch [vascular ring of aorta]
> Hypoplasia of aorta
> Persistent convolutions of aortic arch
> Persistent right aortic arch
> > **Excludes1** hypoplasia of aorta in hypoplastic left heart syndrome (Q23.4)

Q25.5 Atresia of pulmonary artery 🦶🖐

Q25.6 Stenosis of pulmonary artery 🦶🖐
> Supravalvular pulmonary stenosis

CHAPTER 17 (Q00-Q99)

● **Q25.7** **Other congenital malformations of pulmonary artery**

     Q25.71 Coarctation of pulmonary artery 🅒 🄟

     Q25.72 Congenital pulmonary arteriovenous malformation 🅒 🄟
         Congenital pulmonary arteriovenous aneurysm

     Q25.79 Other congenital malformations of pulmonary artery 🅒 🄟
         Aberrant pulmonary artery
         Agenesis of pulmonary artery
         Congenital aneurysm of pulmonary artery
         Congenital anomaly of pulmonary artery
         Hypoplasia of pulmonary artery

   Q25.8 **Other congenital malformations of other great arteries** 🅒 🄟

◨ **Q25.9** **Congenital malformation of great arteries, unspecified** 🅒 🄟

● **Q26** **Congenital malformations of great veins**

   Q26.0 **Congenital stenosis of vena cava** 🅒 🄟
         Congenital stenosis of vena cava (inferior)(superior)

   Q26.1 **Persistent left superior vena cava** 🅒 🄟

   Q26.2 **Total anomalous pulmonary venous connection** 🅒 🄟
         Total anomalous pulmonary venous return [TAPVR], subdiaphragmatic
         Total anomalous pulmonary venous return [TAPVR], supradiaphragmatic

   Q26.3 **Partial anomalous pulmonary venous connection** 🅒 🄟
         Partial anomalous pulmonary venous return

◨ **Q26.4** **Anomalous pulmonary venous connection, unspecified** 🅒 🄟

   Q26.5 **Anomalous portal venous connection**

   Q26.6 **Portal vein-hepatic artery fistula**

   Q26.8 **Other congenital malformations of great veins** 🅒 🄟
         Absence of vena cava (inferior) (superior)
         Azygos continuation of inferior vena cava
         Persistent left posterior cardinal vein
         Scimitar syndrome

◨ **Q26.9** **Congenital malformation of great vein, unspecified** 🅒 🄟
         Congenital anomaly of vena cava (inferior) (superior) NOS

● **Q27** **Other congenital malformations of peripheral vascular system**

     | Excludes2 | anomalies of cerebral and precerebral vessels (Q28.0-Q28.3)
         anomalies of coronary vessels (Q24.5)
         anomalies of pulmonary artery (Q25.5-Q25.7)
         congenital retinal aneurysm (Q14.1)
         hemangioma and lymphangioma (D18.-)

   Q27.0 **Congenital absence and hypoplasia of umbilical artery** 🄟
         Single umbilical artery

   Q27.1 **Congenital renal artery stenosis** 🄟

   Q27.2 **Other congenital malformations of renal artery** 🄟
         Congenital malformation of renal artery NOS
         Multiple renal arteries

● **Q27.3** **Arteriovenous malformation (peripheral)**
         Arteriovenous aneurysm

     | Excludes1 | acquired arteriovenous aneurysm (I77.0)

     | Excludes2 | arteriovenous malformation of cerebral vessels (Q28.2)
         arteriovenous malformation of precerebral vessels (Q28.0)

   ◨ **Q27.30** Arteriovenous malformation, site unspecified 🅒 🄟

   Q27.31 Arteriovenous malformation of vessel of upper limb 🄟

   Q27.32 Arteriovenous malformation of vessel of lower limb 🄟

   Q27.33 Arteriovenous malformation of digestive system vessel 🄟

   Q27.34 Arteriovenous malformation of renal vessel 🄟

   Q27.39 Arteriovenous malformation, other site 🄟

   Q27.4 **Congenital phlebectasia** 🅒 🄟

   Q27.8 **Other specified congenital malformations of peripheral vascular system** 🄟
         Absence of peripheral vascular system
         Atresia of peripheral vascular system
         Congenital aneurysm (peripheral)
         Congenital stricture, artery
         Congenital varix

     | Excludes1 | arteriovenous malformation (Q27.3-)

◨ **Q27.9** **Congenital malformation of peripheral vascular system, unspecified** 🄟
         Anomaly of artery or vein NOS

● **Q28** **Other congenital malformations of circulatory system**

     | Excludes1 | congenital aneurysm NOS (Q27.8)
         congenital coronary aneurysm (Q24.5)
         ruptured cerebral arteriovenous malformation (I60.8)
         ruptured malformation of precerebral vessels (I72.0)

     | Excludes2 | congenital peripheral aneurysm (Q27.8)
         congenital pulmonary aneurysm (Q25.79)
         congenital retinal aneurysm (Q14.1)

   Q28.0 **Arteriovenous malformation of precerebral vessels** 🅒 🄟
         Congenital arteriovenous precerebral aneurysm (nonruptured)

   Q28.1 **Other malformations of precerebral vessels** 🅒 🄟
         Congenital malformation of precerebral vessels NOS
         Congenital precerebral aneurysm (nonruptured)

   Q28.2 **Arteriovenous malformation of cerebral vessels** 🅒 🄟
         Arteriovenous malformation of brain NOS
         Congenital arteriovenous cerebral aneurysm (nonruptured)

   Q28.3 **Other malformations of cerebral vessels** 🅒 🄟
         Congenital cerebral aneurysm (nonruptured)
         Congenital malformation of cerebral vessels NOS
         Developmental venous anomaly

   Q28.8 **Other specified congenital malformations of circulatory system** 🅒 🄟
         Congenital aneurysm, specified site NEC
         Spinal vessel anomaly

◨ **Q28.9** **Congenital malformation of circulatory system, unspecified** 🅒 🄟

N Newborn Age: 0   **P** Pediatric Age: 0–17   **M** Maternity DX: 12–55   **A** Adult Age: 15–124   ♀ Females Only   ♂ Males Only

🅒 Complication\Comorbidity   🄜 Major C\C   🄟 Present on Admission Requirement   🄗 Hospital-Acquired Condition

1347

CONGENITAL MALFORMATIONS OF THE RESPIRATORY SYSTEM (Q30-Q34)

● Q30   Congenital malformations of nose

> **Excludes1**   congenital deviation of nasal septum (Q67.4)

Q30.0   Choanal atresia
> Atresia of nares (anterior) (posterior)
> Congenital stenosis of nares (anterior) (posterior)

Q30.1   Agenesis and underdevelopment of nose
> Congenital absent of nose

Q30.2   Fissured, notched and cleft nose

Q30.3   Congenital perforated nasal septum

Q30.8   Other congenital malformations of nose
> Accessory nose
> Congenital anomaly of nasal sinus wall

■ Q30.9   Congenital malformation of nose, unspecified

● Q31   Congenital malformations of larynx

> **Excludes1**   congenital laryngeal stridor NOS (P28.89)

Q31.0   Web of larynx
> Glottic web of larynx
> Subglottic web of larynx
> Web of larynx NOS

Q31.1   Congenital subglottic stenosis

Q31.2   Laryngeal hypoplasia

Q31.3   Laryngocele

Q31.5   Congenital laryngomalacia

Q31.8   Other congenital malformations of larynx
> Absence of larynx
> Agenesis of larynx
> Atresia of larynx
> Congenital cleft thyroid cartilage
> Congenital fissure of epiglottis
> Congenital stenosis of larynx NEC
> Posterior cleft of cricoid cartilage

■ Q31.9   Congenital malformation of larynx, unspecified

● Q32   Congenital malformations of trachea and bronchus

> **Excludes1**   congenital bronchiectasis (Q33.4)

Q32.0   Congenital tracheomalacia

Q32.1   Other congenital malformations of trachea
> Atresia of trachea
> Congenital anomaly of tracheal cartilage
> Congenital dilatation of trachea
> Congenital malformation of trachea
> Congenital stenosis of trachea
> Congenital tracheocele

Q32.2   Congenital bronchomalacia

Q32.3   Congenital stenosis of bronchus

Q32.4   Other congenital malformations of bronchus
> Absence of bronchus
> Agenesis of bronchus
> Atresia of bronchus
> Congenital diverticulum of bronchus
> Congenital malformation of bronchus NOS

● Q33   Congenital malformations of lung

Q33.0   Congenital cystic lung
> Congenital cystic lung disease
> Congenital honeycomb lung
> Congenital polycystic lung disease

> **Excludes1**   cystic fibrosis (E84.0)
> cystic lung disease, acquired or unspecified (J98.4)

Q33.1   Accessory lobe of lung
> Azygos lobe (fissured), lung

Q33.2   Sequestration of lung

Q33.3   Agenesis of lung
> Congenital absence of lung (lobe)

Q33.4   Congenital bronchiectasis

Q33.5   Ectopic tissue in lung

Q33.6   Congenital hypoplasia and dysplasia of lung

> **Excludes1**   pulmonary hypoplasia associated with short gestation (P28.0)

Q33.8   Other congenital malformations of lung

■ Q33.9   Congenital malformation of lung, unspecified

● Q34   Other congenital malformations of respiratory system

> **Excludes2**   congenital central alveolar hypoventilation syndrome (G47.35)

Q34.0   Anomaly of pleura

Q34.1   Congenital cyst of mediastinum

Q34.8   Other specified congenital malformations of respiratory system
> Atresia of nasopharynx

■ Q34.9   Congenital malformation of respiratory system, unspecified
> Congenital absence of respiratory system
> Congenital anomaly of respiratory system NOS

CLEFT LIP AND CLEFT PALATE (Q35-Q37)

Use additional code to identify associated malformation of the nose (Q30.2)

> **Excludes1**   Robin's syndrome (Q87.0)

● Q35   Cleft palate

> **Includes**   fissure of palate
> palatoschisis

> **Excludes1**   cleft palate with cleft lip (Q37.-)

Q35.1   Cleft hard palate

Q35.3   Cleft soft palate

Q35.5   Cleft hard palate with cleft soft palate

Q35.7   Cleft uvula

■ Q35.9   Cleft palate, unspecified
> Cleft palate NOS

● Q36   Cleft lip

> **Includes**   cheiloschisis
> congenital fissure of lip
> harelip
> labium leporinum

> **Excludes1**   cleft lip with cleft palate (Q37.-)

Q36.0   Cleft lip, bilateral

Q36.1   Cleft lip, median

Q36.9   Cleft lip, unilateral
> Cleft lip NOS

CHAPTER 17 (Q00-Q99)

● Unacceptable Principal Diagnosis   ● Use Additional Character(s)   ■ Unspecified   ▶ Manifestation Code

OGCR Official Guidelines for Coding and Reporting   Excludes 1   Excludes 2   Includes   Use additional   Code first   Code also

Figure 17-3 Cleft palate.

● **Q37 Cleft palate with cleft lip**

> **Includes**   cheilopalatoschisis

Q37.0 Cleft hard palate with bilateral cleft lip 🖾

Q37.1 Cleft hard palate with unilateral cleft lip 🖾
> Cleft hard palate with cleft lip NOS

Q37.2 Cleft soft palate with bilateral cleft lip 🖾

Q37.3 Cleft soft palate with unilateral cleft lip 🖾
> Cleft soft palate with cleft lip NOS

Q37.4 Cleft hard and soft palate with bilateral cleft lip 🖾

Q37.5 Cleft hard and soft palate with unilateral cleft lip 🖾
> Cleft hard and soft palate with cleft lip NOS

■ **Q37.8 Unspecified cleft palate with bilateral cleft lip** 🖾

■ **Q37.9 Unspecified cleft palate with unilateral cleft lip** 🖾
> Cleft palate with cleft lip NOS

OTHER CONGENITAL MALFORMATIONS OF THE DIGESTIVE SYSTEM (Q38-Q45)

● **Q38 Other congenital malformations of tongue, mouth and pharynx**

> **Excludes1**   dentofacial anomalies (M26.-)
> macrostomia (Q18.4)
> microstomia (Q18.5)

Q38.0 Congenital malformations of lips, not elsewhere classified 🖾
> Congenital fistula of lip
> Congenital malformation of lip NOS
> Van der Woude's syndrome

> > **Excludes1**   cleft lip (Q36.-)
> > cleft lip with cleft palate (Q37.-)
> > macrocheilia (Q18.6)
> > microcheilia (Q18.7)

Q38.1 Ankyloglossia 🖾
> *Restricted movement of tongue resulting in speech difficulty*
> Tongue tie

Q38.2 Macroglossia 🖾
> *Excessive size of tongue*
> Congenital hypertrophy of tongue

Q38.3 Other congenital malformations of tongue 🖾
> Aglossia
> Bifid tongue
> Congenital adhesion of tongue
> Congenital fissure of tongue
> Congenital malformation of tongue NOS
> Double tongue
> Hypoglossia
> Hypoplasia of tongue
> Microglossia

Q38.4 Congenital malformations of salivary glands and ducts 🖾
> Atresia of salivary glands and ducts
> Congenital absence of salivary glands and ducts
> Congenital accessory salivary glands and ducts
> Congenital fistula of salivary gland

Q38.5 Congenital malformations of palate, not elsewhere classified 🖾
> Congenital absence of uvula
> Congenital malformation of palate NOS
> Congenital high arched palate

> > **Excludes1**   cleft palate (Q35.-)
> > cleft palate with cleft lip (Q37.-)

Q38.6 Other congenital malformations of mouth 🖾
> Congenital malformation of mouth NOS

Q38.7 Congenital pharyngeal pouch 🖾
> Congenital diverticulum of pharynx

> > **Excludes1**   pharyngeal pouch syndrome (D82.1)

Q38.8 Other congenital malformations of pharynx 🖾
> Congenital malformation of pharynx NOS
> Imperforate pharynx

● **Q39 Congenital malformations of esophagus**

Q39.0 Atresia of esophagus without fistula 🖾🖾
> Atresia of esophagus NOS

Q39.1 Atresia of esophagus with tracheo-esophageal fistula 🖾🖾
> Atresia of esophagus with broncho-esophageal fistula

Q39.2 Congenital tracheo-esophageal fistula without atresia 🖾🖾
> Congenital tracheo-esophageal fistula NOS

Q39.3 Congenital stenosis and stricture of esophagus 🖾🖾

Q39.4 Esophageal web 🖾🖾

Q39.5 Congenital dilatation of esophagus 🖾🖾
> Congenital cardiospasm

Q39.6 Congenital diverticulum of esophagus 🖾🖾
> Congenital esophageal pouch

Q39.8 Other congenital malformations of esophagus 🖾🖾
> Congenital absence of esophagus
> Congenital displacement of esophagus
> Congenital duplication of esophagus

■ **Q39.9 Congenital malformation of esophagus, unspecified** 🖾🖾

● **Q40 Other congenital malformations of upper alimentary tract**

Q40.0 Congenital hypertrophic pyloric stenosis 🖾
> Congenital or infantile constriction
> Congenital or infantile hypertrophy
> Congenital or infantile spasm
> Congenital or infantile stenosis
> Congenital or infantile stricture

Q40.1 Congenital hiatus hernia 🖾
> Congenital displacement of cardia through esophageal hiatus

> > **Excludes1**   congenital diaphragmatic hernia (Q79.0)

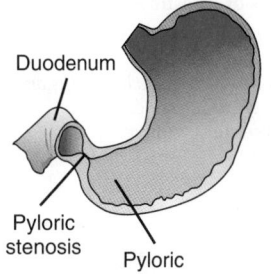

Figure 17-4 Pyloric stenosis.

Duodenum

Pyloric stenosis

Pyloric part of stomach

N Newborn Age: 0   **P** Pediatric Age: 0–17   **M** Maternity DX: 12–55   **A** Adult Age: 15–124   ♀ Females Only   ♂ Males Only

🖾 Complication\Comorbidity   🖾 Major C\C   🖾 Present on Admission Requirement   🖾 Hospital-Acquired Condition

Q40.2 Other specified congenital malformations of stomach
Congenital displacement of stomach
Congenital diverticulum of stomach
Congenital hourglass stomach
Congenital duplication of stomach
Megalogastria
Microgastria

Q40.3 Congenital malformation of stomach, unspecified

Q40.8 Other specified congenital malformations of upper alimentary tract

Q40.9 Congenital malformation of upper alimentary tract, unspecified
Congenital anomaly of upper alimentary tract
Congenital deformity of upper alimentary tract

● **Q41 Congenital absence, atresia and stenosis of small intestine**

Includes   congenital obstruction, occlusion or stricture of small intestine or intestine NOS

Excludes1   cystic fibrosis with intestinal manifestation (E84.11)
meconium ileus NOS (without cystic fibrosis) (P76.0)

Q41.0 Congenital absence, atresia and stenosis of duodenum

Q41.1 Congenital absence, atresia and stenosis of jejunum
Apple peel syndrome
Imperforate jejunum

Q41.2 Congenital absence, atresia and stenosis of ileum

Q41.8 Congenital absence, atresia and stenosis of other specified parts of small intestine

Q41.9 Congenital absence, atresia and stenosis of small intestine, part unspecified
Congenital absence, atresia and stenosis of intestine NOS

● **Q42 Congenital absence, atresia and stenosis of large intestine**

Includes   congenital obstruction, occlusion and stricture of large intestine

Q42.0 Congenital absence, atresia and stenosis of rectum with fistula

Q42.1 Congenital absence, atresia and stenosis of rectum without fistula
Imperforate rectum

Q42.2 Congenital absence, atresia and stenosis of anus with fistula

Q42.3 Congenital absence, atresia and stenosis of anus without fistula
Imperforate anus

Q42.8 Congenital absence, atresia and stenosis of other parts of large intestine

Q42.9 Congenital absence, atresia and stenosis of large intestine, part unspecified

● **Q43 Other congenital malformations of intestine**

Q43.0 Meckel's diverticulum (displaced) (hypertrophic)
Congenital abnormality in which a pouch remains on the lower end of the small intestine
Persistent omphalomesenteric duct
Persistent vitelline duct

Q43.1 Hirschsprung's disease
Developmental disorder of enteric nervous system characterized by absence of ganglion cells in distal colon resulting in functional obstruction.
Aganglionosis
Congenital (aganglionic) megacolon

Q43.2 Other congenital functional disorders of colon
Congenital dilatation of colon

Q43.3 Congenital malformations of intestinal fixation
Congenital omental, anomalous adhesions [bands]
Congenital peritoneal adhesions [bands]
Incomplete rotation of cecum and colon
Insufficient rotation of cecum and colon
Jackson's membrane
Malrotation of colon
Rotation failure of cecum and colon
Universal mesentery

Q43.4 Duplication of intestine

Q43.5 Ectopic anus
Anal opening in abnormal location

Q43.6 Congenital fistula of rectum and anus

Excludes1   congenital fistula of anus with absence, atresia and stenosis (Q42.2)
congenital fistula of rectum with absence, atresia and stenosis (Q42.0)
congenital rectovaginal fistula (Q52.2)
congenital urethrorectal fistula (Q64.7)
pilonidal fistula or sinus (L05.-)

Q43.7 Persistent cloaca
Malformation in which rectum, vagina, and urinary tract form one channel AKA congenital cloaca
Cloaca NOS

Q43.8 Other specified congenital malformations of intestine
Congenital blind loop syndrome
Congenital diverticulitis, colon
Congenital diverticulum, intestine
Dolichocolon
Megaloappendix
Megaloduodenum
Microcolon
Transposition of appendix
Transposition of colon
Transposition of intestine

Q43.9 Congenital malformation of intestine, unspecified

● **Q44 Congenital malformations of gallbladder, bile ducts and liver**

Q44.0 Agenesis, aplasia and hypoplasia of gallbladder
Congenital absence of gallbladder

Q44.1 Other congenital malformations of gallbladder
Congenital malformation of gallbladder NOS
Intrahepatic gallbladder

Q44.2 Atresia of bile ducts

Q44.3 Congenital stenosis and stricture of bile ducts

Q44.4 Choledochal cyst

Q44.5 Other congenital malformations of bile ducts
Accessory hepatic duct
Biliary duct duplication
Congenital malformation of bile duct NOS
Cystic duct duplication

Q44.6   **Cystic disease of liver** 🅲 🅟
Fibrocystic disease of liver

Q44.7   **Other congenital malformations of liver** 🅲 🅟
Accessory liver
Alagille's syndrome
Congenital absence of liver
Congenital hepatomegaly
Congenital malformation of liver NOS

● **Q45**   **Other congenital malformations of digestive system**

> **Excludes2**   congenital diaphragmatic hernia (Q79.0)
> congenital hiatus hernia (Q40.1)

Q45.0   **Agenesis, aplasia and hypoplasia of pancreas** 🅲 🅟
Congenital absence of pancreas

Q45.1   **Annular pancreas** 🅲 🅟

Q45.2   **Congenital pancreatic cyst** 🅲 🅟

Q45.3   **Other congenital malformations of pancreas and pancreatic duct** 🅲 🅟
Accessory pancreas
Congenital malformation of pancreas or pancreatic duct NOS

> **Excludes1**   congenital diabetes mellitus (E10.-)
> cystic fibrosis (E84.0-E84.9)
> fibrocystic disease of pancreas (E84.-)
> neonatal diabetes mellitus (P70.2)

Q45.8   **Other specified congenital malformations of digestive system** 🅟
Absence (complete) (partial) of alimentary tract NOS
Duplication of digestive system
Malposition, congenital of digestive system

▪ Q45.9   **Congenital malformation of digestive system, unspecified** 🅟
Congenital anomaly of digestive system
Congenital deformity of digestive system

CONGENITAL MALFORMATIONS OF GENITAL ORGANS (Q50-Q56)

> **Excludes1**   androgen insensitivity syndrome (E34.5-)
> syndromes associated with anomalies in the number and form of chromosomes (Q90-Q99)

● **Q50**   **Congenital malformations of ovaries, fallopian tubes and broad ligaments**

● Q50.0   **Congenital absence of ovary**

> **Excludes1**   Turner's syndrome (Q96.-)

Q50.01   **Congenital absence of ovary, unilateral** ♀ 🅟

Q50.02   **Congenital absence of ovary, bilateral** ♀ 🅟

Q50.1   **Developmental ovarian cyst** ♀ 🅟

Q50.2   **Congenital torsion of ovary** ♀ 🅟

● Q50.3   **Other congenital malformations of ovary**

Q50.31   **Accessory ovary** ♀ 🅟

Q50.32   **Ovarian streak** ♀ 🅟
Inadequate ovaries with absent follicular and hormonal function
46, XX with streak gonads

Q50.39   **Other congenital malformation of ovary** ♀ 🅟
Congenital malformation of ovary NOS

Q50.4   **Embryonic cyst of fallopian tube** ♀ 🅟
Fimbrial cyst

Q50.5   **Embryonic cyst of broad ligament** ♀ 🅟
Epoophoron cyst
Parovarian cyst

Q50.6   **Other congenital malformations of fallopian tube and broad ligament** ♀ 🅟
Absence of fallopian tube and broad ligament
Accessory fallopian tube and broad ligament
Atresia of fallopian tube and broad ligament
Congenital malformation of fallopian tube or broad ligament NOS

● **Q51**   **Congenital malformations of uterus and cervix**

Q51.0   **Agenesis and aplasia of uterus** ♀ 🅟
Congenital absence of uterus

● Q51.1   **Doubling of uterus with doubling of cervix and vagina**

Q51.10   **Doubling of uterus with doubling of cervix and vagina without obstruction** ♀ 🅟
Doubling of uterus with doubling of cervix and vagina NOS

Q51.11   **Doubling of uterus with doubling of cervix and vagina with obstruction** ♀ 🅟

Q51.2   **Other doubling of uterus** ♀ 🅟
Doubling of uterus NOS
Septate uterus, complete or partial

Q51.3   **Bicornate uterus** ♀ 🅟
Bicornate uterus, complete or partial
Birth defect in which uterus has two separate 'horns' that form top of uterus

Q51.4   **Unicornate uterus** ♀ 🅟
Unicornate uterus with or without a separate uterine horn
Uterus with only one functioning horn
Uterus with half being undeveloped

Q51.5   **Agenesis and aplasia of cervix** ♀ 🅟
Congenital absence of cervix

Q51.6   **Embryonic cyst of cervix** ♀ 🅟

Q51.7   **Congenital fistulae between uterus and digestive and urinary tracts** ♀ 🅟

● Q51.8   **Other congenital malformations of uterus and cervix**

● Q51.81   **Other congenital malformations of uterus**

Q51.810   **Arcuate uterus** ♀ 🅟
Arcuatus uterus

Q51.811   **Hypoplasia of uterus** ♀ 🅟

Q51.818   **Other congenital malformations of uterus** ♀ 🅟
Müllerian anomaly of uterus NEC

● Q51.82   **Other congenital malformations of cervix**

Q51.820   **Cervical duplication** ♀ 🅟

Q51.821   **Hypoplasia of cervix** ♀ 🅟

Q51.828   **Other congenital malformations of cervix** ♀ 🅟

▪ Q51.9   **Congenital malformation of uterus and cervix, unspecified** ♀ 🅟

● **Q52**   **Other congenital malformations of female genitalia**

Q52.0   **Congenital absence of vagina** ♀ 🅟
Vaginal agenesis, total or partial

● Q52.1   **Doubling of vagina**

> **Excludes1**   doubling of vagina with doubling of uterus and cervix (Q51.1-)

▪ Q52.10   **Doubling of vagina, unspecified** ♀ 🅟
Septate vagina NOS

Q52.11   **Transverse vaginal septum** ♀ 🅟

Q52.12   **Longitudinal vaginal septum** ♀ 🅟
Longitudinal vaginal septum with or without obstruction

N Newborn Age: 0   **P** Pediatric Age: 0–17   **M** Maternity DX: 12–55   **A** Adult Age: 15–124   ♀ Females Only   ♂ Males Only

 Complication\Comorbidity   🅜 Major C\C   Present on Admission Requirement   🅗 Hospital-Acquired Condition

1351

CHAPTER 17 (Q00-Q99)

Item 17-1 Testes form in the abdomen of the male and only descend into the scrotum during normal embryonic development. "Ectopic" testes are out of their normal place or "retained" (left behind) in the abdomen. Crypto (hidden) orchism (testicle) is a major risk factor for testicular cancer.

ECTOPIC TESTES	CRYPTORCHID TESTES
Penile	Abdominal
Superficial inguinal	Inguinal
(most common)	Prepubic
Femoral	(most common)

Figure 17-5 Undescended testes and the positions of the testes in various types of cryptorchidism or abnormal paths of descent.

Q52.2 **Congenital rectovaginal fistula** ♀ 🖐
    Excludes1   cloaca (Q43.7)

Q52.3 **Imperforate hymen** ♀ 🖐
    Membrane (hymen) completely closes vaginal orifice

Q52.4 **Other congenital malformations of vagina** ♀ 🖐
    Canal of Nuck cyst, congenital
    Congenital malformation of vagina NOS
    Embryonic vaginal cyst
    Gartner's duct cyst

Q52.5 **Fusion of labia** ♀ 🖐

Q52.6 **Congenital malformation of clitoris** ♀ 🖐

● Q52.7 **Other and unspecified congenital malformations of vulva**
    ◾ Q52.70 **Unspecified congenital malformations of vulva** ♀ 🖐
        Congenital malformation of vulva NOS
    Q52.71 **Congenital absence of vulva** ♀ 🖐
    Q52.79 **Other congenital malformations of vulva** ♀ 🖐
        Congenital cyst of vulva

Q52.8 **Other specified congenital malformations of female genitalia** ♀ 🖐

◾ Q52.9 **Congenital malformation of female genitalia, unspecified** ♀ 🖐

● Q53 **Undescended and ectopic testicle**
   ● Q53.0 **Ectopic testis**
     ◾ Q53.00 **Ectopic testis, unspecified** ♂ 🖐
     Q53.01 **Ectopic testis, unilateral** ♂ 🖐
     Q53.02 **Ectopic testes, bilateral** ♂ 🖐
   ● Q53.1 **Undescended testicle, unilateral**
     ◾ Q53.10 **Unspecified undescended testicle, unilateral** ♂ 🖐
     Q53.11 **Abdominal testis, unilateral** ♂ 🖐
     Q53.12 **Ectopic perineal testis, unilateral** ♂ 🖐

● Q53.2 **Undescended testicle, bilateral**
   ◾ Q53.20 **Undescended testicle, unspecified, bilateral** ♂ 🖐
   Q53.21 **Abdominal testis, bilateral** ♂ 🖐
   Q53.22 **Ectopic perineal testis, bilateral** ♂ 🖐

◾ Q53.9 **Undescended testicle, unspecified** ♂ 🖐
   Cryptorchism NOS

● Q54 **Hypospadias**
   Birth defect of male; urethra opens in abnormal location on shaft
    Excludes1   epispadias (Q64.0)

Q54.0 **Hypospadias, balanic** ♂ 🖐
    Hypospadias, coronal
    Hypospadias, glandular

Q54.1 **Hypospadias, penile** ♂ 🖐

Q54.2 **Hypospadias, penoscrotal** ♂ 🖐

Q54.3 **Hypospadias, perineal** ♂ 🖐

Q54.4 **Congenital chordee** ♂ 🖐
    Chordee without hypospadias

Q54.8 **Other hypospadias** ♂ 🖐
    Hypospadias with intersex state

◾ Q54.9 **Hypospadias, unspecified** ♂ 🖐

● Q55 **Other congenital malformations of male genital organs**
    Excludes1   congenital hydrocele (P83.5)
              hypospadias (Q54.-)

Q55.0 **Absence and aplasia of testis** ♂
    Monorchism

Q55.1 **Hypoplasia of testis and scrotum** ♂
    Fusion of testes

● Q55.2 **Other and unspecified congenital malformations of testis and scrotum**
   ◾ Q55.20 **Unspecified congenital malformations of testis and scrotum** ♂
        Congenital malformation of testis or scrotum NOS
   Q55.21 **Polyorchism** ♂
        Developmental anomaly characterized by presence of more than two testes
   Q55.22 **Retractile testis** ♂ 🖐
   Q55.23 **Scrotal transposition** ♂ 🖐
   Q55.29 **Other congenital malformations of testis and scrotum** ♂

Q55.3 **Atresia of vas deferens** ♂
    Code first any associated cystic fibrosis (E84.-)

Q55.4 **Other congenital malformations of vas deferens, epididymis, seminal vesicles and prostate** ♂
    Absence or aplasia of prostate
    Absence or aplasia of spermatic cord
    Congenital malformation of vas deferens, epididymis, seminal vesicles or prostate NOS

Q55.5 **Congenital absence and aplasia of penis** ♂ 🖐

● Q55.6 **Other congenital malformations of penis**
   Q55.61 **Curvature of penis (lateral)** ♂ 🖐
   Q55.62 **Hypoplasia of penis** ♂ 🖐
        Underdevelopment penis
        Micropenis
   Q55.63 **Congenital torsion of penis** ♂ 🖐
      Excludes1   acquired torsion of penis (N48.82)

● Unacceptable Principal Diagnosis   ● Use Additional Character(s)   ◾ Unspecified   ▶ Manifestation Code

1352   **OGCR**   Official Guidelines for Coding and Reporting   Excludes 1   Excludes 2   Includes   Use additional   Code first   Code also

CHAPTER 17 (Q00-Q99)

Q55.64 **Hidden penis** ♂ 🔍
  Buried penis
  Concealed penis
  Excludes1 acquired buried penis
                (N48.83)

Q55.69 **Other congenital malformation of penis** ♂ 🔍
  Congenital malformation of penis NOS

Q55.7 **Congenital vasocutaneous fistula** ♂
  Abnormal opening between vas deferens and skin

Q55.8 **Other specified congenital malformations of male genital organs** ♂

Q55.9 **Congenital malformation of male genital organ, unspecified** ♂
  Congenital anomaly of male genital organ
  Congenital deformity of male genital organ

● Q56 **Indeterminate sex and pseudohermaphroditism**
  Internal reproductive organs are opposite external physical characteristics.
  Excludes1 46,XX true hermaphrodite (Q99.1)
                androgen insensitivity syndrome (E34.5-)
                chimera 46,XX/46,XY true hermaphrodite
                (Q99.0)
                female pseudohermaphroditism with
                adrenocortical disorder (E25.-)
                pseudohermaphroditism with specified
                chromosomal anomaly (Q96-Q99)
                pure gonadal dysgenesis (Q99.1)

Q56.0 **Hermaphroditism, not elsewhere classified** 🔍
  Ovotestis

Q56.1 **Male pseudohermaphroditism, not elsewhere classified** ♂
  46, XY with streak gonads
  Male pseudohermaphroditism NOS

Q56.2 **Female pseudohermaphroditism, not elsewhere classified** ♀
  Female pseudohermaphroditism NOS

Q56.3 **Pseudohermaphroditism, unspecified** 🔍

Q56.4 **Indeterminate sex, unspecified** 🔍
  Ambiguous genitalia

CONGENITAL MALFORMATIONS OF THE URINARY SYSTEM (Q60-Q64)

● Q60 **Renal agenesis and other reduction defects of kidney**
  Includes congenital absence of kidney
                congenital atrophy of kidney
                infantile atrophy of kidney

Q60.0 **Renal agenesis, unilateral** 🔍🔍
Q60.1 **Renal agenesis, bilateral** 🔍🔍
Q60.2 **Renal agenesis, unspecified** 🔍🔍
Q60.3 **Renal hypoplasia, unilateral** 🔍🔍
Q60.4 **Renal hypoplasia, bilateral** 🔍🔍
Q60.5 **Renal hypoplasia, unspecified** 🔍🔍
Q60.6 **Potter's syndrome** 🔍🔍

● Q61 **Cystic kidney disease**
  Cysts that develop in failing kidney due to end-stage renal disease
  Excludes1 acquired cyst of kidney (N28.1)
                Potter's syndrome (Q60.6)

● Q61.0 **Congenital renal cyst**
  Q61.00 **Congenital renal cyst, unspecified** 🔍🔍
    Cyst of kidney NOS (congenital)
  Q61.01 **Congenital single renal cyst** 🔍🔍
  Q61.02 **Congenital multiple renal cysts** 🔍🔍

● Q61.1 **Polycystic kidney, infantile type**
  Polycystic kidney, autosomal recessive
  Q61.11 **Cystic dilatation of collecting ducts** 🔍🔍
  Q61.19 **Other polycystic kidney, infantile type** 🔍🔍

Q61.2 **Polycystic kidney, adult type** 🔍🔍
  Polycystic kidney, autosomal dominant

Q61.3 **Polycystic kidney, unspecified** 🔍🔍

Q61.4 **Renal dysplasia** 🔍🔍
  Multicystic dysplastic kidney
  Multicystic kidney (development)
  Multicystic kidney disease
  Multicystic renal dysplasia
  Excludes1 polycystic kidney disease
                (Q61.11-Q61.3)

Q61.5 **Medullary cystic kidney** 🔍🔍
  Nephronopthisis
  Sponge kidney NOS

Q61.8 **Other cystic kidney diseases** 🔍🔍
  Fibrocystic kidney
  Fibrocystic renal degeneration or disease

Q61.9 **Cystic kidney disease, unspecified** 🔍🔍
  Meckel-Gruber syndrome

● Q62 **Congenital obstructive defects of renal pelvis and congenital malformations of ureter**

Q62.0 **Congenital hydronephrosis** 🔍🔍

● Q62.1 **Congenital occlusion of ureter**
  Atresia and stenosis of ureter
  Q62.10 **Congenital occlusion of ureter, unspecified** 🔍🔍
  Q62.11 **Congenital occlusion of ureteropelvic junction** 🔍🔍
  Q62.12 **Congenital occlusion of ureterovesical orifice** 🔍🔍

Q62.2 **Congenital megaureter** 🔍🔍
  Congenital dilatation of ureter

● Q62.3 **Other obstructive defects of renal pelvis and ureter**
  Q62.31 **Congenital ureterocele, orthotopic** 🔍🔍
  Q62.32 **Cecoureterocele** 🔍🔍
    Ectopic ureterocele
  Q62.39 **Other obstructive defects of renal pelvis and ureter** 🔍🔍
    Ureteropelvic junction obstruction NOS

Q62.4 **Agenesis of ureter** 🔍
  Congenital absence ureter

Q62.5 **Duplication of ureter** 🔍
  Accessory ureter
  Double ureter

● Q62.6 **Malposition of ureter**
  Q62.60 **Malposition of ureter, unspecified** 🔍
  Q62.61 **Deviation of ureter** 🔍
  Q62.62 **Displacement of ureter** 🔍
  Q62.63 **Anomalous implantation of ureter** 🔍
    Ectopia of ureter
    Ectopic ureter
  Q62.69 **Other malposition of ureter** 🔍

Q62.7 **Congenital vesico-uretero-renal reflux** 🔍

Q62.8 **Other congenital malformations of ureter** 🔍
  Anomaly of ureter NOS

CHAPTER 17 (Q00-Q99)

● **Q63 Other congenital malformations of kidney**

> **Excludes1** congenital nephrotic syndrome (N04.-)

Q63.0 **Accessory kidney** 🔍

Q63.1 **Lobulated, fused and horseshoe kidney** 🔍

Q63.2 **Ectopic kidney** 🔍
> Congenital displaced kidney
> Malrotation of kidney

Q63.3 **Hyperplastic and giant kidney** 🔍
> Compensatory hypertrophy of kidney

Q63.8 **Other specified congenital malformations of kidney** 🔍
> Congenital renal calculi

■ Q63.9 **Congenital malformation of kidney, unspecified** 🔍

● **Q64 Other congenital malformations of urinary system**

Q64.0 **Epispadias** ♂ 🔍
> *Urethral opening somewhere on dorsum of penis*
> **Excludes1** hypospadias (Q54.-)

● Q64.1 **Exstrophy of urinary bladder**
> *Bladder is exposed, inside out, and protrudes through abdominal wall*

■ Q64.10 **Exstrophy of urinary bladder, unspecified** 🔋 🔍
> Ectopia vesicae

Q64.11 **Supravesical fissure of urinary bladder** 🔋 🔍

Q64.12 **Cloacal extrophy of urinary bladder** 🔋 🔍

Q64.19 **Other exstrophy of urinary bladder** 🔋 🔍
> Extroversion of bladder

Q64.2 **Congenital posterior urethral valves** 🔋 🔍

● Q64.3 **Other atresia and stenosis of urethra and bladder neck**

Q64.31 **Congenital bladder neck obstruction** 🔋 🔍
> Congenital obstruction of vesicourethral orifice

Q64.32 **Congenital stricture of urethra** 🔋 🔍

Q64.33 **Congenital stricture of urinary meatus** 🔋 🔍

Q64.39 **Other atresia and stenosis of urethra and bladder neck** 🔋 🔍
> Atresia and stenosis of urethra and bladder neck NOS

Q64.4 **Malformation of urachus** 🔍
> Cyst of urachus
> Patent urachus
> Prolapse of urachus

Q64.5 **Congenital absence of bladder and urethra** 🔍

Q64.6 **Congenital diverticulum of bladder** 🔍

● Q64.7 **Other and unspecified congenital malformations of bladder and urethra**
> **Excludes1** congenital prolapse of bladder (mucosa) (Q79.4)

■ Q64.70 **Unspecified congenital malformation of bladder and urethra** 🔍
> Malformation of bladder or urethra NOS

Q64.71 **Congenital prolapse of urethra** 🔍

Q64.72 **Congenital prolapse of urinary meatus** 🔍

Q64.73 **Congenital urethrorectal fistula** 🔍

Q64.74 **Double urethra** 🔍

Q64.75 **Double urinary meatus** 🔍

Q64.79 **Other congenital malformations of bladder and urethra** 🔍

Q64.8 **Other specified congenital malformations of urinary system** 🔍

■ Q64.9 **Congenital malformation of urinary system, unspecified** 🔍
> Congenital anomaly NOS of urinary system
> Congenital deformity NOS of urinary system

CONGENITAL MALFORMATIONS AND DEFORMATIONS OF THE MUSCULOSKELETAL SYSTEM (Q65-Q79)

● **Q65 Congenital deformities of hip**
> **Excludes1** clicking hip (R29.4)

● Q65.0 **Congenital dislocation of hip, unilateral**

■ Q65.00 **Congenital dislocation of unspecified hip, unilateral** 🔍

Q65.01 **Congenital dislocation of right hip, unilateral** 🔍

Q65.02 **Congenital dislocation of left hip, unilateral** 🔍

Q65.1 **Congenital dislocation of hip, bilateral** 🔍

■ Q65.2 **Congenital dislocation of hip, unspecified** 🔍

● Q65.3 **Congenital partial dislocation of hip, unilateral**

■ Q65.30 **Congenital partial dislocation of unspecified hip, unilateral** 🔍

Q65.31 **Congenital partial dislocation of right hip, unilateral** 🔍

Q65.32 **Congenital partial dislocation of left hip, unilateral** 🔍

Q65.4 **Congenital partial dislocation of hip, bilateral** 🔍

■ Q65.5 **Congenital partial dislocation of hip, unspecified** 🔍

Q65.6 **Congenital unstable hip** 🔍
> Congenital dislocatable hip

● Q65.8 **Other congenital deformities of hip**

Q65.81 **Congenital coxa valga** 🔍

Q65.82 **Congenital coxa vara** 🔍

Q65.89 **Other specified congenital deformities of hip** 🔍
> Anteversion of femoral neck
> Congenital acetabular dysplasia

■ Q65.9 **Congenital deformity of hip, unspecified** 🔍

● **Q66 Congenital deformities of feet**
> **Excludes1** reduction defects of feet (Q72.-)
> valgus deformities (acquired) (M21.0-)
> varus deformities (acquired) (M21.1-)

Q66.0 **Congenital talipes equinovarus** 🔍
> *Heel is turned inward from midline and foot is plantar flexed; AKA clubfoot*

Q66.1 **Congenital talipes calcaneovarus** 🔍
> *Deformity of foot in which heel is turned toward midline of body and anterior of foot is elevated*

Q66.2 **Congenital metatarsus (primus) varus** 🔍
> *Angulation of first metatarsal bone toward midline of body*

Q66.3 **Other congenital varus deformities of feet** 🔍
> Hallux varus, congenital

Q66.4 **Congenital talipes calcaneovalgus** 🔍

● Unacceptable Principal Diagnosis	● Use Additional Character(s)	■ Unspecified	▶ Manifestation Code

OGCR Official Guidelines for Coding and Reporting

| Excludes 1 | Excludes 2 | Includes | Use additional | Code first | Code also |

Item 17-2 **Equinus foot** is a term referring to the hoof of a horse. The deformity is usually congenital or spastic. Talipes equinovarus is referred to as clubfoot. The foot tends to be smaller than normal, with the heel pointing downward and the forefoot turning inward. The heel cord (Achilles tendon) is tight, causing the heel to be drawn up toward the leg.

Figure 17-6 Supination and cavus deformity of forefoot. *(Courtesy Jay Cummings, MD.)* (From Canale: Campbell's Operative Orthopaedics, 10th ed. 2003, Mosby, Inc.)

● **Q66.5 Congenital pes planus**
Congenital flat foot
Congenital rigid flat foot
Congenital spastic (everted) flat foot
> **Excludes1**   pes planus, acquired (M21.4)

■ **Q66.50 Congenital pes planus, unspecified foot** 🔖

Q66.51 Congenital pes planus, right foot 🔖

Q66.52 Congenital pes planus, left foot 🔖

Q66.6 Other congenital valgus deformities of feet 🔖
Inward angulation
Congenital metatarsus valgus

Q66.7 Congenital pes cavus 🔖

● **Q66.8 Other congenital deformities of feet**

■ **Q66.80 Congenital vertical talus deformity, unspecified foot** 🔖

Q66.81 Congenital vertical talus deformity, right foot 🔖

Q66.82 Congenital vertical talus deformity, left foot 🔖

Figure 17-7 Talipes. (From Dorland: Dorland's Illustrated Medical Dictionary, 31st ed. 2007, Saunders, p 1893.)

Q66.89 Other specified congenital deformities of feet 🔖
Congenital asymmetric talipes
Congenital clubfoot NOS
Congenital talipes NOS
Congenital tarsal coalition
Hammer toe, congenital

■ **Q66.9 Congenital deformity of feet, unspecified** 🔖

● **Q67 Congenital musculoskeletal deformities of head, face, spine and chest** 🔖
> **Excludes1**   congenital malformation syndromes classified to Q87.-
> Potter's syndrome (Q60.6)

Q67.0 Congenital facial asymmetry 🔖

Q67.1 Congenital compression facies 🔖

Q67.2 Dolichocephaly 🔖
Long head dimension

Q67.3 Plagiocephaly 🔖
Asymmetric shape of head resulting from irregular closure of cranial sutures

Q67.4 Other congenital deformities of skull, face and jaw 🔖
Congenital depressions in skull
Congenital hemifacial atrophy or hypertrophy
Deviation of nasal septum, congenital
Squashed or bent nose, congenital
> **Excludes1**   dentofacial anomalies [including malocclusion] (M26-)
> syphilitic saddle nose (A50.5)

Q67.5 Congenital deformity of spine 🔖 🔖
Congenital postural scoliosis
Congenital scoliosis NOS
> **Excludes1**   infantile idiopathic scoliosis (M41.0)
> scoliosis due to congenital bony malformation (Q76.3)

Q67.6 Pectus excavatum 🔖
Congenital funnel chest
Funnel-shaped chest depression

Q67.7 Pectus carinatum 🔖
Congenital pigeon chest

Q67.8 Other congenital deformities of chest 🔖 🔖
Congenital deformity of chest wall NOS

● **Q68 Other congenital musculoskeletal deformities**
> **Excludes1**   reduction defects of limb(s) (Q71-Q73)
> **Excludes2**   congenital myotonic chondrodystrophy (G71.13)

Q68.0 Congenital deformity of sternocleidomastoid muscle 🔖
Congenital contracture of sternocleidomastoid (muscle)
Congenital (sternomastoid) torticollis
Sternomastoid tumor (congenital)

Q68.1 Congenital deformity of finger(s) and hand 🔖 🔖
Congenital clubfinger
Spade-like hand (congenital)

Q68.2 Congenital deformity of knee 🔖
Congenital dislocation of knee
Congenital genu recurvatum
Hyperextension of knee resulting from hypermobility

Q68.3 Congenital bowing of femur 🔖
> **Excludes1**   anteversion of femur (neck) (Q65.89)

Q68.4 Congenital bowing of tibia and fibula 🔖

■ **Q68.5 Congenital bowing of long bones of leg, unspecified** 🔖

N Newborn Age: 0   **P** Pediatric Age: 0–17   **M** Maternity DX: 12–55   **A** Adult Age: 15–124   ♀ Females Only   ♂ Males Only
🔖 Complication\Comorbidity   🔖 Major C\C   🔖 Present on Admission Requirement   🔖 Hospital-Acquired Condition

1355

CHAPTER 17 (Q00-Q99)

Figure 17-8 Mild to moderate inbowing of the lower leg. (From Jones KL: Smith's Recognizable Patterns of Human Malformation, 4th ed. Philadelphia, Saunders, 1988, p 671.)

Q68.6 Discoid meniscus

Q68.8 Other specified congenital musculoskeletal deformities ✎
    Congenital deformity of clavicle
    Congenital deformity of elbow
    Congenital deformity of forearm
    Congenital deformity of scapula
    Congenital deformity of wrist
    Congenital dislocation of elbow
    Congenital dislocation of shoulder
    Congenital dislocation of wrist

● **Q69 Polydactyly**
    AKA hyperdactyly, consists of supernumerary fingers or toes

  Q69.0 Accessory finger(s) ✎

  Q69.1 Accessory thumb(s) ✎

  Q69.2 Accessory toe(s) ✎
    Accessory hallux

  ■ **Q69.9 Polydactyly, unspecified** ✎
    Supernumerary digit(s) NOS

● **Q70 Syndactyly**
    Webbing between distal phalanges of adjacent digits

  ● **Q70.0 Fused fingers**
    Complex syndactyly of fingers with synostosis

    ■ **Q70.00 Fused fingers, unspecified hand** ✎

    Q70.01 Fused fingers, right hand ✎

    Q70.02 Fused fingers, left hand ✎

    Q70.03 Fused fingers, bilateral ✎

  ● **Q70.1 Webbed fingers**
    Simple syndactyly of fingers without synostosis

    ■ **Q70.10 Webbed fingers, unspecified hand** ✎

    Q70.11 Webbed fingers, right hand ✎

    Q70.12 Webbed fingers, left hand ✎

    Q70.13 Webbed fingers, bilateral ✎

  ● **Q70.2 Fused toes**
    Complex syndactyly of toes with synostosis

    ■ **Q70.20 Fused toes, unspecified foot** ✎

    Q70.21 Fused toes, right foot ✎

    Q70.22 Fused toes, left foot ✎

    Q70.23 Fused toes, bilateral ✎

  ● **Q70.3 Webbed toes**
    Simple syndactyly of toes without synostosis

    ■ **Q70.30 Webbed toes, unspecified foot** ✎

    Q70.31 Webbed toes, right foot ✎

    Q70.32 Webbed toes, left foot ✎

    Q70.33 Webbed toes, bilateral ✎

Figure 17-9 Polydactyly, congenital duplicated thumb. (From DeLee and Drez's Orthopaedic Sports Medicine, 2nd ed. 2003, Saunders, An Imprint of Elsevier.)

  Q70.4 Polysyndactyly, unspecified ✎
    Excludes1   specified syndactyly of hand and feet - code to specified conditions (Q70.0- - Q70.3-)
    Extra and webbed digits

  ■ **Q70.9 Syndactyly, unspecified** ✎
    Symphalangy NOS

● **Q71 Reduction defects of upper limb**

  ● **Q71.0 Congenital complete absence of upper limb**

    ■ **Q71.00 Congenital complete absence of unspecified upper limb** ✎

    Q71.01 Congenital complete absence of right upper limb ✎

    Q71.02 Congenital complete absence of left upper limb ✎

    Q71.03 Congenital complete absence of upper limb, bilateral ✎

  ● **Q71.1 Congenital absence of upper arm and forearm with hand present**

    ■ **Q71.10 Congenital absence of unspecified upper arm and forearm with hand present** ✎

    Q71.11 Congenital absence of right upper arm and forearm with hand present ✎

    Q71.12 Congenital absence of left upper arm and forearm with hand present ✎

    Q71.13 Congenital absence of upper arm and forearm with hand present, bilateral ✎

  ● **Q71.2 Congenital absence of both forearm and hand**

    ■ **Q71.20 Congenital absence of both forearm and hand, unspecified upper limb** ✎

    Q71.21 Congenital absence of both forearm and hand, right upper limb ✎

    Q71.22 Congenital absence of both forearm and hand, left upper limb ✎

    Q71.23 Congenital absence of both forearm and hand, bilateral ✎

  ● **Q71.3 Congenital absence of hand and finger**

    ■ **Q71.30 Congenital absence of unspecified hand and finger** ✎

    Q71.31 Congenital absence of right hand and finger ✎

    Q71.32 Congenital absence of left hand and finger ✎

    Q71.33 Congenital absence of hand and finger, bilateral ✎

  ● **Q71.4 Longitudinal reduction defect of radius**
    Clubhand (congenital)
    Radial clubhand

    ■ **Q71.40 Longitudinal reduction defect of unspecified radius** ✎

    Q71.41 Longitudinal reduction defect of right radius ✎

    Q71.42 Longitudinal reduction defect of left radius ✎

    Q71.43 Longitudinal reduction defect of radius, bilateral ✎

  ● **Q71.5 Longitudinal reduction defect of ulna**

    ■ **Q71.50 Longitudinal reduction defect of unspecified ulna** ✎

    Q71.51 Longitudinal reduction defect of right ulna ✎

● Unacceptable Principal Diagnosis   ● Use Additional Character(s)   ■ Unspecified   ▶ Manifestation Code
OGCR Official Guidelines for Coding and Reporting   Excludes 1   Excludes 2   Includes   Use additional   Code first   Code also

    Q71.52 Longitudinal reduction defect of left ulna

    Q71.53 Longitudinal reduction defect of ulna, bilateral

● Q71.6 Lobster-claw hand

    Q71.60 Lobster-claw hand, unspecified hand

    Q71.61 Lobster-claw right hand

    Q71.62 Lobster-claw left hand

    Q71.63 Lobster-claw hand, bilateral

● Q71.8 Other reduction defects of upper limb

  ● Q71.81 Congenital shortening of upper limb

    Q71.811 Congenital shortening of right upper limb

    Q71.812 Congenital shortening of left upper limb

    Q71.813 Congenital shortening of upper limb, bilateral

    Q71.819 Congenital shortening of unspecified upper limb

  ● Q71.89 Other reduction defects of upper limb

    Q71.891 Other reduction defects of right upper limb

    Q71.892 Other reduction defects of left upper limb

    Q71.893 Other reduction defects of upper limb, bilateral

    Q71.899 Other reduction defects of unspecified upper limb

● Q71.9 Unspecified reduction defect of upper limb

    Q71.90 Unspecified reduction defect of unspecified upper limb

    Q71.91 Unspecified reduction defect of right upper limb

    Q71.92 Unspecified reduction defect of left upper limb

    Q71.93 Unspecified reduction defect of upper limb, bilateral

● Q72 Reduction defects of lower limb

  ● Q72.0 Congenital complete absence of lower limb

    Q72.00 Congenital complete absence of unspecified lower limb

    Q72.01 Congenital complete absence of right lower limb

    Q72.02 Congenital complete absence of left lower limb

    Q72.03 Congenital complete absence of lower limb, bilateral

  ● Q72.1 Congenital absence of thigh and lower leg with foot present

    Q72.10 Congenital absence of unspecified thigh and lower leg with foot present

    Q72.11 Congenital absence of right thigh and lower leg with foot present

    Q72.12 Congenital absence of left thigh and lower leg with foot present

    Q72.13 Congenital absence of thigh and lower leg with foot present, bilateral

● Q72.2 Congenital absence of both lower leg and foot

    Q72.20 Congenital absence of both lower leg and foot, unspecified lower limb

    Q72.21 Congenital absence of both lower leg and foot, right lower limb

    Q72.22 Congenital absence of both left lower leg and foot, left lower limb

    Q72.23 Congenital absence of both lower leg and foot, bilateral

● Q72.3 Congenital absence of foot and toe(s)

    Q72.30 Congenital absence of unspecified foot and toe(s)

    Q72.31 Congenital absence of right foot and toe(s)

    Q72.32 Congenital absence of left foot and toe(s)

    Q72.33 Congenital absence of foot and toe(s), bilateral

● Q72.4 Longitudinal reduction defect of femur
    Proximal femoral focal deficiency

    Q72.40 Longitudinal reduction defect of unspecified femur

    Q72.41 Longitudinal reduction defect of right femur

    Q72.42 Longitudinal reduction defect of left femur

    Q72.43 Longitudinal reduction defect of femur, bilateral

● Q72.5 Longitudinal reduction defect of tibia

    Q72.50 Longitudinal reduction defect of unspecified tibia

    Q72.51 Longitudinal reduction defect of right tibia

    Q72.52 Longitudinal reduction defect of left tibia

    Q72.53 Longitudinal reduction defect of tibia, bilateral

● Q72.6 Longitudinal reduction defect of fibula

    Q72.60 Longitudinal reduction defect of unspecified fibula

    Q72.61 Longitudinal reduction defect of right fibula

    Q72.62 Longitudinal reduction defect of left fibula

    Q72.63 Longitudinal reduction defect of fibula, bilateral

● Q72.7 Split foot

    Q72.70 Split foot, unspecified lower limb

    Q72.71 Split foot, right lower limb

    Q72.72 Split foot, left lower limb

    Q72.73 Split foot, bilateral

● Q72.8 Other reduction defects of lower limb

  ● Q72.81 Congenital shortening of lower limb

    Q72.811 Congenital shortening of right lower limb

    Q72.812 Congenital shortening of left lower limb

    Q72.813 Congenital shortening of lower limb, bilateral

    Q72.819 Congenital shortening of unspecified lower limb

CHAPTER 17 (Q00-Q99)

● Q72.89 **Other reduction defects of lower limb**
    Q72.891 **Other reduction defects of right lower limb** 🔖
    Q72.892 **Other reduction defects of left lower limb** 🔖
    Q72.893 **Other reduction defects of lower limb, bilateral** 🔖
    ■ Q72.899 **Other reduction defects of unspecified lower limb** 🔖

● Q72.9 **Unspecified reduction defect of lower limb**
    ■ Q72.90 **Unspecified reduction defect of unspecified lower limb** 🔖
    ■ Q72.91 **Unspecified reduction defect of right lower limb** 🔖
    ■ Q72.92 **Unspecified reduction defect of left lower limb** 🔖
    ■ Q72.93 **Unspecified reduction defect of lower limb, bilateral** 🔖

● Q73 **Reduction defects of unspecified limb**
  ■ Q73.0 **Congenital absence of unspecified limb(s)** 🔖
    Amelia NOS

  ■ Q73.1 **Phocomelia, unspecified limb(s)** 🔖
    Phocomelia NOS
    Absence/shortening of long bones primarily as a result of thalidomide

  ■ Q73.8 **Other reduction defects of unspecified limb(s)** 🔖
    Longitudinal reduction deformity of unspecified limb(s)
    Ectromelia of limb NOS
    Gross hypoplasia or aplasia of one or more long bones of limb(s)
    Hemimelia of limb NOS
    Absence of one-half of long bone
    Reduction defect of limb NOS

● Q74 **Other congenital malformations of limb(s)**
   | Excludes1 | polydactyly (Q69.-)
            reduction defect of limb (Q71-Q73)
            syndactyly (Q70.-)

  Q74.0 **Other congenital malformations of upper limb(s), including shoulder girdle** 🔖
    Accessory carpal bones
    Cleidocranial dysostosis
    Congenital pseudarthrosis of clavicle
    Macrodactylia (fingers)
    Madelung's deformity
    Radioulnar synostosis
    Sprengel's deformity
    Triphalangeal thumb

  Q74.1 **Congenital malformation of knee** 🔖
    Congenital absence of patella
    Congenital dislocation of patella
    Congenital genu valgum
    Congenital genu varum
    Rudimentary patella
    | Excludes1 | congenital dislocation of knee (Q68.2)
            congenital genu recurvatum (Q68.2)
            nail patella syndrome (Q87.2)

  Q74.2 **Other congenital malformations of lower limb(s), including pelvic girdle** 🔖
    Congenital fusion of sacroiliac joint
    Congenital malformation of ankle joint
    Congenital malformation of sacroiliac joint
    | Excludes1 | anteversion of femur (neck) (Q65.89)

  Q74.3 **Arthrogryposis multiplex congenita** 🔖🔖

● Q74.8 **Other specified congenital malformations of limb(s)** 🔖
■ Q74.9 **Unspecified congenital malformation of limb(s)** 🔖
    Congenital anomaly of limb(s) NOS

● Q75 **Other congenital malformations of skull and face bones**
  | Excludes1 | congenital malformation of face NOS (Q18.-)
        congenital malformation syndromes classified to Q87.-
        dentofacial anomalies [including malocclusion] (M26.-)
        musculoskeletal deformities of head and face (Q67.0-Q67.4)
        skull defects associated with congenital anomalies of brain such as:
           anencephaly (Q00.0)
           encephalocele (Q01.-)
           hydrocephalus (Q03.-)
           microcephaly (Q02)

  Q75.0 **Craniosynostosis** 🔖
    Premature closure of sutures of skull
    Acrocephaly
    Imperfect fusion of skull
    Oxycephaly
    Trigonocephaly

  Q75.1 **Craniofacial dysostosis** 🔖
    Congential deformity of head
    Crouzon's disease

  Q75.2 **Hypertelorism** 🔖

  Q75.3 **Macrocephaly** 🔖
    Unusually large size of head; AKA megalocephaly

  Q75.4 **Mandibulofacial dysostosis** 🔖
    Franceschetti syndrome
    Treacher Collins syndrome

  Q75.5 **Oculomandibular dysostosis** 🔖
    Ossification of occular and mandibular bones

  Q75.8 **Other specified congenital malformations of skull and face bones** 🔖
    Absence of skull bone, congenital
    Congenital deformity of forehead
    Platybasia

■ Q75.9 **Congenital malformation of skull and face bones, unspecified** 🔖
    Congenital anomaly of face bones NOS
    Congenital anomaly of skull NOS

Item 17–3 Anencephalus is a congenital deformity of the cranial vault. **Craniosynostosis,** also known as craniostenosis and stenocephaly, signifies any form of congenital deformity of the skull that results from the premature closing of the sutures of the skull. **Iniencephaly** is a deformity in which the head and neck are flexed backward to a great extent and the head is very large in comparison to the shortened body.

Figure 17-10 Generalized craniosynostosis in a 4-year-old girl without symptoms or signs of increased intracranial pressure. (From Bell WE, McCormick WF: Increased Intracranial Pressure in Children, 2nd ed. Philadelphia, WB Saunders, 1978, p 116.)

● Unacceptable Principal Diagnosis   ● Use Additional Character(s)   ■ Unspecified   ▶ Manifestation Code

OGCR Official Guidelines for Coding and Reporting | Excludes 1 | | Excludes 2 | Includes   Use additional   Code first   Code also

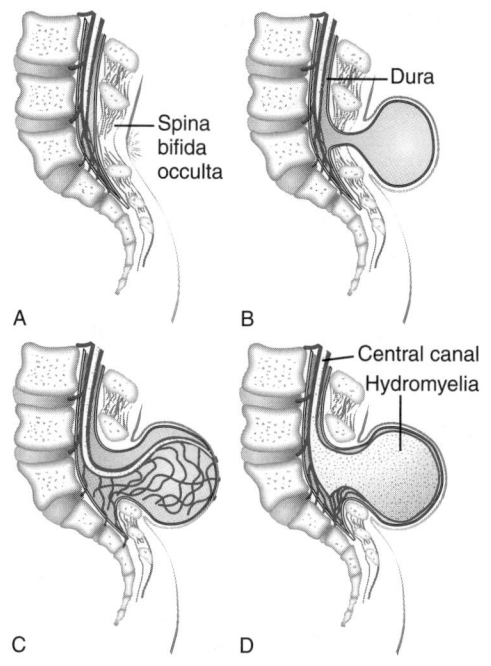

Figure 17-11   A. Spina bifida occulta. **B.** Meningocele.
C. Myelomeningocele. **D.** Myelocystocele (syringomyelocele)
or hydromyelia.

Item 17–4   Spina bifida is a midline spinal defect in which one or
more vertebrae fail to fuse, leaving an opening in the vertebral canal.
When the defect is not visible, it is called spina bifida occulta, and when
it is visible, it is called spina bifida cystica.

● **Q76   Congenital malformations of spine and bony thorax**
   Excludes1   congenital musculoskeletal deformities of
             spine and chest (Q67.5-Q67.8)

Q76.0   Spina bifida occulta 🖰
   Excludes1   meningocele (spinal) (Q05.-)
             spina bifida (aperta) (cystica) (Q05.-)

Q76.1   Klippel-Feil syndrome 🖰
   Cervical fusion syndrome

Q76.2   Congenital spondylolisthesis 🖰
   Congenital spondylolysis
   Excludes1   spondylolisthesis (acquired) (M43.1-)
             spondylolysis (acquired) (M43.0-)

**Q76.3   Congenital scoliosis due to congenital bony
         malformation** 🖰 🖰
   Hemivertebra fusion or failure of segmentation
      with scoliosis

● **Q76.4   Other congenital malformations of spine, not
         associated with scoliosis**
   ● **Q76.41   Congenital kyphosis**
      *Abnormal increase in convexity curvature of
      thoracic spinal column; AKA humpback*
      **Q76.411   Congenital kyphosis, occipito-
               atlanto-axial region** 🖰
      **Q76.412   Congenital kyphosis, cervical
               region** 🖰
      **Q76.413   Congenital kyphosis,
               cervicothoracic region** 🖰
      **Q76.414   Congenital kyphosis, thoracic
               region** 🖰

      **Q76.415   Congenital kyphosis,
               thoracolumbar region** 🖰
   ■ **Q76.419   Congenital kyphosis, unspecified
               region** 🖰
   ● **Q76.42   Congenital lordosis**
      *An abnormal increase in curvature of lumbar
      spine (sway back)*
      **Q76.425   Congenital lordosis,
               thoracolumbar region** 🖰 🖰
      **Q76.426   Congenital lordosis, lumbar
               region** 🖰 🖰
      **Q76.427   Congenital lordosis, lumbosacral
               region** 🖰 🖰
      **Q76.428   Congenital lordosis, sacral and
               sacrococcygeal region** 🖰 🖰
   ■ **Q76.429   Congenital lordosis, unspecified
               region** 🖰 🖰

   **Q76.49   Other congenital malformations of spine,
           not associated with scoliosis** 🖰
      Congenital absence of vertebra NOS
      Congenital fusion of spine NOS
      Congenital malformation of lumbosacral
         (joint) (region) NOS
      Congenital malformation of spine NOS
      Hemivertebra NOS
      Malformation of spine NOS
      Platyspondylisis NOS
      Supernumerary vertebra NOS

Q76.5   Cervical rib 🖰
   Supernumerary rib in cervical region

Q76.6   Other congenital malformations of ribs 🖰 🖰
   Accessory rib
   Congenital absence of rib
   Congenital fusion of ribs
   Congenital malformation of ribs NOS
   Excludes1   short rib syndrome (Q77.2)

Q76.7   Congenital malformation of sternum 🖰 🖰
   Congenital absence of sternum
   Sternum bifidum

**Q76.8   Other congenital malformations of bony
         thorax** 🖰 🖰

■ **Q76.9   Congenital malformation of bony thorax,
         unspecified** 🖰 🖰

● **Q77   Osteochondrodysplasia with defects of growth of tubular
         bones and spine**
   Excludes1   mucopolysaccharidosis (E76.0-E76.3)
   Excludes2   congenital myotonic chondrodystrophy
             (G71.13)

Q77.0   Achondrogenesis 🖰
   Hypochondrogenesis

Q77.1   Thanatophoric short stature 🖰

Q77.2   Short rib syndrome 🖰 🖰
   Asphyxiating thoracic dysplasia [Jeune]

Q77.3   Chondrodysplasia punctata 🖰
   Benign cartilaginous neoplasms
   Excludes1   rhizomelic chondrodysplasia
             punctata (E71.43)

Q77.4   Achondroplasia 🖰 🖰
   *Disturbance of epiphyseal chondroblastic growth and
   maturation, results in dwarfism*
   Hypochondroplasia
   Osteosclerosis congenita

Q77.5   Diastrophic dysplasia 🖰

CHAPTER 17 (Q00-Q99)

N Newborn Age: 0   **P** Pediatric Age: 0–17   **M** Maternity DX: 12–55   **A** Adult Age: 15–124   ♀ Females Only   ♂ Males Only

🖰 Complication\Comorbidity   🖰 Major C\C   🖰 Present on Admission Requirement   🖰 Hospital-Acquired Condition

1359

Q77.6 Chondroectodermal dysplasia 🔖
Defective development of skin, hair, teeth, with polydactyly and defect of cardiac septum
Ellis-van Creveld syndrome

Q77.7 Spondyloepiphyseal dysplasia 🔖

Q77.8 Other osteochondrodysplasia with defects of growth of tubular bones and spine 🔖

🔲 **Q77.9 Osteochondrodysplasia with defects of growth of tubular bones and spine, unspecified** 🔖

⬤ **Q78 Other osteochondrodysplasias**
Disorder of development of bone and cartilage; common cause of dwarfism

> **Excludes2**   congenital myotonic chondrodystrophy (G71.13)

Q78.0 Osteogenesis imperfecta 🔖🔖
Fragilitas ossium
Osteopsathyrosis

Q78.1 Polyostotic fibrous dysplasia 🔖
Albright(-McCune)(-Sternberg) syndrome

Q78.2 Osteopetrosis 🔖🔖
Abnormally dense bone; AKA marble bones disease, ivory bones
Albers-Schönberg syndrome
Osteosclerosis NOS

Q78.3 Progressive diaphyseal dysplasia 🔖
Camurati-Engelmann syndrome

Q78.4 Enchondromatosis 🔖
Thinning of overlying cortex of bone and distorted length
Maffucci's syndrome
Ollier's disease

Q78.5 Metaphyseal dysplasia 🔖
Disturbance in enchondral bone growth, causing ends of shafts to remain larger than normal in circumference
Pyle's syndrome

Q78.6 Multiple congenital exostoses 🔖
Diaphyseal aclasis

Q78.8 Other specified osteochondrodysplasias 🔖
Osteopoikilosis

🔲 **Q78.9 Osteochondrodysplasia, unspecified** 🔖
Chondrodystrophy NOS
AKA skeletal dysplasia (dwarfism) caused by genetic mutations affecting hyaline cartilage capping long bones and vertebrae
Osteodystrophy NOS

⬤ **Q79 Congenital malformations of musculoskeletal system, not elsewhere classified**

> **Excludes2**   congenital (sternomastoid) torticollis (Q68.0)

Q79.0 Congenital diaphragmatic hernia 🔖🔖

> **Excludes1**   congenital hiatus hernia (Q40.1)

Q79.1 Other congenital malformations of diaphragm 🔖🔖
Absence of diaphragm
Congenital malformation of diaphragm NOS
Eventration of diaphragm

Q79.2 Exomphalos 🔖🔖
Abdominal hernia in which part of intestine protrudes at umbilicus; AKA exomphalos and exumbilication
Omphalocele

> **Excludes1**   umbilical hernia (K42.-)

Q79.3 Gastroschisis 🔖🔖
Congenital fissure of anterior abdominal wall often with protrusion of small/large intestine

Q79.4 Prune belly syndrome 🔖🔖🔖
Congenital prolapse of bladder mucosa
Eagle-Barrett syndrome

⬤ **Q79.5 Other congenital malformations of abdominal wall**

> **Excludes1**   umbilical hernia (K42.-)

Q79.51 Congenital hernia of bladder 🔖🔖

Q79.59 Other congenital malformations of abdominal wall 🔖🔖

Q79.6 Ehlers-Danlos syndrome 🔖🔖
Group of inherited disorders of connective tissue; AKA cutis hyperelastica

Q79.8 Other congenital malformations of musculoskeletal system 🔖
Absence of muscle
Absence of tendon
Accessory muscle
Amyotrophia congenita
Congenital constricting bands
Congenital shortening of tendon
Poland syndrome

🔲 **Q79.9 Congenital malformation of musculoskeletal system, unspecified** 🔖
Congenital anomaly of musculoskeletal system NOS
Congenital deformity of musculoskeletal system NOS

OTHER CONGENITAL MALFORMATIONS (Q80-Q89)

⬤ **Q80 Congenital ichthyosis**
Characterized by increased keratinization, resulting in noninflammatory scaling of skin

> **Excludes1**   Refsum's disease (G60.1)

Q80.0 Ichthyosis vulgaris 🔖

Q80.1 X-linked ichthyosis 🔖

Q80.2 Lamellar ichthyosis 🔖
Collodion baby

Q80.3 Congenital bullous ichthyosiform erythroderma 🔖

Q80.4 Harlequin fetus 🔖

Q80.8 Other congenital ichthyosis 🔖

🔲 **Q80.9 Congenital ichthyosis, unspecified** 🔖

⬤ **Q81 Epidermolysis bullosa**
Loosening of epidermis

Q81.0 Epidermolysis bullosa simplex 🔖

> **Excludes1**   Cockayne's syndrome (Q87.1)

Q81.1 Epidermolysis bullosa letalis 🔖
Herlitz' syndrome

Q81.2 Epidermolysis bullosa dystrophica 🔖

Q81.8 Other epidermolysis bullosa 🔖

🔲 **Q81.9 Epidermolysis bullosa, unspecified** 🔖

⬤ **Q82 Other congenital malformations of skin**

> **Excludes1**   acrodermatitis enteropathica (E83.2)
> congenital erythropoietic porphyria (E80.0)
> pilonidal cyst or sinus (L05.-)
> Sturge-Weber (-Dimitri) syndrome (Q85.8)

Q82.0 Hereditary lymphedema 🔖
Characterized by swelling of subcutaneous tissue caused by obstruction of lymphatic vessels and resulting edema of lymph fluid

Q82.1 Xeroderma pigmentosum 🔖
Dry, rough, discolored state of skin, and formation of scaly desquamation

---

⬤ Unacceptable Principal Diagnosis   ⬤ Use Additional Character(s)   🔲 Unspecified   ▶ Manifestation Code

OGCR Official Guidelines for Coding and Reporting   Excludes 1   Excludes 2   Includes   Use additional   Code first   Code also

Q82.2 Mastocytosis 🔖
Characterized by infiltrates of mast cells in tissues/organs
Urticaria pigmentosa
Excludes1   malignant mastocytosis (C96.2)

Q82.3 Incontinentia pigmenti 🔖
Characterized by hyperpigmented cutaneous

Q82.4 Ectodermal dysplasia (anhidrotic) 🔖
Absence/deficiency of tissues/structures, including teeth, hair, nails, and certain glands
Excludes1   Ellis-van Creveld syndrome (Q77.6)

Q82.5 Congenital non-neoplastic nevus 🔖
Birthmark NOS
Flammeus Nevus
Portwine Nevus
Sanguineous Nevus
Strawberry Nevus
Vascular Nevus NOS
Verrucous Nevus
Excludes2   Café au lait spots (L81.3)
lentigo (L81.4)
nevus NOS (D22.-)
araneus nevus (I78.1)
melanocytic nevus (D22.-)
pigmented nevus (D22.-)
spider nevus (I78.1)
stellar nevus (I78.1)

Q82.8 Other specified congenital malformations of skin 🔖
Abnormal palmar creases
Accessory skin tags
Benign familial pemphigus [Hailey-Hailey]
Congenital poikiloderma
Cutis laxa (hyperelastica)
Dermatoglyphic anomalies
Inherited keratosis palmaris et plantaris
Keratosis follicularis [Darier-White]
Excludes1   Ehlers-Danlos syndrome (Q79.6)

🔲 **Q82.9 Congenital malformation of skin, unspecified** 🔖

● **Q83 Congenital malformations of breast**
Excludes2   absence of pectoral muscle (Q79.8)
hypoplasia of breast (N64.82)
micromastia (N64.82)

Q83.0 Congenital absence of breast with absent nipple 🔖

Q83.1 Accessory breast 🔖
Supernumerary breast

Q83.2 Absent nipple 🔖

Q83.3 Accessory nipple 🔖
Supernumerary nipple

Q83.8 Other congenital malformations of breast 🔖

🔲 **Q83.9 Congenital malformation of breast, unspecified** 🔖

● **Q84 Other congenital malformations of integument**
Q84.0 Congenital alopecia 🔖
Congenital atrichosis

Q84.1 Congenital morphological disturbances of hair, not elsewhere classified 🔖
Beaded hair
Monilethrix
Pili annulati
Excludes1   Menkes' kinky hair syndrome (E83.0)

Q84.2 Other congenital malformations of hair 🔖
Congenital hypertrichosis
Congenital malformation of hair NOS
Persistent lanugo

Q84.3 Anonychia 🔖
Absence of nail
Excludes1   nail patella syndrome (Q87.2)

Q84.4 Congenital leukonychia 🔖
Opaque, whitish discoloration of nails; AKA leukopathia unguium

Q84.5 Enlarged and hypertrophic nails 🔖
Congenital onychauxis
Pachyonychia

Q84.6 Other congenital malformations of nails 🔖
Congenital clubnail
Congenital koilonychia
Congenital malformation of nail NOS

Q84.8 Other specified congenital malformations of integument 🔖
Aplasia cutis congenita

🔲 **Q84.9 Congenital malformation of integument, unspecified** 🔖
Congenital anomaly of integument NOS
Congenital deformity of integument NOS

● **Q85 Phakomatoses, not elsewhere classified**
Excludes1   ataxia telangiectasia [Louis-Bar] (G11.3)
familial dysautonomia [Riley-Day] (G90.1)

● **Q85.0 Neurofibromatosis (nonmalignant)**
Developmental changes in nervous system and other structures, with formation of neurofibromas

🔲 **Q85.00 Neurofibromatosis, unspecified**

Q85.01 Neurofibromatosis, type 1
Von Recklinghausen disease

Q85.02 Neurofibromatosis, type 2
Acoustic neurofibromatosis

Q85.03 Schwannomatosis

Q85.09 Other neurofibromatosis

Q85.1 Tuberous sclerosis 🩹🔖
Bourneville's disease
Epiloia

Q85.8 Other phakomatoses, not elsewhere classified 🩹🔖
Peutz-Jeghers Syndrome
Sturge-Weber(-Dimitri) syndrome
von Hippel-Lindau syndrome
Excludes1   Meckel-Gruber syndrome (Q61.9)

🔲 **Q85.9 Phakomatosis, unspecified** 🩹🔖
Hamartosis NOS

● **Q86 Congenital malformation syndromes due to known exogenous causes, not elsewhere classified**
Excludes2   iodine-deficiency-related hypothyroidism (E00-E02)
nonteratogenic effects of substances transmitted via placenta or breast milk (P04.-)

Q86.0 Fetal alcohol syndrome (dysmorphic)

Q86.1 Fetal hydantoin syndrome   N
Meadow's syndrome

Q86.2 Dysmorphism due to warfarin

Q86.8 Other congenital malformation syndromes due to known exogenous causes

CHAPTER 17 (Q00-Q99)

N Newborn Age: 0   **P** Pediatric Age: 0–17   **M** Maternity DX: 12–55   **A** Adult Age: 15–124   ♀ Females Only   ♂ Males Only
🩹 Complication\Comorbidity   🔖 Major C\C   🔖 Present on Admission Requirement   🔖 Hospital-Acquired Condition

1361

● **Q87 Other specified congenital malformation syndromes affecting multiple systems**

Use additional code(s) to identify all associated manifestations

Q87.0 Congenital malformation syndromes predominantly affecting facial appearance 🔖
Acrocephalopolysyndactyly
Acrocephalosyndactyly [Apert]
Cryptophthalmos syndrome
Cyclopia
Goldenhar syndrome
Moebius syndrome
Oro-facial-digital syndrome
Robin syndrome
Whistling face

Q87.1 Congenital malformation syndromes predominantly associated with short stature 🔖🔖
Aarskog syndrome
Cockayne syndrome
De Lange syndrome
Dubowitz syndrome
Noonan syndrome
Prader-Willi syndrome
Robinow-Silverman-Smith syndrome
Russell-Silver syndrome
Seckel syndrome

Excludes1 Ellis-van Creveld syndrome (Q77.6)
Smith-Lemli-Opitz syndrome (E78.72)

Q87.2 Congenital malformation syndromes predominantly involving limbs 🔖🔖
Holt-Oram syndrome
Klippel-Trenaunay-Weber syndrome
Nail patella syndrome
Rubinstein-Taybi syndrome
Sirenomelia syndrome
Thrombocytopenia with absent radius [TAR] syndrome
VATER syndrome

Q87.3 Congenital malformation syndromes involving early overgrowth 🔖🔖
Beckwith-Wiedemann syndrome
Sotos' syndrome
Weaver syndrome

● **Q87.4 Marfan's syndrome**

▪ **Q87.40 Marfan's syndrome, unspecified** 🔖🔖

● **Q87.41 Marfan's syndrome with cardiovascular manifestations**

Q87.410 Marfan's syndrome with aortic dilation 🔖🔖

Q87.418 Marfan's syndrome with other cardiovascular manifestations 🔖🔖

Q87.42 Marfan's syndrome with ocular manifestations 🔖🔖

Q87.43 Marfan's syndrome with skeletal manifestation 🔖🔖

Q87.5 Other congenital malformation syndromes with other skeletal changes 🔖🔖

Q87.8 Other specified congenital malformation syndromes, not elsewhere classified

Excludes1 Zellweger syndrome (E71.510)

Q87.81 Alport syndrome 🔖🔖
Progressive sensorineural hearing loss, progressive pyelonephritis or glomerulonephritis, and ocular defects

Use additional code to identify stage of chronic kidney disease (N18.1-N18.6)

Q87.89 Other specified congenital malformation syndromes, not elsewhere classified 🔖🔖
Laurence-Moon (-Bardet)-Biedl syndrome

● **Q89 Other congenital malformations, not elsewhere classified**

● **Q89.0 Congenital absence and malformations of spleen**

Excludes1 isomerism of atrial appendages (with asplenia or polysplenia) (Q20.6)

Q89.01 Asplenia (congenital) 🔖🔖

Q89.09 Congenital malformations of spleen 🔖🔖
Congenital splenomegaly

Q89.1 Congenital malformations of adrenal gland 🔖

Excludes1 adrenogenital disorders (E25.-)
congenital adrenal hyperplasia (E25.0)

Q89.2 Congenital malformations of other endocrine glands 🔖
Congenital malformation of parathyroid or thyroid gland
Persistent thyroglossal duct
Thyroglossal cyst

Excludes1 congenital goiter (E03.0)
congenital hypothyroidism (E03.1)

Q89.3 Situs inversus 🔖🔖
Lateral transposition of viscera of thorax and abdomen
Dextrocardia with situs inversus
Mirror-image atrial arrangement with situs inversus
Situs inversus or transversus abdominalis
Situs inversus or transversus thoracis
Transposition of abdominal viscera
Transposition of thoracic viscera

Excludes1 dextrocardia NOS (Q24.0)

Q89.4 Conjoined twins 🔖🔖
Craniopagus
Dicephaly
Pygopagus
Thoracopagus

Q89.7 Multiple congenital malformations, not elsewhere classified 🔖
Multiple congenital anomalies NOS
Multiple congenital deformities NOS

Excludes1 congenital malformation syndromes affecting multiple systems (Q87.-)

Q89.8 Other specified congenital malformations 🔖🔖

Use additional code(s) to identify all associated manifestations

▪ **Q89.9 Congenital malformation, unspecified** 🔖
Congenital anomaly NOS
Congenital deformity NOS

● Unacceptable Principal Diagnosis　　🔖 Use Additional Character(s)　　▪ Unspecified　　▶ Manifestation Code
OGCR Official Guidelines for Coding and Reporting　Excludes 1　Excludes 2　Includes　Use additional　Code first　Code also

CHROMOSOMAL ABNORMALITIES, NOT ELSEWHERE CLASSIFIED (Q90-Q99)

Excludes2   mitochondrial metabolic disorders (E88.4-)

● **Q90   Down syndrome**

Use additional code(s) to identify any associated physical conditions and degree of intellectual disabilities (F70-F79)

Q90.0   **Trisomy 21, nonmosaicism (meiotic nondisjunction)** 🗞

Q90.1   **Trisomy 21, mosaicism (mitotic nondisjunction)** 🗞

Q90.2   **Trisomy 21, translocation** 🗞

◼ Q90.9   **Down syndrome, unspecified** 🗞
Trisomy 21 NOS

● **Q91   Trisomy 18 and Trisomy 13**

Q91.0   **Trisomy 18, nonmosaicism (meiotic nondisjunction)** 🞇🗞

Q91.1   **Trisomy 18, mosaicism (mitotic nondisjunction)** 🞇🗞

Q91.2   **Trisomy 18, translocation** 🞇🗞

◼ Q91.3   **Trisomy 18, unspecified** 🞇🗞

Q91.4   **Trisomy 13, nonmosaicism (meiotic nondisjunction)** 🞇🗞

Q91.5   **Trisomy 13, mosaicism (mitotic nondisjunction)** 🞇🗞

Q91.6   **Trisomy 13, translocation** 🞇🗞

◼ Q91.7   **Trisomy 13, unspecified** 🞇🗞

● **Q92   Other trisomies and partial trisomies of the autosomes, not elsewhere classified**

Includes   unbalanced translocations and insertions

Excludes1   trisomies of chromosomes 13, 18, 21 (Q90-Q91)

Q92.0   **Whole chromosome trisomy, nonmosaicism (meiotic nondisjunction)** 🗞

Q92.1   **Whole chromosome trisomy, mosaicism (mitotic nondisjunction)** 🗞

Q92.2   **Partial trisomy** 🗞
Less than whole arm duplicated
Whole arm or more duplicated

Excludes1   partial trisomy due to unbalanced translocation (Q92.5)

Q92.5   **Duplications with other complex rearrangements** 🗞
Partial trisomy due to unbalanced translocations

Code also any associated deletions due to unbalanced translocations, inversions and insertions (Q93.7)

● Q92.6   **Marker chromosomes**
Trisomies due to dicentrics
Trisomies due to extra rings
Trisomies due to isochromosomes
Individual with marker heterochromatin

Q92.61   **Marker chromosomes in normal individual** 🗞

Q92.62   **Marker chromosomes in abnormal individual** 🗞

Q92.7   **Triploidy and polyploidy** 🗞

Q92.8   **Other specified trisomies and partial trisomies of autosomes** 🗞
Duplications identified by fluorescence in situ hybridization (FISH)
Duplications identified by in situ hybridization (ISH)
Duplications seen only at prometaphase

◼ Q92.9   **Trisomy and partial trisomy of autosomes, unspecified** 🗞

● **Q93   Monosomies and deletions from the autosomes, not elsewhere classified**

Q93.0   **Whole chromosome monosomy, nonmosaicism (meiotic nondisjunction)** 🗞

Q93.1   **Whole chromosome monosomy, mosaicism (mitotic nondisjunction)** 🗞

Q93.2   **Chromosome replaced with ring, dicentric or isochromosome** 🗞

Q93.3   **Deletion of short arm of chromosome 4** 🞇🗞
Wolff-Hirschorn syndrome

Q93.4   **Deletion of short arm of chromosome 5** 🞇🗞
Cri-du-chat syndrome

Q93.5   **Other deletions of part of a chromosome** 🞇🗞
Angelman syndrome

Q93.7   **Deletions with other complex rearrangements** 🞇🗞
Deletions due to unbalanced translocations, inversions and insertions

Code also any associated duplications due to unbalanced translocations, inversions and insertions (Q92.5)

● Q93.8   **Other deletions from the autosomes**

Q93.81   **Velo-cardio-facial syndrome** 🞇🗞
Deletion 22q11.2

Q93.88   **Other microdeletions Miller-Dieker syndrome** 🞇🗞
Smith-Magenis syndrome

Q93.89   **Other deletions from the autosomes** 🞇🗞
Deletions identified by fluorescence in situ hybridization (FISH)
Deletions identified by in situ hybridization (ISH)
Deletions seen only at prometaphase

◼ Q93.9   **Deletion from autosomes, unspecified** 🞇🗞

● **Q95   Balanced rearrangements and structural markers, not elsewhere classified**

Includes   Robertsonian and balanced reciprocal translocations and insertions

Q95.0   **Balanced translocation and insertion in normal individual** 🗞

Q95.1   **Chromosome inversion in normal individual** 🗞

Q95.2   **Balanced autosomal rearrangement in abnormal individual** 🗞

Q95.3   **Balanced sex/autosomal rearrangement in abnormal individual** 🗞

Q95.5   **Individual with autosomal fragile site** 🗞

Q95.8   **Other balanced rearrangements and structural markers** 🗞

◼ Q95.9   **Balanced rearrangement and structural marker, unspecified** 🗞

CHAPTER 17 (Q00-Q99)

N Newborn Age: 0   **P** Pediatric Age: 0–17   **M** Maternity DX: 12–55   **A** Adult Age: 15–124   ♀ Females Only   ♂ Males Only

🗞 Complication\Comorbidity   🗞 Major C\C   🗞 Present on Admission Requirement   🗞 Hospital-Acquired Condition

1363

● **Q96 Turner's syndrome**
Caused by missing or incomplete X chromosome affecting growth and sexual development
> **Excludes1**   Noonan syndrome (Q87.1)

Q96.0   Karyotype 45, X ♀

Q96.1   Karyotype 46, X iso (Xq) ♀
    Karyotype 46, isochromosome Xq

Q96.2   Karyotype 46, X with abnormal sex chromosome, except iso (Xq) ♀
    Karyotype 46, X with abnormal sex chromosome, except isochromosome Xq

Q96.3   Mosaicism, 45, X/46, XX or XY ♀

Q96.4   Mosaicism, 45, X/other cell line(s) with abnormal sex chromosome ♀

Q96.8   Other variants of Turner's syndrome ♀

■ Q96.9   Turner's syndrome, unspecified ♀

● **Q97 Other sex chromosome abnormalities, female phenotype, not elsewhere classified**
> **Excludes1**   Turner's syndrome (Q96.-)

Q97.0   Karyotype 47, XXX ♀

Q97.1   Female with more than three X chromosomes ♀

Q97.2   Mosaicism, lines with various numbers of X chromosomes ♀

Q97.3   Female with 46, XY karyotype ♀

Q97.8   Other specified sex chromosome abnormalities, female phenotype ♀

■ Q97.9   Sex chromosome abnormality, female phenotype, unspecified ♀

● **Q98 Other sex chromosome abnormalities, male phenotype, not elsewhere classified**

Q98.0   Klinefelter syndrome karyotype 47, XXY ♂

Q98.1   Klinefelter syndrome, male with more than two X chromosomes ♂

Q98.3   Other male with 46, XX karyotype ♂

■ Q98.4   Klinefelter syndrome, unspecified ♂

Q98.5   Karyotype 47, XYY

Q98.6   Male with structurally abnormal sex chromosome ♂

Q98.7   Male with sex chromosome mosaicism ♂

Q98.8   Other specified sex chromosome abnormalities, male phenotype ♂

■ Q98.9   Sex chromosome abnormality, male phenotype, unspecified ♂

● **Q99 Other chromosome abnormalities, not elsewhere classified**

Q99.0   Chimera 46, XX/46, XY
    Chimera 46, XX/46, XY true hermaphrodite

Q99.1   46, XX true hermaphrodite
    46, XX with streak gonads
    46, XY with streak gonads
    Pure gonadal dysgenesis

Q99.2   Fragile X chromosome
    Fragile X syndrome

Q99.8   Other specified chromosome abnormalities

■ Q99.9   Chromosomal abnormality, unspecified

[handwritten: NOT TO BE USED AS A PRIN DIAG]

[handwritten: when Deb. Dx has been established]

OGCR Section I.B.4.

Signs and symptoms

Codes that describe symptoms and signs, as opposed to diagnoses, are acceptable for reporting purposes when a related definitive diagnosis has not been established (confirmed) by the provider. Chapter 18 of ICD-10-CM, Symptoms, Signs, and Abnormal Clinical and Laboratory Findings, Not Elsewhere Classified (codes R00.0-R99) contains many, but not all codes for symptoms.

Section I.C.18.a. to c.

Symptoms, signs, and abnormal clinical and laboratory findings, not elsewhere classified.

Chapter 18 includes symptoms, signs, abnormal results of clinical or other investigative procedures, and ill-defined conditions regarding which no diagnosis classifiable elsewhere is recorded. Signs and symptoms that point to a specific diagnosis have been assigned to a category in other chapters of the classification.

a. Use of symptom codes

Codes that describe symptoms and signs are acceptable for reporting purposes when a related definitive diagnosis has not been established (confirmed) by the provider.

b. Use of a symptom code with a definitive diagnosis code

Codes for signs and symptoms may be reported in addition to a related definitive diagnosis when the sign or symptom is not routinely associated with that diagnosis, such as the various signs and symptoms associated with complex syndromes. The definitive diagnosis code should be sequenced before the symptom code.

Signs or symptoms that are associated routinely with a disease process should not be assigned as additional codes, unless otherwise instructed by the classification.

c. Combination codes that include symptoms

ICD-10-CM contains a number of combination codes that identify both the definitive diagnosis and common symptoms of that diagnosis. When using one of these combination codes, an additional code should not be assigned for the symptom.

CHAPTER 18

SYMPTOMS, SIGNS AND ABNORMAL CLINICAL AND LABORATORY FINDINGS, NOT ELSEWHERE CLASSIFIED (R00-R99)

Note: This chapter includes symptoms, signs, abnormal results of clinical or other investigative procedures, and ill-defined conditions regarding which no diagnosis classifiable elsewhere is recorded.

Signs and symptoms that point rather definitely to a given diagnosis have been assigned to a category in other chapters of the classification. In general, categories in this chapter include the less well-defined conditions and symptoms that, without the necessary study of the case to establish a final diagnosis, point perhaps equally to two or more diseases or to two or more systems of the body. Practically all categories in the chapter could be designated 'not otherwise specified', 'unknown etiology' or 'transient'. The Alphabetical Index should be consulted to determine which symptoms and signs are to be allocated here and which to other chapters. The residual subcategories, numbered .8, are generally provided for other relevant symptoms that cannot be allocated elsewhere in the classification.

The conditions and signs or symptoms included in categories R00-R94 consist of:
(a) cases for which no more specific diagnosis can be made even after all the facts bearing on the case have been investigated:

(b) signs or symptoms existing at the time of initial encounter that proved to be transient and whose causes could not be determined;
(c) provisional diagnosis in a patient who failed to return for further investigation or care;
(d) cases referred elsewhere for investigation or treatment before the diagnosis was made;
(e) cases in which a more precise diagnosis was not available for any other reason;
(f) certain symptoms, for which supplementary information is provided, that represent important problems in medical care in their own right.

| Excludes2 | abnormal findings on antenatal screening of mother (O28.-)
certain conditions originating in the perinatal period (P04-P96)
signs and symptoms classified in the body system chapters
signs and symptoms of breast (N63, N64.5)

This chapter contains the following blocks:

R00-R09	Symptoms and signs involving the circulatory and respiratory systems
R10-R19	Symptoms and signs involving the digestive system and abdomen
R20-R23	Symptoms and signs involving the skin and subcutaneous tissue
R25-R29	Symptoms and signs involving the nervous and musculoskeletal systems
R30-R39	Symptoms and signs involving the genitourinary system
R40-R46	Symptoms and signs involving cognition, perception, emotional state and behavior
R47-R49	Symptoms and signs involving speech and voice
R50-R69	General symptoms and signs
R70-R79	Abnormal findings on examination of blood, without diagnosis
R80-R82	Abnormal findings on examination of urine, without diagnosis
R83-R89	Abnormal findings on examination of other body fluids, substances and tissues, without diagnosis
R90-R94	Abnormal findings on diagnostic imaging and in function studies, without diagnosis
R97	Abnormal tumor markers
R99	Ill-defined and unknown cause of mortality

SYMPTOMS AND SIGNS INVOLVING THE CIRCULATORY AND RESPIRATORY SYSTEMS (R00-R09)

● **R00 Abnormalities of heart beat**

| Excludes1 | abnormalities originating in the perinatal period (P29.1-)
specified arrhythmias (I47-I49)

■ **R00.0 Tachycardia, unspecified**
Rapid heart rate >100 beats
Rapid heart beat
Sinoauricular tachycardia NOS
Sinus [sinusal] tachycardia NOS

| Excludes1 | neonatal tachycardia (P29.11)
paroxysmal tachycardia (I47.-)

CHAPTER 18 (R00-R99)

◨ **R00.1 Bradycardia, unspecified**
Slow heart rate, <60
Sinoatrial bradycardia
Sinus bradycardia
Slow heart beat
Vagal bradycardia

Use additional code for adverse effect, if applicable, to identify drug (T36-T50 with fifth or sixth character 5)

Excludes1   neonatal bradycardia (P29.12)

R00.2 Palpitations
Awareness of heart beat

R00.8 Other abnormalities of heart beat

◨ **R00.9 Unspecified abnormalities of heart beat**

● **R01 Cardiac murmurs and other cardiac sounds**

Excludes1   cardiac murmurs and sounds originating in the perinatal period (P29.8)

R01.0 Benign and innocent cardiac murmurs
Functional cardiac murmur

◨ **R01.1 Cardiac murmur, unspecified**
Cardiac bruit NOS
Heart murmur NOS

R01.2 Other cardiac sounds
Cardiac dullness, increased or decreased
Precordial friction

OGCR Section I.C.9.a.7.

Hypertension, Transient

Assign code R03.0, Elevated blood pressure reading without diagnosis of hypertension, unless patient has an established diagnosis of hypertension. Assign code O13.-, Gestational [pregnancy-induced] hypertension with significant proteinuria, or O14.-, Pre-eclampsia, for transient hypertension of pregnancy.

● **R03 Abnormal blood-pressure reading, without diagnosis**

R03.0 Elevated blood-pressure reading, without diagnosis of hypertension

Note: This category is to be used to record an episode of elevated blood pressure in a patient in whom no formal diagnosis of hypertension has been made, or as an isolated incidental finding.

MCE: Questionable admission when principal dx

R03.1 Nonspecific low blood-pressure reading

Excludes1   hypotension (I95.-)
maternal hypotension syndrome (O26.5-)
neurogenic orthostatic hypotension (G90.3)

● **R04 Hemorrhage from respiratory passages**

R04.0 Epistaxis
Hemorrhage from nose
Nosebleed

R04.1 Hemorrhage from throat

Excludes2   hemoptysis (R04.2)

R04.2 Hemoptysis ◉
Blood-stained sputum
Cough with hemorrhage

● **R04.8 Hemorrhage from other sites in respiratory passages**

R04.81 Acute idiopathic pulmonary hemorrhage in infants ◉   P
AIPHI
Acute idiopathic hemorrhage in infants over 28 days old

Excludes1   perinatal pulmonary hemorrhage (P26.-)
von Willebrand's disease (D68.0)

R04.89 Hemorrhage from other sites in respiratory passages ◉
Pulmonary hemorrhage NOS

◨ **R04.9 Hemorrhage from respiratory passages, unspecified** ◉

R05 Cough

Excludes1   cough with hemorrhage (R04.2)
smoker's cough (J41.0)

● **R06 Abnormalities of breathing**

Excludes1   acute respiratory distress syndrome (J80)
respiratory arrest (R09.2)
respiratory arrest of newborn (P28.81)
respiratory distress syndrome of newborn (P22.-)
respiratory failure (J96.-)
respiratory failure of newborn (P28.5)

● **R06.0 Dyspnea**

Excludes1   tachypnea NOS (R06.82)
transient tachypnea of newborn (P22.1)

R06.00 Dyspnea, unspecified

R06.01 Orthopnea

R06.02 Shortness of breath

R06.09 Other forms of dyspnea

R06.1 Stridor
Harsh, high-pitched breath sound

Excludes1   congenital laryngeal stridor (P28.89)
laryngismus (stridulus) (J38.5)

R06.2 Wheezing

Excludes1   Asthma (J45.-)

R06.3 Periodic breathing ◉
Cheyne-Stokes breathing
An abnormal pattern of breathing with gradually increasing and decreasing tidal volume with some periods of apnea

R06.4 Hyperventilation

Excludes1   psychogenic hyperventilation (F45.8)

R06.5 Mouth breathing

Excludes2   dry mouth NOS (R68.2)

R06.6 Hiccough

Excludes1   psychogenic hiccough (F45.8)

R06.7 Sneezing

● Unacceptable Principal Diagnosis   ● Use Additional Character(s)   ◨ Unspecified   ▶ Manifestation Code
OGCR Official Guidelines for Coding and Reporting   Excludes 1   Excludes 2   Includes   Use additional   Code first   Code also

● **R06.8**   **Other abnormalities of breathing**

     R06.81   **Apnea, not elsewhere classified**
         Apnea NOS

         | Excludes1 | apnea (of) newborn (P28.4)
                            sleep apnea (G47.3-)
                            sleep apnea of newborn
                               (primary) (P28.3)

     R06.82   **Tachypnea, not elsewhere classified**
         Tachypnea NOS

         | Excludes1 | transitory tachypnea of
                            newborn (P22.1)

     R06.83   **Snoring**

     R06.89   **Other abnormalities of breathing**
         Breath-holding (spells)
         Sighing

■ **R06.9**   **Unspecified abnormalities of breathing**

● **R07**   **Pain in throat and chest**

     | Excludes1 | epidemic myalgia (B33.0)
     | Excludes2 | jaw pain R68.84
                       pain in breast (N64.4)

     R07.0   **Pain in throat**

         | Excludes1 | chronic sore throat (J31.2)
                             sore throat (acute) NOS (J02.9)

         | Excludes2 | dysphagia (R13.1-)
                             pain in neck (M54.2)

     R07.1   **Chest pain on breathing**
         Painful respiration

     R07.2   **Precordial pain**

●   **R07.8**   **Other chest pain**

     R07.81   **Pleurodynia**
         Pleurodynia NOS

         | Excludes1 | epidemic pleurodynia
                             (B33.0)

     R07.82   **Intercostal pain**

     R07.89   **Other chest pain**
         Anterior chest-wall pain NOS

■ **R07.9**   **Chest pain, unspecified**

● **R09**   **Other symptoms and signs involving the circulatory and respiratory system**

     | Excludes1 | acute respiratory distress syndrome (J80)
                       respiratory arrest of newborn (P28.81)
                       respiratory distress syndrome of newborn
                            (P22.0)
                       respiratory failure (J96.-)
                       respiratory failure of newborn (P28.5)

● **R09.0**   **Asphyxia and hypoxemia**

     | Excludes1 | asphyxia due to carbon monoxide
                           (T58.-)
                       asphyxia due to foreign body in
                           respiratory tract (T17.-)
                       birth (intrauterine) asphyxia (P84)
                       hypercapnia (R06.4)
                       hyperventilation (R06.4)
                       traumatic asphyxia (T71-)

     R09.01   **Asphyxia** 🔹

     R09.02   **Hypoxemia**

R09.1   **Pleurisy**
     *Occurs when double membrane (pleura) lining chest
     cavity and lung surface becomes inflamed causing
     sharp pain on inspiration/expiration.*

     | Excludes1 | pleurisy with effusion (J90)

R09.2   **Respiratory arrest** 🔹
     Cardiorespiratory failure

     | Excludes1 | cardiac arrest (I46.-)
                       respiratory arrest of newborn
                           (P28.81)
                       respiratory distress of newborn
                           (P22.0)
                       respiratory failure (J96.-)
                       respiratory failure of newborn
                           (P28.5)
                       respiratory insufficiency (R06.89)
                       respiratory insufficiency of newborn
                           (P28.5)

     MCC: Only if patient discharged alive

R09.3   **Abnormal sputum**
     Abnormal amount of sputum
     Abnormal color of sputum
     Abnormal odor of sputum
     Excessive sputum

     | Excludes1 | blood-stained sputum (R04.2)

● **R09.8**   **Other specified symptoms and signs involving the circulatory and respiratory systems**

     R09.81   **Nasal congestion**

     R09.82   **Postnasal drip**

     R09.89   **Other specified symptoms and signs involving the circulatory and respiratory systems**
         Bruit (arterial)
         Abnormal chest percussion
         Feeling of foreign body in throat
         Friction sounds in chest
         Chest tympany
         Choking sensation
         Rales
            *Wet rattling, clicking, crackling sounds on
              auscultation*
         Weak pulse

         | Excludes2 | foreign body in throat
                           (T17.2-)
                       wheezing (R06.2)

SYMPTOMS AND SIGNS INVOLVING THE DIGESTIVE SYSTEM AND ABDOMEN (R10-R19)

| Excludes1 | congenital or infantile pylorospasm (Q40.0)
                       gastrointestinal hemorrhage (K92.0-K92.2)
                       intestinal obstruction (K56.-)
                       newborn gastrointestinal hemorrhage
                           (P54.0-P54.3)
                       newborn intestinal obstruction (P76.-)
                       pylorospasm (K31.3)
                       signs and symptoms involving the urinary
                           system (R30-R39)
                       symptoms referable to female genital organs
                           (N94.-)
                       symptoms referable to male genital organs
                           male (N48-N50)

N   Newborn Age: 0   **P**   Pediatric Age: 0–17   **M**   Maternity DX: 12–55   **A**   Adult Age: 15–124   ♀   Females Only   ♂   Males Only

🔹   Complication\Comorbidity   🔹   Major C\C   🔹   Present on Admission Requirement   🔹   Hospital-Acquired Condition

1367

● R10   Abdominal and pelvic pain
> **Excludes1** renal colic (N23)
> **Excludes2** dorsalgia (M54.-)
> flatulence and related conditions (R14.-)

R10.0   Acute abdomen
Severe abdominal pain (generalized) (with abdominal rigidity)
> **Excludes1** abdominal rigidity NOS (R19.3)
> generalized abdominal pain NOS (R10.84)
> localized abdominal pain (R10.1-R10.3-)

● R10.1   Pain localized to upper abdomen
◻ R10.10   Upper abdominal pain, unspecified
R10.11   Right upper quadrant pain
R10.12   Left upper quadrant pain
R10.13   Epigastric pain
Dyspepsia
> **Excludes1** functional dyspepsia (K30)

R10.2   Pelvic and perineal pain
> **Excludes1** vulvodynia (N94.81)

● R10.3   Pain localized to other parts of lower abdomen
◻ R10.30   Lower abdominal pain, unspecified
R10.31   Right lower quadrant pain
R10.32   Left lower quadrant pain
R10.33   Periumbilical pain

● R10.8   Other abdominal pain
● R10.81   Abdominal tenderness
Abdominal tenderness NOS
R10.811   Right upper quadrant abdominal tenderness
R10.812   Left upper quadrant abdominal tenderness
R10.813   Right lower quadrant abdominal tenderness
R10.814   Left lower quadrant abdominal tenderness
R10.815   Periumbilic abdominal tenderness
R10.816   Epigastric abdominal tenderness
R10.817   Generalized abdominal tenderness
◻ R10.819   Abdominal tenderness, unspecified site

● R10.82   Rebound abdominal tenderness
R10.821   Right upper quadrant rebound abdominal tenderness
R10.822   Left upper quadrant rebound abdominal tenderness
R10.823   Right lower quadrant rebound abdominal tenderness
R10.824   Left lower quadrant rebound abdominal tenderness
R10.825   Periumbilic rebound abdominal tenderness
R10.826   Epigastric rebound abdominal tenderness
R10.827   Generalized rebound abdominal tenderness
◻ R10.829   Rebound abdominal tenderness, unspecified site

R10.83   Colic   P
Colic NOS
Infantile colic
> **Excludes1** colic in adult and child over 12 months old (R10.84)

R10.84   Generalized abdominal pain
> **Excludes1** generalized abdominal pain associated with acute abdomen (R10.0)

◻ R10.9   Unspecified abdominal pain

● R11   Nausea and vomiting
> **Excludes1** cyclical vomiting associated with migraine (G43.A-)
> excessive vomiting in pregnancy (O21.-)
> hematemesis (K92.0)
> neonatal hematemesis (P54.0)
> newborn vomiting (P92.0-)
> psychogenic vomiting (F50.8)
> vomiting associated with bulimia nervosa (F50.2)
> vomiting following gastrointestinal surgery (K91.0)

● R11.0   Nausea
Nausea NOS
Nausea without vomiting

● R11.1   Vomiting
◻ R11.10   Vomiting, unspecified
Vomiting NOS
R11.11   Vomiting without nausea
R11.12   Projectile vomiting
R11.13   Vomiting of fecal matter
R11.14   Bilious vomiting
Bilious emesis

◻ R11.2   Nausea with vomiting, unspecified
Persistent nausea with vomiting NOS

R12   Heartburn
> **Excludes1** dyspepsia NOS (R10.13)
> functional dyspepsia (K30)

● R13   Aphagia and dysphagia
R13.0   Aphagia
Inability to swallow
> **Excludes1** psychogenic aphagia (F50.9)

● R13.1   Dysphagia
Difficulty swallowing
Code first, if applicable, dysphagia following cerebrovascular disease (I69. with final characters -91)
> **Excludes1** psychogenic dysphagia (F45.8)
◻ R13.10   Dysphagia, unspecified
Difficulty in swallowing NOS
R13.11   Dysphagia, oral phase
R13.12   Dysphagia, oropharyngeal phase
R13.13   Dysphagia, pharyngeal phase
R13.14   Dysphagia, pharyngoesophageal phase
R13.19   Other dysphagia
Cervical dysphagia
Neurogenic dysphagia

CHAPTER 18 (R00-R99)

1368
● Unacceptable Principal Diagnosis   ● Use Additional Character(s)   ◻ Unspecified   ▸ Manifestation Code
OGCR Official Guidelines for Coding and Reporting   Excludes 1   Excludes 2   Includes   Use additional   Code first   Code also

● **R14**   **Flatulence and related conditions**
     Excludes1   psychogenic aerophagy (F45.8)

   R14.0   **Abdominal distension (gaseous)**
      Bloating
      Tympanites (abdominal) (intestinal)

   R14.1   **Gas pain**

   R14.2   **Eructation**
      Belching air from stomach through mouth

   R14.3   **Flatulence**

● **R15**   **Fecal incontinence**
     Includes   encopresis NOS
     Excludes1   fecal incontinence of nonorganic origin
               (F98.1)

   R15.0   **Incomplete defecation**
      Excludes1   constipation (K59.0-)
                 fecal impaction (K56.41)

   R15.1   **Fecal smearing**
      Fecal soiling

   R15.2   **Fecal urgency**

   R15.9   **Full incontinence of feces**
      Fecal incontinence NOS

● **R16**   **Hepatomegaly and splenomegaly, not elsewhere classified**
     Enlargement of liver or spleen

   R16.0   **Hepatomegaly, not elsewhere classified**
      Hepatomegaly NOS

   R16.1   **Splenomegaly, not elsewhere classified**
      Splenomegaly NOS

   R16.2   **Hepatomegaly with splenomegaly, not elsewhere classified**
      Hepatosplenomegaly NOS

■ **R17**   **Unspecified jaundice** 🦠
     Excludes1   neonatal jaundice (P55, P57-P59)

● **R18**   **Ascites**
     Includes   fluid in peritoneal cavity
     Excludes1   ascites in alcoholic cirrhosis (K70.31)
                 ascites in alcoholic hepatitis (K70.11)
                 ascites in toxic liver disease with chronic
                   active hepatitis (K71.51)

   ● **R18.0**   **Malignant ascites** 🦠
      Code first malignancy, such as:
        malignant neoplasm of ovary (C56.-)
        secondary malignant neoplasm of
          retroperitoneum and peritoneum (C78.6)

   R18.8   **Other ascites** 🦠
      Ascites NOS
      Peritoneal effusion (chronic)

● **R19**   **Other symptoms and signs involving the digestive system and abdomen**
     Excludes1   acute abdomen (R10.0)

   ● **R19.0**   **Intra-abdominal and pelvic swelling, mass and lump**
      Excludes1   abdominal distension (gaseous)
                 (R14.-)
                 ascites (R18.-)

     ■ **R19.00**   **Intra-abdominal and pelvic swelling, mass and lump, unspecified site**

     R19.01   **Right upper quadrant abdominal swelling, mass and lump**

     R19.02   **Left upper quadrant abdominal swelling, mass and lump**

     R19.03   **Right lower quadrant abdominal swelling, mass and lump**

     R19.04   **Left lower quadrant abdominal swelling, mass and lump**

     R19.05   **Periumbilic swelling, mass or lump**
       Diffuse or generalized umbilical swelling
         or mass

     R19.06   **Epigastric swelling, mass or lump**

     R19.07   **Generalized intra-abdominal and pelvic swelling, mass and lump**
       Diffuse or generalized intra-abdominal
         swelling or mass NOS
       Diffuse or generalized pelvic swelling or
         mass NOS

     R19.09   **Other intra-abdominal and pelvic swelling, mass and lump**

   ● **R19.1**   **Abnormal bowel sounds**

     R19.11   **Absent bowel sounds**

     R19.12   **Hyperactive bowel sounds**

     R19.15   **Other abnormal bowel sounds**
       Abnormal bowel sounds NOS

   R19.2   **Visible peristalsis**
      Hyperperistalsis

   ● **R19.3**   **Abdominal rigidity**
     Excludes1   abdominal rigidity with severe
                 abdominal pain (R10.0)

     ■ **R19.30**   **Abdominal rigidity, unspecified site**

     R19.31   **Right upper quadrant abdominal rigidity**

     R19.32   **Left upper quadrant abdominal rigidity**

     R19.33   **Right lower quadrant abdominal rigidity**

     R19.34   **Left lower quadrant abdominal rigidity**

     R19.35   **Periumbilic abdominal rigidity**

     R19.36   **Epigastric abdominal rigidity**

     R19.37   **Generalized abdominal rigidity**

   R19.4   **Change in bowel habit**
     Excludes1   constipation (K59.0-)
                 functional diarrhea (K59.1)

   R19.5   **Other fecal abnormalities**
      Abnormal stool color
      Bulky stools
      Mucus in stools
      Occult blood in feces
      Occult blood in stools
     Excludes1   melena (K92.1)
                 neonatal melena (P54.1)

   R19.6   **Halitosis**

   ■ **R19.7**   **Diarrhea, unspecified**
      Diarrhea NOS
     Excludes1   functional diarrhea (K59.1)
                 neonatal diarrhea (P78.3)
                 psychogenic diarrhea (F45.8)

   R19.8   **Other specified symptoms and signs involving the digestive system and abdomen**

N   Newborn Age: 0   **P**   Pediatric Age: 0–17   **M**   Maternity DX: 12–55   **A**   Adult Age: 15–124   ♀   Females Only   ♂   Males Only

🦠   Complication\Comorbidity   🦠   Major C\C   🦠   Present on Admission Requirement   🦠   Hospital-Acquired Condition

1369

CHAPTER 18 (R00-R99)

CHAPTER 18 (R00-R99)

SYMPTOMS AND SIGNS INVOLVING THE SKIN AND SUBCUTANEOUS TISSUE (R20-R23)

Excludes2   symptoms relating to breast (N64.4-N64.5)

● **R20   Disturbances of skin sensation**

Excludes1   dissociative anesthesia and sensory loss (F44.6)
psychogenic disturbances (F45.8)

R20.0   Anesthesia of skin
Loss of sensation

R20.1   Hypoesthesia of skin
Unpleasant abnormal sensation

R20.2   Paresthesia of skin
Abnormal touch sensation, including burning, prickling, often in absence of external stimulus
Formication   Tingling skin
Pins and needles

Excludes1   acroparesthesia (I73.8)

R20.3   Hyperesthesia

R20.8   Other disturbances of skin sensation

■ **R20.9   Unspecified disturbances of skin sensation**

R21   Rash and other nonspecific skin eruption

Includes   rash NOS

Excludes1   specified type of rash- code to condition
vesicular eruption (R23.8)

● **R22   Localized swelling, mass and lump of skin and subcutaneous tissue**

Includes   subcutaneous nodules (localized) (superficial)

Excludes1   abnormal findings on diagnostic imaging (R90-R93)
edema (R60.-)
enlarged lymph nodes (R59.-)
localized adiposity (E65)
swelling of joint (M25.4-)

R22.0   Localized swelling, mass and lump, head

R22.1   Localized swelling, mass and lump, neck

R22.2   Localized swelling, mass and lump, trunk

Excludes1   intra-abdominal or pelvic mass and lump (R19.0-)
intra-abdominal or pelvic swelling (R19.0-)

Excludes2   breast mass and lump (N63)

● **R22.3   Localized swelling, mass and lump, upper limb**

■ **R22.30   Localized swelling, mass and lump, unspecified upper limb**

R22.31   Localized swelling, mass and lump, right upper limb

R22.32   Localized swelling, mass and lump, left upper limb

R22.33   Localized swelling, mass and lump, upper limb, bilateral

● **R22.4   Localized swelling, mass and lump, lower limb**

■ **R22.40   Localized swelling, mass and lump, unspecified lower limb**

R22.41   Localized swelling, mass and lump, right lower limb

R22.42   Localized swelling, mass and lump, left lower limb

R22.43   Localized swelling, mass and lump, lower limb, bilateral

■ **R22.9   Localized swelling, mass and lump, unspecified**

● **R23   Other skin changes**

R23.0   Cyanosis

Excludes1   acrocyanosis (I73.8)
cyanotic attacks of newborn (P28.2)

R23.1   Pallor
Clammy skin

R23.2   Flushing
Excessive blushing

Code first, if applicable, menopausal and female climacteric states (N95.1)

R23.3   Spontaneous ecchymoses
Small hemorrhagic spot of skin; AKA black and blue spot
Petechiae

Excludes1   ecchymoses of newborn (P54.5)
purpura (D69.-)

R23.4   Changes in skin texture
Desquamation of skin   Scaling of skin
Induration of skin

Excludes1   epidermal thickening NOS (L85.9)

R23.8   Other skin changes

■ **R23.9   Unspecified skin changes**

SYMPTOMS AND SIGNS INVOLVING THE NERVOUS AND MUSCULOSKELETAL SYSTEMS (R25-R29)

● **R25   Abnormal involuntary movements**

Excludes1   specific movement disorders (G20-G26)
stereotyped movement disorders (F98.4)
tic disorders (F95.-)

R25.0   Abnormal head movements

■ **R25.1   Tremor, unspecified**

Excludes1   chorea NOS (G25.5)
essential tremor (G25.0)
hysterical tremor (F44.4)
intention tremor (G25.2)

R25.2   Cramp and spasm

Excludes2   carpopedal spasm (R29.0)
charley-horse (M62.831)
infantile spasms (G40.4-)
muscle spasm of back (M62.830)
muscle spasm of calf (M62.831)

R25.3   Fasciculation
Twitching NOS

R25.8   Other abnormal involuntary movements

■ **R25.9   Unspecified abnormal involuntary movements**

● **R26   Abnormalities of gait and mobility**

Excludes1   ataxia NOS (R27.0)
hereditary ataxia (G11.-)
locomotor (syphilitic) ataxia (A52.11)
immobility syndrome (paraplegic) (M62.3)

R26.0   Ataxic gait
Staggering gait

R26.1   Paralytic gait
Spastic gait

R26.2   Difficulty in walking, not elsewhere classified

Excludes1   falling (R29.6)
unsteadiness on feet (R26.81)

● **R26.8   Other abnormalities of gait and mobility**

R26.81   Unsteadiness on feet

R26.89   Other abnormalities of gait and mobility

■ **R26.9   Unspecified abnormalities of gait and mobility**

● Unacceptable Principal Diagnosis   ● Use Additional Character(s)   ■ Unspecified   ▶ Manifestation Code

OGCR   Official Guidelines for Coding and Reporting   Excludes 1   Excludes 2   Includes   Use additional   Code first   Code also

● **R27   Other lack of coordination**
> **Excludes1**   ataxic gait (R26.0)
> hereditary ataxia (G11.-)
> vertigo NOS (R42)

◼ **R27.0   Ataxia, unspecified**
> **Excludes1**   ataxia following cerebrovascular disease (I69. with final characters -93)

R27.8   Other lack of coordination

◼ **R27.9   Unspecified lack of coordination**

● **R29   Other symptoms and signs involving the nervous and musculoskeletal systems**

R29.0   Tetany 🔗
> *Hyperexcitability of nerves and muscles characterized by spasm, twitching, and cramps*
> Carpopedal spasm
> **Excludes1**   hysterical tetany (F44.5)
> neonatal tetany (P71.3)
> parathyroid tetany (E20.9)
> post-thyroidectomy tetany (E89.2)

R29.1   Meningismus 🔗

R29.2   Abnormal reflex
> **Excludes2**   abnormal pupillary reflex (H57.0)
> hyperactive gag reflex (J39.2)
> vasovagal reaction or syncope (R55)

R29.3   Abnormal posture

R29.4   Clicking hip
> **Excludes1**   congenital deformities of hip (Q65.-)

R29.5   Transient paralysis 🔗
> *Code first* any associated spinal cord injury (S14.0, S14.1-, S24.0, S24.1-, S34.0-, S34.1-)
> **Excludes1**   transient ischemic attack (G45.9)

R29.6   Repeated falls
> Falling
> Tendency to fall
> **Excludes2**   at risk for falling (Z91.81)
> history of falling (Z91.81)

> **OGCR**   Section I.C.18.d.
>
> Repeated falls
>
> Code R29.6, Repeated falls, is for use for encounters when a patient has recently fallen and the reason for the fall is being investigated.
>
> Code Z91.81, History of falling, is for use when a patient has fallen in the past and is at risk for future falls. When appropriate, both codes R29.6 and Z91.81 may be assigned together.

● **R29.8   Other symptoms and signs involving the nervous and musculoskeletal systems**

● **R29.81   Other symptoms and signs involving the nervous system**

R29.810   Facial weakness
> Facial droop
> **Excludes1**   Bell's palsy (G51.0)
> facial weakness following cerebrovascular disease (I69. with final characters -92)

R29.818   Other symptoms and signs involving the nervous system

● **R29.89   Other symptoms and signs involving the musculoskeletal system**
> **Excludes2**   pain in limb (M79.6-)

R29.890   Loss of height
> **Excludes1**   osteoporosis (M80-M81)

R29.891   Ocular torticollis
> **Excludes1**   congenital (sterno-mastoid) torticollis Q68.0
> psychogenic torticollis (F45.8)
> spasmodic torticollis (G24.3)
> torticollis due to birth injury (P15.8)
> torticollis NOS M43.6

R29.898   Other symptoms and signs involving the musculoskeletal system

● **R29.9   Unspecified symptoms and signs involving the nervous and musculoskeletal systems**

◼ **R29.90   Unspecified symptoms and signs involving the nervous system**

◼ **R29.91   Unspecified symptoms and signs involving the musculoskeletal system**

SYMPTOMS AND SIGNS INVOLVING THE GENITOURINARY SYSTEM (R30-R39)

● **R30   Pain associated with micturition**
> **Excludes1**   psychogenic pain associated with micturition (F45.8)

R30.0   Dysuria
> *Painful urination*
> Strangury

R30.1   Vesical tenesmus
> *Straining to urinate*

◼ **R30.9   Painful micturition, unspecified**
> Painful urination NOS

● **R31   Hematuria**
> **Excludes1**   hematuria included with underlying conditions, such as:
> acute cystitis with hematuria (N30.01)
> acute prostatitis with hematuria (N41.01)
> recurrent and persistent hematuria in glomerular diseases (N02.-)

R31.0   Gross hematuria

R31.1   Benign essential microscopic hematuria

R31.2   Other microscopic hematuria

◼ **R31.9   Hematuria, unspecified**

◼ **R32   Unspecified urinary incontinence**
> Enuresis NOS
> **Excludes1**   functional urinary incontinence (R39.81)
> nonorganic enuresis (F98.0)
> stress incontinence and other specified urinary incontinence (N39.3-N39.4-)
> urinary incontinence associated with cognitive impairment (R39.81)

N   Newborn Age: 0   **P**   Pediatric Age: 0–17   **M**   Maternity DX: 12–55   **A**   Adult Age: 15–124   ♀ Females Only   ♂ Males Only

🔗 Complication\Comorbidity   🔗 Major C\C   🔗 Present on Admission Requirement   🔗 Hospital-Acquired Condition

CHAPTER 18 (R00-R99)

1371

●**R33   Retention of urine**
> **Excludes1**   psychogenic retention of urine (F45.8)

●**R33.0   Drug induced retention of urine**
> Use additional code for adverse effect, if applicable, to identify drug (T36-T50 with fifth or sixth character 5)

R33.8   Other retention of urine
> *Code first, if applicable, any causal condition, such as:* enlarged prostate (N40.1)

■**R33.9   Retention of urine, unspecified**

R34   Anuria and oliguria
> **Excludes1**   anuria and oliguria complicating abortion or ectopic or molar pregnancy (O00-O07, O08.4)
> anuria and oliguria complicating pregnancy (O26.83-)
> anuria and oliguria complicating the puerperium (O90.4)

●**R35   Polyuria**
> *Passage of excessive volume of urine*
> *Code first, if applicable, any causal condition, such as:* enlarged prostate (N40.1)
> **Excludes1**   psychogenic polyuria (F45.8)

R35.0   Frequency of micturition
> *Discharge or passage of urine; AKA uresis*

R35.1   Nocturia
> *Urinary frequency at night*

R35.8   Other polyuria
> Polyuria NOS

●**R36   Urethral discharge**

R36.0   Urethral discharge without blood

R36.1   Hematospermia ♂
> *Presence of blood in semen*

■**R36.9   Urethral discharge, unspecified**
> Penile discharge NOS
> Urethrorrhea

■**R37   Sexual dysfunction, unspecified**

●**R39   Other and unspecified symptoms and signs involving the genitourinary system**

R39.0   Extravasation of urine 🔗
> *Leakage, discharge*

●**R39.1   Other difficulties with micturition**
> *Code first, if applicable, any causal condition, such as:* enlarged prostate (N40.1)

R39.11   Hesitancy of micturition

R39.12   Poor urinary stream
> Weak urinary steam

R39.13   Splitting of urinary stream

R39.14   Feeling of incomplete bladder emptying

R39.15   Urgency of urination
> **Excludes1**   urge incontinence (N39.41, N39.46)

R39.16   Straining to void

R39.19   Other difficulties with micturition

R39.2   Extrarenal uremia
> Prerenal uremia
> **Excludes1**   uremia NOS (N19)

●**R39.8   Other symptoms and signs involving the genitourinary system**

R39.81   Functional urinary incontinence
> Urinary incontinence due to cognitive impairment, or severe physical disability or immobility
> **Excludes1**   stress incontinence and other specified urinary incontinence (N39.3-N39.4-)
> urinary incontinence NOS (R32)

R39.89   Other symptoms and signs involving the genitourinary system

■**R39.9   Unspecified symptoms and signs involving the genitourinary system**

SYMPTOMS AND SIGNS INVOLVING COGNITION, PERCEPTION, EMOTIONAL STATE AND BEHAVIOR (R40-R46)

> **Excludes1**   symptoms and signs constituting part of a pattern of mental disorder (F01-F99)

●**R40   Somnolence, stupor and coma**
> **Excludes1**   neonatal coma (P91.5)
> somnolence, stupor and coma in diabetes (E08-E13)
> somnolence, stupor and coma in hepatic failure (K72.-)
> somnolence, stupor and coma in hypoglycemia (nondiabetic) (E15)

R40.0   Somnolence
> Drowsiness
> **Excludes1**   coma (R40.2-)

R40.1   Stupor
> *Lowered level of consciousness*
> Catatonic stupor
> Semicoma
> **Excludes1**   catatonic schizophrenia (F20.2)
> coma (R40.2-)
> depressive stupor (F31-F33)
> dissociative stupor (F44.2)
> manic stupor (F30.2)

OGCR   Section I.C.18.e.
> Coma scale
>
> The coma scale codes (R40.2-) can be used in conjunction with traumatic brain injury codes, acute cerebrovascular disease or sequelae of cerebrovascular disease codes. These codes are primarily for use by trauma registries, but they may be used in any setting where this information is collected. The coma scale codes should be sequenced after the diagnosis code(s).
>
> These codes, one from each subcategory, are needed to complete the scale. The 7th character indicates when the scale was recorded. The 7th character should match for all three codes.
>
> At a minimum, report the initial score documented on presentation at your facility. This may be a score from the emergency medicine technician (EMT) or in the emergency department. If desired, a facility may choose to capture multiple coma scale scores.
>
> Assign code R40.24, Glasgow coma scale, total score, when only the total score is documented in the medical record and not the individual score(s).

CHAPTER 18 (R00-R99)

1372

● Unacceptable Principal Diagnosis   ● Use Additional Character(s)   ■ Unspecified   ▶ Manifestation Code

OGCR Official Guidelines for Coding and Reporting   Excludes 1   Excludes 2   Includes   Use additional   Code first   Code also

Glasgow Coma Scale

Eye Opening Response	
• Spontaneous--open with blinking at baseline	4 points
• To verbal stimuli, command, speech	3 points
• To pain only (not applied to face)	2 points
• No response	1 point
Verbal Response	
• Oriented	5 points
• Confused conversation, but able to answer questions	4 points
• Inappropriate words	3 points
• Incomprehensible speech	2 points
• No response	1 point
Motor Response	
• Obeys commands for movement	6 points
• Purposeful movement to painful stimulus	5 points
• Withdraws in response to pain	4 points
• Flexion in response to pain (decorticate posturing)	3 points
• Extension response in response to pain (decerebrate posturing)	2 points
• No response	1 point

Categorization:
Coma: No eye opening, no ability to follow commands, no word verbalizations (3-8)

Head Injury Classification:
Severe Head Injury--GCS score of 8 or less
Moderate Head Injury--GCS score of 9 to 12
Mild head injury--GCS score of 13 to 15

(Adapted from: Advanced Trauma Life Support: Course for Physicians, American College of Surgeons, 1993).
http://www.bt.cdc.gov/masscasualtires/gscale.asp

Figure 18-1

● R40.2　Coma

　　　Code first any associated:
　　　　coma in fracture of skull (S02.-)
　　　　coma in intracranial injury (S06.-)

　　　The appropriate 7th character is to be added to each code from subcategory R40.21-, R40.22-, R40.23-:

0	unspecified time
1	in the field [EMT or ambulance]
2	at arrival to emergency department
3	at hospital admission
4	24 hours or more after hospital admission

　　　Note: A code from each subcategory is required to complete the coma scale.

■ R40.20　Unspecified coma 🕮
　　　Coma NOS
　　　Unconsciousness NOS

● R40.21　Coma scale, eyes open
　　● R40.211　Coma scale, eyes open, never 🕮
　　● R40.212　Coma scale, eyes open, to pain 🕮
　　● R40.213　Coma scale, eyes open, to sound 0, 1, 2, 3, 4 🕮
　　● R40.214　Coma scale, eyes open, spontaneous 0, 1, 2, 3, 4 🕮

● R40.22　Coma scale, best verbal response
　　● R40.221　Coma scale, best verbal response, none 🕮
　　● R40.222　Coma scale, best verbal response, incomprehensible words 🕮
　　● R40.223　Coma scale, best verbal response, inappropriate words 0, 1, 2, 3, 4 🕮
　　● R40.224　Coma scale, best verbal response, confused conversation 0, 1, 2, 3, 4 🕮
　　● R40.225　Coma scale, best verbal response, oriented 0, 1, 2, 3, 4 🕮

● R40.23　Coma scale, best motor response
　　● R40.231　Coma scale, best motor response, none 🕮
　　● R40.232　Coma scale, best motor response, extension 🕮
　　● R40.233　Coma scale, best motor response, abnormal 0, 1, 2, 3, 4 🕮
　　● R40.234　Coma scale, best motor response, flexion withdrawal 🕮
　　● R40.235　Coma scale, best motor response, localizes pain 0, 1, 2, 3, 4 🕮
　　● R40.236　Coma scale, best motor response, obeys commands 0, 1, 2, 3, 4 🕮

● R40.24　Glasgow coma scale, total score
　　　Use codes R40.21- through R40.23- only when the individual score(s) are documented
　　　R40.241　Glasgow coma scale score 13-15
　　　R40.242　Glasgow coma scale score 9-12
　　　R40.243　Glasgow coma scale score 3-8
　　　R40.244　Other coma, without documented Glasgow coma scale score, or with partial score reported

R40.3　Persistent vegetative state 🕮
R40.4　Transient alteration of awareness

● R41　Other symptoms and signs involving cognitive functions and awareness
　　Excludes1　dissociative [conversion] disorders (F44.-)
　　　　　　　mild cognitive impairment, so stated (G31.84)

■ R41.0　Disorientation, unspecified
　　　Confusion NOS　　　　　　　Delirium NOS

R41.1　Anterograde amnesia
R41.2　Retrograde amnesia
R41.3　Other amnesia
　　　Amnesia NOS
　　　Memory loss NOS

　　Excludes1　amnestic disorder due to known physiologic condition (F04)
　　　　　　　amnestic syndrome due to psychoactive substance use (F10-F19 with 5th character .6)
　　　　　　　mild memory disturbance due to known physiological condition (F06.8)
　　　　　　　transient global amnesia (G45.4)

N　Newborn Age: 0　　P　Pediatric Age: 0–17　　M　Maternity DX: 12–55　　A　Adult Age: 15–124　　♀　Females Only　　♂　Males Only
🕮　Complication\Comorbidity　　🕮　Major C\C　　🕮　Present on Admission Requirement　　🕮　Hospital-Acquired Condition

1373

CHAPTER 18 (R00-R99)

R41.4 Neurologic neglect syndrome 🔗

Asomatognosia   Left-sided neglect
Hemi-akinesia   Sensory neglect
Hemi-inattention   Visuospatial neglect
Hemispatial neglect

Excludes1   visuospatial deficit (R41.842)

● R41.8 Other symptoms and signs involving cognitive functions and awareness

R41.81 Age-related cognitive decline   **A**
Senility NOS

R41.82 Altered mental status, unspecified
Change in mental status NOS

Excludes1   altered level of
consciousness (R40.-)
altered mental status due to
known condition - code
to condition
delirium NOS (R41.0)

● R41.83 Borderline intellectual functioning 🔗
IQ level 71 to 84

Excludes1   intellectual disabilities
(F70-F79)

● R41.84 Other specified cognitive deficit

R41.840 Attention and concentration deficit

Excludes1   attention-deficit
hyperactivity disorders
(F90.-)

R41.841 Cognitive communication deficit

R41.842 Visuospatial deficit

R41.843 Psychomotor deficit

R41.844 Frontal lobe and executive function deficit

R41.89 Other symptoms and signs involving cognitive functions and awareness
Anosognosia

R41.9 Unspecified symptoms and signs involving cognitive functions and awareness

R42 Dizziness and giddiness
Light-headedness
Vertigo NOS

Excludes1   vertiginous syndromes (H81.-)
vertigo from infrasound (T75.23)

● R43 Disturbances of smell and taste

R43.0 Anosmia
Absence of sense of smell; AKA anosphresia and olfactory anesthesia

R43.1 Parosmia

R43.2 Parageusia
Perversion of sense of taste or bad taste in mouth; AKA dysgeusia

R43.8 Other disturbances of smell and taste
Mixed disturbance of smell and taste

R43.9 Unspecified disturbances of smell and taste

● R44 Other symptoms and signs involving general sensations and perceptions

Excludes1   alcoholic hallucinations (F1.5)
hallucinations in drug psychosis (F11-F19
with .5)
hallucinations in mood disorders with
psychotic symptoms (F30.2, F31.5,
F32.3, F33.3)
hallucinations in schizophrenia, schizotypal
and delusional disorders (F20-F29)

Excludes2   disturbances of skin sensation (R20.-)

R44.0 Auditory hallucinations 🔗

R44.1 Visual hallucinations

R44.2 Other hallucinations 🔗

R44.3 Hallucinations, unspecified 🔗

R44.8 Other symptoms and signs involving general sensations and perceptions

R44.9 Unspecified symptoms and signs involving general sensations and perceptions

● R45 Symptoms and signs involving emotional state

R45.0 Nervousness
Nervous tension

R45.1 Restlessness and agitation

R45.2 Unhappiness

R45.3 Demoralization and apathy
Excludes1   anhedonia (R45.84)

R45.4 Irritability and anger

R45.5 Hostility

R45.6 Violent behavior

R45.7 State of emotional shock and stress, unspecified

● R45.8 Other symptoms and signs involving emotional state

R45.81 Low self-esteem

R45.82 Worries

R45.83 Excessive crying of child, adolescent or adult

Excludes1   excessive crying of infant
(baby) R68.11

R45.84 Anhedonia
Total loss of feeling of pleasure in pleasurable acts

● R45.85 Homicidal and suicidal ideations
Excludes1   suicide attempt (T14.91)

● R45.850 Homicidal ideations 🔗

R45.851 Suicidal ideations 🔗🔗

R45.86 Emotional lability

R45.87 Impulsiveness

R45.89 Other symptoms and signs involving emotional state

● R46 Symptoms and signs involving appearance and behavior

Excludes1   appearance and behavior in schizophrenia,
schizotypal and delusional disorders
(F20-F29)
mental and behavioral disorders (F01-F99)

R46.0 Very low level of personal hygiene

R46.1 Bizarre personal appearance

R46.2 Strange and inexplicable behavior

R46.3 Overactivity

● Unacceptable Principal Diagnosis   ● Use Additional Character(s)   ■ Unspecified   ▶ Manifestation Code

OGCR Official Guidelines for Coding and Reporting   Excludes 1   Excludes 2   Includes   Use additional   Code first   Code also

R46.4   **Slowness and poor responsiveness**
> **Excludes1**   stupor (R40.1)

R46.5   **Suspiciousness and marked evasiveness**

R46.6   **Undue concern and preoccupation with stressful events**

R46.7   **Verbosity and circumstantial detail obscuring reason for contact**

● R46.8   **Other symptoms and signs involving appearance and behavior**

    ● R46.81   **Obsessive-compulsive behavior**
> **Excludes1**   obsessive-compulsive disorder (F42)

    ● R46.89   **Other symptoms and signs involving appearance and behavior**

SYMPTOMS AND SIGNS INVOLVING SPEECH AND VOICE (R47-R49)

● R47   **Speech disturbances, not elsewhere classified**
> **Excludes1**   autism (F84.0)
> cluttering (F80.81)
> specific developmental disorders of speech and language (F80.-)
> stuttering (F80.81)

● R47.0   **Dysphasia and aphasia**

    R47.01   **Aphasia** 🔗
> **Excludes1**   aphasia following cerebrovascular disease (I69. with final characters -20)
> progressive isolated aphasia (G31.01)

    R47.02   **Dysphasia**
> *Impairment in comprehension of speech, caused by left-sided brain damage*
> **Excludes1**   dysphasia following cerebrovascular disease (I69. with final characters -21)

R47.1   **Dysarthria and anarthria**
> *Motor speech disorder*
> **Excludes1**   dysarthria following cerebrovascular disease (I69. with final characters -22)

● R47.8   **Other speech disturbances**
> **Excludes1**   dysarthria following cerebrovascular disease (I69. with final characters -28)

    R47.81   **Slurred speech**

    ●▶ R47.82   *Fluency disorder in conditions classified elsewhere*
> Stuttering in conditions classified elsewhere
> *Code first underlying disease or condition, such as:*
> Parkinson's disease (G20)
> **Excludes1**   adult onset fluency disorder (F98.5)
> childhood onset fluency disorder (F80.81)
> fluency disorder (stuttering) following cerebrovascular disease (I69. with final characters -23)

    R47.89   **Other speech disturbances**

R47.9   **Unspecified speech disturbances**

● R48   **Dyslexia and other symbolic dysfunctions, not elsewhere classified**
> **Excludes1**   specific developmental disorders of scholastic skills (F81.-)

R48.0   **Dyslexia and alexia**

R48.1   **Agnosia**
> *Loss of ability to recognize objects, persons, sounds, shapes, or smells*
> Astereognosia (astereognosis)
> Autotopagnosia
> **Excludes1**   visual object agnosia (R48.3)

R48.2   **Apraxia**
> *Loss of ability to execute or carry out learned purposeful movements*
> **Excludes1**   apraxia following cerebrovascular disease (I69. with final characters -90)

R48.3   **Visual agnosia**
> Prosopagnosia
> Simultanagnosia (asimultagnosia)

R48.8   **Other symbolic dysfunctions**
> Acalculia
> *Difficulty performing simple mathematical tasks resulting from neurological injury*
> Agraphia

■ R48.9   **Unspecified symbolic dysfunctions**

● R49   **Voice and resonance disorders**
> **Excludes1**   psychogenic voice and resonance disorders (F44.4)

R49.0   **Dysphonia**
> Hoarseness

R49.1   **Aphonia**
> Loss of voice

● R49.2   **Hypernasality and hyponasality**

    R49.21   **Hypernasality**

    R49.22   **Hyponasality**

R49.8   **Other voice and resonance disorders**

■ R49.9   **Unspecified voice and resonance disorder**
> Change in voice NOS
> Resonance disorder NOS

GENERAL SYMPTOMS AND SIGNS (R50-R69)

● R50   **Fever of other and unknown origin**
> **Excludes1**   chills without fever (R68.83)
> febrile convulsions (R56.0-)
> fever of unknown origin during labor (O75.2)
> fever of unknown origin in newborn (P81.9)
> hypothermia due to illness (R68.0)
> malignant hyperthermia due to anesthesia (T88.3)
> puerperal pyrexia NOS (O86.4)

● R50.2   **Drug induced fever**
> Use additional code for adverse effect, if applicable, to identify drug (T36-T50 with fifth or sixth character 5)
> **Excludes1**   postvaccination (postimmunization) fever (R50.83)

CHAPTER 18 (R00-R99)

● **R50.8   Other specified fever**

　● *R50.81   Fever presenting with conditions classified elsewhere*

　　　Code first *underlying condition when associated fever is present, such as with:*
　　　leukemia (C91-C95)
　　　neutropenia (D70.-)
　　　sickle-cell disease (D57.-)

　R50.82   Postprocedural fever

　　　Excludes1   postprocedural infection (T81.4)
　　　posttransfusion fever (R50.84)
　　　postvaccination (postimmunization) fever (R50.83)

　R50.83   Postvaccination fever
　　　Postimmunization fever

　R50.84   Febrile nonhemolytic transfusion reaction
　　　FNHTR
　　　Posttransfusion fever

■ **R50.9   Fever, unspecified**
　　Fever NOS
　　Fever of unknown origin [FUO]
　　Fever with chills
　　Fever with rigors
　　Hyperpyrexia NOS
　　Persistent fever
　　Pyrexia NOS

R51   Headache
　Facial pain NOS

　　Excludes1   atypical face pain (G50.1)
　　migraine and other headache syndromes (G43-G44)
　　trigeminal neuralgia (G50.0)

■ **R52   Pain, unspecified**
　Acute pain NOS　　　　　Pain NOS
　Generalized pain NOS

　　Excludes1   acute and chronic pain, not elsewhere classified (G89.-)
　　localized pain, unspecified type - code to pain by site, such as:
　　　abdomen pain (R10.-)
　　　back pain (M54.9)
　　　breast pain (N64.4)
　　　chest pain (R07.1-R07.9)
　　　ear pain (H92.0-)
　　　eye pain (H57.1)
　　　headache (R51)
　　　joint pain (M25.5-)
　　　limb pain (M79.6-)
　　　lumbar region pain (M54.5)
　　　pelvic and perineal pain (R10.2)
　　　shoulder pain (M25.51-)
　　　spine pain (M54.-)
　　　throat pain (R07.0)
　　　tongue pain (K14.6)
　　　tooth pain (K08.8)
　　　renal colic (N23)
　　pain disorders exclusively related to psychological factors (F45.41)

● **R53   Malaise and fatigue**

　● **R53.0   Neoplastic (malignant) related fatigue**

　　　Code first *associated neoplasm*

R53.1   Weakness
　Asthenia NOS

　　Excludes1   age-related weakness (R54)
　　muscle weakness (M62.8-)
　　senile asthenia (R54)

R53.2   Functional quadriplegia 🔗
　Complete immobility due to severe physical disability or frailty

　　Excludes1   frailty NOS (R54)
　　hysterical paralysis (F44.4)
　　immobility syndrome (M62.3)
　　neurologic quadriplegia (G82.5-)
　　quadriplegia (G82.50)

● **R53.8   Other malaise and fatigue**

　　Excludes1   combat exhaustion and fatigue (F43.0)
　　congenital debility (P96.9)
　　exhaustion and fatigue due to:
　　　depressive episode (F32.-)
　　　excessive exertion (T73.3)
　　　exposure (T73.2)
　　　heat (T67.-)
　　　pregnancy (O26.8-)
　　　recurrent depressive episode (F33)
　　　senile debility (R54)

　R53.81   Other malaise
　　Chronic debility
　　Debility NOS
　　General physical deterioration
　　Malaise NOS
　　Nervous debility

　　　Excludes1   age-related physical debility (R54)

　■ **R53.82   Chronic fatigue, unspecified**
　　Chronic fatigue syndrome NOS

　　　Excludes1   postviral fatigue syndrome (G93.3)

　R53.83   Other fatigue
　　Fatigue NOS　　　　　Lethargy
　　Lack of energy　　　　Tiredness

R54   Age-related physical debility　　　　　　　　　A
　Frailty　　　　　　　Senile asthenia
　Old age　　　　　　 Senile debility
　Senescence

　　Excludes1   age-related cognitive decline (R41.81)
　　senile psychosis (F03)
　　senility NOS (R41.81)

R55   Syncope and collapse
　Blackout
　Fainting
　Vasovagal attack

　　Excludes1   cardiogenic shock (R57.0)
　　carotid sinus syncope (G90.01)
　　heat syncope (T67.1)
　　neurocirculatory asthenia (F45.8)
　　neurogenic orthostatic hypotension (G90.3)
　　orthostatic hypotension (I95.1)
　　postprocedural shock (T81.1-)
　　psychogenic syncope (F48.8)
　　shock NOS (R57.9)
　　shock complicating or following abortion or ectopic or molar pregnancy (O00-O07, O08.3)
　　shock complicating or following labor and delivery (O75.1)
　　Stokes-Adams attack (I45.9)
　　unconsciousness NOS (R40.2-)

● Unacceptable Principal Diagnosis　　　● Use Additional Character(s)　　　■ Unspecified　　　▶ Manifestation Code
OGCR   Official Guidelines for Coding and Reporting　　[Excludes 1]　[Excludes 2]　Includes　Use additional　Code first　Code also

● **R56　Convulsions, not elsewhere classified**
　　Excludes1　dissociative convulsions and seizures (F44.5)
　　　　　　　　epileptic convulsions and seizures (G40.-)
　　　　　　　　newborn convulsions and seizures (P90)

　● **R56.0　Febrile convulsions**

　　　R56.00　Simple febrile convulsions 🔾
　　　　　Febrile convulsion NOS
　　　　　Febrile seizure NOS

　　　R56.01　Complex febrile convulsions 🔾
　　　　　Atypical febrile seizure
　　　　　Complex febrile seizure
　　　　　Complicated febrile seizure
　　　　　Excludes1　status epilepticus (G40.901)

　　R56.1　Post traumatic seizures 🔾
　　　　Excludes1　post traumatic epilepsy (G40.-)

　■ **R56.9　Unspecified convulsions**
　　　　Convulsion disorder　Recurrent convulsions
　　　　Fit NOS　　　　　　Seizure(s) (convulsive) NOS

● **R57　Shock, not elsewhere classified**
　　Excludes1　anaphylactic shock NOS (T78.2)
　　　　　　　　anaphylactic reaction or shock due to
　　　　　　　　　　adverse food reaction (T78.0-)
　　　　　　　　anaphylactic shock due to adverse effect of
　　　　　　　　　　correct drug or medicament properly
　　　　　　　　　　administered (T88.6)
　　　　　　　　anaphylactic shock due to serum (T80.5-)
　　　　　　　　anesthetic shock (T88.3)
　　　　　　　　electric shock (T75.4)
　　　　　　　　obstetric shock (O75.1)
　　　　　　　　postprocedural shock (T81.1-)
　　　　　　　　psychic shock (F43.0)
　　　　　　　　septic shock (R65.21)
　　　　　　　　shock complicating or following ectopic or
　　　　　　　　　　molar pregnancy (O00-O07, O08.3)
　　　　　　　　shock due to lightning (T75.01)
　　　　　　　　traumatic shock (T79.4)
　　　　　　　　toxic shock syndrome (A48.3)

　　R57.0　Cardiogenic shock 🔾
　　　　MCC: Only if patient discharged alive

　　R57.1　Hypovolemic shock 🔾
　　　　Decreased blood volume (loss)
　　　　MCC: Only if patient discharged alive

　　R57.8　Other shock 🔾
　　　　MCC: Only if patient discharged alive

　■ **R57.9　Shock, unspecified** 🔾
　　　　Failure of peripheral circulation NOS
　　　　Resulting in significant blood pressure drop

● **R58　Hemorrhage, not elsewhere classified**
　　Hemorrhage NOS
　　Excludes1　hemorrhage included with underlying
　　　　　　　　　conditions, such as:
　　　　　　　　acute duodenal ulcer with hemorrhage
　　　　　　　　　(K26.0)
　　　　　　　　acute gastritis with bleeding (K29.01)
　　　　　　　　ulcerative enterocolitis with rectal
　　　　　　　　　bleeding (K51.01)

● **R59　Enlarged lymph nodes**
　　Includes　swollen glands
　　Excludes1　lymphadenitis NOS (I88.9)
　　　　　　　　acute lymphadenitis (L04.-)
　　　　　　　　chronic lymphadenitis (I88.1)
　　　　　　　　mesenteric (acute) (chronic) lymphadenitis
　　　　　　　　　(I88.0)

　　R59.0　Localized enlarged lymph nodes

　　R59.1　Generalized enlarged lymph nodes
　　　　Lymphadenopathy NOS

　■ **R59.9　Enlarged lymph nodes, unspecified**

● **R60　Edema, not elsewhere classified**
　　Excludes1　angioneurotic edema (T78.3)
　　　　　　　　ascites (R18.-)
　　　　　　　　cerebral edema (G93.6)
　　　　　　　　cerebral edema due to birth injury (P11.0)
　　　　　　　　edema of larynx (J38.4)
　　　　　　　　edema of nasopharynx (J39.2)
　　　　　　　　edema of pharynx (J39.2)
　　　　　　　　gestational edema (O12.0-)
　　　　　　　　hereditary edema (Q82.0)
　　　　　　　　hydrops fetalis NOS (P83.2)
　　　　　　　　hydrothorax (J94.8)
　　　　　　　　nutritional edema (E40-E46)
　　　　　　　　hydrops fetalis NOS (P83.2)
　　　　　　　　newborn edema (P83.3)
　　　　　　　　pulmonary edema (J81.-)

　　R60.0　Localized edema

　　R60.1　Generalized edema

　■ **R60.9　Edema, unspecified**
　　　　Fluid retention NOS

　R61　Generalized hyperhidrosis
　　　Excessive sweating
　　　Night sweats
　　　Secondary hyperhidrosis
　　　*Code first, if applicable, menopausal and female climacteric
　　　states (N95.1)*
　　　Excludes1　focal (primary) (secondary) hyperhidrosis
　　　　　　　　　(L74.5-)
　　　　　　　　Frey's syndrome (L74.52)
　　　　　　　　localized (primary) (secondary)
　　　　　　　　　hyperhidrosis (L74.5-)

● **R62　Lack of expected normal physiological development in
　　　childhood and adults**
　　　Excludes1　delayed puberty (E30.0)
　　　　　　　　gonadal dysgenesis (Q99.1)
　　　　　　　　hypopituitarism (E23.0)

　　R62.0　Delayed milestone in childhood　　　　　　P
　　　　Delayed attainment of expected physiological
　　　　　developmental stage
　　　　Late talker
　　　　Late walker

　● **R62.5　Other and unspecified lack of expected normal
　　　　physiological development in childhood**
　　　　Excludes1　HIV disease resulting in failure to
　　　　　　　　　thrive (B20)
　　　　　　　　physical retardation due to
　　　　　　　　　malnutrition (E45)

　　　■ **R62.50　Unspecified lack of expected normal
　　　　　physiological development in childhood**　P
　　　　　Infantilism NOS

　　　R62.51　Failure to thrive (child)　　　　　　P
　　　　　Failure to gain weight
　　　　　Excludes1　failure to thrive in child
　　　　　　　　　under 28 days old
　　　　　　　　　(P92.6)

　　　R62.52　Short stature (child)　　　　　　　P
　　　　　Lack of growth　　　　Short stature NOS
　　　　　Physical retardation
　　　　　Excludes1　short stature due to
　　　　　　　　　endocrine disorder
　　　　　　　　　(E34.3)

　　　**R62.59　Other lack of expected normal
　　　　　physiological development in childhood**　P

　　R62.7　Adult failure to thrive　　　　　　　　　A

N Newborn Age: 0　**P** Pediatric Age: 0–17　**M** Maternity DX: 12–55　**A** Adult Age: 15–124　♀ Females Only　♂ Males Only

🔾 Complication\Comorbidity　　🔾 Major C\C　　🔾 Present on Admission Requirement　　🔾 Hospital-Acquired Condition

1377

CHAPTER 18 (R00-R99)

● R63 **Symptoms and signs concerning food and fluid intake**
  Excludes1 bulimia NOS (F50.2)
         eating disorders of nonorganic origin (F50.-)
         malnutrition (E40-E46)

  R63.0 **Anorexia**
       Loss of appetite
       Excludes1 anorexia nervosa (F50.0-)
              loss of appetite of nonorganic origin
              (F50.8)

  R63.1 **Polydipsia**
       Excessive thirst

  R63.2 **Polyphagia**
       Excessive eating   Hyperalimentation NOS

  R63.3 **Feeding difficulties**
       Feeding problem (elderly) (infant) NOS
       Excludes1 feeding problems of newborn (P92.-)
              infant feeding disorder of
              nonorganic origin (F98.2-)

  R63.4 **Abnormal weight loss**

  R63.5 **Abnormal weight gain**
       Excludes1 excessive weight gain in pregnancy
              (O26.0-)
              obesity (E66.-)

  R63.6 **Underweight**
       Use additional code to identify body mass index
       (BMI), if known (Z68.-)
       Excludes1 abnormal weight loss (R63.4)
              anorexia nervosa (F50.0-)
              malnutrition (E40-E46)

  R63.8 **Other symptoms and signs concerning food and
       fluid intake**

R64 **Cachexia** 🔗
    Wasting syndrome
    Code first underlying condition, if known
    Excludes1 abnormal weight loss (R63.4)
           nutritional marasmus (E41)

● R65 **Symptoms and signs specifically associated with systemic
    inflammation and infection**
  ● R65.1 **Systemic inflammatory response syndrome (SIRS)
       of non-infectious origin**
       Code first underlying condition, such as:
           heatstroke (T67.0)
           injury and trauma (S00-T88)
       Excludes1 sepsis - code to infection
              severe sepsis (R65.2)

  ● R65.10 **Systemic inflammatory response syndrome
        (SIRS) of non-infectious origin without
        acute organ dysfunction** 🔗
        Systemic inflammatory response
        syndrome (SIRS) NOS

  ● R65.11 **Systemic inflammatory response syndrome
        (SIRS) of non-infectious origin with acute
        organ dysfunction** 🔗
        Use additional code to identify specific
            acute organ dysfunction, such as:
            acute kidney failure (N17.-)
            acute respiratory failure (J96.0-)
            critical illness myopathy (G72.81)
            critical illness polyneuropathy (G62.81)
            disseminated intravascular
               coagulopathy [DIC] (D65)
            encephalopathy (metabolic) (septic)
               (G93.41)
            hepatic failure (K72.0-)

  ● R65.2 **Severe sepsis**
       Infection with associated acute organ dysfunction
       Sepsis with acute organ dysfunction
       Sepsis with multiple organ dysfunction
       Systemic inflammatory response syndrome
           due to infectious process with acute organ
           dysfunction
       Code first underlying infection, such as:
           infection following a procedure (T81.4)
           infections following infusion, transfusion and
               therapeutic injection (T80.2-)
           puerperal sepsis (O85)
           sepsis following complete or unspecified
               spontaneous abortion (O03.87)
           sepsis following ectopic and molar pregnancy
               (O08.82)
           sepsis following incomplete spontaneous
               abortion (O03.37)
           sepsis following (induced) termination of
               pregnancy (O04.87)
           sepsis NOS A41.9
       Use additional code to identify specific acute
           organ dysfunction, such as:
           acute kidney failure (N17.-)
           acute respiratory failure (J96.0-)
           critical illness myopathy (G72.81)
           critical illness polyneuropathy (G62.81)
           disseminated intravascular coagulopathy [DIC]
               (D65)
           encephalopathy (metabolic) (septic) (G93.41)
           hepatic failure (K72.0-)

  ● R65.20 **Severe sepsis without septic shock** 🔗
        Severe sepsis NOS

  ● R65.21 **Severe sepsis with septic shock** 🔗
        MCC: Only when the principal diagnosis
            is designated as an MCC

OGCR Section I.C.18.g.

SIRS due to Non-Infectious Process

The systemic inflammatory response syndrome (SIRS) can
develop as a result of certain non-infectious disease processes,
such as trauma, malignant neoplasm, or pancreatitis. When
SIRS is documented with a noninfectious condition, and
no subsequent infection is documented, the code for the
underlying condition, such as an injury, should be assigned,
followed by code R65.10, Systemic inflammatory response
syndrome (SIRS) of non-infectious origin without acute organ
dysfunction, or code R65.11, Systemic inflammatory response
syndrome (SIRS) of non-infectious origin with acute organ
dysfunction. If an associated acute organ dysfunction is
documented, the appropriate code(s) for the specific type of
organ dysfunction(s) should be assigned in addition to code
R65.11. If acute organ dysfunction is documented, but it cannot
be determined if the acute organ dysfunction is associated
with SIRS or due to another condition (e.g., directly due to the
trauma), the provider should be queried.

● Unacceptable Principal Diagnosis   ● Use Additional Character(s)   ▮ Unspecified   ▶ Manifestation Code
OGCR Official Guidelines for Coding and Reporting   Excludes 1   Excludes 2   Includes   Use additional   Code first   Code also

CHAPTER 18 (R00-R99)

● **R68**   **Other general symptoms and signs**

   R68.0   **Hypothermia, not associated with low environmental temperature**

     Excludes1   hypothermia NOS (accidental) (T68)
           hypothermia due to anesthesia (T88.51)
           hypothermia due to low environmental temperature (T68)
           newborn hypothermia (P80.-)

   ● **R68.1**   **Nonspecific symptoms peculiar to infancy**

     Excludes1   colic, infantile (R10.83)
           neonatal cerebral irritability (P91.3)
           teething syndrome (K00.7)

     R68.11   **Excessive crying of infant (baby)**   **P**

       Excludes1   excessive crying of child, adolescent, or adult (R45.83)

     R68.12   **Fussy infant (baby)**   **P**
       Irritable infant

     R68.13   **Apparent life threatening event in infant (ALTE)**   **P**
       Apparent life threatening event in newborn

       Code first confirmed diagnosis, *if known*

       Use additional code(s) for associated signs and symptoms if no confirmed diagnosis established, or if signs and symptoms are not associated routinely with confirmed diagnosis, or provide additional information for cause of ALTE

     R68.19   **Other nonspecific symptoms peculiar to infancy**   **P**

   ■ **R68.2**   **Dry mouth, unspecified**

     Excludes1   dry mouth due to dehydration (E86.0)
           dry mouth due to sicca syndrome [Sjögren] (M35.0-)
           salivary gland hyposecretion (K11.7)

   R68.3   **Clubbing of fingers**
     Clubbing of nails

     Excludes1   congenital clubfinger (Q68.1)

   ■ **R68.8**   **Other general symptoms and signs**

     R68.81   **Early satiety**

     R68.82   **Decreased libido**   **A**
       Decreased sexual desire

     R68.83   **Chills (without fever)**
       Chills NOS

       Excludes1   chills with fever (R50.9)

     R68.84   **Jaw pain**
       Mandibular pain
       Maxilla pain

       Excludes1   temporomandibular joint arthralgia (M26.62)

     R68.89   **Other general symptoms and signs**

■ **R69**   **Illness, unspecified**
   Unknown and unspecified cases of morbidity

ABNORMAL FINDINGS ON EXAMINATION OF BLOOD, WITHOUT DIAGNOSIS (R70-R79)

   Excludes1   abnormalities (of)(on):
           abnormal findings on antenatal screening of mother (O28.-)
           coagulation hemorrhagic disorders (D65-D68)
           lipids (E78.-)
           platelets and thrombocytes (D69.-)
           white blood cells classified elsewhere (D70-D72)
           diagnostic abnormal findings classified elsewhere - see Alphabetical Index
           hemorrhagic and hematological disorders of newborn (P50-P61)

● **R70**   **Elevated erythrocyte sedimentation rate and abnormality of plasma viscosity**

   R70.0   **Elevated erythrocyte sedimentation rate**

   R70.1   **Abnormal plasma viscosity**

● **R71**   **Abnormality of red blood cells**

   Excludes1   anemias (D50-D64)
           anemia of premature infant (P61.2)
           benign (familial) polycythemia (D75.0)
           congenital anemias (P61.2-P61.4)
           newborn anemia due to isoimmunization (P55.-)
           polycythemia neonatorum (P61.1)
           polycythemia NOS (D75.1)
           polycythemia vera (D45)
           secondary polycythemia (D75.1)

   R71.0   **Precipitous drop in hematocrit** 🅒
     Drop (precipitous) in hemoglobin
     Drop in hematocrit
       Blood volume that is red blood cells

   R71.8   **Other abnormality of red blood cells**
     Abnormal red-cell morphology NOS
     Abnormal red-cell volume NOS
     Anisocytosis
       Red blood cells of unequal size
     Poikilocytosis
       Red blood cells of abnormal shape

● **R73**   **Elevated blood glucose level**

   Excludes1   diabetes mellitus (E08-E13)
           diabetes mellitus in pregnancy, childbirth and the puerperium (O24.-)
           neonatal disorders (P70.0-P70.2)
           postsurgical hypoinsulinemia (E89.1)

   ● **R73.0**   **Abnormal glucose**

     Excludes1   abnormal glucose in pregnancy (O99.81-)
           diabetes mellitus (E08-E13)
           dysmetabolic syndrome X (E88.81)
           gestational diabetes (O24.4-)
           glycosuria (R81)
           hypoglycemia (E16.2)

     R73.01   **Impaired fasting glucose**
       Elevated fasting glucose

     R73.02   **Impaired glucose tolerance (oral)**
       Elevated glucose tolerance

     R73.09   **Other abnormal glucose**
       Abnormal glucose NOS
       Abnormal non-fasting glucose tolerance
       Latent diabetes
       Prediabetes

   ■ **R73.9**   **Hyperglycemia, unspecified**

CHAPTER 18 (R00-R99)

N Newborn Age: 0   **P** Pediatric Age: 0–17   **M** Maternity DX: 12–55   **A** Adult Age: 15–124   ♀ Females Only   ♂ Males Only

🅒 Complication\Comorbidity   🅜 Major C\C   Present on Admission Requirement   Hospital-Acquired Condition

1379

● **R74**   **Abnormal serum enzyme levels**

     R74.0   **Nonspecific elevation of levels of transaminase and lactic acid dehydrogenase [LDH]**

     R74.8   **Abnormal levels of other serum enzymes**
         Abnormal level of acid phosphatase
         Abnormal level of alkaline phosphatase
         Abnormal level of amylase
         Abnormal level of lipase [triacylglycerol lipase]

     ■ **R74.9**   **Abnormal serum enzyme level, unspecified**

     OGCR   Section I.C.1.2.e and f.

> Patients with inconclusive HIV serology
>
> e. Patients with inconclusive HIV serology, but no definitive diagnosis or manifestations of the illness, may be assigned code R75, Inconclusive laboratory evidence of human immunodeficiency virus [HIV].
>
> f. Previously diagnosed HIV-related illness
>
> Patients with any known prior diagnosis of an HIV-related illness should be coded to B20. Once a patient has developed an HIV-related illness, the patient should always be assigned code B20 on every subsequent admission/encounter. Patients previously diagnosed with any HIV illness (B20) should never be assigned to R75 or Z21, Asymptomatic human immunodeficiency virus [HIV] infection status.

R75   **Inconclusive laboratory evidence of human immunodeficiency virus [HIV]**
     Nonconclusive HIV-test finding in infants

     Excludes1   asymptomatic human immunodeficiency virus [HIV] infection status (Z21)
           human immunodeficiency virus [HIV] disease (B20)

● **R76**   **Other abnormal immunological findings in serum**

     R76.0   **Raised antibody titer**

         Excludes1   isoimmunization in pregnancy (O36.0-O36.1)
              isoimmunization affecting newborn (P55.-)

     ● **R76.1**   **Nonspecific reaction to test for tuberculosis**

         R76.11   **Nonspecific reaction to tuberculin skin test without active tuberculosis**
             Abnormal result of Mantoux test
             PPD positive
             Tuberculin (skin test) positive
             Tuberculin (skin test) reactor

             Excludes1   nonspecific reaction to cell mediated immunity measurement of gamma interferon antigen response without active tuberculosis (R76.12)

         R76.12   **Nonspecific reaction to cell mediated immunity measurement of gamma interferon antigen response without active tuberculosis**
             Nonspecific reaction to QuantiFERON-TB test (QFT) without active tuberculosis

             Excludes1   nonspecific reaction to tuberculin skin test without active tuberculosis (R76.11)
                positive tuberculin skin test (R76.11)

     R76.8   **Other specified abnormal immunological findings in serum**
         Raised level of immunoglobulins NOS

     ■ **R76.9**   **Abnormal immunological finding in serum, unspecified**

● **R77**   **Other abnormalities of plasma proteins**

     Excludes1   disorders of plasma-protein metabolism (E88.0)

     R77.0   **Abnormality of albumin**

     R77.1   **Abnormality of globulin**
         Hyperglobulinemia NOS

     R77.2   **Abnormality of alphafetoprotein**

     R77.8   **Other specified abnormalities of plasma proteins**

     ■ **R77.9**   **Abnormality of plasma protein, unspecified**

● **R78**   **Findings of drugs and other substances, not normally found in blood**

     Use additional code to identify any retained foreign body, if applicable (Z18.-)

     Excludes1   mental or behavioral disorders due to psychoactive substance use (F10-F19)

     R78.0   **Finding of alcohol in blood**

         Use additional external cause code (Y90.-), for detail regarding alcohol level.

     R78.1   **Finding of opiate drug in blood**

     R78.2   **Finding of cocaine in blood**

     R78.3   **Finding of hallucinogen in blood**

     R78.4   **Finding of other drugs of addictive potential in blood**

     R78.5   **Finding of other psychotropic drug in blood**

     R78.6   **Finding of steroid agent in blood**

     ● **R78.7**   **Finding of abnormal level of heavy metals in blood**

         R78.71   **Abnormal lead level in blood**
             Excludes1   lead poisoning (T56.0-)

         R78.79   **Finding of abnormal level of heavy metals in blood**

     ● **R78.8**   **Finding of other specified substances, not normally found in blood**

         R78.81   **Bacteremia** 🔗
             Blood poisoning/bacteremia

             Excludes1   sepsis-code to specified infection (A00-B99)

         R78.89   **Finding of other specified substances, not normally found in blood**
             Finding of abnormal level of lithium in blood

     ■ **R78.9**   **Finding of unspecified substance, not normally found in blood**

● Unacceptable Principal Diagnosis   ● Use Additional Character(s)   ■ Unspecified   ▶ Manifestation Code

OGCR Official Guidelines for Coding and Reporting   Excludes 1   Excludes 2   Includes   Use additional   Code first   Code also

- **R79   Other abnormal findings of blood chemistry**
  Use additional code to identify any retained foreign body, if applicable (Z18.-)
  | **Excludes1** | abnormality of fluid, electrolyte or acid-base balance (E86-E87)
  asymptomatic hyperuricemia (E79.0)
  hyperglycemia NOS (R73.9)
  hypoglycemia NOS (E16.2)
  neonatal hypoglycemia (P70.3-P70.4)
  specific findings indicating disorder of:
    amino-acid metabolism (E70-E72)
    carbohydrate metabolism (E73-E74)
    lipid metabolism (E75.-)

  R79.0   Abnormal level of blood mineral
  Abnormal blood level of cobalt
  Abnormal blood level of copper
  Abnormal blood level of iron
  Abnormal blood level of magnesium
  Abnormal blood level of mineral NEC
  Abnormal blood level of zinc
  | **Excludes1** | abnormal level of lithium (R78.89)
  disorders of mineral metabolism (E83.-)
  neonatal hypomagnesemia (P71.2)
  nutritional mineral deficiency (E58-E61)

  R79.1   Abnormal coagulation profile
  Abnormal or prolonged bleeding time
  Abnormal or prolonged coagulation time
  Abnormal or prolonged partial thromboplastin time [PTT]
  Abnormal or prolonged prothrombin time [PT]
  | **Excludes1** | coagulation defects (D68.-)

- **R79.8   Other specified abnormal findings of blood chemistry**

  R79.81   Abnormal blood-gas level

  R79.82   Elevated C-reactive protein (CRP)

  R79.89   Other specified abnormal findings of blood chemistry

  R79.9   Abnormal finding of blood chemistry, unspecified

ABNORMAL FINDINGS ON EXAMINATION OF URINE, WITHOUT DIAGNOSIS (R80-R82)

| **Excludes1** | abnormal findings on antenatal screening of mother (O28.-)
diagnostic abnormal findings classified elsewhere - see Alphabetical Index
specific findings indicating disorder of:
  amino-acid metabolism (E70-E72)
  carbohydrate metabolism (E73-E74)

- **R80   Proteinuria**
  | **Excludes1** | gestational proteinuria (O12.1-)

  R80.0   Isolated proteinuria
  Idiopathic proteinuria
  | **Excludes1** | isolated proteinuria with specific morphological lesion (N06.-)

  R80.1   Persistent proteinuria, unspecified

  R80.2   Orthostatic proteinuria, unspecified
  Postural proteinuria

  R80.3   Bence Jones proteinuria

  R80.8   Other proteinuria

  R80.9   Proteinuria, unspecified
  Albuminuria NOS

- **R81   Glycosuria**
  | **Excludes1** | renal glycosuria (E74.8)

- **R82   Other and unspecified abnormal findings in urine**
  | **Includes** | chromoabnormalities in urine
  Use additional code to identify any retained foreign body, if applicable (Z18.-)
  | **Excludes2** | hematuria (R31.-)

  R82.0   Chyluria 🔹
  White milky urine
  | **Excludes1** | filarial chyluria (B74.-)

  R82.1   Myoglobinuria 🔹
  Presence of myoglobin (iron containing protein) in urine

  R82.2   Biliuria
  Presence of bile pigments/salts in urine

  R82.3   Hemoglobinuria
  Presence of hemoglobin in urine
  | **Excludes1** | hemoglobinuria due to hemolysis from external causes NEC (D59.6)
  hemoglobinuria due to paroxysmal nocturnal [Marchiafava-Micheli] (D59.5)

  R82.4   Acetonuria
  Ketonuria

  R82.5   Elevated urine levels of drugs, medicaments and biological substances
  Elevated urine levels of catecholamines
  Elevated urine levels of indoleacetic acid
  Elevated urine levels of 17-ketosteroids
  Elevated urine levels of steroids

  R82.6   Abnormal urine levels of substances chiefly nonmedicinal as to source
  Abnormal urine level of heavy metals

  R82.7   Abnormal findings on microbiological examination of urine
  Positive culture findings of urine
  | **Excludes1** | colonization status (Z22.-)

  R82.8   Abnormal findings on cytological and histological examination of urine

- **R82.9   Other and unspecified abnormal findings in urine**

  R82.90   Unspecified abnormal findings in urine

  R82.91   Other chromoabnormalities of urine
  Chromoconversion (dipstick)
  Idiopathic dipstick converts positive for blood with no cellular forms in sediment
  | **Excludes1** | hemoglobinuria (R82.3)
  myoglobinuria (R82.1)

  R82.99   Other abnormal findings in urine
  Cells and casts in urine
  Crystalluria
  Melanuria

CHAPTER 18 (R00-R99)

CHAPTER 18 (R00-R99)

ABNORMAL FINDINGS ON EXAMINATION OF OTHER BODY FLUIDS, SUBSTANCES AND TISSUES, WITHOUT DIAGNOSIS (R83-R89)

> **Excludes1**   abnormal findings on antenatal screening of mother (O28.-)
> diagnostic abnormal findings classified elsewhere - see Alphabetical Index

> **Excludes2**   abnormal findings on examination of blood, without diagnosis (R70-R79)
> abnormal findings on examination of urine, without diagnosis (R80-R82)
> abnormal tumor markers (R97.-)

● **R83**   **Abnormal findings in cerebrospinal fluid**

R83.0   **Abnormal level of enzymes in cerebrospinal fluid**

R83.1   **Abnormal level of hormones in cerebrospinal fluid**

R83.2   **Abnormal level of other drugs, medicaments and biological substances in cerebrospinal fluid**

R83.3   **Abnormal level of substances chiefly nonmedicinal as to source in cerebrospinal fluid**

R83.4   **Abnormal immunological findings in cerebrospinal fluid**

R83.5   **Abnormal microbiological findings in cerebrospinal fluid**
Positive culture findings in cerebrospinal fluid

> **Excludes1**   colonization status (Z22.-)

R83.6   **Abnormal cytological findings in cerebrospinal fluid**

R83.8   **Other abnormal findings in cerebrospinal fluid**
Abnormal chromosomal findings in cerebrospinal fluid

■ **R83.9**   **Unspecified abnormal finding in cerebrospinal fluid**

● **R84**   **Abnormal findings in specimens from respiratory organs and thorax**

> **Includes**   abnormal findings in bronchial washings
> abnormal findings in nasal secretions
> abnormal findings in pleural fluid
> abnormal findings in sputum
> abnormal findings in throat scrapings

> **Excludes1**   blood-stained sputum (R04.2)

R84.0   **Abnormal level of enzymes in specimens from respiratory organs and thorax**

R84.1   **Abnormal level of hormones in specimens from respiratory organs and thorax**

R84.2   **Abnormal level of other drugs, medicaments and biological substances in specimens from respiratory organs and thorax**

R84.3   **Abnormal level of substances chiefly nonmedicinal as to source in specimens from respiratory organs and thorax**

R84.4   **Abnormal immunological findings in specimens from respiratory organs and thorax**

R84.5   **Abnormal microbiological findings in specimens from respiratory organs and thorax**
Positive culture findings in specimens from respiratory organs and thorax

> **Excludes1**   colonization status (Z22.-)

R84.6   **Abnormal cytological findings in specimens from respiratory organs and thorax**

R84.7   **Abnormal histological findings in specimens from respiratory organs and thorax**

R84.8   **Other abnormal findings in specimens from respiratory organs and thorax**
Abnormal chromosomal findings in specimens from respiratory organs and thorax

■ **R84.9**   **Unspecified abnormal finding in specimens from respiratory organs and thorax**

● **R85**   **Abnormal findings in specimens from digestive organs and abdominal cavity**

> **Includes**   abnormal findings in peritoneal fluid
> abnormal findings in saliva

> **Excludes1**   cloudy peritoneal dialysis effluent (R88.0)
> fecal abnormalities (R19.5)

R85.0   **Abnormal level of enzymes in specimens from digestive organs and abdominal cavity**

R85.1   **Abnormal level of hormones in specimens from digestive organs and abdominal cavity**

R85.2   **Abnormal level of other drugs, medicaments and biological substances in specimens from digestive organs and abdominal cavity**

R85.3   **Abnormal level of substances chiefly nonmedicinal as to source in specimens from digestive organs and abdominal cavity**

R85.4   **Abnormal immunological findings in specimens from digestive organs and abdominal cavity**

R85.5   **Abnormal microbiological findings in specimens from digestive organs and abdominal cavity**
Positive culture findings in specimens from digestive organs and abdominal cavity

> **Excludes1**   colonization status (Z22.-)

● **R85.6**   **Abnormal cytological findings in specimens from digestive organs and abdominal cavity**

● **R85.61**   **Abnormal cytologic smear of anus**

> **Excludes1**   abnormal cytological findings in specimens from other digestive organs and abdominal cavity (R85.69)
> carcinoma in situ of anus (histologically confirmed) (D01.3)
> anal intraepithelial neoplasia I [AIN I] (K62.82)
> anal intraepithelial neoplasia II [AIN II] (K62.82)
> anal intraepithelial neoplasia III [AIN III] (D01.3)
> dysplasia (mild) (moderate) of anus (histologically confirmed) (K62.82)
> severe dysplasia of anus (histologically confirmed) (D01.3)

> **Excludes2**   anal high risk human papillomavirus (HPV) DNA test positive (R85.81)
> anal low risk human papillomavirus (HPV) DNA test positive (R85.82)

R85.610   **Atypical squamous cells of undetermined significance on cytologic smear of anus (ASC-US)**

● Unacceptable Principal Diagnosis   ● Use Additional Character(s)   ■ Unspecified   ▶ Manifestation Code

OGCR   Official Guidelines for Coding and Reporting | Excludes 1 | | Excludes 2 | | Includes | | Use additional | | Code first | | Code also |

R85.611   Atypical squamous cells cannot exclude high grade squamous intraepithelial lesion on cytologic smear of anus (ASC-H)

R85.612   Low grade squamous intraepithelial lesion on cytologic smear of anus (LGSIL)

R85.613   High grade squamous intraepithelial lesion on cytologic smear of anus (HGSIL)

R85.614   Cytologic evidence of malignancy on smear of anus

R85.615   Unsatisfactory cytologic smear of anus

> Inadequate sample of cytologic smear of anus

R85.616   Satisfactory anal smear but lacking transformation zone

R85.618   Other abnormal cytological findings on specimens from anus

R85.619   Unspecified abnormal cytological findings in specimens from anus

> Abnormal anal cytology NOS
> Atypical glandular cells of anus NOS

R85.69   Abnormal cytological findings in specimens from other digestive organs and abdominal cavity

R85.7   Abnormal histological findings in specimens from digestive organs and abdominal cavity

● **R85.8**   Other abnormal findings in specimens from digestive organs and abdominal cavity

R85.81   Anal high risk human papillomavirus (HPV) DNA test positive

| Excludes1 | anogenital warts due to human papillomavirus (HPV) (A63.0) condyloma acuminatum (A63.0) |

R85.82   Anal low risk human papillomavirus (HPV) DNA test positive

> Use additional code for associated human papillomavirus (B97.7)

R85.89   Other abnormal findings in specimens from digestive organs and abdominal cavity

> Abnormal chromosomal findings in specimens from digestive organs and abdominal cavity

R85.9   Unspecified abnormal finding in specimens from digestive organs and abdominal cavity

● **R86**   Abnormal findings in specimens from male genital organs

| Includes | abnormal findings in prostatic secretions abnormal findings in semen, seminal fluid abnormal spermatozoa |

| Excludes1 | azoospermia (N46.0-) oligospermia (N46.1-) |

R86.0   Abnormal level of enzymes in specimens from male genital organs ♂

R86.1   Abnormal level of hormones in specimens from male genital organs ♂

R86.2   Abnormal level of other drugs, medicaments and biological substances in specimens from male genital organs ♂

R86.3   Abnormal level of substances chiefly nonmedicinal as to source in specimens from male genital organs ♂

R86.4   Abnormal immunological findings in specimens from male genital organs ♂

R86.5   Abnormal microbiological findings in specimens from male genital organs ♂

> Positive culture findings in specimens from male genital organs

| Excludes1 | colonization status (Z22.-) |

R86.6   Abnormal cytological findings in specimens from male genital organs ♂

R86.7   Abnormal histological findings in specimens from male genital organs ♂

R86.8   Other abnormal findings in specimens from male genital organs ♂

> Abnormal chromosomal findings in specimens from male genital organs

R86.9   Unspecified abnormal finding in specimens from male genital organs ♂

● **R87**   Abnormal findings in specimens from female genital organs

| Includes | abnormal findings in secretion and smears from cervix uteri abnormal findings in secretion and smears from vagina abnormal findings in secretion and smears from vulva |

R87.0   Abnormal level of enzymes in specimens from female genital organs ♀

R87.1   Abnormal level of hormones in specimens from female genital organs ♀

R87.2   Abnormal level of other drugs, medicaments and biological substances in specimens from female genital organs ♀

R87.3   Abnormal level of substances chiefly nonmedicinal as to source in specimens from female genital organs ♀

R87.4   Abnormal immunological findings in specimens from female genital organs ♀

R87.5   Abnormal microbiological findings in specimens from female genital organs ♀

> Positive culture findings in specimens from female genital organs

| Excludes1 | colonization status (Z22.-) |

CHAPTER 18 (R00-R99)

● **R87.6　Abnormal cytological findings in specimens from female genital organs**

● **R87.61　Abnormal cytological findings in specimens from cervix uteri**

> **Excludes1**　abnormal cytological findings in specimens from other female genital organs (R87.69)
> abnormal cytological findings in specimens from vagina (R87.62-)
> carcinoma in situ of cervix uteri (histologically confirmed) (D06.-)
> cervical intraepithelial neoplasia I [CIN I] (N87.0)
> cervical intraepithelial neoplasia II [CIN II] (N87.1)
> cervical intraepithelial neoplasia III [CIN III] (D06.-)
> dysplasia (mild) (moderate) of cervix uteri (histologically confirmed) (N87.-)
> severe dysplasia of cervix uteri (histologically confirmed) (D06.-)

> **Excludes2**　cervical high risk human papillomavirus (HPV) DNA test positive (R87.810)
> cervical low risk human papillomavirus (HPV) DNA test positive (R87.820)

R87.610　Atypical squamous cells of undetermined significance on cytologic smear of cervix (ASC-US) ♀

R87.611　Atypical squamous cells cannot exclude high grade squamous intraepithelial lesion on cytologic smear of cervix (ASC-H) ♀

R87.612　Low grade squamous intraepithelial lesion on cytologic smear of cervix (LGSIL) ♀

R87.613　High grade squamous intraepithelial lesion on cytologic smear of cervix (HGSIL) ♀

R87.614　Cytologic evidence of malignancy on smear of cervix ♀

R87.615　Unsatisfactory cytologic smear of cervix ♀
> Inadequate sample of cytologic smear of cervix

R87.616　Satisfactory cervical smear but lacking transformation zone ♀

R87.618　Other abnormal cytological findings on specimens from cervix uteri ♀

▶ **R87.619　Unspecified abnormal cytological findings in specimens from cervix uteri** ♀
> Abnormal cervical cytology NOS
> Abnormal Papanicolaou smear of cervix NOS
> Abnormal thin preparation smear of cervix NOS
> Atypical endocervical cells of cervix NOS
> Atypical endometrial cells of cervix NOS
> Atypical glandular cells of cervix NOS

● **R87.62　Abnormal cytological findings in specimens from vagina**

> Use additional code to identify acquired absence of uterus and cervix, if applicable (Z90.71-)

> **Excludes1**　abnormal cytological findings in specimens from cervix uteri (R87.61-)
> abnormal cytological findings in specimens from other female genital organs (R87.69)
> carcinoma in situ of vagina (histologically confirmed) (D07.2)
> vaginal intraepithelial neoplasia I [VAIN I] (N89.0)
> vaginal intraepithelial neoplasia II [VAIN II] (N89.1)
> vaginal intraepithelial neoplasia III [VAIN III] (D07.2)
> dysplasia (mild) (moderate) of vagina (histologically confirmed) (N89.-)
> severe dysplasia of vagina (histologically confirmed) (D07.2)

> **Excludes2**　vaginal high risk human papillomavirus (HPV) DNA test positive (R87.811)
> vaginal low risk human papillomavirus (HPV) DNA test positive (R87.821)

R87.620　Atypical squamous cells of undetermined significance on cytologic smear of vagina (ASC-US) ♀

R87.621　Atypical squamous cells cannot exclude high grade squamous intraepithelial lesion on cytologic smear of vagina (ASC-H) ♀

R87.622　Low grade squamous intraepithelial lesion on cytologic smear of vagina (LGSIL) ♀

R87.623　High grade squamous intraepithelial lesion on cytologic smear of vagina (HGSIL) ♀

R87.624　Cytologic evidence of malignancy on smear of vagina ♀

CHAPTER 18 (R00-R99)

● Unacceptable Principal Diagnosis　● Use Additional Character(s)　■ Unspecified　▶ Manifestation Code
1384　OGCR　Official Guidelines for Coding and Reporting　Excludes 1　Excludes 2　Includes　Use additional　Code first　Code also

R87.625 **Unsatisfactory cytologic smear of vagina** ♀
> Inadequate sample of cytologic smear of vagina

R87.628 **Other abnormal cytological findings on specimens from vagina** ♀

R87.629 **Unspecified abnormal cytological findings in specimens from vagina** ♀
> Abnormal Papanicolaou smear of vagina NOS
> Abnormal thin preparation smear of vagina NOS
> Abnormal vaginal cytology NOS
> Atypical endocervical cells of vagina NOS
> Atypical endometrial cells of vagina NOS
> Atypical glandular cells of vagina NOS

R87.69 **Abnormal cytological findings in specimens from other female genital organs** ♀
> Abnormal cytological findings in specimens from female genital organs NOS
>
> **Excludes1**   dysplasia of vulva (histologically confirmed) (N90.0-N90.3)

R87.7 **Abnormal histological findings in specimens from female genital organs** ♀
> **Excludes1**   carcinoma in situ (histologically confirmed) of female genital organs (D06-D07.3)
> cervical intraepithelial neoplasia I [CIN I] (N87.0)
> cervical intraepithelial neoplasia II [CIN II] (N87.1)
> cervical intraepithelial neoplasia III [CIN III] (D06.-)
> dysplasia (mild) (moderate) of cervix uteri (histologically confirmed) (N87.-)
> dysplasia (mild) (moderate) of vagina (histologically confirmed) (N89.-)
> vaginal intraepithelial neoplasia I [VAIN I] (N89.0)
> vaginal intraepithelial neoplasia II [VAIN II] (N89.1)
> vaginal intraepithelial neoplasia III [VAIN III] (D07.2)
> severe dysplasia of cervix uteri (histologically confirmed) (D06.-)
> severe dysplasia of vagina (histologically confirmed) (D07.2)

● **R87.8** **Other abnormal findings in specimens from female genital organs**

● **R87.81** **High risk human papillomavirus (HPV) DNA test positive from female genital organs**
> **Excludes1**   anogenital warts due to human papillomavirus (HPV) (A63.0)
> condyloma acuminatum (A63.0)

R87.810 **Cervical high risk human papillomavirus (HPV) DNA test positive** ♀

R87.811 **Vaginal high risk human papillomavirus (HPV) DNA test positive** ♀

● **R87.82** **Low risk human papillomavirus (HPV) DNA test positive from female genital organs**
> **Use additional** code for associated human papillomavirus (B97.7)

R87.820 **Cervical low risk human papillomavirus (HPV) DNA test positive** ♀

R87.821 **Vaginal low risk human papillomavirus (HPV) DNA test positive** ♀

R87.89 **Other abnormal findings in specimens from female genital organs** ♀
> Abnormal chromosomal findings in specimens from female genital organs

■ **R87.9** **Unspecified abnormal finding in specimens from female genital organs** ♀

● **R88** **Abnormal findings in other body fluids and substances**

R88.0 **Cloudy (hemodialysis) (peritoneal) dialysis effluent**

R88.8 **Abnormal findings in other body fluids and substances**

● **R89** **Abnormal findings in specimens from other organs, systems and tissues**
> **Includes**   abnormal findings in nipple discharge
> abnormal findings in synovial fluid
> abnormal findings in wound secretions

R89.0 **Abnormal level of enzymes in specimens from other organs, systems and tissues**

R89.1 **Abnormal level of hormones in specimens from other organs, systems and tissues**

R89.2 **Abnormal level of other drugs, medicaments and biological substances in specimens from other organs, systems and tissues**

R89.3 **Abnormal level of substances chiefly nonmedicinal as to source in specimens from other organs, systems and tissues**

R89.4 **Abnormal immunological findings in specimens from other organs, systems and tissues**

R89.5 **Abnormal microbiological findings in specimens from other organs, systems and tissues**
> Positive culture findings in specimens from other organs, systems and tissues
>
> **Excludes1**   colonization status (Z22.-)

R89.6 **Abnormal cytological findings in specimens from other organs, systems and tissues**

R89.7 **Abnormal histological findings in specimens from other organs, systems and tissues**

R89.8 **Other abnormal findings in specimens from other organs, systems and tissues**
> Abnormal chromosomal findings in specimens from other organs, systems and tissues

■ **R89.9** **Unspecified abnormal finding in specimens from other organs, systems and tissues**

N Newborn Age: 0   **P** Pediatric Age: 0–17   **M** Maternity DX: 12–55   **A** Adult Age: 15–124   ♀ Females Only   ♂ Males Only

Complication\Comorbidity   Major C\C   Present on Admission Requirement   Hospital-Acquired Condition

1385

ABNORMAL FINDINGS ON DIAGNOSTIC IMAGING AND IN FUNCTION STUDIES, WITHOUT DIAGNOSIS (R90-R94)

Includes
nonspecific abnormal findings on diagnostic imaging by computerized axial tomography [CAT scan]
nonspecific abnormal findings on diagnostic imaging by magnetic resonance imaging [MRI][NMR]
nonspecific abnormal findings on diagnostic imaging by positron emission tomography [PET scan]
nonspecific abnormal findings on diagnostic imaging by thermography
nonspecific abnormal findings on diagnostic imaging by ultrasound [echogram]
nonspecific abnormal findings on diagnostic imaging by X-ray examination

Excludes1
abnormal findings on antenatal screening of mother (O28.-)
diagnostic abnormal findings classified elsewhere - see Alphabetical Index

● **R90**   **Abnormal findings on diagnostic imaging of central nervous system**

     R90.0   **Intracranial space-occupying lesion found on diagnostic imaging of central nervous system**

     ● **R90.8**   **Other abnormal findings on diagnostic imaging of central nervous system**

         R90.81   **Abnormal echoencephalogram**

         ■ **R90.82**   **White matter disease, unspecified**

         R90.89   **Other abnormal findings on diagnostic imaging of central nervous system**
             Other cerebrovascular abnormality found on diagnostic imaging of central nervous system

● **R91**   **Abnormal findings on diagnostic imaging of lung**

     R91.1   **Solitary pulmonary nodule**
         Coin lesion lung
         Solitary pulmonary nodule, subsegmental branch of the bronchial tree

     R91.8   **Other nonspecific abnormal finding of lung field**
         Lung mass NOS found on diagnostic imaging of lung
         Pulmonary infiltrate NOS
         Shadow, lung

● **R92**   **Abnormal and inconclusive findings on diagnostic imaging of breast**

     R92.0   **Mammographic microcalcification found on diagnostic imaging of breast**

         Excludes2   mammographic calcification (calculus) found on diagnostic imaging of breast (R92.1)

     R92.1   **Mammographic calcification found on diagnostic imaging of breast**
         Mammographic calculus found on diagnostic imaging of breast

     R92.2   **Inconclusive mammogram**
         Dense breasts NOS
         Inconclusive mammogram NEC
         Inconclusive mammography due to dense breasts
         Inconclusive mammography NEC

     R92.8   **Other abnormal and inconclusive findings on diagnostic imaging of breast**

● **R93**   **Abnormal findings on diagnostic imaging of other body structures**

     R93.0   **Abnormal findings on diagnostic imaging of skull and head, not elsewhere classified**

         Excludes1   intracranial space-occupying lesion found on diagnostic imaging (R90.0)

     R93.1   **Abnormal findings on diagnostic imaging of heart and coronary circulation**
         Abnormal echocardiogram NOS
         Abnormal heart shadow

     R93.2   **Abnormal findings on diagnostic imaging of liver and biliary tract**
         Nonvisualization of gallbladder

     R93.3   **Abnormal findings on diagnostic imaging of other parts of digestive tract**

     R93.4   **Abnormal findings on diagnostic imaging of urinary organs**
         Filling defect of bladder found on diagnostic imaging
         Filling defect of kidney found on diagnostic imaging
         Filling defect of ureter found on diagnostic imaging

         Excludes1   hypertrophy of kidney (N28.81)

     R93.5   **Abnormal findings on diagnostic imaging of other abdominal regions, including retroperitoneum**

     R93.6   **Abnormal findings on diagnostic imaging of limbs**

         Excludes2   abnormal finding in skin and subcutaneous tissue (R93.8)

     R93.7   **Abnormal findings on diagnostic imaging of other parts of musculoskeletal system**

         Excludes2   abnormal findings on diagnostic imaging of skull (R93.0)

     R93.8   **Abnormal findings on diagnostic imaging of other specified body structures**
         Abnormal finding by radioisotope localization of placenta
         Abnormal radiological finding in skin and subcutaneous tissue
         Mediastinal shift

     R93.9   **Diagnostic imaging inconclusive due to excess body fat of patient**

● **R94**   **Abnormal results of function studies**

     Includes   abnormal results of radionuclide [radioisotope] uptake studies
         abnormal results of scintigraphy

     ● **R94.0**   **Abnormal results of function studies of central nervous system**

         R94.01   **Abnormal electroencephalogram [EEG]**

         R94.02   **Abnormal brain scan**

         R94.09   **Abnormal results of other function studies of central nervous system**

     ● **R94.1**   **Abnormal results of function studies of peripheral nervous system and special senses**

         ● **R94.11**   **Abnormal results of function studies of eye**

             R94.110   **Abnormal electro-oculogram [EOG]**

             R94.111   **Abnormal electroretinogram [ERG]**
                 Abnormal retinal function study

             R94.112   **Abnormal visually evoked potential [VEP]**

             R94.113   **Abnormal oculomotor study**

             R94.118   **Abnormal results of other function studies of eye**

● Unacceptable Principal Diagnosis   ● Use Additional Character(s)   ■ Unspecified   ▶ Manifestation Code

1386   **OGCR** Official Guidelines for Coding and Reporting   Excludes 1   Excludes 2   Includes   Use additional   Code first   Code also

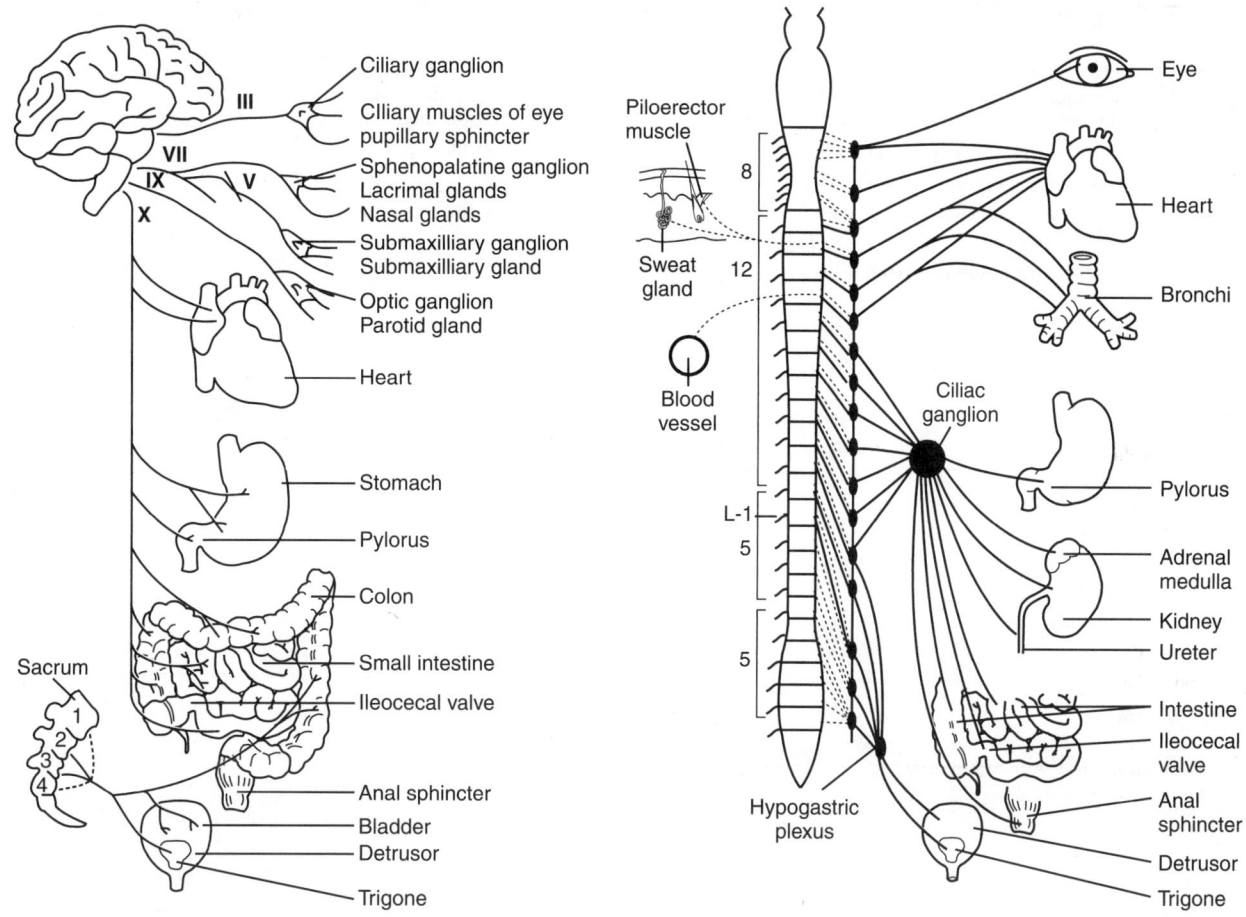

Figure 18-2 **A.** Parasympathetic nervous system. **B.** Sympathetic nervous system. (From Buck CJ: Step-by-Step Medical Coding, St. Louis, WB Saunders, 2010.)

Item 18-1 The **peripheral nervous system** consists of 31 pairs of spinal nerves, 12 pairs of cranial nerves, and the autonomic nerves, which are divided into the parasympathetic and sympathetic nerves. The cranial nerves are: olfactory (I), optic (II), oculomotor (III), trochlear (IV), trigeminal (V), abducens (VI), facial (VII), vestibulocochlear (VIII), glossopharyngeal (IX), vagus (X), accessory (XI), and hypoglossal (XII).

● **R94.12** **Abnormal results of function studies of ear and other special senses**

   R94.120 **Abnormal auditory function study**

   R94.121 **Abnormal vestibular function study**

   R94.128 **Abnormal results of other function studies of ear and other special senses**

● **R94.13** **Abnormal results of function studies of peripheral nervous system**

   ■ **R94.130** **Abnormal response to nerve stimulation, unspecified**

   R94.131 **Abnormal electromyogram [EMG]**

      Excludes1   electromyogram of eye (R94.113)

   R94.138 **Abnormal results of other function studies of peripheral nervous system**

R94.2 **Abnormal results of pulmonary function studies**
   Reduced ventilatory capacity
   Reduced vital capacity

● **R94.3** **Abnormal results of cardiovascular function studies**

   ■ **R94.30** **Abnormal result of cardiovascular function study, unspecified**

   R94.31 **Abnormal electrocardiogram [ECG] [EKG]**
      Excludes1   long QT syndrome (I45.81)

   R94.39 **Abnormal result of other cardiovascular function study**
      Abnormal electrophysiological intracardiac studies
      Abnormal phonocardiogram
      Abnormal vectorcardiogram

R94.4 **Abnormal results of kidney function studies**
   Abnormal renal function test

R94.5 **Abnormal results of liver function studies**

R94.6 **Abnormal results of thyroid function studies**

R94.7 **Abnormal results of other endocrine function studies**
      Excludes2   abnormal glucose (R73.0-)

R94.8 **Abnormal results of function studies of other organs and systems**
   Abnormal basal metabolic rate [BMR]
   Abnormal bladder function test
   Abnormal splenic function test

N Newborn Age: 0   P Pediatric Age: 0–17   M Maternity DX: 12–55   A Adult Age: 15–124   ♀ Females Only   ♂ Males Only

🦎 Complication\Comorbidity   🦎 Major C\C   🦎 Present on Admission Requirement   🦎 Hospital-Acquired Condition

CHAPTER 18 (R00-R99)

ABNORMAL TUMOR MARKERS (R97)

● R97   **Abnormal tumor markers**
Elevated tumor associated antigens [TAA]
Elevated tumor specific antigens [TSA]

R97.0   **Elevated carcinoembryonic antigen [CEA]**

R97.1   **Elevated cancer antigen 125 [CA 125] ♀**

R97.2   **Elevated prostate specific antigen [PSA] ♂**   A
MCE: Questionable admission when principal dx

R97.8   **Other abnormal tumor markers**

ILL-DEFINED AND UNKNOWN CAUSE OF MORTALITY (R99)

▪ R99   **Ill-defined and unknown cause of mortality**
Death (unexplained) NOS
Unspecified cause of mortality

OGCR   Section I.C.18.h.

18.6 Death NOS

Code R99, Ill-defined and unknown cause of mortality, is only for use in the very limited circumstance when a patient who has already died is brought into the emergency department or other healthcare facility and is pronounced dead upon arrival. It does not represent the discharge disposition of death.

● Unacceptable Principal Diagnosis   ● Use Additional Character(s)   ▪ Unspecified   ▶ Manifestation Code

1388   **OGCR**   Official Guidelines for Coding and Reporting   Excludes 1   Excludes 2   Includes   Use additional   Code first   Code also

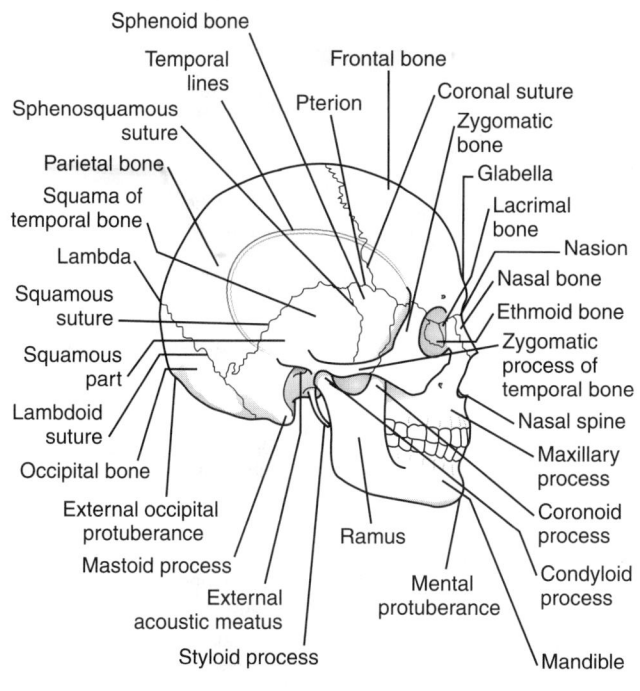

Figure 19-1   Lateral view of skull

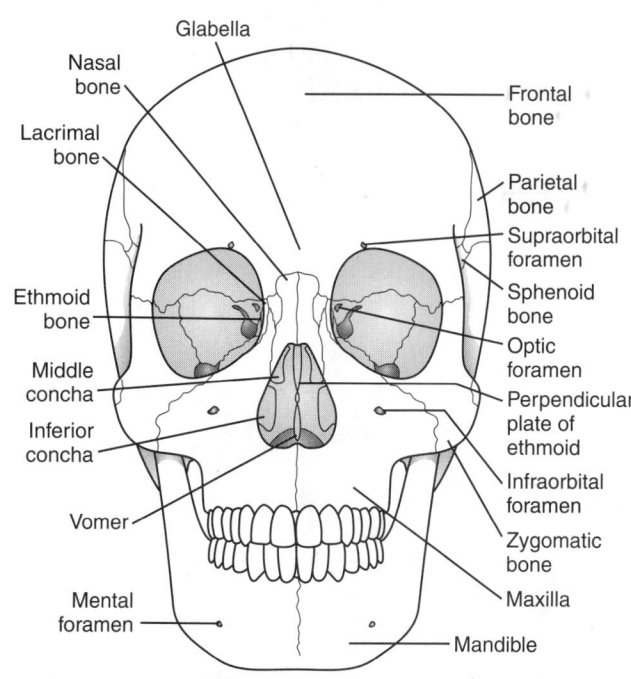

Figure 19-2   Frontal view of skull.

Figure 19-3   Anterior view of vertebral column.

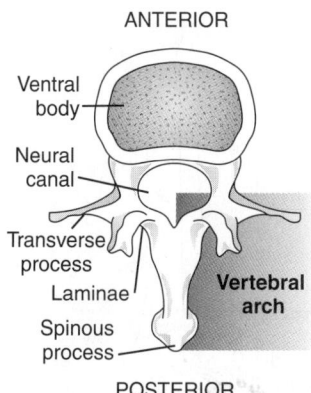

Figure 19-4   Vertebra viewed from above

CHAPTER 19 (S00-T88)

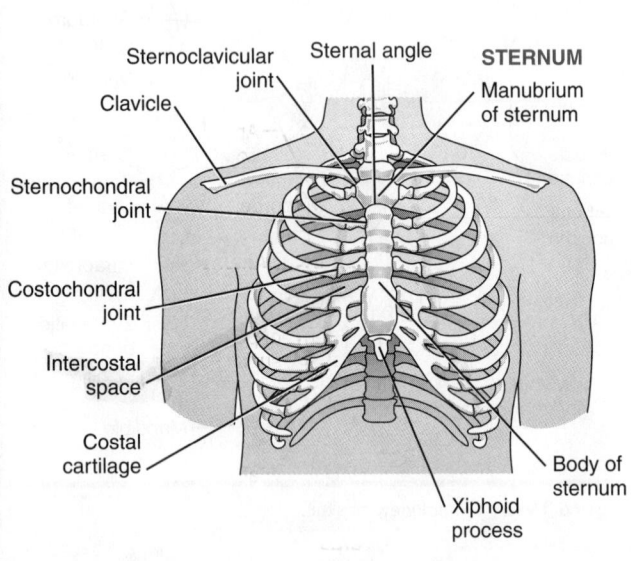

Figure 19-5   Anterior view of rib cage.

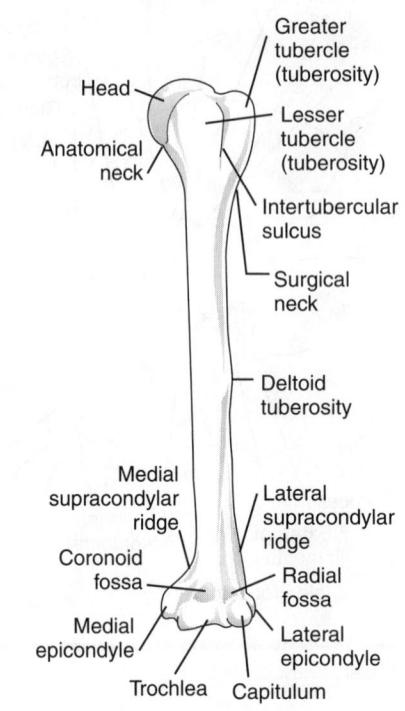

Figure 19-6   Anterior aspect of left humerus.

Figure 19-7   Anterior aspect of left radius and ulna.

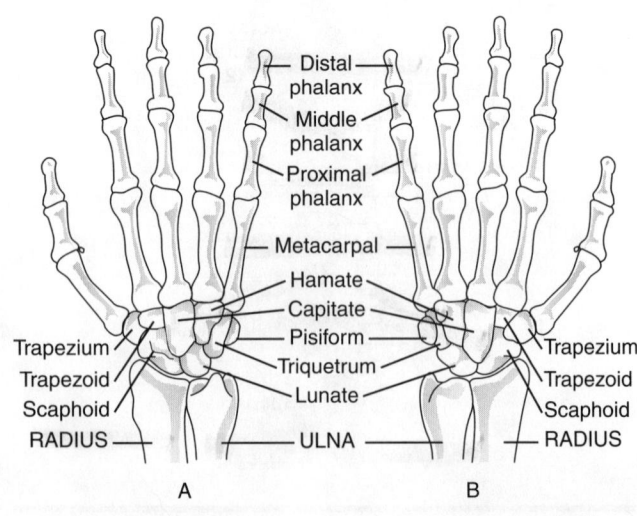

Figure 19-8   Right hand and wrist: **A.** Dorsal surface. **B.** Palmar surface.

● Unacceptable Principal Diagnosis   ● Use Additional Character(s)   ▮ Unspecified   ▶ Manifestation Code

OGCR   Official Guidelines for Coding and Reporting   Excludes 1   Excludes 2   Includes   Use additional   Code first   Code also

1390

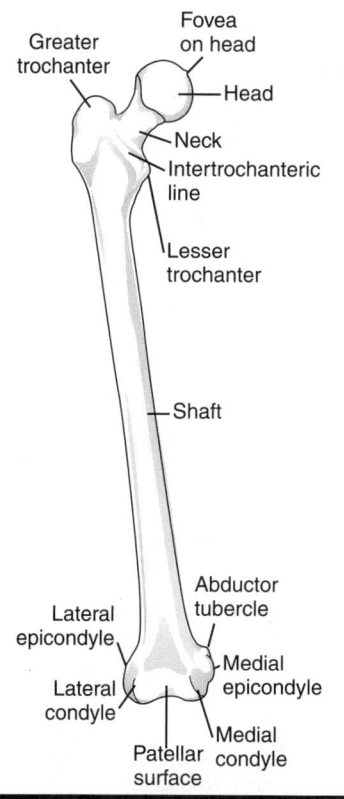

Figure 19-9   Anterior aspect of right femur.

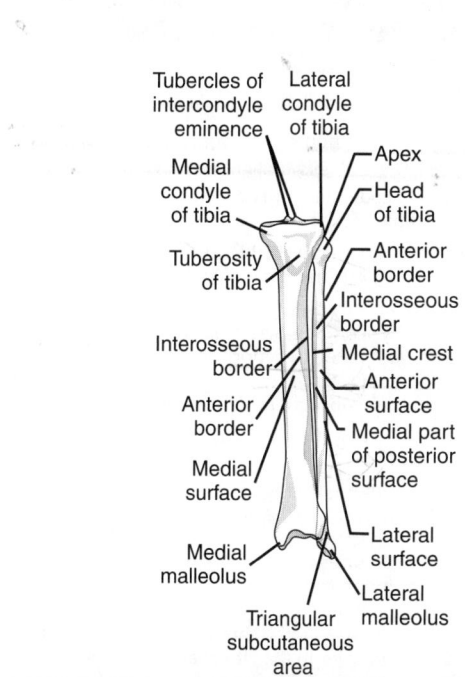

Figure 19-10   Anterior aspect of left tibia and fibula.

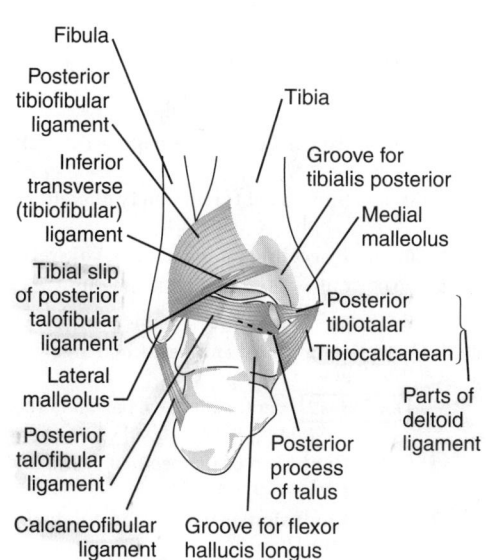

Figure 19-11   Posterior aspect of the left ankle joint.

Figure 19-12   Right foot viewed from above.

CHAPTER 19 (S00-T88)

OGCR Chapter Guidelines are located in **Section I.9.**

CHAPTER 19

INJURY, POISONING AND CERTAIN OTHER CONSEQUENCES OF EXTERNAL CAUSES (S00-T88)

Note: Use secondary code(s) from Chapter 20, External causes of morbidity, to indicate cause of injury. Codes within the T section that include the external cause do not require an additional external cause code.

Use additional code to identify any retained foreign body, if applicable (Z18.-)

Excludes1 birth trauma (P10-P15)
obstetric trauma (O70-O71)

Note: The chapter uses the S-section for coding different types of injuries related to single body regions and the T-section to cover injuries to unspecified body regions as well as poisoning and certain other consequences of external causes.

This chapter contains the following blocks:

S00-S09	Injuries to the head
S10-S19	Injuries to the neck
S20-S29	Injuries to the thorax
S30-S39	Injuries to the abdomen, lower back, lumbar spine, pelvis and external genitals
S40-S49	Injuries to the shoulder and upper arm
S50-S59	Injuries to the elbow and forearm
S60-S69	Injuries to the wrist, hand, and fingers
S70-S79	Injuries to the hip and thigh
S80-S89	Injuries to the knee and lower leg
S90-S99	Injuries to the ankle and foot
T07	Injuries involving multiple body regions
T14	Injury of unspecified body region
T15-T19	Effects of foreign body entering through natural orifice
T20-T32	Burns and corrosions
T20-T25	Burns and corrosions of external body surface, specified by site
T26-T28	Burns and corrosions confined to eye and internal organs
T30-T32	Burns and corrosions of multiple and unspecified body regions
T33-T34	Frostbite
T36-T50	Poisoning by, adverse effect of and underdosing of drugs, medicaments and biological substances
T51-T65	Toxic effects of substances chiefly nonmedicinal as to source
T66-T78	Other and unspecified effects of external causes
T79	Certain early complications of trauma
T80-T88	Complications of surgical and medical care, not elsewhere classified

INJURIES TO THE HEAD (S00-S09)

Includes   injuries of ear
injuries of eye
injuries of face [any part]
injuries of gum
injuries of jaw
injuries of oral cavity
injuries of palate
injuries of periocular area
injuries of scalp
injuries of temporomandibular joint area
injuries of tongue
injuries of tooth

Code also for any associated infection

Excludes2   burns and corrosions (T20-T32)
effects of foreign body in ear (T16)
effects of foreign body in larynx (T17.3)
effects of foreign body in mouth NOS (T18.0)
effects of foreign body in nose (T17.0-T17.1)
effects of foreign body in pharynx (T17.2)
effects of foreign body on external eye (T15.-)
frostbite (T33-T34)
insect bite or sting, venomous (T63.4)

● **S00 Superficial injury of head**

Excludes1   diffuse cerebral contusion (S06.2-)
focal cerebral contusion (S06.3-)
injury of eye and orbit (S05.-)
open wound of head (S01.-)

The appropriate 7th character is to be added to each code from category S00

A	initial encounter
D	subsequent encounter
S	sequela

● **S00.0 Superficial injury of scalp**

●■ **S00.00 Unspecified superficial injury of scalp** D, S ◎

● **S00.01 Abrasion of scalp** D, S ◎

● **S00.02 Blister (nonthermal) of scalp** D, S ◎

● **S00.03 Contusion of scalp** D, S ◎
Bruise of scalp
Hematoma of scalp

● **S00.04 External constriction of part of scalp** D, S ◎

● **S00.05 Superficial foreign body of scalp** D, S ◎
Splinter in the scalp

● **S00.06 Insect bite (nonvenomous) of scalp** D, S ◎

● **S00.07 Other superficial bite of scalp** D, S ◎
Excludes1   open bite of scalp (S01.05)

● **S00.1 Contusion of eyelid and periocular area**
Black eye
Excludes2   contusion of eyeball and orbital tissues (S05.1)

●■ **S00.10 Contusion of unspecified eyelid and periocular area** D, S ◎

● **S00.11 Contusion of right eyelid and periocular area** D, S ◎

● **S00.12 Contusion of left eyelid and periocular area** D, S ◎

● Unacceptable Principal Diagnosis   ● Use Additional Character(s)   ■ Unspecified   ▶ Manifestation Code

OGCR Official Guidelines for Coding and Reporting | Excludes 1 | | Excludes 2 | | Includes | | Use additional | | Code first | | Code also |

● **S00.2   Other and unspecified superficial injuries of eyelid and periocular area**

> **Excludes2**   superficial injury of conjunctiva and cornea (S05.0-)

●■ **S00.20   Unspecified superficial injury of eyelid and periocular area**

S00.201   Unspecified superficial injury of right eyelid and periocular area D, S 🔲

●■ **S00.202   Unspecified superficial injury of left eyelid and periocular area** D, S 🔲

●■ **S00.209   Unspecified superficial injury of unspecified eyelid and periocular area** D, S 🔲

● **S00.21   Abrasion of eyelid and periocular area**

● **S00.211   Abrasion of right eyelid and periocular area** D, S 🔲

● **S00.212   Abrasion of left eyelid and periocular area** D, S 🔲

●■ **S00.219   Abrasion of unspecified eyelid and periocular area** D, S 🔲

● **S00.22   Blister (nonthermal) of eyelid and periocular area**

● **S00.221   Blister (nonthermal) of right eyelid and periocular area** D, S 🔲

● **S00.222   Blister (nonthermal) of left eyelid and periocular area** D, S 🔲

●■ **S00.229   Blister (nonthermal) of unspecified eyelid and periocular area** D, S 🔲

● **S00.24   External constriction of eyelid and periocular area**

● **S00.241   External constriction of right eyelid and periocular area** D, S 🔲

● **S00.242   External constriction of left eyelid and periocular area** D, S 🔲

●■ **S00.249   External constriction of unspecified eyelid and periocular area** D, S 🔲

● **S00.25   Superficial foreign body of eyelid and periocular area**
> Splinter of eyelid and periocular area
> **Excludes2**   retained foreign body in eyelid (H02.81-)

● **S00.251   Superficial foreign body of right eyelid and periocular area** D, S 🔲

● **S00.252   Superficial foreign body of left eyelid and periocular area** D, S 🔲

●■ **S00.259   Superficial foreign body of unspecified eyelid and periocular area** D, S 🔲

● **S00.26   Insect bite (nonvenomous) of eyelid and periocular area**

● **S00.261   Insect bite (nonvenomous) of right eyelid and periocular area** D, S 🔲

● **S00.262   Insect bite (nonvenomous) of left eyelid and periocular area** D, S 🔲

●■ **S00.269   Insect bite (nonvenomous) of unspecified eyelid and periocular area** D, S 🔲

● **S00.27   Other superficial bite of eyelid and periocular area**

> **Excludes1**   open bite of eyelid and periocular area (S01.15)

● **S00.271   Other superficial bite of right eyelid and periocular area** D, S 🔲

● **S00.272   Other superficial bite of left eyelid and periocular area** D, S 🔲

●■ **S00.279   Other superficial bite of unspecified eyelid and periocular area** D, S 🔲

● **S00.3   Superficial injury of nose**

●■ **S00.30   Unspecified superficial injury of nose** D, S 🔲

● **S00.31   Abrasion of nose** D, S 🔲

● **S00.32   Blister (nonthermal) of nose** D, S 🔲

● **S00.33   Contusion of nose** D, S 🔲
> Bruise of nose
> Hematoma of nose

● **S00.34   External constriction of nose** D, S 🔲

● **S00.35   Superficial foreign body of nose** D, S 🔲
> Splinter in the nose

● **S00.36   Insect bite (nonvenomous) of nose** D, S 🔲

● **S00.37   Other superficial bite of nose** D, S 🔲
> **Excludes1**   open bite of nose (S01.25)

● **S00.4   Superficial injury of ear**

● **S00.40   Unspecified superficial injury of ear**

●■ **S00.401   Unspecified superficial injury of right ear** D, S 🔲

●■ **S00.402   Unspecified superficial injury of left ear** D, S 🔲

●■ **S00.409   Unspecified superficial injury of unspecified ear** D, S 🔲

● **S00.41   Abrasion of ear**

● **S00.411   Abrasion of right ear** D, S 🔲

● **S00.412   Abrasion of left ear** D, S 🔲

●■ **S00.419   Abrasion of unspecified ear** D, S 🔲

● **S00.42   Blister (nonthermal) of ear**

● **S00.421   Blister (nonthermal) of right ear** D, S 🔲

● **S00.422   Blister (nonthermal) of left ear** D, S 🔲

●■ **S00.429   Blister (nonthermal) of unspecified ear** D, S 🔲

● **S00.43   Contusion of ear**
> Bruise of ear
> Hematoma of ear

● **S00.431   Contusion of right ear** D, S 🔲

● **S00.432   Contusion of left ear** D, S 🔲

●■ **S00.439   Contusion of unspecified ear** D, S 🔲

● **S00.44   External constriction of ear**

● **S00.441   External constriction of right ear** D, S 🔲

● **S00.442   External constriction of left ear** D, S 🔲

●■ **S00.449   External constriction of unspecified ear** D, S 🔲

CHAPTER 19 (S00-T88)

N Newborn Age: 0   **P** Pediatric Age: 0–17   **M** Maternity DX: 12–55   **A** Adult Age: 15–124   ♀ Females Only   ♂ Males Only

🔲 Complication\Comorbidity   🔲 Major C\C   🔲 Present on Admission Requirement   🔲 Hospital-Acquired Condition

1393

CHAPTER 19 (S00-T88)

● **S00.45 Superficial foreign body of ear**
Splinter in the ear

  ● **S00.451 Superficial foreign body of right ear** D, S

  ● **S00.452 Superficial foreign body of left ear** D, S

  ●■ **S00.459 Superficial foreign body of unspecified ear** D, S

● **S00.46 Insect bite (nonvenomous) of ear**

  ● **S00.461 Insect bite (nonvenomous) of right ear** D, S

  ● **S00.462 Insect bite (nonvenomous) of left ear** D, S

  ●■ **S00.469 Insect bite (nonvenomous) of unspecified ear** D, S

● **S00.47 Other superficial bite of ear**

  Excludes1   open bite of ear (S01.35)

  ● **S00.471 Other superficial bite of right ear** D, S

  ● **S00.472 Other superficial bite of left ear** D, S

  ●■ **S00.479 Other superficial bite of unspecified ear** D, S

● **S00.5 Superficial injury of lip and oral cavity**

  ● **S00.50 Unspecified superficial injury of lip and oral cavity**

    ●■ **S00.501 Unspecified superficial injury of lip** D, S

    ●■ **S00.502 Unspecified superficial injury of oral cavity** D, S

  ● **S00.51 Abrasion of lip and oral cavity**

    ● **S00.511 Abrasion of lip** D, S

    ● **S00.512 Abrasion of oral cavity** D, S

  ● **S00.52 Blister (nonthermal) of lip and oral cavity**

    ● **S00.521 Blister (nonthermal) of lip** D, S

    ● **S00.522 Blister (nonthermal) of oral cavity** D, S

  ● **S00.53 Contusion of lip and oral cavity**

    ● **S00.531 Contusion of lip** D, S
      Bruise of lip
      Hematoma of oral cavity

    ● **S00.532 Contusion of oral cavity** D, S
      Bruise of lip
      Hematoma of oral cavity

  ● **S00.54 External constriction of lip and oral cavity**

    ● **S00.541 External constriction of lip** D, S

    ● **S00.542 External constriction of oral cavity** D, S

  ● **S00.55 Superficial foreign body of lip and oral cavity**

    ● **S00.551 Superficial foreign body of lip** D, S
      Splinter of lip and oral cavity

    ● **S00.552 Superficial foreign body of oral cavity** D, S
      Splinter of lip and oral cavity

● **S00.56 Insect bite (nonvenomous) of lip and oral cavity**

  ● **S00.561 Insect bite (nonvenomous) of lip** D, S

  ● **S00.562 Insect bite (nonvenomous) of oral cavity** D, S

● **S00.57 Other superficial bite of lip and oral cavity**

  ● **S00.571 Other superficial bite of lip** D, S

    Excludes1   open bite of lip (S01.551)

  ● **S00.572 Other superficial bite of oral cavity** D, S

    Excludes1   open bite of oral cavity (S01.552)

● **S00.8 Superficial injury of other parts of head**

  ●■ **S00.80 Unspecified superficial injury of other part of head** D, S

  ● **S00.81 Abrasion of other part of head** D, S

  ● **S00.82 Blister (nonthermal) of other part of head** D, S

  ● **S00.83 Contusion of other part of head** D, S
    Bruise of other part of head
    Hematoma of other part of head

  ● **S00.84 External constriction of other part of head** D, S

  ● **S00.85 Superficial foreign body of other part of head** D, S
    Splinter in other part of head

  ● **S00.86 Insect bite (nonvenomous) of other part of head** D, S

  ● **S00.87 Other superficial bite of other part of head** D, S

    Excludes1   open bite of other part of head (S01.85)

● **S00.9 Superficial injury of unspecified part of head**

  ●■ **S00.90 Unspecified superficial injury of unspecified part of head** D, S

  ●■ **S00.91 Abrasion of unspecified part of head** D, S

  ●■ **S00.92 Blister (nonthermal) of unspecified part of head** D, S

  ●■ **S00.93 Contusion of unspecified part of head** D, S
    Bruise of head
    Hematoma of head

  ●■ **S00.94 External constriction of unspecified part of head** D, S

  ●■ **S00.95 Superficial foreign body of unspecified part of head** D, S
    Splinter of head

  ●■ **S00.96 Insect bite (nonvenomous) of unspecified part of head** D, S

  ●■ **S00.97 Other superficial bite of unspecified part of head** D, S

    Excludes1   open bite of head (S01.95)

● Unacceptable Principal Diagnosis   ● Use Additional Character(s)   ■ Unspecified   ▶ Manifestation Code
OGCR Official Guidelines for Coding and Reporting   Excludes 1   Excludes 2   Includes   Use additional   Code first   Code also

● **S01.32**   **Laceration with foreign body of ear**
   ● **S01.321**   Laceration with foreign body of right ear D, S
   ● **S01.322**   Laceration with foreign body of left ear D, S
   ●■ **S01.329**   Laceration with foreign body of unspecified ear D, S

● **S01.33**   **Puncture wound without foreign body of ear**
   ● **S01.331**   Puncture wound without foreign body of right ear D, S
   ● **S01.332**   Puncture wound without foreign body of left ear D, S
   ●■ **S01.339**   Puncture wound without foreign body of unspecified ear D, S

● **S01.34**   **Puncture wound with foreign body of ear**
   ● **S01.341**   Puncture wound with foreign body of right ear D, S
   ● **S01.342**   Puncture wound with foreign body of left ear D, S
   ●■ **S01.349**   Puncture wound with foreign body of unspecified ear D, S

● **S01.35**   **Open bite of ear**
   Bite of ear NOS
   Excludes1   superficial bite of ear (S00.46, S00.47)
   ● **S01.351**   Open bite of right ear D, S
   ● **S01.352**   Open bite of left ear D, S
   ●■ **S01.359**   Open bite of unspecified ear D, S

● **S01.4**   **Open wound of cheek and temporomandibular area**
  ● **S01.40**   **Unspecified open wound of cheek and temporomandibular area**
   ●■ **S01.401**   Unspecified open wound of right cheek and temporomandibular area D, S
   ●■ **S01.402**   Unspecified open wound of left cheek and temporomandibular area D, S
   ●■ **S01.409**   Unspecified open wound of unspecified cheek and temporomandibular area D, S

  ● **S01.41**   **Laceration without foreign body of cheek and temporomandibular area**
   ● **S01.411**   Laceration without foreign body of right cheek and temporomandibular area D, S
   ● **S01.412**   Laceration without foreign body of left cheek and temporomandibular area D, S
   ●■ **S01.419**   Laceration without foreign body of unspecified cheek and temporomandibular area D, S

  ● **S01.42**   **Laceration with foreign body of cheek and temporomandibular area**
   ● **S01.421**   Laceration with foreign body of right cheek and temporomandibular area D, S
   ● **S01.422**   Laceration with foreign body of left cheek and temporomandibular area D, S
   ●■ **S01.429**   Laceration with foreign body of unspecified cheek and temporomandibular area D, S

● **S01.43**   **Puncture wound without foreign body of cheek and temporomandibular area**
   ● **S01.431**   Puncture wound without foreign body of right cheek and temporomandibular area D, S
   ● **S01.432**   Puncture wound without foreign body of left cheek and temporomandibular area D, S
   ●■ **S01.439**   Puncture wound without foreign body of unspecified cheek and temporomandibular area D, S

● **S01.44**   **Puncture wound with foreign body of cheek and temporomandibular area**
   ● **S01.441**   Puncture wound with foreign body of right cheek and temporomandibular area D, S
   ● **S01.442**   Puncture wound with foreign body of left cheek and temporomandibular area D, S
   ●■ **S01.449**   Puncture wound with foreign body of unspecified cheek and temporomandibular area D, S

● **S01.45**   **Open bite of cheek and temporomandibular area**
   Bite of cheek and temporomandibular area NOS
   Excludes2   superficial bite of cheek and temporomandibular area (S00.86, S00.87)
   ● **S01.451**   Open bite of right cheek and temporomandibular area D, S
   ● **S01.452**   Open bite of left cheek and temporomandibular area D, S
   ●■ **S01.459**   Open bite of unspecified cheek and temporomandibular area D, S

● **S01.5**   **Open wound of lip and oral cavity**
  Excludes2   tooth dislocation (S03.2)
            tooth fracture (S02.5)

  ● **S01.50**   **Unspecified open wound of lip and oral cavity**
   ●■ **S01.501**   Unspecified open wound of lip D, S
   ●■ **S01.502**   Unspecified open wound of oral cavity D, S

  ● **S01.51**   **Laceration of lip and oral cavity without foreign body**
   ● **S01.511**   Laceration without foreign body of lip D, S
   ● **S01.512**   Laceration without foreign body of oral cavity D, S

  ● **S01.52**   **Laceration of lip and oral cavity with foreign body**
   ● **S01.521**   Laceration with foreign body of lip D, S
   ● **S01.522**   Laceration with foreign body of oral cavity D, S

  ● **S01.53**   **Puncture wound of lip and oral cavity without foreign body**
   ● **S01.531**   Puncture wound without foreign body of lip D, S
   ● **S01.532**   Puncture wound without foreign body of oral cavity D, S

● Unacceptable Principal Diagnosis   ● Use Additional Character(s)   ■ Unspecified   ▶ Manifestation Code
OGCR Official Guidelines for Coding and Reporting   Excludes 1   Excludes 2   Includes   Use additional   Code first   Code also

CHAPTER 19 (S00-T88)

● **S01.54 Puncture wound of lip and oral cavity with foreign body**
    ● **S01.541 Puncture wound with foreign body of lip** D, S 🖉
    ● **S01.542 Puncture wound with foreign body of oral cavity** D, S 🖉
● **S01.55 Open bite of lip and oral cavity**
    ● **S01.551 Open bite of lip** D, S 🖉
       Bite of lip NOS
       | Excludes1 | superficial bite of lip (S00.571)
    ● **S01.552 Open bite of oral cavity** D, S 🖉
       Bite of oral cavity NOS
       | Excludes1 | superficial bite of oral cavity (S00.572)

● **S01.8 Open wound of other parts of head**
    ●■ **S01.80 Unspecified open wound of other part of head** D, S 🖉
    ● **S01.81 Laceration without foreign body of other part of head** D, S 🖉
    ● **S01.82 Laceration with foreign body of other part of head** D, S 🖉
    ● **S01.83 Puncture wound without foreign body of other part of head** D, S 🖉
    ● **S01.84 Puncture wound with foreign body of other part of head** D, S 🖉
    ● **S01.85 Open bite of other part of head** D, S 🖉
       Bite of other part of head NOS
       | Excludes1 | superficial bite of other part of head (S00.85)

● **S01.9 Open wound of unspecified part of head**
    ●■ **S01.90 Unspecified open wound of unspecified part of head** D, S 🖉
    ●■ **S01.91 Laceration without foreign body of unspecified part of head** D, S 🖉
    ●■ **S01.92 Laceration with foreign body of unspecified part of head** D, S 🖉
    ●■ **S01.93 Puncture wound without foreign body of unspecified part of head** D, S 🖉
    ●■ **S01.94 Puncture wound with foreign body of unspecified part of head** D, S 🖉
    ●■ **S01.95 Open bite of unspecified part of head** D, S 🖉
       Bite of head NOS
       | Excludes1 | superficial bite of head NOS (S00.97)

● **S02 Fracture of skull and facial bones**

    Note: A fracture not indicated as open or closed should be coded to closed

    The appropriate 7th character is to be added to each code from category S02

A	initial encounter for closed fracture
B	initial encounter for open fracture
D	subsequent encounter for fracture with routine healing
G	subsequent encounter for fracture with delayed healing
K	subsequent encounter for fracture with nonunion
S	sequela

Code also any associated intracranial injury (S06.-)

● **S02.0 Fracture of vault of skull** A, K 🖉, B 🖉, D, G, S 🖉, A, B 🖉
    Fracture of frontal bone
    Fracture of parietal bone

● **S02.1 Fracture of base of skull**
    | Excludes1 | orbit NOS (S02.8)
    | Excludes2 | orbital floor (S02.3-)
    ●■ **S02.10 Unspecified fracture of base of skull** A, K 🖉, B 🖉, D, G, S 🖉, A, B 🖉
    ● **S02.11 Fracture of occiput**
       ● **S02.110 Type I occipital condyle fracture** A, K 🖉, B 🖉, D, G, S 🖉, A, B 🖉
       ● **S02.111 Type II occipital condyle fracture** A, K 🖉, B 🖉, D, G, S 🖉, A, B 🖉
       ● **S02.112 Type III occipital condyle fracture** A, K 🖉, B 🖉, D, G, S 🖉, A, B 🖉
       ●■ **S02.113 Unspecified occipital condyle fracture** A, K 🖉, B 🖉, D, G, S 🖉, A, B 🖉
       ● **S02.118 Other fracture of occiput** A, K 🖉, B 🖉, D, G, S 🖉, A, B 🖉
       ●■ **S02.119 Unspecified fracture of occiput** A, K 🖉, B 🖉, D, G, S 🖉, A, B 🖉
    ● **S02.19 Other fracture of base of skull** A, K 🖉, B 🖉, D, G, S 🖉, A, B 🖉
       Fracture of anterior fossa of base of skull
       Fracture of ethmoid sinus
       Fracture of frontal sinus
       Fracture of middle fossa of base of skull
       Fracture of orbital roof
       Fracture of posterior fossa of base of skull
       Fracture of sphenoid
       Fracture of temporal bone

● **S02.2 Fracture of nasal bones** B, K 🖉, D, G, S 🖉, B 🖉
● **S02.3 Fracture of orbital floor** A, B, K 🖉, D, G, S 🖉, A, B 🖉
    | Excludes1 | orbit NOS (S02.8)
    | Excludes2 | orbital roof (S02.1-)
● **S02.4 Fracture of malar, maxillary and zygoma bones**
    Fracture of superior maxilla
    Fracture of upper jaw (bone)
    Fracture of zygomatic process of temporal bone
    ● **S02.40 Fracture of malar, maxillary and zygoma bones, unspecified**
       ●■ **S02.400 Malar fracture unspecified** A, B, K 🖉, D, G, S 🖉, A, B 🖉
       ●■ **S02.401 Maxillary fracture, unspecified** A, B, K 🖉, D, G, S 🖉, A, B 🖉
       ●■ **S02.402 Zygomatic fracture, unspecified** A, B, K 🖉, D, G, S 🖉, A, B 🖉
    ● **S02.41 LeFort fracture**
       ● **S02.411 LeFort I fracture** A, B, K 🖉, D, G, S 🖉, A, B 🖉
       ● **S02.412 LeFort II fracture** A, B, K 🖉, D, G, S 🖉, A, B 🖉
       ● **S02.413 LeFort III fracture** A, B, K 🖉, D, G, S 🖉, A, B 🖉
    S02.42 Fracture of alveolus of maxilla A, B, K 🖉, D, G, S 🖉, A, B 🖉
● **S02.5 Fracture of tooth (traumatic) Broken tooth** K 🖉, D, G, S 🖉
    | Excludes1 | cracked tooth (nontraumatic) (K03.81)

● **S02.6 Fracture of mandible**
Fracture of lower jaw (bone)

  ● **S02.60 Fracture of mandible of unspecified site**

    ●■ **S02.600 Fracture of unspecified part of body of mandible** A, B, K ✎, D, G, S ✎, A, B ✎

    ●■ **S02.609 Fracture of mandible, unspecified** A, B, K ✎, D, G, S ✎, A, B ✎

  ● **S02.61 Fracture of condylar process of mandible** A, B, K ✎, D, G, S ✎, A, B ✎

  ● **S02.62 Fracture of subcondylar process of mandible** A, B, K ✎, D, G, S ✎, A, B ✎

  ● **S02.63 Fracture of coronoid process of mandible** A, B, K ✎, D, G, S ✎, A, B ✎

  ● **S02.64 Fracture of ramus of mandible** A, B, K ✎, D, G, S ✎, A, B ✎

  ● **S02.65 Fracture of angle of mandible** A, B, K ✎, D, G, S ✎, A, B ✎

  ● **S02.66 Fracture of symphysis of mandible** A, B, K ✎, D, G, S ✎, A, B ✎

  ●■ **S02.67 Fracture of alveolus of mandible** A, B, K ✎, D, G, S ✎, A, B ✎

  ● **S02.69 Fracture of mandible of other specified site** A, B, K ✎, D, G, S ✎, A, B ✎

● **S02.8 Fractures of other specified skull and facial bones** A, B, K ✎, D, G, S ✎, A, B ✎
Fracture of orbit NOS
Fracture of palate

> Excludes1   fracture of orbital floor (S02.3-)
> fracture of orbital roof (S02.1-)

● **S02.9 Fracture of unspecified skull and facial bones**

  ●■ **S02.91 Unspecified fracture of skull** A, K ✎, B ✎, D, G, S ✎, A, B ✎

  ●■ **S02.92 Unspecified fracture of facial bones** A, B, K ✎, D, G, S ✎, A, B ✎

● **S03 Dislocation and sprain of joints and ligaments of head**

> Includes   avulsion of joint (capsule) or ligament of head
> laceration of cartilage, joint (capsule) or ligament of head
> sprain of cartilage, joint (capsule) or ligament of head
> traumatic hemarthrosis of joint or ligament of head
> traumatic rupture of joint or ligament of head
> traumatic subluxation of joint or ligament of head
> traumatic tear of joint or ligament of head

> Code also any associated open wound

> Excludes2   Strain of muscle or tendon of head (S09.1)

The appropriate 7th character is to be added to each code from category S03

> | A | initial encounter |
> | D | subsequent encounter |
> | S | sequela |

● **S03.0 Dislocation of jaw** D, G, S ✎
Dislocation of jaw (cartilage) (meniscus)
Dislocation of mandible
Dislocation of temporomandibular (joint)

● **S03.1 Dislocation of septal cartilage of nose** D, G, S ✎

● **S03.2 Dislocation of tooth** D, G, S ✎

● **S03.4 Sprain of jaw** D, G, S ✎
Sprain of temporomandibular (joint) (ligament)

● **S03.8 Sprain of joints and ligaments of other parts of head** D, G, S ✎

●■ **S03.9 Sprain of joints and ligaments of unspecified parts of head** D, G, S ✎

● **S04 Injury of cranial nerve**
The selection of side should be based on the side of the body being affected

> Code first any associated intracranial injury (S06.-)

> Code also any associated:
> open wound of head (S01.-)
> skull fracture (S02.-)

The appropriate 7th character is to be added to each code from category S04

> | A | initial encounter |
> | D | subsequent encounter |
> | S | sequela |

● **S04.0 Injury of optic nerve and pathways**

> Use additional code to identify any visual field defect or blindness (H53.4-, H54)

  ● **S04.01 Injury of optic nerve**
Injury of 2nd cranial nerve

    ● **S04.011 Injury of optic nerve, right eye** A ✎, D, S ✎

    ● **S04.012 Injury of optic nerve, left eye** A ✎, D, S ✎

    ●■ **S04.019 Injury of optic nerve, unspecified eye** A ✎, D, S ✎
Injury of optic nerve NOS

  ● **S04.02 Injury of optic chiasm** A ✎

  ● **S04.03 Injury of optic tract and pathways**
Injury of optic radiation

    ● **S04.031 Injury of optic tract and pathways, right eye** A ✎, D, S ✎

    ● **S04.032 Injury of optic tract and pathways, left eye** A ✎, D, S ✎

    ●■ **S04.039 Injury of optic tract and pathways, unspecified eye** A ✎, D, S ✎
Injury of optic tract and pathways NOS

  ● **S04.04 Injury of visual cortex**

    ● **S04.041 Injury of visual cortex, right eye** A ✎, D, S ✎

    ● **S04.042 Injury of visual cortex, left eye** A ✎, D, S ✎

    ●■ **S04.049 Injury of visual cortex, unspecified eye** A ✎, D, S ✎
Injury of visual cortex NOS

● **S04.1 Injury of oculomotor nerve**
Injury of 3rd cranial nerve

  ●■ **S04.10 Injury of oculomotor nerve, unspecified side** A ✎, D, S ✎

  ● **S04.11 Injury of oculomotor nerve, right side** A ✎, D, S ✎

  ● **S04.12 Injury of oculomotor nerve, left side** A ✎, D, S ✎

CHAPTER 19 (S00-T88)

- S04.2 **Injury of trochlear nerve**
  Injury of 4th cranial nerve
  - S04.20 **Injury of trochlear nerve, unspecified side**
    A 🐾, D, S 🐾
  - S04.21 **Injury of trochlear nerve, right side** A 🐾, D, S 🐾
  - S04.22 **Injury of trochlear nerve, left side** A 🐾, D, S 🐾

- S04.3 **Injury of trigeminal nerve**
  Injury of 5th cranial nerve
  - S04.30 **Injury of trigeminal nerve, unspecified side** A 🐾, D, S 🐾
  - S04.31 **Injury of trigeminal nerve, right side** A 🐾, D, S 🐾
  - S04.32 **Injury of trigeminal nerve, left side** A 🐾, D, S 🐾

- S04.4 **Injury of abducent nerve**
  Injury of 6th cranial nerve
  - S04.40 **Injury of abducent nerve, unspecified side** A 🐾, D, S 🐾
  - S04.41 **Injury of abducent nerve, right side** A 🐾, D, S 🐾
  - S04.42 **Injury of abducent nerve, left side** A 🐾, D, S 🐾

- S04.5 **Injury of facial nerve**
  Injury of 7th cranial nerve
  - S04.50 **Injury of facial nerve, unspecified side** A 🐾, D, S 🐾
  - S04.51 **Injury of facial nerve, right side** A 🐾, D, S 🐾
  - S04.52 **Injury of facial nerve, left side** A 🐾, D, S 🐾

- S04.6 **Injury of acoustic nerve**
  Injury of auditory nerve
  Injury of 8th cranial nerve
  - S04.60 **Injury of acoustic nerve, unspecified side** A 🐾, D, S 🐾
  - S04.61 **Injury of acoustic nerve, right side** A 🐾, D, S 🐾
  - S04.62 **Injury of acoustic nerve, left side** A 🐾, D, S 🐾

- S04.7 **Injury of accessory nerve**
  Injury of 11th cranial nerve
  - S04.70 **Injury of accessory nerve, unspecified side** A 🐾, D, S 🐾
  - S04.71 **Injury of accessory nerve, right side** A 🐾, D, S 🐾
  - S04.72 **Injury of accessory nerve, left side** A 🐾, D, S 🐾

- S04.8 **Injury of other cranial nerves**
  - S04.81 **Injury of olfactory [1st] nerve**
    - S04.811 **Injury of olfactory [1st] nerve, right side** A 🐾, D, S 🐾
    - S04.812 **Injury of olfactory [1st] nerve, left side** A 🐾, D, S 🐾
    - S04.819 **Injury of olfactory [1st] nerve, unspecified side** A 🐾, D, S 🐾

- S04.89 **Injury of other cranial nerves**
  Injury of vagus [10th] nerve
  - S04.891 **Injury of other cranial nerves, right side** A 🐾, D, S 🐾
  - S04.892 **Injury of other cranial nerves, left side** A 🐾, D, S 🐾
  - S04.899 **Injury of other cranial nerves, unspecified side** A 🐾, D, S 🐾
- S04.9 **Injury of unspecified cranial nerve** A 🐾, D, S 🐾

- S05 **Injury of eye and orbit**
  | **Includes** | open wound of eye and orbit |

Excludes2	2nd cranial [optic] nerve injury (S04.0-)
	3rd cranial [oculomotor] nerve injury (S04.1-)
	open wound of eyelid and periocular area (S01.1-)
	orbital bone fracture (S02.1-, S02.3-, S02.8-)
	superficial injury of eyelid (S00.1-S00.2)

  The appropriate 7th character is to be added to each code from category S05

A	initial encounter
D	subsequent encounter
S	sequela

  - S05.0 **Injury of conjunctiva and corneal abrasion without foreign body**
    | **Excludes1** | foreign body in conjunctival sac (T15.1) |
    | | foreign body in cornea (T15.0) |
    - S05.00 **Injury of conjunctiva and corneal abrasion without foreign body, unspecified eye** D, S 🐾
    - S05.01 **Injury of conjunctiva and corneal abrasion without foreign body, right eye** D, S 🐾
    - S05.02 **Injury of conjunctiva and corneal abrasion without foreign body, left eye** D, S 🐾
  - S05.1 **Contusion of eyeball and orbital tissues**
    Traumatic hyphema
    | **Excludes2** | black eye NOS (S00.1) |
    | | contusion of eyelid and periocular area (S00.1) |
    - S05.10 **Contusion of eyeball and orbital tissues, unspecified eye** D, S 🐾
    - S05.11 **Contusion of eyeball and orbital tissues, right eye** D, S 🐾
    - S05.12 **Contusion of eyeball and orbital tissues, left eye** D, S 🐾
  - S05.2 **Ocular laceration and rupture with prolapse or loss of intraocular tissue**
    - S05.20 **Ocular laceration and rupture with prolapse or loss of intraocular tissue, unspecified eye** A 🐾, D, S 🐾
    - S05.21 **Ocular laceration and rupture with prolapse or loss of intraocular tissue, right eye** A 🐾, D, S 🐾
    - S05.22 **Ocular laceration and rupture with prolapse or loss of intraocular tissue, left eye** A 🐾, D, S 🐾

CHAPTER 19 (S00-T88)

● **S05.3**   **Ocular laceration without prolapse or loss of intraocular tissue**
     Laceration of eye NOS

● ■ **S05.30**   Ocular laceration without prolapse or loss of intraocular tissue, unspecified eye A 🔖, D, S 🔖

● **S05.31**   Ocular laceration without prolapse or loss of intraocular tissue, right eye A 🔖, D, S 🔖

● **S05.32**   Ocular laceration without prolapse or loss of intraocular tissue, left eye A 🔖, D, S 🔖

● **S05.4**   **Penetrating wound of orbit with or without foreign body**

     Excludes2   retained (old) foreign body following penetrating wound in orbit (H05.5-)

● ■ **S05.40**   Penetrating wound of orbit with or without foreign body, unspecified eye A 🔖, D, S 🔖

● **S05.41**   Penetrating wound of orbit with or without foreign body, right eye A 🔖, D, S 🔖

● **S05.42**   Penetrating wound of orbit with or without foreign body, left eye A 🔖, D, S 🔖

● **S05.5**   **Penetrating wound with foreign body of eyeball**

     Excludes2   retained (old) intraocular foreign body (H44.6-, H44.7)

● ■ **S05.50**   Penetrating wound with foreign body of unspecified eyeball A 🔖, D, S 🔖

● **S05.51**   Penetrating wound with foreign body of right eyeball A 🔖, D, S 🔖

● **S05.52**   Penetrating wound with foreign body of left eyeball A 🔖, D, S 🔖

● **S05.6**   **Penetrating wound without foreign body of eyeball**
     Ocular penetration NOS

● ■ **S05.60**   Penetrating wound without foreign body of unspecified eyeball D, S 🔖

● **S05.61**   Penetrating wound without foreign body of right eyeball D, S 🔖

● **S05.62**   Penetrating wound without foreign body of left eyeball D, S 🔖

● **S05.7**   **Avulsion of eye**
     Traumatic enucleation

● ■ **S05.70**   Avulsion of unspecified eye A 🔖, D, S 🔖

● **S05.71**   Avulsion of right eye A 🔖, D, S 🔖

● **S05.72**   Avulsion of left eye A 🔖, D, S 🔖

● **S05.8**   **Other injuries of eye and orbit**
     Lacrimal duct injury

● **S05.8X**   Other injuries of eye and orbit

● **S05.8X1**   Other injuries of right eye and orbit A 🔖, D, S 🔖

● **S05.8X2**   Other injuries of left eye and orbit A 🔖, D, S 🔖

● ■ **S05.8X9**   Other injuries of unspecified eye and orbit A 🔖, D, S 🔖

● **S05.9**   **Unspecified injury of eye and orbit**
     Injury of eye NOS

● ■ **S05.90**   Unspecified injury of unspecified eye and orbit D, S 🔖

● ■ **S05.91**   Unspecified injury of right eye and orbit A 🔖, D, S 🔖

● ■ **S05.92**   Unspecified injury of left eye and orbit A 🔖, D, S 🔖

● **S06**   **Intracranial injury**

     Includes   traumatic brain injury

     Code also any associated:
       open wound of head (S01.-)
       skull fracture (S02.-)

     Excludes1   head injury NOS (S09.90)

     The appropriate 7th character is to be added to each code from category S06

A	initial encounter
D	subsequent encounter
S	sequela

● **S06.0**   **Concussion** D, S 🔖
     Commotio cerebri

     Excludes1   concussion with other intracranial injuries classified in category S06- code to specified intracranial injury

● **S06.0X**   Concussion

● **S06.0X0**   Concussion without loss of consciousness D, S 🔖

● **S06.0X1**   Concussion with loss of consciousness of 30 minutes or less A 🔖, D, S 🔖, A 🔖

● **S06.0X2**   Concussion with loss of consciousness of 31 minutes to 59 minutes A 🔖, D, S 🔖, A 🔖

● **S06.0X3**   Concussion with loss of consciousness of 1 hour to 5 hours 59 minutes A 🔖, D, S 🔖, A 🔖

● **S06.0X4**   Concussion with loss of consciousness of 6 hours to 24 hours A 🔖, D, S 🔖, A 🔖

● **S06.0X5**   Concussion with loss of consciousness greater than 24 hours with return to pre-existing conscious level A 🔖, D, S 🔖, A 🔖

● **S06.0X6**   Concussion with loss of consciousness greater than 24 hours without return to pre-existing conscious level with patient surviving A 🔖, D, S 🔖, A 🔖

● **S06.0X7**   Concussion with loss of consciousness of any duration with death due to brain injury prior to regaining consciousness A 🔖, D, S 🔖, A 🔖

● **S06.0X8**   Concussion with loss of consciousness of any duration with death due to other cause prior to regaining consciousness A 🔖, D, S 🔖, A 🔖

● ■ **S06.0X9**   Concussion with loss of consciousness of unspecified duration A 🔖, D, S 🔖, A 🔖
     Concussion NOS

● Unacceptable Principal Diagnosis   ● Use Additional Character(s)   ■ Unspecified   ▶ Manifestation Code

1400   **OGCR** Official Guidelines for Coding and Reporting | Excludes 1 | | Excludes 2 | | Includes | | Use additional | | Code first | | Code also |

● **S06.1   Traumatic cerebral edema**
Diffuse traumatic cerebral edema
Focal traumatic cerebral edema

  ● **S06.1X   Traumatic cerebral edema**

    ● **S06.1X0   Traumatic cerebral edema without loss of consciousness**
D, S ⬚

> MCC: Only when the principal diagnosis is designated as an MCC

    ● **S06.1X1   Traumatic cerebral edema with loss of consciousness of 30 minutes or less A** ⬚**, D, S** ⬚**, A** ⬚

> MCC: Only when the principal diagnosis is designated as an MCC

    ● **S06.1X2   Traumatic cerebral edema with loss of consciousness of 31 minutes to 59 minutes A** ⬚**, D, S** ⬚**, A** ⬚

> MCC: Only when the principal diagnosis is designated as an MCC

    ● **S06.1X3   Traumatic cerebral edema with loss of consciousness of 1 hour to 5 hours 59 minutes A** ⬚**, D, S** ⬚**, A** ⬚

> MCC: Only when the principal diagnosis is designated as an MCC

    ● **S06.1X4   Traumatic cerebral edema with loss of consciousness of 6 hours to 24 hours A** ⬚**, D, S** ⬚**, A** ⬚

> MCC: Only when the principal diagnosis is designated as an MCC

    ● **S06.1X5   Traumatic cerebral edema with loss of consciousness greater than 24 hours with return to pre-existing conscious level A** ⬚**, D, S** ⬚**, A** ⬚

> MCC: Only when the principal diagnosis is designated as an MCC

    ● **S06.1X6   Traumatic cerebral edema with loss of consciousness greater than 24 hours without return to pre-existing conscious level with patient surviving A** ⬚**, D, S** ⬚**, A** ⬚

> MCC: Only when the principal diagnosis is designated as an MCC

    ● **S06.1X7   Traumatic cerebral edema with loss of consciousness of any duration with death due to brain injury prior to regaining consciousness A** ⬚**, D, S** ⬚**, A** ⬚

> MCC: Only when the principal diagnosis is designated as an MCC

    ● **S06.1X8   Traumatic cerebral edema with loss of consciousness of any duration with death due to other cause prior to regaining consciousness A** ⬚**, D, S** ⬚**, A** ⬚

> MCC: Only when the principal diagnosis is designated as an MCC

    ● ▪ **S06.1X9   Traumatic cerebral edema with loss of consciousness of unspecified duration A** ⬚**, D, S** ⬚**, A** ⬚
Traumatic cerebral edema NOS

> MCC: Only when the principal diagnosis is designated as an MCC

● **S06.2   Diffuse traumatic brain injury**
Diffuse axonal brain injury

> **Excludes1**   traumatic diffuse cerebral edema (S06.1x-)

  ● **S06.2X   Diffuse traumatic brain injury**

    ● **S06.2X0   Diffuse traumatic brain injury without loss of consciousness**
D, S ⬚

    ● **S06.2X1   Diffuse traumatic brain injury with loss of consciousness of 30 minutes or less A** ⬚**, D, S** ⬚**, A** ⬚

    ● **S06.2X2   Diffuse traumatic brain injury with loss of consciousness of 31 minutes to 59 minutes A** ⬚**, D, S** ⬚**, A** ⬚

    ● **S06.2X3   Diffuse traumatic brain injury with loss of consciousness of 1 hour to 5 hours 59 minutes A** ⬚**, D, S** ⬚**, A** ⬚

    ● **S06.2X4   Diffuse traumatic brain injury with loss of consciousness of 6 hours to 24 hours A** ⬚**, D, S** ⬚**, A** ⬚

    ● **S06.2X5   Diffuse traumatic brain injury with loss of consciousness greater than 24 hours with return to pre-existing conscious levels A** ⬚**, D, S** ⬚**, A** ⬚

    ● **S06.2X6   Diffuse traumatic brain injury with loss of consciousness greater than 24 hours without return to pre-existing conscious level with patient surviving A** ⬚**, D, S** ⬚**, A** ⬚

    ● **S06.2X7   Diffuse traumatic brain injury with loss of consciousness of any duration with death due to brain injury prior to regaining consciousness A** ⬚**, D, S** ⬚**, A** ⬚

    ● **S06.2X8   Diffuse traumatic brain injury with loss of consciousness of any duration with death due to other cause prior to regaining consciousness A** ⬚**, D, S** ⬚**, A** ⬚

    ● ▪ **S06.2X9   Diffuse traumatic brain injury with loss of consciousness of unspecified duration A** ⬚**, D, S** ⬚**, A** ⬚
Diffuse traumatic brain injury NOS

N Newborn Age: 0   **P** Pediatric Age: 0–17   **M** Maternity DX: 12–55   **A** Adult Age: 15–124   ♀ Females Only   ♂ Males Only

⬚ Complication\Comorbidity   ⬚ Major C\C   ⬚ Present on Admission Requirement   ⬚ Hospital-Acquired Condition

1401

● **S06.3   Focal traumatic brain injury**

> **Excludes1**   any condition classifiable to
> S06.4-S06.6
> focal cerebral edema (S06.1)

● **S06.30   Unspecified focal traumatic brain injury**

● ■ **S06.300   Unspecified focal traumatic brain injury without loss of consciousness** D, S 🔍

● ■ **S06.301   Unspecified focal traumatic brain injury with loss of consciousness of 30 minutes or less** A 🔍, D, S 🔍, A 🔍

● ■ **S06.302   Unspecified focal traumatic brain injury with loss of consciousness of 31 minutes to 59 minutes** A 🔍, D, S 🔍, A 🔍

● ■ **S06.303   Unspecified focal traumatic brain injury with loss of consciousness of 1 hour to 5 hours 59 minutes** A 🔍, D, S 🔍, A 🔍

● ■ **S06.304   Unspecified focal traumatic brain injury with loss of consciousness of 6 hours to 24 hours** A 🔍, D, S 🔍, A 🔍

● ■ **S06.305   Unspecified focal traumatic brain injury with loss of consciousness greater than 24 hours with return to pre-existing conscious level** A 🔍, D, S 🔍, A 🔍

● ■ **S06.306   Unspecified focal traumatic brain injury with loss of consciousness greater than 24 hours without return to pre-existing conscious level with patient surviving** A 🔍, D, S 🔍, A 🔍

● ■ **S06.307   Unspecified focal traumatic brain injury with loss of consciousness of any duration with death due to brain injury prior to regaining consciousness** A 🔍, D, S 🔍, A 🔍

● ■ **S06.308   Unspecified focal traumatic brain injury with loss of consciousness of any duration with death due to other cause prior to regaining consciousness** A 🔍, D, S 🔍, A 🔍

● ■ **S06.309   Unspecified focal traumatic brain injury with loss of consciousness of unspecified duration** A 🔍, D, S 🔍, A 🔍

> Unspecified focal traumatic brain injury NOS

● **S06.31   Contusion and laceration of right cerebrum**

● **S06.310   Contusion and laceration of right cerebrum without loss of consciousness** A 🔍, D, S 🔍, A 🔍

● **S06.311   Contusion and laceration of right cerebrum with loss of consciousness of 30 minutes or less** A 🔍, D, S 🔍, A 🔍

● **S06.312   Contusion and laceration of right cerebrum with loss of consciousness of 31 minutes to 59 minutes** A 🔍, D, S 🔍, A 🔍

● **S06.313   Contusion and laceration of right cerebrum with loss of consciousness of 1 hour to 5 hours 59 minutes** A 🔍, D, S 🔍, A 🔍

● **S06.314   Contusion and laceration of right cerebrum with loss of consciousness of 6 hours to 24 hours** A 🔍, D, S 🔍, A 🔍

● **S06.315   Contusion and laceration of right cerebrum with loss of consciousness greater than 24 hours with return to pre-existing conscious level** A 🔍, D, S 🔍, A 🔍

● **S06.316   Contusion and laceration of right cerebrum with loss of consciousness greater than 24 hours without return to pre-existing conscious level with patient surviving** A 🔍, D, S 🔍, A 🔍

● **S06.317   Contusion and laceration of right cerebrum with loss of consciousness of any duration with death due to brain injury prior to regaining consciousness** A 🔍, D, S 🔍, A 🔍

● **S06.318   Contusion and laceration of right cerebrum with loss of consciousness of any duration with death due to other cause prior to regaining consciousness** A 🔍, D, S 🔍, A 🔍

● ■ **S06.319   Contusion and laceration of right cerebrum with loss of consciousness of unspecified duration** A 🔍, D, S 🔍, A 🔍

> Contusion and laceration of right cerebrum NOS

● **S06.32   Contusion and laceration of left cerebrum**

● **S06.320   Contusion and laceration of left cerebrum without loss of consciousness** A 🔍, D, S 🔍, A 🔍

● **S06.321   Contusion and laceration of left cerebrum with loss of consciousness of 30 minutes or less** A 🔍, D, S 🔍, A 🔍

● **S06.322   Contusion and laceration of left cerebrum with loss of consciousness of 31 minutes to 59 minutes** A 🔍, D, S 🔍, A 🔍

● **S06.323   Contusion and laceration of left cerebrum with loss of consciousness of 1 hour to 5 hours 59 minutes** A 🔍, D, S 🔍, A 🔍

● **S06.324   Contusion and laceration of left cerebrum with loss of consciousness of 6 hours to 24 hours** A 🔍, D, S 🔍, A 🔍

● **S06.325   Contusion and laceration of left cerebrum with loss of consciousness greater than 24 hours with return to pre-existing conscious level** A 🔍, D, S 🔍, A 🔍

● Unacceptable Principal Diagnosis	● Use Additional Character(s)	■ Unspecified	▶ Manifestation Code
OGCR Official Guidelines for Coding and Reporting	Excludes 1 Excludes 2	Includes Use additional	Code first Code also

● S06.326 Contusion and laceration of left cerebrum with loss of consciousness greater than 24 hours without return to pre-existing conscious level with patient surviving A ⬡, D, S ⬡, A ⬡

● S06.327 Contusion and laceration of left cerebrum with loss of consciousness of any duration with death due to brain injury prior to regaining consciousness A ⬡, D, S ⬡, A ⬡

● S06.328 Contusion and laceration of left cerebrum with loss of consciousness of any duration with death due to other cause prior to regaining consciousness A ⬡, D, S ⬡, A ⬡

●■ S06.329 Contusion and laceration of left cerebrum with loss of consciousness of unspecified duration A ⬡, D, S ⬡, A ⬡
    Contusion and laceration of left cerebrum NOS

● S06.33 Contusion and laceration of cerebrum, unspecified

●■ S06.330 Contusion and laceration of cerebrum, unspecified, without loss of consciousness A ⬡, D, S ⬡, A ⬡

●■ S06.331 Contusion and laceration of cerebrum, unspecified, with loss of consciousness of 30 minutes or less A ⬡, D, S ⬡, A ⬡

●■ S06.332 Contusion and laceration of cerebrum, unspecified, with loss of consciousness of 31 minutes to 59 minutes A ⬡, D, S ⬡, A ⬡

●■ S06.333 Contusion and laceration of cerebrum, unspecified, with loss of consciousness of 1 hour to 5 hours 59 minutes A ⬡, D, S ⬡, A ⬡

●■ S06.334 Contusion and laceration of cerebrum, unspecified, with loss of consciousness of 6 hours to 24 hours A ⬡, D, S ⬡, A ⬡

●■ S06.335 Contusion and laceration of cerebrum, unspecified, with loss of consciousness greater than 24 hours with return to pre-existing conscious level A ⬡, D, S ⬡, A ⬡

●■ S06.336 Contusion and laceration of cerebrum, unspecified, with loss of consciousness greater than 24 hours without return to pre-existing conscious level with patient surviving A ⬡, D, S ⬡, A ⬡

●■ S06.337 Contusion and laceration of cerebrum, unspecified, with loss of consciousness of any duration with death due to brain injury prior to regaining consciousness A ⬡, D, S ⬡, A ⬡

●■ S06.338 Contusion and laceration of cerebrum, unspecified, with loss of consciousness of any duration with death due to other cause prior to regaining consciousness A ⬡, D, S ⬡, A ⬡

●■ S06.339 Contusion and laceration of cerebrum, unspecified, with loss of consciousness of unspecified duration A ⬡, D, S ⬡, A ⬡
    Contusion and laceration of cerebrum NOS

● S06.34 Traumatic hemorrhage of right cerebrum
    Traumatic intracerebral hemorrhage and hematoma of right cerebrum

● S06.340 Traumatic hemorrhage of right cerebrum without loss of consciousness A ⬡, D, S ⬡, A ⬡

● S06.341 Traumatic hemorrhage of right cerebrum with loss of consciousness of 30 minutes or less A ⬡, D, S ⬡, A ⬡

● S06.342 Traumatic hemorrhage of right cerebrum with loss of consciousness of 31 minutes to 59 minutes A ⬡, D, S ⬡, A ⬡

● S06.343 Traumatic hemorrhage of right cerebrum with loss of consciousness of 1 hours to 5 hours 59 minutes A ⬡, D, S ⬡, A ⬡

● S06.344 Traumatic hemorrhage of right cerebrum with loss of consciousness of 6 hours to 24 hours A ⬡, D, S ⬡, A ⬡

● S06.345 Traumatic hemorrhage of right cerebrum with loss of consciousness greater than 24 hours with return to pre-existing conscious level A ⬡, D, S ⬡, A ⬡

● S06.346 Traumatic hemorrhage of right cerebrum with loss of consciousness greater than 24 hours without return to pre-existing conscious level with patient surviving A ⬡, D, S ⬡, A ⬡

● S06.347 Traumatic hemorrhage of right cerebrum with loss of consciousness of any duration with death due to brain injury prior to regaining consciousness A ⬡, D, S ⬡, A ⬡

● S06.348 Traumatic hemorrhage of right cerebrum with loss of consciousness of any duration with death due to other cause prior to regaining consciousness A ⬡, D, S ⬡, A ⬡

●■ S06.349 Traumatic hemorrhage of right cerebrum with loss of consciousness of unspecified duration A ⬡, D, S ⬡, A ⬡
    Traumatic hemorrhage of right cerebrum NOS

N Newborn Age: 0   P Pediatric Age: 0–17   M Maternity DX: 12–55   A Adult Age: 15–124   ♀ Females Only   ♂ Males Only
⬡ Complication\Comorbidity   ■ Major C\C   ⬡ Present on Admission Requirement   ⬡ Hospital-Acquired Condition

1403

CHAPTER 19 (S00-T88)

● **S06.35 Traumatic hemorrhage of left cerebrum**
Traumatic intracerebral hemorrhage and hematoma of left cerebrum

   ● **S06.350 Traumatic hemorrhage of left cerebrum without loss of consciousness** A 🔖, D, S 🔖, A 🔖

   ● **S06.351 Traumatic hemorrhage of left cerebrum with loss of consciousness of 30 minutes or less** A 🔖, D, S 🔖, A 🔖

   ● **S06.352 Traumatic hemorrhage of left cerebrum with loss of consciousness of 31 minutes to 59 minutes** A 🔖, D, S 🔖, A 🔖

   ● **S06.353 Traumatic hemorrhage of left cerebrum with loss of consciousness of 1 hours to 5 hours 59 minutes** A 🔖, D, S 🔖, A 🔖

   ● **S06.354 Traumatic hemorrhage of left cerebrum with loss of consciousness of 6 hours to 24 hours** A 🔖, D, S 🔖, A 🔖

   ● **S06.355 Traumatic hemorrhage of left cerebrum with loss of consciousness greater than 24 hours with return to pre-existing conscious level** A 🔖, D, S 🔖, A 🔖

   ● **S06.356 Traumatic hemorrhage of left cerebrum with loss of consciousness greater than 24 hours without return to pre-existing conscious level with patient surviving** A 🔖, D, S 🔖, A 🔖

   ● **S06.357 Traumatic hemorrhage of left cerebrum with loss of consciousness of any duration with death due to brain injury prior to regaining consciousness** A 🔖, D, S 🔖, A 🔖

   ● **S06.358 Traumatic hemorrhage of left cerebrum with loss of consciousness of any duration with death due to other cause prior to regaining consciousness** A 🔖, D, S 🔖, A 🔖

   ● ▪ **S06.359 Traumatic hemorrhage of left cerebrum with loss of consciousness of unspecified duration** A 🔖, D, S 🔖, A 🔖
Traumatic hemorrhage of left cerebrum NOS

● **S06.36 Traumatic hemorrhage of cerebrum, unspecified**
Traumatic intracerebral hemorrhage and hematoma, unspecified

   ● ▪ **S06.360 Traumatic hemorrhage of cerebrum, unspecified, without loss of consciousness** A 🔖, D, S 🔖, A 🔖

   ● ▪ **S06.361 Traumatic hemorrhage of cerebrum, unspecified, with loss of consciousness of 30 minutes or less** A 🔖, D, S 🔖, A 🔖

   ● ▪ **S06.362 Traumatic hemorrhage of cerebrum, unspecified, with loss of consciousness of 31 minutes to 59 minutes** A 🔖, D, S 🔖, A 🔖

   ● ▪ **S06.363 Traumatic hemorrhage of cerebrum, unspecified, with loss of consciousness of 1 hours to 5 hours 59 minutes** A 🔖, D, S 🔖, A 🔖

   ● ▪ **S06.364 Traumatic hemorrhage of cerebrum, unspecified, with loss of consciousness of 6 hours to 24 hours** A 🔖, D, S 🔖, A 🔖

   ● ▪ **S06.365 Traumatic hemorrhage of cerebrum, unspecified, with loss of consciousness greater than 24 hours with return to pre-existing conscious level** A 🔖, D, S 🔖, A 🔖

   ● ▪ **S06.366 Traumatic hemorrhage of cerebrum, unspecified, with loss of consciousness greater than 24 hours without return to pre-existing conscious level with patient surviving** A 🔖, D, S 🔖, A 🔖

   ● ▪ **S06.367 Traumatic hemorrhage of cerebrum, unspecified, with loss of consciousness of any duration with death due to brain injury prior to regaining consciousness** A 🔖, D, S 🔖, A 🔖

   ● ▪ **S06.368 Traumatic hemorrhage of cerebrum, unspecified, with loss of consciousness of any duration with death due to other cause prior to regaining consciousness** A 🔖, D, S 🔖, A 🔖

   ● ▪ **S06.369 Traumatic hemorrhage of cerebrum, unspecified, with loss of consciousness of unspecified duration** A 🔖, D, S 🔖, A 🔖
Traumatic hemorrhage of cerebrum NOS

● **S06.37 Contusion, laceration, and hemorrhage of cerebellum**

   ● **S06.370 Contusion, laceration, and hemorrhage of cerebellum without loss of consciousness** A 🔖, D, S 🔖, A 🔖

   ● **S06.371 Contusion, laceration, and hemorrhage of cerebellum with loss of consciousness of 30 minutes or less** A 🔖, D, S 🔖, A 🔖

   ● **S06.372 Contusion, laceration, and hemorrhage of cerebellum with loss of consciousness of 31 minutes to 59 minutes** A 🔖, D, S 🔖, A 🔖

   ● **S06.373 Contusion, laceration, and hemorrhage of cerebellum with loss of consciousness of 1 hour to 5 hours 59 minutes** A 🔖, D, S 🔖, A 🔖

● Unacceptable Principal Diagnosis ● Use Additional Character(s) ▪ Unspecified ▶ Manifestation Code

OGCR Official Guidelines for Coding and Reporting Excludes 1 Excludes 2 Includes Use additional Code first Code also

● S06.374   Contusion, laceration, and hemorrhage of cerebellum with loss of consciousness of 6 hours to 24 hours A 🔖, D, S 🔖, A 🔖

● S06.375   Contusion, laceration, and hemorrhage of cerebellum with loss of consciousness greater than 24 hours with return to pre-existing conscious level A 🔖, D, S 🔖, A 🔖

● S06.376   Contusion, laceration, and hemorrhage of cerebellum with loss of consciousness greater than 24 hours without return to pre-existing conscious level with patient surviving A 🔖, D, S 🔖, A 🔖

● S06.377   Contusion, laceration, and hemorrhage of cerebellum with loss of consciousness of any duration with death due to brain injury prior to regaining consciousness A 🔖, D, S 🔖, A 🔖

● S06.378   Contusion, laceration, and hemorrhage of cerebellum with loss of consciousness of any duration with death due to other cause prior to regaining consciousness A 🔖, D, S 🔖, A 🔖

● ■ S06.379   Contusion, laceration, and hemorrhage of cerebellum with loss of consciousness of unspecified duration A 🔖, D, S 🔖, A 🔖

     Contusion, laceration, and hemorrhage of cerebellum NOS

● S06.38   Contusion, laceration, and hemorrhage of brainstem

● S06.380   Contusion, laceration, and hemorrhage of brainstem without loss of consciousness A 🔖, D, S 🔖, A 🔖

● S06.381   Contusion, laceration, and hemorrhage of brainstem with loss of consciousness of 30 minutes or less A 🔖, D, S 🔖, A 🔖

● S06.382   Contusion, laceration, and hemorrhage of brainstem with loss of consciousness of 31 minutes to 59 minutes A 🔖, D, S 🔖, A 🔖

● S06.383   Contusion, laceration, and hemorrhage of brainstem with loss of consciousness of 1 hour to 5 hours 59 minutes A 🔖, D, S 🔖, A 🔖

● S06.384   Contusion, laceration, and hemorrhage of brainstem with loss of consciousness of 6 hours to 24 hours A 🔖, D, S 🔖, A 🔖

● S06.385   Contusion, laceration, and hemorrhage of brainstem with loss of consciousness greater than 24 hours with return to pre-existing conscious level A 🔖, D, S 🔖, A 🔖

● S06.386   Contusion, laceration, and hemorrhage of brainstem with loss of consciousness greater than 24 hours without return to pre-existing conscious level with patient surviving A 🔖, D, S 🔖, A 🔖

● S06.387   Contusion, laceration, and hemorrhage of brainstem with loss of consciousness of any duration with death due to brain injury prior to regaining consciousness A 🔖, D, S 🔖, A 🔖

● S06.388   Contusion, laceration, and hemorrhage of brainstem with loss of consciousness of any duration with death due to other cause prior to regaining consciousness A 🔖, D, S 🔖, A 🔖

● ■ S06.389   Contusion, laceration, and hemorrhage of brainstem with loss of consciousness of unspecified duration A 🔖, D, S 🔖, A 🔖

     Contusion, laceration, and hemorrhage of brainstem NOS

● S06.4   **Epidural hemorrhage**

     Situated outside dura mater

     Extradural hemorrhage NOS

     Intracranial hemorrhage due to trauma

     Extradural hemorrhage (traumatic)

● S06.4X   **Epidural hemorrhage**

● S06.4X0   Epidural hemorrhage without loss of consciousness A 🔖, D, S 🔖, A 🔖

● S06.4X1   Epidural hemorrhage with loss of consciousness of 30 minutes or less A 🔖, D, S 🔖, A 🔖

● S06.4X2   Epidural hemorrhage with loss of consciousness of 31 minutes to 59 minutes A 🔖, D, S 🔖, A 🔖

● S06.4X3   Epidural hemorrhage with loss of consciousness of 1 hour to 5 hours 59 minutes A 🔖, D, S 🔖, A 🔖

● S06.4X4   Epidural hemorrhage with loss of consciousness of 6 hours to 24 hours A 🔖, D, S 🔖, A 🔖

● S06.4X5   Epidural hemorrhage with loss of consciousness greater than 24 hours with return to pre-existing conscious level A 🔖, D, S 🔖, A 🔖

● S06.4X6   Epidural hemorrhage with loss of consciousness greater than 24 hours without return to pre-existing conscious level with patient surviving A 🔖, D, S 🔖, A 🔖

● S06.4X7   Epidural hemorrhage with loss of consciousness of any duration with death due to brain injury prior to regaining consciousness A 🔖, D, S 🔖, A 🔖

CHAPTER 19 (S00-T88)

● S06.4X8   Epidural hemorrhage with loss of consciousness of any duration with death due to other causes prior to regaining consciousness A 🔎, D, S 🔎, A 🔎

●▪ S06.4X9   Epidural hemorrhage with loss of consciousness of unspecified duration A 🔎, D, S 🔎, A 🔎
       Epidural hemorrhage NOS

● S06.5   **Traumatic subdural hemorrhage**

   ● S06.5X   Traumatic subdural hemorrhage

     ● S06.5X0   Traumatic subdural hemorrhage without loss of consciousness A 🔎, D, S 🔎, A 🔎

     ● S06.5X1   Traumatic subdural hemorrhage with loss of consciousness of 30 minutes or less A 🔎, D, S 🔎, A 🔎

     ● S06.5X2   Traumatic subdural hemorrhage with loss of consciousness of 31 minutes to 59 minutes A 🔎, D, S 🔎, A 🔎

     ● S06.5X3   Traumatic subdural hemorrhage with loss of consciousness of 1 hour to 5 hours 59 minutes A 🔎, D, S 🔎, A 🔎

     ● S06.5X4   Traumatic subdural hemorrhage with loss of consciousness of 6 hours to 24 hours A 🔎, D, S 🔎, A 🔎

     ● S06.5X5   Traumatic subdural hemorrhage with loss of consciousness greater than 24 hours with return to pre-existing conscious level A 🔎, D, S 🔎, A 🔎

     ● S06.5X6   Traumatic subdural hemorrhage with loss of consciousness greater than 24 hours without return to pre-existing conscious level with patient surviving A 🔎, D, S 🔎, A 🔎

     ● S06.5X7   Traumatic subdural hemorrhage with loss of consciousness of any duration with death due to brain injury before regaining consciousness A 🔎, D, S 🔎, A 🔎

     ● S06.5X8   Traumatic subdural hemorrhage with loss of consciousness of any duration with death due to other cause before regaining consciousness A 🔎, D, S 🔎, A 🔎

     ●▪ S06.5X9   Traumatic subdural hemorrhage with loss of consciousness of unspecified duration A 🔎, D, S 🔎, A 🔎
       Traumatic subdural hemorrhage NOS

● S06.6   **Traumatic subarachnoid hemorrhage**
     Between arachnoid and pia mater

   ● S06.6X   Traumatic subarachnoid hemorrhage

     ● S06.6X0   Traumatic subarachnoid hemorrhage without loss of consciousness A 🔎, D, S 🔎, A 🔎

     ● S06.6X1   Traumatic subarachnoid hemorrhage with loss of consciousness of 30 minutes or less A 🔎, D, S 🔎, A 🔎

● S06.6X2   Traumatic subarachnoid hemorrhage with loss of consciousness of 31 minutes to 59 minutes A 🔎, D, S 🔎, A 🔎

● S06.6X3   Traumatic subarachnoid hemorrhage with loss of consciousness of 1 hour to 5 hours 59 minutes A 🔎, D, S 🔎, A 🔎

● S06.6X4   Traumatic subarachnoid hemorrhage with loss of consciousness of 6 hours to 24 hours A 🔎, D, S 🔎, A 🔎

● S06.6X5   Traumatic subarachnoid hemorrhage with loss of consciousness greater than 24 hours with return to pre-existing conscious level A 🔎, D, S 🔎, A 🔎

● S06.6X6   Traumatic subarachnoid hemorrhage with loss of consciousness greater than 24 hours without return to pre-existing conscious level with patient surviving A 🔎, D, S 🔎, A 🔎

● S06.6X7   Traumatic subarachnoid hemorrhage with loss of consciousness of any duration with death due to brain injury prior to regaining consciousness A 🔎, D, S 🔎, A 🔎

● S06.6X8   Traumatic subarachnoid hemorrhage with loss of consciousness of any duration with death due to other cause prior to regaining consciousness A 🔎, D, S 🔎, A 🔎

●▪ S06.6X9   Traumatic subarachnoid hemorrhage with loss of consciousness of unspecified duration A 🔎, D, S 🔎, A 🔎
       Traumatic subarachnoid hemorrhage NOS

● S06.8   **Other specified intracranial injuries**

   ● S06.81   Injury of right internal carotid artery, intracranial portion, not elsewhere classified

     ● S06.810   Injury of right internal carotid artery, intracranial portion, not elsewhere classified without loss of consciousness D, S 🔎

     ● S06.811   Injury of right internal carotid artery, intracranial portion, not elsewhere classified with loss of consciousness of 30 minutes or less A 🔎, D, S 🔎, A 🔎

     ● S06.812   Injury of right internal carotid artery, intracranial portion, not elsewhere classified with loss of consciousness of 31 minutes to 59 minutes A 🔎, D, S 🔎, A 🔎

     ● S06.813   Injury of right internal carotid artery, intracranial portion, not elsewhere classified with loss of consciousness of 1 hour to 5 hours 59 minutes A 🔎, D, S 🔎, A 🔎

● Unacceptable Principal Diagnosis   ● Use Additional Character(s)   ▪ Unspecified   ▶ Manifestation Code

OGCR   Official Guidelines for Coding and Reporting   Excludes 1   Excludes 2   Includes   Use additional   Code first   Code also

●S06.814   Injury of right internal carotid artery, intracranial portion, not elsewhere classified with loss of consciousness of 6 hours to 24 hours A 🗪, D, S 🗪, A 🗪

●S06.815   Injury of right internal carotid artery, intracranial portion, not elsewhere classified with loss of consciousness greater than 24 hours with return to pre-existing conscious level A 🗪, D, S 🗪, A 🗪

●S06.816   Injury of right internal carotid artery, intracranial portion, not elsewhere classified with loss of consciousness greater than 24 hours without return to pre-existing conscious level with patient surviving A 🗪, D, S 🗪, A 🗪

●S06.817   Injury of right internal carotid artery, intracranial portion, not elsewhere classified with loss of consciousness of any duration with death due to brain injury prior to regaining consciousness A 🗪, D, S 🗪, A 🗪

●S06.818   Injury of right internal carotid artery, intracranial portion, not elsewhere classified with loss of consciousness of any duration with death due to other cause prior to regaining consciousness A 🗪, D, S 🗪, A 🗪

●■S06.819   Injury of right internal carotid artery, intracranial portion, not elsewhere classified with loss of consciousness of unspecified duration A 🗪, D, S 🗪, A 🗪
         Injury of right internal carotid artery, intracranial portion, not elsewhere classified NOS

●S06.82   Injury of left internal carotid artery, intracranial portion, not elsewhere classified

●S06.820   Injury of left internal carotid artery, intracranial portion, not elsewhere classified without loss of consciousness D, S 🗪

●S06.821   Injury of left internal carotid artery, intracranial portion, not elsewhere classified with loss of consciousness of 30 minutes or less A 🗪, D, S 🗪, A 🗪

●S06.822   Injury of left internal carotid artery, intracranial portion, not elsewhere classified with loss of consciousness of 31 minutes to 59 minutes A 🗪, D, S 🗪, A 🗪

●S06.823   Injury of left internal carotid artery, intracranial portion, not elsewhere classified with loss of consciousness of 1 hour to 5 hours 59 minutes A 🗪, D, S 🗪, A 🗪

●S06.824   Injury of left internal carotid artery, intracranial portion, not elsewhere classified with loss of consciousness of 6 hours to 24 hours A 🗪, D, S 🗪, A 🗪

●S06.825   Injury of left internal carotid artery, intracranial portion, not elsewhere classified with loss of consciousness greater than 24 hours with return to pre-existing conscious level A 🗪, D, S 🗪, A 🗪

●S06.826   Injury of left internal carotid artery, intracranial portion, not elsewhere classified with loss of consciousness greater than 24 hours without return to pre-existing conscious level with patient surviving A 🗪, D, S 🗪, A 🗪

●S06.827   Injury of left internal carotid artery, intracranial portion, not elsewhere classified with loss of consciousness of any duration with death due to brain injury prior to regaining consciousness A 🗪, D, S 🗪, A 🗪

●S06.828   Injury of left internal carotid artery, intracranial portion, not elsewhere classified with loss of consciousness of any duration with death due to other cause prior to regaining consciousness A 🗪, D, S 🗪, A 🗪

●■S06.829   Injury of left internal carotid artery, intracranial portion, not elsewhere classified with loss of consciousness of unspecified duration A 🗪, D, S 🗪, A 🗪
         Injury of left internal carotid artery, intracranial portion, not elsewhere classified NOS

●S06.89   Other specified intracranial injury

●S06.890   Other specified intracranial injury without loss of consciousness D, S 🗪

●S06.891   Other specified intracranial injury with loss of consciousness of 30 minutes or less A 🗪, D, S 🗪, A 🗪

●S06.892   Other specified intracranial injury with loss of consciousness of 31 minutes to 59 minutes A 🗪, D, S 🗪, A 🗪

●S06.893   Other specified intracranial injury with loss of consciousness of 1 hour to 5 hours 59 minutes A 🗪, D, S 🗪, A 🗪

●S06.894   Other specified intracranial injury with loss of consciousness of 6 hours to 24 hours A 🗪, D, S 🗪, A 🗪

●S06.895   Other specified intracranial injury with loss of consciousness greater than 24 hours with return to pre-existing conscious level A 🗪, D, S 🗪, A 🗪

- S06.896 Other specified intracranial injury with loss of consciousness greater than 24 hours without return to pre-existing conscious level with patient surviving A, D, S, A

- S06.897 Other specified intracranial injury with loss of consciousness of any duration with death due to brain injury prior to regaining consciousness A, D, S, A

- S06.898 Other specified intracranial injury with loss of consciousness of any duration with death due to other cause prior to regaining consciousness A, D, S, A

- S06.899 Other specified intracranial injury with loss of consciousness of unspecified duration A, D, S, A

- S06.9 Unspecified intracranial injury
  Brain injury NOS
  Head injury NOS with loss of consciousness
  Excludes1 head injury NOS (S09.90)

  - S06.9X Unspecified intracranial injury
    - S06.9X0 Unspecified intracranial injury without loss of consciousness
    - S06.9X1 Unspecified intracranial injury with loss of consciousness of 30 minutes or less A, D, S, A
    - S06.9X2 Unspecified intracranial injury with loss of consciousness of 31 minutes to 59 minutes A, D, S, A
    - S06.9X3 Unspecified intracranial injury with loss of consciousness of 1 hour to 5 hours 59 minutes A, D, S, A
    - S06.9X4 Unspecified intracranial injury with loss of consciousness of 6 hours to 24 hours A, D, S, A
    - S06.9X5 Unspecified intracranial injury with loss of consciousness greater than 24 hours with return to pre-existing conscious level A, D, S, A
    - S06.9X6 Unspecified intracranial injury with loss of consciousness greater than 24 hours without return to pre-existing conscious level with patient surviving A, D, S, A
    - S06.9X7 Unspecified intracranial injury with loss of consciousness of any duration with death due to brain injury prior to regaining consciousness A, D, S, A
    - S06.9X8 Unspecified intracranial injury with loss of consciousness of any duration with death due to other cause prior to regaining consciousness A, D, S, A
    - S06.9X9 Unspecified intracranial injury with loss of consciousness of unspecified duration A, D, S, A

- S07 Crushing injury of head
  Use additional code for all associated injuries, such as:
  intracranial injuries (S06-)
  skull fractures (S02.-)
  The appropriate 7th character is to be added to each code from category S07

  A initial encounter
  D subsequent encounter
  S sequela

  - S07.0 Crushing injury of face A, D, S, A
  - S07.1 Crushing injury of skull A, D, S, A
  - S07.8 Crushing injury of other parts of head A, D, S, A
  - S07.9 Crushing injury of head, part unspecified A, D, S, A

- S08 Avulsion and traumatic amputation of part of head
  An amputation not identified as partial or complete should be coded to complete
  The appropriate 7th character is to be added to each code from category S08

  A initial encounter
  D subsequent encounter
  S sequela

  - S08.0 Avulsion of scalp D, S
  - S08.1 Traumatic amputation of ear
    - S08.11 Complete traumatic amputation of ear
      - S08.111 Complete traumatic amputation of right ear D, S
      - S08.112 Complete traumatic amputation of left ear D, S
      - S08.119 Complete traumatic amputation of unspecified ear D, S
    - S08.12 Partial traumatic amputation of ear
      - S08.121 Partial traumatic amputation of right ear A, D, S
      - S08.122 Partial traumatic amputation of left ear A, D, S
      - S08.129 Partial traumatic amputation of unspecified ear A, D, S
  - S08.8 Traumatic amputation of other parts of head
    - S08.81 Traumatic amputation of nose
      - S08.811 Complete traumatic amputation of nose D, S
      - S08.812 Partial traumatic amputation of nose D, S
    - S08.89 Traumatic amputation of other parts of head D, S

- S09 Other and unspecified injuries of head
  The appropriate 7th character is to be added to each code from category S09

  A initial encounter
  D subsequent encounter
  S sequela

  - S09.0 Injury of blood vessels of head, not elsewhere classified A, D, S
    Excludes1 injury of cerebral blood vessels (S06.-)
    injury of precerebral blood vessels (S15.-)

● Unacceptable Principal Diagnosis ● Use Additional Character(s) ■ Unspecified ▶ Manifestation Code
OGCR Official Guidelines for Coding and Reporting Excludes 1 Excludes 2 Includes Use additional Code first Code also

● **S09.1 Injury of muscle and tendon of head**

> Code also any associated open wound (S01.-)

> **Excludes2** sprain to joints and ligament of head (S03.9)

● ■ **S09.10 Unspecified injury of muscle and tendon of head** D, S 🔖

>> Injury of muscle and tendon of head NOS

● **S09.11 Strain of muscle and tendon of head** D, S 🔖

● **S09.12 Laceration of muscle and tendon of head** D, S 🔖

● **S09.19 Other specified injury of muscle and tendon of head** D, S 🔖

● **S09.2 Traumatic rupture of ear drum** D, S 🔖

> **Excludes1** traumatic rupture of ear drum due to blast injury (S09.31-)

● ■ **S09.20 Traumatic rupture of unspecified ear drum** A 🔖, D, S 🔖

● **S09.21 Traumatic rupture of right ear drum** A 🔖, D, S 🔖

● **S09.22 Traumatic rupture of left ear drum** A 🔖, D, S 🔖

● **S09.3 Other specified and unspecified injury of middle and inner ear**

> **Excludes1** injury to ear NOS (S09.91-)

> **Excludes2** injury to external ear (S00.4-, S01.3-, S08.1-)

● **S09.30 Unspecified injury of middle and inner ear**

● ■ **S09.301 Unspecified injury of right middle and inner ear** A 🔖, D, S 🔖

● ■ **S09.302 Unspecified injury of left middle and inner ear** A 🔖, D, S 🔖

● ■ **S09.309 Unspecified injury of unspecified middle and inner ear** A 🔖, D, S 🔖

● **S09.31 Primary blast injury of ear**

>> Blast injury of ear NOS

● **S09.311 Primary blast injury of right ear** A 🔖, D, S 🔖

● **S09.312 Primary blast injury of left ear** A 🔖, D, S 🔖

● **S09.313 Primary blast injury of ear, bilateral** A 🔖, D, S 🔖

● ■ **S09.319 Primary blast injury of unspecified ear** A 🔖, D, S 🔖

● **S09.39 Other specified injury of middle and inner ear**

>> Secondary blast injury to ear

● **S09.391 Other specified injury of right middle and inner ear** A 🔖, D, S 🔖

● **S09.392 Other specified injury of left middle and inner ear** A 🔖, D, S 🔖

● ■ **S09.399 Other specified injury of unspecified middle and inner ear** A 🔖, D, S 🔖

● **S09.8 Other specified injuries of head** D, S 🔖

● **S09.9 Unspecified injury of face and head** D, S 🔖

● ■ **S09.90 Unspecified injury of head**

>> Head injury NOS

> **Excludes1** brain injury NOS (S06.9-)
> head injury NOS with loss of consciousness (S06.9-)
> intracranial injury NOS (S06.9-)

● ■ **S09.91 Unspecified injury of ear** D, S 🔖

>> Injury of ear NOS

● ■ **S09.92 Unspecified injury of nose** D, S 🔖

>> Injury of nose NOS

● ■ **S09.93 Unspecified injury of face** D, S 🔖

>> Injury of face NOS

INJURIES TO THE NECK (S10-S19)

> **Includes** injuries of nape
> injuries of supraclavicular region
> injuries of throat

> **Excludes2** burns and corrosions (T20-T32)
> effects of foreign body in esophagus (T18.1)
> effects of foreign body in larynx (T17.3)
> effects of foreign body in pharynx (T17.2)
> effects of foreign body in trachea (T17.4)
> frostbite (T33-T34)
> insect bite or sting, venomous (T63.4)

● **S10 Superficial injury of neck**

> The appropriate 7th character is to be added to each code from category S10

> | | |
> |---|---|
> | A | initial encounter |
> | D | subsequent encounter |
> | S | sequela |

● **S10.0 Contusion of throat** D, S 🔖

>> Contusion of cervical esophagus
>> Contusion of larynx
>> Contusion of pharynx
>> Contusion of trachea

● **S10.1 Other and unspecified superficial injuries of throat**

● ■ **S10.10 Unspecified superficial injuries of throat** D, S 🔖

● **S10.11 Abrasion of throat** D, S 🔖

● **S10.12 Blister (nonthermal) of throat** D, S 🔖

● **S10.14 External constriction of part of throat** D, S 🔖

● **S10.15 Superficial foreign body of throat** D, S 🔖

>> Splinter in the throat

● **S10.16 Insect bite (nonvenomous) of throat** D, S 🔖

● **S10.17 Other superficial bite of throat** D, S 🔖

> **Excludes1** open bite of throat (S11.85)

● **S10.8 Superficial injury of other specified parts of neck**

● ■ **S10.80 Unspecified superficial injury of other specified part of neck** D, S 🔖

● **S10.81 Abrasion of other specified part of neck** D, S 🔖

● **S10.82 Blister (nonthermal) of other specified part of neck** D, S 🔖

● **S10.83 Contusion of other specified part of neck** D, S 🔖

● **S10.84 External constriction of other specified part of neck** D, S 🔖

CHAPTER 19 (S00-T88)

N Newborn Age: 0   **P** Pediatric Age: 0–17   **M** Maternity DX: 12–55   **A** Adult Age: 15–124   ♀ Females Only   ♂ Males Only

🔖 Complication\Comorbidity   🔖 Major C\C   🔖 Present on Admission Requirement   🔖 Hospital-Acquired Condition

1409

- S10.85   **Superficial foreign body of other specified part of neck** D, S
  - Splinter in other part of neck
- S10.86   **Insect bite of other specified part of neck** D, S
- S10.87   **Other superficial bite of other specified part of neck** D, S

  > **Excludes1**   open bite of other specified parts of neck (S11.85)

- S10.9   **Superficial injury of unspecified part of neck**
  - S10.90   **Unspecified superficial injury of unspecified part of neck** D, S
  - S10.91   **Abrasion of unspecified part of neck** D, S
  - S10.92   **Blister (nonthermal) of unspecified part of neck** D, S
  - S10.93   **Contusion of unspecified part of neck** D, S
  - S10.94   **External constriction of unspecified part of neck** D, S
  - S10.95   **Superficial foreign body of unspecified part of neck** D, S
  - S10.96   **Insect bite of unspecified part of neck** D, S
  - S10.97   **Other superficial bite of unspecified part of neck** D, S

- S11   **Open wound of neck**

  Code also any associated:
  - spinal cord injury (S14.0, S14.1-)
  - wound infection

  > **Excludes2**   open fracture of vertebra (S12.- with 7th character B)

  The appropriate 7th character is to be added to each code from category S11

  > A   initial encounter
  > D   subsequent encounter
  > S   sequela

  - S11.0   **Open wound of larynx and trachea**
    - S11.01   **Open wound of larynx**

      > **Excludes2**   open wound of vocal cord (S11.03)

      - S11.011   **Laceration without foreign body of larynx** A, D, S
      - S11.012   **Laceration with foreign body of larynx** A, D, S
      - S11.013   **Puncture wound without foreign body of larynx** A, D, S
      - S11.014   **Puncture wound with foreign body of larynx** A, D, S
      - S11.015   **Open bite of larynx** A, D, S
        - Bite of larynx NOS
      - S11.019   **Unspecified open wound of larynx** A, D, S
    - S11.02   **Open wound of trachea**
      - Open wound of cervical trachea
      - Open wound of trachea NOS

      > **Excludes2**   open wound of thoracic trachea (S27.5-)

      - S11.021   **Laceration without foreign body of trachea** A, D, S
      - S11.022   **Laceration with foreign body of trachea** A, D, S

- S11.023   **Puncture wound without foreign body of trachea** A, D, S
- S11.024   **Puncture wound with foreign body of trachea** A, D, S
- S11.025   **Open bite of trachea** A, D, S
  - Bite of trachea NOS
- S11.029   **Unspecified open wound of trachea** A, D, S
- S11.03   **Open wound of vocal cord**
  - S11.031   **Laceration without foreign body of vocal cord** A, D, S
  - S11.032   **Laceration with foreign body of vocal cord** A, D, S
  - S11.033   **Puncture wound without foreign body of vocal cord** A, D, S
  - S11.034   **Puncture wound with foreign body of vocal cord** A, D, S
  - S11.035   **Open bite of vocal cord** A, D, S
    - Bite of vocal cord NOS
  - S11.039   **Unspecified open wound of vocal cord** A, D, S
- S11.1   **Open wound of thyroid gland**
  - S11.10   **Unspecified open wound of thyroid gland** A, D, S
  - S11.11   **Laceration without foreign body of thyroid gland** A, D, S
  - S11.12   **Laceration with foreign body of thyroid gland** A, D, S
  - S11.13   **Puncture wound without foreign body of thyroid gland** A, D, S
  - S11.14   **Puncture wound with foreign body of thyroid gland** A, D, S
  - S11.15   **Open bite of thyroid gland** A, D, S
    - Bite of thyroid gland NOS
- S11.2   **Open wound of pharynx and cervical esophagus**

  > **Excludes1**   open wound of esophagus NOS (S27.8-)

  - S11.20   **Unspecified open wound of pharynx and cervical esophagus** A, D, S
  - S11.21   **Laceration without foreign body of pharynx and cervical esophagus** A, D, S
  - S11.22   **Laceration with foreign body of pharynx and cervical esophagus** A, D, S
  - S11.23   **Puncture wound without foreign body of pharynx and cervical esophagus** A, D, S
  - S11.24   **Puncture wound with foreign body of pharynx and cervical esophagus** A, D, S
  - S11.25   **Open bite of pharynx and cervical esophagus** A, D, S
    - Bite of pharynx and cervical esophagus NOS
- S11.8   **Open wound of other specified parts of neck**
  - S11.80   **Unspecified open specified wound of other part of neck** D, S
  - S11.81   **Laceration without foreign body of other specified part of neck** D, S
  - S11.82   **Laceration with foreign body of other specified part of neck** D, S

- ●   Unacceptable Principal Diagnosis   ●   Use Additional Character(s)   ■   Unspecified   ▶   Manifestation Code

OGCR   Official Guidelines for Coding and Reporting   Excludes 1   Excludes 2   Includes   Use additional   Code first   Code also

- **S11.83** Puncture wound without foreign body of other specified part of neck D, S
- **S11.84** Puncture wound with foreign body of other specified part of neck D, S
- **S11.85** Open bite of other specified part of neck D, S
  - Bite of other part of neck NOS
  - **Excludes1** superficial bite of other specified part of neck (S10.87)
- **S11.89** Other open wound of other part of neck D, S
- **S11.9** Open wound of unspecified part of neck
  - **S11.90** Unspecified open wound of unspecified part of neck D, S
  - **S11.91** Laceration without foreign body of unspecified part of neck D, S
  - **S11.92** Laceration with foreign body of unspecified part of neck D, S
  - **S11.93** Puncture wound without foreign body of unspecified part of neck D, G, S
  - **S11.94** Puncture wound with foreign body of unspecified part of neck D, G, S
  - **S11.95** Open bite of unspecified part of neck D, G, S
    - Bite of neck NOS
    - **Excludes1** superficial bite of neck (S10.97)

- **S12** Fracture of cervical vertebra and other parts of neck
  - **Note:** A fracture not indicated as displaced or nondisplaced should be coded to displaced
  - A fracture not indicated as open or closed should be coded to closed
  - **Includes** fracture of cervical neural arch
    - fracture of cervical spine
    - fracture of cervical spinous process
    - fracture of cervical transverse process
    - fracture of cervical vertebral arch
    - fracture of neck
  - The appropriate 7th character is to be added to all codes from subcategories S12.0-S12.6

A	initial encounter for closed fracture
B	initial encounter for open fracture
D	subsequent encounter for fracture with routine healing
G	subsequent encounter for fracture with delayed healing
K	subsequent encounter for fracture with nonunion
S	sequela

  - **Code also** any associated cervical spinal cord injury (S14.0, S14.1-)
  - **S12.0** Fracture of first cervical vertebra
    - Atlas
    - **S12.00** Unspecified fracture of first cervical vertebra
      - **S12.000** Unspecified displaced fracture of first cervical vertebra A, K, B, D, G, S, A, B
      - **S12.001** Unspecified nondisplaced fracture of first cervical vertebra A, K, B, D, G, S, A, B
    - **S12.01** Stable burst fracture of first cervical vertebra A, K, B, D, G, S, A, B

- **S12.02** Unstable burst fracture of first cervical vertebra A, K, B, D, G, S, A, B
- **S12.03** Posterior arch fracture of first cervical vertebra
  - **S12.030** Displaced posterior arch fracture of first cervical vertebra A, K, B, D, G, S, A, B
  - **S12.031** Nondisplaced posterior arch fracture of first cervical vertebra A, K, B, D, G, S, A, B
- **S12.04** Lateral mass fracture of first cervical vertebra
  - **S12.040** Displaced lateral mass fracture of first cervical vertebra A, K, B, D, G, S, A, B
  - **S12.041** Nondisplaced lateral mass fracture of first cervical vertebra A, K, B, D, G, S, A, B
- **S12.09** Other fracture of first cervical vertebra
  - **S12.090** Other displaced fracture of first cervical vertebra A, K, B, D, G, S, A, B
  - **S12.091** Other nondisplaced fracture of first cervical vertebra A, K, B, D, G, S, A, B
- **S12.1** Fracture of second cervical vertebra
  - Axis
  - **S12.10** Unspecified fracture of second cervical vertebra
    - **S12.100** Unspecified displaced fracture of second cervical vertebra A, K, B, D, G, S, A, B
    - **S12.101** Unspecified nondisplaced fracture of second cervical vertebra A, K, B, D, G, S, A, B
  - **S12.11** Type II dens fracture
    - **S12.110** Anterior displaced Type II dens fracture A, K, B, D, G, S, A, B
    - **S12.111** Posterior displaced Type II dens fracture A, K, B, D, G, S, A, B
    - **S12.112** Nondisplaced Type II dens fracture A, K, B, D, G, S, A, B
  - **S12.12** Other dens fracture
    - **S12.120** Other displaced dens fracture A, K, B, D, G, S, A, B
    - **S12.121** Other nondisplaced dens fracture A, K, B, D, G, S, A, B
  - **S12.13** Unspecified traumatic spondylolisthesis of second cervical vertebra
    - **S12.130** Unspecified traumatic displaced spondylolisthesis of second cervical vertebra A, K, B, D, G, S, A, B
    - **S12.131** Unspecified traumatic nondisplaced spondylolisthesis of second cervical vertebra A, K, B, D, G, S, A, B
  - **S12.14** Type III traumatic spondylolisthesis of second cervical vertebra A, K, B, D, G, S, A, B

CHAPTER 19 (S00-T88)

CHAPTER 19 (S00-T88)

- S12.15 Other traumatic spondylolisthesis of second cervical vertebra
  - S12.150 Other traumatic displaced spondylolisthesis of second cervical vertebra A, K ⬥, B ⬥, D, G, S ⬥, A, B ⬥
  - S12.151 Other traumatic nondisplaced spondylolisthesis of second cervical vertebra A, K ⬥, B ⬥, D, G, S ⬥, A, B ⬥
- S12.19 Other fracture of second cervical vertebra
  - S12.190 Other displaced fracture of second cervical vertebra A, K ⬥, B ⬥, D, G, S ⬥, A, B ⬥
  - S12.191 Other nondisplaced fracture of second cervical vertebra A, K ⬥, B ⬥, D, G, S ⬥, A, B ⬥
- S12.2 Fracture of third cervical vertebra
  - S12.20 Unspecified fracture of third cervical vertebra
    - S12.200 Unspecified displaced fracture of third cervical vertebra A, K ⬥, B ⬥, D, G, S ⬥, A, B ⬥
    - S12.201 Unspecified nondisplaced fracture of third cervical vertebra A, K ⬥, B ⬥, D, G, S ⬥, A, B ⬥
  - S12.23 Unspecified traumatic spondylolisthesis of third cervical vertebra
    - S12.230 Unspecified traumatic displaced spondylolisthesis of third cervical vertebra A, K ⬥, B ⬥, D, G, S ⬥, A, B ⬥
    - S12.231 Unspecified traumatic nondisplaced spondylolisthesis of third cervical vertebra A, K ⬥, B ⬥, D, G, S ⬥, A, B ⬥
  - S12.24 Type III traumatic spondylolisthesis of third cervical vertebra A, K ⬥, B ⬥, D, G, S ⬥, A, B ⬥
  - S12.25 Other traumatic spondylolisthesis of third cervical vertebra
    - S12.250 Other traumatic displaced spondylolisthesis of third cervical vertebra A, K ⬥, B ⬥, D, G, S ⬥, A, B ⬥
    - S12.251 Other traumatic nondisplaced spondylolisthesis of third cervical vertebra A, K ⬥, B ⬥, D, G, S ⬥, A, B ⬥
  - S12.29 Other fracture of third cervical vertebra
    - S12.290 Other displaced fracture of third cervical vertebra A, K ⬥, B ⬥, D, G, S ⬥, A, B ⬥
    - S12.291 Other nondisplaced fracture of third cervical vertebra A, K ⬥, B ⬥, D, G, S ⬥, A, B ⬥
- S12.3 Fracture of fourth cervical vertebra
  - S12.30 Unspecified fracture of fourth cervical vertebra
    - S12.300 Unspecified displaced fracture of fourth cervical vertebra A, K ⬥, B ⬥, D, G, S ⬥, A, B ⬥
    - S12.301 Unspecified nondisplaced fracture of fourth cervical vertebra A, K ⬥, B ⬥, D, G, S ⬥, A, B ⬥

- S12.33 Unspecified traumatic spondylolisthesis of fourth cervical vertebra
  - S12.330 Unspecified traumatic displaced spondylolisthesis of fourth cervical vertebra A, K ⬥, B ⬥, D, G, S ⬥, A, B ⬥
  - S12.331 Unspecified traumatic nondisplaced spondylolisthesis of fourth cervical vertebra A, K ⬥, B ⬥, D, G, S ⬥, A, B ⬥
- S12.34 Type III traumatic spondylolisthesis of fourth cervical vertebra A, K ⬥, B ⬥, D, G, S ⬥, A, B ⬥
- S12.35 Other traumatic spondylolisthesis of fourth cervical vertebra
  - S12.350 Other traumatic displaced spondylolisthesis of fourth cervical vertebra A, K ⬥, B ⬥, D, G, S ⬥, A, B ⬥
  - S12.351 Other traumatic nondisplaced spondylolisthesis of fourth cervical vertebra A, K ⬥, B ⬥, D, G, S ⬥, A, B ⬥
- S12.39 Other fracture of fourth cervical vertebra
  - S12.390 Other displaced fracture of fourth cervical vertebra A, K ⬥, B ⬥, D, G, S ⬥, A, B ⬥
  - S12.391 Other nondisplaced fracture of fourth cervical vertebra A, K ⬥, B ⬥, D, G, S ⬥, A, B ⬥
- S12.4 Fracture of fifth cervical vertebra
  - S12.40 Unspecified fracture of fifth cervical vertebra
    - S12.400 Unspecified displaced fracture of fifth cervical vertebra A, K ⬥, B ⬥, D, G, S ⬥, A, B ⬥
    - S12.401 Unspecified nondisplaced fracture of fifth cervical vertebra A, K ⬥, B ⬥, D, G, S ⬥, A, B ⬥
  - S12.43 Unspecified traumatic spondylolisthesis of fifth cervical vertebra
    - S12.430 Unspecified traumatic displaced spondylolisthesis of fifth cervical vertebra A, K ⬥, B ⬥, D, G, S ⬥, A, B ⬥
    - S12.431 Unspecified traumatic nondisplaced spondylolisthesis of fifth cervical vertebra A, K ⬥, B ⬥, D, G, S ⬥, A, B ⬥
  - S12.44 Type III traumatic spondylolisthesis of fifth cervical vertebra A, K ⬥, B ⬥, D, G, S ⬥, A, B ⬥
  - S12.45 Other traumatic spondylolisthesis of fifth cervical vertebra
    - S12.450 Other traumatic displaced spondylolisthesis of fifth cervical vertebra A, K ⬥, B ⬥, D, G, S ⬥, A, B ⬥
    - S12.451 Other traumatic nondisplaced spondylolisthesis of fifth cervical vertebra A, K ⬥, B ⬥, D, G, S ⬥, A, B ⬥

● Unacceptable Principal Diagnosis   ● Use Additional Character(s)   ■ Unspecified   ▶ Manifestation Code
OGCR Official Guidelines for Coding and Reporting   Excludes 1   Excludes 2   Includes   Use additional   Code first   Code also

● **S12.49**   Other fracture of fifth cervical vertebra
   ● **S12.490**   Other displaced fracture of fifth cervical vertebra A, K 🌑, B 🌑, D, G, S 🌑, A, B 🌑
   ● **S12.491**   Other nondisplaced fracture of fifth cervical vertebra A, K 🌑, B 🌑, D, G, S 🌑, A, B 🌑

● **S12.5**   Fracture of sixth cervical vertebra
  ● **S12.50**   Unspecified fracture of sixth cervical vertebra
   ● ◼ **S12.500**   Unspecified displaced fracture of sixth cervical vertebra A, K 🌑, B 🌑, D, G, S 🌑, A, B 🌑
   ● ◼ **S12.501**   Unspecified nondisplaced fracture of sixth cervical vertebra A, K 🌑, B 🌑, D, G, S 🌑, A, B 🌑
  ● **S12.53**   Unspecified traumatic spondylolisthesis of sixth cervical vertebra
   ● ◼ **S12.530**   Unspecified traumatic displaced spondylolisthesis of sixth cervical vertebra A, K 🌑, B 🌑, D, G, S 🌑, A, B 🌑
   ● ◼ **S12.531**   Unspecified traumatic nondisplaced spondylolisthesis of sixth cervical vertebra A, K 🌑, B 🌑, D, G, S 🌑, A, B 🌑
  ● **S12.54**   Type III traumatic spondylolisthesis of sixth cervical vertebra A, K 🌑, B 🌑, D, G, S 🌑, A, B 🌑
  ● **S12.55**   Other traumatic spondylolisthesis of sixth cervical vertebra
   ● **S12.550**   Other traumatic displaced spondylolisthesis of sixth cervical vertebra A, K 🌑, B 🌑, D, G, S 🌑, A, B 🌑
   ● **S12.551**   Other traumatic nondisplaced spondylolisthesis of sixth cervical vertebra A, K 🌑, B 🌑, D, G, S 🌑, A, B 🌑
  ● **S12.59**   Other fracture of sixth cervical vertebra
   ● **S12.590**   Other displaced fracture of sixth cervical vertebra A, K 🌑, B 🌑, D, G, S 🌑, A, B 🌑
   ● **S12.591**   Other nondisplaced fracture of sixth cervical vertebra A, K 🌑, B 🌑, D, G, S 🌑, A, B 🌑

● **S12.6**   Fracture of seventh cervical vertebra
  S12.60   Unspecified fracture of seventh cervical vertebra
   ● ◼ **S12.600**   Unspecified displaced fracture of seventh cervical vertebra A, K 🌑, B 🌑, D, G, S 🌑, A, B 🌑
   ● ◼ **S12.601**   Unspecified nondisplaced fracture of seventh cervical vertebra A, K 🌑, B 🌑, D, G, S 🌑, A, B 🌑
  ● **S12.63**   Unspecified traumatic spondylolisthesis of seventh cervical vertebra
   ● ◼ **S12.630**   Unspecified traumatic displaced spondylolisthesis of seventh cervical vertebra A, K 🌑, B 🌑, D, G, S 🌑, A, B 🌑
   ● ◼ **S12.631**   Unspecified traumatic nondisplaced spondylolisthesis of seventh cervical vertebra A, K 🌑, B 🌑, D, G, S 🌑, A, B 🌑

● **S12.64**   Type III traumatic spondylolisthesis of seventh cervical vertebra A, K 🌑, B 🌑, D, G, S 🌑, A, B 🌑
● **S12.65**   Other traumatic spondylolisthesis of seventh cervical vertebra
   ● **S12.650**   Other traumatic displaced spondylolisthesis of seventh cervical vertebra A, K 🌑, B 🌑, D, G, S 🌑, A, B 🌑
   ● **S12.651**   Other traumatic nondisplaced spondylolisthesis of seventh cervical vertebra A, K 🌑, B 🌑, D, G, S 🌑, A, B 🌑
● **S12.69**   Other fracture of seventh cervical vertebra
   ● **S12.690**   Other displaced fracture of seventh cervical vertebra A, K 🌑, B 🌑, D, G, S 🌑, A, B 🌑
   ● **S12.691**   Other nondisplaced fracture of seventh cervical vertebra A, K 🌑, B 🌑, D, G, S 🌑, A, B 🌑

● **S12.8**   Fracture of other parts of neck A 🌑, D, S 🌑, A 🌑

The appropriate 7th character is to be added to code S12.8

A	initial encounter
D	subsequent encounter
S	sequela

Hyoid bone   Thyroid cartilage
Larynx   Trachea

● ◼ **S12.9**   Fracture of neck, unspecified A 🌑, D, S 🌑, A 🌑

The appropriate 7th character is to be added to code S12.9

A	initial encounter
D	subsequent encounter
S	sequela

Fracture of neck NOS
Fracture of cervical spine NOS
Fracture of cervical vertebra NOS

● **S13**   Dislocation and sprain of joints and ligaments at neck level

Includes   avulsion of joint or ligament at neck level
     laceration of cartilage, joint or ligament at neck level
     sprain of cartilage, joint or ligament at neck level
     traumatic hemarthrosis of joint or ligament at neck level
     traumatic rupture of joint or ligament at neck level
     traumatic subluxation of joint or ligament at neck level
     traumatic tear of joint or ligament at neck level

Code also any associated open wound

Excludes2   strain of muscle or tendon at neck level (S16.1)

The appropriate 7th character is to be added to each code from category S13

A	initial encounter
D	subsequent encounter
S	sequela

● **S13.0**   Traumatic rupture of cervical intervertebral disc A 🌑, D, S 🌑, A 🌑

Excludes1   rupture or displacement (nontraumatic) of cervical intervertebral disc NOS (M50.-)

N Newborn Age: 0   **P** Pediatric Age: 0–17   **M** Maternity DX: 12–55   **A** Adult Age: 15–124   ♀ Females Only   ♂ Males Only

🌑 Complication\Comorbidity   🌑 Major C\C   🌑 Present on Admission Requirement   🌑 Hospital-Acquired Condition

1413

● **S13.1**   **Subluxation and dislocation of cervical vertebrae**

Code also any associated:
  open wound of neck (S11.-)
  spinal cord injury (S14.1-)

Excludes2   fracture of cervical vertebrae
    (S12.0-S12.3-)

● **S13.10**   **Subluxation and dislocation of unspecified cervical vertebrae**

●■ **S13.100**   **Subluxation of unspecified cervical vertebrae** A ⬡, D, S ⬡, A ⬡

●■ **S13.101**   **Dislocation of unspecified cervical vertebrae** A ⬡, D, S ⬡, A ⬡

● **S13.11**   **Subluxation and dislocation of C_0/C_1 cervical vertebrae**
  Subluxation and dislocation of atlantooccipital joint
  Subluxation and dislocation of atloidooccipital joint
  Subluxation and dislocation of occipitoatloid joint

● **S13.110**   **Subluxation of C_0/C_1 cervical vertebrae** A ⬡, D, S ⬡, A ⬡

● **S13.111**   **Dislocation of C_0/C_1 cervical vertebrae** A ⬡, D, S ⬡, A ⬡

● **S13.12**   **Subluxation and dislocation of C_1/C_2 cervical vertebrae**
  Subluxation and dislocation of atlantoaxial joint

● **S13.120**   **Subluxation of C_1/C_2 cervical vertebrae** A ⬡, D, S ⬡, A ⬡

● **S13.121**   **Dislocation of C_1/C_2 cervical vertebrae** A ⬡, D, S ⬡, A ⬡

● **S13.13**   **Subluxation and dislocation of C_2/C_3 cervical vertebrae**

● **S13.130**   **Subluxation of C_2/C_3 cervical vertebrae** A ⬡, D, S ⬡, A ⬡

● **S13.131**   **Dislocation of C_2/C_3 cervical vertebrae** A ⬡, D, S ⬡, A ⬡

● **S13.14**   **Subluxation and dislocation of C_3/C_4 cervical vertebrae**

● **S13.140**   **Subluxation of C_3/C_4 cervical vertebrae** A ⬡, D, S ⬡, A ⬡

● **S13.141**   **Dislocation of C_3/C_4 cervical vertebrae** A ⬡, D, S ⬡, A ⬡

● **S13.15**   **Subluxation and dislocation of C_4/C_5 cervical vertebrae**

● **S13.150**   **Subluxation of C_4/C_5 cervical vertebrae** A ⬡, D, S ⬡, A ⬡

● **S13.151**   **Dislocation of C_4/C_5 cervical vertebrae** A ⬡, D, S ⬡, A ⬡

● **S13.16**   **Subluxation and dislocation of C_5/C_6 cervical vertebrae**

● **S13.160**   **Subluxation of C_5/C_6 cervical vertebrae** A ⬡, D, S ⬡, A ⬡

● **S13.161**   **Dislocation of C_5/C_6 cervical vertebrae** A ⬡, D, S ⬡, A ⬡

● **S13.17**   **Subluxation and dislocation of C_6/C_7 cervical vertebrae**

● **S13.170**   **Subluxation of C_6/C_7 cervical vertebrae** A ⬡, D, S ⬡, A ⬡

● **S13.171**   **Dislocation of C_6/C_7 cervical vertebrae** A ⬡, D, S ⬡, A ⬡

● **S13.18**   **Subluxation and dislocation of C_7/T_1 cervical vertebrae**

● **S13.180**   **Subluxation of C_7/T_1 cervical vertebrae** A ⬡, D, S ⬡, A ⬡

● **S13.181**   **Dislocation of C_7/T_1 cervical vertebrae** A ⬡, D, S ⬡, A ⬡

● **S13.2**   **Dislocation of other and unspecified parts of neck**

●■ **S13.20**   **Dislocation of unspecified parts of neck** A ⬡, D, S ⬡, A ⬡

● **S13.29**   **Dislocation of other parts of neck** A ⬡, D, S ⬡, A ⬡

● **S13.4**   **Sprain of ligaments of cervical spine** D, S ⬡
  Sprain of anterior longitudinal (ligament), cervical
  Sprain of atlanto-axial (joints)
  Sprain of atlanto-occipital (joints)
  Whiplash injury of cervical spine

● **S13.5**   **Sprain of thyroid region** D, S ⬡
  Sprain of cricoarytenoid (joint) (ligament)
  Sprain of cricothyroid (joint) (ligament)
  Sprain of thyroid cartilage

● **S13.8**   **Sprain of joints and ligaments of other parts of neck** D, S ⬡

●■ **S13.9**   **Sprain of joints and ligaments of unspecified parts of neck** D, S ⬡

● **S14**   **Injury of nerves and spinal cord at neck level**

Note: Code to highest level of cervical cord injury

Code also any associated:
  fracture of cervical vertebra (S12.0--S12.6.-)
  open wound of neck (S11-)
  transient paralysis (R29.5)

The appropriate 7th character is to be added to each code from category S14

A	initial encounter
D	subsequent encounter
S	sequela

● **S14.0**   **Concussion and edema of cervical spinal cord** A ⬡, D, S ⬡

● **S14.1**   **Other and unspecified injuries of cervical spinal cord**

● **S14.10**   **Unspecified injury of cervical spinal cord**

●■ **S14.101**   **Unspecified injury at C_1 level of cervical spinal cord** A ⬡, D, S ⬡, A ⬡

●■ **S14.102**   **Unspecified injury at C_2 level of cervical spinal cord** A ⬡, D, S ⬡, A ⬡

●■ **S14.103**   **Unspecified injury at C_3 level of cervical spinal cord** A ⬡, D, S ⬡, A ⬡

●■ **S14.104**   **Unspecified injury at C_4 level of cervical spinal cord** A ⬡, D, S ⬡, A ⬡

●■ **S14.105**   **Unspecified injury at C_5 level of cervical spinal cord** A ⬡, D, S ⬡, A ⬡

●■ **S14.106**   **Unspecified injury at C_6 level of cervical spinal cord** A ⬡, D, S ⬡, A ⬡

● Unacceptable Principal Diagnosis   ● Use Additional Character(s)   ■ Unspecified   ▶ Manifestation Code

OGCR   Official Guidelines for Coding and Reporting   Excludes 1   Excludes 2   Includes   Use additional   Code first   Code also

● ■ S14.107 Unspecified injury at C₇ level of cervical spinal cord A ⊗, D, S ⊗, A ⊗

● ■ S14.108 Unspecified injury at C₈ level of cervical spinal cord A ⊗, D, S ⊗

● ■ S14.109 Unspecified injury at unspecified level of cervical spinal cord D, S ⊗

Injury of cervical spinal cord NOS

● S14.11 Complete lesion of cervical spinal cord

● S14.111 Complete lesion at C₁ level of cervical spinal cord A ⊗, D, S ⊗, A ⊗

● S14.112 Complete lesion at C₂ level of cervical spinal cord A ⊗, D, S ⊗, A ⊗

● S14.113 Complete lesion at C₃ level of cervical spinal cord A ⊗, D, S ⊗, A ⊗

● S14.114 Complete lesion at C₄ level of cervical spinal cord A ⊗, D, S ⊗, A ⊗

● S14.115 Complete lesion at C₅ level of cervical spinal cord A ⊗, D, S ⊗, A ⊗

● S14.116 Complete lesion at C₆ level of cervical spinal cord A ⊗, D, S ⊗, A ⊗

● S14.117 Complete lesion at C₇ level of cervical spinal cord A ⊗, D, S ⊗, A ⊗

● S14.118 Complete lesion at C₈ level of cervical spinal cord A ⊗

● ■ S14.119 Complete lesion at unspecified level of cervical spinal cord

● S14.12 Central cord syndrome of cervical spinal cord

● S14.121 Central cord syndrome at C₁ level of cervical spinal cord A ⊗, D, S ⊗, A ⊗

● S14.122 Central cord syndrome at C₂ level of cervical spinal cord A ⊗, D, S ⊗, A ⊗

● S14.123 Central cord syndrome at C₃ level of cervical spinal cord A ⊗, D, S ⊗, A ⊗

● S14.124 Central cord syndrome at C₄ level of cervical spinal cord A ⊗, D, S ⊗, A ⊗

● S14.125 Central cord syndrome at C₅ level of cervical spinal cord A ⊗, D, S ⊗, A ⊗

● S14.126 Central cord syndrome at C₆ level of cervical spinal cord A ⊗, D, S ⊗, A ⊗

● S14.127 Central cord syndrome at C₇ level of cervical spinal cord A ⊗, D, S ⊗, A ⊗

● S14.128 Central cord syndrome at C₈ level of cervical spinal cord A ⊗, D, S ⊗

● ■ S14.129 Central cord syndrome at unspecified level of cervical spinal cord D, S ⊗

● S14.13 Anterior cord syndrome of cervical spinal cord

● S14.131 Anterior cord syndrome at C₁ level of cervical spinal cord A ⊗, D, S ⊗, A ⊗

● S14.132 Anterior cord syndrome at C₂ level of cervical spinal cord A ⊗, D, S ⊗, A ⊗

● S14.133 Anterior cord syndrome at C₃ level of cervical spinal cord A ⊗, D, S ⊗, A ⊗

● S14.134 Anterior cord syndrome at C₄ level of cervical spinal cord A ⊗, D, S ⊗, A ⊗

● S14.135 Anterior cord syndrome at C₅ level of cervical spinal cord A ⊗, D, S ⊗, A ⊗

● S14.136 Anterior cord syndrome at C₆ level of cervical spinal cord A ⊗, D, S ⊗, A ⊗

● S14.137 Anterior cord syndrome at C₇ level of cervical spinal cord A ⊗, D, S ⊗, A ⊗

● S14.138 Anterior cord syndrome at C₈ level of cervical spinal cord A ⊗, D, S ⊗

● ■ S14.139 Anterior cord syndrome at unspecified level of cervical spinal cord D, S ⊗

● S14.14 Brown-Séquard syndrome of cervical spinal cord

● S14.141 Brown-Séquard syndrome at C₁ level of cervical spinal cord A ⊗, D, S ⊗

● S14.142 Brown-Séquard syndrome at C₂ level of cervical spinal cord A ⊗, D, S ⊗

● S14.143 Brown-Séquard syndrome at C₃ level of cervical spinal cord A ⊗, D, S ⊗

● S14.144 Brown-Séquard syndrome at C₄ level of cervical spinal cord A ⊗, D, S ⊗

● S14.145 Brown-Séquard syndrome at C₅ level of cervical spinal cord A ⊗, D, S ⊗

● S14.146 Brown-Séquard syndrome at C₆ level of cervical spinal cord A ⊗, D, S ⊗

● S14.147 Brown-Séquard syndrome at C₇ level of cervical spinal cord A ⊗, D, S ⊗

● S14.148 Brown-Séquard syndrome at C₈ level of cervical spinal cord A ⊗, D, S ⊗

● ■ S14.149 Brown-Séquard syndrome at unspecified level of cervical spinal cord

N Newborn Age: 0   P Pediatric Age: 0–17   M Maternity DX: 12–55   A Adult Age: 15–124   ♀ Females Only   ♂ Males Only

⊗ Complication\Comorbidity   ⊗ Major C\C   ⊗ Present on Admission Requirement   ⊗ Hospital-Acquired Condition

CHAPTER 19 (S00-T88)

● **S14.15 Other incomplete lesions of cervical spinal cord**
Incomplete lesion of cervical spinal cord NOS
Posterior cord syndrome of cervical spinal cord

  ● **S14.151 Other incomplete lesion at C_1 level of cervical spinal cord** A 🔹, D, S 🔹, A 🔹

  ● **S14.152 Other incomplete lesion at C_2 level of cervical spinal cord** A 🔹, D, S 🔹, A 🔹

  ● **S14.153 Other incomplete lesion at C_3 level of cervical spinal cord** A 🔹, D, S 🔹, A 🔹

  ● **S14.154 Other incomplete lesion at C_4 level of cervical spinal cord** A 🔹, D, S 🔹, A 🔹

  ● **S14.155 Other incomplete lesion at C_5 level of cervical spinal cord** A 🔹, D, S 🔹, A 🔹

  ● **S14.156 Other incomplete lesion at C_6 level of cervical spinal cord** A 🔹, D, S 🔹, A 🔹

  ● **S14.157 Other incomplete lesion at C_7 level of cervical spinal cord** A 🔹, D, S 🔹, A 🔹

  ● **S14.158 Other incomplete lesion at C_8 level of cervical spinal cord** A 🔹, D, S 🔹

  ●■ **S14.159 Other incomplete lesion at unspecified level of cervical spinal cord** D, S 🔹

● **S14.2 Injury of nerve root of cervical spine** D, S 🔹

● **S14.3 Injury of brachial plexus** D, S 🔹

● **S14.4 Injury of peripheral nerves of neck** D, S 🔹

● **S14.5 Injury of cervical sympathetic nerves** D, S 🔹

● **S14.8 Injury of other specified nerves of neck** D, S 🔹

●■ **S14.9 Injury of unspecified nerves of neck** D, S 🔹

● **S15 Injury of blood vessels at neck level**

  Code also any associated open wound (S11.-)

  The appropriate 7th character is to be added to each code from category S15

A	initial encounter
D	subsequent encounter
S	sequela

● **S15.0 Injury of carotid artery of neck**
Injury of carotid artery (common) (external) (internal, extracranial portion)
Injury of carotid artery NOS

  Excludes1 injury of internal carotid artery, intracranial portion (S06.8)

  ● **S15.00 Unspecified injury of carotid artery**

    ●■ **S15.001 Unspecified injury of right carotid artery** A 🔹, D, S 🔹

    ●■ **S15.002 Unspecified injury of left carotid artery** A 🔹, D, S 🔹

    ●■ **S15.009 Unspecified injury of unspecified carotid artery** A 🔹, D, S 🔹

● **S15.01 Minor laceration of carotid artery**
Incomplete transection of carotid artery
Laceration of carotid artery NOS
Superficial laceration of carotid artery

  ● **S15.011 Minor laceration of right carotid artery** A 🔹, D, S 🔹

  ● **S15.012 Minor laceration of left carotid artery** A 🔹, D, S 🔹

  ●■ **S15.019 Minor laceration of unspecified carotid artery** A 🔹, D, S 🔹

● **S15.02 Major laceration of carotid artery**
Complete transection of carotid artery
Traumatic rupture of carotid artery

  ● **S15.021 Major laceration of right carotid artery** A 🔹, D, S 🔹

  ● **S15.022 Major laceration of left carotid artery** A 🔹, D, S 🔹

  ●■ **S15.029 Major laceration of unspecified carotid artery** A 🔹, D, S 🔹

● **S15.09 Other specified injury of carotid artery**

  ● **S15.091 Other specified injury of right carotid artery** A 🔹, D, S 🔹

  ● **S15.092 Other specified injury of left carotid artery** A 🔹, D, S 🔹

  ●■ **S15.099 Other specified injury of unspecified carotid artery** A 🔹, D, S 🔹

● **S15.1 Injury of vertebral artery**

  ● **S15.10 Unspecified injury of vertebral artery**

    ●■ **S15.101 Unspecified injury of right vertebral artery** A 🔹, D, S 🔹

    ●■ **S15.102 Unspecified injury of left vertebral artery** A 🔹, D, S 🔹

    ●■ **S15.109 Unspecified injury of unspecified vertebral artery** A 🔹, D, S 🔹

  ● **S15.11 Minor laceration of vertebral artery**
Incomplete transection of vertebral artery
Laceration of vertebral artery NOS
Superficial laceration of vertebral artery

    ● **S15.111 Minor laceration of right vertebral artery** A 🔹, D, S

    ● **S15.112 Minor laceration of left vertebral artery** A 🔹, D, S

    ●■ **S15.119 Minor laceration of unspecified vertebral artery** A 🔹, D, S 🔹

  ● **S15.12 Major laceration of vertebral artery**
Complete transection of vertebral artery
Traumatic rupture of vertebral artery

    ● **S15.121 Major laceration of right vertebral artery** A 🔹, D, S 🔹

    ● **S15.122 Major laceration of left vertebral artery** A 🔹, D, S 🔹

    ●■ **S15.129 Major laceration of unspecified vertebral artery** A 🔹, D, S 🔹

  ● **S15.19 Other specified injury of vertebral artery**

    ● **S15.191 Other specified injury of right vertebral artery** A 🔹, D, S 🔹

    ● **S15.192 Other specified injury of left vertebral artery** A 🔹, D, S 🔹

    ●■ **S15.199 Other specified injury of unspecified vertebral artery** A 🔹, D, S 🔹

● **S15.2   Injury of external jugular vein**
  ● **S15.20   Unspecified injury of external jugular vein**
    ●■ **S15.201   Unspecified injury of right external jugular vein A** 🔴, D, S 🔘
    ●■ **S15.202   Unspecified injury of left external jugular vein A** 🔴, D, S 🔘
    ●■ **S15.209   Unspecified injury of unspecified external jugular vein A** 🔴, D, S 🔘
  ● **S15.21   Minor laceration of external jugular vein**
    Incomplete transection of external jugular vein
    Laceration of external jugular vein NOS
    Superficial laceration of external jugular vein
    ● **S15.211   Minor laceration of right external jugular vein A** 🔴, D, S 🔘
    ● **S15.212   Minor laceration of left external jugular vein A** 🔴, D, S 🔘
    ●■ **S15.219   Minor laceration of unspecified external jugular vein A** 🔴, D, S 🔘
  ● **S15.22   Major laceration of external jugular vein**
    Complete transection of external jugular vein
    Traumatic rupture of external jugular vein
    ● **S15.221   Major laceration of right external jugular vein A** 🔴, D, S 🔘
    ● **S15.222   Major laceration of left external jugular vein A** 🔴, D, S 🔘
    ●■ **S15.229   Major laceration of unspecified external jugular vein A** 🔴, D, S 🔘
  ● **S15.29   Other specified injury of external jugular vein**
    ● **S15.291   Other specified injury of right external jugular vein A** 🔴, D, S 🔘
    ● **S15.292   Other specified injury of left external jugular vein A** 🔴, D, S 🔘
    ●■ **S15.299   Other specified injury of unspecified external jugular vein A** 🔴, D, S 🔘
● **S15.3   Injury of internal jugular vein**
  ● **S15.30   Unspecified injury of internal jugular vein**
    ●■ **S15.301   Unspecified injury of right internal jugular vein A** 🔴, D, S 🔘
    ●■ **S15.302   Unspecified injury of left internal jugular vein A** 🔴, D, S 🔘
    ●■ **S15.309   Unspecified injury of unspecified internal jugular vein A** 🔴, D, S 🔘
  ● **S15.31   Minor laceration of internal jugular vein**
    Incomplete transection of internal jugular vein
    Laceration of internal jugular vein NOS
    Superficial laceration of internal jugular vein
    ● **S15.311   Minor laceration of right internal jugular vein A** 🔴, D, S 🔘
    ● **S15.312   Minor laceration of left internal jugular vein A** 🔴, D, S 🔘
    ●■ **S15.319   Minor laceration of unspecified internal jugular vein A** 🔴, D, S 🔘

● **S15.32   Major laceration of internal jugular vein**
    Complete transection of internal jugular vein
    Traumatic rupture of internal jugular vein
    ● **S15.321   Major laceration of right internal jugular vein A** 🔴, D, S 🔘
    ● **S15.322   Major laceration of left internal jugular vein A** 🔴, D, S 🔘
    ●■ **S15.329   Major laceration of unspecified internal jugular vein A** 🔴, D, S 🔘
  ● **S15.39   Other specified injury of internal jugular vein**
    ● **S15.391   Other specified injury of right internal jugular vein A** 🔴, D, S 🔘
    ● **S15.392   Other specified injury of left internal jugular vein A** 🔴, D, S 🔘
    ●■ **S15.399   Other specified injury of unspecified internal jugular vein A** 🔴, D, S 🔘
● ■ **S15.8   Injury of other specified blood vessels at neck level A** 🔴, D, S 🔘
● ■ **S15.9   Injury of unspecified blood vessel at neck level A** 🔴, D, S 🔘

● **S16   Injury of muscle, fascia and tendon at neck level**
  Code also any associated open wound (S11.-)
  Excludes2   sprain of joint or ligament at neck level (S13.9)
  The appropriate 7th character is to be added to each code from category S16

A	initial encounter
D	subsequent encounter
S	sequela

● **S16.1   Strain of muscle, fascia and tendon at neck level** D, S 🔘
● **S16.2   Laceration of muscle, fascia and tendon at neck level** D, S 🔘
● **S16.8   Other specified injury of muscle, fascia and tendon at neck level** D, S 🔘
● ■ **S16.9   Unspecified injury of muscle, fascia and tendon at neck level** D, S 🔘

● **S17   Crushing injury of neck**
  Use additional code for all associated injuries, such as:
  injury of blood vessels (S15.-)
  open wound of neck (S11.-)
  spinal cord injury (S14.0, S14.1-)
  vertebral fracture (S12.0--S12.3-)

  The appropriate 7th character is to be added to each code from category S17

A	initial encounter
D	subsequent encounter
S	sequela

● **S17.0   Crushing injury of larynx and trachea A** 🔴, D, S 🔘, A 🔘
● **S17.8   Crushing injury of other specified parts of neck A** 🔴, D, S 🔘, A 🔘
● ■ **S17.9   Crushing injury of neck, part unspecified A** 🔴, D, S 🔘, A 🔘

N Newborn Age: 0   **P** Pediatric Age: 0–17   **M** Maternity DX: 12–55   **A** Adult Age: 15–124   ♀ Females Only   ♂ Males Only

🔴 Complication\Comorbidity   🔘 Major C\C   🔘 Present on Admission Requirement   🔘 Hospital-Acquired Condition

1417

● **S19**   **Other and unspecified injuries of neck**

    The appropriate 7th character is to be added to each code from category S19

> A   initial encounter
> D   subsequent encounter
> S   sequela

● **S19.8**   **Other specified injuries of neck**

●■ **S19.80**   **Other specified injuries of unspecified part of neck** D, S 🖐

● **S19.81**   **Other specified injuries of larynx** D, S 🖐

● **S19.82**   **Other specified injuries of cervical trachea** D, S 🖐

> **Excludes2**   other specified injury of thoracic trachea (S27.5-)

● **S19.83**   **Other specified injuries of vocal cord** D, S 🖐

● **S19.84**   **Other specified injuries of thyroid gland** D, S 🖐

● **S19.85**   **Other specified injuries of pharynx and cervical esophagus** D, S 🖐

● **S19.89**   **Other specified injuries of other specified part of neck** D, S 🖐

●■ **S19.9**   **Unspecified injury of neck** D, S 🖐

INJURIES TO THE THORAX (S20-S29)

> **Includes**   injuries of breast
> injuries of chest (wall)
> injuries of interscapular area

> **Excludes2**   burns and corrosions (T20-T32)
> effects of foreign body in bronchus (T17.5)
> effects of foreign body in esophagus (T18.1)
> effects of foreign body in lung (T17.8)
> effects of foreign body in trachea (T17.4)
> frostbite (T33-T34)
> injuries of axilla
> injuries of clavicle
> injuries of scapular region
> injuries of shoulder
> insect bite or sting, venomous (T63.4)

● **S20**   **Superficial injury of thorax**

    The appropriate 7th character is to be added to each code from category S20

> A   initial encounter
> D   subsequent encounter
> S   sequela

● **S20.0**   **Contusion of breast**

●■ **S20.00**   **Contusion of breast, unspecified breast** D, S 🖐

● **S20.01**   **Contusion of right breast** D, S 🖐

● **S20.02**   **Contusion of left breast** D, S 🖐

● **S20.1**   **Other and unspecified superficial injuries of breast**

● **S20.10**   **Unspecified superficial injuries of breast**

●■ **S20.101**   **Unspecified superficial injuries of breast, right breast** D, S 🖐

●■ **S20.102**   **Unspecified superficial injuries of breast, left breast** D, S 🖐

●■ **S20.109**   **Unspecified superficial injuries of breast, unspecified breast** D, S 🖐

● **S20.11**   **Abrasion of breast**

● **S20.111**   **Abrasion of breast, right breast** D, S 🖐

● **S20.112**   **Abrasion of breast, left breast** D, S 🖐

●■ **S20.119**   **Abrasion of breast, unspecified breast** D, S 🖐

● **S20.12**   **Blister (nonthermal) of breast**

● **S20.121**   **Blister (nonthermal) of breast, right breast** D, S 🖐

● **S20.122**   **Blister (nonthermal) of breast, left breast** D, S 🖐

●■ **S20.129**   **Blister (nonthermal) of breast, unspecified breast** D, S 🖐

● **S20.14**   **External constriction of part of breast**

● **S20.141**   **External constriction of part of breast, right breast** D, S 🖐

● **S20.142**   **External constriction of part of breast, left breast** D, S 🖐

●■ **S20.149**   **External constriction of part of breast, unspecified breast** D, S 🖐

● **S20.15**   **Superficial foreign body of breast**
    Splinter in the breast

● **S20.151**   **Superficial foreign body of breast, right breast** D, S 🖐

● **S20.152**   **Superficial foreign body of breast, left breast** D, S 🖐

●■ **S20.159**   **Superficial foreign body of breast, unspecified breast** D, S 🖐

● **S20.16**   **Insect bite (nonvenomous) of breast**

● **S20.161**   **Insect bite (nonvenomous) of breast, right breast** D, S 🖐

● **S20.162**   **Insect bite (nonvenomous) of breast, left breast** D, S 🖐

●■ **S20.169**   **Insect bite (nonvenomous) of breast, unspecified breast** D, S 🖐

● **S20.17**   **Other superficial bite of breast**

> **Excludes1**   open bite of breast (S21.05-)

● **S20.171**   **Other superficial bite of breast, right breast** D, S 🖐

● **S20.172**   **Other superficial bite of breast, left breast** D, S 🖐

●■ **S20.179**   **Other superficial bite of breast, unspecified breast** D, S 🖐

● **S20.2**   **Contusion of thorax**

●■ **S20.20**   **Contusion of thorax, unspecified** D, S 🖐

● **S20.21**   **Contusion of front wall of thorax**

● **S20.211**   **Contusion of right front wall of thorax** D, S 🖐

● **S20.212**   **Contusion of left front wall of thorax** D, S 🖐

●■ **S20.219**   **Contusion of unspecified front wall of thorax** D, S 🖐

● **S20.22**   **Contusion of back wall of thorax**

● **S20.221**   **Contusion of right back wall of thorax** D, S 🖐

● **S20.222**   **Contusion of left back wall of thorax** D, S 🖐

●■ **S20.229**   **Contusion of unspecified back wall of thorax** D, S 🖐

● **S20.3**   Other and unspecified superficial injuries of front wall of thorax

   ● **S20.30**   Unspecified superficial injuries of front wall of thorax

     ● ■ **S20.301**   Unspecified superficial injuries of right front wall of thorax D, S 🖎

     ● ■ **S20.302**   Unspecified superficial injuries of left front wall of thorax D, S 🖎

     ● ■ **S20.309**   Unspecified superficial injuries of unspecified front wall of thorax D, S 🖎

   ● **S20.31**   Abrasion of front wall of thorax

     ● **S20.311**   Abrasion of right front wall of thorax D, S 🖎

     ● **S20.312**   Abrasion of left front wall of thorax D, S 🖎

     ● ■ **S20.319**   Abrasion of unspecified front wall of thorax D, S 🖎

   ● **S20.32**   Blister (nonthermal) of front wall of thorax

     ● **S20.321**   Blister (nonthermal) of right front wall of thorax D, S 🖎

     ● **S20.322**   Blister (nonthermal) of left front wall of thorax D, S 🖎

     ● ■ **S20.329**   Blister (nonthermal) of unspecified front wall of thorax D, S 🖎

   ● **S20.34**   External constriction of front wall of thorax

     ● **S20.341**   External constriction of right front wall of thorax D, S 🖎

     ● **S20.342**   External constriction of left front wall of thorax D, S 🖎

     ● ■ **S20.349**   External constriction of unspecified front wall of thorax D, S 🖎

   ● **S20.35**   Superficial foreign body of front wall of thorax

     Splinter in front wall of thorax

     ● **S20.351**   Superficial foreign body of right front wall of thorax D, S 🖎

     ● **S20.352**   Superficial foreign body of left front wall of thorax D, S 🖎

     ● ■ **S20.359**   Superficial foreign body of unspecified front wall of thorax D, S 🖎

   ● **S20.36**   Insect bite (nonvenomous) of front wall of thorax

     ● **S20.361**   Insect bite (nonvenomous) of right front wall of thorax D, S 🖎

     ● **S20.362**   Insect bite (nonvenomous) of left front wall of thorax D, S 🖎

     ● ■ **S20.369**   Insect bite (nonvenomous) of unspecified front wall of thorax D, S 🖎

   ● **S20.37**   Other superficial bite of front wall of thorax

     | **Excludes1** | open bite of front wall of thorax (S21.14)

     ● **S20.371**   Other superficial bite of right front wall of thorax D, S 🖎

     ● **S20.372**   Other superficial bite of left front wall of thorax D, S 🖎

     ● ■ **S20.379**   Other superficial bite of unspecified front wall of thorax D, S 🖎

● **S20.4**   Other and unspecified superficial injuries of back wall of thorax

   ● **S20.40**   Unspecified superficial injuries of back wall of thorax

     ● ■ **S20.401**   Unspecified superficial injuries of right back wall of thorax D, S 🖎

     ● ■ **S20.402**   Unspecified superficial injuries of left back wall of thorax D, S 🖎

     ● ■ **S20.409**   Unspecified superficial injuries of unspecified back wall of thorax D, S 🖎

   ● **S20.41**   Abrasion of back wall of thorax

     ● **S20.411**   Abrasion of right back wall of thorax D, S 🖎

     ● **S20.412**   Abrasion of left back wall of thorax D, S 🖎

     ● ■ **S20.419**   Abrasion of unspecified back wall of thorax D, S 🖎

   ● **S20.42**   Blister (nonthermal) of back wall of thorax

     ● **S20.421**   Blister (nonthermal) of right back wall of thorax D, S 🖎

     ● **S20.422**   Blister (nonthermal) of left back wall of thorax D, S 🖎

     ● ■ **S20.429**   Blister (nonthermal) of unspecified back wall of thorax D, S 🖎

   ● **S20.44**   External constriction of back wall of thorax

     ● **S20.441**   External constriction of right back wall of thorax D, S 🖎

     ● **S20.442**   External constriction of left back wall of thorax D, S 🖎

     ● ■ **S20.449**   External constriction of unspecified back wall of thorax D, S 🖎

   ● **S20.45**   Superficial foreign body of back wall of thorax

     Splinter of back wall of thorax

     ● **S20.451**   Superficial foreign body of right back wall of thorax D, S 🖎

     ● **S20.452**   Superficial foreign body of left back wall of thorax D, S 🖎

     ● ■ **S20.459**   Superficial foreign body of unspecified back wall of thorax D, S 🖎

   ● **S20.46**   Insect bite (nonvenomous) of back wall of thorax

     ● **S20.461**   Insect bite (nonvenomous) of right back wall of thorax D, S 🖎

     ● **S20.462**   Insect bite (nonvenomous) of left back wall of thorax D, S 🖎

     ● ■ **S20.469**   Insect bite (nonvenomous) of unspecified back wall of thorax D, S 🖎

   ● **S20.47**   Other superficial bite of back wall of thorax

     | **Excludes1** | open bite of back wall of thorax (S21.24)

     ● **S20.471**   Other superficial bite of right back wall of thorax D, S 🖎

     ● **S20.472**   Other superficial bite of left back wall of thorax D, S 🖎

     ● ■ **S20.479**   Other superficial bite of unspecified back wall of thorax D, S 🖎

CHAPTER 19 (S00-T88)

● S20.9   **Superficial injury of unspecified parts of thorax**
   Excludes1   contusion of thorax NOS (S20.20)

●■ S20.90   **Unspecified superficial injury of unspecified parts of thorax** D, S
   Superficial injury of thoracic wall NOS

●■ S20.91   **Abrasion of unspecified parts of thorax** D, S

●■ S20.92   **Blister (nonthermal) of unspecified parts of thorax** D, S

●■ S20.94   **External constriction of unspecified parts of thorax** D, S

●■ S20.95   **Superficial foreign body of unspecified parts of thorax** D, S
   Splinter in thorax NOS

●■ S20.96   **Insect bite (nonvenomous) of unspecified parts of thorax** D, S

●■ S20.97   **Other superficial bite of unspecified parts of thorax** D, S
   Excludes1   open bite of thorax NOS (S21.95)

● **S21   Open wound of thorax**

Code also any associated injury (to) (such as) :
   heart (S26.-)
   intrathoracic organs (S27.-)
   rib fracture (S22.3-, S22.4-)
   spinal cord injury (S24.0-, S24.1-)
   traumatic hemothorax (S27.1)
   traumatic hemopneumothorax (S27.3)
   traumatic pneumothorax (S27.0)
   wound infection

   Excludes1   traumatic amputation (partial) of thorax (S28.1)

The appropriate 7th character is to be added to each code from category S21

A	initial encounter
D	subsequent encounter
S	sequela

● S21.0   **Open wound of breast**

● S21.00   **Unspecified open wound of breast**

●■ S21.001   **Unspecified open wound of right breast** D, S

●■ S21.002   **Unspecified open wound of left breast** D, S

●■ S21.009   **Unspecified open wound of unspecified breast** D, S

● S21.01   **Laceration without foreign body of breast**

● S21.011   **Laceration without foreign body of right breast** D, S

● S21.012   **Laceration without foreign body of left breast** D, S

●■ S21.019   **Laceration without foreign body of unspecified breast** D, S

Item 19–1 Pneumothorax is a collection of gas (positive air pressure) in the pleural space resulting in the lung collapsing. A tension pneumothorax is life-threatening and is a result of air in the pleural space causing a displacement in the mediastinal structures and cardiopulmonary function compromise. A traumatic pneumothorax results from blunt or penetrating injury that disrupts the parietal/visceral pleura. **Hemothorax** is blood or bloody fluid in the pleural cavity as a result of traumatic blood vessel rupture or inflammation of the lungs from pneumonia.

● S21.02   **Laceration with foreign body of breast**

●■ S21.021   **Laceration with foreign body of right breast** D, S

●■ S21.022   **Laceration with foreign body of left breast** D, S

●■ S21.029   **Laceration with foreign body of unspecified breast** D, S

● S21.03   **Puncture wound without foreign body of breast**

●■ S21.031   **Puncture wound without foreign body of right breast** D, S

●■ S21.032   **Puncture wound without foreign body of left breast** D, S

●■ S21.039   **Puncture wound without foreign body of unspecified breast** D, S

● S21.04   **Puncture wound with foreign body of breast**

●■ S21.041   **Puncture wound with foreign body of right breast** D, S

●■ S21.042   **Puncture wound with foreign body of left breast** D, S

●■ S21.049   **Puncture wound with foreign body of unspecified breast** D, S

● S21.05   **Open bite of breast**
   Bite of breast NOS
   Excludes1   superficial bite of breast (S20.17)

●■ S21.051   **Open bite of right breast** D, S

●■ S21.052   **Open bite of left breast** D, S

●■ S21.059   **Open bite of unspecified breast** D, S

● S21.1   **Open wound of front wall of thorax without penetration into thoracic cavity**
   Open wound of chest without penetration into thoracic cavity

● S21.10   **Unspecified open wound of front wall of thorax without penetration into thoracic cavity**

●■ S21.101   **Unspecified open wound of right front wall of thorax without penetration into thoracic cavity** A, D, S

●■ S21.102   **Unspecified open wound of left front wall of thorax without penetration into thoracic cavity** A, D, S

●■ S21.109   **Unspecified open wound of unspecified front wall of thorax without penetration into thoracic cavity** A, D, S

● S21.11   **Laceration without foreign body of front wall of thorax without penetration into thoracic cavity**

● S21.111   **Laceration without foreign body of right front wall of thorax without penetration into thoracic cavity** A, D, S

● S21.112   **Laceration without foreign body of left front wall of thorax without penetration into thoracic cavity** A, D, S

●■ S21.119   **Laceration without foreign body of unspecified front wall of thorax without penetration into thoracic cavity** A, D, S

● S21.12 Laceration with foreign body of front wall of thorax without penetration into thoracic cavity

  ● S21.121 Laceration with foreign body of right front wall of thorax without penetration into thoracic cavity A 🔾, D, S 🔾

  ● S21.122 Laceration with foreign body of left front wall of thorax without penetration into thoracic cavity A 🔾, D, S 🔾

  ● ■ S21.129 Laceration with foreign body of unspecified front wall of thorax without penetration into thoracic cavity A 🔾, D, S 🔾

● S21.13 Puncture wound without foreign body of front wall of thorax without penetration into thoracic cavity

  ● S21.131 Puncture wound without foreign body of right front wall of thorax without penetration into thoracic cavity A 🔾, D, S 🔾

  ● S21.132 Puncture wound without foreign body of left front wall of thorax without penetration into thoracic cavity A 🔾, D, S 🔾

  ● ■ S21.139 Puncture wound without foreign body of unspecified front wall of thorax without penetration into thoracic cavity A 🔾, D, S 🔾

● S21.14 Puncture wound with foreign body of front wall of thorax without penetration into thoracic cavity

  ● S21.141 Puncture wound with foreign body of right front wall of thorax without penetration into thoracic cavity A 🔾, D, S 🔾

  ● S21.142 Puncture wound with foreign body of left front wall of thorax without penetration into thoracic cavity A 🔾, D, S 🔾

  ● ■ S21.149 Puncture wound with foreign body of unspecified front wall of thorax without penetration into thoracic cavity A 🔾, D, S 🔾

● S21.15 Open bite of front wall of thorax without penetration into thoracic cavity
      Bite of front wall of thorax NOS
      Excludes1 superficial bite of front wall of thorax (S20.37)

  ● S21.151 Open bite of right front wall of thorax without penetration into thoracic cavity A 🔾, D, S 🔾

  ● S21.152 Open bite of left front wall of thorax without penetration into thoracic cavity A 🔾, D, S 🔾

  ● ■ S21.159 Open bite of unspecified front wall of thorax without penetration into thoracic cavity A 🔾, D, S 🔾

● S21.2 Open wound of back wall of thorax without penetration into thoracic cavity

  ● S21.20 Unspecified open wound of back wall of thorax without penetration into thoracic cavity

    ● ■ S21.201 Unspecified open wound of right back wall of thorax without penetration into thoracic cavity D, S 🔾

    ● ■ S21.202 Unspecified open wound of left back wall of thorax without penetration into thoracic cavity D, S 🔾

  ● ■ S21.209 Unspecified open wound of unspecified back wall of thorax without penetration into thoracic cavity D, S 🔾

● S21.21 Laceration without foreign body of back wall of thorax without penetration into thoracic cavity

  ● S21.211 Laceration without foreign body of right back wall of thorax without penetration into thoracic cavity D, S 🔾

  ● S21.212 Laceration without foreign body of left back wall of thorax without penetration into thoracic cavity D, S 🔾

  ● ■ S21.219 Laceration without foreign body of unspecified back wall of thorax without penetration into thoracic cavity D, S 🔾

● S21.22 Laceration with foreign body of back wall of thorax without penetration into thoracic cavity

  ● S21.221 Laceration with foreign body of right back wall of thorax without penetration into thoracic cavity D, S 🔾

  ● S21.222 Laceration with foreign body of left back wall of thorax without penetration into thoracic cavity D, S 🔾

  ● ■ S21.229 Laceration with foreign body of unspecified back wall of thorax without penetration into thoracic cavity D, S 🔾

● S21.23 Puncture wound without foreign body of back wall of thorax without penetration into thoracic cavity

  ● S21.231 Puncture wound without foreign body of right back wall of thorax without penetration into thoracic cavity D, S 🔾

  ● S21.232 Puncture wound without foreign body of left back wall of thorax without penetration into thoracic cavity D, S 🔾

  ● ■ S21.239 Puncture wound without foreign body of unspecified back wall of thorax without penetration into thoracic cavity D, S 🔾

● S21.24 Puncture wound with foreign body of back wall of thorax without penetration into thoracic cavity

  ● S21.241 Puncture wound with foreign body of right back wall of thorax without penetration into thoracic cavity D, S 🔾

  ● S21.242 Puncture wound with foreign body of left back wall of thorax without penetration into thoracic cavity D, S 🔾

  ● ■ S21.249 Puncture wound with foreign body of unspecified back wall of thorax without penetration into thoracic cavity D, S 🔾

CHAPTER 19 (S00–T88)

N Newborn Age: 0   P Pediatric Age: 0–17   M Maternity DX: 12–55   A Adult Age: 15–124   ♀ Females Only   ♂ Males Only

🔾 Complication\Comorbidity   🔾 Major C\C   🔾 Present on Admission Requirement   🔾 Hospital-Acquired Condition

● **S21.25　Open bite of back wall of thorax without penetration into thoracic cavity**
Bite of back wall of thorax NOS

> **Excludes1**　superficial bite of back wall of thorax (S20.47)

　● **S21.251　Open bite of right back wall of thorax without penetration into thoracic cavity** D, S 🔖

　● **S21.252　Open bite of left back wall of thorax without penetration into thoracic cavity** D, S 🔖

　●▪ **S21.259　Open bite of unspecified back wall of thorax without penetration into thoracic cavity** D, S 🔖

● **S21.3　Open wound of front wall of thorax with penetration into thoracic cavity**
Open wound of chest with penetration into thoracic cavity

　● **S21.30　Unspecified open wound of front wall of thorax with penetration into thoracic cavity**

　　●▪ **S21.301　Unspecified open wound of right front wall of thorax with penetration into thoracic cavity** A 🔖, D, S 🔖

　　●▪ **S21.302　Unspecified open wound of left front wall of thorax with penetration into thoracic cavity** A 🔖, D, S 🔖

　　●▪ **S21.309　Unspecified open wound of unspecified front wall of thorax with penetration into thoracic cavity** A 🔖, D, S 🔖

　● **S21.31　Laceration without foreign body of front wall of thorax with penetration into thoracic cavity**

　　● **S21.311　Laceration without foreign body of right front wall of thorax with penetration into thoracic cavity** A 🔖, D, S 🔖

　　● **S21.312　Laceration without foreign body of left front wall of thorax with penetration into thoracic cavity** A 🔖, D, S 🔖

　　●▪ **S21.319　Laceration without foreign body of unspecified front wall of thorax with penetration into thoracic cavity** A 🔖, D, S 🔖

　● **S21.32　Laceration with foreign body of front wall of thorax with penetration into thoracic cavity**

　　● **S21.321　Laceration with foreign body of right front wall of thorax with penetration into thoracic cavity** A 🔖, D, S 🔖

　　● **S21.322　Laceration with foreign body of left front wall of thorax with penetration into thoracic cavity** A 🔖, D, S 🔖

　　●▪ **S21.329　Laceration with foreign body of unspecified front wall of thorax with penetration into thoracic cavity** A 🔖, D, S 🔖

● **S21.33　Puncture wound without foreign body of front wall of thorax with penetration into thoracic cavity**

　● **S21.331　Puncture wound without foreign body of right front wall of thorax with penetration into thoracic cavity** A 🔖, D, S 🔖

　● **S21.332　Puncture wound without foreign body of left front wall of thorax with penetration into thoracic cavity** A 🔖, D, S 🔖

　●▪ **S21.339　Puncture wound without foreign body of unspecified front wall of thorax with penetration into thoracic cavity** A 🔖, D, S 🔖

● **S21.34　Puncture wound with foreign body of front wall of thorax with penetration into thoracic cavity**

　● **S21.341　Puncture wound with foreign body of right front wall of thorax with penetration into thoracic cavity** A 🔖, D, S 🔖

　● **S21.342　Puncture wound with foreign body of left front wall of thorax with penetration into thoracic cavity** A 🔖, D, S 🔖

　●▪ **S21.349　Puncture wound with foreign body of unspecified front wall of thorax with penetration into thoracic cavity** A 🔖, D, S 🔖

● **S21.35　Open bite of front wall of thorax with penetration into thoracic cavity**

> **Excludes1**　superficial bite of front wall of thorax (S20.37)

　● **S21.351　Open bite of right front wall of thorax with penetration into thoracic cavity** A 🔖, D, S 🔖

　● **S21.352　Open bite of left front wall of thorax with penetration into thoracic cavity** A 🔖, D, S 🔖

　●▪ **S21.359　Open bite of unspecified front wall of thorax with penetration into thoracic cavity** A 🔖, D, S 🔖

● **S21.4　Open wound of back wall of thorax with penetration into thoracic cavity**

　● **S21.40　Unspecified open wound of back wall of thorax with penetration into thoracic cavity**

　　●▪ **S21.401　Unspecified open wound of right back wall of thorax with penetration into thoracic cavity** A 🔖, D, S 🔖

　　●▪ **S21.402　Unspecified open wound of left back wall of thorax with penetration into thoracic cavity** A 🔖, D, S 🔖

　　●▪ **S21.409　Unspecified open wound of unspecified back wall of thorax with penetration into thoracic cavity** A 🔖, D, S 🔖

　● **S21.41　Laceration without foreign body of back wall of thorax with penetration into thoracic cavity**

　　● **S21.411　Laceration without foreign body of right back wall of thorax with penetration into thoracic cavity** A 🔖, D, S 🔖

● Unacceptable Principal Diagnosis　　● Use Additional Character(s)　　▪ Unspecified　　▶ Manifestation Code

OGCR Official Guidelines for Coding and Reporting　Excludes 1　Excludes 2　Includes　Use additional　Code first　Code also

● S21.412   Laceration without foreign body of left back wall of thorax with penetration into thoracic cavity A 🐾, D, S 🐾

● ■ S21.419   Laceration without foreign body of unspecified back wall of thorax with penetration into thoracic cavity A 🐾, D, S 🐾

● S21.42   Laceration with foreign body of back wall of thorax with penetration into thoracic cavity

● S21.421   Laceration with foreign body of right back wall of thorax with penetration into thoracic cavity A 🐾, D, S 🐾

● S21.422   Laceration with foreign body of left back wall of thorax with penetration into thoracic cavity A 🐾, D, S 🐾

● ■ S21.429   Laceration with foreign body of unspecified back wall of thorax with penetration into thoracic cavity A 🐾, D, S 🐾

● S21.43   Puncture wound without foreign body of back wall of thorax with penetration into thoracic cavity

● S21.431   Puncture wound without foreign body of right back wall of thorax with penetration into thoracic cavity A 🐾, D, S 🐾

● S21.432   Puncture wound without foreign body of left back wall of thorax with penetration into thoracic cavity A 🐾, D, S 🐾

● ■ S21.439   Puncture wound without foreign body of unspecified back wall of thorax with penetration into thoracic cavity A 🐾, D, S 🐾

● S21.44   Puncture wound with foreign body of back wall of thorax with penetration into thoracic cavity

● S21.441   Puncture wound with foreign body of right back wall of thorax with penetration into thoracic cavity A 🐾, D, S 🐾

● S21.442   Puncture wound with foreign body of left back wall of thorax with penetration into thoracic cavity A 🐾, D, S 🐾

● ■ S21.449   Puncture wound with foreign body of unspecified back wall of thorax with penetration into thoracic cavity A 🐾, D, S 🐾

● S21.45   Open bite of back wall of thorax with penetration into thoracic cavity
Bite of back wall of thorax NOS

| **Excludes1** | superficial bite of back wall of thorax (S20.47) |

● S21.451   Open bite of right back wall of thorax with penetration into thoracic cavity A 🐾, D, S 🐾

● S21.452   Open bite of left back wall of thorax with penetration into thoracic cavity A 🐾, D, S 🐾

● ■ S21.459   Open bite of unspecified back wall of thorax with penetration into thoracic cavity A 🐾, D, S 🐾

● S21.9   Open wound of unspecified part of thorax
Open wound of thoracic wall NOS

● ■ S21.90   Unspecified open wound of unspecified part of thorax A 🐾, D, S 🐾

● ■ S21.91   Laceration without foreign body of unspecified part of thorax A 🐾, D, S 🐾

● ■ S21.92   Laceration with foreign body of unspecified part of thorax A 🐾, D, S 🐾

● ■ S21.93   Puncture wound without foreign body of unspecified part of thorax A 🐾, D, S 🐾

● ■ S21.94   Puncture wound with foreign body of unspecified part of thorax A 🐾, D, S 🐾

● ■ S21.95   Open bite of unspecified part of thorax A 🐾, D, S 🐾

| **Excludes1** | superficial bite of thorax (S20.97) |

● S22   Fracture of rib(s), sternum and thoracic spine

Note: A fracture not indicated as displaced or nondisplaced should be coded to displaced

A fracture not indicated as open or closed should be coded to closed

Includes	fracture of thoracic neural arch
	fracture of thoracic spinous process
	fracture of thoracic transverse process
	fracture of thoracic vertebra
	fracture of thoracic vertebral arch

Code first any associated:
injury of intrathoracic organ (S27.-)
spinal cord injury (S24.0-, S24.1-)

Excludes1	transection of thorax (S28.1)
Excludes2	fracture of clavicle (S42.0-)
	fracture of scapula (S42.1-)

The appropriate 7th character is to be added to each code from category S22

A	initial encounter for closed fracture
B	initial encounter for open fracture
D	subsequent encounter for fracture with routine healing
G	subsequent encounter for fracture with delayed healing
K	subsequent encounter for fracture with nonunion
S	sequela

● S22.0   Fracture of thoracic vertebra

● S22.00   Fracture of unspecified thoracic vertebra

● ■ S22.000   Wedge compression fracture of unspecified thoracic vertebra A, K 🐾, B 🐾, D, G, S 🐾, A, B 🐾

● ■ S22.001   Stable burst fracture of unspecified thoracic vertebra A, K 🐾, B 🐾, D, G, S 🐾, A, B 🐾

● ■ S22.002   Unstable burst fracture of unspecified thoracic vertebra A, K 🐾, B 🐾, D, G, S 🐾, A, B 🐾

● ■ S22.008   Other fracture of unspecified thoracic vertebra A, K 🐾, B 🐾, D, G, S 🐾, A, B 🐾

● ■ S22.009   Unspecified fracture of unspecified thoracic vertebra A, K 🐾, B 🐾, D, G, S 🐾, A, B 🐾

N Newborn Age: 0   **P** Pediatric Age: 0–17   **M** Maternity DX: 12–55   **A** Adult Age: 15–124   ♀ Females Only   ♂ Males Only

🐾 Complication\Comorbidity   🐾 Major C\C   🐾 Present on Admission Requirement   🐾 Hospital-Acquired Condition

1423

CHAPTER 19 (S00-T88)

● **S22.01**   Fracture of first thoracic vertebra

   ● **S22.010**   Wedge compression fracture of first thoracic vertebra A, K 🔢, B 🔢, D, G, S 🔢, A, B 🔢

   ● **S22.011**   Stable burst fracture of first thoracic vertebra A, K 🔢, B 🔢, D, G, S 🔢, A, B 🔢

   ● **S22.012**   Unstable burst fracture of first thoracic vertebra A, K 🔢, B 🔢, D, G, S 🔢, A, B 🔢

   ● **S22.018**   Other fracture of first thoracic vertebra A, K 🔢, B 🔢, D, G, S 🔢, A, B 🔢

   ●■ **S22.019**   Unspecified fracture of first thoracic vertebra A, K 🔢, B 🔢, D, G, S 🔢, A, B 🔢

● **S22.02**   Fracture of second thoracic vertebra

   ● **S22.020**   Wedge compression fracture of second thoracic vertebra A, K 🔢, B 🔢, D, G, S 🔢, A, B 🔢

   ● **S22.021**   Stable burst fracture of second thoracic vertebra A, K 🔢, B 🔢, D, G, S 🔢, A, B 🔢

   ● **S22.022**   Unstable burst fracture of second thoracic vertebra A, K 🔢, B 🔢, D, G, S 🔢, A, B 🔢

   ● **S22.028**   Other fracture of second thoracic vertebra A, K 🔢, B 🔢, D, G, S 🔢, A, B 🔢

   ●■ **S22.029**   Unspecified fracture of second thoracic vertebra A, K 🔢, B 🔢, D, G, S 🔢, A, B 🔢

● **S22.03**   Fracture of third thoracic vertebra

   ● **S22.030**   Wedge compression fracture of third thoracic vertebra A, K 🔢, B 🔢, D, G, S 🔢, A, B 🔢

   ● **S22.031**   Stable burst fracture of third thoracic vertebra A, K 🔢, B 🔢, D, G, S 🔢, A, B 🔢

   ● **S22.032**   Unstable burst fracture of third thoracic vertebra A, K 🔢, B 🔢, D, G, S 🔢, A, B 🔢

   ● **S22.038**   Other fracture of third thoracic vertebra A, K 🔢, B 🔢, D, G, S 🔢, A, B 🔢

   ●■ **S22.039**   Unspecified fracture of third thoracic vertebra A, K 🔢, B 🔢, D, G, S 🔢, A, B 🔢

● **S22.04**   Fracture of fourth thoracic vertebra

   ● **S22.040**   Wedge compression fracture of fourth thoracic vertebra A, K 🔢, B 🔢, D, G, S 🔢, A, B 🔢

   ● **S22.041**   Stable burst fracture of fourth thoracic vertebra A, K 🔢, B 🔢, D, G, S 🔢, A, B 🔢

   ● **S22.042**   Unstable burst fracture of fourth thoracic vertebra A, K 🔢, B 🔢, D, G, S 🔢, A, B 🔢

   ● **S22.048**   Other fracture of fourth thoracic vertebra A, K 🔢, B 🔢, D, G, S 🔢, A, B 🔢

   ●■ **S22.049**   Unspecified fracture of fourth thoracic vertebra A, K 🔢, B 🔢, D, G, S 🔢, A, B 🔢

● **S22.05**   Fracture of T_5-T_6 vertebra

   ● **S22.050**   Wedge compression fracture of T_5-T_6 vertebra A, K 🔢, B 🔢, D, G, S 🔢, A, B 🔢

   ● **S22.051**   Stable burst fracture of T_5-T_6 vertebra A, K 🔢, B 🔢, D, G, S 🔢, A, B 🔢

   ● **S22.052**   Unstable burst fracture of T_5-T_6 vertebra A, K 🔢, B 🔢, D, G, S 🔢, A, B 🔢

   ● **S22.058**   Other fracture of T_5-T_6 vertebra A, K 🔢, B 🔢, D, G, S 🔢, A, B 🔢

   ●■ **S22.059**   Unspecified fracture of T_5-T_6 vertebra A, K 🔢, B 🔢, D, G, S 🔢, A, B 🔢

● **S22.06**   Fracture of T_7-T_8 vertebra

   ● **S22.060**   Wedge compression fracture of T_7-T_8 vertebra A, K 🔢, B 🔢, D, G, S 🔢, A, B 🔢

   ● **S22.061**   Stable burst fracture of T_7-T_8 vertebra A, K 🔢, B 🔢, D, G, S 🔢, A, B 🔢

   ● **S22.062**   Unstable burst fracture of T_7-T_8 vertebra A, K 🔢, B 🔢, D, G, S 🔢, A, B 🔢

   ● **S22.068**   Other fracture of T_7-T_8 thoracic vertebra A, K 🔢, B 🔢, D, G, S 🔢, A, B 🔢

   ●■ **S22.069**   Unspecified fracture of T_7-T_8 vertebra A, K 🔢, B 🔢, D, G, S 🔢, A, B 🔢

● **S22.07**   Fracture of T_9-T_{10} vertebra

   ● **S22.070**   Wedge compression fracture of T_9-T_{10} vertebra A, K 🔢, B 🔢, D, G, S 🔢, A, B 🔢

   ● **S22.071**   Stable burst fracture of T_9-T_{10} vertebra A, K 🔢, B 🔢, D, G, S 🔢, A, B 🔢

   ● **S22.072**   Unstable burst fracture of T_9-T_{10} vertebra A, K 🔢, B 🔢, D, G, S 🔢, A, B 🔢

   ● **S22.078**   Other fracture of T_9-T_{10} vertebra A, K 🔢, B 🔢, D, G, S 🔢, A, B 🔢

   ●■ **S22.079**   Unspecified fracture of T_9-T_{10} vertebra A, K 🔢, B 🔢, D, G, S 🔢, A, B 🔢

● **S22.08**   Fracture of T_{11}-T_{12} vertebra

   ● **S22.080**   Wedge compression fracture of T_{11}-T_{12} vertebra A, K 🔢, B 🔢, D, G, S 🔢, A, B 🔢

   ● **S22.081**   Stable burst fracture of T_{11}-T_{12} vertebra A, K 🔢, B 🔢, D, G, S 🔢, A, B 🔢

   ● **S22.082**   Unstable burst fracture of T_{11}-T_{12} vertebra A, K 🔢, B 🔢, D, G, S 🔢, A, B 🔢

   ● **S22.088**   Other fracture of T_{11}-T_{12} vertebra A, K 🔢, B 🔢, D, G, S 🔢, A, B 🔢

   ●■ **S22.089**   Unspecified fracture of T_{11}-T_{12} vertebra A, K 🔢, B 🔢, D, G, S 🔢, A, B 🔢

● Unacceptable Principal Diagnosis   ● Use Additional Character(s)   ■ Unspecified   ▶ Manifestation Code

OGCR Official Guidelines for Coding and Reporting   Excludes 1   Excludes 2   Includes   Use additional   Code first   Code also

- ● **S22.2**   **Fracture of sternum**
  - ●■ **S22.20**   **Unspecified fracture of sternum** A, K 🝱, B 🝱, D, G, S 🝱, A, B 🝱
  - ● **S22.21**   **Fracture of manubrium** A, K 🝱, B 🝱, D, G, S 🝱, A, B 🝱
  - ● **S22.22**   **Fracture of body of sternum** A, K 🝱, B 🝱, D, G, S 🝱, A, B 🝱
  - ● **S22.23**   **Sternal manubrial dissociation** A, K 🝱, B 🝱, D, G, S 🝱, A, B 🝱
  - ● **S22.24**   **Fracture of xiphoid process** A, K 🝱, B 🝱, D, G, S 🝱, A, B 🝱

- ● **S22.3**   **Fracture of one rib**
  - ● **S22.31**   **Fracture of one rib, right side** A, K 🝱, B 🝱, D, G, S 🝱, A, B 🝱
  - ● **S22.32**   **Fracture of one rib, left side** A, K 🝱, B 🝱, D, G, S 🝱, A, B 🝱
  - ●■ **S22.39**   **Fracture of one rib, unspecified side** A, K 🝱, B 🝱, D, G, S 🝱, A, B 🝱

- ● **S22.4**   **Multiple fractures of ribs**
  Fractures of two or more ribs

  | **Excludes1** | flail chest (S22.5-) |
  - ● **S22.41**   **Multiple fractures of ribs, right side** A, K 🝱, B 🝱, D, G, S 🝱, A, B 🝱
  - ● **S22.42**   **Multiple fractures of ribs, left side** A, K 🝱, B 🝱, D, G, S 🝱, A, B 🝱
  - ● **S22.43**   **Multiple fractures of ribs, bilateral** A, K 🝱, B 🝱, D, G, S 🝱, A, B 🝱
  - ●■ **S22.49**   **Multiple fractures of ribs, unspecified side** A, K 🝱, B 🝱, D, G, S 🝱, A, B 🝱

- ● **S22.5**   **Flail chest** K 🝱, A, B 🝱, D, G, S 🝱, A, B 🝱
  Unstable chest due to sternum and/or rib fracture

- ●■ **S22.9**   **Fracture of bony thorax, part unspecified** A, K 🝱, B 🝱, D, G, S 🝱, A, B 🝱

- ● **S23**   **Dislocation and sprain of joints and ligaments of thorax**

  | **Includes** | avulsion of joint or ligament of thorax |

  laceration of cartilage, joint or ligament of thorax

  sprain of cartilage, joint or ligament of thorax

  traumatic hemarthrosis of joint or ligament of thorax

  traumatic rupture of joint or ligament of thorax

  traumatic subluxation of joint or ligament of thorax

  traumatic tear of joint or ligament of thorax

  Code also any associated open wound

  | **Excludes2** | dislocation, sprain of sternoclavicular joint (S43.2, S43.6) |

  strain of muscle or tendon of thorax (S29.01-)

  The appropriate 7th character is to be added to each code from category S23

A	initial encounter
D	subsequent encounter
S	sequela

  - ● **S23.0**   **Traumatic rupture of thoracic intervertebral disc** D, S 🝱

    | **Excludes1** | rupture or displacement (nontraumatic) of thoracic intervertebral disc NOS (M51.- with fifth character 4) |

- ● **S23.1**   **Subluxation and dislocation of thoracic vertebra**

  Code also any associated
  open wound of thorax (S21.-)
  spinal cord injury (S24.0-, S24.1-)

  | **Excludes2** | fracture of thoracic vertebrae (S22.0-) |

  - ● **S23.10**   **Subluxation and dislocation of unspecified thoracic vertebra**
    - ●■ **S23.100**   **Subluxation of unspecified thoracic vertebra** D, S 🝱
    - ●■ **S23.101**   **Dislocation of unspecified thoracic vertebra** D, S 🝱
  - ● **S23.11**   **Subluxation and dislocation of T_1/T_2 thoracic vertebra**
    - ● **S23.110**   **Subluxation of T_1/T_2 thoracic vertebra** D, S 🝱
    - ● **S23.111**   **Dislocation of T_1/T_2 thoracic vertebra** D, S 🝱
  - ● **S23.12**   **Subluxation and dislocation of T_2/T_3-T_3/T_4 thoracic vertebra**
    - ● **S23.120**   **Subluxation of T_2/T_3 thoracic vertebra** D, S 🝱
    - ● **S23.121**   **Dislocation of T_2/T_3 thoracic vertebra** D, S 🝱
    - ● **S23.122**   **Subluxation of T_3/T_4 thoracic vertebra** D, S 🝱
    - ● **S23.123**   **Dislocation of T_3/T_4 thoracic vertebra** D, S 🝱
  - ● **S23.13**   **Subluxation and dislocation of T_4/T_5-T_5/T_6 thoracic vertebra**
    - ● **S23.130**   **Subluxation of T_4/T_5 thoracic vertebra** D, S 🝱
    - ● **S23.131**   **Dislocation of T_4/T_5 thoracic vertebra** D, S 🝱
    - ● **S23.132**   **Subluxation of T_5/T_6 thoracic vertebra** D, S 🝱
    - ● **S23.133**   **Dislocation of T_5/T_6 thoracic vertebra** D, S 🝱
  - ● **S23.14**   **Subluxation and dislocation of T_6/T_7-T_7/T_8 thoracic vertebra**
    - ● **S23.140**   **Subluxation of T_6/T_7 thoracic vertebra** D, S 🝱
    - ● **S23.141**   **Dislocation of T_6/T_7 thoracic vertebra** D, S 🝱
    - ● **S23.142**   **Subluxation of T_7/T_8 thoracic vertebra** D, S 🝱
    - ● **S23.143**   **Dislocation of T_7/T_8 thoracic vertebra** D, S 🝱
  - ● **S23.15**   **Subluxation and dislocation of T_8/T_9-T_9/T_{10} thoracic vertebra**
    - ● **S23.150**   **Subluxation of T_8/T_9 thoracic vertebra** D, S 🝱
    - ● **S23.151**   **Dislocation of T_8/T_9 thoracic vertebra** D, S 🝱
    - ● **S23.152**   **Subluxation of T_9/T_{10} thoracic vertebra** D, S 🝱
    - ● **S23.153**   **Dislocation of T_9/T_{10} thoracic vertebra** D, S 🝱

CHAPTER 19 (S00-T88)

● S23.16　Subluxation and dislocation of T_{10}/T_{11}-T_{11}/T_{12} thoracic vertebra

  ● S23.160　Subluxation of T_{10}/T_{11} thoracic vertebra D, S

  ● S23.161　Dislocation of T_{10}/T_{11} thoracic vertebra D, S

  ● S23.162　Subluxation of T_{11}/T_{12} thoracic vertebra D, S

  ● S23.163　Dislocation of T_{11}/T_{12} thoracic vertebra D, S

● S23.17　Subluxation and dislocation of T_{12}/L_1 thoracic vertebra

  ● S23.170　Subluxation of T_{12}/L_1 thoracic vertebra D, S

  ● S23.171　Dislocation of T_{12}/L_1 thoracic vertebra D, S

● S23.2　Dislocation of other and unspecified parts of thorax

  ●■ S23.20　Dislocation of unspecified part of thorax D, S

  ● S23.29　Dislocation of other parts of thorax D, S

● S23.3　Sprain of ligaments of thoracic spine D, S

● S23.4　Sprain of ribs and sternum

  ● S23.41　Sprain of ribs D, S

  ● S23.42　Sprain of sternum

    ● S23.420　Sprain of sternoclavicular (joint) (ligament) D, S

    ● S23.421　Sprain of chondrosternal joint D, S

    ● S23.428　Other sprain of sternum D, S

    ●■ S23.429　Unspecified sprain of sternum D, S

● S23.8　Sprain of other specified parts of thorax D, S

●■ S23.9　Sprain of unspecified parts of thorax D, S

● S24　Injury of nerves and spinal cord at thorax level

  Note: Code to highest level of thoracic spinal cord injury.

  Code also any associated:
    fracture of thoracic vertebra (S22.0-)
    open wound of thorax (S21.-)
    transient paralysis (R29.5)

  Excludes2　injury of brachial plexus (S14.3)

  The appropriate 7th character is to be added to each code from category S24

A	initial encounter
D	subsequent encounter
S	sequela

● S24.0　Concussion and edema of thoracic spinal cord A, D, S

● S24.1　Other and unspecified injuries of thoracic spinal cord

  ● S24.10　Unspecified injury of thoracic spinal cord

    ●■ S24.101　Unspecified injury at T_1 level of thoracic spinal cord A, D, S, A

    ●■ S24.102　Unspecified injury at T_2-T_6 level of thoracic spinal cord A, D, S, A

    ●■ S24.103　Unspecified injury at T_7-T_{10} level of thoracic spinal cord A, D, S, A

    ●■ S24.104　Unspecified injury at T_{11}-T_{12} level of thoracic spinal cord A, D, S, A

    ●■ S24.109　Unspecified injury at unspecified level of thoracic spinal cord D, S

      Injury of thoracic spinal cord NOS

● S24.11　Complete lesion of thoracic spinal cord

  ● S24.111　Complete lesion at T_1 level of thoracic spinal cord A, D, S, A

  ● S24.112　Complete lesion at T_2-T_6 level of thoracic spinal cord A, D, S, A

  ● S24.113　Complete lesion at T_7-T_{10} level of thoracic spinal cord A, D, S, A

  ● S24.114　Complete lesion at T_{11}-T_{12} level of thoracic spinal cord A, D, S, A

  ●■ S24.119　Complete lesion at unspecified level of thoracic spinal cord D, S

● S24.13　Anterior cord syndrome of thoracic spinal cord

  ● S24.131　Anterior cord syndrome at T_1 level of thoracic spinal cord A, D, S, A

  ● S24.132　Anterior cord syndrome at T_2-T_6 level of thoracic spinal cord A, D, S, A

  ● S24.133　Anterior cord syndrome at T_7-T_{10} level of thoracic spinal cord A, D, S, A

  ● S24.134　Anterior cord syndrome at T_{11}-T_{12} level of thoracic spinal cord A, D, S, A

  ●■ S24.139　Anterior cord syndrome at unspecified level of thoracic spinal cord D, S

● S24.14　Brown-Séquard syndrome of thoracic spinal cord

  ● S24.141　Brown-Séquard syndrome at T_1 level of thoracic spinal cord A, D, S

  ● S24.142　Brown-Séquard syndrome at T_2-T_6 level of thoracic spinal cord A, D, S

  ● S24.143　Brown-Séquard syndrome at T_7-T_{10} level of thoracic spinal cord A, D, S

  ● S24.144　Brown-Séquard syndrome at T_{11}-T_{12} level of thoracic spinal cord A, D, S

  ●■ S24.149　Brown-Séquard syndrome at unspecified level of thoracic spinal cord D, S

● **S24.15 Other incomplete lesions of thoracic spinal cord**
>   Incomplete lesion of thoracic spinal cord NOS
>   Posterior cord syndrome of thoracic spinal cord

   ● **S24.151 Other incomplete lesion at T₁ level of thoracic spinal cord** A 🔷, D, S 🔷, A 🔷

   ● **S24.152 Other incomplete lesion at T₂-T₆ level of thoracic spinal cord** A 🔷, D, S 🔷, A 🔷

   ● **S24.153 Other incomplete lesion at T₇-T₁₀ level of thoracic spinal cord** A 🔷, D, S 🔷, A 🔷

   ● **S24.154 Other incomplete lesion at T₁₁-T₁₂ level of thoracic spinal cord** A 🔷, D, S 🔷, A 🔷

   ●■ **S24.159 Other incomplete lesion at unspecified level of thoracic spinal cord** D, S 🔷

● **S24.2 Injury of nerve root of thoracic spine** D, S 🔷

● **S24.3 Injury of peripheral nerves of thorax** D, S 🔷

● **S24.4 Injury of thoracic sympathetic nervous system** D, S 🔷
>   Injury of cardiac plexus
>   Injury of esophageal plexus
>   Injury of pulmonary plexus
>   Injury of stellate ganglion
>   Injury of thoracic sympathetic ganglion

● **S24.8 Injury of other specified nerves of thorax** D, S 🔷

●■ **S24.9 Injury of unspecified nerve of thorax** D, S 🔷

● **S25 Injury of blood vessels of thorax**
>   The appropriate 7th character is to be added to each code from category S25

> | A | initial encounter |
> | D | subsequent encounter |
> | S | sequela |

>   Code also any associated open wound (S21.-)

● **S25.0 Injury of thoracic aorta**
>   Injury of aorta NOS

   ●■ **S25.00 Unspecified injury of thoracic aorta** A 🔷, D, S 🔷

   ● **S25.01 Minor laceration of thoracic aorta** A 🔷, D, S 🔷
>   Incomplete transection of thoracic aorta
>   Laceration of thoracic aorta NOS
>   Superficial laceration of thoracic aorta

   ● **S25.02 Major laceration of thoracic aorta** A 🔷, D, S 🔷
>   Complete transection of thoracic aorta
>   Traumatic rupture of thoracic aorta

   ● **S25.09 Other specified injury of thoracic aorta** A 🔷, D, S 🔷

● **S25.1 Injury of innominate or subclavian artery**

   ● **S25.10 Unspecified injury of innominate or subclavian artery**

      ●■ **S25.101 Unspecified injury of right innominate or subclavian artery** A 🔷, D, S 🔷

      ●■ **S25.102 Unspecified injury of left innominate or subclavian artery** A 🔷, D, S 🔷

      ●■ **S25.109 Unspecified injury of unspecified innominate or subclavian artery** A 🔷, D, S 🔷

● **S25.11 Minor laceration of innominate or subclavian artery**
>   Incomplete transection of innominate or subclavian artery
>   Laceration of innominate or subclavian artery NOS
>   Superficial laceration of innominate or subclavian artery

   ● **S25.111 Minor laceration of right innominate or subclavian artery** A 🔷, D, S 🔷

   ● **S25.112 Minor laceration of left innominate or subclavian artery** A 🔷, D, S 🔷

   ●■ **S25.119 Minor laceration of unspecified innominate or subclavian artery** A 🔷, D, S 🔷

● **S25.12 Major laceration of innominate or subclavian artery**
>   Complete transection of innominate or subclavian artery
>   Traumatic rupture of innominate or subclavian artery

   ● **S25.121 Major laceration of right innominate or subclavian artery** A 🔷, D, S 🔷

   ● **S25.122 Major laceration of left innominate or subclavian artery** A 🔷, D, S 🔷

   ●■ **S25.129 Major laceration of unspecified innominate or subclavian artery** A 🔷, D, S 🔷

● **S25.19 Other specified injury of innominate or subclavian artery**

   ● **S25.191 Other specified injury of right innominate or subclavian artery** A 🔷, D, S 🔷

   ● **S25.192 Other specified injury of left innominate or subclavian artery** A 🔷, D, S 🔷

   ●■ **S25.199 Other specified injury of unspecified innominate or subclavian artery** A 🔷, D, S 🔷

● **S25.2 Injury of superior vena cava**
>   Injury of vena cava NOS

   ●■ **S25.20 Unspecified injury of superior vena cava** A 🔷, D, S 🔷

   ● **S25.21 Minor laceration of superior vena cava** A 🔷, D, S 🔷
>   Incomplete transection of superior vena cava
>   Laceration of superior vena cava NOS
>   Superficial laceration of superior vena cava

   ● **S25.22 Major laceration of superior vena cava** A 🔷, D, S 🔷
>   Complete transection of superior vena cava
>   Traumatic rupture of superior vena cava

   ● **S25.29 Other specified injury of superior vena cava** A 🔷, D, S 🔷

CHAPTER 19 (S00-T88)

CHAPTER 19 (S00-T88)

- ● S25.3   **Injury of innominate or subclavian vein**
  - ● S25.30   Unspecified injury of innominate or subclavian vein
    - ● ■ S25.301   Unspecified injury of right innominate or subclavian vein A 🔖, D, S 🔖
    - ● ■ S25.302   Unspecified injury of left innominate or subclavian vein A 🔖, D, S 🔖
    - ● ■ S25.309   Unspecified injury of unspecified innominate or subclavian vein A 🔖, D, S 🔖
  - ● S25.31   Minor laceration of innominate or subclavian vein
    Incomplete transection of innominate or subclavian vein
    Laceration of innominate or subclavian vein NOS
    Superficial laceration of innominate or subclavian vein
    - ● S25.311   Minor laceration of right innominate or subclavian vein A 🔖, D, S 🔖
    - ● S25.312   Minor laceration of left innominate or subclavian vein A 🔖, D, S 🔖
    - ● ■ S25.319   Minor laceration of unspecified innominate or subclavian vein A 🔖, D, S 🔖
  - ● S25.32   Major laceration of innominate or subclavian vein
    Complete transection of innominate or subclavian vein
    Traumatic rupture of innominate or subclavian vein
    - ● S25.321   Major laceration of right innominate or subclavian vein A 🔖, D, S 🔖
    - ● S25.322   Major laceration of left innominate or subclavian vein A 🔖, D, S 🔖
    - ● ■ S25.329   Major laceration of unspecified innominate or subclavian vein A 🔖, D, S 🔖
  - ● S25.39   Other specified injury of innominate or subclavian vein
    - ● S25.391   Other specified injury of right innominate or subclavian vein A 🔖, D, S 🔖
    - ● S25.392   Other specified injury of left innominate or subclavian vein A 🔖, D, S 🔖
    - ● ■ S25.399   Other specified injury of unspecified innominate or subclavian vein A 🔖, D, S 🔖
- ● S25.4   **Injury of pulmonary blood vessels**
  - ● S25.40   Unspecified injury of pulmonary blood vessels
    - ● ■ S25.401   Unspecified injury of right pulmonary blood vessels A 🔖, D, S 🔖
    - ● ■ S25.402   Unspecified injury of left pulmonary blood vessels A 🔖, D, S 🔖
    - ● ■ S25.409   Unspecified injury of unspecified pulmonary blood vessels A 🔖, D, S 🔖

- ● S25.41   Minor laceration of pulmonary blood vessels
    Incomplete transection of pulmonary blood vessels
    Laceration of pulmonary blood vessels NOS
    Superficial laceration of pulmonary blood vessels
    - ● S25.411   Minor laceration of right pulmonary blood vessels A 🔖, D, S 🔖
    - ● S25.412   Minor laceration of left pulmonary blood vessels A 🔖, D, S 🔖
    - ● ■ S25.419   Minor laceration of unspecified pulmonary blood vessels A 🔖, D, S 🔖
  - ● S25.42   Major laceration of pulmonary blood vessels
    Complete transection of pulmonary blood vessels
    Traumatic rupture of pulmonary blood vessels
    - ● S25.421   Major laceration of right pulmonary blood vessels A 🔖, D, S 🔖
    - ● S25.422   Major laceration of left pulmonary blood vessels A 🔖, D, S 🔖
    - ● ■ S25.429   Major laceration of unspecified pulmonary blood vessels A 🔖, D, S 🔖
  - ● S25.49   Other specified injury of pulmonary blood vessels
    - ● S25.491   Other specified injury of right pulmonary blood vessels A 🔖, D, S 🔖
    - ● S25.492   Other specified injury of left pulmonary blood vessels A 🔖, D, S 🔖
    - ● ■ S25.499   Other specified injury of unspecified pulmonary blood vessels A 🔖, D, S 🔖
- ● S25.5   **Injury of intercostal blood vessels**
  - ● S25.50   Unspecified injury of intercostal blood vessels
    - ● ■ S25.501   Unspecified injury of intercostal blood vessels, right side A 🔖, D, S 🔖
    - ● ■ S25.502   Unspecified injury of intercostal blood vessels, left side A 🔖, D, S 🔖
    - ● ■ S25.509   Unspecified injury of intercostal blood vessels, unspecified side A 🔖, D, S 🔖
  - ● S25.51   Laceration of intercostal blood vessels
    - ● S25.511   Laceration of intercostal blood vessels, right side A 🔖, D, S 🔖
    - ● S25.512   Laceration of intercostal blood vessels, left side A 🔖, D, S 🔖
    - ● ■ S25.519   Laceration of intercostal blood vessels, unspecified side A 🔖, D, S 🔖

● Unacceptable Principal Diagnosis   ● Use Additional Character(s)   ■ Unspecified   ▶ Manifestation Code

OGCR Official Guidelines for Coding and Reporting   Excludes 1   Excludes 2   Includes   Use additional   Code first   Code also

● S25.59 Other specified injury of intercostal blood vessels
- ● S25.591 Other specified injury of intercostal blood vessels, right side A 🦠, D, S 🦠
- ● S25.592 Other specified injury of intercostal blood vessels, left side A 🦠, D, S 🦠
- ●■ S25.599 Other specified injury of intercostal blood vessels, unspecified side A 🦠, D, S 🦠

● S25.8 Injury of other blood vessels of thorax
  Injury of azygos vein
  Injury of mammary artery or vein
- ● S25.80 Unspecified injury of other blood vessels of thorax
  - ●■ S25.801 Unspecified injury of other blood vessels of thorax, right side A 🦠, D, S 🦠
  - ●■ S25.802 Unspecified injury of other blood vessels of thorax, left side A 🦠, D, S 🦠
  - ●■ S25.809 Unspecified injury of other blood vessels of thorax, unspecified side A 🦠, D, S 🦠
- ● S25.81 Laceration of other blood vessels of thorax
  - ● S25.811 Laceration of other blood vessels of thorax, right side A 🦠, D, S 🦠
  - ● S25.812 Laceration of other blood vessels of thorax, left side A 🦠, D, S 🦠
  - ●■ S25.819 Laceration of other blood vessels of thorax, unspecified side A 🦠, D, S 🦠
- ● S25.89 Other specified injury of other blood vessels of thorax
  - ● S25.891 Other specified injury of other blood vessels of thorax, right side A 🦠, D, S 🦠
  - ● S25.892 Other specified injury of other blood vessels of thorax, left side A 🦠, D, S 🦠
  - ●■ S25.899 Other specified injury of other blood vessels of thorax, unspecified side A 🦠, D, S 🦠

● S25.9 Injury of unspecified blood vessel of thorax
- ●■ S25.90 Unspecified injury of unspecified blood vessel of thorax A 🦠, D, S 🦠
- ●■ S25.91 Laceration of unspecified blood vessel of thorax A 🦠, D, S 🦠
- ●■ S25.99 Other specified injury of unspecified blood vessel of thorax A 🦠, D, S 🦠

● S26 Injury of heart
  The appropriate 7th character is to be added to each code from category S26

A	initial encounter
D	subsequent encounter
S	sequela

  Code also any associated:
    open wound of thorax (S21.-)
    traumatic hemopneumothorax (S27.2)
    traumatic hemothorax (S27.1)
    traumatic pneumothorax (S27.0)

● S26.0 Injury of heart with hemopericardium
  Hemopericardium: effusion of blood within pericardium
- ●■ S26.00 Unspecified injury of heart with hemopericardium A 🦠, D, S 🦠
- ● S26.01 Contusion of heart with hemopericardium A 🦠, D, S 🦠
- ● S26.02 Laceration of heart with hemopericardium
  - ● S26.020 Mild laceration of heart with hemopericardium A 🦠, D, S 🦠
    Laceration of heart without penetration of heart chamber
  - ● S26.021 Moderate laceration of heart with hemopericardium A 🦠, D, S 🦠
    Laceration of heart with penetration of heart chamber
  - ● S26.022 Major laceration of heart with hemopericardium A 🦠, D, S 🦠
    Laceration of heart with penetration of multiple heart chambers
- ● S26.09 Other injury of heart with hemopericardium A 🦠, D, S 🦠

● S26.1 Injury of heart without hemopericardium
  Hemopericardium: effusion of blood within pericardium
- ●■ S26.10 Unspecified injury of heart without hemopericardium A 🦠, D, S 🦠
- ● S26.11 Contusion of heart without hemopericardium A 🦠, D, S 🦠
- ● S26.12 Laceration of heart without hemopericardium A 🦠, D, S 🦠
- ● S26.19 Other injury of heart without hemopericardium A 🦠, D, S 🦠

● S26.9 Injury of heart, unspecified with or without hemopericardium
  Hemopericardium: effusion of blood within pericardium
- ●■ S26.90 Unspecified injury of heart, unspecified with or without hemopericardium A 🦠, D, S 🦠
- ●■ S26.91 Contusion of heart, unspecified with or without hemopericardium A 🦠, D, S 🦠
- ●■ S26.92 Laceration of heart, unspecified with or without hemopericardium A 🦠, D, S 🦠
    Laceration of heart NOS
- ●■ S26.99 Other injury of heart, unspecified with or without hemopericardium A 🦠, D, S 🦠

Item 19–2 Pneumothorax is a collection of gas (positive air pressure) in the pleural space resulting in the lung collapsing. A tension pneumothorax is life-threatening and is a result of air in the pleural space causing a displacement in the mediastinal structures and cardiopulmonary function compromise. A traumatic pneumothorax results from blunt or penetrating injury that disrupts the parietal/visceral pleura. **Hemothorax** is blood or bloody fluid in the pleural cavity as a result of traumatic blood vessel rupture or inflammation of the lungs from pneumonia.

CHAPTER 19 (S00–T88)

● **S27   Injury of other and unspecified intrathoracic organs**

Code also any associated open wound of thorax (S21.-)

Excludes2   injury of cervical esophagus (S10-S19)
injury of trachea (cervical) (S10-S19)

The appropriate 7th character is to be added to each code from category S27

> A   initial encounter
> D   subsequent encounter
> S   sequela

● **S27.0   Traumatic pneumothorax** A, D, S

Excludes1   spontaneous pneumothorax (J93.-)

● **S27.1   Traumatic hemothorax** A, D, S

● **S27.2   Traumatic hemopneumothorax** A, D, S

● **S27.3   Other and unspecified injuries of lung**

  ● **S27.30   Unspecified injury of lung**

    ● ■ **S27.301   Unspecified injury of lung, unilateral** A, D, S

    ● ■ **S27.302   Unspecified injury of lung, bilateral** A, D, S

    ● ■ **S27.309   Unspecified injury of lung, unspecified** A, D, S

  ● **S27.31   Primary blast injury of lung**
Blast injury of lung NOS

    ● **S27.311   Primary blast injury of lung, unilateral** A, D, S

    ● **S27.312   Primary blast injury of lung, bilateral** A, D, S

    ● ■ **S27.319   Primary blast injury of lung, unspecified** A, D, S

  ● **S27.32   Contusion of lung**

    ● **S27.321   Contusion of lung, unilateral** A, D, S

    ● **S27.322   Contusion of lung, bilateral** A, D, S

    ● ■ **S27.329   Contusion of lung, unspecified** A, D, S

  ● **S27.33   Laceration of lung**

    ● **S27.331   Laceration of lung, unilateral** A, D, S

    ● **S27.332   Laceration of lung, bilateral** A, D, S

    ● ■ **S27.339   Laceration of lung, unspecified** A, D, S

  ● **S27.39   Other injuries of lung**
Secondary blast injury of lung

    ● **S27.391   Other injuries of lung, unilateral** A, D, S

    ● **S27.392   Other injuries of lung, bilateral** A, D, S

    ● ■ **S27.399   Other injuries of lung, unspecified** A, D, S

● **S27.4   Injury of bronchus**

  ● **S27.40   Unspecified injury of bronchus**

    ● ■ **S27.401   Unspecified injury of bronchus, unilateral** A, D, S

    ● ■ **S27.402   Unspecified injury of bronchus, bilateral** A, D, S

    ● ■ **S27.409   Unspecified injury of bronchus, unspecified** A, D, S

  ● **S27.41   Primary blast injury of bronchus**
Blast injury of bronchus NOS

    ● **S27.411   Primary blast injury of bronchus, unilateral** A, D, S

    ● **S27.412   Primary blast injury of bronchus, bilateral** A, D, S

    ● ■ **S27.419   Primary blast injury of bronchus, unspecified** A, D, S

  ● **S27.42   Contusion of bronchus**

    ● **S27.421   Contusion of bronchus, unilateral** A, D, S

    ● **S27.422   Contusion of bronchus, bilateral** A, D, S

    ● ■ **S27.429   Contusion of bronchus, unspecified** A, D, S

  ● **S27.43   Laceration of bronchus**

    ● **S27.431   Laceration of bronchus, unilateral** A, D, S

    ● **S27.432   Laceration of bronchus, bilateral** A, D, S

    ● ■ **S27.439   Laceration of bronchus, unspecified** A, D, S

  ● **S27.49   Other injury of bronchus**
Secondary blast injury of bronchus

    ● **S27.491   Other injury of bronchus, unilateral** A, D, S

    ● **S27.492   Other injury of bronchus, bilateral** A, D, S

    ● ■ **S27.499   Other injury of bronchus, unspecified** A, D, S

● **S27.5   Injury of thoracic trachea**

  ● ■ **S27.50   Unspecified injury of thoracic trachea** A, D, S

  ● **S27.51   Primary blast injury of thoracic trachea** A, D, S
Blast injury of thoracic trachea NOS

  ● **S27.52   Contusion of thoracic trachea** A, D, S

  ● **S27.53   Laceration of thoracic trachea** A, D, S

  ● **S27.59   Other injury of thoracic trachea** A, D, S
Secondary blast injury of thoracic trachea

● **S27.6   Injury of pleura**

  ● ■ **S27.60   Unspecified injury of pleura** A, D, S

  ● **S27.63   Laceration of pleura** A, D, S

  ● **S27.69   Other injury of pleura** A, D, S

● **S27.8   Injury of other specified intrathoracic organs**

  ● **S27.80   Injury of diaphragm**

    ● **S27.802   Contusion of diaphragm** A, D, S

    ● **S27.803   Laceration of diaphragm** A, D, S

    ● **S27.808   Other injury of diaphragm** A, D, S

    ● ■ **S27.809   Unspecified injury of diaphragm** A, D, S

  ● **S27.81   Injury of esophagus (thoracic part)**

    ● **S27.812   Contusion of esophagus (thoracic part)** A, D, S

    ● **S27.813   Laceration of esophagus (thoracic part)** A, D, S

● Unacceptable Principal Diagnosis   ● Use Additional Character(s)   ■ Unspecified   ▶ Manifestation Code

OGCR   Official Guidelines for Coding and Reporting | Excludes 1 | | Excludes 2 | Includes   Use additional   Code first   Code also

● S27.818 Other injury of esophagus (thoracic part) A 🔵, D, S 🔘

●🔳 S27.819 Unspecified injury of esophagus (thoracic part) A 🔵, D, S 🔘

● S27.89 Injury of other specified intrathoracic organs
Injury of lymphatic thoracic duct
Injury of thymus gland

● S27.892 Contusion of other specified intrathoracic organs A 🔵, D, S 🔘

● S27.893 Laceration of other specified intrathoracic organs A 🔵, D, S 🔘

● S27.898 Other injury of other specified intrathoracic organs A 🔵, D, S 🔘

●🔳 S27.899 Unspecified injury of other specified intrathoracic organs A 🔵, D, S 🔘

●🔳 S27.9 Injury of unspecified intrathoracic organ A 🔵, D, S 🔘

● S28 Crushing injury of thorax, and traumatic amputation of part of thorax

The appropriate 7th character is to be added to each code from category S28

A	initial encounter
D	subsequent encounter
S	sequela

● S28.0 Crushed chest D, S 🔘

Use additional code for all associated injuries

Excludes1 flail chest (S22.5)

● S28.1 Traumatic amputation (partial) of part of thorax, except breast A 🔵, D, S 🔘

● S28.2 Traumatic amputation of breast

● S28.21 Complete traumatic amputation of breast
Traumatic amputation of breast NOS

● S28.211 Complete traumatic amputation of right breast D, S 🔘

● S28.212 Complete traumatic amputation of left breast D, S 🔘

●🔳 S28.219 Complete traumatic amputation of unspecified breast D, S 🔘

● S28.22 Partial traumatic amputation of breast

● S28.221 Partial traumatic amputation of right breast D, S 🔘

● S28.222 Partial traumatic amputation of left breast D, S 🔘

●🔳 S28.229 Partial traumatic amputation of unspecified breast D, S 🔘

● S29 Other and unspecified injuries of thorax

Code also any associated open wound (S21.-)

The appropriate 7th character is to be added to each code from category S29

A	initial encounter
D	subsequent encounter
S	sequela

● S29.0 Injury of muscle and tendon at thorax level

● S29.00 Unspecified injury of muscle and tendon of thorax

●🔳 S29.001 Unspecified injury of muscle and tendon of front wall of thorax D, S 🔘

●🔳 S29.002 Unspecified injury of muscle and tendon of back wall of thorax D, S 🔘

●🔳 S29.009 Unspecified injury of muscle and tendon of unspecified wall of thorax D, S 🔘

● S29.01 Strain of muscle and tendon of thorax

● S29.011 Strain of muscle and tendon of front wall of thorax D, S 🔘

● S29.012 Strain of muscle and tendon of back wall of thorax D, S 🔘

●🔳 S29.019 Strain of muscle and tendon of unspecified wall of thorax D, S 🔘

● S29.02 Laceration of muscle and tendon of thorax

● S29.021 Laceration of muscle and tendon of front wall of thorax A 🔵, D, S 🔘

● S29.022 Laceration of muscle and tendon of back wall of thorax D, S 🔘

●🔳 S29.029 Laceration of muscle and tendon of unspecified wall of thorax A 🔵, D, S 🔘

● S29.09 Other injury of muscle and tendon of thorax

● S29.091 Other injury of muscle and tendon of front wall of thorax D, S 🔘

● S29.092 Other injury of muscle and tendon of back wall of thorax D, S 🔘

●🔳 S29.099 Other injury of muscle and tendon of unspecified wall of thorax D, S 🔘

● S29.8 Other specified injuries of thorax D, S 🔘

●🔳 S29.9 Unspecified injury of thorax D, S 🔘

INJURIES TO THE ABDOMEN, LOWER BACK, LUMBAR SPINE, PELVIS AND EXTERNAL GENITALS (S30-S39)

Includes injuries to the abdominal wall
injuries to the anus
injuries to the buttock
injuries to the external genitalia
injuries to the flank
injuries to the groin

Excludes2 burns and corrosions (T20-T32)
effects of foreign body in anus and rectum (T18.5)
effects of foreign body in genitourinary tract (T19.-)
effects of foreign body in stomach, small intestine and colon (T18.2-T18.4)
frostbite (T33-T34)
insect bite or sting, venomous (T63.4)

● S30 Superficial injury of abdomen, lower back, pelvis and external genitals

Excludes2 superficial injury of hip (S70.-)

The appropriate 7th character is to be added to each code from category S30

A	initial encounter
D	subsequent encounter
S	sequela

● S30.0 Contusion of lower back and pelvis D, S 🔘
Contusion of buttock

● S30.1 Contusion of abdominal wall D, S 🔘
Contusion of flank
Contusion of groin

● S30.2   Contusion of external genital organs

   ● S30.20   Contusion of unspecified external genital organ

     ● ▪ S30.201   Contusion of unspecified external genital organ, male D, S ⊚

     ● ▪ S30.202   Contusion of unspecified external genital organ, female D, S ⊚

   ● S30.21   Contusion of penis D, S ⊚

   ● S30.22   Contusion of scrotum and testes D, S ⊚

   ● S30.23   Contusion of vagina and vulva D, S ⊚

● S30.3   Contusion of anus D, S ⊚

● S30.8   Other superficial injuries of abdomen, lower back, pelvis and external genitals

   ● S30.81   Abrasion of abdomen, lower back, pelvis and external genitals

     ● S30.810   Abrasion of lower back and pelvis D, S ⊚

     ● S30.811   Abrasion of abdominal wall D, S ⊚

     ● S30.812   Abrasion of penis D, S ⊚

     ● S30.813   Abrasion of scrotum and testes D, S ⊚

     ● S30.814   Abrasion of vagina and vulva D, S ⊚

     ● ▪ S30.815   Abrasion of unspecified external genital organs, male D, S ⊚

     ● ▪ S30.816   Abrasion of unspecified external genital organs, female D, S ⊚

     ● S30.817   Abrasion of anus D, S ⊚

   ● S30.82   Blister (nonthermal) of abdomen, lower back, pelvis and external genitals

     ● S30.820   Blister (nonthermal) of lower back and pelvis D, S ⊚

     ● S30.821   Blister (nonthermal) of abdominal wall D, S ⊚

     ● S30.822   Blister (nonthermal) of penis D, S ⊚

     ● S30.823   Blister (nonthermal) of scrotum and testes D, S ⊚

     ● S30.824   Blister (nonthermal) of vagina and vulva D, S ⊚

     ● ▪ S30.825   Blister (nonthermal) of unspecified external genital organs, male D, S ⊚

     ● ▪ S30.826   Blister (nonthermal) of unspecified external genital organs, female D, S ⊚

     ● S30.827   Blister (nonthermal) of anus D, S ⊚

   ● S30.84   External constriction of abdomen, lower back, pelvis and external genitals

     ● S30.840   External constriction of lower back and pelvis D, S ⊚

     ● S30.841   External constriction of abdominal wall D, S ⊚

     ● S30.842   External constriction of penis D, S ⊚

       Hair tourniquet syndrome of penis

       Use additional cause code to identify the constricting item (W49.0-)

     ● S30.843   External constriction of scrotum and testes D, S ⊚

     ● S30.844   External constriction of vagina and vulva D, S ⊚

     ● ▪ S30.845   External constriction of unspecified external genital organs, male D, S ⊚

     ● ▪ S30.846   External constriction of unspecified external genital organs, female D, S ⊚

   ● S30.85   Superficial foreign body of abdomen, lower back, pelvis and external genitals

       Splinter in the abdomen, lower back, pelvis and external genitals

     ● S30.850   Superficial foreign body of lower back and pelvis D, S ⊚

     ● S30.851   Superficial foreign body of abdominal wall D, S ⊚

     ● S30.852   Superficial foreign body of penis D, S ⊚

     ● S30.853   Superficial foreign body of scrotum and testes D, S ⊚

     ● S30.854   Superficial foreign body of vagina and vulva D, S ⊚

     ● ▪ S30.855   Superficial foreign body of unspecified external genital organs, male D, S ⊚

     ● ▪ S30.856   Superficial foreign body of unspecified external genital organs, female D, S ⊚

     ● S30.857   Superficial foreign body of anus D, S ⊚

   ● S30.86   Insect bite (nonvenomous) of abdomen, lower back, pelvis and external genitals

     ● S30.860   Insect bite (nonvenomous) of lower back and pelvis D, S ⊚

     ● S30.861   Insect bite (nonvenomous) of abdominal wall D, S ⊚

     ● S30.862   Insect bite (nonvenomous) of penis D, S ⊚

     ● S30.863   Insect bite (nonvenomous) of scrotum and testes D, S ⊚

     ● S30.864   Insect bite (nonvenomous) of vagina and vulva D, S ⊚

     ● ▪ S30.865   Insect bite (nonvenomous) of unspecified external genital organs, male D, S ⊚

     ● ▪ S30.866   Insect bite (nonvenomous) of unspecified external genital organs, female D, S ⊚

     ● S30.867   Insect bite (nonvenomous) of anus D, S ⊚

   ● S30.87   Other superficial bite of abdomen, lower back, pelvis and external genitals

     Excludes1   open bite of abdomen, lower back, pelvis and external genitals (S31.05, S31.15, S31.25, S31.35, S31.45, S31.55)

     ● S30.870   Other superficial bite of lower back and pelvis D, S ⊚

     ● S30.871   Other superficial bite of abdominal wall D, S ⊚

● Unacceptable Principal Diagnosis   ● Use Additional Character(s)   ▪ Unspecified   ▶ Manifestation Code

OGCR Official Guidelines for Coding and Reporting   Excludes 1   Excludes 2   Includes   Use additional   Code first   Code also

● S30.872   Other superficial bite of penis
D, S

● S30.873   Other superficial bite of scrotum and testes D, S

● S30.874   Other superficial bite of vagina and vulva D, S

●■ S30.875   Other superficial bite of unspecified external genital organs, male D, S

●■ S30.876   Other superficial bite of unspecified external genital organs, female D, S

● S30.877   Other superficial bite of anus D, S

● S30.9   Unspecified superficial injury of abdomen, lower back, pelvis and external genitals

   ●■ S30.91   Unspecified superficial injury of lower back and pelvis D, S

   ●■ S30.92   Unspecified superficial injury of abdominal wall D, S

   ●■ S30.93   Unspecified superficial injury of penis D, S

   ●■ S30.94   Unspecified superficial injury of scrotum and testes D, S

   ●■ S30.95   Unspecified superficial injury of vagina and vulva D, S

   ●■ S30.96   Unspecified superficial injury of unspecified external genital organs, male D, S

   ●■ S30.97   Unspecified superficial injury of unspecified external genital organs, female D, S

   ●■ S30.98   Unspecified superficial injury of anus D, S

● S31   Open wound of abdomen, lower back, pelvis and external genitals

> Code also any associated:
> spinal cord injury (S24.0, S24.1-, S34.0-, S34.1-)
> wound infection

> | Excludes1 | traumatic amputation of part of abdomen, lower back and pelvis (S38.2-, S38.3) |

> | Excludes2 | open wound of hip (S71.00-S71.02) open fracture of pelvis (S32.1--S32.9 with 7th character B) |

> The appropriate 7th character is to be added to each code from category S31

> | A | initial encounter |
> | D | subsequent encounter |
> | S | sequela |

   ● S31.0   Open wound of lower back and pelvis

     ● S31.00   Unspecified open wound of lower back and pelvis

       ●■ S31.000   Unspecified open wound of lower back and pelvis without penetration into retroperitoneum D, S

> Unspecified open wound of lower back and pelvis NOS

       ●■ S31.001   Unspecified open wound of lower back and pelvis with penetration into retroperitoneum A, D, S

● S31.01   Laceration without foreign body of lower back and pelvis

   ● S31.010   Laceration without foreign body of lower back and pelvis without penetration into retroperitoneum D, S

> Laceration without foreign body of lower back and pelvis NOS

   ● S31.011   Laceration without foreign body of lower back and pelvis with penetration into retroperitoneum A, D, S

● S31.02   Laceration with foreign body of lower back and pelvis

   ● S31.020   Laceration with foreign body of lower back and pelvis without penetration into retroperitoneum D, S

> Laceration with foreign body of lower back and pelvis NOS

   ● S31.021   Laceration with foreign body of lower back and pelvis with penetration into retroperitoneum A, D, S

● S31.03   Puncture wound without foreign body of lower back and pelvis

   ● S31.030   Puncture wound without foreign body of lower back and pelvis without penetration into retroperitoneum D, S

> Puncture wound without foreign body of lower back and pelvis NOS

   ● S31.031   Puncture wound without foreign body of lower back and pelvis with penetration into retroperitoneum A, D, S

● S31.04   Puncture wound with foreign body of lower back and pelvis

   ● S31.040   Puncture wound with foreign body of lower back and pelvis without penetration into retroperitoneum D, S

> Puncture wound with foreign body of lower back and pelvis NOS

   ● S31.041   Puncture wound with foreign body of lower back and pelvis with penetration into retroperitoneum A, D, S

● S31.05   Open bite of lower back and pelvis

> Bite of lower back and pelvis NOS

> | Excludes1 | superficial bite of lower back and pelvis (S30.860, S30.870) |

   ● S31.050   Open bite of lower back and pelvis without penetration into retroperitoneum D, S

> Open bite of lower back and pelvis NOS

   ● S31.051   Open bite of lower back and pelvis with penetration into retroperitoneum A, D, S

N Newborn Age: 0   **P** Pediatric Age: 0–17   **M** Maternity DX: 12–55   **A** Adult Age: 15–124   ♀ Females Only   ♂ Males Only

Complication\Comorbidity   Major C\C   Present on Admission Requirement   Hospital-Acquired Condition

1433

● **S31.1**   **Open wound of abdominal wall without penetration into peritoneal cavity**
Open wound of abdominal wall NOS

> Excludes2   open wound of abdominal wall with penetration into peritoneal cavity (S31.6-)

● **S31.10**   Unspecified open wound of abdominal wall without penetration into peritoneal cavity

  ● ▪ **S31.100**   Unspecified open wound of abdominal wall, right upper quadrant without penetration into peritoneal cavity D, S ✎

  ● ▪ **S31.101**   Unspecified open wound of abdominal wall, left upper quadrant without penetration into peritoneal cavity D, S ✎

  ● ▪ **S31.102**   Unspecified open wound of abdominal wall, epigastric region without penetration into peritoneal cavity D, S ✎

  ● ▪ **S31.103**   Unspecified open wound of abdominal wall, right lower quadrant without penetration into peritoneal cavity D, S ✎

  ● ▪ **S31.104**   Unspecified open wound of abdominal wall, left lower quadrant without penetration into peritoneal cavity D, S ✎

  ● ▪ **S31.105**   Unspecified open wound of abdominal wall, periumbilic region without penetration into peritoneal cavity D, S ✎

  ● ▪ **S31.109**   Unspecified open wound of abdominal wall, unspecified quadrant without penetration into peritoneal cavity D, S ✎
Unspecified open wound of abdominal wall NOS

● **S31.11**   Laceration without foreign body of abdominal wall without penetration into peritoneal cavity

  ● **S31.110**   Laceration without foreign body of abdominal wall, right upper quadrant without penetration into peritoneal cavity D, S ✎

  ● **S31.111**   Laceration without foreign body of abdominal wall, left upper quadrant without penetration into peritoneal cavity D, S ✎

  ● **S31.112**   Laceration without foreign body of abdominal wall, epigastric region without penetration into peritoneal cavity D, S ✎

  ● **S31.113**   Laceration without foreign body of abdominal wall, right lower quadrant without penetration into peritoneal cavity D, S ✎

  ● **S31.114**   Laceration without foreign body of abdominal wall, left lower quadrant without penetration into peritoneal cavity D, S ✎

  ● **S31.115**   Laceration without foreign body of abdominal wall, periumbilic region without penetration into peritoneal cavity D, S ✎

  ● ▪ **S31.119**   Laceration without foreign body of abdominal wall, unspecified quadrant without penetration into peritoneal cavity D, S ✎

● **S31.12**   Laceration with foreign body of abdominal wall without penetration into peritoneal cavity

  ● **S31.120**   Laceration of abdominal wall with foreign body, right upper quadrant without penetration into peritoneal cavity D, S ✎

  ● **S31.121**   Laceration of abdominal wall with foreign body, left upper quadrant without penetration into peritoneal cavity D, S ✎

  ● **S31.122**   Laceration of abdominal wall with foreign body, epigastric region without penetration into peritoneal cavity D, S ✎

  ● **S31.123**   Laceration of abdominal wall with foreign body, right lower quadrant without penetration into peritoneal cavity D, S ✎

  ● **S31.124**   Laceration of abdominal wall with foreign body, left lower quadrant without penetration into peritoneal cavity D, S ✎

  ● **S31.125**   Laceration of abdominal wall with foreign body, periumbilic region without penetration into peritoneal cavity D, S ✎

  ● ▪ **S31.129**   Laceration of abdominal wall with foreign body, unspecified quadrant without penetration into peritoneal cavity D, S ✎

● **S31.13**   Puncture wound of abdominal wall without foreign body without penetration into peritoneal cavity

  ● **S31.130**   Puncture wound of abdominal wall without foreign body, right upper quadrant without penetration into peritoneal cavity D, S ✎

  ● **S31.131**   Puncture wound of abdominal wall without foreign body, left upper quadrant without penetration into peritoneal cavity D, S ✎

  ● **S31.132**   Puncture wound of abdominal wall without foreign body, epigastric region without penetration into peritoneal cavity D, S ✎

  ● **S31.133**   Puncture wound of abdominal wall without foreign body, right lower quadrant without penetration into peritoneal cavity D, S ✎

  ● **S31.134**   Puncture wound of abdominal wall without foreign body, left lower quadrant without penetration into peritoneal cavity D, S ✎

  ● **S31.135**   Puncture wound of abdominal wall without foreign body, periumbilic region without penetration into peritoneal cavity D, S ✎

  ● ▪ **S31.139**   Puncture wound of abdominal wall without foreign body, unspecified quadrant without penetration into peritoneal cavity D, S ✎

● Unacceptable Principal Diagnosis   ● Use Additional Character(s)   ▪ Unspecified   ▶ Manifestation Code

OGCR Official Guidelines for Coding and Reporting   Excludes 1   Excludes 2   Includes   Use additional   Code first   Code also

● **S31.14**   Puncture wound of abdominal wall with foreign body without penetration into peritoneal cavity

    ● **S31.140**   Puncture wound of abdominal wall with foreign body, right upper quadrant without penetration into peritoneal cavity D, S 🖐

    ● **S31.141**   Puncture wound of abdominal wall with foreign body, left upper quadrant without penetration into peritoneal cavity D, S 🖐

    ● **S31.142**   Puncture wound of abdominal wall with foreign body, epigastric region without penetration into peritoneal cavity D, S 🖐

    ● **S31.143**   Puncture wound of abdominal wall with foreign body, right lower quadrant without penetration into peritoneal cavity D, S 🖐

    ● **S31.144**   Puncture wound of abdominal wall with foreign body, left lower quadrant without penetration into peritoneal cavity D, S 🖐

    ● **S31.145**   Puncture wound of abdominal wall with foreign body, periumbilic region without penetration into peritoneal cavity D, S 🖐

    ●■ **S31.149**   Puncture wound of abdominal wall with foreign body, unspecified quadrant without penetration into peritoneal cavity D, S 🖐

● **S31.15**   Open bite of abdominal wall without penetration into peritoneal cavity
     Bite of abdominal wall NOS

     | Excludes1 | superficial bite of abdominal wall (S30.871)

    ● **S31.150**   Open bite of abdominal wall, right upper quadrant without penetration into peritoneal cavity D, S 🖐

    ● **S31.151**   Open bite of abdominal wall, left upper quadrant without penetration into peritoneal cavity D, S 🖐

    ● **S31.152**   Open bite of abdominal wall, epigastric region without penetration into peritoneal cavity D, S 🖐

    ● **S31.153**   Open bite of abdominal wall, right lower quadrant without penetration into peritoneal cavity D, S 🖐

    ● **S31.154**   Open bite of abdominal wall, left lower quadrant without penetration into peritoneal cavity D, S 🖐

    ● **S31.155**   Open bite of abdominal wall, periumbilic region without penetration into peritoneal cavity D, S 🖐

    ●■ **S31.159**   Open bite of abdominal wall, unspecified quadrant without penetration into peritoneal cavity D, S 🖐

● **S31.2**   Open wound of penis

    ●■ **S31.20**   Unspecified open wound of penis D, S 🖐

    ● **S31.21**   Laceration without foreign body of penis D, S 🖐

    ● **S31.22**   Laceration with foreign body of penis D, S 🖐

    ● **S31.23**   Puncture wound without foreign body of penis D, S 🖐

    ● **S31.24**   Puncture wound with foreign body of penis D, S 🖐

    ● **S31.25**   Open bite of penis D, S 🖐
      Bite of penis NOS

      | Excludes1 | superficial bite of penis (S30.862, S30.872)

● **S31.3**   Open wound of scrotum and testes

    ●■ **S31.30**   Unspecified open wound of scrotum and testes D, S 🖐

    ● **S31.31**   Laceration without foreign body of scrotum and testes D, S 🖐

    ● **S31.32**   Laceration with foreign body of scrotum and testes D, S 🖐

    ● **S31.33**   Puncture wound without foreign body of scrotum and testes D, S 🖐

    ● **S31.34**   Puncture wound with foreign body of scrotum and testes D, S 🖐

    ● **S31.35**   Open bite of scrotum and testes D, S 🖐
      Bite of scrotum and testes NOS

      | Excludes1 | superficial bite of scrotum and testes (S30.863, S30.873)

● **S31.4**   Open wound of vagina and vulva

     | Excludes1 | injury to vagina and vulva during delivery (O70.-, O71.4)

    ●■ **S31.40**   Unspecified open wound of vagina and vulva D, S 🖐

    ● **S31.41**   Laceration without foreign body of vagina and vulva D, S 🖐

    ● **S31.42**   Laceration with foreign body of vagina and vulva D, S 🖐

    ● **S31.43**   Puncture wound without foreign body of vagina and vulva D, S 🖐

    ● **S31.44**   Puncture wound with foreign body of vagina and vulva D, S 🖐

    ● **S31.45**   Open bite of vagina and vulva D, S 🖐
      Bite of vagina and vulva NOS

      | Excludes1 | superficial bite of vagina and vulva (S30.864, S30.874)

● **S31.5**   Open wound of unspecified external genital organs

     | Excludes1 | traumatic amputation of external genital organs (S38.21, S38.22)

    ● **S31.50**   Unspecified open wound of unspecified external genital organs

      ●■ **S31.501**   Unspecified open wound of unspecified external genital organs, male D 🖐

      ●■ **S31.502**   Unspecified open wound of unspecified external genital organs, female D 🖐

CHAPTER 19 (S00-T88)

N Newborn Age: 0   **P** Pediatric Age: 0–17   **M** Maternity DX: 12–55   **A** Adult Age: 15–124   ♀ Females Only   ♂ Males Only

 Complication\Comorbidity   🖐 Major C\C   🖐 Present on Admission Requirement   🖐 Hospital-Acquired Condition

1435

● S31.51   Laceration without foreign body of unspecified external genital organs

● ■ S31.511   Laceration without foreign body of unspecified external genital organs, male D ⊘

● ■ S31.512   Laceration without foreign body of unspecified external genital organs, female D ⊘

● S31.52   Laceration with foreign body of unspecified external genital organs

● ■ S31.521   Laceration with foreign body of unspecified external genital organs, male D ⊘

● ■ S31.522   Laceration with foreign body of unspecified external genital organs, female D ⊘

● S31.53   Puncture wound without foreign body of unspecified external genital organs

● ■ S31.531   Puncture wound without foreign body of unspecified external genital organs, male D ⊘

● ■ S31.532   Puncture wound without foreign body of unspecified external genital organs, female D ⊘

● S31.54   Puncture wound with foreign body of unspecified external genital organs

● ■ S31.541   Puncture wound with foreign body of unspecified external genital organs, male D ⊘

● ■ S31.542   Puncture wound with foreign body of unspecified external genital organs, female D ⊘

● S31.55   Open bite of unspecified external genital organs

Bite of unspecified external genital organs NOS

Excludes1   superficial bite of unspecified external genital organs (S30.865, S30.866, S30.875, S30.876)

● ■ S31.551   Open bite of unspecified external genital organs, male D ⊘

● ■ S31.552   Open bite of unspecified external genital organs, female D ⊘

● S31.6   Open wound of abdominal wall with penetration into peritoneal cavity

● S31.60   Unspecified open wound of abdominal wall with penetration into peritoneal cavity

● ■ S31.600   Unspecified open wound of abdominal wall, right upper quadrant with penetration into peritoneal cavity A ⊘, D, S ⊘

● ■ S31.601   Unspecified open wound of abdominal wall, left upper quadrant with penetration into peritoneal cavity A ⊘, D, S ⊘

● ■ S31.602   Unspecified open wound of abdominal wall, epigastric region with penetration into peritoneal cavity A ⊘, D, S ⊘

● ■ S31.603   Unspecified open wound of abdominal wall, right lower quadrant with penetration into peritoneal cavity A ⊘, D, S ⊘

● ■ S31.604   Unspecified open wound of abdominal wall, left lower quadrant with penetration into peritoneal cavity A ⊘, D, S ⊘

● ■ S31.605   Unspecified open wound of abdominal wall, periumbilic region with penetration into peritoneal cavity A ⊘, D, S ⊘

● ■ S31.609   Unspecified open wound of abdominal wall, unspecified quadrant with penetration into peritoneal cavity A ⊘, D, S ⊘

● S31.61   Laceration without foreign body of abdominal wall with penetration into peritoneal cavity

● S31.610   Laceration without foreign body of abdominal wall, right upper quadrant with penetration into peritoneal cavity A ⊘, D, S ⊘

● S31.611   Laceration without foreign body of abdominal wall, left upper quadrant with penetration into peritoneal cavity A ⊘, D, S ⊘

● S31.612   Laceration without foreign body of abdominal wall, epigastric region with penetration into peritoneal cavity A ⊘, D, S ⊘

● S31.613   Laceration without foreign body of abdominal wall, right lower quadrant with penetration into peritoneal cavity A ⊘, D, S ⊘

● S31.614   Laceration without foreign body of abdominal wall, left lower quadrant with penetration into peritoneal cavity A ⊘, D, S ⊘

● S31.615   Laceration without foreign body of abdominal wall, periumbilic region with penetration into peritoneal cavity A ⊘, D, S ⊘

● ■ S31.619   Laceration without foreign body of abdominal wall, unspecified quadrant with penetration into peritoneal cavity A ⊘, D, S ⊘

● S31.62   Laceration with foreign body of abdominal wall with penetration into peritoneal cavity

● S31.620   Laceration with foreign body of abdominal wall, right upper quadrant with penetration into peritoneal cavity A ⊘, D, S ⊘

● S31.621   Laceration with foreign body of abdominal wall, left upper quadrant with penetration into peritoneal cavity A ⊘, D, S ⊘

● S31.622   Laceration with foreign body of abdominal wall, epigastric region with penetration into peritoneal cavity A ⊘, D, S ⊘

● S31.623   Laceration with foreign body of abdominal wall, right lower quadrant with penetration into peritoneal cavity A ⊘, D, S ⊘

● S31.624 Laceration with foreign body of abdominal wall, left lower quadrant with penetration into peritoneal cavity A ⬮, D, S ⬮

● S31.625 Laceration with foreign body of abdominal wall, periumbilic region with penetration into peritoneal cavity A ⬮, D, S ⬮

●■ S31.629 Laceration with foreign body of abdominal wall, unspecified quadrant with penetration into peritoneal cavity A ⬮, D, S ⬮

● S31.63 Puncture wound without foreign body of abdominal wall with penetration into peritoneal cavity

● S31.630 Puncture wound without foreign body of abdominal wall, right upper quadrant with penetration into peritoneal cavity A ⬮, D, S ⬮

● S31.631 Puncture wound without foreign body of abdominal wall, left upper quadrant with penetration into peritoneal cavity A ⬮, D, S ⬮

● S31.632 Puncture wound without foreign body of abdominal wall, epigastric region with penetration into peritoneal cavity A ⬮, D, S ⬮

● S31.633 Puncture wound without foreign body of abdominal wall, right lower quadrant with penetration into peritoneal cavity A ⬮, D, S ⬮

● S31.634 Puncture wound without foreign body of abdominal wall, left lower quadrant with penetration into peritoneal cavity A ⬮, D, S ⬮

● S31.635 Puncture wound without foreign body of abdominal wall, periumbilic region with penetration into peritoneal cavity A ⬮, D, S ⬮

●■ S31.639 Puncture wound without foreign body of abdominal wall, unspecified quadrant with penetration into peritoneal cavity A ⬮, D, S ⬮

● S31.64 Puncture wound with foreign body of abdominal wall with penetration into peritoneal cavity

● S31.640 Puncture wound with foreign body of abdominal wall, right upper quadrant with penetration into peritoneal cavity A ⬮, D, S ⬮

● S31.641 Puncture wound with foreign body of abdominal wall, left upper quadrant with penetration into peritoneal cavity A ⬮, D, S ⬮

● S31.642 Puncture wound with foreign body of abdominal wall, epigastric region with penetration into peritoneal cavity A ⬮, D, S ⬮

● S31.643 Puncture wound with foreign body of abdominal wall, right lower quadrant with penetration into peritoneal cavity A ⬮, D, S ⬮

● S31.644 Puncture wound with foreign body of abdominal wall, left lower quadrant with penetration into peritoneal cavity A ⬮, D, S ⬮

● S31.645 Puncture wound with foreign body of abdominal wall, periumbilic region with penetration into peritoneal cavity A ⬮, D, S ⬮

●■ S31.649 Puncture wound with foreign body of abdominal wall, unspecified quadrant with penetration into peritoneal cavity A ⬮, D, S ⬮

● S31.65 Open bite of abdominal wall with penetration into peritoneal cavity

Excludes1 superficial bite of abdominal wall (S30.861, S30.871)

● S31.650 Open bite of abdominal wall, right upper quadrant with penetration into peritoneal cavity A ⬮, D, S ⬮

● S31.651 Open bite of abdominal wall, left upper quadrant with penetration into peritoneal cavity A ⬮, D, S ⬮

● S31.652 Open bite of abdominal wall, epigastric region with penetration into peritoneal cavity A ⬮, D, S ⬮

● S31.653 Open bite of abdominal wall, right lower quadrant with penetration into peritoneal cavity A ⬮, D, S ⬮

● S31.654 Open bite of abdominal wall, left lower quadrant with penetration into peritoneal cavity A ⬮, D, S ⬮

● S31.655 Open bite of abdominal wall, periumbilic region with penetration into peritoneal cavity A ⬮, D, S ⬮

●■ S31.659 Open bite of abdominal wall, unspecified quadrant with penetration into peritoneal cavity A ⬮, D, S ⬮

- **S31.8 Open wound of other parts of abdomen, lower back and pelvis**
  - **S31.80 Open wound of unspecified buttock**
    - S31.801 Laceration without foreign body of unspecified buttock D, S
    - S31.802 Laceration with foreign body of unspecified buttock D, S
    - S31.803 Puncture wound without foreign body of unspecified buttock D, S
    - S31.804 Puncture wound with foreign body of unspecified buttock D, S
    - S31.805 Open bite of unspecified buttock D, S
      Bite of buttock NOS
      Excludes1 superficial bite of buttock (S30.870)
    - S31.809 Unspecified open wound of unspecified buttock D, S
  - **S31.81 Open wound of right buttock**
    - S31.811 Laceration without foreign body of right buttock D, S
    - S31.812 Laceration with foreign body of right buttock D, S
    - S31.813 Puncture wound without foreign body of right buttock D, S
    - S31.814 Puncture wound with foreign body of right buttock D, S
    - S31.815 Open bite of right buttock D, S
      Bite of right buttock NOS
      Excludes1 superficial bite of buttock (S30.870)
    - S31.819 Unspecified open wound of right buttock D, S
  - **S31.82 Open wound of left buttock**
    - S31.821 Laceration without foreign body of left buttock D, S
    - S31.822 Laceration with foreign body of left buttock D, S
    - S31.823 Puncture wound without foreign body of left buttock D, S
    - S31.824 Puncture wound with foreign body of left buttock D, S
    - S31.825 Open bite of left buttock D, S
      Bite of left buttock NOS
      Excludes1 superficial bite of buttock (S30.870)
    - S31.829 Unspecified open wound of left buttock D, S
  - **S31.83 Open wound of anus**
    - S31.831 Laceration without foreign body of anus D, S
    - S31.832 Laceration with foreign body of anus D, S
    - S31.833 Puncture wound without foreign body of anus D, S
    - S31.834 Puncture wound with foreign body of anus D, S
    - S31.835 Open bite of anus D, S
      Bite of anus NOS
      Excludes1 superficial bite of anus (S30.877)
    - S31.839 Unspecified open wound of anus

- **S32 Fracture of lumbar spine and pelvis**
  Note: A fracture not indicated as displaced or nondisplaced should be coded to displaced
  A fracture not indicated as opened or closed should be coded to closed
  Includes fracture of lumbosacral neural arch
  fracture of lumbosacral spinous process
  fracture of lumbosacral transverse process
  fracture of lumbosacral vertebra
  fracture of lumbosacral vertebral arch
  Code first any associated spinal cord and spinal nerve injury (S34-)
  Excludes1 transection of abdomen (S38.3)
  Excludes2 fracture of hip NOS (S72.0-)
  The appropriate 7th character is to be added to each code from category S32

A	initial encounter for closed fracture
B	initial encounter for open fracture
D	subsequent encounter for fracture with routine healing
G	subsequent encounter for fracture with delayed healing
K	subsequent encounter for fracture with nonunion
S	sequela

  - **S32.0 Fracture of lumbar vertebra**
    Fracture of lumbar spine NOS
    - **S32.00 Fracture of unspecified lumbar vertebra**
      - S32.000 Wedge compression fracture of unspecified lumbar vertebra A, K, B, D, G, S, A, B
      - S32.001 Stable burst fracture of unspecified lumbar vertebra A, K, B, D, G, S, A, B
      - S32.002 Unstable burst fracture of unspecified lumbar vertebra A, K, B, D, G, S, A, B
      - S32.008 Other fracture of unspecified lumbar vertebra A, K, B, D, G, S, A, B
      - S32.009 Unspecified fracture of unspecified lumbar vertebra A, K, B, D, G, S, A, B
    - **S32.01 Fracture of first lumbar vertebra**
      - S32.010 Wedge compression fracture of first lumbar vertebra A, K, B, D, G, S, A, B
      - S32.011 Stable burst fracture of first lumbar vertebra A, K, B, D, G, S, A, B
      - S32.012 Unstable burst fracture of first lumbar vertebra A, K, B, D, G, S, A, B
      - S32.018 Other fracture of first lumbar vertebra A, K, B, D, G, S, A, B
      - S32.019 Unspecified fracture of first lumbar vertebra A, K, B, D, G, S, A, B

CHAPTER 19 (S00-T88)

● **S32.02**   Fracture of second lumbar vertebra

   ● **S32.020**   Wedge compression fracture of second lumbar vertebra A, K 🅒, B 🅒, D, G, S 🅟, A, B 🅗

   ● **S32.021**   Stable burst fracture of second lumbar vertebra A, K 🅒, B 🅒, D, G, S 🅟, A, B 🅗

   ● **S32.022**   Unstable burst fracture of second lumbar vertebra A, K 🅒, B 🅒, D, G, S 🅟, A, B 🅗

   ● **S32.028**   Other fracture of second lumbar vertebra A, K 🅒, B 🅒, D, G, S 🅟, A, B 🅗

   ●◻ **S32.029**   Unspecified fracture of second lumbar vertebra A, K 🅒, B 🅒, D, G, S 🅟, A, B 🅗

● **S32.03**   Fracture of third lumbar vertebra

   ● **S32.030**   Wedge compression fracture of third lumbar vertebra A, K 🅒, B 🅒, D, G, S 🅟, A, B 🅗

   ● **S32.031**   Stable burst fracture of third lumbar vertebra A, K 🅒, B 🅒, D, G, S 🅟, A, B 🅗

   ● **S32.032**   Unstable burst fracture of third lumbar vertebra A, K 🅒, B 🅒, D, G, S 🅟, A, B 🅗

   ● **S32.038**   Other fracture of third lumbar vertebra A, K 🅒, B 🅒, D, G, S 🅟, A, B 🅗

   ●◻ **S32.039**   Unspecified fracture of third lumbar vertebra A, K 🅒, B 🅒, D, G, S 🅟, A, B 🅗

● **S32.04**   Fracture of fourth lumbar vertebra

   ● **S32.040**   Wedge compression fracture of fourth lumbar vertebra A, K 🅒, B 🅒, D, G, S 🅟, A, B 🅗

   ● **S32.041**   Stable burst fracture of fourth lumbar vertebra A, K 🅒, B 🅒, D, G, S 🅟, A, B 🅗

   ● **S32.042**   Unstable burst fracture of fourth lumbar vertebra A, K 🅒, B 🅒, D, G, S 🅟, A, B 🅗

   ● **S32.048**   Other fracture of fourth lumbar vertebra A, K 🅒, B 🅒, D, G, S 🅟, A, B 🅗

   ●◻ **S32.049**   Unspecified fracture of fourth lumbar vertebra A, K 🅒, B 🅒, D, G, S 🅟, A, B 🅗

● **S32.05**   Fracture of fifth lumbar vertebra

   ● **S32.050**   Wedge compression fracture of fifth lumbar vertebra A, K 🅒, B 🅒, D, G, S 🅟, A, B 🅗

   ● **S32.051**   Stable burst fracture of fifth lumbar vertebra A, K 🅒, B 🅒, D, G, S 🅟, A, B 🅗

   ● **S32.052**   Unstable burst fracture of fifth lumbar vertebra A, K 🅒, B 🅒, D, G, S 🅟, A, B 🅗

   ● **S32.058**   Other fracture of fifth lumbar vertebra A, K 🅒, B 🅒, D, G, S 🅟, A, B 🅗

   ●◻ **S32.059**   Unspecified fracture of fifth lumbar vertebra A, K 🅒, B 🅒, D, G, S 🅟, A, B 🅗

● **S32.1**   Fracture of sacrum

   For vertical fractures, code to most medial fracture extension

   Use two codes if both a vertical and transverse fracture are present

   Code also any associated fracture of pelvic ring (S32.8-)

   ●◻ **S32.10**   Unspecified fracture of sacrum A, K 🅒, B 🅒, D, G, S 🅟, A, B 🅗

   ● **S32.11**   Zone I fracture of sacrum

     Vertical sacral ala fracture of sacrum

     ● **S32.110**   Nondisplaced Zone I fracture of sacrum A, K 🅒, B 🅒, D, G, S 🅟, A, B 🅗

     ● **S32.111**   Minimally displaced Zone I fracture of sacrum A, K 🅒, B 🅒, D, G, S 🅟, A, B 🅗

     ● **S32.112**   Severely displaced Zone I fracture of sacrum A, K 🅒, B 🅒, D, G, S 🅟, A, B 🅗

     ●◻ **S32.119**   Unspecified Zone I fracture of sacrum A, K 🅒, B 🅒, D, G, S 🅟, A, B 🅗

   ● **S32.12**   Zone II fracture of sacrum

     Vertical foraminal region fracture of sacrum

     ● **S32.120**   Nondisplaced Zone II fracture of sacrum A, K 🅒, B 🅒, D, G, S 🅟, A, B 🅗

     ● **S32.121**   Minimally displaced Zone II fracture of sacrum A, K 🅒, B 🅒, D, G, S 🅟, A, B 🅗

     ● **S32.122**   Severely displaced Zone II fracture of sacrum A, K 🅒, B 🅒, D, G, S 🅟, A, B 🅗

     ●◻ **S32.129**   Unspecified Zone II fracture of sacrum A, K 🅒, B 🅒, D, G, S 🅟, A, B 🅗

   ● **S32.13**   Zone III fracture of sacrum

     Vertical fracture into spinal canal region of sacrum

     ● **S32.130**   Nondisplaced Zone III fracture of sacrum A, K 🅒, B 🅒, D, G, S 🅟, A, B 🅗

     ● **S32.131**   Minimally displaced Zone III fracture of sacrum A, K 🅒, B 🅒, D, G, S 🅟, A, B 🅗

     ● **S32.132**   Severely displaced Zone III fracture of sacrum A, K 🅒, B 🅒, D, G, S 🅟, A, B 🅗

     ●◻ **S32.139**   Unspecified Zone III fracture of sacrum A, K 🅒, B 🅒, D, G, S 🅟, A, B 🅗

   ● **S32.14**   Type 1 fracture of sacrum A, K 🅒, B 🅒, D, G, S 🅟, A, B 🅗

     Transverse flexion fracture of sacrum without displacement

   ● **S32.15**   Type 2 fracture of sacrum A, K 🅒, B 🅒, D, G, S 🅟, A, B 🅗

     Transverse flexion fracture of sacrum with posterior displacement

   ● **S32.16**   Type 3 fracture of sacrum A, K 🅒, B 🅒, D, G, S 🅟, A, B 🅗

     Transverse extension fracture of sacrum with anterior displacement

CHAPTER 19 (S00-T88)

N Newborn Age: 0   **P** Pediatric Age: 0–17   **M** Maternity DX: 12–55   **A** Adult Age: 15–124   ♀ Females Only   ♂ Males Only

🅒 Complication\Comorbidity   🅒 Major C\C   🅟 Present on Admission Requirement   🅗 Hospital-Acquired Condition

1439

CHAPTER 19 (S00-T88)

● S32.17   Type 4 fracture of sacrum A, K ✪, B ✪, D, G, S ✪, A, B ✪
Transverse segmental comminution of upper sacrum

● S32.19   Other fracture of sacrum A, K ✪, B ✪, D, G, S ✪, A, B ✪

● S32.2   Fracture of coccyx A, K ✪, B ✪, D, G, S ✪, A, B ✪

● S32.3   Fracture of ilium

Excludes1   fracture of ilium with associated disruption of pelvic ring (S32.8-)

● S32.30   Unspecified fracture of ilium

● ■ S32.301   Unspecified fracture of right ilium A, K ✪, B ✪, D, G, S ✪, A, B ✪

● ■ S32.302   Unspecified fracture of left ilium A, K ✪, B ✪, D, G, S ✪, A, B ✪

● ■ S32.309   Unspecified fracture of unspecified ilium A, K ✪, B ✪, D, G, S ✪, A, B ✪

● S32.31   Avulsion fracture of ilium

● S32.311   Displaced avulsion fracture of right ilium A, K ✪, B ✪, D, G, S ✪, A, B ✪

● S32.312   Displaced avulsion fracture of left ilium A, K ✪, B ✪, D, G, S ✪, A, B ✪

● S32.313   Displaced avulsion fracture of unspecified ilium A, K ✪, B ✪, D, G, S ✪, A, B ✪

● S32.314   Nondisplaced avulsion fracture of right ilium A, K ✪, B ✪, D, G, S ✪, A, B ✪

● S32.315   Nondisplaced avulsion fracture of left ilium A, K ✪, B ✪, D, G, S ✪, A, B ✪

● ■ S32.316   Nondisplaced avulsion fracture of unspecified ilium A, K ✪, B ✪, D, G, S ✪, A, B ✪

● S32.39   Other fracture of ilium

● S32.391   Other fracture of right ilium A, K ✪, B ✪, D, G, S ✪, A, B ✪

● S32.392   Other fracture of left ilium A, K ✪, B ✪, D, G, S ✪, A, B ✪

● S32.399   Other fracture of unspecified ilium A, K ✪, B ✪, D, G, S ✪, A, B ✪

● S32.4   Fracture of acetabulum

Code also any associated fracture of pelvic ring (S32.8-)

● S32.40   Unspecified fracture of acetabulum

● ■ S32.401   Unspecified fracture of right acetabulum K ✪, A, B ✪, D, G, S ✪, A, B ✪

● ■ S32.402   Unspecified fracture of left acetabulum K ✪, A, B ✪, D, G, S ✪, A, B ✪

● ■ S32.409   Unspecified fracture of unspecified acetabulum K ✪, A, B ✪, D, G, S ✪, A, B ✪

● S32.41   Fracture of anterior wall of acetabulum

● S32.411   Displaced fracture of anterior wall of right acetabulum K ✪, A, B ✪, D, G, S ✪, A, B ✪

● S32.412   Displaced fracture of anterior wall of left acetabulum K ✪, A, B ✪, D, G, S ✪, A, B ✪

● ■ S32.413   Displaced fracture of anterior wall of unspecified acetabulum K ✪, A, B ✪, D, G, S ✪, A, B ✪

● S32.414   Nondisplaced fracture of anterior wall of right acetabulum K ✪, A, B ✪, D, G, S ✪, A, B ✪

● S32.415   Nondisplaced fracture of anterior wall of left acetabulum K ✪, A, B ✪, D, G, S ✪, A, B ✪

● ■ S32.416   Nondisplaced fracture of anterior wall of unspecified acetabulum K ✪, A, B ✪, D, G, S ✪, A, B ✪

● S32.42   Fracture of posterior wall of acetabulum

● S32.421   Displaced fracture of posterior wall of right acetabulum K ✪, A, B ✪, D, G, S ✪, A, B ✪

● S32.422   Displaced fracture of posterior wall of left acetabulum K ✪, A, B ✪, D, G, S ✪, A, B ✪

● ■ S32.423   Displaced fracture of posterior wall of unspecified acetabulum K ✪, A, B ✪, D, G, S ✪, A, B ✪

● S32.424   Nondisplaced fracture of posterior wall of right acetabulum K ✪, A, B ✪, D, G, S ✪, A, B ✪

● S32.425   Nondisplaced fracture of posterior wall of left acetabulum K ✪, A, B ✪, D, G, S ✪, A, B ✪

● ■ S32.426   Nondisplaced fracture of posterior wall of unspecified acetabulum K ✪, A, B ✪, D, G, S ✪, A, B ✪

● S32.43   Fracture of anterior column [iliopubic] of acetabulum

● S32.431   Displaced fracture of anterior column [iliopubic] of right acetabulum K ✪, A, B ✪, D, G, S ✪, A, B ✪

● S32.432   Displaced fracture of anterior column [iliopubic] of left acetabulum K ✪, A, B ✪, D, G, S ✪, A, B ✪

● ■ S32.433   Displaced fracture of anterior column [iliopubic] of unspecified acetabulum K ✪, A, B ✪, D, G, S ✪, A, B ✪

● S32.434   Nondisplaced fracture of anterior column [iliopubic] of right acetabulum K ✪, A, B ✪, D, G, S ✪, A, B ✪

● S32.435   Nondisplaced fracture of anterior column [iliopubic] of left acetabulum K ✪, A, B ✪, D, G, S ✪, A, B ✪

● ■ S32.436   Nondisplaced fracture of anterior column [iliopubic] of unspecified acetabulum K ✪, A, B ✪, D, G, S ✪, A, B ✪

● Unacceptable Principal Diagnosis   ● Use Additional Character(s)   ■ Unspecified   ▶ Manifestation Code
OGCR   Official Guidelines for Coding and Reporting   Excludes 1   Excludes 2   Includes   Use additional   Code first   Code also

● S32.44   **Fracture of posterior column [ilioischial] of acetabulum**

     ● S32.441   Displaced fracture of posterior column [ilioischial] of right acetabulum K 🦴, A, B 🦴, D, G, S 🦴, A, B 🦴

     ● S32.442   Displaced fracture of posterior column [ilioischial] of left acetabulum K 🦴, A, B 🦴, D, G, S 🦴, A, B 🦴

     ●◼ S32.443   Displaced fracture of posterior column [ilioischial] of unspecified acetabulum K 🦴, A, B 🦴, D, G, S 🦴, A, B 🦴

     ● S32.444   Nondisplaced fracture of posterior column [ilioischial] of right acetabulum K 🦴, A, B 🦴, D, G, S 🦴, A, B 🦴

     ● S32.445   Nondisplaced fracture of posterior column [ilioischial] of left acetabulum K 🦴, A, B 🦴, D, G, S 🦴, A, B 🦴

     ●◼ S32.446   Nondisplaced fracture of posterior column [ilioischial] of unspecified acetabulum K 🦴, A, B 🦴, D, G, S 🦴, A, B 🦴

● S32.45   **Transverse fracture of acetabulum**

     ● S32.451   Displaced transverse fracture of right acetabulum K 🦴, A, B 🦴, D, G, S 🦴, A, B 🦴

     ● S32.452   Displaced transverse fracture of left acetabulum K 🦴, A, B 🦴, D, G, S 🦴, A, B 🦴

     ●◼ S32.453   Displaced transverse fracture of unspecified acetabulum K 🦴, A, B 🦴, D, G, S 🦴, A, B 🦴

     ● S32.454   Nondisplaced transverse fracture of right acetabulum K 🦴, A, B 🦴, D, G, S 🦴, A, B 🦴

     ● S32.455   Nondisplaced transverse fracture of left acetabulum K 🦴, A, B 🦴, D, G, S 🦴, A, B 🦴

     ●◼ S32.456   Nondisplaced transverse fracture of unspecified acetabulum K 🦴, A, B 🦴, D, G, S 🦴, A, B 🦴

● S32.46   **Associated transverse-posterior fracture of acetabulum**

     ● S32.461   Displaced associated transverse-posterior fracture of right acetabulum K 🦴, A, B 🦴, D, G, S 🦴, A, B 🦴

     ● S32.462   Displaced associated transverse-posterior fracture of left acetabulum K 🦴, A, B 🦴, D, G, S 🦴, A, B 🦴

     ●◼ S32.463   Displaced associated transverse-posterior fracture of unspecified acetabulum K 🦴, A, B 🦴, D, G, S 🦴, A, B 🦴

     ● S32.464   Nondisplaced associated transverse-posterior fracture of right acetabulum K 🦴, A, B 🦴, D, G, S 🦴, A, B 🦴

     ● S32.465   Nondisplaced associated transverse-posterior fracture of left acetabulum K 🦴, A, B 🦴, D, G, S 🦴, A, B 🦴

     ●◼ S32.466   Nondisplaced associated transverse-posterior fracture of unspecified acetabulum K 🦴, A, B 🦴, D, G, S 🦴, A, B 🦴

● S32.47   **Fracture of medial wall of acetabulum**

     ● S32.471   Displaced fracture of medial wall of right acetabulum K 🦴, A, B 🦴, D, G, S 🦴, A, B 🦴

     ● S32.472   Displaced fracture of medial wall of left acetabulum K 🦴, A, B 🦴, D, G, S 🦴, A, B 🦴

     ●◼ S32.473   Displaced fracture of medial wall of unspecified acetabulum K 🦴, A, B 🦴, D, G, S 🦴, A, B 🦴

     ● S32.474   Nondisplaced fracture of medial wall of right acetabulum K 🦴, A, B 🦴, D, G, S 🦴, A, B 🦴

     ● S32.475   Nondisplaced fracture of medial wall of left acetabulum K 🦴, A, B 🦴, D, G, S 🦴, A, B 🦴

     ●◼ S32.476   Nondisplaced fracture of medial wall of unspecified acetabulum K 🦴, A, B 🦴, D, G, S 🦴, A, B 🦴

● S32.48   **Dome fracture of acetabulum**

     ● S32.481   Displaced dome fracture of right acetabulum K 🦴, A, B 🦴, D, G, S 🦴, A, B 🦴

     ● S32.482   Displaced dome fracture of left acetabulum K 🦴, A, B 🦴, D, G, S 🦴, A, B 🦴

     ●◼ S32.483   Displaced dome fracture of unspecified acetabulum K 🦴, A, B 🦴, D, G, S 🦴, A, B 🦴

     ● S32.484   Nondisplaced dome fracture of right acetabulum K 🦴, A, B 🦴, D, G, S 🦴, A, B 🦴

     ● S32.485   Nondisplaced dome fracture of left acetabulum K 🦴, A, B 🦴, D, G, S 🦴, A, B 🦴

     ●◼ S32.486   Nondisplaced dome fracture of unspecified acetabulum K 🦴, A, B 🦴, D, G, S 🦴, A, B 🦴

● S32.49   **Other fracture of acetabulum**

     ● S32.491   Other fracture of right acetabulum K 🦴, A, B 🦴, D, G, S 🦴, A, B 🦴

     ● S32.492   Other fracture of left acetabulum K 🦴, A, B 🦴, D, G, S 🦴, A, B 🦴

     ●◼ S32.499   Other fracture of unspecified acetabulum K 🦴, A, B 🦴, D, G, S 🦴, A, B 🦴

● S32.5   **Fracture of pubis**

     | Excludes1 | fracture of pubis with associated disruption of pelvic ring (S32.8-)

● S32.50   **Unspecified fracture of pubis**

     ●◼ S32.501   Unspecified fracture of right pubis A, K 🦴, B 🦴, D, G, S 🦴, A, B 🦴

     ●◼ S32.502   Unspecified fracture of left pubis A, K 🦴, B 🦴, D, G, S 🦴, A, B 🦴

     ●◼ S32.509   Unspecified fracture of unspecified pubis A, K 🦴, B 🦴, D, G, S 🦴, A, B 🦴

N Newborn Age: 0   **P** Pediatric Age: 0–17   **M** Maternity DX: 12–55   **A** Adult Age: 15–124   ♀ Females Only   ♂ Males Only

🦴 Complication\Comorbidity   🦴 Major C\C   🦴 Present on Admission Requirement   🦴 Hospital-Acquired Condition

1441

CHAPTER 19 (S00–T88)

● **S32.51**   **Fracture of superior rim of pubis**
- ● **S32.511**   **Fracture of superior rim of right pubis** A, K 🔒, B 🔒, D, G, S 🔒, B 🔒
- ● **S32.512**   **Fracture of superior rim of left pubis** A, K 🔒, B 🔒, D, G, S 🔒, B 🔒
- ●◼ **S32.519**   **Fracture of superior rim of unspecified pubis** A, K 🔒, B 🔒, D, G, S 🔒, B 🔒

● **S32.59**   **Other specified fracture of pubis**
- ● **S32.591**   **Other specified fracture of right pubis** A, K 🔒, B 🔒, D, G, S 🔒, B 🔒
- ● **S32.592**   **Other specified fracture of left pubis** A, K 🔒, B 🔒, D, G, S 🔒, B 🔒
- ●◼ **S32.599**   **Other specified fracture of unspecified pubis** A, K 🔒, B 🔒, D, G, S 🔒, B 🔒

● **S32.6**   **Fracture of ischium**

> **Excludes1**   fracture of ischium with associated disruption of pelvic ring (S32.8-)

● **S32.60**   **Unspecified fracture of ischium**
- ●◼ **S32.601**   **Unspecified fracture of right ischium** A, K 🔒, B 🔒, D, G, S 🔒, A, B 🔒
- ●◼ **S32.602**   **Unspecified fracture of left ischium** A, K 🔒, B 🔒, D, G, S 🔒, A, B 🔒
- ●◼ **S32.609**   **Unspecified fracture of unspecified ischium** A, K 🔒, B 🔒, D, G, S 🔒, A, B 🔒

● **S32.61**   **Avulsion fracture of ischium**
- ● **S32.611**   **Displaced avulsion fracture of right ischium** A, K 🔒, B 🔒, D, G, S 🔒, A, B 🔒
- ● **S32.612**   **Displaced avulsion fracture of left ischium** A, K 🔒, B 🔒, D, G, S 🔒, A, B 🔒
- ●◼ **S32.613**   **Displaced avulsion fracture of unspecified ischium** A, K 🔒, B 🔒, D, G, S 🔒, A, B 🔒
- ● **S32.614**   **Nondisplaced avulsion fracture of right ischium** A, K 🔒, B 🔒, D, G, S 🔒, A, B 🔒
- ● **S32.615**   **Nondisplaced avulsion fracture of left ischium** A, K 🔒, B 🔒, D, G, S 🔒, A, B 🔒
- ●◼ **S32.616**   **Nondisplaced avulsion fracture of unspecified ischium** A, K 🔒, B 🔒, D, G, S 🔒, A, B 🔒

● **S32.69**   **Other specified fracture of ischium**
- ● **S32.691**   **Other specified fracture of right ischium** A, K 🔒, B 🔒, D, G, S 🔒, A, B 🔒
- ● **S32.692**   **Other specified fracture of left ischium** A, K 🔒, B 🔒, D, G, S 🔒, A, B 🔒
- ●◼ **S32.699**   **Other specified fracture of unspecified ischium** A, K 🔒, B 🔒, D, G, S 🔒, A, B 🔒

● **S32.8**   **Fracture of other parts of pelvis**

> Code also any associated:
> fracture of acetabulum (S32.4-)
> sacral fracture (S32.1-)

● **S32.81**   **Multiple fractures of pelvis with disruption of pelvic ring**
> Multiple pelvic fractures with disruption of pelvic circle
- ● **S32.810**   **Multiple fractures of pelvis with stable disruption of pelvic ring** A, K 🔒, B 🔒, D, G, S 🔒, A, B 🔒
- ● **S32.811**   **Multiple fractures of pelvis with unstable disruption of pelvic ring** A, K 🔒, B 🔒, D, G, S 🔒, A, B 🔒

● **S32.82**   **Multiple fractures of pelvis without disruption of pelvic ring**
> Multiple pelvic fractures without disruption of pelvic circle

● **S32.89**   **Fracture of other parts of pelvis** A, K 🔒, B 🔒, D, G, S 🔒, A, B 🔒

●◼ **S32.9**   **Fracture of unspecified parts of lumbosacral spine and pelvis** A, K 🔒, B 🔒, D, G, S 🔒, A, B 🔒
> Fracture of lumbosacral spine NOS
> Fracture of pelvis NOS

● **S33**   **Dislocation and sprain of joints and ligaments of lumbar spine and pelvis**

> **Includes**   avulsion of joint or ligament of lumbar spine and pelvis
> laceration of cartilage, joint or ligament of lumbar spine and pelvis
> sprain of cartilage, joint or ligament of lumbar spine and pelvis
> traumatic hemarthrosis of joint or ligament of lumbar spine and pelvis
> traumatic rupture of joint or ligament of lumbar spine and pelvis
> traumatic subluxation of joint or ligament of lumbar spine and pelvis
> traumatic tear of joint or ligament of lumbar spine and pelvis

> Code also any associated open wound

> **Excludes1**   nontraumatic rupture or displacement of lumbar intervertebral disc NOS (M51.-)
> obstetric damage to pelvic joints and ligaments (O71.6)

> **Excludes2**   dislocation and sprain of joints and ligaments of hip (S73.-)
> strain of muscle of lower back and pelvis (S39.01-)

The appropriate 7th character is to be added to each code from category S33

A	initial encounter
D	subsequent encounter
S	sequela

● **S33.0**   **Traumatic rupture of lumbar intervertebral disc** D, S 🔒

> **Excludes1**   rupture or displacement (nontraumatic) of lumbar intervertebral disc NOS (M51.- with fifth character 6)

● Unacceptable Principal Diagnosis   ● Use Additional Character(s)   ◼ Unspecified   ▸ Manifestation Code

OGCR Official Guidelines for Coding and Reporting   Excludes 1   Excludes 2   Includes   Use additional   Code first   Code also

● **S33.1   Subluxation and dislocation of lumbar vertebra**

Code also any associated:
    open wound of abdomen, lower back and pelvis
      (S31)
    spinal cord injury (S24.0, S24.1-, S34.0-, S34.1-)

Excludes2   fracture of lumbar vertebrae (S32.0-)

● **S33.10   Subluxation and dislocation of unspecified lumbar vertebra**

     ●▪ **S33.100   Subluxation of unspecified lumbar vertebra** D, S 🖾

     ●▪ **S33.101   Dislocation of unspecified lumbar vertebra** D, S 🖾

● **S33.11   Subluxation and dislocation of L₁/L₂ lumbar vertebra**

     ● **S33.110   Subluxation of L₁/L₂ lumbar vertebra** D, S 🖾

     ● **S33.111   Dislocation of L₁/L₂ lumbar vertebra** D, S 🖾

● **S33.12   Subluxation and dislocation of L₂/L₃ lumbar vertebra**

     ● **S33.120   Subluxation of L₂/L₃ lumbar vertebra** D, S 🖾

     ● **S33.121   Dislocation of L₂/L₃ lumbar vertebra** D, S 🖾

● **S33.13   Subluxation and dislocation of L₃/L₄ lumbar vertebra**

     ● **S33.130   Subluxation of L₃/L₄ lumbar vertebra** D, S 🖾

     ● **S33.131   Dislocation of L₃/L₄ lumbar vertebra** D, S 🖾

● **S33.14   Subluxation and dislocation of L₄/L₅ lumbar vertebra**

     ● **S33.140   Subluxation of L₄/L₅ lumbar vertebra** D, S 🖾

     ● **S33.141   Dislocation of L₄/L₅ lumbar vertebra** D, S 🖾

● **S33.2   Dislocation of sacroiliac and sacrococcygeal joint** D, S 🖾

● **S33.3   Dislocation of other and unspecified parts of lumbar spine and pelvis**

     ●▪ **S33.30   Dislocation of unspecified parts of lumbar spine and pelvis** D, S 🖾

     ●▪ **S33.39   Dislocation of other parts of lumbar spine and pelvis** D, S 🖾

● **S33.4   Traumatic rupture of symphysis pubis** D, S 🖾

● **S33.5   Sprain of ligaments of lumbar spine** D, S 🖾

● **S33.6   Sprain of sacroiliac joint** D, S 🖾

● **S33.8   Sprain of other parts of lumbar spine and pelvis** D, S 🖾

●▪ **S33.9   Sprain of unspecified parts of lumbar spine and pelvis** D, S 🖾

● **S34   Injury of lumbar and sacral spinal cord and nerves at abdomen, lower back and pelvis level**

Note: Code to highest level of lumbar cord injury

The appropriate 7th character is to be added to each code from category S34

A	initial encounter
D	subsequent encounter
S	sequela

Code also any associated:
    fracture of vertebra (S22.0-, S32.0-)
    open wound of abdomen, lower back and pelvis (S31.-)
    transient paralysis (R29.5)

● **S34.0   Concussion and edema of lumbar and sacral spinal cord**

     ● **S34.01   Concussion and edema of lumbar spinal cord** A 🖾

     ● **S34.02   Concussion and edema of sacral spinal cord** A 🖾
        Concussion and edema of conus medullaris

● **S34.1   Other and unspecified injury of lumbar and sacral spinal cord**

     ● **S34.10   Unspecified injury to lumbar spinal cord**

        ●▪ **S34.101   Unspecified injury to L₁ level of lumbar spinal cord** A 🖾, D, S 🖾, A 🖾

        ●▪ **S34.102   Unspecified injury to L₂ level of lumbar spinal cord** A 🖾, D, S 🖾, A 🖾

        ●▪ **S34.103   Unspecified injury to L₃ level of lumbar spinal cord** A 🖾, D, S 🖾, A 🖾

        ●▪ **S34.104   Unspecified injury to L₄ level of lumbar spinal cord** A 🖾, D, S 🖾, A 🖾

        ●▪ **S34.105   Unspecified injury to L₅ level of lumbar spinal cord** A 🖾, D, S 🖾, A 🖾

        ●▪ **S34.109   Unspecified injury to unspecified level of lumbar spinal cord** A 🖾, D, S 🖾, A 🖾

     ● **S34.11   Complete lesion of lumbar spinal cord**

        ● **S34.111   Complete lesion of L₁ level of lumbar spinal cord** A 🖾, D, S 🖾, A 🖾

        ● **S34.112   Complete lesion of L₂ level of lumbar spinal cord** A 🖾, D, S 🖾, A 🖾

        ● **S34.113   Complete lesion of L₃ level of lumbar spinal cord** A 🖾, D, S 🖾, A 🖾

        ● **S34.114   Complete lesion of L₄ level of lumbar spinal cord** A 🖾, D, S 🖾, A 🖾

        ● **S34.115   Complete lesion of L₅ level of lumbar spinal cord** A 🖾, D, S 🖾, A 🖾

        ●▪ **S34.119   Complete lesion of unspecified level of lumbar spinal cord** A 🖾, D, S 🖾, A 🖾

CHAPTER 19 (S00-T88)

● **S34.12 Incomplete lesion of lumbar spinal cord**

     ● **S34.121 Incomplete lesion of L₁ level of lumbar spinal cord** A ☖, D, S ☖, A ☖

     ● **S34.122 Incomplete lesion of L₂ level of lumbar spinal cord** A ☖, D, S ☖, A ☖

     ● **S34.123 Incomplete lesion of L₃ level of lumbar spinal cord** A ☖, D, S ☖, A ☖

     ● **S34.124 Incomplete lesion of L₄ level of lumbar spinal cord** A ☖, D, S ☖, A ☖

     ● **S34.125 Incomplete lesion of L₅ level of lumbar spinal cord** A ☖, D, S ☖, A ☖

     ●■ **S34.129 Incomplete lesion of unspecified level of lumbar spinal cord** A ☖, D, S ☖, A ☖

● **S34.13 Other and unspecified injury to sacral spinal cord**
     Other injury to conus medullaris

     ● **S34.131 Complete lesion of sacral spinal cord** A ☖, D, S ☖, A ☖
         Complete lesion of conus medullaris

     ● **S34.132 Incomplete lesion of sacral spinal cord** A ☖, D, S ☖, A ☖
         Incomplete lesion of conus medullaris

     ●■ **S34.139 Unspecified injury to sacral spinal cord** A ☖, D, S ☖, A ☖
         Unspecified injury of conus medullaris

● **S34.2 Injury of nerve root of lumbar and sacral spine**

     ● **S34.21 Injury of nerve root of lumbar spine** D, S ☖

     ● **S34.22 Injury of nerve root of sacral spine** D, S ☖

● **S34.3 Injury of cauda equina** A ☖, D, S ☖, A ☖

● **S34.4 Injury of lumbosacral plexus** D, S ☖

● **S34.5 Injury of lumbar, sacral and pelvic sympathetic nerves** D, S ☖
     Injury of celiac ganglion or plexus
     Injury of hypogastric plexus
     Injury of mesenteric plexus (inferior) (superior)
     Injury of splanchnic nerve

● **S34.6 Injury of peripheral nerve(s) at abdomen, lower back and pelvis level** D, S ☖

● **S34.8 Injury of other nerves at abdomen, lower back and pelvis level** D, S ☖

●■ **S34.9 Injury of unspecified nerves at abdomen, lower back and pelvis level** D, S ☖

● **S35 Injury of blood vessels at abdomen, lower back and pelvis level**

     The appropriate 7th character is to be added to each code from category S35

A	initial encounter
D	subsequent encounter
S	sequela

     Code also any associated open wound (S31.-)

● **S35.0 Injury of abdominal aorta**
     Excludes1 injury of aorta NOS (S25.0)

     ●■ **S35.00 Unspecified injury of abdominal aorta** A ☖, D, S ☖

● **S35.01 Minor laceration of abdominal aorta** A ☖, D, S ☖
     Incomplete transection of abdominal aorta
     Laceration of abdominal aorta NOS
     Superficial laceration of abdominal aorta

● **S35.02 Major laceration of abdominal aorta** A ☖, D, S ☖
     Complete transection of abdominal aorta
     Traumatic rupture of abdominal aorta

● **S35.09 Other injury of abdominal aorta** A ☖, D, S ☖

● **S35.1 Injury of inferior vena cava**
     Injury of hepatic vein
     Excludes1 injury of vena cava NOS (S25.2)

     ●■ **S35.10 Unspecified injury of inferior vena cava** A ☖, D, S ☖

     ● **S35.11 Minor laceration of inferior vena cava** A ☖, D, S ☖
         Incomplete transection of inferior vena cava
         Laceration of inferior vena cava NOS
         Superficial laceration of inferior vena cava

     ● **S35.12 Major laceration of inferior vena cava** A ☖, D, S ☖
         Complete transection of inferior vena cava
         Traumatic rupture of inferior vena cava

     ● **S35.19 Other injury of inferior vena cava** A ☖, D, S ☖

● **S35.2 Injury of celiac or mesenteric artery and branches**

     ● **S35.21 Injury of celiac artery**

         ● **S35.211 Minor laceration of celiac artery** A ☖, D, S ☖
             Incomplete transection of celiac artery
             Laceration of celiac artery NOS
             Superficial laceration of celiac artery

         ● **S35.212 Major laceration of celiac artery** A ☖, D, S ☖
             Complete transection of celiac artery
             Traumatic rupture of celiac artery

         ● **S35.218 Other injury of celiac artery** A ☖, D, S ☖

         ●■ **S35.219 Unspecified injury of celiac artery** A ☖, D, S ☖

     ● **S35.22 Injury of superior mesenteric artery**

         ● **S35.221 Minor laceration of superior mesenteric artery** A ☖, D, S ☖
             Incomplete transection of superior mesenteric artery
             Laceration of superior mesenteric artery NOS
             Superficial laceration of superior mesenteric artery

         ● **S35.222 Major laceration of superior mesenteric artery** A ☖, D, S ☖
             Complete transection of superior mesenteric artery
             Traumatic rupture of superior mesenteric artery

         ● **S35.228 Other injury of superior mesenteric artery** A ☖, D, S ☖

         ●■ **S35.229 Unspecified injury of superior mesenteric artery** A ☖, D, S ☖

● **S35.23**   **Injury of inferior mesenteric artery**

    ● **S35.231**   **Minor laceration of inferior mesenteric artery** A 🪙, D, S 🪙

       Incomplete transection of inferior mesenteric artery

       Laceration of inferior mesenteric artery NOS

       Superficial laceration of inferior mesenteric artery

    ● **S35.232**   **Major laceration of inferior mesenteric artery** A 🪙, D, S 🪙

       Complete transection of inferior mesenteric artery

       Traumatic rupture of inferior mesenteric artery

    ● **S35.238**   **Other injury of inferior mesenteric artery** A 🪙, D, S 🪙

    ●🔲 **S35.239**   **Unspecified injury of inferior mesenteric artery** A 🪙, D, S 🪙

● **S35.29**   **Injury of branches of celiac and mesenteric artery**

       Injury of gastric artery

       Injury of gastroduodenal artery

       Injury of hepatic artery

       Injury of splenic artery

    ● **S35.291**   **Minor laceration of branches of celiac and mesenteric artery** A 🪙, D, S 🪙

       Incomplete transection of branches of celiac and mesenteric artery

       Laceration of branches of celiac and mesenteric artery NOS

       Superficial laceration of branches of celiac and mesenteric artery

    ● **S35.292**   **Major laceration of branches of celiac and mesenteric artery** A 🪙, D, S 🪙

       Complete transection of branches of celiac and mesenteric artery

       Traumatic rupture of branches of celiac and mesenteric artery

    ● **S35.298**   **Other injury of branches of celiac and mesenteric artery** A 🪙, D, S 🪙

    ●🔲 **S35.299**   **Unspecified injury of branches of celiac and mesenteric artery** A 🪙, D, S 🪙

● **S35.3**   **Injury of portal or splenic vein and branches**

   ● **S35.31**   **Injury of portal vein**

    ● **S35.311**   **Laceration of portal vein** A 🪙, D, S 🪙

    ● **S35.318**   **Other specified injury of portal vein** A 🪙, D, S 🪙

    ●🔲 **S35.319**   **Unspecified injury of portal vein** A 🪙, D, S 🪙

   ● **S35.32**   **Injury of splenic vein**

    ● **S35.321**   **Laceration of splenic vein** A 🪙, D, S 🪙

    ● **S35.328**   **Other specified injury of splenic vein** A 🪙, D, S 🪙

    ●🔲 **S35.329**   **Unspecified injury of splenic vein** A 🪙, D, S 🪙

● **S35.33**   **Injury of superior mesenteric vein**

    ● **S35.331**   **Laceration of superior mesenteric vein** A 🪙, D, S 🪙

    ● **S35.338**   **Other specified injury of superior mesenteric vein** A 🪙, D, S 🪙

    ●🔲 **S35.339**   **Unspecified injury of superior mesenteric vein** A 🪙, D, S 🪙

● **S35.34**   **Injury of inferior mesenteric vein**

    ● **S35.341**   **Laceration of inferior mesenteric vein** A 🪙, D, S 🪙

    ● **S35.348**   **Other specified injury of inferior mesenteric vein** A 🪙, D, S 🪙

    ●🔲 **S35.349**   **Unspecified injury of inferior mesenteric vein** A 🪙, D, S 🪙

● **S35.4**   **Injury of renal blood vessels**

   ● **S35.40**   **Unspecified injury of renal blood vessel**

    ●🔲 **S35.401**   **Unspecified injury of right renal artery** A 🪙, D, S 🪙

    ●🔲 **S35.402**   **Unspecified injury of left renal artery** A 🪙, D, S 🪙

    ●🔲 **S35.403**   **Unspecified injury of unspecified renal artery** A 🪙, D, S 🪙

    ●🔲 **S35.404**   **Unspecified injury of right renal vein** A 🪙, D, S 🪙

    ●🔲 **S35.405**   **Unspecified injury of left renal vein** A 🪙, D, S 🪙

    ●🔲 **S35.406**   **Unspecified injury of unspecified renal vein** A 🪙, D, S 🪙

   ● **S35.41**   **Laceration of renal blood vessel**

    ● **S35.411**   **Laceration of right renal artery** A 🪙, D, S 🪙

    ● **S35.412**   **Laceration of left renal artery** A 🪙, D, S 🪙

    ●🔲 **S35.413**   **Laceration of unspecified renal artery** A 🪙, D, S 🪙

    ● **S35.414**   **Laceration of right renal vein** A 🪙, D, S 🪙

    ● **S35.415**   **Laceration of left renal vein** A 🪙, D, S 🪙

    ●🔲 **S35.416**   **Laceration of unspecified renal vein** A 🪙, D, S 🪙

   ● **S35.49**   **Other specified injury of renal blood vessel**

    ● **S35.491**   **Other specified injury of right renal artery** A 🪙, D, S 🪙

    ● **S35.492**   **Other specified injury of left renal artery** A 🪙, D, S 🪙

    ●🔲 **S35.493**   **Other specified injury of unspecified renal artery** A 🪙, D, S 🪙

    ● **S35.494**   **Other specified injury of right renal vein** A 🪙, D, S 🪙

    ● **S35.495**   **Other specified injury of left renal vein** A 🪙, D, S 🪙

    ●🔲 **S35.496**   **Other specified injury of unspecified renal vein** A 🪙, D, S 🪙

CHAPTER 19 (S00-T88)

N   Newborn Age: 0   P   Pediatric Age: 0–17   M   Maternity DX: 12–55   A   Adult Age: 15–124   ♀   Females Only   ♂   Males Only

🪙   Complication\Comorbidity   🪙   Major C\C   🪙   Present on Admission Requirement   🪙   Hospital-Acquired Condition

● **S35.5 Injury of iliac blood vessels**

●■ **S35.50 Injury of unspecified iliac blood vessel(s)**
A 🗪, D, S 🗪

● **S35.51 Injury of iliac artery or vein**
Injury of hypogastric artery or vein

● **S35.511 Injury of right iliac artery** A 🗪, D, S 🗪

● **S35.512 Injury of left iliac artery** A 🗪, D, S 🗪

●■ **S35.513 Injury of unspecified iliac artery** A 🗪, D, S 🗪

● **S35.514 Injury of right iliac vein** A 🗪, D, S 🗪

● **S35.515 Injury of left iliac vein** A 🗪, D, S 🗪

●■ **S35.516 Injury of unspecified iliac vein** A 🗪, D, S 🗪

● **S35.53 Injury of uterine artery or vein**

● **S35.531 Injury of right uterine artery** A 🗪, D, S 🗪

● **S35.532 Injury of left uterine artery** A 🗪, D, S 🗪

●■ **S35.533 Injury of unspecified uterine artery** A 🗪, D, S 🗪

● **S35.534 Injury of right uterine vein** A 🗪, D, S 🗪

● **S35.535 Injury of left uterine vein** A 🗪, D, S 🗪

●■ **S35.536 Injury of unspecified uterine vein** A 🗪, D, S 🗪

● **S35.59 Injury of other iliac blood vessels** A 🗪, D, S 🗪

● **S35.8 Injury of other blood vessels at abdomen, lower back and pelvis level**
Injury of ovarian artery or vein

● **S35.8X Injury of other blood vessels at abdomen, lower back and pelvis level**

● **S35.8X1 Laceration of other blood vessels at abdomen, lower back and pelvis level** A 🗪, D, S 🗪

● **S35.8X8 Other specified injury of other blood vessels at abdomen, lower back and pelvis level** A 🗪, D, S 🗪

●■ **S35.8X9 Unspecified injury of other blood vessels at abdomen, lower back and pelvis level** A 🗪, D, S 🗪

● **S35.9 Injury of unspecified blood vessel at abdomen, lower back and pelvis level**

●■ **S35.90 Unspecified injury of unspecified blood vessel at abdomen, lower back and pelvis level** A 🗪, D, S 🗪

●■ **S35.91 Laceration of unspecified blood vessel at abdomen, lower back and pelvis level** A 🗪, D, S 🗪

●■ **S35.99 Other specified injury of unspecified blood vessel at abdomen, lower back and pelvis level** A 🗪, D, S 🗪

● **S36 Injury of intra-abdominal organs**
The appropriate 7th character is to be added to each code from category S36

A	initial encounter
D	subsequent encounter
S	sequela

Code also any associated open wound (S31.-)

● **S36.0 Injury of spleen**

●■ **S36.00 Unspecified injury of spleen** A 🗪, D, S 🗪

● **S36.02 Contusion of spleen**

● **S36.020 Minor contusion of spleen** A 🗪, D, S 🗪
Contusion of spleen less than 2 cm

● **S36.021 Major contusion of spleen** A 🗪, D, S 🗪
Contusion of spleen greater than 2 cm

●■ **S36.029 Unspecified contusion of spleen** A 🗪, D, S 🗪

● **S36.03 Laceration of spleen**

● **S36.030 Superficial (capsular) laceration of spleen** A 🗪, D, S 🗪
Laceration of spleen less than 1 cm
Minor laceration of spleen

● **S36.031 Moderate laceration of spleen** A 🗪, D, S 🗪
Laceration of spleen 1 to 3 cm

● **S36.032 Major laceration of spleen** A 🗪, D, S 🗪
Avulsion of spleen
Laceration of spleen greater than 3 cm
Massive laceration of spleen
Multiple moderate lacerations of spleen
Stellate laceration of spleen

●■ **S36.039 Unspecified laceration of spleen** A 🗪, D, S 🗪

● **S36.09 Other injury of spleen** A 🗪, D, S 🗪

● **S36.1 Injury of liver and gallbladder and bile duct**

● **S36.11 Injury of liver**

●■ **S36.112 Contusion of liver** A 🗪, D, S 🗪

●■ **S36.113 Laceration of liver, unspecified degree** A 🗪, D, S 🗪

● **S36.114 Minor laceration of liver** A 🗪, D, S 🗪
Laceration involving capsule only, or, without significant involvement of hepatic parenchyma [i.e., less than 1 cm deep]

● **S36.115 Moderate laceration of liver** A 🗪, D, S 🗪
Laceration involving parenchyma but without major disruption of parenchyma [i.e., less than 10 cm long and less than 3 cm deep]

CHAPTER 19 (S00-T88)

● **S36.116**   Major laceration of liver A 🦠, D, S 🦠
> Laceration with significant disruption of hepatic parenchyma [i.e., greater than 10 cm long and 3 cm deep]
> Multiple moderate lacerations, with or without hematoma
> Stellate laceration of liver

● **S36.118**   Other injury of liver A 🦠, D, S 🦠

●■ **S36.119**   Unspecified injury of liver A 🦠, D, S 🦠

● **S36.12**   Injury of gallbladder

   ● **S36.122**   Contusion of gallbladder A 🦠, D, S 🦠

   ● **S36.123**   Laceration of gallbladder A 🦠, D, S 🦠

   ● **S36.128**   Other injury of gallbladder A 🦠, D, S 🦠

   ●■ **S36.129**   Unspecified injury of gallbladder A 🦠, D, S 🦠

● **S36.13**   Injury of bile duct A 🦠, D, S 🦠

● **S36.2**   Injury of pancreas

   S36.20   Unspecified injury of pancreas

     ●■ **S36.200**   Unspecified injury of head of pancreas A 🦠, D, S 🦠

     ●■ **S36.201**   Unspecified injury of body of pancreas A 🦠, D, S 🦠

     ●■ **S36.202**   Unspecified injury of tail of pancreas A 🦠, D, S 🦠

     ●■ **S36.209**   Unspecified injury of unspecified part of pancreas A 🦠, D, S 🦠

   ● **S36.22**   Contusion of pancreas

     ● **S36.220**   Contusion of head of pancreas A 🦠, D, S 🦠

     ● **S36.221**   Contusion of body of pancreas A 🦠, D, S 🦠

     ● **S36.222**   Contusion of tail of pancreas A 🦠, D, S 🦠

     ●■ **S36.229**   Contusion of unspecified part of pancreas A 🦠, D, S 🦠

   ● **S36.23**   Laceration of pancreas, unspecified degree

     ●■ **S36.230**   Laceration of head of pancreas, unspecified degree A 🦠, D, S 🦠

     ●■ **S36.231**   Laceration of body of pancreas, unspecified degree A 🦠, D, S 🦠

     ●■ **S36.232**   Laceration of tail of pancreas, unspecified degree A 🦠, D, S 🦠

     ●■ **S36.239**   Laceration of unspecified part of pancreas, unspecified degree A 🦠, D, S 🦠

   ● **S36.24**   Minor laceration of pancreas

     ● **S36.240**   Minor laceration of head of pancreas A 🦠, D, S 🦠

     ● **S36.241**   Minor laceration of body of pancreas A 🦠, D, S 🦠

     ● **S36.242**   Minor laceration of tail of pancreas A 🦠, D, S 🦠

     ●■ **S36.249**   Minor laceration of unspecified part of pancreas A 🦠, D, S 🦠

● **S36.25**   Moderate laceration of pancreas

     ● **S36.250**   Moderate laceration of head of pancreas A 🦠, D, S 🦠

     ● **S36.251**   Moderate laceration of body of pancreas A 🦠, D, S 🦠

     ● **S36.252**   Moderate laceration of tail of pancreas A 🦠, D, S 🦠

     ●■ **S36.259**   Moderate laceration of unspecified part of pancreas A 🦠, D, S 🦠

● **S36.26**   Major laceration of pancreas

     ● **S36.260**   Major laceration of head of pancreas A 🦠, D, S 🦠

     ● **S36.261**   Major laceration of body of pancreas A 🦠, D, S 🦠

     ● **S36.262**   Major laceration of tail of pancreas A 🦠, D, S 🦠

     ●■ **S36.269**   Major laceration of unspecified part of pancreas A 🦠, D, S 🦠

● **S36.29**   Other injury of pancreas

     ● **S36.290**   Other injury of head of pancreas A 🦠, D, S 🦠

     ● **S36.291**   Other injury of body of pancreas A 🦠, D, S 🦠

     ● **S36.292**   Other injury of tail of pancreas A 🦠, D, S 🦠

     ●■ **S36.299**   Other injury of unspecified part of pancreas A 🦠, D, S 🦠

● **S36.3**   Injury of stomach

   ●■ **S36.30**   Unspecified injury of stomach A 🦠, D, S 🦠

   ● **S36.32**   Contusion of stomach A 🦠, D, S 🦠

   ● **S36.33**   Laceration of stomach A 🦠, D, S 🦠

   ● **S36.39**   Other injury of stomach A 🦠, D, S 🦠

● **S36.4**   Injury of small intestine

   ● **S36.40**   Unspecified injury of small intestine

     ●■ **S36.400**   Unspecified injury of duodenum A 🦠, D, S 🦠

     ●■ **S36.408**   Unspecified injury of other part of small intestine A 🦠, D, S 🦠

     ●■ **S36.409**   Unspecified injury of unspecified part of small intestine A 🦠, D, S 🦠

   ● **S36.41**   Primary blast injury of small intestine
> Blast injury of small intestine NOS

     ● **S36.410**   Primary blast injury of duodenum A 🦠, D, S 🦠

     ● **S36.418**   Primary blast injury of other part of small intestine A 🦠, D, S 🦠

     ●■ **S36.419**   Primary blast injury of unspecified part of small intestine A 🦠, D, S 🦠

   ● **S36.42**   Contusion of small intestine

     ● **S36.420**   Contusion of duodenum A 🦠, D, S 🦠

     ● **S36.428**   Contusion of other part of small intestine A 🦠, D, S 🦠

     ●■ **S36.429**   Contusion of unspecified part of small intestine A 🦠, D, S 🦠

N Newborn Age: 0   **P** Pediatric Age: 0–17   **M** Maternity DX: 12–55   **A** Adult Age: 15–124   ♀ Females Only   ♂ Males Only

🦠 Complication\Comorbidity   🦠 Major C\C   🦠 Present on Admission Requirement   🦠 Hospital-Acquired Condition

1447

CHAPTER 19 (S00-T88)

● S36.43   Laceration of small intestine
- ● S36.430   Laceration of duodenum A, D, S
- ● S36.438   Laceration of other part of small intestine A, D, S
- ●■ S36.439   Laceration of unspecified part of small intestine A, D, S

● S36.49   Other injury of small intestine
- ● S36.490   Other injury of duodenum A, D, S
- ● S36.498   Other injury of other part of small intestine A, D, S
- ●■ S36.499   Other injury of unspecified part of small intestine A, D, S

● S36.5   Injury of colon

    Excludes2   injury of rectum (S36.6-)

● S36.50   Unspecified injury of colon
- ●■ S36.500   Unspecified injury of ascending [right] colon A, D, S
- ●■ S36.501   Unspecified injury of transverse colon A, D, S
- ●■ S36.502   Unspecified injury of descending [left] colon A, D, S
- ●■ S36.503   Unspecified injury of sigmoid colon A, D, S
- ●■ S36.508   Unspecified injury of other part of colon A, D, S
- ●■ S36.509   Unspecified injury of unspecified part of colon A, D, S

● S36.51   Primary blast injury of colon
    Blast injury of colon NOS
- ● S36.510   Primary blast injury of ascending [right] colon A, D, S
- ● S36.511   Primary blast injury of transverse colon A, D, S
- ● S36.512   Primary blast injury of descending [left] colon A, D, S
- ● S36.513   Primary blast injury of sigmoid colon A, D, S
- ● S36.518   Primary blast injury of other part of colon A, D, S
- ●■ S36.519   Primary blast injury of unspecified part of colon A, D, S

● S36.52   Contusion of colon
- ● S36.520   Contusion of ascending [right] colon A, D, S
- ● S36.521   Contusion of transverse colon A, D, S
- ● S36.522   Contusion of descending [left] colon A, D, S
- ● S36.523   Contusion of sigmoid colon A, D, S
- ● S36.528   Contusion of other part of colon A, D, S
- ●■ S36.529   Contusion of unspecified part of colon A, D, S

● S36.53   Laceration of colon
- ● S36.530   Laceration of ascending [right] colon A, D, S
- ● S36.531   Laceration of transverse colon A, D, S
- ● S36.532   Laceration of descending [left] colon A, D, S
- ● S36.533   Laceration of sigmoid colon A, D, S
- ● S36.538   Laceration of other part of colon A, D, S
- ■ S36.539   Laceration of unspecified part of colon A, D, S

● S36.59   Other injury of colon
    Secondary blast injury of colon
- ● S36.590   Other injury of ascending [right] colon A, D, S
- ● S36.591   Other injury of transverse colon A, D, S
- ● S36.592   Other injury of descending [left] colon A, D, S
- ● S36.593   Other injury of sigmoid colon A, D, S
- ● S36.598   Other injury of other part of colon A, D, S
- ●■ S36.599   Other injury of unspecified part of colon A, D, S

● S36.6   Injury of rectum
- ●■ S36.60   Unspecified injury of rectum A, D, S
- ● S36.61   Primary blast injury of rectum A, D, S
    Blast injury of rectum NOS
- ● S36.62   Contusion of rectum A, D, S
- ● S36.63   Laceration of rectum A, D, S
- ● S36.69   Other injury of rectum A, D, S
    Secondary blast injury of rectum

● S36.8   Injury of other intra-abdominal organs
- ● S36.81   Injury of peritoneum A, D, S
- ● S36.89   Injury of other intra-abdominal organs A
    Injury of retroperitoneum
  - ● S36.892   Contusion of other intra-abdominal organs A, D, S
  - ● S36.893   Laceration of other intra-abdominal organs A, D, S
  - ● S36.898   Other injury of other intra-abdominal organs A, D, S
  - ■ S36.899   Unspecified injury of other intra-abdominal organs A, D, S

● S36.9   Injury of unspecified intra-abdominal organ
- ■ S36.90   Unspecified injury of unspecified intra-abdominal organ A, D, S
- ●■ S36.92   Contusion of unspecified intra-abdominal organ A, D, S
- ●■ S36.93   Laceration of unspecified intra-abdominal organ A, D, S
- ●■ S36.99   Other injury of unspecified intra-abdominal organ A, D, S

●   Unacceptable Principal Diagnosis   ●   Use Additional Character(s)   ■   Unspecified   ▶   Manifestation Code

OGCR   Official Guidelines for Coding and Reporting   Excludes 1   Excludes 2   Includes   Use additional   Code first   Code also

CHAPTER 19 (S00-T88)

● **S37   Injury of urinary and pelvic organs**

> Code also any associated open wound (S31.-)
>
> Excludes1 obstetric trauma to pelvic organs (O71-)
>
> Excludes2 injury of peritoneum (S36.81)
> injury of retroperitoneum (S36.89-)
>
> The appropriate 7th character is to be added to each code from category S37
>
> | | |
> |---|---|
> | A | initial encounter |
> | D | subsequent encounter |
> | S | sequela |

● **S37.0   Injury of kidney**

> Excludes2 acute kidney injury (nontraumatic) (N17.9)

   ● **S37.00   Unspecified injury of kidney**

     ●■ **S37.001   Unspecified injury of right kidney** A 🅒, D, S 🅟

     ●■ **S37.002   Unspecified injury of left kidney** A 🅒, D, S 🅟

     ●■ **S37.009   Unspecified injury of unspecified kidney** A 🅒, D, S 🅟

   ● **S37.01   Minor contusion of kidney**
> Contusion of kidney less than 2 cm
> Contusion of kidney NOS

     ● **S37.011   Minor contusion of right kidney** A 🅒, D, S 🅟

     ● **S37.012   Minor contusion of left kidney** A 🅒, D, S 🅟

     ●■ **S37.019   Minor contusion of unspecified kidney** A 🅒, D, S 🅟

   ● **S37.02   Major contusion of kidney**
> Contusion of kidney greater than 2 cm

     ● **S37.021   Major contusion of right kidney** A 🅒, D, S 🅟

     ● **S37.022   Major contusion of left kidney** A 🅒, D, S 🅟

     ●■ **S37.029   Major contusion of unspecified kidney** A 🅒, D, S 🅟

   ● **S37.03   Laceration of kidney, unspecified degree**

     ●■ **S37.031   Laceration of right kidney, unspecified degree** A 🅒, D, S 🅟

     ●■ **S37.032   Laceration of left kidney, unspecified degree** A 🅒, D, S 🅟

     ●■ **S37.039   Laceration of unspecified kidney, unspecified degree** A 🅒, D, S 🅟

   ● **S37.04   Minor laceration of kidney**
> Laceration of kidney less than 1 cm

     ● **S37.041   Minor laceration of right kidney** A 🅒, D, S 🅟

     ● **S37.042   Minor laceration of left kidney** A 🅒, D, S 🅟

     ●■ **S37.049   Minor laceration of unspecified kidney** A 🅒, D, S 🅟

   ● **S37.05   Moderate laceration of kidney**
> Laceration of kidney 1 to 3 cm

     ● **S37.051   Moderate laceration of right kidney** A 🅒, D, S 🅟

     ● **S37.052   Moderate laceration of left kidney** A 🅒, D, S 🅟

     ●■ **S37.059   Moderate laceration of unspecified kidney** A 🅒, D, S 🅟

● **S37.06   Major laceration of kidney**
> Avulsion of kidney
> Laceration of kidney greater than 3 cm
> Massive laceration of kidney
> Multiple moderate lacerations of kidney
> Stellate laceration of kidney

   ● **S37.061   Major laceration of right kidney** A 🅒, D, S 🅟

   ● **S37.062   Major laceration of left kidney** A 🅒, D, S 🅟

   ●■ **S37.069   Major laceration of unspecified kidney** A 🅒, D, S 🅟

● **S37.09   Other injury of kidney**

   ● **S37.091   Other injury of right kidney** A 🅒, D, S 🅟

   ● **S37.092   Other injury of left kidney** A 🅒, D, S 🅟

   ●■ **S37.099   Other injury of unspecified kidney** A 🅒, D, S 🅟

● **S37.1   Injury of ureter**

   ●■ **S37.10   Unspecified injury of ureter** A 🅒, D, S 🅟

   ● **S37.12   Contusion of ureter** A 🅒, D, S 🅟

   ● **S37.13   Laceration of ureter** A 🅒, D, S 🅟

   ● **S37.19   Other injury of ureter** A 🅒, D, S 🅟

● **S37.2   Injury of bladder**

   ●■ **S37.20   Unspecified injury of bladder** A 🅒, D, S 🅟

   ● **S37.22   Contusion of bladder** A 🅒, D, S 🅟

   ● **S37.23   Laceration of bladder** A 🅒, D, S 🅟

   ● **S37.29   Other injury of bladder** A 🅒, D, S 🅟

● **S37.3   Injury of urethra**

   ●■ **S37.30   Unspecified injury of urethra** A 🅒, D, S 🅟

   ● **S37.32   Contusion of urethra** A 🅒, D, S 🅟

   ● **S37.33   Laceration of urethra** A 🅒, D, S 🅟

   ● **S37.39   Other injury of urethra** A 🅒, D, S 🅟

● **S37.4   Injury of ovary**

   ● **S37.40   Unspecified injury of ovary**

     ●■ **S37.401   Unspecified injury of ovary, unilateral** D 🅟

     ●■ **S37.402   Unspecified injury of ovary, bilateral** D 🅟

     ●■ **S37.409   Unspecified injury of ovary, unspecified** D 🅟

   ● **S37.42   Contusion of ovary**

     ● **S37.421   Contusion of ovary, unilateral** D 🅟

     ● **S37.422   Contusion of ovary, bilateral** D 🅟

     ●■ **S37.429   Contusion of ovary, unspecified** D 🅟

   ● **S37.43   Laceration of ovary**

     ● **S37.431   Laceration of ovary, unilateral** D 🅟

     ● **S37.432   Laceration of ovary, bilateral** D 🅟

     ●■ **S37.439   Laceration of ovary, unspecified** D 🅟

   ● **S37.49   Other injury of ovary**

     ● **S37.491   Other injury of ovary, unilateral** D 🅟

     ● **S37.492   Other injury of ovary, bilateral** D 🅟

     ●■ **S37.499   Other injury of ovary, unspecified** D 🅟

● **S37.5**   **Injury of fallopian tube**
  ● **S37.50**   **Unspecified injury of fallopian tube**
    ● ■ **S37.501**   Unspecified injury of fallopian tube, unilateral D 🖉
    ● ■ **S37.502**   Unspecified injury of fallopian tube, bilateral D 🖉
    ● ■ **S37.509**   Unspecified injury of fallopian tube, unspecified D 🖉
  ● **S37.51**   **Primary blast injury of fallopian tube**
    Blast injury of fallopian tube NOS
    ● **S37.511**   Primary blast injury of fallopian tube, unilateral D 🖉
    ● **S37.512**   Primary blast injury of fallopian tube, bilateral D 🖉
    ● ■ **S37.519**   Primary blast injury of fallopian tube, unspecified D 🖉
  ● **S37.52**   **Contusion of fallopian tube**
    ● **S37.521**   Contusion of fallopian tube, unilateral D 🖉
    ● **S37.522**   Contusion of fallopian tube, bilateral D 🖉
    ● ■ **S37.529**   Contusion of fallopian tube, unspecified D 🖉
  ● **S37.53**   **Laceration of fallopian tube**
    ● **S37.531**   Laceration of fallopian tube, unilateral D 🖉
    ● **S37.532**   Laceration of fallopian tube, bilateral D 🖉
    ● ■ **S37.539**   Laceration of fallopian tube, unspecified D 🖉
  ● **S37.59**   **Other injury of fallopian tube**
    Secondary blast injury of fallopian tube
    ● **S37.591**   Other injury of fallopian tube, unilateral D 🖉
    ● **S37.592**   Other injury of fallopian tube, bilateral D 🖉
    ● ■ **S37.599**   Other injury of fallopian tube, unspecified D 🖉

● **S37.6**   **Injury of uterus**
  | **Excludes1** | injury to gravid uterus (O9A.2-) injury to uterus during delivery (O71.-) |
  ● ■ **S37.60**   Unspecified injury of uterus A 🖉, D 🖉
  ● **S37.62**   Contusion of uterus A 🖉, D 🖉
  ● **S37.63**   Laceration of uterus A 🖉, D 🖉
  ● **S37.69**   Other injury of uterus A 🖉, D 🖉

● **S37.8**   **Injury of other urinary and pelvic organs**
  ● **S37.81**   **Injury of adrenal gland**
    ● **S37.812**   Contusion of adrenal gland A 🖉, D, S 🖉
    ● **S37.813**   Laceration of adrenal gland A 🖉, D, S 🖉
    ● **S37.818**   Other injury of adrenal gland A 🖉, D, S 🖉
    ● ■ **S37.819**   Unspecified injury of adrenal gland A 🖉, D, S 🖉
  ● **S37.82**   **Injury of prostate**
    ● **S37.822**   Contusion of prostate D 🖉
    ● **S37.823**   Laceration of prostate D 🖉
    ● **S37.828**   Other injury of prostate D 🖉
    ● ■ **S37.829**   Unspecified injury of prostate D 🖉

● **S37.89**   **Injury of other urinary and pelvic organ**
  ● **S37.892**   Contusion of other urinary and pelvic organ A 🖉, D, S 🖉
  ● **S37.893**   Laceration of other urinary and pelvic organ A 🖉, D, S 🖉
  ● **S37.898**   Other injury of other urinary and pelvic organ A 🖉, D, S 🖉
  ● ■ **S37.899**   Unspecified injury of other urinary and pelvic organ A 🖉, D, S 🖉

● **S37.9**   **Injury of unspecified urinary and pelvic organ**
  ● ■ **S37.90**   Unspecified injury of unspecified urinary and pelvic organ A 🖉, D, S 🖉
  ● ■ **S37.92**   Contusion of unspecified urinary and pelvic organ A 🖉, D, S 🖉
  ● ■ **S37.93**   Laceration of unspecified urinary and pelvic organ A 🖉, D, S 🖉
  ● ■ **S37.99**   Other injury of unspecified urinary and pelvic organ A 🖉, D, S 🖉

● **S38**   **Crushing injury and traumatic amputation of abdomen, lower back, pelvis and external genitals**
  An amputation not identified as partial or complete should be coded to complete

  The appropriate 7th character is to be added to each code from category S38

A	initial encounter
D	subsequent encounter
S	sequela

● **S38.0**   **Crushing injury of external genital organs**
  Use additional code for any associated injuries
  ● **S38.00**   **Crushing injury of unspecified external genital organs**
    ● ■ **S38.001**   Crushing injury of unspecified external genital organs, male D, S 🖉
    ● ■ **S38.002**   Crushing injury of unspecified external genital organs, female D, S 🖉
  ● **S38.01**   Crushing injury of penis D, S 🖉
  ● **S38.02**   Crushing injury of scrotum and testis D, S 🖉
  ● **S38.03**   Crushing injury of vulva D, S 🖉

● **S38.1**   **Crushing injury of abdomen, lower back, and pelvis** D, S 🖉
  Use additional code for all associated injuries, such as:
  fracture of thoracic or lumbar spine and pelvis (S22.0-, S32.-)
  injury to intra-abdominal organs (S36.-)
  injury to urinary and pelvic organs (S37.-)
  open wound of abdominal wall (S31-)
  spinal cord injury (S34.0, S34.1-)
  | **Excludes2** | crushing injury of external genital organs (S38.2-) |

● **S38.2**   **Traumatic amputation of external genital organs**
  ● **S38.21**   **Traumatic amputation of female external genital organs**
    Traumatic amputation of clitoris
    Traumatic amputation of labium (majus) (minus)
    Traumatic amputation of vulva
    ● **S38.211**   Complete traumatic amputation of female external genital organs D, S 🖉

●   Unacceptable Principal Diagnosis   ●   Use Additional Character(s)   ■   Unspecified   ▶   Manifestation Code

OGCR   Official Guidelines for Coding and Reporting | Excludes 1 | | Excludes 2 | | Includes | | Use additional | | Code first | | Code also |

- S38.212   Partial traumatic amputation of female external genital organs D, S

- S38.22   Traumatic amputation of penis
  - S38.221   Complete traumatic amputation of penis D, S
  - S38.222   Partial traumatic amputation of penis D, S
- S38.23   Traumatic amputation of scrotum and testis
  - S38.231   Complete traumatic amputation of scrotum and testis D, S
  - S38.232   Partial traumatic amputation of scrotum and testis D, S
- S38.3   Transection (partial) of abdomen D, S

- S39   Other and unspecified injuries of abdomen, lower back, pelvis and external genitals

  Code also any associated open wound (S31.-)

  Excludes2   sprain of joints and ligaments of lumbar spine and pelvis (S33.-)

  The appropriate 7th character is to be added to each code from category S39

A	initial encounter
D	subsequent encounter
S	sequela

  - S39.0   Injury of muscle, fascia and tendon of abdomen, lower back and pelvis
    - S39.00   Unspecified injury of muscle, fascia and tendon of abdomen, lower back and pelvis
      - S39.001   Unspecified injury of muscle, fascia and tendon of abdomen D, S
      - S39.002   Unspecified injury of muscle, fascia and tendon of lower back D, S
      - S39.003   Unspecified injury of muscle, fascia and tendon of pelvis D, S
    - S39.01   Strain of muscle, fascia and tendon of abdomen, lower back and pelvis
      - S39.011   Strain of muscle, fascia and tendon of abdomen D, S
      - S39.012   Strain of muscle, fascia and tendon of lower back D, S
      - S39.013   Strain of muscle, fascia and tendon of pelvis D, S
    - S39.02   Laceration of muscle, fascia and tendon of abdomen, lower back and pelvis
      - S39.021   Laceration of muscle, fascia and tendon of abdomen D, S
      - S39.022   Laceration of muscle, fascia and tendon of lower back D, S
      - S39.023   Laceration of muscle, fascia and tendon of pelvis D, S
    - S39.09   Other injury of muscle, fascia and tendon of abdomen, lower back and pelvis
      - S39.091   Other injury of muscle, fascia and tendon of abdomen D, S
      - S39.092   Other injury of muscle, fascia and tendon of lower back D, S
      - S39.093   Other injury of muscle, fascia and tendon of pelvis D, S

  - S39.8   Other specified injuries of abdomen, lower back, pelvis and external genitals
    - S39.81   Other specified injuries of abdomen D, S
    - S39.82   Other specified injuries of lower back D, S
    - S39.83   Other specified injuries of pelvis D, S
    - S39.84   Other specified injuries of external genitals D, S
      - S39.840   Fracture of corpus cavernosum penis D, S
      - S39.848   Other specified injuries of external genitals D, S
  - S39.9   Unspecified injury of abdomen, lower back, pelvis and external genitals
    - S39.91   Unspecified injury of abdomen D, S
    - S39.92   Unspecified injury of lower back D, S
    - S39.93   Unspecified injury of pelvis D, S
    - S39.94   Unspecified injury of external genitals D, S

INJURIES TO THE SHOULDER AND UPPER ARM (S40-S49)

Includes   injuries of axilla injuries of scapular region

Excludes2   burns and corrosions (T20-T32)
frostbite (T33-T34)
injuries of elbow (S50-S59)
insect bite or sting, venomous (T63.4)

- S40   Superficial injury of shoulder and upper arm

  The appropriate 7th character is to be added to each code from category S40

A	initial encounter
D	subsequent encounter
S	sequela

  - S40.0   Contusion of shoulder and upper arm
    - S40.01   Contusion of shoulder
      - S40.011   Contusion of right shoulder D, S
      - S40.012   Contusion of left shoulder D, S
      - S40.019   Contusion of unspecified shoulder D, S
    - S40.02   Contusion of upper arm
      - S40.021   Contusion of right upper arm D, S
      - S40.022   Contusion of left upper arm D, S
      - S40.029   Contusion of unspecified upper arm D, S
  - S40.2   Other superficial injuries of shoulder
    - S40.21   Abrasion of shoulder
      - S40.211   Abrasion of right shoulder D, S
      - S40.212   Abrasion of left shoulder D, S
      - S40.219   Abrasion of unspecified shoulder D, S
    - S40.22   Blister (nonthermal) of shoulder
      - S40.221   Blister (nonthermal) of right shoulder D, S
      - S40.222   Blister (nonthermal) of left shoulder D, S
      - S40.229   Blister (nonthermal) of unspecified shoulder D, S

N   Newborn Age: 0   P   Pediatric Age: 0–17   M   Maternity DX: 12–55   A   Adult Age: 15–124   ♀   Females Only   ♂   Males Only

Complication\Comorbidity   Major C\C   Present on Admission Requirement   Hospital-Acquired Condition

CHAPTER 19 (S00-T88)

● **S40.24** **External constriction of shoulder**
  ● **S40.241** External constriction of right shoulder D, S
  ● **S40.242** External constriction of left shoulder D, S
  ●■ **S40.249** External constriction of unspecified shoulder D, S
● **S40.25** **Superficial foreign body of shoulder**
  Splinter in the shoulder
  ● **S40.251** Superficial foreign body of right shoulder D, S
  ● **S40.252** Superficial foreign body of left shoulder D, S
  ●■ **S40.259** Superficial foreign body of unspecified shoulder D, S
● **S40.26** **Insect bite (nonvenomous) of shoulder**
  ● **S40.261** Insect bite (nonvenomous) of right shoulder D, S
  ● **S40.262** Insect bite (nonvenomous) of left shoulder D, S
  ●■ **S40.269** Insect bite (nonvenomous) of unspecified shoulder D, S
● **S40.27** **Other superficial bite of shoulder**
  Excludes1 open bite of shoulder (S41.05)
  ● **S40.271** Other superficial bite of right shoulder D, S
  ● **S40.272** Other superficial bite of left shoulder D, S
  ●■ **S40.279** Other superficial bite of unspecified shoulder D, S
● **S40.8** **Other superficial injuries of upper arm**
  ● **S40.81** **Abrasion of upper arm**
   ● **S40.811** Abrasion of right upper arm D, S
   ● **S40.812** Abrasion of left upper arm D, S
   ●■ **S40.819** Abrasion of unspecified upper arm D, S
  ● **S40.82** **Blister (nonthermal) of upper arm**
   ● **S40.821** Blister (nonthermal) of right upper arm D, S
   ● **S40.822** Blister (nonthermal) of left upper arm D, S
   ●■ **S40.829** Blister (nonthermal) of unspecified upper arm D, S
  ● **S40.84** **External constriction of upper arm**
   ● **S40.841** External constriction of right upper arm D, S
   ● **S40.842** External constriction of left upper arm D, S
   ●■ **S40.849** External constriction of unspecified upper arm D, S
  ● **S40.85** **Superficial foreign body of upper arm**
   Splinter in the upper arm
   ● **S40.851** Superficial foreign body of right upper arm D, S
   ● **S40.852** Superficial foreign body of left upper arm D, S
   ●■ **S40.859** Superficial foreign body of unspecified upper arm D, S

● **S40.86** **Insect bite (nonvenomous) of upper arm**
  ● **S40.861** Insect bite (nonvenomous) of right upper arm D, S
  ● **S40.862** Insect bite (nonvenomous) of left upper arm D, S
  ●■ **S40.869** Insect bite (nonvenomous) of unspecified upper arm D, S
● **S40.87** **Other superficial bite of upper arm**
  Excludes1 open bite of upper arm (S41.14)
  Excludes2 other superficial bite of shoulder (S40.27-)
  ● **S40.871** Other superficial bite of right upper arm D, S
  ● **S40.872** Other superficial bite of left upper arm D, S
  ●■ **S40.879** Other superficial bite of unspecified upper arm D, S
● **S40.9** **Unspecified superficial injury of shoulder and upper arm**
  ● **S40.91** **Unspecified superficial injury of shoulder**
   ●■ **S40.911** Unspecified superficial injury of right shoulder D, S
   ●■ **S40.912** Unspecified superficial injury of left shoulder D, S
   ●■ **S40.919** Unspecified superficial injury of unspecified shoulder D, S
  ● **S40.92** **Unspecified superficial injury of upper arm**
   ●■ **S40.921** Unspecified superficial injury of right upper arm D, S
   ●■ **S40.922** Unspecified superficial injury of left upper arm D, S
   ●■ **S40.929** Unspecified superficial injury of unspecified upper arm D, S
● **S41** **Open wound of shoulder and upper arm**
  Code also any associated wound infection
  Excludes1 traumatic amputation of shoulder and upper arm (S48.-)
  Excludes2 open fracture of shoulder and upper arm (S42.- with 7th character B or C)
  The appropriate 7th character is to be added to each code from category S41
  A initial encounter
  D subsequent encounter
  S sequela
  ● **S41.0** **Open wound of shoulder**
   ● **S41.00** **Unspecified open wound of shoulder**
    ●■ **S41.001** Unspecified open wound of right shoulder D, S
    ●■ **S41.002** Unspecified open wound of left shoulder D, S
    ●■ **S41.009** Unspecified open wound of unspecified shoulder D, S
   ● **S41.01** **Laceration without foreign body of shoulder**
    ● **S41.011** Laceration without foreign body of right shoulder D, S
    ● **S41.012** Laceration without foreign body of left shoulder D, S
    ●■ **S41.019** Laceration without foreign body of unspecified shoulder D, S

● Unacceptable Principal Diagnosis   ● Use Additional Character(s)   ■ Unspecified   ▶ Manifestation Code
OGCR Official Guidelines for Coding and Reporting   Excludes 1   Excludes 2   Includes   Use additional   Code first   Code also

● **S41.02 Laceration with foreign body of shoulder**
- ● **S41.021** Laceration with foreign body of right shoulder D, S 🔖
- ● **S41.022** Laceration with foreign body of left shoulder D, S 🔖
- ●■ **S41.029** Laceration with foreign body of unspecified shoulder D, S 🔖

● **S41.03 Puncture wound without foreign body of shoulder**
- ● **S41.031** Puncture wound without foreign body of right shoulder D, S 🔖
- ● **S41.032** Puncture wound without foreign body of left shoulder D, S 🔖
- ●■ **S41.039** Puncture wound without foreign body of unspecified shoulder D, S 🔖

● **S41.04 Puncture wound with foreign body of shoulder**
- ● **S41.041** Puncture wound with foreign body of right shoulder D, S 🔖
- ● **S41.042** Puncture wound with foreign body of left shoulder D, S 🔖
- ●■ **S41.049** Puncture wound with foreign body of unspecified shoulder D, S 🔖

● **S41.05 Open bite of shoulder**
Bite of shoulder NOS
> **Excludes1** superficial bite of shoulder (S40.27)
- ● **S41.051** Open bite of right shoulder D, S 🔖
- ● **S41.052** Open bite of left shoulder D, S 🔖
- ●■ **S41.059** Open bite of unspecified shoulder D, S 🔖

● **S41.1 Open wound of upper arm**
- ● **S41.10 Unspecified open wound of upper arm**
  - ●■ **S41.101** Unspecified open wound of right upper arm D, S 🔖
  - ●■ **S41.102** Unspecified open wound of left upper arm D, S 🔖
  - ●■ **S41.109** Unspecified open wound of unspecified upper arm D, S 🔖
- ● **S41.11 Laceration without foreign body of upper arm**
  - ● **S41.111** Laceration without foreign body of right upper arm D, S 🔖
  - ● **S41.112** Laceration without foreign body of left upper arm D, S 🔖
  - ●■ **S41.119** Laceration without foreign body of unspecified upper arm D, S 🔖
- ● **S41.12 Laceration with foreign body of upper arm**
  - ● **S41.121** Laceration with foreign body of right upper arm D, S 🔖
  - ● **S41.122** Laceration with foreign body of left upper arm D, S 🔖
  - ●■ **S41.129** Laceration with foreign body of unspecified upper arm D, S 🔖
- ● **S41.13 Puncture wound without foreign body of upper arm**
  - ● **S41.131** Puncture wound without foreign body of right upper arm D, S 🔖
  - ● **S41.132** Puncture wound without foreign body of left upper arm D, S 🔖

●■ **S41.139** Puncture wound without foreign body of unspecified upper arm D, S 🔖

● **S41.14 Puncture wound with foreign body of upper arm**
- ● **S41.141** Puncture wound with foreign body of right upper arm D, G 🔖
- ● **S41.142** Puncture wound with foreign body of left upper arm D, G 🔖
- ●■ **S41.149** Puncture wound with foreign body of unspecified upper arm D, G 🔖

● **S41.15 Open bite of upper arm**
Bite of upper arm NOS
> **Excludes1** superficial bite of upper arm (S40.87)
- ● **S41.151** Open bite of right upper arm D, G 🔖
- ● **S41.152** Open bite of left upper arm D, G 🔖
- ●■ **S41.159** Open bite of unspecified upper arm D, G 🔖

● **S42 Fracture of shoulder and upper arm**

Note: A fracture not indicated as displaced or nondisplaced should be coded to displaced

A fracture not indicated as open or closed should be coded to closed

> **Excludes1** traumatic amputation of shoulder and upper arm (S48.-)

The appropriate 7th character is to be added to all codes from category S42

Ⓐ	initial encounter for closed fracture
B	initial encounter for open fracture
D	subsequent encounter for fracture with routine healing
G	subsequent encounter for fracture with delayed healing
K	subsequent encounter for fracture with nonunion
P	subsequent encounter for fracture with malunion
S	sequela

● **S42.0 Fracture of clavicle**
- ● **S42.00 Fracture of unspecified part of clavicle**
  - ●■ **S42.001** Fracture of unspecified part of right clavicle B, K, P 🔖, D, G, S 🔖
  - ●■ **S42.002** Fracture of unspecified part of left clavicle B, K, P 🔖, D, G, S 🔖
  - ●■ **S42.009** Fracture of unspecified part of unspecified clavicle B, K, P 🔖, D, G, S 🔖
- ● **S42.01 Fracture of sternal end of clavicle**
  - ● **S42.011** Anterior displaced fracture of sternal end of right clavicle B, K, P 🔖, D, G, S 🔖, B 🔖
  - ● **S42.012** Anterior displaced fracture of sternal end of left clavicle B, K, P 🔖, D, G, S 🔖, B 🔖
  - ●■ **S42.013** Anterior displaced fracture of sternal end of unspecified clavicle B, K, P 🔖, D, G, S 🔖, B 🔖
    Displaced fracture of sternal end of clavicle NOS
  - ● **S42.014** Posterior displaced fracture of sternal end of right clavicle B, K, P 🔖, D, G, S 🔖, B 🔖

● S42.015　Posterior displaced fracture of sternal end of left clavicle B, K, P 🔧, D, G, S 🔧, B 🔧

●■ S42.016　Posterior displaced fracture of sternal end of unspecified clavicle B, K, P 🔧, D, G, S 🔧, B 🔧

● S42.017　Nondisplaced fracture of sternal end of right clavicle B, K, P 🔧, D, G, S 🔧, B 🔧

● S42.018　Nondisplaced fracture of sternal end of left clavicle B, K, P 🔧, D, G, S 🔧, B 🔧

●■ S42.019　Nondisplaced fracture of sternal end of unspecified clavicle B, K, P 🔧, D, G, S 🔧, B 🔧

● S42.02　Fracture of shaft of clavicle

● S42.021　Displaced fracture of shaft of right clavicle B, K, P 🔧, D, G, S 🔧, B 🔧

● S42.022　Displaced fracture of shaft of left clavicle B, K, P 🔧, D, G, S 🔧, B 🔧

●■ S42.023　Displaced fracture of shaft of unspecified clavicle B, K, P 🔧, D, G, S 🔧, B 🔧

● S42.024　Nondisplaced fracture of shaft of right clavicle B, K, P 🔧, D, G, S 🔧, B 🔧

● S42.025　Nondisplaced fracture of shaft of left clavicle B, K, P 🔧, D, G, S 🔧, B 🔧

●■ S42.026　Nondisplaced fracture of shaft of unspecified clavicle B, K, P 🔧, D, G, S 🔧, B 🔧

● S42.03　Fracture of lateral end of clavicle
　　　　　Fracture of acromial end of clavicle

● S42.031　Displaced fracture of lateral end of right clavicle B, K, P 🔧, D, G, S 🔧, B 🔧

● S42.032　Displaced fracture of lateral end of left clavicle B, K, P 🔧, D, G, S 🔧, B 🔧

●■ S42.033　Displaced fracture of lateral end of unspecified clavicle B, K, P 🔧, D, G, S 🔧, B 🔧

● S42.034　Nondisplaced fracture of lateral end of right clavicle B, K, P 🔧, D, G, S 🔧, B 🔧

● S42.035　Nondisplaced fracture of lateral end of left clavicle B, K, P 🔧, D, G, S 🔧, B 🔧

●■ S42.036　Nondisplaced fracture of lateral end of unspecified clavicle B, K, P 🔧, D, G, S 🔧, B 🔧

● S42.1　Fracture of scapula

● S42.10　Fracture of unspecified part of scapula

●■ S42.101　Fracture of unspecified part of scapula, right shoulder B, K, P 🔧, D, G, S 🔧, B 🔧

●■ S42.102　Fracture of unspecified part of scapula, left shoulder B, K, P 🔧, D, G, S 🔧, B 🔧

●■ S42.109　Fracture of unspecified part of scapula, unspecified shoulder B, K, P 🔧, D, G, S 🔧, B 🔧

● S42.11　Fracture of body of scapula

● S42.111　Displaced fracture of body of scapula, right shoulder B, K, P 🔧, D, G, S 🔧, B 🔧

● S42.112　Displaced fracture of body of scapula, left shoulder B, K, P 🔧, D, G, S 🔧, B 🔧

●■ S42.113　Displaced fracture of body of scapula, unspecified shoulder B, K, P 🔧, D, G, S 🔧, B 🔧

● S42.114　Nondisplaced fracture of body of scapula, right shoulder B, K, P 🔧, D, G, S 🔧, B 🔧

● S42.115　Nondisplaced fracture of body of scapula, left shoulder B, K, P 🔧, D, G, S 🔧, B 🔧

●■ S42.116　Nondisplaced fracture of body of scapula, unspecified shoulder B, K, P 🔧, D, G, S 🔧, B 🔧

● S42.12　Fracture of acromial process

● S42.121　Displaced fracture of acromial process, right shoulder B, K, P 🔧, D, G, S 🔧, B 🔧

● S42.122　Displaced fracture of acromial process, left shoulder B, K, P 🔧, D, G, S 🔧, B 🔧

●■ S42.123　Displaced fracture of acromial process, unspecified shoulder B, K, P 🔧, D, G, S 🔧, B 🔧

● S42.124　Nondisplaced fracture of acromial process, right shoulder B, K, P 🔧, D, G, S 🔧, B 🔧

● S42.125　Nondisplaced fracture of acromial process, left shoulder B, K, P 🔧, D, G, S 🔧, B 🔧

●■ S42.126　Nondisplaced fracture, of acromial process, unspecified shoulder B, K, P 🔧, D, G, S 🔧, B 🔧

● S42.13　Fracture of coracoid process

● S42.131　Displaced fracture of coracoid process, right shoulder B, K, P 🔧, D, G, S 🔧, B 🔧

● S42.132　Displaced fracture of coracoid process, left shoulder B, K, P 🔧, D, G, S 🔧, B 🔧

●■ S42.133　Displaced fracture of coracoid process, unspecified shoulder B, K, P 🔧, D, G, S 🔧, B 🔧

● S42.134　Nondisplaced fracture of coracoid process, right shoulder B, K, P 🔧, D, G, S 🔧, B 🔧

● S42.135　Nondisplaced fracture of coracoid process, left shoulder B, K, P 🔧, D, G, S 🔧, B 🔧

●■ S42.136　Nondisplaced fracture of coracoid process, unspecified shoulder B, K, P 🔧, D, G, S 🔧, B 🔧

● **S42.14**   **Fracture of glenoid cavity of scapula**

   ● **S42.141**   Displaced fracture of glenoid cavity of scapula, right shoulder B, K, P, D, G, S, B

   ● **S42.142**   Displaced fracture of glenoid cavity of scapula, left shoulder B, K, P, D, G, S, B

   ● **S42.143**   Displaced fracture of glenoid cavity of scapula, unspecified shoulder B, K, P, D, G, S, B

   ● **S42.144**   Nondisplaced fracture of glenoid cavity of scapula, right shoulder B, K, P, D, G, S, B

   ● **S42.145**   Nondisplaced fracture of glenoid cavity of scapula, left shoulder B, K, P, D, G, S, B

   ● **S42.146**   Nondisplaced fracture of glenoid cavity of scapula, unspecified shoulder B, K, P, D, G, S, B

● **S42.15**   **Fracture of neck of scapula**

   ● **S42.151**   Displaced fracture of neck of scapula, right shoulder B, K, P, D, G, S, B

   ● **S42.152**   Displaced fracture of neck of scapula, left shoulder B, K, P, D, G, S, B

   ● **S42.153**   Displaced fracture of neck of scapula, unspecified shoulder B, K, P, D, G, S, B

   ● **S42.154**   Nondisplaced fracture of neck of scapula, right shoulder B, K, P, D, G, S, B

   ● **S42.155**   Nondisplaced fracture of neck of scapula, left shoulder B, K, P, D, G, S, B

   ● **S42.156**   Nondisplaced fracture of neck of scapula, unspecified shoulder B, K, P, D, G, S, B

● **S42.19**   **Fracture of other part of scapula**

   ● **S42.191**   Fracture of other part of scapula, right shoulder B, K, P, D, G, S, B

   ● **S42.192**   Fracture of other part of scapula, left shoulder B, K, P, D, G, S, B

   ● **S42.199**   Fracture of other part of scapula, unspecified shoulder B, K, P, D, G, S, B

● **S42.2**   **Fracture of upper end of humerus**

   Fracture of proximal end of humerus

   | Excludes2 | fracture of shaft of humerus (S42.3-) physeal fracture of upper end of humerus (S49.0-) |

  ● **S42.20**   **Unspecified fracture of upper end of humerus**

   ● **S42.201**   Unspecified fracture of upper end of right humerus A, K, P, B, D, G, S, A, B

   ● **S42.202**   Unspecified fracture of upper end of left humerus A, K, P, B, D, G, S, A, B

   ● **S42.209**   Unspecified fracture of upper end of unspecified humerus A, K, P, B, D, G, S, A, B

● **S42.21**   **Unspecified fracture of surgical neck of humerus**

   Fracture of neck of humerus NOS

   ● **S42.211**   Unspecified displaced fracture of surgical neck of right humerus A, K, P, B, D, G, S, A, B

   ● **S42.212**   Unspecified displaced fracture of surgical neck of left humerus A, K, P, B, D, G, S, A, B

   ● **S42.213**   Unspecified displaced fracture of surgical neck of unspecified humerus A, K, P, B, D, G, S, A, B

   ● **S42.214**   Unspecified nondisplaced fracture of surgical neck of right humerus A, K, P, B, D, G, S, A, B

   ● **S42.215**   Unspecified nondisplaced fracture of surgical neck of left humerus A, K, P, B, D, G, S, A, B

   ● **S42.216**   Unspecified nondisplaced fracture of surgical neck of unspecified humerus A, K, P, B, D, G, S, A, B

● **S42.22**   **2-part fracture of surgical neck of humerus**

   ● **S42.221**   2-part displaced fracture of surgical neck of right humerus A, K, P, B, D, G, S, A, B

   ● **S42.222**   2-part displaced fracture of surgical neck of left humerus A, K, P, B, D, G, S, A, B

   ● **S42.223**   2-part displaced fracture of surgical neck of unspecified humerus A, K, P, B, D, G, S, A, B

   ● **S42.224**   2-part nondisplaced fracture of surgical neck of right humerus A, K, P, B, D, G, S, A, B

   ● **S42.225**   2-part nondisplaced fracture of surgical neck of left humerus A, K, P, B, D, G, S, A, B

   ● **S42.226**   2-part nondisplaced fracture of surgical neck of unspecified humerus A, K, P, B, D, G, S, A, B

● **S42.23**   **3-part fracture of surgical neck of humerus**

   ● **S42.231**   3-part fracture of surgical neck of right humerus A, K, P, B, D, G, S, A, B

   ● **S42.232**   3-part fracture of surgical neck of left humerus A, K, P, B, D, G, S, A, B

   ● **S42.239**   3-part fracture of surgical neck of unspecified humerus A, K, P, B, D, G, S, A, B

● **S42.24**   **4-part fracture of surgical neck of humerus**

   ● **S42.241**   4-part fracture of surgical neck of right humerus A, K, P, B, D, G, S, A, B

   ● **S42.242**   4-part fracture of surgical neck of left humerus A, K, P, B, D, G, S, A, B

   ● **S42.249**   4-part fracture of surgical neck of unspecified humerus A, K, P, B, D, G, S, A, B

CHAPTER 19 (S00-T88)

● S42.25   Fracture of greater tuberosity of humerus

  ● S42.251   Displaced fracture of greater tuberosity of right humerus
A, K, P 🔷, B 🔷, D, G, S 🔷, A, B 🔷

  ● S42.252   Displaced fracture of greater tuberosity of left humerus
A, K, P 🔷, B 🔷, D, G, S 🔷, A, B 🔷

  ●■ S42.253   Displaced fracture of greater tuberosity of unspecified humerus A, K, P 🔷, B 🔷, D, G, S 🔷, A, B 🔷

  ● S42.254   Nondisplaced fracture of greater tuberosity of right humerus
A, K, P 🔷, B 🔷, D, G, S 🔷, A, B 🔷

  ● S42.255   Nondisplaced fracture of greater tuberosity of left humerus
A, K, P 🔷, B 🔷, D, G, S 🔷, A, B 🔷

  ●■ S42.256   Nondisplaced fracture of greater tuberosity of unspecified humerus A, K, P 🔷, B 🔷, D, G, S 🔷, A, B 🔷

● S42.26   Fracture of lesser tuberosity of humerus

  ● S42.261   Displaced fracture of lesser tuberosity of right humerus
A, K, P 🔷, B 🔷, D, G, S 🔷, A, B 🔷

  ● S42.262   Displaced fracture of lesser tuberosity of left humerus
A, K, P 🔷, B 🔷, D, G, S 🔷, A, B 🔷

  ●■ S42.263   Displaced fracture of lesser tuberosity of unspecified humerus A, K, P 🔷, B 🔷, D, G, S 🔷, A, B 🔷

  ● S42.264   Nondisplaced fracture of lesser tuberosity of right humerus
A, K, P 🔷, B 🔷, D, G, S 🔷, A, B 🔷

  ● S42.265   Nondisplaced fracture of lesser tuberosity of left humerus
A, K, P 🔷, B 🔷, D, G, S 🔷, A, B 🔷

  ●■ S42.266   Nondisplaced fracture of lesser tuberosity of unspecified humerus A, K, P 🔷, B 🔷, D, G, S 🔷, A, B 🔷

● S42.27   Torus fracture of upper end of humerus

The appropriate 7th character is to be added to all codes in subcategory S42.27

A	initial encounter for closed fracture
D	subsequent encounter for fracture with routine healing
G	subsequent encounter for fracture with delayed healing
K	subsequent encounter for fracture with nonunion
P	subsequent encounter for fracture with malunion
S	sequela

  ● S42.271   Torus fracture of upper end of right humerus A, K, P 🔷, D, G, S 🔷, A 🔷

  ● S42.272   Torus fracture of upper end of left humerus A, K, P 🔷, D, G, S 🔷, A 🔷

  ●■ S42.279   Torus fracture of upper end of unspecified humerus A, K, P 🔷, D, G, S 🔷, A 🔷

● S42.29   Other fracture of upper end of humerus
Fracture of anatomical neck of humerus
Fracture of articular head of humerus

  ● S42.291   Other displaced fracture of upper end of right humerus A, K, P 🔷, B 🔷, D, G, S 🔷, A, B 🔷

  ● S42.292   Other displaced fracture of upper end of left humerus A, K, P 🔷, B 🔷, D, G, S 🔷, A, B 🔷

  ●■ S42.293   Other displaced fracture of upper end of unspecified humerus
A, K, P 🔷, B 🔷, D, G, S 🔷, A, B 🔷

  ● S42.294   Other nondisplaced fracture of upper end of right humerus
A, K, P 🔷, B 🔷, D, G, S 🔷, A, B 🔷

  ● S42.295   Other nondisplaced fracture of upper end of left humerus
A, K, P 🔷, B 🔷, D, G, S 🔷, A, B 🔷

  ●■ S42.296   Other nondisplaced fracture of upper end of unspecified humerus A, K, P 🔷, B 🔷, D, G, S 🔷, A, B 🔷

● S42.3   Fracture of shaft of humerus
Fracture of humerus NOS
Fracture of upper arm NOS

Excludes2	physeal fractures of upper end of humerus (S49.0-)
	physeal fractures of lower end of humerus (S49.1-)

● S42.30   Unspecified fracture of shaft of humerus

  ●■ S42.301   Unspecified fracture of shaft of humerus, right arm A, K, P 🔷, B 🔷, D, G, S 🔷, A, B 🔷

  ●■ S42.302   Unspecified fracture of shaft of humerus, left arm A, K, P 🔷, B 🔷, D, G, S 🔷, A, B 🔷

  ●■ S42.309   Unspecified fracture of shaft of humerus, unspecified arm
A, K, P 🔷, B 🔷, D, G, S 🔷, A, B 🔷

● S42.31   Greenstick fracture of shaft of humerus

The appropriate 7th character is to be added to all codes in subcategory S42.31

A	initial encounter for closed fracture
D	subsequent encounter for fracture with routine healing
G	subsequent encounter for fracture with delayed healing
K	subsequent encounter for fracture with nonunion
P	subsequent encounter for fracture with malunion
S	sequela

  ● S42.311   Greenstick fracture of shaft of humerus, right arm A, K, P 🔷, D, G, S 🔷, A 🔷

  ● S42.312   Greenstick fracture of shaft of humerus, left arm A, K, P 🔷, D, G, S 🔷, A 🔷

  ●■ S42.319   Greenstick fracture of shaft of humerus, unspecified arm
A, K, P 🔷, D, G, S 🔷, A 🔷

● Unacceptable Principal Diagnosis   ● Use Additional Character(s)   ■ Unspecified   ▶ Manifestation Code

1456   **OGCR** Official Guidelines for Coding and Reporting   Excludes 1   Excludes 2   Includes   Use additional   Code first   Code also

● **S42.32**   Transverse fracture of shaft of humerus

    ● **S42.321**   Displaced transverse fracture of shaft of humerus, right arm
A, K, P 🦠, B 🦠, D, G, S 🦠, A, B 🦠

    ● **S42.322**   Displaced transverse fracture of shaft of humerus, left arm
A, K, P 🦠, B 🦠, D, G, S 🦠, A, B 🦠

    ●■ **S42.323**   Displaced transverse fracture of shaft of humerus, unspecified arm A, K, P 🦠, B 🦠, D, G, S 🦠, A, B 🦠

    ● **S42.324**   Nondisplaced transverse fracture of shaft of humerus, right arm
A, K, P 🦠, B 🦠, D, G, S 🦠, A, B 🦠

    ● **S42.325**   Nondisplaced transverse fracture of shaft of humerus, left arm
A, K, P 🦠, B 🦠, D, G, S 🦠, A, B 🦠

    ●■ **S42.326**   Nondisplaced transverse fracture of shaft of humerus, unspecified arm A, K, P 🦠, B 🦠, D, G, S 🦠, A, B 🦠

● **S42.33**   Oblique fracture of shaft of humerus

    ● **S42.331**   Displaced oblique fracture of shaft of humerus, right arm
A, K, P 🦠, B 🦠, D, G, S 🦠, A, B 🦠

    ● **S42.332**   Displaced oblique fracture of shaft of humerus, left arm
A, K, P 🦠, B 🦠, D, G, S 🦠, A, B 🦠

    ●■ **S42.333**   Displaced oblique fracture of shaft of humerus, unspecified arm A, K, P 🦠, B 🦠, D, G, S 🦠, A, B 🦠

    ● **S42.334**   Nondisplaced oblique fracture of shaft of humerus, right arm
A, K, P 🦠, B 🦠, D, G, S 🦠, A, B 🦠

    ● **S42.335**   Nondisplaced oblique fracture of shaft of humerus, left arm
A, K, P 🦠, B 🦠, D, G, S 🦠, A, B 🦠

    ●■ **S42.336**   Nondisplaced oblique fracture of shaft of humerus, unspecified arm A, K, P 🦠, B 🦠, D, G, S 🦠, A, B 🦠

● **S42.34**   Spiral fracture of shaft of humerus

    ● **S42.341**   Displaced spiral fracture of shaft of humerus, right arm A, K, P 🦠, B 🦠, D, G, S 🦠, A, B 🦠

    ● **S42.342**   Displaced spiral fracture of shaft of humerus, left arm A, K, P 🦠, B 🦠, D, G, S 🦠, A, B 🦠

    ●■ **S42.343**   Displaced spiral fracture of shaft of humerus, unspecified arm A, K, P 🦠, B 🦠, D, G, S 🦠, A, B 🦠

    ● **S42.344**   Nondisplaced spiral fracture of shaft of humerus, right arm
A, K, P 🦠, B 🦠, D, G, S 🦠, A, B 🦠

    ● **S42.345**   Nondisplaced spiral fracture of shaft of humerus, left arm
A, K, P 🦠, B 🦠, D, G, S 🦠, A, B 🦠

    ●■ **S42.346**   Nondisplaced spiral fracture of shaft of humerus, unspecified arm A, K, P 🦠, B 🦠, D, G, S 🦠, A, B 🦠

● **S42.35**   Comminuted fracture of shaft of humerus

    ● **S42.351**   Displaced comminuted fracture of shaft of humerus, right arm
A, K, P 🦠, B 🦠, D, G, S 🦠, A, B 🦠

    ● **S42.352**   Displaced comminuted fracture of shaft of humerus, left arm
A, K, P 🦠, B 🦠, D, G, S 🦠, A, B 🦠

    ●■ **S42.353**   Displaced comminuted fracture of shaft of humerus, unspecified arm A, K, P 🦠, B 🦠, D, G, S 🦠, A, B 🦠

    ● **S42.354**   Nondisplaced comminuted fracture of shaft of humerus, right arm A, K, P 🦠, B 🦠, D, G, S 🦠, A, B 🦠

    ● **S42.355**   Nondisplaced comminuted fracture of shaft of humerus, left arm A, K, P 🦠, B 🦠, D, G, S 🦠, A, B 🦠

    ●■ **S42.356**   Nondisplaced comminuted fracture of shaft of humerus, unspecified arm A, K, P 🦠, B 🦠, D, G, S 🦠, A, B 🦠

● **S42.36**   Segmental fracture of shaft of humerus

    ● **S42.361**   Displaced segmental fracture of shaft of humerus, right arm
A, K, P 🦠, B 🦠, D, G, S 🦠, A, B 🦠

    ● **S42.362**   Displaced segmental fracture of shaft of humerus, left arm
A, K, P 🦠, B 🦠, D, G, S 🦠, A, B 🦠

    ●■ **S42.363**   Displaced segmental fracture of shaft of humerus, unspecified arm A, K, P 🦠, B 🦠, D, G, S 🦠, A, B 🦠

    ● **S42.364**   Nondisplaced segmental fracture of shaft of humerus, right arm
A, K, P 🦠, B 🦠, D, G, S 🦠, A, B 🦠

    ● **S42.365**   Nondisplaced segmental fracture of shaft of humerus, left arm
A, K, P 🦠, B 🦠, D, G, S 🦠, A, B 🦠

    ●■ **S42.366**   Nondisplaced segmental fracture of shaft of humerus, unspecified arm A, K, P 🦠, B 🦠, D, G, S 🦠, A, B 🦠

● **S42.39**   Other fracture of shaft of humerus

    ● **S42.391**   Other fracture of shaft of right humerus A, K, P 🦠, B 🦠, D, G, S 🦠, A, B 🦠

    ● **S42.392**   Other fracture of shaft of left humerus A, K, P 🦠, B 🦠, D, G, S 🦠, A, B 🦠

    ●■ **S42.399**   Other fracture of shaft of unspecified humerus A, K, P 🦠, B 🦠, D, G, S 🦠, A, B 🦠

● **S42.4**   Fracture of lower end of humerus
Fracture of distal end of humerus

    Excludes2   fracture of shaft of humerus (S42.3-)
physeal fracture of lower end of humerus (S49.1-)

● **S42.40**   Unspecified fracture of lower end of humerus
Fracture of elbow NOS

    ●■ **S42.401**   Unspecified fracture of lower end of right humerus A, K, P 🦠, B 🦠, D, G, S 🦠, A, B 🦠

N   Newborn Age: 0   **P**   Pediatric Age: 0–17   **M**   Maternity DX: 12–55   **A**   Adult Age: 15–124   ♀   Females Only   ♂   Males Only

🦠   Complication\Comorbidity   🦠   Major C\C   🦠   Present on Admission Requirement   🦠   Hospital-Acquired Condition

1457

CHAPTER 19 (S00-T88)

● ■ **S42.402** Unspecified fracture of lower end of left humerus A, K, P 🔾, B 🔾, D, G, S 🔾, A, B 🔾

● ■ **S42.409** Unspecified fracture of lower end of unspecified humerus A, K, P 🔾, B 🔾, D, G, S 🔾, A, B 🔾

● **S42.41** Simple supracondylar fracture without intercondylar fracture of humerus

● **S42.411** Displaced simple supracondylar fracture without intercondylar fracture of right humerus A, K, P 🔾, B 🔾, D, G, S 🔾, A, B 🔾

● **S42.412** Displaced simple supracondylar fracture without intercondylar fracture of left humerus A, K, P 🔾, B 🔾, D, G, S 🔾, A, B 🔾

● ■ **S42.413** Displaced simple supracondylar fracture without intercondylar fracture of unspecified humerus A, K, P 🔾, B 🔾, D, G, S 🔾, A, B 🔾

● **S42.414** Nondisplaced simple supracondylar fracture without intercondylar fracture of right humerus A, K, P 🔾, B 🔾, D, G, S 🔾, A, B 🔾

● **S42.415** Nondisplaced simple supracondylar fracture without intercondylar fracture of left humerus A, K, P 🔾, B 🔾, D, G, S 🔾, A, B 🔾

● ■ **S42.416** Nondisplaced simple supracondylar fracture without intercondylar fracture of unspecified humerus A, K, P 🔾, B 🔾, D, G, S 🔾, A, B 🔾

● **S42.42** Comminuted supracondylar fracture without intercondylar fracture of humerus

● **S42.421** Displaced comminuted supracondylar fracture without intercondylar fracture of right humerus A, K, P 🔾, B 🔾, D, G, S 🔾, A, B 🔾

● **S42.422** Displaced comminuted supracondylar fracture without intercondylar fracture of left humerus A, K, P 🔾, B 🔾, D, G, S 🔾, A, B 🔾

● ■ **S42.423** Displaced comminuted supracondylar fracture without intercondylar fracture of unspecified humerus A, K, P 🔾, B 🔾, D, G, S 🔾, A, B 🔾

● **S42.424** Nondisplaced comminuted supracondylar fracture without intercondylar fracture of right humerus A, K, P 🔾, B 🔾, D, G, S 🔾, A, B 🔾

● **S42.425** Nondisplaced comminuted supracondylar fracture without intercondylar fracture of left humerus A, K, P 🔾, B 🔾, D, G, S 🔾, A, B 🔾

● ■ **S42.426** Nondisplaced comminuted supracondylar fracture without intercondylar fracture of unspecified humerus A, K, P 🔾, B 🔾, D, G, S 🔾, A, B 🔾

● **S42.43** Fracture (avulsion) of lateral epicondyle of humerus

● **S42.431** Displaced fracture (avulsion) of lateral epicondyle of right humerus A, K, P 🔾, B 🔾, D, G, S 🔾, A, B 🔾

● **S42.432** Displaced fracture (avulsion) of lateral epicondyle of left humerus A, K, P 🔾, B 🔾, D, G, S 🔾, A, B 🔾

● ■ **S42.433** Displaced fracture (avulsion) of lateral epicondyle of unspecified humerus A, K, P 🔾, B 🔾, D, G, S 🔾, A, B 🔾

● **S42.434** Nondisplaced fracture (avulsion) of lateral epicondyle of right humerus A, K, P 🔾, B 🔾, D, G, S 🔾, A, B 🔾

● **S42.435** Nondisplaced fracture (avulsion) of lateral epicondyle of left humerus A, K, P 🔾, B 🔾, D, G, S 🔾, A, B 🔾

● ■ **S42.436** Nondisplaced fracture (avulsion) of lateral epicondyle of unspecified humerus A, K, P 🔾, B 🔾, D, G, S 🔾, A, B 🔾

● **S42.44** Fracture (avulsion) of medial epicondyle of humerus

● **S42.441** Displaced fracture (avulsion) of medial epicondyle of right humerus A, K, P 🔾, B 🔾, D, G, S 🔾, A, B 🔾

● **S42.442** Displaced fracture (avulsion) of medial epicondyle of left humerus A, K, P 🔾, B 🔾, D, G, S 🔾, A, B 🔾

● ■ **S42.443** Displaced fracture (avulsion) of medial epicondyle of unspecified humerus A, K, P 🔾, B 🔾, D, G, S 🔾, A, B 🔾

● **S42.444** Nondisplaced fracture (avulsion) of medial epicondyle of right humerus A, K, P 🔾, B 🔾, D, G, S 🔾, A, B 🔾

● **S42.445** Nondisplaced fracture (avulsion) of medial epicondyle of left humerus A, K, P 🔾, B 🔾, D, G, S 🔾, A, B 🔾

● ■ **S42.446** Nondisplaced fracture (avulsion) of medial epicondyle of unspecified humerus A, K, P 🔾, B 🔾, D, G, S 🔾, A, B 🔾

● **S42.447** Incarcerated fracture (avulsion) of medial epicondyle of right humerus A, K, P 🔾, B 🔾, D, G, S 🔾, A, B 🔾

● **S42.448** Incarcerated fracture (avulsion) of medial epicondyle of left humerus A, K, P 🔾, B 🔾, D, G, S 🔾, A, B 🔾

● ■ **S42.449** Incarcerated fracture (avulsion) of medial epicondyle of unspecified humerus A, K, P 🔾, B 🔾, D, G, S 🔾, A, B 🔾

● **S42.45** **Fracture of lateral condyle of humerus**
Fracture of capitellum of humerus

  ● **S42.451** **Displaced fracture of lateral condyle of right humerus**
A, K, P 🔵, B 🔵, D, G, S 🔵, A, B 🔵

  ● **S42.452** **Displaced fracture of lateral condyle of left humerus**
A, K, P 🔵, B 🔵, D, G, S 🔵, A, B 🔵

  ●■ **S42.453** **Displaced fracture of lateral condyle of unspecified humerus**
A, K, P 🔵, B 🔵, D, G, S 🔵, A, B 🔵

  ● **S42.454** **Nondisplaced fracture of lateral condyle of right humerus**
A, K, P 🔵, B 🔵, D, G, S 🔵, A, B 🔵

  ● **S42.455** **Nondisplaced fracture of lateral condyle of left humerus**
A, K, P 🔵, B 🔵, D, G, S 🔵, A, B 🔵

  ●■ **S42.456** **Nondisplaced fracture of lateral condyle of unspecified humerus**
A, K, P 🔵, B 🔵, D, G, S 🔵, A, B 🔵

● **S42.46** **Fracture of medial condyle of humerus**
Trochlea fracture of humerus

  ● **S42.461** **Displaced fracture of medial condyle of right humerus**
A, K, P 🔵, B 🔵, D, G, S 🔵, A, B 🔵

  ● **S42.462** **Displaced fracture of medial condyle of left humerus**
A, K, P 🔵, B 🔵, D, G, S 🔵, A, B 🔵

  ●■ **S42.463** **Displaced fracture of medial condyle of unspecified humerus**
A, K, P 🔵, B 🔵, D, G, S 🔵, A, B 🔵

  ● **S42.464** **Nondisplaced fracture of medial condyle of right humerus**
A, K, P 🔵, B 🔵, D, G, S 🔵, A, B 🔵

  ● **S42.465** **Nondisplaced fracture of medial condyle of left humerus**
A, K, P 🔵, B 🔵, D, G, S 🔵, A, B 🔵

  ●■ **S42.466** **Nondisplaced fracture of medial condyle of unspecified humerus**
A, K, P 🔵, B 🔵, D, G, S 🔵, A, B 🔵

● **S42.47** **Transcondylar fracture of humerus**

  ● **S42.471** **Displaced transcondylar fracture of right humerus** A, K, P 🔵, B 🔵, D, G, S 🔵, A, B 🔵

  ● **S42.472** **Displaced transcondylar fracture of left humerus** A, K, P 🔵, B 🔵, D, G, S 🔵, A, B 🔵

  ●■ **S42.473** **Displaced transcondylar fracture of unspecified humerus**
A, K, P 🔵, B 🔵, D, G, S 🔵, A, B 🔵

  ● **S42.474** **Nondisplaced transcondylar fracture of right humerus**
A, K, P 🔵, B 🔵, D, G, S 🔵, A, B 🔵

  ● **S42.475** **Nondisplaced transcondylar fracture of left humerus**
A, K, P 🔵, B 🔵, D, G, S 🔵, A, B 🔵

  ●■ **S42.476** **Nondisplaced transcondylar fracture of unspecified humerus**
A, K, P 🔵, B 🔵, D, G, S 🔵, A, B 🔵

● **S42.48** **Torus fracture of lower end of humerus**

The appropriate 7th character is to be added to all codes in subcategory S42.48

A	initial encounter for closed fracture
D	subsequent encounter for fracture with routine healing
G	subsequent encounter for fracture with delayed healing
K	subsequent encounter for fracture with nonunion
P	subsequent encounter for fracture with malunion
S	sequela

  ● **S42.481** **Torus fracture of lower end of right humerus** A, K, P 🔵, D, G, S 🔵, A 🔵

  ● **S42.482** **Torus fracture of lower end of left humerus** A, K, P 🔵, D, G, S 🔵, A 🔵

  ●■ **S42.489** **Torus fracture of lower end of unspecified humerus** A, K, P 🔵, D, G, S 🔵, A 🔵

● **S42.49** **Other fracture of lower end of humerus**

  ● **S42.491** **Other displaced fracture of lower end of right humerus** A, K, P 🔵, B 🔵, D, G, S 🔵, A, B 🔵

  ● **S42.492** **Other displaced fracture of lower end of left humerus** A, K, P 🔵, B 🔵, D, G, S 🔵, A, B 🔵

  ●■ **S42.493** **Other displaced fracture of lower end of unspecified humerus**
A, K, P 🔵, B 🔵, D, G, S 🔵, A, B 🔵

  ● **S42.494** **Other nondisplaced fracture of lower end of right humerus**
A, K, P 🔵, B 🔵, D, G, S 🔵, A, B 🔵

  ● **S42.495** **Other nondisplaced fracture of lower end of left humerus**
A, K, P 🔵, B 🔵, D, G, S 🔵, A, B 🔵

  ●■ **S42.496** **Other nondisplaced fracture of lower end of unspecified humerus** A, K, P 🔵, B 🔵

● **S42.9** **Fracture of shoulder girdle, part unspecified**
Fracture of shoulder NOS

  ●■ **S42.90** **Fracture of unspecified shoulder girdle, part unspecified** A, K, P 🔵, B 🔵, D, G, S 🔵, A, B 🔵

  ●■ **S42.91** **Fracture of right shoulder girdle, part unspecified** A, K, P 🔵, B 🔵, D, G, S 🔵, A, B 🔵

  ●■ **S42.92** **Fracture of left shoulder girdle, part unspecified** A, K, P 🔵, B 🔵, D, G, S 🔵, A, B 🔵

N   Newborn Age: 0   **P**   Pediatric Age: 0–17   **M**   Maternity DX: 12–55   **A**   Adult Age: 15–124   ♀   Females Only   ♂   Males Only

🔵 Complication\Comorbidity   🔵 Major C\C   🔵 Present on Admission Requirement   🔵 Hospital-Acquired Condition

1459

CHAPTER 19 (S00-T88)

● **S43 Dislocation and sprain of joints and ligaments of shoulder girdle**

> **Includes**   avulsion of joint or ligament of shoulder girdle
>
> laceration of cartilage, joint or ligament of shoulder girdle
>
> sprain of cartilage, joint or ligament of shoulder girdle
>
> traumatic hemarthrosis of joint or ligament of shoulder girdle
>
> traumatic rupture of joint or ligament of shoulder girdle
>
> traumatic subluxation of joint or ligament of shoulder girdle
>
> traumatic tear of joint or ligament of shoulder girdle

> **Code also** any associated open wound

> **Excludes2**   strain of muscle, fascia and tendon of shoulder and upper arm (S46.-)

> The appropriate 7th character is to be added to each code from category S43

> | | |
> |---|---|
> | A | initial encounter |
> | D | subsequent encounter |
> | S | sequela |

● **S43.0 Subluxation and dislocation of shoulder joint**
> Dislocation of glenohumeral joint
> Subluxation of glenohumeral joint

  ● **S43.00 Unspecified subluxation and dislocation of shoulder joint**
> > Dislocation of humerus NOS
> > Subluxation of humerus NOS

    ●■ **S43.001 Unspecified subluxation of right shoulder joint** D, S 🔄

    ●■ **S43.002 Unspecified subluxation of left shoulder joint** D, S 🔄

    ●■ **S43.003 Unspecified subluxation of unspecified shoulder joint** D, S 🔄

    ●■ **S43.004 Unspecified dislocation of right shoulder joint** D, S 🔄

    ●■ **S43.005 Unspecified dislocation of left shoulder joint** D, S 🔄

    ●■ **S43.006 Unspecified dislocation of unspecified shoulder joint** D, S 🔄

  ● **S43.01 Anterior subluxation and dislocation of humerus**

    ● **S43.011 Anterior subluxation of right humerus** D, S 🔄

    ● **S43.012 Anterior subluxation of left humerus** D, S 🔄

    ●■ **S43.013 Anterior subluxation of unspecified humerus** D, S 🔄

    ● **S43.014 Anterior dislocation of right humerus** D, S 🔄

    ● **S43.015 Anterior dislocation of left humerus** D, S 🔄

    ●■ **S43.016 Anterior dislocation of unspecified humerus** D, S 🔄

  ● **S43.02 Posterior subluxation and dislocation of humerus**

    ● **S43.021 Posterior subluxation of right humerus** D, S 🔄

    ● **S43.022 Posterior subluxation of left humerus** D, S 🔄

    ●■ **S43.023 Posterior subluxation of unspecified humerus** D, S 🔄

    ● **S43.024 Posterior dislocation of right humerus** D, S 🔄

    ● **S43.025 Posterior dislocation of left humerus** D, S 🔄

    ●■ **S43.026 Posterior dislocation of unspecified humerus** D, S 🔄

  ● **S43.03 Inferior subluxation and dislocation of humerus**

    ● **S43.031 Inferior subluxation of right humerus** D, S 🔄

    ● **S43.032 Inferior subluxation of left humerus** D, S 🔄

    ●■ **S43.033 Inferior subluxation of unspecified humerus** D, S 🔄

    ● **S43.034 Inferior dislocation of right humerus** D, S 🔄

    ● **S43.035 Inferior dislocation of left humerus** D, S 🔄

    ●■ **S43.036 Inferior dislocation of unspecified humerus** D, S 🔄

  ● **S43.08 Other subluxation and dislocation of shoulder joint**

    ● **S43.081 Other subluxation of right shoulder joint** D, S 🔄

    ● **S43.082 Other subluxation of left shoulder joint** D, S 🔄

    ●■ **S43.083 Other subluxation of unspecified shoulder joint** D, S 🔄

    ● **S43.084 Other dislocation of right shoulder joint** D, S 🔄

    ● **S43.085 Other dislocation of left shoulder joint** D, S 🔄

    ●■ **S43.086 Other dislocation of unspecified shoulder joint** D, S 🔄

● **S43.1 Subluxation and dislocation of acromioclavicular joint**

  ● **S43.10 Unspecified dislocation of acromioclavicular joint**

    ●■ **S43.101 Unspecified dislocation of right acromioclavicular joint** D, S 🔄

    ●■ **S43.102 Unspecified dislocation of left acromioclavicular joint** D, S 🔄

    ●■ **S43.109 Unspecified dislocation of unspecified acromioclavicular joint** D, S 🔄

  ● **S43.11 Subluxation of acromioclavicular joint**

    ● **S43.111 Subluxation of right acromioclavicular joint** D, S 🔄

    ● **S43.112 Subluxation of left acromioclavicular joint** D, S 🔄

    ●■ **S43.119 Subluxation of unspecified acromioclavicular joint** D, S 🔄

  ● **S43.12 Dislocation of acromioclavicular joint, 100%-200% displacement**

    ● **S43.121 Dislocation of right acromioclavicular joint, 100%-200% displacement** D, S 🔄

    ● **S43.122 Dislocation of left acromioclavicular joint, 100%-200% displacement** D, S 🔄

    ●■ **S43.129 Dislocation of unspecified acromioclavicular joint, 100%-200% displacement** D, S 🔄

● Unacceptable Principal Diagnosis	● Use Additional Character(s)	■ Unspecified	▶ Manifestation Code

OGCR Official Guidelines for Coding and Reporting   Excludes 1   Excludes 2   Includes   Use additional   Code first   Code also

● S43.13   Dislocation of acromioclavicular joint, greater than 200% displacement

     ● S43.131   Dislocation of right acromioclavicular joint, greater than 200% displacement D, S 🏷

     ● S43.132   Dislocation of left acromioclavicular joint, greater than 200% displacement D, S 🏷

     ●■ S43.139   Dislocation of unspecified acromioclavicular joint, greater than 200% displacement D, S 🏷

● S43.14   Inferior dislocation of acromioclavicular joint

     ● S43.141   Inferior dislocation of right acromioclavicular joint D, S 🏷

     ● S43.142   Inferior dislocation of left acromioclavicular joint D, S 🏷

     ●■ S43.149   Inferior dislocation of unspecified acromioclavicular joint D, S 🏷

● S43.15   Posterior dislocation of acromioclavicular joint

     ● S43.151   Posterior dislocation of right acromioclavicular joint D, S 🏷

     ● S43.152   Posterior dislocation of left acromioclavicular joint D, S 🏷

     ●■ S43.159   Posterior dislocation of unspecified acromioclavicular joint D, S 🏷

● S43.2   Subluxation and dislocation of sternoclavicular joint

     ● S43.20   Unspecified subluxation and dislocation of sternoclavicular joint

       ●■ S43.201   Unspecified subluxation of right sternoclavicular joint A 🏷, D, S 🏷, A 🏷

       ●■ S43.202   Unspecified subluxation of left sternoclavicular joint A 🏷, D, S 🏷, A 🏷

       ●■ S43.203   Unspecified subluxation of unspecified sternoclavicular joint A 🏷, D, S 🏷, A 🏷

       ●■ S43.204   Unspecified dislocation of right sternoclavicular joint A 🏷, D, S 🏷, A 🏷

       ●■ S43.205   Unspecified dislocation of left sternoclavicular joint A 🏷, D, S 🏷, A 🏷

       ●■ S43.206   Unspecified dislocation of unspecified sternoclavicular joint A 🏷, D, S 🏷, A 🏷

     ● S43.21   Anterior subluxation and dislocation of sternoclavicular joint

       ● S43.211   Anterior subluxation of right sternoclavicular joint A 🏷, D, S 🏷, A 🏷

       ● S43.212   Anterior subluxation of left sternoclavicular joint A 🏷, D, S 🏷, A 🏷

       ●■ S43.213   Anterior subluxation of unspecified sternoclavicular joint A 🏷, D, S 🏷, A 🏷

     ● S43.214   Anterior dislocation of right sternoclavicular joint A 🏷, D, S 🏷, A 🏷

     ● S43.215   Anterior dislocation of left sternoclavicular joint A 🏷, D, S 🏷, A 🏷

     ●■ S43.216   Anterior dislocation of unspecified sternoclavicular joint A 🏷, D, S 🏷, A 🏷

     ● S43.22   Posterior subluxation and dislocation of sternoclavicular joint

       ● S43.221   Posterior subluxation of right sternoclavicular joint A 🏷, D, S 🏷, A 🏷

       ● S43.222   Posterior subluxation of left sternoclavicular joint A 🏷, D, S 🏷, A 🏷

       ●■ S43.223   Posterior subluxation of unspecified sternoclavicular joint A 🏷, D, S 🏷, A 🏷

       ● S43.224   Posterior dislocation of right sternoclavicular joint A 🏷, D, S 🏷, A 🏷

       ● S43.225   Posterior dislocation of left sternoclavicular joint A 🏷, D, S 🏷, A 🏷

       ●■ S43.226   Posterior dislocation of unspecified sternoclavicular joint A 🏷, D, S 🏷, A 🏷

● S43.3   Subluxation and dislocation of other and unspecified parts of shoulder girdle

     ● S43.30   Subluxation and dislocation of unspecified parts of shoulder girdle

         Dislocation of shoulder girdle NOS
         Subluxation of shoulder girdle NOS

       ●■ S43.301   Subluxation of unspecified parts of right shoulder girdle D, S 🏷

       ●■ S43.302   Subluxation of unspecified parts of left shoulder girdle D, S 🏷

       ●■ S43.303   Subluxation of unspecified parts of unspecified shoulder girdle D, S 🏷

       ●■ S43.304   Dislocation of unspecified parts of right shoulder girdle D, S 🏷

       ●■ S43.305   Dislocation of unspecified parts of left shoulder girdle D, S 🏷

       ●■ S43.306   Dislocation of unspecified parts of unspecified shoulder girdle D, S 🏷

     ● S43.31   Subluxation and dislocation of scapula

       ● S43.311   Subluxation of right scapula D, S 🏷

       ● S43.312   Subluxation of left scapula D, S 🏷

       ●■ S43.313   Subluxation of unspecified scapula D, S 🏷

       ● S43.314   Dislocation of right scapula D, S 🏷

       ● S43.315   Dislocation of left scapula D, S 🏷

       ●■ S43.316   Dislocation of unspecified scapula D, S 🏷

CHAPTER 19 (S00-T88)

- S43.39 Subluxation and dislocation of other parts of shoulder girdle
  - S43.391 Subluxation of other parts of right shoulder girdle D, S
  - S43.392 Subluxation of other parts of left shoulder girdle D, S
  - S43.393 Subluxation of other parts of unspecified shoulder girdle D, S
  - S43.394 Dislocation of other parts of right shoulder girdle D, S
  - S43.395 Dislocation of other parts of left shoulder girdle D, S
  - S43.396 Dislocation of other parts of unspecified shoulder girdle D, S
- S43.4 Sprain of shoulder joint
  - S43.40 Unspecified sprain of shoulder joint
    - S43.401 Unspecified sprain of right shoulder joint D, S
    - S43.402 Unspecified sprain of left shoulder joint D, S
    - S43.409 Unspecified sprain of unspecified shoulder joint D, S
  - S43.41 Sprain of coracohumeral (ligament)
    - S43.411 Sprain of right coracohumeral (ligament) D, S
    - S43.412 Sprain of left coracohumeral (ligament) D, S
    - S43.419 Sprain of unspecified coracohumeral (ligament) D, S
  - S43.42 Sprain of rotator cuff capsule
    - Excludes1 rotator cuff syndrome (complete) (incomplete), not specified as traumatic (M75.1-)
    - Excludes2 injury of tendon of rotator cuff (S46.0-)
    - S43.421 Sprain of right rotator cuff capsule D, S
    - S43.422 Sprain of left rotator cuff capsule D, S
    - S43.429 Sprain of unspecified rotator cuff capsule D, S
  - S43.43 Superior glenoid labrum lesion
    - SLAP lesion
    - S43.431 Superior glenoid labrum lesion of right shoulder D, S
    - S43.432 Superior glenoid labrum lesion of left shoulder D, S
    - S43.439 Superior glenoid labrum lesion of unspecified shoulder D, S
  - S43.49 Other sprain of shoulder joint
    - S43.491 Other sprain of right shoulder joint D, S
    - S43.492 Other sprain of left shoulder joint D, S
    - S43.499 Other sprain of unspecified shoulder joint D, S

- S43.5 Sprain of acromioclavicular joint
  - Sprain of acromioclavicular ligament
  - S43.50 Sprain of unspecified acromioclavicular joint D, S
  - S43.51 Sprain of right acromioclavicular joint D, S
  - S43.52 Sprain of left acromioclavicular joint D, S
- S43.6 Sprain of sternoclavicular joint
  - S43.60 Sprain of unspecified sternoclavicular joint D, S
  - S43.61 Sprain of right sternoclavicular joint D, S
  - S43.62 Sprain of left sternoclavicular joint D, S
- S43.8 Sprain of other specified parts of shoulder girdle
  - S43.80 Sprain of other specified parts of unspecified shoulder girdle D, S
  - S43.81 Sprain of other specified parts of right shoulder girdle D, S
  - S43.82 Sprain of other specified parts of left shoulder girdle D, S
- S43.9 Sprain of unspecified parts of shoulder girdle
  - S43.90 Sprain of unspecified parts of unspecified shoulder girdle D, S
    - Sprain of shoulder girdle NOS
  - S43.91 Sprain of unspecified parts of right shoulder girdle D, S
  - S43.92 Sprain of unspecified parts of left shoulder girdle D, S

- S44 Injury of nerves at shoulder and upper arm level
  - Code also any associated open wound (S41.-)
  - Excludes2 injury of brachial plexus (S14.3-)
  - The appropriate 7th character is to be added to each code from category S44
    - A initial encounter
    - D subsequent encounter
    - S sequela
  - S44.0 Injury of ulnar nerve at upper arm level
    - Excludes1 ulnar nerve NOS (S54.0)
    - S44.00 Injury of ulnar nerve at upper arm level, unspecified arm D, S
    - S44.01 Injury of ulnar nerve at upper arm level, right arm D, S
    - S44.02 Injury of ulnar nerve at upper arm level, left arm D, S
  - S44.1 Injury of median nerve at upper arm level
    - Excludes1 median nerve NOS (S54.1)
    - S44.10 Injury of median nerve at upper arm level, unspecified arm D, S
    - S44.11 Injury of median nerve at upper arm level, right arm D, S
    - S44.12 Injury of median nerve at upper arm level, left arm D, S

● S44.2   Injury of radial nerve at upper arm level
> Excludes1   radial nerve NOS (S54.2)

  ● ■ S44.20   Injury of radial nerve at upper arm level, unspecified arm D, S 🔗

  ● S44.21   Injury of radial nerve at upper arm level, right arm D, S 🔗

  ● S44.22   Injury of radial nerve at upper arm level, left arm D, S 🔗

● S44.3   Injury of axillary nerve

  ● ■ S44.30   Injury of axillary nerve, unspecified arm D, S 🔗

  ● S44.31   Injury of axillary nerve, right arm D, S 🔗

  ● S44.32   Injury of axillary nerve, left arm D, S 🔗

● S44.4   Injury of musculocutaneous nerve

  ● ■ S44.40   Injury of musculocutaneous nerve, unspecified arm D, S 🔗

  ● S44.41   Injury of musculocutaneous nerve, right arm D, S 🔗

  ● S44.42   Injury of musculocutaneous nerve, left arm D, S 🔗

● S44.5   Injury of cutaneous sensory nerve at shoulder and upper arm level

  ● ■ S44.50   Injury of cutaneous sensory nerve at shoulder and upper arm level, unspecified arm D, S 🔗

  ● S44.51   Injury of cutaneous sensory nerve at shoulder and upper arm level, right arm D, S 🔗

  ● S44.52   Injury of cutaneous sensory nerve at shoulder and upper arm level, left arm D, S 🔗

● S44.8   Injury of other nerves at shoulder and upper arm level

  ● S44.8X   Injury of other nerves at shoulder and upper arm level

    ● S44.8X1   Injury of other nerves at shoulder and upper arm level, right arm D, S 🔗

    ● S44.8X2   Injury of other nerves at shoulder and upper arm level, left arm D, S 🔗

    ● ■ S44.8X9   Injury of other nerves at shoulder and upper arm level, unspecified arm D, S 🔗

● S44.9   Injury of unspecified nerve at shoulder and upper arm level

  ● ■ S44.90   Injury of unspecified nerve at shoulder and upper arm level, unspecified arm D, S 🔗

  ● ■ S44.91   Injury of unspecified nerve at shoulder and upper arm level, right arm D, S 🔗

  ● ■ S44.92   Injury of unspecified nerve at shoulder and upper arm level, left arm D, S 🔗

● S45   Injury of blood vessels at shoulder and upper arm level
> Code also any associated open wound (S41.-)
> Excludes2   injury of subclavian artery (S25.1)
> injury of subclavian vein (S25.3)

The appropriate 7th character is to be added to each code from category S45

A	initial encounter
D	subsequent encounter
S	sequela

● S45.0   Injury of axillary artery

  ● S45.00   Unspecified injury of axillary artery

    ● ■ S45.001   Unspecified injury of axillary artery, right side A 🔗, D, S 🔗

    ● ■ S45.002   Unspecified injury of axillary artery, left side A 🔗, D, S 🔗

    ● ■ S45.009   Unspecified injury of axillary artery, unspecified side A 🔗, D, S 🔗

  ● S45.01   Laceration of axillary artery

    ● S45.011   Laceration of axillary artery, right side A 🔗, D, S 🔗

    ● S45.012   Laceration of axillary artery, left side A 🔗, D, S 🔗

    ● ■ S45.019   Laceration of axillary artery, unspecified side A 🔗, D, S 🔗

  ● S45.09   Other specified injury of axillary artery

    ● S45.091   Other specified injury of axillary artery, right side A 🔗, D, S 🔗

    ● S45.092   Other specified injury of axillary artery, left side A 🔗, D, S 🔗

    ● ■ S45.099   Other specified injury of axillary artery, unspecified side A 🔗, D, S 🔗

● S45.1   Injury of brachial artery

  ● S45.10   Unspecified injury of brachial artery

    ● ■ S45.101   Unspecified injury of brachial artery, right side A 🔗, D, S 🔗

    ● ■ S45.102   Unspecified injury of brachial artery, left side A 🔗, D, S 🔗

    ● ■ S45.109   Unspecified injury of brachial artery, unspecified side A 🔗, D, S 🔗

  ● S45.11   Laceration of brachial artery

    ● S45.111   Laceration of brachial artery, right side A 🔗, D, S 🔗

    ● S45.112   Laceration of brachial artery, left side A 🔗, D, S 🔗

    ● ■ S45.119   Laceration of brachial artery, unspecified side A 🔗, D, S 🔗

  ● S45.19   Other specified injury of brachial artery

    ● S45.191   Other specified injury of brachial artery, right side A 🔗, D, S 🔗

    ● S45.192   Other specified injury of brachial artery, left side A 🔗, D, S 🔗

    ● ■ S45.199   Other specified injury of brachial artery, unspecified side A 🔗, D, S 🔗

● S45.2   Injury of axillary or brachial vein

  ● S45.20   Unspecified injury of axillary or brachial vein

    ●■ S45.201   Unspecified injury of axillary or brachial vein, right side A 🦣, D, S 🦣

    ●■ S45.202   Unspecified injury of axillary or brachial vein, left side A 🦣, D, S 🦣

    ●■ S45.209   Unspecified injury of axillary or brachial vein, unspecified side A 🦣, D, S 🦣

  ● S45.21   Laceration of axillary or brachial vein

    ● S45.211   Laceration of axillary or brachial vein, right side A 🦣, D, S 🦣

    ● S45.212   Laceration of axillary or brachial vein, left side A 🦣, D, S 🦣

    ●■ S45.219   Laceration of axillary or brachial vein, unspecified side A 🦣, D, S 🦣

  ● S45.29   Other specified injury of axillary or brachial vein

    ● S45.291   Other specified injury of axillary or brachial vein, right side A 🦣, D, S 🦣

    ● S45.292   Other specified injury of axillary or brachial vein, left side A 🦣, D, S 🦣

    ●■ S45.299   Other specified injury of axillary or brachial vein, unspecified side A 🦣, D, S 🦣

● S45.3   Injury of superficial vein at shoulder and upper arm level

  ● S45.30   Unspecified injury of superficial vein at shoulder and upper arm level

    ●■ S45.301   Unspecified injury of superficial vein at shoulder and upper arm level, right arm A 🦣, D, S 🦣

    ●■ S45.302   Unspecified injury of superficial vein at shoulder and upper arm level, left arm A 🦣, D, S 🦣

    ●■ S45.309   Unspecified injury of superficial vein at shoulder and upper arm level, unspecified arm A 🦣, D, S 🦣

  ● S45.31   Laceration of superficial vein at shoulder and upper arm level

    ● S45.311   Laceration of superficial vein at shoulder and upper arm level, right arm A 🦣, D, S 🦣

    ● S45.312   Laceration of superficial vein at shoulder and upper arm level, left arm A 🦣, D, S 🦣

    ●■ S45.319   Laceration of superficial vein at shoulder and upper arm level, unspecified arm A 🦣, D, S 🦣

  ● S45.39   Other specified injury of superficial vein at shoulder and upper arm level

    ● S45.391   Other specified injury of superficial vein at shoulder and upper arm level, right arm A 🦣, D, S 🦣

    ● S45.392   Other specified injury of superficial vein at shoulder and upper arm level, left arm A 🦣, D, S 🦣

    ●■ S45.399   Other specified injury of superficial vein at shoulder and upper arm level, unspecified arm A 🦣, D, S 🦣

● S45.8   Injury of other specified blood vessels at shoulder and upper arm level

  ● S45.80   Unspecified injury of other specified blood vessels at shoulder and upper arm level

    ●■ S45.801   Unspecified injury of other specified blood vessels at shoulder and upper arm level, right arm A 🦣, D, S 🦣

    ●■ S45.802   Unspecified injury of other specified blood vessels at shoulder and upper arm level, left arm A 🦣, D, S 🦣

    ●■ S45.809   Unspecified injury of other specified blood vessels at shoulder and upper arm level, unspecified arm A 🦣, D, S 🦣

  ● S45.81   Laceration of other specified blood vessels at shoulder and upper arm level

    ● S45.811   Laceration of other specified blood vessels at shoulder and upper arm level, right arm A 🦣, D, S 🦣

    ● S45.812   Laceration of other specified blood vessels at shoulder and upper arm level, left arm A 🦣, D, S 🦣

    ●■ S45.819   Laceration of other specified blood vessels at shoulder and upper arm level, unspecified arm A 🦣, D, S 🦣

  ● S45.89   Other specified injury of other specified blood vessels at shoulder and upper arm level

    ● S45.891   Other specified injury of other specified blood vessels at shoulder and upper arm level, right arm A 🦣, D, S 🦣

    ● S45.892   Other specified injury of other specified blood vessels at shoulder and upper arm level, left arm A 🦣, D, S 🦣

    ●■ S45.899   Other specified injury of other specified blood vessels at shoulder and upper arm level, unspecified arm A 🦣, D, S 🦣

● S45.9   Injury of unspecified blood vessel at shoulder and upper arm level

  ● S45.90   Unspecified injury of unspecified blood vessel at shoulder and upper arm level

    ●■ S45.901   Unspecified injury of unspecified blood vessel at shoulder and upper arm level, right arm A 🦣, D, S 🦣

    ●■ S45.902   Unspecified injury of unspecified blood vessel at shoulder and upper arm level, left arm A 🦣, D, S 🦣

    ●■ S45.909   Unspecified injury of unspecified blood vessel at shoulder and upper arm level, unspecified arm A 🦣, D, S 🦣

● Unacceptable Principal Diagnosis   ● Use Additional Character(s)   ■ Unspecified   ▶ Manifestation Code

OGCR Official Guidelines for Coding and Reporting   Excludes 1   Excludes 2   Includes   Use additional   Code first   Code also

- S45.91   Laceration of unspecified blood vessel at shoulder and upper arm level
  - ● ■ S45.911   Laceration of unspecified blood vessel at shoulder and upper arm level, right arm A 🗇, D, S 🗇
  - ● ■ S45.912   Laceration of unspecified blood vessel at shoulder and upper arm level, left arm A 🗇, D, S 🗇
  - ● ■ S45.919   Laceration of unspecified blood vessel at shoulder and upper arm level, unspecified arm A 🗇, D, S 🗇
- S45.99   Other specified injury of unspecified blood vessel at shoulder and upper arm level
  - ● ■ S45.991   Other specified injury of unspecified blood vessel at shoulder and upper arm level, right arm A 🗇, D, S 🗇
  - ● ■ S45.992   Other specified injury of unspecified blood vessel at shoulder and upper arm level, left arm A 🗇, D, S 🗇
  - ● ■ S45.999   Other specified injury of unspecified blood vessel at shoulder and upper arm level, unspecified arm A 🗇, D, S 🗇

- ● S46   **Injury of muscle, fascia and tendon at shoulder and upper arm level**

  Code also any associated open wound (S41.-)

  Excludes2   injury of muscle, fascia and tendon at elbow (S56.-)
            sprain of joints and ligaments of shoulder girdle (S43.9)

  The appropriate 7th character is to be added to each code from category S46

A	initial encounter
D	subsequent encounter
S	sequela

  - ● S46.0   Injury of muscle(s) and tendon(s) of the rotator cuff of shoulder
    - ● S46.00   Unspecified injury of muscle(s) and tendon(s) of the rotator cuff of shoulder
      - ● ■ S46.001   Unspecified injury of muscle(s) and tendon(s) of the rotator cuff of right shoulder D, S 🗇
      - ● ■ S46.002   Unspecified injury of muscle(s) and tendon(s) of the rotator cuff of left shoulder D, S 🗇
      - ● ■ S46.009   Unspecified injury of muscle(s) and tendon(s) of the rotator cuff of unspecified shoulder D, S 🗇
    - ● S46.01   Strain of muscle(s) and tendon(s) of the rotator cuff of shoulder
      - ● S46.011   Strain of muscle(s) and tendon(s) of the rotator cuff of right shoulder D, S 🗇
      - ● S46.012   Strain of muscle(s) and tendon(s) of the rotator cuff of left shoulder D, S 🗇
      - ● ■ S46.019   Strain of muscle(s) and tendon(s) of the rotator cuff of unspecified shoulder D, S 🗇

  - ● S46.02   Laceration of muscle(s) and tendon(s) of the rotator cuff of shoulder
    - ● S46.021   Laceration of muscle(s) and tendon(s) of the rotator cuff of right shoulder A 🗇, D, S 🗇
    - ● S46.022   Laceration of muscle(s) and tendon(s) of the rotator cuff of left shoulder A 🗇, D, S 🗇
    - ● ■ S46.029   Laceration of muscle(s) and tendon(s) of the rotator cuff of unspecified shoulder A 🗇, D, S 🗇
  - ● S46.09   Other injury of muscle(s) and tendon(s) of the rotator cuff of shoulder
    - ● S46.091   Other injury of muscle(s) and tendon(s) of the rotator cuff of right shoulder D, S 🗇
    - ● S46.092   Other injury of muscle(s) and tendon(s) of the rotator cuff of left shoulder D, S 🗇
    - ● ■ S46.099   Other injury of muscle(s) and tendon(s) of the rotator cuff of unspecified shoulder D, S 🗇
  - ● S46.1   Injury of muscle, fascia and tendon of long head of biceps
    - ● S46.10   Unspecified injury of muscle, fascia and tendon of long head of biceps
      - ● ■ S46.101   Unspecified injury of muscle, fascia and tendon of long head of biceps, right arm D, S 🗇
      - ● ■ S46.102   Unspecified injury of muscle, fascia and tendon of long head of biceps, left arm D, S 🗇
      - ● ■ S46.109   Unspecified injury of muscle, fascia and tendon of long head of biceps, unspecified arm D, S 🗇
    - ● S46.11   Strain of muscle, fascia and tendon of long head of biceps
      - ● S46.111   Strain of muscle, fascia and tendon of long head of biceps, right arm D, S 🗇
      - ● S46.112   Strain of muscle, fascia and tendon of long head of biceps, left arm D, S 🗇
      - ● ■ S46.119   Strain of muscle, fascia and tendon of long head of biceps, unspecified arm D, S 🗇
    - ● S46.12   Laceration of muscle, fascia and tendon of long head of biceps
      - ● S46.121   Laceration of muscle, fascia and tendon of long head of biceps, right arm A 🗇, D, S 🗇
      - ● S46.122   Laceration of muscle, fascia and tendon of long head of biceps, left arm A 🗇, D, S 🗇
      - ● ■ S46.129   Laceration of muscle, fascia and tendon of long head of biceps, unspecified arm A 🗇, D, S 🗇

N Newborn Age: 0   **P** Pediatric Age: 0–17   **M** Maternity DX: 12–55   **A** Adult Age: 15–124   ♀ Females Only   ♂ Males Only

🗇 Complication\Comorbidity   🗇 Major C\C   🗇 Present on Admission Requirement   🗇 Hospital-Acquired Condition

1465

CHAPTER 19 (S00-T88)

● **S46.19** Other injury of muscle, fascia and tendon of long head of biceps

   ● **S46.191** Other injury of muscle, fascia and tendon of long head of biceps, right arm D, S 🔄

   ● **S46.192** Other injury of muscle, fascia and tendon of long head of biceps, left arm D, S 🔄

   ●■ **S46.199** Other injury of muscle, fascia and tendon of long head of biceps, unspecified arm D, S 🔄

● **S46.2** Injury of muscle, fascia and tendon of other parts of biceps

  ● **S46.20** Unspecified injury of muscle, fascia and tendon of other parts of biceps

   ●■ **S46.201** Unspecified injury of muscle, fascia and tendon of other parts of biceps, right arm D, S 🔄

   ●■ **S46.202** Unspecified injury of muscle, fascia and tendon of other parts of biceps, left arm D, S 🔄

   ●■ **S46.209** Unspecified injury of muscle, fascia and tendon of other parts of biceps, unspecified arm D, S 🔄

  ● **S46.21** Strain of muscle, fascia and tendon of other parts of biceps

   ● **S46.211** Strain of muscle, fascia and tendon of other parts of biceps, right arm D, S 🔄

   ● **S46.212** Strain of muscle, fascia and tendon of other parts of biceps, left arm D, S 🔄

   ●■ **S46.219** Strain of muscle, fascia and tendon of other parts of biceps, unspecified arm D, S 🔄

  ● **S46.22** Laceration of muscle, fascia and tendon of other parts of biceps

   ● **S46.221** Laceration of muscle, fascia and tendon of other parts of biceps, right arm A 🔄, D, S 🔄

   ● **S46.222** Laceration of muscle, fascia and tendon of other parts of biceps, left arm A 🔄, D, S 🔄

   ●■ **S46.229** Laceration of muscle, fascia and tendon of other parts of biceps, unspecified arm A 🔄, D, S 🔄

  ● **S46.29** Other injury of muscle, fascia and tendon of other parts of biceps

   ● **S46.291** Other injury of muscle, fascia and tendon of other parts of biceps, right arm D, S 🔄

   ● **S46.292** Other injury of muscle, fascia and tendon of other parts of biceps, left arm D, S 🔄

   ●■ **S46.299** Other injury of muscle, fascia and tendon of other parts of biceps, unspecified arm D, S 🔄

● **S46.3** Injury of muscle, fascia and tendon of triceps

  ● **S46.30** Unspecified injury of muscle, fascia and tendon of triceps

   ●■ **S46.301** Unspecified injury of muscle, fascia and tendon of triceps, right arm D, S 🔄

   ●■ **S46.302** Unspecified injury of muscle, fascia and tendon of triceps, left arm D, S 🔄

   ●■ **S46.309** Unspecified injury of muscle, fascia and tendon of triceps, unspecified arm D, S 🔄

  ● **S46.31** Strain of muscle, fascia and tendon of triceps

   ● **S46.311** Strain of muscle, fascia and tendon of triceps, right arm D, S 🔄

   ● **S46.312** Strain of muscle, fascia and tendon of triceps, left arm D, S 🔄

   ●■ **S46.319** Strain of muscle, fascia and tendon of triceps, unspecified arm D, S 🔄

  ● **S46.32** Laceration of muscle, fascia and tendon of triceps

   ● **S46.321** Laceration of muscle, fascia and tendon of triceps, right arm A 🔄, D, S 🔄

   ● **S46.322** Laceration of muscle, fascia and tendon of triceps, left arm A 🔄, D, S 🔄

   ●■ **S46.329** Laceration of muscle, fascia and tendon of triceps, unspecified arm A 🔄, D, S 🔄

  ● **S46.39** Other injury of muscle, fascia and tendon of triceps

   ● **S46.391** Other injury of muscle, fascia and tendon of triceps, right arm D, S 🔄

   ● **S46.392** Other injury of muscle, fascia and tendon of triceps, left arm D, S 🔄

   ●■ **S46.399** Other injury of muscle, fascia and tendon of triceps, unspecified arm D, S 🔄

● **S46.8** Injury of other muscles, fascia and tendons at shoulder and upper arm level

  ● **S46.80** Unspecified injury of other muscles, fascia and tendons at shoulder and upper arm level

   ●■ **S46.801** Unspecified injury of other muscles, fascia and tendons at shoulder and upper arm level, right arm D, S 🔄

   ●■ **S46.802** Unspecified injury of other muscles, fascia and tendons at shoulder and upper arm level, left arm D, S 🔄

   ●■ **S46.809** Unspecified injury of other muscles, fascia and tendons at shoulder and upper arm level, unspecified arm D, S 🔄

  ● **S46.81** Strain of other muscles, fascia and tendons at shoulder and upper arm level

   ● **S46.811** Strain of other muscles, fascia and tendons at shoulder and upper arm level, right arm D, S 🔄

   ● **S46.812** Strain of other muscles, fascia and tendons at shoulder and upper arm level, left arm D, S 🔄

   ●■ **S46.819** Strain of other muscles, fascia and tendons at shoulder and upper arm level, unspecified arm D, S 🔄

● Unacceptable Principal Diagnosis   ● Use Additional Character(s)   ■ Unspecified   ▶ Manifestation Code

OGCR Official Guidelines for Coding and Reporting   Excludes 1   Excludes 2   Includes   Use additional   Code first   Code also

● **S46.82** Laceration of other muscles, fascia and tendons at shoulder and upper arm level

  ● **S46.821** Laceration of other muscles, fascia and tendons at shoulder and upper arm level, right arm A 🕲, D, S 🕲

  ● **S46.822** Laceration of other muscles, fascia and tendons at shoulder and upper arm level, left arm A 🕲, D, S 🕲

  ●▪ **S46.829** Laceration of other muscles, fascia and tendons at shoulder and upper arm level, unspecified arm A 🕲, D, S 🕲

● **S46.89** Other injury of other muscles, fascia and tendons at shoulder and upper arm level

  ● **S46.891** Other injury of other muscles, fascia and tendons at shoulder and upper arm level, right arm D, S 🕲

  ● **S46.892** Other injury of other muscles, fascia and tendons at shoulder and upper arm level, left arm D, S 🕲

  ●▪ **S46.899** Other injury of other muscles, fascia and tendons at shoulder and upper arm level, unspecified arm D, S 🕲

● **S46.9** Injury of unspecified muscle, fascia and tendon at shoulder and upper arm level

  ● **S46.90** Unspecified injury of unspecified muscle, fascia and tendon at shoulder and upper arm level

    ●▪ **S46.901** Unspecified injury of unspecified muscle, fascia and tendon at shoulder and upper arm level, right arm D, S 🕲

    ●▪ **S46.902** Unspecified injury of unspecified muscle, fascia and tendon at shoulder and upper arm level, left arm D, S 🕲

    ●▪ **S46.909** Unspecified injury of unspecified muscle, fascia and tendon at shoulder and upper arm level, unspecified arm D, S 🕲

  ● **S46.91** Strain of unspecified muscle, fascia and tendon at shoulder and upper arm level

    ●▪ **S46.911** Strain of unspecified muscle, fascia and tendon at shoulder and upper arm level, right arm D, S 🕲

    ●▪ **S46.912** Strain of unspecified muscle, fascia and tendon at shoulder and upper arm level, left arm D, S 🕲

    ●▪ **S46.919** Strain of unspecified muscle, fascia and tendon at shoulder and upper arm level, unspecified arm D, S 🕲

  ● **S46.92** Laceration of unspecified muscle, fascia and tendon at shoulder and upper arm level

    ●▪ **S46.921** Laceration of unspecified muscle, fascia and tendon at shoulder and upper arm level, right arm A 🕲, D, S 🕲

    ●▪ **S46.922** Laceration of unspecified muscle, fascia and tendon at shoulder and upper arm level, left arm A 🕲, D, S 🕲

  ●▪ **S46.929** Laceration of unspecified muscle, fascia and tendon at shoulder and upper arm level, unspecified arm A 🕲, D, S 🕲

● **S46.99** Other injury of unspecified muscle, fascia and tendon at shoulder and upper arm level

  ●▪ **S46.991** Other injury of unspecified muscle, fascia and tendon at shoulder and upper arm level, right arm D, S 🕲

  ●▪ **S46.992** Other injury of unspecified muscle, fascia and tendon at shoulder and upper arm level, left arm D, S 🕲

  ●▪ **S46.999** Other injury of unspecified muscle, fascia and tendon at shoulder and upper arm level, unspecified arm D, S 🕲

● **S47** Crushing injury of shoulder and upper arm

Use additional code for all associated injuries

Excludes2 crushing injury of elbow (S57.0-)

The appropriate 7th character is to be added to each code from category S47

A	initial encounter
D	subsequent encounter
S	sequela

  ● **S47.1** Crushing injury of right shoulder and upper arm D, S 🕲

  ● **S47.2** Crushing injury of left shoulder and upper arm D, S 🕲

  ●▪ **S47.9** Crushing injury of shoulder and upper arm, unspecified arm D, S 🕲

● **S48** Traumatic amputation of shoulder and upper arm

An amputation not identified as partial or complete should be coded to complete

Excludes1 traumatic amputation at elbow level (S58.0)

The appropriate 7th character is to be added to each code from category S48

A	initial encounter
D	subsequent encounter
S	sequela

  ● **S48.0** Traumatic amputation at shoulder joint

    ● **S48.01** Complete traumatic amputation at shoulder joint

      ● **S48.011** Complete traumatic amputation at right shoulder joint A 🕲, D, S 🕲

      ● **S48.012** Complete traumatic amputation at left shoulder joint A 🕲, D, S 🕲

      ●▪ **S48.019** Complete traumatic amputation at unspecified shoulder joint A 🕲, D, S 🕲

    ● **S48.02** Partial traumatic amputation at shoulder joint

      ● **S48.021** Partial traumatic amputation at right shoulder joint A 🕲, D, S 🕲

      ● **S48.022** Partial traumatic amputation at left shoulder joint A 🕲, D, S 🕲

      ●▪ **S48.029** Partial traumatic amputation at unspecified shoulder joint A 🕲, D, S 🕲

● **S48.1**   Traumatic amputation at level between shoulder and elbow

   ● **S48.11**   Complete traumatic amputation at level between shoulder and elbow

      ● **S48.111**   Complete traumatic amputation at level between right shoulder and elbow A 🖸, D, S 🖸

      ● **S48.112**   Complete traumatic amputation at level between left shoulder and elbow A 🖸, D, S 🖸

      ●◾ **S48.119**   Complete traumatic amputation at level between unspecified shoulder and elbow A 🖸, D, S 🖸

   ● **S48.12**   Partial traumatic amputation at level between shoulder and elbow

      ● **S48.121**   Partial traumatic amputation at level between right shoulder and elbow A 🖸, D, S 🖸

      ● **S48.122**   Partial traumatic amputation at level between left shoulder and elbow A 🖸, D, S 🖸

      ●◾ **S48.129**   Partial traumatic amputation at level between unspecified shoulder and elbow A 🖸, D, S 🖸

● **S48.9**   Traumatic amputation of shoulder and upper arm, level unspecified

   ● **S48.91**   Complete traumatic amputation of shoulder and upper arm, level unspecified

      ●◾ **S48.911**   Complete traumatic amputation of right shoulder and upper arm, level unspecified A 🖸, D, S 🖸

      ●◾ **S48.912**   Complete traumatic amputation of left shoulder and upper arm, level unspecified A 🖸, D, S 🖸

      ●◾ **S48.919**   Complete traumatic amputation of unspecified shoulder and upper arm, level unspecified A 🖸, D, S 🖸

   ● **S48.92**   Partial traumatic amputation of shoulder and upper arm, level unspecified

      ●◾ **S48.921**   Partial traumatic amputation of right shoulder and upper arm, level unspecified A 🖸, D, S 🖸

      ●◾ **S48.922**   Partial traumatic amputation of left shoulder and upper arm, level unspecified A 🖸, D, S 🖸

      ●◾ **S48.929**   Partial traumatic amputation of unspecified shoulder and upper arm, level unspecified A 🖸, D, S 🖸

● **S49**   Other and unspecified injuries of shoulder and upper arm

   The appropriate 7th character is to be added to each code from subcategories S49.0 and S49.1

A	initial encounter for closed fracture
D	subsequent encounter for fracture with routine healing
G	subsequent encounter for fracture with delayed healing
K	subsequent encounter for fracture with nonunion
P	subsequent encounter for fracture with malunion
S	sequela

● **S49.0**   Physeal fracture of upper end of humerus

   ● **S49.00**   Unspecified physeal fracture of upper end of humerus

      ●◾ **S49.001**   Unspecified physeal fracture of upper end of humerus, right arm A, K, P 🖸, D, G, S 🖸, A 🖸

      ●◾ **S49.002**   Unspecified physeal fracture of upper end of humerus, left arm A, K, P 🖸, D, G, S 🖸, A 🖸

      ●◾ **S49.009**   Unspecified physeal fracture of upper end of humerus, unspecified arm A, K, P 🖸, D, G, S 🖸, A 🖸

   ● **S49.01**   Salter-Harris Type I physeal fracture of upper end of humerus

      ● **S49.011**   Salter-Harris Type I physeal fracture of upper end of humerus, right arm A, K, P 🖸, D, G, S 🖸, A 🖸

      ● **S49.012**   Salter-Harris Type I physeal fracture of upper end of humerus, left arm A, K, P 🖸, D, G, S 🖸, A 🖸

      ●◾ **S49.019**   Salter-Harris Type I physeal fracture of upper end of humerus, unspecified arm A, K, P 🖸, D, G, S 🖸, A 🖸

   ● **S49.02**   Salter-Harris Type II physeal fracture of upper end of humerus

      ● **S49.021**   Salter-Harris Type II physeal fracture of upper end of humerus, right arm A, K, P 🖸, D, G, S 🖸, A 🖸

      ● **S49.022**   Salter-Harris Type II physeal fracture of upper end of humerus, left arm A, K, P 🖸, D, G, S 🖸, A 🖸

      ●◾ **S49.029**   Salter-Harris Type II physeal fracture of upper end of humerus, unspecified arm A, K, P 🖸, D, G, S 🖸, A 🖸

   ● **S49.03**   Salter-Harris Type III physeal fracture of upper end of humerus

      ● **S49.031**   Salter Harris Type III physeal fracture of upper end of humerus, right arm A, K, P 🖸, D, G, S 🖸, A 🖸

      ● **S49.032**   Salter Harris Type III physeal fracture of upper end of humerus, left arm A, K, P 🖸, D, G, S 🖸, A 🖸

      ●◾ **S49.039**   Salter Harris Type III physeal fracture of upper end of humerus, unspecified arm A, K, P 🖸, D, G, S 🖸, A 🖸

Item 19-3 **SALTER-HARRIS TYPE 1:** epiphysis is completely separated from end of bone, or metaphysic growth plate remains attached to epiphysis

   SALTER-HARRIS TYPE 2: epiphysis and growth plate are partially separated from metaphysis, which is cracked—most common type

   SALTER-HARRIS TYPE 3: fracture occurring through epiphysis and separates part of epiphysis and growth plate from metaphysis fracture, usually at distal end of tibia

   SALTER-HARRIS TYPE 4: fracture runs through epiphysis, across growth plate, into metaphysic, surgery is required to restore joint surface to normal and align growth plate

● Unacceptable Principal Diagnosis	● Use Additional Character(s)
◾ Unspecified	▶ Manifestation Code
OGCR Official Guidelines for Coding and Reporting	Excludes 1 Excludes 2 Includes Use additional Code first Code also

● S49.04   Salter-Harris Type IV physeal fracture of upper end of humerus

　● S49.041   Salter-Harris Type IV physeal fracture of upper end of humerus, right arm A, K, P 🪙, D, G, S 🪙, A 🪙

　● S49.042   Salter-Harris Type IV physeal fracture of upper end of humerus, left arm A, K, P 🪙, D, G, S 🪙, A 🪙

　●■ S49.049   Salter-Harris Type IV physeal fracture of upper end of humerus, unspecified arm A, K, P 🪙, D, G, S 🪙, A 🪙

● S49.09   Other physeal fracture of upper end of humerus

　● S49.091   Other physeal fracture of upper end of humerus, right arm A, K, P 🪙, D, G, S 🪙, A 🪙

　● S49.092   Other physeal fracture of upper end of humerus, left arm A, K, P 🪙, D, G, S 🪙, A 🪙

　●■ S49.099   Other physeal fracture of upper end of humerus, unspecified arm A, K, P 🪙, D, G, S 🪙, A 🪙

● S49.1   Physeal fracture of lower end of humerus

　● S49.10   Unspecified physeal fracture of lower end of humerus

　　●■ S49.101   Unspecified physeal fracture of lower end of humerus, right arm A, K, P 🪙, D, G, S 🪙, A 🪙

　　●■ S49.102   Unspecified physeal fracture of lower end of humerus, left arm A, K, P 🪙, D, G, S 🪙, A 🪙

　　●■ S49.109   Unspecified physeal fracture of lower end of humerus, unspecified arm A, K, P 🪙, D, G, S 🪙, A 🪙

　● S49.11   Salter-Harris Type I physeal fracture of lower end of humerus

　　● S49.111   Salter-Harris Type I physeal fracture of lower end of humerus, right arm A, K, P 🪙, D, G, S 🪙, A 🪙

　　● S49.112   Salter-Harris Type I physeal fracture of lower end of humerus, left arm A, K, P 🪙, D, G, S 🪙, A 🪙

　　●■ S49.119   Salter-Harris Type I physeal fracture of lower end of humerus, unspecified arm A, K, P 🪙, D, G, S 🪙, A 🪙

　● S49.12   Salter-Harris Type II physeal fracture of lower end of humerus

　　● S49.121   Salter-Harris Type II physeal fracture of lower end of humerus, right arm A, K, P 🪙, D, G, S 🪙, A 🪙

　　● S49.122   Salter-Harris Type II physeal fracture of lower end of humerus, left arm A, K, P 🪙, D, G, S 🪙, A 🪙

　　●■ S49.129   Salter-Harris Type II physeal fracture of lower end of humerus, unspecified arm A, K, P 🪙, D, G, S 🪙, A 🪙

● S49.13   Salter Harris Type III physeal fracture of lower end of humerus

　● S49.131   Salter Harris Type III physeal fracture of lower end of humerus, right arm A, K, P 🪙, D, G, S 🪙, A 🪙

　● S49.132   Salter-Harris Type III physeal fracture of lower end of humerus, left arm A, K, P 🪙, D, G, S 🪙, A 🪙

　●■ S49.139   Salter-Harris Type III physeal fracture of lower end of humerus, unspecified arm A, K, P 🪙, D, G, S 🪙, A 🪙

● S49.14   Salter-Harris Type IV physeal fracture of lower end of humerus

　● S49.141   Salter-Harris Type IV physeal fracture of lower end of humerus, right arm A, K, P 🪙, D, G, S 🪙, A 🪙

　● S49.142   Salter-Harris Type IV physeal fracture of lower end of humerus, left arm A, K, P 🪙, D, G, S 🪙, A 🪙

　●■ S49.149   Salter-Harris Type IV physeal fracture of lower end of humerus, unspecified arm A, K, P 🪙, D, G, S 🪙, A 🪙

● S49.19   Other physeal fracture of lower end of humerus

　● S49.191   Other physeal fracture of lower end of humerus, right arm A, K, P 🪙, D, G, S 🪙, A 🪙

　● S49.192   Other physeal fracture of lower end of humerus, left arm A, K, P 🪙, D, G, S 🪙, A 🪙

　● S49.199   Other physeal fracture of lower end of humerus, unspecified arm A, K, P 🪙, D, G, S 🪙, A 🪙

● S49.8   Other specified injuries of shoulder and upper arm

The appropriate 7th character is to be added to each code in subcategory S49.8

A	initial encounter
D	subsequent encounter
S	sequela

　●■ S49.80   Other specified injuries of shoulder and upper arm, unspecified arm D, S 🪙

　● S49.81   Other specified injuries of right shoulder and upper arm D, S 🪙

　● S49.82   Other specified injuries of left shoulder and upper arm D, S 🪙

● S49.9   Unspecified injury of shoulder and upper arm

The appropriate 7th character is to be added to each code in subcategory S49.9

A	initial encounter
D	subsequent encounter
S	sequela

　●■ S49.90   Unspecified injury of shoulder and upper arm, unspecified arm D, S 🪙

　●■ S49.91   Unspecified injury of right shoulder and upper arm D, S 🪙

　●■ S49.92   Unspecified injury of left shoulder and upper arm D, S 🪙

N Newborn Age: 0   **P** Pediatric Age: 0–17   **M** Maternity DX: 12–55   **A** Adult Age: 15–124   ♀ Females Only   ♂ Males Only

🪙 Complication\Comorbidity   🪙 Major C\C   🪙 Present on Admission Requirement   🪙 Hospital-Acquired Condition

1469

INJURIES TO THE ELBOW AND FOREARM (S50-S59)

Excludes2 burns and corrosions (T20-T32)
           frostbite (T33-T34)
           injuries of wrist and hand (S60-S69)
           insect bite or sting, venomous (T63.4)

● S50 Superficial injury of elbow and forearm

Excludes2 superficial injury of wrist and hand (S60.-)

The appropriate 7th character is to be added to each code
from category S50

A	initial encounter
D	subsequent encounter
S	sequela

● S50.0 Contusion of elbow
  ●■ S50.00 Contusion of unspecified elbow D, S
  ● S50.01 Contusion of right elbow D, S
  ● S50.02 Contusion of left elbow D, S

● S50.1 Contusion of forearm
  ●■ S50.10 Contusion of unspecified forearm D, S
  ● S50.11 Contusion of right forearm D, S
  ● S50.12 Contusion of left forearm D, S

● S50.3 Other superficial injuries of elbow
  ● S50.31 Abrasion of elbow
    ● S50.311 Abrasion of right elbow D, S
    ● S50.312 Abrasion of left elbow D, S
    ●■ S50.319 Abrasion of unspecified elbow D, S
  ● S50.32 Blister (nonthermal) of elbow
    ● S50.321 Blister (nonthermal) of right elbow D, S
    ● S50.322 Blister (nonthermal) of left elbow D, S
    ●■ S50.329 Blister (nonthermal) of unspecified elbow D, S
  ● S50.34 External constriction of elbow
    ● S50.341 External constriction of right elbow D, S
    ● S50.342 External constriction of left elbow D, S
    ●■ S50.349 External constriction of unspecified elbow D, S
  ● S50.35 Superficial foreign body of elbow
             Splinter in the elbow
    ● S50.351 Superficial foreign body of right elbow D, S
    ● S50.352 Superficial foreign body of left elbow D, S
    ●■ S50.359 Superficial foreign body of unspecified elbow D, S
  ● S50.36 Insect bite (nonvenomous) of elbow
    ● S50.361 Insect bite (nonvenomous) of right elbow D, S
    ● S50.362 Insect bite (nonvenomous) of left elbow D, S
    ●■ S50.369 Insect bite (nonvenomous) of unspecified elbow D, S

● S50.37 Other superficial bite of elbow
  Excludes1 open bite of elbow (S51.04)
  ● S50.371 Other superficial bite of right elbow D, S
  ● S50.372 Other superficial bite of left elbow D, S
  ●■ S50.379 Other superficial bite of unspecified elbow D, S

● S50.8 Other superficial injuries of forearm
  ● S50.81 Abrasion of forearm
    ● S50.811 Abrasion of right forearm D, S
    ● S50.812 Abrasion of left forearm D, S
    ●■ S50.819 Abrasion of unspecified forearm D, S
  ● S50.82 Blister (nonthermal) of forearm
    ● S50.821 Blister (nonthermal) of right forearm D, S
    ● S50.822 Blister (nonthermal) of left forearm D, S
    ●■ S50.829 Blister (nonthermal) of unspecified forearm D, S
  ● S50.84 External constriction of forearm
    ● S50.841 External constriction of right forearm D, S
    ● S50.842 External constriction of left forearm D, S
    ●■ S50.849 External constriction of unspecified forearm D, S
  ● S50.85 Superficial foreign body of forearm
             Splinter in the forearm
    ● S50.851 Superficial foreign body of right forearm D, S
    ● S50.852 Superficial foreign body of left forearm D, S
    ●■ S50.859 Superficial foreign body of unspecified forearm D, S
  ● S50.86 Insect bite (nonvenomous) of forearm
    ● S50.861 Insect bite (nonvenomous) of right forearm D, S
    ● S50.862 Insect bite (nonvenomous) of left forearm D, S
    ●■ S50.869 Insect bite (nonvenomous) of unspecified forearm D, S
  ● S50.87 Other superficial bite of forearm
    Excludes1 open bite of forearm (S51.84)
    ● S50.871 Other superficial bite of right forearm D, S
    ● S50.872 Other superficial bite of left forearm D, S
    ●■ S50.879 Other superficial bite of unspecified forearm D, S

● S50.9 Unspecified superficial injury of elbow and forearm
  ● S50.90 Unspecified superficial injury of elbow
    ●■ S50.901 Unspecified superficial injury of right elbow D, S
    ●■ S50.902 Unspecified superficial injury of left elbow D, S
    ●■ S50.909 Unspecified superficial injury of unspecified elbow D, S

● Unacceptable Principal Diagnosis   ● Use Additional Character(s)   ■ Unspecified   ▶ Manifestation Code
OGCR Official Guidelines for Coding and Reporting   Excludes 1   Excludes 2   Includes   Use additional   Code first   Code also

● **S50.91** **Unspecified superficial injury of forearm**
- ●■ **S50.911** **Unspecified superficial injury of right forearm** D, S 🔖
- ●■ **S50.912** **Unspecified superficial injury of left forearm** D, S 🔖
- ●■ **S50.919** **Unspecified superficial injury of unspecified forearm** D, S 🔖

● **S51** **Open wound of elbow and forearm**

Code also any associated wound infection

| Excludes1 | open fracture of elbow and forearm (S52.- with open fracture 7th character) traumatic amputation of elbow and forearm (S58.-) |

| Excludes2 | open wound of wrist and hand (S61.-) |

The appropriate 7th character is to be added to each code from category S51

A	initial encounter
D	subsequent encounter
S	sequela

● **S51.0** **Open wound of elbow**
- ● **S51.00** **Unspecified open wound of elbow**
  - ●■ **S51.001** **Unspecified open wound of right elbow** D, S 🔖
  - ●■ **S51.002** **Unspecified open wound of left elbow** D, S 🔖
  - ●■ **S51.009** **Unspecified open wound of unspecified elbow** D, S 🔖
    Open wound of elbow NOS
- ● **S51.01** **Laceration without foreign body of elbow**
  - ● **S51.011** **Laceration without foreign body of right elbow** D, S 🔖
  - ● **S51.012** **Laceration without foreign body of left elbow** D, S 🔖
  - ●■ **S51.019** **Laceration without foreign body of unspecified elbow** D, S 🔖
- ● **S51.02** **Laceration with foreign body of elbow**
  - ● **S51.021** **Laceration with foreign body of right elbow** D, S 🔖
  - ● **S51.022** **Laceration with foreign body of left elbow** D, S 🔖
  - ●■ **S51.029** **Laceration with foreign body of unspecified elbow** D, S 🔖
- ● **S51.03** **Puncture wound without foreign body of elbow**
  - ● **S51.031** **Puncture wound without foreign body of right elbow** D, S 🔖
  - ● **S51.032** **Puncture wound without foreign body of left elbow** D, S 🔖
  - ●■ **S51.039** **Puncture wound without foreign body of unspecified elbow** D, S 🔖
- ● **S51.04** **Puncture wound with foreign body of elbow**
  - ● **S51.041** **Puncture wound with foreign body of right elbow** D, S 🔖
  - ● **S51.042** **Puncture wound with foreign body of left elbow** D, S 🔖
  - ●■ **S51.049** **Puncture wound with foreign body of unspecified elbow** D, S 🔖

● **S51.05** **Open bite of elbow**
Bite of elbow NOS

| Excludes1 | superficial bite of elbow (S50.36, S50.37) |

- ● **S51.051** **Open bite, right elbow** D, S 🔖
- ● **S51.052** **Open bite, left elbow** D, S 🔖
- ●■ **S51.059** **Open bite, unspecified elbow** D, S 🔖

● **S51.8** **Open wound of forearm**

| Excludes2 | open wound of elbow (S51.0-) |

- ● **S51.80** **Unspecified open wound of forearm**
  - ●■ **S51.801** **Unspecified open wound of right forearm** D, S 🔖
  - ●■ **S51.802** **Unspecified open wound of left forearm** D, S 🔖
  - ●■ **S51.809** **Unspecified open wound of unspecified forearm** D, S 🔖
    Open wound of forearm NOS
- ● **S51.81** **Laceration without foreign body of forearm**
  - ● **S51.811** **Laceration without foreign body of right forearm** D, S 🔖
  - ● **S51.812** **Laceration without foreign body of left forearm** D, S 🔖
  - ●■ **S51.819** **Laceration without foreign body of unspecified forearm** D, S 🔖
- ● **S51.82** **Laceration with foreign body of forearm**
  - ● **S51.821** **Laceration with foreign body of right forearm** D, S 🔖
  - ● **S51.822** **Laceration with foreign body of left forearm** D, S 🔖
  - ●■ **S51.829** **Laceration with foreign body of unspecified forearm** D, S 🔖
- ● **S51.83** **Puncture wound without foreign body of forearm**
  - ● **S51.831** **Puncture wound without foreign body of right forearm** D, S 🔖
  - ● **S51.832** **Puncture wound without foreign body of left forearm** D, S 🔖
  - ●■ **S51.839** **Puncture wound without foreign body of unspecified forearm** D, S 🔖
- ● **S51.84** **Puncture wound with foreign body of forearm**
  - ● **S51.841** **Puncture wound with foreign body of right forearm** D, S 🔖
  - ● **S51.842** **Puncture wound with foreign body of left forearm** D, S 🔖
  - ●■ **S51.849** **Puncture wound with foreign body of unspecified forearm** D, S 🔖
- ● **S51.85** **Open bite of forearm**
  Bite of forearm NOS

  | Excludes1 | superficial bite of forearm (S50.86, S50.87) |

  - ● **S51.851** **Open bite of right forearm** D, S 🔖
  - ● **S51.852** **Open bite of left forearm** D, S 🔖
  - ●■ **S51.859** **Open bite of unspecified forearm** D, S 🔖

CHAPTER 19 (S00-T88)

N Newborn Age: 0   **P** Pediatric Age: 0–17   **M** Maternity DX: 12–55   **A** Adult Age: 15–124   ♀ Females Only   ♂ Males Only

🔖 Complication\Comorbidity   🔖 Major C\C   🔖 Present on Admission Requirement   🔖 Hospital-Acquired Condition

1471

CHAPTER 19 (S00–T88)

● **S52**   **Fracture of forearm**

> **Note:** A fracture not identified as displaced or nondisplaced should be coded to displaced
>
> A fracture not designated as open or closed should be coded to closed
>
> The open fracture designations are based on the Gustilo open fracture classification

> | Excludes1 | traumatic amputation of forearm (S58.-) |
> | Excludes2 | fracture at wrist and hand level (S62.-) |

> The appropriate 7th character is to be added to all codes from category S52

> A   initial encounter for closed fracture
> B   initial encounter for open fracture type I or II
>   initial encounter for open fracture NOS
> C   initial encounter for open fracture type IIIA, IIIB, or IIIC
> D   subsequent encounter for closed fracture with routine healing
> E   subsequent encounter for open fracture type I or II with routine healing
> F   subsequent encounter for open fracture type IIIA, IIIB, or IIIC with routine healing
> G   subsequent encounter for closed fracture with delayed healing
> H   subsequent encounter for open fracture type I or II with delayed healing
> J   subsequent encounter for open fracture type IIIA, IIIB, or IIIC with delayed healing
> K   subsequent encounter for closed fracture with nonunion
> M   subsequent encounter for open fracture type I or II with nonunion
> N   subsequent encounter for open fracture type IIIA, IIIB, or IIIC with nonunion
> P   subsequent encounter for closed fracture with malunion
> Q   subsequent encounter for open fracture type I or II with malunion
> R   subsequent encounter for open fracture type IIIA, IIIB, or IIIC with malunion
> S   sequela

● **S52.0**   **Fracture of upper end of ulna**
> Fracture of proximal end of ulna

> | Excludes2 | fracture of elbow NOS (S42.40-) |
> | | fractures of shaft of ulna (S52.2-) |

   ● **S52.00**   **Unspecified fracture of upper end of ulna**

     ●■ **S52.001**   **Unspecified fracture of upper end of right ulna** K, M, N, P, Q, R 🔾, B, C 🔾, D, E, F, G, H, J, S 🔾, B, C 🔾

     ●■ **S52.002**   **Unspecified fracture of upper end of left ulna** K, M, N, P, Q, R 🔾, B, C 🔾, D, E, F, G, H, J, S 🔾, B, C 🔾

     ●■ **S52.009**   **Unspecified fracture of upper end of unspecified ulna** K, M, N, P, Q, R 🔾, B, C 🔾, D, E, F, G, H, J, S 🔾, B, C 🔾

● **S52.01**   **Torus fracture of upper end of ulna**

> The appropriate 7th character is to be added to all codes in subcategory S52.01

> A   initial encounter for closed fracture
> D   subsequent encounter for fracture with routine healing
> G   subsequent encounter for fracture with delayed healing
> K   subsequent encounter for fracture with nonunion
> P   subsequent encounter for fracture with malunion
> S   sequela

   ● **S52.011**   **Torus fracture of upper end of right ulna** A, K, P 🔾, D, G, S 🔾, A 🔾

   ● **S52.012**   **Torus fracture of upper end of left ulna** A, K, P 🔾, D, G, S 🔾, A 🔾

   ●■ **S52.019**   **Torus fracture of upper end of unspecified ulna** A, K, P 🔾, D, G, S 🔾, A 🔾

● **S52.02**   **Fracture of olecranon process without intraarticular extension of ulna**

   ● **S52.021**   **Displaced fracture of olecranon process without intraarticular extension of right ulna** K, M, N, P, Q, R 🔾, B, C 🔾, D, E, F, G, H, J, S 🔾, B, C 🔾

   ● **S52.022**   **Displaced fracture of olecranon process without intraarticular extension of left ulna** K, M, N, P, Q, R 🔾, B, C 🔾, D, E, F, G, H, J, S 🔾, B, C 🔾

   ●■ **S52.023**   **Displaced fracture of olecranon process without intraarticular extension of unspecified ulna** K, M, N, P, Q, R 🔾, B, C 🔾, D, E, F, G, H, J, S 🔾, B, C 🔾

   ● **S52.024**   **Nondisplaced fracture of olecranon process without intraarticular extension of right ulna** K, M, N, P, Q, R 🔾, B, C 🔾, D, E, F, G, H, J, S 🔾, B, C 🔾

   ● **S52.025**   **Nondisplaced fracture of olecranon process without intraarticular extension of left ulna** K, M, N, P, Q, R 🔾, B, C 🔾, D, E, F, G, H, J, S 🔾, B, C 🔾

   ●■ **S52.026**   **Nondisplaced fracture of olecranon process without intraarticular extension of unspecified ulna** K, M, N, P, Q, R 🔾, B, C 🔾, D, E, F, G, H, J, S 🔾, B, C 🔾

● **S52.03**   **Fracture of olecranon process with intraarticular extension of ulna**

   ● **S52.031**   **Displaced fracture of olecranon process with intraarticular extension of right ulna** K, M, N, P, Q, R 🔾, B, C 🔾, D, E, F, G, H, J, S 🔾, B, C 🔾

●   Unacceptable Principal Diagnosis   ●   Use Additional Character(s)   ■   Unspecified   ▶   Manifestation Code

OGCR   Official Guidelines for Coding and Reporting   Excludes 1   Excludes 2   Includes   Use additional   Code first   Code also

- S52.032   **Displaced fracture of olecranon process with intraarticular extension of left ulna** K, M, N, P, Q, R, B, C, D, E, F, G, H, J, S, B, C

- S52.033   **Displaced fracture of olecranon process with intraarticular extension of unspecified ulna** K, M, N, P, Q, R, B, C, D, E, F, G, H, J, S, B, C

- S52.034   **Nondisplaced fracture of olecranon process with intraarticular extension of right ulna** K, M, N, P, Q, R, B, C, D, E, F, G, H, J, S, B, C

- S52.035   **Nondisplaced fracture of olecranon process with intraarticular extension of left ulna** K, M, N, P, Q, R, B, C, D, E, F, G, H, J, S, B, C

- S52.036   **Nondisplaced fracture of olecranon process with intraarticular extension of unspecified ulna** K, M, N, P, Q, R, B, C, D, E, F, G, H, J, S, B, C

- S52.04   **Fracture of coronoid process of ulna**

  - S52.041   **Displaced fracture of coronoid process of right ulna** K, M, N, P, Q, R, B, C, D, E, F, G, H, J, S, B, C

  - S52.042   **Displaced fracture of coronoid process of left ulna** K, M, N, P, Q, R, B, C, D, E, F, G, H, J, S, B, C

  - S52.043   **Displaced fracture of coronoid process of unspecified ulna** K, M, N, P, Q, R, B, C, D, E, F, G, H, J, S, B, C

  - S52.044   **Nondisplaced fracture of coronoid process of right ulna** K, M, N, P, Q, R, B, C, D, E, F, G, H, J, S, B, C

  - S52.045   **Nondisplaced fracture of coronoid process of left ulna** K, M, N, P, Q, R, B, C, D, E, F, G, H, J, S, B, C

  - S52.046   **Nondisplaced fracture of coronoid process of unspecified ulna** K, M, N, P, Q, R, B, C, D, E, F, G, H, J, S, B, C

- S52.09   **Other fracture of upper end of ulna**

  - S52.091   **Other fracture of upper end of right ulna** K, M, N, P, Q, R, B, C, D, E, F, G, H, J, S, B, C

  - S52.092   **Other fracture of upper end of left ulna** K, M, N, P, Q, R, B, C, D, E, F, G, H, J, S, B, C

  - S52.099   **Other fracture of upper end of unspecified ulna** K, M, N, P, Q, R, B, C, D, E, F, G, H, J, S, B, C

- S52.1   **Fracture of upper end of radius**

  Fracture of proximal end of radius

  Excludes2   physeal fractures of upper end of radius (S59.2-)
  fracture of shaft of radius (S52.3-)

  - S52.10   **Unspecified fracture of upper end of radius**

    - S52.101   **Unspecified fracture of upper end of right radius** K, M, N, P, Q, R, B, C, D, E, F, G, H, J, S, B, C

    - S52.102   **Unspecified fracture of upper end of left radius** K, M, N, P, Q, R, B, C, D, E, F, G, H, J, S, B, C

    - S52.109   **Unspecified fracture of upper end of unspecified radius** K, M, N, P, Q, R, B, C, D, E, F, G, H, J, S, B, C

  - S52.11   **Torus fracture of upper end of radius**

    The appropriate 7th character is to be added to all codes in subcategory S52.11

A	initial encounter for closed fracture
D	subsequent encounter for fracture with routine healing
G	subsequent encounter for fracture with delayed healing
K	subsequent encounter for fracture with nonunion
P	subsequent encounter for fracture with malunion
S	sequela

    - S52.111   **Torus fracture of upper end of right radius** A, K, P, D, G, S, A

    - S52.112   **Torus fracture of upper end of left radius** A, K, P, D, G, S, A

    - S52.119   **Torus fracture of upper end of unspecified radius** A, K, P, D, G, S, A

  - S52.12   **Fracture of head of radius**

    - S52.121   **Displaced fracture of head of right radius** K, M, N, P, Q, R, B, C, D, E, F, G, H, J, S, B, C

    - S52.122   **Displaced fracture of head of left radius** K, M, N, P, Q, R, B, C, D, E, F, G, H, J, S, B, C

    - S52.123   **Displaced fracture of head of unspecified radius** K, M, N, P, Q, R, B, C, D, E, F, G, H, J, S, B, C

    - S52.124   **Nondisplaced fracture of head of right radius** K, M, N, P, Q, R, B, C, D, E, F, G, H, J, S, B, C

    - S52.125   **Nondisplaced fracture of head of left radius** K, M, N, P, Q, R, B, C, D, E, F, G, H, J, S, B, C

    - S52.126   **Nondisplaced fracture of head of unspecified radius** K, M, N, P, Q, R, B, C, D, E, F, G, H, J, S, B, C

CHAPTER 19 (S00–T88)

CHAPTER 19 (S00-T88)

● S52.13   Fracture of neck of radius
- ● S52.131   Displaced fracture of neck of right radius K, M, N, P, Q, R 🔧, B, C 🔧, D, E, F, G, H, J, S 🔧, B, C 🔧
- ● S52.132   Displaced fracture of neck of left radius K, M, N, P, Q, R 🔧, B, C 🔧, D, E, F, G, H, J, S 🔧, B, C 🔧
- ●■ S52.133   Displaced fracture of neck of unspecified radius K, M, N, P, Q, R 🔧, B, C 🔧, D, E, F, G, H, J, S 🔧, B, C 🔧
- ● S52.134   Nondisplaced fracture of neck of right radius K, M, N, P, Q, R 🔧, B, C 🔧, D, E, F, G, H, J, S 🔧, B, C 🔧
- ● S52.135   Nondisplaced fracture of neck of left radius K, M, N, P, Q, R 🔧, B, C 🔧, D, E, F, G, H, J, S 🔧, B, C 🔧
- ●■ S52.136   Nondisplaced fracture of neck of unspecified radius K, M, N, P, Q, R 🔧, B, C 🔧, D, E, F, G, H, J, S 🔧, B, C 🔧

● S52.18   Other fracture of upper end of radius
- ● S52.181   Other fracture of upper end of right radius K, M, N, P, Q, R 🔧, B, C 🔧, D, E, F, G, H, J, S 🔧, B, C 🔧
- ● S52.182   Other fracture of upper end of left radius K, M, N, P, Q, R 🔧, B, C 🔧, D, E, F, G, H, J, S 🔧, B, C 🔧
- ●■ S52.189   Other fracture of upper end of unspecified radius K, M, N, P, Q, R 🔧, B, C 🔧, D, E, F, G, H, J, S 🔧, B, C 🔧

● S52.2   Fracture of shaft of ulna
- ● S52.20   Unspecified fracture of shaft of ulna
  Fracture of ulna NOS
  - ●■ S52.201   Unspecified fracture of shaft of right ulna A, K, M, N, P, Q, R 🔧, B, C 🔧, D, E, F, G, H, J, S 🔧, A, B, C 🔧
  - ●■ S52.202   Unspecified fracture of shaft of left ulna A, K, M, N, P, Q, R 🔧, B, C 🔧, D, E, F, G, H, J, S 🔧, A, B, C 🔧
  - ●■ S52.209   Unspecified fracture of shaft of unspecified ulna A, K, M, N, P, Q, R 🔧, B, C 🔧, D, E, F, G, H, J, S 🔧, A, B, C 🔧
- ● S52.21   Greenstick fracture of shaft of ulna

  The appropriate 7th character is to be added to all codes in subcategory S52.21

A	initial encounter for closed fracture
D	subsequent encounter for fracture with routine healing
G	subsequent encounter for fracture with delayed healing
K	subsequent encounter for fracture with nonunion
P	subsequent encounter for fracture with malunion
S	sequela

  - ● S52.211   Greenstick fracture of shaft of right ulna A, K, P 🔧, B, C 🔧, D, G, S 🔧, A 🔧

- ● S52.212   Greenstick fracture of shaft of left ulna A, K, P 🔧, B, C 🔧, D, G, S 🔧, A 🔧
- ●■ S52.219   Greenstick fracture of shaft of unspecified ulna A, K, P 🔧, B, C 🔧, D, G, S 🔧, A 🔧

● S52.22   Transverse fracture of shaft of ulna
- ● S52.221   Displaced transverse fracture of shaft of right ulna A, K, M, N, P, Q, R 🔧, B, C 🔧, D, E, F, G, H, J, S 🔧, A, B, C 🔧
- ● S52.222   Displaced transverse fracture of shaft of left ulna A, K, M, N, P, Q, R 🔧, B, C 🔧, D, E, F, G, H, J, S 🔧, A, B, C 🔧
- ●■ S52.223   Displaced transverse fracture of shaft of unspecified ulna A, K, M, N, P, Q, R 🔧, B, C 🔧, D, E, F, G, H, J, S 🔧, A, B, C 🔧
- ● S52.224   Nondisplaced transverse fracture of shaft of right ulna A, K, M, N, P, Q, R 🔧, B, C 🔧, D, E, F, G, H, J, S 🔧, A, B, C 🔧
- ● S52.225   Nondisplaced transverse fracture of shaft of left ulna A, K, M, N, P, Q, R 🔧, B, C 🔧, D, E, F, G, H, J, S 🔧, A, B, C 🔧
- ●■ S52.226   Nondisplaced transverse fracture of shaft of unspecified ulna A, K, M, N, P, Q, R 🔧, B, C 🔧, D, E, F, G, H, J, S 🔧, A, B, C 🔧

● S52.23   Oblique fracture of shaft of ulna
- ● S52.231   Displaced oblique fracture of shaft of right ulna A, K, M, N, P, Q, R 🔧, B, C 🔧, D, E, F, G, H, J, S 🔧, A, B, C 🔧
- ● S52.232   Displaced oblique fracture of shaft of left ulna A, K, M, N, P, Q, R 🔧, B, C 🔧, D, E, F, G, H, J, S 🔧, A, B, C 🔧
- ●■ S52.233   Displaced oblique fracture of shaft of unspecified ulna A, K, M, N, P, Q, R 🔧, B, C 🔧, D, E, F, G, H, J, S 🔧, A, B, C 🔧
- ● S52.234   Nondisplaced oblique fracture of shaft of right ulna A, K, M, N, P, Q, R 🔧, B, C 🔧, D, E, F, G, H, J, S 🔧, A, B, C 🔧
- ● S52.235   Nondisplaced oblique fracture of shaft of left ulna A, K, M, N, P, Q, R 🔧, B, C 🔧, D, E, F, G, H, J, S 🔧, A, B, C 🔧
- ●■ S52.236   Nondisplaced oblique fracture of shaft of unspecified ulna A, K, M, N, P, Q, R 🔧, B, C 🔧, D, E, F, G, H, J, S 🔧, A, B, C 🔧

● S52.24   Spiral fracture of shaft of ulna
- ● S52.241   Displaced spiral fracture of shaft of ulna, right arm A, K, M, N, P, Q, R 🔧, B, C 🔧, D, E, F, G, H, J, S 🔧, A, B, C 🔧
- ● S52.242   Displaced spiral fracture of shaft of ulna, left arm A, K, M, N, P, Q, R 🔧, B, C 🔧, D, E, F, G, H, J, S 🔧, A, B, C 🔧

● Unacceptable Principal Diagnosis   ● Use Additional Character(s)   ■ Unspecified   ▶ Manifestation Code
OGCR Official Guidelines for Coding and Reporting   Excludes 1   Excludes 2   Includes   Use additional   Code first   Code also

● ■ S52.243   Displaced spiral fracture of shaft of ulna, unspecified arm A, K, M, N, P, Q, R 🕮, B, C 🕮, D, E, F, G, H, J, S 🕮, A, B, C 🕮

● S52.244   Nondisplaced spiral fracture of shaft of ulna, right arm A, K, M, N, P, Q, R 🕮, B, C 🕮, D, E, F, G, H, J, S 🕮, A, B, C 🕮

● S52.245   Nondisplaced spiral fracture of shaft of ulna, left arm A, K, M, N, P, Q, R 🕮, B, C 🕮, D, E, F, G, H, J, S 🕮, A, B, C 🕮

● ■ S52.246   Nondisplaced spiral fracture of shaft of ulna, unspecified arm A, K, M, N, P, Q, R 🕮, B, C 🕮, D, E, F, G, H, J, S 🕮, A, B, C 🕮

● S52.25   Comminuted fracture of shaft of ulna

● S52.251   Displaced comminuted fracture of shaft of ulna, right arm A, K, M, N, P, Q, R 🕮, B, C 🕮, D, E, F, G, H, J, S 🕮, A, B, C 🕮

● S52.252   Displaced comminuted fracture of shaft of ulna, left arm A, K, M, N, P, Q, R 🕮, B, C 🕮, D, E, F, G, H, J, S 🕮, A, B, C 🕮

● ■ S52.253   Displaced comminuted fracture of shaft of ulna, unspecified arm A, K, M, N, P, Q, R 🕮, B, C 🕮, D, E, F, G, H, J, S 🕮, A, B, C 🕮

● S52.254   Nondisplaced comminuted fracture of shaft of ulna, right arm A, K, M, N, P, Q, R 🕮, B, C 🕮, D, E, F, G, H, J, S 🕮, A, B, C 🕮

● S52.255   Nondisplaced comminuted fracture of shaft of ulna, left arm A, K, M, N, P, Q, R 🕮, B, C 🕮, D, E, F, G, H, J, S 🕮, A, B, C 🕮

● ■ S52.256   Nondisplaced comminuted fracture of shaft of ulna, unspecified arm A, K, M, N, P, Q, R 🕮, B, C 🕮, D, E, F, G, H, J, S 🕮, A, B, C 🕮

● S52.26   Segmental fracture of shaft of ulna

● S52.261   Displaced segmental fracture of shaft of ulna, right arm A, K, M, N, P, Q, R 🕮, B, C 🕮, D, E, F, G, H, J, S 🕮, A, B, C 🕮

● S52.262   Displaced segmental fracture of shaft of ulna, left arm A, K, M, N, P, Q, R 🕮, B, C 🕮, D, E, F, G, H, J, S 🕮, A, B, C 🕮

● ■ S52.263   Displaced segmental fracture of shaft of ulna, unspecified arm A, K, M, N, P, Q, R 🕮, B, C 🕮, D, E, F, G, H, J, S 🕮, A, B, C 🕮

● S52.264   Nondisplaced segmental fracture of shaft of ulna, right arm A, K, M, N, P, Q, R 🕮, B, C 🕮, D, E, F, G, H, J, S 🕮, A, B, C 🕮

● S52.265   Nondisplaced segmental fracture of shaft of ulna, left arm A, K, M, N, P, Q, R 🕮, B, C 🕮, D, E, F, G, H, J, S 🕮, A, B, C 🕮

● ■ S52.266   Nondisplaced segmental fracture of shaft of ulna, unspecified arm A, K, M, N, P, Q, R 🕮, B, C 🕮, D, E, F, G, H, J, S 🕮, A, B, C 🕮

● S52.27   Monteggia's fracture of ulna
Fracture of upper shaft of ulna with dislocation of radial head

● S52.271   Monteggia's fracture of right ulna K, M, N, P, Q, R 🕮, B, C 🕮, D, E, F, G, H, J, S 🕮, B, C 🕮

● S52.272   Monteggia's fracture of left ulna K, M, N, P, Q, R 🕮, B, C 🕮, D, E, F, G, H, J, S 🕮, B, C 🕮

● ■ S52.279   Monteggia's fracture of unspecified ulna K, M, N, P, Q, R 🕮, B, C 🕮, D, E, F, G, H, J, S 🕮, B, C 🕮

● S52.28   Bent bone of ulna

● S52.281   Bent bone of right ulna A, K, M, N, P, Q, R 🕮, B, C 🕮, D, E, F, G, H, J, S 🕮, A, B, C 🕮

● S52.282   Bent bone of left ulna A, K, M, N, P, Q, R 🕮, B, C 🕮, D, E, F, G, H, J, S 🕮, A, B, C 🕮

● ■ S52.283   Bent bone of unspecified ulna A, K, M, N, P, Q, R 🕮, B, C 🕮, D, E, F, G, H, J, S 🕮, A, B, C 🕮

● S52.29   Other fracture of shaft of ulna

● S52.291   Other fracture of shaft of right ulna A, K, M, N, P, Q, R 🕮, B, C 🕮, D, E, F, G, H, J, S 🕮, A, B, C 🕮

● S52.292   Other fracture of shaft of left ulna A, K, M, N, P, Q, R 🕮, B, C 🕮, D, E, F, G, H, J, S 🕮, A, B, C 🕮

● ■ S52.299   Other fracture of shaft of unspecified ulna A, K, M, N, P, Q, R 🕮, B, C 🕮, D, E, F, G, H, J, S 🕮, A, B, C 🕮

● S52.3   Fracture of shaft of radius

● S52.30   Unspecified fracture of shaft of radius

● ■ S52.301   Unspecified fracture of shaft of right radius A, K, M, N, P, Q, R 🕮, B, C 🕮, D, E, F, G, H, J, S 🕮, A, B, C 🕮

● ■ S52.302   Unspecified fracture of shaft of left radius A, K, M, N, P, Q, R 🕮, B, C 🕮, D, E, F, G, H, J, S 🕮, A, B, C 🕮

● ■ S52.309   Unspecified fracture of shaft of unspecified radius A, K, M, N, P, Q, R 🕮, B, C 🕮, D, E, F, G, H, J, S 🕮, A, B, C 🕮

● S52.31   Greenstick fracture of shaft of radius

The appropriate 7th character is to be added to all codes in subcategory S52.31

A	initial encounter for closed fracture
D	subsequent encounter for fracture with routine healing
G	subsequent encounter for fracture with delayed healing
K	subsequent encounter for fracture with nonunion
P	subsequent encounter for fracture with malunion
S	sequela

🔾 S52.311   Greenstick fracture of shaft of radius, right arm A, K, P 🕮, D, G, S 🕮, A 🕮

N Newborn Age: 0   **P** Pediatric Age: 0–17   **M** Maternity DX: 12–55   **A** Adult Age: 15–124   ♀ Females Only   ♂ Males Only

🕮 Complication\Comorbidity   🕮 Major C\C   🕮 Present on Admission Requirement   🕮 Hospital-Acquired Condition

1475

● S52.312   Greenstick fracture of shaft of radius, left arm A, K, P 🔧, D, G, S 🔧, A 🔧

●🔲 S52.319   Greenstick fracture of shaft of radius, unspecified arm A, K, P 🔧, D, G, S 🔧, A 🔧

● S52.32   Transverse fracture of shaft of radius

● S52.321   Displaced transverse fracture of shaft of right radius A, K, M, N, P, Q, R 🔧, B, C 🔧, D, E, F, G, H, J, S 🔧, A, B, C 🔧

● S52.322   Displaced transverse fracture of shaft of left radius A, K, M, N, P, Q, R 🔧, B, C 🔧, D, E, F, G, H, J, S 🔧, A, B, C 🔧

●🔲 S52.323   Displaced transverse fracture of shaft of unspecified radius A, K, M, N, P, Q, R 🔧, B, C 🔧, D, E, F, G, H, J, S 🔧, A, B, C 🔧

● S52.324   Nondisplaced transverse fracture of shaft of right radius A, K, M, N, P, Q, R 🔧, B, C 🔧, D, E, F, G, H, J, S 🔧, A, B, C 🔧

● S52.325   Nondisplaced transverse fracture of shaft of left radius A, K, M, N, P, Q, R 🔧, B, C 🔧, D, E, F, G, H, J, S 🔧, A, B, C 🔧

●🔲 S52.326   Nondisplaced transverse fracture of shaft of unspecified radius A, K, M, N, P, Q, R 🔧, B, C 🔧, D, E, F, G, H, J, S 🔧, A, B, C 🔧

● S52.33   Oblique fracture of shaft of radius

● S52.331   Displaced oblique fracture of shaft of right radius A, K, M, N, P, Q, R 🔧, B, C 🔧, D, E, F, G, H, J, S 🔧, A, B, C 🔧

● S52.332   Displaced oblique fracture of shaft of left radius A, K, M, N, P, Q, R 🔧, B, C 🔧, D, E, F, G, H, J, S 🔧, A, B, C 🔧

●🔲 S52.333   Displaced oblique fracture of shaft of unspecified radius A, K, M, N, P, Q, R 🔧, B, C 🔧, D, E, F, G, H, J, S 🔧, A, B, C 🔧

● S52.334   Nondisplaced oblique fracture of shaft of right radius A, K, M, N, P, Q, R 🔧, B, C 🔧, D, E, F, G, H, J, S 🔧, A, B, C 🔧

● S52.335   Nondisplaced oblique fracture of shaft of left radius A, K, M, N, P, Q, R 🔧, B, C 🔧, D, E, F, G, H, J, S 🔧, A, B, C 🔧

●🔲 S52.336   Nondisplaced oblique fracture of shaft of unspecified radius A, K, M, N, P, Q, R 🔧, B, C 🔧, D, E, F, G, H, J, S 🔧, A, B, C 🔧

● S52.34   Spiral fracture of shaft of radius

● S52.341   Displaced spiral fracture of shaft of radius, right arm A, K, M, N, P, Q, R 🔧, B, C 🔧, D, E, F, G, H, J, S 🔧, A, B, C 🔧

● S52.342   Displaced spiral fracture of shaft of radius, left arm A, K, M, N, P, Q, R 🔧, B, C 🔧, D, E, F, G, H, J, S 🔧, A, B, C 🔧

●🔲 S52.343   Displaced spiral fracture of shaft of radius, unspecified arm A, K, M, N, P, Q, R 🔧, B, C 🔧, D, E, F, G, H, J, S 🔧, A, B, C 🔧

● S52.344   Nondisplaced spiral fracture of shaft of radius, right arm A, K, M, N, P, Q, R 🔧, B, C 🔧, D, E, F, G, H, J, S 🔧, A, B, C 🔧

● S52.345   Nondisplaced spiral fracture of shaft of radius, left arm A, K, M, N, P, Q, R 🔧, B, C 🔧, D, E, F, G, H, J, S 🔧, A, B, C 🔧

●🔲 S52.346   Nondisplaced spiral fracture of shaft of radius, unspecified arm A, K, M, N, P, Q, R 🔧, B, C 🔧, D, E, F, G, H, J, S 🔧, A, B, C 🔧

● S52.35   Comminuted fracture of shaft of radius

● S52.351   Displaced comminuted fracture of shaft of radius, right arm A, K, M, N, P, Q, R 🔧, B, C 🔧, D, E, F, G, H, J, S 🔧, A, B, C 🔧

● S52.352   Displaced comminuted fracture of shaft of radius, left arm A, K, M, N, P, Q, R 🔧, B, C 🔧, D, E, F, G, H, J, S 🔧, A, B, C 🔧

●🔲 S52.353   Displaced comminuted fracture of shaft of radius, unspecified arm A, K, M, N, P, Q, R 🔧, B, C 🔧, D, E, F, G, H, J, S 🔧, A, B, C 🔧

● S52.354   Nondisplaced comminuted fracture of shaft of radius, right arm A, K, M, N, P, Q, R 🔧, B, C 🔧, D, E, F, G, H, J, S 🔧, A, B, C 🔧

● S52.355   Nondisplaced comminuted fracture of shaft of radius, left arm A, K, M, N, P, Q, R 🔧, B, C 🔧, D, E, F, G, H, J, S 🔧, A, B, C 🔧

●🔲 S52.356   Nondisplaced comminuted fracture of shaft of radius, unspecified arm A, K, M, N, P, Q, R 🔧, B, C 🔧, D, E, F, G, H, J, S 🔧, A, B, C 🔧

● S52.36   Segmental fracture of shaft of radius

● S52.361   Displaced segmental fracture of shaft of radius, right arm A, K, M, N, P, Q, R 🔧, B, C 🔧, D, E, F, G, H, J, S 🔧, A, B, C 🔧

● S52.362   Displaced segmental fracture of shaft of radius, left arm A, K, M, N, P, Q, R 🔧, B, C 🔧, D, E, F, G, H, J, S 🔧, A, B, C 🔧

●🔲 S52.363   Displaced segmental fracture of shaft of radius, unspecified arm A, K, M, N, P, Q, R 🔧, B, C 🔧, D, E, F, G, H, J, S 🔧, A, B, C 🔧

● S52.364   Nondisplaced segmental fracture of shaft of radius, right arm A, K, M, N, P, Q, R 🔧, B, C 🔧, D, E, F, G, H, J, S 🔧, A, B, C 🔧

● S52.365   Nondisplaced segmental fracture of shaft of radius, left arm A, K, M, N, P, Q, R 🔧, B, C 🔧, D, E, F, G, H, J, S 🔧, A, B, C 🔧

● Unacceptable Principal Diagnosis   ● Use Additional Character(s)   🔲 Unspecified   ▶ Manifestation Code

OGCR Official Guidelines for Coding and Reporting   Excludes 1   Excludes 2   Includes   Use additional   Code first   Code also

● ■ **S52.366**   **Nondisplaced segmental fracture of shaft of radius, unspecified arm** A, K, M, N, P, Q, R 🌑, B, C 🌑, D, E, F, G, H, J, S 🌑, A, B, C 🌑

● **S52.37**   **Galeazzi's fracture**
Fracture of lower shaft of radius with radioulnar joint dislocation

    ● **S52.371**   **Galeazzi's fracture of right radius** A, K, M, N, P, Q, R 🌑, B, C 🌑, D, E, F, G, H, J, S 🌑, A, B, C 🌑

    ● **S52.372**   **Galeazzi's fracture of left radius** A, K, M, N, P, Q, R 🌑, B, C 🌑, D, E, F, G, H, J, S 🌑, A, B, C 🌑

    ● ■ **S52.379**   **Galeazzi's fracture of unspecified radius** A, K, M, N, P, Q, R 🌑, B, C 🌑, D, E, F, G, H, J, S 🌑, A, B, C 🌑

● **S52.38**   **Bent bone of radius**

    ● **S52.381**   **Bent bone of right radius** A, K, M, N, P, Q, R 🌑, B, C 🌑, D, E, F, G, H, J, S 🌑, A, B, C 🌑

    ● **S52.382**   **Bent bone of left radius** A, K, M, N, P, Q, R 🌑, B, C 🌑, D, E, F, G, H, J, S 🌑, A, B, C 🌑

    ● ■ **S52.389**   **Bent bone of unspecified radius** A, K, M, N, P, Q, R 🌑, B, C 🌑, D, E, F, G, H, J, S 🌑, A, B, C 🌑

● **S52.39**   **Other fracture of shaft of radius**

    ● **S52.391**   **Other fracture of shaft of radius, right arm** A, K, M, N, P, Q, R 🌑, B, C 🌑, D, E, F, G, H, J, S 🌑, A, B, C 🌑

    ● **S52.392**   **Other fracture of shaft of radius, left arm** A, K, M, N, P, Q, R 🌑, B, C 🌑, D, E, F, G, H, J, S 🌑, A, B, C 🌑

    ● ■ **S52.399**   **Other fracture of shaft of radius, unspecified arm** A, K, M, N, P, Q, R 🌑, B, C 🌑, D, E, F, G, H, J, S 🌑, A, B, C 🌑

● **S52.5**   **Fracture of lower end of radius**
Fracture of distal end of radius

> **Excludes2**   physeal fractures of lower end of radius (S59.2-)

    ● **S52.50**   **Unspecified fracture of the lower end of radius**

      ● ■ **S52.501**   **Unspecified fracture of the lower end of right radius** A, K, M, N, P, Q, R 🌑, B, C 🌑, D, E, F, G, H, J, S 🌑, A, B, C 🌑

      ● ■ **S52.502**   **Unspecified fracture of the lower end of left radius** A, K, M, N, P, Q, R 🌑, B, C 🌑, D, E, F, G, H, J, S 🌑, A, B, C 🌑

      ● ■ **S52.509**   **Unspecified fracture of the lower end of unspecified radius** A, K, M, N, P, Q, R 🌑, B, C 🌑, D, E, F, G, H, J, S 🌑, A, B, C 🌑

    ● **S52.51**   **Fracture of radial styloid process**

      ● **S52.511**   **Displaced fracture of right radial styloid process** A, K, M, N, P, Q, R 🌑, B, C 🌑, D, E, F, G, H, J, S 🌑, A, B, C 🌑

      ● **S52.512**   **Displaced fracture of left radial styloid process** A, K, M, N, P, Q, R 🌑, B, C 🌑, D, E, F, G, H, J, S 🌑, A, B, C 🌑

      ● ■ **S52.513**   **Displaced fracture of unspecified radial styloid process** A, K, M, N, P, Q, R 🌑, B, C 🌑, D, E, F, G, H, J, S 🌑, A, B, C 🌑

      ● **S52.514**   **Nondisplaced fracture of right radial styloid process** A, K, M, N, P, Q, R 🌑, B, C 🌑, D, E, F, G, H, J, S 🌑, A, B, C 🌑

      ● **S52.515**   **Nondisplaced fracture of left radial styloid process** A, K, M, N, P, Q, R 🌑, B, C 🌑, D, E, F, G, H, J, S 🌑, A, B, C 🌑

      ● ■ **S52.516**   **Nondisplaced fracture of unspecified radial styloid process** A, K, M, N, P, Q, R 🌑, B, C 🌑, D, E, F, G, H, J, S 🌑, A, B, C 🌑

    ● **S52.52**   **Torus fracture of lower end of radius**

The appropriate 7th character is to be added to all codes in subcategory S52.52

A	initial encounter for closed fracture
D	subsequent encounter for fracture with routine healing
G	subsequent encounter for fracture with delayed healing
K	subsequent encounter for fracture with nonunion
P	subsequent encounter for fracture with malunion
S	sequela

      ● **S52.521**   **Torus fracture of lower end of right radius** A, K, P 🌑, D, G, S 🌑, A 🌑

      ● **S52.522**   **Torus fracture of lower end of left radius** A, K, P 🌑, D, G, S 🌑, A 🌑

      ● ■ **S52.529**   **Torus fracture of lower end of unspecified radius** A, K, P 🌑, D, G, S 🌑, A 🌑

    ● **S52.53**   **Colles' fracture**

      ● **S52.531**   **Colles' fracture of right radius** A, K, M, N, P, Q, R 🌑, B, C 🌑, D, E, F, G, H, J, S 🌑, A, B, C 🌑

      ● **S52.532**   **Colles' fracture of left radius** A, K, M, N, P, Q, R 🌑, B, C 🌑, D, E, F, G, H, J, S 🌑, A, B, C 🌑

      ● ■ **S52.539**   **Colles' fracture of unspecified radius** A, K, M, N, P, Q, R 🌑, B, C 🌑, D, E, F, G, H, J, S 🌑, A, B, C 🌑

    ● **S52.54**   **Smith's fracture**

      ● **S52.541**   **Smith's fracture of right radius** A, K, M, N, P, Q, R 🌑, B, C 🌑, D, E, F, G, H, J, S 🌑, A, B, C 🌑

      ● **S52.542**   **Smith's fracture of left radius** A, K, M, N, P, Q, R 🌑, B, C 🌑, D, E, F, G, H, J, S 🌑, A, B, C 🌑

      ● ■ **S52.549**   **Smith's fracture of unspecified radius** A, K, M, N, P, Q, R 🌑, B, C 🌑, D, E, F, G, H, J, S 🌑, A, B, C 🌑

N Newborn Age: 0   **P** Pediatric Age: 0–17   **M** Maternity DX: 12–55   **A** Adult Age: 15–124   ♀ Females Only   ♂ Males Only

🌑 Complication\Comorbidity   🌑 Major C\C   🌑 Present on Admission Requirement   🌑 Hospital-Acquired Condition

1477

CHAPTER 19 (S00-T88)

● S52.55   Other extraarticular fracture of lower end of radius
  ● S52.551   Other extraarticular fracture of lower end of right radius A, K, M, N, P, Q, R ◐, B, C ◐, D, E, F, G, H, J, S ◐, A, B, C ◐
  ● S52.552   Other extraarticular fracture of lower end of left radius A, K, M, N, P, Q, R ◐, B, C ◐, D, E, F, G, H, J, S ◐, A, B, C ◐
  ●■ S52.559   Other extraarticular fracture of lower end of unspecified radius A, K, M, N, P, Q, R ◐, B, C ◐, D, E, F, G, H, J, S ◐, A, B, C ◐

● S52.56   Barton's fracture
  ● S52.561   Barton's fracture of right radius A, K, M, N, P, Q, R ◐, B, C ◐, D, E, F, G, H, J, S ◐, A, B, C ◐
  ● S52.562   Barton's fracture of left radius A, K, M, N, P, Q, R ◐, B, C ◐, D, E, F, G, H, J, S ◐, A, B, C ◐
  ●■ S52.569   Barton's fracture of unspecified radius A, K, M, N, P, Q, R ◐, B, C ◐, D, E, F, G, H, J, S ◐, A, B, C ◐

● S52.57   Other intraarticular fracture of lower end of radius
  ● S52.571   Other intraarticular fracture of lower end of right radius A, K, M, N, P, Q, R ◐, B, C ◐, D, E, F, G, H, J, S ◐, A, B, C ◐
  ● S52.572   Other intraarticular fracture of lower end of left radius A, K, M, N, P, Q, R ◐, B, C ◐, D, E, F, G, H, J, S ◐, A, B, C ◐
  ●■ S52.579   Other intraarticular fracture of lower end of unspecified radius A, K, M, N, P, Q, R ◐, B, C ◐, D, E, F, G, H, J, S ◐, A, B, C ◐

● S52.59   Other fractures of lower end of radius
  ● S52.591   Other fractures of lower end of right radius A, K, M, N, P, Q, R ◐, B, C ◐, D, E, F, G, H, J, S ◐, A, B, C ◐
  ● S52.592   Other fractures of lower end of left radius A, K, M, N, P, Q, R ◐, B, C ◐, D, E, F, G, H, J, S ◐, A, B, C ◐
  ●■ S52.599   Other fractures of lower end of unspecified radius A, K, M, N, P, Q, R ◐, B, C ◐, D, E, F, G, H, J, S ◐, A, B, C ◐

● S52.6   Fracture of lower end of ulna
 ● S52.60   Unspecified fracture of lower end of ulna
  ●■ S52.601   Unspecified fracture of lower end of right ulna A, K, M, N, P, Q, R ◐, B, C ◐, D, E, F, G, H, J, S ◐, A, B, C ◐
  ●■ S52.602   Unspecified fracture of lower end of left ulna A, K, M, N, P, Q, R ◐, B, C ◐, D, E, F, G, H, J, S ◐, A, B, C ◐
  ●■ S52.609   Unspecified fracture of lower end of unspecified ulna A, K, M, N, P, Q, R ◐, B, C ◐, D, E, F, G, H, J, S ◐, A, B, C ◐

● S52.61   Fracture of ulna styloid process
  ● S52.611   Displaced fracture of right ulna styloid process A, K, M, N, P, Q, R ◐, B, C ◐, D, E, F, G, H, J, S ◐, A, B, C ◐
  ● S52.612   Displaced fracture of left ulna styloid process A, K, M, N, P, Q, R ◐, B, C ◐, D, E, F, G, H, J, S ◐, A, B, C ◐
  ●■ S52.613   Displaced fracture of unspecified ulna styloid process A, K, M, N, P, Q, R ◐, B, C ◐, D, E, F, G, H, J, S ◐, A, B, C ◐
  ● S52.614   Nondisplaced fracture of right ulna styloid process A, K, M, N, P, Q, R ◐, B, C ◐, D, E, F, G, H, J, S ◐, A, B, C ◐
  ● S52.615   Nondisplaced fracture of left ulna styloid process A, K, M, N, P, Q, R ◐, B, C ◐, D, E, F, G, H, J, S ◐, A, B, C ◐
  ●■ S52.616   Nondisplaced fracture of unspecified ulna styloid process A, K, M, N, P, Q, R ◐, B, C ◐, D, E, F, G, H, J, S ◐, A, B, C ◐

● S52.62   Torus fracture of lower end of ulna

The appropriate 7th character is to be added to all codes in subcategory S52.62

A	initial encounter for closed fracture
D	subsequent encounter for fracture with routine healing
G	subsequent encounter for fracture with delayed healing
K	subsequent encounter for fracture with nonunion
P	subsequent encounter for fracture with malunion
S	sequela

  ● S52.621   Torus fracture of lower end of right ulna A, K, P ◐, D, G, S ◐, A ◐
  ● S52.622   Torus fracture of lower end of left ulna A, K, P ◐, D, G, S ◐, A ◐
  ●■ S52.629   Torus fracture of lower end of unspecified ulna A, K, P ◐, D, G, S ◐, A ◐

● S52.69   Other fracture of lower end of ulna
  ● S52.691   Other fracture of lower end of right ulna A, K, M, N, P, Q, R ◐, B, C ◐, D, E, F, G, H, J, S ◐, A, B, C ◐
  ● S52.692   Other fracture of lower end of left ulna A, K, M, N, P, Q, R ◐, B, C ◐, D, E, F, G, H, J, S ◐, A, B, C ◐
  ●■ S52.699   Other fracture of lower end of unspecified ulna A, K, M, N, P, Q, R ◐, B, C ◐, D, E, F, G, H, J, S ◐, A, B, C ◐

● S52.9   Unspecified fracture of forearm
  ●■ S52.90   Unspecified fracture of unspecified forearm A, K, M, N, P, Q, R ◐, B, C ◐, D, E, F, G, H, J, S ◐, A, B, C ◐

● Unacceptable Principal Diagnosis   ● Use Additional Character(s)   ■ Unspecified   ▶ Manifestation Code
OGCR Official Guidelines for Coding and Reporting   Excludes 1   Excludes 2   Includes   Use additional   Code first   Code also

● ■ **S52.91 Unspecified fracture of right forearm** A, K, M, N, P, Q, R 🐾, B, C 🐾, D, E, F, G, H, J, S 🐾, A, B, C 🐾

● ■ **S52.92 Unspecified fracture of left forearm** A, K, M, N, P, Q, R 🐾, B, C 🐾, D, E, F, G, H, J, S 🐾, A, B, C 🐾

● **S53 Dislocation and sprain of joints and ligaments of elbow**

> **Includes**   avulsion of joint or ligament of elbow
> laceration of cartilage, joint or ligament of elbow
> sprain of cartilage, joint or ligament of elbow
> traumatic hemarthrosis of joint or ligament of elbow
> traumatic rupture of joint or ligament of elbow
> traumatic subluxation of joint or ligament of elbow
> traumatic tear of joint or ligament of elbow

> Code also any associated open wound

> **Excludes2**   strain of muscle, fascia and tendon at forearm level (S56.-)

> The appropriate 7th character is to be added to each code from category S53

> A   initial encounter
> D   subsequent encounter
> S   sequela

● **S53.0 Subluxation and dislocation of radial head**
Dislocation of radiohumeral joint
Subluxation of radiohumeral joint

> **Excludes1**   Monteggia's fracture-dislocation (S52.27-)

   ● **S53.00 Unspecified subluxation and dislocation of radial head**

     ● ■ **S53.001 Unspecified subluxation of right radial head** D, S 🐾

     ● ■ **S53.002 Unspecified subluxation of left radial head** D, S 🐾

     ● ■ **S53.003 Unspecified subluxation of unspecified radial head** D, S 🐾

     ● ■ **S53.004 Unspecified dislocation of right radial head** D, S 🐾

     ● ■ **S53.005 Unspecified dislocation of left radial head** D, S 🐾

     ● ■ **S53.006 Unspecified dislocation of unspecified radial head** D, S 🐾

   ● **S53.01 Anterior subluxation and dislocation of radial head**
Anteriomedial subluxation and dislocation of radial head

     ● **S53.011 Anterior subluxation of right radial head** D, S 🐾

     ● **S53.012 Anterior subluxation of left radial head** D, S 🐾

     ● ■ **S53.013 Anterior subluxation of unspecified radial head** D, S 🐾

     ● **S53.014 Anterior dislocation of right radial head** D, S 🐾

     ● **S53.015 Anterior dislocation of left radial head** D, S 🐾

     ● ■ **S53.016 Anterior dislocation of unspecified radial head** D, S 🐾

● **S53.02 Posterior subluxation and dislocation of radial head**
Posteriolateral subluxation and dislocation of radial head

   ● **S53.021 Posterior subluxation of right radial head** D, S 🐾

   ● **S53.022 Posterior subluxation of left radial head** D, S 🐾

   ● ■ **S53.023 Posterior subluxation of unspecified radial head** D, S 🐾

   ● **S53.024 Posterior dislocation of right radial head** D, S 🐾

   ● **S53.025 Posterior dislocation of left radial head** D, S 🐾

   ● ■ **S53.026 Posterior dislocation of unspecified radial head** D, S 🐾

● **S53.03 Nursemaid's elbow**

   ● **S53.031 Nursemaid's elbow, right elbow** D, S 🐾

   ● **S53.032 Nursemaid's elbow, left elbow** D, S 🐾

   ● ■ **S53.033 Nursemaid's elbow, unspecified elbow** D, S 🐾

● **S53.09 Other subluxation and dislocation of radial head**

   ● **S53.091 Other subluxation of right radial head** D, S 🐾

   ● **S53.092 Other subluxation of left radial head** D, S 🐾

   ● ■ **S53.093 Other subluxation of unspecified radial head** D, S 🐾

   ● **S53.094 Other dislocation of right radial head** D, S 🐾

   ● **S53.095 Other dislocation of left radial head** D, S 🐾

   ● ■ **S53.096 Other dislocation of unspecified radial head** D, S 🐾

● **S53.1 Subluxation and dislocation of ulnohumeral joint**
Subluxation and dislocation of elbow NOS

> **Excludes1**   dislocation of radial head alone (S53.0-)

   ● **S53.10 Unspecified subluxation and dislocation of ulnohumeral joint**

     ● ■ **S53.101 Unspecified subluxation of right ulnohumeral joint** D, S 🐾

     ● ■ **S53.102 Unspecified subluxation of left ulnohumeral joint** D, S 🐾

     ● ■ **S53.103 Unspecified subluxation of unspecified ulnohumeral joint** D, S 🐾

     ● ■ **S53.104 Unspecified dislocation of right ulnohumeral joint** D, S 🐾

     ● ■ **S53.105 Unspecified dislocation of left ulnohumeral joint** D, S 🐾

     ● ■ **S53.106 Unspecified dislocation of unspecified ulnohumeral joint** D, S 🐾

N Newborn Age: 0   **P** Pediatric Age: 0–17   **M** Maternity DX: 12–55   **A** Adult Age: 15–124   ♀ Females Only   ♂ Males Only

🐾 Complication\Comorbidity   🐾 Major C\C   🐾 Present on Admission Requirement   🐾 Hospital-Acquired Condition

1479

CHAPTER 19 (S00-T88)

● **S53.11** Anterior subluxation and dislocation of ulnohumeral joint

　● **S53.111** Anterior subluxation of right ulnohumeral joint D, S 🔍

　● **S53.112** Anterior subluxation of left ulnohumeral joint D, S 🔍

　●■ **S53.113** Anterior subluxation of unspecified ulnohumeral joint D, S 🔍

　● **S53.114** Anterior dislocation of right ulnohumeral joint D, S 🔍

　● **S53.115** Anterior dislocation of left ulnohumeral joint D, S 🔍

　●■ **S53.116** Anterior dislocation of unspecified ulnohumeral joint D, S 🔍

● **S53.12** Posterior subluxation and dislocation of ulnohumeral joint

　● **S53.121** Posterior subluxation of right ulnohumeral joint D, S 🔍

　● **S53.122** Posterior subluxation of left ulnohumeral joint D, S 🔍

　●■ **S53.123** Posterior subluxation of unspecified ulnohumeral joint D, S 🔍

　● **S53.124** Posterior dislocation of right ulnohumeral joint D, S 🔍

　● **S53.125** Posterior dislocation of left ulnohumeral joint D, S 🔍

　●■ **S53.126** Posterior dislocation of unspecified ulnohumeral joint D, S 🔍

● **S53.13** Medial subluxation and dislocation of ulnohumeral joint

　● **S53.131** Medial subluxation of right ulnohumeral joint D, S 🔍

　● **S53.132** Medial subluxation of left ulnohumeral joint D, S 🔍

　●■ **S53.133** Medial subluxation of unspecified ulnohumeral joint D, S 🔍

　● **S53.134** Medial dislocation of right ulnohumeral joint D, S 🔍

　● **S53.135** Medial dislocation of left ulnohumeral joint D, S 🔍

　●■ **S53.136** Medial dislocation of unspecified ulnohumeral joint D, S 🔍

● **S53.14** Lateral subluxation and dislocation of ulnohumeral joint

　● **S53.141** Lateral subluxation of right ulnohumeral joint D, S 🔍

　● **S53.142** Lateral subluxation of left ulnohumeral joint D, S 🔍

　●■ **S53.143** Lateral subluxation of unspecified ulnohumeral joint D, S 🔍

　● **S53.144** Lateral dislocation of right ulnohumeral joint D, S 🔍

　● **S53.145** Lateral dislocation of left ulnohumeral joint D, S 🔍

　●■ **S53.146** Lateral dislocation of unspecified ulnohumeral joint D, S 🔍

● **S53.19** Other subluxation and dislocation of ulnohumeral joint

　● **S53.191** Other subluxation of right ulnohumeral joint D, S 🔍

　● **S53.192** Other subluxation of left ulnohumeral joint D, S 🔍

　●■ **S53.193** Other subluxation of unspecified ulnohumeral joint D, S 🔍

　● **S53.194** Other dislocation of right ulnohumeral joint D, S 🔍

　● **S53.195** Other dislocation of left ulnohumeral joint D, S 🔍

　●■ **S53.196** Other dislocation of unspecified ulnohumeral joint D, S 🔍

● **S53.2** Traumatic rupture of radial collateral ligament

　| Excludes1 | sprain of radial collateral ligament NOS (S53.43-)

　●■ **S53.20** Traumatic rupture of unspecified radial collateral ligament D, S 🔍

　● **S53.21** Traumatic rupture of right radial collateral ligament D, S 🔍

　● **S53.22** Traumatic rupture of left radial collateral ligament D, S 🔍

● **S53.3** Traumatic rupture of ulnar collateral ligament

　| Excludes1 | sprain of ulnar collateral ligament (S53.44-)

　●■ **S53.30** Traumatic rupture of unspecified ulnar collateral ligament D, S 🔍

　● **S53.31** Traumatic rupture of right ulnar collateral ligament D, S 🔍

　● **S53.32** Traumatic rupture of left ulnar collateral ligament D, S 🔍

● **S53.4** Sprain of elbow

　| Excludes2 | traumatic rupture of radial collateral ligament (S53.2-)
　　　　　　　traumatic rupture of ulnar collateral ligament (S53.3-)

　● **S53.40** Unspecified sprain of elbow

　　●■ **S53.401** Unspecified sprain of right elbow D, S 🔍

　　●■ **S53.402** Unspecified sprain of left elbow D, S 🔍

　　●■ **S53.409** Unspecified sprain of unspecified elbow D, S 🔍
　　　　　　　Sprain of elbow NOS

　● **S53.41** Radiohumeral (joint) sprain

　　● **S53.411** Radiohumeral (joint) sprain of right elbow D, S 🔍

　　● **S53.412** Radiohumeral (joint) sprain of left elbow D, S 🔍

　　●■ **S53.419** Radiohumeral (joint) sprain of unspecified elbow D, S 🔍

　● **S53.42** Ulnohumeral (joint) sprain

　　● **S53.421** Ulnohumeral (joint) sprain of right elbow D, S 🔍

　　● **S53.422** Ulnohumeral (joint) sprain of left elbow D, S 🔍

　　●■ **S53.429** Ulnohumeral (joint) sprain of unspecified elbow D, S 🔍

CHAPTER 19 (S00-T88)

● **S53.43**   Radial collateral ligament sprain

    ● **S53.431**   Radial collateral ligament sprain of right elbow D, S 🔖

    ● **S53.432**   Radial collateral ligament sprain of left elbow D, S 🔖

    ●■ **S53.439**   Radial collateral ligament sprain of unspecified elbow D, S 🔖

● **S53.44**   Ulnar collateral ligament sprain

    ● **S53.441**   Ulnar collateral ligament sprain of right elbow D, S 🔖

    ● **S53.442**   Ulnar collateral ligament sprain of left elbow D, S 🔖

    ●■ **S53.449**   Ulnar collateral ligament sprain of unspecified elbow D, S 🔖

● **S53.49**   Other sprain of elbow

    ● **S53.491**   Other sprain of right elbow D, S 🔖

    ● **S53.492**   Other sprain of left elbow D, S 🔖

    ●■ **S53.499**   Other sprain of unspecified elbow D, S 🔖

● **S54**   **Injury of nerves at forearm level**

    Code also any associated open wound (S51.-)

    Excludes2   injury of nerves at wrist and hand level (S64.-)

    The appropriate 7th character is to be added to each code from category S54

    | | |
    A   initial encounter
    D   subsequent encounter
    S   sequela

● **S54.0**   Injury of ulnar nerve at forearm level
    Injury of ulnar nerve NOS

    ●■ **S54.00**   Injury of ulnar nerve at forearm level, unspecified arm D, S 🔖

    ● **S54.01**   Injury of ulnar nerve at forearm level, right arm D, S 🔖

    ● **S54.02**   Injury of ulnar nerve at forearm level, left arm D, S 🔖

● **S54.1**   Injury of median nerve at forearm level
    Injury of median nerve NOS

    ●■ **S54.10**   Injury of median nerve at forearm level, unspecified arm D, S 🔖

    ● **S54.11**   Injury of median nerve at forearm level, right arm D, S 🔖

    ● **S54.12**   Injury of median nerve at forearm level, left arm D, S 🔖

● **S54.2**   Injury of radial nerve at forearm level
    Injury of radial nerve NOS

    ●■ **S54.20**   Injury of radial nerve at forearm level, unspecified arm D, S 🔖

    ● **S54.21**   Injury of radial nerve at forearm level, right arm D, S 🔖

    ● **S54.22**   Injury of radial nerve at forearm level, left arm D, S 🔖

● **S54.3**   Injury of cutaneous sensory nerve at forearm level

    ●■ **S54.30**   Injury of cutaneous sensory nerve at forearm level, unspecified arm D, S 🔖

    ● **S54.31**   Injury of cutaneous sensory nerve at forearm level, right arm D, S 🔖

    ● **S54.32**   Injury of cutaneous sensory nerve at forearm level, left arm D, S 🔖

● **S54.8**   Injury of other nerves at forearm level

    ● **S54.8X**   Injury of other nerves at forearm level

      ●■ **S54.8X1**   Unspecified injury of other nerves at forearm level, right arm D, S 🔖

      ●■ **S54.8X2**   Unspecified injury of other nerves at forearm level, left arm D, S 🔖

      ●■ **S54.8X9**   Unspecified injury of other nerves at forearm level, unspecified arm D, S 🔖

● **S54.9**   Injury of unspecified nerve at forearm level

    ●■ **S54.90**   Injury of unspecified nerve at forearm level, unspecified arm D, S 🔖

    ●■ **S54.91**   Injury of unspecified nerve at forearm level, right arm D, S 🔖

    ●■ **S54.92**   Injury of unspecified nerve at forearm level, left arm D, S 🔖

● **S55**   **Injury of blood vessels at forearm level**

    Code also any associated open wound (S51.-)

    Excludes2   injury of blood vessels at wrist and hand level (S65.-)
           injury of brachial vessels (S45.1-S45.2)

    The appropriate 7th character is to be added to each code from category S55

    | | |
    A   initial encounter
    D   subsequent encounter
    S   sequela

● **S55.0**   Injury of ulnar artery at forearm level

    ● **S55.00**   Unspecified injury of ulnar artery at forearm level

      ●■ **S55.001**   Unspecified injury of ulnar artery at forearm level, right arm A 🔖, D, S 🔖

      ●■ **S55.002**   Unspecified injury of ulnar artery at forearm level, left arm A 🔖, D, S 🔖

      ●■ **S55.009**   Unspecified injury of ulnar artery at forearm level, unspecified arm A 🔖, D, S 🔖

    ● **S55.01**   Laceration of ulnar artery at forearm level

      ● **S55.011**   Laceration of ulnar artery at forearm level, right arm A 🔖, D, S 🔖

      ● **S55.012**   Laceration of ulnar artery at forearm level, left arm A 🔖, D, S 🔖

      ●■ **S55.019**   Laceration of ulnar artery at forearm level, unspecified arm A 🔖, D, S 🔖

    ● **S55.09**   Other specified injury of ulnar artery at forearm level

      ● **S55.091**   Other specified injury of ulnar artery at forearm level, right arm A 🔖, D, S 🔖

      ● **S55.092**   Other specified injury of ulnar artery at forearm level, left arm A 🔖, D, S 🔖

      ●■ **S55.099**   Other specified injury of ulnar artery at forearm level, unspecified arm A 🔖, D, S 🔖

N Newborn Age: 0   **P** Pediatric Age: 0–17   **M** Maternity DX: 12–55   **A** Adult Age: 15–124   ♀ Females Only   ♂ Males Only

🔖 Complication\Comorbidity   🔖 Major C\C   🔖 Present on Admission Requirement   🔖 Hospital-Acquired Condition

1481

CHAPTER 19 (S00-T88)

- S55.1   **Injury of radial artery at forearm level**
  - S55.10   **Unspecified injury of radial artery at forearm level**
    - S55.101   Unspecified injury of radial artery at forearm level, right arm A, D, S
    - S55.102   Unspecified injury of radial artery at forearm level, left arm A, D, S
    - S55.109   Unspecified injury of radial artery at forearm level, unspecified arm A, D, S
  - S55.11   **Laceration of radial artery at forearm level**
    - S55.111   Laceration of radial artery at forearm level, right arm A, D, S
    - S55.112   Laceration of radial artery at forearm level, left arm A, D, S
    - S55.119   Laceration of radial artery at forearm level, unspecified arm A, D, S
  - S55.19   **Other specified injury of radial artery at forearm level**
    - S55.191   Other specified injury of radial artery at forearm level, right arm A, D, S
    - S55.192   Other specified injury of radial artery at forearm level, left arm A, D, S
    - S55.199   Other specified injury of radial artery at forearm level, unspecified arm A, D, S
- S55.2   **Injury of vein at forearm level**
  - S55.20   **Unspecified injury of vein at forearm level**
    - S55.201   Unspecified injury of vein at forearm level, right arm A, D, S
    - S55.202   Unspecified injury of vein at forearm level, left arm A, D, S
    - S55.209   Unspecified injury of vein at forearm level, unspecified arm A, D, S
  - S55.21   **Laceration of vein at forearm level**
    - S55.211   Laceration of vein at forearm level, right arm A, D, S
    - S55.212   Laceration of vein at forearm level, left arm A, D, S
    - S55.219   Laceration of vein at forearm level, unspecified arm A, D, S
  - S55.29   **Other specified injury of vein at forearm level**
    - S55.291   Other specified injury of vein at forearm level, right arm A, D, S
    - S55.292   Other specified injury of vein at forearm level, left arm A, D, S
    - S55.299   Other specified injury of vein at forearm level, unspecified arm A, D, S

- S55.8   **Injury of other blood vessels at forearm level**
  - S55.80   **Unspecified injury of other blood vessels at forearm level**
    - S55.801   Unspecified injury of other blood vessels at forearm level, right arm A, D, S
    - S55.802   Unspecified injury of other blood vessels at forearm level, left arm A, D, S
    - S55.809   Unspecified injury of other blood vessels at forearm level, unspecified arm A, D, S
  - S55.81   **Laceration of other blood vessels at forearm level**
    - S55.811   Laceration of other blood vessels at forearm level, right arm A, D, S
    - S55.812   Laceration of other blood vessels at forearm level, left arm A, D, S
    - S55.819   Laceration of other blood vessels at forearm level, unspecified arm A, D, S
  - S55.89   **Other specified injury of other blood vessels at forearm level**
    - S55.891   Other specified injury of other blood vessels at forearm level, right arm A, D, S
    - S55.892   Other specified injury of other blood vessels at forearm level, left arm A, D, S
    - S55.899   Other specified injury of other blood vessels at forearm level, unspecified arm A, D, S
- S55.9   **Injury of unspecified blood vessel at forearm level**
  - S55.90   **Unspecified injury of unspecified blood vessel at forearm level**
    - S55.901   Unspecified injury of unspecified blood vessel at forearm level, right arm A, D, S
    - S55.902   Unspecified injury of unspecified blood vessel at forearm level, left arm A, D, S
    - S55.909   Unspecified injury of unspecified blood vessel at forearm level, unspecified arm A, D, S
  - S55.91   **Laceration of unspecified blood vessel at forearm level**
    - S55.911   Laceration of unspecified blood vessel at forearm level, right arm A, D, S
    - S55.912   Laceration of unspecified blood vessel at forearm level, left arm A, D, S
    - S55.919   Laceration of unspecified blood vessel at forearm level, unspecified arm A, D, S

● Unacceptable Principal Diagnosis   ● Use Additional Character(s)   ■ Unspecified   ▶ Manifestation Code

1482   **OGCR**   Official Guidelines for Coding and Reporting   Excludes 1   Excludes 2   Includes   Use additional   Code first   Code also

● S55.99   Other specified injury of unspecified blood vessel at forearm level

  ● ■ S55.991   Other specified injury of unspecified blood vessel at forearm level, right arm A 🗲, D, S 🗲

  ● ■ S55.992   Other specified injury of unspecified blood vessel at forearm level, left arm A 🗲, D, S 🗲

  ● ■ S55.999   Other specified injury of unspecified blood vessel at forearm level, unspecified arm A 🗲, D, S 🗲

● S56   Injury of muscle, fascia and tendon at forearm level

> Code also any associated open wound (S51.-)
>
> **Excludes2**   injury of muscle, fascia and tendon at or below wrist (S66.-)
> sprain of joints and ligaments of elbow (S53.4-)

The appropriate 7th character is to be added to each code from category S56

> A   initial encounter
> D   subsequent encounter
> S   sequela

● S56.0   Injury of flexor muscle, fascia and tendon of thumb at forearm level

  ● S56.00   Unspecified injury of flexor muscle, fascia and tendon of thumb at forearm level

    ● ■ S56.001   Unspecified injury of flexor muscle, fascia and tendon of right thumb at forearm level D, S 🗲

    ● ■ S56.002   Unspecified injury of flexor muscle, fascia and tendon of left thumb at forearm level D, S 🗲

    ● ■ S56.009   Unspecified injury of flexor muscle, fascia and tendon of unspecified thumb at forearm level D, S 🗲

  ● S56.01   Strain of flexor muscle, fascia and tendon of thumb at forearm level

    ● S56.011   Strain of flexor muscle, fascia and tendon of right thumb at forearm level D, S 🗲

    ● S56.012   Strain of flexor muscle, fascia and tendon of left thumb at forearm level D, S 🗲

    ● ■ S56.019   Strain of flexor muscle, fascia and tendon of unspecified thumb at forearm level D, S 🗲

  ● S56.02   Laceration of flexor muscle, fascia and tendon of thumb at forearm level

    ● S56.021   Laceration of flexor muscle, fascia and tendon of right thumb at forearm level A 🗲, D, S 🗲

    ● S56.022   Laceration of flexor muscle, fascia and tendon of left thumb at forearm level A 🗲, D, S 🗲

    ● ■ S56.029   Laceration of flexor muscle, fascia and tendon of unspecified thumb at forearm level A 🗲, D, S 🗲

● S56.09   Other injury of flexor muscle, fascia and tendon of thumb at forearm level

  ● S56.091   Other injury of flexor muscle, fascia and tendon of right thumb at forearm level D, S 🗲

  ● S56.092   Other injury of flexor muscle, fascia and tendon of left thumb at forearm level D, S 🗲

  ● ■ S56.099   Other injury of flexor muscle, fascia and tendon of unspecified thumb at forearm level D, S 🗲

● S56.1   Injury of flexor muscle, fascia and tendon of other and unspecified finger at forearm level

  ● S56.10   Unspecified injury of flexor muscle, fascia and tendon of other and unspecified finger at forearm level

    ● ■ S56.101   Unspecified injury of flexor muscle, fascia and tendon of right index finger at forearm level D, S 🗲

    ● ■ S56.102   Unspecified injury of flexor muscle, fascia and tendon of left index finger at forearm level D, S 🗲

    ● ■ S56.103   Unspecified injury of flexor muscle, fascia and tendon of right middle finger at forearm level D, S 🗲

    ● ■ S56.104   Unspecified injury of flexor muscle, fascia and tendon of left middle finger at forearm level D, S 🗲

    ● ■ S56.105   Unspecified injury of flexor muscle, fascia and tendon of right ring finger at forearm level D, S 🗲

    ● ■ S56.106   Unspecified injury of flexor muscle, fascia and tendon of left ring finger at forearm level D, S 🗲

    ● ■ S56.107   Unspecified injury of flexor muscle, fascia and tendon of right little finger at forearm level D, S 🗲

    ● ■ S56.108   Unspecified injury of flexor muscle, fascia and tendon of left little finger at forearm level D, S 🗲

    ● ■ S56.109   Unspecified injury of flexor muscle, fascia and tendon of unspecified finger at forearm level D, S 🗲

  ● S56.11   Strain of flexor muscle, fascia and tendon of other and unspecified finger at forearm level

    ● S56.111   Strain of flexor muscle, fascia and tendon of right index finger at forearm level D, S 🗲

    ● S56.112   Strain of flexor muscle, fascia and tendon of left index finger at forearm level D, S 🗲

    ● S56.113   Strain of flexor muscle, fascia and tendon of right middle finger at forearm level D, S 🗲

CHAPTER 19 (S00-T88)

● S56.114 Strain of flexor muscle, fascia and tendon of left middle finger at forearm level D, S 🔗

● S56.115 Strain of flexor muscle, fascia and tendon of right ring finger at forearm level D, S 🔗

● S56.116 Strain of flexor muscle, fascia and tendon of left ring finger at forearm level D, S 🔗

● S56.117 Strain of flexor muscle, fascia and tendon of right little finger at forearm level D, S 🔗

● S56.118 Strain of flexor muscle, fascia and tendon of left little finger at forearm level D, S 🔗

●■ S56.119 Strain of flexor muscle, fascia and tendon of finger of unspecified finger at forearm level D, S 🔗

● S56.12 Laceration of flexor muscle, fascia and tendon of other and unspecified finger at forearm level

● S56.121 Laceration of flexor muscle, fascia and tendon of right index finger at forearm level A 🔗, D, S 🔗

● S56.122 Laceration of flexor muscle, fascia and tendon of left index finger at forearm level A 🔗, D, S 🔗

● S56.123 Laceration of flexor muscle, fascia and tendon of right middle finger at forearm level A 🔗, D, S 🔗

● S56.124 Laceration of flexor muscle, fascia and tendon of left middle finger at forearm level A 🔗, D, S 🔗

● S56.125 Laceration of flexor muscle, fascia and tendon of right ring finger at forearm level A 🔗, D, S 🔗

● S56.126 Laceration of flexor muscle, fascia and tendon of left ring finger at forearm level A 🔗, D, S 🔗

● S56.127 Laceration of flexor muscle, fascia and tendon of right little finger at forearm level A 🔗, D, S 🔗

● S56.128 Laceration of flexor muscle, fascia and tendon of left little finger at forearm level A 🔗, D, S 🔗

●■ S56.129 Laceration of flexor muscle, fascia and tendon of unspecified finger at forearm level A 🔗, D, S 🔗

● S56.19 Other injury of flexor muscle, fascia and tendon of other and unspecified finger at forearm level

● S56.191 Other injury of flexor muscle, fascia and tendon of right index finger at forearm level D, S 🔗

● S56.192 Other injury of flexor muscle, fascia and tendon of left index finger at forearm level D, S 🔗

● S56.193 Other injury of flexor muscle, fascia and tendon of right middle finger at forearm level D, S 🔗

● S56.194 Other injury of flexor muscle, fascia and tendon of left middle finger at forearm level D, S 🔗

● S56.195 Other injury of flexor muscle, fascia and tendon of right ring finger at forearm level D, S 🔗

● S56.196 Other injury of flexor muscle, fascia and tendon of left ring finger at forearm level D, S 🔗

● S56.197 Other injury of flexor muscle, fascia and tendon of right little finger at forearm level D, S 🔗

● S56.198 Other injury of flexor muscle, fascia and tendon of left little finger at forearm level D, S 🔗

●■ S56.199 Other injury of flexor muscle, fascia and tendon of unspecified finger at forearm level D, S 🔗

● S56.2 Injury of other flexor muscle, fascia and tendon at forearm level

● S56.20 Unspecified injury of other flexor muscle, fascia and tendon at forearm level

●■ S56.201 Unspecified injury of other flexor muscle, fascia and tendon at forearm level, right arm D, S 🔗

●■ S56.202 Unspecified injury of other flexor muscle, fascia and tendon at forearm level, left arm D, S 🔗

●■ S56.209 Unspecified injury of other flexor muscle, fascia and tendon at forearm level, unspecified arm D, S 🔗

● S56.21 Strain of other flexor muscle, fascia and tendon at forearm level

● S56.211 Strain of other flexor muscle, fascia and tendon at forearm level, right arm D, S 🔗

● S56.212 Strain of other flexor muscle, fascia and tendon at forearm level, left arm D, S 🔗

●■ S56.219 Strain of other flexor muscle, fascia and tendon at forearm level, unspecified arm D, S 🔗

● S56.22 Laceration of other flexor muscle, fascia and tendon at forearm level

● S56.221 Laceration of other flexor muscle, fascia and tendon at forearm level, right arm A 🔗, D, S 🔗

● S56.222 Laceration of other flexor muscle, fascia and tendon at forearm level, left arm A 🔗, D, S 🔗

●■ S56.229 Laceration of other flexor muscle, fascia and tendon at forearm level, unspecified arm A 🔗, D, S 🔗

● S56.29 Other injury of other flexor muscle, fascia and tendon at forearm level

● S56.291 Other injury of other flexor muscle, fascia and tendon at forearm level, right arm D, S 🔗

● S56.292 Other injury of other flexor muscle, fascia and tendon at forearm level, left arm D, S 🔗

●■ S56.299 Other injury of other flexor muscle, fascia and tendon at forearm level, unspecified arm D, S 🔗

● S56.3   Injury of extensor or abductor muscles, fascia and tendons of thumb at forearm level

   ● S56.30   Unspecified injury of extensor or abductor muscles, fascia and tendons of thumb at forearm level

     ●■ S56.301   Unspecified injury of extensor or abductor muscles, fascia and tendons of right thumb at forearm level D, S ⚲

     ●■ S56.302   Unspecified injury of extensor or abductor muscles, fascia and tendons of left thumb at forearm level D, S ⚲

     ●■ S56.309   Unspecified injury of extensor or abductor muscles, fascia and tendons of unspecified thumb at forearm level D, S ⚲

   ● S56.31   Strain of extensor or abductor muscles, fascia and tendons of thumb at forearm level

     ● S56.311   Strain of extensor or abductor muscles, fascia and tendons of right thumb at forearm level D, S ⚲

     ● S56.312   Strain of extensor or abductor muscles, fascia and tendons of left thumb at forearm level D, S ⚲

     ●■ S56.319   Strain of extensor or abductor muscles, fascia and tendons of unspecified thumb at forearm level D, S ⚲

   ● S56.32   Laceration of extensor or abductor muscles, fascia and tendons of thumb at forearm level

     ● S56.321   Laceration of extensor or abductor muscles, fascia and tendons of right thumb at forearm level A ⚲, D, S ⚲

     ● S56.322   Laceration of extensor or abductor muscles, fascia and tendons of left thumb at forearm level A ⚲, D, S ⚲

     ●■ S56.329   Laceration of extensor or abductor muscles, fascia and tendons of unspecified thumb at forearm level A ⚲, D, S ⚲

   ● S56.39   Other injury of extensor or abductor muscles, fascia and tendons of thumb at forearm level

     ● S56.391   Other injury of extensor or abductor muscles, fascia and tendons of right thumb at forearm level D, S ⚲

     ● S56.392   Other injury of extensor or abductor muscles, fascia and tendons of left thumb at forearm level D, S ⚲

     ●■ S56.399   Other injury of extensor or abductor muscles, fascia and tendons of unspecified thumb at forearm level D, S ⚲

● S56.4   Injury of extensor muscle, fascia and tendon of other and unspecified finger at forearm level

   ● S56.40   Unspecified injury of extensor muscle, fascia and tendon of other and unspecified finger at forearm level

     ●■ S56.401   Unspecified injury of extensor muscle, fascia and tendon of right index finger at forearm level D, S ⚲

     ●■ S56.402   Unspecified injury of extensor muscle, fascia and tendon of left index finger at forearm level D, S ⚲

     ●■ S56.403   Unspecified injury of extensor muscle, fascia and tendon of right middle finger at forearm level D, S ⚲

     ●■ S56.404   Unspecified injury of extensor muscle, fascia and tendon of left middle finger at forearm level D, S ⚲

     ●■ S56.405   Unspecified injury of extensor muscle, fascia and tendon of right ring finger at forearm level D, S ⚲

     ●■ S56.406   Unspecified injury of extensor muscle, fascia and tendon of left ring finger at forearm level D, S ⚲

     ●■ S56.407   Unspecified injury of extensor muscle, fascia and tendon of right little finger at forearm level D, S ⚲

     ●■ S56.408   Unspecified injury of extensor muscle, fascia and tendon of left little finger at forearm level D, S ⚲

     ●■ S56.409   Unspecified injury of extensor muscle, fascia and tendon of unspecified finger at forearm level D, S ⚲

   ● S56.41   Strain of extensor muscle, fascia and tendon of other and unspecified finger at forearm level

     ● S56.411   Strain of extensor muscle, fascia and tendon of right index finger at forearm level D, S ⚲

     ● S56.412   Strain of extensor muscle, fascia and tendon of left index finger at forearm level D, S ⚲

     ● S56.413   Strain of extensor muscle, fascia and tendon of right middle finger at forearm level D, S ⚲

     ● S56.414   Strain of extensor muscle, fascia and tendon of left middle finger at forearm level D, S ⚲

     ● S56.415   Strain of extensor muscle, fascia and tendon of right ring finger at forearm level D, S ⚲

     ● S56.416   Strain of extensor muscle, fascia and tendon of left ring finger at forearm level D, S ⚲

     ● S56.417   Strain of extensor muscle, fascia and tendon of right little finger at forearm level D, S ⚲

     ● S56.418   Strain of extensor muscle, fascia and tendon of left little finger at forearm level D, S ⚲

     ●■ S56.419   Strain of extensor muscle, fascia and tendon of finger, unspecified finger at forearm level D, S ⚲

N Newborn Age: 0   **P** Pediatric Age: 0–17   **M** Maternity DX: 12–55   **A** Adult Age: 15–124   ♀ Females Only   ♂ Males Only

⚲ Complication\Comorbidity   ⚲ Major C\C   ⚲ Present on Admission Requirement   ⚲ Hospital-Acquired Condition

1485

CHAPTER 19 (S00-T88)

● S56.42   Laceration of extensor muscle, fascia and tendon of other and unspecified finger at forearm level

   ● S56.421   Laceration of extensor muscle, fascia and tendon of right index finger at forearm level A 🗗, D, S 🗗

   ● S56.422   Laceration of extensor muscle, fascia and tendon of left index finger at forearm level A 🗗, D, S 🗗

   ● S56.423   Laceration of extensor muscle, fascia and tendon of right middle finger at forearm level A 🗗, D, S 🗗

   ● S56.424   Laceration of extensor muscle, fascia and tendon of left middle finger at forearm level A 🗗, D, S 🗗

   ● S56.425   Laceration of extensor muscle, fascia and tendon of right ring finger at forearm level A 🗗, D, S 🗗

   ● S56.426   Laceration of extensor muscle, fascia and tendon of left ring finger at forearm level A 🗗, D, S 🗗

   ● S56.427   Laceration of extensor muscle, fascia and tendon of right little finger at forearm level A 🗗, D, S 🗗

   ● S56.428   Laceration of extensor muscle, fascia and tendon of left little finger at forearm level A 🗗, D, S 🗗

   ●▪ S56.429   Laceration of extensor muscle, fascia and tendon of unspecified finger at forearm level A 🗗, D, S 🗗

● S56.49   Other injury of extensor muscle, fascia and tendon of other and unspecified finger at forearm level

   ● S56.491   Other injury of extensor muscle, fascia and tendon of right index finger at forearm level D, S 🗗

   ● S56.492   Other injury of extensor muscle, fascia and tendon of left index finger at forearm level D, S 🗗

   ● S56.493   Other injury of extensor muscle, fascia and tendon of right middle finger at forearm level D, S 🗗

   ● S56.494   Other injury of extensor muscle, fascia and tendon of left middle finger at forearm level D, S 🗗

   ● S56.495   Other injury of extensor muscle, fascia and tendon of right ring finger at forearm level D, S 🗗

   ● S56.496   Other injury of extensor muscle, fascia and tendon of left ring finger at forearm level D, S 🗗

   ● S56.497   Other injury of extensor muscle, fascia and tendon of right little finger at forearm level D, S 🗗

   ● S56.498   Other injury of extensor muscle, fascia and tendon of left little finger at forearm level D, S 🗗

   ●▪ S56.499   Other injury of extensor muscle, fascia and tendon of unspecified finger at forearm level D, S 🗗

● S56.5   Injury of other extensor muscle, fascia and tendon at forearm level

   ● S56.50   Unspecified injury of other muscle, fascia and tendon at forearm level

     ●▪ S56.501   Unspecified injury of other extensor muscle, fascia and tendon at forearm level, right arm D, S 🗗

     ●▪ S56.502   Unspecified injury of other extensor muscle, fascia and tendon at forearm level, left arm D, S 🗗

     ●▪ S56.509   Unspecified injury of other extensor muscle, fascia and tendon at forearm level, unspecified arm D, S 🗗

   ● S56.51   Strain of other extensor muscle, fascia and tendon at forearm level

     ● S56.511   Strain of other extensor muscle, fascia and tendon at forearm level, right arm D, S 🗗

     ● S56.512   Strain of other extensor muscle, fascia and tendon at forearm level, left arm D, S 🗗

     ●▪ S56.519   Strain of other extensor muscle, fascia and tendon at forearm level, unspecified arm D, S 🗗

   ● S56.52   Laceration of other extensor muscle, fascia and tendon at forearm level

     ● S56.521   Laceration of other extensor muscle, fascia and tendon at forearm level, right arm A 🗗, D, S 🗗

     ● S56.522   Laceration of other extensor muscle, fascia and tendon at forearm level, left arm A 🗗, D, S 🗗

     ●▪ S56.529   Laceration of other extensor muscle, fascia and tendon at forearm level, unspecified arm A 🗗, D, S 🗗

   ● S56.59   Other injury of other extensor muscle, fascia and tendon at forearm level

     ● S56.591   Other injury of other extensor muscle, fascia and tendon at forearm level, right arm D, S 🗗

     ● S56.592   Other injury of other extensor muscle, fascia and tendon at forearm level, left arm D, S 🗗

     ●▪ S56.599   Other injury of other extensor muscle, fascia and tendon at forearm level, unspecified arm D, S 🗗

● S56.8   Injury of other muscles, fascia and tendons at forearm level

   ● S56.80   Unspecified injury of other muscles, fascia and tendons at forearm level

     ●▪ S56.801   Unspecified injury of other muscles, fascia and tendons at forearm level, right arm D, S 🗗

     ●▪ S56.802   Unspecified injury of other muscles, fascia and tendons at forearm level, left arm D, S 🗗

     ●▪ S56.809   Unspecified injury of other muscles, fascia and tendons at forearm level, unspecified arm D, S 🗗

● Unacceptable Principal Diagnosis   ● Use Additional Character(s)   ▪ Unspecified   ▶ Manifestation Code

1486   **OGCR**   Official Guidelines for Coding and Reporting   Excludes 1   Excludes 2   Includes   Use additional   Code first   Code also

● S56.81 **Strain of other muscles, fascia and tendons at forearm level**
- ● S56.811 Strain of other muscles, fascia and tendons at forearm level, right arm D, S
- ● S56.812 Strain of other muscles, fascia and tendons at forearm level, left arm D, S
- ●■ S56.819 Strain of other muscles, fascia and tendons at forearm level, unspecified arm D, S

● S56.82 **Laceration of other muscles, fascia and tendons at forearm level**
- ● S56.821 Laceration of other muscles, fascia and tendons at forearm level, right arm A ⬤, D, S
- ● S56.822 Laceration of other muscles, fascia and tendons at forearm level, left arm A ⬤, D, S
- ●■ S56.829 Laceration of other muscles, fascia and tendons at forearm level, unspecified arm A ⬤, D, S

● S56.89 **Other injury of other muscles, fascia and tendons at forearm level**
- ● S56.891 Other injury of other muscles, fascia and tendons at forearm level, right arm D, S
- ● S56.892 Other injury of other muscles, fascia and tendons at forearm level, left arm D, S
- ●■ S56.899 Other injury of other muscles, fascia and tendons at forearm level, unspecified arm D, S

● S56.9 **Injury of unspecified muscles, fascia and tendons at forearm level**
- ● S56.90 Unspecified injury of unspecified muscles, fascia and tendons at forearm level
  - ●■ S56.901 Unspecified injury of unspecified muscles, fascia and tendons at forearm level, right arm D, S
  - ●■ S56.902 Unspecified injury of unspecified muscles, fascia and tendons at forearm level, left arm D, S
  - ●■ S56.909 Unspecified injury of unspecified muscles, fascia and tendons at forearm level, unspecified arm D, S
- ● S56.91 Strain of unspecified muscles, fascia and tendons at forearm level
  - ●■ S56.911 Strain of unspecified muscles, fascia and tendons at forearm level, right arm D, S
  - ●■ S56.912 Strain of unspecified muscles, fascia and tendons at forearm level, left arm D, S
  - ●■ S56.919 Strain of unspecified muscles, fascia and tendons at forearm level, unspecified arm D, S
- ● S56.92 Laceration of unspecified muscles, fascia and tendons at forearm level
  - ●■ S56.921 Laceration of unspecified muscles, fascia and tendons at forearm level, right arm A ⬤, D, S

- ●■ S56.922 Laceration of unspecified muscles, fascia and tendons at forearm level, left arm A ⬤, D, S
- ●■ S56.929 Laceration of unspecified muscles, fascia and tendons at forearm level, unspecified arm A ⬤, D, S

● S56.99 **Other injury of unspecified muscles, fascia and tendons at forearm level**
- ●■ S56.991 Other injury of unspecified muscles, fascia and tendons at forearm level, right arm D, S
- ●■ S56.992 Other injury of unspecified muscles, fascia and tendons at forearm level, left arm D, S
- ●■ S56.999 Other injury of unspecified muscles, fascia and tendons at forearm level, unspecified arm D, S

● S57 **Crushing injury of elbow and forearm**

Use additional code(s) for all associated injuries

Excludes2 crushing injury of wrist and hand (S67.-)

The appropriate 7th character is to be added to each code from category S57

A	initial encounter
D	subsequent encounter
S	sequela

● S57.0 **Crushing injury of elbow**
- ●■ S57.00 Crushing injury of unspecified elbow D, S
- ● S57.01 Crushing injury of right elbow D, S
- ● S57.02 Crushing injury of left elbow D, S

● S57.8 **Crushing injury of forearm**
- ●■ S57.80 Crushing injury of unspecified forearm D, S
- ● S57.81 Crushing injury of right forearm D, S
- ● S57.82 Crushing injury of left forearm D, S

● S58 **Traumatic amputation of elbow and forearm**

An amputation not identified as partial or complete should be coded to complete

Excludes1 traumatic amputation of wrist and hand (S68.-)

The appropriate 7th character is to be added to each code from category S58

A	initial encounter
D	subsequent encounter
S	sequela

● S58.0 **Traumatic amputation at elbow level**
- ● S58.01 Complete traumatic amputation at elbow level
  - ● S58.011 Complete traumatic amputation at elbow level, right arm A ⬤, D, S
  - ● S58.012 Complete traumatic amputation at elbow level, left arm A ⬤, D, S
  - ●■ S58.019 Complete traumatic amputation at elbow level, unspecified arm A ⬤, D, S

CHAPTER 19 (S00-T88)

● **S58.02** **Partial traumatic amputation at elbow level**

  ● **S58.021** Partial traumatic amputation at elbow level, right arm A 🔩, D, S 🔩

  ● **S58.022** Partial traumatic amputation at elbow level, left arm A 🔩, D, S 🔩

  ● ▪ **S58.029** Partial traumatic amputation at elbow level, unspecified arm A 🔩, D, S 🔩

● **S58.1** **Traumatic amputation at level between elbow and wrist**

  ● **S58.11** **Complete traumatic amputation at level between elbow and wrist**

    ● **S58.111** Complete traumatic amputation at level between elbow and wrist, right arm A 🔩, D, S 🔩

    ● **S58.112** Complete traumatic amputation at level between elbow and wrist, left arm A 🔩, D, S 🔩

    ● ▪ **S58.119** Complete traumatic amputation at level between elbow and wrist, unspecified arm A 🔩, D, S 🔩

  ● **S58.12** **Partial traumatic amputation at level between elbow and wrist**

    ● **S58.121** Partial traumatic amputation at level between elbow and wrist, right arm A 🔩, D, S 🔩

    ● **S58.122** Partial traumatic amputation at level between elbow and wrist, left arm A 🔩, D, S 🔩

    ● ▪ **S58.129** Partial traumatic amputation at level between elbow and wrist, unspecified arm A 🔩, D, S 🔩

● **S58.9** **Traumatic amputation of forearm, level unspecified**

   Excludes1   traumatic amputation of wrist (S68.-)

  ● **S58.91** **Complete traumatic amputation of forearm, level unspecified**

    ● ▪ **S58.911** Complete traumatic amputation of right forearm, level unspecified A 🔩, D, S 🔩

    ● ▪ **S58.912** Complete traumatic amputation of left forearm, level unspecified A 🔩, D, S 🔩

    ● ▪ **S58.919** Complete traumatic amputation of unspecified forearm, level unspecified A 🔩, D, S 🔩

  ● **S58.92** **Partial traumatic amputation of forearm, level unspecified**

    ● ▪ **S58.921** Partial traumatic amputation of right forearm, level unspecified A 🔩, D, S 🔩

    ● ▪ **S58.922** Partial traumatic amputation of left forearm, level unspecified A 🔩, D, S 🔩

    ● ▪ **S58.929** Partial traumatic amputation of unspecified forearm, level unspecified A 🔩, D, S 🔩

● **S59** **Other and unspecified injuries of elbow and forearm**

   Excludes2   other and unspecified injuries of wrist and hand (S69.-)

The appropriate 7th character is to be added to each code from subcategories S59.0, S59.1, and S59.2

A	initial encounter for closed fracture
D	subsequent encounter for fracture with routine healing
G	subsequent encounter for fracture with delayed healing
K	subsequent encounter for fracture with nonunion
P	subsequent encounter for fracture with malunion
S	sequela

● **S59.0** **Physeal fracture of lower end of ulna**

  ● **S59.00** **Unspecified physeal fracture of lower end of ulna**

    ● ▪ **S59.001** Unspecified physeal fracture of lower end of ulna, right arm A, K, P 🔩, D, G, S 🔩

    ● ▪ **S59.002** Unspecified physeal fracture of lower end of ulna, left arm A, K, P 🔩, D, G, S 🔩

    ● ▪ **S59.009** Unspecified physeal fracture of lower end of ulna, unspecified arm A, K, P 🔩, D, G, S 🔩

  ● **S59.01** **Salter-Harris Type I physeal fracture of lower end of ulna**

    ● **S59.011** Salter-Harris Type I physeal fracture of lower end of ulna, right arm A, K, P 🔩, D, G, S 🔩

    ● **S59.012** Salter-Harris Type I physeal fracture of lower end of ulna, left arm A, K, P 🔩, D, G, S 🔩

    ● **S59.019** Salter-Harris Type I physeal fracture of lower end of ulna, unspecified arm A, K, P 🔩, D, G, S 🔩

  ● **S59.02** **Salter-Harris Type II physeal fracture of lower end of ulna**

    ● **S59.021** Salter-Harris Type II physeal fracture of lower end of ulna, right arm A, K, P 🔩, D, G, S 🔩

    ● **S59.022** Salter-Harris Type II physeal fracture of lower end of ulna, left arm A, K, P 🔩, D, G, S 🔩

    ● ▪ **S59.029** Salter-Harris Type II physeal fracture of lower end of ulna, unspecified arm A, K, P 🔩, D, G, S 🔩, A 🔩

Item 19-4 SALTER-HARRIS TYPE 1: epiphysis is completely separated from end of bone, or metaphysic growth plate remains attached to epiphysis

  SALTER-HARRIS TYPE 2: epiphysis and growth plate are partially separated from metaphysis, which is cracked—most common type

  SALTER-HARRIS TYPE 3: fracture occurring through epiphysis and separates part of epiphysis and growth plate from metaphysis fracture, usually at distal end of tibia

  SALTER-HARRIS TYPE 4: fracture runs through epiphysis, across growth plate, into metaphysic, surgery is required to restore joint surface to normal and align growth plate

● Unacceptable Principal Diagnosis   ● Use Additional Character(s)   ▪ Unspecified   ▶ Manifestation Code

OGCR Official Guidelines for Coding and Reporting   Excludes 1   Excludes 2   Includes   Use additional   Code first   Code also

● **S59.03** Salter-Harris Type III physeal fracture of lower end of ulna

    ● **S59.031** Salter-Harris Type III physeal fracture of lower end of ulna, right arm A, K, P 🌑, D, G, S 🔍, A 🔍

    ● **S59.032** Salter-Harris Type III physeal fracture of lower end of ulna, left arm A, K, P 🌑, D, G, S 🔍, A 🔍

    ●■ **S59.039** Salter-Harris Type III physeal fracture of lower end of ulna, unspecified arm A, K, P 🌑, D, G, S 🔍, A 🔍

● **S59.04** Salter-Harris Type IV physeal fracture of lower end of ulna

    ● **S59.041** Salter-Harris Type IV physeal fracture of lower end of ulna, right arm A, K, P 🌑, D, G, S 🔍, A 🔍

    ● **S59.042** Salter-Harris Type IV physeal fracture of lower end of ulna, left arm A, K, P 🌑, D, G, S 🔍, A 🔍

    ●■ **S59.049** Salter-Harris Type IV physeal fracture of lower end of ulna, unspecified arm A, K, P 🌑, D, G, S 🔍, A 🔍

● **S59.09** Other physeal fracture of lower end of ulna

    ● **S59.091** Other physeal fracture of lower end of ulna, right arm A, K, P 🌑, D, G, S 🔍, A 🔍

    ● **S59.092** Other physeal fracture of lower end of ulna, left arm A, K, P 🌑, D, G, S 🔍, A 🔍

    ●■ **S59.099** Other physeal fracture of lower end of ulna, unspecified arm A, K, P 🌑, D, G, S 🔍, A 🔍

● **S59.1** Physeal fracture of upper end of radius

    ● **S59.10** Unspecified physeal fracture of upper end of radius

      ●■ **S59.101** Unspecified physeal fracture of upper end of radius, right arm K, P 🌑, D, G, S 🔍

      ●■ **S59.102** Unspecified physeal fracture of upper end of radius, left arm K, P 🌑, D, G, S 🔍

      ●■ **S59.109** Unspecified physeal fracture of upper end of radius, unspecified arm K, P 🌑, D, G, S 🔍

    ● **S59.11** Salter-Harris Type I physeal fracture of upper end of radius

      ● **S59.111** Salter-Harris Type I physeal fracture of upper end of radius, right arm K, P 🌑, D, G, S 🔍

      ● **S59.112** Salter-Harris Type I physeal fracture of upper end of radius, left arm K, P 🌑, D, G, S 🔍

      ●■ **S59.119** Salter-Harris Type I physeal fracture of upper end of radius, unspecified arm K, P 🌑, D, G, S 🔍

    ● **S59.12** Salter-Harris Type II physeal fracture of upper end of radius

      ● **S59.121** Salter-Harris Type II physeal fracture of upper end of radius, right arm K, P 🌑, D, G, S 🔍

      ● **S59.122** Salter-Harris Type II physeal fracture of upper end of radius, left arm K, P 🌑, D, G, S 🔍

      ●■ **S59.129** Salter-Harris Type II physeal fracture of upper end of radius, unspecified arm K, P 🌑, D, G, S 🔍

    ● **S59.13** Salter-Harris Type III physeal fracture of upper end of radius

      ● **S59.131** Salter-Harris Type III physeal fracture of upper end of radius, right arm K, P 🌑, D, G, S 🔍

      ● **S59.132** Salter-Harris Type III physeal fracture of upper end of radius, left arm K, P 🌑, D, G, S 🔍

      ●■ **S59.139** Salter-Harris Type III physeal fracture of upper end of radius, unspecified arm K, P 🌑, D, G, S 🔍

    ● **S59.14** Salter-Harris Type IV physeal fracture of upper end of radius

      ● **S59.141** Salter-Harris Type IV physeal fracture of upper end of radius, right arm K, P 🌑, D, G, S 🔍

      ● **S59.142** Salter-Harris Type IV physeal fracture of upper end of radius, left arm K, P 🌑, D, G, S 🔍

      ●■ **S59.149** Salter-Harris Type IV physeal fracture of upper end of radius, unspecified arm K, P 🌑, D, G, S 🔍

    ● **S59.19** Other physeal fracture of upper end of radius

      ● **S59.191** Other physeal fracture of upper end of radius, right arm K, P 🌑, D, G, S 🔍

      ● **S59.192** Other physeal fracture of upper end of radius, left arm K, P 🌑, D, G, S 🔍

      ●■ **S59.199** Other physeal fracture of upper end of radius, unspecified arm K, P 🌑, D, G, S 🔍

● **S59.2** Physeal fracture of lower end of radius

    ● **S59.20** Unspecified physeal fracture of lower end of radius

      ●■ **S59.201** Unspecified physeal fracture of lower end of radius, right arm A, K, P 🌑, D, G, S 🔍, A 🔍

      ●■ **S59.202** Unspecified physeal fracture of lower end of radius, left arm A, K, P 🌑, D, G, S 🔍, A 🔍

      ●■ **S59.209** Unspecified physeal fracture of lower end of radius, unspecified arm A, K, P 🌑, D, G, S 🔍, A 🔍

    ● **S59.21** Salter-Harris Type I physeal fracture of lower end of radius

      ● **S59.211** Salter-Harris Type I physeal fracture of lower end of radius, right arm A, K, P 🌑, D, G, S 🔍, A 🔍

      ● **S59.212** Salter-Harris Type I physeal fracture of lower end of radius, left arm A, K, P 🌑, D, G, S 🔍, A 🔍

      ●■ **S59.219** Salter-Harris Type I physeal fracture of lower end of radius, unspecified arm A, K, P 🌑, D, G, S 🔍, A 🔍

N Newborn Age: 0   **P** Pediatric Age: 0–17   **M** Maternity DX: 12–55   **A** Adult Age: 15–124   ♀ Females Only   ♂ Males Only

🌑 Complication\Comorbidity   🔍 Major C\C   🔍 Present on Admission Requirement   🔍 Hospital-Acquired Condition

1489

CHAPTER 19 (S00-T88)

● S59.22   **Salter-Harris Type II physeal fracture of lower end of radius**
- ● S59.221   Salter-Harris Type II physeal fracture of lower end of radius, right arm A, K, P 🖝, D, G, S 🖝, A 🖝
- ● S59.222   Salter-Harris Type II physeal fracture of lower end of radius, left arm A, K, P 🖝, D, G, S 🖝, A 🖝
- ●◼ S59.229   Salter-Harris Type II physeal fracture of lower end of radius, unspecified arm A, K, P 🖝, D, G, S 🖝, A 🖝

● S59.23   **Salter-Harris Type III physeal fracture of lower end of radius**
- ● S59.231   Salter-Harris Type III physeal fracture of lower end of radius, right arm A, K, P 🖝, D, G, S 🖝, A 🖝
- ● S59.232   Salter-Harris Type III physeal fracture of lower end of radius, left arm A, K, P 🖝, D, G, S 🖝, A 🖝
- ●◼ S59.239   Salter-Harris Type III physeal fracture of lower end of radius, unspecified arm A, K, P 🖝, D, G, S 🖝, A 🖝

● S59.24   **Salter-Harris Type IV physeal fracture of lower end of radius**
- ● S59.241   Salter-Harris Type IV physeal fracture of lower end of radius, right arm A, K, P 🖝, D, G, S 🖝, A 🖝
- ● S59.242   Salter-Harris Type IV physeal fracture of lower end of radius, left arm A, K, P 🖝, D, G, S 🖝, A 🖝
- ●◼ S59.249   Salter-Harris Type IV physeal fracture of lower end of radius, unspecified arm A, K, P 🖝, D, G, S 🖝, A 🖝

● S59.29   **Other physeal fracture of lower end of radius**
- ● S59.291   Other physeal fracture of lower end of radius, right arm A, K, P 🖝, D, G, S 🖝, A 🖝
- ● S59.292   Other physeal fracture of lower end of radius, left arm A, K, P 🖝, D, G, S 🖝, A 🖝
- ●◼ S59.299   Other physeal fracture of lower end of radius, unspecified arm A, K, P 🖝, D, G, S 🖝, A 🖝

● S59.8   **Other specified injuries of elbow and forearm**

The appropriate 7th character is to be added to each code in subcategory S59.8

A	initial encounter
D	subsequent encounter
S	sequela

● S59.80   **Other specified injuries of elbow**
- ● S59.801   Other specified injuries of right elbow D, S 🖝
- ● S59.802   Other specified injuries of left elbow D, S 🖝
- ●◼ S59.809   Other specified injuries of unspecified elbow D, S 🖝

● S59.81   **Other specified injuries of forearm**
- ● S59.811   Other specified injuries right forearm D, S 🖝
- ● S59.812   Other specified injuries left forearm D, S 🖝
- ●◼ S59.819   Other specified injuries unspecified forearm D, S 🖝

● S59.9   **Unspecified injury of elbow and forearm**

The appropriate 7th character is to be added to each code in subcategory S59.9

A	initial encounter
D	subsequent encounter
S	sequela

● S59.90   **Unspecified injury of elbow**
- ●◼ S59.901   Unspecified injury of right elbow D, S 🖝
- ●◼ S59.902   Unspecified injury of left elbow D, S 🖝
- ●◼ S59.909   Unspecified injury of unspecified elbow D, S 🖝

● S59.91   **Unspecified injury of forearm**
- ●◼ S59.911   Unspecified injury of right forearm D, S 🖝
- ●◼ S59.912   Unspecified injury of left forearm D, S 🖝
- ●◼ S59.919   Unspecified injury of unspecified forearm D, S 🖝

INJURIES TO THE WRIST, HAND AND FINGERS (S60-S69)

Excludes2   burns and corrosions (T20-T32)
frostbite (T33-T34)
insect bite or sting, venomous (T63.4)

● S60   **Superficial injury of wrist, hand and fingers**

The appropriate 7th character is to be added to each code from category S60

A	initial encounter
D	subsequent encounter
S	sequela

● S60.0   **Contusion of finger without damage to nail**

Excludes1   contusion involving nail (matrix) (S60.1)

● S60.00   **Contusion of unspecified finger without damage to nail** D, S 🖝
Contusion of finger(s) NOS

● S60.01   **Contusion of thumb without damage to nail**
- ● S60.011   Contusion of right thumb without damage to nail D, S 🖝
- ● S60.012   Contusion of left thumb without damage to nail D, S 🖝
- ●◼ S60.019   Contusion of unspecified thumb without damage to nail D, S 🖝

● Unacceptable Principal Diagnosis   ● Use Additional Character(s)   ◼ Unspecified   ▶ Manifestation Code
OGCR Official Guidelines for Coding and Reporting   Excludes 1   Excludes 2   Includes   Use additional   Code first   Code also

- ● S60.02   Contusion of index finger without damage to nail
  - ● S60.021   Contusion of right index finger without damage to nail D, S 🔧
  - ● S60.022   Contusion of left index finger without damage to nail D, S 🔧
  - ●■ S60.029   Contusion of unspecified index finger without damage to nail D, S 🔧
- ● S60.03   Contusion of middle finger without damage to nail
  - ● S60.031   Contusion of right middle finger without damage to nail D, S 🔧
  - ● S60.032   Contusion of left middle finger without damage to nail D, S 🔧
  - ●■ S60.039   Contusion of unspecified middle finger without damage to nail D, S 🔧
- ● S60.04   Contusion of ring finger without damage to nail
  - ● S60.041   Contusion of right ring finger without damage to nail D, S 🔧
  - ● S60.042   Contusion of left ring finger without damage to nail D, S 🔧
  - ●■ S60.049   Contusion of unspecified ring finger without damage to nail D, S 🔧
- ● S60.05   Contusion of little finger without damage to nail
  - ● S60.051   Contusion of right little finger without damage to nail D, S 🔧
  - ● S60.052   Contusion of left little finger without damage to nail D, S 🔧
  - ●■ S60.059   Contusion of unspecified little finger without damage to nail D, S 🔧
- ● S60.1   Contusion of finger with damage to nail
  - ● S60.10   Contusion of unspecified finger with damage to nail D, S 🔧
  - ● S60.11   Contusion of thumb with damage to nail
    - ● S60.111   Contusion of right thumb with damage to nail D, S 🔧
    - ● S60.112   Contusion of left thumb with damage to nail D, S 🔧
    - ●■ S60.119   Contusion of unspecified thumb with damage to nail D, S 🔧
  - ● S60.12   Contusion of index finger with damage to nail
    - ● S60.121   Contusion of right index finger with damage to nail D, S 🔧
    - ● S60.122   Contusion of left index finger with damage to nail D, S 🔧
    - ●■ S60.129   Contusion of unspecified index finger with damage to nail D, S 🔧
  - ● S60.13   Contusion of middle finger with damage to nail
    - ● S60.131   Contusion of right middle finger with damage to nail D, S 🔧
    - ● S60.132   Contusion of left middle finger with damage to nail D, S 🔧
    - ●■ S60.139   Contusion of unspecified middle finger with damage to nail D, S 🔧

- ● S60.14   Contusion of ring finger with damage to nail
  - ● S60.141   Contusion of right ring finger with damage to nail D, S 🔧
  - ● S60.142   Contusion of left ring finger with damage to nail D, S 🔧
  - ●■ S60.149   Contusion of unspecified ring finger with damage to nail D, S 🔧
- ● S60.15   Contusion of little finger with damage to nail
  - ● S60.151   Contusion of right little finger with damage to nail D, S 🔧
  - ● S60.152   Contusion of left little finger with damage to nail D, S 🔧
  - ●■ S60.159   Contusion of unspecified little finger with damage to nail D, S 🔧
- ● S60.2   Contusion of wrist and hand
  - **Excludes2**   contusion of fingers (S60.0-, S60.1-)
  - ● S60.21   Contusion of wrist
    - ● S60.211   Contusion of right wrist D, S 🔧
    - ● S60.212   Contusion of left wrist D, S 🔧
    - ●■ S60.219   Contusion of unspecified wrist D, S 🔧
  - ● S60.22   Contusion of hand
    - ● S60.221   Contusion of right hand D, S 🔧
    - ● S60.222   Contusion of left hand D, S 🔧
    - ●■ S60.229   Contusion of unspecified hand D, S 🔧
- ● S60.3   Other superficial injuries of thumb
  - ● S60.31   Abrasion of thumb
    - ● S60.311   Abrasion of right thumb D, S 🔧
    - ● S60.312   Abrasion of left thumb D, S 🔧
    - ●■ S60.319   Abrasion of unspecified thumb D, S 🔧
  - ● S60.32   Blister (nonthermal) of thumb
    - ● S60.321   Blister (nonthermal) of right thumb D, S 🔧
    - ● S60.322   Blister (nonthermal) of left thumb D, S 🔧
    - ●■ S60.329   Blister (nonthermal) of unspecified thumb D, S 🔧
  - ● S60.34   External constriction of thumb
    Hair tourniquet syndrome of thumb
    Use additional cause code to identify the constricting item (W49.0-)
    - ● S60.341   External constriction of right thumb D, S 🔧
    - ● S60.342   External constriction of left thumb D, S 🔧
    - ●■ S60.349   External constriction of unspecified thumb D, S 🔧
  - ● S60.35   Superficial foreign body of thumb
    Splinter in the thumb
    - ● S60.351   Superficial foreign body of right thumb D, S 🔧
    - ● S60.352   Superficial foreign body of left thumb D, S 🔧
    - ●■ S60.359   Superficial foreign body of unspecified thumb D, S 🔧

N Newborn Age: 0   **P** Pediatric Age: 0–17   **M** Maternity DX: 12–55   **A** Adult Age: 15–124   ♀ Females Only   ♂ Males Only

🔧 Complication\Comorbidity   Major C\C   Present on Admission Requirement   Hospital-Acquired Condition

1491

● **S60.36 Insect bite (nonvenomous) of thumb**
- ● S60.361 Insect bite (nonvenomous) of right thumb D, S
- ● S60.362 Insect bite (nonvenomous) of left thumb D, S
- ●■ S60.369 Insect bite (nonvenomous) of unspecified thumb D, S

● **S60.37 Other superficial bite of thumb**
> **Excludes1** open bite of thumb (S61.05-, S61.15-)
- ● S60.371 Other superficial bite of right thumb D, S
- ● S60.372 Other superficial bite of left thumb D, S
- ●■ S60.379 Other superficial bite of unspecified thumb D, S

● **S60.39 Other superficial injuries of thumb**
- ● S60.391 Other superficial injuries of right thumb D, S
- ● S60.392 Other superficial injuries of left thumb D, S
- ●■ S60.399 Other superficial injuries of unspecified thumb D, S

● **S60.4 Other superficial injuries of other fingers**

● **S60.41 Abrasion of fingers**
- ● S60.410 Abrasion of right index finger D, S
- ● S60.411 Abrasion of left index finger D, S
- ● S60.412 Abrasion of right middle finger D, S
- ● S60.413 Abrasion of left middle finger D, S
- ● S60.414 Abrasion of right ring finger D, S
- ● S60.415 Abrasion of left ring finger D, S
- ● S60.416 Abrasion of right little finger D, S
- ● S60.417 Abrasion of left little finger D, S
- ● S60.418 Abrasion of other finger D, S
  Abrasion of specified finger with unspecified laterality
- ●■ S60.419 Abrasion of unspecified finger D, S

● **S60.42 Blister (nonthermal) of fingers**
- ● S60.420 Blister (nonthermal) of right index finger D, S
- ● S60.421 Blister (nonthermal) of left index finger D, S
- ● S60.422 Blister (nonthermal) of right middle finger D, S
- ● S60.423 Blister (nonthermal) of left middle finger D, S
- ● S60.424 Blister (nonthermal) of right ring finger D, S
- ● S60.425 Blister (nonthermal) of left ring finger D, S
- ● S60.426 Blister (nonthermal) of right little finger D, S

- ● S60.427 Blister (nonthermal) of left little finger D, S
- ● S60.428 Blister (nonthermal) of other finger D, S
  Blister (nonthermal) of specified finger with unspecified laterality
- ●■ S60.429 Blister (nonthermal) of unspecified finger D, S

● **S60.44 External constriction of fingers**
Hair tourniquet syndrome of finger
> Use additional cause code to identify the constricting item (W49.0-)
- ● S60.440 External constriction of right index finger D, S
- ● S60.441 External constriction of left index finger D, S
- ● S60.442 External constriction of right middle finger D, S
- ● S60.443 External constriction of left middle finger D, S
- ● S60.444 External constriction of right ring finger D, S
- ● S60.445 External constriction of left ring finger D, S
- ● S60.446 External constriction of right little finger D, S
- ● S60.447 External constriction of left little finger D, S
- ● S60.448 External constriction of other finger D, S
  External constriction of specified finger with unspecified laterality
- ●■ S60.449 External constriction of unspecified finger

● **S60.45 Superficial foreign body of fingers**
Splinter in the finger(s)
- ● S60.450 Superficial foreign body of right index finger D, S
- ● S60.451 Superficial foreign body of left index finger D, S
- ● S60.452 Superficial foreign body of right middle finger D, S
- ● S60.453 Superficial foreign body of left middle finger D, S
- ● S60.454 Superficial foreign body of right ring finger D, S
- ● S60.455 Superficial foreign body of left ring finger D, S
- ● S60.456 Superficial foreign body of right little finger D, S
- ● S60.457 Superficial foreign body of left little finger D, S
- ● S60.458 Superficial foreign body of other finger D, S
  Superficial foreign body of specified finger with unspecified laterality
- ●■ S60.459 Superficial foreign body of unspecified finger D, S

● Unacceptable Principal Diagnosis ● Use Additional Character(s) ■ Unspecified ▶ Manifestation Code
OGCR Official Guidelines for Coding and Reporting | Excludes 1 | Excludes 2 | Includes | Use additional | Code first | Code also

● **S60.46**   **Insect bite (nonvenomous) of fingers**

   ● **S60.460**   Insect bite (nonvenomous) of right index finger D, S 🔣

   ● **S60.461**   Insect bite (nonvenomous) of left index finger D, S 🔣

   ● **S60.462**   Insect bite (nonvenomous) of right middle finger D, S 🔣

   ● **S60.463**   Insect bite (nonvenomous) of left middle finger D, S 🔣

   ● **S60.464**   Insect bite (nonvenomous) of right ring finger D, S 🔣

   ● **S60.465**   Insect bite (nonvenomous) of left ring finger D, S 🔣

   ● **S60.466**   Insect bite (nonvenomous) of right little finger D, S 🔣

   ● **S60.467**   Insect bite (nonvenomous) of left little finger D, S 🔣

   ● **S60.468**   Insect bite (nonvenomous) of other finger D, S 🔣
       Insect bite (nonvenomous) of specified finger with unspecified laterality

   ●■ **S60.469**   Insect bite (nonvenomous) of unspecified finger D, S 🔣

● **S60.47**   **Other superficial bite of fingers**

   | **Excludes1** | open bite of fingers (S61.25-, S61.35-) |

   ● **S60.470**   Other superficial bite of right index finger D, S 🔣

   ● **S60.471**   Other superficial bite of left index finger D, S 🔣

   ● **S60.472**   Other superficial bite of right middle finger D, S 🔣

   ● **S60.473**   Other superficial bite of left middle finger D, S 🔣

   ● **S60.474**   Other superficial bite of right ring finger D, S 🔣

   ● **S60.475**   Other superficial bite of left ring finger D, S 🔣

   ● **S60.476**   Other superficial bite of right little finger D, S 🔣

   ● **S60.477**   Other superficial bite of left little finger D, S 🔣

   ● **S60.478**   Other superficial bite of other finger D, S 🔣
       Other superficial bite of specified finger with unspecified laterality

   ●■ **S60.479**   Other superficial bite of unspecified finger D, S 🔣

● **S60.5**   **Other superficial injuries of hand**

   | **Excludes2** | superficial injuries of fingers (S60.3-, S60.4-) |

● **S60.51**   **Abrasion of hand**

   ● **S60.511**   Abrasion of right hand D, S 🔣

   ● **S60.512**   Abrasion of left hand D, S 🔣

   ●■ **S60.519**   Abrasion of unspecified hand D, S 🔣

● **S60.52**   **Blister (nonthermal) of hand**

   ● **S60.521**   Blister (nonthermal) of right hand D, S 🔣

   ● **S60.522**   Blister (nonthermal) of left hand D, S 🔣

   ●■ **S60.529**   Blister (nonthermal) of unspecified hand D, S 🔣

● **S60.54**   **External constriction of hand**

   ● **S60.541**   External constriction of right hand D, S 🔣

   ● **S60.542**   External constriction of left hand D, S 🔣

   ●■ **S60.549**   External constriction of unspecified hand D, S 🔣

● **S60.55**   **Superficial foreign body of hand**
       Splinter in the hand

   ● **S60.551**   Superficial foreign body of right hand D, S 🔣

   ● **S60.552**   Superficial foreign body of left hand D, S 🔣

   ●■ **S60.559**   Superficial foreign body of unspecified hand D, S 🔣

● **S60.56**   **Insect bite (nonvenomous) of hand**

   ● **S60.561**   Insect bite (nonvenomous) of right hand D, S 🔣

   ● **S60.562**   Insect bite (nonvenomous) of left hand D, S 🔣

   ●■ **S60.569**   Insect bite (nonvenomous) of unspecified hand D, S 🔣

● **S60.57**   **Other superficial bite of hand**

   | **Excludes1** | open bite of hand (S61.45-) |

   ● **S60.571**   Other superficial bite of hand of right hand D, S 🔣

   ● **S60.572**   Other superficial bite of hand of left hand D, S 🔣

   ●■ **S60.579**   Other superficial bite of hand of unspecified hand D, S 🔣

● **S60.8**   **Other superficial injuries of wrist**

● **S60.81**   **Abrasion of wrist**

   ● **S60.811**   Abrasion of right wrist D, S 🔣

   ● **S60.812**   Abrasion of left wrist D, S 🔣

   ●■ **S60.819**   Abrasion of unspecified wrist D, S 🔣

● **S60.82**   **Blister (nonthermal) of wrist**

   ● **S60.821**   Blister (nonthermal) of right wrist D, S 🔣

   ● **S60.822**   Blister (nonthermal) of left wrist D, S 🔣

   ●■ **S60.829**   Blister (nonthermal) of unspecified wrist D, S 🔣

● **S60.84**   **External constriction of wrist**

   ● **S60.841**   External constriction of right wrist D, S 🔣

   ● **S60.842**   External constriction of left wrist D, S 🔣

   ●■ **S60.849**   External constriction of unspecified wrist D, S 🔣

N Newborn Age: 0   **P** Pediatric Age: 0–17   **M** Maternity DX: 12–55   **A** Adult Age: 15–124   ♀ Females Only   ♂ Males Only

🔣 Complication\Comorbidity   🔣 Major C\C   🔣 Present on Admission Requirement   🔣 Hospital-Acquired Condition

● S60.85 Superficial foreign body of wrist
Splinter in the wrist

   ● S60.851 Superficial foreign body of right wrist D, S 🖉

   ● S60.852 Superficial foreign body of left wrist D, S 🖉

   ●■ S60.859 Superficial foreign body of unspecified wrist D, S 🖉

● S60.86 Insect bite (nonvenomous) of wrist

   ● S60.861 Insect bite (nonvenomous) of right wrist D, S 🖉

   ● S60.862 Insect bite (nonvenomous) of left wrist D, S 🖉

   ●■ S60.869 Insect bite (nonvenomous) of unspecified wrist D, S 🖉

● S60.87 Other superficial bite of wrist

   | Excludes1 | open bite of wrist (S61.55)

   ● S60.871 Other superficial bite of right wrist D, S 🖉

   ● S60.872 Other superficial bite of left wrist D, S 🖉

   ●■ S60.879 Other superficial bite of unspecified wrist D, S 🖉

● S60.9 Unspecified superficial injury of wrist, hand and fingers

  ● S60.91 Unspecified superficial injury of wrist

   ●■ S60.911 Unspecified superficial injury of right wrist D, S 🖉

   ●■ S60.912 Unspecified superficial injury of left wrist D, S 🖉

   ●■ S60.919 Unspecified superficial injury of unspecified wrist D, S 🖉

  ● S60.92 Unspecified superficial injury of hand

   ●■ S60.921 Unspecified superficial injury of right hand D, S 🖉

   ●■ S60.922 Unspecified superficial injury of left hand D, S 🖉

   ●■ S60.929 Unspecified superficial injury of unspecified hand D, S 🖉

  ● S60.93 Unspecified superficial injury of thumb

   ●■ S60.931 Unspecified superficial injury of right thumb D, S 🖉

   ●■ S60.932 Unspecified superficial injury of left thumb D, S 🖉

   ●■ S60.939 Unspecified superficial injury of unspecified thumb D, S 🖉

  ● S60.94 Unspecified superficial injury of other fingers

   ●■ S60.940 Unspecified superficial injury of right index finger D, S 🖉

   ●■ S60.941 Unspecified superficial injury of left index finger D, S 🖉

   ●■ S60.942 Unspecified superficial injury of right middle finger D, S 🖉

   ●■ S60.943 Unspecified superficial injury of left middle finger D, S 🖉

   ●■ S60.944 Unspecified superficial injury of right ring finger D, S 🖉

   ●■ S60.945 Unspecified superficial injury of left ring finger D, S 🖉

   ●■ S60.946 Unspecified superficial injury of right little finger D, S 🖉

   ●■ S60.947 Unspecified superficial injury of left little finger D, S 🖉

   ●■ S60.948 Unspecified superficial injury of other finger D, S 🖉
Unspecified superficial injury of specified finger with unspecified laterality

   ●■ S60.949 Unspecified superficial injury of unspecified finger D, S 🖉

● S61 Open wound of wrist, hand and fingers

Code also any associated wound infection

| Excludes1 | open fracture of wrist, hand and finger (S62.- with 7th character B)
traumatic amputation of wrist and hand (S68.-)

The appropriate 7th character is to be added to each code from category S61

A	initial encounter
D	subsequent encounter
S	sequela

● S61.0 Open wound of thumb without damage to nail

  | Excludes1 | open wound of thumb with damage to nail (S61.1-)

  ● S61.00 Unspecified open wound of thumb without damage to nail

   ●■ S61.001 Unspecified open wound of right thumb without damage to nail D, S 🖉

   ●■ S61.002 Unspecified open wound of left thumb without damage to nail D, S 🖉

   ●■ S61.009 Unspecified open wound of unspecified thumb without damage to nail D, S 🖉

  ● S61.01 Laceration without foreign body of thumb without damage to nail

   ● S61.011 Laceration without foreign body of right thumb without damage to nail D, S 🖉

   ● S61.012 Laceration without foreign body of left thumb without damage to nail D, S 🖉

   ●■ S61.019 Laceration without foreign body of unspecified thumb without damage to nail D, S 🖉

  ● S61.02 Laceration with foreign body of thumb without damage to nail

   ● S61.021 Laceration with foreign body of right thumb without damage to nail D, S 🖉

   ● S61.022 Laceration with foreign body of left thumb without damage to nail D, S 🖉

   ●■ S61.029 Laceration with foreign body of unspecified thumb without damage to nail D, S 🖉

● S61.03   **Puncture wound without foreign body of thumb without damage to nail**

   ● S61.031   **Puncture wound without foreign body of right thumb without damage to nail** D, S 🔖

   ● S61.032   **Puncture wound without foreign body of left thumb without damage to nail** D, S 🔖

   ●■ S61.039   **Puncture wound without foreign body of unspecified thumb without damage to nail** D, S 🔖

● S61.04   **Puncture wound with foreign body of thumb without damage to nail**

   ● S61.041   **Puncture wound with foreign body of right thumb without damage to nail** D, S 🔖

   ● S61.042   **Puncture wound with foreign body of left thumb without damage to nail** D, S 🔖

   ●■ S61.049   **Puncture wound with foreign body of unspecified thumb without damage to nail** D, S 🔖

● S61.05   **Open bite of thumb without damage to nail**
   Bite of thumb NOS

   | **Excludes1** | superficial bite of thumb (S60.36-, S60.37-) |

   ● S61.051   **Open bite of right thumb without damage to nail** D, S 🔖

   ● S61.052   **Open bite of left thumb without damage to nail** D, S 🔖

   ●■ S61.059   **Open bite of unspecified thumb without damage to nail** D, S 🔖

● S61.1   **Open wound of thumb with damage to nail**

  ● S61.10   **Unspecified open wound of thumb with damage to nail**

   ●■ S61.101   **Unspecified open wound of right thumb with damage to nail** D, S 🔖

   ●■ S61.102   **Unspecified open wound of left thumb with damage to nail** D, S 🔖

   ●■ S61.109   **Unspecified open wound of unspecified thumb with damage to nail** D, S 🔖

  ● S61.11   **Laceration without foreign body of thumb with damage to nail**

   ● S61.111   **Laceration without foreign body of right thumb with damage to nail** D, S 🔖

   ● S61.112   **Laceration without foreign body of left thumb with damage to nail** D, S 🔖

   ●■ S61.119   **Laceration without foreign body of unspecified thumb with damage to nail** D, S 🔖

  ● S61.12   **Laceration with foreign body of thumb with damage to nail**

   ● S61.121   **Laceration with foreign body of right thumb with damage to nail** D, S 🔖

   ● S61.122   **Laceration with foreign body of left thumb with damage to nail** D, S 🔖

   ●■ S61.129   **Laceration with foreign body of unspecified thumb with damage to nail** D, S 🔖

● S61.13   **Puncture wound without foreign body of thumb with damage to nail**

   ● S61.131   **Puncture wound without foreign body of right thumb with damage to nail** D, S 🔖

   ● S61.132   **Puncture wound without foreign body of left thumb with damage to nail** D, S 🔖

   ●■ S61.139   **Puncture wound without foreign body of unspecified thumb with damage to nail** D, S 🔖

● S61.14   **Puncture wound with foreign body of thumb with damage to nail**

   ● S61.141   **Puncture wound with foreign body of right thumb with damage to nail** D, S 🔖

   ● S61.142   **Puncture wound with foreign body of left thumb with damage to nail** D, S 🔖

   ●■ S61.149   **Puncture wound with foreign body of unspecified thumb with damage to nail** D, S 🔖

● S61.15   **Open bite of thumb with damage to nail**
   Bite of thumb with damage to nail NOS

   | **Excludes1** | superficial bite of thumb (S60.36-, S60.37-) |

   ● S61.151   **Open bite of right thumb with damage to nail** D, S 🔖

   ● S61.152   **Open bite of left thumb with damage to nail** D, S 🔖

   ●■ S61.159   **Open bite of unspecified thumb with damage to nail** D, S 🔖

● S61.2   **Open wound of other finger without damage to nail**

   | **Excludes1** | open wound of finger involving nail (matrix) (S61.3-) |
   | **Excludes2** | open wound of thumb without damage to nail (S61.0-) |

  ● S61.20   **Unspecified open wound of other finger without damage to nail**

   ●■ S61.200   **Unspecified open wound of right index finger without damage to nail** D, S 🔖

   ●■ S61.201   **Unspecified open wound of left index finger without damage to nail** D, S 🔖

   ●■ S61.202   **Unspecified open wound of right middle finger without damage to nail** D, S 🔖

   ●■ S61.203   **Unspecified open wound of left middle finger without damage to nail** D, S 🔖

   ●■ S61.204   **Unspecified open wound of right ring finger without damage to nail** D, S 🔖

   ●■ S61.205   **Unspecified open wound of left ring finger without damage to nail** D, S 🔖

   ●■ S61.206   **Unspecified open wound of right little finger without damage to nail** D, S 🔖

CHAPTER 19 (S00-T88)

● ◾ S61.207   Unspecified open wound of left little finger without damage to nail D, S 🔍

● ◾ S61.208   Unspecified open wound of other finger without damage to nail D, S 🔍
     Unspecified open wound of specified finger with unspecified laterality without damage to nail

● ◾ S61.209   Unspecified open wound of unspecified finger without damage to nail D, S 🔍

● S61.21   Laceration without foreign body of finger without damage to nail

● S61.210   Laceration without foreign body of right index finger without damage to nail D, S 🔍

● S61.211   Laceration without foreign body of left index finger without damage to nail D, S 🔍

● S61.212   Laceration without foreign body of right middle finger without damage to nail D, S 🔍

● S61.213   Laceration without foreign body of left middle finger without damage to nail D, S 🔍

● S61.214   Laceration without foreign body of right ring finger without damage to nail D, S 🔍

● S61.215   Laceration without foreign body of left ring finger without damage to nail D, S 🔍

● S61.216   Laceration without foreign body of right little finger without damage to nail D, S 🔍

● S61.217   Laceration without foreign body of left little finger without damage to nail D, S 🔍

● S61.218   Laceration without foreign body of other finger without damage to nail D, S 🔍
     Laceration without foreign body of specified finger with unspecified laterality without damage to nail

● ◾ S61.219   Laceration without foreign body of unspecified finger without damage to nail D, S 🔍

● S61.22   Laceration with foreign body of finger without damage to nail

● S61.220   Laceration with foreign body of right index finger without damage to nail D, S 🔍

● S61.221   Laceration with foreign body of left index finger without damage to nail D, S 🔍

● S61.222   Laceration with foreign body of right middle finger without damage to nail D, S 🔍

● S61.223   Laceration with foreign body of left middle finger without damage to nail D, S 🔍

● S61.224   Laceration with foreign body of right ring finger without damage to nail D, S 🔍

● S61.225   Laceration with foreign body of left ring finger without damage to nail D, S 🔍

● S61.226   Laceration with foreign body of right little finger without damage to nail D, S 🔍

● S61.227   Laceration with foreign body of left little finger without damage to nail D, S 🔍

● S61.228   Laceration with foreign body of other finger without damage to nail D, S 🔍
     Laceration with foreign body of specified finger with unspecified laterality without damage to nail

● ◾ S61.229   Laceration with foreign body of unspecified finger without damage to nail D, S 🔍

● S61.23   Puncture wound without foreign body of finger without damage to nail

● S61.230   Puncture wound without foreign body of right index finger without damage to nail D, S 🔍

● S61.231   Puncture wound without foreign body of left index finger without damage to nail D, S 🔍

● S61.232   Puncture wound without foreign body of right middle finger without damage to nail D, S 🔍

● S61.233   Puncture wound without foreign body of left middle finger without damage to nail D, S 🔍

● S61.234   Puncture wound without foreign body of right ring finger without damage to nail D, S 🔍

● S61.235   Puncture wound without foreign body of left ring finger without damage to nail D, S 🔍

● S61.236   Puncture wound without foreign body of right little finger without damage to nail D, S 🔍

● S61.237   Puncture wound without foreign body of left little finger without damage to nail D, S 🔍

● S61.238   Puncture wound without foreign body of other finger without damage to nail D, S 🔍
     Puncture wound without foreign body of specified finger with unspecified laterality without damage to nail

● ◾ S61.239   Puncture wound without foreign body of unspecified finger without damage to nail D, S 🔍

● S61.24   Puncture wound with foreign body of finger without damage to nail

● S61.240   Puncture wound with foreign body of right index finger without damage to nail D, S 🔍

● S61.241   Puncture wound with foreign body of left index finger without damage to nail D, S 🔍

● S61.242   Puncture wound with foreign body of right middle finger without damage to nail D, S 🔍

CHAPTER 19 (S00-T88)

● **S61.243** **Puncture wound with foreign body of left middle finger without damage to nail** D, S ⌾

● **S61.244** **Puncture wound with foreign body of right ring finger without damage to nail** D, S ⌾

● **S61.245** **Puncture wound with foreign body of left ring finger without damage to nail** D, S ⌾

● **S61.246** **Puncture wound with foreign body of right little finger without damage to nail** D, S ⌾

● **S61.247** **Puncture wound with foreign body of left little finger without damage to nail** D, S ⌾

● **S61.248** **Puncture wound with foreign body of other finger without damage to nail** D, S ⌾
     Puncture wound with foreign body of specified finger with unspecified laterality without damage to nail

●■ **S61.249** **Puncture wound with foreign body of unspecified finger without damage to nail** D, S ⌾

● **S61.25** **Open bite of finger without damage to nail**
     Bite of finger without damage to nail NOS

     Excludes1 superficial bite of finger (S60.46-, S60.47-)

● **S61.250** **Open bite of right index finger without damage to nail** D, S ⌾

● **S61.251** **Open bite of left index finger without damage to nail** D, S ⌾

● **S61.252** **Open bite of right middle finger without damage to nail** D, S ⌾

● **S61.253** **Open bite of left middle finger without damage to nail** D, S ⌾

● **S61.254** **Open bite of right ring finger without damage to nail** D, S ⌾

● **S61.255** **Open bite of left ring finger without damage to nail** D, S ⌾

● **S61.256** **Open bite of right little finger without damage to nail** D, S ⌾

● **S61.257** **Open bite of left little finger without damage to nail** D, S ⌾

● **S61.258** **Open bite of other finger without damage to nail** D, S ⌾
     Open bite of specified finger with unspecified laterality without damage to nail

●■ **S61.259** **Open bite of unspecified finger without damage to nail** D, S ⌾

● **S61.3** **Open wound of other finger with damage to nail**

● **S61.30** **Unspecified open wound of finger with damage to nail**

●■ **S61.300** **Unspecified open wound of right index finger with damage to nail** D, S ⌾

●■ **S61.301** **Unspecified open wound of left index finger with damage to nail** D, S ⌾

●■ **S61.302** **Unspecified open wound of right middle finger with damage to nail** D, S ⌾

●■ **S61.303** **Unspecified open wound of left middle finger with damage to nail** D, S ⌾

●■ **S61.304** **Unspecified open wound of right ring finger with damage to nail** D, S ⌾

●■ **S61.305** **Unspecified open wound of left ring finger with damage to nail** D, S ⌾

●■ **S61.306** **Unspecified open wound of right little finger with damage to nail** D, S ⌾

●■ **S61.307** **Unspecified open wound of left little finger with damage to nail** D, S ⌾

●■ **S61.308** **Unspecified open wound of other finger with damage to nail** D, S ⌾
     Unspecified open wound of specified finger with unspecified laterality with damage to nail

●■ **S61.309** **Unspecified open wound of unspecified finger with damage to nail** D, S ⌾

● **S61.31** **Laceration without foreign body of finger with damage to nail**

● **S61.310** **Laceration without foreign body of right index finger with damage to nail** D, S ⌾

● **S61.311** **Laceration without foreign body of left index finger with damage to nail** D, S ⌾

● **S61.312** **Laceration without foreign body of right middle finger with damage to nail** D, S ⌾

● **S61.313** **Laceration without foreign body of left middle finger with damage to nail** D, S ⌾

● **S61.314** **Laceration without foreign body of right ring finger with damage to nail** D, S ⌾

● **S61.315** **Laceration without foreign body of left ring finger with damage to nail** D, S ⌾

● **S61.316** **Laceration without foreign body of right little finger with damage to nail** D, S ⌾

● **S61.317** **Laceration without foreign body of left little finger with damage to nail** D, S ⌾

● **S61.318** **Laceration without foreign body of other finger with damage to nail** D, S ⌾
     Laceration without foreign body of specified finger with unspecified laterality with damage to nail

●■ **S61.319** **Laceration without foreign body of unspecified finger with damage to nail** D, S ⌾

N Newborn Age: 0   **P** Pediatric Age: 0–17   **M** Maternity DX: 12–55   **A** Adult Age: 15–124   ♀ Females Only   ♂ Males Only

⌾ Complication\Comorbidity   ⌾ Major C\C   ⌾ Present on Admission Requirement   ⌾ Hospital-Acquired Condition

1497

CHAPTER 19 (S00-T88)

● **S61.32 Laceration with foreign body of finger with damage to nail**

   ● S61.320 Laceration with foreign body of right index finger with damage to nail D, S

   ● S61.321 Laceration with foreign body of left index finger with damage to nail D, S

   ● S61.322 Laceration with foreign body of right middle finger with damage to nail D, S

   ● S61.323 Laceration with foreign body of left middle finger with damage to nail D, S

   ● S61.324 Laceration with foreign body of right ring finger with damage to nail D, S

   ● S61.325 Laceration with foreign body of left ring finger with damage to nail D, S

   ● S61.326 Laceration with foreign body of right little finger with damage to nail D, S

   ● S61.327 Laceration with foreign body of left little finger with damage to nail D, S

   ● S61.328 Laceration with foreign body of other finger with damage to nail D, S
           Laceration with foreign body of specified finger with unspecified laterality with damage to nail

   ●■ S61.329 Laceration with foreign body of unspecified finger with damage to nail D, S

● **S61.33 Puncture wound without foreign body of finger with damage to nail**

   ● S61.330 Puncture wound without foreign body of right index finger with damage to nail D, S

   ● S61.331 Puncture wound without foreign body of left index finger with damage to nail D, S

   ● S61.332 Puncture wound without foreign body of right middle finger with damage to nail D, S

   ● S61.333 Puncture wound without foreign body of left middle finger with damage to nail D, S

   ● S61.334 Puncture wound without foreign body of right ring finger with damage to nail D, S

   ● S61.335 Puncture wound without foreign body of left ring finger with damage to nail D, S

   ● S61.336 Puncture wound without foreign body of right little finger with damage to nail D, S

   ● S61.337 Puncture wound without foreign body of left little finger with damage to nail D, S

   ● S61.338 Puncture wound without foreign body of other finger with damage to nail D, S
           Puncture wound without foreign body of specified finger with unspecified laterality with damage to nail

   ●■ S61.339 Puncture wound without foreign body of unspecified finger with damage to nail D, S

● **S61.34 Puncture wound with foreign body of finger with damage to nail**

   ● S61.340 Puncture wound with foreign body of right index finger with damage to nail D, S

   ● S61.341 Puncture wound with foreign body of left index finger with damage to nail D, S

   ● S61.342 Puncture wound with foreign body of right middle finger with damage to nail D, S

   ● S61.343 Puncture wound with foreign body of left middle finger with damage to nail D, S

   ● S61.344 Puncture wound with foreign body of right ring finger with damage to nail D, S

   ● S61.345 Puncture wound with foreign body of left ring finger with damage to nail D, S

   ● S61.346 Puncture wound with foreign body of right little finger with damage to nail D, S

   ● S61.347 Puncture wound with foreign body of left little finger with damage to nail D, S

   ● S61.348 Puncture wound with foreign body of other finger with damage to nail D, S
           Puncture wound with foreign body of specified finger with unspecified laterality with damage to nail

   ●■ S61.349 Puncture wound with foreign body of unspecified finger with damage to nail D, S

● **S61.35 Open bite of finger with damage to nail**
     Bite of finger with damage to nail NOS

     | Excludes1 | superficial bite of finger (S60.46-, S60.47-) |

   ● S61.350 Open bite of right index finger with damage to nail D, S

   ● S61.351 Open bite of left index finger with damage to nail D, S

   ● S61.352 Open bite of right middle finger with damage to nail D, S

   ● S61.353 Open bite of left middle finger with damage to nail D, S

   ● S61.354 Open bite of right ring finger with damage to nail D, S

   ● S61.355 Open bite of left ring finger with damage to nail D, S

CHAPTER 19 (S00-T88)

● S61.356   Open bite of right little finger with damage to nail D, S 🕮

● S61.357   Open bite of left little finger with damage to nail D, S 🕮

● S61.358   Open bite of other finger with damage to nail D, S 🕮
       Open bite of specified finger with unspecified laterality with damage to nail

●■ S61.359   Open bite of unspecified finger with damage to nail D, S 🕮

● S61.4   **Open wound of hand**

  ● S61.40   Unspecified open wound of hand

    ●■ S61.401   Unspecified open wound of right hand D, S 🕮

    ●■ S61.402   Unspecified open wound of left hand D, S 🕮

    ●■ S61.409   Unspecified open wound of unspecified hand D, S 🕮

  ● S61.41   Laceration without foreign body of hand

    ● S61.411   Laceration without foreign body of right hand D, S 🕮

    ● S61.412   Laceration without foreign body of left hand D, S 🕮

    ●■ S61.419   Laceration without foreign body of unspecified hand D, S 🕮

  ● S61.42   Laceration with foreign body of hand

    ● S61.421   Laceration with foreign body of right hand D, S 🕮

    ● S61.422   Laceration with foreign body of left hand D, S 🕮

    ●■ S61.429   Laceration with foreign body of unspecified hand D, S 🕮

  ● S61.43   Puncture wound without foreign body of hand

    ● S61.431   Puncture wound without foreign body of right hand D, S 🕮

    ● S61.432   Puncture wound without foreign body of left hand D, S 🕮

    ●■ S61.439   Puncture wound without foreign body of unspecified hand D, S 🕮

  ● S61.44   Puncture wound with foreign body of hand

    ● S61.441   Puncture wound with foreign body of right hand D, S 🕮

    ● S61.442   Puncture wound with foreign body of left hand D, S 🕮

    ●■ S61.449   Puncture wound with foreign body of unspecified hand D, S 🕮

  ● S61.45   Open bite of hand
       Bite of hand NOS

     | Excludes1 | superficial bite of hand (S60.56-, S60.57-)

    ● S61.451   Open bite of right hand D, S 🕮

    ● S61.452   Open bite of left hand D, S 🕮

    ●■ S61.459   Open bite of unspecified hand D, S 🕮

● S61.5   **Open wound of wrist**

  ● S61.50   Unspecified open wound of wrist

    ●■ S61.501   Unspecified open wound of right wrist D, S 🕮

    ●■ S61.502   Unspecified open wound of left wrist D, S 🕮

    ●■ S61.509   Unspecified open wound of unspecified wrist D, S 🕮

  ● S61.51   Laceration without foreign body of wrist

    ● S61.511   Laceration without foreign body of right wrist D, S 🕮

    ● S61.512   Laceration without foreign body of left wrist D, S 🕮

    ●■ S61.519   Laceration without foreign body of unspecified wrist D, S 🕮

  ● S61.52   Laceration with foreign body of wrist

    ● S61.521   Laceration with foreign body of right wrist D, S 🕮

    ● S61.522   Laceration with foreign body of left wrist D, S 🕮

    ●■ S61.529   Laceration with foreign body of unspecified wrist D, S 🕮

  ● S61.53   Puncture wound without foreign body of wrist

    ● S61.531   Puncture wound without foreign body of right wrist D, S 🕮

    ● S61.532   Puncture wound without foreign body of left wrist D, S 🕮

    ●■ S61.539   Puncture wound without foreign body of unspecified wrist D, S 🕮

  ● S61.54   Puncture wound with foreign body of wrist

    ● S61.541   Puncture wound with foreign body of right wrist D, S 🕮

    ● S61.542   Puncture wound with foreign body of left wrist D, S 🕮

    ●■ S61.549   Puncture wound with foreign body of unspecified wrist D, S 🕮

  ● S61.55   Open bite of wrist
       Bite of wrist NOS

     | Excludes1 | superficial bite of wrist (S60.86-, S60.87-)

    ● S61.551   Open bite of right wrist D, S 🕮

    ● S61.552   Open bite of left wrist D, S 🕮

    ●■ S61.559   Open bite of unspecified wrist D, S 🕮

N Newborn Age: 0   **P** Pediatric Age: 0–17   **M** Maternity DX: 12–55   **A** Adult Age: 15–124   ♀ Females Only   ♂ Males Only

🕮 Complication\Comorbidity   🕮 Major C\C   🕮 Present on Admission Requirement   🕮 Hospital-Acquired Condition

1499

● **S62   Fracture at wrist and hand level**

Note: A fracture not indicated as displaced or nondisplaced should be coded to displaced

A fracture not indicated as open or closed should be coded to closed

Excludes1   traumatic amputation of wrist and hand (S68.-)

Excludes2   fracture of distal parts of ulna and radius (S52.-)

The appropriate 7th character is to be added to each code from category S62

A	initial encounter for closed fracture
B	initial encounter for open fracture
D	subsequent encounter for fracture with routine healing
G	subsequent encounter for fracture with delayed healing
K	subsequent encounter for fracture with nonunion
P	subsequent encounter for fracture with malunion
S	sequela

● **S62.0   Fracture of navicular [scaphoid] bone of wrist**

● **S62.00   Unspecified fracture of navicular [scaphoid] bone of wrist**

● ■ **S62.001   Unspecified fracture of navicular [scaphoid] bone of right wrist** B, K, P 🔖, D, G, S 🔖, B 🔖

● ■ **S62.002   Unspecified fracture of navicular [scaphoid] bone of left wrist** B, K, P 🔖, D, G, S 🔖, B 🔖

● ■ **S62.009   Unspecified fracture of navicular [scaphoid] bone of unspecified wrist** B, K, P 🔖, D, G, S 🔖, B 🔖

● **S62.01   Fracture of distal pole of navicular [scaphoid] bone of wrist**
Fracture of volar tuberosity of navicular [scaphoid] bone of wrist

● **S62.011   Displaced fracture of distal pole of navicular [scaphoid] bone of right wrist** B, K, P 🔖, D, G, S 🔖, B 🔖

● **S62.012   Displaced fracture of distal pole of navicular [scaphoid] bone of left wrist** B, K, P 🔖, D, G, S 🔖, B 🔖

● ■ **S62.013   Displaced fracture of distal pole of navicular [scaphoid] bone of unspecified wrist** B, K, P 🔖, D, G, S 🔖, B 🔖

● **S62.014   Nondisplaced fracture of distal pole of navicular [scaphoid] bone of right wrist** B, K, P 🔖, D, G, S 🔖, B 🔖

● **S62.015   Nondisplaced fracture of distal pole of navicular [scaphoid] bone of left wrist** B, K, P 🔖, D, G, S 🔖, B 🔖

● ■ **S62.016   Nondisplaced fracture of distal pole of navicular [scaphoid] bone of unspecified wrist** B, K, P 🔖, D, G, S 🔖, B 🔖

● **S62.02   Fracture of middle third of navicular [scaphoid] bone of wrist**

● **S62.021   Displaced fracture of middle third of navicular [scaphoid] bone of right wrist** B, K, P 🔖, D, G, S 🔖, B 🔖

● **S62.022   Displaced fracture of middle third of navicular [scaphoid] bone of left wrist** B, K, P 🔖, D, G, S 🔖, B 🔖

● ■ **S62.023   Displaced fracture of middle third of navicular [scaphoid] bone of unspecified wrist** B, K, P 🔖, D, G, S 🔖, B 🔖

● **S62.024   Nondisplaced fracture of middle third of navicular [scaphoid] bone of right wrist** B, K, P 🔖, D, G, S 🔖, B 🔖

● **S62.025   Nondisplaced fracture of middle third of navicular [scaphoid] bone of left wrist** B, K, P 🔖, D, G, S 🔖, B 🔖

● ■ **S62.026   Nondisplaced fracture of middle third of navicular [scaphoid] bone of unspecified wrist** B, K, P 🔖, D, G, S 🔖, B 🔖

● **S62.03   Fracture of proximal third of navicular [scaphoid] bone of wrist**

● **S62.031   Displaced fracture of proximal third of navicular [scaphoid] bone of right wrist** B, K, P 🔖, D, G, S 🔖, B 🔖

● **S62.032   Displaced fracture of proximal third of navicular [scaphoid] bone of left wrist** B, K, P 🔖, D, G, S 🔖, B 🔖

● ■ **S62.033   Displaced fracture of proximal third of navicular [scaphoid] bone of unspecified wrist** B, K, P 🔖, D, G, S 🔖, B 🔖

● **S62.034   Nondisplaced fracture of proximal third of navicular [scaphoid] bone of right wrist** B, K, P 🔖, D, G, S 🔖, B 🔖

● **S62.035   Nondisplaced fracture of proximal third of navicular [scaphoid] bone of left wrist** B, K, P 🔖, D, G, S 🔖, B 🔖

● ■ **S62.036   Nondisplaced fracture of proximal third of navicular [scaphoid] bone of unspecified wrist** B, K, P 🔖, D, G, S 🔖, B 🔖

● **S62.1   Fracture of other and unspecified carpal bone(s)**

Excludes2   fracture of scaphoid of wrist (S62.0-)

● **S62.10   Fracture of unspecified carpal bone**
Fracture of wrist NOS

● ■ **S62.101   Fracture of unspecified carpal bone, right wrist** B, K, P 🔖, D, G, S 🔖, B 🔖

● ■ **S62.102   Fracture of unspecified carpal bone, left wrist** B, K, P 🔖, D, G, S 🔖, B 🔖

● ■ **S62.109   Fracture of unspecified carpal bone, unspecified wrist** B, K, P 🔖, D, G, S 🔖, B 🔖

● Unacceptable Principal Diagnosis   ● Use Additional Character(s)   ■ Unspecified   ▶ Manifestation Code
OGCR Official Guidelines for Coding and Reporting   Excludes 1   Excludes 2   Includes   Use additional   Code first   Code also

● **S62.11** Fracture of triquetrum [cuneiform] bone of wrist

  ● **S62.111** Displaced fracture of triquetrum [cuneiform] bone, right wrist B, K, P 🦴, D, G, S 🦴, B 🦴

  ● **S62.112** Displaced fracture of triquetrum [cuneiform] bone, left wrist B, K, P 🦴, D, G, S 🦴, B 🦴

  ●■ **S62.113** Displaced fracture of triquetrum [cuneiform] bone, unspecified wrist B, K, P 🦴, D, G, S 🦴, B 🦴

  ● **S62.114** Nondisplaced fracture of triquetrum [cuneiform] bone, right wrist B, K, P 🦴, D, G, S 🦴, B 🦴

  ● **S62.115** Nondisplaced fracture of triquetrum [cuneiform] bone, left wrist B, K, P 🦴, D, G, S 🦴, B 🦴

  ●■ **S62.116** Nondisplaced fracture of triquetrum [cuneiform] bone, unspecified wrist B, K, P 🦴, D, G, S 🦴, B 🦴

● **S62.12** Fracture of lunate [semilunar]

  ● **S62.121** Displaced fracture of lunate [semilunar], right wrist B, K, P 🦴, D, G, S 🦴, B 🦴

  ● **S62.122** Displaced fracture of lunate [semilunar], left wrist B, K, P 🦴, D, G, S 🦴, B 🦴

  ●■ **S62.123** Displaced fracture of lunate [semilunar], unspecified wrist B, K, P 🦴, D, G, S 🦴, B 🦴

  ● **S62.124** Nondisplaced fracture of lunate [semilunar], right wrist B, K, P 🦴, D, G, S 🦴, B 🦴

  ● **S62.125** Nondisplaced fracture of lunate [semilunar], left wrist B, K, P 🦴, D, G, S 🦴, B 🦴

  ●■ **S62.126** Nondisplaced fracture of lunate [semilunar], unspecified wrist B, K, P 🦴, D, G, S 🦴, B 🦴

● **S62.13** Fracture of capitate [os magnum] bone

  ● **S62.131** Displaced fracture of capitate [os magnum] bone, right wrist B, K, P 🦴, D, G, S 🦴, B 🦴

  ● **S62.132** Displaced fracture of capitate [os magnum] bone, left wrist B, K, P 🦴, D, G, S 🦴, B 🦴

  ●■ **S62.133** Displaced fracture of capitate [os magnum] bone, unspecified wrist B, K, P 🦴, D, G, S 🦴, B 🦴

  ● **S62.134** Nondisplaced fracture of capitate [os magnum] bone, right wrist B, K, P 🦴, D, G, S 🦴, B 🦴

  ● **S62.135** Nondisplaced fracture of capitate [os magnum] bone, left wrist B, K, P 🦴, D, G, S 🦴, B 🦴

  ●■ **S62.136** Nondisplaced fracture of capitate [os magnum] bone, unspecified wrist B, K, P 🦴, D, G, S 🦴, B 🦴

● **S62.14** Fracture of body of hamate [unciform] bone

Fracture of hamate [unciform] bone NOS

  ● **S62.141** Displaced fracture of body of hamate [unciform] bone, right wrist B, K, P 🦴, D, G, S 🦴, B 🦴

● **S62.142** Displaced fracture of body of hamate [unciform] bone, left wrist B, K, P 🦴, D, G, S 🦴, B 🦴

  ●■ **S62.143** Displaced fracture of body of hamate [unciform] bone, unspecified wrist B, K, P 🦴, D, G, S 🦴, B 🦴

  ● **S62.144** Nondisplaced fracture of body of hamate [unciform] bone, right wrist B, K, P 🦴, D, G, S 🦴, B 🦴

  ● **S62.145** Nondisplaced fracture of body of hamate [unciform] bone, left wrist B, K, P 🦴, D, G, S 🦴, B 🦴

  ●■ **S62.146** Nondisplaced fracture of body of hamate [unciform] bone, unspecified wrist B, K, P 🦴, D, G, S 🦴, B 🦴

● **S62.15** Fracture of hook process of hamate [unciform] bone

Fracture of unciform process of hamate [unciform] bone

  ● **S62.151** Displaced fracture of hook process of hamate [unciform] bone, right wrist B, K, P 🦴, D, G, S 🦴, B 🦴

  ● **S62.152** Displaced fracture of hook process of hamate [unciform] bone, left wrist B, K, P 🦴, D, G, S 🦴, B 🦴

  ●■ **S62.153** Displaced fracture of hook process of hamate [unciform] bone, unspecified wrist B, K, P 🦴, D, G, S 🦴, B 🦴

  ● **S62.154** Nondisplaced fracture of hook process of hamate [unciform] bone, right wrist B, K, P 🦴, D, G, S 🦴, B 🦴

  ● **S62.155** Nondisplaced fracture of hook process of hamate [unciform] bone, left wrist B, K, P 🦴, D, G, S 🦴, B 🦴

  ●■ **S62.156** Nondisplaced fracture of hook process of hamate [unciform] bone, unspecified wrist B, K, P 🦴, D, G, S 🦴, B 🦴

● **S62.16** Fracture of pisiform

  ●■ **S62.161** Displaced fracture of pisiform, right wrist B, K, P 🦴, D, G, S 🦴, B 🦴

  ● **S62.162** Displaced fracture of pisiform, left wrist B, K, P 🦴, D, G, S 🦴, B 🦴

  ●■ **S62.163** Displaced fracture of pisiform, unspecified wrist B, K, P 🦴, D, G, S 🦴, B 🦴

  ● **S62.164** Nondisplaced fracture of pisiform, right wrist B, K, P 🦴, D, G, S 🦴, B 🦴

  ● **S62.165** Nondisplaced fracture of pisiform, left wrist B, K, P 🦴, D, G, S 🦴, B 🦴

  ●■ **S62.166** Nondisplaced fracture of pisiform, unspecified wrist B, K, P 🦴, D, G, S 🦴, B 🦴

CHAPTER 19 (S00-T88)

CHAPTER 19 (S00-T88)

● S62.17   Fracture of trapezium [larger multangular]

    ● S62.171   Displaced fracture of trapezium [larger multangular], right wrist B, K, P 🦴, D, G, S 🦴, B 🦴

    ● S62.172   Displaced fracture of trapezium [larger multangular], left wrist B, K, P 🦴, D, G, S 🦴, B 🦴

    ●■ S62.173   Displaced fracture of trapezium [larger multangular], unspecified wrist B, K, P 🦴, D, G, S 🦴, B 🦴

    ● S62.174   Nondisplaced fracture of trapezium [larger multangular], right wrist B, K, P 🦴, D, G, S 🦴, B 🦴

    ● S62.175   Nondisplaced fracture of trapezium [larger multangular], left wrist B, K, P 🦴, D, G, S 🦴, B 🦴

    ●■ S62.176   Nondisplaced fracture of trapezium [larger multangular], unspecified wrist B, K, P 🦴, D, G, S 🦴, B 🦴

● S62.18   Fracture of trapezoid [smaller multangular]

    ● S62.181   Displaced fracture of trapezoid [smaller multangular], right wrist B, K, P 🦴, D, G, S 🦴, B 🦴

    ● S62.182   Displaced fracture of trapezoid [smaller multangular], left wrist B, K, P 🦴, D, G, S 🦴, B 🦴

    ●■ S62.183   Displaced fracture of trapezoid [smaller multangular], unspecified wrist B, K, P 🦴, D, G, S 🦴, B 🦴

    ● S62.184   Nondisplaced fracture of trapezoid [smaller multangular], right wrist B, K, P 🦴, D, G, S 🦴, B 🦴

    ● S62.185   Nondisplaced fracture of trapezoid [smaller multangular], left wrist B, K, P 🦴, D, G, S 🦴, B 🦴

    ●■ S62.186   Nondisplaced fracture of trapezoid [smaller multangular], unspecified wrist B, K, P 🦴, D, G, S 🦴, B 🦴

● S62.2   Fracture of first metacarpal bone

    ● S62.20   Unspecified fracture of first metacarpal bone

       ●■ S62.201   Unspecified fracture of first metacarpal bone, right hand B, K, P 🦴, D, G, S 🦴, B 🦴

       ●■ S62.202   Unspecified fracture of first metacarpal bone, left hand B, K, P 🦴, D, G, S 🦴, B 🦴

       ●■ S62.209   Unspecified fracture of first metacarpal bone, unspecified hand B, K, P 🦴, D, G, S 🦴, B 🦴

    ● S62.21   Bennett's fracture

       ● S62.211   Bennett's fracture, right hand B, K, P 🦴, D, G, S 🦴, B 🦴

       ● S62.212   Bennett's fracture, left hand B, K, P 🦴, D, G, S 🦴, B 🦴

       ●■ S62.213   Bennett's fracture, unspecified hand B, K, P 🦴, D, G, S 🦴, B 🦴

● S62.22   Rolando's fracture

    ● S62.221   Displaced Rolando's fracture, right hand B, K, P 🦴, D, G, S 🦴, B 🦴

    ● S62.222   Displaced Rolando's fracture, left hand B, K, P 🦴, D, G, S 🦴, B 🦴

    ●■ S62.223   Displaced Rolando's fracture, unspecified hand B, K, P 🦴, D, G, S 🦴, B 🦴

    ● S62.224   Nondisplaced Rolando's fracture, right hand B, K, P 🦴, D, G, S 🦴, B 🦴

    ● S62.225   Nondisplaced Rolando's fracture, left hand B, K, P 🦴, D, G, S 🦴, B 🦴

    ●■ S62.226   Nondisplaced Rolando's fracture, unspecified hand B, K, P 🦴, D, G, S 🦴, B 🦴

● S62.23   Other fracture of base of first metacarpal bone

    ● S62.231   Other displaced fracture of base of first metacarpal bone, right hand B, K, P 🦴, D, G, S 🦴, B 🦴

    ● S62.232   Other displaced fracture of base of first metacarpal bone, left hand B, K, P 🦴, D, G, S 🦴, B 🦴

    ●■ S62.233   Other displaced fracture of base of first metacarpal bone, unspecified hand B, K, P 🦴, D, G, S 🦴, B 🦴

    ● S62.234   Other nondisplaced fracture of base of first metacarpal bone, right hand B, K, P 🦴, D, G, S 🦴, B 🦴

    ● S62.235   Other nondisplaced fracture of base of first metacarpal bone, left hand B, K, P 🦴, D, G, S 🦴, B 🦴

    ●■ S62.236   Other nondisplaced fracture of base of first metacarpal bone, unspecified hand B, K, P 🦴, D, G, S 🦴, B 🦴

● S62.24   Fracture of shaft of first metacarpal bone

    ● S62.241   Displaced fracture of shaft of first metacarpal bone, right hand B, K, P 🦴, D, G, S 🦴, B 🦴

    ● S62.242   Displaced fracture of shaft of first metacarpal bone, left hand B, K, P 🦴, D, G, S 🦴, B 🦴

    ●■ S62.243   Displaced fracture of shaft of first metacarpal bone, unspecified hand B, K, P 🦴, D, G, S 🦴, B 🦴

    ● S62.244   Nondisplaced fracture of shaft of first metacarpal bone, right hand B, K, P 🦴, D, G, S 🦴, B 🦴

    ● S62.245   Nondisplaced fracture of shaft of first metacarpal bone, left hand B, K, P 🦴, D, G, S 🦴, B 🦴

    ●■ S62.246   Nondisplaced fracture of shaft of first metacarpal bone, unspecified hand B, K, P 🦴, D, G, S 🦴, B 🦴

● S62.25   Fracture of neck of first metacarpal bone

    ● S62.251   Displaced fracture of neck of first metacarpal bone, right hand B, K, P 🦴, D, G, S 🦴, B 🦴

    ● S62.252   Displaced fracture of neck of first metacarpal bone, left hand B, K, P 🦴, D, G, S 🦴, B 🦴

●   Unacceptable Principal Diagnosis   ●   Use Additional Character(s)   ■   Unspecified   ▶   Manifestation Code

OGCR   Official Guidelines for Coding and Reporting   Excludes 1   Excludes 2   Includes   Use additional   Code first   Code also

● ■ **S62.253** Displaced fracture of neck of first metacarpal bone, unspecified hand B, K, P 🌑, D, G, S 🌑, B 🌑

● **S62.254** Nondisplaced fracture of neck of first metacarpal bone, right hand B, K, P 🌑, D, G, S 🌑, B 🌑

● **S62.255** Nondisplaced fracture of neck of first metacarpal bone, left hand B, K, P 🌑, D, G, S 🌑, B 🌑

● ■ **S62.256** Nondisplaced fracture of neck of first metacarpal bone, unspecified hand B, K, P 🌑, D, G, S 🌑, B 🌑

● **S62.29** Other fracture of first metacarpal bone

● **S62.291** Other fracture of first metacarpal bone, right hand B, K, P 🌑, D, G, S 🌑, B 🌑

● **S62.292** Other fracture of first metacarpal bone, left hand B, K, P 🌑, D, G, S 🌑, B 🌑

● ■ **S62.299** Other fracture of first metacarpal bone, unspecified hand B, K, P 🌑, D, G, S 🌑, B 🌑

● **S62.3** Fracture of other and unspecified metacarpal bone

> **Excludes2**   fracture of first metacarpal bone (S62.2-)

● **S62.30** Unspecified fracture of other metacarpal bone

● ■ **S62.300** Unspecified fracture of second metacarpal bone, right hand B, K, P 🌑, D, G, S 🌑, B 🌑

● ■ **S62.301** Unspecified fracture of second metacarpal bone, left hand B, K, P 🌑, D, G, S 🌑, B 🌑

● ■ **S62.302** Unspecified fracture of third metacarpal bone, right hand B, K, P 🌑, D, G, S 🌑, B 🌑

● ■ **S62.303** Unspecified fracture of third metacarpal bone, left hand B, K, P 🌑, D, G, S 🌑, B 🌑

● ■ **S62.304** Unspecified fracture of fourth metacarpal bone, right hand B, K, P 🌑, D, G, S 🌑, B 🌑

● ■ **S62.305** Unspecified fracture of fourth metacarpal bone, left hand B, K, P 🌑, D, G, S 🌑, B 🌑

● ■ **S62.306** Unspecified fracture of fifth metacarpal bone, right hand B, K, P 🌑, D, G, S 🌑, B 🌑

● ■ **S62.307** Unspecified fracture of fifth metacarpal bone, left hand B, K, P 🌑, D, G, S 🌑, B 🌑

● ■ **S62.308** Unspecified fracture of other metacarpal bone B, K, P 🌑, D, G, S 🌑, B 🌑
Unspecified fracture of specified metacarpal bone with unspecified laterality

● ■ **S62.309** Unspecified fracture of unspecified metacarpal bone B, K, P 🌑, D, G, S 🌑, B 🌑

● **S62.31** Displaced fracture of base of other metacarpal bone

● **S62.310** Displaced fracture of base of second metacarpal bone, right hand B, K, P 🌑, D, G, S 🌑, B 🌑

● **S62.311** Displaced fracture of base of second metacarpal bone, left hand B, K, P 🌑, D, G, S 🌑, B 🌑

● **S62.312** Displaced fracture of base of third metacarpal bone, right hand B, K, P 🌑, D, G, S 🌑, B 🌑

● **S62.313** Displaced fracture of base of third metacarpal bone, left hand B, K, P 🌑, D, G, S 🌑, B 🌑

● **S62.314** Displaced fracture of base of fourth metacarpal bone, right hand B, K, P 🌑, D, G, S 🌑, B 🌑

● **S62.315** Displaced fracture of base of fourth metacarpal bone, left hand B, K, P 🌑, D, G, S 🌑, B 🌑

● **S62.316** Displaced fracture of base of fifth metacarpal bone, right hand B, K, P 🌑, D, G, S 🌑, B 🌑

● **S62.317** Displaced fracture of base of fifth metacarpal bone, left hand B, K, P 🌑, D, G, S 🌑, B 🌑

● **S62.318** Displaced fracture of base of other metacarpal bone B, K, P 🌑, D, G, S 🌑, B 🌑
Displaced fracture of base of specified metacarpal bone with unspecified laterality

● ■ **S62.319** Displaced fracture of base of unspecified metacarpal bone B, K, P 🌑, D, G, S 🌑, B 🌑

● **S62.32** Displaced fracture of shaft of other metacarpal bone

● **S62.320** Displaced fracture of shaft of second metacarpal bone, right hand B, K, P 🌑, D, G, S 🌑, B 🌑

● **S62.321** Displaced fracture of shaft of second metacarpal bone, left hand B, K, P 🌑, D, G, S 🌑, B 🌑

● **S62.322** Displaced fracture of shaft of third metacarpal bone, right hand B, K, P 🌑, D, G, S 🌑, B 🌑

● **S62.323** Displaced fracture of shaft of third metacarpal bone, left hand B, K, P 🌑, D, G, S 🌑, B 🌑

● **S62.324** Displaced fracture of shaft of fourth metacarpal bone, right hand B, K, P 🌑, D, G, S 🌑, B 🌑

● **S62.325** Displaced fracture of shaft of fourth metacarpal bone, left hand B, K, P 🌑, D, G, S 🌑, B 🌑

● **S62.326** Displaced fracture of shaft of fifth metacarpal bone, right hand B, K, P 🌑, D, G, S 🌑, B 🌑

● **S62.327** Displaced fracture of shaft of fifth metacarpal bone, left hand B, K, P 🌑, D, G, S 🌑, B 🌑

● **S62.328** Displaced fracture of shaft of other metacarpal bone B, K, P 🌑, D, G, S 🌑, B 🌑
Displaced fracture of shaft of specified metacarpal bone with unspecified laterality

● ■ **S62.329** Displaced fracture of shaft of unspecified metacarpal bone B, K, P 🌑, D, G, S 🌑, B 🌑

N Newborn Age: 0   **P** Pediatric Age: 0–17   **M** Maternity DX: 12–55   **A** Adult Age: 15–124   ♀ Females Only   ♂ Males Only

🌑 Complication\Comorbidity   🌑 Major C\C   Present on Admission Requirement   🌑 Hospital-Acquired Condition

CHAPTER 19 (S00-T88)

1503

● **S62.33** Displaced fracture of neck of other metacarpal bone

- ● S62.330 Displaced fracture of neck of second metacarpal bone, right hand B, K, P 🔹, D, G, S 🔹, B 🔹
- ● S62.331 Displaced fracture of neck of second metacarpal bone, left hand B, K, P 🔹, D, G, S 🔹, B 🔹
- ● S62.332 Displaced fracture of neck of third metacarpal bone, right hand B, K, P 🔹, D, G, S 🔹, B 🔹
- ● S62.333 Displaced fracture of neck of third metacarpal bone, left hand B, K, P 🔹, D, G, S 🔹, B 🔹
- ● S62.334 Displaced fracture of neck of fourth metacarpal bone, right hand B, K, P 🔹, D, G, S 🔹, B 🔹
- ● S62.335 Displaced fracture of neck of fourth metacarpal bone, left hand B, K, P 🔹, D, G, S 🔹, B 🔹
- ● S62.336 Displaced fracture of neck of fifth metacarpal bone, right hand B, K, P 🔹, D, G, S 🔹, B 🔹
- ● S62.337 Displaced fracture of neck of fifth metacarpal bone, left hand B, K, P 🔹, D, G, S 🔹, B 🔹
- ● S62.338 Displaced fracture of neck of other metacarpal bone B, K, P 🔹, D, G, S 🔹, B 🔹
  Displaced fracture of neck of specified metacarpal bone with unspecified laterality
- ●■ S62.339 Displaced fracture of neck of unspecified metacarpal bone B, K, P 🔹, D, G, S 🔹, B 🔹

● **S62.34** Nondisplaced fracture of base of other metacarpal bone

- ● S62.340 Nondisplaced fracture of base of second metacarpal bone, right hand B, K, P 🔹, D, G, S 🔹, B 🔹
- ● S62.341 Nondisplaced fracture of base of second metacarpal bone, left hand B, K, P 🔹, D, G, S 🔹, B 🔹
- ● S62.342 Nondisplaced fracture of base of third metacarpal bone, right hand B, K, P 🔹, D, G, S 🔹, B 🔹
- ● S62.343 Nondisplaced fracture of base of third metacarpal bone, left hand B, K, P 🔹, D, G, S 🔹, B 🔹
- ● S62.344 Nondisplaced fracture of base of fourth metacarpal bone, right hand B, K, P 🔹, D, G, S 🔹, B 🔹
- ● S62.345 Nondisplaced fracture of base of fourth metacarpal bone, left hand B, K, P 🔹, D, G, S 🔹, B 🔹
- ● S62.346 Nondisplaced fracture of base of fifth metacarpal bone, right hand B, K, P 🔹, D, G, S 🔹, B 🔹
- ● S62.347 Nondisplaced fracture of base of fifth metacarpal bone, left hand B, K, P 🔹, D, G, S 🔹, B 🔹
- ● S62.348 Nondisplaced fracture of base of other metacarpal bone B, K, P 🔹, D, G, S 🔹, B 🔹
  Nondisplaced fracture of base of specified metacarpal bone with unspecified laterality

- ●■ S62.349 Nondisplaced fracture of base of unspecified metacarpal bone B, K, P 🔹, D, G, S 🔹, B 🔹

● **S62.35** Nondisplaced fracture of shaft of other metacarpal bone

- ● S62.350 Nondisplaced fracture of shaft of second metacarpal bone, right hand B, K, P 🔹, D, G, S 🔹, B 🔹
- ● S62.351 Nondisplaced fracture of shaft of second metacarpal bone, left hand B, K, P 🔹, D, G, S 🔹, B 🔹
- ● S62.352 Nondisplaced fracture of shaft of third metacarpal bone, right hand B, K, P 🔹, D, G, S 🔹, B 🔹
- ● S62.353 Nondisplaced fracture of shaft of third metacarpal bone, left hand B, K, P 🔹, D, G, S 🔹, B 🔹
- ● S62.354 Nondisplaced fracture of shaft of fourth metacarpal bone, right hand B, K, P 🔹, D, G, S 🔹, B 🔹
- ● S62.355 Nondisplaced fracture of shaft of fourth metacarpal bone, left hand B, K, P 🔹, D, G, S 🔹, B 🔹
- ● S62.356 Nondisplaced fracture of shaft of fifth metacarpal bone, right hand B, K, P 🔹, D, G, S 🔹, B 🔹
- ● S62.357 Nondisplaced fracture of shaft of fifth metacarpal bone, left hand B, K, P 🔹, D, G, S 🔹, B 🔹
- ● S62.358 Nondisplaced fracture of shaft of other metacarpal bone B, K, P 🔹, D, G, S 🔹, B 🔹
  Nondisplaced fracture of shaft of specified metacarpal bone with unspecified laterality
- ●■ S62.359 Nondisplaced fracture of shaft of unspecified metacarpal bone B, K, P 🔹, D, G, S 🔹, B 🔹

● **S62.36** Nondisplaced fracture of neck of other metacarpal bone

- ● S62.360 Nondisplaced fracture of neck of second metacarpal bone, right hand B, K, P 🔹, D, G, S 🔹, B 🔹
- ● S62.361 Nondisplaced fracture of neck of second metacarpal bone, left hand B, K, P 🔹, D, G, S 🔹, B 🔹
- ● S62.362 Nondisplaced fracture of neck of third metacarpal bone, right hand B, K, P 🔹, D, G, S 🔹, B 🔹
- ● S62.363 Nondisplaced fracture of neck of third metacarpal bone, left hand B, K, P 🔹, D, G, S 🔹, B 🔹
- ● S62.364 Nondisplaced fracture of neck of fourth metacarpal bone, right hand B, K, P 🔹, D, G, S 🔹, B 🔹
- ● S62.365 Nondisplaced fracture of neck of fourth metacarpal bone, left hand B, K, P 🔹, D, G, S 🔹, B 🔹
- ● S62.366 Nondisplaced fracture of neck of fifth metacarpal bone, right hand B, K, P 🔹, D, G, S 🔹, B 🔹
- ● S62.367 Nondisplaced fracture of neck of fifth metacarpal bone, left hand B, K, P 🔹, D, G, S 🔹, B 🔹

● Unacceptable Principal Diagnosis   ● Use Additional Character(s)   ■ Unspecified   ▶ Manifestation Code
OGCR Official Guidelines for Coding and Reporting   Excludes 1   Excludes 2   Includes   Use additional   Code first   Code also

● S62.368   Nondisplaced fracture of neck of other metacarpal bone B, K, P 🅒, D, G, S 🅒, B 🅒
     Nondisplaced fracture of neck of specified metacarpal bone with unspecified laterality

●▪ S62.369   Nondisplaced fracture of neck of unspecified metacarpal bone B, K, P 🅒, D, G, S 🅒, B 🅒

● S62.39   Other fracture of other metacarpal bone

    ● S62.390   Other fracture of second metacarpal bone, right hand B, K, P 🅒, D, G, S 🅒, B 🅒

    ● S62.391   Other fracture of second metacarpal bone, left hand B, K, P 🅒, D, G, S 🅒, B 🅒

    ● S62.392   Other fracture of third metacarpal bone, right hand B, K, P 🅒, D, G, S 🅒, B 🅒

    ● S62.393   Other fracture of third metacarpal bone, left hand B, K, P 🅒, D, G, S 🅒, B 🅒

    ● S62.394   Other fracture of fourth metacarpal bone, right hand B, K, P 🅒, D, G, S 🅒, B 🅒

    ● S62.395   Other fracture of fourth metacarpal bone, left hand B, K, P 🅒, D, G, S 🅒, B 🅒

    ● S62.396   Other fracture of fifth metacarpal bone, right hand B, K, P 🅒, D, G, S 🅒, B 🅒

    ● S62.397   Other fracture of fifth metacarpal bone, left hand B, K, P 🅒, D, G, S 🅒, B 🅒

    ● S62.398   Other fracture of other metacarpal bone B, K, P 🅒, D, G, S 🅒, B 🅒
       Other fracture of specified metacarpal bone with unspecified laterality

    ●▪ S62.399   Other fracture of unspecified metacarpal bone B, K, P 🅒, D, G, S 🅒, B 🅒

● S62.5   Fracture of thumb

   ● S62.50   Fracture of unspecified phalanx of thumb

    ●▪ S62.501   Fracture of unspecified phalanx of right thumb B, K, P 🅒, D, G, S 🅒, B 🅒

    ●▪ S62.502   Fracture of unspecified phalanx of left thumb B, K, P 🅒, D, G, S 🅒, B 🅒

    ●▪ S62.509   Fracture of unspecified phalanx of unspecified thumb B, K, P 🅒, D, G, S 🅒, B 🅒

   ● S62.51   Fracture of proximal phalanx of thumb

    ● S62.511   Displaced fracture of proximal phalanx of right thumb B, K, P 🅒, D, G, S 🅒, B 🅒

    ● S62.512   Displaced fracture of proximal phalanx of left thumb B, K, P 🅒, D, G, S 🅒, B 🅒

    ●▪ S62.513   Displaced fracture of proximal phalanx of unspecified thumb B, K, P 🅒, D, G, S 🅒, B 🅒

● S62.514   Nondisplaced fracture of proximal phalanx of right thumb B, K, P 🅒, D, G, S 🅒, B 🅒

● S62.515   Nondisplaced fracture of proximal phalanx of left thumb B, K, P 🅒, D, G, S 🅒, B 🅒

●▪ S62.516   Nondisplaced fracture of proximal phalanx of unspecified thumb B, K, P 🅒, D, G, S 🅒, B 🅒

● S62.52   Fracture of distal phalanx of thumb

   ● S62.521   Displaced fracture of distal phalanx of right thumb B, K, P 🅒, D, G, S 🅒, B 🅒

   ● S62.522   Displaced fracture of distal phalanx of left thumb B, K, P 🅒, D, G, S 🅒, B 🅒

   ●▪ S62.523   Displaced fracture of distal phalanx of unspecified thumb B, K, P 🅒, D, G, S 🅒, B 🅒

   ● S62.524   Nondisplaced fracture of distal phalanx of right thumb B, K, P 🅒, D, G, S 🅒, B 🅒

   ● S62.525   Nondisplaced fracture of distal phalanx of left thumb B, K, P 🅒, D, G, S 🅒, B 🅒

   ●▪ S62.526   Nondisplaced fracture of distal phalanx of unspecified thumb B, K, P 🅒, D, G, S 🅒, B 🅒

● S62.6   Fracture of other and unspecified finger(s)

   Excludes2   fracture of thumb (S62.5-)

   ● S62.60   Fracture of unspecified phalanx of finger

    ●▪ S62.600   Fracture of unspecified phalanx of right index finger B, K, P 🅒, D, G, S 🅒, B 🅒

    ●▪ S62.601   Fracture of unspecified phalanx of left index finger B, K, P 🅒, D, G, S 🅒, B 🅒

    ●▪ S62.602   Fracture of unspecified phalanx of right middle finger B, K, P 🅒, D, G, S 🅒, B 🅒

    ●▪ S62.603   Fracture of unspecified phalanx of left middle finger B, K, P 🅒, D, G, S 🅒, B 🅒

    ●▪ S62.604   Fracture of unspecified phalanx of right ring finger B, K, P 🅒, D, G, S 🅒, B 🅒

    ●▪ S62.605   Fracture of unspecified phalanx of left ring finger B, K, P 🅒, D, G, S 🅒, B 🅒

    ●▪ S62.606   Fracture of unspecified phalanx of right little finger B, K, P 🅒, D, G, S 🅒, B 🅒

    ●▪ S62.607   Fracture of unspecified phalanx of left little finger B, K, P 🅒, D, G, S 🅒, B 🅒

    ●▪ S62.608   Fracture of unspecified phalanx of other finger B, K, P 🅒, D, G, S 🅒, B 🅒
       Fracture of unspecified phalanx of specified finger with unspecified laterality

    ●▪ S62.609   Fracture of unspecified phalanx of unspecified finger B, K, P 🅒, D, G, S 🅒, B 🅒

N Newborn Age: 0   **P** Pediatric Age: 0–17   **M** Maternity DX: 12–55   **A** Adult Age: 15–124   ♀ Females Only   ♂ Males Only

🅒 Complication\Comorbidity   🅒 Major C\C   🅒 Present on Admission Requirement   🅒 Hospital-Acquired Condition

CHAPTER 19 (S00–T88)

1505

● **S62.61**   Displaced fracture of proximal phalanx of finger

  ● **S62.610**   Displaced fracture of proximal phalanx of right index finger B, K, P ⬟, D, G, S ⬟, B ⬟

  ● **S62.611**   Displaced fracture of proximal phalanx of left index finger B, K, P ⬟, D, G, S ⬟, B ⬟

  ● **S62.612**   Displaced fracture of proximal phalanx of right middle finger B, K, P ⬟, D, G, S ⬟, B ⬟

  ● **S62.613**   Displaced fracture of proximal phalanx of left middle finger B, K, P ⬟, D, G, S ⬟, B ⬟

  ● **S62.614**   Displaced fracture of proximal phalanx of right ring finger B, K, P ⬟, D, G, S ⬟, B ⬟

  ● **S62.615**   Displaced fracture of proximal phalanx of left ring finger B, K, P ⬟, D, G, S ⬟, B ⬟

  ● **S62.616**   Displaced fracture of proximal phalanx of right little finger B, K, P ⬟, D, G, S ⬟, B ⬟

  ● **S62.617**   Displaced fracture of proximal phalanx of left little finger B, K, P ⬟, D, G, S ⬟, B ⬟

  ● **S62.618**   Displaced fracture of proximal phalanx of other finger B, K, P ⬟, D, G, S ⬟, B ⬟

     Displaced fracture of proximal phalanx of specified finger with unspecified laterality

  ●■ **S62.619**   Displaced fracture of proximal phalanx of unspecified finger B, K, P ⬟, D, G, S ⬟, B ⬟

● **S62.62**   Displaced fracture of medial phalanx of finger

  ● **S62.620**   Displaced fracture of medial phalanx of right index finger B, K, P ⬟, D, G, S ⬟, B ⬟

  ● **S62.621**   Displaced fracture of medial phalanx of left index finger B, K, P ⬟, D, G, S ⬟, B ⬟

  ● **S62.622**   Displaced fracture of medial phalanx of right middle finger B, K, P ⬟, D, G, S ⬟, B ⬟

  ● **S62.623**   Displaced fracture of medial phalanx of left middle finger B, K, P ⬟, D, G, S ⬟, B ⬟

  ● **S62.624**   Displaced fracture of medial phalanx of right ring finger B, K, P ⬟, D, G, S ⬟, B ⬟

  ● **S62.625**   Displaced fracture of medial phalanx of left ring finger B, K, P ⬟, D, G, S ⬟, B ⬟

  ● **S62.626**   Displaced fracture of medial phalanx of right little finger B, K, P ⬟, D, G, S ⬟, B ⬟

  ● **S62.627**   Displaced fracture of medial phalanx of left little finger B, K, P ⬟, D, G, S ⬟, B ⬟

  ● **S62.628**   Displaced fracture of medial phalanx of other finger B, K, P ⬟, D, G, S ⬟, B ⬟

     Displaced fracture of medial phalanx of specified finger with unspecified laterality

  ●■ **S62.629**   Displaced fracture of medial phalanx of unspecified finger B, K, P ⬟, D, G, S ⬟, B ⬟

● **S62.63**   Displaced fracture of distal phalanx of finger

  ● **S62.630**   Displaced fracture of distal phalanx of right index finger B, K, P ⬟, D, G, S ⬟, B ⬟

  ● **S62.631**   Displaced fracture of distal phalanx of left index finger B, K, P ⬟, D, G, S ⬟, B ⬟

  ● **S62.632**   Displaced fracture of distal phalanx of right middle finger B, K, P ⬟, D, G, S ⬟, B ⬟

  ● **S62.633**   Displaced fracture of distal phalanx of left middle finger B, K, P ⬟, D, G, S ⬟, B ⬟

  ● **S62.634**   Displaced fracture of distal phalanx of right ring finger B, K, P ⬟, D, G, S ⬟, B ⬟

  ● **S62.635**   Displaced fracture of distal phalanx of left ring finger B, K, P ⬟, D, G, S ⬟, B ⬟

  ● **S62.636**   Displaced fracture of distal phalanx of right little finger B, K, P ⬟, D, G, S ⬟, B ⬟

  ● **S62.637**   Displaced fracture of distal phalanx of left little finger B, K, P ⬟, D, G, S ⬟, B ⬟

  ● **S62.638**   Displaced fracture of distal phalanx of other finger B, K, P ⬟, D, G, S ⬟, B ⬟

     Displaced fracture of distal phalanx of specified finger with unspecified laterality

  ●■ **S62.639**   Displaced fracture of distal phalanx of unspecified finger B, K, P ⬟, D, G, S ⬟, B ⬟

● **S62.64**   Nondisplaced fracture of proximal phalanx of finger

  ● **S62.640**   Nondisplaced fracture of proximal phalanx of right index finger B, K, P ⬟, D, G, S ⬟, B ⬟

  ● **S62.641**   Nondisplaced fracture of proximal phalanx of left index finger B, K, P ⬟, D, G, S ⬟, B ⬟

  ● **S62.642**   Nondisplaced fracture of proximal phalanx of right middle finger B, K, P ⬟, D, G, S ⬟, B ⬟

  ● **S62.643**   Nondisplaced fracture of proximal phalanx of left middle finger B, K, P ⬟, D, G, S ⬟, B ⬟

  ● **S62.644**   Nondisplaced fracture of proximal phalanx of right ring finger B, K, P ⬟, D, G, S ⬟, B ⬟

  ● **S62.645**   Nondisplaced fracture of proximal phalanx of left ring finger B, K, P ⬟, D, G, S ⬟, B ⬟

  ● **S62.646**   Nondisplaced fracture of proximal phalanx of right little finger B, K, P ⬟, D, G, S ⬟, B ⬟

  ● **S62.647**   Nondisplaced fracture of proximal phalanx of left little finger B, K, P ⬟, D, G, S ⬟, B ⬟

● Unacceptable Principal Diagnosis   ● Use Additional Character(s)   ■ Unspecified   ▶ Manifestation Code

OGCR Official Guidelines for Coding and Reporting   Excludes 1   Excludes 2   Includes   Use additional   Code first   Code also

● **S62.648 Nondisplaced fracture of proximal phalanx of other finger** B, K, P 🔩, D, G, S 🔩, B 🔩
   Nondisplaced fracture of proximal phalanx of specified finger with unspecified laterality

●■ **S62.649 Nondisplaced fracture of proximal phalanx of unspecified finger** B, K, P 🔩, D, G, S 🔩, B 🔩

● **S62.65 Nondisplaced fracture of medial phalanx of finger**

● **S62.650 Nondisplaced fracture of medial phalanx of right index finger** B, K, P 🔩, D, G, S 🔩, B 🔩

● **S62.651 Nondisplaced fracture of medial phalanx of left index finger** B, K, P 🔩, D, G, S 🔩, B 🔩

● **S62.652 Nondisplaced fracture of medial phalanx of right middle finger** B, K, P 🔩, D, G, S 🔩, B 🔩

● **S62.653 Nondisplaced fracture of medial phalanx of left middle finger** B, K, P 🔩, D, G, S 🔩, B 🔩

● **S62.654 Nondisplaced fracture of medial phalanx of right ring finger** B, K, P 🔩, D, G, S 🔩, B 🔩

● **S62.655 Nondisplaced fracture of medial phalanx of left ring finger** B, K, P 🔩, D, G, S 🔩, B 🔩

● **S62.656 Nondisplaced fracture of medial phalanx of right little finger** B, K, P 🔩, D, G, S 🔩, B 🔩

● **S62.657 Nondisplaced fracture of medial phalanx of left little finger** B, K, P 🔩, D, G, S 🔩, B 🔩

● **S62.658 Nondisplaced fracture of medial phalanx of other finger** B, K, P 🔩, D, G, S 🔩, B 🔩
   Nondisplaced fracture of medial phalanx of specified finger with unspecified laterality

●■ **S62.659 Nondisplaced fracture of medial phalanx of unspecified finger** B, K, P 🔩, D, G, S 🔩, B 🔩

● **S62.66 Nondisplaced fracture of distal phalanx of finger**

● **S62.660 Nondisplaced fracture of distal phalanx of right index finger** B, K, P 🔩, D, G, S 🔩, B 🔩

● **S62.661 Nondisplaced fracture of distal phalanx of left index finger** B, K, P 🔩, D, G, S 🔩, B 🔩

● **S62.662 Nondisplaced fracture of distal phalanx of right middle finger** B, K, P 🔩, D, G, S 🔩, B 🔩

● **S62.663 Nondisplaced fracture of distal phalanx of left middle finger** B, K, P 🔩, D, G, S 🔩, B 🔩

● **S62.664 Nondisplaced fracture of distal phalanx of right ring finger** B, K, P 🔩, D, G, S 🔩, B 🔩

● **S62.665 Nondisplaced fracture of distal phalanx of left ring finger** B, K, P 🔩, D, G, S 🔩, B 🔩

● **S62.666 Nondisplaced fracture of distal phalanx of right little finger** B, K, P 🔩, D, G, S 🔩, B 🔩

● **S62.667 Nondisplaced fracture of distal phalanx of left little finger** B, K, P 🔩, D, G, S 🔩, B 🔩

● **S62.668 Nondisplaced fracture of distal phalanx of other finger** B, K, P 🔩, D, G, S 🔩, B 🔩
   Nondisplaced fracture of distal phalanx of specified finger with unspecified laterality

●■ **S62.669 Nondisplaced fracture of distal phalanx of unspecified finger** B, K, P 🔩, D, G, S 🔩, B 🔩

● **S62.9 Unspecified fracture of wrist and hand**

●■ **S62.90 Unspecified fracture of unspecified wrist and hand** B, K, P 🔩, D, G, S 🔩, B 🔩

●■ **S62.91 Unspecified fracture of right wrist and hand** B, K, P 🔩, D, G, S 🔩, B 🔩

●■ **S62.92 Unspecified fracture of left wrist and hand** B, K, P 🔩, D, G, S 🔩, B 🔩

● **S63 Dislocation and sprain of joints and ligaments at wrist and hand level**

Includes	avulsion of joint or ligament at wrist and hand level
	laceration of cartilage, joint or ligament at wrist and hand level
	sprain of cartilage, joint or ligament at wrist and hand level
	traumatic hemarthrosis of joint or ligament at wrist and hand level
	traumatic rupture of joint or ligament at wrist and hand level
	traumatic subluxation of joint or ligament at wrist and hand level
	traumatic tear of joint or ligament at wrist and hand level

Code also any associated open wound

Excludes2	strain of muscle, fascia and tendon of wrist and hand (S66.-)

The appropriate 7th character is to be added to each code from category S63

A	initial encounter
D	subsequent encounter
S	sequela

● **S63.0 Subluxation and dislocation of wrist and hand joints**

● **S63.00 Unspecified subluxation and dislocation of wrist and hand**
   Dislocation of carpal bone NOS
   Dislocation of distal end of radius NOS
   Subluxation of carpal bone NOS
   Subluxation of distal end of radius NOS

●■ **S63.001 Unspecified subluxation of right wrist and hand** D, S 🔩

●■ **S63.002 Unspecified subluxation of left wrist and hand** D, S 🔩

●■ **S63.003 Unspecified subluxation of unspecified wrist and hand** D, S 🔩

●■ **S63.004 Unspecified dislocation of right wrist and hand** D, S 🔩

●■ **S63.005 Unspecified dislocation of left wrist and hand** D, S 🔩

●■ **S63.006 Unspecified dislocation of unspecified wrist and hand** D, S 🔩

CHAPTER 19 (S00–T88)

Figure 19-13 Dislocation including displacement and subluxation. (From Grainger & Allison's Diagnostic Radiology: A Textbook of Medical Imaging, 4th ed. 2001, Churchill Livingstone.)

● S63.01 **Subluxation and dislocation of distal radioulnar joint**
- ● S63.011 Subluxation of distal radioulnar joint of right wrist D, S
- ● S63.012 Subluxation of distal radioulnar joint of left wrist D, S
- ● S63.013 Subluxation of distal radioulnar joint of unspecified wrist D, S
- ● S63.014 Dislocation of distal radioulnar joint of right wrist D, S
- ● S63.015 Dislocation of distal radioulnar joint of left wrist D, S
- ● S63.016 Dislocation of distal radioulnar joint of unspecified wrist D, S

● S63.02 **Subluxation and dislocation of radiocarpal joint**
- ● S63.021 Subluxation of radiocarpal joint of right wrist D, S
- ● S63.022 Subluxation of radiocarpal joint of left wrist D, S
- ● S63.023 Subluxation of radiocarpal joint of unspecified wrist D, S
- ● S63.024 Dislocation of radiocarpal joint of right wrist D, S
- ● S63.025 Dislocation of radiocarpal joint of left wrist D, S
- ● S63.026 Dislocation of radiocarpal joint of unspecified wrist D, S

● S63.03 **Subluxation and dislocation of midcarpal joint**
- ● S63.031 Subluxation of midcarpal joint of right wrist D, S
- ● S63.032 Subluxation of midcarpal joint of left wrist D, S
- ● S63.033 Subluxation of midcarpal joint of unspecified wrist D, S
- ● S63.034 Dislocation of midcarpal joint of right wrist D, S

- ● S63.035 Dislocation of midcarpal joint of left wrist D, S
- ● S63.036 Dislocation of midcarpal joint of unspecified wrist D, S

● S63.04 **Subluxation and dislocation of carpometacarpal joint of thumb**
> **Excludes2** interphalangeal subluxation and dislocation of thumb (S63.1-)
- ● S63.041 Subluxation of carpometacarpal joint of right thumb D, S
- ● S63.042 Subluxation of carpometacarpal joint of left thumb D, S
- ● S63.043 Subluxation of carpometacarpal joint of unspecified thumb D, S
- ● S63.044 Dislocation of carpometacarpal joint of right thumb D, S
- ● S63.045 Dislocation of carpometacarpal joint of left thumb D, S
- ● S63.046 Dislocation of carpometacarpal joint of unspecified thumb D, S

● S63.05 **Subluxation and dislocation of other carpometacarpal joint**
> **Excludes2** subluxation and dislocation of carpometacarpal joint of thumb (S63.04-)
- ● S63.051 Subluxation of other carpometacarpal joint of right hand D, S
- ● S63.052 Subluxation of other carpometacarpal joint of left hand D, S
- ● S63.053 Subluxation of other carpometacarpal joint of unspecified hand D, S
- ● S63.054 Dislocation of other carpometacarpal joint of right hand D, S
- ● S63.055 Dislocation of other carpometacarpal joint of left hand D, S
- ● S63.056 Dislocation of other carpometacarpal joint of unspecified hand D, S

● S63.06 **Subluxation and dislocation of metacarpal (bone), proximal end**
- ● S63.061 Subluxation of metacarpal (bone), proximal end of right hand D, S
- ● S63.062 Subluxation of metacarpal (bone), proximal end of left hand D, S
- ● S63.063 Subluxation of metacarpal (bone), proximal end of unspecified hand D, S
- ● S63.064 Dislocation of metacarpal (bone), proximal end of right hand D, S
- ● S63.065 Dislocation of metacarpal (bone), proximal end of left hand D, S
- ● S63.066 Dislocation of metacarpal (bone), proximal end of unspecified hand D, S

● Unacceptable Principal Diagnosis ● Use Additional Character(s) ■ Unspecified ▶ Manifestation Code
OGCR Official Guidelines for Coding and Reporting Excludes 1 Excludes 2 Includes Use additional Code first Code also

CHAPTER 19 (S00-T88)

● **S63.07**   **Subluxation and dislocation of distal end of ulna**

   ● **S63.071**   Subluxation of distal end of right ulna D, S 🔖

   ● **S63.072**   Subluxation of distal end of left ulna D, S 🔖

   ●■ **S63.073**   Subluxation of distal end of unspecified ulna D, S 🔖

   ● **S63.074**   Dislocation of distal end of right ulna D, S 🔖

   ● **S63.075**   Dislocation of distal end of left ulna D, S 🔖

   ●■ **S63.076**   Dislocation of distal end of unspecified ulna D, S 🔖

● **S63.09**   **Other subluxation and dislocation of wrist and hand**

   ● **S63.091**   Other subluxation of right wrist and hand D, S 🔖

   ● **S63.092**   Other subluxation of left wrist and hand D, S 🔖

   ●■ **S63.093**   Other subluxation of unspecified wrist and hand D, S 🔖

   ● **S63.094**   Other dislocation of right wrist and hand D, S 🔖

   ● **S63.095**   Other dislocation of left wrist and hand D, S 🔖

   ●■ **S63.096**   Other dislocation of unspecified wrist and hand D, S 🔖

● **S63.1**   **Subluxation and dislocation of thumb**

   ● **S63.10**   **Unspecified subluxation and dislocation of thumb**

     ●■ **S63.101**   Unspecified subluxation of right thumb D, S 🔖

     ●■ **S63.102**   Unspecified subluxation of left thumb D, S 🔖

     ●■ **S63.103**   Unspecified subluxation of unspecified thumb D, S 🔖

     ●■ **S63.104**   Unspecified dislocation of right thumb D, S 🔖

     ●■ **S63.105**   Unspecified dislocation of left thumb D, S 🔖

     ●■ **S63.106**   Unspecified dislocation of unspecified thumb D, S 🔖

   ● **S63.11**   **Subluxation and dislocation of metacarpophalangeal joint of thumb**

     ● **S63.111**   Subluxation of metacarpophalangeal joint of right thumb D, S 🔖

     ● **S63.112**   Subluxation of metacarpophalangeal joint of left thumb D, S 🔖

     ●■ **S63.113**   Subluxation of metacarpophalangeal joint of unspecified thumb D, S 🔖

     ● **S63.114**   Dislocation of metacarpophalangeal joint of right thumb D, S 🔖

     ● **S63.115**   Dislocation of metacarpophalangeal joint of left thumb D, S 🔖

     ●■ **S63.116**   Dislocation of metacarpophalangeal joint of unspecified thumb D, S 🔖

● **S63.12**   **Subluxation and dislocation of unspecified interphalangeal joint of thumb**

   ●■ **S63.121**   Subluxation of unspecified interphalangeal joint of right thumb D, S 🔖

   ●■ **S63.122**   Subluxation of unspecified interphalangeal joint of left thumb D, S 🔖

   ●■ **S63.123**   Subluxation of unspecified interphalangeal joint of unspecified thumb D, S 🔖

   ●■ **S63.124**   Dislocation of unspecified interphalangeal joint of right thumb D, S 🔖

   ●■ **S63.125**   Dislocation of unspecified interphalangeal joint of left thumb D, S 🔖

   ●■ **S63.126**   Dislocation of unspecified interphalangeal joint of unspecified thumb D, S 🔖

● **S63.13**   **Subluxation and dislocation of proximal interphalangeal joint of thumb**

   ● **S63.131**   Subluxation of proximal interphalangeal joint of right thumb D, S 🔖

   ● **S63.132**   Subluxation of proximal interphalangeal joint of left thumb D, S 🔖

   ●■ **S63.133**   Subluxation of proximal interphalangeal joint of unspecified thumb D, S 🔖

   ● **S63.134**   Dislocation of proximal interphalangeal joint of right thumb D, S 🔖

   ● **S63.135**   Dislocation of proximal interphalangeal joint of left thumb D, S 🔖

   ●■ **S63.136**   Dislocation of proximal interphalangeal joint of unspecified thumb D, S 🔖

● **S63.14**   **Subluxation and dislocation of distal interphalangeal joint of thumb**

   S63.141   Subluxation of distal interphalangeal joint of right thumb D, S 🔖

   ● **S63.142**   Subluxation of distal interphalangeal joint of left thumb D, S 🔖

   ●■ **S63.143**   Subluxation of distal interphalangeal joint of unspecified thumb D, S 🔖

   ● **S63.144**   Dislocation of distal interphalangeal joint of right thumb D, S 🔖

   ● **S63.145**   Dislocation of distal interphalangeal joint of left thumb D, S 🔖

   ●■ **S63.146**   Dislocation of distal interphalangeal joint of unspecified thumb D, S 🔖

N Newborn Age: 0   **P** Pediatric Age: 0–17   **M** Maternity DX: 12–55   **A** Adult Age: 15–124   ♀ Females Only   ♂ Males Only

🔖 Complication\Comorbidity   🔖 Major C\C   🔖 Present on Admission Requirement   🔖 Hospital-Acquired Condition   1509

● **S63.2 Subluxation and dislocation of other finger(s)**

> [Excludes2] subluxation and dislocation of thumb (S63.1-)

● **S63.20 Unspecified subluxation of other finger**

● ■ **S63.200** Unspecified subluxation of right index finger D, S 🔖

● ■ **S63.201** Unspecified subluxation of left index finger D, S 🔖

● ■ **S63.202** Unspecified subluxation of right middle finger D, S 🔖

● ■ **S63.203** Unspecified subluxation of left middle finger D, S 🔖

● ■ **S63.204** Unspecified subluxation of right ring finger D, S 🔖

● ■ **S63.205** Unspecified subluxation of left ring finger D, S 🔖

● ■ **S63.206** Unspecified subluxation of right little finger D, S 🔖

● ■ **S63.207** Unspecified subluxation of left little finger D, S 🔖

● ■ **S63.208** Unspecified subluxation of other finger D, S 🔖
> Unspecified subluxation of specified finger with unspecified laterality

● ■ **S63.209** Unspecified subluxation of unspecified finger D, S 🔖

● **S63.21 Subluxation of metacarpophalangeal joint of finger**

● **S63.210** Subluxation of metacarpophalangeal joint of right index finger D, S 🔖

● **S63.211** Subluxation of metacarpophalangeal joint of left index finger D, S 🔖

● **S63.212** Subluxation of metacarpophalangeal joint of right middle finger D, S 🔖

● **S63.213** Subluxation of metacarpophalangeal joint of left middle finger D, S 🔖

● **S63.214** Subluxation of metacarpophalangeal joint of right ring finger D, S 🔖

● **S63.215** Subluxation of metacarpophalangeal joint of left ring finger D, S 🔖

● **S63.216** Subluxation of metacarpophalangeal joint of right little finger D, S 🔖

● **S63.217** Subluxation of metacarpophalangeal joint of left little finger D, S 🔖

● **S63.218** Subluxation of metacarpophalangeal joint of other finger D, S 🔖
> Subluxation of metacarpophalangeal joint of specified finger with unspecified laterality

● ■ **S63.219** Subluxation of metacarpophalangeal joint of unspecified finger D, S 🔖

● **S63.22 Subluxation of unspecified interphalangeal joint of finger**

● ■ **S63.220** Subluxation of unspecified interphalangeal joint of right index finger D, S 🔖

● ■ **S63.221** Subluxation of unspecified interphalangeal joint of left index finger D, S 🔖

● ■ **S63.222** Subluxation of unspecified interphalangeal joint of right middle finger D, S 🔖

● ■ **S63.223** Subluxation of unspecified interphalangeal joint of left middle finger D, S 🔖

● ■ **S63.224** Subluxation of unspecified interphalangeal joint of right ring finger D, S 🔖

● ■ **S63.225** Subluxation of unspecified interphalangeal joint of left ring finger D, S 🔖

● ■ **S63.226** Subluxation of unspecified interphalangeal joint of right little finger D, S 🔖

● ■ **S63.227** Subluxation of unspecified interphalangeal joint of left little finger D, S 🔖

● ■ **S63.228** Subluxation of unspecified interphalangeal joint of other finger D, S 🔖
> Subluxation of unspecified interphalangeal joint of specified finger with unspecified laterality

● ■ **S63.229** Subluxation of unspecified interphalangeal joint of unspecified finger D, S 🔖

● **S63.23 Subluxation of proximal interphalangeal joint of finger**

● **S63.230** Subluxation of proximal interphalangeal joint of right index finger D, S 🔖

● **S63.231** Subluxation of proximal interphalangeal joint of left index finger D, S 🔖

● **S63.232** Subluxation of proximal interphalangeal joint of right middle finger D, S 🔖

● **S63.233** Subluxation of proximal interphalangeal joint of left middle finger D, S 🔖

● **S63.234** Subluxation of proximal interphalangeal joint of right ring finger D, S 🔖

● **S63.235** Subluxation of proximal interphalangeal joint of left ring finger D, S 🔖

● **S63.236** Subluxation of proximal interphalangeal joint of right little finger D, S 🔖

● **S63.237** Subluxation of proximal interphalangeal joint of left little finger D, S 🔖

● Unacceptable Principal Diagnosis   ● Use Additional Character(s)   ■ Unspecified   ▶ Manifestation Code
OGCR Official Guidelines for Coding and Reporting   [Excludes 1]   [Excludes 2]   Includes   Use additional   Code first   Code also

● S63.238   **Subluxation of proximal interphalangeal joint of other finger** D, S 🔵
    Subluxation of proximal interphalangeal joint of specified finger with unspecified laterality

●■ S63.239   **Subluxation of proximal interphalangeal joint of unspecified finger** D, S 🔵

● S63.24   **Subluxation of distal interphalangeal joint of finger**

    ● S63.240   **Subluxation of distal interphalangeal joint of right index finger** D, S 🔵

    ● S63.241   **Subluxation of distal interphalangeal joint of left index finger** D, S 🔵

    ● S63.242   **Subluxation of distal interphalangeal joint of right middle finger** D, S 🔵

    ● S63.243   **Subluxation of distal interphalangeal joint of left middle finger** D, S 🔵

    ● S63.244   **Subluxation of distal interphalangeal joint of right ring finger** D, S 🔵

    ● S63.245   **Subluxation of distal interphalangeal joint of left ring finger** D, S 🔵

    ● S63.246   **Subluxation of distal interphalangeal joint of right little finger** D, S 🔵

    ● S63.247   **Subluxation of distal interphalangeal joint of left little finger** D, S 🔵

    ● S63.248   **Subluxation of distal interphalangeal joint of other finger** D, S 🔵
       Subluxation of distal interphalangeal joint of specified finger with unspecified laterality

    ●■ S63.249   **Subluxation of distal interphalangeal joint of unspecified finger** D, S 🔵

● S63.25   **Unspecified dislocation of other finger**

    ●■ S63.250   **Unspecified dislocation of right index finger** D, S 🔵

    ●■ S63.251   **Unspecified dislocation of left index finger** D, S 🔵

    ●■ S63.252   **Unspecified dislocation of right middle finger** D, S 🔵

    ●■ S63.253   **Unspecified dislocation of left middle finger** D, S 🔵

    ●■ S63.254   **Unspecified dislocation of right ring finger** D, S 🔵

    ●■ S63.255   **Unspecified dislocation of left ring finger** D, S 🔵

    ●■ S63.256   **Unspecified dislocation of right little finger** D, S 🔵

    ●■ S63.257   **Unspecified dislocation of left little finger** D, S 🔵

●■ S63.258   **Unspecified dislocation of other finger** D, S 🔵
    Unspecified dislocation of specified finger with unspecified laterality

●■ S63.259   **Unspecified dislocation of unspecified finger** D, S 🔵
    Unspecified dislocation of specified finger with unspecified laterality

● S63.26   **Dislocation of metacarpophalangeal joint of finger**

    ● S63.260   **Dislocation of metacarpophalangeal joint of right index finger** D, S 🔵

    ● S63.261   **Dislocation of metacarpophalangeal joint of left index finger** D, S 🔵

    ● S63.262   **Dislocation of metacarpophalangeal joint of right middle finger** D, S 🔵

    ● S63.263   **Dislocation of metacarpophalangeal joint of left middle finger** D, S 🔵

    ● S63.264   **Dislocation of metacarpophalangeal joint of right ring finger** D, S 🔵

    ● S63.265   **Dislocation of metacarpophalangeal joint of left ring finger** D, S 🔵

    ● S63.266   **Dislocation of metacarpophalangeal joint of right little finger** D, S 🔵

    ● S63.267   **Dislocation of metacarpophalangeal joint of left little finger** D, S 🔵

    ● S63.268   **Dislocation of metacarpophalangeal joint of other finger** D, S 🔵
       Dislocation of metacarpophalangeal joint of specified finger with unspecified laterality

    ●■ S63.269   **Dislocation of metacarpophalangeal joint of unspecified finger** D, S 🔵

● S63.27   **Dislocation of unspecified interphalangeal joint of finger**

    ●■ S63.270   **Dislocation of unspecified interphalangeal joint of right index finger** D, S 🔵

    ●■ S63.271   **Dislocation of unspecified interphalangeal joint of left index finger** D, S 🔵

    ●■ S63.272   **Dislocation of unspecified interphalangeal joint of right middle finger** D, S 🔵

    ●■ S63.273   **Dislocation of unspecified interphalangeal joint of left middle finger** D, S 🔵

    ●■ S63.274   **Dislocation of unspecified interphalangeal joint of right ring finger** D, S 🔵

CHAPTER 19 (S00-T88)

N Newborn Age: 0   **P** Pediatric Age: 0–17   **M** Maternity DX: 12–55   **A** Adult Age: 15–124   ♀ Females Only   ♂ Males Only

🔵 Complication\Comorbidity   Major C\C   Present on Admission Requirement   Hospital-Acquired Condition

1511

● ■ **S63.275**   Dislocation of unspecified interphalangeal joint of left ring finger D, S 🔎

● ■ **S63.276**   Dislocation of unspecified interphalangeal joint of right little finger D, S 🔎

● ■ **S63.277**   Dislocation of unspecified interphalangeal joint of left little finger D, S 🔎

● ■ **S63.278**   Dislocation of unspecified interphalangeal joint of other finger D, S 🔎

> Dislocation of unspecified interphalangeal joint of specified finger with unspecified laterality

● ■ **S63.279**   Dislocation of unspecified interphalangeal joint of unspecified finger D, S 🔎

> Dislocation of unspecified interphalangeal joint of specified finger without specified laterality

● **S63.28**   Dislocation of proximal interphalangeal joint of finger

    ● **S63.280**   Dislocation of proximal interphalangeal joint of right index finger D, S 🔎

    ● **S63.281**   Dislocation of proximal interphalangeal joint of left index finger D, S 🔎

    ● **S63.282**   Dislocation of proximal interphalangeal joint of right middle finger D, S 🔎

    ● **S63.283**   Dislocation of proximal interphalangeal joint of left middle finger D, S 🔎

    ● **S63.284**   Dislocation of proximal interphalangeal joint of right ring finger D, S 🔎

    ● **S63.285**   Dislocation of proximal interphalangeal joint of left ring finger D, S 🔎

    ● **S63.286**   Dislocation of proximal interphalangeal joint of right little finger D, S 🔎

    ● **S63.287**   Dislocation of proximal interphalangeal joint of left little finger D, S 🔎

    ● **S63.288**   Dislocation of proximal interphalangeal joint of other finger D, S 🔎

> Dislocation of proximal interphalangeal joint of specified finger with unspecified laterality

    ● ■ **S63.289**   Dislocation of proximal interphalangeal joint of unspecified finger D, S 🔎

● **S63.29**   Dislocation of distal interphalangeal joint of finger

    ● **S63.290**   Dislocation of distal interphalangeal joint of right index finger D, S 🔎

    ● **S63.291**   Dislocation of distal interphalangeal joint of left index finger D, S 🔎

    ● **S63.292**   Dislocation of distal interphalangeal joint of right middle finger D, S 🔎

    ● **S63.293**   Dislocation of distal interphalangeal joint of left middle finger D, S 🔎

    ● **S63.294**   Dislocation of distal interphalangeal joint of right ring finger D, S 🔎

    ● **S63.295**   Dislocation of distal interphalangeal joint of left ring finger D, S 🔎

    ● **S63.296**   Dislocation of distal interphalangeal joint of right little finger D, S 🔎

    ● **S63.297**   Dislocation of distal interphalangeal joint of left little finger D, S 🔎

    ● **S63.298**   Dislocation of distal interphalangeal joint of other finger D, S 🔎

> Dislocation of distal interphalangeal joint of specified finger with unspecified laterality

    ● ■ **S63.299**   Dislocation of distal interphalangeal joint of unspecified finger D, S 🔎

● **S63.3**   Traumatic rupture of ligament of wrist

    ● **S63.30**   Traumatic rupture of unspecified ligament of wrist

      ● ■ **S63.301**   Traumatic rupture of unspecified ligament of right wrist D, S 🔎

      ● ■ **S63.302**   Traumatic rupture of unspecified ligament of left wrist D, S 🔎

      ● ■ **S63.309**   Traumatic rupture of unspecified ligament of unspecified wrist D, S 🔎

    ● **S63.31**   Traumatic rupture of collateral ligament of wrist

      ● **S63.311**   Traumatic rupture of collateral ligament of right wrist D, S 🔎

      ● **S63.312**   Traumatic rupture of collateral ligament of left wrist D, S 🔎

      ● ■ **S63.319**   Traumatic rupture of collateral ligament of unspecified wrist D, S 🔎

    ● **S63.32**   Traumatic rupture of radiocarpal ligament

      ● **S63.321**   Traumatic rupture of right radiocarpal ligament D, S 🔎

      ● **S63.322**   Traumatic rupture of left radiocarpal ligament D, S 🔎

      ● ■ **S63.329**   Traumatic rupture of unspecified radiocarpal ligament D, S 🔎

●   Unacceptable Principal Diagnosis   ●   Use Additional Character(s)   ■   Unspecified   ▶   Manifestation Code

OGCR   Official Guidelines for Coding and Reporting   Excludes 1   Excludes 2   Includes   Use additional   Code first   Code also

● S63.33   Traumatic rupture of ulnocarpal (palmar) ligament

    ● S63.331   Traumatic rupture of right ulnocarpal (palmar) ligament D, S 🔖

    ● S63.332   Traumatic rupture of left ulnocarpal (palmar) ligament D, S 🔖

    ●■ S63.339   Traumatic rupture of unspecified ulnocarpal (palmar) ligament D, S 🔖

● S63.39   Traumatic rupture of other ligament of wrist

    ● S63.391   Traumatic rupture of other ligament of right wrist D, S 🔖

    ● S63.392   Traumatic rupture of other ligament of left wrist D, S 🔖

    ●■ S63.399   Traumatic rupture of other ligament of unspecified wrist D, S 🔖

● S63.4   Traumatic rupture of ligament of finger at metacarpophalangeal and interphalangeal joint(s)

    ● S63.40   Traumatic rupture of unspecified ligament of finger at metacarpophalangeal and interphalangeal joint

      ●■ S63.400   Traumatic rupture of unspecified ligament of right index finger at metacarpophalangeal and interphalangeal joint D, S 🔖

      ●■ S63.401   Traumatic rupture of unspecified ligament of left index finger at metacarpophalangeal and interphalangeal joint D, S 🔖

      ●■ S63.402   Traumatic rupture of unspecified ligament of right middle finger at metacarpophalangeal and interphalangeal joint D, S 🔖

      ●■ S63.403   Traumatic rupture of unspecified ligament of left middle finger at metacarpophalangeal and interphalangeal joint D, S 🔖

      ●■ S63.404   Traumatic rupture of unspecified ligament of right ring finger at metacarpophalangeal and interphalangeal joint D, S 🔖

      ●■ S63.405   Traumatic rupture of unspecified ligament of left ring finger at metacarpophalangeal and interphalangeal joint D, S 🔖

      ●■ S63.406   Traumatic rupture of unspecified ligament of right little finger at metacarpophalangeal and interphalangeal joint D, S 🔖

      ●■ S63.407   Traumatic rupture of unspecified ligament of left little finger at metacarpophalangeal and interphalangeal joint D, S 🔖

      ●■ S63.408   Traumatic rupture of unspecified ligament of other finger at metacarpophalangeal and interphalangeal joint D, S 🔖
         Traumatic rupture of unspecified ligament of specified finger with unspecified laterality at metacarpophalangeal and interphalangeal joint

●■ S63.409   Traumatic rupture of unspecified ligament of unspecified finger at metacarpophalangeal and interphalangeal joint D, S 🔖

● S63.41   Traumatic rupture of collateral ligament of finger at metacarpophalangeal and interphalangeal joint

    ● S63.410   Traumatic rupture of collateral ligament of right index finger at metacarpophalangeal and interphalangeal joint D, S 🔖

    ● S63.411   Traumatic rupture of collateral ligament of left index finger at metacarpophalangeal and interphalangeal joint D, S 🔖

    ● S63.412   Traumatic rupture of collateral ligament of right middle finger at metacarpophalangeal and interphalangeal joint D, S 🔖

    ● S63.413   Traumatic rupture of collateral ligament of left middle finger at metacarpophalangeal and interphalangeal joint D, S 🔖

    ● S63.414   Traumatic rupture of collateral ligament of right ring finger at metacarpophalangeal and interphalangeal joint D, S 🔖

    ● S63.415   Traumatic rupture of collateral ligament of left ring finger at metacarpophalangeal and interphalangeal joint D, S 🔖

    ● S63.416   Traumatic rupture of collateral ligament of right little finger at metacarpophalangeal and interphalangeal joint D, S 🔖

    ● S63.417   Traumatic rupture of collateral ligament of left little finger at metacarpophalangeal and interphalangeal joint D, S 🔖

    ● S63.418   Traumatic rupture of collateral ligament of other finger at metacarpophalangeal and interphalangeal joint D, S 🔖
       Traumatic rupture of collateral ligament of specified finger with unspecified laterality at metacarpophalangeal and interphalangeal joint

    ●■ S63.419   Traumatic rupture of collateral ligament of unspecified finger at metacarpophalangeal and interphalangeal joint D, S 🔖

● S63.42   Traumatic rupture of palmar ligament of finger at metacarpophalangeal and interphalangeal joint

    ● S63.420   Traumatic rupture of palmar ligament of right index finger at metacarpophalangeal and interphalangeal joint D, S 🔖

    ● S63.421   Traumatic rupture of palmar ligament of left index finger at metacarpophalangeal and interphalangeal joint D, S 🔖

    ● S63.422   Traumatic rupture of palmar ligament of right middle finger at metacarpophalangeal and interphalangeal joint D, S 🔖

N Newborn Age: 0   **P** Pediatric Age: 0–17   **M** Maternity DX: 12–55   **A** Adult Age: 15–124   ♀ Females Only   ♂ Males Only

🔖 Complication\Comorbidity   🔖 Major C\C   🔖 Present on Admission Requirement   🔖 Hospital-Acquired Condition

1513

● S63.423   Traumatic rupture of palmar ligament of left middle finger at metacarpophalangeal and interphalangeal joint D, S ✎

● S63.424   Traumatic rupture of palmar ligament of right ring finger at metacarpophalangeal and interphalangeal joint D, S ✎

● S63.425   Traumatic rupture of palmar ligament of left ring finger at metacarpophalangeal and interphalangeal joint D, S ✎

● S63.426   Traumatic rupture of palmar ligament of right little finger at metacarpophalangeal and interphalangeal joint D, S ✎

● S63.427   Traumatic rupture of palmar ligament of left little finger at metacarpophalangeal and interphalangeal joint D, S ✎

● S63.428   Traumatic rupture of palmar ligament of other finger at metacarpophalangeal and interphalangeal joint D, S ✎
     Traumatic rupture of palmar ligament of specified finger with unspecified laterality at metacarpophalangeal and interphalangeal joint

●■ S63.429   Traumatic rupture of palmar ligament of unspecified finger at metacarpophalangeal and interphalangeal joint D, S ✎

● S63.43   Traumatic rupture of volar plate of finger at metacarpophalangeal and interphalangeal joint

● S63.430   Traumatic rupture of volar plate of right index finger at metacarpophalangeal and interphalangeal joint D, S ✎

● S63.431   Traumatic rupture of volar plate of left index finger at metacarpophalangeal and interphalangeal joint D, S ✎

● S63.432   Traumatic rupture of volar plate of right middle finger at metacarpophalangeal and interphalangeal joint D, S ✎

● S63.433   Traumatic rupture of volar plate of left middle finger at metacarpophalangeal and interphalangeal joint D, S ✎

● S63.434   Traumatic rupture of volar plate of right ring finger at metacarpophalangeal and interphalangeal joint D, S ✎

● S63.435   Traumatic rupture of volar plate of left ring finger at metacarpophalangeal and interphalangeal joint D, S ✎

● S63.436   Traumatic rupture of volar plate of right little finger at metacarpophalangeal and interphalangeal joint D, S ✎

● S63.437   Traumatic rupture of volar plate of left little finger at metacarpophalangeal and interphalangeal joint D, S ✎

● S63.438   Traumatic rupture of volar plate of other finger at metacarpophalangeal and interphalangeal joint D, S ✎
     Traumatic rupture of volar plate of specified finger with unspecified laterality at metacarpophalangeal and interphalangeal joint

●■ S63.439   Traumatic rupture of volar plate of unspecified finger at metacarpophalangeal and interphalangeal joint D, S ✎

● S63.49   Traumatic rupture of other ligament of finger at metacarpophalangeal and interphalangeal joint

● S63.490   Traumatic rupture of other ligament of right index finger at metacarpophalangeal and interphalangeal joint D, S ✎

● S63.491   Traumatic rupture of other ligament of left index finger at metacarpophalangeal and interphalangeal joint D, S ✎

● S63.492   Traumatic rupture of other ligament of right middle finger at metacarpophalangeal and interphalangeal joint D, S ✎

● S63.493   Traumatic rupture of other ligament of left middle finger at metacarpophalangeal and interphalangeal joint D, S ✎

● S63.494   Traumatic rupture of other ligament of right ring finger at metacarpophalangeal and interphalangeal joint D, S ✎

● S63.495   Traumatic rupture of other ligament of left ring finger at metacarpophalangeal and interphalangeal joint D, S ✎

● S63.496   Traumatic rupture of other ligament of right little finger at metacarpophalangeal and interphalangeal joint D, S ✎

● S63.497   Traumatic rupture of other ligament of left little finger at metacarpophalangeal and interphalangeal joint D, S ✎

● S63.498   Traumatic rupture of other ligament of other finger at metacarpophalangeal and interphalangeal joint D, S ✎
     Traumatic rupture of ligament of specified finger with unspecified laterality at metacarpophalangeal and interphalangeal joint

●■ S63.499   Traumatic rupture of other ligament of unspecified finger at metacarpophalangeal and interphalangeal joint D, S ✎

● S63.5   Other and unspecified sprain of wrist

● S63.50   Unspecified sprain of wrist

●■ S63.501   Unspecified sprain of right wrist D, S ✎

●■ S63.502   Unspecified sprain of left wrist D, S ✎

●■ S63.509   Unspecified sprain of unspecified wrist D, S ✎

●   Unacceptable Principal Diagnosis   ●   Use Additional Character(s)   ■   Unspecified   ▶   Manifestation Code

OGCR   Official Guidelines for Coding and Reporting   Excludes 1   Excludes 2   Includes   Use additional   Code first   Code also

CHAPTER 19 (S00-T88)

- ● S63.51   Sprain of carpal (joint)
  - ● S63.511   Sprain of carpal joint of right wrist D, S 🔖
  - ● S63.512   Sprain of carpal joint of left wrist D, S 🔖
  - ●■ S63.519   Sprain of carpal joint of unspecified wrist D, S 🔖
- ● S63.52   Sprain of radiocarpal joint
  - Excludes1   traumatic rupture of radiocarpal ligament (S63.32-)
  - ● S63.521   Sprain of radiocarpal joint of right wrist D, S 🔖
  - ● S63.522   Sprain of radiocarpal joint of left wrist D, S 🔖
  - ●■ S63.529   Sprain of radiocarpal joint of unspecified wrist D, S 🔖
- ● S63.59   Other specified sprain of wrist
  - ● S63.591   Other specified sprain of right wrist D, S 🔖
  - ● S63.592   Other specified sprain of left wrist D, S 🔖
  - ●■ S63.599   Other specified sprain of unspecified wrist D, S 🔖
- ● S63.6   Other and unspecified sprain of finger(s)
  - Excludes1   traumatic rupture of ligament of finger at metacarpophalangeal and interphalangeal joint(s) (S63.4-)
  - ● S63.60   Unspecified sprain of thumb
    - ●■ S63.601   Unspecified sprain of right thumb D, S 🔖
    - ●■ S63.602   Unspecified sprain of left thumb D, S 🔖
    - ●■ S63.609   Unspecified sprain of unspecified thumb D, S 🔖
  - ● S63.61   Unspecified sprain of other and unspecified finger(s)
    - ●■ S63.610   Unspecified sprain of right index finger D, S 🔖
    - ●■ S63.611   Unspecified sprain of left index finger D, S 🔖
    - ●■ S63.612   Unspecified sprain of right middle finger D, S 🔖
    - ●■ S63.613   Unspecified sprain of left middle finger D, S 🔖
    - ●■ S63.614   Unspecified sprain of right ring finger D, S 🔖
    - ●■ S63.615   Unspecified sprain of left ring finger D, S 🔖
    - ●■ S63.616   Unspecified sprain of right little finger D, S 🔖
    - ●■ S63.617   Unspecified sprain of left little finger D, S 🔖
    - ●■ S63.618   Unspecified sprain of other finger D, S 🔖
        Unspecified sprain of specified finger with unspecified laterality
    - ●■ S63.619   Unspecified sprain of unspecified finger D, S 🔖

- ● S63.62   Sprain of interphalangeal joint of thumb
  - ● S63.621   Sprain of interphalangeal joint of right thumb D, S 🔖
  - ● S63.622   Sprain of interphalangeal joint of left thumb D, S 🔖
  - ●■ S63.629   Sprain of interphalangeal joint of unspecified thumb D, S 🔖
- ● S63.63   Sprain of interphalangeal joint of other and unspecified finger(s)
  - ● S63.630   Sprain of interphalangeal joint of right index finger D, S 🔖
  - ● S63.631   Sprain of interphalangeal joint of left index finger D, S 🔖
  - ● S63.632   Sprain of interphalangeal joint of right middle finger D, S 🔖
  - ● S63.633   Sprain of interphalangeal joint of left middle finger D, S 🔖
  - ● S63.634   Sprain of interphalangeal joint of right ring finger D, S 🔖
  - ● S63.635   Sprain of interphalangeal joint of left ring finger D, S 🔖
  - ● S63.636   Sprain of interphalangeal joint of right little finger D, S 🔖
  - ● S63.637   Sprain of interphalangeal joint of left little finger D, S 🔖
  - ● S63.638   Sprain of interphalangeal joint of other finger D, S 🔖
  - ●■ S63.639   Sprain of interphalangeal joint of unspecified finger D, S 🔖
- ● S63.64   Sprain of metacarpophalangeal joint of thumb
  - ● S63.641   Sprain of metacarpophalangeal joint of right thumb D, S 🔖
  - ● S63.642   Sprain of metacarpophalangeal joint of left thumb D, S 🔖
  - ●■ S63.649   Sprain of metacarpophalangeal joint of unspecified thumb D, S 🔖
- ● S63.65   Sprain of metacarpophalangeal joint of other and unspecified finger(s)
  - ● S63.650   Sprain of metacarpophalangeal joint of right index finger D, S 🔖
  - ● S63.651   Sprain of metacarpophalangeal joint of left index finger D, S 🔖
  - ● S63.652   Sprain of metacarpophalangeal joint of right middle finger D, S 🔖
  - ● S63.653   Sprain of metacarpophalangeal joint of left middle finger D, S 🔖
  - ● S63.654   Sprain of metacarpophalangeal joint of right ring finger D, S 🔖
  - ● S63.655   Sprain of metacarpophalangeal joint of left ring finger D, S 🔖
  - ● S63.656   Sprain of metacarpophalangeal joint of right little finger D, S 🔖
  - ● S63.657   Sprain of metacarpophalangeal joint of left little finger D, S 🔖
  - ● S63.658   Sprain of metacarpophalangeal joint of other finger D, S 🔖
        Sprain of metacarpophalangeal joint of specified finger with unspecified laterality
  - ●■ S63.659   Sprain of metacarpophalangeal joint of unspecified finger D, S 🔖

CHAPTER 19 (S00-T88)

CHAPTER 19 (S00-T88)

● S63.68   Other sprain of thumb
    ● S63.681   Other sprain of right thumb D, S 🔖
    ● S63.682   Other sprain of left thumb D, S 🔖
    ●■ S63.689   Other sprain of unspecified thumb D, S 🔖

● S63.69   Other sprain of other and unspecified finger(s)
    ● S63.690   Other sprain of right index finger D, S 🔖
    ● S63.691   Other sprain of left index finger D, S 🔖
    ● S63.692   Other sprain of right middle finger D, S 🔖
    ● S63.693   Other sprain of left middle finger D, S 🔖
    ● S63.694   Other sprain of right ring finger D, S 🔖
    ● S63.695   Other sprain of left ring finger D, S 🔖
    ● S63.696   Other sprain of right little finger D, S 🔖
    ● S63.697   Other sprain of left little finger D, S 🔖
    ● S63.698   Other sprain of other finger D, S 🔖
          Other sprain of specified finger with unspecified laterality
    ●■ S63.699   Other sprain of unspecified finger D, S 🔖

● S63.8   Sprain of other part of wrist and hand
    ● S63.8X   Sprain of other part of wrist and hand
       ● S63.8X1   Sprain of other part of right wrist and hand D, S 🔖
       ● S63.8X2   Sprain of other part of left wrist and hand D, S 🔖
       ●■ S63.8X9   Sprain of other part of unspecified wrist and hand D, S 🔖

● S63.9   Sprain of unspecified part of wrist and hand
    ●■ S63.90   Sprain of unspecified part of unspecified wrist and hand D, S 🔖
    ●■ S63.91   Sprain of unspecified part of right wrist and hand D, S 🔖
    ●■ S63.92   Sprain of unspecified part of left wrist and hand D, S 🔖

● S64   Injury of nerves at wrist and hand level

    The appropriate 7th character is to be added to each code from category S64

A	initial encounter
D	subsequent encounter
S	sequela

    Code also any associated open wound (S61.-)

● S64.0   Injury of ulnar nerve at wrist and hand level
    ●■ S64.00   Injury of ulnar nerve at wrist and hand level of unspecified arm D, S 🔖
    ● S64.01   Injury of ulnar nerve at wrist and hand level of right arm D, S 🔖
    ● S64.02   Injury of ulnar nerve at wrist and hand level of left arm D, S 🔖

● S64.1   Injury of median nerve at wrist and hand level
    ●■ S64.10   Injury of median nerve at wrist and hand level of unspecified arm D, S 🔖
    ● S64.11   Injury of median nerve at wrist and hand level of right arm D, S 🔖
    ● S64.12   Injury of median nerve at wrist and hand level of left arm D, S 🔖

● S64.2   Injury of radial nerve at wrist and hand level
    ●■ S64.20   Injury of radial nerve at wrist and hand level of unspecified arm D, S 🔖
    ● S64.21   Injury of radial nerve at wrist and hand level of right arm D, S 🔖
    ● S64.22   Injury of radial nerve at wrist and hand level of left arm D, S 🔖

● S64.3   Injury of digital nerve of thumb
    ●■ S64.30   Injury of digital nerve of unspecified thumb D, S 🔖
    ● S64.31   Injury of digital nerve of right thumb D, S 🔖
    ● S64.32   Injury of digital nerve of left thumb D, S 🔖

● S64.4   Injury of digital nerve of other and unspecified finger
    ●■ S64.40   Injury of digital nerve of unspecified finger D, S 🔖
    ● S64.49   Injury of digital nerve of other finger
       ● S64.490   Injury of digital nerve of right index finger D, S 🔖
       ● S64.491   Injury of digital nerve of left index finger D, S 🔖
       ● S64.492   Injury of digital nerve of right middle finger D, S 🔖
       ● S64.493   Injury of digital nerve of left middle finger D, S 🔖
       ● S64.494   Injury of digital nerve of right ring finger D, S 🔖
       ● S64.495   Injury of digital nerve of left ring finger D, S 🔖
       ● S64.496   Injury of digital nerve of right little finger D, S 🔖
       ● S64.497   Injury of digital nerve of left little finger D, S 🔖
       ● S64.498   Injury of digital nerve of other finger D, S 🔖
          Injury of digital nerve of specified finger with unspecified laterality

● S64.8   Injury of other nerves at wrist and hand level
    ● S64.8X   Injury of other nerves at wrist and hand level
       ● S64.8X1   Injury of other nerves at wrist and hand level of right arm D, S 🔖
       ● S64.8X2   Injury of other nerves at wrist and hand level of left arm D, S 🔖
       ●■ S64.8X9   Injury of other nerves at wrist and hand level of unspecified arm D, S 🔖

● Unacceptable Principal Diagnosis   ● Use Additional Character(s)   ■ Unspecified   ▶ Manifestation Code

OGCR Official Guidelines for Coding and Reporting   Excludes 1   Excludes 2   Includes   Use additional   Code first   Code also

● **S64.9**   **Injury of unspecified nerve at wrist and hand level**

    ●■ **S64.90**   Injury of unspecified nerve at wrist and hand level of unspecified arm D, S 🐾

    ●■ **S64.91**   Injury of unspecified nerve at wrist and hand level of right arm D, S 🐾

    ●■ **S64.92**   Injury of unspecified nerve at wrist and hand level of left arm D, S 🐾

● **S65**   **Injury of blood vessels at wrist and hand level**

    The appropriate 7th character is to be added to each code from category S65

A	initial encounter
D	subsequent encounter
S	sequela

    Code also any associated open wound (S61.-)

● **S65.0**   **Injury of ulnar artery at wrist and hand level**

    ● **S65.00**   Unspecified injury of ulnar artery at wrist and hand level

      ●■ **S65.001**   Unspecified injury of ulnar artery at wrist and hand level of right arm A 🐾, D, S 🐾

      ●■ **S65.002**   Unspecified injury of ulnar artery at wrist and hand level of left arm A 🐾, D, S 🐾

      ●■ **S65.009**   Unspecified injury of ulnar artery at wrist and hand level of unspecified arm A 🐾, D, S 🐾

    ● **S65.01**   Laceration of ulnar artery at wrist and hand level

      ● **S65.011**   Laceration of ulnar artery at wrist and hand level of right arm A 🐾, D, S 🐾

      ● **S65.012**   Laceration of ulnar artery at wrist and hand level of left arm A 🐾, D, S 🐾

      ●■ **S65.019**   Laceration of ulnar artery at wrist and hand level of unspecified arm A 🐾, D, S 🐾

    ● **S65.09**   Other specified injury of ulnar artery at wrist and hand level

      ● **S65.091**   Other specified injury of ulnar artery at wrist and hand level of right arm A 🐾, D, S 🐾

      ● **S65.092**   Other specified injury of ulnar artery at wrist and hand level of left arm A 🐾, D, S 🐾

      ●■ **S65.099**   Other specified injury of ulnar artery at wrist and hand level of unspecified arm A 🐾, D, S 🐾

● **S65.1**   **Injury of radial artery at wrist and hand level**

    ● **S65.10**   Unspecified injury of radial artery at wrist and hand level

      ●■ **S65.101**   Unspecified injury of radial artery at wrist and hand level of right arm A 🐾, D, S 🐾

      ●■ **S65.102**   Unspecified injury of radial artery at wrist and hand level of left arm A 🐾, D, S 🐾

      ●■ **S65.109**   Unspecified injury of radial artery at wrist and hand level of unspecified arm A 🐾, D, S 🐾

● **S65.11**   **Laceration of radial artery at wrist and hand level**

    ● **S65.111**   Laceration of radial artery at wrist and hand level of right arm A 🐾, D, S 🐾

    ● **S65.112**   Laceration of radial artery at wrist and hand level of left arm A 🐾, D, S 🐾

    ●■ **S65.119**   Laceration of radial artery at wrist and hand level of unspecified arm A 🐾, D, S 🐾

● **S65.19**   Other specified injury of radial artery at wrist and hand level

    ● **S65.191**   Other specified injury of radial artery at wrist and hand level of right arm A 🐾, D, S 🐾

    ● **S65.192**   Other specified injury of radial artery at wrist and hand level of left arm A 🐾, D, S 🐾

    ●■ **S65.199**   Other specified injury of radial artery at wrist and hand level of unspecified arm A 🐾, D, S 🐾

● **S65.2**   **Injury of superficial palmar arch**

    ● **S65.20**   Unspecified injury of superficial palmar arch

      ●■ **S65.201**   Unspecified injury of superficial palmar arch of right hand A 🐾, D, S 🐾

      ●■ **S65.202**   Unspecified injury of superficial palmar arch of left hand A 🐾, D, S 🐾

      ●■ **S65.209**   Unspecified injury of superficial palmar arch of unspecified hand A 🐾, D, S 🐾

    ● **S65.21**   Laceration of superficial palmar arch

      ● **S65.211**   Laceration of superficial palmar arch of right hand A 🐾, D, S 🐾

      ● **S65.212**   Laceration of superficial palmar arch of left hand A 🐾, D, S 🐾

      ●■ **S65.219**   Laceration of superficial palmar arch of unspecified hand A 🐾, D, S 🐾

    ● **S65.29**   Other specified injury of superficial palmar arch

      ● **S65.291**   Other specified injury of superficial palmar arch of right hand A 🐾, D, S 🐾

      ● **S65.292**   Other specified injury of superficial palmar arch of left hand A 🐾, D, S 🐾

      ●■ **S65.299**   Other specified injury of superficial palmar arch of unspecified hand A 🐾, D, S 🐾

● **S65.3**   **Injury of deep palmar arch**

    ● **S65.30**   Unspecified injury of deep palmar arch

      ●■ **S65.301**   Unspecified injury of deep palmar arch of right hand A 🐾, D, S 🐾

      ●■ **S65.302**   Unspecified injury of deep palmar arch of left hand A 🐾, D, S 🐾

      ●■ **S65.309**   Unspecified injury of deep palmar arch of unspecified hand A 🐾, D, S 🐾

N Newborn Age: 0   **P** Pediatric Age: 0–17   **M** Maternity DX: 12–55   **A** Adult Age: 15–124   ♀ Females Only   ♂ Males Only

🐾 Complication\Comorbidity   🐾 Major C\C   🐾 Present on Admission Requirement   🐾 Hospital-Acquired Condition

1517

CHAPTER 19 (S00-T88)

● S65.31   Laceration of deep palmar arch

    ● S65.311   Laceration of deep palmar arch of right hand A 🖐, D, S 🖐

    ● S65.312   Laceration of deep palmar arch of left hand A 🖐, D, S 🖐

    ●◼ S65.319   Laceration of deep palmar arch of unspecified hand A 🖐, D, S 🖐

● S65.39   Other specified injury of deep palmar arch

    ● S65.391   Other specified injury of deep palmar arch of right hand A 🖐, D, S 🖐

    ● S65.392   Other specified injury of deep palmar arch of left hand A 🖐, D, S 🖐

    ●◼ S65.399   Other specified injury of deep palmar arch of unspecified hand A 🖐, D, S 🖐

● S65.4   Injury of blood vessel of thumb

    ● S65.40   Unspecified injury of blood vessel of thumb

       ●◼ S65.401   Unspecified injury of blood vessel of right thumb A 🖐, D, S 🖐

       ●◼ S65.402   Unspecified injury of blood vessel of left thumb A 🖐, D, S 🖐

       ●◼ S65.409   Unspecified injury of blood vessel of unspecified thumb A 🖐, D, S 🖐

    ● S65.41   Laceration of blood vessel of thumb

       ● S65.411   Laceration of blood vessel of right thumb A 🖐, D, S 🖐

       ● S65.412   Laceration of blood vessel of left thumb A 🖐, D, S 🖐

       ●◼ S65.419   Laceration of blood vessel of unspecified thumb A 🖐, D, S 🖐

    ● S65.49   Other specified injury of blood vessel of thumb

       ● S65.491   Other specified injury of blood vessel of right thumb A 🖐, D, S 🖐

       ● S65.492   Other specified injury of blood vessel of left thumb A 🖐, D, S 🖐

       ●◼ S65.499   Other specified injury of blood vessel of unspecified thumb A 🖐, D, S 🖐

● S65.5   Injury of blood vessel of other and unspecified finger

    ● S65.50   Unspecified injury of blood vessel of other and unspecified finger

       ●◼ S65.500   Unspecified injury of blood vessel of right index finger A 🖐, D, S 🖐

       ●◼ S65.501   Unspecified injury of blood vessel of left index finger A 🖐, D, S 🖐

       ●◼ S65.502   Unspecified injury of blood vessel of right middle finger A 🖐, D, S 🖐

       ●◼ S65.503   Unspecified injury of blood vessel of left middle finger A 🖐, D, S 🖐

       ●◼ S65.504   Unspecified injury of blood vessel of right ring finger A 🖐, D, S 🖐

       ●◼ S65.505   Unspecified injury of blood vessel of left ring finger A 🖐, D, S 🖐

       ●◼ S65.506   Unspecified injury of blood vessel of right little finger A 🖐, D, S 🖐

       ●◼ S65.507   Unspecified injury of blood vessel of left little finger A 🖐, D, S 🖐

       ●◼ S65.508   Unspecified injury of blood vessel of other finger A 🖐, D, S 🖐

          Unspecified injury of blood vessel of specified finger with unspecified laterality

       ●◼ S65.509   Unspecified injury of blood vessel of unspecified finger A 🖐, D, S 🖐

    ● S65.51   Laceration of blood vessel of other and unspecified finger

       ● S65.510   Laceration of blood vessel of right index finger A 🖐, D, S 🖐

       ● S65.511   Laceration of blood vessel of left index finger A 🖐, D, S 🖐

       ● S65.512   Laceration of blood vessel of right middle finger A 🖐, D, S 🖐

       ● S65.513   Laceration of blood vessel of left middle finger A 🖐, D, S 🖐

       ● S65.514   Laceration of blood vessel of right ring finger A 🖐, D, S 🖐

       ● S65.515   Laceration of blood vessel of left ring finger A 🖐, D, S 🖐

       ● S65.516   Laceration of blood vessel of right little finger A 🖐, D, S 🖐

       ● S65.517   Laceration of blood vessel of left little finger A 🖐, D, S 🖐

       ● S65.518   Laceration of blood vessel of other finger A 🖐, D, S 🖐

          Laceration of blood vessel of specified finger with unspecified laterality

       ●◼ S65.519   Laceration of blood vessel of unspecified finger A 🖐, D, S 🖐

    ● S65.59   Other specified injury of blood vessel of other and unspecified finger

       ● S65.590   Other specified injury of blood vessel of right index finger A 🖐, D, S 🖐

       ● S65.591   Other specified injury of blood vessel of left index finger A 🖐, D, S 🖐

       ● S65.592   Other specified injury of blood vessel of right middle finger A 🖐, D, S 🖐

       ● S65.593   Other specified injury of blood vessel of left middle finger A 🖐, D, S 🖐

       ● S65.594   Other specified injury of blood vessel of right ring finger A 🖐, D, S 🖐

       ● S65.595   Other specified injury of blood vessel of left ring finger A 🖐, D, S 🖐

       ● S65.596   Other specified injury of blood vessel of right little finger A 🖐, D, S 🖐

CHAPTER 19 (S00-T88)

● S65.597   Other specified injury of blood vessel of left little finger A 🩸, D, S 🩹

● S65.598   Other specified injury of blood vessel of other finger A 🩸, D, S 🩹
     Other specified injury of blood vessel of specified finger with unspecified laterality

● ■ S65.599   Other specified injury of blood vessel of unspecified finger A 🩸, D, S 🩹

● S65.8   Injury of other blood vessels at wrist and hand level

   ● S65.80   Unspecified injury of other blood vessels at wrist and hand level

     ● ■ S65.801   Unspecified injury of other blood vessels at wrist and hand level of right arm A 🩸, D, S 🩹

     ● ■ S65.802   Unspecified injury of other blood vessels at wrist and hand level of left arm A 🩸, D, S 🩹

     ● ■ S65.809   Unspecified injury of other blood vessels at wrist and hand level of unspecified arm A 🩸, D, S 🩹

   ● S65.81   Laceration of other blood vessels at wrist and hand level

     ● S65.811   Laceration of other blood vessels at wrist and hand level of right arm A 🩸, D, S 🩹

     ● S65.812   Laceration of other blood vessels at wrist and hand level of left arm A 🩸, D, S 🩹

     ● ■ S65.819   Laceration of other blood vessels at wrist and hand level of unspecified arm A 🩸, D, S 🩹

   ● S65.89   Other specified injury of other blood vessels at wrist and hand level

     ● S65.891   Other specified injury of other blood vessels at wrist and hand level of right arm A 🩸, D, S 🩹

     ● S65.892   Other specified injury of other blood vessels at wrist and hand level of left arm A 🩸, D, S 🩹

     ● ■ S65.899   Other specified injury of other blood vessels at wrist and hand level of unspecified arm A 🩸, D, S 🩹

● S65.9   Injury of unspecified blood vessel at wrist and hand level

   ● S65.90   Unspecified injury of unspecified blood vessel at wrist and hand level

     ● ■ S65.901   Unspecified injury of unspecified blood vessel at wrist and hand level of right arm A 🩸, D, S 🩹

     ● ■ S65.902   Unspecified injury of unspecified blood vessel at wrist and hand level of left arm A 🩸, D, S 🩹

     ● ■ S65.909   Unspecified injury of unspecified blood vessel at wrist and hand level of unspecified arm A 🩸, D, S 🩹

● S65.91   Laceration of unspecified blood vessel at wrist and hand level

   ● ■ S65.911   Laceration of unspecified blood vessel at wrist and hand level of right arm A 🩸, D, S 🩹

   ● ■ S65.912   Laceration of unspecified blood vessel at wrist and hand level of left arm A 🩸, D, S 🩹

   ● ■ S65.919   Laceration of unspecified blood vessel at wrist and hand level of unspecified arm A 🩸, D, S 🩹

● S65.99   Other specified injury of unspecified blood vessel at wrist and hand level

   ● ■ S65.991   Other specified injury of unspecified blood vessel at wrist and hand of right arm A 🩸, D, S 🩹

   ● ■ S65.992   Other specified injury of unspecified blood vessel at wrist and hand of left arm A 🩸, D, S 🩹

   ● ■ S65.999   Other specified injury of unspecified blood vessel at wrist and hand of unspecified arm A 🩸, D, S 🩹

● S66   Injury of muscle, fascia and tendon at wrist and hand level

   Code also any associated open wound (S61.-)

   Excludes2   sprain of joints and ligaments of wrist and hand (S63.-)

   The appropriate 7th character is to be added to each code from category S66

     A   initial encounter
     D   subsequent encounter
     S   sequela

● S66.0   Injury of long flexor muscle, fascia and tendon of thumb at wrist and hand level

   ● S66.00   Unspecified injury of long flexor muscle, fascia and tendon of thumb at wrist and hand level

     ● ■ S66.001   Unspecified injury of long flexor muscle, fascia and tendon of right thumb at wrist and hand level D, S 🩹

     ● ■ S66.002   Unspecified injury of long flexor muscle, fascia and tendon of left thumb at wrist and hand level D, S 🩹

     ● ■ S66.009   Unspecified injury of long flexor muscle, fascia and tendon of unspecified thumb at wrist and hand level D, S 🩹

   ● S66.01   Strain of long flexor muscle, fascia and tendon of thumb at wrist and hand level

     ● S66.011   Strain of long flexor muscle, fascia and tendon of right thumb at wrist and hand level D, S 🩹

     ● S66.012   Strain of long flexor muscle, fascia and tendon of left thumb at wrist and hand level D, S 🩹

     ● ■ S66.019   Strain of long flexor muscle, fascia and tendon of unspecified thumb at wrist and hand level D, S 🩹

N Newborn Age: 0   **P** Pediatric Age: 0–17   **M** Maternity DX: 12–55   **A** Adult Age: 15–124   ♀ Females Only   ♂ Males Only

 Complication\Comorbidity   🩹 Major C\C   🩹 Present on Admission Requirement   🩹 Hospital-Acquired Condition

1519

● **S66.02** Laceration of long flexor muscle, fascia and tendon of thumb at wrist and hand level

● **S66.021** Laceration of long flexor muscle, fascia and tendon of right thumb at wrist and hand level A , D, S

● **S66.022** Laceration of long flexor muscle, fascia and tendon of left thumb at wrist and hand level A , D, S

●■ **S66.029** Laceration of long flexor muscle, fascia and tendon of unspecified thumb at wrist and hand level A , D, S

● **S66.09** Other specified injury of long flexor muscle, fascia and tendon of thumb at wrist and hand level

● **S66.091** Other specified injury of long flexor muscle, fascia and tendon of right thumb at wrist and hand level D, S

● **S66.092** Other specified injury of long flexor muscle, fascia and tendon of left thumb at wrist and hand level D, S

●■ **S66.099** Other specified injury of long flexor muscle, fascia and tendon of unspecified thumb at wrist and hand level D, S

● **S66.1** Injury of flexor muscle, fascia and tendon of other and unspecified finger at wrist and hand level

Excludes2 injury of long flexor muscle, fascia and tendon of thumb at wrist and hand level (S66.0-)

● **S66.10** Unspecified injury of flexor muscle, fascia and tendon of other and unspecified finger at wrist and hand level

●■ **S66.100** Unspecified injury of flexor muscle, fascia and tendon of right index finger at wrist and hand level D, S

●■ **S66.101** Unspecified injury of flexor muscle, fascia and tendon of left index finger at wrist and hand level D, S

●■ **S66.102** Unspecified injury of flexor muscle, fascia and tendon of right middle finger at wrist and hand level D, S

●■ **S66.103** Unspecified injury of flexor muscle, fascia and tendon of left middle finger at wrist and hand level D, S

●■ **S66.104** Unspecified injury of flexor muscle, fascia and tendon of right ring finger at wrist and hand level D, S

●■ **S66.105** Unspecified injury of flexor muscle, fascia and tendon of left ring finger at wrist and hand level D, S

●■ **S66.106** Unspecified injury of flexor muscle, fascia and tendon of right little finger at wrist and hand level D, S

●■ **S66.107** Unspecified injury of flexor muscle, fascia and tendon of left little finger at wrist and hand level D, S

●■ **S66.108** Unspecified injury of flexor muscle, fascia and tendon of other finger at wrist and hand level D, S

Unspecified injury of flexor muscle, fascia and tendon of specified finger with unspecified laterality at wrist and hand level

●■ **S66.109** Unspecified injury of flexor muscle, fascia and tendon of unspecified finger at wrist and hand level D, S

● **S66.11** Strain of flexor muscle, fascia and tendon of other and unspecified finger at wrist and hand level

● **S66.110** Strain of flexor muscle, fascia and tendon of right index finger at wrist and hand level D, S

● **S66.111** Strain of flexor muscle, fascia and tendon of left index finger at wrist and hand level D, S

● **S66.112** Strain of flexor muscle, fascia and tendon of right middle finger at wrist and hand level D, S

● **S66.113** Strain of flexor muscle, fascia and tendon of left middle finger at wrist and hand level D, S

● **S66.114** Strain of flexor muscle, fascia and tendon of right ring finger at wrist and hand level D, S

● **S66.115** Strain of flexor muscle, fascia and tendon of left ring finger at wrist and hand level D, S

● **S66.116** Strain of flexor muscle, fascia and tendon of right little finger at wrist and hand level D, S

● **S66.117** Strain of flexor muscle, fascia and tendon of left little finger at wrist and hand level D, S

● **S66.118** Strain of flexor muscle, fascia and tendon of other finger at wrist and hand level D, S

Strain of flexor muscle, fascia and tendon of specified finger with unspecified laterality at wrist and hand level

●■ **S66.119** Strain of flexor muscle, fascia and tendon of unspecified finger at wrist and hand level D, S

● **S66.12** Laceration of flexor muscle, fascia and tendon of other and unspecified finger at wrist and hand level

● **S66.120** Laceration of flexor muscle, fascia and tendon of right index finger at wrist and hand level A , D, S

● **S66.121** Laceration of flexor muscle, fascia and tendon of left index finger at wrist and hand level A , D, S

● Unacceptable Principal Diagnosis ● Use Additional Character(s) ■ Unspecified ▶ Manifestation Code
OGCR Official Guidelines for Coding and Reporting Excludes 1 Excludes 2 Includes Use additional Code first Code also

● S66.122　Laceration of flexor muscle, fascia and tendon of right middle finger at wrist and hand level A 🔴, D, S 🔵

● S66.123　Laceration of flexor muscle, fascia and tendon of left middle finger at wrist and hand level A 🔴, D, S 🔵

● S66.124　Laceration of flexor muscle, fascia and tendon of right ring finger at wrist and hand level A 🔴, D, S 🔵

● S66.125　Laceration of flexor muscle, fascia and tendon of left ring finger at wrist and hand level A 🔴, D, S 🔵

● S66.126　Laceration of flexor muscle, fascia and tendon of right little finger at wrist and hand level A 🔴, D, S 🔵

● S66.127　Laceration of flexor muscle, fascia and tendon of left little finger at wrist and hand level A 🔴, D, S 🔵

● S66.128　Laceration of flexor muscle, fascia and tendon of other finger at wrist and hand level A 🔴, D, S 🔵
Laceration of flexor muscle, fascia and tendon of specified finger with unspecified laterality at wrist and hand level

●■ S66.129　Laceration of flexor muscle, fascia and tendon of unspecified finger at wrist and hand level A 🔴, D, S 🔵

● S66.19　Other injury of flexor muscle, fascia and tendon of other and unspecified finger at wrist and hand level

● S66.190　Other injury of flexor muscle, fascia and tendon of right index finger at wrist and hand level D, S 🔵

● S66.191　Other injury of flexor muscle, fascia and tendon of left index finger at wrist and hand level D, S 🔵

● S66.192　Other injury of flexor muscle, fascia and tendon of right middle finger at wrist and hand level D, S 🔵

● S66.193　Other injury of flexor muscle, fascia and tendon of left middle finger at wrist and hand level D, S 🔵

● S66.194　Other injury of flexor muscle, fascia and tendon of right ring finger at wrist and hand level D, S 🔵

● S66.195　Other injury of flexor muscle, fascia and tendon of left ring finger at wrist and hand level D, S 🔵

● S66.196　Other injury of flexor muscle, fascia and tendon of right little finger at wrist and hand level D, S 🔵

● S66.197　Other injury of flexor muscle, fascia and tendon of left little finger at wrist and hand level D, S 🔵

● S66.198　Other injury of flexor muscle, fascia and tendon of other finger at wrist and hand level D, S 🔵
Other injury of flexor muscle, fascia and tendon of specified finger with unspecified laterality at wrist and hand level

●■ S66.199　Other injury of flexor muscle, fascia and tendon of unspecified finger at wrist and hand level D, S 🔵

● S66.2　Injury of extensor muscle, fascia and tendon of thumb at wrist and hand level

● S66.20　Unspecified injury of extensor muscle, fascia and tendon of thumb at wrist and hand level

●■ S66.201　Unspecified injury of extensor muscle, fascia and tendon of right thumb at wrist and hand level D, S 🔵

●■ S66.202　Unspecified injury of extensor muscle, fascia and tendon of left thumb at wrist and hand level D, S 🔵

●■ S66.209　Unspecified injury of extensor muscle, fascia and tendon of unspecified thumb at wrist and hand level D, S 🔵

● S66.21　Strain of extensor muscle, fascia and tendon of thumb at wrist and hand level

● S66.211　Strain of extensor muscle, fascia and tendon of right thumb at wrist and hand level D, S 🔵

● S66.212　Strain of extensor muscle, fascia and tendon of left thumb at wrist and hand level D, S 🔵

●■ S66.219　Strain of extensor muscle, fascia and tendon of unspecified thumb at wrist and hand level D, S 🔵

● S66.22　Laceration of extensor muscle, fascia and tendon of thumb at wrist and hand level

● S66.221　Laceration of extensor muscle, fascia and tendon of right thumb at wrist and hand level A 🔴, D, S 🔵

● S66.222　Laceration of extensor muscle, fascia and tendon of left thumb at wrist and hand level A 🔴, D, S 🔵

●■ S66.229　Laceration of extensor muscle, fascia and tendon of unspecified thumb at wrist and hand level A 🔴, D, S 🔵

● S66.29　Other specified injury of extensor muscle, fascia and tendon of thumb at wrist and hand level

● S66.291　Other specified injury of extensor muscle, fascia and tendon of right thumb at wrist and hand level D, S 🔵

● S66.292　Other specified injury of extensor muscle, fascia and tendon of left thumb at wrist and hand level D, S 🔵

●■ S66.299　Other specified injury of extensor muscle, fascia and tendon of unspecified thumb at wrist and hand level D, S 🔵

N Newborn Age: 0　　**P** Pediatric Age: 0–17　　**M** Maternity DX: 12–55　　**A** Adult Age: 15–124　　♀ Females Only　　♂ Males Only

🔴 Complication\Comorbidity　　🔴 Major C\C　　🔵 Present on Admission Requirement　　🔵 Hospital-Acquired Condition

1521

● S66.3   Injury of extensor muscle, fascia and tendon of other and unspecified finger at wrist and hand level

> **Excludes2**   injury of extensor muscle, fascia and tendon of thumb at wrist and hand level (S66.2-)

● S66.30   Unspecified injury of extensor muscle, fascia and tendon of other and unspecified finger at wrist and hand level

● ■ S66.300   Unspecified injury of extensor muscle, fascia and tendon of right index finger at wrist and hand level D, S

● ■ S66.301   Unspecified injury of extensor muscle, fascia and tendon of left index finger at wrist and hand level D, S

● ■ S66.302   Unspecified injury of extensor muscle, fascia and tendon of right middle finger at wrist and hand level D, S

● ■ S66.303   Unspecified injury of extensor muscle, fascia and tendon of left middle finger at wrist and hand level D, S

● ■ S66.304   Unspecified injury of extensor muscle, fascia and tendon of right ring finger at wrist and hand level D, S

● ■ S66.305   Unspecified injury of extensor muscle, fascia and tendon of left ring finger at wrist and hand level D, S

● ■ S66.306   Unspecified injury of extensor muscle, fascia and tendon of right little finger at wrist and hand level D, S

● ■ S66.307   Unspecified injury of extensor muscle, fascia and tendon of left little finger at wrist and hand level D, S

● ■ S66.308   Unspecified injury of extensor muscle, fascia and tendon of other finger at wrist and hand level D, S

> Unspecified injury of extensor muscle, fascia and tendon of specified finger with unspecified laterality at wrist and hand level

● ■ S66.309   Unspecified injury of extensor muscle, fascia and tendon of unspecified finger at wrist and hand level D, S

● S66.31   Strain of extensor muscle, fascia and tendon of other and unspecified finger at wrist and hand level

● S66.310   Strain of extensor muscle, fascia and tendon of right index finger at wrist and hand level D, S

● S66.311   Strain of extensor muscle, fascia and tendon of left index finger at wrist and hand level D, S

● S66.312   Strain of extensor muscle, fascia and tendon of right middle finger at wrist and hand level D, S

● S66.313   Strain of extensor muscle, fascia and tendon of left middle finger at wrist and hand level D, S

● S66.314   Strain of extensor muscle, fascia and tendon of right ring finger at wrist and hand level D, S

● S66.315   Strain of extensor muscle, fascia and tendon of left ring finger at wrist and hand level D, S

● S66.316   Strain of extensor muscle, fascia and tendon of right little finger at wrist and hand level D, S

● S66.317   Strain of extensor muscle, fascia and tendon of left little finger at wrist and hand level D, S

● S66.318   Strain of extensor muscle, fascia and tendon of other finger at wrist and hand level D, S

> Strain of extensor muscle, fascia and tendon of specified finger with unspecified laterality at wrist and hand level

● ■ S66.319   Strain of extensor muscle, fascia and tendon of unspecified finger at wrist and hand level D, S

● S66.32   Laceration of extensor muscle, fascia and tendon of other and unspecified finger at wrist and hand level

● S66.320   Laceration of extensor muscle, fascia and tendon of right index finger at wrist and hand level A, D, S

● S66.321   Laceration of extensor muscle, fascia and tendon of left index finger at wrist and hand level A, D, S

● S66.322   Laceration of extensor muscle, fascia and tendon of right middle finger at wrist and hand level A, D, S

● S66.323   Laceration of extensor muscle, fascia and tendon of left middle finger at wrist and hand level A, D, S

● S66.324   Laceration of extensor muscle, fascia and tendon of right ring finger at wrist and hand level A, D, S

● S66.325   Laceration of extensor muscle, fascia and tendon of left ring finger at wrist and hand level A, D, S

● S66.326   Laceration of extensor muscle, fascia and tendon of right little finger at wrist and hand level A, D, S

● S66.327   Laceration of extensor muscle, fascia and tendon of left little finger at wrist and hand level A, D, S

● **S66.328** **Laceration of extensor muscle, fascia and tendon of other finger at wrist and hand level A** 🔒, D, S 🔒

> Laceration of extensor muscle, fascia and tendon of specified finger with unspecified laterality at wrist and hand level

●■ **S66.329** **Laceration of extensor muscle, fascia and tendon of unspecified finger at wrist and hand level A** 🔒, D, S 🔒

● **S66.39** **Other injury of extensor muscle, fascia and tendon of other and unspecified finger at wrist and hand level**

● **S66.390** **Other injury of extensor muscle, fascia and tendon of right index finger at wrist and hand level** D, S 🔒

● **S66.391** **Other injury of extensor muscle, fascia and tendon of left index finger at wrist and hand level** D, S 🔒

● **S66.392** **Other injury of extensor muscle, fascia and tendon of right middle finger at wrist and hand level** D, S 🔒

● **S66.393** **Other injury of extensor muscle, fascia and tendon of left middle finger at wrist and hand level** D, S 🔒

● **S66.394** **Other injury of extensor muscle, fascia and tendon of right ring finger at wrist and hand level** D, S 🔒

● **S66.395** **Other injury of extensor muscle, fascia and tendon of left ring finger at wrist and hand level** D, S 🔒

● **S66.396** **Other injury of extensor muscle, fascia and tendon of right little finger at wrist and hand level** D, S 🔒

● **S66.397** **Other injury of extensor muscle, fascia and tendon of left little finger at wrist and hand level** D, S 🔒

● **S66.398** **Other injury of extensor muscle, fascia and tendon of other finger at wrist and hand level** D, S 🔒

> Other injury of extensor muscle, fascia and tendon of specified finger with unspecified laterality at wrist and hand level

●■ **S66.399** **Other injury of extensor muscle, fascia and tendon of unspecified finger at wrist and hand level** D, S 🔒

● **S66.4** **Injury of intrinsic muscle, fascia and tendon of thumb at wrist and hand level**

● **S66.40** **Unspecified injury of intrinsic muscle, fascia and tendon of thumb at wrist and hand level**

●■ **S66.401** **Unspecified injury of intrinsic muscle, fascia and tendon of right thumb at wrist and hand level** D, S 🔒

●■ **S66.402** **Unspecified injury of intrinsic muscle, fascia and tendon of left thumb at wrist and hand level** D, S 🔒

●■ **S66.409** **Unspecified injury of intrinsic muscle, fascia and tendon of unspecified thumb at wrist and hand level** D, S 🔒

● **S66.41** **Strain of intrinsic muscle, fascia and tendon of thumb at wrist and hand level**

● **S66.411** **Strain of intrinsic muscle, fascia and tendon of right thumb at wrist and hand level** D, S 🔒

● **S66.412** **Strain of intrinsic muscle, fascia and tendon of left thumb at wrist and hand level** D, S 🔒

●■ **S66.419** **Strain of intrinsic muscle, fascia and tendon of unspecified thumb at wrist and hand level** D, S 🔒

● **S66.42** **Laceration of intrinsic muscle, fascia and tendon of thumb at wrist and hand level**

● **S66.421** **Laceration of intrinsic muscle, fascia and tendon of right thumb at wrist and hand level A** 🔒, D, S 🔒

● **S66.422** **Laceration of intrinsic muscle, fascia and tendon of left thumb at wrist and hand level A** 🔒, D, S 🔒

●■ **S66.429** **Laceration of intrinsic muscle, fascia and tendon of unspecified thumb at wrist and hand level A** 🔒, D, S 🔒

● **S66.49** **Other specified injury of intrinsic muscle, fascia and tendon of thumb at wrist and hand level**

● **S66.491** **Other specified injury of intrinsic muscle, fascia and tendon of right thumb at wrist and hand level** D, S 🔒

● **S66.492** **Other specified injury of intrinsic muscle, fascia and tendon of left thumb at wrist and hand level** D, S 🔒

●■ **S66.499** **Other specified injury of intrinsic muscle, fascia and tendon of unspecified thumb at wrist and hand level** D, S 🔒

CHAPTER 19 (S00-T88)

N Newborn Age: 0   **P** Pediatric Age: 0–17   **M** Maternity DX: 12–55   **A** Adult Age: 15–124   ♀ Females Only   ♂ Males Only

🔒 Complication\Comorbidity   🔒 Major C\C   🔒 Present on Admission Requirement   🔒 Hospital-Acquired Condition

1523

● S66.5 Injury of intrinsic muscle, fascia and tendon of other and unspecified finger at wrist and hand level

> **Excludes2** injury of intrinsic muscle, fascia and tendon of thumb at wrist and hand level (S66.4-)

● S66.50 Unspecified injury of intrinsic muscle, fascia and tendon of other and unspecified finger at wrist and hand level

● ■ S66.500 Unspecified injury of intrinsic muscle, fascia and tendon of right index finger at wrist and hand level D, S

● ■ S66.501 Unspecified injury of intrinsic muscle, fascia and tendon of left index finger at wrist and hand level D, S

● ■ S66.502 Unspecified injury of intrinsic muscle, fascia and tendon of right middle finger at wrist and hand level D, S

● ■ S66.503 Unspecified injury of intrinsic muscle, fascia and tendon of left middle finger at wrist and hand level D, S

● ■ S66.504 Unspecified injury of intrinsic muscle, fascia and tendon of right ring finger at wrist and hand level D, S

● ■ S66.505 Unspecified injury of intrinsic muscle, fascia and tendon of left ring finger at wrist and hand level D, S

● ■ S66.506 Unspecified injury of intrinsic muscle, fascia and tendon of right little finger at wrist and hand level D, S

● ■ S66.507 Unspecified injury of intrinsic muscle, fascia and tendon of left little finger at wrist and hand level D, S

● ■ S66.508 Unspecified injury of intrinsic muscle, fascia and tendon of other finger at wrist and hand level D, S
> Unspecified injury of intrinsic muscle, fascia and tendon of specified finger with unspecified laterality at wrist and hand level

● ■ S66.509 Unspecified injury of intrinsic muscle, fascia and tendon of unspecified finger at wrist and hand level D, S

● S66.51 Strain of intrinsic muscle, fascia and tendon of other and unspecified finger at wrist and hand level

● S66.510 Strain of intrinsic muscle, fascia and tendon of right index finger at wrist and hand level D, S

● S66.511 Strain of intrinsic muscle, fascia and tendon of left index finger at wrist and hand level D, S

● S66.512 Strain of intrinsic muscle, fascia and tendon of right middle finger at wrist and hand level D, S

● S66.513 Strain of intrinsic muscle, fascia and tendon of left middle finger at wrist and hand level D, S

● S66.514 Strain of intrinsic muscle, fascia and tendon of right ring finger at wrist and hand level D, S

● S66.515 Strain of intrinsic muscle, fascia and tendon of left ring finger at wrist and hand level D, S

● S66.516 Strain of intrinsic muscle, fascia and tendon of right little finger at wrist and hand level D, S

● S66.517 Strain of intrinsic muscle, fascia and tendon of left little finger at wrist and hand level D, S

● S66.518 Strain of intrinsic muscle, fascia and tendon of other finger at wrist and hand level D, S
> Strain of intrinsic muscle, fascia and tendon of specified finger with unspecified laterality at wrist and hand level

● ■ S66.519 Strain of intrinsic muscle, fascia and tendon of unspecified finger at wrist and hand level D, S

● S66.52 Laceration of intrinsic muscle, fascia and tendon of other and unspecified finger at wrist and hand level

● S66.520 Laceration of intrinsic muscle, fascia and tendon of right index finger at wrist and hand level A, D, S

● S66.521 Laceration of intrinsic muscle, fascia and tendon of left index finger at wrist and hand level A, D, S

● S66.522 Laceration of intrinsic muscle, fascia and tendon of right middle finger at wrist and hand level A, D, S

● S66.523 Laceration of intrinsic muscle, fascia and tendon of left middle finger at wrist and hand level A, D, S

● S66.524 Laceration of intrinsic muscle, fascia and tendon of right ring finger at wrist and hand level A, D, S

● S66.525 Laceration of intrinsic muscle, fascia and tendon of left ring finger at wrist and hand level A, D, S

● S66.526 Laceration of intrinsic muscle, fascia and tendon of right little finger at wrist and hand level A, D, S

● S66.527 Laceration of intrinsic muscle, fascia and tendon of left little finger at wrist and hand level A, D, S

● Unacceptable Principal Diagnosis   ● Use Additional Character(s)   ■ Unspecified   ▶ Manifestation Code
OGCR Official Guidelines for Coding and Reporting   Excludes 1   Excludes 2   Includes   Use additional   Code first   Code also

● **S66.528**   **Laceration of intrinsic muscle, fascia and tendon of other finger at wrist and hand level A** 🔴,
D, S 🔲

         Laceration of intrinsic muscle, fascia and tendon of specified finger with unspecified laterality at wrist and hand level

● 🔲 **S66.529**   **Laceration of intrinsic muscle, fascia and tendon of unspecified finger at wrist and hand level A** 🔴, D, S 🔲

● **S66.59**   **Other injury of intrinsic muscle, fascia and tendon of other and unspecified finger at wrist and hand level**

● **S66.590**   **Other injury of intrinsic muscle, fascia and tendon of right index finger at wrist and hand level** D, S 🔲

● **S66.591**   **Other injury of intrinsic muscle, fascia and tendon of left index finger at wrist and hand level** D, S 🔲

● **S66.592**   **Other injury of intrinsic muscle, fascia and tendon of right middle finger at wrist and hand level** D, S 🔲

● **S66.593**   **Other injury of intrinsic muscle, fascia and tendon of left middle finger at wrist and hand level** D, S 🔲

● **S66.594**   **Other injury of intrinsic muscle, fascia and tendon of right ring finger at wrist and hand level** D, S 🔲

● **S66.595**   **Other injury of intrinsic muscle, fascia and tendon of left ring finger at wrist and hand level** D, S 🔲

● **S66.596**   **Other injury of intrinsic muscle, fascia and tendon of right little finger at wrist and hand level** D, S 🔲

● **S66.597**   **Other injury of intrinsic muscle, fascia and tendon of left little finger at wrist and hand level** D, S 🔲

● **S66.598**   **Other injury of intrinsic muscle, fascia and tendon of other finger at wrist and hand level** D, S 🔲

         Other injury of intrinsic muscle, fascia and tendon of specified finger with unspecified laterality at wrist and hand level

● 🔲 **S66.599**   **Other injury of intrinsic muscle, fascia and tendon of unspecified finger at wrist and hand level** D, S 🔲

● **S66.8**   **Injury of other specified muscles, fascia and tendons at wrist and hand level**

● **S66.80**   **Unspecified injury of other specified muscles, fascia and tendons at wrist and hand level**

● 🔲 **S66.801**   **Unspecified injury of other specified muscles, fascia and tendons at wrist and hand level, right hand** D, S 🔲

● 🔲 **S66.802**   **Unspecified injury of other specified muscles, fascia and tendons at wrist and hand level, left hand** D, S 🔲

● 🔲 **S66.809**   **Unspecified injury of other specified muscles, fascia and tendons at wrist and hand level, unspecified hand** D, S 🔲

● **S66.81**   **Strain of other specified muscles, fascia and tendons at wrist and hand level**

● **S66.811**   **Strain of other specified muscles, fascia and tendons at wrist and hand level, right hand** D, S 🔲

● **S66.812**   **Strain of other specified muscles, fascia and tendons at wrist and hand level, left hand** D, S 🔲

● 🔲 **S66.819**   **Strain of other specified muscles, fascia and tendons at wrist and hand level, unspecified hand** D, S 🔲

● **S66.82**   **Laceration of other specified muscles, fascia and tendons at wrist and hand level**

● **S66.821**   **Laceration of other specified muscles, fascia and tendons at wrist and hand level, right hand A** 🔴, D, S 🔲

● **S66.822**   **Laceration of other specified muscles, fascia and tendons at wrist and hand level, left hand A** 🔴, D, S 🔲

● 🔲 **S66.829**   **Laceration of other specified muscles, fascia and tendons at wrist and hand level, unspecified hand A** 🔴, D, S 🔲

● **S66.89**   **Other injury of other specified muscles, fascia and tendons at wrist and hand level**

● **S66.891**   **Other injury of other specified muscles, fascia and tendons at wrist and hand level, right hand** D, S 🔲

● **S66.892**   **Other injury of other specified muscles, fascia and tendons at wrist and hand level, left hand** D, S 🔲

● 🔲 **S66.899**   **Other injury of other specified muscles, fascia and tendons at wrist and hand level, unspecified hand** D, S 🔲

N Newborn Age: 0   **P** Pediatric Age: 0–17   **M** Maternity DX: 12–55   **A** Adult Age: 15–124   ♀ Females Only   ♂ Males Only

 Complication\Comorbidity   🔴 Major C\C   🔲 Present on Admission Requirement   🔲 Hospital-Acquired Condition

1525

● **S66.9** **Injury of unspecified muscle, fascia and tendon at wrist and hand level**

  ● **S66.90** **Unspecified injury of unspecified muscle, fascia and tendon at wrist and hand level**

    ●■ **S66.901** Unspecified injury of unspecified muscle, fascia and tendon at wrist and hand level, right hand D, S

    ●■ **S66.902** Unspecified injury of unspecified muscle, fascia and tendon at wrist and hand level, left hand D, S

    ●■ **S66.909** Unspecified injury of unspecified muscle, fascia and tendon at wrist and hand level, unspecified hand D, S

  ● **S66.91** **Strain of unspecified muscle, fascia and tendon at wrist and hand level**

    ●■ **S66.911** Strain of unspecified muscle, fascia and tendon at wrist and hand level, right hand D, S

    ●■ **S66.912** Strain of unspecified muscle, fascia and tendon at wrist and hand level, left hand D, S

    ●■ **S66.919** Strain of unspecified muscle, fascia and tendon at wrist and hand level, unspecified hand D, S

  ● **S66.92** **Laceration of unspecified muscle, fascia and tendon at wrist and hand level**

    ●■ **S66.921** Laceration of unspecified muscle, fascia and tendon at wrist and hand level, right hand A, D, S

    ●■ **S66.922** Laceration of unspecified muscle, fascia and tendon at wrist and hand level, left hand A, D, S

    ●■ **S66.929** Laceration of unspecified muscle, fascia and tendon at wrist and hand level, unspecified hand A, D, S

  ● **S66.99** **Other injury of unspecified muscle, fascia and tendon at wrist and hand level**

    ●■ **S66.991** Other injury of unspecified muscle, fascia and tendon at wrist and hand level, right hand D, S

    ●■ **S66.992** Other injury of unspecified muscle, fascia and tendon at wrist and hand level, left hand D, S

    ●■ **S66.999** Other injury of unspecified muscle, fascia and tendon at wrist and hand level, unspecified hand D, S

● **S67** **Crushing injury of wrist, hand and fingers**

Use additional code for all associated injuries, such as:
fracture of wrist and hand (S62.-)
open wound of wrist and hand (S61.-)

The appropriate 7th character is to be added to each code from category S67

A	initial encounter
D	subsequent encounter
S	sequela

  ● **S67.0** **Crushing injury of thumb**

    ●■ **S67.00** Crushing injury of unspecified thumb D, S

    ● **S67.01** Crushing injury of right thumb D, S

    ● **S67.02** Crushing injury of left thumb D, S

  ● **S67.1** **Crushing injury of other and unspecified finger(s)**

    Excludes2 crushing injury of thumb (S67.0-)

    ●■ **S67.10** Crushing injury of unspecified finger(s) D, S

    ● **S67.19** Crushing injury of other finger(s)

      ● **S67.190** Crushing injury of right index finger D, S

      ● **S67.191** Crushing injury of left index finger D, S

      ● **S67.192** Crushing injury of right middle finger D, S

      ● **S67.193** Crushing injury of left middle finger D, S

      ● **S67.194** Crushing injury of right ring finger D, S

      ● **S67.195** Crushing injury of left ring finger D, S

      ● **S67.196** Crushing injury of right little finger D, S

      ● **S67.197** Crushing injury of left little finger D, S

      ● **S67.198** Crushing injury of other finger D, S
        Crushing injury of specified finger with unspecified laterality

  ● **S67.2** **Crushing injury of hand**

    Excludes2 crushing injury of fingers (S67.1-)
               crushing injury of thumb (S67.0-)

    ●■ **S67.20** Crushing injury of unspecified hand D, S

    ● **S67.21** Crushing injury of right hand D, S

    ● **S67.22** Crushing injury of left hand D, S

  ● **S67.3** **Crushing injury of wrist**

    ●■ **S67.30** Crushing injury of unspecified wrist D, S

    ● **S67.31** Crushing injury of right wrist D, S

    ● **S67.32** Crushing injury of left wrist D, S

● **S67.4**   **Crushing injury of wrist and hand**

> **Excludes1**   crushing injury of hand alone (S67.2-)
> crushing injury of wrist alone (S67.3-)
>
> **Excludes2**   crushing injury of fingers (S67.1-)
> crushing injury of thumb (S67.0-)

   ●■ **S67.40**   Crushing injury of unspecified wrist and hand D, S 🔖

   ● **S67.41**   Crushing injury of right wrist and hand D, S 🔖

   ● **S67.42**   Crushing injury of left wrist and hand D, S 🔖

● **S67.9**   **Crushing injury of unspecified part(s) of wrist, hand and fingers**

   ●■ **S67.90**   Crushing injury of unspecified part(s) of unspecified wrist, hand and fingers D, S 🔖

   ●■ **S67.91**   Crushing injury of unspecified part(s) of right wrist, hand and fingers D, S 🔖

   ●■ **S67.92**   Crushing injury of unspecified part(s) of left wrist, hand and fingers D, S 🔖

● **S68**   **Traumatic amputation of wrist, hand and fingers**

> An amputation not identified as partial or complete should be coded to complete
>
> The appropriate 7th character is to be added to each code from category S68

> | | |
> |---|---|
> | A | initial encounter |
> | D | subsequent encounter |
> | S | sequela |

● **S68.0**   **Traumatic metacarpophalangeal amputation of thumb**

> Traumatic amputation of thumb NOS

   ● **S68.01**   Complete traumatic metacarpophalangeal amputation of thumb

     ● **S68.011**   Complete traumatic metacarpophalangeal amputation of right thumb D, S 🔖

     ● **S68.012**   Complete traumatic metacarpophalangeal amputation of left thumb D, S 🔖

     ●■ **S68.019**   Complete traumatic metacarpophalangeal amputation of unspecified thumb D, S 🔖

   ● **S68.02**   Partial traumatic metacarpophalangeal amputation of thumb

     ● **S68.021**   Partial traumatic metacarpophalangeal amputation of right thumb D, S 🔖

     ● **S68.022**   Partial traumatic metacarpophalangeal amputation of left thumb D, S 🔖

     ●■ **S68.029**   Partial traumatic metacarpophalangeal amputation of unspecified thumb D, S 🔖

● **S68.1**   **Traumatic metacarpophalangeal amputation of other and unspecified finger**

> Traumatic amputation of finger NOS
>
> **Excludes2**   traumatic metacarpophalangeal amputation of thumb (S68.0-)

   ● **S68.11**   Complete traumatic metacarpophalangeal amputation of other and unspecified finger

     ● **S68.110**   Complete traumatic metacarpophalangeal amputation of right index finger D, S 🔖

     ● **S68.111**   Complete traumatic metacarpophalangeal amputation of left index finger D, S 🔖

     ● **S68.112**   Complete traumatic metacarpophalangeal amputation of right middle finger D, S 🔖

     ● **S68.113**   Complete traumatic metacarpophalangeal amputation of left middle finger D, S 🔖

     ● **S68.114**   Complete traumatic metacarpophalangeal amputation of right ring finger D, S 🔖

     ● **S68.115**   Complete traumatic metacarpophalangeal amputation of left ring finger D, S 🔖

     ● **S68.116**   Complete traumatic metacarpophalangeal amputation of right little finger D, S 🔖

     ● **S68.117**   Complete traumatic metacarpophalangeal amputation of left little finger D, S 🔖

     ● **S68.118**   Complete traumatic metacarpophalangeal amputation of other finger D, S 🔖

> Complete traumatic metacarpophalangeal amputation of specified finger with unspecified laterality

     ●■ **S68.119**   Complete traumatic metacarpophalangeal amputation of unspecified finger D, S 🔖

   ● **S68.12**   Partial traumatic metacarpophalangeal amputation of other and unspecified finger

     ● **S68.120**   Partial traumatic metacarpophalangeal amputation of right index finger D, S 🔖

     ● **S68.121**   Partial traumatic metacarpophalangeal amputation of left index finger D, S 🔖

     ● **S68.122**   Partial traumatic metacarpophalangeal amputation of right middle finger D, S 🔖

     ● **S68.123**   Partial traumatic metacarpophalangeal amputation of left middle finger D, S 🔖

     ● **S68.124**   Partial traumatic metacarpophalangeal amputation of right ring finger D, S 🔖

     ● **S68.125**   Partial traumatic metacarpophalangeal amputation of left ring finger D, S 🔖

N Newborn Age: 0   **P** Pediatric Age: 0–17   **M** Maternity DX: 12–55   **A** Adult Age: 15–124   ♀ Females Only   ♂ Males Only

🔖 Complication\Comorbidity   🔖 Major C\C   🔖 Present on Admission Requirement   🔖 Hospital-Acquired Condition

1527

CHAPTER 19 (S00-T88)

● S68.126 Partial traumatic metacarpophalangeal amputation of right little finger D, S ◎

● S68.127 Partial traumatic metacarpophalangeal amputation of left little finger D, S ◎

● S68.128 Partial traumatic metacarpophalangeal amputation of other finger D, S ◎

Partial traumatic metacarpophalangeal amputation of specified finger with unspecified laterality

●■ S68.129 Partial traumatic metacarpophalangeal amputation of unspecified finger D, S ◎

● S68.4 **Traumatic amputation of hand at wrist level**
Traumatic amputation of hand NOS
Traumatic amputation of wrist

● S68.41 Complete traumatic amputation of hand at wrist level

● S68.411 Complete traumatic amputation of right hand at wrist level A ◎, D, S ◎

● S68.412 Complete traumatic amputation of left hand at wrist level A ◎, D, S ◎

●■ S68.419 Complete traumatic amputation of unspecified hand at wrist level A ◎, D, S ◎

● S68.42 Partial traumatic amputation of hand at wrist level

● S68.421 Partial traumatic amputation of right hand at wrist level A ◎, D, S ◎

● S68.422 Partial traumatic amputation of left hand at wrist level A ◎, D, S ◎

●■ S68.429 Partial traumatic amputation of unspecified hand at wrist level A ◎, D, S ◎

● S68.5 **Traumatic transphalangeal amputation of thumb**
Traumatic interphalangeal joint amputation of thumb

● S68.51 Complete traumatic transphalangeal amputation of thumb

● S68.511 Complete traumatic transphalangeal amputation of right thumb D, S ◎

● S68.512 Complete traumatic transphalangeal amputation of left thumb D, S ◎

●■ S68.519 Complete traumatic transphalangeal amputation of unspecified thumb D, S ◎

● S68.52 Partial traumatic transphalangeal amputation of thumb

● S68.521 Partial traumatic transphalangeal amputation of right thumb D, S ◎

● S68.522 Partial traumatic transphalangeal amputation of left thumb D, S ◎

●■ S68.529 Partial traumatic transphalangeal amputation of unspecified thumb D, S ◎

● S68.6 **Traumatic transphalangeal amputation of other and unspecified finger**

● S68.61 Complete traumatic transphalangeal amputation of other and unspecified finger(s)

● S68.610 Complete traumatic transphalangeal amputation of right index finger D, S ◎

● S68.611 Complete traumatic transphalangeal amputation of left index finger D, S ◎

● S68.612 Complete traumatic transphalangeal amputation of right middle finger D, S ◎

● S68.613 Complete traumatic transphalangeal amputation of left middle finger D, S ◎

● S68.614 Complete traumatic transphalangeal amputation of right ring finger D, S ◎

● S68.615 Complete traumatic transphalangeal amputation of left ring finger D, S ◎

● S68.616 Complete traumatic transphalangeal amputation of right little finger D, S ◎

● S68.617 Complete traumatic transphalangeal amputation of left little finger D, S ◎

● S68.618 Complete traumatic transphalangeal amputation of other finger D, S ◎

Complete traumatic transphalangeal amputation of specified finger with unspecified laterality

●■ S68.619 Complete traumatic transphalangeal amputation of unspecified finger D, S ◎

● S68.62 Partial traumatic transphalangeal amputation of other and unspecified finger

● S68.620 Partial traumatic transphalangeal amputation of right index finger D, S ◎

● S68.621 Partial traumatic transphalangeal amputation of left index finger D, S ◎

● S68.622 Partial traumatic transphalangeal amputation of right middle finger D, S ◎

● S68.623 Partial traumatic transphalangeal amputation of left middle finger D, S ◎

● S68.624 Partial traumatic transphalangeal amputation of right ring finger D, S ◎

● S68.625 Partial traumatic transphalangeal amputation of left ring finger D, S ◎

● S68.626 Partial traumatic transphalangeal amputation of right little finger D, S ◎

● Unacceptable Principal Diagnosis   ● Use Additional Character(s)   ■ Unspecified   ▶ Manifestation Code

OGCR Official Guidelines for Coding and Reporting   Excludes 1   Excludes 2   Includes   Use additional   Code first   Code also

● S68.627   **Partial traumatic transphalangeal amputation of left little finger** D, S 🔲

● S68.628   **Partial traumatic transphalangeal amputation of other finger** D, S 🔲
     Partial traumatic transphalangeal amputation of specified finger with unspecified laterality

● ■ S68.629   **Partial traumatic transphalangeal amputation of unspecified finger** D, S 🔲

● **S68.7**   **Traumatic transmetacarpal amputation of hand**

   ● **S68.71**   **Complete traumatic transmetacarpal amputation of hand**

     ● S68.711   **Complete traumatic transmetacarpal amputation of right hand** A 🔲, D, S 🔲

     ● S68.712   **Complete traumatic transmetacarpal amputation of left hand** A 🔲, D, S 🔲

     ● ■ S68.719   **Complete traumatic transmetacarpal amputation of unspecified hand** A 🔲, D, S 🔲

   ● **S68.72**   **Partial traumatic transmetacarpal amputation of hand**

     ● S68.721   **Partial traumatic transmetacarpal amputation of right hand** A 🔲, D, S 🔲

     ● S68.722   **Partial traumatic transmetacarpal amputation of left hand** A 🔲, D, S 🔲

     ● ■ S68.729   **Partial traumatic transmetacarpal amputation of unspecified hand** A 🔲, D, S 🔲

● **S69**   **Other and unspecified injuries of wrist, hand and finger(s)**

   The appropriate 7th character is to be added to each code from category S69

A	initial encounter
D	subsequent encounter
S	sequela

   ● **S69.8**   **Other specified injuries of wrist, hand and finger(s)**

     ● ■ **S69.80**   **Other specified injuries of unspecified wrist, hand and finger(s)** D, S 🔲

     ● **S69.81**   **Other specified injuries of right wrist, hand and finger(s)** D, S 🔲

     ● **S69.82**   **Other specified injuries of left wrist, hand and finger(s)** D, S 🔲

   ● **S69.9**   **Unspecified injury of wrist, hand and finger(s)**

     ● ■ **S69.90**   **Unspecified injury of unspecified wrist, hand and finger(s)** D, S 🔲

     ● ■ **S69.91**   **Unspecified injury of right wrist, hand and finger(s)** D, S 🔲

     ● ■ **S69.92**   **Unspecified injury of left wrist, hand and finger(s)** D, S 🔲

INJURIES TO THE HIP AND THIGH (S70-S79)

Excludes2	burns and corrosions (T20-T32)
	frostbite (T33-T34)
	snake bite (T63.0-)
	venomous insect bite or sting (T63.4-)

● **S70**   **Superficial injury of hip and thigh**

   The appropriate 7th character is to be added to each code from category S70

A	initial encounter
D	subsequent encounter
S	sequela

   ● **S70.0**   **Contusion of hip**

     ● ■ **S70.00**   **Contusion of unspecified hip** D, S 🔲

     ● **S70.01**   **Contusion of right hip** D, S 🔲

     ● **S70.02**   **Contusion of left hip** D, S 🔲

   ● **S70.1**   **Contusion of thigh**

     ● ■ **S70.10**   **Contusion of unspecified thigh** D, S 🔲

     ● **S70.11**   **Contusion of right thigh** D, S 🔲

     ● **S70.12**   **Contusion of left thigh** D, S 🔲

   ● **S70.2**   **Other superficial injuries of hip**

     ● **S70.21**   **Abrasion of hip**

       ● S70.211   **Abrasion, right hip** D, S 🔲

       ● S70.212   **Abrasion, left hip** D, S 🔲

       ● ■ S70.219   **Abrasion, unspecified hip** D, S 🔲

     ● **S70.22**   **Blister (nonthermal) of hip**

       ● S70.221   **Blister (nonthermal), right hip** D, S 🔲

       ● S70.222   **Blister (nonthermal), left hip** D, S 🔲

       ● ■ S70.229   **Blister (nonthermal), unspecified hip** D, S 🔲

     ● **S70.24**   **External constriction of hip**

       ● S70.241   **External constriction, right hip** D, S 🔲

       ● S70.242   **External constriction, left hip** D, S 🔲

       ● ■ S70.249   **External constriction, unspecified hip** D, S 🔲

     ● **S70.25**   **Superficial foreign body of hip**
       Splinter in the hip

       ● S70.251   **Superficial foreign body, right hip** D, S 🔲

       ● S70.252   **Superficial foreign body, left hip** D, S 🔲

       ● ■ S70.259   **Superficial foreign body, unspecified hip** D, S 🔲

     ● **S70.26**   **Insect bite (nonvenomous) of hip**

       ● S70.261   **Insect bite (nonvenomous), right hip** D, S 🔲

       ● S70.262   **Insect bite (nonvenomous), left hip** D, S 🔲

       ● ■ S70.269   **Insect bite (nonvenomous), unspecified hip** D, S 🔲

N   Newborn Age: 0   **P**   Pediatric Age: 0–17   **M**   Maternity DX: 12–55   **A**   Adult Age: 15–124   ♀   Females Only   ♂   Males Only

🔲   Complication\Comorbidity   🔲   Major C\C   🔲   Present on Admission Requirement   🔲   Hospital-Acquired Condition

● S70.27   Other superficial bite of hip
    Excludes1   open bite of hip (S71.05-)
    ● S70.271   Other superficial bite of hip, right hip D, S 🔍
    ● S70.272   Other superficial bite of hip, left hip D, S 🔍
    ●■ S70.279   Other superficial bite of hip, unspecified hip D, S 🔍

● S70.3   Other superficial injuries of thigh
    ● S70.31   Abrasion of thigh
        ● S70.311   Abrasion, right thigh D, S 🔍
        ● S70.312   Abrasion, left thigh D, S 🔍
        ●■ S70.319   Abrasion, unspecified thigh D, S 🔍
    ● S70.32   Blister (nonthermal) of thigh
        ● S70.321   Blister (nonthermal), right thigh D, S 🔍
        ● S70.322   Blister (nonthermal), left thigh D, S 🔍
        ●■ S70.329   Blister (nonthermal), unspecified thigh D, S 🔍
    ● S70.34   External constriction of thigh
        ● S70.341   External constriction, right thigh D, S 🔍
        ● S70.342   External constriction, left thigh D, S 🔍
        ●■ S70.349   External constriction, unspecified thigh D, S 🔍
    ● S70.35   Superficial foreign body of thigh
        Splinter in the thigh
        ● S70.351   Superficial foreign body, right thigh D, S 🔍
        ● S70.352   Superficial foreign body, left thigh D, S 🔍
        ●■ S70.359   Superficial foreign body, unspecified thigh D, S 🔍
    ● S70.36   Insect bite (nonvenomous) of thigh
        ● S70.361   Insect bite (nonvenomous), right thigh D, S 🔍
        ● S70.362   Insect bite (nonvenomous), left thigh D, S 🔍
        ●■ S70.369   Insect bite (nonvenomous), unspecified thigh D, S 🔍
    ● S70.37   Other superficial bite of thigh
        Excludes1   open bite of thigh (S71.15)
        ● S70.371   Other superficial bite of right thigh D, S 🔍
        ● S70.372   Other superficial bite of left thigh D, S 🔍
        ●■ S70.379   Other superficial bite of unspecified thigh D, S 🔍

● S70.9   Unspecified superficial injury of hip and thigh
    ● S70.91   Unspecified superficial injury of hip
        ●■ S70.911   Unspecified superficial injury of right hip D, S 🔍
        ●■ S70.912   Unspecified superficial injury of left hip D, S 🔍
        ●■ S70.919   Unspecified superficial injury of unspecified hip D, S 🔍

● S70.92   Unspecified superficial injury of thigh
    ●■ S70.921   Unspecified superficial injury of right thigh D, S 🔍
    ●■ S70.922   Unspecified superficial injury of left thigh D, S 🔍
    ●■ S70.929   Unspecified superficial injury of unspecified thigh D, S 🔍

● S71   Open wound of hip and thigh
    Code also any associated wound infection
    Excludes1   open fracture of hip and thigh (S72.-)
                traumatic amputation of hip and thigh (S78.-)
    Excludes2   bite of venomous animal (T63.-)
                open wound of ankle, foot and toes (S91.-)
                open wound of knee and lower leg (S81.-)

    The appropriate 7th character is to be added to each code from category S71

    | A | initial encounter |
    | D | subsequent encounter |
    | S | sequela |

    ● S71.0   Open wound of hip
        ● S71.00   Unspecified open wound of hip
            ●■ S71.001   Unspecified open wound, right hip D, S 🔍
            ●■ S71.002   Unspecified open wound, left hip D, S 🔍
            ●■ S71.009   Unspecified open wound, unspecified hip D, S 🔍
        ● S71.01   Laceration without foreign body of hip
            ● S71.011   Laceration without foreign body, right hip D, S 🔍
            ● S71.012   Laceration without foreign body, left hip D, S 🔍
            ●■ S71.019   Laceration without foreign body, unspecified hip D, S 🔍
        ● S71.02   Laceration with foreign body of hip
            ● S71.021   Laceration with foreign body, right hip D, S 🔍
            ● S71.022   Laceration with foreign body, left hip D, S 🔍
            ●■ S71.029   Laceration with foreign body, unspecified hip D, S 🔍
        ● S71.03   Puncture wound without foreign body of hip
            ● S71.031   Puncture wound without foreign body, right hip D, S 🔍
            ● S71.032   Puncture wound without foreign body, left hip D, S 🔍
            ●■ S71.039   Puncture wound without foreign body, unspecified hip D, S 🔍
        ● S71.04   Puncture wound with foreign body of hip
            ● S71.041   Puncture wound with foreign body, right hip D, S 🔍
            ● S71.042   Puncture wound with foreign body, left hip D, S 🔍
            ●■ S71.049   Puncture wound with foreign body, unspecified hip D, S 🔍

● Unacceptable Principal Diagnosis   ● Use Additional Character(s)   ■ Unspecified   ▶ Manifestation Code
OGCR   Official Guidelines for Coding and Reporting   Excludes 1   Excludes 2   Includes   Use additional   Code first   Code also

● **S71.05   Open bite of hip**
    Bite of hip NOS
    Excludes1 superficial bite of hip
    (S70.26, S70.27)

    ● **S71.051   Open bite, right hip** D, S ◔

    ● **S71.052   Open bite, left hip** D, S ◔

    ●◼ **S71.059   Open bite, unspecified hip**
        D, S ◔

● **S71.1   Open wound of thigh**

    ● **S71.10   Unspecified open wound of thigh**

        ●◼ **S71.101   Unspecified open wound, right
            thigh** D, S ◔

        ●◼ **S71.102   Unspecified open wound, left
            thigh** D, S ◔

        ●◼ **S71.109   Unspecified open wound,
            unspecified thigh** D, S ◔

    ● **S71.11   Laceration without foreign body of thigh**

        ● **S71.111   Laceration without foreign body,
            right thigh** D, S ◔

        ● **S71.112   Laceration without foreign body,
            left thigh** D, S ◔

        ●◼ **S71.119   Laceration without foreign body,
            unspecified thigh** D, S ◔

    ● **S71.12   Laceration with foreign body of thigh**

        ● **S71.121   Laceration with foreign body,
            right thigh** D, S ◔

        ● **S71.122   Laceration with foreign body, left
            thigh** D, S ◔

        ●◼ **S71.129   Laceration with foreign body,
            unspecified thigh** D, S ◔

    ● **S71.13   Puncture wound without foreign body of
        thigh**

        ● **S71.131   Puncture wound without foreign
            body, right thigh** D, S ◔

        ● **S71.132   Puncture wound without foreign
            body, left thigh** D, S ◔

        ●◼ **S71.139   Puncture wound without foreign
            body, unspecified thigh** D, S ◔

    ● **S71.14   Puncture wound with foreign body of
        thigh**

        ● **S71.141   Puncture wound with foreign
            body, right thigh** D, S ◔

        ● **S71.142   Puncture wound with foreign
            body, left thigh** D, S ◔

        ●◼ **S71.149   Puncture wound with foreign
            body, unspecified thigh** D, S ◔

    ● **S71.15   Open bite of thigh**
        Bite of thigh NOS
        Excludes1 superficial bite of thigh
        (S70.37-)

        ● **S71.151   Open bite, right thigh** D, S ◔

        ● **S71.152   Open bite, left thigh** D, S ◔

        ●◼ **S71.159   Open bite, unspecified thigh**
            D, S ◔

● **S72   Fracture of femur**

    Note: A fracture not indicated as displaced or
    nondisplaced should be coded to displaced

    A fracture not indicated as open or closed should be
    coded to closed

    The open fracture designations are based on the
    Gustilo open fracture classification

    Excludes1 traumatic amputation of hip and thigh
    (S78.-)

    Excludes2 fracture of lower leg and ankle (S82.-)
    fracture of foot (S92.-)
    periprosthetic fracture of prosthetic implant
    of hip (T84.040, T84.041)

    The appropriate 7th character is to be added to all codes
    from category S72

A	initial encounter for open fracture
B	initial encounter for open fracture type I or II
initial encounter for open fracture NOS
C	initial encounter for open fracture type IIIA, IIIB,
or IIIC
D	subsequent encounter for closed fracture with
routine healing
E	subsequent encounter for open fracture type I or
II with routine healing
F	subsequent encounter for open fracture type
IIIA, IIIB, or IIIC with routine healing
G	subsequent encounter for closed fracture with
delayed healing
H	subsequent encounter for open fracture type I or
II with delayed healing
J	subsequent encounter for open fracture type
IIIA, IIIB, or IIIC with delayed healing
K	subsequent encounter for closed fracture with
nonunion
M	subsequent encounter for open fracture type I or
II with nonunion
N	subsequent encounter for open fracture type
IIIA, IIIB, or IIIC with nonunion
P	subsequent encounter for closed fracture with
malunion
Q	subsequent encounter for open fracture type I or
II with malunion
R	subsequent encounter for open fracture type
IIIA, IIIB, or IIIC with malunion
S	sequela

● **S72.0   Fracture of head and neck of femur**
    Excludes2 physeal fracture of upper end of femur
    (S79.0-)

    ● **S72.00   Fracture of unspecified part of neck of
        femur**
        Fracture of hip NOS
        Fracture of neck of femur NOS

        ●◼ **S72.001   Fracture of unspecified part of
            neck of right femur**
            K, M, N, P, Q, R ◔, A, B, C ◔,
            D, E, F, G, H, J, S ◔, A, B, C ◔

        ●◼ **S72.002   Fracture of unspecified part of
            neck of left femur**
            K, M, N, P, Q, R ◔, A, B, C ◔,
            D, E, F, G, H, J, S ◔, A, B, C ◔

        ●◼ **S72.009   Fracture of unspecified part of
            neck of unspecified femur**
            K, M, N, P, Q, R ◔, A, B, C ◔,
            D, E, F, G, H, J, S ◔, A, B, C ◔

N Newborn Age: 0   **P** Pediatric Age: 0–17   **M** Maternity DX: 12–55   **A** Adult Age: 15–124   ♀ Females Only   ♂ Males Only

◔ Complication\Comorbidity   ◔ Major C\C   ◔ Present on Admission Requirement   ◔ Hospital-Acquired Condition

CHAPTER 19 (S00-T88)

1531

CHAPTER 19 (S00-T88)

● **S72.01 Unspecified intracapsular fracture of femur**
 Subcapital fracture of femur

● ● **S72.011 Unspecified intracapsular fracture of right femur**
 K, M, N, P, Q, R ⬡, A, B, C ⬡, D, E, F, G, H, J, S ⬡, A, B, C ⬡

● ● **S72.012 Unspecified intracapsular fracture of left femur**
 K, M, N, P, Q, R ⬡, A, B, C ⬡, D, E, F, G, H, J, S ⬡, A, B, C ⬡

● ● **S72.019 Unspecified intracapsular fracture of unspecified femur**
 K, M, N, P, Q, R ⬡, A, B, C ⬡, D, E, F, G, H, J, S ⬡, A, B, C ⬡

● **S72.02 Fracture of epiphysis (separation) (upper) of femur**
 Transepiphyseal fracture of femur
 Fracture and separation across growth plate

 Excludes1 capital femoral epiphyseal fracture (pediatric) of femur (S79.01-)
 Salter-Harris Type I physeal fracture of upper end of femur (S79.01-)

● **S72.021 Displaced fracture of epiphysis (separation) (upper) of right femur** K, M, N, P, Q, R ⬡, A, B, C ⬡, D, E, F, G, H, J, S ⬡, A, B, C ⬡

● **S72.022 Displaced fracture of epiphysis (separation) (upper) of left femur** K, M, N, P, Q, R ⬡, A, B, C ⬡, D, E, F, G, H, J, S ⬡, A, B, C ⬡

● ● **S72.023 Displaced fracture of epiphysis (separation) (upper) of unspecified femur**
 K, M, N, P, Q, R ⬡, A, B, C ⬡, D, E, F, G, H, J, S ⬡, A, B, C ⬡

● **S72.024 Nondisplaced fracture of epiphysis (separation) (upper) of right femur** K, M, N, P, Q, R ⬡, A, B, C ⬡, D, E, F, G, H, J, S ⬡, A, B, C ⬡

● **S72.025 Nondisplaced fracture of epiphysis (separation) (upper) of left femur** K, M, N, P, Q, R ⬡, A, B, C ⬡, D, E, F, G, H, J, S ⬡, A, B, C ⬡

● ● **S72.026 Nondisplaced fracture of epiphysis (separation) (upper) of unspecified femur**
 K, M, N, P, Q, R ⬡, A, B, C ⬡, D, E, F, G, H, J, S ⬡, A, B, C ⬡

● **S72.03 Midcervical fracture of femur**
 Transcervical fracture of femur NOS

● **S72.031 Displaced midcervical fracture of right femur** K, M, N, P, Q, R ⬡, A, B, C ⬡, D, E, F, G, H, J, S ⬡, A, B, C ⬡

● **S72.032 Displaced midcervical fracture of left femur** K, M, N, P, Q, R ⬡, A, B, C ⬡, D, E, F, G, H, J, S ⬡, A, B, C ⬡

● ● **S72.033 Displaced midcervical fracture of unspecified femur**
 K, M, N, P, Q, R ⬡, A, B, C ⬡, D, E, F, G, H, J, S ⬡, A, B, C ⬡

● **S72.034 Nondisplaced midcervical fracture of right femur**
 K, M, N, P, Q, R ⬡, A, B, C ⬡, D, E, F, G, H, J, S ⬡, A, B, C ⬡

● **S72.035 Nondisplaced midcervical fracture of left femur**
 K, M, N, P, Q, R ⬡, A, B, C ⬡, D, E, F, G, H, J, S ⬡, A, B, C ⬡

● ● **S72.036 Nondisplaced midcervical fracture of unspecified femur**
 K, M, N, P, Q, R ⬡, A, B, C ⬡, D, E, F, G, H, J, S ⬡, A, B, C ⬡

● **S72.04 Fracture of base of neck of femur**
 Cervicotrochanteric fracture of femur

● **S72.041 Displaced fracture of base of neck of right femur**
 K, M, N, P, Q, R ⬡, A, B, C ⬡, D, E, F, G, H, J, S ⬡, A, B, C ⬡

● **S72.042 Displaced fracture of base of neck of left femur**
 K, M, N, P, Q, R ⬡, A, B, C ⬡, D, E, F, G, H, J, S ⬡, A, B, C ⬡

● ● **S72.043 Displaced fracture of base of neck of unspecified femur**
 K, M, N, P, Q, R ⬡, A, B, C ⬡, D, E, F, G, H, J, S ⬡, A, B, C ⬡

● **S72.044 Nondisplaced fracture of base of neck of right femur**
 K, M, N, P, Q, R ⬡, A, B, C ⬡, D, E, F, G, H, J, S ⬡, A, B, C ⬡

● **S72.045 Nondisplaced fracture of base of neck of left femur**
 K, M, N, P, Q, R ⬡, A, B, C ⬡, D, E, F, G, H, J, S ⬡, A, B, C ⬡

● ● **S72.046 Nondisplaced fracture of base of neck of unspecified femur**
 K, M, N, P, Q, R ⬡, A, B, C ⬡, D, E, F, G, H, J, S ⬡, A, B, C ⬡

● **S72.05 Unspecified fracture of head of femur**
 Fracture of head of femur NOS

● ● **S72.051 Unspecified fracture of head of right femur** K, M, N, P, Q, R ⬡, A, B, C ⬡, D, E, F, G, H, J, S ⬡, A, B, C ⬡

● ● **S72.052 Unspecified fracture of head of left femur** K, M, N, P, Q, R ⬡, A, B, C ⬡, D, E, F, G, H, J, S ⬡, A, B, C ⬡

● ● **S72.059 Unspecified fracture of head of unspecified femur**
 K, M, N, P, Q, R ⬡, A, B, C ⬡, D, E, F, G, H, J, S ⬡, A, B, C ⬡

● **S72.06 Articular fracture of head of femur**

● **S72.061 Displaced articular fracture of head of right femur**
 K, M, N, P, Q, R ⬡, A, B, C ⬡, D, E, F, G, H, J, S ⬡, A, B, C ⬡

● **S72.062 Displaced articular fracture of head of left femur**
 K, M, N, P, Q, R ⬡, A, B, C ⬡, D, E, F, G, H, J, S ⬡, A, B, C ⬡

● ● **S72.063 Displaced articular fracture of head of unspecified femur**
 K, M, N, P, Q, R ⬡, A, B, C ⬡, D, E, F, G, H, J, S ⬡, A, B, C ⬡

● Unacceptable Principal Diagnosis   ● Use Additional Character(s)   ⬛ Unspecified   ▶ Manifestation Code
OGCR Official Guidelines for Coding and Reporting   Excludes 1   Excludes 2   Includes   Use additional   Code first   Code also

● S72.064   **Nondisplaced articular fracture of head of right femur**
K, M, N, P, Q, R 🦠, A, B, C 🦠, D, E, F, G, H, J, S 🦠, A, B, C 🦠

● S72.065   **Nondisplaced articular fracture of head of left femur**
K, M, N, P, Q, R 🦠, A, B, C 🦠, D, E, F, G, H, J, S 🦠, A, B, C 🦠

● ◼ S72.066   **Nondisplaced articular fracture of head of unspecified femur**
K, M, N, P, Q, R 🦠, A, B, C 🦠, D, E, F, G, H, J, S 🦠, A, B, C 🦠

● S72.09   **Other fracture of head and neck of femur**

  ● S72.091   **Other fracture of head and neck of right femur** K, M, N, P, Q, R 🦠, A, B, C 🦠, D, E, F, G, H, J, S 🦠, A, B, C 🦠

  ● S72.092   **Other fracture of head and neck of left femur** K, M, N, P, Q, R 🦠, A, B, C 🦠, D, E, F, G, H, J, S 🦠, A, B, C 🦠

  ● ◼ S72.099   **Other fracture of head and neck of unspecified femur**
K, M, N, P, Q, R 🦠, A, B, C 🦠, D, E, F, G, H, J, S 🦠, A, B, C 🦠

● **S72.1   Pertrochanteric fracture**
Fracture extending close to, but not into, joint

  ● S72.10   **Unspecified trochanteric fracture of femur**
Fracture of trochanter NOS

    ● ◼ S72.101   **Unspecified trochanteric fracture of right femur** K, M, N, P, Q, R 🦠, A, B, C 🦠, D, E, F, G, H, J, S 🦠, A, B, C 🦠

    ● ◼ S72.102   **Unspecified trochanteric fracture of left femur** K, M, N, P, Q, R 🦠, A, B, C 🦠, D, E, F, G, H, J, S 🦠, A, B, C 🦠

    ● ◼ S72.109   **Unspecified trochanteric fracture of unspecified femur**
K, M, N, P, Q, R 🦠, A, B, C 🦠, D, E, F, G, H, J, S 🦠, A, B, C 🦠

  ● S72.11   **Fracture of greater trochanter of femur**

    ● S72.111   **Displaced fracture of greater trochanter of right femur**
K, M, N, P, Q, R 🦠, A, B, C 🦠, D, E, F, G, H, J, S 🦠, A, B, C 🦠

    ● S72.112   **Displaced fracture of greater trochanter of left femur**
K, M, N, P, Q, R 🦠, A, B, C 🦠, D, E, F, G, H, J, S 🦠, A, B, C 🦠

    ● ◼ S72.113   **Displaced fracture of greater trochanter of unspecified femur**
K, M, N, P, Q, R 🦠, A, B, C 🦠, D, E, F, G, H, J, S 🦠, A, B, C 🦠

    ● S72.114   **Nondisplaced fracture of greater trochanter of right femur**
K, M, N, P, Q, R 🦠, A, B, C 🦠, D, E, F, G, H, J, S 🦠, A, B, C 🦠

    ● S72.115   **Nondisplaced fracture of greater trochanter of left femur**
K, M, N, P, Q, R 🦠, A, B, C 🦠, D, E, F, G, H, J, S 🦠, A, B, C 🦠

    ● ◼ S72.116   **Nondisplaced fracture of greater trochanter of unspecified femur**
K, M, N, P, Q, R 🦠, A, B, C 🦠, D, E, F, G, H, J, S 🦠, A, B, C 🦠

● S72.12   **Fracture of lesser trochanter of femur**

  ● S72.121   **Displaced fracture of lesser trochanter of right femur**
K, M, N, P, Q, R 🦠, A, B, C 🦠, D, E, F, G, H, J, S 🦠, A, B, C 🦠

  ● S72.122   **Displaced fracture of lesser trochanter of left femur**
K, M, N, P, Q, R 🦠, A, B, C 🦠, D, E, F, G, H, J, S 🦠, A, B, C 🦠

  ● ◼ S72.123   **Displaced fracture of lesser trochanter of unspecified femur**
K, M, N, P, Q, R 🦠, A, B, C 🦠, D, E, F, G, H, J, S 🦠, A, B, C 🦠

  ● S72.124   **Nondisplaced fracture of lesser trochanter of right femur**
K, M, N, P, Q, R 🦠, A, B, C 🦠, D, E, F, G, H, J, S 🦠, A, B, C 🦠

  ● S72.125   **Nondisplaced fracture of lesser trochanter of left femur**
K, M, N, P, Q, R 🦠, A, B, C 🦠, D, E, F, G, H, J, S 🦠, A, B, C 🦠

  ● ◼ S72.126   **Nondisplaced fracture of lesser trochanter of unspecified femur**
K, M, N, P, Q, R 🦠, A, B, C 🦠, D, E, F, G, H, J, S 🦠, A, B, C 🦠

● S72.13   **Apophyseal fracture of femur**
Pertaining to articulations between articular facets of adjacent vertebrae

    Excludes1   chronic (nontraumatic) slipped upper femoral epiphysis (M93.0-)

  ● S72.131   **Displaced apophyseal fracture of right femur** K, M, N, P, Q, R 🦠, A, B, C 🦠, D, E, F, G, H, J, S 🦠, A, B, C 🦠

  ● S72.132   **Displaced apophyseal fracture of left femur** K, M, N, P, Q, R 🦠, A, B, C 🦠, D, E, F, G, H, J, S 🦠, A, B, C 🦠

  ● ◼ S72.133   **Displaced apophyseal fracture of unspecified femur**
K, M, N, P, Q, R 🦠, A, B, C 🦠, D, E, F, G, H, J, S 🦠, A, B, C 🦠

  ● S72.134   **Nondisplaced apophyseal fracture of right femur**
K, M, N, P, Q, R 🦠, A, B, C 🦠, D, E, F, G, H, J, S 🦠, A, B, C 🦠

  ● S72.135   **Nondisplaced apophyseal fracture of left femur**
K, M, N, P, Q, R 🦠, A, B, C 🦠, D, E, F, G, H, J, S 🦠, A, B, C 🦠

  ● ◼ S72.136   **Nondisplaced apophyseal fracture of unspecified femur**
K, M, N, P, Q, R 🦠, A, B, C 🦠, D, E, F, G, H, J, S 🦠, A, B, C 🦠

● S72.14   **Intertrochanteric fracture of femur**

  ● S72.141   **Displaced intertrochanteric fracture of right femur**
K, M, N, P, Q, R 🦠, A, B, C 🦠, D, E, F, G, H, J, S 🦠, A, B, C 🦠

  ● S72.142   **Displaced intertrochanteric fracture of left femur**
K, M, N, P, Q, R 🦠, A, B, C 🦠, D, E, F, G, H, J, S 🦠, A, B, C 🦠

  ● ◼ S72.143   **Displaced intertrochanteric fracture of unspecified femur**
K, M, N, P, Q, R 🦠, A, B, C 🦠, D, E, F, G, H, J, S 🦠, A, B, C 🦠

N Newborn Age: 0   **P** Pediatric Age: 0–17   **M** Maternity DX: 12–55   **A** Adult Age: 15–124   ♀ Females Only   ♂ Males Only

🦠 Complication\Comorbidity   🦠 Major C\C   🦠 Present on Admission Requirement   🦠 Hospital-Acquired Condition

1533

- S72.144 Nondisplaced intertrochanteric fracture of right femur
  K, M, N, P, Q, R ✪, A, B, C ✪, D, E, F, G, H, J, S ✪, A, B, C ✪

- S72.145 Nondisplaced intertrochanteric fracture of left femur
  K, M, N, P, Q, R ✪, A, B, C ✪, D, E, F, G, H, J, S ✪, A, B, C ✪

- ■ S72.146 Nondisplaced intertrochanteric fracture of unspecified femur
  K, M, N, P, Q, R ✪, A, B, C ✪, D, E, F, G, H, J, S ✪, A, B, C ✪

- S72.2 Subtrochanteric fracture of femur
  Subtrochanteric: inferior to trochanter

  - S72.21 Displaced subtrochanteric fracture of right femur K, M, N, P, Q, R ✪, A, B, C ✪, D, E, F, G, H, J, S ✪, A, B, C ✪

  - S72.22 Displaced subtrochanteric fracture of left femur K, M, N, P, Q, R ✪, A, B, C ✪, D, E, F, G, H, J, S ✪, A, B, C ✪

  - ■ S72.23 Displaced subtrochanteric fracture of unspecified femur K, M, N, P, Q, R ✪, A, B, C ✪, D, E, F, G, H, J, S ✪, A, B, C ✪

  - S72.24 Nondisplaced subtrochanteric fracture of right femur K, M, N, P, Q, R ✪, A, B, C ✪, D, E, F, G, H, J, S ✪, A, B, C ✪

  - S72.25 Nondisplaced subtrochanteric fracture of left femur K, M, N, P, Q, R ✪, A, B, C ✪, D, E, F, G, H, J, S ✪, A, B, C ✪

  - ■ S72.26 Nondisplaced subtrochanteric fracture of unspecified femur K, M, N, P, Q, R ✪, A, B, C ✪, D, E, F, G, H, J, S ✪, A, B, C ✪

- S72.3 Fracture of shaft of femur

  - S72.30 Unspecified fracture of shaft of femur

    - ■ S72.301 Unspecified fracture of shaft of right femur K, M, N, P, Q, R ✪, A, B, C ✪, D, E, F, G, H, J, S ✪, A, B, C ✪

    - ■ S72.302 Unspecified fracture of shaft of left femur K, M, N, P, Q, R ✪, A, B, C ✪, D, E, F, G, H, J, S ✪, A, B, C ✪

    - ■ S72.309 Unspecified fracture of shaft of unspecified femur
      K, M, N, P, Q, R ✪, A, B, C ✪, D, E, F, G, H, J, S ✪, A, B, C ✪

  - S72.32 Transverse fracture of shaft of femur

    - S72.321 Displaced transverse fracture of shaft of right femur K, M, N, P, Q, R ✪, A, B, C ✪, D, E, F, G, H, J, S ✪, A, B, C ✪

    - S72.322 Displaced transverse fracture of shaft of left femur K, M, N, P, Q, R ✪, A, B, C ✪, D, E, F, G, H, J, S ✪, A, B, C ✪

    - ■ S72.323 Displaced transverse fracture of shaft of unspecified femur
      K, M, N, P, Q, R ✪, A, B, C ✪, D, E, F, G, H, J, S ✪, A, B, C ✪

    - S72.324 Nondisplaced transverse fracture of shaft of right femur
      K, M, N, P, Q, R ✪, A, B, C ✪, D, E, F, G, H, J, S ✪, A, B, C ✪

    - S72.325 Nondisplaced transverse fracture of shaft of left femur
      K, M, N, P, Q, R ✪, A, B, C ✪, D, E, F, G, H, J, S ✪, A, B, C ✪

- ■ S72.326 Nondisplaced transverse fracture of shaft of unspecified femur
  K, M, N, P, Q, R ✪, A, B, C ✪, D, E, F, G, H, J, S ✪, A, B, C ✪

- S72.33 Oblique fracture of shaft of femur

  - S72.331 Displaced oblique fracture of shaft of right femur
    K, M, N, P, Q, R ✪, A, B, C ✪, D, E, F, G, H, J, S ✪, A, B, C ✪

  - S72.332 Displaced oblique fracture of shaft of left femur
    K, M, N, P, Q, R ✪, A, B, C ✪, D, E, F, G, H, J, S ✪, A, B, C ✪

  - ■ S72.333 Displaced oblique fracture of shaft of unspecified femur
    K, M, N, P, Q, R ✪, A, B, C ✪, D, E, F, G, H, J, S ✪, A, B, C ✪

  - S72.334 Nondisplaced oblique fracture of shaft of right femur
    K, M, N, P, Q, R ✪, A, B, C ✪, D, E, F, G, H, J, S ✪, A, B, C ✪

  - S72.335 Nondisplaced oblique fracture of shaft of left femur
    K, M, N, P, Q, R ✪, A, B, C ✪, D, E, F, G, H, J, S ✪, A, B, C ✪

  - ■ S72.336 Nondisplaced oblique fracture of shaft of unspecified femur
    K, M, N, P, Q, R ✪, A, B, C ✪, D, E, F, G, H, J, S ✪, A, B, C ✪

- S72.34 Spiral fracture of shaft of femur

  - S72.341 Displaced spiral fracture of shaft of right femur K, M, N, P, Q, R ✪, A, B, C ✪, D, E, F, G, H, J, S ✪, A, B, C ✪

  - S72.342 Displaced spiral fracture of shaft of left femur K, M, N, P, Q, R ✪, A, B, C ✪, D, E, F, G, H, J, S ✪, A, B, C ✪

  - ■ S72.343 Displaced spiral fracture of shaft of unspecified femur
    K, M, N, P, Q, R ✪, A, B, C ✪, D, E, F, G, H, J, S ✪, A, B, C ✪

  - S72.344 Nondisplaced spiral fracture of shaft of right femur
    K, M, N, P, Q, R ✪, A, B, C ✪, D, E, F, G, H, J, S ✪, A, B, C ✪

  - S72.345 Nondisplaced spiral fracture of shaft of left femur
    K, M, N, P, Q, R ✪, A, B, C ✪, D, E, F, G, H, J, S ✪, A, B, C ✪

  - ■ S72.346 Nondisplaced spiral fracture of shaft of unspecified femur
    K, M, N, P, Q, R ✪, A, B, C ✪, D, E, F, G, H, J, S ✪, A, B, C ✪

- S72.35 Comminuted fracture of shaft of femur

  - S72.351 Displaced comminuted fracture of shaft of right femur
    K, M, N, P, Q, R ✪, A, B, C ✪, D, E, F, G, H, J, S ✪, A, B, C ✪

  - S72.352 Displaced comminuted fracture of shaft of left femur
    K, M, N, P, Q, R ✪, A, B, C ✪, D, E, F, G, H, J, S ✪, A, B, C ✪

  - ■ S72.353 Displaced comminuted fracture of shaft of unspecified femur
    K, M, N, P, Q, R ✪, A, B, C ✪, D, E, F, G, H, J, S ✪, A, B, C ✪

- Unacceptable Principal Diagnosis   ● Use Additional Character(s)   ■ Unspecified   ▶ Manifestation Code

OGCR Official Guidelines for Coding and Reporting   Excludes 1   Excludes 2   Includes   Use additional   Code first   Code also

● S72.354   Nondisplaced comminuted fracture of shaft of right femur K, M, N, P, Q, R 🩺, A, B, C 🩺, D, E, F, G, H, J, S 🩺, A, B, C 🩺

● S72.355   Nondisplaced comminuted fracture of shaft of left femur K, M, N, P, Q, R 🩺, A, B, C 🩺, D, E, F, G, H, J, S 🩺, A, B, C 🩺

●■ S72.356   Nondisplaced comminuted fracture of shaft of unspecified femur K, M, N, P, Q, R 🩺, A, B, C 🩺, D, E, F, G, H, J, S 🩺, A, B, C 🩺

● S72.36   Segmental fracture of shaft of femur

  ● S72.361   Displaced segmental fracture of shaft of right femur K, M, N, P, Q, R 🩺, A, B, C 🩺, D, E, F, G, H, J, S 🩺, A, B, C 🩺

  ● S72.362   Displaced segmental fracture of shaft of left femur K, M, N, P, Q, R 🩺, A, B, C 🩺, D, E, F, G, H, J, S 🩺, A, B, C 🩺

  ●■ S72.363   Displaced segmental fracture of shaft of unspecified femur K, M, N, P, Q, R 🩺, A, B, C 🩺, D, E, F, G, H, J, S 🩺, A, B, C 🩺

  ● S72.364   Nondisplaced segmental fracture of shaft of right femur K, M, N, P, Q, R 🩺, A, B, C 🩺, D, E, F, G, H, J, S 🩺, A, B, C 🩺

  ● S72.365   Nondisplaced segmental fracture of shaft of left femur K, M, N, P, Q, R 🩺, A, B, C 🩺, D, E, F, G, H, J, S 🩺, A, B, C 🩺

  ●■ S72.366   Nondisplaced segmental fracture of shaft of unspecified femur K, M, N, P, Q, R 🩺, A, B, C 🩺, D, E, F, G, H, J, S 🩺, A, B, C 🩺

● S72.39   Other fracture of shaft of femur

  ● S72.391   Other fracture of shaft of right femur K, M, N, P, Q, R 🩺, A, B, C 🩺, D, E, F, G, H, J, S 🩺, A, B, C 🩺

  ● S72.392   Other fracture of shaft of left femur K, M, N, P, Q, R 🩺, A, B, C 🩺, D, E, F, G, H, J, S 🩺, A, B, C 🩺

  ●■ S72.399   Other fracture of shaft of unspecified femur K, M, N, P, Q, R 🩺, A, B, C 🩺, D, E, F, G, H, J, S 🩺, A, B, C 🩺

● S72.4   Fracture of lower end of femur

Fracture of distal end of femur

> **Excludes2**   fracture of shaft of femur (S72.3-)
> physeal fracture of lower end of femur (S79.1-)

● S72.40   Unspecified fracture of lower end of femur

  ●■ S72.401   Unspecified fracture of lower end of right femur A, K, M, N, P, Q, R 🩺, B, C 🩺, D, E, F, G, H, J, S 🩺, A, B, C 🩺

  ●■ S72.402   Unspecified fracture of lower end of left femur A, K, M, N, P, Q, R 🩺, B, C 🩺, D, E, F, G, H, J, S 🩺, A, B, C 🩺

●■ S72.409   Unspecified fracture of lower end of unspecified femur A, K, M, N, P, Q, R 🩺, B, C 🩺, D, E, F, G, H, J, S 🩺, A, B, C 🩺

● S72.41   Unspecified condyle fracture of lower end of femur

Condyle fracture of femur NOS

  ●■ S72.411   Displaced unspecified condyle fracture of lower end of right femur A, K, M, N, P, Q, R 🩺, B, C 🩺, D, E, F, G, H, J, S 🩺, A, B, C 🩺

  ●■ S72.412   Displaced unspecified condyle fracture of lower end of left femur A, K, M, N, P, Q, R 🩺, B, C 🩺, D, E, F, G, H, J, S 🩺, A, B, C 🩺

  ●■ S72.413   Displaced unspecified condyle fracture of lower end of unspecified femur A, K, M, N, P, Q, R 🩺, B, C 🩺, D, E, F, G, H, J, S 🩺, A, B, C 🩺

  ●■ S72.414   Nondisplaced unspecified condyle fracture of lower end of right femur A, K, M, N, P, Q, R 🩺, B, C 🩺, D, E, F, G, H, J, S 🩺, A, B, C 🩺

  ●■ S72.415   Nondisplaced unspecified condyle fracture of lower end of left femur A, K, M, N, P, Q, R 🩺, B, C 🩺, D, E, F, G, H, J, S 🩺, A, B, C 🩺

  ●■ S72.416   Nondisplaced unspecified condyle fracture of lower end of unspecified femur A, K, M, N, P, Q, R 🩺, B, C 🩺, D, E, F, G, H, J, S 🩺, A, B, C 🩺

● S72.42   Fracture of lateral condyle of femur

  ● S72.421   Displaced fracture of lateral condyle of right femur A, K, M, N, P, Q, R 🩺, B, C 🩺, D, E, F, G, H, J, S 🩺, A, B, C 🩺

  ● S72.422   Displaced fracture of lateral condyle of left femur A, K, M, N, P, Q, R 🩺, B, C 🩺, D, E, F, G, H, J, S 🩺, A, B, C 🩺

  ●■ S72.423   Displaced fracture of lateral condyle of unspecified femur A, K, M, N, P, Q, R 🩺, B, C 🩺, D, E, F, G, H, J, S 🩺, A, B, C 🩺

  ● S72.424   Nondisplaced fracture of lateral condyle of right femur A, K, M, N, P, Q, R 🩺, B, C 🩺, D, E, F, G, H, J, S 🩺, A, B, C 🩺

  ● S72.425   Nondisplaced fracture of lateral condyle of left femur A, K, M, N, P, Q, R 🩺, B, C 🩺, D, E, F, G, H, J, S 🩺, A, B, C 🩺

  ●■ S72.426   Nondisplaced fracture of lateral condyle of unspecified femur A, K, M, N, P, Q, R 🩺, B, C 🩺, D, E, F, G, H, J, S 🩺, A, B, C 🩺

CHAPTER 19 (S00-T88)

● **S72.43**   **Fracture of medial condyle of femur**

  ● **S72.431**   Displaced fracture of medial condyle of right femur A, K, M, N, P, Q, R 🔄, B, C 🔄, D, E, F, G, H, J, S 🔄, A, B, C 🔄

  ● **S72.432**   Displaced fracture of medial condyle of left femur A, K, M, N, P, Q, R 🔄, B, C 🔄, D, E, F, G, H, J, S 🔄, A, B, C 🔄

  ●■ **S72.433**   Displaced fracture of medial condyle of unspecified femur A, K, M, N, P, Q, R 🔄, B, C 🔄, D, E, F, G, H, J, S 🔄, A, B, C 🔄

  ● **S72.434**   Nondisplaced fracture of medial condyle of right femur A, K, M, N, P, Q, R 🔄, B, C 🔄, D, E, F, G, H, J, S 🔄, A, B, C 🔄

  ● **S72.435**   Nondisplaced fracture of medial condyle of left femur A, K, M, N, P, Q, R 🔄, B, C 🔄, D, E, F, G, H, J, S 🔄, A, B, C 🔄

  ●■ **S72.436**   Nondisplaced fracture of medial condyle of unspecified femur A, K, M, N, P, Q, R 🔄, B, C 🔄, D, E, F, G, H, J, S 🔄, A, B, C 🔄

● **S72.44**   **Fracture of lower epiphysis (separation) of femur**

   Excludes1   Salter-Harris Type I physeal fracture of lower end of femur (S79.11-)

  ● **S72.441**   Displaced fracture of lower epiphysis (separation) of right femur A, K, M, N, P, Q, R 🔄, B, C 🔄, D, E, F, G, H, J, S 🔄, A, B, C 🔄

  ● **S72.442**   Displaced fracture of lower epiphysis (separation) of left femur A, K, M, N, P, Q, R 🔄, B, C 🔄, D, E, F, G, H, J, S 🔄, A, B, C 🔄

  ●■ **S72.443**   Displaced fracture of lower epiphysis (separation) of unspecified femur A, K, M, N, P, Q, R 🔄, B, C 🔄, D, E, F, G, H, J, S 🔄, A, B, C 🔄

  ● **S72.444**   Nondisplaced fracture of lower epiphysis (separation) of right femur A, K, M, N, P, Q, R 🔄, B, C 🔄, D, E, F, G, H, J, S 🔄, A, B, C 🔄

  ● **S72.445**   Nondisplaced fracture of lower epiphysis (separation) of left femur A, K, M, N, P, Q, R 🔄, B, C 🔄, D, E, F, G, H, J, S 🔄, A, B, C 🔄

  ●■ **S72.446**   Nondisplaced fracture of lower epiphysis (separation) of unspecified femur A, K, M, N, P, Q, R 🔄, B, C 🔄, D, E, F, G, H, J, S 🔄, A, B, C 🔄

● **S72.45**   **Supracondylar fracture without intracondylar extension of lower end of femur**

   Supracondylar fracture of lower end of femur NOS

   Excludes1   supracondylar fracture with intracondylar extension of lower end of femur (S72.46-)

  ● **S72.451**   Displaced supracondylar fracture without intracondylar extension of lower end of right femur A, K, M, N, P, Q, R 🔄, B, C 🔄, D, E, F, G, H, J, S 🔄, A, B, C 🔄

  ● **S72.452**   Displaced supracondylar fracture without intracondylar extension of lower end of left femur A, K, M, N, P, Q, R 🔄, B, C 🔄, D, E, F, G, H, J, S 🔄, A, B, C 🔄

  ●■ **S72.453**   Displaced supracondylar fracture without intracondylar extension of lower end of unspecified femur A, K, M, N, P, Q, R 🔄, B, C 🔄, D, E, F, G, H, J, S 🔄, A, B, C 🔄

  ● **S72.454**   Nondisplaced supracondylar fracture without intracondylar extension of lower end of right femur A, K, M, N, P, Q, R 🔄, B, C 🔄, D, E, F, G, H, J, S 🔄, A, B, C 🔄

  ● **S72.455**   Nondisplaced supracondylar fracture without intracondylar extension of lower end of left femur A, K, M, N, P, Q, R 🔄, B, C 🔄, D, E, F, G, H, J, S 🔄, A, B, C 🔄

  ●■ **S72.456**   Nondisplaced supracondylar fracture without intracondylar extension of lower end of unspecified femur A, K, M, N, P, Q, R 🔄, B, C 🔄, D, E, F, G, H, J, S 🔄, A, B, C 🔄

● **S72.46**   **Supracondylar fracture with intracondylar extension of lower end of femur**

   Excludes1   supracondylar fracture without intracondylar extension of lower end of femur (S72.45-)

  ● **S72.461**   Displaced supracondylar fracture with intracondylar extension of lower end of right femur A, K, M, N, P, Q, R 🔄, B, C 🔄, D, E, F, G, H, J, S 🔄, A, B, C 🔄

  ● **S72.462**   Displaced supracondylar fracture with intracondylar extension of lower end of left femur A, K, M, N, P, Q, R 🔄, B, C 🔄, D, E, F, G, H, J, S 🔄, A, B, C 🔄

  ●■ **S72.463**   Displaced supracondylar fracture with intracondylar extension of lower end of unspecified femur A, K, M, N, P, Q, R 🔄, B, C 🔄, D, E, F, G, H, J, S 🔄, A, B, C 🔄

● S72.464 **Nondisplaced supracondylar fracture with intracondylar extension of lower end of right femur A, K, M, N, P, Q, R 🍀, B, C 🍀, D, E, F, G, H, J, S 🍀, A, B, C 🍀**

● S72.465 **Nondisplaced supracondylar fracture with intracondylar extension of lower end of left femur A, K, M, N, P, Q, R 🍀, B, C 🍀, D, E, F, G, H, J, S 🍀, A, B, C 🍀**

● ■ S72.466 **Nondisplaced supracondylar fracture with intracondylar extension of lower end of unspecified femur A, K, M, N, P, Q, R 🍀, B, C 🍀, D, E, F, G, H, J, S 🍀, A, B, C 🍀**

● S72.47 **Torus fracture of lower end of femur**

The appropriate 7th character is to be added to all codes in subcategory S72.47

A	initial encounter for closed fracture
D	subsequent encounter for fracture with routine healing
G	subsequent encounter for fracture with delayed healing
K	subsequent encounter for fracture with nonunion
P	subsequent encounter for fracture with malunion
S	sequela

● S72.471 **Torus fracture of lower end of right femur A, K, P 🍀, 🍀, D, G, S 🍀, A 🍀**

● S72.472 **Torus fracture of lower end of left femur A, K, P 🍀, 🍀, D, G, S 🍀, A 🍀**

● ■ S72.479 **Torus fracture of lower end of unspecified femur A, K, P 🍀, 🍀, D, G, S 🍀, A 🍀**

● S72.49 **Other fracture of lower end of femur**

● S72.491 **Other fracture of lower end of right femur A, K, M, N, P, Q, R 🍀, B, C 🍀, D, E, F, G, H, J, S 🍀, A, B, C 🍀**

● S72.492 **Other fracture of lower end of left femur A, K, M, N, P, Q, R 🍀, B, C 🍀, D, E, F, G, H, J, S 🍀, A, B, C 🍀**

● ■ S72.499 **Other fracture of lower end of unspecified femur A, K, M, N, P, Q, R 🍀, B, C 🍀, D, E, F, G, H, J, S 🍀, A, B, C 🍀**

● S72.8 **Other fracture of femur**

● S72.8X **Other fracture of femur**

● S72.8X1 **Other fracture of right femur K, M, N, P, Q, R 🍀, A, B, C 🍀, D, E, F, G, H, J, S 🍀, A, B, C 🍀**

● S72.8X2 **Other fracture of left femur K, M, N, P, Q, R 🍀, A, B, C 🍀, D, E, F, G, H, J, S 🍀, A, B, C 🍀**

● ■ S72.8X9 **Other fracture of unspecified femur K, M, N, P, Q, R 🍀, A, B, C 🍀, D, E, F, G, H, J, S 🍀, A, B, C 🍀**

● S72.9 **Unspecified fracture of femur**
Fracture of thigh NOS
Fracture of upper leg NOS

Excludes1	fracture of hip NOS (S72.00-, S72.01-)

● ■ S72.90 **Unspecified fracture of unspecified femur K, M, N, P, Q, R 🍀, A, B, C 🍀, D, E, F, G, H, J, S 🍀, A, B, C 🍀**

● ■ S72.91 **Unspecified fracture of right femur K, M, N, P, Q, R 🍀, A, B, C 🍀, D, E, F, G, H, J, S 🍀, A, B, C 🍀**

● ■ S72.92 **Unspecified fracture of left femur K, M, N, P, Q, R 🍀, A, B, C 🍀, D, E, F, G, H, J, S 🍀, A, B, C 🍀**

● S73 **Dislocation and sprain of joint and ligaments of hip**

Includes	avulsion of joint or ligament of hip
	laceration of cartilage, joint or ligament of hip
	sprain of cartilage, joint or ligament of hip
	traumatic hemarthrosis of joint or ligament of hip
	traumatic rupture of joint or ligament of hip
	traumatic subluxation of joint or ligament of hip
	traumatic tear of joint or ligament of hip

Code also any associated open wound

Excludes2	strain of muscle, fascia and tendon of hip and thigh (S76.-)

The appropriate 7th character is to be added to each code from category S73

A	initial encounter
D	subsequent encounter
S	sequela

● S73.0 **Subluxation and dislocation of hip**
Out of position

Excludes2	dislocation and subluxation of hip prosthesis (T84.020, T84.021)

● S73.00 **Unspecified subluxation and dislocation of hip**
Dislocation of hip NOS
Subluxation of hip NOS

● ■ S73.001 **Unspecified subluxation of right hip A 🍀, D, S 🍀, A 🍀**

● ■ S73.002 **Unspecified subluxation of left hip A 🍀, D, S 🍀, A 🍀**

● ■ S73.003 **Unspecified subluxation of unspecified hip A 🍀, D, S 🍀, A 🍀**

● ■ S73.004 **Unspecified dislocation of right hip A 🍀, D, S 🍀, A 🍀**

● ■ S73.005 **Unspecified dislocation of left hip A 🍀, D, S 🍀, A 🍀**

● ■ S73.006 **Unspecified dislocation of unspecified hip A 🍀, D, S 🍀, A 🍀**

● S73.01 **Posterior subluxation and dislocation of hip**

● S73.011 **Posterior subluxation of right hip A 🍀, D, S 🍀, A 🍀**

● S73.012 **Posterior subluxation of left hip A 🍀, D, S 🍀, A 🍀**

● ■ S73.013 **Posterior subluxation of unspecified hip A 🍀, D, S 🍀, A 🍀**

● S73.014 **Posterior dislocation of right hip A 🍀, D, S 🍀, A 🍀**

● S73.015 **Posterior dislocation of left hip A 🍀, D, S 🍀, A 🍀**

● ■ S73.016 **Posterior dislocation of unspecified hip A 🍀, D, S 🍀, A 🍀**

CHAPTER 19 (S00-T88)

● **S73.02　Obturator subluxation and dislocation of hip**
　　● S73.021　Obturator subluxation of right hip A 🐾, D, S 🐾, A 🐾
　　● S73.022　Obturator subluxation of left hip A 🐾, D, S 🐾, A 🐾
　　●■ S73.023　Obturator subluxation of unspecified hip A 🐾, D, S 🐾, A 🐾
　　● S73.024　Obturator dislocation of right hip A 🐾, D, S 🐾, A 🐾
　　● S73.025　Obturator dislocation of left hip A 🐾, D, S 🐾, A 🐾
　　●■ S73.026　Obturator dislocation of unspecified hip A 🐾, D, S 🐾, A 🐾

● **S73.03　Other anterior dislocation of hip**
　　● S73.031　Other anterior subluxation of right hip A 🐾, D, S 🐾, A 🐾
　　● S73.032　Other anterior subluxation of left hip A 🐾, D, S 🐾, A 🐾
　　●■ S73.033　Other anterior subluxation of unspecified hip A 🐾, D, S 🐾, A 🐾
　　● S73.034　Other anterior dislocation of right hip A 🐾, D, S 🐾, A 🐾
　　● S73.035　Other anterior dislocation of left hip A 🐾, D, S 🐾, A 🐾
　　●■ S73.036　Other anterior dislocation of unspecified hip A 🐾, D, S 🐾, A 🐾

● **S73.04　Central dislocation of hip**
　　● S73.041　Central subluxation of right hip A 🐾, D, S 🐾, A 🐾
　　● S73.042　Central subluxation of left hip A 🐾, D, S 🐾, A 🐾
　　●■ S73.043　Central subluxation of unspecified hip A 🐾, D, S 🐾, A 🐾
　　● S73.044　Central dislocation of right hip A 🐾, D, S 🐾, A 🐾
　　● S73.045　Central dislocation of left hip A 🐾, D, S 🐾, A 🐾
　　●■ S73.046　Central dislocation of unspecified hip A 🐾, D, S 🐾, A 🐾

● **S73.1　Sprain of hip**
　● **S73.10　Unspecified sprain of hip**
　　●■ S73.101　Unspecified sprain of right hip D, S 🐾
　　●■ S73.102　Unspecified sprain of left hip D, S 🐾
　　●■ S73.109　Unspecified sprain of unspecified hip D, S 🐾
　● **S73.11　Iliofemoral ligament sprain of hip**
　　● S73.111　Iliofemoral ligament sprain of right hip D, S 🐾
　　● S73.112　Iliofemoral ligament sprain of left hip D, S 🐾
　　●■ S73.119　Iliofemoral ligament sprain of unspecified hip D, S 🐾
　● **S73.12　Ischiocapsular (ligament) sprain of hip**
　　● S73.121　Ischiocapsular ligament sprain of right hip D, S 🐾
　　● S73.122　Ischiocapsular ligament sprain of left hip D, S 🐾
　　●■ S73.129　Ischiocapsular ligament sprain of unspecified hip D, S 🐾

● **S73.19　Other sprain of hip**
　　● S73.191　Other sprain of right hip D, S 🐾
　　● S73.192　Other sprain of left hip D, S 🐾
　　●■ S73.199　Other sprain of unspecified hip D, S 🐾

● **S74　Injury of nerves at hip and thigh level**

Code also any associated open wound (S71.-)

Excludes2　injury of nerves at ankle and foot level (S94.-)
　　　　　injury of nerves at lower leg level (S84.-)

The appropriate 7th character is to be added to each code from category S74

> A　initial encounter
> D　subsequent encounter
> S　sequela

● **S74.0　Injury of sciatic nerve at hip and thigh level**
　　●■ S74.00　Injury of sciatic nerve at hip and thigh level, unspecified leg D, S 🐾
　　● S74.01　Injury of sciatic nerve at hip and thigh level, right leg D, S 🐾
　　● S74.02　Injury of sciatic nerve at hip and thigh level, left leg D, S 🐾

● **S74.1　Injury of femoral nerve at hip and thigh level**
　　●■ S74.10　Injury of femoral nerve at hip and thigh level, unspecified leg D, S 🐾
　　● S74.11　Injury of femoral nerve at hip and thigh level, right leg D, S 🐾
　　● S74.12　Injury of femoral nerve at hip and thigh level, left leg D, S 🐾

● **S74.2　Injury of cutaneous sensory nerve at hip and thigh level**
　　●■ S74.20　Injury of cutaneous sensory nerve at hip and thigh level, unspecified leg D, S 🐾
　　● S74.21　Injury of cutaneous sensory nerve at hip and high level, right leg D, S 🐾
　　● S74.22　Injury of cutaneous sensory nerve at hip and thigh level, left leg D, S 🐾

● **S74.8　Injury of other nerves at hip and thigh level**
　● **S74.8X　Injury of other nerves at hip and thigh level**
　　● S74.8X1　Injury of other nerves at hip and thigh level, right leg D, S 🐾
　　● S74.8X2　Injury of other nerves at hip and thigh level, left leg D, S 🐾
　　●■ S74.8X9　Injury of other nerves at hip and thigh level, unspecified leg D, S 🐾

● **S74.9　Injury of unspecified nerve at hip and thigh level**
　　●■ S74.90　Injury of unspecified nerve at hip and thigh level, unspecified leg D, S 🐾
　　●■ S74.91　Injury of unspecified nerve at hip and thigh level, right leg D, S 🐾
　　●■ S74.92　Injury of unspecified nerve at hip and thigh level, left leg D, S 🐾

● Unacceptable Principal Diagnosis　● Use Additional Character(s)　■ Unspecified　▶ Manifestation Code
OGCR　Official Guidelines for Coding and Reporting　Excludes 1　Excludes 2　Includes　Use additional　Code first　Code also

● **S75   Injury of blood vessels at hip and thigh level**

> Code also any associated open wound (S71.-)
>
> Excludes2   injury of blood vessels at lower leg level (S85.-)
> injury of popliteal artery (S85.0)
>
> The appropriate 7th character is to be added to each code from category S75
>
> A   initial encounter
> D   subsequent encounter
> S   sequela

● **S75.0   Injury of femoral artery**

   ● **S75.00   Unspecified injury of femoral artery**

      ● **S75.001   Unspecified injury of femoral artery, right leg** A 🖾, D, S 🖾

      ● **S75.002   Unspecified injury of femoral artery, left leg** A 🖾, D, S 🖾

      ● **S75.009   Unspecified injury of femoral artery, unspecified leg** A 🖾, D, S 🖾

   ● **S75.01   Minor laceration of femoral artery**
> Incomplete transection of femoral artery
> Laceration of femoral artery NOS
> Superficial laceration of femoral artery

      ● **S75.011   Minor laceration of femoral artery, right leg** A 🖾, D, S 🖾

      ● **S75.012   Minor laceration of femoral artery, left leg** A 🖾, D, S 🖾

      ● **S75.019   Minor laceration of femoral artery, unspecified leg** A 🖾, D, S 🖾

   ● **S75.02   Major laceration of femoral artery**
> Complete transection of femoral artery
> Traumatic rupture of femoral artery

      ● **S75.021   Major laceration of femoral artery, right leg** A 🖾, D, S 🖾

      ● **S75.022   Major laceration of femoral artery, left leg** A 🖾, D, S 🖾

      ● **S75.029   Major laceration of femoral artery, unspecified leg** A 🖾, D, S 🖾

   ● **S75.09   Other specified injury of femoral artery**

      ● **S75.091   Other specified injury of femoral artery, right leg** A 🖾, D, S 🖾

      ● **S75.092   Other specified injury of femoral artery, left leg** A 🖾, D, S 🖾

      ● **S75.099   Other specified injury of femoral artery, unspecified leg** A 🖾, D, S 🖾

● **S75.1   Injury of femoral vein at hip and thigh level**

   ● **S75.10   Unspecified injury of femoral vein at hip and thigh level**

      ● **S75.101   Unspecified injury of femoral vein at hip and thigh level, right leg** A 🖾, D, S 🖾

      ● **S75.102   Unspecified injury of femoral vein at hip and thigh level, left leg** A 🖾, D, S 🖾

      ● **S75.109   Unspecified injury of femoral vein at hip and thigh level, unspecified leg** A 🖾, D, S 🖾

   ● **S75.11   Minor laceration of femoral vein at hip and thigh level**
> Incomplete transection of femoral vein at hip and thigh level
> Laceration of femoral vein at hip and thigh level NOS
> Superficial laceration of femoral vein at hip and thigh level

      ● **S75.111   Minor laceration of femoral vein at hip and thigh level, right leg** A 🖾, D, S 🖾

      ● **S75.112   Minor laceration of femoral vein at hip and thigh level, left leg** A 🖾, D, S 🖾

      ● **S75.119   Minor laceration of femoral vein at hip and thigh level, unspecified leg** A 🖾, D, S 🖾

   ● **S75.12   Major laceration of femoral vein at hip and thigh level**
> Complete transection of femoral vein at hip and thigh level
> Traumatic rupture of femoral vein at hip and thigh level

      ● **S75.121   Major laceration of femoral vein at hip and thigh level, right leg** A 🖾, D, S 🖾

      ● **S75.122   Major laceration of femoral vein at hip and thigh level, left leg** A 🖾, D, S 🖾

      ● **S75.129   Major laceration of femoral vein at hip and thigh level, unspecified leg** A 🖾, D, S 🖾

   ● **S75.19   Other specified injury of femoral vein at hip and thigh level**

      ● **S75.191   Other specified injury of femoral vein at hip and thigh level, right leg** A 🖾, D, S 🖾

      ● **S75.192   Other specified injury of femoral vein at hip and thigh level, left leg** A 🖾, D, S 🖾

      ● **S75.199   Other specified injury of femoral vein at hip and thigh level, unspecified leg** A 🖾, D, S 🖾

● **S75.2   Injury of greater saphenous vein at hip and thigh level**

> Excludes1   greater saphenous vein NOS (S85.3)

   ● **S75.20   Unspecified injury of greater saphenous vein at hip and thigh level**

      ● **S75.201   Unspecified injury of greater saphenous vein at hip and thigh level, right leg** A 🖾, D, S 🖾

      ● **S75.202   Unspecified injury of greater saphenous vein at hip and thigh level, left leg** A 🖾, D, S 🖾

      ● **S75.209   Unspecified injury of greater saphenous vein at hip and thigh level, unspecified leg** A 🖾, D, S 🖾

N Newborn Age: 0   P Pediatric Age: 0–17   M Maternity DX: 12–55   A Adult Age: 15–124   ♀ Females Only   ♂ Males Only

🖾 Complication\Comorbidity   🖾 Major C\C   🖾 Present on Admission Requirement   🖾 Hospital-Acquired Condition

● S75.21 **Minor laceration of greater saphenous vein at hip and thigh level**
    Incomplete transection of greater saphenous vein at hip and thigh level
    Laceration of greater saphenous vein at hip and thigh level NOS
    Superficial laceration of greater saphenous vein at hip and thigh level

  ● S75.211 **Minor laceration of greater saphenous vein at hip and thigh level, right leg** A 🦴, D, S 🦴

  ● S75.212 **Minor laceration of greater saphenous vein at hip and thigh level, left leg** A 🦴, D, S 🦴

  ●■ S75.219 **Minor laceration of greater saphenous vein at hip and thigh level, unspecified leg** A 🦴, D, S 🦴

● S75.22 **Major laceration of greater saphenous vein at hip and thigh level**
    Complete transection of greater saphenous vein at hip and thigh level
    Traumatic rupture of greater saphenous vein at hip and thigh level

  ● S75.221 **Major laceration of greater saphenous vein at hip and thigh level, right leg** A 🦴, D, S 🦴

  ● S75.222 **Major laceration of greater saphenous vein at hip and thigh level, left leg** A 🦴, D, S 🦴

  ●■ S75.229 **Major laceration of greater saphenous vein at hip and thigh level, unspecified leg** A 🦴, D, S 🦴

● S75.29 **Other specified injury of greater saphenous vein at hip and thigh level**

  ● S75.291 **Other specified injury of greater saphenous vein at hip and thigh level, right leg** A 🦴, D, S 🦴

  ● S75.292 **Other specified injury of greater saphenous vein at hip and thigh level, left leg** A 🦴, D, S 🦴

  ●■ S75.299 **Other specified injury of greater saphenous vein at hip and thigh level, unspecified leg** A 🦴, D, S 🦴

● S75.8 **Injury of other blood vessels at hip and thigh level**

  ● S75.80 **Unspecified injury of other blood vessels at hip and thigh level**

    ●■ S75.801 **Unspecified injury of other blood vessels at hip and thigh level, right leg** A 🦴, D, S 🦴

    ●■ S75.802 **Unspecified injury of other blood vessels at hip and thigh level, left leg** A 🦴, D, S 🦴

    ●■ S75.809 **Unspecified injury of other blood vessels at hip and thigh level, unspecified leg** A 🦴, D, S 🦴

● S75.81 **Laceration of other blood vessels at hip and thigh level**

  ● S75.811 **Laceration of other blood vessels at hip and thigh level, right leg** A 🦴, D, S 🦴

  ● S75.812 **Laceration of other blood vessels at hip and thigh level, left leg** A 🦴, D, S 🦴

  ●■ S75.819 **Laceration of other blood vessels at hip and thigh level, unspecified leg** A 🦴, D, S 🦴

● S75.89 **Other specified injury of other blood vessels at hip and thigh level**

  ● S75.891 **Other specified injury of other blood vessels at hip and thigh level, right leg** A 🦴, D, S 🦴

  ● S75.892 **Other specified injury of other blood vessels at hip and thigh level, left leg** A 🦴, D, S 🦴

  ●■ S75.899 **Other specified injury of other blood vessels at hip and thigh level, unspecified leg** A 🦴, D, S 🦴

● S75.9 **Injury of unspecified blood vessel at hip and thigh level**

  ● S75.90 **Unspecified injury of unspecified blood vessel at hip and thigh level**

    ●■ S75.901 **Unspecified injury of unspecified blood vessel at hip and thigh level, right leg** A 🦴, D, S 🦴

    ●■ S75.902 **Unspecified injury of unspecified blood vessel at hip and thigh level, left leg** A 🦴, D, S 🦴

    ●■ S75.909 **Unspecified injury of unspecified blood vessel at hip and thigh level, unspecified leg** A 🦴, D, S 🦴

  ● S75.91 **Laceration of unspecified blood vessel at hip and thigh level**

    ●■ S75.911 **Laceration of unspecified blood vessel at hip and thigh level, right leg** A 🦴, D, S 🦴

    ●■ S75.912 **Laceration of unspecified blood vessel at hip and thigh level, left leg** A 🦴, D, S 🦴

    ●■ S75.919 **Laceration of unspecified blood vessel at hip and thigh level, unspecified leg** A 🦴, D, S 🦴

  ● S75.99 **Other specified injury of unspecified blood vessel at hip and thigh level**

    ●■ S75.991 **Other specified injury of unspecified blood vessel at hip and thigh level, right leg** A 🦴, D, S 🦴

    ●■ S75.992 **Other specified injury of unspecified blood vessel at hip and thigh level, left leg** A 🦴, D, S 🦴

    ●■ S75.999 **Other specified injury of unspecified blood vessel at hip and thigh level, unspecified leg** A 🦴, D, S 🦴

● Unacceptable Principal Diagnosis   ● Use Additional Character(s)   ■ Unspecified   ▶ Manifestation Code
OGCR Official Guidelines for Coding and Reporting   Excludes 1   Excludes 2   Includes   Use additional   Code first   Code also

● **S76 Injury of muscle, fascia and tendon at hip and thigh level**

> Code also any associated open wound (S71.-)

> Excludes2   injury of muscle, fascia and tendon at lower leg level (S86)
> sprain of joint and ligament of hip (S73.1)

The appropriate 7th character is to be added to each code from category S76

A	initial encounter
D	subsequent encounter
S	sequela

● **S76.0 Injury of muscle, fascia and tendon of hip**

● **S76.00 Unspecified injury of muscle, fascia and tendon of hip**

● ■ S76.001 Unspecified injury of muscle, fascia and tendon of right hip D, S 🔖

● ■ S76.002 Unspecified injury of muscle, fascia and tendon of left hip D, S 🔖

● ■ S76.009 Unspecified injury of muscle, fascia and tendon of unspecified hip D, S 🔖

● **S76.01 Strain of muscle, fascia and tendon of hip**

● S76.011 Strain of muscle, fascia and tendon of right hip D, S 🔖

● S76.012 Strain of muscle, fascia and tendon of left hip D, S 🔖

● ■ S76.019 Strain of muscle, fascia and tendon of unspecified hip D, S 🔖

● **S76.02 Laceration of muscle, fascia and tendon of hip**

● S76.021 Laceration of muscle, fascia and tendon of right hip A 🔖, D, S 🔖

● S76.022 Laceration of muscle, fascia and tendon of left hip A 🔖, D, S 🔖

● ■ S76.029 Laceration of muscle, fascia and tendon of unspecified hip A 🔖, D, S 🔖

● **S76.09 Other specified injury of muscle, fascia and tendon of hip**

● S76.091 Other specified injury of muscle, fascia and tendon of right hip D, S 🔖

● S76.092 Other specified injury of muscle, fascia and tendon of left hip D, S 🔖

● ■ S76.099 Other specified injury of muscle, fascia and tendon of unspecified hip D, S 🔖

● **S76.1 Injury of quadriceps muscle, fascia and tendon**
Injury of patellar ligament (tendon)

● **S76.10 Unspecified injury of quadriceps muscle, fascia and tendon**

● ■ S76.101 Unspecified injury of right quadriceps muscle, fascia and tendon D, S 🔖

● ■ S76.102 Unspecified injury of left quadriceps muscle, fascia and tendon D, S 🔖

● ■ S76.109 Unspecified injury of unspecified quadriceps muscle, fascia and tendon D, S 🔖

● **S76.11 Strain of quadriceps muscle, fascia and tendon**

● S76.111 Strain of right quadriceps muscle, fascia and tendon D, S 🔖

● S76.112 Strain of left quadriceps muscle, fascia and tendon D, S 🔖

● ■ S76.119 Strain of unspecified quadriceps muscle, fascia and tendon D, S 🔖

● **S76.12 Laceration of quadriceps muscle, fascia and tendon**

● S76.121 Laceration of right quadriceps muscle, fascia and tendon A 🔖, D, S 🔖

● S76.122 Laceration of left quadriceps muscle, fascia and tendon A 🔖, D, S 🔖

● ■ S76.129 Laceration of unspecified quadriceps muscle, fascia and tendon A 🔖, D, S 🔖

● **S76.19 Other specified injury of quadriceps muscle, fascia and tendon**

● S76.191 Other specified injury of right quadriceps muscle, fascia and tendon D, S 🔖

● S76.192 Other specified injury of left quadriceps muscle, fascia and tendon D, S 🔖

● ■ S76.199 Other specified injury of unspecified quadriceps muscle, fascia and tendon D, S 🔖

● **S76.2 Injury of adductor muscle, fascia and tendon of thigh**

● ■ **S76.20 Unspecified injury of adductor muscle, fascia and tendon of thigh**

● ■ S76.201 Unspecified injury of adductor muscle, fascia and tendon of right thigh D, S 🔖

● ■ S76.202 Unspecified injury of adductor muscle, fascia and tendon of left thigh D, S 🔖

● ■ S76.209 Unspecified injury of adductor muscle, fascia and tendon of unspecified thigh D, S 🔖

● **S76.21 Strain of adductor muscle, fascia and tendon of thigh**

● S76.211 Strain of adductor muscle, fascia and tendon of right thigh D, S 🔖

● S76.212 Strain of adductor muscle, fascia and tendon of left thigh D, S 🔖

● ■ S76.219 Strain of adductor muscle, fascia and tendon of unspecified thigh D, S 🔖

● **S76.22 Laceration of adductor muscle, fascia and tendon of thigh**

● S76.221 Laceration of adductor muscle, fascia and tendon of right thigh A 🔖, D, S 🔖

● S76.222 Laceration of adductor muscle, fascia and tendon of left thigh A 🔖, D, S 🔖

● ■ S76.229 Laceration of adductor muscle, fascia and tendon of unspecified thigh A 🔖, D, S 🔖

CHAPTER 19 (S00-T88)

● S76.29   Other injury of adductor muscle, fascia and tendon of thigh

     ● S76.291   Other injury of adductor muscle, fascia and tendon of right thigh D, S 🔊

     ● S76.292   Other injury of adductor muscle, fascia and tendon of left thigh D, S 🔊

     ●■ S76.299   Other injury of adductor muscle, fascia and tendon of unspecified thigh D, S 🔊

● S76.3   Injury of muscle, fascia and tendon of the posterior muscle group at thigh level

     ● S76.30   Unspecified injury of muscle, fascia and tendon of the posterior muscle group at thigh level

       ●■ S76.301   Unspecified injury of muscle, fascia and tendon of the posterior muscle group at thigh level, right thigh D, S 🔊

       ●■ S76.302   Unspecified injury of muscle, fascia and tendon of the posterior muscle group at thigh level, left thigh D, S 🔊

       ●■ S76.309   Unspecified injury of muscle, fascia and tendon of the posterior muscle group at thigh level, unspecified thigh D, S 🔊

     ● S76.31   Strain of muscle, fascia and tendon of the posterior muscle group at thigh level

       ● S76.311   Strain of muscle, fascia and tendon of the posterior muscle group at thigh level, right thigh D, S 🔊

       ● S76.312   Strain of muscle, fascia and tendon of the posterior muscle group at thigh level, left thigh D, S 🔊

       ●■ S76.319   Strain of muscle, fascia and tendon of the posterior muscle group at thigh level, unspecified thigh D, S 🔊

     ● S76.32   Laceration of muscle, fascia and tendon of the posterior muscle group at thigh level

       ● S76.321   Laceration of muscle, fascia and tendon of the posterior muscle group at thigh level, right thigh A 🔊, D, S 🔊

       ● S76.322   Laceration of muscle, fascia and tendon of the posterior muscle group at thigh level, left thigh A 🔊, D, S 🔊

       ●■ S76.329   Laceration of muscle, fascia and tendon of the posterior muscle group at thigh level, unspecified thigh A 🔊, D, S 🔊

     ● S76.39   Other specified injury of muscle, fascia and tendon of the posterior muscle group at thigh level

       ● S76.391   Other specified injury of muscle, fascia and tendon of the posterior muscle group at thigh level, right thigh D, S 🔊

● S76.392   Other specified injury of muscle, fascia and tendon of the posterior muscle group at thigh level, left thigh D, S 🔊

●■ S76.399   Other specified injury of muscle, fascia and tendon of the posterior muscle group at thigh level, unspecified thigh D, S 🔊

● S76.8   Injury of other specified muscles, fascia and tendons at thigh level

     ● S76.80   Unspecified injury of other specified muscles, fascia and tendons at thigh level

       ●■ S76.801   Unspecified injury of other specified muscles, fascia and tendons at thigh level, right thigh D, S 🔊

       ●■ S76.802   Unspecified injury of other specified muscles, fascia and tendons at thigh level, left thigh D, S 🔊

       ●■ S76.809   Unspecified injury of other specified muscles, fascia and tendons at thigh level, unspecified thigh D, S 🔊

     ● S76.81   Strain of other specified specified muscles, fascia and tendons at thigh level

       ● S76.811   Strain of other specified muscles, fascia and tendons at thigh level, right thigh D, S 🔊

       ● S76.812   Strain of other specified muscles, fascia and tendons at thigh level, left thigh D, S 🔊

       ●■ S76.819   Strain of other specified muscles, fascia and tendons at thigh level, unspecified thigh D, S 🔊

     ● S76.82   Laceration of other specified muscles, fascia and tendons at thigh level

       ● S76.821   Laceration of other specified muscles, fascia and tendons at thigh level, right thigh A 🔊, D, S 🔊

       ● S76.822   Laceration of other specified muscles, fascia and tendons at thigh level, left thigh A 🔊, D, S 🔊

       ●■ S76.829   Laceration of other specified muscles, fascia and tendons at thigh level, unspecified thigh A 🔊, D, S 🔊

     ● S76.89   Other injury of other specified muscles, fascia and tendons at thigh level

       ● S76.891   Other injury of other specified muscles, fascia and tendons at thigh level, right thigh D, S 🔊

       ● S76.892   Other injury of other specified muscles, fascia and tendons at thigh level, left thigh D, S 🔊

       ●■ S76.899   Other injury of other specified muscles, fascia and tendons at thigh level, unspecified thigh D, S 🔊

CHAPTER 19 (S00-T88)

● Unacceptable Principal Diagnosis   ● Use Additional Character(s)   ■ Unspecified   ▶ Manifestation Code
OGCR Official Guidelines for Coding and Reporting   Excludes 1   Excludes 2   Includes   Use additional   Code first   Code also

- S76.9   **Injury of unspecified muscles, fascia and tendons at thigh level**
  - S76.90   **Unspecified injury of unspecified muscles, fascia and tendons at thigh level**
    - S76.901   Unspecified injury of unspecified muscles, fascia and tendons at thigh level, right thigh D, S
    - S76.902   Unspecified injury of unspecified muscles, fascia and tendons at thigh level, left thigh D, S
    - S76.909   Unspecified injury of unspecified muscles, fascia and tendons at thigh level, unspecified thigh D, S
  - S76.91   **Strain of unspecified muscles, fascia and tendons at thigh level**
    - S76.911   Strain of unspecified muscles, fascia and tendons at thigh level, right thigh D, S
    - S76.912   Strain of unspecified muscles, fascia and tendons at thigh level, left thigh D, S
    - S76.919   Strain of unspecified muscles, fascia and tendons at thigh level, unspecified thigh D, S
  - S76.92   **Laceration of unspecified muscles, fascia and tendons at thigh level**
    - S76.921   Laceration of unspecified muscles, fascia and tendons at thigh level, right thigh A, D, S
    - S76.922   Laceration of unspecified muscles, fascia and tendons at thigh level, left thigh A, D, S
    - S76.929   Laceration of unspecified muscles, fascia and tendons at thigh level, unspecified thigh A, D, S
  - S76.99   **Other specified injury of unspecified muscles, fascia and tendons at thigh level**
    - S76.991   Other specified injury of unspecified muscles, fascia and tendons at thigh level, right thigh D, S
    - S76.992   Other specified injury of unspecified muscles, fascia and tendons at thigh level, left thigh D, S
    - S76.999   Other specified injury of unspecified muscles, fascia and tendons at thigh level, unspecified thigh D, S

- S77   **Crushing injury of hip and thigh**

  Use additional code(s) for all associated injuries

  | Excludes2 | crushing injury of ankle and foot (S97.-) |
  | | crushing injury of lower leg (S87.-) |

  The appropriate 7th character is to be added to each code from category S77

A	initial encounter
D	subsequent encounter
S	sequela

- S77.0   **Crushing injury of hip**
  - S77.00   Crushing injury of unspecified hip A, D, S, A
  - S77.01   Crushing injury of right hip A, D, S, A
  - S77.02   Crushing injury of left hip A, D, S, A
- S77.1   **Crushing injury of thigh**
  - S77.10   Crushing injury of unspecified thigh A, D, S, A
  - S77.11   Crushing injury of right thigh A, D, S, A
  - S77.12   Crushing injury of left thigh A, D, S, A
- S77.2   **Crushing injury of hip with thigh**
  - S77.20   Crushing injury of unspecified hip with thigh D, S
  - S77.21   Crushing injury of right hip with thigh D, S
  - S77.22   Crushing injury of left hip with thigh D, S

- S78   **Traumatic amputation of hip and thigh**

  An amputation not identified as partial or complete should be coded to complete

  | Excludes1 | traumatic amputation of knee (S88.0-) |

  The appropriate 7th character is to be added to each code from category S78

A	initial encounter
D	subsequent encounter
S	sequela

- S78.0   **Traumatic amputation at hip joint**
  - S78.01   **Complete traumatic amputation at hip joint**
    - S78.011   Complete traumatic amputation at right hip joint A, D, S
    - S78.012   Complete traumatic amputation at left hip joint A, D, S
    - S78.019   Complete traumatic amputation at unspecified hip joint A, D, S
  - S78.02   **Partial traumatic amputation at hip joint**
    - S78.021   Partial traumatic amputation at right hip joint A, D, S
    - S78.022   Partial traumatic amputation at left hip joint A, D, S
    - S78.029   Partial traumatic amputation at unspecified hip joint A, D, S
- S78.1   **Traumatic amputation at level between hip and knee**

  | Excludes1 | traumatic amputation of knee (S88.0-) |

  - S78.11   **Complete traumatic amputation at level between hip and knee**
    - S78.111   Complete traumatic amputation at level between right hip and knee A, D, S
    - S78.112   Complete traumatic amputation at level between left hip and knee A, D, S
    - S78.119   Complete traumatic amputation at level between unspecified hip and knee A, D, S

CHAPTER 19 (S00–T88)

● S78.12   Partial traumatic amputation at level between hip and knee

   ● S78.121   Partial traumatic amputation at level between right hip and knee A 🔵, D, S 🔵

   ● S78.122   Partial traumatic amputation at level between left hip and knee A 🔵, D, S 🔵

   ●■ S78.129   Partial traumatic amputation at level between unspecified hip and knee A 🔵, D, S 🔵

● S78.9   Traumatic amputation of hip and thigh, level unspecified

   ● S78.91   Complete traumatic amputation of hip and thigh, level unspecified

      ●■ S78.911   Complete traumatic amputation of right hip and thigh, level unspecified A 🔵, D, S 🔵

      ●■ S78.912   Complete traumatic amputation of left hip and thigh, level unspecified A 🔵, D, S 🔵

      ●■ S78.919   Complete traumatic amputation of unspecified hip and thigh, level unspecified A 🔵, D, S 🔵

   ● S78.92   Partial traumatic amputation of hip and thigh, level unspecified

      ●■ S78.921   Partial traumatic amputation of right hip and thigh, level unspecified A 🔵, D, S 🔵

      ●■ S78.922   Partial traumatic amputation of left hip and thigh, level unspecified A 🔵, D, S 🔵

      ●■ S78.929   Partial traumatic amputation of unspecified hip and thigh, level unspecified A 🔵, D, S 🔵

● S79   Other and unspecified injuries of hip and thigh

   Note: A fracture not indicated as open or closed should be coded to closed

   The appropriate 7th character is to be added to each code from subcategories S79.0 and S79.1

A	initial encounter for closed fracture
D	subsequent encounter for fracture with routine healing
G	subsequent encounter for fracture with delayed healing
K	subsequent encounter for fracture with nonunion
P	subsequent encounter for fracture with malunion
S	sequela

   ● S79.0   Physeal fracture of upper end of femur
      [Excludes1] apophyseal fracture of upper end of femur (S72.13-)
                   nontraumatic slipped upper femoral epiphysis (M93.0-)

      ● S79.00   Unspecified physeal fracture of upper end of femur

         ●■ S79.001   Unspecified physeal fracture of upper end of right femur K, P 🔵, A 🔵, D, G, S 🔵

         ●■ S79.002   Unspecified physeal fracture of upper end of left femur K, P 🔵, A 🔵, D, G, S 🔵, A 🔵

         ●■ S79.009   Unspecified physeal fracture of upper end of unspecified femur K, P 🔵, A 🔵, D, G, S 🔵, A 🔵

Item 19–5   SALTER-HARRIS TYPE 1: epiphysis is completely separated from end of bone, or metaphysic growth plate remains attached to epiphysis
   SALTER-HARRIS TYPE 2: epiphysis and growth plate are partially separated from metaphysis, which is cracked—most common type
   SALTER-HARRIS TYPE 3: fracture occurring through epiphysis and separates part of epiphysis and growth plate from metaphysis fracture, usually at distal end of tibia
   SALTER-HARRIS TYPE 4: fracture runs through epiphysis, across growth plate, into metaphysic, surgery is required to restore joint surface to normal and align growth plate

   ● S79.01   Salter-Harris Type I physeal fracture of upper end of femur
      Acute on chronic slipped capital femoral epiphysis (traumatic)
      Acute slipped capital femoral epiphysis (traumatic)
      Capital femoral epiphyseal fracture
      [Excludes1] chronic slipped upper femoral epiphysis (nontraumatic) (M93.02-)

      ● S79.011   Salter-Harris Type I physeal fracture of upper end of right femur K, P 🔵, A 🔵, D, G, S 🔵, A 🔵

      ● S79.012   Salter-Harris Type I physeal fracture of upper end of left femur K, P 🔵, A 🔵, D, G, S 🔵, A 🔵

      ●■ S79.019   Salter-Harris Type I physeal fracture of upper end of unspecified femur K, P 🔵, A 🔵, D, G, S 🔵, A 🔵

   ● S79.09   Other physeal fracture of upper end of femur

      ● S79.091   Other physeal fracture of upper end of right femur K, P 🔵, A 🔵, D, G, S 🔵, A 🔵

      ● S79.092   Other physeal fracture of upper end of left femur K, P 🔵, A 🔵, D, G, S 🔵, A 🔵

      ●■ S79.099   Other physeal fracture of upper end of unspecified femur K, P 🔵, A 🔵, D, G, S 🔵, A 🔵

● S79.1   Physeal fracture of lower end of femur

   ● S79.10   Unspecified physeal fracture of lower end of femur

      ●■ S79.101   Unspecified physeal fracture of lower end of right femur A, K, P 🔵, D, G, S 🔵, A 🔵

      ●■ S79.102   Unspecified physeal fracture of lower end of left femur A, K, P 🔵, D, G, S 🔵, A 🔵

      ●■ S79.109   Unspecified physeal fracture of lower end of unspecified femur A, K, P 🔵, D, G, S 🔵, A 🔵

● Unacceptable Principal Diagnosis   ● Use Additional Character(s)   ■ Unspecified   ▶ Manifestation Code
OGCR Official Guidelines for Coding and Reporting   [Excludes 1] [Excludes 2] Includes Use additional Code first Code also

● S79.11   Salter-Harris Type I physeal fracture of lower end of femur

  ● S79.111   Salter-Harris Type I physeal fracture of lower end of right femur A, K, P 🔴, D, G, S ⚪, A ⚪

  ● S79.112   Salter-Harris Type I physeal fracture of lower end of left femur A, K, P 🔴, D, G, S ⚪, A ⚪

  ●◼ S79.119   Salter-Harris Type I physeal fracture of lower end of unspecified femur A, K, P 🔴, D, G, S ⚪, A ⚪

● S79.12   Salter-Harris Type II physeal fracture of lower end of femur

  ● S79.121   Salter-Harris Type II physeal fracture of lower end of right femur A, K, P 🔴, D, G, S ⚪, A ⚪

  ● S79.122   Salter-Harris Type II physeal fracture of lower end of left femur A, K, P 🔴, D, G, S ⚪, A ⚪

  ●◼ S79.129   Salter-Harris Type II physeal fracture of lower end of unspecified femur A, K, P 🔴, D, G, S ⚪, A ⚪

● S79.13   Salter-Harris Type III physeal fracture of lower end of femur

  ● S79.131   Salter-Harris Type III physeal fracture of lower end of right femur A, K, P 🔴, D, G, S ⚪, A ⚪

  ● S79.132   Salter-Harris Type III physeal fracture of lower end of left femur A, K, P 🔴, D, G, S ⚪, A ⚪

  ●◼ S79.139   Salter-Harris Type III physeal fracture of lower end of unspecified femur A, K, P 🔴, D, G, S ⚪, A ⚪

● S79.14   Salter-Harris Type IV physeal fracture of lower end of femur

  ● S79.141   Salter-Harris Type IV physeal fracture of lower end of right femur A, K, P 🔴, D, G, S ⚪, A ⚪

  ● S79.142   Salter-Harris Type IV physeal fracture of lower end of left femur A, K, P 🔴, D, G, S ⚪, A ⚪

  ●◼ S79.149   Salter-Harris Type IV physeal fracture of lower end of unspecified femur A, K, P 🔴, D, G, S ⚪, A ⚪

● S79.19   Other physeal fracture of lower end of femur

  ● S79.191   Other physeal fracture of lower end of right femur A, K, P 🔴, D, G, S ⚪, A ⚪

  ● S79.192   Other physeal fracture of lower end of left femur A, K, P 🔴, D, G, S ⚪, A ⚪

  ●◼ S79.199   Other physeal fracture of lower end of unspecified femur A, K, P 🔴, D, G, S ⚪, A ⚪

● S79.8   Other specified injuries of hip and thigh

The appropriate 7th character is to be added to each code in subcategory S79.8

A	initial encounter
D	subsequent encounter
S	sequela

  ● S79.81   Other specified injuries of hip

    ● S79.811   Other specified injuries of right hip D, S ⚪

    ● S79.812   Other specified injuries of left hip D, S ⚪

    ●◼ S79.819   Other specified injuries of unspecified hip D, S ⚪

  ● S79.82   Other specified injuries of thigh

    ● S79.821   Other specified injuries of right thigh D, S ⚪

    ● S79.822   Other specified injuries of left thigh D, S ⚪

    ●◼ S79.829   Other specified injuries of unspecified thigh D, S ⚪

● S79.9   Unspecified injury of hip and thigh

The appropriate 7th character is to be added to each code in subcategory S79.9

A	initial encounter
D	subsequent encounter
S	sequela

  ● S79.91   Unspecified injury of hip

    ●◼ S79.911   Unspecified injury of right hip D, S ⚪

    ●◼ S79.912   Unspecified injury of left hip D, S ⚪

    ●◼ S79.919   Unspecified injury of unspecified hip D, S ⚪

  ● S79.92   Unspecified injury of thigh

    ●◼ S79.921   Unspecified injury of right thigh D, S ⚪

    ●◼ S79.922   Unspecified injury of left thigh D, S ⚪

    ●◼ S79.929   Unspecified injury of unspecified thigh D, S ⚪

INJURIES TO THE KNEE AND LOWER LEG (S80-S89)

Excludes2	burns and corrosions (T20-T32)
	frostbite (T33-T34)
	injuries of ankle and foot, except fracture of ankle and malleolus (S90-S99)
	insect bite or sting, venomous (T63.4)

● S80   Superficial injury of knee and lower leg

Excludes2	superficial injury of ankle and foot (S90.-)

The appropriate 7th character is to be added to each code from category S80

A	initial encounter
D	subsequent encounter
S	sequela

  ● S80.0   Contusion of knee

    ●◼ S80.00   Contusion of unspecified knee D, S ⚪

    ● S80.01   Contusion of right knee D, S ⚪

    ● S80.02   Contusion of left knee D, S ⚪

N Newborn Age: 0   **P** Pediatric Age: 0–17   **M** Maternity DX: 12–55   **A** Adult Age: 15–124   ♀ Females Only   ♂ Males Only

🔴 Complication\Comorbidity   ⚪ Major C\C   ⚪ Present on Admission Requirement   ⚪ Hospital-Acquired Condition

1545

- S80.1   Contusion of lower leg
  - S80.10   Contusion of unspecified lower leg D, S
  - S80.11   Contusion of right lower leg D, S
  - S80.12   Contusion of left lower leg D, S
- S80.2   Other superficial injuries of knee
  - S80.21   Abrasion of knee
    - S80.211   Abrasion, right knee D, S
    - S80.212   Abrasion, left knee D, S
    - S80.219   Abrasion, unspecified knee D, S
  - S80.22   Blister (nonthermal) of knee
    - S80.221   Blister (nonthermal), right knee D, S
    - S80.222   Blister (nonthermal), left knee D, S
    - S80.229   Blister (nonthermal), unspecified knee D, S
  - S80.24   External constriction of knee
    - S80.241   External constriction, right knee D, S
    - S80.242   External constriction, left knee D, S
    - S80.249   External constriction, unspecified knee D, S
  - S80.25   Superficial foreign body of knee
    Splinter in the knee
    - S80.251   Superficial foreign body, right knee D, S
    - S80.252   Superficial foreign body, left knee D, S
    - S80.259   Superficial foreign body, unspecified knee D, S
  - S80.26   Insect bite (nonvenomous) of knee
    - S80.261   Insect bite (nonvenomous), right knee D, S
    - S80.262   Insect bite (nonvenomous), left knee D, S
    - S80.269   Insect bite (nonvenomous), unspecified knee D, S
  - S80.27   Other superficial bite of knee
    Excludes1   open bite of knee (S81.05-)
    - S80.271   Other superficial bite of right knee D, S
    - S80.272   Other superficial bite of left knee D, S
    - S80.279   Other superficial bite of unspecified knee D, S
- S80.8   Other superficial injuries of lower leg
  - S80.81   Abrasion of lower leg
    - S80.811   Abrasion, right lower leg D, S
    - S80.812   Abrasion, left lower leg D, S
    - S80.819   Abrasion, unspecified lower leg D, S

- S80.82   Blister (nonthermal) of lower leg
  - S80.821   Blister (nonthermal), right lower leg D, S
  - S80.822   Blister (nonthermal), left lower leg D, S
  - S80.829   Blister (nonthermal), unspecified lower leg D, S
- S80.84   External constriction of lower leg
  - S80.841   External constriction, right lower leg D, S
  - S80.842   External constriction, left lower leg D, S
  - S80.849   External constriction, unspecified lower leg D, S
- S80.85   Superficial foreign body of lower leg
  Splinter in the lower leg
  - S80.851   Superficial foreign body, right lower leg D, S
  - S80.852   Superficial foreign body, left lower leg D, S
  - S80.859   Superficial foreign body, unspecified lower leg D, S
- S80.86   Insect bite (nonvenomous) of lower leg
  - S80.861   Insect bite (nonvenomous), right lower leg D, S
  - S80.862   Insect bite (nonvenomous), left lower leg D, S
  - S80.869   Insect bite (nonvenomous), unspecified lower leg D, S
- S80.87   Other superficial bite of lower leg
  Excludes1   open bite of lower leg (S81.85-)
  - S80.871   Other superficial bite, right lower leg D, S
  - S80.872   Other superficial bite, left lower leg D, S
  - S80.879   Other superficial bite, unspecified lower leg D, S
- S80.9   Unspecified superficial injury of knee and lower leg
  - S80.91   Unspecified superficial injury of knee
    - S80.911   Unspecified superficial injury of right knee D, S
    - S80.912   Unspecified superficial injury of left knee D, S
    - S80.919   Unspecified superficial injury of unspecified knee D, S
  - S80.92   Unspecified superficial injury of lower leg
    - S80.921   Unspecified superficial injury of right lower leg D, S
    - S80.922   Unspecified superficial injury of left lower leg D, S
    - S80.929   Unspecified superficial injury of unspecified lower leg D, S

- Unacceptable Principal Diagnosis   - Use Additional Character(s)   Unspecified   Manifestation Code
OGCR Official Guidelines for Coding and Reporting   Excludes 1   Excludes 2   Includes   Use additional   Code first   Code also

CHAPTER 19 (S00-T88)

● **S81   Open wound of knee and lower leg**

    <u>Code also</u> any associated wound infection

    | Excludes1 | open fracture of knee and lower leg (S82.-)

                     traumatic amputation of lower leg (S88.-)

    | Excludes2 | open wound of ankle and foot (S91.-)

    The appropriate 7th character is to be added to each code from category S81

    | A   initial encounter
    | D   subsequent encounter
    | S   sequela

● **S81.0   Open wound of knee**

   ● **S81.00   Unspecified open wound of knee**

     ●■ **S81.001   Unspecified open wound, right knee** D, S 🔍

     ●■ **S81.002   Unspecified open wound, left knee** D, S 🔍

     ●■ **S81.009   Unspecified open wound, unspecified knee** D, S 🔍

   ● **S81.01   Laceration without foreign body of knee**

     ● **S81.011   Laceration without foreign body, right knee** D, S 🔍

     ● **S81.012   Laceration without foreign body, left knee** D, S 🔍

     ●■ **S81.019   Laceration without foreign body, unspecified knee** D, S 🔍

   ● **S81.02   Laceration with foreign body of knee**

     ● **S81.021   Laceration with foreign body, right knee** D, S 🔍

     ● **S81.022   Laceration with foreign body, left knee** D, S 🔍

     ●■ **S81.029   Laceration with foreign body, unspecified knee** D, S 🔍

   ● **S81.03   Puncture wound without foreign body of knee**

     ● **S81.031   Puncture wound without foreign body, right knee** D, S 🔍

     ● **S81.032   Puncture wound without foreign body, left knee** D, S 🔍

     ●■ **S81.039   Puncture wound without foreign body, unspecified knee** D, S 🔍

   ● **S81.04   Puncture wound with foreign body of knee**

     ● **S81.041   Puncture wound with foreign body, right knee** D, S 🔍

     ● **S81.042   Puncture wound with foreign body, left knee** D, S 🔍

     ●■ **S81.049   Puncture wound with foreign body, unspecified knee** D, S 🔍

   ● **S81.05   Open bite of knee**

     Bite of knee NOS

     | Excludes1 | superficial bite of knee (S80.27-)

     ● **S81.051   Open bite, right knee** D, S 🔍

     ● **S81.052   Open bite, left knee** D, S 🔍

     ●■ **S81.059   Open bite, unspecified knee** D, S 🔍

● **S81.8   Open wound of lower leg**

   ● **S81.80   Unspecified open wound of lower leg**

     ●■ **S81.801   Unspecified open wound, right lower leg** D, S 🔍

     ●■ **S81.802   Unspecified open wound, left lower leg** D, S 🔍

     ●■ **S81.809   Unspecified open wound, unspecified lower leg** D, S 🔍

   ● **S81.81   Laceration without foreign body of lower leg**

     ● **S81.811   Laceration without foreign body, right lower leg** D, S 🔍

     ● **S81.812   Laceration without foreign body, left lower leg** D, S 🔍

     ●■ **S81.819   Laceration without foreign body, unspecified lower leg** D, S 🔍

   ● **S81.82   Laceration with foreign body of lower leg**

     ● **S81.821   Laceration with foreign body, right lower leg** D, S 🔍

     ● **S81.822   Laceration with foreign body, left lower leg** D, S 🔍

     ●■ **S81.829   Laceration with foreign body, unspecified lower leg** D, S 🔍

   ● **S81.83   Puncture wound without foreign body of lower leg**

     ● **S81.831   Puncture wound without foreign body, right lower leg** D, S 🔍

     ● **S81.832   Puncture wound without foreign body, left lower leg** D, S 🔍

     ●■ **S81.839   Puncture wound without foreign body, unspecified lower leg** D, S 🔍

   ● **S81.84   Puncture wound with foreign body of lower leg**

     ● **S81.841   Puncture wound with foreign body, right lower leg** D, S 🔍

     ● **S81.842   Puncture wound with foreign body, left lower leg** D, S 🔍

     ●■ **S81.849   Puncture wound with foreign body, unspecified lower leg** D, S 🔍

   ● **S81.85   Open bite of lower leg**

     Bite of lower leg NOS

     | Excludes1 | superficial bite of lower leg (S80.86-, S80.87-)

     ● **S81.851   Open bite, right lower leg** D, S 🔍

     ● **S81.852   Open bite, left lower leg** D, S 🔍

     ●■ **S81.859   Open bite, unspecified lower leg** D, S 🔍

CHAPTER 19 (S00-T88)

N Newborn Age: 0   **P** Pediatric Age: 0–17   **M** Maternity DX: 12–55   **A** Adult Age: 15–124   ♀ Females Only   ♂ Males Only

🔍 Complication\Comorbidity   🔍 Major C\C   🔍 Present on Admission Requirement   🔍 Hospital-Acquired Condition

1547

● **S82   Fracture of lower leg, including ankle**

Note: A fracture not indicated as displaced or nondisplaced should be coded to displaced

A fracture not indicated as open or closed should be coded to closed

The open fracture designations are based on the Gustilo open fracture classification

Includes	fracture of malleolus
Excludes1	traumatic amputation of lower leg (S88.-)
Excludes2	fracture of foot, except ankle (S92.-)
	periprosthetic fracture of prosthetic implant of knee (T84.042, T84.043)

The appropriate 7th character is to be added to all codes from category S82

A   initial encounter for open fracture
B   initial encounter for open fracture type I or II initial encounter for open fracture NOS
C   initial encounter for open fracture type IIIA, IIIB, or IIIC
D   subsequent encounter for closed fracture with routine healing
E   subsequent encounter for open fracture type I or II with routine healing
F   subsequent encounter for open fracture type IIIA, IIIB, or IIIC with routine healing
G   subsequent encounter for closed fracture with delayed healing
H   subsequent encounter for open fracture type I or II with delayed healing
J   subsequent encounter for open fracture type IIIA, IIIB, or IIIC with delayed healing
K   subsequent encounter for closed fracture with nonunion
M   subsequent encounter for open fracture type I or II with nonunion
N   subsequent encounter for open fracture type IIIA, IIIB, or IIIC with nonunion
P   subsequent encounter for closed fracture with malunion
Q   subsequent encounter for open fracture type I or II with malunion
R   subsequent encounter for open fracture type IIIA, IIIB, or IIIC with malunion
S   sequela

● **S82.0   Fracture of patella**
Knee cap

● **S82.00   Unspecified fracture of patella**

●■ **S82.001   Unspecified fracture of right patella** A, B, C, K, M, N, P, Q, R ✪, D, E, F, G, H, J, S ✪, A, B, C ✪

●■ **S82.002   Unspecified fracture of left patella** A, B, C, K, M, N, P, Q, R ✪, D, E, F, G, H, J, S ✪, A, B, C ✪

●■ **S82.009   Unspecified fracture of unspecified patella** A, B, C, K, M, N, P, Q, R ✪, D, E, F, G, H, J, S ✪, A, B, C ✪

● **S82.01   Osteochondral fracture of patella**

● **S82.011   Displaced osteochondral fracture of right patella** A, B, C, K, M, N, P, Q, R ✪, D, E, F, G, H, J, S ✪, A, B, C ✪

● **S82.012   Displaced osteochondral fracture of left patella** A, B, C, K, M, N, P, Q, R ✪, D, E, F, G, H, J, S ✪, A, B, C ✪

●■ **S82.013   Displaced osteochondral fracture of unspecified patella** A, B, C, K, M, N, P, Q, R ✪, D, E, F, G, H, J, S ✪, A, B, C ✪

● **S82.014   Nondisplaced osteochondral fracture of right patella** A, B, C, K, M, N, P, Q, R ✪, D, E, F, G, H, J, S ✪, A, B, C ✪

● **S82.015   Nondisplaced osteochondral fracture of left patella** A, B, C, K, M, N, P, Q, R ✪, D, E, F, G, H, J, S ✪, A, B, C ✪

●■ **S82.016   Nondisplaced osteochondral fracture of unspecified patella** A, B, C, K, M, N, P, Q, R ✪, D, E, F, G, H, J, S ✪, A, B, C ✪

● **S82.02   Longitudinal fracture of patella**

● **S82.021   Displaced longitudinal fracture of right patella** A, B, C, K, M, N, P, Q, R ✪, D, E, F, G, H, J, S ✪, A, B, C ✪

● **S82.022   Displaced longitudinal fracture of left patella** A, B, C, K, M, N, P, Q, R ✪, D, E, F, G, H, J, S ✪, A, B, C ✪

●■ **S82.023   Displaced longitudinal fracture of unspecified patella** A, B, C, K, M, N, P, Q, R ✪, D, E, F, G, H, J, S ✪, A, B, C ✪

● **S82.024   Nondisplaced longitudinal fracture of right patella** A, B, C, K, M, N, P, Q, R ✪, D, E, F, G, H, J, S ✪, A, B, C ✪

● **S82.025   Nondisplaced longitudinal fracture of left patella** A, B, C, K, M, N, P, Q, R ✪, D, E, F, G, H, J, S ✪, A, B, C ✪

●■ **S82.026   Nondisplaced longitudinal fracture of unspecified patella** A, B, C, K, M, N, P, Q, R ✪, D, E, F, G, H, J, S ✪, A, B, C ✪

● **S82.03   Transverse fracture of patella**

● **S82.031   Displaced transverse fracture of right patella** A, B, C, K, M, N, P, Q, R ✪, D, E, F, G, H, J, S ✪, A, B, C ✪

● **S82.032   Displaced transverse fracture of left patella** A, B, C, K, M, N, P, Q, R ✪, D, E, F, G, H, J, S ✪, A, B, C ✪

●■ **S82.033   Displaced transverse fracture of unspecified patella** A, B, C, K, M, N, P, Q, R ✪, D, E, F, G, H, J, S ✪, A, B, C ✪

- S82.034   Nondisplaced transverse fracture of right patella A, B, C, K, M, N, P, Q, R 🔸, D, E, F, G, H, J, S 🔸, A, B, C 🔸
- S82.035   Nondisplaced transverse fracture of left patella A, B, C, K, M, N, P, Q, R 🔸, D, E, F, G, H, J, S 🔸, A, B, C 🔸
- ■ S82.036   Nondisplaced transverse fracture of unspecified patella A, B, C, K, M, N, P, Q, R 🔸, D, E, F, G, H, J, S 🔸, A, B, C 🔸

- S82.04   **Comminuted fracture of patella**
  - S82.041   Displaced comminuted fracture of right patella A, B, C, K, M, N, P, Q, R 🔸, D, E, F, G, H, J, S 🔸, A, B, C 🔸
  - S82.042   Displaced comminuted fracture of left patella A, B, C, K, M, N, P, Q, R 🔸, D, E, F, G, H, J, S 🔸, A, B, C 🔸
  - ■ S82.043   Displaced comminuted fracture of unspecified patella A, B, C, K, M, N, P, Q, R 🔸, D, E, F, G, H, J, S 🔸, A, B, C 🔸
  - S82.044   Nondisplaced comminuted fracture of right patella A, B, C, K, M, N, P, Q, R 🔸, D, E, F, G, H, J, S 🔸, A, B, C 🔸
  - S82.045   Nondisplaced comminuted fracture of left patella A, B, C, K, M, N, P, Q, R 🔸, D, E, F, G, H, J, S 🔸, A, B, C 🔸
  - ■ S82.046   Nondisplaced comminuted fracture of unspecified patella A, B, C, K, M, N, P, Q, R 🔸, D, E, F, G, H, J, S 🔸, A, B, C 🔸

- S82.09   **Other fracture of patella**
  - S82.091   Other fracture of right patella A, B, C, K, M, N, P, Q, R 🔸, D, E, F, G, H, J, S 🔸, A, B, C 🔸
  - S82.092   Other fracture of left patella A, B, C, K, M, N, P, Q, R 🔸, D, E, F, G, H, J, S 🔸, A, B, C 🔸
  - ■ S82.099   Other fracture of unspecified patella A, B, C, K, M, N, P, Q, R 🔸, D, E, F, G, H, J, S 🔸, A, B, C 🔸

- S82.1   **Fracture of upper end of tibia**
  Fracture of proximal end of tibia

Excludes2	fracture of shaft of tibia (S82.2-)
	physeal fracture of upper end of tibia (S89.0-)

  - S82.10   **Unspecified fracture of upper end of tibia**
    - ■ S82.101   Unspecified fracture of upper end of right tibia A, K, M, N, P, Q, R 🔸, B, C 🔸, D, E, F, G, H, J, S 🔸, A, B, C 🔸
    - ■ S82.102   Unspecified fracture of upper end of left tibia A, K, M, N, P, Q, R 🔸, B, C 🔸, D, E, F, G, H, J, S 🔸, A, B, C 🔸
    - ■ S82.109   Unspecified fracture of upper end of unspecified tibia A, K, M, N, P, Q, R 🔸, B, C 🔸, D, E, F, G, H, J, S 🔸, A, B, C 🔸

- S82.11   **Fracture of tibial spine**
  - S82.111   Displaced fracture of right tibial spine A, K, M, N, P, Q, R 🔸, B, C 🔸, D, E, F, G, H, J, S 🔸, A, B, C 🔸
  - S82.112   Displaced fracture of left tibial spine A, K, M, N, P, Q, R 🔸, B, C 🔸, D, E, F, G, H, J, S 🔸, A, B, C 🔸
  - ■ S82.113   Displaced fracture of unspecified tibial spine A, K, M, N, P, Q, R 🔸, B, C 🔸, D, E, F, G, H, J, S 🔸, A, B, C 🔸
  - S82.114   Nondisplaced fracture of right tibial spine A, K, M, N, P, Q, R 🔸, B, C 🔸, D, E, F, G, H, J, S 🔸, A, B, C 🔸
  - S82.115   Nondisplaced fracture of left tibial spine A, K, M, N, P, Q, R 🔸, B, C 🔸, D, E, F, G, H, J, S 🔸, A, B, C 🔸
  - ■ S82.116   Nondisplaced fracture of unspecified tibial spine A, K, M, N, P, Q, R 🔸, B, C 🔸, D, E, F, G, H, J, S 🔸, A, B, C 🔸

- S82.12   **Fracture of lateral condyle of tibia**
  - S82.121   Displaced fracture of lateral condyle of right tibia A, K, M, N, P, Q, R 🔸, B, C 🔸, D, E, F, G, H, J, S 🔸, A, B, C 🔸
  - S82.122   Displaced fracture of lateral condyle of left tibia A, K, M, N, P, Q, R 🔸, B, C 🔸, D, E, F, G, H, J, S 🔸, A, B, C 🔸
  - ■ S82.123   Displaced fracture of lateral condyle of unspecified tibia A, K, M, N, P, Q, R 🔸, B, C 🔸, D, E, F, G, H, J, S 🔸, A, B, C 🔸
  - S82.124   Nondisplaced fracture of lateral condyle of right tibia A, K, M, N, P, Q, R 🔸, B, C 🔸, D, E, F, G, H, J, S 🔸, A, B, C 🔸
  - S82.125   Nondisplaced fracture of lateral condyle of left tibia A, K, M, N, P, Q, R 🔸, B, C 🔸, D, E, F, G, H, J, S 🔸, A, B, C 🔸
  - ■ S82.126   Nondisplaced fracture of lateral condyle of unspecified tibia A, K, M, N, P, Q, R 🔸, B, C 🔸, D, E, F, G, H, J, S 🔸, A, B, C 🔸

- S82.13   **Fracture of medial condyle of tibia**
  - S82.131   Displaced fracture of medial condyle of right tibia A, K, M, N, P, Q, R 🔸, B, C 🔸, D, E, F, G, H, J, S 🔸, A, B, C 🔸
  - S82.132   Displaced fracture of medial condyle of left tibia A, K, M, N, P, Q, R 🔸, B, C 🔸, D, E, F, G, H, J, S 🔸, A, B, C 🔸
  - ■ S82.133   Displaced fracture of medial condyle of unspecified tibia A, K, M, N, P, Q, R 🔸, B, C 🔸, D, E, F, G, H, J, S 🔸, A, B, C 🔸

CHAPTER 19 (S00-T88)

N   Newborn Age: 0   P   Pediatric Age: 0–17   M   Maternity DX: 12–55   A   Adult Age: 15–124   ♀ Females Only   ♂ Males Only
🔸 Complication\Comorbidity   🔸 Major C\C   🔸 Present on Admission Requirement   🔸 Hospital-Acquired Condition
1549

● S82.134   Nondisplaced fracture of medial condyle of right tibia A, K, M, N, P, Q, R ✪, B, C ✪, D, E, F, G, H, J, S ✪, A, B, C ✪

● S82.135   Nondisplaced fracture of medial condyle of left tibia A, K, M, N, P, Q, R ✪, B, C ✪, D, E, F, G, H, J, S ✪, A, B, C ✪

● ◼ S82.136   Nondisplaced fracture of medial condyle of unspecified tibia A, K, M, N, P, Q, R ✪, B, C ✪, D, E, F, G, H, J, S ✪, A, B, C ✪

● S82.14   Bicondylar fracture of tibia
Fracture of tibial plateau NOS

● S82.141   Displaced bicondylar fracture of right tibia A, K, M, N, P, Q, R ✪, B, C ✪, D, E, F, G, H, J, S ✪, A, B, C ✪

● S82.142   Displaced bicondylar fracture of left tibia A, K, M, N, P, Q, R ✪, B, C ✪, D, E, F, G, H, J, S ✪, A, B, C ✪

● ◼ S82.143   Displaced bicondylar fracture of unspecified tibia A, K, M, N, P, Q, R ✪, B, C ✪, D, E, F, G, H, J, S ✪, A, B, C ✪

● S82.144   Nondisplaced bicondylar fracture of right tibia A, K, M, N, P, Q, R ✪, B, C ✪, D, E, F, G, H, J, S ✪, A, B, C ✪

● S82.145   Nondisplaced bicondylar fracture of left tibia A, K, M, N, P, Q, R ✪, B, C ✪, D, E, F, G, H, J, S ✪, A, B, C ✪

● ◼ S82.146   Nondisplaced bicondylar fracture of unspecified tibia A, K, M, N, P, Q, R ✪, B, C ✪, D, E, F, G, H, J, S ✪, A, B, C ✪

● S82.15   Fracture of tibial tuberosity

● S82.151   Displaced fracture of right tibial tuberosity A, K, M, N, P, Q, R ✪, B, C ✪, D, E, F, G, H, J, S ✪, A, B, C ✪

● S82.152   Displaced fracture of left tibial tuberosity A, K, M, N, P, Q, R ✪, B, C ✪, D, E, F, G, H, J, S ✪, A, B, C ✪

● ◼ S82.153   Displaced fracture of unspecified tibial tuberosity A, K, M, N, P, Q, R ✪, B, C ✪, D, E, F, G, H, J, S ✪, A, B, C ✪

● S82.154   Nondisplaced fracture of right tibial tuberosity A, K, M, N, P, Q, R ✪, B, C ✪, D, E, F, G, H, J, S ✪, A, B, C ✪

● S82.155   Nondisplaced fracture of left tibial tuberosity A, K, M, N, P, Q, R ✪, B, C ✪, D, E, F, G, H, J, S ✪, A, B, C ✪

● ◼ S82.156   Nondisplaced fracture of unspecified tibial tuberosity A, K, M, N, P, Q, R ✪, B, C ✪, D, E, F, G, H, J, S ✪, A, B, C ✪

● S82.16   Torus fracture of upper end of tibia
The appropriate 7th character is to be added to all codes in subcategory S82.16

A	initial encounter for closed fracture
D	subsequent encounter for fracture with routine healing
G	subsequent encounter for fracture with delayed healing
K	subsequent encounter for fracture with nonunion
P	subsequent encounter for fracture with malunion
S	sequela

● S82.161   Torus fracture of upper end of right tibia A, K, P ✪, D, G, S ✪, A ✪

● S82.162   Torus fracture of upper end of left tibia A, K, P ✪, D, G, S ✪, A ✪

● ◼ S82.169   Torus fracture of upper end of unspecified tibia A, K, P ✪, D, G, S ✪, A ✪

● S82.19   Other fracture of upper end of tibia

● S82.191   Other fracture of upper end of right tibia A, K, M, N, P, Q, R ✪, B, C ✪, D, E, F, G, H, J, S ✪, A, B, C ✪

● S82.192   Other fracture of upper end of left tibia A, K, M, N, P, Q, R ✪, B, C ✪, D, E, F, G, H, J, S ✪, A, B, C ✪

● ◼ S82.199   Other fracture of upper end of unspecified tibia A, K, M, N, P, Q, R ✪, B, C ✪, D, E, F, G, H, J, S ✪, A, B, C ✪

● S82.2   Fracture of shaft of tibia

● S82.20   Unspecified fracture of shaft of tibia
Fracture of tibia NOS

● ◼ S82.201   Unspecified fracture of shaft of right tibia A, K, M, N, P, Q, R ✪, B, C ✪, D, E, F, G, H, J, S ✪, A, B, C ✪

● ◼ S82.202   Unspecified fracture of shaft of left tibia A, K, M, N, P, Q, R ✪, B, C ✪, D, E, F, G, H, J, S ✪, A, B, C ✪

● ◼ S82.209   Unspecified fracture of shaft of unspecified tibia A, K, M, N, P, Q, R ✪, B, C ✪, D, E, F, G, H, J, S ✪, A, B, C ✪

● S82.22   Transverse fracture of shaft of tibia

● S82.221   Displaced transverse fracture of shaft of right tibia A, K, M, N, P, Q, R ✪, B, C ✪, D, E, F, G, H, J, S ✪, A, B, C ✪

● S82.222   Displaced transverse fracture of shaft of left tibia A, K, M, N, P, Q, R ✪, B, C ✪, D, E, F, G, H, J, S ✪, A, B, C ✪

● ◼ S82.223   Displaced transverse fracture of shaft of unspecified tibia A, K, M, N, P, Q, R ✪, B, C ✪, D, E, F, G, H, J, S ✪, A, B, C ✪

● Unacceptable Principal Diagnosis   ● Use Additional Character(s)   ◼ Unspecified   ▸ Manifestation Code

OGCR   Official Guidelines for Coding and Reporting   Excludes 1   Excludes 2   Includes   Use additional   Code first   Code also

- ● S82.224 Nondisplaced transverse fracture of shaft of right tibia A, K, M, N, P, Q, R 🔶, B, C 🔶, D, E, F, G, H, J, S 🔶, A, B, C 🔶
- ● S82.225 Nondisplaced transverse fracture of shaft of left tibia A, K, M, N, P, Q, R 🔶, B, C 🔶, D, E, F, G, H, J, S 🔶, A, B, C 🔶
- ●■ S82.226 Nondisplaced transverse fracture of shaft of unspecified tibia A, K, M, N, P, Q, R 🔶, B, C 🔶, D, E, F, G, H, J, S 🔶, A, B, C 🔶
- ● S82.23 Oblique fracture of shaft of tibia
  - ● S82.231 Displaced oblique fracture of shaft of right tibia A, K, M, N, P, Q, R 🔶, B, C 🔶, D, E, F, G, H, J, S 🔶, A, B, C 🔶
  - ● S82.232 Displaced oblique fracture of shaft of left tibia A, K, M, N, P, Q, R 🔶, B, C 🔶, D, E, F, G, H, J, S 🔶, A, B, C 🔶
  - ●■ S82.233 Displaced oblique fracture of shaft of unspecified tibia A, K, M, N, P, Q, R 🔶, B, C 🔶, D, E, F, G, H, J, S 🔶, A, B, C 🔶
  - ● S82.234 Nondisplaced oblique fracture of shaft of right tibia A, K, M, N, P, Q, R 🔶, B, C 🔶, D, E, F, G, H, J, S 🔶, A, B, C 🔶
  - ● S82.235 Nondisplaced oblique fracture of shaft of left tibia A, K, M, N, P, Q, R 🔶, B, C 🔶, D, E, F, G, H, J, S 🔶, A, B, C 🔶
  - ●■ S82.236 Nondisplaced oblique fracture of shaft of unspecified tibia A, K, M, N, P, Q, R 🔶, B, C 🔶, D, E, F, G, H, J, S 🔶, A, B, C 🔶
- ● S82.24 Spiral fracture of shaft of tibia
  Toddler fracture
  - ● S82.241 Displaced spiral fracture of shaft of right tibia A, K, M, N, P, Q, R 🔶, B, C 🔶, D, E, F, G, H, J, S 🔶, A, B, C 🔶
  - ● S82.242 Displaced spiral fracture of shaft of left tibia A, K, M, N, P, Q, R 🔶, B, C 🔶, D, E, F, G, H, J, S 🔶, A, B, C 🔶
  - ●■ S82.243 Displaced spiral fracture of shaft of unspecified tibia A, K, M, N, P, Q, R 🔶, B, C 🔶, D, E, F, G, H, J, S 🔶, A, B, C 🔶
  - ● S82.244 Nondisplaced spiral fracture of shaft of right tibia A, K, M, N, P, Q, R 🔶, B, C 🔶, D, E, F, G, H, J, S 🔶, A, B, C 🔶
  - ● S82.245 Nondisplaced spiral fracture of shaft of left tibia A, K, M, N, P, Q, R 🔶, B, C 🔶, D, E, F, G, H, J, S 🔶, A, B, C 🔶
  - ●■ S82.246 Nondisplaced spiral fracture of shaft of unspecified tibia A, K, M, N, P, Q, R 🔶, B, C 🔶, D, E, F, G, H, J, S 🔶, A, B, C 🔶

- ● S82.25 Comminuted fracture of shaft of tibia
  - ● S82.251 Displaced comminuted fracture of shaft of right tibia A, K, M, N, P, Q, R 🔶, B, C 🔶, D, E, F, G, H, J, S 🔶, A, B, C 🔶
  - ● S82.252 Displaced comminuted fracture of shaft of left tibia A, K, M, N, P, Q, R 🔶, B, C 🔶, D, E, F, G, H, J, S 🔶, A, B, C 🔶
  - ●■ S82.253 Displaced comminuted fracture of shaft of unspecified tibia A, K, M, N, P, Q, R 🔶, B, C 🔶, D, E, F, G, H, J, S 🔶, A, B, C 🔶
  - ● S82.254 Nondisplaced comminuted fracture of shaft of right tibia A, K, M, N, P, Q, R 🔶, B, C 🔶, D, E, F, G, H, J, S 🔶, A, B, C 🔶
  - ● S82.255 Nondisplaced comminuted fracture of shaft of left tibia A, K, M, N, P, Q, R 🔶, B, C 🔶, D, E, F, G, H, J, S 🔶, A, B, C 🔶
  - ●■ S82.256 Nondisplaced comminuted fracture of shaft of unspecified tibia A, K, M, N, P, Q, R 🔶, B, C 🔶, D, E, F, G, H, J, S 🔶, A, B, C 🔶
- ● S82.26 Segmental fracture of shaft of tibia
  - ● S82.261 Displaced segmental fracture of shaft of right tibia A, K, M, N, P, Q, R 🔶, B, C 🔶, D, E, F, G, H, J, S 🔶, A, B, C 🔶
  - ● S82.262 Displaced segmental fracture of shaft of left tibia A, K, M, N, P, Q, R 🔶, B, C 🔶, D, E, F, G, H, J, S 🔶, A, B, C 🔶
  - ●■ S82.263 Displaced segmental fracture of shaft of unspecified tibia A, K, M, N, P, Q, R 🔶, B, C 🔶, D, E, F, G, H, J, S 🔶, A, B, C 🔶
  - ● S82.264 Nondisplaced segmental fracture of shaft of right tibia A, K, M, N, P, Q, R 🔶, B, C 🔶, D, E, F, G, H, J, S 🔶, A, B, C 🔶
  - ● S82.265 Nondisplaced segmental fracture of shaft of left tibia A, K, M, N, P, Q, R 🔶, B, C 🔶, D, E, F, G, H, J, S 🔶, A, B, C 🔶
  - ●■ S82.266 Nondisplaced segmental fracture of shaft of unspecified tibia A, K, M, N, P, Q, R 🔶, B, C 🔶, D, E, F, G, H, J, S 🔶, A, B, C 🔶
- ● S82.29 Other fracture of shaft of tibia
  - ● S82.291 Other fracture of shaft of right tibia A, K, M, N, P, Q, R 🔶, B, C 🔶, D, E, F, G, H, J, S 🔶, A, B, C 🔶
  - ● S82.292 Other fracture of shaft of left tibia A, K, M, N, P, Q, R 🔶, B, C 🔶, D, E, F, G, H, J, S 🔶, A, B, C 🔶
  - ●■ S82.299 Other fracture of shaft of unspecified tibia A, K, M, N, P, Q, R 🔶, B, C 🔶, D, E, F, G, H, J, S 🔶, A, B, C 🔶

CHAPTER 19 (S00-T88)

N Newborn Age: 0   P Pediatric Age: 0–17   M Maternity DX: 12–55   A Adult Age: 15–124   ♀ Females Only   ♂ Males Only
🔶 Complication\Comorbidity   🔶 Major C\C   🔶 Present on Admission Requirement   🔶 Hospital-Acquired Condition

1551

● **S82.3 Fracture of lower end of tibia**

> | Excludes1 | bimalleolar fracture of lower leg (S82.84-)
> fracture of medial malleolus alone (S82.5-)
> Maisonneuve's fracture (S82.86-)
> pilon fracture of distal tibia (S82.87-)
> trimalleolar fractures of lower leg (S82.85-)

● **S82.30 Unspecified fracture of lower end of tibia**

  ● ■ **S82.301 Unspecified fracture of lower end of right tibia** B, C, K, M, N, P, Q, R ⬡, D, E, F, G, H, J, S ⬡, B, C ⬡

  ● ■ **S82.302 Unspecified fracture of lower end of left tibia** B, C, K, M, N, P, Q, R ⬡, D, E, F, G, H, J, S ⬡, B, C ⬡

  ● ■ **S82.309 Unspecified fracture of lower end of unspecified tibia** B, C, K, M, N, P, Q, R ⬡, D, E, F, G, H, J, S ⬡, B, C ⬡

● **S82.31 Torus fracture of lower end of tibia**

The appropriate 7th character is to be added to all codes in subcategory S82.31

A	initial encounter for closed fracture
D	subsequent encounter for fracture with routine healing
G	subsequent encounter for fracture with delayed healing
K	subsequent encounter for fracture with nonunion
P	subsequent encounter for fracture with malunion
S	sequela

  ● **S82.311 Torus fracture of lower end of right tibia** A, K, P ⬡, D, G, S ⬡, A ⬡

  ● **S82.312 Torus fracture of lower end of left tibia** A, K, P ⬡, D, G, S ⬡, A ⬡

  ● ■ **S82.319 Torus fracture of lower end of unspecified tibia** A, K, P ⬡, D, G, S ⬡, A ⬡

● **S82.39 Other fracture of lower end of tibia**

  ● **S82.391 Other fracture of lower end of right tibia** B, C, K, M, N, P, Q, R ⬡, D, E, F, G, H, J, S ⬡, B, C ⬡

  ● **S82.392 Other fracture of lower end of left tibia** B, C, K, M, N, P, Q, R ⬡, D, E, F, G, H, J, S ⬡, B, C ⬡

  ● ■ **S82.399 Other fracture of lower end of unspecified tibia** B, C, K, M, N, P, Q, R ⬡, D, E, F, G, H, J, S ⬡, B, C ⬡

● **S82.4 Fracture of shaft of fibula**

> | Excludes2 | fracture of lateral malleolus alone (S82.6-)

● **S82.40 Unspecified fracture of shaft of fibula**

  ● ■ **S82.401 Unspecified fracture of shaft of right fibula** K, M, N, P, Q, R ⬡, B, C ⬡, D, E, F, G, H, J, S ⬡, B, C ⬡

  ● ■ **S82.402 Unspecified fracture of shaft of left fibula** K, M, N, P, Q, R ⬡, B, C ⬡, D, E, F, G, H, J, S ⬡, B, C ⬡

  ● ■ **S82.409 Unspecified fracture of shaft of unspecified fibula** K, M, N, P, Q, R ⬡, B, C ⬡, D, E, F, G, H, J, S ⬡, B, C ⬡

● **S82.42 Transverse fracture of shaft of fibula**

  ● **S82.421 Displaced transverse fracture of shaft of right fibula** K, M, N, P, Q, R ⬡, B, C ⬡, D, E, F, G, H, J, S ⬡, B, C ⬡

  ● **S82.422 Displaced transverse fracture of shaft of left fibula** K, M, N, P, Q, R ⬡, B, C ⬡, D, E, F, G, H, J, S ⬡, B, C ⬡

  ● ■ **S82.423 Displaced transverse fracture of shaft of unspecified fibula** K, M, N, P, Q, R ⬡, B, C ⬡, D, E, F, G, H, J, S ⬡, B, C ⬡

  ● **S82.424 Nondisplaced transverse fracture of shaft of right fibula** K, M, N, P, Q, R ⬡, B, C ⬡, D, E, F, G, H, J, S ⬡, B, C ⬡

  ● **S82.425 Nondisplaced transverse fracture of shaft of left fibula** K, M, N, P, Q, R ⬡, B, C ⬡, D, E, F, G, H, J, S ⬡, B, C ⬡

  ● ■ **S82.426 Nondisplaced transverse fracture of shaft of unspecified fibula** K, M, N, P, Q, R ⬡, B, C ⬡, D, E, F, G, H, J, S ⬡, B, C ⬡

● **S82.43 Oblique fracture of shaft of fibula**

  ● **S82.431 Displaced oblique fracture of shaft of right fibula** K, M, N, P, Q, R ⬡, B, C ⬡, D, E, F, G, H, J, S ⬡, B, C ⬡

  ● **S82.432 Displaced oblique fracture of shaft of left fibula** K, M, N, P, Q, R ⬡, B, C ⬡, D, E, F, G, H, J, S ⬡, B, C ⬡

  ● ■ **S82.433 Displaced oblique fracture of shaft of unspecified fibula** K, M, N, P, Q, R ⬡, B, C ⬡, D, E, F, G, H, J, S ⬡, B, C ⬡

  ● **S82.434 Nondisplaced oblique fracture of shaft of right fibula** K, M, N, P, Q, R ⬡, B, C ⬡, D, E, F, G, H, J, S ⬡, B, C ⬡

  ● **S82.435 Nondisplaced oblique fracture of shaft of left fibula** K, M, N, P, Q, R ⬡, B, C ⬡, D, E, F, G, H, J, S ⬡, B, C ⬡

  ● ■ **S82.436 Nondisplaced oblique fracture of shaft of unspecified fibula** K, M, N, P, Q, R ⬡, B, C ⬡, D, E, F, G, H, J, S ⬡, B, C ⬡

● Unacceptable Principal Diagnosis   ● Use Additional Character(s)   ■ Unspecified   ▶ Manifestation Code

OGCR Official Guidelines for Coding and Reporting   Excludes 1   Excludes 2   Includes   Use additional   Code first   Code also

● **S82.44**   **Spiral fracture of shaft of fibula**

  ● **S82.441**   **Displaced spiral fracture of shaft of right fibula** K, M, N, P, Q, R, B, C, D, E, F, G, H, J, S, B, C

  ● **S82.442**   **Displaced spiral fracture of shaft of left fibula** K, M, N, P, Q, R, B, C, D, E, F, G, H, J, S, B, C

  ●■ **S82.443**   **Displaced spiral fracture of shaft of unspecified fibula** K, M, N, P, Q, R, B, C, D, E, F, G, H, J, S, B, C

  ● **S82.444**   **Nondisplaced spiral fracture of shaft of right fibula** K, M, N, P, Q, R, B, C, D, E, F, G, H, J, S, B, C

  ● **S82.445**   **Nondisplaced spiral fracture of shaft of left fibula** K, M, N, P, Q, R, B, C, D, E, F, G, H, J, S, B, C

  ●■ **S82.446**   **Nondisplaced spiral fracture of shaft of unspecified fibula** K, M, N, P, Q, R, B, C, D, E, F, G, H, J, S, B, C

● **S82.45**   **Comminuted fracture of shaft of fibula**

  ● **S82.451**   **Displaced comminuted fracture of shaft of right fibula** K, M, N, P, Q, R, B, C, D, E, F, G, H, J, S, B, C

  ● **S82.452**   **Displaced comminuted fracture of shaft of left fibula** K, M, N, P, Q, R, B, C, D, E, F, G, H, J, S, B, C

  ●■ **S82.453**   **Displaced comminuted fracture of shaft of unspecified fibula** K, M, N, P, Q, R, B, C, D, E, F, G, H, J, S, B, C

  ● **S82.454**   **Nondisplaced comminuted fracture of shaft of right fibula** K, M, N, P, Q, R, B, C, D, E, F, G, H, J, S, B, C

  ● **S82.455**   **Nondisplaced comminuted fracture of shaft of left fibula** K, M, N, P, Q, R, B, C, D, E, F, G, H, J, S, B, C

  ●■ **S82.456**   **Nondisplaced comminuted fracture of shaft of unspecified fibula** K, M, N, P, Q, R, B, C, D, E, F, G, H, J, S, B, C

● **S82.46**   **Segmental fracture of shaft of fibula**

  ● **S82.461**   **Displaced segmental fracture of shaft of right fibula** K, M, N, P, Q, R, B, C, D, E, F, G, H, J, S, B, C

  ● **S82.462**   **Displaced segmental fracture of shaft of left fibula** K, M, N, P, Q, R, B, C, D, E, F, G, H, J, S, B, C

  ●■ **S82.463**   **Displaced segmental fracture of shaft of unspecified fibula** K, M, N, P, Q, R, B, C, D, E, F, G, H, J, S, B, C

  ● **S82.464**   **Nondisplaced segmental fracture of shaft of right fibula** K, M, N, P, Q, R, B, C, D, E, F, G, H, J, S, B, C

  ● **S82.465**   **Nondisplaced segmental fracture of shaft of left fibula** K, M, N, P, Q, R, B, C, D, E, F, G, H, J, S, B, C

  ●■ **S82.466**   **Nondisplaced segmental fracture of shaft of unspecified fibula** K, M, N, P, Q, R, B, C, D, E, F, G, H, J, S, B, C

● **S82.49**   **Other fracture of shaft of fibula**

  ● **S82.491**   **Other fracture of shaft of right fibula** K, M, N, P, Q, R, B, C, D, E, F, G, H, J, S, B, C

  ● **S82.492**   **Other fracture of shaft of left fibula** K, M, N, P, Q, R, B, C, D, E, F, G, H, J, S, B, C

  ●■ **S82.499**   **Other fracture of shaft of unspecified fibula** K, M, N, P, Q, R, B, C, D, E, F, G, H, J, S, B, C

● **S82.5**   **Fracture of medial malleolus**

  | **Excludes1** | pilon fracture of distal tibia (S82.87-)
Salter-Harris type III of lower end of tibia (S89.13-)
Salter-Harris type IV of lower end of tibia (S89.14-) |

  ● **S82.51**   **Displaced fracture of medial malleolus of right tibia** B, C, K, M, N, P, Q, R, D, E, F, G, H, J, S, B, C

  ● **S82.52**   **Displaced fracture of medial malleolus of left tibia** B, C, K, M, N, P, Q, R, D, E, F, G, H, J, S, B, C

  ●■ **S82.53**   **Displaced fracture of medial malleolus of unspecified tibia** B, C, K, M, N, P, Q, R, D, E, F, G, H, J, S, B, C

  ● **S82.54**   **Nondisplaced fracture of medial malleolus of right tibia** B, C, K, M, N, P, Q, R, D, E, F, G, H, J, S, B, C

  ● **S82.55**   **Nondisplaced fracture of medial malleolus of left tibia** B, C, K, M, N, P, Q, R, D, E, F, G, H, J, S, B, C

  ●■ **S82.56**   **Nondisplaced fracture of medial malleolus of unspecified tibia** B, C, K, M, N, P, Q, R, D, E, F, G, H, J, S, B, C

● **S82.6**   **Fracture of lateral malleolus**

  | **Excludes1** | pilon fracture of distal tibia (S82.87-) |

  ● **S82.61**   **Displaced fracture of lateral malleolus of right fibula** B, C, K, M, N, P, Q, R, D, E, F, G, H, J, S, B, C

  ● **S82.62**   **Displaced fracture of lateral malleolus of left fibula** B, C, K, M, N, P, Q, R, D, E, F, G, H, J, S, B, C

  ●■ **S82.63**   **Displaced fracture of lateral malleolus of unspecified fibula** B, C, K, M, N, P, Q, R, D, E, F, G, H, J, S, B, C

  ● **S82.64**   **Nondisplaced fracture of lateral malleolus of right fibula** B, C, K, M, N, P, Q, R, D, E, F, G, H, J, S, B, C

  ● **S82.65**   **Nondisplaced fracture of lateral malleolus of left fibula** B, C, K, M, N, P, Q, R, D, E, F, G, H, J, S, B, C

  ●■ **S82.66**   **Nondisplaced fracture of lateral malleolus of unspecified fibula** B, C, K, M, N, P, Q, R, D, E, F, G, H, J, S, B, C

N Newborn Age: 0   **P** Pediatric Age: 0–17   **M** Maternity DX: 12–55   **A** Adult Age: 15–124   ♀ Females Only   ♂ Males Only

Complication\Comorbidity   Major C\C   Present on Admission Requirement   Hospital-Acquired Condition

1553

CHAPTER 19 (S00-T88)

- **S82.8   Other fractures of lower leg**
  - **S82.81   Torus fracture of upper end of fibula**

    The appropriate 7th character is to be added to all codes in subcategory S82.81

A	initial encounter for closed fracture
D	subsequent encounter for fracture with routine healing
G	subsequent encounter for fracture with delayed healing
K	subsequent encounter for fracture with nonunion
P	subsequent encounter for fracture with malunion
S	sequela

    - **S82.811   Torus fracture of upper end of right fibula K, P**, D, G, S
    - **S82.812   Torus fracture of upper end of left fibula K, P**, D, G, S
    - **S82.819   Torus fracture of upper end of unspecified fibula K, P**, D, G, S

  - **S82.82   Torus fracture of lower end of fibula**

    The appropriate 7th character is to be added to all codes in subcategory S82.82

A	initial encounter for closed fracture
D	subsequent encounter for fracture with routine healing
G	subsequent encounter for fracture with delayed healing
K	subsequent encounter for fracture with nonunion
P	subsequent encounter for fracture with malunion
S	sequela

    - **S82.821   Torus fracture of lower end of right fibula K, P**, D, G, S
    - **S82.822   Torus fracture of lower end of left fibula K, P**, D, G, S
    - **S82.829   Torus fracture of lower end of unspecified fibula K, P**, D, G, S

  - **S82.83   Other fracture of upper and lower end of fibula**
    - **S82.831   Other fracture of upper and lower end of right fibula K, M, N, P, Q, R**, B, C, D, E, F, G, H, J, S, B, C
    - **S82.832   Other fracture of upper and lower end of left fibula K, M, N, P, Q, R**, B, C, D, E, F, G, H, J, S, B, C
    - **S82.839   Other fracture of upper and lower end of unspecified fibula K, M, N, P, Q, R**, B, C, D, E, F, G, H, J, S, B, C

- **S82.84   Bimalleolar fracture of lower leg**
  - **S82.841   Displaced bimalleolar fracture of right lower leg B, C, K, M, N, P, Q, R**, D, E, F, G, H, J, S, B, C
  - **S82.842   Displaced bimalleolar fracture of left lower leg B, C, K, M, N, P, Q, R**, D, E, F, G, H, J, S, B, C
  - **S82.843   Displaced bimalleolar fracture of unspecified lower leg B, C, K, M, N, P, Q, R**, D, E, F, G, H, J, S, B, C
  - **S82.844   Nondisplaced bimalleolar fracture of right lower leg B, C, K, M, N, P, Q, R**, D, E, F, G, H, J, S, B, C
  - **S82.845   Nondisplaced bimalleolar fracture of left lower leg B, C, K, M, N, P, Q, R**, D, E, F, G, H, J, S, B, C
  - **S82.846   Nondisplaced bimalleolar fracture of unspecified lower leg B, C, K, M, N, P, Q, R**, D, E, F, G, H, J, S, B, C

- **S82.85   Trimalleolar fracture of lower leg**
  - **S82.851   Displaced trimalleolar fracture of right lower leg B, C, K, M, N, P, Q, R**, D, E, F, G, H, J, S, B, C
  - **S82.852   Displaced trimalleolar fracture of left lower leg B, C, K, M, N, P, Q, R**, D, E, F, G, H, J, S, B, C
  - **S82.853   Displaced trimalleolar fracture of unspecified lower leg B, C, K, M, N, P, Q, R**, D, E, F, G, H, J, S, B, C
  - **S82.854   Nondisplaced trimalleolar fracture of right lower leg B, C, K, M, N, P, Q, R**, D, E, F, G, H, J, S, B, C
  - **S82.855   Nondisplaced trimalleolar fracture of left lower leg B, C, K, M, N, P, Q, R**, D, E, F, G, H, J, S, B, C
  - **S82.856   Nondisplaced trimalleolar fracture of unspecified lower leg B, C, K, M, N, P, Q, R**, D, E, F, G, H, J, S, B, C

- **S82.86   Maisonneuve's fracture**
  - **S82.861   Displaced Maisonneuve's fracture of right leg K, M, N, P, Q, R**, B, C, D, E, F, G, H, J, S, B, C
  - **S82.862   Displaced Maisonneuve's fracture of left leg K, M, N, P, Q, R**, B, C, D, E, F, G, H, J, S, B, C

● ■ S82.863   Displaced Maisonneuve's fracture of unspecified leg K, M, N, P, Q, R 🐾, B, C 🐾, D, E, F, G, H, J, S 🐾, B, C 🐾

● S82.864   Nondisplaced Maisonneuve's fracture of right leg K, M, N, P, Q, R 🐾, B, C 🐾, D, E, F, G, H, J, S 🐾, B, C 🐾

● S82.865   Nondisplaced Maisonneuve's fracture of left leg K, M, N, P, Q, R 🐾, B, C 🐾, D, E, F, G, H, J, S 🐾, B, C 🐾

● ■ S82.866   Nondisplaced Maisonneuve's fracture of unspecified leg K, M, N, P, Q, R 🐾, B, C 🐾, D, E, F, G, H, J, S 🐾, B, C 🐾

● S82.87   Pilon fracture of tibia

● S82.871   Displaced pilon fracture of right tibia B, C, K, M, N, P, Q, R 🐾, D, E, F, G, H, J, S 🐾, B, C 🐾

● S82.872   Displaced pilon fracture of left tibia B, C, K, M, N, P, Q, R 🐾, D, E, F, G, H, J, S 🐾, B, C 🐾

● ■ S82.873   Displaced pilon fracture of unspecified tibia B, C, K, M, N, P, Q, R 🐾, D, E, F, G, H, J, S 🐾, B, C 🐾

● S82.874   Nondisplaced pilon fracture of right tibia B, C, K, M, N, P, Q, R 🐾, D, E, F, G, H, J, S 🐾, B, C 🐾

● S82.875   Nondisplaced pilon fracture of left tibia B, C, K, M, N, P, Q, R 🐾, D, E, F, G, H, J, S 🐾, B, C 🐾

● ■ S82.876   Nondisplaced pilon fracture of unspecified tibia B, C, K, M, N, P, Q, R 🐾, D, E, F, G, H, J, S 🐾, B, C 🐾

● S82.89   Other fractures of lower leg
Fracture of ankle NOS

● S82.891   Other fracture of right lower leg B, C, K, M, N, P, Q, R 🐾, D, E, F, G, H, J, S 🐾, B, C 🐾

● S82.892   Other fracture of left lower leg B, C, K, M, N, P, Q, R 🐾, D, E, F, G, H, J, S 🐾, B, C 🐾

● ■ S82.899   Other fracture of unspecified lower leg B, C, K, M, N, P, Q, R 🐾, D, E, F, G, H, J, S 🐾, B, C 🐾

● S82.9   Unspecified fracture of lower leg

● ■ S82.90   Unspecified fracture of unspecified lower leg A, K, M, N, P, Q, R 🐾, B, C 🐾, D, E, F, G, H, J, S 🐾, A, B, C 🐾

● ■ S82.91   Unspecified fracture of right lower leg A, K, M, N, P, Q, R 🐾, B, C 🐾, D, E, F, G, H, J, S 🐾, A, B, C 🐾

● ■ S82.92   Unspecified fracture of left lower leg A, K, M, N, P, Q, R 🐾, B, C 🐾, D, E, F, G, H, J, S 🐾, A, B, C 🐾

● S83   Dislocation and sprain of joints and ligaments of knee

| Includes | avulsion of joint or ligament of knee |

laceration of cartilage, joint or ligament of knee
sprain of cartilage, joint or ligament of knee
traumatic hemarthrosis of joint or ligament of knee
traumatic rupture of joint or ligament of knee
traumatic subluxation of joint or ligament of knee
traumatic tear of joint or ligament of knee

Code also any associated open wound

Excludes1   derangement of patella (M22.0-M22.3)
injury of patellar ligament (tendon) (S76.1-)
internal derangement of knee (M23.-)
old dislocation of knee (M24.36)
pathological dislocation of knee (M24.36)
recurrent dislocation of knee (M22.0)

Excludes2   strain of muscle, fascia and tendon of lower leg (S86.-)

The appropriate 7th character is to be added to each code from category S83

A	initial encounter
D	subsequent encounter
S	sequela

● S83.0   Subluxation and dislocation of patella

● S83.00   Unspecified subluxation and dislocation of patella

● ■ S83.001   Unspecified subluxation of right patella D, S 🐾

● ■ S83.002   Unspecified subluxation of left patella D, S 🐾

● ■ S83.003   Unspecified subluxation of unspecified patella D, S 🐾

● ■ S83.004   Unspecified dislocation of right patella D, S 🐾

● ■ S83.005   Unspecified dislocation of left patella D, S 🐾

● ■ S83.006   Unspecified dislocation of unspecified patella D, S 🐾

● S83.01   Lateral subluxation and dislocation of patella

● S83.011   Lateral subluxation of right patella D, S 🐾

● S83.012   Lateral subluxation of left patella D, S 🐾

● ■ S83.013   Lateral subluxation of unspecified patella D, S 🐾

● S83.014   Lateral dislocation of right patella D, S 🐾

● S83.015   Lateral dislocation of left patella D, S 🐾

● ■ S83.016   Lateral dislocation of unspecified patella D, S 🐾

N Newborn Age: 0   **P** Pediatric Age: 0–17   **M** Maternity DX: 12–55   **A** Adult Age: 15–124   ♀ Females Only   ♂ Males Only

🐾 Complication\Comorbidity   🐾 Major C\C   🐾 Present on Admission Requirement   🐾 Hospital-Acquired Condition

1555

● **S83.09**   Other subluxation and dislocation of patella

   ● **S83.091**   Other subluxation of right patella D, S 🔍

   ● **S83.092**   Other subluxation of left patella D, S 🔍

   ●■ **S83.093**   Other subluxation of unspecified patella D, S 🔍

   ● **S83.094**   Other dislocation of right patella D, S 🔍

   ● **S83.095**   Other dislocation of left patella D, S 🔍

   ●■ **S83.096**   Other dislocation of unspecified patella D, S 🔍

● **S83.1**   Subluxation and dislocation of knee

   Excludes2   instability of knee prosthesis (T84.022, T84.023)

  ● **S83.10**   Unspecified subluxation and dislocation of knee

   ●■ **S83.101**   Unspecified subluxation of right knee D, S 🔍

   ●■ **S83.102**   Unspecified subluxation of left knee D, S 🔍

   ●■ **S83.103**   Unspecified subluxation of unspecified knee D, S 🔍

   ●■ **S83.104**   Unspecified dislocation of right knee D, S 🔍

   ●■ **S83.105**   Unspecified dislocation of left knee D, S 🔍

   ●■ **S83.106**   Unspecified dislocation of unspecified knee D, S 🔍

  ● **S83.11**   Anterior subluxation and dislocation of proximal end of tibia

    Posterior subluxation and dislocation of distal end of femur

   ● **S83.111**   Anterior subluxation of proximal end of tibia, right knee D, S 🔍

   ● **S83.112**   Anterior subluxation of proximal end of tibia, left knee D, S 🔍

   ●■ **S83.113**   Anterior subluxation of proximal end of tibia, unspecified knee D, S 🔍

   ● **S83.114**   Anterior dislocation of proximal end of tibia, right knee D, S 🔍

   ● **S83.115**   Anterior dislocation of proximal end of tibia, left knee D, S 🔍

   ●■ **S83.116**   Anterior dislocation of proximal end of tibia, unspecified knee D, S 🔍

  ● **S83.12**   Posterior subluxation and dislocation of proximal end of tibia

    Anterior dislocation of distal end of femur

   ● **S83.121**   Posterior subluxation of proximal end of tibia, right knee D, S 🔍

   ● **S83.122**   Posterior subluxation of proximal end of tibia, left knee D, S 🔍

   ●■ **S83.123**   Posterior subluxation of proximal end of tibia, unspecified knee D, S 🔍

   ● **S83.124**   Posterior dislocation of proximal end of tibia, right knee D, S 🔍

   ● **S83.125**   Posterior dislocation of proximal end of tibia, left knee D, S 🔍

   ●■ **S83.126**   Posterior dislocation of proximal end of tibia, unspecified knee D, S 🔍

● **S83.13**   Medial subluxation and dislocation of proximal end of tibia

   ● **S83.131**   Medial subluxation of proximal end of tibia, right knee D, S 🔍

   ● **S83.132**   Medial subluxation of proximal end of tibia, left knee D, S 🔍

   ●■ **S83.133**   Medial subluxation of proximal end of tibia, unspecified knee D, S 🔍

   ● **S83.134**   Medial dislocation of proximal end of tibia, right knee D, S 🔍

   ● **S83.135**   Medial dislocation of proximal end of tibia, left knee D, S 🔍

   ●■ **S83.136**   Medial dislocation of proximal end of tibia, unspecified knee D, S 🔍

● **S83.14**   Lateral subluxation and dislocation of proximal end of tibia

   ● **S83.141**   Lateral subluxation of proximal end of tibia, right knee D, S 🔍

   ● **S83.142**   Lateral subluxation of proximal end of tibia, left knee D, S 🔍

   ●■ **S83.143**   Lateral subluxation of proximal end of tibia, unspecified knee D, S 🔍

   ● **S83.144**   Lateral dislocation of proximal end of tibia, right knee D, S 🔍

   ● **S83.145**   Lateral dislocation of proximal end of tibia, left knee D, S 🔍

   ●■ **S83.146**   Lateral dislocation of proximal end of tibia, unspecified knee D, S 🔍

● **S83.19**   Other subluxation and dislocation of knee

   ● **S83.191**   Other subluxation of right knee D, S 🔍

   ● **S83.192**   Other subluxation of left knee D, S 🔍

   ●■ **S83.193**   Other subluxation of unspecified knee D, S 🔍

   ● **S83.194**   Other dislocation of right knee D, S 🔍

   ● **S83.195**   Other dislocation of left knee D, S 🔍

   ●■ **S83.196**   Other dislocation of unspecified knee D, S 🔍

● **S83.2**   Tear of meniscus, current injury

   Excludes1   old bucket-handle tear (M23.2)

  ● **S83.20**   Tear of unspecified meniscus, current injury

    Tear of meniscus of knee NOS

   ●■ **S83.200**   Bucket-handle tear of unspecified meniscus, current injury, right knee D, S 🔍

   ●■ **S83.201**   Bucket-handle tear of unspecified meniscus, current injury, left knee D, S 🔍

   ●■ **S83.202**   Bucket-handle tear of unspecified meniscus, current injury, unspecified knee D, S 🔍

   ●■ **S83.203**   Other tear of unspecified meniscus, current injury, right knee D, S 🔍

   ●■ **S83.204**   Other tear of unspecified meniscus, current injury, left knee D, S 🔍

● Unacceptable Principal Diagnosis   ● Use Additional Character(s)   ■ Unspecified   ▶ Manifestation Code

1556   **OGCR** Official Guidelines for Coding and Reporting   Excludes 1   Excludes 2   Includes   Use additional   Code first   Code also

CHAPTER 19 (S00-T88)

● ■ **S83.205**   Other tear of unspecified meniscus, current injury, unspecified knee D, S

● ■ **S83.206**   Unspecified tear of unspecified meniscus, current injury, right knee D, S

● ■ **S83.207**   Unspecified tear of unspecified meniscus, current injury, left knee D, S

● ■ **S83.209**   Unspecified tear of unspecified meniscus, current injury, unspecified knee D, S

● **S83.21**   Bucket-handle tear of medial meniscus, current injury

     ● **S83.211**   Bucket-handle tear of medial meniscus, current injury, right knee D, S

     ● **S83.212**   Bucket-handle tear of medial meniscus, current injury, left knee D, S

     ● ■ **S83.219**   Bucket-handle tear of medial meniscus, current injury, unspecified knee D, S

● **S83.22**   Peripheral tear of medial meniscus, current injury

     ● **S83.221**   Peripheral tear of medial meniscus, current injury, right knee D, S

     ● **S83.222**   Peripheral tear of medial meniscus, current injury, left knee D, S

     ● ■ **S83.229**   Peripheral tear of medial meniscus, current injury, unspecified knee D, S

● **S83.23**   Complex tear of medial meniscus, current injury

     ● **S83.231**   Complex tear of medial meniscus, current injury, right knee D, S

     ● **S83.232**   Complex tear of medial meniscus, current injury, left knee D, S

     ● ■ **S83.239**   Complex tear of medial meniscus, current injury, unspecified knee D, S

● **S83.24**   Other tear of medial meniscus, current injury

     ● **S83.241**   Other tear of medial meniscus, current injury, right knee D, S

     ● **S83.242**   Other tear of medial meniscus, current injury, left knee D, S

     ● ■ **S83.249**   Other tear of medial meniscus, current injury, unspecified knee D, S

● **S83.25**   Bucket-handle tear of lateral meniscus, current injury

     ● **S83.251**   Bucket-handle tear of lateral meniscus, current injury, right knee D, S

     ● **S83.252**   Bucket-handle tear of lateral meniscus, current injury, left knee D, S

     ● ■ **S83.259**   Bucket-handle tear of lateral meniscus, current injury, unspecified knee D, S

● **S83.26**   Peripheral tear of lateral meniscus, current injury

     ● **S83.261**   Peripheral tear of lateral meniscus, current injury, right knee D, S

     ● **S83.262**   Peripheral tear of lateral meniscus, current injury, left knee D, S

     ● ■ **S83.269**   Peripheral tear of lateral meniscus, current injury, unspecified knee D, S

● **S83.27**   Complex tear of lateral meniscus, current injury

     ● **S83.271**   Complex tear of lateral meniscus, current injury, right knee D, S

     ● **S83.272**   Complex tear of lateral meniscus, current injury, left knee D, S

     ● ■ **S83.279**   Complex tear of lateral meniscus, current injury, unspecified knee D, S

● **S83.28**   Other tear of lateral meniscus, current injury

     ● **S83.281**   Other tear of lateral meniscus, current injury, right knee D, S

     ● **S83.282**   Other tear of lateral meniscus, current injury, left knee D, S

     ● ■ **S83.289**   Other tear of lateral meniscus, current injury, unspecified knee D, S

● **S83.3**   Tear of articular cartilage of knee, current

     ● ■ **S83.30**   Tear of articular cartilage of unspecified knee, current D, S

     ● **S83.31**   Tear of articular cartilage of right knee, current D, S

     ● **S83.32**   Tear of articular cartilage of left knee, current D, S

● **S83.4**   Sprain of collateral ligament of knee

     ● **S83.40**   Sprain of unspecified collateral ligament of knee

         ● ■ **S83.401**   Sprain of unspecified collateral ligament of right knee D, S

         ● ■ **S83.402**   Sprain of unspecified collateral ligament of left knee D, S

         ● ■ **S83.409**   Sprain of unspecified collateral ligament of unspecified knee D, S

     ● **S83.41**   Sprain of medial collateral ligament of knee

         Sprain of tibial collateral ligament

         ● **S83.411**   Sprain of medial collateral ligament of right knee D, S

         ● **S83.412**   Sprain of medial collateral ligament of left knee D, S

         ● ■ **S83.419**   Sprain of medial collateral ligament of unspecified knee D, S

     ● **S83.42**   Sprain of lateral collateral ligament of knee

         Sprain of fibular collateral ligament

         ● **S83.421**   Sprain of lateral collateral ligament of right knee D, S

         ● **S83.422**   Sprain of lateral collateral ligament of left knee D, S

         ● ■ **S83.429**   Sprain of lateral collateral ligament of unspecified knee D, S

N Newborn Age: 0   **P** Pediatric Age: 0–17   **M** Maternity DX: 12–55   **A** Adult Age: 15–124   ♀ Females Only   ♂ Males Only

Complication\Comorbidity   Major C\C   Present on Admission Requirement   Hospital-Acquired Condition

1557

- S83.5   Sprain of cruciate ligament of knee
  - S83.50   Sprain of unspecified cruciate ligament of knee
    - S83.501   Sprain of unspecified cruciate ligament of right knee D, S
    - S83.502   Sprain of unspecified cruciate ligament of left knee D, S
    - S83.509   Sprain of unspecified cruciate ligament of unspecified knee D, S
  - S83.51   Sprain of anterior cruciate ligament of knee
    - S83.511   Sprain of anterior cruciate ligament of right knee D, S
    - S83.512   Sprain of anterior cruciate ligament of left knee D, S
    - S83.519   Sprain of anterior cruciate ligament of unspecified knee D, S
  - S83.52   Sprain of posterior cruciate ligament of knee
    - S83.521   Sprain of posterior cruciate ligament of right knee D, S
    - S83.522   Sprain of posterior cruciate ligament of left knee D, S
    - S83.529   Sprain of posterior cruciate ligament of unspecified knee D, S
- S83.6   Sprain of the superior tibiofibular joint and ligament
  - S83.60   Sprain of the superior tibiofibular joint and ligament, unspecified knee D, S
  - S83.61   Sprain of the superior tibiofibular joint and ligament, right knee D, S
  - S83.62   Sprain of the superior tibiofibular joint and ligament, left knee D, S
- S83.8   Sprain of other specified parts of knee
  - S83.8X   Sprain of other specified parts of knee
    - S83.8X1   Sprain of other specified parts of right knee D, S
    - S83.8X2   Sprain of other specified parts of left knee D, S
    - S83.8X9   Sprain of other specified parts of unspecified knee D, S
- S83.9   Sprain of unspecified site of knee
  - S83.90   Sprain of unspecified site of unspecified knee D, S
  - S83.91   Sprain of unspecified site of right knee D, S
  - S83.92   Sprain of unspecified site of left knee D, S

- S84   Injury of nerves at lower leg level

  Code also any associated open wound (S81.-)

  Excludes2   injury of nerves at ankle and foot level (S94.-)

  The appropriate 7th character is to be added to each code from category S84

A	initial encounter
D	subsequent encounter
S	sequela

  - S84.0   Injury of tibial nerve at lower leg level
    - S84.00   Injury of tibial nerve at lower leg level, unspecified leg D, S
    - S84.01   Injury of tibial nerve at lower leg level, right leg D, S
    - S84.02   Injury of tibial nerve at lower leg level, left leg D, S
  - S84.1   Injury of peroneal nerve at lower leg level
    - S84.10   Injury of peroneal nerve at lower leg level, unspecified leg D, S
    - S84.11   Injury of peroneal nerve at lower leg level, right leg D, S
    - S84.12   Injury of peroneal nerve at lower leg level, left leg D, S
  - S84.2   Injury of cutaneous sensory nerve at lower leg level
    - S84.20   Injury of cutaneous sensory nerve at lower leg level, unspecified leg D, S
    - S84.21   Injury of cutaneous sensory nerve at lower leg level, right leg D, S
    - S84.22   Injury of cutaneous sensory nerve at lower leg level, left leg D, S
  - S84.8   Injury of other nerves at lower leg level
    - S84.80   Injury of other nerves at lower leg level
      - S84.801   Injury of other nerves at lower leg level, right leg D, S
      - S84.802   Injury of other nerves at lower leg level, left leg D, S
      - S84.809   Injury of other nerves at lower leg level, unspecified leg D, S
  - S84.9   Injury of unspecified nerve at lower leg level
    - S84.90   Injury of unspecified nerve at lower leg level, unspecified leg D, S
    - S84.91   Injury of unspecified nerve at lower leg level, right leg D, S
    - S84.92   Injury of unspecified nerve at lower leg level, left leg D, S

- S85   Injury of blood vessels at lower leg level

  Code also any associated open wound (S81.-)

  Excludes2   injury of blood vessels at ankle and foot level (S95.-)

  The appropriate 7th character is to be added to each code from category S85

A	initial encounter
D	subsequent encounter
S	sequela

  - S85.0   Injury of popliteal artery
    - S85.00   Unspecified injury of popliteal artery
      - S85.001   Unspecified injury of popliteal artery, right leg A, D, S

● Unacceptable Principal Diagnosis   ● Use Additional Character(s)   ■ Unspecified   ▶ Manifestation Code

OGCR Official Guidelines for Coding and Reporting   Excludes 1   Excludes 2   Includes   Use additional   Code first   Code also

● ■ **S85.002** Unspecified injury of popliteal artery, left leg A 🐾, D, S 🐾

● ■ **S85.009** Unspecified injury of popliteal artery, unspecified leg A 🐾, D, S 🐾

● **S85.01** Laceration of popliteal artery

  ● **S85.011** Laceration of popliteal artery, right leg A 🐾, D, S 🐾

  ● **S85.012** Laceration of popliteal artery, left leg A 🐾, D, S 🐾

  ● ■ **S85.019** Laceration of popliteal artery, unspecified leg A 🐾, D, S 🐾

● **S85.09** Other specified injury of popliteal artery

  ● **S85.091** Other specified injury of popliteal artery, right leg A 🐾, D, S 🐾

  ● **S85.092** Other specified injury of popliteal artery, left leg A 🐾, D, S 🐾

  ● ■ **S85.099** Other specified injury of popliteal artery, unspecified leg A 🐾, D, S 🐾

● **S85.1** Injury of tibial artery

● **S85.10** Unspecified injury of unspecified tibial artery

  Injury of tibial artery NOS

  ● ■ **S85.101** Unspecified injury of unspecified tibial artery, right leg A 🐾, D, S 🐾

  ● ■ **S85.102** Unspecified injury of unspecified tibial artery, left leg A 🐾, D, S 🐾

  ● ■ **S85.109** Unspecified injury of unspecified tibial artery, unspecified leg A 🐾, D, S 🐾

● **S85.11** Laceration of unspecified tibial artery

  ● ■ **S85.111** Laceration of unspecified tibial artery, right leg A 🐾, D, S 🐾

  ● ■ **S85.112** Laceration of unspecified tibial artery, left leg A 🐾, D, S 🐾

  ● ■ **S85.119** Laceration of unspecified tibial artery, unspecified leg A 🐾, D, S 🐾

● **S85.12** Other specified injury of unspecified tibial artery

  ● ■ **S85.121** Other specified injury of unspecified tibial artery, right leg A 🐾, D, S 🐾

  ● ■ **S85.122** Other specified injury of unspecified tibial artery, left leg A 🐾, D, S 🐾

  ● ■ **S85.129** Other specified injury of unspecified tibial artery, unspecified leg A 🐾, D, S 🐾

● **S85.13** Unspecified injury of anterior tibial artery

  ● ■ **S85.131** Unspecified injury of anterior tibial artery, right leg A 🐾, D, S 🐾

  ● ■ **S85.132** Unspecified injury of anterior tibial artery, left leg A 🐾, D, S 🐾

  ● ■ **S85.139** Unspecified injury of anterior tibial artery, unspecified leg A 🐾, D, S 🐾

● **S85.14** Laceration of anterior tibial artery

  ● **S85.141** Laceration of anterior tibial artery, right leg A 🐾, D, S 🐾

  ● **S85.142** Laceration of anterior tibial artery, left leg A 🐾, D, S 🐾

  ● ■ **S85.149** Laceration of anterior tibial artery, unspecified leg A 🐾, D, S 🐾

● **S85.15** Other specified injury of anterior tibial artery

  ● **S85.151** Other specified injury of anterior tibial artery, right leg A 🐾, D, S 🐾

  ● **S85.152** Other specified injury of anterior tibial artery, left leg A 🐾, D, S 🐾

  ● ■ **S85.159** Other specified injury of anterior tibial artery, unspecified leg A 🐾, D, S 🐾

● **S85.16** Unspecified injury of posterior tibial artery

  ● ■ **S85.161** Unspecified injury of posterior tibial artery, right leg A 🐾, D, S 🐾

  ● ■ **S85.162** Unspecified injury of posterior tibial artery, left leg A 🐾, D, S 🐾

  ● ■ **S85.169** Unspecified injury of posterior tibial artery, unspecified leg A 🐾, D, S 🐾

● **S85.17** Laceration of posterior tibial artery

  ● **S85.171** Laceration of posterior tibial artery, right leg A 🐾, D, S 🐾

  ● **S85.172** Laceration of posterior tibial artery, left leg A 🐾, D, S 🐾

  ● ■ **S85.179** Laceration of posterior tibial artery, unspecified leg A 🐾, D, S 🐾

● **S85.18** Other specified injury of posterior tibial artery

  ● **S85.181** Other specified injury of posterior tibial artery, right leg A 🐾, D, S 🐾

  ● **S85.182** Other specified injury of posterior tibial artery, left leg A 🐾, D, S 🐾

  ● ■ **S85.189** Other specified injury of posterior tibial artery, unspecified leg A 🐾, D, S 🐾

● **S85.2** Injury of peroneal artery

● **S85.20** Unspecified injury of peroneal artery

  ● ■ **S85.201** Unspecified injury of peroneal artery, right leg A 🐾, D, S 🐾

  ● ■ **S85.202** Unspecified injury of peroneal artery, left leg A 🐾, D, S 🐾

  ● ■ **S85.209** Unspecified injury of peroneal artery, unspecified leg A 🐾, D, S 🐾

● **S85.21** Laceration of peroneal artery

  ● **S85.211** Laceration of peroneal artery, right leg A 🐾, D, S 🐾

  ● **S85.212** Laceration of peroneal artery, left leg A 🐾, D, S 🐾

  ● ■ **S85.219** Laceration of peroneal artery, unspecified leg A 🐾, D, S 🐾

N Newborn Age: 0 **P** Pediatric Age: 0–17 **M** Maternity DX: 12–55 **A** Adult Age: 15–124 ♀ Females Only ♂ Males Only

🐾 Complication\Comorbidity 🐾 Major C\C 🐾 Present on Admission Requirement 🐾 Hospital-Acquired Condition

1559

CHAPTER 19 (S00-T88)

● S85.29   Other specified injury of peroneal artery
  ● S85.291   Other specified injury of peroneal artery, right leg A 🦠, D, S 🦠
  ● S85.292   Other specified injury of peroneal artery, left leg A 🦠, D, S 🦠
  ●◼ S85.299   Other specified injury of peroneal artery, unspecified leg A 🦠, D, S 🦠

● S85.3   Injury of greater saphenous vein at lower leg level
  Injury of greater saphenous vein NOS
  Injury of saphenous vein NOS

  ● S85.30   Unspecified injury of greater saphenous vein at lower leg level
    ●◼ S85.301   Unspecified injury of greater saphenous vein at lower leg level, right leg A 🦠, D, S 🦠
    ●◼ S85.302   Unspecified injury of greater saphenous vein at lower leg level, left leg A 🦠, D, S 🦠
    ●◼ S85.309   Unspecified injury of greater saphenous vein at lower leg level, unspecified leg A 🦠, D, S 🦠

  ● S85.31   Laceration of greater saphenous vein at lower leg level
    ● S85.311   Laceration of greater saphenous vein at lower leg level, right leg A 🦠, D, S 🦠
    ● S85.312   Laceration of greater saphenous vein at lower leg level, left leg A 🦠, D, S 🦠
    ●◼ S85.319   Laceration of greater saphenous vein at lower leg level, unspecified leg A 🦠, D, S 🦠

  ● S85.39   Other specified injury of greater saphenous vein at lower leg level
    ● S85.391   Other specified injury of greater saphenous vein at lower leg level, right leg A 🦠, D, S 🦠
    ● S85.392   Other specified injury of greater saphenous vein at lower leg level, left leg A 🦠, D, S 🦠
    ●◼ S85.399   Other specified injury of greater saphenous vein at lower leg level, unspecified leg A 🦠, D, S 🦠

● S85.4   Injury of lesser saphenous vein at lower leg level
  ● S85.40   Unspecified injury of lesser saphenous vein at lower leg level
    ●◼ S85.401   Unspecified injury of lesser saphenous vein at lower leg level, right leg A 🦠, D, S 🦠
    ●◼ S85.402   Unspecified injury of lesser saphenous vein at lower leg level, left leg A 🦠, D, S 🦠
    ●◼ S85.409   Unspecified injury of lesser saphenous vein at lower leg level, unspecified leg A 🦠, D, S 🦠

● S85.41   Laceration of lesser saphenous vein at lower leg level
  ● S85.411   Laceration of lesser saphenous vein at lower leg level, right leg A 🦠, D, S 🦠
  ● S85.412   Laceration of lesser saphenous vein at lower leg level, left leg A 🦠, D, S 🦠
  ●◼ S85.419   Laceration of lesser saphenous vein at lower leg level, unspecified leg A 🦠, D, S 🦠

● S85.49   Other specified injury of lesser saphenous vein at lower leg level
  ● S85.491   Other specified injury of lesser saphenous vein at lower leg level, right leg A 🦠, D, S 🦠
  ● S85.492   Other specified injury of lesser saphenous vein at lower leg level, left leg A 🦠, D, S 🦠
  ●◼ S85.499   Other specified injury of lesser saphenous vein at lower leg level, unspecified leg A 🦠, D, S 🦠

● S85.5   Injury of popliteal vein
  ● S85.50   Unspecified injury of popliteal vein
    ●◼ S85.501   Unspecified injury of popliteal vein, right leg A 🦠, D, S 🦠
    ●◼ S85.502   Unspecified injury of popliteal vein, left leg A 🦠, D, S 🦠
    ●◼ S85.509   Unspecified injury of popliteal vein, unspecified leg A 🦠, D, S 🦠

  ● S85.51   Laceration of popliteal vein
    ● S85.511   Laceration of popliteal vein, right leg A 🦠, D, S 🦠
    ● S85.512   Laceration of popliteal vein, left leg A 🦠, D, S 🦠
    ●◼ S85.519   Laceration of popliteal vein, unspecified leg A 🦠, D, S 🦠

  ● S85.59   Other specified injury of popliteal vein
    ● S85.591   Other specified injury of popliteal vein, right leg A 🦠, D, S 🦠
    ● S85.592   Other specified injury of popliteal vein, left leg A 🦠, D, S 🦠
    ●◼ S85.599   Other specified injury of popliteal vein, unspecified leg A 🦠, D, S 🦠

● S85.8   Injury of other blood vessels at lower leg level
  ● S85.80   Unspecified injury of other blood vessels at lower leg level
    ●◼ S85.801   Unspecified injury of other blood vessels at lower leg level, right leg A 🦠, D, S 🦠
    ●◼ S85.802   Unspecified injury of other blood vessels at lower leg level, left leg A 🦠, D, S 🦠
    ●◼ S85.809   Unspecified injury of other blood vessels at lower leg level, unspecified leg A 🦠, D, S 🦠

● Unacceptable Principal Diagnosis   ● Use Additional Character(s)   ◼ Unspecified   ▶ Manifestation Code
OGCR Official Guidelines for Coding and Reporting   Excludes 1   Excludes 2   Includes   Use additional   Code first   Code also

● **S85.81**   Laceration of other blood vessels at lower
leg level

  ● **S85.811**   Laceration of other blood vessels
at lower leg level, right leg A 🗘,
D, S 🗘

  ● **S85.812**   Laceration of other blood vessels
at lower leg level, left leg A 🗘,
D, S 🗘

  ● ■ **S85.819**   Laceration of other blood vessels
at lower leg level, unspecified leg
A 🗘, D, S 🗘

● **S85.89**   Other specified injury of other blood
vessels at lower leg level

  ● **S85.891**   Other specified injury of other
blood vessels at lower leg level,
right leg A 🗘, D, S 🗘

  ● **S85.892**   Other specified injury of other
blood vessels at lower leg level,
left leg A 🗘, D, S 🗘

  ● ■ **S85.899**   Other specified injury of other
blood vessels at lower leg level,
unspecified leg A 🗘, D, S 🗘

● **S85.9**   Injury of unspecified blood vessel at lower leg
level

  ● **S85.90**   Unspecified injury of unspecified blood
vessel at lower leg level

    ● ■ **S85.901**   Unspecified injury of unspecified
blood vessel at lower leg level,
right leg A 🗘, D, S 🗘

    ● ■ **S85.902**   Unspecified injury of unspecified
blood vessel at lower leg level,
left leg A 🗘, D, S 🗘

    ● ■ **S85.909**   Unspecified injury of unspecified
blood vessel at lower leg level,
unspecified leg A 🗘, D, S 🗘

  ● **S85.91**   Laceration of unspecified blood vessel at
lower leg level

    ● ■ **S85.911**   Laceration of unspecified blood
vessel at lower leg level, right leg
A 🗘, D, S 🗘

    ● ■ **S85.912**   Laceration of unspecified blood
vessel at lower leg level, left leg
A 🗘, D, S 🗘

    ● ■ **S85.919**   Laceration of unspecified blood
vessel at lower leg level,
unspecified leg A 🗘, D, S 🗘

  ● **S85.99**   Other specified injury of unspecified
blood vessel at lower leg level

    ● ■ **S85.991**   Other specified injury of
unspecified blood vessel at lower
leg level, right leg A 🗘, D, S 🗘

    ● ■ **S85.992**   Other specified injury of
unspecified blood vessel at lower
leg level, left leg A 🗘, D, S 🗘

    ● ■ **S85.999**   Other specified injury of
unspecified blood vessel at lower
leg level, unspecified leg A 🗘,
D, S 🗘

● **S86**   Injury of muscle, fascia and tendon at lower leg level

  Code also any associated open wound (S81.-)

  Excludes2   injury of muscle, fascia and tendon at ankle
(S96.-)

    injury of patellar ligament (tendon) (S76.1-)

    sprain of joints and ligaments of knee (S83.-)

The appropriate 7th character is to be added to each code
from category S86

A	initial encounter
D	subsequent encounter
S	sequela

● **S86.0**   Injury of Achilles tendon

  ● **S86.00**   Unspecified injury of Achilles tendon

    ● ■ **S86.001**   Unspecified injury of right
Achilles tendon D, S 🗘

    ● ■ **S86.002**   Unspecified injury of left
Achilles tendon D, S 🗘

    ● ■ **S86.009**   Unspecified injury of unspecified
Achilles tendon D, S 🗘

  ● **S86.01**   Strain of Achilles tendon

    ● **S86.011**   Strain of right Achilles tendon
D, S 🗘

    ● **S86.012**   Strain of left Achilles tendon
D, S 🗘

    ● ■ **S86.019**   Strain of unspecified Achilles
tendon D, S 🗘

  ● **S86.02**   Laceration of Achilles tendon

    ● **S86.021**   Laceration of right Achilles
tendon A 🗘, D, S 🗘

    ● **S86.022**   Laceration of left Achilles tendon
A 🗘, D, S 🗘

    ● ■ **S86.029**   Laceration of unspecified
Achilles tendon A 🗘, D, S 🗘

  ● **S86.09**   Other specified injury of Achilles tendon

    ● **S86.091**   Other specified injury of right
Achilles tendon D, S 🗘

    ● **S86.092**   Other specified injury of left
Achilles tendon D, S 🗘

    ● ■ **S86.099**   Other specified injury of
unspecified Achilles tendon
D, S 🗘

● **S86.1**   Injury of other muscle(s) and tendon(s) of
posterior muscle group at lower leg level

  ● **S86.10**   Unspecified injury of other muscle(s) and
tendon(s) of posterior muscle group at
lower leg level

    ● ■ **S86.101**   Unspecified injury of other
muscle(s) and tendon(s) of
posterior muscle group at lower
leg level, right leg D, S 🗘

    ● ■ **S86.102**   Unspecified injury of other
muscle(s) and tendon(s) of
posterior muscle group at lower
leg level, left leg D, S 🗘

    ● ■ **S86.109**   Unspecified injury of other
muscle(s) and tendon(s) of
posterior muscle group at lower
leg level, unspecified leg D, S 🗘

N Newborn Age: 0   **P** Pediatric Age: 0–17   **M** Maternity DX: 12–55   **A** Adult Age: 15–124   ♀ Females Only   ♂ Males Only

🗘 Complication\Comorbidity   🗘 Major C\C   🗘 Present on Admission Requirement   🗘 Hospital-Acquired Condition

1561

● S86.11   Strain of other muscle(s) and tendon(s) of posterior muscle group at lower leg level

     ● S86.111   Strain of other muscle(s) and tendon(s) of posterior muscle group at lower leg level, right leg D, S 🔊

     ● S86.112   Strain of other muscle(s) and tendon(s) of posterior muscle group at lower leg level, left leg D, S 🔊

     ●■ S86.119   Strain of other muscle(s) and tendon(s) of posterior muscle group at lower leg level, unspecified leg D, S 🔊

● S86.12   Laceration of other muscle(s) and tendon(s) of posterior muscle group at lower leg level

     ● S86.121   Laceration of other muscle(s) and tendon(s) of posterior muscle group at lower leg level, right leg A 🔊, D, S 🔊

     ● S86.122   Laceration of other muscle(s) and tendon(s) of posterior muscle group at lower leg level, left leg A 🔊, D, S 🔊

     ●■ S86.129   Laceration of other muscle(s) and tendon(s) of posterior muscle group at lower leg level, unspecified leg A 🔊, D, S 🔊

● S86.19   Other injury of other muscle(s) and tendon(s) of posterior muscle group at lower leg level

     ● S86.191   Other injury of other muscle(s) and tendon(s) of posterior muscle group at lower leg level, right leg D, S 🔊

     ● S86.192   Other injury of other muscle(s) and tendon(s) of posterior muscle group at lower leg level, left leg D, S 🔊

     ●■ S86.199   Other injury of other muscle(s) and tendon(s) of posterior muscle group at lower leg level, unspecified leg D, S 🔊

● S86.2   Injury of muscle(s) and tendon(s) of anterior muscle group at lower leg level

   ● S86.20   Unspecified injury of muscle(s) and tendon(s) of anterior muscle group at lower leg level

     ●■ S86.201   Unspecified injury of muscle(s) and tendon(s) of anterior muscle group at lower leg level, right leg D, S 🔊

     ●■ S86.202   Unspecified injury of muscle(s) and tendon(s) of anterior muscle group at lower leg level, left leg D, S 🔊

     ●■ S86.209   Unspecified injury of muscle(s) and tendon(s) of anterior muscle group at lower leg level, unspecified leg D, S 🔊

● S86.21   Strain of muscle(s) and tendon(s) of anterior muscle group at lower leg level

     ● S86.211   Strain of muscle(s) and tendon(s) of anterior muscle group at lower leg level, right leg D, S 🔊

     ● S86.212   Strain of muscle(s) and tendon(s) of anterior muscle group at lower leg level, left leg D, S 🔊

     ●■ S86.219   Strain of muscle(s) and tendon(s) of anterior muscle group at lower leg level, unspecified leg D, S 🔊

● S86.22   Laceration of muscle(s) and tendon(s) of anterior muscle group at lower leg level

     ● S86.221   Laceration of muscle(s) and tendon(s) of anterior muscle group at lower leg level, right leg A 🔊, D, S 🔊

     ● S86.222   Laceration of muscle(s) and tendon(s) of anterior muscle group at lower leg level, left leg A 🔊, D, S 🔊

     ●■ S86.229   Laceration of muscle(s) and tendon(s) of anterior muscle group at lower leg level, unspecified leg A 🔊, D, S 🔊

● S86.29   Other injury of muscle(s) and tendon(s) of anterior muscle group at lower leg level

     ● S86.291   Other injury of muscle(s) and tendon(s) of anterior muscle group at lower leg level, right leg D, S 🔊

     ● S86.292   Other injury of muscle(s) and tendon(s) of anterior muscle group at lower leg level, left leg D, S 🔊

     ●■ S86.299   Other injury of muscle(s) and tendon(s) of anterior muscle group at lower leg level, unspecified leg D, S 🔊

● S86.3   Injury of muscle(s) and tendon(s) of peroneal muscle group at lower leg level

   ● S86.30   Unspecified injury of muscle(s) and tendon(s) of peroneal muscle group at lower leg level

     ●■ S86.301   Unspecified injury of muscle(s) and tendon(s) of peroneal muscle group at lower leg level, right leg D, S 🔊

     ●■ S86.302   Unspecified injury of muscle(s) and tendon(s) of peroneal muscle group at lower leg level, left leg D, S 🔊

     ●■ S86.309   Unspecified injury of muscle(s) and tendon(s) of peroneal muscle group at lower leg level, unspecified leg D, S 🔊

   ● S86.31   Strain of muscle(s) and tendon(s) of peroneal muscle group at lower leg level

     ● S86.311   Strain of muscle(s) and tendon(s) of peroneal muscle group at lower leg level, right leg D, S 🔊

     ● S86.312   Strain of muscle(s) and tendon(s) of peroneal muscle group at lower leg level, left leg D, S 🔊

     ●■ S86.319   Strain of muscle(s) and tendon(s) of peroneal muscle group at lower leg level, unspecified leg D, S 🔊

●   Unacceptable Principal Diagnosis   ●   Use Additional Character(s)   ■   Unspecified   ▶   Manifestation Code

OGCR   Official Guidelines for Coding and Reporting   Excludes 1   Excludes 2   Includes   Use additional   Code first   Code also

- **S86.32** Laceration of muscle(s) and tendon(s) of peroneal muscle group at lower leg level
  - **S86.321** Laceration of muscle(s) and tendon(s) of peroneal muscle group at lower leg level, right leg A 🔴, D, S 🔵
  - **S86.322** Laceration of muscle(s) and tendon(s) of peroneal muscle group at lower leg level, left leg A 🔴, D, S 🔵
  - **S86.329** Laceration of muscle(s) and tendon(s) of peroneal muscle group at lower leg level, unspecified leg A 🔴, D, S 🔵
- **S86.39** Other injury of muscle(s) and tendon(s) of peroneal muscle group at lower leg level
  - **S86.391** Other injury of muscle(s) and tendon(s) of peroneal muscle group at lower leg level, right leg D, S 🔵
  - **S86.392** Other injury of muscle(s) and tendon(s) of peroneal muscle group at lower leg level, left leg D, S 🔵
  - **S86.399** Other injury of muscle(s) and tendon(s) of peroneal muscle group at lower leg level, unspecified leg D, S 🔵
- **S86.8** Injury of other muscles and tendons at lower leg level
  - **S86.80** Unspecified injury of other muscles and tendons at lower leg level
    - **S86.801** Unspecified injury of other muscle(s) and tendon(s) at lower leg level, right leg D, S 🔵
    - **S86.802** Unspecified injury of other muscle(s) and tendon(s) at lower leg level, left leg D, S 🔵
    - **S86.809** Unspecified injury of other muscle(s) and tendon(s) at lower leg level, unspecified leg D, S 🔵
  - **S86.81** Strain of other muscles and tendons at lower leg level
    - **S86.811** Strain of other muscle(s) and tendon(s) at lower leg level, right leg D, S 🔵
    - **S86.812** Strain of other muscle(s) and tendon(s) at lower leg level, left leg D, S 🔵
    - **S86.819** Strain of other muscle(s) and tendon(s) at lower leg level, unspecified leg D, S 🔵
  - **S86.82** Laceration of other muscles and tendons at lower leg level
    - **S86.821** Laceration of other muscle(s) and tendon(s) at lower leg level, right leg A 🔴, D, S 🔵
    - **S86.822** Laceration of other muscle(s) and tendon(s) at lower leg level, left leg A 🔴, D, S 🔵
    - **S86.829** Laceration of other muscle(s) and tendon(s) at lower leg level, unspecified leg A 🔴, D, S 🔵
- **S86.89** Other injury of other muscles and tendons at lower leg level
  - **S86.891** Other injury of other muscle(s) and tendon(s) at lower leg level, right leg D, S 🔵
  - **S86.892** Other injury of other muscle(s) and tendon(s) at lower leg level, left leg D, S 🔵
  - **S86.899** Other injury of other muscle(s) and tendon(s) at lower leg level, unspecified leg D, S 🔵
- **S86.9** Injury of unspecified muscle and tendon at lower leg level
  - **S86.90** Unspecified injury of unspecified muscle and tendon at lower leg level
    - **S86.901** Unspecified injury of unspecified muscle(s) and tendon(s) at lower leg level, right leg D, S 🔵
    - **S86.902** Unspecified injury of unspecified muscle(s) and tendon(s) at lower leg level, left leg D, S 🔵
    - **S86.909** Unspecified injury of unspecified muscle(s) and tendon(s) at lower leg level, unspecified leg D, S 🔵
  - **S86.91** Strain of unspecified muscle and tendon at lower leg level
    - **S86.911** Strain of unspecified muscle(s) and tendon(s) at lower leg level, right leg D, S 🔵
    - **S86.912** Strain of unspecified muscle(s) and tendon(s) at lower leg level, left leg D, S 🔵
    - **S86.919** Strain of unspecified muscle(s) and tendon(s) at lower leg level, unspecified leg D, S 🔵
  - **S86.92** Laceration of unspecified muscle and tendon at lower leg level
    - **S86.921** Laceration of unspecified muscle(s) and tendon(s) at lower leg level, right leg A 🔴, D, S 🔵
    - **S86.922** Laceration of unspecified muscle(s) and tendon(s) at lower leg level, left leg A 🔴, D, S 🔵
    - **S86.929** Laceration of unspecified muscle(s) and tendon(s) at lower leg level, unspecified leg A 🔴, D, S 🔵
  - **S86.99** Other injury of unspecified muscle and tendon at lower leg level
    - **S86.991** Other injury of unspecified muscle(s) and tendon(s) at lower leg level, right leg D, S 🔵
    - **S86.992** Other injury of unspecified muscle(s) and tendon(s) at lower leg level, left leg D, S 🔵
    - **S86.999** Other injury of unspecified muscle(s) and tendon(s) at lower leg level, unspecified leg D, S 🔵

CHAPTER 19 (S00-T88)

● S87   Crushing injury of lower leg

    Use additional code(s) for all associated injuries

    Excludes2   crushing injury of ankle and foot (S97.-)

    The appropriate 7th character is to be added to each code from category S87

      A   initial encounter
      D   subsequent encounter
      S   sequela

  ● S87.0   Crushing injury of knee

   ● S87.00   Crushing injury of unspecified knee D, S

   ● S87.01   Crushing injury of right knee D, S

   ● S87.02   Crushing injury of left knee D, S

  ● S87.8   Crushing injury of lower leg

   ● S87.80   Crushing injury of unspecified lower leg D, S

   ● S87.81   Crushing injury of right lower leg D, S

   ● S87.82   Crushing injury of left lower leg D, S

● S88   Traumatic amputation of lower leg

    An amputation not identified as partial or complete should be coded to complete

    Excludes1   traumatic amputation of ankle and foot (S98.-)

    The appropriate 7th character is to be added to each code from category S88

      A   initial encounter
      D   subsequent encounter
      S   sequela

  ● S88.0   Traumatic amputation at knee level

   ● S88.01   Complete traumatic amputation at knee level

    ● S88.011   Complete traumatic amputation at knee level, right lower leg A, D, S

    ● S88.012   Complete traumatic amputation at knee level, left lower leg A, D, S

    ● S88.019   Complete traumatic amputation at knee level, unspecified lower leg A, D, S

   ● S88.02   Partial traumatic amputation at knee level

    ● S88.021   Partial traumatic amputation at knee level, right lower leg A, D, S

    ● S88.022   Partial traumatic amputation at knee level, left lower leg A, D, S

    ● S88.029   Partial traumatic amputation at knee level, unspecified lower leg A, D, S

  ● S88.1   Traumatic amputation at level between knee and ankle

   ● S88.11   Complete traumatic amputation at level between knee and ankle

    ● S88.111   Complete traumatic amputation at level between knee and ankle, right lower leg A, D, S

    ● S88.112   Complete traumatic amputation at level between knee and ankle, left lower leg A, D, S

    ● S88.119   Complete traumatic amputation at level between knee and ankle, unspecified lower leg A, D, S

   ● S88.12   Partial traumatic amputation at level between knee and ankle

    ● S88.121   Partial traumatic amputation at level between knee and ankle, right lower leg A, D, S

    ● S88.122   Partial traumatic amputation at level between knee and ankle, left lower leg A, D, S

    ● S88.129   Partial traumatic amputation at level between knee and ankle, unspecified lower leg A, D, S

  ● S88.9   Traumatic amputation of lower leg, level unspecified

   ● S88.91   Complete traumatic amputation of lower leg, level unspecified

    ● S88.911   Complete traumatic amputation of right lower leg, level unspecified A, D, S

    ● S88.912   Complete traumatic amputation of left lower leg, level unspecified A, D, S

    ● S88.919   Complete traumatic amputation of unspecified lower leg, level unspecified A, D, S

   ● S88.92   Partial traumatic amputation of lower leg, level unspecified

    ● S88.921   Partial traumatic amputation of right lower leg, level unspecified A, D, S

    ● S88.922   Partial traumatic amputation of left lower leg, level unspecified A, D, S

    ● S88.929   Partial traumatic amputation of unspecified lower leg, level unspecified A, D, S

● S89   Other and unspecified injuries of lower leg

    Note: A fracture not indicated as open or closed should be coded to closed

    Excludes2   other and unspecified injuries of ankle and foot (S99.-)

    The appropriate 7th character is to be added to each code from subcategories S89.0, S89.1, S89.2, and S89.3

      A   initial encounter for closed fracture
      D   subsequent encounter for fracture with routine healing
      G   subsequent encounter for fracture with delayed healing
      K   subsequent encounter for fracture with nonunion
      P   subsequent encounter for fracture with malunion
      S   sequela

  ● S89.0   Physeal fracture of upper end of tibia

   ● S89.00   Unspecified physeal fracture of upper end of tibia

    ● S89.001   Unspecified physeal fracture of upper end of right tibia A, K, P, D, G, S, A

    ● S89.002   Unspecified physeal fracture of upper end of left tibia A, K, P, D, G, S, A

    ● S89.009   Unspecified physeal fracture of upper end of unspecified tibia A, K, P, D, G, S, A

● Unacceptable Principal Diagnosis   ● Use Additional Character(s)   ■ Unspecified   ▶ Manifestation Code

OGCR Official Guidelines for Coding and Reporting   Excludes 1   Excludes 2   Includes   Use additional   Code first   Code also

● S89.01   Salter-Harris Type I physeal fracture of upper end of tibia

    ● S89.011   Salter-Harris Type I physeal fracture of upper end of right tibia A, K, P 🦠, D, G, S 🦠, A 🦠

    ● S89.012   Salter-Harris Type I physeal fracture of upper end of left tibia A, K, P 🦠, D, G, S 🦠, A 🦠

    ●■ S89.019   Salter-Harris Type I physeal fracture of upper end of unspecified tibia A, K, P 🦠, D, G, S 🦠, A 🦠

● S89.02   Salter-Harris Type II physeal fracture of upper end of tibia

    ● S89.021   Salter-Harris Type II physeal fracture of upper end of right tibia A, K, P 🦠, D, G, S 🦠, A 🦠

    ● S89.022   Salter-Harris Type II physeal fracture of upper end of left tibia A, K, P 🦠, D, G, S 🦠, A 🦠

    ●■ S89.029   Salter-Harris Type II physeal fracture of upper end of unspecified tibia A, K, P 🦠, D, G, S 🦠, A 🦠

● S89.03   Salter-Harris Type III physeal fracture of upper end of tibia

    ● S89.031   Salter-Harris Type III physeal fracture of upper end of right tibia A, K, P 🦠, D, G, S 🦠, A 🦠

    ● S89.032   Salter-Harris Type III physeal fracture of upper end of left tibia A, K, P 🦠, D, G, S 🦠, A 🦠

    ●■ S89.039   Salter-Harris Type III physeal fracture of upper end of unspecified tibia A, K, P 🦠, D, G, S 🦠, A 🦠

● S89.04   Salter-Harris Type IV physeal fracture of upper end of tibia

    ● S89.041   Salter-Harris Type IV physeal fracture of upper end of right tibia A, K, P 🦠, D, G, S 🦠, A 🦠

    ● S89.042   Salter-Harris Type IV physeal fracture of upper end of left tibia A, K, P 🦠, D, G, S 🦠, A 🦠

    ●■ S89.049   Salter-Harris Type IV physeal fracture of upper end of unspecified tibia A, K, P 🦠, D, G, S 🦠, A 🦠

● S89.09   Other physeal fracture of upper end of tibia

    ● S89.091   Other physeal fracture of upper end of right tibia A, K, P 🦠, D, G, S 🦠, A 🦠

    ● S89.092   Other physeal fracture of upper end of left tibia A, K, P 🦠, D, G, S 🦠, A 🦠

    ●■ S89.099   Other physeal fracture of upper end of unspecified tibia A, K, P 🦠, D, G, S 🦠, A 🦠

● S89.1   Physeal fracture of lower end of tibia

   ● S89.10   Unspecified physeal fracture of lower end of tibia

    ●■ S89.101   Unspecified physeal fracture of lower end of right tibia K, P 🦠, D, G, S 🦠

    ●■ S89.102   Unspecified physeal fracture of lower end of left tibia K, P 🦠, D, G, S 🦠

    ●■ S89.109   Unspecified physeal fracture of lower end of unspecified tibia K, P 🦠, D, G, S 🦠

● S89.11   Salter-Harris Type I physeal fracture of lower end of tibia

    ● S89.111   Salter-Harris Type I physeal fracture of lower end of right tibia K, P 🦠, D, G, S 🦠

    ● S89.112   Salter-Harris Type I physeal fracture of lower end of left tibia K, P 🦠, D, G, S 🦠

    ●■ S89.119   Salter-Harris Type I physeal fracture of lower end of unspecified tibia K, P 🦠, D, G, S 🦠

● S89.12   Salter-Harris Type II physeal fracture of lower end of tibia

    ● S89.121   Salter-Harris Type II physeal fracture of lower end of right tibia K, P 🦠, D, G, S 🦠

    ● S89.122   Salter-Harris Type II physeal fracture of lower end of left tibia K, P 🦠, D, G, S 🦠

    ●■ S89.129   Salter-Harris Type II physeal fracture of lower end of unspecified tibia K, P 🦠, D, G, S 🦠

● S89.13   Salter-Harris Type III physeal fracture of lower end of tibia

    | **Excludes1** | fracture of medial malleolus (adult) (S82.5-)

    ● S89.131   Salter-Harris Type III physeal fracture of lower end of right tibia K, P 🦠, D, G, S 🦠

    ● S89.132   Salter-Harris Type III physeal fracture of lower end of left tibia K, P 🦠, D, G, S 🦠

    ●■ S89.139   Salter-Harris Type III physeal fracture of lower end of unspecified tibia K, P 🦠, D, G, S 🦠

● S89.14   Salter-Harris Type IV physeal fracture of lower end of tibia

    | **Excludes1** | fracture of medial malleolus (adult) (S82.5-)

    ● S89.141   Salter-Harris Type IV physeal fracture of lower end of right tibia K, P 🦠, D, G, S 🦠

    ● S89.142   Salter-Harris Type IV physeal fracture of lower end of left tibia K, P 🦠, D, G, S 🦠

    ●■ S89.149   Salter-Harris Type IV physeal fracture of lower end of unspecified tibia K, P 🦠, D, G, S 🦠

● S89.19   Other physeal fracture of lower end of tibia

    ● S89.191   Other physeal fracture of lower end of right tibia K, P 🦠, D, G, S 🦠

    ● S89.192   Other physeal fracture of lower end of left tibia K, P 🦠, D, G, S 🦠

    ●■ S89.199   Other physeal fracture of lower end of unspecified tibia K, P 🦠, D, G, S 🦠

CHAPTER 19 (S00-T88)

N Newborn Age: 0   **P** Pediatric Age: 0–17   **M** Maternity DX: 12–55   **A** Adult Age: 15–124   ♀ Females Only   ♂ Males Only

🦠 Complication\Comorbidity   🦠 Major C\C   🦠 Present on Admission Requirement   🦠 Hospital-Acquired Condition

1565

● **S89.2**   **Physeal fracture of upper end of fibula**
   ● **S89.20**   Unspecified physeal fracture of upper end of fibula
     ●■ **S89.201**   Unspecified physeal fracture of upper end of right fibula K, P, D, G, S
     ●■ **S89.202**   Unspecified physeal fracture of upper end of left fibula K, P, D, G, S
     ●■ **S89.209**   Unspecified physeal fracture of upper end of unspecified fibula K, P, D, G, S

   ● **S89.21**   Salter-Harris Type I physeal fracture of upper end of fibula
     ● **S89.211**   Salter-Harris Type I physeal fracture of upper end of right fibula K, P, D, G, S
     ● **S89.212**   Salter-Harris Type I physeal fracture of upper end of left fibula K, P, D, G, S
     ●■ **S89.219**   Salter-Harris Type I physeal fracture of upper end of unspecified fibula K, P, D, G, S

   ● **S89.22**   Salter-Harris Type II physeal fracture of upper end of fibula
     ● **S89.221**   Salter-Harris Type II physeal fracture of upper end of right fibula K, P, D, G, S
     ● **S89.222**   Salter-Harris Type II physeal fracture of upper end of left fibula K, P, D, G, S
     ●■ **S89.229**   Salter-Harris Type II physeal fracture of upper end of unspecified fibula K, P, D, G, S

   ● **S89.29**   Other physeal fracture of upper end of fibula
     ● **S89.291**   Other physeal fracture of upper end of right fibula K, P, D, G, S
     ● **S89.292**   Other physeal fracture of upper end of left fibula K, P, D, G, S
     ●■ **S89.299**   Other physeal fracture of upper end of unspecified fibula K, P, D, G, S

● **S89.3**   **Physeal fracture of lower end of fibula**
   ● **S89.30**   Unspecified physeal fracture of lower end of fibula
     ●■ **S89.301**   Unspecified physeal fracture of lower end of right fibula K, P, D, G, S
     ●■ **S89.302**   Unspecified physeal fracture of lower end of left fibula K, P, D, G, S
     ●■ **S89.309**   Unspecified physeal fracture of lower end of unspecified fibula K, P, D, G, S

   ● **S89.31**   Salter-Harris Type I physeal fracture of lower end of fibula
     ● **S89.311**   Salter-Harris Type I physeal fracture of lower end of right fibula K, P, D, G, S
     ● **S89.312**   Salter-Harris Type I physeal fracture of lower end of left fibula K, P, D, G, S
     ●■ **S89.319**   Salter-Harris Type I physeal fracture of lower end of unspecified fibula K, P, D, G, S

   ● **S89.32**   Salter-Harris Type II physeal fracture of lower end of fibula
     ● **S89.321**   Salter-Harris Type II physeal fracture of lower end of right fibula K, P, D, G, S
     ● **S89.322**   Salter-Harris Type II physeal fracture of lower end of left fibula K, P, D, G, S
     ●■ **S89.329**   Salter-Harris Type II physeal fracture of lower end of unspecified fibula K, P, D, G, S

   ● **S89.39**   Other physeal fracture of lower end of fibula
     ● **S89.391**   Other physeal fracture of lower end of right fibula K, P, D, G, S
     ● **S89.392**   Other physeal fracture of lower end of left fibula K, P, D, G, S
     ●■ **S89.399**   Other physeal fracture of lower end of unspecified fibula K, P, D, G, S

● **S89.8**   **Other specified injuries of lower leg**
   The appropriate 7th character is to be added to each code in subcategory S89.8

A	initial encounter
D	subsequent encounter
S	sequela

   ●■ **S89.80**   Other specified injuries of unspecified lower leg D, S
   ● **S89.81**   Other specified injuries of right lower leg D, S
   ● **S89.82**   Other specified injuries of left lower leg D, S

● **S89.9**   **Unspecified injury of lower leg**
   The appropriate 7th character is to be added to each code in subcategory S89.9

A	initial encounter
D	subsequent encounter
S	sequela

   ●■ **S89.90**   Unspecified injury of unspecified lower leg D, S
   ●■ **S89.91**   Unspecified injury of right lower leg D, S
   ●■ **S89.92**   Unspecified injury of left lower leg D, S

INJURIES TO THE ANKLE AND FOOT (S90-S99)

Excludes2   burns and corrosions (T20-T32)
                fracture of ankle and malleolus (S82.-)
                frostbite (T33-T34)
                insect bite or sting, venomous (T63.4)

● **S90**   **Superficial injury of ankle, foot and toes**
   The appropriate 7th character is to be added to each code from category S90

A	initial encounter
D	subsequent encounter
S	sequela

   ● **S90.0**   **Contusion of ankle**
     ●■ **S90.00**   Contusion of unspecified ankle D, S
     ● **S90.01**   Contusion of right ankle D, S
     ● **S90.02**   Contusion of left ankle D, S

● Unacceptable Principal Diagnosis   ● Use Additional Character(s)   ■ Unspecified   ▶ Manifestation Code

1566   **OGCR** Official Guidelines for Coding and Reporting | Excludes 1 | | Excludes 2 | | Includes | | Use additional | | Code first | | Code also |

● **S90.1**   **Contusion of toe without damage to nail**
- ● **S90.11**   Contusion of great toe without damage to nail
  - ● **S90.111**   Contusion of right great toe without damage to nail D, S 🔍
  - ● **S90.112**   Contusion of left great toe without damage to nail D, S 🔍
  - ●■ **S90.119**   Contusion of unspecified great toe without damage to nail D, S 🔍
- ● **S90.12**   Contusion of lesser toe without damage to nail
  - ● **S90.121**   Contusion of right lesser toe(s) without damage to nail D, S 🔍
  - ● **S90.122**   Contusion of left lesser toe(s) without damage to nail D, S 🔍
  - ●■ **S90.129**   Contusion of unspecified lesser toe(s) without damage to nail D, S 🔍
    Contusion of toe NOS

● **S90.2**   **Contusion of toe with damage to nail**
- ● **S90.21**   Contusion of great toe with damage to nail
  - ● **S90.211**   Contusion of right great toe with damage to nail D, S 🔍
  - ● **S90.212**   Contusion of left great toe with damage to nail D, S 🔍
  - ●■ **S90.219**   Contusion of unspecified great toe with damage to nail D, S 🔍
- ● **S90.22**   Contusion of lesser toe with damage to nail
  - ● **S90.221**   Contusion of right lesser toe(s) with damage to nail D, S 🔍
  - ● **S90.222**   Contusion of left lesser toe(s) with damage to nail D, S 🔍
  - ●■ **S90.229**   Contusion of unspecified lesser toe(s) with damage to nail D, S 🔍

● **S90.3**   **Contusion of foot**
> **Excludes2**   contusion of toes (S90.1-, S90.2-)
- ●■ **S90.30**   Contusion of unspecified foot D, S 🔍
  Contusion of foot NOS
- ● **S90.31**   Contusion of right foot D, S 🔍
- ● **S90.32**   Contusion of left foot D, S 🔍

● **S90.4**   **Other superficial injuries of toe**
- ● **S90.41**   Abrasion of toe
  - ● **S90.411**   Abrasion, right great toe D, S 🔍
  - ● **S90.412**   Abrasion, left great toe D, S 🔍
  - ●■ **S90.413**   Abrasion, unspecified great toe D, S 🔍
  - ● **S90.414**   Abrasion, right lesser toe(s) D, S 🔍
  - ● **S90.415**   Abrasion, left lesser toe(s) D, S 🔍
  - ●■ **S90.416**   Abrasion, unspecified lesser toe(s) D, S 🔍
- ● **S90.42**   Blister (nonthermal) of toe
  - ● **S90.421**   Blister (nonthermal), right great toe D, S 🔍
  - ● **S90.422**   Blister (nonthermal), left great toe D, S 🔍
  - ●■ **S90.423**   Blister (nonthermal), unspecified great toe D, S 🔍
  - ● **S90.424**   Blister (nonthermal), right lesser toe(s) D, S 🔍
  - ● **S90.425**   Blister (nonthermal), left lesser toe(s) D, S 🔍
  - ●■ **S90.426**   Blister (nonthermal), unspecified lesser toe(s) D, S 🔍
- ● **S90.44**   External constriction of toe
  Hair tourniquet syndrome of toe
  - ● **S90.441**   External constriction, right great toe D, S 🔍
  - ● **S90.442**   External constriction, left great toe D, S 🔍
  - ●■ **S90.443**   External constriction, unspecified great toe D, S 🔍
  - ● **S90.444**   External constriction, right lesser toe(s) D, S 🔍
  - ● **S90.445**   External constriction, left lesser toe(s) D, S 🔍
  - ●■ **S90.446**   External constriction, unspecified lesser toe(s) D, S 🔍
- ● **S90.45**   Superficial foreign body of toe
  Splinter in the toe
  - ● **S90.451**   Superficial foreign body, right great toe D, S 🔍
  - ● **S90.452**   Superficial foreign body, left great toe D, S 🔍
  - ●■ **S90.453**   Superficial foreign body, unspecified great toe D, S 🔍
  - ● **S90.454**   Superficial foreign body, right lesser toe(s) D, S 🔍
  - ● **S90.455**   Superficial foreign body, left lesser toe(s) D, S 🔍
  - ●■ **S90.456**   Superficial foreign body, unspecified lesser toe(s)
- ● **S90.46**   Insect bite (nonvenomous) of toe
  - ● **S90.461**   Insect bite (nonvenomous), right great toe D, S 🔍
  - ● **S90.462**   Insect bite (nonvenomous), left great toe D, S 🔍
  - ●■ **S90.463**   Insect bite (nonvenomous), unspecified great toe D, S 🔍
  - ● **S90.464**   Insect bite (nonvenomous), right lesser toe(s) D, S 🔍
  - ● **S90.465**   Insect bite (nonvenomous), left lesser toe(s) D, S 🔍
  - ●■ **S90.466**   Insect bite (nonvenomous), unspecified lesser toe(s)
- ● **S90.47**   Other superficial bite of toe
  > **Excludes1**   open bite of toe (S91.15-, S91.25-)
  - ● **S90.471**   Other superficial bite of right great toe D, S 🔍
  - ● **S90.472**   Other superficial bite of left great toe D, S 🔍
  - ●■ **S90.473**   Other superficial bite of unspecified great toe D, S 🔍
  - ● **S90.474**   Other superficial bite of right lesser toe(s) D, S 🔍
  - ● **S90.475**   Other superficial bite of left lesser toe(s) D, S 🔍
  - ●■ **S90.476**   Other superficial bite of unspecified lesser toe(s)

N Newborn Age: 0   **P** Pediatric Age: 0–17   **M** Maternity DX: 12–55   **A** Adult Age: 15–124   ♀ Females Only   ♂ Males Only

🔍 Complication\Comorbidity   🔍 Major C\C   🔍 Present on Admission Requirement   🔍 Hospital-Acquired Condition

1567

CHAPTER 19 (S00-T88)

CHAPTER 19 (S00-T88)

● **S90.5   Other superficial injuries of ankle**
  ● **S90.51   Abrasion of ankle**
    ● S90.511   Abrasion, right ankle D, S
    ● S90.512   Abrasion, left ankle D, S
    ●■ S90.519   Abrasion, unspecified ankle D, S
  ● **S90.52   Blister (nonthermal) of ankle**
    ● S90.521   Blister (nonthermal), right ankle D, S
    ● S90.522   Blister (nonthermal), left ankle D, S
    ●■ S90.529   Blister (nonthermal), unspecified ankle D, S
  ● **S90.54   External constriction of ankle**
    ● S90.541   External constriction, right ankle D, S
    ● S90.542   External constriction, left ankle D, S
    ●■ S90.549   External constriction, unspecified ankle D, S
  ● **S90.55   Superficial foreign body of ankle**
    Splinter in the ankle
    ● S90.551   Superficial foreign body, right ankle D, S
    ● S90.552   Superficial foreign body, left ankle D, S
    ●■ S90.559   Superficial foreign body, unspecified ankle D, S
  ● **S90.56   Insect bite (nonvenomous) of ankle**
    ● S90.561   Insect bite (nonvenomous), right ankle D, S
    ● S90.562   Insect bite (nonvenomous), left ankle D, S
    ●■ S90.569   Insect bite (nonvenomous), unspecified ankle D, S
  ● **S90.57   Other superficial bite of ankle**
    Excludes1   open bite of ankle (S91.05-)
    ● S90.571   Other superficial bite of ankle, right ankle D, S
    ● S90.572   Other superficial bite of ankle, left ankle D, S
    ●■ S90.579   Other superficial bite of ankle, unspecified ankle D, S

● **S90.8   Other superficial injuries of foot**
  ● **S90.81   Abrasion of foot**
    ● S90.811   Abrasion, right foot D, S
    ● S90.812   Abrasion, left foot D, S
    ●■ S90.819   Abrasion, unspecified foot D, S
  ● **S90.82   Blister (nonthermal) of foot**
    ● S90.821   Blister (nonthermal), right foot D, S
    ● S90.822   Blister (nonthermal), left foot D, S
    ●■ S90.829   Blister (nonthermal), unspecified foot D, S

● **S90.84   External constriction of foot**
    ● S90.841   External constriction, right foot D, S
    ● S90.842   External constriction, left foot D, S
    ●■ S90.849   External constriction, unspecified foot D, S
● **S90.85   Superficial foreign body of foot**
    Splinter in the foot
    ● S90.851   Superficial foreign body, right foot D, S
    ● S90.852   Superficial foreign body, left foot D, S
    ●■ S90.859   Superficial foreign body, unspecified foot D, S
● **S90.86   Insect bite (nonvenomous) of foot**
    ● S90.861   Insect bite (nonvenomous), right foot D, S
    ● S90.862   Insect bite (nonvenomous), left foot D, S
    ●■ S90.869   Insect bite (nonvenomous), unspecified foot D, S
● **S90.87   Other superficial bite of foot**
    Excludes1   open bite of foot (S91.35-)
    ● S90.871   Other superficial bite of right foot D, S
    ● S90.872   Other superficial bite of left foot D, S
    ●■ S90.879   Other superficial bite of unspecified foot D, S
● **S90.9   Unspecified superficial injury of ankle, foot and toe**
  ● **S90.91   Unspecified superficial injury of ankle**
    ●■ S90.911   Unspecified superficial injury of right ankle D, S
    ●■ S90.912   Unspecified superficial injury of left ankle D, S
    ●■ S90.919   Unspecified superficial injury of unspecified ankle D, S
  ● **S90.92   Unspecified superficial injury of foot**
    ●■ S90.921   Unspecified superficial injury of right foot D, S
    ●■ S90.922   Unspecified superficial injury of left foot D, S
    ●■ S90.929   Unspecified superficial injury of unspecified foot D, S
  S90.93   Unspecified superficial injury of toes
    ●■ S90.931   Unspecified superficial injury of right great toe D, S
    ●■ S90.932   Unspecified superficial injury of left great toe D, S
    ●■ S90.933   Unspecified superficial injury of unspecified great toe D, S
    ●■ S90.934   Unspecified superficial injury of right lesser toe(s) D, S
    ●■ S90.935   Unspecified superficial injury of left lesser toe(s) D, S
    ●■ S90.936   Unspecified superficial injury of unspecified lesser toe(s) D, S

● Unacceptable Principal Diagnosis   ● Use Additional Character(s)   ■ Unspecified   ▶ Manifestation Code
OGCR Official Guidelines for Coding and Reporting   Excludes 1   Excludes 2   Includes   Use additional   Code first   Code also

● S91 Open wound of ankle, foot and toes

Code also any associated wound infection

Excludes1 open fracture of ankle, foot and toes (S92.-
with 7th character B)
traumatic amputation of ankle and foot
(S98.-)

The appropriate 7th character is to be added to each code
from category S91

A   initial encounter
D   subsequent encounter
S   sequela

● S91.0 Open wound of ankle

● S91.00 Unspecified open wound of ankle

● S91.001 Unspecified open wound, right
ankle D, S

● S91.002 Unspecified open wound, left
ankle D, S

● S91.009 Unspecified open wound,
unspecified ankle D, S

● S91.01 Laceration without foreign body of ankle

● S91.011 Laceration without foreign body,
right ankle D, S

● S91.012 Laceration without foreign body,
left ankle D, S

● S91.019 Laceration without foreign body,
unspecified ankle D, S

● S91.02 Laceration with foreign body of ankle

● S91.021 Laceration with foreign body,
right ankle D, S

● S91.022 Laceration with foreign body, left
ankle D, S

● S91.029 Laceration with foreign body,
unspecified ankle D, S

● S91.03 Puncture wound without foreign body of
ankle

● S91.031 Puncture wound without foreign
body, right ankle D, S

● S91.032 Puncture wound without foreign
body, left ankle D, S

● S91.039 Puncture wound without foreign
body, unspecified ankle D, S

● S91.04 Puncture wound with foreign body of
ankle

● S91.041 Puncture wound with foreign
body, right ankle D, S

● S91.042 Puncture wound with foreign
body, left ankle D, S

● S91.049 Puncture wound with foreign
body, unspecified ankle D, S

● S91.05 Open bite of ankle

Excludes1 superficial bite of ankle
(S90.56-, S90.57-)

● S91.051 Open bite, right ankle D, S

● S91.052 Open bite, left ankle D, S

● S91.059 Open bite, unspecified ankle
D, S

● S91.1 Open wound of toe without damage to nail

● S91.10 Unspecified open wound of toe without
damage to nail

● S91.101 Unspecified open wound of right
great toe without damage to nail
D, S

● S91.102 Unspecified open wound of left
great toe without damage to nail
D, S

● S91.103 Unspecified open wound of
unspecified great toe without
damage to nail D, S

● S91.104 Unspecified open wound of right
lesser toe(s) without damage to
nail D, S

● S91.105 Unspecified open wound of left
lesser toe(s) without damage to
nail D, S

● S91.106 Unspecified open wound of
unspecified lesser toe(s) without
damage to nail D, S

● S91.109 Unspecified open wound of
unspecified toe(s) without
damage to nail D, S

● S91.11 Laceration without foreign body of toe
without damage to nail

● S91.111 Laceration without foreign body
of right great toe without damage
to nail D, S

● S91.112 Laceration without foreign body
of left great toe without damage
to nail D, S

● S91.113 Laceration without foreign body
of unspecified great toe without
damage to nail D, S

● S91.114 Laceration without foreign body
of right lesser toe(s) without
damage to nail D, S

● S91.115 Laceration without foreign body
of left lesser toe(s) without
damage to nail D, S

● S91.116 Laceration without foreign body
of unspecified lesser toe(s)
without damage to nail D, S

● S91.119 Laceration without foreign body
of unspecified toe without
damage to nail D, S

● S91.12 Laceration with foreign body of toe
without damage to nail

● S91.121 Laceration with foreign body of
right great toe without damage to
nail D, S

● S91.122 Laceration with foreign body of
left great toe without damage to
nail D, S

● S91.123 Laceration with foreign body of
unspecified great toe without
damage to nail D, S

● S91.124 Laceration with foreign body of
right lesser toe(s) without
damage to nail D, S

● S91.125 Laceration with foreign body of
left lesser toe(s) without damage
to nail D, S

● S91.126 Laceration with foreign body of
unspecified lesser toe(s) without
damage to nail D, S

● S91.129 Laceration with foreign body of
unspecified toe(s) without
damage to nail D, S

● **S91.13**   Puncture wound without foreign body of toe without damage to nail

    ● **S91.131**   Puncture wound without foreign body of right great toe without damage to nail D, S 🔍

    ● **S91.132**   Puncture wound without foreign body of left great toe without damage to nail D, S 🔍

    ●◼ **S91.133**   Puncture wound without foreign body of unspecified great toe without damage to nail D, S 🔍

    ● **S91.134**   Puncture wound without foreign body of right lesser toe(s) without damage to nail D, S 🔍

    ● **S91.135**   Puncture wound without foreign body of left lesser toe(s) without damage to nail D, S 🔍

    ●◼ **S91.136**   Puncture wound without foreign body of unspecified lesser toe(s) without damage to nail D, S 🔍

    ●◼ **S91.139**   Puncture wound without foreign body of unspecified toe(s) without damage to nail D, S 🔍

● **S91.14**   Puncture wound with foreign body of toe without damage to nail

    ● **S91.141**   Puncture wound with foreign body of right great toe without damage to nail D, S 🔍

    ● **S91.142**   Puncture wound with foreign body of left great toe without damage to nail D, S 🔍

    ●◼ **S91.143**   Puncture wound with foreign body of unspecified great toe without damage to nail D, S 🔍

    ● **S91.144**   Puncture wound with foreign body of right lesser toe(s) without damage to nail D, S 🔍

    ● **S91.145**   Puncture wound with foreign body of left lesser toe(s) without damage to nail D, S 🔍

    ●◼ **S91.146**   Puncture wound with foreign body of unspecified lesser toe(s) without damage to nail D, S 🔍

    ●◼ **S91.149**   Puncture wound with foreign body of unspecified toe(s) without damage to nail D, S 🔍

● **S91.15**   Open bite of toe without damage to nail
      Bite of toe NOS

    Excludes1   superficial bite of toe (S90.46-, S90.47-)

    ● **S91.151**   Open bite of right great toe without damage to nail D, S 🔍

    ● **S91.152**   Open bite of left great toe without damage to nail D, S 🔍

    ●◼ **S91.153**   Open bite of unspecified great toe without damage to nail D, S 🔍

    ● **S91.154**   Open bite of right lesser toe(s) without damage to nail D, S 🔍

    ● **S91.155**   Open bite of left lesser toe(s) without damage to nail D, S 🔍

    ●◼ **S91.156**   Open bite of unspecified lesser toe(s) without damage to nail D, S 🔍

    ●◼ **S91.159**   Open bite of unspecified toe(s) without damage to nail D, S 🔍

● **S91.2**   Open wound of toe with damage to nail

   ● **S91.20**   Unspecified open wound of toe with damage to nail

    ●◼ **S91.201**   Unspecified open wound of right great toe with damage to nail D, S 🔍

    ●◼ **S91.202**   Unspecified open wound of left great toe with damage to nail D, S 🔍

    ●◼ **S91.203**   Unspecified open wound of unspecified great toe with damage to nail D, S 🔍

    ●◼ **S91.204**   Unspecified open wound of right lesser toe(s) with damage to nail D, S 🔍

    ●◼ **S91.205**   Unspecified open wound of left lesser toe(s) with damage to nail D, S 🔍

    ●◼ **S91.206**   Unspecified open wound of unspecified lesser toe(s) with damage to nail D, S 🔍

    ●◼ **S91.209**   Unspecified open wound of unspecified toe(s) with damage to nail D, S 🔍

   ● **S91.21**   Laceration without foreign body of toe with damage to nail

    ● **S91.211**   Laceration without foreign body of right great toe with damage to nail D, S 🔍

    ● **S91.212**   Laceration without foreign body of left great toe with damage to nail D, S 🔍

    ●◼ **S91.213**   Laceration without foreign body of unspecified great toe with damage to nail D, S 🔍

    ● **S91.214**   Laceration without foreign body of right lesser toe(s) with damage to nail D, S 🔍

    ● **S91.215**   Laceration without foreign body of left lesser toe(s) with damage to nail D, S 🔍

    ●◼ **S91.216**   Laceration without foreign body of unspecified lesser toe(s) with damage to nail D, S 🔍

    ●◼ **S91.219**   Laceration without foreign body of unspecified toe(s) with damage to nail D, S 🔍

   ● **S91.22**   Laceration with foreign body of toe with damage to nail

    ● **S91.221**   Laceration with foreign body of right great toe with damage to nail D, S 🔍

    ● **S91.222**   Laceration with foreign body of left great toe with damage to nail D, S 🔍

● Unacceptable Principal Diagnosis   ● Use Additional Character(s)   ◼ Unspecified   ▶ Manifestation Code

OGCR Official Guidelines for Coding and Reporting   Excludes 1   Excludes 2   Includes   Use additional   Code first   Code also

CHAPTER 19 (S00-T88)

● ■ S91.223 Laceration with foreign body of unspecified great toe with damage to nail D, S ⊗

● S91.224 Laceration with foreign body of right lesser toe(s) with damage to nail D, S ⊗

● S91.225 Laceration with foreign body of left lesser toe(s) with damage to nail D, S ⊗

● ■ S91.226 Laceration with foreign body of unspecified lesser toe(s) with damage to nail D, S ⊗

● ■ S91.229 Laceration with foreign body of unspecified toe(s) with damage to nail D, S ⊗

● S91.23 Puncture wound without foreign body of toe with damage to nail

● S91.231 Puncture wound without foreign body of right great toe with damage to nail D, S ⊗

● S91.232 Puncture wound without foreign body of left great toe with damage to nail D, S ⊗

● ■ S91.233 Puncture wound without foreign body of unspecified great toe with damage to nail D, S ⊗

● S91.234 Puncture wound without foreign body of right lesser toe(s) with damage to nail D, S ⊗

● S91.235 Puncture wound without foreign body of left lesser toe(s) with damage to nail D, S ⊗

● ■ S91.236 Puncture wound without foreign body of unspecified lesser toe(s) with damage to nail D, S ⊗

● ■ S91.239 Puncture wound without foreign body of unspecified toe(s) with damage to nail D, S ⊗

● S91.24 Puncture wound with foreign body of toe with damage to nail

● S91.241 Puncture wound with foreign body of right great toe with damage to nail D, S ⊗

● S91.242 Puncture wound with foreign body of left great toe with damage to nail D, S ⊗

● ■ S91.243 Puncture wound with foreign body of unspecified great toe with damage to nail D, S ⊗

● S91.244 Puncture wound with foreign body of right lesser toe(s) with damage to nail D, S ⊗

● S91.245 Puncture wound with foreign body of left lesser toe(s) with damage to nail D, S ⊗

● ■ S91.246 Puncture wound with foreign body of unspecified lesser toe(s) with damage to nail D, S ⊗

● ■ S91.249 Puncture wound with foreign body of unspecified toe(s) with damage to nail D, S ⊗

● S91.25 Open bite of toe with damage to nail
Bite of toe with damage to nail NOS
| Excludes1 | superficial bite of toe (S90.46-, S90.47-)

● S91.251 Open bite of right great toe with damage to nail D, S ⊗

● S91.252 Open bite of left great toe with damage to nail D, S ⊗

● ■ S91.253 Open bite of unspecified great toe with damage to nail D, S ⊗

● S91.254 Open bite of right lesser toe(s) with damage to nail D, S ⊗

● S91.255 Open bite of left lesser toe(s) with damage to nail D, S ⊗

● ■ S91.256 Open bite of unspecified lesser toe(s) with damage to nail D, S ⊗

● ■ S91.259 Open bite of unspecified toe(s) with damage to nail D, S ⊗

● S91.3 Open wound of foot

● S91.30 Unspecified open wound of foot

● ■ S91.301 Unspecified open wound, right foot D, S ⊗

● ■ S91.302 Unspecified open wound, left foot D, S ⊗

● ■ S91.309 Unspecified open wound, unspecified foot D, S ⊗

● S91.31 Laceration without foreign body of foot

● S91.311 Laceration without foreign body, right foot D, S ⊗

● S91.312 Laceration without foreign body, left foot D, S ⊗

● ■ S91.319 Laceration without foreign body, unspecified foot D, S ⊗

● S91.32 Laceration with foreign body of foot

● S91.321 Laceration with foreign body, right foot D, S ⊗

● S91.322 Laceration with foreign body, left foot D, S ⊗

● ■ S91.329 Laceration with foreign body, unspecified foot D, S ⊗

● S91.33 Puncture wound without foreign body of foot

● S91.331 Puncture wound without foreign body, right foot D, S ⊗

● S91.332 Puncture wound without foreign body, left foot D, S ⊗

● ■ S91.339 Puncture wound without foreign body, unspecified foot D, S ⊗

● S91.34 Puncture wound with foreign body of foot

● S91.341 Puncture wound with foreign body, right foot D, S ⊗

● S91.342 Puncture wound with foreign body, left foot D, S ⊗

● ■ S91.349 Puncture wound with foreign body, unspecified foot D, S ⊗

● S91.35 Open bite of foot
| Excludes1 | superficial bite of foot (S90.86-, S90.87-)

● S91.351 Open bite, right foot D, S ⊗

● S91.352 Open bite, left foot D, S ⊗

● ■ S91.359 Open bite, unspecified foot D, S ⊗

N Newborn Age: 0   **P** Pediatric Age: 0–17   **M** Maternity DX: 12–55   **A** Adult Age: 15–124   ♀ Females Only   ♂ Males Only

⊗ Complication\Comorbidity   ⊗ Major C\C   ⊗ Present on Admission Requirement   ⊗ Hospital-Acquired Condition

CHAPTER 19 (S00-T88)

1571

● S92 **Fracture of foot and toe, except ankle**

> **Note:** A fracture not indicated as displaced or nondisplaced should be coded to displaced
>
> A fracture not indicated as open or closed should be coded to closed

> **Excludes1** traumatic amputation of ankle and foot (S98.-)

> **Excludes2** fracture of ankle (S82.-)
> fracture of malleolus (S82.-)

The appropriate 7th character is to be added to each code from category S92

A	initial encounter for closed fracture
B	initial encounter for open fracture
D	subsequent encounter for fracture with routine healing
G	subsequent encounter for fracture with delayed healing
K	subsequent encounter for fracture with nonunion
P	subsequent encounter for fracture with malunion
S	sequela

● S92.0 **Fracture of calcaneus**
> Heel bone   Os calcis

● S92.00 **Unspecified fracture of calcaneus**

●■ S92.001 Unspecified fracture of right calcaneus B, K, P, D, G, S, B

●■ S92.002 Unspecified fracture of left calcaneus B, K, P, D, G, S, B

●■ S92.009 Unspecified fracture of unspecified calcaneus B, K, P, D, G, S, B

● S92.01 **Fracture of body of calcaneus**

● S92.011 Displaced fracture of body of right calcaneus B, K, P, D, G, S, B

● S92.012 Displaced fracture of body of left calcaneus B, K, P, D, G, S, B

●■ S92.013 Displaced fracture of body of unspecified calcaneus B, K, P, D, G, S, B

● S92.014 Nondisplaced fracture of body of right calcaneus B, K, P, D, G, S, B

● S92.015 Nondisplaced fracture of body of left calcaneus B, K, P, D, G, S, B

●■ S92.016 Nondisplaced fracture of body of unspecified calcaneus B, K, P, D, G, S, B

● S92.02 **Fracture of anterior process of calcaneus**

● S92.021 Displaced fracture of anterior process of right calcaneus B, K, P, D, G, S, B

● S92.022 Displaced fracture of anterior process of left calcaneus B, K, P, D, G, S, B

●■ S92.023 Displaced fracture of anterior process of unspecified calcaneus B, K, P, D, G, S, B

● S92.024 Nondisplaced fracture of anterior process of right calcaneus B, K, P, D, G, S, B

● S92.025 Nondisplaced fracture of anterior process of left calcaneus B, K, P, D, G, S, B

●■ S92.026 Nondisplaced fracture of anterior process of unspecified calcaneus B, K, P, D, G, S, B

● S92.03 **Avulsion fracture of tuberosity of calcaneus**

● S92.031 Displaced avulsion fracture of tuberosity of right calcaneus B, K, P, D, G, S, B

● S92.032 Displaced avulsion fracture of tuberosity of left calcaneus B, K, P, D, G, S, B

●■ S92.033 Displaced avulsion fracture of tuberosity of unspecified calcaneus B, K, P, D, G, S, B

● S92.034 Nondisplaced avulsion fracture of tuberosity of right calcaneus B, K, P, D, G, S, B

● S92.035 Nondisplaced avulsion fracture of tuberosity of left calcaneus B, K, P, D, G, S, B

●■ S92.036 Nondisplaced avulsion fracture of tuberosity of unspecified calcaneus B, K, P, D, G, S, B

● S92.04 **Other fracture of tuberosity of calcaneus**

● S92.041 Displaced other fracture of tuberosity of right calcaneus B, K, P, D, G, S, B

● S92.042 Displaced other fracture of tuberosity of left calcaneus B, K, P, D, G, S, B

●■ S92.043 Displaced other fracture of tuberosity of unspecified calcaneus B, K, P, D, G, S, B

● S92.044 Nondisplaced other fracture of tuberosity of right calcaneus B, K, P, D, G, S, B

● S92.045 Nondisplaced other fracture of tuberosity of left calcaneus B, K, P, D, G, S, B

●■ S92.046 Nondisplaced other fracture of tuberosity of unspecified calcaneus B, K, P, D, G, S, B

● S92.05 **Other extraarticular fracture of calcaneus**

● S92.051 Displaced other extraarticular fracture of right calcaneus B, K, P, D, G, S, B

● S92.052 Displaced other extraarticular fracture of left calcaneus B, K, P, D, G, S, B

●■ S92.053 Displaced other extraarticular fracture of unspecified calcaneus B, K, P, D, G, S, B

● S92.054 Nondisplaced other extraarticular fracture of right calcaneus B, K, P, D, G, S, B

● S92.055 Nondisplaced other extraarticular fracture of left calcaneus B, K, P, D, G, S, B

●■ S92.056 Nondisplaced other extraarticular fracture of unspecified calcaneus B, K, P, D, G, S, B

● **S92.06**   **Intraarticular fracture of calcaneus**

   ● **S92.061**   Displaced intraarticular fracture of right calcaneus B, K, P 🅒, D, G, S 🅢, B 🅗

   ● **S92.062**   Displaced intraarticular fracture of left calcaneus B, K, P 🅒, D, G, S 🅢, B 🅗

   ●■ **S92.063**   Displaced intraarticular fracture of unspecified calcaneus B, K, P 🅒, D, G, S 🅢, B 🅗

   ● **S92.064**   Nondisplaced intraarticular fracture of right calcaneus B, K, P 🅒, D, G, S 🅢, B 🅗

   ● **S92.065**   Nondisplaced intraarticular fracture of left calcaneus B, K, P 🅒, D, G, S 🅢, B 🅗

   ●■ **S92.066**   Nondisplaced intraarticular fracture of unspecified calcaneus B, K, P 🅒, D, G, S 🅢, B 🅗

● **S92.1**   **Fracture of talus**
   Astragalus

  ● **S92.10**   **Unspecified fracture of talus**

   ●■ **S92.101**   Unspecified fracture of right talus B, K, P 🅒, D, G, S 🅢, B 🅗

   ●■ **S92.102**   Unspecified fracture of left talus B, K, P 🅒, D, G, S 🅢, B 🅗

   ●■ **S92.109**   Unspecified fracture of unspecified talus B, K, P 🅒, D, G, S 🅢, B 🅗

  ● **S92.11**   **Fracture of neck of talus**

   ● **S92.111**   Displaced fracture of neck of right talus B, K, P 🅒, D, G, S 🅢, B 🅗

   ● **S92.112**   Displaced fracture of neck of left talus B, K, P 🅒, D, G, S 🅢, B 🅗

   ●■ **S92.113**   Displaced fracture of neck of unspecified talus B, K, P 🅒, D, G, S 🅢, B 🅗

   ● **S92.114**   Nondisplaced fracture of neck of right talus B, K, P 🅒, D, G, S 🅢, B 🅗

   ● **S92.115**   Nondisplaced fracture of neck of left talus B, K, P 🅒, D, G, S 🅢, B 🅗

   ●■ **S92.116**   Nondisplaced fracture of neck of unspecified talus B, K, P 🅒, D, G, S 🅢, B 🅗

  ● **S92.12**   **Fracture of body of talus**

   ● **S92.121**   Displaced fracture of body of right talus B, K, P 🅒, D, G, S 🅢, B 🅗

   ● **S92.122**   Displaced fracture of body of left talus B, K, P 🅒, D, G, S 🅢, B 🅗

   ●■ **S92.123**   Displaced fracture of body of unspecified talus B, K, P 🅒, D, G, S 🅢, B 🅗

   ● **S92.124**   Nondisplaced fracture of body of right talus B, K, P 🅒, D, G, S 🅢, B 🅗

   ● **S92.125**   Nondisplaced fracture of body of left talus B, K, P 🅒, D, G, S 🅢, B 🅗

   ●■ **S92.126**   Nondisplaced fracture of body of unspecified talus B, K, P 🅒, D, G, S 🅢, B 🅗

● **S92.13**   **Fracture of posterior process of talus**

   ● **S92.131**   Displaced fracture of posterior process of right talus B, K, P 🅒, D, G, S 🅢, B 🅗

   ● **S92.132**   Displaced fracture of posterior process of left talus B, K, P 🅒, D, G, S 🅢, B 🅗

   ●■ **S92.133**   Displaced fracture of posterior process of unspecified talus B, K, P 🅒, D, G, S 🅢, B 🅗

   ● **S92.134**   Nondisplaced fracture of posterior process of right talus B, K, P 🅒, D, G, S 🅢, B 🅗

   ● **S92.135**   Nondisplaced fracture of posterior process of left talus B, K, P 🅒, D, G, S 🅢, B 🅗

   ●■ **S92.136**   Nondisplaced fracture of posterior process of unspecified talus B, K, P 🅒, D, G, S 🅢, B 🅗

● **S92.14**   **Dome fracture of talus**

   Excludes1   osteochondritis dissecans (M93.2)

   ● **S92.141**   Displaced dome fracture of right talus B, K, P 🅒, D, G, S 🅢, B 🅗

   ● **S92.142**   Displaced dome fracture of left talus B, K, P 🅒, D, G, S 🅢, B 🅗

   ●■ **S92.143**   Displaced dome fracture of unspecified talus B, K, P 🅒, D, G, S 🅢, B 🅗

   ● **S92.144**   Nondisplaced dome fracture of right talus B, K, P 🅒, D, G, S 🅢, B 🅗

   ● **S92.145**   Nondisplaced dome fracture of left talus B, K, P 🅒, D, G, S 🅢, B 🅗

   ●■ **S92.146**   Nondisplaced dome fracture of unspecified talus B, K, P 🅒, D, G, S 🅢, B 🅗

● **S92.15**   **Avulsion fracture (chip fracture) of talus**

   ● **S92.151**   Displaced avulsion fracture (chip fracture) of right talus B, K, P 🅒, D, G, S 🅢, B 🅗

   ● **S92.152**   Displaced avulsion fracture (chip fracture) of left talus B, K, P 🅒, D, G, S 🅢, B 🅗

   ●■ **S92.153**   Displaced avulsion fracture (chip fracture) of unspecified talus B, K, P 🅒, D, G, S 🅢, B 🅗

   ● **S92.154**   Nondisplaced avulsion fracture (chip fracture) of right talus B, K, P 🅒, D, G, S 🅢, B 🅗

   ● **S92.155**   Nondisplaced avulsion fracture (chip fracture) of left talus B, K, P 🅒, D, G, S 🅢, B 🅗

   ●■ **S92.156**   Nondisplaced avulsion fracture (chip fracture) of unspecified talus B, K, P 🅒, D, G, S 🅢, B 🅗

● **S92.19**   **Other fracture of talus**

   ● **S92.191**   Other fracture of right talus B, K, P 🅒, D, G, S 🅢, B 🅗

   ● **S92.192**   Other fracture of left talus B, K, P 🅒, D, G, S 🅢, B 🅗

   ●■ **S92.199**   Other fracture of unspecified talus B, K, P 🅒, D, G, S 🅢, B 🅗

N Newborn Age: 0   **P** Pediatric Age: 0–17   **M** Maternity DX: 12–55   **A** Adult Age: 15–124   ♀ Females Only   ♂ Males Only

🅒 Complication\Comorbidity   🅜 Major C\C   🅢 Present on Admission Requirement   🅗 Hospital-Acquired Condition

1573

CHAPTER 19 (S00-T88)

● S92.2   Fracture of other and unspecified tarsal bone(s)

  ● S92.20   Fracture of unspecified tarsal bone(s)

    ●■ S92.201   Fracture of unspecified tarsal bone(s) of right foot B, K, P ✪, D, G, S ✪, B ✪

    ●■ S92.202   Fracture of unspecified tarsal bone(s) of left foot B, K, P ✪, D, G, S ✪, B ✪

    ●■ S92.209   Fracture of unspecified tarsal bone(s) of unspecified foot B, K, P ✪, D, G, S ✪, B ✪

  ● S92.21   Fracture of cuboid bone

    ● S92.211   Displaced fracture of cuboid bone of right foot B, K, P ✪, D, G, S ✪, B ✪

    ● S92.212   Displaced fracture of cuboid bone of left foot B, K, P ✪, D, G, S ✪, B ✪

    ●■ S92.213   Displaced fracture of cuboid bone of unspecified foot B, K, P ✪, D, G, S ✪, B ✪

    ● S92.214   Nondisplaced fracture of cuboid bone of right foot B, K, P ✪, D, G, S ✪, B ✪

    ● S92.215   Nondisplaced fracture of cuboid bone of left foot B, K, P ✪, D, G, S ✪, B ✪

    ●■ S92.216   Nondisplaced fracture of cuboid bone of unspecified foot B, K, P ✪, D, G, S ✪, B ✪

  ● S92.22   Fracture of lateral cuneiform

    ● S92.221   Displaced fracture of lateral cuneiform of right foot B, K, P ✪, D, G, S ✪, B ✪

    ● S92.222   Displaced fracture of lateral cuneiform of left foot B, K, P ✪, D, G, S ✪, B ✪

    ●■ S92.223   Displaced fracture of lateral cuneiform of unspecified foot B, K, P ✪, D, G, S ✪, B ✪

    ● S92.224   Nondisplaced fracture of lateral cuneiform of right foot B, K, P ✪, D, G, S ✪, B ✪

    ● S92.225   Nondisplaced fracture of lateral cuneiform of left foot B, K, P ✪, D, G, S ✪, B ✪

    ●■ S92.226   Nondisplaced fracture of lateral cuneiform of unspecified foot B, K, P ✪, D, G, S ✪, B ✪

  ● S92.23   Fracture of intermediate cuneiform

    ● S92.231   Displaced fracture of intermediate cuneiform of right foot B, K, P ✪, D, G, S ✪, B ✪

    ● S92.232   Displaced fracture of intermediate cuneiform of left foot B, K, P ✪, D, G, S ✪, B ✪

    ●■ S92.233   Displaced fracture of intermediate cuneiform of unspecified foot B, K, P ✪, D, G, S ✪, B ✪

    ● S92.234   Nondisplaced fracture of intermediate cuneiform of right foot B, K, P ✪, D, G, S ✪, B ✪

    ● S92.235   Nondisplaced fracture of intermediate cuneiform of left foot B, K, P ✪, D, G, S ✪, B ✪

    ●■ S92.236   Nondisplaced fracture of intermediate cuneiform of unspecified foot B, K, P ✪, D, G, S ✪, B ✪

  ● S92.24   Fracture of medial cuneiform

    ● S92.241   Displaced fracture of medial cuneiform of right foot B, K, P ✪, D, G, S ✪, B ✪

    ● S92.242   Displaced fracture of medial cuneiform of left foot B, K, P ✪, D, G, S ✪, B ✪

    ●■ S92.243   Displaced fracture of medial cuneiform of unspecified foot B, K, P ✪, D, G, S ✪, B ✪

    ● S92.244   Nondisplaced fracture of medial cuneiform of right foot B, K, P ✪, D, G, S ✪, B ✪

    ● S92.245   Nondisplaced fracture of medial cuneiform of left foot B, K, P ✪, D, G, S ✪, B ✪

    ●■ S92.246   Nondisplaced fracture of medial cuneiform of unspecified foot B, K, P ✪, D, G, S ✪, B ✪

  ● S92.25   Fracture of navicular [scaphoid] of foot

    ● S92.251   Displaced fracture of navicular [scaphoid] of right foot B, K, P ✪, D, G, S ✪, B ✪

    ● S92.252   Displaced fracture of navicular [scaphoid] of left foot B, K, P ✪, D, G, S ✪, B ✪

    ●■ S92.253   Displaced fracture of navicular [scaphoid] of unspecified foot B, K, P ✪, D, G, S ✪, B ✪

    ● S92.254   Nondisplaced fracture of navicular [scaphoid] of right foot B, K, P ✪, D, G, S ✪, B ✪

    ● S92.255   Nondisplaced fracture of navicular [scaphoid] of left foot B, K, P ✪, D, G, S ✪, B ✪

    ●■ S92.256   Nondisplaced fracture of navicular [scaphoid] of unspecified foot B, K, P ✪, D, G, S ✪, B ✪

● S92.3   Fracture of metatarsal bone(s)

  ● S92.30   Fracture of unspecified metatarsal bone(s)

    ●■ S92.301   Fracture of unspecified metatarsal bone(s), right foot B, K, P ✪, D, G, S ✪, B ✪

    ●■ S92.302   Fracture of unspecified metatarsal bone(s), left foot B, K, P ✪, D, G, S ✪, B ✪

    ●■ S92.309   Fracture of unspecified metatarsal bone(s), unspecified foot B, K, P ✪, D, G, S ✪, B ✪

  ● S92.31   Fracture of first metatarsal bone

    ● S92.311   Displaced fracture of first metatarsal bone, right foot B, K, P ✪, D, G, S ✪, B ✪

    ● S92.312   Displaced fracture of first metatarsal bone, left foot B, K, P ✪, D, G, S ✪, B ✪

● ■ S92.313   Displaced fracture of first metatarsal bone, unspecified foot
B, K, P 🖰, D, G, S 🖰, B 🖰

● S92.314   Nondisplaced fracture of first metatarsal bone, right foot
B, K, P 🖰, D, G, S 🖰, B 🖰

● S92.315   Nondisplaced fracture of first metatarsal bone, left foot
B, K, P 🖰, D, G, S 🖰, B 🖰

● ■ S92.316   Nondisplaced fracture of first metatarsal bone, unspecified foot
B, K, P 🖰, D, G, S 🖰, B 🖰

● S92.32   Fracture of second metatarsal bone

● S92.321   Displaced fracture of second metatarsal bone, right foot
B, K, P 🖰, D, G, S 🖰, B 🖰

● S92.322   Displaced fracture of second metatarsal bone, left foot
B, K, P 🖰, D, G, S 🖰, B 🖰

● ■ S92.323   Displaced fracture of second metatarsal bone, unspecified foot
B, K, P 🖰, D, G, S 🖰, B 🖰

● S92.324   Nondisplaced fracture of second metatarsal bone, right foot
B, K, P 🖰, D, G, S 🖰, B 🖰

● S92.325   Nondisplaced fracture of second metatarsal bone, left foot
B, K, P 🖰, D, G, S 🖰, B 🖰

● ■ S92.326   Nondisplaced fracture of second metatarsal bone, unspecified foot
B, K, P 🖰, D, G, S 🖰, B 🖰

● S92.33   Fracture of third metatarsal bone

● S92.331   Displaced fracture of third metatarsal bone, right foot
B, K, P 🖰, D, G, S 🖰, B 🖰

● S92.332   Displaced fracture of third metatarsal bone, left foot
B, K, P 🖰, D, G, S 🖰, B 🖰

● ■ S92.333   Displaced fracture of third metatarsal bone, unspecified foot
B, K, P 🖰, D, G, S 🖰, B 🖰

● S92.334   Nondisplaced fracture of third metatarsal bone, right foot
B, K, P 🖰, D, G, S 🖰, B 🖰

● S92.335   Nondisplaced fracture of third metatarsal bone, left foot
B, K, P 🖰, D, G, S 🖰, B 🖰

● ■ S92.336   Nondisplaced fracture of third metatarsal bone, unspecified foot
B, K, P 🖰, D, G, S 🖰, B 🖰

● S92.34   Fracture of fourth metatarsal bone

● S92.341   Displaced fracture of fourth metatarsal bone, right foot
B, K, P 🖰, D, G, S 🖰, B 🖰

● S92.342   Displaced fracture of fourth metatarsal bone, left foot
B, K, P 🖰, D, G, S 🖰, B 🖰

● S92.343   Displaced fracture of fourth metatarsal bone, unspecified foot
B, K, P 🖰, D, G, S 🖰, B 🖰

● ■ S92.344   Nondisplaced fracture of fourth metatarsal bone, right foot
B, K, P 🖰, D, G, S 🖰, B 🖰

● S92.345   Nondisplaced fracture of fourth metatarsal bone, left foot
B, K, P 🖰, D, G, S 🖰, B 🖰

● ■ S92.346   Nondisplaced fracture of fourth metatarsal bone, unspecified foot
B, K, P 🖰, D, G, S 🖰, B 🖰

● S92.35   Fracture of fifth metatarsal bone

● S92.351   Displaced fracture of fifth metatarsal bone, right foot
B, K, P 🖰, D, G, S 🖰, B 🖰

● S92.352   Displaced fracture of fifth metatarsal bone, left foot
B, K, P 🖰, D, G, S 🖰, B 🖰

● ■ S92.353   Displaced fracture of fifth metatarsal bone, unspecified foot
B, K, P 🖰, D, G, S 🖰, B 🖰

● S92.354   Nondisplaced fracture of fifth metatarsal bone, right foot
B, K, P 🖰, D, G, S 🖰, B 🖰

● S92.355   Nondisplaced fracture of fifth metatarsal bone, left foot
B, K, P 🖰, D, G, S 🖰, B 🖰

● ■ S92.356   Nondisplaced fracture of fifth metatarsal bone, unspecified foot
B, K, P 🖰, D, G, S 🖰, B 🖰

● S92.4   Fracture of great toe

● S92.40   Unspecified fracture of great toe

● ■ S92.401   Displaced unspecified fracture of right great toe K, P 🖰, D, G, S 🖰

● ■ S92.402   Displaced unspecified fracture of left great toe K, P 🖰, D, G, S 🖰

● ■ S92.403   Displaced unspecified fracture of unspecified great toe K, P 🖰, D, G, S 🖰

● ■ S92.404   Nondisplaced unspecified fracture of right great toe K, P 🖰, D, G, S 🖰

● ■ S92.405   Nondisplaced unspecified fracture of left great toe K, P 🖰, D, G, S 🖰

● ■ S92.406   Nondisplaced unspecified fracture of unspecified great toe K, P 🖰, D, G, S 🖰

● S92.41   Fracture of proximal phalanx of great toe

● S92.411   Displaced fracture of proximal phalanx of right great toe K, P 🖰, D, G, S 🖰

● S92.412   Displaced fracture of proximal phalanx of left great toe K, P 🖰, D, G, S 🖰

● ■ S92.413   Displaced fracture of proximal phalanx of unspecified great toe K, P 🖰, D, G, S 🖰

● S92.414   Nondisplaced fracture of proximal phalanx of right great toe K, P 🖰, D, G, S 🖰

● S92.415   Nondisplaced fracture of proximal phalanx of left great toe K, P 🖰, D, G, S 🖰

● ■ S92.416   Nondisplaced fracture of proximal phalanx of unspecified great toe K, P 🖰, D, G, S 🖰

N Newborn Age: 0   **P** Pediatric Age: 0–17   **M** Maternity DX: 12–55   **A** Adult Age: 15–124   ♀ Females Only   ♂ Males Only

🖰 Complication\Comorbidity   🖰 Major C\C   🖰 Present on Admission Requirement   🖰 Hospital-Acquired Condition

1575

CHAPTER 19 (S00-T88)

● S92.42   Fracture of distal phalanx of great toe

  ● S92.421   Displaced fracture of distal phalanx of right great toe K, P 🔍, D, G, S 🔍

  ● S92.422   Displaced fracture of distal phalanx of left great toe K, P 🔍, D, G, S 🔍

  ●■ S92.423   Displaced fracture of distal phalanx of unspecified great toe K, P 🔍, D, G, S 🔍

  ● S92.424   Nondisplaced fracture of distal phalanx of right great toe K, P 🔍, D, G, S 🔍

  ● S92.425   Nondisplaced fracture of distal phalanx of left great toe K, P 🔍, D, G, S 🔍

  ●■ S92.426   Nondisplaced fracture of distal phalanx of unspecified great toe K, P 🔍, D, G, S 🔍

● S92.49   Other fracture of great toe

  ● S92.491   Other fracture of right great toe K, P 🔍, D, G, S 🔍

  ● S92.492   Other fracture of left great toe K, P 🔍, D, G, S 🔍

  ●■ S92.499   Other fracture of unspecified great toe K, P 🔍, D, G, S 🔍

● S92.5   Fracture of lesser toe(s)

 ● S92.50   Unspecified fracture of lesser toe(s)

  ●■ S92.501   Displaced unspecified fracture of right lesser toe(s) K, P 🔍, D, G, S 🔍

  ●■ S92.502   Displaced unspecified fracture of left lesser toe(s) K, P 🔍, D, G, S 🔍

  ●■ S92.503   Displaced unspecified fracture of unspecified lesser toe(s) K, P 🔍, D, G, S 🔍

  ●■ S92.504   Nondisplaced unspecified fracture of right lesser toe(s) K, P 🔍, D, G, S 🔍

  ●■ S92.505   Nondisplaced unspecified fracture of left lesser toe(s) K, P 🔍, D, G, S 🔍

  ●■ S92.506   Nondisplaced unspecified fracture of unspecified lesser toe(s) K, P 🔍, D, G, S 🔍

 ● S92.51   Fracture of proximal phalanx of lesser toe(s)

  ● S92.511   Displaced fracture of proximal phalanx of right lesser toe(s) K, P 🔍, D, G, S 🔍

  ● S92.512   Displaced fracture of proximal phalanx of left lesser toe(s) K, P 🔍, D, G, S 🔍

  ●■ S92.513   Displaced fracture of proximal phalanx of unspecified lesser toe(s) K, P 🔍, D, G, S 🔍

  ● S92.514   Nondisplaced fracture of proximal phalanx of right lesser toe(s) K, P 🔍, D, G, S 🔍

  ● S92.515   Nondisplaced fracture of proximal phalanx of left lesser toe(s) K, P 🔍, D, G, S 🔍

  ●■ S92.516   Nondisplaced fracture of proximal phalanx of unspecified lesser toe(s) K, P 🔍, D, G, S 🔍

● S92.52   Fracture of medial phalanx of lesser toe(s)

  ● S92.521   Displaced fracture of medial phalanx of right lesser toe(s) K, P 🔍, D, G, S 🔍

  ● S92.522   Displaced fracture of medial phalanx of left lesser toe(s) K, P 🔍, D, G, S 🔍

  ●■ S92.523   Displaced fracture of medial phalanx of unspecified lesser toe(s) K, P 🔍, D, G, S 🔍

  ● S92.524   Nondisplaced fracture of medial phalanx of right lesser toe(s) K, P 🔍, D, G, S 🔍

  ● S92.525   Nondisplaced fracture of medial phalanx of left lesser toe(s) K, P 🔍, D, G, S 🔍

  ●■ S92.526   Nondisplaced fracture of medial phalanx of unspecified lesser toe(s) K, P 🔍, D, G, S 🔍

● S92.53   Fracture of distal phalanx of lesser toe(s)

  ● S92.531   Displaced fracture of distal phalanx of right lesser toe(s) K, P 🔍, D, G, S 🔍

  ● S92.532   Displaced fracture of distal phalanx of left lesser toe(s) K, P 🔍, D, G, S 🔍

  ●■ S92.533   Displaced fracture of distal phalanx of unspecified lesser toe(s) K, P 🔍, D, G, S 🔍

  ● S92.534   Nondisplaced fracture of distal phalanx of right lesser toe(s) K, P 🔍, D, G, S 🔍

  ● S92.535   Nondisplaced fracture of distal phalanx of left lesser toe(s) K, P 🔍, D, G, S 🔍

  ●■ S92.536   Nondisplaced fracture of distal phalanx of unspecified lesser toe(s) K, P 🔍, D, G, S 🔍

● S92.59   Other fracture of lesser toe(s)

  ● S92.591   Other fracture of right lesser toe(s) K, P 🔍, D, G, S 🔍

  ● S92.592   Other fracture of left lesser toe(s) K, P 🔍, D, G, S 🔍

  ●■ S92.599   Other fracture of unspecified lesser toe(s) K, P 🔍, D, G, S 🔍

● S92.9   Unspecified fracture of foot and toe

 ● S92.90   Unspecified fracture of foot

  ●■ S92.901   Unspecified fracture of right foot B, K, P 🔍, D, G, S 🔍, B 🔍

  ●■ S92.902   Unspecified fracture of left foot B, K, P 🔍, D, G, S 🔍, B 🔍

  ●■ S92.909   Unspecified fracture of unspecified foot B, K, P 🔍, D, G, S 🔍, B 🔍

 ● S92.91   Unspecified fracture of toe

  ●■ S92.911   Unspecified fracture of right toe(s) K, P 🔍, D, G, S 🔍

  ●■ S92.912   Unspecified fracture of left toe(s) K, P 🔍, D, G, S 🔍

  ●■ S92.919   Unspecified fracture of unspecified toe(s) K, P 🔍, D, G, S 🔍

● S93   **Dislocation and sprain of joints and ligaments at ankle, foot and toe level**

     Includes   avulsion of joint or ligament of ankle, foot and toe

         laceration of cartilage, joint or ligament of ankle, foot and toe

         sprain of cartilage, joint or ligament of ankle, foot and toe

         traumatic hemarthrosis of joint or ligament of ankle, foot and toe

         traumatic rupture of joint or ligament of ankle, foot and toe

         traumatic subluxation of joint or ligament of ankle, foot and toe

         traumatic tear of joint or ligament of ankle, foot and toe

     Code also any associated open wound

     Excludes2   strain of muscle and tendon of ankle and foot (S96.-)

     The appropriate 7th character is to be added to each code from category S93

> A   initial encounter
> D   subsequent encounter
> S   sequela

● S93.0   **Subluxation and dislocation of ankle joint**
     Subluxation and dislocation of astragalus
     Subluxation and dislocation of fibula, lower end
     Subluxation and dislocation of talus
     Subluxation and dislocation of tibia, lower end

    ● S93.01   Subluxation of right ankle joint D, S 🦠

    ● S93.02   Subluxation of left ankle joint D, S 🦠

    ● ■ S93.03   Subluxation of unspecified ankle joint D, S 🦠

    ● S93.04   Dislocation of right ankle joint D, S 🦠

    ● S93.05   Dislocation of left ankle joint D, S 🦠

    ● ■ S93.06   Dislocation of unspecified ankle joint D, S 🦠

● S93.1   **Subluxation and dislocation of toe**

    ● S93.10   Unspecified subluxation and dislocation of toe
        Dislocation of toe NOS
        Subluxation of toe NOS

       ● ■ S93.101   Unspecified subluxation of right toe(s) D, S 🦠

       ● ■ S93.102   Unspecified subluxation of left toe(s) D, S 🦠

       ● ■ S93.103   Unspecified subluxation of unspecified toe(s) D, S 🦠

       ● ■ S93.104   Unspecified dislocation of right toe(s) D, S 🦠

       ● ■ S93.105   Unspecified dislocation of left toe(s) D, S 🦠

       ● ■ S93.106   Unspecified dislocation of unspecified toe(s) D, S 🦠

    ● S93.11   Dislocation of interphalangeal joint

       ● S93.111   Dislocation of interphalangeal joint of right great toe D, S 🦠

       ● S93.112   Dislocation of interphalangeal joint of left great toe D, S 🦠

       ● ■ S93.113   Dislocation of interphalangeal joint of unspecified great toe D, S 🦠

       ● S93.114   Dislocation of interphalangeal joint of right lesser toe(s) D, S 🦠

       ● S93.115   Dislocation of interphalangeal joint of left lesser toe(s) D, S 🦠

       ● ■ S93.116   Dislocation of interphalangeal joint of unspecified lesser toe(s) D, S 🦠

       ● ■ S93.119   Dislocation of interphalangeal joint of unspecified toe(s) D, S 🦠

    ● S93.12   Dislocation of metatarsophalangeal joint

       ● S93.121   Dislocation of metatarsophalangeal joint of right great toe D, S 🦠

       ● S93.122   Dislocation of metatarsophalangeal joint of left great toe D, S 🦠

       ● ■ S93.123   Dislocation of metatarsophalangeal joint of unspecified great toe D, S 🦠

       ● S93.124   Dislocation of metatarsophalangeal joint of right lesser toe(s) D, S 🦠

       ● S93.125   Dislocation of metatarsophalangeal joint of left lesser toe(s) D, S 🦠

       ● ■ S93.126   Dislocation of metatarsophalangeal joint of unspecified lesser toe(s) D, S 🦠

       ● ■ S93.129   Dislocation of metatarsophalangeal joint of unspecified toe(s) D, S 🦠

    ● S93.13   Subluxation of interphalangeal joint

       ● S93.131   Subluxation of interphalangeal joint of right great toe D, S 🦠

       ● S93.132   Subluxation of interphalangeal joint of left great toe D, S 🦠

       ● ■ S93.133   Subluxation of interphalangeal joint of unspecified great toe D, S 🦠

       ● S93.134   Subluxation of interphalangeal joint of right lesser toe(s) D, S 🦠

       ● S93.135   Subluxation of interphalangeal joint of left lesser toe(s) D, S 🦠

       ● ■ S93.136   Subluxation of interphalangeal joint of unspecified lesser toe(s) D, S 🦠

       ● ■ S93.139   Subluxation of interphalangeal joint of unspecified toe(s) D, S 🦠

    ● S93.14   Subluxation of metatarsophalangeal joint

       ● S93.141   Subluxation of metatarsophalangeal joint of right great toe D, S 🦠

       ● S93.142   Subluxation of metatarsophalangeal joint of left great toe D, S 🦠

       ● ■ S93.143   Subluxation of metatarsophalangeal joint of unspecified great toe D, S 🦠

       ● S93.144   Subluxation of metatarsophalangeal joint of right lesser toe(s) D, S 🦠

       ● S93.145   Subluxation of metatarsophalangeal joint of left lesser toe(s) D, S 🦠

       ● ■ S93.146   Subluxation of metatarsophalangeal joint of unspecified lesser toe(s) D, S 🦠

       ● ■ S93.149   Subluxation of metatarsophalangeal joint of unspecified toe(s) D, S 🦠

CHAPTER 19 (S00-T88)

- **S93.3 Subluxation and dislocation of foot**
  - **Excludes2** dislocation of toe (S93.1-)
  - **S93.30 Unspecified subluxation and dislocation of foot**
    - Dislocation of foot NOS
    - Subluxation of foot NOS
    - **S93.301** Unspecified subluxation of right foot D, S
    - **S93.302** Unspecified subluxation of left foot D, S
    - **S93.303** Unspecified subluxation of unspecified foot D, S
    - **S93.304** Unspecified dislocation of right foot D, S
    - **S93.305** Unspecified dislocation of left foot D, S
    - **S93.306** Unspecified dislocation of unspecified foot D, S
  - **S93.31 Subluxation and dislocation of tarsal joint**
    - **S93.311** Subluxation of tarsal joint of right foot D, S
    - **S93.312** Subluxation of tarsal joint of left foot D, S
    - **S93.313** Subluxation of tarsal joint of unspecified foot D, S
    - **S93.314** Dislocation of tarsal joint of right foot D, S
    - **S93.315** Dislocation of tarsal joint of left foot D, S
    - **S93.316** Dislocation of tarsal joint of unspecified foot D, S
  - **S93.32 Subluxation and dislocation of tarsometatarsal joint**
    - **S93.321** Subluxation of tarsometatarsal joint of right foot D, S
    - **S93.322** Subluxation of tarsometatarsal joint of left foot D, S
    - **S93.323** Subluxation of tarsometatarsal joint of unspecified foot D, S
    - **S93.324** Dislocation of tarsometatarsal joint of right foot D, S
    - **S93.325** Dislocation of tarsometatarsal joint of left foot D, S
    - **S93.326** Dislocation of tarsometatarsal joint of unspecified foot D, S
  - **S93.33 Other subluxation and dislocation of foot**
    - **S93.331** Other subluxation of right foot D, S
    - **S93.332** Other subluxation of left foot D, S
    - **S93.333** Other subluxation of unspecified foot D, S
    - **S93.334** Other dislocation of right foot D, S
    - **S93.335** Other dislocation of left foot D, S
    - **S93.336** Other dislocation of unspecified foot D, S

- **S93.4 Sprain of ankle**
  - *Injury to ligaments when one or more is stretched/torn*
  - **Excludes2** injury of Achilles tendon (S86.0-)
  - **S93.40 Sprain of unspecified ligament of ankle**
    - Sprain of ankle NOS
    - Sprained ankle NOS
    - **S93.401** Sprain of unspecified ligament of right ankle D, S
    - **S93.402** Sprain of unspecified ligament of left ankle D, S
    - **S93.409** Sprain of unspecified ligament of unspecified ankle D, S
  - **S93.41 Sprain of calcaneofibular ligament**
    - **S93.411** Sprain of calcaneofibular ligament of right ankle D, S
    - **S93.412** Sprain of calcaneofibular ligament of left ankle D, S
    - **S93.419** Sprain of calcaneofibular ligament of unspecified ankle D, S
  - **S93.42 Sprain of deltoid ligament**
    - **S93.421** Sprain of deltoid ligament of right ankle D, S
    - **S93.422** Sprain of deltoid ligament of left ankle D, S
    - **S93.429** Sprain of deltoid ligament of unspecified ankle D, S
  - **S93.43 Sprain of tibiofibular ligament**
    - **S93.431** Sprain of tibiofibular ligament of right ankle D, S
    - **S93.432** Sprain of tibiofibular ligament of left ankle D, S
    - **S93.439** Sprain of tibiofibular ligament of unspecified ankle D, S
  - **S93.49 Sprain of other ligament of ankle**
    - Sprain of internal collateral ligament
    - Sprain of talofibular ligament
    - **S93.491** Sprain of other ligament of right ankle D, S
    - **S93.492** Sprain of other ligament of left ankle D, S
    - **S93.499** Sprain of other ligament of unspecified ankle D, S

- **S93.5 Sprain of toe**
  - **S93.50 Unspecified sprain of toe**
    - **S93.501** Unspecified sprain of right great toe D, S
    - **S93.502** Unspecified sprain of left great toe D, S
    - **S93.503** Unspecified sprain of unspecified great toe D, S
    - **S93.504** Unspecified sprain of right lesser toe(s) D, S
    - **S93.505** Unspecified sprain of left lesser toe(s) D, S
    - **S93.506** Unspecified sprain of unspecified lesser toe(s) D, S
    - **S93.509** Unspecified sprain of unspecified toe(s) D, S

- Unacceptable Principal Diagnosis
- Use Additional Character(s)
- Unspecified
- Manifestation Code
- **OGCR** Official Guidelines for Coding and Reporting
- Excludes 1
- Excludes 2
- Includes
- Use additional
- Code first
- Code also

● **S93.51**   Sprain of interphalangeal joint of toe

    ● **S93.511**   Sprain of interphalangeal joint of right great toe D, S 🔖

    ● **S93.512**   Sprain of interphalangeal joint of left great toe D, S 🔖

    ●■ **S93.513**   Sprain of interphalangeal joint of unspecified great toe D, S 🔖

    ● **S93.514**   Sprain of interphalangeal joint of right lesser toe(s) D, S 🔖

    ● **S93.515**   Sprain of interphalangeal joint of left lesser toe(s) D, S 🔖

    ●■ **S93.516**   Sprain of interphalangeal joint of unspecified lesser toe(s) D, S 🔖

    ●■ **S93.519**   Sprain of interphalangeal joint of unspecified toe(s) D, S 🔖

● **S93.52**   Sprain of metatarsophalangeal joint of toe

    ● **S93.521**   Sprain of metatarsophalangeal joint of right great toe D, S 🔖

    ● **S93.522**   Sprain of metatarsophalangeal joint of left great toe D, S 🔖

    ●■ **S93.523**   Sprain of metatarsophalangeal joint of unspecified great toe D, S 🔖

    ● **S93.524**   Sprain of metatarsophalangeal joint of right lesser toe(s) D, S 🔖

    ● **S93.525**   Sprain of metatarsophalangeal joint of left lesser toe(s) D, S 🔖

    ●■ **S93.526**   Sprain of metatarsophalangeal joint of unspecified lesser toe(s) D, S 🔖

    ●■ **S93.529**   Sprain of metatarsophalangeal joint of unspecified toe(s) D, S 🔖

● **S93.6**   Sprain of foot

    Excludes2   sprain of metatarsophalangeal joint of toe (S93.52-)
               sprain of toe (S93.5-)

    ● **S93.60**   Unspecified sprain of foot

       ●■ **S93.601**   Unspecified sprain of right foot D, S 🔖

       ●■ **S93.602**   Unspecified sprain of left foot D, S 🔖

       ●■ **S93.609**   Unspecified sprain of unspecified foot D, S 🔖

    ● **S93.61**   Sprain of tarsal ligament of foot

       ● **S93.611**   Sprain of tarsal ligament of right foot D, S 🔖

       ● **S93.612**   Sprain of tarsal ligament of left foot D, S 🔖

       ●■ **S93.619**   Sprain of tarsal ligament of unspecified foot D, S 🔖

    ● **S93.62**   Sprain of tarsometatarsal ligament of foot

       ● **S93.621**   Sprain of tarsometatarsal ligament of right foot D, S 🔖

       ● **S93.622**   Sprain of tarsometatarsal ligament of left foot D, S 🔖

       ●■ **S93.629**   Sprain of tarsometatarsal ligament of unspecified foot D, S 🔖

● **S93.69**   Other sprain of foot

    ● **S93.691**   Other sprain of right foot D, S 🔖

    ● **S93.692**   Other sprain of left foot D, S 🔖

    ●■ **S93.699**   Other sprain of unspecified foot D, S 🔖

● **S94**   Injury of nerves at ankle and foot level

    The appropriate 7th character is to be added to each code from category S94

       A   initial encounter
       D   subsequent encounter
       S   sequela

    Code also any associated open wound (S91.-)

    ● **S94.0**   Injury of lateral plantar nerve

       ●■ **S94.00**   Injury of lateral plantar nerve, unspecified leg D, S 🔖

       ● **S94.01**   Injury of lateral plantar nerve, right leg D, S 🔖

       ● **S94.02**   Injury of lateral plantar nerve, left leg D, S 🔖

    ● **S94.1**   Injury of medial plantar nerve

       ●■ **S94.10**   Injury of medial plantar nerve, unspecified leg D, S 🔖

       ● **S94.11**   Injury of medial plantar nerve, right leg D, S 🔖

       ● **S94.12**   Injury of medial plantar nerve, left leg D, S 🔖

    ● **S94.2**   Injury of deep peroneal nerve at ankle and foot level

       Injury of terminal, lateral branch of deep peroneal nerve

       ●■ **S94.20**   Injury of deep peroneal nerve at ankle and foot level, unspecified leg D, S 🔖

       ● **S94.21**   Injury of deep peroneal nerve at ankle and foot level, right leg D, S 🔖

       ● **S94.22**   Injury of deep peroneal nerve at ankle and foot level, left leg D, S 🔖

    ● **S94.3**   Injury of cutaneous sensory nerve at ankle and foot level

       ●■ **S94.30**   Injury of cutaneous sensory nerve at ankle and foot level, unspecified leg D, S 🔖

       ● **S94.31**   Injury of cutaneous sensory nerve at ankle and foot level, right leg D, S 🔖

       ● **S94.32**   Injury of cutaneous sensory nerve at ankle and foot level, left leg D, S 🔖

    ● **S94.8**   Injury of other nerves at ankle and foot level

       ● **S94.8X**   Injury of other nerves at ankle and foot level

          ● **S94.8X1**   Injury of other nerves at ankle and foot level, right leg D, S 🔖

          ● **S94.8X2**   Injury of other nerves at ankle and foot level, left leg D, S 🔖

          ●■ **S94.8X9**   Injury of other nerves at ankle and foot level, unspecified leg D, S 🔖

    ● **S94.9**   Injury of unspecified nerve at ankle and foot level

       ●■ **S94.90**   Injury of unspecified nerve at ankle and foot level, unspecified leg D, S 🔖

       ●■ **S94.91**   Injury of unspecified nerve at ankle and foot level, right leg D, S 🔖

       ●■ **S94.92**   Injury of unspecified nerve at ankle and foot level, left leg D, S 🔖

CHAPTER 19 (S00–T88)

N   Newborn Age: 0   **P**   Pediatric Age: 0–17   **M**   Maternity DX: 12–55   **A**   Adult Age: 15–124   ♀   Females Only   ♂   Males Only

🔖 Complication\Comorbidity   🔖 Major C\C   Present on Admission Requirement   🔖 Hospital-Acquired Condition

1579

● **S95   Injury of blood vessels at ankle and foot level**

> Code also any associated open wound (S91.-)

> **Excludes2**   injury of posterior tibial artery and vein (S85.1-, S85.8-)

> The appropriate 7th character is to be added to each code from category S95

> A   initial encounter
> D   subsequent encounter
> S   sequela

● **S95.0   Injury of dorsal artery of foot**

  ● **S95.00   Unspecified injury of dorsal artery of foot**

    ●■ **S95.001**   Unspecified injury of dorsal artery of right foot A ✪, D, S ✪

    ●■ **S95.002**   Unspecified injury of dorsal artery of left foot A ✪, D, S ✪

    ●■ **S95.009**   Unspecified injury of dorsal artery of unspecified foot A ✪, D, S ✪

  ● **S95.01   Laceration of dorsal artery of foot**

    ● **S95.011**   Laceration of dorsal artery of right foot A ✪, D, S ✪

    ● **S95.012**   Laceration of dorsal artery of left foot A ✪, D, S ✪

    ●■ **S95.019**   Laceration of dorsal artery of unspecified foot A ✪, D, S ✪

  ● **S95.09   Other specified injury of dorsal artery of foot**

    ● **S95.091**   Other specified injury of dorsal artery of right foot A ✪, D, S ✪

    ● **S95.092**   Other specified injury of dorsal artery of left foot A ✪, D, S ✪

    ●■ **S95.099**   Other specified injury of dorsal artery of unspecified foot A ✪, D, S ✪

● **S95.1   Injury of plantar artery of foot**

  ● **S95.10   Unspecified injury of plantar artery of foot**

    ●■ **S95.101**   Unspecified injury of plantar artery of right foot A ✪, D, S ✪

    ●■ **S95.102**   Unspecified injury of plantar artery of left foot A ✪, D, S ✪

    ●■ **S95.109**   Unspecified injury of plantar artery of unspecified foot A ✪, D, S ✪

  ● **S95.11   Laceration of plantar artery of foot**

    ● **S95.111**   Laceration of plantar artery of right foot A ✪, D, S ✪

    ● **S95.112**   Laceration of plantar artery of left foot A ✪, D, S ✪

    ●■ **S95.119**   Laceration of plantar artery of unspecified foot A ✪, D, S ✪

  ● **S95.19   Other specified injury of plantar artery of foot**

    ● **S95.191**   Other specified injury of plantar artery of right foot A ✪, D, S ✪

    ● **S95.192**   Other specified injury of plantar artery of left foot A ✪, D, S ✪

    ●■ **S95.199**   Other specified injury of plantar artery of unspecified foot A ✪, D, S ✪

● **S95.2   Injury of dorsal vein of foot**

  ● **S95.20   Unspecified injury of dorsal vein of foot**

    ●■ **S95.201**   Unspecified injury of dorsal vein of right foot A ✪, D, S ✪

    ●■ **S95.202**   Unspecified injury of dorsal vein of left foot A ✪, D, S ✪

    ●■ **S95.209**   Unspecified injury of dorsal vein of unspecified foot A ✪, D, S ✪

  ● **S95.21   Laceration of dorsal vein of foot**

    ● **S95.211**   Laceration of dorsal vein of right foot A ✪, D, S ✪

    ● **S95.212**   Laceration of dorsal vein of left foot A ✪, D, S ✪

    ●■ **S95.219**   Laceration of dorsal vein of unspecified foot A ✪, D, S ✪

  ● **S95.29   Other specified injury of dorsal vein of foot**

    ● **S95.291**   Other specified injury of dorsal vein of right foot A ✪, D, S ✪

    ● **S95.292**   Other specified injury of dorsal vein of left foot A ✪, D, S ✪

    ●■ **S95.299**   Other specified injury of dorsal vein of unspecified foot A ✪, D, S ✪

● **S95.8   Injury of other blood vessels at ankle and foot level**

  ● **S95.80   Unspecified injury of other blood vessels at ankle and foot level**

    ●■ **S95.801**   Unspecified injury of other blood vessels at ankle and foot level, right leg A ✪, D, S ✪

    ●■ **S95.802**   Unspecified injury of other blood vessels at ankle and foot level, left leg A ✪, D, S ✪

    ●■ **S95.809**   Unspecified injury of other blood vessels at ankle and foot level, unspecified leg A ✪, D, S ✪

  ● **S95.81   Laceration of other blood vessels at ankle and foot level**

    ● **S95.811**   Laceration of other blood vessels at ankle and foot level, right leg A ✪, D, S ✪

    ● **S95.812**   Laceration of other blood vessels at ankle and foot level, left leg A ✪, D, S ✪

    ●■ **S95.819**   Laceration of other blood vessels at ankle and foot level, unspecified leg A ✪, D, S ✪

  ● **S95.89   Other specified injury of other blood vessels at ankle and foot level**

    ● **S95.891**   Other specified injury of other blood vessels at ankle and foot level, right leg A ✪, D, S ✪

    ● **S95.892**   Other specified injury of other blood vessels at ankle and foot level, left leg A ✪, D, S ✪

    ●■ **S95.899**   Other specified injury of other blood vessels at ankle and foot level, unspecified leg A ✪, D, S ✪

● Unacceptable Principal Diagnosis   ● Use Additional Character(s)   ■ Unspecified   ▶ Manifestation Code

1580   **OGCR** Official Guidelines for Coding and Reporting   Excludes 1   Excludes 2   Includes   Use additional   Code first   Code also

- **S95.9**   **Injury of unspecified blood vessel at ankle and foot level**
  - **S95.90**   Unspecified injury of unspecified blood vessel at ankle and foot level
    - **S95.901**   Unspecified injury of unspecified blood vessel at ankle and foot level, right leg A 🍪, D, S 🐚
    - **S95.902**   Unspecified injury of unspecified blood vessel at ankle and foot level, left leg A 🍪, D, S 🐚
    - **S95.909**   Unspecified injury of unspecified blood vessel at ankle and foot level, unspecified leg A 🍪, D, S 🐚
  - **S95.91**   Laceration of unspecified blood vessel at ankle and foot level
    - **S95.911**   Laceration of unspecified blood vessel at ankle and foot level, right leg A 🍪, D, S 🐚
    - **S95.912**   Laceration of unspecified blood vessel at ankle and foot level, left leg A 🍪, D, S 🐚
    - **S95.919**   Laceration of unspecified blood vessel at ankle and foot level, unspecified leg A 🍪, D, S 🐚
  - **S95.99**   Other specified injury of unspecified blood vessel at ankle and foot level
    - **S95.991**   Other specified injury of unspecified blood vessel at ankle and foot level, right leg A 🍪, D, S 🐚
    - **S95.992**   Other specified injury of unspecified blood vessel at ankle and foot level, left leg A 🍪, D, S 🐚
    - **S95.999**   Other specified injury of unspecified blood vessel at ankle and foot level, unspecified leg A 🍪, D, S 🐚

- **S96**   **Injury of muscle and tendon at ankle and foot level**

  Code also any associated open wound (S91.-)

  Excludes2   injury of Achilles tendon (S86.0-)
  sprain of joints and ligaments of ankle and foot (S93.-)

  The appropriate 7th character is to be added to each code from category S96

A	initial encounter
D	subsequent encounter
S	sequela

  - **S96.0**   Injury of muscle and tendon of long flexor muscle of toe at ankle and foot level
    - **S96.00**   Unspecified injury of muscle and tendon of long flexor muscle of toe at ankle and foot level
      - **S96.001**   Unspecified injury of muscle and tendon of long flexor muscle of toe at ankle and foot level, right foot D, S 🐚
      - **S96.002**   Unspecified injury of muscle and tendon of long flexor muscle of toe at ankle and foot level, left foot D, S 🐚
      - **S96.009**   Unspecified injury of muscle and tendon of long flexor muscle of toe at ankle and foot level, unspecified foot D, S 🐚

  - **S96.01**   Strain of muscle and tendon of long flexor muscle of toe at ankle and foot level
    - **S96.011**   Strain of muscle and tendon of long flexor muscle of toe at ankle and foot level, right foot D, S 🐚
    - **S96.012**   Strain of muscle and tendon of long flexor muscle of toe at ankle and foot level, left foot D, S 🐚
    - **S96.019**   Strain of muscle and tendon of long flexor muscle of toe at ankle and foot level, unspecified foot D, S 🐚
  - **S96.02**   Laceration of muscle and tendon of long flexor muscle of toe at ankle and foot level
    - **S96.021**   Laceration of muscle and tendon of long flexor muscle of toe at ankle and foot level, right foot A 🍪, D, S 🐚
    - **S96.022**   Laceration of muscle and tendon of long flexor muscle of toe at ankle and foot level, left foot A 🍪, D, S 🐚
    - **S96.029**   Laceration of muscle and tendon of long flexor muscle of toe at ankle and foot level, unspecified foot A 🍪, D, S 🐚
  - **S96.09**   Other injury of muscle and tendon of long flexor muscle of toe at ankle and foot level
    - **S96.091**   Other injury of muscle and tendon of long flexor muscle of toe at ankle and foot level, right foot D, S 🐚
    - **S96.092**   Other injury of muscle and tendon of long flexor muscle of toe at ankle and foot level, left foot D, S 🐚
    - **S96.099**   Other injury of muscle and tendon of long flexor muscle of toe at ankle and foot level, unspecified foot D, S 🐚
  - **S96.1**   Injury of muscle and tendon of long extensor muscle of toe at ankle and foot level
    - **S96.10**   Unspecified injury of muscle and tendon of long extensor muscle of toe at ankle and foot level
      - **S96.101**   Unspecified injury of muscle and tendon of long extensor muscle of toe at ankle and foot level, right foot D, S 🐚
      - **S96.102**   Unspecified injury of muscle and tendon of long extensor muscle of toe at ankle and foot level, left foot D, S 🐚
      - **S96.109**   Unspecified injury of muscle and tendon of long extensor muscle of toe at ankle and foot level, unspecified foot D, S 🐚

N Newborn Age: 0   **P** Pediatric Age: 0–17   **M** Maternity DX: 12–55   **A** Adult Age: 15–124   ♀ Females Only   ♂ Males Only

🍪 Complication\Comorbidity   Major C\C   Present on Admission Requirement   Hospital-Acquired Condition

CHAPTER 19 (S00-T88)

1581

CHAPTER 19 (S00-T88)

● S96.11   Strain of muscle and tendon of long extensor muscle of toe at ankle and foot level

  ● S96.111   Strain of muscle and tendon of long extensor muscle of toe at ankle and foot level, right foot D, S

  ● S96.112   Strain of muscle and tendon of long extensor muscle of toe at ankle and foot level, left foot D, S

  ●■ S96.119   Strain of muscle and tendon of long extensor muscle of toe at ankle and foot level, unspecified foot D, S

● S96.12   Laceration of muscle and tendon of long extensor muscle of toe at ankle and foot level

  ● S96.121   Laceration of muscle and tendon of long extensor muscle of toe at ankle and foot level, right foot A, D, S

  ● S96.122   Laceration of muscle and tendon of long extensor muscle of toe at ankle and foot level, left foot A, D, S

  ●■ S96.129   Laceration of muscle and tendon of long extensor muscle of toe at ankle and foot level, unspecified foot A, D, S

● S96.19   Other specified injury of muscle and tendon of long extensor muscle of toe at ankle and foot level

  ● S96.191   Other specified injury of muscle and tendon of long extensor muscle of toe at ankle and foot level, right foot D, S

  ● S96.192   Other specified injury of muscle and tendon of long extensor muscle of toe at ankle and foot level, left foot D, S

  ●■ S96.199   Other specified injury of muscle and tendon of long extensor muscle of toe at ankle and foot level, unspecified foot D, S

● S96.2   Injury of intrinsic muscle and tendon at ankle and foot level

  ● S96.20   Unspecified injury of intrinsic muscle and tendon at ankle and foot level

    ●■ S96.201   Unspecified injury of intrinsic muscle and tendon at ankle and foot level, right foot D, S

    ●■ S96.202   Unspecified injury of intrinsic muscle and tendon at ankle and foot level, left foot D, S

    ●■ S96.209   Unspecified injury of intrinsic muscle and tendon at ankle and foot level, unspecified foot D, S

  ● S96.21   Strain of intrinsic muscle and tendon at ankle and foot level

    ● S96.211   Strain of intrinsic muscle and tendon at ankle and foot level, right foot D, S

    ● S96.212   Strain of intrinsic muscle and tendon at ankle and foot level, left foot D, S

    ●■ S96.219   Strain of intrinsic muscle and tendon at ankle and foot level, unspecified foot D, S

● S96.22   Laceration of intrinsic muscle and tendon at ankle and foot level

  ● S96.221   Laceration of intrinsic muscle and tendon at ankle and foot level, right foot A, D, S

  ● S96.222   Laceration of intrinsic muscle and tendon at left ankle and foot level, left foot A, D, S

  ●■ S96.229   Laceration of intrinsic muscle and tendon at ankle and foot level, unspecified foot A, D, S

● S96.29   Other specified injury of intrinsic muscle and tendon at ankle and foot level

  ● S96.291   Other specified injury of intrinsic muscle and tendon at ankle and foot level, right foot D, S

  ● S96.292   Other specified injury of intrinsic muscle and tendon at ankle and foot level, left foot D, S

  ●■ S96.299   Other specified injury of intrinsic muscle and tendon at ankle and foot level, unspecified foot D, S

● S96.8   Injury of other specified muscles and tendons at ankle and foot level

  ● S96.80   Unspecified injury of other specified muscles and tendons at ankle and foot level

    ●■ S96.801   Unspecified injury of other specified muscles and tendons at ankle and foot level, right foot D, S

    ●■ S96.802   Unspecified injury of other specified muscles and tendons at ankle and foot level, left foot D, S

    ●■ S96.809   Unspecified injury of other specified muscles and tendons at ankle and foot level, unspecified foot D, S

  ● S96.81   Strain of other specified muscles and tendons at ankle and foot level

    ● S96.811   Strain of other specified muscles and tendons at ankle and foot level, right foot D, S

    ● S96.812   Strain of other specified muscles and tendons at ankle and foot level, left foot D, S

    ●■ S96.819   Strain of other specified muscles and tendons at ankle and foot level, unspecified foot D, S

  ● S96.82   Laceration of other specified muscles and tendons at ankle and foot level

    ● S96.821   Laceration of other specified muscles and tendons at ankle and foot level, right foot A, D, S

    ● S96.822   Laceration of other specified muscles and tendons at ankle and foot level, left foot A, D, S

    ●■ S96.829   Laceration of other specified muscles and tendons at ankle and foot level, unspecified foot A, D, S

● Unacceptable Principal Diagnosis   ● Use Additional Character(s)   ■ Unspecified   ▶ Manifestation Code

1582   **OGCR** Official Guidelines for Coding and Reporting   Excludes 1   Excludes 2   Includes   Use additional   Code first   Code also

- ● **S96.89** Other specified injury of other specified muscles and tendons at ankle and foot level
  - ● **S96.891** Other specified injury of other specified muscles and tendons at ankle and foot level, right foot D, S 🖉
  - ● **S96.892** Other specified injury of other specified muscles and tendons at ankle and foot level, left foot D, S 🖉
  - ●■ **S96.899** Other specified injury of other specified muscles and tendons at ankle and foot level, unspecified foot D, S 🖉
- ● **S96.9** Injury of unspecified muscle and tendon at ankle and foot level
  - ● **S96.90** Unspecified injury of unspecified muscle and tendon at ankle and foot level
    - ●■ **S96.901** Unspecified injury of unspecified muscle and tendon at ankle and foot level, right foot D, S 🖉
    - ●■ **S96.902** Unspecified injury of unspecified muscle and tendon at ankle and foot level, left foot D, S 🖉
    - ●■ **S96.909** Unspecified injury of unspecified muscle and tendon at ankle and foot level, unspecified foot D, S 🖉
  - ● **S96.91** Strain of unspecified muscle and tendon at ankle and foot level
    - ●■ **S96.911** Strain of unspecified muscle and tendon at ankle and foot level, right foot D, S 🖉
    - ●■ **S96.912** Strain of unspecified muscle and tendon at ankle and foot level, left foot D, S 🖉
    - ●■ **S96.919** Strain of unspecified muscle and tendon at ankle and foot level, unspecified foot D, S 🖉
  - ● **S96.92** Laceration of unspecified muscle and tendon at ankle and foot level
    - ●■ **S96.921** Laceration of unspecified muscle and tendon at ankle and foot level, right foot A 🖉, D, S 🖉
    - ●■ **S96.922** Laceration of unspecified muscle and tendon at ankle and foot level, left foot A 🖉, D, S 🖉
    - ●■ **S96.929** Laceration of unspecified muscle and tendon at ankle and foot level, unspecified foot A 🖉, D, S 🖉
  - ● **S96.99** Other specified injury of unspecified muscle and tendon at ankle and foot level
    - ●■ **S96.991** Other specified injury of unspecified muscle and tendon at ankle and foot level, right foot D, S 🖉
    - ●■ **S96.992** Other specified injury of unspecified muscle and tendon at ankle and foot level, left foot D, S 🖉
    - ●■ **S96.999** Other specified injury of unspecified muscle and tendon at ankle and foot level, unspecified foot D, S 🖉

- ● **S97** Crushing injury of ankle and foot

  Use additional code(s) for all associated injuries

  The appropriate 7th character is to be added to each code from category S97

A	initial encounter
D	subsequent encounter
S	sequela

  - ● **S97.0** Crushing injury of ankle
    - ●■ **S97.00** Crushing injury of unspecified ankle D, S 🖉
    - ● **S97.01** Crushing injury of right ankle D, S 🖉
    - ● **S97.02** Crushing injury of left ankle D, S 🖉
  - ● **S97.1** Crushing injury of toe
    - ● **S97.10** Crushing injury of unspecified toe(s)
      - ●■ **S97.101** Crushing injury of unspecified right toe(s) D, S 🖉
      - ●■ **S97.102** Crushing injury of unspecified left toe(s) D, S 🖉
      - ●■ **S97.109** Crushing injury of unspecified toe(s) D, S 🖉
        Crushing injury of toe NOS
    - ● **S97.11** Crushing injury of great toe
      - ● **S97.111** Crushing injury of right great toe D, S 🖉
      - ● **S97.112** Crushing injury of left great toe D, S 🖉
      - ●■ **S97.119** Crushing injury of unspecified great toe D, S 🖉
    - ● **S97.12** Crushing injury of lesser toe(s)
      - ● **S97.121** Crushing injury of right lesser toe(s) D, S 🖉
      - ● **S97.122** Crushing injury of left lesser toe(s) D, S 🖉
      - ●■ **S97.129** Crushing injury of lesser toe(s), unspecified toe(s) D, S 🖉
  - ● **S97.8** Crushing injury of foot
    - ●■ **S97.80** Crushing injury of foot, unspecified side D, S 🖉
      Crushing injury of foot NOS
    - ● **S97.81** Crushing injury of right foot D, S 🖉
    - ● **S97.82** Crushing injury of left foot D, S 🖉

- ● **S98** Traumatic amputation of ankle and foot

  An amputation not identified as partial or complete should be coded to complete

  The appropriate 7th character is to be added to each code from category S98

A	initial encounter
D	subsequent encounter
S	sequela

  - ● **S98.0** Traumatic amputation of foot at ankle level
    - ● **S98.01** Complete traumatic amputation of foot at ankle level
      - ● **S98.011** Complete traumatic amputation of right foot at ankle level A 🖉, D, S 🖉
      - ● **S98.012** Complete traumatic amputation of left foot at ankle level A 🖉, D, S 🖉
      - ●■ **S98.019** Complete traumatic amputation of unspecified foot at ankle level A 🖉, D, S 🖉

N Newborn Age: 0   **P** Pediatric Age: 0–17   **M** Maternity DX: 12–55   **A** Adult Age: 15–124   ♀ Females Only   ♂ Males Only

🖉 Complication\Comorbidity   🖉 Major C\C   🖉 Present on Admission Requirement   🖉 Hospital-Acquired Condition

1583

CHAPTER 19 (S00-T88)

● S98.02   **Partial traumatic amputation of foot at ankle level**

  ● S98.021   **Partial traumatic amputation of right foot at ankle level A** 🔾, D, S 🔾

  ● S98.022   **Partial traumatic amputation of left foot at ankle level A** 🔾, D, S 🔾

  ● ■ S98.029   **Partial traumatic amputation of unspecified foot at ankle level A** 🔾, D, S 🔾

● S98.1   **Traumatic amputation of one toe**

 ● S98.11   **Complete traumatic amputation of great toe**

  ● S98.111   **Complete traumatic amputation of right great toe** D, S 🔾

  ● S98.112   **Complete traumatic amputation of left great toe** D, S 🔾

  ● ■ S98.119   **Complete traumatic amputation of unspecified great toe** D, S 🔾

 ● S98.12   **Partial traumatic amputation of great toe**

  ● S98.121   **Partial traumatic amputation of right great toe** D, S 🔾

  ● S98.122   **Partial traumatic amputation of left great toe** D, S 🔾

  ● ■ S98.129   **Partial traumatic amputation of unspecified great toe** D, S 🔾

 ● S98.13   **Complete traumatic amputation of one lesser toe**
     Traumatic amputation of toe NOS

  ● S98.131   **Complete traumatic amputation of one right lesser toe** D, S 🔾

  ● S98.132   **Complete traumatic amputation of one left lesser toe** D, S 🔾

  ● ■ S98.139   **Complete traumatic amputation of one unspecified lesser toe** D, S 🔾

 ● S98.14   **Partial traumatic amputation of one lesser toe**

  ● S98.141   **Partial traumatic amputation of one right lesser toe** D, S 🔾

  ● S98.142   **Partial traumatic amputation of one left lesser toe** D, S 🔾

  ● ■ S98.149   **Partial traumatic amputation of one unspecified lesser toe** D, S 🔾

● S98.2   **Traumatic amputation of two or more lesser toes**

 ● S98.21   **Complete traumatic amputation of two or more lesser toes**

  ● S98.211   **Complete traumatic amputation of two or more right lesser toes** D, S 🔾

  ● S98.212   **Complete traumatic amputation of two or more left lesser toes** D, S 🔾

  ● ■ S98.219   **Complete traumatic amputation of two or more unspecified lesser toes** D, S 🔾

● S98.22   **Partial traumatic amputation of two or more lesser toes**

  ● S98.221   **Partial traumatic amputation of two or more right lesser toes** D, S 🔾

  ● S98.222   **Partial traumatic amputation of two or more left lesser toes** D, S 🔾

  ● ■ S98.229   **Partial traumatic amputation of two or more unspecified lesser toes** D, S 🔾

● S98.3   **Traumatic amputation of midfoot**

 ● S98.31   **Complete traumatic amputation of midfoot**

  ● S98.311   **Complete traumatic amputation of right midfoot A** 🔾, D, S 🔾

  ● S98.312   **Complete traumatic amputation of left midfoot A** 🔾, D, S 🔾

  ● ■ S98.319   **Complete traumatic amputation of unspecified midfoot A** 🔾, D, S 🔾

 ● S98.32   **Partial traumatic amputation of midfoot**

  ● S98.321   **Partial traumatic amputation of right midfoot A** 🔾, D, S 🔾

  ● S98.322   **Partial traumatic amputation of left midfoot A** 🔾, D, S 🔾

  ● ■ S98.329   **Partial traumatic amputation of unspecified midfoot A** 🔾, D, S 🔾

● S98.9   **Traumatic amputation of foot, level unspecified**

 ● S98.91   **Complete traumatic amputation of foot, level unspecified**

  ● S98.911   **Complete traumatic amputation of right foot, level unspecified A** 🔾, D, S 🔾

  ● S98.912   **Complete traumatic amputation of left foot, level unspecified A** 🔾, D, S 🔾

  ● ■ S98.919   **Complete traumatic amputation of unspecified foot, level unspecified A** 🔾, D, S 🔾

 ● S98.92   **Partial traumatic amputation of foot, level unspecified**

  ● ■ S98.921   **Partial traumatic amputation of right foot, level unspecified A** 🔾, D, S 🔾

  ● ■ S98.922   **Partial traumatic amputation of left foot, level unspecified A** 🔾, D, S 🔾

  ● ■ S98.929   **Partial traumatic amputation of unspecified foot, level unspecified A** 🔾, D, S 🔾

● S99   **Other and unspecified injuries of ankle and foot**

   The appropriate 7th character is to be added to each code from category S99

A	initial encounter
D	subsequent encounter
S	sequela

 ● S99.8   **Other specified injuries of ankle and foot**

  ● S99.81   **Other specified injuries of ankle**

   ● S99.811   **Other specified injuries of right ankle** D, S 🔾

● Unacceptable Principal Diagnosis   ● Use Additional Character(s)   ■ Unspecified   ▶ Manifestation Code

OGCR Official Guidelines for Coding and Reporting   Excludes 1   Excludes 2   Includes   Use additional   Code first   Code also

● S99.812   Other specified injuries of left ankle D, S ⬡

●■ S99.819   Other specified injuries of unspecified ankle D, S ⬡

● S99.82   Other specified injuries of foot

● S99.821   Other specified injuries of right foot D, S ⬡

● S99.822   Other specified injuries of left foot D, S ⬡

●■ S99.829   Other specified injuries of unspecified foot D, S ⬡

● S99.9   Unspecified injury of ankle and foot

● S99.91   Unspecified injury of ankle

●■ S99.911   Unspecified injury of right ankle D, S ⬡

●■ S99.912   Unspecified injury of left ankle D, S ⬡

●■ S99.919   Unspecified injury of unspecified ankle D, S ⬡

● S99.92   Unspecified injury of foot

●■ S99.921   Unspecified injury of right foot D, S ⬡

●■ S99.922   Unspecified injury of left foot D, S ⬡

●■ S99.929   Unspecified injury of unspecified foot D, S ⬡

INJURY, POISONING AND CERTAIN OTHER CONSEQUENCES OF EXTERNAL CAUSES (T07-T88)

INJURIES INVOLVING MULTIPLE BODY REGIONS (T07)

Excludes1	burns and corrosions (T20-T32)
	frostbite (T33-T34)
	insect bite or sting, venomous (T63.4)
	sunburn (L55.-)

■ T07   Unspecified multiple injuries

Excludes1   injury NOS (T14)

INJURY OF UNSPECIFIED BODY REGION (T14)

● T14   Injury of unspecified body region

Excludes1   multiple unspecified injuries (T07)

T14.8   Other injury of unspecified body region

Abrasion NOS	Fracture NOS
Contusion NOS	Skin injury NOS
Crush injury NOS	Vascular injury NOS

● T14.9   Unspecified injury

■ T14.90   Injury, unspecified
Injury NOS

T14.91   Suicide attempt
Attempted suicide NOS

EFFECTS OF FOREIGN BODY ENTERING THROUGH NATURAL ORIFICE (T15-T19)

Excludes2	foreign body accidentally left in operation wound (T81.5-)
	foreign body in penetrating wound - see open wound by body region
	residual foreign body in soft tissue (M79.5)
	splinter, without open wound - see superficial injury by body region

● T15   Foreign body on external eye

Excludes2	foreign body in penetrating wound of orbit and eye ball (S05.4-, S05.5-)
	open wound of eyelid and periocular area (S01.1-)
	retained foreign body in eyelid (H02.8-)
	retained (old) foreign body in penetrating wound of orbit and eye ball (H05.5-, H44.6-, H44.7-)
	superficial foreign body of eyelid and periocular area (S00.25-)

The appropriate 7th character is to be added to each code from category T15

A	initial encounter
D	subsequent encounter
S	sequela

● T15.0   Foreign body in cornea

●■ T15.00   Foreign body in cornea, unspecified eye D, S ⬡

● T15.01   Foreign body in cornea, right eye D, S ⬡

● T15.02   Foreign body in cornea, left eye D, S ⬡

● T15.1   Foreign body in conjunctival sac

●■ T15.10   Foreign body in conjunctival sac, unspecified eye D, S ⬡

● T15.11   Foreign body in conjunctival sac, right eye D, S ⬡

● T15.12   Foreign body in conjunctival sac, left eye D, S ⬡

● T15.8   Foreign body in other and multiple parts of external eye
Foreign body in lacrimal punctum

●■ T15.80   Foreign body in other and multiple parts of external eye, unspecified eye D, S ⬡

● T15.81   Foreign body in other and multiple parts of external eye, right eye D, S ⬡

● T15.82   Foreign body in other and multiple parts of external eye, left eye D, S ⬡

● T15.9   Foreign body on external eye, part unspecified

●■ T15.90   Foreign body on external eye, part unspecified, unspecified eye D, S ⬡

●■ T15.91   Foreign body on external eye, part unspecified, right eye D, S ⬡

●■ T15.92   Foreign body on external eye, part unspecified, left eye D, S ⬡

CHAPTER 19 (S00-T88)

● **T16**   **Foreign body in ear**

    Includes   foreign body in auditory canal

    The appropriate 7th character is to be added to each code from category T16

> A   initial encounter
> D   subsequent encounter
> S   sequela

   ● **T16.1**   **Foreign body in right ear** D, S ✎

   ● **T16.2**   **Foreign body in left ear** D, S ✎

   ●◼ **T16.9**   **Foreign body in ear, unspecified ear** D, S ✎

● **T17**   **Foreign body in respiratory tract**

    The appropriate 7th character is to be added to each code from category T17

> A   initial encounter
> D   subsequent encounter
> S   sequela

   ● **T17.0**   **Foreign body in nasal sinus** D, S ✎

   ● **T17.1**   **Foreign body in nostril** D, S ✎
      Foreign body in nose NOS

   ● **T17.2**   **Foreign body in pharynx** D, S ✎
      Foreign body in nasopharynx
      Foreign body in throat NOS

     ● **T17.20**   **Unspecified foreign body in pharynx**

       ●◼ **T17.200**   **Unspecified foreign body in pharynx causing asphyxiation** D, S ✎

       ●◼ **T17.208**   **Unspecified foreign body in pharynx causing other injury** D, S ✎

     ● **T17.21**   **Gastric contents in pharynx**
       Aspiration of gastric contents into pharynx
       Vomitus in pharynx

       ● **T17.210**   **Gastric contents in pharynx causing asphyxiation** D, S ✎

       ● **T17.218**   **Gastric contents in pharynx causing other injury** D, S ✎

     ● **T17.22**   **Food in pharynx**
       Bones in pharynx
       Seeds in pharynx

       ● **T17.220**   **Food in pharynx causing asphyxiation** D, S ✎

       ● **T17.228**   **Food in pharynx causing other injury** D, S ✎

     ● **T17.29**   **Other foreign object in pharynx**

       ● **T17.290**   **Other foreign object in pharynx causing asphyxiation** D, S ✎

       ● **T17.298**   **Other foreign object in pharynx causing other injury** D, S ✎

   ● **T17.3**   **Foreign body in larynx**

     ● **T17.30**   **Unspecified foreign body in larynx**

       ●◼ **T17.300**   **Unspecified foreign body in larynx causing asphyxiation** D, S ✎

       ●◼ **T17.308**   **Unspecified foreign body in larynx causing other injury** D, S ✎

● **T17.31**   **Gastric contents in larynx**
    Aspiration of gastric contents into larynx
    Vomitus in larynx

   ● **T17.310**   **Gastric contents in larynx causing asphyxiation** D, S ✎

   ● **T17.318**   **Gastric contents in larynx causing other injury** D, S ✎

● **T17.32**   **Food in larynx**
    Bones in larynx
    Seeds in larynx

   ● **T17.320**   **Food in larynx causing asphyxiation** D, S ✎

   ● **T17.328**   **Food in larynx causing other injury** D, S ✎

● **T17.39**   **Other foreign object in larynx**

   ● **T17.390**   **Other foreign object in larynx causing asphyxiation** D, S ✎

   ● **T17.398**   **Other foreign object in larynx causing other injury** D, S ✎

● **T17.4**   **Foreign body in trachea**

   ● **T17.40**   **Unspecified foreign body in trachea**

     ●◼ **T17.400**   **Unspecified foreign body in trachea causing asphyxiation** A ✎, D, S ✎

     ●◼ **T17.408**   **Unspecified foreign body in trachea causing other injury** A ✎, D, S ✎

   ● **T17.41**   **Gastric contents in trachea**
      Aspiration of gastric contents into trachea
      Vomitus in trachea

     ● **T17.410**   **Gastric contents in trachea causing asphyxiation** A ✎, D, S ✎

     ● **T17.418**   **Gastric contents in trachea causing other injury** A ✎, D, S ✎

   ● **T17.42**   **Food in trachea**
      Bones in trachea
      Seeds in trachea

     ● **T17.420**   **Food in trachea causing asphyxiation** A ✎, D, S ✎

     ● **T17.428**   **Food in trachea causing other injury** A ✎, D, S ✎

   ● **T17.49**   **Other foreign object in trachea**

     ● **T17.490**   **Other foreign object in trachea causing asphyxiation** A ✎, D, S ✎

     ● **T17.498**   **Other foreign object in trachea causing other injury** A ✎, D, S ✎

● **T17.5**   **Foreign body in bronchus**

   ● **T17.50**   **Unspecified foreign body in bronchus**

     ●◼ **T17.500**   **Unspecified foreign body in bronchus causing asphyxiation** A ✎, D, S ✎

     ●◼ **T17.508**   **Unspecified foreign body in bronchus causing other injury** A ✎, D, S ✎

● Unacceptable Principal Diagnosis   ● Use Additional Character(s)   ◼ Unspecified   ▶ Manifestation Code

OGCR   Official Guidelines for Coding and Reporting | Excludes 1 | | Excludes 2 | | Includes | | Use additional | | Code first | | Code also |

● **T17.51 Gastric contents in bronchus**
Aspiration of gastric contents into bronchus
Vomitus in bronchus

   ● **T17.510 Gastric contents in bronchus causing asphyxiation A** 🔵, D, S �—

   ● **T17.518 Gastric contents in bronchus causing other injury A** 🔵, D, S �—

● **T17.52 Food in bronchus**
Bones in bronchus
Seeds in bronchus

   ● **T17.520 Food in bronchus causing asphyxiation A** 🔵, D, S �—

   ● **T17.528 Food in bronchus causing other injury A** 🔵, D, S �—

● **T17.59 Other foreign object in bronchus**

   ● **T17.590 Other foreign object in bronchus causing asphyxiation A** 🔵, D, S �—

   ● **T17.598 Other foreign object in bronchus causing other injury A** 🔵, D, S �—

● **T17.8 Foreign body in other parts of respiratory tract**
Foreign body in bronchioles
Foreign body in lung

   ● **T17.80 Unspecified foreign body in other parts of respiratory tract**

     ● ■ **T17.800 Unspecified foreign body in other parts of respiratory tract causing asphyxiation A** 🔵, D, S �—

     ● ■ **T17.808 Unspecified foreign body in other parts of respiratory tract causing other injury A** 🔵, D, S �—

   ● **T17.81 Gastric contents in other parts of respiratory tract**
Aspiration of gastric contents into other parts of respiratory tract
Vomitus in other parts of respiratory tract

     ● **T17.810 Gastric contents in other parts of respiratory tract causing asphyxiation A** 🔵, D, S �—

     ● **T17.818 Gastric contents in other parts of respiratory tract causing other injury A** 🔵, D, S �—

   ● **T17.82 Food in other parts of respiratory tract**
Bones in other parts of respiratory tract
Seeds in other parts of respiratory tract

     ● **T17.820 Food in other parts of respiratory tract causing asphyxiation A** 🔵, D, S �—

     ● **T17.828 Food in other parts of respiratory tract causing other injury A** 🔵, D, S �—

   ● **T17.89 Other foreign object in other parts of respiratory tract**

     ● **T17.890 Other foreign object in other parts of respiratory tract causing asphyxiation A** 🔵, D, S �—

     ● **T17.898 Other foreign object in other parts of respiratory tract causing other injury A** 🔵, D, S �—

● **T17.9 Foreign body in respiratory tract, part unspecified**

   ● **T17.90 Unspecified foreign body in respiratory tract, part unspecified**

     ● ■ **T17.900 Unspecified foreign body in respiratory tract, part unspecified causing asphyxiation** D, S �—

     ● ■ **T17.908 Unspecified foreign body in respiratory tract, part unspecified causing other injury** D, S �—

   ● **T17.91 Gastric contents in respiratory tract, part unspecified**
Aspiration of gastric contents into respiratory tract, part unspecified
Vomitus in trachea respiratory tract, part unspecified

     ● ■ **T17.910 Gastric contents in respiratory tract, part unspecified causing asphyxiation** D, S �—

     ● ■ **T17.918 Gastric contents in respiratory tract, part unspecified causing other injury** D, S �—

   ● **T17.92 Food in respiratory tract, part unspecified**
Bones in respiratory tract, part unspecified
Seeds in respiratory tract, part unspecified

     ● ■ **T17.920 Food in respiratory tract, part unspecified causing asphyxiation** D, S �—

     ● ■ **T17.928 Food in respiratory tract, part unspecified causing other injury** D, S �—

   ● **T17.99 Other foreign object in respiratory tract, part unspecified**

     ● ■ **T17.990 Other foreign object in respiratory tract, part unspecified in causing asphyxiatio** D, S �—

     ● ■ **T17.998 Other foreign object in respiratory tract, part unspecified causing other injur** D, S �—

● **T18 Foreign body in alimentary tract**

   | **Excludes2** | foreign body in pharynx (T17.2-) |

The appropriate 7th character is to be added to each code from category T18

A	initial encounter
D	subsequent encounter
S	sequela

● **T18.0 Foreign body in mouth** D, S �—

● **T18.1 Foreign body in esophagus**

   | **Excludes2** | foreign body in respiratory tract (T17.-) |

   ● **T18.10 Unspecified foreign body in esophagus**

     ● ■ **T18.100 Unspecified foreign body in esophagus causing compression of trachea** D, S �—
Unspecified foreign body in esophagus causing obstruction of respiration

     ● ■ **T18.108 Unspecified foreign body in esophagus causing other injury** D, S �—

N Newborn Age: 0   **P** Pediatric Age: 0–17   **M** Maternity DX: 12–55   **A** Adult Age: 15–124   ♀ Females Only   ♂ Males Only

🔵 Complication\Comorbidity   🔵 Major C\C   �— Present on Admission Requirement   🔵 Hospital-Acquired Condition

1587

● **T18.11**   **Gastric contents in esophagus** D, S 🔖
     Vomitus in esophagus

     ● **T18.110**   **Gastric contents in esophagus causing compression of trachea** D, S 🔖
         Gastric contents in esophagus causing obstruction of respiration

     ● **T18.118**   **Gastric contents in esophagus causing other injury** D, S 🔖

● **T18.12**   **Food in esophagus**
     Bones in esophagus
     Seeds in esophagus

     ● **T18.120**   **Food in esophagus causing compression of trachea** D, S 🔖
         Food in esophagus causing obstruction of respiration

     ● **T18.128**   **Food in esophagus causing other injury** D, S 🔖

● **T18.19**   **Other foreign object in esophagus**

     ● **T18.190**   **Other foreign object in esophagus causing compression of trachea** D, S 🔖
         Other foreign body in esophagus causing obstruction of respiration

     ● **T18.198**   **Other foreign object in esophagus causing other injury** D, S 🔖

● **T18.2**   **Foreign body in stomach** D, S 🔖

● **T18.3**   **Foreign body in small intestine** D, S 🔖

● **T18.4**   **Foreign body in colon** D, S 🔖

● **T18.5**   **Foreign body in anus and rectum** D, S 🔖
     Foreign body in rectosigmoid (junction)

● **T18.8**   **Foreign body in other parts of alimentary tract** D, S 🔖

●■ **T18.9**   **Foreign body of alimentary tract, part unspecified** D, S 🔖
     Foreign body in digestive system NOS
     Swallowed foreign body NOS

● **T19**   **Foreign body in genitourinary tract**

   | Excludes2 | complications due to implanted mesh (T83.7-)
     mechanical complications of contraceptive device (intrauterine) (vaginal) (T83.3-)
     presence of contraceptive device (intrauterine) (vaginal) (Z97.5)

The appropriate 7th character is to be added to each code from category T19

A	initial encounter
D	subsequent encounter
S	sequela

● **T19.0**   **Foreign body in urethra** D, S 🔖

● **T19.1**   **Foreign body in bladder** D, S 🔖

● **T19.2**   **Foreign body in vulva and vagina** D, S 🔖

● **T19.3**   **Foreign body in uterus** D, S 🔖

● **T19.4**   **Foreign body in penis** D, S 🔖

● **T19.8**   **Foreign body in other parts of genitourinary tract** D, S 🔖

●■ **T19.9**   **Foreign body in genitourinary tract, part unspecified** D, S 🔖

BURNS AND CORROSIONS (T20-T32)

| Includes | burns (thermal) from electrical heating appliances
     burns (thermal) from electricity
     burns (thermal) from flame
     burns (thermal) from friction
     burns (thermal) from hot air and hot gases
     burns (thermal) from hot objects
     burns (thermal) from lightning
     burns (thermal) from radiation chemical
     burn [corrosion] (external) (internal) scalds

| Excludes2 | erythema [dermatitis] ab igne (L59.0)
     radiation-related disorders of the skin and subcutaneous tissue (L55-L59)
     sunburn (L55.-)

A   B

Figure 19-14   A. 2nd degree burn. B. 3rd degree burn. (From Cummings: Otolaryngology: Head & Neck Surgery, 4th ed. 2005, Mosby.)

OGCR   Section I.C.19.d.

Burns and Corrosions

The ICD-10-CM makes a distinction between burn and corrosions. The burn codes are for thermal burns, except sunburns, that come from a heat source, such as a fire or hot appliance. The burn codes are also for burns resulting from electricity and radiation. Corrosions are burns due to chemicals. The guidelines for burns and corrosions are the same.

Current burns (T20-T25) are classified by depth, extent and by agent (X code). Burns are classified by depth as first degree (erythema), second degree (blistering), and third degree (full-thickness involvement). Burns of the eye and internal organs (T26-T28) are classified by site, but not by degree.

1) Sequencing of burn and related condition codes

Sequence first the code that reflects the highest degree of burn when more than one burn is present.

a. When the reason for the admission or encounter is for treatment of external multiple burns, sequence first the code that reflects the burn of the highest degree.

b. When a patient has both internal and external burns, the circumstances of admission govern the selection of the principal diagnosis or first-listed diagnosis.

c. When a patient is admitted for burn injuries and other related conditions such as smoke inhalation and/or respiratory failure, the circumstances of admission govern the selection of the principal or first-listed diagnosis.

2) Burns of the same local site

Classify burns of the same local site (three-character category level, T20-T28) but of different degrees to the subcategory identifying the highest degree recorded in the diagnosis.

1588

● Unacceptable Principal Diagnosis   ● Use Additional Character(s)   ■ Unspecified   ▶ Manifestation Code

OGCR Official Guidelines for Coding and Reporting | Excludes 1 | | Excludes 2 | | Includes | | Use additional | | Code first | | Code also |

BURNS AND CORROSIONS OF EXTERNAL BODY SURFACE, SPECIFIED BY SITE (T20-T25)

Includes   burns and corrosions of first degree [erythema]

burns and corrosions of second degree [blisters][epidermal loss]

burns and corrosions of third degree [deep necrosis of underlying tissue] [full-thickness skin loss]

Use additional code from category T31 or T32 to identify extent of body surface involved

- ● **T20** **Burn and corrosion of head, face, and neck**

    Excludes2   burn and corrosion of ear drum (T28.41, T28.91)

    burn and corrosion of eye and adnexa (T26.-)

    burn and corrosion of mouth and pharynx (T28.0)

    The appropriate 7th character is to be added to each code from category T20

A	initial encounter
D	subsequent encounter
S	sequela

- ● **T20.0** **Burn of unspecified degree of head, face, and neck**

    Use additional external cause code to identify the source, place and intent of the burn (X00-X19, X75-X77, X96-X98, Y92)

    - ●■ **T20.00** Burn of unspecified degree of head, face, and neck, unspecified site D, S

    - ● **T20.01** Burn of unspecified degree of ear [any part, except ear drum]

        Excludes2   burn of ear drum (T28.41-)

        - ●■ **T20.011** Burn of unspecified degree of right ear [any part, except ear drum] D, S

        - ●■ **T20.012** Burn of unspecified degree of left ear [any part, except ear drum] D, S

        - ●■ **T20.019** Burn of unspecified degree of unspecified ear [any part, except ear drum] D, S

    - ●■ **T20.02** Burn of unspecified degree of lip(s) D, S
    - ●■ **T20.03** Burn of unspecified degree of chin D, S
    - ●■ **T20.04** Burn of unspecified degree of nose (septum) D, S
    - ●■ **T20.05** Burn of unspecified degree of scalp [any part] D, S
    - ●■ **T20.06** Burn of unspecified degree of forehead and cheek D, S
    - ●■ **T20.07** Burn of unspecified degree of neck D, S
    - ●■ **T20.09** Burn of unspecified degree of multiple sites of head, face, and neck D, S

- ● **T20.1** **Burn of first degree of head, face, and neck**

    Use additional external cause code to identify the source, place and intent of the burn (X00-X19, X75-X77, X96-X98, Y92)

    - ●■ **T20.10** Burn of first degree of head, face, and neck, unspecified site D, S

    - ● **T20.11** Burn of first degree of ear [any part, except ear drum]

        Excludes2   burn of ear drum (T28.41-)

        - ● **T20.111** Burn of first degree of right ear [any part, except ear drum] D, S

        - ● **T20.112** Burn of first degree of left ear [any part, except ear drum] D, S

        - ●■ **T20.119** Burn of first degree of unspecified ear [any part, except ear drum] D, S

    - ● **T20.12** Burn of first degree of lip(s) D, S
    - ● **T20.13** Burn of first degree of chin D, S
    - ● **T20.14** Burn of first degree of nose (septum) D, S
    - ● **T20.15** Burn of first degree of scalp [any part] D, S
    - ● **T20.16** Burn of first degree of forehead and cheek D, S
    - ● **T20.17** Burn of first degree of neck D, S
    - ● **T20.19** Burn of first degree of multiple sites of head, face, and neck D, S

- ● **T20.2** **Burn of second degree of head, face, and neck**

    Use additional external cause code to identify the source, place and intent of the burn (X00-X19, X75-X77, X96-X98, Y92)

    - ●■ **T20.20** Burn of second degree of head, face, and neck, unspecified site D, S

    - ● **T20.21** Burn of second degree of ear [any part, except ear drum]

        Excludes2   burn of ear drum (T28.41-)

        - ● **T20.211** Burn of second degree of right ear [any part, except ear drum] D, S

        - ● **T20.212** Burn of second degree of left ear [any part, except ear drum] D, S

        - ●■ **T20.219** Burn of second degree of unspecified ear [any part, except ear drum] D, S

    - ● **T20.22** Burn of second degree of lip(s) D, S
    - ● **T20.23** Burn of second degree of chin D, S
    - ● **T20.24** Burn of second degree of nose (septum) D, S
    - ● **T20.25** Burn of second degree of scalp [any part] D, S
    - ● **T20.26** Burn of second degree of forehead and cheek D, S
    - ● **T20.27** Burn of second degree of neck D, S
    - ● **T20.29** Burn of second degree of multiple sites of head, face, and neck D, S

- ● **T20.3** **Burn of third degree of head, face, and neck**

    Use additional external cause code to identify the source, place and intent of the burn (X00-X19, X75-X77, X96-X98, Y92)

    - ●■ **T20.30** Burn of third degree of head, face, and neck, unspecified site A, D, S, A

    - ● **T20.31** Burn of third degree of ear [any part, except ear drum]

        Excludes2   burn of ear drum (T28.41-)

        - ● **T20.311** Burn of third degree of right ear [any part, except ear drum] A, D, S, A

        - ● **T20.312** Burn of third degree of left ear [any part, except ear drum] A, D, S, A

        - ●■ **T20.319** Burn of third degree of unspecified ear [any part, except ear drum] A, D, S, A

N Newborn Age: 0   **P** Pediatric Age: 0–17   **M** Maternity DX: 12–55   **A** Adult Age: 15–124   ♀ Females Only   ♂ Males Only

Complication\Comorbidity   Major C\C   Present on Admission Requirement   Hospital-Acquired Condition

1589

CHAPTER 19 (S00-T88)

● T20.32   Burn of third degree of lip(s) A ✪, D, S ✪, A ✪

● T20.33   Burn of third degree of chin A ✪, D, S ✪, A ✪

● T20.34   Burn of third degree of nose (septum) A ✪, D, S ✪, A ✪

● T20.35   Burn of third degree of scalp [any part] A ✪, D, S ✪, A ✪

● T20.36   Burn of third degree of forehead and cheek A ✪, D, S ✪, A ✪

● T20.37   Burn of third degree of neck A ✪, D, S ✪, A ✪

● T20.39   Burn of third degree of multiple sites of head, face, and neck A ✪, D, S ✪, A ✪

● T20.4   Corrosion of unspecified degree of head, face, and neck

Code first (T51-T65) to identify chemical and intent

Use additional external cause code to identify place (Y92)

●●■ T20.40   Corrosion of unspecified degree of head, face, and neck, unspecified site D, S ✪

●● T20.41   Corrosion of unspecified degree of ear [any part, except ear drum]

     Excludes2   corrosion of ear drum (T28.91-)

●●■ T20.411   Corrosion of unspecified degree of right ear [any part, except ear drum] D, S ✪

●●■ T20.412   Corrosion of unspecified degree of left ear [any part, except ear drum] D, S ✪

●●■ T20.419   Corrosion of unspecified degree of unspecified ear [any part, except ear drum] D, S ✪

●●■ T20.42   Corrosion of unspecified degree of lip(s) D, S ✪

●●■ T20.43   Corrosion of unspecified degree of chin D, S ✪

●●■ T20.44   Corrosion of unspecified degree of nose (septum) D, S ✪

●●■ T20.45   Corrosion of unspecified degree of scalp [any part] D, S ✪

●●■ T20.46   Corrosion of unspecified degree of forehead and cheek D, S ✪

●●■ T20.47   Corrosion of unspecified degree of neck D, S ✪

●●■ T20.49   Corrosion of unspecified degree of multiple sites of head, face, and neck D, S ✪

● T20.5   Corrosion of first degree of head, face, and neck

Code first (T51-T65) to identify chemical and intent

Use additional external cause code to identify place (Y92)

●●■ T20.50   Corrosion of first degree of head, face, and neck, unspecified site D, S ✪

● T20.51   Corrosion of first degree of ear [any part, except ear drum]

     Excludes2   corrosion of ear drum (T28.91-)

●● T20.511   Corrosion of first degree of right ear [any part, except ear drum] D, S ✪

●● T20.512   Corrosion of first degree of left ear [any part, except ear drum] D, S ✪

●●■ T20.519   Corrosion of first degree of unspecified ear [any part, except ear drum] D, S ✪

●● T20.52   Corrosion of first degree of lip(s) D, S ✪

●● T20.53   Corrosion of first degree of chin D, S ✪

●● T20.54   Corrosion of first degree of nose (septum) D, S ✪

●● T20.55   Corrosion of first degree of scalp [any part] D, S ✪

●● T20.56   Corrosion of first degree of cheek D, S ✪

●● T20.57   Corrosion of first degree of neck D, S ✪

●● T20.59   Corrosion of first degree of multiple sites of head, face, and neck D, S ✪

● T20.6   Corrosion of second degree of head, face, and neck

Code first (T51-T65) to identify chemical and intent

Use additional external cause code to identify place (Y92)

●●■ T20.60   Corrosion of second degree of head, face, and neck, unspecified site D, S ✪

● T20.61   Corrosion of second degree of ear [any part, except ear drum]

     Excludes2   corrosion of ear drum (T28.91-)

●● T20.611   Corrosion of second degree of right ear [any part, except ear drum] D, S ✪

●● T20.612   Corrosion of second degree of left ear [any part, except ear drum] D, S ✪

●●■ T20.619   Corrosion of second degree of unspecified ear [any part, except ear drum] D, S ✪

●● T20.62   Corrosion of second degree of lip(s) D, S ✪

●● T20.63   Corrosion of second degree of chin D, S ✪

●● T20.64   Corrosion of second degree of nose (septum) D, S ✪

●● T20.65   Corrosion of second degree of scalp [any part] D, S ✪

●● T20.66   Corrosion of second degree of forehead and cheek D, S ✪

●● T20.67   Corrosion of second degree of neck D, S ✪

●● T20.69   Corrosion of second degree of multiple sites of head, face, and neck D, S ✪

● T20.7   Corrosion of third degree of head, face, and neck

Code first (T51-T65) to identify chemical and intent

Use additional external cause code to identify place (Y92)

●●■ T20.70   Corrosion of third degree of head, face, and neck, unspecified site A ✪, D, S ✪, A ✪

● T20.71   Corrosion of third degree of ear [any part, except ear drum]

     Excludes2   corrosion of ear drum (T28.91-)

●● T20.711   Corrosion of third degree of right ear [any part, except ear drum] A ✪, D, S ✪, A ✪

● Unacceptable Principal Diagnosis   ● Use Additional Character(s)   ■ Unspecified   ▶ Manifestation Code

OGCR   Official Guidelines for Coding and Reporting   Excludes 1   Excludes 2   Includes   Use additional   Code first   Code also

●● **T20.712** Corrosion of third degree of left ear [any part, except ear drum] **A** 🪙, D, S 🪙, A 🪙

●●■ **T20.719** Corrosion of third degree of unspecified ear [any part, except ear drum] A 🪙, D, S 🪙, A 🪙

●● **T20.72** Corrosion of third degree of lip(s) A 🪙, D, S 🪙, A 🪙

●● **T20.73** Corrosion of third degree of chin A 🪙, D, S 🪙, A 🪙

●● **T20.74** Corrosion of third degree of nose (septum) A 🪙, D, S 🪙, A 🪙

●● **T20.75** Corrosion of third degree of scalp [any part] A 🪙, D, S 🪙, A 🪙

●● **T20.76** Corrosion of third degree of forehead and cheek A 🪙, D, S 🪙, A 🪙

●● **T20.77** Corrosion of third degree of neck A 🪙, D, S 🪙, A 🪙

●● **T20.79** Corrosion of third degree of multiple sites of head, face, and neck A 🪙, D, S 🪙, A 🪙

● **T21** **Burn and corrosion of trunk**

> **Includes**   burns and corrosion of hip region
>
> **Excludes2**   burns and corrosion of:
>   axilla (T22.- with fifth character 4)
>   scapular region (T22.- with fifth character 6)
>   shoulder (T22. with fifth character 5)
>
> The appropriate 7th character is to be added to each code from category T21
>
> | A | initial encounter |
> |---|---|
> | D | subsequent encounter |
> | S | sequela |

● **T21.0** **Burn of unspecified degree of trunk**

> **Use additional** external cause code to identify the source, place and intent of the burn (X00-X19, X75-X77, X96-X98, Y92)

●■ **T21.00** Burn of unspecified degree of trunk, unspecified site D, S 🪙

●■ **T21.01** Burn of unspecified degree of chest wall D, S 🪙
  Burn of of unspecified degree of breast

●■ **T21.02** Burn of unspecified degree of abdominal wall D, S 🪙
  Burn of unspecified degree of flank
  Burn of unspecified degree of groin

●■ **T21.03** Burn of unspecified degree of upper back D, S 🪙
  Burn of unspecified degree of interscapular region

●■ **T21.04** Burn of unspecified degree of lower back D, S 🪙

●■ **T21.05** Burn of unspecified degree of buttock D, S 🪙
  Burn of unspecified degree of anus

●■ **T21.06** Burn of unspecified degree of male genital region D, S 🪙
  Burn of unspecified degree of penis
  Burn of unspecified degree of scrotum
  Burn of unspecified degree of testis

●■ **T21.07** Burn of unspecified degree of female genital region D, S 🪙
  Burn of unspecified degree of labium (majus) (minus)
  Burn of unspecified degree of perineum
  Burn of unspecified degree of vulva
  > **Excludes2**   burn of vagina (T28.3)

●■ **T21.09** Burn of unspecified degree of other site of trunk D, S 🪙

● **T21.1** **Burn of first degree of trunk**

> **Use additional** external cause code to identify the source, place and intent of the burn (X00-X19, X75-X77, X96-X98, Y92)

●■ **T21.10** Burn of first degree of trunk, unspecified site D, S 🪙

● **T21.11** Burn of first degree of chest wall D, S 🪙
  Burn of first degree of breast

● **T21.12** Burn of first degree of abdominal wall D, S 🪙
  Burn of first degree of flank
  Burn of first degree of groin

● **T21.13** Burn of first degree of upper back D, S 🪙
  Burn of first degree of interscapular region

● **T21.14** Burn of first degree of lower back D, S 🪙

● **T21.15** Burn of first degree of buttock D, S 🪙
  Burn of first degree of anus

● **T21.16** Burn of first degree of male genital region D, S 🪙
  Burn of first degree of penis
  Burn of first degree of scrotum
  Burn of first degree of testis

● **T21.17** Burn of first degree of female genital region D, S 🪙
  Burn of first degree of labium (majus) (minus)
  Burn of first degree of perineum
  Burn of first degree of vulva
  > **Excludes2**   burn of vagina (T28.3)

● **T21.19** Burn of first degree of other site of trunk D, S 🪙

● **T21.2** **Burn of second degree of trunk**

> **Use additional** external cause code to identify the source, place and intent of the burn (X00-X19, X75-X77, X96-X98, Y92)

●■ **T21.20** Burn of second degree of trunk, unspecified site D, S 🪙

● **T21.21** Burn of second degree of chest wall D, S 🪙
  Burn of second degree of breast

● **T21.22** Burn of second degree of abdominal wall D, S 🪙
  Burn of second degree of flank
  Burn of second degree of groin

● **T21.23** Burn of second degree of upper back D, S 🪙
  Burn of second degree of interscapular region

● **T21.24** Burn of second degree of lower back D, S 🪙

● **T21.25** Burn of second degree of buttock D, S 🪙
  Burn of second degree of anus

CHAPTER 19 (S00-T88)

● T21.26   **Burn of second degree of male genital region** D, S
     Burn of second degree of penis
     Burn of second degree of scrotum
     Burn of second degree of testis

● T21.27   **Burn of second degree of female genital region** D, S
     Burn of second degree of labium (majus) (minus)
     Burn of second degree of perineum
     Burn of second degree of vulva
     | Excludes2 | burn of vagina (T28.3)

● T21.29   **Burn of second degree of other site of trunk** D, S

● T21.3   **Burn of third degree of trunk**

     Use additional external cause code to identify the source, place and intent of the burn (X00-X19, X75-X77, X96-X98, Y92)

● T21.30   **Burn of third degree of trunk, unspecified site** A, D, S, A

● T21.31   **Burn of third degree of chest wall** A, D, S, A
     Burn of third degree of breast

● T21.32   **Burn of third degree of abdominal wall** A, D, S, A
     Burn of third degree of flank
     Burn of third degree of groin

● T21.33   **Burn of third degree of upper back** A, D, S, A
     Burn of third degree of interscapular region

● T21.34   **Burn of third degree of lower back** A, D, S, A

● T21.35   **Burn of third degree of buttock** A, D, S, A
     Burn of third degree of anus

● T21.36   **Burn of third degree of male genital region** A, D, S, A
     Burn of third degree of penis
     Burn of third degree of scrotum
     Burn of third degree of testis

● T21.37   **Burn of third degree of female genital region** A, D, S, A
     Burn of third degree of labium (majus) (minus)
     Burn of third degree of perineum
     Burn of third degree of vulva
     | Excludes2 | burn of vagina (T28.3)

● T21.39   **Burn of third degree of other site of trunk** A, D, S, A

● T21.4   **Corrosion of unspecified degree of trunk**

     Code first (T51-T65) to identify chemical and intent

     Use additional external cause code to identify place (Y92)

● T21.40   **Corrosion of unspecified degree of trunk, unspecified site** D, S

● T21.41   **Corrosion of unspecified degree of chest wall** D, S
     Corrosion of unspecified degree of breast

● T21.42   **Corrosion of unspecified degree of abdominal wall** D, S
     Corrosion of unspecified degree of flank
     Corrosion of unspecified degree of groin

● T21.43   **Corrosion of unspecified degree of upper back** D, S
     Corrosion of unspecified degree of interscapular region

● T21.44   **Corrosion of unspecified degree of lower back** D, S

● T21.45   **Corrosion of unspecified degree of buttock** D, S
     Corrosion of unspecified degree of anus

● T21.46   **Corrosion of unspecified degree of male genital region** D, S
     Corrosion of unspecified degree of penis
     Corrosion of unspecified degree of scrotum
     Corrosion of unspecified degree of testis

● T21.47   **Corrosion of unspecified degree of female genital region** D, S
     Corrosion of unspecified degree of labium (majus) (minus)
     Corrosion of unspecified degree of perineum
     Corrosion of unspecified degree of vulva
     | Excludes2 | corrosion of vagina (T28.8)

● T21.49   **Corrosion of unspecified degree of other site of trunk** D, S

● T21.5   **Corrosion of first degree of trunk**

     Code first (T51-T65) to identify chemical and intent

     Use additional external cause code to identify place (Y92)

● T21.50   **Corrosion of first degree of trunk, unspecified site** D, S

● T21.51   **Corrosion of first degree of chest wall** D, S
     Corrosion of first degree of breast

● T21.52   **Corrosion of first degree of abdominal wall** D, S
     Corrosion of first degree of flank
     Corrosion of first degree of groin

● T21.53   **Corrosion of first degree of upper back** D, S
     Corrosion of first degree of interscapular region

● T21.54   **Corrosion of first degree of lower back** D, S

● T21.55   **Corrosion of first degree of buttock** D, S
     Corrosion of first degree of anus

● T21.56   **Corrosion of first degree of male genital region** D, S
     Corrosion of first degree of penis
     Corrosion of first degree of scrotum
     Corrosion of first degree of testis

● T21.57   **Corrosion of first degree of female genital region** D, S
     Corrosion of first degree of labium (majus) (minus)
     Corrosion of first degree of perineum
     Corrosion of first degree of vulva
     | Excludes2 | corrosion of vagina (T28.8)

● T21.59   **Corrosion of first degree of other site of trunk** D, S

● T21.6   **Corrosion of second degree of trunk**

     Code first (T51-T65) to identify chemical and intent

     Use additional external cause code to identify place (Y92)

● T21.60   **Corrosion of second degree of trunk, unspecified site** D, S

● T21.61   **Corrosion of second degree of chest wall** D, S
     Corrosion of second degree of breast

● Unacceptable Principal Diagnosis   ● Use Additional Character(s)   ■ Unspecified   ▶ Manifestation Code

OGCR Official Guidelines for Coding and Reporting | Excludes 1 | | Excludes 2 | | Includes | | Use additional | | Code first | | Code also |

●●T21.62   **Corrosion of second degree of abdominal wall** D, S
    Corrosion of second degree of flank
    Corrosion of second degree of groin

●●T21.63   **Corrosion of second degree of upper back** D, S
    Corrosion of second degree of interscapular region

●●T21.64   **Corrosion of second degree of lower back** D, S

●●T21.65   **Corrosion of second degree of buttock** D, S
    Corrosion of second degree of anus

●●T21.66   **Corrosion of second degree of male genital region** D, S
    Corrosion of second degree of penis
    Corrosion of second degree of scrotum
    Corrosion of second degree of testis

●●T21.67   **Corrosion of second degree of female genital region** D, S
    Corrosion of second degree of labium (majus) (minus)
    Corrosion of second degree of perineum
    Corrosion of second degree of vulva
    Excludes2   corrosion of vagina (T28.8)

●●T21.69   **Corrosion of second degree of other site of trunk** D, S

●T21.7   **Corrosion of third degree of trunk**
    Code first (T51-T65) *to identify chemical and intent*
    Use additional external cause code to identify place (Y92)

●●■T21.70   **Corrosion of third degree of trunk, unspecified site** A, D, S, A

●●T21.71   **Corrosion of third degree of chest wall** A, D, S, A
    Corrosion of third degree of breast

●●T21.72   **Corrosion of third degree of abdominal wall** A, D, S, A
    Corrosion of third degree of flank
    Corrosion of third degree of groin

●●T21.73   **Corrosion of third degree of upper back** A, D, S, A
    Corrosion of third degree of interscapular region

●●T21.74   **Corrosion of third degree of lower back** A, D, S, A

●●T21.75   **Corrosion of third degree of buttock** A, D, S, A
    Corrosion of third degree of anus

●●T21.76   **Corrosion of third degree of male genital region** A, D, S, A
    Corrosion of third degree of penis
    Corrosion of third degree of scrotum
    Corrosion of third degree of testis

●●T21.77   **Corrosion of third degree of female genital region** A, D, S, A
    Corrosion of third degree of labium (majus) (minus)
    Corrosion of third degree of perineum
    Corrosion of third degree of vulva
    Excludes2   corrosion of vagina (T28.8)

●●T21.79   **Corrosion of third degree of other site of trunk** A, D, S, A

●T22   **Burn and corrosion of shoulder and upper limb, except wrist and hand**
    Excludes2   burn and corrosion of interscapular region (T21.-)
                 burn and corrosion of wrist and hand (T23.-)

The appropriate 7th character is to be added to each code from category T22

A	initial encounter
D	subsequent encounter
S	sequela

●●■T22.0   **Burn of unspecified degree of shoulder and upper limb, except wrist and hand**
    Use additional external cause code to identify the source, place and intent of the burn (X00-X19, X75-X77, X96-X98, Y92)

●●■T22.00   **Burn of unspecified degree of shoulder and upper limb, except wrist and hand, unspecified site** D, S

●T22.01   **Burn of unspecified degree of forearm**

●■T22.011   **Burn of unspecified degree of right forearm** D, S

●■T22.012   **Burn of unspecified degree of left forearm** D, S

●■T22.019   **Burn of unspecified degree of unspecified forearm** D, S

●T22.02   **Burn of unspecified degree of elbow**

●■T22.021   **Burn of unspecified degree of right elbow** D, S

●■T22.022   **Burn of unspecified degree of left elbow** D, S

●■T22.029   **Burn of unspecified degree of unspecified elbow** D, S

●T22.03   **Burn of unspecified degree of upper arm**

●■T22.031   **Burn of unspecified degree of right upper arm** D, S

●■T22.032   **Burn of unspecified degree of left upper arm** D, S

●■T22.039   **Burn of unspecified degree of unspecified upper arm** D, S

●T22.04   **Burn of unspecified degree of axilla**

●■T22.041   **Burn of unspecified degree of right axilla** D, S

●■T22.042   **Burn of unspecified degree of left axilla** D, S

●■T22.049   **Burn of unspecified degree of unspecified axilla** D, S

●T22.05   **Burn of unspecified degree of shoulder**

●■T22.051   **Burn of unspecified degree of right shoulder** D, S

●■T22.052   **Burn of unspecified degree of left shoulder** D, S

●■T22.059   **Burn of unspecified degree of unspecified shoulder** D, S

●T22.06   **Burn of unspecified degree of scapular region**

●■T22.061   **Burn of unspecified degree of right scapular region** D, S

●■T22.062   **Burn of unspecified degree of left scapular region** D, S

●■T22.069   **Burn of unspecified degree of unspecified scapular region** D, S

CHAPTER 19 (S00-T88)

● **T22.09** Burn of unspecified degree of multiple sites of shoulder and upper limb, except wrist and hand

   ● ◾ **T22.091** Burn of unspecified degree of multiple sites of right shoulder and upper limb, except wrist and hand D, S 🔖

   ● ◾ **T22.092** Burn of unspecified degree of multiple sites of left shoulder and upper limb, except wrist and hand D, S 🔖

   ● ◾ **T22.099** Burn of unspecified degree of multiple sites of unspecified shoulder and upper limb, except wrist and hand D, S 🔖

● **T22.1 Burn of first degree of shoulder and upper limb, except wrist and hand**

   Use additional external cause code to identify the source, place and intent of the burn (X00-X19, X75-X77, X96-X98, Y92)

  ● ◾ **T22.10** Burn of first degree of shoulder and upper limb, except wrist and hand, unspecified site D, S 🔖

  ● **T22.11** Burn of first degree of forearm

   ● **T22.111** Burn of first degree of right forearm D, S 🔖

   ● **T22.112** Burn of first degree of left forearm D, S 🔖

   ● ◾ **T22.119** Burn of first degree of unspecified forearm D, S 🔖

  ● **T22.12** Burn of first degree of elbow

   ● **T22.121** Burn of first degree of right elbow D, S 🔖

   ● **T22.122** Burn of first degree of left elbow D, S 🔖

   ● ◾ **T22.129** Burn of first degree of unspecified elbow D, S 🔖

  ● **T22.13** Burn of first degree of upper arm

   ● **T22.131** Burn of first degree of right upper arm D, S 🔖

   ● **T22.132** Burn of first degree of left upper arm D, S 🔖

   ● ◾ **T22.139** Burn of first degree of unspecified upper arm D, S 🔖

  ● **T22.14** Burn of first degree of axilla

   ● **T22.141** Burn of first degree of right axilla D, S 🔖

   ● **T22.142** Burn of first degree of left axilla D, S 🔖

   ● ◾ **T22.149** Burn of first degree of unspecified axilla D, S 🔖

  ● **T22.15** Burn of first degree of shoulder

   ● **T22.151** Burn of first degree of right shoulder D, S 🔖

   ● **T22.152** Burn of first degree of left shoulder D, S 🔖

   ● ◾ **T22.159** Burn of first degree of unspecified shoulder D, S 🔖

● **T22.16** Burn of first degree of scapular region

   ● **T22.161** Burn of first degree of right scapular region D, S 🔖

   ● **T22.162** Burn of first degree of left scapular region D, S 🔖

   ● ◾ **T22.169** Burn of first degree of unspecified scapular region D, S 🔖

● **T22.19** Burn of first degree of multiple sites of shoulder and upper limb, except wrist and hand

   ● **T22.191** Burn of first degree of multiple sites of right shoulder and upper limb, except wrist and hand D, S 🔖

   ● **T22.192** Burn of first degree of multiple sites of left shoulder and upper limb, except wrist and hand D, S 🔖

   ● ◾ **T22.199** Burn of first degree of multiple sites of unspecified shoulder and upper limb, except wrist and hand D, S 🔖

● **T22.2** Burn of second degree of shoulder and upper limb, except wrist and hand

   Use additional external cause code to identify the source, place and intent of the burn (X00-X19, X75-X77, X96-X98, Y92)

  ● ◾ **T22.20** Burn of second degree of shoulder and upper limb, except wrist and hand, unspecified site D, S 🔖

  ● **T22.21** Burn of second degree of forearm

   ● **T22.211** Burn of second degree of right forearm D, S 🔖

   ● **T22.212** Burn of second degree of left forearm D, S 🔖

   ● ◾ **T22.219** Burn of second degree of unspecified forearm D, S 🔖

  ● **T22.22** Burn of second degree of elbow

   ● **T22.221** Burn of second degree of right elbow D, S 🔖

   ● **T22.222** Burn of second degree of left elbow D, S 🔖

   ● ◾ **T22.229** Burn of second degree of unspecified elbow D, S 🔖

  ● **T22.23** Burn of second degree of upper arm

   ● **T22.231** Burn of second degree of right upper arm D, S 🔖

   ● **T22.232** Burn of second degree of left upper arm D, S 🔖

   ● ◾ **T22.239** Burn of second degree of unspecified upper arm D, S 🔖

  ● **T22.24** Burn of second degree of axilla

   ● **T22.241** Burn of second degree of right axilla D, S 🔖

   ● **T22.242** Burn of second degree of left axilla D, S 🔖

   ● ◾ **T22.249** Burn of second degree of unspecified axilla D, S 🔖

● Unacceptable Principal Diagnosis	● Use Additional Character(s)	◾ Unspecified	▶ Manifestation Code
OGCR Official Guidelines for Coding and Reporting	Excludes 1 Excludes 2	Includes Use additional	Code first Code also

● **T22.25 Burn of second degree of shoulder**
- ● **T22.251** Burn of second degree of right shoulder D, S
- ● **T22.252** Burn of second degree of left shoulder D, S
- ●■ **T22.259** Burn of second degree of unspecified shoulder D, S

● **T22.26 Burn of second degree of scapular region**
- ● **T22.261** Burn of second degree of right scapular region D, S
- ● **T22.262** Burn of second degree of left scapular region D, S
- ●■ **T22.269** Burn of second degree of unspecified scapular region D, S

● **T22.29 Burn of second degree of multiple sites of shoulder and upper limb, except wrist and hand**
- ● **T22.291** Burn of second degree of multiple sites of right shoulder and upper limb, except wrist and hand D, S
- ● **T22.292** Burn of second degree of multiple sites of left shoulder and upper limb, except wrist and hand D, S
- ●■ **T22.299** Burn of second degree of multiple sites of unspecified shoulder and upper limb, except wrist and hand D, S

● **T22.3 Burn of third degree of shoulder and upper limb, except wrist and hand**

> Use additional external cause code to identify the source, place and intent of the burn (X00-X19, X75-X77, X96-X98, Y92)

- ●■ **T22.30** Burn of third degree of shoulder and upper limb, except wrist and hand, unspecified site A, D, S, A

● **T22.31 Burn of third degree of forearm**
- ● **T22.311** Burn of third degree of right forearm A, D, S, A
- ● **T22.312** Burn of third degree of left forearm A, D, S, A
- ●■ **T22.319** Burn of third degree of unspecified forearm A, D, S, A

● **T22.32 Burn of third degree of elbow**
- ● **T22.321** Burn of third degree of right elbow A, D, S, A
- ● **T22.322** Burn of third degree of left elbow A, D, S, A
- ●■ **T22.329** Burn of third degree of unspecified elbow A, D, S, A

● **T22.33 Burn of third degree of upper arm**
- ● **T22.331** Burn of third degree of right upper arm A, D, S, A
- ● **T22.332** Burn of third degree of left upper arm A, D, S, A
- ●■ **T22.339** Burn of third degree of unspecified upper arm A, D, S, A

● **T22.34 Burn of third degree of axilla**
- ● **T22.341** Burn of third degree of right axilla A, D, S, A
- ● **T22.342** Burn of third degree of left axilla A, D, S, A
- ●■ **T22.349** Burn of third degree of unspecified axilla A, D, S, A

● **T22.35 Burn of third degree of shoulder**
- ● **T22.351** Burn of third degree of right shoulder A, D, S, A
- ● **T22.352** Burn of third degree of left shoulder A, D, S, A
- ●■ **T22.359** Burn of third degree of unspecified shoulder A, D, S, A

● **T22.36 Burn of third degree of scapular region**
- ● **T22.361** Burn of third degree of right scapular region A, D, S, A
- ● **T22.362** Burn of third degree of left scapular region A, D, S, A
- ●■ **T22.369** Burn of third degree of unspecified scapular region A, D, S, A

● **T22.39 Burn of third degree of multiple sites of shoulder and upper limb, except wrist and hand**
- ● **T22.391** Burn of third degree of multiple sites of right shoulder and upper limb, except wrist and hand A, D, S, A
- ● **T22.392** Burn of third degree of multiple sites of left shoulder and upper limb, except wrist and hand A, D, S, A
- ●■ **T22.399** Burn of third degree of multiple sites of unspecified shoulder and upper limb, except wrist and hand A, D, S, A

● **T22.4 Corrosion of unspecified degree of shoulder and upper limb, except wrist and hand**

> *Code first (T51-T65) to identify chemical and intent*
>
> Use additional external cause code to identify place (Y92)

- ●●■ **T22.40** Corrosion of unspecified degree of shoulder and upper limb, except wrist and hand, unspecified site D, S

● **T22.41 Corrosion of unspecified degree of forearm**
- ●●■ **T22.411** Corrosion of unspecified degree of right forearm D, S
- ●●■ **T22.412** Corrosion of unspecified degree of left forearm D, S
- ●●■ **T22.419** Corrosion of unspecified degree of unspecified forearm D, S

● **T22.42 Corrosion of unspecified degree of elbow**
- ●●■ **T22.421** Corrosion of unspecified degree of right elbow D, S
- ●●■ **T22.422** Corrosion of unspecified degree of left elbow D, S
- ●●■ **T22.429** Corrosion of unspecified degree of unspecified elbow D, S

N Newborn Age: 0   **P** Pediatric Age: 0–17   **M** Maternity DX: 12–55   **A** Adult Age: 15–124   ♀ Females Only   ♂ Males Only

Complication\Comorbidity   Major C\C   Present on Admission Requirement   Hospital-Acquired Condition

1595

CHAPTER 19 (S00-T88)

CHAPTER 19 (S00-T88)

● **T22.43** Corrosion of unspecified degree of upper arm
- ●●■ **T22.431** Corrosion of unspecified degree of right upper arm D, S 🔄
- ●●■ **T22.432** Corrosion of unspecified degree of left upper arm D, S 🔄
- ●●■ **T22.439** Corrosion of unspecified degree of unspecified upper arm D, S 🔄

● **T22.44** Corrosion of unspecified degree of axilla
- ●●■ **T22.441** Corrosion of unspecified degree of right axilla D, S 🔄
- ●●■ **T22.442** Corrosion of unspecified degree of left axilla D, S 🔄
- ●●■ **T22.449** Corrosion of unspecified degree of unspecified axilla D, S 🔄

● **T22.45** Corrosion of unspecified degree of shoulder
- ●●■ **T22.451** Corrosion of unspecified degree of right shoulder D, S 🔄
- ●●■ **T22.452** Corrosion of unspecified degree of left shoulder D, S 🔄
- ●●■ **T22.459** Corrosion of unspecified degree of unspecified shoulder D, S 🔄

● **T22.46** Corrosion of unspecified degree of scapular region
- ●●■ **T22.461** Corrosion of unspecified degree of right scapular region D, S 🔄
- ●●■ **T22.462** Corrosion of unspecified degree of left scapular region D, S 🔄
- ●●■ **T22.469** Corrosion of unspecified degree of unspecified scapular region D, S 🔄

● **T22.49** Corrosion of unspecified degree of multiple sites of shoulder and upper limb, except wrist and hand
- ●●■ **T22.491** Corrosion of unspecified degree of multiple sites of right shoulder and upper limb, except wrist and hand D, S 🔄
- ●●■ **T22.492** Corrosion of unspecified degree of multiple sites of left shoulder and upper limb, except wrist and hand D, S 🔄
- ●●■ **T22.499** Corrosion of unspecified degree of multiple sites of unspecified shoulder and upper limb, except wrist and hand D, S 🔄

● **T22.5** Corrosion of first degree of shoulder and upper limb, except wrist and hand

     Code first (T51-T65) to identify chemical and intent

     Use additional external cause code to identify place (Y92)

- ●●■ **T22.50** Corrosion of first degree of shoulder and upper limb, except wrist and hand unspecified site D, S 🔄
- ● **T22.51** Corrosion of first degree of forearm
  - ●● **T22.511** Corrosion of first degree of right forearm D, S 🔄
  - ●● **T22.512** Corrosion of first degree of left forearm D, S 🔄
  - ●●■ **T22.519** Corrosion of first degree of unspecified forearm D, S 🔄

● **T22.52** Corrosion of first degree of elbow
- ●● **T22.521** Corrosion of first degree of right elbow D, S 🔄
- ●● **T22.522** Corrosion of first degree of left elbow D, S 🔄
- ●●■ **T22.529** Corrosion of first degree of unspecified elbow D, S 🔄

● **T22.53** Corrosion of first degree of upper arm
- ●● **T22.531** Corrosion of first degree of right upper arm D, S 🔄
- ●● **T22.532** Corrosion of first degree of left upper arm D, S 🔄
- ●●■ **T22.539** Corrosion of first degree of unspecified upper arm D, S 🔄

● **T22.54** Corrosion of first degree of axilla
- ●● **T22.541** Corrosion of first degree of right axilla D, S 🔄
- ●● **T22.542** Corrosion of first degree of left axilla D, S 🔄
- ●●■ **T22.549** Corrosion of first degree of unspecified axilla D, S 🔄

● **T22.55** Corrosion of first degree of shoulder
- ●● **T22.551** Corrosion of first degree of right shoulder D, S 🔄
- ●● **T22.552** Corrosion of first degree of left shoulder D, S 🔄
- ●●■ **T22.559** Corrosion of first degree of unspecified shoulder D, S 🔄

● **T22.56** Corrosion of first degree of scapular region
- ●● **T22.561** Corrosion of first degree of right scapular region D, S 🔄
- ●● **T22.562** Corrosion of first degree of left scapular region D, S 🔄
- ●●■ **T22.569** Corrosion of first degree of unspecified scapular region D, S 🔄

● **T22.59** Corrosion of first degree of multiple sites of shoulder and upper limb, except wrist and hand
- ●● **T22.591** Corrosion of first degree of multiple sites of right shoulder and upper limb, except wrist and hand D, S 🔄
- ●● **T22.592** Corrosion of first degree of multiple sites of left shoulder and upper limb, except wrist and hand D, S 🔄
- ●●■ **T22.599** Corrosion of first degree of multiple sites of unspecified shoulder and upper limb, except wrist and hand D, S 🔄

● **T22.6** Corrosion of second degree of shoulder and upper limb, except wrist and hand

     Code first (T51-T65) to identify chemical and intent

     Use additional external cause code to identify place (Y92)

- ●●■ **T22.60** Corrosion of second degree of shoulder and upper limb, except wrist and hand, unspecified site D, S 🔄

● Unacceptable Principal Diagnosis   ● Use Additional Character(s)   ■ Unspecified   ▶ Manifestation Code

OGCR Official Guidelines for Coding and Reporting   Excludes 1   Excludes 2   Includes   Use additional   Code first   Code also

● **T22.61**   Corrosion of second degree of forearm
  ● ● **T22.611**   Corrosion of second degree of right forearm D, S 🖢
  ● ● **T22.612**   Corrosion of second degree of left forearm D, S 🖢
  ● ● ■ **T22.619**   Corrosion of second degree of unspecified forearm D, S 🖢

● **T22.62**   Corrosion of second degree of elbow
  ● ● **T22.621**   Corrosion of second degree of right elbow D, S 🖢
  ● ● **T22.622**   Corrosion of second degree of left elbow D, S 🖢
  ● ● ■ **T22.629**   Corrosion of second degree of unspecified elbow D, S 🖢

● **T22.63**   Corrosion of second degree of upper arm
  ● ● **T22.631**   Corrosion of second degree of right upper arm D, S 🖢
  ● ● **T22.632**   Corrosion of second degree of left upper arm D, S 🖢
  ● ● ■ **T22.639**   Corrosion of second degree of unspecified upper arm D, S 🖢

● **T22.64**   Corrosion of second degree of axilla
  ● ● **T22.641**   Corrosion of second degree of right axilla D, S 🖢
  ● ● **T22.642**   Corrosion of second degree of left axilla D, S 🖢
  ● ● ■ **T22.649**   Corrosion of second degree of unspecified axilla D, S 🖢

● **T22.65**   Corrosion of second degree of shoulder
  ● ● **T22.651**   Corrosion of second degree of right shoulder D, S 🖢
  ● ● **T22.652**   Corrosion of second degree of left shoulder D, S 🖢
  ● ● ■ **T22.659**   Corrosion of second degree of unspecified shoulder D, S 🖢

● **T22.66**   Corrosion of second degree of scapular region
  ● ● **T22.661**   Corrosion of second degree of right scapular region D, S 🖢
  ● ● **T22.662**   Corrosion of second degree of left scapular region D, S 🖢
  ● ● ■ **T22.669**   Corrosion of second degree of unspecified scapular region D, S 🖢

● **T22.69**   Corrosion of second degree of multiple sites of shoulder and upper limb, except wrist and hand
  ● ● **T22.691**   Corrosion of second degree of multiple sites of right shoulder and upper limb, except wrist and hand D, S 🖢
  ● ● **T22.692**   Corrosion of second degree of multiple sites of left shoulder and upper limb, except wrist and hand D, S 🖢
  ● ● ■ **T22.699**   Corrosion of second degree of multiple sites of unspecified shoulder and upper limb, except wrist and hand D, S 🖢

● **T22.7**   Corrosion of third degree of shoulder and upper limb, except wrist and hand
  Code first (T51-T65) to identify chemical and intent
  Use additional external cause code to identify place (Y92)
  ● ● ■ **T22.70**   Corrosion of third degree of shoulder and upper limb, except wrist and hand, unspecified site A 🖢, D, S 🖢, A 🖢

  ● **T22.71**   Corrosion of third degree of forearm
    ● ● **T22.711**   Corrosion of third degree of right forearm A 🖢, D, S 🖢, A 🖢
    ● ● **T22.712**   Corrosion of third degree of left forearm A 🖢, D, S 🖢, A 🖢
    ● ● ■ **T22.719**   Corrosion of third degree of unspecified forearm A 🖢, D, S 🖢, A 🖢

  ● **T22.72**   Corrosion of third degree of elbow
    ● ● **T22.721**   Corrosion of third degree of right elbow A 🖢, D, S 🖢, A 🖢
    ● ● **T22.722**   Corrosion of third degree of left elbow A 🖢, D, S 🖢, A 🖢
    ● ● ■ **T22.729**   Corrosion of third degree of unspecified elbow A 🖢, D, S 🖢, A 🖢

  ● **T22.73**   Corrosion of third degree of upper arm
    ● ● **T22.731**   Corrosion of third degree of right upper arm A 🖢, D, S 🖢, A 🖢
    ● ● **T22.732**   Corrosion of third degree of left upper arm A 🖢, D, S 🖢, A 🖢
    ● ● ■ **T22.739**   Corrosion of third degree of unspecified upper arm A 🖢, D, S 🖢, A 🖢

  ● **T22.74**   Corrosion of third degree of axilla
    ● ● **T22.741**   Corrosion of third degree of right axilla A 🖢, D, S 🖢, A 🖢
    ● ● **T22.742**   Corrosion of third degree of left axilla A 🖢, D, S 🖢, A 🖢
    ● ● ■ **T22.749**   Corrosion of third degree of unspecified axilla A 🖢, D, S 🖢, A 🖢

  ● **T22.75**   Corrosion of third degree of shoulder
    ● ● **T22.751**   Corrosion of third degree of right shoulder A 🖢, D, S 🖢, A 🖢
    ● ● **T22.752**   Corrosion of third degree of left shoulder A 🖢, D, S 🖢, A 🖢
    ● ● ■ **T22.759**   Corrosion of third degree of unspecified shoulder A 🖢, D, S 🖢, A 🖢

  ● **T22.76**   Corrosion of third degree of scapular region
    ● ● **T22.761**   Corrosion of third degree of right scapular region A 🖢, D, S 🖢, A 🖢
    ● ● **T22.762**   Corrosion of third degree of left scapular region A 🖢, D, S 🖢, A 🖢
    ● ● ■ **T22.769**   Corrosion of third degree of unspecified scapular region A 🖢, D, S 🖢, A 🖢

N Newborn Age: 0   **P** Pediatric Age: 0–17   **M** Maternity DX: 12–55   **A** Adult Age: 15–124   ♀ Females Only   ♂ Males Only

🖢 Complication\Comorbidity   🖢 Major C\C   Present on Admission Requirement   🖢 Hospital-Acquired Condition

1597

CHAPTER 19 (S00-T88)

● **T22.79** Corrosion of third degree of multiple sites of shoulder and upper limb, except wrist and hand

●● **T22.791** Corrosion of third degree of multiple sites of right shoulder and upper limb, except wrist and hand A 🖑, D, S 🖑, A 🖑

●● **T22.792** Corrosion of third degree of multiple sites of left shoulder and upper limb, except wrist and hand A 🖑, D, S 🖑, A 🖑

●●■ **T22.799** Corrosion of third degree of multiple sites of unspecified shoulder and upper limb, except wrist and hand A 🖑, D, S 🖑, A 🖑

● **T23** Burn and corrosion of wrist and hand

The appropriate 7th character is to be added to each code from category T23

A	initial encounter
D	subsequent encounter
S	sequela

● **T23.0** Burn of unspecified degree of wrist and hand

Use additional external cause code to identify the source, place and intent of the burn (X00-X19, X75-X77, X96-X98, Y92)

● **T23.00** Burn of unspecified degree of hand, unspecified site

●■ **T23.001** Burn of unspecified degree of right hand, unspecified site D, S 🖑

●■ **T23.002** Burn of unspecified degree of left hand, unspecified site D, S 🖑

●■ **T23.009** Burn of unspecified degree of unspecified hand, unspecified site D, S 🖑

● **T23.01** Burn of unspecified degree of thumb (nail)

●■ **T23.011** Burn of unspecified degree of right thumb (nail) D, S 🖑

●■ **T23.012** Burn of unspecified degree of left thumb (nail) D, S 🖑

●■ **T23.019** Burn of unspecified degree of unspecified thumb (nail) D, S 🖑

● **T23.02** Burn of unspecified degree of single finger (nail) except thumb

●■ **T23.021** Burn of unspecified degree of single right finger (nail) except thumb D, S 🖑

●■ **T23.022** Burn of unspecified degree of single left finger (nail) except thumb D, S 🖑

●■ **T23.029** Burn of unspecified degree of unspecified single finger (nail) except thumb D, S 🖑

● **T23.03** Burn of unspecified degree of multiple fingers (nail), not including thumb

●■ **T23.031** Burn of unspecified degree of multiple right fingers (nail), not including thumb D, S 🖑

●■ **T23.032** Burn of unspecified degree of multiple left fingers (nail), not including thumb D, S 🖑

●■ **T23.039** Burn of unspecified degree of unspecified multiple fingers (nail), not including thumb D, S 🖑

● **T23.04** Burn of unspecified degree of multiple fingers (nail), including thumb

●■ **T23.041** Burn of unspecified degree of multiple right fingers (nail), including thumb D, S 🖑

●■ **T23.042** Burn of unspecified degree of multiple left fingers (nail), including thumb D, S 🖑

●■ **T23.049** Burn of unspecified degree of unspecified multiple fingers (nail), including thumb D, S 🖑

● **T23.05** Burn of unspecified degree of palm

●■ **T23.051** Burn of unspecified degree of right palm D, S 🖑

●■ **T23.052** Burn of unspecified degree of left palm D, S 🖑

●■ **T23.059** Burn of unspecified degree of unspecified palm D, S 🖑

● **T23.06** Burn of unspecified degree of back of hand

●■ **T23.061** Burn of unspecified degree of back of right hand D, S 🖑

●■ **T23.062** Burn of unspecified degree of back of left hand D, S 🖑

●■ **T23.069** Burn of unspecified degree of back of unspecified hand D, S 🖑

● **T23.07** Burn of unspecified degree of wrist

●■ **T23.071** Burn of unspecified degree of right wrist D, S 🖑

●■ **T23.072** Burn of unspecified degree of left wrist D, S 🖑

●■ **T23.079** Burn of unspecified degree of unspecified wrist D, S 🖑

● **T23.09** Burn of unspecified degree of multiple sites of wrist and hand

●■ **T23.091** Burn of unspecified degree of multiple sites of right wrist and hand D, S 🖑

●■ **T23.092** Burn of unspecified degree of multiple sites of left wrist and hand D, S 🖑

●■ **T23.099** Burn of unspecified degree of multiple sites of unspecified wrist and hand D, S 🖑

● **T23.1** Burn of first degree of wrist and hand

Use additional external cause code to identify the source, place and intent of the burn (X00-X19, X75-X77, X96-X98, Y92)

● **T23.10** Burn of first degree of hand, unspecified site

●■ **T23.101** Burn of first degree of right hand, unspecified site D, S 🖑

●■ **T23.102** Burn of first degree of left hand, unspecified site D, S 🖑

●■ **T23.109** Burn of first degree of unspecified hand, unspecified site D, S 🖑

● **T23.11** Burn of first degree of thumb (nail)

● **T23.111** Burn of first degree of right thumb (nail) D, S 🖑

● **T23.112** Burn of first degree of left thumb (nail) D, S 🖑

●■ **T23.119** Burn of first degree of unspecified thumb (nail) D, S 🖑

● Unacceptable Principal Diagnosis   ● Use Additional Character(s)   ■ Unspecified   ▶ Manifestation Code

OGCR Official Guidelines for Coding and Reporting   Excludes 1   Excludes 2   Includes   Use additional   Code first   Code also

● **T23.12** **Burn of first degree of single finger (nail) except thumb**

   ● **T23.121** Burn of first degree of single right finger (nail) except thumb D, S ◎

   ● **T23.122** Burn of first degree of single left finger (nail) except thumb D, S ◎

   ●■ **T23.129** Burn of first degree of unspecified single finger (nail) except thumb D, S ◎

● **T23.13** **Burn of first degree of multiple fingers (nail), not including thumb**

   ● **T23.131** Burn of first degree of multiple right fingers (nail), not including thumb D, S ◎

   ● **T23.132** Burn of first degree of multiple left fingers (nail), not including thumb D, S ◎

   ●■ **T23.139** Burn of first degree of unspecified multiple fingers (nail), not including thumb D, S ◎

● **T23.14** **Burn of first degree of multiple fingers (nail), including thumb**

   ● **T23.141** Burn of first degree of multiple right fingers (nail), including thumb D, S ◎

   ● **T23.142** Burn of first degree of multiple left fingers (nail), including thumb D, S ◎

   ●■ **T23.149** Burn of first degree of unspecified multiple fingers (nail), including thumb D, S ◎

● **T23.15** **Burn of first degree of palm**

   ● **T23.151** Burn of first degree of right palm D, S ◎

   ● **T23.152** Burn of first degree of left palm D, S ◎

   ●■ **T23.159** Burn of first degree of unspecified palm D, S ◎

● **T23.16** **Burn of first degree of back of hand**

   ● **T23.161** Burn of first degree of back of right hand D, S ◎

   ● **T23.162** Burn of first degree of back of left hand D, S ◎

   ●■ **T23.169** Burn of first degree of back of unspecified hand D, S ◎

● **T23.17** **Burn of first degree of wrist**

   ● **T23.171** Burn of first degree of right wrist D, S ◎

   ● **T23.172** Burn of first degree of left wrist D, S ◎

   ●■ **T23.179** Burn of first degree of unspecified wrist D, S ◎

● **T23.19** **Burn of first degree of multiple sites of wrist and hand**

   ● **T23.191** Burn of first degree of multiple sites of right wrist and hand D, S ◎

   ● **T23.192** Burn of first degree of multiple sites of left wrist and hand D, S ◎

   ●■ **T23.199** Burn of first degree of multiple sites of unspecified wrist and hand D, S ◎

● **T23.2** **Burn of second degree of wrist and hand**

   Use additional external cause code to identify the source, place and intent of the burn (X00-X19, X75-X77, X96-X98, Y92)

   ● **T23.20** Burn of second degree of hand, unspecified site

     ●■ **T23.201** Burn of second degree of right hand, unspecified site D, S ◎

     ●■ **T23.202** Burn of second degree of left hand, unspecified site D, S ◎

     ●■ **T23.209** Burn of second degree of unspecified hand, unspecified site D, S ◎

   ● **T23.21** Burn of second degree of thumb (nail)

     ● **T23.211** Burn of second degree of right thumb (nail) D, S ◎

     ● **T23.212** Burn of second degree of left thumb (nail) D, S ◎

     ●■ **T23.219** Burn of second degree of unspecified thumb (nail) D, S ◎

   ● **T23.22** Burn of second degree of single finger (nail) except thumb

     ● **T23.221** Burn of second degree of single right finger (nail) except thumb D, S ◎

     ● **T23.222** Burn of second degree of single left finger (nail) except thumb D, S ◎

     ●■ **T23.229** Burn of second degree of unspecified single finger (nail) except thumb D, S ◎

   ● **T23.23** Burn of second degree of multiple fingers (nail), not including thumb

     ● **T23.231** Burn of second degree of multiple right fingers (nail), not including thumb D, S ◎

     ● **T23.232** Burn of second degree of multiple left fingers (nail), not including thumb D, S ◎

     ●■ **T23.239** Burn of second degree of unspecified multiple fingers (nail), not including thumb D, S ◎

   ● **T23.24** Burn of second degree of multiple fingers (nail), including thumb

     ● **T23.241** Burn of second degree of multiple right fingers (nail), including thumb D, S ◎

     ● **T23.242** Burn of second degree of multiple left fingers (nail), including thumb D, S ◎

     ●■ **T23.249** Burn of second degree of unspecified multiple fingers (nail), including thumb D, S ◎

   ● **T23.25** Burn of second degree of palm

     ● **T23.251** Burn of second degree of right palm D, S ◎

     ● **T23.252** Burn of second degree of left palm D, S ◎

     ●■ **T23.259** Burn of second degree of unspecified palm D, S ◎

CHAPTER 19 (S00-T88)

● T23.26   Burn of second degree of back of hand

   ● T23.261   Burn of second degree of back of right hand D, S

   ● T23.262   Burn of second degree of back of left hand D, S

   ● ■ T23.269   Burn of second degree of back of unspecified hand D, S

● T23.27   Burn of second degree of wrist

   ● T23.271   Burn of second degree of right wrist D, S

   ● T23.272   Burn of second degree of left wrist D, S

   ● ■ T23.279   Burn of second degree of unspecified wrist D, S

● T23.29   Burn of second degree of multiple sites of wrist and hand

   ● T23.291   Burn of second degree of multiple sites of right wrist and hand D, S

   ● T23.292   Burn of second degree of multiple sites of left wrist and hand D, S

   ● ■ T23.299   Burn of second degree of multiple sites of unspecified wrist and hand D, S

● T23.3   Burn of third degree of wrist and hand

   Use additional external cause code to identify the source, place and intent of the burn (X00-X19, X75-X77, X96-X98, Y92)

● T23.30   Burn of third degree of hand, unspecified site

   ● ■ T23.301   Burn of third degree of right hand, unspecified site A, D, S, A

   ● ■ T23.302   Burn of third degree of left hand, unspecified site A, D, S, A

   ● ■ T23.309   Burn of third degree of unspecified hand, unspecified site A, D, S, A

● T23.31   Burn of third degree of thumb (nail)

   ● T23.311   Burn of third degree of right thumb (nail) A, D, S, A

   ● T23.312   Burn of third degree of left thumb (nail) A, D, S, A

   ● ■ T23.319   Burn of third degree of unspecified thumb (nail) A, D, S, A

● T23.32   Burn of third degree of single finger (nail) except thumb

   ● T23.321   Burn of third degree of single right finger (nail) except thumb A, D, S, A

   ● T23.322   Burn of third degree of single left finger (nail) except thumb A, D, S, A

   ● ■ T23.329   Burn of third degree of unspecified single finger (nail) except thumb A, D, S, A

● T23.33   Burn of third degree of multiple fingers (nail), not including thumb

   ● T23.331   Burn of third degree of multiple right fingers (nail), not including thumb A, D, S, A

   ● T23.332   Burn of third degree of multiple left fingers (nail), not including thumb A, D, S, A

   ● ■ T23.339   Burn of third degree of unspecified multiple fingers (nail), not including thumb A, D, S, A

● T23.34   Burn of third degree of multiple fingers (nail), including thumb

   ● T23.341   Burn of third degree of multiple right fingers (nail), including thumb A, D, S, A

   ● T23.342   Burn of third degree of multiple left fingers (nail), including thumb A, D, S, A

   ● ■ T23.349   Burn of third degree of unspecified multiple fingers (nail), including thumb A, D, S, A

● T23.35   Burn of third degree of palm

   ● T23.351   Burn of third degree of right palm A, D, S, A

   ● T23.352   Burn of third degree of left palm A, D, S, A

   ● ■ T23.359   Burn of third degree of unspecified palm A, D, S, A

● T23.36   Burn of third degree of back of hand

   ● T23.361   Burn of third degree of back of right hand A, D, S, A

   ● T23.362   Burn of third degree of back of left hand A, D, S, A

   ● ■ T23.369   Burn of third degree of back of unspecified hand A, D, S, A

● T23.37   Burn of third degree of wrist

   ● T23.371   Burn of third degree of right wrist A, D, S, A

   ● T23.372   Burn of third degree of left wrist A, D, S, A

   ● ■ T23.379   Burn of third degree of unspecified wrist A, D, S, A

● T23.39   Burn of third degree of multiple sites of wrist and hand

   ● T23.391   Burn of third degree of multiple sites of right wrist and hand A, D, S, A

   ● T23.392   Burn of third degree of multiple sites of left wrist and hand A, D, S, A

   ● ■ T23.399   Burn of third degree of multiple sites of unspecified wrist and hand A, D, S, A

● Unacceptable Principal Diagnosis	● Use Additional Character(s)	■ Unspecified	▶ Manifestation Code
OGCR Official Guidelines for Coding and Reporting	Excludes 1 Excludes 2	Includes Use additional	Code first Code also

●**T23.4 Corrosion of unspecified degree of wrist and hand**

Code first (T51-T65) to identify chemical and intent

Use additional external cause code to identify place (Y92)

●**T23.40 Corrosion of unspecified degree of hand, unspecified site**

●●■**T23.401 Corrosion of unspecified degree of right hand, unspecified site** D, S ◉

●●■**T23.402 Corrosion of unspecified degree of left hand, unspecified site** D, S ◉

●●■**T23.409 Corrosion of unspecified degree of unspecified hand, unspecified site** D, S ◉

●**T23.41 Corrosion of unspecified degree of thumb (nail)**

●●**T23.411 Corrosion of unspecified degree of right thumb (nail)** D, S ◉

●●**T23.412 Corrosion of unspecified degree of left thumb (nail)** D, S ◉

●●**T23.419 Corrosion of unspecified degree of unspecified thumb (nail)** D, S ◉

●**T23.42 Corrosion of unspecified degree of single finger (nail) except thumb**

●●■**T23.421 Corrosion of unspecified degree of single right finger (nail) except thumb** D, S ◉

●●■**T23.422 Corrosion of unspecified degree of single left finger (nail) except thumb** D, S ◉

●●■**T23.429 Corrosion of unspecified degree of unspecified single finger (nail) except thumb** D, S ◉

●**T23.43 Corrosion of unspecified degree of multiple fingers (nail), not including thumb**

●●■**T23.431 Corrosion of unspecified degree of multiple right fingers (nail), not including thumb** D, S ◉

●●■**T23.432 Corrosion of unspecified degree of multiple left fingers (nail), not including thumb** D, S ◉

●●■**T23.439 Corrosion of unspecified degree of unspecified multiple fingers (nail), not including thumb** D, S ◉

●**T23.44 Corrosion of unspecified degree of multiple fingers (nail), including thumb**

●●■**T23.441 Corrosion of unspecified degree of multiple right fingers (nail), including thumb** D, S ◉

●●■**T23.442 Corrosion of unspecified degree of multiple left fingers (nail), including thumb** D, S ◉

●●■**T23.449 Corrosion of unspecified degree of unspecified multiple fingers (nail), including thumb** D, S ◉

●**T23.45 Corrosion of unspecified degree of palm**

●●■**T23.451 Corrosion of unspecified degree of right palm** D, S ◉

●●■**T23.452 Corrosion of unspecified degree of left palm** D, S ◉

●●■**T23.459 Corrosion of unspecified degree of unspecified palm** D, S ◉

●**T23.46 Corrosion of unspecified degree of back of hand**

●●■**T23.461 Corrosion of unspecified degree of back of right hand** D, S ◉

●●■**T23.462 Corrosion of unspecified degree of back of left hand** D, S ◉

●●■**T23.469 Corrosion of unspecified degree of back of unspecified hand** D, S ◉

●**T23.47 Corrosion of unspecified degree of wrist**

●●■**T23.471 Corrosion of unspecified degree of right wrist** D, S ◉

●●■**T23.472 Corrosion of unspecified degree of left wrist** D, S ◉

●●■**T23.479 Corrosion of unspecified degree of unspecified wrist** D, S ◉

●**T23.49 Corrosion of unspecified degree of multiple sites of wrist and hand**

●●■**T23.491 Corrosion of unspecified degree of multiple sites of right wrist and hand** D, S ◉

●●■**T23.492 Corrosion of unspecified degree of multiple sites of left wrist and hand** D, S ◉

●●■**T23.499 Corrosion of unspecified degree of multiple sites of unspecified wrist and hand** D, S ◉

●**T23.5 Corrosion of first degree of wrist and hand**

Code first (T51-T65) to identify chemical and intent

Use additional external cause code to identify place (Y92)

●**T23.50 Corrosion of first degree of hand, unspecified site**

●●■**T23.501 Corrosion of first degree of right hand, unspecified site** D, S ◉

●●■**T23.502 Corrosion of first degree of left hand, unspecified site** D, S ◉

●●■**T23.509 Corrosion of first degree of unspecified hand, unspecified site** D, S ◉

●**T23.51 Corrosion of first degree of thumb (nail)**

●●**T23.511 Corrosion of first degree of right thumb (nail)** D, S ◉

●●**T23.512 Corrosion of first degree of left thumb (nail)** D, S ◉

●●■**T23.519 Corrosion of first degree of unspecified thumb (nail)** D, S ◉

●**T23.52 Corrosion of first degree of single finger (nail) except thumb**

●●**T23.521 Corrosion of first degree of single right finger (nail) except thumb** D, S ◉

●●**T23.522 Corrosion of first degree of single left finger (nail) except thumb** D, S ◉

●●■**T23.529 Corrosion of first degree of unspecified single finger (nail) except thumb** D, S ◉

●**T23.53 Corrosion of first degree of multiple fingers (nail), not including thumb**

●●**T23.531 Corrosion of first degree of multiple right fingers (nail), not including thumb** D, S ◉

●● **T23.532** Corrosion of first degree of multiple left fingers (nail), not including thumb D, S ◌

●● **T23.539** Corrosion of first degree of unspecified multiple fingers (nail), not including thumb D, S ◌

● **T23.54** Corrosion of first degree of multiple fingers (nail), including thumb

●● **T23.541** Corrosion of first degree of multiple right fingers (nail), including thumb D, S ◌

●● **T23.542** Corrosion of first degree of multiple left fingers (nail), including thumb D, S ◌

●●■ **T23.549** Corrosion of first degree of unspecified multiple fingers (nail), including thumb D, S ◌

● **T23.55** Corrosion of first degree of palm

●● **T23.551** Corrosion of first degree of right palm D, S ◌

●● **T23.552** Corrosion of first degree of left palm D, S ◌

●●■ **T23.559** Corrosion of first degree of unspecified palm D, S ◌

● **T23.56** Corrosion of first degree of back of hand

●● **T23.561** Corrosion of first degree of back of right hand D, S ◌

●● **T23.562** Corrosion of first degree of back of left hand D, S ◌

●●■ **T23.569** Corrosion of first degree of back of unspecified hand D, S ◌

● **T23.57** Corrosion of first degree of wrist

●● **T23.571** Corrosion of first degree of right wrist D, S ◌

●● **T23.572** Corrosion of first degree of left wrist D, S ◌

●●■ **T23.579** Corrosion of first degree of unspecified wrist D, S ◌

● **T23.59** Corrosion of first degree of multiple sites of wrist and hand

●● **T23.591** Corrosion of first degree of multiple sites of right wrist and hand D, S ◌

●● **T23.592** Corrosion of first degree of multiple sites of left wrist and hand D, S ◌

●●■ **T23.599** Corrosion of first degree of multiple sites of unspecified wrist and hand D, S ◌

● **T23.6** Corrosion of second degree of wrist and hand

Code first (T51-T65) *to identify chemical and intent*

Use additional external cause code to identify place (Y92)

● **T23.60** Corrosion of second degree of hand, unspecified site

●●■ **T23.601** Corrosion of second degree of right hand, unspecified site D, S ◌

●●■ **T23.602** Corrosion of second degree of left hand, unspecified site D, S ◌

●●■ **T23.609** Corrosion of second degree of unspecified hand, unspecified site D, S ◌

● **T23.61** Corrosion of second degree of thumb (nail)

●● **T23.611** Corrosion of second degree of right thumb (nail) D, S ◌

●● **T23.612** Corrosion of second degree of left thumb (nail) D, S ◌

●●■ **T23.619** Corrosion of second degree of unspecified thumb (nail) D, S ◌

● **T23.62** Corrosion of second degree of single finger (nail) except thumb

●● **T23.621** Corrosion of second degree of single right finger (nail) except thumb D, S ◌

●● **T23.622** Corrosion of second degree of single left finger (nail) except thumb D, S ◌

●●■ **T23.629** Corrosion of second degree of unspecified single finger (nail) except thumb D, S ◌

● **T23.63** Corrosion of second degree of multiple fingers (nail), not including thumb

●● **T23.631** Corrosion of second degree of multiple right fingers (nail), not including thumb D, S ◌

●● **T23.632** Corrosion of second degree of multiple left fingers (nail), not including thumb D, S ◌

●●■ **T23.639** Corrosion of second degree of unspecified multiple fingers (nail), not including thumb D, S ◌

● **T23.64** Corrosion of second degree of multiple fingers (nail), including thumb

●● **T23.641** Corrosion of second degree of multiple right fingers (nail), including thumb D, S ◌

●● **T23.642** Corrosion of second degree of multiple left fingers (nail), including thumb D, S ◌

●●■ **T23.649** Corrosion of second degree of unspecified multiple fingers (nail), including thumb D, S ◌

● **T23.65** Corrosion of second degree of palm

●● **T23.651** Corrosion of second degree of right palm D, S ◌

●● **T23.652** Corrosion of second degree of left palm D, S ◌

●●■ **T23.659** Corrosion of second degree of unspecified palm D, S ◌

● **T23.66** Corrosion of second degree of back of hand

●● **T23.661** Corrosion of second degree back of right hand D, S ◌

●● **T23.662** Corrosion of second degree back of left hand D, S ◌

●●■ **T23.669** Corrosion of second degree back of unspecified hand D, S ◌

● **T23.67** Corrosion of second degree of wrist

●● **T23.671** Corrosion of second degree of right wrist D, S ◌

●● **T23.672** Corrosion of second degree of left wrist D, S ◌

●●■ **T23.679** Corrosion of second degree of unspecified wrist D, S ◌

● Unacceptable Principal Diagnosis   ● Use Additional Character(s)   ■ Unspecified   ▶ Manifestation Code

1602   **OGCR** Official Guidelines for Coding and Reporting   Excludes 1   Excludes 2   Includes   Use additional   Code first   Code also

● **T23.69** Corrosion of second degree of multiple sites of wrist and hand

   ●● **T23.691** Corrosion of second degree of multiple sites of right wrist and hand D, S 🔖

   ●● **T23.692** Corrosion of second degree of multiple sites of left wrist and hand D, S 🔖

   ●●◻ **T23.699** Corrosion of second degree of multiple sites of unspecified wrist and hand D, S 🔖

● **T23.7** Corrosion of third degree of wrist and hand

   Code first (T51-T65) *to identify chemical and intent*

   Use additional external cause code to identify place (Y92)

  ● **T23.70** Corrosion of third degree of hand, unspecified site

   ●●◻ **T23.701** Corrosion of third degree of right hand, unspecified site A 🔖, D, S 🔖, A 🔖

   ●●◻ **T23.702** Corrosion of third degree of left hand, unspecified site A 🔖, D, S 🔖, A 🔖

   ●●◻ **T23.709** Corrosion of third degree of unspecified hand, unspecified site A 🔖, D, S 🔖, A 🔖

  ● **T23.71** Corrosion of third degree of thumb (nail)

   ●● **T23.711** Corrosion of third degree of right thumb (nail) A 🔖, D, S 🔖, A 🔖

   ●● **T23.712** Corrosion of third degree of left thumb (nail) A 🔖, D, S 🔖, A 🔖

   ●●◻ **T23.719** Corrosion of third degree of unspecified thumb (nail) A 🔖, D, S 🔖, A 🔖

  ● **T23.72** Corrosion of third degree of single finger (nail) except thumb

   ●● **T23.721** Corrosion of third degree of single right finger (nail) except thumb A 🔖, D, S 🔖, A 🔖

   ●● **T23.722** Corrosion of third degree of single left finger (nail) except thumb A 🔖, D, S 🔖, A 🔖

   ●●◻ **T23.729** Corrosion of third degree of unspecified single finger (nail) except thumb A 🔖, D, S 🔖, A 🔖

  ● **T23.73** Corrosion of third degree of multiple fingers (nail), not including thumb

   ●● **T23.731** Corrosion of third degree of multiple right fingers (nail), not including thumb A 🔖, D, S 🔖, A 🔖

   ●● **T23.732** Corrosion of third degree of multiple left fingers (nail), not including thumb A 🔖, D, S 🔖, A 🔖

   ●●◻ **T23.739** Corrosion of third degree of unspecified multiple fingers (nail), not including thumb A 🔖, D, S 🔖, A 🔖

  ● **T23.74** Corrosion of third degree of multiple fingers (nail), including thumb

   ●● **T23.741** Corrosion of third degree of multiple right fingers (nail), including thumb A 🔖, D, S 🔖, A 🔖

   ●● **T23.742** Corrosion of third degree of multiple left fingers (nail), including thumb A 🔖, D, S 🔖, A 🔖

   ●●◻ **T23.749** Corrosion of third degree of unspecified multiple fingers (nail), including thumb A 🔖, D, S 🔖, A 🔖

  ● **T23.75** Corrosion of third degree of palm

   ●● **T23.751** Corrosion of third degree of right palm A 🔖, D, S 🔖, A 🔖

   ●● **T23.752** Corrosion of third degree of left palm A 🔖, D, S 🔖, A 🔖

   ●●◻ **T23.759** Corrosion of third degree of unspecified palm A 🔖, D, S 🔖, A 🔖

  ● **T23.76** Corrosion of third degree of back of hand

   ●● **T23.761** Corrosion of third degree of back of right hand A 🔖, D, S 🔖, A 🔖

   ●● **T23.762** Corrosion of third degree of back of left hand A 🔖, D, S 🔖, A 🔖

   ●●◻ **T23.769** Corrosion of third degree of back of unspecified hand A 🔖, D, S 🔖, A 🔖

  ● **T23.77** Corrosion of third degree of wrist

   ●● **T23.771** Corrosion of third degree of right wrist A 🔖, D, S 🔖, A 🔖

   ●● **T23.772** Corrosion of third degree of left wrist A 🔖, D, S 🔖, A 🔖

   ●●◻ **T23.779** Corrosion of third degree of unspecified wrist A 🔖, D, S 🔖, A 🔖

  ● **T23.79** Corrosion of third degree of multiple sites of wrist and hand

   ●● **T23.791** Corrosion of third degree of multiple sites of right wrist and hand A 🔖, D, S 🔖, A 🔖

   ●● **T23.792** Corrosion of third degree of multiple sites of left wrist and hand A 🔖, D, S 🔖, A 🔖

   ●●◻ **T23.799** Corrosion of third degree of multiple sites of unspecified wrist and hand A 🔖, D, S 🔖, A 🔖

● **T24** Burn and corrosion of lower limb, except ankle and foot

   Excludes2   burn and corrosion of ankle and foot (T25.-)
                     burn and corrosion of hip region (T21.-)

   The appropriate 7th character is to be added to each code from category T24

A	initial encounter
D	subsequent encounter
S	sequela

  ● **T24.0** Burn of unspecified degree of lower limb, except ankle and foot

   Use additional external cause code to identify the source, place and intent of the burn (X00-X19, X75-X77, X96-X98, Y92)

  ● **T24.00** Burn of unspecified degree of unspecified site of lower limb, except ankle and foot

   ●◻ **T24.001** Burn of unspecified degree of unspecified site of right lower limb, except ankle and foot D, S 🔖

● ■ **T24.002** Burn of unspecified degree of unspecified site of left lower limb, except ankle and foot D, S 🔖

● ■ **T24.009** Burn of unspecified degree of unspecified site of unspecified lower limb, except ankle and foot D, S 🔖

● **T24.01** Burn of unspecified degree of thigh

　● ■ **T24.011** Burn of unspecified degree of right thigh D, S 🔖

　● ■ **T24.012** Burn of unspecified degree of left thigh D, S 🔖

　● ■ **T24.019** Burn of unspecified degree of unspecified thigh D, S 🔖

● **T24.02** Burn of unspecified degree of knee

　● ■ **T24.021** Burn of unspecified degree of right knee D, S 🔖

　● ■ **T24.022** Burn of unspecified degree of left knee D, S 🔖

　● ■ **T24.029** Burn of unspecified degree of unspecified knee D, S 🔖

● **T24.03** Burn of unspecified degree of lower leg

　● ■ **T24.031** Burn of unspecified degree of right lower leg D, S 🔖

　● ■ **T24.032** Burn of unspecified degree of left lower leg D, S 🔖

　● ■ **T24.039** Burn of unspecified degree of unspecified lower leg D, S 🔖

● **T24.09** Burn of unspecified degree of multiple sites of lower limb, except ankle and foot

　● ■ **T24.091** Burn of unspecified degree of multiple sites of right lower limb, except ankle and foot D, S 🔖

　● ■ **T24.092** Burn of unspecified degree of multiple sites of left lower limb, except ankle and foot D, S 🔖

　● ■ **T24.099** Burn of unspecified degree of multiple sites of unspecified lower limb, except ankle and foot D, S 🔖

● **T24.1** Burn of first degree of lower limb, except ankle and foot

　Use additional external cause code to identify the source, place and intent of the burn (X00-X19, X75-X77, X96-X98, Y92)

　● **T24.10** Burn of first degree of unspecified site of lower limb, except ankle and foot

　　● ■ **T24.101** Burn of first degree of unspecified site of right lower limb, except ankle and foot D, S 🔖

　　● ■ **T24.102** Burn of first degree of unspecified site of left lower limb, except ankle and foot D, S 🔖

　　● ■ **T24.109** Burn of first degree of unspecified site of unspecified lower limb, except ankle and foot D, S 🔖

● **T24.11** Burn of first degree of thigh

　● **T24.111** Burn of first degree of right thigh D, S 🔖

　● **T24.112** Burn of first degree of left thigh D, S 🔖

　● ■ **T24.119** Burn of first degree of unspecified thigh D, S 🔖

● **T24.12** Burn of first degree of knee

　● **T24.121** Burn of first degree of right knee D, S 🔖

　● **T24.122** Burn of first degree of left knee D, S 🔖

　● ■ **T24.129** Burn of first degree of unspecified knee D, S 🔖

● **T24.13** Burn of first degree of lower leg

　● **T24.131** Burn of first degree of right lower leg D, S 🔖

　● **T24.132** Burn of first degree of left lower leg D, S 🔖

　● ■ **T24.139** Burn of first degree of unspecified lower leg D, S 🔖

● **T24.19** Burn of first degree of multiple sites of lower limb, except ankle and foot

　● **T24.191** Burn of first degree of multiple sites of right lower limb, except ankle and foot D, S 🔖

　● **T24.192** Burn of first degree of multiple sites of left lower limb, except ankle and foot D, S 🔖

　● ■ **T24.199** Burn of first degree of multiple sites of unspecified lower limb, except ankle and foot D, S 🔖

● **T24.2** Burn of second degree of lower limb, except ankle and foot

　Use additional external cause code to identify the source, place and intent of the burn (X00-X19, X75-X77, X96-X98, Y92)

　● **T24.20** Burn of second degree of unspecified site of lower limb, except ankle and foot

　　● ■ **T24.201** Burn of second degree of unspecified site of right lower limb, except ankle and foot D, S 🔖

　　● ■ **T24.202** Burn of second degree of unspecified site of left lower limb, except ankle and foot D, S 🔖

　　● ■ **T24.209** Burn of second degree of unspecified site of unspecified lower limb, except ankle and foot D, S 🔖

● **T24.21** Burn of second degree of thigh

　● **T24.211** Burn of second degree of right thigh D, S 🔖

　● **T24.212** Burn of second degree of left thigh D, S 🔖

　● ■ **T24.219** Burn of second degree of unspecified thigh D, S 🔖

● **T24.22** Burn of second degree of knee

　● **T24.221** Burn of second degree of right knee D, S 🔖

　● **T24.222** Burn of second degree of left knee D, S 🔖

　● ■ **T24.229** Burn of second degree of unspecified knee D, S 🔖

● Unacceptable Principal Diagnosis　　● Use Additional Character(s)　　■ Unspecified　　▶ Manifestation Code

OGCR Official Guidelines for Coding and Reporting　　Excludes 1　　Excludes 2　　Includes　　Use additional　　Code first　　Code also

● **T24.23**   **Burn of second degree of lower leg**

     ● **T24.231**   **Burn of second degree of right lower leg** D, S 🗓

     ● **T24.232**   **Burn of second degree of left lower leg** D, S 🗓

     ●■ **T24.239**   **Burn of second degree of unspecified lower leg** D, S 🗓

● **T24.29**   **Burn of second degree of multiple sites of lower limb, except ankle and foot**

     ● **T24.291**   **Burn of second degree of multiple sites of right lower limb, except ankle and foot** D, S 🗓

     ● **T24.292**   **Burn of second degree of multiple sites of left lower limb, except ankle and foot** D, S 🗓

     ●■ **T24.299**   **Burn of second degree of multiple sites of unspecified lower limb, except ankle and foot** D, S 🗓

● **T24.3**   **Burn of third degree of lower limb, except ankle and foot**

     Use additional external cause code to identify the source, place and intent of the burn (X00-X19, X75-X77, X96-X98, Y92)

     ● **T24.30**   **Burn of third degree of unspecified site of lower limb, except ankle and foot**

         ●■ **T24.301**   **Burn of third degree of unspecified site of right lower limb, except ankle and foot** A 🗓, D, S 🗓, A 🗓

         ●■ **T24.302**   **Burn of third degree of unspecified site of left lower limb, except ankle and foot** A 🗓, D, S 🗓, A 🗓

         ●■ **T24.309**   **Burn of third degree of unspecified site of unspecified lower limb, except ankle and foot** A 🗓, D, S 🗓, A 🗓

     ● **T24.31**   **Burn of third degree of thigh**

         ● **T24.311**   **Burn of third degree of right thigh** A 🗓, D, S 🗓, A 🗓

         ● **T24.312**   **Burn of third degree of left thigh** A 🗓, D, S 🗓, A 🗓

         ●■ **T24.319**   **Burn of third degree of unspecified thigh** A 🗓, D, S 🗓, A 🗓

     ● **T24.32**   **Burn of third degree of knee**

         ● **T24.321**   **Burn of third degree of right knee** A 🗓, D, S 🗓, A 🗓

         ● **T24.322**   **Burn of third degree of left knee** A 🗓, D, S 🗓, A 🗓

         ●■ **T24.329**   **Burn of third degree of unspecified knee** A 🗓, D, S 🗓, A 🗓

     ● **T24.33**   **Burn of third degree of lower leg**

         ● **T24.331**   **Burn of third degree of right lower leg** A 🗓, D, S 🗓, A 🗓

         ● **T24.332**   **Burn of third degree of left lower leg** A 🗓, D, S 🗓, A 🗓

         ●■ **T24.339**   **Burn of third degree of unspecified lower leg** A 🗓, D, S 🗓, A 🗓

● **T24.39**   **Burn of third degree of multiple sites of lower limb, except ankle and foot**

     ● **T24.391**   **Burn of third degree of multiple sites of right lower limb, except ankle and foot** A 🗓, D, S 🗓, A 🗓

     ● **T24.392**   **Burn of third degree of multiple sites of left lower limb, except ankle and foot** A 🗓, D, S 🗓, A 🗓

     ●■ **T24.399**   **Burn of third degree of multiple sites of unspecified lower limb, except ankle and foot** A 🗓, D, S 🗓, A 🗓

● **T24.4**   **Corrosion of unspecified degree of lower limb, except ankle and foot**

     Code first (T51-T65) *to identify chemical and intent*

     Use additional external cause code to identify place (Y92)

     ● **T24.40**   **Corrosion of unspecified degree of unspecified site of lower limb, except ankle and foot**

         ●●■ **T24.401**   **Corrosion of unspecified degree of unspecified site of right lower limb, except ankle and foot** D, S 🗓

         ●●■ **T24.402**   **Corrosion of unspecified degree of unspecified site of left lower limb, except ankle and foot** D, S 🗓

         ●●■ **T24.409**   **Corrosion of unspecified degree of unspecified site of unspecified lower limb, except ankle and foot** D, S 🗓

     ● **T24.41**   **Corrosion of unspecified degree of thigh**

         ●●■ **T24.411**   **Corrosion of unspecified degree of right thigh** D, S 🗓

         ●●■ **T24.412**   **Corrosion of unspecified degree of left thigh** D, S 🗓

         ●●■ **T24.419**   **Corrosion of unspecified degree of unspecified thigh** D, S 🗓

     ● **T24.42**   **Corrosion of unspecified degree of knee**

         ●●■ **T24.421**   **Corrosion of unspecified degree of right knee** D, S 🗓

         ●●■ **T24.422**   **Corrosion of unspecified degree of left knee** D, S 🗓

         ●●■ **T24.429**   **Corrosion of unspecified degree of unspecified knee** D, S 🗓

     ● **T24.43**   **Corrosion of unspecified degree of lower leg**

         ●●■ **T24.431**   **Corrosion of unspecified degree of right lower leg** D, S 🗓

         ●●■ **T24.432**   **Corrosion of unspecified degree of left lower leg** D, S 🗓

         ●●■ **T24.439**   **Corrosion of unspecified degree of unspecified lower leg** D, S 🗓

     ● **T24.49**   **Corrosion of unspecified degree of multiple sites of lower limb, except ankle and foot**

         ●●■ **T24.491**   **Corrosion of unspecified degree of multiple sites of right lower limb, except ankle and foot** D, S 🗓

         ●●■ **T24.492**   **Corrosion of unspecified degree of multiple sites of left lower limb, except ankle and foot** D, S 🗓

N Newborn Age: 0   **P** Pediatric Age: 0–17   **M** Maternity DX: 12–55   **A** Adult Age: 15–124   ♀ Females Only   ♂ Males Only

🗓 Complication\Comorbidity   🗓 Major C\C   🗓 Present on Admission Requirement   🗓 Hospital-Acquired Condition

1605

CHAPTER 19 (S00-T88)

CHAPTER 19 (S00-T88)

● ● ▪ **T24.499** Corrosion of unspecified degree of multiple sites of unspecified lower limb, except ankle and foot
D, S 🔖

● **T24.5** Corrosion of first degree of lower limb, except ankle and foot

  Code first (T51-T65) *to identify chemical and intent*

  Use additional external cause code to identify place (Y92)

  ● **T24.50** Corrosion of first degree of unspecified site of lower limb, except ankle and foot

    ● ● ▪ **T24.501** Corrosion of first degree of unspecified site of right lower limb, except ankle and foot D, S 🔖

    ● ● ▪ **T24.502** Corrosion of first degree of unspecified site of left lower limb, except ankle and foot D, S 🔖

    ● ● ▪ **T24.509** Corrosion of first degree of unspecified site of unspecified lower limb, except ankle and foot D, S 🔖

  ● **T24.51** Corrosion of first degree of thigh

    ● ● **T24.511** Corrosion of first degree of right thigh D, S 🔖

    ● ● **T24.512** Corrosion of first degree of left thigh D, S 🔖

    ● ● ▪ **T24.519** Corrosion of first degree of unspecified thigh D, S 🔖

  ● **T24.52** Corrosion of first degree of knee

    ● ● **T24.521** Corrosion of first degree of right knee D, S 🔖

    ● ● **T24.522** Corrosion of first degree of left knee D, S 🔖

    ● ● ▪ **T24.529** Corrosion of first degree of unspecified knee D, S 🔖

  ● **T24.53** Corrosion of first degree of lower leg

    ● ● **T24.531** Corrosion of first degree of right lower leg D, S 🔖

    ● ● **T24.532** Corrosion of first degree of left lower leg D, S 🔖

    ● ● ▪ **T24.539** Corrosion of first degree of unspecified lower leg D, S 🔖

  ● **T24.59** Corrosion of first degree of multiple sites of lower limb, except ankle and foot

    ● ● **T24.591** Corrosion of first degree of multiple sites of right lower limb, except ankle and foot D, S 🔖

    ● ● **T24.592** Corrosion of first degree of multiple sites of left lower limb, except ankle and foot D, S 🔖

    ● ● ▪ **T24.599** Corrosion of first degree of multiple sites of unspecified lower limb, except ankle and foot D, S 🔖

● **T24.6** Corrosion of second degree of lower limb, except ankle and foot

  Code first (T51-T65) *to identify chemical and intent*

  Use additional external cause code to identify place (Y92)

  ● **T24.60** Corrosion of second degree of unspecified site of lower limb, except ankle and foot

    ● ● ▪ **T24.601** Corrosion of second degree of unspecified site of right lower limb, except ankle and foot D, S 🔖

    ● ● ▪ **T24.602** Corrosion of second degree of unspecified site of left lower limb, except ankle and foot D, S 🔖

    ● ● ▪ **T24.609** Corrosion of second degree of unspecified site of unspecified lower limb, except ankle and foot D, S 🔖

  ● **T24.61** Corrosion of second degree of thigh

    ● ● **T24.611** Corrosion of second degree of right thigh D, S 🔖

    ● ● **T24.612** Corrosion of second degree of left thigh D, S 🔖

    ● ● ▪ **T24.619** Corrosion of second degree of unspecified thigh D, S 🔖

  ● **T24.62** Corrosion of second degree of knee

    ● ● **T24.621** Corrosion of second degree of right knee D, S 🔖

    ● ● **T24.622** Corrosion of second degree of left knee D, S 🔖

    ● ● ▪ **T24.629** Corrosion of second degree of unspecified knee D, S 🔖

  ● **T24.63** Corrosion of second degree of lower leg

    ● ● **T24.631** Corrosion of second degree of right lower leg D, S 🔖

    ● ● **T24.632** Corrosion of second degree of left lower leg D, S 🔖

    ● ● ▪ **T24.639** Corrosion of second degree of unspecified lower leg D, S 🔖

  ● **T24.69** Corrosion of second degree of multiple sites of lower limb, except ankle and foot

    ● ● **T24.691** Corrosion of second degree of multiple sites of right lower limb, except ankle and foot D, S 🔖

    ● ● **T24.692** Corrosion of second degree of multiple sites of left lower limb, except ankle and foot D, S 🔖

    ● ● ▪ **T24.699** Corrosion of second degree of multiple sites of unspecified lower limb, except ankle and foot D, S 🔖

● **T24.7** Corrosion of third degree of lower limb, except ankle and foot

  Code first (T51-T65) *to identify chemical and intent*

  Use additional external cause code to identify place (Y92)

  ● **T24.70** Corrosion of third degree of unspecified site of lower limb, except ankle and foot

    ● ● ▪ **T24.701** Corrosion of third degree of unspecified site of right lower limb, except ankle and foot A 🔖, D, S 🔖, A 🔖

    ● ● ▪ **T24.702** Corrosion of third degree of unspecified site of left lower limb, except ankle and foot A 🔖, D, S 🔖, A 🔖

    ● ● ▪ **T24.709** Corrosion of third degree of unspecified site of unspecified lower limb, except ankle and foot A 🔖, D, S 🔖, A 🔖

● Unacceptable Principal Diagnosis   ● Use Additional Character(s)   ▪ Unspecified   ▶ Manifestation Code

OGCR Official Guidelines for Coding and Reporting   Excludes 1   Excludes 2   Includes   Use additional   Code first   Code also

● **T24.71** Corrosion of third degree of thigh

  ●● **T24.711** Corrosion of third degree of right thigh A 🔖, D, S 🔖, A 🔖

  ●● **T24.712** Corrosion of third degree of left thigh A 🔖, D, S 🔖, A 🔖

  ●●▫ **T24.719** Corrosion of third degree of unspecified thigh A 🔖, D, S 🔖, A 🔖

● **T24.72** Corrosion of third degree of knee

  ●● **T24.721** Corrosion of third degree of right knee A 🔖, D, S 🔖, A 🔖

  ●● **T24.722** Corrosion of third degree of left knee A 🔖, D, S 🔖, A 🔖

  ●●▫ **T24.729** Corrosion of third degree of unspecified knee A 🔖, D, S 🔖, A 🔖

● **T24.73** Corrosion of third degree of lower leg

  ●● **T24.731** Corrosion of third degree of right lower leg A 🔖, D, S 🔖, A 🔖

  ●● **T24.732** Corrosion of third degree of left lower leg A 🔖, D, S 🔖, A 🔖

  ●●▫ **T24.739** Corrosion of third degree of unspecified lower leg A 🔖, D, S 🔖, A 🔖

● **T24.79** Corrosion of third degree of multiple sites of lower limb, except ankle and foot

  ●● **T24.791** Corrosion of third degree of multiple sites of right lower limb, except ankle and foot A 🔖, D, S 🔖, A 🔖

  ●● **T24.792** Corrosion of third degree of multiple sites of left lower limb, except ankle and foot A 🔖, D, S 🔖, A 🔖

  ●●▫ **T24.799** Corrosion of third degree of multiple sites of unspecified lower limb, except ankle and foot A 🔖, D, S 🔖, A 🔖

● **T25**   **Burn and corrosion of ankle and foot**

    The appropriate 7th character is to be added to each code from category T25

A	initial encounter
D	subsequent encounter
S	sequela

● **T25.0**   Burn of unspecified degree of ankle and foot

    <mark>Use additional</mark> external cause code to identify the source, place and intent of the burn (X00-X19, X75-X77, X96-X98, Y92)

  ● **T25.01** Burn of unspecified degree of ankle

    ●▫ **T25.011** Burn of unspecified degree of right ankle D, S 🔖

    ●▫ **T25.012** Burn of unspecified degree of left ankle D, S 🔖

    ●▫ **T25.019** Burn of unspecified degree of unspecified ankle D, S 🔖

  ● **T25.02** Burn of unspecified degree of foot

    Excludes2   burn of unspecified degree of toe(s) (nail) (T25.03-)

    ●▫ **T25.021** Burn of unspecified degree of right foot D, S 🔖

    ●▫ **T25.022** Burn of unspecified degree of left foot D, S 🔖

    ●▫ **T25.029** Burn of unspecified degree of unspecified foot D, S 🔖

  ● **T25.03** Burn of unspecified degree of toe(s) (nail)

    ●▫ **T25.031** Burn of unspecified degree of right toe(s) (nail) D, S 🔖

    ●▫ **T25.032** Burn of unspecified degree of left toe(s) (nail) D, S 🔖

    ●▫ **T25.039** Burn of unspecified degree of unspecified toe(s) (nail) D, S 🔖

  ● **T25.09** Burn of unspecified degree of multiple sites of ankle and foot

    ●▫ **T25.091** Burn of unspecified degree of multiple sites of right ankle and foot D, S 🔖

    ●▫ **T25.092** Burn of unspecified degree of multiple sites of left ankle and foot D, S 🔖

    ●▫ **T25.099** Burn of unspecified degree of multiple sites of unspecified ankle and foot D, S 🔖

● **T25.1**   Burn of first degree of ankle and foot

    <mark>Use additional</mark> external cause code to identify the source, place and intent of the burn (X00-X19, X75-X77, X96-X98, Y92)

  ● **T25.11** Burn of first degree of ankle

    ● **T25.111** Burn of first degree of right ankle D, S 🔖

    ● **T25.112** Burn of first degree of left ankle D, S 🔖

    ●▫ **T25.119** Burn of first degree of unspecified ankle D, S 🔖

  ● **T25.12** Burn of first degree of foot

    Excludes2   burn of first degree of toe(s) (nail) (T25.13-)

    ● **T25.121** Burn of first degree of right foot D, S 🔖

    ● **T25.122** Burn of first degree of left foot D, S 🔖

    ●▫ **T25.129** Burn of first degree of unspecified foot D, S 🔖

  ● **T25.13** Burn of first degree of toe(s) (nail)

    ● **T25.131** Burn of first degree of right toe(s) (nail) D, S 🔖

    ● **T25.132** Burn of first degree of left toe(s) (nail) D, S 🔖

    ●▫ **T25.139** Burn of first degree of unspecified toe(s) (nail) D, S 🔖

  ● **T25.19** Burn of first degree of multiple sites of ankle and foot

    ● **T25.191** Burn of first degree of multiple sites of right ankle and foot D, S 🔖

    ● **T25.192** Burn of first degree of multiple sites of left ankle and foot D, S 🔖

    ●▫ **T25.199** Burn of first degree of multiple sites of unspecified ankle and foot D, S 🔖

CHAPTER 19 (S00-T88)

● **T25.2   Burn of second degree of ankle and foot**

    Use additional external cause code to identify the source, place and intent of the burn (X00-X19, X75-X77, X96-X98, Y92)

    ● **T25.21   Burn of second degree of ankle**

       ● **T25.211   Burn of second degree of right ankle** D, S 🔏

       ● **T25.212   Burn of second degree of left ankle** D, S 🔏

       ●■ **T25.219   Burn of second degree of unspecified ankle** D, S 🔏

    ● **T25.22   Burn of second degree of foot**

       Excludes2   burn of second degree of toe(s) (nail) (T25.23-)

       ● **T25.221   Burn of second degree of right foot** D, S 🔏

       ● **T25.222   Burn of second degree of left foot** D, S 🔏

       ●■ **T25.229   Burn of second degree of unspecified foot** D, S 🔏

    ● **T25.23   Burn of second degree of toe(s) (nail)**

       ● **T25.231   Burn of second degree of right toe(s) (nail)** D, S 🔏

       ● **T25.232   Burn of second degree of left toe(s) (nail)** D, S 🔏

       ●■ **T25.239   Burn of second degree of unspecified toe(s) (nail)** D, S 🔏

    ● **T25.29   Burn of second degree of multiple sites of ankle and foot**

       ● **T25.291   Burn of second degree of multiple sites of right ankle and foot** D, S 🔏

       ● **T25.292   Burn of second degree of multiple sites of left ankle and foot** D, S 🔏

       ●■ **T25.299   Burn of second degree of multiple sites of unspecified ankle and foot** D, S 🔏

● **T25.3   Burn of third degree of ankle and foot**

    Use additional external cause code to identify the source, place and intent of the burn (X00-X19, X75-X77, X96-X98, Y92)

    ● **T25.31   Burn of third degree of ankle**

       ● **T25.311   Burn of third degree of right ankle** A 🔏, D, S 🔏, A 🔏

       ● **T25.312   Burn of third degree of left ankle** A 🔏, D, S 🔏, A 🔏

       ●■ **T25.319   Burn of third degree of unspecified ankle** A 🔏, D, S 🔏, A 🔏

    ● **T25.32   Burn of third degree of foot**

       Excludes2   burn of third degree of toe(s) (nail) (T25.33-)

       ● **T25.321   Burn of third degree of right foot** A 🔏, D, S 🔏, A 🔏

       ● **T25.322   Burn of third degree of left foot** A 🔏, D, S 🔏, A 🔏

       ●■ **T25.329   Burn of third degree of unspecified foot** A 🔏, D, S 🔏, A 🔏

● **T25.33   Burn of third degree of toe(s) (nail)**

    ● **T25.331   Burn of third degree of right toe(s) (nail)** A 🔏, D, S 🔏, A 🔏

    ● **T25.332   Burn of third degree of left toe(s) (nail)** A 🔏, D, S 🔏, A 🔏

    ●■ **T25.339   Burn of third degree of unspecified toe(s) (nail)** A 🔏, D, S 🔏, A 🔏

● **T25.39   Burn of third degree of multiple sites of ankle and foot**

    ● **T25.391   Burn of third degree of multiple sites of right ankle and foot** A 🔏, D, S 🔏, A 🔏

    ● **T25.392   Burn of third degree of multiple sites of left ankle and foot** A 🔏, D, S 🔏, A 🔏

    ● **T25.399   Burn of third degree of multiple sites of unspecified ankle and foot** A 🔏, D, S 🔏, A 🔏

● **T25.4   Corrosion of unspecified degree of ankle and foot**

    Code first (T51-T65) to identify chemical and intent

    Use additional external cause code to identify place (Y92)

    ● **T25.41   Corrosion of unspecified degree of ankle**

       ●●■ **T25.411   Corrosion of unspecified degree of right ankle** D, S 🔏

       ●●■ **T25.412   Corrosion of unspecified degree of left ankle** D, S 🔏

       ●●■ **T25.419   Corrosion of unspecified degree of unspecified ankle** D, S 🔏

    ● **T25.42   Corrosion of unspecified degree of foot**

       Excludes2   corrosion of unspecified degree of toe(s) (nail) (T25.43-)

       ●●■ **T25.421   Corrosion of unspecified degree of right foot** D, S 🔏

       ●●■ **T25.422   Corrosion of unspecified degree of left foot** D, S 🔏

       ●●■ **T25.429   Corrosion of unspecified degree of unspecified foot** D, S 🔏

    ● **T25.43   Corrosion of unspecified degree of toe(s) (nail)**

       ●●■ **T25.431   Corrosion of unspecified degree of right toe(s) (nail)** D, S 🔏

       ●●■ **T25.432   Corrosion of unspecified degree of left toe(s) (nail)** D, S 🔏

       ●●■ **T25.439   Corrosion of unspecified degree of unspecified toe(s) (nail)** D, S 🔏

    ● **T25.49   Corrosion of unspecified degree of multiple sites of ankle and foot**

       ●●■ **T25.491   Corrosion of unspecified degree of multiple sites of right ankle and foot** D, S 🔏

       ●●■ **T25.492   Corrosion of unspecified degree of multiple sites of left ankle and foot** D, S 🔏

       ●●■ **T25.499   Corrosion of unspecified degree of multiple sites of unspecified ankle and foot** D, S 🔏

● Unacceptable Principal Diagnosis   ● Use Additional Character(s)   ■ Unspecified   ▶ Manifestation Code

OGCR Official Guidelines for Coding and Reporting   Excludes 1   Excludes 2   Includes   Use additional   Code first   Code also

● **T25.5**   **Corrosion of first degree of ankle and foot**

    Code first (T51-T65) *to identify chemical and intent*

    Use additional external cause code to identify place (Y92)

   ● **T25.51**   Corrosion of first degree of ankle

     ● ● **T25.511**   Corrosion of first degree of right ankle D, S

     ● ● **T25.512**   Corrosion of first degree of left ankle D, S

     ● ● ■ **T25.519**   Corrosion of first degree of unspecified ankle D, S

   ● **T25.52**   Corrosion of first degree of foot

     | Excludes2 | corrosion of first degree of toe(s) (nail) (T25.53-)

     ● ● **T25.521**   Corrosion of first degree of right foot D, S

     ● ● **T25.522**   Corrosion of first degree of left foot D, S

     ● ● ■ **T25.529**   Corrosion of first degree of unspecified foot D, S

   ● **T25.53**   Corrosion of first degree of toe(s) (nail)

     ● ● **T25.531**   Corrosion of first degree of right toe(s) (nail) D, S

     ● ● **T25.532**   Corrosion of first degree of left toe(s) (nail) D, S

     ● ● ■ **T25.539**   Corrosion of first degree of unspecified toe(s) (nail) D, S

   ● **T25.59**   Corrosion of first degree of multiple sites of ankle and foot

     ● ● **T25.591**   Corrosion of first degree of multiple sites of right ankle and foot D, S

     ● ● **T25.592**   Corrosion of first degree of multiple sites of left ankle and foot D, S

     ● ● ■ **T25.599**   Corrosion of first degree of multiple sites of unspecified ankle and foot D, S

● **T25.6**   **Corrosion of second degree of ankle and foot**

    Code first (T51-T65) *to identify chemical and intent*

    Use additional external cause code to identify place (Y92)

   ● **T25.61**   Corrosion of second degree of ankle

     ● ● **T25.611**   Corrosion of second degree of right ankle D, S

     ● ● **T25.612**   Corrosion of second degree of left ankle D, S

     ● ● ■ **T25.619**   Corrosion of second degree of unspecified ankle D, S

   ● **T25.62**   Corrosion of second degree of foot

     | Excludes2 | corrosion of second degree of toe(s) (nail) (T25.63-)

     ● ● **T25.621**   Corrosion of second degree of right foot D, S

     ● ● **T25.622**   Corrosion of second degree of left foot D, S

     ● ● ■ **T25.629**   Corrosion of second degree of unspecified foot D, S

● **T25.63**   Corrosion of second degree of toe(s) (nail)

     ● ● **T25.631**   Corrosion of second degree of right toe(s) (nail) D, S

     ● ● **T25.632**   Corrosion of second degree of left toe(s) (nail) D, S

     ● ● ■ **T25.639**   Corrosion of second degree of unspecified toe(s) (nail) D, S

   ● **T25.69**   Corrosion of second degree of multiple sites of ankle and foot

     ● ● **T25.691**   Corrosion of second degree of right ankle and foot D, S

     ● ● **T25.692**   Corrosion of second degree of left ankle and foot D, S

     ● ● ■ **T25.699**   Corrosion of second degree of unspecified ankle and foot D, S

● **T25.7**   **Corrosion of third degree of ankle and foot**

    Code first (T51-T65) *to identify chemical and intent*

    Use additional external cause code to identify place (Y92)

   ● **T25.71**   Corrosion of third degree of ankle

     ● ● **T25.711**   Corrosion of third degree of right ankle A, D, S, A

     ● ● **T25.712**   Corrosion of third degree of left ankle A, D, S, A

     ● ● ■ **T25.719**   Corrosion of third degree of unspecified ankle A, D, S, A

   ● **T25.72**   Corrosion of third degree of foot

     | Excludes2 | corrosion of third degree of toe(s) (nail) (T25.73-)

     ● ● **T25.721**   Corrosion of third degree of right foot A, D, S, A

     ● ● **T25.722**   Corrosion of third degree of left foot A, D, S, A

     ● ● ■ **T25.729**   Corrosion of third degree of unspecified foot A, D, S, A

   ● **T25.73**   Corrosion of third degree of toe(s) (nail)

     ● ● **T25.731**   Corrosion of third degree of right toe(s) (nail) A, D, S, A

     ● ● **T25.732**   Corrosion of third degree of left toe(s) (nail) A, D, S, A

     ● ● ■ **T25.739**   Corrosion of third degree of unspecified toe(s) (nail) A, D, S, A

   ● **T25.79**   Corrosion of third degree of multiple sites of ankle and foot

     ● ● **T25.791**   Corrosion of third degree of multiple sites of right ankle and foot A, D, S, A

     ● ● **T25.792**   Corrosion of third degree of multiple sites of left ankle and foot A, D, S, A

     ● ● ■ **T25.799**   Corrosion of third degree of multiple sites of unspecified ankle and foot A, D, S, A

N Newborn Age: 0   **P** Pediatric Age: 0–17   **M** Maternity DX: 12–55   **A** Adult Age: 15–124   ♀ Females Only   ♂ Males Only

Complication\Comorbidity   Major C\C   Present on Admission Requirement   Hospital-Acquired Condition

1609

BURNS AND CORROSIONS CONFINED TO EYE AND INTERNAL ORGANS (T26-T28)

● **T26**   **Burn and corrosion confined to eye and adnexa**

The appropriate 7th character is to be added to each code from category T26

> A   initial encounter
> D   subsequent encounter
> S   sequela

● **T26.0**   **Burn of eyelid and periocular area**

Use additional external cause code to identify the source, place and intent of the burn (X00-X19, X75-X77, X96-X98, Y92)

●■ **T26.00**   **Burn of unspecified eyelid and periocular area** D, S 🗞

● **T26.01**   **Burn of right eyelid and periocular area** D, S 🗞

● **T26.02**   **Burn of left eyelid and periocular area** D, S 🗞

● **T26.1**   **Burn of cornea and conjunctival sac**

Use additional external cause code to identify the source, place and intent of the burn (X00-X19, X75-X77, X96-X98, Y92)

●■ **T26.10**   **Burn of cornea and conjunctival sac, unspecified eye** D, S 🗞

● **T26.11**   **Burn of cornea and conjunctival sac, right eye** D, S 🗞

● **T26.12**   **Burn of cornea and conjunctival sac, left eye** D, S 🗞

● **T26.2**   **Burn with resulting rupture and destruction of eyeball**

Use additional external cause code to identify the source, place and intent of the burn (X00-X19, X75-X77, X96-X98, Y92)

●■ **T26.20**   **Burn with resulting rupture and destruction of unspecified eyeball** A 🗞, D, S 🗞, A 🗞

● **T26.21**   **Burn with resulting rupture and destruction of right eyeball** A 🗞, D, S 🗞, A 🗞

● **T26.22**   **Burn with resulting rupture and destruction of left eyeball** A 🗞, D, S 🗞, A 🗞

● **T26.3**   **Burns of other specified parts of eye and adnexa**

Use additional external cause code to identify the source, place and intent of the burn (X00-X19, X75-X77, X96-X98, Y92)

●■ **T26.30**   **Burns of other specified parts of unspecified eye and adnexa** D, S 🗞

● **T26.31**   **Burns of other specified parts of right eye and adnexa** D, S 🗞

● **T26.32**   **Burns of other specified parts of left eye and adnexa** D, S 🗞

● **T26.4**   **Burn of eye and adnexa, part unspecified**

Use additional external cause code to identify the source, place and intent of the burn (X00-X19, X75-X77, X96-X98, Y92)

●■ **T26.40**   **Burn of unspecified eye and adnexa, part unspecified** D, S 🗞

●■ **T26.41**   **Burn of right eye and adnexa, part unspecified** D, S 🗞

●■ **T26.42**   **Burn of left eye and adnexa, part unspecified** D, S 🗞

● **T26.5**   **Corrosion of eyelid and periocular area**

Code first (T51-T65) to identify chemical and intent

Use additional external cause code to identify place (Y92)

●●■ **T26.50**   **Corrosion of unspecified eyelid and periocular area** D, S 🗞

●● **T26.51**   **Corrosion of right eyelid and periocular area** D, S 🗞

●● **T26.52**   **Corrosion of left eyelid and periocular area** D, S 🗞

● **T26.6**   **Corrosion of cornea and conjunctival sac**

Code first (T51-T65) to identify chemical and intent

Use additional external cause code to identify place (Y92)

●●■ **T26.60**   **Corrosion of cornea and conjunctival sac, unspecified eye** D, S 🗞

●● **T26.61**   **Corrosion of cornea and conjunctival sac, right eye** D, S 🗞

●● **T26.62**   **Corrosion of cornea and conjunctival sac, left eye** D, S 🗞

● **T26.7**   **Corrosion with resulting rupture and destruction of eyeball**

Code first (T51-T65) to identify chemical and intent

Use additional external cause code to identify place (Y92)

●●■ **T26.70**   **Corrosion with resulting rupture and destruction of unspecified eyeball** A 🗞, D, S 🗞, A 🗞

●● **T26.71**   **Corrosion with resulting rupture and destruction of right eyeball** A 🗞, D, S 🗞, A 🗞

●● **T26.72**   **Corrosion with resulting rupture and destruction of left eyeball** A 🗞, D, S 🗞, A 🗞

● **T26.8**   **Corrosions of other specified parts of eye and adnexa**

Code first (T51-T65) to identify chemical and intent

Use additional external cause code to identify place (Y92)

●●■ **T26.80**   **Corrosions of other specified parts of unspecified eye and adnexa** D, S 🗞

●● **T26.81**   **Corrosions of other specified parts of right eye and adnexa** D, S 🗞

●● **T26.82**   **Corrosions of other specified parts of left eye and adnexa** D, S 🗞

● **T26.9**   **Corrosion of eye and adnexa, part unspecified**

Code first (T51-T65) to identify chemical and intent

Use additional external cause code to identify place (Y92)

●●■ **T26.90**   **Corrosion of unspecified eye and adnexa, part unspecified** D, S 🗞

●●■ **T26.91**   **Corrosion of right eye and adnexa, part unspecified** D, S 🗞

●●■ **T26.92**   **Corrosion of left eye and adnexa, part unspecified** D, S 🗞

● Unacceptable Principal Diagnosis   ● Use Additional Character(s)   ■ Unspecified   ▶ Manifestation Code

1610   **OGCR** Official Guidelines for Coding and Reporting   Excludes 1   Excludes 2   Includes   Use additional   Code first   Code also

● **T27**   **Burn and corrosion of respiratory tract**

> Use additional external cause code to identify the source and intent of the burn (X00- X19, X75-X77, X96-X98)
>
> Use additional external cause code to identify place (Y92)
>
> The appropriate 7th character is to be added to each code from category T27

> | | |
> |---|---|
> | A | initial encounter |
> | D | subsequent encounter |
> | S | sequela |

● **T27.0**   **Burn of larynx and trachea** A 🗫, D, S 🗫, A 🗫

● **T27.1**   **Burn involving larynx and trachea with lung** A 🗫, D, S 🗫, A 🗫

● **T27.2**   **Burn of other parts of respiratory tract** A 🗫, D, S 🗫, A 🗫
> Burn of thoracic cavity

●●■ **T27.3**   **Burn of respiratory tract, part unspecified** A 🗫, D, S 🗫, A 🗫

> *Code first (T51-T65) to identify chemical and intent for codes T27.4-T27.7*

● **T27.4**   **Corrosion of larynx and trachea** A 🗫, D, S 🗫, A 🗫

● **T27.5**   **Corrosion involving larynx and trachea with lung** A 🗫, D, S 🗫, A 🗫

● **T27.6**   **Corrosion of other parts of respiratory tract** A 🗫, D, S 🗫, A 🗫

●●■ **T27.7**   **Corrosion of respiratory tract, part unspecified** A 🗫, D, S 🗫, A 🗫

● **T28**   **Burn and corrosion of other internal organs**

> Use additional external cause code to identify the source and intent of the burn (X00- X19, X75-X77, X96-X98)
>
> Use additional external cause code to identify place (Y92)
>
> The appropriate 7th character is to be added to each code from category T28

> | | |
> |---|---|
> | A | initial encounter |
> | D | subsequent encounter |
> | S | sequela |

● **T28.0**   **Burn of mouth and pharynx** D, S 🗫

● **T28.1**   **Burn of esophagus** A 🗫, D, S 🗫, A 🗫

● **T28.2**   **Burn of other parts of alimentary tract** A 🗫, D, S 🗫, A 🗫

● **T28.3**   **Burn of internal genitourinary organs** D, S 🗫

● **T28.4**   **Burns of other and unspecified internal organs**

    ●■ **T28.40**   **Burn of unspecified internal organ** D, S 🗫

    ● **T28.41**   **Burn of ear drum**

       ● **T28.411**   **Burn of right ear drum** D, S 🗫

       ● **T28.412**   **Burn of left ear drum** D, S 🗫

       ●■ **T28.419**   **Burn of unspecified ear drum** D, S 🗫

    ●● **T28.49**   **Burn of other internal organ** D, S 🗫

> *Code first (T51-T65) to identify chemical and intent for T28.5-T28.9-*

● **T28.5**   **Corrosion of mouth and pharynx** D, S 🗫

● **T28.6**   **Corrosion of esophagus** A 🗫, D, S 🗫, A 🗫

● **T28.7**   **Corrosion of other parts of alimentary tract** A 🗫, D, S 🗫, A 🗫

● **T28.8**   **Corrosion of internal genitourinary organs** D, S 🗫

● **T28.9**   **Corrosions of other and unspecified internal organs**

    ●■ **T28.90**   **Corrosions of unspecified internal organs** D, S 🗫

    ● **T28.91**   **Corrosions of ear drum**

       ● **T28.911**   **Corrosions of right ear drum** D, S 🗫

       ● **T28.912**   **Corrosions of left ear drum** D, S 🗫

       ● **T28.919**   **Corrosions of unspecified ear drum** D, S 🗫

    ● **T28.99**   **Corrosions of other internal organs** D, S 🗫

BURNS AND CORROSIONS OF MULTIPLE AND UNSPECIFIED BODY REGIONS (T30-T32)

● **T30**   **Burn and corrosion, body region unspecified**

    ■ **T30.0**   **Burn of unspecified body region, unspecified degree**
> This code is not for inpatient use. Code to specified site and degree of burns
> Burn NOS
> Multiple burns NOS

    ■ **T30.4**   **Corrosion of unspecified body region, unspecified degree**
> This code is not for inpatient use. Code to specified site and degree of corrosion
> Corrosion NOS
> Multiple corrosion NOS

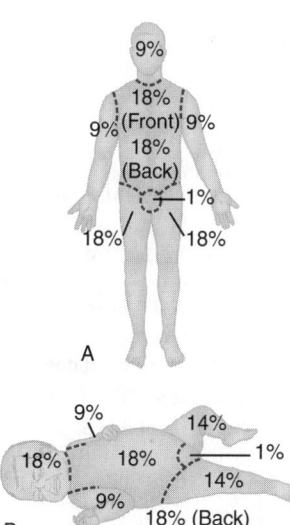

A

B

Figure 19-15   Rule of nines: percentages of total body area. (From Marx: Rosen's Emergency Medicine: Concepts and Clinical Practice, 6th ed. 2006, Mosby.)

OGCR Section I.C.19.d.5.

> **Assign separate code for each burn site**
>
> When coding burns, assign separate codes for each burn site. Category T30, Burn and corrosion, body region unspecified is extremely vague and should rarely be used.

CHAPTER 19 (S00-T88)

OGCR See Section III.C.19.d.

● **T31 Burns classified according to extent of body surface involved**

> This category is to be used as the primary code only when the site of the burn is unspecified. It should be used as a supplementary code with categories T20-T25 when the site is specified.

T31.0 Burns involving less than 10% of body surface

● **T31.1 Burns involving 10-19% of body surface**

> **T31.10 Burns involving 10-19% of body surface with 0% to 9% third degree burns 🜨 🜨**
> > Burns involving 10-19% of body surface NOS
>
> **T31.11 Burns involving 10-19% of body surface with 10-19% third degree burns 🜨 🜨**

● **T31.2 Burns involving 20-29% of body surface**

> **T31.20 Burns involving 20-29% of body surface with 0% to 9% third degree burns 🜨 🜨**
> > Burns involving 20-29% of body surface NOS
>
> **T31.21 Burns involving 20-29% of body surface with 10-19% third degree burns 🜨 🜨**
>
> **T31.22 Burns involving 20-29% of body surface with 20-29% third degree burns 🜨 🜨**

● **T31.3 Burns involving 30-39% of body surface**

> **T31.30 Burns involving 30-39% of body surface with 0% to 9% third degree burns 🜨 🜨**
> > Burns involving 30-39% of body surface NOS
>
> **T31.31 Burns involving 30-39% of body surface with 10-19% third degree burns 🜨 🜨**
>
> **T31.32 Burns involving 30-39% of body surface with 20-29% third degree burns 🜨 🜨**
>
> **T31.33 Burns involving 30-39% of body surface with 30-39% third degree burns 🜨 🜨**

● **T31.4 Burns involving 40-49% of body surface**

> **T31.40 Burns involving 40-49% of body surface with 0% to 9% third degree burns 🜨**
> > Burns involving 40-49% of body surface NOS
>
> **T31.41 Burns involving 40-49% of body surface with 10-19% third degree burns 🜨 🜨**
>
> **T31.42 Burns involving 40-49% of body surface with 20-29% third degree burns 🜨 🜨**
>
> **T31.43 Burns involving 40-49% of body surface with 30-39% third degree burns 🜨 🜨**
>
> **T31.44 Burns involving 40-49% of body surface with 40-49% third degree burns 🜨 🜨**

● **T31.5 Burns involving 50-59% of body surface**

> **T31.50 Burns involving 50-59% of body surface with 0% to 9% third degree burns 🜨 🜨**
> > Burns involving 50-59% of body surface NOS
>
> **T31.51 Burns involving 50-59% of body surface with 10-19% third degree burns 🜨 🜨**
>
> **T31.52 Burns involving 50-59% of body surface with 20-29% third degree burns 🜨 🜨**
>
> **T31.53 Burns involving 50-59% of body surface with 30-39% third degree burns 🜨 🜨**
>
> **T31.54 Burns involving 50-59% of body surface with 40-49% third degree burns 🜨 🜨**
>
> **T31.55 Burns involving 50-59% of body surface with 50-59% third degree burns 🜨 🜨**

● **T31.6 Burns involving 60-69% of body surface**

> **T31.60 Burns involving 60-69% of body surface with 0% to 9% third degree burns 🜨 🜨**
> > Burns involving 60-69% of body surface NOS
>
> **T31.61 Burns involving 60-69% of body surface with 10-19% third degree burns 🜨 🜨**
>
> **T31.62 Burns involving 60-69% of body surface with 20-29% third degree burns 🜨 🜨**
>
> **T31.63 Burns involving 60-69% of body surface with 30-39% third degree burns 🜨 🜨**
>
> **T31.64 Burns involving 60-69% of body surface with 40-49% third degree burns 🜨 🜨**
>
> **T31.65 Burns involving 60-69% of body surface with 50-59% third degree burns 🜨 🜨**
>
> **T31.66 Burns involving 60-69% of body surface with 60-69% third degree burns 🜨 🜨**

● **T31.7 Burns involving 70-79% of body surface**

> **T31.70 Burns involving 70-79% of body surface with 0% to 9% third degree burns 🜨 🜨**
> > Burns involving 70-79% of body surface NOS
>
> **T31.71 Burns involving 70-79% of body surface with 10-19% third degree burns 🜨 🜨**
>
> **T31.72 Burns involving 70-79% of body surface with 20-29% third degree burns 🜨 🜨**
>
> **T31.73 Burns involving 70-79% of body surface with 30-39% third degree burns 🜨 🜨**
>
> **T31.74 Burns involving 70-79% of body surface with 40-49% third degree burns 🜨 🜨**
>
> **T31.75 Burns involving 70-79% of body surface with 50-59% third degree burns 🜨 🜨**
>
> **T31.76 Burns involving 70-79% of body surface with 60-69% third degree burns 🜨 🜨**
>
> **T31.77 Burns involving 70-79% of body surface with 70-79% third degree burns 🜨 🜨**

● **T31.8 Burns involving 80-89% of body surface**

> **T31.80 Burns involving 80-89% of body surface with 0% to 9% third degree burns 🜨 🜨**
> > Burns involving 80-89% of body surface NOS
>
> **T31.81 Burns involving 80-89% of body surface with 10-19% third degree burns 🜨 🜨**
>
> **T31.82 Burns involving 80-89% of body surface with 20-29% third degree burns 🜨 🜨**
>
> **T31.83 Burns involving 80-89% of body surface with 30-39% third degree burns 🜨 🜨**
>
> **T31.84 Burns involving 80-89% of body surface with 40-49% third degree burns 🜨 🜨**
>
> **T31.85 Burns involving 80-89% of body surface with 50-59% third degree burns 🜨 🜨**
>
> **T31.86 Burns involving 80-89% of body surface with 60-69% third degree burns 🜨 🜨**
>
> **T31.87 Burns involving 80-89% of body surface with 70-79% third degree burns 🜨 🜨**
>
> **T31.88 Burns involving 80-89% of body surface with 80-89% third degree burns 🜨 🜨**

● **T31.9 Burns involving 90% or more of body surface**

    T31.90   Burns involving 90% or more of body surface with 0% to 9% third degree burns 🅒 🅟
                Burns involving 90% or more of body surface NOS

    T31.91   Burns involving 90% or more of body surface with 10-19% third degree burns 🅒 🅟

    T31.92   Burns involving 90% or more of body surface with 20-29% third degree burns 🅒 🅟

    T31.93   Burns involving 90% or more of body surface with 30-39% third degree burns 🅒 🅟

    T31.94   Burns involving 90% or more of body surface with 40-49% third degree burns 🅒 🅟

    T31.95   Burns involving 90% or more of body surface with 50-59% third degree burns 🅒 🅟

    T31.96   Burns involving 90% or more of body surface with 60-69% third degree burns 🅒 🅟

    T31.97   Burns involving 90% or more of body surface with 70-79% third degree burns 🅒 🅟

    T31.98   Burns involving 90% or more of body surface with 80-89% third degree burns 🅒 🅟

    T31.99   Burns involving 90% or more of body surface with 90% or more third degree burns 🅒 🅟

● **T32 Corrosions classified according to extent of body surface involved**

    Note: This category is to be used as the primary code only when the site of the corrosion is unspecified. It may be used as a supplementary code with categories T20-T25 when the site is specified.

    T32.0 Corrosions involving less than 10% of body surface

● **T32.1 Corrosions involving 10-19% of body surface**

    T32.10   Corrosions involving 10-19% of body surface with 0% to 9% third degree corrosion 🅒 🅟
                Corrosions involving 10-19% of body surface NOS

    T32.11   Corrosions involving 10-19% of body surface with 10-19% third degree corrosion 🅒 🅟

● **T32.2 Corrosions involving 20-29% of body surface**

    T32.20   Corrosions involving 20-29% of body surface with 0% to 9% third degree corrosion 🅒 🅟

    T32.21   Corrosions involving 20-29% of body surface with 10-19% third degree corrosion 🅒 🅟

    T32.22   Corrosions involving 20-29% of body surface with 20-29% third degree corrosion 🅒 🅟

● **T32.3 Corrosions involving 30-39% of body surface**

    T32.30   Corrosions involving 30-39% of body surface with 0% to 9% third degree corrosion 🅒 🅟

    T32.31   Corrosions involving 30-39% of body surface with 10-19% third degree corrosion 🅒 🅟

    T32.32   Corrosions involving 30-39% of body surface with 20-29% third degree corrosion 🅒 🅟

    T32.33   Corrosions involving 30-39% of body surface with 30-39% third degree corrosion 🅒 🅟

● **T32.4 Corrosions involving 40-49% of body surface**

    T32.40   Corrosions involving 40-49% of body surface with 0% to 9% third degree corrosion 🅒 🅟

    T32.41   Corrosions involving 40-49% of body surface with 10-19% third degree corrosion 🅒 🅟

    T32.42   Corrosions involving 40-49% of body surface with 20-29% third degree corrosion 🅒 🅟

    T32.43   Corrosions involving 40-49% of body surface with 30-39% third degree corrosion 🅒 🅟

    T32.44   Corrosions involving 40-49% of body surface with 40-49% third degree corrosion 🅒 🅟

● **T32.5 Corrosions involving 50-59% of body surface**

    T32.50   Corrosions involving 50-59% of body surface with 0% to 9% third degree corrosion 🅒 🅟

    T32.51   Corrosions involving 50-59% of body surface with 10-19% third degree corrosion 🅒 🅟

    T32.52   Corrosions involving 50-59% of body surface with 20-29% third degree corrosion 🅒 🅟

    T32.53   Corrosions involving 50-59% of body surface with 30-39% third degree corrosion 🅒 🅟

    T32.54   Corrosions involving 50-59% of body surface with 40-49% third degree corrosion 🅒 🅟

    T32.55   Corrosions involving 50-59% of body surface with 50-59% third degree corrosion 🅒 🅟

● **T32.6 Corrosions involving 60-69% of body surface**

    T32.60   Corrosions involving 60-69% of body surface with 0% to 9% third degree corrosion 🅒 🅟

    T32.61   Corrosions involving 60-69% of body surface with 10-19% third degree corrosion 🅒 🅟

    T32.62   Corrosions involving 60-69% of body surface with 20-29% third degree corrosion 🅒 🅟

    T32.63   Corrosions involving 60-69% of body surface with 30-39% third degree corrosion 🅒 🅟

    T32.64   Corrosions involving 60-69% of body surface with 40-49% third degree corrosion 🅒 🅟

    T32.65   Corrosions involving 60-69% of body surface with 50-59% third degree corrosion 🅒 🅟

    T32.66   Corrosions involving 60-69% of body surface with 60-69% third degree corrosion 🅒 🅟

N Newborn Age: 0   **P** Pediatric Age: 0–17   **M** Maternity DX: 12–55   **A** Adult Age: 15–124   ♀ Females Only   ♂ Males Only

🅒 Complication\Comorbidity   Major C\C   Present on Admission Requirement   Hospital-Acquired Condition

1613

CHAPTER 19 (S00-T88)

● **T32.7**   Corrosions involving 70-79% of body surface

     T32.70   Corrosions involving 70-79% of body surface with 0% to 9% third degree corrosion 🔾 🔾

     T32.71   Corrosions involving 70-79% of body surface with 10-19% third degree corrosion 🔾 🔾

     T32.72   Corrosions involving 70-79% of body surface with 20-29% third degree corrosion 🔾 🔾

     T32.73   Corrosions involving 70-79% of body surface with 30-39% third degree corrosion 🔾 🔾

     T32.74   Corrosions involving 70-79% of body surface with 40-49% third degree corrosion 🔾 🔾

     T32.75   Corrosions involving 70-79% of body surface with 50-59% third degree corrosion 🔾 🔾

     T32.76   Corrosions involving 70-79% of body surface with 60-69% third degree corrosion 🔾 🔾

     T32.77   Corrosions involving 70-79% of body surface with 70-79% third degree corrosion 🔾 🔾

● **T32.8**   Corrosions involving 80-89% of body surface

     T32.80   Corrosions involving 80-89% of body surface with 0% to 9% third degree corrosion 🔾 🔾

     T32.81   Corrosions involving 80-89% of body surface with 10-19% third degree corrosion 🔾 🔾

     T32.82   Corrosions involving 80-89% of body surface with 20-29% third degree corrosion 🔾 🔾

     T32.83   Corrosions involving 80-89% of body surface with 30-39% third degree corrosion 🔾 🔾

     T32.84   Corrosions involving 80-89% of body surface with 40-49% third degree corrosion 🔾 🔾

     T32.85   Corrosions involving 80-89% of body surface with 50-59% third degree corrosion 🔾 🔾

     T32.86   Corrosions involving 80-89% of body surface with 60-69% third degree corrosion 🔾 🔾

     T32.87   Corrosions involving 80-89% of body surface with 70-79% third degree corrosion 🔾 🔾

     T32.88   Corrosions involving 80-89% of body surface with 80-89% third degree corrosion 🔾 🔾

● **T32.9**   Corrosions involving 90% or more of body surface

     T32.90   Corrosions involving 90% or more of body surface with 0% to 9% third degree corrosion 🔾 🔾

     T32.91   Corrosions involving 90% or more of body surface with 10-19% third degree corrosion 🔾 🔾

     T32.92   Corrosions involving 90% or more of body surface with 20-29% third degree corrosion 🔾 🔾

     T32.93   Corrosions involving 90% or more of body surface with 30-39% third degree corrosion 🔾 🔾

     T32.94   Corrosions involving 90% or more of body surface with 40-49% third degree corrosion 🔾 🔾

     T32.95   Corrosions involving 90% or more of body surface with 50-59% third degree corrosion 🔾 🔾

     T32.96   Corrosions involving 90% or more of body surface with 60-69% third degree corrosion 🔾 🔾

     T32.97   Corrosions involving 90% or more of body surface with 70-79% third degree corrosion 🔾 🔾

     T32.98   Corrosions involving 90% or more of body surface with 80-89% third degree corrosion 🔾 🔾

     T32.99   Corrosions involving 90% or more of body surface with 90% or more third degree corrosion 🔾 🔾

FROSTBITE (T33-T34)

| Excludes2 | hypothermia and other effects of reduced temperature (T68, T69.-) |

● **T33**   Superficial frostbite

    | Includes | frostbite with partial thickness skin loss |

    The appropriate 7th character is to be added to each code from category T33

     A   initial encounter
     D   subsequent encounter
     S   sequela

● **T33.0**   Superficial frostbite of head

   ● **T33.01**   Superficial frostbite of ear

     ● **T33.011**   Superficial frostbite of right ear A 🔾, D, S 🔾, A 🔾

     ● **T33.012**   Superficial frostbite of left ear A 🔾, D, S 🔾, A 🔾

     ● ■ **T33.019**   Superficial frostbite of unspecified ear A 🔾, D, S 🔾, A 🔾

   ● **T33.02**   Superficial frostbite of nose A 🔾, D, S 🔾, A 🔾

   ● **T33.09**   Superficial frostbite of other part of head A 🔾, D, S 🔾, A 🔾

● **T33.1**   Superficial frostbite of neck A 🔾, D, S 🔾, A 🔾

● **T33.2**   Superficial frostbite of thorax A 🔾, D, S 🔾, A 🔾

● **T33.3**   Superficial frostbite of abdominal wall, lower back and pelvis A 🔾, D, S 🔾, A 🔾

● **T33.4**   Superficial frostbite of arm

    | Excludes2 | superficial frostbite of wrist and hand (T33.5-) |

   ● ■ **T33.40**   Superficial frostbite of unspecified arm A 🔾, D, S 🔾, A 🔾

   ● **T33.41**   Superficial frostbite of right arm A 🔾, D, S 🔾, A 🔾

   ● **T33.42**   Superficial frostbite of left arm A 🔾, D, S 🔾, A 🔾

● Unacceptable Principal Diagnosis   ● Use Additional Character(s)   ■ Unspecified   ▶ Manifestation Code

1614   **OGCR** Official Guidelines for Coding and Reporting | Excludes 1 | | Excludes 2 | | Includes | | Use additional | | Code first | | Code also |

- **T33.5 Superficial frostbite of wrist, hand, and fingers**
  - **T33.51 Superficial frostbite of wrist**
    - **T33.511 Superficial frostbite of right wrist** A, D, S, A
    - **T33.512 Superficial frostbite of left wrist** A, D, S, A
    - **T33.519 Superficial frostbite of unspecified wrist** A, D, S, A
  - **T33.52 Superficial frostbite of hand**
    - **Excludes2** superficial frostbite of fingers (T33.53-)
    - **T33.521 Superficial frostbite of right hand** A, D, S, A
    - **T33.522 Superficial frostbite of left hand** A, D, S, A
    - **T33.529 Superficial frostbite of unspecified hand** A, D, S, A
  - **T33.53 Superficial frostbite of finger(s)**
    - **T33.531 Superficial frostbite of right finger(s)** A, D, S, A
    - **T33.532 Superficial frostbite of left finger(s)** A, D, S, A
    - **T33.539 Superficial frostbite of unspecified finger(s)** A, D, S, A
- **T33.6 Superficial frostbite of hip and thigh**
  - **T33.60 Superficial frostbite of unspecified hip and thigh** A, D, S, A
  - **T33.61 Superficial frostbite of right hip and thigh** A, D, S, A
  - **T33.62 Superficial frostbite of left hip and thigh** A, D, S, A
- **T33.7 Superficial frostbite of knee and lower leg**
  - **Excludes2** superficial frostbite of ankle and foot (T33.8-)
  - **T33.70 Superficial frostbite of unspecified knee and lower leg** A, D, S, A
  - **T33.71 Superficial frostbite of right knee and lower leg** A, D, S, A
  - **T33.72 Superficial frostbite of left knee and lower leg** A, D, S, A
- **T33.8 Superficial frostbite of ankle, foot, and toe(s)**
  - **T33.81 Superficial frostbite of ankle**
    - **T33.811 Superficial frostbite of right ankle** A, D, S, A
    - **T33.812 Superficial frostbite of left ankle** A, D, S, A
    - **T33.819 Superficial frostbite of unspecified ankle** A, D, S, A
  - **T33.82 Superficial frostbite of foot**
    - **T33.821 Superficial frostbite of right foot** A, D, S, A
    - **T33.822 Superficial frostbite of left foot** A, D, S, A
    - **T33.829 Superficial frostbite of unspecified foot** A, D, S, A

- **T33.83 Superficial frostbite of toe(s)**
  - **T33.831 Superficial frostbite of right toe(s)** A, D, S, A
  - **T33.832 Superficial frostbite of left toe(s)** A, D, S, A
  - **T33.839 Superficial frostbite of unspecified toe(s)** A, D, S, A
- **T33.9 Superficial frostbite of other and unspecified sites**
  - **T33.90 Superficial frostbite of unspecified sites** A, D, S, A
    Superficial frostbite NOS
  - **T33.99 Superficial frostbite of other sites** A, D, S, A
    Superficial frostbite of leg NOS
    Superficial frostbite of trunk NOS
- **T34 Frostbite with tissue necrosis**

  The appropriate 7th character is to be added to each code from category T34

A	initial encounter
D	subsequent encounter
S	sequela

  - **T34.0 Frostbite with tissue necrosis of head**
    - **T34.01 Frostbite with tissue necrosis of ear**
      - **T34.011 Frostbite with tissue necrosis of right ear** A, D, S, A
      - **T34.012 Frostbite with tissue necrosis of left ear** A, D, S, A
      - **T34.019 Frostbite with tissue necrosis of unspecified ear** A, D, S, A
    - **T34.02 Frostbite with tissue necrosis of nose** A, D, S, A
    - **T34.09 Frostbite with tissue necrosis of other part of head** A, D, S, A
  - **T34.1 Frostbite with tissue necrosis of neck** A, D, S, A
  - **T34.2 Frostbite with tissue necrosis of thorax** A, D, S, A
  - **T34.3 Frostbite with tissue necrosis of abdominal wall, lower back and pelvis** A, D, S, A
  - **T34.4 Frostbite with tissue necrosis of arm**
    - **Excludes2** frostbite with tissue necrosis of wrist and hand (T34.5-)
    - **T34.40 Frostbite with tissue necrosis of unspecified arm** A, D, S, A
    - **T34.41 Frostbite with tissue necrosis of right arm** A, D, S, A
    - **T34.42 Frostbite with tissue necrosis of left arm** A, D, S, A
  - **T34.5 Frostbite with tissue necrosis of wrist, hand, and finger(s)**
    - **T34.51 Frostbite with tissue necrosis of wrist**
      - **T34.511 Frostbite with tissue necrosis of right wrist** A, D, S, A
      - **T34.512 Frostbite with tissue necrosis of left wrist** A, D, S, A
      - **T34.519 Frostbite with tissue necrosis of unspecified wrist** A, D, S, A

CHAPTER 19 (S00-T88)

● T34.52   Frostbite with tissue necrosis of hand
    Excludes2   frostbite with tissue necrosis of finger(s) (T34.53-)
    ● T34.521   Frostbite with tissue necrosis of right hand A 🔒, D, S 🔒, A 🔒
    ● T34.522   Frostbite with tissue necrosis of left hand A 🔒, D, S 🔒, A 🔒
    ● ■ T34.529   Frostbite with tissue necrosis of unspecified hand A 🔒, D, S 🔒, A 🔒

● T34.53   Frostbite with tissue necrosis of finger(s)
    ● T34.531   Frostbite with tissue necrosis of right finger(s) A 🔒, D, S 🔒, A 🔒
    ● T34.532   Frostbite with tissue necrosis of left finger(s) A 🔒, D, S 🔒, A 🔒
    ● ■ T34.539   Frostbite with tissue necrosis of unspecified finger(s) A 🔒, D, S 🔒, A 🔒

● T34.6   Frostbite with tissue necrosis of hip and thigh
    ● ■ T34.60   Frostbite with tissue necrosis of unspecified hip and thigh A 🔒, D, S 🔒, A 🔒
    ● T34.61   Frostbite with tissue necrosis of right hip and thigh A 🔒, D, S 🔒, A 🔒
    ● T34.62   Frostbite with tissue necrosis of left hip and thigh A 🔒, D, S 🔒, A 🔒

● T34.7   Frostbite with tissue necrosis of knee and lower leg
    Excludes2   frostbite with tissue necrosis of ankle and foot (T34.8-)
    ● ■ T34.70   Frostbite with tissue necrosis of unspecified knee and lower leg A 🔒, D, S 🔒, A 🔒
    ● T34.71   Frostbite with tissue necrosis of right knee and lower leg A 🔒, D, S 🔒, A 🔒
    ● T34.72   Frostbite with tissue necrosis of left knee and lower leg A 🔒, D, S 🔒, A 🔒

● T34.8   Frostbite with tissue necrosis of ankle, foot, and toe(s)
    ● T34.81   Frostbite with tissue necrosis of ankle
        ● T34.811   Frostbite with tissue necrosis of right ankle A 🔒, D, S 🔒, A 🔒
        ● T34.812   Frostbite with tissue necrosis of left ankle A 🔒, D, S 🔒, A 🔒
        ● ■ T34.819   Frostbite with tissue necrosis of unspecified ankle A 🔒, D, S 🔒, A 🔒
    ● T34.82   Frostbite with tissue necrosis of foot
        ● T34.821   Frostbite with tissue necrosis of right foot A 🔒, D, S 🔒, A 🔒
        ● T34.822   Frostbite with tissue necrosis of left foot A 🔒, D, S 🔒, A 🔒
        ● ■ T34.829   Frostbite with tissue necrosis of unspecified foot A 🔒, D, S 🔒, A 🔒
    ● T34.83   Frostbite with tissue necrosis of toe(s)
        ● T34.831   Frostbite with tissue necrosis of right toe(s) A 🔒, D, S 🔒, A 🔒
        ● T34.832   Frostbite with tissue necrosis of left toe(s) A 🔒, D, S 🔒, A 🔒
        ● ■ T34.839   Frostbite with tissue necrosis of unspecified toe(s) A 🔒, D, S 🔒, A 🔒

● T34.9   Frostbite with tissue necrosis of other and unspecified sites
    ● ■ T34.90   Frostbite with tissue necrosis of unspecified sites A 🔒, D, S 🔒, A 🔒
        Frostbite with tissue necrosis NOS
    ● T34.99   Frostbite with tissue necrosis of other sites A 🔒, D, S 🔒, A 🔒
        Frostbite with tissue necrosis of leg NOS
        Frostbite with tissue necrosis of trunk NOS

OGCR   See Guidelines Section I.C.19.e.

POISONING BY, ADVERSE EFFECTS OF AND UNDERDOSING OF DRUGS, MEDICAMENTS AND BIOLOGICAL SUBSTANCES (T36-T50)

Includes   adverse effect of correct substance properly administered
poisoning by overdose of substance
poisoning by wrong substance given or taken in error
underdosing by (inadvertently) (deliberately) taking less substance than prescribed or instructed

Code first, for adverse effects, the nature of the adverse effect, such as:
adverse effect NOS (T88.7)
aspirin gastritis (K29.-)
blood disorders (D56-D76)
contact dermatitis (L23-L25)
dermatitis due to substances taken internally (L27.-)
nephropathy (N14.0-N14.2)

Note: The drug giving rise to the adverse effect should be identified by use of codes from categories T36-T50 with fifth or sixth character 5.

Use additional code(s) to specify:
manifestations of poisoning
underdosing or failure in dosage during medical and surgical care (Y63.6, Y63.8-Y63.9)
underdosing of medication regimen (Z91.12-, Z91.13-)

Excludes1   toxic reaction to local anesthesia in pregnancy (O29.3-)

Excludes2   abuse and dependence of psychoactive substances (F10-F19)
abuse of non-dependence-producing substances (F55.-)
drug reaction and poisoning affecting newborn (P00-P96)
pathological drug intoxication (inebriation) (F10-F19)

● T36   Poisoning by, adverse effect of and underdosing of systemic antibiotics
    Excludes1   antineoplastic antibiotics (T45.1-)
    locally applied antibiotic NEC (T49.0)
    topically used antibiotic for ear, nose and throat (T49.6)
    topically used antibiotic for eye (T49.5)

    The appropriate 7th character is to be added to each code from category T36

    | A | initial encounter |
    | D | subsequent encounter |
    | S | sequela |

    ● T36.0   Poisoning by, adverse effect of and underdosing of penicillins
        ● T36.0X   Poisoning by, adverse effect of and underdosing of penicillins
            ● T36.0X1   Poisoning by penicillins, accidental (unintentional) D, S 🔒
                Poisoning by penicillins NOS

● Unacceptable Principal Diagnosis   ● Use Additional Character(s)   ■ Unspecified   ▶ Manifestation Code

1616   OGCR   Official Guidelines for Coding and Reporting | Excludes 1 | | Excludes 2 | | Includes | | Use additional | | Code first | | Code also |

● **T36.0X2 Poisoning by penicillins, intentional self-harm** D, S 🔗

● **T36.0X3 Poisoning by penicillins, assault** D, S 🔗

● **T36.0X4 Poisoning by penicillins, undetermined** D, S 🔗

● **T36.0X5 Adverse effect of penicillins** D, S 🔗

● **T36.0X6 Underdosing of penicillins** D, S 🔗

● **T36.1 Poisoning by, adverse effect of and underdosing of cephalosporins and other betalactam antibiotics**

  ● **T36.1X Poisoning by, adverse effect of and underdosing of cephalosporins and other beta-lactam antibiotics**

    ● **T36.1X1 Poisoning by cephalosporins and other beta-lactam antibiotics, accidental (unintentional)** D, S 🔗
        Poisoning by cephalosporins and other beta-lactam antibiotics NOS

    ● **T36.1X2 Poisoning by cephalosporins and other beta-lactam antibiotics, intentional self-harm** D, S 🔗

    ● **T36.1X3 Poisoning by cephalosporins and other beta-lactam antibiotics, assault** D, S 🔗

    ● **T36.1X4 Poisoning by cephalosporins and other beta-lactam antibiotics, undetermined** D, S 🔗

    ● **T36.1X5 Adverse effect of cephalosporins and other beta-lactam antibiotics** D, S 🔗

    ● **T36.1X6 Underdosing of cephalosporins and other beta-lactam antibiotics** D, S 🔗

● **T36.2 Poisoning by, adverse effect of and underdosing of chloramphenicol group**

  ● **T36.2X Poisoning by, adverse effect of and underdosing of chloramphenicol group**

    ● **T36.2X1 Poisoning by chloramphenicol group, accidental (unintentional)** D, S 🔗
        Poisoning by chloramphenicol group NOS

    ● **T36.2X2 Poisoning by chloramphenicol group, intentional self-harm** D, S 🔗

    ● **T36.2X3 Poisoning by chloramphenicol group, assault** D, S 🔗

    ● **T36.2X4 Poisoning by chloramphenicol group, undetermined** D, S 🔗

    ● **T36.2X5 Adverse effect of chloramphenicol group** A, D, S 🔗

    ● **T36.2X6 Underdosing of chloramphenicol group** D, S 🔗

● **T36.3 Poisoning by, adverse effect of and underdosing of macrolides**

  ● **T36.3X Poisoning by, adverse effect of and underdosing of macrolides**

    ● **T36.3X1 Poisoning by macrolides, accidental (unintentional)** D, S 🔗
        Poisoning by macrolides NOS

    ● **T36.3X2 Poisoning by macrolides, intentional self-harm** D, S 🔗

● **T36.3X3 Poisoning by macrolides, assault** D, S 🔗

● **T36.3X4 Poisoning by macrolides, undetermined** D, S 🔗

● **T36.3X5 Adverse effect of macrolides** D, S 🔗

● **T36.3X6 Underdosing of macrolides** D, S 🔗

● **T36.4 Poisoning by, adverse effect of and underdosing of tetracyclines**

  ● **T36.4X Poisoning by, adverse effect of and underdosing of tetracyclines**

    ● **T36.4X1 Poisoning by tetracyclines, accidental (unintentional)** D, S 🔗
        Poisoning by tetracyclines NOS

    ● **T36.4X2 Poisoning by tetracyclines, intentional self-harm** D, S 🔗

    ● **T36.4X3 Poisoning by tetracyclines, assault** D, S 🔗

    ● **T36.4X4 Poisoning by tetracyclines, undetermined** D, S 🔗

    ● **T36.4X5 Adverse effect of tetracyclines** D, S 🔗

    ● **T36.4X6 Underdosing of tetracyclines** A, D, S 🔗

● **T36.5 Poisoning by, adverse effect of and underdosing of aminoglycosides**
    Poisoning by, adverse effect of and underdosing of streptomycin

  ● **T36.5X Poisoning by, adverse effect of and underdosing of aminoglycosides**

    ● **T36.5X1 Poisoning by aminoglycosides, accidental (unintentional)** D, S 🔗
        Poisoning by aminoglycosides NOS

    ● **T36.5X2 Poisoning by aminoglycosides, intentional self-harm** D, S 🔗

    ● **T36.5X3 Poisoning by aminoglycosides, assault** D, S 🔗

    ● **T36.5X4 Poisoning by aminoglycosides, undetermined** D, S 🔗

    ● **T36.5X5 Adverse effect of aminoglycosides** D, S 🔗

    ● **T36.5X6 Underdosing of aminoglycosides** A, D, S 🔗

● **T36.6 Poisoning by, adverse effect of and underdosing of rifampicins**

  ● **T36.6X Poisoning by, adverse effect of and underdosing of rifampicins**

    ● **T36.6X1 Poisoning by rifampicins, accidental (unintentional)** D, S 🔗
        Poisoning by rifampicins NOS

    ● **T36.6X2 Poisoning by rifampicins, intentional self-harm** D, S 🔗

    ● **T36.6X3 Poisoning by rifampicins, assault** D, S 🔗

    ● **T36.6X4 Poisoning by rifampicins, undetermined** D, S 🔗

    ● **T36.6X5 Adverse effect of rifampicins** D, S 🔗

    ● **T36.6X6 Underdosing of rifampicins** A, D, S 🔗

CHAPTER 19 (S00-T88)

N Newborn Age: 0   **P** Pediatric Age: 0–17   **M** Maternity DX: 12–55   **A** Adult Age: 15–124   ♀ Females Only   ♂ Males Only

🔗 Complication\Comorbidity   🔗 Major C\C   🔗 Present on Admission Requirement   🔗 Hospital-Acquired Condition

1617

● **T36.7 Poisoning by, adverse effect of and underdosing of antifungal antibiotics, systemically used**

  ● **T36.7X Poisoning by, adverse effect of and underdosing of antifungal antibiotics, systemically used**

    ● **T36.7X1 Poisoning by antifungal antibiotics, systemically used, accidental (unintentional)** D, S 🔖
         Poisoning by antifungal antibiotics, systemically used NOS

    ● **T36.7X2 Poisoning by antifungal antibiotics, systemically used, intentional self-harm** D, S 🔖

    ● **T36.7X3 Poisoning by antifungal antibiotics, systemically used, assault** D, S 🔖

    ● **T36.7X4 Poisoning by antifungal antibiotics, systemically used, undetermined** D, S 🔖

    ● **T36.7X5 Adverse effect of antifungal antibiotics, systemically used** D, S 🔖

    ● **T36.7X6 Underdosing of antifungal antibiotics, systemically used** A, D, S 🔖

● **T36.8 Poisoning by, adverse effect of and underdosing of other systemic antibiotics**

  ● **T36.8X Poisoning by, adverse effect of and underdosing of other systemic antibiotics**

    ● **T36.8X1 Poisoning by other systemic antibiotics, accidental (unintentional)** D, S 🔖
         Poisoning by other systemic antibiotics NOS

    ● **T36.8X2 Poisoning by other systemic antibiotics, intentional self-harm** D, S 🔖

    ● **T36.8X3 Poisoning by other systemic antibiotics, assault** D, S 🔖

    ● **T36.8X4 Poisoning by other systemic antibiotics, undetermined** D, S 🔖

    ● **T36.8X5 Adverse effect of other systemic antibiotics** D, S 🔖

    ● **T36.8X6 Underdosing of other systemic antibiotics** A, D, S 🔖

● **T36.9 Poisoning by, adverse effect of and underdosing of unspecified systemic antibiotic**

  ● ◼ **T36.91 Poisoning by unspecified systemic antibiotic, accidental (unintentional)** D, S 🔖
         Poisoning by systemic antibiotic NOS

  ● ◼ **T36.92 Poisoning by unspecified systemic antibiotic, intentional self-harm** D, S 🔖

  ● ◼ **T36.93 Poisoning by unspecified systemic antibiotic, assault** D, S 🔖

  ● ◼ **T36.94 Poisoning by unspecified systemic antibiotic, undetermined** D, S 🔖

  ● ◼ **T36.95 Adverse effect of unspecified systemic antibiotic** D, S 🔖

  ● ◼ **T36.96 Underdosing of unspecified systemic antibiotic** A, D, S 🔖

● **T37 Poisoning by, adverse effect of and underdosing of other systemic anti-infectives and antiparasitics**

  | Excludes1 | anti-infectives topically used for ear, nose and throat (T49.6-)
     anti-infectives topically used for eye (T49.5-)
     locally applied anti-infectives NEC (T49.0-)

The appropriate 7th character is to be added to each code from category T37

A	initial encounter
D	subsequent encounter
S	sequela

● **T37.0 Poisoning by, adverse effect of and underdosing of sulfonamides**

  ● **T37.0X Poisoning by, adverse effect of and underdosing of sulfonamides**

    ● **T37.0X1 Poisoning by sulfonamides, accidental (unintentional)** D, S 🔖
         Poisoning by sulfonamides NOS

    ● **T37.0X2 Poisoning by sulfonamides, intentional self-harm** D, S 🔖

    ● **T37.0X3 Poisoning by sulfonamides, assault** D, S 🔖

    ● **T37.0X4 Poisoning by sulfonamides, undetermined** D, S 🔖

    ● **T37.0X5 Adverse effect of sulfonamides** D, S 🔖

    ● **T37.0X6 Underdosing of sulfonamides** A, D, S 🔖

● **T37.1 Poisoning by, adverse effect of and underdosing of antimycobacterial drugs**

  | Excludes1 | rifampicins (T36.6-) streptomycin (T36.5-)

  ● **T37.1X Poisoning by, adverse effect of and underdosing of antimycobacterial drugs**

    ● **T37.1X1 Poisoning by antimycobacterial drugs, accidental (unintentional)** D, S 🔖
         Poisoning by antimycobacterial drugs NOS

    ● **T37.1X2 Poisoning by antimycobacterial drugs, intentional self-harm** D, S 🔖

    ● **T37.1X3 Poisoning by antimycobacterial drugs, assault** D, S 🔖

    ● **T37.1X4 Poisoning by antimycobacterial drugs, undetermined** D, S 🔖

    ● **T37.1X5 Adverse effect of antimycobacterial drugs** D, S 🔖

    ● **T37.1X6 Underdosing of antimycobacterial drugs** A, D, S 🔖

● **T37.2 Poisoning by, adverse effect of and underdosing of antimalarials and drugs acting on other blood protozoa**

  | Excludes1 | hydroxyquinoline derivatives (T37.8-)

  ● **T37.2X Poisoning by, adverse effect of and underdosing of antimalarials and drugs acting on other blood protozoa**

    ● **T37.2X1 Poisoning by antimalarials and drugs acting on other blood protozoa, accidental (unintentional)** D, S 🔖
         Poisoning by antimalarials and drugs acting on other blood protozoa NOS

● Unacceptable Principal Diagnosis   ● Use Additional Character(s)   ◼ Unspecified   ▸ Manifestation Code

OGCR Official Guidelines for Coding and Reporting | Excludes 1 | | Excludes 2 | | Includes | | Use additional | | Code first | | Code also |

● T37.2X2　Poisoning by antimalarials and drugs acting on other blood protozoa, intentional self-harm D, S ⊘

● T37.2X3　Poisoning by antimalarials and drugs acting on other blood protozoa, assault D, S ⊘

● T37.2X4　Poisoning by antimalarials and drugs acting on other blood protozoa, undetermined D, S ⊘

● T37.2X5　Adverse effect of antimalarials and drugs acting on other blood protozoa D, S ⊘

● T37.2X6　Underdosing of antimalarials and drugs acting on other blood protozoa A, D, S ⊘

● T37.3　Poisoning by, adverse effect of and underdosing of other antiprotozoal drugs

● T37.3X　Poisoning by, adverse effect of and underdosing of other antiprotozoal drugs

● T37.3X1　Poisoning by other antiprotozoal drugs, accidental (unintentional) D, S ⊘
　　　　　　Poisoning by other antiprotozoal drugs NOS

● T37.3X2　Poisoning by other antiprotozoal drugs, intentional self-harm D, S ⊘

● T37.3X3　Poisoning by other antiprotozoal drugs, assault D, S ⊘

● T37.3X4　Poisoning by other antiprotozoal drugs, undetermined D, S ⊘

● T37.3X5　Adverse effect of other antiprotozoal drugs D, S ⊘

● T37.3X6　Underdosing of other antiprotozoal drugs A, D, S ⊘

● T37.4　Poisoning by, adverse effect of and underdosing of anthelminthics

● T37.4X　Poisoning by, adverse effect of and underdosing of anthelminthics

● T37.4X1　Poisoning by anthelminthics, accidental (unintentional) D, S ⊘
　　　　　　Poisoning by anthelminthics NOS

● T37.4X2　Poisoning by anthelminthics, intentional self-harm D, S ⊘

● T37.4X3　Poisoning by anthelminthics, assault D, S ⊘

● T37.4X4　Poisoning by anthelminthics, undetermined D, S ⊘

● T37.4X5　Adverse effect of anthelminthics D, S ⊘

● T37.4X6　Underdosing of anthelminthics A, D, S ⊘

● T37.5　Poisoning by, adverse effect of and underdosing of antiviral drugs

　　　| Excludes1 |　amantadine (T42.8-)
　　　　　　　　　cytarabine (T45.1-)

● T37.5X　Poisoning by, adverse effect of and underdosing of antiviral drugs

● T37.5X1　Poisoning by antiviral drugs, accidental (unintentional) D, S ⊘
　　　　　　Poisoning by antiviral drugs NOS

● T37.5X2　Poisoning by antiviral drugs, intentional self-harm D, S ⊘

● T37.5X3　Poisoning by antiviral drugs, assault D, S ⊘

● T37.5X4　Poisoning by antiviral drugs, undetermined D, S ⊘

● T37.5X5　Adverse effect of antiviral drugs D, S ⊘

● T37.5X6　Underdosing of antiviral drugs A, D, S ⊘

● T37.8　Poisoning by, adverse effect of and underdosing of other specified systemic anti-infectives and antiparasitics
　　　Poisoning by, adverse effect of and underdosing of hydroxyquinoline derivatives

　　　| Excludes1 |　antimalarial drugs (T37.2-)

● T37.8X　Poisoning by, adverse effect of and underdosing of other specified systemic anti-infectives and antiparasitics

● T37.8X1　Poisoning by other specified systemic anti-infectives and antiparasitics, accidental (unintentional) D, S ⊘
　　　　　　Poisoning by other specified systemic anti-infectives and antiparasitics NOS

● T37.8X2　Poisoning by other specified systemic anti-infectives and antiparasitics, intentional self-harm D, S ⊘

● T37.8X3　Poisoning by other specified systemic anti-infectives and antiparasitics, assault D, S ⊘

● T37.8X4　Poisoning by other specified systemic anti-infectives and antiparasitics, undetermined D, S ⊘

● T37.8X5　Adverse effect of other specified systemic anti-infectives and antiparasitics D, S ⊘

● T37.8X6　Underdosing of other specified systemic anti-infectives and antiparasitics A, D, S ⊘

● T37.9　Poisoning by, adverse effect of and underdosing of unspecified systemic anti-infective and antiparasitics

●■ T37.91　Poisoning by unspecified systemic anti-infective and antiparasitics, accidental (unintentional) D, S ⊘
　　　　　　Poisoning by, adverse effect of and underdosing of systemic anti-infective and antiparasitics NOS

●■ T37.92　Poisoning by unspecified systemic anti-infective and antiparasitics, intentional self-harm D, S ⊘

●■ T37.93　Poisoning by unspecified systemic anti-infective and antiparasitics, assault D, S ⊘

●■ T37.94　Poisoning by unspecified systemic anti-infective and antiparasitics, undetermined D, S ⊘

●■ T37.95　Adverse effect of unspecified systemic anti-infective and antiparasitic D, S ⊘

●■ T37.96　Underdosing of unspecified systemic anti-infectives and antiparasitics A, D, S ⊘

CHAPTER 19 (S00-T88)

CHAPTER 19 (S00-T88)

● **T38** **Poisoning by, adverse effect of and underdosing of hormones and their synthetic substitutes and antagonists, not elsewhere classified**

| Excludes1 | mineralocorticoids and their antagonists (T50.0-)
oxytocic hormones (T48.0-)
parathyroid hormones and derivatives (T50.9-) |

The appropriate 7th character is to be added to each code from category T38

A   initial encounter
D   subsequent encounter
S   sequela

● **T38.0** **Poisoning by, adverse effect of and underdosing of glucocorticoids and synthetic analogues**

| Excludes1 | glucocorticoids, topically used (T49.-) |

● **T38.0X** **Poisoning by, adverse effect of and underdosing of glucocorticoids and synthetic analogues**

● **T38.0X1** **Poisoning by glucocorticoids and synthetic analogues, accidental (unintentional)** D, S 🔍
Poisoning by glucocorticoids and synthetic analogues NOS

● **T38.0X2** **Poisoning by glucocorticoids and synthetic analogues, intentional self-harm** D, S 🔍

● **T38.0X3** **Poisoning by glucocorticoids and synthetic analogues, assault** D, S 🔍

● **T38.0X4** **Poisoning by glucocorticoids and synthetic analogues, undetermined** D, S 🔍

● **T38.0X5** **Adverse effect of glucocorticoids and synthetic analogues** D, S 🔍

● **T38.0X6** **Underdosing of glucocorticoids and synthetic analogues** A, D, S 🔍

● **T38.1** **Poisoning by, adverse effect of and underdosing of thyroid hormones and substitutes**

● **T38.1X** **Poisoning by, adverse effect of and underdosing of thyroid hormones and substitutes**

● **T38.1X1** **Poisoning by thyroid hormones and substitutes, accidental (unintentional)** D, S 🔍
Poisoning by thyroid hormones and substitutes NOS

● **T38.1X2** **Poisoning by thyroid hormones and substitutes, intentional self-harm** D, S 🔍

● **T38.1X3** **Poisoning by thyroid hormones and substitutes, assault** D, S 🔍

● **T38.1X4** **Poisoning by thyroid hormones and substitutes, undetermined** D, S 🔍

● **T38.1X5** **Adverse effect of thyroid hormones and substitutes** D, S 🔍

● **T38.1X6** **Underdosing of thyroid hormones and substitutes** A, D, S 🔍

● **T38.2** **Poisoning by, adverse effect of and underdosing of antithyroid drugs**

● **T38.2X** **Poisoning by, adverse effect of and underdosing of antithyroid drugs**

● **T38.2X1** **Poisoning by antithyroid drugs, accidental (unintentional)** D, S 🔍
Poisoning by antithyroid drugs NOS

● **T38.2X2** **Poisoning by antithyroid drugs, intentional self-harm** D, S 🔍

● **T38.2X3** **Poisoning by antithyroid drugs, assault** D, S 🔍

● **T38.2X4** **Poisoning by antithyroid drugs, undetermined** D, S 🔍

● **T38.2X5** **Adverse effect of antithyroid drugs** D, S 🔍

● **T38.2X6** **Underdosing of antithyroid drugs** A, D, S 🔍

● **T38.3** **Poisoning by, adverse effect of and underdosing of insulin and oral hypoglycemic [antidiabetic] drugs**

● **T38.3X** **Poisoning by, adverse effect of and underdosing of insulin and oral hypoglycemic [antidiabetic] drugs**

● **T38.3X1** **Poisoning by insulin and oral hypoglycemic [antidiabetic] drugs, accidental (unintentional)** D, S 🔍
Poisoning by insulin and oral hypoglycemic [antidiabetic] drugs NOS

● **T38.3X2** **Poisoning by insulin and oral hypoglycemic [antidiabetic] drugs, intentional self-harm** D, S 🔍

● **T38.3X3** **Poisoning by insulin and oral hypoglycemic [antidiabetic] drugs, assault** D, S 🔍

● **T38.3X4** **Poisoning by insulin and oral hypoglycemic [antidiabetic] drugs, undetermined** D, S 🔍

● **T38.3X5** **Adverse effect of insulin and oral hypoglycemic [antidiabetic] drugs** D, S 🔍

● **T38.3X6** **Underdosing of insulin and oral hypoglycemic [antidiabetic] drugs** A, D, S 🔍

● **T38.4** **Poisoning by, adverse effect of and underdosing of oral contraceptives**
Poisoning by, adverse effect of and underdosing of multiple- and single-ingredient oral contraceptive preparations

● **T38.4X** **Poisoning by, adverse effect of and underdosing of oral contraceptives**

● **T38.4X1** **Poisoning by oral contraceptives, accidental (unintentional)** D, S 🔍
Poisoning by oral contraceptives NOS

● **T38.4X2** **Poisoning by oral contraceptives, intentional self-harm** D, S 🔍

● **T38.4X3** **Poisoning by oral contraceptives, assault** D, S 🔍

● **T38.4X4** **Poisoning by oral contraceptives, undetermined** D, S 🔍

● **T38.4X5** **Adverse effect of oral contraceptives** D, S 🔍

● **T38.4X6** **Underdosing of oral contraceptives** A, D, S 🔍

● Unacceptable Principal Diagnosis   ● Use Additional Character(s)   ▪ Unspecified   ▸ Manifestation Code

1620   OGCR   Official Guidelines for Coding and Reporting   Excludes 1   Excludes 2   Includes   Use additional   Code first   Code also

● **T38.5 Poisoning by, adverse effect of and underdosing of other estrogens and progestogens**
     Poisoning by, adverse effect of and underdosing of estrogens and progestogens mixtures and substitutes

     ● **T38.5X Poisoning by, adverse effect of and underdosing of other estrogens and progestogens**

         ● **T38.5X1 Poisoning by other estrogens and progestogens, accidental (unintentional)** D, S 🔖
             Poisoning by other estrogens and progestogens NOS

         ● **T38.5X2 Poisoning by other estrogens and progestogens, intentional self-harm** D, S 🔖

         ● **T38.5X3 Poisoning by other estrogens and progestogens, assault** D, S 🔖

         ● **T38.5X4 Poisoning by other estrogens and progestogens, undetermined** D, S 🔖

         ● **T38.5X5 Adverse effect of other estrogens and progestogens** D, S 🔖

         ● **T38.5X6 Underdosing of other estrogens and progestogens** A, D, S 🔖

● **T38.6 Poisoning by, adverse effect of and underdosing of antigonadotrophins, antiestrogens, antiandrogens, not elsewhere classified**
     Poisoning by, adverse effect of and underdosing of tamoxifen

     ● **T38.6X Poisoning by, adverse effect of and underdosing of antigonadotrophins, antiestrogens, antiandrogens, not elsewhere classified**

         ● **T38.6X1 Poisoning by antigonadotrophins, antiestrogens, antiandrogens, not elsewhere classified, accidental (unintentional)** D, S 🔖
             Poisoning by antigonadotrophins, antiestrogens, antiandrogens, not elsewhere classified NOS

         ● **T38.6X2 Poisoning by antigonadotrophins, antiestrogens, antiandrogens, not elsewhere classified, intentional self-harm** D, S 🔖

         ● **T38.6X3 Poisoning by antigonadotrophins, antiestrogens, antiandrogens, not elsewhere classified, assault** D, S 🔖

         ● **T38.6X4 Poisoning by antigonadotrophins, antiestrogens, antiandrogens, not elsewhere classified, undetermined** D, S 🔖

         ● **T38.6X5 Adverse effect of antigonadotrophins, antiestrogens, antiandrogens, not elsewhere classified** D, S 🔖

         ● **T38.6X6 Underdosing of antigonadotrophins, antiestrogens, antiandrogens, not elsewhere classified** A, D, S 🔖

● **T38.7 Poisoning by, adverse effect of and underdosing of androgens and anabolic congeners**

     ● **T38.7X Poisoning by, adverse effect of and underdosing of androgens and anabolic congeners**

         ● **T38.7X1 Poisoning by androgens and anabolic congeners, accidental (unintentional)** D, S 🔖
             Poisoning by androgens and anabolic congeners NOS

         ● **T38.7X2 Poisoning by androgens and anabolic congeners, intentional self-harm** D, S 🔖

         ● **T38.7X3 Poisoning by androgens and anabolic congeners, assault** D, S 🔖

         ● **T38.7X4 Poisoning by androgens and anabolic congeners, undetermined** D, S 🔖

         ● **T38.7X5 Adverse effect of androgens and anabolic congeners** D, S 🔖

         ● **T38.7X6 Underdosing of androgens and anabolic congeners** A, D, S 🔖

● **T38.8 Poisoning by, adverse effect of and underdosing of other and unspecified hormones and synthetic substitutes**

     ● **T38.80 Poisoning by, adverse effect of and underdosing of unspecified hormones and synthetic substitutes**

         ●■ **T38.801 Poisoning by unspecified hormones and synthetic substitutes, accidental (unintentional)** D, S 🔖
             Poisoning by unspecified hormones and synthetic substitutes NOS

         ●■ **T38.802 Poisoning by unspecified hormones and synthetic substitutes, intentional self-harm** D, S 🔖

         ●■ **T38.803 Poisoning by unspecified hormones and synthetic substitutes, assault** D, S 🔖

         ●■ **T38.804 Poisoning by unspecified hormones and synthetic substitutes, undetermined** D, S 🔖

         ●■ **T38.805 Adverse effect of unspecified hormones and synthetic substitutes** D, S 🔖

         ●■ **T38.806 Underdosing of unspecified hormones and synthetic substitutes** A, D, S 🔖

     ● **T38.81 Poisoning by, adverse effect of and underdosing of anterior pituitary [adenohypophyseal] hormones**

         ● **T38.811 Poisoning by anterior pituitary [adenohypophyseal] hormones, accidental (unintentional)** D, S 🔖
             Poisoning by anterior pituitary [adenohypophyseal] hormones NOS

         ● **T38.812 Poisoning by anterior pituitary [adenohypophyseal] hormones, intentional self-harm** D, S 🔖

         ● **T38.813 Poisoning by anterior pituitary [adenohypophyseal] hormones, assault** D, S 🔖

N Newborn Age: 0   **P** Pediatric Age: 0–17   **M** Maternity DX: 12–55   **A** Adult Age: 15–124   ♀ Females Only   ♂ Males Only

🔖 Complication\Comorbidity   🔖 Major C\C   🔖 Present on Admission Requirement   🔖 Hospital-Acquired Condition

1621

● T38.814   Poisoning by anterior pituitary [adenohypophyseal] hormones, undetermined D, S

● T38.815   Adverse effect of anterior pituitary [adenohypophyseal] hormones D, S

● T38.816   Underdosing of anterior pituitary [adenohypophyseal] hormones A, D, S

● T38.89   Poisoning by, adverse effect of and underdosing of other hormones and synthetic substitutes

    ● T38.891   Poisoning by other hormones and synthetic substitutes, accidental (unintentional) D, S
        Poisoning by other hormones and synthetic substitutes NOS

    ● T38.892   Poisoning by other hormones and synthetic substitutes, intentional self-harm D, S

    ● T38.893   Poisoning by other hormones and synthetic substitutes, assault D, S

    ● T38.894   Poisoning by other hormones and synthetic substitutes, undetermined D, S

    ● T38.895   Adverse effect of other hormones and synthetic substitutes D, S

    ● T38.896   Underdosing of other hormones and synthetic substitutes A, D, S

● T38.9   Poisoning by, adverse effect of and underdosing of other and unspecified hormone antagonists

   ● T38.90   Poisoning by, adverse effect of and underdosing of unspecified hormone antagonists

    ●■ T38.901   Poisoning by unspecified hormone antagonists, accidental (unintentional) D, S
        Poisoning by unspecified hormone antagonists NOS

    ●■ T38.902   Poisoning by unspecified hormone antagonists, intentional self-harm D, S

    ●■ T38.903   Poisoning by unspecified hormone antagonists, assault D, S

    ●■ T38.904   Poisoning by unspecified hormone antagonists, undetermined D, S

    ●■ T38.905   Adverse effect of unspecified hormone antagonists D, S

    ●■ T38.906   Underdosing of unspecified hormone antagonists A, D, S

   ● T38.99   Poisoning by, adverse effect of and underdosing of other hormone antagonists

    ● T38.991   Poisoning by other hormone antagonists, accidental (unintentional) D, S
        Poisoning by other hormone antagonists NOS

    ● T38.992   Poisoning by other hormone antagonists, intentional self-harm D, S

    ● T38.993   Poisoning by other hormone antagonists, assault D, S

● T38.994   Poisoning by other hormone antagonists, undetermined D, S

● T38.995   Adverse effect of other hormone antagonists D, S

● T38.996   Underdosing of other hormone antagonists A, D, S

● T39   Poisoning by, adverse effect of and underdosing of nonopioid analgesics, antipyretics and antirheumatics

    The appropriate 7th character is to be added to each code from category T39

> A   initial encounter
> D   subsequent encounter
> S   sequela

● T39.0   Poisoning by, adverse effect of and underdosing of salicylates

   ● T39.01   Poisoning by, adverse effect of and underdosing of aspirin
        Poisoning by, adverse effect of and underdosing of acetylsalicylic acid

    ● T39.011   Poisoning by aspirin, accidental (unintentional) D, S

    ● T39.012   Poisoning by aspirin, intentional self-harm D, S

    ● T39.013   Poisoning by aspirin, assault D, S

    ● T39.014   Poisoning by aspirin, undetermined D, S

    ● T39.015   Adverse effect of aspirin D, S

    ● T39.016   Underdosing of aspirin A, D, S

   ● T39.09   Poisoning by, adverse effect of and underdosing of other salicylates

    ● T39.091   Poisoning by salicylates, accidental (unintentional) D, S
        Poisoning by salicylates NOS

    ● T39.092   Poisoning by salicylates, intentional self-harm D, S

    ● T39.093   Poisoning by salicylates, assault D, S

    ● T39.094   Poisoning by salicylates, undetermined D, S

    ● T39.095   Adverse effect of salicylates D, S

    ● T39.096   Underdosing of salicylates A, D, S

● T39.1   Poisoning by, adverse effect of and underdosing of 4-Aminophenol derivatives

   ● T39.1X   Poisoning by, adverse effect of and underdosing of 4-Aminophenol derivatives

    ● T39.1X1   Poisoning by 4-Aminophenol derivatives, accidental (unintentional)
        Poisoning by 4-Aminophenol derivatives NOS

    ● T39.1X2   Poisoning by 4-Aminophenol derivatives, intentional self-harm D, S

    ● T39.1X3   Poisoning by 4-Aminophenol derivatives, assault D, S

    ● T39.1X4   Poisoning by 4-Aminophenol derivatives, undetermined D, S

● Unacceptable Principal Diagnosis   ● Use Additional Character(s)   ■ Unspecified   ▶ Manifestation Code

OGCR Official Guidelines for Coding and Reporting | Excludes 1 | | Excludes 2 | Includes   Use additional   Code first   Code also

● **T39.1X5 Adverse effect of 4-Aminophenol derivatives** D, S 🗘

● **T39.1X6 Underdosing of 4-Aminophenol derivatives** A, D, S 🗘

● **T39.2 Poisoning by, adverse effect of and underdosing of pyrazolone derivatives**

  ● **T39.2X Poisoning by, adverse effect of and underdosing of pyrazolone derivatives**

    ● **T39.2X1 Poisoning by pyrazolone derivatives, accidental (unintentional)** D, S 🗘
      Poisoning by pyrazolone derivatives NOS

    ● **T39.2X2 Poisoning by pyrazolone derivatives, intentional self-harm** D, S 🗘

    ● **T39.2X3 Poisoning by pyrazolone derivatives, assault** D, S 🗘

    ● **T39.2X4 Poisoning by pyrazolone derivatives, undetermined** D, S 🗘

    ● **T39.2X5 Adverse effect of pyrazolone derivatives** D, S 🗘

    ● **T39.2X6 Underdosing of pyrazolone derivatives** A, D, S 🗘

● **T39.3 Poisoning by, adverse effect of and underdosing of other nonsteroidal anti-inflammatory drugs [NSAID]**

  ● **T39.31 Poisoning by, adverse effect of and underdosing of propionic acid derivatives**
    Poisoning by, adverse effect of and underdosing of fenoprofen
    Poisoning by, adverse effect of and underdosing of flurbiprofen
    Poisoning by, adverse effect of and underdosing of ibuprofen
    Poisoning by, adverse effect of and underdosing of ketoprofen
    Poisoning by, adverse effect of and underdosing of naproxen
    Poisoning by, adverse effect of and underdosing of oxaprozin

    ● **T39.311 Poisoning by propionic acid derivatives, accidental (unintentional)** D, S 🗘

    ● **T39.312 Poisoning by propionic acid derivatives, intentional self-harm** D, S 🗘

    ● **T39.313 Poisoning by propionic acid derivatives, assault** D, S 🗘

    ● **T39.314 Poisoning by propionic acid derivatives, undetermined** D, S 🗘

    ● **T39.315 Adverse effect of propionic acid derivatives** D, S 🗘

    ● **T39.316 Underdosing of propionic acid derivatives** A, D, S 🗘

  ● **T39.39 Poisoning by, adverse effect of and underdosing of other nonsteroidal anti-inflammatory drugs [NSAID]**

    ● **T39.391 Poisoning by other nonsteroidal anti-inflammatory drugs [NSAID], accidental (unintentional)** D, S 🗘
      Poisoning by other nonsteroidal anti-inflammatory drugs NOS

● **T39.392 Poisoning by other nonsteroidal anti-inflammatory drugs [NSAID], intentional self-harm** D, S 🗘

● **T39.393 Poisoning by other nonsteroidal anti-inflammatory drugs [NSAID], assault** D, S 🗘

● **T39.394 Poisoning by other nonsteroidal anti-inflammatory drugs [NSAID], undetermined** D, S 🗘

● **T39.395 Adverse effect of other nonsteroidal anti-inflammatory drugs [NSAID]** D, S 🗘

● **T39.396 Underdosing of other nonsteroidal anti-inflammatory drugs [NSAID]** A, D, S 🗘

● **T39.4 Poisoning by, adverse effect of and underdosing of antirheumatics, not elsewhere classified**

  Excludes1 poisoning by, adverse effect of and underdosing of glucocorticoids (T38.0-)
    poisoning by, adverse effect of and underdosing of salicylates (T39.0-)

  ● **T39.4X Poisoning by, adverse effect of and underdosing of antirheumatics, not elsewhere classified**

    ● **T39.4X1 Poisoning by antirheumatics, not elsewhere classified, accidental (unintentional)** D, S 🗘
      Poisoning by antirheumatics, not elsewhere classified NOS

    ● **T39.4X2 Poisoning by antirheumatics, not elsewhere classified, intentional self-harm** D, S 🗘

    ● **T39.4X3 Poisoning by antirheumatics, not elsewhere classified, assault** D, S 🗘

    ● **T39.4X4 Poisoning by antirheumatics, not elsewhere classified, undetermined** D, S 🗘

    ● **T39.4X5 Adverse effect of antirheumatics, not elsewhere classified** D, S 🗘

    ● **T39.4X6 Underdosing of antirheumatics, not elsewhere classified** A, D, S 🗘

● **T39.8 Poisoning by, adverse effect of and underdosing of other nonopioid analgesics and antipyretics, not elsewhere classified**

  ● **T39.8X Poisoning by, adverse effect of and underdosing of other nonopioid analgesics and antipyretics, not elsewhere classified**

    ● **T39.8X1 Poisoning by other nonopioid analgesics and antipyretics, not elsewhere classified, accidental (unintentional)** D, S 🗘
      Poisoning by other nonopioid analgesics and antipyretics, not elsewhere classified NOS

    ● **T39.8X2 Poisoning by other nonopioid analgesics and antipyretics, not elsewhere classified, intentional self-harm** D, S 🗘

N Newborn Age: 0   **P** Pediatric Age: 0–17   **M** Maternity DX: 12–55   **A** Adult Age: 15–124   ♀ Females Only   ♂ Males Only

🗘 Complication\Comorbidity   🗘 Major C\C   ■ Present on Admission Requirement   🗘 Hospital-Acquired Condition

1623

● **T39.8X3** **Poisoning by other nonopioid analgesics and antipyretics, not elsewhere classified, assault** D, S 🖉

● **T39.8X4** **Poisoning by other nonopioid analgesics and antipyretics, not elsewhere classified, undetermined** D, S 🖉

● **T39.8X5** **Adverse effect of other nonopioid analgesics and antipyretics, not elsewhere classified** D, S 🖉

● **T39.8X6** **Underdosing of other nonopioid analgesics and antipyretics, not elsewhere classified** A, D, S 🖉

● **T39.9** **Poisoning by, adverse effect of and underdosing of unspecified nonopioid analgesic, antipyretic and antirheumatic**

● ■ **T39.91** **Poisoning by unspecified nonopioid analgesic, antipyretic and antirheumatic, accidental (unintentional)** D, S 🖉
  Poisoning by nonopioid analgesic, antipyretic and antirheumatic NOS

● ■ **T39.92** **Poisoning by unspecified nonopioid analgesic, antipyretic and antirheumatic, intentional self-harm** D, S 🖉

● ■ **T39.93** **Poisoning by unspecified nonopioid analgesic, antipyretic and antirheumatic, assault** D, S 🖉

● ■ **T39.94** **Poisoning by unspecified nonopioid analgesic, antipyretic and antirheumatic, undetermined** D, S 🖉

● ■ **T39.95** **Adverse effect of unspecified nonopioid analgesic, antipyretic and antirheumatic** D, S 🖉

● ■ **T39.96** **Underdosing of unspecified nonopioid analgesic, antipyretic and antirheumatic** A, D, S 🖉

● **T40** **Poisoning by, adverse effect of and underdosing of narcotics and psychodysleptics [hallucinogens]**

Excludes2 drug dependence and related mental and behavioral disorders due to psychoactive substance use (F10.-F19.-)

The appropriate 7th character is to be added to each code from category T40

A	initial encounter
D	subsequent encounter
S	sequela

● **T40.0** **Poisoning by, adverse effect of and underdosing of opium**

● **T40.0X** **Poisoning by, adverse effect of and underdosing of opium**

T40.0X1 **Poisoning by opium, accidental (unintentional)** D, S 🖉
  Poisoning by opium NOS

● **T40.0X2** **Poisoning by opium, intentional self-harm** D, S 🖉

● **T40.0X3** **Poisoning by opium, assault** D, S 🖉

● **T40.0X4** **Poisoning by opium, undetermined** D, S 🖉

● **T40.0X5** **Adverse effect of opium** D, S 🖉

● **T40.0X6** **Underdosing of opium** A, D, S 🖉

● **T40.1** **Poisoning by and adverse effect of heroin**

● **T40.1X** **Poisoning by and adverse effect of heroin**

● **T40.1X1** **Poisoning by heroin, accidental (unintentional)** D, S 🖉
  Poisoning by heroin NOS

● **T40.1X2** **Poisoning by heroin, intentional self-harm** D, S 🖉

● **T40.1X3** **Poisoning by heroin, assault** D, S 🖉

● **T40.1X4** **Poisoning by heroin, undetermined** D, S 🖉

● **T40.1X5** **Adverse effect of heroin** D, S 🖉

● **T40.2** **Poisoning by, adverse effect of and underdosing of other opioids**

● **T40.2X** **Poisoning by, adverse effect of and underdosing of other opioids**

● **T40.2X1** **Poisoning by other opioids, accidental (unintentional)** D, S 🖉
  Poisoning by other opioids NOS

● **T40.2X2** **Poisoning by other opioids, intentional self-harm** D, S 🖉

● **T40.2X3** **Poisoning by other opioids, assault** D, S 🖉

● **T40.2X4** **Poisoning by other opioids, undetermined** D, S 🖉

● **T40.2X5** **Adverse effect of other opioids** D, S 🖉

● **T40.2X6** **Underdosing of other opioids** A, D, S 🖉

● **T40.3** **Poisoning by, adverse effect of and underdosing of methadone**

● **T40.3X** **Poisoning by, adverse effect of and underdosing of methadone**

● **T40.3X1** **Poisoning by methadone, accidental (unintentional)** D, S 🖉
  Poisoning by methadone NOS

● **T40.3X2** **Poisoning by methadone, intentional self-harm** D, S 🖉

● **T40.3X3** **Poisoning by methadone, assault** D, S 🖉

● **T40.3X4** **Poisoning by methadone, undetermined** D, S 🖉

● **T40.3X5** **Adverse effect of methadone** D, S 🖉

● **T40.3X6** **Underdosing of methadone** A, D, S 🖉

● **T40.4** **Poisoning by, adverse effect of and underdosing of other synthetic narcotics**

● **T40.4X** **Poisoning by, adverse effect of and underdosing of other synthetic narcotics** D, S 🖉

● **T40.4X1** **Poisoning by other synthetic narcotics, accidental (unintentional)** D, S 🖉
  Poisoning by other synthetic narcotics NOS

● **T40.4X2** **Poisoning by other synthetic narcotics, intentional self-harm** D, S 🖉

● Unacceptable Principal Diagnosis   ● Use Additional Character(s)   ■ Unspecified   ▶ Manifestation Code
OGCR Official Guidelines for Coding and Reporting   Excludes 1   Excludes 2   Includes   Use additional   Code first   Code also

● T40.4X3   Poisoning by other synthetic narcotics, assault D, S 🗌

● T40.4X4   Poisoning by other synthetic narcotics, undetermined D, S 🗌

● T40.4X5   Adverse effect of other synthetic narcotics D, S 🗌

● T40.4X6   Underdosing of other synthetic narcotics A, D, S 🗌

● T40.5   Poisoning by, adverse effect of and underdosing of cocaine

   ● T40.5X   Poisoning by, adverse effect of and underdosing of cocaine

     ● T40.5X1   Poisoning by cocaine, accidental (unintentional) D, S 🗌
           Poisoning by cocaine NOS

     ● T40.5X2   Poisoning by cocaine, intentional self-harm D, S 🗌

     ● T40.5X3   Poisoning by cocaine, assault D, S 🗌

     ● T40.5X4   Poisoning by cocaine, undetermined D, S 🗌

     ● T40.5X5   Adverse effect of cocaine D, S 🗌

     ● T40.5X6   Underdosing of cocaine A, D, S 🗌

● T40.6   Poisoning by, adverse effect of and underdosing of other and unspecified narcotics

   ● T40.60   Poisoning by, adverse effect of and underdosing of unspecified narcotics

     ● ◼ T40.601   Poisoning by unspecified narcotics, accidental (unintentional) D, S 🗌
           Poisoning by narcotics NOS

     ● ◼ T40.602   Poisoning by unspecified narcotics, intentional self-harm D, S 🗌

     ● ◼ T40.603   Poisoning by unspecified narcotics, assault D, S 🗌

     ● ◼ T40.604   Poisoning by unspecified narcotics, undetermined D, S 🗌

     ● ◼ T40.605   Adverse effect of unspecified narcotics D, S 🗌

     ● ◼ T40.606   Underdosing of unspecified narcotics A, D, S 🗌

   ● T40.69   Poisoning by, adverse effect of and underdosing of other narcotics

     ● T40.691   Poisoning by other narcotics, accidental (unintentional) D, S 🗌
           Poisoning by other narcotics NOS

     ● T40.692   Poisoning by other narcotics, intentional self-harm D, S 🗌

     ● T40.693   Poisoning by other narcotics, assault D, S 🗌

     ● T40.694   Poisoning by other narcotics, undetermined D, S 🗌

     ● T40.695   Adverse effect of other narcotics D, S 🗌

     ● T40.696   Underdosing of other narcotics A, D, S 🗌

● T40.7   Poisoning by, adverse effect of and underdosing of cannabis (derivatives)

   ● T40.7X   Poisoning by, adverse effect of and underdosing of cannabis (derivatives)

     ● T40.7X1   Poisoning by cannabis (derivatives), accidental (unintentional) D, S 🗌
           Poisoning by cannabis NOS

     ● T40.7X2   Poisoning by cannabis (derivatives), intentional self-harm D, S 🗌

     ● T40.7X3   Poisoning by cannabis (derivatives), assault D, S 🗌

     ● T40.7X4   Poisoning by cannabis (derivatives), undetermined D, S 🗌

     ● T40.7X5   Adverse effect of cannabis (derivatives) D, S 🗌

     ● T40.7X6   Underdosing of cannabis (derivatives) A, D, S 🗌

● T40.8   Poisoning by and adverse effect of lysergide [LSD]

   ● T40.8X   Poisoning by and adverse effect of lysergide [LSD]

     ● T40.8X1   Poisoning by lysergide [LSD], accidental (unintentional) D, S 🗌
           Poisoning by lysergide [LSD] NOS

     ● T40.8X2   Poisoning by lysergide [LSD], intentional self-harm D, S 🗌

     ● T40.8X3   Poisoning by lysergide [LSD], assault D, S 🗌

     ● T40.8X4   Poisoning by lysergide [LSD], undetermined D, S 🗌

     ● T40.8X5   Adverse effect of lysergide [LSD] D, S 🗌

● T40.9   Poisoning by, adverse effect of and underdosing of other and unspecified psychodysleptics [hallucinogens]

   ● T40.90   Poisoning by, adverse effect of and underdosing of unspecified psychodysleptics [hallucinogens]

     ● ◼ T40.901   Poisoning by unspecified psychodysleptics [hallucinogens], accidental (unintentional) D, S 🗌

     ● ◼ T40.902   Poisoning by unspecified psychodysleptics [hallucinogens], intentional self-harm D, S 🗌

     ● ◼ T40.903   Poisoning by unspecified psychodysleptics [hallucinogens], assault D, S 🗌

     ● ◼ T40.904   Poisoning by unspecified psychodysleptics [hallucinogens], undetermined D, S 🗌

     ● ◼ T40.905   Adverse effect of unspecified psychodysleptics [hallucinogens] D, S 🗌

     ● ◼ T40.906   Underdosing of unspecified psychodysleptics A, D, S 🗌

N Newborn Age: 0   **P** Pediatric Age: 0–17   **M** Maternity DX: 12–55   **A** Adult Age: 15–124   ♀ Females Only   ♂ Males Only

🔧 Complication\Comorbidity   🔧 Major C\C   🗌 Present on Admission Requirement   🗌 Hospital-Acquired Condition

1625

CHAPTER 19 (S00-T88)

● **T40.99** **Poisoning by, adverse effect of and underdosing of other psychodysleptics [hallucinogens]**

   ● **T40.991** **Poisoning by other psychodysleptics [hallucinogens], accidental (unintentional)** D, S 🔧

      Poisoning by other psychodysleptics [hallucinogens] NOS

   ● **T40.992** **Poisoning by other psychodysleptics [hallucinogens], intentional self-harm** D, S 🔧

   ● **T40.993** **Poisoning by other psychodysleptics [hallucinogens], assault** D, S 🔧

   ● **T40.994** **Poisoning by other psychodysleptics [hallucinogens], undetermined** D, S 🔧

   ● **T40.995** **Adverse effect of other psychodysleptics [hallucinogens]** D, S 🔧

   ● **T40.996** **Underdosing of other psychodysleptics** A, D, S 🔧

● **T41** **Poisoning by, adverse effect of and underdosing of anesthetics and therapeutic gases**

   Excludes1 benzodiazepines (T42.4-)
           cocaine (T40.5-)
           complications of anesthesia during pregnancy (O29.-)
           complications of anesthesia during labor and delivery (O74.-)
           complications of anesthesia during the puerperium (O89.-) opioids (T40.0-T40.2-)

   The appropriate 7th character is to be added to each code from category T41

      A   initial encounter
      D   subsequent encounter
      S   sequela

● **T41.0** **Poisoning by, adverse effect of and underdosing of inhaled anesthetics**

   Excludes1 oxygen (T41.5-)

   ● **T41.0X** **Poisoning by, adverse effect of and underdosing of inhaled anesthetics**

     ● **T41.0X1** **Poisoning by inhaled anesthetics, accidental (unintentional)** D, S 🔧
        Poisoning by inhaled anesthetics NOS

     ● **T41.0X2** **Poisoning by inhaled anesthetics, intentional self-harm** D, S 🔧

     ● **T41.0X3** **Poisoning by inhaled anesthetics, assault** D, S 🔧

     ● **T41.0X4** **Poisoning by inhaled anesthetics, undetermined** D, S 🔧

     ● **T41.0X5** **Adverse effect of inhaled anesthetics** D, S 🔧

     ● **T41.0X6** **Underdosing of inhaled anesthetics** A, D, S 🔧

● **T41.1** **Poisoning by, adverse effect of and underdosing of intravenous anesthetics**

   Poisoning by, adverse effect of and underdosing of thiobarbiturates

   ● **T41.1X** **Poisoning by, adverse effect of and underdosing of intravenous anesthetics**

     ● **T41.1X1** **Poisoning by intravenous anesthetics, accidental (unintentional)** D, S 🔧
        Poisoning by intravenous anesthetics NOS

     ● **T41.1X2** **Poisoning by intravenous anesthetics, intentional self-harm** D, S 🔧

     ● **T41.1X3** **Poisoning by intravenous anesthetics, assault** D, S 🔧

     ● **T41.1X4** **Poisoning by intravenous anesthetics, undetermined** D, S 🔧

     ● **T41.1X5** **Adverse effect of intravenous anesthetics** D, S 🔧

     ● **T41.1X6** **Underdosing of intravenous anesthetics** A, D, S 🔧

● **T41.2** **Poisoning by, adverse effect of and underdosing of other and unspecified general anesthetics**

   ● **T41.20** **Poisoning by, adverse effect of and underdosing of unspecified general anesthetics**

     ●■ **T41.201** **Poisoning by unspecified general anesthetics, accidental (unintentional)** D, S 🔧
        Poisoning by general anesthetics NOS

     ●■ **T41.202** **Poisoning by unspecified general anesthetics, intentional self-harm** D, S 🔧

     ●■ **T41.203** **Poisoning by unspecified general anesthetics, assault** D, S 🔧

     ●■ **T41.204** **Poisoning by unspecified general anesthetics, undetermined** D, S 🔧

     ●■ **T41.205** **Adverse effect of unspecified general anesthetics** D, S 🔧

     ●■ **T41.206** **Underdosing of unspecified general anesthetics** A, D, S 🔧

   ● **T41.29** **Poisoning by, adverse effect of and underdosing of other general anesthetics**

     ● **T41.291** **Poisoning by other general anesthetics, accidental (unintentional)** D, S 🔧
        Poisoning by other general anesthetics NOS

     ● **T41.292** **Poisoning by other general anesthetics, intentional self-harm** D, S 🔧

     ● **T41.293** **Poisoning by other general anesthetics, assault** D, S 🔧

     ● **T41.294** **Poisoning by other general anesthetics, undetermined** D, S 🔧

     ● **T41.295** **Adverse effect of other general anesthetics** D, S 🔧

     ● **T41.296** **Underdosing of other general anesthetics** A, D, S 🔧

● Unacceptable Principal Diagnosis   ● Use Additional Character(s)   ■ Unspecified   ▶ Manifestation Code

1626   **OGCR** Official Guidelines for Coding and Reporting   Excludes 1   Excludes 2   Includes   Use additional   Code first   Code also

● **T41.3** **Poisoning by, adverse effect of and underdosing of local anesthetics**
Cocaine (topical)

Excludes2   poisoning by cocaine used as a central nervous system stimulant (T40.5x1-T40.5x4)

● **T41.3X** **Poisoning by, adverse effect of and underdosing of local anesthetics**

  ● **T41.3X1** **Poisoning by local anesthetics, accidental (unintentional)** D, S 🔍
Poisoning by local anesthetics NOS

  ● **T41.3X2** **Poisoning by local anesthetics, intentional self-harm** D, S 🔍

  ● **T41.3X3** **Poisoning by local anesthetics, assault** D, S 🔍

  ● **T41.3X4** **Poisoning by local anesthetics, undetermined** D, S 🔍

  ● **T41.3X5** **Adverse effect of local anesthetics** D, S 🔍

  ● **T41.3X6** **Underdosing of local anesthetics** A, D, S 🔍

● **T41.4** **Poisoning by, adverse effect of and underdosing of unspecified anesthetic**

  ●■ **T41.41** **Poisoning by unspecified anesthetic, accidental (unintentional)** D, S 🔍
Poisoning by anesthetic NOS

  ●■ **T41.42** **Poisoning by unspecified anesthetic, intentional self-harm** D, S 🔍

  ●■ **T41.43** **Poisoning by unspecified anesthetic, assault** D, S 🔍

  ●■ **T41.44** **Poisoning by unspecified anesthetic, undetermined** D, S 🔍

  ●■ **T41.45** **Adverse effect of unspecified anesthetic** D, S 🔍

  ●■ **T41.46** **Underdosing of unspecified anesthetics** A, D, S 🔍

● **T41.5** **Poisoning by, adverse effect of and underdosing of therapeutic gases**

  ● **T41.5X** **Poisoning by, adverse effect of and underdosing of therapeutic gases**

   ● **T41.5X1** **Poisoning by therapeutic gases, accidental (unintentional)** D, S 🔍
Poisoning by therapeutic gases NOS

   ● **T41.5X2** **Poisoning by therapeutic gases, intentional self-harm** D, S 🔍

   ● **T41.5X3** **Poisoning by therapeutic gases, assault** D, S 🔍

   ● **T41.5X4** **Poisoning by therapeutic gases, undetermined** D, S 🔍

   ● **T41.5X5** **Adverse effect of therapeutic gases** D, S 🔍

   ● **T41.5X6** **Underdosing of therapeutic gases** A, D, S 🔍

● **T42** **Poisoning by, adverse effect of and underdosing of antiepileptic, sedative-hypnotic and antiparkinsonism drugs**

Excludes2   drug dependence and related mental and behavioral disorders due to psychoactive substance use (F10.--F19.-)

The appropriate 7th character is to be added to each code from category T42

A	initial encounter
D	subsequent encounter
S	sequela

● **T42.0** **Poisoning by, adverse effect of and underdosing of hydantoin derivatives**

  ● **T42.0X** **Poisoning by, adverse effect of and underdosing of hydantoin derivatives**

   ● **T42.0X1** **Poisoning by hydantoin derivatives, accidental (unintentional)** D, S 🔍
Poisoning by hydantoin derivatives NOS

   ● **T42.0X2** **Poisoning by hydantoin derivatives, intentional self-harm** D, S 🔍

   ● **T42.0X3** **Poisoning by hydantoin derivatives, assault** D, S 🔍

   ● **T42.0X4** **Poisoning by hydantoin derivatives, undetermined** D, S 🔍

   ● **T42.0X5** **Adverse effect of hydantoin derivatives** D, S 🔍

   ● **T42.0X6** **Underdosing of hydantoin derivatives** A, D, S 🔍

● **T42.1** **Poisoning by, adverse effect of and underdosing of iminostilbenes**
Poisoning by, adverse effect of and underdosing of carbamazepine

  ● **T42.1X** **Poisoning by, adverse effect of and underdosing of iminostilbenes** D, S 🔍

   ● **T42.1X1** **Poisoning by iminostilbenes, accidental (unintentional)** D, S 🔍
Poisoning by iminostilbenes NOS

   ● **T42.1X2** **Poisoning by iminostilbenes, intentional self-harm** D, S 🔍

   ● **T42.1X3** **Poisoning by iminostilbenes, assault** D, S 🔍

   ● **T42.1X4** **Poisoning by iminostilbenes, undetermined** D, S 🔍

   ● **T42.1X5** **Adverse effect of iminostilbenes** D, S 🔍

   ● **T42.1X6** **Underdosing of iminostilbenes** A, D, S 🔍

● **T42.2** **Poisoning by, adverse effect of and underdosing of succinimides and oxazolidinediones**

  ● **T42.2X** **Poisoning by, adverse effect of and underdosing of succinimides and oxazolidinediones**

   ● **T42.2X1** **Poisoning by succinimides and oxazolidinediones, accidental (unintentional)** D, S 🔍
Poisoning by succinimides and oxazolidinediones NOS

CHAPTER 19 (S00-T88)

● **T42.2X2** **Poisoning by succinimides and oxazolidinediones, intentional self-harm** D, S 🔖

● **T42.2X3** **Poisoning by succinimides and oxazolidinediones, assault** D, S 🔖

● **T42.2X4** **Poisoning by succinimides and oxazolidinediones, undetermined** D, S 🔖

● **T42.2X5** **Adverse effect of succinimides and oxazolidinediones** D, S 🔖

● **T42.2X6** **Underdosing of succinimides and oxazolidinediones** A, D, S 🔖

● **T42.3** **Poisoning by, adverse effect of and underdosing of barbiturates**

| Excludes1 | poisoning by, adverse effect of and underdosing of thiobarbiturates (T41.1-) |

● **T42.3X** **Poisoning by, adverse effect of and underdosing of barbiturates**

● **T42.3X1** **Poisoning by barbiturates, accidental (unintentional)** D, S 🔖
Poisoning by barbiturates NOS

● **T42.3X2** **Poisoning by barbiturates, intentional self-harm** D, S 🔖

● **T42.3X3** **Poisoning by barbiturates, assault** D, S 🔖

● **T42.3X4** **Poisoning by barbiturates, undetermined** D, S 🔖

● **T42.3X5** **Adverse effect of barbiturates** D, S 🔖

● **T42.3X6** **Underdosing of barbiturates** A, D, S 🔖

● **T42.4** **Poisoning by, adverse effect of and underdosing of benzodiazepines**

● **T42.4X** **Poisoning by, adverse effect of and underdosing of benzodiazepines**

● **T42.4X1** **Poisoning by benzodiazepines, accidental (unintentional)** D, S 🔖
Poisoning by benzodiazepines NOS

● **T42.4X2** **Poisoning by benzodiazepines, intentional self-harm** D, S 🔖

● **T42.4X3** **Poisoning by benzodiazepines, assault** D, S 🔖

● **T42.4X4** **Poisoning by benzodiazepines, undetermined** D, S 🔖

● **T42.4X5** **Adverse effect of benzodiazepines** D, S 🔖

● **T42.4X6** **Underdosing of benzodiazepines** A, D, S 🔖

● **T42.5** **Poisoning by, adverse effect of and underdosing of mixed antiepileptics**

● **T42.5X** **Poisoning by, adverse effect of and underdosing of antiepileptics**

● **T42.5X1** **Poisoning by mixed antiepileptics, accidental (unintentional)** D, S 🔖
Poisoning by mixed antiepileptics NOS

● **T42.5X2** **Poisoning by mixed antiepileptics, intentional self-harm** D, S 🔖

● **T42.5X3** **Poisoning by mixed antiepileptics, assault** D, S 🔖

● **T42.5X4** **Poisoning by mixed antiepileptics, undetermined** D, S 🔖

● **T42.5X5** **Adverse effect of mixed antiepileptics** D, S 🔖

● **T42.5X6** **Underdosing of mixed antiepileptics** A, D, S 🔖

● **T42.6** **Poisoning by, adverse effect of and underdosing of other antiepileptic and sedative-hypnotic drugs**
Poisoning by, adverse effect of and underdosing of methaqualone
Poisoning by, adverse effect of and underdosing of valproic acid

| Excludes1 | poisoning by, adverse effect of and underdosing of carbamazepine (T42.1-) |

● **T42.6X** **Poisoning by, adverse effect of and underdosing of other antiepileptic and sedative-hypnotic drugs**

● **T42.6X1** **Poisoning by other antiepileptic and sedative-hypnotic drugs, accidental (unintentional)** D, S 🔖
Poisoning by other antiepileptic and sedative-hypnotic drugs NOS

● **T42.6X2** **Poisoning by other antiepileptic and sedative-hypnotic drugs, intentional self-harm** D, S 🔖

● **T42.6X3** **Poisoning by other antiepileptic and sedative-hypnotic drugs, assault** D, S 🔖

● **T42.6X4** **Poisoning by other antiepileptic and sedative-hypnotic drugs, undetermined** D, S 🔖

● **T42.6X5** **Adverse effect of other antiepileptic and sedative-hypnotic drugs** D, S 🔖

● **T42.6X6** **Underdosing of other antiepileptic and sedative-hypnotic drugs** A, D, S 🔖

● **T42.7** **Poisoning by, adverse effect of and underdosing of unspecified antiepileptic and sedative-hypnotic drugs**

● ■ **T42.71** **Poisoning by unspecified antiepileptic and sedative-hypnotic drugs, accidental (unintentional)** D, S 🔖
Poisoning by antiepileptic and sedative-hypnotic drugs NOS

● ■ **T42.72** **Poisoning by unspecified antiepileptic and sedative-hypnotic drugs, intentional self-harm** D, S 🔖

● ■ **T42.73** **Poisoning by unspecified antiepileptic and sedative-hypnotic drugs, assault** D, S 🔖

● ■ **T42.74** **Poisoning by unspecified antiepileptic and sedative-hypnotic drugs, undetermined** D, S 🔖

● ■ **T42.75** **Adverse effect of unspecified antiepileptic and sedative-hypnotic drugs** D, S 🔖

● ■ **T42.76** **Underdosing of unspecified antiepileptic and sedative-hypnotic drugs** A, D, S 🔖

● Unacceptable Principal Diagnosis   ● Use Additional Character(s)   ■ Unspecified   ▶ Manifestation Code

1628   OGCR Official Guidelines for Coding and Reporting | Excludes 1 | | Excludes 2 | Includes   Use additional   Code first   Code also

●T42.8　Poisoning by, adverse effect of and underdosing of antiparkinsonism drugs and other central muscle-tone depressants
>　Poisoning by, adverse effect of and underdosing of amantadine

　●T42.8X　Poisoning by, adverse effect of and underdosing of antiparkinsonism drugs and other central muscle-tone depressants

　　●T42.8X1　Poisoning by antiparkinsonism drugs and other central muscle-tone depressants, accidental (unintentional) D, S 🔍
>　　　Poisoning by antiparkinsonism drugs and other central muscle-tone depressants NOS

　　●T42.8X2　Poisoning by antiparkinsonism drugs and other central muscle-tone depressants, intentional self-harm D, S 🔍

　　●T42.8X3　Poisoning by antiparkinsonism drugs and other central muscle-tone depressants, assault D, S 🔍

　　●T42.8X4　Poisoning by antiparkinsonism drugs and other central muscle-tone depressants, undetermined D, S 🔍

　　●T42.8X5　Adverse effect of antiparkinsonism drugs and other central muscle-tone depressants D, S 🔍

　　●T42.8X6　Underdosing of antiparkinsonism drugs and other central muscle-tone depressants A, D, S 🔍

●T43　Poisoning by, adverse effect of and underdosing of psychotropic drugs, not elsewhere classified

　Excludes1　appetite depressants (T50.5-)
　　　barbiturates (T42.3-)
　　　benzodiazepines (T42.4-)
　　　methaqualone (T42.6-)
　　　psychodysleptics [hallucinogens] (T40.7-T40.9-)

　Excludes2　drug dependence and related mental and behavioral disorders due to psychoactive substance use (F10.--F19.-)

　The appropriate 7th character is to be added to each code from category T43

> A　initial encounter
> D　subsequent encounter
> S　sequela

　●T43.0　Poisoning by, adverse effect of and underdosing of tricyclic and tetracyclic antidepressants

　　●T43.01　Poisoning by, adverse effect of and underdosing of tricyclic antidepressants

　　　●T43.011　Poisoning by tricyclic antidepressants, accidental (unintentional) D, S 🔍
>　　　　Poisoning by tricyclic antidepressants NOS

　　　●T43.012　Poisoning by tricyclic antidepressants, intentional self-harm D, S 🔍

　　　●T43.013　Poisoning by tricyclic antidepressants, assault D, S 🔍

●T43.014　Poisoning by tricyclic antidepressants, undetermined D, S 🔍

●T43.015　Adverse effect of tricyclic antidepressants D, S 🔍

●T43.016　Underdosing of tricyclic antidepressants A, D, S 🔍

●T43.02　Poisoning by, adverse effect of and underdosing of tetracyclic antidepressants

　●T43.021　Poisoning by tetracyclic antidepressants, accidental (unintentional) D, S 🔍
>　　Poisoning by tetracyclic antidepressants NOS

　●T43.022　Poisoning by tetracyclic antidepressants, intentional self-harm D, S 🔍

　●T43.023　Poisoning by tetracyclic antidepressants, assault D, S 🔍

　●T43.024　Poisoning by tetracyclic antidepressants, undetermined D, S 🔍

　●T43.025　Adverse effect of tetracyclic antidepressants D, S 🔍

　●T43.026　Underdosing of tetracyclic antidepressants A, D, S 🔍

●T43.1　Poisoning by, adverse effect of and underdosing of monoamine-oxidase-inhibitor antidepressants

　●T43.1X　Poisoning by, adverse effect of and underdosing of monoamine-oxidase-inhibitor antidepressants

　　●T43.1X1　Poisoning by monoamine-oxidase-inhibitor antidepressants, accidental (unintentional) D, S 🔍
>　　　Poisoning by monoamine-oxidase-inhibitor antidepressants NOS

　　●T43.1X2　Poisoning by monoamine-oxidase-inhibitor antidepressants, intentional self-harm D, S 🔍

　　●T43.1X3　Poisoning by monoamine-oxidase-inhibitor antidepressants, assault D, S 🔍

　　●T43.1X4　Poisoning by monoamine-oxidase-inhibitor antidepressants, undetermined D, S 🔍

　　●T43.1X5　Adverse effect of monoamine-oxidase-inhibitor antidepressants D, S 🔍

　　●T43.1X6　Underdosing of monoamine-oxidase-inhibitor antidepressants A, D, S 🔍

●T43.2　Poisoning by, adverse effect of and underdosing of other and unspecified antidepressants

　●T43.20　Poisoning by, adverse effect of and underdosing of unspecified antidepressants

　　●■T43.201　Poisoning by unspecified antidepressants, accidental (unintentional) D, S 🔍
>　　　Poisoning by antidepressants NOS

CHAPTER 19 (S00-T88)

● ▪ T43.202 Poisoning by unspecified
             antidepressants, intentional
             self-harm D, S 🔍

● ▪ T43.203 Poisoning by unspecified
             antidepressants, assault D, S 🔍

● ▪ T43.204 Poisoning by unspecified
             antidepressants, undetermined
             D, S 🔍

● ▪ T43.205 Adverse effect of unspecified
             antidepressants D, S 🔍

● ▪ T43.206 Underdosing of unspecified
             antidepressants A, D, S 🔍

● T43.21 Poisoning by, adverse effect of and
          underdosing of selective serotonin and
          norepinephrine reuptake inhibitors
            Poisoning by, adverse effect of
              and underdosing of SSNRI
              antidepressants

  ● T43.211 Poisoning by selective serotonin
             and norepinephrine reuptake
             inhibitors, accidental
             (unintentional) D, S 🔍

  ● T43.212 Poisoning by selective serotonin
             and norepinephrine reuptake
             inhibitors, intentional self-harm
             D, S 🔍

  ● T43.213 Poisoning by selective serotonin
             and norepinephrine reuptake
             inhibitors, assault D, S 🔍

  ● T43.214 Poisoning by selective serotonin
             and norepinephrine reuptake
             inhibitors, undetermined D, S 🔍

  ● T43.215 Adverse effect of selective
             serotonin and norepinephrine
             reuptake inhibitors D, S 🔍

  ● T43.216 Underdosing of selective
             serotonin and norepinephrine
             reuptake inhibitors A, D, S 🔍

● T43.22 Poisoning by, adverse effect of and
          underdosing of selective serotonin
          reuptake inhibitors
            Poisoning by, adverse effect of and
              underdosing of SSRI antidepressants

  ● T43.221 Poisoning by selective serotonin
             reuptake inhibitors, accidental
             (unintentional) D, S 🔍

  ● T43.222 Poisoning by selective serotonin
             reuptake inhibitors, intentional
             self-harm D, S 🔍

  ● T43.223 Poisoning by selective serotonin
             reuptake inhibitors, assault
             D, S 🔍

  ● T43.224 Poisoning by selective serotonin
             reuptake inhibitors,
             undetermined D, S 🔍

  ● T43.225 Adverse effect of selective
             serotonin reuptake inhibitors
             D, S 🔍

  ● T43.226 Underdosing of selective
             serotonin reuptake inhibitors
             A, D, S 🔍

● T43.29 Poisoning by, adverse effect of and
          underdosing of other antidepressants

  ● T43.291 Poisoning by other
             antidepressants, accidental
             (unintentional) D, S 🔍
               Poisoning by other
                 antidepressants NOS

  ● T43.292 Poisoning by other
             antidepressants, intentional
             self- harm D, S 🔍

  ● T43.293 Poisoning by other
             antidepressants, assault D, S 🔍

  ● T43.294 Poisoning by other
             antidepressants, undetermined
             D, S 🔍

  ● T43.295 Adverse effect of other
             antidepressants D, S 🔍

  ● T43.296 Underdosing of other
             antidepressants A, D, S 🔍

● T43.3 Poisoning by, adverse effect of and underdosing of
         phenothiazine antipsychotics and neuroleptics

  ● T43.3X Poisoning by, adverse effect of
            and underdosing of phenothiazine
            antipsychotics and neuroleptics

    ● T43.3X1 Poisoning by phenothiazine
               antipsychotics and neuroleptics,
               accidental (unintentional) D, S 🔍
                 Poisoning by phenothiazine
                   antipsychotics and
                   neuroleptics NOS

    ● T43.3X2 Poisoning by phenothiazine
               antipsychotics and neuroleptics,
               intentional self-harm D, S 🔍

    ● T43.3X3 Poisoning by phenothiazine
               antipsychotics and neuroleptics,
               assault D, S 🔍

    ● T43.3X4 Poisoning by phenothiazine
               antipsychotics and neuroleptics,
               undetermined D, S 🔍

    ● T43.3X5 Adverse effect of phenothiazine
               antipsychotics and neuroleptics
               D, S 🔍

    ● T43.3X6 Underdosing of phenothiazine
               antipsychotics and neuroleptics
               A, D, S 🔍

● T43.4 Poisoning by, adverse effect of and underdosing of
         butyrophenone and thiothixene neuroleptics

  ● T43.4X Poisoning by, adverse effect of and
            underdosing of butyrophenone and
            thiothixene neuroleptics

    ● T43.4X1 Poisoning by butyrophenone and
               thiothixene neuroleptics,
               accidental (unintentional) D, S 🔍
                 Poisoning by butyrophenone
                   and thiothixene
                   neuroleptics NOS

    ● T43.4X2 Poisoning by butyrophenone and
               thiothixene neuroleptics,
               intentional self-harm D, S 🔍

    ● T43.4X3 Poisoning by butyrophenone and
               thiothixene neuroleptics, assault
               D, S 🔍

● Unacceptable Principal Diagnosis   ● Use Additional Character(s)   ▪ Unspecified   ▶ Manifestation Code

OGCR Official Guidelines for Coding and Reporting | Excludes 1 | | Excludes 2 | | Includes | | Use additional | | Code first | | Code also |

● T43.4X4 Poisoning by butyrophenone and thiothixene neuroleptics, undetermined D, S ◎

● T43.4X5 Adverse effect of butyrophenone and thiothixene neuroleptics D, S ◎

● T43.4X6 Underdosing of butyrophenone and thiothixene neuroleptics A, D, S ◎

● T43.5 Poisoning by, adverse effect of and underdosing of other and unspecified antipsychotics and neuroleptics

Excludes1   poisoning by, adverse effect of and underdosing of rauwolfia (T46.5-)

● T43.50 Poisoning by, adverse effect of and underdosing of unspecified antipsychotics and neuroleptics

● ■ T43.501 Poisoning by unspecified antipsychotics and neuroleptics, accidental (unintentional) D, S ◎
Poisoning by antipsychotics and neuroleptics NOS

● ■ T43.502 Poisoning by unspecified antipsychotics and neuroleptics, intentional self-harm D, S ◎

● ■ T43.503 Poisoning by unspecified antipsychotics and neuroleptics, assault D, S ◎

● ■ T43.504 Poisoning by unspecified antipsychotics and neuroleptics, undetermined D, S ◎

● ■ T43.505 Adverse effect of unspecified antipsychotics and neuroleptics D, S ◎

● ■ T43.506 Underdosing of unspecified antipsychotics and neuroleptics A, D, S ◎

● T43.59 Poisoning by, adverse effect of and underdosing of other antipsychotics and neuroleptics

● T43.591 Poisoning by other antipsychotics and neuroleptics, accidental (unintentional) D, S ◎
Poisoning by other antipsychotics and neuroleptics NOS

● T43.592 Poisoning by other antipsychotics and neuroleptics, intentional self-harm D, S ◎

● T43.593 Poisoning by other antipsychotics and neuroleptics, assault D, S ◎

● T43.594 Poisoning by other antipsychotics and neuroleptics, undetermined D, S ◎

● T43.595 Adverse effect of other antipsychotics and neuroleptics D, S ◎

● T43.596 Underdosing of other antipsychotics and neuroleptics A, D, S ◎

● T43.6 Poisoning by, adverse effect of and underdosing of psychostimulants

Excludes1   poisoning by, adverse effect of and underdosing of cocaine (T40.5-)

● T43.60 Poisoning by, adverse effect of and underdosing of unspecified psychostimulant

● ■ T43.601 Poisoning by unspecified psychostimulants, accidental (unintentional) D, S ◎
Poisoning by psychostimulants NOS

● ■ T43.602 Poisoning by unspecified psychostimulants, intentional self-harm D, S ◎

● ■ T43.603 Poisoning by unspecified psychostimulants, assault D, S ◎

● ■ T43.604 Poisoning by unspecified psychostimulants, undetermined D, S ◎

● ■ T43.605 Adverse effect of unspecified psychostimulants D, S ◎

● ■ T43.606 Underdosing of unspecified psychostimulants A, D, S ◎

● T43.61 Poisoning by, adverse effect of and underdosing of caffeine

● T43.611 Poisoning by caffeine, accidental (unintentional) D, S ◎
Poisoning by caffeine NOS

● T43.612 Poisoning by caffeine, intentional self-harm D, S ◎

● T43.613 Poisoning by caffeine, assault D, S ◎

● T43.614 Poisoning by caffeine, undetermined D, S ◎

● T43.615 Adverse effect of caffeine D, S ◎

● T43.616 Underdosing of caffeine A, D, S ◎

● T43.62 Poisoning by, adverse effect of and underdosing of amphetamines
Poisoning by, adverse effect of and underdosing of methamphetamines

● T43.621 Poisoning by amphetamines, accidental (unintentional) D, S ◎
Poisoning by amphetamines NOS

● T43.622 Poisoning by amphetamines, intentional self-harm D, S ◎

● T43.623 Poisoning by amphetamines, assault D, S ◎

● T43.624 Poisoning by amphetamines, undetermined D, S ◎

● T43.625 Adverse effect of amphetamines D, S ◎

● T43.626 Underdosing of amphetamines A, D, S ◎

● T43.63 Poisoning by, adverse effect of and underdosing of methylphenidate

● T43.631 Poisoning by methylphenidate, accidental (unintentional) D, S ◎
Poisoning by methylphenidate NOS

● T43.632 Poisoning by methylphenidate, intentional self-harm D, S ◎

CHAPTER 19 (S00-T88)

● **T43.633 Poisoning by methylphenidate, assault** D, S 🔍

● **T43.634 Poisoning by methylphenidate, undetermined** D, S 🔍

● **T43.635 Adverse effect of methylphenidate** D, S 🔍

● **T43.636 Underdosing of methylphenidate** A, D, S 🔍

● **T43.69 Poisoning by, adverse effect of and underdosing of other psychostimulants**

● **T43.691 Poisoning by other psychostimulants, accidental (unintentional)** D, S 🔍
Poisoning by other psychostimulants NOS

● **T43.692 Poisoning by other psychostimulants, intentional self-harm** D, S 🔍

● **T43.693 Poisoning by other psychostimulants, assault** D, S 🔍

● **T43.694 Poisoning by other psychostimulants, undetermined** D, S 🔍

● **T43.695 Adverse effect of other psychostimulants** D, S 🔍

● **T43.696 Underdosing of other psychostimulants** A, D, S 🔍

● **T43.8 Poisoning by, adverse effect of and underdosing of other psychotropic drugs**

● **T43.8X Poisoning by, adverse effect of and underdosing of other psychotropic drugs**

● **T43.8X1 Poisoning by other psychotropic drugs, accidental (unintentional)** D, S 🔍
Poisoning by other psychotropic drugs NOS

● **T43.8X2 Poisoning by other psychotropic drugs, intentional self-harm** D, S 🔍

● **T43.8X3 Poisoning by other psychotropic drugs, assault** D, S 🔍

● **T43.8X4 Poisoning by other psychotropic drugs, undetermined** D, S 🔍

● **T43.8X5 Adverse effect of other psychotropic drugs** D, S 🔍

● **T43.8X6 Underdosing of other psychotropic drugs** A, D, S 🔍

● **T43.9 Poisoning by, adverse effect of and underdosing of unspecified psychotropic drug**

● ■ **T43.91 Poisoning by unspecified psychotropic drug, accidental (unintentional)** D, S 🔍
Poisoning by psychotropic drug NOS

● ■ **T43.92 Poisoning by unspecified psychotropic drug, intentional self-harm** D, S 🔍

● ■ **T43.93 Poisoning by unspecified psychotropic drug, assault** D, S 🔍

● ■ **T43.94 Poisoning by unspecified psychotropic drug, undetermined** D, S 🔍

● ■ **T43.95 Adverse effect of unspecified psychotropic drug** D, S 🔍

● ■ **T43.96 Underdosing of unspecified psychotropic drug** A, D, S 🔍

● **T44 Poisoning by, adverse effect of and underdosing of drugs primarily affecting the autonomic nervous system**

The appropriate 7th character is to be added to each code from category T44

A	initial encounter
D	subsequent encounter
S	sequela

● **T44.0 Poisoning by, adverse effect of and underdosing of anticholinesterase agents**

● **T44.0X Poisoning by, adverse effect of and underdosing of anticholinesterase agents**

● **T44.0X1 Poisoning by anticholinesterase agents, accidental (unintentional)** D, S 🔍
Poisoning by anticholinesterase agents NOS

● **T44.0X2 Poisoning by anticholinesterase agents, intentional self-harm** D, S 🔍

● **T44.0X3 Poisoning by anticholinesterase agents, assault** D, S 🔍

● **T44.0X4 Poisoning by anticholinesterase agents, undetermined** D, S 🔍

● **T44.0X5 Adverse effect of anticholinesterase agents** D, S 🔍

● **T44.0X6 Underdosing of anticholinesterase agents** A, D, S 🔍

● **T44.1 Poisoning by, adverse effect of and underdosing of other parasympathomimetics [cholinergics]**

● **T44.1X Poisoning by, adverse effect of and underdosing of other parasympathomimetics [cholinergics]**

● **T44.1X1 Poisoning by other parasympathomimetics [cholinergics], accidental (unintentional)** D, S 🔍
Poisoning by other parasympathomimetics [cholinergics] NOS

● **T44.1X2 Poisoning by other parasympathomimetics [cholinergics], intentional self-harm** D, S 🔍

● **T44.1X3 Poisoning by other parasympathomimetics [cholinergics], assault** D, S 🔍

● **T44.1X4 Poisoning by other parasympathomimetics [cholinergics], undetermined** D, S 🔍

● **T44.1X5 Adverse effect of other parasympathomimetics [cholinergics]** D, S 🔍

● **T44.1X6 Underdosing of other parasympathomimetics** A, D, S 🔍

● **T44.2 Poisoning by, adverse effect of and underdosing of ganglionic blocking drugs**

● **T44.2X Poisoning by, adverse effect of and underdosing of ganglionic blocking drugs**

● **T44.2X1 Poisoning by ganglionic blocking drugs, accidental (unintentional)** D, S 🔍
Poisoning by ganglionic blocking drugs NOS

● **T44.2X2 Poisoning by ganglionic blocking drugs, intentional self-harm** D, S 🔍

● Unacceptable Principal Diagnosis   ● Use Additional Character(s)   ■ Unspecified   ▶ Manifestation Code
OGCR Official Guidelines for Coding and Reporting | Excludes 1 | | Excludes 2 | Includes Use additional Code first Code also

● **T44.2X3** Poisoning by ganglionic blocking drugs, assault D, S 🔖

● **T44.2X4** Poisoning by ganglionic blocking drugs, undetermined D, S 🔖

● **T44.2X5** Adverse effect of ganglionic blocking drugs D, S 🔖

● **T44.2X6** Underdosing of ganglionic blocking drugs A, D, S 🔖

● **T44.3** Poisoning by, adverse effect of and underdosing of other parasympatholytics [anticholinergics and antimuscarinics] and spasmolytics
> Poisoning by, adverse effect of and underdosing of papaverine

  ● **T44.3X** Poisoning by, adverse effect of and underdosing of other parasympatholytics [anticholinergics and antimuscarinics] and spasmolytics

    ● **T44.3X1** Poisoning by other parasympatholytics [anticholinergics and antimuscarinics] and spasmolytics, accidental (unintentional) D, S 🔖
> Poisoning by other parasympatholytics [anticholinergics and antimuscarinics] and spasmolytics NOS

    ● **T44.3X2** Poisoning by other parasympatholytics [anticholinergics and antimuscarinics] and spasmolytics, intentional self-harm D, S 🔖

    ● **T44.3X3** Poisoning by other parasympatholytics [anticholinergics and antimuscarinics] and spasmolytics, assault D, S 🔖

    ● **T44.3X4** Poisoning by other parasympatholytics [anticholinergics and antimuscarinics] and spasmolytics, undetermined D, S 🔖

    ● **T44.3X5** Adverse effect of other parasympatholytics [anticholinergics and antimuscarinics] and spasmolytics D, S 🔖

    ● **T44.3X6** Underdosing of other parasympatholytics [anticholinergics and antimuscarinics] and spasmolytics A, D, S 🔖

● **T44.4** Poisoning by, adverse effect of and underdosing of predominantly alpha-adrenoreceptor agonists
> Poisoning by, adverse effect of and underdosing of metaraminol

  ● **T44.4X** Poisoning by, adverse effect of and underdosing of predominantly alpha-adrenoreceptor agonists

    ● **T44.4X1** Poisoning by predominantly alpha-adrenoreceptor agonists, accidental (unintentional) D, S 🔖
> Poisoning by predominantly alpha-adrenoreceptor agonists NOS

● **T44.4X2** Poisoning by predominantly alpha-adrenoreceptor agonists, intentional self-harm D, S 🔖

● **T44.4X3** Poisoning by predominantly alpha-adrenoreceptor agonists, assault D, S 🔖

● **T44.4X4** Poisoning by predominantly alpha-adrenoreceptor agonists, undetermined D, S 🔖

● **T44.4X5** Adverse effect of predominantly alpha-adrenoreceptor agonists D, S 🔖

● **T44.4X6** Underdosing of predominantly alpha-adrenoreceptor agonists A, D, S 🔖

● **T44.5** Poisoning by, adverse effect of and underdosing of predominantly beta-adrenoreceptor agonists
> **Excludes1**   poisoning by, adverse effect of and underdosing of beta-adrenoreceptor agonists used in asthma therapy (T48.6-)

  ● **T44.5X** Poisoning by, adverse effect of and underdosing of predominantly beta-adrenoreceptor agonists

    ● **T44.5X1** Poisoning by predominantly beta-adrenoreceptor agonists, accidental (unintentional) D, S 🔖
> Poisoning by predominantly beta-adrenoreceptor agonists NOS

    ● **T44.5X2** Poisoning by predominantly beta-adrenoreceptor agonists, intentional self-harm D, S 🔖

    ● **T44.5X3** Poisoning by predominantly beta-adrenoreceptor agonists, assault D, S 🔖

    ● **T44.5X4** Poisoning by predominantly beta-adrenoreceptor agonists, undetermined D, S 🔖

    ● **T44.5X5** Adverse effect of predominantly beta-adrenoreceptor agonists D, S 🔖

    ● **T44.5X6** Underdosing of predominantly beta-adrenoreceptor agonists A, D, S 🔖

● **T44.6** Poisoning by, adverse effect of and underdosing of alpha-adrenoreceptor antagonists
> **Excludes1**   poisoning by, adverse effect of and underdosing of ergot alkaloids (T48.0)

  ● **T44.6X** Poisoning by, adverse effect of and underdosing of alpha-adrenoreceptor antagonists

    ● **T44.6X1** Poisoning by alpha-adrenoreceptor antagonists, accidental (unintentional) D, S 🔖
> Poisoning by alpha-adrenoreceptor antagonists NOS

    ● **T44.6X2** Poisoning by alpha-adrenoreceptor antagonists, intentional self-harm D, S 🔖

    ● **T44.6X3** Poisoning by alpha-adrenoreceptor antagonists, assault D, S 🔖

● T44.6X4 Poisoning by alpha-
adrenoreceptor antagonists,
undetermined D, S 🔬

● T44.6X5 Adverse effect of alpha-
adrenoreceptor antagonists
D, S 🔬

● T44.6X6 Underdosing of alpha-
adrenoreceptor antagonists
A, D, S 🔬

● T44.7 Poisoning by, adverse effect of and underdosing of
beta-adrenoreceptor antagonists

● T44.7X Poisoning by, adverse effect of and
underdosing of beta-adrenoreceptor
antagonists

● T44.7X1 Poisoning by beta-adrenoreceptor
antagonists, accidental
(unintentional) D, S 🔬
Poisoning by beta-
adrenoreceptor antagonists
NOS

● T44.7X2 Poisoning by beta-adrenoreceptor
antagonists, intentional self-harm
D, S 🔬

● T44.7X3 Poisoning by beta-adrenoreceptor
antagonists, assault D, S 🔬

● T44.7X4 Poisoning by beta-adrenoreceptor
antagonists, undetermined D, S 🔬

● T44.7X5 Adverse effect of beta-
adrenoreceptor antagonists
D, S 🔬

● T44.7X6 Underdosing of beta-
adrenoreceptor antagonists
A, D, S 🔬

● T44.8 Poisoning by, adverse effect of and underdosing of
centrally-acting and adrenergic-neuron- blocking
agents

Excludes1   poisoning by, adverse effect of and
underdosing of clonidine (T46.5)
poisoning by, adverse effect of and
underdosing of guanethidine
(T46.5)

● T44.8X Poisoning by, adverse effect of and
underdosing of centrally-acting and
adrenergic-neuron-blocking agents

● T44.8X1 Poisoning by centrally-acting and
adrenergic-neuron-blocking
agents, accidental (unintentional)
D, S 🔬
Poisoning by centrally-acting
and adrenergic-neuron-
blocking agents NOS

● T44.8X2 Poisoning by centrally-acting and
adrenergic-neuron-blocking
agents, intentional self-harm
D, S 🔬

● T44.8X3 Poisoning by centrally-acting and
adrenergic-neuron-blocking
agents, assault D, S 🔬

● T44.8X4 Poisoning by centrally-acting and
adrenergic-neuron-blocking
agents, undetermined D, S 🔬

● T44.8X5 Adverse effect of centrally-acting
and adrenergic-neuron-blocking
agents D, S 🔬

● T44.8X6 Underdosing of centrally-acting
and adrenergic-neuron-blocking
agents A, D, S 🔬

● T44.9 Poisoning by, adverse effect of and underdosing of
other and unspecified drugs primarily affecting the
autonomic nervous system
Poisoning by, adverse effect of and underdosing
of drug stimulating both alpha and beta-
adrenoreceptors

● T44.90 Poisoning by, adverse effect of and
underdosing of unspecified drugs
primarily affecting the autonomic nervous
system

●■ T44.901 Poisoning by unspecified drugs
primarily affecting the autonomic
nervous system, accidental
(unintentional) D, S 🔬
Poisoning by unspecified drugs
primarily affecting the
autonomic nervous system
NOS

●■ T44.902 Poisoning by unspecified drugs
primarily affecting the autonomic
nervous system, intentional
self-harm D, S 🔬

●■ T44.903 Poisoning by unspecified drugs
primarily affecting the autonomic
nervous system, assault D, S 🔬

●■ T44.904 Poisoning by unspecified drugs
primarily affecting the autonomic
nervous system, undetermined
D, S 🔬

●■ T44.905 Adverse effect of unspecified
drugs primarily affecting the
autonomic nervous system
D, S 🔬

●■ T44.906 Underdosing of unspecified
drugs primarily affecting the
autonomic nervous system
A, D, S 🔬

● T44.99 Poisoning by, adverse effect of and
underdosing of other drugs primarily
affecting the autonomic nervous system

● T44.991 Poisoning by other drug
primarily affecting the autonomic
nervous system, accidental
(unintentional) D, S 🔬
Poisoning by other drugs
primarily affecting the
autonomic nervous system
NOS

● T44.992 Poisoning by other drug
primarily affecting the autonomic
nervous system, intentional
self-harm D, S 🔬

● T44.993 Poisoning by other drug
primarily affecting the autonomic
nervous system, assault D, S 🔬

● T44.994 Poisoning by other drug
primarily affecting the autonomic
nervous system, undetermined
D, S 🔬

● T44.995 Adverse effect of other drug
primarily affecting the autonomic
nervous system D, S 🔬

● T44.996 Underdosing of other drug
primarily affecting the autonomic
nervous system A, D, S 🔬

● Unacceptable Principal Diagnosis   ● Use Additional Character(s)   ■ Unspecified   ▶ Manifestation Code
OGCR Official Guidelines for Coding and Reporting   Excludes 1   Excludes 2   Includes   Use additional   Code first   Code also

● **T45 Poisoning by, adverse effect of and underdosing of primarily systemic and hematological agents, not elsewhere classified**

The appropriate 7th character is to be added to each code from category T45

A	initial encounter
D	subsequent encounter
S	sequela

● **T45.0 Poisoning by, adverse effect of and underdosing of antiallergic and antiemetic drugs**

> **Excludes1**   poisoning by, adverse effect of and underdosing of phenothiazine-based neuroleptics (T43.3)

● **T45.0X Poisoning by, adverse effect of and underdosing of antiallergic and antiemetic drugs**

● **T45.0X1 Poisoning by antiallergic and antiemetic drugs, accidental (unintentional)** D, S
> Poisoning by antiallergic and antiemetic drugs NOS

● **T45.0X2 Poisoning by antiallergic and antiemetic drugs, intentional self-harm** D, S

● **T45.0X3 Poisoning by antiallergic and antiemetic drugs, assault** D, S

● **T45.0X4 Poisoning by antiallergic and antiemetic drugs, undetermined** D, S

● **T45.0X5 Adverse effect of antiallergic and antiemetic drugs** D, S

● **T45.0X6 Underdosing of antiallergic and antiemetic drugs** A, D, S

● **T45.1 Poisoning by, adverse effect of and underdosing of antineoplastic and immunosuppressive drugs**

> **Excludes1**   poisoning by, adverse effect of and underdosing of tamoxifen (T38.6)

● **T45.1X Poisoning by, adverse effect of and underdosing of antineoplastic and immunosuppressive drugs**

● **T45.1X1 Poisoning by antineoplastic and immunosuppressive drugs, accidental (unintentional)** D, S
> Poisoning by antineoplastic and immunosuppressive drugs NOS

● **T45.1X2 Poisoning by antineoplastic and immunosuppressive drugs, intentional self-harm** D, S

● **T45.1X3 Poisoning by antineoplastic and immunosuppressive drugs, assault** D, S

● **T45.1X4 Poisoning by antineoplastic and immunosuppressive drugs, undetermined** D, S

● **T45.1X5 Adverse effect of antineoplastic and immunosuppressive drugs** D, S

● **T45.1X6 Underdosing of antineoplastic and immunosuppressive drugs** A, D, S

● **T45.2 Poisoning by, adverse effect of and underdosing of vitamins**

> **Excludes2**   poisoning by, adverse effect of and underdosing of nicotinic acid (derivatives) (T46.7)
> poisoning by, adverse effect of and underdosing of iron (T45.4)
> poisoning by, adverse effect of and underdosing of vitamin K (T45.7)

● **T45.2X Poisoning by, adverse effect of and underdosing of vitamins**

● **T45.2X1 Poisoning by vitamins, accidental (unintentional)** D, S
> Poisoning by vitamins NOS

● **T45.2X2 Poisoning by vitamins, intentional self-harm** D, S

● **T45.2X3 Poisoning by vitamins, assault** D, S

● **T45.2X4 Poisoning by vitamins, undetermined** D, S

● **T45.2X5 Adverse effect of vitamins** D, S

● **T45.2X6 Underdosing of vitamins** A, D, S

> **Excludes1**   vitamin deficiencies (E50-E56)

● **T45.3 Poisoning by, adverse effect of and underdosing of enzymes**

● **T45.3X Poisoning by, adverse effect of and underdosing of enzymes**

● **T45.3X1 Poisoning by enzymes, accidental (unintentional)** D, S
> Poisoning by enzymes NOS

● **T45.3X2 Poisoning by enzymes, intentional self-harm** D, S

● **T45.3X3 Poisoning by enzymes, assault** D, S

● **T45.3X4 Poisoning by enzymes, undetermined** D, S

● **T45.3X5 Adverse effect of enzymes** D, S

● **T45.3X6 Underdosing of enzymes** A, D, S

● **T45.4 Poisoning by, adverse effect of and underdosing of iron and its compounds**

● **T45.4X Poisoning by, adverse effect of and underdosing of iron and its compounds**

● **T45.4X1 Poisoning by iron and its compounds, accidental (unintentional)** D, S
> Poisoning by iron and its compounds NOS

● **T45.4X2 Poisoning by iron and its compounds, intentional self-harm** D, S

● **T45.4X3 Poisoning by iron and its compounds, assault** D, S

● **T45.4X4 Poisoning by iron and its compounds, undetermined** D, S

● **T45.4X5 Adverse effect of iron and its compounds** D, S

● **T45.4X6 Underdosing of iron and its compounds** A, D, S

> **Excludes1**   iron deficiency (E61.1)

CHAPTER 19 (S00-T88)

N   Newborn Age: 0   P   Pediatric Age: 0–17   M   Maternity DX: 12–55   A   Adult Age: 15–124   ♀ Females Only   ♂ Males Only

 Complication\Comorbidity   Major C\C   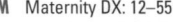 Present on Admission Requirement   Hospital-Acquired Condition

CHAPTER 19 (S00-T88)

● **T45.5** **Poisoning by, adverse effect of and underdosing of anticoagulants and antithrombotic drugs**

  ● **T45.51** **Poisoning by, adverse effect of and underdosing of anticoagulants**

    T45.511 **Poisoning by anticoagulants, accidental (unintentional)** D, S ◎
      Poisoning by anticoagulants NOS

    ● **T45.512** **Poisoning by anticoagulants, intentional self-harm** D, S ◎

    ● **T45.513** **Poisoning by anticoagulants, assault** D, S ◎

    ● **T45.514** **Poisoning by anticoagulants, undetermined** D, S ◎

    ● **T45.515** **Adverse effect of anticoagulants** D, S ◎

    ● **T45.516** **Underdosing of anticoagulants** A, D, S ◎

  ● **T45.52** **Poisoning by, adverse effect of and underdosing of antithrombotic drugs**
    Poisoning by, adverse effect of and underdosing of antiplatelet drugs

    | Excludes2 | poisoning by, adverse effect of and underdosing of aspirin (T39.01-) poisoning by, adverse effect of and underdosing of acetylsalicylic acid (T39.01-) |

    ● **T45.521** **Poisoning by antithrombotic drugs, accidental (unintentional)** D, S ◎
      Poisoning by antithrombotic drug NOS

    ● **T45.522** **Poisoning by antithrombotic drugs, intentional self-harm** D, S ◎

    ● **T45.523** **Poisoning by antithrombotic drugs, assault** D, S ◎

    ● **T45.524** **Poisoning by antithrombotic drugs, undetermined** D, S ◎

    ● **T45.525** **Adverse effect of antithrombotic drugs** D, S ◎

    ● **T45.526** **Underdosing of antithrombotic drugs** A, D, S ◎

● **T45.6** **Poisoning by, adverse effect of and underdosing of fibrinolysis-affecting drugs**

  ● **T45.60** **Poisoning by, adverse effect of and underdosing of unspecified fibrinolysis-affecting drugs**

    ●■ **T45.601** **Poisoning by unspecified fibrinolysis-affecting drugs, accidental (unintentional)** D, S ◎
      Poisoning by fibrinolysis-affecting drug NOS

    ●■ **T45.602** **Poisoning by unspecified fibrinolysis-affecting drugs, intentional self-harm** D, S ◎

    ●■ **T45.603** **Poisoning by unspecified fibrinolysis-affecting drugs, assault** D, S ◎

    ●■ **T45.604** **Poisoning by unspecified fibrinolysis-affecting drugs, undetermined** D, S ◎

    ●■ **T45.605** **Adverse effect of unspecified fibrinolysis-affecting drugs** D, S ◎

    ●■ **T45.606** **Underdosing of unspecified fibrinolysis-affecting drugs** A, D, S ◎

  ● **T45.61** **Poisoning by, adverse effect of and underdosing of thrombolytic drugs**

    ● **T45.611** **Poisoning by thrombolytic drug, accidental (unintentional)** D, S ◎
      Poisoning by thrombolytic drug NOS

    ● **T45.612** **Poisoning by thrombolytic drug, intentional self-harm** D, S ◎

    ● **T45.613** **Poisoning by thrombolytic drug, assault** D, S ◎

    ● **T45.614** **Poisoning by thrombolytic drug, undetermined** D, S ◎

    ● **T45.615** **Adverse effect of thrombolytic drugs** D, S ◎

    ● **T45.616** **Underdosing of thrombolytic drugs** A, D, S ◎

  ● **T45.62** **Poisoning by, adverse effect of and underdosing of hemostatic drugs**

    ● **T45.621** **Poisoning by hemostatic drug, accidental (unintentional)** D, S ◎
      Poisoning by hemostatic drug NOS

    ● **T45.622** **Poisoning by hemostatic drug, intentional self-harm** D, S ◎

    ● **T45.623** **Poisoning by hemostatic drug, assault** D, S ◎

    ● **T45.624** **Poisoning by hemostatic drug, undetermined** D, S ◎

    ● **T45.625** **Adverse effect of hemostatic drug** D, S ◎

    ● **T45.626** **Underdosing of hemostatic drugs** A, D, S ◎

  ● **T45.69** **Poisoning by, adverse effect of and underdosing of other fibrinolysis-affecting drugs**

    ● **T45.691** **Poisoning by other fibrinolysis-affecting drugs, accidental (unintentional)** D, S ◎
      Poisoning by other fibrinolysis-affecting drug NOS

    ● **T45.692** **Poisoning by other fibrinolysis-affecting drugs, intentional self-harm** D, S ◎

    ● **T45.693** **Poisoning by other fibrinolysis-affecting drugs, assault** D, S ◎

    ● **T45.694** **Poisoning by other fibrinolysis-affecting drugs, undetermined** D, S ◎

    ● **T45.695** **Adverse effect of other fibrinolysis-affecting drugs** D, S ◎

    ● **T45.696** **Underdosing of other fibrinolysis-affecting drugs** A, D, S ◎

● **T45.7**   Poisoning by, adverse effect of and underdosing of anticoagulant antagonists, vitamin K and other coagulants

  ● **T45.7X**   Poisoning by, adverse effect of and underdosing of anticoagulant antagonists, vitamin K and other coagulants

    ● **T45.7X1**   Poisoning by anticoagulant antagonists, vitamin K and other coagulants, accidental (unintentional) D, S
         Poisoning by anticoagulant antagonists, vitamin K and other coagulants NOS

    ● **T45.7X2**   Poisoning by anticoagulant antagonists, vitamin K and other coagulants, intentional self-harm D, S

    ● **T45.7X3**   Poisoning by anticoagulant antagonists, vitamin K and other coagulants, assault D, S

    ● **T45.7X4**   Poisoning by anticoagulant antagonists, vitamin K and other coagulants, undetermined D, S

    ● **T45.7X5**   Adverse effect of anticoagulant antagonists, vitamin K and other coagulants D, S

    ● **T45.7X6**   Underdosing of anticoagulant antagonist, vitamin K and other coagulants A, D, S
         Excludes1   vitamin K deficiency (E56.1)

● **T45.8**   Poisoning by, adverse effect of and underdosing of other primarily systemic and hematological agents
     Poisoning by, adverse effect of and underdosing of liver preparations and other antianemic agents
     Poisoning by, adverse effect of and underdosing of natural blood and blood products
     Poisoning by, adverse effect of and underdosing of plasma substitute
     Excludes2   poisoning by, adverse effect of and underdosing of immunoglobulin (T50.Z1)
         poisoning by, adverse effect of and underdosing of iron (T45.4)
         transfusion reactions (T80.-)

  ● **T45.8X**   Poisoning by, adverse effect of and underdosing of other primarily systemic and hematological agents

    ● **T45.8X1**   Poisoning by other primarily systemic and hematological agents, accidental (unintentional) D, S
         Poisoning by other primarily systemic and hematological agents NOS

    ● **T45.8X2**   Poisoning by other primarily systemic and hematological agents, intentional self-harm D, S

    ● **T45.8X3**   Poisoning by other primarily systemic and hematological agents, assault D, S

    ● **T45.8X4**   Poisoning by other primarily systemic and hematological agents, undetermined D, S

● **T45.8X5**   Adverse effect of other primarily systemic and hematological agents D, S

● **T45.8X6**   Underdosing of other primarily systemic and hematological agents A, D, S

● **T45.9**   Poisoning by, adverse effect of and underdosing of unspecified primarily systemic and hematological agent

  ● ■ **T45.91**   Poisoning by unspecified primarily systemic and hematological agent, accidental (unintentional) D, S
         Poisoning by primarily systemic and hematological agent NOS

  ● ■ **T45.92**   Poisoning by unspecified primarily systemic and hematological agent, intentional self-harm D, S

  ● ■ **T45.93**   Poisoning by unspecified primarily systemic and hematological agent, assault D, S

  ● ■ **T45.94**   Poisoning by unspecified primarily systemic and hematological agent, undetermined D, S

  ● ■ **T45.95**   Adverse effect of unspecified primarily systemic and hematological agent D, S

  ● ■ **T45.96**   Underdosing of unspecified primarily systemic and hematological agent A, D, S

● **T46**   Poisoning by, adverse effect of and underdosing of agents primarily affecting the cardiovascular system
     Excludes1   poisoning by, adverse effect of and underdosing of metaraminol (T44.4)

     The appropriate 7th character is to be added to each code from category T46

A	initial encounter
D	subsequent encounter
S	sequela

● **T46.0**   Poisoning by, adverse effect of and underdosing of cardiac-stimulant glycosides and drugs of similar action

  ● **T46.0X**   Poisoning by, adverse effect of and underdosing of cardiac-stimulant glycosides and drugs of similar action

    ● **T46.0X1**   Poisoning by cardiac-stimulant glycosides and drugs of similar action, accidental (unintentional) D, S
         Poisoning by cardiac-stimulant glycosides and drugs of similar action NOS

    ● **T46.0X2**   Poisoning by cardiac-stimulant glycosides and drugs of similar action, intentional self-harm D, S

    ● **T46.0X3**   Poisoning by cardiac-stimulant glycosides and drugs of similar action, assault D, S

    ● **T46.0X4**   Poisoning by cardiac-stimulant glycosides and drugs of similar action, undetermined D, S

    ● **T46.0X5**   Adverse effect of cardiac-stimulant glycosides and drugs of similar action D, S

    ● **T46.0X6**   Underdosing of cardiac-stimulant glycosides and drugs of similar action A, D, S

CHAPTER 19 (S00-T88)

● **T46.1 Poisoning by, adverse effect of and underdosing of calcium-channel blockers**

  ● **T46.1X Poisoning by, adverse effect of and underdosing of calcium-channel blockers**

    ● **T46.1X1 Poisoning by calcium-channel blockers, accidental (unintentional)** D, S 🔍

        Poisoning by calcium-channel blockers NOS

    ● **T46.1X2 Poisoning by calcium-channel blockers, intentional self-harm** D, S 🔍

    ● **T46.1X3 Poisoning by calcium-channel blockers, assault** D, S 🔍

    ● **T46.1X4 Poisoning by calcium-channel blockers, undetermined** D, S 🔍

    ● **T46.1X5 Adverse effect of calcium-channel blockers** D, S 🔍

    ● **T46.1X6 Underdosing of calcium-channel blockers** A, D, S 🔍

● **T46.2 Poisoning by, adverse effect of and underdosing of other antidysrhythmic drugs, not elsewhere classified**

    Excludes1   poisoning by, adverse effect of and underdosing of beta-adrenoreceptor antagonists (T44.7-)

  ● **T46.2X Poisoning by, adverse effect of and underdosing of other antidysrhythmic drugs**

    ● **T46.2X1 Poisoning by other antidysrhythmic drugs, accidental (unintentional)** D, S 🔍

        Poisoning by other antidysrhythmic drugs NOS

    ● **T46.2X2 Poisoning by other antidysrhythmic drugs, intentional self-harm** D, S 🔍

    ● **T46.2X3 Poisoning by other antidysrhythmic drugs, assault** D, S 🔍

    ● **T46.2X4 Poisoning by other antidysrhythmic drugs, undetermined** D, S 🔍

    ● **T46.2X5 Adverse effect of other antidysrhythmic drugs** D, S 🔍

    ● **T46.2X6 Underdosing of other antidysrhythmic drugs** A, D, S 🔍

● **T46.3 Poisoning by, adverse effect of and underdosing of coronary vasodilators**

    Poisoning by, adverse effect of and underdosing of dipyridamole

    Excludes1   poisoning by, adverse effect of and underdosing of calcium-channel blockers (T46.1)

  ● **T46.3X Poisoning by, adverse effect of and underdosing of coronary vasodilators**

    ● **T46.3X1 Poisoning by coronary vasodilators, accidental (unintentional)** D, S 🔍

        Poisoning by coronary vasodilators NOS

    ● **T46.3X2 Poisoning by coronary vasodilators, intentional self-harm** D, S 🔍

● **T46.3X3 Poisoning by coronary vasodilators, assault** D, S 🔍

● **T46.3X4 Poisoning by coronary vasodilators, undetermined** D, S 🔍

● **T46.3X5 Adverse effect of coronary vasodilators** D, S 🔍

● **T46.3X6 Underdosing of coronary vasodilators** A, D, S 🔍

● **T46.4 Poisoning by, adverse effect of and underdosing of angiotensin-converting-enzyme inhibitors**

  ● **T46.4X Poisoning by, adverse effect of and underdosing of angiotensin-converting-enzyme inhibitors**

    ● **T46.4X1 Poisoning by angiotensin-converting-enzyme inhibitors, accidental (unintentional)** D, S 🔍

        Poisoning by angiotensin-converting-enzyme inhibitors NOS

    ● **T46.4X2 Poisoning by angiotensin-converting-enzyme inhibitors, intentional self-harm** D, S 🔍

    ● **T46.4X3 Poisoning by angiotensin-converting-enzyme inhibitors, assault** D, S 🔍

    ● **T46.4X4 Poisoning by angiotensin-converting-enzyme inhibitors, undetermined** D, S 🔍

    ● **T46.4X5 Adverse effect of angiotensin-converting-enzyme inhibitors** D, S 🔍

    ● **T46.4X6 Underdosing of angiotensin-converting-enzyme inhibitors** A, D, S 🔍

● **T46.5 Poisoning by, adverse effect of and underdosing of other antihypertensive drugs**

    Excludes2   poisoning by, adverse effect of and underdosing of beta-adrenoreceptor antagonists (T44.7)

    poisoning by, adverse effect of and underdosing of calcium-channel blockers (T46.1)

    poisoning by, adverse effect of and underdosing of diuretics (T50.0-T50.2)

  ● **T46.5X Poisoning by, adverse effect of and underdosing of other antihypertensive drugs**

    ● **T46.5X1 Poisoning by other antihypertensive drugs, accidental (unintentional)** D, S 🔍

        Poisoning by other antihypertensive drugs NOS

    ● **T46.5X2 Poisoning by other antihypertensive drugs, intentional self-harm** D, S 🔍

    ● **T46.5X3 Poisoning by other antihypertensive drugs, assault** D, S 🔍

    ● **T46.5X4 Poisoning by other antihypertensive drugs, undetermined** D, S 🔍

    ● **T46.5X5 Adverse effect of other antihypertensive drugs** D, S 🔍

    ● **T46.5X6 Underdosing of other antihypertensive drugs** A, D, S 🔍

● Unacceptable Principal Diagnosis   ● Use Additional Character(s)   ■ Unspecified   ▶ Manifestation Code

OGCR Official Guidelines for Coding and Reporting   Excludes 1   Excludes 2   Includes   Use additional   Code first   Code also

● T46.6   **Poisoning by, adverse effect of and underdosing of antihyperlipidemic and antiarteriosclerotic drugs**

   ● T46.6X   **Poisoning by, adverse effect of and underdosing of antihyperlipidemic and antiarteriosclerotic drugs**

     ● T46.6X1   **Poisoning by antihyperlipidemic and antiarteriosclerotic drugs, accidental (unintentional)** D, S 🔊
            Poisoning by antihyperlipidemic and antiarteriosclerotic drugs NOS

     ● T46.6X2   **Poisoning by antihyperlipidemic and antiarteriosclerotic drugs, intentional self-harm** D, S 🔊

     ● T46.6X3   **Poisoning by antihyperlipidemic and antiarteriosclerotic drugs, assault** D, S 🔊

     ● T46.6X4   **Poisoning by antihyperlipidemic and antiarteriosclerotic drugs, undetermined** D, S 🔊

     ● T46.6X5   **Adverse effect of antihyperlipidemic and antiarteriosclerotic drugs** D, S 🔊

     ● T46.6X6   **Underdosing of antihyperlipidemic and antiarteriosclerotic drugs** A, D, S 🔊

● T46.7   **Poisoning by, adverse effect of and underdosing of peripheral vasodilators**
     Poisoning by, adverse effect of and underdosing of nicotinic acid (derivatives)

     | Excludes1 | poisoning by, adverse effect of and underdosing of papaverine (T44.3)

   ● T46.7X   **Poisoning by, adverse effect of and underdosing of peripheral vasodilators**

     ● T46.7X1   **Poisoning by peripheral vasodilators, accidental (unintentional)** D, S 🔊
            Poisoning by peripheral vasodilators NOS

     ● T46.7X2   **Poisoning by peripheral vasodilators, intentional self-harm** D, S 🔊

     ● T46.7X3   **Poisoning by peripheral vasodilators, assault** D, S 🔊

     ● T46.7X4   **Poisoning by peripheral vasodilators, undetermined** D, S 🔊

     ● T46.7X5   **Adverse effect of peripheral vasodilators** D, S 🔊

     ● T46.7X6   **Underdosing of peripheral vasodilators** A, D, S 🔊

● T46.8   **Poisoning by, adverse effect of and underdosing of antivaricose drugs, including sclerosing agents**

   ● T46.8X   **Poisoning by, adverse effect of and underdosing of antivaricose drugs, including sclerosing agents**

     ● T46.8X1   **Poisoning by antivaricose drugs, including sclerosing agents, accidental (unintentional)** D, S 🔊
            Poisoning by antivaricose drugs, including sclerosing agents NOS

     ● T46.8X2   **Poisoning by antivaricose drugs, including sclerosing agents, intentional self-harm** D, S 🔊

     ● T46.8X3   **Poisoning by antivaricose drugs, including sclerosing agents, assault** D, S 🔊

     ● T46.8X4   **Poisoning by antivaricose drugs, including sclerosing agents, undetermined** D, S 🔊

     ● T46.8X5   **Adverse effect of antivaricose drugs, including sclerosing agents** D, S 🔊

     ● T46.8X6   **Underdosing of antivaricose drugs, including sclerosing agents** A, D, S 🔊

● T46.9   **Poisoning by, adverse effect of and underdosing of other and unspecified agents primarily affecting the cardiovascular system**

   ● T46.90   **Poisoning by, adverse effect of and underdosing of unspecified agents primarily affecting the cardiovascular system**

     ●■ T46.901   **Poisoning by unspecified agents primarily affecting the cardiovascular system, accidental (unintentional)** D, S 🔊

     ●■ T46.902   **Poisoning by unspecified agents primarily affecting the cardiovascular system, intentional self-harm** D, S 🔊

     ●■ T46.903   **Poisoning by unspecified agents primarily affecting the cardiovascular system, assault** D, S 🔊

     ●■ T46.904   **Poisoning by unspecified agents primarily affecting the cardiovascular system, undetermined** D, S 🔊

     ●■ T46.905   **Adverse effect of unspecified agents primarily affecting the cardiovascular system** D, S 🔊

     ●■ T46.906   **Underdosing of unspecified agents primarily affecting the cardiovascular system** A, D, S 🔊

   ● T46.99   **Poisoning by, adverse effect of and underdosing of other agents primarily affecting the cardiovascular system**

     ● T46.991   **Poisoning by other agents primarily affecting the cardiovascular system, accidental (unintentional)** D, S 🔊

     ● T46.992   **Poisoning by other agents primarily affecting the cardiovascular system, intentional self-harm** D, S 🔊

     ● T46.993   **Poisoning by other agents primarily affecting the cardiovascular system, assault** D, S 🔊

     ● T46.994   **Poisoning by other agents primarily affecting the cardiovascular system, undetermined** D, S 🔊

     ● T46.995   **Adverse effect of other agents primarily affecting the cardiovascular system** D, S 🔊

     ● T46.996   **Underdosing of other agents primarily affecting the cardiovascular system** A, D, S 🔊

CHAPTER 19 (S00-T88)

N Newborn Age: 0   **P** Pediatric Age: 0–17   **M** Maternity DX: 12–55   **A** Adult Age: 15–124   ♀ Females Only   ♂ Males Only

🔊 Complication\Comorbidity   🔊 Major C\C   🔊 Present on Admission Requirement   🔊 Hospital-Acquired Condition

1639

● **T47   Poisoning by, adverse effect of and underdosing of agents primarily affecting the gastrointestinal system**

The appropriate 7th character is to be added to each code from category T47

> A   initial encounter
> D   subsequent encounter
> S   sequela

● **T47.0   Poisoning by, adverse effect of and underdosing of histamine H2-receptor blockers**

● **T47.0X   Poisoning by, adverse effect of and underdosing of histamine H2-receptor blockers**

● **T47.0X1   Poisoning by histamine H2-receptor blockers, accidental (unintentional)** D, S 🔍
> Poisoning by histamine H2-receptor blockers NOS

● **T47.0X2   Poisoning by histamine H2-receptor blockers, intentional self-harm** D, S 🔍

● **T47.0X3   Poisoning by histamine H2-receptor blockers, assault** D, S 🔍

● **T47.0X4   Poisoning by histamine H2-receptor blockers, undetermined** D, S 🔍

● **T47.0X5   Adverse effect of histamine H2-receptor blockers** D, S 🔍

● **T47.0X6   Underdosing of histamine H2-receptor blockers** A, D, S 🔍

● **T47.1   Poisoning by, adverse effect of and underdosing of other antacids and anti-gastric-secretion drugs**

● **T47.1X   Poisoning by, adverse effect of and underdosing of other antacids and anti-gastric-secretion drugs**

● **T47.1X1   Poisoning by other antacids and anti-gastric-secretion drugs, accidental (unintentional)** D, S 🔍
> Poisoning by other antacids and anti-gastric-secretion drugs NOS

● **T47.1X2   Poisoning by other antacids and anti-gastric-secretion drugs, intentional self-harm** D, S 🔍

● **T47.1X3   Poisoning by other antacids and anti-gastric-secretion drugs, assault** D, S 🔍

● **T47.1X4   Poisoning by other antacids and anti-gastric-secretion drugs, undetermined** D, S 🔍

● **T47.1X5   Adverse effect of other antacids and anti-gastric-secretion drugs** D, S 🔍

● **T47.1X6   Underdosing of other antacids and anti-gastric-secretion drugs** A, D, S 🔍

● **T47.2   Poisoning by, adverse effect of and underdosing of stimulant laxatives**

● **T47.2X   Poisoning by, adverse effect of and underdosing of stimulant laxatives**

● **T47.2X1   Poisoning by stimulant laxatives, accidental (unintentional)** D, S 🔍
> Poisoning by stimulant laxatives NOS

● **T47.2X2   Poisoning by stimulant laxatives, intentional self-harm** D, S 🔍

● **T47.2X3   Poisoning by stimulant laxatives, assault** D, S 🔍

● **T47.2X4   Poisoning by stimulant laxatives, undetermined** D, S 🔍

● **T47.2X5   Adverse effect of stimulant laxatives** D, S 🔍

● **T47.2X6   Underdosing of stimulant laxatives** A, D, S 🔍

● **T47.3   Poisoning by, adverse effect of and underdosing of saline and osmotic laxatives**

● **T47.3X   Poisoning by and adverse effect of saline and osmotic laxatives**

● **T47.3X1   Poisoning by saline and osmotic laxatives, accidental (unintentional)** D, S 🔍
> Poisoning by saline and osmotic laxatives NOS

● **T47.3X2   Poisoning by saline and osmotic laxatives, intentional self-harm** D, S 🔍

● **T47.3X3   Poisoning by saline and osmotic laxatives, assault** D, S 🔍

● **T47.3X4   Poisoning by saline and osmotic laxatives, undetermined** D, S 🔍

● **T47.3X5   Adverse effect of saline and osmotic laxatives** D, S 🔍

● **T47.3X6   Underdosing of saline and osmotic laxatives** A, D, S 🔍

● **T47.4   Poisoning by, adverse effect of and underdosing of other laxatives**

● **T47.4X   Poisoning by, adverse effect of and underdosing of other laxatives**

● **T47.4X1   Poisoning by other laxatives, accidental (unintentional)** D, S 🔍
> Poisoning by other laxatives NOS

● **T47.4X2   Poisoning by other laxatives, intentional self-harm** D, S 🔍

● **T47.4X3   Poisoning by other laxatives, assault** D, S 🔍

● **T47.4X4   Poisoning by other laxatives, undetermined** D, S 🔍

● **T47.4X5   Adverse effect of other laxatives** D, S 🔍

● **T47.4X6   Underdosing of other laxatives** A, D, S 🔍

● **T47.5   Poisoning by, adverse effect of and underdosing of digestants**

● **T47.5X   Poisoning by, adverse effect of and underdosing of digestants**

● **T47.5X1   Poisoning by digestants, accidental (unintentional)** D, S 🔍
> Poisoning by digestants NOS

● **T47.5X2   Poisoning by digestants, intentional self-harm** D, S 🔍

● **T47.5X3   Poisoning by digestants, assault** D, S 🔍

● **T47.5X4   Poisoning by digestants, undetermined** D, S 🔍

● **T47.5X5   Adverse effect of digestants** D, S 🔍

● **T47.5X6   Underdosing of digestants** A, D, S 🔍

● Unacceptable Principal Diagnosis   ● Use Additional Character(s)   ■ Unspecified   ▶ Manifestation Code

OGCR   Official Guidelines for Coding and Reporting   Excludes 1   Excludes 2   Includes   Use additional   Code first   Code also

● T47.6   Poisoning by, adverse effect of and underdosing of antidiarrheal drugs

    Excludes2   poisoning by, adverse effect of and underdosing of systemic antibiotics and other anti-infectives (T36-T37)

   ● T47.6X   Poisoning by, adverse effect of and underdosing of antidiarrheal drugs

     ● T47.6X1   Poisoning by antidiarrheal drugs, accidental (unintentional) D, S 🔖
        Poisoning by antidiarrheal drugs NOS

     ● T47.6X2   Poisoning by antidiarrheal drugs, intentional self-harm D, S 🔖

     ● T47.6X3   Poisoning by antidiarrheal drugs, assault D, S 🔖

     ● T47.6X4   Poisoning by antidiarrheal drugs, undetermined D, S 🔖

     ● T47.6X5   Adverse effect of antidiarrheal drugs D, S 🔖

     ● T47.6X6   Underdosing of antidiarrheal drugs A, D, S 🔖

● T47.7   Poisoning by, adverse effect of and underdosing of emetics

   ● T47.7X   Poisoning by, adverse effect of and underdosing of emetics

     ● T47.7X1   Poisoning by emetics, accidental (unintentional) D, S 🔖
        Poisoning by emetics NOS

     ● T47.7X2   Poisoning by emetics, intentional self-harm D, S 🔖

     ● T47.7X3   Poisoning by emetics, assault D, S 🔖

     ● T47.7X4   Poisoning by emetics, undetermined D, S 🔖

     ● T47.7X5   Adverse effect of emetics D, S 🔖

     ● T47.7X6   Underdosing of emetics A, D, S 🔖

● T47.8   Poisoning by, adverse effect of and underdosing of other agents primarily affecting gastrointestinal system

   ● T47.8X   Poisoning by, adverse effect of and underdosing of other agents primarily affecting gastrointestinal system

     ● T47.8X1   Poisoning by other agents primarily affecting gastrointestinal system, accidental (unintentional) D, S 🔖
        Poisoning by other agents primarily affecting gastrointestinal system NOS

     ● T47.8X2   Poisoning by other agents primarily affecting gastrointestinal system, intentional self-harm D, S 🔖

     ● T47.8X3   Poisoning by other agents primarily affecting gastrointestinal system, assault D, S 🔖

     ● T47.8X4   Poisoning by other agents primarily affecting gastrointestinal system, undetermined D, S 🔖

     ● T47.8X5   Adverse effect of other agents primarily affecting gastrointestinal system D, S 🔖

     ● T47.8X6   Underdosing of other agents primarily affecting gastrointestinal system A, D, S 🔖

● T47.9   Poisoning by, adverse effect of and underdosing of unspecified agents primarily affecting the gastrointestinal system

   ●■ T47.91   Poisoning by unspecified agents primarily affecting the gastrointestinal system, accidental (unintentional) D, S 🔖
        Poisoning by agents primarily affecting the gastrointestinal system NOS

   ●■ T47.92   Poisoning by unspecified agents primarily affecting the gastrointestinal system, intentional self-harm D, S 🔖

   ●■ T47.93   Poisoning by unspecified agents primarily affecting the gastrointestinal system, assault D, S 🔖

   ●■ T47.94   Poisoning by unspecified agents primarily affecting the gastrointestinal system, undetermined D, S 🔖

   ●■ T47.95   Adverse effect of unspecified agents primarily affecting the gastrointestinal system D, S 🔖

   ●■ T47.96   Underdosing of unspecified agents primarily affecting the gastrointestinal system A, D, S 🔖

● T48   Poisoning by, adverse effect of and underdosing of agents primarily acting on smooth and skeletal muscles and the respiratory system

   The appropriate 7th character is to be added to each code from category T48

A	initial encounter
D	subsequent encounter
S	sequela

   ● T48.0   Poisoning by, adverse effect of and underdosing of oxytocic drugs

     Excludes1   poisoning by, adverse effect of and underdosing of estrogens, progestogens and antagonists (T38.4-T38.6)

    ● T48.0X   Poisoning by, adverse effect of and underdosing of oxytocic drugs

     ● T48.0X1   Poisoning by oxytocic drugs, accidental (unintentional) D, S 🔖
        Poisoning by oxytocic drugs NOS

     ● T48.0X2   Poisoning by oxytocic drugs, intentional self-harm D, S 🔖

     ● T48.0X3   Poisoning by oxytocic drugs, assault D, S 🔖

     ● T48.0X4   Poisoning by oxytocic drugs, undetermined D, S 🔖

     ● T48.0X5   Adverse effect of oxytocic drugs D, S 🔖

     ● T48.0X6   Underdosing of oxytocic drugs A, D, S 🔖

CHAPTER 19 (S00-T88)

● **T48.1** Poisoning by, adverse effect of and underdosing of skeletal muscle relaxants [neuromuscular blocking agents]

  ● **T48.1X** Poisoning by, adverse effect of and underdosing of skeletal muscle relaxants [neuromuscular blocking agents]

    ● **T48.1X1** Poisoning by skeletal muscle relaxants [neuromuscular blocking agents], accidental (unintentional) D, S 🚫
      Poisoning by skeletal muscle relaxants [neuromuscular blocking agents] NOS

    ● **T48.1X2** Poisoning by skeletal muscle relaxants [neuromuscular blocking agents], intentional self-harm D, S 🚫

    ● **T48.1X3** Poisoning by skeletal muscle relaxants [neuromuscular blocking agents], assault D, S 🚫

    ● **T48.1X4** Poisoning by skeletal muscle relaxants [neuromuscular blocking agents], undetermined D, S 🚫

    ● **T48.1X5** Adverse effect of skeletal muscle relaxants [neuromuscular blocking agents] D, S 🚫

    ● **T48.1X6** Underdosing of skeletal muscle relaxants [neuromuscular blocking agents] A, D, S 🚫

● **T48.2** Poisoning by, adverse effect of and underdosing of other and unspecified drugs acting on muscles

  ● **T48.20** Poisoning by, adverse effect of and underdosing of unspecified drugs acting on muscles

    ●■ **T48.201** Poisoning by unspecified drugs acting on muscles, accidental (unintentional) D, S 🚫
      Poisoning by unspecified drugs acting on muscles NOS

    ●■ **T48.202** Poisoning by unspecified drugs acting on muscles, intentional self-harm D, S 🚫

    ●■ **T48.203** Poisoning by unspecified drugs acting on muscles, assault D, S 🚫

    ●■ **T48.204** Poisoning by unspecified drugs acting on muscles, undetermined D, S 🚫

    ●■ **T48.205** Adverse effect of unspecified drugs acting on muscles D, S 🚫

    ●■ **T48.206** Underdosing of unspecified drugs acting on muscles A, D, S 🚫

  ● **T48.29** Poisoning by, adverse effect of and underdosing of other drugs acting on muscles

    ● **T48.291** Poisoning by other drugs acting on muscles, accidental (unintentional) D, S 🚫
      Poisoning by other drugs acting on muscles NOS

    ● **T48.292** Poisoning by other drugs acting on muscles, intentional self-harm D, S 🚫

    ● **T48.293** Poisoning by other drugs acting on muscles, assault D, S 🚫

    ● **T48.294** Poisoning by other drugs acting on muscles, undetermined D, S 🚫

    ● **T48.295** Adverse effect of other drugs acting on muscles D, S 🚫

    ● **T48.296** Underdosing of other drugs acting on muscles A, D, S 🚫

● **T48.3** Poisoning by, adverse effect of and underdosing of antitussives

  ● **T48.3X** Poisoning by, adverse effect of and underdosing of antitussives

    ● **T48.3X1** Poisoning by antitussives, accidental (unintentional) D, S 🚫
      Poisoning by antitussives NOS

    ● **T48.3X2** Poisoning by antitussives, intentional self-harm D, S 🚫

    ● **T48.3X3** Poisoning by antitussives, assault D, S 🚫

    ● **T48.3X4** Poisoning by antitussives, undetermined D, S 🚫

    ● **T48.3X5** Adverse effect of antitussives D, S 🚫

    ● **T48.3X6** Underdosing of antitussives A, D, S 🚫

● **T48.4** Poisoning by, adverse effect of and underdosing of expectorants

  ● **T48.4X** Poisoning by, adverse effect of and underdosing of expectorants

    ● **T48.4X1** Poisoning by expectorants, accidental (unintentional) D, S 🚫
      Poisoning by expectorants NOS

    ● **T48.4X2** Poisoning by expectorants, intentional self-harm D, S 🚫

    ● **T48.4X3** Poisoning by expectorants, assault D, S 🚫

    ● **T48.4X4** Poisoning by expectorants, undetermined D, S 🚫

    ● **T48.4X5** Adverse effect of expectorants D, S 🚫

    ● **T48.4X6** Underdosing of expectorants A, D, S 🚫

● **T48.5** Poisoning by, adverse effect of and underdosing of other anti-common-cold drugs
  Poisoning by, adverse effect of and underdosing of decongestants

Excludes2	poisoning by, adverse effect of and underdosing of antipyretics, NEC (T39.9-)

    poisoning by, adverse effect of and underdosing of non-steroidal antiinflammatory drugs (T39.3-)

    poisoning by, adverse effect of and underdosing of salicylates (T39.0-)

  ● **T48.5X** Poisoning by, adverse effect of and underdosing of other anti-common-cold drugs

    ● **T48.5X1** Poisoning by other anti-common-cold drugs, accidental (unintentional) D, S 🚫
      Poisoning by other anti-common-cold drugs NOS

    ● **T48.5X2** Poisoning by other anti-common-cold drugs, intentional self-harm D, S 🚫

● Unacceptable Principal Diagnosis   ● Use Additional Character(s)   ■ Unspecified   ▶ Manifestation Code

1642   **OGCR** Official Guidelines for Coding and Reporting   Excludes 1   Excludes 2   Includes   Use additional   Code first   Code also

● T48.5X3 Poisoning by other anti-common-cold drugs, assault D, S 🔖

● T48.5X4 Poisoning by other anti-common-cold drugs, undetermined D, S 🔖

● T48.5X5 Adverse effect of other anti-common-cold drugs D, S 🔖

● T48.5X6 Underdosing of other anti-common-cold drugs A, D, S 🔖

● T48.6 Poisoning by, adverse effect of and underdosing of antiasthmatics, not elsewhere classified
Poisoning by, adverse effect of and underdosing of beta-adrenoreceptor agonists used in asthma therapy

Excludes1   poisoning by, adverse effect of and underdosing of beta-adrenoreceptor agonists not used in asthma therapy (T44.5)
poisoning by, adverse effect of and underdosing of anterior pituitary [adenohypophyseal] hormones (T38.8)

● T48.6X Poisoning by, adverse effect of and underdosing of antiasthmatics

● T48.6X1 Poisoning by antiasthmatics, accidental (unintentional) D, S 🔖
Poisoning by antiasthmatics NOS

● T48.6X2 Poisoning by antiasthmatics, intentional self-harm D, S 🔖

● T48.6X3 Poisoning by antiasthmatics, assault D, S 🔖

● T48.6X4 Poisoning by antiasthmatics, undetermined D, S 🔖

● T48.6X5 Adverse effect of antiasthmatics D, S 🔖

● T48.6X6 Underdosing of antiasthmatics A, D, S 🔖

● T48.9 Poisoning by, adverse effect of and underdosing of other and unspecified agents primarily acting on the respiratory system

● T48.90 Poisoning by, adverse effect of and underdosing of unspecified agents primarily acting on the respiratory system

● ■ T48.901 Poisoning by unspecified agents primarily acting on the respiratory system, accidental (unintentional) D, S 🔖

● ■ T48.902 Poisoning by unspecified agents primarily acting on the respiratory system, intentional self-harm D, S 🔖

● ■ T48.903 Poisoning by unspecified agents primarily acting on the respiratory system, assault D, S 🔖

● ■ T48.904 Poisoning by unspecified agents primarily acting on the respiratory system, undetermined D, S 🔖

● ■ T48.905 Adverse effect of unspecified agents primarily acting on the respiratory system D, S 🔖

● ■ T48.906 Underdosing of unspecified agents primarily acting on the respiratory system A, D, S 🔖

● T48.99 Poisoning by, adverse effect of and underdosing of other agents primarily acting on the respiratory system

● T48.991 Poisoning by other agents primarily acting on the respiratory system, accidental (unintentional) D, S 🔖

● T48.992 Poisoning by other agents primarily acting on the respiratory system, intentional self-harm D, S 🔖

● T48.993 Poisoning by other agents primarily acting on the respiratory system, assault D, S 🔖

● T48.994 Poisoning by other agents primarily acting on the respiratory system, undetermined D, S 🔖

● T48.995 Adverse effect of other agents primarily acting on the respiratory system D, S 🔖

● T48.996 Underdosing of other agents primarily acting on the respiratory system A, D, S 🔖

● T49 Poisoning by, adverse effect of and underdosing of topical agents primarily affecting skin and mucous membrane and by ophthalmological, otorhinolaryngological and dental drugs

Includes   poisoning by, adverse effect of and underdosing of glucocorticoids, topically used

The appropriate 7th character is to be added to each code from category T49

A   initial encounter
D   subsequent encounter
S   sequela

● T49.0 Poisoning by, adverse effect of and underdosing of local antifungal, anti-infective and anti-inflammatory drugs

● T49.0X Poisoning by, adverse effect of and underdosing of local antifungal, anti-infective and anti-inflammatory drugs

● T49.0X1 Poisoning by local antifungal, anti-infective and anti-inflammatory drugs, accidental (unintentional) D, S 🔖
Poisoning by local antifungal, anti-infective and anti-inflammatory drugs NOS

● T49.0X2 Poisoning by local antifungal, anti-infective and anti-inflammatory drugs, intentional self-harm D, S 🔖

● T49.0X3 Poisoning by local antifungal, anti-infective and anti-inflammatory drugs, assault D, S 🔖

● T49.0X4 Poisoning by local antifungal, anti-infective and anti-inflammatory drugs, undetermined D, S 🔖

● T49.0X5 Adverse effect of local antifungal, anti-infective and anti-inflammatory drugs D, S 🔖

● T49.0X6 Underdosing of local antifungal, anti-infective and anti-inflammatory drugs A, D, S 🔖

- T49.1 Poisoning by, adverse effect of and underdosing of antipruritics
  - T49.1X Poisoning by, adverse effect of and underdosing of antipruritics
    - T49.1X1 Poisoning by antipruritics, accidental (unintentional) D, S
      Poisoning by antipruritics NOS
    - T49.1X2 Poisoning by antipruritics, intentional self-harm D, S
    - T49.1X3 Poisoning by antipruritics, assault D, S
    - T49.1X4 Poisoning by antipruritics, undetermined D, S
    - T49.1X5 Adverse effect of antipruritics D, S
    - T49.1X6 Underdosing of antipruritics A, D, S
- T49.2 Poisoning by, adverse effect of and underdosing of local astringents and local detergents
  - T49.2X Poisoning by, adverse effect of and underdosing of local astringents and local detergents
    - T49.2X1 Poisoning by local astringents and local detergents, accidental (unintentional) D, S
      Poisoning by local astringents and local detergents NOS
    - T49.2X2 Poisoning by local astringents and local detergents, intentional self-harm D, S
    - T49.2X3 Poisoning by local astringents and local detergents, assault D, S
    - T49.2X4 Poisoning by local astringents and local detergents, undetermined D, S
    - T49.2X5 Adverse effect of local astringents and local detergents D, S
    - T49.2X6 Underdosing of local astringents and local detergents A, D, S
- T49.3 Poisoning by, adverse effect of and underdosing of emollients, demulcents and protectants
  - T49.3X Poisoning by, adverse effect of and underdosing of emollients, demulcents and protectants
    - T49.3X1 Poisoning by emollients, demulcents and protectants, accidental (unintentional) D, S
      Poisoning by emollients, demulcents and protectants NOS
    - T49.3X2 Poisoning by emollients, demulcents and protectants, intentional self-harm D, S
    - T49.3X3 Poisoning by emollients, demulcents and protectants, assault D, S
    - T49.3X4 Poisoning by emollients, demulcents and protectants, undetermined D, S
    - T49.3X5 Adverse effect of emollients, demulcents and protectants D, S
    - T49.3X6 Underdosing of emollients, demulcents and protectants A, D, S

- T49.4 Poisoning by, adverse effect of and underdosing of keratolytics, keratoplastics, and other hair treatment drugs and preparations
  - T49.4X Poisoning by, adverse effect of and underdosing of keratolytics, keratoplastics, and other hair treatment drugs and preparations D, S
    - T49.4X1 Poisoning by keratolytics, keratoplastics, and other hair treatment drugs and preparations, accidental (unintentional) D, S
      Poisoning by keratolytics, keratoplastics, and other hair treatment drugs and preparations NOS
    - T49.4X2 Poisoning by keratolytics, keratoplastics, and other hair treatment drugs and preparations, intentional self-harm D, S
    - T49.4X3 Poisoning by keratolytics, keratoplastics, and other hair treatment drugs and preparations, assault D, S
    - T49.4X4 Poisoning by keratolytics, keratoplastics, and other hair treatment drugs and preparations, undetermined D, S
    - T49.4X5 Adverse effect of keratolytics, keratoplastics, and other hair treatment drugs and preparations D, S
    - T49.4X6 Underdosing of keratolytics, keratoplastics, and other hair treatment drugs and preparations A, D, S
- T49.5 Poisoning by, adverse effect of and underdosing of ophthalmological drugs and preparations
  - T49.5X Poisoning by, adverse effect of and underdosing of ophthalmological drugs and preparations
    - T49.5X1 Poisoning by ophthalmological drugs and preparations, accidental (unintentional) D, S
      Poisoning by ophthalmological drugs and preparations NOS
    - T49.5X2 Poisoning by ophthalmological drugs and preparations, intentional self-harm D, S
    - T49.5X3 Poisoning by ophthalmological drugs and preparations, assault D, S
    - T49.5X4 Poisoning by ophthalmological drugs and preparations, undetermined D, S
    - T49.5X5 Adverse effect of ophthalmological drugs and preparations D, S
    - T49.5X6 Underdosing of ophthalmological drugs and preparations A, D, S

- Unacceptable Principal Diagnosis   Use Additional Character(s)   Unspecified   Manifestation Code
OGCR Official Guidelines for Coding and Reporting   Excludes 1   Excludes 2   Includes   Use additional   Code first   Code also

● **T49.6** Poisoning by, adverse effect of and underdosing of otorhinolaryngological drugs and preparations

  ● **T49.6X** Poisoning by, adverse effect of and underdosing of otorhinolaryngological drugs and preparations

    ● **T49.6X1** Poisoning by otorhinolaryngological drugs and preparations, accidental (unintentional) D, S

       Poisoning by otorhinolaryngological drugs and preparations NOS

    ● **T49.6X2** Poisoning by otorhinolaryngological drugs and preparations, intentional self-harm D, S

    ● **T49.6X3** Poisoning by otorhinolaryngological drugs and preparations, assault D, S

    ● **T49.6X4** Poisoning by otorhinolaryngological drugs and preparations, undetermined D, S

    ● **T49.6X5** Adverse effect of otorhinolaryngological drugs and preparations D, S

    ● **T49.6X6** Underdosing of otorhinolaryngological drugs and preparations A, D, S

● **T49.7** Poisoning by, adverse effect of and underdosing of dental drugs, topically applied

  ● **T49.7X** Poisoning by, adverse effect of and underdosing of dental drugs, topically applied

    ● **T49.7X1** Poisoning by dental drugs, topically applied, accidental (unintentional) D, S

       Poisoning by dental drugs, topically applied NOS

    ● **T49.7X2** Poisoning by dental drugs, topically applied, intentional self-harm D, S

    ● **T49.7X3** Poisoning by dental drugs, topically applied, assault D, S

    ● **T49.7X4** Poisoning by dental drugs, topically applied, undetermined D, S

    ● **T49.7X5** Adverse effect of dental drugs, topically applied D, S

    ● **T49.7X6** Underdosing of dental drugs, topically applied A, D, S

● **T49.8** Poisoning by, adverse effect of and underdosing of other topical agents

     Poisoning by, adverse effect of and underdosing of spermicides

  ● **T49.8X** Poisoning by, adverse effect of and underdosing of other topical agents

    ● **T49.8X1** Poisoning by other topical agents, accidental (unintentional) D, S

       Poisoning by other topical agents NOS

    ● **T49.8X2** Poisoning by other topical agents, intentional self-harm D, S

    ● **T49.8X3** Poisoning by other topical agents, assault D, S

    ● **T49.8X4** Poisoning by other topical agents, undetermined D, S

    ● **T49.8X5** Adverse effect of other topical agents D, S

    ● **T49.8X6** Underdosing of other topical agents A, D, S

● **T49.9** Poisoning by, adverse effect of and underdosing of unspecified topical agent

  ● ■ **T49.91** Poisoning by unspecified topical agent, accidental (unintentional) D, S

  ● ■ **T49.92** Poisoning by unspecified topical agent, intentional self-harm D, S

  ● ■ **T49.93** Poisoning by unspecified topical agent, assault D, S

  ● ■ **T49.94** Poisoning by unspecified topical agent, undetermined D, S

  ● ■ **T49.95** Adverse effect of unspecified topical agent D, S

  ● ■ **T49.96** Underdosing of unspecified topical agent A, D, S

T50 Poisoning by, adverse effect of and underdosing of diuretics and other and unspecified drugs, medicaments and biological substances

     The appropriate 7th character is to be added to each code from category T50

A	initial encounter
D	subsequent encounter
S	sequela

● **T50.0** Poisoning by, adverse effect of and underdosing of mineralocorticoids and their antagonists

  ● **T50.0X** Poisoning by, adverse effect of and underdosing of mineralocorticoids and their antagonists

    ● **T50.0X1** Poisoning by mineralocorticoids and their antagonists, accidental (unintentional) D, S

       Poisoning by mineralocorticoids and their antagonists NOS

    ● **T50.0X2** Poisoning by mineralocorticoids and their antagonists, intentional self-harm D, S

    ● **T50.0X3** Poisoning by mineralocorticoids and their antagonists, assault D, S

    ● **T50.0X4** Poisoning by mineralocorticoids and their antagonists, undetermined D, S

    ● **T50.0X5** Adverse effect of mineralocorticoids and their antagonists D, S

    ● **T50.0X6** Underdosing of mineralocorticoids and their antagonists A, D, S

N Newborn Age: 0   **P** Pediatric Age: 0–17   **M** Maternity DX: 12–55   **A** Adult Age: 15–124   ♀ Females Only   ♂ Males Only

Complication\Comorbidity   Major C\C   Present on Admission Requirement   Hospital-Acquired Condition   1645

CHAPTER 19 (S00-T88)

CHAPTER 19 (S00-T88)

● **T50.1 Poisoning by, adverse effect of and underdosing of loop [high-ceiling] diuretics**
  ● **T50.1X Poisoning by, adverse effect of and underdosing of loop [high-ceiling] diuretics**
    ● **T50.1X1 Poisoning by loop [high-ceiling] diuretics, accidental (unintentional)** D, S
      Poisoning by loop [high-ceiling] diuretics NOS
    ● **T50.1X2 Poisoning by loop [high-ceiling] diuretics, intentional self-harm** D, S
    ● **T50.1X3 Poisoning by loop [high-ceiling] diuretics, assault** D, S
    ● **T50.1X4 Poisoning by loop [high-ceiling] diuretics, undetermined** D, S
    ● **T50.1X5 Adverse effect of loop [high-ceiling] diuretics** D, S
    ● **T50.1X6 Underdosing of loop [high-ceiling] diuretics** A, D, S

● **T50.2 Poisoning by, adverse effect of and underdosing of carbonic-anhydrase inhibitors, benzothiadiazides and other diuretics**
    Poisoning by, adverse effect of and underdosing of acetazolamide
  ● **T50.2X Poisoning by, adverse effect of and underdosing of carbonic-anhydrase inhibitors, benzothiadiazides and other diuretics** D, S
    ● **T50.2X1 Poisoning by carbonic-anhydrase inhibitors, benzothiadiazides and other diuretics, accidental (unintentional)** D, S
      Poisoning by carbonic-anhydrase inhibitors, benzothiadiazides and other diuretics NOS
    ● **T50.2X2 Poisoning by carbonic-anhydrase inhibitors, benzothiadiazides and other diuretics, intentional self-harm** D, S
    ● **T50.2X3 Poisoning by carbonic-anhydrase inhibitors, benzothiadiazides and other diuretics, assault** D, S
    ● **T50.2X4 Poisoning by carbonic-anhydrase inhibitors, benzothiadiazides and other diuretics, undetermined** D, S
    ● **T50.2X5 Adverse effect of carbonic-anhydrase inhibitors, benzothiadiazides and other diuretics** D, S
    ● **T50.2X6 Underdosing of carbonic-anhydrase inhibitors, benzothiadiazides and other diuretics** A, D, S

● **T50.3 Poisoning by, adverse effect of and underdosing of electrolytic, caloric and water-balance agents**
    Poisoning by, adverse effect of and underdosing of oral rehydration salts
  ● **T50.3X Poisoning by, adverse effect of and underdosing of electrolytic, caloric and water-balance agents**
    ● **T50.3X1 Poisoning by electrolytic, caloric and water-balance agents, accidental (unintentional)** D, S
      Poisoning by electrolytic, caloric and water-balance agents NOS

● **T50.3X2 Poisoning by electrolytic, caloric and water-balance agents, intentional self-harm** D, S
● **T50.3X3 Poisoning by electrolytic, caloric and water-balance agents, assault** D, S
● **T50.3X4 Poisoning by electrolytic, caloric and water-balance agents, undetermined** D, S
● **T50.3X5 Adverse effect of electrolytic, caloric and water-balance agents** D, S
● **T50.3X6 Underdosing of electrolytic, caloric and water-balance agents** A, D, S

● **T50.4 Poisoning by, adverse effect of and underdosing of drugs affecting uric acid metabolism**
  ● **T50.4X Poisoning by, adverse effect of and underdosing of drugs affecting uric acid metabolism**
    ● **T50.4X1 Poisoning by drugs affecting uric acid metabolism, accidental (unintentional)** D, S
      Poisoning by drugs affecting uric acid metabolism NOS
    ● **T50.4X2 Poisoning by drugs affecting uric acid metabolism, intentional self-harm** D, S
    ● **T50.4X3 Poisoning by drugs affecting uric acid metabolism, assault** D, S
    ● **T50.4X4 Poisoning by drugs affecting uric acid metabolism, undetermined** D, S
    ● **T50.4X5 Adverse effect of drugs affecting uric acid metabolism** D, S
    ● **T50.4X6 Underdosing of drugs affecting uric acid metabolism** A, D, S

● **T50.5 Poisoning by, adverse effect of and underdosing of appetite depressants**
  ● **T50.5X Poisoning by, adverse effect of and underdosing of appetite depressants**
    ● **T50.5X1 Poisoning by appetite depressants, accidental (unintentional)** D, S
      Poisoning by appetite depressants NOS
    ● **T50.5X2 Poisoning by appetite depressants, intentional self-harm** D, S
    ● **T50.5X3 Poisoning by appetite depressants, assault** D, S
    ● **T50.5X4 Poisoning by appetite depressants, undetermined** D, S
    ● **T50.5X5 Adverse effect of appetite depressants** D, S
    ● **T50.5X6 Underdosing of appetite depressants** A, D, S

● **T50.6 Poisoning by, adverse effect of and underdosing of antidotes and chelating agents**
    Poisoning by, adverse effect of and underdosing of alcohol deterrents
  ● **T50.6X Poisoning by, adverse effect of and underdosing of antidotes and chelating agents**

● Unacceptable Principal Diagnosis   ● Use Additional Character(s)   ■ Unspecified   ▶ Manifestation Code
OGCR Official Guidelines for Coding and Reporting   Excludes 1   Excludes 2   Includes   Use additional   Code first   Code also

- ● **T50.6X1** Poisoning by antidotes and chelating agents, accidental (unintentional) D, S 🖰
  - Poisoning by antidotes and chelating agents NOS
- ● **T50.6X2** Poisoning by antidotes and chelating agents, intentional self-harm D, S 🖰
- ● **T50.6X3** Poisoning by antidotes and chelating agents, assault D, S 🖰
- ● **T50.6X4** Poisoning by antidotes and chelating agents, undetermined D, S 🖰
- ● **T50.6X5** Adverse effect of antidotes and chelating agents D, S 🖰
- ● **T50.6X6** Underdosing of antidotes and chelating agents A, D, S 🖰

- ● **T50.7** Poisoning by, adverse effect of and underdosing of analeptics and opioid receptor antagonists
  - ● **T50.7X** Poisoning by, adverse effect of and underdosing of analeptics and opioid receptor antagonists
    - ● **T50.7X1** Poisoning by analeptics and opioid receptor antagonists, accidental (unintentional) D, S 🖰
      - Poisoning by analeptics and opioid receptor antagonists NOS
    - ● **T50.7X2** Poisoning by analeptics and opioid receptor antagonists, intentional self-harm D, S 🖰
    - ● **T50.7X3** Poisoning by analeptics and opioid receptor antagonists, assault D, S 🖰
    - ● **T50.7X4** Poisoning by analeptics and opioid receptor antagonists, undetermined D, S 🖰
    - ● **T50.7X5** Adverse effect of analeptics and opioid receptor antagonists D, S 🖰
    - ● **T50.7X6** Underdosing of analeptics and opioid receptor antagonists A, D, S 🖰

- ● **T50.8** Poisoning by, adverse effect of and underdosing of diagnostic agents
  - ● **T50.8X** Poisoning by, adverse effect of and underdosing of diagnostic agents
    - ● **T50.8X1** Poisoning by diagnostic agents, accidental (unintentional) D, S 🖰
      - Poisoning by diagnostic agents NOS
    - ● **T50.8X2** Poisoning by diagnostic agents, intentional self-harm D, S 🖰
    - ● **T50.8X3** Poisoning by diagnostic agents, assault D, S 🖰
    - ● **T50.8X4** Poisoning by diagnostic agents, undetermined D, S 🖰
    - ● **T50.8X5** Adverse effect of diagnostic agents D, S 🖰
    - ● **T50.8X6** Underdosing of diagnostic agents A, D, S 🖰

- ● **T50.A** Poisoning by, adverse effect of and underdosing of bacterial vaccines
  - ● **T50.A1** Poisoning by, adverse effect of and underdosing of pertussis vaccine, including combinations with a pertussis component
    - ● **T50.A11** Poisoning by pertussis vaccine, including combinations with a pertussis component, accidental (unintentional) D, S 🖰
    - ● **T50.A12** Poisoning by pertussis vaccine, including combinations with a pertussis component, intentional self-harm D, S 🖰
    - ● **T50.A13** Poisoning by pertussis vaccine, including combinations with a pertussis component, assault D, S 🖰
    - ● **T50.A14** Poisoning by pertussis vaccine, including combinations with a pertussis component, undetermined D, S 🖰
    - ● **T50.A15** Adverse effect of pertussis vaccine, including combinations with a pertussis component D, S 🖰
    - ● **T50.A16** Underdosing of pertussis vaccine, including combinations with a pertussis component A, D, S 🖰
  - ● **T50.A2** Poisoning by, adverse effect of and underdosing of mixed bacterial vaccines without a pertussis component
    - ● **T50.A21** Poisoning by mixed bacterial vaccines without a pertussis component, accidental (unintentional) D, S 🖰
    - ● **T50.A22** Poisoning by mixed bacterial vaccines without a pertussis component, intentional self-harm D, S 🖰
    - ● **T50.A23** Poisoning by mixed bacterial vaccines without a pertussis component, assault D, S 🖰
    - ● **T50.A24** Poisoning by mixed bacterial vaccines without a pertussis component, undetermined D, S 🖰
    - ● **T50.A25** Adverse effect of mixed bacterial vaccines without a pertussis component D, S 🖰
    - ● **T50.A26** Underdosing of mixed bacterial vaccines without a pertussis component A, D, S 🖰
  - ● **T50.A9** Poisoning by, adverse effect of and underdosing of other bacterial vaccines
    - ● **T50.A91** Poisoning by other bacterial vaccines, accidental (unintentional) D, S 🖰
    - ● **T50.A92** Poisoning by other bacterial vaccines, intentional self-harm D, S 🖰
    - ● **T50.A93** Poisoning by other bacterial vaccines, assault D, S 🖰
    - ● **T50.A94** Poisoning by other bacterial vaccines, undetermined D, S 🖰
    - ● **T50.A95** Adverse effect of other bacterial vaccines D, S 🖰
    - ● **T50.A96** Underdosing of other bacterial vaccines A, D, S 🖰

N Newborn Age: 0   **P** Pediatric Age: 0–17   **M** Maternity DX: 12–55   **A** Adult Age: 15–124   ♀ Females Only   ♂ Males Only

🖰 Complication\Comorbidity   🖰 Major C\C   🖰 Present on Admission Requirement   🖰 Hospital-Acquired Condition

1647

● **T50.B** Poisoning by, adverse effect of and underdosing of viral vaccines
- ● **T50.B1** Poisoning by, adverse effect of and underdosing of smallpox vaccines
  - ● **T50.B11** Poisoning by smallpox vaccines, accidental (unintentional) D, S
  - ● **T50.B12** Poisoning by smallpox vaccines, intentional self-harm D, S
  - ● **T50.B13** Poisoning by smallpox vaccines, assault D, S
  - ● **T50.B14** Poisoning by smallpox vaccines, undetermined D, S
  - ● **T50.B15** Adverse effect of smallpox vaccines D, S
  - ● **T50.B16** Underdosing of smallpox vaccines A, D, S
- ● **T50.B9** Poisoning by, adverse effect of and underdosing of other viral vaccines
  - ● **T50.B91** Poisoning by other viral vaccines, accidental (unintentional) D, S
  - ● **T50.B92** Poisoning by other viral vaccines, intentional self-harm D, S
  - ● **T50.B93** Poisoning by other viral vaccines, assault D, S
  - ● **T50.B94** Poisoning by other viral vaccines, undetermined D, S
  - ● **T50.B95** Adverse effect of other viral vaccines D, S
  - ● **T50.B96** Underdosing of other viral vaccines A, D, S

● **T50.Z** Poisoning by, adverse effect of and underdosing of other vaccines and biological substances
- ● **T50.Z1** Poisoning by, adverse effect of and underdosing of immunoglobulin
  - ● **T50.Z11** Poisoning by immunoglobulin, accidental (unintentional) D, S
  - ● **T50.Z12** Poisoning by immunoglobulin, intentional self-harm D, S
  - ● **T50.Z13** Poisoning by immunoglobulin, assault D, S
  - ● **T50.Z14** Poisoning by immunoglobulin, undetermined D, S
  - ● **T50.Z15** Adverse effect of immunoglobulin D, S
  - ● **T50.Z16** Underdosing of immunoglobulin A, D, S
- ● **T50.Z9** Poisoning by, adverse effect of and underdosing of other vaccines and biological substances
  - ● **T50.Z91** Poisoning by other vaccines and biological substances, accidental (unintentional) D, S
  - ● **T50.Z92** Poisoning by other vaccines and biological substances, intentional self-harm D, S

● **T50.Z93** Poisoning by other vaccines and biological substances, assault D, S
● **T50.Z94** Poisoning by other vaccines and biological substances, undetermined D, S
● **T50.Z95** Adverse effect of other vaccines and biological substances D, S
● **T50.Z96** Underdosing of other vaccines and biological substances A, D, S

● **T50.9** Poisoning by, adverse effect of and underdosing of other and unspecified drugs, medicaments and biological substances
- ● **T50.90** Poisoning by, adverse effect of and underdosing of unspecified drugs, medicaments and biological substances
  - ●■ **T50.901** Poisoning by unspecified drugs, medicaments and biological substances, accidental (unintentional)
  - ●■ **T50.902** Poisoning by unspecified drugs, medicaments and biological substances, intentional self-harm
  - ●■ **T50.903** Poisoning by unspecified drugs, medicaments and biological substances, assault
  - ●■ **T50.904** Poisoning by unspecified drugs, medicaments and biological substances, undetermined
  - ●■ **T50.905** Adverse effect of unspecified drugs, medicaments and biological substances
  - ●■ **T50.906** Underdosing of unspecified drugs, medicaments and biological substances
- ● **T50.99** Poisoning by, adverse effect of and underdosing of other drugs, medicaments and biological substances
  - ● **T50.991** Poisoning by other drugs, medicaments and biological substances, accidental (unintentional)
  - ● **T50.992** Poisoning by other drugs, medicaments and biological substances, intentional self-harm
  - ● **T50.993** Poisoning by other drugs, medicaments and biological substances, assault
  - ● **T50.994** Poisoning by other drugs, medicaments and biological substances, undetermined
  - ● **T50.995** Adverse effect of other drugs, medicaments and biological substances
  - ● **T50.996** Underdosing of other drugs, medicaments and biological substances

● Unacceptable Principal Diagnosis   ● Use Additional Character(s)   ■ Unspecified   ▶ Manifestation Code
OGCR Official Guidelines for Coding and Reporting   Excludes 1   Excludes 2   Includes   Use additional   Code first   Code also

TOXIC EFFECTS OF SUBSTANCES CHIEFLY NONMEDICINAL AS TO SOURCE (T51-T65)

Note: When no intent is indicated code to accidental. Undetermined intent is only for use when there is specific documentation in the record that the intent of the toxic effect cannot be determined

Use additional code(s): for all associated manifestations of toxic effect, such as:
respiratory conditions due to external agents (J60-J70)
personal history of foreign body fully removed (Z87.821)
to identify any retained foreign body, if applicable (Z18.-)

Excludes1 contact with and (suspected) exposure to toxic substances (Z77.-)

● **T51** **Toxic effect of alcohol**

The appropriate 7th character is to be added to each code from category T51

> A   initial encounter
> D   subsequent encounter
> S   sequela

● **T51.0** **Toxic effect of ethanol**
    Toxic effect of ethyl alcohol

> **Excludes2** acute alcohol intoxication or 'hangover' effects (F10.129, F10.229, F10.929)
> drunkenness (F10.129, F10.229, F10.929)
> pathological alcohol intoxication (F10.129, F10.229, F10.929)

  ● **T51.0X** **Toxic effect of ethanol**

    ● **T51.0X1** **Toxic effect of ethanol, accidental (unintentional)** D, S
        Toxic effect of ethanol NOS

    ● **T51.0X2** **Toxic effect of ethanol, intentional self-harm** D, S

    ● **T51.0X3** **Toxic effect of ethanol, assault** D, S

    ● **T51.0X4** **Toxic effect of ethanol, undetermined** A, D, S

● **T51.1** **Toxic effect of methanol**
    Toxic effect of methyl alcohol

  ● **T51.1X** **Toxic effect of methanol**

    ● **T51.1X1** **Toxic effect of methanol, accidental (unintentional)** D, S
        Toxic effect of methanol NOS

    ● **T51.1X2** **Toxic effect of methanol, intentional self-harm** D, S

    ● **T51.1X3** **Toxic effect of methanol, assault** D, S

    ● **T51.1X4** **Toxic effect of methanol, undetermined** D, S

● **T51.2** **Toxic effect of 2-Propanol**
    Toxic effect of isopropyl alcohol

  ● **T51.2X** **Toxic effect of 2-Propanol**

    ● **T51.2X1** **Toxic effect of 2-Propanol, accidental (unintentional)** D, S
        Toxic effect of 2-Propanol NOS

    ● **T51.2X2** **Toxic effect of 2-Propanol, intentional self-harm** D, S

    ● **T51.2X3** **Toxic effect of 2-Propanol, assault** D, S

    ● **T51.2X4** **Toxic effect of 2-Propanol, undetermined** D, S

● **T51.3** **Toxic effect of fusel oil**
    Toxic effect of amyl alcohol
    Toxic effect of butyl [1-butanol] alcohol
    Toxic effect of propyl [1-propanol] alcohol

  ● **T51.3X** **Toxic effect of fusel oil**

    ● **T51.3X1** **Toxic effect of fusel oil, accidental (unintentional)** D, S
        Toxic effect of fusel oil NOS

    ● **T51.3X2** **Toxic effect of fusel oil, intentional self-harm** D, S

    ● **T51.3X3** **Toxic effect of fusel oil, assault** D, S

    ● **T51.3X4** **Toxic effect of fusel oil, undetermined** D, S

● **T51.8** **Toxic effect of other alcohols**

  ● **T51.8X** **Toxic effect of other alcohols**

    ● **T51.8X1** **Toxic effect of other alcohols, accidental (unintentional)** D, S
        Toxic effect of other alcohols NOS

    ● **T51.8X2** **Toxic effect of other alcohols, intentional self-harm** D, S

    ● **T51.8X3** **Toxic effect of other alcohols, assault** D, S

    ● **T51.8X4** **Toxic effect of other alcohols, undetermined** D, S

● **T51.9** **Toxic effect of unspecified alcohol**

  ●■ **T51.91** **Toxic effect of unspecified alcohol, accidental (unintentional)** D, S

  ●■ **T51.92** **Toxic effect of unspecified alcohol, intentional self-harm** D, S

  ●■ **T51.93** **Toxic effect of unspecified alcohol, assault** D, S

  ●■ **T51.94** **Toxic effect of unspecified alcohol, undetermined** D, S

● **T52** **Toxic effect of organic solvents**

> **Excludes1** halogen derivatives of aliphatic and aromatic hydrocarbons (T53.-)

The appropriate 7th character is to be added to each code from category T52

> A   initial encounter
> D   subsequent encounter
> S   sequela

● **T52.0** **Toxic effects of petroleum products**
    Toxic effects of gasoline [petrol]
    Toxic effects of kerosene [paraffin oil]
    Toxic effects of paraffin wax
    Toxic effects of ether petroleum
    Toxic effects of naphtha petroleum
    Toxic effects of spirit petroleum

  ● **T52.0X** **Toxic effects of petroleum products**

    ● **T52.0X1** **Toxic effect of petroleum products, accidental (unintentional)** D, S
        Toxic effects of petroleum products NOS

    ● **T52.0X2** **Toxic effect of petroleum products, intentional self-harm** D, S

    ● **T52.0X3** **Toxic effect of petroleum products, assault** D, S

    ● **T52.0X4** **Toxic effect of petroleum products, undetermined** D, S

CHAPTER 19 (S00-T88)

● **T52.1   Toxic effects of benzene**

> Excludes1 homologues of benzene (T52.2)
> nitroderivatives and
> aminoderivatives of benzene
> and its homologues (T65.3)

● **T52.1X   Toxic effects of benzene**

● **T52.1X1   Toxic effect of benzene, accidental (unintentional)** D, S
Toxic effects of benzene NOS

● **T52.1X2   Toxic effect of benzene, intentional self-harm** D, S

● **T52.1X3   Toxic effect of benzene, assault** D, S

● **T52.1X4   Toxic effect of benzene, undetermined** D, S

● **T52.2   Toxic effects of homologues of benzene**
Toxic effects of toluene [methylbenzene]
Toxic effects of xylene [dimethylbenzene]

● **T52.2X   Toxic effects of homologues of benzene**

● **T52.2X1   Toxic effect of homologues of benzene, accidental (unintentional)** D, S
Toxic effects of homologues of benzene NOS

● **T52.2X2   Toxic effect of homologues of benzene, intentional self-harm** D, S

● **T52.2X3   Toxic effect of homologues of benzene, assault** D, S

● **T52.2X4   Toxic effect of homologues of benzene, undetermined** D, S

● **T52.3   Toxic effects of glycols**

● **T52.3X   Toxic effects of glycols**

● **T52.3X1   Toxic effect of glycols, accidental (unintentional)** D, S
Toxic effects of glycols NOS

● **T52.3X2   Toxic effect of glycols, intentional self-harm** D, S

● **T52.3X3   Toxic effect of glycols, assault** D, S

● **T52.3X4   Toxic effect of glycols, undetermined** D, S

● **T52.4   Toxic effects of ketones**

● **T52.4X   Toxic effects of ketones**

● **T52.4X1   Toxic effect of ketones, accidental (unintentional)** D, S
Toxic effects of ketones NOS

● **T52.4X2   Toxic effect of ketones, intentional self-harm** D, S

● **T52.4X3   Toxic effect of ketones, assault** D, S

● **T52.4X4   Toxic effect of ketones, undetermined** D, S

● **T52.8   Toxic effects of other organic solvents**

● **T52.8X   Toxic effects of other organic solvents**

● **T52.8X1   Toxic effect of other organic solvents, accidental (unintentional)** D, S
Toxic effects of other organic solvents NOS

● **T52.8X2   Toxic effect of other organic solvents, intentional self-harm** D, S

● **T52.8X3   Toxic effect of other organic solvents, assault** D, S

● **T52.8X4   Toxic effect of other organic solvents, undetermined** D, S

● **T52.9   Toxic effects of unspecified organic solvent**

● ■ **T52.91   Toxic effect of unspecified organic solvent, accidental (unintentional)** D, S

● ■ **T52.92   Toxic effect of unspecified organic solvent, intentional self-harm** D, S

● ■ **T52.93   Toxic effect of unspecified organic solvent, assault** D, S

● ■ **T52.94   Toxic effect of unspecified organic solvent, undetermined** D, S

● **T53   Toxic effect of halogen derivatives of aliphatic and aromatic hydrocarbons**

> The appropriate 7th character is to be added to each code from category T53

> | A | initial encounter |
> | D | subsequent encounter |
> | S | sequela |

● **T53.0   Toxic effects of carbon tetrachloride**
Toxic effects of tetrachloromethane

● **T53.0X   Toxic effects of carbon tetrachloride**

● **T53.0X1   Toxic effect of carbon tetrachloride, accidental (unintentional)** D, S
Toxic effects of carbon tetrachloride NOS

● **T53.0X2   Toxic effect of carbon tetrachloride, intentional self- harm** D, S

● **T53.0X3   Toxic effect of carbon tetrachloride, assault** D, S

● **T53.0X4   Toxic effect of carbon tetrachloride, undetermined** D, S

● **T53.1   Toxic effects of chloroform**
Toxic effects of trichloromethane

● **T53.1X   Toxic effects of chloroform**

● **T53.1X1   Toxic effect of chloroform, accidental (unintentional)** D, S
Toxic effects of chloroform NOS

● **T53.1X2   Toxic effect of chloroform, intentional self-harm** D, S

● **T53.1X3   Toxic effect of chloroform, assault** D, S

● **T53.1X4   Toxic effect of chloroform, undetermined** D, S

● **T53.2   Toxic effects of trichloroethylene**
Toxic effects of trichloroethene

● **T53.2X   Toxic effects of trichloroethylene**

● **T53.2X1   Toxic effect of trichloroethylene, accidental (unintentional)** D, S
Toxic effects of trichloroethylene NOS

● **T53.2X2   Toxic effect of trichloroethylene, intentional self-harm** D, S

● **T53.2X3   Toxic effect of trichloroethylene, assault** D, S

● **T53.2X4   Toxic effect of trichloroethylene, undetermined** D, S

● Unacceptable Principal Diagnosis   ● Use Additional Character(s)   ■ Unspecified   ▶ Manifestation Code

OGCR Official Guidelines for Coding and Reporting   Excludes 1   Excludes 2   Includes   Use additional   Code first   Code also

● **T53.3**   **Toxic effects of tetrachloroethylene**
Toxic effects of perchloroethylene
Toxic effect of tetrachloroethene

   ● **T53.3X**   **Toxic effects of tetrachloroethylene**

     ● **T53.3X1**   **Toxic effect of tetrachloroethylene, accidental (unintentional)** D, S
Toxic effects of tetrachloroethylene NOS

     ● **T53.3X2**   **Toxic effect of tetrachloroethylene, intentional self-harm** D, S

     ● **T53.3X3**   **Toxic effect of tetrachloroethylene, assault** D, S

     ● **T53.3X4**   **Toxic effect of tetrachloroethylene, undetermined** D, S

● **T53.4**   **Toxic effects of dichloromethane**
Toxic effects of methylene chloride

   ● **T53.4X**   **Toxic effects of dichloromethane**

     ● **T53.4X1**   **Toxic effect of dichloromethane, accidental (unintentional)** D, S
Toxic effects of dichloromethane NOS

     ● **T53.4X2**   **Toxic effect of dichloromethane, intentional self-harm** D, S

     ● **T53.4X3**   **Toxic effect of dichloromethane, assault** D, S

     ● **T53.4X4**   **Toxic effect of dichloromethane, undetermined** D, S

● **T53.5**   **Toxic effects of chlorofluorocarbons**

   ● **T53.5X**   **Toxic effects of chlorofluorocarbons**

     ● **T53.5X1**   **Toxic effect of chlorofluorocarbons, accidental (unintentional)** D, S
Toxic effects of chlorofluorocarbons NOS

     ● **T53.5X2**   **Toxic effect of chlorofluorocarbons, intentional self-harm** D, S

     ● **T53.5X3**   **Toxic effect of chlorofluorocarbons, assault** D, S

     ● **T53.5X4**   **Toxic effect of chlorofluorocarbons, undetermined** D, S

● **T53.6**   **Toxic effects of other halogen derivatives of aliphatic hydrocarbons**

   ● **T53.6X**   **Toxic effects of other halogen derivatives of aliphatic hydrocarbons**

     ● **T53.6X1**   **Toxic effect of other halogen derivatives of aliphatic hydrocarbons, accidental (unintentional)** D, S
Toxic effects of other halogen derivatives of aliphatic hydrocarbons NOS

     ● **T53.6X2**   **Toxic effect of other halogen derivatives of aliphatic hydrocarbons, intentional self-harm** D, S

     ● **T53.6X3**   **Toxic effect of other halogen derivatives of aliphatic hydrocarbons, assault** D, S

     ● **T53.6X4**   **Toxic effect of other halogen derivatives of aliphatic hydrocarbons, undetermined** D, S

● **T53.7**   **Toxic effects of other halogen derivatives of aromatic hydrocarbons**

   ● **T53.7X**   **Toxic effects of other halogen derivatives of aromatic hydrocarbons**

     ● **T53.7X1**   **Toxic effect of other halogen derivatives of aromatic hydrocarbons, accidental (unintentional)** D, S
Toxic effects of other halogen derivatives of aromatic hydrocarbons NOS

     ● **T53.7X2**   **Toxic effect of other halogen derivatives of aromatic hydrocarbons, intentional self-harm** D, S

     ● **T53.7X3**   **Toxic effect of other halogen derivatives of aromatic hydrocarbons, assault** D, S

     ● **T53.7X4**   **Toxic effect of other halogen derivatives of aromatic hydrocarbons, undetermined** D, S

● **T53.9**   **Toxic effects of unspecified halogen derivatives of aliphatic and aromatic hydrocarbons**

   ●■ **T53.91**   Toxic effect of unspecified halogen derivatives of aliphatic and aromatic hydrocarbons, accidental (unintentional) D, S

   ●■ **T53.92**   Toxic effect of unspecified halogen derivatives of aliphatic and aromatic hydrocarbons, intentional self-harm D, S

   ●■ **T53.93**   Toxic effect of unspecified halogen derivatives of aliphatic and aromatic hydrocarbons, assault D, S

   ●■ **T53.94**   Toxic effect of unspecified halogen derivatives of aliphatic and aromatic hydrocarbons, undetermined D, S

● **T54**   **Toxic effect of corrosive substances**

The appropriate 7th character is to be added to each code from category T54

A	initial encounter
D	subsequent encounter
S	sequela

● **T54.0**   **Toxic effects of phenol and phenol homologues**

   ● **T54.0X**   **Toxic effects of phenol and phenol homologues**

     ● **T54.0X1**   **Toxic effect of phenol and phenol homologues, accidental (unintentional)** D, S
Toxic effects of phenol and phenol homologues NOS

     ● **T54.0X2**   **Toxic effect of phenol and phenol homologues, intentional self-harm** D, S

     ● **T54.0X3**   **Toxic effect of phenol and phenol homologues, assault** D, S

     ● **T54.0X4**   **Toxic effect of phenol and phenol homologues, undetermined** D, S

N Newborn Age: 0   **P** Pediatric Age: 0–17   **M** Maternity DX: 12–55   **A** Adult Age: 15–124   ♀ Females Only   ♂ Males Only
Complication\Comorbidity   Major C\C   Present on Admission Requirement   Hospital-Acquired Condition

1651

CHAPTER 19 (S00-T88)

● **T54.1   Toxic effects of other corrosive organic compounds**

  ● **T54.1X   Toxic effects of other corrosive organic compounds**

    ● **T54.1X1   Toxic effect of other corrosive organic compounds, accidental (unintentional)** D, S 🔎
      Toxic effects of other corrosive organic compounds NOS

    ● **T54.1X2   Toxic effect of other corrosive organic compounds, intentional self-harm** D, S 🔎

    ● **T54.1X3   Toxic effect of other corrosive organic compounds, assault** D, S 🔎

    ● **T54.1X4   Toxic effect of other corrosive organic compounds, undetermined** D, S 🔎

● **T54.2   Toxic effects of corrosive acids and acid-like substances**
  Toxic effects of hydrochloric acid
  Toxic effects of sulfuric acid

  ● **T54.2X   Toxic effects of corrosive acids and acid-like substances**

    ● **T54.2X1   Toxic effect of corrosive acids and acid-like substances, accidental (unintentional)** D, S 🔎
      Toxic effects of corrosive acids and acid-like substances NOS

    ● **T54.2X2   Toxic effect of corrosive acids and acid-like substances, intentional self-harm** D, S 🔎

    ● **T54.2X3   Toxic effect of corrosive acids and acid-like substances, assault** D, S 🔎

    ● **T54.2X4   Toxic effect of corrosive acids and acid-like substances, undetermined** D, S 🔎

● **T54.3   Toxic effects of corrosive alkalis and alkali-like substances**
  Toxic effects of potassium hydroxide
  Toxic effects of sodium hydroxide

  ● **T54.3X   Toxic effects of corrosive alkalis and alkali-like substances**

    ● **T54.3X1   Toxic effect of corrosive alkalis and alkali-like substances, accidental (unintentional)** D, S 🔎
      Toxic effects of corrosive alkalis and alkali-like substances NOS

    ● **T54.3X2   Toxic effect of corrosive alkalis and alkali-like substances, intentional self-harm** D, S 🔎

    ● **T54.3X3   Toxic effect of corrosive alkalis and alkali-like substances, assault** D, S 🔎

    ● **T54.3X4   Toxic effect of corrosive alkalis and alkali-like substances, undetermined** D, S 🔎

● **T54.9   Toxic effects of unspecified corrosive substance**

  ●■ **T54.91   Toxic effect of unspecified corrosive substance, accidental (unintentional)** D, S 🔎

  ●■ **T54.92   Toxic effect of unspecified corrosive substance, intentional self-harm** D, S 🔎

  ●■ **T54.93   Toxic effect of unspecified corrosive substance, assault** D, S 🔎

  ●■ **T54.94   Toxic effect of unspecified corrosive substance, undetermined** D, S 🔎

● **T55   Toxic effect of soaps and detergents**

The appropriate 7th character is to be added to each code from category T55

> A   initial encounter
> D   subsequent encounter
> S   sequela

  ● **T55.0   Toxic effect of soaps**

    ● **T55.0X   Toxic effect of soaps**

      ● **T55.0X1   Toxic effect of soaps, accidental (unintentional)** D, S 🔎
        Toxic effect of soaps NOS

      ● **T55.0X2   Toxic effect of soaps, intentional self-harm** D, S 🔎

      ● **T55.0X3   Toxic effect of soaps, assault** D, S 🔎

      ● **T55.0X4   Toxic effect of soaps, undetermined** D, S 🔎

  ● **T55.1   Toxic effect of detergents**

    ● **T55.1X   Toxic effect of detergents**

      ● **T55.1X1   Toxic effect of detergents, accidental (unintentional)** D, S 🔎
        Toxic effect of detergents NOS

      ● **T55.1X2   Toxic effect of detergents, intentional self-harm** D, S 🔎

      ● **T55.1X3   Toxic effect of detergents, assault** D, S 🔎

      ● **T55.1X4   Toxic effect of detergents, undetermined** D, S 🔎

● **T56   Toxic effect of metals**

> **Includes**   toxic effects of fumes and vapors of metals
> toxic effects of metals from all sources, except medicinal substances

> Use additional code to identify any retained metal foreign body, if applicable (Z18.0-, T18.1-)

> **Excludes1**   arsenic and its compounds (T57.0)
> manganese and its compounds (T57.2)

The appropriate 7th character is to be added to each code from category T56

> A   initial encounter
> D   subsequent encounter
> S   sequela

  ● **T56.0   Toxic effects of lead and its compounds**

    ● **T56.0X   Toxic effects of lead and its compounds**

      ● **T56.0X1   Toxic effect of lead and its compounds, accidental (unintentional)** D, S 🔎
        Toxic effects of lead and its compounds NOS

      ● **T56.0X2   Toxic effect of lead and its compounds, intentional self-harm** D, S 🔎

      ● **T56.0X3   Toxic effect of lead and its compounds, assault** D, S 🔎

      ● **T56.0X4   Toxic effect of lead and its compounds, undetermined** D, S 🔎

CHAPTER 19 (S00-T88)

● Unacceptable Principal Diagnosis   ● Use Additional Character(s)   ■ Unspecified   ▶ Manifestation Code

1652   **OGCR** Official Guidelines for Coding and Reporting   Excludes 1   Excludes 2   Includes   Use additional   Code first   Code also

- ● **T56.1**   Toxic effects of mercury and its compounds
  - ● **T56.1X**   Toxic effects of mercury and its compounds
    - ● **T56.1X1**   Toxic effect of mercury and its compounds, accidental (unintentional) D, S 🔲
      Toxic effects of mercury and its compounds NOS
    - ● **T56.1X2**   Toxic effect of mercury and its compounds, intentional self-harm D, S 🔲
    - ● **T56.1X3**   Toxic effect of mercury and its compounds, assault D, S 🔲
    - ● **T56.1X4**   Toxic effect of mercury and its compounds, undetermined D, S 🔲
- ● **T56.2**   Toxic effects of chromium and its compounds
  - ● **T56.2X**   Toxic effects of chromium and its compounds
    - ● **T56.2X1**   Toxic effect of chromium and its compounds, accidental (unintentional) D, S 🔲
      Toxic effects of chromium and its compounds NOS
    - ● **T56.2X2**   Toxic effect of chromium and its compounds, intentional self-harm D, S 🔲
    - ● **T56.2X3**   Toxic effect of chromium and its compounds, assault D, S 🔲
    - ● **T56.2X4**   Toxic effect of chromium and its compounds, undetermined D, S 🔲
- ● **T56.3**   Toxic effects of cadmium and its compounds
  - ● **T56.3X**   Toxic effects of cadmium and its compounds
    - ● **T56.3X1**   Toxic effect of cadmium and its compounds, accidental (unintentional) D, S 🔲
      Toxic effects of cadmium and its compounds NOS
    - ● **T56.3X2**   Toxic effect of cadmium and its compounds, intentional self-harm D, S 🔲
    - ● **T56.3X3**   Toxic effect of cadmium and its compounds, assault D, S 🔲
    - ● **T56.3X4**   Toxic effect of cadmium and its compounds, undetermined D, S 🔲
- ● **T56.4**   Toxic effects of copper and its compounds
  - ● **T56.4X**   Toxic effects of copper and its compounds
    - ● **T56.4X1**   Toxic effect of copper and its compounds, accidental (unintentional) D, S 🔲
      Toxic effects of copper and its compounds NOS
    - ● **T56.4X2**   Toxic effect of copper and its compounds, intentional self-harm D, S 🔲
    - ● **T56.4X3**   Toxic effect of copper and its compounds, assault D, S 🔲
    - ● **T56.4X4**   Toxic effect of copper and its compounds, undetermined D, S 🔲

- ● **T56.5**   Toxic effects of zinc and its compounds
  - ● **T56.5X**   Toxic effects of zinc and its compounds
    - ● **T56.5X1**   Toxic effect of zinc and its compounds, accidental (unintentional) D, S 🔲
      Toxic effects of zinc and its compounds NOS
    - ● **T56.5X2**   Toxic effect of zinc and its compounds, intentional self-harm D, S 🔲
    - ● **T56.5X3**   Toxic effect of zinc and its compounds, assault D, S 🔲
    - ● **T56.5X4**   Toxic effect of zinc and its compounds, undetermined D, S 🔲
- ● **T56.6**   Toxic effects of tin and its compounds
  - ● **T56.6X**   Toxic effects of tin and its compounds
    - ● **T56.6X1**   Toxic effect of tin and its compounds, accidental (unintentional) D, S 🔲
      Toxic effects of tin and its compounds NOS
    - ● **T56.6X2**   Toxic effect of tin and its compounds, intentional self-harm D, S 🔲
    - ● **T56.6X3**   Toxic effect of tin and its compounds, assault D, S 🔲
    - ● **T56.6X4**   Toxic effect of tin and its compounds, undetermined D, S 🔲
- ● **T56.7**   Toxic effects of beryllium and its compounds
  - ● **T56.7X**   Toxic effects of beryllium and its compounds
    - ● **T56.7X1**   Toxic effect of beryllium and its compounds, accidental (unintentional) D, S 🔲
      Toxic effects of beryllium and its compounds NOS
    - ● **T56.7X2**   Toxic effect of beryllium and its compounds, intentional self-harm D, S 🔲
    - ● **T56.7X3**   Toxic effect of beryllium and its compounds, assault D, S 🔲
    - ● **T56.7X4**   Toxic effect of beryllium and its compounds, undetermined D, S 🔲
- ● **T56.8**   Toxic effects of other metals
  - ● **T56.81**   Toxic effect of thallium
    - ● **T56.811**   Toxic effect of thallium, accidental (unintentional) D, S 🔲
      Toxic effect of thallium NOS
    - ● **T56.812**   Toxic effect of thallium, intentional self-harm D, S 🔲
    - ● **T56.813**   Toxic effect of thallium, assault D, S 🔲
    - ● **T56.814**   Toxic effect of thallium, undetermined D, S 🔲
  - ● **T56.89**   Toxic effects of other metals
    - ● **T56.891**   Toxic effect of other metals, accidental (unintentional) D, S 🔲
      Toxic effects of other metals NOS
    - ● **T56.892**   Toxic effect of other metals, intentional self-harm D, S 🔲
    - ● **T56.893**   Toxic effect of other metals, assault D, S 🔲
    - ● **T56.894**   Toxic effect of other metals, undetermined D, S 🔲

N Newborn Age: 0   **P** Pediatric Age: 0–17   **M** Maternity DX: 12–55   **A** Adult Age: 15–124   ♀ Females Only   ♂ Males Only

🔲 Complication\Comorbidity   🔲 Major C\C   🔲 Present on Admission Requirement   🔲 Hospital-Acquired Condition

1653

CHAPTER 19 (S00-T88)

● T56.9   Toxic effects of unspecified metal

    ●■ T56.91   Toxic effect of unspecified metal, accidental (unintentional) D, S

    ●■ T56.92   Toxic effect of unspecified metal, intentional self-harm D, S

    ●■ T56.93   Toxic effect of unspecified metal, assault D, S

    ●■ T56.94   Toxic effect of unspecified metal, undetermined D, S

● T57   Toxic effect of other inorganic substances

    The appropriate 7th character is to be added to each code from category T57

      A   initial encounter
      D   subsequent encounter
      S   sequela

    ● T57.0   Toxic effect of arsenic and its compounds

      ● T57.0X   Toxic effect of arsenic and its compounds

        ● T57.0X1   Toxic effect of arsenic and its compounds, accidental (unintentional) D, S
          Toxic effect of arsenic and its compounds NOS

        ● T57.0X2   Toxic effect of arsenic and its compounds, intentional self-harm D, S

        ● T57.0X3   Toxic effect of arsenic and its compounds, assault D, S

        ● T57.0X4   Toxic effect of arsenic and its compounds, undetermined D, S

    ● T57.1   Toxic effect of phosphorus and its compounds

      Excludes1   organophosphate insecticides (T60.0)

      ● T57.1X   Toxic effect of phosphorus and its compounds

        ● T57.1X1   Toxic effect of phosphorus and its compounds, accidental (unintentional) D, S
          Toxic effect of phosphorus and its compounds NOS

        ● T57.1X2   Toxic effect of phosphorus and its compounds, intentional self-harm D, S

        ● T57.1X3   Toxic effect of phosphorus and its compounds, assault D, S

        ● T57.1X4   Toxic effect of phosphorus and its compounds, undetermined D, S

    ● T57.2   Toxic effect of manganese and its compounds

      ● T57.2X   Toxic effect of manganese and its compounds

        ● T57.2X1   Toxic effect of manganese and its compounds, accidental (unintentional) D, S
          Toxic effect of manganese and its compounds NOS

        ● T57.2X2   Toxic effect of manganese and its compounds, intentional self-harm D, S

        ● T57.2X3   Toxic effect of manganese and its compounds, assault D, S

        ● T57.2X4   Toxic effect of manganese and its compounds, undetermined D, S

● T57.3   Toxic effect of hydrogen cyanide

    ● T57.3X   Toxic effect of hydrogen cyanide

      ● T57.3X1   Toxic effect of hydrogen cyanide, accidental (unintentional) D, S
        Toxic effect of hydrogen cyanide NOS

      ● T57.3X2   Toxic effect of hydrogen cyanide, intentional self-harm D, S

      ● T57.3X3   Toxic effect of hydrogen cyanide, assault D, S

      ● T57.3X4   Toxic effect of hydrogen cyanide, undetermined D, S

● T57.8   Toxic effect of other specified inorganic substances

    ● T57.8X   Toxic effect of other specified inorganic substances

      ● T57.8X1   Toxic effect of other specified inorganic substances, accidental (unintentional) D, S
        Toxic effect of other specified inorganic substances NOS

      ● T57.8X2   Toxic effect of other specified inorganic substances, intentional self-harm D, S

      ● T57.8X3   Toxic effect of other specified inorganic substances, assault D, S

      ● T57.8X4   Toxic effect of other specified inorganic substances, undetermined D, S

● T57.9   Toxic effect of unspecified inorganic substance

    ●■ T57.91   Toxic effect of unspecified inorganic substance, accidental (unintentional) D, S

    ●■ T57.92   Toxic effect of unspecified inorganic substance, intentional self-harm D, S

    ●■ T57.93   Toxic effect of unspecified inorganic substance, assault D, S

    ●■ T57.94   Toxic effect of unspecified inorganic substance, undetermined D, S

● T58   Toxic effect of carbon monoxide

    Includes   asphyxiation from carbon monoxide
        toxic effect of carbon monoxide from all sources

    The appropriate 7th character is to be added to each code from category T58

      A   initial encounter
      D   subsequent encounter
      S   sequela

    ● T58.0   Toxic effect of carbon monoxide from motor vehicle exhaust
      Toxic effect of exhaust gas from gas engine
      Toxic effect of exhaust gas from motor pump

      ● T58.01   Toxic effect of carbon monoxide from motor vehicle exhaust, accidental (unintentional) D, S

      ● T58.02   Toxic effect of carbon monoxide from motor vehicle exhaust, intentional self-harm D, S

      ● T58.03   Toxic effect of carbon monoxide from motor vehicle exhaust, assault D, S

      ● T58.04   Toxic effect of carbon monoxide from motor vehicle exhaust, undetermined D, S

● Unacceptable Principal Diagnosis   ● Use Additional Character(s)   ■ Unspecified   ▶ Manifestation Code

OGCR Official Guidelines for Coding and Reporting | Excludes 1 | | Excludes 2 | | Includes | | Use additional | | Code first | | Code also |

● **T58.1   Toxic effect of carbon monoxide from utility gas**
     Toxic effect of acetylene
     Toxic effect of gas NOS used for lighting, heating, cooking
     Toxic effect of water gas

   ● **T58.11   Toxic effect of carbon monoxide from utility gas, accidental (unintentional)** D, S 🔖

   ● **T58.12   Toxic effect of carbon monoxide from utility gas, intentional self-harm** D, S 🔖

   ● **T58.13   Toxic effect of carbon monoxide from utility gas, assault** D, S 🔖

   ● **T58.14   Toxic effect of carbon monoxide from utility gas, undetermined** D, S 🔖

● **T58.2   Toxic effect of carbon monoxide from incomplete combustion of other domestic fuels**
     Toxic effect of carbon monoxide from incomplete combustion of coal, coke, kerosene, wood

   ● **T58.2X   Toxic effect of carbon monoxide from incomplete combustion of other domestic fuels**

     ● **T58.2X1   Toxic effect of carbon monoxide from incomplete combustion of other domestic fuels, accidental (unintentional)** D, S 🔖

     ● **T58.2X2   Toxic effect of carbon monoxide from incomplete combustion of other domestic fuels, intentional self-harm** D, S 🔖

     ● **T58.2X3   Toxic effect of carbon monoxide from incomplete combustion of other domestic fuels, assault** D, S 🔖

     ● **T58.2X4   Toxic effect of carbon monoxide from incomplete combustion of other domestic fuels, undetermined** D, S 🔖

● **T58.8   Toxic effect of carbon monoxide from other source**
     Toxic effect of carbon monoxide from blast furnace gas
     Toxic effect of carbon monoxide from fuels in industrial use
     Toxic effect of carbon monoxide from kiln vapor

   ● **T58.8X   Toxic effect of carbon monoxide from other source**

     ● **T58.8X1   Toxic effect of carbon monoxide from other source, accidental (unintentional)** D, S 🔖

     ● **T58.8X2   Toxic effect of carbon monoxide from other source, intentional self-harm** D, S 🔖

     ● **T58.8X3   Toxic effect of carbon monoxide from other source, assault** D, S 🔖

     ● **T58.8X4   Toxic effect of carbon monoxide from other source, undetermined** D, S 🔖

● **T58.9   Toxic effect of carbon monoxide from unspecified source**

   ●■ **T58.91   Toxic effect of carbon monoxide from unspecified source, accidental (unintentional)** D, S 🔖

   ●■ **T58.92   Toxic effect of carbon monoxide from unspecified source, intentional self-harm** D, S 🔖

   ●■ **T58.93   Toxic effect of carbon monoxide from unspecified source, assault** D, S 🔖

   ●■ **T58.94   Toxic effect of carbon monoxide from unspecified source, undetermined** D, S 🔖

● **T59   Toxic effect of other gases, fumes and vapors**

   | **Includes** | aerosol propellants |
   | **Excludes1** | chlorofluorocarbons (T53.5) |

   The appropriate 7th character is to be added to each code from category T59

A	initial encounter
D	subsequent encounter
S	sequela

● **T59.0   Toxic effect of nitrogen oxides**

   ● **T59.0X   Toxic effect of nitrogen oxides**

     ● **T59.0X1   Toxic effect of nitrogen oxides, accidental (unintentional)** D, S 🔖
       Toxic effect of nitrogen oxides NOS

     ● **T59.0X2   Toxic effect of nitrogen oxides, intentional self-harm** D, S 🔖

     ● **T59.0X3   Toxic effect of nitrogen oxides, assault** D, S 🔖

     ● **T59.0X4   Toxic effect of nitrogen oxides, undetermined** D, S 🔖

● **T59.1   Toxic effect of sulfur dioxide**

   ● **T59.1X   Toxic effect of sulfur dioxide**

     ● **T59.1X1   Toxic effect of sulfur dioxide, accidental (unintentional)** D, S 🔖
       Toxic effect of sulfur dioxide NOS

     ● **T59.1X2   Toxic effect of sulfur dioxide, intentional self-harm** D, S 🔖

     ● **T59.1X3   Toxic effect of sulfur dioxide, assault** D, S 🔖

     ● **T59.1X4   Toxic effect of sulfur dioxide, undetermined** D, S 🔖

● **T59.2   Toxic effect of formaldehyde**

   ● **T59.2X   Toxic effect of formaldehyde**

     ● **T59.2X1   Toxic effect of formaldehyde, accidental (unintentional)** D, S 🔖
       Toxic effect of formaldehyde NOS

     ● **T59.2X2   Toxic effect of formaldehyde, intentional self-harm** D, S 🔖

     ● **T59.2X3   Toxic effect of formaldehyde, assault** D, S 🔖

     ● **T59.2X4   Toxic effect of formaldehyde, undetermined** D, S 🔖

● **T59.3   Toxic effect of lacrimogenic gas**
     Toxic effect of tear gas

   ● **T59.3X   Toxic effect of lacrimogenic gas**

     ● **T59.3X1   Toxic effect of lacrimogenic gas, accidental (unintentional)** D, S 🔖
       Toxic effect of lacrimogenic gas NOS

     ● **T59.3X2   Toxic effect of lacrimogenic gas, intentional self-harm** D, S 🔖

     ● **T59.3X3   Toxic effect of lacrimogenic gas, assault** D, S 🔖

     ● **T59.3X4   Toxic effect of lacrimogenic gas, undetermined** D, S 🔖

● **T59.4   Toxic effect of chlorine gas**

   ● **T59.4X   Toxic effect of chlorine gas**

     ● **T59.4X1   Toxic effect of chlorine gas, accidental (unintentional)** D, S 🔖
       Toxic effect of chlorine gas NOS

N Newborn Age: 0   **P** Pediatric Age: 0–17   **M** Maternity DX: 12–55   **A** Adult Age: 15–124   ♀ Females Only   ♂ Males Only

🔖 Complication\Comorbidity   🔖 Major C\C   🔖 Present on Admission Requirement   🔖 Hospital-Acquired Condition

1655

CHAPTER 19 (S00-T88)

● T59.4X2   Toxic effect of chlorine gas, intentional self-harm D, S 🔍

● T59.4X3   Toxic effect of chlorine gas, assault D, S 🔍

● T59.4X4   Toxic effect of chlorine gas, undetermined D, S 🔍

● T59.5   Toxic effect of fluorine gas and hydrogen fluoride

   ● T59.5X   Toxic effect of fluorine gas and hydrogen fluoride

     ● T59.5X1   Toxic effect of fluorine gas and hydrogen fluoride, accidental (unintentional) D, S 🔍
         Toxic effect of fluorine gas and hydrogen fluoride NOS

     ● T59.5X2   Toxic effect of fluorine gas and hydrogen fluoride, intentional self-harm D, S 🔍

     ● T59.5X3   Toxic effect of fluorine gas and hydrogen fluoride, assault D, S 🔍

     ● T59.5X4   Toxic effect of fluorine gas and hydrogen fluoride, undetermined D, S 🔍

● T59.6   Toxic effect of hydrogen sulfide

   ● T59.6X   Toxic effect of hydrogen sulfide

     ● T59.6X1   Toxic effect of hydrogen sulfide, accidental (unintentional) D, S 🔍
         Toxic effect of hydrogen sulfide NOS

     ● T59.6X2   Toxic effect of hydrogen sulfide, intentional self-harm D, S 🔍

     ● T59.6X3   Toxic effect of hydrogen sulfide, assault D, S 🔍

     ● T59.6X4   Toxic effect of hydrogen sulfide, undetermined D, S 🔍

● T59.7   Toxic effect of carbon dioxide

   ● T59.7X   Toxic effect of carbon dioxide

     ● T59.7X1   Toxic effect of carbon dioxide, accidental (unintentional) D, S 🔍
         Toxic effect of carbon dioxide NOS

     ● T59.7X2   Toxic effect of carbon dioxide, intentional self-harm D, S 🔍

     ● T59.7X3   Toxic effect of carbon dioxide, assault D, S 🔍

     ● T59.7X4   Toxic effect of carbon dioxide, undetermined D, S 🔍

● T59.8   Toxic effect of other specified gases, fumes and vapors

   ● T59.81   Toxic effect of smoke
     Smoke inhalation

     | Excludes2 | toxic effect of cigarette (tobacco) smoke (T65.22-) |

     ● T59.811   Toxic effect of smoke, accidental (unintentional) D, S 🔍
         Toxic effect of smoke NOS

     ● T59.812   Toxic effect of smoke, intentional self-harm D, S 🔍

     ● T59.813   Toxic effect of smoke, assault D, S 🔍

     ● T59.814   Toxic effect of smoke, undetermined D, S 🔍

● T59.89   Toxic effect of other specified gases, fumes and vapors

   ● ■ T59.891   Toxic effect of other specified gases, fumes and vapors, accidental (unintentional) D, S 🔍

   ● ■ T59.892   Toxic effect of other specified gases, fumes and vapors, intentional self-harm D, S 🔍

   ● ■ T59.893   Toxic effect of other specified gases, fumes and vapors, assault D, S 🔍

   ● ■ T59.894   Toxic effect of other specified gases, fumes and vapors, undetermined D, S 🔍

● T59.9   Toxic effect of unspecified gases, fumes and vapors

   ● T59.91   Toxic effect of unspecified gases, fumes and vapors, accidental (unintentional) D, S 🔍

   ● T59.92   Toxic effect of unspecified gases, fumes and vapors, intentional self-harm D, S 🔍

   ● T59.93   Toxic effect of unspecified gases, fumes and vapors, assault D, S 🔍

   ● T59.94   Toxic effect of unspecified gases, fumes and vapors, undetermined D, S 🔍

● T60   Toxic effect of pesticides

   | Includes | toxic effect of wood preservatives |

   The appropriate 7th character is to be added to each code from category T60

A	initial encounter
D	subsequent encounter
S	sequela

● T60.0   Toxic effect of organophosphate and carbamate insecticides

   ● T60.0X   Toxic effect of organophosphate and carbamate insecticides

     ● T60.0X1   Toxic effect of organophosphate and carbamate insecticides, accidental (unintentional) D, S 🔍
         Toxic effect of organophosphate and carbamate insecticides NOS

     ● T60.0X2   Toxic effect of organophosphate and carbamate insecticides, intentional self-harm D, S 🔍

     ● T60.0X3   Toxic effect of organophosphate and carbamate insecticides, assault D, S 🔍

     ● T60.0X4   Toxic effect of organophosphate and carbamate insecticides, undetermined D, S 🔍

● T60.1   Toxic effect of halogenated insecticides

   | Excludes1 | chlorinated hydrocarbon (T53.-) |

   ● T60.1X   Toxic effect of halogenated insecticides

     ● T60.1X1   Toxic effect of halogenated insecticides, accidental (unintentional) D, S 🔍
         Toxic effect of halogenated insecticides NOS

     ● T60.1X2   Toxic effect of halogenated insecticides, intentional self-harm D, S 🔍

     ● T60.1X3   Toxic effect of halogenated insecticides, assault D, S 🔍

     ● T60.1X4   Toxic effect of halogenated insecticides, undetermined D, S 🔍

● Unacceptable Principal Diagnosis   ● Use Additional Character(s)   ■ Unspecified   ▶ Manifestation Code

OGCR   Official Guidelines for Coding and Reporting   Excludes 1   Excludes 2   Includes   Use additional   Code first   Code also

- ● **T60.2** Toxic effect of other insecticides
  - ● **T60.2X** Toxic effect of other insecticides
    - ● **T60.2X1** Toxic effect of other insecticides, accidental (unintentional) D, S 🔖
      Toxic effect of other insecticides NOS
    - ● **T60.2X2** Toxic effect of other insecticides, intentional self-harm D, S 🔖
    - ● **T60.2X3** Toxic effect of other insecticides, assault D, S 🔖
    - ● **T60.2X4** Toxic effect of other insecticides, undetermined D, S 🔖
- ● **T60.3** Toxic effect of herbicides and fungicides
  - ● **T60.3X** Toxic effect of herbicides and fungicides
    - ● **T60.3X1** Toxic effect of herbicides and fungicides, accidental (unintentional) D, S 🔖
      Toxic effect of herbicides and fungicides NOS
    - ● **T60.3X2** Toxic effect of herbicides and fungicides, intentional self-harm D, S 🔖
    - ● **T60.3X3** Toxic effect of herbicides and fungicides, assault D, S 🔖
    - ● **T60.3X4** Toxic effect of herbicides and fungicides, undetermined D, S 🔖
- ● **T60.4** Toxic effect of rodenticides
  - **Excludes1**   strychnine and its salts (T65.1)
    thallium (T56.81-)
  - ● **T60.4X** Toxic effect of rodenticides
    - ● **T60.4X1** Toxic effect of rodenticides, accidental (unintentional) D, S 🔖
      Toxic effect of rodenticides NOS
    - ● **T60.4X2** Toxic effect of rodenticides, intentional self-harm D, S 🔖
    - ● **T60.4X3** Toxic effect of rodenticides, assault D, S 🔖
    - ● **T60.4X4** Toxic effect of rodenticides, undetermined D, S 🔖
- ● **T60.8** Toxic effect of other pesticides
  - ● **T60.8X** Toxic effect of other pesticides
    - ● **T60.8X1** Toxic effect of other pesticides, accidental (unintentional) D, S 🔖
      Toxic effect of other pesticides NOS
    - ● **T60.8X2** Toxic effect of other pesticides, intentional self-harm D, S 🔖
    - ● **T60.8X3** Toxic effect of other pesticides, assault D, S 🔖
    - ● **T60.8X4** Toxic effect of other pesticides, undetermined D, S 🔖
- ● **T60.9** Toxic effect of unspecified pesticide
  - ● ▣ **T60.91** Toxic effect of unspecified pesticide, accidental (unintentional) D, S 🔖
  - ● ▣ **T60.92** Toxic effect of unspecified pesticide, intentional self-harm D, S 🔖
  - ● ▣ **T60.93** Toxic effect of unspecified pesticide, assault D, S 🔖
  - ● ▣ **T60.94** Toxic effect of unspecified pesticide, undetermined D, S 🔖

- ● **T61** Toxic effect of noxious substances eaten as seafood
  - **Excludes1**   allergic reaction to food, such as:
    anaphylactic reaction or shock due to adverse food reaction (T78.0-)
    dermatitis (L23.6, L25.4, L27.2)
    gastroenteritis (noninfective) (K52.2)
    anaphylactic shock (T78.02, T78.05)
    bacterial foodborne intoxications (A05.-)
    toxic effect of food contaminants, such as:
    aflatoxin and other mycotoxins (T64)
    cyanides (T65.0-)
    harmful algae bloom (T65.82-)
    hydrogen cyanide (T57.3-)
    mercury (T56.1-)
    red tide (T65.82-)

  The appropriate 7th character is to be added to each code from category T61

A	initial encounter
D	subsequent encounter
S	sequela

  - ● **T61.0** Ciguatera fish poisoning
    - ● **T61.01** Ciguatera fish poisoning, accidental (unintentional) D, S 🔖
    - ● **T61.02** Ciguatera fish poisoning, intentional self-harm D, S 🔖
    - ● **T61.03** Ciguatera fish poisoning, assault D, S 🔖
    - ● **T61.04** Ciguatera fish poisoning, undetermined D, S 🔖
  - ● **T61.1** Scombroid fish poisoning
    Histamine-like syndrome
    - ● **T61.11** Scombroid fish poisoning, accidental (unintentional) D, S 🔖
    - ● **T61.12** Scombroid fish poisoning, intentional self-harm D, S 🔖
    - ● **T61.13** Scombroid fish poisoning, assault D, S 🔖
    - ● **T61.14** Scombroid fish poisoning, undetermined D, S 🔖
  - ● **T61.7** Other fish and shellfish poisoning
    - ● **T61.77** Other fish poisoning
      - ● **T61.771** Other fish poisoning, accidental (unintentional) D, S 🔖
      - ● **T61.772** Other fish poisoning, intentional self-harm D, S 🔖
      - ● **T61.773** Other fish poisoning, assault D, S 🔖
      - ● **T61.774** Other fish poisoning, undetermined D, S 🔖
    - ● **T61.78** Other shellfish poisoning
      - ● **T61.781** Other shellfish poisoning, accidental (unintentional) D, S 🔖
      - ● **T61.782** Other shellfish poisoning, intentional self-harm D, S 🔖
      - ● **T61.783** Other shellfish poisoning, assault D, S 🔖
      - ● **T61.784** Other shellfish poisoning, undetermined D, S 🔖
  - ● **T61.8** Toxic effect of other seafood
    - ● **T61.8X** Toxic effect of other seafood
      - ● **T61.8X1** Toxic effect of other seafood, accidental (unintentional) D, S 🔖
      - ● **T61.8X2** Toxic effect of other seafood, intentional self-harm D, S 🔖

CHAPTER 19 (S00-T88)

N Newborn Age: 0   **P** Pediatric Age: 0–17   **M** Maternity DX: 12–55   **A** Adult Age: 15–124   ♀ Females Only   ♂ Males Only
🔖 Complication\Comorbidity   🔖 Major C\C   🔖 Present on Admission Requirement   🔖 Hospital-Acquired Condition
1657

- T61.8X3   Toxic effect of other seafood, assault D, S
- T61.8X4   Toxic effect of other seafood, undetermined D, S
- T61.9   Toxic effect of unspecified seafood
  - T61.91   Toxic effect of unspecified seafood, accidental (unintentional) D, S
  - T61.92   Toxic effect of unspecified seafood, intentional self-harm D, S
  - T61.93   Toxic effect of unspecified seafood, assault D, S
  - T61.94   Toxic effect of unspecified seafood, undetermined D, S

- T62   Toxic effect of other noxious substances eaten as food

  Excludes1   allergic reaction to food, such as:
  > anaphylactic shock (reaction) due to adverse food reaction (T78.0-)
  > dermatitis (L23.6, L25.4, L27.2)
  > gastroenteritis (noninfective) (K52.2)
  > bacterial food borne intoxications (A05.-)
  > toxic effect of food contaminants, such as:
  > aflatoxin and other mycotoxins (T64)
  > cyanides (T65.0-)
  > hydrogen cyanide (T57.3-)
  > mercury (T56.1-)

  The appropriate 7th character is to be added to each code from category T62

A	initial encounter
D	subsequent encounter
S	sequela

  - T62.0   Toxic effect of ingested mushrooms
    - T62.0X   Toxic effect of ingested mushrooms
      - T62.0X1   Toxic effect of ingested mushrooms, accidental (unintentional) D, S
        Toxic effect of ingested mushrooms NOS
      - T62.0X2   Toxic effect of ingested mushrooms, intentional self-harm D, S
      - T62.0X3   Toxic effect of ingested mushrooms, assault D, S
      - T62.0X4   Toxic effect of ingested mushrooms, undetermined D, S
  - T62.1   Toxic effect of ingested berries
    - T62.1X   Toxic effect of ingested berries
      - T62.1X1   Toxic effect of ingested berries, accidental (unintentional) D, S
        Toxic effect of ingested berries NOS
      - T62.1X2   Toxic effect of ingested berries, intentional self-harm D, S
      - T62.1X3   Toxic effect of ingested berries, assault D, S
      - T62.1X4   Toxic effect of ingested berries, undetermined D, S
  - T62.2   Toxic effect of other ingested (parts of) plant(s)
    - T62.2X   Toxic effect of other ingested (parts of) plant(s)
      - T62.2X1   Toxic effect of other ingested (parts of) plant(s), accidental (unintentional) D, S
        Toxic effect of other ingested (parts of) plant(s) NOS

- T62.2X2   Toxic effect of other ingested (parts of) plant(s), intentional self-harm D, S
- T62.2X3   Toxic effect of other ingested (parts of) plant(s), assault D, S
- T62.2X4   Toxic effect of other ingested (parts of) plant(s), undetermined D, S
- T62.8   Toxic effect of other specified noxious substances eaten as food
  - T62.8X   Toxic effect of other specified noxious substances eaten as food
    - T62.8X1   Toxic effect of other specified noxious substances eaten as food, accidental (unintentional) D, S
      Toxic effect of other specified noxious substances eaten as food NOS
    - T62.8X2   Toxic effect of other specified noxious substances eaten as food, intentional self-harm D, S
    - T62.8X3   Toxic effect of other specified noxious substances eaten as food, assault D, S
    - T62.8X4   Toxic effect of other specified noxious substances eaten as food, undetermined D, S
- T62.9   Toxic effect of unspecified noxious substance eaten as food
  - T62.91   Toxic effect of unspecified noxious substance eaten as food, accidental (unintentional) D, S
    Toxic effect of unspecified noxious substance eaten as food NOS
  - T62.92   Toxic effect of unspecified noxious substance eaten as food, intentional self-harm D, S
  - T62.93   Toxic effect of unspecified noxious substance eaten as food, assault D, S
  - T62.94   Toxic effect of unspecified noxious substance eaten as food, undetermined D, S

- T63   Toxic effect of contact with venomous animals and plants

  Includes   bite or touch of venomous animal
  > pricked or stuck by thorn or leaf

  Excludes2   ingestion of toxic animal or plant (T61.-, T62.-)

  The appropriate 7th character is to be added to each code from category T63

A	initial encounter
D	subsequent encounter
S	sequela

  - T63.0   Toxic effect of snake venom
    - T63.00   Toxic effect of unspecified snake venom
      - T63.001   Toxic effect of unspecified snake venom, accidental (unintentional) D, S
        Toxic effect of unspecified snake venom NOS
      - T63.002   Toxic effect of unspecified snake venom, intentional self-harm D, S
      - T63.003   Toxic effect of unspecified snake venom, assault D, S
      - T63.004   Toxic effect of unspecified snake venom, undetermined D, S

● Unacceptable Principal Diagnosis   ● Use Additional Character(s)   ■ Unspecified   ▶ Manifestation Code

1658   OGCR Official Guidelines for Coding and Reporting   Excludes 1   Excludes 2   Includes   Use additional   Code first   Code also

● **T63.01**   Toxic effect of rattlesnake venom
    ● **T63.011**   Toxic effect of rattlesnake venom, accidental (unintentional) D, S ◎
        Toxic effect of rattlesnake venom NOS
    ● **T63.012**   Toxic effect of rattlesnake venom, intentional self-harm D, S ◎
    ● **T63.013**   Toxic effect of rattlesnake venom, assault D, S ◎
    ● **T63.014**   Toxic effect of rattlesnake venom, undetermined D, S ◎

● **T63.02**   Toxic effect of coral snake venom
    ● **T63.021**   Toxic effect of coral snake venom, accidental (unintentional) D, S ◎
        Toxic effect of coral snake venom NOS
    ● **T63.022**   Toxic effect of coral snake venom, intentional self-harm D, S ◎
    ● **T63.023**   Toxic effect of coral snake venom, assault D, S ◎
    ● **T63.024**   Toxic effect of coral snake venom, undetermined D, S ◎

● **T63.03**   Toxic effect of taipan venom
    ● **T63.031**   Toxic effect of taipan venom, accidental (unintentional) D, S ◎
        Toxic effect of taipan venom NOS
    ● **T63.032**   Toxic effect of taipan venom, intentional self-harm D, S ◎
    ● **T63.033**   Toxic effect of taipan venom, assault D, S ◎
    ● **T63.034**   Toxic effect of taipan venom, undetermined D, S ◎

● **T63.04**   Toxic effect of cobra venom
    ● **T63.041**   Toxic effect of cobra venom, accidental (unintentional) D, S ◎
        Toxic effect of cobra venom NOS
    ● **T63.042**   Toxic effect of cobra venom, intentional self-harm D, S ◎
    ● **T63.043**   Toxic effect of cobra venom, assault D, S ◎
    ● **T63.044**   Toxic effect of cobra venom, undetermined D, S ◎

● **T63.06**   Toxic effect of venom of other North and South American snake
    ● **T63.061**   Toxic effect of venom of other North and South American snake, accidental (unintentional) D, S ◎
        Toxic effect of venom of other North and South American snake NOS
    ● **T63.062**   Toxic effect of venom of other North and South American snake, intentional self-harm D, S ◎
    ● **T63.063**   Toxic effect of venom of other North and South American snake, assault D, S ◎
    ● **T63.064**   Toxic effect of venom of other North and South American snake, undetermined D, S ◎

● **T63.07**   Toxic effect of venom of other Australian snake
    ● **T63.071**   Toxic effect of venom of other Australian snake, accidental (unintentional) D, S ◎
        Toxic effect of venom of other Australian snake NOS
    ● **T63.072**   Toxic effect of venom of other Australian snake, intentional self-harm D, S ◎
    ● **T63.073**   Toxic effect of venom of other Australian snake, assault D, S ◎
    ● **T63.074**   Toxic effect of venom of other Australian snake, undetermined D, S ◎

● **T63.08**   Toxic effect of venom of other African and Asian snake
    ● **T63.081**   Toxic effect of venom of other African and Asian snake, accidental (unintentional) D, S ◎
        Toxic effect of venom of other African and Asian snake NOS
    ● **T63.082**   Toxic effect of venom of other African and Asian snake, intentional self-harm D, S ◎
    ● **T63.083**   Toxic effect of venom of other African and Asian snake, assault D, S ◎
    ● **T63.084**   Toxic effect of venom of other African and Asian snake, undetermined D, S ◎

● **T63.09**   Toxic effect of venom of other snake
    ● **T63.091**   Toxic effect of venom of other snake, accidental (unintentional) D, S ◎
        Toxic effect of venom of other snake NOS
    ● **T63.092**   Toxic effect of venom of other snake, intentional self-harm D, S ◎
    ● **T63.093**   Toxic effect of venom of other snake, assault D, S ◎
    ● **T63.094**   Toxic effect of venom of other snake, undetermined D, S ◎

● **T63.1**   Toxic effect of venom of other reptiles
    ● **T63.11**   Toxic effect of venom of gila monster
        ● **T63.111**   Toxic effect of venom of gila monster, accidental (unintentional) D, S ◎
            Toxic effect of venom of gila monster NOS
        ● **T63.112**   Toxic effect of venom of gila monster, intentional self-harm D, S ◎
        ● **T63.113**   Toxic effect of venom of gila monster, assault D, S ◎
        ● **T63.114**   Toxic effect of venom of gila monster, undetermined D, S ◎

N Newborn Age: 0   **P** Pediatric Age: 0–17   **M** Maternity DX: 12–55   **A** Adult Age: 15–124   ♀ Females Only   ♂ Males Only

◎ Complication\Comorbidity   ◎ Major C\C   ◎ Present on Admission Requirement   ◎ Hospital-Acquired Condition

CHAPTER 19 (S00-T88)

1659

● **T63.12**   **Toxic effect of venom of other venomous lizard**
- ● **T63.121**   Toxic effect of venom of other venomous lizard, accidental (unintentional) D, S
  - Toxic effect of venom of other venomous lizard NOS
- ● **T63.122**   Toxic effect of venom of other venomous lizard, intentional self-harm D, S
- ● **T63.123**   Toxic effect of venom of other venomous lizard, assault D, S
- ● **T63.124**   Toxic effect of venom of other venomous lizard, undetermined D, S

● **T63.19**   **Toxic effect of venom of other reptiles**
- ● **T63.191**   Toxic effect of venom of other reptiles, accidental (unintentional) D, S
  - Toxic effect of venom of other reptiles NOS
- ● **T63.192**   Toxic effect of venom of other reptiles, intentional self-harm D, S
- ● **T63.193**   Toxic effect of venom of other reptiles, assault D, S
- ● **T63.194**   Toxic effect of venom of other reptiles, undetermined D, S

● **T63.2**   **Toxic effect of venom of scorpion**
- ● **T63.2X**   **Toxic effect of venom of scorpion**
  - ● **T63.2X1**   Toxic effect of venom of scorpion, accidental (unintentional) D, S
    - Toxic effect of venom of scorpion NOS
  - ● **T63.2X2**   Toxic effect of venom of scorpion, intentional self-harm D, S
  - ● **T63.2X3**   Toxic effect of venom of scorpion, assault D, S
  - ● **T63.2X4**   Toxic effect of venom of scorpion, undetermined D, S

● **T63.3**   **Toxic effect of venom of spider**
- ● **T63.30**   **Toxic effect of unspecified spider venom**
  - ●■ **T63.301**   Toxic effect of unspecified spider venom, accidental (unintentional) D, S
  - ●■ **T63.302**   Toxic effect of unspecified spider venom, intentional self-harm D, S
  - ●■ **T63.303**   Toxic effect of unspecified spider venom, assault D, S
  - ●■ **T63.304**   Toxic effect of unspecified spider venom, undetermined D, S
- ● **T63.31**   **Toxic effect of venom of black widow spider**
  - ● **T63.311**   Toxic effect of venom of black widow spider, accidental (unintentional) D, S
  - ● **T63.312**   Toxic effect of venom of black widow spider, intentional self-harm D, S
  - ● **T63.313**   Toxic effect of venom of black widow spider, assault D, S
  - ● **T63.314**   Toxic effect of venom of black widow spider, undetermined D, S

● **T63.32**   **Toxic effect of venom of tarantula**
- ● **T63.321**   Toxic effect of venom of tarantula, accidental (unintentional) D, S
- ● **T63.322**   Toxic effect of venom of tarantula, intentional self-harm D, S
- ● **T63.323**   Toxic effect of venom of tarantula, assault D, S
- ● **T63.324**   Toxic effect of venom of tarantula, undetermined D, S

● **T63.33**   **Toxic effect of venom of brown recluse spider**
- ● **T63.331**   Toxic effect of venom of brown recluse spider, accidental (unintentional) D, S
- ● **T63.332**   Toxic effect of venom of brown recluse spider, intentional self-harm D, S
- ● **T63.333**   Toxic effect of venom of brown recluse spider, assault D, S
- ● **T63.334**   Toxic effect of venom of brown recluse spider, undetermined D, S

● **T63.39**   **Toxic effect of venom of other spider**
- ● **T63.391**   Toxic effect of venom of other spider, accidental (unintentional) D, S
- ● **T63.392**   Toxic effect of venom of other spider, intentional self-harm D, S
- ● **T63.393**   Toxic effect of venom of other spider, assault D, S
- ● **T63.394**   Toxic effect of venom of other spider, undetermined D, S

● **T63.4**   **Toxic effect of venom of other arthropods**
- ● **T63.41**   **Toxic effect of venom of centipedes and venomous millipedes**
  - ● **T63.411**   Toxic effect of venom of centipedes and venomous millipedes, accidental (unintentional) D, S
  - ● **T63.412**   Toxic effect of venom of centipedes and venomous millipedes, intentional self-harm D, S
  - ● **T63.413**   Toxic effect of venom of centipedes and venomous millipedes, assault D, S
  - ● **T63.414**   Toxic effect of venom of centipedes and venomous millipedes, undetermined D, S
- ● **T63.42**   **Toxic effect of venom of ants**
  - ● **T63.421**   Toxic effect of venom of ants, accidental (unintentional) D, S
  - ● **T63.422**   Toxic effect of venom of ants, intentional self-harm D, S
  - ● **T63.423**   Toxic effect of venom of ants, assault D, S
  - ● **T63.424**   Toxic effect of venom of ants, undetermined D, S

● Unacceptable Principal Diagnosis   ● Use Additional Character(s)   ■ Unspecified   ▶ Manifestation Code

OGCR Official Guidelines for Coding and Reporting   Excludes 1   Excludes 2   Includes   Use additional   Code first   Code also

● **T63.43 Toxic effect of venom of caterpillars**
- ● **T63.431** Toxic effect of venom of caterpillars, accidental (unintentional) D, S 🔍
- ● **T63.432** Toxic effect of venom of caterpillars, intentional self-harm D, S 🔍
- ● **T63.433** Toxic effect of venom of caterpillars, assault D, S 🔍
- ● **T63.434** Toxic effect of venom of caterpillars, undetermined D, S 🔍

● **T63.44 Toxic effect of venom of bees**
- ● **T63.441** Toxic effect of venom of bees, accidental (unintentional) D, S 🔍
- ● **T63.442** Toxic effect of venom of bees, intentional self-harm D, S 🔍
- ● **T63.443** Toxic effect of venom of bees, assault D, S 🔍
- ● **T63.444** Toxic effect of venom of bees, undetermined D, S 🔍

● **T63.45 Toxic effect of venom of hornets**
- ● **T63.451** Toxic effect of venom of hornets, accidental (unintentional) D, S 🔍
- ● **T63.452** Toxic effect of venom of hornets, intentional self-harm D, S 🔍
- ● **T63.453** Toxic effect of venom of hornets, assault D, S 🔍
- ● **T63.454** Toxic effect of venom of hornets, undetermined D, S 🔍

● **T63.46 Toxic effect of venom of wasps**
Toxic effect of yellow jacket
- ● **T63.461** Toxic effect of venom of wasps, accidental (unintentional) D, S 🔍
- ● **T63.462** Toxic effect of venom of wasps, intentional self-harm D, S 🔍
- ● **T63.463** Toxic effect of venom of wasps, assault D, S 🔍
- ● **T63.464** Toxic effect of venom of wasps, undetermined D, S 🔍

● **T63.48 Toxic effect of venom of other arthropod**
- ● **T63.481** Toxic effect of venom of other arthropod, accidental (unintentional) D, S 🔍
- ● **T63.482** Toxic effect of venom of other arthropod, intentional self-harm D, S 🔍
- ● **T63.483** Toxic effect of venom of other arthropod, assault D, S 🔍
- ● **T63.484** Toxic effect of venom of other arthropod, undetermined D, S 🔍

● **T63.5 Toxic effect of contact with venomous fish**
> **Excludes2**   poisoning by ingestion of fish (T61-)
● **T63.51 Toxic effect of contact with stingray**
- ● **T63.511** Toxic effect of contact with stingray, accidental (unintentional) D, S 🔍
- ● **T63.512** Toxic effect of contact with stingray, intentional self-harm D, S 🔍
- ● **T63.513** Toxic effect of contact with stingray, assault D, S 🔍
- ● **T63.514** Toxic effect of contact with stingray, undetermined D, S 🔍

● **T63.59 Toxic effect of contact with other venomous fish**
- ● **T63.591** Toxic effect of contact with other venomous fish, accidental (unintentional) D, S 🔍
- ● **T63.592** Toxic effect of contact with other venomous fish, intentional self-harm D, S 🔍
- ● **T63.593** Toxic effect of contact with other venomous fish, assault D, S 🔍
- ● **T63.594** Toxic effect of contact with other venomous fish, undetermined D, S 🔍

● **T63.6 Toxic effect of contact with other venomous marine animals**
> **Excludes1**   sea-snake venom (T63.09)
> **Excludes2**   poisoning by ingestion of shellfish (T61.78-)
● **T63.61 Toxic effect of contact with Portugese Man-o-war**
Toxic effect of contact with bluebottle
- ● **T63.611** Toxic effect of contact with Portugese Man-o-war, accidental (unintentional) D, S 🔍
- ● **T63.612** Toxic effect of contact with Portugese Man-o-war, intentional self-harm D, S 🔍
- ● **T63.613** Toxic effect of contact with Portugese Man-o-war, assault D, S 🔍
- ● **T63.614** Toxic effect of contact with Portugese Man-o-war, undetermined D, S 🔍

● **T63.62 Toxic effect of contact with other jellyfish**
- ● **T63.621** Toxic effect of contact with other jellyfish, accidental (unintentional) D, S 🔍
- ● **T63.622** Toxic effect of contact with other jellyfish, intentional self-harm D, S 🔍
- ● **T63.623** Toxic effect of contact with other jellyfish, assault D, S 🔍
- ● **T63.624** Toxic effect of contact with other jellyfish, undetermined D, S 🔍

● **T63.63 Toxic effect of contact with sea anemone**
- ● **T63.631** Toxic effect of contact with sea anemone, accidental (unintentional) D, S 🔍
- ● **T63.632** Toxic effect of contact with sea anemone, intentional self-harm D, S 🔍
- ● **T63.633** Toxic effect of contact with sea anemone, assault D, S 🔍
- ● **T63.634** Toxic effect of contact with sea anemone, undetermined D, S 🔍

CHAPTER 19 (S00-T88)

N Newborn Age: 0   **P** Pediatric Age: 0–17   **M** Maternity DX: 12–55   **A** Adult Age: 15–124   ♀ Females Only   ♂ Males Only

🔍 Complication\Comorbidity   🔍 Major C\C   🔍 Present on Admission Requirement   🔍 Hospital-Acquired Condition

1661

● **T63.69** Toxic effect of contact with other venomous marine animals

   ● **T63.691** Toxic effect of contact with other venomous marine animals, accidental (unintentional) D, S ⊚

   ● **T63.692** Toxic effect of contact with other venomous marine animals, intentional self-harm D, S ⊚

   ● **T63.693** Toxic effect of contact with other venomous marine animals, assault D, S ⊚

   ● **T63.694** Toxic effect of contact with other venomous marine animals, undetermined D, S ⊚

● **T63.7** Toxic effect of contact with venomous plant

  ● **T63.71** Toxic effect of contact with venomous marine plant

   ● **T63.711** Toxic effect of contact with venomous marine plant, accidental (unintentional) D, S ⊚

   ● **T63.712** Toxic effect of contact with venomous marine plant, intentional self-harm D, S ⊚

   ● **T63.713** Toxic effect of contact with venomous marine plant, assault D, S ⊚

   ● **T63.714** Toxic effect of contact with venomous marine plant, undetermined D, S ⊚

  ● **T63.79** Toxic effect of contact with other venomous plant

   ● **T63.791** Toxic effect of contact with other venomous plant, accidental (unintentional) D, S ⊚

   ● **T63.792** Toxic effect of contact with other venomous plant, intentional self-harm D, S ⊚

   ● **T63.793** Toxic effect of contact with other venomous plant, assault D, S ⊚

   ● **T63.794** Toxic effect of contact with other venomous plant, undetermined D, S ⊚

● **T63.8** Toxic effect of contact with other venomous animals

  ● **T63.81** Toxic effect of contact with venomous frog

    | Excludes1 | contact with nonvenomous frog (W62.0) |

   ● **T63.811** Toxic effect of contact with venomous frog, accidental (unintentional) D, S ⊚

   ● **T63.812** Toxic effect of contact with venomous frog, intentional self-harm D, S ⊚

   ● **T63.813** Toxic effect of contact with venomous frog, assault D, S ⊚

   ● **T63.814** Toxic effect of contact with venomous frog, undetermined D, S ⊚

  ● **T63.82** Toxic effect of contact with venomous toad

    | Excludes1 | contact with nonvenomous toad (W62.1) |

   ● **T63.821** Toxic effect of contact with venomous toad, accidental (unintentional) D, S ⊚

   ● **T63.822** Toxic effect of contact with venomous toad, intentional self-harm D, S ⊚

   ● **T63.823** Toxic effect of contact with venomous toad, assault D, S ⊚

   ● **T63.824** Toxic effect of contact with venomous toad, undetermined D, S ⊚

  ● **T63.83** Toxic effect of contact with other venomous amphibian

    | Excludes1 | contact with nonvenomous amphibian (W62.9) |

   ● **T63.831** Toxic effect of contact with other venomous amphibian, accidental (unintentional) D, S ⊚

   ● **T63.832** Toxic effect of contact with other venomous amphibian, intentional self-harm D, S ⊚

   ● **T63.833** Toxic effect of contact with other venomous amphibian, assault D, S ⊚

   ● **T63.834** Toxic effect of contact with other venomous amphibian, undetermined D, S ⊚

  ● **T63.89** Toxic effect of contact with other venomous animals

   ● **T63.891** Toxic effect of contact with other venomous animals, accidental (unintentional) D, S ⊚

   ● **T63.892** Toxic effect of contact with other venomous animals, intentional self-harm D, S ⊚

   ● **T63.893** Toxic effect of contact with other venomous animals, assault D, S ⊚

   ● **T63.894** Toxic effect of contact with other venomous animals, undetermined D, S ⊚

● **T63.9** Toxic effect of contact with unspecified venomous animal

  ●■ **T63.91** Toxic effect of contact with unspecified venomous animal, accidental (unintentional) D, S ⊚

  ●■ **T63.92** Toxic effect of contact with unspecified venomous animal, intentional self-harm D, S ⊚

  ●■ **T63.93** Toxic effect of contact with unspecified venomous animal, assault D, S ⊚

  ●■ **T63.94** Toxic effect of contact with unspecified venomous animal, undetermined D, S ⊚

● **T64** Toxic effect of aflatoxin and other mycotoxin food contaminants

The appropriate 7th character is to be added to each code from category T64

A	initial encounter
D	subsequent encounter
S	sequela

● **T64.0** Toxic effect of aflatoxin

  ● **T64.01** Toxic effect of aflatoxin, accidental (unintentional) D, S ⊚

  ● **T64.02** Toxic effect of aflatoxin, intentional self-harm D, S ⊚

  ● **T64.03** Toxic effect of aflatoxin, assault D, S ⊚

  ● **T64.04** Toxic effect of aflatoxin, undetermined D, S ⊚

● Unacceptable Principal Diagnosis   ● Use Additional Character(s)   ■ Unspecified   ▸ Manifestation Code

OGCR Official Guidelines for Coding and Reporting | Excludes 1 | | Excludes 2 | Includes   Use additional   Code first   Code also

● **T64.8**   **Toxic effect of other mycotoxin food contaminants**

    ● **T64.81**   **Toxic effect of other mycotoxin food contaminants, accidental (unintentional)** D, S 🗎

    ● **T64.82**   **Toxic effect of other mycotoxin food contaminants, intentional self-harm** D, S 🗎

    ● **T64.83**   **Toxic effect of other mycotoxin food contaminants, assault** D, S 🗎

    ● **T64.84**   **Toxic effect of other mycotoxin food contaminants, undetermined** D, S 🗎

● **T65**   **Toxic effect of other and unspecified substances**

    The appropriate 7th character is to be added to each code from category T65

       | | |
       A   initial encounter
       D   subsequent encounter
       S   sequela

    ● **T65.0**   **Toxic effect of cyanides**

       Excludes1   hydrogen cyanide (T57.3-)

     ● **T65.0X**   **Toxic effect of cyanides**

       ● **T65.0X1**   **Toxic effect of cyanides, accidental (unintentional)** D, S 🗎
          Toxic effect of cyanides NOS

       ● **T65.0X2**   **Toxic effect of cyanides, intentional self-harm** D, S 🗎

       ● **T65.0X3**   **Toxic effect of cyanides, assault** D, S 🗎

       ● **T65.0X4**   **Toxic effect of cyanides, undetermined** D, S 🗎

    ● **T65.1**   **Toxic effect of strychnine and its salts**

     ● **T65.1X**   **Toxic effect of strychnine and its salts**

       ● **T65.1X1**   **Toxic effect of strychnine and its salts, accidental (unintentional)** D, S 🗎
          Toxic effect of strychnine and its salts NOS

       ● **T65.1X2**   **Toxic effect of strychnine and its salts, intentional self-harm** D, S 🗎

       ● **T65.1X3**   **Toxic effect of strychnine and its salts, assault** D, S 🗎

       ● **T65.1X4**   **Toxic effect of strychnine and its salts, undetermined** D, S 🗎

    ● **T65.2**   **Toxic effect of tobacco and nicotine**

       Excludes2   nicotine dependence (F17.-)

     ● **T65.21**   **Toxic effect of chewing tobacco**

       ● **T65.211**   **Toxic effect of chewing tobacco, accidental (unintentional)** D, S 🗎
          Toxic effect of chewing tobacco NOS

       ● **T65.212**   **Toxic effect of chewing tobacco, intentional self-harm** D, S 🗎

       ● **T65.213**   **Toxic effect of chewing tobacco, assault** D, S 🗎

       ● **T65.214**   **Toxic effect of chewing tobacco, undetermined** D, S 🗎

     ● **T65.22**   **Toxic effect of tobacco cigarettes**
       Toxic effect of tobacco smoke

       Use additional code for exposure to second hand tobacco smoke (Z57.31, Z77.22)

       ● **T65.221**   **Toxic effect of tobacco cigarettes, accidental (unintentional)** D, S 🗎
          Toxic effect of tobacco cigarettes NOS

       ● **T65.222**   **Toxic effect of tobacco cigarettes, intentional self-harm** D, S 🗎

       ● **T65.223**   **Toxic effect of tobacco cigarettes, assault** D, S 🗎

       ● **T65.224**   **Toxic effect of tobacco cigarettes, undetermined** D, S 🗎

     ● **T65.29**   **Toxic effect of other tobacco and nicotine**

       ● **T65.291**   **Toxic effect of other tobacco and nicotine, accidental (unintentional)** D, S 🗎
          Toxic effect of other tobacco and nicotine NOS

       ● **T65.292**   **Toxic effect of other tobacco and nicotine, intentional self-harm** D, S 🗎

       ● **T65.293**   **Toxic effect of other tobacco and nicotine, assault** D, S 🗎

       ● **T65.294**   **Toxic effect of other tobacco and nicotine, undetermined** D, S 🗎

    ● **T65.3**   **Toxic effect of nitroderivatives and aminoderivatives of benzene and its homologues**
       Toxic effect of anilin [benzenamine]
       Toxic effect of nitrobenzene
       Toxic effect of trinitrotoluene

     ● **T65.3X**   **Toxic effect of nitroderivatives and aminoderivatives of benzene and its homologues**

       ● **T65.3X1**   **Toxic effect of nitroderivatives and aminoderivatives of benzene and its homologues, accidental (unintentional)** D, S 🗎
          Toxic effect of nitroderivatives and aminoderivatives of benzene and its homologues NOS

       ● **T65.3X2**   **Toxic effect of nitroderivatives and aminoderivatives of benzene and its homologues, intentional self-harm** D, S 🗎

       ● **T65.3X3**   **Toxic effect of nitroderivatives and aminoderivatives of benzene and its homologues, assault** D, S 🗎

       ● **T65.3X4**   **Toxic effect of nitroderivatives and aminoderivatives of benzene and its homologues, undetermined** D, S 🗎

● **T65.4**   **Toxic effect of carbon disulfide**
  ● **T65.4X**   **Toxic effect of carbon disulfide**
   ● **T65.4X1**   **Toxic effect of carbon disulfide, accidental (unintentional)** D, S 🔖
     Toxic effect of carbon disulfide NOS
   ● **T65.4X2**   **Toxic effect of carbon disulfide, intentional self-harm** D, S 🔖
   ● **T65.4X3**   **Toxic effect of carbon disulfide, assault** D, S 🔖
   ● **T65.4X4**   **Toxic effect of carbon disulfide, undetermined** D, S 🔖

● **T65.5**   **Toxic effect of nitroglycerin and other nitric acids and esters**
  Toxic effect of 1,2,3-Propanetriol trinitrate
  ● **T65.5X**   **Toxic effect of nitroglycerin and other nitric acids and esters**
   ● **T65.5X1**   **Toxic effect of nitroglycerin and other nitric acids and esters, accidental (unintentional)** D, S 🔖
     Toxic effect of nitroglycerin and other nitric acids and esters NOS
   ● **T65.5X2**   **Toxic effect of nitroglycerin and other nitric acids and esters, intentional self-harm** D, S 🔖
   ● **T65.5X3**   **Toxic effect of nitroglycerin and other nitric acids and esters, assault** D, S 🔖
   ● **T65.5X4**   **Toxic effect of nitroglycerin and other nitric acids and esters, undetermined** D, S 🔖

● **T65.6**   **Toxic effect of paints and dyes, not elsewhere classified**
  ● **T65.6X**   **Toxic effect of paints and dyes, not elsewhere classified**
   ● **T65.6X1**   **Toxic effect of paints and dyes, not elsewhere classified, accidental (unintentional)** D, S 🔖
     Toxic effect of paints and dyes NOS
   ● **T65.6X2**   **Toxic effect of paints and dyes, not elsewhere classified, intentional self-harm** D, S 🔖
   ● **T65.6X3**   **Toxic effect of paints and dyes, not elsewhere classified, assault** D, S 🔖
   ● **T65.6X4**   **Toxic effect of paints and dyes, not elsewhere classified, undetermined** D, S 🔖

● **T65.8**   **Toxic effect of other specified substances**
  ● **T65.81**   **Toxic effect of latex**
   ● **T65.811**   **Toxic effect of latex, accidental (unintentional)** D, S 🔖
     Toxic effect of latex NOS
   ● **T65.812**   **Toxic effect of latex, intentional self-harm** D, S 🔖
   ● **T65.813**   **Toxic effect of latex, assault** D, S 🔖
   ● **T65.814**   **Toxic effect of latex, undetermined** D, S 🔖

● **T65.82**   **Toxic effect of harmful algae and algae toxins**
  Toxic effect of (harmful) algae bloom NOS
  Toxic effect of blue-green algae bloom
  Toxic effect of brown tide
  Toxic effect of cyanobacteria bloom
  Toxic effect of Florida red tide
  Toxic effect of pfiesteria piscicida
  Toxic effect of red tide
  ● **T65.821**   **Toxic effect of harmful algae and algae toxins, accidental (unintentional)** D, S 🔖
     Toxic effect of harmful algae and algae toxins NOS
  ● **T65.822**   **Toxic effect of harmful algae and algae toxins, intentional self-harm** D, S 🔖
  ● **T65.823**   **Toxic effect of harmful algae and algae toxins, assault** D, S 🔖
  ● **T65.824**   **Toxic effect of harmful algae and algae toxins, undetermined** D, S 🔖

● **T65.83**   **Toxic effect of fiberglass**
  ● **T65.831**   **Toxic effect of fiberglass, accidental (unintentional)** D, S 🔖
     Toxic effect of fiberglass NOS
  ● **T65.832**   **Toxic effect of fiberglass, intentional self-harm** D, S 🔖
  ● **T65.833**   **Toxic effect of fiberglass, assault** D, S 🔖
  ● **T65.834**   **Toxic effect of fiberglass, undetermined** D, S 🔖

● **T65.89**   **Toxic effect of other specified substances**
  ● **T65.891**   **Toxic effect of other specified substances, accidental (unintentional)** D, S 🔖
     Toxic effect of other specified substances NOS
  ● **T65.892**   **Toxic effect of other specified substances, intentional self-harm** D, S 🔖
  ● **T65.893**   **Toxic effect of other specified substances, assault** D, S 🔖
  ● **T65.894**   **Toxic effect of other specified substances, undetermined** D, S 🔖

● **T65.9**   **Toxic effect of unspecified substance**
  ●▪ **T65.91**   **Toxic effect of unspecified substance, accidental (unintentional)** D, S 🔖
     Poisoning NOS
  ●▪ **T65.92**   **Toxic effect of unspecified substance, intentional self-harm** D, S 🔖
  ●▪ **T65.93**   **Toxic effect of unspecified substance, assault** D, S 🔖
  ●▪ **T65.94**   **Toxic effect of unspecified substance, undetermined** D, S 🔖

OTHER AND UNSPECIFIED EFFECTS OF EXTERNAL CAUSES (T66-T78)

● ■ **T66 Radiation sickness, unspecified** D, S 🔖

> **Excludes1**   specified adverse effects of radiation, such as:
> > burns (T20-T31)
> > leukemia (C91-C95)
> > radiation gastroenteritis and colitis (K52.0)
> > radiation pneumonitis (J70.0)
> > radiation related disorders of the skin and subcutaneous tissue (L55-L59)
> > sunburn (L55.-)

> The appropriate 7th character is to be added to code T66
> | | |
> |---|---|
> | A | initial encounter |
> | D | subsequent encounter |
> | S | sequela |

● **T67 Effects of heat and light**

> **Excludes1**   erythema [dermatitis] ab igne (L59.0)
> > malignant hyperpyrexia due to anesthesia (T88.3)
> > radiation-related disorders of the skin and subcutaneous tissue (L55-L59)

> **Excludes2**   burns (T20-T31)
> > sunburn (L55.-)
> > sweat disorder due to heat (L74-L75)

> The appropriate 7th character is to be added to each code from category T67
> | | |
> |---|---|
> | A | initial encounter |
> | D | subsequent encounter |
> | S | sequela |

● **T67.0 Heatstroke and sunstroke A** 🔖**, D, S** 🔖**, A** 🔖
> > Heat apoplexy
> > Heat pyrexia
> > Siriasis
> > Thermoplegia
> > Use additional code(s) to identify any associated complications of heatstroke, such as:
> > > coma and stupor (R40.-)
> > > systemic inflammatory response syndrome (R65.1-)

● **T67.1 Heat syncope** D, S 🔖
> > Heat collapse

● **T67.2 Heat cramp** D, S 🔖

● **T67.3 Heat exhaustion, anhydrotic** D, S 🔖
> > Heat prostration due to water depletion
> > **Excludes1**   heat exhaustion due to salt depletion (T67.4)

● **T67.4 Heat exhaustion due to salt depletion** D, S 🔖
> > Heat prostration due to salt (and water) depletion

● ■ **T67.5 Heat exhaustion, unspecified** D, S 🔖
> > Heat prostration NOS

● **T67.6 Heat fatigue, transient** D, S 🔖

● **T67.7 Heat edema** D, S 🔖

● **T67.8 Other effects of heat and light** D, S 🔖

● ■ **T67.9 Effect of heat and light, unspecified** D, S 🔖

● **T68 Hypothermia** D, S 🔖
> > Accidental hypothermia
> > Hypothermia NOS

> Use additional code to identify source of exposure:
> > Exposure to excessive cold of man-made origin (W93)
> > Exposure to excessive cold of natural origin (X31)

> **Excludes1**   hypothermia following anesthesia (T88.51)
> > hypothermia not associated with low environmental temperature (R68.0)
> > hypothermia of newborn (P80.-)

> **Excludes2**   frostbite (T33-T34)

> The appropriate 7th character is to be added to code T68
> | | |
> |---|---|
> | A | initial encounter |
> | D | subsequent encounter |
> | S | sequela |

● **T69 Other effects of reduced temperature**

> Use additional code to identify source of exposure:
> > Exposure to excessive cold of man-made origin (W93)
> > Exposure to excessive cold of natural origin (X31)

> **Excludes2**   frostbite (T33-T34)

> The appropriate 7th character is to be added to each code from category T69
> | | |
> |---|---|
> | A | initial encounter |
> | D | subsequent encounter |
> | S | sequela |

● **T69.0 Immersion hand and foot**

> ● **T69.01 Immersion hand**

> > ● **T69.011 Immersion hand, right hand** D, S 🔖

> > ● **T69.012 Immersion hand, left hand** D, S 🔖

> > ● ■ **T69.019 Immersion hand, unspecified hand** D, S 🔖

> ● **T69.02 Immersion foot**
> > Trench foot

> > ● **T69.021 Immersion foot, right foot A** 🔖**, D, S** 🔖**, A** 🔖

> > ● **T69.022 Immersion foot, left foot A** 🔖**, D, S** 🔖**, A** 🔖

> > ● ■ **T69.029 Immersion foot, unspecified foot A** 🔖**, D, S** 🔖**, A** 🔖

● **T69.1 Chilblains** D, S 🔖

● **T69.8 Other specified effects of reduced temperature** D, S 🔖

● ■ **T69.9 Effect of reduced temperature, unspecified** D, S 🔖

● **T70 Effects of air pressure and water pressure**

> The appropriate 7th character is to be added to each code from category T70
> | | |
> |---|---|
> | A | initial encounter |
> | D | subsequent encounter |
> | S | sequela |

● **T70.0 Otitic barotrauma** D, S 🔖
> > Aero-otitis media
> > Effects of change in ambient atmospheric pressure or water pressure on ears

● **T70.1 Sinus barotrauma** D, S 🔖
> > Aerosinusitis
> > Effects of change in ambient atmospheric pressure on sinuses

---

N Newborn Age: 0   P Pediatric Age: 0–17   M Maternity DX: 12–55   A Adult Age: 15–124   ♀ Females Only   ♂ Males Only

🔖 Complication\Comorbidity   🔖 Major C\C   🔖 Present on Admission Requirement   🔖 Hospital-Acquired Condition

● **T70.2** **Other and unspecified effects of high altitude**

> Excludes2   polycythemia due to high altitude (D75.1)

  ● ■ **T70.20**   Unspecified effects of high altitude D, S

  ● **T70.29**   Other effects of high altitude D, S
> Alpine sickness
> Anoxia due to high altitude
> Barotrauma NOS
> Hypobaropathy
> Mountain sickness

● **T70.3**   Caisson disease [decompression sickness] A, D, S, A
> Compressed-air disease
> Diver's palsy or paralysis

● **T70.4**   Effects of high-pressure fluids D, S
> Hydraulic jet injection (industrial)
> Pneumatic jet injection (industrial)
> Traumatic jet injection (industrial)

● **T70.8**   Other effects of air pressure and water pressure D, S

● ■ **T70.9**   Effect of air pressure and water pressure, unspecified D, S

● **T71**   **Asphyxiation**
> Mechanical suffocation
> Traumatic suffocation

> Excludes1   acute respiratory distress (syndrome) (J80)
> anoxia due to high altitude (T70.2)
> asphyxia NOS (R09.01)
> asphyxia from carbon monoxide (T58.-)
> asphyxia from inhalation of food or foreign body (T17.-)
> asphyxia from other gases, fumes and vapors (T59.-)
> respiratory distress (syndrome) in newborn (P22.-)

> The appropriate 7th character is to be added to each code from category T71

> | | |
> |---|---|
> | A | initial encounter |
> | D | subsequent encounter |
> | S | sequela |

● **T71.1**   **Asphyxiation due to mechanical threat to breathing**
> Suffocation due to mechanical threat to breathing

  ● **T71.11**   **Asphyxiation due to smothering under pillow**

    ● **T71.111**   **Asphyxiation due to smothering under pillow, accidental A, D, S, A**
> Asphyxiation due to smothering under pillow NOS

    ● **T71.112**   **Asphyxiation due to smothering under pillow, intentional self-harm A, D, S, A**

    ● **T71.113**   **Asphyxiation due to smothering under pillow, assault A, D, S, A**

    ● **T71.114**   **Asphyxiation due to smothering under pillow, undetermined A, D, S, A**

  ● **T71.12**   **Asphyxiation due to plastic bag**

    ● **T71.121**   **Asphyxiation due to plastic bag, accidental A, D, S, A**
> Asphyxiation due to plastic bag NOS

    ● **T71.122**   **Asphyxiation due to plastic bag, intentional self-harm A, D, S, A**

    ● **T71.123**   **Asphyxiation due to plastic bag, assault A, D, S, A**

    ● **T71.124**   **Asphyxiation due to plastic bag, undetermined A, D, S, A**

  ● **T71.13**   **Asphyxiation due to being trapped in bed linens**

    ● **T71.131**   **Asphyxiation due to being trapped in bed linens, accidental A, D, S, A**
> Asphyxiation due to being trapped in bed linens NOS

    ● **T71.132**   **Asphyxiation due to being trapped in bed linens, intentional self-harm A, D, S, A**

    ● **T71.133**   **Asphyxiation due to being trapped in bed linens, assault A, D, S, A**

    ● **T71.134**   **Asphyxiation due to being trapped in bed linens, undetermined A, D, S, A**

  ● **T71.14**   **Asphyxiation due to smothering under another person's body (in bed)**

    ● **T71.141**   **Asphyxiation due to smothering under another person's body (in bed), accidental A, D, S, A**
> Asphyxiation due to smothering under another person's body (in bed) NOS

    ● **T71.143**   **Asphyxiation due to smothering under another person's body (in bed), assault A, D, S, A**

    ● **T71.144**   **Asphyxiation due to smothering under another person's body (in bed), undetermined A, D, S, A**

  ● **T71.15**   **Asphyxiation due to smothering in furniture**

    ● **T71.151**   **Asphyxiation due to smothering in furniture, accidental A, D, S, A**
> Asphyxiation due to smothering in furniture NOS

    ● **T71.152**   **Asphyxiation due to smothering in furniture, intentional self-harm A, D, S, A**

    ● **T71.153**   **Asphyxiation due to smothering in furniture, assault A, D, S, A**

    ● **T71.154**   **Asphyxiation due to smothering in furniture, undetermined A, D, S, A**

● Unacceptable Principal Diagnosis   ● Use Additional Character(s)   ■ Unspecified   ▶ Manifestation Code

OGCR Official Guidelines for Coding and Reporting   Excludes 1   Excludes 2   Includes   Use additional   Code first   Code also

●**T71.16 Asphyxiation due to hanging**
Hanging by window shade cord

Use additional code for any associated
injuries, such as:
crushing injury of neck (S17.-)
fracture of cervical vertebrae
(S12.0-S12.2-)
open wound of neck (S11.-)

●**T71.161 Asphyxiation due to hanging,
accidental A** 🔴, D, S 🔵, A 🔵
Asphyxiation due to hanging
NOS
Hanging NOS

●**T71.162 Asphyxiation due to hanging,
intentional self-harm A** 🔴,
D, S 🔵, A 🔵

●**T71.163 Asphyxiation due to hanging,
assault A** 🔴, D, S 🔵, A 🔵

●**T71.164 Asphyxiation due to hanging,
undetermined A** 🔴, D, S 🔵, A 🔵

●**T71.19 Asphyxiation due to mechanical**
Threat to breathing due to other causes

●**T71.191 Asphyxiation due to mechanical
threat to breathing due to other
causes, accidental A** 🔴, D, S 🔵,
A 🔵
Asphyxiation due to other
causes NOS

●**T71.192 Asphyxiation due to mechanical
threat to breathing due to other
causes, intentional self-harm
A** 🔴, D, S 🔵, A 🔵

●**T71.193 Asphyxiation due to mechanical
threat to breathing due to other
causes, assault A** 🔴, D, S 🔵, A 🔵

●**T71.194 Asphyxiation due to mechanical
threat to breathing due to other
causes, undetermined A** 🔴,
D, S 🔵, A 🔵

●**T71.2 Asphyxiation due to systemic oxygen deficiency
due to low oxygen content in ambient air**
Suffocation due to systemic oxygen deficiency due
to low oxygen content in ambient air

●■**T71.20 Asphyxiation due to systemic oxygen
deficiency due to low oxygen content in
ambient air due to unspecified cause A** 🔴,
D, S 🔵

●**T71.21 Asphyxiation due to cave-in or falling
earth A** 🔴, D, S 🔵

Use additional code for any associated
cataclysm (X34-X38)

●**T71.22 Asphyxiation due to being trapped in a car
trunk**

●**T71.221 Asphyxiation due to being trapped
in a car trunk, accidental A** 🔴,
D, S 🔵

●**T71.222 Asphyxiation due to being
trapped in a car trunk, intentional
self-harm A** 🔴, D, S 🔵

●**T71.223 Asphyxiation due to being
trapped in a car trunk, assault
A** 🔴, D, S 🔵

●**T71.224 Asphyxiation due to being
trapped in a car trunk,
undetermined A** 🔴, D, S 🔵

●**T71.23 Asphyxiation due to being trapped in a
(discarded) refrigerator**

●**T71.231 Asphyxiation due to being
trapped in a (discarded)
refrigerator, accidental A** 🔴,
D, S 🔵

●**T71.232 Asphyxiation due to being trapped
in a (discarded) refrigerator,
intentional self-harm A** 🔴, D, S 🔵

●**T71.233 Asphyxiation due to being
trapped in a (discarded)
refrigerator, assault A** 🔴, D, S 🔵

●**T71.234 Asphyxiation due to being
trapped in a (discarded)
refrigerator, undetermined A** 🔴,
D, S 🔵

●**T71.29 Asphyxiation due to being trapped in
other low oxygen environment A** 🔴,
D, S 🔵

●■**T71.9 Asphyxiation due to unspecified cause A** 🔴,
D, S 🔵, A 🔵
Suffocation (by strangulation) due to unspecified
cause
Suffocation NOS
Systemic oxygen deficiency due to low oxygen
content in ambient air due to unspecified
cause
Systemic oxygen deficiency due to mechanical
threat to breathing due to unspecified cause
Traumatic asphyxia NOS

●**T73 Effects of other deprivation**
The appropriate 7th character is to be added to each code
from category T73

A   initial encounter
D   subsequent encounter
S   sequela

●**T73.0 Starvation** D, S 🔵
Deprivation of food

●**T73.1 Deprivation of water** D, S 🔵

●**T73.2 Exhaustion due to exposure** D, S 🔵

●**T73.3 Exhaustion due to excessive exertion** D, S 🔵
Exhaustion due to overexertion

●**T73.8 Other effects of deprivation** D, S 🔵

●■**T73.9 Effect of deprivation, unspecified** D, S 🔵

●**T74 Adult and child abuse, neglect and other maltreatment,
confirmed**
Use additional code, if applicable, to identify any
associated current injury
external cause code to identify perpetrator, if known
(Y07.-)

Excludes1   abuse and maltreatment in pregnancy
(O9A.3-, O9A.4-, O9A.5-)
adult and child maltreatment, suspected
(T76.-)

The appropriate 7th character is to be added to each code
from category T74

A   initial encounter
D   subsequent encounter
S   sequela

●**T74.0 Neglect or abandonment, confirmed**

●**T74.01 Adult neglect or abandonment, confirmed
A** 🔴, D, S 🔵

●**T74.02 Child neglect or abandonment, confirmed
A** 🔴, D, S 🔵

N Newborn Age: 0   **P** Pediatric Age: 0–17   **M** Maternity DX: 12–55   **A** Adult Age: 15–124   ♀ Females Only   ♂ Males Only

🔴 Complication\Comorbidity   🔵 Major C\C   🔵 Present on Admission Requirement   🔵 Hospital-Acquired Condition

1667

● T74.1   **Physical abuse, confirmed**
> Excludes2   sexual abuse (T74.2-)

　● T74.11   **Adult physical abuse, confirmed A** 🔎**,**
　　　　　　　D, S 🔎

　● T74.12   **Child physical abuse, confirmed A** 🔎**,**
　　　　　　　D, S 🔎

> Excludes2   shaken infant syndrome
> (T74.4)

● T74.2   **Sexual abuse, confirmed**
　　　Rape, confirmed
　　　Sexual assault, confirmed

　● T74.21   **Adult sexual abuse, confirmed A** 🔎**, D, S** 🔎

　● T74.22   **Child sexual abuse, confirmed A** 🔎**, D, S** 🔎

● T74.3   **Psychological abuse, confirmed**

　● T74.31   **Adult psychological abuse, confirmed**
　　　　　　　D, S 🔎

　● T74.32   **Child psychological abuse, confirmed A** 🔎**,**
　　　　　　　D, S 🔎

● T74.4   **Shaken infant syndrome A** 🔎**, D, S** 🔎

● T74.9   **Unspecified maltreatment, confirmed**

　●■ T74.91   **Unspecified adult maltreatment, confirmed**
　　　　　　　A 🔎**, D, S** 🔎

　●■ T74.92   **Unspecified child maltreatment, confirmed**
　　　　　　　A 🔎**, D, S** 🔎

● T75   **Other and unspecified effects of other external causes**
> Excludes1   adverse effects NEC (T78.-)
> Excludes2   burns (electric) (T20-T31)

　The appropriate 7th character is to be added to each code
　from category T75

> | | |
> |---|---|
> | A | initial encounter |
> | D | subsequent encounter |
> | S | sequela |

● T75.0   **Effects of lightning**
　　　Struck by lightning

　●■ T75.00   **Unspecified effects of lightning D, S** 🔎
　　　　　　　Struck by lightning NOS

　● T75.01   **Shock due to being struck by lightning**
　　　　　　　D, S 🔎

　● T75.09   **Other effects of lightning D, S** 🔎

> Use additional code for other effects of
> lightning

●■ T75.1   **Unspecified effects of drowning and nonfatal**
　　　　submersion A 🔎**, D, S** 🔎**, A** 🔎
　　　Immersion

> Excludes1   specified effects of drowning code to
> effects

● T75.2   **Effects of vibration**

　●■ T75.20   **Unspecified effects of vibration D, S** 🔎

　● T75.21   **Pneumatic hammer syndrome D, S** 🔎

　● T75.22   **Traumatic vasospastic syndrome D, S** 🔎

　● T75.23   **Vertigo from infrasound D, S** 🔎
> Excludes1   vertigo NOS (R42)

　● T75.29   **Other effects of vibration D, S** 🔎

● T75.3   **Motion sickness D, S** 🔎
　　　Airsickness   Travel sickness
　　　Seasickness

> Use additional external cause code to identify
> vehicle or type of motion (Y92.81-, Y93.5-)

● T75.4   **Electrocution D, S** 🔎
　　　Shock from electric current
　　　Shock from electroshock gun (taser)

● T75.8   **Other specified effects of external causes**

　● T75.81   **Effects of abnormal gravitation [G] forces**
　　　　　　　D, S 🔎

　● T75.82   **Effects of weightlessness D, S** 🔎

　● T75.89   **Other specified effects of external causes**
　　　　　　　D, S 🔎

● T76   **Adult and child abuse, neglect and other maltreatment,**
　　　suspected

> Use additional code, if applicable, to identify any
> associated current injury

> Excludes1   adult and child maltreatment, confirmed
> (T74.-)
> suspected abuse and maltreatment in
> pregnancy (O9A.3-, O9A.4-, O9A.5-)
> suspected adult physical and sexual abuse,
> ruled out (Z04.71)
> suspected child physical and sexual abuse,
> ruled out (Z04.72)

　The appropriate 7th character is to be added to each code
　from category T76

> | | |
> |---|---|
> | A | initial encounter |
> | D | subsequent encounter |
> | S | sequela |

● T76.0   **Neglect or abandonment, suspected**

　● T76.01   **Adult neglect or abandonment, suspected**
　　　　　　　A 🔎**, D, S** 🔎

　● T76.02   **Child neglect or abandonment, suspected**
　　　　　　　A 🔎**, D, S** 🔎

● T76.1   **Physical abuse, suspected**

　● T76.11   **Adult physical abuse, suspected A** 🔎**,**
　　　　　　　D, S 🔎

　● T76.12   **Child physical abuse, suspected A** 🔎**,**
　　　　　　　D, S 🔎

● T76.2   **Sexual abuse, suspected**
　　　Rape, suspected
　　　Sexual abuse, suspected
> Excludes1   alleged abuse, ruled out (Z04.7)

　● T76.21   **Adult sexual abuse, suspected A** 🔎**, D, S** 🔎

　● T76.22   **Child sexual abuse, suspected A** 🔎**, D, S** 🔎

● T76.3   **Psychological abuse, suspected**

　● T76.31   **Adult psychological abuse, suspected**
　　　　　　　D, S 🔎

　● T76.32   **Child psychological abuse, suspected A** 🔎**,**
　　　　　　　D, S 🔎

● T76.9   **Unspecified maltreatment, suspected**

　●■ T76.91   **Unspecified adult maltreatment, suspected**
　　　　　　　A 🔎**, D, S** 🔎

　●■ T76.92   **Unspecified child maltreatment, suspected**
　　　　　　　A 🔎**, D, S** 🔎

● Unacceptable Principal Diagnosis　　● Use Additional Character(s)　　■ Unspecified　　▶ Manifestation Code

OGCR   Official Guidelines for Coding and Reporting　　Excludes 1　Excludes 2　Includes　Use additional　Code first　Code also

● **T78   Adverse effects, not elsewhere classified**

     Excludes2   complications of surgical and medical care NEC (T80-T88)

     The appropriate 7th character is to be added to each code from category T78

     | | |
     A   initial encounter
     D   subsequent encounter
     S   sequela

● **T78.0   Anaphylactic reaction due to food**
     Anaphylactic reaction due to adverse food reaction
     Anaphylactic shock or reaction due to nonpoisonous foods
     Anaphylactoid reaction due to food

     ●■ **T78.00   Anaphylactic reaction due to unspecified food** A , D, S

     ● **T78.01   Anaphylactic reaction due to peanuts** A , D, S

     ● **T78.02   Anaphylactic reaction due to shellfish (crustaceans)** A , D, S

     ● **T78.03   Anaphylactic reaction due to other fish** A , D, S

     ● **T78.04   Anaphylactic reaction due to fruits and vegetables** A , D, S

     ● **T78.05   Anaphylactic reaction due to tree nuts and seeds** A , D, S
         Excludes1   anaphylactic reaction due to peanuts (T78.01)

     ● **T78.06   Anaphylactic reaction due to food additives** A , D, S

     ● **T78.07   Anaphylactic reaction due to milk and dairy products** A , D, S

     ● **T78.08   Anaphylactic reaction due to eggs** A , D, S

     ● **T78.09   Anaphylactic reaction due to other food products** A , D, S

● **T78.1   Other adverse food reactions, not elsewhere classified** D, S

     Use additional code to identify the type of reaction

     Excludes1   anaphylactic reaction or shock due to adverse food reaction (T78.0-)
         anaphylactic reaction due to food (T78.0-)
         bacterial food borne intoxications (A05.-)

     Excludes2   allergic and dietetic gastroenteritis and colitis (K52.2)
         allergic rhinitis due to food (J30.5)
         dermatitis due to food in contact with skin (L23.6, L24.6, L25.4)
         dermatitis due to ingested food (L27.2)

●■ **T78.2   Anaphylactic shock, unspecified** A , D, S
     Occurs when allergic response triggers large quantities of histamines, prostaglandins, leukotrienes resulting in systemic vasodilation
     Allergic shock
     Anaphylactic reaction
     Anaphylaxis

     Excludes1   anaphylactic reaction or shock due to adverse effect of correct medicinal substance properly administered (T88.6)
         anaphylactic reaction or shock due to adverse food reaction (T78.0-)
         anaphylactic reaction or shock due to serum (T80.5-)

● **T78.3   Angioneurotic edema** D, S
     Allergic angioedema
     Giant urticaria
     Vascular disorder resulting from abnormalities of autonomic nervous system fibers supplying blood vessels
     Quincke's edema

     Excludes1   serum urticaria (T80.6-)
         urticaria (L50.-)

● **T78.4   Other and unspecified allergy** D, S

     Excludes1   specified types of allergic reaction such as:
         allergic diarrhea (K52.2)
         allergic gastroenteritis and colitis (K52.2)
         dermatitis (L23-L25, L27.-)
         hay fever (J30.1)

     ● **T78.40   Allergy, unspecified** D, S
         Allergic reaction NOS
         Hypersensitivity NOS

     ● **T78.41   Arthus phenomenon** D, S
         Arthus reaction

     ● **T78.49   Other allergy** D, S

● **T78.8   Other adverse effects, not elsewhere classified** D, S

CERTAIN EARLY COMPLICATIONS OF TRAUMA (T79)

● **T79   Certain early complications of trauma, not elsewhere classified**

     Excludes2   acute respiratory distress syndrome (J80)
         complications occurring during or following medical procedures (T80-T88)
         complications of surgical and medical care NEC (T80-T88)
         newborn respiratory distress syndrome (P22.0)

     The appropriate 7th character is to be added to each code from category T79

     | | |
     A   initial encounter
     D   subsequent encounter
     S   sequela

● **T79.0   Air embolism (traumatic)** A , D, S

     Excludes1   air embolism complicating:
         abortion or ectopic or molar pregnancy (O00-O07, O08.2)
         pregnancy, childbirth and the puerperium (O88.0)
         air embolism following:
         infusion, transfusion, and therapeutic injection (T80.0)
         procedure NEC (T81.7-)

CHAPTER 19 (S00-T88)

N Newborn Age: 0   **P** Pediatric Age: 0–17   **M** Maternity DX: 12–55   **A** Adult Age: 15–124   ♀ Females Only   ♂ Males Only

 Complication\Comorbidity   Major C\C   Present on Admission Requirement   Hospital-Acquired Condition

1669

● **T79.1 Fat embolism (traumatic) A** 🔖**, D, S** 🔖

> **Excludes1**   fat embolism complicating:
> abortion or ectopic or molar
>   pregnancy (O00-O07, O08.2)
> pregnancy, childbirth and the
>   puerperium (O88.8)

● **T79.2 Traumatic secondary and recurrent hemorrhage
and seroma A** 🔖**, D, S** 🔖

● **T79.4 Traumatic shock A** 🔖**, D, S** 🔖
> Shock (immediate) (delayed) following injury

> **Excludes1**   anaphylactic shock due to adverse
>   food reaction (T78.0-)
> anaphylactic shock due to correct
>   medicinal substance properly
>   administered (T88.6)
> anaphylactic shock due to serum
>   (T80.5-)
> anaphylactic shock NOS (T78.2)
> anesthetic shock (T88.2)
> electric shock (T75.4)
> nontraumatic shock NEC (R57.-)
> obstetric shock (O75.1)
> postprocedural shock (T81.1-)
> septic shock (R65.21)
> shock complicating abortion or
>   ectopic or molar pregnancy
>   (O00-O07, O08.3)
> shock due to lightning (T75.01)
> shock NOS (R57.9)

● **T79.5 Traumatic anuria A** 🔖**, D, S** 🔖
> Crush syndrome
> Renal failure following crushing

● **T79.6 Traumatic ischemia of muscle D, S** 🔖
> Traumatic rhabdomyolysis
> Volkmann's ischemic contracture

> **Excludes2**   anterior tibial syndrome (M76.8)
> compartment syndrome (traumatic)
>   (T79.A-)
> nontraumatic ischemia of muscle
>   (M62.2-)

● **T79.7 Traumatic subcutaneous emphysema A** 🔖**, D, S** 🔖

> **Excludes1**   emphysema NOS (J43)
> emphysema (subcutaneous)
>   resulting from a procedure
>   (T81.82)

● **T79.A Traumatic compartment syndrome**

> **Excludes1**   fibromyalgia (M79.7)
> nontraumatic compartment
>   syndrome (M79.A-)
> traumatic ischemic infarction of
>   muscle (T79.6)

●■ **T79.A0 Compartment syndrome, unspecified A** 🔖**,
D, S** 🔖
> Compartment syndrome NOS

● **T79.A1 Traumatic compartment syndrome of
upper extremity**
> Traumatic compartment syndrome of
>   shoulder, arm, forearm, wrist, hand,
>   and fingers

> ● **T79.A11 Traumatic compartment
> syndrome of right upper
> extremity A** 🔖**, D, S** 🔖

> ● **T79.A12 Traumatic compartment syndrome
> of left upper extremity A** 🔖**,
> D, S** 🔖

> ●■ **T79.A19 Traumatic compartment
> syndrome of unspecified upper
> extremity A** 🔖**, D, S** 🔖

● **T79.A2 Traumatic compartment syndrome of
lower extremity**
> Traumatic compartment syndrome of hip,
>   buttock, thigh, leg, foot, and toes

> ● **T79.A21 Traumatic compartment
> syndrome of right lower
> extremity A** 🔖**, D, S** 🔖

> ● **T79.A22 Traumatic compartment syndrome
> of left lower extremity A** 🔖**,
> D, S** 🔖

> ●■ **T79.A29 Traumatic compartment
> syndrome of unspecified lower
> extremity A** 🔖**, D, S** 🔖

● **T79.A3 Traumatic compartment syndrome of
abdomen A** 🔖**, D, S** 🔖

● **T79.A9 Traumatic compartment syndrome of other
sites A** 🔖**, D, S** 🔖

● **T79.8 Other early complications of trauma D, S** 🔖

●■ **T79.9 Unspecified early complication of trauma D, S** 🔖

COMPLICATIONS OF SURGICAL AND MEDICAL CARE, NOT ELSEWHERE CLASSIFIED (T80-T88)

Use additional code for adverse effect, if applicable, to
identify drug (T36-T50 with fifth or sixth character 5)

Use additional code(s) to identify the specified condition
resulting from the complication.

Use additional code to identify devices involved and
details of circumstances (Y62-Y82)

Excludes2   any encounters with medical care for
> postprocedural conditions in which no
> complications are present, such as:
> artificial opening status (Z93.-)
> closure of external stoma (Z43.-)
> fitting and adjustment of external
>   prosthetic device (Z44.-)
> burns and corrosions from local applications
>   and irradiation (T20-T32)
> complications of surgical procedures
>   during pregnancy, childbirth and the
>   puerperium (O00-O9A)
> mechanical complication of respirator
>   [ventilator] (J95.850)
> poisoning and toxic effects of drugs and
>   chemicals (T36-T65 with fifth or sixth
>   character 1-4 or 6)
> postprocedural fever (R50.82)
> specified complications classified elsewhere,
>   such as:
> cerebrospinal fluid leak from spinal
>   puncture (G97.0)
> colostomy malfunction (K94.0-)
> disorders of fluid and electrolyte
>   imbalance (E86- E87)
> functional disturbances following cardiac
>   surgery (I97.0-I97.1)
> intraoperative and postprocedural
>   complications of specified body
>   systems (D78.-, E36.-, E89.-, G97.3-,
>   G97.4, H59.3-, H59.-, H95.2-, H95.3,
>   I97.4-, I97.5, J95.6-, J95.7, K91.6-, L76.-,
>   M96.-, N99.-)
> ostomy complications (J95.0-, K94-,
>   N99.5-)
> postgastric surgery syndromes (K91.1)
> postlaminectomy syndrome NEC (M96.1)
> postmastectomy lymphedema syndrome
>   (I97.2)
> postsurgical blind-loop syndrome (K91.2)
> ventilator associated pneumonia (J95.851)

CHAPTER 19 (S00-T88)

● Unacceptable Principal Diagnosis   ● Use Additional Character(s)   ■ Unspecified   ▶ Manifestation Code

OGCR Official Guidelines for Coding and Reporting   Excludes 1   Excludes 2   Includes   Use additional   Code first   Code also

● **T80   Complications following infusion, transfusion and therapeutic injection**

> **Includes**   complications following perfusion

> **Excludes2**   bone marrow transplant rejection (T86.01)
> febrile nonhemolytic transfusion reaction (R50.84)
> fluid overload due to transfusion (E87.71)
> posttransfusion purpura (D69.51)
> transfusion associated circulatory overload (TACO) (E87.71)
> transfusion (red blood cell) associated hemochromatosis (E83.111)
> transfusion related acute lung injury (TRALI) (J95.84)

The appropriate 7th character is to be added to each code from category T80

> A   initial encounter
> D   subsequent encounter
> S   sequela

● **T80.0   Air embolism following infusion, transfusion and therapeutic injection** A 🔾, D, S 🔾, A 🔾

● **T80.1   Vascular complications following infusion, transfusion and therapeutic injection** A 🔾, D, S 🔾

> **Use additional** code to identify the vascular complication

> **Excludes2**   extravasation of vesicant agent (T80.81-)
> infiltration of vesicant agent (T80.81-)
> vascular complications specified as due to prosthetic devices, implants and grafts (T82.8-T83.8, T84.8-, T85.8)
> postprocedural vascular complications (T81.7-)

● **T80.2   Infections following infusion, transfusion and therapeutic injection**

> **Use additional** code to identify the specific infection, such as:
> sepsis (A41.9)

> **Use additional** code (R65.2-) to identify severe sepsis, if applicable

> **Excludes2**   infections specified as due to prosthetic devices, implants and grafts (T82.6-T82.7, T83.5-T83.6, T84.5-T84.7, T85.7)
> postprocedural infections (T81.4)

● **T80.21   Infection due to central venous catheter**

● **T80.211   Bloodstream infection due to central venous catheter** D, S 🔾, A 🔾

> Catheter-related bloodstream infection (CRBSI) NOS
> Central line-associated bloodstream infection (CLABSI)
> Bloodstream infection due to Hickman catheter
> Bloodstream infection due to peripherally inserted central catheter (PICC)
> Bloodstream infection due to portacath (port-a-cath)
> Bloodstream infection due to triple lumen catheter
> Bloodstream infection due to umbilical venous catheter

● **T80.212   Local infection due to central venous catheter** D, S 🔾, A 🔾

> Exit or insertion site infection
> Local infection due to Hickman catheter
> Local infection due to peripherally inserted central catheter (PICC)
> Local infection due to portacath (port-a-cath)
> Local infection due to triple lumen catheter
> Local infection due to umbilical venous catheter
> Port or reservoir infection
> Tunnel infection

● **T80.218   Other infection due to central venous catheter** D, S 🔾, A 🔾

> Other central line-associated infection
> Other infection due to Hickman catheter
> Other infection due to peripherally inserted central catheter (PICC)
> Other infection due to portacath (port-a-cath)
> Other infection due to triple lumen catheter
> Other infection due to umbilical venous catheter

● ■ **T80.219   Unspecified infection due to central venous catheter** D, S 🔾, A 🔾

> Central line-associated infection NOS
> Unspecified infection due to Hickman catheter
> Unspecified infection due to peripherally inserted central catheter (PICC)
> Unspecified infection due to portacath (port-a-cath)
> Unspecified infection due to triple lumen catheter
> Unspecified infection due to umbilical venous catheter

● **T80.22   Acute infection following transfusion, infusion, or injection of blood and blood products**

● **T80.29   Infection following other infusion, transfusion and therapeutic injection** A 🔾, D, S 🔾

● **T80.3   ABO incompatibility reaction due to transfusion of blood or blood products**

> **Excludes1**   minor blood group antigens reactions (Duffy) (E) (K(ell)) (Kidd) (Lewis) (M) (N) (P) (S) (T80.A)

● **T80.30   ABO incompatibility reaction due to transfusion of blood or blood products, unspecified** A 🔾, D, S 🔾, A 🔾

> ABO incompatibility blood transfusion NOS
> Reaction to ABO incompatibility from transfusion NOS

● **T80.31** **ABO incompatibility with hemolytic transfusion reaction**

  ● **T80.310** **ABO incompatibility with acute hemolytic transfusion reaction A** 🗈, D, S 🗈, A 🗈
    ABO incompatibility with hemolytic transfusion reaction less than 24 hours after transfusion
    Acute hemolytic transfusion reaction (AHTR) due to ABO incompatibility

  ● **T80.311** **ABO incompatibility with delayed hemolytic transfusion reaction A** 🗈, D, S 🗈, A 🗈
    ABO incompatibility with hemolytic transfusion reaction 24 hours or more after transfusion
    Delayed hemolytic transfusion reaction (DHTR) due to ABO incompatibility

  ●■ **T80.319** **ABO incompatibility with hemolytic transfusion reaction, unspecified A** 🗈, D, S 🗈, A 🗈
    ABO incompatibility with hemolytic transfusion reaction at unspecified time after transfusion
    Hemolytic transfusion reaction (HTR) due to ABO incompatibility NOS

● **T80.39** **Other ABO incompatibility reaction due to transfusion of blood or blood products A** 🗈, D, S 🗈, A 🗈
  Delayed serologic transfusion reaction (DSTR) from ABO incompatibility
  Other ABO incompatible blood transfusion
  Other reaction to ABO incompatible blood transfusion

● **T80.4** **Rh incompatibility reaction due to transfusion of blood or blood products**
  Reaction due to incompatibility of Rh antigens (C) (c) (D) (E) (e)

●■ **T80.40** **Rh incompatibility reaction due to transfusion of blood or blood products, unspecified A** 🗈, D, S 🗈
  Reaction due to Rh factor in transfusion NOS
  Rh incompatible blood transfusion NOS

● **T80.41** **Rh incompatibility with hemolytic transfusion reaction**

  ● **T80.410** **Rh incompatibility with acute hemolytic transfusion reaction A** 🗈, D, S 🗈
    Acute hemolytic transfusion reaction (AHTR) due to Rh incompatibility
    Rh incompatibility with hemolytic transfusion reaction less than 24 hours after transfusion

  ● **T80.411** **Rh incompatibility with delayed hemolytic transfusion reaction A** 🗈, D, S 🗈
    Delayed hemolytic transfusion reaction (DHTR) due to Rh incompatibility
    Rh incompatibility with hemolytic transfusion reaction 24 hours or more after transfusion

  ●■ **T80.419** **Rh incompatibility with hemolytic transfusion reaction, unspecified A** 🗈, D, S 🗈
    Rh incompatibility with hemolytic transfusion reaction at unspecified time after transfusion
    Hemolytic transfusion reaction (HTR) due to Rh incompatibility NOS

● **T80.49** **Other Rh incompatibility reaction due to transfusion of blood or blood products A** 🗈, D, S 🗈
  Delayed serologic transfusion reaction (DSTR) from Rh incompatibility
  Other reaction to Rh incompatible blood transfusion

● **T80.A** **Non-ABO incompatibility reaction due to transfusion of blood or blood products**
  Reaction due to incompatibility of minor antigens (Duffy) (Kell) (Kidd) (Lewis) (M) (N) (P) (S)

● **T80.A0** **Non-ABO incompatibility reaction due to transfusion of blood or blood products, unspecified A** 🗈, D, S 🗈
  Non-ABO antigen incompatibility reaction from transfusion NOS

● **T80.A1** **Non-ABO incompatibility with hemolytic transfusion reaction**

  ● **T80.A10** **Non-ABO incompatibility with acute hemolytic transfusion reaction A** 🗈, D, S 🗈
    Acute hemolytic transfusion reaction (AHTR) due to non-ABO incompatibility
    Non-ABO incompatibility with hemolytic transfusion reaction less than 24 hours after transfusion

  ● **T80.A11** **Non-ABO incompatibility with delayed hemolytic transfusion reaction A** 🗈, D, S 🗈
    Delayed hemolytic transfusion reaction (DHTR) due to non-ABO incompatibility
    Non-ABO incompatibility with hemolytic transfusion reaction 24 or more hours after transfusion

  ●■ **T80.A19** **Non-ABO incompatibility with hemolytic transfusion reaction, unspecified A** 🗈, D, S 🗈
    Hemolytic transfusion reaction (HTR) due to non-ABO incompatibility NOS
    Non-ABO incompatibility with hemolytic transfusion reaction at unspecified time after transfusion

● **T80.A9** **Other non-ABO incompatibility reaction due to transfusion of blood or blood products A** 🗈, D, S 🗈
  Delayed serologic transfusion reaction (DSTR) from non-ABO incompatibility
  Other reaction to non-ABO incompatible blood transfusion

1672

● Unacceptable Principal Diagnosis   ● Use Additional Character(s)   ■ Unspecified   ▶ Manifestation Code

OGCR Official Guidelines for Coding and Reporting   Excludes 1   Excludes 2   Includes   Use additional   Code first   Code also

● **T80.5**   **Anaphylactic reaction due to serum**
     Allergic reaction due to serum
     Anaphylactic shock due to serum
     Anaphylactoid reaction due to serum
     Anaphylaxis due to serum

     Excludes1   ABO incompatibility reaction due to transfusion of blood or blood products (T80.3-)
             allergic reaction or shock NOS (T78.2)
             anaphylactic reaction or shock NOS (T78.2)
             anaphylactic reaction or shock due to adverse effect of correct medicinal substance properly administered (T88.6)
             other serum reaction (T80.6-)

     ● **T80.51**   **Anaphylactic reaction due to administration of blood and blood products** D, S

     ● **T80.52**   **Anaphylactic reaction due to vaccination** D, S

     ● **T80.59**   **Anaphylactic reaction due to other serum** D, S

● **T80.6**   **Other serum reactions**
     Intoxication by serum   Serum sickness
     Protein sickness   Serum urticaria
     Serum rash

     Excludes2   serum hepatitis (B16.-)

     ● **T80.61**   **Other serum reaction due to administration of blood and blood products** D, S

     ● **T80.62**   **Other serum reaction due to vaccination** D, S

     ● **T80.69**   **Other serum reaction due to other serum** D, S

● **T80.8**   **Other complications following infusion, transfusion and therapeutic injection**

     ● **T80.81**   **Extravasation of vesicant agent**
          Infiltration of vesicant agent

         ● **T80.810**   **Extravasation of vesicant antineoplastic chemotherapy** A, D, S
             Infiltration of vesicant antineoplastic chemotherapy

         ● **T80.818**   **Extravasation of other vesicant agent** A, D, S
             Infiltration of other vesicant agent

     ● **T80.89**   **Other complications following infusion, transfusion and therapeutic injection** D, S
          Delayed serologic transfusion reaction (DSTR), unspecified incompatibility

          Use additional code to identify graft-versus-host reaction, if applicable, (D89.81-)

● **T80.9**   **Unspecified complication following infusion, transfusion and therapeutic injection**

     ● ■ **T80.90**   **Unspecified complication following infusion and therapeutic injection** D, S

     ● **T80.91**   **Hemolytic transfusion reaction, unspecified incompatibility**

         Excludes1   ABO incompatibility with hemolytic transfusion reaction (T80.31-)
             Non-ABO incompatibility with hemolytic transfusion reaction (T80.A1-)
             Rh incompatibility with hemolytic transfusion reaction (T80.41-)

         ● ■ **T80.910**   **Acute hemolytic transfusion reaction, unspecified incompatibility** A, D, S

         ● ■ **T80.911**   **Delayed hemolytic transfusion reaction, unspecified incompatibility** A, D, S

         ● ■ **T80.919**   **Hemolytic transfusion reaction, unspecified incompatibility, unspecified as acute or delayed** A, D, S
             Hemolytic transfusion reaction NOS

     ● ■ **T80.92**   **Unspecified transfusion reaction** D, S
          Transfusion reaction NOS

● **T81**   **Complications of procedures, not elsewhere classified**

     Use additional code for adverse effect, if applicable, to identify drug (T36-T50 with fifth or sixth character 5)

     Excludes2   complications following immunization (T88.0-T88.1)
             complications following infusion, transfusion and therapeutic injection (T80.-)
             complications of transplanted organs and tissue (T86.-)
             poisoning and toxic effects of drugs and chemicals (T36-T65 with fifth or sixth character 1-4 or 6)
             specified complications classified elsewhere, such as:
                complication of prosthetic devices, implants and grafts (T82-T85)
                dermatitis due to drugs and medicaments (L23.3, L24.4, L25.1, L27.0-L27.1)
                endosseous dental implant failure (M27.6-)
                floppy iris syndrome (IFIS) (intraoperative) H21.81
                intraoperative and postprocedural complications of specific body system (D78.-, E36.-, E89.-, G97.3-, G97.4, H59.3-, H59.-, H95.2-, H95.3, I97.4-, I97.5, J95, K91-, L76.-, M96.-, N99.-)
                ostomy complications (J95.0-, K94.-, N99.5-)
                plateau iris syndrome (post-iridectomy) (postprocedural) H21.82

The appropriate 7th character is to be added to each code from category T81

A	initial encounter
D	subsequent encounter
S	sequela

● **T81.1   Postprocedural shock**
Shock during or resulting from a procedure, not elsewhere classified

> Excludes1   anaphylactic shock NOS (T78.2)
> anaphylactic shock due to correct substance properly administered (T88.6)
> anaphylactic shock due to serum (T80.5-)
> anesthetic shock (T88.2)
> electric shock (T75.4)
> obstetric shock (O75.1)
> septic shock (R65.21)
> shock following abortion or ectopic or molar pregnancy (O00-O07, O08.3)
> traumatic shock (T79.4)

●■ **T81.10   Postprocedural shock unspecified** D, S
Collapse NOS during or resulting from a procedure, not elsewhere classified
Postprocedural failure of peripheral circulation
Postprocedural shock NOS

● **T81.11   Postprocedural cardiogenic shock** D, S

● **T81.12   Postprocedural septic shock** D, S
Postprocedural endotoxic shock during or resulting from a procedure, not elsewhere classified
Postprocedural gram-negative shock during or resulting from a procedure, not elsewhere classified

> *Code first* underlying infection

> Use additional code, to identify any associated acute organ dysfunction, if applicable

● **T81.19   Other postprocedural shock** D, S
Postprocedural hypovolemic shock

● **T81.3   Disruption of wound, not elsewhere classified**
Disruption of any suture materials or other closure methods

> Excludes1   breakdown (mechanical) of permanent sutures (T85.612)
> displacement of permanent sutures (T85.622)
> disruption of cesarean delivery wound (O90.0)
> disruption of perineal obstetric wound (O90.1)
> mechanical complication of permanent sutures NEC (T85.692)

● **T81.30   Disruption of wound, unspecified** A, D, S
Disruption of wound NOS

● **T81.31   Disruption of external operation (surgical) wound, not elsewhere classified** A, D, S

> Excludes1   dehiscence of amputation stump (T87.81)
Dehiscence of operation wound NOS
Disruption of operation wound NOS
Disruption or dehiscence of closure of cornea
Disruption or dehiscence of closure of mucosa
Disruption or dehiscence of closure of skin and subcutaneous tissue
Full-thickness skin disruption or dehiscence
Superficial disruption or dehiscence of operation wound

● **T81.32   Disruption of internal operation (surgical) wound, not elsewhere classified** A, D, S
Deep disruption or dehiscence of operation wound NOS
Disruption or dehiscence of closure of internal organ or other internal tissue
Disruption or dehiscence of closure of muscle or muscle flap
Disruption or dehiscence of closure of ribs or rib cage
Disruption or dehiscence of closure of skull or craniotomy
Disruption or dehiscence of closure of sternum or sternotomy
Disruption or dehiscence of closure of tendon or ligament
Disruption or dehiscence of closure of superficial or muscular fascia

● **T81.33   Disruption of traumatic injury wound repair** A, D, S
Disruption or dehiscence of closure of traumatic laceration (external) (internal)

● **T81.4   Infection following a procedure** A, D, S, A
Intra-abdominal abscess following a procedure
Postprocedural infection, not elsewhere classified
Sepsis following a procedure
Stitch abscess following a procedure
Subphrenic abscess following a procedure
Wound abscess following a procedure

> Use additional code to identify infection

> Use additional code (R65.2-) to identify severe sepsis, if applicable

> Excludes1   obstetric surgical wound infection (O86.0)
> postprocedural fever NOS (R50.82)
> postprocedural retroperitoneal abscess (K68.11)

> Excludes2   bleb associated endophthalmitis (H59.4-)
> infection due to infusion, transfusion and therapeutic injection (T80.2-)
> infection due to prosthetic devices, implants and grafts (T82.6-T82.7, T83.5-T83.6, T84.5-T84.7, T85.7)

● **T81.5   Complications of foreign body accidentally left in body following procedure**

● **T81.50   Unspecified complication of foreign body accidentally left in body following procedure**

●■ **T81.500   Unspecified complication of foreign body accidentally left in body following surgical operation** A, D, S, A

● Unacceptable Principal Diagnosis   ● Use Additional Character(s)   ■ Unspecified   ▶ Manifestation Code
OGCR Official Guidelines for Coding and Reporting   Excludes 1   Excludes 2   Includes   Use additional   Code first   Code also

● ■ T81.501   Unspecified complication of foreign body accidentally left in body following infusion or transfusion A 🦠, D, S 🦠, A 🦠

● ■ T81.502   Unspecified complication of foreign body accidentally left in body following kidney dialysis A 🦠, D, S 🦠, A 🦠

● ■ T81.503   Unspecified complication of foreign body accidentally left in body following injection or immunization A 🦠, D, S 🦠, A 🦠

● ■ T81.504   Unspecified complication of foreign body accidentally left in body following endoscopic examination A 🦠, D, S 🦠, A 🦠

● ■ T81.505   Unspecified complication of foreign body accidentally left in body following heart catheterization A 🦠, D, S 🦠, A 🦠

● ■ T81.506   Unspecified complication of foreign body accidentally left in body following aspiration, puncture or other catheterization A 🦠, D, S 🦠, A 🦠

● ■ T81.507   Unspecified complication of foreign body accidentally left in body following removal of catheter or packing A 🦠, D, S 🦠, A 🦠

● ■ T81.508   Unspecified complication of foreign body accidentally left in body following other procedure A 🦠, D, S 🦠, A 🦠

● ■ T81.509   Unspecified complication of foreign body accidentally left in body following unspecified procedure A 🦠, D, S 🦠, A 🦠

● T81.51   Adhesions due to foreign body accidentally left in body following procedure

    ● T81.510   Adhesions due to foreign body accidentally left in body following surgical operation A 🦠, D, S 🦠, A 🦠

    ● T81.511   Adhesions due to foreign body accidentally left in body following infusion or transfusion A 🦠, D, S 🦠, A 🦠

    ● T81.512   Adhesions due to foreign body accidentally left in body following kidney dialysis A 🦠, D, S 🦠, A 🦠

    ● T81.513   Adhesions due to foreign body accidentally left in body following injection or immunization A 🦠, D, S 🦠, A 🦠

    ● T81.514   Adhesions due to foreign body accidentally left in body following endoscopic examination A 🦠, D, S 🦠, A 🦠

    ● T81.515   Adhesions due to foreign body accidentally left in body following heart catheterization A 🦠, D, S 🦠, A 🦠

    ● T81.516   Adhesions due to foreign body accidentally left in body following aspiration, puncture or other catheterization A 🦠, D, S 🦠, A 🦠

● T81.517   Adhesions due to foreign body accidentally left in body following removal of catheter or packing A 🦠, D, S 🦠, A 🦠

● T81.518   Adhesions due to foreign body accidentally left in body following other procedure A 🦠, D, S 🦠, A 🦠

● ■ T81.519   Adhesions due to foreign body accidentally left in body following unspecified procedure A 🦠, D, S 🦠, A 🦠

● T81.52   Obstruction due to foreign body accidentally left in body following procedure

    ● T81.520   Obstruction due to foreign body accidentally left in body following surgical operation A 🦠, D, S 🦠, A 🦠

    ● T81.521   Obstruction due to foreign body accidentally left in body following infusion or transfusion A 🦠, D, S 🦠, A 🦠

    ● T81.522   Obstruction due to foreign body accidentally left in body following kidney dialysis A 🦠, D, S 🦠, A 🦠

    ● T81.523   Obstruction due to foreign body accidentally left in body following injection or immunization A 🦠, D, S 🦠, A 🦠

    ● T81.524   Obstruction due to foreign body accidentally left in body following endoscopic examination A 🦠, D, S 🦠, A 🦠

    ● T81.525   Obstruction due to foreign body accidentally left in body following heart catheterization A 🦠, D, S 🦠, A 🦠

    ● T81.526   Obstruction due to foreign body accidentally left in body following aspiration, puncture or other catheterization A 🦠, D, S 🦠, A 🦠

    ● T81.527   Obstruction due to foreign body accidentally left in body following removal of catheter or packing A 🦠, D, S 🦠, A 🦠

    ● T81.528   Obstruction due to foreign body accidentally left in body following other procedure A 🦠, D, S 🦠, A 🦠

    ● ■ T81.529   Obstruction due to foreign body accidentally left in body following unspecified procedure A 🦠, D, S 🦠, A 🦠

● T81.53   Perforation due to foreign body accidentally left in body following procedure

    ● T81.530   Perforation due to foreign body accidentally left in body following surgical operation A 🦠, D, S 🦠, A 🦠

    ● T81.531   Perforation due to foreign body accidentally left in body following infusion or transfusion A 🦠, D, S 🦠, A 🦠

N Newborn Age: 0   **P** Pediatric Age: 0–17   **M** Maternity DX: 12–55   **A** Adult Age: 15–124   ♀ Females Only   ♂ Males Only

🦠 Complication\Comorbidity   🦠 Major C\C   🦠 Present on Admission Requirement   🦠 Hospital-Acquired Condition

1675

● T81.532 Perforation due to foreign body accidentally left in body following kidney dialysis A, D, S, A

● T81.533 Perforation due to foreign body accidentally left in body following injection or immunization A, D, S, A

● T81.534 Perforation due to foreign body accidentally left in body following endoscopic examination A, D, S, A

● T81.535 Perforation due to foreign body accidentally left in body following heart catheterization A, D, S, A

● T81.536 Perforation due to foreign body accidentally left in body following aspiration, puncture or other catheterization A, D, S, A

● T81.537 Perforation due to foreign body accidentally left in body following removal of catheter or packing A, D, S, A

● T81.538 Perforation due to foreign body accidentally left in body following other procedure A, D, S, A

●■ T81.539 Perforation due to foreign body accidentally left in body following unspecified procedure A, D, S, A

● T81.59 Other complications of foreign body accidentally left in body following procedure

Excludes2 obstruction or perforation due to prosthetic devices and implants intentionally left in body (T82.0-T82.5, T83.0-T83.4, T83.7, T84.0-T84.4, T85.0-T85.6)

● T81.590 Other complications of foreign body accidentally left in body following surgical operation A, D, S, A

● T81.591 Other complications of foreign body accidentally left in body following infusion or transfusion A, D, S, A

● T81.592 Other complications of foreign body accidentally left in body following kidney dialysis A, D, S, A

● T81.593 Other complications of foreign body accidentally left in body following injection or immunization A, D, S, A

● T81.594 Other complications of foreign body accidentally left in body following endoscopic examination A, D, S, A

● T81.595 Other complications of foreign body accidentally left in body following heart catheterization A, D, S, A

● T81.596 Other complications of foreign body accidentally left in body following aspiration, puncture or other catheterization A, D, S, A

● T81.597 Other complications of foreign body accidentally left in body following removal of catheter or packing A, D, S, A

● T81.598 Other complications of foreign body accidentally left in body following other procedure A, D, S, A

●■ T81.599 Other complications of foreign body accidentally left in body following unspecified procedure A, D, S, A

● T81.6 Acute reaction to foreign substance accidentally left during a procedure

Excludes2 complications of foreign body accidentally left in body cavity or operation wound following procedure (T81.5-)

●■ T81.60 Unspecified acute reaction to foreign substance accidentally left during a procedure A, D, S, A

● T81.61 Aseptic peritonitis due to foreign substance accidentally left during a procedure A, D, S, A
Chemical peritonitis

● T81.69 Other acute reaction to foreign substance accidentally left during a procedure A, D, S, A

● T81.7 Vascular complications following a procedure, not elsewhere classified
Air embolism following procedure NEC
Phlebitis or thrombophlebitis resulting from a procedure

Excludes1 embolism complicating abortion or ectopic or molar pregnancy (O00-O07, O08.2)
embolism complicating pregnancy, childbirth and the puerperium (O88.-)
traumatic embolism (T79.0)

Excludes2 embolism due to prosthetic devices, implants and grafts (T82.8, T83.8, T84.8-, T85.8)
embolism following infusion, transfusion and therapeutic injection (T80.0)

● T81.71 Complication of artery following a procedure, not elsewhere classified

● T81.710 Complication of mesenteric artery following a procedure, not elsewhere classified A, D, S

● T81.711 Complication of renal artery following a procedure, not elsewhere classified A, D, S

● T81.718 Complication of other artery following a procedure, not elsewhere classified A, D, S

●■ T81.719 Complication of unspecified artery following a procedure, not elsewhere classified A, D, S

● T81.72 Complication of vein following a procedure, not elsewhere classified A, D, S

● Unacceptable Principal Diagnosis   ● Use Additional Character(s)   ■ Unspecified   ▶ Manifestation Code
OGCR Official Guidelines for Coding and Reporting   Excludes 1   Excludes 2   Includes   Use additional   Code first   Code also

● **T81.8**   **Other complications of procedures, not elsewhere classified**
> Excludes2   hypothermia following anesthesia (T88.51)
> malignant hyperpyrexia due to anesthesia (T88.3)

   ● **T81.81**   **Complication of inhalation therapy** D, S 🔧

   ● **T81.82**   **Emphysema (subcutaneous) resulting from a procedure** D, S 🔧

   ● **T81.83**   **Persistent postprocedural fistula A** 🔧, D, S 🔧

   ● **T81.89**   **Other complications of procedures, not elsewhere classified** D, S 🔧
> Use additional code to specify complication, such as:
> postprocedural delirium (F05)

● ■ **T81.9**   **Unspecified complication of procedure** D, S 🔧

● **T82**   **Complications of cardiac and vascular prosthetic devices, implants and grafts**
> Excludes2   failure and rejection of transplanted organs and tissue (T86.-)

> The appropriate 7th character is to be added to each code from category T82

> | | |
> | --- | --- |
> | A | initial encounter |
> | D | subsequent encounter |
> | S | sequela |

● **T82.0**   **Mechanical complication of heart valve prosthesis**
> Mechanical complication of artificial heart valve
> Excludes1   mechanical complication of biological heart valve graft (T82.22-)

   ● **T82.01**   **Breakdown (mechanical) of heart valve prosthesis A** 🔧, D, S 🔧

   ● **T82.02**   **Displacement of heart valve prosthesis A** 🔧, D, S 🔧
> Malposition of heart valve prosthesis

   ● **T82.03**   **Leakage of heart valve prosthesis A** 🔧, D, S 🔧

   ● **T82.09**   **Other mechanical complication of heart valve prosthesis A** 🔧, D, S 🔧
> Obstruction (mechanical) of heart valve prosthesis
> Perforation of heart valve prosthesis
> Protrusion of heart valve prosthesis

● **T82.1**   **Mechanical complication of cardiac electronic device**

   ● **T82.11**   **Breakdown (mechanical) of cardiac electronic device**

     ● **T82.110**   **Breakdown (mechanical) of cardiac electrode A** 🔧, D, S 🔧

     ● **T82.111**   **Breakdown (mechanical) of cardiac pulse generator (battery) A** 🔧, D, S 🔧

     ● **T82.118**   **Breakdown (mechanical) of other cardiac electronic device A** 🔧, D, S 🔧

     ● ■ **T82.119**   **Breakdown (mechanical) of unspecified cardiac electronic device A** 🔧, D, S 🔧

   ● **T82.12**   **Displacement of cardiac electronic device**
> Malposition of cardiac electronic device

     ● **T82.120**   **Displacement of cardiac electrode A** 🔧, D, S 🔧

     ● **T82.121**   **Displacement of cardiac pulse generator (battery) A** 🔧, D, S 🔧

     ● **T82.128**   **Displacement of other cardiac electronic device A** 🔧, D, S 🔧

     ● ■ **T82.129**   **Displacement of unspecified cardiac electronic device A** 🔧, D, S 🔧

   ● **T82.19**   **Other mechanical complication of cardiac electronic device**
> Leakage of cardiac electronic device
> Obstruction of cardiac electronic device
> Perforation of cardiac electronic device
> Protrusion of cardiac electronic device

     ● **T82.190**   **Other mechanical complication of cardiac electrode A** 🔧, D, S 🔧

     ● **T82.191**   **Other mechanical complication of cardiac pulse generator (battery) A** 🔧, D, S 🔧

     ● **T82.198**   **Other mechanical complication of other cardiac electronic device A** 🔧, D, S 🔧

     ● ■ **T82.199**   **Other mechanical complication of unspecified cardiac device A** 🔧, D, S 🔧

● **T82.2**   **Mechanical complication of coronary artery bypass graft and biological heart valve graft**
> Excludes1   mechanical complication of artificial heart valve prosthesis (T82.0-)

   ● **T82.21**   **Mechanical complication of coronary artery bypass graft**

     ● **T82.211**   **Breakdown (mechanical) of coronary artery bypass graft A** 🔧, D, S 🔧

     ● **T82.212**   **Displacement of coronary artery bypass graft A** 🔧, D, S 🔧
> Malposition of coronary artery bypass graft

     ● **T82.213**   **Leakage of coronary artery bypass graft A** 🔧, D, S 🔧

     ● **T82.218**   **Other mechanical complication of coronary artery bypass graft A** 🔧, D, S 🔧
> Obstruction, mechanical of coronary artery bypass graft
> Perforation of coronary artery bypass graft
> Protrusion of coronary artery bypass graft

   ● **T82.22**   **Mechanical complication of biological heart valve graft**

     ● **T82.221**   **Breakdown (mechanical) of biological heart valve graft A** 🔧, D, S 🔧

     ● **T82.222**   **Displacement of biological heart valve graft A** 🔧, D, S 🔧
> Malposition of biological heart valve graft

     ● **T82.223**   **Leakage of biological heart valve graft A** 🔧, D, S 🔧

     ● **T82.228**   **Other mechanical complication of biological heart valve graft A** 🔧, D, S 🔧
> Obstruction of biological heart valve graft
> Perforation of biological heart valve graft
> Protrusion of biological heart valve graft

CHAPTER 19 (S00-T88)

N Newborn Age: 0	**P** Pediatric Age: 0–17	**M** Maternity DX: 12–55	**A** Adult Age: 15–124	♀ Females Only	♂ Males Only
🔧 Complication\Comorbidity	🔧 Major C\C	🔧 Present on Admission Requirement	🔧 Hospital-Acquired Condition		

● **T82.3 Mechanical complication of other vascular grafts**
  ● **T82.31 Breakdown (mechanical) of other vascular grafts**
    ● **T82.310 Breakdown (mechanical) of aortic (bifurcation) graft (replacement)** A, D, S
    ● **T82.311 Breakdown (mechanical) of carotid arterial graft (bypass)** A, D, S
    ● **T82.312 Breakdown (mechanical) of femoral arterial graft (bypass)** A, D, S
    ● **T82.318 Breakdown (mechanical) of other vascular grafts** A, D, S
    ●■ **T82.319 Breakdown (mechanical) of unspecified vascular grafts** A, D, S
  ● **T82.32 Displacement of other vascular grafts**
    Malposition of other vascular grafts
    ● **T82.320 Displacement of aortic (bifurcation) graft (replacement)** A, D, S
    ● **T82.321 Displacement of carotid arterial graft (bypass)** A, D, S
    ● **T82.322 Displacement of femoral arterial graft (bypass)** A, D, S
    ● **T82.328 Displacement of other vascular grafts** A, D, S
    ●■ **T82.329 Displacement of unspecified vascular grafts** A, D, S
  ● **T82.33 Leakage of other vascular grafts**
    ● **T82.330 Leakage of aortic (bifurcation) graft (replacement)** A, D, S
    ● **T82.331 Leakage of carotid arterial graft (bypass)** A, D, S
    ● **T82.332 Leakage of femoral arterial graft (bypass)** A, D, S
    ● **T82.338 Leakage of other vascular grafts** A, D, S
    ●■ **T82.339 Leakage of unspecified vascular graft** A, D, S
  ● **T82.39 Other mechanical complication of other vascular grafts**
    Obstruction (mechanical) of other vascular grafts
    Perforation of other vascular grafts
    Protrusion of other vascular grafts
    ● **T82.390 Other mechanical complication of aortic (bifurcation) graft (replacement)** A, D, S
    ● **T82.391 Other mechanical complication of carotid arterial graft (bypass)** A, D, S
    ● **T82.392 Other mechanical complication of femoral arterial graft (bypass)** A, D, S
    ● **T82.398 Other mechanical complication of other vascular grafts** A, D, S
    ●■ **T82.399 Other mechanical complication of unspecified vascular grafts** A, D, S

● **T82.4 Mechanical complication of vascular dialysis catheter**
  Mechanical complication of hemodialysis catheter
  Excludes1 mechanical complication of intraperitoneal dialysis catheter (T85.62)
  ● **T82.41 Breakdown (mechanical) of vascular dialysis catheter** A, D, S
  ● **T82.42 Displacement of vascular dialysis catheter** A, D, S
    Malposition of vascular dialysis catheter
  ● **T82.43 Leakage of vascular dialysis catheter** A, D, S
  ● **T82.49 Other complication of vascular dialysis catheter** A, D, S
    Obstruction (mechanical) of vascular dialysis catheter
    Perforation of vascular dialysis catheter
    Protrusion of vascular dialysis catheter
● **T82.5 Mechanical complication of other cardiac and vascular devices and implants**
  Excludes2 mechanical complication of epidural and subdural infusion catheter (T85.61)
  ● **T82.51 Breakdown (mechanical) of other cardiac and vascular devices and implants**
    ● **T82.510 Breakdown (mechanical) of surgically created arteriovenous fistula** A, D, S
    ● **T82.511 Breakdown (mechanical) of surgically created arteriovenous shunt** A, D, S
    ● **T82.512 Breakdown (mechanical) of artificial heart** A, D, S
    ● **T82.513 Breakdown (mechanical) of balloon (counterpulsation) device** A, D, S
    ● **T82.514 Breakdown (mechanical) of infusion catheter** A, D, S
    ● **T82.515 Breakdown (mechanical) of umbrella device** A, D, S
    ● **T82.518 Breakdown (mechanical) of other cardiac and vascular devices and implants** A, D, S
    ●■ **T82.519 Breakdown (mechanical) of unspecified cardiac and vascular devices and implants** A, D, S
  ● **T82.52 Displacement of other cardiac and vascular devices and implants**
    Malposition of other cardiac and vascular devices and implants
    ● **T82.520 Displacement of surgically created arteriovenous fistula** A, D, S
    ● **T82.521 Displacement of surgically created arteriovenous shunt** A, D, S
    ● **T82.522 Displacement of artificial heart** A, D, S
    ● **T82.523 Displacement of balloon (counterpulsation) device** A, D, S
    ● **T82.524 Displacement of infusion catheter** A, D, S

● Unacceptable Principal Diagnosis ● Use Additional Character(s) ■ Unspecified ▶ Manifestation Code
OGCR Official Guidelines for Coding and Reporting | Excludes 1 | Excludes 2 | Includes | Use additional | Code first | Code also

● T82.525　Displacement of umbrella device A 🐾, D, S 🐾

● T82.528　Displacement of other cardiac and vascular devices and implants A 🐾, D, S 🐾

●■ T82.529　Displacement of unspecified cardiac and vascular devices and implants A 🐾, D, S 🐾

● T82.53　Leakage of other cardiac and vascular devices and implants

● T82.530　Leakage of surgically created arteriovenous fistula A 🐾, D, S 🐾

● T82.531　Leakage of surgically created arteriovenous shunt A 🐾, D, S 🐾

● T82.532　Leakage of artificial heart A 🐾, D, S 🐾

● T82.533　Leakage of balloon (counterpulsation) device A 🐾, D, S 🐾

● T82.534　Leakage of infusion catheter A 🐾, D, S 🐾

● T82.535　Leakage of umbrella device A 🐾, D, S 🐾

● T82.538　Leakage of other cardiac and vascular devices and implants A 🐾, D, S 🐾

●■ T82.539　Leakage of unspecified cardiac and vascular devices and implants A 🐾, D, S 🐾

● T82.59　Other mechanical complication of other cardiac and vascular devices and implants
　　Obstruction (mechanical) of other cardiac and vascular devices and implants
　　Perforation of other cardiac and vascular devices and implants
　　Protrusion of other cardiac and vascular devices and implants

● T82.590　Other mechanical complication of surgically created arteriovenous fistula A 🐾, D, S 🐾

● T82.591　Other mechanical complication of surgically created arteriovenous shunt A 🐾, D, S 🐾

● T82.592　Other mechanical complication of artificial heart A 🐾, D, S 🐾

● T82.593　Other mechanical complication of balloon (counterpulsation) device A 🐾, D, S 🐾

● T82.594　Other mechanical complication of infusion catheter A 🐾, D, S 🐾

● T82.595　Other mechanical complication of umbrella device A 🐾, D, S 🐾

● T82.598　Other mechanical complication of other cardiac and vascular devices and implants A 🐾, D, S 🐾

●■ T82.599　Other mechanical complication of unspecified cardiac and vascular devices and implants A 🐾, D, S 🐾

● T82.6　Infection and inflammatory reaction due to cardiac valve prosthesis A 🐾, D, S 🐾

　　Use additional code to identify infection

● T82.7　Infection and inflammatory reaction due to other cardiac and vascular devices, implants and grafts A 🐾, D, S 🐾

　　Use additional code to identify infection

● T82.8　Other specified complications of cardiac and vascular prosthetic devices, implants and grafts

● T82.81　Embolism of cardiac and vascular prosthetic devices, implants and grafts

● T82.817　Embolism of cardiac prosthetic devices, implants and grafts A 🐾, D, S 🐾

● T82.818　Embolism of vascular prosthetic devices, implants and grafts A 🐾, D, S 🐾

● T82.82　Fibrosis of cardiac and vascular prosthetic devices, implants and grafts

● T82.827　Fibrosis of cardiac prosthetic devices, implants and grafts A 🐾, D, S 🐾

● T82.828　Fibrosis of vascular prosthetic devices, implants and grafts A 🐾, D, S 🐾

● T82.83　Hemorrhage of cardiac and vascular prosthetic devices, implants and grafts

● T82.837　Hemorrhage of cardiac prosthetic devices, implants and grafts A 🐾, D, S 🐾

● T82.838　Hemorrhage of vascular prosthetic devices, implants and grafts A 🐾, D, S 🐾

● T82.84　Pain from cardiac and vascular prosthetic devices, implants and grafts

● T82.847　Pain from cardiac prosthetic devices, implants and grafts A 🐾, D, S 🐾

● T82.848　Pain from vascular prosthetic devices, implants and grafts A 🐾, D, S 🐾

● T82.85　Stenosis of cardiac and vascular prosthetic devices, implants and grafts

● T82.857　Stenosis of cardiac prosthetic devices, implants and grafts A 🐾, D, S 🐾

● T82.858　Stenosis of vascular prosthetic devices, implants and grafts A 🐾, D, S 🐾

● T82.86　Thrombosis of cardiac and vascular prosthetic devices, implants and grafts

● T82.867　Thrombosis of cardiac prosthetic devices, implants and grafts A 🐾, D, S 🐾

● T82.868　Thrombosis of vascular prosthetic devices, implants and grafts A 🐾, D, S 🐾

● T82.89　Other specified complication of cardiac and vascular prosthetic devices, implants and grafts

● T82.897　Other specified complication of cardiac prosthetic devices, implants and grafts A 🐾, D, S 🐾

● T82.898　Other specified complication of vascular prosthetic devices, implants and grafts A 🐾, D, S 🐾

●■ T82.9　Unspecified complication of cardiac and vascular prosthetic device, implant and graft A 🐾, D, S 🐾

N Newborn Age: 0　　**P** Pediatric Age: 0–17　　**M** Maternity DX: 12–55　　**A** Adult Age: 15–124　　♀ Females Only　　♂ Males Only

🐾 Complication\Comorbidity　　🐾 Major C\C　　🐾 Present on Admission Requirement　　🐾 Hospital-Acquired Condition

CHAPTER 19 (S00–T88)

1679

● **T83 Complications of genitourinary prosthetic devices, implants and grafts**

> **Excludes2**   failure and rejection of transplanted organs and tissue (T86.-)

The appropriate 7th character is to be added to each code from category T83

> A   initial encounter
> D   subsequent encounter
> S   sequela

● **T83.0 Mechanical complication of urinary (indwelling) catheter**

> **Excludes2**   complications of stoma of urinary tract (N99.5-)

● **T83.01 Breakdown (mechanical) of urinary (indwelling) catheter**

     ● **T83.010 Breakdown (mechanical) of cystostomy catheter A** 🜲, D, S 🜲

     ● **T83.018 Breakdown (mechanical) of other indwelling urethral catheter** D, S 🜲

● **T83.02 Displacement of urinary (indwelling) catheter**

> Malposition of urinary (indwelling) catheter

     ● **T83.020 Displacement of cystostomy catheter A** 🜲, D, S 🜲

     ● **T83.028 Displacement of other indwelling urethral catheter** D, S 🜲

● **T83.03 Leakage of urinary (indwelling) catheter**

     ● **T83.030 Leakage of cystostomy catheter A** 🜲, D, S 🜲

     ● **T83.038 Leakage of other indwelling urethral catheter**

● **T83.09 Other mechanical complication of urinary (indwelling) catheter**

> Obstruction (mechanical) of urinary (indwelling) catheter
> Perforation of urinary (indwelling) catheter
> Protrusion of urinary (indwelling) catheter

     ● **T83.090 Other mechanical complication of cystostomy catheter A** 🜲, D, S 🜲

     ● **T83.098 Other mechanical complication of other indwelling urethral catheter** D, S 🜲

● **T83.1 Mechanical complication of other urinary devices and implants**

● **T83.11 Breakdown (mechanical) of other urinary devices and implants**

     ● **T83.110 Breakdown (mechanical) of urinary electronic stimulator device A** 🜲, D, S 🜲

     ● **T83.111 Breakdown (mechanical) of urinary sphincter implant A** 🜲, D, S 🜲

     ● **T83.112 Breakdown (mechanical) of urinary stent A** 🜲, D, S 🜲

     ● **T83.118 Breakdown (mechanical) of other urinary devices and implants A** 🜲, D, S 🜲

● **T83.12 Displacement of other urinary devices and implants**

> Malposition of other urinary devices and implants

     ● **T83.120 Displacement of urinary electronic stimulator device A** 🜲, D, S 🜲

     ● **T83.121 Displacement of urinary sphincter implant A** 🜲, D, S 🜲

     ● **T83.122 Displacement of urinary stent A** 🜲, D, S 🜲

     ● **T83.128 Displacement of other urinary devices and implants A** 🜲, D, S 🜲

● **T83.19 Other mechanical complication of other urinary devices and implants**

> Leakage of other urinary devices and implants
> Obstruction (mechanical) of other urinary devices and implants
> Perforation of other urinary devices and implants
> Protrusion of other urinary devices and implants

     ● **T83.190 Other mechanical complication of urinary electronic stimulator device A** 🜲, D, S 🜲

     ● **T83.191 Other mechanical complication of urinary sphincter implant A** 🜲, D, S 🜲

     ● **T83.192 Other mechanical complication of urinary stent A** 🜲, D, S 🜲

     ● **T83.198 Other mechanical complication of other urinary devices and implants A** 🜲, D, S 🜲

● **T83.2 Mechanical complication of graft of urinary organ**

     ● **T83.21 Breakdown (mechanical) of graft of urinary organ A** 🜲, D, S 🜲

     ● **T83.22 Displacement of graft of urinary organ A** 🜲, D, S 🜲

> Malposition of graft of urinary organ

     ● **T83.23 Leakage of graft of urinary organ A** 🜲, D, S 🜲

     ● **T83.29 Other mechanical complication of graft of urinary organ A** 🜲, D, S 🜲

> Obstruction (mechanical) of graft of urinary organ
> Perforation of graft of urinary organ
> Protrusion of graft of urinary organ

● **T83.3 Mechanical complication of intrauterine contraceptive device**

     ● **T83.31 Breakdown (mechanical) of intrauterine contraceptive device** D, S 🜲

     ● **T83.32 Displacement of intrauterine contraceptive device** D, S 🜲

> Malposition of intrauterine contraceptive device

     ● **T83.39 Other mechanical complication of intrauterine contraceptive device** D, S 🜲

> Leakage of intrauterine contraceptive device
> Obstruction (mechanical) of intrauterine contraceptive device
> Perforation of intrauterine contraceptive device
> Protrusion of intrauterine contraceptive device

● Unacceptable Principal Diagnosis   ● Use Additional Character(s)   ■ Unspecified   ▶ Manifestation Code

OGCR Official Guidelines for Coding and Reporting   Excludes 1   Excludes 2   Includes   Use additional   Code first   Code also

● **T83.4 Mechanical complication of other prosthetic devices, implants and grafts of genital tract**

  ● **T83.41 Breakdown (mechanical) of other prosthetic devices, implants and grafts of genital tract**

    ● **T83.410 Breakdown (mechanical) of penile (implanted) prosthesis A** 🔵, D, S 🔵

    ● **T83.418 Breakdown (mechanical) of other prosthetic devices, implants and grafts of genital tract A** 🔵, D, S 🔵

  ● **T83.42 Displacement of other prosthetic devices, implants and grafts of genital tract**
    Malposition of other prosthetic devices, implants and grafts of genital tract

    ● **T83.420 Displacement of penile (implanted) prosthesis A** 🔵, D, S 🔵

    ● **T83.428 Displacement of other prosthetic devices, implants and grafts of genital tract A** 🔵, D, S 🔵

  ● **T83.49 Other mechanical complication of other prosthetic devices, implants and grafts of genital tract**
    Leakage of other prosthetic devices, implants and grafts of genital tract
    Obstruction, mechanical of other prosthetic devices, implants and grafts of genital tract
    Perforation of other prosthetic devices, implants and grafts of genital tract
    Protrusion of other prosthetic devices, implants and grafts of genital tract

    ● **T83.490 Other mechanical complication of penile (implanted) prosthesis A** 🔵, D, S 🔵

    ● **T83.498 Other mechanical complication of other prosthetic devices, implants and grafts of genital tract A** 🔵, D, S 🔵

● **T83.5 Infection and inflammatory reaction due to prosthetic device, implant and graft in urinary system**
    Use additional code to identify infection

  ● **T83.51 Infection and inflammatory reaction due to indwelling urinary catheter A** 🔵, D, S 🔵, A 🔵

    Excludes2   complications of stoma of urinary tract (N99.5-)

  ● **T83.59 Infection and inflammatory reaction due to prosthetic device, implant and graft in urinary system A** 🔵, D, S 🔵

● **T83.6 Infection and inflammatory reaction due to prosthetic device, implant and graft in genital tract A** 🔵, D, S 🔵
    Use additional code to identify infection

● **T83.7 Complications due to implanted mesh and other prosthetic materials**

  ● **T83.71 Erosion of implanted mesh and other prosthetic materials to surrounding organ or tissue**

    ● **T83.711 Erosion of implanted vaginal mesh and other prosthetic materials to surrounding organ or tissue**
      Erosion of implanted vaginal mesh and other prosthetic materials into pelvic floor muscles

    ● **T83.718 Erosion of other implanted mesh and other prosthetic materials to surrounding organ or tissue**

  ● **T83.72 Exposure of implanted mesh and other prosthetic materials into surrounding organ or tissue**

    ● **T83.721 Exposure of implanted vaginal mesh and other prosthetic materials into vagina**
      Exposure of implanted vaginal mesh and other prosthetic materials through vaginal wall

    ● **T83.728 Exposure of other implanted mesh and other prosthetic materials to surrounding organ or tissue**

● **T83.8 Other specified complications of genitourinary prosthetic devices, implants and grafts**

  ● **T83.81 Embolism of genitourinary prosthetic devices, implants and grafts A** 🔵, D, S 🔵

  ● **T83.82 Fibrosis of genitourinary prosthetic devices, implants and grafts A** 🔵, D, S 🔵

  ● **T83.83 Hemorrhage of genitourinary prosthetic devices, implants and grafts A** 🔵, D, S 🔵

  ● **T83.84 Pain from genitourinary prosthetic devices, implants and grafts A** 🔵, D, S 🔵

  ● **T83.85 Stenosis of genitourinary prosthetic devices, implants and grafts A** 🔵, D, S 🔵

  ● **T83.86 Thrombosis of genitourinary prosthetic devices, implants and grafts A** 🔵, D, S 🔵

  ● **T83.89 Other specified complication of genitourinary prosthetic devices, implants and grafts A** 🔵, D, S 🔵

●■ **T83.9 Unspecified complication of genitourinary prosthetic device, implant and graft A** 🔵, D, S 🔵

● **T84 Complications of internal orthopedic prosthetic devices, implants and grafts**

    Excludes2   failure and rejection of transplanted organs and tissues (T86.-)
        fracture of bone following insertion of orthopedic implant, joint prosthesis or bone plate (M96.6)

    The appropriate 7th character is to be added to each code from category T84

    A initial encounter
    D subsequent encounter
    S sequela

● **T84.0 Mechanical complication of internal joint prosthesis**

  ● **T84.01 Broken internal joint prosthesis**
    Breakage (fracture) of prosthetic joint
    Broken prosthetic joint implant

    Excludes1   periprosthetic joint implant fracture (T84.04)

    ● **T84.010 Broken internal right hip prosthesis A** 🔵, D, S 🔵

    ● **T84.011 Broken internal left hip prosthesis A** 🔵, D, S 🔵

    ● **T84.012 Broken internal right knee prosthesis A** 🔵, D, S 🔵

    ● **T84.013 Broken internal left knee prosthesis A** 🔵, D, S 🔵

    ● **T84.018 Broken internal joint prosthesis, other site A** 🔵, D, S 🔵

      Use additional code to identify the joint (Z96.6-)

    ●■ **T84.019 Broken internal joint prosthesis, unspecified site A** 🔵, D, S 🔵

● **T84.02**   **Dislocation of internal joint prosthesis**
Instability of internal joint prosthesis
Subluxation of internal joint prosthesis

  ● **T84.020**   **Dislocation of internal right hip prosthesis A** 🦴, D, S 🦴

  ● **T84.021**   **Dislocation of internal left hip prosthesis A** 🦴, D, S 🦴

  ● **T84.022**   **Instability of internal right knee prosthesis A** 🦴, D, S 🦴

  ● **T84.023**   **Instability of internal left knee prosthesis A** 🦴, D, S 🦴

  ● **T84.028**   **Dislocation of other internal joint prosthesis A** 🦴, D, S 🦴

     Use additional code to identify the joint (Z96.6-)

  ● ■ **T84.029**   **Dislocation of unspecified internal joint prosthesis A** 🦴, D, S 🦴

● **T84.03**   **Mechanical loosening of internal prosthetic joint**
Aseptic loosening of prosthetic joint

  ● **T84.030**   **Mechanical loosening of internal right hip prosthetic joint A** 🦴, D, S 🦴

  ● **T84.031**   **Mechanical loosening of internal left hip prosthetic joint A** 🦴, D, S 🦴

  ● **T84.032**   **Mechanical loosening of internal right knee prosthetic joint A** 🦴, D, S 🦴

  ● **T84.033**   **Mechanical loosening of internal left knee prosthetic joint A** 🦴, D, S 🦴

  ● **T84.038**   **Mechanical loosening of other internal prosthetic joint A** 🦴, D, S 🦴

     Use additional code to identify the joint (Z96.6-)

  ● ■ **T84.039**   **Mechanical loosening of unspecified internal prosthetic joint A** 🦴, D, S 🦴

● **T84.04**   **Periprosthetic fracture around internal prosthetic joint**

     | Excludes2 | breakage (fracture) of prosthetic joint (T84.01)

  ● **T84.040**   **Periprosthetic fracture around internal prosthetic right hip joint A** 🦴, D, S 🦴

  ● **T84.041**   **Periprosthetic fracture around internal prosthetic left hip joint A** 🦴, D, S 🦴

  ● **T84.042**   **Periprosthetic fracture around internal prosthetic right knee joint A** 🦴, D, S 🦴

  ● **T84.043**   **Periprosthetic fracture around internal prosthetic left knee joint A** 🦴, D, S 🦴

  ● **T84.048**   **Periprosthetic fracture around other internal prosthetic joint A** 🦴, D, S 🦴

     Use additional code to identify the joint (Z96.6-)

  ● ■ **T84.049**   **Periprosthetic fracture around unspecified internal prosthetic joint A** 🦴, D, S 🦴

● **T84.05**   **Periprosthetic osteolysis of internal prosthetic joint**

     Use additional code to identify major osseous defect, if applicable (M89.7-)

  ● **T84.050**   **Periprosthetic osteolysis of internal prosthetic right hip joint A** 🦴, D, S 🦴

  ● **T84.051**   **Periprosthetic osteolysis of internal prosthetic left hip joint A** 🦴, D, S 🦴

  ● **T84.052**   **Periprosthetic osteolysis of internal prosthetic right knee joint A** 🦴, D, S 🦴

  ● **T84.053**   **Periprosthetic osteolysis of internal prosthetic left knee joint A** 🦴, D, S 🦴

  ● **T84.058**   **Periprosthetic osteolysis of other internal prosthetic joint A** 🦴, D, S 🦴

     Use additional code to identify the joint (Z96.6-)

  ● ■ **T84.059**   **Periprosthetic osteolysis of unspecified internal prosthetic joint A** 🦴, D, S 🦴

● **T84.06**   **Wear of articular bearing surface of internal prosthetic joint**

  ● **T84.060**   **Wear of articular bearing surface of internal prosthetic right hip joint A** 🦴, D, S 🦴

  ● **T84.061**   **Wear of articular bearing surface of internal prosthetic left hip joint A** 🦴, D, S 🦴

  ● **T84.062**   **Wear of articular bearing surface of internal prosthetic right knee joint A** 🦴, D, S 🦴

  ● **T84.063**   **Wear of articular bearing surface of internal prosthetic left knee joint A** 🦴, D, S 🦴

  ● **T84.068**   **Wear of articular bearing surface of other internal prosthetic joint A** 🦴, D, S 🦴

     Use additional code to identify the joint (Z96.6-)

  ● ■ **T84.069**   **Wear of articular bearing surface of unspecified internal prosthetic joint A** 🦴, D, S 🦴

● **T84.09**   **Other mechanical complication of internal joint prosthesis**
Prosthetic joint implant failure NOS

  ● **T84.090**   **Other mechanical complication of internal right hip prosthesis A** 🦴, D, S 🦴

  ● **T84.091**   **Other mechanical complication of internal left hip prosthesis A** 🦴, D, S 🦴

  ● **T84.092**   **Other mechanical complication of internal right knee prosthesis A** 🦴, D, S 🦴

  ● **T84.093**   **Other mechanical complication of internal left knee prosthesis A** 🦴, D, S 🦴

  ● **T84.098**   **Other mechanical complication of other internal joint prosthesis A** 🦴, D, S 🦴

     Use additional code to identify the joint (Z96.6-)

  ● ■ **T84.099**   **Other mechanical complication of unspecified internal joint prosthesis A** 🦴, D, S 🦴

● **T84.1　Mechanical complication of internal fixation device of bones of limb**

> | Excludes2 | mechanical complication of internal fixation device of bones of feet (T84.2-) |

> mechanical complication of internal fixation device of bones of fingers (T84.2-)
> mechanical complication of internal fixation device of bones of hands (T84.2-)
> mechanical complication of internal fixation device of bones of toes (T84.2-)

● **T84.11　Breakdown (mechanical) of internal fixation device of bones of limb**

　● **T84.110　Breakdown (mechanical) of internal fixation device of right humerus** A 🝰, D, S 🝰

　● **T84.111　Breakdown (mechanical) of internal fixation device of left humerus** A 🝰, D, S 🝰

　● **T84.112　Breakdown (mechanical) of internal fixation device of bone of right forearm** A 🝰, D, S 🝰

　● **T84.113　Breakdown (mechanical) of internal fixation device of bone of left forearm** A 🝰, D, S 🝰

　● **T84.114　Breakdown (mechanical) of internal fixation device of right femur** A 🝰, D, S 🝰

　● **T84.115　Breakdown (mechanical) of internal fixation device of left femur** A 🝰, D, S 🝰

　● **T84.116　Breakdown (mechanical) of internal fixation device of bone of right lower leg** A 🝰, D, S 🝰

　● **T84.117　Breakdown (mechanical) of internal fixation device of bone of left lower leg** A 🝰, D, S 🝰

　●■ **T84.119　Breakdown (mechanical) of internal fixation device of unspecified bone of limb** A 🝰, D, S 🝰

● **T84.12　Displacement of internal fixation device of bones of limb**

> Malposition of internal fixation device of bones of limb

　● **T84.120　Displacement of internal fixation device of right humerus** A 🝰, D, S 🝰

　● **T84.121　Displacement of internal fixation device of left humerus** A 🝰, D, S 🝰

　● **T84.122　Displacement of internal fixation device of bone of right forearm** A 🝰, D, S 🝰

　● **T84.123　Displacement of internal fixation device of bone of left forearm** A 🝰, D, S 🝰

　● **T84.124　Displacement of internal fixation device of right femur** A 🝰, D, S 🝰

　● **T84.125　Displacement of internal fixation device of left femur** A 🝰, D, S 🝰

● **T84.126　Displacement of internal fixation device of bone of right lower leg** A 🝰, D, S 🝰

● **T84.127　Displacement of internal fixation device of bone of left lower leg** A 🝰, D, S 🝰

●■ **T84.129　Displacement of internal fixation device of unspecified bone of limb** A 🝰, D, S 🝰

● **T84.19　Other mechanical complication of internal fixation device of bones of limb**

> Obstruction (mechanical) of internal fixation device of bones of limb
> Perforation of internal fixation device of bones of limb
> Protrusion of internal fixation device of bones of limb

　● **T84.190　Other mechanical complication of internal fixation device of right humerus** A 🝰, D, S 🝰

　● **T84.191　Other mechanical complication of internal fixation device of left humerus** A 🝰, D, S 🝰

　● **T84.192　Other mechanical complication of internal fixation device of bone of right forearm** A 🝰, D, S 🝰

　● **T84.193　Other mechanical complication of internal fixation device of bone of left forearm** A 🝰, D, S 🝰

　● **T84.194　Other mechanical complication of internal fixation device of right femur** A 🝰, D, S 🝰

　● **T84.195　Other mechanical complication of internal fixation device of left femur** A 🝰, D, S 🝰

　● **T84.196　Other mechanical complication of internal fixation device of bone of right lower leg** A 🝰, D, S 🝰

　● **T84.197　Other mechanical complication of internal fixation device of bone of left lower leg** A 🝰, D, S 🝰

　●■ **T84.199　Other mechanical complication of internal fixation device of unspecified bone of limb** A 🝰, D, S 🝰

● **T84.2　Mechanical complication of internal fixation device of other bones**

　● **T84.21　Breakdown (mechanical) of internal fixation device of other bones**

　　● **T84.210　Breakdown (mechanical) of internal fixation device of bones of hand and fingers** A 🝰, D, S 🝰

　　● **T84.213　Breakdown (mechanical) of internal fixation device of bones of foot and toes** A 🝰, D, S 🝰

　　● **T84.216　Breakdown (mechanical) of internal fixation device of vertebrae** A 🝰, D, S 🝰

　　● **T84.218　Breakdown (mechanical) of internal fixation device of other bones** A 🝰, D, S 🝰

N Newborn Age: 0　　**P** Pediatric Age: 0–17　　**M** Maternity DX: 12–55　　**A** Adult Age: 15–124　　♀ Females Only　　♂ Males Only

🝰 Complication\Comorbidity　　🝰 Major C\C　　🝰 Present on Admission Requirement　　🝰 Hospital-Acquired Condition

1683

● **T84.22   Displacement of internal fixation device of other bones**

Malposition of internal fixation device of other bones

  ● **T84.220   Displacement of internal fixation device of bones of hand and fingers A** 🗘, D, S 🗘

  ● **T84.223   Displacement of internal fixation device of bones of foot and toes A** 🗘, D, S 🗘

  ● **T84.226   Displacement of internal fixation device of vertebrae A** 🗘, D, S 🗘

  ● **T84.228   Displacement of internal fixation device of other bones A** 🗘, D, S 🗘

● **T84.29   Other mechanical complication of internal fixation device of other bones**

Obstruction (mechanical) of internal fixation device of other bones

Perforation of internal fixation device of other bones

Protrusion of internal fixation device of other bones

  ● **T84.290   Other mechanical complication of internal fixation device of bones of hand and fingers A** 🗘, D, S 🗘

  ● **T84.293   Other mechanical complication of internal fixation device of bones of foot and toes A** 🗘, D, S 🗘

  ● **T84.296   Other mechanical complication of internal fixation device of vertebrae A** 🗘, D, S 🗘

  ● **T84.298   Other mechanical complication of internal fixation device of other bones A** 🗘, D, S 🗘

● **T84.3   Mechanical complication of other bone devices, implants and grafts**

Excludes2   other complications of bone graft (T86.83-)

● **T84.31   Breakdown (mechanical) of other bone devices, implants and grafts**

  ● **T84.310   Breakdown (mechanical) of electronic bone stimulator A** 🗘, D, S 🗘

  ● **T84.318   Breakdown (mechanical) of other bone devices, implants and grafts A** 🗘, D, S 🗘

● **T84.32   Displacement of other bone devices, implants and grafts**

Malposition of other bone devices, implants and grafts

  ● **T84.320   Displacement of electronic bone stimulator A** 🗘, D, S 🗘

  ● **T84.328   Displacement of other bone devices, implants and grafts A** 🗘, D, S 🗘

● **T84.39   Other mechanical complication of other bone devices, implants and grafts**

Obstruction (mechanical) of other bone devices, implants and grafts

Perforation of other bone devices, implants and grafts

Protrusion of other bone devices, implants and grafts

  ● **T84.390   Other mechanical complication of electronic bone stimulator A** 🗘, D, S 🗘

  ● **T84.398   Other mechanical complication of other bone devices, implants and grafts A** 🗘, D, S 🗘

● **T84.4   Mechanical complication of other internal orthopedic devices, implants and grafts**

● **T84.41   Breakdown (mechanical) of other internal orthopedic devices, implants and grafts**

  ● **T84.410   Breakdown (mechanical) of muscle and tendon graft A** 🗘, D, S 🗘

  ● **T84.418   Breakdown (mechanical) of other internal orthopedic devices, implants and grafts A** 🗘, D, S 🗘

● **T84.42   Displacement of other internal orthopedic devices, implants and grafts**

Malposition of other internal orthopedic devices, implants and grafts

  ● **T84.420   Displacement of muscle and tendon graft A** 🗘, D, S 🗘

  ● **T84.428   Displacement of other internal orthopedic devices, implants and grafts A** 🗘, D, S 🗘

● **T84.49   Other mechanical complication of other internal orthopedic devices, implants and grafts**

Mechanical complication of other internal orthopedic devices, implants and grafts NOS

Obstruction (mechanical) of other internal orthopedic devices, implants and grafts

Perforation of other internal orthopedic devices, implants and grafts

Protrusion of other internal orthopedic devices, implants and grafts

  ● **T84.490   Other mechanical complication of muscle and tendon graft A** 🗘, D, S 🗘

  ● **T84.498   Other mechanical complication of other internal orthopedic devices, implants and grafts A** 🗘, D, S 🗘

● **T84.5   Infection and inflammatory reaction due to internal joint prosthesis**

Use additional code to identify infection

● ■ **T84.50   Infection and inflammatory reaction due to unspecified internal joint prosthesis A** 🗘, D, S 🗘

  ● **T84.51   Infection and inflammatory reaction due to internal right hip prosthesis A** 🗘, D, S 🗘

  ● **T84.52   Infection and inflammatory reaction due to internal left hip prosthesis A** 🗘, D, S 🗘

  ● **T84.53   Infection and inflammatory reaction due to internal right knee prosthesis A** 🗘, D, S 🗘

- ● T84.54   Infection and inflammatory reaction due to internal left knee prosthesis A 🐾, D, S 🐾
- ● T84.59   Infection and inflammatory reaction due to other internal joint prosthesis A 🐾, D, S 🐾
- ● T84.6   Infection and inflammatory reaction due to internal fixation device

  <u>Use additional</u> code to identify infection

  - ●■ T84.60   Infection and inflammatory reaction due to internal fixation device of unspecified site A 🐾, D, S 🐾, A 🐾
  - ● T84.61   Infection and inflammatory reaction due to internal fixation device of arm
    - ● T84.610   Infection and inflammatory reaction due to internal fixation device of right humerus A 🐾, D, S 🐾, A 🐾
    - ● T84.611   Infection and inflammatory reaction due to internal fixation device of left humerus A 🐾, D, S 🐾, A 🐾
    - ● T84.612   Infection and inflammatory reaction due to internal fixation device of right radius A 🐾, D, S 🐾, A 🐾
    - ● T84.613   Infection and inflammatory reaction due to internal fixation device of left radius A 🐾, D, S 🐾, A 🐾
    - ● T84.614   Infection and inflammatory reaction due to internal fixation device of right ulna A 🐾, D, S 🐾, A 🐾
    - ● T84.615   Infection and inflammatory reaction due to internal fixation device of left ulna A 🐾, D, S 🐾, A 🐾
    - ●■ T84.619   Infection and inflammatory reaction due to internal fixation device of unspecified bone of arm A 🐾, D, S 🐾, A 🐾
  - ● T84.62   Infection and inflammatory reaction due to internal fixation device of leg
    - ● T84.620   Infection and inflammatory reaction due to internal fixation device of right femur A 🐾, D, S 🐾
    - ● T84.621   Infection and inflammatory reaction due to internal fixation device of left femur A 🐾, D, S 🐾
    - ● T84.622   Infection and inflammatory reaction due to internal fixation device of right tibia A 🐾, D, S 🐾
    - ● T84.623   Infection and inflammatory reaction due to internal fixation device of left tibia A 🐾, D, S 🐾
    - ● T84.624   Infection and inflammatory reaction due to internal fixation device of right fibula A 🐾, D, S 🐾
    - ● T84.625   Infection and inflammatory reaction due to internal fixation device of left fibula A 🐾, D, S 🐾
    - ●■ T84.629   Infection and inflammatory reaction due to internal fixation device of unspecified bone of leg A 🐾, D, S 🐾

- ● T84.63   Infection and inflammatory reaction due to internal fixation device of spine A 🐾, D, S 🐾, A 🐾
- ● T84.69   Infection and inflammatory reaction due to internal fixation device of other site A 🐾, D, S 🐾, A 🐾
- ● T84.7   Infection and inflammatory reaction due to other internal orthopedic prosthetic devices, implants and grafts A 🐾, D, S 🐾, A 🐾

  <u>Use additional</u> code to identify infection

- ● T84.8   Other specified complications of internal orthopedic prosthetic devices, implants and grafts
  - ● T84.81   Embolism due to internal orthopedic prosthetic devices, implants and grafts A 🐾, D, S 🐾
  - ● T84.82   Fibrosis due to internal orthopedic prosthetic devices, implants and grafts A 🐾, D, S 🐾
  - ● T84.83   Hemorrhage due to internal orthopedic prosthetic devices, implants and grafts A 🐾, D, S 🐾
  - ● T84.84   Pain due to internal orthopedic prosthetic devices, implants and grafts A 🐾, D, S 🐾
  - ● T84.85   Stenosis due to internal orthopedic prosthetic devices, implants and grafts A 🐾, D, S 🐾
  - ● T84.86   Thrombosis due to internal orthopedic prosthetic devices, implants and grafts A 🐾, D, S 🐾
  - ● T84.89   Other specified complication of internal orthopedic prosthetic devices, implants and grafts A 🐾, D, S 🐾
- ●■ T84.9   Unspecified complication of internal orthopedic prosthetic device, implant and graft A 🐾, D, S 🐾
- ● T85   Complications of other internal prosthetic devices, implants and grafts

  | Excludes2 | failure and rejection of transplanted organs and tissue (T86.-) |

  The appropriate 7th character is to be added to each code from category T85

A	initial encounter
D	subsequent encounter
S	sequela

  - ● T85.0   Mechanical complication of ventricular intracranial (communicating) shunt
    - ● T85.01   Breakdown (mechanical) of ventricular intracranial (communicating) shunt A 🐾, D, S 🐾
    - ● T85.02   Displacement of ventricular intracranial (communicating) shunt A 🐾, D, S 🐾

      Malposition of ventricular intracranial (communicating) shunt
    - ● T85.03   Leakage of ventricular intracranial (communicating) shunt A 🐾, D, S 🐾
    - ● T85.09   Other mechanical complication of ventricular intracranial (communicating) shunt A 🐾, D, S 🐾

      Obstruction (mechanical) of ventricular intracranial (communicating) shunt

      Perforation of ventricular intracranial (communicating) shunt

      Protrusion of ventricular intracranial (communicating) shunt

● **T85.1** **Mechanical complication of implanted electronic stimulator of nervous system**

● **T85.11** **Breakdown (mechanical) of implanted electronic stimulator of nervous system**

● **T85.110** Breakdown (mechanical) of implanted electronic neurostimulator (electrode) of brain A 🔾, D, S 🔾

● **T85.111** Breakdown (mechanical) of implanted electronic neurostimulator (electrode) of peripheral nerve A 🔾, D, S 🔾

● **T85.112** Breakdown (mechanical) of implanted electronic neurostimulator (electrode) of spinal cord A 🔾, D, S 🔾

● **T85.118** Breakdown (mechanical) of other implanted electronic stimulator of nervous system A 🔾, D, S 🔾

● **T85.12** **Displacement of implanted electronic stimulator of nervous system**
Malposition of implanted electronic stimulator of nervous system

● **T85.120** Displacement of implanted electronic neurostimulator (electrode) of brain A 🔾, D, S 🔾

● **T85.121** Displacement of implanted electronic neurostimulator (electrode) of peripheral nerve A 🔾, D, S 🔾

● **T85.122** Displacement of implanted electronic neurostimulator (electrode) of spinal cord A 🔾, D, S 🔾

● **T85.128** Displacement of other implanted electronic stimulator of nervous system A 🔾, D, S 🔾

● **T85.19** **Other mechanical complication of implanted electronic stimulator of nervous system**
Leakage of implanted electronic stimulator of nervous system
Obstruction (mechanical) of implanted electronic stimulator of nervous system
Perforation of implanted electronic stimulator of nervous system
Protrusion of implanted electronic stimulator of nervous system

● **T85.190** Other mechanical complication of implanted electronic neurostimulator (electrode) of brain A 🔾, D, S 🔾

● **T85.191** Other mechanical complication of implanted electronic neurostimulator (electrode) of peripheral nerve A 🔾, D, S 🔾

● **T85.192** Other mechanical complication of implanted electronic neurostimulator (electrode) of spinal cord A 🔾, D, S 🔾

● **T85.199** Other mechanical complication of other implanted electronic stimulator of nervous system A 🔾, D, S 🔾

● **T85.2** **Mechanical complication of intraocular lens**

● **T85.21** **Breakdown (mechanical) of intraocular lens** A 🔾, D, S 🔾

● **T85.22** **Displacement of intraocular lens** A 🔾, D, S 🔾
Malposition of intraocular lens

● **T85.29** **Other mechanical complication of intraocular lens** A 🔾, D, S 🔾
Obstruction (mechanical) of intraocular lens
Perforation of intraocular lens
Protrusion of intraocular lens

● **T85.3** **Mechanical complication of other ocular prosthetic devices, implants and grafts**
Excludes2 other complications of corneal graft (T86.84-)

● **T85.31** **Breakdown (mechanical) of other ocular prosthetic devices, implants and grafts**

● **T85.310** Breakdown (mechanical) of prosthetic orbit of right eye A 🔾, D, S 🔾

● **T85.311** Breakdown (mechanical) of prosthetic orbit of left eye A 🔾, D, S 🔾

● **T85.318** Breakdown (mechanical) of other ocular prosthetic devices, implants and grafts D, S 🔾

● **T85.32** **Displacement of other ocular prosthetic devices, implants and grafts**
Malposition of other ocular prosthetic devices, implants and grafts

● **T85.320** Displacement of prosthetic orbit of right eye A 🔾, D, S 🔾

● **T85.321** Displacement of prosthetic orbit of left eye A 🔾, D, S 🔾

● **T85.328** Displacement of other ocular prosthetic devices, implants and grafts A 🔾, D, S 🔾

● **T85.39** **Other mechanical complication of other ocular prosthetic devices, implants and grafts**
Obstruction (mechanical) of other ocular prosthetic devices, implants and grafts
Perforation of other ocular prosthetic devices, implants and grafts
Protrusion of other ocular prosthetic devices, implants and grafts

● **T85.390** Other mechanical complication of prosthetic orbit of right eye A 🔾, D, S 🔾

● **T85.391** Other mechanical complication of prosthetic orbit of left eye A 🔾, D, S 🔾

● **T85.398** Other mechanical complication of other ocular prosthetic devices, implants and grafts D, S 🔾

● Unacceptable Principal Diagnosis ● Use Additional Character(s) ■ Unspecified ▶ Manifestation Code
OGCR Official Guidelines for Coding and Reporting Excludes 1 Excludes 2 Includes Use additional Code first Code also

● **T85.4 Mechanical complication of breast prosthesis and implant**

　● **T85.41 Breakdown (mechanical) of breast prosthesis and implant** A 🦠, D, S 🦠

　● **T85.42 Displacement of breast prosthesis and implant** A 🦠, D, S 🦠
　　　Malposition of breast prosthesis and implant

　● **T85.43 Leakage of breast prosthesis and implant** A 🦠, D, S 🦠

　● **T85.44 Capsular contracture of breast implant** A 🦠, D, S 🦠

　● **T85.49 Other mechanical complication of breast prosthesis and implant** A 🦠, D, S 🦠
　　　Obstruction (mechanical) of breast prosthesis and implant
　　　Perforation of breast prosthesis and implant
　　　Protrusion of breast prosthesis and implant

● **T85.5 Mechanical complication of gastrointestinal prosthetic devices, implants and grafts**

　● **T85.51 Breakdown (mechanical) of gastrointestinal prosthetic devices, implants and grafts**

　　● **T85.510 Breakdown (mechanical) of bile duct prosthesis** A 🦠, D, S 🦠

　　● **T85.511 Breakdown (mechanical) of esophageal anti-reflux device** A 🦠, D, S 🦠

　　● **T85.518 Breakdown (mechanical) of other gastrointestinal prosthetic devices, implants and grafts** A 🦠, D, S 🦠

　● **T85.52 Displacement of gastrointestinal prosthetic devices, implants and grafts**
　　　Malposition of gastrointestinal prosthetic devices, implants and grafts

　　● **T85.520 Displacement of bile duct prosthesis** A 🦠, D, S 🦠

　　● **T85.521 Displacement of esophageal anti-reflux device** A 🦠, D, S 🦠

　　● **T85.528 Displacement of other gastrointestinal prosthetic devices, implants and grafts** A 🦠, D, S 🦠

　● **T85.59 Other mechanical complication of gastrointestinal prosthetic devices, implants and**
　　　Obstruction, mechanical of gastrointestinal prosthetic devices, implants and grafts
　　　Perforation of gastrointestinal prosthetic devices, implants and grafts
　　　Protrusion of gastrointestinal prosthetic devices, implants and grafts

　　● **T85.590 Other mechanical complication of bile duct prosthesis** A 🦠, D, S 🦠

　　● **T85.591 Other mechanical complication of esophageal anti-reflux device** A 🦠, D, S 🦠

　　● **T85.598 Other mechanical complication of other gastrointestinal prosthetic devices, implants and grafts** A 🦠, D, S 🦠

● **T85.6 Mechanical complication of other specified internal and external prosthetic devices, implants and grafts**

　● **T85.61 Breakdown (mechanical) of other specified internal prosthetic devices, implants and grafts**

　　● **T85.610 Breakdown (mechanical) of epidural and subdural infusion catheter** A 🦠, D, S 🦠

　　● **T85.611 Breakdown (mechanical) of intraperitoneal dialysis catheter** A 🦠, D, S 🦠

　　　Excludes1　mechanical complication of vascular dialysis catheter (T82.4-)

　　● **T85.612 Breakdown (mechanical) of permanent sutures** A 🦠, D, S 🦠

　　　Excludes1　mechanical complication of permanent (wire) suture used in bone repair (T84.1-T84.2)

　　● **T85.613 Breakdown (mechanical) of artificial skin graft and decellularized allodermis** A 🦠, D, S 🦠
　　　Failure of artificial skin graft and decellularized allodermis
　　　Non-adherence of artificial skin graft and decellularized allodermis
　　　Poor incorporation of artificial skin graft and decellularized allodermis
　　　Shearing of artificial skin graft and decellularized allodermis

　　● **T85.614 Breakdown (mechanical) of insulin pump** A 🦠, D, S 🦠

　　● **T85.618 Breakdown (mechanical) of other specified internal prosthetic devices, implants and grafts** A 🦠, D, S 🦠

　● **T85.62 Displacement of other specified internal prosthetic devices, implants and grafts**
　　　Malposition of other specified internal prosthetic devices, implants and grafts

　　● **T85.620 Displacement of epidural and subdural infusion catheter** A 🦠, D, S 🦠

　　● **T85.621 Displacement of intraperitoneal dialysis catheter** A 🦠, D, S 🦠

　　　Excludes1　mechanical complication of vascular dialysis catheter (T82.4-)

● T85.622 Displacement of permanent sutures A 🔗, D, S 🔗

> Excludes1 mechanical complication of permanent (wire) suture used in bone repair (T84.1-T84.2)

● T85.623 Displacement of artificial skin graft and decellularized allodermis A 🔗, D, S 🔗
> Dislodgement of artificial skin graft and decellularized allodermis
> Displacement of artificial skin graft and decellularized allodermis

● T85.624 Displacement of insulin pump A 🔗, D, S 🔗

● T85.628 Displacement of other specified internal prosthetic devices, implants and grafts A 🔗, D, S 🔗

● T85.63 Leakage of other specified internal prosthetic devices, implants and grafts

● T85.630 Leakage of epidural and subdural infusion catheter A 🔗, D, S 🔗

● T85.631 Leakage of intraperitoneal dialysis catheter A 🔗, D, S 🔗

> Excludes1 mechanical complication of vascular dialysis catheter (T82.4)

● T85.633 Leakage of insulin pump A 🔗, D, S 🔗

● T85.638 Leakage of other specified internal prosthetic devices, implants and grafts A 🔗, D, S 🔗

● T85.69 Other mechanical complication of other specified internal prosthetic devices, implants and grafts
> Obstruction, mechanical of other specified internal prosthetic devices, implants and grafts
> Perforation of other specified internal prosthetic devices, implants and grafts
> Protrusion of other specified internal prosthetic devices, implants and grafts

● T85.690 Other mechanical complication of epidural and subdural infusion catheter A 🔗, D, S 🔗

● T85.691 Other mechanical complication of intraperitoneal dialysis catheter A 🔗, D, S 🔗

> Excludes1 mechanical complication of vascular dialysis catheter (T82.4)

● T85.692 Other mechanical complication of permanent sutures A 🔗, D, S 🔗

> Excludes1 mechanical complication of permanent (wire) suture used in bone repair (T84.1-T84.2)

● T85.693 Other mechanical complication of artificial skin graft and decellularized allodermis A 🔗, D, S 🔗

● T85.694 Other mechanical complication of insulin pump A 🔗, D, S 🔗

● T85.698 Other mechanical complication of other specified internal prosthetic devices, implants and grafts A 🔗, D, S 🔗
> Mechanical complication of nonabsorbable surgical material NOS

● T85.7 Infection and inflammatory reaction due to other internal prosthetic devices, implants and grafts
> Use additional code to identify infection

● T85.71 Infection and inflammatory reaction due to peritoneal dialysis catheter A 🔗, D, S 🔗

● T85.72 Infection and inflammatory reaction due to insulin pump A 🔗, D, S 🔗

● T85.79 Infection and inflammatory reaction due to other internal prosthetic devices, implants and grafts A 🔗, D, S 🔗

● T85.8 Other specified complications of internal prosthetic devices, implants and grafts, not elsewhere classified

● T85.81 Embolism due to internal prosthetic devices, implants and grafts, not elsewhere classified A 🔗, D, S 🔗

● T85.82 Fibrosis due to internal prosthetic devices, implants and grafts, not elsewhere classified A 🔗, D, S 🔗

● T85.83 Hemorrhage due to internal prosthetic devices, implants and grafts, not elsewhere classified A 🔗, D, S 🔗

● T85.84 Pain due to internal prosthetic devices, implants and grafts, not elsewhere classified A 🔗, D, S 🔗

● T85.85 Stenosis due to internal prosthetic devices, implants and grafts, not elsewhere classified A 🔗, D, S 🔗

● T85.86 Thrombosis due to internal prosthetic devices, implants and grafts, not elsewhere classified A 🔗, D, S 🔗

● T85.89 Other specified complication of internal prosthetic devices, implants and grafts, not elsewhere classified A 🔗, D, S 🔗

●■ T85.9 Unspecified complication of internal prosthetic device, implant and graft D, S 🔗
> Complication of internal prosthetic device, implant and graft NOS

● Unacceptable Principal Diagnosis   ● Use Additional Character(s)   ■ Unspecified   ▶ Manifestation Code

OGCR Official Guidelines for Coding and Reporting   Excludes 1   Excludes 2   Includes   Use additional   Code first   Code also

● **T86**   **Complications of transplanted organs and tissue**

Use additional code to identify other transplant complications, such as:
graft-versus-host disease (D89.81-)
malignancy associated with organ transplant (C80.2)
post-transplant lymphoproliferative disorders (PTLD) (D47.Z1)

● **T86.0**   **Complications of bone marrow transplant**

◻ **T86.00**   Unspecified complication of bone marrow transplant 🦠

T86.01   Bone marrow transplant rejection 🦠

T86.02   Bone marrow transplant failure 🦠

T86.03   Bone marrow transplant infection 🦠

T86.09   Other complications of bone marrow transplant 🦠

● **T86.1**   **Complications of kidney transplant**

◻ **T86.10**   Unspecified complication of kidney transplant 🦠

T86.11   Kidney transplant rejection 🦠

T86.12   Kidney transplant failure 🦠

T86.13   Kidney transplant infection 🦠

Use additional code to specify infection

T86.19   Other complication of kidney transplant 🦠

OGCR   Section I.C.19.g.3.

> Organ Transplant Complications
>
> Transplant Complications
>
> (a) Transplant complications other than kidney
>
> Codes under category T86, Complications of transplanted organs and tissues, are for use for both complications and rejection of transplanted organs. A transplant complication code is only assigned if the complication affects the function of the transplanted organ. Two codes are required to fully describe a transplant complication: the appropriate code from category T86 and a secondary code that identifies the complication.
>
> Pre-existing conditions or conditions that develop after the transplant are not coded as complications unless they affect the function of the transplanted organs.
>
> See I.C.21 for transplant organ removal status
>
> See I.C.2 for malignant neoplasm associated with transplanted organ.

● **T86.2**   **Complications of heart transplant**

| Excludes1 | complication of:
artificial heart device (T82.5)
heart-lung transplant (T86.3)

◻ **T86.20**   Unspecified complication of heart transplant 🦠

T86.21   Heart transplant rejection 🦠

T86.22   Heart transplant failure 🦠

T86.23   Heart transplant infection 🦠

Use additional code to specify infection

● **T86.29**   Other complications of heart transplant

T86.290   Cardiac allograft vasculopathy 🦠

| Excludes1 | atherosclerosis of coronary arteries (I25.75-, I25.76-, I25.81-)

T86.298   Other complications of heart transplant 🦠

● **T86.3**   **Complications of heart-lung transplant**

◻ **T86.30**   Unspecified complication of heart-lung transplant 🦠

T86.31   Heart-lung transplant rejection 🦠

T86.32   Heart-lung transplant failure 🦠

T86.33   Heart-lung transplant infection 🦠

Use additional code to specify infection

T86.39   Other complications of heart-lung transplant 🦠

● **T86.4**   **Complications of liver transplant**

◻ **T86.40**   Unspecified complication of liver transplant 🦠

T86.41   Liver transplant rejection 🦠

T86.42   Liver transplant failure 🦠

T86.43   Liver transplant infection 🦠

Use additional code to identify infection, such as:
Cytomegalovirus (CMV) infection (B25.-)

T86.49   Other complications of liver transplant 🦠

● **T86.5**   **Complications of stem cell transplant**

Complications from stem cells from peripheral blood
Complications from stem cells from umbilical cord

● **T86.8**   **Complications of other transplanted organs and tissues**

● **T86.81**   **Complications of lung transplant**

| Excludes1 | complication of heart-lung transplant (T86.3-)

T86.810   Lung transplant rejection 🦠

T86.811   Lung transplant failure 🦠

T86.812   Lung transplant infection 🦠

Use additional code to specify infection

T86.818   Other complications of lung transplant 🦠

◻ **T86.819**   Unspecified complication of lung transplant 🦠

● **T86.82**   **Complications of skin graft (allograft) (autograft)**

| Excludes2 | complication of artificial skin graft (T85.64)

T86.820   Skin graft (allograft) rejection 🦠

T86.821   Skin graft (allograft) (autograft) failure 🦠

T86.822   Skin graft (allograft) (autograft) infection 🦠

Use additional code to specify infection

T86.828   Other complications of skin graft (allograft) (autograft) 🦠

● ◻ **T86.829**   Unspecified complication of skin graft (allograft) (autograft) 🦠

N   Newborn Age: 0   **P**   Pediatric Age: 0–17   **M**   Maternity DX: 12–55   **A**   Adult Age: 15–124   ♀   Females Only   ♂   Males Only

🦠   Complication\Comorbidity   🦠   Major C\C   🦠   Present on Admission Requirement   🦠   Hospital-Acquired Condition

CHAPTER 19 (S00-T88)

- ● T86.83   **Complications of bone graft**
  - Excludes2   mechanical complications of bone graft (T84.3-)
  - T86.830   **Bone graft rejection** 🖝
  - T86.831   **Bone graft failure** 🖝
  - T86.832   **Bone graft infection** 🖝
    - Use additional code to specify infection
  - T86.838   **Other complications of bone graft** 🖝
  - ◼ T86.839   **Unspecified complication of bone graft** 🖝
- ● T86.84   **Complications of corneal transplant**
  - Excludes2   mechanical complications of corneal graft (T85.3-)
  - T86.840   **Corneal transplant rejection** 🖝
  - T86.841   **Corneal transplant failure** 🖝
  - T86.842   **Corneal transplant infection** 🖝
    - Use additional code to specify infection
  - T86.848   **Other complications of corneal transplant** 🖝
  - ◼ T86.849   **Unspecified complication of corneal transplant** 🖝
- ● T86.85   **Complication of intestine transplant**
  - T86.850   **Intestine transplant rejection** 🖝
  - T86.851   **Intestine transplant failure** 🖝
  - T86.852   **Intestine transplant infection** 🖝
    - Use additional code to specify infection
  - T86.858   **Other complications of intestine transplant** 🖝
  - ◼ T86.859   **Unspecified complication of intestine transplant** 🖝
- ● T86.89   **Complications of other transplanted tissue**
  - Transplant failure or rejection of pancreas
  - T86.890   **Other transplanted tissue rejection** 🖝
  - T86.891   **Other transplanted tissue failure** 🖝
  - T86.892   **Other transplanted tissue infection** 🖝
    - Use additional code to specify infection
  - T86.898   **Other complications of other transplanted tissue** 🖝
  - ◼ T86.899   **Unspecified complication of other transplanted tissue** 🖝
- ● T86.9   **Complication of unspecified transplanted organ and tissue**
  - ◼ T86.90   **Unspecified complication of unspecified transplanted organ and tissue** 🖝
  - ◼ T86.91   **Unspecified transplanted organ and tissue rejection** 🖝
  - ◼ T86.92   **Unspecified transplanted organ and tissue failure** 🖝
  - ◼ T86.93   **Unspecified transplanted organ and tissue infection** 🖝
    - Use additional code to specify infection
  - ◼ T86.99   **Other complications of unspecified transplanted organ and tissue** 🖝

- ● T87   **Complications peculiar to reattachment and amputation**
  - ● T87.0   **Complications of reattached (part of) upper extremity**
    - ● T87.0X   **Complications of reattached (part of) upper extremity**
      - T87.0X1   **Complications of reattached (part of) right upper extremity** 🖝
      - T87.0X2   **Complications of reattached (part of) left upper extremity** 🖝
      - ◼ T87.0X9   **Complications of reattached (part of) unspecified upper extremity** 🖝
  - ● T87.1   **Complications of reattached (part of) lower extremity**
    - ● T87.1X   **Complications of reattached (part of) lower extremity**
      - T87.1X1   **Complications of reattached (part of) right lower extremity** 🖝
      - T87.1X2   **Complications of reattached (part of) left lower extremity** 🖝
      - ◼ T87.1X9   **Complications of reattached (part of) unspecified lower extremity** 🖝
  - T87.2   **Complications of other reattached body part** 🖝
  - ● T87.3   **Neuroma of amputation stump**
    - ● ◼ T87.30   **Neuroma of amputation stump, unspecified extremity**
    - T87.31   **Neuroma of amputation stump, right upper extremity**
    - T87.32   **Neuroma of amputation stump, left upper extremity**
    - T87.33   **Neuroma of amputation stump, right lower extremity**
    - T87.34   **Neuroma of amputation stump, left lower extremity**
  - ● T87.4   **Infection of amputation stump**
    - ◼ T87.40   **Infection of amputation stump, unspecified extremity** 🖝
    - T87.41   **Infection of amputation stump, right upper extremity** 🖝
    - T87.42   **Infection of amputation stump, left upper extremity** 🖝
    - T87.43   **Infection of amputation stump, right lower extremity** 🖝
    - T87.44   **Infection of amputation stump, left lower extremity** 🖝
  - ● T87.5   **Necrosis of amputation stump**
    - ◼ T87.50   **Necrosis of amputation stump, unspecified extremity**
    - T87.51   **Necrosis of amputation stump, right upper extremity**
    - T87.52   **Necrosis of amputation stump, left upper extremity**
    - T87.53   **Necrosis of amputation stump, right lower extremity**
    - T87.54   **Necrosis of amputation stump, left lower extremity**

● Unacceptable Principal Diagnosis   ● Use Additional Character(s)   ◼ Unspecified   ▶ Manifestation Code

OGCR Official Guidelines for Coding and Reporting | Excludes 1 | | Excludes 2 | | Includes | | Use additional | | Code first | | Code also |

● **T87.8   Other complications of amputation stump**

  ● **T87.81   Dehiscence of amputation stump**

  ● **T87.89   Other complications of amputation stump**
     Amputation stump contracture
     Amputation stump contracture of next
        proximal joint
     Amputation stump flexion
     Amputation stump edema
     Amputation stump hematoma

     | Excludes2 | phantom limb syndrome
             (G54.6-G54.7)

  ■ **T87.9   Unspecified complications of amputation stump**

● **T88   Other complications of surgical and medical care, not elsewhere classified**

   | Excludes2 | complication following infusion, transfusion
         and therapeutic injection (T80.-)
         complication following procedure NEC
           (T81.-)
         complications of anesthesia in labor and
           delivery (O74.-)
         complications of anesthesia in pregnancy
           (O29.-)
         complications of anesthesia in puerperium
           (O89.-)
         complications of devices, implants and
           grafts (T82-T85)
         complications of obstetric surgery and
           procedure (O75.4)
         dermatitis due to drugs and medicaments
           (L23.3, L24.4, L25.1, L27.0-L27.1)
         poisoning and toxic effects of drugs and
           chemicals (T36-T65 with fifth or sixth
           character 1-4 or 6)
         specified complications classified elsewhere

   The appropriate 7th character is to be added to each code
     from category T88

     | A   initial encounter
     | D   subsequent encounter
     | S   sequela |

● **T88.0   Infection following immunization A** 🔖, D, S 🔖
     Sepsis following immunization

● **T88.1   Other complications following immunization, not elsewhere classified A** 🔖, D, S 🔖
     Generalized vaccinia
     Rash following immunization

     | Excludes1 | vaccinia not from vaccine (B08.011)
     | Excludes2 | anaphylactic shock due to serum
             (T80.5-)
          other serum reactions (T80.6-)
          postimmunization arthropathy
            (M02.2)
          postimmunization encephalitis
            (G04.02)
          postimmunization fever (R50.83)

●● **T88.2   Shock due to anesthesia A** 🔖, D, S 🔖

     Use additional code for adverse effect, if
        applicable, to identify drug (T41.- with fifth
        or sixth character 5)

     | Excludes1 | complications of anesthesia (in):
            labor and delivery (O74.-)
            pregnancy (O29.-)
            puerperium (O89.-)
            postprocedural shock NOS
              (T81.1-)

●● **T88.3   Malignant hyperthermia due to anesthesia A** 🔖, D, S 🔖

     Use additional code for adverse effect, if
        applicable, to identify drug (T41.- with fifth
        or sixth character 5)

● **T88.4   Failed or difficult intubation** D, S 🔖

● **T88.5   Other complications of anesthesia**

     Use additional code for adverse effect, if
        applicable, to identify drug (T41.- with fifth
        or sixth character 5)

    T88.51   Hypothermia following anesthesia D, S 🔖

    T88.52   Failed moderate sedation during procedure D, S 🔖
       Failed conscious sedation during
          procedure

       | Excludes2 | personal history of failed
              moderate sedation
              (Z92.83)

    T88.59   Other complications of anesthesia D, S 🔖

●● **T88.6   Anaphylactic reaction due to adverse effect of correct drug or medicament properly administered A** 🔖, D, S 🔖
     Anaphylactic shock due to adverse effect of
        correct drug or medicament properly
        administered
     Anaphylactoid reaction NOS

     Use additional code for adverse effect, if
        applicable, to identify drug (T41.- with fifth
        or sixth character 5)

     | Excludes1 | anaphylactic reaction due to serum
             (T80.5-)
          anaphylactic shock or reaction due to
            adverse food reaction (T78.0-)

●●■ **T88.7   Unspecified adverse effect of drug or medicament** D, S 🔖
     Drug hypersensitivity NOS
     Drug reaction NOS

     Use additional code for adverse effect, if
        applicable, to identify drug (T41.- with fifth
        or sixth character 5)

     | Excludes1 | specified adverse effects of drugs
             and medicaments (A00-R94 and
             T80-T88.6, T88.8)

● **T88.8   Other specified complications of surgical and medical care, not elsewhere classified** D, S 🔖

     Use additional code to identify the complication

●■ **T88.9   Complication of surgical and medical care, unspecified** D, S 🔖

N   Newborn Age: 0   **P**   Pediatric Age: 0–17   **M**   Maternity DX: 12–55   **A**   Adult Age: 15–124   ♀   Females Only   ♂   Males Only

🔖   Complication\Comorbidity   🔖   Major C\C   🔖   Present on Admission Requirement   🔖   Hospital-Acquired Condition

1691

OGCR See Guidelines, Section I.20.

CHAPTER 20

EXTERNAL CAUSES OF MORBIDITY
(V00-Y99)

Note: This chapter permits the classification of environmental events and circumstances as the cause of injury, and other adverse effects. Where a code from this section is applicable, it is intended that it shall be used secondary to a code from another chapter of the Classification indicating the nature of the condition. Most often, the condition will be classifiable to Chapter 19, Injury, poisoning and certain other consequences of external causes (S00-T88). Other conditions that may be stated to be due to external causes are classified in Chapters I to XVIII. For these conditions, codes from Chapter 20 should be used to provide additional information as to the cause of the condition.

This chapter contains the following blocks:

V00-X58	Accidents
V00-V99	Transport accidents
V00-V09	Pedestrian injured in transport accident
V10-V19	Pedal cycle rider injured in transport accident
V20-V29	Motorcycle rider injured in transport accident
V30-V39	Occupant of three-wheeled motor vehicle injured in transport accident
V40-V49	Car occupant injured in transport accident
V50-V59	Occupant of pick-up truck or van injured in transport accident
V60-V69	Occupant of heavy transport vehicle injured in transport accident
V70-V79	Bus occupant injured in transport accident
V80-V89	Other land transport accidents
V90-V94	Water transport accidents
V95-V97	Air and space transport accidents
V98-V99	Other and unspecified transport accidents
W00-X58	Other external causes of accidental injury
W00-W19	Slipping, tripping, stumbling and falls
W20-W49	Exposure to inanimate mechanical forces
W50-W64	Exposure to animate mechanical forces
W65-W74	Accidental non-transport drowning and submersion
W85-W99	Exposure to electric current, radiation and extreme ambient air temperature and pressure
X00-X08	Exposure to smoke, fire and flames
X10-X19	Contact with heat and hot substances
X30-X39	Exposure to forces of nature
X52, X58	Accidental exposure to other specified factors
X71-X83	Intentional self-harm
X92-Y08	Assault
Y21-Y33	Event of undetermined intent
Y35-Y38	Legal intervention, operations of war, military operations, and terrorism
Y62-Y84	Complications of medical and surgical care
Y62-Y69	Misadventures to patients during surgical and medical care
Y70-Y82	Medical devices associated with adverse incidents in diagnostic and therapeutic use
Y83-Y84	Surgical and other medical procedures as the cause of abnormal reaction of the patient, or of later complication, without mention of misadventure at the time of the procedure
Y90-Y99	Supplementary factors related to causes of morbidity classified elsewhere

ACCIDENTS (V00-X58)

TRANSPORT ACCIDENTS (V00-V99)

Note: This section is structured in 12 groups. Those relating to land transport accidents (V01- V89) reflect the victim's mode of transport and are subdivided to identify the victim's 'counterpart' or the type of event. The vehicle of which the injured person is an occupant is identified in the first two characters since it is seen as the most important factor to identify for prevention purposes. A transport accident is one in which the vehicle involved must be moving or running or in use for transport purposes at the time of the accident.

Use additional code to identify:
Airbag injury (W22.1)
Type of street or road (Y92.4-)
Use of cellular telephone and other electronic equipment at the time of the transport accident (Y93.C-)

Excludes1 agricultural vehicles in stationary use or maintenance (W31.-)
assault by crashing of motor vehicle (Y03.-)
automobile or motor cycle in stationary use or maintenance - code to type of accident
crashing of motor vehicle, undetermined intent (Y32)
intentional self-harm by crashing of motor vehicle (X82)

Excludes2 transport accidents due to cataclysm (X34-X38)

Note: Definitions of transport vehicles:

(a) A transport accident is any accident involving a device designed primarily for, or used at the time primarily for, conveying persons or good from one place to another.

(b) A public highway [trafficway] or street is the entire width between property lines (or other boundary lines) of land open to the public as a matter of right or custom for purposes of moving persons or property from one place to another. A roadway is that part of the public highway designed, improved and customarily used for vehicular traffic.

(c) A traffic accident is any vehicle accident occurring on the public highway [i.e. originating on, terminating on, or involving a vehicle partially on the highway]. A vehicle accident is assumed to have occurred on the public highway unless another place is specified, except in the case of accidents involving only off-road motor vehicles, which are classified as nontraffic accidents unless the contrary is stated.

(d) A nontraffic accident is any vehicle accident that occurs entirely in any place other than a public highway.

(e) A pedestrian is any person involved in an accident who was not at the time of the accident riding in or on a motor vehicle, railway train, streetcar or animal-drawn or other vehicle, or on a pedal cycle or animal. This includes, a person changing a tire or working on a parked car. It also includes the use of a pedestrian conveyance such as a baby carriage, ice-skates, roller skates, a skateboard, nonmotorized or motorized wheelchair, motorized mobility scooter, or nonmotorized scooter.

(f) A driver is an occupant of a transport vehicle who is operating or intending to operate it.

● Unacceptable Principal Diagnosis ● Use Additional Character(s) ■ Unspecified ▶ Manifestation Code

OGCR Official Guidelines for Coding and Reporting | Excludes 1 | Excludes 2 | Includes | Use additional | Code first | Code also

(g) A passenger is any occupant of a transport vehicle other than the driver, except a person traveling on the outside of the vehicle.

(h) A person on the outside of a vehicle is any person being transported by a vehicle but not occupying the space normally reserved for the driver or passengers, or the space intended for the transport of property. This includes the body, bumper, fender, roof, running board or step of a vehicle.

(i) A pedal cycle is any land transport vehicle operated solely by nonmotorized pedals including a bicycle or tricycle.

(j) A pedal cyclist is any person riding a pedal cycle or in a sidecar or trailer attached to a pedal cycle.

(k) A motorcycle is a two-wheeled motor vehicle with one or two riding saddles and sometimes with a third wheel for the support of a sidecar. The sidecar is considered part of the motorcycle.

(l) A motorcycle rider is any person riding a motorcycle or in a sidecar or trailer attached to the motorcycle.

(m) A three-wheeled motor vehicle is a motorized tricycle designed primarily for on-road use. This includes a motor-driven tricycle, a motorized rickshaw, or a three-wheeled motor car.

(n) A car [automobile] is a four-wheeled motor vehicle designed primarily for carrying up to 7 persons. A trailer being towed by the car is considered part of the car.

(o) A pick-up truck or van is a four or six-wheeled motor vehicle designed for carrying passengers as well as property or cargo weighing less than the local limit for classification as a heavy goods vehicle, and not requiring a special driver's license. This includes a minivan and a sport-utility vehicle (SUV).

(p) A heavy transport vehicle is a motor vehicle designed primarily for carrying property, meeting local criteria for classification as a heavy goods vehicle in terms of weight and requiring a special driver's license.

(q) A bus (coach) is a motor vehicle designed or adapted primarily for carrying more than 10 passengers, and requiring a special driver's license.

(r) A railway train or railway vehicle is any device, with or without freight or passenger cars coupled to it, designed for traffic on a railway track. This includes subterranean (subways) or elevated trains.

(s) A streetcar is a device designed and used primarily for transporting passengers within a municipality, running on rails, usually subject to normal traffic control signals, and operated principally on a right-of-way that forms part of the roadway. This includes a tram or trolley that runs on rails. A trailer being towed by a streetcar is considered part of the streetcar.

(t) A special vehicle mainly used on industrial premises is a motor vehicle designed primarily for use within the buildings and premises of industrial or commercial establishments. This includes battery-powered trucks, forklifts, coal-cars in a coal mine, logging cars and trucks used in mines or quarries.

(u) A special vehicle mainly used in agriculture is a motor vehicle designed specifically for use in farming and agriculture (horticulture), to work the land, tend and harvest crops and transport materials on the farm. This includes harvesters, farm machinery and tractor and trailers.

(v) A special construction vehicle is a motor vehicle designed specifically for use on construction and demolition sites. This includes bulldozers, diggers, earth levellers, dump trucks, backhoes, front-end loaders, pavers, and mechanical shovels.

(w) A special all-terrain vehicle is a motor vehicle of special design to enable it to negotiate over rough or soft terrain, snow or sand. This includes snow mobiles, all-terrain vehicles (ATV), and dune buggies. It does not include passenger vehicle designated as sport utility vehicles. (SUV)

(w) A watercraft is any device designed for transporting passengers or goods on water. This includes motor or sail boats, ships, and hovercraft.

(x) An aircraft is any device for transporting passengers or goods in the air. This includes hot-air balloons, gliders, helicopters and airplanes.

(y) A military vehicle is any motorized vehicle operating on a public roadway owned by the military and being operated by a member of the military.

PEDESTRIAN INJURED IN TRANSPORT ACCIDENT (V00-V09)

Includes	person changing tire on transport vehicle person examining engine of vehicle broken down in (on side of) road
Excludes1	fall due to non-transport collision with other person (W03) pedestrian on foot falling (slipping) on ice and snow (W00.-) struck or bumped by another person (W51)

● **V00 Pedestrian conveyance accident**

Use additional place of occurrence and activity external cause codes, if known (Y92.-, Y93.-)

Excludes1	collision with another person without fall (W51) fall due to person on foot colliding with another person on foot (W03) fall from non-moving wheelchair, nonmotorized scooter and motorized mobility scooter without collision (W05.-) pedestrian (conveyance) collision with other land transport vehicle (V01-V09) pedestrian on foot falling (slipping) on ice and snow (W00.-)

The appropriate 7th character is to be added to each code from category V00

A	initial encounter
D	subsequent encounter
S	sequela

● **V00.0 Pedestrian on foot injured in collision with pedestrian conveyance**

    ● **V00.01 Pedestrian on foot injured in collision with roller-skater** S 🔖

    ● **V00.02 Pedestrian on foot injured in collision with skateboarder** S 🔖

    ● **V00.09 Pedestrian on foot injured in collision with other pedestrian conveyance** S 🔖

● **V00.1 Rolling-type pedestrian conveyance accident**

Excludes1	accident with babystroller (V00.82-) accident with wheelchair (powered) (V00.81-) accident with motorized mobility scooter (V00.83-)

    ● **V00.11 In-line roller-skate accident**

        ● **V00.111 Fall from in-line roller-skates** A, D, S 🔖

        ● **V00.112 In-line roller-skater colliding with stationary object** A, D, S 🔖

● **V00.118 Other in-line roller-skate accident** A, D, S

> **Excludes1** roller-skater collision with other land transport vehicle (V01-V09 with 5th character 1)

● **V00.12 Non-in-line roller-skate accident**

● **V00.121 Fall from non-in-line roller-skates** A, D, S

● **V00.122 Non-in-line roller-skater colliding with stationary object** A, D, S

● **V00.128 Other non-in-line roller-skating accident** A, D, S

> **Excludes1** roller-skater collision with other land transport vehicle (V01-V09 with 5th character 1)

● **V00.13 Skateboard accident**

● **V00.131 Fall from skateboard** A, D, S

● **V00.132 Skateboarder colliding with stationary object** A, D, S

● **V00.138 Other skateboard accident** A, D, S

> **Excludes1** skateboarder collision with other land transport vehicle (V01-V09 with 5th character 2)

● **V00.14 Scooter (nonmotorized) accident**

> **Excludes1** motorscooter accident (V20-V29)

● **V00.141 Fall from scooter (nonmotorized)** A, D, S

● **V00.142 Scooter (nonmotorized) colliding with stationary object** A, D, S

● **V00.148 Other scooter (nonmotorized) accident** A, D, S

> **Excludes1** scooter (non-motorized) collision with other land transport vehicle (V01-V09 with fifth character 9)

● **V00.15 Heelies accident**
Rolling shoe
Wheeled shoe
Wheelies accident

● **V00.151 Fall from heelies** A, D, S

● **V00.152 Heelies colliding with stationary object** A, D, S

● **V00.158 Other heelies accident** A, D, S

● **V00.18 Accident on other rolling-type pedestrian conveyance**

● **V00.181 Fall from other rolling-type pedestrian conveyance** S

● **V00.182 Pedestrian on other rolling-type pedestrian conveyance colliding with stationary object** S

● **V00.188 Other accident on other rolling-type pedestrian conveyance** S

● **V00.2 Gliding-type pedestrian conveyance accident**

● **V00.21 Ice-skates accident**

● **V00.211 Fall from ice-skates** S

● **V00.212 Ice-skater colliding with stationary object** S

● **V00.218 Other ice-skates accident** S

> **Excludes1** ice-skater collision with other land transport vehicle (V01-V09 with 5th digit 9)

● **V00.22 Sled accident**

● **V00.221 Fall from sled** S

● **V00.222 Sledder colliding with stationary object** S

● **V00.228 Other sled accident** S

> **Excludes1** sled collision with other land transport vehicle (V01-V09 with 5th digit 9)

● **V00.28 Other gliding-type pedestrian conveyance accident**

● **V00.281 Fall from other gliding-type pedestrian conveyance** S

● **V00.282 Pedestrian on other gliding-type pedestrian conveyance colliding with stationary object** S

● **V00.288 Other accident on other gliding-type pedestrian conveyance** S

> **Excludes1** gliding-type pedestrian conveyance collision with other land transport vehicle (V01-V09 with 5th digit 9)

● **V00.3 Flat-bottomed pedestrian conveyance accident**

● **V00.31 Snowboard accident**

● **V00.311 Fall from snowboard** A, D, S

● **V00.312 Snowboarder colliding with stationary object** A, D, S

● **V00.318 Other snowboard accident** A, D, S

> **Excludes1** snowboarder collision with other land transport vehicle (V01-V09 with 5th digit 9)

CHAPTER 20 (V01-Y99)

● Unacceptable Principal Diagnosis ● Use Additional Character(s) ■ Unspecified ▶ Manifestation Code
OGCR Official Guidelines for Coding and Reporting Excludes 1 Excludes 2 Includes Use additional Code first Code also

● **V00.32 Snow-ski accident**
  ● **V00.321 Fall from snow-skis** A, D, S 🔖
  ● **V00.322 Snow-skier colliding with stationary object** A, D, S 🔖
  ● **V00.328 Other snow-ski accident** A, D, S 🔖

    | Excludes1 | snow-skier collision with other land transport vehicle (V01-V09 with 5th digit 9) |

● **V00.38 Other flat-bottomed pedestrian conveyance accident**
  ● **V00.381 Fall from other flat-bottomed pedestrian conveyance** S 🔖
  ● **V00.382 Pedestrian on other flat-bottomed pedestrian conveyance colliding with stationary object** S 🔖
  ● **V00.388 Other accident on other flat-bottomed pedestrian conveyance** S 🔖

● **V00.8 Accident on other pedestrian conveyance**
  ● **V00.81 Accident with wheelchair (powered)**
    ● **V00.811 Fall from moving wheelchair (powered)** S 🔖

      | Excludes1 | fall from non-moving wheelchair (W05.0) |

    ● **V00.812 Wheelchair (powered) colliding with stationary object** S 🔖
    ● **V00.818 Other accident with wheelchair (powered)** S 🔖
  ● **V00.82 Accident with babystroller**
    ● **V00.821 Fall from babystroller** S 🔖
    ● **V00.822 Babystroller colliding with stationary object** S 🔖
    ● **V00.828 Other accident with babystroller** S 🔖
  ● **V00.83 Accident with motorized mobility scooter**
    ● **V00.831 Fall from motorized mobility scooter**

      | Excludes1 | fall from non-moving motorized mobility scooter (W05.2) |

    ● **V00.832 Motorized mobility scooter colliding with stationary object**
    ● **V00.838 Other accident with motorized mobility scooter**

● **V00.89 Accident on other pedestrian conveyance**
  ● **V00.891 Fall from other pedestrian conveyance** S 🔖
  ● **V00.892 Pedestrian on other pedestrian conveyance colliding with stationary object** S 🔖
  ● **V00.898 Other accident on other pedestrian conveyance** S 🔖

    | Excludes1 | other pedestrian (conveyance) collision with other land transport vehicle (V01-V09 with 5th digit 9) |

● **V01 Pedestrian injured in collision with pedal cycle**

  The appropriate 7th character is to be added to each code from category V01

A	initial encounter
D	subsequent encounter
S	sequela

  ● **V01.0 Pedestrian injured in collision with pedal cycle in nontraffic accident**
    ● **V01.00 Pedestrian on foot injured in collision with pedal cycle in nontraffic accident** A, D, S 🔖

      Pedestrian NOS injured in collision with pedal cycle in nontraffic accident

    ● **V01.01 Pedestrian on roller-skates injured in collision with pedal cycle in nontraffic accident** A, D, S 🔖
    ● **V01.02 Pedestrian on skateboard injured in collision with pedal cycle in nontraffic accident** A, D, S 🔖
    ● **V01.09 Pedestrian with other conveyance injured in collision with pedal cycle in nontraffic accident** A, D, S 🔖

      Pedestrian with babystroller injured in collision with pedal cycle in nontraffic accident

      Pedestrian in wheelchair (powered) injured in collision with pedal cycle in nontraffic accident

      Pedestrian in motorized mobility scooter injured in collision with pedal cycle in nontraffic accident

      Pedestrian on ice-skates injured in collision with pedal cycle in nontraffic accident

      Pedestrian on nonmotorized scooter injured in collision with pedal cycle in nontraffic accident

      Pedestrian on sled injured in collision with pedal cycle in nontraffic accident

      Pedestrian on snowboard injured in collision with pedal cycle in nontraffic accident

      Pedestrian on snow-skis injured in collision with pedal cycle in nontraffic accident

CHAPTER 20 (V01-Y99)

CHAPTER 20 (V01-Y99)

● **V01.1** **Pedestrian injured in collision with pedal cycle in traffic accident**

  ● **V01.10** **Pedestrian on foot injured in collision with pedal cycle in traffic accident** A, D, S ✎

     Pedestrian NOS injured in collision with pedal cycle in traffic accident

  ● **V01.11** **Pedestrian on roller-skates injured in collision with pedal cycle in traffic accident** A, D, S ✎

  ● **V01.12** **Pedestrian on skateboard injured in collision with pedal cycle in traffic accident** A, D, S ✎

  ● **V01.19** **Pedestrian with other conveyance injured in collision with pedal cycle in traffic accident** A, D, S ✎

     Pedestrian with babystroller injured in collision with pedal cycle in traffic accident

     Pedestrian in wheelchair (powered) injured in collision with pedal cycle in traffic accident

     Pedestrian in motorized mobility scooter injured in collision with pedal cycle in traffic accident

     Pedestrian on ice-skates injured in collision with pedal cycle in traffic accident

     Pedestrian on nonmotorized scooter injured in collision with pedal cycle in traffic accident

     Pedestrian on sled injured in collision with pedal cycle in traffic accident

     Pedestrian on snowboard injured in collision with pedal cycle in traffic accident

     Pedestrian on snow-skis injured in collision with pedal cycle in traffic accident

● **V01.9** **Pedestrian injured in collision with pedal cycle, unspecified whether traffic or nontraffic accident**

  ●■ **V01.90** **Pedestrian on foot injured in collision with pedal cycle, unspecified whether traffic or nontraffic accident** A, D, S ✎

     Pedestrian NOS injured in collision with pedal cycle, unspecified whether traffic or nontraffic accident

  ●■ **V01.91** **Pedestrian on roller-skates injured in collision with pedal cycle, unspecified whether traffic or nontraffic accident** A, D, S ✎

  ●■ **V01.92** **Pedestrian on skateboard injured in collision with pedal cycle, unspecified whether traffic or nontraffic accident** A, D, S ✎

●■ **V01.99** **Pedestrian with other conveyance injured in collision with pedal cycle, unspecified whether traffic or nontraffic accident** A, D, S ✎

  Pedestrian with babystroller injured in collision with pedal cycle, unspecified whether traffic or nontraffic accident

  Pedestrian in wheelchair (powered) injured in collision with pedal cycle, unspecified whether traffic or nontraffic accident

  Pedestrian in motorized mobility scooter injured in collision with pedal cycle, unspecified whether traffic or nontraffic accident

  Pedestrian on ice-skates injured in collision with pedal cycle unspecified, whether traffic or nontraffic accident

  Pedestrian on nonmotorized scooter injured in collision with pedal cycle, unspecified whether traffic or nontraffic accident

  Pedestrian on sled injured in collision with pedal cycle unspecified, whether traffic or nontraffic accident

  Pedestrian on snowboard injured in collision with pedal cycle, unspecified whether traffic or nontraffic accident

  Pedestrian on snow-skis injured in collision with pedal cycle, unspecified whether traffic or nontraffic accident

● **V02** **Pedestrian injured in collision with two- or three-wheeled motor vehicle**

  The appropriate 7th character is to be added to each code from category V02

A	initial encounter
D	subsequent encounter
S	sequela

● **V02.0** **Pedestrian injured in collision with two- or three-wheeled motor vehicle in nontraffic accident**

  ● **V02.00** **Pedestrian on foot injured in collision with two- or three-wheeled motor vehicle in nontraffic accident** A, D, S ✎

     Pedestrian NOS injured in collision with two- or three-wheeled motor vehicle in nontraffic accident

  ● **V02.01** **Pedestrian on roller-skates injured in collision with two- or three-wheeled motor vehicle in nontraffic accident** A, D, S ✎

  ● **V02.02** **Pedestrian on skateboard injured in collision with two- or three-wheeled motor vehicle in nontraffic accident** A, D, S ✎

● Unacceptable Principal Diagnosis   ● Use Additional Character(s)   ■ Unspecified   ▶ Manifestation Code

OGCR Official Guidelines for Coding and Reporting   Excludes 1   Excludes 2   Includes   Use additional   Code first   Code also

● **V02.09 Pedestrian with other conveyance injured in collision with two- or three-wheeled motor vehicle in nontraffic accident** A, D, S 🔖

     Pedestrian with babystroller injured in collision with two- or three-wheeled motor vehicle in nontraffic accident

     Pedestrian on ice-skates injured in collision with two- or three-wheeled motor vehicle in nontraffic accident

     Pedestrian in wheelchair (powered) injured in collision with two- or three-wheeled motor vehicle in nontraffic accident

     Pedestrian in motorized mobility scooter injured in collision with two- or three-wheeled motor vehicle in nontraffic accident

     Pedestrian on nonmotorized scooter injured in collision with two- or three-wheeled motor vehicle in nontraffic accident

     Pedestrian on sled injured in collision with two- or three-wheeled motor vehicle in nontraffic accident

     Pedestrian on snowboard injured in collision with two- or three-wheeled motor vehicle in nontraffic accident

     Pedestrian on snow-skis injured in collision with two- or three-wheeled motor vehicle in nontraffic accident

● **V02.1 Pedestrian injured in collision with two- or three-wheeled motor vehicle in traffic accident**

  ● **V02.10 Pedestrian on foot injured in collision with two- or three-wheeled motor vehicle in traffic accident** A, D, S 🔖

     Pedestrian NOS injured in collision with two- or three-wheeled motor vehicle in traffic accident

  ● **V02.11 Pedestrian on roller-skates injured in collision with two- or three-wheeled motor vehicle in traffic accident** A, D, S 🔖

  ● **V02.12 Pedestrian on skateboard injured in collision with two- or three-wheeled motor vehicle in traffic accident** A, D, S 🔖

  ● **V02.19 Pedestrian with other conveyance injured in collision with two- or three-wheeled motor vehicle in traffic accident** A, D, S 🔖

     Pedestrian with babystroller injured in collision with two- or three-wheeled motor vehicle in traffic accident

     Pedestrian in wheelchair (powered) injured in collision with two- or three-wheeled motor vehicle in traffic accident

     Pedestrian in motorized mobility scooter injured in collision with two- or three-wheeled motor vehicle in traffic accident

     Pedestrian on ice-skates injured in collision with two- or three-wheeled motor vehicle in traffic accident

     Pedestrian on nonmotorized scooter injured in collision with two- or three-wheeled motor vehicle in traffic accident

     Pedestrian on sled injured in collision with two- or three-wheeled motor vehicle in traffic accident

     Pedestrian on snowboard injured in collision with two- or three-wheeled motor vehicle in traffic accident

     Pedestrian on snow-skis injured in collision with two- or three-wheeled motor vehicle in traffic accident

● **V02.9 Pedestrian injured in collision with two- or three-wheeled motor vehicle, unspecified whether traffic or nontraffic accident**

  ● ■ **V02.90 Pedestrian on foot injured in collision with two- or three-wheeled motor vehicle, unspecified whether traffic or nontraffic accident** A, D, S 🔖

     Pedestrian NOS injured in collision with two- or three-wheeled motor vehicle, unspecified whether traffic or nontraffic accident

  ● ■ **V02.91 Pedestrian on roller-skates injured in collision with two- or three-wheeled motor vehicle, unspecified whether traffic or nontraffic accident** A, D, S 🔖

  ● ■ **V02.92 Pedestrian on skateboard injured in collision with two- or three-wheeled motor vehicle, unspecified whether traffic or nontraffic accident** A, D, S 🔖

  ● ■ **V02.99 Pedestrian with other conveyance injured in collision with two- or three-wheeled motor vehicle, unspecified whether traffic or nontraffic accident** A, D, S 🔖

     Pedestrian with babystroller injured in collision with two- or three-wheeled motor vehicle, unspecified whether traffic or nontraffic accident

     Pedestrian in wheelchair (powered) injured in collision with two- or three-wheeled motor vehicle, unspecified whether traffic or nontraffic accident

     Pedestrian in motorized mobility scooter injured in collision with two- or three-wheeled motor vehicle, unspecified whether traffic or nontraffic accident

     Pedestrian on ice-skates injured in collision with two- or three-wheeled motor vehicle, unspecified whether traffic or nontraffic accident

     Pedestrian on nonmotorized scooter injured in collision with two- or three-wheeled motor vehicle, unspecified whether traffic or nontraffic accident

     Pedestrian on sled injured in collision with two- or three-wheeled motor vehicle, unspecified whether traffic or nontraffic accident

     Pedestrian on snowboard injured in collision with two- or three-wheeled motor vehicle, unspecified whether traffic or nontraffic accident

     Pedestrian on snow-skis injured in collision with two- or three-wheeled motor vehicle, unspecified whether traffic or nontraffic accident

CHAPTER 20 (V01–Y99)

N Newborn Age: 0   **P** Pediatric Age: 0–17   **M** Maternity DX: 12–55   **A** Adult Age: 15–124   ♀ Females Only   ♂ Males Only

🔖 Complication\Comorbidity   🔖 Major C\C   🔖 Present on Admission Requirement   🔖 Hospital-Acquired Condition

1697

● **V03 Pedestrian injured in collision with car, pick-up truck or van**

The appropriate 7th character is to be added to each code from category V03

> A initial encounter
> D subsequent encounter
> S sequela

● **V03.0 Pedestrian injured in collision with car, pick-up truck or van in nontraffic accident**

　● **V03.00 Pedestrian on foot injured in collision with car, pick-up truck or van in nontraffic accident** A, D, S
　　Pedestrian NOS injured in collision with car, pick-up truck or van in nontraffic accident

　● **V03.01 Pedestrian on roller-skates injured in collision with car, pick-up truck or van in nontraffic accident** A, D, S

　● **V03.02 Pedestrian on skateboard injured in collision with car, pick-up truck or van in nontraffic accident** A, D, S

　● **V03.09 Pedestrian with other conveyance injured in collision with car, pick-up truck or van in nontraffic accident** A, D, S
　　Pedestrian with babystroller injured in collision with car, pick-up truck or van in nontraffic accident
　　Pedestrian in wheelchair (powered) injured in collision with car, pick-up truck or van in nontraffic accident
　　Pedestrian in motorized mobility scooter injured in collision with car, pick-up truck or van in nontraffic accident
　　Pedestrian on ice-skates injured in collision with car, pick-up truck or van in nontraffic accident
　　Pedestrian on nonmotorized scooter injured in collision with car, pick-up truck or van in nontraffic accident
　　Pedestrian on sled injured in collision with car, pick-up truck or van in nontraffic accident
　　Pedestrian on snowboard injured in collision with car, pick-up truck or van in nontraffic accident
　　Pedestrian on snow-skis injured in collision with car, pick-up truck or van in nontraffic accident

● **V03.1 Pedestrian injured in collision with car, pick-up truck or van in traffic accident**

　● **V03.10 Pedestrian on foot injured in collision with car, pick-up truck or van in traffic accident** A, D, S
　　Pedestrian NOS injured in collision with car, pick-up truck or van in traffic accident

　● **V03.11 Pedestrian on roller-skates injured in collision with car, pick-up truck or van in traffic accident** A, D, S

　● **V03.12 Pedestrian on skateboard injured in collision with car, pick-up truck or van in traffic accident** A, D, S

　● **V03.19 Pedestrian with other conveyance injured in collision with car, pick-up truck or van in traffic accident** A, D, S
　　Pedestrian with babystroller injured in collision with car, pick-up truck or van in traffic accident
　　Pedestrian in wheelchair (powered) injured in collision with car, pick-up truck or van in traffic accident
　　Pedestrian in motorized mobility scooter injured in collision with car, pick-up truck or van in traffic accident
　　Pedestrian on ice-skates injured in collision with car, pick-up truck or van in traffic accident
　　Pedestrian on nonmotorized scooter injured in collision with car, pick-up truck or van in traffic accident
　　Pedestrian on sled injured in collision with car, pick-up truck or van in traffic accident
　　Pedestrian on snowboard injured in collision with car, pick-up truck or van in traffic accident
　　Pedestrian on snow-skis injured in collision with car, pick-up truck or van in traffic accident

● **V03.9 Pedestrian injured in collision with car, pick-up truck or van, unspecified whether traffic or nontraffic accident**

　●■ **V03.90 Pedestrian on foot injured in collision with car, pick-up truck or van, unspecified whether traffic or nontraffic accident** A, D, S
　　Pedestrian NOS injured in collision with car, pick-up truck or van, unspecified whether traffic or nontraffic accident

　●■ **V03.91 Pedestrian on roller-skates injured in collision with car, pick-up truck or van, unspecified whether traffic or nontraffic accident** A, D, S

　●■ **V03.92 Pedestrian on skateboard injured in collision with car, pick-up truck or van, unspecified whether traffic or nontraffic accident** A, D, S

● Unacceptable Principal Diagnosis　● Use Additional Character(s)　■ Unspecified　▶ Manifestation Code
OGCR Official Guidelines for Coding and Reporting　Excludes 1　Excludes 2　Includes　Use additional　Code first　Code also

● ■ **V03.99 Pedestrian with other conveyance injured in collision with car, pick-up truck or van, unspecified whether traffic or nontraffic accident** A, D, S 🖾

   Pedestrian with babystroller injured in collision with car, pick-up truck or van, unspecified whether traffic or nontraffic accident

   Pedestrian in wheelchair (powered) injured in collision with car, pick-up truck or van, unspecified whether traffic or nontraffic accident

   Pedestrian in motorized mobility scooter injured in collision with car, pick-up truck or van, unspecified whether traffic or nontraffic accident

   Pedestrian on ice-skates injured in collision with car, pick-up truck or van, unspecified whether traffic or nontraffic accident

   Pedestrian on nonmotorized scooter injured in collision with car, pick-up truck or van, unspecified whether traffic or nontraffic accident

   Pedestrian on sled injured in collision with car, pick-up truck or van in nontraffic accident

   Pedestrian on snowboard injured in collision with car, pick-up truck or van, unspecified whether traffic or nontraffic accident

   Pedestrian on snow-skis injured in collision with car, pick-up truck or van, unspecified whether traffic or nontraffic accident

● **V04   Pedestrian injured in collision with heavy transport vehicle or bus**

   | Excludes1 | pedestrian injured in collision with military vehicle (V09.01, V09.21) |

   The appropriate 7th character is to be added to each code from category V04

A	initial encounter
D	subsequent encounter
S	sequela

● **V04.0   Pedestrian injured in collision with heavy transport vehicle or bus in nontraffic accident**

● **V04.00   Pedestrian on foot injured in collision with heavy transport vehicle or bus in nontraffic accident** A, D, S 🖾

   Pedestrian NOS injured in collision with heavy transport vehicle or bus in nontraffic accident

● **V04.01   Pedestrian on roller-skates injured in collision with heavy transport vehicle or bus in nontraffic accident** A, D, S 🖾

● **V04.02   Pedestrian on skateboard injured in collision with heavy transport vehicle or bus in nontraffic accident** A, D, S 🖾

● **V04.09   Pedestrian with other conveyance injured in collision with heavy transport vehicle or bus in nontraffic accident** A, D, S 🖾

   Pedestrian with babystroller injured in collision with heavy transport vehicle or bus in nontraffic accident

   Pedestrian in wheelchair (powered) injured in collision with heavy transport vehicle or bus in nontraffic accident

   Pedestrian in motorized mobility scooter injured in collision with heavy transport vehicle or bus in nontraffic accident

   Pedestrian on ice-skates injured in collision with heavy transport vehicle or bus in nontraffic accident

   Pedestrian on nonmotorized scooter injured in collision with heavy transport vehicle or bus in nontraffic accident

   Pedestrian on sled injured in collision with heavy transport vehicle or bus in nontraffic accident

   Pedestrian on snowboard injured in collision with heavy transport vehicle or bus in nontraffic accident

   Pedestrian on snow-skis injured in collision with heavy transport vehicle or bus in nontraffic accident

● **V04.1   Pedestrian injured in collision with heavy transport vehicle or bus in traffic accident**

● **V04.10   Pedestrian on foot injured in collision with heavy transport vehicle or bus in traffic accident** A, D, S 🖾

   Pedestrian NOS injured in collision with heavy transport vehicle or bus in traffic accident

● **V04.11   Pedestrian on roller-skates injured in collision with heavy transport vehicle or bus in traffic accident** A, D, S 🖾

● **V04.12   Pedestrian on skateboard injured in collision with heavy transport vehicle or bus in traffic accident** A, D, S 🖾

● **V04.19   Pedestrian with other conveyance injured in collision with heavy transport vehicle or bus in traffic accident** A, D, S 🖾

   Pedestrian with babystroller injured in collision with heavy transport vehicle or bus in traffic accident

   Pedestrian in wheelchair (powered) injured in collision with heavy transport vehicle or bus in traffic accident

   Pedestrian in motorized mobility scooter injured in collision with heavy transport vehicle or bus in traffic accident

   Pedestrian on ice-skates injured in collision with heavy transport vehicle or bus in traffic accident

   Pedestrian on nonmotorized scooter injured in collision with heavy transport vehicle or bus in traffic accident

   Pedestrian on sled injured in collision with heavy transport vehicle or bus in traffic accident

   Pedestrian on snowboard injured in collision with heavy transport vehicle or bus in traffic accident

   Pedestrian on snow-skis injured in collision with heavy transport vehicle or bus in traffic accident

● V04.9   **Pedestrian injured in collision with heavy transport vehicle or bus, unspecified whether traffic or nontraffic accident**

  ● ■ V04.90   **Pedestrian on foot injured in collision with heavy transport vehicle or bus, unspecified whether traffic or nontraffic accident** A, D, S 🔖

      Pedestrian NOS injured in collision with heavy transport vehicle or bus, unspecified whether traffic or nontraffic accident

  ● ■ V04.91   **Pedestrian on roller-skates injured in collision with heavy transport vehicle or bus, unspecified whether traffic or nontraffic accident** A, D, S 🔖

  ● ■ V04.92   **Pedestrian on skateboard injured in collision with heavy transport vehicle or bus, unspecified whether traffic or nontraffic accident** A, D, S 🔖

  ● ■ V04.99   **Pedestrian with other conveyance injured in collision with heavy transport vehicle or bus, unspecified whether traffic or nontraffic accident** A, D, S 🔖

      Pedestrian with babystroller injured in collision with heavy transport vehicle or bus, unspecified whether traffic or nontraffic accident

      Pedestrian in wheelchair (powered) injured in collision with heavy transport vehicle or bus, unspecified whether traffic or nontraffic accident

      Pedestrian in motorized mobility scooter injured in collision with heavy transport vehicle or bus, unspecified whether traffic or nontraffic accident

      Pedestrian on ice-skates injured in collision with heavy transport vehicle or bus, unspecified whether traffic or nontraffic accident

      Pedestrian on nonmotorized scooter injured in collision with heavy transport vehicle or bus, unspecified whether traffic or nontraffic accident

      Pedestrian on sled injured in collision with heavy transport vehicle or bus, unspecified whether traffic or nontraffic accident

      Pedestrian on snowboard injured in collision with heavy transport vehicle or bus, unspecified whether traffic or nontraffic accident

      Pedestrian on snow-skis injured in collision with heavy transport vehicle or bus, unspecified whether traffic or nontraffic accident

● V05   **Pedestrian injured in collision with railway train or railway vehicle**

The appropriate 7th character is to be added to each code from category V05

> A   initial encounter
> D   subsequent encounter
> S   sequela

● V05.0   **Pedestrian injured in collision with railway train or railway vehicle in nontraffic accident**

  ● V05.00   **Pedestrian on foot injured in collision with railway train or railway vehicle in nontraffic accident** A, D, S 🔖

      Pedestrian NOS injured in collision with railway train or railway vehicle in nontraffic accident

  ● V05.01   **Pedestrian on roller-skates injured in collision with railway train or railway vehicle in nontraffic accident** A, D, S 🔖

  ● V05.02   **Pedestrian on skateboard injured in collision with railway train or railway vehicle in nontraffic accident** A, D, S 🔖

  ● V05.09   **Pedestrian with other conveyance injured in collision with railway train or railway vehicle in nontraffic accident** A, D, S 🔖

      Pedestrian with babystroller injured in collision with railway train or railway vehicle in nontraffic accident

      Pedestrian in wheelchair (powered) injured in collision with railway train or railway vehicle in nontraffic accident

      Pedestrian in motorized mobility scooter injured in collision with railway train or railway vehicle in nontraffic accident

      Pedestrian on ice-skates injured in collision with railway train or railway vehicle in nontraffic accident

      Pedestrian on nonmotorized scooter injured in collision with railway train or railway vehicle in nontraffic accident

      Pedestrian on sled injured in collision with railway train or railway vehicle in nontraffic accident

      Pedestrian on snowboard injured in collision with railway train or railway vehicle in nontraffic accident

      Pedestrian on snow-skis injured in collision with railway train or railway vehicle in nontraffic accident

● Unacceptable Principal Diagnosis   ● Use Additional Character(s)   ■ Unspecified   ▶ Manifestation Code

OGCR   Official Guidelines for Coding and Reporting   Excludes 1   Excludes 2   Includes   Use additional   Code first   Code also

● **V05.1** **Pedestrian injured in collision with railway train or railway vehicle in traffic accident**

  ● **V05.10** **Pedestrian on foot injured in collision with railway train or railway vehicle in traffic accident** A, D, S 🖑

    Pedestrian NOS injured in collision with railway train or railway vehicle in traffic accident

  ● **V05.11** **Pedestrian on roller-skates injured in collision with railway train or railway vehicle in traffic accident** A, D, S 🖑

  ● **V05.12** **Pedestrian on skateboard injured in collision with railway train or railway vehicle in traffic accident** A, D, S 🖑

  ● **V05.19** **Pedestrian with other conveyance injured in collision with railway train or railway vehicle in traffic accident** A, D, S 🖑

    Pedestrian with babystroller injured in collision with railway train or railway vehicle in traffic accident

    Pedestrian in wheelchair (powered) injured in collision with railway train or railway vehicle in traffic accident

    Pedestrian in motorized mobility scooter injured in collision with railway train or railway vehicle in traffic accident

    Pedestrian on ice-skates injured in collision with railway train or railway vehicle in traffic accident

    Pedestrian on nonmotorized scooter injured in collision with railway train or railway vehicle in traffic accident

    Pedestrian on sled injured in collision with railway train or railway vehicle in traffic accident

    Pedestrian on snowboard injured in collision with railway train or railway vehicle in traffic accident

    Pedestrian on snow-skis injured in collision with railway train or railway vehicle in traffic accident

● **V05.9** **Pedestrian injured in collision with railway train or railway vehicle, unspecified whether traffic or nontraffic accident**

  ●■ **V05.90** **Pedestrian on foot injured in collision with railway train or railway vehicle, unspecified whether traffic or nontraffic accident** A, D, S 🖑

    Pedestrian NOS injured in collision with railway train or railway vehicle, unspecified whether traffic or nontraffic accident

  ●■ **V05.91** **Pedestrian on roller-skates injured in collision with railway train or railway vehicle, unspecified whether traffic or nontraffic accident** A, D, S 🖑

  ●■ **V05.92** **Pedestrian on skateboard injured in collision with railway train or railway vehicle, unspecified whether traffic or nontraffic accident** A, D, S 🖑

●■ **V05.99** **Pedestrian with other conveyance injured in collision with railway train or railway vehicle, unspecified whether traffic or nontraffic accident** A, D, S 🖑

    Pedestrian with babystroller injured in collision with railway train or railway vehicle, unspecified whether traffic or nontraffic

    Pedestrian in wheelchair (powered) injured in collision with railway train or railway vehicle, unspecified whether traffic or nontraffic

    Pedestrian in motorized mobility scooter injured in collision with railway train or railway vehicle, unspecified whether traffic or nontraffic

    Pedestrian on ice-skates injured in collision with railway train or railway vehicle, unspecified whether traffic or nontraffic

    Pedestrian on nonmotorized scooter injured in collision with railway train or railway vehicle, unspecified whether traffic or nontraffic

    Pedestrian on sled injured in collision with railway train or railway vehicle, unspecified whether traffic or nontraffic

    Pedestrian on snowboard injured in collision with railway train or railway vehicle, unspecified whether traffic or nontraffic

    Pedestrian on snow-skis injured in collision with railway train or railway vehicle, unspecified whether traffic or nontraffic

● **V06** **Pedestrian injured in collision with other nonmotor vehicle**

  Includes   collision with animal-drawn vehicle, animal being ridden, nonpowered streetcar

  Excludes1   pedestrian injured in collision with pedestrian conveyance (V00.0-)

The appropriate 7th character is to be added to each code from category V06

> A   initial encounter
> D   subsequent encounter
> S   sequela

● **V06.0** **Pedestrian injured in collision with other nonmotor vehicle in nontraffic accident**

  ● **V06.00** **Pedestrian on foot injured in collision with other nonmotor vehicle in nontraffic accident** A, D, S 🖑

    Pedestrian NOS injured in collision with other nonmotor vehicle in nontraffic accident

  ● **V06.01** **Pedestrian on roller-skates injured in collision with other nonmotor vehicle in nontraffic accident** A, D, S 🖑

  ● **V06.02** **Pedestrian on skateboard injured in collision with other nonmotor vehicle in nontraffic accident** A, D, S 🖑

N Newborn Age: 0   **P** Pediatric Age: 0–17   **M** Maternity DX: 12–55   **A** Adult Age: 15–124   ♀ Females Only   ♂ Males Only

🖎 Complication\Comorbidity   🖎 Major C\C   🖑 Present on Admission Requirement   🖎 Hospital-Acquired Condition

1701

● V06.09   **Pedestrian with other conveyance injured in collision with other nonmotor vehicle in nontraffic accident** A, D, S 🔖

Pedestrian with babystroller injured in collision with other nonmotor vehicle in nontraffic accident

Pedestrian in wheelchair (powered) injured in collision with other nonmotor vehicle in nontraffic accident

Pedestrian in motorized mobility scooter injured in collision with other nonmotor vehicle in nontraffic accident

Pedestrian on ice-skates injured in collision with other nonmotor vehicle in nontraffic accident

Pedestrian on nonmotorized scooter injured in collision with other nonmotor vehicle in nontraffic accident

Pedestrian on sled injured in collision with other nonmotor vehicle in nontraffic accident

Pedestrian on snowboard injured in collision with other nonmotor vehicle in nontraffic accident

Pedestrian on snow-skis injured in collision with other nonmotor vehicle in nontraffic accident

● **V06.1**   **Pedestrian injured in collision with other nonmotor vehicle in traffic accident**

● V06.10   **Pedestrian on foot injured in collision with other nonmotor vehicle in traffic accident** A, D, S 🔖

Pedestrian NOS injured in collision with other nonmotor vehicle in traffic accident

● V06.11   **Pedestrian on roller-skates injured in collision with other nonmotor vehicle in traffic accident** A, D, S 🔖

● V06.12   **Pedestrian on skateboard injured in collision with other nonmotor vehicle in traffic accident** A, D, S 🔖

● V06.19   **Pedestrian with other conveyance injured in collision with other nonmotor vehicle in traffic accident** A, D, S 🔖

Pedestrian with babystroller injured in collision with other nonmotor vehicle in nontraffic accident

Pedestrian in wheelchair (powered) injured in collision with other nonmotor vehicle in traffic accident

Pedestrian in motorized mobility scooter injured in collision with other nonmotor vehicle in traffic accident

Pedestrian on ice-skates injured in collision with other nonmotor vehicle in traffic accident

Pedestrian on nonmotorized scooter injured in collision with other nonmotor vehicle in traffic accident

Pedestrian on sled injured in collision with other nonmotor vehicle in traffic accident

Pedestrian on snowboard injured in collision with other nonmotor vehicle in traffic accident

Pedestrian on snow-skis injured in collision with other nonmotor vehicle in traffic accident

● V06.9   **Pedestrian injured in collision with other nonmotor vehicle, unspecified whether traffic or nontraffic accident**

●■ V06.90   **Pedestrian on foot injured in collision with other nonmotor vehicle, unspecified whether traffic or nontraffic accident** A, D, S 🔖

Pedestrian NOS injured in collision with other nonmotor vehicle, unspecified whether traffic or nontraffic accident

●■ V06.91   **Pedestrian on roller-skates injured in collision with other nonmotor vehicle, unspecified whether traffic or nontraffic accident** A, D, S 🔖

●■ V06.92   **Pedestrian on skateboard injured in collision with other nonmotor vehicle, unspecified whether traffic or nontraffic accident** A, D, S 🔖

●■ V06.99   **Pedestrian with other conveyance injured in collision with other nonmotor vehicle, unspecified whether traffic or nontraffic accident** A, D, S 🔖

Pedestrian with babystroller injured in collision with other nonmotor vehicle, unspecified whether traffic or nontraffic accident

Pedestrian in wheelchair (powered) injured in collision with other nonmotor vehicle, unspecified whether traffic or nontraffic accident

Pedestrian in motorized mobility scooter injured in collision with other nonmotor vehicle, unspecified whether traffic or nontraffic accident

Pedestrian on ice-skates injured in collision with other nonmotor vehicle, unspecified whether traffic or nontraffic accident

Pedestrian on nonmotorized scooter injured in collision with other nonmotor vehicle, unspecified whether traffic or nontraffic accident

Pedestrian on sled injured in collision with other nonmotor vehicle, unspecified whether traffic or nontraffic accident

Pedestrian on snowboard injured in collision with other nonmotor vehicle, unspecified whether traffic or nontraffic accident

Pedestrian on snow-skis injured in collision with other nonmotor vehicle, unspecified whether traffic or nontraffic accident

● **V09**   **Pedestrian injured in other and unspecified transport accidents**

The appropriate 7th character is to be added to each code from category V09

A	initial encounter
D	subsequent encounter
S	sequela

● **V09.0**   **Pedestrian injured in nontraffic accident involving other and unspecified motor vehicles**

●■ V09.00   **Pedestrian injured in nontraffic accident involving unspecified motor vehicles** A, D, S 🔖

● V09.01   **Pedestrian injured in nontraffic accident involving military vehicle** A, D, S 🔖

●   Unacceptable Principal Diagnosis   ● Use Additional Character(s)   ■ Unspecified   ▶ Manifestation Code

OGCR   Official Guidelines for Coding and Reporting | Excludes 1 | | Excludes 2 | | Includes | | Use additional | | Code first | | Code also |

● V09.09   Pedestrian injured in nontraffic accident involving other motor vehicles A, D, S 🖐
          Pedestrian injured in nontraffic accident by special vehicle

●■ V09.1   Pedestrian injured in unspecified nontraffic accident A, D, S 🖐

● V09.2   Pedestrian injured in traffic accident involving other and unspecified motor vehicles

   ●■ V09.20   Pedestrian injured in traffic accident involving unspecified motor vehicles A, D, S 🖐

   ● V09.21   Pedestrian injured in traffic accident involving military vehicle A, D, S 🖐

   ● V09.29   Pedestrian injured in traffic accident involving other motor vehicles A, D, S 🖐

●■ V09.3   Pedestrian injured in unspecified traffic accident A, D, S 🖐

●■ V09.9   Pedestrian injured in unspecified transport accident A, D, S 🖐

PEDAL CYCLE RIDER INJURED IN TRANSPORT ACCIDENT (V10-V19)

Includes	any non-motorized vehicle, excluding an animal-drawn vehicle, or a sidecar or trailer attached to the pedal cycle
Excludes2	rupture of pedal cycle tire (W37.0)

● V10   Pedal cycle rider injured in collision with pedestrian or animal

Excludes1	pedal cycle rider collision with animal-drawn vehicle or animal being ridden (Vl6.-)

The appropriate 7th character is to be added to each code from category V10

A	initial encounter
D	subsequent encounter
S	sequela

● V10.0   Pedal cycle driver injured in collision with pedestrian or animal in nontraffic accident A, D, S 🖐

● V10.1   Pedal cycle passenger injured in collision with pedestrian or animal in nontraffic accident A, D, S 🖐

●■ V10.2   Unspecified pedal cyclist injured in collision with pedestrian or animal in nontraffic accident A, D, S 🖐

● V10.3   Person boarding or alighting a pedal cycle injured in collision with pedestrian or animal A, D, S 🖐

● V10.4   Pedal cycle driver injured in collision with pedestrian or animal in traffic accident A, D, S 🖐

● V10.5   Pedal cycle passenger injured in collision with pedestrian or animal in traffic accident A, D, S 🖐

●■ V10.9   Unspecified pedal cyclist injured in collision with pedestrian or animal in traffic accident A, D, S 🖐

● V11   Pedal cycle rider injured in collision with other pedal cycle

The appropriate 7th character is to be added to each code from category V11

A	initial encounter
D	subsequent encounter
S	sequela

● V11.0   Pedal cycle driver injured in collision with other pedal cycle in nontraffic accident A, D, S 🖐

● V11.1   Pedal cycle passenger injured in collision with other pedal cycle in nontraffic accident A, D, S 🖐

●■ V11.2   Unspecified pedal cyclist injured in collision with other pedal cycle in nontraffic accident A, D, S 🖐

● V11.3   Person boarding or alighting a pedal cycle injured in collision with other pedal cycle A, D, S 🖐

● V11.4   Pedal cycle driver injured in collision with other pedal cycle in traffic accident A, D, S 🖐

● V11.5   Pedal cycle passenger injured in collision with other pedal cycle in traffic accident A, D, S 🖐

●■ V11.9   Unspecified pedal cyclist injured in collision with other pedal cycle in traffic accident A, D, S 🖐

● V12   Pedal cycle rider injured in collision with two- or three-wheeled motor vehicle

The appropriate 7th character is to be added to each code from category V12

A	initial encounter
D	subsequent encounter
S	sequela

● V12.0   Pedal cycle driver injured in collision with two- or three-wheeled motor vehicle in nontraffic accident A, D, S 🖐

● V12.1   Pedal cycle passenger injured in collision with two- or three-wheeled motor vehicle in nontraffic accident A, D, S 🖐

●■ V12.2   Unspecified pedal cyclist injured in collision with two- or three-wheeled motor vehicle in nontraffic accident A, D, S 🖐

● V12.3   Person boarding or alighting a pedal cycle injured in collision with two- or three-wheeled motor vehicle A, D, S 🖐

● V12.4   Pedal cycle driver injured in collision with two- or three-wheeled motor vehicle in traffic accident A, D, S 🖐

● V12.5   Pedal cycle passenger injured in collision with two- or three-wheeled motor vehicle in traffic accident A, D, S 🖐

●■ V12.9   Unspecified pedal cyclist injured in collision with two- or three-wheeled motor vehicle in traffic accident A, D, S 🖐

● V13   Pedal cycle rider injured in collision with car, pick-up truck or van

The appropriate 7th character is to be added to each code from category V13

A	initial encounter
D	subsequent encounter
S	sequela

● V13.0   Pedal cycle driver injured in collision with car, pick-up truck or van in nontraffic accident A, D, S 🖐

● V13.1   Pedal cycle passenger injured in collision with car, pick-up truck or van in nontraffic accident A, D, S 🖐

●■ V13.2   Unspecified pedal cyclist injured in collision with car, pick-up truck or van in nontraffic accident A, D, S 🖐

● V13.3   Person boarding or alighting a pedal cycle injured in collision with car, pick-up truck or van A, D, S 🖐

● V13.4   Pedal cycle driver injured in collision with car, pick-up truck or van in traffic accident A, D, S 🖐

CHAPTER 20 (V01-Y99)

● V13.5   **Pedal cycle passenger injured in collision with car, pick-up truck or van in traffic accident** A, D, S 🖉

●■ V13.9   **Unspecified pedal cyclist injured in collision with car, pick-up truck or van in traffic accident** A, D, S 🖉

● V14   **Pedal cycle rider injured in collision with heavy transport vehicle or bus**

> **Excludes1**   pedal cycle rider injured in collision with military vehicle (V19.81)

> The appropriate 7th character is to be added to each code from category V14

A	initial encounter
D	subsequent encounter
S	sequela

● V14.0   **Pedal cycle driver injured in collision with heavy transport vehicle or bus in nontraffic accident** A, D, S 🖉

● V14.1   **Pedal cycle passenger injured in collision with heavy transport vehicle or bus in nontraffic accident** A, D, S 🖉

●■ V14.2   **Unspecified pedal cyclist injured in collision with heavy transport vehicle or bus in nontraffic accident** A, D, S 🖉

● V14.3   **Person boarding or alighting a pedal cycle injured in collision with heavy transport vehicle or bus** A, D, S 🖉

● V14.4   **Pedal cycle driver injured in collision with heavy transport vehicle or bus in traffic accident** A, D, S 🖉

● V14.5   **Pedal cycle passenger injured in collision with heavy transport vehicle or bus in traffic accident** A, D, S 🖉

●■ V14.9   **Unspecified pedal cyclist injured in collision with heavy transport vehicle or bus in traffic accident** A, D, S 🖉

● V15   **Pedal cycle rider injured in collision with railway train or railway vehicle**

> The appropriate 7th character is to be added to each code from category V15

A	initial encounter
D	subsequent encounter
S	sequela

● V15.0   **Pedal cycle driver injured in collision with railway train or railway vehicle in nontraffic accident** A, D, S 🖉

● V15.1   **Pedal cycle passenger injured in collision with railway train or railway vehicle in nontraffic accident** A, D, S 🖉

●■ V15.2   **Unspecified pedal cyclist injured in collision with railway train or railway vehicle in nontraffic accident** A, D, S 🖉

● V15.3   **Person boarding or alighting a pedal cycle injured in collision with railway train or railway vehicle** A, D, S 🖉

● V15.4   **Pedal cycle driver injured in collision with railway train or railway vehicle in traffic accident** A, D, S 🖉

● V15.5   **Pedal cycle passenger injured in collision with railway train or railway vehicle in traffic accident** A, D, S 🖉

●■ V15.9   **Unspecified pedal cyclist injured in collision with railway train or railway vehicle in traffic accident** A, D, S 🖉

● V16   **Pedal cycle rider injured in collision with other nonmotor vehicle**

> **Includes**   collision with animal-drawn vehicle, animal being ridden, streetcar

> The appropriate 7th character is to be added to each code from category V16

A	initial encounter
D	subsequent encounter
S	sequela

● V16.0   **Pedal cycle driver injured in collision with other nonmotor vehicle in nontraffic accident** A, D, S 🖉

● V16.1   **Pedal cycle passenger injured in collision with other nonmotor vehicle in nontraffic accident** A, D, S 🖉

●■ V16.2   **Unspecified pedal cyclist injured in collision with other nonmotor vehicle in nontraffic accident** A, D, S 🖉

● V16.3   **Person boarding or alighting a pedal cycle injured in collision with other nonmotor vehicle in nontraffic accident** A, D, S 🖉

● V16.4   **Pedal cycle driver injured in collision with other nonmotor vehicle in traffic accident** A, D, S 🖉

● V16.5   **Pedal cycle passenger injured in collision with other nonmotor vehicle in traffic accident** A, D, S 🖉

●■ V16.9   **Unspecified pedal cyclist injured in collision with other nonmotor vehicle in traffic accident** A, D, S 🖉

● V17   **Pedal cycle rider injured in collision with fixed or stationary object**

> The appropriate 7th character is to be added to each code from category V17

A	initial encounter
D	subsequent encounter
S	sequela

● V17.0   **Pedal cycle driver injured in collision with fixed or stationary object in nontraffic accident** A, D, S 🖉

● V17.1   **Pedal cycle passenger injured in collision with fixed or stationary object in nontraffic accident** A, D, S 🖉

●■ V17.2   **Unspecified pedal cyclist injured in collision with fixed or stationary object in nontraffic accident** A, D, S 🖉

● V17.3   **Person boarding or alighting a pedal cycle injured in collision with fixed or stationary object** A, D, S 🖉

● V17.4   **Pedal cycle driver injured in collision with fixed or stationary object in traffic accident** A, D, S 🖉

● V17.5   **Pedal cycle passenger injured in collision with fixed or stationary object in traffic accident** A, D, S 🖉

●■ V17.9   **Unspecified pedal cyclist injured in collision with fixed or stationary object in traffic accident** A, D, S 🖉

● **V18　Pedal cycle rider injured in noncollision transport accident**

>　**Includes**　fall or thrown from pedal cycle (without antecedent collision)
>　　　　overturning pedal cycle NOS
>　　　　overturning pedal cycle without collision

>　The appropriate 7th character is to be added to each code from category V18

>　　A　initial encounter
>　　D　subsequent encounter
>　　S　sequela

● **V18.0　Pedal cycle driver injured in noncollision transport accident in nontraffic accident** A, D, S

● **V18.1　Pedal cycle passenger injured in noncollision transport accident in nontraffic accident** A, D, S

● ■ **V18.2　Unspecified pedal cyclist injured in noncollision transport accident in nontraffic accident** A, D, S

● **V18.3　Person boarding or alighting a pedal cycle injured in noncollision transport accident** A, D, S

● **V18.4　Pedal cycle driver injured in noncollision transport accident in traffic accident** A, D, S

● **V18.5　Pedal cycle passenger injured in noncollision transport accident in traffic accident** A, D, S

● ■ **V18.9　Unspecified pedal cyclist injured in noncollision transport accident in traffic accident** A, D, S

● **V19　Pedal cycle rider injured in other and unspecified transport accidents**

>　The appropriate 7th character is to be added to each code from category V19

>　　A　initial encounter
>　　D　subsequent encounter
>　　S　sequela

● **V19.0　Pedal cycle driver injured in collision with other and unspecified motor vehicles in nontraffic accident**

● ■ **V19.00　Pedal cycle driver injured in collision with unspecified motor vehicles in nontraffic accident** A, D, S

● **V19.09　Pedal cycle driver injured in collision with other motor vehicles in nontraffic accident** A, D, S

● **V19.1　Pedal cycle passenger injured in collision with other and unspecified motor vehicles in nontraffic accident**

● ■ **V19.10　Pedal cycle passenger injured in collision with unspecified motor vehicles in nontraffic accident** A, D, S

● **V19.19　Pedal cycle passenger injured in collision with other motor vehicles in nontraffic accident** A, D, S

● **V19.2　Unspecified pedal cyclist injured in collision with other and unspecified motor vehicles in nontraffic accident**

● ■ **V19.20　Unspecified pedal cyclist injured in collision with unspecified motor vehicles in nontraffic accident** A, D, S
>　　Pedal cycle collision NOS, nontraffic

● ■ **V19.29　Unspecified pedal cyclist injured in collision with other motor vehicles in nontraffic accident** A, D, S

● ■ **V19.3　Pedal cyclist (driver) (passenger) injured in unspecified nontraffic accident** A, D, S
>　Pedal cycle accident NOS, nontraffic
>　Pedal cyclist injured in nontraffic accident NOS

● **V19.4　Pedal cycle driver injured in collision with other and unspecified motor vehicles in traffic accident**

● ■ **V19.40　Pedal cycle driver injured in collision with unspecified motor vehicles in traffic accident** A, D, S

● **V19.49　Pedal cycle driver injured in collision with other motor vehicles in traffic accident** A, D, S

● **V19.5　Pedal cycle passenger injured in collision with other and unspecified motor vehicles in traffic accident**

● ■ **V19.50　Pedal cycle passenger injured in collision with unspecified motor vehicles in traffic accident** A, D, S

● **V19.59　Pedal cycle passenger injured in collision with other motor vehicles in traffic accident** A, D, S

● **V19.6　Unspecified pedal cyclist injured in collision with other and unspecified motor vehicles in traffic accident**

● ■ **V19.60　Unspecified pedal cyclist injured in collision with unspecified motor vehicles in traffic accident** A, D, S
>　　Pedal cycle collision NOS (traffic)

● ■ **V19.69　Unspecified pedal cyclist injured in collision with other motor vehicles in traffic accident** A, D, S

● **V19.8　Pedal cyclist (driver) (passenger) injured in other specified transport accidents**

● **V19.81　Pedal cyclist (driver) (passenger) injured in transport accident with military vehicle** A, D, S

● **V19.88　Pedal cyclist (driver) (passenger) injured in other specified transport accidents** A, D, S

● ■ **V19.9　Pedal cyclist (driver) (passenger) injured in unspecified traffic accident** A, D, S
>　Pedal cycle accident NOS

MOTORCYCLE RIDER INJURED IN TRANSPORT ACCIDENT (V20-V29)

>　**Includes**　moped motorcycle with sidecar motorized bicycle motor scooter

>　**Excludes1**　three-wheeled motor vehicle (V30-V39)

● **V20　Motorcycle rider injured in collision with pedestrian or animal**

>　**Excludes1**　motorcycle rider collision with animal-drawn vehicle or animal being ridden (V26.-)

>　The appropriate 7th character is to be added to each code from category V20

>　　A　initial encounter
>　　D　subsequent encounter
>　　S　sequela

● **V20.0　Motorcycle driver injured in collision with pedestrian or animal in nontraffic accident** A, D, S

● **V20.1　Motorcycle passenger injured in collision with pedestrian or animal in nontraffic accident** A, D, S

● ■ **V20.2** **Unspecified motorcycle rider injured in collision with pedestrian or animal in nontraffic accident** A, D, S 🗸

● **V20.3** **Person boarding or alighting a motorcycle injured in collision with pedestrian or animal** A, D, S 🗸

● **V20.4** **Motorcycle driver injured in collision with pedestrian or animal in traffic accident** A, D, S 🗸

● **V20.5** **Motorcycle passenger injured in collision with pedestrian or animal in traffic accident** A, D, S 🗸

● ■ **V20.9** **Unspecified motorcycle rider injured in collision with pedestrian or animal in traffic accident** A, D, S 🗸

● **V21** **Motorcycle rider injured in collision with pedal cycle**

The appropriate 7th character is to be added to each code from category V21

A	initial encounter
D	subsequent encounter
S	sequela

● **V21.0** **Motorcycle driver injured in collision with pedal cycle in nontraffic accident** A, D, S 🗸

● **V21.1** **Motorcycle passenger injured in collision with pedal cycle in nontraffic accident** A, D, S 🗸

● ■ **V21.2** **Unspecified motorcycle rider injured in collision with pedal cycle in nontraffic accident** A, D, S 🗸

● **V21.3** **Person boarding or alighting a motorcycle injured in collision with pedal cycle** A, D, S 🗸

● **V21.4** **Motorcycle driver injured in collision with pedal cycle in traffic accident** A, D, S 🗸

● **V21.5** **Motorcycle passenger injured in collision with pedal cycle in traffic accident** A, D, S 🗸

● ■ **V21.9** **Unspecified motorcycle rider injured in collision with pedal cycle in traffic accident** A, D, S 🗸

● **V22** **Motorcycle rider injured in collision with two- or three-wheeled motor vehicle**

The appropriate 7th character is to be added to each code from category V22

A	initial encounter
D	subsequent encounter
S	sequela

● **V22.0** **Motorcycle driver injured in collision with two- or three-wheeled motor vehicle in nontraffic accident** A, D, S 🗸

● **V22.1** **Motorcycle passenger injured in collision with two- or three-wheeled motor vehicle in nontraffic accident** A, D, S 🗸

● ■ **V22.2** **Unspecified motorcycle rider injured in collision with two- or three-wheeled motor vehicle in nontraffic accident** A, D, S 🗸

● **V22.3** **Person boarding or alighting a motorcycle injured in collision with two- or three-wheeled motor vehicle** A, D, S 🗸

● **V22.4** **Motorcycle driver injured in collision with two- or three-wheeled motor vehicle in traffic accident** A, D, S 🗸

● **V22.5** **Motorcycle passenger injured in collision with two- or three-wheeled motor vehicle in traffic accident** A, D, S 🗸

● ■ **V22.9** **Unspecified motorcycle rider injured in collision with two- or three-wheeled motor vehicle in traffic accident** A, D, S 🗸

● **V23** **Motorcycle rider injured in collision with car, pick-up truck or van**

The appropriate 7th character is to be added to each code from category V23

A	initial encounter
D	subsequent encounter
S	sequela

● **V23.0** **Motorcycle driver injured in collision with car, pick-up truck or van in nontraffic accident** A, D, S 🗸

● **V23.1** **Motorcycle passenger injured in collision with car, pick-up truck or van in nontraffic accident** A, D, S 🗸

● ■ **V23.2** **Unspecified motorcycle rider injured in collision with car, pick-up truck or van in nontraffic accident** A, D, S 🗸

● **V23.3** **Person boarding or alighting a motorcycle injured in collision with car, pick-up truck or van** A, D, S 🗸

● **V23.4** **Motorcycle driver injured in collision with car, pick-up truck or van in traffic accident** A, D, S 🗸

● **V23.5** **Motorcycle passenger injured in collision with car, pick-up truck or van in traffic accident** A, D, S 🗸

● ■ **V23.9** **Unspecified motorcycle rider injured in collision with car, pick-up truck or van in traffic accident** A, D, S 🗸

● **V24** **Motorcycle rider injured in collision with heavy transport vehicle or bus**

> **Excludes1**   motorcycle rider injured in collision with military vehicle (V29.81)

The appropriate 7th character is to be added to each code from category V24

A	initial encounter
D	subsequent encounter
S	sequela

● **V24.0** **Motorcycle driver injured in collision with heavy transport vehicle or bus in nontraffic accident** A, D, S 🗸

● **V24.1** **Motorcycle passenger injured in collision with heavy transport vehicle or bus in nontraffic accident** A, D, S 🗸

● ■ **V24.2** **Unspecified motorcycle rider injured in collision with heavy transport vehicle or bus in nontraffic accident** A, D, S 🗸

● **V24.3** **Person boarding or alighting a motorcycle injured in collision with heavy transport vehicle or bus** A, D, S 🗸

● **V24.4** **Motorcycle driver injured in collision with heavy transport vehicle or bus in traffic accident** A, D, S 🗸

● **V24.5** **Motorcycle passenger injured in collision with heavy transport vehicle or bus in traffic accident** A, D, S 🗸

● ■ **V24.9** **Unspecified motorcycle rider injured in collision with heavy transport vehicle or bus in traffic accident** A, D, S 🗸

● Unacceptable Principal Diagnosis   ● Use Additional Character(s)   ■ Unspecified   ▶ Manifestation Code

OGCR Official Guidelines for Coding and Reporting | Excludes 1 | | Excludes 2 | | Includes | | Use additional | | Code first | | Code also |

● **V25   Motorcycle rider injured in collision with railway train or railway vehicle**

> The appropriate 7th character is to be added to each code from category V25

> A   initial encounter
> D   subsequent encounter
> S   sequela

● **V25.0**   Motorcycle driver injured in collision with railway train or railway vehicle in nontraffic accident A, D, S

● **V25.1**   Motorcycle passenger injured in collision with railway train or railway vehicle in nontraffic accident A, D, S

●■ **V25.2**   Unspecified motorcycle rider injured in collision with railway train or railway vehicle in nontraffic accident A, D, S

● **V25.3**   Person boarding or alighting a motorcycle injured in collision with railway train or railway vehicle A, D, S

● **V25.4**   Motorcycle driver injured in collision with railway train or railway vehicle in traffic accident A, D, S

● **V25.5**   Motorcycle passenger injured in collision with railway train or railway vehicle in traffic accident A, D, S

●■ **V25.9**   Unspecified motorcycle rider injured in collision with railway train or railway vehicle in traffic accident A, D, S

● **V26   Motorcycle rider injured in collision with other nonmotor vehicle**

> **Includes**   collision with animal-drawn vehicle, animal being ridden, streetcar

> The appropriate 7th character is to be added to each code from category V26

> A   initial encounter
> D   subsequent encounter
> S   sequela

● **V26.0**   Motorcycle driver injured in collision with other nonmotor vehicle in nontraffic accident A, D, S

● **V26.1**   Motorcycle passenger injured in collision with other nonmotor vehicle in nontraffic accident A, D, S

●■ **V26.2**   Unspecified motorcycle rider injured in collision with other nonmotor vehicle in nontraffic accident A, D, S

● **V26.3**   Person boarding or alighting a motorcycle injured in collision with other nonmotor vehicle A, D, S

● **V26.4**   Motorcycle driver injured in collision with other nonmotor vehicle in traffic accident A, D, S

● **V26.5**   Motorcycle passenger injured in collision with other nonmotor vehicle in traffic accident A, D, S

●■ **V26.9**   Unspecified motorcycle rider injured in collision with other nonmotor vehicle in traffic accident A, D, S

● **V27   Motorcycle rider injured in collision with fixed or stationary object**

> The appropriate 7th character is to be added to each code from category V27

> A   initial encounter
> D   subsequent encounter
> S   sequela

● **V27.0**   Motorcycle driver injured in collision with fixed or stationary object in nontraffic accident A, D, S

● **V27.1**   Motorcycle passenger injured in collision with fixed or stationary object in nontraffic accident A, D, S

●■ **V27.2**   Unspecified motorcycle rider injured in collision with fixed or stationary object in nontraffic accident A, D, S

● **V27.3**   Person boarding or alighting a motorcycle injured in collision with fixed or stationary object A, D, S

● **V27.4**   Motorcycle driver injured in collision with fixed or stationary object in traffic accident A, D, S

● **V27.5**   Motorcycle passenger injured in collision with fixed or stationary object in traffic accident A, D, S

●■ **V27.9**   Unspecified motorcycle rider injured in collision with fixed or stationary object in traffic accident A, D, S

● **V28   Motorcycle rider injured in noncollision transport accident**

> **Includes**   fall or thrown from motorcycle (without antecedent collision)
> overturning motorcycle NOS
> overturning motorcycle without collision

> The appropriate 7th character is to be added to each code from category V28

> A   initial encounter
> D   subsequent encounter
> S   sequela

● **V28.0**   Motorcycle driver injured in noncollision transport accident in nontraffic accident A, D, S

● **V28.1**   Motorcycle passenger injured in noncollision transport accident in nontraffic accident A, D, S

●■ **V28.2**   Unspecified motorcycle rider injured in noncollision transport accident in nontraffic accident A, D, S

● **V28.3**   Person boarding or alighting a motorcycle injured in noncollision transport accident A, D, S

● **V28.4**   Motorcycle driver injured in noncollision transport accident in traffic accident A, D, S

● **V28.5**   Motorcycle passenger injured in noncollision transport accident in traffic accident A, D, S

●■ **V28.9**   Unspecified motorcycle rider injured in noncollision transport accident in traffic accident A, D, S

CHAPTER 20 (V01-Y99)

● **V29   Motorcycle rider injured in other and unspecified transport accidents**

> The appropriate 7th character is to be added to each code from category V29

> | A | initial encounter |
> |---|---|
> | D | subsequent encounter |
> | S | sequela |

● **V29.0   Motorcycle driver injured in collision with other and unspecified motor vehicles in nontraffic accident**

● ■ **V29.00   Motorcycle driver injured in collision with unspecified motor vehicles in nontraffic accident** A, D, S

● **V29.09   Motorcycle driver injured in collision with other motor vehicles in nontraffic accident** A, D, S

● **V29.1   Motorcycle passenger injured in collision with other and unspecified motor vehicles in nontraffic accident**

● ■ **V29.10   Motorcycle passenger injured in collision with unspecified motor vehicles in nontraffic accident** A, D, S

● **V29.19   Motorcycle passenger injured in collision with other motor vehicles in nontraffic accident** A, D, S

● **V29.2   Unspecified motorcycle rider injured in collision with other and unspecified motor vehicles in nontraffic accident**

● ■ **V29.20   Unspecified motorcycle rider injured in collision with unspecified motor vehicles in nontraffic accident** A, D, S
> Motorcycle collision NOS, nontraffic

● ■ **V29.29   Unspecified motorcycle rider injured in collision with other motor vehicles in nontraffic accident** A, D, S

● ■ **V29.3   Motorcycle rider (driver) (passenger) injured in unspecified nontraffic accident** A, D, S
> Motorcycle accident NOS, nontraffic
> Motorcycle rider injured in nontraffic accident NOS

● **V29.4   Motorcycle driver injured in collision with other and unspecified motor vehicles in traffic accident**

● ■ **V29.40   Motorcycle driver injured in collision with unspecified motor vehicles in traffic accident** A, D, S

● **V29.49   Motorcycle driver injured in collision with other motor vehicles in traffic accident** A, D, S

● **V29.5   Motorcycle passenger injured in collision with other and unspecified motor vehicles in traffic accident**

● ■ **V29.50   Motorcycle passenger injured in collision with unspecified motor vehicles in traffic accident** A, D, S

● **V29.59   Motorcycle passenger injured in collision with other motor vehicles in traffic accident** A, D, S

● **V29.6   Unspecified motorcycle rider injured in collision with other and unspecified motor vehicles in traffic accident**

● ■ **V29.60   Unspecified motorcycle rider injured in collision with unspecified motor vehicles in traffic accident** A, D, S
> Motorcycle collision NOS (traffic)

● ■ **V29.69   Unspecified motorcycle rider injured in collision with other motor vehicles in traffic accident** A, D, S

● **V29.8   Motorcycle rider (driver) (passenger) injured in other specified transport accidents**

● **V29.81   Motorcycle rider (driver) (passenger) injured in transport accident with military vehicle** A, D, S

● **V29.88   Motorcycle rider (driver) (passenger) injured in other specified transport accidents** A, D, S

● ■ **V29.9   Motorcycle rider (driver) (passenger) injured in unspecified traffic accident** A, D, S
> Motorcycle accident NOS

OCCUPANT OF THREE-WHEELED MOTOR VEHICLE INJURED IN TRANSPORT ACCIDENT (V30-V39)

> | Includes | motorized tricycle |
> |---|---|
> | | motorized rickshaw |
> | | three-wheeled motor car |

> | Excludes1 | all-terrain vehicles (V86.-) |
> |---|---|
> | | motorcycle with sidecar (V20-V29) |
> | | vehicle designed primarily for off-road use (V86.-) |

● **V30   Occupant of three-wheeled motor vehicle injured in collision with pedestrian or animal**

> | Excludes1 | three-wheeled motor vehicle collision with animal-drawn vehicle or animal being ridden (V36.-) |
> |---|---|

> The appropriate 7th character is to be added to each code from category V30

> | A | initial encounter |
> |---|---|
> | D | subsequent encounter |
> | S | sequela |

● **V30.0   Driver of three-wheeled motor vehicle injured in collision with pedestrian or animal in nontraffic accident** A, D, S

● **V30.1   Passenger in three-wheeled motor vehicle injured in collision with pedestrian or animal in nontraffic accident** A, D, S

● **V30.2   Person on outside of three-wheeled motor vehicle injured in collision with pedestrian or animal in nontraffic accident** A, D, S

● ■ **V30.3   Unspecified occupant of three-wheeled motor vehicle injured in collision with pedestrian or animal in nontraffic accident** A, D, S

● **V30.4   Person boarding or alighting a three-wheeled motor vehicle injured in collision with pedestrian or animal** A, D, S

● **V30.5   Driver of three-wheeled motor vehicle injured in collision with pedestrian or animal in traffic accident** A, D, S

● **V30.6   Passenger in three-wheeled motor vehicle injured in collision with pedestrian or animal in traffic accident** A, D, S

● **V30.7   Person on outside of three-wheeled motor vehicle injured in collision with pedestrian or animal in traffic accident** A, D, S

● ■ **V30.9   Unspecified occupant of three-wheeled motor vehicle injured in collision with pedestrian or animal in traffic accident** A, D, S

● Unacceptable Principal Diagnosis   ● Use Additional Character(s)   ■ Unspecified   ▶ Manifestation Code

1708   **OGCR** Official Guidelines for Coding and Reporting   Excludes 1   Excludes 2   Includes   Use additional   Code first   Code also

● **V31** **Occupant of three-wheeled motor vehicle injured in collision with pedal cycle**

    The appropriate 7th character is to be added to each code from category V31

> A   initial encounter
> D   subsequent encounter
> S   sequela

● **V31.0** Driver of three-wheeled motor vehicle injured in collision with pedal cycle in nontraffic accident A, D, S 🖐

● **V31.1** Passenger in three-wheeled motor vehicle injured in collision with pedal cycle in nontraffic accident A, D, S 🖐

● **V31.2** Person on outside of three-wheeled motor vehicle injured in collision with pedal cycle in nontraffic accident A, D, S 🖐

●■ **V31.3** Unspecified occupant of three-wheeled motor vehicle injured in collision with pedal cycle in nontraffic accident A, D, S 🖐

● **V31.4** Person boarding or alighting a three-wheeled motor vehicle injured in collision with pedal cycle A, D, S 🖐

● **V31.5** Driver of three-wheeled motor vehicle injured in collision with pedal cycle in traffic accident A, D, S 🖐

● **V31.6** Passenger in three-wheeled motor vehicle injured in collision with pedal cycle in traffic accident A, D, S 🖐

● **V31.7** Person on outside of three-wheeled motor vehicle injured in collision with pedal cycle in traffic accident A, D, S 🖐

●■ **V31.9** Unspecified occupant of three-wheeled motor vehicle injured in collision with pedal cycle in traffic accident A, D, S 🖐

● **V32** **Occupant of three-wheeled motor vehicle injured in collision with two- or three-wheeled motor vehicle**

    The appropriate 7th character is to be added to each code from category V32

> A   initial encounter
> D   subsequent encounter
> S   sequela

● **V32.0** Driver of three-wheeled motor vehicle injured in collision with two- or three-wheeled motor vehicle in nontraffic accident A, D, S 🖐

● **V32.1** Passenger in three-wheeled motor vehicle injured in collision with two- or three-wheeled motor vehicle in nontraffic accident A, D, S 🖐

● **V32.2** Person on outside of three-wheeled motor vehicle injured in collision with two- or three-wheeled motor vehicle in nontraffic accident A, D, S 🖐

●■ **V32.3** Unspecified occupant of three-wheeled motor vehicle injured in collision with two- or three-wheeled motor vehicle in nontraffic accident A, D, S 🖐

● **V32.4** Person boarding or alighting a three-wheeled motor vehicle injured in collision with two- or three-wheeled motor vehicle A, D, S 🖐

● **V32.5** Driver of three-wheeled motor vehicle injured in collision with two- or three-wheeled motor vehicle in traffic accident A, D, S 🖐

● **V32.6** Passenger in three-wheeled motor vehicle injured in collision with two- or three-wheeled motor vehicle in traffic accident A, D, S 🖐

● **V32.7** Person on outside of three-wheeled motor vehicle injured in collision with two- or three-wheeled motor vehicle in traffic accident A, D, S 🖐

●■ **V32.9** Unspecified occupant of three-wheeled motor vehicle injured in collision with two- or three-wheeled motor vehicle in traffic accident A, D, S 🖐

● **V33** **Occupant of three-wheeled motor vehicle injured in collision with car, pick-up truck or van**

    The appropriate 7th character is to be added to each code from category V33

> A   initial encounter
> D   subsequent encounter
> S   sequela

● **V33.0** Driver of three-wheeled motor vehicle injured in collision with car, pick-up truck or van in nontraffic accident A, D, S 🖐

● **V33.1** Passenger in three-wheeled motor vehicle injured in collision with car, pick-up truck or van in nontraffic accident A, D, S 🖐

● **V33.2** Person on outside of three-wheeled motor vehicle injured in collision with car, pick-up truck or van in nontraffic accident A, D, S 🖐

●■ **V33.3** Unspecified occupant of three-wheeled motor vehicle injured in collision with car, pick-up truck or van in nontraffic accident A, D, S 🖐

● **V33.4** Person boarding or alighting a three-wheeled motor vehicle injured in collision with car, pick-up truck or van A, D, S 🖐

● **V33.5** Driver of three-wheeled motor vehicle injured in collision with car, pick-up truck or van in traffic accident A, D, S 🖐

● **V33.6** Passenger in three-wheeled motor vehicle injured in collision with car, pick-up truck or van in traffic accident A, D, S 🖐

● **V33.7** Person on outside of three-wheeled motor vehicle injured in collision with car, pick-up truck or van in traffic accident A, D, S 🖐

●■ **V33.9** Unspecified occupant of three-wheeled motor vehicle injured in collision with car, pick-up truck or van in traffic accident A, D, S 🖐

● **V34** **Occupant of three-wheeled motor vehicle injured in collision with heavy transport vehicle or bus**

> **Excludes1**   occupant of three-wheeled motor vehicle injured in collision with military vehicle (V39.81)

    The appropriate 7th character is to be added to each code from category V34

> A   initial encounter
> D   subsequent encounter
> S   sequela

● **V34.0** Driver of three-wheeled motor vehicle injured in collision with heavy transport vehicle or bus in nontraffic accident A, D, S 🖐

● **V34.1** Passenger in three-wheeled motor vehicle injured in collision with heavy transport vehicle or bus in nontraffic accident A, D, S 🖐

● **V34.2** Person on outside of three-wheeled motor vehicle injured in collision with heavy transport vehicle or bus in nontraffic accident A, D, S 🖐

●■ **V34.3** Unspecified occupant of three-wheeled motor vehicle injured in collision with heavy transport vehicle or bus in nontraffic accident A, D, S 🖐

N Newborn Age: 0   **P** Pediatric Age: 0–17   **M** Maternity DX: 12–55   **A** Adult Age: 15–124   ♀ Females Only   ♂ Males Only

🖐 Complication\Comorbidity   Major C\C   Present on Admission Requirement   Hospital-Acquired Condition

1709

CHAPTER 20 (V01-Y99)

- V34.4 Person boarding or alighting a three-wheeled motor vehicle injured in collision with heavy transport vehicle or bus A, D, S

- V34.5 Driver of three-wheeled motor vehicle injured in collision with heavy transport vehicle or bus in traffic accident A, D, S

- V34.6 Passenger in three-wheeled motor vehicle injured in collision with heavy transport vehicle or bus in traffic accident A, D, S

- V34.7 Person on outside of three-wheeled motor vehicle injured in collision with heavy transport vehicle or bus in traffic accident A, D, S

- V34.9 Unspecified occupant of three-wheeled motor vehicle injured in collision with heavy transport vehicle or bus in traffic accident A, D, S

- V35 Occupant of three-wheeled motor vehicle injured in collision with railway train or railway vehicle

   The appropriate 7th character is to be added to each code from category V35

A	initial encounter
D	subsequent encounter
S	sequela

- V35.0 Driver of three-wheeled motor vehicle injured in collision with railway train or railway vehicle in nontraffic accident A, D, S

- V35.1 Passenger in three-wheeled motor vehicle injured in collision with railway train or railway vehicle in nontraffic accident A, D, S

- V35.2 Person on outside of three-wheeled motor vehicle injured in collision with railway train or railway vehicle in nontraffic accident A, D, S

- V35.3 Unspecified occupant of three-wheeled motor vehicle injured in collision with railway train or railway vehicle in nontraffic accident A, D, S

- V35.4 Person boarding or alighting a three-wheeled motor vehicle injured in collision with railway train or railway vehicle

- V35.5 Driver of three-wheeled motor vehicle injured in collision with railway train or railway vehicle in traffic accident A, D, S

- V35.6 Passenger in three-wheeled motor vehicle injured in collision with railway train or railway vehicle in traffic accident A, D, S

- V35.7 Person on outside of three-wheeled motor vehicle injured in collision with railway train or railway vehicle in traffic accident A, D, S

- V35.9 Unspecified occupant of three-wheeled motor vehicle injured in collision with railway train or railway vehicle in traffic accident A, D, S

- V36 Occupant of three-wheeled motor vehicle injured in collision with other nonmotor vehicle

   Includes collision with animal-drawn vehicle, animal being ridden, streetcar

   The appropriate 7th character is to be added to each code from category V36

A	initial encounter
D	subsequent encounter
S	sequela

- V36.0 Driver of three-wheeled motor vehicle injured in collision with other nonmotor vehicle in nontraffic accident A, D, S

- V36.1 Passenger in three-wheeled motor vehicle injured in collision with other nonmotor vehicle in nontraffic accident A, D, S

- V36.2 Person on outside of three-wheeled motor vehicle injured in collision with other nonmotor vehicle in nontraffic accident A, D, S

- V36.3 Unspecified occupant of three-wheeled motor vehicle injured in collision with other nonmotor vehicle in nontraffic accident A, D, S

- V36.4 Person boarding or alighting a three-wheeled motor vehicle injured in collision with other nonmotor vehicle A, D, S

- V36.5 Driver of three-wheeled motor vehicle injured in collision with other nonmotor vehicle in traffic accident A, D, S

- V36.6 Passenger in three-wheeled motor vehicle injured in collision with other nonmotor vehicle in traffic accident A, D, S

- V36.7 Person on outside of three-wheeled motor vehicle injured in collision with other nonmotor vehicle in traffic accident A, D, S

- V36.9 Unspecified occupant of three-wheeled motor vehicle injured in collision with other nonmotor vehicle in traffic accident A, D, S

- V37 Occupant of three-wheeled motor vehicle injured in collision with fixed or stationary object

   The appropriate 7th character is to be added to each code from category V37

A	initial encounter
D	subsequent encounter
S	sequela

- V37.0 Driver of three-wheeled motor vehicle injured in collision with fixed or stationary object in nontraffic accident A, D, S

- V37.1 Passenger in three-wheeled motor vehicle injured in collision with fixed or stationary object in nontraffic accident A, D, S

- V37.2 Person on outside of three-wheeled motor vehicle injured in collision with fixed or stationary object in nontraffic accident A, D, S

- V37.3 Unspecified occupant of three-wheeled motor vehicle injured in collision with fixed or stationary object in nontraffic accident A, D, S

- V37.4 Person boarding or alighting a three-wheeled motor vehicle injured in collision with fixed or stationary object A, D, S

- V37.5 Driver of three-wheeled motor vehicle injured in collision with fixed or stationary object in traffic accident A, D, S

- V37.6 Passenger in three-wheeled motor vehicle injured in collision with fixed or stationary object in traffic accident A, D, S

- V37.7 Person on outside of three-wheeled motor vehicle injured in collision with fixed or stationary object in traffic accident A, D, S

- V37.9 Unspecified occupant of three-wheeled motor vehicle injured in collision with fixed or stationary object in traffic accident A, D, S

● Unacceptable Principal Diagnosis   ● Use Additional Character(s)   ■ Unspecified   ▶ Manifestation Code

1710   **OGCR** Official Guidelines for Coding and Reporting   Excludes 1   Excludes 2   Includes   Use additional   Code first   Code also

● **V38 Occupant of three-wheeled motor vehicle injured in noncollision transport accident**

> | Includes | fall or thrown from three-wheeled motor vehicle
> overturning of three-wheeled motor vehicle NOS
> overturning of three-wheeled motor vehicle without collision |

> The appropriate 7th character is to be added to each code from category V38

> | A | initial encounter |
> |---|---|
> | D | subsequent encounter |
> | S | sequela |

● **V38.0 Driver of three-wheeled motor vehicle injured in noncollision transport accident in nontraffic accident** A, D, S ⓗ

● **V38.1 Passenger in three-wheeled motor vehicle injured in noncollision transport accident in nontraffic accident** A, D, S ⓗ

● **V38.2 Person on outside of three-wheeled motor vehicle injured in noncollision transport accident in nontraffic accident** A, D, S ⓗ

●■ **V38.3 Unspecified occupant of three-wheeled motor vehicle injured in noncollision transport accident in nontraffic accident** A, D, S ⓗ

● **V38.4 Person boarding or alighting a three-wheeled motor vehicle injured in noncollision transport accident** A, D, S ⓗ

● **V38.5 Driver of three-wheeled motor vehicle injured in noncollision transport accident in traffic accident** A, D, S ⓗ

● **V38.6 Passenger in three-wheeled motor vehicle injured in noncollision transport accident in traffic accident** A, D, S ⓗ

● **V38.7 Person on outside of three-wheeled motor vehicle injured in noncollision transport accident in traffic accident** A, D, S ⓗ

●■ **V38.9 Unspecified occupant of three-wheeled motor vehicle injured in noncollision transport accident in traffic accident** A, D, S ⓗ

● **V39 Occupant of three-wheeled motor vehicle injured in other and unspecified transport accidents**

> The appropriate 7th character is to be added to each code from category V39

> | A | initial encounter |
> |---|---|
> | D | subsequent encounter |
> | S | sequela |

● **V39.0 Driver of three-wheeled motor vehicle injured in collision with other and unspecified motor vehicles in nontraffic accident**

●■ **V39.00 Driver of three-wheeled motor vehicle injured in collision with unspecified motor vehicles in nontraffic accident** A, D, S ⓗ

● **V39.09 Driver of three-wheeled motor vehicle injured in collision with other motor vehicles in nontraffic accident** A, D, S ⓗ

● **V39.1 Passenger in three-wheeled motor vehicle injured in collision with other and unspecified motor vehicles in nontraffic accident**

●■ **V39.10 Passenger in three-wheeled motor vehicle injured in collision with unspecified motor vehicles in nontraffic accident** A, D, S ⓗ

● **V39.19 Passenger in three-wheeled motor vehicle injured in collision with other motor vehicles in nontraffic accident** A, D, S ⓗ

● **V39.2 Unspecified occupant of three-wheeled motor vehicle injured in collision with other and unspecified motor vehicles in nontraffic accident**

●■ **V39.20 Unspecified occupant of three-wheeled motor vehicle injured in collision with unspecified motor vehicles in nontraffic accident** A, D, S ⓗ
> Collision NOS involving three-wheeled motor vehicle, nontraffic

●■ **V39.29 Unspecified occupant of three-wheeled motor vehicle injured in collision with other motor vehicles in nontraffic accident** A, D, S ⓗ

●■ **V39.3 Occupant (driver) (passenger) of three-wheeled motor vehicle injured in unspecified nontraffic accident** A, D, S ⓗ
> Accident NOS involving three-wheeled motor vehicle, nontraffic
> Occupant of three-wheeled motor vehicle injured in nontraffic accident NOS

● **V39.4 Driver of three-wheeled motor vehicle injured in collision with other and unspecified motor vehicles in traffic accident**

●■ **V39.40 Driver of three-wheeled motor vehicle injured in collision with unspecified motor vehicles in traffic accident** A, D, S ⓗ

● **V39.49 Driver of three-wheeled motor vehicle injured in collision with other motor vehicles in traffic accident** A, D, S ⓗ

● **V39.5 Passenger in three-wheeled motor vehicle injured in collision with other and unspecified motor vehicles in traffic accident**

●■ **V39.50 Passenger in three-wheeled motor vehicle injured in collision with unspecified motor vehicles in traffic accident** A, D, S ⓗ

● **V39.59 Passenger in three-wheeled motor vehicle injured in collision with other motor vehicles in traffic accident** A, D, S ⓗ

● **V39.6 Unspecified occupant of three-wheeled motor vehicle injured in collision with other and unspecified motor vehicles in traffic accident**

●■ **V39.60 Unspecified occupant of three-wheeled motor vehicle injured in collision with unspecified motor vehicles in traffic accident** A, D, S ⓗ
> Collision NOS involving three-wheeled motor vehicle (traffic)

●■ **V39.69 Unspecified occupant of three-wheeled motor vehicle injured in collision with other motor vehicles in traffic accident** A, D, S ⓗ

● **V39.8 Occupant (driver) (passenger) of three-wheeled motor vehicle injured in other specified transport accidents**

● **V39.81 Occupant (driver) (passenger) of three-wheeled motor vehicle injured in transport accident with military vehicle** A, D, S ⓗ

● **V39.89 Occupant (driver) (passenger) of three-wheeled motor vehicle injured in other specified transport accidents** A, D, S ⓗ

●■ **V39.9 Occupant (driver) (passenger) of three-wheeled motor vehicle injured in unspecified traffic accident** A, D, S ⓗ
> Accident NOS involving three-wheeled motor vehicle

N Newborn Age: 0   **P** Pediatric Age: 0–17   **M** Maternity DX: 12–55   **A** Adult Age: 15–124   ♀ Females Only   ♂ Males Only

ⓒ Complication\Comorbidity   ⓜ Major C\C   ⓗ Present on Admission Requirement   ⓗ Hospital-Acquired Condition

CAR OCCUPANT INJURED IN TRANSPORT ACCIDENT (V40-V49)

Includes   a four-wheeled motor vehicle designed primarily for carrying passengers
                automobile (pulling a trailer or camper)

Excludes1   bus (V50-V59)
                minibus (V50-V59)
                minivan (V50-V59)
                motorcoach (V70-V79)
                pick-up truck (V50-V59)
                sport utility vehicle (SUV) (V50-V59)

● **V40 Car occupant injured in collision with pedestrian or animal**

Excludes1 car collision with animal-drawn vehicle or animal being ridden (V46.-)

The appropriate 7th character is to be added to each code from category V40

A   initial encounter
D   subsequent encounter
S   sequela

● **V40.0** Car driver injured in collision with pedestrian or animal in nontraffic accident A, D, S

● **V40.1** Car passenger injured in collision with pedestrian or animal in nontraffic accident A, D, S

● **V40.2** Person on outside of car injured in collision with pedestrian or animal in nontraffic accident A, D, S

●■ **V40.3** Unspecified car occupant injured in collision with pedestrian or animal in nontraffic accident A, D, S

● **V40.4** Person boarding or alighting a car injured in collision with pedestrian or animal A, D, S

● **V40.5** Car driver injured in collision with pedestrian or animal in traffic accident A, D, S

● **V40.6** Car passenger injured in collision with pedestrian or animal in traffic accident A, D, S

● **V40.7** Person on outside of car injured in collision with pedestrian or animal in traffic accident A, D, S

●■ **V40.9** Unspecified car occupant injured in collision with pedestrian or animal in traffic accident A, D, S

● **V41 Car occupant injured in collision with pedal cycle**

The appropriate 7th character is to be added to each code from category V41

A   initial encounter
D   subsequent encounter
S   sequela

● **V41.0** Car driver injured in collision with pedal cycle in nontraffic accident A, D, S

● **V41.1** Car passenger injured in collision with pedal cycle in nontraffic accident A, D, S

● **V41.2** Person on outside of car injured in collision with pedal cycle in nontraffic accident A, D, S

●■ **V41.3** Unspecified car occupant injured in collision with pedal cycle in nontraffic accident A, D, S

● **V41.4** Person boarding or alighting a car injured in collision with pedal cycle A, D, S

● **V41.5** Car driver injured in collision with pedal cycle in traffic accident A, D, S

● **V41.6** Car passenger injured in collision with pedal cycle in traffic accident A, D, S

● **V41.7** Person on outside of car injured in collision with pedal cycle in traffic accident A, D, S

●■ **V41.9** Unspecified car occupant injured in collision with pedal cycle in traffic accident A, D, S

● **V42 Car occupant injured in collision with two- or three-wheeled motor vehicle**

The appropriate 7th character is to be added to each code from category V42

A   initial encounter
D   subsequent encounter
S   sequela

● **V42.0** Car driver injured in collision with two- or three-wheeled motor vehicle in nontraffic accident A, D, S

● **V42.1** Car passenger injured in collision with two- or three-wheeled motor vehicle in nontraffic accident A, D, S

● **V42.2** Person on outside of car injured in collision with two- or three-wheeled motor vehicle in nontraffic accident A, D, S

●■ **V42.3** Unspecified car occupant injured in collision with two- or three-wheeled motor vehicle in nontraffic accident A, D, S

● **V42.4** Person boarding or alighting a car injured in collision with two- or three- wheeled motor vehicle A, D, S

● **V42.5** Car driver injured in collision with two- or three-wheeled motor vehicle in traffic accident A, D, S

● **V42.6** Car passenger injured in collision with two- or three-wheeled motor vehicle in traffic accident A, D, S

● **V42.7** Person on outside of car injured in collision with two- or three-wheeled motor vehicle in traffic accident A, D, S

●■ **V42.9** Unspecified car occupant injured in collision with two- or three-wheeled motor vehicle in traffic accident A, D, S

● **V43 Car occupant injured in collision with car, pick-up truck or van**

The appropriate 7th character is to be added to each code from category V43

A   initial encounter
D   subsequent encounter
S   sequela

● **V43.0** Car driver injured in collision with car, pick-up truck or van in nontraffic accident

● **V43.01** Car driver injured in collision with sport utility vehicle in nontraffic accident A, D, S

● **V43.02** Car driver injured in collision with other type car in nontraffic accident A, D, S

● **V43.03** Car driver injured in collision with pick-up truck in nontraffic accident A, D, S

● **V43.04** Car driver injured in collision with van in nontraffic accident A, D, S

● **V43.1** Car passenger injured in collision with car, pick-up truck or van in nontraffic accident

● **V43.11** Car passenger injured in collision with sport utility vehicle in nontraffic accident A, D, S

● **V43.12** Car passenger injured in collision with other type car in nontraffic accident A, D, S

● **V43.13** Car passenger injured in collision with pick-up in nontraffic accident A, D, S

● **V43.14** Car passenger injured in collision with van in nontraffic accident A, D, S

● Unacceptable Principal Diagnosis   ● Use Additional Character(s)   ■ Unspecified   ▶ Manifestation Code
OGCR Official Guidelines for Coding and Reporting   Excludes 1   Excludes 2   Includes   Use additional   Code first   Code also

CHAPTER 20 (V01-Y99)

● **V43.2** Person on outside of car injured in collision with car, pick-up truck or van in nontraffic accident

  ● **V43.21** Person on outside of car injured in collision with sport utility vehicle in nontraffic accident A, D, S 🔖

  ● **V43.22** Person on outside of car injured in collision with other type car in nontraffic accident A, D, S 🔖

  ● **V43.23** Person on outside of car injured in collision with pick-up truck in nontraffic accident A, D, S 🔖

  ● **V43.24** Person on outside of car injured in collision with van in nontraffic accident A, D, S 🔖

● **V43.3** Unspecified car occupant injured in collision with car, pick-up truck or van in nontraffic accident

  ●■ **V43.31** Unspecified car occupant injured in collision with sport utility vehicle in nontraffic accident A, D, S 🔖

  ●■ **V43.32** Unspecified car occupant injured in collision with other type car in nontraffic accident A, D, S 🔖

  ●■ **V43.33** Unspecified car occupant injured in collision with pick-up truck in nontraffic accident A, D, S 🔖

  ●■ **V43.34** Unspecified car occupant injured in collision with van in nontraffic accident A, D, S 🔖

● **V43.4** Person boarding or alighting a car injured in collision with car, pick-up truck or van

  ● **V43.41** Person boarding or alighting a car injured in collision with sport utility vehicle A, D, S 🔖

  ● **V43.42** Person boarding or alighting a car injured in collision with other type car A, D, S 🔖

  ● **V43.43** Person boarding or alighting a car injured in collision with pick-up truck A, D, S 🔖

  ● **V43.44** Person boarding or alighting a car injured in collision with van A, D, S 🔖

● **V43.5** Car driver injured in collision with car, pick-up truck or van in traffic accident

  ● **V43.51** Car driver injured in collision with sport utility vehicle in traffic accident A, D, S 🔖

  ● **V43.52** Car driver injured in collision with other type car in traffic accident A, D, S 🔖

  ● **V43.53** Car driver injured in collision with pick-up truck in traffic accident A, D, S 🔖

  ● **V43.54** Car driver injured in collision with van in traffic accident A, D, S 🔖

● **V43.6** Car passenger injured in collision with car, pick-up truck or van in traffic accident

  ● **V43.61** Car passenger injured in collision with sport utility vehicle in traffic accident A, D, S 🔖

  ● **V43.62** Car passenger injured in collision with other type car in traffic accident A, D, S 🔖

  ● **V43.63** Car passenger injured in collision with pick-up truck in traffic accident A, D, S 🔖

  ● **V43.64** Car passenger injured in collision with van in traffic accident A, D, S 🔖

● **V43.7** Person on outside of car injured in collision with car, pick-up truck or van in traffic accident

  ● **V43.71** Person on outside of car injured in collision with sport utility vehicle in traffic accident A, D, S 🔖

  ● **V43.72** Person on outside of car injured in collision with other type car in traffic accident A, D, S 🔖

  ● **V43.73** Person on outside of car injured in collision with pick-up truck in traffic accident A, D, S 🔖

  ● **V43.74** Person on outside of car injured in collision with van in traffic accident A, D, S 🔖

● **V43.9** Unspecified car occupant injured in collision with car, pick-up truck or van in traffic accident

  ●■ **V43.91** Unspecified car occupant injured in collision with sport utility vehicle in traffic accident A, D, S 🔖

  ●■ **V43.92** Unspecified car occupant injured in collision with other type car in traffic accident A, D, S 🔖

  ●■ **V43.93** Unspecified car occupant injured in collision with pick-up truck in traffic accident A, D, S 🔖

  ●■ **V43.94** Unspecified car occupant injured in collision with van in traffic accident A, D, S 🔖

● **V44** Car occupant injured in collision with heavy transport vehicle or bus

  Excludes1   car occupant injured in collision with military vehicle (V49.81)

  The appropriate 7th character is to be added to each code from category V44

A	initial encounter
D	subsequent encounter
S	sequela

● **V44.0** Car driver injured in collision with heavy transport vehicle or bus in nontraffic accident A, D, S 🔖

● **V44.1** Car passenger injured in collision with heavy transport vehicle or bus in nontraffic accident A, D, S 🔖

● **V44.2** Person on outside of car injured in collision with heavy transport vehicle or bus in nontraffic accident A, D, S 🔖

●■ **V44.3** Unspecified car occupant injured in collision with heavy transport vehicle or bus in nontraffic accident A, D, S 🔖

● **V44.4** Person boarding or alighting a car injured in collision with heavy transport vehicle or bus A, D, S 🔖

● **V44.5** Car driver injured in collision with heavy transport vehicle or bus in traffic accident A, D, S 🔖

● **V44.6** Car passenger injured in collision with heavy transport vehicle or bus in traffic accident A, D, S 🔖

● **V44.7** Person on outside of car injured in collision with heavy transport vehicle or bus in traffic accident A, D, S 🔖

●■ **V44.9** Unspecified car occupant injured in collision with heavy transport vehicle or bus in traffic accident A, D, S 🔖

CHAPTER 20 (V01–Y99)

● **V45**   **Car occupant injured in collision with railway train or railway vehicle**

> The appropriate 7th character is to be added to each code from category V45

> | A | initial encounter |
> |---|---|
> | D | subsequent encounter |
> | S | sequela |

- ● V45.0   Car driver injured in collision with railway train or railway vehicle in nontraffic accident A, D, S 🗎

- ● V45.1   Car passenger injured in collision with railway train or railway vehicle in nontraffic accident A, D, S 🗎

- ● V45.2   Person on outside of car injured in collision with railway train or railway vehicle in nontraffic accident A, D, S 🗎

- ●■ V45.3   Unspecified car occupant injured in collision with railway train or railway vehicle in nontraffic accident A, D, S 🗎

- ● V45.4   Person boarding or alighting a car injured in collision with railway train or railway vehicle A, D, S 🗎

- ● V45.5   Car driver injured in collision with railway train or railway vehicle in traffic accident A, D, S 🗎

- ● V45.6   Car passenger injured in collision with railway train or railway vehicle in traffic accident A, D, S 🗎

- ● V45.7   Person on outside of car injured in collision with railway train or railway vehicle in traffic accident A, D, S 🗎

- ●■ V45.9   Unspecified car occupant injured in collision with railway train or railway vehicle in traffic accident A, D, S 🗎

● **V46**   **Car occupant injured in collision with other nonmotor vehicle**

> **Includes**   collision with animal-drawn vehicle, animal being ridden, streetcar

> The appropriate 7th character is to be added to each code from category V46

> | A | initial encounter |
> |---|---|
> | D | subsequent encounter |
> | S | sequela |

- ● V46.0   Car driver injured in collision with other nonmotor vehicle in nontraffic accident A, D, S 🗎

- ● V46.1   Car passenger injured in collision with other nonmotor vehicle in nontraffic accident A, D, S 🗎

- ● V46.2   Person on outside of car injured in collision with other nonmotor vehicle in nontraffic accident A, D, S 🗎

- ●■ V46.3   Unspecified car occupant injured in collision with other nonmotor vehicle in nontraffic accident A, D, S 🗎

- ● V46.4   Person boarding or alighting a car injured in collision with other nonmotor vehicle A, D, S 🗎

- ● V46.5   Car driver injured in collision with other nonmotor vehicle in traffic accident A, D, S 🗎

- ● V46.6   Car passenger injured in collision with other nonmotor vehicle in traffic accident A, D, S 🗎

- ● V46.7   Person on outside of car injured in collision with other nonmotor vehicle in traffic accident A, D, S 🗎

- ●■ V46.9   Unspecified car occupant injured in collision with other nonmotor vehicle in traffic accident A, D, S 🗎

● **V47**   **Car occupant injured in collision with fixed or stationary object**

> The appropriate 7th character is to be added to each code from category V47

> | A | initial encounter |
> |---|---|
> | D | subsequent encounter |
> | S | sequela |

- ● V47.0   Car driver injured in collision with fixed or stationary object in nontraffic accident

  - ● V47.01   Driver of sport utility vehicle injured in collision with fixed or stationary object in nontraffic accident A, D, S 🗎

  - ● V47.02   Driver of other type car injured in collision with fixed or stationary object in nontraffic accident A, D, S 🗎

- ● V47.1   Car passenger injured in collision with fixed or stationary object in nontraffic accident

  - ● V47.11   Passenger of sport utility vehicle injured in collision with fixed or stationary object in nontraffic accident A, D, S 🗎

  - ● V47.12   Passenger of other type car injured in collision with fixed or stationary object in nontraffic accident A, D, S 🗎

- ● V47.2   Person on outside of car injured in collision with fixed or stationary object in nontraffic accident A, D, S 🗎

- ● V47.3   Unspecified car occupant injured in collision with fixed or stationary object in nontraffic accident

  - ●■ V47.31   Unspecified occupant of sport utility vehicle injured in collision with fixed or stationary object in nontraffic accident A, D, S 🗎

  - ●■ V47.32   Unspecified occupant of other type car injured in collision with fixed or stationary object in nontraffic accident A, D, S 🗎

- ● V47.4   Person boarding or alighting a car injured in collision with fixed or stationary object A, D, S 🗎

- ● V47.5   Car driver injured in collision with fixed or stationary object in traffic accident

  - ● V47.51   Driver of sport utility vehicle injured in collision with fixed or stationary object in traffic accident A, D, S 🗎

  - ● V47.52   Driver of other type car injured in collision with fixed or stationary object in traffic accident A, D, S 🗎

- ● V47.6   Car passenger injured in collision with fixed or stationary object in traffic accident

  - ● V47.61   Passenger of sport utility vehicle injured in collision with fixed or stationary object in traffic accident A, D, S 🗎

  - ● V47.62   Passenger of other type car injured in collision with fixed or stationary object in traffic accident A, D, S 🗎

- ● V47.7   Person on outside of car injured in collision with fixed or stationary object in traffic accident A, D, S 🗎

- ● V47.9   Unspecified car occupant injured in collision with fixed or stationary object in traffic accident

  - ●■ V47.91   Unspecified occupant of sport utility vehicle injured in collision with fixed or stationary object in traffic accident A, D, S 🗎

  - ●■ V47.92   Unspecified occupant of other type car injured in collision with fixed or stationary object in traffic accident A, D, S 🗎

● Unacceptable Principal Diagnosis   ● Use Additional Character(s)   ■ Unspecified   ▶ Manifestation Code

OGCR   Official Guidelines for Coding and Reporting   Excludes 1   Excludes 2   Includes   Use additional   Code first   Code also

● **V48 Car occupant injured in noncollision transport accident**

> | **Includes** | overturning car NOS |
> |---|---|
> | | overturning car without collision |

>   The appropriate 7th character is to be added to each code
>   from category V48

> | A | initial encounter |
> |---|---|
> | D | subsequent encounter |
> | S | sequela |

- ● **V48.0 Car driver injured in noncollision transport accident in nontraffic accident** A, D, S 🔖
- ● **V48.1 Car passenger injured in noncollision transport accident in nontraffic accident** A, D, S 🔖
- ● **V48.2 Person on outside of car injured in noncollision transport accident in nontraffic accident** A, D, S 🔖
- ●■ **V48.3 Unspecified car occupant injured in noncollision transport accident in nontraffic accident** A, D, S 🔖
- ● **V48.4 Person boarding or alighting a car injured in noncollision transport accident** A, D, S 🔖
- ● **V48.5 Car driver injured in noncollision transport accident in traffic accident** A, D, S 🔖
- ● **V48.6 Car passenger injured in noncollision transport accident in traffic accident** A, D, S 🔖
- ● **V48.7 Person on outside of car injured in noncollision transport accident in traffic accident** A, D, S 🔖
- ●■ **V48.9 Unspecified car occupant injured in noncollision transport accident in traffic accident** A, D, S 🔖

● **V49 Car occupant injured in other and unspecified transport accidents**

>   The appropriate 7th character is to be added to each code
>   from category V49

> | A | initial encounter |
> |---|---|
> | D | subsequent encounter |
> | S | sequela |

- ● **V49.0 Driver injured in collision with other and unspecified motor vehicles in nontraffic accident**
    - ●■ **V49.00 Driver injured in collision with unspecified motor vehicles in nontraffic accident** A, D, S 🔖
    - ● **V49.09 Driver injured in collision with other motor vehicles in nontraffic accident** A, D, S 🔖
- ● **V49.1 Passenger injured in collision with other and unspecified motor vehicles in nontraffic accident**
    - ●■ **V49.10 Passenger injured in collision with unspecified motor vehicles in nontraffic accident** A, D, S 🔖
    - ● **V49.19 Passenger injured in collision with other motor vehicles in nontraffic accident** A, D, S 🔖
- ● **V49.2 Unspecified car occupant injured in collision with other and unspecified motor vehicles in nontraffic accident**
    - ●■ **V49.20 Unspecified car occupant injured in collision with unspecified motor vehicles in nontraffic accident** A, D, S 🔖
          Car collision NOS, nontraffic
    - ●■ **V49.29 Unspecified car occupant injured in collision with other motor vehicles in nontraffic accident** A, D, S 🔖
- ● **V49.3 Car occupant (driver) (passenger) injured in unspecified nontraffic accident** A, D, S 🔖
          Car accident NOS, nontraffic
          Car occupant injured in nontraffic accident NOS

- ● **V49.4 Driver injured in collision with other and unspecified motor vehicles in traffic accident**
    - ●■ **V49.40 Driver injured in collision with unspecified motor vehicles in traffic accident** A, D, S 🔖
    - ● **V49.49 Driver injured in collision with other motor vehicles in traffic accident** A, D, S 🔖
- ● **V49.5 Passenger injured in collision with other and unspecified motor vehicles in traffic accident**
    - ●■ **V49.50 Passenger injured in collision with unspecified motor vehicles in traffic accident** A, D, S 🔖
    - ● **V49.59 Passenger injured in collision with other motor vehicles in traffic accident** A, D, S 🔖
- ● **V49.6 Unspecified car occupant injured in collision with other and unspecified motor vehicles in traffic accident**
    - ●■ **V49.60 Unspecified car occupant injured in collision with unspecified motor vehicles in traffic accident** A, D, S 🔖
          Car collision NOS (traffic)
    - ●■ **V49.69 Unspecified car occupant injured in collision with other motor vehicles in traffic accident** A, D, S 🔖
- ● **V49.8 Car occupant (driver) (passenger) injured in other specified transport accidents**
    - ● **V49.81 Car occupant (driver) (passenger) injured in transport accident with military vehicle** A, D, S 🔖
    - ● **V49.88 Car occupant (driver) (passenger) injured in other specified transport accidents** A, D, S 🔖
- ●■ **V49.9 Car occupant (driver) (passenger) injured in unspecified traffic accident** A, D, S 🔖
          Car accident NOS

OCCUPANT OF PICK-UP TRUCK OR VAN INJURED IN TRANSPORT ACCIDENT (V50-V59)

> | **Includes** | a four- or six-wheel motor vehicle designed primarily for carrying passengers and property but weighing less than the local limit for classification as a heavy goods vehicle |
> |---|---|
> | | minibus |
> | | minivan |
> | | sport utility vehicle (SUV) |
> | | truck |
> | | van |

> | **Excludes1** | heavy transport vehicle (V60-V69) |
> |---|---|

● **V50 Occupant of pick-up truck or van injured in collision with pedestrian or animal**

> | **Excludes1** | pick-up truck or van collision with animal-drawn vehicle or animal being ridden (V56.-) |
> |---|---|

>   The appropriate 7th character is to be added to each code
>   from category V50

> | A | initial encounter |
> |---|---|
> | D | subsequent encounter |
> | S | sequela |

- ● **V50.0 Driver of pick-up truck or van injured in collision with pedestrian or animal in nontraffic accident** A, D, S 🔖
- ● **V50.1 Passenger in pick-up truck or van injured in collision with pedestrian or animal in nontraffic accident** A, D, S 🔖

N Newborn Age: 0   **P** Pediatric Age: 0–17   **M** Maternity DX: 12–55   **A** Adult Age: 15–124   ♀ Females Only   ♂ Males Only

🔖 Complication\Comorbidity   🔖 Major C\C   🔖 Present on Admission Requirement   🔖 Hospital-Acquired Condition

● V50.2   Person on outside of pick-up truck or van injured in collision with pedestrian or animal in nontraffic accident A, D, S ✍

●■ V50.3   Unspecified occupant of pick-up truck or van injured in collision with pedestrian or animal in nontraffic accident A, D, S ✍

● V50.4   Person boarding or alighting a pick-up truck or van injured in collision with pedestrian or animal A, D, S ✍

● V50.5   Driver of pick-up truck or van injured in collision with pedestrian or animal in traffic accident A, D, S ✍

● V50.6   Passenger in pick-up truck or van injured in collision with pedestrian or animal in traffic accident A, D, S ✍

● V50.7   Person on outside of pick-up truck or van injured in collision with pedestrian or animal in traffic accident A, D, S ✍

●■ V50.9   Unspecified occupant of pick-up truck or van injured in collision with pedestrian or animal in traffic accident A, D, S ✍

● **V51**   **Occupant of pick-up truck or van injured in collision with pedal cycle**

> The appropriate 7th character is to be added to each code from category V51

> | | |
> |---|---|
> | A | initial encounter |
> | D | subsequent encounter |
> | S | sequela |

● V51.0   Driver of pick-up truck or van injured in collision with pedal cycle in nontraffic accident A, D, S ✍

● V51.1   Passenger in pick-up truck or van injured in collision with pedal cycle in nontraffic accident A, D, S ✍

● V51.2   Person on outside of pick-up truck or van injured in collision with pedal cycle in nontraffic accident A, D, S ✍

●■ V51.3   Unspecified occupant of pick-up truck or van injured in collision with pedal cycle in nontraffic accident A, D, S ✍

● V51.4   Person boarding or alighting a pick-up truck or van injured in collision with pedal cycle A, D, S ✍

● V51.5   Driver of pick-up truck or van injured in collision with pedal cycle in traffic accident A, D, S ✍

● V51.6   Passenger in pick-up truck or van injured in collision with pedal cycle in traffic accident A, D, S ✍

● V51.7   Person on outside of pick-up truck or van injured in collision with pedal cycle in traffic accident A, D, S ✍

●■ V51.9   Unspecified occupant of pick-up truck or van injured in collision with pedal cycle in traffic accident A, D, S ✍

● **V52**   **Occupant of pick-up truck or van injured in collision with two- or three-wheeled motor vehicle**

> The appropriate 7th character is to be added to each code from category V52

> | | |
> |---|---|
> | A | initial encounter |
> | D | subsequent encounter |
> | S | sequela |

● V52.0   Driver of pick-up truck or van injured in collision with two- or three-wheeled motor vehicle in nontraffic accident A, D, S ✍

● V52.1   Passenger in pick-up truck or van injured in collision with two- or three-wheeled motor vehicle in nontraffic accident A, D, S ✍

● V52.2   Person on outside of pick-up truck or van injured in collision with two- or three-wheeled motor vehicle in nontraffic accident A, D, S ✍

●■ V52.3   Unspecified occupant of pick-up truck or van injured in collision with two- or three-wheeled motor vehicle in nontraffic accident A, D, S ✍

● V52.4   Person boarding or alighting a pick-up truck or van injured in collision with two- or three-wheeled motor vehicle A, D, S ✍

● V52.5   Driver of pick-up truck or van injured in collision with two- or three-wheeled motor vehicle in traffic accident A, D, S ✍

● V52.6   Passenger in pick-up truck or van injured in collision with two- or three-wheeled motor vehicle in traffic accident A, D, S ✍

● V52.7   Person on outside of pick-up truck or van injured in collision with two- or three-wheeled motor vehicle in traffic accident A, D, S ✍

●■ V52.9   Unspecified occupant of pick-up truck or van injured in collision with two- or three-wheeled motor vehicle in traffic accident A, D, S ✍

● **V53**   **Occupant of pick-up truck or van injured in collision with car, pick-up truck or van**

> The appropriate 7th character is to be added to each code from category V53

> | | |
> |---|---|
> | A | initial encounter |
> | D | subsequent encounter |
> | S | sequela |

● V53.0   Driver of pick-up truck or van injured in collision with car, pick-up truck or van in nontraffic accident A, D, S ✍

● V53.1   Passenger in pick-up truck or van injured in collision with car, pick-up truck or van in nontraffic accident A, D, S ✍

● V53.2   Person on outside of pick-up truck or van injured in collision with car, pick-up truck or van in nontraffic accident A, D, S ✍

●■ V53.3   Unspecified occupant of pick-up truck or van injured in collision with car, pick-up truck or van in nontraffic accident A, D, S ✍

● V53.4   Person boarding or alighting a pick-up truck or van injured in collision with car, pick-up truck or van A, D, S ✍

● V53.5   Driver of pick-up truck or van injured in collision with car, pick-up truck or van in traffic accident A, D, S ✍

● V53.6   Passenger in pick-up truck or van injured in collision with car, pick-up truck or van in traffic accident A, D, S ✍

● V53.7   Person on outside of pick-up truck or van injured in collision with car, pick-up truck or van in traffic accident A, D, S ✍

●■ V53.9   Unspecified occupant of pick-up truck or van injured in collision with car, pick-up truck or van in traffic accident A, D, S ✍

CHAPTER 20 (V01-Y99)

● Unacceptable Principal Diagnosis   ● Use Additional Character(s)   ■ Unspecified   ▶ Manifestation Code

OGCR Official Guidelines for Coding and Reporting   Excludes 1   Excludes 2   Includes   Use additional   Code first   Code also

● **V54**   **Occupant of pick-up truck or van injured in collision with heavy transport vehicle or bus**

> **Excludes1**   occupant of pick-up truck or van injured in collision with military vehicle (V59.81)

> The appropriate 7th character is to be added to each code from category V54

> | | |
> |---|---|
> | A | initial encounter |
> | D | subsequent encounter |
> | S | sequela |

● **V54.0**   Driver of pick-up truck or van injured in collision with heavy transport vehicle or bus in nontraffic accident A, D, S

● **V54.1**   Passenger in pick-up truck or van injured in collision with heavy transport vehicle or bus in nontraffic accident A, D, S

● **V54.2**   Person on outside of pick-up truck or van injured in collision with heavy transport vehicle or bus in nontraffic accident A, D, S

●■ **V54.3**   Unspecified occupant of pick-up truck or van injured in collision with heavy transport vehicle or bus in nontraffic accident A, D, S

● **V54.4**   Person boarding or alighting a pick-up truck or van injured in collision with heavy transport vehicle or bus A, D, S

● **V54.5**   Driver of pick-up truck or van injured in collision with heavy transport vehicle or bus in traffic accident A, D, S

● **V54.6**   Passenger in pick-up truck or van injured in collision with heavy transport vehicle or bus in traffic accident A, D, S

● **V54.7**   Person on outside of pick-up truck or van injured in collision with heavy transport vehicle or bus in traffic accident A, D, S

●■ **V54.9**   Unspecified occupant of pick-up truck or van injured in collision with heavy transport vehicle or bus in traffic accident A, D, S

● **V55**   **Occupant of pick-up truck or van injured in collision with railway train or railway vehicle**

> The appropriate 7th character is to be added to each code from category V55

> | | |
> |---|---|
> | A | initial encounter |
> | D | subsequent encounter |
> | S | sequela |

● **V55.0**   Driver of pick-up truck or van injured in collision with railway train or railway vehicle in nontraffic accident A, D, S

● **V55.1**   Passenger in pick-up truck or van injured in collision with railway train or railway vehicle in nontraffic accident A, D, S

● **V55.2**   Person on outside of pick-up truck or van injured in collision with railway train or railway vehicle in nontraffic accident A, D, S

●■ **V55.3**   Unspecified occupant of pick-up truck or van injured in collision with railway train or railway vehicle in nontraffic accident A, D, S

● **V55.4**   Person boarding or alighting a pick-up truck or van injured in collision with railway train or railway vehicle A, D, S

● **V55.5**   Driver of pick-up truck or van injured in collision with railway train or railway vehicle in traffic accident A, D, S

● **V55.6**   Passenger in pick-up truck or van injured in collision with railway train or railway vehicle in traffic accident A, D, S

● **V55.7**   Person on outside of pick-up truck or van injured in collision with railway train or railway vehicle in traffic accident A, D, S

●■ **V55.9**   Unspecified occupant of pick-up truck or van injured in collision with railway train or railway vehicle in traffic accident A, D, S

● **V56**   **Occupant of pick-up truck or van injured in collision with other nonmotor vehicle**

> **Includes**   collision with animal-drawn vehicle, animal being ridden, streetcar

> The appropriate 7th character is to be added to each code from category V56

> | | |
> |---|---|
> | A | initial encounter |
> | D | subsequent encounter |
> | S | sequela |

● **V56.0**   Driver of pick-up truck or van injured in collision with other nonmotor vehicle in nontraffic accident A, D, S

● **V56.1**   Passenger in pick-up truck or van injured in collision with other nonmotor vehicle in nontraffic accident A, D, S

● **V56.2**   Person on outside of pick-up truck or van injured in collision with other nonmotor vehicle in nontraffic accident A, D, S

●■ **V56.3**   Unspecified occupant of pick-up truck or van injured in collision with other nonmotor vehicle in nontraffic accident A, D, S

● **V56.4**   Person boarding or alighting a pick-up truck or van injured in collision with other nonmotor vehicle A, D, S

● **V56.5**   Driver of pick-up truck or van injured in collision with other nonmotor vehicle in traffic accident A, D, S

● **V56.6**   Passenger in pick-up truck or van injured in collision with other nonmotor vehicle in traffic accident A, D, S

● **V56.7**   Person on outside of pick-up truck or van injured in collision with other nonmotor vehicle in traffic accident A, D, S

●■ **V56.9**   Unspecified occupant of pick-up truck or van injured in collision with other nonmotor vehicle in traffic accident A, D, S

● **V57**   **Occupant of pick-up truck or van injured in collision with fixed or stationary object**

> The appropriate 7th character is to be added to each code from category V57

> | | |
> |---|---|
> | A | initial encounter |
> | D | subsequent encounter |
> | S | sequela |

● **V57.0**   Driver of pick-up truck or van injured in collision with fixed or stationary object in nontraffic accident A, D, S

● **V57.1**   Passenger in pick-up truck or van injured in collision with fixed or stationary object in nontraffic accident A, D, S

● **V57.2**   Person on outside of pick-up truck or van injured in collision with fixed or stationary object in nontraffic accident A, D, S

●■ **V57.3**   Unspecified occupant of pick-up truck or van injured in collision with fixed or stationary object in nontraffic accident A, D, S

● **V57.4**   Person boarding or alighting a pick-up truck or van injured in collision with fixed or stationary object A, D, S

N Newborn Age: 0   **P** Pediatric Age: 0–17   **M** Maternity DX: 12–55   **A** Adult Age: 15–124   ♀ Females Only   ♂ Males Only

   Complication\Comorbidity   Major C\C   Present on Admission Requirement   Hospital-Acquired Condition

1717

● **V57.5** Driver of pick-up truck or van injured in collision with fixed or stationary object in traffic accident A, D, S 📋

● **V57.6** Passenger in pick-up truck or van injured in collision with fixed or stationary object in traffic accident A, D, S 📋

● **V57.7** Person on outside of pick-up truck or van injured in collision with fixed or stationary object in traffic accident A, D, S 📋

●🔲 **V57.9** Unspecified occupant of pick-up truck or van injured in collision with fixed or stationary object in traffic accident A, D, S 📋

● **V58** Occupant of pick-up truck or van injured in noncollision transport accident

> **Includes**   overturning pick-up truck or van NOS
> overturning pick-up truck or van without collision

The appropriate 7th character is to be added to each code from category V58

> A   initial encounter
> D   subsequent encounter
> S   sequela

● **V58.0** Driver of pick-up truck or van injured in noncollision transport accident in nontraffic accident A, D, S 📋

● **V58.1** Passenger in pick-up truck or van injured in noncollision transport accident in nontraffic accident A, D, S 📋

● **V58.2** Person on outside of pick-up truck or van injured in noncollision transport accident in nontraffic accident A, D, S 📋

●🔲 **V58.3** Unspecified occupant of pick-up truck or van injured in noncollision transport accident in nontraffic accident A, D, S 📋

● **V58.4** Person boarding or alighting a pick-up truck or van injured in noncollision transport accident A, D, S 📋

● **V58.5** Driver of pick-up truck or van injured in noncollision transport accident in traffic accident A, D, S 📋

● **V58.6** Passenger in pick-up truck or van injured in noncollision transport accident in traffic accident A, D, S 📋

● **V58.7** Person on outside of pick-up truck or van injured in noncollision transport accident in traffic accident A, D, S 📋

●🔲 **V58.9** Unspecified occupant of pick-up truck or van injured in noncollision transport accident in traffic accident A, D, S 📋

● **V59** Occupant of pick-up truck or van injured in other and unspecified transport accidents

The appropriate 7th character is to be added to each code from category V59

> A   initial encounter
> D   subsequent encounter
> S   sequela

● **V59.0** Driver of pick-up truck or van injured in collision with other and unspecified motor vehicles in nontraffic accident

●🔲 **V59.00** Driver of pick-up truck or van injured in collision with unspecified motor vehicles in nontraffic accident A, D, S 📋

● **V59.09** Driver of pick-up truck or van injured in collision with other motor vehicles in nontraffic accident A, D, S 📋

● **V59.1** Passenger in pick-up truck or van injured in collision with other and unspecified motor vehicles in nontraffic accident

●🔲 **V59.10** Passenger in pick-up truck or van injured in collision with unspecified motor vehicles in nontraffic accident A, D, S 📋

● **V59.19** Passenger in pick-up truck or van injured in collision with other motor vehicles in nontraffic accident A, D, S 📋

● **V59.2** Unspecified occupant of pick-up truck or van injured in collision with other and unspecified motor vehicles in nontraffic accident

●🔲 **V59.20** Unspecified occupant of pick-up truck or van injured in collision with unspecified motor vehicles in nontraffic accident A, D, S 📋
> Collision NOS involving pick-up truck or van, nontraffic

●🔲 **V59.29** Unspecified occupant of pick-up truck or van injured in collision with other motor vehicles in nontraffic accident A, D, S 📋

●🔲 **V59.3** Occupant (driver) (passenger) of pick-up truck or van injured in unspecified nontraffic accident A, D, S 📋
> Accident NOS involving pick-up truck or van, nontraffic
> Occupant of pick-up truck or van injured in nontraffic accident NOS

● **V59.4** Driver of pick-up truck or van injured in collision with other and unspecified motor vehicles in traffic accident

●🔲 **V59.40** Driver of pick-up truck or van injured in collision with unspecified motor vehicles in traffic accident A, D, S 📋

● **V59.49** Driver of pick-up truck or van injured in collision with other motor vehicles in traffic accident A, D, S 📋

● **V59.5** Passenger in pick-up truck or van injured in collision with other and unspecified motor vehicles in traffic accident

●🔲 **V59.50** Passenger in pick-up truck or van injured in collision with unspecified motor vehicles in traffic accident A, D, S 📋

● **V59.59** Passenger in pick-up truck or van injured in collision with other motor vehicles in traffic accident A, D, S 📋

● **V59.6** Unspecified occupant of pick-up truck or van injured in collision with other and unspecified motor vehicles in traffic accident

●🔲 **V59.60** Unspecified occupant of pick-up truck or van injured in collision with unspecified motor vehicles in traffic accident A, D, S 📋
> Collision NOS involving pick-up truck or van (traffic)

●🔲 **V59.69** Unspecified occupant of pick-up truck or van injured in collision with other motor vehicles in traffic accident A, D, S 📋

● **V59.8** Occupant (driver) (passenger) of pick-up truck or van injured in other specified transport accidents

● **V59.81** Occupant (driver) (passenger) of pick-up truck or van injured in transport accident with military vehicle A, D, S 📋

● **V59.88** Occupant (driver) (passenger) of pick-up truck or van injured in other specified transport accidents A, D, S 📋

●🔲 **V59.9** Occupant (driver) (passenger) of pick-up truck or van injured in unspecified traffic accident A, D, S 📋
> Accident NOS involving pick-up truck or van

● Unacceptable Principal Diagnosis   ● Use Additional Character(s)   🔲 Unspecified   ▶ Manifestation Code

1718   **OGCR** Official Guidelines for Coding and Reporting   Excludes 1   Excludes 2   Includes   Use additional   Code first   Code also

OCCUPANT OF HEAVY TRANSPORT VEHICLE INJURED IN TRANSPORT ACCIDENT (V60-V69)

Includes	18 wheeler
	armored car
	panel truck
Excludes1	bus
	motorcoach

● **V60** Occupant of heavy transport vehicle injured in collision with pedestrian or animal

　Excludes1　heavy transport vehicle collision with animal-drawn vehicle or animal being ridden (V66.-)

The appropriate 7th character is to be added to each code from category V60

A	initial encounter
D	subsequent encounter
S	sequela

● **V60.0** Driver of heavy transport vehicle injured in collision with pedestrian or animal in nontraffic accident A, D, S

● **V60.1** Passenger in heavy transport vehicle injured in collision with pedestrian or animal in nontraffic accident A, D, S

● **V60.2** Person on outside of heavy transport vehicle injured in collision with pedestrian or animal in nontraffic accident A, D, S

●■ **V60.3** Unspecified occupant of heavy transport vehicle injured in collision with pedestrian or animal in nontraffic accident A, D, S

● **V60.4** Person boarding or alighting a heavy transport vehicle injured in collision with pedestrian or animal A, D, S

● **V60.5** Driver of heavy transport vehicle injured in collision with pedestrian or animal in traffic accident A, D, S

● **V60.6** Passenger in heavy transport vehicle injured in collision with pedestrian or animal in traffic accident A, D, S

● **V60.7** Person on outside of heavy transport vehicle injured in collision with pedestrian or animal in traffic accident A, D, S

●■ **V60.9** Unspecified occupant of heavy transport vehicle injured in collision with pedestrian or animal in traffic accident A, D, S

● **V61** Occupant of heavy transport vehicle injured in collision with pedal cycle

The appropriate 7th character is to be added to each code from category V61

A	initial encounter
D	subsequent encounter
S	sequela

● **V61.0** Driver of heavy transport vehicle injured in collision with pedal cycle in nontraffic accident A, D, S

● **V61.1** Passenger in heavy transport vehicle injured in collision with pedal cycle in nontraffic accident A, D, S

● **V61.2** Person on outside of heavy transport vehicle injured in collision with pedal cycle in nontraffic accident A, D, S

●■ **V61.3** Unspecified occupant of heavy transport vehicle injured in collision with pedal cycle in nontraffic accident A, D, S

● **V61.4** Person boarding or alighting a heavy transport vehicle injured in collision with pedal cycle while boarding or alighting A, D, S

● **V61.5** Driver of heavy transport vehicle injured in collision with pedal cycle in traffic accident A, D, S

● **V61.6** Passenger in heavy transport vehicle injured in collision with pedal cycle in traffic accident A, D, S

● **V61.7** Person on outside of heavy transport vehicle injured in collision with pedal cycle in traffic accident A, D, S

●■ **V61.9** Unspecified occupant of heavy transport vehicle injured in collision with pedal cycle in traffic accident A, D, S

● **V62** Occupant of heavy transport vehicle injured in collision with two- or three-wheeled motor vehicle

The appropriate 7th character is to be added to each code from category V62

A	initial encounter
D	subsequent encounter
S	sequela

● **V62.0** Driver of heavy transport vehicle injured in collision with two- or three-wheeled motor vehicle in nontraffic accident A, D, S

● **V62.1** Passenger in heavy transport vehicle injured in collision with two- or three-wheeled motor vehicle in nontraffic accident A, D, S

● **V62.2** Person on outside of heavy transport vehicle injured in collision with two- or three-wheeled motor vehicle in nontraffic accident A, D, S

●■ **V62.3** Unspecified occupant of heavy transport vehicle injured in collision with two- or three-wheeled motor vehicle in nontraffic accident A, D, S

● **V62.4** Person boarding or alighting a heavy transport vehicle injured in collision with two- or three-wheeled motor vehicle A, D, S

● **V62.5** Driver of heavy transport vehicle injured in collision with two- or three-wheeled motor vehicle in traffic accident A, D, S

● **V62.6** Passenger in heavy transport vehicle injured in collision with two- or three-wheeled motor vehicle in traffic accident A, D, S

● **V62.7** Person on outside of heavy transport vehicle injured in collision with two- or three-wheeled motor vehicle in traffic accident A, D, S

●■ **V62.9** Unspecified occupant of heavy transport vehicle injured in collision with two- or three-wheeled motor vehicle in traffic accident A, D, S

● **V63** Occupant of heavy transport vehicle injured in collision with car, pick-up truck or van

The appropriate 7th character is to be added to each code from category V63

A	initial encounter
D	subsequent encounter
S	sequela

● **V63.0** Driver of heavy transport vehicle injured in collision with car, pick-up truck or van in nontraffic accident A, D, S

● **V63.1** Passenger in heavy transport vehicle injured in collision with car, pick-up truck or van in nontraffic accident A, D, S

N Newborn Age: 0　P Pediatric Age: 0–17　M Maternity DX: 12–55　A Adult Age: 15–124　♀ Females Only　♂ Males Only　　Complication\Comorbidity　　Major C\C　　Present on Admission Requirement　　Hospital-Acquired Condition

CHAPTER 20 (V01-Y99)

1719

● V63.2 **Person on outside of heavy transport vehicle injured in collision with car, pick-up truck or van in nontraffic accident** A, D, S 🖉

●■ V63.3 **Unspecified occupant of heavy transport vehicle injured in collision with car, pick-up truck or van in nontraffic accident** A, D, S 🖉

● V63.4 **Person boarding or alighting a heavy transport vehicle injured in collision with car, pick-up truck or van** A, D, S 🖉

● V63.5 **Driver of heavy transport vehicle injured in collision with car, pick-up truck or van in traffic accident** A, D, S 🖉

● V63.6 **Passenger in heavy transport vehicle injured in collision with car, pick-up truck or van in traffic accident** A, D, S 🖉

● V63.7 **Person on outside of heavy transport vehicle injured in collision with car, pick-up truck or van in traffic accident** A, D, S 🖉

●■ V63.9 **Unspecified occupant of heavy transport vehicle injured in collision with car, pick-up truck or van in traffic accident** A, D, S 🖉

● V64 **Occupant of heavy transport vehicle injured in collision with heavy transport vehicle or bus**

> | Excludes1 | occupant of heavy transport vehicle injured in collision with military vehicle (V69.81) |
> |---|---|

The appropriate 7th character is to be added to each code from category V64

A	initial encounter
D	subsequent encounter
S	sequela

● V64.0 **Driver of heavy transport vehicle injured in collision with heavy transport vehicle or bus in nontraffic accident** A, D, S 🖉

● V64.1 **Passenger in heavy transport vehicle injured in collision with heavy transport vehicle or bus in nontraffic accident** A, D, S 🖉

● V64.2 **Person on outside of heavy transport vehicle injured in collision with heavy transport vehicle or bus in nontraffic accident** A, D, S 🖉

●■ V64.3 **Unspecified occupant of heavy transport vehicle injured in collision with heavy transport vehicle or bus in nontraffic accident** A, D, S 🖉

● V64.4 **Person boarding or alighting a heavy transport vehicle injured in collision with heavy transport vehicle or bus while boarding or alighting** A, D, S 🖉

● V64.5 **Driver of heavy transport vehicle injured in collision with heavy transport vehicle or bus in traffic accident** A, D, S 🖉

● V64.6 **Passenger in heavy transport vehicle injured in collision with heavy transport vehicle or bus in traffic accident** A, D, S 🖉

● V64.7 **Person on outside of heavy transport vehicle injured in collision with heavy transport vehicle or bus in traffic accident** A, D, S 🖉

●■ V64.9 **Unspecified occupant of heavy transport vehicle injured in collision with heavy transport vehicle or bus in traffic accident** A, D, S 🖉

● V65 **Occupant of heavy transport vehicle injured in collision with railway train or railway vehicle**

The appropriate 7th character is to be added to each code from category V65

A	initial encounter
D	subsequent encounter
S	sequela

● V65.0 **Driver of heavy transport vehicle injured in collision with railway train or railway vehicle in nontraffic accident** A, D, S 🖉

● V65.1 **Passenger in heavy transport vehicle injured in collision with railway train or railway vehicle in nontraffic accident** A, D, S 🖉

● V65.2 **Person on outside of heavy transport vehicle injured in collision with railway train or railway vehicle in nontraffic accident** A, D, S 🖉

●■ V65.3 **Unspecified occupant of heavy transport vehicle injured in collision with railway train or railway vehicle in nontraffic accident** A, D, S 🖉

● V65.4 **Person boarding or alighting a heavy transport vehicle injured in collision with railway train or railway vehicle** A, D, S 🖉

● V65.5 **Driver of heavy transport vehicle injured in collision with railway train or railway vehicle in traffic accident** A, D, S 🖉

● V65.6 **Passenger in heavy transport vehicle injured in collision with railway train or railway vehicle in traffic accident** A, D, S 🖉

● V65.7 **Person on outside of heavy transport vehicle injured in collision with railway train or railway vehicle in traffic accident** A, D, S 🖉

●■ V65.9 **Unspecified occupant of heavy transport vehicle injured in collision with railway train or railway vehicle in traffic accident** A, D, S 🖉

● V66 **Occupant of heavy transport vehicle injured in collision with other nonmotor vehicle**

> | Includes | collision with animal-drawn vehicle, animal being ridden, streetcar |
> |---|---|

The appropriate 7th character is to be added to each code from category V66

A	initial encounter
D	subsequent encounter
S	sequela

● V66.0 **Driver of heavy transport vehicle injured in collision with other nonmotor vehicle in nontraffic accident** A, D, S 🖉

● V66.1 **Passenger in heavy transport vehicle injured in collision with other nonmotor vehicle in nontraffic accident** A, D, S 🖉

● V66.2 **Person on outside of heavy transport vehicle injured in collision with other nonmotor vehicle in nontraffic accident** A, D, S 🖉

●■ V66.3 **Unspecified occupant of heavy transport vehicle injured in collision with other nonmotor vehicle in nontraffic accident** A, D, S 🖉

● V66.4 **Person boarding or alighting a heavy transport vehicle injured in collision with other nonmotor vehicle** A, D, S 🖉

● V66.5 **Driver of heavy transport vehicle injured in collision with other nonmotor vehicle in traffic accident** A, D, S 🖉

● Unacceptable Principal Diagnosis   ● Use Additional Character(s)   ■ Unspecified   ▶ Manifestation Code

OGCR Official Guidelines for Coding and Reporting   Excludes 1   Excludes 2   Includes   Use additional   Code first   Code also

● V66.6   Passenger in heavy transport vehicle injured in collision with other nonmotor vehicle in traffic accident A, D, S 🔖

● V66.7   Person on outside of heavy transport vehicle injured in collision with other nonmotor vehicle in traffic accident A, D, S 🔖

●🔲 V66.9   Unspecified occupant of heavy transport vehicle injured in collision with other nonmotor vehicle in traffic accident A, D, S 🔖

● **V67**   **Occupant of heavy transport vehicle injured in collision with fixed or stationary object**

> The appropriate 7th character is to be added to each code from category V67

> | A | initial encounter |
> |---|---|
> | D | subsequent encounter |
> | S | sequela |

● V67.0   Driver of heavy transport vehicle injured in collision with fixed or stationary object in nontraffic accident A, D, S 🔖

● V67.1   Passenger in heavy transport vehicle injured in collision with fixed or stationary object in nontraffic accident A, D, S 🔖

● V67.2   Person on outside of heavy transport vehicle injured in collision with fixed or stationary object in nontraffic accident A, D, S 🔖

●🔲 V67.3   Unspecified occupant of heavy transport vehicle injured in collision with fixed or stationary object in nontraffic accident A, D, S 🔖

● V67.4   Person boarding or alighting a heavy transport vehicle injured in collision with fixed or stationary object A, D, S 🔖

● V67.5   Driver of heavy transport vehicle injured in collision with fixed or stationary object in traffic accident A, D, S 🔖

● V67.6   Passenger in heavy transport vehicle injured in collision with fixed or stationary object in traffic accident A, D, S 🔖

● V67.7   Person on outside of heavy transport vehicle injured in collision with fixed or stationary object in traffic accident A, D, S 🔖

●🔲 V67.9   Unspecified occupant of heavy transport vehicle injured in collision with fixed or stationary object in traffic accident A, D, S 🔖

● **V68**   **Occupant of heavy transport vehicle injured in noncollision transport accident**

> **Includes**   overturning heavy transport vehicle NOS
> overturning heavy transport vehicle without collision

> The appropriate 7th character is to be added to each code from category V68

> | A | initial encounter |
> |---|---|
> | D | subsequent encounter |
> | S | sequela |

● V68.0   Driver of heavy transport vehicle injured in noncollision transport accident in nontraffic accident A, D, S 🔖

● V68.1   Passenger in heavy transport vehicle injured in noncollision transport accident in nontraffic accident A, D, S 🔖

● V68.2   Person on outside of heavy transport vehicle injured in noncollision transport accident in nontraffic accident A, D, S 🔖

●🔲 V68.3   Unspecified occupant of heavy transport vehicle injured in noncollision transport accident in nontraffic accident A, D, S 🔖

● V68.4   Person boarding or alighting a heavy transport vehicle injured in noncollision transport accident A, D, S 🔖

● V68.5   Driver of heavy transport vehicle injured in noncollision transport accident in traffic accident A, D, S 🔖

● V68.6   Passenger in heavy transport vehicle injured in noncollision transport accident in traffic accident A, D, S 🔖

● V68.7   Person on outside of heavy transport vehicle injured in noncollision transport accident in traffic accident A, D, S 🔖

●🔲 V68.9   Unspecified occupant of heavy transport vehicle injured in noncollision transport accident in traffic accident

● **V69**   **Occupant of heavy transport vehicle injured in other and unspecified transport accidents**

> The appropriate 7th character is to be added to each code from category V69

> | A | initial encounter |
> |---|---|
> | D | subsequent encounter |
> | S | sequela |

● V69.0   Driver of heavy transport vehicle injured in collision with other and unspecified motor vehicles in nontraffic accident

     ●🔲 V69.00   Driver of heavy transport vehicle injured in collision with unspecified motor vehicles in nontraffic accident A, D, S 🔖

     ● V69.09   Driver of heavy transport vehicle injured in collision with other motor vehicles in nontraffic accident A, D, S 🔖

● V69.1   Passenger in heavy transport vehicle injured in collision with other and unspecified motor vehicles in nontraffic accident

     ●🔲 V69.10   Passenger in heavy transport vehicle injured in collision with unspecified motor vehicles in nontraffic accident A, D, S 🔖

     ● V69.19   Passenger in heavy transport vehicle injured in collision with other motor vehicles in nontraffic accident A, D, S 🔖

● V69.2   Unspecified occupant of heavy transport vehicle injured in collision with other and unspecified motor vehicles in nontraffic accident

     ●🔲 V69.20   Unspecified occupant of heavy transport vehicle injured in collision with unspecified motor vehicles in nontraffic accident A, D, S 🔖
       Collision NOS involving heavy transport vehicle, nontraffic

     ●🔲 V69.29   Unspecified occupant of heavy transport vehicle injured in collision with other motor vehicles in nontraffic accident A, D, S 🔖

● V69.3   Occupant (driver) (passenger) of heavy transport vehicle injured in unspecified nontraffic accident A, D, S 🔖

     Accident NOS involving heavy transport vehicle, nontraffic
     Occupant of heavy transport vehicle injured in nontraffic accident NOS

N Newborn Age: 0   **P** Pediatric Age: 0–17   **M** Maternity DX: 12–55   **A** Adult Age: 15–124   ♀ Females Only   ♂ Males Only

🔖 Complication\Comorbidity   🔖 Major C\C   🔖 Present on Admission Requirement   🔖 Hospital-Acquired Condition

1721

CHAPTER 20 (V01-Y99)

CHAPTER 20 (V01-Y99)

● V69.4   Driver of heavy transport vehicle injured in collision with other and unspecified motor vehicles in traffic accident

    ●■ V69.40   Driver of heavy transport vehicle injured in collision with unspecified motor vehicles in traffic accident A, D, S 🔖

      ● V69.49   Driver of heavy transport vehicle injured in collision with other motor vehicles in traffic accident A, D, S 🔖

● V69.5   Passenger in heavy transport vehicle injured in collision with other and unspecified motor vehicles in traffic accident

    ●■ V69.50   Passenger in heavy transport vehicle injured in collision with unspecified motor vehicles in traffic accident A, D, S 🔖

      ● V69.59   Passenger in heavy transport vehicle injured in collision with other motor vehicles in traffic accident A, D, S 🔖

● V69.6   Unspecified occupant of heavy transport vehicle injured in collision with other and unspecified motor vehicles in traffic accident

    ●■ V69.60   Unspecified occupant of heavy transport vehicle injured in collision with unspecified motor vehicles in traffic accident A, D, S 🔖

               Collision NOS involving heavy transport vehicle (traffic)

    ●■ V69.69   Unspecified occupant of heavy transport vehicle injured in collision with other motor vehicles in traffic accident A, D, S 🔖

● V69.8   Occupant (driver) (passenger) of heavy transport vehicle injured in other specified transport accidents

      ● V69.81   Occupant (driver) (passenger) of heavy transport vehicle injured in transport accidents with military vehicle A, D, S 🔖

      ● V69.88   Occupant (driver) (passenger) of heavy transport vehicle injured in other specified transport accidents A, D, S 🔖

●■ V69.9   Occupant (driver) (passenger) of heavy transport vehicle injured in unspecified traffic accident A, D, S 🔖

           Accident NOS involving heavy transport vehicle

BUS OCCUPANT INJURED IN TRANSPORT ACCIDENT (V70-V79)

Includes	motorcoach
Excludes1	minibus (V50-V59)

● V70   Bus occupant injured in collision with pedestrian or animal

Excludes1	bus collision with animal-drawn vehicle or animal being ridden (V76.-)

The appropriate 7th character is to be added to each code from category V70

A	initial encounter
D	subsequent encounter
S	sequela

   ● V70.0   Driver of bus injured in collision with pedestrian or animal in nontraffic accident A, D, S 🔖

   ● V70.1   Passenger on bus injured in collision with pedestrian or animal in nontraffic accident A, D, S 🔖

   ● V70.2   Person on outside of bus injured in collision with pedestrian or animal in nontraffic accident A, D, S 🔖

   ●■ V70.3   Unspecified occupant of bus injured in collision with pedestrian or animal in nontraffic accident A, D, S 🔖

   ● V70.4   Person boarding or alighting from bus injured in collision with pedestrian or animal A, D, S 🔖

   ● V70.5   Driver of bus injured in collision with pedestrian or animal in traffic accident A, D, S 🔖

   ● V70.6   Passenger on bus injured in collision with pedestrian or animal in traffic accident A, D, S 🔖

   ● V70.7   Person on outside of bus injured in collision with pedestrian or animal in traffic accident A, D, S 🔖

   ●■ V70.9   Unspecified occupant of bus injured in collision with pedestrian or animal in traffic accident A, D, S 🔖

● V71   Bus occupant injured in collision with pedal cycle

The appropriate 7th character is to be added to each code from category V71

A	initial encounter
D	subsequent encounter
S	sequela

   ● V71.0   Driver of bus injured in collision with pedal cycle in nontraffic accident A, D, S 🔖

   ● V71.1   Passenger on bus injured in collision with pedal cycle in nontraffic accident A, D, S 🔖

   ● V71.2   Person on outside of bus injured in collision with pedal cycle in nontraffic accident A, D, S 🔖

   ●■ V71.3   Unspecified occupant of bus injured in collision with pedal cycle in nontraffic accident A, D, S 🔖

   ● V71.4   Person boarding or alighting from bus injured in collision with pedal cycle A, D, S 🔖

   ● V71.5   Driver of bus injured in collision with pedal cycle in traffic accident A, D, S 🔖

   ● V71.6   Passenger on bus injured in collision with pedal cycle in traffic accident A, D, S 🔖

   ● V71.7   Person on outside of bus injured in collision with pedal cycle in traffic accident A, D, S 🔖

   ●■ V71.9   Unspecified occupant of bus injured in collision with pedal cycle in traffic accident A, D, S 🔖

● V72   Bus occupant injured in collision with two- or three-wheeled motor vehicle

The appropriate 7th character is to be added to each code from category V72

A	initial encounter
D	subsequent encounter
S	sequela

   ● V72.0   Driver of bus injured in collision with two- or three-wheeled motor vehicle in nontraffic accident A, D, S 🔖

   ● V72.1   Passenger on bus injured in collision with two- or three-wheeled motor vehicle in nontraffic accident A, D, S 🔖

   ● V72.2   Person on outside of bus injured in collision with two- or three-wheeled motor vehicle in nontraffic accident A, D, S 🔖

   ●■ V72.3   Unspecified occupant of bus injured in collision with two- or three-wheeled motor vehicle in nontraffic accident A, D, S 🔖

   ● V72.4   Person boarding or alighting from bus injured in collision with two- or three-wheeled motor vehicle A, D, S 🔖

● Unacceptable Principal Diagnosis   ● Use Additional Character(s)   ■ Unspecified   ▶ Manifestation Code

OGCR   Official Guidelines for Coding and Reporting   Excludes 1   Excludes 2   Includes   Use additional   Code first   Code also

● V72.5   Driver of bus injured in collision with two- or three-wheeled motor vehicle in traffic accident
A, D, S ⊛

● V72.6   Passenger on bus injured in collision with two- or three-wheeled motor vehicle in traffic accident
A, D, S ⊛

● V72.7   Person on outside of bus injured in collision with two- or three-wheeled motor vehicle in traffic accident A, D, S ⊛

●■ V72.9   Unspecified occupant of bus injured in collision with two- or three-wheeled motor vehicle in traffic accident A, D, S ⊛

● V73   Bus occupant injured in collision with car, pick-up truck or van

> The appropriate 7th character is to be added to each code from category V73

> | A | initial encounter |
> |---|---|
> | D | subsequent encounter |
> | S | sequela |

● V73.0   Driver of bus injured in collision with car, pick-up truck or van in nontraffic accident A, D, S ⊛

● V73.1   Passenger on bus injured in collision with car, pick-up truck or van in nontraffic accident
A, D, S ⊛

● V73.2   Person on outside of bus injured in collision with car, pick-up truck or van in nontraffic accident
A, D, S ⊛

●■ V73.3   Unspecified occupant of bus injured in collision with car, pick-up truck or van in nontraffic accident
A, D, S ⊛

● V73.4   Person boarding or alighting from bus injured in collision with car, pick-up truck or van A, D, S ⊛

● V73.5   Driver of bus injured in collision with car, pick-up truck or van in traffic accident A, D, S ⊛

● V73.6   Passenger on bus injured in collision with car, pick-up truck or van in traffic accident A, D, S ⊛

● V73.7   Person on outside of bus injured in collision with car, pick-up truck or van in traffic accident
A, D, S ⊛

●■ V73.9   Unspecified occupant of bus injured in collision with car, pick-up truck or van in traffic accident
A, D, S ⊛

● V74   Bus occupant injured in collision with heavy transport vehicle or bus

> **Excludes1**   bus occupant injured in collision with military vehicle (V79.81)

> The appropriate 7th character is to be added to each code from category V74

> | A | initial encounter |
> |---|---|
> | D | subsequent encounter |
> | S | sequela |

● V74.0   Driver of bus injured in collision with heavy transport vehicle or bus in nontraffic accident
A, D, S ⊛

● V74.1   Passenger on bus injured in collision with heavy transport vehicle or bus in nontraffic accident
A, D, S ⊛

● V74.2   Person on outside of bus injured in collision with heavy transport vehicle or bus in nontraffic accident A, D, S ⊛

●■ V74.3   Unspecified occupant of bus injured in collision with heavy transport vehicle or bus in nontraffic accident A, D, S ⊛

● V74.4   Person boarding or alighting from bus injured in collision with heavy transport vehicle or bus
A, D, S ⊛

● V74.5   Driver of bus injured in collision with heavy transport vehicle or bus in traffic accident
A, D, S ⊛

● V74.6   Passenger on bus injured in collision with heavy transport vehicle or bus in traffic accident
A, D, S ⊛

● V74.7   Person on outside of bus injured in collision with heavy transport vehicle or bus in traffic accident
A, D, S ⊛

●■ V74.9   Unspecified occupant of bus injured in collision with heavy transport vehicle or bus in traffic accident A, D, S ⊛

● V75   Bus occupant injured in collision with railway train or railway vehicle

> The appropriate 7th character is to be added to each code from category V75

> | A | initial encounter |
> |---|---|
> | D | subsequent encounter |
> | S | sequela |

● V75.0   Driver of bus injured in collision with railway train or railway vehicle in nontraffic accident
A, D, S ⊛

● V75.1   Passenger on bus injured in collision with railway train or railway vehicle in nontraffic accident
A, D, S ⊛

● V75.2   Person on outside of bus injured in collision with railway train or railway vehicle in nontraffic accident A, D, S ⊛

●■ V75.3   Unspecified occupant of bus injured in collision with railway train or railway vehicle in nontraffic accident A, D, S ⊛

● V75.4   Person boarding or alighting from bus injured in collision with railway train or railway vehicle
A, D, S ⊛

● V75.5   Driver of bus injured in collision with railway train or railway vehicle in traffic accident
A, D, S ⊛

● V75.6   Passenger on bus injured in collision with railway train or railway vehicle in traffic accident
A, D, S ⊛

● V75.7   Person on outside of bus injured in collision with railway train or railway vehicle in traffic accident
A, D, S ⊛

●■ V75.9   Unspecified occupant of bus injured in collision with railway train or railway vehicle in traffic accident A, D, S ⊛

● V76   Bus occupant injured in collision with other nonmotor vehicle

> **Includes**   collision with animal-drawn vehicle, animal being ridden, streetcar

> The appropriate 7th character is to be added to each code from category V76

> | A | initial encounter |
> |---|---|
> | D | subsequent encounter |
> | S | sequela |

● V76.0   Driver of bus injured in collision with other nonmotor vehicle in nontraffic accident A, D, S ⊛

● V76.1   Passenger on bus injured in collision with other nonmotor vehicle in nontraffic accident A, D, S ⊛

CHAPTER 20 (V01-Y99)

N Newborn Age: 0   **P** Pediatric Age: 0–17   **M** Maternity DX: 12–55   **A** Adult Age: 15–124   ♀ Females Only   ♂ Males Only

⊛ Complication\Comorbidity   ⊛ Major C\C   ⊛ Present on Admission Requirement   ⊛ Hospital-Acquired Condition

1723

CHAPTER 20 (V01-Y99)

● V76.2 Person on outside of bus injured in collision with other nonmotor vehicle in nontraffic accident A, D, S 🔖

●■ V76.3 Unspecified occupant of bus injured in collision with other nonmotor vehicle in nontraffic accident A, D, S 🔖

● V76.4 Person boarding or alighting from bus injured in collision with other nonmotor vehicle A, D, S 🔖

● V76.5 Driver of bus injured in collision with other nonmotor vehicle in traffic accident A, D, S 🔖

● V76.6 Passenger on bus injured in collision with other nonmotor vehicle in traffic accident A, D, S 🔖

● V76.7 Person on outside of bus injured in collision with other nonmotor vehicle in traffic accident A, D, S 🔖

●■ V76.9 Unspecified occupant of bus injured in collision with other nonmotor vehicle in traffic accident A, D, S 🔖

● V77 Bus occupant injured in collision with fixed or stationary object

> The appropriate 7th character is to be added to each code from category V77

> | A | initial encounter |
> | D | subsequent encounter |
> | S | sequela |

● V77.0 Driver of bus injured in collision with fixed or stationary object in nontraffic accident A, D, S 🔖

● V77.1 Passenger on bus injured in collision with fixed or stationary object in nontraffic accident A, D, S 🔖

● V77.2 Person on outside of bus injured in collision with fixed or stationary object in nontraffic accident A, D, S 🔖

●■ V77.3 Unspecified occupant of bus injured in collision with fixed or stationary object in nontraffic accident A, D, S 🔖

● V77.4 Person boarding or alighting from bus injured in collision with fixed or stationary object A, D, S 🔖

● V77.5 Driver of bus injured in collision with fixed or stationary object in traffic accident A, D, S 🔖

● V77.6 Passenger on bus injured in collision with fixed or stationary object in traffic accident A, D, S 🔖

● V77.7 Person on outside of bus injured in collision with fixed or stationary object in traffic accident A, D, S 🔖

●■ V77.9 Unspecified occupant of bus injured in collision with fixed or stationary object in traffic accident A, D, S 🔖

● V78 Bus occupant injured in noncollision transport accident

> | Includes | overturning bus NOS |
> | | overturning bus without collision |

> The appropriate 7th character is to be added to each code from category V78

> | A | initial encounter |
> | D | subsequent encounter |
> | S | sequela |

● V78.0 Driver of bus injured in noncollision transport accident in nontraffic accident A, D, S 🔖

● V78.1 Passenger on bus injured in noncollision transport accident in nontraffic accident A, D, S 🔖

● V78.2 Person on outside of bus injured in noncollision transport accident in nontraffic accident A, D, S 🔖

●■ V78.3 Unspecified occupant of bus injured in noncollision transport accident in nontraffic accident A, D, S 🔖

● V78.4 Person boarding or alighting from bus injured in noncollision transport accident A, D, S 🔖

● V78.5 Driver of bus injured in noncollision transport accident in traffic accident A, D, S 🔖

● V78.6 Passenger on bus injured in noncollision transport accident in traffic accident A, D, S 🔖

● V78.7 Person on outside of bus injured in noncollision transport accident in traffic accident A, D, S 🔖

●■ V78.9 Unspecified occupant of bus injured in noncollision transport accident in traffic accident A, D, S 🔖

● V79 Bus occupant injured in other and unspecified transport accidents

> The appropriate 7th character is to be added to each code from category V79

> | A | initial encounter |
> | D | subsequent encounter |
> | S | sequela |

● V79.0 Driver of bus injured in collision with other and unspecified motor vehicles in nontraffic accident

●■ V79.00 Driver of bus injured in collision with unspecified motor vehicles in nontraffic accident A, D, S 🔖

● V79.09 Driver of bus injured in collision with other motor vehicles in nontraffic accident A, D, S 🔖

● V79.1 Passenger on bus injured in collision with other and unspecified motor vehicles in nontraffic accident

●■ V79.10 Passenger on bus injured in collision with unspecified motor vehicles in nontraffic accident A, D, S 🔖

● V79.19 Passenger on bus injured in collision with other motor vehicles in nontraffic accident A, D, S 🔖

● V79.2 Unspecified bus occupant injured in collision with other and unspecified motor vehicles in nontraffic accident

●■ V79.20 Unspecified bus occupant injured in collision with unspecified motor vehicles in nontraffic accident A, D, S 🔖
    Bus collision NOS, nontraffic

●■ V79.29 Unspecified bus occupant injured in collision with other motor vehicles in nontraffic accident A, D, S 🔖

●■ V79.3 Bus occupant (driver) (passenger) injured in unspecified nontraffic accident A, D, S 🔖
    Bus accident NOS, nontraffic
    Bus occupant injured in nontraffic accident NOS

● V79.4 Driver of bus injured in collision with other and unspecified motor vehicles in traffic accident

●■ V79.40 Driver of bus injured in collision with unspecified motor vehicles in traffic accident A, D, S 🔖

● V79.49 Driver of bus injured in collision with other motor vehicles in traffic accident A, D, S 🔖

● Unacceptable Principal Diagnosis   ● Use Additional Character(s)   ■ Unspecified   ▶ Manifestation Code
OGCR Official Guidelines for Coding and Reporting   [Excludes 1] [Excludes 2] [Includes] [Use additional] [Code first] [Code also]

● V79.5   **Passenger on bus injured in collision with other and unspecified motor vehicles in traffic accident**

   ●■ V79.50   **Passenger on bus injured in collision with unspecified motor vehicles in traffic accident** A, D, S 🔍

   ● V79.59   **Passenger on bus injured in collision with other motor vehicles in traffic accident** A, D, S 🔍

● V79.6   **Unspecified bus occupant injured in collision with other and unspecified motor vehicles in traffic accident**

   ●■ V79.60   **Unspecified bus occupant injured in collision with unspecified motor vehicles in traffic accident** A, D, S 🔍
      Bus collision NOS (traffic)

   ●■ V79.69   **Unspecified bus occupant injured in collision with other motor vehicles in traffic accident** A, D, S 🔍

● V79.8   **Bus occupant (driver) (passenger) injured in other specified transport accidents**

   ● V79.81   **Bus occupant (driver) (passenger) injured in transport accidents with military vehicle** A, D, S 🔍

   ● V79.88   **Bus occupant (driver) (passenger) injured in other specified transport accidents** A, D, S 🔍

●■ V79.9   **Bus occupant (driver) (passenger) injured in unspecified traffic accident** A, D, S 🔍
    Bus accident NOS

OTHER LAND TRANSPORT ACCIDENTS (V80-V89)

● **V80**   **Animal-rider or occupant of animal-drawn vehicle injured in transport accident**

   The appropriate 7th character is to be added to each code from category V80

A	initial encounter
D	subsequent encounter
S	sequela

● V80.0   **Animal-rider or occupant of animal drawn vehicle injured by fall from or being thrown from animal or animal-drawn vehicle in noncollision accident**

   ● V80.01   **Animal-rider injured by fall from or being thrown from animal in noncollision accident**

     ● V80.010   **Animal-rider injured by fall from or being thrown from horse in noncollision accident** A, D, S 🔍

     ● V80.018   **Animal-rider injured by fall from or being thrown from other animal in noncollision accident** A, D, S 🔍

   ● V80.02   **Occupant of animal-drawn vehicle injured by fall from or being thrown from animal-drawn vehicle in noncollision accident** A, D, S 🔍
      Overturning animal-drawn vehicle NOS
      Overturning animal-drawn vehicle without collision

● V80.1   **Animal-rider or occupant of animal-drawn vehicle injured in collision with pedestrian or animal**

Excludes1	animal-rider or animal-drawn vehicle collision with animal-drawn vehicle or animal being ridden (V80.7)

   ● V80.11   **Animal-rider injured in collision with pedestrian or animal** A, D, S 🔍

   ● V80.12   **Occupant of animal-drawn vehicle injured in collision with pedestrian or animal** A, D, S 🔍

● V80.2   **Animal-rider or occupant of animal-drawn vehicle injured in collision with pedal cycle**

   ● V80.21   **Animal-rider injured in collision with pedal cycle** A, D, S 🔍

   ● V80.22   **Occupant of animal-drawn vehicle injured in collision with pedal cycle** A, D, S 🔍

● V80.3   **Animal-rider or occupant of animal-drawn vehicle injured in collision with two- or three-wheeled motor vehicle**

   ● V80.31   **Animal-rider injured in collision with two- or three-wheeled motor vehicle** A, D, S 🔍

   ● V80.32   **Occupant of animal-drawn vehicle injured in collision with two- or three-wheeled motor vehicle** A, D, S 🔍

● V80.4   **Animal-rider or occupant of animal-drawn vehicle injured in collision with car, pick-up truck, van, heavy transport vehicle or bus**

Excludes1	animal-rider injured in collision with military vehicle (V80.910) occupant of animal-drawn vehicle injured in collision with military vehicle (V80.920)

   ● V80.41   **Animal-rider injured in collision with car, pick-up truck, van, heavy transport vehicle or bus** A, D, S 🔍

   ● V80.42   **Occupant of animal-drawn vehicle injured in collision with car, pick-up truck, van, heavy transport vehicle or bus** A, D, S 🔍

● V80.5   **Animal-rider or occupant of animal-drawn vehicle injured in collision with other specified motor vehicle**

   ● V80.51   **Animal-rider injured in collision with other specified motor vehicle** A, D, S 🔍

   ● V80.52   **Occupant of animal-drawn vehicle injured in collision with other specified motor vehicle** A, D, S 🔍

● V80.6   **Animal-rider or occupant of animal-drawn vehicle injured in collision with railway train or railway vehicle**

   ● V80.61   **Animal-rider injured in collision with railway train or railway vehicle** A, D, S 🔍

   ● V80.62   **Occupant of animal-drawn vehicle injured in collision with railway train or railway vehicle** A, D, S 🔍

● V80.7   **Animal-rider or occupant of animal-drawn vehicle injured in collision with other nonmotor vehicles**

   ● V80.71   **Animal-rider or occupant of animal-drawn vehicle injured in collision with animal being ridden**

     ● V80.710   **Animal-rider injured in collision with other animal being ridden** A, D, S 🔍

     ● V80.711   **Occupant of animal-drawn vehicle injured in collision with animal being ridden** A, D, S 🔍

● **V80.72** **Animal-rider or occupant of animal-drawn vehicle injured in collision with other animal-drawn vehicle**

    ● **V80.720** **Animal-rider injured in collision with animal-drawn vehicle** A, D, S ✪

    ● **V80.721** **Occupant of animal-drawn vehicle injured in collision with other animal-drawn vehicle** A, D, S ✪

● **V80.73** **Animal-rider or occupant of animal-drawn vehicle injured in collision with streetcar**

    ● **V80.730** **Animal-rider injured in collision with streetcar** A, D, S ✪

    ● **V80.731** **Occupant of animal-drawn vehicle injured in collision with streetcar** A, D, S ✪

● **V80.79** **Animal-rider or occupant of animal-drawn vehicle injured in collision with other nonmotor vehicles**

    ● **V80.790** **Animal-rider injured in collision with other nonmotor vehicles** A, D, S ✪

    ● **V80.791** **Occupant of animal-drawn vehicle injured in collision with other nonmotor vehicles** A, D, S ✪

● **V80.8** **Animal-rider or occupant of animal-drawn vehicle injured in collision with fixed or stationary object**

    ● **V80.81** **Animal-rider injured in collision with fixed or stationary object** A, D, S ✪

    ● **V80.82** **Occupant of animal-drawn vehicle injured in collision with fixed or stationary object** A, D, S ✪

● **V80.9** **Animal-rider or occupant of animal-drawn vehicle injured in other and unspecified transport accidents**

    ● **V80.91** **Animal-rider injured in other and unspecified transport accidents**

        ● **V80.910** **Animal-rider injured in transport accident with military vehicle** A, D, S ✪

        ● **V80.918** **Animal-rider injured in other transport accident** A, D, S ✪

        ●■ **V80.919** **Animal-rider injured in unspecified transport accident** A, D, S ✪
            Animal rider accident NOS

    ● **V80.92** **Occupant of animal-drawn vehicle injured in other and unspecified transport accidents**

        ● **V80.920** **Occupant of animal-drawn vehicle injured in transport accident with military vehicle** A, D, S ✪

        ● **V80.928** **Occupant of animal-drawn vehicle injured in other transport accident** A, D, S ✪

        ●■ **V80.929** **Occupant of animal-drawn vehicle injured in unspecified transport accident** A, D, S ✪
            Animal-drawn vehicle accident NOS

● **V81** **Occupant of railway train or railway vehicle injured in transport accident**

    Includes   derailment of railway train or railway vehicle
             person on outside of train

    Excludes1   streetcar (V82.-)

    The appropriate 7th character is to be added to each code from category V81

        A   initial encounter
        D   subsequent encounter
        S   sequela

● **V81.0** **Occupant of railway train or railway vehicle injured in collision with motor vehicle in nontraffic accident** A, D, S ✪

    Excludes1   occupant of railway train or railway vehicle injured due to collision with military vehicle (V81.83)

● **V81.1** **Occupant of railway train or railway vehicle injured in collision with motor vehicle in traffic accident** A, D, S ✪

    Excludes1   occupant of railway train or railway vehicle injured due to collision with military vehicle (V81.83)

● **V81.2** **Occupant of railway train or railway vehicle injured in collision with or hit by rolling stock** A, D, S ✪

● **V81.3** **Occupant of railway train or railway vehicle injured in collision with other object** A, D, S ✪
    Railway collision NOS

● **V81.4** **Person injured while boarding or alighting from railway train or railway vehicle** A, D, S ✪

● **V81.5** **Occupant of railway train or railway vehicle injured by fall in railway train or railway vehicle** A, D, S ✪

● **V81.6** **Occupant of railway train or railway vehicle injured by fall from railway train or railway vehicle** A, D, S ✪

● **V81.7** **Occupant of railway train or railway vehicle injured in derailment without antecedent collision** A, D, S ✪

● **V81.8** **Occupant of railway train or railway vehicle injured in other specified railway accidents**

    ● **V81.81** **Occupant of railway train or railway vehicle injured due to explosion or fire on train** A, D, S ✪

    ● **V81.82** **Occupant of railway train or railway vehicle injured due to object falling onto train** A, D, S ✪
        Occupant of railway train or railway vehicle injured due to falling earth onto train
        Occupant of railway train or railway vehicle injured due to falling rocks onto train
        Occupant of railway train or railway vehicle injured due to falling snow onto train
        Occupant of railway train or railway vehicle injured due to falling trees onto train

    ● **V81.83** **Occupant of railway train or railway vehicle injured due to collision with military vehicle** A, D, S ✪

    ● **V81.89** **Occupant of railway train or railway vehicle injured due to other specified railway accident** A, D, S ✪

●■ **V81.9** **Occupant of railway train or railway vehicle injured in unspecified railway accident** A, D, S ✪
    Railway accident NOS

● Unacceptable Principal Diagnosis   ● Use Additional Character(s)   ■ Unspecified   ▶ Manifestation Code

OGCR Official Guidelines for Coding and Reporting   Excludes 1   Excludes 2   Includes   Use additional   Code first   Code also

● **V82 Occupant of powered streetcar injured in transport accident**

Includes	interurban electric car
	person on outside of streetcar
	tram (car)
	trolley (car)

Excludes1	bus (V70-V79)
	motorcoach (V70-V79)
	nonpowered streetcar (V76.-)
	train (V81.-)

The appropriate 7th character is to be added to each code from category V82

A	initial encounter
D	subsequent encounter
S	sequela

● **V82.0 Occupant of streetcar injured in collision with motor vehicle in nontraffic accident** A, D, S 🦢

● **V82.1 Occupant of streetcar injured in collision with motor vehicle in traffic accident** A, D, S 🦢

● **V82.2 Occupant of streetcar injured in collision with or hit by rolling stock** A, D, S 🦢

● **V82.3 Occupant of streetcar injured in collision with other object** A, D, S 🦢

Excludes1	collision with animal-drawn vehicle or animal being ridden (V82.8)

● **V82.4 Person injured while boarding or alighting from streetcar** A, D, S 🦢

● **V82.5 Occupant of streetcar injured by fall in streetcar** A, D, S 🦢

Excludes1	fall in streetcar:
	while boarding or alighting (V82.4)
	with antecedent collision (V82.0-V82.3)

● **V82.6 Occupant of streetcar injured by fall from streetcar** A, D, S 🦢

Excludes1	fall from streetcar:
	while boarding or alighting (V82.4)
	with antecedent collision (V82.0-V82.3)

● **V82.7 Occupant of streetcar injured in derailment without antecedent collision** A, D, S 🦢

Excludes1	occupant of streetcar injured in derailment with antecedent collision (V82.0-V82.3)

● **V82.8 Occupant of streetcar injured in other specified transport accidents** A, D, S 🦢
Streetcar collision with military vehicle
Streetcar collision with train or nonmotor vehicles

●■ **V82.9 Occupant of streetcar injured in unspecified traffic accident** A, D, S 🦢
Streetcar accident NOS

● **V83 Occupant of special vehicle mainly used on industrial premises injured in transport accident**

Includes	battery-powered airport passenger vehicle
	battery-powered truck (baggage) (mail)
	coal-car in mine
	forklift (truck)
	logging car
	self-propelled industrial truck
	station baggage truck (powered)
	tram, truck, or tub (powered) in mine or quarry

Excludes1	special construction vehicles (V85.-)
	special industrial vehicle in stationary use or maintenance (W31.-)

The appropriate 7th character is to be added to each code from category V83

A	initial encounter
D	subsequent encounter
S	sequela

● **V83.0 Driver of special industrial vehicle injured in traffic accident** A, D, S 🦢

● **V83.1 Passenger of special industrial vehicle injured in traffic accident** A, D, S 🦢

● **V83.2 Person on outside of special industrial vehicle injured in traffic accident** A, D, S 🦢

●■ **V83.3 Unspecified occupant of special industrial vehicle injured in traffic accident** A, D, S 🦢

● **V83.4 Person injured while boarding or alighting from special industrial vehicle** A, D, S 🦢

● **V83.5 Driver of special industrial vehicle injured in nontraffic accident** A, D, S 🦢

● **V83.6 Passenger of special industrial vehicle injured in nontraffic accident** A, D, S 🦢

● **V83.7 Person on outside of special industrial vehicle injured in nontraffic accident** A, D, S 🦢

●■ **V83.9 Unspecified occupant of special industrial vehicle injured in nontraffic accident** A, D, S 🦢
Special-industrial-vehicle accident NOS

● **V84 Occupant of special vehicle mainly used in agriculture injured in transport accident**

Includes	self-propelled farm machinery
	tractor (and trailer)

Excludes1	animal-powered farm machinery accident (W30.8-)
	contact with combine harvester (W30.0)
	special agricultural vehicle in stationary use or maintenance (W30.-)

The appropriate 7th character is to be added to each code from category V84

A	initial encounter
D	subsequent encounter
S	sequela

● **V84.0 Driver of special agricultural vehicle injured in traffic accident** A, D, S 🦢

● **V84.1 Passenger of special agricultural vehicle injured in traffic accident** A, D, S 🦢

● **V84.2 Person on outside of special agricultural vehicle injured in traffic accident** A, D, S 🦢

●■ **V84.3 Unspecified occupant of special agricultural vehicle injured in traffic accident** A, D, S 🦢

● **V84.4 Person injured while boarding or alighting from special agricultural vehicle** A, D, S 🦢

● **V84.5 Driver of special agricultural vehicle injured in nontraffic accident** A, D, S 🦢

CHAPTER 20 (V01-Y99)

N Newborn Age: 0   **P** Pediatric Age: 0–17   **M** Maternity DX: 12–55   **A** Adult Age: 15–124   ♀ Females Only   ♂ Males Only

🦢 Complication\Comorbidity   🦢 Major C\C   🦢 Present on Admission Requirement   🦢 Hospital-Acquired Condition

1727

● V84.6 **Passenger of special agricultural vehicle injured in nontraffic accident** A, D, S 🔖

● V84.7 **Person on outside of special agricultural vehicle injured in nontraffic accident** A, D, S 🔖

●■ V84.9 **Unspecified occupant of special agricultural vehicle injured in nontraffic accident** A, D, S 🔖
     Special-agricultural vehicle accident NOS

● V85 **Occupant of special construction vehicle injured in transport accident**

   Includes   bulldozer
             digger
             dump truck
             earth-leveller
             mechanical shovel
             road-roller

   Excludes1   special industrial vehicle (V83.-)
             special construction vehicle in stationary use or maintenance (W31.-)

The appropriate 7th character is to be added to each code from category V85

   A   initial encounter
   D   subsequent encounter
   S   sequela

● V85.0 **Driver of special construction vehicle injured in traffic accident** A, D, S 🔖

● V85.1 **Passenger of special construction vehicle injured in traffic accident** A, D, S 🔖

● V85.2 **Person on outside of special construction vehicle injured in traffic accident** A, D, S 🔖

●■ V85.3 **Unspecified occupant of special construction vehicle injured in traffic accident** A, D, S 🔖

● V85.4 **Person injured while boarding or alighting from special construction vehicle** A, D, S 🔖

● V85.5 **Driver of special construction vehicle injured in nontraffic accident** A, D, S 🔖

● V85.6 **Passenger of special construction vehicle injured in nontraffic accident** A, D, S 🔖

● V85.7 **Person on outside of special construction vehicle injured in nontraffic accident** A, D, S 🔖

●■ V85.9 **Unspecified occupant of special construction vehicle injured in nontraffic accident** A, D, S 🔖
     Special-construction-vehicle accident NOS

● V86 **Occupant of special all-terrain or other off-road motor vehicle, injured in transport accident**

   Excludes1   special all-terrain vehicle in stationary use or maintenance (W31.-)
             sport-utility vehicle (V50-V59)
             three-wheeled motor vehicle designed for on-road use (V30-V39)

The appropriate 7th character is to be added to each code from category V86

   A   initial encounter
   D   subsequent encounter
   S   sequela

● V86.0 **Driver of special all-terrain or other off-road motor vehicle injured in traffic accident**

   ● V86.01 **Driver of ambulance or fire engine injured in traffic accident** A, D, S 🔖

   ● V86.02 **Driver of snowmobile injured in traffic accident** A, D, S 🔖

   ● V86.03 **Driver of dune buggy injured in traffic accident** A, D, S 🔖

   ● V86.04 **Driver of military vehicle injured in traffic accident** A, D, S 🔖

   ● V86.09 **Driver of other off-road special all-terrain or other off-road vehicle injured in traffic accident** A, D, S 🔖
       Driver of dirt bike injured in traffic accident
       Driver of go cart injured in traffic accident
       Driver of golf cart injured in traffic accident

● V86.1 **Passenger of special all-terrain or other off-road motor vehicle injured in traffic accident**

   ● V86.11 **Passenger of ambulance or fire engine injured in traffic accident** A, D, S 🔖

   ● V86.12 **Passenger of snowmobile injured in traffic accident** A, D, S 🔖

   ● V86.13 **Passenger of dune buggy injured in traffic accident** A, D, S 🔖

   ● V86.14 **Passenger of military vehicle injured in traffic accident** A, D, S 🔖

   ● V86.19 **Passenger of other off-road special all-terrain or other off-road off-road motor vehicle injured in traffic accident** A, D, S 🔖
       Passenger of dirt bike injured in traffic accident
       Passenger of go cart injured in traffic accident
       Passenger of golf cart injured in traffic accident

● V86.2 **Person on outside of special all-terrain or other off-road motor vehicle injured in traffic accident**

   ● V86.21 **Person on outside of ambulance or fire engine injured in traffic accident** A, D, S 🔖

   ● V86.22 **Person on outside of snowmobile injured in traffic accident** A, D, S 🔖

   ● V86.23 **Person on outside of dune buggy injured in traffic accident** A, D, S 🔖

   ● V86.24 **Person on outside of military vehicle injured in traffic accident** A, D, S 🔖

   ● V86.29 **Person on outside of other special all-terrain or other off-road motor vehicle injured in traffic accident** A, D, S 🔖
       Person on outside of dirt bike injured in traffic accident
       Person on outside of go cart in traffic accident
       Person on outside of golf cart injured in traffic accident

● V86.3 **Unspecified occupant of special all-terrain or other off-road motor vehicle injured in traffic accident**

   ●■ V86.31 **Unspecified occupant of ambulance or fire engine injured in traffic accident** A, D, S 🔖

   ●■ V86.32 **Unspecified occupant of snowmobile injured in traffic accident** A, D, S 🔖

   ●■ V86.33 **Unspecified occupant of dune buggy injured in traffic accident** A, D, S 🔖

   ●■ V86.34 **Unspecified occupant of military vehicle injured in traffic accident** A, D, S 🔖

   ●■ V86.39 **Unspecified occupant of other special all-terrain or other off-road motor vehicle injured in traffic accident** A, D, S 🔖
       Unspecified occupant of dirt bike injured in traffic accident
       Unspecified occupant of go cart injured in traffic accident
       Unspecified occupant of golf cart injured in traffic accident

● Unacceptable Principal Diagnosis   ● Use Additional Character(s)   ■ Unspecified   ▶ Manifestation Code
OGCR Official Guidelines for Coding and Reporting   Excludes 1   Excludes 2   Includes   Use additional   Code first   Code also

● **V86.4** **Person injured while boarding or alighting from special all-terrain or other off-road motor vehicle**

  ● **V86.41** **Person injured while boarding or alighting from ambulance or fire engine** A, D, S 🔲

  ● **V86.42** **Person injured while boarding or alighting from snowmobile** A, D, S 🔲

  ● **V86.43** **Person injured while boarding or alighting from dune buggy** A, D, S 🔲

  ● **V86.44** **Person injured while boarding or alighting from military vehicle** A, D, S 🔲

  ● **V86.49** **Person injured while boarding or alighting from other special all-terrain or other off-road motor vehicle** A, D, S 🔲
    Person injured while boarding or alighting from dirt bike
    Person injured while boarding or alighting from go cart
    Person injured while boarding or alighting from golf cart

● **V86.5** **Driver of special all-terrain or other off-road motor vehicle injured in nontraffic accident**

  ● **V86.51** **Driver of ambulance or fire engine injured in nontraffic accident** A, D, S 🔲

  ● **V86.52** **Driver of snowmobile injured in nontraffic accident** A, D, S 🔲

  ● **V86.53** **Driver of dune buggy injured in nontraffic accident** A, D, S 🔲

  ● **V86.54** **Driver of military vehicle injured in nontraffic accident** A, D, S 🔲

  ● **V86.59** **Driver of other off-road special all-terrain or other off-road motor vehicle injured in nontraffic accident** A, D, S 🔲
    Driver of dirt bike injured in nontraffic accident
    Driver of go cart injured in nontraffic accident
    Driver of golf cart injured in nontraffic accident

● **V86.6** **Passenger of special all-terrain or other off-road motor vehicle injured in nontraffic accident**

  ● **V86.61** **Passenger of ambulance or fire engine injured in nontraffic accident** A, D, S 🔲

  ● **V86.62** **Passenger of snowmobile injured in nontraffic accident** A, D, S 🔲

  ● **V86.63** **Passenger of dune buggy injured in nontraffic accident** A, D, S 🔲

  ● **V86.64** **Passenger of military vehicle injured in nontraffic accident** A, D, S 🔲

  ● **V86.69** **Passenger of other special all-terrain or other off-road vehicle injured in nontraffic accident** A, D, S 🔲
    Passenger of dirt bike injured in nontraffic accident
    Passenger of go cart injured in nontraffic accident
    Passenger of golf cart injured in nontraffic accident

● **V86.7** **Person on outside of special all-terrain or other off-road motor vehicle injured in nontraffic accident**

  ● **V86.71** **Person on outside of ambulance or fire engine injured in nontraffic accident** A, D, S 🔲

  ● **V86.72** **Person on outside of snowmobile injured in nontraffic accident** A, D, S 🔲

  ● **V86.73** **Person on outside of dune buggy injured in nontraffic accident** A, D, S 🔲

  ● **V86.74** **Person on outside of military vehicle injured in nontraffic accident** A, D, S 🔲

  ● **V86.79** **Person on outside of other special all-terrain or other off-road motor vehicles injured in nontraffic accident** A, D, S 🔲
    Person on outside of dirt bike injured in nontraffic accident
    Person on outside of go cart injured in nontraffic accident
    Person on outside of golf cart injured in nontraffic accident

● **V86.9** **Unspecified occupant of special all-terrain or other off-road motor vehicle injured in nontraffic accident**

  ● 🔲 **V86.91** **Unspecified occupant of ambulance or fire engine injured in nontraffic accident** A, D, S 🔲

  ● 🔲 **V86.92** **Unspecified occupant of snowmobile injured in nontraffic accident** A, D, S 🔲

  ● 🔲 **V86.93** **Unspecified occupant of dune buggy injured in nontraffic accident** A, D, S 🔲

  ● 🔲 **V86.94** **Unspecified occupant of military vehicle injured in nontraffic accident** A, D, S 🔲

  ● 🔲 **V86.99** **Unspecified occupant of other off-road special all-terrain or other off-road motor vehicle injured in nontraffic accident** A, D, S 🔲
    All-terrain motor-vehicle accident NOS
    Off-road motor-vehicle accident NOS
    Other motor-vehicle accident NOS
    Unspecified occupant of dirt bike injured in nontraffic accident
    Unspecified occupant of go cart injured in nontraffic accident
    Unspecified occupant of golf cart injured in nontraffic accident
    Unspecified occupant of race car injured in nontraffic accident

● **V87** **Traffic accident of specified type but victim's mode of transport unknown**

> **Excludes1** collision involving:
>   pedal cycle (V10-V19)
>   pedestrian (V01-V09)

The appropriate 7th character is to be added to each code from category V87

> A　initial encounter
> D　subsequent encounter
> S　sequela

● **V87.0** **Person injured in collision between car and two- or three-wheeled powered vehicle (traffic)** A, D, S 🔲

● **V87.1** **Person injured in collision between other motor vehicle and two- or three-wheeled motor vehicle (traffic)** A, D, S 🔲

● **V87.2** **Person injured in collision between car and pick-up truck or van (traffic)** A, D, S 🔲

● **V87.3** **Person injured in collision between car and bus (traffic)** A, D, S 🔲

● **V87.4** **Person injured in collision between car and heavy transport vehicle (traffic)** A, D, S 🔲

● **V87.5** **Person injured in collision between heavy transport vehicle and bus (traffic)** A, D, S 🔲

● **V87.6** **Person injured in collision between railway train or railway vehicle and car (traffic)** A, D, S 🔲

● **V87.7** **Person injured in collision between other specified motor vehicles (traffic)** A, D, S 🔲

N Newborn Age: 0　　**P** Pediatric Age: 0–17　　**M** Maternity DX: 12–55　　**A** Adult Age: 15–124　　♀ Females Only　　♂ Males Only

🔲 Complication\Comorbidity　　🔲 Major C\C　　🔲 Present on Admission Requirement　　🔲 Hospital-Acquired Condition

1729

● **V87.8**   **Person injured in other specified noncollision transport accidents involving motor vehicle (traffic)** A, D, S 🖉

● **V87.9**   **Person injured in other specified (collision) (noncollision) transport accidents involving nonmotor vehicle (traffic)** A, D, S 🖉

● **V88**   **Nontraffic accident of specified type but victim's mode of transport unknown**

> Excludes1   collision involving:
> > pedal cycle (V10-V19)
> > pedestrian (V01-V09)

> The appropriate 7th character is to be added to each code from category V88

> | | |
> |---|---|
> | A | initial encounter |
> | D | subsequent encounter |
> | S | sequela |

● **V88.0**   **Person injured in collision between car and two- or three-wheeled motor vehicle, nontraffic** A, D, S 🖉

● **V88.1**   **Person injured in collision between other motor vehicle and two- or three-wheeled motor vehicle, nontraffic** A, D, S 🖉

● **V88.2**   **Person injured in collision between car and pick-up truck or van, nontraffic** A, D, S 🖉

● **V88.3**   **Person injured in collision between car and bus, nontraffic** A, D, S 🖉

● **V88.4**   **Person injured in collision between car and heavy transport vehicle, nontraffic** A, D, S 🖉

● **V88.5**   **Person injured in collision between heavy transport vehicle and bus, nontraffic** A, D, S 🖉

● **V88.6**   **Person injured in collision between railway train or railway vehicle and car, nontraffic** A, D, S 🖉

● **V88.7**   **Person injured in collision between other specified motor vehicle, nontraffic** A, D, S 🖉

● **V88.8**   **Person injured in other specified noncollision transport accidents involving motor vehicle, nontraffic** A, D, S 🖉

● **V88.9**   **Person injured in other specified (collision) (noncollision) transport accidents involving nonmotor vehicle, nontraffic** A, D, S 🖉

● **V89**   **Motor- or nonmotor-vehicle accident, type of vehicle unspecified**

> The appropriate 7th character is to be added to each code from category V89

> | | |
> |---|---|
> | A | initial encounter |
> | D | subsequent encounter |
> | S | sequela |

● ◼ **V89.0**   **Person injured in unspecified motor-vehicle accident, nontraffic** A, D, S 🖉
> Motor-vehicle accident NOS, nontraffic

● ◼ **V89.1**   **Person injured in unspecified nonmotor-vehicle accident, nontraffic** A, D, S 🖉
> Nonmotor-vehicle accident NOS (nontraffic)

● ◼ **V89.2**   **Person injured in unspecified motor-vehicle accident, traffic** A, D, S 🖉
> Motor-vehicle accident [MVA] NOS
> Road (traffic) accident [RTA] NOS

● ◼ **V89.3**   **Person injured in unspecified nonmotor-vehicle accident, traffic** A, D, S 🖉
> Nonmotor-vehicle traffic accident NOS

● ◼ **V89.9**   **Person injured in unspecified vehicle accident** A, D, S 🖉
> Collision NOS

WATER TRANSPORT ACCIDENTS (V90-V94)

● **V90**   **Drowning and submersion due to accident to watercraft**

> Excludes1   civilian water transport accident involving military watercraft (V94.81-)
> > fall into water not from watercraft (W16.-)
> > military watercraft accident in military or war operations (Y36.0-, Y37.0-)
> > water-transport–related drowning or submersion without accident to watercraft (V92.-)

> The appropriate 7th character is to be added to each code from category V90

> | | |
> |---|---|
> | A | initial encounter |
> | D | subsequent encounter |
> | S | sequela |

● **V90.0**   **Drowning and submersion due to watercraft overturning**

  ● **V90.00**   **Drowning and submersion due to merchant ship overturning** A, D, S 🖉

  ● **V90.01**   **Drowning and submersion due to passenger ship overturning** A, D, S 🖉
> Drowning and submersion due to ferry-boat overturning
> Drowning and submersion due to liner overturning

  ● **V90.02**   **Drowning and submersion due to fishing boat overturning** A, D, S 🖉

  ● **V90.03**   **Drowning and submersion due to other powered watercraft overturning** A, D, S 🖉
> Drowning and submersion due to hovercraft (on open water) overturning
> Drowning and submersion due to jet ski overturning

  ● **V90.04**   **Drowning and submersion due to sailboat overturning** A, D, S 🖉

  ● **V90.05**   **Drowning and submersion due to canoe or kayak overturning** A, D, S 🖉

  ● **V90.06**   **Drowning and submersion due to (nonpowered) inflatable craft overturning** A, D, S 🖉

  ● **V90.08**   **Drowning and submersion due to other unpowered watercraft overturning** A, D, S 🖉
> Drowning and submersion due to windsurfer overturning

  ● ◼ **V90.09**   **Drowning and submersion due to unspecified watercraft overturning** A, D, S 🖉
> Drowning and submersion due to boat NOS overturning
> Drowning and submersion due to ship NOS overturning
> Drowning and submersion due to watercraft NOS overturning

● **V90.1**   **Drowning and submersion due to watercraft sinking**

  ● **V90.10**   **Drowning and submersion due to merchant ship sinking** A, D, S 🖉

  ● **V90.11**   **Drowning and submersion due to passenger ship sinking** A, D, S 🖉
> Drowning and submersion due to ferry-boat sinking
> Drowning and submersion due to liner sinking

● Unacceptable Principal Diagnosis   ● Use Additional Character(s)   ◼ Unspecified   ▶ Manifestation Code

OGCR Official Guidelines for Coding and Reporting   Excludes 1   Excludes 2   Includes   Use additional   Code first   Code also

● **V90.12** Drowning and submersion due to fishing boat sinking A, D, S 🔗

● **V90.13** Drowning and submersion due to other powered watercraft sinking A, D, S 🔗
    Drowning and submersion due to hovercraft (on open water) sinking
    Drowning and submersion due to jet ski sinking

● **V90.14** Drowning and submersion due to sailboat sinking A, D, S 🔗

● **V90.15** Drowning and submersion due to canoe or kayak sinking A, D, S 🔗

● **V90.16** Drowning and submersion due to (nonpowered) inflatable craft sinking A, D, S 🔗

● **V90.18** Drowning and submersion due to other unpowered watercraft sinking A, D, S 🔗

● ■ **V90.19** Drowning and submersion due to unspecified watercraft sinking A, D, S 🔗
    Drowning and submersion due to boat NOS sinking
    Drowning and submersion due to ship NOS sinking
    Drowning and submersion due to watercraft NOS sinking

● **V90.2** Drowning and submersion due to falling or jumping from burning watercraft

● **V90.20** Drowning and submersion due to falling or jumping from burning merchant ship A, D, S 🔗

● **V90.21** Drowning and submersion due to falling or jumping from burning passenger ship A, D, S 🔗
    Drowning and submersion due to falling or jumping from burning ferry-boat
    Drowning and submersion due to falling or jumping from burning liner

● **V90.22** Drowning and submersion due to falling or jumping from burning fishing boat A, D, S 🔗

● **V90.23** Drowning and submersion due to falling or jumping from other burning powered watercraft A, D, S 🔗
    Drowning and submersion due to falling and jumping from burning hovercraft (on open water)
    Drowning and submersion due to falling and jumping from burning jet ski

● **V90.24** Drowning and submersion due to falling or jumping from burning sailboat A, D, S 🔗

● **V90.25** Drowning and submersion due to falling or jumping from burning canoe or kayak A, D, S 🔗

● **V90.26** Drowning and submersion due to falling or jumping from burning (nonpowered) inflatable craft A, D, S 🔗

● **V90.27** Drowning and submersion due to falling or jumping from burning water-skis A, D, S 🔗

● **V90.28** Drowning and submersion due to falling or jumping from other burning unpowered watercraft A, D, S 🔗
    Drowning and submersion due to falling and jumping from burning surf-board
    Drowning and submersion due to falling and jumping from burning windsurfer

● ■ **V90.29** Drowning and submersion due to falling or jumping from unspecified burning watercraft A, D, S 🔗
    Drowning and submersion due to falling or jumping from burning boat NOS
    Drowning and submersion due to falling or jumping from burning ship NOS
    Drowning and submersion due to falling or jumping from burning watercraft NOS

● **V90.3** Drowning and submersion due to falling or jumping from crushed watercraft

● **V90.30** Drowning and submersion due to falling or jumping from crushed merchant ship A, D, S 🔗

● **V90.31** Drowning and submersion due to falling or jumping from crushed passenger ship A, D, S 🔗
    Drowning and submersion due to falling and jumping from crushed ferry-boat
    Drowning and submersion due to falling and jumping from crushed liner

● **V90.32** Drowning and submersion due to falling or jumping from crushed fishing boat A, D, S 🔗

● **V90.33** Drowning and submersion due to falling or jumping from other crushed powered watercraft A, D, S 🔗
    Drowning and submersion due to falling and jumping from crushed hovercraft
    Drowning and submersion due to falling and jumping from crushed jet ski

● **V90.34** Drowning and submersion due to falling or jumping from crushed sailboat A, D, S 🔗

● **V90.35** Drowning and submersion due to falling or jumping from crushed canoe or kayak A, D, S 🔗

● **V90.36** Drowning and submersion due to falling or jumping from crushed (nonpowered) inflatable craft A, D, S 🔗

● **V90.37** Drowning and submersion due to falling or jumping from crushed water-skis A, D, S 🔗

● **V90.38** Drowning and submersion due to falling or jumping from other crushed unpowered watercraft A, D, S 🔗
    Drowning and submersion due to falling and jumping from crushed surf-board
    Drowning and submersion due to falling and jumping from crushed windsurfer

N Newborn Age: 0   **P** Pediatric Age: 0–17   **M** Maternity DX: 12–55   **A** Adult Age: 15–124   ♀ Females Only   ♂ Males Only

🔗 Complication\Comorbidity   🔗 Major C\C   🔗 Present on Admission Requirement   🔗 Hospital-Acquired Condition

1731

● ■ **V90.39** **Drowning and submersion due to falling or jumping from crushed unspecified watercraft** A, D, S 🔊

> Drowning and submersion due to falling and jumping from crushed boat NOS
>
> Drowning and submersion due to falling and jumping from crushed ship NOS
>
> Drowning and submersion due to falling and jumping from crushed watercraft NOS

● **V90.8** **Drowning and submersion due to other accident to watercraft**

● **V90.80** **Drowning and submersion due to other accident to merchant ship** A, D, S 🔊

● **V90.81** **Drowning and submersion due to other accident to passenger ship** A, D, S 🔊

> Drowning and submersion due to other accident to ferry-boat
>
> Drowning and submersion due to other accident to liner

● **V90.82** **Drowning and submersion due to other accident to fishing boat** A, D, S 🔊

● **V90.83** **Drowning and submersion due to other accident to other powered watercraft** A, D, S 🔊

> Drowning and submersion due to other accident to hovercraft (on open water)
>
> Drowning and submersion due to other accident to jet ski

● **V90.84** **Drowning and submersion due to other accident to sailboat** A, D, S 🔊

● **V90.85** **Drowning and submersion due to other accident to canoe or kayak** A, D, S 🔊

● **V90.86** **Drowning and submersion due to other accident to (nonpowered) inflatable craft** A, D, S 🔊

● **V90.87** **Drowning and submersion due to other accident to water-skis** A, D, S 🔊

● **V90.88** **Drowning and submersion due to other accident to other unpowered watercraft** A, D, S 🔊

> Drowning and submersion due to other accident to surf-board
>
> Drowning and submersion due to other accident to windsurfer

● ■ **V90.89** **Drowning and submersion due to other accident to unspecified watercraft** A, D, S 🔊

> Drowning and submersion due to other accident to boat NOS
>
> Drowning and submersion due to other accident to ship NOS
>
> Drowning and submersion due to other accident to watercraft NOS

● **V91** **Other injury due to accident to watercraft**

> **Includes**   any injury except drowning and submersion as a result of an accident to watercraft
>
> **Excludes1**   civilian water transport accident involving military watercraft (V94.81-)
> military watercraft accident in military or war operations (Y36, Y37-)
>
> **Excludes2**   drowning and submersion due to accident to watercraft (V90.-)

The appropriate 7th character is to be added to each code from category V91

> A   initial encounter
> D   subsequent encounter
> S   sequela

● **V91.0** **Burn due to watercraft on fire**

> **Excludes1**   burn from localized fire or explosion on board ship without accident to watercraft (V93.-)

● **V91.00** **Burn due to merchant ship on fire** A, D, S 🔊

● **V91.01** **Burn due to passenger ship on fire** A, D, S 🔊

> Burn due to ferry-boat on fire
>
> Burn due to liner on fire

● **V91.02** **Burn due to fishing boat on fire** A, D, S 🔊

● **V91.03** **Burn due to other powered watercraft on fire** A, D, S 🔊

> Burn due to hovercraft (on open water) on fire
>
> Burn due to jet ski on fire

● **V91.04** **Burn due to sailboat on fire** A, D, S 🔊

● **V91.05** **Burn due to canoe or kayak on fire** A, D, S 🔊

● **V91.06** **Burn due to (nonpowered) inflatable craft on fire** A, D, S 🔊

● **V91.07** **Burn due to water-skis on fire** A, D, S 🔊

● **V91.08** **Burn due to other unpowered watercraft on fire** A, D, S 🔊

● ■ **V91.09** **Burn due to unspecified watercraft on fire** A, D, S 🔊

> Burn due to boat NOS on fire
>
> Burn due to ship NOS on fire
>
> Burn due to watercraft NOS on fire

● **V91.1** **Crushed between watercraft and other watercraft or other object due to collision**

> Crushed by lifeboat after abandoning ship in a collision
>
> **Note:** Select the specified type of watercraft that the victim was on at the time of the collision.

● **V91.10** **Crushed between merchant ship and other watercraft or other object due to collision** A, D, S 🔊

● **V91.11** **Crushed between passenger ship and other watercraft or other object due to collision** A, D, S 🔊

> Crushed between ferry-boat and other watercraft or other object due to collision
>
> Crushed between liner and other watercraft or other object due to collision

● **V91.12   Crushed between fishing boat and other watercraft or other object due to collision** A, D, S 🖾

● **V91.13   Crushed between other powered watercraft and other watercraft or other object due to collision** A, D, S 🖾
     Crushed between hovercraft (on open water) and other watercraft or other object due to collision
     Crushed between jet ski and other watercraft or other object due to collision

● **V91.14   Crushed between sailboat and other watercraft or other object due to collision** A, D, S 🖾

● **V91.15   Crushed between canoe or kayak and other watercraft or other object due to collision** A, D, S 🖾

● **V91.16   Crushed between (nonpowered) inflatable craft and other watercraft or other object due to collision** A, D, S 🖾

● **V91.18   Crushed between other unpowered watercraft and other watercraft or other object due to collision** A, D, S 🖾
     Crushed between surfboard and other watercraft or other object due to collision
     Crushed between windsurfer and other watercraft or other object due to collision

●■ **V91.19   Crushed between unspecified watercraft and other watercraft or other object due to collision** A, D, S 🖾
     Crushed between boat NOS and other watercraft or other object due to collision
     Crushed between ship NOS and other watercraft or other object due to collision
     Crushed between watercraft NOS and other watercraft or other object due to collision

● **V91.2   Fall due to collision between watercraft and other watercraft or other object**
     Fall while remaining on watercraft after collision

     Note: Select the specified type of watercraft that the victim was on at the time of the collision.

     | Excludes1 | crushed between watercraft and other watercraft and other object due to collision (V91.1-)
                 drowning and submersion due to falling from crushed watercraft (V90.3-)

● **V91.20   Fall due to collision between merchant ship and other watercraft or other object** A, D, S 🖾

● **V91.21   Fall due to collision between passenger ship and other watercraft or other object** A, D, S 🖾
     Fall due to collision between ferry-boat and other watercraft or other object
     Fall due to collision between liner and other watercraft or other object

● **V91.22   Fall due to collision between fishing boat and other watercraft or other object** A, D, S 🖾

● **V91.23   Fall due to collision between other powered watercraft and other watercraft or other object** A, D, S 🖾
     Fall due to collision between hovercraft (on open water) and other watercraft or other object
     Fall due to collision between jet ski and other watercraft or other object

● **V91.24   Fall due to collision between sailboat and other watercraft or other object** A, D, S 🖾

● **V91.25   Fall due to collision between canoe or kayak and other watercraft or other object** A, D, S 🖾

● **V91.26   Fall due to collision between (nonpowered) inflatable craft and other watercraft or other object** A, D, S 🖾

●■ **V91.29   Fall due to collision between unspecified watercraft and other watercraft or other object** A, D, S 🖾
     Fall due to collision between boat NOS and other watercraft or other object
     Fall due to collision between ship NOS and other watercraft or other object
     Fall due to collision between watercraft NOS and other watercraft or other object

● **V91.3   Hit or struck by falling object due to accident to watercraft**
     Hit or struck by falling object (part of damaged watercraft or other object) after falling or jumping from damaged watercraft

     | Excludes2 | drowning or submersion due to fall or jumping from damaged watercraft (V90.2-, V90.3-)

● **V91.30   Hit or struck by falling object due to accident to merchant ship** A, D, S 🖾

● **V91.31   Hit or struck by falling object due to accident to passenger ship** A, D, S 🖾
     Hit or struck by falling object due to accident to ferry-boat
     Hit or struck by falling object due to accident to liner

● **V91.32   Hit or struck by falling object due to accident to fishing boat** A, D, S 🖾

● **V91.33   Hit or struck by falling object due to accident to other powered watercraft** A, D, S 🖾
     Hit or struck by falling object due to accident to hovercraft (on open water)
     Hit or struck by falling object due to accident to jet ski

● **V91.34   Hit or struck by falling object due to accident to sailboat** A, D, S 🖾

● **V91.35   Hit or struck by falling object due to accident to canoe or kayak** A, D, S 🖾

● **V91.36   Hit or struck by falling object due to accident to (nonpowered) inflatable craft** A, D, S 🖾

N Newborn Age: 0   **P** Pediatric Age: 0–17   **M** Maternity DX: 12–55   **A** Adult Age: 15–124   ♀ Females Only   ♂ Males Only

🖾 Complication\Comorbidity   🖾 Major C\C   🖾 Present on Admission Requirement   🖾 Hospital-Acquired Condition   1733

● **V91.37** **Hit or struck by falling object due to accident to water-skis** A, D, S 🔖
   Hit by water-skis after jumping off of waterskis

● **V91.38** **Hit or struck by falling object due to accident to other unpowered watercraft** A, D, S 🔖
   Hit or struck by surf-board after falling off damaged surf-board
   Hit or struck by object after falling off damaged windsurfer

●■ **V91.39** **Hit or struck by falling object due to accident to unspecified watercraft** A, D, S 🔖
   Hit or struck by falling object due to accident to boat NOS
   Hit or struck by falling object due to accident to ship NOS
   Hit or struck by falling object due to accident to watercraft NOS

● **V91.8** **Other injury due to other accident to watercraft**

● **V91.80** **Other injury due to other accident to merchant ship** A, D, S 🔖

● **V91.81** **Other injury due to other accident to passenger ship** A, D, S 🔖
   Other injury due to other accident to ferry-boat
   Other injury due to other accident to liner

● **V91.82** **Other injury due to other accident to fishing boat** A, D, S 🔖

● **V91.83** **Other injury due to other accident to other powered watercraft** A, D, S 🔖
   Other injury due to other accident to hovercraft (on open water)
   Other injury due to other accident to jet ski

● **V91.84** **Other injury due to other accident to sailboat** A, D, S 🔖

● **V91.85** **Other injury due to other accident to canoe or kayak** A, D, S 🔖

● **V91.86** **Other injury due to other accident to (nonpowered) inflatable craft** A, D, S 🔖

● **V91.87** **Other injury due to other accident to water-skis** A, D, S 🔖

● **V91.88** **Other injury due to other accident to other unpowered watercraft** A, D, S 🔖
   Other injury due to other accident to surf-board
   Other injury due to other accident to windsurfer

●■ **V91.89** **Other injury due to other accident to unspecified watercraft** A, D, S 🔖
   Other injury due to other accident to boat NOS
   Other injury due to other accident to ship NOS
   Other injury due to other accident to watercraft NOS

● **V92** **Drowning and submersion due to accident on board watercraft, without accident to watercraft**

   Excludes1 civilian water transport accident involving military watercraft (V94.81-)
   drowning or submersion due to accident to watercraft (V90-V91)
   drowning or submersion of diver who voluntarily jumps from boat not involved in an accident (W16.711, W16.721)
   fall into water without watercraft (W16.-)
   military watercraft accident in military or war operations (Y36, Y37)

   The appropriate 7th character is to be added to each code from category V92

A	initial encounter
D	subsequent encounter
S	sequela

● **V92.0** **Drowning and submersion due to fall off watercraft**
   Drowning and submersion due to fall from gangplank of watercraft
   Drowning and submersion due to fall overboard watercraft

   Excludes2 hitting head on object or bottom of body of water due to fall from watercraft (V94.0-)

● **V92.00** **Drowning and submersion due to fall off merchant ship** A, D, S 🔖

● **V92.01** **Drowning and submersion due to fall off passenger ship** A, D, S 🔖
   Drowning and submersion due to fall off ferry-boat
   Drowning and submersion due to fall off liner

● **V92.02** **Drowning and submersion due to fall off fishing boat** A, D, S 🔖

● **V92.03** **Drowning and submersion due to fall off other powered watercraft** A, D, S 🔖
   Drowning and submersion due to fall off hovercraft (on open water)
   Drowning and submersion due to fall off jet ski

● **V92.04** **Drowning and submersion due to fall off sailboat** A, D, S 🔖

● **V92.05** **Drowning and submersion due to fall off canoe or kayak** A, D, S 🔖

● **V92.06** **Drowning and submersion due to fall off (nonpowered) inflatable craft** A, D, S 🔖

● **V92.07** **Drowning and submersion due to fall off water-skis** A, D, S 🔖

   Excludes1 drowning and submersion due to falling off burning water-skis (V90.27)
   drowning and submersion due to falling off crushed water-skis (V90.37)
   hit by boat while water-skiing NOS (V94.x)

● Unacceptable Principal Diagnosis   ● Use Additional Character(s)   ■ Unspecified   ▶ Manifestation Code
OGCR Official Guidelines for Coding and Reporting   Excludes 1   Excludes 2   Includes   Use additional   Code first   Code also

- ● **V92.08 Drowning and submersion due to fall off other unpowered watercraft** A, D, S 🖐
  - Drowning and submersion due to fall off surf-board
  - Drowning and submersion due to fall off windsurfer

  > **Excludes1** drowning and submersion due to fall off burning unpowered watercraft (V90.28)
  > drowning and submersion due to fall off crushed unpowered watercraft (V90.38)
  > drowning and submersion due to fall off damaged unpowered watercraft (V90.88)
  > drowning and submersion due to rider of nonpowered watercraft being hit by other watercraft (V94...)
  > other injury due to rider of nonpowered watercraft being hit by other watercraft (V94...)

- ●🔲 **V92.09 Drowning and submersion due to fall off unspecified watercraft** A, D, S 🖐
  - Drowning and submersion due to fall off boat NOS
  - Drowning and submersion due to fall off ship
  - Drowning and submersion due to fall off watercraft NOS

- ● **V92.1 Drowning and submersion due to being thrown overboard by motion of watercraft**

  > **Excludes1** drowning and submersion due to fall off surf-board (V92.08)
  > drowning and submersion due to fall off water-skis (V92.07)
  > drowning and submersion due to fall off windsurfer (V92.08)

  - ● **V92.10 Drowning and submersion due to being thrown overboard by motion of merchant ship** A, D, S 🖐
  - ● **V92.11 Drowning and submersion due to being thrown overboard by motion of passenger ship** A, D, S 🖐
    - Drowning and submersion due to being thrown overboard by motion of ferry-boat
    - Drowning and submersion due to being thrown overboard by motion of liner
  - ● **V92.12 Drowning and submersion due to being thrown overboard by motion of fishing boat** A, D, S 🖐
  - ● **V92.13 Drowning and submersion due to being thrown overboard by motion of other powered watercraft** A, D, S 🖐
    - Drowning and submersion due to being thrown overboard by motion of hovercraft
  - ● **V92.14 Drowning and submersion due to being thrown overboard by motion of sailboat** A, D, S 🖐
  - ● **V92.15 Drowning and submersion due to being thrown overboard by motion of canoe or kayak** A, D, S 🖐

- ● **V92.16 Drowning and submersion due to being thrown overboard by motion of (nonpowered) inflatable craft** A, D, S 🖐
- ●🔲 **V92.19 Drowning and submersion due to being thrown overboard by motion of unspecified watercraft** A, D, S 🖐
  - Drowning and submersion due to being thrown overboard by motion of boat NOS
  - Drowning and submersion due to being thrown overboard by motion of ship NOS
  - Drowning and submersion due to being thrown overboard by motion of watercraft NOS

- ● **V92.2 Drowning and submersion due to being washed overboard from watercraft**

  Code first any associated cataclysm (X37.0-)

  - ● **V92.20 Drowning and submersion due to being washed overboard from merchant ship** A, D, S 🖐
  - ● **V92.21 Drowning and submersion due to being washed overboard from passenger ship** A, D, S 🖐
    - Drowning and submersion due to being washed overboard from ferry-boat
    - Drowning and submersion due to being washed overboard from liner
  - ● **V92.22 Drowning and submersion due to being washed overboard from fishing boat** A, D, S 🖐
  - ● **V92.23 Drowning and submersion due to being washed overboard from other powered watercraft** A, D, S 🖐
    - Drowning and submersion due to being washed overboard from hovercraft (on open water)
    - Drowning and submersion due to being washed overboard from jet ski
  - ● **V92.24 Drowning and submersion due to being washed overboard from sailboat** A, D, S 🖐
  - ● **V92.25 Drowning and submersion due to being washed overboard from canoe or kayak** A, D, S 🖐
  - ● **V92.26 Drowning and submersion due to being washed overboard from (nonpowered) inflatable craft** A, D, S 🖐
  - ● **V92.27 Drowning and submersion due to being washed overboard from water-skis** A, D, S 🖐

    > **Excludes1** drowning and submersion due to fall off water-skis (V92.07)

  - ● **V92.28 Drowning and submersion due to being washed overboard from other unpowered watercraft** A, D, S 🖐
    - Drowning and submersion due to being washed overboard from surf-board
    - Drowning and submersion due to being washed overboard from windsurfer
  - ●🔲 **V92.29 Drowning and submersion due to being washed overboard from unspecified watercraft** A, D, S 🖐
    - Drowning and submersion due to being washed overboard from boat NOS
    - Drowning and submersion due to being washed overboard from ship NOS
    - Drowning and submersion due to being washed overboard from watercraft NOS

V93   Other injury due to accident on board watercraft, without accident to watercraft

> **Excludes1**   civilian water transport accident involving military watercraft (V94.81-)
> other injury due to accident to watercraft (V91.-)
> military watercraft accident in military or war operations (Y36, Y37-)

> **Excludes2**   drowning and submersion due to accident on board watercraft, without accident to watercraft (V92.-)

The appropriate 7th character is to be added to each code from category V93

A	initial encounter
D	subsequent encounter
S	sequela

● **V93.0   Burn due to localized fire on board watercraft**

> **Excludes1**   burn due to watercraft on fire (V91.0-)

● **V93.00   Burn due to localized fire on board merchant vessel** A, D, S ◎

● **V93.01   Burn due to localized fire on board passenger vessel** A, D, S ◎
> Burn due to localized fire on board ferry-boat
> Burn due to localized fire on board liner

● **V93.02   Burn due to localized fire on board fishing boat** A, D, S ◎

● **V93.03   Burn due to localized fire on board other powered watercraft** A, D, S ◎
> Burn due to localized fire on board hovercraft
> Burn due to localized fire on board jet ski

● **V93.04   Burn due to localized fire on board sailboat** A, D, S ◎

●■ **V93.09   Burn due to localized fire on board unspecified watercraft** A, D, S ◎
> Burn due to localized fire on board boat NOS
> Burn due to localized fire on board ship NOS
> Burn due to localized fire on board watercraft NOS

● **V93.1   Other burn on board watercraft**
> Burn due to source other than fire on board watercraft

> **Excludes1**   burn due to watercraft on fire (V91.0-)

● **V93.10   Other burn on board merchant vessel** A, D, S ◎

● **V93.11   Other burn on board passenger vessel** A, D, S ◎
> Other burn on board ferry-boat
> Other burn on board liner

● **V93.12   Other burn on board fishing boat** A, D, S ◎

● **V93.13   Other burn on board other powered watercraft** A, D, S ◎
> Other burn on board hovercraft
> Other burn on board jet ski

● **V93.14   Other burn on board sailboat** A, D, S ◎

●■ **V93.19   Other burn on board unspecified watercraft** A, D, S ◎
> Other burn on board boat NOS
> Other burn on board ship NOS
> Other burn on board watercraft NOS

● **V93.2   Heat exposure on board watercraft**

> **Excludes1**   exposure to man-made heat not aboard watercraft (W92)
> exposure to natural heat while on board watercraft (X30)
> exposure to sunlight while on board watercraft (X32)

> **Excludes2**   burn due to fire on board watercraft (V93.0-)

● **V93.20   Heat exposure on board merchant ship** A, D, S ◎

● **V93.21   Heat exposure on board passenger ship** A, D, S ◎
> Heat exposure on board ferry-boat
> Heat exposure on board liner

● **V93.22   Heat exposure on board fishing boat** A, D, S ◎

● **V93.23   Heat exposure on board other powered watercraft** A, D, S ◎
> Heat exposure on board hovercraft

● **V93.24   Heat exposure on board sailboat** A, D, S ◎

●■ **V93.29   Heat exposure on board unspecified watercraft** A, D, S ◎
> Heat exposure on board boat NOS
> Heat exposure on board ship NOS
> Heat exposure on board watercraft NOS

● **V93.3   Fall on board watercraft**

> **Excludes1**   fall due to collision of watercraft (V91.2-)

● **V93.30   Fall on board merchant ship** A, D, S ◎

● **V93.31   Fall on board passenger ship** A, D, S ◎
> Fall on board ferry-boat
> Fall on board liner

● **V93.32   Fall on board fishing boat** A, D, S ◎

● **V93.33   Fall on board other powered watercraft** A, D, S ◎
> Fall on board hovercraft (on open water)
> Fall on board jet ski

● **V93.34   Fall on board sailboat** A, D, S ◎

● **V93.35   Fall on board canoe or kayak** A, D, S ◎

● **V93.36   Fall on board (nonpowered) inflatable craft** A, D, S ◎

● **V93.38   Fall on board other unpowered watercraft** A, D, S ◎

●■ **V93.39   Fall on board unspecified watercraft** A, D, S ◎
> Fall on board boat NOS
> Fall on board ship NOS
> Fall on board watercraft NOS

● **V93.4   Struck by falling object on board watercraft**
> Hit by falling object on board watercraft

> **Excludes1**   struck by falling object due to accident to watercraft (V91.3)

● **V93.40   Struck by falling object on merchant ship** A, D, S ◎

● **V93.41   Struck by falling object on passenger ship** A, D, S ◎
> Struck by falling object on ferry-boat
> Struck by falling object on liner

● **V93.42   Struck by falling object on fishing boat** A, D, S ◎

● **V93.43   Struck by falling object on other powered watercraft** A, D, S ◎
> Struck by falling object on hovercraft

● Unacceptable Principal Diagnosis   ● Use Additional Character(s)   ■ Unspecified   ▶ Manifestation Code

OGCR Official Guidelines for Coding and Reporting   Excludes 1   Excludes 2   Includes   Use additional   Code first   Code also

● **V93.44 Struck by falling object on sailboat** A, D, S 🔖

● **V93.48 Struck by falling object on other unpowered watercraft** A, D, S 🔖

●■ **V93.49 Struck by falling object on unspecified watercraft** A, D, S 🔖

● **V93.5 Explosion on board watercraft**
　Boiler explosion on steamship

　Excludes2   fire on board watercraft (V93.0-)

● **V93.50 Explosion on board merchant ship** A, D, S 🔖

● **V93.51 Explosion on board passenger ship** A, D, S 🔖
　Explosion on board ferry-boat
　Explosion on board liner

● **V93.52 Explosion on board fishing boat** A, D, S 🔖

● **V93.53 Explosion on board other powered watercraft** A, D, S 🔖
　Explosion on board hovercraft
　Explosion on board jet ski

● **V93.54 Explosion on board sailboat** A, D, S 🔖

●■ **V93.59 Explosion on board unspecified watercraft** A, D, S 🔖
　Explosion on board boat NOS
　Explosion on board ship NOS
　Explosion on board watercraft NOS

● **V93.6 Machinery accident on board watercraft**

　Excludes1   machinery explosion on board watercraft (V93.4-)
　machinery fire on board watercraft (V93.0-)

● **V93.60 Machinery accident on board merchant ship** A, D, S 🔖

● **V93.61 Machinery accident on board passenger ship** A, D, S 🔖
　Machinery accident on board ferry-boat
　Machinery accident on board liner

● **V93.62 Machinery accident on board fishing boat** A, D, S 🔖

● **V93.63 Machinery accident on board other powered watercraft** A, D, S 🔖
　Machinery accident on board hovercraft

● **V93.64 Machinery accident on board sailboat** A, D, S 🔖

●■ **V93.69 Machinery accident on board unspecified watercraft** A, D, S 🔖
　Machinery accident on board boat NOS
　Machinery accident on board ship NOS
　Machinery accident on board watercraft NOS

● **V93.8 Other injury due to other accident on board watercraft**
　Accidental poisoning by gases or fumes on watercraft

● **V93.80 Other injury due to other accident on board merchant ship** A, D, S 🔖

● **V93.81 Other injury due to other accident on board passenger ship** A, D, S 🔖
　Other injury due to other accident on board ferry-boat
　Other injury due to other accident on board liner

● **V93.82 Other injury due to other accident on board fishing boat** A, D, S 🔖

● **V93.83 Other injury due to other accident on board other powered watercraft** A, D, S 🔖
　Other injury due to other accident on board hovercraft
　Other injury due to other accident on board jet ski

● **V93.84 Other injury due to other accident on board sailboat** A, D, S 🔖

● **V93.85 Other injury due to other accident on board canoe or kayak** A, D, S 🔖

● **V93.86 Other injury due to other accident on board (nonpowered) inflatable craft** A, D, S 🔖

● **V93.87 Other injury due to other accident on board water-skis** A, D, S 🔖
　Hit or struck by object while waterskiing

● **V93.88 Other injury due to other accident on board other unpowered watercraft** A, D, S 🔖
　Hit or struck by object while surfing
　Hit or struck by object while on board windsurfer

●■ **V93.89 Other injury due to other accident on board unspecified watercraft** A, D, S 🔖
　Other injury due to other accident on board boat NOS
　Other injury due to other accident on board ship NOS
　Other injury due to other accident on board watercraft NOS

● **V94 Other and unspecified water transport accidents**

　Excludes1   military watercraft accidents in military or war operations (Y36, Y37)

　The appropriate 7th character is to be added to each code from category V94

A	initial encounter
D	subsequent encounter
S	sequela

● **V94.0 Hitting object or bottom of body of water due to fall from watercraft** A, D, S 🔖

　Excludes2   drowning and submersion due to fall from watercraft (V92.0-)

● **V94.1 Bather struck by watercraft**
　Swimmer hit by watercraft

● **V94.11 Bather struck by powered watercraft** A, D, S 🔖

● **V94.12 Bather struck by nonpowered watercraft** A, D, S 🔖

● **V94.2 Rider of nonpowered watercraft struck by other watercraft**

● **V94.21 Rider of nonpowered watercraft struck by other nonpowered watercraft** A, D, S 🔖
　Canoer hit by other nonpowered watercraft
　Surfer hit by other nonpowered watercraft
　Windsurfer hit by other nonpowered watercraft

● **V94.22 Rider of nonpowered watercraft struck by powered watercraft** A, D, S 🔖
　Canoer hit by motorboat
　Surfer hit by motorboat
　Windsurfer hit by motorboat

N Newborn Age: 0   **P** Pediatric Age: 0–17   **M** Maternity DX: 12–55   **A** Adult Age: 15–124   ♀ Females Only   ♂ Males Only

🔖 Complication\Comorbidity   🔖 Major C\C   🔖 Present on Admission Requirement   🔖 Hospital-Acquired Condition

1737

● **V94.3 Injury to rider of (inflatable) watercraft being pulled behind other watercraft**

     ● **V94.31 Injury to rider of (inflatable) recreational watercraft being pulled behind other watercraft** A, D, S 🔊

         Injury to rider of inner-tube pulled behind motor boat

     ● **V94.32 Injury to rider of non-recreational watercraft being pulled behind other watercraft** A, D, S 🔊

         Injury to occupant of dingy being pulled behind boat or ship

         Injury to occupant of life-raft being pulled behind boat or ship

● **V94.4 Injury to barefoot water-skier** A, D, S 🔊

     Injury to person being pulled behind boat or ship

● **V94.8 Other water transport accident**

     ● **V94.81 Water transport accident involving military watercraft**

         ● **V94.810 Civilian watercraft involved in water transport accident with military watercraft** A, D, S 🔊

            Passenger on civilian watercraft injured due to accident with military watercraft

         ● **V94.811 Civilian in water injured by military watercraft** A, D, S 🔊

         ● **V94.818 Other water transport accident involving military watercraft** A, D, S 🔊

     ● **V94.89 Other water transport accident** A, D, S 🔊

● ◾ **V94.9 Unspecified water transport accident** A, D, S 🔊

     Water transport accident NOS

AIR AND SPACE TRANSPORT ACCIDENTS (V95-V97)

> **Excludes1**   military aircraft accidents in military or war operations (Y36, Y37)

● **V95 Accident to powered aircraft causing injury to occupant**

     The appropriate 7th character is to be added to each code from category V95

A	initial encounter
D	subsequent encounter
S	sequela

● **V95.0 Helicopter accident injuring occupant**

     ● ◾ **V95.00 Unspecified helicopter accident injuring occupant** A, D, S 🔊

     ● **V95.01 Helicopter crash injuring occupant** A, D, S 🔊

     ● **V95.02 Forced landing of helicopter injuring occupant** A, D, S 🔊

     ● **V95.03 Helicopter collision injuring occupant** A, D, S 🔊

         Helicopter collision with any object, fixed, movable or moving

     ● **V95.04 Helicopter fire injuring occupant** A, D, S 🔊

     ● **V95.05 Helicopter explosion injuring occupant** A, D, S 🔊

     ● **V95.09 Other helicopter accident injuring occupant** A, D, S 🔊

● **V95.1 Ultralight, microlight or powered-glider accident injuring occupant**

     ● ◾ **V95.10 Unspecified ultralight, microlight or powered-glider accident injuring occupant** A, D, S 🔊

     ● **V95.11 Ultralight, microlight or powered-glider crash injuring occupant** A, D, S 🔊

     ● **V95.12 Forced landing of ultralight, microlight or powered-glider injuring occupant** A, D, S 🔊

     ● **V95.13 Ultralight, microlight or powered-glider collision injuring occupant** A, D, S 🔊

         Ultralight, microlight or powered-glider collision with any object, fixed, movable or moving

     ● **V95.14 Ultralight, microlight or powered-glider fire injuring occupant** A, D, S 🔊

     ● **V95.15 Ultralight, microlight or powered-glider explosion injuring occupant** A, D, S 🔊

     ● **V95.19 Other ultralight, microlight or powered-glider accident injuring occupant** A, D, S 🔊

● **V95.2 Other private fixed-wing aircraft accident injuring occupant**

     ● ◾ **V95.20 Unspecified accident to other private fixed-wing aircraft, injuring occupant** A, D, S 🔊

     ● **V95.21 Other private fixed-wing aircraft crash injuring occupant** A, D, S 🔊

     ● **V95.22 Forced landing of other private fixed-wing aircraft injuring occupant** A, D, S 🔊

     ● **V95.23 Other private fixed-wing aircraft collision injuring occupant** A, D, S 🔊

         Other private fixed-wing aircraft collision with any object, fixed, movable or moving

     ● **V95.24 Other private fixed-wing aircraft fire injuring occupant** A, D, S 🔊

     ● **V95.25 Other private fixed-wing aircraft explosion injuring occupant** A, D, S 🔊

     ● **V95.29 Other accident to other private fixed-wing aircraft injuring occupant** A, D, S 🔊

● **V95.3 Commercial fixed-wing aircraft accident injuring occupant**

     ● ◾ **V95.30 Unspecified accident to commercial fixed-wing aircraft injuring occupant** A, D, S 🔊

     ● **V95.31 Commercial fixed-wing aircraft crash injuring occupant** A, D, S 🔊

     ● **V95.32 Forced landing of commercial fixed-wing aircraft injuring occupant** A, D, S 🔊

     ● **V95.33 Commercial fixed-wing aircraft collision injuring occupant** A, D, S 🔊

         Commercial fixed-wing aircraft collision with any object, fixed, movable or moving

     ● **V95.34 Commercial fixed-wing aircraft fire injuring occupant** A, D, S 🔊

     ● **V95.35 Commercial fixed-wing aircraft explosion injuring occupant** A, D, S 🔊

     ● **V95.39 Other accident to commercial fixed-wing aircraft injuring occupant** A, D, S 🔊

● Unacceptable Principal Diagnosis   ● Use Additional Character(s)   ◾ Unspecified   ◾ Manifestation Code

OGCR Official Guidelines for Coding and Reporting   Excludes 1   Excludes 2   Includes   Use additional   Code first   Code also

● **V95.4   Spacecraft accident injuring occupant**

  ● ■ **V95.40   Unspecified spacecraft accident injuring occupant** A, D, S 🖉

  ● **V95.41   Spacecraft crash injuring occupant** A, D, S 🖉

  ● **V95.42   Forced landing of spacecraft injuring occupant** A, D, S 🖉

  ● **V95.43   Spacecraft collision injuring occupant** A, D, S 🖉

    Spacecraft collision with any object, fixed, moveable or moving

  ● **V95.44   Spacecraft fire injuring occupant** A, D, S 🖉

  ● **V95.45   Spacecraft explosion injuring occupant** A, D, S 🖉

  ● **V95.49   Other spacecraft accident injuring occupant** A, D, S 🖉

● **V95.8   Other powered aircraft accidents injuring occupant** A, D, S 🖉

● ■ **V95.9   Unspecified aircraft accident injuring occupant** A, D, S 🖉

    Aircraft accident NOS
    Air transport accident NOS

● **V96   Accident to nonpowered aircraft causing injury to occupant**

  The appropriate 7th character is to be added to each code from category V96

A	initial encounter
D	subsequent encounter
S	sequela

● **V96.0   Balloon accident injuring occupant**

  ● ■ **V96.00   Unspecified balloon accident injuring occupant** A, D, S 🖉

  ● **V96.01   Balloon crash injuring occupant** A, D, S 🖉

  ● **V96.02   Forced landing of balloon injuring occupant** A, D, S 🖉

  ● **V96.03   Balloon collision injuring occupant** A, D, S 🖉

    Balloon collision with any object, fixed, moveable or moving

  ● **V96.04   Balloon fire injuring occupant** A, D, S 🖉

  ● **V96.05   Balloon explosion injuring occupant** A, D, S 🖉

  ● **V96.09   Other balloon accident injuring occupant** A, D, S 🖉

● **V96.1   Hang-glider accident injuring occupant**

  ● ■ **V96.10   Unspecified hang-glider accident injuring occupant** A, D, S 🖉

  ● **V96.11   Hang-glider crash injuring occupant** A, D, S 🖉

  ● **V96.12   Forced landing of hang-glider injuring occupant** A, D, S 🖉

  ● **V96.13   Hang-glider collision injuring occupant** A, D, S 🖉

    Hang-glider collision with any object, fixed, moveable or moving

  ● **V96.14   Hang-glider fire injuring occupant** A, D, S 🖉

  ● **V96.15   Hang-glider explosion injuring occupant** A, D, S 🖉

  ● **V96.19   Other hang-glider accident injuring occupant** A, D, S 🖉

● **V96.2   Glider (nonpowered) accident injuring occupant**

  ● ■ **V96.20   Unspecified glider (nonpowered) accident injuring occupant** A, D, S 🖉

  ● **V96.21   Glider (nonpowered) crash injuring occupant** A, D, S 🖉

  ● **V96.22   Forced landing of glider (nonpowered) injuring occupant** A, D, S 🖉

  ● **V96.23   Glider (nonpowered) collision injuring occupant** A, D, S 🖉

    Glider (nonpowered) collision with any object, fixed, moveable or moving

  ● **V96.24   Glider (nonpowered) fire injuring occupant** A, D, S 🖉

  ● **V96.25   Glider (nonpowered) explosion injuring occupant** A, D, S 🖉

  ● **V96.29   Other glider (nonpowered) accident injuring occupant** A, D, S 🖉

● **V96.8   Other nonpowered-aircraft accidents injuring occupant** A, D, S 🖉

    Kite carrying a person accident injuring occupant

● ■ **V96.9   Unspecified nonpowered-aircraft accident injuring occupant** A, D, S 🖉

    Nonpowered-aircraft accident NOS

● **V97   Other specified air transport accidents**

  The appropriate 7th character is to be added to each code from category V97

A	initial encounter
D	subsequent encounter
S	sequela

● **V97.0   Occupant of aircraft injured in other specified air transport accidents** A, D, S 🖉

    Fall in, on or from aircraft in air transport accident

    Excludes1   accident while boarding or alighting aircraft (V97.1)

● **V97.1   Person injured while boarding or alighting from aircraft** A, D, S 🖉

● **V97.2   Parachutist accident**

  ● **V97.21   Parachutist entangled in object** A, D, S 🖉

    Parachutist landing in tree

  ● **V97.22   Parachutist injured on landing** A, D, S 🖉

  ● **V97.29   Other parachutist accident** A, D, S 🖉

● **V97.3   Person on ground injured in air transport accident**

  ● **V97.31   Hit by object falling from aircraft** A, D, S 🖉

    Hit by crashing aircraft
    Injured by aircraft hitting house
    Injured by aircraft hitting car

  ● **V97.32   Injured by rotating propeller** A, D, S 🖉

  ● **V97.33   Sucked into jet engine** A, D, S 🖉

  ● **V97.39   Other injury to person on ground due to air transport accident** A, D, S 🖉

● **V97.8   Other air transport accidents, not elsewhere classified**

    Excludes1   aircraft accident NOS (V95.9)
        exposure to changes in air pressure during ascent or descent (W94.-)

  ● **V97.81   Air transport accident involving military aircraft**

    ● **V97.810   Civilian aircraft involved in air transport accident with military aircraft** A, D, S 🖉

      Passenger in civilian aircraft injured due to accident with military aircraft

    ● **V97.811   Civilian injured by military aircraft** A, D, S 🖉

● **V97.818 Other air transport accident involving military aircraft**
A, D, S

● **V97.89 Other air transport accidents, not elsewhere classified** A, D, S
Injury from machinery on aircraft

OTHER AND UNSPECIFIED TRANSPORT ACCIDENTS (V98-V99)

Excludes1   vehicle accident, type of vehicle unspecified (V89.-)

● **V98 Other specified transport accidents**

The appropriate 7th character is to be added to each code from category V98

A	initial encounter
D	subsequent encounter
S	sequela

● **V98.0 Accident to, on or involving cable-car, not on rails**
A, D, S
Caught or dragged by cable-car, not on rails
Fall or jump from cable-car, not on rails
Object thrown from or in cable-car, not on rails

● **V98.1 Accident to, on or involving land-yacht** A, D, S

● **V98.2 Accident to, on or involving ice yacht** A, D, S

● **V98.3 Accident to, on or involving ski lift** A, D, S
Accident to, on or involving ski chair-lift
Accident to, on or involving ski-lift with gondola

● **V98.8 Other specified transport accidents** A, D, S

● ■ **V99 Unspecified transport accident** A, D, S

The appropriate 7th character is to be added to code V99

A	initial encounter
D	subsequent encounter
S	sequela

OTHER EXTERNAL CAUSES OF ACCIDENTAL INJURY (W00-X58)

SLIPPING, TRIPPING, STUMBLING AND FALLS (W00-W19)

Excludes1   assault involving a fall (Y01-Y02)
fall (in) (from):
    animal (V80.-)
    machinery (in operation) (W28-W31)
    transport vehicle (V01-V99)
intentional self-harm involving a fall (X80-X81)

Excludes2   at risk for fall (history of fall) Z91.81
fall (in) (from):
    burning building (X00.-)
    into fire (X00-X04, X08-X09)

● **W00 Fall due to ice and snow**

Includes   pedestrian on foot falling (slipping) on ice and snow

Excludes1   fall on (from) ice and snow involving pedestrian conveyance (V00.-)
fall from stairs and steps not due to ice and snow (W10.-)

The appropriate 7th character is to be added to each code from category W00

A	initial encounter
D	subsequent encounter
S	sequela

● **W00.0 Fall on same level due to ice and snow** S

● **W00.1 Fall from stairs and steps due to ice and snow** S

● **W00.2 Other fall from one level to another due to ice and snow** S

● ■ **W00.9 Unspecified fall due to ice and snow** S

● **W01 Fall on same level from slipping, tripping and stumbling**

Includes   fall on moving sidewalk

Excludes1   fall due to bumping (striking) against object (W18.0-)
fall in shower or bathtub (W18.2-)
fall on same level NOS (W18.30)
fall on same level from slipping, tripping and stumbling due to ice or snow (W00.0)
fall off or from toilet (W18.1-)
slipping, tripping and stumbling NOS (W18.40)
slipping, tripping and stumbling without falling (W18.4-)

The appropriate 7th character is to be added to each code from category W01

A	initial encounter
D	subsequent encounter
S	sequela

● **W01.0 Fall on same level from slipping, tripping and stumbling without subsequent striking against object** S
Falling over animal

● **W01.1 Fall on same level from slipping, tripping and stumbling with subsequent striking against object**

● ■ **W01.10 Fall on same level from slipping, tripping and stumbling with subsequent striking against unspecified object** S

● **W01.11 Fall on same level from slipping, tripping and stumbling with subsequent striking against sharp object**

● **W01.110 Fall on same level from slipping, tripping and stumbling with subsequent striking against sharp glass** S

● **W01.111 Fall on same level from slipping, tripping and stumbling with subsequent striking against power tool or machine** S

● **W01.118 Fall on same level from slipping, tripping and stumbling with subsequent striking against other sharp object** S

● ■ **W01.119 Fall on same level from slipping, tripping and stumbling with subsequent striking against unspecified sharp object** S

● **W01.19 Fall on same level from slipping, tripping and stumbling with subsequent striking against other object**

● **W01.190 Fall on same level from slipping, tripping and stumbling with subsequent striking against furniture** S

● **W01.198 Fall on same level from slipping, tripping and stumbling with subsequent striking against other object** S

● Unacceptable Principal Diagnosis   ● Use Additional Character(s)   ■ Unspecified   ▶ Manifestation Code

OGCR   Official Guidelines for Coding and Reporting | Excludes 1 | | Excludes 2 | | Includes | | Use additional | | Code first | | Code also |

● **W03 Other fall on same level due to collision with another person** A, D, S 🔳

     Fall due to non-transport collision with other person

     | **Excludes1** | collision with another person without fall (W51)
                     crushed or pushed by a crowd or human stampede (W52)
                     fall involving pedestrian conveyance (V00-V09)
                     fall due to ice or snow (W00)
                     fall on same level NOS (W18.30)

     The appropriate 7th character is to be added to code W03

     | A | initial encounter |
     | D | subsequent encounter |
     | S | sequela |

● **W04 Fall while being carried or supported by other persons** S 🔳

     Accidentally dropped while being carried

     The appropriate 7th character is to be added to code W04

     | A | initial encounter |
     | D | subsequent encounter |
     | S | sequel |

● **W05 Fall from non-moving wheelchair, nonmotorized scooter and motorized mobility scooter**

     | **Excludes1** | fall from moving wheelchair (powered) (V00.811)
                     fall from moving motorized mobility scooter (V08.831)
                     fall from nonmotorized scooter (V08.841)

     The appropriate 7th character is to be added to each code from category W05

     | A | initial encounter |
     | D | subsequent encounter |
     | S | sequela |

   ● **W05.0 Fall from non-moving wheelchair** S 🔳
   ● **W05.1 Fall from non-moving nonmotorized scooter** S 🔳
   ● **W05.2 Fall from non-moving motorized mobility scooter** S 🔳

● **W06 Fall from bed** S 🔳

     The appropriate 7th character is to be added to code W06

     | A | initial encounter |
     | D | subsequent encounter |
     | S | sequela |

● **W07 Fall from chair** S 🔳

     The appropriate 7th character is to be added to code W07

     | A | initial encounter |
     | D | subsequent encounter |
     | S | sequela |

● **W08 Fall from other furniture** S 🔳

     The appropriate 7th character is to be added to code W08

     | A | initial encounter |
     | D | subsequent encounter |
     | S | sequela |

● **W09 Fall on and from playground equipment**

     | **Excludes1** | fall involving recreational machinery (W31)

     The appropriate 7th character is to be added to each code from category W09

     | A | initial encounter |
     | D | subsequent encounter |
     | S | sequela |

   ● **W09.0 Fall on or from playground slide** A, D, S 🔳
   ● **W09.1 Fall from playground swing** A, D, S 🔳
   ● **W09.2 Fall on or from jungle gym** A, D, S 🔳
   ● **W09.8 Fall on or from other playground equipment** A, D, S 🔳

● **W10 Fall on and from stairs and steps**

     | **Excludes1** | fall from stairs and steps due to ice and snow (W00.1)

     The appropriate 7th character is to be added to each code from category W10

     | A | initial encounter |
     | D | subsequent encounter |
     | S | sequela |

   ● **W10.0 Fall (on) (from) escalator** S 🔳
   ● **W10.1 Fall (on) (from) sidewalk curb** S 🔳
   ● **W10.2 Fall (on) (from) incline** S 🔳
       Fall (on) (from) ramp
   ● **W10.8 Fall (on) (from) other stairs and steps** S 🔳
   ●■ **W10.9 Fall (on) (from) unspecified stairs and steps** S 🔳

● **W11 Fall on and from ladder** S 🔳

     The appropriate 7th character is to be added to code W11

     | A | initial encounter |
     | D | subsequent encounter |
     | S | sequela |

● **W12 Fall on and from scaffolding** S 🔳

     The appropriate 7th character is to be added to code W12

     | A | initial encounter |
     | D | subsequent encounter |
     | S | sequela |

● **W13 Fall from, out of or through building or structure**

     The appropriate 7th character is to be added to each code from category W13

     | A | initial encounter |
     | D | subsequent encounter |
     | S | sequela |

   ● **W13.0 Fall from, out of or through balcony** S 🔳
       Fall from, out of or through railing
   ● **W13.1 Fall from, out of or through bridge** S 🔳
   ● **W13.2 Fall from, out of or through roof** S 🔳
   ● **W13.3 Fall through floor** S 🔳
   ● **W13.4 Fall from, out of or through window** S 🔳

     | **Excludes2** | fall with subsequent striking against sharp glass (W01.110)

   ● **W13.8 Fall from, out of or through other building or structure** S 🔳
       Fall from, out of or through viaduct
       Fall from, out of or through wall
       Fall from, out of or through flag-pole

CHAPTER 20 (V01-Y99)

CHAPTER 20 (V01-Y99)

● **W13.9 Fall from, out of or through building, not otherwise specified** S 🔊

> **Excludes1**   collapse of a building or structure (W20.-)
> fall or jump from burning building or structure (X00.-)

● **W14 Fall from tree** S 🔊

The appropriate 7th character is to be added to code W14

> A   initial encounter
> D   subsequent encounter
> S   sequela

● **W15 Fall from cliff** A, D, S 🔊

The appropriate 7th character is to be added to code W15

> A   initial encounter
> D   subsequent encounter
> S   sequela

● **W16 Fall, jump or diving into water**

> **Excludes1**   accidental non-watercraft drowning and submersion not involving fall (W65-W74)
> effects of air pressure from diving (W94.-)
> fall into water from watercraft (V90-V94)
> hitting an object or against bottom when falling from watercraft (V94.0)

> **Excludes2**   striking or hitting diving board (W21.3)

The appropriate 7th character is to be added to each code from category W16

> A   initial encounter
> D   subsequent encounter
> S   sequela

● **W16.0 Fall into swimming pool**
    Fall into swimming pool NOS

> **Excludes1**   fall into empty swimming pool (W17.3)

   ● **W16.01 Fall into swimming pool striking water surface**

     ● **W16.011 Fall into swimming pool striking water surface causing drowning and submersion** S 🔊

> **Excludes1**   drowning and submersion while in swimming pool without fall (W67)

     ● **W16.012 Fall into swimming pool striking water surface causing other injury** S 🔊

   ● **W16.02 Fall into swimming pool striking bottom**

     ● **W16.021 Fall into swimming pool striking bottom causing drowning and submersion** S 🔊

> **Excludes1**   drowning and submersion while in swimming pool without fall (W67)

     ● **W16.022 Fall into swimming pool striking bottom causing other injury** S 🔊

● **W16.03 Fall into swimming pool striking wall**

   ● **W16.031 Fall into swimming pool striking wall causing drowning and submersion** S 🔊

> **Excludes1**   drowning and submersion while in swimming pool without fall (W67)

   ● **W16.032 Fall into swimming pool striking wall causing other injury** S 🔊

● **W16.1 Fall into natural body of water**
    Fall into lake
    Fall into open sea
    Fall into river
    Fall into stream

   ● **W16.11 Fall into natural body of water striking water surface**

     ● **W16.111 Fall into natural body of water striking water surface causing drowning and submersion** S 🔊

> **Excludes1**   drowning and submersion while in natural body of water without fall (W69)

     ● **W16.112 Fall into natural body of water striking water surface causing other injury** S 🔊

   ● **W16.12 Fall into natural body of water striking bottom**

     ● **W16.121 Fall into natural body of water striking bottom causing drowning and submersion** S 🔊

> **Excludes1**   drowning and submersion while in natural body of water without fall (W69)

     ● **W16.122 Fall into natural body of water striking bottom causing other injury** S 🔊

   ● **W16.13 Fall into natural body of water striking side**

     ● **W16.131 Fall into natural body of water striking side causing drowning and submersion** S 🔊

> **Excludes1**   drowning and submersion while in natural body of water without fall (W69)

     ● **W16.132 Fall into natural body of water striking side causing other injury** S 🔊

● Unacceptable Principal Diagnosis   ● Use Additional Character(s)   ■ Unspecified   ▶ Manifestation Code

OGCR   Official Guidelines for Coding and Reporting   Excludes 1   Excludes 2   Includes   Use additional   Code first   Code also

● **W16.2 Fall in (into) filled bathtub or bucket of water**

   ● **W16.21 Fall in (into) filled bathtub**

       | Excludes1 | fall into empty bathtub (W18.2)

      ● **W16.211 Fall in (into) filled bathtub causing drowning and submersion** S 🗫

          | Excludes1 | drowning and submersion while in filled bathtub without fall (W65)

      ● **W16.212 Fall in (into) filled bathtub causing other injury** S 🗫

   ● **W16.22 Fall in (into) bucket of water**

      ● **W16.221 Fall in (into) bucket of water causing drowning and submersion** S 🗫

      ● **W16.222 Fall in (into) bucket of water causing other injury** S 🗫

● **W16.3 Fall into other water**
       Fall into fountain
       Fall into reservoir

   ● **W16.31 Fall into other water striking water surface**

      ● **W16.311 Fall into other water striking water surface causing drowning and submersion** S 🗫

          | Excludes1 | drowning and submersion while in other water without fall (W73)

      ● **W16.312 Fall into other water striking water surface causing other injury** S 🗫

   ● **W16.32 Fall into other water striking bottom**

      ● **W16.321 Fall into other water striking bottom causing drowning and submersion** S 🗫

          | Excludes1 | drowning and submersion while in other water without fall (W73)

      ● **W16.322 Fall into other water striking bottom causing other injury** S 🗫

   ● **W16.33 Fall into other water striking wall**

      ● **W16.331 Fall into other water striking wall causing drowning and submersion** S 🗫

          | Excludes1 | drowning and submersion while in other water without fall (W73)

      ● **W16.332 Fall into other water striking wall causing other injury** S 🗫

● **W16.4 Fall into unspecified water**

   ●■ **W16.41 Fall into unspecified water causing drowning and submersion** S 🗫

   ●■ **W16.42 Fall into unspecified water causing other injury** S 🗫

● **W16.5 Jumping or diving into swimming pool**

   ● **W16.51 Jumping or diving into swimming pool striking water surface**

      ● **W16.511 Jumping or diving into swimming pool striking water surface causing drowning and submersion** S 🗫

          | Excludes1 | drowning and submersion while in swimming pool without jumping or diving (W67)

      ● **W16.512 Jumping or diving into swimming pool striking water surface causing other injury** S 🗫

   ● **W16.52 Jumping or diving into swimming pool striking bottom**

      ● **W16.521 Jumping or diving into swimming pool striking bottom causing drowning and submersion** S 🗫

          | Excludes1 | drowning and submersion while in swimming pool without jumping or diving (W67)

      ● **W16.522 Jumping or diving into swimming pool striking bottom causing other injury** S 🗫

   ● **W16.53 Jumping or diving into swimming pool striking wall**

      ● **W16.531 Jumping or diving into swimming pool striking wall causing drowning and submersion** S 🗫

          | Excludes1 | drowning and submersion while in swimming pool without jumping or diving (W67)

      ● **W16.532 Jumping or diving into swimming pool striking wall causing other injury** S 🗫

CHAPTER 20 (V01-Y99)

● **W16.6 Jumping or diving into natural body of water**
    Jumping or diving into lake
    Jumping or diving into open sea
    Jumping or diving into river
    Jumping or diving into stream

  ● **W16.61 Jumping or diving into natural body of water striking water surface**

    ● **W16.611 Jumping or diving into natural body of water striking water surface causing drowning and submersion** S ✎

       Excludes1   drowning and submersion while in natural body of water without jumping or diving (W69)

    ● **W16.612 Jumping or diving into natural body of water striking water surface causing other injury** S ✎

  ● **W16.62 Jumping or diving into natural body of water striking bottom**

    ● **W16.621 Jumping or diving into natural body of water striking bottom causing drowning and submersion** S ✎

       Excludes1   drowning and submersion while in natural body of water without jumping or diving (W69)

    ● **W16.622 Jumping or diving into natural body of water striking bottom causing other injury** S ✎

● **W16.7 Jumping or diving from boat**

     Excludes1   fall from boat into water - see watercraft accident (V90-V94)

  ● **W16.71 Jumping or diving from boat striking water surface**

    ● **W16.711 Jumping or diving from boat striking water surface causing drowning and submersion** S ✎

    ● **W16.712 Jumping or diving from boat striking water surface causing other injury** S ✎

  ● **W16.72 Jumping or diving from boat striking bottom**

    ● **W16.721 Jumping or diving from boat striking bottom causing drowning and submersion** S ✎

    ● **W16.722 Jumping or diving from boat striking bottom causing other injury** S ✎

● **W16.8 Jumping or diving into other water**
    Jumping or diving into fountain
    Jumping or diving into reservoir

  ● **W16.81 Jumping or diving into other water striking water surface**

    ● **W16.811 Jumping or diving into other water striking water surface causing drowning and submersion** S ✎

       Excludes1   drowning and submersion while in other water without jumping or diving (W73)

    ● **W16.812 Jumping or diving into other water striking water surface causing other injury** S ✎

  ● **W16.82 Jumping or diving into other water striking bottom**

    ● **W16.821 Jumping or diving into other water striking bottom causing drowning and submersion** S ✎

       Excludes1   drowning and submersion while in other water without jumping or diving (W73)

    ● **W16.822 Jumping or diving into other water striking bottom causing other injury** S ✎

  ● **W16.83 Jumping or diving into other water striking wall**

    ● **W16.831 Jumping or diving into other water striking wall causing drowning and submersion** S ✎

       Excludes1   drowning and submersion while in other water without jumping or diving (W73)

    ● **W16.832 Jumping or diving into other water striking wall causing other injury** S ✎

● **W16.9 Jumping or diving into unspecified water**

  ●■ **W16.91 Jumping or diving into unspecified water causing drowning and submersion** S ✎

  ●■ **W16.92 Jumping or diving into unspecified water causing other injury** S ✎

● **W17 Other fall from one level to another**

    The appropriate 7th character is to be added to each code from category W17

A	initial encounter
D	subsequent encounter
S	sequela

● **W17.0 Fall into well** A, D, S ✎

● **W17.1 Fall into storm drain or manhole** A, D, S ✎

● **W17.2 Fall into hole** S ✎
    Fall into pit

● **W17.3 Fall into empty swimming pool** S ✎

     Excludes1   fall into filled swimming pool (W16.0-)

● **W17.4 Fall from dock** S ✎

●   Unacceptable Principal Diagnosis   ●   Use Additional Character(s)   ■   Unspecified   ▶   Manifestation Code

OGCR   Official Guidelines for Coding and Reporting   Excludes 1   Excludes 2   Includes   Use additional   Code first   Code also

- **W17.8 Other fall from one level to another**
  - **W17.81 Fall down embankment (hill)** S
  - **W17.82 Fall from (out of) grocery cart** S
    - Fall due to grocery cart tipping over
  - **W17.89 Other fall from one level to another** S
    - Fall from cherry picker
    - Fall from lifting device
    - Fall from mobile elevated work platform [MEWP]
    - Fall from sky lift

- **W18 Other slipping, tripping and stumbling and falls**

  The appropriate 7th character is to be added to each code from category W18

A	initial encounter
D	subsequent encounter
S	sequela

  - **W18.0 Fall due to bumping against object**
    - Striking against object with subsequent fall
    - **Excludes1**   fall on same level due to slipping, tripping, or stumbling with subsequent striking against object (W01.1-)
    - **W18.00 Striking against unspecified object with subsequent fall** S
    - **W18.01 Striking against sports equipment with subsequent fall** S
    - **W18.02 Striking against glass with subsequent fall** S
    - **W18.09 Striking against other object with subsequent fall** S
  - **W18.1 Fall from or off toilet**
    - **W18.11 Fall from or off toilet without subsequent striking against object** S
      - Fall from (off) toilet NOS
    - **W18.12 Fall from or off toilet with subsequent striking against object** S
  - **W18.2 Fall in (into) shower or empty bathtub** S
    - **Excludes1**   fall in full bathtub causing drowning or submersion (W16.21-)
  - **W18.3 Other and unspecified fall on same level**
    - **W18.30 Fall on same level, unspecified** S
    - **W18.31 Fall on same level due to stepping on an object** S
      - Fall on same level due to stepping on an animal
      - **Excludes1**   slipping, tripping and stumbling without fall due to stepping on animal (W18.41)
    - **W18.39 Other fall on same level** S
  - **W18.4 Slipping, tripping and stumbling without falling**
    - **Excludes1**   collision with another person without fall (W51)
    - **W18.40 Slipping, tripping and stumbling without falling, unspecified** S
    - **W18.41 Slipping, tripping and stumbling without falling due to stepping on object** S
      - Slipping, tripping and stumbling without falling due to stepping on animal
      - **Excludes1**   slipping, tripping and stumbling with fall due to stepping on animal (W18.31)

  - **W18.42 Slipping, tripping and stumbling without falling due to stepping into hole or opening** S
  - **W18.43 Slipping, tripping and stumbling without falling due to stepping from one level to another** S
  - **W18.49 Other slipping, tripping and stumbling without falling** S

- **W19 Unspecified fall** S
  - Accidental fall NOS

  The appropriate 7th character is to be added to code W19

A	initial encounter
D	subsequent encounter
S	sequela

EXPOSURE TO INANIMATE MECHANICAL FORCES (W20-W49)

Excludes1   assault (X91-Y08)
contact or collision with animals or persons (W50-W64)
exposure to inanimate mechanical forces involving military or war operations (Y36.-, Y37.-)
intentional self-harm (X70-X83)

- **W20 Struck by thrown, projected or falling object**

  Code first any associated:
  cataclysm (X34-X39)
  lightning strike (T75.00)

  Excludes1   falling object in:
  machinery accident (W24, W28-W31)
  transport accident (V01-V99)
  object set in motion by:
  explosion (W35-W40)
  firearm (W32-W34)
  struck by thrown sports equipment (W21.-)

  The appropriate 7th character is to be added to each code from category W20

A	initial encounter
D	subsequent encounter
S	sequela

  - **W20.0 Struck by falling object in cave-in** S
    - **Excludes2**   asphyxiation due to cave-in (T71.21)
  - **W20.1 Struck by object due to collapse of building** S
    - **Excludes1**   struck by object due to collapse of burning building (X00.2, X02.2)
  - **W20.8 Other cause of strike by thrown, projected or falling object** S
    - **Excludes1**   struck by thrown sports equipment (W21.-)

- **W21 Striking against or struck by sports equipment**
  - **Excludes1**   assault with sports equipment (Y08.0-)
    striking against or struck by sports equipment with subsequent fall (W18.01)

  The appropriate 7th character is to be added to each code from category W21

A	initial encounter
D	subsequent encounter
S	sequela

  - **W21.0 Struck by hit or thrown ball**
    - **W21.00 Struck by hit or thrown ball, unspecified type** A, D, S

N   Newborn Age: 0   P   Pediatric Age: 0–17   M   Maternity DX: 12–55   A   Adult Age: 15–124   ♀ Females Only   ♂ Males Only

Complication\Comorbidity   Major C\C   Present on Admission Requirement   Hospital-Acquired Condition

CHAPTER 20 (V01-Y99)

- W21.01 **Struck by football** A, D, S 🔖
- W21.02 **Struck by soccer ball** A, D, S 🔖
- W21.03 **Struck by baseball** A, D, S 🔖
- W21.04 **Struck by golf ball** A, D, S 🔖
- W21.05 **Struck by basketball** A, D, S 🔖
- W21.06 **Struck by volleyball** A, D, S 🔖
- W21.07 **Struck by softball** A, D, S 🔖
- W21.09 **Struck by other hit or thrown ball** A, D, S 🔖
- W21.1 **Struck by bat, racquet or club**
  - W21.11 **Struck by baseball bat** A, D, S 🔖
  - W21.12 **Struck by tennis racquet** A, D, S 🔖
  - W21.13 **Struck by golf club** A, D, S 🔖
  - W21.19 **Struck by other bat, racquet or club** A, D, S 🔖
- W21.2 **Struck by hockey stick or puck**
  - W21.21 **Struck by hockey stick**
    - W21.210 **Struck by ice hockey stick** A, D, S 🔖
    - W21.211 **Struck by field hockey stick** A, D, S 🔖
  - W21.22 **Struck by hockey puck**
    - W21.220 **Struck by ice hockey puck** A, D, S 🔖
    - W21.221 **Struck by field hockey puck** A, D, S 🔖
- W21.3 **Struck by sports foot wear**
  - W21.31 **Struck by shoe cleats** A, D, S 🔖
    Stepped on by shoe cleats
  - W21.32 **Struck by skate blades** A, D, S 🔖
    Skated over by skate blades
  - W21.39 **Struck by other sports foot wear** A, D, S 🔖
- W21.4 **Striking against diving board** A, D, S 🔖
  Use additional code for subsequent falling into water, if applicable (W16.-)
- W21.8 **Striking against or struck by other sports equipment**
  - W21.81 **Striking against or struck by football helmet** A, D, S 🔖
  - W21.89 **Striking against or struck by other sports equipment** A, D, S 🔖
- W21.9 **Striking against or struck by unspecified sports equipment** A, D, S 🔖
- W22 **Striking against or struck by other objects**

  | Excludes1 | striking against or struck by object with subsequent fall (W18.09) |

  The appropriate 7th character is to be added to each code from category W22

A	initial encounter
D	subsequent encounter
S	sequela

  - W22.0 **Striking against stationary object**

    | Excludes1 | striking against stationary sports equipment (W21.8) |

    - W22.01 **Walked into wall** S 🔖
    - W22.02 **Walked into lamppost** S 🔖

- W22.03 **Walked into furniture** S 🔖
- W22.04 **Striking against wall of swimming pool**
  - W22.041 **Striking against wall of swimming pool causing drowning and submersion** S 🔖

    | Excludes1 | drowning and submersion while swimming without striking against wall (W67) |

  - W22.042 **Striking against wall of swimming pool causing other injury** S 🔖
- W22.09 **Striking against other stationary object** S 🔖
- W22.1 **Striking against or struck by automobile airbag**
  - W22.10 **Striking against or struck by unspecified automobile airbag** S 🔖
  - W22.11 **Striking against or struck by driver side automobile airbag** S 🔖
  - W22.12 **Striking against or struck by front passenger side automobile airbag** S 🔖
  - W22.19 **Striking against or struck by other automobile airbag** S 🔖
- W22.8 **Striking against or struck by other objects** S 🔖
  Striking against or struck by object NOS

  | Excludes1 | struck by thrown, projected or falling object (W20.-) |

- W23 **Caught, crushed, jammed or pinched in or between objects**

Excludes1	injury caused by cutting or piercing instruments (W25-W27)
	injury caused by firearms malfunction (W32.1, W33.1-, W34.1-)
	injury caused by lifting and transmission devices (W24.-)
	injury caused by machinery (W28-W31)
	injury caused by nonpowered hand tools (W27.-)
	injury caused by transport vehicle being used as a means of transportation (V01-V99)
	injury caused by struck by thrown, projected or falling object (W20.-)

  The appropriate 7th character is to be added to each code from category W23

A	initial encounter
D	subsequent encounter
S	sequela

  - W23.0 **Caught, crushed, jammed, or pinched between moving objects** S 🔖
  - W23.1 **Caught, crushed, jammed, or pinched between stationary objects** S 🔖

● Unacceptable Principal Diagnosis   ● Use Additional Character(s)   ■ Unspecified   ▶ Manifestation Code

OGCR Official Guidelines for Coding and Reporting | Excludes 1 | | Excludes 2 | | Includes | | Use additional | | Code first | | Code also |

● **W24 Contact with lifting and transmission devices, not elsewhere classified**

> **Excludes1**   transport accidents (V01-V99)

> The appropriate 7th character is to be added to each code from category W24
>
> | | |
> |---|---|
> | A | initial encounter |
> | D | subsequent encounter |
> | S | sequela |

● **W24.0 Contact with lifting devices, not elsewhere classified** S 🖐
> Contact with chain hoist
> Contact with drive belt
> Contact with pulley (block)

● **W24.1 Contact with transmission devices, not elsewhere classified** A, D, S 🖐
> Contact with transmission belt or cable

● **W25 Contact with sharp glass** S 🖐

> *Code first* any associated:
> injury due to flying glass from explosion or firearm discharge (W32-W40)
> transport accident (V00-V99)

> **Excludes1**   fall on same level due to slipping, tripping and stumbling with subsequent striking against sharp glass (W01.10)
> striking against sharp glass with subsequent fall (W18.02)

> The appropriate 7th character is to be added to code W25
>
> | | |
> |---|---|
> | A | initial encounter |
> | D | subsequent encounter |
> | S | sequela |

● **W26 Contact with knife, sword or dagger**

> The appropriate 7th character is to be added to each code from category W26
>
> | | |
> |---|---|
> | A | initial encounter |
> | D | subsequent encounter |
> | S | sequela |

● **W26.0 Contact with knife** S 🖐
> **Excludes1**   contact with electric knife (W29.1)

● **W26.1 Contact with sword or dagger** S 🖐

● **W27 Contact with nonpowered hand tool**

> The appropriate 7th character is to be added to each code from category W27
>
> | | |
> |---|---|
> | A | initial encounter |
> | D | subsequent encounter |
> | S | sequela |

● **W27.0 Contact with workbench tool** S 🖐
> Contact with auger
> Contact with axe
> Contact with chisel
> Contact with handsaw
> Contact with screwdriver

● **W27.1 Contact with garden tool** S 🖐
> Contact with hoe
> Contact with nonpowered lawn mower
> Contact with pitchfork
> Contact with rake

● **W27.2 Contact with scissors** S 🖐

● **W27.3 Contact with needle (sewing)** S 🖐
> **Excludes1**   contact with hypodermic needle (W46.-)

● **W27.4 Contact with kitchen utensil** S 🖐
> Contact with fork
> Contact with ice-pick
> Contact with can-opener NOS

● **W27.5 Contact with paper-cutter** S 🖐

● **W27.8 Contact with other nonpowered hand tool** S 🖐
> Contact with nonpowered sewing machine
> Contact with shovel

● **W28 Contact with powered lawn mower** S 🖐
> Powered lawn mower (commercial) (residential)

> **Excludes1**   contact with nonpowered lawn mower (W27.1)

> **Excludes2**   exposure to electric current (W86.-)

> The appropriate 7th character is to be added to code W28
>
> | | |
> |---|---|
> | A | initial encounter |
> | D | subsequent encounter |
> | S | sequela |

● **W29 Contact with other powered hand tools and household machinery**

> **Excludes1**   contact with commercial machinery (W31.82)
> contact with hot household appliance (X15)
> contact with nonpowered hand tool (W27.-)
> exposure to electric current (W86)

> The appropriate 7th character is to be added to each code from category W29
>
> | | |
> |---|---|
> | A | initial encounter |
> | D | subsequent encounter |
> | S | sequela |

● **W29.0 Contact with powered kitchen appliance** S 🖐
> Contact with blender
> Contact with can-opener
> Contact with garbage disposal
> Contact with mixer

● **W29.1 Contact with electric knife** S 🖐

● **W29.2 Contact with other powered household machinery** S 🖐
> Contact with electric fan
> Contact with powered dryer (clothes) (powered) (spin)
> Contact with washing-machine
> Contact with sewing machine

● **W29.3 Contact with powered garden and outdoor hand tools and machinery** S 🖐
> Contact with chainsaw
> Contact with edger
> Contact with garden cultivator (tiller)
> Contact with hedge trimmer
> Contact with other powered garden tool
> **Excludes1**   contact with powered lawn mower (W28)

● **W29.4 Contact with nail gun** S 🖐

● **W29.8 Contact with other powered powered hand tools and household machinery** S 🖐
> Contact with do-it-yourself tool NOS

CHAPTER 20 (V01-Y99)

● **W30   Contact with agricultural machinery**

> **Includes**   animal-powered farm machine

> **Excludes1**   agricultural transport vehicle accident (V01-V99)
> explosion of grain store (W40.8)
> exposure to electric current (W86.-)

The appropriate 7th character is to be added to each code from category W30

> A   initial encounter
> D   subsequent encounter
> S   sequela

● **W30.0   Contact with combine harvester** A, D, S
> Contact with reaper
> Contact with thresher

● **W30.1   Contact with power take-off devices (PTO)** A, D, S

● **W30.2   Contact with hay derrick** A, D, S

● **W30.3   Contact with grain storage elevator** A, D, S
> **Excludes1**   explosion of grain store (W40.8)

● **W30.8   Contact with other specified agricultural machinery**

  ● **W30.81   Contact with agricultural transport vehicle in stationary use** A, D, S
> Contact with agricultural transport vehicle under repair, not on public roadway
> **Excludes1**   agricultural transport vehicle accident (V01-V99)

  ● **W30.89   Contact with other specified agricultural machinery** A, D, S

● ■ **W30.9   Contact with unspecified agricultural machinery** A, D, S
> Contact with farm machinery NOS

● **W31   Contact with other and unspecified machinery**

> **Excludes1**   contact with agricultural machinery (W30.-)
> contact with machinery in transport under own power or being towed by a vehicle (V01-V99)
> exposure to electric current (W86)

The appropriate 7th character is to be added to each code from category W31

> A   initial encounter
> D   subsequent encounter
> S   sequela

● **W31.0   Contact with mining and earth-drilling machinery** A, D, S
> Contact with bore or drill (land) (seabed)
> Contact with shaft hoist
> Contact with shaft lift
> Contact with undercutter

● **W31.1   Contact with metalworking machines** A, D, S
> Contact with abrasive wheel
> Contact with forging machine
> Contact with lathe
> Contact with mechanical shears
> Contact with metal drilling machine
> Contact with milling machine
> Contact with power press
> Contact with rolling-mill
> Contact with metal sawing machine

● **W31.2   Contact with powered woodworking and forming machines** A, D, S
> Contact with band saw
> Contact with bench saw
> Contact with circular saw
> Contact with molding machine
> Contact with overhead plane
> Contact with powered saw
> Contact with radial saw
> Contact with sander
> **Excludes1**   nonpowered woodworking tools (W27.0)

● **W31.3   Contact with prime movers** A, D, S
> Contact with gas turbine
> Contact with internal combustion engine
> Contact with steam engine
> Contact with water driven turbine

● **W31.8   Contact with other specified machinery**

  ● **W31.81   Contact with recreational machinery** A, D, S
> Contact with roller-coaster

  ● **W31.82   Contact with other commercial machinery** A, D, S
> Contact with commercial electric fan
> Contact with commercial kitchen appliances
> Contact with commercial powered dryer (clothes) (powered) (spin)
> Contact with commercial washing-machine
> Contact with commercial sewing machine
> **Excludes1**   contact with household machinery (W29.-)
> contact with powered lawn mower (W28)

  ● **W31.83   Contact with special construction vehicle in stationary use** A, D, S
> Contact with special construction vehicle under repair, not on public roadway
> **Excludes1**   special construction vehicle accident (V01-V99)

  ● **W31.89   Contact with other specified machinery** A, D, S

● ■ **W31.9   Contact with unspecified machinery** A, D, S
> Contact with machinery NOS

● Unacceptable Principal Diagnosis   ● Use Additional Character(s)   ■ Unspecified   ▶ Manifestation Code

OGCR Official Guidelines for Coding and Reporting   Excludes 1   Excludes 2   Includes   Use additional   Code first   Code also

●W32 **Accidental handgun discharge and malfunction**

Includes   accidental discharge and malfunction of gun for single hand use
accidental discharge and malfunction of pistol
accidental discharge and malfunction of revolver
handgun discharge and malfunction NOS

Excludes1   accidental airgun discharge and malfunction (W34.010, W34.110)
accidental BB gun discharge and malfunction (W34.010, W34.110)
accidental pellet gun discharge and malfunction (W34.010, W34.110)
accidental shotgun discharge and malfunction (W33.01, W33.11)
assault by handgun discharge (X93)
handgun discharge involving legal intervention (Y35.0-)
handgun discharge involving military or war operations (Y36.4-)
intentional self-harm by handgun discharge (X72)
Very pistol discharge and malfunction (W34.09, W34.19)

The appropriate 7th character is to be added to each code from category W32

A   initial encounter
D   subsequent encounter
S   sequela

W32.0 **Accidental handgun discharge** A, D, S

W32.1 **Accidental handgun malfunction** A, D, S
Injury due to explosion of handgun (parts)
Injury due to malfunction of mechanism or component of handgun
Injury due to recoil of handgun
Powder burn from handgun

●W33 **Accidental rifle, shotgun and larger firearm discharge and malfunction**

Includes   rifle, shotgun and larger firearm discharge and malfunction NOS

Excludes1   accidental airgun discharge and malfunction (W34.010, W34.110)
accidental BB gun discharge and malfunction (W34.010, W34.110)
accidental handgun discharge and malfunction (W32-)
accidental pellet gun discharge and malfunction (W34.010, W34.110)
assault by rifle, shotgun and larger firearm discharge (X94)
firearm discharge involving legal intervention (Y35.0-)
firearm discharge involving military or war operations (Y36.4-)
intentional self-harm by rifle, shotgun and larger firearm discharge (X73)

The appropriate 7th character is to be added to each code from category W33

A   initial encounter
D   subsequent encounter
S   sequela

●W33.0 **Accidental rifle, shotgun and larger firearm discharge**

●■W33.00 **Accidental discharge of unspecified larger firearm** A, D, S
Discharge of unspecified larger firearm NOS

●W33.01 **Accidental discharge of shotgun**
A, D, S
Discharge of shotgun NOS

●W33.02 **Accidental discharge of hunting rifle**
A, D, S
Discharge of hunting rifle NOS

●W33.03 **Accidental discharge of machine gun**
A, D, S
Discharge of machine gun NOS

●W33.09 **Accidental discharge of other larger firearm** A, D, S
Discharge of other larger firearm NOS

●W33.1 **Accidental rifle, shotgun and larger firearm malfunction**
Injury due to explosion of rifle, shotgun and larger firearm (parts)
Injury due to malfunction of mechanism or component of rifle, shotgun and larger firearm
Injury due to piercing, cutting, crushing or pinching due to (by) slide trigger mechanism, scope or other gun part
Injury due to recoil of rifle, shotgun and larger firearm
Powder burn from rifle, shotgun and larger firearm

●■W33.10 **Accidental malfunction of unspecified larger firearm** A, D, S
Malfunction of unspecified larger firearm NOS

●W33.11 **Accidental malfunction of shotgun**
A, D, S
Malfunction of shotgun NOS

●W33.12 **Accidental malfunction of hunting rifle**
A, D, S
Malfunction of hunting rifle NOS

●W33.13 **Accidental malfunction of machine gun**
A, D, S
Malfunction of machine gun NOS

●W33.19 **Accidental malfunction of other larger firearm** A, D, S
Malfunction of other larger firearm NOS

●W34 **Accidental discharge and malfunction from other and unspecified firearms and guns**

The appropriate 7th character is to be added to each code from category W34

A   initial encounter
D   subsequent encounter
S   sequela

●W34.0 **Accidental discharge from other and unspecified firearms and guns**

●■W34.00 **Accidental discharge from unspecified firearms or gun** A, D, S
Discharge from firearm NOS
Gunshot wound NOS
Shot NOS

●W34.01 **Accidental discharge of gas, air or spring-operated guns**

●W34.010 **Accidental discharge of airgun**
A, D, S
Accidental discharge of BB gun
Accidental discharge of pellet gun

●W34.011 **Accidental discharge of paintball gun** A, D, S
Accidental injury due to paintball discharge

CHAPTER 20 (V01-Y99)

● **W34.018** Accidental discharge of other gas, air or spring-operated gun A, D, S 🔖

● **W34.09** Accidental discharge from other specified firearms A, D, S 🔖
　Accidental discharge from Very pistol [flare]

● **W34.1** Accidental malfunction from other and unspecified firearms and guns

● ■ **W34.10** Accidental malfunction from unspecified firearms or gun A, D, S 🔖
　Firearm malfunction NOS

● **W34.11** Accidental malfunction of gas, air or spring-operated guns

● **W34.110** Accidental malfunction of airgun A, D, S 🔖
　Accidental malfunction of BB gun
　Accidental malfunction of pellet gun

● **W34.111** Accidental malfunction of paintball gun A, D, S 🔖
　Accidental injury due to paintball gun malfunction

● **W34.118** Accidental malfunction of other gas, air or spring-operated gun A, D, S 🔖

● **W34.19** Accidental malfunction from other specified firearms A, D, S 🔖
　Accidental malfunction from Very pistol [flare]

● **W35** Explosion and rupture of boiler A, D, S 🔖

| Excludes1 | explosion and rupture of boiler on watercraft (V93.4) |

The appropriate 7th character is to be added to code W35

A	initial encounter
D	subsequent encounter
S	sequela

● **W36** Explosion and rupture of gas cylinder

The appropriate 7th character is to be added to each code from category W36

A	initial encounter
D	subsequent encounter
S	sequela

● **W36.1** Explosion and rupture of aerosol can A, D, S 🔖

● **W36.2** Explosion and rupture of air tank A, D, S 🔖

● **W36.3** Explosion and rupture of pressurized-gas tank A, D, S 🔖

● **W36.8** Explosion and rupture of other gas cylinder A, D, S 🔖

● ■ **W36.9** Explosion and rupture of unspecified gas cylinder A, D, S 🔖

● **W37** Explosion and rupture of pressurized tire, pipe or hose

The appropriate 7th character is to be added to each code from category W37

A	initial encounter
D	subsequent encounter
S	sequela

● **W37.0** Explosion of bicycle tire A, D, S 🔖

● **W37.8** Explosion and rupture of other pressurized tire, pipe or hose A, D, S 🔖

● **W38** Explosion and rupture of other specified pressurized devices A, D, S 🔖

The appropriate 7th character is to be added to code W38

A	initial encounter
D	subsequent encounter
S	sequela

● **W39** Discharge of firework S 🔖

The appropriate 7th character is to be added to code W39

A	initial encounter
D	subsequent encounter
S	sequela

● **W40** Explosion of other materials

Excludes1	assault by explosive material (X96)
	explosion involving legal intervention (Y35.1-)
	explosion involving military or war operations (Y36.0-, Y36.2-)
	intentional self-harm by explosive material (X75)

The appropriate 7th character is to be added to each code from category W40

A	initial encounter
D	subsequent encounter
S	sequela

● **W40.0** Explosion of blasting material S 🔖
　Explosion of blasting cap
　Explosion of detonator
　Explosion of dynamite
　Explosion of explosive (any) used in blasting operations

● **W40.1** Explosion of explosive gases S 🔖
　Explosion of acetylene
　Explosion of butane
　Explosion of coal gas
　Explosion in mine NOS
　Explosion of explosive gas
　Explosion of fire damp
　Explosion of gasoline fumes
　Explosion of methane
　Explosion of propane

● **W40.8** Explosion of other specified explosive materials S 🔖
　Explosion in dump NOS
　Explosion in factory NOS
　Explosion in grain store
　Explosion in munitions

| Excludes1 | explosion involving legal intervention (Y35.1-) |
| | explosion involving military or war operations (Y36.0-, Y36.2-) |

● ■ **W40.9** Explosion of unspecified explosive materials S 🔖
　Explosion NOS

● **W42** Exposure to noise

The appropriate 7th character is to be added to each code from category W42

A	initial encounter
D	subsequent encounter
S	sequela

● **W42.0** Exposure to supersonic waves A, D, S 🔖

● **W42.9** Exposure to other noise A, D, S 🔖
　Exposure to sound waves NOS

● Unacceptable Principal Diagnosis　　● Use Additional Character(s)　　■ Unspecified　　▶ Manifestation Code

OGCR Official Guidelines for Coding and Reporting　　Excludes 1　　Excludes 2　　Includes　　Use additional　　Code first　　Code also

● **W45 Foreign body or object entering through skin**

> **Excludes2**   contact with hand tools (nonpowered)
> (powered) (W27-W29)
> contact with knife, sword or dagger (W26.-)
> contact with sharp glass (W25.-)
> struck by objects (W20-W22)

The appropriate 7th character is to be added to each code from category W45

> A   initial encounter
> D   subsequent encounter
> S   sequela

● **W45.0 Nail entering through skin** S 🔖

● **W45.1 Paper entering through skin** S 🔖
> Paper cut

● **W45.2 Lid of can entering through skin** S 🔖

● **W45.8 Other foreign body or object entering through skin** S 🔖
> Splinter in skin NOS

● **W46 Contact with hypodermic needle**

The appropriate 7th character is to be added to each code from category W46

> A   initial encounter
> D   subsequent encounter
> S   sequela

● **W46.0 Contact with hypodermic needle** S 🔖
> Hypodermic needle stick NOS

● **W46.1 Contact with contaminated hypodermic needle** S 🔖

● **W49 Exposure to other inanimate mechanical forces**

> **Includes**   exposure to abnormal gravitational [G]
> forces exposure to inanimate mechanical
> forces NEC

> **Excludes1**   exposure to inanimate mechanical forces
> involving military or war operations
> (Y36.-, Y37.-)

The appropriate 7th character is to be added to each code from category W49

> A   initial encounter
> D   subsequent encounter
> S   sequela

● **W49.0 Item causing external constriction**

> ● **W49.01 Hair causing external constriction** A, D, S 🔖

> ● **W49.02 String or thread causing external constriction** A, D, S 🔖

> ● **W49.03 Rubber band causing external constriction** A, D, S 🔖

> ● **W49.04 Ring or other jewelry causing external constriction** A, D, S 🔖

> ● **W49.09 Other item causing external constriction** A, D, S 🔖

● **W49.9 Exposure to other inanimate mechanical forces** A, D, S 🔖

EXPOSURE TO ANIMATE MECHANICAL FORCES (W50-W64)

> **Excludes1**   toxic effect of contact with venomous
> animals and plants (T63.-)

● **W50 Accidental hit, strike, kick, twist, bite or scratch by another person**

> **Includes**   hit, strike, kick, twist, bite, or scratch by
> another person NOS

> **Excludes1**   assault by bodily force (Y04)
> struck by objects (W20-W22)

The appropriate 7th character is to be added to each code from category W50

> A   initial encounter
> D   subsequent encounter
> S   sequela

● **W50.0 Accidental hit or strike by another person** S 🔖
> Hit or strike by another person NOS

● **W50.1 Accidental kick by another person** S 🔖
> Kick by another person NOS

● **W50.2 Accidental twist by another person** S 🔖
> Twist by another person NOS

● **W50.3 Accidental bite by another person** A, D, S 🔖
> Human bite
> Bite by another person NOS

● **W50.4 Accidental scratch by another person** S 🔖
> Scratch by another person NOS

● **W51 Accidental striking against or bumped into by another person** S 🔖

> **Excludes1**   assault by striking against or bumping into
> by another person (Y04.2)
> fall due to collision with another person (W03)

The appropriate 7th character is to be added to code W51

> A   initial encounter
> D   subsequent encounter
> S   sequela

● **W52 Crushed, pushed or stepped on by crowd or human stampede** A, D, S 🔖
> Crushed, pushed or stepped on by crowd or human
> stampede with or without fall

The appropriate 7th character is to be added to code W52

> A   initial encounter
> D   subsequent encounter
> S   sequela

● **W53 Contact with rodent**

> **Includes**   contact with saliva, feces or urine of rodent

The appropriate 7th character is to be added to each code from category W53

> A   initial encounter
> D   subsequent encounter
> S   sequela

● **W53.0 Contact with mouse**

> ● **W53.01 Bitten by mouse** S 🔖

> ● **W53.09 Other contact with mouse** S 🔖

● **W53.1 Contact with rat**

> ● **W53.11 Bitten by rat** S 🔖

> ● **W53.19 Other contact with rat** S 🔖

CHAPTER 20 (V01-Y99)

- ● W53.2   Contact with squirrel
    - ● W53.21   Bitten by squirrel S 🔊
    - ● W53.29   Other contact with squirrel S 🔊
- ● W53.8   Contact with other rodent
    - ● W53.81   Bitten by other rodent S 🔊
    - ● W53.89   Other contact with other rodent S 🔊

- ● W54   Contact with dog

    | Includes | contact with saliva, feces or urine of dog |

    The appropriate 7th character is to be added to each code from category W54

    | A | initial encounter |
    | D | subsequent encounter |
    | S | sequela |

    - ● W54.0   Bitten by dog S 🔊
    - ● W54.1   Struck by dog S 🔊
        Knocked over by dog
    - ● W54.8   Other contact with dog S 🔊

- ● W55   Contact with other mammals

    | Includes | contact with saliva, feces or urine of mammal |

    | Excludes1 | animal being ridden - see transport accidents |
    | | bitten or struck by dog (W54) |
    | | bitten or struck by rodent (W53.-) |
    | | contact with marine mammals (W56.x-) |

    The appropriate 7th character is to be added to each code from category W55

    | A | initial encounter |
    | D | subsequent encounter |
    | S | sequela |

    - ● W55.0   Contact with cat
        - ● W55.01   Bitten by cat S 🔊
        - ● W55.03   Scratched by cat S 🔊
        - ● W55.09   Other contact with cat S 🔊
    - ● W55.1   Contact with horse
        - ● W55.11   Bitten by horse S 🔊
        - ● W55.12   Struck by horse S 🔊
        - ● W55.19   Other contact with horse S 🔊
    - ● W55.2   Contact with cow
        Contact with bull
        - ● W55.21   Bitten by cow S 🔊
        - ● W55.22   Struck by cow S 🔊
            Gored by bull
        - ● W55.29   Other contact with cow S 🔊
    - ● W55.3   Contact with other hoof stock
        Contact with goats
        Contact with sheep
        - ● W55.31   Bitten by other hoof stock S 🔊
        - ● W55.32   Struck by other hoof stock S 🔊
            Gored by goat
            Gored by ram
        - ● W55.39   Other contact with other hoof stock S 🔊
    - ● W55.4   Contact with pig
        - ● W55.41   Bitten by pig S 🔊
        - ● W55.42   Struck by pig S 🔊
        - ● W55.49   Other contact with pig S 🔊

- ● W55.5   Contact with raccoon
    - ● W55.51   Bitten by raccoon S 🔊
    - ● W55.52   Struck by raccoon S 🔊
    - ● W55.59   Other contact with raccoon S 🔊
- ● W55.8   Contact with other mammals
    - ● W55.81   Bitten by other mammals S 🔊
    - ● W55.82   Struck by other mammals S 🔊
    - ● W55.89   Other contact with other mammals S 🔊

- ● W56   Contact with nonvenomous marine animal

    | Excludes1 | contact with venomous marine animal (T63.-) |

    The appropriate 7th character is to be added to each code from category W56

    | A | initial encounter |
    | D | subsequent encounter |
    | S | sequela |

    - ● W56.0   Contact with dolphin
        - ● W56.01   Bitten by dolphin S 🔊
        - ● W56.02   Struck by dolphin S 🔊
        - ● W56.09   Other contact with dolphin S 🔊
    - ● W56.1   Contact with sea lion
        - ● W56.11   Bitten by sea lion S 🔊
        - ● W56.12   Struck by sea lion S 🔊
        - ● W56.19   Other contact with sea lion S 🔊
    - ● W56.2   Contact with orca
        Contact with killer whale
        - ● W56.21   Bitten by orca S 🔊
        - ● W56.22   Struck by orca S 🔊
        - ● W56.29   Other contact with orca S 🔊
    - ● W56.3   Contact with other marine mammals
        - ● W56.31   Bitten by other marine mammals S 🔊
        - ● W56.32   Struck by other marine mammals S 🔊
        - ● W56.39   Other contact with other marine mammals S 🔊
    - ● W56.4   Contact with shark
        - ● W56.41   Bitten by shark S 🔊
        - ● W56.42   Struck by shark S 🔊
        - ● W56.49   Other contact with shark S 🔊
    - ● W56.5   Contact with other fish
        - ● W56.51   Bitten by other fish S 🔊
        - ● W56.52   Struck by other fish S 🔊
        - ● W56.59   Other contact with other fish S 🔊
    - ● W56.8   Contact with other nonvenomous marine animals
        - ● W56.81   Bitten by other nonvenomous marine animals S 🔊
        - ● W56.82   Struck by other nonvenomous marine animals S 🔊
        - ● W56.89   Other contact with other nonvenomous marine animals S 🔊

- ● W57   Bitten or stung by nonvenomous insect and other nonvenomous arthropods S 🔊

    | Excludes1 | contact with venomous insects and arthropods (T63.2-, T63.3-, T63.4-) |

    The appropriate 7th character is to be added to code W57

    | A | initial encounter |
    | D | subsequent encounter |
    | S | sequela |

● Unacceptable Principal Diagnosis   ● Use Additional Character(s)   ■ Unspecified   ▶ Manifestation Code

OGCR   Official Guidelines for Coding and Reporting   Excludes 1   Excludes 2   Includes   Use additional   Code first   Code also

● **W58 Contact with crocodile or alligator**

    The appropriate 7th character is to be added to each code from category W58

A	initial encounter
D	subsequent encounter
S	sequela

    ● **W58.0 Contact with alligator**
        ● **W58.01 Bitten by alligator** S 🦠
        ● **W58.02 Struck by alligator** S 🦠
        ● **W58.03 Crushed by alligator** S 🦠
        ● **W58.09 Other contact with alligator** S 🦠
    ● **W58.1 Contact with crocodile**
        ● **W58.11 Bitten by crocodile** S 🦠
        ● **W58.12 Struck by crocodile** S 🦠
        ● **W58.13 Crushed by crocodile** S 🦠
        ● **W58.19 Other contact with crocodile** S 🦠

● **W59 Contact with other nonvenomous reptiles**

Excludes1	contact with venomous reptile (T63.0-, T63.1-)

    The appropriate 7th character is to be added to each code from category W59

A	initial encounter
D	subsequent encounter
S	sequela

    ● **W59.0 Contact with nonvenomous lizards**
        ● **W59.01 Bitten by nonvenomous lizards** S 🦠
        ● **W59.02 Struck by nonvenomous lizards** S 🦠
        ● **W59.09 Other contact with nonvenomous lizards** S 🦠
                Exposure to nonvenomous lizards
    ● **W59.1 Contact with nonvenomous snakes**
        ● **W59.11 Bitten by nonvenomous snake** S 🦠
        ● **W59.12 Struck by nonvenomous snake** S 🦠
        ● **W59.13 Crushed by nonvenomous snake** S 🦠
        ● **W59.19 Other contact with nonvenomous snake** S 🦠
    ● **W59.2 Contact with turtles**
Excludes1	contact with tortoises (W59.8-)
        ● **W59.21 Bitten by turtle** S 🦠
        ● **W59.22 Struck by turtle** S 🦠
        ● **W59.29 Other contact with turtle** S 🦠
                Exposure to turtles
    ● **W59.8 Contact with other nonvenomous reptiles**
        ● **W59.81 Bitten by other nonvenomous reptiles** S 🦠
        ● **W59.82 Struck by other nonvenomous reptiles** S 🦠
        ● **W59.83 Crushed by other nonvenomous reptiles** S 🦠
        ● **W59.89 Other contact with other nonvenomous reptiles** S 🦠

● **W60 Contact with nonvenomous plant thorns and spines and sharp leaves** S 🦠

Excludes1	contact with venomous plants (T63.x-)

    The appropriate 7th character is to be added to code W60

A	initial encounter
D	subsequent encounter
S	sequela

● **W61 Contact with birds (domestic) (wild)**

Includes	contact with excreta of birds

    The appropriate 7th character is to be added to each code from category W61

A	initial encounter
D	subsequent encounter
S	sequela

    ● **W61.0 Contact with parrot**
        ● **W61.01 Bitten by parrot** S 🦠
        ● **W61.02 Struck by parrot** S 🦠
        ● **W61.09 Other contact with parrot** S 🦠
                Exposure to parrots
    ● **W61.1 Contact with macaw**
        ● **W61.11 Bitten by macaw** S 🦠
        ● **W61.12 Struck by macaw** S 🦠
        ● **W61.19 Other contact with macaw** S 🦠
                Exposure to macaws
    ● **W61.2 Contact with other psittacines**
        ● **W61.21 Bitten by other psittacines** S 🦠
        ● **W61.22 Struck by other psittacines** S 🦠
        ● **W61.29 Other contact with other psittacines** S 🦠
                Exposure to other psittacines
    ● **W61.3 Contact with chicken**
        ● **W61.32 Struck by chicken** S 🦠
        ● **W61.33 Pecked by chicken** S 🦠
        ● **W61.39 Other contact with chicken** S 🦠
                Exposure to chickens
    ● **W61.4 Contact with turkey**
        ● **W61.42 Struck by turkey** S 🦠
        ● **W61.43 Pecked by turkey** S 🦠
        ● **W61.49 Other contact with turkey** S 🦠
    ● **W61.5 Contact with goose**
        ● **W61.51 Bitten by goose** S 🦠
        ● **W61.52 Struck by goose** S 🦠
        ● **W61.59 Other contact with goose** S 🦠
    ● **W61.6 Contact with duck**
        ● **W61.61 Bitten by duck** S 🦠
        ● **W61.62 Struck by duck** S 🦠
        ● **W61.69 Other contact with duck** S 🦠
    ● **W61.9 Contact with other birds**
        ● **W61.91 Bitten by other birds** S 🦠
        ● **W61.92 Struck by other birds** S 🦠
        ● **W61.99 Other contact with other birds** S 🦠
                Contact with bird NOS

● **W62 Contact with nonvenomous amphibians**

Excludes1	contact with venomous amphibians (T63.81-R63.83)

    The appropriate 7th character is to be added to each code from category W62

A	initial encounter
D	subsequent encounter
S	sequela

    ● **W62.0 Contact with nonvenomous frogs** S 🦠
    ● **W62.1 Contact with nonvenomous toads** S 🦠
    ● **W62.9 Contact with other nonvenomous amphibians** S 🦠

CHAPTER 20 (V01-Y99)

N Newborn Age: 0   **P** Pediatric Age: 0–17   **M** Maternity DX: 12–55   **A** Adult Age: 15–124   ♀ Females Only   ♂ Males Only

🦠 Complication\Comorbidity   🦠 Major C\C   🦠 Present on Admission Requirement   🦠 Hospital-Acquired Condition

1753

● **W64 Exposure to other animate mechanical forces** S 🔖

    | **Includes** | exposure to nonvenomous animal NOS |

    | **Excludes1** | contact with venomous animal (T63.-) |

    The appropriate 7th character is to be added to code W64

        A   initial encounter
        D   subsequent encounter
        S   sequela

ACCIDENTAL NON-TRANSPORT DROWNING AND SUBMERSION (W65-W74)

    | **Excludes1** | accidental drowning and submersion due to fall into water (W16.-) |
    | | accidental drowning and submersion due to water transport accident (V90.-, V92.-) |

    | **Excludes2** | accidental drowning and submersion due to cataclysm (X34-X39) |

● **W65 Accidental drowning and submersion while in bathtub** S 🔖

    | **Excludes1** | accidental drowning and submersion due to fall in (into) bathtub (W16.211) |

    The appropriate 7th character is to be added to code W65

        A   initial encounter
        D   subsequent encounter
        S   sequela

● **W67 Accidental drowning and submersion while in swimming pool** S 🔖

    | **Excludes1** | accidental drowning and submersion due to fall into swimming pool (W16.011, W16.021, W16.031) |
    | | accidental drowning and submersion due to striking into wall of swimming pool (W22.041) |

    The appropriate 7th character is to be added to code W67

        A   initial encounter
        D   subsequent encounter
        S   sequela

● **W69 Accidental drowning and submersion while in natural water** S 🔖

    Accidental drowning and submersion while in lake
    Accidental drowning and submersion while in open sea
    Accidental drowning and submersion while in river
    Accidental drowning and submersion while in stream

    | **Excludes1** | accidental drowning and submersion due to fall into natural body of water (W16.111, W16.121, W16.131) |

    The appropriate 7th character is to be added to code W69

        A   initial encounter
        D   subsequent encounter
        S   sequela

● **W73 Other specified cause of accidental non-transport drowning and submersion** S 🔖

    Accidental drowning and submersion while in quenching tank
    Accidental drowning and submersion while in reservoir

    | **Excludes1** | accidental drowning and submersion due to fall into other water (W16.311, W16.321, W16.331) |

    The appropriate 7th character is to be added to code W73

        A   initial encounter
        D   subsequent encounter
        S   sequela

●■ **W74 Unspecified cause of accidental drowning and submersion** S 🔖

    Drowning NOS

    The appropriate 7th character is to be added to code W74

        A   initial encounter
        D   subsequent encounter
        S   sequela

EXPOSURE TO ELECTRIC CURRENT, RADIATION AND EXTREME AMBIENT AIR TEMPERATURE AND PRESSURE (W85-W99)

    | **Excludes1** | exposure to: |
    | | failure in dosage of radiation or temperature during surgical and medical care (Y63.2-Y63.5) |
    | | lightning (T75.0-) |
    | | natural cold (X31) |
    | | natural heat (X30) |
    | | natural radiation NOS (X39) |
    | | radiological procedure and radiotherapy (Y84.2) |
    | | sunlight (X32) |

● **W85 Exposure to electric transmission lines** S 🔖

    Broken power line

    The appropriate 7th character is to be added to code W85

        A   initial encounter
        D   subsequent encounter
        S   sequela

● **W86 Exposure to other specified electric current**

    The appropriate 7th character is to be added to each code from category W86

        A   initial encounter
        D   subsequent encounter
        S   sequela

● **W86.0 Exposure to domestic wiring and appliances** S 🔖

● **W86.1 Exposure to industrial wiring, appliances and electrical machinery** S 🔖

    Exposure to conductors
    Exposure to control apparatus
    Exposure to electrical equipment and machinery
    Exposure to transformers

● Unacceptable Principal Diagnosis   ● Use Additional Character(s)   ■ Unspecified   ▶ Manifestation Code

OGCR Official Guidelines for Coding and Reporting   Excludes 1   Excludes 2   Includes   Use additional   Code first   Code also

- **W86.8 Exposure to other electric current** S 🔍
  - Exposure to wiring and appliances in or on farm (not farmhouse)
  - Exposure to wiring and appliances outdoors
  - Exposure to wiring and appliances in or on public building
  - Exposure to wiring and appliances in or on residential institutions
  - Exposure to wiring and appliances in or on schools

- **W88 Exposure to ionizing radiation**

  | **Excludes1** | exposure to sunlight (X32) |

  The appropriate 7th character is to be added to each code from category W88

A	initial encounter
D	subsequent encounter
S	sequela

  - **W88.0 Exposure to X-rays** S 🔍
  - **W88.1 Exposure to radioactive isotopes** S 🔍
  - **W88.8 Exposure to other ionizing radiation** S 🔍

- **W89 Exposure to man-made visible and ultraviolet light**

  | **Includes** | exposure to welding light (arc) |
  | **Excludes2** | exposure to sunlight (X32) |

  The appropriate 7th character is to be added to each code from category W89

A	initial encounter
D	subsequent encounter
S	sequela

  - **W89.0 Exposure to welding light (arc)** A, D, S 🔍
  - **W89.1 Exposure to tanning bed** A, D, S 🔍
  - **W89.8 Exposure to other man-made visible and ultraviolet light** A, D, S 🔍
  - **W89.9 Exposure to unspecified man-made visible and ultraviolet light** A, D, S 🔍

- **W90 Exposure to other nonionizing radiation**

  | **Excludes1** | exposure to sunlight (X32) |

  The appropriate 7th character is to be added to each code from category W90

A	initial encounter
D	subsequent encounter
S	sequela

  - **W90.0 Exposure to radiofrequency** S 🔍
  - **W90.1 Exposure to infrared radiation** S 🔍
  - **W90.2 Exposure to laser radiation** S 🔍
  - **W90.8 Exposure to other nonionizing radiation** S 🔍

- **W92 Exposure to excessive heat of man-made origin** S 🔍

  The appropriate 7th character is to be added to code W92

A	initial encounter
D	subsequent encounter
S	sequela

- **W93 Exposure to excessive cold of man-made origin**

  The appropriate 7th character is to be added to each code from category W93

A	initial encounter
D	subsequent encounter
S	sequela

  - **W93.0 Contact with or inhalation of dry ice**
    - **W93.01 Contact with dry ice** S 🔍
    - **W93.02 Inhalation of dry ice** S 🔍
  - **W93.1 Contact with or inhalation of liquid air**
    - **W93.11 Contact with liquid air** S 🔍
      - Contact with liquid hydrogen
      - Contact with liquid nitrogen
    - **W93.12 Inhalation of liquid air** S 🔍
      - Inhalation of liquid hydrogen
      - Inhalation of liquid nitrogen
  - **W93.2 Prolonged exposure in deep freeze unit or refrigerator** S 🔍
  - **W93.8 Exposure to other excessive cold of man-made origin** S 🔍

- **W94 Exposure to high and low air pressure and changes in air pressure**

  The appropriate 7th character is to be added to each code from category W94

A	initial encounter
D	subsequent encounter
S	sequela

  - **W94.0 Exposure to prolonged high air pressure** S 🔍
  - **W94.1 Exposure to prolonged low air pressure**
    - **W94.11 Exposure to residence or prolonged visit at high altitude** S 🔍
    - **W94.12 Exposure to other prolonged low air pressure** S 🔍
  - **W94.2 Exposure to rapid changes in air pressure during ascent**
    - **W94.21 Exposure to reduction in atmospheric pressure while surfacing from deep-water diving** S 🔍
    - **W94.22 Exposure to reduction in atmospheric pressure while surfacing from underground** S 🔍
    - **W94.23 Exposure to sudden change in air pressure in aircraft during ascent** S 🔍
    - **W94.29 Exposure to other rapid changes in air pressure during ascent** S 🔍
  - **W94.3 Exposure to rapid changes in air pressure during descent**
    - **W94.31 Exposure to sudden change in air pressure in aircraft during ascent or descent** S 🔍
    - **W94.32 Exposure to high air pressure from rapid descent in water** S 🔍
    - **W94.39 Exposure to other rapid changes in air pressure during descent** S 🔍

- **W99 Exposure to other man-made environmental factors** S 🔍

  The appropriate 7th character is to be added to code W99

A	initial encounter
D	subsequent encounter
S	sequela

N Newborn Age: 0   **P** Pediatric Age: 0–17   **M** Maternity DX: 12–55   **A** Adult Age: 15–124   ♀ Females Only   ♂ Males Only

🔍 Complication\Comorbidity   🔍 Major C\C   🔍 Present on Admission Requirement   🔍 Hospital-Acquired Condition

1755

CHAPTER 20 (V01–Y99)

EXPOSURE TO SMOKE, FIRE AND FLAMES (X00-X08)

Excludes1   arson (X97)

Excludes2   explosions (W35-W40)
     lightning (T75.0-)
     transport accident (V01-V99)

● **X00 Exposure to uncontrolled fire in building or structure**

     Includes   conflagration in building or structure

     Code first any associated cataclysm

     Excludes2   exposure to ignition or melting of nightwear (X05)
       exposure to ignition or melting of other clothing and apparel (X06-)
       exposure to other specified smoke, fire and flames (X08.-)

     The appropriate 7th character is to be added to each code from category X00

     A   initial encounter
     D   subsequent encounter
     S   sequela

● **X00.0 Exposure to flames in uncontrolled fire in building or structure** A, D, S 🔍

● **X00.1 Exposure to smoke in uncontrolled fire in building or structure** A, D, S 🔍

● **X00.2 Injury due to collapse of burning building or structure in uncontrolled fire** A, D, S 🔍

     Excludes1   injury due to collapse of building not on fire (W20.1)

● **X00.3 Fall from burning building or structure in uncontrolled fire** A, D, S 🔍

● **X00.4 Hit by object from burning building or structure in uncontrolled fire** A, D, S 🔍

● **X00.5 Jump from burning building or structure in uncontrolled fire** A, D, S 🔍

● **X00.8 Other exposure to uncontrolled fire in building or structure** A, D, S 🔍

● **X01 Exposure to uncontrolled fire, not in building or structure**

     Includes   exposure to forest fire

     The appropriate 7th character is to be added to each code from category X01

     A   initial encounter
     D   subsequent encounter
     S   sequela

● **X01.0 Exposure to flames in uncontrolled fire, not in building or structure** S 🔍

● **X01.1 Exposure to smoke in uncontrolled fire, not in building or structure** S 🔍

● **X01.3 Fall due to uncontrolled fire, not in building or structure** S 🔍

● **X01.4 Hit by object due to uncontrolled fire, not in building or structure** S 🔍

● **X01.8 Other exposure to uncontrolled fire, not in building or structure** S 🔍

● **X02 Exposure to controlled fire in building or structure**

     Includes   exposure to fire in fireplace exposure to fire in stove

     The appropriate 7th character is to be added to each code from category X02

     A   initial encounter
     D   subsequent encounter
     S   sequela

● **X02.0 Exposure to flames in controlled fire in building or structure** A, D, S 🔍

● **X02.1 Exposure to smoke in controlled fire in building or structure** A, D, S 🔍

● **X02.2 Injury due to collapse of burning building or structure in controlled fire** A, D, S 🔍

     Excludes1   injury due to collapse of building not on fire (W20.1)

● **X02.3 Fall from burning building or structure in controlled fire** A, D, S 🔍

● **X02.4 Hit by object from burning building or structure in controlled fire** A, D, S 🔍

● **X02.5 Jump from burning building or structure in controlled fire** A, D, S 🔍

● **X02.8 Other exposure to controlled fire in building or structure** D, S 🔍

● **X03 Exposure to controlled fire, not in building or structure**

     Includes   exposure to bon fire exposure to camp fire exposure to trash fire

     The appropriate 7th character is to be added to each code from category X03

     A   initial encounter
     D   subsequent encounter
     S   sequela

● **X03.0 Exposure to flames in controlled fire, not in building or structure** A, D, S 🔍

● **X03.1 Exposure to smoke in controlled fire, not in building or structure** A, D, S 🔍

● **X03.3 Fall due to controlled fire, not in building or structure** A, D, S 🔍

● **X03.4 Hit by object due to controlled fire, not in building or structure** A, D, S 🔍

● **X03.8 Other exposure to controlled fire, not in building or structure** A, D, S 🔍

● **X04 Exposure to ignition of highly flammable material** A, D, S 🔍

     Exposure to ignition of gasoline
     Exposure to ignition of kerosene
     Exposure to ignition of petrol

     Excludes2   exposure to ignition or melting of nightwear (X05)
       exposure to ignition or melting of other clothing and apparel (X06)

     The appropriate 7th character is to be added to code X04

     A   initial encounter
     D   subsequent encounter
     S   sequela

● Unacceptable Principal Diagnosis   ● Use Additional Character(s)   ■ Unspecified   ▶ Manifestation Code

OGCR Official Guidelines for Coding and Reporting | Excludes 1 | Excludes 2 | Includes | Use additional | Code first | Code also |

● **X05   Exposure to ignition or melting of nightwear** A, D, S 🔳

     Excludes2   exposure to uncontrolled fire in building or structure (X00.-)
             exposure to uncontrolled fire, not in building or structure (X01.-)
             exposure to controlled fire in building or structure (X02.-)
             exposure to controlled fire, not in building or structure (X03.-)
             exposure to ignition of highly flammable materials (X04.-)

     The appropriate 7th character is to be added to code X05

A	initial encounter
D	subsequent encounter
S	sequela

● **X06   Exposure to ignition or melting of other clothing and apparel**

     Excludes2   exposure to uncontrolled fire in building or structure (X00.-)
             exposure to uncontrolled fire, not in building or structure (X01.-)
             exposure to controlled fire in building or structure (X02.-)
             exposure to controlled fire, not in building or structure (X03.-)
             exposure to ignition of highly flammable materials (X04.-)

     The appropriate 7th character is to be added to each code from category X06

A	initial encounter
D	subsequent encounter
S	sequela

  ● **X06.0   Exposure to ignition of plastic jewelry** S 🔳

  ● **X06.1   Exposure to melting of plastic jewelry** S 🔳

  ● **X06.2   Exposure to ignition of other clothing and apparel** S 🔳

  ● **X06.3   Exposure to melting of other clothing and apparel** S 🔳

● **X08   Exposure to other specified smoke, fire and flames**

     The appropriate 7th character is to be added to each code from category X08

A	initial encounter
D	subsequent encounter
S	sequela

  ● **X08.0   Exposure to bed fire**
       Exposure to mattress fire

  ●🔳 **X08.00   Exposure to bed fire due to unspecified burning material** S 🔳

  ● **X08.01   Exposure to bed fire due to burning cigarette** S 🔳

  ● **X08.09   Exposure to bed fire due to other burning material** S 🔳

  ● **X08.1   Exposure to sofa fire**

  ●🔳 **X08.10   Exposure to sofa fire due to unspecified burning material** S 🔳

  ● **X08.11   Exposure to sofa fire due to burning cigarette** S 🔳

  ● **X08.19   Exposure to sofa fire due to other burning material** S 🔳

  ● **X08.2   Exposure to other furniture fire**

  ●🔳 **X08.20   Exposure to other furniture fire due to unspecified burning material** S 🔳

  ● **X08.21   Exposure to other furniture fire due to burning cigarette** S 🔳

  ● **X08.29   Exposure to other furniture fire due to other burning material** S 🔳

  ● **X08.8   Exposure to other specified smoke, fire and flames** S 🔳

CONTACT WITH HEAT AND HOT SUBSTANCES (X10-X19)

     Excludes1   exposure to excessive natural heat (X30)
             exposure to fire and flames (X00-X09)

● **X10   Contact with hot drinks, food, fats and cooking oils**

     The appropriate 7th character is to be added to each code from category X10

A	initial encounter
D	subsequent encounter
S	sequela

  ● **X10.0   Contact with hot drinks** S 🔳

  ● **X10.1   Contact with hot food** S 🔳

  ● **X10.2   Contact with fats and cooking oils** S 🔳

● **X11   Contact with hot tap-water**

     Includes   contact with boiling tap-water
             contact with boiling water NOS

     Excludes1   contact with water heated on stove (X12)

     The appropriate 7th character is to be added to each code from category X11

A	initial encounter
D	subsequent encounter
S	sequela

  ● **X11.0   Contact with hot water in bath or tub** S 🔳

     Excludes1   contact with running hot water in bath or tub (X11.1)

  ● **X11.1   Contact with running hot water** S 🔳
       Contact with hot water running out of hose
       Contact with hot water running out of tap

  ● **X11.8   Contact with other hot tap-water** S 🔳
       Contact with hot water in bucket
       Contact with hot tap-water NOS

● **X12   Contact with other hot fluids** S 🔳
     Contact with water heated on stove

     Excludes1   hot (liquid) metals (X18)

     The appropriate 7th character is to be added to code X12

A	initial encounter
D	subsequent encounter
S	sequela

● **X13   Contact with steam and other hot vapors**

     The appropriate 7th character is to be added to each code from category X13

A	initial encounter
D	subsequent encounter
S	sequela

  ● **X13.0   Inhalation of steam and other hot vapors** S 🔳

  ● **X13.1   Other contact with steam and other hot vapors** S 🔳

N Newborn Age: 0   **P** Pediatric Age: 0–17   **M** Maternity DX: 12–55   **A** Adult Age: 15–124   ♀ Females Only   ♂ Males Only

🔳 Complication\Comorbidity   🔳 Major C\C   🔳 Present on Admission Requirement   🔳 Hospital-Acquired Condition

1757

● **X14　Contact with hot air and other hot gases**

> The appropriate 7th character is to be added to each code from category X14

> | A | initial encounter |
> | D | subsequent encounter |
> | S | sequela |

- ● **X14.0　Inhalation of hot air and gases** S
- ● **X14.1　Other contact with hot air and other hot gases** S

● **X15　Contact with hot household appliances**

> **Excludes1**　contact with heating appliances (X16)
> contact with powered household appliances (W29.-)
> exposure to controlled fire in building or structure due to household appliance (X02.8)
> exposure to household appliances electrical current (W86.0)

> The appropriate 7th character is to be added to each code from category X15

> | A | initial encounter |
> | D | subsequent encounter |
> | S | sequela |

- ● **X15.0　Contact with hot stove (kitchen)** S
- ● **X15.1　Contact with hot toaster** S
- ● **X15.2　Contact with hotplate** S
- ● **X15.3　Contact with hot saucepan or skillet** S
- ● **X15.8　Contact with other hot household appliances** S
  > Contact with cooker
  > Contact with kettle
  > Contact with light bulbs

● **X16　Contact with hot heating appliances, radiators and pipes** S

> **Excludes1**　contact with powered appliances (W29.-)
> exposure to controlled fire in building or structure due to appliance (X02.8)
> exposure to industrial appliances electrical current (W86.1)

> The appropriate 7th character is to be added to code X16

> | A | initial encounter |
> | D | subsequent encounter |
> | S | sequela |

● **X17　Contact with hot engines, machinery and tools** S

> **Excludes1**　contact with hot heating appliances, radiators and pipes (X16)
> contact with hot household appliances (X15)

> The appropriate 7th character is to be added to code X17

> | A | initial encounter |
> | D | subsequent encounter |
> | S | sequela |

● **X18　Contact with other hot metals** S
> Contact with liquid metal

> The appropriate 7th character is to be added to code X18

> | A | initial encounter |
> | D | subsequent encounter |
> | S | sequela |

● **X19　Contact with other heat and hot substances** S

> **Excludes1**　objects that are not normally hot, e.g., an object made hot by a house fire (X00-X09)

> The appropriate 7th character is to be added to code X19

> | A | initial encounter |
> | D | subsequent encounter |
> | S | sequela |

EXPOSURE TO FORCES OF NATURE (X30-X39)

● **X30　Exposure to excessive natural heat** S
> Exposure to excessive heat as the cause of sunstroke
> Exposure to heat NOS

> **Excludes1**　excessive heat of man-made origin (W92)
> exposure to man-made radiation (W89)
> exposure to sunlight (X32)
> exposure to tanning bed (W89)

> The appropriate 7th character is to be added to code X30

> | A | initial encounter |
> | D | subsequent encounter |
> | S | sequela |

● **X31　Exposure to excessive natural cold** S
> Excessive cold as the cause of chilblains NOS
> Excessive cold as the cause of immersion foot or hand
> Exposure to cold NOS
> Exposure to weather conditions

> **Excludes1**　cold of man-made origin (W93.-)
> contact with or inhalation of:
> dry ice (W93.-)
> liquefied gas (W93.-)

> The appropriate 7th character is to be added to code X31

> | A | initial encounter |
> | D | subsequent encounter |
> | S | sequela |

● **X32　Exposure to sunlight** S

> **Excludes1**　radiation-related disorders of the skin and subcutaneous tissue (L55-L59)
> man-made radiation (tanning bed) (W89)

> The appropriate 7th character is to be added to code X32

> | A | initial encounter |
> | D | subsequent encounter |
> | S | sequela |

● **X34　Earthquake** S

> **Excludes2**　tidal wave (tsunami) due to earthquake (X37.41)

> The appropriate 7th character is to be added to code X34

> | A | initial encounter |
> | D | subsequent encounter |
> | S | sequela |

● **X35　Volcanic eruption** S

> **Excludes2**　tidal wave (tsunami) due to volcanic eruption (X37.41)

> The appropriate 7th character is to be added to code X35

> | A | initial encounter |
> | D | subsequent encounter |
> | S | sequela |

● Unacceptable Principal Diagnosis　　● Use Additional Character(s)　　■ Unspecified　　▶ Manifestation Code

OGCR　Official Guidelines for Coding and Reporting　　| Excludes 1 | Excludes 2 | Includes | Use additional | Code first | Code also |

● **X36   Avalanche, landslide and other earth movements**

    | Includes | victim of mudslide of cataclysmic nature
    | Excludes1 | earthquake (X34)
    | Excludes2 | transport accident involving collision with avalanche or landslide not in motion (V01-V99)

    The appropriate 7th character is to be added to each code from category X36

A	initial encounter
D	subsequent encounter
S	sequela

● **X36.0   Collapse of dam or man-made structure causing earth movement** S

● **X36.1   Avalanche, landslide, or mudslide** S

● **X37   Cataclysmic storm**

    The appropriate 7th character is to be added to each code from category X37

A	initial encounter
D	subsequent encounter
S	sequela

● **X37.0   Hurricane** S
     Storm surge   Typhoon

● **X37.1   Tornado** S
     Cyclone   Twister

● **X37.2   Blizzard (snow) (ice)** S

● **X37.3   Dust storm** S

● **X37.4   Tidalwave** S

     ● **X37.41   Tidal wave due to earthquake or volcanic eruption** S
        Tidal wave NOS
        Tsunami

     ● **X37.42   Tidal wave due to storm** S

     ● **X37.43   Tidal wave due to landslide** S

● **X37.8   Other cataclysmic storms** S
     Cloudburst
     Torrential rain
     | Excludes2 | flood (X38)

● **X37.9   Unspecified cataclysmic storm** S
     Storm NOS
     | Excludes1 | collapse of dam or man-made structure causing earth movement (X39.0)

● **X38   Flood** S
    Flood arising from remote storm
    Flood of cataclysmic nature arising from melting snow
    Flood resulting directly from storm
    | Excludes1 | collapse of dam or man-made structure causing earth movement (X39.0)
        tidal wave NOS (X37.41)
        tidal wave caused by storm (X37.2)

    The appropriate 7th character is to be added to code X38

A	initial encounter
D	subsequent encounter
S	sequela

● **X39   Exposure to other forces of nature**

    The appropriate 7th character is to be added to each code from category X39

A	initial encounter
D	subsequent encounter
S	sequela

● **X39.0   Exposure to natural radiation**
    | Excludes1 | contact with and (suspected) exposure to radon and other naturally occuring radiation (Z77.122)
        exposure to man-made radiation (W88-W90)
        exposure to sunlight (X32)

    ● **X39.01   Exposure to radon** S

    ● **X39.08   Exposure to other natural radiation** S

● **X39.8   Other exposure to forces of nature** A, D, S

ACCIDENTAL EXPOSURE TO OTHER SPECIFIED FACTORS (X52, X58)

● **X52   Prolonged stay in weightless environment** A, D, S
    Weightlessness in spacecraft (simulator)

    The appropriate 7th character is to be added to code X52

A	initial encounter
D	subsequent encounter
S	sequela

● **X58   Exposure to other specified factors** A, D, S
    Accident NOS
    Exposure NOS

    The appropriate 7th character is to be added to code X58

A	initial encounter
D	subsequent encounter
S	sequela

INTENTIONAL SELF-HARM (X71-X83)

Purposely self-inflicted injury
Suicide (attempted)

● **X71   Intentional self-harm by drowning and submersion**

    The appropriate 7th character is to be added to each code from category X71

A	initial encounter
D	subsequent encounter
S	sequela

● **X71.0   Intentional self-harm by drowning and submersion while in bathtub** S

● **X71.1   Intentional self-harm by drowning and submersion while in swimming pool** S

● **X71.2   Intentional self-harm by drowning and submersion after jump into swimming pool** S

● **X71.3   Intentional self-harm by drowning and submersion in natural water** S

● **X71.8   Other intentional self-harm by drowning and submersion** S

● **X71.9   Intentional self-harm by drowning and submersion, unspecified** S

CHAPTER 20 (V01-Y99)

● X72   **Intentional self-harm by handgun discharge** S 🔊
     Intentional self-harm by gun for single hand use
     Intentional self-harm by pistol
     Intentional self-harm by revolver

> | **Excludes1** | Very pistol (X74.8) |
> |---|---|

     The appropriate 7th character is to be added to code X72

> | A | initial encounter |
> |---|---|
> | D | subsequent encounter |
> | S | sequela |

● X73   **Intentional self-harm by rifle, shotgun and larger firearm discharge**

> | **Excludes1** | airgun (X74.01) |
> |---|---|

     The appropriate 7th character is to be added to each code from category X73

> | A | initial encounter |
> |---|---|
> | D | subsequent encounter |
> | S | sequela |

    ● X73.0   **Intentional self-harm by shotgun discharge** S 🔊
    ● X73.1   **Intentional self-harm by hunting rifle discharge** S 🔊
    ● X73.2   **Intentional self-harm by machine gun discharge** S 🔊
    ● X73.8   **Intentional self-harm by other larger firearm discharge** S 🔊
    ●■ X73.9   **Intentional self-harm by unspecified larger firearm discharge** S 🔊

● X74   **Intentional self-harm by other and unspecified firearm and gun discharge**

     The appropriate 7th character is to be added to each code from category X74

> | A | initial encounter |
> |---|---|
> | D | subsequent encounter |
> | S | sequela |

    ● X74.0   **Intentional self-harm by gas, air or spring-operated guns**
      ● X74.01   **Intentional self-harm by airgun** S 🔊
        Intentional self-harm by BB gun discharge
        Intentional self-harm by pellet gun discharge
      ● X74.02   **Intentional self-harm by paintball gun** S 🔊
      ●■ X74.09   **Intentional self-harm by other gas, air or spring-operated gun** S 🔊
    ● X74.8   **Intentional self-harm by other firearm discharge** S 🔊
        Intentional self-harm by Very pistol [flare] discharge
    ● X74.9   **Intentional self-harm by unspecified firearm discharge** S 🔊

● X75   **Intentional self-harm by explosive material** S 🔊

     The appropriate 7th character is to be added to code X75

> | A | initial encounter |
> |---|---|
> | D | subsequent encounter |
> | S | sequela |

● X76   **Intentional self-harm by smoke, fire and flames** S 🔊

     The appropriate 7th character is to be added to code X76

> | A | initial encounter |
> |---|---|
> | D | subsequent encounter |
> | S | sequela |

● X77   **Intentional self-harm by steam, hot vapors and hot objects**

     The appropriate 7th character is to be added to each code from category X77

> | A | initial encounter |
> |---|---|
> | D | subsequent encounter |
> | S | sequela |

    ● X77.0   **Intentional self-harm by steam or hot vapors** S 🔊
    ● X77.1   **Intentional self-harm by hot tap water** S 🔊
    ● X77.2   **Intentional self-harm by other hot fluids** S 🔊
    ● X77.3   **Intentional self-harm by hot household appliances** S 🔊
    ● X77.8   **Intentional self-harm by other hot objects** S 🔊
    ●■ X77.9   **Intentional self-harm by unspecified hot objects** S 🔊

● X78   **Intentional self-harm by sharp object**

     The appropriate 7th character is to be added to each code from category X78

> | A | initial encounter |
> |---|---|
> | D | subsequent encounter |
> | S | sequela |

    ● X78.0   **Intentional self-harm by sharp glass** S 🔊
    ● X78.1   **Intentional self-harm by knife** S 🔊
    ● X78.2   **Intentional self-harm by sword or dagger** S 🔊
    ● X78.8   **Intentional self-harm by other sharp object** S 🔊
    ●■ X78.9   **Intentional self-harm by unspecified sharp object** S 🔊

● X79   **Intentional self-harm by blunt object** S 🔊

     The appropriate 7th character is to be added to code X79

> | A | initial encounter |
> |---|---|
> | D | subsequent encounter |
> | S | sequela |

● X80   **Intentional self-harm by jumping from a high place** S 🔊
     Intentional fall from one level to another

     The appropriate 7th character is to be added to code X80

> | A | initial encounter |
> |---|---|
> | D | subsequent encounter |
> | S | sequela |

● X81   **Intentional self-harm by jumping or lying in front of moving object**

     The appropriate 7th character is to be added to each code from category X81

> | A | initial encounter |
> |---|---|
> | D | subsequent encounter |
> | S | sequela |

    ● X81.0   **Intentional self-harm by jumping or lying in front of motor vehicle** S 🔊
    ● X81.1   **Intentional self-harm by jumping or lying in front of (subway) train** S 🔊
    ● X81.8   **Intentional self-harm by jumping or lying in front of other moving object** S 🔊

● Unacceptable Principal Diagnosis   ● Use Additional Character(s)   ■ Unspecified   ▶ Manifestation Code

   OGCR Official Guidelines for Coding and Reporting | Excludes 1 | | Excludes 2 | | Includes | | Use additional | | Code first | | Code also |

● **X82 Intentional self-harm by crashing of motor vehicle**

> The appropriate 7th character is to be added to each code from category X82

> | A | initial encounter |
> |---|---|
> | D | subsequent encounter |
> | S | sequela |

● **X82.0 Intentional collision of motor vehicle with other motor vehicle** S 🔖

● **X82.1 Intentional collision of motor vehicle with train** S 🔖

● **X82.2 Intentional collision of motor vehicle with tree** S 🔖

● **X82.8 Other intentional self-harm by crashing of motor vehicle** S 🔖

● **X83 Intentional self-harm by other specified means**

> **Excludes1**   intentional self-harm by poisoning or contact with toxic substance - see Table of Drugs and Chemicals

> The appropriate 7th character is to be added to each code from category X83

> | A | initial encounter |
> |---|---|
> | D | subsequent encounter |
> | S | sequela |

● **X83.0 Intentional self-harm by crashing of aircraft** S 🔖

● **X83.1 Intentional self-harm by electrocution** S 🔖

● **X83.2 Intentional self-harm by exposure to extremes of cold** S 🔖

● **X83.8 Intentional self-harm by other specified means** S 🔖

ASSAULT (X92-Y08)

> **Includes**   homicide injuries inflicted by another person with intent to injure or kill, by any means

> **Excludes1**   injuries due to legal intervention (Y35.-)
> injuries due to operations of war (Y36.-)
> injuries due to terrorism (Y38.-)

● **X92 Assault by drowning and submersion**

> The appropriate 7th character is to be added to each code from category X92

> | A | initial encounter |
> |---|---|
> | D | subsequent encounter |
> | S | sequela |

● **X92.0 Assault by drowning and submersion while in bathtub**

● **X92.1 Assault by drowning and submersion while in swimming pool**

● **X92.2 Assault by drowning and submersion after push into swimming pool**

● **X92.3 Assault by drowning and submersion in natural water**

● **X92.8 Other assault by drowning and submersion**

●■ **X92.9 Assault by drowning and submersion, unspecified**

● **X93 Assault by handgun discharge**

> Assault by discharge of gun for single hand use
> Assault by discharge of pistol
> Assault by discharge of revolver

> **Excludes1**   Very pistol (X95.8)

> The appropriate 7th character is to be added to code X93

> | A | initial encounter |
> |---|---|
> | D | subsequent encounter |
> | S | sequela |

● **X94 Assault by rifle, shotgun and larger firearm discharge**

> **Excludes1**   airgun (X95.01)

> The appropriate 7th character is to be added to each code from category X94

> | A | initial encounter |
> |---|---|
> | D | subsequent encounter |
> | S | sequela |

● **X94.0 Assault by shotgun**

● **X94.1 Assault by hunting rifle**

● **X94.2 Assault by machine gun**

● **X94.8 Assault by other larger firearm discharge**

●■ **X94.9 Assault by unspecified larger firearm discharge**

● **X95 Assault by other and unspecified firearm and gun discharge**

> The appropriate 7th character is to be added to each code from category X95

> | A | initial encounter |
> |---|---|
> | D | subsequent encounter |
> | S | sequela |

● **X95.0 Assault by gas, air or spring-operated guns**

  ● **X95.01 Assault by airgun discharge**
> Assault by BB gun discharge
> Assault by pellet gun discharge

  ● **X95.02 Assault by paintball gun discharge**

  ● **X95.09 Assault by other gas, air or spring-operated gun**

● **X95.8 Assault by other firearm discharge**
> Assault by very pistol [flare] discharge

●■ **X95.9 Assault by unspecified firearm discharge**

● **X96 Assault by explosive material**

> **Excludes1**   incendiary device (X97)
> terrorism involving explosive material (Y38.2-)

> The appropriate 7th character is to be added to each code from category X96

> | A | initial encounter |
> |---|---|
> | D | subsequent encounter |
> | S | sequela |

● **X96.0 Assault by antipersonnel bomb**
> **Excludes1**   antipersonnel bomb use in military or war (Y36.2-)

● **X96.1 Assault by gasoline bomb**

● **X96.2 Assault by letter bomb**

● **X96.3 Assault by fertilizer bomb**

● **X96.4 Assault by pipe bomb**

● **X96.8 Assault by other specified explosive**

●■ **X96.9 Assault by unspecified explosive**

N Newborn Age: 0   **P** Pediatric Age: 0–17   **M** Maternity DX: 12–55   **A** Adult Age: 15–124   ♀ Females Only   ♂ Males Only

🔖 Complication\Comorbidity   Major C\C   🔖 Present on Admission Requirement   🔖 Hospital-Acquired Condition

1761

CHAPTER 20 (V01-Y99)

● **X97 Assault by smoke, fire and flames**
Assault by arson
Assault by cigarettes
Assault by incendiary device

The appropriate 7th character is to be added to code X97

A initial encounter
D subsequent encounter
S sequela

● **X98 Assault by steam, hot vapors and hot objects**

The appropriate 7th character is to be added to each code from category X98

A initial encounter
D subsequent encounter
S sequela

● **X98.0 Assault by steam or hot vapors**
● **X98.1 Assault by hot tap water**
● **X98.2 Assault by hot fluids**
● **X98.3 Assault by hot household appliances**
● **X98.8 Assault by other hot objects**
●■ **X98.9 Assault by unspecified hot objects**

● **X99 Assault by sharp object**
Excludes1 assault by strike by sports equipment (Y08.0-)

The appropriate 7th character is to be added to each code from category X99

A initial encounter
D subsequent encounter
S sequela

● **X99.0 Assault by sharp glass**
● **X99.1 Assault by knife**
● **X99.2 Assault by sword or dagger**
● **X99.8 Assault by other sharp object**
●■ **X99.9 Assault by unspecified sharp object**
Assault by stabbing NOS

● **Y00 Assault by blunt object**
Excludes1 assault by strike by sports equipment (Y08.0)

The appropriate 7th character is to be added to code Y00

A initial encounter
D subsequent encounter
S sequela

● **Y01 Assault by pushing from high place**

The appropriate 7th character is to be added to code Y01

A initial encounter
D subsequent encounter
S sequela

● **Y02 Assault by pushing or placing victim in front of moving object**

The appropriate 7th character is to be added to each code from category Y02

A initial encounter
D subsequent encounter
S sequela

● **Y02.0 Assault by pushing or placing victim in front of motor vehicle**
● **Y02.1 Assault by pushing or placing victim in front of (subway) train**
● **Y02.8 Assault by pushing or placing victim in front of other moving object**

● **Y03 Assault by crashing of motor vehicle**

The appropriate 7th character is to be added to each code from category Y03

A initial encounter
D subsequent encounter
S sequela

● **Y03.0 Assault by being hit or run over by motor vehicle**
● **Y03.8 Other assault by crashing of motor vehicle**

● **Y04 Assault by bodily force**
Excludes1 assault by:
submersion (X92.-)
use of weapon (X93-X95, X99, Y00)

The appropriate 7th character is to be added to each code from category Y04

A initial encounter
D subsequent encounter
S sequela

● **Y04.0 Assault by unarmed brawl or fight**
● **Y04.1 Assault by human bite**
● **Y04.2 Assault by strike against or bumped into by another person**
● **Y04.8 Assault by other bodily force**
Assault by bodily force NOS

OGCR Section I.C.19.f.

Adult and child abuse, neglect and other maltreatment

Sequence first the appropriate code from categories T74.- or T76.- for abuse, neglect and other maltreatment, followed by any accompanying mental health or injury code(s).

If the documentation in the medical record states abuse or neglect it is coded as confirmed. It is coded as suspected if it is documented as suspected.

For cases of confirmed abuse or neglect an external cause code from the assault section (X92-Y08) should be added to identify the cause of any physical injuries. A perpetrator code (Y07) should be added when the perpetrator of the abuse is known. For suspected cases of abuse or neglect, do not report external cause or perpetrator code.

If a suspected case of abuse, neglect or mistreatment is ruled out during an encounter code Z04.71, Encounter for examination and observation following alleged physical adult abuse, ruled out, or code Z04.72, Encounter for examination and observation following alleged child physical abuse, ruled out, should be used, not a code from T76.

If a suspected case of alleged rape or sexual abuse is ruled out during an encounter code Z04.41, Encounter for examination and observation following alleged physical adult abuse, ruled out, or code Z04.42, Encounter for examination and observation following alleged rape or sexual abuse, ruled out, should be used, not a code from T76.

● Unacceptable Principal Diagnosis ● Use Additional Character(s) ■ Unspecified ▶ Manifestation Code
OGCR Official Guidelines for Coding and Reporting | Excludes 1 | Excludes 2 | Includes | Use additional | Code first | Code also

● **Y07   Perpetrator of assault, maltreatment and neglect**

     Note: Codes from this category are for use only in cases of confirmed abuse (T74.-)

     Selection of the correct perpetrator code is based on the relationship between the perpetrator and the victim

     Includes   perpetrator of abandonment
                    perpetrator of emotional neglect
                    perpetrator of mental cruelty
                    perpetrator of physical abuse
                    perpetrator of physical neglect
                    perpetrator of sexual abuse
                    perpetrator of torture

● **Y07.0   Spouse or partner, perpetrator of maltreatment and neglect**

     Spouse or partner, perpetrator of maltreatment and neglect against spouse or partner

     Y07.01   Husband, perpetrator of maltreatment and neglect ♂   **A**

     Y07.02   Wife, perpetrator of maltreatment and neglect ♀

     Y07.03   Male partner, perpetrator of maltreatment and neglect ♂

     Y07.04   Female partner, perpetrator of maltreatment and neglect ♀

● **Y07.1   Parent (adoptive) (biological), perpetrator of maltreatment and neglect**

     Y07.11   Biological father, perpetrator of maltreatment and neglect ♂   **A**

     Y07.12   Biological mother, perpetrator of maltreatment and neglect ♀

     Y07.13   Adoptive father, perpetrator of maltreatment and neglect ♂   **A**

     Y07.14   Adoptive mother, perpetrator of maltreatment and neglect ♀

● **Y07.4   Other family member, perpetrator of maltreatment and neglect**

     ● **Y07.41   Sibling, perpetrator of maltreatment and neglect**

         Excludes1   stepsibling, perpetrator of maltreatment and neglect (Y07.435, Y07.436)

         Y07.410   Brother, perpetrator of maltreatment and neglect ♂

         Y07.411   Sister, perpetrator of maltreatment and neglect ♀

     ● **Y07.42   Foster parent, perpetrator of maltreatment and neglect**

         Y07.420   Foster father, perpetrator of maltreatment and neglect ♂   **A**

         Y07.421   Foster mother, perpetrator of maltreatment and neglect ♀

     ● **Y07.43   Stepparent or stepsibling, perpetrator of maltreatment and neglect**

         Y07.430   Stepfather, perpetrator of maltreatment and neglect ♂   **A**

         Y07.432   Male friend of parent (co-residing in household), perpetrator of maltreatment and neglect ♂

         Y07.433   Stepmother, perpetrator of maltreatment and neglect ♀

         Y07.434   Female friend of parent (co-residing in household), perpetrator of maltreatment and neglect ♀

         Y07.435   Stepbrother, perpetrator or maltreatment and neglect ♂

         Y07.436   Stepsister, perpetrator of maltreatment and neglect ♀

     ● **Y07.49   Other family member, perpetrator of maltreatment and neglect**

         Y07.490   Male cousin, perpetrator of maltreatment and neglect ♂

         Y07.491   Female cousin, perpetrator of maltreatment and neglect ♀

         Y07.499   Other family member, perpetrator of maltreatment and neglect

● **Y07.5   Non-family member, perpetrator of maltreatment and neglect**

     ■ **Y07.50   Unspecified non-family member, perpetrator of maltreatment and neglect**

     ● **Y07.51   Daycare provider, perpetrator of maltreatment and neglect**

         Y07.510   At-home childcare provider, perpetrator of maltreatment and neglect   **A**

         Y07.511   Daycare center childcare provider, perpetrator of maltreatment and neglect   **A**

         Y07.512   At-home adultcare provider, perpetrator of maltreatment and neglect   **A**

         Y07.513   Adultcare center provider, perpetrator of maltreatment and neglect   **A**

         ■ **Y07.519   Unspecified daycare provider, perpetrator of maltreatment and neglect**

     ● **Y07.52   Healthcare provider, perpetrator of maltreatment and neglect**

         Y07.521   Mental health provider, perpetrator of maltreatment and neglect

         Y07.528   Other therapist or healthcare provider, perpetrator of maltreatment and neglect

            Nurse perpetrator of maltreatment and neglect

            Occupational therapist perpetrator of maltreatment and neglect

            Physical therapist perpetrator of maltreatment and neglect

            Speech therapist perpetrator of maltreatment and neglect

         ■ **Y07.529   Unspecified healthcare provider, perpetrator of maltreatment and neglect**

     Y07.53   Teacher or instructor, perpetrator of maltreatment and neglect

         Coach, perpetrator of maltreatment and neglect

     Y07.59   Other non-family member, perpetrator of maltreatment and neglect

● ■ **Y07.9   Unspecified perpetrator of maltreatment and neglect**

N Newborn Age: 0   **P** Pediatric Age: 0–17   **M** Maternity DX: 12–55   **A** Adult Age: 15–124   ♀ Females Only   ♂ Males Only

🄲 Complication\Comorbidity   🄼 Major C\C   Present on Admission Requirement   Hospital-Acquired Condition

1763

CHAPTER 20 (V01–Y99)

CHAPTER 20 (V01-Y99)

● **Y08   Assault by other specified means**

> The appropriate 7th character is to be added to each code from category Y08

A	initial encounter
D	subsequent encounter
S	sequela

  ● **Y08.0   Assault by strike by sport equipment**

    ● **Y08.01   Assault by strike by hockey stick**

    ● **Y08.02   Assault by strike by baseball bat**

    ● **Y08.09   Assault by strike by other specified type of sport equipment**

  ● **Y08.8   Assault by other specified means**

    ● **Y08.81   Assault by crashing of aircraft**

    ● **Y08.89   Assault by other specified means**

● **Y09   Assault by unspecified means**

> Assassination (attempted) NOS
> Homicide (attempted) NOS
> Manslaughter (attempted) NOS
> Murder (attempted) NOS

EVENT OF UNDETERMINED INTENT (Y21-Y33)

> Undetermined intent is only for use when there is specific documentation in the record that the intent of the injury cannot be determined. If no such documentation is present, code to accidental (unintentional)

● **Y21   Drowning and submersion, undetermined intent**

> The appropriate 7th character is to be added to each code from category Y21

A	initial encounter
D	subsequent encounter
S	sequela

  ● **Y21.0   Drowning and submersion while in bathtub, undetermined intent** S 🔗

  ● **Y21.1   Drowning and submersion after fall into bathtub, undetermined intent** S 🔗

  ● **Y21.2   Drowning and submersion while in swimming pool, undetermined intent** S 🔗

  ● **Y21.3   Drowning and submersion after fall into swimming pool, undetermined intent** S 🔗

  ● **Y21.4   Drowning and submersion in natural water, undetermined intent** S 🔗

  ● **Y21.8   Other drowning and submersion, undetermined intent** S 🔗

  ●■ **Y21.9   Unspecified drowning and submersion, undetermined intent** S 🔗

● **Y22   Handgun discharge, undetermined intent** A, D, S 🔗

> Discharge of gun for single hand use, undetermined intent
> Discharge of pistol, undetermined intent
> Discharge of revolver, undetermined intent

> **Excludes2**   very pistol (Y24.8)

> The appropriate 7th character is to be added to code Y22

A	initial encounter
D	subsequent encounter
S	sequela

● **Y23   Rifle, shotgun and larger firearm discharge, undetermined intent**

> **Excludes2**   airgun (Y24.0)

> The appropriate 7th character is to be added to each code from category Y23

A	initial encounter
D	subsequent encounter
S	sequela

  ● **Y23.0   Shotgun discharge, undetermined intent** A, D, S 🔗

  ● **Y23.1   Hunting rifle discharge, undetermined intent** A, D, S 🔗

  ● **Y23.2   Military firearm discharge, undetermined intent** A, D, S 🔗

  ● **Y23.3   Machine gun discharge, undetermined intent** A, D, S 🔗

  ● **Y23.8   Other larger firearm discharge, undetermined intent** A, D, S 🔗

  ●■ **Y23.9   Unspecified larger firearm discharge, undetermined intent** A, D, S 🔗

● **Y24   Other and unspecified firearm discharge, undetermined intent**

> The appropriate 7th character is to be added to each code from category Y24

A	initial encounter
D	subsequent encounter
S	sequela

  ● **Y24.0   Airgun discharge, undetermined intent** A, D, S 🔗
> BB gun discharge, undetermined intent
> Pellet gun discharge, undetermined intent

  ● **Y24.8   Other firearm discharge, undetermined intent** A, D, S 🔗
> Paintball gun discharge, undetermined intent
> Very pistol [flare] discharge, undetermined intent

  ●■ **Y24.9   Unspecified firearm discharge, undetermined intent** A, D, S 🔗

● **Y25   Contact with explosive material, undetermined intent** A, D, S 🔗

> The appropriate 7th character is to be added to code Y25

A	initial encounter
D	subsequent encounter
S	sequela

● **Y26   Exposure to smoke, fire and flames, undetermined intent** S 🔗

> The appropriate 7th character is to be added to code Y26

A	initial encounter
D	subsequent encounter
S	sequela

● **Y27   Contact with steam, hot vapors and hot objects, undetermined intent**

> The appropriate 7th character is to be added to each code from category Y27

A	initial encounter
D	subsequent encounter
S	sequela

  ● **Y27.0   Contact with steam and hot vapors, undetermined intent** S 🔗

  ● **Y27.1   Contact with hot tap water, undetermined intent** S 🔗

● Unacceptable Principal Diagnosis   ● Use Additional Character(s)   ■ Unspecified   ▶ Manifestation Code

OGCR Official Guidelines for Coding and Reporting   Excludes 1   Excludes 2   Includes   Use additional   Code first   Code also

● **Y27.2** Contact with hot fluids, undetermined intent S 🔍

● **Y27.3** Contact with hot household appliance, undetermined intent S 🔍

● **Y27.8** Contact with other hot objects, undetermined intent S 🔍

●◼ **Y27.9** Contact with unspecified hot objects, undetermined intent S 🔍

● **Y28** Contact with sharp object, undetermined intent

The appropriate 7th character is to be added to each code from category Y28

A	initial encounter
D	subsequent encounter
S	sequela

● **Y28.0** Contact with sharp glass, undetermined intent S 🔍

● **Y28.1** Contact with knife, undetermined intent S 🔍

● **Y28.2** Contact with sword or dagger, undetermined intent S 🔍

● **Y28.8** Contact with other sharp object, undetermined intent S 🔍

●◼ **Y28.9** Contact with unspecified sharp object, undetermined intent S 🔍

● **Y29** Contact with blunt object, undetermined intent S 🔍

The appropriate 7th character is to be added to code Y29

A	initial encounter
D	subsequent encounter
S	sequela

● **Y30** Falling, jumping or pushed from a high place, undetermined intent S 🔍

Victim falling from one level to another, undetermined intent

The appropriate 7th character is to be added to code Y30

A	initial encounter
D	subsequent encounter
S	sequela

● **Y31** Falling, lying or running before or into moving object, undetermined intent S 🔍

The appropriate 7th character is to be added to code Y31

A	initial encounter
D	subsequent encounter
S	sequela

● **Y32** Crashing of motor vehicle, undetermined intent S 🔍

The appropriate 7th character is to be added to code Y32

A	initial encounter
D	subsequent encounter
S	sequela

● **Y33** Other specified events, undetermined intent S 🔍

The appropriate 7th character is to be added to code Y33

A	initial encounter
D	subsequent encounter
S	sequela

LEGAL INTERVENTION, OPERATIONS OF WAR, MILITARY OPERATIONS, AND TERRORISM (Y35-Y38)

● **Y35** Legal intervention

Includes	any injury sustained as a result of an encounter with any law enforcement official, serving in any capacity at the time of the encounter, whether on-duty or off-duty. Includes injury to law enforcement official, suspect and bystander

The appropriate 7th character is to be added to each code from category Y35

A	initial encounter
D	subsequent encounter
S	sequela

● **Y35.0** Legal intervention involving firearm discharge

● **Y35.00** Legal intervention involving unspecified firearm discharge

Legal intervention involving gunshot wound

Legal intervention involving shot NOS

●◼ **Y35.001** Legal intervention involving unspecified firearm discharge, law enforcement official injured A, D, S 🔍

●◼ **Y35.002** Legal intervention involving unspecified firearm discharge, bystander injured A, D, S 🔍

●◼ **Y35.003** Legal intervention involving unspecified firearm discharge, suspect injured A, D, S 🔍

● **Y35.01** Legal intervention involving injury by machine gun

● **Y35.011** Legal intervention involving injury by machine gun, law enforcement official injured A, D, S 🔍

● **Y35.012** Legal intervention involving injury by machine gun, bystander injured A, D, S 🔍

● **Y35.013** Legal intervention involving injury by machine gun, suspect injured A, D, S 🔍

● **Y35.02** Legal intervention involving injury by handgun

● **Y35.021** Legal intervention involving injury by handgun, law enforcement official injured A, D, S 🔍

● **Y35.022** Legal intervention involving injury by handgun, bystander injured A, D, S 🔍

● **Y35.023** Legal intervention involving injury by handgun, suspect injured A, D, S 🔍

● **Y35.03** Legal intervention involving injury by rifle pellet

● **Y35.031** Legal intervention involving injury by rifle pellet, law enforcement official injured A, D, S 🔍

● **Y35.032** Legal intervention involving injury by rifle pellet, bystander injured A, D, S 🔍

CHAPTER 20 (V01-Y99)

● **Y35.033** Legal intervention involving injury by rifle pellet, suspect injured A, D, S 🔗

● **Y35.04** Legal intervention involving injury by rubber bullet

  ● **Y35.041** Legal intervention involving injury by rubber bullet, law enforcement official injured A, D, S 🔗

  ● **Y35.042** Legal intervention involving injury by rubber bullet, bystander injured A, D, S 🔗

  ● **Y35.043** Legal intervention involving injury by rubber bullet, suspect injured A, D, S 🔗

● **Y35.09** Legal intervention involving other firearm discharge

  ● **Y35.091** Legal intervention involving other firearm discharge, law enforcement official injured A, D, S 🔗

  ● **Y35.092** Legal intervention involving other firearm discharge, bystander injured A, D, S 🔗

  ● **Y35.093** Legal intervention involving other firearm discharge, suspect injured A, D, S 🔗

● **Y35.1** Legal intervention involving explosives

  ● **Y35.10** Legal intervention involving unspecified explosives

    ●■ **Y35.101** Legal intervention involving unspecified explosives, law enforcement official injured A, D, S 🔗

    ●■ **Y35.102** Legal intervention involving unspecified explosives, bystander injured A, D, S 🔗

    ●■ **Y35.103** Legal intervention involving unspecified explosives, suspect injured A, D, S 🔗

  ● **Y35.11** Legal intervention involving injury by dynamite

    ● **Y35.111** Legal intervention involving injury by dynamite, law enforcement official injured A, D, S 🔗

    ● **Y35.112** Legal intervention involving injury by dynamite, bystander injured A, D, S 🔗

    ● **Y35.113** Legal intervention involving injury by dynamite, suspect injured A, D, S 🔗

  ● **Y35.12** Legal intervention involving injury by explosive shell

    ● **Y35.121** Legal intervention involving injury by explosive shell, law enforcement official injured A, D, S 🔗

    ● **Y35.122** Legal intervention involving injury by explosive shell, bystander injured A, D, S 🔗

    ● **Y35.123** Legal intervention involving injury by explosive shell, suspect injured A, D, S 🔗

● **Y35.19** Legal intervention involving other explosives
Legal intervention involving injury by grenade
Legal intervention involving injury by mortar bomb

  ● **Y35.191** Legal intervention involving other explosives, law enforcement official injured A, D, S 🔗

  ● **Y35.192** Legal intervention involving other explosives, bystander injured A, D, S 🔗

  ● **Y35.193** Legal intervention involving other explosives, suspect injured A, D, S 🔗

● **Y35.2** Legal intervention involving gas
Legal intervention involving asphyxiation by gas
Legal intervention involving poisoning by gas

  ● **Y35.20** Legal intervention involving unspecified gas

    ●■ **Y35.201** Legal intervention involving unspecified gas, law enforcement official injured A, D, S 🔗

    ●■ **Y35.202** Legal intervention involving unspecified gas, bystander injured A, D, S 🔗

    ●■ **Y35.203** Legal intervention involving unspecified gas, suspect injured A, D, S 🔗

  ● **Y35.21** Legal intervention involving injury by tear gas

    ● **Y35.211** Legal intervention involving injury by tear gas, law enforcement official injured A, D, S 🔗

    ● **Y35.212** Legal intervention involving injury by tear gas, bystander injured A, D, S 🔗

    ● **Y35.213** Legal intervention involving injury by tear gas, suspect injured A, D, S 🔗

  ● **Y35.29** Legal intervention involving other gas

    ● **Y35.291** Legal intervention involving other gas, law enforcement official injured A, D, S 🔗

    ● **Y35.292** Legal intervention involving other gas, bystander injured A, D, S 🔗

    ● **Y35.293** Legal intervention involving other gas, suspect injured A, D, S 🔗

● **Y35.3** Legal intervention involving blunt objects
Legal intervention involving being hit or struck by blunt object

  ● **Y35.30** Legal intervention involving unspecified blunt objects

    ●■ **Y35.301** Legal intervention involving unspecified blunt objects, law enforcement official injured A, D, S 🔗

    ●■ **Y35.302** Legal intervention involving unspecified blunt objects, bystander injured A, D, S 🔗

    ●■ **Y35.303** Legal intervention involving unspecified blunt objects, suspect injured A, D, S 🔗

● Unacceptable Principal Diagnosis   ● Use Additional Character(s)   ■ Unspecified   ▶ Manifestation Code

OGCR Official Guidelines for Coding and Reporting   Excludes 1   Excludes 2   Includes   Use additional   Code first   Code also

● Y35.31   Legal intervention involving baton

  ● Y35.311   **Legal intervention involving baton, law enforcement official injured** A, D, S 🔖

  ● Y35.312   **Legal intervention involving baton, bystander injured** A, D, S 🔖

  ● Y35.313   **Legal intervention involving baton, suspect injured** A, D, S 🔖

● Y35.39   **Legal intervention involving other blunt objects**

  ● Y35.391   **Legal intervention involving other blunt objects, law enforcement official injured** A, D, S 🔖

  ● Y35.392   **Legal intervention involving other blunt objects, bystander injured** A, D, S 🔖

  ● Y35.393   **Legal intervention involving other blunt objects, suspect injured** A, D, S 🔖

● Y35.4   **Legal intervention involving sharp objects**
  Legal intervention involving being cut by sharp objects
  Legal intervention involving being stabbed by sharp objects

  ● Y35.40   **Legal intervention involving unspecified sharp objects**

    ● ■ Y35.401   **Legal intervention involving unspecified sharp objects, law enforcement official injured** A, D, S 🔖

    ● ■ Y35.402   **Legal intervention involving unspecified sharp objects, bystander injured** A, D, S 🔖

    ● ■ Y35.403   **Legal intervention involving unspecified sharp objects, suspect injured** A, D, S 🔖

  ● Y35.41   **Legal intervention involving bayonet**

    ● Y35.411   **Legal intervention involving bayonet, law enforcement official injured** A, D, S 🔖

    ● Y35.412   **Legal intervention involving bayonet, bystander injured** A, D, S 🔖

    ● Y35.413   **Legal intervention involving bayonet, suspect injured** A, D, S 🔖

  ● Y35.49   **Legal intervention involving other sharp objects**

    ● Y35.491   **Legal intervention involving other sharp objects, law enforcement official injured** A, D, S 🔖

    ● Y35.492   **Legal intervention involving other sharp objects, bystander injured** A, D, S 🔖

    ● Y35.493   **Legal intervention involving other sharp objects, suspect injured** A, D, S 🔖

● Y35.8   **Legal intervention involving other specified means**

  ● Y35.81   **Legal intervention involving manhandling**

    ● Y35.811   **Legal intervention involving manhandling, law enforcement official injured** A, D, S 🔖

    ● Y35.812   **Legal intervention involving manhandling, bystander injured** A, D, S 🔖

    ● Y35.813   **Legal intervention involving manhandling, suspect injured** A, D, S 🔖

  ● Y35.89   **Legal intervention involving other specified means**

    ● Y35.891   **Legal intervention involving other specified means, law enforcement official injured** A, D, S 🔖

    ● Y35.892   **Legal intervention involving other specified means, bystander injured** A, D, S 🔖

    ● Y35.893   **Legal intervention involving other specified means, suspect injured** A, D, S 🔖

● Y35.9   **Legal intervention, means unspecified**

  ● ■ Y35.91   **Legal intervention, means unspecified, law enforcement official injured** A, D, S 🔖

  ● ■ Y35.92   **Legal intervention, means unspecified, bystander injured** A, D, S 🔖

  ● ■ Y35.93   **Legal intervention, means unspecified, suspect injured** A, D, S 🔖

● Y36   **Operations of war**

Includes	injuries to military personnel and civilians caused by war, civil insurrection, and peacekeeping missions
Excludes1	injury to military personnel occurring during peacetime military operations (Y37.-)
	military vehicles involved in transport accidents with non-military vehicle during peacetime (V09.01, V09.21, V19.81, V29.81, V39.81, V49.81, V59.81, V69.81, V79.81)

The appropriate 7th character is to be added to each code from category Y36

A	initial encounter
D	subsequent encounter
S	sequela

● Y36.0   **War operations involving explosion of marine weapons**
  Weapons and military watercraft

  ● Y36.00   **War operations involving explosion of unspecified marine weapon**
    War operations involving underwater blast NOS

    ● ■ Y36.000   **War operations involving explosion of unspecified marine weapon, military personnel** A, D, S 🔖

    ● ■ Y36.001   **War operations involving explosion of unspecified marine weapon, civilian** A, D, S 🔖

  ● Y36.01   **War operations involving explosion of depth-charge**

    ● Y36.010   **War operations involving explosion of depth-charge, military personnel** A, D, S 🔖

    ● Y36.011   **War operations involving explosion of depth-charge, civilian** A, D, S 🔖

● **Y36.02** War operations involving explosion of marine mine
　　War operations involving explosion of marine mine, at sea or in harbor

　● **Y36.020** War operations involving explosion of marine mine, military personnel A, D, S 🔖

　● **Y36.021** War operations involving explosion of marine mine, civilian A, D, S 🔖

● **Y36.03** War operations involving explosion of sea-based artillery shell

　● **Y36.030** War operations involving explosion of sea-based artillery shell, military personnel A, D, S 🔖

　● **Y36.031** War operations involving explosion of sea-based artillery shell, civilian A, D, S 🔖

● **Y36.04** War operations involving explosion of torpedo

　● **Y36.040** War operations involving explosion of torpedo, military personnel A, D, S 🔖

　● **Y36.041** War operations involving explosion of torpedo, civilian A, D, S 🔖

● **Y36.05** War operations involving accidental detonation of onboard marine weapons

　● **Y36.050** War operations involving accidental detonation of onboard marine weapons, military personnel A, D, S 🔖

　● **Y36.051** War operations involving accidental detonation of onboard marine weapons, civilian A, D, S 🔖

● **Y36.09** War operations involving explosion of other marine weapons

　● **Y36.090** War operations involving explosion of other marine weapons, military personnel A, D, S 🔖

　● **Y36.091** War operations involving explosion of other marine weapons, civilian A, D, S 🔖

● **Y36.1** War operations involving destruction of aircraft

　● ▪ **Y36.10** War operations involving unspecified destruction of aircraft

　　● ▪ **Y36.100** War operations involving unspecified destruction of aircraft, military personnel A, D, S 🔖

　　● ▪ **Y36.101** War operations involving unspecified destruction of aircraft, civilian A, D, S 🔖

● **Y36.11** War operations involving destruction of aircraft due to enemy fire or explosives
　　War operations involving destruction of aircraft due to air to air missile
　　War operations involving destruction of aircraft due to explosive placed on aircraft
　　War operations involving destruction of aircraft due to rocket propelled grenade [RPG]
　　War operations involving destruction of aircraft due to small arms fire
　　War operations involving destruction of aircraft due to surface to air missile

　● **Y36.110** War operations involving destruction of aircraft due to enemy fire or explosives, military personnel A, D, S 🔖

　● **Y36.111** War operations involving destruction of aircraft due to enemy fire or explosives, civilian A, D, S 🔖

● **Y36.12** War operations involving destruction of aircraft due to collision with other aircraft

　● **Y36.120** War operations involving destruction of aircraft due to collision with other aircraft, military personnel A, D, S 🔖

　● **Y36.121** War operations involving destruction of aircraft due to collision with other aircraft, civilian A, D, S 🔖

● **Y36.13** War operations involving destruction of aircraft due to onboard fire

　● **Y36.130** War operations involving destruction of aircraft due to onboard fire, military personnel A, D, S 🔖

　● **Y36.131** War operations involving destruction of aircraft due to onboard fire, civilian A, D, S 🔖

● **Y36.14** War operations involving destruction of aircraft due to accidental detonation of onboard munitions and explosives

　● **Y36.140** War operations involving destruction of aircraft due to accidental detonation of onboard munitions and explosives, military personnel A, D, S 🔖

　● **Y36.141** War operations involving destruction of aircraft due to accidental detonation of onboard munitions and explosives, civilian A, D, S 🔖

● **Y36.19** War operations involving other destruction of aircraft

　● **Y36.190** War operations involving other destruction of aircraft, military personnel A, D, S 🔖

　● **Y36.191** War operations involving other destruction of aircraft, civilian A, D, S 🔖

● Unacceptable Principal Diagnosis　　● Use Additional Character(s)　　▪ Unspecified　　▶ Manifestation Code

OGCR Official Guidelines for Coding and Reporting　│Excludes 1│　│Excludes 2│　Includes　Use additional　Code first　Code also

● Y36.2   **War operations involving other explosions and fragments**

    Excludes1   war operations involving explosion of aircraft (Y36.1-)

         war operations involving explosion of marine weapons (Y36.0-)

         war operations involving explosion of nuclear weapons (Y36.5-)

         war operations involving explosion occurring after cessation of hostilities (Y36.8-)

● Y36.20   **War operations involving unspecified explosion and fragments**

     War operations involving air blast NOS

     War operations involving blast NOS

     War operations involving blast fragments NOS

     War operations involving blast wave NOS

     War operations involving blast wind NOS

     War operations involving explosion NOS

     War operations involving explosion of bomb NOS

    ●■ Y36.200   **War operations involving unspecified explosion and fragments, military personnel** A, D, S 🔖

    ●■ Y36.201   **War operations involving unspecified explosion and fragments, civilian** A, D, S 🔖

● Y36.21   **War operations involving explosion of aerial bomb**

    ● Y36.210   **War operations involving explosion of aerial bomb, military personnel** A, D, S 🔖

    ● Y36.211   **War operations involving explosion of aerial bomb, civilian** A, D, S 🔖

● Y36.22   **War operations involving explosion of guided missile**

    ● Y36.220   **War operations involving explosion of guided missile, military personnel** A, D, S 🔖

    ● Y36.221   **War operations involving explosion of guided missile, civilian** A, D, S 🔖

● Y36.23   **War operations involving explosion of improvised explosive device [IED]**

     War operations involving explosion of person-borne improvised explosive device [IED]

     War operations involving explosion of vehicle-borne improvised explosive device [IED]

     War operations involving explosion of roadside improvised explosive device [IED]

    ● Y36.230   **War operations involving explosion of improvised explosive device [IED], military personnel** A, D, S 🔖

    ● Y36.231   **War operations involving explosion of improvised explosive device [IED], civilian** A, D, S 🔖

● Y36.24   **War operations involving explosion due to accidental detonation and discharge of own munitions or munitions launch device**

    ● Y36.240   **War operations involving explosion due to accidental detonation and discharge of own munitions or munitions launch device, military personnel** A, D, S 🔖

    ● Y36.241   **War operations involving explosion due to accidental detonation and discharge of own munitions or munitions launch device, civilian** A, D, S 🔖

● Y36.25   **War operations involving fragments from munitions**

    ● Y36.250   **War operations involving fragments from munitions, military personnel** A, D, S 🔖

    ● Y36.251   **War operations involving fragments from munitions, civilian** A, D, S 🔖

● Y36.26   **War operations involving fragments of improvised explosive device [IED]**

     War operations involving fragments of person-borne improvised explosive device [IED]

     War operations involving fragments of vehicle-borne improvised explosive device [IED]

     War operations involving fragments of roadside improvised explosive device [IED]

    ● Y36.260   **War operations involving fragments of improvised explosive device [IED], military personnel** A, D, S 🔖

    ● Y36.261   **War operations involving fragments of improvised explosive device [IED], civilian** A, D, S 🔖

● Y36.27   **War operations involving fragments from weapons**

    ● Y36.270   **War operations involving fragments from weapons, military personnel** A, D, S 🔖

    ● Y36.271   **War operations involving fragments from weapons, civilian** A, D, S 🔖

● Y36.29   **War operations involving other explosions and fragments**

     War operations involving explosion of grenade

     War operations involving explosions of land mine

     War operations involving shrapnel NOS

    ● Y36.290   **War operations involving other explosions and fragments, military personnel** A, D, S 🔖

    ● Y36.291   **War operations involving other explosions and fragments, civilian** A, D, S 🔖

N Newborn Age: 0   **P** Pediatric Age: 0–17   **M** Maternity DX: 12–55   **A** Adult Age: 15–124   ♀ Females Only   ♂ Males Only

🔖 Complication\Comorbidity   🔖 Major C\C   🔖 Present on Admission Requirement   🔖 Hospital-Acquired Condition

1769

CHAPTER 20 (V01-Y99)

● **Y36.3   War operations involving fires, conflagrations and hot substances**
War operations involving smoke, fumes, and heat from fires, conflagrations and hot substances

> **Excludes1**   war operations involving fires and conflagrations aboard military aircraft (Y36.1-)
> war operations involving fires and conflagrations aboard military watercraft (Y36.0-)
> war operations involving fires and conflagrations caused indirectly by conventional weapons (Y36.2-)
> war operations involving fires and thermal effects of nuclear weapons (Y36.53-)

● **Y36.30   War operations involving unspecified fire, conflagration and hot substance**

● ▪ **Y36.300   War operations involving unspecified fire, conflagration and hot substance, military personnel** A, D, S 🖐

● ▪ **Y36.301   War operations involving unspecified fire, conflagration and hot substance, civilian** A, D, S 🖐

● **Y36.31   War operations involving gasoline bomb**
War operations involving incendiary bomb
War operations involving petrol bomb

● **Y36.310   War operations involving gasoline bomb, military personnel** A, D, S 🖐

● **Y36.311   War operations involving gasoline bomb, civilian** A, D, S 🖐

● **Y36.32   War operations involving incendiary bullet**

● **Y36.320   War operations involving incendiary bullet, military personnel** A, D, S 🖐

● **Y36.321   War operations involving incendiary bullet, civilian** A, D, S 🖐

● **Y36.33   War operations involving flamethrower**

● **Y36.330   War operations involving flamethrower, military personnel** A, D, S 🖐

● **Y36.331   War operations involving flamethrower, civilian** A, D, S 🖐

● **Y36.39   War operations involving other fires, conflagrations and hot substances**

● **Y36.390   War operations involving other fires, conflagrations and hot substances, military personnel** A, D, S 🖐

● **Y36.391   War operations involving other fires, conflagrations and hot substances, civilian** A, D, S 🖐

● **Y36.4   War operations involving firearm discharge and other forms of conventional warfare**

● **Y36.41   War operations involving rubber bullets**

● **Y36.410   War operations involving rubber bullets, military personnel** A, D, S 🖐

● **Y36.411   War operations involving rubber bullets, civilian** A, D, S 🖐

● **Y36.42   War operations involving firearms pellets**

● **Y36.420   War operations involving firearms pellets, military personnel** A, D, S 🖐

● **Y36.421   War operations involving firearms pellets, civilian** A, D, S 🖐

● **Y36.43   War operations involving other firearms discharge**
War operations involving bullets NOS

> **Excludes1**   war operations involving munitions fragments (Y36.25-)
> war operations involving incendiary bullets (Y36.32-)

● **Y36.430   War operations involving other firearms discharge, military personnel** A, D, S 🖐

● **Y36.431   War operations involving other firearms discharge, civilian** A, D, S 🖐

● **Y36.44   War operations involving unarmed hand to hand combat**

> **Excludes1**   war operations involving combat using blunt or piercing object (Y36.45-)
> war operations involving intentional restriction of air and airway (Y36.46-)
> war operations involving unintentional restriction of air and airway (Y36.47-)

● **Y36.440   War operations involving unarmed hand to hand combat, military personnel** A, D, S 🖐

● **Y36.441   War operations involving unarmed hand to hand combat, civilian** A, D, S 🖐

● **Y36.45   War operations involving combat using blunt or piercing object**

● **Y36.450   War operations involving combat using blunt or piercing object, military personnel** A, D, S 🖐

● **Y36.451   War operations involving combat using blunt or piercing object, civilian** A, D, S 🖐

● **Y36.46   War operations involving intentional restriction of air and airway**

● **Y36.460   War operations involving intentional restriction of air and airway, military personnel** A, D, S 🖐

● **Y36.461   War operations involving intentional restriction of air and airway, civilian** A, D, S 🖐

● **Y36.47   War operations involving unintentional restriction of air and airway**

● **Y36.470   War operations involving unintentional restriction of air and airway, military personnel** A, D, S 🖐

● **Y36.471   War operations involving unintentional restriction of air and airway, civilian** A, D, S 🖐

● Unacceptable Principal Diagnosis   ● Use Additional Character(s)   ▪ Unspecified   ▶ Manifestation Code

OGCR Official Guidelines for Coding and Reporting | Excludes 1 | | Excludes 2 | Includes   Use additional   Code first   Code also

● **Y36.49**   **War operations involving other forms of conventional warfare**

  ● **Y36.490**   **War operations involving other forms of conventional warfare, military personnel** A, D, S 🔒

  ● **Y36.491**   **War operations involving other forms of conventional warfare, civilian** A, D, S 🔒

● **Y36.5**   **War operations involving nuclear weapons**
    War operations involving dirty bomb NOS

 ● **Y36.50**   **War operations involving unspecified effect of nuclear weapon**

  ●▪ **Y36.500**   **War operations involving unspecified effect of nuclear weapon, military personnel** A, D, S 🔒

  ●▪ **Y36.501**   **War operations involving unspecified effect of nuclear weapon, civilian** A, D, S 🔒

 ● **Y36.51**   **War operations involving direct blast effect of nuclear weapon**
    War operations involving blast pressure of nuclear weapon

  ● **Y36.510**   **War operations involving direct blast effect of nuclear weapon, military personnel** A, D, S 🔒

  ● **Y36.511**   **War operations involving direct blast effect of nuclear weapon, civilian** A, D, S 🔒

 ● **Y36.52**   **War operations involving indirect blast effect of nuclear weapon**
    War operations involving being thrown by blast of nuclear weapon
    War operations involving being struck or crushed by blast debris of nuclear weapon

  ● **Y36.520**   **War operations involving indirect blast effect of nuclear weapon, military personnel** A, D, S 🔒

  ● **Y36.521**   **War operations involving indirect blast effect of nuclear weapon, civilian** A, D, S 🔒

 ● **Y36.53**   **War operations involving thermal radiation effect of nuclear weapon**
    War operations involving direct heat from nuclear weapon
    War operation involving fireball effects from nuclear weapon

  ● **Y36.530**   **War operations involving thermal radiation effect of nuclear weapon, military personnel** A, D, S 🔒

  ● **Y36.531**   **War operations involving thermal radiation effect of nuclear weapon, civilian** A, D, S 🔒

 ● **Y36.54**   **War operation involving nuclear radiation effects of nuclear weapon**
    War operation involving acute radiation exposure from nuclear weapon
    War operation involving exposure to immediate ionizing radiation from nuclear weapon
    War operation involving fallout exposure from nuclear weapon
    War operation involving secondary effects of nuclear weapons

  ● **Y36.540**   **War operation involving nuclear radiation effects of nuclear weapon, military personnel** A, D, S 🔒

  ● **Y36.541**   **War operation involving nuclear radiation effects of nuclear weapon, civilian** A, D, S 🔒

 ● **Y36.59**   **War operation involving other effects of nuclear weapons**

  ● **Y36.590**   **War operation involving other effects of nuclear weapons, military personnel** A, D, S 🔒

  ● **Y36.591**   **War operation involving other effects of nuclear weapons, civilian** A, D, S 🔒

● **Y36.6**   **War operations involving biological weapons**

 ● **Y36.6X**   **War operations involving biological weapons**

  ● **Y36.6X0**   **War operations involving biological weapons, military personnel** A, D, S 🔒

  ● **Y36.6X1**   **War operations involving biological weapons, civilian** A, D, S 🔒

● **Y36.7**   **War operations involving chemical weapons and other forms of unconventional warfare**

    Excludes 1   war operations involving incendiary devices (Y36.3-, Y36.5-)

 ● **Y36.7X**   **War operations involving chemical weapons and other forms of unconventional warfare**

  ● **Y36.7X0**   **War operations involving chemical weapons and other forms of unconventional warfare, military personnel** A, D, S 🔒

  ● **Y36.7X1**   **War operations involving chemical weapons and other forms of unconventional warfare, civilian** A, D, S 🔒

● **Y36.8**   **War operations occurring after cessation of hostilities**
    War operations classifiable to categories Y36.0-Y36.8 but occurring after cessation of hostilities

 ● **Y36.81**   **Explosion of mine placed during war operations but exploding after cessation of hostilities**

  ● **Y36.810**   **Explosion of mine placed during war operations but exploding after cessation of hostilities, military personnel** A, D, S 🔒

  ● **Y36.811**   **Explosion of mine placed during war operations but exploding after cessation of hostilities, civilian** A, D, S 🔒

 ● **Y36.82**   **Explosion of bomb placed during war operations but exploding after cessation of hostilities**

  ● **Y36.820**   **Explosion of bomb placed during war operations but exploding after cessation of hostilities, military personnel** A, D, S 🔒

  ● **Y36.821**   **Explosion of bomb placed during war operations but exploding after cessation of hostilities, civilian** A, D, S 🔒

● Y36.88   Other war operations occurring after cessation of hostilities

   ● Y36.880   Other war operations occurring after cessation of hostilities, military personnel A, D, S 🔖

   ● Y36.881   Other war operations occurring after cessation of hostilities, civilian A, D, S 🔖

● Y36.89   Unspecified war operations occurring after cessation of hostilities

   ●■ Y36.890   Unspecified war operations occurring after cessation of hostilities, military personnel A, D, S 🔖

   ●■ Y36.891   Unspecified war operations occurring after cessation of hostilities, civilian A, D, S 🔖

● Y36.9   Other and unspecified war operations

   ●■ Y36.90   War operations, unspecified A, D, S 🔖

   ●■ Y36.91   War operations involving unspecified weapon of mass destruction [WMD] A, D, S 🔖

   ● Y36.92   War operations involving friendly fire A, D, S 🔖

● Y37   Military operations

| Includes | Injuries to military personnel and civilians occurring during peacetime on military property and during routine military exercises and operations |

Excludes 1	military aircraft involved in aircraft accident with civilian aircraft (V97.81-)
	military vehicles involved in transport accident with civilian vehicle (V09.01, V09.21, V19.81, V29.81, V39.81, V49.81, V59.81, V69.81, V79.81)
	military watercraft involved in water transport accident with civilian watercraft (V94.81-)
	war operations (Y36.-)

The appropriate 7th character is to be added to each code from category Y37

> A   initial encounter
> D   subsequent encounter
> S   sequela

● Y37.0   Military operations involving explosion of marine weapons

   ● Y37.00   Military operations involving explosion of unspecified marine weapon
      Military operations involving underwater blast NOS

      ●■ Y37.000   Military operations involving explosion of unspecified marine weapon, military personnel A, D, S 🔖

      ●■ Y37.001   Military operations involving explosion of unspecified marine weapon, civilian A, D, S 🔖

● Y37.01   Military operations involving explosion of depth-charge

   ● Y37.010   Military operations involving explosion of depth-charge, military personnel A, D, S 🔖

   ● Y37.011   Military operations involving explosion of depth-charge, civilian A, D, S 🔖

● Y37.02   Military operations involving explosion of marine mine
      Military operations involving explosion of marine mine, at sea or in harbor

   ● Y37.020   Military operations involving explosion of marine mine, military personnel A, D, S 🔖

   ● Y37.021   Military operations involving explosion of marine mine, civilian A, D, S 🔖

● Y37.03   Military operations involving explosion of sea-based artillery shell

   ● Y37.030   Military operations involving explosion of sea-based artillery shell, military personnel A, D, S 🔖

   ● Y37.031   Military operations involving explosion of sea-based artillery shell, civilian A, D, S 🔖

● Y37.04   Military operations involving explosion of torpedo

   ● Y37.040   Military operations involving explosion of torpedo, military personnel A, D, S 🔖

   ● Y37.041   Military operations involving explosion of torpedo, civilian A, D, S 🔖

● Y37.05   Military operations involving accidental detonation of onboard marine weapons

   ● Y37.050   Military operations involving accidental detonation of onboard marine weapons, military personnel A, D, S 🔖

   ● Y37.051   Military operations involving accidental detonation of onboard marine weapons, civilian A, D, S 🔖

● Y37.09   Military operations involving explosion of other marine weapons

   ● Y37.090   Military operations involving explosion of other marine weapons, military personnel A, D, S 🔖

   ● Y37.091   Military operations involving explosion of other marine weapons, civilian A, D, S 🔖

● Y37.1   Military operations involving destruction of aircraft

   ● Y37.10   Military operations involving unspecified destruction of aircraft

      ●■ Y37.100   Military operations involving unspecified destruction of aircraft, military personnel A, D, S 🔖

      ●■ Y37.101   Military operations involving unspecified destruction of aircraft, civilian A, D, S 🔖

● Unacceptable Principal Diagnosis   ● Use Additional Character(s)   ■ Unspecified   ▶ Manifestation Code

OGCR   Official Guidelines for Coding and Reporting | Excludes 1 | | Excludes 2 | | Includes | | Use additional | | Code first | | Code also |

● **Y37.11 Military operations involving destruction of aircraft due to enemy fire or explosives**
    Military operations involving destruction of aircraft due to air to air missile
    Military operations involving destruction of aircraft due to explosive placed on aircraft
    Military operations involving destruction of aircraft due to rocket propelled grenade [RPG]
    Military operations involving destruction of aircraft due to small arms fire
    Military operations involving destruction of aircraft due to surface to air missile

   ● **Y37.110 Military operations involving destruction of aircraft due to enemy fire or explosives, military personnel** A, D, S 🖉

   ● **Y37.111 Military operations involving destruction of aircraft due to enemy fire or explosives, civilian** A, D, S 🖉

● **Y37.12 Military operations involving destruction of aircraft due to collision with other aircraft**

   ● **Y37.120 Military operations involving destruction of aircraft due to collision with other aircraft, military personnel** A, D, S 🖉

   ● **Y37.121 Military operations involving destruction of aircraft due to collision with other aircraft, civilian** A, D, S 🖉

● **Y37.13 Military operations involving destruction of aircraft due to onboard fire**

   ● **Y37.130 Military operations involving destruction of aircraft due to onboard fire, military personnel** A, D, S 🖉

   ● **Y37.131 Military operations involving destruction of aircraft due to onboard fire, civilian** A, D, S 🖉

● **Y37.14 Military operations involving destruction of aircraft due to accidental detonation of onboard munitions and explosives**

   ● **Y37.140 Military operations involving destruction of aircraft due to accidental detonation of onboard munitions and explosives, military personnel** A, D, S 🖉

   ● **Y37.141 Military operations involving destruction of aircraft due to accidental detonation of onboard munitions and explosives, civilian** A, D, S 🖉

● **Y37.19 Military operations involving other destruction of aircraft**

   ● **Y37.190 Military operations involving other destruction of aircraft, military personnel** A, D, S 🖉

   ● **Y37.191 Military operations involving other destruction of aircraft, civilian** A, D, S 🖉

● **Y37.2 Military operations involving other explosions and fragments**

   Excludes1 military operations involving explosion of aircraft (Y37.1-)
            military operations involving explosion of marine weapons (Y37.0-)
            military operations involving explosion of nuclear weapons (Y37.5-)

● **Y37.20 Military operations involving unspecified explosion and fragments**
    Military operations involving air blast NOS
    Military operations involving blast NOS
    Military operations involving blast fragments NOS
    Military operations involving blast wave NOS
    Military operations involving blast wind NOS
    Military operations involving explosion NOS
    Military operations involving explosion of bomb NOS

   ● ■ **Y37.200 Military operations involving unspecified explosion and fragments, military personnel** A, D, S 🖉

   ● ■ **Y37.201 Military operations involving unspecified explosion and fragments, civilian** A, D, S 🖉

● **Y37.21 Military operations involving explosion of aerial bomb**

   ● **Y37.210 Military operations involving explosion of aerial bomb, military personnel** A, D, S 🖉

   ● **Y37.211 Military operations involving explosion of aerial bomb, civilian** A, D, S 🖉

● **Y37.22 Military operations involving explosion of guided missile**

   ● **Y37.220 Military operations involving explosion of guided missile, military personnel** A, D, S 🖉

   ● **Y37.221 Military operations involving explosion of guided missile, civilian** A, D, S 🖉

● **Y37.23 Military operations involving explosion of improvised explosive device [IED]**
    Military operations involving explosion of person-borne improvised explosive device [IED]
    Military operations involving explosion of vehicle-borne improvised explosive device [IED]
    Military operations involving explosion of roadside improvised explosive device [IED]

   ● **Y37.230 Military operations involving explosion of improvised explosive device [IED], military personnel** A, D, S 🖉

   ● **Y37.231 Military operations involving explosion of improvised explosive device [IED], civilian** A, D, S 🖉

CHAPTER 20 (V01-Y99)

N Newborn Age: 0   **P** Pediatric Age: 0–17   **M** Maternity DX: 12–55   **A** Adult Age: 15–124   ♀ Females Only   ♂ Males Only

🖉 Complication\Comorbidity   🖉 Major C\C   🖉 Present on Admission Requirement   🖉 Hospital-Acquired Condition   **1773**

CHAPTER 20 (V01-Y99)

● **Y37.24** **Military operations involving explosion due to accidental detonation and discharge of own munitions or munitions launch device**

   ● **Y37.240** **Military operations involving explosion due to accidental detonation and discharge of own munitions or munitions launch device, military personnel** A, D, S

   ● **Y37.241** **Military operations involving explosion due to accidental detonation and discharge of own munitions or munitions launch device, civilian** A, D, S

● **Y37.25** **Military operations involving fragments from munitions**

   ● **Y37.250** **Military operations involving fragments from munitions, military personnel** A, D, S

   ● **Y37.251** **Military operations involving fragments from munitions, civilian** A, D, S

● **Y37.26** **Military operations involving fragments of improvised explosive device [IED]**

   Military operations involving fragments of person-borne improvised explosive device [IED]

   Military operations involving fragments of vehicle-borne improvised explosive device [IED]

   Military operations involving fragments of roadside improvised explosive device [IED]

   ● **Y37.260** **Military operations involving fragments of improvised explosive device [IED], military personnel** A, D, S

   ● **Y37.261** **Military operations involving fragments of improvised explosive device [IED], civilian** A, D, S

● **Y37.27** **Military operations involving fragments from weapons**

   ● **Y37.270** **Military operations involving fragments from weapons, military personnel** A, D, S

   ● **Y37.271** **Military operations involving fragments from weapons, civilian** A, D, S

● **Y37.29** **Military operations involving other explosions and fragments**

   Military operations involving explosion of grenade

   Military operations involving explosions of land mine

   Military operations involving shrapnel NOS

   ● **Y37.290** **Military operations involving other explosions and fragments, military personnel** A, D, S

   ● **Y37.291** **Military operations involving other explosions and fragments, civilian** A, D, S

● **Y37.3** **Military operations involving fires, conflagrations and hot substances**

Military operations involving smoke, fumes, and heat from fires, conflagrations and hot substances

   Excludes1   military operations involving fires and conflagrations aboard military aircraft (Y37.1-)

            military operations involving fires and conflagrations aboard military watercraft (Y37.0-)

            military operations involving fires and conflagrations caused indirectly by conventional weapons (Y37.2-)

            military operations involving fires and thermal effects of nuclear weapons (Y36.53-)

● **Y37.30** **Military operations involving unspecified fire, conflagration and hot substance**

   ●■ **Y37.300** **Military operations involving unspecified fire, conflagration and hot substance, military personnel** A, D, S

   ●■ **Y37.301** **Military operations involving unspecified fire, conflagration and hot substance, civilian** A, D, S

● **Y37.31** **Military operations involving gasoline bomb**

Military operations involving incendiary bomb

Military operations involving petrol bomb

   ● **Y37.310** **Military operations involving gasoline bomb, military personnel** A, D, S

   ● **Y37.311** **Military operations involving gasoline bomb, civilian** A, D, S

● **Y37.32** **Military operations involving incendiary bullet**

   ● **Y37.320** **Military operations involving incendiary bullet, military personnel** A, D, S

   ● **Y37.321** **Military operations involving incendiary bullet, civilian** A, D, S

● **Y37.33** **Military operations involving flamethrower**

   ● **Y37.330** **Military operations involving flamethrower, military personnel** A, D, S

   ● **Y37.331** **Military operations involving flamethrower, civilian** A, D, S

● **Y37.39** **Military operations involving other fires, conflagrations and hot substances**

   ● **Y37.390** **Military operations involving other fires, conflagrations and hot substances, military personnel** A, D, S

   ● **Y37.391** **Military operations involving other fires, conflagrations and hot substances, civilian** A, D, S

● Unacceptable Principal Diagnosis   ● Use Additional Character(s)   ■ Unspecified   ▶ Manifestation Code

OGCR Official Guidelines for Coding and Reporting   Excludes 1   Excludes 2   Includes   Use additional   Code first   Code also

● **Y37.4**   **Military operations involving firearm discharge and other forms of conventional warfare**
- ● **Y37.41**   **Military operations involving rubber bullets**
  - ● **Y37.410**   **Military operations involving rubber bullets, military personnel** A, D, S 🗞
  - ● **Y37.411**   **Military operations involving rubber bullets, civilian** A, D, S 🗞
- ● **Y37.42**   **Military operations involving firearms pellets**
  - ● **Y37.420**   **Military operations involving firearms pellets, military personnel** A, D, S 🗞
  - ● **Y37.421**   **Military operations involving firearms pellets, civilian** A, D, S 🗞
- ● **Y37.43**   **Military operations involving other firearms discharge**
  Military operations involving bullets NOS
Excludes1	military operations involving munitions fragments (Y37.25-)
	military operations involving incendiary bullets (Y37.32-)
  - ● **Y37.430**   **Military operations involving other firearms discharge, military personnel** A, D, S 🗞
  - ● **Y37.431**   **Military operations involving other firearms discharge, civilian** A, D, S 🗞
- ● **Y37.44**   **Military operations involving unarmed hand to hand combat**
Excludes1	military operations involving combat using blunt or piercing object (Y37.45-)
	military operations involving intentional restriction of air and airway (Y37.46-)
	military operations involving unintentional restriction of air and airway (Y37.47-)
  - ● **Y37.440**   **Military operations involving unarmed hand to hand combat, military personnel** A, D, S 🗞
  - ● **Y37.441**   **Military operations involving unarmed hand to hand combat, civilian** A, D, S 🗞
- ● **Y37.45**   **Military operations involving combat using blunt or piercing object**
  - ● **Y37.450**   **Military operations involving combat using blunt or piercing object, military personnel** A, D, S 🗞
  - ● **Y37.451**   **Military operations involving combat using blunt or piercing object, civilian** A, D, S 🗞

- ● **Y37.46**   **Military operations involving intentional restriction of air and airway**
  - ● **Y37.460**   **Military operations involving intentional restriction of air and airway, military personnel** A, D, S 🗞
  - ● **Y37.461**   **Military operations involving intentional restriction of air and airway, civilian** A, D, S 🗞
- ● **Y37.47**   **Military operations involving unintentional restriction of air and airway**
  - ● **Y37.470**   **Military operations involving unintentional restriction of air and airway, military personnel** A, D, S 🗞
  - ● **Y37.471**   **Military operations involving unintentional restriction of air and airway, civilian** A, D, S 🗞
- ● **Y37.49**   **Military operations involving other forms of conventional warfare**
  - ● **Y37.490**   **Military operations involving other forms of conventional warfare, military personnel** A, D, S 🗞
  - ● **Y37.491**   **Military operations involving other forms of conventional warfare, civilian** A, D, S 🗞
● **Y37.5**   **Military operations involving nuclear weapons**
  Military operation involving dirty bomb NOS
- ● **Y37.50**   **Military operations involving unspecified effect of nuclear weapon**
  - ●■ **Y37.500**   **Military operations involving unspecified effect of nuclear weapon, military personnel** A, D, S 🗞
  - ●■ **Y37.501**   **Military operations involving unspecified effect of nuclear weapon, civilian** A, D, S 🗞
- ● **Y37.51**   **Military operations involving direct blast effect of nuclear weapon**
  Military operations involving blast pressure of nuclear weapon
  - ● **Y37.510**   **Military operations involving direct blast effect of nuclear weapon, military personnel** A, D, S 🗞
  - ● **Y37.511**   **Military operations involving direct blast effect of nuclear weapon, civilian** A, D, S 🗞
- ● **Y37.52**   **Military operations involving indirect blast effect of nuclear weapon**
  Military operations involving being thrown by blast of nuclear weapon
  Military operations involving being struck or crushed by blast debris of nuclear weapon
  - ● **Y37.520**   **Military operations involving indirect blast effect of nuclear weapon, military personnel** A, D, S 🗞
  - ● **Y37.521**   **Military operations involving indirect blast effect of nuclear weapon, civilian** A, D, S 🗞

CHAPTER 20 (V01–Y99)

N   Newborn Age: 0   **P**   Pediatric Age: 0–17   **M**   Maternity DX: 12–55   **A**   Adult Age: 15–124   ♀   Females Only   ♂   Males Only

🗞 Complication\Comorbidity   🗞 Major C\C   🗞 Present on Admission Requirement   🗞 Hospital-Acquired Condition

1775

CHAPTER 20 (V01–Y99)

● **Y37.53** **Military operations involving thermal radiation effect of nuclear weapon**
    Military operations involving direct heat from nuclear weapon
    Military operation involving fireball effects from nuclear weapon

  ● **Y37.530** **Military operations involving thermal radiation effect of nuclear weapon, military personnel** A, D, S 🔊

  ● **Y37.531** **Military operations involving thermal radiation effect of nuclear weapon, civilian** A, D, S 🔊

● **Y37.54** **Military operation involving nuclear radiation effects of nuclear weapon**
    Military operation involving acute radiation exposure from nuclear weapon
    Military operation involving exposure to immediate ionizing radiation from nuclear weapon
    Military operation involving fallout exposure from nuclear weapon
    Military operation involving secondary effects of nuclear weapons

  ● **Y37.540** **Military operation involving nuclear radiation effects of nuclear weapon, military personnel** A, D, S 🔊

  ● **Y37.541** **Military operation involving nuclear radiation effects of nuclear weapon, civilian** A, D, S 🔊

● **Y37.59** **Military operation involving other effects of nuclear weapons**

  ● **Y37.590** **Military operation involving other effects of nuclear weapons, military personnel** A, D, S 🔊

  ● **Y37.591** **Military operation involving other effects of nuclear weapons, civilian** A, D, S 🔊

● **Y37.6** **Military operations involving biological weapons**

  ● **Y37.6X** **Military operations involving biological weapons**

    ● **Y37.6X0** **Military operations involving biological weapons, military personnel** A, D, S 🔊

    ● **Y37.6X1** **Military operations involving biological weapons, civilian** A, D, S 🔊

● **Y37.7** **Military operations involving chemical weapons and other forms of unconventional warfare**

  | Excludes1 | military operations involving incendiary devices (Y36.3-, Y36.5-)

  ● **Y37.7X** **Military operations involving chemical weapons and other forms of unconventional warfare**

    ● **Y37.7X0** **Military operations involving chemical weapons and other forms of unconventional warfare, military personnel** A, D, S 🔊

    ● **Y37.7X1** **Military operations involving chemical weapons and other forms of unconventional warfare, civilian** A, D, S 🔊

● **Y37.9** **Other and unspecified military operations**

  ●■ **Y37.90** **Military operations, unspecified** A, D, S 🔊

  ●■ **Y37.91** **Military operations involving unspecified weapon of mass destruction [WMD]** A, D, S 🔊

  ● **Y37.92** **Military operations involving friendly fire** A, D, S 🔊

● **Y38** **Terrorism**
    These codes are for use to identify injuries resulting from the unlawful use of force or violence against persons or property to intimidate or coerce a government, the civilian population, or any segment thereof, in furtherance of political or social objective

    Use additional code for place of occurrence (Y92.-)

    The appropriate 7th character is to be added to each code from category Y38

    | A | initial encounter |
    | D | subsequent encounter |
    | S | sequela |

● **Y38.0** **Terrorism involving explosion of marine weapons**
    Terrorism involving depth-charge
    Terrorism involving marine mine
    Terrorism involving mine NOS, at sea or in harbor
    Terrorism involving sea-based artillery shell
    Terrorism involving torpedo
    Terrorism involving underwater blast

  ● **Y38.0X** **Terrorism involving explosion of marine weapons**

    ● **Y38.0X1** **Terrorism involving explosion of marine weapons, public safety official injured** A, D, S 🔊

    ● **Y38.0X2** **Terrorism involving explosion of marine weapons, civilian injured** A, D, S 🔊

    ● **Y38.0X3** **Terrorism involving explosion of marine weapons, terrorist injured** A, D, S 🔊

● **Y38.1** **Terrorism involving destruction of aircraft**
    Terrorism involving aircraft burned
    Terrorism involving aircraft exploded
    Terrorism involving aircraft being shot down
    Terrorism involving aircraft used as a weapon

  ● **Y38.1X** **Terrorism involving destruction of aircraft**

    ● **Y38.1X1** **Terrorism involving destruction of aircraft, public safety official injured** A, D, S 🔊

    ● **Y38.1X2** **Terrorism involving destruction of aircraft, civilian injured** A, D, S 🔊

    ● **Y38.1X3** **Terrorism involving destruction of aircraft, terrorist injured** A, D, S 🔊

● Unacceptable Principal Diagnosis   ● Use Additional Character(s)   ■ Unspecified   ▶ Manifestation Code

OGCR Official Guidelines for Coding and Reporting | Excludes 1 | | Excludes 2 | Includes   Use additional   Code first   Code also

● **Y38.2 Terrorism involving other explosions and fragments**
Terrorism involving antipersonnel (fragments) bomb
Terrorism involving blast NOS
Terrorism involving explosion NOS
Terrorism involving explosion of breech block
Terrorism involving explosion of cannon block
Terrorism involving explosion (fragments) of artillery shell
Terrorism involving explosion (fragments) of bomb
Terrorism involving explosion (fragments) of grenade
Terrorism involving explosion (fragments) of guided missile
Terrorism involving explosion (fragments) of land mine
Terrorism involving explosion of mortar bomb
Terrorism involving explosion of munitions
Terrorism involving explosion (fragments) of rocket
Terrorism involving explosion (fragments) of shell
Terrorism involving shrapnel
Terrorism involving mine NOS, on land

> **Excludes1** terrorism involving explosion of nuclear weapon (Y38.5)
> terrorism involving suicide bomber (Y38.81)

● **Y38.2X Terrorism involving other explosions and fragments**

  ● **Y38.2X1 Terrorism involving other explosions and fragments, public safety official injured** A, D, S

  ● **Y38.2X2 Terrorism involving other explosions and fragments, civilian injured** A, D, S

  ● **Y38.2X3 Terrorism involving other explosions and fragments, terrorist injured** A, D, S

● **Y38.3 Terrorism involving fires, conflagration and hot substances**
Terrorism involving conflagration NOS
Terrorism involving fire NOS
Terrorism involving petrol bomb

> **Excludes1** terrorism involving fire or heat of nuclear weapon (Y38.5)

● **Y38.3X Terrorism involving fires, conflagration and hot substances**

  ● **Y38.3X1 Terrorism involving fires, conflagration and hot substances, public safety official injured** A, D, S

  ● **Y38.3X2 Terrorism involving fires, conflagration and hot substances, civilian injured** A, D, S

  ● **Y38.3X3 Terrorism involving fires, conflagration and hot substances, terrorist injured** A, D, S

● **Y38.4 Terrorism involving firearms**
Terrorism involving carbine bullet
Terrorism involving machine gun bullet
Terrorism involving pellets (shotgun)
Terrorism involving pistol bullet
Terrorism involving rifle bullet
Terrorism involving rubber (rifle) bullet

● **Y38.4X Terrorism involving firearms**

  ● **Y38.4X1 Terrorism involving firearms, public safety official injured** A, D, S

  ● **Y38.4X2 Terrorism involving firearms, civilian injured** A, D, S

  ● **Y38.4X3 Terrorism involving firearms, terrorist injured** A, D, S

● **Y38.5 Terrorism involving nuclear weapons**
Terrorism involving blast effects of nuclear weapon
Terrorism involving exposure to ionizing radiation from nuclear weapon
Terrorism involving fireball effect of nuclear weapon
Terrorism involving heat from nuclear weapon

● **Y38.5X Terrorism involving nuclear weapons**

  ● **Y38.5X1 Terrorism involving nuclear weapons, public safety official injured** A, D, S

  ● **Y38.5X2 Terrorism involving nuclear weapons, civilian injured** A, D, S

  ● **Y38.5X3 Terrorism involving nuclear weapons, terrorist injured** A, D, S

● **Y38.6 Terrorism involving biological weapons**
Terrorism involving anthrax
Terrorism involving cholera
A serious, often deadly, infectious disease of small intestine
Terrorism involving smallpox

● **Y38.6X Terrorism involving biological weapons**

  ● **Y38.6X1 Terrorism involving biological weapons, public safety official injured** A, D, S

  ● **Y38.6X2 Terrorism involving biological weapons, civilian injured** A, D, S

  ● **Y38.6X3 Terrorism involving biological weapons, terrorist injured** A, D, S

● **Y38.7 Terrorism involving chemical weapons**
Terrorism involving gases, fumes, chemicals
Terrorism involving hydrogen cyanide
Terrorism involving phosgene
Terrorism involving sarin

● **Y38.7X Terrorism involving chemical weapons**

  ● **Y38.7X1 Terrorism involving chemical weapons, public safety official injured** A, D, S

  ● **Y38.7X2 Terrorism involving chemical weapons, civilian injured** A, D, S

  ● **Y38.7X3 Terrorism involving chemical weapons, terrorist injured** A, D, S

● **Y38.8 Terrorism involving other and unspecified means**

  ●■ **Y38.80 Terrorism involving unspecified means** A, D, S
  Terrorism NOS

  ● **Y38.81 Terrorism involving suicide bomber**

    ● **Y38.811 Terrorism involving suicide bomber, public safety official injured** A, D, S

    ● **Y38.812 Terrorism involving suicide bomber, civilian injured** A, D, S

  ● **Y38.89 Terrorism involving other means**
  Terrorism involving drowning and submersion
  Terrorism involving lasers
  Terrorism involving piercing or stabbing instruments

    ● **Y38.891 Terrorism involving other means, public safety official injured** A, D, S

N Newborn Age: 0   **P** Pediatric Age: 0–17   **M** Maternity DX: 12–55   **A** Adult Age: 15–124   ♀ Females Only   ♂ Males Only

Complication\Comorbidity   Major C\C   Present on Admission Requirement   Hospital-Acquired Condition

CHAPTER 20 (V01-Y99)

● Y38.892 **Terrorism involving other means, civilian injured** A, D, S 🔖

● Y38.893 **Terrorism involving other means, terrorist injured** A, D, S 🔖

● Y38.9 **Terrorism, secondary effects**

Note: This code is for use to identify conditions occurring subsequent to a terrorist attack not those that are due to the initial terrorist attack.

● Y38.9X **Terrorism, secondary effects**

● Y38.9X1 **Terrorism, secondary effects, public safety official injured** A, D, S 🔖

● Y38.9X2 **Terrorism, secondary effects, civilian injured categories** A, D, S 🔖

COMPLICATIONS OF MEDICAL AND SURGICAL CARE (Y62-Y84)

| **Includes** | complications of medical devices surgical and medical procedures as the cause of abnormal reaction of the patient, or of later complication, without mention of misadventure at the time of the procedure |

MISADVENTURES TO PATIENTS DURING SURGICAL AND MEDICAL CARE (Y62-Y69)

| **Excludes2** | breakdown or malfunctioning of medical device (during procedure) (after implantation) (ongoing use) (Y70-Y82) surgical and medical procedures as the cause of abnormal reaction of the patient, without mention of misadventure at the time of the procedure (Y83-Y84) |

● Y62 **Failure of sterile precautions during surgical and medical care**

Y62.0 **Failure of sterile precautions during surgical operation**

Y62.1 **Failure of sterile precautions during infusion or transfusion**

Y62.2 **Failure of sterile precautions during kidney dialysis and other perfusion**

Y62.3 **Failure of sterile precautions during injection or immunization**

Y62.4 **Failure of sterile precautions during endoscopic examination**

Y62.5 **Failure of sterile precautions during heart catheterization**

Y62.6 **Failure of sterile precautions during aspiration, puncture and other catheterization**

Y62.8 **Failure of sterile precautions during other surgical and medical care**

■ Y62.9 **Failure of sterile precautions during unspecified surgical and medical care**

● Y63 **Failure in dosage during surgical and medical care**

| **Excludes2** | accidental overdose of drug or wrong drug given in error (T36-T50) |

Y63.0 **Excessive amount of blood or other fluid given during transfusion or infusion**

Y63.1 **Incorrect dilution of fluid used during infusion**

Y63.2 **Overdose of radiation given during therapy**

Y63.3 **Inadvertent exposure of patient to radiation during medical care**

Y63.4 **Failure in dosage in electroshock or insulin-shock therapy**

Y63.5 **Inappropriate temperature in local application and packing**

Y63.6 **Underdosing and nonadministration of necessary drug, medicament or biological substance**

Y63.8 **Failure in dosage during other surgical and medical care**

■ Y63.9 **Failure in dosage during unspecified surgical and medical care**

● Y64 **Contaminated medical or biological substances**

Y64.0 **Contaminated medical or biological substance, transfused or infused**

Y64.1 **Contaminated medical or biological substance, injected or used for immunization**

Y64.8 **Contaminated medical or biological substance administered by other means**

■ Y64.9 **Contaminated medical or biological substance administered by unspecified means**

Administered contaminated medical or biological substance NOS

● Y65 **Other misadventures during surgical and medical care**

Y65.0 **Mismatched blood in transfusion**

Y65.1 **Wrong fluid used in infusion**

Y65.2 **Failure in suture or ligature during surgical operation**

Y65.3 **Endotracheal tube wrongly placed during anesthetic procedure**

Y65.4 **Failure to introduce or to remove other tube or instrument**

● Y65.5 **Performance of wrong procedure (operation)**

● Y65.51 **Performance of wrong procedure (operation) on correct patient**

Wrong device implanted into correct surgical site

| **Excludes1** | performance of correct procedure (operation) on wrong side or body part (Y65.53) |

MCE: Wrong procedure performed

● Y65.52 **Performance of procedure (operation) on patient not scheduled for surgery**

Performance of procedure (operation) intended for another patient

Performance of procedure (operation) on wrong patient

MCE: Wrong procedure performed

● Y65.53 **Performance of correct procedure (operation) on wrong side or body part**

Performance of correct procedure (operation) on wrong side

Performance of correct procedure (operation) on wrong site

MCE: Wrong procedure performed

Y65.8 **Other specified misadventures during surgical and medical care**

● Unacceptable Principal Diagnosis   ● Use Additional Character(s)   ■ Unspecified   ▸ Manifestation Code

OGCR Official Guidelines for Coding and Reporting | Excludes 1 | | Excludes 2 | | Includes | | Use additional | | Code first | | Code also |

Y66   **Nonadministration of surgical and medical care**
Premature cessation of surgical and medical care

> **Excludes1**   DNR status (Z66)
> palliative care (Z51.5)

Y69   **Unspecified misadventure during surgical and medical care**

**MEDICAL DEVICES ASSOCIATED WITH ADVERSE INCIDENTS
IN DIAGNOSTIC AND THERAPEUTIC USE (Y70-Y82)**

> **Includes**   breakdown or malfunction of medical devices (during use) (after implantation) (ongoing use)

> **Excludes1**   misadventure to patients during surgical and medical care, classifiable to (Y62-Y69)
> later complications following use of medical devices without breakdown or malfunctioning of device (Y83-Y84)

Y70   **Anesthesiology devices associated with adverse incidents**

Y70.0   Diagnostic and monitoring anesthesiology devices associated with adverse incidents

Y70.1   Therapeutic (nonsurgical) and rehabilitative anesthesiology devices associated with adverse incidents

Y70.2   Prosthetic and other implants, materials and accessory anesthesiology devices associated with adverse incidents

Y70.3   Surgical instruments, materials and anesthesiology devices (including sutures) associated with adverse incidents

Y70.8   Miscellaneous anesthesiology devices associated with adverse incidents, not elsewhere classified

Y71   **Cardiovascular devices associated with adverse incidents**

Y71.0   Diagnostic and monitoring cardiovascular devices associated with adverse incidents

Y71.1   Therapeutic (nonsurgical) and rehabilitative cardiovascular devices associated with adverse incidents

Y71.2   Prosthetic and other implants, materials and accessory cardiovascular devices associated with adverse incidents

Y71.3   Surgical instruments, materials and cardiovascular devices (including sutures) associated with adverse incidents

Y71.8   Miscellaneous cardiovascular devices associated with adverse incidents, not elsewhere classified

Y72   **Otorhinolaryngological devices associated with adverse incidents**

Y72.0   Diagnostic and monitoring otorhinolaryngological devices associated with adverse incidents

Y72.1   Therapeutic (nonsurgical) and rehabilitative otorhinolaryngological devices associated with adverse incidents

Y72.2   Prosthetic and other implants, materials and accessory otorhinolaryngological devices associated with adverse incidents

Y72.3   Surgical instruments, materials and otorhinolaryngological devices (including sutures) associated with adverse incidents

Y72.8   Miscellaneous otorhinolaryngological devices associated with adverse incidents, not elsewhere classified

Y73   **Gastroenterology and urology devices associated with adverse incidents**

Y73.0   Diagnostic and monitoring gastroenterology and urology devices associated with adverse incidents

Y73.1   Therapeutic (nonsurgical) and rehabilitative gastroenterology and urology devices associated with adverse incidents

Y73.2   Prosthetic and other implants, materials and accessory gastroenterology and urology devices associated with adverse incidents

Y73.3   Surgical instruments, materials and gastroenterology and urology devices (including sutures) associated with adverse incidents

Y73.8   Miscellaneous gastroenterology and urology devices associated with adverse incidents, not elsewhere classified

Y74   **General hospital and personal-use devices associated with adverse incidents**

Y74.0   Diagnostic and monitoring general hospital and personal-use devices associated with adverse incidents

Y74.1   Therapeutic (nonsurgical) and rehabilitative general hospital and personal-use devices associated with adverse incidents

Y74.2   Prosthetic and other implants, materials and accessory general hospital and personal-use devices associated with adverse incidents

Y74.3   Surgical instruments, materials and general hospital and personal-use devices (including sutures) associated with adverse incidents

Y74.8   Miscellaneous general hospital and personal-use devices associated with adverse incidents, not elsewhere classified

Y75   **Neurological devices associated with adverse incidents**

Y75.0   Diagnostic and monitoring neurological devices associated with adverse incidents

Y75.1   Therapeutic (nonsurgical) and rehabilitative neurological devices associated with adverse incidents

Y75.2   Prosthetic and other implants, materials and neurological devices associated with adverse incidents

Y75.3   Surgical instruments, materials and neurological devices (including sutures) associated with adverse incidents

Y75.8   Miscellaneous neurological devices associated with adverse incidents, not elsewhere classified

Y76   **Obstetric and gynecological devices associated with adverse incidents**

Y76.0   Diagnostic and monitoring obstetric and gynecological devices associated with adverse incidents ♀

Y76.1   Therapeutic (nonsurgical) and rehabilitative obstetric and gynecological devices associated with adverse incidents ♀

Y76.2   Prosthetic and other implants, materials and accessory obstetric and gynecological devices associated with adverse incidents ♀

Y76.3   Surgical instruments, materials and obstetric and gynecological devices (including sutures) associated with adverse incidents ♀

Y76.8   Miscellaneous obstetric and gynecological devices associated with adverse incidents, not elsewhere classified ♀

N Newborn Age: 0   **P** Pediatric Age: 0–17   **M** Maternity DX: 12–55   **A** Adult Age: 15–124   ♀ Females Only   ♂ Males Only

Complication\Comorbidity   Major C\C   Present on Admission Requirement   Hospital-Acquired Condition

1779

CHAPTER 20 (V01-Y99)

● Y77   Ophthalmic devices associated with adverse incidents

   Y77.0   Diagnostic and monitoring ophthalmic devices associated with adverse incidents

   Y77.1   Therapeutic (nonsurgical) and rehabilitative ophthalmic devices associated with adverse incidents

   Y77.2   Prosthetic and other implants, materials and accessory ophthalmic devices associated with adverse incidents

   Y77.3   Surgical instruments, materials and ophthalmic devices (including sutures) associated with adverse incidents

   Y77.8   Miscellaneous ophthalmic devices associated with adverse incidents, not elsewhere classified

● Y78   Radiological devices associated with adverse incidents

   Y78.0   Diagnostic and monitoring radiological devices associated with adverse incidents

   Y78.1   Therapeutic (nonsurgical) and rehabilitative radiological devices associated with adverse incidents

   Y78.2   Prosthetic and other implants, materials and accessory radiological devices associated with adverse incidents

   Y78.3   Surgical instruments, materials and radiological devices (including sutures) associated with adverse incidents

   Y78.8   Miscellaneous radiological devices associated with adverse incidents, not elsewhere classified

● Y79   Orthopedic devices associated with adverse incidents

   Y79.0   Diagnostic and monitoring orthopedic devices associated with adverse incidents

   Y79.1   Therapeutic (nonsurgical) and rehabilitative orthopedic devices associated with adverse incidents

   Y79.2   Prosthetic and other implants, materials and accessory orthopedic devices associated with adverse incidents

   Y79.3   Surgical instruments, materials and orthopedic devices (including sutures) associated with adverse incidents

   Y79.8   Miscellaneous orthopedic devices associated with adverse incidents, not elsewhere classified

● Y80   Physical medicine devices associated with adverse incidents

   Y80.0   Diagnostic and monitoring physical medicine devices associated with adverse incidents

   Y80.1   Therapeutic (nonsurgical) and rehabilitative physical medicine devices associated with adverse incidents

   Y80.2   Prosthetic and other implants, materials and accessory physical medicine devices associated with adverse incidents

   Y80.3   Surgical instruments, materials and physical medicine devices (including sutures) associated with adverse incidents

   Y80.8   Miscellaneous physical medicine devices associated with adverse incidents, not elsewhere classified

● Y81   General- and plastic-surgery devices associated with adverse incidents

   Y81.0   Diagnostic and monitoring general- and plastic-surgery devices associated with adverse incidents

   Y81.1   Therapeutic (nonsurgical) and rehabilitative general- and plastic-surgery devices associated with adverse incidents

   Y81.2   Prosthetic and other implants, materials and accessory general- and plastic-surgery devices associated with adverse incidents

   Y81.3   Surgical instruments, materials and general- and plastic-surgery devices (including sutures) associated with adverse incidents

   Y81.8   Miscellaneous general- and plastic-surgery devices associated with adverse incidents, not elsewhere classified

● Y82   Other and unspecified medical devices associated with adverse incidents

   Y82.8   Other medical devices associated with adverse incidents

   ■ Y82.9   Unspecified medical devices associated with adverse incidents

---

SURGICAL AND OTHER MEDICAL PROCEDURES AS THE CAUSE OF ABNORMAL REACTION OF THE PATIENT, OR OF LATER COMPLICATION, WITHOUT MENTION OF MISADVENTURE AT THE TIME OF THE PROCEDURE (Y83-Y84)

   Excludes1 misadventures to patients during surgical and medical care, classifiable to (Y62-Y69)

● Y83   Surgical operation and other surgical procedures as the cause of abnormal reaction of the patient, or of later complication, without mention of misadventure at the time of the procedure

   Y83.0   Surgical operation with transplant of whole organ as the cause of abnormal reaction of the patient, or of later complication, without mention of misadventure at the time of the procedure

   Y83.1   Surgical operation with implant of artificial internal device as the cause of abnormal reaction of the patient, or of later complication, without mention of misadventure at the time of the procedure

   Y83.2   Surgical operation with anastomosis, bypass or graft as the cause of abnormal reaction of the patient, or of later complication, without mention of misadventure at the time of the procedure

   Y83.3   Surgical operation with formation of external stoma as the cause of abnormal reaction of the patient, or of later complication, without mention of misadventure at the time of the procedure

   Y83.4   Other reconstructive surgery as the cause of abnormal reaction of the patient, or of later complication, without mention of misadventure at the time of the procedure

   Y83.5   Amputation of limb(s) as the cause of abnormal reaction of the patient, or of later complication, without mention of misadventure at the time of the procedure

   Y83.6   Removal of other organ (partial) (total) as the cause of abnormal reaction of the patient, or of later complication, without mention of misadventure at the time of the procedure

   Y83.8   Other surgical procedures as the cause of abnormal reaction of the patient, or of later complication, without mention of misadventure at the time of the procedure

   ■ Y83.9   Surgical procedure, unspecified as the cause of abnormal reaction of the patient, or of later complication, without mention of misadventure at the time of the procedure

● Unacceptable Principal Diagnosis   ● Use Additional Character(s)   ■ Unspecified   ▶ Manifestation Code

OGCR   Official Guidelines for Coding and Reporting | Excludes 1 | | Excludes 2 | | Includes | | Use additional | | Code first | | Code also |

● **Y84**   **Other medical procedures as the cause of abnormal reaction of the patient, or of later complication, without mention of misadventure at the time of the procedure**

     Y84.0   Cardiac catheterization as the cause of abnormal reaction of the patient, or of later complication, without mention of misadventure at the time of the procedure

     Y84.1   Kidney dialysis as the cause of abnormal reaction of the patient, or of later complication, without mention of misadventure at the time of the procedure

     Y84.2   Radiological procedure and radiotherapy as the cause of abnormal reaction of the patient, or of later complication, without mention of misadventure at the time of the procedure

     Y84.3   Shock therapy as the cause of abnormal reaction of the patient, or of later complication, without mention of misadventure at the time of the procedure

     Y84.4   Aspiration of fluid as the cause of abnormal reaction of the patient, or of later complication, without mention of misadventure at the time of the procedure

     Y84.5   Insertion of gastric or duodenal sound as the cause of abnormal reaction of the patient, or of later complication, without mention of misadventure at the time of the procedure

     Y84.6   Urinary catheterization as the cause of abnormal reaction of the patient, or of later complication, without mention of misadventure at the time of the procedure

     Y84.7   Blood-sampling as the cause of abnormal reaction of the patient, or of later complication, without mention of misadventure at the time of the procedure

     Y84.8   Other medical procedures as the cause of abnormal reaction of the patient, or of later complication, without mention of misadventure at the time of the procedure

     ■ **Y84.9**   Medical procedure, unspecified as the cause of abnormal reaction of the patient, or of later complication, without mention of misadventure at the time of the procedure

---

SUPPLEMENTARY FACTORS RELATED TO CAUSES OF MORBIDITY CLASSIFIED ELSEWHERE (Y90-Y99)

     Note: These categories may be used to provide supplementary information concerning causes of morbidity. They are not to be used for single-condition coding.

● **Y90**   **Evidence of alcohol involvement determined by blood alcohol level**

     Code first any associated alcohol related disorders (F10)

     Y90.0   Blood alcohol level of less than 20 mg/100 ml

     Y90.1   Blood alcohol level of 20-39 mg/100 ml

     Y90.2   Blood alcohol level of 40-59 mg/100 ml

     Y90.3   Blood alcohol level of 60-79 mg/100 ml

     Y90.4   Blood alcohol level of 80-99 mg/100 ml

     Y90.5   Blood alcohol level of 100-119 mg/100 ml

     Y90.6   Blood alcohol level of 120-199 mg/100 ml

     Y90.7   Blood alcohol level of 200-239 mg/100 ml

     Y90.8   Blood alcohol level of 240 mg/100 ml or more

     Y90.9   Presence of alcohol in blood, level not specified

---

OGCR   Section I.C.20.b.

20.9 Place of Occurrence

Place of Occurrence Guideline

Codes from category Y92, Place of occurrence of the external cause, are secondary codes for use after other external cause codes to identify the location of the patient at the time of injury or other condition.

A place of occurrence code is used only once, at the initial encounter for treatment. No 7th characters are used for Y92. Only one code from Y92 should be recorded on a medical record. A place of occurrence code should be used in conjunction with an activity code, Y93.

Do not use place of occurrence code Y92.9 if the place is not stated or is not applicable.

● **Y92**   **Place of occurrence of the external cause**

     The following category is for use, when relevant, to identify the place of occurrence of the external cause. Use in conjunction with an activity code.

     Place of occurrence should be recorded only at the initial encounter for treatment

     ● **Y92.0**   **Non-institutional (private) residence as the place of occurrence of the external cause**

         Excludes1   abandoned or derelict house (Y92.89)
                   home under construction but not yet occupied (Y92.6-)
                   institutional place of residence (Y92.1-)

         ● **Y92.00**   Unspecified non-institutional (private) residence as the place of occurrence of the external cause

            ■ **Y92.000**   Kitchen of unspecified non-institutional (private) residence as the place of occurrence of the external cause

            ■ **Y92.001**   Dining room of unspecified non-institutional (private) residence as the place of occurrence of the external cause

            ■ **Y92.002**   Bathroom of unspecified non-institutional private) residence single-family (private) house as the place of occurrence of the external cause

            ■ **Y92.003**   Bedroom of unspecified non-institutional (private) residence as the place of occurrence of the external cause

            ■ **Y92.007**   Garden or yard of unspecified non-institutional (private) residence as the place of occurrence of the external cause

            ■ **Y92.008**   Other place in unspecified non-institutional (private) residence as the place of occurrence of the external cause

            ■ **Y92.009**   Unspecified place in unspecified non-institutional (private) residence as the place of occurrence of the external cause

                 Home (NOS) as the place of occurrence of the external cause

---

N   Newborn Age: 0   **P**   Pediatric Age: 0–17   **M**   Maternity DX: 12–55   **A**   Adult Age: 15–124   ♀   Females Only   ♂   Males Only

🔍   Complication\Comorbidity   🔍   Major C\C   🔍   Present on Admission Requirement   🔍   Hospital-Acquired Condition

1781

● **Y92.01 Single-family non-institutional (private) house as the place of occurrence of the external cause**
Farmhouse as the place of occurrence of the external cause

Excludes1   barn (Y92.71)
chicken coop or hen house (Y92.72)
farm field (Y92.73)
orchard (Y92.74)
single family mobile home or trailer (Y92.02-)
slaughter house (Y92.86)

Y92.010   Kitchen of single-family (private) house as the place of occurrence of the external cause

Y92.011   Dining room of single-family (private) house as the place of occurrence of the external cause

Y92.012   Bathroom of single-family (private) house as the place of occurrence of the external cause

Y92.013   Bedroom of single-family (private) house as the place of occurrence of the external cause

Y92.014   Private driveway to single-family (private) house as the place of occurrence of the external cause

Y92.015   Private garage of single-family (private) house as the place of occurrence of the external cause

Y92.016   Swimming pool in single-family (private) house or garden as the place of occurrence of the external cause

Y92.017   Garden or yard in single-family (private) house as the place of occurrence of the external cause

Y92.018   Other place in single-family (private) house as the place of occurrence of the external cause

Y92.019   Unspecified place in single-family (private) house as the place of occurrence of the external cause

● **Y92.02 Mobile home as the place of occurrence of the external cause**

Y92.020   Kitchen in mobile home as the place of occurrence of the external cause

Y92.021   Dining room in mobile home as the place of occurrence of the external cause

Y92.022   Bathroom in mobile home as the place of occurrence of the external cause

Y92.023   Bedroom in mobile home as the place of occurrence of the external cause

Y92.024   Driveway of mobile home as the place of occurrence of the external cause

Y92.025   Garage of mobile home as the place of occurrence of the external cause

Y92.026   Swimming pool of mobile home as the place of occurrence of the external cause

Y92.027   Garden or yard of mobile home as the place of occurrence of the external cause

Y92.028   Other place in mobile home as the place of occurrence of the external cause

Y92.029   Unspecified place in mobile home as the place of occurrence of the external cause

● **Y92.03 Apartment as the place of occurrence of the external cause**
Condominium as the place of occurrence of the external cause
Co-op apartment as the place of occurrence of the external cause

Y92.030   Kitchen in apartment as the place of occurrence of the external cause

Y92.031   Bathroom in apartment as the place of occurrence of the external cause

Y92.032   Bedroom in apartment as the place of occurrence of the external cause

Y92.038   Other place in apartment as the place of occurrence of the external cause

Y92.039   Unspecified place in apartment as the place of occurrence of the external cause

● **Y92.04 Boarding-house as the place of occurrence of the external cause**

Y92.040   Kitchen in boarding-house as the place of occurrence of the external cause

Y92.041   Bathroom in boarding-house as the place of occurrence of the external cause

Y92.042   Bedroom in boarding-house as the place of occurrence of the external cause

Y92.043   Driveway of boarding-house as the place of occurrence of the external cause

Y92.044   Garage of boarding-house as the place of occurrence of the external cause

Y92.045   Swimming pool of boarding-house as the place of occurrence of the external cause

Y92.046   Garden or yard of boarding-house as the place of occurrence of the external cause

Y92.048   Other place in boarding-house as the place of occurrence of the external cause

Y92.049   Unspecified place in boarding-house as the place of occurrence of the external cause

● Unacceptable Principal Diagnosis   ● Use Additional Character(s)   ■ Unspecified   ▶ Manifestation Code
OGCR Official Guidelines for Coding and Reporting   Excludes 1   Excludes 2   Includes   Use additional   Code first   Code also

● **Y92.09 Other non-institutional residence as the place of occurrence of the external cause**

   Y92.090   Kitchen in other non-institutional residence as the place of occurrence of the external cause

   Y92.091   Bathroom in other non-institutional residence as the place of occurrence of the external cause

   Y92.092   Bedroom in other non-institutional residence as the place of occurrence of the external cause

   Y92.093   Driveway of other non-institutional residence as the place of occurrence of the external cause

   Y92.094   Garage of other non-institutional residence as the place of occurrence of the external cause

   Y92.095   Swimming pool of other non-institutional residence as the place of occurrence of the external cause

   Y92.096   Garden or yard of other non-institutional residence as the place of occurrence of the external cause

   Y92.098   Other place in other non-institutional residence as the place of occurrence of the external cause

   Y92.099   Unspecified place in other non-institutional residence as the place of occurrence of the external cause

● **Y92.1 Institutional (nonprivate) residence as the place of occurrence of the external cause**

   Y92.10   Unspecified residential institution as the place of occurrence of the external cause

●   Y92.11   Children's home and orphanage as the place of occurrence of the external cause

   Y92.110   Kitchen in children's home and orphanage as the place of occurrence of the external cause

   Y92.111   Bathroom in children's home and orphanage as the place of occurrence of the external cause

   Y92.112   Bedroom in children's home and orphanage as the place of occurrence of the external cause

   Y92.113   Driveway of children's home and orphanage as the place of occurrence of the external cause

   Y92.114   Garage of children's home and orphanage as the place of occurrence of the external cause

   Y92.115   Swimming pool of children's home and orphanage as the place of occurrence of the external cause

   Y92.116   Garden or yard of children's home and orphanage as the place of occurrence of the external cause

   Y92.118   Other place in children's home and orphanage as the place of occurrence of the external cause

   Y92.119   Unspecified place in children's home and orphanage as the place of occurrence of the external cause

● **Y92.12 Nursing home as the place of occurrence of the external cause**

   Home for the sick as the place of occurrence of the external cause

   Hospice as the place of occurrence of the external cause

   Y92.120   Kitchen in nursing home as the place of occurrence of the external cause

   Y92.121   Bathroom in nursing home as the place of occurrence of the external cause

   Y92.122   Bedroom in nursing home as the place of occurrence of the external cause

   Y92.123   Driveway of nursing home as the place of occurrence of the external cause

   Y92.124   Garage of nursing home as the place of occurrence of the external cause

   Y92.125   Swimming pool of nursing home as the place of occurrence of the external cause

   Y92.126   Garden or yard of nursing home as the place of occurrence of the external cause

   Y92.128   Other place in nursing home as the place of occurrence of the external cause

   Y92.129   Unspecified place in nursing home as the place of occurrence of the external cause

● **Y92.13 Military base as the place of occurrence of the external cause**

   Excludes1   military training grounds (Y92.83)

   Y92.130   Kitchen on military base as the place of occurrence of the external cause

   Y92.131   Mess hall on military base as the place of occurrence of the external cause

   Y92.133   Barracks on military base as the place of occurrence of the external cause

   Y92.135   Garage on military base as the place of occurrence of the external cause

   Y92.136   Swimming pool on military base as the place of occurrence of the external cause

   Y92.137   Garden or yard on military base as the place of occurrence of the external cause

   Y92.138   Other place on military base as the place of occurrence of the external cause

   Y92.139   Unspecified place military base as the place of occurrence of the external cause

● **Y92.14** Prison as the place of occurrence of the external cause

     Y92.140 Kitchen in prison as the place of occurrence of the external cause

     Y92.141 Dining room in prison as the place of occurrence of the external cause

     Y92.142 Bathroom in prison as the place of occurrence of the external cause

     Y92.143 Cell of prison as the place of occurrence of the external cause

     Y92.146 Swimming pool of prison as the place of occurrence of the external cause

     Y92.147 Courtyard of prison as the place of occurrence of the external cause

     Y92.148 Other place in prison as the place of occurrence of the external cause

     ▪ Y92.149 Unspecified place in prison as the place of occurrence of the external cause

● **Y92.15** Reform school as the place of occurrence of the external cause

     Y92.150 Kitchen in reform school as the place of occurrence of the external cause

     Y92.151 Dining room in reform school as the place of occurrence of the external cause

     Y92.152 Bathroom in reform school as the place of occurrence of the external cause

     Y92.153 Bedroom in reform school as the place of occurrence of the external cause

     Y92.154 Driveway of reform school as the place of occurrence of the external cause

     Y92.155 Garage of reform school as the place of occurrence of the external cause

     Y92.156 Swimming pool of reform school as the place of occurrence of the external cause

     Y92.157 Garden or yard of reform school as the place of occurrence of the external cause

     Y92.158 Other place in reform school as the place of occurrence of the external cause

     ▪ Y92.159 Unspecified place in reform school as the place of occurrence of the external cause

● **Y92.16** School dormitory as the place of occurrence of the external cause

     Excludes1   reform school as the place of occurrence of the external cause (Y92.15-)
                 school buildings and grounds as the place of occurrence of the external cause (Y92.2-)
                 school sports and athletic areas as the place of occurrence of the external cause (Y92.3-)

     Y92.160 Kitchen in school dormitory as the place of occurrence of the external cause

     Y92.161 Dining room in school dormitory as the place of occurrence of the external cause

     Y92.162 Bathroom in school dormitory as the place of occurrence of the external cause

     Y92.163 Bedroom in school dormitory as the place of occurrence of the external cause

     Y92.168 Other place in school dormitory as the place of occurrence of the external cause

     ▪ Y92.169 Unspecified place in school dormitory as the place of occurrence of the external cause

● **Y92.19** Other specified residential institution as the place of occurrence of the external cause

     Y92.190 Kitchen in other specified residential institution as the place of occurrence of the external cause

     Y92.191 Dining room in other specified residential institution as the place of occurrence of the external cause

     Y92.192 Bathroom in other specified residential institution as the place of occurrence of the external cause

     Y92.193 Bedroom in other specified residential institution as the place of occurrence of the external cause

     Y92.194 Driveway of other specified residential institution as the place of occurrence of the external cause

     Y92.195 Garage of other specified residential institution as the place of occurrence of the external cause

     Y92.196 Pool of other specified residential institution as the place of occurrence of the external cause

     Y92.197 Garden or yard of other specified residential institution as the place of occurrence of the external cause

     Y92.198 Other place in other specified residential institution as the place of occurrence of the external cause

     ▪ Y92.199 Unspecified place in other specified residential institution as the place of occurrence of the external cause

● Unacceptable Principal Diagnosis   ◗ Use Additional Character(s)   ▪ Unspecified   ▸ Manifestation Code

OGCR Official Guidelines for Coding and Reporting   Excludes 1   Excludes 2   Includes   Use additional   Code first   Code also

● **Y92.2   School, other institution and public administrative area as the place of occurrence of the external cause**
Building and adjacent grounds used by the general public or by a particular group of the public

Excludes1   building under construction as the place of occurrence of the external cause (Y92.6)
residential institution as the place of occurrence of the external cause (Y92.1)
school dormitory as the place of occurrence of the external cause (Y92.16-)
sports and athletics area of schools as the place of occurrence of the external cause (Y92.3-)

● **Y92.21   School (private) (public) (state) as the place of occurrence of the external cause**

Y92.210   Daycare center as the place of occurrence of the external cause 🕮

Y92.211   Elementary school as the place of occurrence of the external cause 🕮
Kindergarten as the place of occurrence of the external cause

Y92.212   Middle school as the place of occurrence of the external cause 🕮

Y92.213   High school as the place of occurrence of the external cause 🕮

Y92.214   College as the place of occurrence of the external cause 🕮
University as the place of occurrence of the external cause

Y92.215   Trade school as the place of occurrence of the external cause 🕮

Y92.218   Other school as the place of occurrence of the external cause 🕮

■ Y92.219   Unspecified school as the place of occurrence of the external cause 🕮

Y92.22   Religious institution as the place of occurrence of the external cause 🕮
Church as the place of occurrence of the external cause
Mosque as the place of occurrence of the external cause
Synagogue as the place of occurrence of the external cause

● **Y92.23   Hospital as the place of occurrence of the external cause**

Excludes1   ambulatory (outpatient) health services establishments (Y92.53-)
home for the sick as the place of occurrence of the external cause (Y92.12-)
hospice as the place of occurrence of the external cause (Y92.12-)
nursing home as the place of occurrence of the external cause (Y92.12-)

Y92.230   Patient room in hospital as the place of occurrence of the external cause

Y92.231   Patient bathroom in hospital as the place of occurrence of the external cause

Y92.232   Corridor of hospital as the place of occurrence of the external cause

Y92.233   Cafeteria of hospital as the place of occurrence of the external cause

Y92.234   Operating room of hospital as the place of occurrence of the external cause

Y92.238   Other place in hospital as the place of occurrence of the external cause

■ Y92.239   Unspecified place in hospital as the place of occurrence of the external cause

● **Y92.24   Public administrative building as the place of occurrence of the external cause**

Y92.240   Courthouse as the place of occurrence of the external cause 🕮

Y92.241   Library as the place of occurrence of the external cause 🕮

Y92.242   Post office as the place of occurrence of the external cause 🕮

Y92.243   City hall as the place of occurrence of the external cause 🕮

Y92.248   Other public administrative building as the place of occurrence of the external cause 🕮

● **Y92.25   Cultural building as the place of occurrence of the external cause**

Y92.250   Art gallery as the place of occurrence of the external cause 🕮

Y92.251   Museum as the place of occurrence of the external cause 🕮

Y92.252 Music hall as the place of occurrence of the external cause

Y92.253 Opera house as the place of occurrence of the external cause

Y92.254 Theater (live) as the place of occurrence of the external cause

Y92.258 Other cultural public building as the place of occurrence of the external cause

Y92.26 Movie house or cinema as the place of occurrence of the external cause

Y92.29 Other specified public building as the place of occurrence of the external cause

Assembly hall as the place of occurrence of the external cause
Clubhouse as the place of occurrence of the external cause

● Y92.3 Sports and athletics area as the place of occurrence of the external cause

● Y92.31 Athletic court as the place of occurrence of the external cause

Excludes1 tennis court in private home or garden (Y92.09)

Y92.310 Basketball court as the place of occurrence of the external cause

Y92.311 Squash court as the place of occurrence of the external cause

Y92.312 Tennis court as the place of occurrence of the external cause

Y92.318 Other athletic court as the place of occurrence of the external cause

● Y92.32 Athletic field as the place of occurrence of the external cause

Y92.320 Baseball field as the place of occurrence of the external cause

Y92.321 Football field as the place of occurrence of the external cause

Y92.322 Soccer field as the place of occurrence of the external cause

Y92.328 Other athletic field as the place of occurrence of the external cause

Cricket field as the place of occurrence of the external cause
Hockey field as the place of occurrence of the external cause

● Y92.33 Skating rink as the place of occurrence of the external cause

Y92.330 Ice skating rink (indoor) (outdoor) as the place of occurrence of the external cause

Y92.331 Roller skating rink as the place of occurrence of the external cause

Y92.34 Swimming pool (public) as the place of occurrence of the external cause

Excludes1 swimming pool in private home or garden (Y92.016)

Y92.39 Other specified sports and athletic area as the place of occurrence of the external cause

Golf-course as the place of occurrence of the external cause
Gymnasium as the place of occurrence of the external cause
Riding-school as the place of occurrence of the external cause
Stadium as the place of occurrence of the external cause

● Y92.4 Street, highway and other paved roadways as the place of occurrence of the external cause

Excludes1 private driveway of residence (Y92.0x4, Y92.1x3)

● Y92.41 Street and highway as the place of occurrence of the external cause

■ Y92.410 Unspecified street and highway as the place of occurrence of the external cause

Road NOS as the place of occurrence of the external cause

Y92.411 Interstate highway as the place of occurrence of the external cause

Freeway as the place of occurrence of the external cause
Motorway as the place of occurrence of the external cause

Y92.412 Parkway as the place of occurrence of the external cause

Y92.413 State road as the place of occurrence of the external cause

Y92.414 Local residential or business street as the place of occurrence of the external cause

Y92.415 Exit ramp or entrance ramp of street or highway as the place of occurrence of the external cause

● Y92.48 Other paved roadways as the place of occurrence of the external cause

Y92.480 Sidewalk as the place of occurrence of the external cause

Y92.481 Parking lot as the place of occurrence of the external cause

Y92.482 Bike path as the place of occurrence of the external cause

Y92.488 Other paved roadways as the place of occurrence of the external cause

● Unacceptable Principal Diagnosis   ● Use Additional Character(s)   ■ Unspecified   ▶ Manifestation Code

OGCR Official Guidelines for Coding and Reporting | Excludes 1 | | Excludes 2 | | Includes | | Use additional | | Code first | | Code also |

● **Y92.5**   **Trade and service area as the place of occurrence of the external cause**

    Excludes1   garage in private home (Y92.015)
                schools and other public
                administration buildings (Y92.2-)

● **Y92.51**   **Private commercial establishments as the place of occurrence of the external cause**

    Y92.510   **Bank as the place of occurrence of the external cause** 🖐

    Y92.511   **Restaurant or café as the place of occurrence of the external cause** 🖐

    Y92.512   **Supermarket, store or market as the place of occurrence of the external cause** 🖐

    Y92.513   **Shop (commercial) as the place of occurrence of the external cause** 🖐

● **Y92.52**   **Service areas as the place of occurrence of the external cause**

    Y92.520   **Airport as the place of occurrence of the external cause** 🖐

    Y92.521   **Bus station as the place of occurrence of the external cause** 🖐

    Y92.522   **Railway station as the place of occurrence of the external cause** 🖐

    Y92.523   **Highway rest stop as the place of occurrence of the external cause** 🖐

    Y92.524   **Gas station as the place of occurrence of the external cause** 🖐

       Petroleum station as the place of occurrence of the external cause

       Service station as the place of occurrence of the external cause

● **Y92.53**   **Ambulatory health services establishments as the place of occurrence of the external cause**

    Y92.530   **Ambulatory surgery center as the place of occurrence of the external cause** 🖐

       Outpatient surgery center, including that connected with a hospital as the place of occurrence of the external cause

       Same day surgery center, including that connected with a hospital as the place of occurrence of the external cause

    Y92.531   **Health care provider office as the place of occurrence of the external cause** 🖐

       Physician office as the place of occurrence of the external cause

    Y92.532   **Urgent care center as the place of occurrence of the external cause** 🖐

    Y92.538   **Other ambulatory health services establishments as the place of occurrence of the external cause** 🖐

● **Y92.59**   **Other trade areas as the place of occurrence of the external cause** 🖐

       Office building as the place of occurrence of the external cause

       Casino as the place of occurrence of the external cause

       Garage (commercial) as the place of occurrence of the external cause

       Hotel as the place of occurrence of the external cause

       Radio or television station as the place of occurrence of the external cause

       Shopping mall as the place of occurrence of the external cause

       Warehouse as the place of occurrence of the external cause

● **Y92.6**   **Industrial and construction area as the place of occurrence of the external cause**

    Y92.61   **Building [any] under construction as the place of occurrence of the external cause** 🖐

    Y92.62   **Dock or shipyard as the place of occurrence of the external cause** 🖐

       Dockyard as the place of occurrence of the external cause

       Dry dock as the place of occurrence of the external cause

       Shipyard as the place of occurrence of the external cause

    Y92.63   **Factory as the place of occurrence of the external cause** 🖐

       Factory building as the place of occurrence of the external cause

       Factory premises as the place of occurrence of the external cause

       Industrial yard as the place of occurrence of the external cause

    Y92.64   **Mine or pit as the place of occurrence of the external cause** 🖐

       Mine as the place of occurrence of the external cause

    Y92.65   **Oil rig as the place of occurrence of the external cause** 🖐

       Pit (coal) (gravel) (sand) as the place of occurrence of the external cause

    Y92.69   **Other specified industrial and construction area as the place of occurrence of the external cause** 🖐

       Gasworks as the place of occurrence of the external cause

       Power-station (coal) (nuclear) (oil) as the place of occurrence of the external cause

       Tunnel under construction as the place of occurrence of the external cause

       Workshop as the place of occurrence of the external cause

● **Y92.7**   **Farm as the place of occurrence of the external cause**

       Ranch as the place of occurrence of the external cause

    Excludes1   farmhouse and home premises of farm (Y92.01-)

    Y92.71   **Barn as the place of occurrence of the external cause** 🖐

    Y92.72   **Chicken coop as the place of occurrence of the external cause** 🖐

       Hen house as the place of occurrence of the external cause

N Newborn Age: 0   **P** Pediatric Age: 0–17   **M** Maternity DX: 12–55   **A** Adult Age: 15–124   ♀ Females Only   ♂ Males Only

🖐 Complication\Comorbidity   🖐 Major C\C   🖐 Present on Admission Requirement   🖐 Hospital-Acquired Condition

1787

Y92.73   Farm field as the place of occurrence of the external cause ✎

Y92.74   Orchard as the place of occurrence of the external cause ✎

Y92.79   Other farm location as the place of occurrence of the external cause ✎

● Y92.8   Other places as the place of occurrence of the external cause

   ● Y92.81   Transport vehicle as the place of occurrence of the external cause

      Excludes1   transport accidents (V00-V99)

      Y92.810   Car as the place of occurrence of the external cause ✎

      Y92.811   Bus as the place of occurrence of the external cause ✎

      Y92.812   Truck as the place of occurrence of the external cause ✎

      Y92.813   Airplane as the place of occurrence of the external cause ✎

      Y92.814   Boat as the place of occurrence of the external cause ✎

      Y92.815   Train as the place of occurrence of the external cause ✎

      Y92.816   Subway car as the place of occurrence of the external cause ✎

      Y92.818   Other transport vehicle as the place of occurrence of the external cause ✎

   ● Y92.82   Wilderness area

      Y92.820   Desert as the place of occurrence of the external cause ✎

      Y92.821   Forest as the place of occurrence of the external cause ✎

      Y92.828   Other wilderness area as the place of occurrence of the external cause ✎
               Swamp as the place of occurrence of the external cause
               Mountain as the place of occurrence of the external cause
               Marsh as the place of occurrence of the external cause
               Prairie as the place of occurrence of the external cause

   ● Y92.83   Recreation area as the place of occurrence of the external cause

      Y92.830   Public park as the place of occurrence of the external cause ✎

      Y92.831   Amusement park as the place of occurrence of the external cause ✎

      Y92.832   Beach as the place of occurrence of the external cause ✎
               Seashore as the place of occurrence of the external cause

      Y92.833   Campsite as the place of occurrence of the external cause ✎

      Y92.834   Zoological garden (zoo) as the place of occurrence of the external cause ✎

      Y92.838   Other recreation area as the place of occurrence of the external cause ✎

   Y92.84   Military training ground as the place of occurrence of the external cause ✎

   Y92.85   Railroad track as the place of occurrence of the external cause ✎

   Y92.86   Slaughter house as the place of occurrence of the external cause ✎

   Y92.89   Other specified places as the place of occurrence of the external cause ✎
            Derelict house as the place of occurrence of the external cause

■ Y92.9   Unspecified place or not applicable ✎

   OGCR   See Section I.C.20.c.

   Activity code

● Y93   Activity codes

   Note: Category Y93 is provided for use to indicate the activity of the person seeking healthcare for an injury or health condition, such as a heart attack while shoveling snow, which resulted from, or was contributed to, by the activity. These codes are appropriate for use for both acute injuries, such as those from chapter 19, and conditions that are due to the long-term, cumulative effects of an activity, such as those from chapter 13. They are also appropriate for use with external cause codes for cause and intent if identifying the activity provides additional information on the event. These codes should be used in conjunction with codes for external cause status (Y99) and place of occurrence (Y92).

   This section contains the following broad activity categories:

      Y93.0   Activities involving walking and running

      Y93.1   Activities involving water and water craft

      Y93.2   Activities involving ice and snow

      Y93.3   Activities involving climbing, rappelling, and jumping off

      Y93.4   Activities involving dancing and other rhythmic movement

      Y93.5   Activities involving other sports and athletics played individually

      Y93.6   Activities involving other sports and athletics played as a team or group

      Y93.7   Activities involving other specified sports and athletics

      Y93.A   Activities involving other cardiorespiratory exercise

      Y93.B   Activities involving other muscle strengthening exercises

      Y93.C   Activities involving computer technology and electronic devices

      Y93.D   Activities involving arts and handcrafts

      Y93.E   Activities involving personal hygiene and interior property and clothing maintenance

      Y93.F   Activities involving caregiving

      Y93.G   Activities involving food preparation, cooking and grilling

● Unaccceptable Principal Diagnosis   ● Use Additional Character(s)   ■ Unspecified   ▶ Manifestation Code

OGCR   Official Guidelines for Coding and Reporting   Excludes 1   Excludes 2   Includes   Use additional   Code first   Code also

Y93.H   Activities involving exterior property and land maintenance, building and construction

Y93.I   Activities involving roller coasters and other types of external motion

Y93.J   Activities involving playing musical instrument

Y93.K   Activities involving animal care

Y93.8   Activities, other specified

Y93.9   Activity, unspecified

● **Y93.0   Activities involving walking and running**

> Excludes1   Activity, walking an animal (Y93.K1)
> Activity, walking or running on a treadmill (Y93.A1)

Y93.01   Activity, walking, marching and hiking
Activity, walking, marching and hiking on level or elevated terrain

> Excludes1   activity, mountain climbing (Y93.31)

Y93.02   Activity, running

● **Y93.1   Activities involving water and water craft**

> Excludes1   activities involving ice (Y93.2-)

Y93.11   Activity, swimming

Y93.12   Activity, springboard and platform diving

Y93.13   Activity, water polo

Y93.14   Activity, water aerobics and water exercise

Y93.15   Activity, underwater diving and snorkeling
Activity, SCUBA diving

Y93.16   Activity, rowing, canoeing, kayaking, rafting and tubing
Activity, canoeing, kayaking, rafting and tubing in calm and turbulent water

Y93.17   Activity, water skiing and wake boarding

Y93.18   Activity, surfing, windsurfing and boogie boarding
Activity, water sliding

Y93.19   Activity, other involving water and watercraft
Activity involving water NOS
Activity, parasailing
Activity, water survival training and testing

● **Y93.2   Activities involving ice and snow**

> Excludes1   activity, shoveling ice and snow (Y93.H1)

Y93.21   Activity, ice skating
Activity, figure skating (singles) (pairs)
Activity, ice dancing

> Excludes1   activity, ice hockey (Y93.22)

Y93.22   Activity, ice hockey

Y93.23   Activity, snow (alpine) (downhill) skiing, snow boarding, sledding, tobogganing and snow tubing

> Excludes1   activity, cross country skiing (Y93.24)

Y93.24   Activity, cross country skiing
Activity, nordic skiing

Y93.29   Activity, other activity involving ice and snow
Activity, activity involving ice and snow NOS

● **Y93.3   Activities involving climbing, rappelling and jumping off**

> Excludes1   activity, hiking on level or elevated terrain (Y93.01)
> activity, jumping rope (Y93.56)
> activity, trampoline jumping (Y93.44)

Y93.31   Activity, mountain climbing, rock climbing and wall climbing

Y93.32   Activity, rappelling

Y93.33   Activity, BASE jumping
Activity, building, Antenna, Span, Earth jumping

Y93.34   Activity, bungee jumping

Y93.35   Activity, hang gliding

Y93.39   Activity, other activity involving climbing, rappelling and jumping off

● **Y93.4   Activities involving dancing and other rhythmic movement**

> Excludes1   activity, martial arts (Y93.75)

Y93.41   Activity, dancing

Y93.42   Activity, yoga

Y93.43   Activity, gymnastics
Activity, rhythmic gymnastics

> Excludes1   activity, trampolining (Y93.44)

Y93.44   Activity, trampolining

Y93.45   Activity, cheerleading

Y93.49   Activity, other involving dancing and other rhythmic movements

● **Y93.5   Activities involving other sports and athletics played individually**

> Excludes1   activity, dancing (Y93.41)
> activity, gymnastic (Y93.43)
> activity, trampolining (Y93.44)
> activity, yoga (Y93.42)

Y93.51   Activity, roller skating (inline) and skateboarding

Y93.52   Activity, horseback riding

Y93.53   Activity, golf

Y93.54   Activity, bowling

Y93.55   Activity, bike riding

Y93.56   Activity, jumping rope

Y93.57   Activity, non-running track and field events

> Excludes1   activity, running (any form) (Y93.02)

Y93.59   Activity, other involving other sports and athletics played individually

> Excludes1   activities involving climbing, rappelling, and jumping (Y93.3-)
> activities involving ice and snow (Y93.2-)
> activities involving walking and running (Y93.0-)
> activities involving water and watercraft (Y93.1-)

● **Y93.6 Activities involving other sports and athletics played as a team or group**

> **Excludes1**   activity, ice hockey (Y93.22)
> activity, water polo (Y93.13)

Y93.61 Activity, American tackle football
Activity, football NOS

Y93.62 Activity, American flag or touch football

Y93.63 Activity, rugby

Y93.64 Activity, baseball
Activity, softball

Y93.65 Activity, lacrosse and field hockey

Y93.66 Activity, soccer

Y93.67 Activity, basketball

Y93.68 Activity, volleyball (beach) (court)

Y93.6A Activity, physical games generally associated with school recess, summer camp and children   P
Activity, capture the flag
Activity, dodge ball
Activity, four square
Activity, kickball

Y93.69 Activity, other involving other sports and athletics played as a team or group
Cricket

● **Y93.7 Activities involving other specified sports and athletics**

Y93.71 Activity, boxing

Y93.72 Activity, wrestling

Y93.73 Activity, racquet and hand sports
Activity, handball
Activity, racquetball
Activity, squash
Activity, tennis

Y93.74 Activity, frisbee
Activity, ultimate frisbee

Y93.75 Activity, martial arts
Activity, combatives

Y93.79 Activity, other specified sports and athletics

> **Excludes1**   sports and athletics activities specified in categories Y93.0-Y93.6

● **Y93.A Activities involving other cardiorespiratory exercise**
Activities involving physical training

Y93.A1 Activity, exercise machines primarily for cardiorespiratory conditioning
Activity, elliptical and stepper machines
Activity, stationary bike
Activity, treadmill

Y93.A2 Activity, calisthenics
Activity, jumping jacks
Activity, warm up and cool down

Y93.A3 Activity, aerobic and step exercise

Y93.A4 Activity, circuit training

Y93.A5 Activity, obstacle course
Activity, challenge course
Activity, confidence course

Y93.A6 Activity, grass drills
Activity, guerilla drills

Y93.A9 Activity, other involving other cardiorespiratory exercise

> **Excludes1**   activities involving cardiorespiratory exercise specified in categories Y93.0-Y93.7

● **Y93.B Activity involving other muscle strengthening exercises**

Y93.B1 Activity, exercise machines primarily for muscle strengthening

Y93.B2 Activity, push-ups, pull-ups, sit-ups

Y93.B3 Activity, free weights
Activity, barbells
Activity, dumbbells

Y93.B4 Activity, pilates

Y93.B9 Activity, other involving other muscle strengthening exercises

> **Excludes1**   activities involving muscle strengthening specified in categories Y93.0-Y93.A

● **Y93.C Activities involving computer technology and electronic devices**

> **Excludes1**   activity, electronic musical keyboard or instruments (Y93.J-)

Y93.C1 Activity, computer keyboarding
Activity, electronic game playing using keyboard or other stationary device

Y93.C2 Activity, hand held interactive electronic device
Activity, cellular telephone and communication device
Activity, electronic game playing using interactive device

> **Excludes1**   activity, electronic game playing using keyboard or other stationary device (Y93.C1)

Y93.C9 Activity, other involving computer technology and electronic devices

● **Y93.D Activities involving arts and handcrafts**

> **Excludes1**   activities involving playing musical instrument (Y93.J-)

Y93.D1 Knitting and crocheting

Y93.D2 Sewing

Y93.D3 Furniture building and finishing
Furniture repair

Y93.D9 Activity, other involving arts and handcrafts

● **Y93.E Activities involving personal hygiene and interior property and clothing maintenance**

> **Excludes1**   activities involving cooking and grilling (Y93.G-)
> activities involving exterior property and land maintenance, building and construction (Y93.H-)
> activity involving caregiving (Y93.F-)
> activity, dishwashing (Y93.G1)
> activity, food preparation (Y93.G1)
> activity, gardening (Y93.H2)

Y93.E1 Activity, personal bathing and showering

Y93.E2 Activity, laundry

Y93.E3 Activity, vacuuming

Y93.E4 Activity, ironing

Y93.E5 Activity, floor mopping and cleaning

● Unacceptable Principal Diagnosis   ◑ Use Additional Character(s)   ■ Unspecified   ▶ Manifestation Code

OGCR Official Guidelines for Coding and Reporting   Excludes 1   Excludes 2   Includes   Use additional   Code first   Code also

Y93.E6   **Activity, residential relocation**
    Activity, packing up and unpacking involved in moving to a new residence

Y93.E8   **Activity, other personal hygiene activity**

Y93.E9   **Activity, other household maintenance**

● **Y93.F**   **Activities involving person providing caregiving**
    Activity involving the provider of caregiving

    Y93.F1   **Activity, caregiving involving bathing**

    Y93.F2   **Activity, caregiving involving lifting**

    Y93.F9   **Activity, other caregiving**

● **Y93.G**   **Activities involving food preparation, cooking and grilling**

    Y93.G1   **Activity, food preparation and clean up**
       Activity, dishwashing

    Y93.G2   **Activity, grilling and smoking food**

    Y93.G3   **Activity, cooking and baking**
       Activity, use of stove, oven and microwave oven

    Y93.G9   **Activity, other activity involving cooking and grilling**

● **Y93.H**   **Activities involving property and land maintenance, building and construction**

    Y93.H1   **Activity, digging, shoveling and raking**
       Activity, dirt digging
       Activity, raking leaves
       Activity, snow shoveling

    Y93.H2   **Activity, gardening and landscaping**
       Activity, pruning, trimming shrubs, weeding

    Y93.H3   **Activity, building and construction**

    Y93.H9   **Activity, other activity involving property and land maintenance, building and construction**

● **Y93.I**   **Activities involving roller coasters and other types of external motion**

    Y93.I1   **Activity, rollercoaster riding**

    Y93.I9   **Activity, other involving external motion**

● **Y93.J**   **Activities involving playing musical instrument**
    Activity involving playing electric musical instrument

    Y93.J1   **Activity, piano playing**
       Activity, musical keyboard (electronic) playing

    Y93.J2   **Activity, drum and other percussion instrument playing**

    Y93.J3   **Activity, string instrument playing**

    Y93.J4   **Activity, winds and brass instrument playing**

● **Y93.K**   **Activities involving animal care**
    Excludes1   activity, horseback riding (Y93.52)

    Y93.K1   **Activity, walking an animal**

    Y93.K2   **Activity, milking an animal**

    Y93.K3   **Activity, grooming and shearing an animal**

    Y93.K9   **Activity, other activity involving animal care**

● **Y93.8**   **Other activity**

    Y93.81   **Activity, refereeing a sports activity**

    Y93.82   **Activity, spectator at an event**

    Y93.83   **Activity, rough housing and horseplay**

    Y93.84   **Activity, sleeping**

    Y93.89   **Activity, other specified**

● **Y93.9**   **Activity, unspecified**

    Y95   **Nosocomial condition**

● **Y99**   **External cause status**

    Note: A single code from category Y99 should be used in conjunction with the external cause code(s) assigned to a record to indicate the status of the person at the time the event occurred.

    Y99.0   **Civilian activity done for income or pay**
       Civilian activity done for financial or other compensation
       Excludes1   military activity (Y99.1)
             volunteer activity (Y99.2)

    Y99.1   **Military activity**
       Excludes1   activity of off duty military personnel (Y99.8)

    Y99.2   **Volunteer activity**
       Excludes1   activity of child or other family member assisting in compensated work of other family member (Y99.8)

    Y99.8   **Other external cause status**
       Activity NEC
       Activity of child or other family member assisting in compensated work of other family member
       Hobby not done for income
       Leisure activity
       Off-duty activity of military personnel
       Recreation or sport not for income or while a student
       Student activity
       Excludes1   civilian activity done for income or compensation (Y99.0)
               military activity (Y99.1)

■ **Y99.9**   **Unspecified external cause status**

N   Newborn Age: 0   P   Pediatric Age: 0–17   M   Maternity DX: 12–55   A   Adult Age: 15–124   ♀ Females Only   ♂ Males Only

Complication\Comorbidity   Major C\C   Present on Admission Requirement   Hospital-Acquired Condition

OGCR See Guidelines, Section II.C.21.

CHAPTER 21

FACTORS INFLUENCING HEALTH STATUS AND CONTACT WITH HEALTH SERVICES (Z00-Z99)

Note: Z codes represent reasons for encounters. A corresponding procedure code must accompany a Z code if a procedure is performed. Categories Z00-Z99 are provided for occasions when circumstances other than a disease, injury or external cause classifiable to categories A00-Y89 are recorded as 'diagnoses' or 'problems.' This can arise in two main ways:

(a) When a person who may or may not be sick encounters the health services for some specific purpose, such as to receive limited care or service for a current condition, to donate an organ or tissue, to receive prophylactic vaccination (immunization), or to discuss a problem which is in itself not a disease or injury.

(b) When some circumstance or problem is present which influences the person's health status but is not in itself a current illness or injury.

This chapter contains the following blocks:

Z00-Z13	Persons encountering health services for examination
Z14-Z15	Genetic carrier and genetic susceptibility to disease
Z16	Resistance to antimicrobial drugs
Z17	Estrogen receptor status
Z18	Retained foreign body fragments
Z20-Z28	Persons with potential health hazards related to communicable diseases
Z30-Z39	Persons encountering health services in circumstances related to reproduction
Z40-Z53	Encounters for other specific health care
Z55-Z65	Persons with potential health hazards related to socioeconomic and psychosocial circumstances
Z66	Do not resuscitate status
Z67	Blood type
Z68	Body mass index (BMI)
Z69-Z76	Persons encountering health services in other circumstances
Z77-Z99	Persons with potential health hazards related to family and personal history and certain conditions influencing health status

PERSONS ENCOUNTERING HEALTH SERVICES FOR EXAMINATIONS (Z00-Z13)

Note: Nonspecific abnormal findings disclosed at the time of these examinations are classified to categories R70-R94.

Excludes1 examinations related to pregnancy and reproduction (Z30-Z36, Z39.-)

● **Z00 Encounter for general examination without complaint, suspected or reported diagnosis**

Excludes1 encounter for examination for administrative purposes (Z02.-)

Excludes2 encounter for pre-procedural examinations (Z01.81-)
special screening examinations (Z11-Z13)

● **Z00.0 Encounter for general adult medical examination**
Encounter for adult periodic examination (annual) (physical) and any associated laboratory and radiologic examinations

Excludes1 encounter for examination of sign or symptom - code to sign or symptom
general health check-up of infant or child (Z00.12.-)

❶● **Z00.00 Encounter for general adult medical examination without abnormal findings** 🔍 A
Encounter for adult health check-up NOS

❶● **Z00.01 Encounter for general adult medical examination with abnormal findings** 🔍 A
Use additional code to identify abnormal findings

● **Z00.1 Encounter for newborn, infant and child health examinations**

● **Z00.11 Newborn health examination**
Health check for child under 29 days old
Use additional code to identify any abnormal findings
Excludes1 health check for child over 28 days old (Z00.12-)

❶● **Z00.110 Health examination for newborn under 8 days old** 🔍 N
Health check for newborn under 8 days old

❶● **Z00.111 Health examination for newborn 8 to 28 days old** 🔍 N
Health check for newborn 8 to 28 days old
Newborn weight check

● **Z00.12 Encounter for routine child health examination**
Encounter for development testing of infant or child
Health check (routine) for child over 28 days old
Excludes1 health check for child under 29 days old (Z0.11-)
health supervision of foundling or other healthy infant or child (Z76.1-Z76.2)
newborn health examination (Z00.11-)

❶● **Z00.121 Encounter for routine child health examination with abnormal findings** 🔍 P
Use additional code to identify abnormal findings

❶● **Z00.129 Encounter for routine child health examination without abnormal findings** 🔍 P
Encounter for routine child health examination NOS

❶● **Z00.2 Encounter for examination for period of rapid growth in childhood** 🔍 P

❶● **Z00.3 Encounter for examination for adolescent development state** 🔍 P
Encounter for puberty development state

❶● **Z00.5 Encounter for examination of potential donor of organ and tissue** 🔍

❶ **Z00.6 Encounter for examination for normal comparison and control in clinical research program** 🔍
Examination of participant or control in clinical research program

● Unacceptable Principal Diagnosis   ● Use Additional Character(s)   ■ Unspecified   ▶ Manifestation Code
OGCR Official Guidelines for Coding and Reporting   Excludes 1   Excludes 2   Includes   Use additional   Code first   Code also
❶ First Listed   ❶/❷ First Listed or Secondary   ❷ Secondary Only

● **Z00.7   Encounter for examination for period of delayed growth in childhood**

     ❶● **Z00.70   Encounter for examination for period of delayed growth in childhood without abnormal findings** 🔍   **P**

     ❶● **Z00.71   Encounter for examination for period of delayed growth in childhood with abnormal findings** 🔍   **P**

         Use additional code to identify abnormal findings

❶● **Z00.8   Encounter for other general examination** 🔍

         Encounter for health examination in population surveys

● **Z01   Encounter for other special examination without complaint, suspected or reported diagnosis**

     Includes   routine examination of specific system

     Note: Codes from category Z01 represent the reason for the encounter. A separate procedure code is required to identify any examinations or procedures performed.

     Excludes1   encounter for examination for administrative purposes (Z02.-)
         encounter for examination for suspected conditions, proven not to exist (Z03.-)
         encounter for laboratory and radiologic examinations as a component of general medical examinations (Z00.0-)
         encounter for laboratory, radiologic and imaging examinations for sign(s) and symptom(s) - code to the sign(s) or symptom(s)

     Excludes2   screening examinations (Z11-Z13)

● **Z01.0   Encounter for examination of eyes and vision**

     Excludes1   examination for driving license (Z02.4)

     ❶ **Z01.00   Encounter for examination of eyes and vision without abnormal findings** 🔍
         Encounter for examination of eyes and vision NOS

     ❶ **Z01.01   Encounter for examination of eyes and vision with abnormal findings** 🔍
         Use additional code to identify abnormal findings

● **Z01.1   Encounter for examination of ears and hearing**

     ❶● **Z01.10   Encounter for examination of ears and hearing without abnormal findings** 🔍
         Encounter for examination of ears and hearing NOS

     ● **Z01.11   Encounter for examination of ears and hearing with abnormal findings**

         ❶● **Z01.110   Encounter for hearing examination following failed hearing screening** 🔍

         ❶● **Z01.118   Encounter for examination of ears and hearing with other abnormal findings** 🔍
             Use additional code to identify abnormal findings

     ❶● **Z01.12   Encounter for hearing conservation and treatment** 🔍

● **Z01.2   Encounter for dental examination and cleaning**

     ❶● **Z01.20   Encounter for dental examination and cleaning without abnormal findings** 🔍
         Encounter for dental examination and cleaning NOS

     ❶● **Z01.21   Encounter for dental examination and cleaning with abnormal findings** 🔍
         Use additional code to identify abnormal findings

● **Z01.3   Encounter for examination of blood pressure**

     ❶● **Z01.30   Encounter for examination of blood pressure without abnormal findings** 🔍
         Encounter for examination of blood pressure NOS

     ❶● **Z01.31   Encounter for examination of blood pressure with abnormal findings** 🔍
         Use additional code to identify abnormal findings

● **Z01.4   Encounter for gynecological examination**

     Excludes2   pregnancy examination or test (Z32.0-)
         routine examination for contraceptive maintenance (Z30.4-)

     ● **Z01.41   Encounter for routine gynecological examination**
         Encounter for general gynecological examination with or without cervical smear
         Encounter for gynecological examination (general) (routine) NOS
         Encounter for pelvic examination (annual) (periodic)

         Use additional code:
         for screening for human papillomavirus, if applicable (Z11.51)
         for screening vaginal pap smear, if applicable (Z12.72)
         to identify acquired absence of uterus, if applicable (Z90.71-)

         Excludes1   gynecologic examination status-post hysterectomy for malignant condition (Z08)
             screening cervical pap smear not a part of a routine gynecological examination (Z12.4)

         ❶ **Z01.411   Encounter for gynecological examination (general) (routine) with abnormal findings** ♀ 🔍

         ❶ **Z01.419   Encounter for gynecological examination (general) (routine) without abnormal findings** ♀ 🔍
             Use additional code to identify abnormal findings

     ❶ **Z01.42   Encounter for cervical smear to confirm findings of recent normal smear following initial abnormal smear** ♀ 🔍

N   Newborn Age: 0   **P**   Pediatric Age: 0–17   **M**   Maternity DX: 12–55   **A**   Adult Age: 15–124   ♀   Females Only   ♂   Males Only

🔍   Complication\Comorbidity   🔍   Major C\C   🔍   Present on Admission Requirement   🔍   Hospital-Acquired Condition

1793

CHAPTER 21 (Z00–Z99)

CHAPTER 21 (Z00-Z99)

● **Z01.8 Encounter for other specified special examinations**

  ● **Z01.81 Encounter for preprocedural examinations**
    Encounter for preoperative examinations
    Encounter for radiological and
        imaging examinations as part of
        preprocedural examination

    ❶ **Z01.810 Encounter for preprocedural
        cardiovascular examination**

    ❶ **Z01.811 Encounter for preprocedural
        respiratory examination**

    ❶● **Z01.812 Encounter for preprocedural
        laboratory examination**
        Blood and urine tests prior to
            treatment or procedure

    ❶● **Z01.818 Encounter for other
        preprocedural examination**
        Encounter for preprocedural
            examination NOS
        Encounter for examinations
            prior to antineoplastic
            chemotherapy

  ❶● **Z01.82 Encounter for allergy testing**
        Excludes1   encounter for antibody
            response examination
            (Z01.84)

  ❶● **Z01.83 Encounter for blood typing**
        Encounter for Rh typing

  ❶● **Z01.84 Encounter for antibody response
        examination**
        Encounter for immunity status testing
        Excludes1   encounter for allergy testing
            (Z01.82)

  ❶● **Z01.89 Encounter for other specified special
        examinations** *Routine testing in
            absence of S+S, diagnoses*

● **Z02 Encounter for administrative examination**

  ❶● **Z02.0 Encounter for examination for admission to
        educational institution**
        Encounter for examination for admission to
            preschool (education)
        Encounter for examination for re-admission to
            school following illness or medical treatment

  ❶ **Z02.1 Encounter for pre-employment examination**

  ❶● **Z02.2 Encounter for examination for admission to
        residential institution**
        Excludes1   examination for admission to prison
            (Z02.89)

  ❶ **Z02.3 Encounter for examination for recruitment to
        armed forces**

  ❶● **Z02.4 Encounter for examination for driving license**

  ❶● **Z02.5 Encounter for examination for participation in
        sport**
        Excludes1   blood-alcohol and blood-drug test
            (Z02.83)

  ❶● **Z02.6 Encounter for examination for insurance
        purposes**

  ● **Z02.7 Encounter for issue of medical certificate**
        Excludes1   encounter for general medical
            examination (Z00-Z01,
            Z02.0-Z02.6, Z02.8-Z02.9)

    ❶● **Z02.71 Encounter for disability determination**
        Encounter for issue of medical certificate
            of incapacity
        Encounter for issue of medical certificate
            of invalidity

    ❶● **Z02.79 Encounter for issue of other medical
        certificate**

[handwritten left margin: Preprocedural Evaluations Only and assign a code for the condition to describe the reason for surgery as an additional diagnoses - Code also any findings related to the pre-op evaluation]

● **Z02.8 Encounter for other administrative examinations**

  ❶ **Z02.81 Encounter for paternity testing**

  ❶● **Z02.82 Encounter for adoption services**

  ❶ **Z02.83 Encounter for blood-alcohol and blood-
        drug test**

        Use additional code for findings of
            alcohol or drugs in blood (R78.-)

  ❶● **Z02.89 Encounter for other administrative
        examinations**
        Encounter for examination for admission
            to prison
        Encounter for examination for admission
            to summer camp
        Encounter for immigration examination
        Encounter for naturalization examination
        Encounter for premarital examination
        Excludes1   health supervision of
            foundling or other
            healthy infant or child
            (Z76.1-Z76.2)

❶●■ **Z02.9 Encounter for administrative examinations,
        unspecified**

OGCR Section II.C.21.c.6.

21.2.2. Observation

There are two observation Z code categories. They are for use in very limited circumstances when a person is being observed for a suspected condition that is ruled out. The observation codes are not for use if an injury or illnesses or any signs or symptoms related to the suspected condition are present. In such cases the diagnosis/symptom code is used with the corresponding external cause code.

The observation codes are to be used as principal diagnosis only. Additional codes may be used in addition to the observation code but only if they are unrelated to the suspected condition being observed.

Codes from subcategory Z03.7 Encounter for suspected maternal and fetal conditions ruled out, may either be used as a first listed or as an additional code assignment depending on the case. They are for use in very limited circumstances on a maternal record when an encounter is for a suspected maternal or fetal condition that is ruled out during that encounter (for example, a maternal or fetal condition may be suspected due to an abnormal test result). These codes should not be used when the condition is confirmed. In those cases, the confirmed condition should be coded. In addition, these codes are not for use if an illness or any signs or symptoms related to the suspected condition or problem are present. In such cases the diagnosis/symptom code is used.

Additional codes may be used in addition to the code from subcategory Z03.7, but only if they are unrelated to the suspected condition being evaluated.

Codes from subcategory Z03.7 may not be used for encounters for antenatal screening of mother. *See Section I.C.21. Screening.*

For encounters for suspected fetal condition that are inconclusive following testing and evaluation, assign the appropriate code from category O35, O36, O40 or O41.

The observation Z code categories:

Z03 Encounter for medical observation for suspected diseases and conditions ruled out

Z04 Encounter for examination and observation for other reasons

Except: Z04.9, Encounter for examination and observation for unspecified reason

---

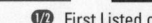

● Unacceptable Principal Diagnosis   ● Use Additional Character(s)   ■ Unspecified   ▶ Manifestation Code

OGCR Official Guidelines for Coding and Reporting | Excludes 1 | | Excludes 2 | Includes   Use additional   Code first   Code also

❶ First Listed   ❶/❷ First Listed or Secondary   ❷ Secondary Only

● **Z03**   **Encounter for medical observation for suspected diseases and conditions ruled out**

This category is to be used when a person without a diagnosis is suspected of having an abnormal condition, without signs or symptoms, which requires study, but after examination and observation, is ruled out. This category is also for use for administrative and legal observation status.

> **Excludes1**   contact with and (suspected) exposures hazardous to health (Z77.-)
> newborn observation for suspected condition, ruled out (P00-P04)
> person with feared complaint in whom no diagnosis is made (Z71.1)
> signs or symptoms under study - code to signs or symptoms

❶ **Z03.6**   **Encounter for observation for suspected toxic effect from ingested substance ruled out** 🔍

Encounter for observation for suspected adverse effect from drug

Encounter for observation for suspected poisoning

● **Z03.7**   **Encounter for suspected maternal and fetal conditions ruled out**

Encounter for suspected maternal and fetal conditions not found

> **Excludes1**   known or suspected fetal anomalies affecting management of mother, not ruled out (O26.-, O35.-, O36.-, O40.-, O41.-)

❶● **Z03.71**   **Encounter for suspected problem with amniotic cavity and membrane ruled out** ♀ 🔍   **M**

Encounter for suspected oligohydramnios ruled out

Encounter for suspected polyhydramnios ruled out

❶● **Z03.72**   **Encounter for suspected placental problem ruled out** ♀ 🔍   **M**

❶● **Z03.73**   **Encounter for suspected fetal anomaly ruled out** ♀ 🔍   **M**

❶● **Z03.74**   **Encounter for suspected problem with fetal growth ruled out** ♀ 🔍   **M**

❶● **Z03.75**   **Encounter for suspected cervical shortening ruled out** ♀ 🔍   **M**

❶● **Z03.79**   **Encounter for other suspected maternal and fetal conditions ruled out** ♀ 🔍   **M**

● **Z03.8**   **Encounter for observation for other suspected diseases and conditions ruled out**

● **Z03.81**   **Encounter for observation for suspected exposure to biological agents ruled out**

❶ **Z03.810**   **Encounter for observation for suspected exposure to anthrax ruled out** 🔍

❶ **Z03.818**   **Encounter for observation for suspected exposure to other biological agents ruled out** 🔍

❶ **Z03.89**   **Encounter for observation for other suspected diseases and conditions ruled out** 🔍

● **Z04**   **Encounter for examination and observation for other reasons**

> **Includes**   encounter for examination for medicolegal reasons

This category is to be used when a person without a diagnosis is suspected of having an abnormal condition, without signs or symptoms, which requires study, but after examination and observation, is ruled-out. This category is also for use for administrative and legal observation status.

❶ **Z04.1**   **Encounter for examination and observation following transport accident** 🔍

> **Excludes1**   encounter for examination and observation following work accident (Z04.2)

❶ **Z04.2**   **Encounter for examination and observation following work accident** 🔍

❶ **Z04.3**   **Encounter for examination and observation following other accident** 🔍

● **Z04.4**   **Encounter for examination and observation following alleged rape**

Encounter for examination and observation of victim following alleged rape

Encounter for examination and observation of victim following alleged sexual abuse

❶ **Z04.41**   **Encounter for examination and observation following alleged adult rape** 🔍   **A**

Suspected adult rape, ruled out

Suspected adult sexual abuse, ruled out

❶ **Z04.42**   **Encounter for examination and observation following alleged child rape** 🔍   **P**

Suspected child rape, ruled out

Suspected child sexual abuse, ruled out

❶ **Z04.6**   **Encounter for general psychiatric examination, requested by authority** 🔍

● **Z04.7**   **Encounter for examination and observation following alleged physical abuse**

❶ **Z04.71**   **Encounter for examination and observation following alleged adult physical abuse** 🔍   **A**

Suspected adult physical abuse, ruled out

> **Excludes1**   confirmed case of adult physical abuse (T74.-)
> encounter for examination and observation following alleged adult sexual abuse (Z04.41)
> suspected case of adult physical abuse, not ruled out (T76.-)

❶ **Z04.72**   **Encounter for examination and observation following alleged child physical abuse** 🔍   **P**

Suspected child physical abuse, ruled out

> **Excludes1**   confirmed case of child physical abuse (T74.-)
> encounter for examination and observation following alleged child sexual abuse (Z04.42)
> suspected case of child physical abuse, not ruled out (T76.-)

CHAPTER 21 (Z00-Z99)

---

❶ ● **Z04.8   Encounter for examination and observation for other specified reasons** 🔍

> Encounter for examination and observation for request for expert evidence

½ ● ■ **Z04.9   Encounter for examination and observation for unspecified reason** 🔍

> Encounter for observation NOS

OGCR   See Section II.C.21.c.7.

The follow-up codes are used to explain continuing surveillance following completed treatment of a disease, condition, or injury. They imply that the condition has been fully treated and no longer exists. They should not be confused with aftercare codes, or injury codes with 7th character "D," that explain ongoing care of a healing condition or its sequelae. Follow-up codes may be used in conjunction with history codes to provide the full picture of the healed condition and its treatment. The follow-up code is sequenced first, followed by the history code.

A follow-up code may be used to explain multiple visits. Should a condition be found to have recurred on the follow-up visit, then the code for the condition should be assigned as an additional diagnosis.

The follow-up Z code categories:

Z08   Encounter for follow-up examination after completed treatment for malignant neoplasm

Z09   Encounter for follow-up examination after completed treatment for conditions other than malignant neoplasm

Z39   Encounter for maternal postpartum care and examination

½ ● **Z08   Encounter for follow-up examination after completed treatment for malignant neoplasm** 🔍

> Medical surveillance following completed treatment

> Use additional code to identify any acquired absence of organs (Z90.-)

> Use additional code to identify the personal history of malignant neoplasm (Z85.-)

> **Excludes1**   aftercare following medical care (Z43-Z49, Z51)

½ ● **Z09   Encounter for follow-up examination after completed treatment for conditions other than malignant neoplasm** 🔍

> Medical surveillance following completed treatment

> Use additional code to identify any applicable history of disease code (Z86.-. Z87.-)

> **Excludes1**   aftercare following medical care (Z43-Z49, Z51)
> surveillance of contraception (Z30.4-)
> surveillance of prosthetic and other medical devices (Z44-Z46)

● **Z11   Encounter for screening for infectious and parasitic diseases**

> Screening is the testing for disease or disease precursors in asymptomatic individuals so that early detection and treatment can be provided for those who test positive for the disease.

> **Excludes1**   encounter for diagnostic examination - code to sign or symptom

½ ● **Z11.0   Encounter for screening for intestinal infectious diseases** 🔍

OGCR   Section II.C.21.c.5.

Screening

Screening is the testing for disease or disease precursors in seemingly well individuals so that early detection and treatment can be provided for those who test positive for the disease (e.g., screening mammogram).

The testing of a person to rule out or confirm a suspected diagnosis because the patient has some sign or symptom is a diagnostic examination, not a screening. In these cases, the sign or symptom is used to explain the reason for the test.

A screening code may be a first listed code if the reason for the visit is specifically the screening exam. It may also be used as an additional code if the screening is done during an office visit for other health problems. A screening code is not necessary if the screening is inherent to a routine examination, such as a pap smear done during a routine pelvic examination.

Should a condition be discovered during the screening then the code for the condition may be assigned as an additional diagnosis.

The Z code indicates that a screening exam is planned. A procedure code is required to confirm that the screening was performed.

The screening Z codes / categories:

Z11   Encounter for screening for infectious and parasitic diseases

Z12   Encounter for screening for malignant neoplasms

Z13   Encounter for screening for other diseases and disorders
 Except: Z13.9, Encounter for screening, unspecified

Z36   Encounter for antenatal screening for mother

½ ● **Z11.1   Encounter for screening for respiratory tuberculosis** 🔍

½ ● **Z11.2   Encounter for screening for other bacterial diseases** 🔍

½ ● **Z11.3   Encounter for screening for infections with a predominantly sexual mode of transmission** 🔍

> **Excludes2**   encounter for screening for human immunodeficiency virus [HIV] (Z11.4)
> encounter for screening for human papillomavirus (Z11.51)

½ ● **Z11.4   Encounter for screening for human immunodeficiency virus [HIV]** 🔍

● **Z11.5   Encounter for screening for other viral diseases**

> **Excludes2**   encounter for screening for viral intestinal disease (Z11.0)

½ ● **Z11.51   Encounter for screening for human papillomavirus (HPV)** 🔍

½ ● **Z11.59   Encounter for screening for other viral diseases** 🔍

½ ● **Z11.6   Encounter for screening for other protozoal diseases and helminthiases** 🔍

> *Diseases or infestations caused by parasitic worms*

> **Excludes2**   encounter for screening for protozoal intestinal disease (Z11.0)

½ ● **Z11.8   Encounter for screening for other infectious and parasitic diseases** 🔍

> Encounter for screening for chlamydia
> Encounter for screening for rickettsial
> Encounter for screening for spirochetal
> Encounter for screening for mycoses

½ ● ■ **Z11.9   Encounter for screening for infectious and parasitic diseases, unspecified** 🔍

● Unacceptable Principal Diagnosis   ● Use Additional Character(s)   ■ Unspecified   ▶ Manifestation Code
OGCR Official Guidelines for Coding and Reporting   Excludes 1   Excludes 2   Includes   Use additional   Code first   Code also
❶ First Listed   ½ First Listed or Secondary   ❷ Secondary Only

●**Z12 Encounter for screening for malignant neoplasms**
Screening is the testing for disease or disease precursors in asymptomatic individuals so that early detection and treatment can be provided for those who test positive for the disease.

Use additional code to identify any family history of malignant neoplasm (Z80.-)

Excludes1   encounter for diagnostic examination - code to sign or symptom

1/2 ● **Z12.0 Encounter for screening for malignant neoplasm of stomach** 🖉

● **Z12.1 Encounter for screening for malignant neoplasm of intestinal tract**

1/2 ● ■ **Z12.10 Encounter for screening for malignant neoplasm of intestinal tract, unspecified** 🖉

1/2 ● **Z12.11 Encounter for screening for malignant neoplasm of colon** 🖉
Encounter for screening colonoscopy NOS

1/2 ● **Z12.12 Encounter for screening for malignant neoplasm of rectum** 🖉

1/2 ● **Z12.13 Encounter for screening for malignant neoplasm of small intestine** 🖉

1/2 ● **Z12.2 Encounter for screening for malignant neoplasm of respiratory organs** 🖉

● **Z12.3 Encounter for screening for malignant neoplasm of breast**

1/2 ● **Z12.31 Encounter for screening mammogram for malignant neoplasm of breast** 🖉

Excludes1   inconclusive mammogram (R92.2)

1/2 ● **Z12.39 Encounter for other screening for malignant neoplasm of breast** 🖉

1/2 ● **Z12.4 Encounter for screening for malignant neoplasm of cervix ♀** 🖉
Encounter for screening pap smear for malignant neoplasm of cervix

Excludes1   encounter for screening for human papillomavirus (Z11.51)
when screening is part of general gynecological examination (Z01.4-)

1/2 **Z12.5 Encounter for screening for malignant neoplasm of prostate ♂** 🖉

1/2 ● **Z12.6 Encounter for screening for malignant neoplasm of bladder** 🖉

● **Z12.7 Encounter for screening for malignant neoplasm of other genitourinary organs**

1/2 ● **Z12.71 Encounter for screening for malignant neoplasm of testis ♂** 🖉

1/2 ● **Z12.72 Encounter for screening for malignant neoplasm of vagina ♀** 🖉
Vaginal pap smear status - post hysterectomy for non-malignant condition

Use additional code to identify acquired absence of uterus (Z90.71-)

Excludes1   vaginal pap smear status - post hysterectomy for malignant conditions (Z08)

1/2 ● **Z12.73 Encounter for screening for malignant neoplasm of ovary ♀** 🖉

1/2 ● **Z12.79 Encounter for screening for malignant neoplasm of other genitourinary organs** 🖉

● **Z12.8 Encounter for screening for malignant neoplasm of other sites**

1/2 ● **Z12.81 Encounter for screening for malignant neoplasm of oral cavity** 🖉

1/2 ● **Z12.82 Encounter for screening for malignant neoplasm of nervous system** 🖉

1/2 ● **Z12.83 Encounter for screening for malignant neoplasm of skin** 🖉

1/2 ● **Z12.89 Encounter for screening for malignant neoplasm of other sites** 🖉

1/2 ● ■ **Z12.9 Encounter for screening for malignant neoplasm, site unspecified** 🖉

● **Z13 Encounter for screening for other diseases and disorders**
Screening is the testing for disease or disease precursors in asymptomatic individuals so that early detection and treatment can be provided for those who test positive for the disease.

Excludes1   encounter for diagnostic examination - code to sign or symptom

1/2 ● **Z13.0 Encounter for screening for diseases of the blood and blood-forming organs and certain disorders involving the immune mechanism** 🖉

1/2 ● **Z13.1 Encounter for screening for diabetes mellitus** 🖉

● **Z13.2 Encounter for screening for nutritional, metabolic and other endocrine disorders**

1/2 ● **Z13.21 Encounter for screening for nutritional disorder** 🖉

● **Z13.22 Encounter for screening for metabolic disorder**

1/2 ● **Z13.220 Encounter for screening for lipoid disorders** 🖉
Encounter for screening for cholesterol level
Encounter for screening for hypercholesterolemia
Encounter for screening for hyperlipidemia

1/2 ● **Z13.228 Encounter for screening for other metabolic disorders** 🖉

1/2 ● **Z13.29 Encounter for screening for other suspected endocrine disorder** 🖉

Excludes1   encounter for screening for diabetes mellitus (Z13.1)

1/2 ● **Z13.4 Encounter for screening for certain developmental disorders in childhood** 🖉   P
Encounter for screening for developmental handicaps in early childhood

Excludes1   routine development testing of infant or child (Z00.1-)

1/2 ● **Z13.5 Encounter for screening for eye and ear disorders** 🖉

Excludes2   encounter for general hearing examination (Z01.1-)
encounter for general vision examination (Z01.0-)

1/2 ● **Z13.6 Encounter for screening for cardiovascular disorders** 🖉

● **Z13.7 Encounter for screening for genetic and chromosomal anomalies**

Excludes1   genetic testing for procreative management (Z31.4-)

1/2 ● **Z13.71 Encounter for nonprocreative screening for genetic disease carrier status** 🖉

1/2 ● **Z13.79 Encounter for other screening for genetic and chromosomal anomalies** 🖉

N   Newborn Age: 0   P   Pediatric Age: 0–17   M   Maternity DX: 12–55   A   Adult Age: 15–124   ♀   Females Only   ♂   Males Only

🖉   Complication\Comorbidity   🖉   Major C\C   🖉   Present on Admission Requirement   🖉   Hospital-Acquired Condition

● **Z13.8 Encounter for screening for other specified diseases and disorders**

> Excludes2   screening for malignant neoplasms (Z12.-)

● **Z13.81 Encounter for screening for digestive system disorders**

12 ● **Z13.810 Encounter for screening for upper gastrointestinal disorder** ⊚

12 ● **Z13.811 Encounter for screening for lower gastrointestinal disorder** ⊚

> Excludes1   encounter for screening for intestinal infectious disease (Z11.0)

12 ● **Z13.818 Encounter for screening for other digestive system disorders** ⊚

● **Z13.82 Encounter for screening for musculoskeletal disorder**

12 ● **Z13.820 Encounter for screening for osteoporosis** ⊚

12 ● **Z13.828 Encounter for screening for other musculoskeletal disorder** ⊚

12 ● **Z13.83 Encounter for screening for respiratory disorder NEC** ⊚

> Excludes1   encounter for screening for respiratory tuberculosis (Z11.1)

12 ● **Z13.84 Encounter for screening for dental disorders** ⊚

● **Z13.85 Encounter for screening for nervous system disorders**

12 ● **Z13.850 Encounter for screening for traumatic brain injury** ⊚

12 ● **Z13.858 Encounter for screening for other nervous system disorders** ⊚

12 ● **Z13.88 Encounter for screening for disorder due to exposure to contaminants** ⊚

> Excludes1   those exposed to contaminants without suspected disorders (Z57-Z77.-)

12 ● **Z13.89 Encounter for screening for other disorder** ⊚
> Encounter for screening for genitourinary disorders

❷ ● ■ **Z13.9 Encounter for screening, unspecified** ⊚

GENETIC CARRIER AND GENETIC SUSCEPTIBILITY TO DISEASE (Z14-Z15)

● **Z14 Genetic carrier**

● **Z14.0 Hemophilia A carrier**

12 ● **Z14.01 Asymptomatic hemophilia A carrier** ⊚

12 ● **Z14.02 Symptomatic hemophilia A carrier** ⊚

12 ● **Z14.1 Cystic fibrosis carrier** ⊚

12 ● **Z14.8 Genetic carrier of other disease** ⊚

● **Z15 Genetic susceptibility to disease**

> Excludes1   chromosomal anomalies (Q90-Q99)

> Includes   confirmed abnormal gene

> Use additional code, if applicable, for any associated family history of the disease (Z80-Z84)

● **Z15.0 Genetic susceptibility to malignant neoplasm**

> *Code first if applicable, any current malignant neoplasm (C00-C75, C81-C96)*

> Use additional code, if applicable, for any personal history of malignant neoplasm (Z85.-)

❷ ● **Z15.01 Genetic susceptibility to malignant neoplasm of breast** ⊚

❷ ● **Z15.02 Genetic susceptibility to malignant neoplasm of ovary** ♀ ⊚

❷ ● **Z15.03 Genetic susceptibility to malignant neoplasm of prostate** ♂ ⊚

❷ ● **Z15.04 Genetic susceptibility to malignant neoplasm of endometrium** ♀ ⊚

❷ ● **Z15.09 Genetic susceptibility to other malignant neoplasm** ⊚

● **Z15.8 Genetic susceptibility to other disease**

❷ ● **Z15.81 Genetic susceptibility to multiple endocrine neoplasia [MEN]** ⊚

> Excludes1   multiple endocrine neoplasia [MEN] syndromes (E31.2-)

❷ ● **Z15.89 Genetic susceptibility to other disease** ⊚

RESISTANCE TO ANTIMICROBIAL DRUGS (Z16)

● **Z16 Resistance to antimicrobial drugs**

> **Note:** The codes in this category are provided for use as additional codes to identify the resistance and non-responsiveness of a condition to antimicrobial drugs.

> *Code first the infection*

> Excludes1   Methicillin resistant Staphylococcus aureus infection (A49.02)
> Methicillin resistant Staphylococcus aureus infection in diseases classified elsewhere (B95.62)
> Methicillin resistant Staphylococcus aureus pneumonia (J15.212)
> Sepsis due to Methicillin resistant Staphylococcus aureus (A41.02)

● **Z16.1 Resistance to beta lactam antibiotics**

❷ ■ **Z16.10 Resistance to unspecified beta lactam antibiotics**

❷ **Z16.11 Resistance to penicillins**
> Resistance to amoxicillin
> Resistance to ampicillin

❷ **Z16.12 Extended spectrum beta lactamase (ESBL) resistance**

❷ **Z16.19 Resistance to other specified beta lactam antibiotics**
> Resistance to cephalosporins

● **Z16.2 Resistance to other antibiotics**

❷ ■ **Z16.20 Resistance to unspecified antibiotic**
> Resistance to antibiotics NOS

❷ **Z16.21 Resistance to vancomycin**

❷ **Z16.22 Resistance to vancomycin related antibiotics**

❷ **Z16.23 Resistance to quinolones and fluoroquinolones**

❷ **Z16.24   Resistance to multiple antibiotics**

❷ **Z16.29   Resistance to other single specified antibiotic**
Resistance to aminoglycosides
Resistance to macrolides
Resistance to sulfonamides
Resistance to tetracyclines

● **Z16.3   Resistance to other antimicrobial drugs**

| **Excludes1** | resistance to antibiotics (Z16.1-, Z16.2-) |

❷ ■ **Z16.30   Resistance to unspecified antimicrobial drugs**
Drug resistance NOS

❷ **Z16.31   Resistance to antiparasitic drug(s)**
Resistance to quinine and related compounds

❷ **Z16.32   Resistance to antifungal drug(s)**

❷ **Z16.33   Resistance to antiviral drug(s)**

● **Z16.34   Resistance to antimycobacterial drug(s)**
Resistance to tuberculostatics

❷ **Z16.341   Resistance to single antimycobacterial drug**
Resistance to antimycobacterial drug NOS

❷ **Z16.342   Resistance to multiple antimycobacterial drugs**

❷ **Z16.35   Resistance to multiple antimicrobial drugs**

| **Excludes1** | Resistance to multiple antibiotics only (Z16.24) |

❷ **Z16.39   Resistance to other specified antimicrobial drug**

ESTROGEN RECEPTOR STATUS (Z17)

● **Z17   Estrogen receptor status**
Code first malignant neoplasm of breast (C50.-)

⑫● **Z17.0   Estrogen receptor positive status [ER+]** 🔖

⑫● **Z17.1   Estrogen receptor negative status [ER-]** 🔖

RETAINED FOREIGN BODY FRAGMENTS (Z18)

● **Z18   Retained foreign body fragments**

Includes	embedded fragment (status)
	embedded splinter (status)
	retained foreign body status

Excludes1	artificial joint prosthesis status (Z96.6-)
	foreign body accidentally left during a procedure (T81.5-)
	foreign body entering through orifice (T15-T19)
	in situ cardiac device (Z95.-)
	organ or tissue replaced by means other than transplant (Z96.-, Z97.-)
	organ or tissue replaced by transplant (Z94.-)
	personal history of retained foreign body fully removed Z87.821
	superficial foreign body (non-embedded splinter) - code to superficial foreign body, by site

● **Z18.0   Retained radioactive fragments**

⑫● **Z18.01   Retained depleted uranium fragments** 🔖

⑫● **Z18.09   Other retained radioactive fragments** 🔖
Other retained depleted isotope fragments
Retained nontherapeutic radioactive fragments

● **Z18.1   Retained metal fragments**

| **Excludes1** | retained radioactive metal fragments (Z18.01-Z18.09) |

⑫●■ **Z18.10   Retained metal fragments, unspecified** 🔖
Retained metal fragment NOS

⑫● **Z18.11   Retained magnetic metal fragments** 🔖

⑫● **Z18.12   Retained nonmagnetic metal fragments** 🔖

⑫●● **Z18.2   Retained plastic fragments** 🔖
Acrylics fragments
Diethylhexylphthalates fragments
Isocyanate fragments

● **Z18.3   Retained organic fragments**

⑫● **Z18.31   Retained animal quills or spines** 🔖

⑫● **Z18.32   Retained tooth** 🔖

⑫● **Z18.33   Retained wood fragments** 🔖

⑫● **Z18.39   Other retained organic fragments** 🔖

● **Z18.8   Other specified retained foreign body**

⑫● **Z18.81   Retained glass fragments** 🔖

⑫● **Z18.83   Retained stone or crystalline fragments** 🔖
Retained concrete or cement fragments

⑫● **Z18.89   Other specified retained foreign body fragments** 🔖

⑫● **Z18.9   Retained foreign body fragments, unspecified material** 🔖

PERSONS WITH POTENTIAL HEALTH HAZARDS RELATED TO COMMUNICABLE DISEASES (Z20-Z28)

● **Z20   Contact with and (suspected) exposure to communicable diseases**

| **Excludes1** | carrier of infectious disease (Z22.-) |
| | diagnosed current infectious or parasitic disease - see Alphabetic Index |

| **Excludes2** | personal history of infectious and parasitic diseases (Z86.1-) |

● **Z20.0   Contact with and (suspected) exposure to intestinal infectious diseases**

⑫ **Z20.01   Contact with and (suspected) exposure to intestinal infectious diseases due to Escherichia coli (E. coli)**

⑫● **Z20.09   Contact with and (suspected) exposure to other intestinal infectious diseases**

⑫● **Z20.1   Contact with and (suspected) exposure to tuberculosis**

⑫● **Z20.2   Contact with and (suspected) exposure to infections with a predominantly sexual mode of transmission**

⑫● **Z20.3   Contact with and (suspected) exposure to rabies**

⑫● **Z20.4   Contact with and (suspected) exposure to rubella**

⑫ **Z20.5   Contact with and (suspected) exposure to viral hepatitis**

⑫ **Z20.6   Contact with and (suspected) exposure to human immunodeficiency virus [HIV]**

| **Excludes1** | asymptomatic human immunodeficiency virus [HIV] HIV infection status (Z21) |

⑫● **Z20.7   Contact with and (suspected) exposure to pediculosis, acariasis and other infestations**

N Newborn Age: 0   **P** Pediatric Age: 0–17   **M** Maternity DX: 12–55   **A** Adult Age: 15–124   ♀ Females Only   ♂ Males Only

🔖 Complication\Comorbidity   🔖 Major C\C   🔖 Present on Admission Requirement   🔖 Hospital-Acquired Condition

1799

● **Z20.8** **Contact with and (suspected) exposure to other communicable diseases**

　● **Z20.81** **Contact with and (suspected) exposure to other bacterial communicable diseases**

　　⑫● **Z20.810** **Contact with and (suspected) exposure to anthrax**

　　⑫● **Z20.811** **Contact with and (suspected) exposure to meningococcus**

　　⑫● **Z20.818** **Contact with and (suspected) exposure to other bacterial communicable diseases**

　● **Z20.82** **Contact with and (suspected) exposure to other viral communicable diseases**

　　⑫● **Z20.820** **Contact with and (suspected) exposure to varicella**

　　⑫● **Z20.828** **Contact with and (suspected) exposure to other viral communicable diseases**

　⑫● **Z20.89** **Contact with and (suspected) exposure to other communicable diseases**

⑫●■ **Z20.9** **Contact with and (suspected) exposure to unspecified communicable disease**

⑫ **Z21** **Asymptomatic human immunodeficiency virus [HIV] infection status**
HIV positive NOS

Code first Human immunodeficiency virus [HIV] disease complicating pregnancy, childbirth and the puerperium, if applicable (O98.7-)

Excludes1 acquired immunodeficiency syndrome (B20)
contact with human immunodeficiency virus [HIV] (Z20.6)
exposure to human immunodeficiency virus [HIV] (Z20.6)
human immunodeficiency virus [HIV] disease (B20)
inconclusive laboratory evidence of human immunodeficiency virus [HIV] (R75)

MCE: Questionable admission when principal dx

● **Z22** **Carrier of infectious disease**

Includes colonization status
suspected carrier

⑫● **Z22.0** **Carrier of typhoid** 🔍

⑫● **Z22.1** **Carrier of other intestinal infectious diseases** 🔍

⑫● **Z22.2** **Carrier of diphtheria** 🔍

● **Z22.3** **Carrier of other specified bacterial diseases**

　⑫● **Z22.31** **Carrier of bacterial disease due to meningococci** 🔍

　● **Z22.32** **Carrier of bacterial disease due to staphylococci**

　　⑫● **Z22.321** **Carrier or suspected carrier of Methicillin susceptible Staphylococcus aureus** 🔍
MSSA colonization

　　⑫● **Z22.322** **Carrier or suspected carrier of Methicillin resistant Staphylococcus aureus** 🔍
MRSA colonization

　⑫ **Z22.33** **Carrier of bacterial disease due to streptococci**

　　● **Z22.330** **Carrier of Group B streptococcus** 🔍

　　● **Z22.338** **Carrier of other streptococcus** 🔍

　⑫● **Z22.39** **Carrier of other specified bacterial diseases** 🔍

⑫● **Z22.4** **Carrier of infections with a predominantly sexual mode of transmission** 🔍

● **Z22.5** **Carrier of viral hepatitis**

　⑫●■ **Z22.50** **Carrier of unspecified viral hepatitis** 🔍

　⑫● **Z22.51** **Carrier of viral hepatitis B** 🔍
Hepatitis B surface antigen [HBsAg] carrier

　⑫● **Z22.52** **Carrier of viral hepatitis C** 🔍

　⑫● **Z22.59** **Carrier of other viral hepatitis** 🔍

⑫● **Z22.6** **Carrier of human T-lymphotropic virus type-1 [HTLV-1] infection** 🔍

⑫● **Z22.8** **Carrier of other infectious diseases** 🔍

⑫●■ **Z22.9** **Carrier of infectious disease, unspecified** 🔍

⑫● **Z23** **Encounter for immunization** 🔍

Code first any routine childhood examination

Note: Procedure codes are required to identify the types of immunizations given.

● **Z28** **Immunization not carried out and underimmunization status**

Includes vaccination not carried out

● **Z28.0** **Immunization not carried out because of contraindication**

　⑫● **Z28.01** **Immunization not carried out because of acute illness of patient** 🔍

　⑫● **Z28.02** **Immunization not carried out because of chronic illness or condition of patient** 🔍

　⑫● **Z28.03** **Immunization not carried out because of immune compromised state of patient** 🔍

　⑫● **Z28.04** **Immunization not carried out because of patient allergy to vaccine or component** 🔍

　⑫● **Z28.09** **Immunization not carried out because of other contraindication** 🔍

⑫● **Z28.1** **Immunization not carried out because of patient decision for reasons of belief or group pressure** 🔍
Immunization not carried out because of religious belief

● **Z28.2** **Immunization not carried out because of patient decision for other and unspecified reason**

　⑫●■ **Z28.20** **Immunization not carried out because of patient decision for unspecified reason** 🔍

　⑫● **Z28.21** **Immunization not carried out because of patient refusal** 🔍

　⑫● **Z28.29** **Immunization not carried out because of patient decision for other reason** 🔍

⑫● **Z28.3** **Underimmunization status** 🔍
Delinquent immunization status
Lapsed immunization schedule status

● **Z28.8** **Immunization not carried out for other reason**

　⑫● **Z28.81** **Immunization not carried out due to patient having had the disease** 🔍

　⑫● **Z28.82** **Immunization not carried out because of caregiver refusal** 🔍
Immunization not carried out because of guardian refusal
Immunization not carried out because of parent refusal

Excludes1 immunization not carried out because of caregiver refusal because of religious belief (Z28.1)

　⑫● **Z28.89** **Immunization not carried out for other reason** 🔍

⑫●■ **Z28.9** **Immunization not carried out for unspecified reason** 🔍

● Unacceptable Principal Diagnosis	🔘 Use Additional Character(s)	■ Unspecified	▶ Manifestation Code

OGCR Official Guidelines for Coding and Reporting　| Excludes 1 | Excludes 2 | Includes | Use additional | Code first | Code also |

❶ First Listed　⑫ First Listed or Secondary　❷ Secondary Only

PERSONS ENCOUNTERING HEALTH SERVICES IN CIRCUMSTANCES RELATED TO REPRODUCTION (Z30-Z39)

● **Z30   Encounter for contraceptive management**

　● **Z30.0   Encounter for general counseling and advice on contraception**

　　● **Z30.01   Encounter for initial prescription of contraceptives**

　　　| Excludes1 | encounter for surveillance of contraceptives (Z30.4-) |

　　　🔟● **Z30.011   Encounter for initial prescription of contraceptive pills** ♀ 🅿

　　　🔟● **Z30.012   Encounter for prescription of emergency contraception** ♀ 🅿
　　　　　Encounter for postcoital contraception

　　　🔟● **Z30.013   Encounter for initial prescription of injectable contraceptive** ♀ 🅿

　　　🔟● **Z30.014   Encounter for initial prescription of intrauterine contraceptive device** ♀ 🅿

　　　　　| Excludes1 | encounter for insertion of intrauterine contraceptive device (Z30.430, Z30.432) |

　　　🔟● **Z30.018   Encounter for initial prescription of other contraceptives** ♀ 🅿

　　　🔟●■ **Z30.019   Encounter for initial prescription of contraceptives, unspecified** ♀ 🅿

　　🔟● **Z30.02   Counseling and instruction in natural family planning to avoid pregnancy** 🅿

　　🔟● **Z30.09   Encounter for other general counseling and advice on contraception** 🅿
　　　　Encounter for family planning advice NOS

　🔟● **Z30.2   Encounter for sterilization** 🅿

　● **Z30.4   Encounter for surveillance of contraceptives**

　　🔟●■ **Z30.40   Encounter for surveillance of contraceptives, unspecified** 🅿

　　🔟● **Z30.41   Encounter for surveillance of contraceptive pills** ♀ 🅿
　　　　Encounter for repeat prescription for contraceptive pill

　　🔟● **Z30.42   Encounter for surveillance of injectable contraceptive** ♀ 🅿

　　● **Z30.43   Encounter for surveillance of intrauterine contraceptive device**

　　　🔟● **Z30.430   Encounter for insertion of intrauterine contraceptive device** ♀ 🅿

　　　🔟● **Z30.431   Encounter for routine checking of intrauterine contraceptive device** ♀ 🅿

　　　🔟● **Z30.432   Encounter for removal of intrauterine contraceptive device** ♀ 🅿

　　　🔟● **Z30.433   Encounter for removal and reinsertion of intrauterine contraceptive device** ♀ 🅿
　　　　　Encounter for replacement of intrauterine contraceptive device

　　🔟● **Z30.49   Encounter for surveillance of other contraceptives** ♀ 🅿

　🔟● **Z30.8   Encounter for other contraceptive management** ♀ 🅿
　　　Encounter for postvasectomy sperm count
　　　Encounter for routine examination for contraceptive maintenance

　　　| Excludes1 | sperm count following sterilization reversal (Z31.42) |
　　　| | sperm count for fertility testing (Z31.41) |

　🔟●■ **Z30.9   Encounter for contraceptive management, unspecified** 🅿

● **Z31   Encounter for procreative management**

Excludes1	complications associated with artificial fertilization (N98.-)
	female infertility (N97.-)
	male infertility (N46.-)

　🔟● **Z31.0   Encounter for reversal of previous sterilization** 🅿

　● **Z31.4   Encounter for procreative investigation and testing**

　　| Excludes1 | postvasectomy sperm count (Z30.8) |

　　🔟● **Z31.41   Encounter for fertility testing** 🅿
　　　　Encounter for fallopian tube patency testing
　　　　Encounter for sperm count for fertility testing

　　🔟● **Z31.42   Aftercare following sterilization reversal** 🅿
　　　　Sperm count following sterilization reversal

　　● **Z31.43   Encounter for genetic testing of female for procreative management**

　　　Use additional code for recurrent pregnancy loss, if applicable (N96, O26.2-)

　　　| Excludes1 | nonprocreative genetic testing (Z13.7-) |

　　　🔟● **Z31.430   Encounter of female for testing for genetic disease carrier status for procreative management** ♀ 🅿

　　　🔟● **Z31.438   Encounter for other genetic testing of female for procreative management** ♀ 🅿

　　● **Z31.44   Encounter for genetic testing of male for procreative management**

　　　| Excludes1 | nonprocreative genetic testing (Z13.7-) |

　　　🔟● **Z31.440   Encounter of male for testing for genetic disease carrier status for procreative management** ♂ 🅿

　　　🔟● **Z31.441   Encounter for testing of male partner of patient with recurrent pregnancy loss** ♂ 🅿   **A**

　　　🔟● **Z31.448   Encounter for other genetic testing of male for procreative management** ♂ 🅿   **A**

　　🔟● **Z31.49   Encounter for other procreative investigation and testing** 🅿

　🔟● **Z31.5   Encounter for genetic counseling** 🅿

CHAPTER 21 (Z00-Z99)

N Newborn Age: 0   **P** Pediatric Age: 0–17   **M** Maternity DX: 12–55   **A** Adult Age: 15–124   ♀ Females Only   ♂ Males Only

🅒 Complication\Comorbidity   🅜 Major C\C   🅟 Present on Admission Requirement   🅗 Hospital-Acquired Condition

1801

● **Z31.6** **Encounter for general counseling and advice on procreation**

ⓥ ● **Z31.61** **Procreative counseling and advice using natural family planning** 🔖

ⓥ ● **Z31.62** **Encounter for fertility preservation counseling** 🔖
Encounter for fertility preservation counseling prior to cancer therapy
Encounter for fertility preservation counseling prior to surgical removal of gonads

ⓥ ● **Z31.69** **Encounter for other general counseling and advice on procreation** 🔖

● **Z31.8** **Encounter for other procreative management**

❶ ● **Z31.81** **Encounter for male factor infertility in female patient** ♀ 🔖

❶ ● **Z31.82** **Encounter for Rh incompatibility status** ♀ 🔖

❶ ● **Z31.83** **Encounter for assisted reproductive fertility procedure cycle** ♀ 🔖
Patient undergoing in vitro fertilization cycle

Use additional code to identify the type of infertility

Excludes1 pre-cycle diagnosis and testing - code to reason for encounter

❶ ● **Z31.84** **Encounter for fertility preservation procedure** 🔖
Encounter for fertility preservation procedure prior to cancer therapy
Encounter for fertility preservation procedure prior to surgical removal of gonads

ⓥ ● **Z31.89** **Encounter for other procreative management** 🔖

ⓥ ● **Z31.9** **Encounter for procreative management, unspecified** 🔖

● **Z32** **Encounter for pregnancy test and childbirth and childcare instruction**

● **Z32.0** **Encounter for pregnancy test**

ⓥ **Z32.00** **Encounter for pregnancy test, result unknown** ♀
Encounter for pregnancy test NOS

ⓥ **Z32.01** **Encounter for pregnancy test, result positive** ♀ 🔖   M

ⓥ **Z32.02** **Encounter for pregnancy test, result negative** ♀ 🔖

ⓥ ● **Z32.2** **Encounter for childbirth instruction** 🔖

ⓥ ● **Z32.3** **Encounter for childcare instruction** 🔖
Encounter for prenatal or postpartum childcare instruction

● **Z33** **Pregnant state**

❷ ● **Z33.1** **Pregnant state, incidental** ♀ 🔖   M
Pregnant state NOS

Excludes1 complications of pregnancy (O00-O9A)

❶ **Z33.2** **Encounter for elective termination of pregnancy** ♀   M

Excludes1 early fetal death with retention of dead fetus (O02.1)
late fetal death (O36.4)
spontaneous abortion (O03)

● **Z34** **Encounter for supervision of normal pregnancy**

Excludes1 any complication of pregnancy (O00-O9A)
encounter for pregnancy test (Z32.0-)
encounter for supervision of high risk pregnancy (O09.-)

● **Z34.0** **Encounter for supervision of normal first pregnancy**

❶ ● ■ **Z34.00** **Encounter for supervision of normal first pregnancy, unspecified trimester** ♀ 🔖   M

❶ ● **Z34.01** **Encounter for supervision of normal first pregnancy, first trimester** ♀ 🔖   M

❶ ● **Z34.02** **Encounter for supervision of normal first pregnancy, second trimester** ♀ 🔖   M

❶ ● **Z34.03** **Encounter for supervision of normal first pregnancy, third trimester** ♀ 🔖   M

● **Z34.8** **Encounter for supervision of other normal pregnancy**

❶ ● ■ **Z34.80** **Encounter for supervision of other normal pregnancy, unspecified trimester** ♀ 🔖   M

❶ ● **Z34.81** **Encounter for supervision of other normal pregnancy, first trimester** ♀ 🔖   M

❶ ● **Z34.82** **Encounter for supervision of other normal pregnancy, second trimester** ♀ 🔖   M

❶ ● **Z34.83** **Encounter for supervision of other normal pregnancy, third trimester** ♀ 🔖   M

● **Z34.9** **Encounter for supervision of normal pregnancy, unspecified**

❶ ● ■ **Z34.90** **Encounter for supervision of normal pregnancy, unspecified, unspecified trimester** ♀ 🔖   M

❶ ● ■ **Z34.91** **Encounter for supervision of normal pregnancy, unspecified, first trimester** ♀ 🔖   M

❶ ● ■ **Z34.92** **Encounter for supervision of normal pregnancy, unspecified, second trimester** ♀ 🔖   M

❶ ● ■ **Z34.93** **Encounter for supervision of normal pregnancy, unspecified, third trimester** ♀ 🔖   M

ⓥ ● **Z36** **Encounter for antenatal screening of mother** ♀ 🔖   M

Excludes1 abnormal findings on antenatal screening of mother (O28.-)
diagnostic examination - code to sign or symptom
encounter for suspected maternal and fetal conditions ruled out (Z03.7-)
suspected fetal condition affecting management of pregnancy - code to condition in Chapter 15

Excludes2 genetic counseling and testing (Z31.43-, Z31.5)
routine prenatal care (Z34)

● **Z3A** **Weeks of gestation**

Note: Codes from category Z3A are for use, only on the maternal record, to indicate the weeks of gestation of the pregnancy.

Code first complications of pregnancy, childbirth and the puerperium (O00-O9A)

● **Z3A.0** **Weeks of gestation of pregnancy, unspecified or less than 10 weeks**

❷ **Z3A.00** **Weeks of gestation of pregnancy not specified**

❷ **Z3A.01** **Less than 8 weeks gestation of pregnancy**

❷ **Z3A.08** **8 weeks gestation of pregnancy**

❷ **Z3A.09** **9 weeks gestation of pregnancy**

● Unacceptable Principal Diagnosis   ● Use Additional Character(s)   ■ Unspecified   ▶ Manifestation Code

OGCR Official Guidelines for Coding and Reporting   Excludes 1   Excludes 2   Includes   Use additional   Code first   Code also

❶ First Listed   ⓥ First Listed or Secondary   ❷ Secondary Only

● **Z3A.1 Weeks of gestation of pregnancy, weeks 10-19**
     ❷ Z3A.10   10 weeks gestation of pregnancy
     ❷ Z3A.11   11 weeks gestation of pregnancy
     ❷ Z3A.12   12 weeks gestation of pregnancy
     ❷ Z3A.13   13 weeks gestation of pregnancy
     ❷ Z3A.14   14 weeks gestation of pregnancy
     ❷ Z3A.15   15 weeks gestation of pregnancy
     ❷ Z3A.16   16 weeks gestation of pregnancy
     ❷ Z3A.17   17 weeks gestation of pregnancy
     ❷ Z3A.18   18 weeks gestation of pregnancy
     ❷ Z3A.19   19 weeks gestation of pregnancy

● **Z3A.2 Weeks of gestation of pregnancy, weeks 20-29**
     ❷ Z3A.20   20 weeks gestation of pregnancy
     ❷ Z3A.21   21 weeks gestation of pregnancy
     ❷ Z3A.22   22 weeks gestation of pregnancy
     ❷ Z3A.23   23 weeks gestation of pregnancy
     ❷ Z3A.24   24 weeks gestation of pregnancy
     ❷ Z3A.25   25 weeks gestation of pregnancy
     ❷ Z3A.26   26 weeks gestation of pregnancy
     ❷ Z3A.27   27 weeks gestation of pregnancy
     ❷ Z3A.28   28 weeks gestation of pregnancy
     ❷ Z3A.29   29 weeks gestation of pregnancy

● **Z3A.3 Weeks of gestation of pregnancy, weeks 30-39**
     ❷ Z3A.30   30 weeks gestation of pregnancy
     ❷ Z3A.31   31 weeks gestation of pregnancy
     ❷ Z3A.32   32 weeks gestation of pregnancy
     ❷ Z3A.33   33 weeks gestation of pregnancy
     ❷ Z3A.34   34 weeks gestation of pregnancy
     ❷ Z3A.35   35 weeks gestation of pregnancy
     ❷ Z3A.36   36 weeks gestation of pregnancy
     ❷ Z3A.37   37 weeks gestation of pregnancy
     ❷ Z3A.38   38 weeks gestation of pregnancy
     ❷ Z3A.39   39 weeks gestation of pregnancy

● **Z3A.4 Weeks of gestation of pregnancy, weeks 40 or greater**
     ❷ Z3A.40   40 weeks gestation of pregnancy
     ❷ Z3A.41   41 weeks gestation of pregnancy
     ❷ Z3A.42   42 weeks gestation of pregnancy
     ❷ Z3A.49   Greater than 42 weeks gestation of pregnancy

● **Z37   Outcome of delivery**
     This category is intended for use as an additional code to identify the outcome of delivery on the mother's record. It is not for use on the newborn record.
     Excludes1   stillbirth (P95)
❷● **Z37.0   Single live birth** ♀ 🅗   **M**
❷● **Z37.1   Single stillbirth** ♀ 🅗   **M**
❷● **Z37.2   Twins, both liveborn** ♀ 🅗   **M**
❷● **Z37.3   Twins, one liveborn and one stillborn** ♀ 🅗   **M**
❷● **Z37.4   Twins, both stillborn** ♀ 🅗   **M**
● **Z37.5   Other multiple births, all liveborn**
     ❷●■ **Z37.50   Multiple births, unspecified, all liveborn** ♀   **M**
     ❷● **Z37.51   Triplets, all liveborn** ♀ 🅗   **M**
     ❷● **Z37.52   Quadruplets, all liveborn** ♀ 🅗   **M**
     ❷● **Z37.53   Quintuplets, all liveborn** ♀ 🅗   **M**
     ❷● **Z37.54   Sextuplets, all liveborn** ♀ 🅗   **M**
     ❷● **Z37.59   Other multiple births, all liveborn** ♀ 🅗   **M**

● **Z37.6   Other multiple births, some liveborn**
     ❷●■ **Z37.60   Multiple births, unspecified, some liveborn** ♀   **M**
     ❷● **Z37.61   Triplets, some liveborn** ♀ 🅗   **M**
     ❷● **Z37.62   Quadruplets, some liveborn** ♀ 🅗   **M**
     ❷● **Z37.63   Quintuplets, some liveborn** ♀ 🅗   **M**
     ❷● **Z37.64   Sextuplets, some liveborn** ♀ 🅗   **M**
     ❷● **Z37.69   Other multiple births, some liveborn** ♀ 🅗   **M**
❷● **Z37.7   Other multiple births, all stillborn** ♀ 🅗   **M**
❷●■ **Z37.9   Outcome of delivery, unspecified** ♀ 🅗   **M**
     Multiple birth NOS
     Single birth NOS

● **Z38   Liveborn infants according to place of birth and type of delivery**
     This category is for use as the principal code on the initial record of a newborn baby. It is to be used for the initial birth record only. It is not to be used on the mother's record.
     ● **Z38.0   Single liveborn infant, born in hospital**
       Single liveborn infant, born in birthing center or other health care facility
       ❶ **Z38.00   Single liveborn infant, delivered vaginally** 🅗   **N**
       ❶ **Z38.01   Single liveborn infant, delivered by cesarean** 🅗   **N**
     ❶● **Z38.1   Single liveborn infant, born outside hospital** 🅗   **N**
     ❶■ **Z38.2   Single liveborn infant, unspecified as to place of birth** 🅗   **N**
       Single liveborn infant NOS
     ● **Z38.3   Twin liveborn infant, born in hospital**
       ❶ **Z38.30   Twin liveborn infant, delivered vaginally** 🅗   **N**
       ❶ **Z38.31   Twin liveborn infant, delivered by cesarean** 🅗   **N**
     ❶● **Z38.4   Twin liveborn infant, born outside hospital** 🅗   **N**
     ❶■ **Z38.5   Twin liveborn infant, unspecified as to place of birth** 🅗   **N**
     ● **Z38.6   Other multiple liveborn infant, born in hospital**
       ❶ **Z38.61   Triplet liveborn infant, delivered vaginally** 🅗   **N**
       ❶ **Z38.62   Triplet liveborn infant, delivered by cesarean** 🅗   **N**
       ❶ **Z38.63   Quadruplet liveborn infant, delivered vaginally** 🅗   **N**
       ❶ **Z38.64   Quadruplet liveborn infant, delivered by cesarean** 🅗   **N**
       ❶ **Z38.65   Quintuplet liveborn infant, delivered vaginally** 🅗   **N**
       ❶ **Z38.66   Quintuplet liveborn infant, delivered by cesarean** 🅗   **N**
       ❶ **Z38.68   Other multiple liveborn infant, delivered vaginally** 🅗   **N**
       ❶ **Z38.69   Other multiple liveborn infant, delivered by cesarean** 🅗   **N**
     ❶● **Z38.7   Other multiple liveborn infant, born outside hospital** 🅗   **N**
     ❶■ **Z38.8   Other multiple liveborn infant, unspecified as to place of birth** 🅗   **N**

N Newborn Age: 0   **P** Pediatric Age: 0–17   **M** Maternity DX: 12–55   **A** Adult Age: 15–124   ♀ Females Only   ♂ Males Only

🅒 Complication\Comorbidity   ◆ Major C\C   🅗 Present on Admission Requirement   🅗 Hospital-Acquired Condition

1803

CHAPTER 21 (Z00-Z99)

● **Z39 Encounter for maternal postpartum care and examination**

❶ **Z39.0 Encounter for care and examination of mother immediately after delivery** ♀ 🔍   **M**

Care and observation in uncomplicated cases when the delivery occurs outside a healthcare facility

    Excludes1   care for postpartum complication - see Alphabetic index

❶● **Z39.1 Encounter for care and examination of lactating mother** ♀ 🔍   **M**

Encounter for supervision of lactation

    Excludes1   disorders of lactation (O92.-)

❶● **Z39.2 Encounter for routine postpartum follow-up** ♀ 🔍 **M**

ENCOUNTERS FOR OTHER SPECIFIC HEALTH CARE (Z40-Z53)

Categories Z40-Z53 are intended for use to indicate a reason for care. They may be used for patients who have already been treated for a disease or injury, but who are receiving aftercare or prophylactic care, or care to consolidate the treatment, or to deal with a residual state

    Excludes2   follow-up examination for medical surveillance after treatment (Z08-Z09)

● **Z40 Encounter for prophylactic surgery**

    Excludes1   organ donations (Z52.-)

therapeutic organ removal - code to condition

● **Z40.0 Encounter for prophylactic surgery for risk factors related to malignant neoplasms**

Admission for prophylactic organ removal

Use additional code to identify risk factor

🔢 **Z40.00 Encounter for prophylactic removal of unspecified organ** 🔍

🔢 **Z40.01 Encounter for prophylactic removal of breast** 🔍

🔢 **Z40.02 Encounter for prophylactic removal of ovary** ♀ 🔍

🔢 **Z40.09 Encounter for prophylactic removal of other organ** 🔍

🔢● **Z40.8 Encounter for other prophylactic surgery** 🔍

🔢●◼ **Z40.9 Encounter for prophylactic surgery, unspecified** 🔍

● **Z41 Encounter for procedures for purposes other than remedying health state**

🔢 **Z41.1 Encounter for cosmetic surgery** 🔍

Encounter for cosmetic breast implant
Encounter for cosmetic procedure

    Excludes1   encounter for plastic and reconstructive surgery following medical procedure or healed injury (Z42.-)

encounter for post-mastectomy breast implantation (Z42.1)

🔢 **Z41.2 Encounter for routine and ritual male circumcision** ♂ 🔍

🔢● **Z41.3 Encounter for ear piercing** 🔍

🔢● **Z41.8 Encounter for other procedures for purposes other than remedying health state** 🔍

🔢●◼ **Z41.9 Encounter for procedure for purposes other than remedying health state, unspecified** 🔍

● **Z42 Encounter for plastic and reconstructive surgery following medical procedure or healed injury**

    Excludes1   encounter for cosmetic plastic surgery (Z41.1)

encounter for plastic surgery for treatment of current injury - code to relevent injury

❶ **Z42.1 Encounter for breast reconstruction following mastectomy** 🔍   **A**

    Excludes1   deformity and disproportion of reconstructed breast (N65.1-)

❶ **Z42.8 Encounter for other plastic and reconstructive surgery following medical procedure or healed injury** 🔍

● **Z43 Encounter for attention to artificial openings**

    Includes   closure of artificial openings

passage of sounds or bougies through artificial openings
reforming artificial openings
removal of catheter from artificial openings
toilet or cleansing of artificial openings

    Excludes1   artificial opening status only, without need for care (Z93.-)

complications of external stoma (J95.0-, K94.-, N99.5-)

    Excludes2   fitting and adjustment of prosthetic and other devices (Z44-Z46)

🔢 **Z43.0 Encounter for attention to tracheostomy** 🔍

🔢 **Z43.1 Encounter for attention to gastrostomy** 🔗🔍

🔢 **Z43.2 Encounter for attention to ileostomy** 🔍

🔢 **Z43.3 Encounter for attention to colostomy** 🔍

🔢 **Z43.4 Encounter for attention to other artificial openings of digestive tract** 🔍

🔢 **Z43.5 Encounter for attention to cystostomy** 🔍

🔢 **Z43.6 Encounter for attention to other artificial openings of urinary tract** 🔍

Encounter for attention to nephrostomy
Encounter for attention to ureterostomy
Encounter for attention to urethrostomy

🔢 **Z43.7 Encounter for attention to artificial vagina** 🔍

🔢 **Z43.8 Encounter for attention to other artificial openings** 🔍

🔢●◼ **Z43.9 Encounter for attention to unspecified artificial opening** 🔍

● **Z44 Encounter for fitting and adjustment of external prosthetic device**

    Includes   removal or replacement of external prosthetic device

    Excludes1   malfunction or other complications of device - see Alphabetical Index

presence of prosthetic device (Z97.-)

● **Z44.0 Encounter for fitting and adjustment of artificial arm**

● **Z44.00 Encounter for fitting and adjustment of unspecified artificial arm**

🔢◼ **Z44.001 Encounter for fitting and adjustment of unspecified right artificial arm** 🔍

🔢◼ **Z44.002 Encounter for fitting and adjustment of unspecified left artificial arm** 🔍

🔢◼ **Z44.009 Encounter for fitting and adjustment of unspecified artificial arm, unspecified arm** 🔍

● Unacceptable Principal Diagnosis   ● Use Additional Character(s)   ◼ Unspecified   ▶ Manifestation Code

OGCR Official Guidelines for Coding and Reporting   Excludes 1   Excludes 2   Includes   Use additional   Code first   Code also

❶ First Listed   🔢 First Listed or Secondary   ❷ Secondary Only

● **Z44.01** **Encounter for fitting and adjustment of complete artificial arm**

    ½ **Z44.011** Encounter for fitting and adjustment of complete right artificial arm

    ½ **Z44.012** Encounter for fitting and adjustment of complete left artificial arm

    ½ ▪ **Z44.019** Encounter for fitting and adjustment of complete artificial arm, unspecified arm

● **Z44.02** **Encounter for fitting and adjustment of partial artificial arm**

    ½ **Z44.021** Encounter for fitting and adjustment of partial artificial right arm

    ½ **Z44.022** Encounter for fitting and adjustment of partial artificial left arm

    ½ ▪ **Z44.029** Encounter for fitting and adjustment of partial artificial arm, unspecified arm

● **Z44.1** **Encounter for fitting and adjustment of artificial leg**

    ● **Z44.10** Encounter for fitting and adjustment of unspecified artificial leg

     ½ ▪ **Z44.101** Encounter for fitting and adjustment of unspecified right artificial leg

     ½ ▪ **Z44.102** Encounter for fitting and adjustment of unspecified left artificial leg

     ½ ▪ **Z44.109** Encounter for fitting and adjustment of unspecified artificial leg, unspecified leg

    ● **Z44.11** Encounter for fitting and adjustment of complete artificial leg

     ½ **Z44.111** Encounter for fitting and adjustment of complete right artificial leg

     ½ **Z44.112** Encounter for fitting and adjustment of complete left artificial leg

     ½ ▪ **Z44.119** Encounter for fitting and adjustment of complete artificial leg, unspecified leg

    ● **Z44.12** Encounter for fitting and adjustment of partial artificial leg

     ½ **Z44.121** Encounter for fitting and adjustment of partial artificial right leg

     ½ **Z44.122** Encounter for fitting and adjustment of partial artificial left leg

     ½ ▪ **Z44.129** Encounter for fitting and adjustment of partial artificial leg, unspecified leg

● **Z44.2** **Encounter for fitting and adjustment of artificial eye**

    | Excludes1 | mechanical complication of ocular prosthesis (T85.3)

    ½ ▪ **Z44.20** Encounter for fitting and adjustment of artificial eye, unspecified

    ½ **Z44.21** Encounter for fitting and adjustment of artificial right eye

    ½ **Z44.22** Encounter for fitting and adjustment of artificial left eye

● **Z44.3** **Encounter for fitting and adjustment of external breast prosthesis**

    | Excludes1 | complications of breast implant (T85.4-)
       encounter for adjustment or removal of breast implant (Z45.81-)
       encounter for initial breast implant insertion for cosmetic breast augmentation (Z41.1)
       encounter for breast reconstruction following mastectomy (Z42.1)

    ½ ▪ **Z44.30** Encounter for fitting and adjustment of external breast prosthesis, unspecified breast ♀

    ½ **Z44.31** Encounter for fitting and adjustment of external right breast prosthesis ♀

    ½ **Z44.32** Encounter for fitting and adjustment of external left breast prosthesis ♀

½ ● **Z44.8** Encounter for fitting and adjustment of other external prosthetic devices

½ ● ▪ **Z44.9** Encounter for fitting and adjustment of unspecified external prosthetic device

● **Z45** **Encounter for adjustment and management of implanted device**

    Includes   removal or replacement of implanted device
    | Excludes1 | malfunction or other complications of device - see Alphabetical Index
       presence of prosthetic and other devices (Z95-Z97)
    | Excludes2 | encounter for fitting and adjustment of non-implanted device (Z46.-)

● **Z45.0** **Encounter for adjustment and management of cardiac device**

    ● **Z45.01** Encounter for adjustment and management of cardiac pacemaker

     | Excludes1 | encounter for adjustment and management of automatic implantable cardiac defibrillator with synchronous cardiac pacemaker (Z45.02)

     ½ **Z45.010** Encounter for checking and testing of cardiac pacemaker pulse generator [battery]
       Encounter for replacing cardiac pacemaker pulse generator [battery]
       MCE: Questionable admission when principal dx

     ½ **Z45.018** Encounter for adjustment and management of other part of cardiac pacemaker
       MCE: Questionable admission when principal dx

    ½ **Z45.02** Encounter for adjustment and management of automatic implantable cardiac defibrillator
       Encounter for adjustment and management of automatic implantable cardiac defibrillator with synchronous cardiac pacemaker
       MCE: Questionable admission when principal dx

    ½ **Z45.09** Encounter for adjustment and management of other cardiac device
       MCE: Questionable admission when principal dx

CHAPTER 21 (Z00-Z99)

🔢 **Z45.1** Encounter for adjustment and management of infusion pump 🔖

🔢 **Z45.2** Encounter for adjustment and management of vascular access device 🔖
Encounter for adjustment and management of vascular catheters

> **Excludes1** encounter for adjustment and management of renal dialysis catheter (Z49.01)

● **Z45.3** Encounter for adjustment and management of implanted devices of the special senses

🔢 **Z45.31** Encounter for adjustment and management of implanted visual substitution device 🔖

● **Z45.32** Encounter for adjustment and management of implanted hearing device

> **Excludes1** encounter for fitting and adjustment of hearing aide (Z46.1)

🔢 **Z45.320** Encounter for adjustment and management of bone conduction device 🔖

🔢 **Z45.321** Encounter for adjustment and management of cochlear device 🔖

🔢 **Z45.328** Encounter for adjustment and management of other implanted hearing device 🔖

● **Z45.4** Encounter for adjustment and management of implanted nervous system device

🔢 **Z45.41** Encounter for adjustment and management of cerebrospinal fluid drainage device 🔖
Encounter for adjustment and management of cerebral ventricular (communicating) shunt

🔢 **Z45.42** Encounter for adjustment and management of neuropacemaker (brain) (peripheral nerve) (spinal cord) 🔖

🔢 **Z45.49** Encounter for adjustment and management of other implanted nervous system device 🔖

● **Z45.8** Encounter for adjustment and management of other implanted devices

● **Z45.81** Encounter for adjustment or removal of breast implant
Encounter for elective implant exchange (different material) (different size)
Encounter removal of tissue expander without synchronous insertion of permanent implant

> **Excludes1** complications of breast implant (T85.4-)
encounter for initial breast implant insertion for cosmetic breast augmentation (Z41.1)
encounter for breast reconstruction following mastectomy (Z42.1)

🔢 **Z45.811** Encounter for adjustment or removal of right breast implant ♀ 🔖

🔢 **Z45.812** Encounter for adjustment or removal of left breast implant ♀ 🔖

🔢 **Z45.819** Encounter for adjustment or removal of unspecified breast implant ♀ 🔖

🔢● **Z45.82** Encounter for adjustment or removal of myringotomy device (stent) (tube) 🔖

🔢● **Z45.89** Encounter for adjustment and management of other implanted devices 🔖

🔢●■ **Z45.9** Encounter for adjustment and management of unspecified implanted device 🔖

● **Z46** Encounter for fitting and adjustment of other devices
Includes removal or replacement of other device
Excludes1 malfunction or other complications of device - see Alphabetical Index
Excludes2 encounter for fitting and management of implanted devices (Z45.-)
issue of repeat prescription only (Z76.0)
presence of prosthetic and other devices (Z95-Z97)

🔢● **Z46.0** Encounter for fitting and adjustment of spectacles and contact lenses 🔖

🔢● **Z46.1** Encounter for fitting and adjustment of hearing aid 🔖

> **Excludes1** encounter for adjustment and management of implanted hearing device (Z45.32-)

🔢 **Z46.2** Encounter for fitting and adjustment of other devices related to nervous system and special senses 🔖

> **Excludes2** encounter for adjustment and management of implanted nervous system device (Z45.4-)
encounter for adjustment and management of implanted visual substitution device (Z45.31)

🔢 **Z46.3** Encounter for fitting and adjustment of dental prosthetic device 🔖
Encounter for fitting and adjustment of dentures

🔢● **Z46.4** Encounter for fitting and adjustment of orthodontic device 🔖

● **Z46.5** Encounter for fitting and adjustment of other gastrointestinal appliance and device

> **Excludes1** encounter for attention to artificial openings of digestive tract (Z43.1-Z43.4)

🔢● **Z46.51** Encounter for fitting and adjustment of gastric lap band 🔖

🔢● **Z46.59** Encounter for fitting and adjustment of other gastrointestinal appliance and device 🔖

🔢● **Z46.6** Encounter for fitting and adjustment of urinary device 🔖

> **Excludes2** attention to artificial openings of urinary tract (Z43.5, Z43.6)

● **Z46.8** Encounter for fitting and adjustment of other specified devices

🔢● **Z46.81** Encounter for fitting and adjustment of insulin pump 🔖
Encounter for insulin pump instruction and training
Encounter for insulin pump titration

🔢 **Z46.82** Encounter for fitting and adjustment of non-vascular catheter 🔖

🔢● **Z46.89** Encounter for fitting and adjustment of other specified devices 🔖
Encounter for fitting and adjustment of wheelchair

Ⅴ⑫● ■ **Z46.9 Encounter for fitting and adjustment of unspecified device** ✎

● **Z47 Orthopedic aftercare**

> **Excludes1** aftercare for healing fracture - code to fracture with 7th character D

Ⅴ⑫ **Z47.1 Aftercare following joint replacement surgery** ✎

> Use additional code to identify the joint (Z96.6-)

Ⅴ⑫ **Z47.2 Encounter for removal of internal fixation device** ✎

> **Excludes1** encounter for adjustment of internal fixation device for fracture treatment - code to fracture with appropriate 7th character
> encounter for removal of external fixation device - code to fracture with 7th character D
> infection or inflammatory reaction to internal fixation device (T84.6-)
> mechanical complication of internal fixation device (T84.1-)

● **Z47.3 Aftercare following explantation of joint prosthesis**

> Aftercare following explantation of joint prosthesis, staged procedure
> Encounter for joint prosthesis insertion following prior explantation of joint prosthesis

Ⅴ⑫ **Z47.31 Aftercare following explantation of shoulder joint prosthesis**

> **Excludes1** acquired absence of shoulder joint following prior explantation of shoulder joint prosthesis (Z89.23-)
> shoulder joint prosthesis explantation status (Z89.23-)

Ⅴ⑫ **Z47.32 Aftercare following explantation of hip joint prosthesis**

> **Excludes1** acquired absence of hip joint following prior explantation of hip joint prosthesis (Z89.62-)
> hip joint prosthesis explantation status (Z89.62-)

Ⅴ⑫ **Z47.33 Aftercare following explantation of knee joint prosthesis**

> **Excludes1** acquired absence of knee joint following prior explantation of knee prosthesis (Z89.52-)
> knee joint prosthesis explantation status (Z89.52-)

● **Z47.8 Encounter for other orthopedic aftercare**

Ⅴ⑫ **Z47.81 Encounter for orthopedic aftercare following surgical amputation** ✎

> Use additional code to identify the limb amputated (Z89.-)

Ⅴ⑫ **Z47.82 Encounter for orthopedic aftercare following scoliosis surgery** ✎

Ⅴ⑫ **Z47.89 Encounter for other orthopedic aftercare** ✎

● **Z48 Encounter for other postprocedural aftercare**

> **Excludes1** encounter for follow-up examination after completed treatment (Z08-Z09)
> **Excludes2** encounter for attention to artificial openings (Z43.-)
> encounter for fitting and adjustment of prosthetic and other devices (Z44-Z46)

● **Z48.0 Encounter for attention to dressings, sutures and drains**

> **Excludes1** encounter for planned postprocedural wound closure (Z48.1)

Ⅴ⑫● **Z48.00 Encounter for change or removal of nonsurgical wound dressing** ✎

> Encounter for change or removal of wound dressing NOS

Ⅴ⑫● **Z48.01 Encounter for change or removal of surgical wound dressing** ✎

Ⅴ⑫● **Z48.02 Encounter for removal of sutures** ✎

> Encounter for removal of staples

Ⅴ⑫ **Z48.03 Encounter for change or removal of drains** ✎

Ⅴ⑫ **Z48.1 Encounter for planned postprocedural wound closure** ✎

> **Excludes1** encounter for attention to dressings and sutures (Z48.0-)

● **Z48.2 Encounter for aftercare following organ transplant**

Ⅴ⑫● **Z48.21 Encounter for aftercare following heart transplant** 🅒 ✎

> MCC: Only when the principal diagnosis is designated as a CC

Ⅴ⑫● **Z48.22 Encounter for aftercare following kidney transplant** 🅒 ✎

> MCC: Only when the principal diagnosis is designated as a CC

Ⅴ⑫● **Z48.23 Encounter for aftercare following liver transplant** 🅒 ✎

> MCC: Only when the principal diagnosis is designated as a CC

Ⅴ⑫● **Z48.24 Encounter for aftercare following lung transplant** 🅒 ✎

> MCC: Only when the principal diagnosis is designated as a CC

● **Z48.28 Encounter for aftercare following multiple organ transplant**

Ⅴ⑫● **Z48.280 Encounter for aftercare following heart-lung transplant** 🅒 ✎

> MCC: Only when the principal diagnosis is designated as a CC

Ⅴ⑫● **Z48.288 Encounter for aftercare following multiple organ transplant** ✎

● **Z48.29 Encounter for aftercare following other organ transplant**

Ⅴ⑫● **Z48.290 Encounter for aftercare following bone marrow transplant** 🅒 ✎

> MCC: Only when the principal diagnosis is designated as a CC

Ⅴ⑫● **Z48.298 Encounter for aftercare following other organ transplant** ✎

CHAPTER 21 (Z00-Z99)

CHAPTER 21 (Z00-Z99)

⑫ Z48.3 Aftercare following surgery for neoplasm 🔍
Use additional code to identify the neoplasm

● **Z48.8 Encounter for other specified postprocedural aftercare**

● **Z48.81 Encounter for surgical aftercare following surgery on specified body systems**
These codes identify the body system requiring aftercare. They are for use in conjunction with other aftercare codes to fully explain the aftercare encounter. The condition treated should also be coded if still present.

Excludes1   aftercare for injury - code the injury with 7th character D
aftercare following surgery for neoplasm (Z48.3)

Excludes2   aftercare following organ transplant (Z48.2-)
orthopedic aftercare (Z47.-)

⑫ **Z48.810 Encounter for surgical aftercare following surgery on the sense organs** 🔍

⑫ **Z48.811 Encounter for surgical aftercare following surgery on the nervous system** 🔍

Excludes2   encounter for surgical aftercare following surgery on the sense organs (Z48.810)

⑫ **Z48.812 Encounter for surgical aftercare following surgery on the circulatory system** 🔍

⑫ **Z48.813 Encounter for surgical aftercare following surgery on the respiratory system** 🔍

⑫ **Z48.814 Encounter for surgical aftercare following surgery on the teeth or oral cavity** 🔍

⑫ **Z48.815 Encounter for surgical aftercare following surgery on the digestive system** 🔍

⑫ **Z48.816 Encounter for surgical aftercare following surgery on the genitourinary system** 🔍

Excludes1   encounter for aftercare following sterilization reversal (Z31.42)

⑫ **Z48.817 Encounter for surgical aftercare following surgery on the skin and subcutaneous tissue** 🔍

⑫ **Z48.89 Encounter for other specified surgical aftercare** 🔍

● **Z49 Encounter for care involving renal dialysis**
Code also associated end stage renal disease (N18.6)

● **Z49.0 Preparatory care for renal dialysis**
Encounter for dialysis instruction and training

⑫ **Z49.01 Encounter for fitting and adjustment of extracorporeal dialysis catheter** 🔍
Removal or replacement of renal dialysis catheter
Toilet or cleansing of renal dialysis catheter

⑫● **Z49.02 Encounter for fitting and adjustment of peritoneal dialysis catheter** 🔍

● **Z49.3 Encounter for adequacy testing for dialysis**

⑫● **Z49.31 Encounter for adequacy testing for hemodialysis** 🔍

⑫● **Z49.32 Encounter for adequacy testing for peritoneal dialysis** 🔍
Encounter for peritoneal equilibration test

● **Z51 Encounter for other aftercare**
Code also condition requiring care

Excludes1   follow-up examination after treatment (Z08-Z09)

❶ **Z51.0 Encounter for antineoplastic radiation therapy** 🔍

● **Z51.1 Encounter for antineoplastic chemotherapy and immunotherapy**

Excludes2   encounter for chemotherapy and immunotherapy for nonneoplastic condition--code to condition

❶ **Z51.11 Encounter for antineoplastic chemotherapy** 🔍

❶ **Z51.12 Encounter for antineoplastic immunotherapy** 🔍

⑫● **Z51.5 Encounter for palliative care** 🔍

● **Z51.8 Encounter for other specified aftercare**

Excludes1   holiday relief care (Z75.5)

⑫ **Z51.81 Encounter for therapeutic drug level monitoring** 🔍
Code also any long-term (current) drug therapy (Z79.-)

Excludes1   encounter for blood-drug test for administrative or medicolegal reasons (Z02.83)

⑫● **Z51.89 Encounter for other specified aftercare** 🔍

● **Z52 Donors of organs and tissues**
Includes   autologous and other living donors
Excludes1   cadaveric donor - omit code
examination of potential donor (Z00.5)

● **Z52.0 Blood donor**

● **Z52.00 Unspecified blood donor**

❶● **Z52.000 Unspecified donor, whole blood** 🔍

❶● **Z52.001 Unspecified donor, stem cells** 🔍

❶● **Z52.008 Unspecified donor, other blood** 🔍

● **Z52.01 Autologous blood donor**

❶● **Z52.010 Autologous donor, whole blood** 🔍

❶● **Z52.011 Autologous donor, stem cells** 🔍

❶● **Z52.018 Autologous donor, other blood** 🔍

● Unacceptable Principal Diagnosis   ● Use Additional Character(s)   ■ Unspecified   ▶ Manifestation Code
OGCR Official Guidelines for Coding and Reporting   Excludes 1   Excludes 2   Includes   Use additional   Code first   Code also
❶ First Listed   ⑫ First Listed or Secondary   ❷ Secondary Only

● **Z52.09**   **Other blood donor**
     Volunteer donor

     ❶● **Z52.090**   **Other blood donor, whole blood** 🔖

     ❶● **Z52.091**   **Other blood donor, stem cells** 🔖

     ❶● **Z52.098**   **Other blood donor, other blood** 🔖

● **Z52.1**   **Skin donor**

     ❶■ **Z52.10**   **Skin donor, unspecified** 🔖

     ❶ **Z52.11**   **Skin donor, autologous** 🔖

     ❶ **Z52.19**   **Skin donor, other** 🔖

● **Z52.2**   **Bone donor**

     ❶■ **Z52.20**   **Bone donor, unspecified** 🔖

     ❶ **Z52.21**   **Bone donor, autologous** 🔖

     ❶ **Z52.29**   **Bone donor, other** 🔖

❶ **Z52.3**   **Bone marrow donor** 🔖

❶ **Z52.4**   **Kidney donor** 🔖

❶ **Z52.5**   **Cornea donor** 🔖

❶ **Z52.6**   **Liver donor** 🔖

● **Z52.8**   **Donor of other specified organs or tissues**

     ● **Z52.81**   **Egg (Oocyte) donor**

         ❶● **Z52.810**   **Egg (Oocyte) donor under age 35, anonymous recipient** ♀ 🔖
         Egg donor under age 35 NOS

         ❶● **Z52.811**   **Egg (Oocyte) donor under age 35, designated recipient** ♀ 🔖

         ❶● **Z52.812**   **Egg (Oocyte) donor age 35 and over, anonymous recipient** ♀ 🔖
         Egg donor age 35 and over NOS

         ❶● **Z52.813**   **Egg (Oocyte) donor age 35 and over, designated recipient** ♀ 🔖

         ❶●■ **Z52.819**   **Egg (Oocyte) donor, unspecified** ♀ 🔖

     ❶ **Z52.89**   **Donor of other specified organs or tissues** 🔖

❶■ **Z52.9**   **Donor of unspecified organ or tissue** 🔖
     Donor NOS

● **Z53**   **Persons encountering health services for specific procedures and treatment, not carried out**

     ● **Z53.0**   **Procedure and treatment not carried out because of contraindication**

         ①②● **Z53.01**   **Procedure and treatment not carried out due to patient smoking** 🔖

         ①②● **Z53.09**   **Procedure and treatment not carried out because of other contraindication** 🔖

     ①②● **Z53.1**   **Procedure and treatment not carried out because of patient's decision for reasons of belief and group pressure** 🔖

     ● **Z53.2**   **Procedure and treatment not carried out because of patient's decision for other and unspecified reasons**

         ①②●■ **Z53.20**   **Procedure and treatment not carried out because of patient's decision for unspecified reasons** 🔖

         ①②● **Z53.21**   **Procedure and treatment not carried out due to patient leaving prior to being seen by health care provider** 🔖

         ①②● **Z53.29**   **Procedure and treatment not carried out because of patient's decision for other reasons** 🔖

①②● **Z53.8**   **Procedure and treatment not carried out for other reasons** 🔖

①②●■ **Z53.9**   **Procedure and treatment not carried out, unspecified reason** 🔖

PERSONS WITH POTENTIAL HEALTH HAZARDS RELATED TO SOCIOECONOMIC AND PSYCHOSOCIAL CIRCUMSTANCES (Z55-Z65)

● **Z55**   **Problems related to education and literacy**

     Excludes1   disorders of psychological development (F80-F89)

     ①②● **Z55.0**   **Illiteracy and low-level literacy** 🔖

     ①②● **Z55.1**   **Schooling unavailable and unattainable** 🔖

     ①②● **Z55.2**   **Failed school examinations** 🔖

     ①②● **Z55.3**   **Underachievement in school** 🔖

     ①②● **Z55.4**   **Educational maladjustment and discord with teachers and classmates** 🔖

     ①②● **Z55.8**   **Other problems related to education and literacy** 🔖
     Problems related to inadequate teaching

     ①②●■ **Z55.9**   **Problems related to education and literacy, unspecified** 🔖
     Academic problems NOS

● **Z56**   **Problems related to employment and unemployment**

     Excludes2   occupational exposure to risk factors (Z57.-)   problems related to housing and economic circumstances (Z59.-)

     ①②●■ **Z56.0**   **Unemployment, unspecified** 🔖

     ①②● **Z56.1**   **Change of job** 🔖   **A**

     ①②● **Z56.2**   **Threat of job loss** 🔖

     ①②● **Z56.3**   **Stressful work schedule** 🔖

     ①②● **Z56.4**   **Discord with boss and workmates** 🔖

     ①②● **Z56.5**   **Uncongenial work environment** 🔖
     Difficult conditions at work

     ①②● **Z56.6**   **Other physical and mental strain related to work** 🔖

     ● **Z56.8**   **Other problems related to employment**

         ①②● **Z56.81**   **Sexual harassment on the job** 🔖

         ①②● **Z56.82**   **Military deployment status** 🔖
         Individual (civilian or military) currently deployed in theater or in support of military war, peacekeeping and humanitarian operations

         ①②● **Z56.89**   **Other problems related to employment** 🔖

     ①②●■ **Z56.9**   **Unspecified problems related to employment** 🔖
     Occupational problems NOS

● **Z57**   **Occupational exposure to risk factors**

     ①②● **Z57.0**   **Occupational exposure to noise** 🔖

     ①②● **Z57.1**   **Occupational exposure to radiation** 🔖

     ①②● **Z57.2**   **Occupational exposure to dust** 🔖

     ● **Z57.3**   **Occupational exposure to other air contaminants**

         ①②● **Z57.31**   **Occupational exposure to environmental tobacco smoke** 🔖

         Excludes2   exposure to environmental tobacco smoke (Z77.22)

         ①②● **Z57.39**   **Occupational exposure to other air contaminants** 🔖

     ①②● **Z57.4**   **Occupational exposure to toxic agents in agriculture** 🔖
     Occupational exposure to solids, liquids, gases or vapors in agriculture

---

N   Newborn Age: 0   **P**   Pediatric Age: 0–17   **M**   Maternity DX: 12–55   **A**   Adult Age: 15–124   ♀   Females Only   ♂   Males Only

🔖   Complication\Comorbidity   🔖   Major C\C   🔖   Present on Admission Requirement   🔖   Hospital-Acquired Condition

1809

1/2 ● **Z57.5 Occupational exposure to toxic agents in other industries** 🔍
　　　Occupational exposure to solids, liquids, gases or vapors in other industries

1/2 ● **Z57.6 Occupational exposure to extreme temperature** 🔍

1/2 ● **Z57.7 Occupational exposure to vibration** 🔍

1/2 ● **Z57.8 Occupational exposure to other risk factors** 🔍

1/2 ● ■ **Z57.9 Occupational exposure to unspecified risk factor** 🔍

● **Z59 Problems related to housing and economic circumstances**
　　　Excludes2 problems related to upbringing (Z62.-)

1/2 ● **Z59.0 Homelessness** 🔍

1/2 ● **Z59.1 Inadequate housing** 🔍
　　　Lack of heating
　　　Restriction of space
　　　Technical defects in home preventing adequate care
　　　Unsatisfactory surroundings
　　　Excludes1 problems related to the natural and physical environment (Z77.1-)

1/2 ● **Z59.2 Discord with neighbors, lodgers and landlord** 🔍

1/2 ● **Z59.3 Problems related to living in residential institution** 🔍
　　　Boarding-school resident
　　　Excludes1 institutional upbringing (Z62.2)

1/2 ● **Z59.4 Lack of adequate food and safe drinking water** 🔍
　　　Inadequate drinking water supply
　　　Excludes1 effects of hunger (T73.0)
　　　　　　　　　inappropriate diet or eating habits (Z72.4)
　　　　　　　　　malnutrition (E40-E46)

1/2 ● **Z59.5 Extreme poverty** 🔍

1/2 ● **Z59.6 Low income** 🔍

1/2 ● **Z59.7 Insufficient social insurance and welfare support** 🔍

1/2 ● **Z59.8 Other problems related to housing and economic circumstances** 🔍
　　　Foreclosure on loan
　　　Isolated dwelling
　　　Problems with creditors

1/2 ● ■ **Z59.9 Problem related to housing and economic circumstances, unspecified** 🔍

● **Z60 Problems related to social environment**

1/2 ● **Z60.0 Problems of adjustment to life-cycle transitions** 🔍
　　　Empty nest syndrome
　　　Phase of life problem
　　　Problem with adjustment to retirement [pension]

1/2 ● **Z60.2 Problems related to living alone** 🔍

1/2 ● **Z60.3 Acculturation difficulty** 🔍
　　　Problem with migration
　　　Problem with social transplantation

1/2 ● **Z60.4 Social exclusion and rejection** 🔍
　　　Exclusion and rejection on the basis of personal characteristics, such as unusual physical appearance, illness or behavior.
　　　Excludes1 target of adverse discrimination such as for racial or religious reasons (Z60.5)

1/2 ● **Z60.5 Target of (perceived) adverse discrimination and persecution** 🔍
　　　Excludes1 social exclusion and rejection (Z60.4)

1/2 ● **Z60.8 Other problems related to social environment** 🔍

1/2 ● ■ **Z60.9 Problem related to social environment, unspecified** 🔍

● **Z62 Problems related to upbringing**
　　　Includes current and past negative life events in childhood
　　　　　　current and past problems of a child related to upbringing
　　　Excludes2 maltreatment syndrome (T74.-)
　　　　　　　　problems related to housing and economic circumstances (Z59.-)

1/2 ● **Z62.0 Inadequate parental supervision and control** 🔍

1/2 ● **Z62.1 Parental overprotection** 🔍

● **Z62.2 Upbringing away from parents**
　　　Excludes1 problems with boarding school (Z59.3)

1/2 ● **Z62.21 Child in welfare custody** 🔍　　　　P
　　　Child in care of non-parental family member
　　　Child in foster care
　　　Excludes2 problem for parent due to child in welfare custody (Z63.5)

1/2 ● **Z62.22 Institutional upbringing** 🔍
　　　Child living in orphanage or group home

1/2 ● **Z62.29 Other upbringing away from parents** 🔍

1/2 ● **Z62.3 Hostility towards and scapegoating of child** 🔍　　P

1/2 ● **Z62.6 Inappropriate (excessive) parental pressure** 🔍

● **Z62.8 Other specified problems related to upbringing**

● **Z62.81 Personal history of abuse in childhood**

1/2 ● **Z62.810 Personal history of physical and sexual abuse in childhood** 🔍
　　　Excludes1 current child physical abuse (T74.12, T76.12)
　　　　　　　　current child sexual abuse (T74.22, T76.22)

1/2 ● **Z62.811 Personal history of psychological abuse in childhood** 🔍
　　　Excludes1 current child psychological abuse (T74.32, T76.32)

1/2 ● **Z62.812 Personal history of neglect in childhood** 🔍
　　　Excludes1 current child neglect (T74.02, T76.02)

1/2 ● ■ **Z62.819 Personal history of unspecified abuse in childhood** 🔍
　　　Excludes1 current child abuse NOS (T74.92, T76.92)

● **Z62.82 Parent-child conflict**

1/2 ● **Z62.820 Parent-biological child conflict** 🔍
　　　Parent-child problem NOS

1/2 ● **Z62.821 Parent-adopted child conflict** 🔍

1/2 ● **Z62.822 Parent-foster child conflict** 🔍

● **Z62.89 Other specified problems related to upbringing**

1/2 ● **Z62.890 Parent-child estrangement NEC** 🔍

1/2 ● **Z62.891 Sibling rivalry** 🔍

1/2 ● **Z62.898 Other specified problems related to upbringing** 🔍

1/2 ● ■ **Z62.9 Problem related to upbringing, unspecified** 🔍

CHAPTER 21 (Z00-Z99)

● **Z63** **Other problems related to primary support group, including family circumstances**

    Excludes2   maltreatment syndrome (T74.-, T76)
            parent-child problems (Z62.-)
            problems related to negative life events in childhood (Z62.-)
            problems related to upbringing (Z62.-)

  ① ● **Z63.0** **Problems in relationship with spouse or partner**

      Excludes1   counseling for spousal or partner abuse problems (Z69.1)
              counseling related to sexual attitude, behavior, and orientation (Z70.-)

  ① ● **Z63.1** **Problems in relationship with in-laws**

  ● **Z63.3** **Absence of family member**

      Excludes1   absence of family member due to disappearance and death (Z63.4)
              absence of family member due to separation and divorce (Z63.5)

    ① ● **Z63.31** **Absence of family member due to military deployment**
        Individual or family affected by other family member being on military deployment

        Excludes1   family disruption due to return of family member from military deployment (Z63.71)

    ① ● **Z63.32** **Other absence of family member**

  ① ● **Z63.4** **Disappearance and death of family member**
      Assumed death of family member
      Bereavement

  ① ● **Z63.5** **Disruption of family by separation and divorce**
      Marital estrangement

  ① ● **Z63.6** **Dependent relative needing care at home**

  ● **Z63.7** **Other stressful life events affecting family and household**

    ① ● **Z63.71** **Stress on family due to return of family member from military deployment**
        Individual or family affected by family member having returned from military deployment (current or past conflict)

    ① ● **Z63.72** **Alcoholism and drug addiction in family**

    ① ● **Z63.79** **Other stressful life events affecting family and household**
        Anxiety (normal) about sick person in family
        Health problems within family
        Ill or disturbed family member
        Isolated family

  ① ● **Z63.8** **Other specified problems related to primary support group**
      Family discord NOS
      Family estrangement NOS
      High expressed emotional level within family
      Inadequate family support NOS
      Inadequate or distorted communication within family

  ① ● ■ **Z63.9** **Problem related to primary support group, unspecified**
      Relationship disorder NOS

● **Z64** **Problems related to certain psychosocial circumstances**

  ① ● **Z64.0** **Problems related to unwanted pregnancy** ♀   **M**

  ① ● **Z64.1** **Problems related to multiparity** ♀

  ① ● **Z64.4** **Discord with counselors**
      Discord with probation officer
      Discord with social worker

● **Z65** **Problems related to other psychosocial circumstances**

  ① ● **Z65.0** **Conviction in civil and criminal proceedings without imprisonment**

  ① ● **Z65.1** **Imprisonment and other incarceration**

  ① ● **Z65.2** **Problems related to release from prison**

  ① ● **Z65.3** **Problems related to other legal circumstances**
      Arrest
      Child custody or support proceedings
      Litigation
      Prosecution

  ① ● **Z65.4** **Victim of crime and terrorism**
      Victim of torture

  ① ● **Z65.5** **Exposure to disaster, war and other hostilities**   **A**

      Excludes1   target of perceived discrimination or persecution (Z60.5)

  ① ● **Z65.8** **Other specified problems related to psychosocial circumstances**

  ① ● ■ **Z65.9** **Problem related to unspecified psychosocial circumstances**

DO NOT RESUSCITATE STATUS (Z66)

❷ ● **Z66** **Do not resuscitate**
    DNR status

BLOOD TYPE (Z67)

● **Z67** **Blood type**

  ● **Z67.1** **Type A blood**
    ❷ ● **Z67.10** **Type A blood, Rh positive**
    ❷ ● **Z67.11** **Type A blood, Rh negative**

  ● **Z67.2** **Type B blood**
    ❷ ● **Z67.20** **Type B blood, Rh positive**
    ❷ ● **Z67.21** **Type B blood, Rh negative**

  ● **Z67.3** **Type AB blood**
    ❷ ● **Z67.30** **Type AB blood, Rh positive**
    ❷ ● **Z67.31** **Type AB blood, Rh negative**

  ● **Z67.4** **Type O blood**
    ❷ ● **Z67.40** **Type O blood, Rh positive**
    ❷ ● **Z67.41** **Type O blood, Rh negative**

  ● **Z67.9** **Unspecified blood type**
    ❷ ● **Z67.90** **Unspecified blood type, Rh positive**
    ❷ ● ■ **Z67.91** **Unspecified blood type, Rh negative**

BODY MASS INDEX [BMI] (Z68)

● **Z68** **Body mass index [BMI]**
    Kilograms per meters squared

    Note: BMI adult codes are for use for persons 21 years of age or older.

           BMI pediatric codes are for use for persons 2-20 years of age. These percentiles are based on the growth charts published by the Centers for Disease Control and Prevention (CDC)

  ❷ ● **Z68.1** **Body mass index (BMI) 19 or less, adult**   **A**

● Z68.2   Body mass index (BMI) 20-29, adult
  ❷● Z68.20   Body mass index (BMI) 20.0-20.9, adult 🔗 A
  ❷● Z68.21   Body mass index (BMI) 21.0-21.9, adult 🔗 A
  ❷● Z68.22   Body mass index (BMI) 22.0-22.9, adult 🔗 A
  ❷● Z68.23   Body mass index (BMI) 23.0-23.9, adult 🔗 A
  ❷● Z68.24   Body mass index (BMI) 24.0-24.9, adult 🔗 A
  ❷● Z68.25   Body mass index (BMI) 25.0-25.9, adult 🔗 A
  ❷● Z68.26   Body mass index (BMI) 26.0-26.9, adult 🔗 A
  ❷● Z68.27   Body mass index (BMI) 27.0-27.9, adult 🔗 A
  ❷● Z68.28   Body mass index (BMI) 28.0-28.9, adult 🔗 A
  ❷● Z68.29   Body mass index (BMI) 29.0-29.9, adult 🔗 A

● Z68.3   Body mass index (BMI) 30-39, adult
  ❷● Z68.30   Body mass index (BMI) 30.0-30.9, adult 🔗 A
  ❷● Z68.31   Body mass index (BMI) 31.0-31.9, adult 🔗 A
  ❷● Z68.32   Body mass index (BMI) 32.0-32.9, adult 🔗 A
  ❷● Z68.33   Body mass index (BMI) 33.0-33.9, adult 🔗 A
  ❷● Z68.34   Body mass index (BMI) 34.0-34.9, adult 🔗 A
  ❷● Z68.35   Body mass index (BMI) 35.0-35.9, adult 🔗 A
  ❷● Z68.36   Body mass index (BMI) 36.0-36.9, adult 🔗 A
  ❷● Z68.37   Body mass index (BMI) 37.0-37.9, adult 🔗 A
  ❷● Z68.38   Body mass index (BMI) 38.0-38.9, adult 🔗 A
  ❷● Z68.39   Body mass index (BMI) 39.0-39.9, adult 🔗 A

● Z68.4   Body mass index (BMI) 40 or greater, adult
  ❷● Z68.41 Body mass index (BMI) 40.0-44.9, adult 🔗 A
  ❷● Z68.42 Body mass index (BMI) 45.0-49.9, adult 🔗 A
  ❷● Z68.43 Body mass index (BMI) 50-59.9, adult 🔗 A
  ❷● Z68.44 Body mass index (BMI) 60.0-69.9, adult 🔗 A
  ❷● Z68.45 Body mass index (BMI) 70 or greater, adult 🔗 A

● Z68.5   Body mass index (BMI) pediatric
  ❷● Z68.51   Body mass index (BMI) pediatric, less than 5th percentile for age 🔗 P
  ❷● Z68.52   Body mass index (BMI) pediatric, 5th percentile to less than 85th percentile for age 🔗 P
  ❷● Z68.53   Body mass index (BMI) pediatric, 85th percentile to less than 95th percentile for age 🔗 P
  ❷● Z68.54   Body mass index (BMI) pediatric, greater than or equal to 95th percentile for age 🔗 P

PERSONS ENCOUNTERING HEALTH SERVICES IN OTHER CIRCUMSTANCES (Z69-Z76)

● Z69   Encounter for mental health services for victim and perpetrator of abuse

  Includes   counseling for victims and perpetrators of abuse

  ● Z69.0   Encounter for mental health services for child abuse problems

    ● Z69.01   Encounter for mental health services for parental child abuse

      ①❷ Z69.010   Encounter for mental health services for victim of parental child abuse 🔗 P

      ①❷● Z69.011   Encounter for mental health services for perpetrator of parental child abuse 🔗

        Excludes1   encounter for mental health services for non-parental child abuse (Z69.02-)

    ● Z69.02   Encounter for mental health services for non-parental child abuse

      ①❷ Z69.020   Encounter for mental health services for victim of non-parental child abuse 🔗 P

      ①❷● Z69.021   Encounter for mental health services for perpetrator of non-parental child abuse 🔗

  ● Z69.1   Encounter for mental health services for spousal or partner abuse problems

    ①❷● Z69.11   Encounter for mental health services for victim of spousal or partner abuse 🔗

    ①❷● Z69.12   Encounter for mental health services for perpetrator of spousal or partner abuse 🔗

  ● Z69.8   Encounter for mental health services for victim or perpetrator of other abuse

    ①❷● Z69.81   Encounter for mental health services for victim of other abuse 🔗
      Encounter for rape victim counseling

    ①❷● Z69.82   Encounter for mental health services for perpetrator of other abuse 🔗

● Z70   Counseling related to sexual attitude, behavior and orientation

  Includes   encounter for mental health services for sexual attitude, behavior and orientation

  Excludes2   contraceptive or procreative counseling (Z30-Z31)

  ①❷● Z70.0   Counseling related to sexual attitude 🔗

  ①❷● Z70.1   Counseling related to patient's sexual behavior and orientation 🔗
    Patient concerned regarding impotence
    Patient concerned regarding non-responsiveness
    Patient concerned regarding promiscuity
    Patient concerned regarding sexual orientation

  ①❷● Z70.2   Counseling related to sexual behavior and orientation of third party 🔗
    Advice sought regarding sexual behavior and orientation of child
    Advice sought regarding sexual behavior and orientation of partner
    Advice sought regarding sexual behavior and orientation of spouse

  ①❷● Z70.3   Counseling related to combined concerns regarding sexual attitude, behavior and orientation 🔗

  ①❷● Z70.8   Other sex counseling 🔗
    Encounter for sex education

  ①❷● ■ Z70.9   Sex counseling, unspecified 🔗

● Z71   Persons encountering health services for other counseling and medical advice, not elsewhere classified

  Excludes2   contraceptive or procreation counseling (Z30-Z31)
    sex counseling (Z70.-)

  ①❷● Z71.0   Person encountering health services to consult on behalf of another person 🔗
    Person encountering health services to seek advice or treatment for non-attending third party

    Excludes2   anxiety (normal) about sick person in family (Z63.7)
      expectant (adoptive) parent(s) pre-birth pediatrician visit (Z76.81)

● Unacceptable Principal Diagnosis   ● Use Additional Character(s)   ■ Unspecified   ▶ Manifestation Code
OGCR Official Guidelines for Coding and Reporting   Excludes 1   Excludes 2   Includes   Use additional   Code first   Code also
❶ First Listed   ①② First Listed or Secondary   ❷ Secondary Only

⑫● **Z71.1** **Person with feared health complaint in whom no diagnosis is made** 🔖
> Person encountering health services with feared condition which was not demonstrated
> Person encountering health services in which problem was normal state
> 'Worried well'
>> **Excludes1**   medical observation for suspected diseases and conditions proven not to exist (Z03.-)

⑫● **Z71.2** **Person consulting for explanation of examination or test findings** 🔖

⑫● **Z71.3** **Dietary counseling and surveillance** 🔖
> Use additional code for any associated underlying medical condition
> Use additional code to identify body mass index (BMI), if known (Z68.-)

● **Z71.4** **Alcohol abuse counseling and surveillance**
> Use additional code for alcohol abuse or dependence (F10.-)

⑫● **Z71.41** **Alcohol abuse counseling and surveillance of alcoholic** 🔖

⑫● **Z71.42** **Counseling for family member of alcoholic** 🔖
> Counseling for significant other, partner, or friend of alcoholic

● **Z71.5** **Drug abuse counseling and surveillance**
> Use additional code for drug abuse or dependence (F11-F16, F18-F19)

⑫● **Z71.51** **Drug abuse counseling and surveillance of drug abuser** 🔖

⑫● **Z71.52** **Counseling for family member of drug abuser** 🔖
> Counseling for significant other, partner, or friend of drug abuser

⑫● **Z71.6** **Tobacco abuse counseling** 🔖
> Use additional code for nicotine dependence (F17.-)

⑫● **Z71.7** **Human immunodeficiency virus [HIV] counseling** 🔖

● **Z71.8** **Other specified counseling**
>> **Excludes2**   counseling for contraception (Z30.0-)
>> counseling for genetics (Z31.5)
>> counseling for procreative management (Z31.6-)

⑫● **Z71.81** **Spiritual or religious counseling** 🔖

⑫● **Z71.89** **Other specified counseling** 🔖

⑫●■ **Z71.9** **Counseling, unspecified** 🔖
> Encounter for medical advice NOS

● **Z72** **Problems related to lifestyle**
>> **Excludes2**   problems related to life-management difficulty (Z73.-)
>> problems related to socioeconomic and psychosocial circumstances (Z55-Z65)

⑫● **Z72.0** **Tobacco use** 🔖
> Tobacco use NOS
>> **Excludes1**   history of tobacco dependence (Z87.891)
>> nicotine dependence (F17.2-)
>> tobacco dependence (F17.2-)
>> tobacco use during pregnancy (O99.33-)

⑫● **Z72.3** **Lack of physical exercise** 🔖

⑫● **Z72.4** **Inappropriate diet and eating habits** 🔖
>> **Excludes1**   behavioral eating disorders of infancy or childhood (F98.2.-F98.3)
>> eating disorders (F50.-)
>> lack of adequate food (Z59.4)
>> malnutrition and other nutritional deficiencies (E40-E64)

● **Z72.5** **High risk sexual behavior**
> Promiscuity
>> **Excludes1**   paraphilias (F65)

⑫● **Z72.51** **High risk heterosexual behavior** 🔖

⑫● **Z72.52** **High risk homosexual behavior** 🔖

⑫● **Z72.53** **High risk bisexual behavior** 🔖

⑫● **Z72.6** **Gambling and betting** 🔖
>> **Excludes1**   compulsive or pathological gambling (F63.0)

● **Z72.8** **Other problems related to lifestyle**

● **Z72.81** **Antisocial behavior**
>> **Excludes1**   conduct disorders (F91.-)

⑫ **Z72.810** **Child and adolescent antisocial behavior** 🔖   **P**
> Antisocial behavior (child) (adolescent) without manifest psychiatric disorder
> Delinquency NOS
> Group delinquency
> Offenses in the context of gang membership
> Stealing in company with others
> Truancy from school

⑫ **Z72.811** **Adult antisocial behavior** 🔖   **A**
> Adult antisocial behavior without manifest psychiatric disorder

● **Z72.82** **Problems related to sleep**

⑫ **Z72.820** **Sleep deprivation**
> Lack of adequate sleep
>> **Excludes1**   insomnia (G47.0-)

⑫ **Z72.821** **Inadequate sleep hygiene** 🔖
> Bad sleep habits
> Irregular sleep habits
> Unhealthy sleep wake schedule
>> **Excludes1**   insomnia (F51.0-, G47.0-)

⑫● **Z72.89** **Other problems related to lifestyle** 🔖
> Self-damaging behavior

⑫●■ **Z72.9** **Problem related to lifestyle, unspecified** 🔖

● **Z73** **Problems related to life management difficulty**
>> **Excludes2**   problems related to socioeconomic and psychosocial circumstances (Z55-Z65)

⑫● **Z73.0** **Burn-out** 🔖

⑫● **Z73.1** **Type A behavior pattern** 🔖

⑫● **Z73.2** **Lack of relaxation and leisure** 🔖

⑫● **Z73.3** **Stress, not elsewhere classified** 🔖
> Physical and mental strain NOS
>> **Excludes1**   stress related to employment or unemployment (Z56.-)

⑫● **Z73.4** **Inadequate social skills, not elsewhere classified** 🔖

⑫● **Z73.5** **Social role conflict, not elsewhere classified** 🔖

⑫● **Z73.6** **Limitation of activities due to disability** 🔖
>> **Excludes1**   care-provider dependency (Z74.-)

CHAPTER 21 (Z00-Z99)

N Newborn Age: 0   **P** Pediatric Age: 0–17   **M** Maternity DX: 12–55   **A** Adult Age: 15–124   ♀ Females Only   ♂ Males Only

 Complication\Comorbidity   🔖 Major C\C   🔖 Present on Admission Requirement   🔖 Hospital-Acquired Condition

1813

CHAPTER 21 (Z00-Z99)

● **Z73.8 Other problems related to life management difficulty**

  ● **Z73.81 Behavioral insomnia of childhood**

    ⑫● **Z73.810 Behavioral insomnia of childhood, sleep-onset association type** 🔍   P

    ⑫● **Z73.811 Behavioral insomnia of childhood, limit setting type** 🔍   P

    ⑫● **Z73.812 Behavioral insomnia of childhood, combined type** 🔍   P

    ⑫●■ **Z73.819 Behavioral insomnia of childhood, unspecified type** 🔍   P

  ⑫● **Z73.82 Dual sensory impairment** 🔍

  ⑫● **Z73.89 Other problems related to life management difficulty** 🔍

● ⑫●■ **Z73.9 Problem related to life management difficulty, unspecified** 🔍

● **Z74 Problems related to care provider dependency**

    | **Excludes2** | dependence on enabling machines or devices NEC (Z99.-)

  ● **Z74.0 Reduced mobility**

    ⑫● **Z74.01 Bed confinement status** 🔍
         Bedridden

    ⑫● **Z74.09 Other reduced mobility**
         Chairridden
         Reduced mobility NOS

        | **Excludes2** | wheelchair dependence (Z99.3)

  ⑫● **Z74.1 Need for assistance with personal care** 🔍

  ⑫● **Z74.2 Need for assistance at home and no other household member able to render care** 🔍

  ⑫● **Z74.3 Need for continuous supervision** 🔍

  ⑫● **Z74.8 Other problems related to care provider dependency** 🔍

  ⑫●■ **Z74.9 Problem related to care provider dependency, unspecified** 🔍

● **Z75 Problems related to medical facilities and other health care**

  ⑫● **Z75.0 Medical services not available in home**

        | **Excludes1** | no other household member able to render care (Z74.2)

  ⑫● **Z75.1 Person awaiting admission to adequate facility elsewhere**

  ⑫● **Z75.2 Other waiting period for investigation and treatment**

  ⑫● **Z75.3 Unavailability and inaccessibility of health care facilities**

        | **Excludes1** | bed unavailable (Z75.1)

  ⑫● **Z75.4 Unavailability and inaccessibility of other helping agencies**

  ⑫● **Z75.5 Holiday relief care** 🔍

  ⑫● **Z75.8 Other problems related to medical facilities and other health care**

  ⑫●■ **Z75.9 Unspecified problem related to medical facilities and other health care**

● **Z76 Persons encountering health services in other circumstances**

  ⑫● **Z76.0 Encounter for issue of repeat prescription** 🔍
     Encounter for issue of repeat prescription for appliance
     Encounter for issue of repeat prescription for medicaments
     Encounter for issue of repeat prescription for spectacles

        | **Excludes2** | issue of medical certificate (Z02.7) repeat prescription for contraceptive (Z30.4-)

  ❶ **Z76.1 Encounter for health supervision and care of foundling** 🔍

  ❶● **Z76.2 Encounter for health supervision and care of other healthy infant and child** 🔍   P
     Encounter for medical or nursing care or supervision of healthy infant under circumstances such as adverse socioeconomic conditions at home
     Encounter for medical or nursing care or supervision of healthy infant under circumstances such as awaiting foster or adoptive placement
     Encounter for medical or nursing care or supervision of healthy infant under circumstances such as maternal illness
     Encounter for medical or nursing care or supervision of healthy infant under circumstances such as number of children at home preventing or interfering with normal care

  ⑫ **Z76.3 Healthy person accompanying sick person** 🔍

  ⑫ **Z76.4 Other boarder to healthcare facility** 🔍

        | **Excludes1** | homelessness (Z59.0)

  ⑫ **Z76.5 Malingerer [conscious simulation]** 🔍
     Person feigning illness (with obvious motivation)

        | **Excludes1** | factitious disorder (F68.1-) peregrinating patient (F68.1-)

  ● **Z76.8 Persons encountering health services in other specified circumstances**

    ⑫● **Z76.81 Expectant parent(s) prebirth pediatrician visit** 🔍
         Pre-adoption pediatrician visit for adoptive parent(s)

    ⑫● **Z76.82 Awaiting organ transplant status** 🔍
         Patient waiting for organ availability

    ⑫● **Z76.89 Persons encountering health services in other specified circumstances** 🔍
         Persons encountering health services NOS

PERSONS WITH POTENTIAL HEALTH HAZARDS RELATED TO FAMILY AND PERSONAL HISTORY AND CERTAIN CONDITIONS INFLUENCING HEALTH STATUS (Z77-Z99)

Code also any follow-up examination (Z08-Z09)

● **Z77   Other contact with and (suspected) exposures hazardous to health**

> **Includes**   contact with and (suspected) exposures to potential hazards to health
>
> **Excludes2**   contact with and (suspected) exposure to communicable diseases (Z20.-)
> exposure to (parental) (environmental) tobacco smoke in the perinatal period (P96.81)
> newborn (suspected to be) affected by noxious substances transmitted via placenta or breast milk (P04.-)
> occupational exposure to risk factors (Z57.-)
> retained foreign body (Z18.-)
> retained foreign body fully removed (Z87.821)
> toxic effects of substances chiefly nonmedicinal as to source (T51-T65)

● **Z77.0   Contact with and (suspected) exposure to hazardous, chiefly nonmedicinal, chemicals**

  ● **Z77.01   Contact with and (suspected) exposure to hazardous metals**

   ⑫● **Z77.010   Contact with and (suspected) exposure to arsenic**

   ⑫● **Z77.011   Contact with and (suspected) exposure to lead** 🔍

   ⑫● **Z77.012   Contact with and (suspected) exposure to uranium**

   > **Excludes1**   retained depleted uranium fragments (Z18.01)

   ⑫● **Z77.018   Contact with and (suspected) exposure to other hazardous metals**
   > Contact with and (suspected) exposure to chromium compounds
   > Contact with and (suspected) exposure to nickel dust

  ● **Z77.02   Contact with and (suspected) exposure to hazardous aromatic compounds**

   ⑫● **Z77.020   Contact with and (suspected) exposure to aromatic amines**

   ⑫● **Z77.021   Contact with and (suspected) exposure to benzene**

   ⑫● **Z77.028   Contact with and (suspected) exposure to other hazardous aromatic compounds**
   > Aromatic dyes NOS
   > Polycyclic aromatic hydrocarbons

  ● **Z77.09   Contact with and (suspected) exposure to other hazardous, chiefly nonmedicinal, chemicals**

   ⑫● **Z77.090   Contact with and (suspected) exposure to asbestos** 🔍

   ⑫● **Z77.098   Contact with and (suspected) exposure to other hazardous, chiefly nonmedicinal, chemicals**
   > Dyes NOS

● **Z77.1   Contact with and (suspected) exposure to environmental pollution and hazards in the physical environment**

  ● **Z77.11   Contact with and (suspected) exposure to environmental pollution**

   ⑫● **Z77.110   Contact with and (suspected) exposure to air pollution** 🔍

   ⑫● **Z77.111   Contact with and (suspected) exposure to water pollution** 🔍

   ⑫● **Z77.112   Contact with and (suspected) exposure to soil pollution** 🔍

   ⑫● **Z77.118   Contact with and (suspected) exposure to other environmental pollution** 🔍

  ● **Z77.12   Contact with and (suspected) exposure to hazards in the physical environment**

   ⑫● **Z77.120   Contact with and (suspected) exposure to mold (toxic)**

   ⑫● **Z77.121   Contact with and (suspected) exposure to harmful algae and algae toxins** 🔍
   > Contact with and (suspected) exposure to (harmful) algae bloom NOS
   > Contact with and (suspected) exposure to blue-green algae bloom
   > Contact with and (suspected) exposure to brown tide
   > Contact with and (suspected) exposure to cyanobacteria bloom
   > Contact with and (suspected) exposure to Florida red tide
   > Contact with and (suspected) exposure to pfiesteria piscicida
   > Contact with and (suspected) exposure to red tide

   ⑫● **Z77.122   Contact with and (suspected) exposure to noise** 🔍

   ⑫● **Z77.123   Contact with and (suspected) exposure to radon and other naturally occuring radiation** 🔍

   > **Excludes2**   radiation exposure as the cause of a confirmed condition (W88-W90, X39.0-)
   > radiation sickness NOS (T66)

   ⑫● **Z77.128   Contact with and (suspected) exposure to other hazards in the physical environment** 🔍

CHAPTER 21 (Z00-Z99)

CHAPTER 21 (Z00-Z99)

● **Z77.2 Contact with and (suspected) exposure to other hazardous substances**

⑫● **Z77.21 Contact with and (suspected) exposure to potentially hazardous body fluids** 🖊

⑫● **Z77.22 Contact with and (suspected) exposure to environmental tobacco smoke (acute) (chronic)** 🖊

Exposure to second hand tobacco smoke (acute) (chronic)
Passive smoking (acute) (chronic)

| Excludes1 | nicotine dependence (F17.-) tobacco use (Z72.0) |

| Excludes2 | occupational exposure to environmental tobacco smoke (Z57.31) |

⑫● **Z77.29 Contact with and (suspected) exposure to other hazardous substances**

⑫● **Z77.9 Other contact with and (suspected) exposures hazardous to health** 🖊

● **Z78 Other specified health status**

| Excludes2 | asymptomatic human immunodeficiency virus [HIV] infection status (Z21) postprocedural status (Z93- Z99) sex reassignment status (Z87.890) |

⑫● **Z78.0 Asymptomatic menopausal state ♀** 🖊   **A**

Menopausal state NOS
Postmenopausal status NOS

| Excludes2 | symptomatic menopausal state (N95.1) |

⑫● **Z78.1 Physical restraint status**

| Excludes1 | physical restraint due to a procedure - omit code |

⑫● **Z78.9 Other specified health status**

● **Z79 Long term (current) drug therapy**

| Includes | long term (current) drug use for prophylactic purposes |

Code also any therapeutic drug level monitoring (Z51.81)

| Excludes2 | drug abuse and dependence (F11-F19) drug use complicating pregnancy, childbirth, and the puerperium (O99.32-) |

● **Z79.0 Long term (current) use of anticoagulants and antithrombotics/antiplatelets**

| Excludes2 | long term (current) use of aspirin (Z79.82) |

⑫ **Z79.01 Long term (current) use of anticoagulants** 🖊

⑫● **Z79.02 Long term (current) use of antithrombotics/antiplatelets** 🖊

⑫● **Z79.1 Long term (current) use of non-steroidal anti-inflammatories (NSAID)** 🖊

| Excludes2 | long term (current) use of aspirin (Z79.82) |

⑫● **Z79.2 Long term (current) use of antibiotics** 🖊

⑫ **Z79.3 Long term (current) use of hormonal contraceptives** 🖊

Long term (current) use of birth control pill or patch

⑫ **Z79.4 Long term (current) use of insulin** 🖊

● **Z79.5 Long term (current) use of steroids**

⑫● **Z79.51 Long term (current) use of inhaled steroids** 🖊

⑫● **Z79.52 Long term (current) use of systemic steroids** 🖊

● **Z79.8 Other long term (current) drug therapy**

● **Z79.81 Long term (current) use of agents affecting estrogen receptors and estrogen levels**

Code first, if applicable:
malignant neoplasm of breast (C50.-)
malignant neoplasm of prostate (C61)

Use additional code, if applicable, to identify:
estrogen receptor positive status (Z17.0)
family history of breast cancer (Z80.3)
genetic susceptibility to malignant neoplasm (cancer) (Z15.0-)
personal history of breast cancer (Z85.3)
personal history of prostate cancer (Z85.46)
postmenopausal status (Z78.0)

| Excludes1 | hormone replacement therapy (postmenopausal) (Z79.890) |

⑫● **Z79.810 Long term (current) use of selective estrogen receptor modulators (SERMs)** 🖊

Long term (current) use of raloxifene (Evista)
Long term (current) use of tamoxifen (Nolvadex)
Long term (current) use of toremifene (Fareston)

⑫● **Z79.811 Long term (current) use of aromatase inhibitors** 🖊

Long term (current) use of anastrozole (Arimidex)
Long term (current) use of exemestane (Aromasin)
Long term (current) use of letrozole (Femara)

⑫● **Z79.818 Long term (current) use of other agents affecting estrogen receptors and estrogen levels** 🖊

Long term (current) use of estrogen receptor downregulators
Long term (current) use of fulvestrant (Faslodex)
Long term (current) use of gonadotropin-releasing hormone (GnRH) agonist
Long term (current) use of goserelin acetate (Zoladex)
Long term (current) use of leuprolide acetate (leuprorelin) (Lupron)
Long term (current) use of megestrol acetate (Megace)

⑫ **Z79.82 Long term (current) use of aspirin** 🖊

⑫● **Z79.83 Long term (current) use of bisphosphonates**

● Unacceptable Principal Diagnosis   ● Use Additional Character(s)   ■ Unspecified   ▶ Manifestation Code

OGCR Official Guidelines for Coding and Reporting   Excludes 1   Excludes 2   Includes   Use additional   Code first   Code also

❶ First Listed   ⑫ First Listed or Secondary   ❷ Secondary Only

● **Z79.89**   **Other long term (current) drug therapy**
    ⑫● **Z79.890**   Hormone replacement therapy (postmenopausal) ♀ 🔍
    ⑫● **Z79.891**   Long term (current) use of opiate analgesic 🔍
         Long term (current) use of methadone for pain management

Excludes1	methodone use NOS (F11.2-) use of methodone for treatment of heroin addiction (F11.2-)

    ⑫● **Z79.899**   Other long term (current) drug therapy 🔍

● **Z80**   **Family history of primary malignant neoplasm**
    ⑫● **Z80.0**   **Family history of malignant neoplasm of digestive organs** 🔍
       Conditions classifiable to C15-C26
    ⑫● **Z80.1**   **Family history of malignant neoplasm of trachea, bronchus and lung** 🔍
       Conditions classifiable to C33-C34
    ⑫● **Z80.2**   **Family history of malignant neoplasm of other respiratory and intrathoracic organs** 🔍
       Conditions classifiable to C30-C32, C37-C39
    ⑫● **Z80.3**   **Family history of malignant neoplasm of breast** 🔍
       Conditions classifiable to C50.-
    ● **Z80.4**   **Family history of malignant neoplasm of genital organs**
       Conditions classifiable to C51-C63
      ⑫● **Z80.41**   **Family history of malignant neoplasm of ovary** ♀ 🔍
      ⑫● **Z80.42**   **Family history of malignant neoplasm of prostate** ♂ 🔍
      ⑫● **Z80.43**   **Family history of malignant neoplasm of testis** ♂ 🔍
      ⑫● **Z80.49**   **Family history of malignant neoplasm of other genital organs** 🔍
    ● **Z80.5**   **Family history of malignant neoplasm of urinary tract**
       Conditions classifiable to C64-C68
      ⑫● **Z80.51**   **Family history of malignant neoplasm of kidney** 🔍
      ⑫● **Z80.52**   **Family history of malignant neoplasm of bladder** 🔍
      ⑫● **Z80.59**   **Family history of malignant neoplasm of other urinary tract organ** 🔍
    ⑫● **Z80.6**   **Family history of leukemia** 🔍
       Conditions classifiable to C91-C95
    ⑫● **Z80.7**   **Family history of other malignant neoplasms of lymphoid, hematopoietic and related tissues** 🔍
       Conditions classifiable to C81-C90, C96.-
    ⑫● **Z80.8**   **Family history of malignant neoplasm of other organs or systems** 🔍
       Conditions classifiable to C00-C14, C40-C49, C69-C79
    ⑫● ■ **Z80.9**   **Family history of malignant neoplasm, unspecified** 🔍
       Conditions classifiable to C80.1

● **Z81**   **Family history of mental and behavioral disorders**
    ⑫● **Z81.0**   **Family history of intellectual disabilities** 🔍
       Conditions classifiable to F70-F79
    ⑫● **Z81.1**   **Family history of alcohol abuse and dependence** 🔍
       Conditions classifiable to F10.-
    ⑫● **Z81.2**   **Family history of tobacco abuse and dependence** 🔍
       Conditions classifiable to F17.-
    ⑫● **Z81.3**   **Family history of other psychoactive substance abuse and dependence** 🔍
       Conditions classifiable to F11-F16, F18-F19
    ⑫● **Z81.4**   **Family history of other substance abuse and dependence** 🔍
       Conditions classifiable to F55
    ⑫● **Z81.8**   **Family history of other mental and behavioral disorders** 🔍
       Conditions classifiable elsewhere in F01-F99

● **Z82**   **Family history of certain disabilities and chronic diseases (leading to disablement)**
    ⑫● **Z82.0**   **Family history of epilepsy and other diseases of the nervous system** 🔍
       Conditions classifiable to G00-G99
    ⑫● **Z82.1**   **Family history of blindness and visual loss** 🔍
       Conditions classifiable to H54.-
    ⑫● **Z82.2**   **Family history of deafness and hearing loss** 🔍
       Conditions classifiable to H90-H91
    ⑫● **Z82.3**   **Family history of stroke** 🔍
       Conditions classifiable to I60-I64
    ● **Z82.4**   **Family history of ischemic heart disease and other diseases of the circulatory system**
       Conditions classifiable to I00-I52, I65-I99
      ⑫● **Z82.41**   **Family history of sudden cardiac death** 🔍
      ⑫● **Z82.49**   **Family history of ischemic heart disease and other diseases of the circulatory system** 🔍
    ⑫● **Z82.5**   **Family history of asthma and other chronic lower respiratory diseases** 🔍
       Conditions classifiable to J40-J47

Excludes2	family history of other diseases of the respiratory system (Z83.6)

    ● **Z82.6**   **Family history of arthritis and other diseases of the musculoskeletal system and connective tissue**
       Conditions classifiable to M00-M99
      ⑫● **Z82.61**   **Family history of arthritis** 🔍
      ⑫● **Z82.62**   **Family history of osteoporosis** 🔍
      ⑫● **Z82.69**   **Family history of other diseases of the musculoskeletal system and connective tissue** 🔍
    ● **Z82.7**   **Family history of congenital malformations, deformations and chromosomal abnormalities**
       Conditions classifiable to Q00-Q99
      ⑫● **Z82.71**   **Family history of polycystic kidney** 🔍
      ⑫● **Z82.79**   **Family history of other congenital malformations, deformations and chromosomal abnormalities** 🔍
    ⑫● **Z82.8**   **Family history of other disabilities and chronic diseases leading to disablement, not elsewhere classified** 🔍

[handwritten notes:] Z80-Z87 History Codes maybe used as secondary codes if impact on current care of family history

● **Z83   Family history of other specific disorders**

> **Excludes2**   contact with and (suspected) exposure to communicable disease in the family (Z20.-)

⑫● **Z83.0   Family history of human immunodeficiency virus [HIV] disease** 🔍
>   Conditions classifiable to B20

⑫● **Z83.1   Family history of other infectious and parasitic diseases** 🔍
>   Conditions classifiable to A00-B19, B25-B94, B99

⑫● **Z83.2   Family history of diseases of the blood and blood-forming organs and certain disorders involving the immune mechanism** 🔍
>   Conditions classifiable to D50-D89

⑫● **Z83.3   Family history of diabetes mellitus** 🔍
>   Conditions classifiable to E08-E13

● **Z83.4   Family history of other endocrine, nutritional and metabolic diseases**
>   Conditions classifiable to E00-E07, E15-E88

⑫● **Z83.41   Family history of multiple endocrine neoplasia [MEN] syndrome** 🔍

⑫● **Z83.49   Family history of other endocrine, nutritional and metabolic diseases** 🔍

● **Z83.5   Family history of eye and ear disorders**

● **Z83.51   Family history of eye disorders**
>   Conditions classifiable to H00-H53, H55-H59

> **Excludes2**   family history of blindness and visual loss (Z82.1)

⑫● **Z83.511   Family history of glaucoma** 🔍

⑫● **Z83.518   Family history of other specified eye disorder** 🔍

⑫ **Z83.52   Family history of ear disorders** 🔍
>   Conditions classifiable to H60-H83, H92-H95

> **Excludes2**   family history of deafness and hearing loss (Z82.2)

⑫● **Z83.6   Family history of other diseases of the respiratory system** 🔍
>   Conditions classifiable to J00-J39, J60-J99

> **Excludes2**   family history of asthma and other chronic lower respiratory diseases (Z82.5)

● **Z83.7   Family history of diseases of the digestive system**
>   Conditions classifiable to K00-K93

⑫● **Z83.71   Family history of colonic polyps** 🔍

> **Excludes1**   family history of malignant neoplasm of digestive organs (Z80.0)

⑫● **Z83.79   Family history of other diseases of the digestive system** 🔍

● **Z84   Family history of other conditions**

⑫● **Z84.0   Family history of diseases of the skin and subcutaneous tissue** 🔍
>   Conditions classifiable to L00-L99

⑫● **Z84.1   Family history of disorders of kidney and ureter** 🔍
>   Conditions classifiable to N00-N29

⑫● **Z84.2   Family history of other diseases of the genitourinary system** 🔍
>   Conditions classifiable to N30-N99

⑫● **Z84.3   Family history of consanguinity** 🔍

● **Z84.8   Family history of other specified conditions**

⑫● **Z84.81   Family history of carrier of genetic disease** 🔍

⑫● **Z84.89   Family history of other specified conditions** 🔍

● **Z85   Personal history of malignant neoplasm**

> *Code first any follow-up examination after treatment of malignant neoplasm (Z08)*

> Use additional code to identify:
>   alcohol use and dependence (F10.-)
>   exposure to environmental tobacco smoke (Z77.22)
>   history of tobacco use (Z87.891)
>   occupational exposure to environmental tobacco smoke (Z57.31)
>   tobacco dependence (F17.-)
>   tobacco use (Z72.0)

> **Excludes2**   personal history of benign neoplasm (Z86.01-)
>   personal history of carcinoma-in-situ (Z86.00-)

● **Z85.0   Personal history of malignant neoplasm of digestive organs**

⑫● ■ **Z85.00   Personal history of malignant neoplasm of unspecified digestive organ** 🔍

⑫● **Z85.01   Personal history of malignant neoplasm of esophagus** 🔍
>   Conditions classifiable to C15

● **Z85.02   Personal history of malignant neoplasm of stomach**

⑫● **Z85.020   Personal history of malignant carcinoid tumor of stomach** 🔍
>   Conditions classifiable to C7A.092

⑫● **Z85.028   Personal history of other malignant neoplasm of stomach** 🔍
>   Conditions classifiable to C16

● **Z85.03   Personal history of malignant neoplasm of large intestine**

⑫● **Z85.030   Personal history of malignant carcinoid tumor of large intestine** 🔍
>   Conditions classifiable to C7A.022-C7A.025, C7A.029

⑫● **Z85.038   Personal history of other malignant neoplasm of large intestine** 🔍
>   Conditions classifiable to C18

● **Z85.04   Personal history of malignant neoplasm of rectum, rectosigmoid junction, and anus**

⑫● **Z85.040   Personal history of malignant carcinoid tumor of rectum** 🔍
>   Conditions classifiable to C7A.026

⑫● **Z85.048   Personal history of other malignant neoplasm of rectum, rectosigmoid junction, and anus** 🔍
>   Conditions classifiable to C19-C21

● ● **Z85.05** **Personal history of malignant neoplasm of liver** 🔲
      Conditions classifiable to C22

● **Z85.06** **Personal history of malignant neoplasm of small intestine**

  1/2 ● **Z85.060** **Personal history of malignant carcinoid tumor of small intestine** 🔲
      Conditions classifiable to C7A.01-

  1/2 ● **Z85.068** **Personal history of other malignant neoplasm of small intestine** 🔲
      Conditions classifiable to C17

1/2 ● **Z85.07** **Personal history of malignant neoplasm of pancreas** 🔲
      Conditions classifiable to C25

● ● **Z85.09** **Personal history of malignant neoplasm of other digestive organs** 🔲

● **Z85.1** **Personal history of malignant neoplasm of trachea, bronchus and lung**

 ● **Z85.11** **Personal history of malignant neoplasm of bronchus and lung**

  1/2 ● **Z85.110** **Personal history of malignant carcinoid tumor of bronchus and lung**
      Conditions classifiable to C7A.090

  1/2 ● **Z85.118** **Personal history of other malignant neoplasm of bronchus and lung** 🔲
      Conditions classifiable to C34

 1/2 ● **Z85.12** **Personal history of malignant neoplasm of trachea** 🔲
      Conditions classifiable to C33

● **Z85.2** **Personal history of malignant neoplasm of other respiratory and intrathoracic organs**

 1/2 ● ■ **Z85.20** **Personal history of malignant neoplasm of unspecified respiratory organ** 🔲

 1/2 ● **Z85.21** **Personal history of malignant neoplasm of larynx** 🔲
      Conditions classifiable to C32

 1/2 ● **Z85.22** **Personal history of malignant neoplasm of nasal cavities, middle ear, and accessory sinuses** 🔲
      Conditions classifiable to C30-C31

 ● **Z85.23** **Personal history of malignant neoplasm of thymus**

  1/2 ● **Z85.230** **Personal history of malignant carcinoid tumor of thymus** 🔲
      Conditions classifiable to C7A.091

  1/2 ● **Z85.238** **Personal history of other malignant neoplasm of thymus** 🔲
      Conditions classifiable to C37

 1/2 ● **Z85.29** **Personal history of malignant neoplasm of other respiratory and intrathoracic organs** 🔲

● ● **Z85.3** **Personal history of malignant neoplasm of breast** 🔲
      Conditions classifiable to C50.-

● **Z85.4** **Personal history of malignant neoplasm of genital organs**
      Conditions classifiable to C51-C63

 1/2 ● ■ **Z85.40** **Personal history of malignant neoplasm of unspecified female genital organ** ♀ 🔲

 1/2 ● **Z85.41** **Personal history of malignant neoplasm of cervix uteri** ♀ 🔲

 1/2 ● **Z85.42** **Personal history of malignant neoplasm of other parts of uterus** ♀ 🔲

 1/2 ● **Z85.43** **Personal history of malignant neoplasm of ovary** ♀ 🔲

 1/2 ● **Z85.44** **Personal history of malignant neoplasm of other female genital organs** ♀ 🔲

 1/2 ● ■ **Z85.45** **Personal history of malignant neoplasm of unspecified male genital organ** ♂ 🔲

 1/2 ● **Z85.46** **Personal history of malignant neoplasm of prostate** ♂ 🔲

 1/2 ● **Z85.47** **Personal history of malignant neoplasm of testis** ♂ 🔲

 1/2 ● **Z85.48** **Personal history of malignant neoplasm of epididymis** ♂ 🔲

 1/2 ● **Z85.49** **Personal history of malignant neoplasm of other male genital organs** ♂ 🔲

● **Z85.5** **Personal history of malignant neoplasm of urinary tract**
      Conditions classifiable to C64-C68

 1/2 ● ■ **Z85.50** **Personal history of malignant neoplasm of unspecified urinary tract organ** 🔲

 1/2 ● **Z85.51** **Personal history of malignant neoplasm of bladder** 🔲

 ● **Z85.52** **Personal history of malignant neoplasm of kidney**

   | **Excludes1** | personal history of malignant neoplasm of renal pelvis (Z85.53) |

  1/2 ● **Z85.520** **Personal history of malignant carcinoid tumor of kidney** 🔲
      Conditions classifiable to C7A.093

  1/2 ● **Z85.528** **Personal history of other malignant neoplasm of kidney** 🔲
      Conditions classifiable to C64

 1/2 ● **Z85.53** **Personal history of malignant neoplasm of renal pelvis** 🔲

 1/2 ● **Z85.54** **Personal history of malignant neoplasm of ureter** 🔲

 1/2 ● **Z85.59** **Personal history of malignant neoplasm of other urinary tract organ** 🔲

1/2 ● **Z85.6** **Personal history of leukemia** 🔲
      Conditions classifiable to C91-C95

   | **Excludes1** | leukemia in remission C91.0-C95.9 with 5th character 1 |

● **Z85.7** **Personal history of other malignant neoplasms of lymphoid, hematopoietic and related tissues**

 1/2 ● **Z85.71** **Personal history of Hodgkin lymphoma** 🔲
      Conditions classifiable to C81

 1/2 ● **Z85.72** **Personal history of non-Hodgkin lymphomas** 🔲
      Conditions classifiable to C82-C85

CHAPTER 21 (Z00-Z99)

N Newborn Age: 0   **P** Pediatric Age: 0–17   **M** Maternity DX: 12–55   **A** Adult Age: 15–124   ♀ Females Only   ♂ Males Only

🔲 Complication\Comorbidity   🔲 Major C\C   🔲 Present on Admission Requirement   🔲 Hospital-Acquired Condition

1819

CHAPTER 21 (Z00-Z99)

(V2)● **Z85.79** **Personal history of other malignant neoplasms of lymphoid, hematopoietic and related tissues** 🖉
Conditions classifiable to C88-C90, C96

Excludes1   multiple myeloma in
remission (C90.01)
plasma cell leukemia in
remission (C90.11)
plasmacytoma in remission
(C90.21)

● **Z85.8 Personal history of malignant neoplasms of other organs and systems**
Conditions classifiable to C00-C14, C40-C49, C69-C79, C7A.098

● **Z85.81 Personal history of malignant neoplasm of lip, oral cavity, and pharynx**

(V2)● **Z85.810** **Personal history of malignant neoplasm of tongue** 🖉

(V2)● **Z85.818** **Personal history of malignant neoplasm of other sites of lip, oral cavity, and pharynx** 🖉

(V2)●■ **Z85.819** **Personal history of malignant neoplasm of unspecified site of lip, oral cavity, and pharynx** 🖉

● **Z85.82 Personal history of malignant neoplasm of skin**

(V2)● **Z85.820** **Personal history of malignant melanoma of skin** 🖉
Conditions classifiable to C43

(V2)●● **Z85.821** **Personal history of Merkel cell carcinoma** 🖉
Conditions classifiable to C4A

(V2)●● **Z85.828** **Personal history of other malignant neoplasm of skin** 🖉
Conditions classifiable to C44

● **Z85.83 Personal history of malignant neoplasm of bone and soft tissue**

(V2)●● **Z85.830** **Personal history of malignant neoplasm of bone** 🖉

(V2)●● **Z85.831** **Personal history of malignant neoplasm of soft tissue** 🖉

Excludes2   personal history
of malignant
neoplasm of
skin (Z85.82-)

● **Z85.84 Personal history of malignant neoplasm of eye and nervous tissue**

(V2)●● **Z85.840** **Personal history of malignant neoplasm of eye** 🖉

(V2)●● **Z85.841** **Personal history of malignant neoplasm of brain** 🖉

(V2)●● **Z85.848** **Personal history of malignant neoplasm of other parts of nervous tissue** 🖉

● **Z85.85 Personal history of malignant neoplasm of endocrine glands**

(V2)●● **Z85.850** **Personal history of malignant neoplasm of thyroid** 🖉

(V2)●● **Z85.858** **Personal history of malignant neoplasm of other endocrine glands** 🖉

(V2)●● **Z85.89 Personal history of malignant neoplasm of other organs and systems** 🖉

(V2)●■ **Z85.9 Personal history of malignant neoplasm, unspecified** 🖉
Conditions classifiable to C7A.00, C80.1

● **Z86 Personal history of certain other diseases**
Code first any follow-up examination after treatment (Z09)

● **Z86.0 Personal history of in-situ and benign neoplasms and neoplasms of uncertain behavior**

Excludes2   personal history of malignant
neoplasms (Z85.-)

● **Z86.00 Personal history of in-situ neoplasm**

(V2)● **Z86.000** **Personal history of in-situ neoplasm of breast** 🖉

(V2)● **Z86.001** **Personal history of in-situ neoplasm of cervix uteri** ♀ 🖉

(V2)● **Z86.008** **Personal history of in-situ neoplasm of other site** 🖉

● **Z86.01 Personal history of benign neoplasm**

(V2)● **Z86.010** **Personal history of colonic polyps** 🖉

(V2)● **Z86.011** **Personal history of benign neoplasm of the brain** 🖉

(V2)● **Z86.012** **Personal history of benign carcinoid tumor** 🖉

(V2)● **Z86.018** **Personal history of other benign neoplasm** 🖉

(V2)● **Z86.03 Personal history of neoplasm of uncertain behavior** 🖉

● **Z86.1 Personal history of infectious and parasitic diseases**
Conditions classifiable to A00-B89, B99

Excludes1   personal history of infectious
diseases specific to a body
system sequelae of infectious
and parasitic diseases (B90-B94)

(V2)● **Z86.11 Personal history of tuberculosis** 🖉

(V2)● **Z86.12 Personal history of poliomyelitis** 🖉

(V2)● **Z86.13 Personal history of malaria** 🖉

(V2)● **Z86.14 Personal history of Methicillin resistant Staphylococcus aureus infection** 🖉
Personal history of MRSA infection

(V2)● **Z86.19 Personal history of other infectious and parasitic diseases** 🖉

(V2)● **Z86.2 Personal history of diseases of the blood and blood-forming organs and certain disorders involving the immune mechanism** 🖉
Conditions classifiable to D50-D89

● **Z86.3 Personal history of endocrine, nutritional and metabolic diseases**
Conditions classifiable to E00-E88

(V2)● **Z86.31 Personal history of diabetic foot ulcer** 🖉

Excludes2   current diabetic foot ulcer
(E08.621, E09.621,
E10.621, E11.621,
E13.621)

(V2)● **Z86.32 Personal history of gestational diabetes** 🖉
Personal history of conditions classifiable to O24.4-

Excludes1   gestational diabetes mellitus
in current pregnancy
(O24.4-)

(V2)● **Z86.39 Personal history of other endocrine, nutritional and metabolic disease** 🖉

● Unacceptable Principal Diagnosis   ● Use Additional Character(s)   ■ Unspecified   ▶ Manifestation Code
OGCR Official Guidelines for Coding and Reporting   Excludes 1   Excludes 2   Includes   Use additional   Code first   Code also
❶ First Listed   (V2) First Listed or Secondary   ❷ Secondary Only

● **Z86.5　Personal history of mental and behavioral disorders**
Conditions classifiable to F40-F59

1/2 ● **Z86.51　Personal history of combat and operational stress reaction** 🔖　　　　　　**A**

1/2 ● **Z86.59　Personal history of other mental and behavioral disorders** 🔖

● **Z86.6　Personal history of diseases of the nervous system and sense organs**
Conditions classifiable to G00-G99, H00-H95

1/2 ● **Z86.61　Personal history of infections of the central nervous system** 🔖
Personal history of encephalitis
Personal history of meningitis

1/2 ● **Z86.69　Personal history of other diseases of the nervous system and sense organs** 🔖

● **Z86.7　Personal history of diseases of the circulatory system**
Conditions classifiable to I00-I99

Excludes2　old myocardial infarction (I25.2)
personal history of anaphylactic shock (Z87.892)
postmyocardial infarction syndrome (I24.1)

● **Z86.71　Personal history of venous thrombosis and embolism**

1/2 ● **Z86.711　Personal history of pulmonary embolism** 🔖

1/2 ● **Z86.718　Personal history of other venous thrombosis and embolism** 🔖

1/2 ● **Z86.72　Personal history of thrombophlebitis** 🔖

1/2 ● **Z86.73　Personal history of transient ischemic attack (TIA), and cerebral infarction without residual deficits** 🔖
Personal history of prolonged reversible ischemic neurological deficit (PRIND)
Personal history of stroke NOS without residual deficits

Excludes1　personal history of traumatic brain injury (Z87.820)
sequelae of cerebrovascular disease (I69.-)

1/2 ● **Z86.74　Personal history of sudden cardiac arrest** 🔖
Personal history of sudden cardiac death successfully resuscitated

1/2 ● **Z86.79　Personal history of other diseases of the circulatory system** 🔖

● **Z87　Personal history of other diseases and conditions**
Code first any follow-up examination after treatment (Z09)

● **Z87.0　Personal history of diseases of the respiratory system**
Conditions classifiable to J00-J99

1/2 ● **Z87.01　Personal history of pneumonia (recurrent)** 🔖

1/2 ● **Z87.09　Personal history of other diseases of the respiratory system** 🔖

● **Z87.1　Personal history of diseases of the digestive system**
Conditions classifiable to K00-K93

1/2 ● **Z87.11　Personal history of peptic ulcer disease** 🔖

1/2 ● **Z87.19　Personal history of other diseases of the digestive system** 🔖

1/2 ● **Z87.2　Personal history of diseases of the skin and subcutaneous tissue** 🔖
Conditions classifiable to L00-L99

Excludes2　personal history of diabetic foot ulcer (Z86.31)

● **Z87.3　Personal history of diseases of the musculoskeletal system and connective tissue**
Conditions classifiable to M00-M99

Excludes2　personal history of (healed) traumatic fracture (Z87.81)

● **Z87.31　Personal history of (healed) nontraumatic fracture**

1/2 ● **Z87.310　Personal history of (healed) osteoporosis fracture** 🔖
Personal history of (healed) fragility fracture
Personal history of (healed) collapsed vertebra due to osteoporosis

1/2 ● **Z87.311　Personal history of (healed) other pathological fracture** 🔖
Personal history of (healed) collapsed vertebra NOS

Excludes2　personal history of osteoporosis fracture (Z87.310)

1/2 ● **Z87.312　Personal history of (healed) stress fracture** 🔖
Personal history of (healed) fatigue fracture

1/2 ● **Z87.39　Personal history of other diseases of the musculoskeletal system and connective tissue** 🔖

● **Z87.4　Personal history of diseases of genitourinary system**
Conditions classifiable to N00-N99

● **Z87.41　Personal history of dysplasia of the female genital tract**

Excludes1　personal history of malignant neoplasm of female genital tract (Z85.40-Z85.44)

1/2 ● **Z87.410　Personal history of cervical dysplasia** ♀ 🔖

1/2 ● **Z87.411　Personal history of vaginal dysplasia** ♀ 🔖

1/2 ● **Z87.412　Personal history of vulvar dysplasia** ♀ 🔖

1/2 ● **Z87.42　Personal history of other diseases of the female genital tract** ♀ 🔖

● **Z87.43　Personal history of diseases of male genital organs**

1/2 ● **Z87.430　Personal history of prostatic dysplasia** 🔖

Excludes1　personal history of malignant neoplasm of prostate (Z85.46)

1/2 ● **Z87.438　Personal history of other diseases of male genital organs** 🔖

N　Newborn Age: 0　　**P**　Pediatric Age: 0–17　　**M**　Maternity DX: 12–55　　**A**　Adult Age: 15–124　　♀　Females Only　　♂　Males Only

🔖 Complication\Comorbidity　　🔖 Major C\C　　🔖 Present on Admission Requirement　　🔖 Hospital-Acquired Condition

CHAPTER 21 (Z00-Z99)

● **Z87.44**   **Personal history of diseases of urinary system**

     Excludes1   personal history of malignant neoplasm of cervix uteri (Z85.41)

1/2 ● **Z87.440**   **Personal history of urinary (tract) infections** 🔲

1/2 ● **Z87.441**   **Personal history of nephrotic syndrome** 🔲

1/2 ● **Z87.442**   **Personal history of urinary calculi** 🔲

     Personal history of kidney stones

1/2 ● **Z87.448**   **Personal history of other diseases of urinary system** 🔲

● **Z87.5**   **Personal history of complications of pregnancy, childbirth and the puerperium**

     Conditions classifiable to O00-O9A

     Excludes2   recurrent pregnancy loss (N96)

1/2 ● **Z87.51**   **Personal history of pre-term labor** ♀ 🔲

     Excludes1   current pregnancy with history of pre-term labor (O09.21-)

1/2 ● **Z87.59**   **Personal history of other complications of pregnancy, childbirth and the puerperium** ♀ 🔲

     Personal history of trophoblastic disease

● **Z87.7**   **Personal history of (corrected) congenital malformations**

     Conditions classifiable to Q00-Q89 that have been repaired or corrected

     Excludes1   congenital malformations that have been partially corrected or repair but which still require medical treatment - code to condition

     Excludes2   other postprocedural states (Z98.-)
     personal history of medical treatment (Z92.-)
     presence of cardiac and vascular implants and grafts (Z95.-)
     presence of other devices (Z97.-)
     presence of other functional implants (Z96.-)
     transplanted organ and tissue status (Z94.-)

● **Z87.71**   **Personal history of (corrected) congenital malformations of genitourinary system**

1/2 ● **Z87.710**   **Personal history of (corrected) hypospadias** ♂ 🔲

1/2 ● **Z87.718**   **Personal history of other specified (corrected) congenital malformations of genitourinary system** 🔲

● **Z87.72**   **Personal history of (corrected) congenital malformations of nervous system and sense organs**

1/2 ● **Z87.720**   **Personal history of (corrected) congenital malformations of eye** 🔲

1/2 ● **Z87.721**   **Personal history of (corrected) congenital malformations of ear** 🔲

1/2 ● **Z87.728**   **Personal history of other specified (corrected) congenital malformations of nervous system and sense organs** 🔲

● **Z87.73**   **Personal history of (corrected) congenital malformations of digestive system**

1/2 ● **Z87.730**   **Personal history of (corrected) cleft lip and palate** 🔲

1/2 ● **Z87.738**   **Personal history of other specified (corrected) congenital malformations of digestive system** 🔲

1/2 ● **Z87.74**   **Personal history of (corrected) congenital malformations of heart and circulatory system** 🔲

1/2 ● **Z87.75**   **Personal history of (corrected) congenital malformations of respiratory system** 🔲

1/2 ● **Z87.76**   **Personal history of (corrected) congenital malformations of integument, limbs and musculoskeletal system** 🔲

● **Z87.79**   **Personal history of other (corrected) congenital malformations**

1/2 ● **Z87.790**   **Personal history of (corrected) congenital malformations of face and neck** 🔲

1/2 ● **Z87.798**   **Personal history of other (corrected) congenital malformations** 🔲

● **Z87.8**   **Personal history of other specified conditions**

     Excludes2   personal history of self harm (Z91.5)

1/2 ● **Z87.81**   **Personal history of (healed) traumatic fracture** 🔲

     Excludes2   personal history of (healed) nontraumatic fracture (Z87.31-)

● **Z87.82**   **Personal history of other (healed) physical injury and trauma**

     Conditions classifiable to S00-T88, except traumatic fractures

1/2 ● **Z87.820**   **Personal history of traumatic brain injury** 🔲

     Excludes1   personal history of transient ischemic attack (TIA), and cerebral infarction without residual deficits (Z86.73)

1/2 ● **Z87.821**   **Personal history of retained foreign body fully removed** 🔲

1/2 ● **Z87.828**   **Personal history of other (healed) physical injury and trauma** 🔲

● **Z87.89**   **Personal history of other specified conditions**

1/2 **Z87.890**   **Personal history of sex reassignment**

1/2 ● **Z87.891**   **Personal history of nicotine dependence** 🔲

     Excludes1   current nicotine dependence (F17.2-)

●   Unacceptable Principal Diagnosis   ●   Use Additional Character(s)   🔲   Unspecified   ▶   Manifestation Code

OGCR   Official Guidelines for Coding and Reporting   Excludes 1   Excludes 2   Includes   Use additional   Code first   Code also

❶   First Listed   1/2   First Listed or Secondary   ❷   Secondary Only

⑫● **Z87.892 Personal history of anaphylaxis** 🔍

      Code also allergy status such as:
         allergy status to drugs, medicaments and biological substances (Z88.-)
         allergy status, other than to drugs and biological substances (Z91.0-)

⑫● **Z87.898 Personal history of other specified conditions** 🔍

● **Z88 Allergy status to drugs, medicaments and biological substances**

    Excludes2   allergy status, other than to drugs and biological substances (Z91.0-)

⑫● **Z88.0 Allergy status to penicillin** 🔍

⑫● **Z88.1 Allergy status to other antibiotic agents status** 🔍

⑫● **Z88.2 Allergy status to sulfonamides status** 🔍

⑫● **Z88.3 Allergy status to other anti-infective agents status** 🔍

⑫● **Z88.4 Allergy status to anesthetic agent status** 🔍

⑫● **Z88.5 Allergy status to narcotic agent status** 🔍

⑫● **Z88.6 Allergy status to analgesic agent status** 🔍

⑫● **Z88.7 Allergy status to serum and vaccine status** 🔍

⑫● **Z88.8 Allergy status to other drugs, medicaments and biological substances status** 🔍

⑫●■ **Z88.9 Allergy status to unspecified drugs, medicaments and biological substances status** 🔍

● **Z89 Acquired absence of limb**

    Includes   amputation status
            postprocedural loss of limb
            post-traumatic loss of limb

    Excludes1   acquired deformities of limbs (M20-M21)
            congenital absence of limbs (Q71-Q73)

● **Z89.0 Acquired absence of thumb and other finger(s)**

● **Z89.01 Acquired absence of thumb**

⑫● **Z89.011 Acquired absence of right thumb** 🔍

⑫● **Z89.012 Acquired absence of left thumb** 🔍

⑫●■ **Z89.019 Acquired absence of unspecified thumb** 🔍

● **Z89.02 Acquired absence of other finger(s)**

    Excludes2   acquired absence of thumb (Z89.01-)

⑫● **Z89.021 Acquired absence of right finger(s)** 🔍

⑫● **Z89.022 Acquired absence of left finger(s)** 🔍

⑫●■ **Z89.029 Acquired absence of unspecified finger(s)** 🔍

● **Z89.1 Acquired absence of hand and wrist**

● **Z89.11 Acquired absence of hand**

⑫● **Z89.111 Acquired absence of right hand** 🔍

⑫● **Z89.112 Acquired absence of left hand** 🔍

⑫●■ **Z89.119 Acquired absence of unspecified hand** 🔍

● **Z89.12 Acquired absence of wrist**
      Disarticulation at wrist

⑫● **Z89.121 Acquired absence of right wrist** 🔍

⑫● **Z89.122 Acquired absence of left wrist** 🔍

⑫●■ **Z89.129 Acquired absence of unspecified wrist** 🔍

● **Z89.2 Acquired absence of upper limb above wrist**

● **Z89.20 Acquired absence of upper limb, unspecified level**

⑫●■ **Z89.201 Acquired absence of right upper limb, unspecified level** 🔍

⑫●■ **Z89.202 Acquired absence of left upper limb, unspecified level** 🔍

⑫●■ **Z89.209 Acquired absence of unspecified upper limb, unspecified level** 🔍
      Acquired absence of arm NOS

● **Z89.21 Acquired absence of upper limb below elbow**

⑫● **Z89.211 Acquired absence of right upper limb below elbow** 🔍

⑫● **Z89.212 Acquired absence of left upper limb below elbow** 🔍

⑫●■ **Z89.219 Acquired absence of unspecified upper limb below elbow** 🔍

● **Z89.22 Acquired absence of upper limb above elbow**
      Disarticulation at elbow

⑫● **Z89.221 Acquired absence of right upper limb above elbow** 🔍

⑫● **Z89.222 Acquired absence of left upper limb above elbow** 🔍

⑫●■ **Z89.229 Acquired absence of unspecified upper limb above elbow** 🔍

● **Z89.23 Acquired absence of shoulder**
      Acquired absence of shoulder joint following explantation of shoulder joint prosthesis, with or without presence of antibiotic-impregnated cement spacer

⑫● **Z89.231 Acquired absence of right shoulder** 🔍

⑫● **Z89.232 Acquired absence of left shoulder** 🔍

⑫●■ **Z89.239 Acquired absence of unspecified shoulder** 🔍

● **Z89.4 Acquired absence of toe(s), foot, and ankle**

● **Z89.41 Acquired absence of great toe**

⑫● **Z89.411 Acquired absence of right great toe** 🔍

⑫● **Z89.412 Acquired absence of left great toe** 🔍

⑫●■ **Z89.419 Acquired absence of unspecified great toe** 🔍

● **Z89.42 Acquired absence of other toe(s)**

    Excludes2   acquired absence of great toe (Z89.41-)

⑫● **Z89.421 Acquired absence of other right toe(s)** 🔍

⑫● **Z89.422 Acquired absence of other left toe(s)** 🔍

⑫●■ **Z89.429 Acquired absence of other toe(s), unspecified side** 🔍

N Newborn Age: 0   **P** Pediatric Age: 0–17   **M** Maternity DX: 12–55   **A** Adult Age: 15–124   ♀ Females Only   ♂ Males Only

🔍 Complication\Comorbidity   🔍 Major C\C   🔍 Present on Admission Requirement   🔍 Hospital-Acquired Condition

1823

CHAPTER 21 (Z00-Z99)

CHAPTER 21 (Z00-Z99)

- Z89.43   Acquired absence of foot
  - ⑫ Z89.431   Acquired absence of right foot 🔍
  - ⑫ Z89.432   Acquired absence of left foot 🔍
  - ⑫● Z89.439   Acquired absence of unspecified foot 🔍
- Z89.44   Acquired absence of ankle
  Disarticulation of ankle
  - ⑫● Z89.441   Acquired absence of right ankle 🔍
  - ⑫● Z89.442   Acquired absence of left ankle 🔍
  - ⑫●■ Z89.449   Acquired absence of unspecified ankle 🔍
- Z89.5   Acquired absence of leg below knee
  - Z89.51   Acquired absence of leg below knee
    - ⑫● Z89.511   Acquired absence of right leg below knee 🔍
    - ⑫● Z89.512   Acquired absence of left leg below knee 🔍
    - ⑫● Z89.519   Acquired absence of unspecified leg below knee 🔍
  - Z89.52   Acquired absence of knee
    Acquired absence of knee joint following explantation of knee joint prosthesis, with or without presence of antibiotic-impregnated cement spacer
    - ⑫● Z89.521   Acquired absence of right knee 🔍
    - ⑫● Z89.522   Acquired absence of left knee 🔍
    - ⑫● Z89.529   Acquired absence of unspecified knee 🔍
- Z89.6   Acquired absence of leg above knee
  - Z89.61   Acquired absence of leg above knee
    Acquired absence of leg NOS
    Disarticulation at knee
    - ⑫● Z89.611   Acquired absence of right leg above knee 🔍
    - ⑫● Z89.612   Acquired absence of left leg above knee 🔍
    - ⑫●■ Z89.619   Acquired absence of unspecified leg above knee 🔍
  - Z89.62   Acquired absence of hip
    Acquired absence of hip joint following explantation of hip joint prosthesis, with or without presence of antibiotic-impregnated cement spacer
    Disarticulation at hip
    - ⑫● Z89.621   Acquired absence of right hip joint 🔍
    - ⑫● Z89.622   Acquired absence of left hip joint 🔍
    - ⑫●■ Z89.629   Acquired absence of unspecified hip joint 🔍
- ⑫●■ Z89.9   Acquired absence of limb, unspecified 🔍
- ● Z90   Acquired absence of organs, not elsewhere classified
  - **Includes**   postprocedural or post-traumatic loss of body part NEC
  - **Excludes1**   congenital absence - see Alphabetical Index
  - **Excludes2**   postprocedural absence of endocrine glands (E89.-)
  - ● Z90.0   Acquired absence of part of head and neck
    - ⑫● Z90.01   Acquired absence of eye 🔍
    - ⑫● Z90.02   Acquired absence of larynx 🔍

- ⑫● Z90.09   Acquired absence of other part of head and neck 🔍
  Acquired absence of nose
  - **Excludes2**   teeth (K08.1)
- ● Z90.1   Acquired absence of breast and nipple
  - ⑫ Z90.10   Acquired absence of unspecified breast and nipple 🔍
  - ⑫ Z90.11   Acquired absence of right breast and nipple 🔍
  - ⑫ Z90.12   Acquired absence of left breast and nipple 🔍
  - ⑫ Z90.13   Acquired absence of bilateral breasts and nipples 🔍
- ⑫● Z90.2   Acquired absence of lung [part of] 🔍
- ⑫● Z90.3   Acquired absence of stomach [part of] 🔍
- ● Z90.4   Acquired absence of other specified parts of digestive tract
  - ● Z90.41   Acquired absence of pancreas
    Use additional code to identify any associated:
    insulin use (Z79.4)
    diabetes mellitus, postpancreatectomy (E13.-)
    - ⑫● Z90.410   Acquired total absence of pancreas 🔍
      Acquired absence of pancreas NOS
    - ⑫● Z90.411   Acquired partial absence of pancreas 🔍
  - ⑫● Z90.49   Acquired absence of other specified parts of digestive tract 🔍
- ⑫● Z90.5   Acquired absence of kidney 🔍
- ⑫● Z90.6   Acquired absence of other parts of urinary tract 🔍
  Acquired absence of bladder
- ● Z90.7   Acquired absence of genital organ(s)
  - **Excludes1**   personal history of sex reassignment (Z87.890)
  - **Excludes2**   female genital mutilation status (N90.81-)
  - ● Z90.71   Acquired absence of cervix and uterus
    - ⑫● Z90.710   Acquired absence of both cervix and uterus ♀ 🔍
      Acquired absence of uterus NOS
      Status post total hysterectomy
    - ⑫● Z90.711   Acquired absence of uterus with remaining cervical stump ♀ 🔍
      Status post partial hysterectomy with remaining cervical stump
    - ⑫● Z90.712   Acquired absence of cervix with remaining uterus ♀ 🔍
  - ● Z90.72   Acquired absence of ovaries
    - ⑫● Z90.721   Acquired absence of ovaries, unilateral ♀
    - ⑫● Z90.722   Acquired absence of ovaries, bilateral ♀
  - ⑫● Z90.79   Acquired absence of other genital organ(s) 🔍
- ● Z90.8   Acquired absence of other organs
  - ⑫● Z90.81   Acquired absence of spleen 🔍
  - ⑫● Z90.89   Acquired absence of other organs 🔍

● Unacceptable Principal Diagnosis   ● Use Additional Character(s)   ■ Unspecified   ▶ Manifestation Code
OGCR   Official Guidelines for Coding and Reporting   Excludes 1   Excludes 2   Includes   Use additional   Code first   Code also
❶ First Listed   ⑫ First Listed or Secondary   ❷ Secondary Only

● **Z91   Personal risk factors, not elsewhere classified**

> **Excludes2**   contact with and (suspected) exposures hazardous to health (Z77.-)
> exposure to pollution and other problems related to physical environment (Z77.1-)
> occupational exposure to risk factors (Z57.-)
> personal history of physical injury and trauma (Z87.81, Z87.82-)

● **Z91.0   Allergy status, other than to drugs and biological substances**

> **Excludes2**   allergy status to drugs, medicaments, and biological substances (Z88.-)

  ● **Z91.01   Food allergy status**

> **Excludes2**   food additives allergy status (Z91.02)

    ⑫● **Z91.010   Allergy to peanuts** 🔖

    ⑫● **Z91.011   Allergy to milk products** 🔖

> **Excludes1**   lactose intolerance (E73.-)

    ⑫● **Z91.012   Allergy to eggs** 🔖

    ⑫● **Z91.013   Allergy to seafood** 🔖
Allergy to shellfish
Allergy to octopus or squid ink

    ⑫● **Z91.018   Allergy to other foods** 🔖
Allergy to nuts other than peanuts

  ⑫● **Z91.02   Food additives allergy status** 🔖

  ● **Z91.03   Insect allergy status**

    ⑫● **Z91.030   Bee allergy status** 🔖

    ⑫● **Z91.038   Other insect allergy status** 🔖

  ● **Z91.04   Nonmedicinal substance allergy status**

    ⑫● **Z91.040   Latex allergy status** 🔖
Latex sensitivity status

    ⑫● **Z91.041   Radiographic dye allergy status** 🔖
Allergy status to contrast media used for diagnostic X-ray procedure

    ⑫● **Z91.048   Other nonmedicinal substance allergy status** 🔖

  ⑫● **Z91.09   Other allergy status, other than to drugs and biological substances** 🔖

● **Z91.1   Patient's noncompliance with medical treatment and regimen**

  ❷● **Z91.11   Patient's noncompliance with dietary regimen** 🔖

  ● **Z91.12   Patient's intentional underdosing of medication regimen**

> *Code first* underdosing of medication (T36-T50) with fifth or sixth character 6

> **Excludes1**   adverse effect of prescribed drug taken as directed - code to adverse effect
> poisoning (overdose) - code to poisoning

    ❷● **Z91.120   Patient's intentional underdosing of medication regimen due to financial hardship** 🔖

    ❷● **Z91.128   Patient's intentional underdosing of medication regimen for other reason** 🔖

● **Z91.13   Patient's unintentional underdosing of medication regimen**

> *Code first* underdosing of medication (T36-T50) with fifth or sixth character 6

> **Excludes1**   adverse effect of prescribed drug taken as directed - code to adverse effect
> poisoning (overdose) - code to poisoning

  ❷● **Z91.130   Patient's unintentional underdosing of medication regimen due to age-related debility** 🔖

  ❷● **Z91.138   Patient's unintentional underdosing of medication regimen for other reason** 🔖

  ❷● **Z91.14   Patient's other noncompliance with medication regimen** 🔖
Patient's underdosing of medication NOS

  ⑫● **Z91.15   Patient's noncompliance with renal dialysis** 🔖

  ❷● **Z91.19   Patient's noncompliance with other medical treatment and regimen** 🔖

● **Z91.4   Personal history of psychological trauma, not elsewhere classified**

  ● **Z91.41   Personal history of adult abuse**

> **Excludes2**   personal history of abuse in childhood (Z62.81-)

    ❷● **Z91.410   Personal history of adult physical and sexual abuse** 🔖   **A**

> **Excludes1**   current adult physical abuse (T74.11, T76.11)
> current adult sexual abuse (T74.21, T76.11)

    ❷● **Z91.411   Personal history of adult psychological abuse** 🔖   **A**

    ❷● **Z91.412   Personal history of adult neglect** 🔖   **A**

> **Excludes1**   current adult neglect (T74.01, T76.01)

    ❷● **Z91.419   Personal history of unspecified adult abuse** 🔖   **A**

  ❷● **Z91.49   Other personal history of psychological trauma, not elsewhere classified** 🔖

❷● **Z91.5   Personal history of self-harm** 🔖
Personal history of parasuicide
Personal history of self-poisoning
Personal history of suicide attempt

● **Z91.8   Other specified personal risk factors, not elsewhere classified**

  ❷● **Z91.81   History of falling** 🔖
At risk for falling

  ⑫● **Z91.82   Personal history of military deployment** 🔖
Individual (civilian or military) with past history of military war, peacekeeping and humanitarian deployment (current or past conflict)
Returned from military deployment

N Newborn Age: 0   **P** Pediatric Age: 0–17   **M** Maternity DX: 12–55   **A** Adult Age: 15–124   ♀ Females Only   ♂ Males Only

🔖 Complication\Comorbidity   🔖 Major C\C   Present on Admission Requirement   🔖 Hospital-Acquired Condition

1825

⑫● **Z91.83**   **Wandering in diseases classified elsewhere** 🔍

> *Code first* underlying disorder such as:
> Alzheimer's disease (G30-)
> autism or pervasive developmental
> disorder (F84-)
> intellectual disabilities (F70-F79)
> unspecified dementia with behavioral
> disturbance (F03.9-)

❷● **Z91.89**   **Other specified personal risk factors, not elsewhere classified** 🔍

● **Z92**   **Personal history of medical treatment**

> **Excludes2**   postprocedural states (Z98.-)

❷● **Z92.0**   **Personal history of contraception** 🔍

> **Excludes1**   counseling or management of current
> contraceptive practices (Z30.-)
> long term (current) use of
> contraception (Z79.3)
> presence of (intrauterine)
> contraceptive device (Z97.5)

● **Z92.2**   **Personal history of drug therapy**

> **Excludes2**   long term (current) drug therapy
> (Z79.-)

⑫● **Z92.21**   **Personal history of antineoplastic chemotherapy** 🔍

⑫● **Z92.22**   **Personal history of monoclonal drug therapy** 🔍

⑫● **Z92.23**   **Personal history of estrogen therapy** 🔍

● **Z92.24**   **Personal history of steroid therapy**

     ⑫● **Z92.240**   **Personal history of inhaled steroid therapy** 🔍

     ⑫● **Z92.241**   **Personal history of systemic steroid therapy** 🔍
> Personal history of steroid
> therapy NOS

⑫● **Z92.25**   **Personal history of immunosupression therapy** 🔍

> **Excludes2**   personal history of steroid
> therapy (Z92.24)

⑫● **Z92.29**   **Personal history of other drug therapy** 🔍

❷● **Z92.3**   **Personal history of irradiation** 🔍
> Personal history of exposure to therapeutic radiation

> **Excludes1**   exposure to radiation in the physical
> environment (Z77.12)
> occupational exposure to radiation
> (Z57.1)

● **Z92.8**   **Personal history of other medical treatment**

❷● **Z92.81**   **Personal history of extracorporeal membrane oxygenation (ECMO)** 🔍

⑫● **Z92.82**   **Status post administration of tPA (rtPA) in a different facility within the last 24 hours prior to admission to current facility** 🔍

> *Code first* condition requiring tPA
> administration, such as:
> acute cerebral infarction (I63.-)
> acute myocardial infarction (I21.-, I22.-)

⑫● **Z92.83**   **Personal history of failed moderate sedation** 🔍
> Personal history of failed conscious
> sedation

> **Excludes2**   failed moderate sedation
> during procedure
> (T88.52)

❷● **Z92.89**   **Personal history of other medical treatment** 🔍

● **Z93**   **Artificial opening status**

> **Excludes1**   artificial openings requiring attention or
> management (Z43.-)
> complications of external stoma (J95.0-,
> K94.-, N99.5-)

❷● **Z93.0**   **Tracheostomy status** 🔍

❷● **Z93.1**   **Gastrostomy status** 🔍

❷● **Z93.2**   **Ileostomy status** 🔍

❷● **Z93.3**   **Colostomy status** 🔍

❷● **Z93.4**   **Other artificial openings of gastrointestinal tract status** 🔍

● **Z93.5**   **Cystostomy status**

     ❷●■ **Z93.50**   **Unspecified cystostomy status** 🔍

     ❷● **Z93.51**   **Cutaneous-vesicostomy status** 🔍

     ❷● **Z93.52**   **Appendico-vesicostomy status** 🔍

     ❷● **Z93.59**   **Other cystostomy status** 🔍

❷● **Z93.6**   **Other artificial openings of urinary tract status** 🔍
> Nephrostomy status
> Ureterostomy status
> Urethrostomy status

❷● **Z93.8**   **Other artificial opening status** 🔍

❷●■ **Z93.9**   **Artificial opening status, unspecified** 🔍

● **Z94**   **Transplanted organ and tissue status**

> **Includes**   organ or tissue replaced by heterogenous or
> homogenous transplant

> **Excludes1**   complications of transplanted organ or
> tissue - see Alphabetical Index

> **Excludes2**   presence of vascular grafts (Z95.-)

❷● **Z94.0**   **Kidney transplant status** 🔒 🔍

❷● **Z94.1**   **Heart transplant status** 🔒 🔍

> **Excludes1**   artificial heart status (Z95.811)
> heart-valve replacement status
> (Z95.2-Z95.4)

❷● **Z94.2**   **Lung transplant status** 🔒 🔍

❷● **Z94.3**   **Heart and lungs transplant status** 🔒 🔍
> MCC: Only when the principal diagnosis is
> designated as a CC

❷● **Z94.4**   **Liver transplant status** 🔒 🔍

❷● **Z94.5**   **Skin transplant status** 🔍
> Autogenous skin transplant status

❷● **Z94.6**   **Bone transplant status** 🔍

❷● **Z94.7**   **Corneal transplant status** 🔍

● **Z94.8**   **Other transplanted organ and tissue status**

     ❷● **Z94.81**   **Bone marrow transplant status** 🔒 🔍

     ❷● **Z94.82**   **Intestine transplant status** 🔒 🔍

     ❷● **Z94.83**   **Pancreas transplant status** 🔒 🔍

     ❷● **Z94.84**   **Stem cells transplant status** 🔒 🔍

     ❷● **Z94.89**   **Other transplanted organ and tissue status** 🔍

❷●■ **Z94.9**   **Transplanted organ and tissue status, unspecified** 🔍

● Unacceptable Principal Diagnosis   ● Use Additional Character(s)   ■ Unspecified   ▶ Manifestation Code

OGCR   Official Guidelines for Coding and Reporting   Excludes 1   Excludes 2   Includes   Use additional   Code first   Code also

❶ First Listed   ⑫ First Listed or Secondary   ❷ Secondary Only

●**Z95 Presence of cardiac and vascular implants and grafts**

    Excludes1   complications of cardiac and vascular devices, implants and grafts (T82.-)

❷● **Z95.0 Presence of cardiac pacemaker** 🔖

    Excludes1   adjustment or management of cardiac pacemaker (Z45.0)
                  presence of automatic (implantable) cardiac defibrillator with synchronous cardiac pacemaker Z95.810

❷● **Z95.1 Presence of aortocoronary bypass graft** 🔖

❷● **Z95.2 Presence of prosthetic heart valve** 🔖
        Presence of heart valve NOS

❷● **Z95.3 Presence of xenogenic heart valve** 🔖

❷● **Z95.4 Presence of other heart-valve replacement** 🔖

❷● **Z95.5 Presence of coronary angioplasty implant and graft** 🔖

    Excludes1   coronary angioplasty status without implant and graft (Z98.61)

● **Z95.8 Presence of other cardiac and vascular implants and grafts**

  ● **Z95.81 Presence of other cardiac implants and grafts**

    ❷● **Z95.810 Presence of automatic (implantable) cardiac defibrillator** 🔖
           Presence of automatic (implantable) cardiac defibrillator with synchronous cardiac pacemaker

    ❷● **Z95.811 Presence of heart assist device** 🔖🔖

    ❷● **Z95.812 Presence of fully implantable artificial heart** 🔖

    ❷● **Z95.818 Presence of other cardiac implants and grafts** 🔖

  ● **Z95.82 Presence of other vascular implants and grafts**

    ❷● **Z95.820 Peripheral vascular angioplasty status with implants and grafts** 🔖

        Excludes1   peripheral vascular angioplasty without implant and graft (Z98.62)

    ❷● **Z95.828 Presence of other vascular implants and grafts** 🔖
           Presence of intravascular prosthesis NEC

❷● ■ **Z95.9 Presence of cardiac and vascular implant and graft, unspecified** 🔖

●**Z96 Presence of other functional implants**

    Excludes2   complications of internal prosthetic devices, implants and grafts (T82-T85)
            fitting and adjustment of prosthetic and other devices (Z44-Z46)

❷● **Z96.0 Presence of urogenital implants** 🔖

❷● **Z96.1 Presence of intraocular lens** 🔖
        Presence of pseudophakia

●**Z96.2 Presence of otological and audiological implants**

  ❷● ■ **Z96.20 Presence of otological and audiological implant, unspecified**

  ❷● **Z96.21 Cochlear implant status**

  ❷● **Z96.22 Myringotomy tube(s) status**

  ❷● **Z96.29 Presence of other otological and audiological implants**
        Presence of bone-conduction hearing device
        Presence of eustachian tube stent
        Stapes replacement

❷● **Z96.3 Presence of artificial larynx**

●**Z96.4 Presence of endocrine implants**

  ❷● **Z96.41 Presence of insulin pump (external) (internal)** 🔖

  ❷● **Z96.49 Presence of other endocrine implants** 🔖

❷● **Z96.5 Presence of tooth-root and mandibular implants**

●**Z96.6 Presence of orthopedic joint implants**

  ❷● ■ **Z96.60 Presence of unspecified orthopedic joint implant** 🔖

  ●**Z96.61 Presence of artificial shoulder joint**

    ❷● **Z96.611 Presence of right artificial shoulder joint** 🔖

    ❷● **Z96.612 Presence of left artificial shoulder joint** 🔖

    ❷● ■ **Z96.619 Presence of unspecified artificial shoulder joint** 🔖

  ●**Z96.62 Presence of artificial elbow joint**

    ❷● **Z96.621 Presence of right artificial elbow joint** 🔖

    ❷● **Z96.622 Presence of left artificial elbow joint** 🔖

    ❷● ■ **Z96.629 Presence of unspecified artificial elbow joint** 🔖

  ●**Z96.63 Presence of artificial wrist joint**

    ❷● **Z96.631 Presence of right artificial wrist joint** 🔖

    ❷● **Z96.632 Presence of left artificial wrist joint** 🔖

    ❷● ■ **Z96.639 Presence of unspecified artificial wrist joint** 🔖

  ●**Z96.64 Presence of artificial hip joint**
        Hip-joint replacement (partial) (total)

    ❷● **Z96.641 Presence of right artificial hip joint** 🔖

    ❷● **Z96.642 Presence of left artificial hip joint** 🔖

    ❷● **Z96.643 Presence of artificial hip joint, bilateral** 🔖

    ❷● ■ **Z96.649 Presence of unspecified artificial hip joint** 🔖

  ●**Z96.65 Presence of artificial knee joint**

    ❷● **Z96.651 Presence of right artificial knee joint** 🔖

    ❷● **Z96.652 Presence of left artificial knee joint** 🔖

    ❷● **Z96.653 Presence of artificial knee joint, bilateral** 🔖

    ❷● ■ **Z96.659 Presence of unspecified artificial knee joint** 🔖

● **Z96.66** Presence of artificial ankle joint

    ❷● **Z96.661** Presence of right artificial ankle joint 🔍

    ❷● **Z96.662** Presence of left artificial ankle joint 🔍

    ❷●■ **Z96.669** Presence of unspecified artificial ankle joint 🔍

● **Z96.69** Presence of other orthopedic joint implants

    ❷● **Z96.691** Finger-joint replacement of right hand 🔍

    ❷● **Z96.692** Finger-joint replacement of left hand 🔍

    ❷● **Z96.693** Finger-joint replacement, bilateral 🔍

    ❷● **Z96.698** Presence of other orthopedic joint implants 🔍

❷● **Z96.7** Presence of other bone and tendon implants 🔍
    Presence of skull plate

● **Z96.8** Presence of other specified functional implants

    ❷● **Z96.81** Presence of artificial skin 🔍

    ❷● **Z96.89** Presence of other specified functional implants 🔍

❷●■ **Z96.9** Presence of functional implant, unspecified 🔍

● **Z97** **Presence of other devices**

    Excludes1 complications of internal prosthetic devices, implants and grafts (T82-T85)
           fitting and adjustment of prosthetic and other devices (Z44-Z46)

    Excludes2 presence of cerebrospinal fluid drainage device (Z98.2)

❷● **Z97.0** Presence of artificial eye 🔍

● **Z97.1** Presence of artificial limb (complete) (partial)

    ❷●■ **Z97.10** Presence of artificial limb (complete) (partial), unspecified 🔍

    ❷● **Z97.11** Presence of artificial right arm (complete) (partial) 🔍

    ❷● **Z97.12** Presence of artificial left arm (complete) (partial) 🔍

    ❷● **Z97.13** Presence of artificial right leg (complete) (partial) 🔍

    ❷● **Z97.14** Presence of artificial left leg (complete) (partial) 🔍

    ❷● **Z97.15** Presence of artificial arms, bilateral (complete) (partial) 🔍

    ❷● **Z97.16** Presence of artificial legs, bilateral (complete) (partial) 🔍

❷● **Z97.2** Presence of dental prosthetic device (complete) (partial) 🔍
    Presence of dentures (complete) (partial)

❷● **Z97.3** Presence of spectacles and contact lenses

❷● **Z97.4** Presence of external hearing-aid

❷● **Z97.5** Presence of (intrauterine) contraceptive device ♀ 🔍

    Excludes1 checking, reinsertion or removal of contraceptive device (Z30.43)

❷● **Z97.8** Presence of other specified devices 🔍

● **Z98** **Other postprocedural states**

    Excludes2 aftercare (Z43-Z49, Z51)
           follow-up medical care (Z08-Z09)
           postprocedural complication - see Alphabetical Index

❷● **Z98.0** Intestinal bypass and anastomosis status 🔍

    Excludes2 bariatric surgery status (Z98.84)
           gastric bypass status (Z98.84)
           obesity surgery status (Z98.84)

❷● **Z98.1** Arthrodesis status 🔍

❷● **Z98.2** Presence of cerebrospinal fluid drainage device 🔍
    Presence of CSF shunt

❷● **Z98.3** Post therapeutic collapse of lung status 🔍

    Code first underlying disease

● **Z98.4** Cataract extraction status

    Use additional code to identify intraocular lens implant status (Z96.1)

    Excludes1 aphakia (H27.0)

    ❷● **Z98.41** Cataract extraction status, right eye 🔍

    ❷● **Z98.42** Cataract extraction status, left eye 🔍

    ❷●■ **Z98.49** Cataract extraction status, unspecified eye 🔍

● **Z98.5** Sterilization status

    Excludes1 female infertility (N97.-)
           male infertility (N46.-)

    ❷● **Z98.51** Tubal ligation status ♀ 🔍

    ❷● **Z98.52** Vasectomy status ♂ 🔍   **A**

● **Z98.6** Angioplasty status

    ❷● **Z98.61** Coronary angioplasty status 🔍

        Excludes1 coronary angioplasty status with implant and graft (Z95.5)

    ❷● **Z98.62** Peripheral vascular angioplasty status 🔍

        Excludes1 peripheral vascular angioplasty status with implant and graft (Z95.820)

● **Z98.8** Other specified postprocedural states

    ● **Z98.81** Dental procedure status

        ❷● **Z98.810** Dental sealant status 🔍

        ❷● **Z98.811** Dental restoration status 🔍
            Dental crown status
            Dental fillings status

        ❷● **Z98.818** Other dental procedure status 🔍

    ❷● **Z98.82** Breast implant status 🔍

        Excludes1 breast implant removal status (Z98.86)

    ❷● **Z98.83** Filtering (vitreous) bleb after glaucoma surgery status 🔍

        Excludes1 inflammation (infection) of postprocedural bleb (H59.4-)

    ❷● **Z98.84** Bariatric surgery status 🔍
        Gastric banding status
        Gastric bypass status for obesity
        Obesity surgery status

        Excludes1 bariatric surgery status complicating pregnancy, childbirth, or the puerperium (O99.84)

        Excludes2 intestinal bypass and anastomosis status (Z98.0)

CHAPTER 21 (Z00-Z99)

● Unacceptable Principal Diagnosis   ● Use Additional Character(s)   ■ Unspecified   ▶ Manifestation Code

OGCR Official Guidelines for Coding and Reporting   Excludes 1   Excludes 2   Includes   Use additional   Code first   Code also

❶ First Listed   ❶/❷ First Listed or Secondary   ❷ Secondary Only

❷● **Z98.85** **Transplanted organ removal status** 🔖
Transplanted organ previously removed due to complication, failure, rejection or infection

> | Excludes1 | encounter for removal of transplanted organ -code to complication of transplanted organ (T86.-)

❷● **Z98.86** **Personal history of breast implant removal** 🔖

● **Z98.87** **Personal history of in utero procedure**

     ❷● **Z98.870** **Personal history of in utero procedure during pregnancy** ♀ 🔖

> | Excludes2 | complications from in utero procedure for current pregnancy (O35.7) supervision of current pregnancy with history of in utero procedure during previous pregnancy (O09.82-)

     ❷● **Z98.871** **Personal history of in utero procedure while a fetus** 🔖

❷● **Z98.89** **Other specified postprocedural states** 🔖
Personal history of surgery, not elsewhere classified

● **Z99** **Dependence on enabling machines and devices, not elsewhere classified**

> | Excludes1 | cardiac pacemaker status (Z95.0)

❷● **Z99.0** **Dependence on aspirator** 🔖

● **Z99.1** **Dependence on respirator**
Dependence on ventilator

     ❷ **Z99.11** **Dependence on respirator [ventilator] status** 🔖🔖

     ❶ **Z99.12** **Encounter for respirator [ventilator] dependence during power failure** 🔖🔖

> | Excludes1 | mechanical complication of respirator [ventilator] (J95.850)

❷● **Z99.2** **Dependence on renal dialysis** 🔖
Hemodialysis status
Peritoneal dialysis status
Presence of arteriovenous shunt for dialysis
Renal dialysis status NOS

> | Excludes1 | encounter for fitting and adjustment of dialysis catheter (Z49.0-) noncompliance with renal dialysis (Z91.15)

❷● **Z99.3** **Dependence on wheelchair** 🔖
Wheelchair confinement status

Code first cause of dependence, such as:
muscular dystrophy (G71.0)
obesity (E66.-)

● **Z99.8** **Dependence on other enabling machines and devices**

     ❷● **Z99.81** **Dependence on supplemental oxygen** 🔖
Dependence on long-term oxygen

     ❷● **Z99.89** **Dependence on other enabling machines and devices** 🔖
Dependence on machine or device NOS

N Newborn Age: 0   **P** Pediatric Age: 0–17   **M** Maternity DX: 12–55   **A** Adult Age: 15–124   ♀ Females Only   ♂ Males Only

🔖 Complication\Comorbidity   🔖 Major C\C   🔖 Present on Admission Requirement   🔖 Hospital-Acquired Condition   **1829**

CHAPTER 21 (Z00-Z99)

Master the ICD-9-CM and ICD-10-CM/PCS
with these easy-to-use textbooks.

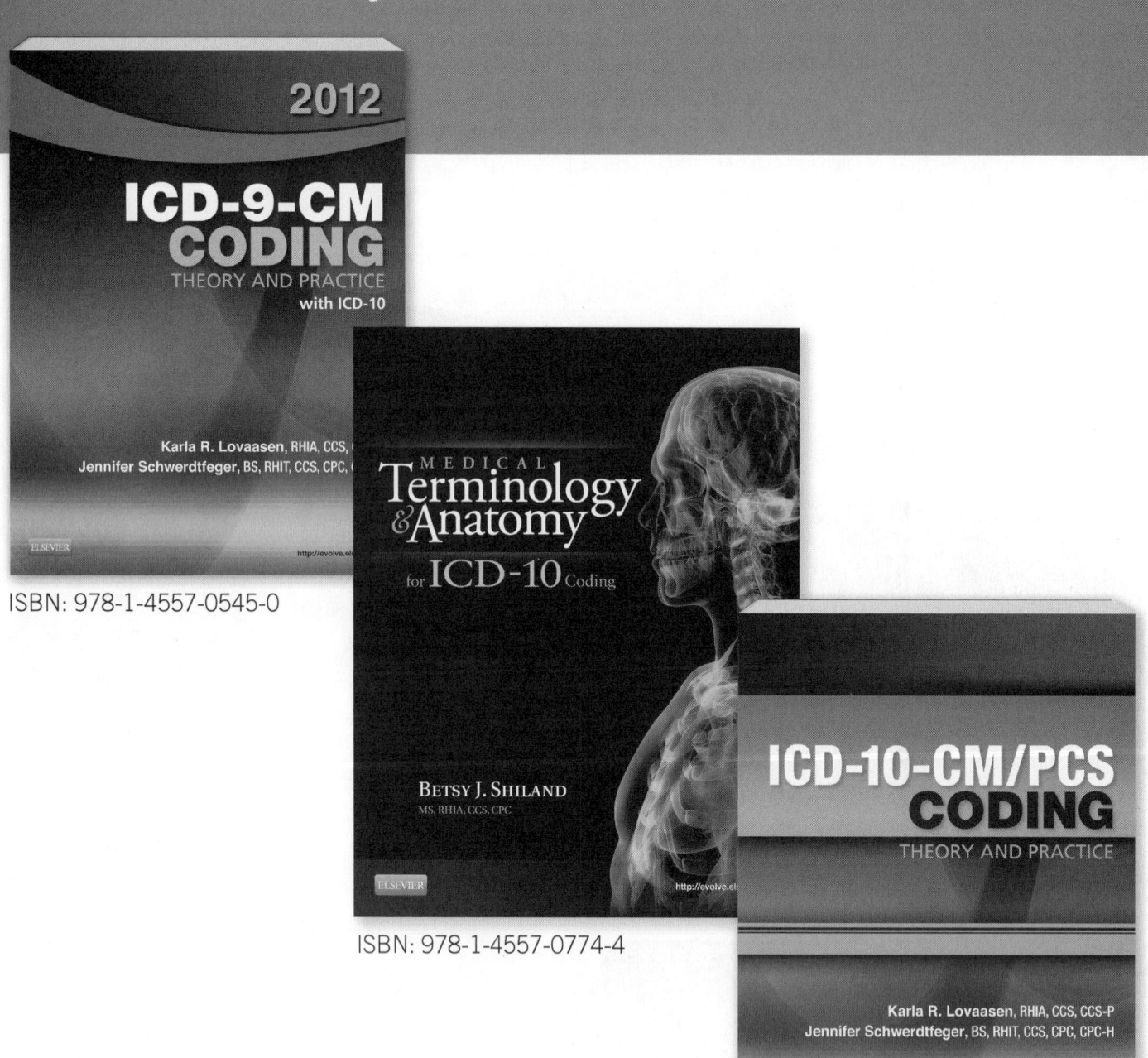

ISBN: 978-1-4557-0545-0

ISBN: 978-1-4557-0774-4

ISBN: 978-1-4557-0795-9

Trust Carol J. Buck and Elsevier
to take you through the levels of coding success

Step 4:
Professional Resources

Step 3:
Certify

With the resources you need for every level of coding success, Carol J. Buck and Elsevier are with you every step of your coding career. From beginning to advanced, from the classroom to the workplace, from application to certification, the Step Series products are your guides to greater opportunities and successful career advancement.

Step 2:
Practice

Step 1:
Learn

Keep climbing with the most trusted name in medical coding.

Author and Educator
Carol J. Buck, MS, CPC, CPC-H, CCS-P

3-00

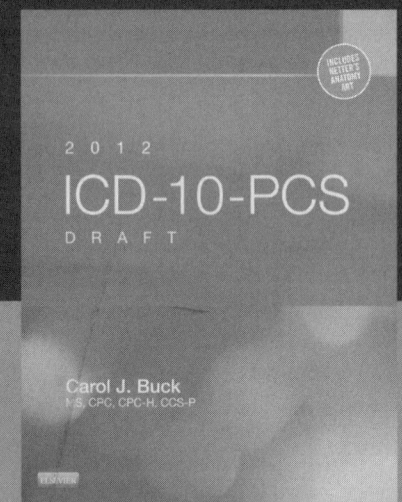